Kaplan's Cardiac Anesthesia

Kaplan's Cardiac Anesthesia

FIFTH EDITION

EDITOR

Joel A. Kaplan, MD, CPE, FACC

Dean Emeritus, School of Medicine
Former Chancellor, Health Sciences Center
Professor of Clinical Anesthesiology
University of Louisville School of Medicine
Louisville, Kentucky

Professor, Clinical Anesthesiology
University of California, San Diego, School of Medicine
San Diego, California

ASSOCIATE EDITORS

David L. Reich, MD

Horace W. Goldsmith Professor and Chair
Department of Anesthesiology
Mount Sinai School of Medicine
New York, New York

Carol L. Lake, MD, MBA, MPH

Chief Executive Officer
Verefi Technologies, Inc.
Elizabethtown, Pennsylvania

Steven N. Konstadt, MD, MBA, FACC

Professor and Chair, Department of Anesthesiology
Maimonides Medical Center
Brooklyn, New York

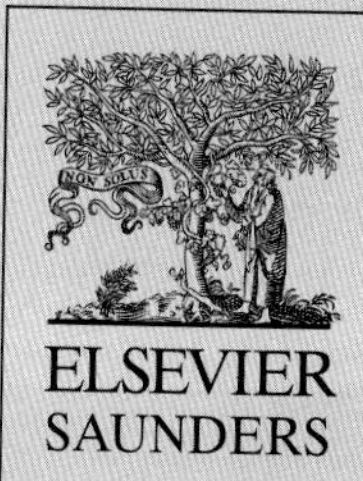

ELSEVIER
SAUNDERS

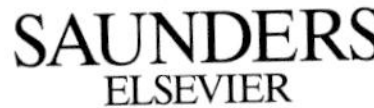

SAUNDERS
ELSEVIER

1600 John F. Kennedy Blvd.
Suite 1800
Philadelphia, PA 19103-2899

ISBN 1-4160-0253-7
ISBN 978-1416-00253-6

Kaplan's Cardiac Anesthesia
Fifth Edition

Notice

Knowledge and best practice in this field are constantly changing. As new research and experience broaden our knowledge, changes in practice, treatment, and drug therapy may become necessary or appropriate. Readers are advised to check the most current information provided (i) on procedures or (ii) by the manufacturer of each product to be administered, to verify the recommended dose or formula, the method and duration of administration, and contraindications. It is the responsibility of the practitioner, relying on their own experience and knowledge of the patient, to take all appropriate safety precautions. To the fullest extent of the law, neither the Publisher nor the Authors assume any liability for any injury and/or damage to persons or property arising out of or related to any use of the material contained in this book.

Library of Congress Cataloging-in-Publication Data

Kaplan's cardiac anesthesia / [edited by] Joel A. Kaplan . . . [et al.].–5th ed.
p. ; cm.
Includes bibliographical references and index.
ISBN 1-4160-0253-7
1. Anesthesia in cardiology. 2. Heart—Surgery. I. Kaplan, Joel A.
[DNLM: 1. Anesthesia. 2. Cardiac Surgical Procedures. 3. Heart–drug effects. WO 245 C267 2006]
RD87.3.C37C363 2006
617.9′67412—dc22

2005050029

Publisher: Natasha Andjelkovic
Developmental Editor: Arlene Chappelle
Publishing Services Manager: Tina Rebane
Senior Project Manager: Mary Anne Folcher
Design Direction: Karen O'Keefe Owens
Marketing Manager: Emily Christie

Printed in the United States of America

Last digit is the print number 9 8 7 6 5 4 3 2 1

To my loving wife, Norma, on the occasion of our fortieth wedding anniversary.

JAK

CONTRIBUTORS

David H. Adams, MD
Marie-Josée and Henry R. Kravis Professor
Department of Cardiothoracic Surgery
Mount Sinai School of Medicine
Chairman
Department of Cardiothoracic Surgery
Mount Sinai Medical Center
New York, New York
2: Milestones in Cardiac Surgery
4: The Future of Cardiac Surgery and Anesthesia

Ahmad Adi, MD
Staff Anesthesiologist
Department of Cardiothoracic Anesthesiology
The Cleveland Clinic
Cleveland, Ohio
5: Cardiac Physiology

Lishan Aklog, MD
Assistant Professor
Department of Cardiothoracic Surgery
Mount Sinai Medical Center
New York, New York
21: Minimally Invasive Cardiac Surgery

Michael J. Andritsos, MD
Instructor
Department of Anesthesiology
Washington University School of Medicine
St. Louis, Missouri
13: Cardiac Electrophysiology: Diagnosis and Treatment

Ani C. Anyanwu, MD, FRCS
Clinical Fellow in Cardiothoracic Surgery
Department of Cardiothoracic Surgery
Mount Sinai Medical Center
New York, New York
4: The Future of Cardiac Surgery and Anesthesia

James M. Bailey, MD, PhD
Clinical Associate Professor
Department of Anesthesiology
Emory University School of Medicine
Atlanta, Georgia
33: Postoperative Cardiovascular Management

Daniel Bainbridge, MD, FRCPC
Assistant Professor
Department of Anesthesia and Perioperative Medicine
The University of Western Ontario
Active Staff Anesthesiologist
Department of Anesthesia and Perioperative Medicine
London Health Sciences Centre—University Hospital
London, Ontario, Canada
32: Postoperative Cardiac Recovery and Outcomes

Paul G. Barash, MD
Professor of Anesthesiology
Yale University School of Medicine
Attending Anesthesiologist
Yale–New Haven Hospital
New Haven, Connecticut
4: The Future of Cardiac Surgery and Anesthesia

Victor C. Baum, MD
Professor of Anesthesiology and Pediatrics
Director of Cardiac Anesthesia
Department of Anesthesiology
University of Virginia School of Medicine
Charlottesville, Virginia
22: Congenital Heart Disease in Adults

Elliott Bennett-Guerrero, MD
Associate Professor
Department of Anesthesiology
Duke University Medical Center
Director of Perioperative Clinical Research
Duke Clinical Research Institute
Durham, North Carolina
8: Systemic Inflammation

Dan E. Berkowitz, MD
Associate Professor, Department of Anesthesiology and Critical Care Medicine
Assistant Professor, Department of Biomedical Engineering
The Johns Hopkins University School of Medicine
Anesthesiologist
The Johns Hopkins Hospital
Baltimore, Maryland
9: Pharmacology of Anesthetic Drugs

T. Andrew Bowdle, MD, PhD
Professor of Anesthesiology and Pharmaceutics
Chief, Division of Cardiothoracic Anesthesiology
Department of Anesthesiology
University of Washington School of Medicine
Seattle, Washington
40: Reducing Errors in Cardiac Anesthesiology

John F. Butterworth IV, MD
Robert K. Stoelting Professor and Chair
Department of Anesthesia
Indiana University School of Medicine
Anesthesiologist
Clarian University Hospital
Indianapolis, Indiana
10: Cardiovascular Pharmacology

Alfonso Casta, MD
Lecturer in Anaesthesia
Department of Anaesthesia
Harvard Medical School
Senior Associate in Cardiac Anesthesia
Department of Anesthesiology, Perioperative and Pain Medicine
Children's Hospital Boston
Boston, Massachusetts
26: Anesthesia for Heart, Lung, and Heart-Lung Transplantation

Charles E. Chambers, MD
Professor of Medicine and Radiology
Pennsylvania State University School of Medicine
Director, Cardiac Catheterization Laboratories
Milton S. Hershey Medical Center
Hershey, Pennsylvania
12: The Cardiac Catheterization Laboratory: Diagnostic and Therapeutic Procedures in the Adult Patient

Mark A. Chaney, MD
Associate Professor
Director of Cardiac Anesthesia
Department of Anesthesia and Critical Care
University of Chicago Hospitals
Chicago, Illinois
37: Pain Management for the Postoperative Cardiac Patient

Davy C. H. Cheng, MD, MSc, FRCPC
Professor and Chair
Department of Anesthesia and Perioperative Medicine
The University of Western Ontario
Chief
Department of Anesthesia and Perioperative Medicine
London Health Sciences Centre
St. Joseph's Health Care London
London, Ontario, Canada
32: Postoperative Cardiac Recovery and Outcomes

Albert T. Cheung, MD
Professor
Department of Anesthesiology and Critical Care Medicine
University of Pennsylvania School of Medicine
Philadelphia, Pennsylvania
23: Thoracic Aortic Disease

John L. Chow, MD, MS
Assistant Professor
Divisions of Cardiovascular Anesthesia and Critical Care Medicine
Department of Anesthesia
Stanford University School of Medicine
Stanford, California
28: Cardiopulmonary Bypass and the Anesthesiologist

David J. Cook, MD
Professor
Department of Anesthesiology
Mayo Clinic College of Medicine
Rochester, Minnesota
20: Valvular Heart Disease: Replacement and Repair

Marianne Coutu, MD, FRCSC
Assistant Professor
Cardiac Surgery Department
University of Sherbrooke Medical Center
Fleurimont, Quebec, Canada
21: Minimally Invasive Cardiac Surgery

Karen B. Domino, MD, MPH
Professor of Anesthesiology
Chair, ASA Committee on Professional Liability
University of Washington School of Medicine
Seattle, Washington
40: Reducing Errors in Cardiac Anesthesiology

Marcel E. Durieux, MD, PhD
Professor, Department of Anesthesiology
Clinical Professor, Department of Neurological Surgery
University of Virginia Medical Center
Charlottesville, Virginia
Professor, Department of Anesthesiology, Pain Management, and Home Ventilation
University Hospital
Maastricht, The Netherlands
7: Molecular Cardiovascular Medicine

Harvey L. Edmonds, Jr., PhD
Director of Cardiovascular Services
Surgical Monitoring Associates, Inc.
Bala Cynwyd, Pennsylvania
17: Central Nervous System Monitoring

Mark L. Edwards, MBChB, FANZCA
Assistant Professor of Anesthesiology
Division of Cardiothoracic Anesthesiology
Department of Anesthesiology
University of Washington School of Medicine
Seattle, Washington
40: Reducing Errors in Cardiac Anesthesiology

Mitchell Faddis, MD, PhD
Associate Professor of Medicine
Cardiovascular Division
Department of Internal Medicine
Washington University School of Medicine
St. Louis, Missouri
13: Cardiac Electrophysiology: Diagnosis and Treatment

Farzan Filsoufi, MD
Assistant Professor
Director, Cardiac Valve Center
Department of Cardiothoracic Surgery
Mount Sinai Medical Center
New York, New York
2: Milestones in Cardiac Surgery

Gregory W. Fischer, MD
Instructor in Anesthesiology
Department of Anesthesiology
Mount Sinai School of Medicine
New York, New York
27: New Approaches to the Surgical Treatment of End-Stage Heart Failure

Lee A. Fleisher, MD, FACC
Robert D. Dripps Professor and Chair
Department of Anesthesia and Critical Care
University of Pennsylvania School of Medicine
Philadelphia, Pennsylvania
11: Assessment of Cardiac Risk and the Cardiology Consultation: Examining, Imaging, Optimizing, and Recommending

Valentin Fuster, MD, PhD
Professor of Cardiology
Mount Sinai School of Medicine
Director
Weiner Cardiovascular Institute and Kravis Center for Cardiovascular Health
Mount Sinai Medical Center
New York, New York
3: The Future of Cardiology

Dean T. Giacobbe, MD
Fellow in Cardiothoracic Anesthesiology
University of Pennsylvania School of Medicine
Philadelphia, Pennsylvania
36: Long-Term Complications and Management

Leanne Groban, MD
Associate Professor
Department of Anesthesiology
Wake Forest University School of Medicine
Winston-Salem, North Carolina
10: Cardiovascular Pharmacology

Hilary P. Grocott, MD, FRCPC
Associate Professor
Department of Anesthesiology
Duke University Medical Center
Durham, North Carolina
30: Organ Protection during Cardiopulmonary Bypass

Kelly L. Grogan, MD
Assistant Professor
Department of Anesthesiology and Critical Care Medicine
The Johns Hopkins University School of Medicine
Anesthesiologist
The Johns Hopkins Hospital
Baltimore, Maryland
9: Pharmacology of Anesthetic Drugs

Eugene A. Hessel II, MD, FACS
Professor, Anesthesiology and Surgery (Cardiothoracic)
University of Kentucky College of Medicine
Attending Anesthesiologist
Chandler University of Kentucky Medical Center
Lexington, Kentucky
1: Evolution of Cardiac Anesthesia and Surgery

Thomas L. Higgins, MD, MBA, FACC
Associate Professor of Medicine and Anesthesiology
Tufts University School of Medicine
Boston, Massachusetts
Chief, Critical Care Division
Departments of Medicine, Surgery and Anesthesiology
Bay State Medical Center
Springfield, Massachusetts
34: Postoperative Respiratory Care

Zak Hillel, MD, PhD
Professor of Clinical Anesthesiology
Columbia University College of Physicians and Surgeons
Director of Cardiac Anesthesia
St. Luke's–Roosevelt Hospital Center
New York, New York
5: Cardiac Physiology

Roberta L. Hines, MD
Nicholas M. Greene Professor of Anesthesiology
Professor and Chair
Department of Anesthesiology
Yale University School of Medicine
Chief of Anesthesia
Yale-New Haven Hospital
New Haven, Connecticut
5: Cardiac Physiology
31: Discontinuing Cardiopulmonary Bypass

Charles W. Hogue, Jr., MD
Associate Professor
Department of Anesthesiology and Critical Care Medicine
Washington School of Medicine
St. Louis, Missouri
13: Cardiac Electrophysiology: Diagnosis and Treatment

Jiri Horak, MD
Assistant Professor
Department of Anesthesiology and Critical Care
University of Pennsylvania School of Medicine
Philadelphia, Pennsylvania
11: Assessment of Cardiac Risk and the Cardiology Consultation: Examining, Imaging, Optimizing, and Recommending

Jay Horrow, MD, FAHA
Professor and Chairman
Department of Anesthesiology
Drexel University School of Medicine
Professor of Epidemiology and Biostatistics
Drexel University School of Public Health
Hahnemann University Hospital
Philadelphia, Pennsylvania
29: Transfusion Medicine and Coagulation Disorders

Philippe R. Housmans, MD, PhD
Professor
Department of Anesthesiology
Mayo Clinic College of Medicine
Rochester, Minnesota
20: Valvular Heart Disease: Replacement and Repair

Ivan Iglesias, MD
Assistant Professor
Department of Anesthesia and Perioperative Medicine
The University of Western Ontario
London Health Sciences Centre–University Hospital
London, Ontario, Canada
35: Central Nervous System Dysfunction after Cardiopulmonary Bypass

Brian Johnson, MD
Associate Staff Anesthesiologist
Department of General Anesthesiology
The Cleveland Clinic
Cleveland, Ohio
5: Cardiac Physiology

Ronald A. Kahn, MD
Associate Professor
Department of Anesthesiology and Surgery
Mount Sinai School of Medicine
Divisional Director, Vascular Anesthesiology
Mount Sinai Medical Center
New York, New York
15: Intraoperative Echocardiography

Max Kanevsky, MD, PhD
Assistant Professor of Anesthesia
Division of Cardiovascular Anesthesia
Department of Anesthesia
Stanford University School of Medicine
Stanford, California
28: Cardiopulmonary Bypass and the Anesthesiologist

Joel A. Kaplan, MD, CPE
Dean Emeritus, School of Medicine
Former Chancellor, Health Sciences Center
Professor of Anesthesiology
University of Louisville School of Medicine
Louisville, Kentucky
Professor, Clinical Anesthesiology
University of California, San Diego, School of Medicine
San Diego, California
5: Cardiac Physiology
14: Monitoring of the Heart and Vascular System
19: Anesthesia for Myocardial Revascularization
29: Transfusion Medicine and Coagulation Disorders
31: Discontinuing Cardiopulmonary Bypass

Steven N. Konstadt, MD, FACC
Professor and Chairman
Department of Anesthesiology
Maimonides Medical Center
New York, New York
15: Intraoperative Echocardiography

Mark Kozak, MD
Associate Professor of Medicine
Department of Medicine
Pennsylvania State University School of Medicine
Staff Cardiologist
Department of Medicine/Cardiology
Milton S. Hershey Medical Center
Hershey, Pennsylvania
12: The Cardiac Catheterization Laboratory: Diagnostic and Therapeutic Procedures in the Adult Patient

Jerrold H. Levy, MD
Professor of Anesthesiology
Emory University School of Medicine
Director of Cardiothoracic Anesthesia
Deputy Chair, Research
Department of Anesthesiology Emory Healthcare
Atlanta, Georgia
33: Postoperative Cardiovascular Management

Michael G. Licina, MD
Staff Anesthesiologist
Department of Cardiothoracic Anesthesiology
The Cleveland Clinic
Cleveland, Ohio
5: Cardiac Physiology

Martin J. London, MD
Professor of Clinical Anesthesia
Department of Anesthesia and Perioperative Care
University of California, San Francisco
Attending Anesthesiologist
San Francisco Veterans Affairs Medical Center
San Francisco, California
19: Anesthesia for Myocardial Revascularization

Michael J. Mercincavage, MAd
Financial Administrator
Department of Clinical Effectiveness and Quality Improvement
University of Pennsylvania Health System
Philadelphia, Pennsylvania
39: Evaluating Quality in Cardiovascular Surgery

Alexander J. Mittnacht, MD
Assistant Professor
Department of Anesthesiology
Mount Sinai School of Medicine
Assistant Attending
Department of Cardiothoracic Anesthesiology
Mount Sinai Hospital
New York, New York
14: Monitoring of the Heart and Vascular System
19: Anesthesia for Myocardial Revascularization

Christina T. Mora-Mangano, MD
Professor of Anesthesia
Stanford University Medical Center
Stanford, California
28: Cardiopulmonary Bypass and the Anesthesiologist

Pedro R. Moreno, MD, FACC
Associate Professor of Medicine/Cardiology
Director, Interventional Cardiology Research
Mount Sinai School of Medicine
New York, New York
3: The Future of Cardiology

J. Paul Mounsey, BM, BCh, PhD
Associate Professor of Medicine
Department of Internal Medicine, Cardiovascular Division
University of Virginia
Charlottesville, Virginia
7: Molecular Cardiovascular Medicine

John M. Murkin, MD, FRCPC
Professor
Consultant and Director of Cardiac Anesthesia
Department of Anesthesia and Perioperative Medicine
The University of Western Ontario
London Health Sciences Centre–University Hospital
London, Ontario, Canada
35: Central Nervous System Dysfunction after Cardiopulmonary Bypass

Andrew W. Murray, MD
Assistant Professor
Department of Anesthesiology
University of Pittsburgh
University of Pittsburgh Medical Center
Presbyterian University Hospital
Pittsburgh, Pennsylvania
26: Anesthesia for Heart, Lung, and Heart-Lung Transplantation

Michael J. Murray, MD
Professor of Anesthesiology
Mayo Clinic College of Medicine
Dean Emeritus
Mayo School of Health Sciences
Chair, Department of Anesthesiology
Mayo Clinic
Jacksonville, Florida
36: Long-Term Complications and Management

Howard J. Nathan, MD
Professor and Vice Chair (Research)
Department of Anesthesiology
University of Ottawa Heart Institute
Ottawa, Ontario, Canada
6: Coronary Physiology and Atherosclerosis

Gregory A. Nuttall, MD
Associate Professor
Department of Anesthesiology
Mayo Clinic College of Medicine
Rochester, Minnesota
24: Uncommon Cardiac Diseases

Daniel Nyhan, MD
Professor and Chief of Cardiac Anesthesia
Department of Anesthesiology and Critical Care Medicine
Associate Professor, Department of Surgery
The Johns Hopkins University School of Medicine
Anesthesiologist
The Johns Hopkins Hospital
Baltimore, Maryland
9: Pharmacology of Anesthetic Drugs

Edward R. M. O'Brien, MD, FRCPC, FACC
Associate Professor of Medicine (Cardiology) and Biochemistry
University of Ottawa
CIHR-Medtronic Research Chair
University of Ottawa Heart Institute
Ottawa, Ontario, Canada
6: Coronary Physiology and Atherosclerosis

William C. Oliver, Jr., MD
Associate Professor
Department of Anesthesiology
Mayo Clinic College of Medicine
Rochester, Minnesota
24: Uncommon Cardiac Diseases

Enrique J. Pantin, MD
Assistant Professor of Anesthesiology
Department of Anesthesia
University of Medicine and Dentistry of New Jersey
Chief, Section of Intraoperative Echocardiography
Chief, Section of Pediatric Anesthesia
Robert Wood Johnson University Hospital
New Brunswick, New Jersey
23: Thoracic Aortic Disease

Joseph J. Quinlan, MD
Associate Professor
Department of Anesthesiology
University of Pittsburgh
Chief Anesthesiologist
University of Pittsburgh Medical Center
Presbyterian University Hospital
Pittsburgh, Pennsylvania
26: Anesthesia for Heart, Lung, and Heart-Lung Transplantation

James G. Ramsay, MD
Professor
Director, Anesthesiology Critical Care
Department of Anesthesiology
Emory University School of Medicine
Anesthesiology Service Chief
Emory University Hospital
Atlanta, Georgia
33: Postoperative Cardiovascular Management

Kent H. Rehfeldt, MD
Assistant Professor
Department of Anesthesiology
Mayo Clinic College of Medicine
Rochester, Minnesota
20: Vascular Heart Disease: Replacement and Repair

David L. Reich, MD
Horace W. Goldsmith
Professor and Chair
Department of Anesthesiology
Mount Sinai School of Medicine
New York, New York
14: Monitoring of the Heart and Vascular System

Bryan J. Robertson, MD
Staff Cardiologist
Allegheny General Hospital
Pittsburgh Cardiology Associates
Pittsburgh, Pennsylvania
12: The Cardiac Catheterization Laboratory: Diagnostic and Therapeutic Procedures in the Adult Patient

Roger L. Royster, MD, FACC
Professor and Executive Vice Chair
Department of Anesthesiology
Wake Forest University School of Medicine
Cardiac Anesthesiologist
Wake Forest University Baptist Medical Center
Winston-Salem, North Carolina
10: Cardiovascular Pharmacology

Marc A. Rozner, PhD, MD
Associate Professor
Departments of Anesthesiology and Cardiology
Associate Anesthesiologist
Department of Anesthesiology and Pain Medicine
University of Texas
M. D. Anderson Cancer Center
Adjunct Assistant Professor of Integrative Biology and Pharmacology
University of Texas Houston Health Science Center
Houston, Texas
25: Cardiac Pacing and Electroversion

Sacha P. Salzberg, MD
Postdoctoral Research Fellow
Department of Cardiothoracic Surgery
Mount Sinai Medical Center
New York, New York
2: Milestones in Cardiac Surgery

Javier Sanz, MD
Instructor
Clinical MR/CT Program
Wiener Cardiovascular Institute and Kravis Center for Cardiovascular Health
Mount Sinai Medical Center
New York, New York
3: The Future of Cardiology

Robert Savage, MD
Staff Anesthesiologist
Department of Cardiothoracic Anesthesiology
The Cleveland Clinic Foundation
Cleveland, Ohio
5: Cardiac Physiology

Joseph Silio Savino, MD
Associate Professor
Department of Anesthesiology and Critical Care
University of Pennsylvania School of Medicine
Vice Chairman for Strategic Planning and Clinical Operations
Section Chief
Cardiovascular Thoracic Anesthesia and Critical Care
Department of Anesthesiology and Critical Care
University of Pennsylvania Health System
Philadelphia, Pennsylvania
16: Decision Making and Perioperative Echocardiography
39: Evaluating Quality in Cardiovascular Surgery

Alan Jay Schwartz, MD, MSEd
Clinical Professor of Anesthesiology
Department of Anesthesiology and Critical Care Medicine
University of Pennsylvania
Senior Anesthesiologist
Pediatric Anesthesiology Fellowship Director and Director of Education
Children's Hospital of Philadelphia
Philadelphia, Pennsylvania
41: Cardiac Anesthesia: Training, Qualifications, Teaching, and Learning

Jack S. Shanewise, MD, FASE
Associate Professor of Clinical Anesthesiology
Director, Division of Cardiothoracic Anesthesiology
Department of Anesthesiology
Columbia University College of Physicians and Surgeons
Chief of Cardiac Anesthesia
Columbia-Presbyterian Hospital
New York, New York
31: Discontinuing Cardiopulmonary Bypass

Stanton K. Shernan, MD
Assistant Professor of Anesthesia
Department of Anesthesiology, Perioperative and Pain Medicine
Harvard Medical School
Director of Cardiac Anesthesia
Brigham and Women's Hospital
Boston, Massachusetts
15: Intraoperative Echocardiography

Linda Shore-Lesserson, MD
Associate Professor
Department of Anesthesiology
Mount Sinai Medical School
Chief, Division of Cardiothoracic Anesthesiology
Director, Fellowship in Cardiothoracic Anesthesiology
Mount Sinai Medical Center
New York, New York
18: Coagulation Monitoring

Thomas F. Slaughter, MD
Professor of Anesthesiology
Department of Anesthesiology
Section on Cardiothoracic Anesthesiology
Wake Forest University School of Medicine
Winston-Salem, North Carolina
10: Cardiovascular Pharmacology

Bruce D. Spiess, MD, FAHA
Professor of Anesthesiology and Emergency Medicine
Department of Anesthesia
Director of Research
Department of Anesthesiology
VCU–Medical College of Virginia
Richmond, Virginia
29: Transfusion Medicine and Coagulation Disorders

Mark Stafford-Smith, MD, CM, FRCPC
Associate Professor
Department of Anesthesiology
Duke University Medical Center
Durham, North Carolina
30: Organ Protection during Cardiopulmonary Bypass

Marc E. Stone, MD
Assistant Professor
Department of Anesthesiology
Mount Sinai School of Medicine
Attending Physician
Director of Education, Cardiothoracic Anesthesiology
Mount Sinai Medical Center
New York, New York
27: New Approaches to the Surgical Treatment of End-Stage Heart Failure

Cephas P. Swamidoss, MD, MS, MPH
Associate Professor of Clinical Anesthesiology
Department of Anesthesia
Weill Cornell Medical College
Assistant Attending Anesthesiologist
New York–Presbyterian Hospital
New York, New York
4: The Future of Cardiac Surgery and Anesthesia

Kenichi Tanaka, MD
Assistant Professor of Anesthesiology
Department of Anesthesiology
Emory University School of Medicine
Atlanta, Georgia
Attending Physician
Department of Anesthesiology
Veterans Affairs Medical Center
Decatur, Georgia
33: Postoperative Cardiovascular Management

Daniel M. Thys, MD
Professor of Clinical Anesthesiology
Columbia University College of Physicians and Surgeons
Chairman, Department of Anesthesiology
St. Luke's–Roosevelt Hospital Center
New York, New York
5: Cardiac Physiology

Mark F. Trankina, MD
Associate Professor
University of Alabama School of Medicine
Staff Anesthesiologist
St. Vincent's Hospital
Birmingham, Alabama
25: Cardiac Pacing and Electroversion

Juan F. Viles-Gonzalez, MD
Research Fellow
Cardiovascular Biology
Wiener Cardiovascular Institute and Kravis Center for Cardiovascular Health
Mount Sinai School of Medicine
New York, New York
3: The Future of Cardiology

Stuart Joel Weiss, MD, PhD
Associate Professor
Department of Anesthesiology and Critical Care
University of Pennsylvania School of Medicine
Philadelphia, Pennsylvania
16: Decision-Making and Perioperative Transesophageal Echocardiography

Jean-Pierre Yared, MD
Medical Director, Cardiovascular Intensive Care Unit
Department of Cardiac Anesthesiology and Critical Care
The Cleveland Clinic Foundation
Cleveland, Ohio
34: Postoperative Respiratory Care

James R. Zaidan, MD, MBA
Professor and Chair
Associate Dean for Graduate Medical Education
Emory University School of Medicine
Department of Anesthesiology
Atlanta, Georgia
38: Financial Aspects of Patient Care

David A. Zvara, MD
Associate Professor of Cardiothoracic Anesthesiology
Department of Anesthesiology
Wake Forest University School of Medicine
Winston-Salem, North Carolina
10: Cardiovascular Pharmacology

PREFACE

The fifth edition of *Cardiac Anesthesia* has been written to further improve the anesthetic management of the patient with cardiac disease undergoing cardiac or noncardiac surgery. Since publication of the first edition in 1979, continued advances in this field have made it the leading subspeciality in anesthesiology. In order to maintain its place as the standard reference textbook, this edition has been completely revised, expanded, and updated throughout to reflect the ongoing changes in cardiovascular care. Significant contributions to the text have been made by leading cardiologists and cardiac surgeons to fully cover the broader aspects of the total care of the cardiac patient.

The introductory section has been added to recognize the fiftieth anniversary of the first successful open-heart surgical procedure performed using cardiopulmonary bypass, by John H. Gibbon, Jr., MD, at Jefferson Hospital in Philadelphia on May 6, 1953. This great pioneer was my surgical professor when I was a medical student at Jefferson, from 1964 to 1968, and it was on his surgical service that I first became interested in the perioperative care of cardiac patients. It was my good fortune to have observed some of the early care and to have participated in advancing some of the management of cardiac surgical patients. I have invited other leaders in the field to detail the past, update information on the present level of care, and predict the future care and strategies for patients with cardiovascular disease.

After the introductory section, the content of *Kaplan's Cardiac Anesthesia* ranges from the basic sciences through translational medicine to the clinical care of the sickest cardiac patients. The final section emphasizes quality of care, training standards, and reducing errors in the practice of cardiac anesthesia. Because of the large volume of material, tables, and figures, several teaching aids have been added to this edition to help highlight the most important information. The Key Points in each chapter are listed on the first page and serve as an outline of the content, and Teaching Boxes have been included with many of the "take-home messages."

The text is organized into eight sections: (I) Past, Present, and Future; (II) Cardiovascular Physiology, Pharmacology, and Molecular Biology, including the latest cardiovascular molecular medicine; (III) Preoperative Evaluation, with expanded sections on interventional cardiology and the electrophysiology laboratory; (IV) Monitoring, including a new chapter on decision making based on transesophageal echocardiography; (V) Anesthetic Techniques for Cardiac Surgical Procedures, with new chapters on minimally invasive surgery and treatment of end-stage heart failure; (VI) Extracorporeal Circulation, with an emphasis on organ protection; (VII) Postoperative Care, with the latest material on pain management; and (VIII) Practice Management. The emphasis throughout is on using the latest scientific developments to guide proper therapeutic interventions in the perioperative period.

Kaplan's Cardiac Anesthesia was written by the acknowledged experts in each specific area or related specialties. It is the most authoritative and up-to-date collection of material in the field. Each chapter aims to provide the scientific foundation in the area as well as the clinical basis for practice. All of the chapters have been coordinated in an effort to maximize their clinical utility. Whenever possible, material has been integrated from the fields of anesthesiology, cardiology, cardiac surgery, and pharmacology to present a complete clinical picture. Thus, this edition should serve as the definitive text for cardiac anesthesia residents, fellows, attendings, cardiologists, cardiac surgeons, intensivists, and others interested in the management of the patient with cardiac disease for either cardiac or noncardiac surgery.

This edition should also further facilitate the application of the techniques and procedures that have been learned in cardiac surgical operating rooms to cardiac patients undergoing noncardiac surgery. These patients compose a larger group than those undergoing cardiac surgery, and they are often sicker and at higher risk, since their underlying cardiac disease is not corrected by the operative procedure. Cardiac anesthesiologists are increasingly applying their skills to improve outcomes for these patients.

The publication of the first edition of *Cardiac Anesthesia* solidified the foundation of the subspecialty and was followed by other textbooks and a journal in the field. In addition, many cardiac anesthesiologists have become leaders in academic medicine, serving as deans, vice presidents, and chancellors. These developments reflect the maturity of the field, the excellence of our practitioners, and the wide contributions anesthesiologists have always made to medicine. This edition is being published at a time when many changes are taking place in our speciality and all of medicine. There is a great need to continue to produce excellent specialists in anesthesiology in order to be able to care for the expanding pool of elderly and sick patients. It is hoped that *Kaplan's Cardiac Anesthesia* will contribute to the education of these future outstanding clinicians, educators, and researchers.

The editors gratefully acknowledge the contributions made by the authors of each of the chapters. They are the dedicated experts who have made the field of cardiac anesthesia what it is today and are the teachers of our young colleagues practicing anesthesiology around the world. This book would not have been possible without their hard work and expertise.

Joel A. Kaplan, MD, CPE, FACC
Editor

CONTENTS

Color plates precede Section I.

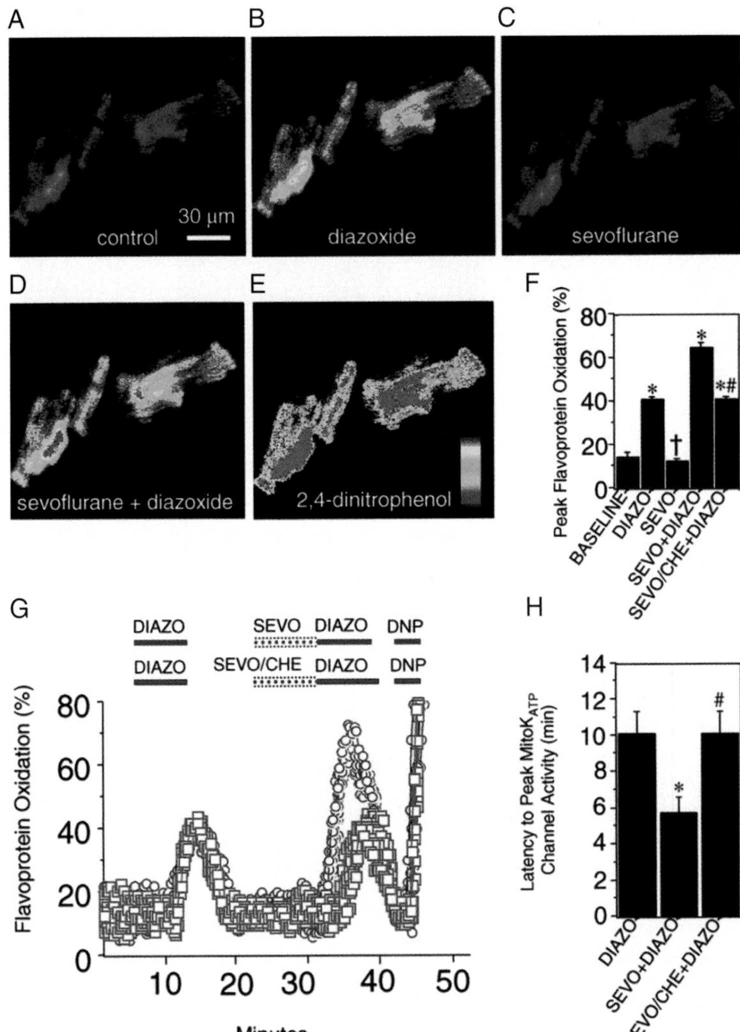

Figure 9–13 Effect of sevoflurane (SEVO) (2.8% [vol/vol]) on diazoxide (DIAZO)-induced flavoprotein oxidation in myocytes excited at 480 nm. Similar results were obtained for isoflurane. An artificial color scale was used to visualize the relative intensity of emitted fluorescence at 530 nm (dark blue indicates reduced flavoproteins; red indicates fully oxidized flavoproteins). (*A*) At baseline. (*B*) At 100 μm DIAZO (same cells). (*C*) At 2 MAC SEVO. (*D*) At 100 μm DIAZO preceded by 2 MAC SEVO. Red color indicates intense local oxidation by mitochondrial clusters. (*E*) At 100 μm 2,4-dinitrophenol (DNP). (*F*) Mean percentages of peak flavoprotein fluorescence depending on the drugs exposed to myocytes. **P* < 0.0001 versus baseline or SEVO + DIAZO versus DIAZO alone. #*P* not significantly different from DIAZO. †*P* not significantly different from baseline. SEVO/CHE indicates concomitant treatment of myocytes with SEVO and chelerythrine (CHE) at 2 μm before exposure to DIAZO. (*G*) Time-lapse analysis of alterations in fluorescence intensity in individual myocytes expressed as percentage of DNP-induced fluorescence (see text). The blue squares and red circles indicate values from eight different experiments. (*H*) Latency to peak activation of mitoK$_{ATP}$ channels in response to the various treatment regimens. **P* < 0.001 versus DIAZO. #*P* not significant versus DIAZO. Data are mean ± SD.[100]

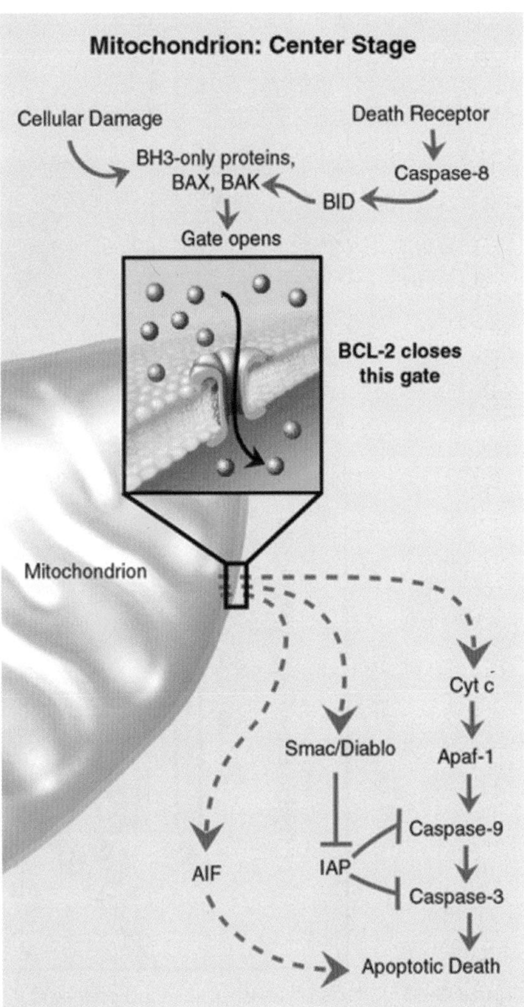

Figure 9–14 Center stage in apoptosis. In this view, numerous cell-death stimuli work through the mitochondria. They cause proapoptotic members of the BCL-2 family, such as BAX and BAK, to either open new pores or modify existing channels in the mitochondrial membrane, releasing cytochrome *c* and other proteins that lead to caspase activation and cell death. BCL-2 itself, which is antiapoptotic, somehow blocks the pore or channel opening.[500]

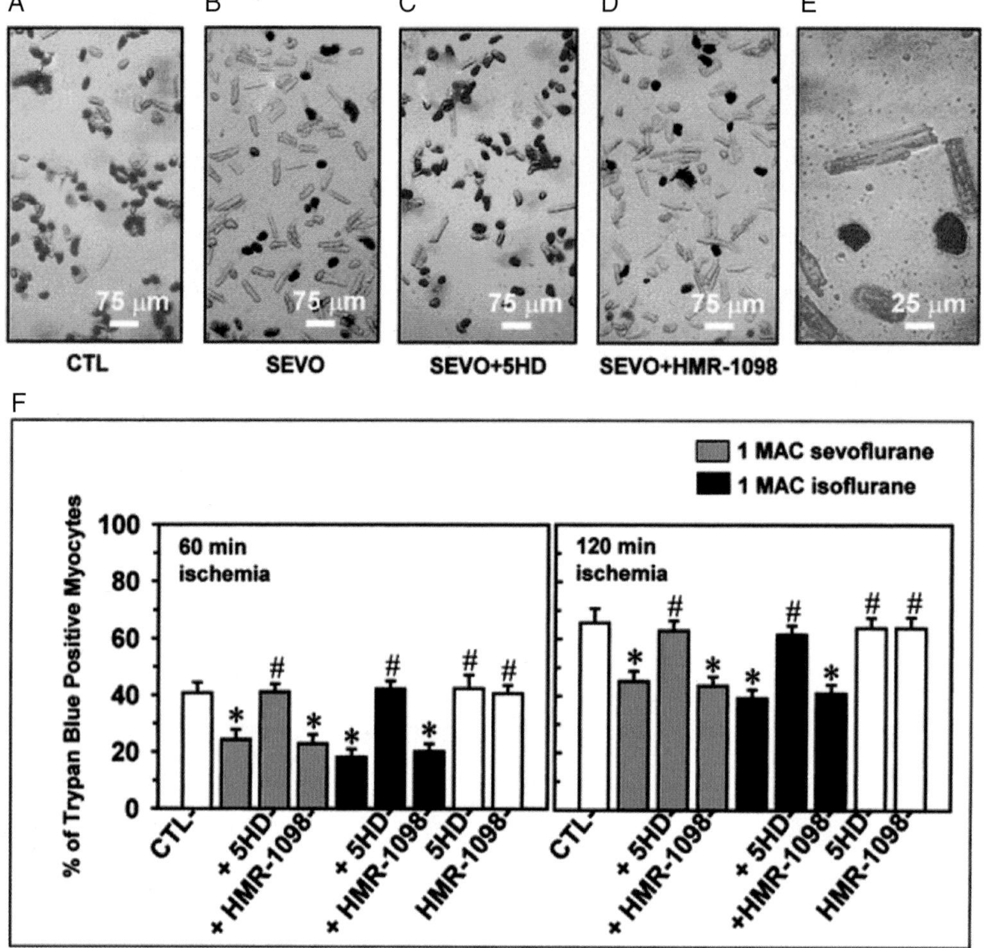

Figure 9–15 Effects of the specific mitochondrial K_{ATP} (mitoK_{ATP}) channel blocker 5-hydroxy-decanoate (5HD) and the specific sarcolemmal K_{ATP} (sarcK_{ATP}) channel blocker HMR-1098 on sevoflurane (SEVO)- and isoflurane (ISO)-mediated protection at 1 MAC against 60 or 120 minutes of ischemia in myocytes as assessed by trypan blue staining. (*A*) Control myocytes after 60 min of ischemia. Myocytes staining dark blue indicate irreversible cell damage. (*B*) Myocytes exposed to SEVO before ischemia. Most myocytes retain their rod-shaped morphology. (*C*) Myocytes exposed to 5HD and SEVO before ischemia. The protective effect of SEVO is abolished. (*D*) Myocytes exposed to HMR-1098 and SEVO before ischemia. The protection by SEVO is unaffected. (*E*) Representative trypan blue–positive and –negative myocytes after exposure to ischemia seen at higher magnification. (*F*) Trypan blue–positive myocytes are indicated as percentage of total viable myocytes before ischemia. CTL indicates control group and represents myocytes exposed to 60 or 120 min of ischemia alone. Data are mean ± SD. *$P < 0.0001$ versus respective CTL. #*P* not significant versus respective CTL.[100]

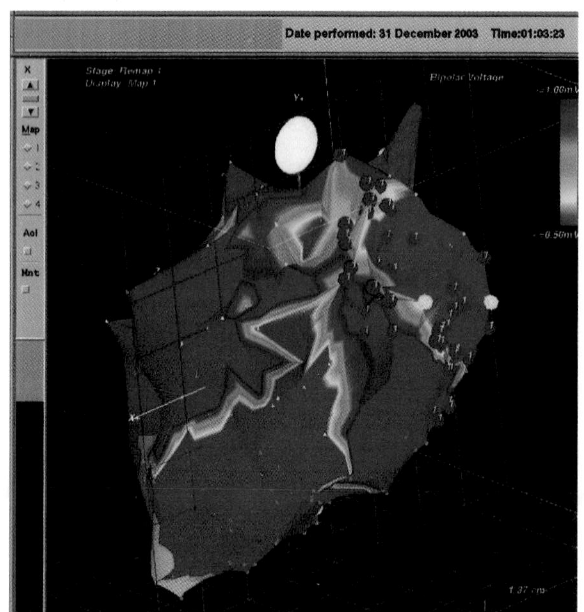

Figure 13–28 Electroanatomic mapping to guide catheter ablation of ventricular tachycardia. An electroanatomical map of the left ventricle of a patient with an ischemic cardiomyopathy complicated by ventricular tachycardia is shown. The posterolateral aspect of the left ventricle is displayed with color coding for the size of the ventricular electrograms recorded from the endocardial surface. Regions of myocardial scar are plotted in red corresponding to electrograms of less than 0.5 mV, and regions of viable myocardium corresponding to electrograms greater than 1.0 mV are plotted in purple. Border zones around myocardial scars are in between these regions. One border zone in this patient represents the location of "exit sites" for multiple forms of hemodynamically unstable ventricular tachycardia. Catheter ablation at sites plotted as red circles resulted in disruption of all forms of ventricular tachycardia.

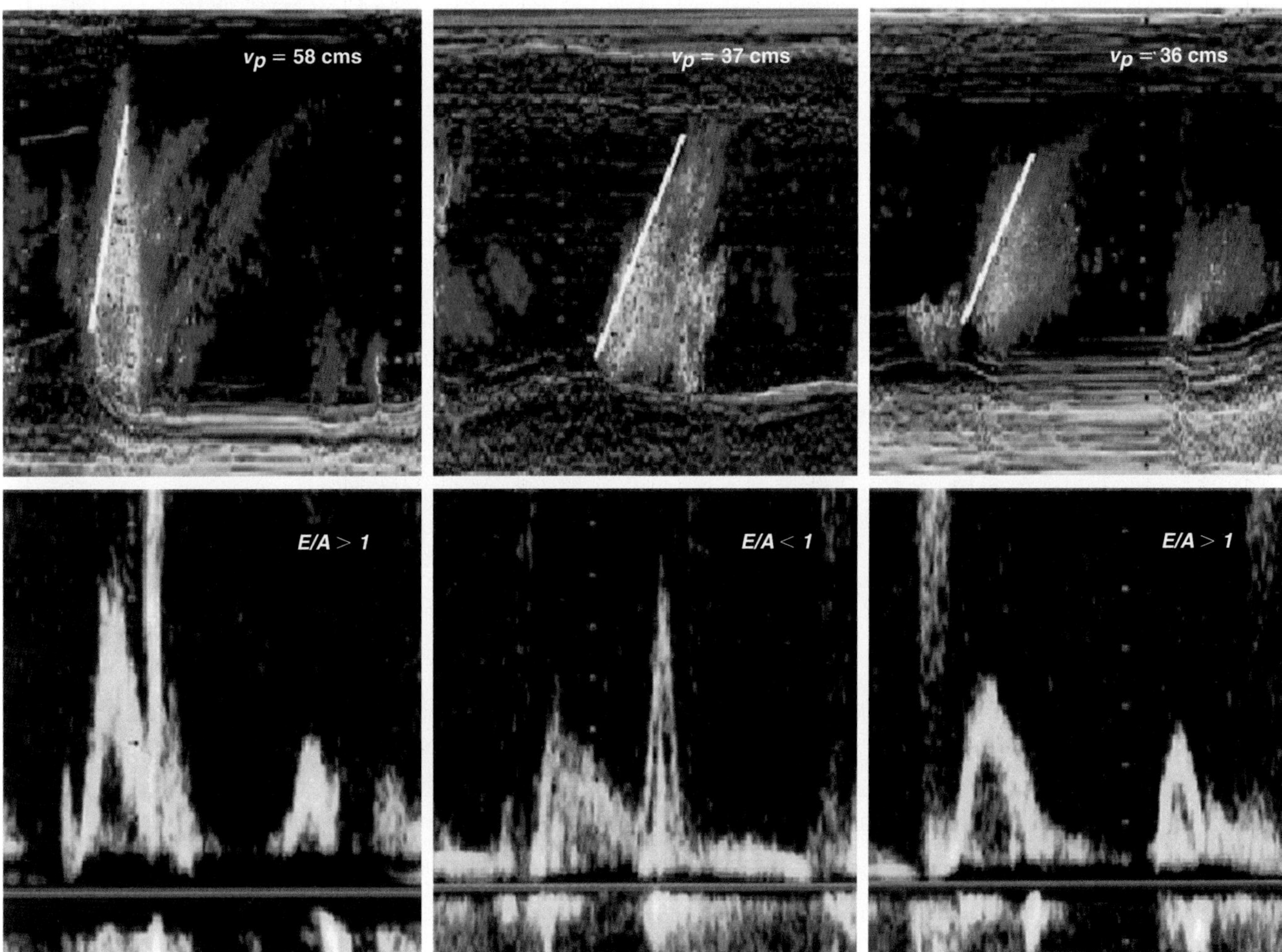

Figure 15–14 Color M-mode Doppler and pulsed-wave Doppler images of left ventricular filling. *Left*, Normal filling pattern (vp = 58 cm/sec, E/A > 1). *Middle*, Delayed relaxation (DR) filling pattern (vp = 37 cm/sec, E/A < 1). *Right*, Pseudo-normal (PN) filling pattern (vp = 36 cm/sec, E/A > 1). (Reproduced with permission from De Meya S, De Sutterb J, Vierendeelsa J, Verdoncka P: Diastolic filling and pressure imaging: Taking advantage of the information in a colour M-mode Doppler image. Eur J Echocardiogr 2:219, 2001, with permission from the European society of Cardiology.)

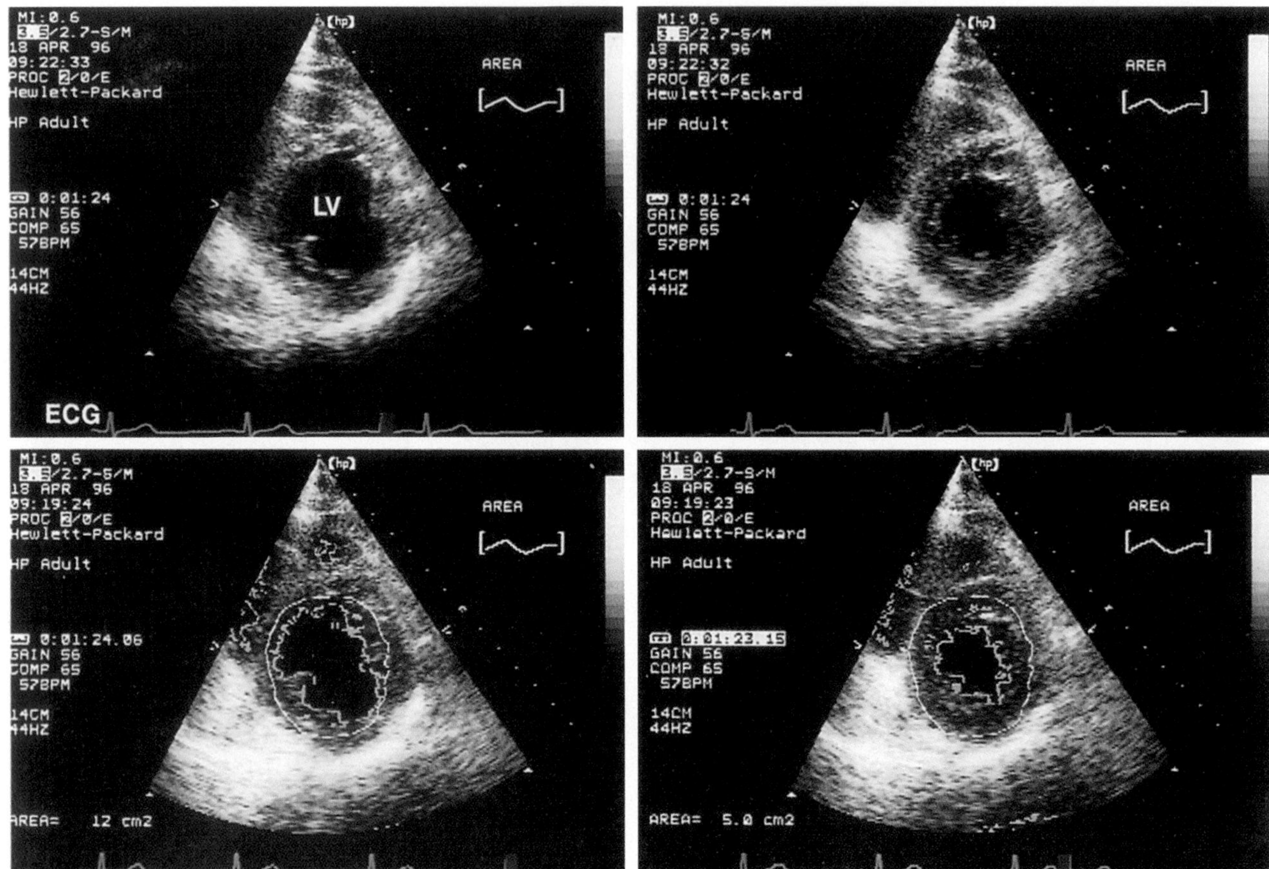

Figure 15–18 Automated endocardial tracking derived from the analysis of integrated backscattered ultrasound signals from the interface between blood pool and myocardium. All four stop-frame transthoracic echocardiographic images display the short-axis profile of the left ventricle (LV) at the level of the papillary muscles with anterior structures near the apex of the sector and the patient's left positioned on the right side of the image. An electrocardiographic (ECG) trace is depicted in green and interrupted at the point of acquisition of the stop-frame image. Depth calibrations are at 1.0-cm intervals. *Upper left panel:* Diastolic stop-frame image of the short-axis image of the LV cavity demonstrates distinct endocardial margins. *Lower left panel:* Diastolic stop frame image of the LV (corresponding to *upper left panel*) with superimposed user-defined region of interest (blue closed loop). Automated endocardial tracking is depicted by light brown-colored contours and closely follows the endocardial contours depicted in the *upper left panel. Upper right panel:* Systolic stop-frame image of the short-axis image of the LV cavity demonstrates clear delineation of the endocardium. *Lower right panel:* Systolic stop-frame image of the LV (corresponding to *upper right panel* with superimposed user-defined region of interest (blue closed loop). Automated endocardial tracking is depicted by light brown-colored contours of the blood pool myocardial interface, which closely follows the endocardium depicted in the upper right panel. (From Louie EK, Louie DS: New echocardiographic technology: Does it add to clinical decision making? Semin Cardiothorac Vasc Anesth 1:16, 1997.)

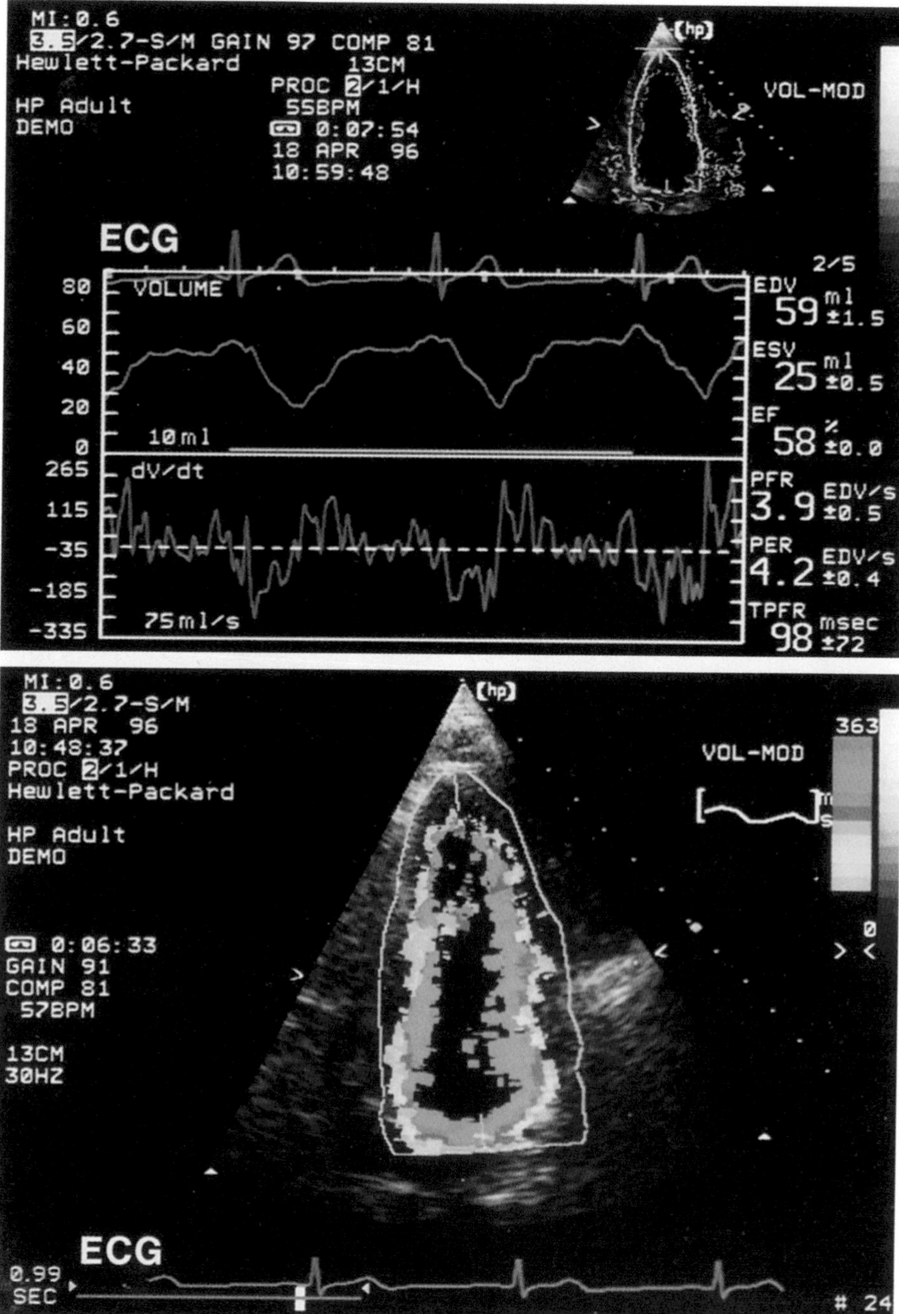

Figure 15–19 Derived indices of global and regional systolic left ventricular function from automated endocardial tracking of integrated backscattered ultrasound signals. The miniature B-mode image in the *upper right hand corner of the upper panel* (transthoracic echocardiographic apical four-chamber view) displays the image of the left ventricle along with the user-defined region of interest (blue closed loop that includes a semiautomated determination of the mitral annular plane and the left ventricular long axis). The light brown trace indicates the tracking of the left ventricular endocardium and the mitral annular plane. The apical four-chamber image permits derivation of left ventricular volumes by a single-plane modified Simpson formula. Depth calibrations are at 1.0-cm intervals. Derived parameters are presented as time varying graphics (green traces) below the electrocardiogram (ECG). The instantaneous time varying volume curve for the left ventricle is represented by the *upper trace* and permits derivation of the average left ventricular end-diastolic volume (59 + 1.5 mL), end-systolic volume (25 + 0.5 mL), and ejection fraction (58 + 0.0 percent). The *lower trace* represents the first derivative (dV/dt) of the volume curve and permits measurement of the peak left ventricular diastolic filling rate (3.9 + 0.5 end-diastolic volumes/sec), peak systolic ejection rate (4.2 + 0.4 end-diastolic volumes/sec), and the time from the QRS to the peak filling rate (98 + 72 msec). *Lower panel:* Color-encoded isochronal maps of systolic endocardial excursion are mapped onto the B-mode echocardiographic image of the transthoracic apical four-chamber view of the left ventricle. The blue closed loop represents the user-defined region of interest. The color scale (*upper right corner*) represents isochronal intervals beginning with the initial 33-msec interval following the QRS (orange) and successively progressing at 33-msec intervals through shades of yellow, green, and blue. The concentric rings of color superimposed on the B-mode echocardiographic image of this normal left ventricle represent successive isochronal maps of the inward excursion of the endocardium during systole. The width of any given color zone represents the magnitude of endocardial excursion at that particular segment of the left ventricle for the specified isochronal interval. Qualitative and quantitative assessment of regional systolic function is possible from such images. Equivalent isochronal maps of diastolic endocardial motion could also be constructed to assess global and regional left ventricular filling patterns.

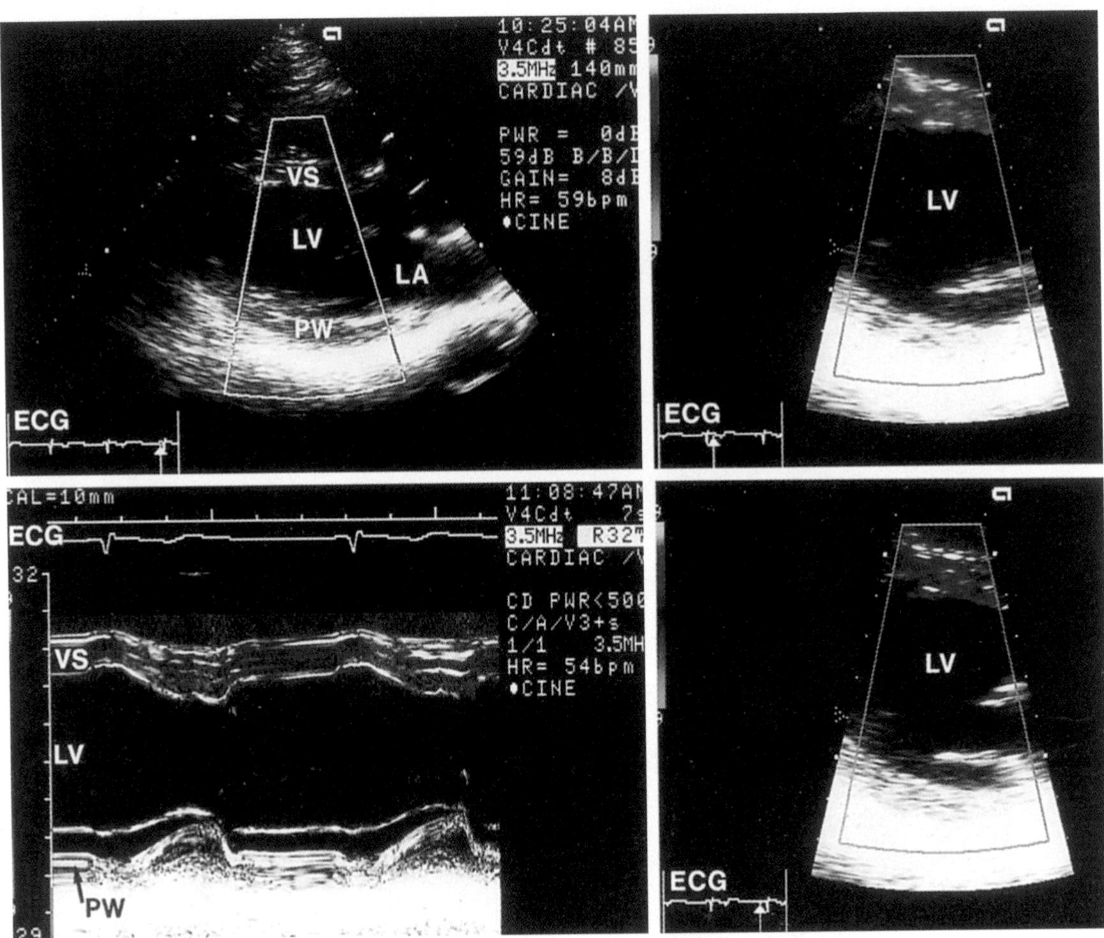

Figure 15–20 Color Doppler myocardial velocity mapping. *Upper left panel:* Stop-frame diastolic image from a cine loop of the transthoracic parasternal long-axis image of the left ventricle (LV) and left atrium (LA). The ventricular septum (VS) and left ventricular posterior walls (PW) are clearly imaged. Timing of the stop frame is indicated by the *arrow* referenced to the electrocardiogram (ECG) in the *lower left corner of the panel*. The quadrilateral region of interest superimposed on the B-mode image is redisplayed in the upper and lower right panels. Depth calibrations are at 5-cm intervals (bright dots) and 1-cm intervals (subdued dots). *Upper right panel:* Early systolic stop-frame image from the transthoracic parasternal long-axis image of the LV with superimposed color Doppler myocardial velocity mapping. Myocardial velocities relative to the transducer (located at the apex of the sector) range from shades of blue (9 cm/sec directed away from the transducer) to shades of red (9 cm/sec directed toward the transducer) as depicted by the color bar on the *left side of the panel*. Note the ventricular septum is encoded blue as it contracts toward the center of the LV (away from the transducer) and the posterior wall is encoded red as it contracts toward the center of the LV (toward the transducer). *Lower right panel*: The display format is the same as in the upper right panel except a late diastolic stop-frame image is shown. Now the left ventricular septum is moving outward (encoded red for motion towards the transducer) and the posterior wall is also moving away from the center of the left ventricle (encoded blue for motion away from the transducer). *Lower left panel*: M-mode echocardiogram at the level of the chordae tendineae targeted from a transthoracic parasternal long-axis view of the LV (such as that portrayed in the *upper left panel*). The superimposed color Doppler map of myocardial velocities is derived from a transducer located at the top of the M-mode image. The VS and PW are clearly delineated and the simultaneous ECG is provided for timing purposes. Depth calibrations are at 1.0-cm intervals and time calibrations are at 200-msec intervals (minor divisions). The VS is encoded blue during systole, because it is moving toward the center of the LV and away from the transducer and red during diastole when it is moving away from the center of the LV and toward the transducer. The PW shows a reciprocal pattern of color Doppler myocardial velocity mapping, which is less well demonstrated in this image. The inherently high sampling rate of the dedicated single M-mode Doppler sampling beam permits high temporal resolution of the myocardial velocity map.

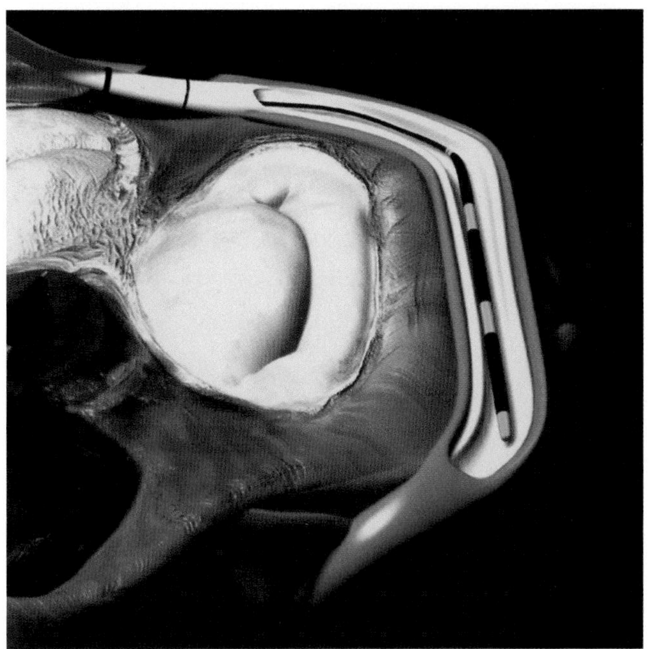

Figure 20–32 Effect of annuloplasty device on mitral annular geometry. The annuloplasty device decreases the distance between the anterior and posterior annulus, increasing leaflet coaptation. (From Liddicoat JR, MacNiell BD, Gillinov AM, et al: Percutaneous mitral valve repair: A feasibility study in a bovine model of acute ischemic mitral regurgitation. Catheter Cardiovasc Interv 60:411, 2003.)

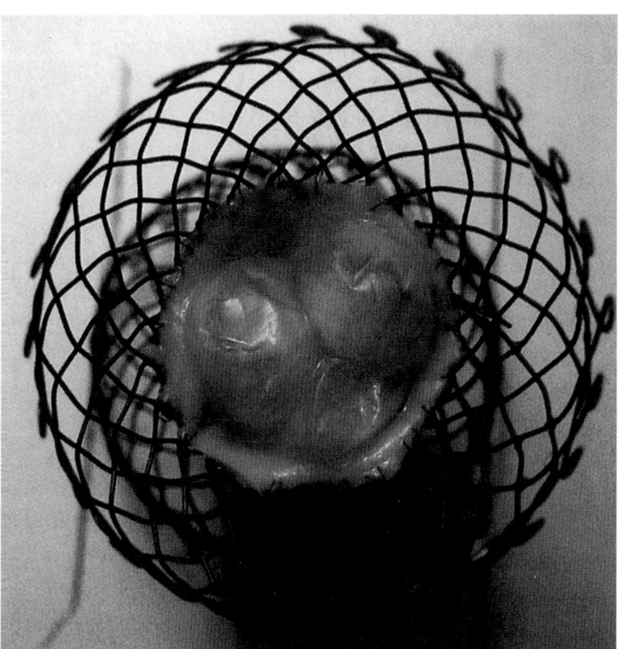

Figure 20–33 A front view of the stent, showing the pulmonary valve in the closed position, as seen from the ventricular side. (From Boudjemline Y, Agnoletti G, Bonnet D, et al: Percutaneous pulmonary valve replacement in a large right ventricular outflow tract. J Am Coll Cardiol 43:1082, 2004.)

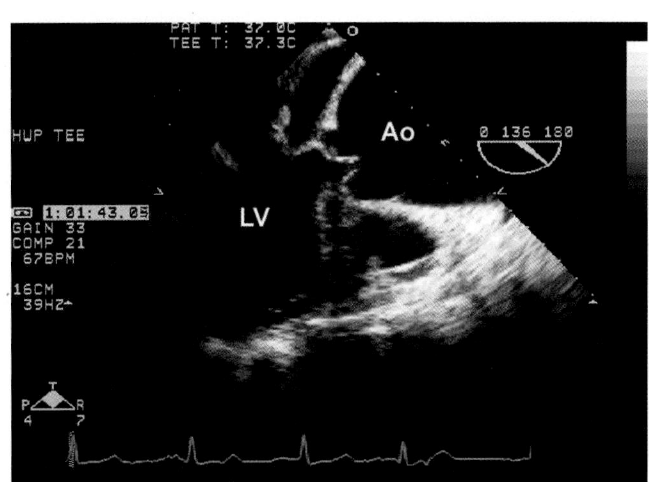

A

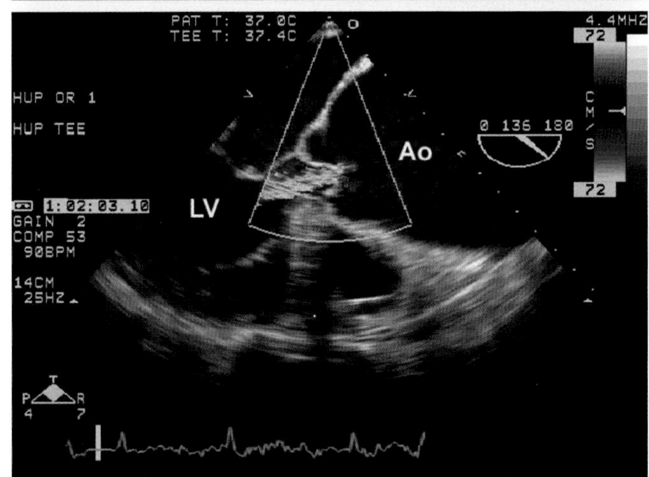

B

Figure 23–1 TEE mid-esophageal long-axis images of the aortic valve demonstrating aneurysmal dilation of the aortic root and ascending aorta (*A*). Doppler color flow imaging (*B*) demonstrating severe aortic regurgitation caused by outward tethering of the aortic valve cusps by the aortic aneurysm. LV = left ventricle; Ao = aorta.

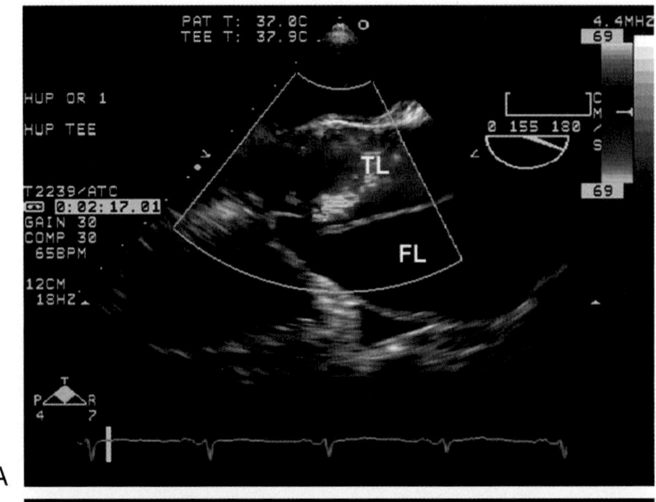

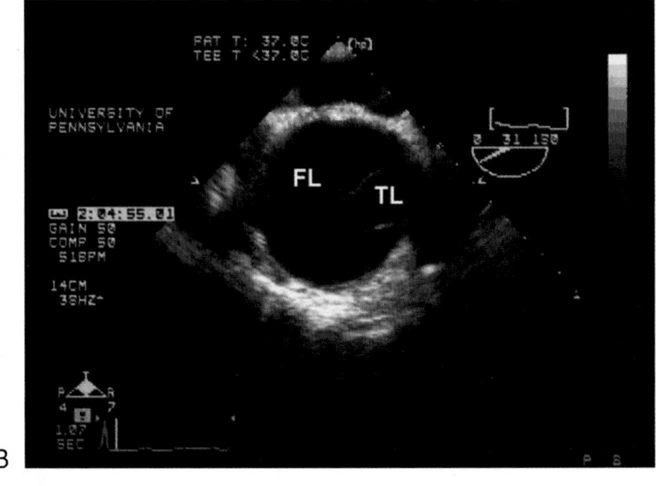

Figure 23–26 TEE mid-esophageal long-axis image of the aortic valve (*A*) and short-axis image of the ascending aorta (*B*) in a patient with a type A aortic dissection. An intimal flap separating the true lumen (TL) of the aorta with the false lumen (FL) was demonstrated in the aortic root and ascending aorta. Extension of the dissection into the aortic root may cause aortic regurgitation or coronary insufficiency.

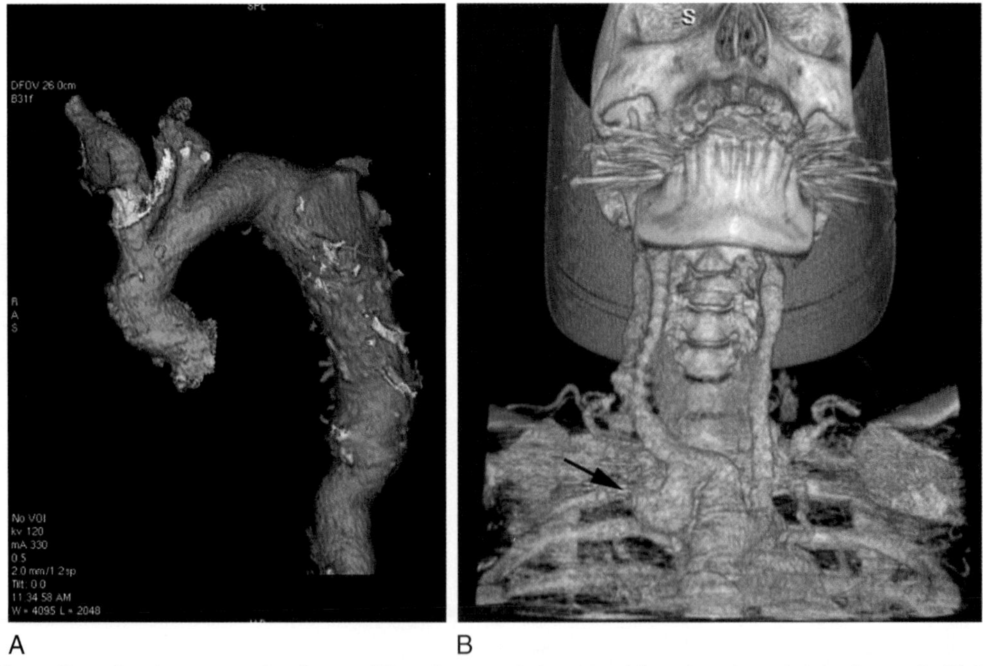

Figure 23–29 Three-dimensional reconstruction from a CT angiogram of the aorta (*A*) and aortic arch branch vessels (*B*) from a patient with Takayasu's arteritis. The reconstructions demonstrated aneurysmal dilation of the descending thoracic aorta, proximal innominate artery, and both subclavian arteries. The left and right (*arrow*) subclavian arteries were occluded distal to the aneurysm.

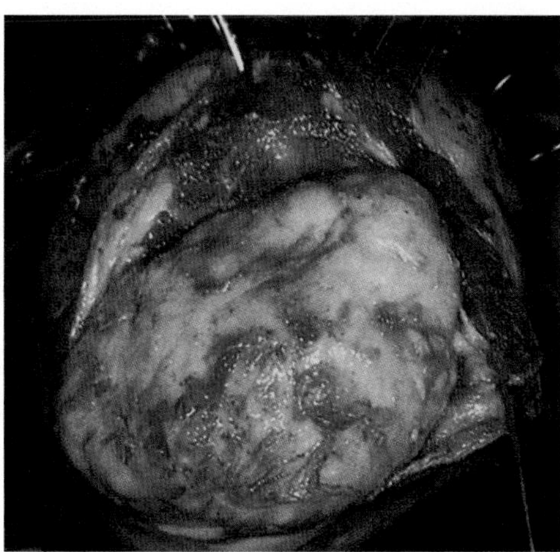

Figure 24–3 Dissection of ventricular fibroma (patient 12; patient's head is at top). (Reprinted with permission from Cho JM, Danielson GK, Puga FJ, et al: Surgical resection of ventricular cardiac fibromas: Early and late results. Ann Thorac Surg 76:1933, 2003.)

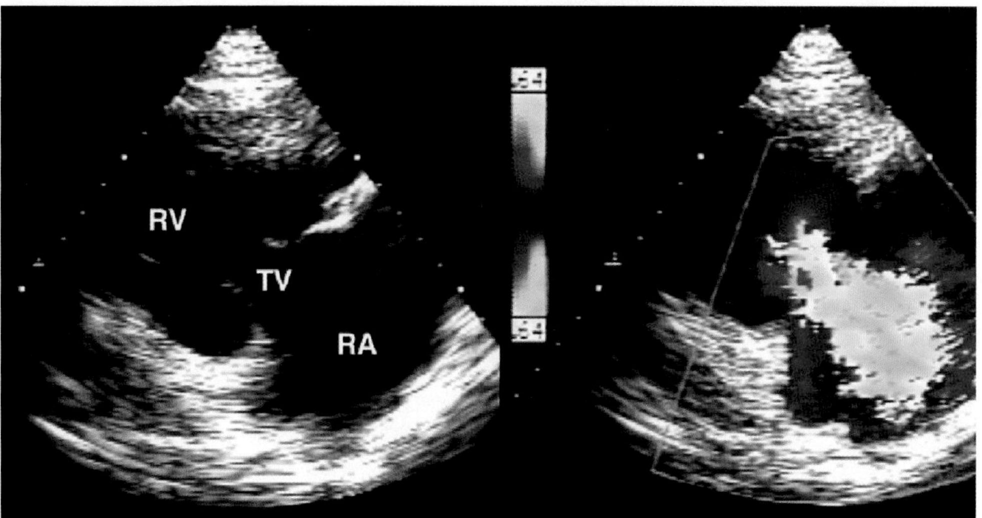

Figure 24–4 Echocardiogram of a patient with carcinoid heart disease displaying the right ventricle (RV), tricuspid valve (TV), and right atrium (RA) showing thickening and tethering of the TV due to carcinoid plaque (*left*) resulting in poor coaptation of the TV leaflets with severe tricuspid regurgitation demonstrated by the large color jet in the RA with ventricular systole (*right*). (Reprinted with permission from Oh JK, Seward JB, Tajik AJ: The Echo Manual, 2nd edition. Philadelphia, Lippincott Williams & Wilkins, 1999; © Mayo Foundation, Click RL, Olson LJ, Edwards WD, et al, Mayo Clinic, Department of Cardiovascular Diseases, Rochester, MN 55905: Echocardiography and systemic diseases. J Am Soc Echocardiogr 7:201, 1994, Fig. 13–7.)

Figure 24–5 Photograph of a pulmonary valve excised from a patient with carcinoid heart disease showing carcinoid plaques that have caused cusp thickening and annular constriction (leading to stenosis) and cusp retraction with a fixed triangular orifice (leading to regurgitation). Carcinoid plaques in the pulmonary artery sinuses behind the cusps have produced irregular ridges that simulate coronary artery ostia (*arrows*). (Reprinted with permission from Oh JK, Seward JB, Tajik AJ: The Echo Manual, 2nd edition. Philadelphia, Lippincott Williams & Wilkins, 1999; © Mayo Foundation, Click RL, Olson LJ, Edwards WD, et al, Mayo Clinic, Department of Cardiovascular Diseases, Rochester, MN 55905: Echocardiography and systemic diseases. J Am Soc Echocardiogr 7:201, 1994, Fig. 13–6.)

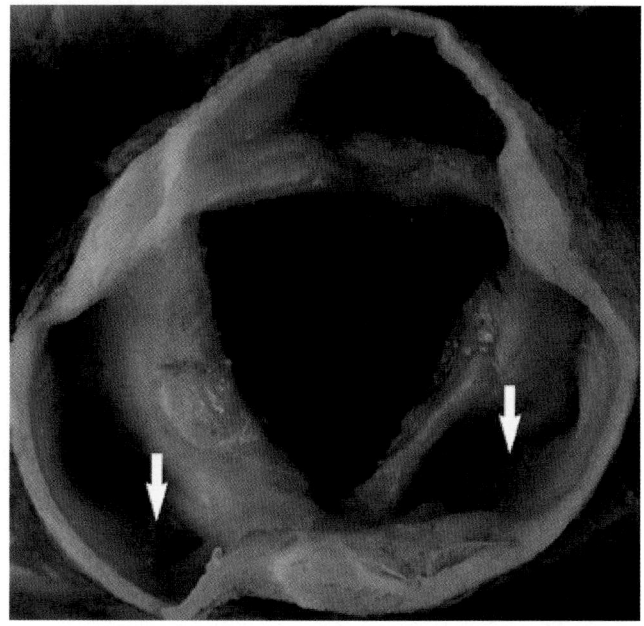

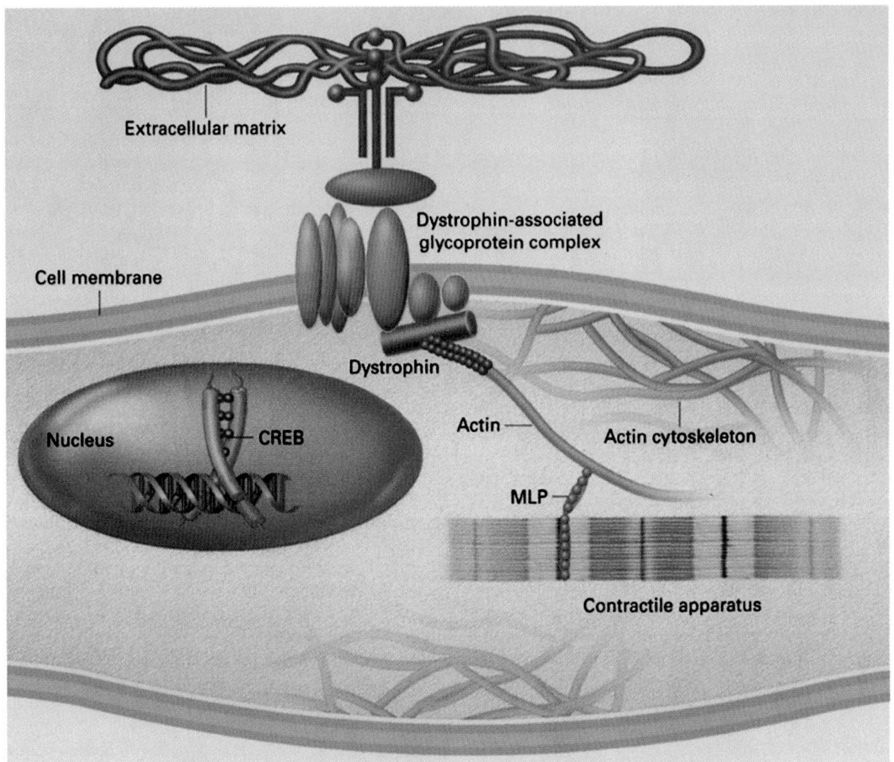

Figure 24–6 A cardiac myocyte and the molecules that have been implicated in dilated cardiomyopathy. (Reprinted with permission from Leiden JM: The genetics of dilated cardiomyopathy—Emerging clues to the puzzle. N Engl J Med 337;1080, 1997.)

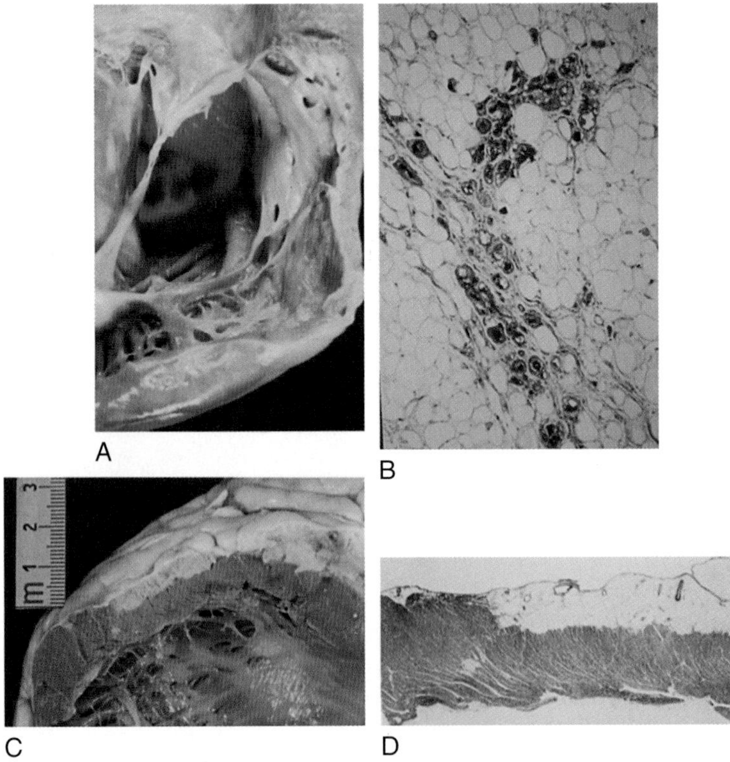

Figure 24–19 *(A)* Histologic view at high magnification of surviving degenerated right ventricular myocytes in the setting of extensive fatty replacement and tiny interstitial fibrosis. *(B)* Gross *(C)* and histologic *(D)* sections of the anterior left ventricular wall showing striking subepicardial fatty infiltration and fibrosis. (Reprinted with permission from Corrado D, Basso C, Thiene G, et al: Spectrum of clinicopathologic manifestations of arrhythmogenic right ventricular cardiomyopathy/dysplasia: A multicenter study. J Am Coll Cardiol 30:1517, 1997.)

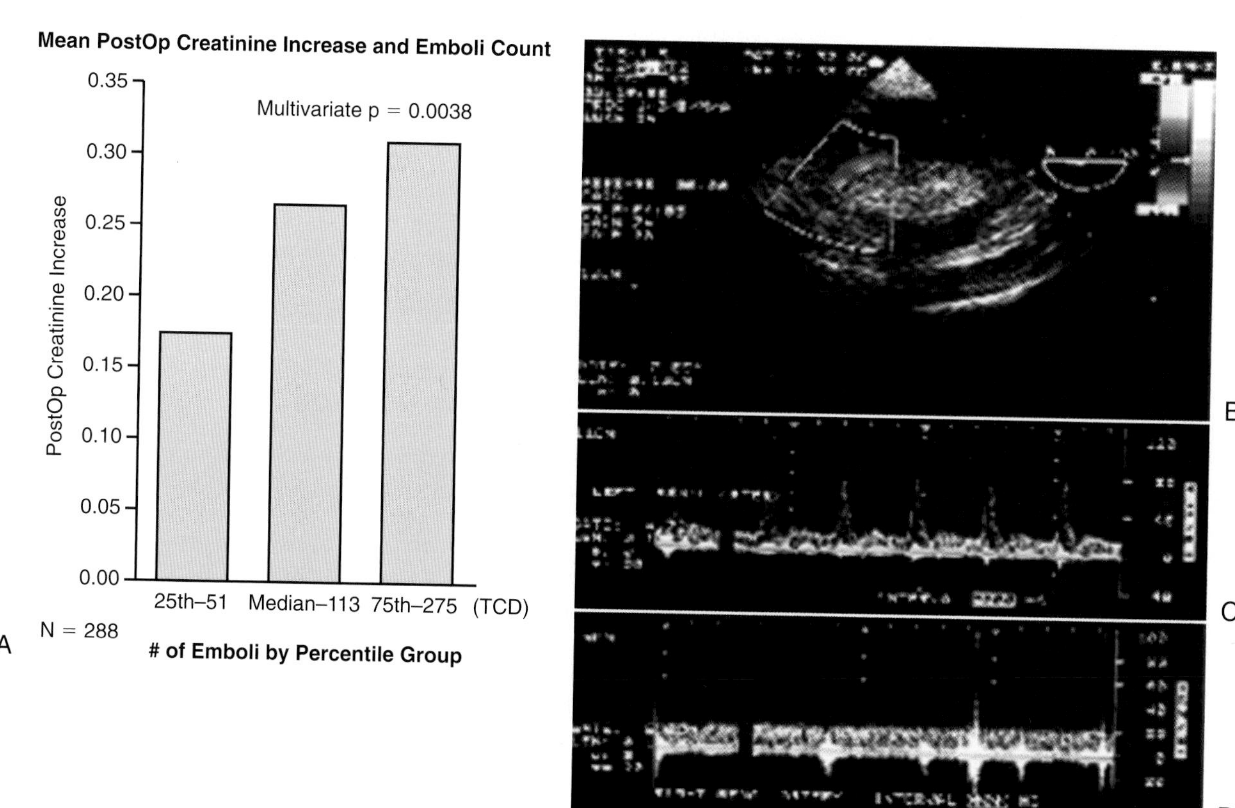

Figure 30–5 *(A)* Intraoperative arterial emboli counts, as estimated by transcranial Doppler scanning of the middle cerebral artery, are directly associated with a rise in the serum level of creatinine after coronary artery bypass surgery. *(B)* Intraoperative renal monitoring for emboli is possible by TEE imaging of the left renal artery. *(C)* Pulsed-wave Doppler renal artery monitoring before bypass demonstrates pulsatile flow and no evidence of emboli. *(D)* Doppler signals during bypass reveal nonpulsatile flow with intermittent emboli. See also Color Plates. (*A*, adapted from Sreeram GM, Grocott HP, White WD, et al: Transcranial Doppler emboli count predicts rise in creatinine after coronary artery bypass graft surgery. J Cardiothorac Vasc Anesth 18:548, 2004.)

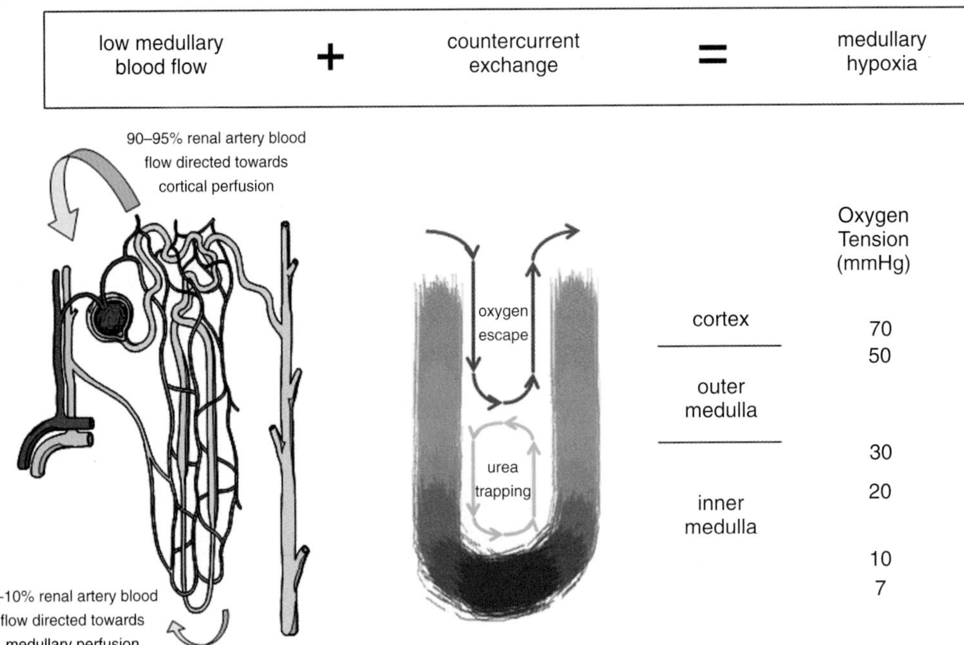

Figure 30–6 Normally sluggish blood flow in the renal medulla facilitates the countercurrent exchange mechanism that maintains the medullary urea gradient necessary for water reabsorption. However, this characteristic of the renal microcirculation also permits an oxygen diffusion shunt to occur, and combined with metabolic demands from active tubular reabsorption, it contributes to the precarious physiology of renal perfusion, including low medullary PO_2, also known as medullary hypoxia (7 to 10 mm Hg). Medullary hypoxia is exaggerated by hypovolemia or hemorrhage because reduced medullary blood flow, increased countercurrent exchange, and increased tubular solute reabsorption are associated with these conditions.

Part I

PAST, PRESENT, AND FUTURE

Chapter 1

EVOLUTION OF CARDIAC ANESTHESIA AND SURGERY*

Eugene A. Hessel II, MD, FACS

The more extensive a man's knowledge, of what has been done, the greater will be his power of knowing what to do.

Benjamin Disraeli, 1804–1881

Those who cannot remember the past are condemned to repeat it.

Santayana, *Life of Reason*

In the continual remembrance of a glorious past, individuals and nations find their inspiration.

Sir William Osler, 1849–1919

Why examine the past? As W. Bruce Fye's (past president of American College of Cardiology) appropriately titled essay suggests, medical history is a valuable tool to help us frame the present and predict the future.[1] First, it tells us of our heritage, of how we got to where we are. Second, it helps us appreciate what we have today and to place our practice in perspective. Third, it provides clues to the characteristics of successful persons and of the discovery process. Finally, it may inspire us to add to the rich history of our profession.

Cardiac surgery, and hence cardiac anesthesia, is remarkably young, nearly their entire history having occurred in slightly over the past 100 years, and the most important advances have occurred within the lifetime of currently practicing physicians. Many of the participants are either still living or left personal accounts of these events, and original publications are readily available. The reader may be surprised by how recent in origin are the procedures that are taken for granted today. In 1936, there was no known surgical treatment for congenital (CHD) or valvular heart disease (VHD). In the summer of 1944, there was no surgical palliation available for cyanotic CHD. At the start of 1952, open cardiac surgery was not possible. In January 1960, there was no satisfactory prosthetic valve available, no implantable pacemaker, and no closed-chest massage, and infant heart surgery was very risky. In early 1967, direct coronary artery surgery was a rarity and saphenous vein bypass surgery was unheard of, as were human heart transplantation and surgical therapy of tricuspid atresia and hypoplastic left heart syndrome. Intra-aortic balloon pumping, cardioplegia, monitoring of heparin dosing, balloon-tipped pulmonary artery catheters (PACs), high-dose narcotic anesthesia, dopamine, dobutamine, and prostaglandin therapy were not yet available. In 1984, internal mammary artery (IMA) grafting was not generally practiced, nor was monitoring by pulse oximetry, capnography, or transesophageal echocardiography (TEE). Propofol, aprotinin, amrinone, and adenosine were not available, and nitric oxide was considered to be only an environmental toxin.

Writing history is always subjective. The author makes decisions as to what is important and what should be included. There is also the problem of priority. Options include who first conceived of a technique, who discovered or perfected it in the laboratory, who first attempted to use it (but failed), who first successfully applied it clinically, who first published it, or who popularized the practice. Often two or more persons introduced a new procedure or therapy at nearly the same time and possibly (it is often difficult to know for certain) independently and unaware of the other's work. In some secondary sources, the dating is confused because an author has used the date of publication rather than the date of the procedure. In this chapter, the latter was used and the original paper was consulted when there was ambiguity. This author also readily acknowledges an orientation to the history involving North America and especially the United States. This is not meant to ignore the tremendous contributions made by workers in many other countries, often antedating advances made in the United States.

The history of cardiac anesthesia is intimately related to other advances in science, medicine, and cardiac surgery. Cardiac anesthesia is obviously closely connected to the developments in cardiac surgery. Usually this was a matter of anesthesiologists responding and adapting to the special needs and requirements of cardiac surgery, but sometimes advances in cardiac anesthesia were enabling to cardiac surgery (e.g., TEE and narcotic anesthesia). Both subspecialties are clearly influenced by advances in cardiology and pharmacology. The relations between surgery and cardiology have been both supportive and enabling, and competitive. The detailed diagnoses of CHD or coronary artery disease (CAD) were of limited significance prior to the availability of surgical therapy, while surgical treatment usually required more precise diagnosis. The competition between cardiology and surgery in the management of obstructive CAD has been largely beneficial, stimulating improvement in both fields. Likewise, cardiac anesthesia and cardiology have been mutually supportive. The uses of cardiovascular drugs, PACs, and TEE are just three examples.

*Some of this chapter was originally published as part of the author's chapter (Chapter 1) in Estafanous FG, Barash PG, Reves JG (eds): Cardiac Anesthesia: Principles and Clinical Practice, 2nd edition. Philadelphia, Lippincott, Williams, & Wilkins, 2001, pp 3–25 (used with permission) and in an article written by the author in the ASA Newsletter (October 2001;65:5–9) (used with permission). (A copy of the full text of the article can be obtained from ASA, 520 N. Northwest Highway, Park Ridge, IL 60068-2573.)

Table 1–1 **Timeline of Cardiac Anesthesia, Surgery, and Medicine**

Era	Cardiac Surgery	Cardiology, Cardiopulmonary Bypass, and Other Contributions From Science	Anesthesia and Cardiac Anesthesia
1628–1938: The beginnings	1896: Suture cardiac wound (Rehn) 1925: Mitral commissurotomy (Souttar)	1628: Function of the heart described (Harvey) 1895: Discovery of x-rays (Roentgen) [NOBEL] 1903: ECG (Einthoven) [NOBEL] 1900–1915: Blood typing and transfusion (Landsteiner et al) 1916–1938: Heparin (McLean, Best) 1936: *Atlas of Congenital Heart Disease* (Maude Abbott) 1937–1939: Protamine neutralization (Chargaft, Olson, Jopes)	1845–1847: Inhalation anesthesia (Long, Wells, Morton, Snow, Simpson) 1899: Endotracheal ventilation for thoracic surgery (Matas) 1924: To-and-fro CO_2 absorber (Waters) 1930: Circle system (Sword) 1933: Cyclopropane 1934: Thiopental (Lundy)
1938–1952: Closed heart surgery develops	1938: Ligate PDA (Gross) [LASKER] 1944: Resect coarctation (Crafoord) 1944: Systemic-PA shunt (Blalock and Tausig) [LASKER] 1947–1949: Pulmonary valvotomy (Sellors, Brock) and infundibulectomy (Sellors, Brock) 1947: Internal defibrillation (Beck) 1948: Mitral commissurotomy (Bailey, Harken, Brock) 1950: IMA implant (Vineberg) 1952: Aortic valvotomy (Bailey) 1952: Ball valve in descending aorta (Hufnagel) 1952: Pulmonary valvotomy with right heart bypass (Dodril)	1941: Cardiac catheterization (Forssmann in 1929, Cournand and Richards in 1941) [NOBEL] 1948: Start of Framingham Heart Study 1950: Transvenous pacing (Bigelow, Callaghan, Hopps) 1950: Antifoam (Clark) 1952: First prospective randomized clinical study (streptomycin for tuberculosis) 1952: External pacemaker (Zoll) [LASKER]	1942: Curare 1946: First article on cardiac anesthesia (Harmel and Lamont) 1949: Succinylcholine 1950: Plastic IV cannula (Mayo Clinic) 1951: Anesthesia for mitral commissurotomy (Keown) 1952: Copper kettle (Morris) 1952: Cardiotachoscope (Himmelstein)
1952–1960: Open heart surgery appears	1952: Close ASD with atrial well (Gross) 1952: Close ASD with hypothermia (Lewis) 1953: Close ASD with heart-lung machine (Gibbon) [LASKER] 1954: OHS with cross-circulation (Lillehei) [LASKER] 1955: Series of OHS with heart-lung machine (Kirklin, Lillehei) 1958: Glenn shunt 1958: Senning procedure	1953: Structure of DNA (Watson and Crick) [NOBEL and LASKER] 1953: Seldinger technique of percutaneous vascular access 1956: External defibrillation (Zoll) [LASKER] 1957: Epicardial pacemaker (Lillehei) 1957: Median sternotomy (Julian) 1957: Moderate hypothermia (Sealy)	1954: Anesthesia for hypothermia (Keown) 1955: EEG monitoring (Mayo Clinic) 1956: First textbook on cardiac anesthesia (Keown) 1957: Articles on anesthesia for CPB (multiple)

Table 1–1 **Timeline of Cardiac Anesthesia, Surgery, and Medicine**—(Continued)

Era	Cardiac Surgery	Cardiology, Cardiopulmonary Bypass, and Other Contributions From Science	Anesthesia and Cardiac Anesthesia
		1959: Femoral cannulation (Lillehei) 1959: Deep hypothermic circulatory arrest (Drew) 1959: Selective coronary angiography (Sones) [LASKER] 1959: *Journal of Thoracic and Cardiovascular Surgery* 1959–60: Transseptal left heart catheterization (Ross, Cope, Brockenbrough, and Braunwald)	
1960–1970: Rapid advances	1960: AV replacement with ball valve (Harken); MV replacement with ball valve (Starr) 1963: Mustard procedure for TGA (Mustard) 1967: Aortocoronary CABG (Favaloro) 1967: Heart transplantation (Barnard) 1968: Multivessel CABG (Johnson) 1968: Internal mammary artery for CABG (Green) 1968: Fontan procedure (Fontan)	1960: Closed chest massage (Kouwenhoven) [LASKER] 1960: Implantable pacemaker (Cardack and Greatbatch) 1960: Hemodilution prime (Zuhdi) 1961: Coronary care units (Julian) 1962: β-Blockers (Black) 1963: M-mode echo (Edler and Hertz 1954 [LASKER], Joyner and Reid 1963, Feigenbaum 1972) 1965: Drug therapy ("anti-impulse") of aortic dissection (Wheat) 1965: DHCA for infant surgery (Dillard, et al) 1966: Balloon septostomy (Rashkind) 1966: Hardshell bubble oxygenator/heat exchanger (DeWall) 1967: IABP (Kantrowitz) 1967–1971: Mobile coronary care, Medic One (Pantridge and Geddes; Cobb, et al)	1963: Monitoring left atrial pressure (Kirklin, Theye) 1967: Anesthesia for surgery for coronary artery disease (Wynands) 1969: Narcotic (morphine) cardiac anesthesia (Lowenstein)
1970–1980: More advances	1970: Tilting disc prosthetic heart valve (Bjork) 1970: Tissue valves (glutaraldehyde-preserved stented heterografts) (Carpentier, Ionescu, Hancock) 1975: Arterial switch operation for TGA (Jatene)	1970: PAC (Swan, Ganz, Forrester) 1970: Calcium channel blockers 1970s: Microfiltration during CPB 1973: Cold potassium cardioplegia (Gay and Ebert)	1972–3: PAC monitoring in cardiac surgery and anesthesia (Civetta and Gabel, Lappas) 1972 1972: Association of Cardiac Anesthesiologists 1976: Monitoring V_5 (Kaplan) 1976: Nitroglycerin infusions (Kaplan)

Table continued on following page

Table 1–1 Timeline of Cardiac Anesthesia, Surgery, and Medicine—(Continued)

Era	Cardiac Surgery	Cardiology, Cardiopulmonary Bypass, and Other Contributions From Science	Anesthesia and Cardiac Anesthesia
	1978–1981: St. Jude valve (Nicoloff) 1979–1981: Norwood procedure for HLHS (Norwood)	1973: Transvenous endocardial biopsy (Caves) 1974: Dopamine 1975: Dobutamine 1975: Heparin monitoring by ACT (Bull) 1975: Microporous membrane oxygenators 1976: PGE_2 for keeping ductus open (Olley) 1976: HMG-CoA inhibitors (Statins) (Endo) 1977: ACE inhibitors (Cushman and Ondettia) 1979–1983: Thrombolytic therapy for AMI (Rentrop, Kennedy, et al)	1978: Founding SCA (Marino, Burges, Peuler) 1978: High-dose fentanyl anesthesia (Stanley et al) 1979: First modern textbook on cardiac anesthesia (Kaplan)
1980–1990	1980: Mitral annuloplasty rings (Carpentier) leads to resurgence of MV repair 1981–1985: Explosive growth in cardiac transplantation 1981: First heart-lung transplant (Reitz) 1982: First total artificial heart (de Vries) 1985–1986: Cleveland Clinic's superior long-term results with IMA grafts (Lyttle, Loop) lead to general use of IMA as conduit of choice 1987: Stentless valves (David)	1980: Cyclosporin (Shumway) 1980: AICD (Mirowski et al) 1980–1996: Transcatheter procedures 1981: Inflammatory response to CPB (Kirklin) 1982: PDE-III inhibitor inotropic agents 1980s: Common employment of membrane oxygenators, centrifugal pumps, and retrograde cardioplegia 1987: NO is EDRF (Ignarro, Moncado) [NOBEL] 1987: Aprotinin (Royston et al) 1988: CSF drainage for spinal cord protection (McCullough)	1980: M-mode TEE (Matsumoto and Oka) 1981: PAC detects myocardial ischemia (Kaplan) 1982: Alpha-stat ABG management (Ream) 1982: Two-dimensional TEE 1983: Isoflurane steal (Reiz) 1983: Direct measure cerebral blood flow during CPB (Reves, Hendricksen) 1985: Impact of myocardial ischemia on outcome (Slogoff and Keats) 1986: Cerebral protection with barbiturates (Nussmeier and Slogoff) 1987: Journal of Cardiothoracic Anesthesia (Kaplan) 1987: Color flow TEE 1989: Choice of anesthetic agent does not affect outcome (Slogoff et al, Tuman)
1990–2000	1991–1997: Off-pump CABG (Benetti, Buffalo, Subramanian) 1991: Warm heart surgery (Lichtenstein) Fast tracking 1996: Heart-Port "port access" surgery (Stevens, Pompili, et al)	1990: Heparin-coated circuits 1990: Retrograde cerebral perfusion (Ueda) 1991: Endovascular grafts for abdominal aortic surgery (Parodi and Palmaz) 1991: Modified ultrafiltration (MUF) (Elliott and Naik) 1992: Epivascular scanning for atherosclerosis detection (Kouchoukos)	1994: SCA and *Anesthesia Analgesia* affiliate 1996: Beta blockers for noncardiac surgery (Mangano) 1998: First examination in perioperative TEE

Table 1–1 **Timeline of Cardiac Anesthesia, Surgery, and Medicine—**(Continued)

Era	Cardiac Surgery	Cardiology, Cardiopulmonary Bypass, and Other Contributions From Science	Anesthesia and Cardiac Anesthesia
		1992–1994: Use of NO to treat pulmonary hypertension 1994: "Bare" coronary stents approved by FDA 1995: GP IIb/IIIa blockers 1998: Augmented venous return	
2000–present: The 21st century	Heart failure surgery Genetic manipulation, stem cell implantation Robotic surgery	2003: Drug-eluting coronary stents approved by FDA 2003 (April14): Human Genome Project completed (F. Collins et al) Percutaneous repair of MR and replacement of AV Direct thrombin inhibitors for CPB Minimization of CPB circuits	Myocardial preconditioning by anesthetic agents Transfusions: good or bad? 2004: "Journal-within-a-journal" (SCA and *Anesthesia and Analgesia*)

NOBEL = Nobel Prize; LASKER = Lasker Prize.

Thus, it is difficult to discuss the evolution of cardiac anesthesia in a vacuum without noting what was going on in these various other fields. Table 1–1 notes some of the seminal advances in these various fields. A detailed history of cardiac surgery is found in Chapter 2, in an earlier chapter by this author,[2] and in several other illuminating articles and texts.[3-9] Several recent articles and books review the history of cardiology.[1,10-14] The evolutions of cardiac anesthesia and surgery are also closely tied with that of cardiopulmonary bypass (CPB).

CARDIAC ANESTHESIA TIMELINE

The early pioneers in cardiac surgery readily acknowledged the important role played by anesthesiologists.[15] In their first paper on the systemic–to–pulmonary artery shunt, Alfred Blalock and Helen Taussig mentioned by name the anesthesiologists involved in each case,[16] as did Potts et al[17] and Sellors[18] in their early case reports. In his Harvey Lecture delivered in November 1945, Blalock offered as proof of the skill of the anesthesiologists, Austin Lamont and Merel Harmel, who worked with him, "that there have been no deaths during the operation on the 55 patients."[19] In referring to his aortopulmonary anastomosis operation, Potts stated that "in an operation of this type, expert anesthesia is essential." But perhaps Russell C. Brock (later Lord Brock) expressed it most eloquently in his Alexander Simpson-Smith lecture given at the Medical Society of London on June 15, 1949, while discussing closed surgery for tetralogy of Fallot: "It is a type of surgery that is not for the lone operator.... Teamwork is of course essential in the operating theatre, where in addition to the surgical and nursing assistants, the anaesthetist plays a part of fundamental importance which deserves a special tribute."[20]

Unfortunately, little has been written on the history of cardiac anesthesia. Although Meade addressed a section on anesthesia in his *A History of Thoracic Surgery*, cardiac anesthesia was not mentioned.[3] Kenneth Keown, in the 1963 edition of his textbook on cardiac anesthesia,[21] and Carol Lake, in her textbook on pediatric cardiac anesthesia,[22] have included brief chapters on the history of cardiac anesthesia, whereas Jim Arens[23] and Earl Wynands[24] have written articles on the subject. The latter, written by one of the pioneering cardiac anesthesiologists in North America, is a rich review that emphasizes the contributions of Canadian anesthetists and contains numerous personal memories of the participants as well as of the author. Finally, Arthur Keats, another one of the pioneers in the development of this subspecialty, reflected on his personal perspective on its development in his 1983 Rovenstine Lecture,[25] as did Edward Lowenstein in his 2003 Abbott Lecture.[26] Table 1–2 lists some of the notable developments and contributions in cardiac anesthesia.[27-67]

Early Developments in Anesthesia for Thoracic Surgery

Before cardiac surgery, and hence cardiac anesthesia, could begin, fundamental advances in supporting patients during thoracic surgery had to be accomplished. This history of thoracic anesthesia has been thoroughly reviewed by L. Rendell-Baker[68] and J. Kaplan[69] and to a lesser degree by Richard Meade[3] and S. L. Johnson.[4] Of course, the pivotal advance was the introduction of anesthesia itself in the late 1840s. However, the next major challenge to thoracic surgery was how to ventilate the patient when the chest was open. Some ingenious approaches were explored, such as placing the patient's head in a positive-pressure box (Brauer in 1904 and Murphy in 1905) or operating within a negative-pressure

Table 1–2 Notable Contributions in Cardiac Anesthesia

	Date	Event	Anesthesiologist	Location	Reference
1.	1946	First paper on cardiac anesthesia	M. H. Harmel and A. Lamont	Johns Hopkins Hospital	27
2.	1950	Plastic IV cannula	D. J. Massa, J. S. Lundy et al	Mayo Clinic	28
3.	1951	Anesthesia for mitral commissurotomy	K. K. Keown	Philadelphia	29
4.	1952	Cardiotachoscope	A. Himmelstein	New York	30
5.	1954	Esophageal stethoscope	C. Smith	Hospital for Sick Children, Toronto	31
6.	1954	Anesthesia for cardiac surgery under hypothermia	K. K. Keown	Philadelphia	32
7.	1956	First textbook on cardiac anesthesia	K. K. Keown	Philadelphia	33
8.	1957	Anesthesia for cardiopulmonary bypass	E. A. Gain D. Mendelsohn et al R. T. Patrick et al K. K. Keown	U Alberta Cleveland Mayo Clinic Philadelphia	34 35 36 37
9.	1955	EEG monitoring during cardiopulmonary bypass	R. A. Theye	Mayo Clinic	38
10.	1963	Monitoring left atrial pressure	R. A. Theye and J. W. Kirklin	Mayo Clinic	39
11.	1967	First paper on anesthesia for coronary artery surgery (Vineberg procedure)	J. E. Wynands et al	Montreal	40
12.	1969	Narcotic (morphine) anesthesia	E. Lowenstein et al	Massachusetts General Hospital	41
13.	1972	Pulmonary artery catheter monitoring during cardiac surgery and cannulation of right internal jugular vein	J. M. Civetta and J. C. Gabel D. Lappas et al	Massachusetts General Hospital	42 43
14.	1976	Monitoring V_5 lead for detecting myocardial ischemia	J. A. Kaplan	Emory University	44
15.	1976	Nitroglycerin infusions to treat myocardial ischemia	J. A. Kaplan	Emory University	45
16.	1978	Founding, Society of Cardiovascular Anesthesiologists	Robert Marino, first president		46
17.	1978	High-dose fentanyl anesthesia	T. H. Stanley et al	University Utah	47
18.	1979	First modern American textbook on cardiac anesthesia	J. A. Kaplan, editor	Emory University	48
19.	1980	M-mode transesophageal echocardiography monitoring	M. Matsumoto and Y. Yoka	Albert Einstein	49
20.	1981	Pulmonary artery catheter to detect myocardial ischemia	J. A. Kaplan	Emory University	50
21.	1982	Alpha-stat blood gas management	A. K. Ream et al	Stanford University	51
22.	1982	Two-dimensional transesophageal echocardiography monitoring	M. K. Cahalan, P. Kremer, M. Roizen	University of California at San Francisco	52 53
23.	1983	Isoflurane steal described	S. Reiz	Umea, Sweden	54
24.	1983	Direct measurement of cerebral blood flow during cardiopulmonary bypass	J. G. Reves et al L. H. Hendricksen et al	University Alabama Copenhagen	55, 56 57
25.	1985	Impact of myocardial ischemia on outcome	S. Slogoff and A. Keats	Texas Heart Institute	58
26.	1986	Cerebral protection with barbiturates	N. A. Nussemeier and S. Slogoff	Texas Heart Institute	59
27.	1987	First issue of the *Journal of Cardiothoracic Anesthesia*	J. A. Kaplan, editor		
28.	1987	Color-flow transesophageal echocardiography	N. P. deBruijn et al	Duke University	60
29	1987	Aprotinin reduces perioperative bleeding	D. Royston, W. Van Oeveren et al	England, Holland	61, 62
30.	1989	Anesthetic agent per se does not affect outcome	K. Tuman et al S. Slogoff and A. S. Keats	Rush University Texas Heart Institute	63 64
31.	1996	Practice guidelines for transesophageal echocardiography (TEE)	ASA and SCA		65
32.	1998	First examination in perioperative TEE	National Board of Echocardiography	United States of America	
33.	1999	Guidelines for comprehensive intraoperative TEE examination	ASE and SCA		66
34.	2002	Guidelines for training in perioperative TEE	ASE and SCA		67

chamber with only the patient's head outside (Sauerbruch in 1904); for a while, even into the 1940s, positive-pressure ventilation via a tight-fitting mask was used, particularly for children. The solution, however, was endotracheal ventilation. The first elective oral endotracheal intubation for anesthesia was performed by the Scottish surgeon William Macewan in 1878. In 1888, the American surgeon Joseph O'Dwyer designed metal endotracheal tubes with a conical tip to occlude the larynx and added a bellows device to provide positive-pressure ventilation. This was first used and advocated as the best means of preventing pulmonary collapse during thoracic surgery by the surgeon Rudolph Matas of New Orleans in about 1899. In 1919, Ivan Magill of Britain introduced blind nasal endotracheal intubation using red rubber "Magill tubes," and in 1926, Arthur Guedel of Indianapolis introduced cuffed endotracheal tubes. Although direct vision laryngoscope-aided intubation was slowly adopted in the 1920s, the Miller and Macintosh blades were not introduced until the early 1940s.

In 1924, Ralph Waters at the University of Wisconsin introduced his to-and-fro carbon dioxide absorber utilizing soda lime granules. This was favored by many cardiac anesthesiologists until the mid 1950s, although Brian Sword had introduced his circle system with valves and in-circuit carbon dioxide absorber, removing the canister from the patient's face in 1930. Ayre introduced his T-piece in 1937, and G. Jackson Rees, his modification, in 1950.

The first important new anesthetic agent after ether, chloroform, and nitrous oxide was cyclopropane, which was introduced to clinical anesthesia by Ralph Waters in 1933 and was adopted by many cardiac anesthesiologists as an induction, if not maintenance, agent of choice. Its major drawback was its flammability, which led to its ready replacement when halothane became available in the late 1950s. In 1952, Lucien Morris invented the copper kettle, permitting more precise quantification of anesthetic dosing. Later in that decade, the temperature-compensated agent-specific vaporizers ("TEC") were introduced by Cyprane Limited of England.

In 1934, John Lundy of the Mayo Clinic introduced thiopental into the practice of anesthesia, and for many years, it was used as a maintenance agent as well as an induction agent. In 1942, Griffith and Johnson of Montreal first used curare, and Stephens used it to facilitate thoracic surgery in 1947. Succinylcholine became available in 1949.

Mechanical ventilators were developed as early as 1907 (Draeger "Pulmotor"). Crafoord introduced his commercially available Spiropulsator in 1940, and Blease introduced the "pulmoflator" after World War II. However, the use of ventilators in the operating room was not readily accepted until the late 1950s, and "modern" intensive care unit (ICU)–type ventilators (e.g., Bennett, Bird) did not appear until the 1960s.

Although a few recovery rooms were established before World War II and an Anesthesia Study Commission report published in 1947 suggested that recovery rooms could improve outcome, they did not become common until the mid 1950s. Surgical ICUs, greatly spurred by the advent of cardiac surgery, did not develop until the early 1960s.[70,71]

Early Cardiac Anesthesia

Little is known about the anesthesia provided during early cardiac surgical operations. Ellis in 1975[72] reviewed the anesthetic management of Sir Henry Souttar's patient who underwent mitral commissurotomy in 1925.[73] He states anesthesia was administered by a surgeon, Eric Lindsay (although in a letter written to Brian Blades 30 years after the event, Souttar gives credit to his anesthetist, John Challis[5]). The patient was premedicated with morphine and atropine, induced with "ACE" (a combination of absolute alcohol, chloroform, and ether), and maintained with ether administered via an endotracheal catheter. The patient apparently breathed spontaneously throughout the procedure. Blood pressure was monitored about every 5 minutes.

In 1994, Anthony Dobell[74] outlined the anesthetic management of the patient in whom Robert Gross first ligated a patent ductus arteriosus (PDA) in 1938. Anesthesia was provided by a nurse anesthetist (Betty "Bess" Lank) who used a tight-fitting shrunken (with alcohol) adult mask strapped to the child's face. Monitoring included a finger on the superficial temporal pulse. The anesthetic agent used was cyclopropane. Blood was available but not needed.[75] For Clarence Crafoord's first coarctation repairs accomplished in 1944, anesthesia consisted of cyclopropane–nitrous oxide administered via an air-tight endotracheal tube using controlled ventilation provided by a "spiropulsator" respirator.[76]

On November 29, 1944, Austin Lamont, director of anesthesia, and his "resident" Merel Harmel, in his eleventh month of anesthesia training (Merel Harmel, personal communication), provided anesthesia for Alfred Blalock's first (and successful) "Blalock-Taussig" (subclavian–to–pulmonary artery) shunt (the "blue baby" operation) at Johns Hopkins Hospital[16,27,77] (Fig. 1–1). Blalock, professor of surgery at Hopkins, was partially responsible for developing this anesthesia team when, in 1941, apparently recognizing that advances in cardiac and thoracic surgery would require a significantly higher level of support than that provided by surgeon-directed nurse anesthetists (a lesson that Gibbon had to relearn 10 years later), he encouraged Lamont, then an instructor in surgery at Hopkins, to develop a more professional level of anesthesia expertise in the Department of Surgery. Lamont thereupon obtained anesthesia residency training under Ralph Waters at the University of Wisconsin in Madison and additional training under Emery Rovenstine in New York and then returned as director of anesthesia at Hopkins in 1943.[78]

Between 1946 and 1950, the first papers on cardiac anesthesia appeared, reviewing the challenging experience of providing anesthesia for severely cyanotic and debilitated children undergoing systemic–to–pulmonary artery shunt operations.[27,79-82] Again, the words of Lord Brock came to mind: "(these) operations . . . involve considerable anxiety (and) demand the work and attention of an enthusiastic, loyal, and courageous team."[20] It is hard to overestimate the anxiety produced in contemplating anesthetizing for the first time one of these nearly moribund children (often with virtually no exercise tolerance, bedridden, and suffering from repeated hypoxic spells) for this radically new operation. Common themes in these reports included heavy premedication (morphine and scopolamine), induction and maintenance with cyclopropane (with or without a little ether), and endotracheal intubation (a few tried mask only early in their experience but quickly abandoned this for endotracheal intubation because of problems with maintaining ventilation, despite the concerns about postintubation airway problems in children). Most used controlled ventilation (with or without use of curare). The Waters to-and-fro carbon dioxide–absorbing canister closed system was usually used. Monitoring methods were not detailed, nor was fluid management discussed except to warn against fluid

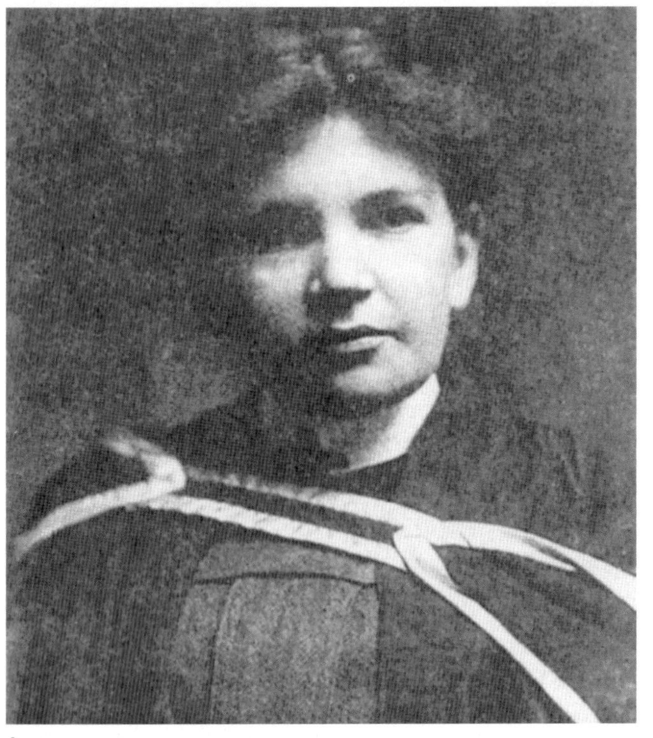

A

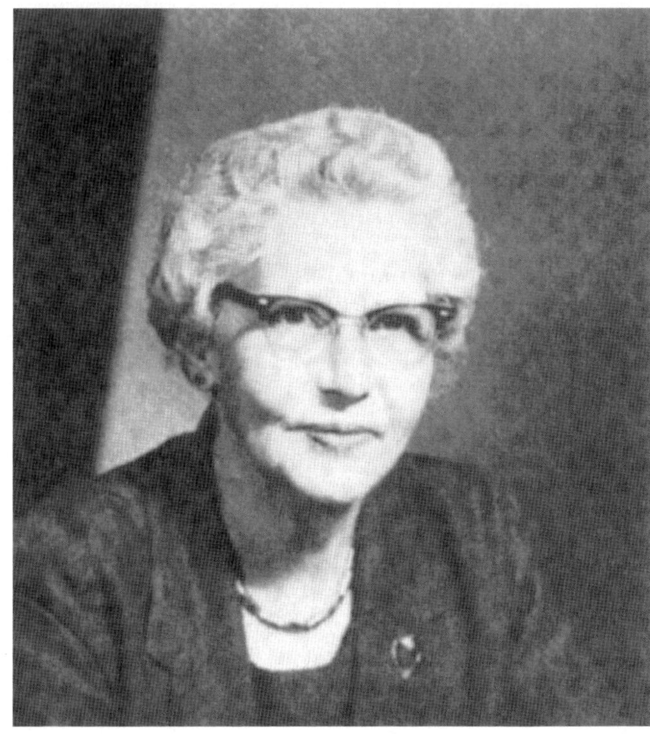

B

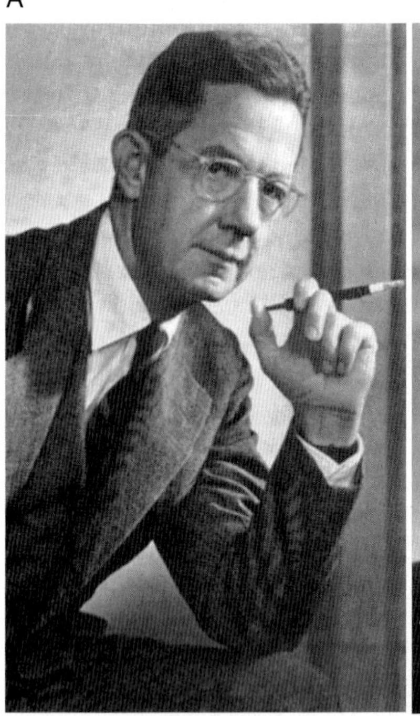

C

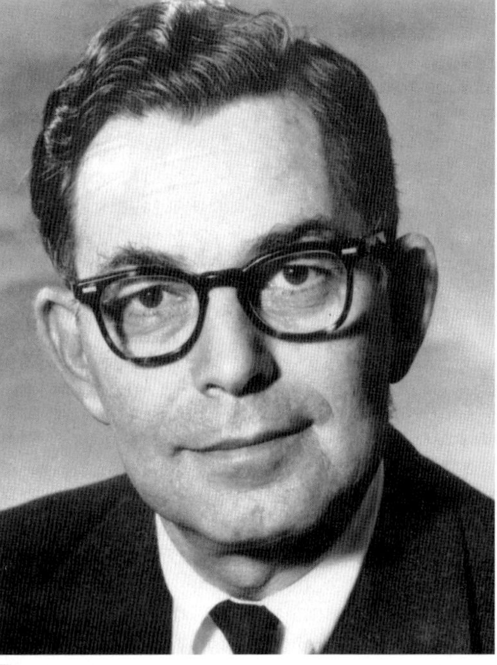

D

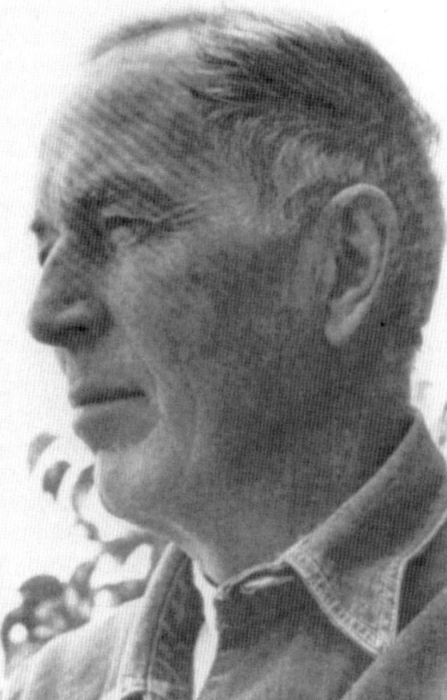

E

Figure 1–1 The Blalock-Taussig shunt ("blue baby") operation. A team effort. (*A*) Maude Abbott, pathoanatomist, McGill University. Her pioneering studies of the nature of congenital heart disease leading up to the publication of her book *Atlas of Congenital Heart Disease* in 1936 provided a basis for Helen Taussig's clinical studies of congenital heart disease. (*B*) Helen Taussig, pediatric cardiologist, Johns Hopkins Hospital, suggested to Blalock that his experimental subclavian-to-pulmonary shunt could palliate hypoxemia in children with tetralogy of Fallot, and she referred patients to him. She anticipated the use of drugs to keep patent ductuses open to palliate neonates with cyanotic heart disease, subsequently described by the Toronto group in 1976. (*C*) Alfred Blalock, surgeon, Johns Hopkins, performed the first systemic–to–pulmonary artery shunt operation for a "blue baby" on November 29, 1944. (*D*) Merel Harmel, anesthesia resident, and (*E*) Austin Lamont, anesthesia attending, provided anesthesia for this first and subsequent shunt procedures. In 1946, they published the first paper on cardiac anesthesia. (*A* and *B* are from Westaby and Bosher,[9] with permission of the author; *C* is from Shumaker[8] with permission; *D* is from Wood Library–Museum of Anesthesiology, with permission; *E* is from Muravchick and Rosenberg, Anesthesiology,[78] American Society of Anesthesiologists, with permission.)

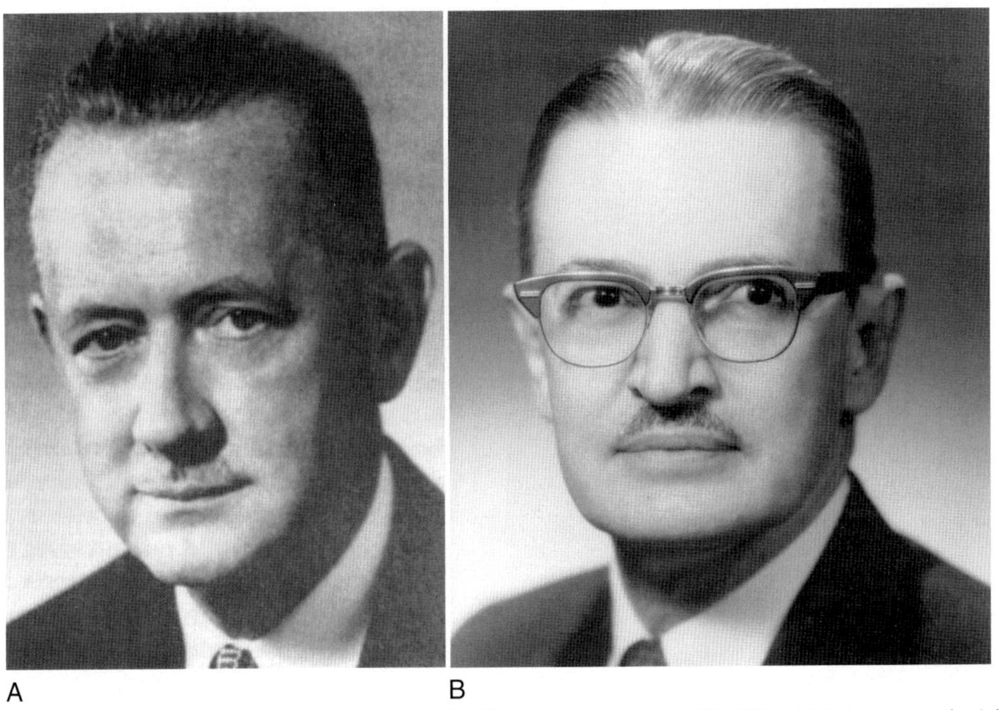

Figure 1–2 The Children's Memorial Hospital in Chicago team. (*A*) Willis Potts, surgeon, and (*B*) William McQuiston, anesthesiologist at Children's Memorial Hospital in Chicago, introduced mild hypothermia as adjunct and reported remarkably excellent results in their first 1000 cases between 1946 and 1956. (*A* is from Shumaker,[8] with permission; *B* is from Wood Library–Museum of Anesthesiology, with permission.)

overloading. Usually, a cannula was placed in the saphenous vein of the ankle and plasma was administered. In Harmel and Lamont's[27] report of Blalock's first 103 cases at Johns Hopkins Hospital (10 weeks to 20 years old), the mortality rate was 23%. In William McQuiston's[82] report of Willis Potts'[17] first 236 shunt cases at Children's Memorial Hospital in Chicago, the mortality rate was 13%, but the mortality rate in the 135 patients between 3 and 16 years of age in whom a shunt was actually constructed was only 3% (Fig. 1–2). These remarkable results were achieved without the "benefit" of electrocardiographic (ECG) monitoring, arterial and central venous catheters, monitoring of pulse oximetry and end-tidal CO_2, "modern" inhalation agents, narcotics, muscle relaxants, antibiotics, ICUs, or even recovery rooms. In May 1948, the Chicago group began using mild surface-induced hypothermia ("refrigeration") (rectal temperature of 92°–93°F) in these cyanotic children and observed a decreased incidence of cerebral hypoxia and cerebral death (2.5% versus 7% and 4%, respectively, in historical controls) in shunted patients and a reduced mortality (14% versus 54%) in those in whom a shunt could not be constructed.[82] This was the first clinical use of hypothermia in cardiac surgery, a technique that would reappear on many occasions in the future. Alvin Harris[80] in San Francisco described a somewhat different anesthetic technique in 25 children, using rectal avertin to induce basal narcosis and maintaining the patients with nitrous/oxygen, curare, and morphine sulfate (later to be called "balanced anesthesia"), although this technique did not appear to be well accepted at that time.[83]

Robert M. Smith of Boston Children's Hospital[83] and E. M. Papper and Thomas McDermott at Babies Hospital in New York City[84] reviewed the pathophysiology and anesthetic management of patients with PDA, coarctation of the aorta, pulmonic stenosis, and vascular rings as well as those with tetralogy of Fallot. Papper and McDermott emphasized the benefits of endotracheal intubation (although M. H. Adelman[85] reported his successful use of mask ventilation during surgery for PDA). By 1950, the Boston Children's Hospital group (Gross and Smith) reported a mortality rate of 1% in 455 children operated upon for PDA and 8.5% in 155 children operated upon for coarctation.[83] The Chicago Memorial Children's Hospital group (Potts, McQuiston, and Baffes[86]) reported the results in their first 1000 operations for CHD as of February 1955; the mortality in surgery for isolated pulmonic stenosis (61 patients) was 1.6%, 0% for PDA (347 patients), and 4% for coarctation of the aorta (52 patients). Again, these were achieved without the "benefits" of modern anesthesia technology.

Kenneth Keown provided anesthesia for Charles Bailey's[87] first successful closed mitral commissurotomy on June 10, 1948 (Fig. 1–3). It followed four prior failures; 5 of their next 10 patients also died. These were difficult times; they were treating desperately ill patients while developing a whole new type of surgery and anesthesia. But they persisted, and over the next 8 years, they performed more than 2000 cases, and the mortality rate fell to 7.5%. In 1951, Keown published the first paper on providing anesthesia for mitral commissurotomy,[29] and reports from other groups appeared shortly thereafter.[88-92] Moderate premedication including phenobarbital and morphine or meperidine was usually recommended. All groups emphasized the importance of using the lightest possible anesthesia but different agents were used to accomplish this. An extreme example of light anesthesia was the technique of C. E. Wasmuth at the Cleveland Clinic. He used nitrous oxide (80% to 50%) in oxygen supplemented with small amounts of thiopental, morphine, or meperidine and local infiltration of the intercostal incision and insisted that the patient respond to questioning throughout the procedure (but

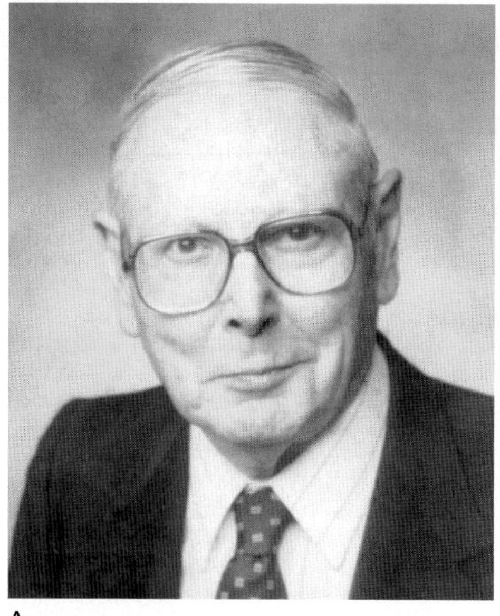

A

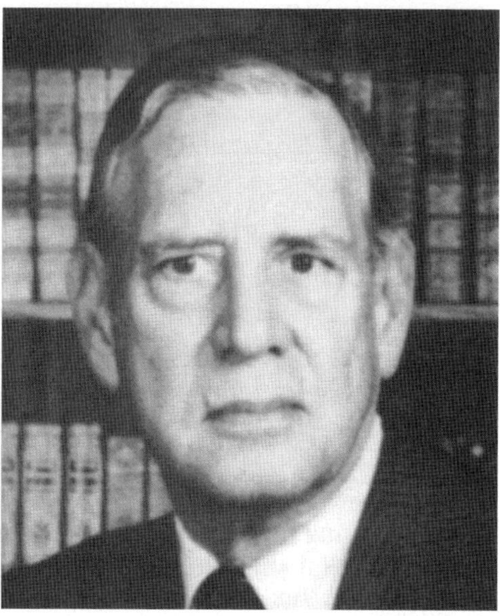

B

Figure 1–3 Early mitral commissurotomy team. (*A*) Charles Bailey, surgeon, and (*B*) Kenneth Keown, Anesthesiologist, Hahnemann Medical College, Philadelphia, accomplished the first successful mitral commissurotomy in June 1948 and helped popularize this procedure. Keown published the first paper on anesthesia for mitral commissurotomy in 1951 and the first textbook on cardiac anesthesia in 1956. (*A* is from Westaby and Bosher,[9] with permission; *B* is from Wood Library–Museum of Anesthesiology, with permission.)

they denied pain and had no recall!).[89] All used endotracheal intubation, often with topical anesthesia; however, there was considerable controversy as to whether ventilation should be merely assisted (to avoid the possible negative impact of controlled ventilation on right ventricular function) or controlled, as well as regarding the pros and cons of using muscle relaxants such as curare[90,91] or infusions of succinylcholine.[92] Two authors recommended use of mechanical ventilators to provide reliable ventilation and "free up the anesthesiologist's hands for other exceedingly important duties."[89,90] Notably, the Swedes had been using ventilators during cardiac surgery since the late 1930s.[76] In the earliest report, Keown advocated running an infusion of procaine throughout the case to reduce arrhythmias,[29] but this was not adopted by most subsequent authors. Continuous ECG monitoring was used by all, some with use of an oscilloscope.[88,89] All started large-bore intravenous access and had blood available including blood pumps and means of giving intra-arterial transfusions, but all emphasized the need to minimize fluid and blood administration to avoid fluid overload. Keown[29] even advocated removing the venous cannula at the end of the case (if the patient was stable) "to avoid the temptation to give excessive fluids." All patients were extubated at the end of the case but given supplemental oxygen postoperatively. Several groups used paravertebral or intercostal nerve blocks for postoperative analgesia. All authors emphasized the need to move the patient and change their positions slowly and gently, while they were under anesthesia or emerging, to avoid hemodynamic instability.

Perhaps an even more daunting task was providing anesthesia for patients with severe aortic regurgitation undergoing insertion of a prosthetic ball valve in the descending aorta by Charles Huffnagel of Georgetown University (with temporary exclusion of a segment of the descending aorta without benefit of left heart bypass or CPB). This was first performed in September 1952.[93] The anesthetic management of these patients was described by John A. O'Donnell and Thomas F. McDermott in 1955.[94] All 42 of their patients were in medically irreversible congestive heart failure (CHF), and 40% had intractable angina pectoris with 10 to 20 attacks a day. After discovering early in their experience that these patients did not tolerate a depth of general anesthesia to permit endotracheal intubation, thereafter they intubated these patients with topical anesthesia and then induced very light general anesthesia with a small dose of thiopental and maintained them on nitrous oxide and oxygen supplemented with intravenous morphine or small amounts of ether. Systolic arterial pressure was kept above 100 mm Hg with phenylephrine if needed. Continuous ECG monitoring by oscilloscope and recorder was employed with a cardiologist present. Two 15-gauge intravenous needles were placed. The radial artery was surgically exposed, not for monitoring but to use if needed to withdraw blood to treat extreme hypertension during aortic cross-clamping or to administer intra-arterial transfusion in the case of catastrophic hemorrhage. Blood transfusion replaced blood loss (average, 800 mL), and an electrical defibrillator was always available. The arterial pressure (measured by auscultation in the upper extremities) did not rise as much as anticipated, and in some not at all, with aortic cross-clamping. There were nine hospital deaths (20%); three died during surgery from cardiac arrest or ventricular fibrillation before, during, or following valve insertion, while four died suddenly 5 to 9 days postoperatively after an apparently uncomplicated recovery.

In 1954, S. J. Evelyn and I. Mackay reviewed their anesthetic techniques and results with cardiac anesthesia in 820 cases performed at the Toronto General Hospital.[95] Their hospital mortality rates were remarkable: tetralogy of Fallot (shunts) (342 patients), 6%; PDA (133 patients), 0%; coarctation (29 patients), 0%; and mitral valve surgery (260 patients), 6%.

Little has been written about the anesthesia used in the early cases of direct-vision open heart surgery with moderate surface-induced hypothermia.[96,97] John F. Lewis et al[98] indi-

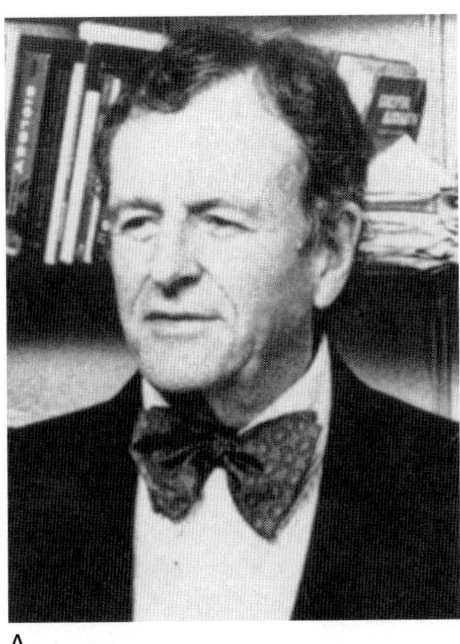

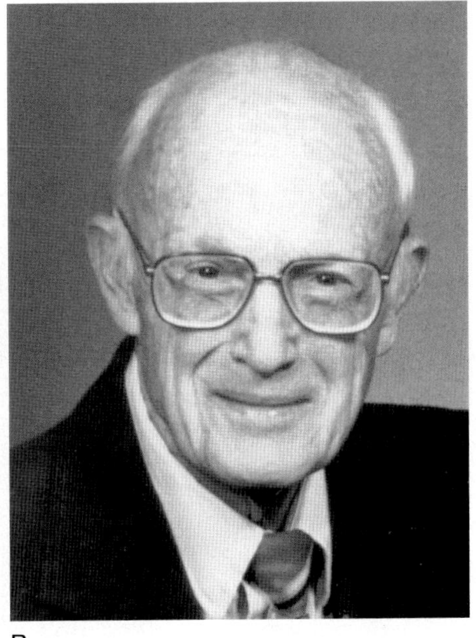

Figure 1–4 Early Denver cardiac surgery team. (*A*) Henry Swan, surgeon, and (*B*) Robert Virtue, anesthesiologist, advanced the use of brief periods of circulatory arrest during moderate hypothermia to permit direct vision open heart surgery in the early and mid 1950s. (*A* is from Shumacker,[8] with permission from the author; *B* is from Wood Library–Museum of Anesthesiology, with permission.)

cated that anesthesia was induced with thiopental and curare, patients were intubated, and ECG and rectal temperature were monitored. Henry Swan et al[97] indicated that anesthesia was also induced with thiopental and maintained with cyclopropane and ether, or ether alone. In 1954, the Hahnemann group (Kenneth Keown, Charles Bailey, and others) reported their early animal and clinical experience.[99] Keown expounded on anesthetic principles and technique. They used endotracheal cyclopropane anesthesia with ECG monitoring. Shivering (often only detectable by ECG) was treated with small doses of thiopental, and procaine infusions were used to combat arrhythmias.[32]

In Denver, Robert W. Virtue with Henry Swan (Fig. 1–4) (and others) amplified their anesthetic management a little in a 1955 report of their first 100 cases done using hypothermia.[100] Monitoring included ECG, EEG, blood pressure by auscultation (although this was not measured in 12% of cases and could not be obtained in one third of patients below 35° C and in two thirds by 33°–31° C). Patients were given an "ordinary" anesthesia. Ether was the preferred agent ("second plane, third stage"), supplemented with curare. They suggested that anesthetizing these patients was a "two-man job," with one devoting full attention to maintenance of hyperventilation to deliberately achieve a respiratory alkalosis that they thought reduced the incidence of ventricular fibrillation. They measured right atrial pH (measured at patient's temperature) just before arrest and aimed for it to be greater than 7.5 ("alpha-stat" management). Two plastic cannulas were placed in arm veins, and all blood loss was replaced with at least equal amounts of blood. Postarrest, 100% oxygen was administered with nitrous oxide (50%) added if needed. Patients were extubated when breathing adequately, apparently often before they awakened. Ventricular fibrillation occurred in 15%, and although two thirds were resuscitated, only 20% survived, whereas six of the seven experiencing cardiac arrest survived. Postoperative hemorrhagic shock (versus cardiac failure) posed a difficult diagnostic problem. Average duration of circulatory arrest was 5 minutes (range, 2 to 10 minutes). Only 1 of 36 (3%) with favorable lesions (e.g., secundum atrial septal defect [ASD], isolated pulmonary valvular or infundibular stenosis) died, while six of the eight (75%) with primum ASD or ventricular septal defect (VSD) died. Eight of 10 with tetralogy (undergoing only relief of their pulmonary stenosis) survived.

In 1957, B. A. Sellick in London,[101] and in 1959, A. W. Conn et al at the Hospital for Sick Children in Toronto,[102] reviewed their anesthetic techniques for direct-vision surgery using only hypothermia. Sellick used nitrous oxide with oxygen plus ether and complete relaxation with curare after thiopental and succinylcholine for induction and intubation, while Conn et al used the same agents but without muscle relaxation except for intubation. By 1959, Conn (Fig. 1–5) had switched to using halothane. In Conn et al's paper, a detailed section on monitoring appeared for the first time. Monitoring included a multichannel recorder and oscilloscope, ECG, EEG, and the availability of transducers for direct pressure monitoring, although blood pressure was usually monitored with a Collens oscillometer. They also reported flooding the surgical field with carbon dioxide to minimize the risk of air embolization. Neither Sellick's nor Conn's groups had a death in their 32 and 63 patients, respectively.

Anesthesia for Early Cardiac Surgery Using Cardiopulmonary Bypass

Anesthesia for John Gibbon's[103] first successful case using an artificial heart-lung machine for total CPB to close an ASD was provided by a nurse anesthetist, Katherine Rawlins. It consisted of 2 g of thiopental and manually assisted endotracheal ventilation (Fig. 1–6). The endotracheal tube had apparently been placed by a physician because nurses were not allowed

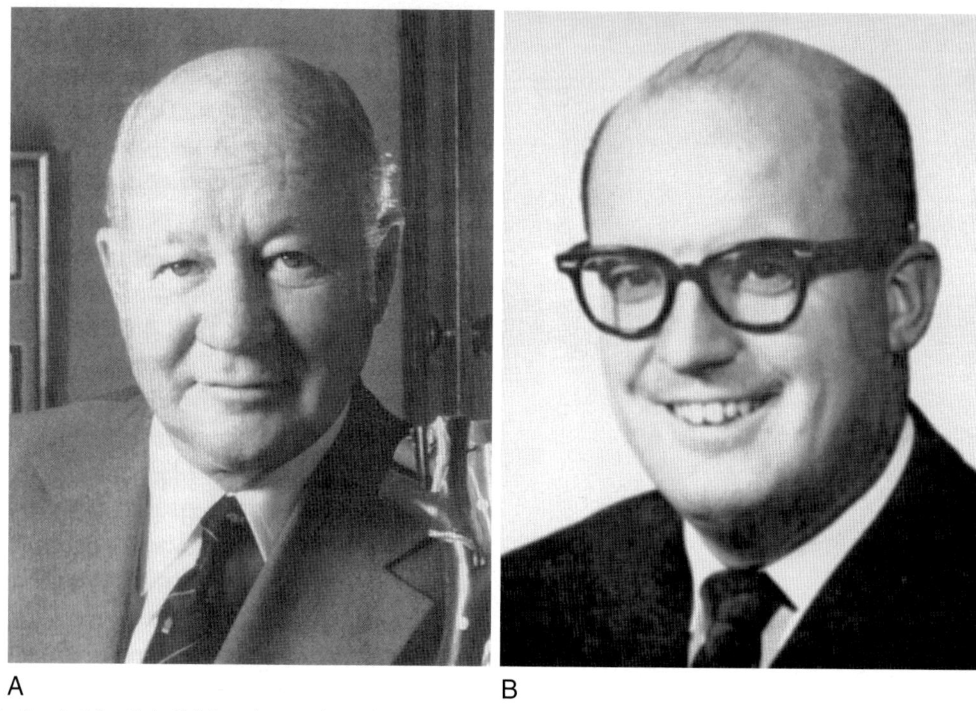

Figure 1–5 Early Hospital for Sick Children (Toronto) cardiac surgery team. (*A*) William Mustard, surgeon, and (*B*) A. W. Conn, anesthesiologist, Hospital for Sick Children in Toronto, reported remarkable success closing atrial septal defects without using cardiopulmonary bypass during moderate hypothermia. Mustard reported early attempts at cardiopulmonary bypass using biologic (monkey) lungs for infant surgery and in 1963 introduced his interatrial venous transposition operation ("Mustard procedure") for transposition of the great arteries. (*A* is from Shumaker,[8] with permission; *B* is from Wood Library–Museum of Anesthesiology, with permission.)

to do such a procedure at that time (per A. B. Tarrow: "First successful open-heart operation using the heart-lung machine," Wood Library-Museum Tape No. LD0054, 1992). Direct blood pressure readings were made via a needle inserted in the right brachial artery that was connected to a mercury manometer. The veins in both ankles were cannulated for administration of intravenous fluids. The patient was quite light at the conclusion of the operation and an hour later, when returned to her bed in the hospital ward, was awake, recognizing people and talking.[104] According to Anthony Dobell, who was a surgery resident under Gibbon at that time (and subsequently became chief of cardiac surgery at the Royal Victoria Hospital in Montreal): "A major factor in the deaths of the children was poor ventilation prior to going on CPB. There were no physician anesthesiologists at Jefferson at that time and of course mechanical ventilators had not been developed (sic). Some of the children were already moribund by the time they were connected to the heart-lung machine. Thus at Jefferson, lack of expertise in anesthesia, pediatric cardiology and cardiac pathology all played a part in the initial failures."[7] This was apparently recognized by Gibbon, who 2 years later facilitated the recruitment of two clinically and academically experienced anesthesiologists to Jefferson (per A. B. Tarrow as cited above). Harris Shumacker,[105] a close personal friend and a pioneering cardiac surgeon himself, has written an intimate biography of John H. Gibbon, Jr., and these early experiences.

For C. Walton Lillehei's early cases of cardiac surgery using controlled cross-circulation (in which the patient's parent served as the heart-lung "machine"), the patients were induced with nitrous oxide–cyclopropane and then maintained on thiopental and curare while the donors (parents) were induced and maintained with thiopental and curare. During bypass, the donors were hyperventilated (2 to 3 times normal) to induce a respiratory alkalosis to counterbalance the metabolic acidosis that regularly occurred during the low-flow (34 to 40 mL/kg/min) perfusion of the patient. There was no mention of monitoring, invasive catheters, or fluid management other than blood administration. In the first eight patients who underwent closure of VSDs (5 months to 5 years of age), the average time "on bypass" was 14 minutes (range, 9 to 28 minutes); six survived.[106] According to James Arens,[23] Fred van Bergen and Joe Buckley administered anesthesia to the patient while Jim Matthews and Earl Schultz cared for the father donor for the first successful case (Fig. 1–7).

In 1956, right in the middle of the time that extracorporeal perfusion was being introduced, Kenneth K. Keown of Hahnemann Medical College, who provided anesthesia for Charles Bailey, published the first textbook on anesthesia for surgery of the heart.[33] This book provides an insight into the nature of cardiac anesthesia at that time. As a testimony to the teamwork that had developed between cardiac surgeons and cardiac anesthesiologists, he listed the prominent teams practicing at that time (Table 1–3). He also summarized the expected mortality rates for the various procedures performed at that time (Table 1–4). He emphasized the role of the anesthesiologist in ensuring that the patient was ready for surgery, the use of checklists for equipment and supplies, and the avoidance of shortcuts. He also listed what he hoped would be coming in the near future: a more ideal inhalation anesthetic (potent, rapid acting, nonirritating, nonexplosive), mechanical ventilators, arterial catheters with Po_2 and pH measurement, and a practical mechanical heart-lung machine. All were achieved before the end of that decade.

Anesthesiologists Robert Patrick, R. A. Theye, and Emerson Moffitt along with physiologists/cardiologists H. J. C. Swan (of

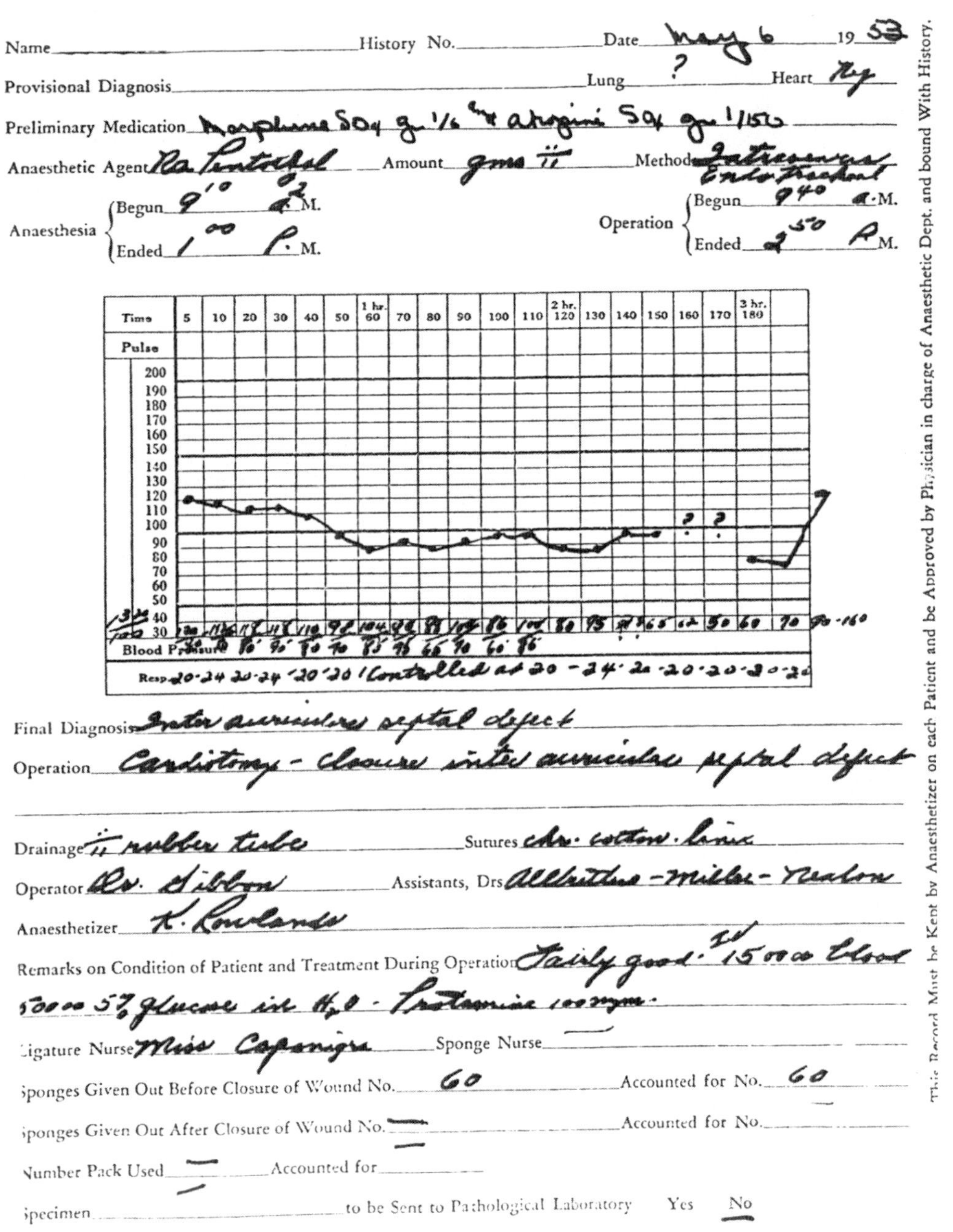

Form 123

ANAESTHESIA RECORD
JEFFERSON HOSPITAL
PHILADELPHIA, PA.

Name ______ History No. ______ Date May 6 19 53

Provisional Diagnosis ______ Lung ? Heart Neg

Preliminary Medication Morphine SO4 gr 1/6 & atropine SO4 gr 1/150

Anaesthetic Agent Na Pentothal Amount gms ii Method Intravenous Endotracheal

Anaesthesia: Begun 9:10 A.M. Ended 1:00 P.M.

Operation: Begun 9:40 A.M. Ended 2:50 P.M.

Time	5	10	20	30	40	50	1 hr. 60	70	80	90	100	110	2 hr. 120	130	140	150	160	170	3 hr. 180

Pulse 200 190 180 170 160 150 140 130 120 110 100 90 80 70 60 50 40 30

Blood Pressure

Resp 20-24 20-24 20-20 Controlled at 20-24 20-20-20-20-20

Final Diagnosis Inter auricular septal defect

Operation Cardiotomy - closure inter auricular septal defect

Drainage #14 rubber tube Sutures chr. cotton. linen

Operator Dr. Gibbon Assistants, Drs Allbritten - Miller - Nealon

Anaesthetizer K. Rowlands

Remarks on Condition of Patient and Treatment During Operation Fairly good. 1500 cc blood 500 cc 5% glucose in H2O - Protamine 100 mgm.

Ligature Nurse Miss Capanigra Sponge Nurse ______

Sponges Given Out Before Closure of Wound No. 60 Accounted for No. 60

Sponges Given Out After Closure of Wound No. — Accounted for No. ______

Number Pack Used — Accounted for ______

Specimen ______ to be Sent to Pathological Laboratory Yes No

This Record Must be Kept by Anaesthetizer on each Patient and be Approved by Physician in charge of Anaesthetic Dept. and bound With History.

Figure 1–6 Anesthetic record for the first successful use of a mechanical heart-lung machine for total cardiopulmonary bypass to close an atrial septal defect by John Gibbon, Jr., on May 6, 1953, at Jefferson Hospital, Philadelphia. (Copy of record courtesy of Arthur B. Tarrow, MD, 2002, with permission from A. B. Tarrow and the Wood Library–Museum of Anesthesiology.)

PAC fame) and Earl Wood participated on the team led by surgeon John Kirklin at the Mayo Clinic in the laboratory investigation and subsequent conduct of the first successful series of cardiac operations using a mechanical heart-lung machine (Mayo-Gibbon) in the spring of 1955[107,108] (Fig. 1–8). Over the next 4 years, they and several other groups reviewed their initial experience at delivering anesthesia care for patients undergoing cardiac surgery using mechanical heart-lung machines.[34-37,109-111] These reports reflect major differences of opinion regarding the optimal oxygenator, flow rates, lung management, control of arterial pressure, and need to add carbon dioxide or anesthesia to the extracorporeal circuit during CPB. The degree of management, intervention, and monitoring ranged from the detailed protocol at the Mayo Clinic[36] to the minimalist approach at Baylor/Texas Children's Hospital in Houston (Denton Cooley and Arthur Keats)[110] (Fig. 1–9). The former resembled modern-day practice: flows were kept at about 2.4 L/min/M^2 (60 to 200 mL/kg/min), and a volatile anesthetic was administered via a vaporizer on the oxygenator. Intra-arterial pressure, venous pressure, rectal temperature, EEG, ECG, inline venous saturation, and arterial blood gases were monitored. Fluid and blood balances were

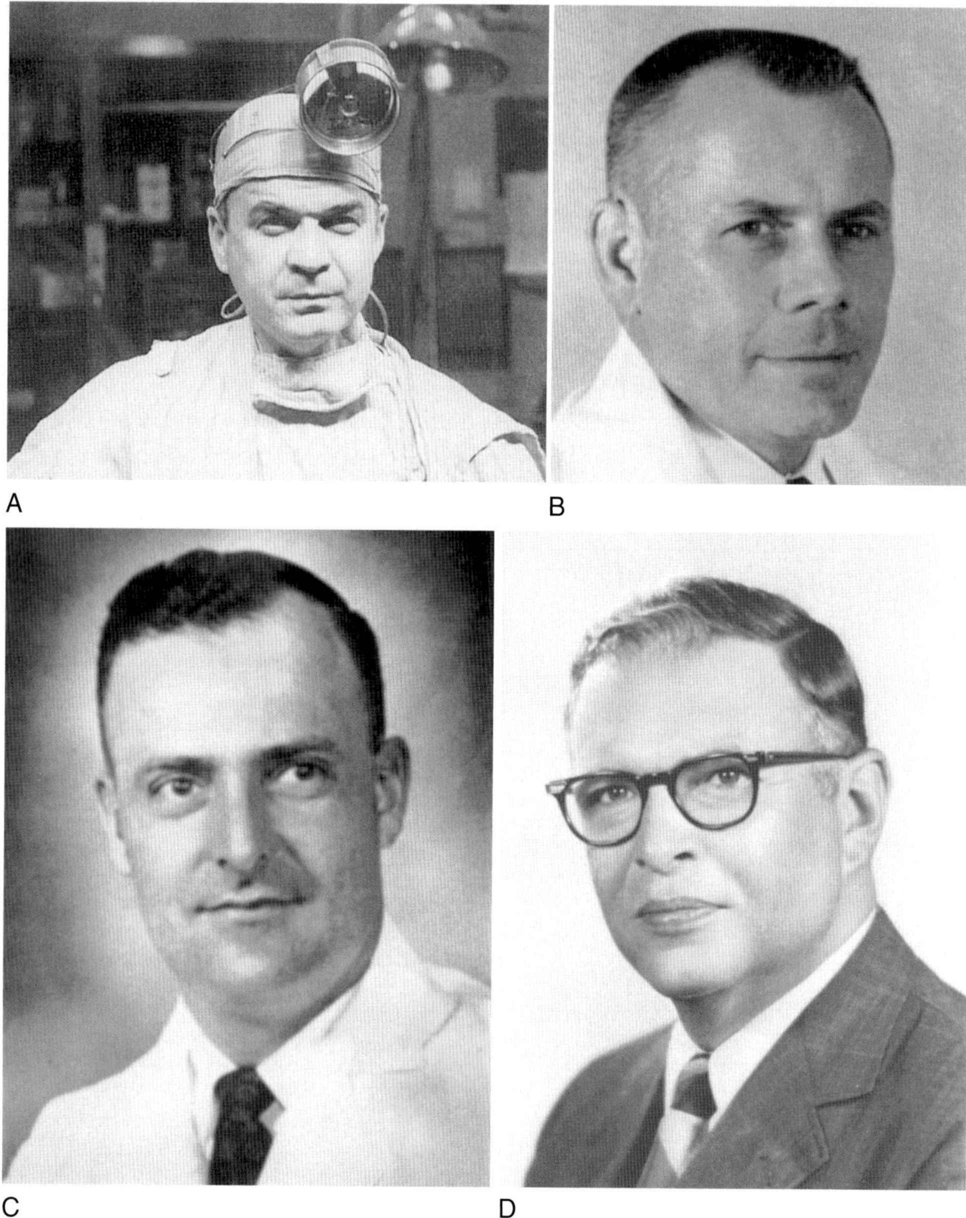

Figure 1–7 University of Minnesota cross-circulation team. The first successful closure of a ventricular septal defect was performed using controlled cross-circulation (the patient's parent served as the heart-lung machine) at the University of Minnesota, April 20, 1954. (*A*) C. Walton Lillehei, surgeon, Fred van Bergen (*B*), and Joe Buckley (*C*) provided anesthesia for the patient, while Jim Mathews (*D*) and Earl Schultz (not shown) anesthetized the parent. Lillehei and his team went on to make many contributions to the development of cardiac surgery. (*A* is from Westaby and Bosher,[9] with permission from the author; *B, C,* and *D* are from Wood Library–Museum of Anesthesiology, with permission.)

meticulously monitored, and a written, detailed protocol for step-by-step management was published. Vasopressor drugs and resuscitation drugs were readied for administration.[36] At the other extreme was the practice in Houston (Cooley and Keats). They monitored only one lead of the ECG (not invasive arterial pressure, venous pressure, EEG, or temperature), ran flows at between 35 (adults) and 50 (infants) mL/kg/min, and administered only D-tubocurarine during bypass (with no recall observed). However, their mean duration of CPB was only 13 minutes.[110] Some attributed the amnesia to cerebral hypoperfusion (due to low Pa_{CO_2} and low-flow rates) and found that patients rarely awakened during CPB without anesthesia when flows were 35 to 40 mL/kg/min but invariably awakened with flows of 60 mL/kg/min (which was treated with small amounts of barbiturates and narcotics).[34] The Mayo Clinic group observed no EEG changes during their high-flow CPB,[36,38] whereas the University of Minnesota group observed severely abnormal EEG changes during their low-flow CPB,[109] although no gross neurologic abnormalities were noted postbypass. However, their bypass times were also usually very short (average, 14 minutes; range, 8 to 17 for first seven cases).[112] All favored using minimal anesthesia and expected patients to be awake and extubated at the end of the procedure.

At the end of the 1950s, Mason Sones introduced direct coronary angiography, a procedure that would have a momentous impact on the future of cardiac surgery and anesthesia.[113]

Table 1–3 Early Cardiac Surgery and Anesthesia Teams*

Surgeon	Anesthesiologist(s)	Location
C. P. Bailey	K. K. Keown	Philadelphia
A. Blalock	M. H. Harmel and A. Lamont	Johns Hopkins Hospital
R. C. Brock	E. H. Rink and Lucas	London
D. B. Effler	D. E. Hale and J. F. Vijon	Cleveland Clinic
D. E. Harken	L. D. Vandam	Boston
C. A. Hufnagel	T. F. McDermott	Georgetown University
E. B. Kay	D. Mendelsohn	Cleveland
J. W. Kirklin	R. T. Patrick and R. A. Theye	Mayo Clinic
C. W. Lillehei	F. H. VanBergen	University of Minnesota
D. W. G. Murray	S. J. Evelyn	Toronto
W. J. Potts	W. O. McQuiston	Chicago Children's
T. H. Sellors	B. A. Sellick and Brown	London
H. Swan	R. W. Virtue	Denver
R. Varco	J. J. Buckley	University of Minnesota

*Modified from Keown KK, 1956, p. 8.[33]

Table 1–4 Estimated Mortality Associated With Cardiac Surgery, 1956†‡

Congenital	
Tetralogy of Fallot (shunts)	12%
Tetralogy of Fallot (Brock-Sellors procedure)	"lower"
Pulmonic stenosis (isolated)	5%
Atrial septal defect, secundum	12%
Atrial septal defect, primum	60%
Atrial septal defect with partial anomalous venous return	12%
Patent ductus arteriosus	2½–3%
Aortic stenosis	7%
Acquired	
Mitral stenosis	7½%
Aortic stenosis	15%
Mitral regurgitation	12%
Aortic regurgitation	25%
Coronary artery surgery (Vineberg, Beck procedures)	20%
Pericardiectomy	5%

†All closed procedures or with moderate hypothermia; none with cardiopulmonary bypass.
‡Modified from Keown KK, 1956, p. 13-14.[33]

The 1960s

The 1960s featured an explosive growth in the volume and breadth of cardiac surgery, which included heart-valve replacement,[114,115] advanced surgery for CHD, especially in infants,[116-118] human heart transplantation,[119] and coronary artery bypass grafting (CABG).[120,121] This required many more cardiac anesthesiologists with new knowledge and skills. Closed chest massage was introduced in 1960,[122] as were permanent implantable pacemakers[123] and hemodilution prime.[124] Monitoring of left atrial pressure became common and gave new insight into the discrepancies between right- and left-heart function.[39] The appearance of surgical ICUs and ICU ventilators offered a new venue for the anesthesiologist, while the introduction of the intra-aortic balloon pump in 1967 offered a new approach ("mechanical circulatory assist") for the treatment of perioperative cardiac failure.[125] Deep hypothermic circulatory arrest (DHCA) was reintroduced (especially for surgery on infants) and offered further challenges to the cardiac anesthesiologist.[118,126]

Halothane was first introduced into anesthesia practice in 1957, but there was initial hesitation to use it for cardiac surgery because of concern about its myocardial and respiratory effects. However, the desire to use a potent nonexplosive agent led the groups at the Mayo Clinic[127] and Indiana University[128] to explore the use of low concentrations (<0.8% to 1.0%) in 50% nitrous oxide for adults and children undergoing open and closed cardiac surgery. Thereafter, this agent rapidly replaced most other agents and became the anesthetic of choice for cardiac surgery until the landmark article by Lowenstein et al at the Massachusetts General Hospital (MGH) in 1969.[41] In that article, they indicated they had used high-dose morphine (0.5 to 3 mg/kg) as the main anesthetic in 1100 patients because it was devoid of myocardial depression, and hence they considered it to be the agent of choice in patients with minimal cardiac reserve (e.g., end-stage valvular and CAD). This was rapidly adopted by others, and high-dose narcotic–oxygen–muscle relaxant came to be known as the "cardiac anesthetic." Mainly morphine was used for the next 10 years until it was replaced by the synthetic narcotics, initially fentanyl in doses of 50 to 100 μg/kg, as popularized in the United States by Theodore H. Stanley of the University of Utah.[47] Fentanyl overcame some of the limitations of high-dose morphine including vasodilation and need for blood volume expansion.

Lowenstein has vividly described the challenges of cardiac anesthesia in the 1960s in his splendid chapter in a book on the history of the anesthesia department at MGH.[129] He

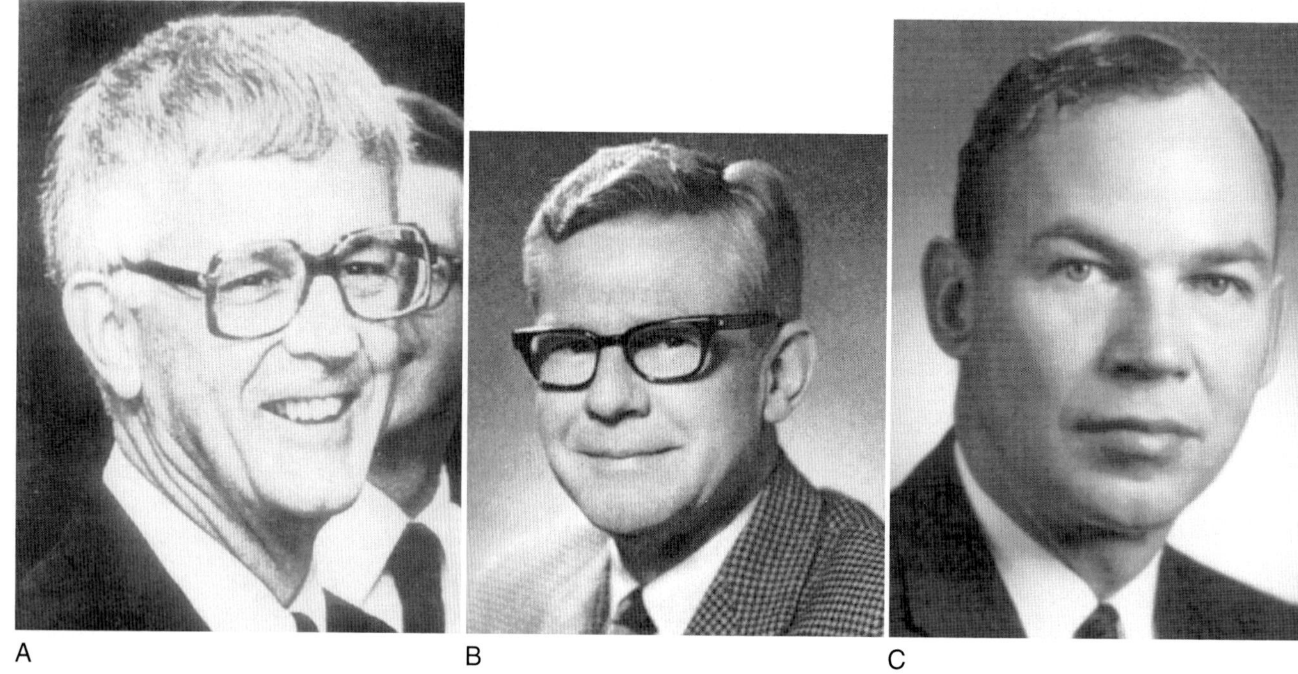

Figure 1–8 The sophisticated Mayo Clinic team initiated the first successful series of open heart surgeries using a modified (Mayo) Gibbon heart lung machine in the spring of 1955 following extensive laboratory evaluation. (*A*) John Kirklin, surgeon, and (*B*) Robert Patrick and (*C*) R. A. Theye, anesthesiologists. Emerson Moffit participated as an anesthesia fellow and subsequently became a leader in cardiac anesthesia at the Mayo Clinic (see Fig. 1–10). H. J. C. Swan (of pulmonary artery catheter fame and Earl Wood (physiologist/cardiologist) (not shown) were also key members of that innovative team. (*A* is from Westaby and Bosher,[9] with permission from the author; *B* and *C* are from Wood Library–Museum of Anesthesiology, with permission.)

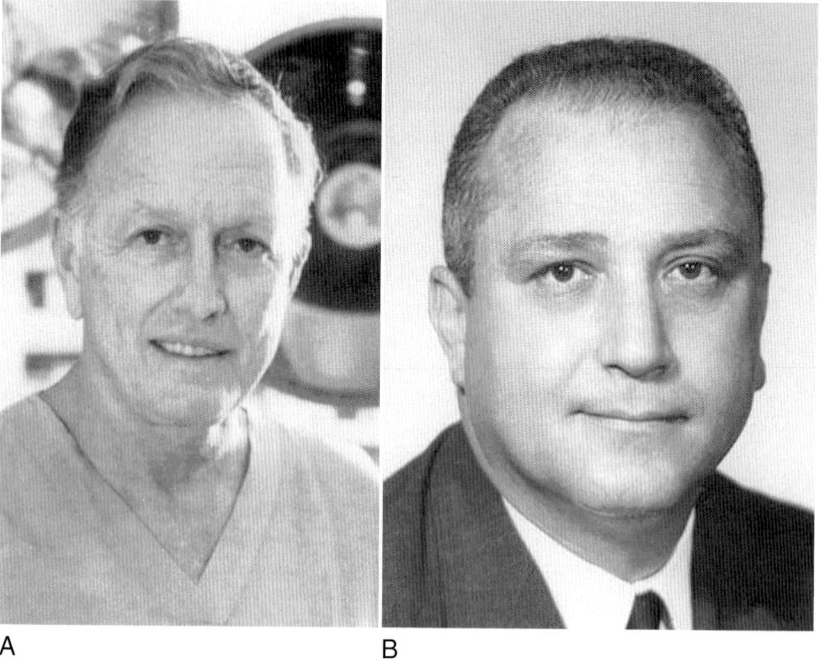

Figure 1–9 The Texas Heart Institute cardiac surgery team. (*A*) Denton Cooley, surgeon, and (*B*) Arthur Keats, anesthesiologist, started their famous open heart surgery program in the mid 1950s; both have gone on to make many contributions to cardiac surgery and anesthesia, respectively. (*A* is from Westaby and Bosher,[9] with permission from the author; *B* is from Wood Library–Museum of Anesthesiology, with permission.)

recalled that 3 of the 10 patients managed during his first rotation on the cardiac anesthesia rotation as a resident in 1962 arrested during induction. James Arens has also described the challenges of cardiac anesthesia in that era. In 1966, when he started work at the Ochsner Clinic, "the heart room was hell—no one wanted to work there."[23]

In 1967, J. Earl Wynands of Montreal published the first article on the anesthetic management of patients with CAD undergoing revascularization (Vineberg procedure).[40] This was followed by an article by John F. Viljoen of the Cleveland Clinic based on experience with 1500 IMA implant procedures.[130] Both emphasized the desirability of generous premedication, adequate depth of anesthesia, invasive monitoring of arterial and central venous pressures, frequent measurements of arterial blood gases and serum potassium, and postoperative endotracheal ventilation with adequate analgesia and sedation for 4 to 24 hours and close cardiovascular surveillance in the ICU. Wynands emphasized the importance of maintaining arterial pressures close to baseline and keeping hematocrit around 40%. By 1970, Wynands reported a hospital mortality of only 1.3% in their last 78 patients despite the fact that one third had angina at rest.[131] Donald Effler, the chief of cardiac surgery at the Cleveland Clinic, attributed much of the improved results to anesthetic management.[132] Viljoen advocated intermittent administration of nitroglycerin intramuscularly,[130] and in 1976, Joel A. Kaplan, then at Emory University, introduced the use of nitroglycerin infusions during coronary artery surgery.[45]

The 1970s

Recognizing the importance of integrating cardiology into the practice of anesthesiology, a symposium on this topic, edited by Arthur Keats, was published in the August 1970 issue of *Anesthesiology*.[133] There was a similar symposium reported in the July 2004 issue of the *British Journal of Anaesthesia*.[134]

In that same month, H. J. C. Swan and William Ganz in Los Angeles introduced their PAC,[135] and cardiac anesthesiologists were quick to bring it into the operating room, permitting more precise hemodynamic monitoring and intervention.[42,43] Joel Kaplan advocated the importance of cardiac anesthesiologists to surgeons and anesthesiology residents. He popularized the use of the V_5 lead[44] and the PAC to detect myocardial ischemia[50] and nitroglycerin infusions to treat it.[45] In 1979, Kaplan edited the first edition of this first modern comprehensive textbook on cardiac anesthesia, which became the standard reference in the specialty. Fellowships in cardiac anesthesia appeared and attracted many residents who became future leaders in this subspecialty. In 1972, the Association of Cardiac Anesthesiologists was founded,[23,129] followed in 1978 by the Society of Cardiovascular Anesthesiologists (SCA).[46]

Meanwhile, important advances were occurring in cardiac surgery and medicine. Cold potassium cardioplegia was introduced in 1973,[136] objective monitoring of heparin and its reversal by the activated coagulation time (ACT) in 1975,[137,138] the use of prostaglandin infusions to palliate critically ill cyanotic infants in 1976[139] (a therapy anticipated by Helen Taussig years earlier[140]), and percutaneous transluminal coronary angioplasty in 1977.[141] The arterial switch operation was first successfully accomplished in 1975[142]; in 1979, William Norwood introduced his staged repair of hypoplastic left-heart syndrome.[143] Tilting disc valves (e.g., Bjork-Shiley[144,145]) and bioprostheses (e.g., stent-mounted valves[146,147]) gradually displaced Starr-Edwards ball valves during this time.

The 1980s

With the introduction of cyclosporine to combat rejection in 1980,[148] the number of heart transplants performed grew from about 100 per year to 2400 per year in the next 5 years. The first artificial heart was implanted in 1982,[149,150] and although it failed as a permanent device, it opened the way for powerful assist devices and the development of more effective total artificial hearts that continues to the present time. IMAs became the bypass graft of choice for coronary artery bypass,[151,152] and mitral valve repair gained acceptance.[153,154] Better understanding and modulation of the pathophysiology of CPB were being achieved, and cardiac anesthesiologists were intimately involved in much of this work.

The Alabama group drew attention to the systemic inflammatory response to CPB in 1981,[155] and this led to the serendipitous discovery of the benefits of aprotinin in reducing blood loss during CPB by David Royston and others in 1987.[61,62,156]

An article by Allen Ream et al at Stanford in 1982 led to a rethinking of proper management of P_{CO_2} and pH during hypothermic CPB[51] and led to the near-complete shift from pH-stat to alpha-stat management during that decade. In 1983 through 1984, the groups at the University of Alabama and in Copenhagen[55-57] reported for the first time studies on cerebral blood flow during clinical CPB, which spurred multiple subsequent studies on the incidence, etiology, and efforts to reduce perioperative neurologic dysfunction. This was amplified by a seminal study from the Texas Heart Institute in which Nancy Nussmeier and Stephen Slogoff demonstrated that the use of high-dose thiopental (to produce isoelectric EEG; average dose, about 40 mg/kg) reduced the rate of postoperative neuropsychiatric dysfunction following open ventricle operations,[59] although the general applicability of these data has subsequently been challenged. By the end of the decade, membrane oxygenators had nearly replaced bubble oxygenators, and centrifugal pumps were gaining in popularity.

In 1983, a paper by Sebastian Reiz of Umea, Sweden, raised concern about the risk of coronary steal with isoflurane[54] and led to a flurry of experimental and clinical studies on this topic. Today, volatile anesthetics are considered cardioprotective[157,158] (see Chapters 9 and 19). A perhaps more provocative and influential study appeared 2 years later in which Stephen Slogoff and Arthur Keats of the Texas Heart Institute in Houston documented the frequency of intraoperative myocardial ischemia during coronary artery surgery and showed that it was associated with postoperative myocardial infarction.[58] They also showed that an anesthesiologist (the infamous anesthesiologist #7) can have an impact (negative) on the incidence of this problem. This paper helped initiate the intense study of perioperative ischemia—its causes and methods to prevent it, which continue to the present day. In 1989, two papers occurred side-by-side, again one from Slogoff and Keats at the Texas Heart Institute and the other from Kenneth Tuman et al at Rush-Presbyterian-St. Luke's Medical Center in Chicago, documenting in large prospective studies (more than 1000 patients in each study) what cardiac anesthesiologists had been saying since 1946: that the choice of anesthetic agents, per se, did not significantly affect outcome.[63,64] Studies, however, are reexamining this proposition (De Hert et al[158]).

Perhaps of greatest impact on the subspecialty in the 1980s was the contribution of cardiac anesthesiologists to the introduction of M-mode and two-dimensional TEE to cardiology and anesthesia in 1980.[49,52,53] It was quickly applied to cardiac surgery and helped to further define the subspecialty of cardiac anesthesiology. In 1987, Kaplan started the first journal devoted to cardiothoracic anesthesia: *Journal of Cardiothoracic Anesthesia*[159] (*Vascular* was added to the title in 1991), and in the same year, nitric oxide was identified as the endothelium-derived relaxing factor.[160]

The 1990s to the Present

Major changes have occurred in cardiac surgery during the past 15 years that have required adaptive changes by cardiac anesthesiologists, many of whom have contributed to the development, application, and evaluation of these techniques, including "fast-tracking," warm bypass, retrograde cerebral perfusion, augmented venous return, heparin-coated circuits, modified ultrafiltration, minimized heart-lung machines/extracorporeal circuits, minimal access and "port access" valve surgery, off-pump coronary artery surgery, stentless valves, valve repair, transmyocardial laser, surgery for heart failure including implantation of partial and total artificial hearts, more aggressive neonatal surgery, use of nitric oxide in the operating room and ICU, and the beginning of robotic surgery. The apparent increased prevalence and/or recognition of heparin-induced thrombocytopenia and thrombosis (HITT) has stimulated cardiac anesthesiologists to become involved in novel approaches for the conduct of CPB in these patients.

The emphasis on evidenced-based medicine and public awareness and interest in outcome[161] ("report card medicine"[162]) and changes in the economics and in the "business of medicine," managed care, commercialization of medical practice, and open competition have all required change and adaptation by the subspecialty. The reduced availability of public funds for research and education has put stress on research and development capabilities. Drug and equipment manufacturers play an increasing role in sponsoring research and educational activities, introducing the potential for bias.[163]

Despite this, much productive research is ongoing. Three weeks before Gibbon successfully used total CPB, Watson and Crick published their seminal paper on the structure of DNA (the "double helix").[164] Clearly these two events have radically changed cardiac medicine. Although the impact of the latter has taken more time, it is likely to ultimately be more profound. Almost exactly 50 years later, the Human Genome Project was completed.[165] Cardiac anesthesiologists are actively studying the application of these developments.

Major research contributions have been made and continue to be added in such diverse areas as the pathophysiology of CPB, including the systemic inflammation response, neurologic consequences of cardiac surgery, alpha-stat versus pH-stat blood gas management during hypothermia, perioperative myocardial ischemia, molecular cardiovascular medicine,[166] anesthetic myocardial preconditioning,[157] deep hypothermia with or without circulatory arrest in both adults and children, retrograde cerebral perfusion, evaluation of new cardiovascular and anesthetic drugs, changes in coagulation associated with CPB including its monitoring and modulation with drugs, the role (and dangers) of transfusion therapy, the application and improvement of information provided by TEE, the application of central neuroaxial blockade to cardiac surgical patients, "fast-tracking," and the benefits of early extubation.[167,168] Cardiac anesthesiologists have also made important contributions in the area of risk assessment and outcomes research and have been instrumental in initiating large multicenter collaborative research projects to study outcome and assess methods of improving outcomes in cardiac surgery.

In collaboration with echocardiologists (and the American Society for Echocardiology), cardiac anesthesiologists (through the SCA) and American Society of Anesthesiologists (ASA) developed "Practice Guidelines for Perioperative TEE" in 1996.[65] In 1999, "Guidelines for Comprehensive Intraoperative TEE Examination" was written,[66] and in 2002, "Guidelines for Training and Periop TEE" appeared.[67] Cardiovascular anesthesiologists also contributed to the formation of the National Board of Echocardiography, culminating with the administration of the first examination in perioperative TEE in 1998, and in 2000, with efforts to obtain certification of anesthesiologists in perioperative TEE. In 2000, SCA submitted an application to the Accreditation Council for Graduate Medical Education (ACGME) for accreditation of resident education programs in the subspecialty of cardiothoracic anesthesia.

SPECIAL ASPECTS IN THE EVOLUTION OF CARDIAC ANESTHESIA

Monitoring

Monitoring receives much attention in modern anesthesia practice as evidenced by basic monitoring standards and practice guidelines (e.g., for PAC and TEE) issued by the ASA. However, as noted previously, in articles on cardiac anesthesia up until the mid 1950s, monitoring was rarely mentioned, if at all. Obviously, these anesthesiologists heavily depended upon their five senses (awareness and clinical acumen, color of the skin, pupillary size, and a finger on the pulse), behavior that the modern anesthesiologist could usefully emulate.

The first "new" monitor to be introduced was the ECG. Studies using paper recorders during adult[169] and pediatric[170] surgery were reported by cardiologists in 1939 and 1948. However, apparently ECG monitoring was not commonly practiced[171] until the advent of closed mitral commissurotomy, during which arrhythmias were a major problem and all early reports mentioned use of ECG monitoring. Initially, this was accomplished using ordinary diagnostic ECG machines with paper recorders; but in the early 1950s, oscilloscopic monitors were introduced to facilitate continuous ECG monitoring.[30,88,89] A major advance in ECG monitoring occurred in 1976 when Joel Kaplan advocated the use of the V_5 lead to detect myocardial ischemia in patients with CAD.[44]

With the introduction of CPB in the mid 1950s, sphygmomanometry could no longer provide reliable arterial pressure monitoring, and use of invasive arterial catheters (at least during CPB) not only for pressure monitoring but also for arterial blood gas monitoring was introduced. Initially, these were often placed in the radial artery via cutdown by the surgeon, and it was not until the late 1960s that anesthesiologists began to place these lines percutaneously. Blood gas analysis was a difficult and time-consuming process and hence infrequently performed until the late 1950s, when Clark, Severinghaus, and Astrup introduced their PO_2, PCO_2, and pH electrodes.[172] Even then, it took a few years until blood gas analysis was commonplace.

A major theme of early experiences with surgery using CPB was difficulty in assessing blood volume status and evaluating ventricular function postbypass. Soon thereafter, monitoring of venous pressure (initially from catheters placed in arm veins and external jugular veins, but then from central lines placed via the groin or arm veins or placed directly into the right atrium at time of surgery) was introduced. However, as early as 1963, the Mayo Clinic group called attention to the frequent discrepancies between central venous (right atrial) and left atrial pressures and described placing catheters directly into the left atrium to monitor function and filling of the left heart.[39] Subsequent authors emphasized the importance of monitoring left atrial pressure in this manner in cardiac surgical patients.[173,174] The monitoring of cardiac patients was revolutionized in 1970 when Swan, Ganz, and Forrester introduced their balloon-tipped PAC.[135] Kaplan helped popularize the use of the PAC during cardiac surgery[175] and emphasized its role in the early diagnosis of myocardial ischemia.[50] Not only did the PAC allow estimation of the left atrial pressure but it also provided access to mixed venous blood for oxygen analysis, and in 1972, it was modified to permit the monitoring of cardiac output by thermodilution. Although the Mayo Clinic group and a few others had monitored cardiac output and identified its prognostic importance and usefulness as a guide to therapy from the dawn of cardiac surgery, cardiac output was difficult to measure and was not generally used until thermodilution via PACs became available. In 1959, the Johns Hopkins Hospital group identified mixed venous oxygen as their most useful indicator of prognosis following cardiac surgery.[176] Although cardiac anesthesiologists were among the first and strongest proponents of the use of the PAC, they were also among the first to point out its limitations[177] and to indicate that not all cardiac surgical patients required a PAC.[178,179]

The Mayo Clinic group from 1955 used EEG monitoring during CPB, and they advocated its value as a monitor of anesthetic depth as well as integrity of cerebral perfusion.[38] Others concurred,[180] but early on skepticism was raised.[181,182] It is interesting that this debate is still unresolved 50 years later.

Transesophageal Echocardiography

TEE has had a profound effect on the practice of cardiac anesthesiology in the past two decades, and, conversely, anesthesiologists played a key role in the introduction of this modality to the practice of cardiogy.[183] Paul Barash of Yale was among the first to apply echocardiography in anesthesiology when he evaluated the effects of halothane on ventricular function in children using transthoracic M-mode echocardiography.[184] Transesophageal Doppler was first described in 1971, and transesophageal M-mode in 1976. In 1980, Masayuki Matsumoto and Yasu Oka at Albert Einstein College of Medicine in the Bronx perceived the future of TEE in cardiac anesthesia when they described the use of M-mode TEE for continuous monitoring of left ventricular function in 21 patients during cardiac surgery.[49] However, M-mode TEE was difficult to interpret except by the extremely sophisticated clinician. Although some primitive two-dimensional TEE scanners were described between 1977 and 1980, it was not until Souquet, Schluter, and Hanrath[185] introduced their phased-array transducer system mounted on the end of a gastroscope that TEE became a practical reality. In the early 1980s, Peter Hanrath brought prototypes to the Mayo Clinic and the University of California in San Francisco (UCSF). A cardiology fellow from Hanrath's group in Germany, P. Kremer, joined anesthesiologists Michael Cahalan and Michael Roizen at UCSF, and at the 1982 meeting of the ASA, they started the TEE "revolution" when they presented their results in monitoring cardiac and vascular surgery patients with this new TEE probe, describing its usefulness in assessing filling and function of the left ventricle, myocardial ischemia, and intracardiac air.[52,53] Cucchiara et al[186] at the Mayo Clinic described its usefulness in detecting air embolism during neurosurgery, while the UCSF group described its superiority over ECG in detecting myocardial ischemia.[187] In 1987, Cahalan et al[188] and Fiona Clements and Norbert deBruijn at Duke University[189] wrote review articles on the use of TEE in anesthesiology. In 1986, Hewlett-Packard introduced color flow Doppler with TEE, and in 1987, deBruijn et al at Duke University reviewed their early experience with this new technology.[60] In that same year, pulsed-wave Doppler was added to TEE, while in 1989, biplane probes first became available. The SCA has played a key role in the development of perioperative TEE. In collaboration with the ASA, they developed the Practice Guidelines for Perioperative TEE in 1996, and in collaboration with the American Society of Echocardiography, they helped initiate the first examination in perioperative TEE, which was administered by the National Board of Echocardiography in 1998. Today, use of TEE is one of the defining characteristics of a cardiac anesthesiologist.

Cardiac Anesthesia Becomes a Subspecialty

It is difficult to identify a precise time when this occurred. In a sense it began with Harmel and Lamont's care of Blalock's blue babies in late 1944 leading to the first paper on cardiac anesthesia in 1946,[27] or with the publishing of the first textbook on cardiac anesthesia by Keown in 1956.[33] Some could argue that because the subspecialty is not recognized by the American Board of Anesthesiology or the American Board of Medical Specialties it is not a subspecialty. However, Lowenstein has convincingly supported his conclusion that cardiac anesthesia fulfills Ralph Waters' (the first academic anesthesiologist in the United States) requirements of a specialty: men and women, publications, and organizations that accept its subspecialty status.[26] This is because of the special knowledge, skills, and activities required of anesthesiologists who attend to these patients. In the beginning, this consisted of the intimate knowledge of the pathophysiology of CHD and how various anesthetic techniques interacted with this pathophysiology.[83] Later, the pathophysiology of VHD and CAD was added.[131] After that was knowledge of the entirely new techniques that surgeons used to manage these patients: initially hypothermia, then CPB and all of its nuances, including DHCA, coronary perfusion, cardioplegia, and retrograde cerebral perfusion. In recent years, this has included minimally invasive techniques such as "port access" (Heart-Port) surgery.[190] "Advanced" monitoring techniques, not usually used in noncardiac anesthesia at the time they were introduced, were on the list of new skills and knowledge required of the cardiac anesthesiologist. These included ECG; EEG; arterial, central venous, and left atrial pressures; next, the PAC; and, most recently, TEE. Intimate knowledge of blood coagulation and anticoagulation and the administration of blood products (often in large quantities) and of various drugs used to modify coagulation was required. Finally, a thorough understanding of the pathophysiology of abnormal hemodynamic states and manipulation with potent and often novel hemodynamically active agents and mechanical assist devices was required. It is apparent that much of this is eventually transferred and adopted into the general practice of noncardiac anesthesia.

To gain all of this knowledge and skill, residents began to seek special training (fellowships) in cardiac anesthesia in the 1970s. One of the first such programs, if not the first, was started at MGH in 1971,[129] and soon thereafter at the University of Pennsylvania, Emory University, University of

Table 1–5 Presidents of Society of Cardiovascular Anesthesiologists

1979	Robert J. Marino	New Orleans, LA
1979–1981	Gerald J. Reves	University of Alabama (later at Duke University)
1981–1983	Fawzy G Estafanous	Cleveland Clinic
1983–1985	Joel A. Kaplan	Emory University (later at Mount Sinai School of Medicine, NYC; then University of Louisville)
1985–1987	Paul G. Barash	Yale University
1987–1989	George E. Burgess III	Baton Rouge, LA
1989–1991	J. Earl Wynands	University of Ottawa (formally McGill University)
1991–1993	John L. Waller	Emory University
1993–1995	Alan J. Schwartz	Medical College of Pennsylvania
1995–1997	Michael F. Roizen	University of Chicago
1997–1999	Richard Davis	University of Oregon
1999–2001	Daniel M. Thys	Columbia University
2001–2003	Roger Moore	Deborah Heart and Lung Center, Browns Mills, NJ
2003–2005	Glen Gravlee	Ohio State University
2005–2007	James Ramsay	Emory University

Alabama, Texas Heart Institute, Stanford University, and the Cleveland Clinic, to name only a few. These were important "incubators" for future cardiac anesthesiologists. Also, modern encyclopedic textbooks on cardiac anesthesia began to appear, starting with the first edition of this text, edited by Joel Kaplan in 1979, and cardiac anesthesiologists began to meet together to share their experience, ideas, and problems. In 1972, the Association of Cardiac Anesthesiologists was founded with Brian Dalton as president, Emerson Moffitt as vice president, and Edward Lowenstein as secretary.[23,129] Because the latter organization limited its membership to 50, the SCA was established in 1978 by Robert Marino, George Burgess, and Martin Peuler, young cardiac anesthesiologists at the Oschner Clinic[46] (Table 1–5). The SCA quickly became the leading subspecialty society in the entire specialty of anesthesiology, with a membership of about 7200, representing 65 countries.[191] In 1987, a new journal appeared devoted to the subspecialty, the *Journal of Cardiothoracic Anesthesia,* introduced by Joel Kaplan. In 1994, the International Anesthesia Research Society (IARS) and the SCA joined in developing a section on cardiovascular anesthesia in the journal *Anesthesia and Analgesia.*[192]

Another somewhat unique characteristic of the subspecialty of cardiac anesthesia was the concept of a team. Brock spoke of this in his previously mentioned lecture in 1949,[20] and Keown listed such teams in 1956[33] (see Table 1–3). The surgeon was no longer able to oversee the whole procedure. Dodds, in his 1961 paper "The Anaesthetist's Role in Open Heart Surgery," emphasized the role of the anesthetist in caring for the patient and overseeing perfusion during CPB so that the surgeon could concentrate on the problems involved in correcting the cardiac defects.[193] Cardiac anesthesiologists also continued to care for these patients in the early postoperative period, and cardiac surgery and cardiac anesthesia played important roles in the development of surgical intensive care units.[70] Lowenstein described the importance of the interaction of surgeons, cardiologists, and anesthesiologists in research, clinical care, and education in the development of the cardiac anesthesia and surgery programs at MGH.[129]

Maturation of the Subspecialty: Leadership and Professionalism

The past two decades have witnessed remarkable growth of this subspecialty in terms of prominence and scientific contributions. Some of the latter have been mentioned earlier. Many cardiac anesthesiologists have became chairs of anesthesia departments and a few, deans, and some have been promoted to dean or vice president of a medical center or university. During the past decade, six cardiac anesthesiologists served as dean of a medical school (124 schools) at the same time. Cardiac anesthesiologists have also been officers and presidents of the ASA, presidents of the American Board of Anesthesiology, editors of the journal *Anesthesiology,* received the ASA Excellence in Research and the Distinguished Service Awards, and given the Rovenstine and Sheldon Lectures.

Cardiac anesthesiologists play active roles in the Society of Thoracic Surgeons, the American Society of Echocardiography, and the American College of Cardiology/American Heart Association (e.g., committees to develop guidelines for perioperative cardiovascular evaluation for noncardiac surgery and for management of arrhythmias); serve as editors or associate editors of the major anesthesia journals and as reviewers for many nonanesthesia journals; and organize and direct major annual workshops on CPB, TEE, and neurologic complications of cardiac surgery.

However, Lowenstein argues that another unique characteristic of the practice of medicine in general and of cardiac anesthesia in particular is *professionalism.* A profession is an occupation that has been granted many privileges by society in exchange for an obligation to benefit society. This includes not only responsibilities to individual patients but also, in Lowenstein's opinion, what he calls *civic professionalism.*[26] Professionalism can readily be eroded and must be protected. As Braunwald has pointed out,[11] although subspecialization has enormous benefits with greater technical expertise and improved patient care, teaching, and research, it also fragments the practice of medicine. "Who is left to oversee and integrate the care of the (cardiac) patient?", he asks. Skilled specialists can perform remarkable procedures but may not always pay equal attention to the more fundamental question of whether the procedure should be performed in the first place. The response of the leaders of this subspecialty has always been: *we* should. Kenneth Keown, in his textbook on cardiac anesthesia in 1956, stated that anesthesiologists should be physicians first and be involved in surgical decision making.[37] Carl Hug thoroughly amplified these themes in his 1999 Rovenstine lecture entitled "Patient Values, Hippocrates, Science and Technology: What We (Physicians) Can Do Versus What We Should Do for the Patient,"[194] and Lowenstein, in his 2003 Abbott Lecture, addressed what physicians can, and in his opinion, what they should do in the realm of "civic professionalism."[26]

SOME OF THE GREAT PIONEERS IN CARDIAC ANESTHESIA†

It is always hazardous to propose a major list of contributors—one is bound to overlook important persons and alienate others and therefore must expect criticism. Despite these concerns, the author wishes to emphasize a number of individuals who have made major and, importantly, long-term contributions to the practice of and education in cardiac anesthesia (and often to anesthesia in general as well).

H. Merel Harmel, along with his mentor, *Austin Lamont* (see Fig. 1–1), provided anesthesia for most of Alfred Blalock's early shunt procedures. Harmel gave anesthesia for Blalock's first case during the eleventh month of his anesthesia training (Merel Harmel, personal communication). Harmel and Lamont then published the first paper on cardiac anesthesia in 1946.[27] Harmel also received formal residency training in anesthesiology under Ralph Waters in Wisconsin[78] and in 1968 became chair of anesthesiology at the first of four different medical schools, most recently at Duke University, where he still teaches. In 1947, Lamont joined Robert Dripps at the University of Pennsylvania,‡ where he played an important role in advancing academic anesthesia and the founding of the Association of University Anesthetists (now termed Anesthesiologists) in 1953.[78]

Kenneth K. Keown,[195] as previously mentioned, provided anesthesia for Charles Bailey's (see Fig. 1–3) first successful mitral commissurotomy in 1948 while a first-year faculty member at Hahnemann Medical College, where he continued to direct cardiac anesthesia until 1957. His and Bailey's work was featured in a *Time* magazine article in 1953. In 1951, he published the first paper on anesthesia for mitral commissurotomy,[29] and in 1956, the first textbook on cardiac anesthesia.[33] He was an early proponent of the use of lidocaine to suppress cardiac arrhythmias during surgery[196,197] and published early papers on anesthesia for cardiac catheterization in infants and children,[198] during hypothermia for cardiac surgery,[32,99] and for open heart surgery.[37] In 1957, he returned to his home state to become founding chair of the Department of Anesthesiology at the University of Missouri–Columbia. There he made his greatest contribution by urging and finally winning recognition of anesthesiology as an independent specialty of medicine and departmental status in the medical schools.[199] He served as first vice president of the ASA (1960–1961), chairman of the board of trustees of the IARS (1967), and chairman of the Section of Anesthesiology of the American Medical Association (1964–1965).

Arthur S. Keats was an early collaborator with Denton Cooley when they started their work in pediatric open heart surgery at the Texas Heart Institute in the mid 1950s (see Fig. 1–9) and where he still works. Arens has listed some of Keats' early contributions to cardiac anesthesia.[23] Keats published early papers on providing anesthesia for CPB in children[110] and the use of succinylcholine[200] and was an early advocate of, and demonstrated the safety of, endotracheal intubation in children and the hemodynamic effects of controlled ventilation. In 1970, he edited the first symposium on the integration of cardiology into anesthesia[133] and in 1984 presented his Rovenstine Lecture, which provided an insightful view of the early history of cardiac anesthesia and lessons he learned over his first 30 years of cardiac anesthesia practice. Later he presented an iconoclastic paper on anesthesia mortality in his 1990 Sheldon Lecture[201] (and his skepticism has been supported by a review published 12 years later[202]). In 1985 and 1989, he co-authored seminal articles with Stephen Slogoff on the significance and pathogenesis of perioperative myocardial ischemia and the absence of effect of choice of anesthetic agent on outcome of cardiac surgery.[58,64,203]

Perhaps of even greater significance are his contributions to the entire specialty of anesthesiology. He was the editor-in-chief of *Anesthesiology* (1970–1973) and president of the American Board of Anesthesiology (1975–1972), where he was responsible for revamping and modifying the written and oral board examinations and introducing the in-training examination in anesthesiology.

As an anesthesia resident, *Emerson A. Moffitt* was a member of the pioneering team at the Mayo Clinic (laboratory and subsequent clinical work) led by John Kirklin, which introduced reproducibly successful open heart surgery using a heart-lung machine in 1955.[36,107] While at the Mayo Clinic, he conducted and published many sophisticated studies on the pathophysiology of CPB[204-206] and summarized the anesthetic care of cardiac patients.[111] He subsequently became chief of anesthesia at Saint Mary's Hospital (the principal cardiac surgery hospital at the Mayo Clinic). In the early 1960s, he collaborated with surgeon Dwight McGoon in a remarkable series of 100 aortic valve replacements without a death[207] (Fig. 1–10). In 1972, he was one of the co-founders of the Association of Cardiac Anesthesiologists and in that same year became chairman of anesthesiology at Dalhousie University in Nova Scotia.

After a sabbatical with H. J. C. Swan in Los Angeles (1979–1980), he embarked on numerous sophisticated studies on the impact of various anesthetic techniques on the balance of myocardial oxygen demand and supply during clinical cardiac anesthesia using coronary sinus catheters between 1980 and 1992. Summarizing some of this work, in 1986 he, with Dhun Sethna, published two review articles covering the coronary circulation and the effects of anesthesia on it in *Anesthesia and Analgesia*.[208,209] He also was chair of the board of trustees of the IARS and the Association of Canadian University Departments of Anaesthesia and an associate editor of *Anesthesia and Analgesia* and the *Canadian Anaesthetists Society Journal*.

J. Earl Wynands provided anesthesia to Vineberg's patients undergoing IMA implant operation, and in 1967, he wrote the first article on providing anesthesia for patients undergoing the Vineberg procedure[40] (Fig. 1–11). He was co-founder of the Association of Cardiac Anesthesiologists and president of the SCA from 1987 to 1989. He has contributed many important articles to the literature and trained many cardiac anesthesiologists. In 1996, he published a well-illustrated and informative paper on the contributions of Canadian anesthesiologists to the subspecialty, much of it based on his personal recollection.[24] He is one of the few anesthesiologists to receive the Order of Canada.

†For a personal insight into some of these pioneers, the interested reader is referred to the Wood Library-Museum of the ASA Living History Series videotapes: No. LH0077—Robert W. Virtue. Interview by Phillip Bromage, Feb 1982; No. LH0024—Merel Harmel. Interview by Philip Bromarge and Robert Virtue, 1983; No. LH 0032—Arthur Keats. Interview by M. T. "Pepper" Jenkins, 1978; and No. LH0033—Kenneth Keown. Interview by Noel Lawson, 1982.

‡This partnership subsequently broke up in 1946 when Blalock rejected Lamont's proposal to establish a "professional" physician-delivered anesthesia and academic program in anesthesiology at Johns Hopkins. Lamont left Johns Hopkins and then joined Robert Dripps at the Hospital of the University of Pennsylvania (see Ref. 78).

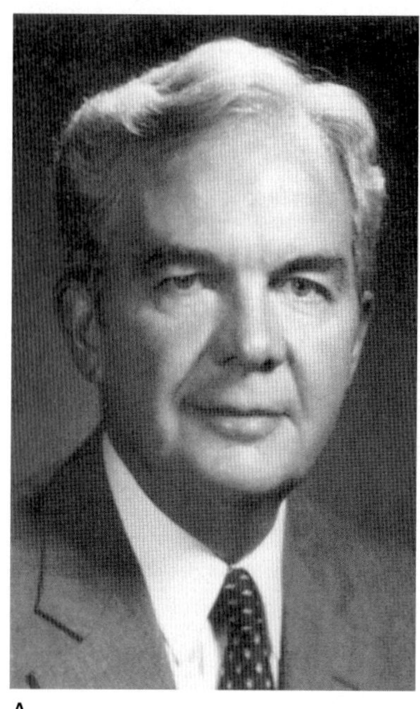
A
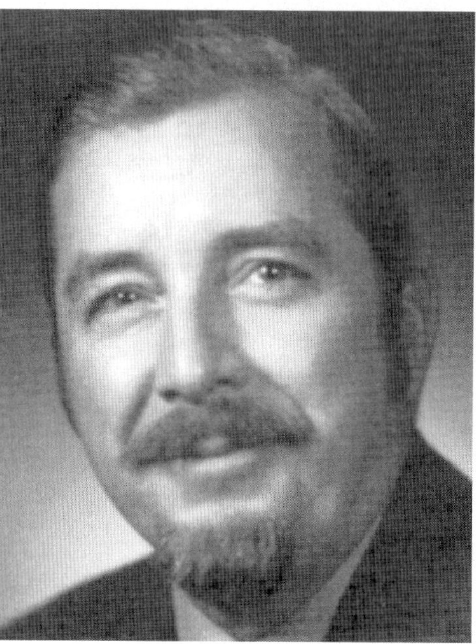
B

Figure 1–10 Master Mayo Clinic team. (*A*) Dwight McGoon, surgeon, and (*B*) Emerson Moffitt, anesthesiologist. In 1965 they reported a series of 100 consecutive aortic valve replacements without a death. Both have made many important contributions to their respective subspecialties. (*A* is from Westaby and Bosher,[9] with permission from the author; *B* is from Wood Library–Museum of Anesthesiology, with permission.)

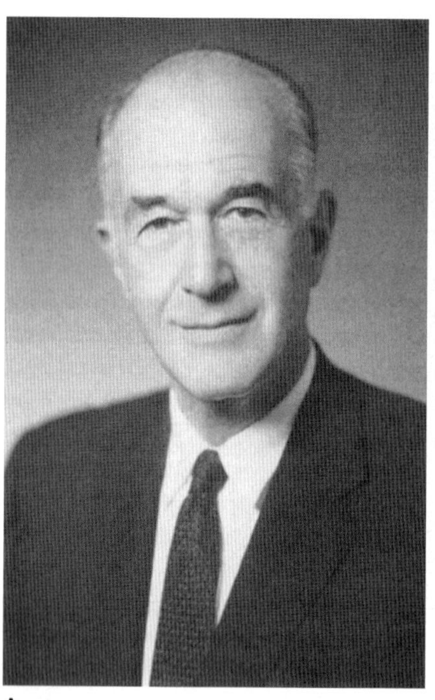
A
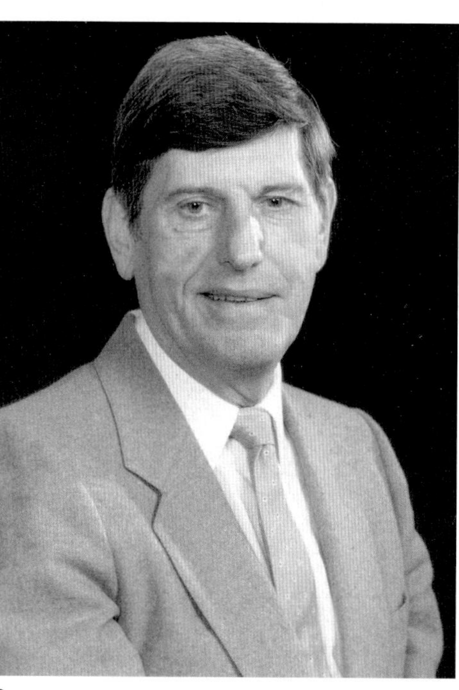
B

Figure 1–11 Early surgery for coronary artery disease. (*A*) Arthur Vineberg, surgeon, McGill University, Montreal, began experimental development of his internal mammary artery implant operation in 1946 and applied it clinically in the early 1950s. Only after Mason Sones (cardiologist, Cleveland Clinic) demonstrated patency of these grafts did the operation become popular. (*B*) J. Earl Wynands provided anesthesia for these procedures by Vineberg in the 1960s and wrote the first paper on this topic in 1967, reporting remarkably good results in 1970. He went on to make many other contributions to the subspecialty. (*A* is from Shumaker,[8] with permission; *B* is from Wood Library–Museum of Anesthesiology, with permission.)

Edward Lowenstein (Fig. 1–12) is considered by many to be the father of academic cardiac anesthesia. In 1969, he became the first chief of the first academic cardiac anesthesia group (CAG) (devoted exclusively to anesthetic management of cardiac surgical patients).[129] In 1969, he was the first author in their landmark article that introduced high-dose narcotic (morphine) anesthesia.[41] Interestingly, their abstract was rejected for presentation at the annual meeting of the ASA.[210] In 1976, he and John Bland published an experimental study demonstrating the benefits of inhalation anesthesia (halothane) on myocardial ischemia.[211] This may have been the first demonstration of myocardial preconditioning by a volatile anesthetic (although at that time they attributed the benefits to favorable effects on the balance of myocardial oxygen supply and demand). In 1972, he helped establish the Association of Cardiac Anesthesiologists (founding secretary), and in 1974, he organized the first ASA Refresher Course in Cardiac Anesthesia.[129] In 1993, as chair of the Publications Committee, he helped negotiate the relationship between *Anesthesia and Analgesia* (IARS) and the SCA.[192]

In recent years, he has done graduate studies in ethics and now serves in the Division of Medical Ethics of the Harvard Medical School. His Abbott Lecture at the 25th Annual Meeting of the SCA on professionalism and ethics reflects this interest.[26] In 1971, the CAG at MGH established one of the first 1-year fellowship programs in cardiac anesthesia. Of those who finished during the next 12 years, 15 became professors, 12 became chairs of departments, and 12 have led

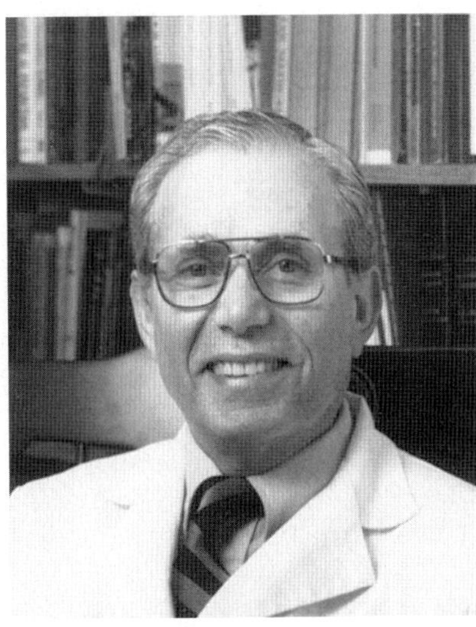

Figure 1–12 Edward Lowenstein, "father of academic cardiac anesthesiology" and director of one of the first cardiac anesthesia groups (1969), initiated one of the first 1-year cardiac anesthesia fellowship programs (1971) at the Massachusetts General Hospital, Boston. He, along with other members of this group, introduced high-dose narcotic anesthesia (1969), and he is now a leader in ethics and professionalism in anesthesia. (Photograph courtesy of E. Lowenstein.)

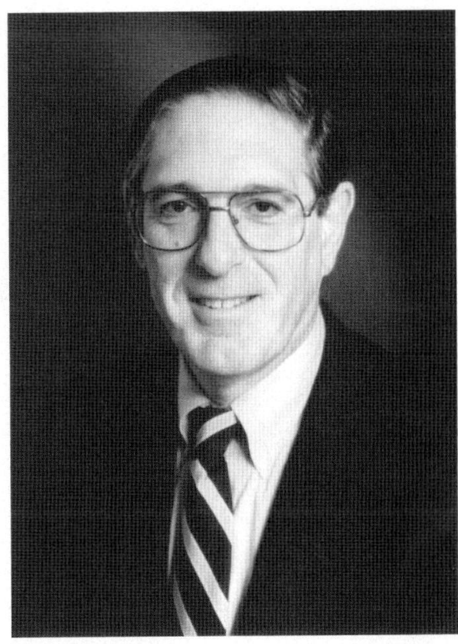

Figure 1–13 Joel A. Kaplan, "promoter" of cardiac anesthesia, emphasized the importance of the subspecialty to surgeons, cardiologists, and anesthesiologists and popularized the use of pulmonary artery catheters, nitroglycerin infusions, and monitoring the V_5 lead. He edited the first modern encyclopedic textbooks *Cardiac Anesthesia* (1979), *Thoracic Anesthesia* (1983), and *Vascular Anesthesia* (1991), and the first journal devoted to cardiothoracic anesthesia (1987). He was a cardiac anesthesia program director (Emory), department chairman (Mount Sinai, NY), and, most recently, Dean of the School of Medicine, Chancellor of the Health Sciences Center, and Executive Vice President of the University of Louisville (Louisville, KY). (Photograph courtesy of J. Kaplan.)

anesthetic groups.[129] Many of the leaders in the subspecialty are graduates of this program.

In 1976, 1 year after becoming new staff members at the Oschner Clinic where they were expected to provide cardiac anesthesia, *Robert Marino and George E. Burgess III*, along with colleague Martin Peuler, contacted the Association of Cardiac Anesthesiologists about membership but were turned down because of its limited membership. So, after surveying their colleagues, they decided to form a new society open to anyone interested in cardiovascular anesthesia, and in November 1978, the SCA was established with Marino as the first president. Their aim was the promulgation of the subspecialty through education and exchange of ideas, starting with the first annual meeting in 1979 (50 attended) and a newsletter beginning in May of that same year.[46] Burgess became its sixth president (see Table 1–5). Both have remained active (currently on the Board of Directors) in nurturing this society, which now has more than 7200 members, with more than 1000 attending its annual meeting.

Joel A. Kaplan (Fig. 1–13), the editor of this text, deserves much credit for the popularity and status of this subspecialty. Starting out as a young faculty member at Emory University, he "sold" the importance and value of cardiac anesthesiologists to surgeons and cardiologists and anesthesia residents at various institutions and meetings. This text, which he edits, first came out in 1979, was the first modern encyclopedic textbook in cardiac anesthesia, and set the standard against which all other texts in the subspecialty are measured. His name almost became synonymous with the PAC (see the logo on the fourth edition of this textbook and on earlier issues of the journal he edits). He helped introduce intravenous nitroglycerin infusions[45] and monitoring of the V_5 lead[44] to the subspecialty. In 1987, he started the first journal devoted to the subspecialty: *Journal of Cardiothoracic* (and subsequently added: *Vascular*) *Anesthesia*. He was the fourth president of the SCA (1983 to 1985), and in recognition of his knowledge and his skills as a communicator, he presented a refresher course lecture on cardiac anesthesia for more than 10 years at the annual meeting of the ASA. He moved from Emory to become chair of anesthesiology at Mount Sinai School of Medicine, and then to Louisville, Kentucky, where he was Dean of the School of Medicine and leader of the university's Health Science Center.

J. Gerald Reves (Fig. 1–14) started his career in cardiac anesthesia with William Lell at the University of Alabama. In 1984, he published a landmark study of cerebral blood flow during CPB,[56] which ushered in a career-long investigation of the cerebral effects of CPB and many other studies by his group. He became director of cardiac anesthesia at Duke University, where he developed one of the strongest clinical, research, and fellowship programs in cardiac anesthesia. Subsequently, as department chairman, he developed similarly strong programs in many other subspecialties of anesthesia. Recently, he became dean of the Medical University of South Carolina in Charleston. He was the second president of the SCA, first associate editor-in-chief for cardiovascular anesthesia of the journal *Anesthesia and Analgesia* (in 1994), and one of the editors of a major textbook in cardiac anesthesia. However, in the author's opinion, his greatest contribution to the subspecialty has been his strong advocacy of full status for the subspecialty and championing strong clinical and research-oriented fellowship training.

Michael K. Cahalan (Fig. 1–15) is largely responsible for introducing TEE to cardiology in the United States and for popularizing its use in anesthesiology.[52,53] He authored one of the first review articles on the subject[188] and has played crucial roles in developing ASA/SCA guidelines for perioperative TEE,[65] the American Society of Echocardiography/SCA guidelines for performing a basic perioperative TEE examination,[66]

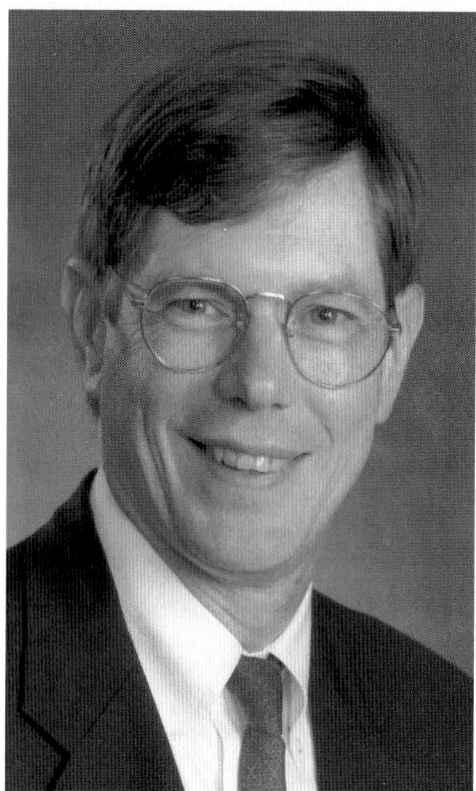

Figure 1–14 J. Gerald Reves, a strong proponent of academic cardiac anesthesia, was an early student of the effects of cardiopulmonary bypass on the central nervous system. He built a strong academic anesthesia program (expert clinical care, outstanding research, academic fellowship training) at Duke University. He has been a strong advocate of special training and formal recognition of cardiac anesthesiologists. He is now a dean of the Medical University of South Carolina. (Photograph courtesy of Wood Library–Museum of Anesthesiology.)

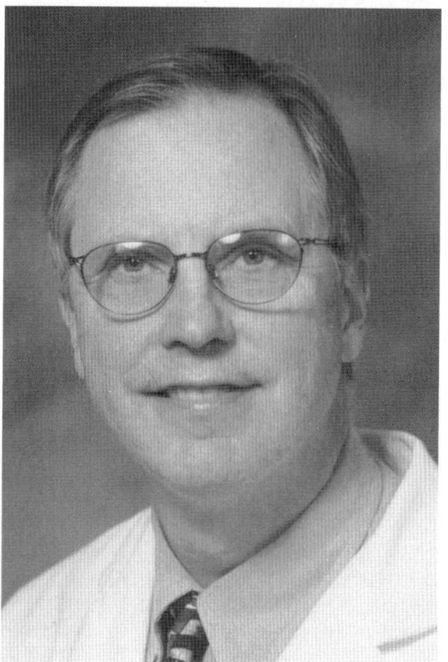

Figure 1–15 Michael K. Cahalan, "father of perioperative transesophageal echocardiography" (TEE), pioneered exploration of the use of TEE perioperatively at the University of California in San Francisco in 1982. He helped to introduce this modality to cardiologists, surgeons, and anesthesiologists. He also helped lead the subspecialty into collaboration with echocardiologists with the development of postgraduate courses, guidelines, and certifying examinations in perioperative TEE. (Photograph courtesy of M. K. Cahalan.)

and for training in perioperative TEE.[67] He contributed much to the acceptance of cardiac anesthesiologists as qualified echocardiographers by cardiologists and to nurturing collaboration with echocardiologists and the American Society of Echocardiography. He produced one of the first educational CD-ROMs on TEE, is a multiple repeat ASA refresher course lecturer on this topic, and is currently chairman of the Department of Anesthesiology at the University of Utah.

Dennis T. Mangano (Fig. 1–16) could be considered the father of multicenter collaborative trials in cardiac anesthesia and the epidemiology of perioperative cardiac morbidity. This began with important publications on the role of pulmonary artery catheterization in cardiac surgery[178] and perioperative ECG monitoring, the effect of perioperative myocardial ischemia during noncardiac surgery on postoperative cardiac morbidity,[212] and a review article on perioperative cardiac morbidity[213] based on careful studies of his patients in San Francisco. In the late 1980s, he initiated the Multi-Center Study of Perioperative Ischemia Research Group (MCSPI), which includes more than 80 medical centers throughout the United States, Canada, Europe, and the Ischemia Research and Education Foundation Investigators, permitting the prospective enrollment and study of thousands of patients. These may have been modeled after the multicenter studies being conducted by cardiologists. This has helped launch the career of many young cardiac anesthesia investigators and has resulted in numerous important publications. Among the most notable were the study on the profound benefits of prophylactic β-blockade on patients undergoing noncardiac surgery,[214] which launched its general acceptance into medical practice; the study of the incidence of neurologic complications of CPB,[215] which reawakened interest in the problem in the general medical and nonmedical community; and the study of the roles of acadesine[216] and of aspirin[217] in reducing

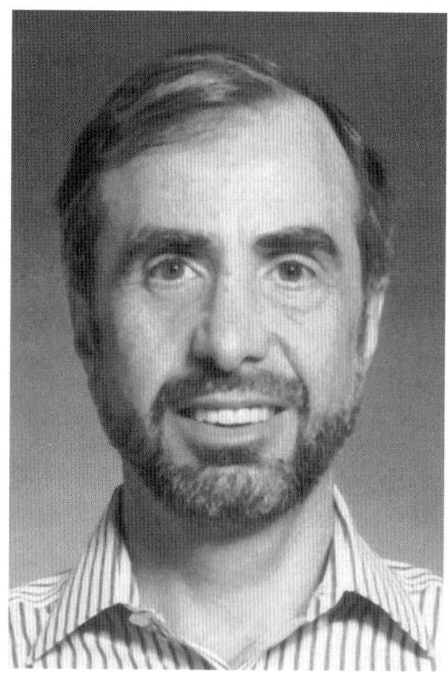

Figure 1–16 Dennis T. Mangano, "father of multicenter studies in cardiac anesthesia," drew attention to perioperative cardiac morbidity and conducted studies that led to the acceptance of the use of prophylactic β-adrenergic–blocking agents during noncardiac surgery. (Photograph courtesy of D. Mangano.)

Table 1–6 Changes Over the Past 45 Years in Cardiac Anesthesia	Keown's Textbook (1956)	Kaplan's Textbook (Fifth Edition, 2006)
Coauthors	0	94
Chapters	20	41
Pages	109	1411
Words	32,000	1,100,000
References	115	11,913
Size	$5^3/_4 \times 8^5/_8 \times {}^1/_2$ in	$8^5/_8 \times 11^1/_4 \times 2^1/_2$ in
Weight	12 oz	nearly 8 lb

New chapters and topics in Kaplan's Fifth Edition

Future of cardiology, cardiothoracic surgery, and cardiac anesthesia
Advances in coronary pathophysiology
Molecular cardiovascular medicine
Systemic inflammation with surgery and cardiopulmonary bypass
New cardiovascular drugs
Assessment of cardiac risk
Cardiac interventional laboratory
Cardiac electrophysiology laboratory
Transesophageal echocardiography and other cardiovascular monitors
Clinical decision making with transesophageal echocardiography
Minimally invasive and robotic cardiac surgery
Implantable cardiac defibrillators
Ventricular assist devices and artificial hearts
Postoperative cardiac outcomes
Business of running the operating rooms and intensive care units
Quality of care in cardiac surgery
Decreasing errors in cardiac anesthesia

perioperative morbidity following coronary artery surgery. Many of these articles have appeared in nonanesthesia journals (e.g., *New England Journal of Medicine* and *Journal of the American Medical Association*), which has helped raise the stature of cardiac anesthesia in the nonanesthesia medical community. He has nurtured the careers of many cardiac anesthesiologists.

CONCLUDING COMMENTS

One way of measuring the progress in cardiac anesthesia is to compare the latest edition of this textbook with the first textbook in cardiac anesthesia published nearly 50 years ago by Keown[33] (Table 1–6). Another way is to look at the number of participants. In 1970, Dalton identified fewer than 50 anesthesiologists concentrating on cardiac anesthesia in the United States and Canada.[26,129] There are currently more than 7200 members of the SCA from around the world.

Cardiac anesthesia has made innumerable contributions to the general practice of anesthesia as well as cardiac medicine and surgery. Some of these include ECG monitoring; use of arterial, central venous, and pulmonary artery catheters and hemodynamic data; perioperative TEE; and the use of arterial blood gases and acid-base analysis. Cardiac anesthesiologists led the way in involving anesthesiologists in postoperative care and participated in the development of intensive respiratory and surgical care units and critical care laboratories ("stat labs")[218] and, conversely, with introducing the methods and philosophy of critical care into the operating room. The introduction of the use of many new cardiovascular drugs (e.g., inotropic agents, vasodilators, vasopressors, antiarrhythmics, antifibrinolytics, direct thrombin inhibitors, and new hemostatic agents) into the operating room environment and general anesthesia care was largely accomplished by cardiac anesthesiologists. Cardiac anesthesiologists were largely responsible for identifying the incidence, significance, role of tachycardia, and methods to reduce perioperative myocardial ischemia (especially the use of β-adrenergic–blocking agents), in providing guidance in the preoperative assessment and perioperative management of cardiac patients undergoing noncardiac surgery, and in reassessing the role and benefits of preoperative laboratory testing. Many cardiac anesthesiologists have made extremely important contributions to the specialty of anesthesiology. Three examples stand out: Austin Lamont was a driving force for the development of academic anesthesia and the founding of the Association of University Anesthetists (Anesthesiologists). Kenneth Keown played a major role in facilitating the reorganization of the independent specialty status of anesthesia in organized medicine and in medical schools. Arthur Keats modernized the examination system of the ABA and introduced the in-training examination.

Several authors have examined the nature of discovery and evolution of medicine in general and of cardiac medicine and surgery in particular.[2,11,219-224] Julius Comroe's monograph *Retrospectroscope. Insights Into Medical Discovery*[222] is particularly illuminating. Gott identified four common attributes of the great innovators in cardiac surgery: brilliance, determination, creativity, and courage.[7] However, when mentioning progress, the patients should not be forgotten. This is best expressed by Westaby's comment after reviewing the clinical course of Barney Miller, the first patient to receive a Jarvik artificial heart: "We should remember that without the consent of many courageous patients, the great advances in cardiac surgery could not occur."[9]

What can be learned from this review of the history of cardiac anesthesia? To paraphrase Eugene Braunwald's recent essay on the history of cardiology,[11] it is observed first that achievements and progress did not develop de novo; they were built on many decades of research, usually by basic scientists and engineers. Second, they came from interdisciplinary collaborations that included physiologists, cardiologists, surgeons, and anesthesiologists, people working in laboratories and clinics, and people from academia, industry, and private practice. Third, they often involve international participation with leadership provided from many different countries.

There are a number of relevant observations to be made from a review of the history of cardiac surgery and anesthesiology.

1. Serendipity often comes into play. Examples include the discovery of heparin (McLean was looking for a *coagulant*[225,226]), protamine reversal of heparin (Chargoff and Olson were trying to *prolong the action* of heparin[227]), selective coronary angiography (Sones was performing an aortic root arteriogram when the catheter inadvertently slipped into the coronary artery), closed chest massage (Kouwenhoven and Jude noted a pressure rise when the defibrillator paddles were applied), and aprotinin (while trying to block the inflammatory response to CPB, the investigators noted that the surgical fields were surprisingly dry).
2. Beware of rejecting new ideas and the danger of "conventional wisdom" and "expert" opinion. The early rejection of surgery on the heart by Billroth, the idea of

cardiac catheterization (Forssmann was fired by his chief of surgery after demonstrating its feasibility[1]), and the general rejection of Kolessov's and Green's IMA–coronary artery anastomosis are just a few of many examples.

3. Youth does not preclude innovative success and in fact tends to foster it. McLean was a medical student when he discovered heparin,[225,226] and Gross was a surgery resident when he first successfully ligated a PDA. Forssmann was also a surgical resident when he first successfully performed right heart catheterization (on himself). Harmel was a resident when he provided anesthesia for Dr. Blalock's first shunt operations and when he and Lamont wrote the first paper on cardiac anesthesia. Keown was a first-year faculty member when he anesthetized Bailey's first successful mitral commissurotomy patient. Gibbon constructed his first successful heart-lung machine while still in training. However, advanced age is not a limitation: William Kouwenhoven was a 75-year-old retired engineer when he developed and introduced closed chest massage, and Lowell Edwards was a retired engineer when he collaborated with surgeon Albert Starr to develop and introduce their phenomenally successfully prosthetic heart valves in the early 1960s.
4. The importance of laboratory work in providing a foundation for clinical success.[11] Most of the great clinical advances, for example, ligation of PDA, resection of coarctation, creation of the subclavian–to–pulmonary artery shunt, IMA implantation, artificial valves, and artificial hearts, were preceded by extensive laboratory investigation. Further, as pointed out by Comroe, many of these clinical advances were dependent on basic science research, much of which had no apparent practical application at the time that it was performed.[221]
5. A creative environment and supportive basic science and laboratory research are important. Currently, the pressure of clinical work, the reduction in support for basic and clinical research in academic centers, and perhaps a desire for personal wealth have eroded leadership in new science and new advances. As a subspecialty, this issue needs to be addressed to ameliorate these limitations.
6. The importance of challenging the status quo, the "standard of care" (e.g., hypothermia, cold cardioplegia, prolonged intubation), and of reexamining discarded ideas and methods (e.g., potassium cardiac arrest, mitral annuloplasty, off-pump CABG, radial artery grafts, homograft valves, the Ross procedure, etc.).
7. The great cardiac anesthesiologists of the past (and present) have contributed much more to anesthesia than just to their subspecialty. They have been productive citizens of anesthesia, medicine, and society, and they should be emulated.
8. Finally, anesthesiologists all "stand on the shoulders of giants."

If the reader becomes overly impressed with the accomplishments and outcomes achieved with current "modern" cardiac surgery and anesthesia, recall some of the remarkably good results of our predecessors. In their 1956 report of their first 1000 cases of surgery for CHD at Chicago's Memorial Children's Hospital, Potts and McQuiston (surgeon and anesthesiologist, respectively) reported no deaths in their 347 children (28 days to 16 years of age) undergoing closure of a PDA.[86] In 1959, Conn[102] reported 63 consecutive secundum ASDs closed with aid of hypothermia and inflow occlusion at the Hospital for Sick Children in Toronto without a fatality. In 1970, Wynands et al[131] reported only one death in their last 78 patients undergoing a Vineberg procedure in Montreal, even though one third had rest angina and this operation did not result in immediate improvement in coronary perfusion. Perhaps most striking of all was the report by Dwight McGoon and Emerson Moffitt (surgeon and anesthesiologist) of the Mayo Clinic of their first 100 aortic valve replacements with a Starr-Edwards valve performed between February 1963 and December 1964 with *no* deaths.[207] This was all done prior to the availability of CABG, cardioplegia, PACs, and TEE.

In closing this brief history of cardiac surgery and anesthesia, listen to Lord Brock: "These operations . . . are tiring and anxious procedures involving much care, responsibility and hard work. Fortunately they have their happier side and we are in large part recompensated for the long and difficult hours by seeing the almost miraculous change in the children themselves and in witnessing the joy and relief of the parents when they see their children running about happily and without effort like other children."[20] The modern anesthesiologist is perhaps jaded by daily miracles that they do not recognize.

According to John Kirklin on the occasion of the 25th anniversary of open heart surgery at the Mayo Clinic: "We could, of course . . . rejoice in our accomplishments, and accept the idea that nature sets certain limits to everything, including cardiac surgery. Billroth expressed such a view in 1897 when he said that cardiac surgery had reached the limits set by nature. Those in 1954 who urged aborting the pump-oxygenator effort must have had a similar notion. Not the passage of time but the efforts of many people have proven the idea to be wrong at both points in time. I believe that acceptance of such an idea today would also be wrong."[108]

Finally, as Paul Dudley White, America's first academic cardiologist, stated: by studying medical history "we acquire a better perspective of our own place in history with the humbling realization of our role as merely a link in the long chain of the acquisition and application of medical knowledge."[1] Undoubtedly much, if not all, of what constitutes the knowledge and practice of cardiac anesthesia today will be replaced in the future, and what is done today will also "become history."

REFERENCES

1. Fye WB: President's Page. Medical history: A valuable tool to help us frame the present and predict the future. J Am Coll Cardiol 41:346, 2003
2. Hessel EA II: History of cardiac surgery and anesthesia. *In* Estafanous FG, Barash PG, Reves JG (eds): Cardiac Anesthesia: Principles and Clinical Practice, 2nd edition. Philadelphia, Lippincott, Williams, & Wilkins, 2001, p 3
3. Meade RH: A History of Thoracic Surgery. Springfield, IL, Charles C Thomas, 1961
4. Johnson SL: The History of Cardiac Surgery: 1896-1955. Baltimore, The Johns Hopkins Press, 1970
5. Litwak RS: The growth of cardiac surgery: Historical notes. *In* Harken DE (ed): Cardiac Surgery, I. Cardiovasc Clin 3:5, 1971
6. Kirklin JW: Technical and scientific advances in cardiac surgery over the past 25 years. Ann Thorac Surg 49:26, 1990
7. Gott VL: And it happened during our lifetime.... Ann Thorac Surg 55:1057, 1993
8. Shumacker HB Jr: The evolution of cardiac surgery. Bloomington, IN, Indiana University Press, 1992
9. Westaby S, Bosher C: Landmarks in Cardiac Surgery. Oxford, Isis Medical Media, 1998
10. Mehta NJ, Khan IA: Cardiology's 10 greatest discoveries of the 20th century. Texas Heart Inst J 229:164, 002

11. Braunwald E: Cardiology: The past, present, and the future (The Simon Dock Lecture). J Am Coll Cardiol 42:2031, 2003
12. Fye WB: American Cardiology: The History of a Specialty and Its College. Baltimore, MD, Johns Hopkins University Press, 1996
13. Ryan TJ: The coronary angiogram and its seminal contributions to cardiovascular medicine over five decades. Circulation 106:752, 2002
14. Meyer RA: History of ultrasound in cardiology. J Ultrasound Med 23:1, 2004
15. Hessel EA II: Cardiac anesthesia timeline. ASA Newsletter 65:5, 2001
16. Blalock A, Taussig HB: The surgical treatment of malformations of the heart in which there is pulmonary stenosis or pulmonary atresia. JAMA 138:189, 1945
17. Potts WJ, Smith S, Gibson S: Anastomosis of the aorta to a pulmonary artery. Certain types in congenital heart disease. JAMA 132:627, 1946
18. Sellors TH: Surgery of pulmonary stenosis. A case in which the pulmonary valve was successfully divided. Lancet 1:988, 1948
19. Blalock A: Physiopathology and surgical treatment of congenital cardiovascular defects (Harvey Lecture November 15, 1945). Bull NY Acad Med 22:57, 1946
20. Brock RC: The surgery of pulmonic stenosis. (The Alexander Simpson-Smith Lecture). BMJ 2:399, 1949
21. Keown KK: Anesthesia for Surgery of the Heart, 2nd edition. Springfield, IL, Charles C Thomas, 1963
22. Lake CL: History of pediatric cardiac anesthesia. *In* Lake CL (ed): Pediatric Cardiac Anesthesia, 3rd edition. Stanford, CT, Appleton and Lange, 1998, p 1
23. Arens JF: Three decades of cardiac anesthesia. Mt Sinai J Med 52:516, 1985
24. Wynands JE: History of cardiac anaesthesia. The contribution of Canadian anaesthetists to the evolution of cardiac surgery. Can J Anaesth 43:518, 1996
25. Keats AS: The Rovenstine Lecture, 1983: Cardiovascular anesthesia: Perceptions and perspectives. Anesthesiology 60:467, 1984
26. Lowenstein E: Cardiac anesthesiology, professionalism and ethics: A microcosm of anesthesiology and medicine. Anesth Analg 98:927, 2004
27. Harmel MH, Lamont A: Anesthesia in the surgical treatment of congenital pulmonic stenosis. Anesthesiology 7:477, 1946
28. Massa DJ, Lundy JS, Faulconer A, et al: A plastic needle. Proc Staff Meet Mayo Clin 25:413, 1950
29. Keown KK, Grove DD, Roth HS: Anesthesia for commissurotomy for mitral stenosis. Preliminary report. JAMA 146:446, 1951
30. Himmelstein A, Scheiner M: The cardiotachoscope. Anesthesiology 13:62, 1952
31. Smith C: An endo-esophageal stethoscope. Anesthesiology 15:566, 1954
32. Keown KK, Bailey CP, Downing DF, et al: Hypothermia as an adjunct to the anesthetic management of the cyanotic patient for intracardiac surgery. Anesth Analg 33:213, 1954
33. Keown KK: Anesthesia for Surgery of the Heart. Springfield, IL, Charles C Thomas, 1956
34. Gain EA: Anaesthetic experiences using extracorporeal circulation for open heart surgery. Can Anaesth Soc J 4:419, 1957
35. Mendelsohn D, MacKrell TN, MacLachlan MA, et al: Experiences using the pump-oxygenator for open cardiac surgery in man. Anesthesiology 18:223, 1957
36. Patrick RT, Theye RA, Moffitt EA: Studies in extracorporeal circulation. V. Anesthesia and supportive care during intracardiac surgery with the Gibbon-type pump-oxygenator. Anesthesiology 18:673, 1957
37. Keown KK, Gilman RA, Bailey CP: Open heart surgery: Anesthesia and surgical experience. JAMA 165:781, 1957
38. Theye RA, Patrick RT, Kirklin JW: The electroencephalogram in patients undergoing open intracardiac operations with the aid of extracorporeal circulation. J Thorac Surg 34:709, 1957
39. Kirklin JW, Theye RA: Cardiac performance after open intracardiac surgery. Circulation 28:1061, 1963
40. Wynands JE, Sheridan CA, Kelkar K: Coronary artery disease and anaesthesia (experience in 120 patients for revascularization of the heart). Can Anaesth Soc J 14:382, 1967
41. Lowenstein E, Hallowell P, Levine FH, et al: Cardiovascular response to large doses of intravenous morphine in man. N Engl J Med 281:1389, 1969
42. Civetta JM, Gabel JC: Flow directed-pulmonary artery catheterization in surgical patients: indications and modification of technique. Ann Surg 176:753, 1972
43. Lappas D, Lell WA, Gabel JC, et al: Indirect measurement of left-atrial pressure in surgical patients—Pulmonary-capillary wedge pressure and pulmonary-artery diastolic pressure compared with left-atrial pressure. Anesthesiology 38:394, 1973
44. Kaplan JA, King SB: The precordial electrocardiographic lead (V_5) in patients who have coronary-artery disease. Anesthesiology 45:570, 1976
45. Kaplan JA, Dunbar RW, Jones EL: Nitroglycerin infusion during coronary-artery surgery. Anesthesiology 45:14, 1976
46. Marino RJ, Burgess GE III: The history of SCA. 25th Annual Meeting of the Society of Cardiovascular Anesthesiologists. Program booklet page 25, SCA, Richmond, VA, 2003
47. Stanley TH, Webster LR: Anesthetic requirements and cardiovascular effects of fentanyl-oxygen and fentanyl-diazapam-oxygen anesthesia in man. Anesth Analg 57:411, 1978
48. Kaplan JA (ed): Cardiac Anesthesia. Philadelphia, WB Saunders, 1979
49. Matsumoto M, Oka Y, Strom J, et al: Application of transesophageal echocardiography to continuous intraoperative monitoring of left ventricular performance. Am J Cardiol 46:95, 1980
50. Kaplan JA, Wells PH: Early diagnoses of myocardial ischemia using the pulmonary artery catheter. Anesth Analg 60:789, 1981
51. Ream AK, Reitz BA, Silverberg G: Temperature correction of PCO_2 and pH in estimating acid-base status: An example of the emperor's new clothes? Anesthesiology 56:41, 1982
52. Cahalan MK, Kremer P, Schiller NB, et al: Intraoperative monitoring with two-dimensional transesophageal echocardiography (abstract). Anesthesiology 57:A, 1982
53. Roizen MF, Kremer P, Cahalan M, et al: Monitoring with transesophageal echocardiography: patients undergoing supraceliac aortic occlusion (abstract). Anesthesiology 57:A, 1982
54. Reiz S, Balfors E, Sorensen MB, et al: Isoflurane: A powerful coronary vasodilator in patients with coronary artery disease. Anesthesiology 59:91, 1983
55. McKay RD, Reves JG, Karp RB, et al: Effects of cardiopulmonary bypass on cerebral blood flow (abstract) Anesth Analg 62:274, 1983
56. Govier AV, Reves JG, McKay RD, et al: Factors and their influence on regional cerebral blood flow during nonpulsatile cardiopulmonary bypass. Ann Thorac Surg 38:592, 1984
57. Henriksen L, Hjelms E, Lindeburgh T: Brain hyperperfusion during cardiac operations. Cerebral blood flow measured in man by intra-arterial injection of xenon-133: Evidence suggestive of intraoperative microembolism. J Thorac Cardiovasc Surg 86:202, 1983
58. Slogoff S, Keats AS: Does perioperative myocardial ischemia lead to postoperative myocardial infarctions? Anesthesiology 62:107, 1985
59. Nussmeier NA, Arlund C, Slogoff S: Neuropsychiatric complications after cardiopulmonary bypass: Cerebral protection by a barbiturate. Anesthesiology 64:165, 1986
60. deBruijn NP, Clements FM, Kisslo JA: Intraoperative color-flow mapping: Initial experience. Anesth Analg 66:386, 1987
61. Royston D, Bidstrup BD, Taylor KM, et al: Effect of aprotinin on need for blood transfusion after repeat open heart surgery. Lancet 2:1289, 1987
62. Van Oeveren W, Jansen NJG, Bidstrup BP, et al: Effects of aprotinin on hemostatic mechanisms during cardiopulmonary bypass. Ann Thorac Surg 44:640, 1987
63. Tuman KJ, McCarthy RJ, Spiess BD, et al: Does choice of anesthetic agent significantly affect outcome of coronary artery surgery? Anesthesiology 70:199, 1989
64. Slogoff S, Keats AS: Randomized trial of primary anesthetic agents on outcome of coronary artery bypass operations. Anesthesiology 70:179, 1989
65. Practice guidelines for perioperative echocardiography. A report by the American Society of Anesthesiologists and the Society of Cardiovascular Anesthesiologists task force on transesophageal echocardiography. Anesthesiology 84:986, 1996
66. Shanewise JS, Cheung AT, Aronson S, et al: ASE/SCA Guidelines for performing a comprehensive intraoperative multiplane transesophageal echocardiography examination. Anesth Analg 89:870, 1999
67. Cahalan MK, Abel M, Goldman M, et al: American Society of Echocardiography and Society of Cardiovascular Anesthesiologists Task Force guidelines for training in perioperative echocardiography. Anesth Analg 94:1384, 2002
68. Rendell-Baker L: History of thoracic anesthesia. *In* Mushin WW (ed): Thoracic Anesthesia. Philadelphia, FA Davis, 1963, p 598
69. Kaplan JA: History of thoracic anesthesia. *In* Kaplan JA (ed): Thoracic Anesthesia. Churchill Livingstone, 1983, New York, pp 3–9
70. Hilberman M: The evolution of intensive care units. Crit Care Med 3:159, 1975
71. Calverley RK: Anesthesia as a specialty. Past, present, future. *In* Barash PG, Cullen BF, Stoelting RK (eds): Clinical Anesthesia, 3rd edition. Philadelphia Lippincott-Raven, 1997
72. Ellis RH: The first transauricular mitral valvotomy. An account to mark the fiftieth anniversary of the operation. Anaesthesia 30:374, 1975

73. Souttar HS: The surgical treatment of mitral stenosis. Br Med J 2:603, 1925
74. Dobell ARC: The ductus and the coarctation. Ann Thorac Surg 57:246, 1994
75. Gross RE, Hubbard JP: Surgical ligation of a patent ductus arteriosus. JAMA 112:729, 1939
76. Crafoord C, Nylin G: Congenital coarctation of the aorta and its surgical treatment. J Thorac Surg 14:347, 1945
77. Nuland SB: A triumph of twentieth-century medicine: Helen Taussig and the blue-baby operation. *In* Nuland SB (ed). Doctors: The Biography of Medicine. New York, Vintage Books-Random House, 1988, p 422
78. Muravchick S, Rosenberg H: Austin Lamont and the evolution of modern academic American anesthesiology. Anesthesiology 84:436, 1996
79. Rink EH, Helliwell PJ, Hutton AM: Anaesthesia for operations for the relief of congenital pulmonary stenosis. Guys Hosp Rep 97:48, 1948
80. Harris AJ: The management of anesthesia for congenital heart operations in children. Anesthesiology 11:328, 1950
81. McQuiston WO: Anesthetic problems in cardiac surgery in children. Anesthesiology 10:590, 1949
82. McQuiston WO: Anesthesia in cardiac surgery. Observations on three hundred sixty-two cases. Arch Surg 61:892, 1950
83. Smith RM: Circulatory factors affecting anesthesia in surgery for congenital heart disease. Anesthesiology 13:38, 1952
84. Papper EM, McDermott F: Anesthesia in cardiac surgery. Surg Clinic NA 32:655, 1952
85. Adelman MH: Anesthesia in surgery of the patent ductus arteriosus. Anesthesiology 9:42, 1948
86. Potts WJ, McQuiston WO, Baffes TG: Causes of death in one thousand operations for congenital heart disease. Arch Surg 73:508, 1956
87. Bailey CP: The surgical treatment of mitral stenosis (mitral commissurotomy). Dis Chest 15:377, 1949
88. Artusio JF Jr: Anesthetic management of the rheumatic cardiac for mitral valvulotomy. The Bull NY Acad Med 29:684, 1953
89. Wasmuth CE: Anesthesia for mitral commissurotomy. Cleve Clin Q 171:737, 1953
90. Preston FS: Anaesthesia for mitral valvotomy. Br J Anaesth 25:299, 1953
91. Pender JW: Anesthesia for mitral commissurotomy. Anesthesiology 14:77, 1953
92. Little DM, Sutton GC: Succinylcholine-nitrous oxide anaesthesia for mitral commissurotomy. Can Anaesth Soc J 2:156, 1955
93. Hufnagel CA, Harvey WP: The surgical correction of aortic regurgitation: Preliminary report. Bull Georgetown Univ Med Center 6:3.1953
94. O'Donnell JA, McDermott F: Anesthetic problems of surgical correction of aortic insufficiency. Anesthesiology 16:343, 1955
95. Evelyn SJ, Mackay I: Anesthetic for cardiac surgery. Anesth Analg 33:186, 1954
96. Lewis FJ, Taufic M: Closure of arterial septal defects with aid of hypothermia: Experimental accomplishments and the report of one successful case. Surgery 33:52, 1953
97. Swan H, Zeavin I, Blount SG Jr, et al: Surgery by direct vision in the open heart during hypothermia. JAMA 153:1081, 1953
98. Lewis JF, Varco RL, Taufic M: Repair of atrial septal defects in man under direct vision with the aid of hypothermia. Surgery 36:538, 1954
99. Downing DR, Cookson BA, Keown KK, et al: Hypothermia in cardiac surgery. J Pediatr 44:134, 1954
100. Swan H, Virtue RW, Blount SG Jr, et al: Hypothermia in surgery. Analysis of clinical cases. Ann Surg 142:382, 1955
101. Sellick BA: A method of hypothermia for open heart surgery. Lancet 1:443, 1957
102. Conn AW, Allan D, Junkin CI: Anaesthesia with hypothermia for closure of atrial septal defects in children. Can Anaesth Soc J 6:327, 1959
103. Gibbon JH Jr: Application of a mechanical heart and lung apparatus to cardiac surgery. Minnesota Med 37:171, 1954
104. Romaine-Davis A: John Gibbon and His Heart-Lung Machine. Philadelphia, University of Pensylvania Press, 1991
105. Schumacker HB Jr: A Dream of the Heart: The Life of John H. Gibbon, Jr., Father of the Heart-Long Machine. Santa Barbara, CA, Fithain Press, 1999
106. Lillehei CW, Cohen M, Warden HE, et al: The results of direct vision closure of ventricular septal defects in eight patients by means of controlled cross circulation. Surg Gynecol Obstet 43:1980, 1955
107. Kirklin JW, Dushane JW, Patrick RT, et al: Intracardiac surgery with the aid of a mechanical pump-oxygenator system (Gibbon type): Report of eight cases. Proc Staff Meetings Mayo Clin 30:201, 1955
108. Kirklin JW: Open heart surgery at the Mayo Clinic. The 25th Anniversary. Mayo Clin Proc 55:339, 1980
109. Mathews JH, Buckley JJ, Van Bergen FH: Acute effect of low-flow extracorporeal circulation on cerebral physiology (abstract). Anesthesiology 18:169, 1957
110. Keats AS, Kurosu Y, Telford J, et al: Anesthetic problems in cardiopulmonary bypass for open heart surgery: Experiences with 200 patients. Anesthesiology 19:501, 1958
111. Moffitt EA, Theye RA: Management of anesthesia, perfusion and supportive care during open intracardiac operations and extracorporeal circulation. Br J Anaesth 31:441, 1959
112. Lillehei CW, DeWall RA, Read RC, et al: Direct vision intracardiac surgery in man using a simple, disposable artificial oxygenator. Dis Chest 29:1, 1956
113. Sones FM Jr, Shirey EK, Proudfit L, et al: Cine-coronary arteriography (abstract). Circulation 20:773, 1959
114. Starr A, Edwards ML: Mitral replacement: Clinical experience with a ball-valve prosthesis. Ann Surg 154:726, 1961
115. Starr A, Edwards ML, McCord CW, et al: Aortic valve replacement. Clinical experience with a semirigid ball-valve prosthesis. Circulation 27:779, 1963
116. Mustard WT: Successful two-stage correction of transposition of the great vessels. Surgery 55:469, 1964
117. Fontan F, Baudet E: Surgical repair of tricuspid atresia. Thorax 26:2408, 1971
118. Dillard DH, Mohri H, Hessel EA, et al: Correction of total anomalous pulmonary venous drainage in infants using hypothermia and total circulatory arrest. Circulation 35/36(suppl I):I-105, 1967
119. Barnard CN: The operation. A human cardiac transplant: An interim report of a successful operation performed at Groote Schuur Hospital, Cape Town. S Afr Med J 41:1271, 1967
120. Favaloro RG: Saphenous vein autograft replacement of severe segmental coronary artery occlusion. Ann Thorac Surg 5:334, 1968
121. Johnson WD, Flemma RJ, Lepley D, et al: Extended treatment of severe coronary artery disease: A total surgical approach. Ann Surg 170:460, 1969
122. Kouwenhoven WB, Jude JR, Knickerbocker GG: Closed-chest cardiac management. JAMA 173:1064, 1960
123. Chardack WM, Gage AA, Greatbatch W: A transistorized implantable pacemaker for the long-term correction of complete heart block. Surgery 48:643, 1960
124. Zuhdi N, McCollough B, Carey J, et al: Double-helical reservoir heart-lung machine. Designed for hypothermic perfusion primed with 5% glucose in water inducing hypothermia. Arch Surg 82:166, 1961
125. Kantrowitz A, Tjonneland S, Freed PS, et al: Initial clinical experience with intraaortic balloon pumping in cardiogenic shock. JAMA 203:113, 1968
126. Barratt-Boyes BG, Simpson MN, Neutze JM: Intracardiac surgery in neonates and infants under deep hypothermia. Circulation 61/62(suppl III):III-71, 1970
127. Dawson B, Theye RA, Kirklin JW: Halothane in open cardiac operations: A technique for use with extracorporeal circulation. Anesth Analg 39:59, 1960
128. Taylor C, Stoelting VK: Halothane (fluothane) anaesthesia for pediatric cardiac surgery. Can Anaesth Soc J 8:247, 1961
129. Lowenstein E: A journey of the heart: Cardiac anesthesia. *In* Kitz RJ (ed): This Is No Humbug. Reminiscences of the Department of Anesthesia at the Massachusetts General Hospital—A History. Boston, 2003, p 269
130. Viljoen JF: Anaesthesia for internal mammary implant surgery. Anaesthesia 23:515, 1968
131. Wynands JE, Sheridan CA, Batra MS, et al: Coronary artery disease. Anesthesiology 33:260, 1970
132. Effler DB: Anesthesia in revascularization surgery: A new advance (editorial). J Thorac Cardiovasc Surg 56:163, 1968
133. Keats AS (ed): Symposium on cardiology and anesthesiology. Anesthesiology 33:125, 1970
134. Cardiovascular Disease in Anesthesia and Critical Care. Postgraduate issue. BJA 93:1, 2004
135. Swan HJC, Ganz W, Forrester J, et al: Catheterization of the heart in man with use of a flow-directed balloon-tipped catheter. N Engl J Med 283:447, 1970
136. Gay WA Jr, Ebert PA: Functional, metabolic, and morphologic effects of potassium-induced cardioplegia. Surgery 74:284, 1973
137. Bull BS, Korpmon RA, Huse WM, et al: Heparin therapy during extracorporeal circulation. I. Problems inherent in existing heparin protocols. J Thorac Cardiovasc Surg 69:674, 1975
138. Bull BS, Huse WM, Brauer FS, et al: Heparin therapy during extracorporeal circulation. II. The use of a dose-response curve to individualize heparin and protamine dosage. J Thorac Cardiovasc Surg 69:685, 1975

139. Olley PM, Coceani F, Bodach E: E-type prostaglandins. A new emergency therapy for certain cyanotic congenital heart malformations. Circulation 53:728, 1976
140. Taussig HB: On the evaluation of our knowledge of congenital malformations of the heart (The T. Duckett Jones Memorial Lecture). Circulation 31:768, 1965
141. Gruntzig A: Transluminal dilitation of coronary-artery stenosis. Lancet 2:263, 1978
142. Jatene AD, Fontes VF, Paulista DP, et al: Anatomic correction of transposition of the great vessels. J Thorac Cardiovasc Surg 72:364, 1976
143. Norwood WI, Lang P, Castaneda AR, et al: Experience with operations for hypoplastic left heart syndrome. J Thorac Cardiovasc Surg 82:511, 1981
144. Bjork VO: The central flow tilting disc valve prosthesis (Bjork-Shiley) for mitral valve replacement. Scand J Thorac Cardiovasc Surg 4:15.1970
145. Bjork VO, Holmgren A, Olin C, et al: Clinical and hemodynamic results of aortic valve replacement with the Bjork-Shiley tilting disc valve prosthesis. Scand J Thorac Cardiovasc Surg 5:177, 1971
146. Hannah H, Reis RL: Current status of porcine heterograft prosthesis. A 5-year appraisal. Circulation 54(suppl III) III-27, 1976
147. Ionescu MI, Tandon AP, Mary DAS, et al: Heart valve replacement with the Ionescu-Shiley pericardial xenograft. J Thorac Cardiovasc Surg 73:31, 1977
148. Oyer PE, Stinson EB, Jamieson SW, et al: One-year experience with cyclosporin-A in clinical heart transplantation. Heart Transplant 1:285, 1982
149. DeVries WC, Anderson JL, Joyce LD, et al: Clinical use of the total artificial heart. N Engl J Med 310:273, 1984
150. Pace NL, Mathews MM, Stanley TH: Anesthetic management of the first permanent orthotopic prosthetic cardiac replacement (total artificial heart) in man. Anesth Analg 63:685, 1984
151. Lytle BW, Loop FD, Cosgrove DM, et al: Long-term (5 to 12 years) serial studies of internal mammary artery and saphenous vein coronary bypass grafts. J Thorac Cardiovasc Surg 89:248, 1985
152. Loop FD, Lytle BW, Cosgrove DM, et al: Influence of the internal-mammary-artery graft on the 10-year survival and other cardiac events. N Engl J Med 314:1, 1986
153. Carpentier A, Chauvaud S, Fabiani JM, et al: Reconstructive surgery of mitral valve incompetence. Ten-year appraisal. J Thorac Cardiovas Surg 79:338, 1980
154. Carpentier A: Cardiac valve surgery: The "French Connection." J Thorac Cardiovasc Surg 86:323, 1983
155. Chenoweth DE, Cooper SW, Hugli TE, et al: Complement activation during cardiopulmonary bypass. N Engl J Med 304:497, 1981
156. Royston D: High-dose aprotinin therapy: A review of the first five-years experience (review article). J Cardiothorac Vasc Anesth 6:76, 1992
157. Tanaka K, Ludwig LM, Kersten JR, et al: Mechanisms of cardioprotection by volatile anesthetics. Anesthesiology 100:707, 2004
158. De Hert SG, Van der Linden PJ, Cromheecke S, et al: Choice of primary anesthetic regimen can influence intensive care unit length of stay after coronary surgery with cardiopulmonary bypass. Anesthesiology 101:9, 2004
159. Kaplan JA: Cardiothoracic anesthesia: The subspecialty speaks out. J Cardiothorac Anesth 1:1, 1987
160. Ignarro LJ, Buga GM, Wood KS, et al: Endothelium-derived relaxing factor produced and released from artery and vein is nitric oxide. Proc Natl Acad Sci USA 84:9265, 1987
161. Burack JH, Impellizzeri P, Hormel P, et al: Public reporting of surgical mortality: A survey of New York State cardiac surgeons. Ann Thorac Surg 68:1195, 1999
162. Green J, Wintfeld N: Report cards on cardiac surgeons: Assessing the New York State approach. N Engl J Med 332:1229, 1995
163. Bhandari M, Busse JW, Jackowski D, et al: Association between industry funding and statistically significant pro-industry findings in medical and surgical randomized trials. CMA 170:477, 2004
164. Watson JD, Crick FHC: A structure for deoxyribose nucleic acid. Nature 171:737, 1953
165. Austin CP: The impact of the completed human genome sequence on the development of novel therapeutics for human disease. Annu Rev Med 55:1, 2004
166. Bello EA, Schwinn DA: Molecular biology and medicine: A primer for the clinician. Anesthesiology 85:1462, 1996
167. Myles PS, Daly DJ, Djaiani G, et al: A systematic review of the safety and effectiveness of fast-track cardiac anesthesia. Anesthesiology 99:982, 2003
168. Barash PG, Lescovich F, Katz JD, et al: Early extubation following pediatric cardiothoracic operation. A viable alternative. Ann Thorac Surg 29:228, 1980
169. Feil H, Rossman PL: Electrocardiographic observations in cardiac surgery. Ann Intern Med 13:402, 1939
170. Ziegler RF: The cardiac mechanism during anesthesia and operation in patients with congenital heart disease and cyanosis. Bull Johns Hopkins Hosp 33:237, 1948
171. Smith RM, Wiley HP: Evaluation of electrocardiography during congenital heart surgery. Anesthesiology 18:398, 1957
172. Severinghaus JW, Astrup PB: pH and acid-base balance measurements. Int Anesth Clin 37:55, 1999
173. Fishman NH, Hutchinson JC, Roe BB: Controlled atrial hypertension: A method for supporting cardiac output following open heart surgery. J Thorac Cardiovasc Surg 52:777, 1966
174. Sarin CL, Yalav E, Clement AJ, et al: The necessity for measurement of left atrial pressure after cardiac surgery. Thorax 75:185, 1970
175 Waller JL, Johnson SP, Kaplan JA: Usefulness of pulmonary artery catheter during aortocoronary bypass surgery (abstract). Anesth Analg 61:221, 1982
176. Boyd AD, Tremblay RE, Spencer FC, et al: Estimation of cardiac output soon after intracardiac surgery with cardiopulmonary bypass. Ann Surg 150:613, 1959
177. Pace NL: A critique of flow-directed pulmonary arterial catheterization. Anesthesiology 47:455, 1977
178. Mangano DT: Monitoring pulmonary arterial pressure in coronary artery disease. Anesthesiology 53:364, 1980
179. Tuman KJ, McCarthy RJ, Spiess BD, et al: Effects of pulmonary artery catheterization on outcome in patients undergoing coronary artery surgery. Anesthesiology 70:199, 1989
180. Stephen CR, Bourgeois-Gavardin M, Dent S, et al: Anesthetic management in open-heart surgery: Electroencephalo-graphic and metabolic findings in 81 patients. Anesth Analg 38:198, 1959
181. Coons RE, Keats AS, Cooley DA: Significance of electroencephalographic changes occurring during cardiopulmonary bypass. Anesthesiology 20:804, 1959
182. Davenport HT, Arfel G, Sanchez FR: The electroencephalogram in patients undergoing open heart surgery with heart-lung machine. Anesthesiology 20:674, 1959
183. Seward JB: Transesophageal echocardiography. Past, present, future. *In* Freeman WK, Seward JB, Khandheria (eds): Transesophageal Echocardiography. Boston, Little, Brown and Co, 1994, p 1
184. Barash PG, Glanz S, Katz JD, et al: Ventricular function in children during halothane anesthesia: An echocardiographic evaluation. Anesthesiology 49:79, 1978
185. Schluter M, Langenstein BA, Polster J, et al: Transesophageal cross-sectional echocardiography with a phased-array transducer system. Technique and initial clinical results. Br Heart J 48:67, 1982
186. Cucchiara RF, Nugent M, Seward JB, et al: Air embolism in upright neurosurgical patients: detection and localization by two-dimensional transesophageal echocardiography. Anesthesiology 60:353, 1984
187. Smith JS, Cahalan MF, Benfiel DJ, et al: Intraoperative detection of myocardial ischemia in high-risk patients: Electrocardiography versus two-dimensional transesophageal echocardiography. Circulation 72:1015, 1985
188. Cahalan MK, Litt L, Botvinick EH, et al: Advances in noninvasive cardiovascular imaging: implication for the anesthesiologist. Anesthesiology 66:356, 1987
189. Clements FM, deBruijn NP: Perioperative evaluation of regional wall motion by transesophageal two-dimensional echocardiography. Anesth Analg 66:249, 1987
190. Siegel LC, St Goar FG, Stevens JH, et al: Monitoring considerations for post-access surgery. Circulation 96:562, 1987
191. Hogue CW, Tuman KJ, Gravlee G: Cardiovascular anesthesia: The Society of Cardiovascular Anesthesiologists, its journal and new opportunities. Anesth Analg 98:1200, 2004
192. Lowenstein B, Miller RD: The International Anesthesia Research Society and the Society of Cardiovascular Anesthesiologists: A new partnership. Anesth Analg 78:1, 1994
193. Dodds WA, Graves HB, Nixon JE, et al: The anaesthetist's role in open heart surgery. Can Anaesth Soc J 8:239, 1961
194. Hug CC Jr: Rovenstine Lecture. Patient values. Hippocrates, science and technology: What we (physicians) can do *versus* what we should do for the patient. Anesthesiology 93:556–564, 2000
195. Rosenberg H, Axelrod JF: Kenneth K: Keown, MD: Pioneer of cardiac anesthesiology. J Cardiothorac Vasc Anesth 8:577, 1994
196. Hitchock P, Keown KK: Lidocaine in cardiac arrhythmias (abstract). Fed Proc 17:378, 1958
197. Hitchock P, Keown KK: The management of cardiac arrhythmias during cardiac surgery. So Med J 52:702, 1959

198. Keown KK, Fisher SM, Downing DF, et al: Anesthesia for cardiac catheterization in infants and children. Anesthesiology 18:270, 1957
199. Keown KK: Status of anesthesiology, 1965 (chairman's address). JAMA 95:761, 1966
200. Telford J, Keats AS: Succinylcholine in cardiovascular surgery in infants and children. Anesthesiology 18:841, 1958
201. Keats AS: Anesthesia mortality in perspective (T. H. Sheldon Lecture). Anesth Analg 71:113, 1990
202. Lagasse RS: Anesthesia safety: Model or myth? A review of the published literature and analysis of current original data. Anesthesiology 97:160, 2002
203. Slogoff S, Keats AS: Further observations in perioperative myocardial ischemia. Anesthesiology 65:539, 1988
204. Moffitt EA, Patrick RT, Swan HJC, et al: A study of blood flow, venous blood oxygen saturation, blood pressure and peripheral vascular resistance during total body perfusion. Anesthesiology 20:18, 1959
205. Moffitt EA, Kirklin JW, Theye RA: Physiologic changes during whole-body perfusion in tetralogy of Fallot. J Thorac Cardiovasc Surg 44:180, 1962
206. McGoon DC, Moffitt EA, Theye RA, et al: Physiologic studies during high flow normothermic whole body perfusion. J Thorac Cardiovasc Surg 39:275, 1960
207. McGoon DC, Pestana C, Moffitt EA: Decreased risk of aortic valve surgery. Arch Surg 91:779, 1965
208. Sethna DH, Moffitt EA: An appreciation of the coronary circulation. Anesth Analg 65:264, 1986
209. Moffitt EA, Sethna DA: The coronary circulation and myocardial oxygenation in coronary artery disease. Effect of anesthesia. Anesth Analg 65:395, 1986
210. Lowenstein E: The birth of opioid anesthesia. Anesthesiology 100:1013, 2004
211. Bland JHL, Lowenstein E: Halothane induced decrease in experimental myocardial ischemia in the non-failing heart. Anesthesiology 45:287, 1976
212. Mangano DT, Browner WS, Hollenberg M, et al: Association of perioperative myocardial ischemia with cardiac morbidity and mortality in men undergoing noncardiac surgery. N Engl J Med 323:1781, 1990
213. Mangano DT: Perioperative cardiac morbidity. Anesthesiology 72:153, 1990
214. Mangano DT, Layug EL, Wallace A, et al: Effect of atenolol on mortality and cardiovascular morbidity after noncardiac surgery. N Engl J Med 335:1713, 1996
215. Roach GW, Kanchuger M, Mangano CM, et al: Adverse neurologic outcomes after coronary artery surgery. N Engl J Med 335:1857, 1996
216. Mangano DT: Effects of acadesine on myocardial infarction, stroke and death following surgery. A meta-analysis of the 5 international randomized trials. JAMA 277:325, 1997
217. Mangano DT: Aspirin and mortality from coronary bypass surgery. N Engl J Med 347:1309, 2002
218. Lowenstein E: Measure it and they will come: The acute care laboratory. *In* Kitz RT (ed): This Is No Humbug. Reminiscences of the Department of Anesthesia at the Massachusetts General Hospital—A History. Boston, 2003, p 331
219. Gibbon JH Jr: The inquiring mind (editorial). Ann Surg 130:137, 1949
220. Blalock A: The nature of discovery. Ann Surg 144:289, 1956
221. Comroe JH Jr, Dripps RD: Ben Franklin and open heart surgery. Circ Res 35:661, 1974
222. Comroe JH Jr: Retrospectroscope. Insights Into Medical Discovery. Meno Park, CA, VonGher Press, 1977
223. Shires GT: The fourth surgical renaissance? Ann Surg 192:269, 1980
224. Spencer FC: Intellectual creativity in thoracic surgeons. J Thorac Cardiovasc Surg 86:163, 1983
225. Couch NP: About heparin, or . . . whatever happened to Jay McLean? J Vasc Surg 10:1, 1989
226. Baird RJ: "Give us the tools . . . ." The story of heparin, as told by sketches from the likes of William Howell, Jay McLean, Charles Best and Gordon Murray. J Vasc Surg 11:4, 1990
227. Chargaff E, Olson KB: Studies on the chemistry of blood coagulation. IV. Studies on the action of heparin and other anticoagulants. The influence of protamine on the anticoagulant effect in vitro. J Biol Chem 122:153, 1937

Chapter 2

MILESTONES IN CARDIAC SURGERY

Sacha P. Salzberg, MD • Farzan Filsoufi, MD • David H. Adams, MD

As early as the 18th and early 19th centuries, the heart was considered the noblest organ within the human body. At that point in time the heart was deemed unsuitable for surgery. This is best reflected by Billroth, one of the most prominent surgeons of the 19th century: ". . . attempting any kind of procedure on the heart would be prostitution of the surgical art."[1] He also stated, "A surgeon who would attempt such an operation (cardiac suture) should lose the respect of his colleagues . . . ."[1] Similarly, in 1896, Paget from Great Britain predicted that ". . . surgery of the heart has probably reached the limits set by nature to all surgery; no new method, no new discovery, can overcome the natural difficulties that attend a wound of the heart."[2]

Progress in a variety of areas in medicine, including anatomy, physiology, and pharmacology, has contributed to the development of the surgical specialties, including cardiac surgery. It was not until the introduction of anesthetic agents, such as ether and chloroform in the mid 19th century, that the performance of major surgical procedures became a reality. The development of intratracheal insufflation by Meltzer in 1909[3] paved the way for future cardiothoracic operations by maintaining ventilatory exchange and expansion of the lungs. Finally, it was the development of cardiopulmonary bypass (CPB) in the mid 20th century that allowed surgeons to gain access into the cavities of the heart and to perform procedures in a bloodless field. In this chapter, the landmark events and milestones in cardiac surgery are reviewed. In addition, it is essential to emphasize that milestones alone are not sufficient; it is the continuous collaboration of a multitude of brilliant minds and the stepwise evolution of pioneering techniques and procedures that have brought cardiac surgery to its present status.

THE EARLY DAYS: BEFORE CARDIOPULMONARY BYPASS

Trauma and Heart Wounds

The first operations involving the mediastinum were related to trauma. In 1893, Williams from Chicago was the first to surgically suture the pericardium in a patient following a penetrating stab wound. Three years later, Rehn from Germany successfully repaired a right ventricular stab wound (Table 2–1). Over a period of 10 years, Rehn performed 124 cases of cardiac suture with a recovery rate of 40%. It was his landmark report of this consecutive series with an excellent success rate, for that time, that moved cardiac surgery into the realm of possibility.[4] In the United States, Hill was the first surgeon to repair a cardiac injury. Complex cardiac surgery became a reality with the advent of the second world war, when Harken reported a series of 100 soldiers in whom he had removed intracardiac foreign bodies.[5]

Valve Surgery

In addition to chest trauma and stab wounds, valvular heart disease (VHD) secondary to rheumatic fever was the dominant cause of heart disease in the early 20th century. Following Rehn's report,[4] several internists suggested that mitral stenosis might be relieved by surgery. It was Brunton who sparked a storm of controversy in 1902 with his "Preliminary Note on the Possibility of Treating Mitral Stenosis by Surgical Methods."[6] Brunton's suggestion, although premature, was correct and ultimately would come to fruition. In 1913, it was Doyen who unsuccessfully attempted to relieve what he believed to be congenital pulmonary stenosis. That same year Tuffier reported the first attempt to surgically treat severe aortic stenosis by digital aortic valve invagination into the valvular orifice.[7] This was successful, and the patient survived for at least 12 years. Two decades would pass after Brunton's statement before mitral stenosis would be reconsidered for surgical treatment.

In 1923, at Boston's Peter Bent Brigham Hospital, the distinguished physician Levine collaborated with the chief of surgery, Cutler, who successfully operated on a 12-year-old child with mitral stenosis. Using a knife inserted via the left ventricle, Cutler incised the mitral valve with the intent of rendering it slightly incompetent. In 1925, Souttar of London performed another landmark operation on a 19-year-old girl with mitral stenosis in which endotracheal intubation was used.[8] This permitted transpleural exposure and facilitated left atrial entrance so that digital dilatation of the stenotic mitral valve could be performed. In 1948, Bailey in Philadelphia, Harken in Boston, and Brock in London independently replicated Souttar's operation, not knowing of the others' activities, making closed commissurotomy into a reality.[9,10] Performed mainly with digital guidance, the operations often were more ingenious than effective.

In the 1950s, several techniques of repair for mitral regurgitation were attempted. In 1954, Bailey used a patch of pericardium to correct mitral regurgitation.[11] Davila et al[12] described the concept of circumferential suture of the mitral annulus in 1955 to reduce the size of the annulus. In 1956, the technique of annular plication at the posteromedial commissure using transatrial sutures was reported by Nichols.[13] Hufnagel[14] was the first to successfully implant a self-contained ball valve in a patient with severe aortic incompetence in the descending thoracic aorta in 1952. Without CPB, the prosthetic valve had to be placed in the descending

Table 2–1 Prior to Cardiopulmonary Bypass

Name	Year	Location	Accomplishment
Rehn	1896	Frankfurt	Repair after trauma
Brunton	1902	England	Suggestion of surgical correction of mitral stenosis (MS)
Meltzer, Auer	1909	New York	Artificial ventilation
Levine, Cutler, Mackenzie	1923	Boston	First operation for MS
Souttar	1925	London	Digital dilatation in MS
Gross	1938	Boston	Ligation of patent ductus arteriosus
Blalock, Taussig	1944	Nashville	Palliative shunt for tetralogy of Fallot
Harken	1944	Europe	Removed foreign bodies during the war
Gross, Craaford	1945	Boston, Stockholm	Surgical correction of coarctation of aorta (COA)
Bailey Harken Brock	1948	Philadelphia Boston London	Digital dilatation for MS
Bigelow	1950	Toronto	Hypothermia decreasing total body oxygen consumption for surgery on pulmonary valve stenosis and atrial septal defect
Hufnagel	1952	Washington, DC	Self-contained caged-ball valve implanted into descending thoracic aorta

thoracic aorta leading to unfavorable hemodynamics and a suboptimal outcome, but heralding a new era for prosthetic valve implantation in humans. This ball-valve prototype became the design for valves used in the open-heart era.

Myocardial Revascularization

In 1935, Beck from Cleveland[15] created a procedure in which he grafted a pectoralis muscle onto the pericardium in an attempt to increase the blood flow to the ischemic myocardium through the development of collateral circulation. In a similar attempt in 1946, Vineberg from Canada developed surgical procedures in order to directly increase the blood supply to the myocardium.[16] This procedure consisted of implanting the free end of an internal mammary artery (IMA) directly into the myocardium. No attempt was made at this time to anastomose the IMA to any coronary artery. During the next 15 years, this operation was performed successfully in several hundred patients. Experimentally, however, Demikhov from the former Soviet Union completed a direct IMA graft anastomosis in 1952, in an animal model. In 1957, Bailey from Philadelphia and Longmire from Los Angeles were the first to successfully conduct coronary endarterectomies on human patients.[17]

Aortic Surgery

Early attempts at surgical correction of aortic aneurysms consisted of the interruption of arterial flow by either ligation or the stimulation of thrombosis. These procedures met with variable success, depending on the position of the aneurysm and the extent of collateral circulation. Further innovative measures used to achieve thrombosis of the aneurysms included intravascular application of electric current and cellophane wrapping, with or without other irritating materials. Gurin first attempted a surgical intervention with aortic fenestration, in order to treat a malperfusion syndrome in 1935. In the late 1940s, Abbott from England and Paulin advanced the surgical treatment by wrapping the aorta with cellophane to prevent aortic rupture. During the same period, it was Harris and Shumaker[18] who first reported the surgical excision of a descending thoracic aneurysm. Meanwhile, Dubost et al[19] in Paris were the first to use a homograft to replace an abdominal aortic aneurysm.

MODERN CARDIAC SURGERY: CARDIOPULMONARY BYPASS AND MYOCARDIAL PROTECTION

Despite the ingenuity of closed cardiac operations, the management of more complicated lesions required direct vision. Because only brief intracardiac exposure would be possible with normothermic vena caval occlusion, the use of hypothermia to prolong this period was explored in the late 1940s by Bigelow et al.[20] They documented in animals that hypothermia reduced the total body oxygen consumption in proportion to the temperature drop.[21] These data made it possible for surgeons to repair the first directly visualized pulmonary valve stenosis and atrial septal defects (ASDs) in 1952.

In 1953, a landmark event in cardiac surgery occurred when Gibbon[22] successfully closed an ASD in an 18-year-old girl using CPB (Table 2–2). The idea that CPB might be developed had its origin in 1931, when Gibbon witnessed the collapse of a patient due to a massive pulmonary embolism after a general surgical operation. While the patient deteriorated, Gibbon searched for ways to help. To no avail, the patient then underwent a closed pulmonary embolectomy, a so-called Trendelenburg operation, by Churchill. Nineteen years of research preceded Gibbon's success, much of the effort having been conducted with his wife.[22] It was also the collaboration with Watson from IBM, who was intrigued and fascinated by Gibbon's work, that led to the development of a heart-lung machine, containing a rotating vertical cylinder oxygenator and a modified DeBakey rotary pump.[22] To those who witnessed this achievement, as well as the rest of the world, the case was absolutely astounding. Subsequently, in 1953, Gibbon operated on two additional patients, two young girls, both

Table 2–2 Cardiopulmonary Bypass

Name	Year	Location	Accomplishment
McLean	1915	Baltimore	Heparin
Best	1933	Toronto	Heparin purified and used in research
Kolff	1944	Leiden	Membrane lung
Boerema	1950	Amsterdam	Extracorporeal heat exchanger
Gibbon	1953	Philadelphia	Atrial septal defect closure
Lillehei, DeWall, Kirklin	1954	Minnesota	Parabiotic oxygenator and improved bubble oxygenator
Gollan	1950s	Ohio	Hypothermia and hemodilution in animals

Table 2–3 Myocardial Protection

Name	Year	Location	Accomplishment
Melrose	1955	London	Cardiac arrest with potassium citrate
Shumway	1960	Palo Alto	Topical cardiac cooling
Hölscher, Bretschneider, Kirsch	1964	Germany	Reexamined chemical cardioplegia (CC)
Braimbridge, Hearse	1975	London	Cold (4°C) CC formulation
Buckberg, Follette	1979	Los Angelas	Potassium-blood (CC)
Menasche	1986	Paris	Potassium-magnesium-blood (CC)
Menasche	1990	Paris	Retrograde cardioplegia

about 5 years of age, with alleged ASDs. Because of the diagnostic imprecision, both cases turned out to be very difficult, and Gibbon, upset by these failures, declared a moratorium on open-heart surgery with his heart-lung machine.

Kirklin from Minnesota constructed an improved version of the Gibbon pump-oxygenator and in March 1955 successfully performed an intracardiac operation.[23] In August 1954, Lillehei, also in Minnesota,[24] performed his first open-heart operation in which he connected the patient's parent to the patient with plastic tubing as a living oxygenator, creating a cross-circulation between the two individuals. The method was successful, but the possibility of donor complications and limitations of the method to pediatric cases made Lillehei assign a research fellow, DeWall, to the development of a more suitable pump-oxygenator.[25] DeWall's success was aided by the earlier work of Clark, who had reported the use of a bubble oxygenator in 1950 with effective debubbling capability. Beginning in May 1955, it was DeWall's bubble oxygenators that made Lillehei's extraordinary cardiac surgery program possible.

Another essential issue that emerged was the necessity of providing myocardial protection in conjunction with a bloodless operative field (Table 2–3). In 1955, Melrose et al[26] facilitated their goal of direct-vision cardiac surgery when they arrested the heart with potassium citrate. This technique was abandoned because of extensive and irreversible myocardial damage, and it would be years until elective cardiac arrest would be explored again. In the interim, the earlier work of Bigelow (1950) provided the basis for perfusion root cardiac cooling (Gott and Cross, 1957) and topical cardiac cooling (Shumway, 1959). Chemical myocardial arrest (cardioplegic solution) was reexamined by a number of German investigators in the 1960s. Hölscher, Bretschneider, and Kirsch independently developed different formulations, which were used clinically as early as 1964. In London, Braimbridge, a basic scientist, and Hearse combined their efforts, resulting in a chemical cardioplegia solution that retained an essentially extracellular ionic character. Introduced clinically in 1975, the cold (4°C) chemical cardioplegia formulation was widely adopted.[27] Shumway and Lower used Swan's principle of hypothermic arrest and effectively used methods of topical cardiac hypothermia in the 1960s, marking a significant improvement in myocardial protection.[28] Further studies revealed that topical hypothermia alone was insufficient to minimize intraoperative ischemic injury.[29,30] In the late 1970s and early 1980s, Follette et al[31] introduced cold hyperkalemic blood cardioplegia. In 1979, Buckberg introduced a similar concept, in which he proposed the use of potassium-enriched blood, which improved buffering and oxygenating capacities of the solution.[32]

In 1984, Atkins combined hypothermia and ventricular fibrillation and produced successful results for coronary revascularization. Two years later, Murray demonstrated the advantages of using intermittent ischemia and reperfusion, which enabled the heart to withstand longer periods of arrest. In 1991, Lichtenstein and Salerno reported the use of continuous warm blood cardioplegia.[33] Meanwhile, in the 1980s, Menasche et al[34] emboldened the Lichtenstein and Salerno approach in their use of whole blood enriched with potassium and magnesium. They also introduced the concept of retro-

Table 2–4 Valve Surgery

Name	Year	Location	Accomplishment
Murray	1955	Canada	Homograft in the descending thoracic aorta.
Braunwald	1959	Bethesda	Mitral valve replacement
Harken	1960	Boston	Aortic valve replacement
Duran, Gunning	1964	Oxford	Aortic valve stent-mounted xenograft
Binet, Carpentier	1965	Paris	Formalin-preserved frame-mounted porcine xenograft
Carpentier	1968	Paris	Mitral valve repair using prosthetic annuloplasty rings
Carpentier	1996	Paris	Thoracoscopic mitral valve repair

grade cardioplegia delivery through the coronary sinus, which is currently used in adult cardiac surgery[35] (see Chapters 28 and 30).

VALVE SURGERY

Prosthetic Valve Replacement

Nina Braunwald implanted a polyurethane mechanical prosthesis in the mitral position in 1959 at the National Institutes of Health. In 1960, Harken was the first to successfully perform an aortic valve replacement (AVR) with a subcoronary implantation of a caged-ball valve prosthesis, basing the valve design on Hufnagel's ball-valve concept[36-38] (Table 2–4). Since prosthetic valves appeared, many designs had to be withdrawn from the market due to structural deficiencies or high postoperative complication rates. Starr and Edwards[39] were the first to successfully implant a caged-ball valve with good long-term results in 1960. The Starr-Edwards valve became the most popular valve, being implanted in patients with valvular heart disease for nearly two decades. However, this valve was associated with a high transvalvular gradient as well as a high thromboembolic event rate. In the late 1960s, further research activities led to the use of pyrolytic carbon, a hemocompatible material, in the construction of mechanical valves. This significant technological advance facilitated the development of a new generation of valves with improved hemodynamic performances and a lower profile, such as the pivotal monoleaflet discs (Björk-Shiley in 1969) and bileaflet winglet valves (St. Jude Medical Center in 1977).

Homografts, Xenografts, and Bioprosthetic Valves

In 1955, Murray[40] inserted an aortic homograft in the descending thoracic aorta of a patient with aortic regurgitation. In 1962, Ross and Barratt-Boyes reported the first implantation of a homograft in the aortic position. While remarkably effective, the availability of homograft aortic valves was a problem that precipitated exploration into the field of xenotransplantation. In 1964, Duran and Gunning performed the first clinical aortic valve replacement in Oxford, with a stent-mounted freeze-dried xenograft valve bioprosthesis.[41] A year later in Paris, Binet, Carpentier, and colleagues reported their early experience with a formalin-preserved frame-mounted porcine xenograft valve bioprosthesis.[42] However, within a few years, the formalin-preserved xenograft valve bioprosthesis failed and required replacement. Carpentier then devoted his attention to the chemical bases of valve degeneration and preservation. He found glutaraldehyde to be the most suitable and durable way to fix tissues and decrease or even eliminate the immunogenicity and subsequent inflammatory response to this foreign body.

Carpentier et al[43] reported the first successful xenograft valve replacement in 1965. In 1967, glutaraldehyde became commercially available and was used as a means of effectively fixing biological tissues. This led to the broad commercial availability of biological valves and the development of new prostheses such as the Carpentier-Edwards, Hancock, and Angell-Shiley valves in the 1970s.[44] Despite their limited durability, secondary to structural valve deterioration, these prostheses were implanted in large numbers of elderly patients due to the lack of need for postoperative anticoagulation. In 1967, Ross reported the use of a pulmonary autograft in the aortic position (Ross procedure).[82]

Mitral Valve Repair

It was Lillehei et al in 1957[45] who reported the first suture mitral annuloplasty by placing heavy silk sutures in the dilated area of the mitral annulus. In 1959, Merendino et al[46] reported the concept of posteromedial annuloplasty. Subsequently, Kay et al,[47] Wooler et al,[48] and Reed et al[49] described other techniques of annuloplasty, but none of them were able to provide good long-term results and were therefore abandoned. In 1960, McGoon et al,[50] from the Mayo Clinic, reported the resection-plication of the posterior leaflet for the treatment of mitral valve insufficiency due to leaflet prolapse. In 1968, Carpentier[83] reported the first use of a prosthetic ring to perform a remodeling annuloplasty. During the next two decades, additional repair techniques were developed to broaden the application of reconstructive valve surgery for patients with mitral valve disease.[51] In the mid 1990s, research efforts further focused on the development of minimally invasive cardiac procedures. In 1996, Carpentier et al[52] performed the first videoscopic mitral valve repair through a right minithoracotomy. Carpentier et al[53] and Mohr et al[54] also performed the first mitral valve repair using robotic assistance in 1998 (see Chapters 20 and 21).

MYOCARDIAL REVASCULARIZATION

It was only when coronary arteriography was accidentally discovered at the Cleveland Clinic by Sones in 1958[55] that a

Table 2–5 **Myocardial Revascularization**

Name	Year	Location	Accomplishment
Carrel	1910	Lyon	Suggestion of coronary artery bypass surgery with blood vessel conduits
Bailey	1955	Philadelphia	Excision of a left ventricular aneurysm, with no cardiopulmonary bypass
Effler, Favaloro	1958	Cleveland	Initiation to coronary artery bypass surgery
Cooley	1958	Houston	Excision of a left ventricular aneurysm, with cardiopulmonary bypass
Jatene	1985	Brazil	Combination of left ventricular aneurysm excision with reconstruction of the ventricular cavity to reduce volume overload.

rational basis for surgical myocardial revascularization with a coronary artery bypass grafting (CABG) procedure was established by Effler and Favaloro[56] (Table 2–5). With the development of the heart-lung machine, Sabiston[57] was the first to use a saphenous vein graft as a bypass conduit from the ascending aorta to the distal right coronary artery in 1962. This procedure was further refined by DeBakey, Dennis, Green, and Garrett.[58] In an attempt to treat anginal symptoms, in 1964, Kolessov[59] was the first to perform an internal mammary graft anastomosis to a coronary artery. In the 1980s, CABG became one of the most performed surgical procedures in the United States and the gold standard therapy in patients with multivessel coronary artery disease. Despite excellent results, neurologic complications and systemic inflammatory response after CABG with CPB have led to the development of less invasive surgical approaches. Throughout the past decade, technical improvements including the development of stabilizing platforms, positioning devices, and coronary occluder-shunts have made off-pump coronary artery bypass grafting (OPCAB) procedures an alternative to conventional CABG with CPB (see Chapters 19 and 21).

A major complication of myocardial infarction is the formation of a left ventricular aneurysm. The first excisions of a left ventricular aneurysm were performed before CPB by Bailey et al[60] in 1955 and 3 years later by Cooley et al[61] using CPB. An important contribution was reported in 1985 by Jatene from Brazil when he combined left ventricular aneurysm excision with reconstruction of the ventricular cavity to reduce volume overload.[62] Additional improvements to this procedure were achieved with a more geometrical approach to ventricular reconstruction by Dor et al.[63]

AORTIC SURGERY (DISSECTION AND ANEURYSMS)

Cooley and DeBakey were the real pioneers in defining replacement of the ascending aorta in 1956[64] (Table 2–6). The first group to combine aortic valve repair and insertion of an allograft in a patient with Marfan syndrome was Mueller et al in 1960.[65] Attention then shifted to the development of several suitable artificial conduits. Vinyon-N cloth was the first fabric tissue to be used by Blakemore and Voorhees.[66] When DeBakey discovered Dacron in a Houston department store, few people thought that this would actually become the material for the conduit of choice, as an artificial replacement of the aorta.[67] The availability of both synthetic vascular grafts and CPB with profound hypothermia made possible the excision and replacement of the ascending, transverse arch, and thoracoabdominal aortic aneurysms and dissections.[68] In 1968, Bentall and De Bono[69] were the first to use a composite valve-graft conduit to replace the aortic root and ascending aorta. The coronary arteries were sewn to orifices that were created in the tube graft. The remaining aorta was wrapped tightly around the tube graft, creating an inclusion cylinder arrangement. In 1981, to facilitate coronary blood flow, following aortic root replacement, Cabrol et al[70] advocated the use of an 8- to 10-mm Dacron graft. These pioneering procedures using modern low-profile mechanical valves and hemostatic collagen or gelatin-impregnated woven Dacron grafts have led to several variations of this procedure that are still used today. Cerebral protection and aortic arch surgery are fields in which significant progress has been made over the past few years, especially by Griepp et al,[71,72] who developed the trifurcated graft for antegrade cerebral perfusion (see Chapter 23).

CARDIAC TRANSPLANTATION

Cardiac transplantation has been established as an effective therapy for patients with end-stage heart failure. Research began with the experiments of Carrel and Guthrie in 1905 when they attempted heterotransplantation of the heart and heart/lungs in animals[73] (Table 2–7). In 1933, Mann from the Mayo Clinic performed heterotopic cardiac transplantation and concluded that rejection was due to a biological factor. Demikhov was the first to carry out heterotopic transplantation of the heart (1940) and heart and lungs (1946). However, his prodigious efforts became widely known only when his 1960 monograph, "Experimental Transplantation of Vital Organs," was translated from Russian into English.[74]

The cardiac transplantation method used today was developed at Stanford by Angell and Shumway,[75] who commented that the idea evolved from one of their myocardial protection (topical cooling) experiments, in which with 1 hour of aortic cross-clamping on CPB, it was decided to remove the heart and then resuture it into position. Subsequently, they used the hearts of donor dogs and performed allotransplants, a remarkable effort that was carried out before chemical immunosuppression was available. Although early mortality was high due to rejection, efforts principally by Shumway's group and Reemtsma from Tulane improved the ability to diagnose and immunologically manage this devastating complication. It was the advent of immunosuppression that heralded a new era in this field. Reemtsma from Tulane, first, and then Blumenstock from Cooperstown used methotrexate to prolong survival after transplantation in dogs. By the mid 1960s, CPB, myocardial protection, and postoperative care

Table 2–6 Aortic Surgery

Name	Year	Location	Accomplishment
Matas	1902	New Orleans	Suturing aneurysmal sac from within
Carrel	1910	Lyon	Excision of aortic aneurysms and vascular graft interposition
Gross	1948	Russia	Resection of aortic segments and interposition with homograft
Voorhees	1952	New York	Cloth utilization for vascular grafts
DeBakey, Cooley	1953	Houston	Successful resection and homograft replacement of a descending thoracic aneurysm
Borst Griepp	1964 1975	Hannover New York	Excision and replacement of ascending, transverse arch and thoracoabdominal aortic aneurysms and dissections with synthetic vascular grafts and profound perfusion hypothermia

Table 2–7 Heart Transplantation

Name	Year	Location	Accomplishment
Carrel, Guthrie	1905	Lyon	Cardiac and pulmonary heterotransplantation in animals
Mann	1933	Mayo Clinic, Minnesota	Heterotopic cardiac transplantation
Demikhov	1940 1946	Soviet Union	Heterotopic transplantation of the heart (1940) and heart/lungs (1946)
Angell, Shumway	1960	Palo Alto, CA	Allotransplants in dogs
Barnard	1967	Capetown	Heart transplant

had improved considerably. The basis for clinical transplantation had been established, even though there remained huge logistical and legal issues to be surmounted.

In 1967, a 50-year-old male South African patient was taken to the operating room by Barnard, where he received the heart of a 25-year-old woman who had had a fatal automobile accident, leaving her brain dead. The patient was started on basic immunosuppressive therapy in the operating room and made a swift recovery. However, on day 13 after the initial transplantation, the patient developed pneumonia, from which he never recovered. This successful transplant stirred many debates. Even before the death in South Africa, a panel of specialists gathered in New York to debate the moral and ethical issues linked to this achievement. Opinions ranged from outrage to optimism. Within the first year after Barnard's success, more than 100 transplants by more than 50 different surgical teams were performed.[76] However, with only 15% of patients surviving 1 year after the procedure, enthusiasm for heart transplantation waned by the end of 1971.

Rejection being the major cause of failure, research efforts were redirected again into diagnosing and treating this condition. It was the Stanford group who developed an antilymphocytic serum; this was a home-made rabbit anti-human thymocyte globulin and was used to treat acute rejection. Initially, there were only clinical markers for rejection, but it was the transvenous endomyocardial biopsy, developed in 1972, that allowed clinicians to histologically assess, and follow, transplant recipients. It was the Stanford team who also introduced routine T-cell monitoring to better titrate any immunosuppressive regimen and to limit toxic effects. The advent of cyclosporine, first discovered by Borel in Switzerland in 1973, had a significant impact on survival rates after heart transplantations. It was first used in renal transplantation in 1978.

In addition to better donor organ preservation and immunosuppression, the improvements in preoperative and postoperative care led to the widespread adoption of cardiac transplantation. In Great Britain, English at Papworth and Yacoub at Harefield developed successful and productive transplant programs.[84,85] Subsequently, the limiting factor of donor organ shortage became painfully apparent to the surgical community. Meanwhile, pediatric transplantation developed under the strong influence of Bailey,[86] especially in neonates with hypoplastic left heart syndrome (see Chapter 26).

CARDIAC ASSIST DEVICES

In 1954, Dennis' group from Brooklyn first used a pump-oxygenator to support a nonsurgical patient in severe heart failure[77] (Table 2–8). In 1961, the concept of afterload reduction using "arterial counterpulsation" was first described by Harken[87] and further developed into the intra-aortic balloon pump by Moulopoulos[88] in Cleveland.

In 1956, Kolff and Akutsu[89] both reported their experience with a total artificial heart implantation in an animal. The National Heart, Lung, and Blood Institute began the Artificial Heart Program in 1964. It started with the development of mechanical devices for short- and then long-term circulatory support. At the time, the available devices required patients to be tethered to bulky external power sources, which severely restricted mobility and independence. In 1969, Cooley performed the first successful bridge-to-transplantation in a patient.

In the 1970s, engineering efforts focused on developing miniaturized pneumatic devices. It was in 1974 that the Artificial Heart Program turned their development efforts toward

Table 2–8 **Cardiac Assist Devices**

Name	Year	Location	Accomplishment
Dennis	1954	Brooklyn	Pump-oxygenator to support a nonsurgical patient in cardiac failure
Harken	1961	Boston	Afterload reduction using "arterial counterpulsation"
Spencer DeBakey	Early 1960s	Houston	Left ventricular assist device use in post-cardiac surgical patients
Cooley, Demikhov	1937	Houston, Russia	Artificial heart development
Kolff, Akutsu	1958	Utah	Reported total artificial heart implantation in an animal
Kolff	1982	Utah	Clinical implantation of a total artificial heart

Table 2–9 **Arrhythmia Surgery**

Name	Year	Location	Accomplishment
Durrer, McGoon, Sealy	1967	Amsterdam, United States	Atrioventricular conduction occurred over an accessory pathway in patients with Wolff-Parkinson-White syndrome, which permitted operative management of the syndrome.
Cox	1982	United States	Cut and sew maze

totally implantable devices. The 1980s marked the first implantation of a pneumatic total artificial heart (Jarvik-7-100) by DeVries. Shortly thereafter, Copeland described a long-term survivor who had received a total artificial heart, as a bridge to cardiac transplantation.

In view of the dramatic complications such as thromboembolism, severe infections, and very low survival rates, the enthusiasm for the total artificial heart faltered. In 1991 the Food and Drug Administration initiated a moratorium on the use of the Jarvik heart. Two years later, however, the FDA gave a new investigational device exemption for a total artificial heart. In 1994, the FDA approved the use of a left ventricular assist device with an external power source as a bridge to transplantation.[78] In 1999, the landmark REMATCH (Randomized Evaluation of Mechanical Assistance for the Treatment of Congestive Heart Failure) trial established left ventricular assist device therapy as a real part of the treatment for patients with terminal heart failure.[78] In the past decade, miniaturization, creation of biocompatible surfaces, and device engineering have led to the invention of many new devices, such as the new DeBakey VAD (Micromedtech Inc.), the Jarvik 2000 (Jarvik Heart Inc.), the HeartMate VE (Thoratec Inc.), and the Incor (Berlin Heart). These are microaxial devices in which an impeller accelerates the blood through the pump. Fluid dynamics play a crucial role here, as the aim has been to minimize friction and subsequent hemolysis. The expected increase in patients with end-stage heart failure during the coming years will certainly broaden the application of this new technology (see Chapter 27).

ARRHYTHMIA SURGERY

In 1967, Durrer[79] from Amsterdam documented by intraoperative mapping in patients with the Wolff-Parkinson-White syndrome that atrioventricular conduction occurred over an accessory pathway (Table 2–9). Employment of Durrer's mapping approach permitted operative management of arrhythmias (Dwight McGoon, Will Sealy; United States). Guiraudon from Paris reported a new technique of encircling endomyocardial ventriculotomy to treat malignant ventricular arrhythmias.[80] In the 1980s, Cox from St. Louis developed a surgical procedure to cure atrial fibrillation based on the electrophysiologic understanding of this disease. This surgical procedure created an electrical maze in the atria. The atrial incisions prevent reentry and allow sinus impulses to activate the entire atrial myocardium.[81] During the 1990s, this procedure was further modified and simplified, leading to the development of the modified maze procedure, restoring sinus rhythm with the use of different types of energy sources to create atrial lesions (see Chapter 13).

REFERENCES

1. Rose E: Herztamponade. Deutsche Zeitschrift fuer Chirurgie 20:329, 1884
2. Paget S: Surgery of the Chest. London, John Wright, 1896, p 121
3. Meltzer SJ: Continuous respiration without respiratory movement. J Exp Med 11:622, 1909
4. Rehn L: Ueber penetrierende herzwunden und herznaht. Arch Klin Chir 55:315, 1897
5. Harken DE: Foreign bodies in and in relation to the thoracic blood vessels and heart, I: Techniques for approaching and removing foreign bodies from the chambers of the heart. Surg Gynecol Obstet 83:117, 1946
6. Brunton L: Preliminary note on the possibility of treating mitral stenosis by surgical methods. Lancet 1:352, 1902
7. Tuffier T: La Chirurgie du Coeur. Rapports. Proces Verbaux et Discussion 1, 1921
8. Souttar H: The surgical treatment of mitral stenosis. Br Med J 2:603, 1925
9. Johnson L: The History of Cardiac Surgery 1896–1955. Baltimore, The Johns Hopkins University Press, 1970, p 87
10. Westaby SBC: Landmarks in Cardiac Surgery. Oxford, Oxford University Press, 1997
11. Bailey CP, Jamison WL, Bakst AE, et al: The surgical correction of mitral insufficiency by the use of pericardial grafts. J Thorac Surg 28:551, 1954
12. Davila JC, Glover RP, Trout RG, et al: Circumferential suture of the mitral ring: A method for the surgical correction of mitral insufficiency. J Thorac Surg 30:531, 1955; discussion, 560, 1955
13. Nichols HT: Mitral insufficiency: Treatment by polar cross-fusion of the mitral annulus fibrosis. J Thorac Surg 33:102, 1957

14. Hufnagel CA: The surgical correction of aortic insufficiency: A preliminary report. Bull Georgetown Univ Med Ctr 6:60, 1952
15. Beck C: The development of a new blood supply to the heart by operation. Ann Surg 102:802, 1935
16. Vineberg AM: Internal mammary coronary anastomosis in the surgical treatment of coronary artery insufficiency. Can Med Assoc J 64:204, 1951
17. Longmire WP Jr, Cannon JA, Kattus AA: Direct-vision coronary endarterectomy for angina pectoris. N Engl J Med 259:993, 1958
18. Harris J, Shumacker HB Jr: Cure of dissecting aneurysm of thoracic aorta by total excision. AMA Arch Surg 73:991, 1956
19. Dubost C, Allary M, Oeconomos N: Resection of an aneurysm of the abdominal aorta: Reestablishment of the continuity by a preserved human arterial graft, with result after five months. AMA Arch Surg 64:405, 1952
20. Bigelow WG, Callaghan JC, Hopps JA: General hypothermia for experimental intracardiac surgery: the use of electrophrenic respirations, an artificial pacemaker for cardiac standstill, and radio-frequency rewarming in general hypothermia. Trans Meet Am Surg Assoc Am Surg Assoc 68:211, 1950
21. Bigelow WG, Lindsay WK, et al: Oxygen transport and utilization in dogs at low body temperatures. Am J Physiol 160:125, 1950
22. Gibbon JH Jr: The development of the heart-lung apparatus. Am J Surg 135:608, 1978
23. Kirklin JW, Dushane JW, Patrick RT, et al: Intracardiac surgery with the aid of a mechanical pump-oxygenator system (Gibbon type): report of eight cases. Mayo Clin Proc 30:201, 1955
24. Warden HE, Cohen M, Read RC, et al: Controlled cross circulation for open intracardiac surgery: Physiologic studies and results of creation and closure of ventricular septal defects. J Thorac Surg 28:331, 1954; discussion, 341, 1954
25. Warden HE, Dewall RA, Read RC, et al: Total cardiac by-pass utilizing continuous perfusion from reservoir of oxygenated blood. Proc Soc Exp Biol Med 90:246, 1955
26. Melrose DG, Dreyer B, Bentall HH, et al: Elective cardiac arrest. Lancet 269:21, 1955
27. Hearse DJ, Jynge P, Braimbridge MV: Protection of the Ischemic Myocardium. New York, Raven, 1981
28. Stewart BD, Virtue RW, Swan H: Cardiac arrest and ventricular fibrillation: experimental study in dogs with acute hypoxia and hypercapnia and in dogs with chronic hypoxia. AMA Arch Surg 66:703, 1953
29. Hurley EJ, Lower RR, Dong E Jr, et al: Clinical experience with local hypothermia in elective cardiac arrest. J Thorac Cardiovasc Surg 47:50, 1964
30. Caranna LJ, Neustein HB, Swan H: Pathologic changes in experimental hypothermia. Arch Surg 82:147, 1961
31. Follette D, Fey K, Mulder D, et al: Prolonged safe aortic clamping by combining membrane stabilization, multidose cardioplegia, and appropriate pH reperfusion. J Thorac Cardiovasc Surg 74:682, 1977
32. Follette DM, Steed DL, Foglia R, et al: Advantages of intermittent blood cardioplegia over intermittent ischemia during prolonged hypothermic aortic clamping. Circulation 58:I-200, 1978
33. Salerno TA, Houck JP, Barrozo CA, et al: Retrograde continuous warm blood cardioplegia: A new concept in myocardial protection. Ann Thorac Surg 51:245, 1991
34. Menasche P, Grousset C, Gauduel Y, et al: Enhancement of cardioplegic protection with the free-radical scavenger peroxidase. Circulation 74:III-138, 1986
35. Menasche P, Subayi JB, Piwnica A: Retrograde coronary sinus cardioplegia for aortic valve operations: A clinical report on 500 patients. Ann Thorac Surg 49:556, 1990; discussion 563, 1990
36. Hufnagel CA: Basic concepts of cardiac and vascular reconstruction. Georgetown Med Bull 14:88, 1960
37. Harken DE, Taylor WJ, Lefemine AA, et al: Aortic valve replacement with a caged ball valve. Am J Cardiol 9:292, 1962
38. Braunwald NS, Cooper T, Morrow AG: Complete replacement of the mitral valve. Successful clinical application of a flexible polyurethane prosthesis. J Thorac Cardiovasc Surg 40:1, 1960
39. Starr A, Edwards ML: Mitral replacement: Clinical experience with a ball-valve prosthesis. Ann Surg 154:726, 1961
40. Murray G: Homologous aortic-valve-segment transplants as surgical treatment for aortic and mitral insufficiency. Angiology 7:466, 1956
41. Duran CM: [Homotransplants of the aortic valve. Technique and results]. Ann Chir Thorac Cardiovasc 25:488, 1964
42. Binet JP, Carpentier A, Langlois J, et al: [Implantation of heterogenic valves in the treatment of aortic cardiopathies]. C R Acad Sci Hebd Seances Acad Sci D 261:5733, 1965
43. Carpentier A, Guilmet D, Dubost C: Aortic mitral and tricuspid valve replacement with frame-mounted aortic heterografts. Thoraxchir Vask Chir 16:615, 1968
44. Carpentier A, Deloche A, Relland J, et al: Six-year follow-up of glutaraldehyde-preserved heterografts. With particular reference to the treatment of congenital valve malformations. J Thorac Cardiovasc Surg 68:771, 1974
45. Lillehei CW, Gott VL, Dewall RA, et al: The surgical treatment of stenotic or regurgitant lesions of the mitral and aortic valves by direct vision utilizing a pump-oxygenator. J Thorac Surg 35:154, 1958
46. Merendino KA, Thomas GI, Jesseph JE, et al: The open correction of rheumatic mitral regurgitation and/or stenosis with special reference to regurgitation treated by posteromedial annuloplasty utilizing a pump-oxygenator. Ann Surg 150:5, 1959
47. Kay EB, Nogueira C, Head LR, et al: Surgical treatment of mitral insufficiency. J Thorac Surg 36:677, 1958
48. Wooler GH, Nixon PG, Grimshaw VA, et al: Experiences with the repair of the mitral valve in mitral incompetence. Thorax 17:49, 1962
49. Reed GE, Tice DA, Clauss RH: Asymmetric exaggerated mitral annuloplasty: repair of mitral insufficiency with hemodynamic predictability. J Thorac Cardiovasc Surg 49:752, 1965
50. Ellis FH Jr, Frye RL, McGoon DC: Results of reconstructive operations for mitral insufficiency due to ruptured chordae tendineae. Surgery 59:165, 1966
51. Carpentier A, Deloche A, Dauptain J, et al: A new reconstructive operation for correction of mitral and tricuspid insufficiency. J Thorac Cardiovasc Surg 61:1, 1971
52. Carpentier A, Loulmet D, Le Bret E, et al: [Open heart operation under video surgery and minithoracotomy. First case (mitral valvuloplasty) operated with success]. C R Acad Sci III 319:219, 1996
53. Carpentier A, Loulmet D, Aupecle B, et al: Computer-assisted cardiac surgery. Lancet 353:379, 1999
54. Mohr FW, Falk V, Diegeler A, et al: Computer-enhanced "robotic" cardiac surgery: Experience in 148 patients. J Thorac Cardiovasc Surg 121:842, 2001
55. Sones FM Jr: Cine-coronary arteriography. Ohio Med 58:1018, 1962
56. Effler DB: A new era of coronary artery surgery. Surg Gynecol Obstet 123:1310, 1966
57. Sabiston DC Jr: Surgery of the coronary circulation. J R Coll Surg Edinb 8:105, 1963
58. DeBakey ME, McCollum CH 3rd: Coronary artery bypass procedures. Comprehens Ther 1:14, 1975
59. Kolessov VI: Mammary artery-coronary artery anastomosis as method of treatment for angina pectoris. J Thorac Cardiovasc Surg 54:535, 1967
60. Bailey CP, Bolton HE, Nichols H, et al: Ventriculoplasty for cardiac aneurysm. J Thorac Surg 35:37, 1958; discussion 64, 1958
61. Cooley DA, Henly WS, Amad KH, et al: Ventricular aneurysm following myocardial infarction: Results of surgical treatment. Ann Surg 150:595, 1959
62. Jatene AD: Left ventricular aneurysmectomy. Resection or reconstruction. J Thorac Cardiovasc Surg 89:321, 1985
63. Dor V, Saab M, Coste P, et al: Left ventricular aneurysm: A new surgical approach. Thorac Cardiovasc Surg 37:11, 1989
64. DeBakey ME, Cooley DA: Successful resection of aneurysm of thoracic aorta and replacement by graft. JAMA 152:673, 1953
65. Muller WH Jr, Warren WD, Dammann JF Jr, et al: Surgical relief of aortic insufficiency by direct operation on the aortic valve. Circulation 21:587, 1960
66. Blakemore AH, Voorhees AB Jr: The use of tubes constructed from Vinyon N cloth in bridging arterial defects experimental and clinical. Ann Surg 140:324, 1954
67. Debakey ME, Jordan GL Jr, Abbott JP, et al: The fate of Dacron vascular grafts. Arch Surg 89:757, 1964
68. Griepp RB, Stinson EB, Hollingsworth JF, et al: Prosthetic replacement of the aortic arch. J Thorac Cardiovasc Surg 70:1051, 1975
69. Bentall H, De Bono A: A technique for complete replacement of the ascending aorta. Thorax 23:338, 1968
70. Cabrol C, Pavie A, Gandjbakhch I, et al: Complete replacement of the ascending aorta with reimplantation of the coronary arteries: New surgical approach. J Thorac Cardiovasc Surg 81:309, 1981
71. Griepp EB, Griepp RB: Cerebral consequences of hypothermic circulatory arrest in adults. J Card Surg 7:134, 1992
72. Spielvogel D, Strauch JT, Minanov OP, et al: Aortic arch replacement using a trifurcated graft and selective cerebral antegrade perfusion. Ann Thorac Surg 74:S1810, 2002; discussion S1825, 2002
73. Carrel A, Guthrie C: Uniterminal and biterminal venous transplantations. Gynecol Obstet 2:266, 1906

74. Baevskii RM, Demikhov VP, Sharovskaia NM: [Assessment of the status of the circulatory system in dogs with transplanted heart]. Biull Eksp Biol Med 65:119, 1968
75. Angell WW, Shumway NE: Resuscitative storage of the cadaver heart transplant. Surg Forum 17:224, 1966
76. Clark DA, Schroeder JS, Griepp RB, et al: Cardiac transplantation in man. Review of first three years' experience. Am J Med 54:563, 1973
77. Newman MH, Stuckey JH, Levowitz BS, et al: Complete and partial perfusion of animal and human subjects with the pump-oxygenator: A study of factors yielding consistent survival, successful application to one case. Surgery 38:30, 1955
78. Rose EA, Moskowitz AJ, Packer M, et al: The REMATCH trial: Rationale, design, and end points. Randomized Evaluation of Mechanical Assistance for the Treatment of Congestive Heart Failure. Ann Thorac Surg 67:723, 1999
79. Durrer D, Roos JP: Epicardial excitation of the ventricles in a patient with Wolff-Parkinson-White syndrome (type B). Circulation 35:15, 1967
80. Guiraudon GM, Ofiesh JG, Kaushik R: Extended vertical transatrial septal approach to the mitral valve. Ann Thorac Surg 52:1058, 1991; discussion 1060, 1991
81. Cox JL, Schuessler RB, Cain ME, et al: Surgery for atrial fibrillation. Semin Thorac Cardiovasc Surg 1:67, 19891
82. Ross DN: Replacement of aortic and mitral valves with a pulmonary autograft. Cancer 2:956, 1967
83. Carpentier A: Cardiac valve surgery. J Thorac Cardiovasc Surg 86:323, 1987
84. English TA: Heart transplantation—1979. Trans Hunter Soc 37, 38:143, 1978–1980
85. Yacoub MH, Reid CJ, Al-Khadimi RN, et al: Cardiac transplantation: The London Experience. Z Kardiol 74(Suppl 6):45, 1985
86. Bailey LL, Takeuchi Y, Williams WG, et al: Surgical management of congenital cardiovascular anomalies with the use of profound hypothermia and circulatory arrest. J Thorac Cardiovasc Surg 71:485, 1976
87. Harken D, Clauss R, Birtwell W, et al: Assisted circulation: The arterial counterpulsator. J Thorac Cardiovasc Surg 41:447, 1961
88. Moulopoulos SD: Diastolic balloon pumping in the aorta. Am Heart J 63:669, 1962
89. Kolff WJ, Blazer R: The artificial heart. Trans Am Soc Artif Int Organs 7:59, 1956

Chapter 3

THE FUTURE OF CARDIOLOGY

Javier Sanz, MD • Valentin Fuster, MD, PhD • Juan F. Viles-Gonzalez, MD • Pedro R. Moreno, MD

KEY POINTS

1. The absolute mortality and morbidity rates of cardiovascular disorders are going to increase in relation to the aging of the population and the high prevalence of risk factors for atherothrombotic disease. Heart failure and atrial fibrillation are expected to be the new epidemics.
2. The largest potential impact will come from the appropriate application of effective preventive measures.
3. The identification of a variety of biomarkers and their physiologic significance will allow for a more refined stratification of risk in different clinical settings.
4. Newer imaging modalities (in particular, computed tomography and magnetic resonance imaging) will aid in the earlier diagnosis and improved evaluation of multiple cardiovascular disorders.
5. The genomics/proteomics revolution will provide significant knowledge on the mechanisms of disease and eventually allow for personalized medicine (assessment of the individual risk and potential effects of interventions).
6. Newer drugs for a variety of diseases are going to become available in the near future and contribute to improved survival.
7. The number of percutaneous interventions (for coronary artery disease, arrhythmias, congenital heart disease, valvular abnormalities) will continue to rise, and this may result in a reduction in indications for surgical procedures.
8. Tissue engineering and genetic and cell therapy are the most promising future modalities to provide a definitive cure for cardiovascular disease.

The second half of the 20th century witnessed an impressive accrual of knowledge and technologic progress in the field of cardiovascular medicine. Notable advances included the recognition of the importance of prevention (with the identification of well-defined risk factors for atherosclerosis), a deeper understanding of the pathophysiology of atherothrombotic disease (ATD), the development of diagnostic tools (e.g., coronary angiography, echocardiography), and a variety of therapeutic options such as cardiovascular drugs (β-blockers, angiotensin-converting enzyme inhibitors [ACEIs], statins, aspirin, clopidogrel, thrombolytics, glycoprotein IIb/IIIa inhibitors, low-molecular-weight heparins), percutaneous coronary interventions (PCIs) (angioplasty, stenting), electrical devices (pacemakers, defibrillators), and cardiac surgical procedures (coronary artery bypass grafting [CABG], valve replacement, and heart transplantation). These innovations have completely transformed the daily practice of cardiovascular medicine throughout the world. Similar changes are expected to occur in the next 50 years as a result of significant modifications in patients' characteristics, better knowledge of the genetic and molecular bases of disease, refinements in risk stratification, and more specialized preventive, diagnostic, and therapeutic modalities. Such developments will likely revolutionize medical practice in general and the approach to cardiovascular disease (CVD) in particular. Cardiovascular professionals, especially those beginning their clinical or academic careers, should be aware of the demands and challenges they must meet in the near future. Several areas of current research are anticipated to generate new advances of substantial impact during the next few years. The following pages provide a general overview and predict possible scenarios for the short- and mid-term future.

SIGNIFICANCE OF CARDIOVASCULAR DISEASE AND DEMOGRAPHICS

CVD affects almost 65 million individuals in the United States (20% of the population). Of these, approximately 40% are seniors (≥65 years). CVD is the leading cause of mortality, causing almost 40% of all deaths, surpassing the next five deadly diseases combined. Half of the coronary artery disease (CAD) deaths are due to myocardial infarction (MI). Every 30 seconds there is a new MI in America. During the time spent reading this paragraph, one person died from CVD in the United States. The economic impact is equally huge, with an estimated annual cost of more than $350 billion.[1] These breathtaking figures do not apply exclusively to the industrialized world: CVD is also the leading cause of death worldwide, accounting for more than 17 million deaths every year.[2,3] Although the elderly are at increased risk, this pandemic affects all layers in the community and all ethnic groups.[3] More women than men die every year due to CVD (particularly from CAD), contradicting the common disbelief of a lesser burden for females.[1]

During the next 50 years, variations in the U.S. demographics will result from a combination of changes in mortality, fertility, and migration patterns. Although difficult to predict, no major modifications are expected in the latter two elements. Life expectancy of the already existing U.S. population will therefore be the most influential factor in patients' demographics.[4] With the steady increase in life expectancy achieved during the 20th century, which is likely to continue, the American population is becoming progressively older. More importantly, the large generation of "baby-boomers" will reach their senior age in the next 20 years (2010s and 2020s), and by 2050 there will be about 80 million seniors[5] (Fig. 3–1). The relative importance of CVD is even higher in the elderly, with 84% of all cardiovascular deaths occurring in patients 65 years or older.[4] Despite the impressive 60% decrease in age-adjusted mortality rates related to CVD achieved during the prior century,[6] the absolute number of deaths attributable to heart disease is projected to increase

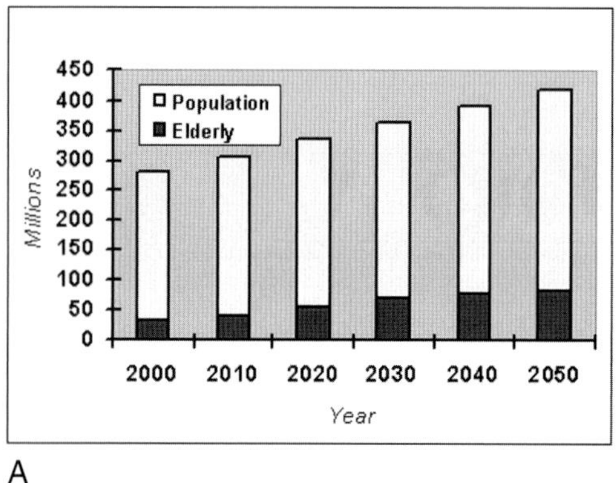

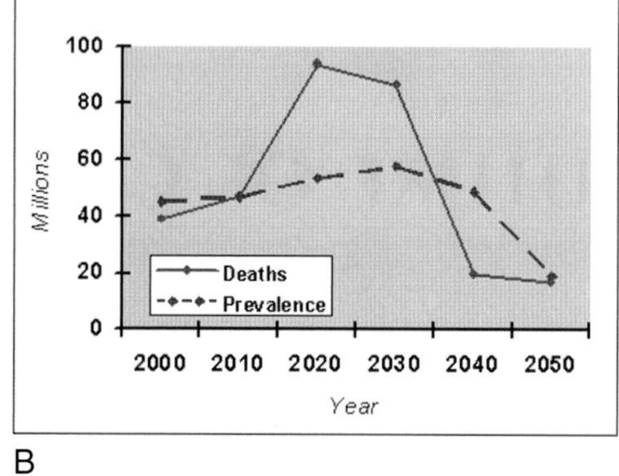

Figure 3–1 (*A*) Projected total population and number of older people (≥65 years) for the first half of the 21st century in the United States. A steady growth in the population as well as in the proportion of elderly individuals can be anticipated. (*B*) Projected mortality and prevalence of cardiovascular disease in the first half of the 21st century. In the first quarter of the century, prevalence and particularly mortality will increase as a result of the aging and growth of the population. This may be followed by substantial decreases if current and future preventive and therapeutic measures are effective (see text).

by more than 100%.[4] In this context, it appears that mortality has been delayed rather than decreased. It will probably take several decades before there is a substantial drop in absolute mortality rates. The prevalence of chronic CVD will also be augmented, not only in relation to the aging of the population but also due to the increase in risk factors (see later) and improvements in survival of patients who would have died in the past. Together with more common interventions, a parallel rise in costs will follow, particularly during the first quarter of the 21st century.[7]

Cardiovascular specialists will encounter larger numbers of elderly patients in the near future. A variety of physiologic changes occur in the aging cardiovascular system, including increased vascular and myocardial stiffness, left ventricular hypertrophy with slowed relaxation, diminished β-adrenoceptor responsiveness, autonomic dysfunction, and overall impaired cardiovascular reserve.[8] These patients carry a higher atherosclerotic burden and more frequent cardiovascular risk factors, such as arterial hypertension (HTN) and diabetes mellitus (DM). Altogether, this will result in an increased prevalence of CHD, stroke, heart failure (HF), degenerative valvular disease, and atrial fibrillation. Additionally, the elderly have more associated morbid conditions, are more likely to be multimedicated, and are more prone to adverse drug reactions and to complications with therapeutic interventions such as thrombolysis, angioplasty, or surgery.[9-13] As a result, older patients with different cardiovascular disorders are frequently undertreated.[6] Despite their higher baseline risk, the elderly gain substantial benefit from adequate interventions, often superior to their younger counterparts.[14,15] Aged patients have traditionally been underrepresented in clinical trials, and, as it has been noted, the practice of evidence-based medicine in this subgroup is particularly difficult.[8] It is essential to continue current efforts to identify the optimal therapeutic approaches for this population, which are likely to be similar to those with demonstrated efficacy in the younger patients.[16-18]

RISK STRATIFICATION AND DIAGNOSIS

Major Risk Factors

Box 3–1 shows the major risk factors that contribute to enhanced development and/or progression of ATD. Although well recognized, these risk factors are far from being under control (Fig. 3–2), and for many, the prevalence is growing. More than 50% of Americans have elevated total cholesterol levels; 50 million have HTN, the main predisposing factor for stroke and HF, and the international prevalence approaches 700 million.[1,2] Although the number of smokers has decreased in the United States, it keeps growing in developing countries and is anticipated to reach 500 million worldwide by 2025.[2] Diabetes mellitus (DM) is a CAD equivalent, with a cardiovascular risk for asymptomatic diabetics as high as for nondiabetics with a prior MI. In addition, DM portends an

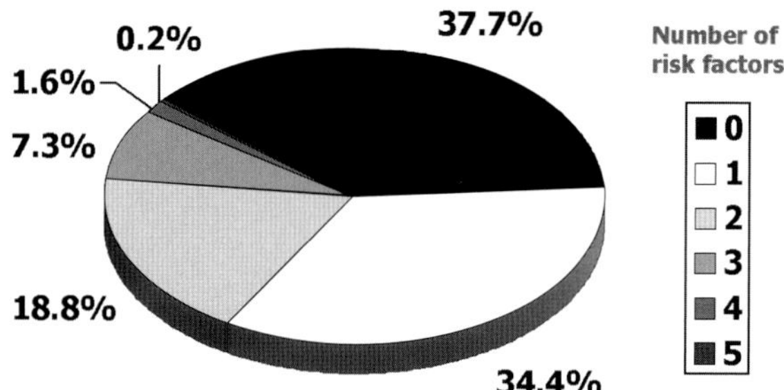

Figure 3–2 Prevalence of major risk factors for cardiovascular disease in the United States. As noted in the figure, more than 60% of the American population has at least one self-reported risk factor. (Data from Greenlund et al: Arch Intern Med 164:181, 2004.)

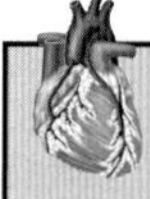

BOX 3–1 ***Major Independent Risk Factors for the Development and Progression of Atherosclerotic Disease***[19,28]

- Advancing age
- Elevated blood pressure
- Diabetes mellitus
- Cigarette smoking
- Elevated total (and LDL) cholesterol
- Decreased HDL cholesterol
- Obesity (particularly abdominal)
- Physical inactivity
- Family history of premature CHD

LDL = low-density lipoprotein; HDL = high-density lipoprotein; CHD = coronary heart disease.

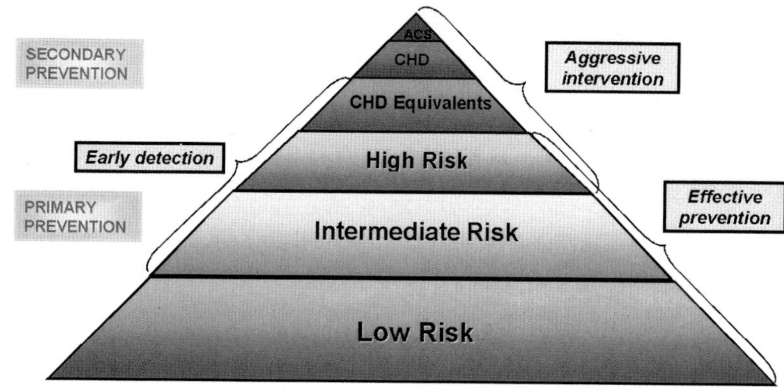

Figure 3–3 "Prevention pyramid" showing risk distribution in the community. Although certain subgroups of subjects have substantially elevated risk profiles, the majority of events (in absolute terms) occur in the low-intermediate risk categories, which comprise the majority of the population. ACS = acute coronary syndromes; CHD = coronary heart disease. (Modified from Fuster V et al: Circulation 99:1132, 1999.)

unfavorable prognosis after an acute coronary syndrome (ACS) and less benefit from different therapeutic modalities.[12,19-21] It is estimated that approximately 17 million Americans are diabetic. The age-adjusted prevalence of DM has almost tripled in the past 40 years and it will further increase during the next decades, both in the United States and worldwide.[22] Most importantly, type 2 DM is an emerging epidemic among children and young adults.[6] A similar situation is noted for obesity, the main determinant for the development of type 2 DM, with more than 60% of adults and 15% of children being overweight.[1] An estimated 60% of the world population (including adolescents) do not engage in sufficient physical activity.[6] Excess risk associated with elevated blood levels of triglycerides may represent independent prognostic value[23] or an association with other atherogenic lipid particles. Hypertriglyceridemia and low high-density lipoprotein (HDL) are part of the *metabolic syndrome*, a constellation of metabolic abnormalities that also comprises HTN, abdominal obesity, impaired fasting glucose, and DM and that affects 47 million Americans.[19,24] These figures point out the paramount importance of cardiovascular prevention (see later).

Major risk factors account for more than 80% of excess risk for premature CAD and, accordingly, equations for risk calculation have been developed.[25-27] Although clinically useful, they are encumbered by several limitations.[28] First, there is large interindividual variability within a particular risk group. Furthermore, using these scores, a substantial proportion of individuals fall into the category of intermediate risk. Because of the risk distribution in the community (Fig. 3–3), asymptomatic subjects with subclinical disease and/or predisposing factors account for the vast majority of the population. Millions of individuals are categorized as intermediate-risk, even though only a proportion of them will eventually develop clinically relevant CVD. This points to the necessity of finding additional markers that can aid in refining risk stratification and predicting individual risk (Fig. 3–4). Such an approach is of crucial importance for planning future cost-effective interventions (see Chapter 11).

Biomarkers

Acute coronary events are frequently secondary to the rupture of an atherosclerotic "vulnerable" plaque with superimposed thrombosis. The concept of plaque vulnerability has been challenged by increasing evidence of the systemic nature of atherosclerosis. Instead, the term "vulnerable patient" appears more appropriate, as some individuals show abnormalities in the blood that predispose them to the development of ATD and its complications.[29] The constellations of metabolic, immune, and hematologic abnormalities associated with ATD affect the vascular system globally. Similarly, a cascade of neurohormonal changes accompanies different cardiac diseases. A variety of serum markers that reflect metabolic, thrombotic, inflammatory, neuroendocrine, hemodynamic, or oxidative processes have been identified or are under active investigation (Tables 3–1 and 3–2), showing great potential in the diagnosis and estimation of prognosis. The ultimate goal is to identify biomarkers that are easily and reproducibly measured, with the ability to provide independent additional information over traditional risk factors, in the settings of both primary and secondary prevention, and in large groups of the population.

Many serum markers reflect different aspects of the metabolic status of the individual. High total cholesterol or low-density lipoprotein (LDL) cholesterol levels are well-known risk factors for the development and progression of ATD. However, they may be too rudimentary for a refined assessment.[30] Several subfractions of blood lipids classified according to their size and/or density are associated with elevated risk and are being evaluated as potential markers for clinical application (see Table 3–1). Evidence of altered glucose metabolism precedes overt DM and can be used to identify individuals with higher risk or higher prevalence of subclini-

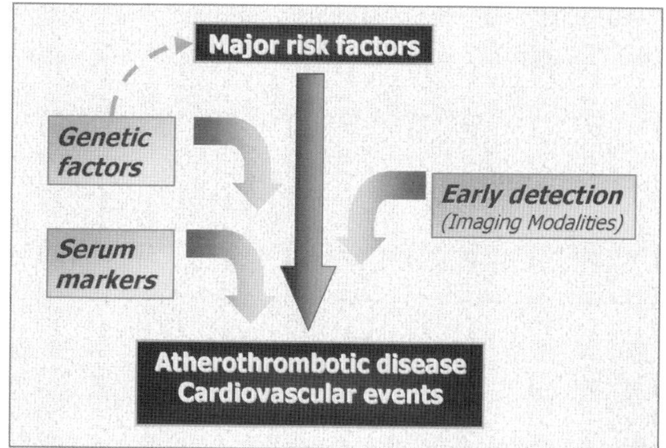

Figure 3–4 Overall strategy for the future prediction of risk of developing cardiovascular disorders. Major risk factors will continue to be the basis for stratification. However, this will be refined by the inclusion of genetic factors (influencing the development of disease or risk factors themselves), measurement of a variety of serum markers, and early detection of subclinical disease with different imaging modalities.

Table 3–1 Traditional and New Biomarkers in Atherothrombotic Disease

Lipids	Inflammatory	Prothrombotic	Metabolic	Infectious	Oxidative	Other
Triglycerides Small, dense LDL particles Large VLDL Small HDL IDL Apolipoproteins: A-I (decreased), B, C-III, E Lipoprotein-associated phospholipase A2 Lipoprotein(a)	hsCRP Interleukins (IL-1, -6, -10, -18) Serum Amyloid A Tumor necrosis factor α Adhesion molecules (ICAM-1, VCAM-1, P-selectin) MMP-9 Pregnancy-associated plasma protein A CD40 ligand Heat-shock protein Leukocyte count Myeloperoxidase FAS/FAS ligand	Fibrinogen Factors V, VII, VIII, XIII, von Willebrand D dimer Plasminogen Tissue plasminogen activator, plasminogen activator inhibitor Circulating tissue factor Protein S, C, thrombomodulin, antithrombin III (decreased) Blood viscosity	Plasma insulin Insulin resistance Impaired fasting glucose Impaired glucose tolerance Leptin Homocysteine	*Chlamydia pneumoniae* Herpes simplex virus Cytomegalovirus *Helicobacter pylori* Influenza Circulating bacterial endotoxin	Oxidized LDL Antibodies against oxidized LDL Modified tyrosines Glutathione, glutathione-peroxidase F-2 isoprostane	Psychosocial factors Ethnic factors Nitric oxide metabolites Asymmetric dimethylarginine Circulating nonesterified fatty acids

LDL = low-density lipoprotein; VLDL = very low-density lipoprotein; HDL = high-density lipoprotein; IDL = intermediate-density lipoprotein; hsCRP = high-sensitivity C-reactive protein; ICAM-1 = intercellular adhesion molecule; VCAM-1 = vascular cell adhesion molecule; MMP-9 = matrix metalloproteinase-9.

Table 3–2 Biomarkers Associated With a Variety of Cardiac and Hemodynamic Disorders

Neuroendocrine Activation	Oxidative Stress	Inflammatory
ANP	Malondialdehyde	Interleukin-6
BNP	Lipid peroxides	Tumor necrosis factor
N-terminal-pro-ANP	Glutathione peroxidase	FAS/FAS ligand
N-terminal-pro-BNP Renin activity Angiotensin II Aldosterone Nitric oxide cGMP Adrenomedullin Endothelin-1 Norepinephrine Epinephrine	Adrenolutin	

ANP = atrial natriuretic peptide; BNP = brain natriuretic peptide; cGMP = cyclic guanosine monophosphate.

cal atherosclerosis.[31-33] Increased levels of leptin, a protein secreted by adipocytes that is involved in appetite regulation, obesity, and insulin resistance, are also associated with increased cardiovascular risk.[34] Homocysteine is a metabolite of the amino acid methionine with toxic, proinflammatory, and prothrombotic properties. Increased plasma levels correlate with a higher incidence of CAD, particularly in patients with renal insufficiency.[35]

Another group of novel risk factors includes markers of a sustained prothrombotic or inflammatory state, both of which are intimately interrelated. Increased concentrations of procoagulant factors and/or markers of ongoing clot formation are associated with higher risk for cardiovascular events.[36] A similar association is observed with a number of inflammatory markers. High-sensitivity C-reactive protein (hsCRP) has the most cumulative evidence for discriminatory capacity in different settings. Traditionally considered a nonspecific acute-phase reactant, hsCRP is also a marker of low-grade vascular inflammation. Plasma concentrations of hsCRP have demonstrated a significant, dose-response relationship with the probability of coronary events, stroke, peripheral vascular disease, and sudden cardiac death, independent of other major risk factors (including the metabolic syndrome).[37-39] It is also useful for the prediction of recurrent events in those with diabetes, angina, MI, vascular disease in other territories, or after coronary artery stenting.[40-45] The hsCRP can be used to place patients with intermediate risk in a higher or lower category[46] and to identify subjects who will benefit the most with primary or secondary prevention measures.[42,47,48] Plasma levels have shown inconsistent correlations with measurements of subclinical atherosclerosis, suggesting that they indicate disease activity rather than merely plaque burden.[37] In summary, hsCRP is currently the most appealing alternative to traditional risk factors for risk stratification and the most plausible candidate for prompt widespread use in the population.[38]

The potential role for several microorganisms in the development of atherosclerotic lesions or their complication has not been confirmed in trials, and it has been suggested that an associated inflammatory response might be the pathophysiologic link between infection and atherosclerosis.[49-52] Future studies will undoubtedly contribute to further understanding of the role, if any, of infectious agents in CVD.

Indicators of hemodynamic status and neurohormonal activation comprise a different category of biomarkers. Adrenomedullin, a peptide with vasodilator and natriuretic properties released from a variety of tissues, may be an independent prognostic factor in HF.[53] Other natriuretic peptides are synthesized in the myocardium and released in response to myocardial stretching or increased wall tension. Atrial natriuretic peptide (ANP) is produced in the atria, whereas brain natriuretic peptide (BNP) originates mainly in the ventricles. They are synthesized as prohormones and subsequently split into the active hormones and N-terminal fragments. Both peptides, particularly BNP, are currently the most useful hemodynamic markers.[54] In subjects with ACSs, high levels of BNP or N-terminal pro-BNP are predictors of increased risk of death or subsequent HF on follow-up, and they may also be useful in guiding therapy.[55-57] In the setting of HF, natriuretic peptides have already shown potential for the detection of systolic and diastolic dysfunction or structural heart disease in general,[58,59] the diagnosis of HF in patients with dyspnea,[60] the prediction and monitoring of response to treatment,[61,62] therapeutic decision-making,[63,64] or prognosis estimation.[65] An elevated level of these peptides is a marker of increased overall cardiovascular risk, even in asymptomatic individuals, independent of traditional risk factors.[66]

It is likely that in the next few years the molecular roles as well as the prognostic significance and relative importance of many of these new biomarkers will be elucidated. This will allow for more sophisticated algorithms for risk stratification in the setting of both primary and secondary prevention in CAD and in other cardiovascular disorders. With improved refinements in assessing each individual's risk, cost-effective interventions and further reductions in events will follow. An important application for these newer biomarkers will be the estimation of perioperative cardiac risk in subjects undergoing both cardiac and noncardiac surgery. Preliminary results suggest that both hsCRP and BNP measured preoperatively can be used to predict surgical benefit or perioperative cardiovascular and infectious complications[67-71] (see Chapters 11, 32, 39, and 40).

Imaging Techniques

An alternative approach for the early diagnosis of CVD is the use of imaging modalities that can detect and ideally quantify the burden of subclinical disease. The results of such tests in asymptomatic subjects may prompt aggressive risk factor modification or additional interventions. In subjects with known CVD, they may be used as a tool of further risk stratification, follow-up, or guidance of therapy. Atherosclerosis in other territories is a surrogate of CAD; it is therefore not surprising that increased intima-media thickness of the aorta or carotid or femoral arteries as measured by ultrasound is correlated with higher risk of cardiovascular events.[72,73]

The noninvasive visualization of the coronary arteries has been a long pursued ambition driven by the realization of its enormous impact in the daily management of CAD. Because many acute coronary events originate from minimally stenotic plaques, it would be important to identify those plaques with anatomopathologic characteristics associated with high risk.[74] Several techniques, such as intravascular ultrasound, thermography, optical coherence tomography, and near-infrared spectroscopy, have been developed in an attempt to detect different markers of vulnerability.[75] They are, however, limited by their invasive nature. In the past few years, two techniques have emerged with the potential to offer a reasonable alternative to invasive catheterization. The early application of computed tomography (CT) for the imaging of the heart was for the detection of coronary calcium, a specific marker of atherosclerosis.[76] Electron beam CT (EBCT) and multislice CT (MSCT) reliably detect and quantify the amount of coronary calcification. In asymptomatic individuals, the risk of coronary events on follow-up increases proportionally with the calcium score.[77-79] This is independent of traditional risk factors, and therefore the test may be particularly useful in subjects with intermediate risk.[80] Alternative applications of calcium imaging may include monitoring the response to therapy[81] or evaluation of aortic valve disease.[82] Significant recent technological advances, particularly for MSCT, make this the most solid modality for noninvasive, contrast-enhanced coronary angiography (Fig. 3–5), with good diagnostic accuracy in the detection of significant coronary stenoses.[83-85] In addition, nonstenotic lesions can be visualized and initial steps have been taken toward plaque characterization.[86,87] Newer and improved scanner generations are already available, and in the next few years more and more patients will likely benefit from these imaging modalities. A reduced need for invasive diagnostic catheterizations may be forecast, although the improved detection of early or asymptomatic disease may finally result in more coronary interventions.

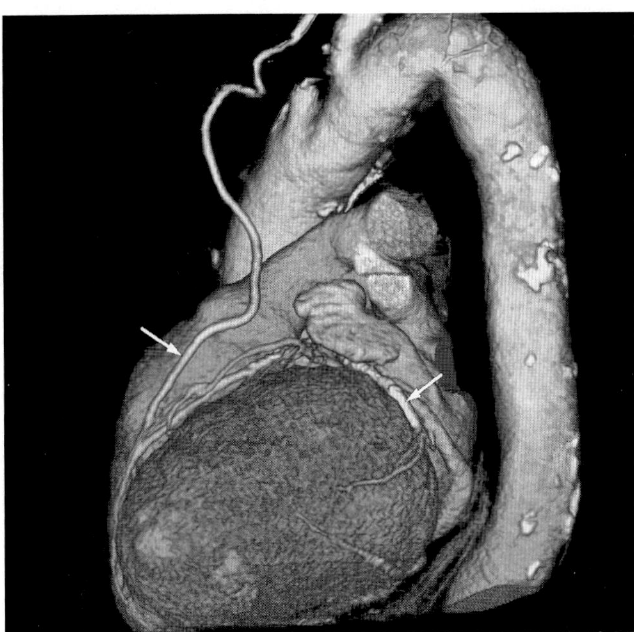

Figure 3–5 Three-dimensional volume-rendered reconstruction of a coronary multislice computed tomography angiogram in a patient with a history of percutaneous and surgical revascularization. A patent left internal mammary artery bypass graft can be seen (*left arrow*), anastomosing to the distal left anterior descending artery. Additionally, a stent is noted in the left circumflex artery (*right arrow*), and multiple calcified plaques are present along the descending thoracic aorta.

Widespread use of CT, however, may be restricted by its high radiation as well as limited diagnostic capability in cases of significant calcification or metallic artifacts (as in the presence of stents). In this regard, magnetic resonance imaging (MRI) may emerge as the technique of choice in the mid-term future. Current results are promising although improvements in spatial and temporal resolution are still needed.[88] MRI offers many other advantages and is probably the technique with higher capabilities for the diagnosis of CAD. Magnetic resonance angiography of different territories is a well-established modality of routine use in many centers. Additionally, MRI has excellent ability for the detection and characterization of atherosclerotic plaques, including the coronary tree, as well as thrombosis.[89-92] It is feasible to use MRI to screen large

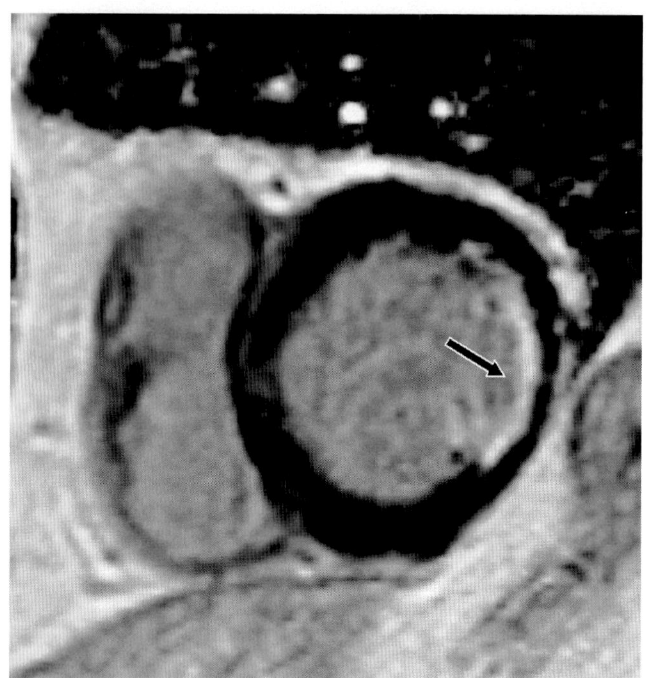

Figure 3–6 Magnetic resonance delayed enhancement imaging demonstrating a subendocardial lateral myocardial infarction (*arrow*, bright signal). The transmural extent can be easily quantified.

groups of patients and to obtain measures of plaque burden that correlate with traditional risk factors.[93] In patients receiving lipid-lowering therapy, it is possible to detect and quantify reductions in plaque size.[94,95] In the study of cardiac disease, the versatility of this technique allows for the evaluation of multiple physiopathologic aspects in one single examination.[96,97]

MRI is the gold standard for the evaluation of ventricular mass, volume, and function.[98] Stress-induced changes in myocardial perfusion or function have good sensitivity and specificity for the diagnosis of coronary artery stenoses.[99-101] In the setting of preoperative evaluation, stress MRI is a useful tool for the prediction of surgical cardiovascular complications.[102] In addition, MRI is superior to other imaging modalities for the visualization of an MI (Fig. 3–6) after the administration of gadolinium contrast agents (delayed hyperenhancement).[103-105] Several reports have demonstrated that the transmural extent of hyperenhancement in CAD correlates inversely with the probability of functional recovery after revascularization[106,107] or medical treatment.[108] Interestingly, small infarctions occurring after surgical revascularization (and which may explain the lack of functional recovery in some segments) are readily detected with MRI.[109] Newer sequences and contrast agents promise to increase the ability to detect atherosclerotic lesions and ischemia.[110,111] In addition, MRI spectroscopy, a technique that allows for noninvasive quantification of myocardial metabolites, holds promise in the diagnosis of different myocardial diseases.[112]

An emerging and exciting field of imaging is aimed at the visualization of biologic processes at the molecular and cellular level. Molecular imaging agents can be created by attaching a target-specific ligand (e.g., an antibody or an enzyme substrate) to another component (microbubbles, fluorochromes, magnetic compounds, or radioisotopes) that can be imaged with the appropriate technique. The new contrast agent is designed to detect a specific metabolic pathway or molecule, and, on some occasions, even be activated by it[113] (Fig. 3–7). In the field of CVD, initial reports using MRI, positron emission tomography (PET), and ultrasound or near-infrared spectroscopy have demonstrated the possibility to detect fibrin, oxidized lipids, expression of endothelial adhesion molecules, monocyte recruitment, apoptosis, or neoangiogenesis[113] (see Chapters 11, 15, and 16).

Because of the specific strengths and weaknesses of different imaging approaches, there is a current movement toward the development of fusion technologies, combining imaging modalities in a single machine. In this regard, the PET-CT scanner is already a reality and others will emerge in the near future. Similarly, improved image postprocessing techniques will enable the creation of interactive three-dimensional maps of the heart or the whole cardiovascular system combining data from different modalities. Real-time reconstructions of such maps with the ability to guide physicians during interventional or surgical procedures may become available soon.[114]

Genetics

One of the cornerstones of medical progress will be a deeper knowledge of genetic determinants of normal and disease physiology. The completion of the Human Genome Project in 2003 with the entire sequencing of the human genome was an important landmark. As a result, the foundation for a thorough understanding of gene structure, function, and interactions (genomics), as well as their resulting products (proteomics), has been achieved. While humans share 99.9% of their DNA sequences, the 0.1% variability probably explains much of the interindividual differences in susceptibility for disease or its complications, as well as response to therapy.[115] As an example, it is estimated that 40% to 60% of the variance of CAD can be explained by genetic differences.[116] To date, hundreds of thousands of different genetic mutations have been recognized, and many polymorphisms leading to cardiovascular disorders identified. The cardiovascular disorders that have been linked to genetic abnormalities range from the development of risk factors to the predisposition for multiple cardiac diseases, such as MI, HF, arrhythmias, and cardiomyopathies (Table 3–3).

A novel medical area arising from the genomics/proteomics revolution is pharmacogenomics. This discipline is devoted to the identification of those genetic traits linked to beneficial, harmful, or absent responses to particular drugs, as well as pharmacologic interactions.[117] As an example, a mutation in hepatic microsomal enzymes is associated with an increased risk for bleeding complications in subjects treated with warfarin.[118] Similar mutations have been identified that can predict the degree of response or the risk of adverse effects to a variety of cardiovascular drugs such as statins, ACEI, or digoxin.[119]

The initial optimism derived from the identification of many of these polymorphisms has been tempered by the realization of the complex interaction among multiple genetic traits, molecular pathways, and environmental factors, eventually resulting in the clinical manifestation of a disease or the effect of a drug. This is particularly true for common diseases, such as CAD or DM, in which multiple genes and factors are involved. These intricate relations will be elucidated over many years. Nonetheless, the ultimate goal of the genetics/genomics revolution is the provision of truly personalized

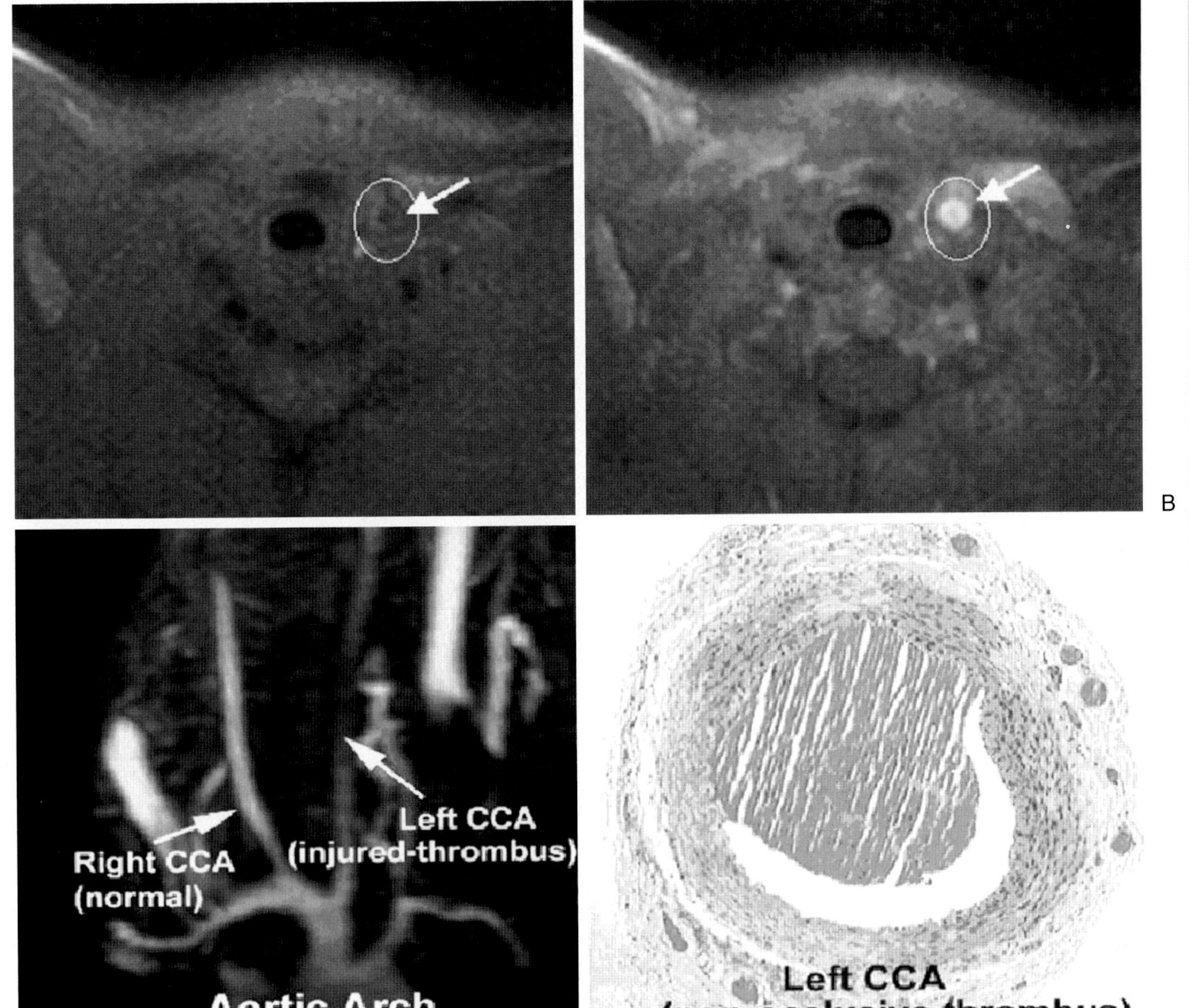

Figure 3–7 In vivo "molecular imaging" of experimentally induced thrombus in porcine carotid arteries using a fibrin-targeted MRI contrast agent. (*A*) Precontrast T1-weighted image of left injured common carotid artery (CCA, *arrow*), where the thrombus cannot readily be detected. (*B*) A dramatic contrast enhancement of the thrombus is noted (*arrow*) after the fibrin-targeted contrast agent injection. Note that the contralateral uninjured CCA does not show any enhancement. (*C*) A contrast-enhanced MR angiogram shows the patency of the right uninjured CCA (normal) and the decreased flow in the injured (thrombosed) left CCA. (*D*) Corresponding histologic (H&E stained) section of the left injured CCA. (Images courtesy of Dr. M. Sirol and Dr. Z. Fayad, Mount Sinai Hospital.)

medical care based on the genetic profile of the individual. In the near future it will be possible to perform genetic testing for a variety of monogenic cardiovascular disorders, particularly in subjects with a strong family history. In a mid-term projection, with the development of large genetic and population databases, the ability to screen an individual for a large number of genetic mutations, allowing for the early diagnosis of silent diseases, an extremely refined estimate of risk, or guidance of therapy on a personalized basis, may be achieved. Eventually there may be a device with a patient's complete genetic information, enabling physicians to determine the exact preventive or therapeutic measure that will be effective (and to what extent) for each person.[114]

PRIMARY PREVENTION

Despite the exciting and attractive new therapeutic modalities that may await in the future, probably the biggest impact in the reduction of morbidity and mortality secondary to CVD in the general population will come from appropriate use of currently available knowledge. An aggressive treatment of risk factors can reduce excess risk by 30% to 50%.[28] Millions of people in the intermediate-risk category can benefit from adequate application of well-defined lifestyle-related and pharmacologic interventions, in the setting of both primary and secondary prevention. One of the major challenges that health care professionals will face in forthcoming years will be to

Table 3–3 **Proteins With Abnormal Synthesis/Function Secondary to Genetic Disorders That Have Been Associated With Cardiovascular Disease and Risk Factors**

Disease	Gene Products
Dyslipidemia	LDL receptor, apolipoproteins, ABC transporters, cholesterol ester transfer protein, hepatic lipase, upstream transcription factor-1
Hypertension	Mineralocorticoids, mineralocorticoid receptors, sodium channels, α_2-receptors, β_1-receptors, angiotensin-converting enzyme, angiotensin II receptor, α-adducin
Diabetes	PPAR-γ, PPAR-γ coactivator, nuclear respiratory factor, insulin, insulin receptor, cytotoxic T-lymphocyte antigen-4, lipoprotein lipase
Obesity	Leptin, leptin receptor, pro-opiomelanocortin
ATD/CHD	Paraoxonase-1, lamin-A, matrix metalloproteinase-9, factor VII, factor V, prothrombin, thrombospondin, plasminogen activator inhibitor, limphotoxin-α, connexin 37, stromelysin, toll-like receptor, phosphodieasterase 4D, 5-lipooxygenase, 5-lipo-oxygenase activating protein, cytochrome P450 epoxygenase, myocyte enhancer factor 2A
Hypertrophic cardiomyopathy	Troponins, actin, myosin, myosin-binding protein, α-tropomyosin, titin
Dilated cardiomyopathy	Dystrophin, troponins, myosin, actin, desmin, lamin A, lamin C, sodium channel
Heart failure	α_2-receptors, β_1-receptors, β_2-receptors
Arrhythmias	Sodium, potassium and calcium channels, ryanodine receptor

ATD = atherothrombotic disease; CHD = coronary heart disease; LDL = low-density lipoprotein; PPAR = peroxisome proliferator-activated receptors.

ensure the universal availability of such options for those at risk. In addition, it will be paramount to devote specific efforts to the initiation of preventive measures (particularly regarding lifestyle) at an early age, as many risk factors develop during childhood.

Approximately 30% of subjects with HTN are not aware of their condition, and an additional 36% are either not treated or uncontrolled.[1] Less than half of those qualifying for lipid-lowering therapy actually receive any treatment.[1] A decrease in 5% of systolic blood pressure or total cholesterol (approximately 7 mm Hg and 15 mg/dL, respectively) would be associated with an approximately 25% reduction in the risk of cardiovascular events.[120] It is estimated that one of every three diabetics is not diagnosed.[121] Apart from strict metabolic control, the use of medications with proved beneficial effects on CAD, such as statins or ACEIs, is advantageous in these patients.[122,123]

Cessation of smoking decreases the risk of CAD by 50% after 1 year.[1] A nicotine vaccine, which leads to the formation of nicotine-binding antibodies preventing its interaction with the nicotine receptor, is undergoing initial human trials.[124] Rimonabant, a selective cannabinoid type 1 receptor blocker, has proved useful for discontinuation of smoking habit or weight loss.[125] If confirmed in further studies, this or similar drugs may have enormous impact in risk factor management.

An adequate dietary intake of antioxidant vitamins is associated with decreased cardiovascular risk.[126] The hypothesis that supplementary amounts might reduce the incidence of cardiovascular events has to date been disappointing.[127] Ongoing trials will answer the question of whether multivitamin supplements and high folate intake, which can decrease plasma concentrations of homocysteine, also reduce cardiovascular risk. Aspirin can also be an effective preventive measure for asymptomatic high-risk subjects.[128]

Novel lines of research for the management of CAD are evolving. Statins are currently the most widely used drugs, reducing plaque size in parallel with their ability to lower LDL.[95] Newer agents, such as ezetimibe, an inhibitor of cholesterol absorption in the intestine, can induce further decreases.[129] Even small increases in plasmatic HDL, probably the most potent endogenous antiatherogenic agent, lead to significant reductions in cardiovascular risk, making it a particularly desirable pharmacologic target.[130] Inhibitors of cholesterol ester transfer protein, which is involved in reverse cholesterol transport and HDL catabolism, raise HDL and have already been tested in clinical trials.[131] Recombinant apolipoprotein A-I (apoA-I), a component of HDL, can be given intravenously and preliminary results are encouraging.[132] Alternatively, production of apoA-I and A-II can be enhanced by agonists of the peroxisome proliferator-activated receptors (PPARs), which are also involved in the regulation of a variety of atherogenesis-related processes. PPAR agonists include statins, fibrates, glitazones, and newer selective agents that have proved effective in causing plaque regression in experimental models.[94]

Plaque neovascularization, metalloproteinase activity, and leukocyte infiltration are all factors related to plaque instability. Drugs inhibiting these processes are in a preclinical stage of development.[133-135] Tissue factor, the most potent thrombogenic component of the plaque core, is released by macrophages undergoing apoptotic death. Inhibitors of tissue factor or apoptosis are other attractive targets for future therapies.[136,137] In a broader perspective, many processes associated with aging (including HTN, DM, atherosclerosis, impaired myocardial performance, and so on) appear to be related to glycation and oxidation of proteins that result in extensive cross-linking of extracellular matrix components. New therapies directed at breaking these links have shown promising results in preclinical studies, and if they hold true, they could provide a compelling approach to simultaneously address multiple components of CVD and perhaps aging itself.[138]

THERAPY AND SECONDARY PREVENTION

Therapy for Coronary Artery Disease

In the 20th century, impressive increases in the survival of patients presenting with an MI were shown, particularly in relation to the development of coronary care units and the early application of reperfusion therapies. These achievements are, however, overshadowed by the fact that more than 300,000 persons still die every year in the United States before they can receive appropriate treatment. If clinicians want to further reduce mortality, it will be imperative to implement health policies that ensure universal and rapid availability of resources for patients suffering an acute coronary syndrome. Current efforts include educational campaigns for the prompt recognition of symptoms and improvements in the time to treatment (such as public-access defibrillation, portable telemetry monitors, or accessibility to specialized centers).[139-142]

The importance of antithrombotic therapy was realized in the past century with the generalization of the use of aspirin, heparin, and fibrinolytics. Additional antiplatelet agents, such as clopidogrel, low-molecular-weight heparins, and the family of glycoprotein IIb/IIIa inhibitors, have joined the armamentarium of drugs for CAD.[143-145] Newer antithrombotic agents have theoretical advantages and may extend the benefits of current therapies. Direct thrombin inhibitors interfere with the "pleiotropic" effects of thrombin, including platelet aggregation and secretion, synthesis of mediators of thrombus formation, proliferation of fibroblasts, and mitogenesis of smooth muscle cells. A randomized trial using aspirin plus oral ximelagatran, a representative member of this class, for the secondary prevention after MI demonstrated that the combination was more effective than aspirin alone.[146] Factor Xa inhibitors are a different family of antithrombotics with potential advantages over low-molecular-weight heparins.[147] Two different drugs, pentasaccharide and DX-9065a, have been tested already in different clinical settings such as unstable angina[148] or in combination with reperfusion strategies.[149,150] The drug-eluting stents, with their significantly reduced rates of restenosis, may prove a revolution in revascularization therapy.[151] Larger studies with longer follow-up and the evaluation of efficacy in a variety of settings (such as DM) will be needed to confirm the potential of these devices. Interestingly, a meta-analysis has shown that they do not improve mid-term mortality rates,[151] again emphasizing the importance of risk factors control and secondary prevention measures in the care of these patients.

As in the case of primary prevention, appropriate use of well-known therapies (such as aspirin, β-blockers, or ACEIs) could avoid thousands of premature deaths every year.[152,153] For patients undergoing surgery, β-blockers (and probably also statins) have the ability to prevent perioperative cardiovascular events, and present data suggest they are largely underused.[154,155] Current efforts such as interactive quality control tools appear to improve adherence to clinical guidelines.[153]

Despite these foreseeable advances, the aforementioned therapies are aimed at slowing or at best halting the progression and/or complications of the disease, but, once established, the cardiac damage is currently irreversible. A major breakthrough may arise from cell and genetic therapies (see later) with the potential to regenerate myocardial tissue and, for the first time, to achieve complete normalization of cardiac function and a real cure for this common disease.

Therapy for Heart Failure

There are 5 million Americans with HF, which is accompanied by a 20% mortality rate in 1 year.[1] This condition is the most common diagnosis in hospitalized elderly patients.[6] With the aging of the population and prolonged survival for a variety of cardiomyopathies (particularly CAD), HF is expected to reach epidemic proportions in the next decades.[156] Beneficial therapies (such as ACEIs or β-blockers) are directed to the attenuation of the neuroendocrine activation associated with HF. Similarly, based on the underlying molecular, metabolic, and immune events accompanying HF, newer agents are in various stages of development. For some, such as vasopeptidase inhibitors,[157] endothelin antagonists,[158,159] or anticytokine agents,[160] preliminary results have been disappointing. More promising have been levosimendan (a calcium sensitizer with inotropic and vasodilator properties),[161] tolvaptan (a vasopressin antagonist),[162] or nesiritide (recombinant BNP).[163] An earlier phase of investigation included drugs directed to the improvement of myocardial metabolic profile or the decrease of apoptosis.[164,165]

In the past few years, there has been an impressive expansion in the use of electrical devices for HF patients. The remarkable improvements in survival associated with automatic implantable defibrillators have resulted in continuously expanding indications.[166] There is also growing evidence of the beneficial effects of ventricular pacing and cardiac resynchronization in patients with systolic dysfunction.[167] In sum, an exponential rise in the number of patients who will benefit from these devices, which will become increasingly sophisticated, can be anticipated (see Chapters 13, 25, and 27).

Nonetheless, as in the case of CAD, these approaches are far from curative. For many patients with advanced disease, the only current therapeutic option is heart transplantation. In the United States, less than 5% of patients who could benefit from it actually receive an organ, and the demand is going to increase. Artificial hearts may be a solution for the future, as technologic advances continue to improve the results of these devices.[168] An appealing alternative that could similarly overcome the lack of donors might be xenotransplantation (most likely using porcine hearts), if several limitations related to immunologic and logistic barriers can be solved.[169] However, the most exciting possibilities will likely come from gene and cell therapy (see later).

Therapy for Valvular Heart Disease

After the control of rheumatic heart disease in the antibiotic era, aortic stenosis (of degenerative origin) and mitral regurgitation (in the setting of cardiomyopathy, particularly CAD) will remain the most prevalent valvular abnormalities, and common problems encountered by cardiovascular specialists. There is some evidence of common pathogenic mechanisms between CAD and the degenerative changes leading to aortic stenosis (AS). Treatments with beneficial effects on CAD may prove useful for AS, allowing for a medical treatment at least in part for the patients.[170] Advances in prostheses design are leading to improved durability and safety profile for those in whom replacement is needed.[171] In addition, some of the newer antithrombotics have the potential to facilitate the management of such patients.[172]

As the field of cardiac intervention continues to grow, percutaneous myocardial revascularization, closure of certain congenital heart defects, and balloon valvuloplasty for both aortic and mitral stenosis are routine practice in many centers. Expanding this approach, percutaneous strategies for valvular replacement or repair are being developed. Preliminary results of implantation of aortic and pulmonary prostheses, as well as valve repair for mitral insufficiency in humans, have been reported.[173-175] In the longer term, a promising approach may come from tissue engineering (see later) generating biologically active artificial valves. This valvular "transplant" might overcome many of the limitations of current prostheses, such as durability, long-term need for anticoagulation, or increased risk of endocarditis.

Therapy for Arrhythmias

Improved understanding of the genetic, molecular, and electrophysiologic mechanisms contributing to the triggering and perpetuation of arrhythmias will result in better and safer antiarrhythmic drugs (particularly for the prevention of sudden cardiac death) as well as a broader range of curative ablation procedures. As mentioned, the number of implanted electrical devices with a variety of functions (pacing, programmed stimulation, defibrillation, and so on) will increase in the near future.[176]

Atrial fibrillation (AF) deserves special consideration. Associated with aging, HTN, and increased prevalence of cardiac diseases, it will become one of the cardiovascular epidemics of the present century.[177] Today, more than 2 million Americans have AF or atrial flutter.[1] Several groups have developed a variety of catheter-based techniques with the potential to cure this disorder, at least in selected groups of patients.[178-180] In addition, new antiarrhythmic drugs with selectivity for atrial tissue are under evaluation.[181] Much of the morbidity and mortality of atrial fibrillation derives from the high risk of embolic events and the need for chronic anticoagulation. For those patients in whom maintenance of sinus rhythm is not possible or not indicated, newer antithrombotics promise to generate significant improvements in the management of this arrhythmia.[182] Ximelagatran has already proved as effective as warfarin and probably safer in subjects with nonrheumatic AF, with the added advantage of not requiring regular coagulation monitoring.[183] Additional trials to evaluate its efficacy in other settings are warranted (see Chapters 10, 13, and 29).

Therapy for Congenital Heart Disease

Traditionally considered a field for only pediatric specialists, the survival in many congenital cardiac abnormalities is improving dramatically. In the near future, physicians will treat more adults with corrected congenital heart diseases, and they will need to be familiar with the pathophysiology and therapeutic options for these disorders.[184] It is also expected that many of them will require additional interventional or surgical procedures during follow-up (see Chapter 22). Earlier diagnoses, aided by imaging techniques or genetic testing, will be followed in some cases by prenatal treatment, including intrauterine interventions[185] or genetic therapy (see later).

Genetic Therapy

In general terms, genetic therapies for cardiovascular medicine are currently aimed at enhancing the activity of endogenous systems with proangiogenic, inotropic, or protective (antiapoptotic, antioxidant, anti-inflammatory) properties. This can be achieved through either the delivery of genes whose function is abnormally diminished in the patient or blocking others (or their transcript products) with deleterious effects.[186] Different diseases may require different approaches. As an example, a patient with idiopathic dilated cardiomyopathy may benefit from therapies improving contractility, whereas a subject with chronic angina and normal function may require proangiogenic factors to increase myocardial perfusion. The variety of possible routes for gene delivery into the myocardium includes intrapericardial, intracoronary, intramural (into the vessel wall through direct injection or via coated stents/prostheses), and intramyocardial (transepicardial or transendocardial). Genes can be transported by viral or nonviral vectors, with the former showing currently more potential for sustained expression of the delivered gene.[187]

A variety of genes with proangiogenic properties, such as those encoding vascular endothelial growth factor (VEGF) or fibroblast growth factor, have already been used in phase I and II human trials of myocardial and limb ischemia, and preliminary results are encouraging.[188-191] HF is associated with downregulation and loss of function of β-adrenergic receptors, as well as abnormal handling of intracellular calcium. Genetic approaches addressing these anomalies are being evaluated in preclinical studies.[192-195] Protective therapy can be applied to the myocardium (for instance, to decrease reperfusion injury)[196] and to prevent accelerated atherosclerosis in venous grafts or intrastent restenosis.[197,198] In the field of arrhythmias, several monogenic disorders such as the long QT syndrome may be curable by replacing the defective genes. In addition, preliminary work shows that the transfer of specific genes can modify the electrophysiologic properties of cardiac cells.[199] This approach has already been used in a preclinical model of AF, in which gene delivery at the level of the atrioventricular node resulted in slowed conduction and ventricular rate control.[200] Genetic therapy may be of use in the management of risk factors for ATD, such as DM[201] or hypercholesterolemia (e.g., intravenous injection of a vector carrying the gene for apoA-1 results in increased liver production of HDL).[202] Other potential applications include local delivery to individual atherosclerotic lesions, replacement of abnormal proteins in genetic cardiomyopathies, or even early treatment of congenital heart disease.[187]

In the future, targeted gene transfer to specific areas (e.g., to injured endothelium or degraded collagen via specific receptors) may be possible, solving the issue of invasive local delivery. A number of these strategies might be useful even before the event occurs, leading to the concept of "preemptive" gene therapy. Ideally, some of these genes could remain dormant and their transcription would be activated only under the pathologic conditions (e.g., hypoxia).[187]

Cell Therapy

An old paradigm in cardiac biology assumed that from shortly after birth to senescence the heart has a relatively stable number of cardiomyocytes, implying that myocyte regeneration had little role in cardiac homeostasis. In the few past years, a growing body of evidence documented the existence of cycling ventricular myocytes in the normal and pathologic (post–acute MI and chronic HF) mammalian heart in several species, including humans.[203,204] The origin of these replicating cardiomyocytes remains controversial. There is evidence that extracardiac precursor cells derived from the bone marrow can migrate and locate the myocardium.[205,206] In addition, multipotent resident cardiac stem cells, with the ability to give rise to myocytes, smooth muscle, and endothelial cells, have been isolated from the human heart.[207] It appears that there is indeed an intrinsic mechanism for myocardial repair, but it seems to be inefficient. A number of cell transplantation therapies to enhance this mechanism of "self-repair" are under current investigation. The implications are huge, and potential applications include regeneration of postinfarction scar, induction of neovessels, or restoration of contractile function, among others. As in the case of genetic therapy, a variety of methods for delivery are available.[208]

Cells of embryonic origin are attractive, but ethical problems involved in their use need to be addressed. Preliminary data on transplantation of skeletal myoblasts have shown improvements in cardiac function and functional class, but a potential proarrhythmogenic effect has been noted.[209] The largest experience to date has been with bone marrow–derived mesenchymal stem cells, which also have pluripotent properties.[210] Clinical trials using this approach have demonstrated its feasibility and resulted in promising improvements in myocardial function and viability.[211-213] Preclinical data on cardiac stem cells have shown impressive results on myocardial regeneration.[207] An alternative approach consists of creating a local stimulus for homing, proliferation, and/or differentiation of progenitor cells, using cytokines such as granulocyte colony–stimulating factor, hepatocyte growth factor, or insulin-like growth factor, alone or in combination with the cells.[214-216] Multiple issues remain to be solved, such as the optimal cell lineage, fate after transplantation, dosing, route of administration, or replication/differentiation patterns. Nonetheless, a new era of cardiovascular therapy has started and holds promise in bringing, for the first time, real cures to a variety of common disorders.

Tissue Engineering

This emerging field is devoted to the construction of biological substitutes for a variety of tissues or even whole organs, in order to restore, maintain, or improve the tissue function. Such biologically active implants would overcome the limitations of current prosthetic devices that include thrombogenicity, neointimal proliferation, limited durability, or inability to grow, providing a complete restitution of the injured component.[217] To date, it has been shown that it is feasible to seed endothelial cells (or their progenitors) onto prosthetic vascular grafts or modified biomaterials or even to construct whole grafts by superimposed layers of fibroblasts, collagen, smooth muscle, and endothelial cells. These conduits resemble native vessels in that they are metabolically and biochemically active, and preliminary results suggest long-term patency.[218] Alternatively, cells can be implanted on absorbable scaffolds that can be shaped in different ways to generate more complex structures, such as neopulmonary arteries or cardiac valves.[219,220] Sheets of viable, beating cardiomyocytes have been developed on biodegradable scaffolds.[221] These advances open the possibility for the future construction of an entire bioengineered heart that may obviate the need for organ donors.

Therapies Based on Nanotechnology

Nanotechnology, a discipline dedicated to the creation of structures in the nanometer scale by the manipulation of individual atoms or molecules, also has an enormous potential for medical applications.[222] Some of these constructs may show "intelligent" properties, with the ability to be activated in greater or lesser degree in response to environmental factors or tissue enzymes. Possible applications include the development of targeted contrast agents (see Imaging Techniques) or implantable, sustained drug-delivery systems with more predictable release. Minuscule biosensors with the ability to continuously monitor plasma or tissue levels of different substances (e.g., glucose or lactate) may constitute a valuable tool for the diagnosis, follow-up, or intraoperative care of patients.[222] In the distant future, it may be possible to administer microrobots that will continue to circulate in the blood pool, monitor substance concentrations and metabolic activities of thousands of processes, and even participate in tissue repair.[114]

CONCLUSIONS AND IMPLICATIONS FOR CARDIOVASCULAR SPECIALISTS

In the short term, there will be an increase in the prevalence of CVD in parallel with the aging of the population and the prolonged survival for many cardiovascular disorders (Fig. 3–8). Major advances will occur in the field of primary and secondary prevention, with the identification of genetic and biochemical markers of risk that will improve the ability to identify those patients more prone to events or to benefit from interventions. This field will be complemented by the progress in imaging technologies that will also be useful for earlier diagnosis, as well as the evaluation of the effects of treatment. The development of newer and more effective pharmacologic, electrical, and interventional therapies will continue to improve survival in a variety of CVDs. Major efforts will be needed to expand the beneficial effects of current and future knowledge, through appropriate health policies, to the majority of the population. This can lead, in the mid term, to the decrease in the worldwide burden of CVD after the successful application of preventive and therapeutic measures.

In a longer perspective, the very optimistic dream of achieving a cure for CVD may become a reality, particularly if the promising prospects of regenerative genetic and cell therapy fully materialize in the next decades. For those individuals with a specific disorder, the damaged tissue might simply be healed or replaced by endogenous mechanisms or autologous transplants, obviating the need for chronic or palliative therapy. Even further in time, it may be possible, with extensive understanding of the genetic and molecular processes implicated in the development or progression of disease, to evaluate with one single blood or DNA test the sus-

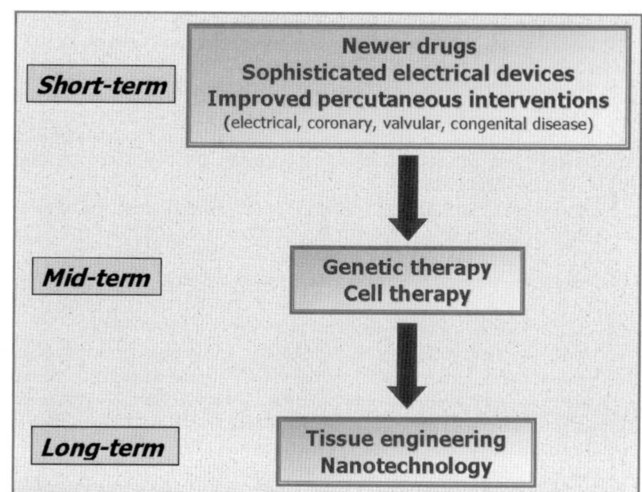

Figure 3–8 Overview of foreseeable therapeutic advances in cardiovascular medicine in coming years.

ceptibility of an individual for thousands of different conditions even before any of them develop, triggering the application of adequate preventive interventions. In such a day, CVD may become an ailment of the past, although this is beyond the most optimistic view of the authors.

In the first half of the 21st century, the combination of more elderly people, improved survival, growing numbers of interventions, and more frequent medical visits will lead to an increased demand for cardiovascular specialists.[223] A reasonable estimate is that the need for physicians will double in the next 50 years.[4] A shortage in health care professionals is likely to occur, particularly when the "baby-boomers" abandon the workforce and become seniors. It is therefore important to continue to recruit new physicians and to stimulate them to participate in cardiovascular prevention and care. Subspecialization is expected to be a requirement in light of the broadening of knowledge and technologic developments. However, a solid global understanding of the physiopathology, diagnosis, and treatment of CVD, with a particular emphasis on early detection and prevention, will continue to be fundamental for the new cardiovascular specialists.[223]

Acknowledgments

Dr. Sanz's work is supported by a research grant from the Spanish Society of Cardiology ("Beca para la Formación en Investigación Post-Residencia").

REFERENCES

1. American Heart Association: Heart Disease and Stroke Statistics—2004 Update. Dallas, TX, American Heart Association, 2003
2. Bonow RO, Smaha LA, Smith SC Jr, et al: World Heart Day 2002: The international burden of cardiovascular disease: Responding to the emerging global epidemic. Circulation 106:1602, 2002
3. Yusuf S, Reddy S, Ounpuu S, et al: Global burden of cardiovascular diseases: Part II: Variations in cardiovascular disease by specific ethnic groups and geographic regions and prevention strategies. Circulation 104:2855, 2001
4. Foot DK, Lewis RP, Pearson TA, et al: Demographics and cardiology, 1950-2050. J Am Coll Cardiol 35:1067, 2000
5. U.S. Census Bureau: Available at http://www.census.gov/ipc/www/usinterimproj/natprojtab02a.pdf. Accessed October 12, 2004
6. Beller GA: Coronary heart disease in the first 30 years of the 21st century: Challenges and opportunities: The 33rd Annual James B. Herrick Lecture of the Council on Clinical Cardiology of the American Heart Association. Circulation 103:2428, 2001
7. Steinwachs DM, Collins-Nakai RL, Cohn LH, et al: The future of cardiology: Utilization and costs of care. J Am Coll Cardiol 35:1092, 2000
8. Priebe H-J: The aged cardiovascular risk patient. Br J Anaesth 85:763, 2000
9. Gurwitz JH, Field TS, Harrold LR, et al: Incidence and preventability of adverse drug events among older persons in the ambulatory setting. JAMA 289:1107, 2003
10. Pirmohamed M, James S, Meakin S, et al: Adverse drug reactions as cause of admission to hospital: Prospective analysis of 18 820 patients. BMJ 329:15, 2004
11. Alfonso F, Azcona L, Perez-Vizcayno MJ, et al: Initial results and long-term clinical and angiographic implications of coronary stenting in elderly patients. Am J Cardiol 83:1483, 1999
12. Eagle KA, Berger PB, Calkins H, et al: ACC/AHA guideline update for perioperative cardiovascular evaluation for noncardiac surgery—executive summary: A report of the American College of Cardiology/American Heart Association Task Force on Practice Guidelines (Committee to Update the 1996 Guidelines on Perioperative Cardiovascular Evaluation for Noncardiac Surgery). J Am Coll Cardiol 39:542, 2002
13. Barnett SD, Halpin LS, Speir AM, et al: Postoperative complications among octogenarians after cardiovascular surgery. Ann Thorac Surg 76:726, 2003
14. Alter DA, Manuel DG, Gunraj N, et al: Age, risk-benefit trade-offs, and the projected effects of evidence-based therapies. Am J Med 116:540, 2004
15. Stenestrand U, Wallentin L: Fibrinolytic therapy in patients 75 years and older with ST-segment-elevation myocardial infarction: One-year follow-up of a large prospective cohort. Arch Intern Med 163:965, 2003
16. Bridges CR, Edwards FH, Peterson ED, et al: Cardiac surgery in nonagenarians and centenarians. J Am Coll Surg 197:347, 2003
17. Chauhan MS, Kuntz RE, Ho KKL, et al: Coronary artery stenting in the aged. J Am Coll Cardiol 37:856, 2001
18. Graham MM, Ghali WA, Faris PD, et al: Survival after coronary revascularization in the elderly. Circulation 105:2378, 2002
19. Executive Summary of The Third Report of the National Cholesterol Education Program (NCEP) Expert Panel on Detection, Evaluation, and Treatment of High Blood Cholesterol In Adults (Adult Treatment Panel III). JAMA 285:2486, 2001
20. Juul AB, Wetterslev J, Kofoed-Enevoldsen A: Long-term postoperative mortality in diabetic patients undergoing major non-cardiac surgery. Eur J Anaesthesiol 21:523, 2004
21. Mehran R, Dangas GD, Kobayashi Y, et al: Short- and long-term results after multivessel stenting in diabetic patients. J Am Coll Cardiol 43:1348, 2004
22. Howard BV, Rodriguez BL, Bennett PH, et al: Prevention Conference VI: Diabetes and cardiovascular disease: Writing Group I: Epidemiology. Circulation 105:132e, 2002
23. Cullen P: Evidence that triglycerides are an independent coronary heart disease risk factor. Am J Cardiol 86:943, 2000
24. Ford ES, Giles WH, Dietz WH: Prevalence of the metabolic syndrome among US adults: Findings from the Third National Health and Nutrition Examination Survey. JAMA 287:356, 2002
25. Khot UN, Khot MB, Bajzer CT, et al: Prevalence of conventional risk factors in patients with coronary heart disease. JAMA 290:898, 2003
26. Assmann G, Cullen P, Schulte H: Simple scoring scheme for calculating the risk of acute coronary events based on the 10-year follow-up of the Prospective Cardiovascular Munster (PROCAM) Study. Circulation 105:310, 2002
27. Wilson PWF, D'Agostino RB, Levy D, et al: Prediction of coronary heart disease using risk factor categories. Circulation 97:1837, 1998
28. Grundy SM, Pasternak R, Greenland P, et al: Assessment of cardiovascular risk by use of multiple-risk-factor assessment equations: A statement for healthcare professionals from the American Heart Association and the American College of Cardiology. Circulation 100:1481, 1999.
29. Naghavi M, Libby P, Falk E, et al: From vulnerable plaque to vulnerable patient: A call for new definitions and risk assessment strategies: Part II. Circulation 108:1772, 2003
30. Carmena R, Duriez P, Fruchart J-C: Atherogenic lipoprotein particles in atherosclerosis. Circulation 109:III-2, 2004
31. Meigs JB, Larson MG, D'Agostino RB, et al: Coronary artery calcification in type 2 diabetes and insulin resistance: The Framingham Offspring Study. Diabetes Care 25:1313, 2002
32. Rubins HB, Robins SJ, Collins D, et al: Diabetes, plasma insulin, and cardiovascular disease: Subgroup analysis from the Department of Veterans Affairs High-Density Lipoprotein Intervention Trial (VA-HIT). Arch Intern Med 162:2597, 2002
33. Reilly MP, Wolfe ML, Rhodes T, et al: Measures of insulin resistance add incremental value to the clinical diagnosis of metabolic syndrome in association with coronary atherosclerosis. Circulation 110:803, 2004
34. Wallace AM, McMahon AD, Packard CJ, et al: Plasma leptin and the risk of cardiovascular disease in the West of Scotland Coronary Prevention Study (WOSCOPS). Circulation 104:3052, 2001
35. Wald DS, Law M, Morris JK: Homocysteine and cardiovascular disease: Evidence on causality from a meta-analysis. BMJ 325:1202, 2002
36. Bogaty P, Poirier P, Simard S, et al: Biological profiles in subjects with recurrent acute coronary events compared with subjects with long-standing stable angina. Circulation 103:3062, 2001
37. Pearson TA, Mensah GA, Alexander RW, et al: Markers of inflammation and cardiovascular disease: Application to clinical and public health practice: A statement for healthcare professionals from the Centers for Disease Control and Prevention and the American Heart Association. Circulation 107:499, 2003
38. Ridker PM, Wilson PW, Grundy SM: Should C-reactive protein be added to metabolic syndrome and to assessment of global cardiovascular risk? Circulation 109:2818, 2004
39. Ridker PM, Brown NJ, Vaughan DE, et al: Established and emerging plasma biomarkers in the prediction of first atherothrombotic events. Circulation 109:IV, 2004

40. Schulze MB, Rimm EB, Li T, et al: C-reactive protein and incident cardiovascular events among men with diabetes. Diabetes Care 27:889, 2004
41. Lindahl B, Toss H, Siegbahn A, et al: Markers of myocardial damage and inflammation in relation to long-term mortality in unstable coronary artery disease. FRISC Study Group. Fragmin during Instability in Coronary Artery Disease. N Engl J Med 343:1139, 2000
42. Ridker PM, Rifai N, Pfeffer MA, et al: Long-term effects of pravastatin on plasma concentration of C-reactive protein. Circulation 100:230, 1999
43. Zairis MN, Ambrose JA, Manousakis SJ, et al: The impact of plasma levels of C-reactive protein, lipoprotein (a) and homocysteine on the long-term prognosis after successful coronary stenting: The Global Evaluation of New Events and Restenosis After Stent Implantation Study. J Am Coll Cardiol 40:1375, 2002
44. Rossi E, Biasucci LM, Citterio F, et al: Risk of myocardial infarction and angina in patients with severe peripheral vascular disease: Predictive role of C-reactive protein. Circulation 105:800, 2002
45. Di Napoli M, Papa F, Bocola V: C-reactive protein in ischemic stroke: An independent prognostic factor. Stroke 32:917, 2001
46. Ridker PM, Rifai N, Rose L, et al: Comparison of C-reactive protein and low-density lipoprotein cholesterol levels in the prediction of first cardiovascular events. N Engl J Med 347:1557, 2002
47. Ridker PM, Cushman M, Stampfer MJ, et al: Inflammation, aspirin, and the risk of cardiovascular disease in apparently healthy men. N Engl J Med 336:973, 1997
48. Ridker PM, Rifai N, Clearfield M, et al: Measurement of C-reactive protein for the targeting of statin therapy in the primary prevention of acute coronary events. N Engl J Med 344:1959, 2001
49. Haider AW, Wilson PWF, Larson MG, et al: The association of seropositivity to Helicobacter pylori, Chlamydia pneumoniae, and cytomegalovirus with risk of cardiovascular disease: A prospective study. J Am Coll Cardiol 40:1408, 2002
50. Smieja M, Gnarpe J, Lonn E, et al: Multiple infections and subsequent cardiovascular events in the Heart Outcomes Prevention Evaluation (HOPE) Study. Circulation 107:251, 2003
51. Danesh J, Whincup P, Lewington S, et al: Chlamydia pneumoniae IgA titres and coronary heart disease. Prospective study and meta-analysis. Eur Heart J 23:371, 2002
52. Zhu J, Quyyumi AA, Norman JE, et al: Cytomegalovirus in the pathogenesis of atherosclerosis: The role of inflammation as reflected by elevated C-reactive protein levels. J Am Coll Cardiol 34:1738, 1999
53. Pousset F, Masson F, Chavirovskaia O, et al: Plasma adrenomedullin, a new independent predictor of prognosis in patients with chronic heart failure. Eur Heart J 21:1009, 2000
54. Latini R, Masson S, Anand I, et al: The comparative prognostic value of plasma neurohormones at baseline in patients with heart failure enrolled in Val-HeFT. Eur Heart J 25:292, 2004
55. Jernberg T, James S, Lindahl B, et al: NT-proBNP in unstable coronary artery disease—Experiences from the FAST, GUSTO IV and FRISC II trials. Eur J Heart Fail 6:319, 2004
56. Mega JL, Morrow DA, de Lemos JA, et al: B-type natriuretic peptide at presentation and prognosis in patients with ST-segment elevation myocardial infarction: An ENTIRE-TIMI-23 substudy. J Am Coll Cardiol 44:335, 2004
57. Jernberg T, Lindahl B, Siegbahn A, et al: N-terminal pro-brain natriuretic peptide in relation to inflammation, myocardial necrosis, and the effect of an invasive strategy in unstable coronary artery disease. J Am Coll Cardiol 42:1909, 2003
58. Nakamura M, Endo H, Nasu M, et al: Value of plasma B type natriuretic peptide measurement for heart disease screening in a Japanese population. Heart 87:131, 2002
59. Maisel AS, Koon J, Krishnaswamy P, et al: Utility of B-natriuretic peptide as a rapid, point-of-care test for screening patients undergoing echocardiography to determine left ventricular dysfunction. Am Heart J 141:367, 2001
60. Maisel AS, Krishnaswamy P, Nowak RM, et al: Rapid measurement of B-type natriuretic peptide in the emergency diagnosis of heart failure. N Engl J Med 347:161, 2002
61. Gackowski A, Isnard R, Golmard J-L, et al: Comparison of echocardiography and plasma B-type natriuretic peptide for monitoring the response to treatment in acute heart failure. Eur Heart J 25:1788, 2004
62. Richards AM, Doughty R, Nicholls MG, et al: Neurohumoral prediction of benefit from carvedilol in ischemic left ventricular dysfunction. Circulation 99:786, 1999
63. Troughton RW, Frampton CM, Yandle TG, et al: Treatment of heart failure guided by plasma aminoterminal brain natriuretic peptide (N-BNP) concentrations. The Lancet 355:1126, 2000
64. Mueller C, Scholer A, Laule-Kilian K, et al: Use of B-type natriuretic peptide in the evaluation and management of acute dyspnea. N Engl J Med 350:647, 2004
65. Anand IS, Fisher LD, Chiang Y-T, et al: Changes in brain natriuretic peptide and norepinephrine over time and mortality and morbidity in the Valsartan Heart Failure Trial (Val-HeFT). Circulation 107:1278, 2003
66. Wang TJ, Larson MG, Levy D, et al: Plasma natriuretic peptide levels and the risk of cardiovascular events and death. N Engl J Med 350:655, 2004
67. Biancari F, Lahtinen J, Lepojarvi S, et al: Preoperative C-reactive protein and outcome after coronary artery bypass surgery. Ann Thorac Surg 76:2007, 2003
68. Boeken U, Feindt P, Zimmermann N, et al: Increased preoperative C-reactive protein (CRP)-values without signs of an infection and complicated course after cardiopulmonary bypass (CPB)-operations. Eur J Cardio-Thorac Surg 13:541, 1998
69. Fransen EJ, Maessen JG, Elenbaas TWO, et al: Increased preoperative C-reactive protein plasma levels as a risk factor for postoperative infections. Ann Thorac Surg 67:134, 1999
70. Chello M, Mastroroberto P, Perticone F, et al: Plasma levels of atrial and brain natriuretic peptides as indicators of recovery of left ventricular systolic function after coronary artery bypass. Eur J Cardio-Thorac Surg 20:140, 2001
71. Saribulbul O, Alat I, Coskun S, et al: The role of brain natriuretic peptide in the prediction of cardiac performance in coronary artery bypass grafting. Tex Heart Inst J 30:298, 2003
72. O'Leary DH, Polak JF, Kronmal RA, et al: Carotid artery intima and media thickness as a risk factor for myocardial infarction and stroke in older adults. N Engl J Med 340:14, 1999
73. van der Meer IM, Bots ML, Hofman A, et al: Predictive value of noninvasive measures of atherosclerosis for incident myocardial infarction: The Rotterdam Study. Circulation 109:1089, 2004
74. Naghavi M, Libby P, Falk E, et al: From vulnerable plaque to vulnerable patient: A call for new definitions and risk assessment strategies: Part I. Circulation 108:1664, 2003
75. Fayad ZA, Fuster V: Clinical imaging of the high-risk or vulnerable atherosclerotic plaque. Circ Res 89:305, 2001
76. O'Rourke RA, Brundage BH, Froelicher VF, et al: American College of Cardiology/American Heart Association Expert Consensus Document on electron-beam computed tomography for the diagnosis and prognosis of coronary artery disease. J Am Coll Cardiol 36:326, 2000
77. Kondos GT, Hoff JA, Sevrukov A, et al: Electron-beam tomography, coronary artery calcium and cardiac events: A 37-month follow-up of 5635 initially asymptomatic low- to intermediate-risk adults. Circulation 107:2571, 2003
78. O'Malley PG, Taylor AJ, Jackson JL, et al: Prognostic value of coronary electron-beam computed tomography for coronary heart disease events in asymptomatic populations. Am J Cardiol 85:945, 2000
79. Greenland P, LaBree L, Azen SP, et al: Coronary artery calcium score combined with Framingham score for risk prediction in asymptomatic individuals. JAMA 291:210, 2004
80. Greenland P, Gaziano JM: Clinical practice. Selecting asymptomatic patients for coronary computed tomography or electrocardiographic exercise testing. N Engl J Med 349:465, 2003
81. Callister TQ, Raggi P, Cooil B, et al: Effect of HMG-CoA reductase inhibitors on coronary artery disease as assessed by electron-beam computed tomography. N Engl J Med 339:1972, 1998
82. Messika-Zeitoun D, Aubry MC, Detaint D, et al: Evaluation and clinical implications of aortic valve calcification measured by electron-beam computed tomography. Circulation 110:356, 2004
83. Ropers D, Baum U, Pohle K, et al: Detection of coronary artery stenoses with thin-slice multi-detector row spiral computed tomography and multiplanar reconstruction. Circulation 107:664, 2003
84. Mollet NR, Cademartiri F, Nieman K, et al: Multislice spiral computed tomography coronary angiography in patients with stable angina pectoris. J Am Coll Cardiol 43:2265, 2004
85. Martuscelli E, Romagnoli A, D'Eliseo A, et al: Accuracy of thin-slice computed tomography in the detection of coronary stenoses. Eur Heart J 25:1043, 2004
86. Leber AW, Knez A, Becker A, et al: Accuracy of multidetector spiral computed tomography in identifying and differentiating the composition of coronary atherosclerotic plaques: A comparative study with intracoronary ultrasound. J Am Coll Cardiol 43:1241, 2004
87. Viles-Gonzalez JF, Poon M, Sanz J, et al: In vivo 16-slice, multidetector-row computed tomography for the assessment of experimental atherosclerosis: Comparison with magnetic resonance imaging and histopathology. Circulation 110:1467, 2004

88. Kim WY, Danias PG, Stuber M, et al: Coronary magnetic resonance angiography for the detection of coronary stenoses. N Engl J Med 345:1863, 2001
89. Fayad ZA, Nahar T, Fallon JT, et al: In vivo magnetic resonance evaluation of atherosclerotic plaques in the human thoracic aorta: A comparison with transesophageal echocardiography. Circulation 101:2503, 2000
90. Kramer CM, Cerilli LA, Hagspiel K, et al: Magnetic resonance imaging identifies the fibrous cap in atherosclerotic abdominal aortic aneurysm. Circulation 109:1016, 2004
91. Fayad ZA, Fuster V, Fallon JT, et al: Noninvasive in vivo human coronary artery lumen and wall imaging using black-blood magnetic resonance imaging. Circulation 102:506, 2000
92. Corti R, Osende JI, Fayad ZA, et al: In vivo noninvasive detection and age definition of arterial thrombus by MRI. J Am Coll Cardiol 39:1366, 2002
93. Taniguchi H, Momiyama Y, Fayad ZA, et al: In vivo magnetic resonance evaluation of associations between aortic atherosclerosis and both risk factors and coronary artery disease in patients referred for coronary angiography. Am Heart J 148:137, 2004
94. Corti R, Osende JI, Fallon JT, et al: The selective paroxysmal proliferator-activated receptor-gamma agonist has an additive effect on plaque regression in combination with simvastatin in experimental atherosclerosis: In vivo study by high-resolution magnetic resonance imaging. J Am Coll Cardiol 43:464, 2004
95. Corti R, Fuster V, Fayad ZA, et al: Lipid lowering by simvastatin induces regression of human atherosclerotic lesions: Two years' follow-up by high-resolution noninvasive magnetic resonance imaging. Circulation 106:2884, 2002
96. Plein S, Ridgway JP, Jones TR, et al: Coronary artery disease: Assessment with a comprehensive MR imaging protocol—initial results. Radiology 225:300, 2002
97. Poon M, Fuster V, Fayad Z: Cardiac magnetic resonance imaging: A "one-stop-shop" evaluation of myocardial dysfunction. Curr Opin Cardiol 17:663, 2002
98. Rajappan K, Bellenger NG, Anderson L, et al: The role of cardiovascular magnetic resonance in heart failure. Eur J Heart Fail 2:241, 2000
99. Giang TH, Nanz D, Coulden R, et al: Detection of coronary artery disease by magnetic resonance myocardial perfusion imaging with various contrast medium doses: First European multi-centre experience. Eur Heart J 25:1657, 2004
100. Paetsch I, Jahnke C, Wahl A, et al: Comparison of dobutamine stress magnetic resonance, adenosine stress magnetic resonance, and adenosine stress magnetic resonance perfusion. Circulation 110:835, 2004
101. Nagel E, Lehmkuhl HB, Bocksch W, et al: Noninvasive diagnosis of ischemia-induced wall motion abnormalities with the use of high-dose dobutamine stress MRI: Comparison with dobutamine stress echocardiography. Circulation 99:763, 1999
102. Rerkpattanapipat P, Morgan TM, Neagle CM, et al: Assessment of preoperative cardiac risk with magnetic resonance imaging. Am J Cardiol 90:416, 2002
103. Klein C, Nekolla SG, Bengel FM, et al: Assessment of myocardial viability with contrast-enhanced magnetic resonance imaging: Comparison with positron emission tomography. Circulation 105:162, 2002
104. Nelson C, McCrohon J, Khafagi F, et al: Impact of scar thickness on the assessment of viability using dobutamine echocardiography and thallium single-photon emission computed tomography: A comparison with contrast-enhanced magnetic resonance imaging. J Am Coll Cardiol 43:1248, 2004
105. Wagner A, Mahrholdt H, Holly TA, et al: Contrast-enhanced MRI and routine single photon emission computed tomography (SPECT) perfusion imaging for detection of subendocardial myocardial infarcts: An imaging study. Lancet 361:374, 2003
106. Kim RJ, Wu E, Rafael A, et al: The use of contrast-enhanced magnetic resonance imaging to identify reversible myocardial dysfunction. N Engl J Med 343:1445, 2000
107. Selvanayagam JB, Kardos A, Francis JM, et al: Value of delayed-enhancement cardiovascular magnetic resonance imaging in predicting myocardial viability after surgical revascularization. Circulation 110:1535, 2004
108. Bello D, Shah DJ, Farah GM, et al: Gadolinium cardiovascular magnetic resonance predicts reversible myocardial dysfunction and remodeling in patients with heart failure undergoing beta-blocker therapy. Circulation 108:1945, 2003
109. Selvanayagam JB, Kardos A, Francis JM, et al: Value of delayed-enhancement cardiovascular magnetic resonance imaging in predicting myocardial viability after surgical revascularization. Circulation 110:1535, 2004
110. Fieno DS, Shea SM, Li Y, et al: Myocardial perfusion imaging based on the blood oxygen level-dependent effect using T2-prepared steady-state free-precession magnetic resonance imaging. Circulation 110:1284, 2004
111. Sirol M, Itskovich VV, Mani V, et al: Lipid-rich atherosclerotic plaques detected by gadofluorine-enhanced in vivo magnetic resonance imaging. Circulation 109:2890, 2004
112. Bottomley PA, Weiss RG: Non-invasive magnetic-resonance detection of creatine depletion in non-viable infarcted myocardium. Lancet 351:714, 1998
113. Jaffer FA, Weissleder R: Seeing within: Molecular imaging of the cardiovascular system. Circ Res 94:433, 2004
114. Flower J, Dreifus LS, Bove AA, et al: Technological advances and the next 50 years of cardiology. J Am Coll Cardiol 35:81B, 2000
115. Collins FS, McKusick VA: Implications of the Human Genome Project for medical science. JAMA 285:540, 2001
116. Lusis AJ, Fogelman AM, Fonarow GC: Genetic basis of atherosclerosis: Part I: New genes and pathways. Circulation 110:1868, 2004
117. Evans WE, McLeod HL: Pharmacogenomics—Drug disposition, drug targets, and side effects. N Engl J Med 348:538, 2003
118. Higashi MK, Veenstra DL, Kondo LM, et al: Association between CYP2C9 genetic variants and anticoagulation-related outcomes during warfarin therapy. JAMA 287:1690, 2002
119. Nabel EG: Cardiovascular disease. N Engl J Med 349:60, 2003
120. Emberson J, Whincup P, Morris R, et al: Evaluating the impact of population and high-risk strategies for the primary prevention of cardiovascular disease. Eur Heart J 25:484, 2004
121. Harris MI, Flegal KM, Cowie CC, et al: Prevalence of diabetes, impaired fasting glucose, and impaired glucose tolerance in U.S. adults. The Third National Health and Nutrition Examination Survey, 1988-1994. Diabetes Care 21:518, 1998
122. Snow V, Aronson MD, Hornbake ER, et al: Lipid control in the management of type 2 diabetes mellitus: A clinical practice guideline from the American College of Physicians. Ann Intern Med 140:644, 2004
123. Effects of ramipril on cardiovascular and microvascular outcomes in people with diabetes mellitus: Results of the HOPE study and MICRO-HOPE substudy. Lancet 355:253, 2000
124. Hall W: The prospects for immunotherapy in smoking cessation. Lancet 360:1089, 2002
125. Cleland JGF, Ghosh J, Freemantle N, et al: Clinical trials update and cumulative meta-analyses from the American College of Cardiology: WATCH, SCD-HeFT, DINAMIT, CASINO, INSPIRE, STRATUS-U.S., RIO-Lipids and cardiac resynchronisation therapy in heart failure. Eur J Heart Fail 6:501, 2004
126. Khaw K-T, Bingham S, Welch A, et al: Relation between plasma ascorbic acid and mortality in men and women in EPIC-Norfolk prospective study: A prospective population study. Lancet 357:657, 2001
127. MRC/BHF Heart Protection Study of antioxidant vitamin supplementation in 20536 high-risk individuals: A randomised placebo-controlled trial. Lancet 360:23, 2002
128. Pearson TA, Blair SN, Daniels SR, et al: AHA Guidelines for Primary Prevention of Cardiovascular Disease and Stroke: 2002 Update: Consensus Panel Guide to Comprehensive Risk Reduction for Adult Patients Without Coronary or Other Atherosclerotic Vascular Diseases. Circulation 106:388, 2002
129. Ballantyne CM, Houri J, Notarbartolo A, et al: Effect of ezetimibe coadministered with atorvastatin in 628 patients with primary hypercholesterolemia: A prospective, randomized, double-blind trial. Circulation 107:2409, 2003
130. Gotto AM Jr, Brinton EA: Assessing low levels of high-density lipoprotein cholesterol as a risk factor in coronary heart disease: A working group report and update. J Am Coll Cardiol 43:717, 2004
131. Brousseau ME, Schaefer EJ, Wolfe ML, et al: Effects of an inhibitor of cholesteryl ester transfer protein on HDL cholesterol. N Engl J Med 350:1505, 2004
132. Nissen SE, Tsunoda T, Tuzcu EM, et al: Effect of recombinant ApoA-I Milano on coronary atherosclerosis in patients with acute coronary syndromes: A randomized controlled trial. JAMA 290:2292, 2003
133. Moulton KS, Vakili K, Zurakowski D, et al: Inhibition of plaque neovascularization reduces macrophage accumulation and progression of advanced atherosclerosis. PNAS 100:4736, 2003
134. Lutters BC, Leeuwenburgh MA, Appeldoorn CC, et al: Blocking endothelial adhesion molecules: A potential therapeutic strategy to combat atherogenesis. Curr Opin Lipidol 15:545, 2004
135. Eriksson EE: Mechanisms of leukocyte recruitment to atherosclerotic lesions: Future prospects. Curr Opin Lipidol 15:553, 2004
136. Badimon JJ, Lettino M, Toschi V, et al: Local inhibition of tissue factor reduces the thrombogenicity of disrupted human atherosclerotic plaques: Effects of tissue factor pathway inhibitor on plaque thrombogenicity under flow conditions. Circulation 99:1780, 1999

137. Hutter R, Valdiviezo C, Sauter BV, et al: Caspase-3 and tissue factor expression in lipid-rich plaque macrophages: Evidence for apoptosis as link between inflammation and atherothrombosis. Circulation 109:2001, 2004
138. Susic D, Varagic J, Ahn J, et al: Crosslink breakers: A new approach to cardiovascular therapy. Curr Opin Cardiol 19:336, 2004
139. Andersen HR, Nielsen TT, Vesterlund T, et al: Danish multicenter randomized study on fibrinolytic therapy versus acute coronary angioplasty in acute myocardial infarction: Rationale and design of the Danish Trial in Acute Myocardial Infarction-2 (DANAMI-2). Am Heart J 146:234, 2003
140. Steg PG, Bonnefoy E, Chabaud S, et al: Impact of time to treatment on mortality after prehospital fibrinolysis or primary angioplasty: Data from the CAPTIM randomized clinical trial. Circulation 108:2851, 2003
141. The Public Access Defibrillation Trial Investigators: Public-access defibrillation and survival after out-of-hospital cardiac arrest. N Engl J Med 351:637, 2004
142. Wellens HJJ, Gorgels AP, de Munter H: Cardiac arrest outside of a hospital: How can we improve results of resuscitation? Circulation 107:1948, 2003
143. The Clopidogrel in Unstable Angina to Prevent Recurrent Events Trial Investigators: Effects of clopidogrel in addition to aspirin in patients with acute coronary syndromes without ST-segment elevation. N Engl J Med 345:494, 2001
144. Wong GC, Giugliano RP, Antman EM: Use of low-molecular-weight heparins in the management of acute coronary artery syndromes and percutaneous coronary intervention. JAMA 289:331, 2003
145. Boersma E, Harrington RA, Moliterno DJ, et al: Platelet glycoprotein IIb/IIIa inhibitors in acute coronary syndromes: A meta-analysis of all major randomised clinical trials. Lancet 359:189, 2002
146. Wallentin L, Wilcox RG, Weaver WD, et al: Oral ximelagatran for secondary prophylaxis after myocardial infarction: The ESTEEM randomised controlled trial. Lancet 362:789, 2003
147. Shimbo D, Osende J, Chen J, et al: Antithrombotic effects of DX-9065a, a direct factor Xa inhibitor: A comparative study in humans versus low-molecular-weight heparin. Thromb Haemost 88:733, 2002
148. Simoons ML, Bobbink IWG, Boland J, et al: A dose-finding study of fondaparinux in patients with non-ST-segment elevation acute coronary syndromes: The Pentasaccharide in Unstable Angina (PENTUA) study. J Am Coll Cardiol 43:2183, 2004
149. Coussement PK, Bassand JP, Convens C, et al: A synthetic factor-Xa inhibitor (ORG31540/SR9017A) as an adjunct to fibrinolysis in acute myocardial infarction. The PENTALYSE study. Eur Heart J 22:1716, 2001
150. Alexander JH, Dyke CK, Yang H, et al: Initial experience with factor-Xa inhibition in percutaneous coronary intervention: The XaNADU-PCI Pilot. J Thromb Haemost 2:234, 2004
151. Babapulle MN, Joseph L, Belisle P, et al: A hierarchical Bayesian meta-analysis of randomised clinical trials of drug-eluting stents. Lancet 364:583, 2004
152. Hennekens CH: Increasing burden of cardiovascular disease: Current knowledge and future directions for research on risk factors. Circulation 97:1095, 1998
153. LaBresh KA, Ellrodt AG, Gliklich R, et al: Get with the guidelines for cardiovascular secondary prevention: Pilot results. Arch Intern Med 164:203, 2004
154. Lindenauer PK, Fitzgerald J, Hoople N, et al: The potential preventability of postoperative myocardial infarction: Underuse of perioperative {beta}-adrenergic blockade. Arch Intern Med 164:762, 2004
155. Lindenauer PK, Pekow P, Wang K, et al: Lipid-lowering therapy and in-hospital mortality following major noncardiac surgery. JAMA 291:2092, 2004
156. Braunwald E: Cardiology: The past, the present, and the future. J Am Coll Cardiol 42:2031, 2003
157. Packer M, Califf RM, Konstam MA, et al: Comparison of omapatrilat and enalapril in patients with chronic heart failure: The Omapatrilat Versus Enalapril Randomized Trial of Utility in Reducing Events (OVERTURE). Circulation 106:920, 2002
158. O'Connor CM, Gattis WA, Adams J, et al: Tezosentan in patients with acute heart failure and acute coronary syndromes: Results of the Randomized Intravenous Tezosentan Study (RITZ-4). J Am Coll Cardiol 41:1452, 2003
159. Anand PI, McMurray PJ, Cohn PJN, et al: Long-term effects of darusentan on left-ventricular remodeling and clinical outcomes in the EndothelinA Receptor Antagonist Trial in Heart Failure (EARTH): Randomised, double-blind, placebo-controlled trial. Lancet 364:347, 2004
160. Mann DL, McMurray JJV, Packer M, et al: Targeted anticytokine therapy in patients with chronic heart failure: Results of the Randomized Etanercept Worldwide Evaluation (RENEWAL). Circulation 109:1594, 2004
161. Follath F, Cleland JGF, Just H, et al: Efficacy and safety of intravenous levosimendan compared with dobutamine in severe low-output heart failure (the LIDO study): A randomised double-blind trial. Lancet 360:196, 2002
162. Gheorghiade M, Gattis WA, O'Connor CM, et al: Effects of tolvaptan, a vasopressin antagonist, in patients hospitalized with worsening heart failure: A randomized controlled trial. JAMA 291:1963, 2004
163. Publication Committee for the VMAC Investigators: Intravenous nesiritide vs nitroglycerin for treatment of decompensated congestive heart failure: A randomized controlled trial. JAMA 287:1531, 2002
164. Nikolaidis LA, Elahi D, Hentosz T, et al: Recombinant glucagon-like peptide-1 increases myocardial glucose uptake and improves left ventricular performance in conscious dogs with pacing-induced dilated cardiomyopathy. Circulation 110:955, 2004
165. Chandrashekhar Y, Sen S, Anway R, et al: Long-term caspase inhibition ameliorates apoptosis, reduces myocardial troponin-I cleavage, protects left ventricular function, and attenuates remodeling in rats with myocardial infarction. J Am Coll Cardiol 43:295, 2004
166. Epstein AE: An update on implantable cardioverter-defibrillator guidelines. Curr Opin Cardiol 19:23, 2004
167. McAlister FA, Ezekowitz JA, Wiebe N, et al: Systematic review: Cardiac resynchronization in patients with symptomatic heart failure. Ann Intern Med 141:381, 2004
168. Copeland JG, Smith RG, Arabia FA, et al: Cardiac Replacement with a total artificial heart as a bridge to transplantation. N Engl J Med 351:859, 2004
169. Platt J, DiSesa V, Gail D, et al: Recommendations of the National Heart, Lung, and Blood Institute Heart and Lung Xenotransplantation Working Group. Circulation 106:1043, 2002
170. Rosenhek R, Rader F, Loho N, et al: Statins but not angiotensin-converting enzyme inhibitors delay progression of aortic stenosis. Circulation 110:1291, 2004
171. Bach DS: Choice of prosthetic heart valves: Update for the next generation. J Am Coll Cardiol 42:1717, 2003
172. Schlitt A, Buerke M, Hauroeder B, et al: Fondaparinux and enoxaparin in comparison to unfractionated heparin in preventing thrombus formation on mechanical heart valves in an ex vivo rabbit model. Thromb Haemost 90:245, 2003
173. Cribier A, Eltchaninoff H, Bash A, et al: Percutaneous transcatheter implantation of an aortic valve prosthesis for calcific aortic stenosis: First human case description. Circulation 106:3006, 2002
174. Bonhoeffer P, Boudjemline Y, Qureshi SA, et al: Percutaneous insertion of the pulmonary valve. J Am Coll Cardiol 39:1664, 2002
175. Percutaneous Mitral Valve Repair Using the Edge-to-Edge Technique: Phase I U.S. Trial Results. Presented at Annual Scientific Sessions of the American College of Cardiology, New Orleans, March 7, 2004
176. Wellens HJ: Cardiac arrhythmias: The quest for a cure: A historical perspective. J Am Coll Cardiol 44:1155, 2004
177. Steinberg JS: Atrial fibrillation: An emerging epidemic? Heart 90:239, 2004
178. Chen S-A, Hsieh M-H, Tai C-T, et al: Initiation of atrial fibrillation by ectopic beats originating from the pulmonary veins: Electrophysiological characteristics, pharmacological responses, and effects of radiofrequency ablation. Circulation 100:1879, 1999
179. Oral H, Knight BP, Tada H, et al: Pulmonary vein isolation for paroxysmal and persistent atrial fibrillation. Circulation 105:1077, 2002
180. Pappone C, Oreto G, Rosanio S, et al: Atrial electroanatomic remodeling after circumferential radiofrequency pulmonary vein ablation: Efficacy of an anatomic approach in a large cohort of patients with atrial fibrillation. Circulation 104:2539, 2001
181. Blaauw Y, Gogelein H, Tieleman RG, et al: "Early" class III drugs for the treatment of atrial fibrillation: Efficacy and atrial selectivity of AVE0118 in remodeled atria of the goat. Circulation 110:1717, 2004
182. The Atrial Fibrillation Follow-up Investigation of Rhythm Management (AFFIRM) Investigators: A comparison of rate control and rhythm control in patients with atrial fibrillation. N Engl J Med 347:1825, 2002
183. Olsson SB: Stroke prevention with the oral direct thrombin inhibitor ximelagatran compared with warfarin in patients with non-valvular atrial fibrillation (SPORTIF III): Randomised controlled trial. Lancet 362:1691, 2003
184. Hoffman JIE, Kaplan S, Liberthson RR: Prevalence of congenital heart disease. Am Heart J 147:425, 2004
185. Tworetzky W, Wilkins-Haug L, Jennings RW, et al: Balloon dilation of severe aortic stenosis in the fetus: potential for prevention of hypoplastic left heart syndrome: Candidate selection, technique, and results of successful intervention. Circulation 110:2125, 2004
186. Melo LG, Pachori AS, Kong D, et al: Gene and cell-based therapies for heart disease. FASEB J 18:648, 2004

187. Yla-Herttuala S, Martin JF: Cardiovascular gene therapy. Lancet 355:213, 2000
188. Losordo DW, Vale PR, Hendel RC, et al: Phase 1/2 placebo-controlled, double-blind, dose-escalating trial of myocardial vascular endothelial growth factor 2 gene transfer by catheter delivery in patients with chronic myocardial ischemia. Circulation 105:2012, 2002
189. Vale PR, Losordo DW, Milliken CE, et al: Randomized, single-blind, placebo-controlled pilot study of catheter-based myocardial gene transfer for therapeutic angiogenesis using left ventricular electromechanical mapping in patients with chronic myocardial ischemia. Circulation 103:2138, 2001
190. Grines CL, Watkins MW, Helmer G, et al: Angiogenic Gene Therapy (AGENT) Trial in patients with stable angina pectoris. Circulation 105:1291, 2002
191. Rajagopalan S, Mohler ER III, Lederman RJ, et al: Regional angiogenesis with vascular endothelial growth factor in peripheral arterial disease: A phase II randomized, double-blind, controlled study of adenoviral delivery of vascular endothelial growth factor 121 in patients with disabling intermittent claudication. Circulation 108:1933, 2003
192. Shah AS, Lilly RE, Kypson AP, et al: Intracoronary adenovirus-mediated delivery and overexpression of the {beta}2-adrenergic receptor in the heart: Prospects for molecular ventricular assistance. Circulation 101:408, 2000
193. Roth DM, Bayat H, Drumm JD, et al: Adenylyl cyclase increases survival in cardiomyopathy. Circulation 105:1989, 2002
194. del Monte F, Williams E, Lebeche D, et al: Improvement in survival and cardiac metabolism after gene transfer of sarcoplasmic reticulum Ca(2+)-ATPase in a rat model of heart failure. Circulation 104:1424, 2001
195. del Monte F, Harding SE, Dec GW, et al: Targeting phospholamban by gene transfer in human heart failure. Circulation 105:904, 2002
196. Melo LG, Agrawal R, Zhang L, et al: Gene therapy strategy for long-term myocardial protection using adeno-associated virus-mediated delivery of heme oxygenase gene. Circulation 105:602, 2002
197. Mann MJ, Whittemore AD, Donaldson MC, et al: Ex-vivo gene therapy of human vascular bypass grafts with E2F decoy: The PREVENT single-centre, randomised, controlled trial. The Lancet 354:1493, 1999
198. Muhs A, Heublein B, Schletter J, et al: Preclinical evaluation of inducible nitric oxide synthase lipoplex gene therapy for inhibition of stent-induced vascular neointimal lesion formation. Hum Gene Ther 14:375, 2003
199. Nuss HB, Marban E, Johns DC: Overexpression of a human potassium channel suppresses cardiac hyperexcitability in rabbit ventricular myocytes. J Clin Invest 103:889, 1999
200. Donahue JK, Heldman AW, Fraser H, et al: Focal modification of electrical conduction in the heart by viral gene transfer. Nat Med 6:1395, 2000
201. Yechoor V, Chan L: Gene therapy progress and prospects: Gene therapy for diabetes mellitus. Gene Ther 2004
202. Tangirala RK, Tsukamoto K, Chun SH, et al: Regression of atherosclerosis induced by liver-directed gene transfer of apolipoprotein A-I in mice. Circulation 100:1816, 1999
203. Beltrami AP, Urbanek K, Kajstura J, et al: Evidence that human cardiac myocytes divide after myocardial infarction. N Engl J Med 344:1750, 2001
204. Kajstura J, Leri A, Finato N, et al: Myocyte proliferation in end-stage cardiac failure in humans. Proc Natl Acad Sci U S A 95:8801, 1998
205. Asahara T, Masuda H, Takahashi T, et al: Bone marrow origin of endothelial progenitor cells responsible for postnatal vasculogenesis in physiological and pathological neovascularization. Circ Res 85:221, 1999
206. Quaini F, Urbanek K, Beltrami AP, et al: Chimerism of the transplanted heart. N Engl J Med 346:5, 2002
207. Beltrami AP, Barlucchi L, Torella D, et al: Adult cardiac stem cells are multipotent and support myocardial regeneration. Cell 114:763, 2003
208. Mathur A, Martin JF: Stem cells and repair of the heart. Lancet 364:183, 2004
209. Menasche P, Hagege AA, Vilquin JT, et al: Autologous skeletal myoblast transplantation for severe postinfarction left ventricular dysfunction. J Am Coll Cardiol 41:1078, 2003
210. Jiang Y, Jahagirdar BN, Reinhardt RL, et al: Pluripotency of mesenchymal stem cells derived from adult marrow. Nature 418:41, 2002
211. Assmus B, Schachinger V, Teupe C, et al: Transplantation of Progenitor Cells and Regeneration Enhancement in Acute Myocardial Infarction (TOPCARE-AMI). Circulation 106:3009, 2002
212. Britten MB, Abolmaali ND, Assmus B, et al: Infarct Remodeling After Intracoronary Progenitor Cell Treatment in Patients With Acute Myocardial Infarction (TOPCARE-AMI): Mechanistic insights from serial contrast-enhanced magnetic resonance imaging. Circulation 108:2212, 2003
213. Wollert KC, Meyer GP, Lotz J, et al: Intracoronary autologous bone-marrow cell transfer after myocardial infarction: The BOOST randomised controlled clinical trial. The Lancet 364:141, 2004
214. Welch S, Plank D, Witt S, et al: Cardiac-specific IGF-1 expression attenuates dilated cardiomyopathy in tropomodulin-overexpressing transgenic mice. Circ Res 90:641, 2002
215. Kang H-J, Kim H-S, Zhang S-Y, et al: Effects of intracoronary infusion of peripheral blood stem-cells mobilised with granulocyte-colony stimulating factor on left ventricular systolic function and restenosis after coronary stenting in myocardial infarction: The MAGIC cell randomised clinical trial. Lancet 363:751, 2004
216. Nakamura T, Mizuno S, Matsumoto K, et al: Myocardial protection from ischemia/reperfusion injury by endogenous and exogenous HGF. J Clin Invest 106:1511, 2000
217. Nugent HM, Edelman ER: Tissue engineering therapy for cardiovascular disease. Circ Res 92:1068, 2003
218. Deutsch M, Meinhart J, Fischlein T, et al: Clinical autologous in vitro endothelialization of infrainguinal ePTFE grafts in 100 patients: A 9-year experience. Surgery 126:847, 1999
219. Shinoka T, Shum-Tim D, Ma PX, et al: Creation of viable pulmonary artery autografts through tissue engineering. J Thorac Cardiovasc Surg 115:536-545; discussion 545, 1998.
220. Shinoka T: Tissue engineered heart valves: Autologous cell seeding on biodegradable polymer scaffold. Artif Organs 26:402, 2002
221. Shimizu T, Yamato M, Isoi Y, et al: Fabrication of pulsatile cardiac tissue grafts using a novel 3-dimensional cell sheet manipulation technique and temperature-responsive cell culture surfaces. Circ Res 90:40e, 2002
222. Thrall JH: Nanotechnology and medicine. Radiology 230:315, 2004
223. Fuster V, Hirshfeld J, John W, et al: Working group 8: Defining the different types of cardiovascular specialists and developing a new model for training general clinical cardiologists. J Am Coll Cardiol 44:267, 2004

Chapter 4

THE FUTURE OF CARDIAC SURGERY AND ANESTHESIA

Ani C. Anyanwu, MD* • David H. Adams, MD* • Cephas P. Swamidoss, MD† • Paul G. Barash, MD†

The Future of Cardiac Surgery

KEY POINTS

1. The future of cardiac surgery is closely related to the future of cardiology.
2. The relative decrease in demand for coronary artery surgery is largely a reflection of increasing use of percutaneous coronary revascularization. In contrast, the need for valvular heart surgery is likely to rise in the immediate future.
3. Heart failure is increasing in epidemic proportions and is likely to lead to a large increase in the surgical workload in future years.
4. The early 21st century has witnessed a change in the characteristics of patients undergoing cardiac surgery (they are older and sicker), and this factor is likely to have the greatest impact on cardiac anesthesiologists.
5. Surgical treatment of coronary artery disease is likely to move in the direction of off-pump coronary artery bypass and minimally invasive surgery and the use of multiple arterial grafts and include the treatment of ischemic mitral regurgitation.
6. There has been a resurgence of interest in surgery for atrial fibrillation due to the availability of technology that allows surgeons to perform ablation of the pathways around the pulmonary venous inflow.
7. Increased utilization of surgical and anesthesia services will outpace the rate of overall population growth in the future.
8. Economic forces such as regionalization of care, alternative recovery models, and cost reduction measures will affect the use and availability of new cardiac surgical procedures.
9. A consensus has emerged for the need to establish reliable, reproducible measures of health care performance.
10. The role of cardiac anesthesiologists will continue to be defined by forces frequently outside of the specialty, such as hospital administrators, patients' desires, and legislative mandates.

The future of cardiac surgery is closely related to the future of cardiology (see Chapter 3). Because of advances in diagnosis, better medical management, and changing epidemiology and prognosis of cardiovascular disease, the indications for surgical therapy have evolved considerably since the 1980s. However, the greatest determinant of future cardiac surgical practice is the rapidly expanding arena of interventional cardiology. Several diseases that were the domain of surgery can now be managed with percutaneous interventions. The scope and practice of cardiac surgery have evolved considerably since the 1950s (see Chapters 1 and 2) and will continue to evolve in response to these changes in epidemiology and cardiac diagnosis and management. New surgical procedures are being developed while some procedures have become obsolete. For example, in the 1980s, endoventricular resections formed the mainstay of treatment for intractable ventricular arrhythmias, but these procedures are rarely used and have been superseded by new pharmacologic agents and implantable defibrillators. In contrast, chronic atrial fibrillation (AF) encountered in surgical patients, which was regarded as untreatable in the 1980s, is now treated with surgical ablation (see Chapter 13). Changes in surgical practice have obvious implications for cardiac anesthesiology. The developments in cardiac surgery that are most likely to impact on the cardiac anesthesiologist are the changing demand, changing patients, evolution of new surgical techniques, and reduced invasiveness of surgery.

*The Future of Cardiac Surgery
†The Future of Cardiac Anesthesia

DEMAND FOR CARDIAC SURGERY

About 800,000 adult cardiac operations are performed annually worldwide, the majority being operations to treat ischemic or valvular heart disease. Many developed countries are experiencing a relative decrease in surgery for ischemic heart disease, while the reverse pattern is seen in developing countries, with an increase in surgery for ischemic heart disease. The Society of Thoracic Surgeons in the United States reported a decline in isolated coronary artery bypass graft (CABG) procedures from approximately 200,000 in 1997 to an average of 150,000 per year for 1998 to 2003.[1] The relative decrease in demand for CABG surgery is largely a reflection of increasing application of percutaneous coronary revascularization. Drug-eluting stents have been further reducing referrals for CABG surgery, as they are believed to provide better long-term palliation for coronary artery stenosis and therefore compete with the sustainable long-term palliation that was hitherto only achieved with surgery.[2] Whether the drug-eluting stents will indeed provide superior long-term relief from cardiac events is uncertain as meta-analysis of early randomized trials did not show any survival advantage or reduction in myocardial infarction (MI) with drug elution compared with bare metal stents.[3] If it emerges that these stents delay rather than prevent in-stent stenosis, surgeons may experience a rebound increase in CABG referrals in the future. Although increasing primary preventative measures, and the use of cholesterol-lowering drugs and aspirin, may reduce the incidence and severity of coronary artery disease (CAD), these will probably not affect the demand for coronary revascularization in the immediate future. In the longer term, these primary preventative measures will increasingly yield benefit, and the prevalence of surgically relevant CAD will probably decline. Novel approaches to treat CAD such as angiogenesis are also under development and if successful will further reduce the need for CABG surgery.

In contrast, the need for valvular heart surgery is likely to rise in the immediate future. With improved hygiene and primary health care, rheumatic heart disease is now rare in most developed and many developing countries. With the exception of ischemic mitral regurgitation (MR), there are now no effective primary health measures for preventing most valvular disease (the etiology being largely degenerative or idiopathic). These valve pathologies will likely increase in prevalence and will continue to dominate the future practice of valve surgery. In contrast, rheumatic valvular disease continues to decline in prevalence. Valve patients are therefore older and will have more comorbidities than had been the case in the early era of valve surgery. With the present ability to perform valve reparative surgery with low operative risk and good outcomes, increasing numbers of asymptomatic patients will be referred for surgical treatment. It is now recognized that the traditional practice of waiting for ventricular dilatation prior to recommending valve surgery is detrimental to long-term outcomes because changes associated with ventricular dilatation and remodeling are often irreversible.[4,5] Future guidelines on the indications for surgical treatment in valve disease are being developed and are likely to lower thresholds for surgical intervention. Finally, the shift toward increasing use of bioprosthetic valves in the late 1990s is likely to result in an increased number of patients presenting for valve reoperations over the next decade.

One area likely to experience an increase in surgical workload is surgery for heart failure (HF). HF is increasing in epidemic proportions, and for many patients, there is no effective palliation of symptoms. Ventricular restoration procedures and mitral repair for advanced cardiomyopathy are being increasingly used. Artificial heart programs will likely witness expansion with the advent of newer devices for bridging or destination therapy.

CHANGING PATIENTS

This is the aspect of future cardiac surgical practice that is likely to have the greatest impact on the cardiac anesthesiologist. The early 2000s witnessed a change in the characteristics of patients undergoing cardiac surgery. Patients are older, have worse cardiac disease (poorer target vessels, poorer ventricular function), and have more comorbidity (severe vascular disease, renal disease, obesity, advanced respiratory disease). For example, in patients undergoing isolated CABG in the United Kingdom between 1993 and 2003, the proportion of patients above the age of 75 increased from 2% to 10% with increases also seen in the incidence of diabetes, renal failure, and HF and an overall yearly increased inoperative risk as predicted by the euroSCORE method.[6] Many surgeons have observed a similar trend.

Furthermore, because of advances in surgical, anesthetic, and perioperative care, the boundaries of cardiac surgery are continually extended to accommodate patients who would have previously been regarded as inoperable; such patients are usually very high risk and present special challenges to the cardiac anesthesiologist. Indeed, in many centers it is becoming rare for patients to be refused surgery because of comorbidity or advanced age. Surgical procedures are also becoming more complex, requiring longer periods of cardiopulmonary bypass (CPB) and myocardial ischemia, which pose additional management demands on the anesthesiologist. The modern era of cardioplegic protection enables surgeons to undertake complex reparative surgery where previously they would have either declared the patient inoperable or performed the minimal procedure that would allow survival (rather than the best long-term benefit) of the patient.

Reoperative surgery is also on the rise. The explosion of cardiac surgery in the 1980s and early 1990s has produced a cohort of millions of surviving patients worldwide who have had previous cardiac surgery. As most cardiac surgery is palliative rather than definitive, increasing numbers of surviving patients present yearly for reoperative surgery (e.g., for endocarditis, replacement of degenerated biological valves, and repeat CABG surgery). The low-risk "routine" cardiac surgery patient is increasingly becoming a rarity; in the future, few patients will be "routine" and most will pose unique anesthetic and surgical challenges.

Advances in cardiologic treatment also paradoxically present new burdens to the cardiac surgeon and anesthesiologist. Many patients who would otherwise have died following acute MI now survive with severe left ventricular dysfunction, making them higher risk for surgical intervention. Furthermore, by selecting out those patients with the most favorable disease for percutaneous intervention, patients referred for surgery are rarely straightforward and generally have advanced or complex disease. Multiple stents from previous interventions occasionally present technical problems in finding a suitable area for anastomosis in subsequent CABG operations. Prevalent use of potent antiplatelet agents increases the hemorrhagic complications of surgery. If percutaneous valve technology becomes a clinical reality, it is likely that the simple valve defects will be selected out for percutaneous intervention, leaving the complex valves for surgical intervention and thus further filtering out the low-risk or "straightforward" patient from the cardiac surgical practice (see Chapters 11 and 12).

EXPANDING SURGICAL APPROACHES

Ischemic Heart Disease

Surgical treatment of CAD has not changed substantially in the past 10 years. Although there have been changes in intraoperative surgical management (e.g., myocardial preservation and use of off-pump [OPCAB] surgery), the essential operation has not changed since the 1980s. The predominant operation in the early 2000s remains internal mammary artery (IMA) grafting to the left anterior descending coronary artery, with aortocoronary saphenous vein grafting to other target vessels (see Chapters 19 and 20). Although the use of multiple arterial grafts was widely promoted in the 1990s, the uptake remains low. Results on multiple arterial grafting are promising and show the long-term benefit of bilateral IMA grafting and encouraging mid-term results with other arterial grafts.[7-9] Many surgeons are gradually adopting multiple arterial grafting and, as long-term data emerge over the next few years, the application of arterial grafting is likely to become more widespread. Adjunctive surgical procedures for ischemic heart disease, notably mitral valve annuloplasty for ischemic MR and left ventricular remodeling for akinetic or dyskinetic segments, are likely to be performed more frequently following recognition of better long-term results compared with revascularization alone.[10,11] Ischemic MR will also be a likely area of further development, especially as it is now appreciated that annuloplasty alone (the current treatment) does not provide a lasting cure in up to 50% of patients.[12] New asymmetric annuloplasty rings that support the restricted posterior leaflet (which causes the regurgitation) are already in use and should delay the occurrence of recurrent regurgitation. Procedures to support the ventricular wall (thus preventing further retraction of the already restricted posterior leaflet) are under current investigation.

Valvular Heart Disease

With the declining frequency of CABG surgery, it is likely that most centers will experience a relative or absolute increase in valvular heart surgery.[13] The likely changes in heart valve surgery in the future will probably reflect an increase in valve-conserving approaches and an increase in the use of bioprosthetic valves. Valve repair surgery, particularly of the mitral valve, is increasing in frequency. The Society of Thoracic Surgeons (STS) database records a doubling in the number of mitral valve repairs between 1999 and 2003, from 4000 to 8000 procedures, with mitral repair constituting more than half of all mitral valve operations in 2003 compared with a third in 1999.[1] The procedures for mitral valve repair are now well established, and it is likely their application will continue to expand.[14] Techniques for repair of the aortic valve are less well developed and have been less reproducible. Reports[15,16] have been encouraging, and with further development and refinement of techniques, repair of the aortic valve may become more widely practiced.[17] Valve placement will remain for those valves that are not repairable. Increasingly, most patients and surgeons are opting for bioprosthetic valves because of superior longevity of present-generation pericardial valves, lower risk associated with valve replacement, and increased appreciation of the morbidity associated with anticoagulation.[18,19] Surgery on the tricuspid valve (mainly repair) is also increasing and has doubled in frequency since 2000.[1] This trend is likely to continue and is a reflection of the appreciation of the inferior long-term outcome associated with deteriorating tricuspid regurgitation, if left untreated in patients undergoing mitral valve surgery[20,21] (see Chapter 20).

Alternatives to conventional surgical treatment are being explored. Devices that may allow mitral repair without CPB are currently under investigation and may become available for use within this decade. Tissue-engineered valves are also a possible prospect for the future. Several percutaneous options to surgical valve repair and replacement are being developed and are in trial. Early clinical experience with percutaneous repair of regurgitant mitral valves has resulted in reduction in MR and some improvement in symptoms, but most patients had significant residual regurgitation.[22] Based on current understanding of the pathology and pathophysiology of mitral and aortic valve disease, it is unlikely that percutaneous approaches can reproduce similar functional results (near-complete reversal of stenosis or regurgitation in a majority of patients) to that seen with surgical repair or replacement. However, as the technology develops, patients may be prepared to accept a less-perfect result, with the option of future surgery if required, in preference to cardiac surgery (as is currently seen with percutaneous treatment of CAD). These developments will further reduce referrals for valve repair surgery and may complicate subsequent surgical management of these valves if required.

Heart Failure

HF probably provides the greatest potential for expansion within cardiac surgery. Unfortunately, this has been the case since the 1970s, with little increase in the proportion of HF patients who can be treated surgically. Despite huge research investment, there are yet no available surgical treatments that can be widely applied to the hundreds of thousands of patients worldwide who die of HF every year. Transplantation remains the most effective form of surgery for HF, but because of high mortality and morbidity, restricted availability of donors, and only modest survival benefit over medical therapy, application of transplantation is restricted to a tiny minority.[23]

Several alternative approaches to treating HF have been proposed since the 1970s, including cardiomyoplasty, ventricular assist devices (VADs), total artificial hearts, and partial left ventriculectomy (Batista operation), but none has yielded sustainable improvement in survival and quality of life.[24] Some novel approaches have been developed in the past 10 years, but they remain largely confined to experimental studies and presently do not have significant clinical promise (Table 4–1). Once the heart dilates and symptoms of HF appear, the prognosis is poor with 5-year survival below 50% regardless of surgical treatment applied. At this stage, surgery cannot reverse the adverse ventricular modeling. Edmunds[5] is skeptical about the role of surgery in treatment of HF, a situation he likened to "reading tarot cards." The most worthwhile

Table 4–1 Novel Approaches to Treating Heart Failure With Factors Limiting Their Clinical Application

Xenotransplantation	Survival beyond 100 days has not been achieved in pig-to-primate models, and acute xenograft rejection has not been overcome.[25]
Myocardial restraint devices	Animal and human studies suggest that although these devices may help slow the progression of ventricular dilatation, they seem not to offer benefit in the already dilated and remodeled ventricle with established chronic heart failure.[26]
Injection of bone marrow–derived stem cells or skeletal myoblasts	Unresolved issues involve optimum cell type to be used, cell dosage, method of delivery, and whether new myocytes form functional units.[27]

surgical interventions for the immediate future remain conventional surgical techniques including coronary revascularization, remodeling of post-MI ventricles (such as Dor's approach), and mitral valve repair.

One area where expansion in HF surgery may be seen in the near future is the use of new-generation VADs for destination therapy.[28] Randomized trials have shown that VADs yield better survival compared with medical treatment in selected patients who are not suitable for transplantation.[29] Although survival is better, high morbidity (mainly infectious, thromboembolic, and bleeding complications) limits benefits in quality of life. Indeed, this high morbidity prevents wider applicability of destination therapy for the majority of HF patients who need it the most, as they are elderly or have severe comorbid disease, such that the risks of surgery outweigh the potential benefits. As device technology and patient management protocols improve, the use of mechanical replacement devices for destination therapy and as an alternative to transplantation may become routine. Newer devices such as axial flow pumps, total implantable devices, and new-generation artificial hearts are under evaluation (see Chapter 27).

Other Techniques

There has been a resurgence in interest in AF surgery because of availability of technology that allows surgeons to perform ablation around the atrial venous inflows without the added complexity and morbidity associated with the original "cut and sew" Maze procedure.[30] These procedures are relatively simple to apply and do not unduly prolong the operation. This type of surgery is increasingly becoming routine in patients undergoing cardiac operations who have a prior history of AF (see Chapter 13).

The management of thoracic aortic disease is also evolving with incorporation of endovascular approaches. Unique problems posed by anatomy of the thoracic aorta and its branches, the often nondiscrete nature of aneurysmal disease (absence of aneurysm neck), and uncertain clinical benefit have limited the feasibility and application of these endovascular techniques.[31] However, as anatomic and technologic barriers are overcome, their use will become more widespread as endovascular therapies have considerably less morbidity compared with open aortic surgery (see Chapter 23).

REDUCED INVASIVENESS

There has been a surge in minimally invasive approaches to conventional cardiac procedures. These approaches present unique challenges to the cardiac anesthesiologist and surgeon. Although there is little direct evidence that these minimally invasive techniques are directly beneficial to the patient, compared with conventional techniques, minimally invasive cardiac surgery is here to stay and its applications are likely to expand in the future. The expansion of minimally invasive surgery is largely driven by advances in technology, commercial pressure, media promotion, demands by patients, adoption by cardiologists of new techniques, and need to provide "new" operations to compete with other cardiology advances. The latter is very important because with the severe competition between surgery and percutaneous interventional cardiology, patients generally opt for less invasive forms of therapy (even when they may compromise efficacy). To compete with percutaneous therapy, surgery must not only be effective but also be less invasive, carry less morbidity, and be less disruptive to the patient's quality of life. If cardiac surgeons continue to perform essentially the same operations they performed 30 years ago, it is unlikely that the specialty will survive the onslaught of modern high-technology nonsurgical therapies. The goals for the future include delivery of effective surgical treatments that are less traumatic to the patient and allow minimal hospital stays with shorter periods of postoperative convalescence. Modifications in anesthetic management and approaches to perioperative analgesia are crucial to achieving this goal (see Chapters 19 and 21).

Off-Pump and Beating Heart Surgery

The sudden growth of OPCAB surgery witnessed in the late 1990s has somewhat slowed, with about 20% of coronary artery operations performed without CPB in 2003.[6] This is largely explained because only a minority of existing surgeons who experimented with off-pump techniques in the 1990s persisted with the technique. However, as the technique is now well established, increasing numbers of surgical residents are acquiring the techniques of OPCAB surgery[32,33]; as these residents become practicing surgeons, the frequency of OPCAB is likely to witness another (more gradual) increase. Five- to 10-year data on outcomes and graft patency with OPCAB will emerge in the next few years. If these show sustainable benefits, then OPCAB surgery may challenge conventional CABG as the gold standard, because the adverse effects of CPB (although minimal in most patients) are well accepted (see Chapter 19).

The late 1990s also experienced a renewed interest in beating heart surgery (cardiac surgery without myocardial ischemia). Some surgeons have returned to performing valve operations without cardioplegia, a procedure largely abandoned in the early 1980s when safe cardioplegia emerged. Beating heart surgery is achieved by avoiding aortic clamping or by continuous antegrade or retrograde blood perfusion during clamping. The rationale for this practice is that by avoiding myocardial ischemia, the insult of surgery on the myocardium is reduced, resulting in better postoperative cardiac outcomes. Proponents argue that it is a more physiologic approach and is preferable to ischemic arrest in dilated or hypertrophic ventricles, which may tolerate ischemia poorly.[34,35] Beating heart surgery is also a useful technique in reoperations, particularly in the setting of patent arterial grafts.

Minimally Invasive Approaches

The popularization of the MIDCAB operation (minimally invasive direct coronary artery bypass) in the mid 1990s marked the beginning of the era of minimally invasive cardiac surgery. The procedure was widely embraced by both the media and cardiac surgeons as the beginning of a new future, with predictions that in the 21st century many CABG operations would be performed as ambulatory procedures with same-day or next-day discharge and patients returning to full activity within 1 week.[36] Ten years later, however, only a negligible number of coronary artery operations are performed through a minimally invasive approach. Indeed, very few MIDCAB operations are currently performed, even though it is now possible to perform multivessel revascularization through a small thoracotomy.[37] Similarly, few surgeons perform heart valve surgery through a limited sternotomy or small thoracotomy or endoscopically, even though studies with mid-term follow-up have demonstrated the safety and efficacy of minimally invasive and endoscopic valve surgery[38,39] (see Chapters 19 through 21).

It is not clear why minimally invasive cardiac surgery has not been more widely embraced; however, it may be because it uproots basic concepts of surgery that many regard as sacrosanct such as the importance of palpation and tactile feedback, adequate and wide exposure, and safety first.[40] In contradistinction to OPCAB surgery, which has been widely adopted at many centers, most of the world experience and published data on minimally invasive valve surgery remain restricted to few centers. However, if valve surgery is to expand to the asymptomatic patient (as is likely the case in the future) or if surgery is to become a realistic alternative to percutaneous valve technology (which may soon be available), it has to be performed with limited trauma and disruption to the patient. Asymptomatic patients and their cardiologists will likely seek surgeons who can perform a reliable operation with minimal trauma. Serious valve surgery programs are therefore likely to increase the application of minimally invasive surgery in the future, to survive the increasingly stiff competition in the world of cardiac surgery.

Robotics

The goal of totally endoscopic cardiac surgery has been made achievable by robotic technology.[41] Totally endoscopic coronary operations and mitral valve operations, among others, have now been undertaken with robotic assistance. While the technology is still being developed and evaluated, basic techniques and feasibility have been established.[42] Robotic surgery is currently limited to a minority of cardiac centers, and some are skeptical as to whether application of robotic technology will become widespread or practical.[40] Two major questions will determine the expansion of robotic technology in the future (assuming the technique is shown to be safe, reproducible, and applicable to a majority of patients). First, if surgeons have been resistant to embracing simpler minimally invasive approaches, such as reduced sternotomy, will they adopt robotic techniques? And second, will the technology be affordable and logistically adoptable by all cardiac surgical centers, or will it remain exclusive to a minority? Whether robotic surgery will be the future of cardiac surgery is uncertain, but robotics will no doubt have some future role in the cardiac surgery armamentarium (see Chapter 21).

Awake Surgery

Awake cardiac surgery was pioneered in Turkey by Karagoz and colleagues in 1998.[43] They reported their experience with the first 137 patients.[44] Although the technique was initially applied only to MIDCAB procedures, the technique has been extended to OPCAB operations via sternotomy[44,45] and also to valve procedures requiring CPB.[46] The use of awake surgery has expanded to several centers, mainly in Europe and Asia, with proponents claiming that it allows ultrafast tracking and earlier mobilization and discharge of patients. Although Zenati and Paiste performed the first procedure in United States in 2000,[47] the technique has generally not expanded in use in North America.

The anesthesiology community has met these developments with skepticism, with a leading cardiac anesthesiologist describing awake cardiac surgery as "risky business" and a "marketing tool" and advising that "there is no place for this trick in the cardiac anesthesiologist's armamentarium."[48] The reality, however, is that patient wishes and perceptions are increasingly driving health care delivery and physicians will strive to make health care delivery more patient friendly (which indeed was the founding basis of anesthesiology). If a patient's perception of an ideal cardiac operation is walking into a hospital, lying awake on a table having a robotic operation, having dinner that evening, and going home the next afternoon, then it is likely that is what will be provided and that awake surgery, despite its drawbacks, will necessarily become part of the technique of at least some cardiac anesthesiologists (even if for the wrong reasons).

Although most surgeons and anesthesiologists will probably not embrace awake surgery, it is likely that in the future an increasing number of innovators, particularly proponents of robotic and minimally invasive surgery, will adopt this approach in a bid to provide the utopia of a truly ultra–minimally invasive operation that can offer patients an acceptable alternative to percutaneous cardiac intervention. Paradoxically, although many surgeons and anesthesiologists may frown at this prospect, it may well be this development that will ultimately ensure the survival of cardiac surgery (and, by extension, cardiac anesthesiology) in this increasingly competitive world of health care provision. Such developments may seem far-fetched, but it is difficult to conceive that, in 50 years' time, in order to replace a 2-cm heart valve it will still be necessary to make 30-cm incisions, divide the sternum, and expose the whole heart, as was done in the 1960s. Surgeons of the future may well look back at this era as the medieval days of cardiac surgery.

RANDOMIZED TRIALS THAT WILL AFFECT CARDIAC SURGERY

Several important multicenter trials involving cardiac surgery are in progress and will have significant influence on the future of the specialty. The Surgical Treatment for Ischemic Heart Failure (STITCH) trial[49] is an international multicenter study randomizing patients with HF due to ischemic heart disease to medical therapy, CABG surgery alone, or CABG surgery and surgical ventricular restoration. This trial will report by 2008 and should define the role of surgical ventricular restoration. The Acorn CorCap trial randomized 300 patients with dilated cardiomyopathy to receive the Acorn CorCap cardiac support device, either in isolation or in combination with mitral valve surgery, with controls receiving medical management or isolated mitral valve replacement.[50] The CorCap is a proprietary mesh wrap that is implanted around the heart to provide external support, thereby reducing ventricular wall stress and possibly promoting reverse remodeling. Enrollment in this trial is complete, and early results presented at the 2004 American Heart Association meeting are promising, with 1-year follow-up showing reduction in progressive left ventricular dilatation and some improvement in quality of life.[51] As medium-term follow-up data from this trial emerge, the clinical role for this device will be determined. Other HF trials in progress include the Randomized Evaluation of the Novacor LVAS in a Non-Transplant Population (RELIANT), which compares the Novacor LVAS with the Heartmate XVE device for destination therapy (see Chapter 27).

Several trials of coronary revascularization are also being undertaken. One of the most ambitious is the Future Revascularization Evaluation in Patients with Diabetes Mellitus: Optimal Management of Multivessel Disease (FREEDOM) trial, which is a $25 million international multicenter trial funded by the National Heart, Lung, and Blood Institute (NHLBI).[52] This trial started recruitment in 2005 and aims to randomize 2,400 diabetic patients with multivessel CAD to CABG or percutaneous coronary intervention (PCI). FREEDOM is the first major CABG versus PCI trial that will include the use of drug-eluting stents. The trial is expected to close in 2010. Several smaller trials are also under way in various aspects of CABG. Long-term results from trials evaluating OPCAB surgery and multiple arterial grafting should begin to emerge by the end of the decade.

The Future of Cardiac Anesthesia

EMERGING FACE OF CARDIAC ANESTHESIA

Changes in Clinical Practice

The myriad changes in cardiology and cardiothoracic surgery have implications for the clinical practice of cardiac anesthesia. The implementation of fast-tracking protocols and the use of minimally invasive techniques have led to greater involvement of the cardiac anesthesiologist in perioperative care, enlarging the scope of clinical practice (see Chapters 14 through 31 for details of anesthetic management). To achieve maximal success, careful selection of those patients best suited to minimally invasive techniques or those patients who would most benefit from fast-tracking protocols is necessary.

A better understanding by administrators of the background, tools, and training of cardiac anesthesiologists has led to an increasing call for their involvement in the perioperative period. In this way, interprofessional accountability is increased, leading to a situation in which cardiologists, cardiothoracic surgeons, and anesthesiologists sublimate their individual professional goals to a common goal of maximizing patient care and quality in the setting of limited resources. Although initial selection criteria are primarily in the domain of the cardiologist and the cardiothoracic surgeon, the final decision is increasingly being made in conjunction with the cardiac anesthesiologist, who brings to the table an understanding of issues involving the intensive care unit (ICU). For instance, patients with diffuse myocardial disease may not be suitable candidates for minimally invasive techniques. Patients with poor preoperative myocardial function or multiple comorbidities may not benefit, or may even suffer, from involvement in fast-tracking protocols. Anesthesiologists, long involved in risk stratification, are able to incorporate their knowledge of risk into patient suitability, monitoring, and medications (see Chapter 11).

There has also been a greater involvement of the cardiac anesthesiologist during the postoperative period (see Chapters 32 to 37). Immediate postoperative management of mechanical ventilation with techniques to promote early extubation facilitates advancing the patient to later stages of recovery. In the late postoperative period, the expertise that cardiac anesthesiologists have in pain management is needed to expedite the recovery of the cardiac surgical patient. Pain relief adequate to facilitate postdischarge patient functioning is mandatory for optimal recovery. Increasingly, cardiac anesthesiologists are being consulted to provide pain management that will expedite recovery after cardiac surgery. These two areas, ICU management and pain management, have made cardiac anesthesiologists an integral part of the patient care team, rather than marginalizing them to care limited to the operating room. As the movement toward increased accountability for patient services continues to grow,[53] cardiac anesthesiologists will be called on to further enhance their value in order to maintain this integral position in patient care.

Although there were initial concerns about the potential decrease in volume relating to cardiology procedures, the change under way will in all likelihood bring an increased patient volume to anesthesiologists *outside* of the operating room. This expanded volume can enable cardiac anesthesiologists to maintain economic viability in an era of decreased resource utilization. Although these cardiology procedures are less invasive, they often require either deep sedation or a general anesthesia in addition to diagnostic transesophageal echocardiography (TEE) and hemodynamic monitoring to be successfully completed (see Chapters 12 and 13).

Cost Reduction Measures

Surgical outcomes, as defined by a decreased need for inotropic support, decreased perioperative bleeding, and decreased hypothermia, have improved due to the refinement of surgical techniques, new blood conservation strategies, new pharmacologic and anesthetic therapy, and the use of next-generation cardioplegia solutions. Changes in postoperative care have attempted to keep stride with these changes, leading to an emerging national benchmark postoperative length of stay (LOS) for routine coronary artery bypass graft (CABG) patients of less than 24 hours in the ICU and a 4- to 6-day total hospital stay. Routine postoperative care is the single greatest contributor to CABG costs, greater than costs incurred by the operating room, medical supplies, laboratory, pharmacy, radiology, and anesthesiology services. In curbing these expenses, savings can be generated (see Chapters 32 and 38). Decreases in LOS have led to new expectations and practices in the form of expediting critical care. Findings by the Medicare Cooperative Cardiovascular Project (CCP), a Health Care Financing Administration (HCFA [now Centers for Medicare and Medicaid Services])-sponsored initiative to profile national practice patterns and outcomes for major cardiac diagnosis-related groups (DRGs) and to create benchmarks of performance based on the results garnered from the top 10% of hospitals nationwide, indicate that, of the 796 hospitals profiled, only 80 programs fell within the top 10% of the benchmark for average LOS for routine CABG.[54]

Another technique advocated to decrease ICU LOS centers is "fast-tracking," with the use of short-acting anesthetics, early extubation, and "reassurance" techniques in the ICU. Elective extubation within 1 hour of arrival in the ICU in patients with short cardiopulmonary bypass (CPB) times (<50 minutes) and without sustained systemic hypothermia (<32°C) has been determined to be safe. Methods associated with reducing LOS in step-down units include the implementation of aggressive activity protocols (AAPs) and the creation of discharge holding areas. Because ICU costs associated with CABG surgery account for an estimated 12% of total perioperative cardiac costs, any decrease in ICU utilization contributes to a significant decrease in expenditures. When the economic ramifications of early tracheal extubation are analyzed, total costs per CABG surgery are decreased by 25%, primarily in nursing and ICU costs.[55] Further evaluation shows that department cost savings were 23% for ICU nursing and supplies, 11% for floor nursing and supplies, and 12% for respiratory therapy resources. There have been concerns expressed that fast-track techniques may be associated with a higher rate of morbidity. However, meta-analyses by Myles et al[56] and Cheng et al[57] found that there is no evidence of increased mortality or morbidity rates with fast-track cardiac anesthesia techniques that use lower opioid dose regimens compared with traditional high-dose opioid techniques (see Chapters 9, 11, 19, 21, 32, 34, 37, and 39).

Alternative Recovery Models

Other attempts to decrease cost in the perioperative period have focused on recovery of the patient in facilities other than the ICU.[58] Suggestions to achieve this goal include the creation of AAPs and alternative facilities of care. Preliminary data indicate that AAPs may lead to decreased average LOS. The goal with this practice is to facilitate movement of the patient through the health care system. By walking patients five to six times per day or increasing their self-function in activities of daily living, providers are able to decrease the time to reach prescribed performance standards for transfer to the next stage of care. Integral to the implementation of AAPs is the use of prophylactic medications to prevent the most common complications, including β-blockade (for AF), H_2 antagonists (for postoperative nausea and vomiting), and steroid therapy (for pericardial inflammation and pain).[59]

Eligibility criteria for inclusion in AAPs often mirror those set for early extubation protocols, broadly defined as hemodynamic stability and minimal chest tube drainage. Preoperative assignment is made into a low- or high-risk group for perioperative complications. Those patients in the low-risk group are assigned to AAPs; whereas those in the high-risk group are pushed to achieve greater activity levels than might otherwise be expected given their risk category. In this fashion, two benchmarks for LOS are created: one for the AAP group and one for the slow-to-recover group; however, both benchmarks are being created at levels improved from traditional norms. Exclusion criteria in those centers testing AAPs vary but may include the use of support devices (intra-aortic balloon pump [IABP], femoral artery monitors) or vasoactive medications (epinephrine, dopamine, dobutamine); however, even these criteria are being challenged. In essence, this technique accelerates the time frame for currently prescribed recovery goals. Changing the roles, responsibilities, and expectations, in addition to the number of nursing and allied health staff, is integral to the success of this new model. This higher level of acuity requires greater nursing facility with such areas as advanced respiratory care, pain management, and working with patients with support devices (chest tubes, pacemakers, feeding tubes, Foley catheters), in addition to the responsibilities they are already trained to handle.

NEWER TECHNOLOGIES AND TECHNIQUES IN CARDIAC ANESTHESIOLOGY

Technologic advances permit information transfer in real-time. *Telemedicine* is defined as the use of electronic communications and information technologies to provide and support clinical care at a distance.[60] While in-person interaction with patients is preferable, telemedicine can be used as an adjunctive therapeutic modality, a method to extend the timeframe of therapeutic contact, and an alternative when in-person contact is not possible. Although many of the legal, financial, and ethical issues are still being discussed and have yet to be laid to rest, the role of telemedicine is gaining importance in medicine. The effect of a multiple-site ICU telemedicine program on clinical and economic outcomes was studied.[61] The researchers found that the use of telemedicine-based, remote intensivists was associated with improved clinical outcomes and hospital financial performance. Similarly, the use of technology to improve access to real-time reading of radiographic studies for patients in rural areas has gained popularity.[62] With the continued proliferation of cardiac surgery programs and the increased demand for, but limited supply of, TEE-proficient/certified cardiac anesthesiologists, it is not difficult to imagine the use of such technology to improve access to TEE skills (see Chapters 15, 16, and 41).

Health Policy and Public Accountability

Increasingly, policy initiatives have been instituted to prove competency, ensure standards of quality and patient safety, and provide public accountability. For instance, the Leapfrog Group,[63,64] a business roundtable collaboration of large employers and insurers, implemented evidence-based referral standards for five surgical conditions, including CABG and percutaneous coronary interventions, to ensure that patients with high-risk conditions are treated in hospitals with the best outcomes.

Since the late 1970s, the American Board of Medical Specialties (ABMS) has evaluated the effectiveness of the relationship between board certification, focusing primarily on initial certification, and patient care outcomes. In a systematic review of the literature on studies published between 1966 and 1999, only 5% of the studies used research methods that were appropriate to assess the research question and, among these, more than half supported a positive relationship between board certification status and clinical outcomes.[65] Despite the controversial question and results, a survey showed that certification and maintenance of certification are highly desirable to the public, the public would prefer that physicians are able to demonstrate skills and competencies to member boards of the ABMS, and that physicians should be evaluated more frequently than any ABMS member currently requires.[66]

Transesophageal Echocardiography Certification

The introduction of new technologies in the practice of medicine brings up issues of training, certification, and credentialing. The ABMS states that "the intent of certification is to provide assurance to the public that a physician specialist who is certified has successfully completed an approved educational program and an evaluation process that includes an examination designed to assess the knowledge, skills, and experience required to provide quality patient care in that specialty."[67] Although echocardiography has been in clinical use since the 1970s, it is still a relatively new technique in the practice of anesthesiology. Although its clinical benefits are established, problems surrounding training, certification, and credentialing remain. An editorial in 1974 described the growing demand for echocardiography information by cardiologists, yet deplored the paucity of adequately trained echocardiographers.[68] A similar situation exists today among cardiac anesthesiologists. Many cardiac surgeons and cardiac surgery programs rely on TEE for intraoperative decision-making, yet only a minority of anesthesiologists have had formal education in the technique. Morewood et al[69] surveyed members of the Society of Cardiovascular Anesthesiologists (SCA) and found that although 94% of respondents practiced in institutions that use perioperative TEE, less than 30% had formalized training, only 17% passed a certification examination, and more than 50% said that their institution did not have specific credentialing criteria. Some experts have suggested that TEE can be safely and effectively learned on the job, provided that an expert mentor is available to ensure that essential information is not missed.[70]

In the early 1990s, both the American Society of Echocardiography and the SCA began to independently establish guidelines and test for certification in TEE.[71] After cooperative discussions between the two groups, the National Board of Echocardiography (NBE) was formed in 1998 with the purpose of developing standards and administering examinations in the field of perioperative transesophageal echocardiography (PTE). The National Board of Medical Examiners was retained to administer the examination. In 2002, the American College of Cardiology and the American Heart Association were asked by a multidisciplinary task force to revise their 1990 joint document on clinical competence in adult echocardiography. This revised document was developed with SCA collaboration, endorsed by the SCA, and published in 2003.[72] At a future date, the NBE envisions developing a separate certification process for perioperative TEE (see Chapters 15 and 41).

Cardiothoracic Anesthesiology Fellowship Accreditation

In 1997, the SCA recommended pursuit of Accreditation Council for Graduate Medical Education (ACGME) accreditation of advanced training in cardiothoracic anesthesiology. A primary impetus to the initial recommendation was the lack of uniformity in the exposure of trainees to the many facets of cardiothoracic anesthesiology, including exposure to perioperative echocardiography. In 2000, the SCA submitted a proposal for accreditation to the ACGME. The board of directors of the SCA undertook this initiative to clearly delineate the broad base of clinical didactic and research activities that constitute optimal training, with the belief that approval by the ACGME would provide the public with a stamp of approval and ensure patient quality of care. This effort is for accreditation of subspecialty training, not subspecialty board certification in cardiothoracic anesthesiology (see Chapter 41).

Policy and Public Accountability

Legislators and public policy officials have long stated that the rise in health care costs must be controlled but not at the expense of quality of care.[73] Reform efforts have reduced health care costs, but many questions remain regarding the quality of care that accompanies this cost reduction. Although the reform proposals differ, one consensus has emerged—the need to establish reliable, reproducible measures of health care performance. To that end, the concept of health care report cards has emerged.[74] In its current use, a health care report card refers to any effort that quantifies or qualifies specific indicators or criteria to establish comparative estimations of the value of health care. These indicators, for example, take the form of time to hospital discharge, cost of services, mortality rates, delivery of preventive services, and patient satisfaction. The key to understanding the role of health care report cards is an appreciation of their comparative nature. Since the 1990s, the use of report cards has dramatically changed the pace and process of health care reform and affected providers, insurers, regulators, and patients.

The publication of report cards that purport to reflect quality of health care provider performance is rapidly becoming more common and more controversial.[75] The nascent use of health care report cards is fraught with difficulties.[76] The perceptions exist that data sources are inaccurate and that there are no well-defined measures of quality of care. Information used to evaluate performance is generally obtained from computerized administrative databases or medical records. Such sources contain incorrect, misleading, or incomplete data. The administrative databases were originally designed to facilitate accurate and timely payment to providers, with the added benefit of compiling demographic and clinical data related to patient encounters. These databases, however, contain many errors in the coding system of diagnoses, conditions, procedures, and treatments. The use of medical records may provide a good source of clinical information, but the cost associated with retrieval, the subjectivity of interpretation of test results, and the potential for overstatement of medical record notations to justify a hospital stay (or to satisfy insurance requirements) also limit their utility.

Although a number of risk adjustment systems are in use, there exists little proof that these systems are valid or reliable.[77] Risk adjustment using regression models is a statistical method of "leveling the playing field" to account for baseline differences so that the influence of care can be quantified. Unlike the automotive or computer industries, which have specifications for quality production of services, the health care industry must deal with more uncertainty and individuality in the form of patients and their diseases. The incorporation of risk stratification must be made into ongoing studies of clinical outcome (see Chapters 11, 32, and 39).

CONCLUSION

Increasingly, medicine is forced to respond to elements outside its control. This chapter enumerated some of the issues that cardiothoracic surgeons and cardiac anesthesiologists will confront over future decades. Each field has undergone major changes over the past decade. Cardiac anesthesia does not stand alone but rather is intricately linked to the changes occurring in both cardiology and cardiothoracic surgery. In fact, the changes have been so profound that, as pointed out by Mangano,[78] the NHBLI initiated an 18-month effort to develop recommendations for the future of perioperative medicine.

REFERENCES

1. The Society of Thoracic Surgeons: National Adult Cardiac Surgery Database. 2004. Available at: www.sts.org. Accessed: January 5, 2005

2. Ferreira AC, Peter AA, Salerno TA, et al: Clinical impact of drug-eluting stents in changing referral practices for coronary surgical revascularization in a tertiary care center. Ann Thorac Surg 75:485, 2003
3. Babapulle MN, Joseph L, Belisle P, et al: A hierarchical Bayesian meta-analysis of randomised clinical trials of drug-eluting stents. Lancet 364:583, 2004
4. Borer JS, Kupfer K: Mitral regurgitation: Current treatment options and their selection. Curr Treat Options Cardiovasc Med 6:509, 2004
5. Edmunds LH Jr: Reading tarot cards. Surg Clin North Am 84:323, 2004
6. Keogh BE, Kinsman R: Fifth National Adult Cardiac Surgical Database Report 2003. Henley-on-Thames, Dendrite, 2004
7. Taggart DP, D'Amico R, Altman DG: Effect of arterial revascularisation on survival: A systematic review of studies comparing bilateral and single internal mammary arteries. Lancet 358:870, 2001
8. Zacharias A, Habib RH, Schwann TA, et al: Improved survival with radial artery versus vein conduits in coronary bypass surgery with left internal thoracic artery to left anterior descending artery grafting. Circulation 109:1489, 2004
9. Tatoulis J, Buxton BF, Fuller JA: Patencies of 2127 arterial to coronary conduits over 15 years. Ann Thorac Surg 77:93, 2004
10. Aklog L, Filsoufi F, Flores KQ, et al: Does coronary artery bypass grafting alone correct moderate ischemic mitral regurgitation? Circulation 104(suppl I):I-68, 2001
11. Dor V: Surgical remodeling of left ventricle. Surg Clin North Am 84:27, 2004
12. McGee EC, Gillinov AM, Blackstone EH, et al: Recurrent mitral regurgitation after annuloplasty for functional ischemic mitral regurgitation. J Thorac Cardiovasc Surg 128:916, 2004
13. Northrup WF III, Emery RW, Nicoloff DM, et al: Opposite trends in coronary artery and valve surgery in a large multisurgeon practice, 1979. Ann Thorac Surg 77:488, 2004
14. Adams DH, Filsoufi F: Another chapter in an enlarging book: Repair of degenerative mitral valves. J Thorac Cardiovasc Surg 125:1197, 2003
15. Langer F, Aicher D, Kissinger A, et al: Aortic valve repair using a differentiated surgical strategy. Circulation 110(suppl I):II-67, 2004
16. Minakata K, Schaff HV, Zehr KJ, et al: Is repair of aortic valve regurgitation a safe alternative to valve replacement? J Thorac Cardiovasc Surg 127:645, 2004
17. Yacoub MH, Cohn LH: Novel approaches to cardiac valve repair: From structure to function: Part II. Circulation 109:1064, 2004
18. von Oppell UO, Zilla P: Prosthetic heart valves: Why biological? J Long Term Eff Med Implants 11:105, 2001
19. Puvimanasinghe JP, Takkenberg JJ, Edwards MB, et al: Comparison of outcomes after aortic valve replacement with a mechanical valve or a bioprosthesis using microsimulation. Heart 90:1172, 2004
20. Dreyfus GD, Corbi PJ, Chan KM, et al: Secondary tricuspid regurgitation or dilatation: Which should be the criteria for surgical repair? Ann Thorac Surg 79:127, 2005
21. Gold JP: When should tricuspid valve replacement/repair accompany mitral valve surgery? Adv Cardiol 41:133, 2004
22. Vahanian A, Acar C: Percutaneous valve procedures: What is the future? Curr Opin Cardiol 20:100, 2005
23. Anyanwu A, Treasure T: Prognosis after heart transplantation: Transplants alone cannot be the solution for end-stage heart failure. BMJ 326:509, 2003
24. Vitali E, Colombo T, Fratto P, et al: Surgical therapy in advanced heart failure. Am J Cardiol 91:88F, 2003
25. Hoerbelt R, Madsen JC: Feasibility of xenotransplantation. Surg Clin North Am 84:289, 2004
26. Gorman RC, Jackson BM, Gorman JH: The potential role of ventricular compressive therapy. Surg Clin North Am 84:45, 2004
27. Taylor DA: Cell-based myocardial repair: How should we proceed? Int J Cardiol 95(suppl 1):S8, 2004
28. Westaby S: Ventricular assist devices as destination therapy. Surg Clin North Am 84:91, 2004
29. Rose EA, Gelijns AC, Moskowitz AJ, et al: Long-term mechanical left ventricular assistance for end-stage heart failure. N Engl J Med 345:1435, 2001
30. Navia JL, Gillinov AM, McCarthy PM: Curative surgery for atrial fibrillation. Current status and minimally invasive approaches. Minerva Cardioangiol 52:155, 2004
31. Bush RL, Lin PH, Lumsden AB: Endovascular treatment of the thoracic aorta. Vasc Endovascular Surg 37:399, 2003
32. Jenkins D, Al Ruzzeh S, Khan S, et al: Multivessel off-pump coronary artery bypass grafting can be taught to trainee surgeons. J Card Surg 18:419, 2003
33. Caputo M, Bryan AJ, Capoun R, et al: The evolution of training in off-pump coronary surgery in a single institution. Ann Thorac Surg 74:S1403, 2002
34. Matsumoto Y, Watanabe G, Endo M, et al: Efficacy and safety of on-pump beating heart surgery for valvular disease. Ann Thorac Surg 74:678, 2002
35. Gersak B, Sutlic Z: Aortic and mitral valve surgery on the beating heart is lowering cardiopulmonary bypass and aortic cross-clamp time. Heart Surg Forum 5:182, 2002
36. Elbeery JR, Chitwood WR Jr: Minimally invasive cardiac surgery. Heart surgery for the 21st century. N C Med J 58:374, 1997
37. Srivastava SP, Patel KN, Skantharaja R, et al: Off-pump complete revascularization through a left lateral thoracotomy (ThoraCAB): The first 200 cases. Ann Thorac Surg 76:46, 2003
38. Casselman FP, Van Slycke S, Wellens F, et al: Mitral valve surgery can now routinely be performed endoscopically. Circulation 108(suppl I):I-I48, 2003
39. Mihaljevic T, Cohn LH, Unic D, et al: One thousand minimally invasive valve operations: Early and late results. Ann Surg 240:529, 2004
40. Robicsek F: Robotic cardiac surgery: Quo vadis? J Thorac Cardiovasc Surg 126:623, 2003
41. Kypson AP, Nifong LW, Chitwood WR Jr: Robotic cardiac surgery. J Long Term Eff Med Implants 13:451, 2003
42. Boyd WD, Stahl KD: The Janus syndrome: A perspective on a new era of computer-enhanced robotic cardiac surgery. J Thorac Cardiovasc Surg 126:625, 2003
43. Karagoz HY, Sonmez B, Bakkaloglu B, et al: Coronary artery bypass grafting in the conscious patient without endotracheal general anesthesia. Ann Thorac Surg 70:91, 2000
44. Karagoz HY, Kurtoglu M, Bakkaloglu B, et al: Coronary artery bypass grafting in the awake patient: Three years' experience in 137 patients. J Thorac Cardiovasc Surg 125:1401, 2003
45. Aybek T, Kessler P, Khan MF, et al: Operative techniques in awake coronary artery bypass grafting. J Thorac Cardiovasc Surg 125:1394, 2003
46. Schachner T, Bonatti J, Balogh D, et al: Aortic valve replacement in the conscious patient under regional anesthesia without endotracheal intubation. J Thorac Cardiovasc Surg 125:1526, 2003
47. Zenati MA, Paiste J, Williams JP, et al: Minimally invasive coronary bypass without general endotracheal anesthesia. Ann Thorac Surg 72:1380, 2001
48. Mangano CT: Risky business. J Thorac Cardiovasc Surg 125:1204, 2003
49. The Surgical Treatment for Ischemic Heart Failure (STITCH) Trial. 2005. Available at: www.stitchtrial.org. Accessed: April 19, 2005
50. Mann DL, Acker MA, Jessup M, et al: Rationale, design, and methods for a pivotal randomized clinical trial for the assessment of a cardiac support device in patients with New York Heart Association Class III-IV heart failure. J Card Fail 10:185, 2004
51. Late-breaking clinical trials abstracts. Circulation 111:1725, 2005
52. Future Revascularization Evaluation in Patients with Diabetes Mellitus: Optimal Management of Multivessel Disease. 2005. Available at: www.clinicaltrials.gov/ct/gui/show/NCT00086450. Accessed: April 19, 2005.
53. Mark DB, Hlatky MA: Medical economics and the assessment of value in cardiovascular medicine (Part II). Circulation 106:626, 2002
54. Ellerbeck EF, Jencks SF, Radford MJ, et al: Quality of care for Medicare patients with acute myocardial infarction: A four-state pilot study from the Cooperative Cardiovascular Project. JAMA 273:1509, 1995
55. Cheng DC, Karski J, Peniston C, et al: Early tracheal extubation after CABG surgery reduces costs and improves resource use: A prospective randomized controlled trial. Anesthesiology 85:1300, 1996
56. Myles PL, Daly DJ, Djaiaini G, et al: A systematic review of the safety and effectiveness of fast-track cardiac anesthesia. Anesthesiology 99:982, 2003
57. Cheng DC, Bainbridge D, Martin JE, et al: Does off-pump coronary artery bypass reduce mortality, morbidity, and resource utilization? Anesthesiology 102:188, 2005
58. Aps C: Fast-tracking in cardiac surgery. Br J Hosp Med 54:139, 1995
59. Jesurum JT, Alexander WA, Anderson JJ, et al: Fast-track recovery after aortocoronary bypass surgery. Semin Periop Nurs 5:12, 1996
60. Ad Hoc Committee: American Association of Cardiovascular and Pulmonary Rehabilitation Telemedicine position statement. J Cardiopulm Rehab 21:261, 2001
61. Breslow MJ, Rosenfeld BA, Doerfler M, et al: Effect of a multiple-site intensive care unit telemedicine program on clinical and economic outcomes: An alternative paradigm for intensivist staffing. Crit Care Med 32:31, 2004
62. Wang DZ: Telemedicine: The solution to provide rural stroke coverage and the answer to the shortage of stroke neurologists and radiologists (editorial comment). Stroke 34:2957, 2003
63. The Leapfrog Group: Available at: http://www.leapfroggroup.org/FactSheets/EHR_FactSheet.PDF. Accessed: August 14, 2004
64. Rogowski JA, Horbar JD, Staiger DO, et al: Indirect vs direct hospital quality indicators for very low birth weight infants. JAMA 291:202, 2004
65. Sharp LK, Bashook PG, Lipsky MS, et al: Specialty board certification and clinical outcomes: The missing link. Acad Med 77:534, 2002

66. Brennan TA, Horwitz RI, Duffy FD, et al: The role of physician specialty board certification status in the quality movement. JAMA 292:1038, 2004
67. American Board of Medical Specialties: Annual Report and Reference Handbook, Evanston, Ill, 2001
68. Feigenbaum H: Educational problems in echocardiography. Am J Cardiol 34:741, 1974
69. Morewood GH, Gallagher ME, Conlay LA: Current practice patterns for perioperative TEE in the United States (abstract). Anesth Analg 92:SCA94, 2001
70. Cahalan M, Foster E: Training in TEE: In the lab or on the job? Anesth Analg 81:217, 1995
71. Pearlman AS: ASExam: The end of the beginning. J Am Soc Echocardiogr 10:14, 1997
72. Quinones MA, Douglas PS, Foster E, et al: ACC/AHA clinical competence statement on echocardiography. J Am Coll Cardiol 41:687, 2003
73. Fleming ST: The relationship between the cost and quality of hospital care: A review of the literature. Med Care Rev 47:487, 1990
74. Swamidoss CP, Brull SJ, Watrous G, et al: Health-care report cards and implications for anesthesia. Anesthesiology 88:809, 1998
75. Epstein A: Performance reports on quality: Prototypes, problems and prospects. N Engl J Med 333:57, 1995
76. Hannan EL, Wu C, Ryan TJ, et al: Do hospitals and surgeons with higher coronary artery bypass graft surgery volumes still have lower risk-adjusted mortality rates? Circulation 108:795, 2003
77. Iezzoni LI, Ash AS, Coffman GA, et al: Predicting in-hospital mortality: A comparison of severity measurement approaches. Med Care 347, 1992
78. Mangano DT: Perioperative medicine: NHLBI Working Group deliberations and recommendations. J Cardiothorac Vasc Anesth 18:1, 2004

Part II

CARDIOVASCULAR PHYSIOLOGY, PHARMACOLOGY, AND MOLECULAR BIOLOGY

Chapter 5

CARDIAC PHYSIOLOGY

Brian Johnson, MD • Ahmad Adi, MD • Michael G. Licina, MD • Zak Hillel, MD, PhD • Daniel M. Thys, MD • Roberta L. Hines, MD • Joel A. Kaplan, MD

KEY POINTS

1. Heart rate, preload, afterload, and contractility determine the cardiac output. Alterations in one or more of the determinants of cardiovascular performance directly affect the integrity of the circulation.
2. Phases of the cardiac cycle are best displayed in a pressure-volume diagram/loop.
3. Diastology has recently become the most important focus of cardiac physiology.
4. Diastole consists of isovolumic relaxation, passive ventricular filling, and active or atrial filling.
5. The stroke volume is the difference between the end-diastolic volume and the end-systolic volume. The ejection fraction is the stroke volume divided by the end-diastolic volume.
6. The end-diastolic pressure-volume relation is the preferred load-independent measurement of myocardial contractility.
7. The heart rate affects cardiac output, stroke volume, coronary artery filling, and myocardial contractility.
8. There are marked physiologic differences between the right and left ventricles.
9. Pressure-volume loops can be used to demonstrate the differences between systolic and diastolic failure.
10. The Frank-Starling relationship and the pressure-volume loop are both clinically useful physiologic tools.

A thorough knowledge of the principles of cardiovascular physiology is the foundation for the practice of cardiovascular anesthesia. It serves as the basis of understanding the pathophysiologic mechanisms of cardiac disease as well as the patient's pharmacologic and surgical management.

To assess the physiologic basis for cardiac dysfunction, a systematic inspection of the elements that determine cardiac output (CO) is required. These intrinsic factors—heart rate (HR)/rhythm, preload, contractility, and afterload—are co-dependent such that abnormality in one often results in altered function in the others. This complex interaction is intrinsically designed to regulate beat-to-beat changes in the cardiovascular system, thereby adapting to changes in physiologic demands.

Heart rate, preload, afterload, and contractility determine CO, which, in turn, when combined with peripheral arterial resistance, determines arterial pressure for organ perfusion. Similarly, the arterial system contributes to ventricular afterload, and these interactions influence mechanoreceptors in the carotid artery and aortic arch providing feedback signals to higher levels in the central nervous system (medullary and vasomotor center). These centers then modulate venous return, HR, contractility, and arterial resistance[1] (Fig. 5–1).

The heart's primary function is to deliver sufficient oxygenated blood to meet the metabolic requirements of the peripheral tissues. Under normal circumstances, the heart acts as a servant by varying the CO in accordance with total tissue needs.[2] Tissue needs may vary with exercise, heart disease, trauma, surgery, or administration of drugs. Although tissue needs regulate circulatory requirements, the heart can become a limiting factor, particularly in patients with cardiac disease. In this regard, it is important to differentiate circulatory function from cardiac and myocardial function.[3]

Circulatory function refers to the function of the entire circulatory system, including the heart, blood vessels, and blood volume. Failure of any one of these can lead to significant circulatory dysfunction. For example, hypovolemia can lead to circulatory failure or shock in the presence of normal blood vessels and a normal heart.

Cardiac function includes the function of the myocardium, valves, conduction tissue, and supporting structures. Dysfunction of any of these can lead to cardiac and circulatory failure. The myocardium can be entirely normal, but the heart can fail due to valvular insufficiency.

Myocardial function depends on the cardiac muscle itself and its blood supply. Myocardial failure can result from actual muscle damage or myocardial ischemia, leading to inadequate muscle function. Obviously, myocardial dysfunction can produce cardiac failure and circulatory disturbances.

The focus of this chapter is on the heart's function as a pump. The various determinants of its pumping function are reviewed and, where applicable, newer clinical measurements of ventricular function are discussed.

CARDIAC CYCLE

The cardiac cycle of the left ventricle (LV) begins as excitation of the myocardium, which results in a sequence of mechanical events that lead to a pressure gradient being developed, ejection of the stroke volume (SV), and forward flow of blood through the body. These phases can be discussed based on the electrical activity, intracardiac pressures, intracardiac volumes, opening and closing of the cardiac valves, or the flow of blood into the peripheral circulation. Most practical of these is the relationship of pressure to volume over the course of the cycle. In this regard, systole represents the rapid increase in intracardiac pressure followed by the rapid decrease in volume. Diastole, on the other hand, represents first a rapid decrease in pressure followed by an increase in volume. An alternative to this approach is to exclude any temporal element

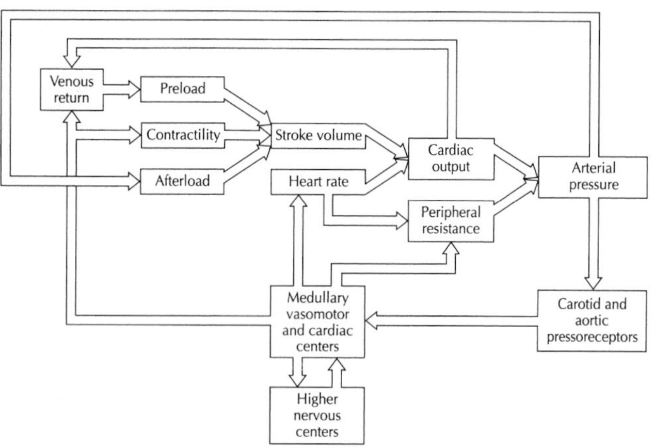

Figure 5–1 Interactions controlling the intact circulation. Changes in one or more of the determinants of cardiovascular performance directly affect the integrity of the circulation. Such interdependence must be considered whenever analyzing or treating hemodynamic disturbances. (Adapted from Badke FR, O'Rourke RA: Cardiovascular physiology. *In* Stein JH [ed]: Internal Medicine. Boston, Little, Brown, 1983, pp 407–423.)

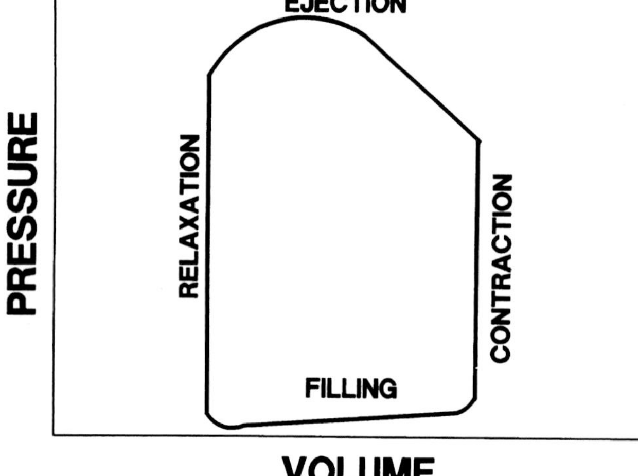

Figure 5–2 Phases of the cardiac cycle displayed in a pressure-volume diagram.

and to study the relation of pressure to volume in the framework of a pressure-volume diagram (Fig. 5–2). In this diagram, the pressure is typically displayed on the vertical axis and the volume on the horizontal axis. This yields a pressure-volume loop of four distinct phases over the course of one contraction: isovolumic contraction, ventricular ejection (rapid and slow), isovolumic relaxation, and filling (rapid and diastasis).

Phases of the Cardiac Cycle

Isovolumic Contraction Phase

This phase represents the first portion of systolic activity of the myocardial muscle (Box 5–1). It occurs just after the QRS complex on the electrocardiogram (ECG), when individual myocardial fibers begin to shorten. As the contraction continues, the ventricular pressure increases rapidly, exceeding atrial pressure and forcing the atrioventricular (AV) valve to close due to the reversed pressure gradient. While the AV valve closes, it also balloons up into the atrium and causes the chordal apparatus to tense, holding the coaptation point at its optimal position thus preventing regurgitation.[4] This now forms a sealed chamber (ventricle) because the AV valve has closed and the semilunar valves have yet to open. This is represented as contraction in Figure 5–2. The ventricle continues to alter shape without changing its volume, thereby resulting in increased pressure. In awake canine hearts, the ventricle has been shown to change into an ellipse. This shape seems to be volume dependent, and at lower volumes the shape during contraction is spherical.[5]

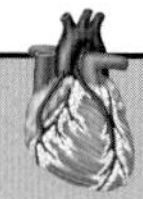

BOX 5–1 ***The Phases of the Cardiac Cycle Consist of***

- Isovolumic contraction
- Ejection
- Isovolumic relaxation
- Diastolic filling

Early work by Frank[6] has shown that tension (T) developed by cardiac muscle is determined by the initial length (L) or stretch of the muscle. In isolated muscles, the optimal tension developed is known as L_{max}. At muscle lengths below or above L_{max}, the developed tension is less than maximal (Fig. 5–3). Advances in laboratory study of muscle have shown that the primary determinant of developed tension is not total muscle length but sarcomere length (SL).[7] Although the SL-T relationship is similar to the L-T relationship, small differences, such as the absence of a descending limb, are present.[8]

In intact hearts, the equivalent of the L-T relationship is the pressure-volume relationship measured during the isovolumic phase of contraction.[9] This pressure is determined by Laplace's law, which states that

$$P = T/r \qquad (1)$$

where P is the developed pressure, T is the wall tension, and r is the radius of the ventricle. This equation shows that the radius and tension of the ventricle determine the pressure, not the volume of the ventricle. The effects of change in the end-diastolic volume (EDV) are attenuated by the three-dimensional nature of the ventricle, and the pressure gradient created is mostly from the effect of wall tension and radius. When the EDV increases by 50% (from 100 to 150 mL), the radius of the ventricle increases only 14% (from 3.17 to 3.63

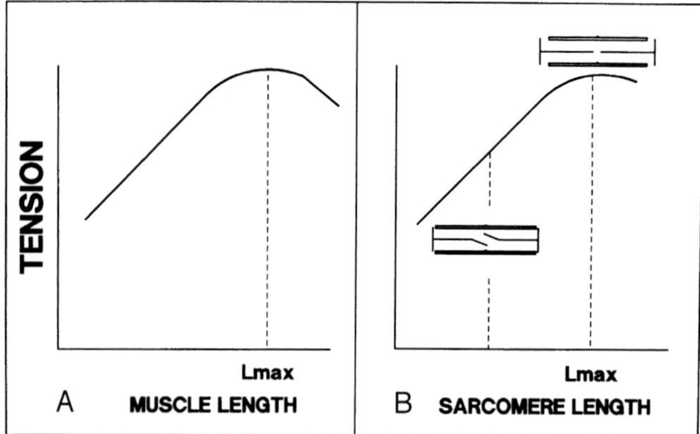

Figure 5–3 *(A)* Length-tension diagram for an isolated cardiac muscle. L_{max} = optimal length of an isolated muscle as maximal tension is developed. *(B)* Sarcomere length-tension diagram. At L_{max}, the thick and thin filaments overlap perfectly.

cm). If this small change in radius or SL leads to changes in pressure, then the SL-T relationship must be sensitive to small changes. In fact, the SL-T relationship for cardiac muscle is very steep and a change in SL of 0.7 (1.6 to 2.3) mm yields a change from near zero to maximum wall tension. With increased contractility, the slope of the SL-T relationship is shifted left and any given SL will give a higher developed tension and increased pressure. The same is true for maximal changes in tension over time (dT/dt) and pressure over time (dP/dt).[10]

Ejection Phase

As soon as the developed pressure exceeds that of the resting pressure of the aorta or pulmonary artery, the semilunar valves open and the ejection phase begins. This correlates to ejection in Figure 5–2. The actual opening of the valves is due to the movement of blood across the valve leaflets caused by the pressure gradient. The ejection phase leads to a marked decrease in ventricular volume and a slight increase in pressure initially that rapidly decreases to the dicrotic notch pressure. The equalization of the pressure gradient between the ventricular and aortic pressures signals the end of the ejection phase and allows closure of the semilunar valves. This is the point of smallest ventricular size and volume, also known as the end-systolic volume (ESV). This ESV is greatly dependent on the contractile state of the ventricle and the properties of the vascular system.

Nearly two decades after the work of Frank was published about L-T relationships, Paterson and Starling[11] reported their results on ejecting mammalian hearts. They noted that at a constant aortic pressure the SV varied directly with the EDV. This is the Starling relationship, which differs from the Frank relationship in that it depends not only on the SL-T but also on the interaction among muscle force, velocity, and length. These relationships have been studied at length in the isolated heart muscle.[12-14]

The relationship among muscle force, velocity, and length is not readily applied to the clinical setting, due to the extreme difficulty of obtaining measurements in intact hearts.[15] In clinical practice, these difficulties lead to use of the EDV and ESV, which are relatively easy to measure. The difference between these two is the SV (Fig. 5–4):

$$SV = EDV - ESV \tag{2}$$

In addition, by using the SV equation divided by the EDV, ejection fraction (EF) can be obtained.

$$EF = (EDV - ESV)/EDV \tag{3}$$

$$EF = SV/EDV \tag{4}$$

EF is a well-known estimation of global cardiac function that is used worldwide. It allows application of the Starling principle in the study of cardiac function based on changes in EDV as they relate to SV. The use of transesophageal echocardiography (TEE) has greatly enhanced the clinician's ability to directly visualize EDV and ESV using biplane apical and single-plane ellipsoidal methods (see Chapters 15 and 16).[16,17]

Isovolumic Relaxation Phase

The biochemical process of isovolumic relaxation begins to occur before the blood has even stopped flowing out of the ventricle and is an energy-consuming process. The term *relaxation phase* refers to the period immediately following closure of the semilunar valves. It is a phase in which the ventricle undergoes a rapid decrease in pressure and no change in

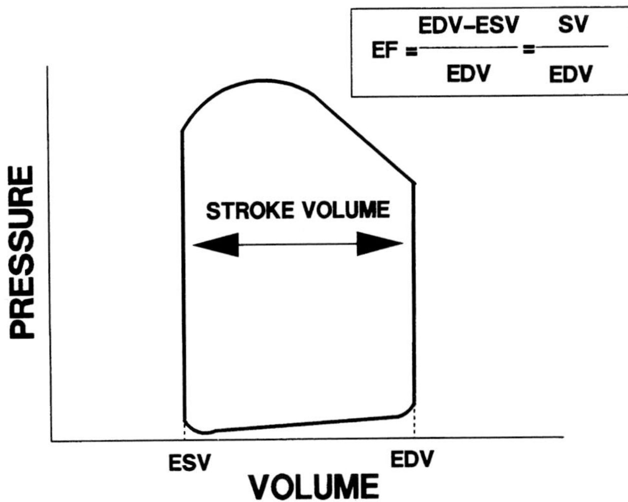

Figure 5–4 Pressure-volume diagram indicating end-diastolic volume (EDV), end-systolic volume (ESV), stroke volume (SV), and the equation for ejection fraction (EF).

volume, returning to the precontractile configuration.[18] Over the past several years, many important questions have arisen regarding this phase of the cycle. As advances in cardiac imaging have continued to progress, the importance of this phase has become better understood (see diastolic function discussion later and Chapters 14 and 15). The prevailing load on the heart, the inactivation of the actin-myosin cross-links, and spatial and temporal nonuniformity are so integral to the previous contraction phase that the effects of diastolic function are becoming more prominent within clinical practice[19,20] (Table 5–1).

Filling Phase (Diastolic Filling)

As the relaxation phase continues, the ventricular pressure continues to drop. At the same time, the atria are receiving blood flow from the pulmonary veins (left atrium [LA]) or the superior and inferior vena cava (right atrium [RA]), thus

Table 5–1 Determinants of Relaxation in the Intact Heart

Loading
Internal restoring forces (cardiac fiber)
External restoring forces (intact heart)
Configurational loading: end-ejection pressure-volume relation
Hemodynamic loading (cardiocirculatory system)
Arterial impedance
Transmission of pressure wave in the coronary circulation
Laplace relationship during rapid filling phase, pericardium, right ventricular hemodynamics
Inactivation
Metabolic control: coronary circulation
Neurohumoral control: catecholamines
Drugs
Nonuniformity
Spatial and temporal distribution of force and loading inactivation

experiencing rises in pressure and volume, shown as filling in Figure 5–2. As the atrial pressure rises and ventricular pressure drops, a crossover point is reached where the AV valves open and blood flows down the pressure gradient into the ventricle. There are two phases to this flow: (1) a rapid phase based solely on the pressure gradient and (2) a slower active phase based on the contraction of the atria (atrial kick). During this filling, the ventricular volume increases rapidly and yet the ventricular pressure changes very little, if at all, in the normal heart. This is measured by the end-diastolic pressure-volume relation (EDPVR), which describes ventricular distensibility and has a strong relationship to the compliance of the ventricle, extrinsic factors, and the determinants of ventricular relaxation (Table 5–2). This process continues until the next electrical signal, which starts the contraction phase again.

DIASTOLIC FUNCTION

Diastology, or the study of diastolic function, has become the most important focus of cardiac physiology in the past few years. Diastolic dysfunction has been seen in 40% to 50% of patients with congestive heart failure (CHF) despite normal systolic function.[21,22] This led to a shift in thinking about cardiac function not only as the typical systolic factors of contractile force, ejection of SV, and generation of CO, but as diastolic factors as well. The use of transthoracic echocardiography (TTE) and TEE has greatly improved this knowledge of diastole by showing the actual real-time activities in the heart, as related to filling pressures, shape, and relaxation. It is now possible to relate diastolic dysfunction, which is increased impedance to ventricular filling, to structural and pathologic causes of CHF[23] (Table 5–3). Failure of the right ventricle (RV) can contribute to left-sided diastolic dysfunction by increasing cardiac pressures, which causes decreased relaxation of the myocardium yielding decreased myocardial distensibility. The LV is dependent on multiple factors for its diastolic function[24] (Fig. 5–5). These factors are discussed later and related to echocardiographic and Doppler findings commonly seen in relation to them. Newer measurements of diastolic function are discussed later in this chapter.

Table 5–2 Determinants of Left Ventricular Distensibility

Extrinsic Factors
Pericardium
Right ventricle
Intrapleural and mediastinal pressures
Coronary vascular volume
Physical Properties of the Left Ventricle
Ventricular geometry
Volume
Wall thickness
Composition of ventricular wall (scar, amyloid)
Myocardial Relaxation
Load
Inactivation
Spatial and temporal nonuniformity

Table 5–3 Conditions Involving Diastolic Heart Failure*

Conditions	Mechanisms of Diastolic Dysfunction
Mitral or tricuspid stenosis	Increased resistance to atrial emptying
Constrictive pericarditis	Increased resistance to ventricular inflow, with decreased ventricular diastolic capacity
Restrictive cardiomyopathies (amyloidosis, hemochromatosis, diffuse fibrosis)	Increased resistance to ventricular inflow
Obliterative cardiomyopathy (endocardial fibroelastosis, Loeffler's syndrome)	Increased resistance to ventricular inflow
Ischemic heart disease	Postinfarction scarring and hypertrophy (remodeling)
Flash pulmonary edema, dyspnea during angina	Diastolic calcium overload
Impaired myocardial relaxation	Increased resistance to ventricular inflow
Hypertrophic heart disease (hypertrophic cardiomyopathy, chronic hypertension, aortic stenosis)	Impaired myocardial relaxation Diastolic calcium overload Increased resistance to ventricular inflow due to thick chamber walls, altered collagen matrix Activation of renin-angiotensin system
Volume overload (aortic or mitral regurgitation, arteriovenous fistula)	Increased diastolic volume relative to ventricular capacity Myocardial hypertrophy, fibrosis
Dilated cardiomyopathy	Impaired myocardial relaxation Diastolic calcium overload Myocardial fibrosis or scar

From Grossman W: Diastolic dysfunction in congestive heart failure. N Engl J Med 325:1557, 1991.
*Diastolic heart failure is defined as increased resistance to filling of one or both cardiac ventricles.

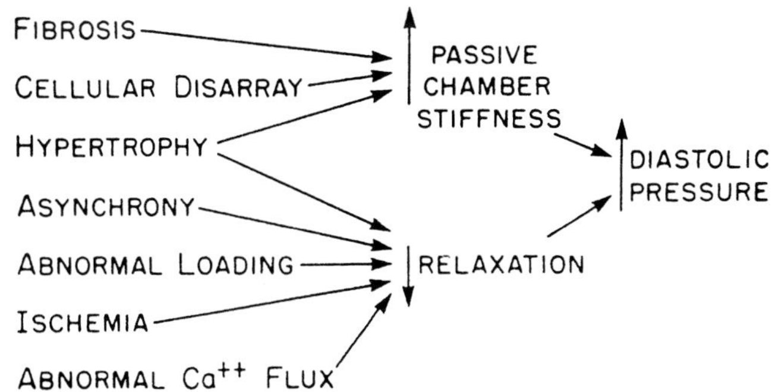

Figure 5–5 Factors responsible for increased chamber stiffness and decreased relaxation that culminate in diastolic dysfunction and increased LV diastolic pressure. Note that ventricular hypertrophy affects both stiffness and relaxation, increasing the risk of diastolic dysfunction. (From Stauffer JC, Gaasch WH: Recognition and treatment of left ventricular dysfunction. Prog Cardiovasc Dis 32:319, 1990.)

Table 5–4 **Factors Influencing Left Ventricular Relaxation**

Factor	Rate
Load	
Early systolic	Slower
Late systolic	Faster
Positive inotropes	
Catecholamines	Faster
Amrinone, milrinone	Faster
Digoxin	Slower
Calcium	Unchanged
Negative inotropes	
Propranolol	Slower
Heart rate increase	Faster
Preload (moderate rise)	Unchanged
Demand ischemia	Slower

Determinants of Diastolic Function

Myocardial Relaxation

Relaxation of the myocardium is the first step in the physiologic process of diastole (see Fig. 5–2). It begins during the end of the previous systolic contraction and is intimately related to systolic forces. It is also key in the determination of the length and amount of early passive ventricular filling. Relaxation relies heavily on the use of energy and ATP to drive the calcium from the cell into the sarcoplasmic reticulum. This energy-dependent process is controlled by myriad regulatory proteins and by numerous clinical factors (Table 5–4). Failure of relaxation leads to rapid Ca^{++} overload, particularly at increased levels of stimulating frequency.[25] This may explain the diastolic dysfunction associated with the use of pacemakers set at high rates[26] (Fig. 5–6).

The primary determinant of ventricular isovolumic relaxation is the peak negative pressure drop in the ventricle during relaxation measured by taking the first derivative of the LV pressure tracing. This can be measured by accurate invasive micromanometer pressure transducers in the LV. The time constant of relaxation (tau), which is a measure of relative relaxation, is obtained by taking the peak negative pressure drop and relating it to the monoexponential decay of relaxation to the level of about 5 mm Hg. The fact that an arbitrary value is used for the low end of decay may lead to some inducible error.[27] By relating this drop in pressure to time, tau is less afterload and contractility dependent than negative peak pressure alone.[28] In a clinical study comparing hypertrophic cardiomyopathy (HOCM) patients (i.e., diastolic dysfunction) with normal control patients, Kato et al found increases in tau and left ventricular end-diastolic pressure (LVEDP) in HOCM patients. These increases in tau and LVEDP were discovered by using noninvasive tissue Doppler to determine the peak negative myocardial velocity gradient, which is a noninvasive index of diastolic function.[29] The continued development of advanced technologies in tissue imaging and measurement is leading to further understanding of diastolic function and its relationship to pathology.

PASSIVE VENTRICULAR FILLING

The first phase of filling starts with the opening of the MV and the flow of blood down the newly generated pressure gradient from the LA into the LV. The rate of flow has both a rapid rate and slow rate as the pressure gradient approaches equilibration. Diastasis is the period of no flow across the MV after the conclusion of passive filling and immediately prior to atrial systole. The main determinants of transmitral flow

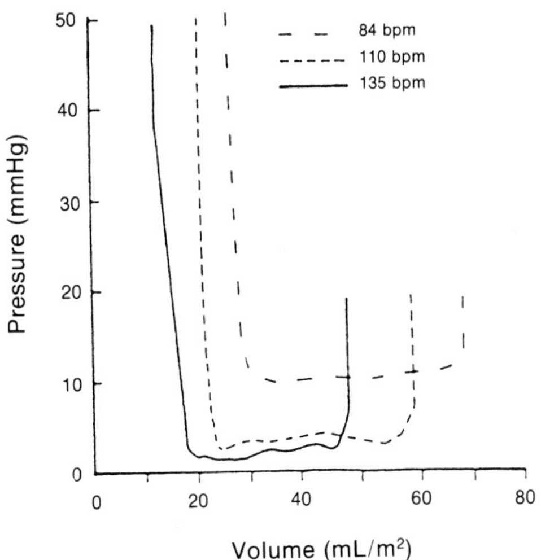

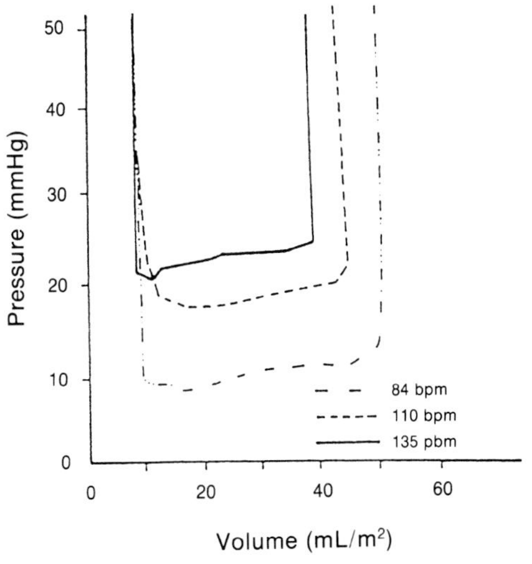

Figure 5–6 Response of LV diastolic pressure and volume at different paced heart rates in a patient with normal coronary arteries *(left)* and in a patient with coronary artery disease *(right)*. In the normal patient, diastolic pressure and volume decreased with increasing heart rate. In the patient with coronary artery disease, volume decreased but diastolic pressure increased twofold with increasing heart rate. (From Aroesty JM, McKay RG, Heller GV, et al: Simultaneous assessment of left ventricular systolic and diastolic dysfunction during pacing-induced ischemia. Circulation 71:889, 1985.)

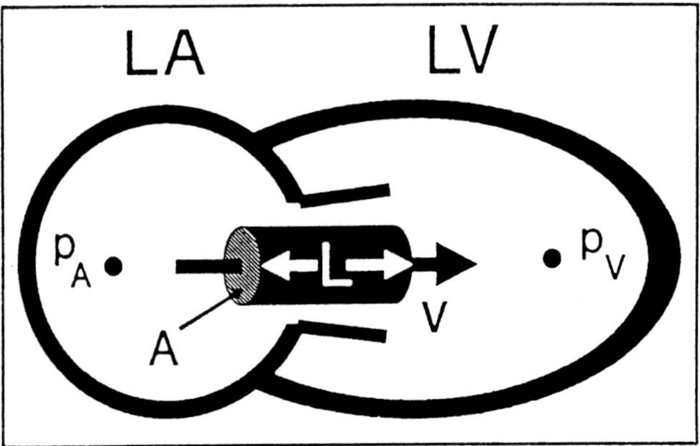

Figure 5–7 Diagram of transmitral blood flow velocity (V). A blood cylinder with area A and length L is accelerated by the pressure difference between left atrial (LA) pressure (P_A) and left ventricular (LV) pressure (P_V). (From Thomas JD, Newell JB, Choong CYP, et al: Physical and physiological determinants of transmitral velocity: Numerical analysis. Am J Physiol 260:H1718, 1991.)

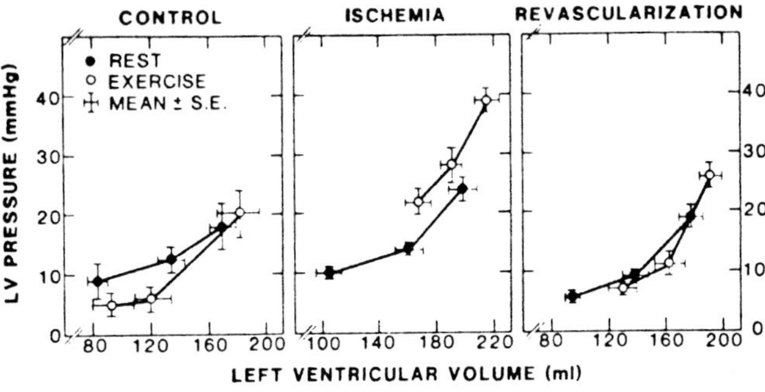

Figure 5–8 Average of the coordinates of the diastolic pressure-volume relationship at three diastolic points in three groups of patients at rest and during exercise. The *middle* and *right panels* represent the same patient group before and after myocardial revascularization, respectively. *(Middle)* Note that exercise shifted the pressure-volume relationship upward to the left during exercise. *(Right)* This sign of diastolic dysfunction had disappeared during postoperative exercise. (From Carroll JD, Hess OM, Hirzel HO, et al: Left ventricular systolic and diastolic function in coronary artery disease: Effects of revascularization on exercise-induced ischemia. Circulation 72:119, 1985.)

are the LV compliance (stiffness) and the rate of rise of the transmitral gradient (Fig. 5–7). High-pressure gradients will accelerate the flow rate, while decreasing compliance (i.e., high LVEDP) will decrease the flow rate.[30] Additional factors such as MV recoil, ventricular diastolic suction, and pericardial constraints can all lead to changes in the passive flow of blood[31,32] (Table 5–5). Firstenberg et al[33] showed that the intraventricular pressure gradient developed by relaxation had direct correlation with filling and eventual systolic function. Many disease states can contribute to increasing stiffness of the ventricle and thus affect the amount of passive filling that can occur during the early phase of diastole. In aging, angina, CAD, and HOCM, myocardial stiffness is greatly increased, thus impairing inflow into the ventricle.[22,34-36] Numerous drugs and cardiac revascularization can all improve dysfunction or reduce exercise-induced stiffness[37,38] (Fig. 5–8). For example, studies have shown an increase in angiotensin-converting enzyme (ACE) in concentric cardiac hypertrophy from hypertension, thus leading to the increased use of ACE inhibitors as a treatment for both cardiac and vascular reasons.[39]

ATRIAL OR ACTIVE FILLING

Atrial contraction, or "atrial kick," occurs at the end of diastole just prior to the closing of the MV and after passive flow has reached the diastasis. Normally, greater than 75% of flow occurs during the passive portion of diastole. In the presence of severe diastolic dysfunction, this normal relationship cannot take place and the atrial kick becomes essential to maintain SV and cardiac output. The atrial kick continues to compensate for decreased LV compliance (increase in LVEDP) and LV filling is initially maintained. Eventually, the increased pressures overcome the capacity of the LA to contribute to the total LV volume, and the atrium assumes a very passive role and becomes dilated. If normal sinus rhythm is not maintained, the atrial kick cannot function in its supportive role, and further CHF occurs rapidly. Reestablishment of normal sinus rhythm by cardioversion or sequential pacing can reverse the CHF symptoms.[40]

Table 5–5 Effect of the Determinants of the Transmitral Pressure Gradient on Transmitral Blood Flow Velocity

Determinant	Change in Peak Transmitral Blood Flow Velocity
High atrial pressure	Increase
Slow ventricular relaxation	Small decrease
Increased myocardial stiffness	Decrease
Increased systolic function	Unchanged

Modified from Thomas JD: Assessment of diastolic heart failure by echocardiography. Heart Failure 7:195, 1991.

Relating Echocardiography to Diastolic Function

The relationship between the stages of diastolic function and findings on both TEE and TTE has greatly enhanced the study and importance of diastolic function (Box 5–2). It is the emergence of these technologies that has led to the inclusion of the following descriptions of echocardiographic means of noninvasively measuring diastolic function. Using TTE and TEE in combination with Doppler techniques has made it possible via indirect means to obtain LV filling patterns.[22,41,42] The most commonly accepted means of analyzing the flow patterns are via the Doppler transmitral flow and the pulmonary vein flow. Newer modes of measurement using tissue Doppler and color M-mode are leading to further insights into diastolic function.

Transmitral flow patterns are the first method, which is performed by placing a pulsed-wave Doppler signal in the area between the MV leaflet tips. Two waves are obtained: first the

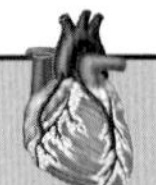
BOX 5–2 ***Diastolic Function Can Be Measured Clinically by Use of***

- Transmitral pulsed-wave Doppler flow patterns
- Pulmonary vein two-dimensional Doppler flow patterns
- Color M-mode Doppler echocardiography

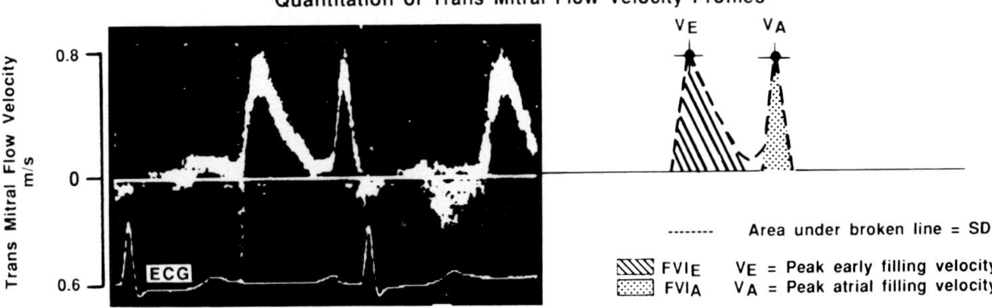

Figure 5–9 Transmitral flow-velocity profile and diagrammatic representation of its quantification.

E wave, which represents the early passive flow across the mitral valve; and second, the A wave, which represents atrial systole (Fig. 5–9). The small area of no flow between the E and A waves represents the diastasis. By comparing the ratios of these two waves, it is possible to form a view of diastolic function. The ratios change with disease and age to yield several patterns, which represent different stages of failure. In early diastolic failure, the E/A wave ratio becomes less than 1, and the waves reverse with the E wave being shorter than the A wave; this is known as the delayed relaxation pattern. As failure progresses, the waves become pseudonormalized; that is, the E/A ratio reverts to the normal pattern of greater than 1. However, the E/A ratio in the pseudonormalized pattern will revert to the delayed relaxation pattern with a preload-reducing Valsalva maneuver. The final stage of failure as seen via the MV shows a high, rapidly decelerating E wave with a small A wave; this pattern is known as the restrictive pattern. The use of these patterns on Doppler imaging allows for the staging of diastolic failure from a mild form to a more severe form. In fact, the restrictive pattern of diastolic dysfunction is associated with poor outcome and increased mortality.[41,42]

The use of pulmonary vein two-dimensional Doppler is becoming more common.[43] It must be interpreted with the data from transmitral flow studies. The normal pulmonary vein flow is a high double-peak systolic flow with a smaller shorter peak diastolic flow and a small flow reversal during atrial contraction. When looking at this in the pseudonormalization stage of failure, a blunting of the systolic flow in the pulmonary vein and a higher diastolic flow are seen, leading to the interpretation of actual diastolic failure and not a normal pattern. These Doppler waves, along with other echocardiographic information, show a good correlation to diastolic function (see Chapter 15).

Color M-mode and *tissue Doppler* are the newest tools with which to evaluate ventricular diastolic dysfunction. These new Doppler applications have been shown to provide an accurate estimation of LV relaxation independent of preload conditions. These modalities are used not only for diagnostic purposes but also for establishing prognosis and evaluating the effect of therapeutic intervention.[41-43]

In contrast to standard pulsed-wave Doppler, which provides the temporal distribution of blood flow velocities in a specific location, color M-mode Doppler echocardiography provides the spatiotemporal distribution of these velocities across a vertical line. Thus, the information displayed in a color M-mode recording of the LV inflow is comparable to the tracing of multiple simultaneous pulsed-wave Doppler from the mitral orifice to the apex (Fig. 15–15). This figure demonstrates the typical pattern displayed by normal patients in sinus rhythm. A first wave corresponds to the early filling (E wave), and atrial contractions are manifested by the second wave (A wave). The slope of the color wavefront is the velocity at which flow propagates within the ventricle (Vp). In normal ventricles, the spatial position of the maximal velocity is closer to the ventricle than the apex, suggesting that intraventricular pressure gradient during the early filling E wave produces a suction force that accelerates flow beyond the mitral orifice. The recoil of the apex produces the suction mechanism drawing blood from the mid and basal portions of the heart during early diastole. These gradients are markedly reduced in ischemia and cardiomyopathy.[44,45]

Doppler ultrasound has been used for the measurement of blood flow velocities across intravascular structures using red blood cells, which reflect low-amplitude Doppler signals and relatively high velocity. In contrast, moving tissue (i.e., myocardium) reflects low velocities and high-amplitude Doppler signals. To display these tissue velocities, two alterations in the Doppler signal processing are required: (1) bypass the high-pass filter and (2) use a lower gain amplification to eliminate the weaker signals. Thus, tissue Doppler echocardiography (TDE) can be used in different acoustic windows to quantify myocardial velocities in multiple segments of the myocardium. Typical display will show a velocity signal directed toward the LV centroid during systole (Sm) and two signals directed away during diastole early (Em) and late (Am) (Fig. 15–16).

In a normal young patient, the TDE velocities resemble the mitral inflow velocity and they change the same way with age. What makes TDE a better diagnostic tool is its ability to differentiate between restrictive cardiomyopathy and constrictive pericarditis; Em will be normal or high in patients with constrictive pericarditis who have normal systolic function.[45] It has also been found that TDE is very sensitive in detecting rejection in heart transplant patients.[43]

SYSTOLIC FUNCTION

Systolic function is the period existing between closure of the MV and the start of contraction to the end of ejection of blood from the heart. The primary purpose of systole is the ejection of blood into the circulation via the generation of a pressure gradient. Systolic function has been used to determine outcome and therapeutic effectiveness for years. The use of TEE in the operating room allows for the evaluation of function during cardiac surgery, leading to better real-time treatment to improve the outcome of patients. What was once a tool of cardiologists has now become a tool of the anesthesiologist in the operating room/intensive care unit (see Chapters 15, 16, 19, 31, and 33).

Cardiac Output

CO is the amount of blood flowing into the circulation per minute. It reflects not only the condition of the heart but also the entire vascular system and is subject to the autoregulatory systems of the vasculature and tissues.[46] CO may not adjust to the requirements of the tissues in the presence of severe cardiac failure, leading to multiorgan system failure. The equation for CO is listed below and involves HR and SV.

$$CO = SV \times HR \quad (5)$$

The primary determinants for CO are the HR and the SV. It is also dependent on many other secondary factors, including venous return, systemic vascular resistance, peripheral oxygen use, total blood volume, respiration, and body position. Normal range of CO is between 5 and 6 L/min in a 70-kg man, with an SV of 60 to 90 mL per beat and an HR of 80 beats per minute. CO is highly variable in the normal healthy individual, being able to increase up to 25 to 30 L/min during situations of high metabolic demand.

The cardiac index (CI) is used to compare different sizes of individuals and is now part of routine clinical practice. This is done by correcting the standard CO equation for body surface area (BSA).

$$CI = (SV \times HR)/BSA \quad (6)$$

$$CI = CO/BSA \quad (7)$$

Normal values are 2.5 to 3.5 L/min/m^2 for the normal 70-kg man. By correcting for BSA, it is then possible to compare patients at a common level of function, despite differences in body habitus (see Chapter 14 for a detailed discussion of measurement techniques for CO).

Stroke Volume

The SV is the amount of blood ejected by the ventricle with each single contraction. Within the pressure-volume relationship, the SV is readily recognized as the difference between the EDV and the ESV (see Fig. 5–4). The determinants of SV are analogous to those of the force-velocity-length measurements in isolated muscle preparations: preload, afterload, and contractility. Although these variables have a very clear meaning in reference to isolated muscles, their exact significance is much more ambiguous in the intact heart.

Preload

DEFINITION

Preload is equal to the ventricular wall stress at end-diastole. It is determined by ventricular EDV, end-diastolic pressure (EDP), and wall thickness. The interaction of these factors is expressed by the Laplace equation. To apply the preload principle to clinical practice, the following adjustments can be made:

1. *Substituting ventricular volumes for preload stress.* Changes in preload are usually not expressed by changes in stress but by changes in ventricular EDV. In clinical practice, ventricular volumes appear to most closely approximate muscle fiber length. In normal humans, a straight-line relationship has been demonstrated between EDV and SV.[47]
2. *Substituting ventricular pressures for ventricular volumes.* Ventricular pressures are often substituted for ventricular volumes when assessing the filling conditions of the ventricle. In humans, an LVEDV of 70 to 100 mL/m^2 generates an EDP of 12 mm Hg, provided the distensibility of the ventricle is normal. Clinically, left atrial pressure (LAP), pulmonary artery occlusion or capillary wedge pressure (PAOP or PCWP), pulmonary artery diastolic pressure (PADP), right atrial pressure (RAP), and central venous pressure (CVP) are often used as substitutes for LVEDP and LVEDV. Their accuracy in predicting LV preload is determined by the distensibility properties of the ventricle, the integrity of the mitral valve, the presence of normal pulmonary conditions, the integrity of the pulmonic and tricuspid valves, and RV function.

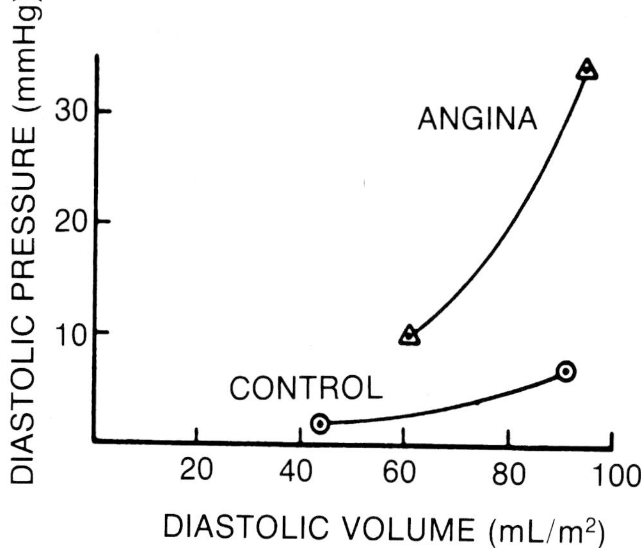

Figure 5–10 LV diastolic pressure-volume relationship during an attack of variant angina. The more than threefold rise in diastolic pressure that occurred during the anginal attack was due to decreased compliance, which shifted the diastolic pressure-volume curve upward. (From Gaasch WH, Apstein CS, Levine HJ: Diastolic properties of the left ventricle. *In* Levine HJ, Gaasch WH [eds]: The Ventricle. Boston, Martinus Nijhoff Publishing, 1985, p 143.)

The assumption that ventricular distensibility is normal is not a valid assumption in many patients with cardiac disease. With coronary artery disease (CAD) or aortic disease, diastolic function is often altered so that small increases in ventricular volume can produce large changes in ventricular pressure (Fig. 5–10).

DETERMINANTS

Factors affecting the preload of the heart include the total blood volume, body position, intrathoracic pressure, intrapericardial pressure, venous tone, pumping action of skeletal muscles, and the atrial contribution to ventricular filling.[48-50]

The total blood volume is about 70 to 75 mL/kg and is distributed between intrathoracic (15%) and extrathoracic (85%) compartments. The extrathoracic blood volume is divided among veins (70%), arteries (10%), and capillaries (5%). More blood can be stored in the venous system because the venous compliance or capacitance is about 20 times larger than arterial. Changes in total blood volume thus mostly affect venous blood volume. Compliance (C) is defined by the ratio of the change in volume (dV) over change in pressure (dP). Venous pressure can be increased by infusion of blood or fluids into the venous reservoir or by decreasing venous com-

Table 5–6 **Causes of Perioperative Ventricular Hypovolemia**
Diminished Intravascular Volume
Surgical bleeding
Extravasation
Excessive diuresis
Reduced fluid intake
Reduced Venous Return
Increased capacitance (consider: anesthetic, vasodilators, sympatholytics)
Increased resistance to venous flow (consider: PEEP, acute pulmonary HTN, PE, atrial masses, tamponade, univentricular failure)

PEEP = positive end-expiratory pressure; HTN = hypertension; PE = pulmonary embolism.

Table 5–7 **Perioperative Ventricular Hypervolemia**
Causes
Regurgitant valvular heart lesions
Ischemic heart disease
Viral and idiopathic cardiomyopathy
Chronic pulmonary and systemic hypertension
End-stage stenotic valvular lesions
Consequences
Increase in wall tension
Increase in myocardial oxygen consumption
Reduced contractility
Management Goals
Vasodilators (consider nitroglycerin, nitroprusside, hydralazine, ACE inhibitors)
Diuretics
Inotropic support
Ventricular assist devices
Surgery when applicable

ACE = angiotensin-converting enzyme.

pliance. Venomotor tone is controlled by local, regional, and central autonomic nervous mechanisms and pharmacologic interventions on the muscles of the vessel wall. Neural mechanisms enhance venous tone during muscular exercise, anxiety, and marked hypotension. Common causes of changing preload are decreases or increases in blood volume (Tables 5–6 and 5–7).

The venous pressure gradient between the peripheral and central parts of the venous system causes blood to be returned to the right heart and fill the RV during diastole until RVEDV is reached at end-diastole. The pulmonary circulation, like the venous system, is a low-pressure, high-compliance system. The pulmonary venous pressure is determined by the combined effects of pulmonary blood flow, postcapillary venous tone, intrapulmonary pressure, and impedance to LA/LV inflow (atrial tumors, mitral valve disease, LV dysfunction with elevation of LVEDP) (see RV function discussion later).

Large increases in HR decrease the duration of diastole and, hence, can lower preload. Synchronous atrial contraction makes a significant contribution to LV preload. This is best seen when a patient develops a nodal rhythm. There are often 10% to 30% decreases in blood pressure (BP) and CO with loss of the atrial contraction. The hemodynamic effect of loss of this contribution to preload is most severe in patients with decreased LV compliance (aortic stenosis or idiopathic hypertrophic subaortic stenosis) (see Chapter 20).

MEASUREMENT

The LVEDV is difficult to measure clinically, and measurements have only recently become possible with techniques such as echocardiography, ventriculography, radionuclide scans, and conductance catheters, all of which can be used in the operating room or the intensive care unit. TEE has been extensively used to measure LV areas as an approximation of LV volumes; however, it is limited by its two-dimensionality. Some studies have found a good correlation between areas and volumes, and have also shown that in surgical patients, EDV derived from a single plane is a significant determinant of SV.[51,52]

The LVEDP can be measured with placement of a catheter into the LA. The LA catheter is commonly inserted surgically through one of the pulmonary veins. The LAP provides a good approximation of LVEDP, provided the mitral valve is normal (Fig. 5–11).[53] The most common technique for the estimation of LVEDP during cardiac surgery is the placement of a pulmonary artery catheter (PAC).[54] The PCWP usually provides a good approximation of LVEDP. Marked alterations in airway pressure, such as occur during the use of high levels of positive end-expiratory pressure (PEEP), may disturb the relationship between the PCWP and LAP.[55] Depending on the compliance of the pulmonary parenchyma, either part or all of the airway pressure may be transmitted to the PAC. This must be considered when evaluating LV filling pressure with the PAC in patients receiving mechanical ventilation and PEEP. When the catheter cannot be advanced into the wedge position, the PADP may be used to estimate the LVEDP. It is usually quite accurate unless the pulmonary vascular resistance (PVR) is markedly elevated. The CVP provides the poorest estimate of LVEDP, although it is frequently used in patients with good function of the RV and LV. When cardiac disease is characterized by disparate RV and LV functions, the CVP may be misleading as an indicator of LVEDP.[56] It is important to remember that LV and RV preload and function curves are not always equal or even parallel.[57] However, the CVP is a reasonably good reflection of RV preload. It accurately reflects RVEDV in most cases, unless a change in RV compliance occurs with events such as an RV infarction.

Afterload

DEFINITION

Afterload is the second major determinant of the mechanical properties of cardiac muscle fibers and performance of the intact heart (Box 5–3). Afterload can be considered either as the stress imposed on the ventricular wall during systole or as the arterial impedance to the ejection of SV.

WALL STRESS

Afterload defined as systolic ventricular wall stress is the burden that the RV or LV wall has to shoulder for ejecting its

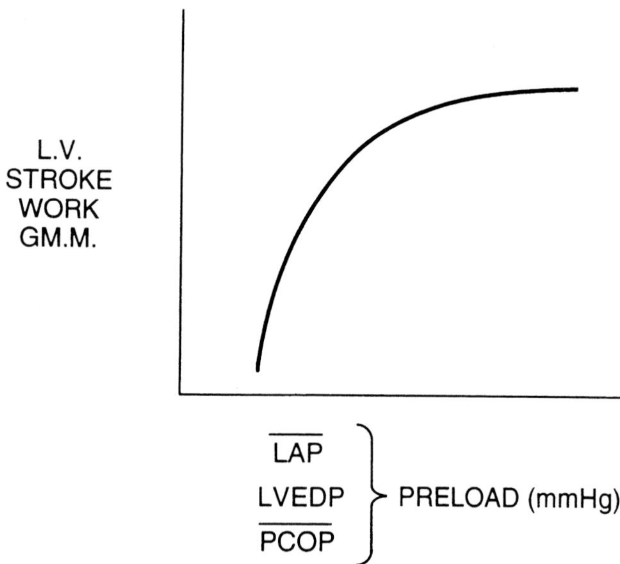

Figure 5–11 The Frank-Starling relation of chamber diastolic length (represented as left ventricular end-diastolic pressure [LVEDP], pulmonary capillary occlusion pressure [PCOP], or left atrial pressure [LAP]) and ventricular performance (cardiac output [CO], stroke volume [SV], cardiac index [CI], left ventricular [LV] stroke work). With increasing diastolic muscle-fiber length, that is, preload, both LV and right ventricular performance can increase steadily. However, once the limit of preload reserve is reached, myocardial performance cannot be enhanced further by augmenting SV.

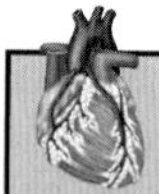

BOX 5–3 *Measurements of Afterload Are*

- Wall stress
- Impedance
- Effective arterial elastance
- Systolic intraventricular pressure
- Systemic vascular resistance
- Pulmonary vascular resistance

SV. This stress can be expressed and quantified by the Laplace equation:

$$\sigma = \frac{P \cdot r}{2h} \tag{8}$$

where σ is the stress (dynes·cm^{-2}), P the pressure generated by the LV throughout systole, and r and h the corresponding radius and thickness of RV or LV wall.

It is convenient to consider wall stress at specific moments of the ejection phase (e.g., at the start of ejection, at peak ventricular pressure, and at end-systole). Stress at end-systole is used because it heralds the end of LV force development in the cardiac cycle beyond which muscle fibers stop shortening.[58] There also exists an inverse relationship between velocity of circumferential fiber shortening (V_{cf}) and LV end-systolic stress ($stress_{ES}$) (Fig. 5–12).

IMPEDANCE

Afterload can also be considered as the external or extracardiac forces (impedance) present in the systemic circulation that oppose ventricular ejection and pulsatile flow. Because the LV is coupled to the systemic circulation through the open aortic valve, the pulsatile flow (SV) and pressure generated by the LV will be hindered by the compliance and resistance of the arterial system. These are determined by the physical properties of the aorta and its side branches (viscoelastic properties and diameter) and by the properties of their content (blood).[59] The amplitude of the components (harmonics) of the pressure and flow waves that travel down the arterial tree will be modified, and the sequence of appearance of pressure and flow waves (phase angle) altered. The ratio of pressure to flow at a given frequency is the impedance for that frequency. Its units are dynes/sec/cm^{-5}. The overall spectrum of ratios and phases determines overall impedance. The impedance at a particular vascular cross-section is termed *input impedance* (e.g., aortic input impedance is the ratio of the pressure moduli to flow moduli at the aortic root).[60,61] Input impedance is affected by reflected waves coming from more distal parts of the circulation. Vasoactive pharmacologic interventions may also modify vascular impedance. When the ratio of pressure to flow is determined at zero frequency (nonpulsatile or steady flow), resistance is obtained. The SVR clinically obtained as the ratio of the pressure differential between mean arterial pressure (MAP) and RAP or CVP and CO is an oversimplified version of the resistance calculated at zero-frequency impedance and does not take the pulsatile nature of blood flow into consideration.[58] It is based on the circulatory analog of Ohm's law:

$$Q = P/R \tag{9}$$

or

$$P = Q \times R \tag{10}$$

that determines that the pressure (P) generated during the ejection of a given flow (Q) is proportional to that flow and to the resistance (R) encountered by that flow. This resistance is mainly determined by arteriolar resistance (SVR) so that

$$SVR = [MAP - RAP]/CO \tag{11}$$

There also exists an inverse relationship between CO and SVR. Rearrangement of the SVR equation so that (MAP – RAP) = CO × SVR shows that identical MAP levels can exist under conditions of high CO and low SVR or under conditions of low CO and high SVR. The shift from a low CO/high SVR condition to a more favorable high CO/low SVR condition can be achieved by the use of vasodilators. The rationale of the treatment of LV or RV failure by afterload reduction is based on this principle. Increasing SVR will shift RV or LV function curves downward, and decreasing SVR will shift the curves upward[62] (Fig. 5–13).

EFFECTIVE ARTERIAL ELASTANCE

This definition of afterload also takes the coupling of the LV to the arterial system into consideration. However, rather than looking at the pressure-to-volume ratio in a dynamic setting, it captures this relationship at end-systole (E_{ES}). The effective arterial elastance (E_a) is a measure of afterload that describes a mechanical characteristic of the vascular system. It is based on the observation that for any bolus of blood (SV) ejected into the arterial system, a pressure will be generated. If the SV is larger, the pressure will be higher. When various values of SV versus end-systolic pressure (ESP) are plotted, a linear relation is obtained: the *effective arterial elastance.* The slope of this relation is steep when the afterload is high, flatter when the afterload is low. Because the slope (E_a) of the arterial end-systolic pressure-volume relationship (AESPVR) does not change much with arterial compliance but does change sub-

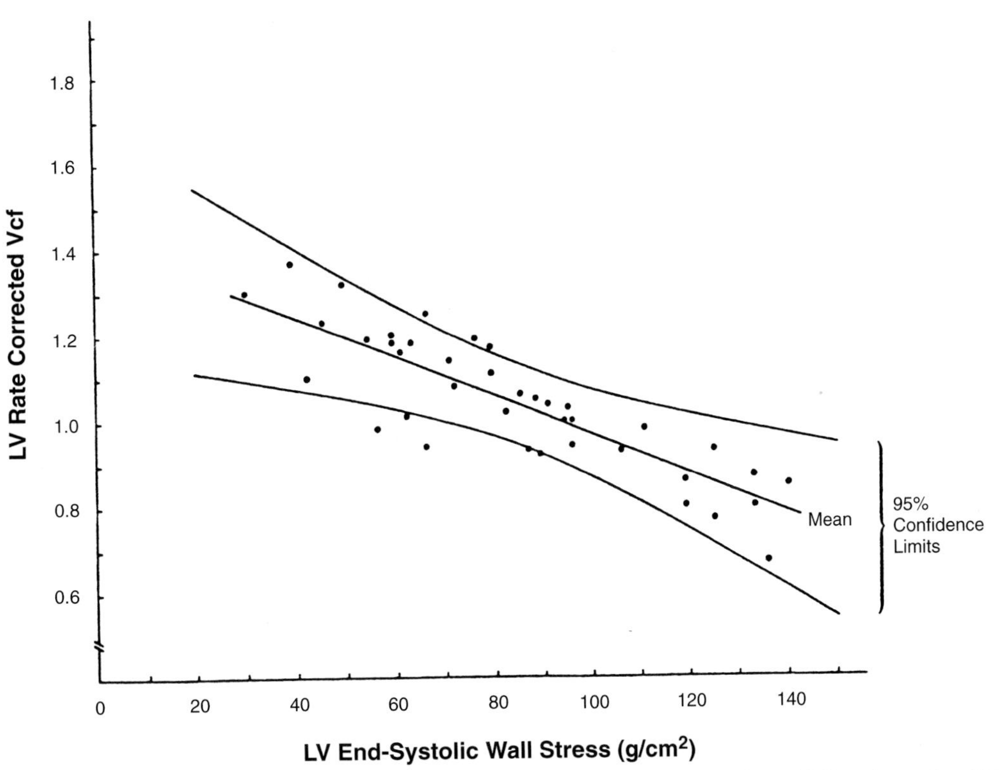

Figure 5–12 Inverse relationship between LV end-systolic stress ($stress_{ES}$) and LV velocity of circumferential fiber shortening (V_{cf}). (From Lang RM, Borow KM, Neuman A, Janzen D: Systemic vascular resistance: An unreliable index of left ventricular afterload. Circulation 74:1114, 1986.)

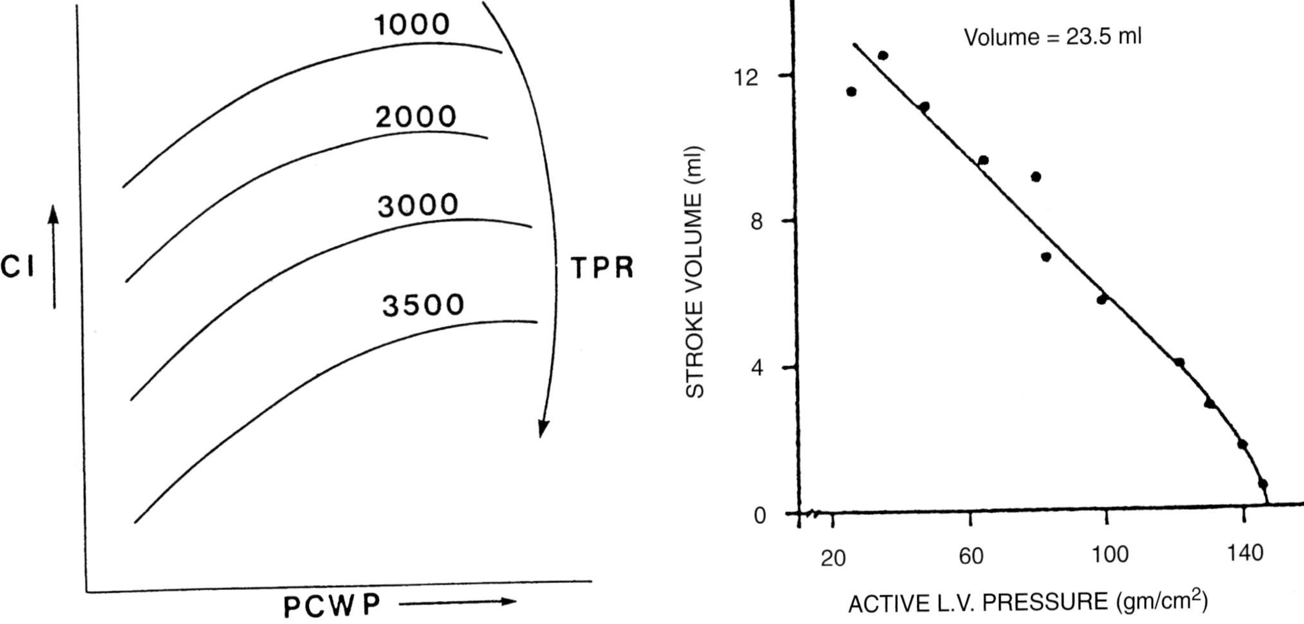

Figure 5–13 A family of Frank-Starling curves is demonstrated with the cardiac index (CI) on the vertical axis and the pulmonary capillary wedge pressure (PCWP) on the horizontal axis. As total peripheral resistance (TPR) is increased from 1000 toward 3500 dynes/sec/cm^{-5}, the curves are shifted down to the right. (From Braunwald E: Determinants and assessment of cardiac function. N Engl J Med 296:86, 1977.)

Figure 5–14 Inverse relationship between left ventricular (LV) pressure and stroke volume during contractions with increasing LV systolic pressure in the isotonically contracting left ventricle of the dog, at constant LV end-diastolic volume (23.5 mL). (Reproduced from Burns JW, Covell JW, Ross J Jr: Mechanics of isotonic left ventricular contractions. Am J Physiol 224:725, 1973.)

stantially with changes in SVR, it is reasonable to consider E_a as an index of vascular resistance and of afterload.[63]

SYSTOLIC INTRAVENTRICULAR PRESSURE

Intraventricular pressure is an important component of afterload (Fig. 5–14) and an inverse relationship exists between SV and LV pressure. When the systolic arterial pressure suddenly increases, as after cross-clamping of the thoracic aorta, SV initially decreases and then normalizes through a compensatory increase in LVEDV or heterometric autoregulation (Fig. 5–15). Later, the initial increase in EDV is followed by an increase in cardiac contractility while LVEDV and LVEDP normalize.

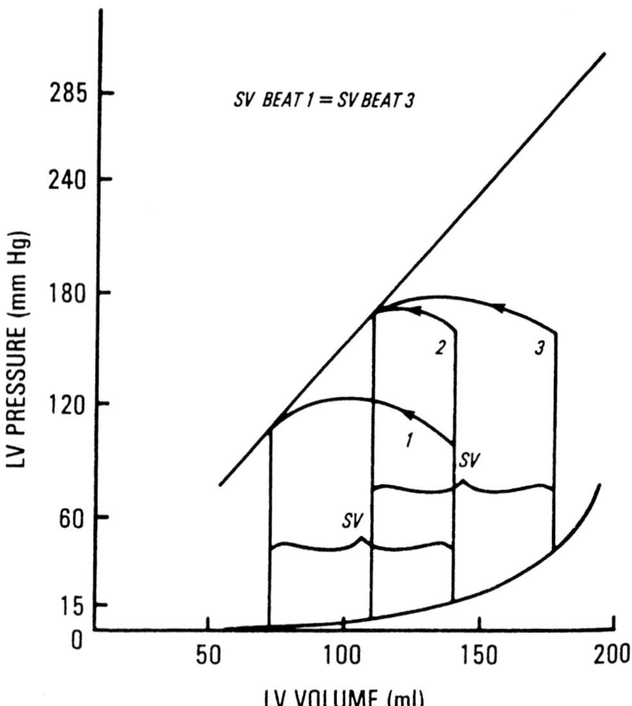

Figure 5–15 When LV pressure suddenly increases, stroke volume (SV) drops initially (SV_1 to SV_2). Later, the first adjustment consists of an increase in LV end-diastolic volume with normalization of SV (SV_2 to SV_3 = SV_1), which is a compensation (heterometric autoregulation) that occurs through the Starling mechanism. (Reproduced from Ross J Jr: The cardiac pump. *In* West JB [ed]: Physiologic Basis of Medical Practice. Baltimore, Williams & Wilkins, 1991.)

This phenomenon is called the *Anrep phenomenon*, and the adaptive mechanism that explains it is called *homeometric autoregulation*.[64,65]

Assuming an MAP of 80 mm Hg, an RAP of 10 mm Hg, and a CO of 5 L/min, SVR amounts to 14 mm Hg/L/min or Wood units. SVR can also be expressed by the more fundamental, but less convenient, dynes·sec·cm^{-5} units by multiplying the Wood units by 79.9. Normal values for SVR are in the range of 900 to 1500 dynes·sec·cm^{-5}. In clinical practice, SVR is the most commonly used index of afterload. However, when comparing the influence of various pressor agents on SVR and end-systolic stress, Lang et al[58] observed that, compared with end-systolic stress, SVR consistently underestimates drug-induced decreases in afterload and overestimates drug-induced increases in afterload.

Contractility

Definition

The third determinant of SV is contractility. Contractility is an intrinsic property of the cardiac cell that defines the amount of work that the heart can perform at a given load. Contractility is primarily determined by the availability of intracellular Ca^{++}. With depolarization of the cardiac cell, a small amount of Ca^{++} enters the cell and triggers the release of additional Ca^{++} from intracellular storage sites (sarcoplasmic reticulum). The Ca^{++} binds to troponin, tropomyosin is displaced from the active binding site on actin, and actin-myosin crossbridges are formed.[66] All agents with positive inotropic properties, such as the catecholamines, have in common that they increase intracellular Ca^{++}, whereas negative inotropes have the opposite effect (Table 5–8).

Table 5–8 Factors Affecting Contractility

Factors Increasing Contractility
Sympathetic stimulation—direct increases of the force of contraction, as well as indirect increases due to increased heart rate (rate treppe effect, or Bowditch phenomenon)
Parasympathetic inhibition producing increased heart rate
Administration of positive inotropic drugs such as digitalis
Factors Decreasing Contractility
Parasympathetic stimulation—decreased rate effect
Sympathetic inhibition via withdrawal of catecholamines or blockade of adrenergic receptors
Administration of β-adrenergic–blocking drugs, slow calcium channel blockers, or other myocardial depressants
Myocardial ischemia and infarction
Intrinsic myocardial diseases such as cardiomyopathies
Hypoxia and acidosis

Determinants

The large number of methods developed to measure contractility in the intact heart suggest that it is difficult to measure. Indices of contractility can be classified according to the phase of the cardiac cycle during which they are obtained.

Isovolumic Contraction Phase Indices. Isovolumic phase indices are obtained during the isovolumic phase of the contraction prior to the opening of the aortic valve. The paradigm of such indices is dP/dt. It is obtained by placing a catheter with a micromanometer at its tip into the LV. The LV pressure is continuously sampled while an electronic differentiator calculates the first derivative of pressures, or dP/dt (mm Hg/sec). The highest value of dP/dt, or peak dP/dt, is considered proportional to contractility. Because the heart's developed tension, or pressure, is dependent on the initial length of the cardiac muscle, it is predictable that dP/dt will be preload dependent.

Ejection Phase Indices. The standard ejection phase index of contractility is the EF:

$$EF = SV/EDV \qquad (12)$$

With the increasing availability of noninvasive cardiac imaging techniques, ejection phase indices are widely used in clinical practice. One of the reasons for their widespread use is that a clear association between EF and prognosis has been found. Mock et al demonstrated that in medically treated patients with CAD, those with a low EF had a worse prognosis regardless of the number of affected coronary vessels.[67]

Load-Independent Indices. Because traditional indices of contractility are load dependent, different approaches to the quantification of the contractile properties of the heart have been explored. In one such approach, Suga et al[68,69] studied instantaneous pressure and volume in the canine heart. The ratio of ventricular pressure over volume is the ventricular elastance, which varies throughout the cardiac cycle (*time-varying elastance*). For each cardiac cycle, Suga et al[68,69] defined the maximal value of this ratio as the end-systolic elastance (E_{ES}) and the point at which it was reached as the end-systolic

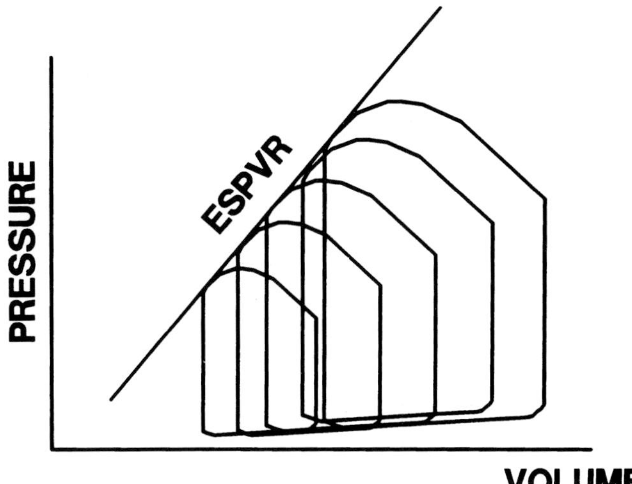

Figure 5–16 The end-systolic pressure-volume relationship (ESPVR) is obtained by connecting all the end-systolic points measured during a rapid decrease in preload.

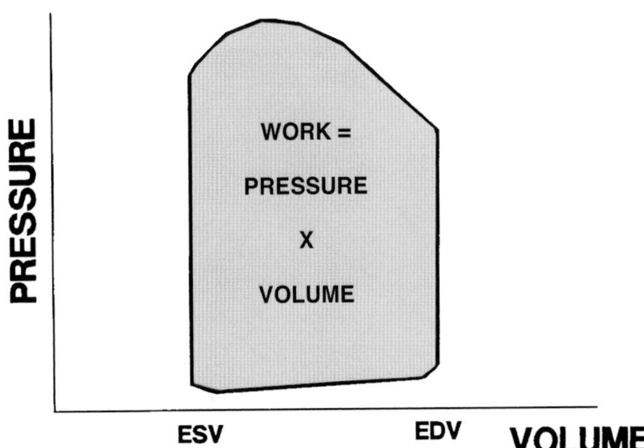

Figure 5–18 Mechanical work is equal to the product of pressure and volume. ESV = end-systolic volume; EDV = end-diastolic volume.

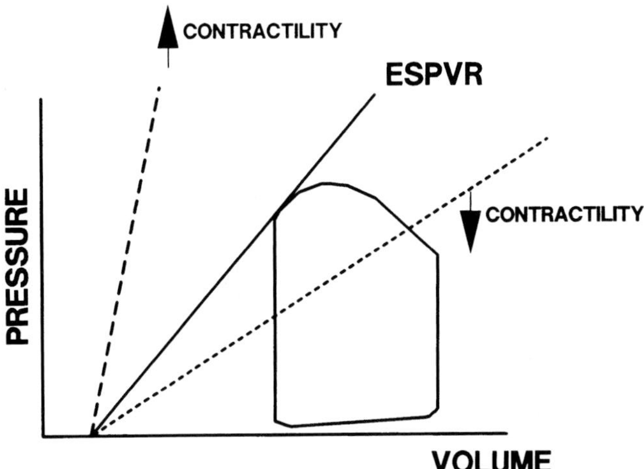

Figure 5–17 The slope of the ESPVR line is proportional to contractility; it is steeper at higher contractility and flatter at lower contractility.

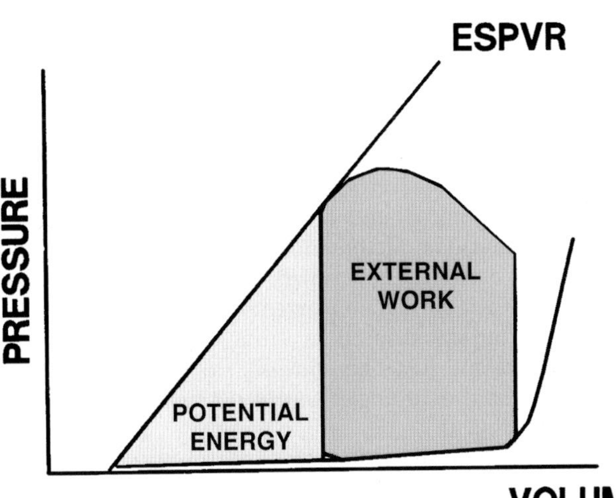

Figure 5–19 The total oxygen consumption of the heart is equal to the sum of the oxygen required for mechanical work and the end-systolic elastic potential energy. ESPVR = end-systolic pressure-volume relation.

point. They further noted that with rapid decreases in preload, all consecutive end-systolic points were positioned on a single straight line, known as the end-systolic pressure-volume relation (ESPVR) (Fig. 5–16). The slope of this line (E_{ES}) is proportional to contractility; it is steeper at higher contractility and flatter at lower contractility (Fig. 5–17).

The ESPVR concept provides such a useful framework for analysis of ventricular function that it warrants in-depth study. In addition, with the introduction of new technology, such as echocardiography and conductance catheters, the ability to continuously measure ventricular volumes is rapidly becoming a reality.[70-72]

The ESPVR can also yield some information about myocardial energy and oxygen utilization. Suga et al[73] discovered that the area inside the pressure-volume loop related proportionally to the amount of mechanical work performed inside the heart. They took the ESPVR and extrapolated the line to a theoretical zero volume. As seen in Figure 5–19, this creates a triangle on the left side of the graph that relates to the basal metabolic and coupling energy requirements of the myocardium. Inotropes increase both contractility (increase the slope of the ESPVR) and all portions of myocardial oxygen consumption[74] (Fig. 5–20).

Another measure of contractility shown to be somewhat independent of loading factors has been preload-recruitable stroke work (PRSW).[75-77] The measurement of PRSW was first demonstrated in 1985, as the relationship between the LV stroke work and the EDV.[75] A linear relationship obtained from plotting EDV and LV stroke work appears to be related to contractility that is independent (within physiologic ranges) of preload and afterload.[75-77]

The newest measurement of contractility makes great use of TDE to describe regional LV function. Vogel et al described a technique of using TDE to determine the isovolumic myocardial acceleration (IVA). IVA is simple measurement of the rate of acceleration of the myocardial tissues taken by sampling the peak and basal velocities then dividing them by their time interval.[78] While not yet ready for clinical practice, this method shows great promise in yielding a load-independent minimally invasive method for determining contractility.

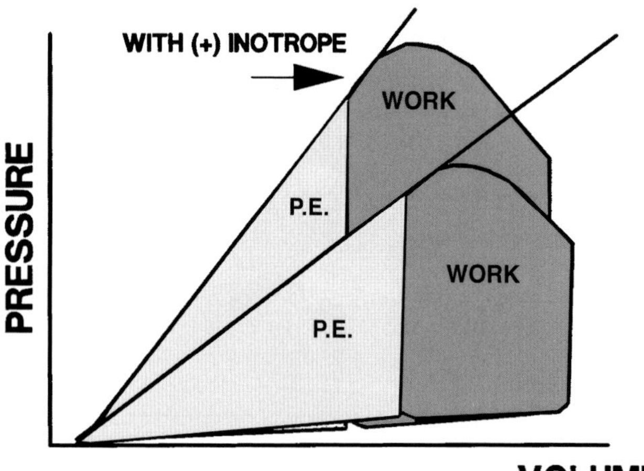

Figure 5–20 The administration of a positive inotrope results not only in increased mechanical work but also in increased potential energy (PE).

Heart Rate

The second major determinate of CO is HR. It is one of the most variable determinants of overall cardiac function. It also has great importance to all portions of the cardiac cycle. The HR is controlled by multiple systems, such as the cardiac conduction system, central nervous system, and autonomic nervous system, which respond via complex pathways to changes in the internal and external conditions. Besides the neural and hormonal factors, many pharmacologic controls are available as well. The primary determinant of HR lies within the cardiac conduction system—the rate of slow depolarization of the sinoatrial node at the junction of the superior vena cava and RA. This intrinsic rhythm operates even without standard neurologic controls as shown in the heart transplant recipient.

Neural mechanisms exert some control over the natural HR in the intact heart by altering conduction velocity at the AV node. Signals from autonomic receptors in the circulation are transmitted to the brain stem where adjustments are made to increase HR via the sympathetic system or decrease HR via the vagal system. The normal heart with a typical resting HR of 70 beats/minute is controlled predominantly by vagal tone.[79,80] The loss of vagal tone leads to a faster HR as seen in denervated hearts.[81,82] The loss of the vagal system also decreased responsiveness to atropine and other chronotropic substances, especially in aging, failing hearts.[81,82]

An interesting relationship is the fact that HR itself can increase the contractility of the heart (Table 5–9). This is known as the treppe or step (Bowditch) phenomenon, which shows that at increased HRs, the slope of the ESPVR increases in a stepwise fashion related to the increased rate[83,84] (Fig. 5–21). This increase is thought to be due to increases in the level of intracellular calcium. Therefore, as described earlier, the increased calcium allows for increased excitation/contraction coupling and increased contractility. This buildup of calcium can cause calcium overload during tachycardic situations, leading to failure.

Table 5–9 Effect of Increasing Heart Rate on Cardiac Function

Shortening of systole
Shortening of diastole
Decreased left ventricular myocardial perfusion time
Decrease in ventricular filling
Rate-dependent change in stroke volume
Rate-dependent change in cardiac output
Rate-dependent positive inotropic effect

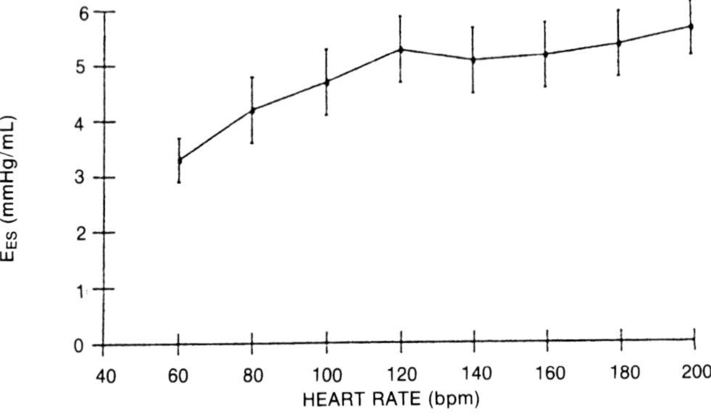

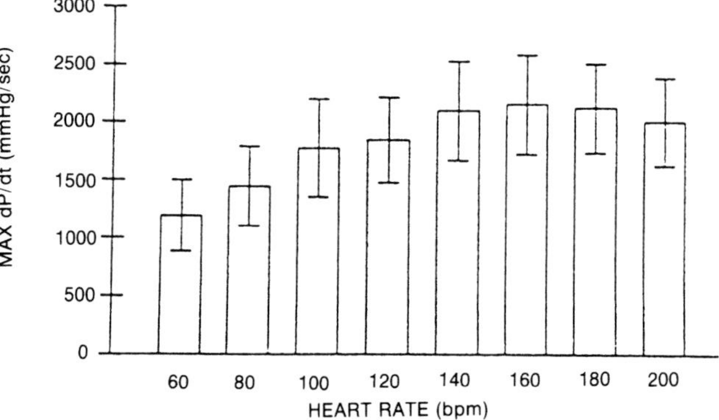

Figure 5–21 Relationship between heart rate and the slope of the ESPVR (*top;* bars are standard errors) and effect of heart rate on peak changes in tension over time (dP/dt) *(bottom)*. (Modified from Maughan WL, Sunagawa K, Burkhoff D, et al: Effect of heart rate on the canine end-systolic pressure-volume relationship. Circulation 72:654, 1985.)

RIGHT VENTRICULAR FUNCTION

The contractile pattern, as well as the afterload presented to each ventricle (i.e., RV versus LV), results in marked physiologic differences between the ventricles (Box 5–4). In contrast to the LV, which has a relatively simple and unified mechanism of contraction (by coaxial shortening), RV contraction occurs in three distinct phases. Initially, the spiral muscles contract, resulting in a downward movement of the tricuspid valve and shortening of the longitudinal axis of the RV chamber. This is followed by movement of the RV free wall

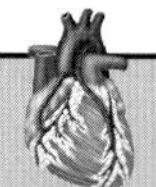

BOX 5–4 ***In Comparison to the Left Ventricle, the Right Ventricle Is***

- More complex with phases of contraction
- Better suited to eject large volumes of blood
- More sensitive to afterload
- Less sensitive to preload

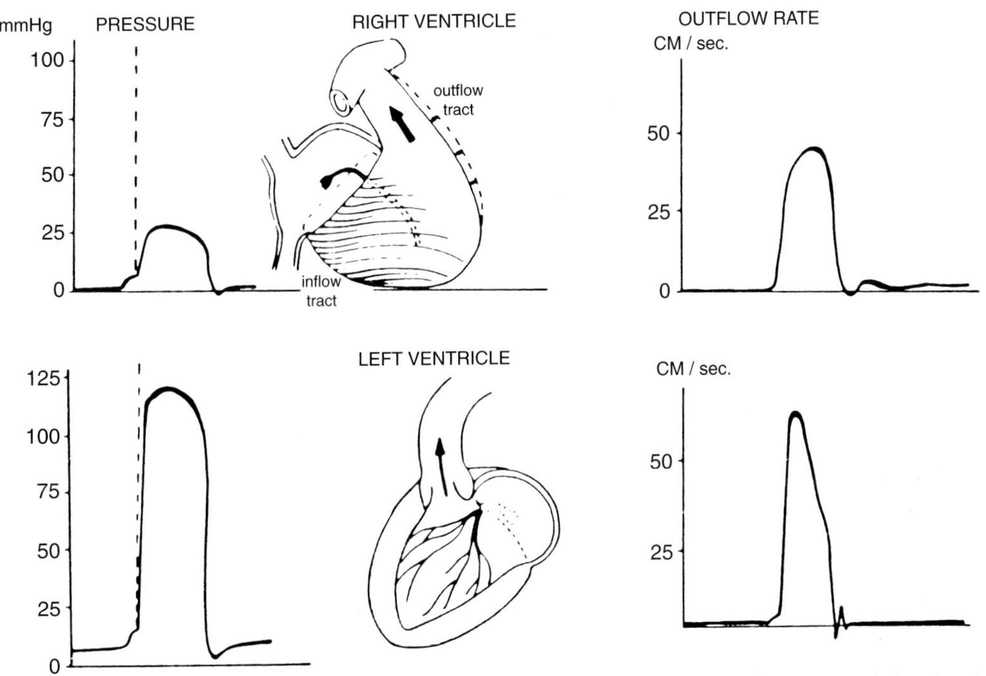

Figure 5–22 Comparison of pressure and ejection rate patterns of right and left ventricles. (From Rushmer RF, et al: Functional anatomy of cardiac contraction. *In* Rushmer RF [ed]: Structure and Function of the Cardiovascular System. Philadelphia, WB Saunders Company, 1972, pp 33-69.)

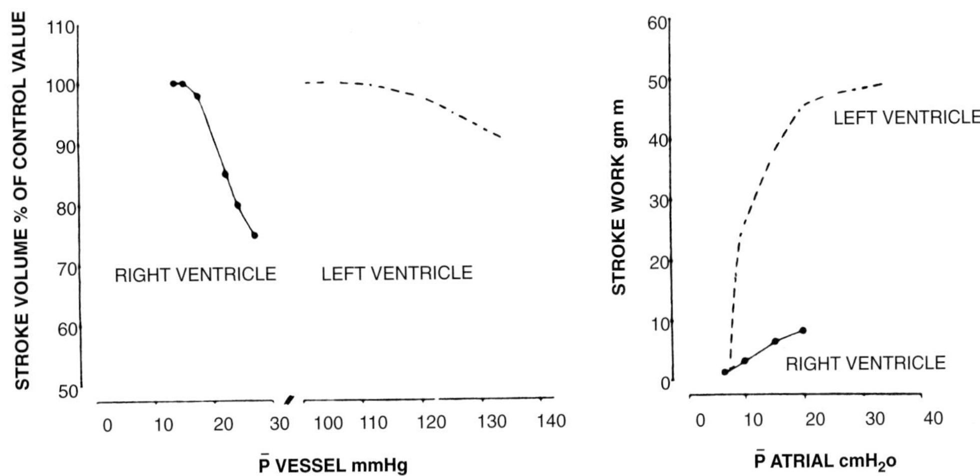

Figure 5–23 Varying effects of afterload and preload seen in ventricular function curves from the right and left ventricles. The RV output is more afterload dependent and less preload dependent than the LV. (From McFadden ER, Braunwald E: Cor pulmonale and pulmonary thromboembolism. *In* Braunwald E [ed]: Textbook of Cardiovascular Medicine. Philadelphia, WB Saunders Company, 1980, pp 1643–1680.)

inward toward the intraventricular septum (IVS). Because the RV free wall has limited muscular power, alterations in or failure of the IVS to contract normally will disturb the systolic function of the RV to a *much greater* degree than does a loss of RV free wall contractility. Finally, the third phase of RV contraction occurs when LV contraction imposes a "wringer" action, further augmenting overall RV contraction.[85]

The characteristics of RV ejection reflect the inability of this thin-walled chamber to withstand any acute increases in afterload. The velocity of RV ejection increases more gradually, peaks later, and decreases more slowly than LV ejection (Fig. 5–22). Although the RV is ideally suited to eject large volumes of blood (with minimal amounts of shortening), it is unable to withstand the development of high intraventricular pressures. If the normal RV is subjected to an acute increase in intraventricular pressure (as a result of an increased RV afterload), a several-fold increase in RV wall tension is observed. Any acute increases in RV afterload lead to increases in both EDV and transmural pressure.[86]

Global RV function is exquisitely sensitive to the impedance offered by the pulmonary vasculature. The significance of alteration in PVR (RV afterload), as a determinant of RV function, has been demonstrated by numerous investigators. In comparison with the LV, which maintains a constant output over a relatively wide range of afterloads, the RV output abruptly decreases with even small increases in afterload[87] (Fig. 5–23). Under normal conditions of RV function, any increase in afterload is accompanied by a substantial decrease in RVEF.[88] However, normal RV contractile function is usually maintained until the mean PAP is 40 mm Hg or greater.[89] Conversely, the RV appears to be less preload dependent than the LV (i.e., for a given preload, a smaller increase in SV is seen in the RV). In addition, the factors that govern the preload of each chamber are different. Flow to the right heart is dependent on the pressure difference between the intrathoracic and extrathoracic venous beds. However, the major determinant of LV preload is pulmonary venous drainage and is, therefore, independent of changes in intrathoracic pressure.

VENTRICULAR INTERACTION

Ventricular interaction is a process that is vital to the integration of heart and lung function. This relationship occurs both during systole and diastole and is a result of an intimate anatomic association between the RV and LV (Box 5–5). The major physiologic impact of this ventricular interaction relates to (1) the effect of the distention of one ventricle on the other and (2) the contribution of LV contraction to the development of RV systolic pressure. Factors that contribute to normal ventricular interaction include the IVS, pericardium, and shared coronary blood flow.

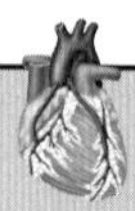

BOX 5–5 *Ventricular Interaction Is*

- A process vital to integration of the heart and lung function
- Affected by the intraventricular septum (IVS), pericardium, and shared coronary blood flow
- Able to produce "ventricular interference" when IVS location and geometry are altered
- Important to the diastolic pressure-volume relationship of both ventricles

The IVS is a thick muscular wall that separates the LV and RV. Anatomically, the fibers of the IVS appear to be a continuation of fibers from the LV free wall. As a result, the IVS is usually considered functionally part of the LV. The normal radius of curvature of the IVS is concave toward the LV and convex toward the RV. However, the systolic pressure gradient produced across the IVS regulates its ultimate location with respect to each ventricle. Normally, the pressure gradient between the ventricles creates a dominant axial force on the septal surface of the LV and, therefore, the IVS moves toward and with the RV.[90]

Taylor et al and other investigators have shown the importance of the position of the IVS in developing parallel shifts of the diastolic pressure-volume relationships of both ventricles under altered loading conditions.[91] In a canine preparation, the LV was progressively distended by increasing aliquots of blood (50 mL), and increased RV diastolic pressures were observed. Similarly, removal of blood from the RV reduced LV pressures. This relationship may have direct clinical importance as defined by the work of Laver et al,[92] who adopted the term "ventricular interference" or "ventricular interdependence" to describe the importance of IVS location and geometry in maintaining normal cardiac performance. Ordinarily, increases in the PCWP, which are associated with a decreased CO, are diagnostic of LV failure. However, under certain circumstances, such as increased PAPs or increased RV end-diastolic volume (RVEDV) and pressure (RVEDP), the IVS shifts into the LV cavity. Consequently, an increased PCWP and decreased CO are noted as a result of acute RV failure and a secondary decrease in LV filling:

$$\uparrow \text{PAP} \rightarrow \uparrow \text{RVEDV and} \uparrow \text{RVEDP} \rightarrow \text{shift of IVS} \rightarrow$$
$$\downarrow \text{CO} \leftarrow \uparrow \text{PCWP} \leftarrow \downarrow \text{LV volume}$$

In this situation, rather than acting in concert with the LV, the IVS is physiologically associated with the RV, resulting in an "internal tamponade." These alterations in the geometry and location of the IVS are the primary determinants of the pressure-volume characteristics of each ventricle, regardless of the presence or absence of the pericardium. Echocardiographic studies have shown that with increasing LV volume, with an intact pericardium, the IVS is shifted into the RV cavity, resulting in an increase in RV diastolic pressure.[93] Conversely, RV volume overload has been shown to cause abnormal septal wall motion.[94] This occurs secondary to a reduction in the transseptal gradient accompanied by a diastolic flattening and encroachment of the septum into the LV cavity. RV volume overload results in alteration of the diastolic pressure, shape, and performance of the LV.[95]

The pericardium functions to further reinforce the interdependence and the effect of volume-pressure alterations between the ventricles. Several studies have demonstrated the ability of the pericardium to impose a restriction on dilation of the RV and LV in situations of volume and pressure loading.[96] In these studies, increased RV pressure or volume resulted in smaller LV dimensions with the pericardium intact compared with postpericardiotomy. Following pericardiotomy, the main determinant of diastolic pressure-volume relationships was the contractile property of the myocardial wall.

When acute alterations in arterial and venous pressures affect all four cardiac chambers simultaneously and equally, such that total cardiac volume is increased, pericardial restraint rather than shifting of the IVS may be the predominant mechanism mediating changes in the passive diastolic properties of both ventricles.[97] However, when acute increases in preload and afterload affect one ventricle independent of the contralateral ventricle, such as in acute pulmonary embolism, the resultant effects on the diastolic pressure-volume relationship of the contralateral ventricle are dependent on pericardial restraint in addition to loading conditions produced by both internal (shifting of the septum) and external (peripheral circulatory impedance) factors.[98,99]

The importance of alterations in RV function has been demonstrated in a variety of clinical settings. Abnormalities of RV performance may occur (1) as a primary event, (2) secondary to LV failure, or (3) secondary to alterations in the mechanisms of ventricular interaction.[100] Clinically, the measurement that is most frequently used to quantify RV function is the right ventricular ejection fraction (RVEF) (see Chapter 14). Decreases in overall RV performance (as measured by RVEF) may be associated with (1) RV ischemia, (2) RV infarction, (3) pressure overload (acute or chronic), (4) volume overload (acute or chronic), and (5) alterations in the contractile performance of the RV from nonischemic etiologies (particularly during cardiac surgery).

LV failure is the most common cause of RV dysfunction occurring as a result of passive increases in PAPs. The hemodynamics associated with this scenario occur as a result of an increased RV afterload and decreased RVEF and SV. RV pressure overload secondary to LV failure is accompanied by LV systolic dysfunction and *increases* in LV end-diastolic dimension and volume (LVEDV).

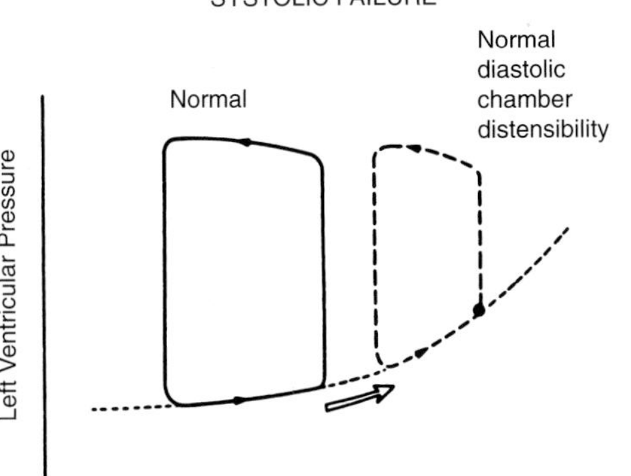

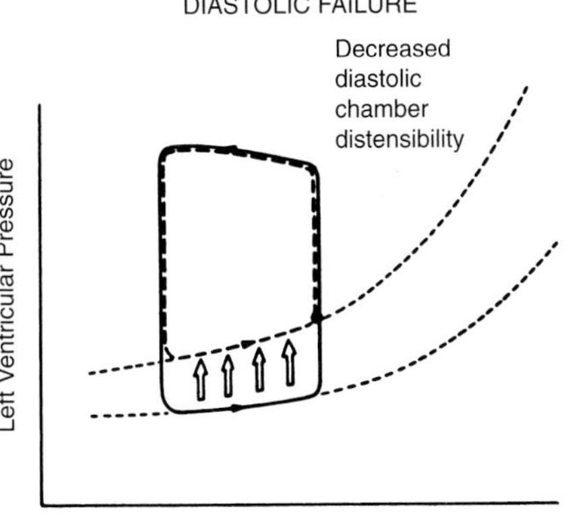

Figure 5–24 *(Left)* A schematized left ventricular (LV) pressure-volume loop from a patient with primary systolic failure. A normal LV pressure-volume loop *(solid loop)* is shown on the left portion of the curve, whereas the transition to systolic failure *(dashed loop)* is shown on the right portion of the curve. Systolic failure is manifest as an increase in LV end-systolic volume and as a reduction in the extent of shortening (stroke volume). LV end-diastolic pressure is increased because LV volume is increased. As indicated by the *arrow*, the diastolic portion of the pressure-volume loop has simply shifted to the right along the same diastolic pressure-volume relation. No change in the distensibility of the left ventricle has occurred. *(Right)* An LV pressure-volume loop from a patient with primary diastolic failure *(dashed loop)*. Note that the LV end-diastolic pressure is the same as that in the patient with primary systolic failure, as denoted by the filled circle (•) on the pressure-volume loops. However, in the *right panel*, this is related to an upward shift of the LV diastolic pressure-volume relation *(arrows)*. This indicates a decrease in LV diastolic distensibility, such that a higher diastolic pressure is required to achieve the same diastolic volume. In this patient, no change in end-diastolic volume or systolic shortening has occurred. (From Lorell BH: Left ventricular diastolic pressure-volume relations: Understanding and managing congestive heart failure. Heart Failure 4:206, 1988.)

CONCLUSION

The study of cardiac physiology is far from finished.[101,102] Physiologists and clinicians are constantly making advances into the realm of defining the individual parameters of LV and RV diastolic and systolic function. As they continue this quest, the development of new technologies is helping delineate clinical applications. The pressure-volume loop has been added to the Frank-Starling relationship as clinically useful cardiovascular physiologic tools.[101] Figure 5–24 shows the contrasting changes seen with pressure-volume loops in patients with systolic versus diastolic heart failure. The uses of advanced imaging technologies (especially TEE), faster computers, smaller equipment, and less invasive devices are greatly enhancing the clinician's ability to care for cardiac patients. The continued development of 3D echocardiography will someday provide the ability to actually see the volume relationships in the heart in real time.

REFERENCES

1. Badke FR, O'Rourke RA: Cardiovascular physiology. *In* Stein JH (ed): Internal Medicine. Boston, Little, Brown, 1983, pp 407–423
2. Guyton AC: Regulation of cardiac output. N Engl J Med 227:805, 1967
3. Braunwald E: Determinants and assessment of cardiac function. N Engl J Med 296:86, 1977
4. Grayzel J: The cardiac cycle. J Cardiothorac Vasc Anesth 5:649, 1991
5. Rankin JS, McHale PA, Arentzen CE, et al: The three-dimensional dynamic geometry of the left ventricle in the conscious dog. Circ Res 39:304, 1976
6. Frank O: Zur dynamik des herzmuskels. Z Biol 32:370, 1895
7. Ter Keurs HEDJ, Rijnsburger WH, van Heuningen R, et al: Tension development and sarcomere length in rat cardiac trabeculae. Evidence of length-dependent activation. Circ Res 46:703, 1980
8. Jewell BR: A reexamination of the influence of muscle length on myocardial performance. Circ Res 40:221, 1977
9. Kentish JC: The length-tension relation in the myocardium and its cellular basis. Heart Failure 4:125, 1988
10. Lakatta EG, Jewell BR: Length-dependent activation; its effects on the length-tension relation in cat ventricular muscle. Circ Res 40:251, 1977
11. Paterson S, Starling EH: On the mechanical factors which determine the output of the ventricles. J Physiol 48:357, 1914
12. Brutsaert DL, Sonnenblick EH: Force-velocity-length relations in the contractile elements in heart muscle of the cat. Circ Res 24:137, 1969
13. Forman R, Ford LE, Sonnenblick EH: Effect of muscle length on the force-velocity relationship of tetanized cardiac muscle. Circ Res 31:195, 1972
14. Katz AM: Physiology of the Heart. 3rd ed. Philadelphia, Lippincott, Williams & Wilkins, 2001
15. Peterson KL, Uther JH, Shabetai R, et al: Assessment of left ventricular performance in man. Instantaneous tension-velocity-length relations obtained with the aid of an electromagnetic velocity catheter in the ascending aorta. Circulation 47:924, 1973
16. McGowan JH, Cleland JG: Reliability of reporting LV systolic function by echocardiography: A systematic review of 3 methods. Am Heart J 146:388, 2003
17. Schiller NB: Ejection fraction by echocardiography. Am Heart J 146:380, 2003
18. Brutsaert DL, Housmans PR, Goethals MA: Dual control of relaxation. Its role in ventricular function in the mammalian heart. Circ Res 47:637, 1980
19. Brutsaert DL, Rademakers FE, Sys SU: Triple control of relaxation. Its role in the ventricular function in the mammalian heart. Circulation 69:190, 1984
20. Brutsaert DL, Rademakers FE, Sys SU, et al: Analysis of relaxation in the evaluation of ventricular function of the heart. Prog Cardiovasc Dis 28:143, 1985
21. Redfield MM, Jacobsen SJ, Burnett JC, et al: Burden of systolic and diastolic ventricular dysfunction in the community: Appreciating the scope of the epidemic. JAMA 289:194, 2003
22. Groban L: Diastolic dysfunction in the elderly. J Cardiothorac Vasc Anesth 19:228, 2005
23. Grossman W: Diastolic dysfunction in congestive heart failure. N Engl J Med 325:1557, 1991
24. Stauffer JC, Gaasch WH: Recognition and treatment of left ventricular dysfunction. Prog Cardiovasc Dis 32:319, 1990
25. Gwathmey JK, Slawaky MT, Hajjar RT, et al: Role of intracellular calcium handling in force-interval relationships of human ventricular myocardium. J Clin Invest 85:1599, 1990
26. Aroesty JM, McKay RG, Heller GV, et al: Simultaneous assessment of left ventricular systolic and diastolic dysfunction during pacing-induced ischemia. Circulation 71:889, 1985
27. Weiss JL, Fredericksen JW, Weisfeldt ML: Hemodynamic determinants of the time-course of fall in canine left ventricular pressure. J Clin Invest 58:751, 1976

28. Gilbert JC, Glantz SA: Determinants of left ventricular filling and of the diastolic pressure-volume relation. Circ Res 64:827, 1989
29. Kato T, Noda A, Ilawa H, et al: Myocardial velocity gradient as a non-invasively determined index of left ventricular diastolic dysfunction in patients with hypertrophic cardiomyopathy. J Am Coll Cardiol 42:278, 2003
30. Thomas JD, Newell JB, Choong CYP, Weyman AE: Physical and physiological determinants of transmitral velocity: Numerical analysis. Am J Physiol 260:H1718, 1991
31. Hori M, Yellin EL, Sonnenblick EH: Left ventricular diastolic suction as a mechanism of ventricular filling. Jpn Circ J 46:124, 1982
32. Spadaro J, Bing OHL, Gaasch WH, Weintraub RM: Pericardial modulation of right and left ventricular diastolic interaction. Circ Res 48:233, 1981
33. Firstenberg MS, Greenberg NL, Main ML, et al: Determinants of diastolic myocardial tissue Doppler velocities: Influence of relaxation and preload. J Appl Physiol 90:299, 2001
34. Bonow RO, Bacharach SL, Green MV, et al: Impaired diastolic filling in patients with coronary artery disease: Assessment with radionuclide angiography. Circulation 64:315, 1981
35. Redfield MM: Understanding diastolic heart failure. N Engl J Med 350:1930, 2004
36. King DL: Diastolic heart failure: Abnormalities in active relaxation and passive stiffness of the left ventricle. N Eng J Med 351:1143, 2004
37. Carroll JD, Lang RM, Neumann AL, et al: The differential effects of positive inotropic and vasodilator therapy on diastolic properties in patients with congestive cardiomyopathies. Circulation 74:815, 1986
38. Carroll JD, Hess OM, Hirzel HO, et al: Left ventricular systolic and diastolic function in coronary artery disease: Effects of revascularization on exercise-induced ischemia. Circulation 72:119, 1985
39. Schunkert H, Dzau VJ, Tang SS, et al: Increased rat cardiac angiotensin-converting enzyme activity and mRNA expression in pressure overload ventricular hypertrophy: Effects on coronary resistance, contractility and relaxation. J Clin Invest 86:1913, 1990
40. Lorell BH: Left ventricular diastolic pressure-volume relations: Understanding and managing congestive heart failure. Heart Failure 4:206, 1988
41. Maurer MS, Spevack D, Birkhoff D, et al: Diastolic dysfunction diagnosed by Doppler echocardiography. J Am Coll Cardiol 44:1543-1549, 2004
42. Zile MR, Brutsaert DL: New concepts in diastolic dysfunction and diastolic heart failure. Part I: Diagnosis, prognosis, and measurements of diastolic function. Circulation 105:1387, 2002
43. Weyman AE: The year in echocardiography. J Am Coll Cardiol 45:448, 2005
44. Brun P, Tribouilloy C, Duval A, et al: Left ventricular flow propagation during early filling is related to wall relaxation: A color M-mode Doppler analysis. J Am Coll Cardiol 20:420, 1992
45. DeMaya S, DeSutterb J, Vierendeelsa J, et al: Diastolic filling and pressure imaging: Taking advantage of the information in a color M-mode Doppler image. Eur J Echocardiol 2:219-233, 2001
46. Guyton AC, Coleman TG, Granger HJ: Circulation: Overall regulation. Annu Rev Physiol 34:13, 1972
47. Nixon JV, Murray RG, Leonard PD, et al: Effect of large variations in preload on left ventricular performance characteristics in normal subjects. Circulation 65:698, 1982
48. Luce JM: The cardiovascular effects of mechanical ventilation and positive end-expiratory pressure. JAMA 252:807, 1984
49. Lake CL: Anesthesia and pericardial disease. Anesth Analg 62:431, 1983
50. Ross J, Sobel BE: Regulation of cardiac contraction. Annu Rev Physiol 34:47, 1972
51. Thys DM, Hillel Z, Goldman ME, et al: Comparison of hemodynamic indices derived by invasive monitoring and two-dimensional echocardiography. Anesthesiology 67:630, 1987
52. Clements FM, Harpole DH, Quill T, et al: Estimation of left ventricular volume and ejection fraction by two-dimensional transesophageal echocardiography: Comparison of short-axis imaging and simultaneous radionuclide angiography. Br J Anaesth 64:331, 1990
53. Humphrey CB, Oury JH, Virgill RW, et al: An analysis of direct and indirect measurement of left atrial filling pressures. J Thorac Cardiovasc Surg 41:643, 1976
54. Swan HJC, Ganz W, Forrester JS, et al: Catheterization of the heart in man with the use of a flow-directed balloon-tip catheter. N Engl J Med 283:447, 1970
55. Lorzman J, Powers SR, Older T, et al: Correlation of pulmonary wedge and left atrial pressure: A study in the patient receiving positive end-expiratory pressure ventilation. Arch Surg 109:270, 1974
56. Civetta JM, Cagel JC, Laver MB: Disparate ventricular function in surgical patients. Surg Forum 22:136, 1971
57. Sarnoff SJ, Berglund E: Ventricular function. I. Starling's law of the heart studied by means of simultaneous right and left ventricular function curves in the dog. Circulation 9:706, 1954
58. Lang RM, Borow KM, Neuman A, Janzen D: Systemic vascular resistance: An unreliable index of left ventricular afterload. Circulation 74:1114, 1986
59. Milnor WR: Hemodynamics. *In* Milnor WR (ed): Vascular Impedance. Baltimore, Williams and Wilkins, 1982
60. Noordergraaf A, Melbin J: Ventricular afterload: A succinct yet comprehensive definition. Am Heart J 95:545, 1978
61. Nichols WW, Conti CR, Walker WE, et al: Input impedance of the systemic circulation in man. Circ Res 40:451, 1977
62. Kaplan JA: Vasodilators and combined inotrope and vasodilator therapy for the low-output syndrome. *In* Kaplan JA (ed): Cardiac Anesthesia: Cardiovascular Pharmacology. Orlando, FL, Grune & Stratton, 1983
63. Sunagawa K, Maugham WL, Burkhoff D, Sagawa K: Left ventricular interaction with arterial load studied in isolated canine ventricle. Am J Physiol 245:H773, 1983
64. Burns JW, Covell JW, Ross J Jr: Mechanics of isotonic left ventricular contractions. Am J Physiol 224:725, 1973
65. Monroe RG, Gamble WJ, LaFarge CG, et al: The Anrep effect reconsidered. J Clin Invest 51:2573, 1972
66. Krueger JW: Fundamental mechanisms that govern cardiac function: A short review of sarcomere mechanics. Heart Failure 4:137, 1988
67. Mock MB, Ringqvist I, Fisher LD, et al: Survival of medically treated patients in the Coronary Artery Surgery Study (CASS) registry. Circulation 66:562, 1982
68. Suga H, Sagawa K, Shoukas AA: Load independence of the instantaneous pressure-volume ratio of the canine left ventricle and effects of epinephrine and heart rate on the ratio. Circ Res 32:314, 1973
69. Suga H, Sagawa K: Instantaneous pressure-volume relationships and their ratio in the excised, supported canine left ventricle. Circ Res 35:117, 1974
70. Kass DA, Maughan WL: From Emax to pressure-volume relations: A broader view. Circulation 77:1203, 1988
71. Kass DA, Yamazaki T, Burkhoff D, et al: Determination of left ventricular end-systolic pressure-volume relationships by conductance (volume) catheter technique. Circulation 73:586, 1986
72. Schreuder JJ, Biervliet JD, van der Velde ET, et al: Systolic and diastolic pressure-volume relationships during cardiac surgery. J Cardiothoracic Vasc Anesth 5:539, 1991
73. Suga H, Hayashi T, Shirahata M: Ventricular systolic pressure-volume area as predictor of cardiac oxygen consumption. Am J Physiol 240:H39, 1981
74. Nozawa T, Yasumura Y, Futaki S, et al: Efficiency of energy transfer from pressure-volume area to external mechanical work increases with contractile state and decreases with afterload in the left ventricle of the anesthetized closed-chest dog. Circulation 77:1116, 1988
75. Glower DD, Spratt JA, Snow NK, et al: Linearity of the Frank-Starling relationship in the intact heart: The concept of preload-recruitable stroke work. Circulation 71:944, 1985
76. Feneley MP, Skelton TN, Kisslo KB, et al: Comparison of preload-recruitable stroke work, end-systolic pressure-volume and dP/dt_{max}-end-diastolic volume relations as indexes of left ventricular contractile performance in patients undergoing routine cardiac catheterization. J Am Coll Cardiol 19:1522, 1992
77. Pagel PS, Kampine JP, Schmeling WT, et al: Comparison of end-systolic pressure-length relations and preload-recruitable stroke work as indices of myocardial contractility in the conscious anesthetized, chronically instrumented dog. Anesthesiology 73:278, 1990.
78. Vogel M, Cheung MM, Li J, et al: Noninvasive assessment of LV force-frequency relationships using tissue Doppler-derived isovolumic acceleration. Circulation 107:1647-1652, 2003
79. Higgins CB, Vatner SF, Braunwald E: Parasympathetic control of the heart. Pharmacol Rev 25:119, 1973
80. Sutton JR, Cole A, Gunning J, et al: Control of heart rate in healthy young men. Lancet 2:1398, 1967
81. Cannom DS, Graham AF, Harrison DC: Electrophysiological studies in the denervated transplanted human heart: Response to atrial pacing and atropine. Circ Res 32:268, 1973
82. McLaughlin PR, Kleinman JH, Martin RP, et al: The effects of exercise and atrial pacing on left ventricular volume and contractility in patients with innervated and denervated hearts. Circulation 58:476, 1978
83. Maughan WL, Sunagawa K, Burkhoff D, et al: Effect of heart rate on the canine end-systolic pressure-volume relationship. Circulation 72:654, 1985

84. Ross J Jr: The cardiac pump. *In* West JB (ed): Physiologic Basis of Medical Practice. Baltimore, Williams & Wilkins, 1991, section 2
85. Rushmer RF, et al: Functional anatomy of cardiac contraction. *In* Rushmer RF (ed): Structure and Function of the Cardiovascular System. Philadelphia, WB Saunders Company, 1972, pp 33–69
86. Stein PD, Sabbath HH, Auler DT, et al: Performance of the failing and non-failing right ventricle of patients with pulmonary hypertension. Am J Cardiol 44:1050, 1979
87. McFadden ER, Braunwald E: Cor pulmonale and pulmonary thromboembolism. *In* Braunwald E (ed): Textbook of Cardiovascular Medicine. Philadelphia, WB Saunders, 1980, pp 1643–1680
88. Weber KT, Janicki JS, Shroff S, et al: Contractile mechanisms and interaction of the right and left ventricles. Am J Cardiol 47:680, 1981
89. Weber K, Janicki J, Shroff S, et al: The right ventricle: Physiologic and pathophysiologic considerations. Crit Care Med 11:323, 1983
90. Jardin F, Farcot JC, Boisanti C, et al: Influence of positive end-expiratory pressure on left ventricular performance. N Engl J Med 304:387, 1981
91. Taylor RR, Covell JW, Sonnenblick EH, et al: Dependence of ventricular distensibility effect on filling of the opposite ventricle. Am J Physiol 218:711, 1967
92. Laver MB, Stauss WH, Robost GM: Herbert Shubin Memorial Lectures. Right and left ventricular geometry: Adjustments during acute respiratory failure. Crit Care Med 7:509, 1975
93. Meyer RA, Schwartz DC, Ben Zing G, Kaplan S: Ventricular septum in right ventricular volume overload: An echocardiographic study. Am J Cardiol 330:349, 1972
94. Brinker J, Weiss J, Lappi D, et al: Leftward septal displacement during right ventricular loading in man. Circulation 61:626, 1980
95. Bemis CE, Serur JR, Borkenhagen D, et al: Influences of right ventricular filling pressure on left ventricular pressure and dimension. Circ Res 34:498, 1974
96. Spadro J, Bing O, Gaasch W, et al: Pericardial modulation of right and left ventricular diastolic interaction. Circ Res 48:233, 1985
97. Molaug M, Geiran O, Stokland O, et al: Dynamics of the interventricular septum and free ventricular walls during blood volume expansion and selective right ventricular volume loading in dogs. Acta Physiol Scand 116:245, 1982
98. Dell'Italia LJ, Walsh RA: Right ventricular diastolic pressure-volume relations and regional dimensions during acute alterations in loading conditions. Circulation 77:1276, 1988
99. Feneley MP, Olsen CO, Glower DD, et al: Effect of acutely increased right ventricular afterload on work output from the left ventricle in conscious dogs. Systolic ventricular interaction. Circ Res 65:135, 1989
100. Dell'Italia L: The right ventricle: Anatomy, physiology and clinical implications. Curr Probl Cardiol 16:659, 1991
101. Katz A: Ernest Henry Starling: His predecessors and the "law of the heart." Circulation 106:2986, 2002
102. Carabello B: Evolution of the study of left ventricular function: Everything old is new again. Circulation 105:2701, 2002

Chapter 6

CORONARY PHYSIOLOGY AND ATHEROSCLEROSIS

Edward R. M. O'Brien, MD • Howard J. Nathan, MD

KEY POINTS

1. To safely care for patients with coronary artery disease in the perioperative period, the clinician must understand how the coronary circulation functions in health and disease.
2. Coronary endothelium modulates myocardial blood flow by producing factors that relax or contract the underlying vascular smooth muscle.
3. Vascular endothelial cells help maintain the fluidity of blood by elaborating anticoagulant, fibrinolytic, and antiplatelet substances.
4. One of the earliest changes in coronary artery disease, preceding the appearance of stenoses, is the loss of the vasoregulatory and antithrombotic functions of the endothelium.
5. The mean systemic arterial pressure and not the diastolic pressure may be the most useful and reliable measure of coronary perfusion pressure in the clinical setting.
6. Although sympathetic activation increases myocardial oxygen demand, activation of α-adrenergic receptors causes coronary vasoconstriction.
7. It is unlikely that one substance alone (e.g., adenosine) provides the link between myocardial metabolism and myocardial blood flow under a variety of conditions.
8. As coronary perfusion pressure decreases, the inner layers of myocardium nearest the left ventricular cavity are the first to become ischemic and display impaired relaxation and contraction.
9. The progression of an atherosclerotic lesion is similar to the process of wound healing.
10. Lipid-lowering therapy can help restore endothelial function and prevent coronary events.

When caring for patients with coronary artery disease (CAD), the anesthesiologist must prevent or minimize myocardial ischemia by maintaining optimal conditions for perfusion of the heart. This goal can be achieved only with an understanding of the many factors that determine myocardial blood flow in both health and disease. This chapter begins with an overview of the structure and function of coronary arteries. Rapid progress has been made in the past several decades in the understanding of the physiology of blood vessels, particularly the role of the endothelium in maintaining flow. Following this overview is an analysis of the major determinants of coronary blood flow. Physiologic or pharmacologic interventions alter myocardial flow by their effects on these factors. The section on coronary pressure-flow relationships explains the important concepts of autoregulation and coronary reserve. Studies of the coronary circulation are sometimes misinterpreted because of an inadequate understanding of the complex interrelationships among the heart, the coronary circulation, and the peripheral circulation. The discussion of pathophysiology begins with a description of the process of atherosclerosis and the current understanding of how this disease evolves and causes clinical events. Next, the anatomy and hemodynamic effects of a coronary stenosis are explained. Coronary collateral function and development are reviewed here. These concepts are the basis of predicting how significantly the stenoses seen on angiography impair myocardial perfusion. The topic of the final section is the pathophysiology of myocardial ischemia. Here, the concepts learned in the preceding sections are applied in an analysis of clinical ischemic syndromes. The final section highlights future directions in the treatment of CAD.

ANATOMY AND PHYSIOLOGY OF BLOOD VESSELS

The coronary vasculature has been traditionally divided into three functional groups: large conductance vessels visible on coronary angiography, which offer little resistance to blood flow; small resistance vessels ranging in size from about 250 to 10 μm in diameter; and veins. Although it has been taught that arterioles (precapillary vessels <50 μm in size) account for most of the coronary resistance, studies indicate that under resting conditions, 45% to 50% of total coronary vascular resistance resides in vessels larger than 100 μm in diameter[1-3] (Fig. 6–1). This may be due, in part, to the relatively great length of the small arteries. During intense pharmacologic dilation, the proportion of total coronary vascular resistance due to larger arteries and veins is even greater.[2] The regulation of tone in coronary arteries larger than 100 μm in diameter plays an important role in delivering adequate myocardial perfusion.[4] One of the early changes in CAD is a diminished ability of the endothelium of epicardial coronary arteries to dilate in response to increased flow (see Endothelium-Derived Relaxing Factors). Advances in technology have enabled measurement, in the beating heart, of diameters of coronary vessels as small as 15 μm. It is becoming evident that, in response to a given intervention, different size classes of coronary vessels can change diameter with different intensity or even in opposite directions.[5,6] This heterogeneity of response according to vessel size would be an important consideration in predicting the effects of vasoactive agents on myocardial perfusion. For example, a drug that dilated large vessels and collaterals but not arterioles would be beneficial to patients with CAD (see Coronary Steal).

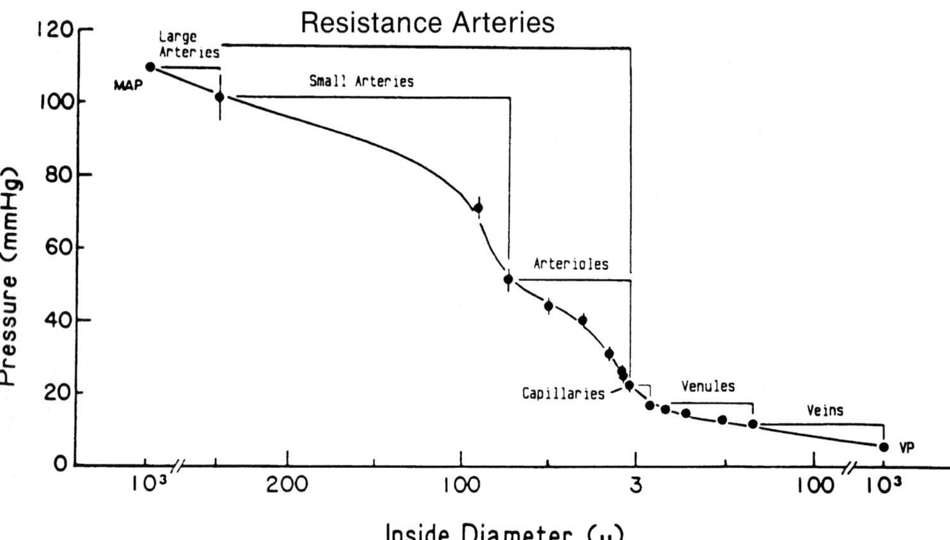

Figure 6–1 Pressure drop through the hamster cheek pouch circulation illustrates the resistance and nomenclature of various portions of the vascular bed. The important contribution of small arteries to vascular resistance is clearly shown here. Similar observations have been made in the coronary circulation. MAP = mean arterial pressure; VP = venous pressure. Error bars indicate SE. (From Davis MJ, Ferrer PN, Gore RW: Vascular anatomy and hydrostatic pressure profile in the hamster cheek pouch. Am J Physiol 250:H291, 1986.)

Normal Artery Wall

The arterial lumen is lined by a monolayer of endothelial cells that overlies smooth muscle cells (Fig. 6–2). The inner layer of smooth muscle cells, known as the intima, is circumscribed by the internal elastic lamina. Between the internal elastic lamina and external elastic lamina is another layer of smooth muscle cells, the media. Outside the external elastic lamina is an adventitia that is sparsely populated by cells and microvessels of the vasa vasorum.

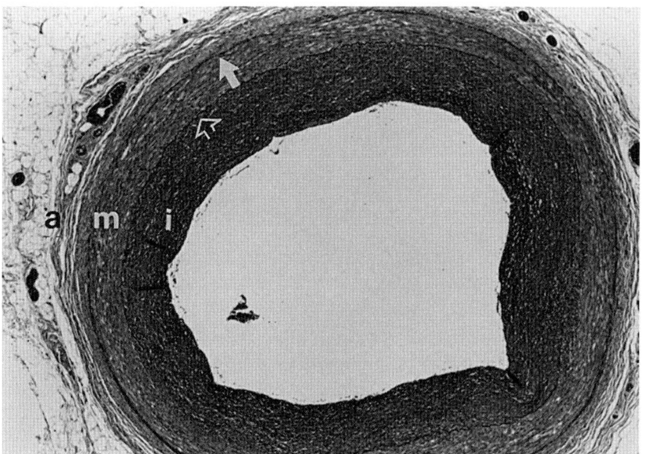

Figure 6–2 Normal human coronary artery of a 32-year-old woman. The intima (i) and media (m) are composed of smooth muscle cells. The adventitia (a) consists of a loose collection of adipocytes, fibroblasts, vasa vasorum, and nerves. The media is separated from the intima by the internal elastic lamina *(open arrow)* and the adventitia by the external elastic lamina *(closed arrow)*. (Movat's pentachrome-stained slide, original magnification × 6.6.)

Intima

Traditionally, the intima has been considered the most important layer of the artery wall.[7] At birth, the intima is only a potential space. As part of the normal development of many large arteries, smooth muscle cells invade this space and form a neointima. This diffuse form of intimal thickening consists of several layers of smooth muscle cells and connective tissue. The thickness of the intima may vary. For convenience, the intima/media ratio is often measured, and the normal range is 0.1 to 1.0. How this benign intima forms is not well understood. Presumably, the intima represents a physiologic adaptation to changes in arterial flow and wall tension. The intima is made up of two distinct layers.[8] As seen on electron microscopy, the inner layer subjacent to the luminal endothelium contains an abundance of proteoglycan ground substance. Smooth muscle cells found in this layer are usually distributed as isolated cells in a sea of matrix, rather than in contiguous layers. A few macrophages may also be found in this layer underneath the endothelial monolayer. The outer, musculoelastic layer of the intima is adjacent to the internal elastic lamina and contains smooth muscle cells and elastic fibers.

Media

In normal adult arteries, several smooth muscle cell subpopulations with distinct lineages exist within the media.[9] These diverse cell populations likely fulfill different functions in order to maintain homeostasis in the artery wall. For example, in response to pressure elevations, increases in smooth muscle cell mass and extracellular matrix may be required. Alternatively, for arteries to be able to stretch both longitudinally and circumferentially, smooth muscle cells with variable orientations of cytoskeletal fibers must be present. These distinct cell types may be important not only in health but also in disease. In certain experimental models of neointimal formation, proliferation and inward migration of subpopulations of medial smooth muscle cells occur.[10] The biologic determinants of medial smooth muscle cell diversity are unknown.[11]

Adventitia

The adventitia, the outermost layer of the artery wall, normally consists of a sparse collection of fibroblasts, microvessels (vasa vasorum), nerves, and few inflammatory cells. The majority of the vasa vasorum that nourish the inner layers of the artery wall originates in the adventitia. Traditionally, the adventitia has been ignored and is not thought to play a role in vascular lesion formation. However, as explained later, there is experimental evidence to support the concept that adventitial fibroblasts differentiate into myofibroblasts. After injury, these myofibroblasts may migrate inward to participate in lesion development.[12,13]

Transmembrane and Transcellular Communication

Blood vessels respond to a multitude of neural, humoral, and mechanical stimuli in fulfilling their role in homeostasis. When norepinephrine, released from adrenergic nerve terminals in the adventitia, binds to receptors on the vascular smooth muscle cell membrane, a series of events take place, culminating in a change in vessel diameter. Much progress has been made in understanding this transmembrane signaling since the discovery of cyclic adenosine monophosphate (cAMP) in the late 1950s. Hormones circulating in the blood must interact with receptors on endothelial cells before the message reaches the vascular smooth muscle cells. The mechanism of communication between cells has been one of the central themes of biologic research in the last decades. Future understanding of cardiovascular disease will likely be based on identification of abnormalities of the molecules involved in transmembrane and transcellular communication. A brief introduction to these topics is provided here.

Figure 6–3 illustrates examples of pathways of transmembrane signaling. Up to five components can be involved: receptor, G protein, effector producing a second messenger, phosphorylation of regulator protein, and the consequent change in cell behavior. G proteins (guanine nucleotide binding regulatory proteins) are made up of three subunits (α, β, γ) and float in the cell membrane. On contact with a ligand-receptor complex, guanosine diphosphate (GDP) on the α subunit is replaced by guanosine triphosphate (GTP). The activated α subunit then dissociates from the β-γ complex and can interact with several membrane targets (Fig. 6–3*B*). For example, β-receptor activation results in the activation of G_s (s = stimulate), which stimulates the synthesis of cAMP by adenylyl cyclase. Muscarinic receptor activation activates a G_i (i = inhibit) protein that inhibits adenylyl cyclase. A single G protein can interact with more than one effector. In this way the G protein can be a branch point for the regulation of multiple effectors in response to a single signal. These proteins have already been implicated in human disease: Cholera toxin covalently modifies G_s so that it becomes persistently active in stimulating adenylyl cyclase in intestinal epithelial cells, likely causing the severe diarrhea of cholera.

Several second-messenger systems have been characterized. G_s can directly enhance conductance through calcium channels, with the increased intracellular calcium acting as second messenger. The cyclic nucleotides, cAMP and cyclic guanosine monophosphate (cGMP), act as second messengers. Their intracellular action is terminated when they are cleaved by phosphodiesterase enzymes, which, in turn, are also regulated by stimuli and second messengers. The breakdown products of membrane phosphoinositide constitute another, more recently recognized, set of second messengers.[14] In response to

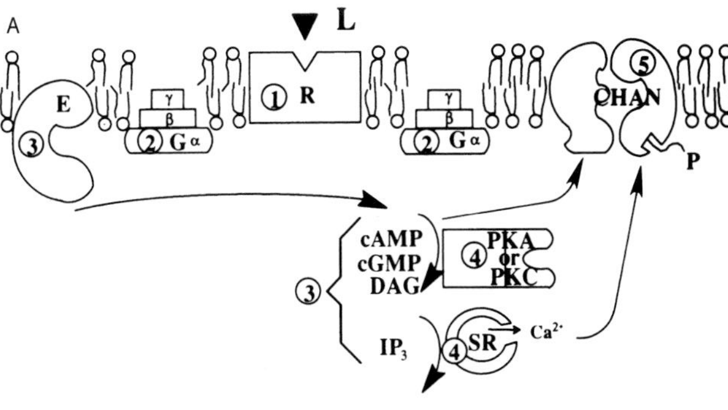

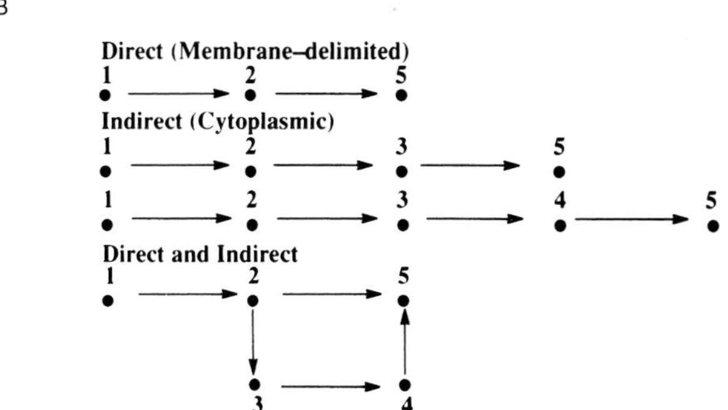

Figure 6–3 Steps in the process whereby hormone-receptor binding results in a change in cell behavior. In this example, the final result is the opening of an ion channel. *(A)* A hormone or ligand (L) binds to a receptor (R) embedded in the cell membrane. The receptor-ligand complex interacts with G protein (G) floating in the membrane, resulting in activation of the α subunit (Ga). The activated α subunit can then follow different pathways *(B)*. Effector enzymes in the membrane (E), such as adenylyl cyclase, cyclic guanosine monophosphate (cGMP), phospholipase C, or phospholipase A_2, change the cytoplasmic concentration of their "messengers": cyclic adenosine monophosphate (cAMP), cGMP, diacylglycerol (DAG), and inositol-1,4,5-triphosphate (IP_3). These soluble molecules activate protein kinase A or C (PKA, PKC), or release Ca^{++} from sarcoplasmic reticulum (SR). Subsequently, cell behavior is changed by phosphorylation of an ionic channel on the cell membrane (CHAN) or by release of Ca^{++} from SR. *(B)* Several pathways coupling receptor activation to final effect are illustrated. It is likely that multiple pathways are activated concomitantly, both facilitatory and inhibitory. In this way, the final response can be determined by the sum of the effects of several stimuli. (*A, B,* From Brown AM, Birnbaumer L: Ionic channels and their regulation by G-protein subunits. Annu Rev Physiol 52:197, 1990.)

agonists such as vasopressin, G protein is activated, leading to activation of the membrane-associated enzyme phospholipase C. This enzyme cleaves phosphatidylinositol-4,5-biphosphate on the inner leaflet of the plasma membrane, producing inositol-1,4,5-triphosphate (IP_3) and diacylglycerol (DAG). Both are second messengers. IP_3 diffuses through the cytoplasm and mobilizes calcium from intracellular stores. DAG remains within the plasma membrane and activates protein kinase C, which modulates cellular activity by phosphorylating intracellular proteins. In many cell types, activation of the same receptors that control phosphoinositide breakdown also results in the liberation of arachidonate and/or eicosanoids (prostaglandins, leukotrienes, and thromboxanes). The resultant change in cell behavior can be the opening of an ion channel, contraction or relaxation of smooth muscle, secretory activity, or initiation of cell division (see Chapter 7).

Endothelium

Although the vascular endothelium was once thought of as an inert lining for blood vessels, it is more accurately characterized as a very active, distributed organ with many biologic functions. It has synthetic (Table 6–1) and metabolic (Table 6–2) capabilities and contains receptors for a variety of vasoactive substances (Table 6–3). Functions of the endothelium that may play an important role in the pathophysiology of ischemic heart disease are discussed.

Endothelium-Derived Relaxing Factors

The first vasoactive endothelial substance to be discovered was prostacyclin (PGI_2), a product of the cyclooxygenase pathway of arachidonic acid metabolism (Fig. 6–4 and Box 6–1).[15] The production of PGI_2 is activated by shear stress, pulsatility of flow, hypoxia, and a variety of vasoactive mediators. Upon production it leaves the endothelial cell and acts in the local environment to cause relaxation of the underlying smooth muscle or to inhibit platelet aggregation. Both actions are mediated by the stimulation of adenylyl cyclase in the target cell to produce cAMP.

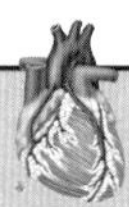

BOX 6–1 *Endothelium-Derived Relaxing and Contracting Factors*

Healthy endothelial cells have an important role in modulating coronary tone by producing

Vascular Muscle Relaxing Factors

- Prostacyclin
- Nitric oxide
- Hyperpolarizing factor

Vascular Muscle Contracting Factors

- Prostaglandin H_2
- Thromboxane A_2
- Endothelin

In 1980, Furchgott and Zawadzki[16] observed that the presence of an intact endothelium was necessary for acetylcholine-induced vasodilation. Since that time it has been shown that many physiologic stimuli cause vasodilation by stimulating the release of a labile, diffusible, nonprostanoid molecule termed "endothelium-derived relaxing factor" (EDRF) (see Fig. 6–4), now known to be nitric oxide (NO). NO is the basis of a widespread paracrine signal transduction mechanism whereby one cell type can modulate the behavior of adjacent cells of a different type.[17,18] NO is a very small lipophilic molecule that can readily diffuse across biologic membranes and into the cytosol of nearby cells. The half-life of the molecule is less than 5 seconds so that only the local environment can be affected. NO is synthesized from the amino acid l-arginine by NO synthase (NOS). In vascular endothelium, the enzyme (eNOS or NOS3) is always present (constitutive) and resides in the cytoplasm. Its function depends on the presence of Ca^{++} and calmodulin as well as tetrahydrobiopterin. Serine phosphorylation is important for prolonged activity. The enzyme is activated in response to receptor occupancy or physical stimulation (see Table 6–3). When NO diffuses into the cytosol of the target cell, it binds with the heme group of soluble guanylate cyclase, resulting in a 50- to 200-fold increase in production of cGMP, its second messenger. If the target cells are vascular smooth muscle cells, vasodilation

Table 6–1 Substances Produced by Vascular Endothelium

Antithrombotic Substances	Procoagulants
Prostacyclin	von Willebrand factor
Antithrombin III	Collagen
Plasminogen activator	Fibronectin
Protein C	Thromboplastin
α_2-Macroglobulin	Thrombospondin
Glycosaminoglycans (heparin)	Plasminogen inhibitors Platelet-activating factor Thromboxane A_2

From Bassenge E, Busse R: Endothelial modulation of coronary tone. Prog Cardiovasc Dis 30:349, 1988.

Table 6–2 Vasoactive Substances Processed by Vascular Endothelium

Uptake and Metabolism	Enzymatic Conversion or Degradation
Norepinephrine	Angiotensin I to angiotensin II (ACE)
Serotonin	Angiotensin II to angiotensin III (angiotensinase)
Prostaglandins (E_1, E_2, $E_{2\alpha}$)	Bradykinin degradation (ACE)
Leukotrienes	Substance P degradation
Adenosine	

ACE = angiotensin-converting enzyme.
From Bassenge E, Busse R: Endothelial modulation of coronary tone. Prog Cardiovasc Dis 30:349, 1988.

Table 6–3 Stimulators of Endothelium-Mediated Vasodilation

Transmitters	ADP
Acetylcholine	Adenosine
Norepinephrine	Serotonin
Peptides	Thrombin
Angiotensin	Trypsin
Bradykinin	**Local Hormones**
Vasopressin	Histamine
Oxytocin	Platelet-activating factor
Substance P	**Physicochemical Stimuli**
Vasoactive intestinal peptide	Shear stress (flow)
Calcitonin gene–related peptide	Mechanical stress (pulsatility)
Platelet or Blood Components	Hypoxia
ATP	

ATP = adenosine triphosphate; ADP = adenosine diphosphate.
Modified from Bassenge E, Busse R: Endothelial modulation of coronary tone. Prog Cardiovasc Dis 30:349, 1988.

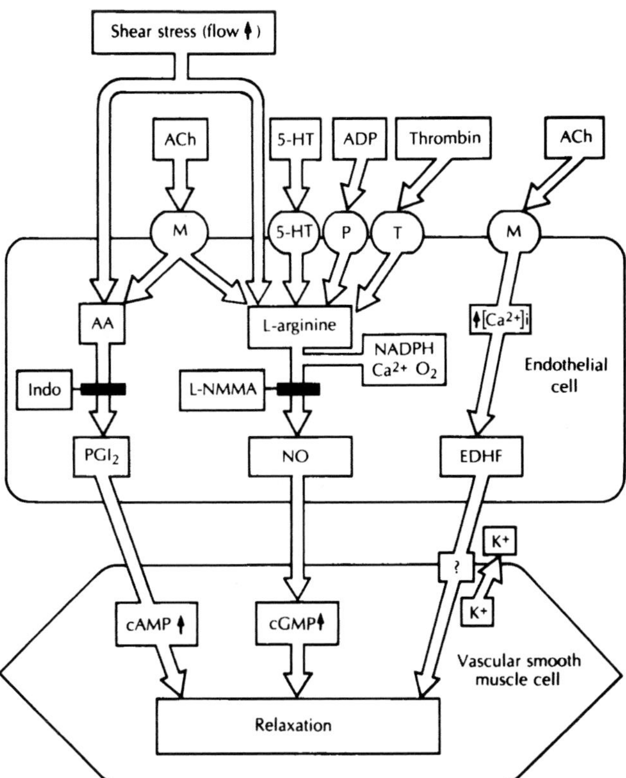

Figure 6–4 The production of endothelium-derived vasodilator substances. Prostacyclin (PGI_2) is produced via the cyclooxygenase pathway of arachidonic acid (AA) metabolism, which can be blocked by indomethacin (Indo) and aspirin. PGI_2 stimulates smooth muscle adenylyl cyclase and increases cyclic adenosine monophosphate (cAMP) production, which cause relaxation. Endothelium-derived relaxing factor (EDRF), now known to be nitric oxide (NO), is produced by the action of NO synthase on L-arginine in the presence of reduced nicotinamide adenine dinucleotide phosphate (NADPH), oxygen (O_2), and calcium and calmodulin. This process can be blocked by arginine analogs like N^G-monomethyl-L-arginine (LNMMA). NO combines with guanylate cyclase in the smooth muscle cell to stimulate production of cyclic guanosine monophosphate (cGMP), which results in relaxation. Less well characterized is an endothelium-derived factor, which hyperpolarizes the smooth muscle membrane (EDHF) and probably acts via activation of potassium (K^+) channels. ACh = acetylcholine; M = muscarinic receptor; 5-HT = serotonin; ADP = adenosine diphosphate; P = purinergic receptor; T = thrombin receptor. (From Rubanyi GM: Endothelium, platelets, and coronary vasospasm. Coron Artery Dis 1:645, 1990.)

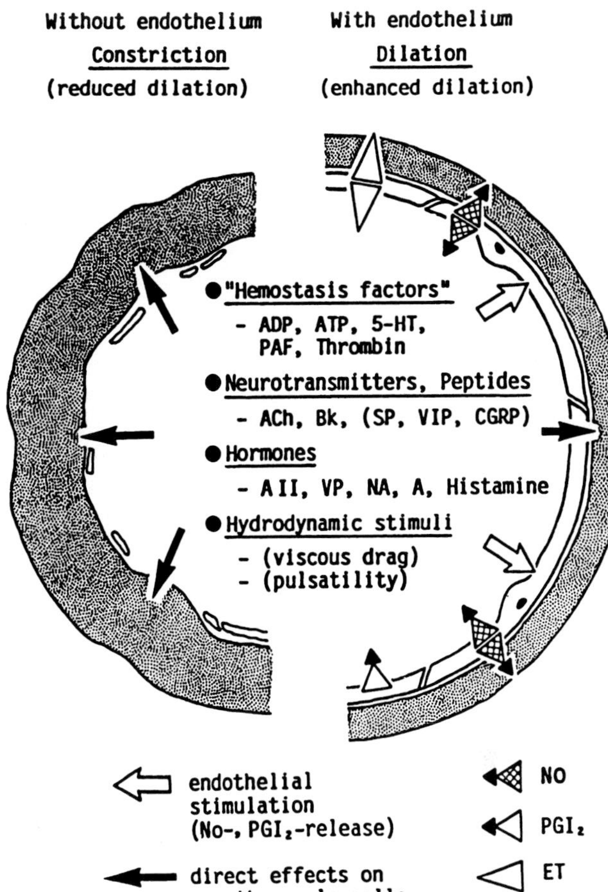

Figure 6–5 The role of endothelium in the control of coronary tone. Intact endothelium has an important modulatory role in the effect of numerous factors on vascular smooth muscle. In the absence of a functional endothelium (mechanical trauma, atherosclerosis), many factors act directly on smooth muscle to cause constriction *(left side)*. Under normal conditions *(right side)*, the release of NO (endothelium-derived relaxing factor [EDRF]) and prostacyclin (PGI_2) stimulated by these same factors can attenuate constriction or cause dilation. PGI_2 release is predominantly into the lumen, whereas EDRF release is similar on both the luminal and abluminal sides. Substances in parentheses elicit only vasodilation. ADP = adenosine monophosphate; ATP = adenosine triphosphate; 5-HT = serotonin; PAF = platelet-activating factor; ACh = acetylcholine; BK = bradykinin; SP = substance P; VIP = vasoactive intestinal polypeptide; CGRP = calcitonin gene–related peptide; AII = angiotensin II; VP = vasopressin; NA = norepinephrine; A = adenosine; ET = endothelin. (From Bassenge E, Heusch G: Endothelial and neurohumoral control of coronary blood flow in health and disease. Rev Physiol Biochem Pharmacol 116:77, 1990.)

occurs; if the target cells are platelets, adhesion and aggregation are inhibited. In vascular smooth muscle, cGMP leads to activation of protein kinase G, which phosphorylates various intracellular target proteins, including the myosin light-chain regulatory subunit and proteins that control intracellular calcium.[19]

It is likely that NO is the final common effector molecule of nitrovasodilators (including sodium nitroprusside and organic nitrates such as nitroglycerin). The cardiovascular system is in a constant state of active vasodilation that is dependent on the generation of NO. The molecule is more important in controlling vascular tone in veins and arteries compared with arterioles. When the microcirculation dilates in response to metabolic myocardial demand (e.g., exercise), increased flow through epicardial coronary arteries increases shear stress at the endothelium. This leads to release of NO, which causes vascular smooth muscle relaxation and dilation of the conductance vessels, thereby facilitating the increase in flow. The importance of the loss of this mechanism in atherosclerosis is underlined by the fact that in this situation more than 50% of the resistance to flow in the coronary circulation resides in vessels larger than 100 μm in diameter (see Fig. 6–1). Abnormalities in the ability of the endothelium to produce NO likely play a role in diseases such as diabetes, atherosclerosis, and hypertension.[20,21] The venous circulation of humans seems to have a lower basal release of NO and an increased sensitivity to nitrovasodilators compared with the arterial side of the circulation.[22]

Many agents, such as acetylcholine and norepinephrine, can cause contraction when applied directly to the vascular smooth muscle membrane instead of relaxation, which occurs when it is applied to the intact endothelium (Fig. 6–5). The net effect of neural or humoral stimuli depends on a combination of direct effects mediated by binding to vascular smooth muscle receptors and indirect effects due to the ligand binding to endothelial receptors causing NO release from the endothelium. In the presence of healthy endothelium, vasodilation usually predominates. When the endothelium is absent (e.g., injured vessel) or diseased (e.g., atherosclerosis), vasoconstriction may be the net effect. NO has important roles in neurohumoral regulation of vascular tone, in preventing intravascular platelet aggregation, and in the structural adaptation of blood vessels to the demands of blood flow and pressure. Knowledge of its role in inflammation and atherosclerosis is rapidly expanding.

In addition to prostacyclin and NO, another, less well understood, pathway for receptor-mediated or mechanically induced endothelium-derived vasodilation exists that is associated with smooth muscle hyperpolarization. Both epoxyeicosatrienoic acid (a metabolite of cytochrome P450) and H_2O_2 have been suggested as possible endothelium-derived hyperpolarizing factors (EDHFs).[23,24] Smooth muscle relaxation is a result of hyperpolarization of the myocyte, which leads to decreased intracellular calcium concentration. EDHF-mediated vasodilation can be blocked by inhibition of calcium-dependent potassium channels. EDHF may have an important vasodilator role in the human coronary microcirculation.[25]

Endothelium-Derived Contracting Factors

Contracting factors produced by the endothelium include prostaglandin H_2, thromboxane A_2 (via cyclooxygenase), and the peptide endothelin. Endothelin is a potent vasoconstrictor peptide (100-fold more potent than norepinephrine) with remarkable similarities to the toxin of the burrowing asp.[26] Both have potent coronary constrictor activity to which the strong cardiac toxicity and lethality of the toxin are attributed.[27] Three closely related 21-amino-acid peptides have been identified: endothelin-1 (ET-1), ET-2, and ET-3. The primary product of vascular endothelium is ET-1, which is synthesized from prepro-endothelin-1 within vascular endothelial cells by the action of endothelin-converting enzymes. It is not stored but rather rapidly synthesized in response to stimuli such as ischemia, hypoxia, and shear stress and released predominantly abluminally (toward the underlying smooth muscle).[28] In vascular smooth muscle cells, ET-1 binds to specific membrane receptors (ET_A) and, via phospholipase C, induces an increase in intracellular calcium resulting in long-lasting contractions.[29] It is also linked via a G_i protein to voltage-operated calcium channels. This peptide has a greater vasoconstricting potency than any other cardiovascular hormone, and in pharmacologic doses it can abolish coronary flow, leading to ventricular fibrillation and death.[30] Another receptor subtype, ET_B, is expressed by both smooth muscle and endothelium and binds ET-1 and ET-3 equally well (Fig. 6–6). When isolated vessels are perfused with ET-1, there is an initial NO-mediated vasodilation due to binding with ET_B receptors on the endothelial cells followed by contraction due to binding of ET-1 to ET_A receptors on the vascular smooth muscle membrane. Studies with bosentan, a combined oral ET_A/ET_B receptor antagonist, have demonstrated that endothelin exerts a basal coronary vasoconstrictor tone in humans.[31] There is evidence that endothelin may play a role in the pathophysiology of pulmonary and arterial hypertension, atherosclerosis, myocardial ischemic syndromes, and heart failure.[28] Clinical trials of bosentan in patients with congestive heart failure[32] and hypertension have shown promise, but hepatic side effects have limited the dose to less than 500 mg daily, with the primary indication being severe pulmonary hypertension.[33]

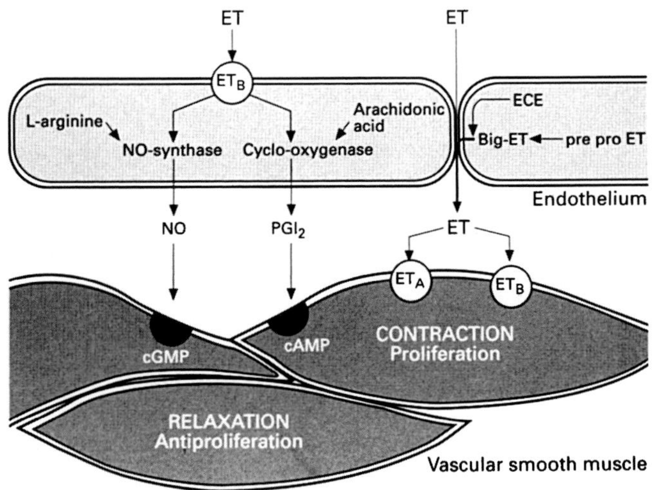

Figure 6–6 Endothelin (ET) released abluminally interacts with ET_A and ET_B receptors on vascular smooth muscle to cause contraction. Activators of ET_B receptors on endothelial cells cause vasodilation. ECE = endothelin-converting enzyme; PGI_2 = prostacyclin; cGMP = cyclic guanosine monophosphate; cAMP = cyclic adenosine monophosphate. (Reprinted from Luscher TF: Do we need endothelin antagonists? Cardiovasc Res 29:2089, 1997. Reproduced with permission of Elsevier Science-NL, Sara Burgerhartstraat 25, 1055 KV Amsterdam, the Netherlands.)

Endothelial Inhibition of Platelets

A primary function of endothelium is to maintain the fluidity of blood. This is achieved by the synthesis and release of anticoagulant (e.g., thrombomodulin, protein C), fibrinolytic (e.g., tissue-type plasminogen activator), and platelet inhibitory (e.g., PGI_2, NO) substances (Box 6–2).[34] Mediators released from aggregating platelets stimulate the release of NO and PGI_2 from intact endothelium, which act together to increase blood flow and decrease platelet adhesion and aggregation (Fig. 6–7), thereby flushing away microthrombi and maintaining the patency of the vessel.

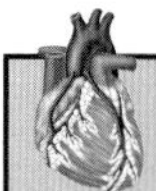

BOX 6–2 *Endothelial Inhibition of Platelets*

Healthy endothelial cells have a role in maintaining the fluidity of blood by producing

- Anticoagulant factors: protein C and thrombomodulin
- Fibrinolytic factor: tissue-type plasminogen activator
- Platelet inhibitory substances: prostacyclin and nitric oxide

With vital roles in modulating the tone of vascular smooth muscle, inhibiting platelets, and processing circulating chemicals, it seems clear that endothelial cell dysfunction would cause or contribute to ischemic syndromes. There is evidence of endothelial dysfunction in atherosclerosis, hyperlipidemia, diabetes, and hypertension.[35] Procedures such as coronary artery surgery and angioplasty disrupt the endothelium. The role of endothelium in the pathophysiology of myocardial ischemia is discussed (see Dynamic Stenosis).

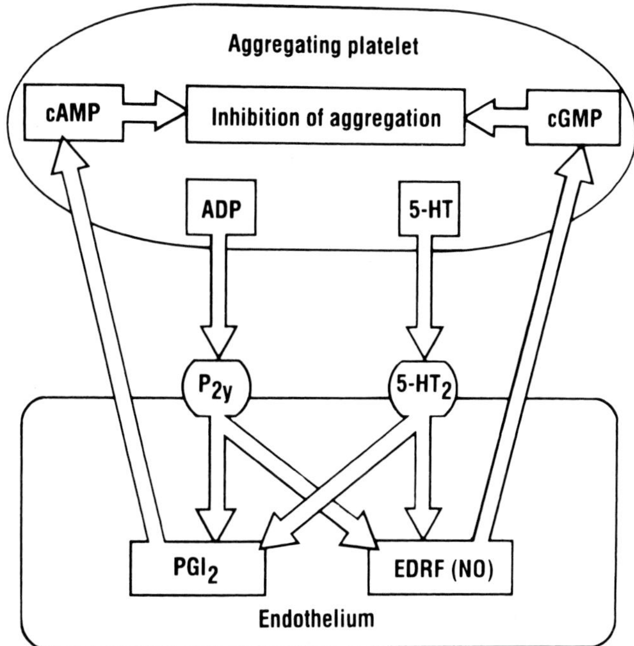

Figure 6–7 Inhibition of platelet adhesion and aggregation by intact endothelium. Aggregating platelets release adenosine diphosphate (ADP) and serotonin (5-HT), which stimulate the synthesis and release of prostacyclin (PGI_2) and endothelium-derived relaxing factor (EDRF; nitric oxide [NO]), which diffuse back to the platelets and inhibit further adhesion and aggregation and can cause disaggregation. PGI_2 and EDRF act synergistically by increasing platelet cyclic adenosine monophosphate (cAMP) and cyclic guanosine monophosphate (cGMP), respectively. By inhibiting platelets and also increasing blood flow by causing vasodilation, PGI_2 and EDRF can flush away microthrombi and prevent thrombosis of intact vessels. P_{2y} = purinergic receptor. (From Rubanyi GM: Endothelium, platelets, and coronary vasospasm. Coron Artery Dis 1:645, 1990.)

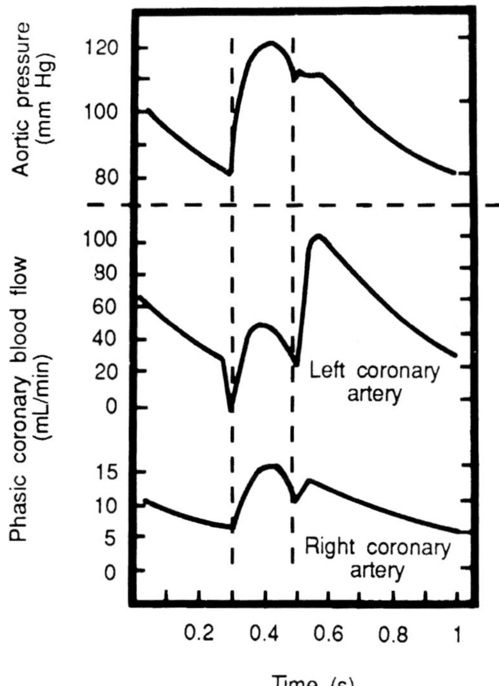

Figure 6–8 Blood flow in the left and right coronary arteries. The right ventricle is perfused throughout the cardiac cycle. Flow to the left ventricle is largely confined to diastole. (From Berne RM, Levy MN: Special circulations. *In* Berne RM, Levy MN [eds]: Physiology. St. Louis, CV Mosby, 1988, pp 540–560.)

DETERMINANTS OF CORONARY BLOOD FLOW

Under normal conditions, there are four major determinants of coronary blood flow: perfusion pressure, myocardial extravascular compression, myocardial metabolism, and neurohumoral control. Changes in myocardial perfusion caused by different interventions can be explained by analyzing the effects of those interventions on these four factors.

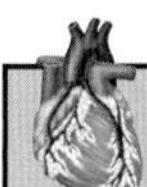

BOX 6–3 ***Determinants of Coronary Blood Flow***

The primary determinants of coronary blood flow are
- Perfusion pressure
- Myocardial extravascular compression
- Myocardial metabolism
- Neurohumoral control

Perfusion Pressure and Myocardial Compression

Coronary blood flow is proportional to the pressure gradient across the coronary circulation (Box 6–3). This gradient is calculated by subtracting downstream coronary pressure from the pressure in the root of the aorta. The determination of downstream pressure is complicated because the intramural coronary vessels are compressed with each heartbeat.

During systole, the heart throttles its own blood supply. The force of systolic myocardial compression is greatest in the subendocardial layers, where it approximates intraventricular pressure. Resistance due to extravascular compression increases with blood pressure, heart rate, contractility, and preload. Because it is difficult to measure intramyocardial pressure, the relative importance of these factors is controversial.[36,37] Flow is impeded both by direct compression and by shear caused by twisting of vessels as the heart contracts. Myocardial extravascular compression is less in the right ventricle, where pressures are lower and coronary perfusion persists during systole (Fig. 6–8). In pathologic conditions associated with pulmonary hypertension, right coronary blood flow assumes a phasic pattern similar to left coronary flow. Under normal conditions, extravascular compression contributes only a small component (10% to 25%) to total coronary vascular resistance. When the coronary vessels are dilated by pharmacologic agents such as dipyridamole or during ischemia, the effects of extravascular compression on myocardial perfusion become more important (see Transmural Blood Flow).

With each contraction, the intramural vessels are squeezed and blood is expelled forward into the coronary sinus and retrograde into the epicardial arteries. The large coronary arteries on the epicardial surface act as capacitors, charging with blood during systole and expelling blood into the coronary circulation during diastole.[38] Coronary capacitance likely explains the findings of Bellamy,[39] who reported that flow in the proximal left anterior descending coronary artery of the dog ceased when arterial pressure decreased below 45 mm Hg. It was suggested that flow throughout the coronary circulation stopped at pressures far in excess of the pressure at the coronary sinus. This pressure at which flow stopped was termed *critical closing pressure* or *zero-flow pressure* (P_{zf}). This had important implications in the calculation of coronary resistance because the effective downstream pressure would be P_{zf} and not the much lower coronary venous pressure. This is analogous to a stream with a waterfall, where flow rate over the waterfall depends on the drop from the source to the waterfall edge and is unaffected by the distance to the bottom of the falls. It was later suggested that flow through the intramural coronary vessels continues after coronary inflow near the ostia (measured by Bellamy[39]) has ceased.[40,41] There is evidence that antegrade movement of red blood cells in 20-μm arterioles continues until coronary pressure is a few mmHg higher than coronary sinus pressure.[42] Thus, the concept of a critical closing pressure greatly in excess of coronary sinus pressure is probably not valid in the coronary circulation.

Although the true downstream pressure of the coronary circulation is likely close to the coronary sinus pressure, other choices may be more appropriate in clinical circumstances. In patients with CAD, the subendocardial layers of the left ventricle are at greatest risk of ischemia and necrosis (see Transmural Blood Flow). Because this layer is perfused mostly when the aortic valve is closed, the most appropriate measure of the driving pressure for flow here is the average pressure in the aortic root during diastole. This can be approximated by aortic diastolic or mean pressure. Pressures monitored in peripheral arteries by routine methods in clinical settings can differ from central aortic readings. This is due to distortion of the pressure waveform as it is propagated through the arterial tree and inaccuracies associated with the hydraulic and electronic components of the monitoring system. Under these conditions, the mean arterial pressure may be the most reliable measure of coronary driving pressure. The true downstream pressure of the left ventricular subendocardium is the left ventricular diastolic pressure, which can be estimated by pulmonary artery occlusion pressure. When the right ventricle is at risk of ischemia (e.g., severe pulmonary hypertension), right ventricular diastolic pressure or central venous pressure may be a more appropriate choice for downstream pressure.

Myocardial Metabolism

Myocardial blood flow, like flow in the brain and skeletal muscle, is primarily under metabolic control. Even when the heart is cut off from external control mechanisms (neural and humoral factors), its ability to match blood flow to its metabolic requirements is almost unaffected.[35] Because coronary venous oxygen tension is normally 15 to 20 mm Hg, there is only a small amount of oxygen available through increased extraction. A major increase in cardiac oxygen consumption (MV_{O_2}), beyond the normal resting value of 80 to 100 mLO_2/100 g of myocardium, can occur only if oxygen delivery is increased by augmentation of coronary blood flow. Normally, flow and metabolism are closely matched so that over a wide range of oxygen consumption coronary sinus oxygen saturation changes little.[43]

Despite intensive research over the past several decades, the mediator or mediators linking myocardial metabolism so effectively to myocardial blood flow are still unknown. Hypotheses of metabolic control propose that vascular tone is linked either to a substrate that is depleted, such as oxygen or adenosine triphosphate (ATP), or to the accumulation of a metabolite such as CO_2 or hydrogen ion (Box 6–4). Adenosine has been proposed in both categories. Feigl[43] has proposed six criteria for a chemical transmitter between the cardiac myocyte and the coronary vascular smooth muscle cell.

1. The transmitter is released under appropriate conditions and can be recovered from the tissue under those conditions.
2. Transmitter substance infused into the target tissue should faithfully mimic physiologic activation.
3. The biochemical apparatus for production of the proposed transmitter is present in the tissue in an appropriate location.
4. A mechanism for inactivation and/or uptake of the transmitter is present at an appropriate location in the tissue.
5. The action of various inhibitors and blocking agents on synthesis, release, target-organ receptor function, or transmitter inactivation should have effects consistent with the hypothesis. Blocking agents should give the same effect whether the transmitter is released physiologically or artificially applied.
6. Quantitative studies should indicate that the amount and time course of transmitter release under physiologic conditions are appropriate to give the indicated effect.

Many potential mediators of metabolic regulation have been proposed.[44] Although NO has a role in many coronary vasoregulatory pathways, it does not fulfill the role of metabolic regulator as blockade of NOS does not alter the increase in myocardial blood flow associated with an increase in myocardial oxygen demand.[45] The arguments for oxygen, carbon dioxide, and adenosine are briefly examined.

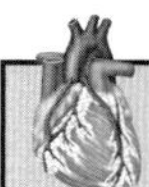

BOX 6–4 ***Myocardial Metabolism***

Several molecules have been proposed as the link between myocardial metabolism and myocardial blood flow including
- Oxygen
- Carbon dioxide
- Adenosine

Current evidence suggests that a combination of local factors act together, each with differing importance during rest, exercise, and ischemia, to match myocardial oxygen delivery to demand.

Oxygen

For oxygen to regulate coronary flow through a direct vascular action, the coronary smooth muscle would have to be more sensitive to lack of oxygen than the working cardiocytes. Coronary microvessels in vitro do not relax until P_{O_2} is below 5 mm Hg, a level well below the average P_{O_2} of 20 mm Hg in cardiac muscle cytosol.[46,47] With myocardial oxygen consumption held constant, increases in arterial oxygen content cause coronary flow to decrease while decreases in arterial oxygen content cause flow to increase. These changes could explain only 40% of the increase in flow observed with tachycardia.[48] It is undecided whether the constancy of myocardial oxygen tension is the cause or the consequence of the excellent match between myocardial metabolism and myocardial blood flow.[49]

Carbon Dioxide

The end product of substrate oxidation is CO_2, the formation of which is directly related to the level of cardiac work. Carbon dioxide is highly diffusible and can easily reach coronary smooth muscle cells. Unfortunately, it is very difficult to separate the effects on coronary tone of increasing CO_2 from concomitant increases in other metabolites. Broten et al[48] pump-perfused the left main coronary artery of dogs and used an oxygenator in the perfusion circuit to alter coronary arterial PCO_2 and PO_2 at a constant level of myocardial metabolism. Increases in arterial and coronary sinus PCO_2 caused increases in coronary blood flow in the absence of changes in myocardial oxygen consumption. Interestingly, there was a synergistic action of PCO_2 and PO_2: The increase in flow with elevation of PCO_2 was much greater at low PO_2 and vice versa. The effect of increasing CO_2, however, could not completely account for flow changes associated with an increase in myocardial oxygen consumption.

Adenosine

Adenosine is a powerful coronary vasodilator via its activation of receptors on vascular endothelium and smooth muscle. In 1963, both Berne[50] and Gerlach et al[51] independently demonstrated the production of adenosine in ischemic heart muscle. They hypothesized that the release of adenosine may serve as a feedback signal inducing coronary vasodilation and augmenting coronary blood flow in proportion to myocardial metabolic needs. Initially it was suggested that adenosine formation was coupled to myocardial oxygen tension.[50] To explain metabolic regulation by adenosine under both normoxic and ischemic conditions, a substrate theory has been proposed whereby adenosine production is linked to the cardiac energy state by the regulation of cytosolic AMP concentration.[52] According to this theory, increases in cardiac work lead to a fall in ATP potential, which results in a quantitatively appropriate change in cytosolic AMP concentration, leading to increased adenosine release. In this way the rate of adenosine production is determined by the myocardial oxygen supply/demand ratio. It is likely that adenosine causes coronary arteriolar dilation through stimulation of A_1 receptors directly coupled to ATP-sensitive K^+ (K^+_{ATP}) channels and A_2 receptor–mediated elevation of cAMP/protein kinase A, which leads to vasodilation in part by opening of K^+_{ATP} channels.[53,54]

Evidence against the adenosine hypothesis is accumulating. Adenosine deaminase is an enzyme that, when introduced in sufficient quantity into the myocardium, can significantly reduce the interstitial concentration of adenosine. Aminophylline and theophylline interfere with the coronary dilating effects of adenosine by acting on the receptor on vascular smooth muscle. Experiments using these agents to inhibit adenosine effect have shown that resting coronary blood flow, exercise-induced coronary dilation, autoregulation, and reactive hyperemia are largely unrelated to adenosine.[55-58] Measuring coronary microvessel diameters in beating hearts in situ, Kanatsuka et al[5] found that when MVO_2 was doubled by pacing, vessels between 40 and 380 μm dilated; whereas when a similar increase in flow was induced by the infusion of adenosine or dipyridamole at constant MVO_2, only vessels smaller than 150 μm dilated. Although adenosine does not seem to have an important role in metabolic regulation in the normal heart, adenosine blockade has been shown to cause a decrease in blood flow to hypoperfused myocardium sufficient to decrease systolic segment shortening.[59] Adenosine may have other important roles in ischemia where there is evidence of a cardioprotective action.[60,61]

Current evidence suggests that a combination of local factors act together, perhaps with differing importance in different situations, to match myocardial oxygen delivery to demand. The extreme difficulty of designing an experiment that can distinguish the effects of individual factors on coronary blood flow suggests that the exact mechanism of metabolic coronary regulation will not soon be elucidated.

Neural and Humoral Control

Neural Control

The role of neural control in the regulation of myocardial blood flow is difficult to study because sympathetic or parasympathetic activation can cause profound changes in heart rate, blood pressure, and contractility. The resulting changes in coronary tone, mediated by metabolic regulation, can mask the concomitant direct effects of autonomic nerves on coronary smooth muscle. Studies of isolated vessels have given results that contradict in vivo studies in part because of damage to the endothelium during preparation. Despite these difficulties, there is much interest in exploring the role of autonomic control, because it is implicated in the pathogenesis of myocardial ischemia.

CORONARY INNERVATION

The heart is supplied with branches of the sympathetic and parasympathetic divisions of the autonomic nervous system. Thicker vagal fibers end in the adventitia of coronary vessels, whereas fine nonmedullated sympathetic fibers end on vascular smooth muscle cells.[62] Large and small coronary arteries and veins are richly innervated. The sympathetic nerves to the heart and coronary vessels arise from the superior, middle, and inferior cervical sympathetic ganglia and the first four thoracic ganglia. The stellate ganglion (formed when the inferior cervical and first thoracic ganglia merge) is a major source of cardiac sympathetic innervation. The vagi supply the heart with efferent cholinergic nerves.

PARASYMPATHETIC CONTROL

Vagal stimulation causes bradycardia, decreased contractility, and lower blood pressure. The resultant fall in MVO_2 causes a metabolically mediated coronary vasoconstriction. When myocardial metabolism is held constant, however, cholinergic coronary dilation is consistently observed in response to exogenous acetylcholine, electrical vagal stimulation, and reflex activation through baroreceptors, chemoreceptors, and ventricular receptors.[35,43,63] These effects can be abolished by atropine.

In patients with angiographically normal coronary arteries, the response to intracoronary acetylcholine injection is predominantly dilation; whereas in atherosclerotic segments of epicardial arteries, constriction is observed.[64-66] Acetylcholine injected intraluminally binds to muscarinic receptors on the endothelium and stimulates the release of NO, which causes smooth muscle dilation. Acetylcholine is not normally found circulating in the blood but is released from vagal fibers and reaches the coronary smooth muscle from the adventitial side. Surprisingly, activation of muscarinic receptors on vascular smooth muscle cells causes constriction. Parasympathetic stimulation normally causes coronary vasodilation. This response depends on the ability of the coronary endothelium to elaborate NO and perhaps also EDHF (see earlier).[67,68] Parasympathetic control has not been shown to be important in the initiation of myocardial ischemia.

β-ADRENERGIC CORONARY DILATION

β-Receptor activation causes dilation of both large and small coronary vessels even in the absence of changes in blood flow.[35,43] Studies in animals indicate that both β_1- and β_2-receptors are present throughout the coronary circulation but that β_1-receptors predominate in the conductance vessels, whereas β_2-receptors predominate in the resistance vessels. Mature canine coronary collaterals respond similarly to the conductance vessels.[69,70] β-Adrenergic coronary dilation may improve the speed and accuracy of coronary blood flow regulation during exercise.[71]

α-ADRENERGIC CORONARY CONSTRICTION

Activation of the sympathetic nerves to the heart results in increases in heart rate, contractility, and blood pressure, which lead to a marked, metabolically mediated increase in coronary blood flow (Box 6–5). This suggested to early investigators that the effect of sympathetic coronary innervation is vasodilation. More recent investigation has revealed that the direct effect of sympathetic stimulation is coronary vasoconstriction, which is in competition with the metabolically mediated dilation of exercise or excitement. Whether adrenergic coronary constriction is powerful enough to further diminish blood flow in ischemic myocardium or if it can have some beneficial effect in the distribution of myocardial blood flow is controversial.

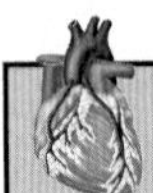

BOX 6–5 *α-Adrenergic Coronary Constriction*

Sympathetic activation causes increased heart rate, contractility, and blood pressure, leading to a marked metabolically mediated increase in coronary blood flow. Surprisingly, the direct effect of sympathetic stimulation on the coronary vessels is vasoconstriction, sufficient to restrict the increase in blood flow and increase oxygen extraction.

CLASSIFICATION

α-Adrenergic receptors can be classified anatomically as presynaptic or postsynaptic and according to their pharmacologic properties as α_1 and α_2 (Table 6–4). The receptors can be further divided into subtypes according to their signal transduction mechanism (G protein subtype) and second messenger (adenylyl cyclase, phospholipase C, etc.).[72]

PRESYNAPTIC α-RECEPTORS

α-Receptors on cardiac sympathetic nerve terminals mediate feedback inhibition of neuronal norepinephrine release. Both α_1- and α_2-receptors seem to be involved because exercise-induced increases in heart rate and contractility can be potentiated by either idazoxan (α_2-blockade) or prazocin (α_1-blockade).[73]

CARDIAC MUSCLE CELLS

Activation of myocardial α_1-receptors results in a positive inotropic effect that, in contrast to β-receptor activation, is associated with prolongation of contraction. Although normally of minor functional importance, this effect may serve as an inotropic reserve mechanism when β-receptor–mediated inotropy is impaired (e.g., hypothyroidism, cardiac failure, chronic propranolol treatment).[74] The importance of this mechanism in humans is uncertain. An increase in inotropy due to stimulation of myocardial α-receptors would result in increased $MV O_2$ and a metabolically mediated coronary dilation.

CORONARY ENDOTHELIUM

Binding of norepinephrine to α_2-receptors on vascular endothelium stimulates the release of NO, which acts to relax vascular smooth muscle. The endothelium can also act to limit the effect of norepinephrine by metabolizing it. In these ways the endothelium modulates the direct constrictive effects of α-adrenergic activation. Abnormal endothelial function in atherosclerosis may predispose to excessive α-adrenergic constriction and is implicated in the pathogenesis of myocardial ischemia (see Dynamic Stenosis).

CORONARY RESISTANCE

The magnitude of α-adrenergic vasoconstriction that occurs in the coronary bed is small compared with that which occurs in the skin and skeletal muscle. In the presence of β-blockade, intense sympathetic stimulation results in only a 20% to 30% increase in coronary resistance.[75] Mohrman and Feigl[76] examined the effect of sympathetic activation on coronary flow in the absence of β-blockade. The net effect of α-receptor vaso-

Table 6–4 Classification of α-Adrenergic Receptor Subtypes in the Heart*

Selective Agonists	Selective Antagonists	Effects of Activation
α_1		
Phenylephrine Methoxamine	Prazosin	*Presynaptic:* feedback inhibition of norepinephrine release *Postsynaptic:* coronary vasoconstriction, increase in myocardial inotropism, arrhythmias
α_2		
Clonidine Azepexole BHT 920 UK 14, 304	Yohimbine Rauwolscine Idazoxan	*Presynaptic:* feedback inhibition of norepinephrine release *Postsynaptic:* coronary vasoconstriction, arrhythmias (?)

Modified from Heusch G: Alpha-adrenergic mechanisms in myocardial ischemia. Circulation 81:1, 1990, by permission of the American Heart Association.

*Norepinephrine is a nonselective agonist. Phentolamine and phenoxybenzamine are nonselective antagonists. Phenylephrine also causes β-receptor activation.

constriction was to restrict the metabolically related flow increase by 30%, thereby increasing oxygen extraction and decreasing coronary sinus oxygen content.

Epicardial coronary diameter changes little during sympathetic stimulation.[77] α_1-Adrenergic and α_2-adrenergic receptors are found throughout the coronary circulation; however, α_1 seem to be more important in the large epicardial vessels, whereas α_2 predominates in small coronary vessels less than 100 μm in diameter.[78] Studies of mature coronary collateral vessels in dogs have generally failed to provide evidence of α-receptor–mediated vasoconstriction.[79] Following heart transplantation, patients demonstrated a lesser increase in myocardial blood flow after a cold pressor test in denervated regions of the heart.[80] The authors argue that this was not due to increased myocardial metabolism secondary to myocardial β-receptor activation. They suggest that sympathetic innervation has an important role in coronary vessel dilation during stress.

EXERCISE

α-Adrenergic coronary constrictor tone during exercise is exerted predominantly by circulating catecholamines.[81] Numerous studies indicate that myocardial blood flow during exercise is limited by α vasoconstriction.[35] In a study of exercising dogs, Huang and Feigl found that despite an increase in total coronary flow in an α-blocked region of myocardium, flow to the inner, subendocardial layer was diminished.[82] These results suggest a beneficial effect of α-adrenergic coronary constriction on the distribution of blood flow within the myocardium.

MYOCARDIAL ISCHEMIA

Buffington and Feigl[83] demonstrated the persistence of α-adrenergic coronary vasoconstriction distal to a moderate coronary stenosis during norepinephrine infusion. Investigations in dogs have demonstrated that, as coronary reserve is depleted by increasing stenosis severity, the response to sympathetic stimulation shifts from a metabolically induced coronary dilation to coronary constriction.[84,85] These observations suggest that sympathetic coronary vasoconstriction limits coronary blood flow even during myocardial ischemia, when autoregulatory reserve is exhausted (see Coronary Reserve). There is no consensus as to the importance of α_1- versus α_2-receptors in ischemic myocardium.[35] Using constant flow coronary perfusion in anesthetized dogs, Nathan and Feigl[86] compared the transmural distribution of myocardial blood flow in α-blocked and intact regions of myocardium during hypoperfusion. Surprisingly, α-blockade diverted blood flow from the subendocardium to the subepicardium. This suggests that α vasoconstriction had limited flow more in the subepicardium, thereby producing an anti-steal effect and improved perfusion of the more vulnerable inner layers of the left ventricle. Chilian and Ackell[87] found similar results in exercising dogs with an artificial coronary stenosis. On the other hand, work from Heusch and colleagues[88,89] demonstrated improved subendocardial perfusion distal to a severe coronary stenosis with α_2-receptor blockade. This controversy is unresolved.[90] α-Receptor blockers have not been shown to have a role in the treatment of myocardial ischemia in patients with CAD.

STUDIES IN HUMANS

Studies indicate that there is little α-adrenoceptor–mediated tone in resting humans.[91] Clinical studies have failed to provide convincing evidence that α-adrenergic coronary constriction plays an important role in Prinzmetal's variant angina (angina with ST-segment elevation at rest).[92] During sympathetic activation, however, there is evidence that α vasoconstriction can precipitate myocardial ischemia by further narrowing diseased coronary arteries. This has been shown during isometric exercise, during dynamic exercise, and with the cold pressor test (see Dynamic Stenosis).[93-98]

Humoral Control

A complete understanding of the effects of circulating substances on the coronary vessels would require determining their effects on large versus small coronary vessels while separating direct effects on coronary vessels from changes in tone mediated by changes in myocardial metabolism. This is further complicated by the critical role of an intact vascular endothelium in modulating these responses (see Endothelium). Some of the better-studied agents are discussed briefly.

The peptide hormones include vasopressin (AVP), atrial natriuretic peptide (ANP), vasoactive intestinal peptide, neuropeptide Y, and calcitonin gene–related peptide.[44] Of these, AVP and ANP have been the most studied. It has been demonstrated in dogs that AVP, in concentrations 3 to 30 times those found in stressed patients, can cause vasoconstriction sufficient to produce myocardial ischemia.[99] In large coronary arteries, the dilator response (via NO) likely exceeded the constrictor response.[35] In physiologic concentrations, AVP acts primarily as an antidiuretic hormone with little effect on the coronary circulation. ANP can cause endothelium-dependent coronary dilation but is not known to have significant vascular effects in physiologic concentrations.[100]

Angiotensin-converting enzyme (ACE) is present on vascular endothelium and converts angiotensin I to angiotensin II (AII), which causes coronary vasoconstriction. AII also facilitates the release of norepinephrine from presynaptic adrenergic nerve terminals. ACE inactivates bradykinin, which can attenuate vasoconstriction via NO stimulation. Thus, ACE inhibition can reduce coronary tone by suppressing AII formation and degrading bradykinin and perhaps also by decreasing norepinephrine release. Despite these theoretical considerations, ACE inhibition has not been shown to be of benefit in human myocardial ischemia other than through control of afterload.[101]

PGI_2 and thromboxane (TxA_2) are synthesized from arachidonic acid in a reaction catalyzed by cyclooxygenase. PGI_2 is synthesized in the vascular endothelium and, in addition to inhibiting platelet aggregation, induces vasodilation (see Endothelium-Derived Relaxing Factors). TxA_2 is mainly synthesized in platelets and causes platelet aggregation and vasoconstriction in the presence of damaged vascular endothelium. In response to TxA_2 the intact endothelium releases NO, causing both vasodilation and platelet disaggregation, a mechanism to maintain patency of normal vessels (see Endothelial Inhibition of Platelets). Unlike platelets, the vascular endothelium can synthesize proteins de novo, and thus cyclooxygenase acetylation via aspirin administration has a lesser effect in reducing vascular PGI_2 than platelet TxA_2. Other than in platelet-vessel interactions and inflammation, prostaglandins are not known to have an important role in the regulation of coronary blood flow.[35] Serotonin (5-HT) is another platelet product that can cause endothelium-dependent dilation of coronary arterial vessels smaller than 100 μm but causes constriction of larger epicardial coronary arteries.[102]

Histamine receptors are present in the coronary vessels. H_1-receptors are located on vascular smooth muscle cells of large and small coronary arteries and mediate vasoconstriction. H_2-receptors are located on smooth muscle cells of arterioles and mediate vasodilation. H_1-receptors are also located on vascular endothelium and can mediate vasodilation via stimulation of NO release. In patients with vasospastic angina and endothelial dysfunction, administration of exogenous histamine can cause vasospasm.[54,103]

CORONARY PRESSURE-FLOW RELATIONS

Autoregulation

Autoregulation is the tendency for organ blood flow to remain constant despite changes in arterial perfusion pressure.[104] Autoregulation can maintain flow to myocardium served by stenotic coronary arteries despite low perfusion pressure distal to the obstruction. This is a local mechanism of control and can be observed in isolated, denervated hearts. If MVO_2 is fixed, coronary blood flow remains relatively constant between mean arterial pressures of 60 to 140 mm Hg. At a given cardiac workload, the level of flow (determined by metabolic regulation) is maintained constant over a broad range of pressure by autoregulation (Fig. 6–9).

To study autoregulation, coronary perfusion pressure must be varied while holding MVO_2 constant. This is difficult in the heart because changing aortic pressure changes both the perfusion pressure for the coronary arteries and the afterload of the left ventricle. Thus, changes in aortic pressure inevitably change MVO_2. This problem is overcome by cannulating the coronary arteries and perfusing them with a pump. However, even when heart rate and aortic pressure are held constant, MVO_2 changes with changing coronary pressure. This is because myocardial contractility and metabolism increase when coronary pressure is raised above the normal autoperfused level. This phenomenon is known as the Gregg effect and may be explained by the "garden hose" hypothesis of Lochner, whereby engorgement of the coronary vasculature elongates the myocardial sarcomere length during diastole and contractile strength is increased due to the Frank-Starling mechanism (for a detailed review see Feigl[43] and Gregg[105]).

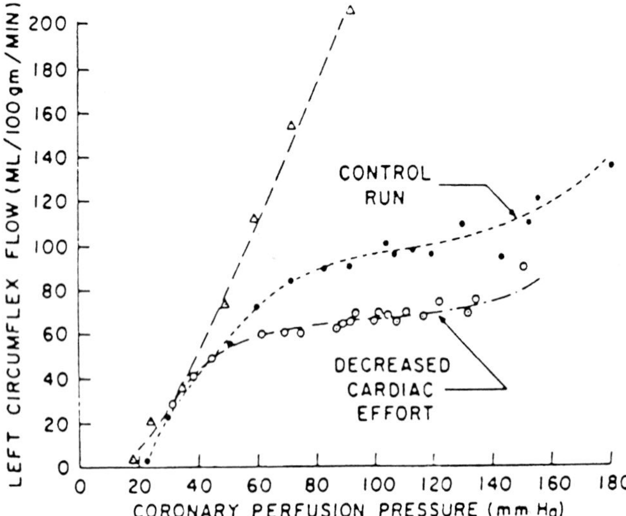

Figure 6–9 Autoregulation at two levels of myocardial oxygen consumption. Pressure in the cannulated left circumflex artery was varied independently of aortic pressure. When pressures were suddenly raised or lowered from 40 mm Hg, flow instantaneously increased with pressure *(steep line, open triangles)*. With time, flow decreases to the steady-state level determined by oxygen consumption *(open* and *closed circles)*. The vertical distance from the steady-state (autoregulating) line to the instantaneous pressure-flow line is the autoregulatory flow reserve (see text). (From Mosher P, Ross J Jr, McFate PA, Shaw RF: Control of coronary blood flow by an autoregulatory mechanism. Circ Res 14:250, 1964.)

In addition to the Gregg effect, two other issues complicate studies of autoregulation: collateral flow and myocardial oxygen extraction. If pressure is lowered in the left coronary artery and not in the right, there is a pressure gradient for flow from the right to left coronary artery via collateral vessels. Flow measured proximally in the left coronary artery then underestimates flow reaching the myocardium. Normal coronary sinus oxygen tension (CSO_2) is below 20 mm Hg. Dole and Nuno observed that autoregulation was effective when CSO_2 was below 25 mm Hg but was completely lost when CSO_2 exceeded 32 mm Hg. Autoregulation can be intensified by vasoconstriction (increased oxygen extraction) and attenuated by vasodilation (decreased oxygen extraction).[106,107] The degradation of autoregulation with α-receptor blockade suggests a benefit of adrenergic coronary vasoconstriction.[108]

Early reports indicated that autoregulation is less effective in the right ventricle than the left. Now it has been suggested that increases in right coronary pressures may produce large changes in MVO_2, perhaps due to an exaggerated Gregg effect. When changes in myocardial metabolism are taken into account, autoregulation in the right and left ventricles is similar.[109,110]

Quantitation of the degree of autoregulation must involve a comparison of the observed change in vascular resistance to the change in resistance that would have occurred in the absence of flow autoregulation. Some degree of autoregulation exists when the relative change in flow ($\Delta F/F$) is less than the relative change in pressure ($\Delta P/P$). From these definitions, Dole has derived an autoregulation index that can be used to quantify the effects of different agents on coronary autoregulation.[107,111]

Three theories have been proposed to explain coronary autoregulation: the tissue pressure theory, the myogenic theory, and the metabolic theory.[112] The tissue pressure hypothesis proposes that changes in perfusion pressure result in directionally similar changes in capillary filtration and therefore tissue pressure. In this way extravascular resistance would oppose changes in flow with changes in perfusion pressure. Experimental evidence has shown, however, that there is no relationship between the degree of autoregulation and the magnitude of change in tissue pressure. Arterial smooth muscle contracts in response to augmented intraluminal pressure; this is known as the myogenic response. This response has been demonstrated in coronary arterioles in the presence and absence of functioning endothelium.[113] The argument for myogenic regulation of coronary flow is that myocardial metabolic changes are not rapid enough to explain large decreases in resistance following coronary occlusions for one or two heartbeats. However, myocardial metabolic events have been shown to occur during the course of a single cardiac contraction.[114] The metabolic theory of autoregulation proposes that coronary arteriolar tone is determined by the balance of myocardial oxygen supply and demand. An increase in flow above the requirements of metabolism would wash out metabolites or cause accumulation of substrates, and this would be the signal for an appropriate change in coronary tone. Although metabolic regulation and autoregulation are separate phenomena, they may therefore have a common underlying mechanism. Metabolic regulation was discussed earlier (see Myocardial Metabolism). For an instructive, three-dimensional, graphic analysis of the interrelations among coronary artery pressure, myocardial metabolism, and coronary blood flow, see Feigl et al.[115]

Coronary Reserve

Myocardial ischemia causes intense coronary vasodilation. Following a 10- to 30-second coronary occlusion, restoration of perfusion pressure is accompanied by a marked increase in coronary flow. This large increase in flow, which can be five or six times resting flow in the dog, is termed *reactive hyperemia.* The repayment volume is greater than the debt volume (Fig. 6–10). There is, however, no overpayment of the oxygen debt because oxygen extraction falls during the hyperemia.[116] The presence of high coronary flows when coronary venous oxygen content is high suggests that mediators other than oxygen are responsible for this metabolically induced vasodilation.[43] The difference between resting coronary blood flow and peak flow during reactive hyperemia represents the autoregulatory coronary flow reserve: the further capacity of the arteriolar bed to dilate in response to ischemia. Figure 6–9 shows the flow reserve is the vertical distance from the autoregulating pressure-flow curve (open or closed circles) to the nonautoregulating curve (triangles). The reserve is greater at higher perfusing pressure and lower MVO_2. Unlike cannula-perfused preparations in which these data are obtained, in the clinical setting increases in pressure increase both perfusing pressure and MVO_2. Reactive hyperemia responses have been used in animals and humans to estimate coronary reserve in conditions such as obstructive coronary disease, aortic stenosis, and left ventricular hypertrophy (see Critical Stenosis).[117-119] The myocardial fractional flow reserve (FFR) is calculated by dividing the pressure in a coronary vessel distal to a stenosis during maximal pharmacologic dilation by the aortic root pressure. This ratio can be easily measured in the angiography suite and has been recommended as a useful index of the functional severity of coronary stenoses of intermediate morphologic severity on angiography, as well as a measure of residual obstruction following interventions.[120,121]

It has been generally accepted that the coronary resistance vessels are maximally dilated when coronary perfusion pressure is reduced sufficiently to cause myocardial ischemia. In fact, agents such as adenosine, carbochromen, and dipyridamole can cause further increases in coronary flow in the presence of intense ischemia, when autoregulatory reserve is believed to be exhausted. This pharmacologic vasodilator reserve is greater than the autoregulatory vasodilator reserve. If flow to ischemic myocardium can be increased by pharmacologic dilation of resistance vessels, the use of these agents should reverse ischemic dysfunction and metabolism. Arteriolar dilators have, in general, not been found to be beneficial during myocardial ischemia. Coronary blood flow in the different layers of the ventricle must be reviewed to understand why (Box 6–6).

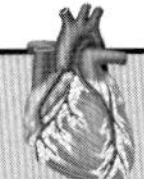

BOX 6–6 ***Transmural Blood Flow***

- When coronary perfusion pressure is inadequate, the inner third of the left ventricular wall is the first region to become ischemic or necrotic.
- During systole, intramyocardial pressure is highest in the inner layers of the ventricle, and this restricts perfusion to that region.
- In eccentric hypertrophy, this effect is exaggerated, and the subendocardium is at increased risk of ischemia.

Transmural Blood Flow

It is well known that when coronary perfusion pressure is inadequate, the inner one third to one quarter of the left ventricular wall is the first region to become ischemic or necrotic.[122] This increased vulnerability of the subendocardium may be due to an increased demand for perfusion or a decreased supply, compared with the outer layers. There has been extensive study of the transmural distribution of oxygen consumption, utilization of oxidizable substrates, activity of glycolytic and mitochondrial enzymes, tissue contents of endogenous substrates, high-energy phosphates, lactate, isoforms of contractile proteins, and fiber stress and fiber shortening. In general, these studies indicate that if such differences exist between the layers of the left ventricle, they are unlikely to exceed 10% to 20%.[43,123] It is likely that preferential underperfusion of the subendocardium is the primary determinant of its increased vulnerability.

Regional blood flow in the myocardium is usually determined using radioactive microspheres. These plastic beads, labeled with a radioisotope, are injected into the bloodstream. The assumption is that they mix uniformly with blood and are distributed in proportion to blood flow, as if they were red blood cells.[124] Because they are rigid and larger than red cells (9- or 15-μm diameters are usually chosen), they are trapped in the microcirculation. At the end of an experiment, the heart

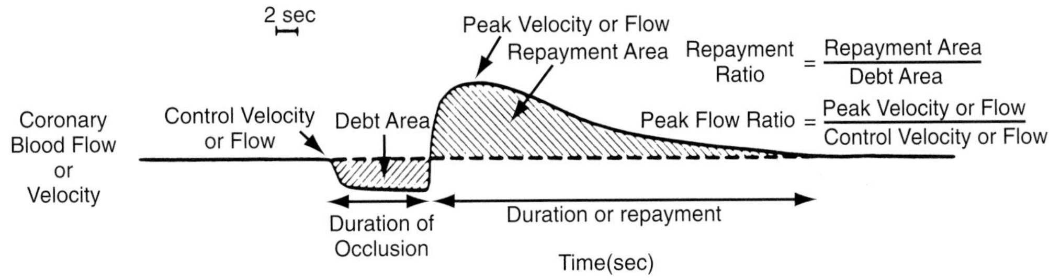

Figure 6–10 Schematic diagram of the reactive hyperemic response to a 10-second coronary occlusion. (From Marcus ML: Metabolic regulation of coronary blood flow. *In* Marcus ML [ed]: The Coronary Circulation in Health and Disease. New York, McGraw-Hill, 1983, pp 65–92. Reproduced with permission of The McGraw-Hill Companies.)

can be divided into small blocks and the amount of radioactivity in each piece measured in a gamma counter. The blood flow to each block of tissue is proportional to the number of microspheres in each piece, which can be determined from its radioactivity. By using different radioisotopes as labels, several sets of microspheres can be injected during an experiment, giving "snapshots" of what flow was at the time of each injection. It is difficult to reduce the variability of the technique below 10%.[43,125] Using this technique, subendocardial blood flow is found to be about 10% greater than subepicardial blood flow under normal circumstances. This gives a normal subendocardial/subepicardial or inner/outer (I/O) blood flow ratio of 1:10. This ratio is maintained at normal perfusing pressures even at heart rates above 200 beats/min.

If coronary pressure is gradually reduced, autoregulation is exhausted and flow decreases in the inner layers of the left ventricle before it begins to decrease in the outer layers (Fig. 6–11). This indicates that there is less flow reserve in the subendocardium than in the subepicardium. The limits of autoregulation depend on the level of cardiac work (see Autoregulation) and on the experimental conditions. In conscious dogs, the mean coronary pressure at which evidence of subendocardial ischemia appeared was 38 mm Hg at a heart rate of 100 beats/min and increased to 61 mm Hg at 200 beats/min. Subepicardial flow during tachycardia did not fall even at pressures as low as 33 mm Hg.[126] Because subepicardial flow is rarely inadequate, a subendocardial/subepicardial blood flow ratio close to 1.0 indicates adequate subendocardial flow and an appropriate matching of myocardial oxygen supply to oxygen demand. For this reason, the I/O ratio is often used as a measure of the adequacy of myocardial blood flow.

Three mechanisms have been proposed to explain the decreased coronary reserve in the subendocardium: differential systolic intramyocardial pressure, differential diastolic intramyocardial pressure, and interactions between systole

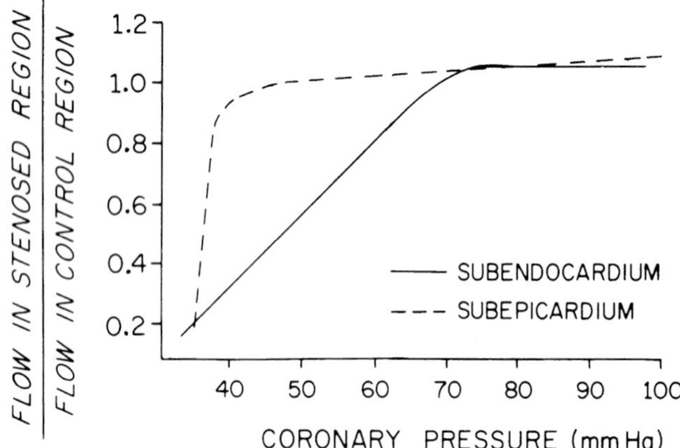

Figure 6–11 Pressure-flow relationships of the subepicardial and subendocardial thirds of the left ventricle in anesthetized dogs. In the subendocardium, autoregulation is exhausted and flow becomes pressure dependent when pressure distal to a stenosis falls below 70 mm Hg. In the subepicardium, autoregulation persists until perfusion pressure falls below 40 mm Hg. Autoregulatory coronary reserve is less in the subendocardium. (Redrawn from Guyton RA, McClenathan JH, Newman GE, Michaelis LL: Significance of subendocardial ST segment elevation caused by coronary stenosis in the dog. Am J Cardiol 40:373, 1977.)

and diastole. Because the force of systolic myocardial compression is greatest in the inner layers of the ventricle and is low at the subepicardium, it was believed that the outer layers of the heart were perfused throughout the cardiac cycle while the subendocardium was perfused only during diastole. The subendocardium would have to obtain its entire flow during only a portion of the cycle and, therefore, would have to have a lower resistance. Studies suggesting that there may be very little systolic flow even to the outer layers argue against this explanation.[127] The second mechanism is based on the high coronary pressures observed when coronary flow has ceased during a long diastole, P_{zf} (see Perfusion Pressure).[39] The shape of the pressure-flow relation during a long diastole suggests that P_{zf} is higher in the subendocardium. This means that perfusion pressure for the subendocardium is lower in diastole compared with the outer layers of myocardium. Available evidence suggests that P_{zf} is not high in any layer and unlikely to be more than 2 to 3 mm Hg higher in the subendocardium than in the subepicardium.[127] Hoffman[127] and Hoffman and Spaan[109] proposed an interaction between systole and diastole as the explanation for the increased vulnerability of the subendocardium to ischemia. During systole, intramyocardial pressure is high enough throughout most of the ventricular wall to squeeze blood out of the intramural vessels and into the extramural coronary veins and arteries. Because the compressive force is greatest in the subendocardium, vessels here are the narrowest at end-systole. At the beginning of diastole, blood is directed first to vessels with the lowest resistance, then to the larger vessels in the subepicardium, and last to the most narrowed vessels in the subendocardium. In this way, should the duration of diastole or the diastolic perfusion pressure be reduced, the subendocardial muscle would receive the least flow. Spaan[36] presents an interesting analysis of the interaction between arterial pressure and force of contraction as an intramyocardial pump. Although this theory is compatible with existing evidence, support for it remains indirect until it becomes possible to measure phasic pressures and flows in separate layers of myocardium.

When the left ventricle hypertrophies in response to a pressure load (aortic stenosis, hypertension), myofibrillar growth outstrips the capillary network, resulting in decreased capillary density and increased diffusion distances. The net effect is to reduce coronary autoregulatory reserve.[128] The transmural gradient of reserve is exaggerated as well, so that the subendocardium is at increased risk of ischemia in the hypertrophied heart compared with normal.[129]

In addition to the transmural gradient of coronary reserve from outer to inner layer of the left ventricle, there is marked variation of reserve between small regions of myocardium within a layer.[130] This heterogeneity of flow reserve may explain why pharmacologic reserve exceeds autoregulatory reserve (see Coronary Reserve). During hypoperfusion regional myocardial blood flow is decreased, but in all layers some small pieces of muscle have no flow reserve left while adjacent pieces can have substantial reserve. Fewer pieces retain reserve in the subendocardium than in the subepicardium. The increase in flow in response to an infusion of adenosine is due to increased flow in the small regions with reserve, with no change in the adjacent fully dilated regions.[131-133] These findings suggest that ischemia causes maximal coronary vasodilation and that increases in flow with adenosine or dipyridamole are due to dilation of vessels in nonischemic regions. Contrasting evidence is provided by Duncker and Bache,[54] who used a balloon occluder to simulate a coronary stenosis in exercising dogs. The occluder was adjusted to maintain distal coronary pressure constant at 43 mm Hg. During exercise, an intracoronary infusion of adenosine increased blood flow to all myocardial layers and improved regional systolic segment shortening. Although this is evidence of vasodilator reserve in ischemic myocardium, the constant distal pressure preparation does not faithfully mimic a coronary stenosis because it makes transmural steal impossible (see Coronary Steal). In general, pharmacologic dilation of resistance vessels has the potential to worsen ischemia by producing coronary steal. Dilation of larger penetrating vessels (50 to 500 μm in diameter) with nitrovasodilators could preferentially decrease resistance to blood flow to the subendocardium, and this may, in addition to favorable effects on the systemic circulation, explain the usefulness of nitrates in the treatment of angina.[54]

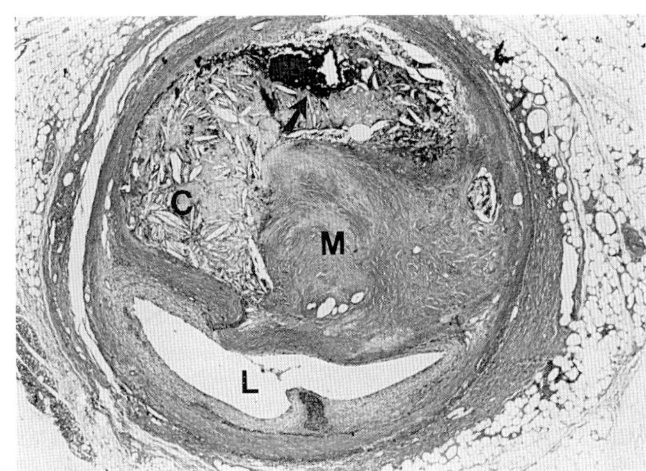

Figure 6–12 Atherosclerotic human coronary artery of an 80-year-old man. There is severe narrowing of the central arterial lumen (L). The intima consists of a complex collection of cells, extracellular matrix (M), and a necrotic core with cholesterol (C) deposits. Rupture of plaque microvessels has resulted in intraplaque hemorrhage *(arrow)* at the base of the necrotic core. (Movat's pentachrome-stained slide, original magnification ×40.)

ATHEROSCLEROSIS

The atherosclerotic lesion consists of an excessive accumulation of smooth muscle cells in the intima, with quantitative and qualitative changes in the noncellular connective tissue components of the artery wall and intracellular and extracellular deposition of lipoproteins and mineral components (e.g., calcium) (Box 6–7). By definition, *atherosclerosis* is a combination of "atherosis" and "sclerosis." The latter term, *sclerosis*, refers to the hard collagenous material that accumulates in lesions and is usually more voluminous than the pultaceous "gruel" of the atheroma (Fig. 6–12).

Stary[134] noted that the earliest detectable change in the evolution of coronary atherosclerosis in young people was the accumulation of intracellular lipid in the subendothelial region, giving rise to lipid-filled macrophages or "foam cells." Grossly, a collection of foam cells may give the artery wall the appearance of a "fatty streak." In general, fatty streaks are covered by a layer of intact endothelium and are not characterized by excessive smooth muscle cell accumulation. At later stages of atherogenesis, extracellular lipoproteins accumulate in the musculoelastic layer of the intima, eventually forming an avascular core of lipid-rich debris that is separated from the central arterial lumen by a fibrous cap of collagenous material. Foam cells are not usually seen deep within the atheromatous core, but are frequently found at the periphery of the lipid core.

Atherogenesis

Certain human arteries are more prone to develop atherosclerosis than others. For example, the coronary, renal, and internal carotid arteries, as well as some areas of the aorta, are known to be common sites for lesion formation.[134] In the Pathobiological Determinants of Atherosclerosis in Youth (PDAY) study, the aorta and right coronary arteries of 1378 young people aged 15 to 34 years who died as a result of trauma were studied.[135] Two-dimensional maps of lipid-laden fatty streaks and fibrous plaques were made for each vessel. Although atherosclerosis is usually clinically silent until middle age or later, these investigators found that the disease process begins in adolescence or childhood. Moreover, fatty streaks and fibrous plaques do not occur randomly in the circulation, but follow a well-defined distribution pattern. For example, in the right coronary artery fatty streaks were found with the highest probability in the proximal 2 cm of this vessel, which closely parallels the distribution of raised fibrous lesions. However, in the abdominal aorta, where aortic lesions are commonly found, the high prevalence of fatty streaks did not always correlate with the prevalence of raised fibrous lesions. Therefore, at least in the aorta, the role of childhood fatty streaks in the development of adult fibrous lesions is uncertain.

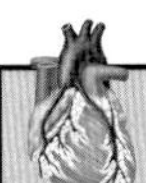

BOX 6–7 ***Atherosclerosis***

- The atherosclerotic process begins in childhood and adolescence.
- The progression of an atherosclerotic lesion has many similarities to the process of wound healing.
- Inflammation, lipid infiltration, and smooth muscle proliferation have important roles in atherogenesis.
- Impairment of endothelial function is an early consequence of atherosclerosis.
- Lipid-lowering therapy can help restore endothelial function and prevent coronary events.

The atherogenic stimuli that promote the progression of early lesions to clinically relevant stenoses are not known. The development of CAD is associated with various risk factors. Dyslipidemias, hypertension, diabetes mellitus, cigarette smoking, and a family history of premature CAD are known to correlate with premature vascular disease. The association between lipid disorders and atherogenesis is best understood and is discussed below. Unfortunately, little is known about how the remaining risk factors may contribute to lesion development.

Historically, there are two classic theories of atherogenesis. According to von Rokitansky's[136] thrombogenic (or encrustation) theory, fibrin is the initiating factor in lesion development. Later, Duguid[137] expanded on this theory by suggesting that atherosclerosis is the result of altered fibrinolysis, whereas more recent studies have documented the overexpression of prothrombotic factors, such as plasminogen activator inhibitor-1, in atherosclerotic plaques.[138] Alternatively, in 1856, Virchow's[139] inhibition (or insudation) theory proposed that atherosclerotic lesions were the result of altered vessel wall permeability. Variations of this theory have been suggested by others and all support the concept that the accumulation of various plasma components, including lipoproteins, may be important during lesion formation. For example, Ross and Glomset[140] blended the concepts of these original hypotheses into the "response-to-injury" hypothesis, in which both lipid infiltration and thrombus formation play important roles in atherogenesis. Similarly, Schwartz and colleagues[141] compared arterial narrowing in atherosclerotic arteries with the process of wound healing. This perspective has advantages, as it allows a multifactorial process such as atherosclerosis to be broken down into components of a more completely understood process such as the biology of a skin wound. For example, wound healing of any form begins with the formation of a clot (fibrin- and fibronectin-containing gel) that fills the wound and provides a provisional matrix for inflammatory cells, fibroblasts, and newly formed microvessels.[142,143] This is followed by the proliferation and migration of fibroblasts into the wound.[144] By day 7 after injury, microvessels grow into the base of the wound and form granulation tissue. As the wound matures and undergoes contracture, these blood vessels regress and fibroblasts disappear. Following resorption of microvessels, tissue hypoxia develops and likely plays a role in the completion of the final scarring process.[145] As discussed below, there is now ample evidence to suggest that many similar events take place during arterial wound healing; however, as atherosclerosis is a chronic process, it is likely that vascular lesion formation involves indolent levels of inflammation with ongoing cycles of injury and repair over many years.[142,146,147]

Arterial Wall Inflammation

A number of studies have demonstrated the presence of monocytes/macrophages and T lymphocytes in the arteries of not only advanced lesions but also early atherosclerotic lesions of young adults.[148,149] Moreover, in experimental atherosclerosis, leukocyte infiltration into the vascular wall is known to precede smooth muscle cell hyperplasia.[150] Once inside the artery wall, mononuclear cells may play several important roles in lesion development. For example, monocytes may transform into macrophages and become involved in the local oxidation of low-density lipoproteins (LDLs) and accumulation of oxidized LDLs. Alternatively, macrophages in the artery wall may act as a rich source of factors that, for example, promote cell proliferation, migration, or the breakdown of local tissue barriers. The latter process of local tissue degradation may be very important for the initiation of acute coronary artery syndromes as loss of arterial wall integrity may lead to plaque fissuring or rupture.[151]

Normally, the endothelium exhibits a low affinity for circulating leukocytes. The transmigration of leukocytes into the artery wall must occur as a facilitated process. The release of proinflammatory cytokines such as interleukin-1 may promote the expression of leukocyte adhesive molecules.[152] For simplicity, the interaction between leukocytes and the endothelium can be considered to involve three steps.[153] First, leukocytes in the bloodstream must loosely associate and roll along the endothelium, a process that is mediated by selectins expressed on endothelial cells.[152] Second, firm adhesion of these leukocytes to endothelial cells occurs via the interaction between integrins, such as $\alpha_4\beta_1$ (also known as very late antigen-4, or VLA-4), expressed on leukocytes, and counter-receptors, such as vascular cell adhesion molecule-1, or VCAM-1, on endothelial cells.[154] Finally, the transmigration of leukocytes into the subendothelial space is mediated by various migration-inducing factors, such as monocyte chemoattractant protein-1, or MCP-1.[155]

Dysfunction, discontinuity, or injury of the endothelial cell monolayer has been postulated to play a significant role in facilitating the transmigration of leukocytes into the intima and the development of intimal hyperplasia. However, the premise that regrowth of a healthy endothelium limits neointimal accumulation is inconsistent with the results of several independent lines of investigation. For example, in experimental models smooth muscle cell proliferation is not increased in arterial regions devoid of an endothelium.[156] Moreover, restoration of the endothelium, as might be achieved by seeding endothelial cells back into a denuded artery, does not decrease neointimal accumulation after vascular interventions.[157] The presence of an endothelium in the central lumen of an artery and resistance to intimal growth do not appear to be inextricably linked. Finally, it is important to note that the endothelium is not restricted to the central lumen, as the artery wall is also invested with a rich supply of microvessels (i.e., vasa vasorum).[158-161] The vasa vasorum are likely another portal of entry for inflammatory cells into the artery wall, particularly because the expression of certain adhesion molecules is more abundant in the endothelium lining these microvessels than that of the central arterial lumen.[162]

Role of Lipoproteins in Lesion Formation

The clinical and experimental evidence linking dyslipidemias with atherogenesis is well established and need not be reviewed here. However, the exact mechanisms by which lipid moieties contribute to the pathogenesis of atherosclerosis remain elusive. Although the simple concept of cholesterol accumulating in artery walls until flow is obstructed may be correct in certain animal models, this theory is not correct for human arteries.

Much of the pioneering work in understanding cholesterol metabolism is based on seminal observations by Brown and Goldstein.[163] The work of these two investigators focused on LDL, the so-called bad form of cholesterol, and the absence (or deficient forms) of the LDL receptor that are seen in familial hypercholesterolemia (FH). Patients with FH have high levels of LDL cholesterol and have accelerated forms of atherosclerosis as cholesterol moieties enter the cell via an alternate route. In the absence of a functional LDL receptor, LDL cholesterol is oxidized and taken up by scavenger receptors of monocytes and macrophages resident within the artery wall. Steinberg[164] integrated these data into a theory of atherogenesis that highlights the central role of LDL oxidation and the formation of lipid-laden monocytes in fatty streaks.

One of the major consequences of cholesterol accumulation in the artery wall is thought to be the impairment of endothelial function. The endothelium is more than a physical barrier between the bloodstream and the artery wall. Under normal conditions, the endothelium is capable of modulating vascular tone (e.g., via NO), thrombogenicity, fibrinolysis, platelet function, and inflammation. In the presence of traditional risk factors, particularly dyslipidemias, these protective endothelial functions are reduced or lost. It is important to note that the loss of these endothelium-derived functions may occur in the presence or absence of an underlying atherosclerotic plaque and may simply imply that atherogenesis has begun. Aggressive attempts to normalize atherosclerotic risk factors (e.g., diet and lipid-lowering therapies) may markedly attenuate endothelial dysfunction, even in the presence of extensive atherosclerosis. A number of clinical studies demonstrate dramatic improvements in endothelial function, as well as cardiovascular morbidity and mortality, with the use of inhibitors of 3-hydroxy-3-methylglutaryl coenzyme A (HMG-CoA) reductase, or "statins."[165-167] Future studies may help clarify the exact mechanisms by which dyslipidemias (and other risk factors) alter endothelial function.

Smooth Muscle Cell Proliferation, Migration, and Arterial Remodeling

The dominant cell type in atherosclerotic lesions is the smooth muscle cell, and as lesions progress the number of smooth muscle cells in the artery wall tends to increase. Therefore, smooth muscle replication must occur at some time during atherogenesis. Perhaps the first line of evidence that cell replication occurs in human arteries is from the observation that atherosclerotic plaques contain monoclonal cell populations. Elegant studies by Benditt and Benditt[168] demonstrated that groups (or clones) of cells that arise from a single progenitor cell are present in tissue from atherosclerotic coronary arteries of women who were deficient in glucose-6-phosphate dehydrogenase (G6PD). As G6PD is an X-chromosome–linked enzyme that has two isoforms, cells would express only one isoform, with the other isoform being suppressed on the inactivated X chromosome. Groups of cells in an atherosclerotic plaque that contain only one isoform of G6PD are likely the result of proliferation of a single progenitor cell. Murry et al[169] studied the monoclonality of atherosclerotic plaques using X chromosome inactivation patterns. Using the polymerase chain reaction, they examined the monoclonality of plaques according to the methylation pattern of the human androgen receptor gene, a highly polymorphic locus on the X chromosome for which 90% of women are heterozygous. These investigators noted that diseased and normal arteries contain monoclonal populations (or patches) of cells. They speculated that the monoclonality of plaques might be due to expansion of a preexisting monoclonal patch of cells, rather than mutation or selection of individual cells in the artery wall.

Little is known about when and why cells proliferate in the artery wall. However, it is known that early in life there is a rapid expansion in neointimal smooth muscle cell mass. Sims et al described the accumulation of intimal smooth muscle cells in the left anterior descending coronary artery of neonates.[170,171] Using electron microscopy, these investigators demonstrated interruptions in the internal elastic lamina in coronary arteries where a neointima had formed. These interruptions in the internal elastic lamina are not present in all human arteries. Indeed, the internal mammary artery, which typically is devoid of atherosclerosis, has an intact internal elastic lamina. It has been suggested that medial smooth muscle cells migrate inward through breaks in the internal elastic lamina to expand and form a neointima. The frequency and degree of smooth muscle cell replication in adult coronary arteries have been examined by various investigators. The majority of these studies have demonstrated very low replication rates in tissue from both normal and diseased arteries.[172-175] Whether these low cell replication rates are sufficient to gradually result in advanced lesions or if sporadic bursts of replication occur in response to injury is unknown. Finally, it is recognized that programmed cell death, or apoptosis, occurs in the artery wall.[176] The accumulation of cells in the artery wall is a function of not only cell proliferation but also apoptosis.

The role of smooth muscle cell migration in adult CAD is poorly understood. It has been suggested, however, that like fibroblasts that migrate into the base of a wound, arterial wall smooth muscle cells migrate inward to expand plaque mass. Smooth muscle cell migration into the intima has been studied in various animal models of neointimal formation (e.g., rat carotid artery model).[11] The majority of these models demonstrate the inward migration of medial smooth muscle cells after normal arteries are subjected to balloon injury. A number of growth factors (e.g., platelet-derived growth factor) have been shown to play an important role in facilitating smooth muscle cell migration in these models.[177-179] Unfortunately, the clinical relevance of these experimental observations remains to be clarified, as the milieu for cell migration in complex human lesions appears to be very different from that of normal animal arteries that are subjected to injury. More information is required regarding the factors that regulate smooth muscle cell migration, as well as why smooth muscle cells differ in their propensity to migrate after injury.

Finally, it is important to point out that the buildup of atherosclerotic plaque does not always translate into the formation of arterial obstructions.[142] For example, Glagov et al[180] noted that human vessels can accumulate massive amounts of atherosclerotic plaque without encroaching on the central arterial lumen. Instead, abluminal expansion of the artery wall may occur until 40% of the area encompassed by the internal elastic lamina is occupied by plaque; thereafter, no further enlargement may occur, and luminal narrowing may ensue. While this form of compensatory enlargement is referred to as "remodeling," the term is confusing as it holds different meaning in different contexts (Fig. 6–13).[180-182] For example, remodeling has also been used to describe the arterial response to changes in blood flow (e.g., during pregnancy or in the neonatal period) or pressure (e.g., hypertension).[183] In addition, remodeling has been invoked as a key component of the response to arterial injury—however, with quite a different meaning.[184] In animal models of arterial injury as well as studies of human coronary arteries that have undergone angioplasty (or percutaneous transluminal coronary angioplasty [PTCA]), "shrinkage" or constrictive remodeling of the artery wall is a major determinant of luminal narrowing, whereas neointimal formation plays a minor role in this process.[185-192]

How arterial wall constriction is accomplished or why some but not all arteries undergo compensatory dilatation in order to preserve lumen area is incompletely understood.[193-195] Blood flow and shear stress are known to play a critical role in remodeling. The response of arteries to chronic alterations in blood flow is endothelium dependent.[196,197] For example, Langille and O'Donnell[196] demonstrated in rabbit carotid arteries that decreased blood flow results in narrowing of the vessel diameter that is unchanged with papaverine and likely due to structural changes in the artery wall. However, when the endothelium is removed from these vessels, the response to reduced blood flow is abolished. In atherosclerotic arteries that contain a rich network of endothelial cell–lined microvessels or vasa vasorum, the role of the endothelium in regulating remodeling may be very important.[198-200]

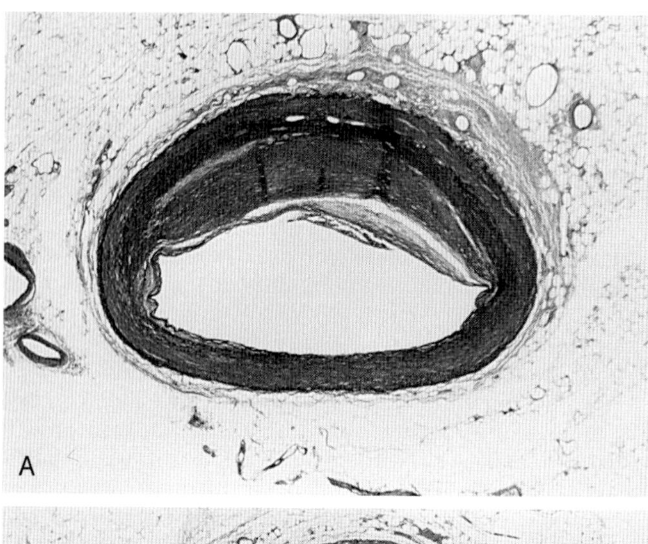

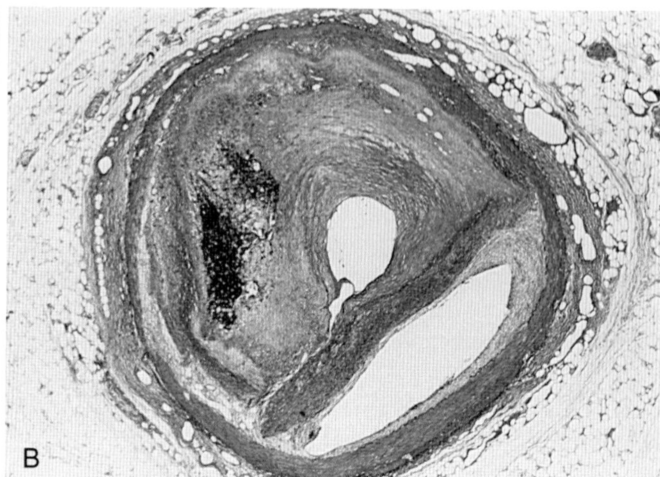

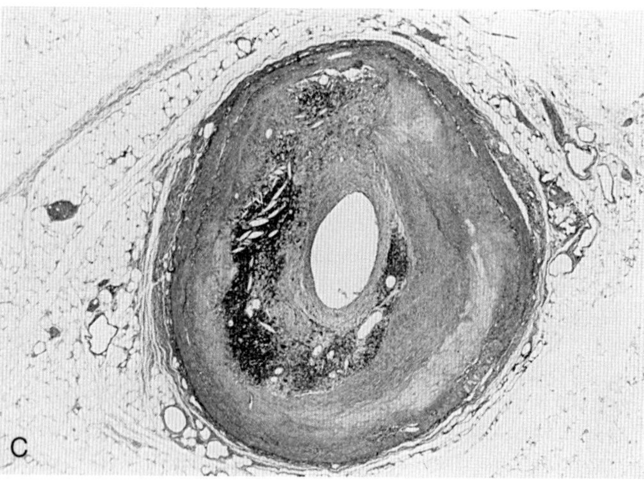

Figure 6–13 Arterial remodeling. Serial sections, proximal *(A)*, mid *(B)*, and distal *(C)*, of an atherosclerotic human left circumflex coronary artery (Movat's pentachrome-stained slide, original magnification ×40). There is narrowing of the central arterial lumen in the mid and distal sections; however, the total arterial area of these sections is also larger than that of the proximal section. The ability of arteries to undergo compensatory enlargement is referred to as *arterial remodeling*.

PATHOPHYSIOLOGY OF CORONARY BLOOD FLOW

Coronary Artery Stenoses and Plaque Rupture

Coronary atherosclerosis is a chronic disease that develops over decades, remaining clinically silent for prolonged periods of time (Box 6–8). Clinical manifestations of CAD occur when the atherosclerotic plaque mass encroaches on the vessel lumen and obstructs coronary blood flow causing angina. Alternatively, cracks or fissures may develop in the atherosclerotic lesions and result in acute thromboses that cause unstable angina or myocardial infarction.

Patients with stable angina typically have lesions with smooth borders on angiography. Only a minority of coronary lesions are concentric, with most having a complex geometry varying in shape over their length. Eccentric stenoses, with a remaining pliable, musculoelastic arc of normal wall, can vary in diameter and resistance in response to changes in vasomotor tone or intraluminal pressure. The majority of human coronary stenoses are compliant.[201] The intima of the normal portion of the vessel wall is often thickened, making endothelial dysfunction probable (see Dynamic Stenosis). In contrast, patients with unstable angina usually have lesions characterized by overhanging edges, scalloped or irregular borders, or multiple irregularities. These complicated stenoses likely represent ruptured plaque or partially occlusive thrombus or both.[202] On angiography these lesions may appear segmental, confined to a short segment of an otherwise normal proximal coronary artery. At autopsy, however, the most common pathologic finding is *diffuse* vessel involvement with superimposed segmental obstruction of greater severity.[203] In a diffusely narrowed vessel, even modest progression of luminal narrowing can be significant. In such an artery, rating the significance of the obstruction by the percentage of diameter reduction relative to adjacent vessel segments underestimates its physiologic importance.[204,205] Therefore, understanding the characteristics of atherosclerotic plaques is of central importance to the management of acute coronary artery syndromes.

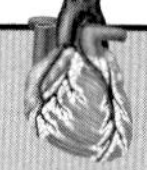

BOX 6–8 *Pathophysiology of Coronary Blood Flow*

- In the majority of patients experiencing a myocardial infarction, the coronary occlusion occurs at the site of <50% stenosis.
- Plaque rupture leads to incremental growth of coronary stenoses and can cause coronary events.
- Plaque rupture occurs at the shoulder of the plaque where inflammatory cells are found.

The intuitive notion that the severity of coronary artery stenoses should correlate with the risk of complications from CAD has been disproved by several key investigations. Ambrose et al[206] reviewed the coronary angiograms of 38 patients who had had a Q-wave myocardial infarction in the interval between serial studies. On the preinfarct angiograms, the mean percentage stenosis at the coronary segment that was later responsible for infarction was only 34%. Similarly, Little et al[207] reviewed the coronary angiograms of 42 patients who also had this procedure performed at an interval prior to and after myocardial infarction. Total occlusion of a previously patent artery was observed in 29 patients; yet for 19 of these occluded arteries, the degree of stenosis was less than 50% on the initial angiogram. Therefore, although the revascularization of arteries with critical stenoses in target lesions is appropriately indicated in order to reduce symptoms and myocardial ischemia, the risk of further cardiac events remains because atherosclerosis is a diffuse process, and mild or modest angiographic stenoses are more likely to result in subsequent myocardial infarction than are severe stenoses.

With this background comes the problem of predicting which arterial segments with minimal angiographic disease will later develop new critical stenoses. Clues to the answer for this question are emerging from careful pathologic studies of lesions by Davies and Thomas.[208] Superficial intimal injury (plaque erosions) and intimal tears of variable depth (plaque fissures) with overlying microscopic mural thrombosis are commonly found in atherosclerotic plaques. In the absence of obstructive luminal thrombosis, these intimal injuries do not cause clinical events. However, disruption of the fibrous cap, or plaque rupture, is a more serious event that typically results in the formation of clinically significant arterial thromboses. From autopsy studies it is known that rupture-prone plaques tend to have a thin, friable fibrous cap.[209] The site of plaque rupture is thought to be the shoulder of the plaque, where substantial numbers of mononuclear inflammatory cells are commonly found.[210] The mechanisms responsible for the local accumulation of these cells at this location in the plaque are unknown; presumably, monocyte chemotactic factors, the expression of leukocyte cell adhesion molecules, and specific cytokines are involved.[162,211] Moreover, macrophages in plaques have been shown to express factors such as stromelysin, which promote the breakdown of the extracellular matrix and thereby weaken the structural integrity of the plaque.[151] Currently, no effective strategies have been designed to limit the possibility of plaque rupture; however, as discussed later, aggressive lipid-lowering therapy may be a helpful preventative measure.

Hemodynamics

If accurate angiographic assessment of the geometry of a coronary stenosis is made, hydrodynamic principles can be used to estimate the physiologic significance of the obstruction.[212] Energy is lost when blood flows through a stenosis because of entrance effects, frictional losses in the stenotic segment, and separation losses due to turbulence as blood exits the stenosis (Fig. 6–14). The equation relating stenosis geometry to hemodynamic severity is:

$$\Delta P = fQ + sQ^2$$

where ΔP is the pressure drop across the stenosis, Q is the volume flow of blood, f is a factor accounting for frictional effects, and s accounts for separation effects. Based on the Poiseuille law for laminar flow:

$$f = \frac{8\pi\eta\, LA_n}{A_s^2}$$

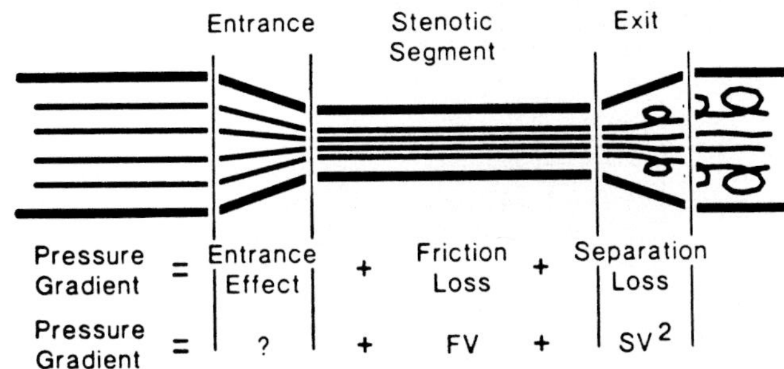

Figure 6–14 Sources of energy loss across a stenosis. Equations that (accurately) predict the pressure gradient across a stenosis usually ignore entrance effects. Frictional losses are proportional to blood velocity but are usually not important except in very long stenoses. Separation losses, due to turbulence as blood exits the stenosis, increase with the square of blood velocity and account for more than 75% of energy loss. V = blood velocity; F = friction coefficient (Poiseuille); S = separation coefficient (see text). (From Marcus ML: The physiologic effects of a coronary stenosis. *In* Marcus ML [ed]: The Coronary Circulation in Health and Disease. New York, McGraw-Hill, 1983, pp 242–269. Reproduced with permission of The McGraw-Hill Companies.)

where η is the blood viscosity, L is stenosis length, A_n is the cross-sectional area of the normal vessel, and A_s is the cross-sectional area of the stenosis. The separation or turbulence factor is

$$s = \frac{\rho k}{2}\left(\frac{A_n}{A_s} - 1\right)^2$$

where ρ is blood density and *k* is an experimentally determined coefficient. Thus, frictional losses are directly proportional to the first power of stenosis length but are inversely proportional to the square of the area (or fourth power of diameter). Separation losses are particularly prominent because they increase with the square of flow. Even at resting flows, more than 75% of energy loss is due to this turbulence when blood exits the stenosis. Except for very long stenoses, the frictional term can be neglected.[201] Thus, the amount of energy loss or pressure drop across the obstruction increases exponentially as flow rate increases. For this reason, exercise, anemia, and arteriolar vasodilator drugs (e.g., dipyridamole) are poorly tolerated in the presence of a severe stenosis. Figure 6–15 illustrates that although resting flow is unaffected until coronary diameter is reduced by more than 80%, maximal flow begins to fall when diameter is reduced by 50%.

Resting flow in Figure 6–15 remains constant as lumen diameter decreases because the coronary arterioles progressively dilate, thereby reducing the resistance of the distal coronary bed sufficiently to compensate for the resistance of the stenosis. As the severity of the stenosis increases further, the arteriolar bed can no longer compensate and flow begins to fall. As stenosis severity increases, distal perfusion pressure falls, arterioles dilate to maintain flow until autoregulation is exhausted (in the subendocardium first), and flow becomes pressure dependent. As illustrated (see Fig. 6–9), the distal pressure (or stenosis diameter) at which flow becomes pressure dependent is lower at low levels of myocardial metabolism (MVO_2). The interpretation of normal resting flow can be difficult in the presence of CAD. A coronary artery supplying blood through collaterals to a large mass of myocardium requires high resting flow rates, and even a mild stenosis may be flow limiting.

The frequently used term *critical stenosis* is usually defined as a coronary constriction sufficient to prevent an increase in

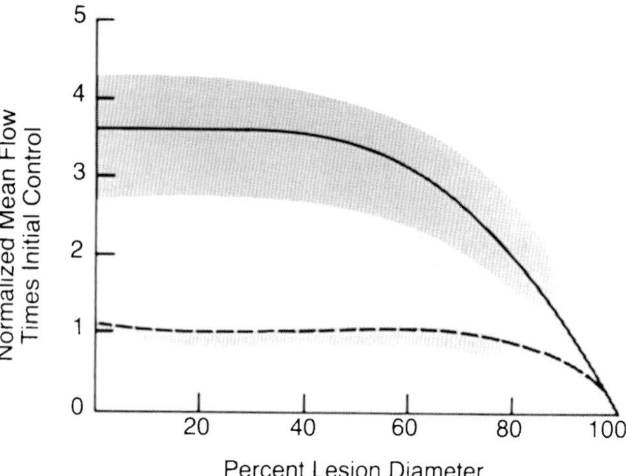

Figure 6–15 Effect of increasing stenosis severity at resting and maximal coronary flows. At rest, lumen diameter must be reduced by more than 80% before flow decreases. Because pressure drop across a stenosis increases exponentially with blood velocity, maximal coronary flow is restricted by a 50% diameter reduction. (From Gould KL, Lipscomb K: Effect of coronary stenoses on coronary flow reserve and resistance. Am J Cardiol 34:48, 1974.)

flow over resting values in response to increased myocardial oxygen demands.[213] This is a greater degree of obstruction than an angiographically significant stenosis, which is usually defined as a reduction in cross-sectional area of 75%, which is equivalent to a 50% decrease in the diameter of a concentric stenosis.[204] A critical stenosis is demonstrated experimentally by blunting or abolishing reactive hyperemia (see Autoregulation). This is evidence that autoregulation has been exhausted in at least the inner layer of myocardium (see Transmural Blood Flow). It should be noted that the critical nature of the stenosis is relative to the resting MVO_2. If oxygen demand decreases, some coronary autoregulatory reserve is recovered and the stenosis is no longer critical. The failure to recognize this fact has led to misinterpretation of studies designed to demonstrate coronary steal (see later).

Coronary Collaterals

Coronary collaterals are anastomotic connections, without an intervening capillary bed, between different coronary arteries or between branches of the same artery. In the normal human heart, these vessels are small and have little or no functional role. In patients with CAD well-developed coronary collateral vessels may play a critical role in preventing death and myocardial infarction. Individual differences in the capability of developing a sufficient collateral circulation is a determinant of the vulnerability of the myocardium to coronary occlusive disease.[214] There is great interspecies variation in the ability of the collateral circulation to support myocardial perfusion after acute coronary occlusion: Pigs and rats have very little collateral circulation and infarct almost all the area at risk, whereas dogs and cats with better collateralization infarct less than 75% of the area at risk.[215] In the guinea pig, collaterals are so well developed that coronary occlusion does not even decrease myocardial blood flow. There are also differences in the location of collateral vessels. In dogs collaterals develop in a narrow subepicardial zone, at the border of the potentially ischemic region, whereas in pigs a dense subendocardial plexus develops in response to coronary occlusion. In the presence of coronary disease, humans exhibit a small number of large epicardial collateral vessels and numerous small subendocardial vessels.

In response to coronary occlusion, native coronary collateral vessels do not passively stretch but undergo an active growth process that within 8 weeks, in the dog, can restore perfusion sufficient to support normal myocardial function even during exercise. Human collaterals have a tortuous corkscrew-like pattern visible on angiography. This may be due to an embryonal pattern of vascular development where longitudinal growth of smooth muscle cells occurs at the same time as radial growth. In the nongrowing adult heart, this increase in length results in tortuosity.[216] There is much interest in discovering the factors that control collateral vessel growth in the hope of providing therapy for patients who cannot be revascularized otherwise. *Arteriogenesis* refers to the transformation of preexisting collateral arterioles into functional arteries with a thick muscular coat and the acquisition of viscoelastic and vasomotor properties.[217] Fujita and Tambara[218] provide an overview of the process: a high-grade coronary stenosis decreases distal intra-arterial pressure, resulting in an increased pressure gradient across the preexisting collateral network. Increased collateral blood flow results in increased shear stress at the endothelium, which upregulates cell adhesion molecules. Upregulation leads to adherence of monocytes, which transform into macrophages, and the production and release of growth factors such as granulocyte macrophage colony-stimulating factor (GM-CSF), monocyte chemoattractant protein-1 (MCP-1), and basic fibroblast growth factor (bFGF). Angiogenesis is not directly related to collateral vessel development but refers to the proliferation, migration, and tube formation of capillaries in the central area of ischemic regions.[219] The development of a treatment to promote collateral growth in patients with intractable CAD is currently a subject of intense investigation.

Evidence in dogs suggests that mature coronary collaterals respond differently to neurohumoral stimulation than normal coronary arteries. Collaterals do not constrict in response to α-receptor activation but do dilate in response to β_1- or β_2-agonists. They constrict in response to prostaglandin $F_{2\alpha}$ ($PGF_{2\alpha}$) and angiotensin II, but less so than do normal vessels. Remarkably, collateral vessels constrict in response to vasopressin to a much greater extent than normal vessels. In vivo studies in dogs indicate that levels of vasopressin present during stress (hemorrhage, cardiopulmonary bypass) can diminish flow to collateral-dependent myocardium. This finding is likely due both to constriction of collateral vessels as well as enhanced vasoconstriction of the resistance vessels in the collateral-dependent myocardium.[79] It is possible that the endothelial cells of both types of vessels are dysfunctional.[220] Relaxation in response to nitroglycerin is enhanced. This is a further mechanism for the beneficial effects of nitroglycerin in CAD. The deleterious effects of coronary arteriolar dilators such as adenosine and dipyridamole are discussed later (see Coronary Steal).

It has been estimated that, in humans, perfusion via collaterals can equal perfusion via a vessel with a 90% diameter obstruction.[221] Although coronary collateral flow can be sufficient to preserve structure and resting myocardial function, muscle dependent on collateral flow usually becomes ischemic when oxygen demand rises above resting levels.[222] It is possible that evidence from patients with angina underestimates collateral function of the population of all patients with CAD.

Perhaps individuals with coronary obstructions but excellent collateralization remain asymptomatic and are not studied.

Pathogenesis of Myocardial Ischemia

Ischemia is the condition of oxygen deprivation accompanied by inadequate removal of metabolites consequent to reduced perfusion.[223] Clinically, myocardial ischemia is a decrease in the blood flow supply/demand ratio resulting in impaired function. There is no universally accepted "gold standard" for the presence of myocardial ischemia. In practice, symptoms, anatomic findings, and evidence of myocardial dysfunction must be combined before concluding that myocardial ischemia is present.[224] Conclusive evidence of anaerobic metabolism in the setting of reduced coronary blood flow (relative to demand) would be convincing. Such evidence is extremely difficult to obtain, even in experimental preparations.

Determinants of Myocardial Oxygen Supply/Demand Ratio

An increase in myocardial oxygen requirement beyond the capacity of the coronary circulation to deliver oxygen results in myocardial ischemia (Box 6–9). This is the most common mechanism leading to ischemic episodes in chronic stable angina and during exercise testing. Intraoperatively, the anesthesiologist must measure and control the determinants of myocardial oxygen consumption and protect the patient from "demand" ischemia. The major determinants of myocardial oxygen consumption are heart rate, myocardial contractility, and wall stress (chamber pressure × radius/wall thickness). Shortening, activation, and basal metabolic requirements are minor determinants of MVO_2 (Fig. 6–16).

An increase in heart rate can reduce subendocardial perfusion by shortening diastole. Coronary perfusion pressure may fall due to reduced systemic pressure or increased left ventricular end-diastolic pressure. With the onset of ischemia, perfusion may be further compromised by delayed ventricular relaxation (decreased subendocardial perfusion time) and decreased diastolic compliance (increased left ventricular end-diastolic pressure). Anemia and hypoxia can also compromise delivery of oxygen to the myocardium. Several indices of myocardial oxygen supply/demand ratio have been proposed to guide therapy. The rate-pressure product (heart rate × systolic blood pressure) gives a good estimate of MVO_2 but does not correlate well with ischemia. A patient with a systolic pressure of 160 and heart rate of 70 has a much lower likelihood of ischemia than does a patient with a pressure of 70 and rate of 160, although both have a rate-pressure product of 11,200. The ratio of the diastolic pressure-time index (DPTI) to the systolic pressure-time index (SPTI) was devised to estimate subendocardial perfusion and takes into account determinants of oxygen delivery (Fig. 6–17).[225-228] When blood oxygen content was included, the index became a good predictor of endocardial flow in animals with normal coronary arteries. The ratio of mean arterial pressure/heart rate has been proposed as a correlate of myocardial ischemia.[229] In dogs with moderate-to-severe coronary stenoses, systolic shortening was best with high pressures and low heart rate and worst with low pressure and high heart rate. None of these indices has proven to be reliable in the clinical setting. Their major value is to bring attention to the important variables determining the supply/demand ratio. These variables should be measured (or estimated) and controlled individually.

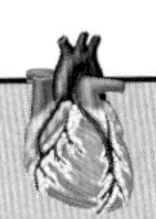

BOX 6–9 *Determinants of Myocardial Oxygen Supply/Demand Ratio*

The major determinants of myocardial oxygen consumption are

- Heart rate
- Myocardial contractility
- Wall stress (chamber pressure × radius/wall thickness)

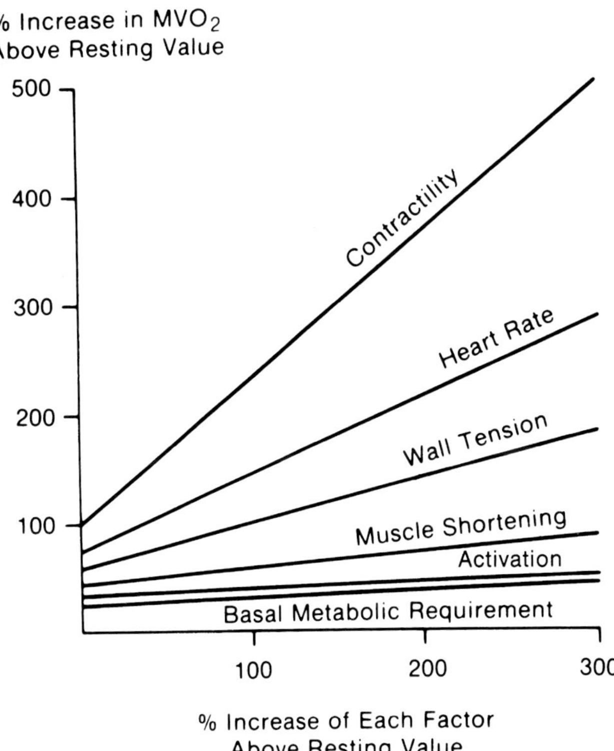

Figure 6–16 Relative importance of variables that determine myocardial oxygen consumption (MVO_2). Each line roughly approximates the effect of manipulating one variable without changing the others. Most interventions cause changes in several of the variables at the same time. The importance of contractility, which is difficult to monitor in practice, is apparent. (From Marcus ML: Metabolic regulation of coronary blood flow. *In* Marcus ML [ed]: The Coronary Circulation in Health and Disease. New York, McGraw-Hill, 1983, pp 65–92. Reproduced with permission of The McGraw-Hill Companies.)

Dynamic Stenosis

Patients with CAD can have variable exercise tolerance during the day and between days. Ambulatory monitoring of the electrocardiogram has demonstrated that ST-segment changes indicative of myocardial ischemia, in the absence of changes in oxygen demand, are common.[230] These findings are explained by variations over time in the severity of the obstruction to blood flow imposed by coronary stenoses.

Although the term *hardening of the arteries* suggests rigid, narrowed vessels, in fact most stenoses are eccentric and have a remaining arc of compliant tissue (Fig. 6–18). A modest amount (10%) of shortening of the muscle in the compliant

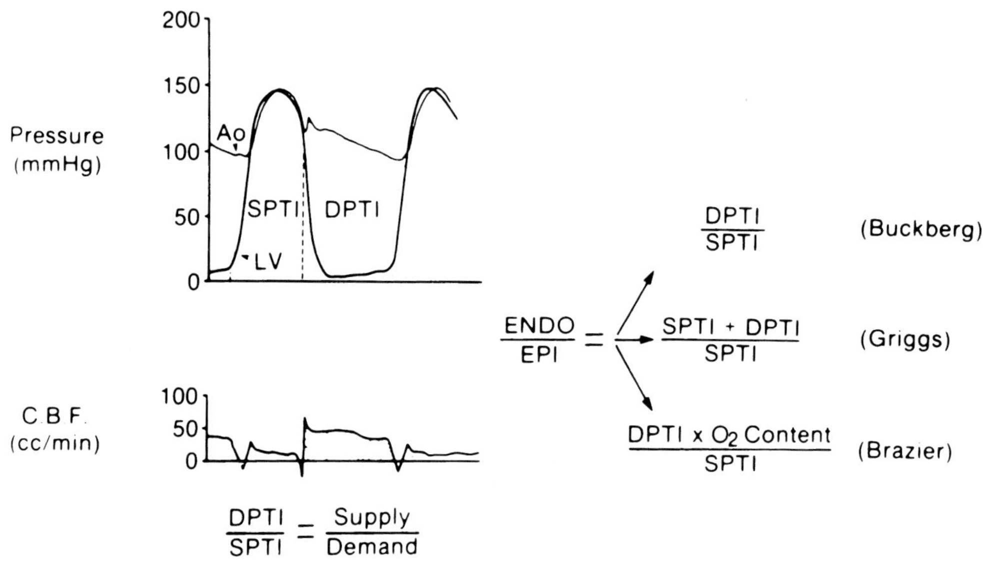

Figure 6–17 Three indices, proposed to predict the adequacy of subendocardial perfusion in normal dogs, illustrate the variables determining myocardial oxygen supply and demand. The systolic pressure-time index (SPTI) relates to oxygen demand. The diastolic pressure-time index (DPTI) relates to the supply of coronary blood flow (CBF) to the inner layers of the left ventricle. Arterial oxygen content (O_2 content) is important when there are large changes in hematocrit. Ao = aortic pressure; LV = left ventricular pressure; ENDO = subendocardial layer of left ventricle; EPI = subepicardial layer of the left ventricle. (From Hoffman JIE, Buckberg GD: Transmural variations in myocardial perfusion. *In* Yu PN, Goodwin JF [eds]: Progress in Cardiology. Philadelphia, Lea & Febiger, 1976, p 37.)

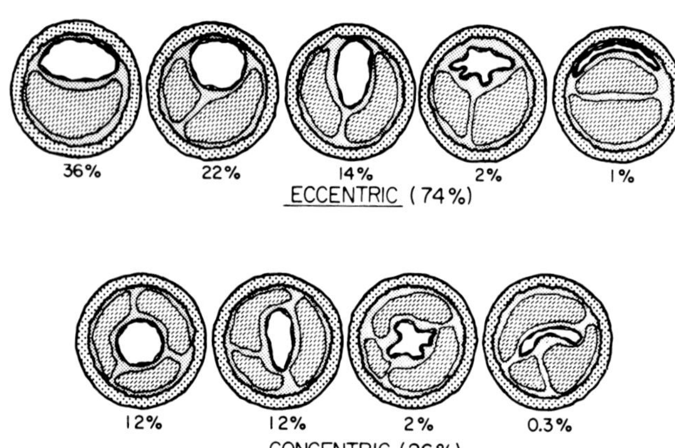

Figure 6–18 Drawings and incidence of the various types of structure of stenoses observed in human coronary artery specimens. In almost three quarters of vessels with greater than 50% narrowing, the residual arterial lumen was eccentric and partially circumscribed by an arc of normal arterial wall. In such lesions, a fall in intraluminal pressure or an increase in vasomotor tone can cause lumen diameter to decrease further, sufficiently to precipitate myocardial ischemia. (From Brown BG, Bolson EL, Dodge HT: Dynamic mechanisms in human coronary stenosis. Circulation 70:917, 1984; redrawn from Freudenberg H, Lichtlen PR: The normal wall segment in coronary stenoses—a postmortem study. Z Kardiol 70:863, 1981.)

region of the vessel can cause dramatic changes in lumen caliber.[201] This was part of Prinzmetal's original proposal to explain coronary spasm. Maseri et al[231] suggest that the term *spasm* be reserved for "situations where coronary constriction is both focal, sufficiently profound to cause transient coronary occlusion, and is responsible for reversible attacks of angina at rest" (i.e., variant angina). Although this syndrome is rare, lesser degrees of obstruction in response to vasoconstrictor stimuli are very common among patients with CAD.

Sympathetic tone can be increased by the cold pressor test (immersing the arm in ice water) or by isometric handgrip testing. In response to this maneuver, coronary resistance decreased in normal subjects but increased in patients with coronary disease, some of whom experienced angina.[232] This increase in resistance appears to be mediated by α-receptors because it can be prevented by phentolamine. Studies using quantitative coronary angiography have documented reductions in caliber in diseased vessels in contrast to dilation of vessels in normal subjects. [98,233] Zeiher et al [233] showed that the same vessel segments that constricted with the cold pressor test also constricted in response to an infusion of acetylcholine. Because the normal, dilatory response to acetylcholine is dependent on intact endothelium, these findings suggest that the abnormal response of stenotic coronary arteries is due to endothelial dysfunction.

Animal models of coronary vasospasm demonstrate that enhanced vascular smooth muscle reactivity may also underlie vasospasm.[234] Rho, a GTP-binding protein, sensitizes vascular smooth muscle cells to calcium by inhibiting myosin phosphatase activity through an effector protein called Rho-kinase. Upregulation of this pathway may be a mechanism of coronary vasospasm. Interestingly, Rho-kinase inhibitors have been shown to block agonist-induced vasoconstriction of internal thoracic artery segments from patients undergoing coronary artery surgery.[235]

It has also been noted that, in patients with coronary disease, some of the angiographically normal appearing segments also respond abnormally.[66,236] It seems likely that, during the development of coronary atherosclerosis, endothelial dysfunction precedes the appearance of visible stenoses. In patients with angiographically smooth coronary arteries, Vita et al[237] found that an abnormal response to acetylcholine was correlated with serum cholesterol, male gender, age, and family history of coronary disease. The normal dilation of epicardial coronary arteries in response to increased blood flow (shear stress) has been shown to be absent in atherosclerotic vessels.[238] In addition, it has been demonstrated that patients with coronary disease respond to serotonin with coronary vasoconstriction instead of the normal vasodilatory response.[239,240] The concentrations of serotonin used were within the range found in coronary sinus blood of patients with coronary disease. Very high concentrations of serotonin may be found on the endothelium at the site of aggregating platelets.[239] All of these findings point to the central role of endothelial dysfunction in the abnormal coronary vasomotion of patients with atherosclerosis (see Endothelium).[241]

Coronary Steal

Steal occurs when the perfusion pressure for a vasodilated vascular bed (in which flow is pressure dependent) is lowered by vasodilation in a parallel vascular bed, both beds usually being distal to a stenosis. Two kinds of coronary steal are illustrated: collateral and transmural (Fig. 6–19).

Collateral steal in which one vascular bed (R_3), distal to an occluded vessel, is dependent on collateral flow from a vascular bed (R_2) supplied by a stenotic artery is shown (Fig. 6–19*A*). Because collateral resistance is high, the R_3 arterioles are dilated to maintain flow in the resting condition (autoregulation). Dilation of the R_2 arterioles increases flow across the stenosis R_1 and decreases pressure P_2. If R_3 resistance cannot further decrease sufficiently, flow there decreases, producing or worsening ischemia in the collateral-dependent bed. The values of all of the resistances, including collaterals, and the baseline myocardial metabolic state determine how powerful the vasodilator stimulus must be to produce ischemia in the collateral bed. Failure to recognize this has confounded studies of vasodilator drugs. If collateral vessels are very well developed or MVO_2 is low, sufficient autoregulatory reserve may remain in the collateral-dependent bed to maintain adequate myocardial blood flow even with the administration of a moderately powerful vasodilator.

Transmural steal is illustrated (Fig. 6–19*B*). Normally, vasodilator reserve is less in the subendocardium (see Transmural Blood Flow). In the presence of a stenosis, flow may become pressure dependent in the subendocardium while autoregulation is maintained in the subepicardium. This is illustrated (see Fig. 6–11), where at a perfusion pressure of 50 mm Hg, flow has fallen in the subendocardium while the subepicardium retains autoregulatory reserve. Dilation of the subepicardial arterioles, R_2, then increases flow across the stenosis (R_1), causing P_2 to fall and resulting in decreased flow to the subendocardium as subepicardial flow increases.

The term *steal* is most appropriate when the vasodilation is caused by a pharmacologic agent (adenosine, dipyridamole) producing "luxury" flow (beyond metabolic requirements) in the vascular bed with coronary reserve (R_2). The same redistribution of blood flow also occurs during exercise in response to metabolically mediated vasodilation. The study of coronary steal demonstrates well the complex interrelationships among the determinants of myocardial blood flow.

FUTURE DIRECTIONS

There is a major need to not only identify but also treat the nonstenotic plaque that is prone to rupture. Although angiography is ideal for imaging the lumen of arteries, it provides little information about the atherosclerotic process within the vessel wall. Unfortunately, newer imaging techniques, such as intravascular ultrasound and electron beam computer tomography, have yet to evolve as practical predictive modalities that can be used to manage patients at risk for acute coronary syndromes secondary to plaque rupture. Interestingly, clues to the biology of plaque rupture are indirectly emerging from clinical trials with statins, in that these trials show very modest reductions in the angiographic degree of vessel stenoses but consistently demonstrate a significant decrease in acute ischemic events. For example, in the West of Scotland Coronary Prevention Study,[242] the use of pravastatin as a primary prevention strategy in hypercholesterolemic men produced a 31% risk reduction for nonfatal myocardial infarction and coronary heart disease death. Similarly, in the Scandinavian Simvastatin Survival Study (4S),[243] the likelihood of developing angina and myocardial infarction and the need for revascularization procedures in patients with hypercholesterolemia and known CAD were dramatically reduced in patients treated with the statin simvastatin. There is much interest in explor-

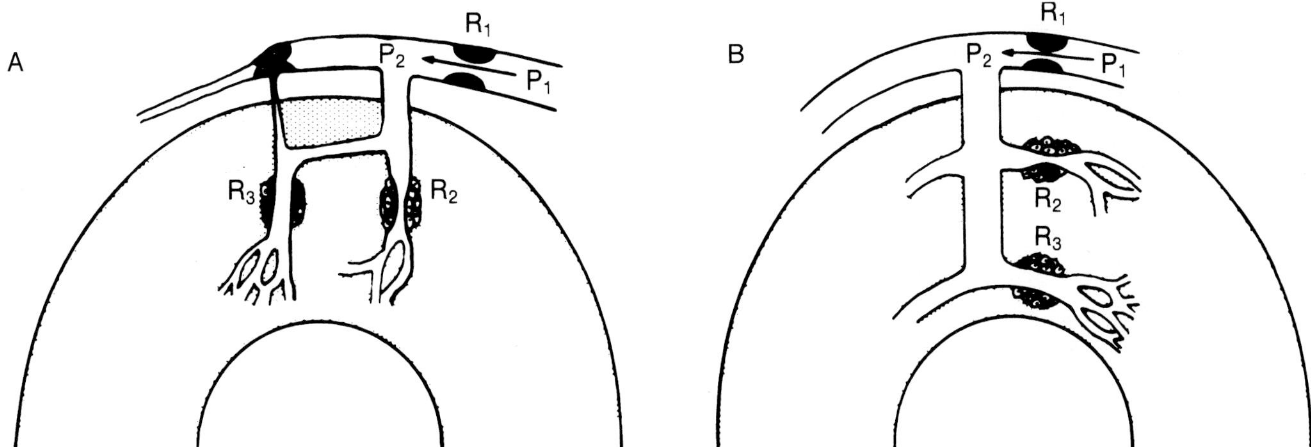

Figure 6–19 Conditions for coronary steal between different areas of the heart (collateral steal *[A]*) and between the subendocardial and the subepicardial layers of the left ventricle (transmural steal *[B]*). See text for detailed description. R_1 = stenosis resistance; P_1 = aortic pressure; P_2 = pressure distal to the stenosis; R_2 and R_3 = resistance of autoregulating and pressure-dependent vascular beds, respectively. (From Epstein SE, Cannon RO, Talbot TL: Hemodynamic principles in the control of coronary blood flow. Am J Cardiol 56:4E, 1985.)

ing the apparent pleotrophic effects of statins that extend beyond lipid lowering.[244,245]

There is also much to be learned about the factors that modulate arterial remodeling. In some instances, arteries are able to accommodate for the accumulation of plaque mass; whereas in others, only a limited degree of remodeling may occur. Inadequate remodeling is particularly important after coronary interventional procedures, as studies using intravascular ultrasound estimate that approximately two thirds of luminal narrowing after angioplasty is due to shrinkage (or contracture) of the artery wall.[246] With the expanding use of intracoronary metallic stents that hold the artery open like an intraluminal scaffold, the problem of arterial wall contracture has been minimized. Moreover, the use of drug-coated stents appears to have reduced further the risk of developing stenosis within a stent (or in-stent restenosis).[247,248] Presumably, the accumulation of blood-borne cells or the inward migration of arterial wall cells is involved in stent stenosis; however, this problem is only now beginning to be studied in detail.[249,250]

There is also a growing need to better understand the role of vascular progenitor cells in lesion formation.[251] Studies suggest that endothelial and smooth muscle cells appear to be derived from multiple sources such as circulating stem and progenitor cells, as well as tissue-resident progenitor cell populations.[251,252] Vascular cell transdifferentiation (or "plasticity") refers to the ability of a mature cell to acquire some or all of the characteristics of another mature cell. Transdifferentiation of endothelial cells into smooth muscle cells used to be largely a speculative concept. However, several studies now support the concept that the endothelium itself is the source of at least some artery wall smooth muscle cells.[253-256] While there is much interest in the potential involvement of vascular progenitor cells in angiogenesis and vascular repair, scattered reports of their potential involvement in the pathogenesis of human diseases are also emerging. For example, observations from organ transplantations highlight the involvement of a blood-borne population of human vascular cells in lesion formation.[257] Circulating progenitor cells may also be essential for maintaining vascular wall homeostasis. For example, patients with known risk factors for CAD have diminished levels of circulating endothelial progenitor cells (EPCs).[258,259] Moreover, circulating EPC levels are lower in patients who develop in-stent restenosis compared with patients with patent stents or an absence of CAD.[250] Hence, taken together, the emerging data suggest that vascular progenitor cells may play a critical role, not only in maintaining the artery wall but also in ensuring that appropriate repair mechanisms occur in the face of injury. Therapeutic strategies that target EPC mobilization, homing, and differentiation may prove beneficial. Indeed, it is well recognized that statins increase the abundance of circulating EPC, and perhaps this, in part, explains the overall benefit of this drug class on stabilizing the artery wall and reducing acute ischemic events.[260,261] While more data are required before the biology of vascular progenitor cells is more completely understood, these insights signal an important change in the understanding of the pathogenesis of a wide variety of vascular lesions and may lead to novel treatment strategies for the populations at risk.

REFERENCES

1. Zweifach BW, Lipowsky HH: Pressure-flow relations in blood and lymph microcirculation. *In* Berne R, Sperelakis N (eds): Handbook of Physiology, Section 2: The Cardiovascular System, Volume III, Microcirculation. Baltimore, Williams & Wilkins, 1984, pp 251–307
2. Marcus ML, Chilian WM, Kanatsuka H, et al: Understanding the coronary circulation through studies at the microvascular level. Circulation 82:1, 1990
3. Mulvany MJ, Aalkjaer C: Structure and function of small arteries. Physiol Rev 70:921, 1990
4. Merkus D, Chilian WM, Stepp DW: Functional characteristics of the coronary microcirculation. Herz 24:496, 1999
5. Kanatsuka H, Lamping KG, Eastham CL, et al: Comparison of the effects of increased myocardial oxygen consumption and adenosine on the coronary microvascular resistance. Circ Res 65:1296, 1989
6. Chilian WM, Layne SM, Eastham CL, et al: Heterogeneous microvascular coronary alpha-adrenergic vasoconstriction. Circ Res 64:376, 1989
7. Schwartz SM, deBlois D, O'Brien ER: The intima: Soil for atherosclerosis and restenosis. Circ Res 77:445, 1995
8. Stary HC, Blankenhorn DH, Chandler AB, et al: A definition of the intima of human arteries and of its atherosclerosis-prone regions. Circulation 85:391, 1992
9. Frid MG, Moiseeva EP, Stenmark KR: Multiple phenotypically distinct smooth muscle cell populations exist in the adult and developing bovine pulmonary arterial media in vivo. Circ Res 75:669, 1994
10. Clowes AW, Clowes MM, Reidy MA: Kinetics of cellular proliferation after arterial injury. I. Smooth muscle growth in the absence of endothelium. Lab Invest 49:327, 1983
11. Clowes AW, Schwartz SM: Significance of quiescent smooth muscle migration in the injured rat carotid artery. Circ Res 56:139, 1985
12. Shi Y, O'Brien J, Fard A, et al: Adventitial myofibroblasts contribute to neointimal formation in injured porcine coronary arteries. Circulation 94:1655, 1996
13. Scott NA, Cipolla GD, Ross CE, et al: Identification of a potential role for the adventitia in vascular lesion formation after balloon overstretch injury of porcine coronary arteries. Circulation 93:2178, 1996
14. Rana RS, Hokin LE: Role of phosphoinositides in transmembrane signaling. Physiol Rev 70:115, 1990
15. Moncada S, Higgs EA, Vane JR: Human arterial and venous tissues generate prostacyclin (prostaglandin X), a potent inhibitor of platelet aggregation. Lancet I:18, 1977
16. Furchgott RF, Zawadzki JV: The obligatory role of endothelial cells in the relaxation of arterial smooth muscle by acetylcholine. Nature 288:373, 1980
17. Ignarro LJ: Nitric oxide. A novel signal transduction mechanism for transcellular communication. Hypertension 16:477, 1990
18. Ignarro LJ: Biological actions and properties of endothelium-derived nitric oxide formed and released from artery and vein. Circ Res 65:1, 1989
19. Lincoln TM, Dey N, Sellak H: Invited review: cGMP-dependent protein kinase signaling mechanisms in smooth muscle: From the regulation of tone to gene expression. J Appl Physiol 91:1421, 2001
20. Moncada S, Palmer RMJ, Higgs EA: Nitric oxide: Physiology, pathophysiology, and pharmacology. Pharmacol Rev 43:109, 1991
21. Harrison DG, Cai H: Endothelial control of vasomotion and nitric oxide production. Cardiol Clin 21:289, 2003
22. Vallance P, Collier J, Moncada S: Nitric oxide synthesized from L-arginine mediates endothelium-dependent dilatation in human veins. Physiol Rev 23:1053, 1989
23. Miura H, Bosnjak JJ, Ning G, et al: Role for hydrogen peroxide in flow-induced dilation of human coronary arterioles. Circ Res 92: e31-e40, 2003
24. Busse R, Edwards G, Feletou M, et al: EDHF: Bringing the concepts together. Trends Pharmacol Sci 23:374, 2002
25. Miura H, Wachtel RE, Liu Y, et al: Flow-induced dilation of human coronary arterioles: Important role of Ca(2+)-activated K(+) channels. Circulation 103:1992, 2001
26. Miyauchi T, Tomobe Y, Shiba R, et al: Involvement of endothelin in the regulation of human vascular tonus. Potent vasoconstrictor effect and existence in endothelial cells. Circulation 81:1874, 1990
27. Lee SY, Lee CY, Chen YM, et al: Coronary vasospasm as the primary cause of death due to the venom of the burrowing asp, Atractaspis engaddensis. Toxicon 24:285, 1986
28. Goodwin AT, Yacoub MH: Role of endogenous endothelin on coronary flow in health and disease. Coron Artery Dis 12:517, 2001
29. Hirata Y, Yoshimi H, Takata S: Cellular mechanism of action by a novel vasoconstrictor endothelin in cultured rat vascular smooth muscle cells. Biochem Biophys Res Commun 154:868, 1988
30. Clozel J-P, Clozel M: Effects of endothelin on the coronary vascular bed in open-chest dogs. Circ Res 65:1193, 1989
31. Wenzel RR, Fleisch M, Shaw S, et al: Hemodynamic and coronary effects of the endothelin antagonist bosentan in patients with coronary artery disease. Circulation 98:2235, 1998

32. Mylona P, Cleland JG: Update of REACH-1 and MERIT-HF clinical trials in heart failure. Cardio.net Editorial Team. Eur J Heart Fail 1:197, 1999
33. Humbert M, Sitbon O, Simonneau G: Treatment of pulmonary arterial hypertension. N Engl J Med 351:1425, 2004.
34. Hoak JC: The endothelium, platelets, and coronary vasospasm. Adv Intern Med 34:353, 1989
35. Bassenge E, Heusch G: Endothelial and neurohumoral control of coronary blood flow in health and disease. Rev Physiol Biochem Pharmacol 116:77, 1990
36. Spaan JA: Mechanical determinants of myocardial perfusion. Basic Res Cardiol 90:89, 1995
37. Westerhof N: Physiological hypotheses—intramyocardial pressure. A new concept, suggestions for measurement. Basic Res Cardiol 85:105, 1990
38. Mates RE, Klocke FJ, Canty JM Jr: Coronary capacitance. Progr Cardiovasc Dis 1, 1988
39. Bellamy RF: Diastolic coronary artery pressure-flow relations in the dog. Circ Res 43:92, 1978
40. Eng C, Jentzer JH, Kirk ES: The effects of coronary capacitance on the interpretation of diastolic pressure-flow relationships. Circ Res 50:334, 1982
41. Messina LM, Hanley FL, Uhlig PN, et al: Effects of pressure gradients between branches of the left coronary artery on the pressure axis intercept and the shape of steady-state circumflex pressure-flow relations in dogs. Circ Res 56:11, 1985
42. Kanatsuka H, Ashikawa K, Suzuki T, et al: Diameter change and pressure-red blood cell velocity relations in coronary microvessels during long diastoles in the canine left ventricle. Circ Res 66:503, 1990
43. Feigl EO: Coronary physiology. Physiol Rev 63:1, 1983
44. Hoffman JI, Piedimonte G, Maxwell AJ, et al: Aspects of coronary vasomotor regulation. Adv Exp Med Biol 381:135, 1995
45. Tune JD, Richmond KN, Gorman MW, et al: Control of coronary blood flow during exercise. Exp Biol Med (Maywood) 227:238, 2002
46. Gellai M, Norton JM, Detar R: Evidence for direct control of coronary vascular tone by oxygen. Circ Res 32:279, 1973
47. Weiss HR, Neubauer JA, Lipp JA: Quantitative determination of regional oxygen consumption in the dog heart. Circ Res 42:394, 1978
48. Broten TP, Romson JL, Fullerton DA, et al: Synergistic action of myocardial oxygen and carbon dioxide in controlling coronary blood flow. Circ Res 68:531, 1991
49. Spaan JA, Dankelman J: Theoretical analysis of coronary blood flow and tissue oxygen pressure-control. Adv Exp Med Biol 346:189, 1993
50. Berne RM: Cardiac nucleotides in hypoxia: Possible role in regulation of coronary blood flow. Am J Physiol 204:317, 1963
51. Gerlach E, Deuticke B, Dreisbach RH: Der Nucleotid-Abbau im Herzmuskel bei Sauerstoffmangel und seine mogliche Bedeutung fur die Coronardurchblutung. Naturwissenschaften 6:228, 1963
52. Olsson RA, Bunger R: Metabolic control of coronary blood flow. Prog Cardiovasc Dis 29:369, 1987
53. Standen NB, Quayle JM: K+ channel modulation in arterial smooth muscle. Acta Physiol Scand 164:549, 1998
54. Duncker DJ, Bache RJ: Regulation of coronary vasomotor tone under normal conditions and during acute myocardial hypoperfusion. Pharmacol Ther 86:87, 2000
55. Kroll K, Feigl EO: Adenosine is unimportant in controlling coronary blood flow in unstressed dog hearts. Am J Physiol 249:H1176, 1985
56. Bache RJ, Dai X, Schwarts JS, et al: Role of adenosine in coronary vasodilation during exercise. Circ Res 62:846, 1988
57. Dole WP, Yamada N, Bishop VS, et al: Role of adenosine in coronary blood flow regulation after reductions in perfusion pressure. Circ Res 56:517, 1985
58. Saito D, Steinhard CR, Nixon DG, et al: Intracoronary adenosine deaminase reduces canine myocardial reactive hyperemia. Circ Res 49:1262, 1981
59. Laxson DD, Homans DC, Bache RJ: Inhibition of adenosine-mediated coronary vasodilation exacerbates myocardial ischemia during exercise. Am J Physiol 265:H1471, 1993
60. Baxter GF: Role of adenosine in delayed preconditioning of myocardium. Cardiovasc Res 55:483, 2002
61. Zaugg M, Lucchinetti E, Uecker M, et al: Anaesthetics and cardiac preconditioning. Part I. Signalling and cytoprotective mechanisms. Br J Anaesth 91:551, 2003
62. Woollard HH: The innervation of the heart. J Anat Physiol 60:345, 1926
63. Van Winkle DM, Feigl EO: Acetylcholine causes coronary vasodilation in dogs and baboons. Circ Res 65:1580, 1989
64. Horio Y, Yasue H, Okumura K, et al: Effects of intracoronary injection of acetylcholine on coronary arterial hemodynamics and diameter. Am J Cardiol 62:887, 1988
65. Hodgson JMB, Marshall JJ: Direct vasoconstriction and endothelium-dependent vasodilation: Mechanisms of acetylcholine effects on coronary flow and arterial diameter in patients with nonstenotic coronary arteries. Circulation 79:1043, 1989
66. Ludmer PL, Selwyn AP, Shook TL, et al: Paradoxical vasoconstriction induced by acetylcholine in the atherosclerotic coronary arteries. N Engl J Med 315:1046, 1986
67. Feigl EO: EDRF—a protective factor? Nature 331:490, 1988
68. Feigl EO: Neural control of coronary blood flow. J Vasc Res 35:85, 1998
69. Feldman RD, Christy JP, Paul ST, et al: β-Adrenergic receptors on canine coronary collateral vessels: characterization and function. Am J Physiol 257:H1634, 1989
70. Mosher P, Ross J Jr, McFate PA, et al: Control of coronary blood flow by an autoregulatory mechanism. Circ Res 14:250, 1964
71. Gorman MW, Tune JD, Richmond KN, et al: Feedforward sympathetic coronary vasodilation in exercising dogs. J Appl Physiol 89:1892, 2000
72. Holtz J: Alpha-adrenoceptor subtypes in the coronary circulation. Basic Res Cardiol 85(suppl 1):81, 1990
73. Guth BD, Thaulow E, Heusch G, et al: Myocardial effects of selective alpha-adrenoceptor blockade during exercise in dogs. Circ Res 66:1703, 1990
74. Heusch G: Alpha-adrenergic mechanisms in myocardial ischemia. Circulation 81:1, 1990
75. Kelley KO, Feigl EO: Segmental alpha-receptor-mediated vasoconstriction in the canine coronary circulation. Circ Res 43:908, 1978
76. Mohrman DE, Feigl EO: Competition between sympathetic vasoconstriction and metabolic vasodilation in the canine coronary circulation. Circ Res 42:79, 1978
77. Heusch G, Deussen A: Nifedipine prevents sympathetic vasoconstriction distal to severe coronary stenoses. J Cardiovasc Pharmacol 6:378, 1984
78. Chilian WM: Adrenergic vasomotion in the coronary microcirculation. Basic Res Cardiol 85(suppl 1):111, 1990
79. Harrison DG, Sellke FW, Quillen JE: Neurohumoral regulation of coronary collateral vasomotor tone. Basic Res Cardiol 85(suppl 1):121, 1990
80. DiCarli MF, Tobes MC, Mangner T, et al: Effects of cardiac sympathetic innervation on coronary blood flow. N Engl J Med 336:1208, 1997
81. Chilian WM, Harrison DG, Haws CW, et al: Adrenergic coronary tone during submaximal exercise in the dog is produced by circulating catecholamines. Evidence for adrenergic denervation supersensitivity in the myocardium but not in coronary vessels. Circ Res 58:68, 1986
82. Huang AH, Feigl EO: Adrenergic coronary vasoconstriction helps maintain uniform transmural blood flow distribution during exercise. Circ Res 62:286, 1988
83. Buffington CW, Feigl EO: Adrenergic coronary vasoconstriction in the presence of coronary stenosis in the dog. Circ Res 48:416, 1981
84. Heusch G, Deussen A: The effects of cardiac sympathetic nerve stimulation on the perfusion of stenotic coronary arteries in the dog. Circ Res 53:8, 1983
85. Bassenge E, Walter P, Doutheil U: Wirkungsmumkehr der adrenergischen Coronargefassreakton in Abhangigkeit vom Coronargefasstonus. Pflugers Arch 297:146, 1967
86. Nathan HJ, Feigl EO: Adrenergic coronary vasoconstriction lessens transmural steal during coronary hypoperfusion. Am J Physiol 250:H645, 1986
87. Chilian WM, Ackell PH: Transmural differences in sympathetic coronary constriction during exercise in the presence of coronary stenosis. Circ Res 62:216, 1988
88. Seitelberger R, Guth BD, Heusch G, et al: Intracoronary $alpha_2$-adrenergic receptor blockade attenuates ischemia in conscious dogs during exercise. Circ Res 62:436, 1988
89. Baumgart D, Heusch G: Neuronal control of coronary blood flow. Basic Res Cardiol 90:142, 1995
90. Feigl EO: Adrenergic control of transmural coronary blood flow. Basic Res Cardiol 85(suppl 1):167, 1990
91. Hodgson JMB, Cohen MD, Szentpetery S, et al: Effects of regional alpha- and beta-blockade on resting and hyperemic coronary blood flow in conscious, unstressed humans. Circulation 79:797, 1989
92. Chierchia S, Davies G, Berkenboom G, et al: Alpha-adrenergic receptors and coronary spasm: an elusive link. Circulation 69:8, 1984
93. Brown BG, Lee AB, Bolson EL, et al: Reflex constriction of significant coronary stenosis as a mechanism contributing to ischemic left ventricular dysfunction during isometric exercise. Circulation 70:18, 1984
94. Berkenboom G, Unger P: Alpha-adrenergic coronary constriction in effort angina. Basic Res Cardiol 85(suppl 1):359, 1990
95. Berkenboom GM, Abramowicz M, Vandermoten P, et al: Role of alpha-adrenergic coronary tone in exercise induced angina pectoris. Am J Cardiol 57:195, 1986

96. Gage JE, Hess OM, Murakami T, et al: Vasoconstriction of stenotic coronary arteries during dynamic exercise in patients with classic angina pectoris: Reversibility by nitroglycerin. Circulation 73:865, 1986
97. Chilian WM, Layne SM: Coronary microvascular responses to reductions in perfusion pressure. Evidence for persistent arteriolar vasomotor tone during coronary hypoperfusion. Circ Res 66:1227, 1990
98. Nabel EG, Ganz P, Gordon JB, et al: Dilation of normal and constriction of atherosclerotic coronary arteries caused by the cold pressor test. Circulation 77:43, 1988
99. Maturi MF, Martin SE, Markle D, et al: Production of myocardial ischemia in dogs by constriction of nondiseased small vessels. Circulation 83:2111, 1991
100. Chu A, Morris K, Kuehl W, et al: Effects of atrial natriuretic peptide on the coronary arterial vasculature in humans. Circulation 80:1627, 1989
101. Linder C, Heusch G: ACE-inhibitors for the treatment of myocardial ischemia? Cardiovasc Drugs Ther 4:1375, 1990
102. Lamping KG, Kanatsuka H, Eastham CL, et al: Nonuniform vasomotor responses of the coronary microcirculation to serotonin and vasopressin. Circ Res 65:343, 1989
103. Ginsburg R, Bristow MR, Kantrowitz N, et al: Histamine provocation of clinical coronary artery spasm: Implications concerning pathogenesis of variant angina pectoris. Am Heart J 102:819, 1981
104. Johnson PC: Autoregulation of blood flow. Circ Res 59:483, 1986
105. Gregg DE: Effect of coronary perfusion pressure or coronary flow on oxygen usage of the myocardium. Circ Res 13:497, 1963
106. Dole WP, Nuno DW: Myocardial oxygen tension determines the degree and pressure range of coronary autoregulation. Circ Res 59:202, 1986
107. Dole WP: Autoregulation of the coronary circulation. Prog Cardiovasc Dis 29:293, 1987
108. Jones CE, Liang IYS, Gwirtz PA: Effects of alpha-adrenergic blockade on coronary autoregulation in dogs. Am J Physiol 253:H365, 1987
109. Hoffman JIE, Spaan JA: Pressure-flow relations in coronary circulation. Physiol Rev 70:331, 1990
110. Feigl EO: Coronary autoregulation. J Hypertens Suppl 7: S55; discussion, 1989
111. Hickey RF, Sybert PE, Verrier ED, et al: Effects of halothane, enflurane, and isoflurane on coronary blood flow, autoregulation, and coronary vascular reserve in the canine heart. Anesthesiology 68:21, 1988
112. Sestier FJ, Mildenberger RR, Klassen GA: Role of autoregulation in spatial and temporal perfusion heterogeneity of canine myocardium. Am J Physiol 235:H64, 1978
113. Kuo L, Chilian WM, Davis MJ: Coronary arteriolar myogenic response is independent of endothelium. Circ Res 66:860, 1990
114. Fossel ET, Morgan HE, Ingwall JS: Measurement of changes in high-energy phosphates in the cardiac cycle by using 31P nuclear magnetic resonance. Proc Natl Acad Sci USA 77:3654, 1980
115. Feigl EO, Neat GW, Huang AH: Interrelations between coronary artery pressure, myocardial metabolism and coronary blood flow. J Mol Cell Cardiol 22:375, 1990
116. Ruiter JH, Spaan JAE, Laird JD: Transient oxygen uptake during myocardial reactive hyperemia in the dog. Am J Physiol 235:H87, 1978
117. Marcus ML: Metabolic regulation of coronary blood flow. *In* Marcus ML (eds): The Coronary Circulation in Health and Disease. New York, McGraw-Hill, 1983, pp 65–92
118. Bourdarias JP: Coronary reserve: Concept and physiological variations. Eur Heart J 16(suppl I):2, 1995
119. Nitenberg A, Antony I: Coronary vascular reserve in humans: A critical review of methods of evaluation and of interpretation of the results. Eur Heart J 16(suppl I):7, 1995
120. Kern MJ: Coronary physiology revisited: Practical insights from the cardiac catheterization laboratory. Circulation 101:1344, 2000
121. Aude YW, Garza L: How to prevent unnecessary coronary interventions: Identifying lesions responsible for ischemia in the cath lab. Curr Opin Cardiol 18:394, 2003
122. Hoffman JIE: Transmural myocardial perfusion. Prog Cardiovasc Dis 29:429, 1987
123. van der Vusse GJ, Arts T, Glatz JFC, et al: Transmural differences in energy metabolism of the left ventricular myocardium: Fact or fiction? J Mol Cell Cardiol 22:23, 1990
124. Bassingthwaighte JB, Malone MA, Moffett TC, et al: Validity of microsphere depositions for regional myocardial flows. Am J Physiol 253:H184, 1987
125. Buckberg GD, Luck JC, Payne DB, et al: Some sources of error in measuring regional blood flow with radioactive microspheres. J Appl Physiol 31:598, 1971
126. Canty JM Jr, Giglia J, Kandath D: Effect of tachycardia on regional function and transmural myocardial perfusion during graded coronary pressure reduction in conscious dogs. Circulation 82:1815, 1990
127. Hoffman JIE: Transmural myocardial perfusion. *In* Kajiya F, Klassen GA, Spaan JAE, Hoffman JIE (eds): Coronary Circulation—Basic Mechanism and Clinical Relevance. Tokyo, Springer-Verlag, 1990, pp 141–152
128. Harrison DG, Florentine MS, Brooks LA, et al: The effect of hypertension and left ventricular hypertrophy on the lower range of coronary autoregulation. Circulation 77:1108, 1988
129. Tomanek RJ: Response of the coronary vasculature to myocardial hypertrophy. J Am Coll Cardiol 15:528, 1990
130. Hoffman JI: Heterogeneity of myocardial blood flow. Basic Res Cardiol 90:103, 1995
131. Coggins DL, Flynn AE, Austin RE, et al: Nonuniform loss of regional flow reserve during myocardial ischemia in dogs. Circ Res 67:253, 1990
132. Pantely GA, Bristow JD, Swenson LJ, et al: Incomplete coronary vasodilation during myocardial ischemia in swine. Am J Physiol 249:638, 1985
133. Aversano T, Becker LC: Persistence of coronary vasodilator reserve despite functionally significant flow reduction. Am J Physiol 248:H403, 1985
134. Stary HC: Evolution and progression of atherosclerotic lesions in coronary arteries of children and young adults. Arteriosclerosis 9(suppl 1): I-19, 1989
135. PDAY Research Group: Relationship of atherosclerosis in young men to serum lipoprotein cholesterol concentrations and smoking: A preliminary report from the Pathobiological Determinants of Atherosclerosis in Youth. JAMA 264:3018, 1990
136. von Rokitansky C: A Manual of Pathological Anatomy. London, The Sydenham Society, 1852
137. Duguid JB: Thrombosis as a factor in atherogenesis. J Pathol Bacteriol 58:207, 1946
138. Schneiderman J, Sawdey MS, Keeton MR, et al: Increased type 1 plasminogen activator inhibitor gene expression in atherosclerotic human arteries. Proc Natl Acad Sci USA 89:6998, 1992
139. Virchow R: Gesammelte Abhandlungen zur wissenschaftlichen Medicin, Phlogose und Thrombose im Gefassystem. Berlin, Meidinger Sohn and Co, 1856, pp 458–463
140. Ross R, Glomset JA: The pathogenesis of atherosclerosis. N Engl J Med 295:369, 1976
141. Schwartz SM, Murry CE, O'Brien ER: Vessel wall response to injury. Sci Med 3:12, 1996
142. Dvorak HF, Harvey VS, Estrella P, et al: Fibrin-containing gels induce angiogenesis. Implications for tumor stroma generation and wound healing. Lab Invest 57:673, 1987
143. Hunt TK, Knighton DR, Thakral KK, et al: Studies on inflammation and wound healing: Angiogenesis and collagen synthesis stimulated in vivo by resident and activated wound macrophage. Surgery 96:48, 1984
144. Gabbiani G: The biology of the myofibroblast. Kidney Int 41:530, 1996
145. Dvorak HF: Tumors: Wounds that do not heal. Similarities between tumor stroma generation and wound healing. N Engl J Med 315:1650, 1986
146. Ross R: The pathogenesis of atherosclerosis: A perspective for the 1990s. Nature 362:801, 1993
147. Munro JM, Cotran RS: The pathogenesis of atherosclerosis: Atherogenesis and inflammation. Lab Invest 58:249, 1988
148. Jonasson L, Holm J, Skalli O, et al: Regional accumulations of T cells, macrophages, and smooth muscle cells in the human atherosclerotic plaque. Arteriosclerosis 6:131, 1986
149. Katsuda S, Boyd HC, Fligner C, et al: Human atherosclerosis: Immunocytochemical analysis of the cell composition of lesions of young adults. Am J Pathol 140:907, 1992
150. Prescott MF, McBride CK, Court M: Development of intimal lesions after leukocyte migration into the vascular wall. Am J Pathol 135:835, 1989
151. Henney AM, Wakeley PR, Davies MJ, et al: Localization of stromelysin gene expression in atherosclerotic plaques by in situ hybridization. Proc Natl Acad Sci USA 88:8154, 1991
152. Bevilacqua MP, Slengelin S, Gimbrone MAJ, et al: Endothelial leukocyte adhesion molecule 1: An inducible receptor for neutrophils related to complement regulatory proteins and lectins. Science 243:1160, 1989
153. Springer TA: Traffic signals for lymphocyte recirculation and leukocyte emigration: The multistep paradigm. Cell 76:301, 1994
154. Osborn L, Hession C, Tizard R, et al: Direct expression cloning of vascular cell adhesion molecules 1, a cytokine-induced endothelial protein that binds to lymphocytes. Cell 59:1203, 1989
155. Nelken NA, Coughlin SR, Gordon D, et al: Monocyte chemoattractant protein-1 in human atheromatous plaques. J Clin Invest 88:1121, 1991
156. Reidy MA, Silver M: Endothelial regeneration. Lack of intimal proliferation after defined injury to rat aorta. Am J Pathol 118:173, 1985

157. Conte MS, Choudhry RP, Shirakowa M, et al: Endothelial cell seeding fails to attenuate intimal thickening in balloon-injured rabbit arteries. J Vasc Surg 21:413, 1995
158. Winternitz MC, Thomas RM, LeCompte PM: The Biology of Arteriosclerosis. Springfield, IL, Charles C Thomas, 1938
159. Barger AC, Beeuwkes R, Lainey LL, et al: Hypothesis: Vasa vasorum and neovascularization of human coronary arteries. N Engl J Med 310:175, 1984
160. O'Brien ER, Garvin MR, Dev R, et al: Angiogenesis in human coronary atherosclerotic plaques. Am J Pathol 145:883, 1994
161. Pels K, Labinaz M, O'Brien ER: Arterial wall neovascularization: Potential role in atherosclerosis and restenosis. Japan Circ J 35:241, 1997.
162. O'Brien KD, McDonald TO, Chait A, et al: Neovascular expression of E-selectin intercellular adhesion molecule-1, and vascular cell adhesion molecule-1 in human atherosclerosis and their relation to intimal leukocyte content. Circulation 93:672, 1996
163. Brown MS, Goldstein JL: A receptor-mediated pathway for cholesterol homeostasis. Science 232:34, 1986
164. Steinberg D: Antioxidant vitamins and coronary heart disease. N Engl J Med 328:1444, 1993
165. The Scandinavian Simvastatin Survival Study Group: Randomised trial of cholesterol lowering in 4444 patients with coronary heart disease: The Scandinavian Simvastatin Survival Study (4S). Lancet 344:1383, 1994
166. Treasure CB, Klein JL, Weintraub WS: Beneficial effects of cholesterol-lowering therapy on the coronary endothelium in patients with coronary artery disease. N Engl J Med 332:481, 1995
167. Anderson TJ, Meredith IT, Yeung AC, et al: The effect of cholesterol-lowering and antioxidant therapy on endothelium-dependent coronary vasomotion. N Engl J Med 332:488, 1995
168. Benditt EP, Benditt JM: Evidence for a monoclonal origin of human atherosclerotic plaques. Proc Natl Acad Sci USA 70:1753, 1973
169. Murry CE, Gipaya CT, Bartosek T, et al: Monoclonality of smooth muscle cells in human atherosclerosis. Am J Pathol 151:697, 1997
170. Sims FH, Gavin JB, Vanderwee MA: The intima of human coronary arteries. Am Heart J 118:32, 1989
171. Sims FH, Gavin JB: The early development of intimal thickening of human coronary arteries. Coron Artery Dis 1:205, 1990
172. Gordon D, Reidy MA, Benditt EP, et al: Cell proliferation in human coronary arteries. Proc Natl Acad Sci USA 87:4600, 1990
173. O'Brien ER, Alpers CE, Stewart DK, et al: Proliferation in primary and restenotic coronary atherectomy tissue: Implications for antiproliferative therapy. Circ Res 73:223, 1993
174. Villaschi S, Spagnoli LG: Autoradiographic and ultrastructural studies on the human fibroatheromatous plaque. Atherosclerosis 48:95, 1983
175. Spagnoli LG, Villaschi S, Neri L, et al: Autoradiographic studies of the smooth muscle cells in human arteries. Artery Wall 7:107, 1981
176. Bennett MR, Evan GI, Schwartz SM: Apoptosis of human vascular smooth muscle cells derived from normal vessels and coronary atherosclerotic plaques. J Clin Invest 95:2266, 1995
177. Lindner V, Olson NE, Clowes AW, et al: Heparin inhibits smooth muscle cell proliferation in injured rat arteries by displacing basic fibroblast growth factor. J Clin Invest 90:2044, 1992
178. Jackson CL, Raines EW, Ross R, et al: Role of endogenous platelet-derived growth factor in arterial smooth muscle cell migration after balloon catheter injury. Arterioscler Thromb 13:1218, 1993
179. Reidy MA, Irvin C, Lindner V: Migration of arterial wall cells. Expression of plasminogen activators and inhibitors in injured rat arteries. Circ Res 78:405, 1996
180. Glagov S, Weisenberg E, Zarins CK, et al: Compensatory enlargement of human atherosclerotic coronary arteries. N Engl J Med 316:1371, 1987
181. Folkow B: Physiological aspects of primary hypertension. Physiol Rev 62:347, 1982
182. Jamal A, Bendeck M, Langille BL: Structural changes and recovery of function after arterial injury. Arterioscler Thromb 12:307, 1992
183. Folkow B: "Structural factor" in primary and secondary hypertension. Hypertension 16:89, 1990
184. Isner JM: Vascular remodeling: Honey, I think I shrunk the artery. Circ 89:2937, 1994
185. Lafont A, Guzman LA, Whitlow PL, et al: Restenosis after experimental angioplasty. Intimal, medial, and adventitial changes associated with constrictive remodeling. Circ Res 76:996, 1995
186. Kakuta T, Currier JW, Haudenschild CC, et al: Differences in compensatory vessel enlargement, not intimal formation, account for restenosis following angioplasty in the hypercholesterolemic rabbit model. Circulation 89:2809, 1994
187. Post MJ, Borst C, Kuntz RE: The relative importance of arterial remodeling compared with intimal hyperplasia in lumen renarrowing after balloon angioplasty. A study in the normal rabbit and the hypercholesterolemic Yucatan micropig. Circulation 89:2816, 1994
188. Pasterkamp G, Borst C, Post MJ, et al: Atherosclerotic arterial remodeling in the superficial femoral artery. Individual variation in local compensatory enlargement response. Circulation 93:1818, 1996
189. Kimura T, Kaburagi S, Tamura T, et al: Remodeling of human coronary arteries undergoing coronary angioplasty or atherectomy. Circulation 96:475, 1999
190. Luo H, Nishioka T, Eigler NL, et al: Coronary artery restenosis after balloon angioplasty in humans is associated with circumferential coronary artery constriction. Arterioscler Thromb Vasc Biol 16:1393, 1999
191. Mintz GS, Popma JJ, Pichard AD, et al: Arterial remodeling after coronary angioplasty. A serial intravascular ultrasound study. Circulation 94:35, 1996
192. Pasterkamp G, de Kleijn D, Borst C: Arterial remodeling in atherosclerosis, restenosis and after alteration of blood flow: Potential mechanisms and clinical implications. Cardiovasc Res 45:843, 2000
193. Schwartz SM, Murry CE, O'Brien ER: Vessel wall response to injury. Sci Med 3:12, 1996
194. Shi Y, Pieniek M, Fard A, et al: Adventitial remodeling after coronary artery injury. Circulation 93:340, 1996
195. Bryant SR, Bjercke RJ, Erichsen DA, et al: Vascular remodeling in response to altered blood flow is mediated by fibroblast growth factor-2. Circ Res 84:323, 1999
196. Langille BL, O'Donnell F: Reductions in arterial diameter produced by chronic diseases in blood flow are endothelium-dependent. Science 231:405, 1986
197. Jamal A, Bendeck M, Langille BL: Structural changes and recovery of function after arterial injury. Arterioscler Thromb 12:307, 1992
198. Koester W: Endarteritis and arteritis. Berl Klin Wochenschr 13:454, 1876
199. Geiringer E: Intimal vascularization and atherosclerosis. J Pathol Bacteriol 63:201, 1951
200. Heistad DH, Armstrong ML: Blood flow through vasa vasorum of coronary arteries in atherosclerotic monkeys. Arteriosclerosis 6:326, 1986
201. Brown BG, Bolson EL, Dodge HT: Dynamic mechanisms in human coronary stenosis. Circulation 70:917, 1984
202. Levin DC, Gardiner GA: Coronary arteriography. *In* Braunwald E (ed): Heart Disease, 3rd edition. Philadelphia, WB Saunders, 1988, pp 268–310
203. Arnett EN, Isner JM, Redwood DR, et al: Coronary artery narrowing in coronary heart disease: Comparison of cineangiographic and necropsy findings. Ann Intern Med 91:350, 1979
204. Wilson RF: Assessing the severity of coronary artery stenoses. N Engl J Med 334:1735, 1996
205. Marcus ML: The physiologic effects of a coronary stenosis. *In* Marcus ML (ed): The Coronary Circulation in Health and Disease. New York, McGraw-Hill, 1983, pp 242–269
206. Ambrose JA, Tannenbaum MA, Alexopoulos D, et al: Angiographic progression of coronary artery disease and the development of myocardial infarction. J Am Coll Cardiol 12:56, 1988
207. Little WC, Constantinescu M, Applegate RJ, et al: Can coronary angiography predict the site of a subsequent myocardial infarction in patients with mild-to-moderate coronary artery disease? Circulation 78:1157, 1988
208. Davies MJ, Thomas AC: Plaque fissuring—The cause of acute myocardial infarction, sudden ischemic death, and crescendo angina. Br Heart J 53:363, 1985
209. Richardson PD, Davies MJ, Born GV: Influence of plaque configuration and stress distribution on fissuring of coronary atherosclerotic plaques. Lancet 2:941, 1989
210. Van der Wal AC, Becker AE, van der Loos CM, et al: Site of intimal rupture or erosion of thrombosed coronary atherosclerotic plaque is characterized by an inflammatory process irrespective of the dominant plaque morphology. Circulation 89:36, 1994
211. Libby P, Hansson GK: Involvement of the immune system in human atherogenesis: Current knowledge and unanswered questions. Lab Invest 64:5, 1991
212. Demer L, Gould KL, Kirkeeide R: Assessing stenosis severity; Coronary flow reserve, collateral function, quantitative coronary arteriography, positron imaging, and digital subtraction angiography. A review and analysis. Progr Cardiovasc Dis 307, 1988
213. Gould KL, Lipscomb K, Hamilton GW: Physiologic basis for assessing critical coronary stenosis. Am J Cardiol 33:87, 1974
214. Koerselman J, van der Graf Y, De Jaegere PP, et al: Coronary collaterals: An important and underexposed aspect of coronary artery disease. Circulation 107:2507, 2003
215. Schaper W, Gorge G, Winkler B, et al: The collateral circulation of the heart. Progr Cardiovasc Dis 57, 1988

216. Schaper W: Biological and molecular biological aspects of angiogenesis in coronary collateral development. *In* Nakamura M, Vanhoutte PM (eds): Coronary Circulation in Physiological and Pathophysiological States. Tokyo, Springer-Verlag, 1991, pp 21–27
217. Conway EM, Collen D, Carmeliet P: Molecular mechanisms of blood vessel growth. Cardiovasc Res 49:507, 2001
218. Fujita M, Tambara K: Recent insights into human coronary collateral development. Heart 90:246, 2004
219. Carmeliet P: Mechanisms of angiogenesis and arteriogenesis. Nat Med 6:389, 2000
220. Sellke FW, Quillen JE, Brooks LA, et al: Endothelial modulation of the coronary vasculature in vessels perfused via mature collaterals. Circulation 81:1938, 1990
221. Verani MS: The functional significance of coronary collateral vessels: Anecdote confronts science. Cathet Cardiovasc Diagn 9:333, 1983
222. Marcus ML: The coronary collateral circulation. *In* Marcus ML (ed): The Coronary Circulation in Health and Disease. New York, McGraw-Hill, 1983, pp 221–241
223. Braunwald E, Sobel BE: Coronary blood flow and myocardial ischemia. *In* Braunwald E (ed): Heart Disease, 3rd edition. Philadelphia, WB Saunders, 1988, pp 1191–1221
224. Hlatky MA, Mark DB, Califf RM, et al: Angina, myocardial ischemia and coronary disease: Gold standards, operational definitions and correlations. J Clin Epidemiol 42:381, 1989
225. Hoffman JIE, Buckberg GD: Transmural variations in myocardial perfusion. *In* Yu PN, Goodwin JF (eds): Progress in Cardiology. Philadelphia, Lea & Febiger, 1976, p 37
226. Buckberg GD, Fixler DE, Archie JP, et al: Experimental subendocardial ischemia in dogs with normal coronary arteries. Circ Res 30:67, 1972
227. Griggs DM, Nakamura Y: Effects of coronary constriction on myocardial distribution of Iodoantipyrine-I-131. Am J Physiol 215:1082, 1968
228. Brazier J, Cooper N, Buckberg GD: The adequacy of subendocardial oxygen delivery: The interaction of determinants of flow, arterial oxygen content and myocardial oxygen need. Circulation 49:968, 1974
229. Buffington CW: Hemodynamic determinants of ischemic myocardial dysfunction in the presence of coronary stenosis in dogs. Anesthesiology 63:651, 1985
230. Stone PH: Mechanisms of silent myocardial ischemia: Implications for selection of optimal therapy. Adv Cardiol 37:328, 1990
231. Maseri A, Newman C, Davies G: Coronary vasomotor tone: A heterogeneous entity. Eur Heart J 10(suppl F):2, 1989
232. Malacoff RF, Mudge GH, Holman BL, et al: Effect of cold pressor test on regional myocardial blood flow in patients with coronary artery disease. Am Heart J 106:78, 1983
233. Zeiher AM, Drexler H, Wollschlaeger H, et al: Coronary vasomotion in response to sympathetic stimulation in humans: Importance of the functional integrity of the endothelium. J Am Coll Cardiol 14:1181, 1989
234. Konidala S, Gutterman DD: Coronary vasospasm and the regulation of coronary blood flow. Prog Cardiovasc Dis 46:349, 2004
235. Batchelor TJ, Sadaba JR, Ishola A, et al: Rho-kinase inhibitors prevent agonist-induced vasospasm in human internal mammary artery. Br J Pharmacol 132:302, 2001
236. Werns SW, Walton JA, Hsia HH: Evidence of endothelial dysfunction in angiographically normal coronary arteries of patients with coronary artery disease. Circulation 79:287, 1989
237. Vita JA, Treasure CB, Nabel EG, et al: Coronary vasomotor response to acetylcholine relates to risk factors for coronary artery disease. Circulation 81:491, 1990
238. Nabel EG, Selwyn AP, Ganz P: Large coronary arteries in humans are responsive to changing blood flow: An endothelium-dependent mechanism that fails in patients with atherosclerosis. J Am Coll Cardiol 16:349, 1990
239. Golino P, Piscione F, Willerson JT, et al: Divergent effects of serotonin on coronary artery dimensions and blood flow in patients with coronary atherosclerosis and control patients. N Engl J Med 324:641, 1991
240. McFadden EP, Clarke JG, Davies GJ, et al: Effect of intracoronary serotonin on coronary vessels in patients with stable angina and patients with variant angina. N Engl J Med 324:648, 1991
241. Golino P, Maseri A: Serotonin receptors in human coronary arteries. Circulation 90:1573, 1994
242. Shepherd J, Cobbe SM, Ford I, et al: Prevention of coronary heart disease with pravastatin in men with hypercholesterolemia. West of Scotland Coronary Prevention Study Group. N Engl J Med 333:1301, 1995
243. Burke AP, Farb A, Malcolm GT, et al: Coronary risk factors and plaque morphology in men with coronary disease who died suddenly. N Engl J Med 336:1276, 1997
244. Schonbeck U, Libby P: Inflammation, immunity, and HMG-CoA reductase inhibitors: Statins as antiinflammatory agents? Circulation 109(suppl II), 2004
245. Halcox JPJ, Deanfield JE: Beyond the laboratory: Clinical implications for statin pleiotropy. Circulation 109(suppl II), 2004
246. Mintz GS, Popma JJ, Pichard AD, et al: Arterial remodeling after coronary angioplasty. A serial intravascular ultrasound study. Circulation 94:35, 1996
247. Kimura T, Yokoi H, Nakagawa Y, et al: Three-year follow-up after implementation of metallic coronary artery stents. N Engl J Med 334:561, 1996
248. Froeschl M, Olsen S, Ma X, et al: Current understanding of in-stent restenosis and the potential benefit of drug-eluting stents. Curr Drug Targets Cardiovasc Haematol Disord 4:103, 2004
249. Kearney M, Pieczek A, Haley L, et al: Histopathology of in-stent restenosis in patients with peripheral artery disease. Circulation 95:1998, 1997
250. Hibbert B, Chen Y-X, O'Brien ER: c-Kit-immunopositive vascular progenitor cells populate human coronary in-stent restenosis but not primary atherosclerotic lesions. Am J Physiol (Heart Circ Physiol) 287:H518, 2004
251. Hibbert B, Olsen S, O'Brien ER: Involvement of progenitor cells in vascular repair. Trends Cardiovasc Med 13:322, 2003
252. Majka SM, Jackson KA, Kienstra KA, et al: Distinct progenitor populations in skeletal muscle are bone marrow derived and exhibit different cell fates during vascular regeneration. J Clin Invest 111:71, 2003
253. deRuiter MC, Poelmann RE, VanMunsteren JC, et al: Embryonic endothelial cells transdifferentiate into mesenchymal cells expressing smooth muscle actins in vivo and in vitro. Circ Res 80:444, 1997
254. Hall SM, Hislop AA, Pierce CM, et al: Prenatal origins of human intrapulmonary arteries: Formation and smooth muscle maturation. Am J Respir Cell Mol Biol 23:194, 2000
255. Frid MG, Kale VA, Stenmark KR: Mature vascular endothelium can give rise to smooth muscle cells via endothelial-mesenchymal transdifferentiation: In vitro analysis. Circ Res 90:1189, 2002
256. Ishisaki A, Hayashi H, Li A-J, et al: Human umbilical vein endothelium-derived cells retain potential to differentiate into smooth muscle-like cells. J Biol Chem 278:1303, 2003
257. Quaini F, Urbanek K, Beltrami AP, et al: Chimerism of the transplanted heart. N Engl J Med 346:5, 2002
258. Hill JM, Zalos G, Halcox JP, et al: Circulating endothelial progenitor cells, vascular function, and cardiovascular risk. N Engl J Med 348:593, 2003
259. Vasa M, Fichtlscherer S, Aicher A, et al: Number and migratory activity of circulating endothelial progenitor cells inversely correlate with risk factors for coronary artery disease. Circ Res 89:e1, 2001
260. Vasa M, Fichtlscherer S, Adler K, et al: Increase in circulating endothelial progenitor cells by statin therapy in patients with stable coronary artery disease. Circulation 103:2885, 2001
261. Walter DH, Rittig K, Bahlmann FH, et al: Statin therapy accelerates reendothelialization: A novel effect involving mobilization and incorporation of bone marrow-derived endothelial progenitor cells. Circulation 105:3017, 2002

Chapter 7
MOLECULAR CARDIOVASCULAR MEDICINE

Marcel E. Durieux, MD, PhD • Paul Mounsey, MD

KEY POINTS

1. The rapid development of molecular biology techniques has greatly expanded the understanding of cardiac functioning and is beginning to be applied clinically.
2. Cardiac ion channels form the machinery behind the cardiac rhythm; cardiac membrane receptors regulate cardiac function.
3. Sodium, potassium, and calcium channels are the main types involved in the cardiac action potential. Many subtypes exist and their molecular structures are known in some detail, allowing a molecular explanation for such phenomena as voltage sensing, ion selectivity, and inactivation.
4. Muscarinic and adrenergic receptors, both of the G protein–coupled receptor class, are the main regulators of cardiac function.
5. Adenosine plays important roles in myocardial preconditioning through an action on ATP-regulated K channels and is an effective antiarrhythmic drug by its action on G protein–coupled adenosine receptors.
6. Volatile anesthetics significantly affect calcium channels and muscarinic receptors.
7. Cardiovascular diagnosis through molecular techniques and treatment through gene therapy have not yet become standard practice but offer potential for future clinical options.

The past decades have witnessed what may well be termed a revolution in the biomedical sciences, as molecular methodologies have suddenly jumped onto the clinical scene. Molecular biology originated in the 1950s, its birth most commonly identified with the description of the structure of deoxyribonucleic acid (DNA) by Watson and Crick.[1] For many years after, it was practiced almost exclusively in the research laboratory. Much of this research involved the laborious process of cloning: the identification of DNA molecules encoding specific proteins. Although at the time most people in the field realized that these advances would one day be of immense importance to clinical medicine, the exact place they would take was unclear.

Not generally appreciated was the rapidity with which molecular biology would advance. Now, five decades since the discovery of the structure of DNA, the human genome has been sequenced completely. Techniques for manipulating nucleic acids have been simplified enormously, and for many routine procedures kits are now available. The development of the polymerase chain reaction (PCR), a technique of remarkable simplicity and flexibility, has dramatically increased the speed with which many molecular biology procedures can be performed; in addition, it has allowed the invention of many new ones. Novel techniques are directed at screening large amounts of genetic material for changes associated with disease states. As a result of these and other developments, molecular biology has far advanced beyond cloning, and its techniques are now used routinely to study the expression and functioning of proteins in health and disease.

Cardiovascular medicine has been a major beneficiary of these advances. Not only have the electrophysiologic and pump functions of the heart been placed on a firm molecular footing, but for a number of disease states the pathophysiology has been determined, allowing progress in therapeutic development. Importantly, there is no indication that the pace of progress in molecular biology has slowed. If anything, the opposite is the case, and more dramatic advances may be expected in the years to come. Thus, techniques such as gene therapy may become available as therapeutic options in cardiac disease.

In this chapter, the most important aspects of molecular cardiovascular medicine are surveyed, with specific emphasis on medical issues relevant to the anesthesiologist. The myocyte membrane signaling proteins are of primary importance in this respect, and the two major classes—membrane channels and membrane receptors—are discussed. Simply stated, the channels form the machinery behind the cardiac rhythm, whereas the receptors are involved in regulation of cardiac function. This is, of course, an overgeneralization, as close interactions among the various systems exist. In fact, these interactions have stimulated some of the more exciting areas of investigation in molecular cardiovascular medicine. In each of these sections, a brief overview of the general properties of the class of proteins is provided, and examples specific to the cardiovascular system are discussed. Each section ends with a discussion of some clinical correlations.

The actions of anesthetics on these systems are also described. This area is one of active investigation. Much detail remains to be filled in, but it is clear now that anesthetics, at clinically relevant concentrations, interact with a number of cardiac signaling systems. Although it is too early to completely explain the cardiac side effects of the various anesthetics through these mechanisms, there is no doubt that such interactions can be of significant clinical relevance. Considering the rapid pace of research in this area, rather than attempting to be all-inclusive, two examples for which a significant body of information is available, and where clinical relevance appears likely, are emphasized. These examples are (1) the cardiac Ca^{++} channels and (2) the muscarinic acetylcholine receptors.

The final section looks ahead toward several developments that are not yet actual clinical practice but that may be anticipated in the not-too-distant future.

In addition to providing an overview of the current state of knowledge, this chapter demonstrates a few of the many methodologies that have been used to obtain these results, in order to enable the reader to access the current literature with more ease.

MACHINERY BEHIND THE CARDIAC RHYTHM: ION CHANNELS

The cardiac action potential results from the flow of ions through ion channels, which are the membrane-bound proteins that form the structural basis of cardiac electrical excitability. In response to changes in electrical potential across the cell membrane, ion channels open to allow the passive flux of ions into or out of the cell along their electrochemical gradients. Ion flux results in a flow of current, which displaces the cell membrane potential toward the potential at which the electrochemical gradient for the ion is zero, called the equilibrium potential (E) for the ion. Depolarization of the cell could, in principle, result from an inward cation current or an outward anion current; for repolarization the reverse is true. In excitable cells, action potentials are mainly caused by the flow of cation currents. Membrane depolarization results principally from the flow of Na^+ down its electrochemical gradient (E_{Na} is around +50 mV), whereas repolarization results from the outward flux of K^+ down its electrochemical gradient (E_K is around −90 mV). Opening and closing of multiple ion channels of a single type results in an individual ionic current. The integrated activity of many different ionic currents, each activated over precisely regulated potential ranges and at different times in the cardiac cycle, results in the cardiac action potential. Ion channels are usually highly (but not uniquely) *selective* for a single ion (e.g., K^+ channels, Na^+ channels). Channels may *rectify*, that is, pass current in one direction across the membrane more easily than the other. Electrical and chemical stimuli, which lead to opening and closing of the channel, cause a conformational change in the channel molecule (*gating*). The rate of change of channel conformation (*gating kinetics*) may be very rapid, in which case the channel will open (*activate*) almost immediately (e.g., Na^+ channels), or relatively slow, which will result in a delay in channel activation (e.g., delayed rectifier K^+ channels). After activation, ion channels may stay open until closed by another stimulus (e.g., repolarization of the membrane) or may close (*inactivate*) in the face of a continued stimulus. Inactivated channels will usually not reopen on repeat stimulation until they have recovered from inactivation (Box 7–1).

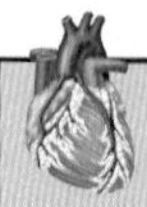

BOX 7–1 *Properties of Ion Channels*

- Ion selectivity
- Rectification (passing current more easily in one direction than the other)
- Gating (mechanism for opening and closing the channel):
  - Activation (opening)
  - Inactivation (closing)

Patch Clamping

The exciting developments in the understanding of the molecular physiology of the cardiac action potential that have occurred in the past 25 years have resulted from the development and implementation of *patch clamping*, which allows recording of ion flow through individual channel molecules, *voltage clamping* of isolated cardiac cells, and from the *cloning and heterologous expression* of ion channel genes. Comparison of ionic currents recorded in isolated myocytes with currents recorded from cells expressing ion channel genes has resulted in the identification of many of the ion channel molecules that underlie the cardiac action potential.

The development of the voltage clamp technique in the early 1950s, and its application to multicellular preparations of cardiac muscle, allowed identification of the major ionic currents that underlie the cardiac action potential. The whole cell currents recorded by the technique were smooth waveforms derived from summation of the activity of thousands of ion channels, and many different patterns of events at the single-channel level, arising from more than one molecular species, can summate to produce identical whole cell current waveforms. Patch clamping allows resolution of events at the single-channel level. In this technique small patches of cell membrane (≈1 μm²) are isolated electrically and physically in the tip of a glass micropipette.[2] Single-channel events can then be resolved because there are only a few ion channel molecules present in the patch. Current flowing across the patch typically jumps between well-defined values corresponding to sudden opening or closing of the ion-conducting pore (Fig. 7–1*A*). The whole cell current will be the sum of the currents through all of the individual channels in the cell membrane; summation of the current flowing through a single channel

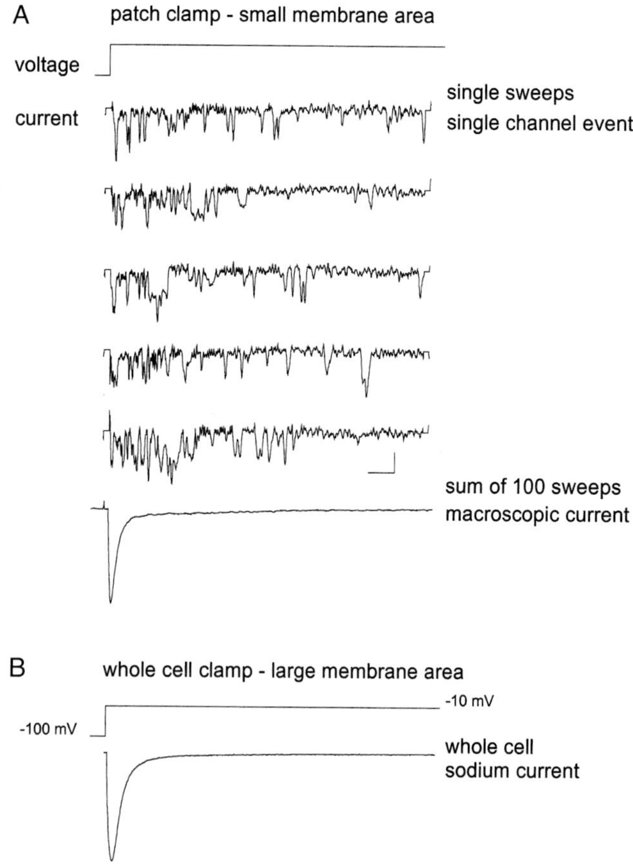

Figure 7–1 Voltage clamp recordings from muscle Na^+ channels. *(A)* Patch clamp recordings. Individual Na^+ channel openings are recorded as short-lived downward deflections. Note that openings are concentrated in the first part of the trace. The *upper five traces* represent a single depolarizing clamp pulse. The sum of 100 such pulses *(bottom trace)* re-creates the whole cell current *(B)*.

during repeated stimuli will reproduce the macroscopic whole cell current (Fig. 7–1*A*, *B*). As channel opening and closing in response to a stimulus is a stochastic phenomenon, the regulation of ion flow, whether resulting from a change in membrane potential or from interaction with regulator molecules, is usually achieved by increasing the *probability* that the channel will be open. Thus, in Figure 7–1, which shows records from human cardiac muscle Na^+ channels, the channels open *(activate)* a few milliseconds after depolarization, because the *probability* that the channel will be open increases. Similarly, as the channels spontaneously close (*inactivate*), the open probability decreases.

An ion current with distinct electrical and pharmacologic properties indicates the presence of a population of identical ion channel molecules. Application of molecular techniques has allowed the identification of many ion channel molecules and thus a better understanding of the currents that underlie the cardiac action potential. An evolving area is tailoring of pharmacologic agents that interact with specific channel types to shape the action potential.

Electrical Events Underlying the Cardiac Action Potential

Figure 7–2 shows a diagram of a cardiac action potential with a summary of the ionic currents flowing during each phase. As far as has been determined, the probable molecular identity of the ion channels that underlie these currents is also given. The biophysical properties of these currents are examined first; subsequent sections focus on possible molecular mechanisms underlying the biophysical phenomena.

Resting Membrane Potential and the Role of I_{K1}

The resting cardiac membrane potential is maintained close to the equilibrium potential for potassium (E_K) by a background, inwardly rectifying, highly selective K^+ current (I_{K1}).[3] Under physiologic conditions, the E_K is around −90 mV, and displacement of the membrane potential from this value should result in inward or outward current through I_{K1}, thus returning the membrane potential toward E_K. However, although I_{K1} passes significant *inward* current at potentials negative to E_K, at positive potentials the channels display inward rectification (i.e., they pass inward current more easily than outward current), which limits outward current flow and reduces the tendency for I_{K1} to hyperpolarize the membrane. This situation has obvious significance for an excitable cell; inward rectification allows the initiation of action potentials and limits cellular K^+ loss during the action potential. I_{K1} is large in ventricular cells, smaller in atrial cells, and almost absent in nodal tissue.[4] This finding explains why ventricular cells rest near E_K and have a high threshold for excitation, atrial cells have a more positive resting potential, and nodal cells have no defined resting potential.

Phase 0: The Rapid Upstroke of the Cardiac Action Potential

The rapid upstroke of the cardiac action potential (phase 0) is caused by the flow of a large inward Na^+ current (I_{Na}) (Box 7–2).[5] I_{Na} is activated by depolarization of the sarcolemma to a threshold potential of −65 to −70 mV. I_{Na} activation, and

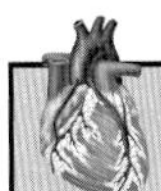

BOX 7–2 *Cardiac Action Potential*

- Phase 0 (rapid upstroke): primarily Na^+ channel opening
- Phase 1 (early rapid repolarization): inactivation of Na^+ current, opening of K^+ channels
- Phase 2 (plateau phase): balance between K^+ currents and Ca^{++} currents
- Phase 3 (final rapid repolarizations): activation of Ca^{++} channels
- Phase 4 (diastolic depolarization): balance between Na^+ and K^+ currents

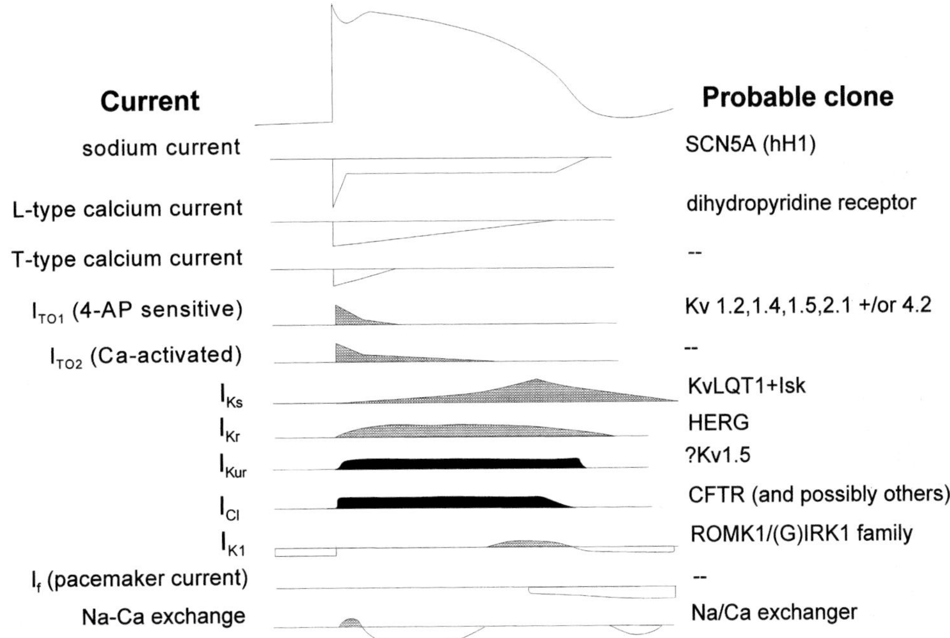

Figure 7–2 Ionic currents underlying the cardiac action potential. Currents are listed on the left, and the ion channel genes encoding the currents are listed on the right. 4-AP = 4-aminopyridine; CFTR = cystic fibrosis transmembrane regulator. (From Roden DM, Lazzarra R, Rosen R, et al, for the SADS Foundation Task Force on LQTS: Multiple mechanisms in the long QT syndrome: Current knowledge, gaps and future directions. Circulation 94:1996, 1996.)

hence the action potential, is an all-or-nothing response. Subthreshold depolarizations have only local effects on the membrane. After the threshold for activation of fast Na^+ channels is exceeded, Na^+ channels open (i.e., I_{Na} activates) and Na^+ ions enter the cell down their electrochemical gradient. This results in displacement of the membrane potential toward the equilibrium potential for Na^+ ions, around +50 mV. I_{Na} activation is transient, lasting at most 1 to 2 milliseconds because, simultaneous with activation, a second, slightly slower conformational change in the channel molecule occurs (inactivation), which closes the ion pore in the face of continued membrane depolarization (see Fig. 7–1, *A, B*). The channel cannot open again until it has recovered from inactivation (i.e., regained its resting conformation), a process that requires repolarization to the resting potential for a defined period of time. The channels cycle through three states: *resting* (and available for activation), *open*, and *inactivated*. While the channel is inactivated, it is absolutely refractory to repeated stimulation. Stimuli that occur during recovery from inactivation will result in opening of fewer Na^+ channels (because not all have recovered), and the resulting action potential will have a reduced maximal rate of depolarization and reduced conduction velocity. Na^+ channels do not need to open to become inactivated. If the resting membrane potential depolarizes for a time, inactivation will occur in some channels and subsequent stimulation will result in an action potential of reduced amplitude and conduction velocity.

Phase 1: Early Rapid Repolarization

The early rapid repolarization phase of the action potential, which follows immediately after phase 0, results both from rapid inactivation of the majority of the Na^+ current and from activation of a transient outward current (I_{TO}), carried mainly by K^+ ions. On depolarization of the membrane, I_{TO} opens rapidly, over about 20 milliseconds, before spontaneously inactivating. I_{TO} comprises two separate currents: the rapidly inactivating I_{TO1}, which is activated by depolarization and blocked by 4-aminopyridine, and the slowly inactivating I_{TO2}, which is activated by elevated intracellular Ca^{++} (possibly explaining the observation that action potential duration tends to decrease with rapid heart rates and hypercalcemia)[6-8] (Fig. 7–3).

In addition to its effect on phase 1, I_{TO}, in combination with the delayed rectifier potassium currents (I_{Kr} and I_{Ks}) and I_{K1}, also contributes to membrane repolarization. Potentially, arrhythmogenic prolongation of the action potential in myocardial cells recovered from patients with myocardial hypertrophy,[9] congestive cardiomyopathy,[6] and from the border zone of myocardial infarction[10] appears to result from depression of I_{TO}.

Phases 2 and 3: The Plateau Phase and Final Rapid Repolarization

The action potential plateau and final rapid repolarization are mediated by a balance between the slow inward current and outward, predominantly K^+, currents. During the plateau phase, membrane conductance to all ions falls and very little current flows. Potassium conductance is low because of inward rectification of I_{K1} (i.e., inward current passes more easily than outward current), so very little outward current flows despite the large outward electrochemical gradient for K^+ ions and the delayed onset of the outwardly rectifying K^+ currents (I_{Ks}, I_{Kr}, and I_{Kur}). The resulting small outward current is balanced by inward current, predominantly through L-type

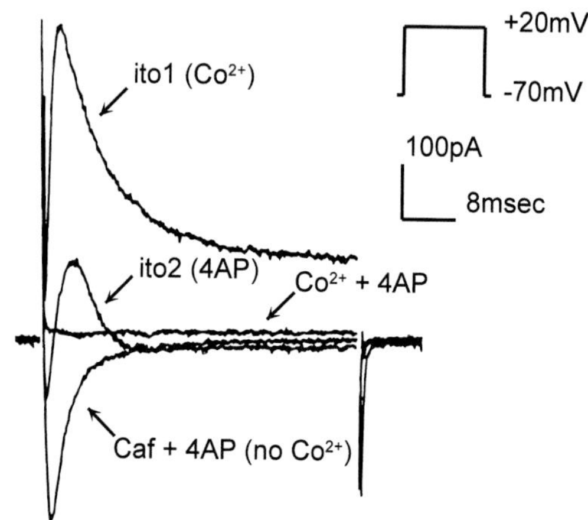

Figure 7–3 Voltage clamp recordings from an atrial myocyte showing pharmacologic separation of I_{TO1} (ito1) and I_{TO2} (ito2). In the presence of cobalt ions, only I_{TO1} is seen. When cobalt is omitted and 4-aminopyridine (4-AP) is added, I_{TO2} is revealed. Caffeine (Caf) eliminates I_{TO2}, leaving the underlying inward calcium current. In the presence of both 4-aminopyridine and cobalt ions, all outward currents are inhibited. (From Wang Z, Fermini B, Nattel S: Delayed rectifier outward current and repolarization in human atrial myocytes. Circ Res 73:276, 1993.)

Ca^{++} channels ($I_{Ca\text{-}L}$) but also via a slowly inactivating population of Na^+ channels, and a small inward flux of chloride (Cl^-) ions, possibly carried by the cardiac variant of the ATP-dependent cystic fibrosis transmembrane regulator (CFTR) channel (abnormalities of which underlie cystic fibrosis).[11,12] Phase 3, regenerative rapid repolarization, results from time-dependent inactivation of L-type Ca^{++} current and increasing outward current through delayed rectifier K^+ channels. The net membrane current becomes outward and the cell repolarizes.

SLOW INWARD CA++ CURRENT

The slow inward current ($I_{Ca\text{-}L}$) is activated by depolarization of the cell to potentials less negative than −40 to −50 mV. In ventricular and atrial myocytes and in Purkinje fibers, $I_{Ca\text{-}L}$ is activated by the regenerative depolarization caused by I_{Na} during phase 0 of the action potential. $I_{Ca\text{-}L}$ does not contribute significantly to phase 0 because, in comparison to I_{Na}, it activates much more slowly (over about 10 milliseconds) and is smaller in amplitude. $I_{Ca\text{-}L}$ also inactivates slowly and therefore contributes the major inward current during the plateau of the action potential. $I_{Ca\text{-}L}$ flows through L-type (long-lasting) Ca^{++} channels, which are sensitive to block by dihydropyridines (e.g., nifedipine), and activation of contraction is related to the magnitude of the resulting calcium influx.[13] The gating of $I_{Ca\text{-}L}$ is generally similar to I_{Na} in that channel opening and closing are dependent on membrane potential and time. Ca^{++} channels are also, importantly, dynamically regulated by the autonomic nervous system.[14,15] β-Agonists activate $I_{Ca\text{-}L}$ (and hence increase myocardial contractility) indirectly by activating adenylyl cyclase via a guanosine triphosphate (GTP)-binding protein G_s (Fig. 7–4). The resulting increase in intracellular cyclic adenosine monophosphate (cAMP) activates protein kinase A (PKA), which phosphorylates the Ca^{++} channel. Phosphorylated channels open in response to membrane depolarization; nonphosphorylated channels do not, so the effect of β-adrenergic stimulation is to increase the number of functional channels. The electrophysiologic effect of this is illustrated in Figure 7–5, which shows enhancement of the slow inward current by elevation of the adenosine

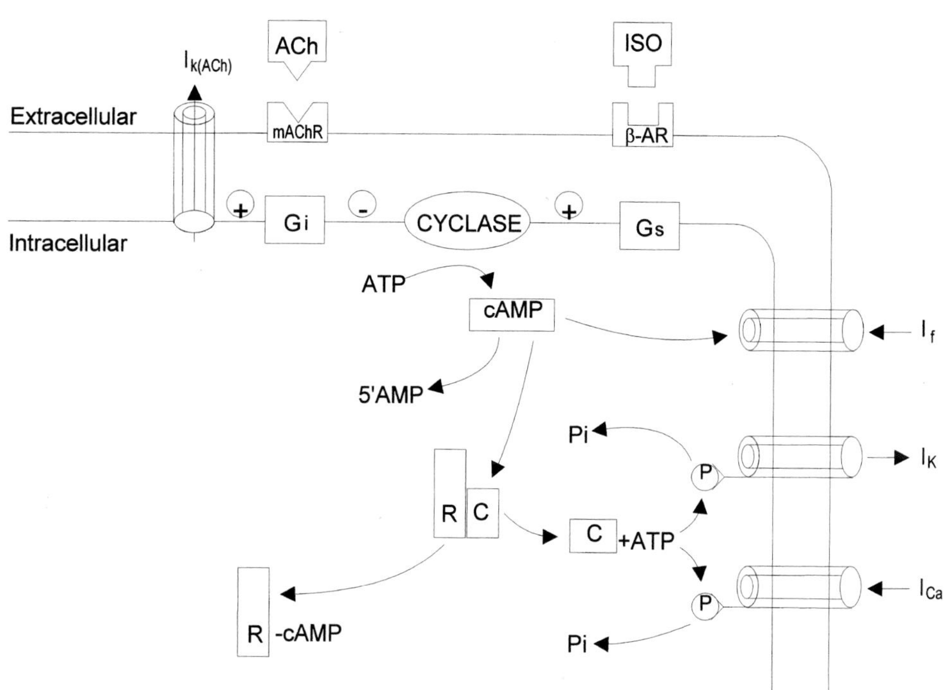

Figure 7–4 Autonomic regulation of ion currents. ACh = acetylcholine; mAChR = M2 muscarinic receptor; ISO = isoproterenol; β-AR = β-adrenergic receptor; Gi and Gs = guanosine triphosphate–binding proteins; CYCLASE = adenylyl cyclase; ATP = adenosine triphosphate; cAMP = cyclic adenosine monophosphate; 5′AMP = adenosine 5′-monophosphate; Pi = pyrophosphate; R and C = regulatory and catalytic subunits, respectively, of protein kinase A. For further discussion, see text.

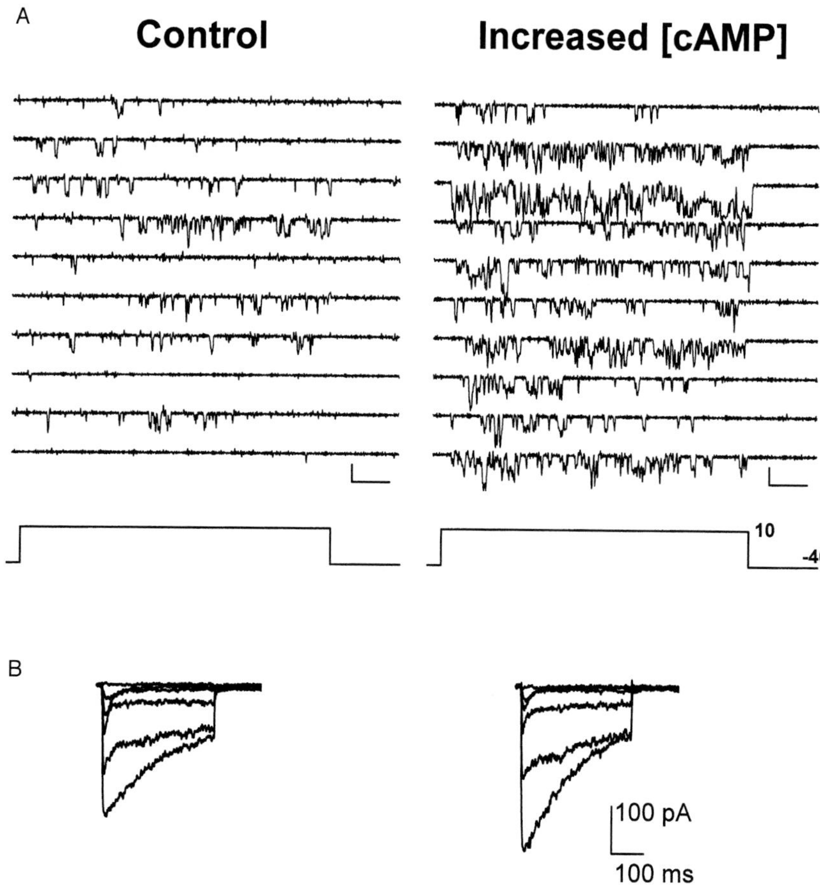

Figure 7–5 Effects of elevated cyclic adenosine monophosphate (cAMP) on cardiac calcium channels. *(A)* Single-channel recordings. *(B)* Whole cell currents. *Left panels* are control recordings; *right panels* show the effect of elevation of intracellular cAMP (in this case induced by exposure to parathyroid hormone). Note the increased probability of channel opening and resulting increase in whole cell current in the presence of elevated cAMP. *(A, B,* Modified from Rampe D, Lacerda AE, Dage RC, Brown AM: Parathyroid hormone: An endogenous modulator of cardiac calcium channels. Am J Physiol 261[6 Pt 2]:H1945, 1991.)

monophosphate (AMP) level in single-channel Ca^{++} channels and in intact cells. β-Adrenergic effects on $I_{Ca\text{-}L}$ are antagonized by acetylcholine, which, in myocardial cells, activates M_2 muscarinic receptors and inhibits adenylyl cyclase through activation of the GTP-binding protein G_i.

In the relatively depolarized pacemaker cells, which lack I_{K1}, I_{Na} is inactivated and the slow inward current is solely responsible for the upstroke of the action potential. $I_{Ca\text{-}L}$ can also generate slowly propagated action potentials in diseased or damaged myocardial cells in which I_{Na} has been inactivated by depolarization. These *slow responses*, which may occur in the border zone of myocardial infarctions, are important because they may cause the slow conduction necessary to produce reentrant arrhythmias.

DELAYED RECTIFIER K^+ CURRENTS

Delayed rectifier K^+ channels are present in all cardiac myocytes. They open slowly (over 200 to 300 milliseconds) after depolarization of the membrane to the plateau level (−10 mV and greater), producing a K^+-selective outward current, I_K. I_K does not inactivate on prolonged depolarization (unlike I_{Na} and $I_{Ca\text{-}L}$), and the channels close on repolarization of the membrane. Unlike I_{K1}, I_K displays outward rectification; that is, it passes outward current more easily than inward current. This is the expected behavior for a K^+-selective channel because both the concentration and electrical gradients for potassium are outward. Thus, for any depolarizing displacement of membrane potential from E_K, the driving force will be larger in an outward direction. Similar to $I_{Ca\text{-}L}$, I_K is under autonomic control (see Fig. 7–4). β-Adrenergic stimulation enhances I_K by a mechanism similar to that of the enhancement of $I_{Ca\text{-}L}$, thus ensuring repolarization of the cell in the face of increased inward Ca^{++} current.[16]

Three components of I_K, carried by different channel molecules, can be distinguished. A rapidly activating component, I_{Kr}, is blocked by the compound E4031 (a class III antiarrhythmic agent), which leaves a slower activating component, I_{Ks}, unaffected.[17] Figure 7–6 also emphasizes the importance of I_K in the regulation of repolarization, and hence, of action potential duration. A third component, the ultra-rapidly activated delayed rectifier, I_{Kur}, can be distinguished in atrial (but not ventricular) myocytes.[18] This additional repolarizing current explains in part the enhancement of repolarization in atrial myocardium compared with ventricle and Purkinje fibers.

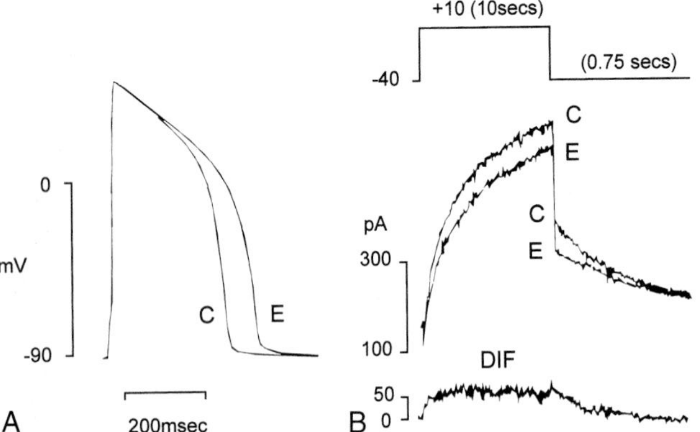

Figure 7–6 *(A)* Effect on action potential duration of blockade of I_{Kr} by E4031 in isolated guinea pig ventricular myocytes. After application of E4031, outward repolarizing currents are inhibited and action potential duration is increased. *(B)* Voltage clamp records showing separation of I_{Kr} and I_{Ks} by E4031. The control delayed rectifier K^+ current (C) is partially inhibited by E4031 (E), and the difference between the two currents (DIF) represents I_{Ks}. *(A, B,* From Sanguinetti MC, Jurkiewicz NK: Two components of cardiac delayed rectifier K^+ current. Differential sensitivity to block by class III antiarrhythmic agents. J Gen Physiol 96:195, 1990. Reproduced from The Journal of General Physiology by copyright permission of The Rockefeller University Press.)

REPOLARIZATION IN DIFFERENT CARDIAC TISSUE TYPES

Phase 3 repolarization in atrium and pacemaker tissues, but not in ventricular myocardium, is also enhanced by the presence of a large outward repolarizing K^+ current [$I_{K(ACh)}$].[19,20] This potential independent current is activated indirectly by stimulation of muscarinic (M2-type) receptors by acetylcholine or purinergic (A-type) receptors by adenosine.[21] This channel is potential independent and is activated via binding of an activated, membrane-bound GTP-binding protein (G_i), as is discussed later.[22]

There is variability in action potential duration between cells in the normal ventricle.[23] There is a gradient in action potential duration across the myocardium (from epicardium to endocardium), and specialized mid-myocardial cells (M cells) have been identified, which exhibit prolongation of action potential duration at slow stimulation rates, possibly as a result of a decrease in I_{Ks}.

Phase 4: Diastolic Depolarization and I_f

Phase 4 diastolic depolarization, or normal automaticity, is a normal feature of cardiac cells in the sinus and atrioventricular (AV) nodes, but subsidiary pacemaker activity is also observed in the His-Purkinje system and in some specialized atrial and ventricular myocardial cells (see Chapter 13). Pacemaker discharge from the sinus node normally predominates because the rate of diastolic depolarization in the sinoatrial (SA) node is faster than in other pacemaker tissues. Pacemaker activity results from a slow net gain of positive charge, which depolarizes the cell from its maximal diastolic potential to threshold.

Pacemaker cells in the sinus node are relatively depolarized, with a maximal diastolic potential of −60 to −70 mV and a threshold potential of −40 mV. Rapid regenerative depolarization (phase 0) is dependent on opening of T-type and then L-type Ca^{++} channels. Repolarization is dependent on activation of delayed rectifier K channels, and the maximum diastolic potential is around −80 mV. Pacemaker channels are activated by hyperpolarization to this potential and produce a slow inward Na current, I_f (see Fig. 7–2). This flows against slowly inactivating delayed rectifier K^+ currents and results in diastolic depolarization.[24] Because the current is nonselective among cations, its reversal potential lies between E_K and E_{Na}, at around −10 mV, and activation of I_f will tend to depolarize the cell toward this value. Similar to $I_{Ca\text{-}L}$, I_f is under autonomic control (see Fig. 7–4) through GTP-dependent binding proteins G_s and G_i, which regulate cAMP production by adenylyl cyclase.[25-27] β-Adrenergic stimulation shifts the voltage dependence of activation of I_f to more depolarized potentials, so for any hyperpolarizing stimulus, more I_f will be activated and diastolic depolarization will be enhanced. Acetylcholine has the opposite effect (Fig. 7–7).

Molecular Biology of Ion Channels

The preceding sections have focused on the electrical events that underlie cardiac electrical excitability and on the identification of cardiac ionic currents on the basis of their biophysical properties. Subsequent sections examine the molecular physiology of these electrical phenomena. The first step in understanding the molecular physiology of cardiac electrical excitability is to identify the ion channel proteins responsible for the ionic currents. Figure 7–2 gives the current status

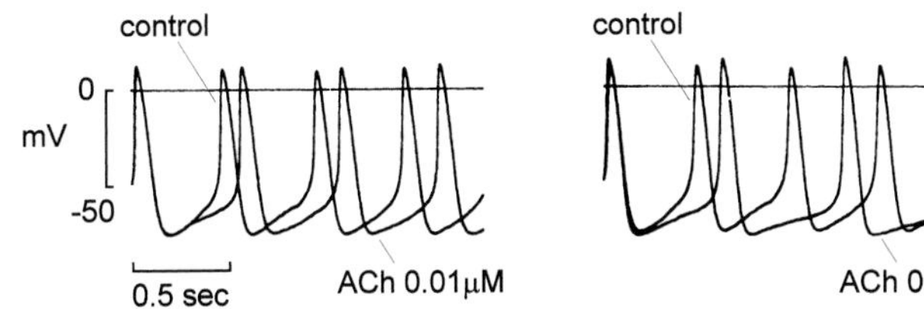

Figure 7–7 Effect of acetylcholine on spontaneous pacemaker activity in isolated sinoatrial (SA) node cells. Pacemaker activity in control solution is compared with activity in increasing doses of ACh. Note the slowing of diastolic depolarization and resultant slowing of heart rate. (From DiFrancesco D: Current I and the neuronal modulation of heart rate. *In* Zipes DP, Jaliffe J [eds]: Cardiac Electrophysiology From Cell to Bedside. Philadelphia, WB Saunders Company, 1990, p 28.)

of knowledge of the probable clone underlying each of the cardiac ionic currents. There are firm molecular candidates for voltage-gated Na^+ and L-type Ca^{++} channels. Similarly, channel molecules with properties similar to delayed rectifier K^+ channels, the 4-aminopyridine–sensitive component of I_{TO}, the inward rectifier I_{K1}, the ligand-gated K^+ channel $I_{K(ACh)}$, and the pacemaker current I_f have been cloned. Figure 7–8 shows diagrams of the predicted membrane topology of some of these channels. Voltage-gated Na^+, Ca^{++}, and K^+ channels exist as conglomerates of molecules, consisting of a large α subunit and several accessory subunits (labeled β, δ, and γ in Fig. 7–8). The α subunit alone is usually sufficient to induce channel activity in biologic membranes, but its activity is modulated by the presence of the accessory subunits. The diagrams in Figure 7–8 were deduced from hydrophobicity analysis of the primary structure of the major channel polypeptides. Regions of the polypeptides predicted to span the membrane are those that contain a high concentration of hydrophobic amino acids, whereas peptides linking these transmembrane sections are hydrophilic. Na^+ and Ca^{++} channel α subunits (Fig. 7–8, *A* and *B*) are strikingly similar, each consisting of four homologous transmembrane domains (labeled I to IV), linked by cytoplasmic peptides. Each homologous domain contains six linked membrane-spanning segments (labeled S1 to S6). These large polypeptides, containing more than 2000 amino acids, form a tetrameric structure and generate Na^+ or Ca^{++} channel activity in biologic membranes. Voltage-gated K^+ channel α subunits by contrast are much smaller (Fig. 7–8*C*), having a single transmembrane domain with six membrane-spanning segments, an arrangement similar to one of the individual domains of Na^+ and Ca^{++} channels. In order to produce K^+ channel activity, four molecules are noncovalently linked in the membrane to produce a tetrameric structure, similar to an Na^+ or a Ca^{++} channel. The structure of the inwardly rectifying K^+ channel molecules, I_{K1} and $I_{K(ACh)}$, is dissimilar from other K^+ channels (Fig. 7–8*C*). The molecules are much less complex, having only two membrane-spanning segments, although these segments share considerable homology with the S5 and S6 segments of the classic voltage-gated K^+ channel.

Voltage-gated ion channel activity requires that the channel molecule should sense and respond to changes in membrane potential, form an ion-selective membrane pore, and (in some cases) inactivate despite continuing depolarization. The molecular mechanisms for these phenomena are examined in separate sections later.

Molecular Mechanisms

Voltage Sensor

Channel proteins respond to changes in electrical potential across the cell membrane by conformational changes (*gating*), which result from electrostatic interactions between charged portions of the molecule and the membrane electric field (Box 7–3). Gating of the channel is associated with a measurable flow of electrical charge through the membrane lipid bilayer (called *gating current*), as a zone of the molecule rich in electrical charge moves within the membrane.[28] This charge movement is linked to opening of the channel pore. The voltage sensor of voltage-dependent ion channels resides in the mobile S4 membrane-spanning segments, α-helical structures unusually rich in positively charged amino acids.[29] At rest, each of the positive charges in the S4 segment is balanced by fixed negative charges in other segments of the molecule. The resting membrane potential (negative inside) forces the (mobile) positive charges inward and the fixed negative charges outward. This dynamic equilibrium holds the channel pore closed. Upon depolarization the force pulling the positive charge inward is relieved; positive charges (the S4 segments) are repelled outward and assume new partners with the fixed negative membrane charges. This charge movement comprises the *gating current*. If the depolarizing stimulus is short, repolarization of the membrane is followed by a gating current of equal and opposite magnitude as the S4 segment relaxes to its original position. If the depolarizing stimulus is prolonged, however, the movement of the S4 segments induces a conformational change in the channel molecule, which prohibits easy return to baseline. This conformational change in the channel molecule is manifested as activation (or channel opening), and this is closely coupled to channel closing (or inactivation, see below) in channels that inactivate. Thus, small changes in the membrane electric field cause conformational changes in the channel molecule, which result in opening (and closing) of the channel pore. An S4 segment rich in positive charge is a remarkably consistent feature of voltage-gated ion channels from a variety of different species and with a variety of ion selectivities. The dependence of channel activation on membrane potential is proportional to the density of positive charge in the S4 segment.

Ion Channel Pore and Selectivity Filter

The presence of four homologous domains in voltage-gated Na^+ and Ca^{++} channels suggests that basic ion channel architecture consists of a transmembrane pore surrounded by the four homologous domains arranged symmetrically (see Fig. 7–8). The membrane-spanning segments each form an α helix so that the walls of the pore will be derived from α-helical segments from each of the four domains. A pore formed from four such α helices would have limiting dimen-

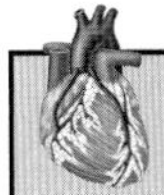

BOX 7–3 ***Molecular Mechanisms of Ion Channels***

- Voltage sensor
- Gating mechanism (activation and inactivation)
- Ion pore
- Selectivity filter

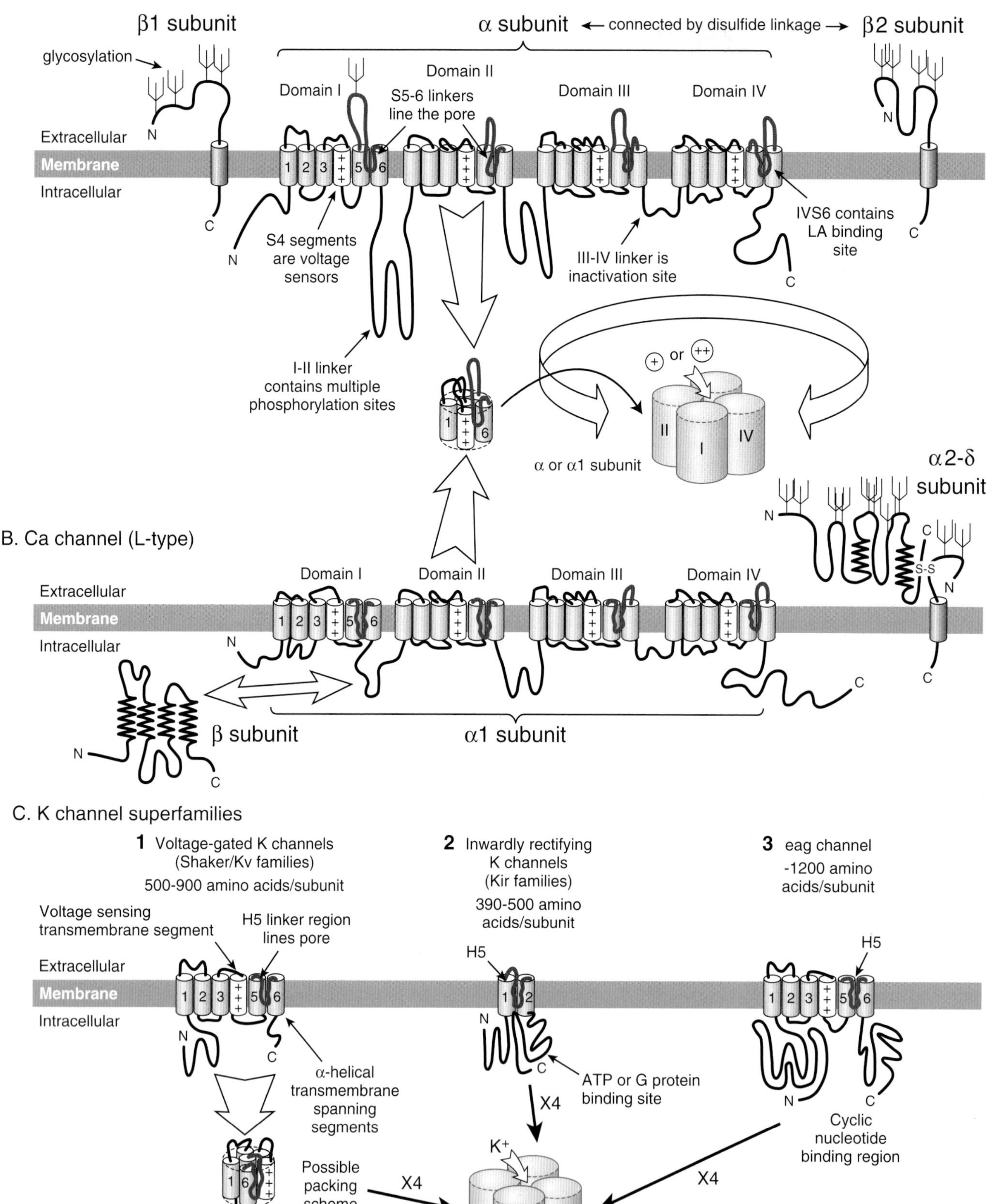

Figure 7–8 Diagrams of ion channel molecular structure. *(A)* Na^+ channel. *(B)* Ca^{++} channel. *(C)* K^+ channels. ATP = adenosine triphosphate. For further discussion, see text.

sions of 3 by 5 Angstrom units, similar to the size inferred for the Na^+ channel pore by measurement of the permeability of cations of different sizes.[30,31]

The selectivity filter is formed by the S5 and S6 membrane-spanning segments of each domain along with their peptide linker.[32] As emphasized in Figure 7–8, unlike the hydrophilic extracellular linkers between other membrane-spanning segments, the S5/S6 linker is sufficiently hydrophobic to place it (at least partially) within the membrane lipid bilayer. The channel pore is lined both by the S5/S6 linker and the S5 and S6 membrane-spanning segments. Point mutations in the S5/S6 linker have dramatic effects on channel ion selectivity and reduce channel conductance to its primary ion. Extensive site-directed mutagenesis experiments of the S5/S6 linkers from a variety of channels suggest that they form a funnel that allows the passage of a specific ion into the pore. In Na^+ channels, selectivity is imposed by two rings of negatively charged amino acids at the outer mouth of the funnel, which collect Na^+ ions for transmission into the cell.[33]

Channel Inactivation

Inactivation gating is the process by which ion channels close in the face of continuing depolarization. Inactivation is characteristic of voltage-gated Na^+ and Ca^{++} channels and the K^+ channels underlying I_{TO}. Inactivation begins after activation gating, as a second, slower conformational change in the molecule that halts the ion flux through the channel. Inactivation gating is thus closely coupled to activation gating, and ionic current flows only while both the activation and inactivation gates are open simultaneously. In Na^+ channels, the inactivation gate is formed by the intracellular peptide linker between homologous domains III and IV[34] (Fig. 7–9*A*). This peptide is postulated to act as a hinged lid, which moves upward to plug the ion pore (and thus halt current flow) shortly after membrane depolarization.[29] In order for the channel to recover from inactivation (i.e., to be ready to open in response to a new depolarizing stimulus), the III/IV linker peptide must resume its resting position, a process that requires hyperpolarization of the membrane to the resting potential for a finite period of time. Site-directed mutagenesis of the III/IV linker peptide has revealed a trio of hydrophobic amino acid residues (isoleucine [I], phenylalanine [F], and methionine [M]), near to the domain III end of the peptide that are crucial for normal channel inactivation. Replacement of just one of these residues (the phenylalanine) almost completely removes inactivation. These residues are postulated to latch

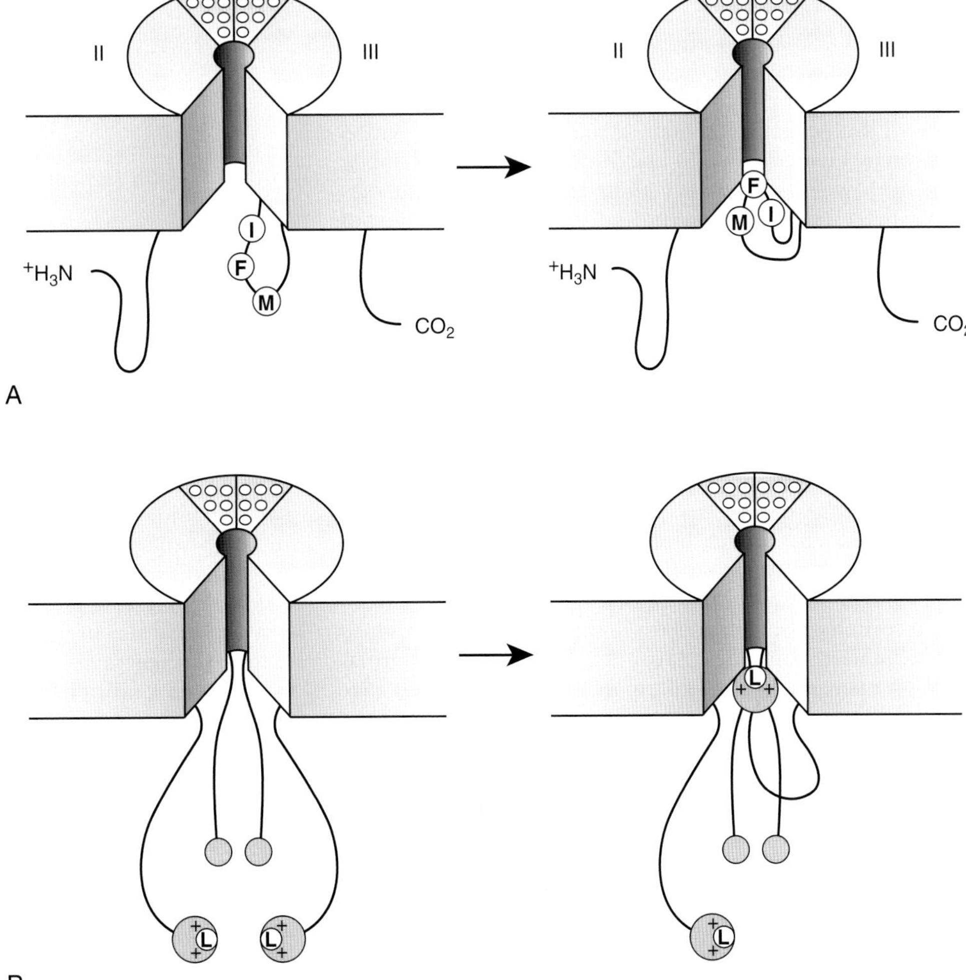

Figure 7–9 Mechanism of inactivation of Na^+ and K^+ channels. *(A)* The hinged-lid mechanism of Na^+ channel inactivation. *(B)* The ball-and-chain mechanism of K^+ channel inactivation. For further discussion, see text. (*A, B,* From Catterall WA: Structure and function of voltage-gated ion channels. Annu Rev Biochem 64:493, 1995. With permission, from the Annual Review of Biochemistry, Volume 64, © 1995, by Annual Reviews, Inc.)

onto a receptor in the channel pore to close the channel. The molecular basis of inactivation in K^+ channels is rather different from Na^+ channels. Since the four domains of K^+ channels are formed by noncovalently linked molecules, there are no interdomain linkers to plug the channel pore. In K^+ channels, a picture of an N-terminal ball-and-chain mechanism has emerged[35] (Fig. 7–9*B*). The terminal 20 or so amino acids are very hydrophobic and are postulated to swing up and attach to the open pore. The next few amino acids contain a number of positively charged residues that draw the whole N-terminal end up to the membrane. These two domains act as a ball. The remaining amino acids, up to the beginning of the transmembrane S1 segment, act as a chain. If the chain is made longer, inactivation is slower, and vice versa.

Molecular Biology of Voltage-Gated Na^+ Channels

Voltage-gated Na^+ channels with similar general structure, of four homologous domains linked by intracellular and extracellular peptides, have been cloned from a wide variety of tissues.[5] Human Na^+ channel isoforms identified to date include hH1 (the cardiac isoform, a product of the *SCN5A* gene) and hSKM1 (the skeletal muscle isoform, a product of the *SCN4A* gene) and several brain and neuronal isoforms. There are important structural and functional differences, however, between muscle and neuronal channels. Neuronal channels have a long I/II linker peptide that contains five short amino acid sequences (called consensus sites), which are substrates for phosphorylation by cAMP-dependent protein kinase. This 200-amino-acid sequence, which is deleted in cardiac and skeletal muscle channels, allows the possibility of regulation of neuronal channel activity by β-adrenergic receptors. All Na^+ channels contain a site for phosphorylation by protein kinase C in the inactivation gate (III/IV linker sequence), which allows regulation of all Na^+ channel isoforms by α_1-adrenergic receptors. Gating schemes are not identical in all kinds of Na^+ channels. Cardiac and skeletal muscle channels have distinctly different kinds of inactivation gating than do neuronal channels. Macroscopic cardiac Na^+ currents decay more slowly than do neuronal currents, and they decay with two components. At the single-channel level, the difference lies in the ability for muscle Na^+ channels to reopen after initially closing so that they sometimes manifest prolonged bursts of openings. Records of channel activity during cardiac action potentials confirm that Na^+ channel openings occur during the plateau, producing a late Na^+ current. This contributes, along with Ca^{++} currents, to the characteristic prolongation of the cardiac action potential, which allows protracted entry of Ca^{++}.

Expression of Na^+ channel α subunit is sufficient to induce Na^+ currents, but in order to reproduce currents with normal gating properties, coexpression of one or more of three auxiliary β subunits is usually necessary. β Subunits have been identified as small (around 200 amino acids) peptides with a single predicted transmembrane domain that copurifies with the α subunits. Brain channels require the β_1, β_2, and β_3 subunits for normal gating properties. Muscle channels use only β_1 and β_3 subunits. Coexpression of β subunit(s) with neuronal or skeletal muscle α subunits results in Na^+ currents of increased amplitude that decay more quickly. In contrast, coexpression of the β subunit does not affect cardiac Na^+ current kinetics, which are rapid when the α subunit is expressed alone. Coexpression of the β subunit, however, enhances channel expression.

Effects of Lidocaine

Local anesthetic agents block the conduction of nerve impulses by blocking neuronal Na^+ channels. Their antiarrhythmic action results from blockade of cardiac Na^+ channels. Local anesthetic block is use dependent; that is, the degree of block increases as stimulation rate increases, an effect that results from a reduction in the number of channels available for opening after membrane depolarization. The exact molecular mechanism of their action remains unresolved, but two possible theories have emerged. The first, the *modulated receptor* theory, states that the affinity of the Na^+ channel for binding lidocaine depends on the conformational state of the Na^+ channel protein.[36,37] The inactivated form was thought to be most avid, the open state next most avid, and the closed or resting state the least avid; that is, the affinity of the receptor is *modulated* by the gating state of the channel, and hyperpolarized Na^+ channels bind less drug than depolarized ones. The drug-bound inactivation gate was also postulated to display abnormal kinetics. In the second hypothesis, the *guarded/trapped receptor* model, the affinity of the channel protein stays constant regardless of the kinetic state.[38] Rather, the drug is allowed to access the binding site only when the channel is open. The drug binds to its receptor site and is trapped there by the inactivation gate. The drug-binding site is available only after the activation gate opens (the receptor is *guarded* by the gate), and the inactivation gate must be open for the drug to exit (the drug is *trapped* by the gate). In either event, the effect of lidocaine is to suppress Na^+ current amplitude. This effect is dose dependent but also much more marked at higher stimulation rates. Local anesthetics bind to the Na^+ channel pore in the S6 membrane-spanning segment of domain IV, and mutation of a few critical residues in this region renders the channel insensitive to local anesthetics.[39]

Molecular Biology of Voltage-Gated Ca^{++} Channels

Voltage-gated Ca^{++} channels share the same tetrameric structure as Na^+ channels, but there are important structural differences. These are related to the diversity of function of Ca^{++} channels, which serve not only to depolarize the cell but also to supply precise amounts of Ca^{++} for regulation of subcellular processes. Voltage-gated Ca^{++} channels may be classified electrophysiologically into low-voltage-activated (T type) and high-voltage-activated (L type, the predominant muscle isoform, dihydropyridine sensitive, and N type, the neuronal isoform).[40] Other high-voltage-activated isoforms (P, Q, and R types) have also been identified on the basis of toxin sensitivities. Ca^{++} channels have a complex subunit structure with α_2, δ, β, and γ subunits identified in addition to the α_1 pore-forming unit (see Fig. 7–8*B*). The α_2 and δ subunits form a membrane-bound disulfide-linked dimer, $\alpha_2\delta$. The γ subunit is also membrane bound. The β subunit is intracellular and contains many phosphorylation sites. Coexpression of the cardiac pore-forming α_1 subunit with its accessory subunits results in enhanced current amplitude and accelerated activation ($\alpha_2\gamma$ and β), enhanced dihydropyridine binding suggesting an increase in the number of channels (β), and enhanced inactivation rate (β). Coexpression of the γ subunit has little effect on cardiac channels.

Molecular Biology of Voltage-Gated K^+ Channels

Deducing the molecular identity of voltage-gated K^+ channels in human myocardium is complex. Several K^+ channel genes have been cloned, and because K^+ channels are formed from noncovalently linked tetramers, multiple possible arrays of different channel molecules are possible.[41] A further level of complexity is added by accessory channel subunits, which can have dramatic effects on channel function. The nomenclature of K^+ channels is based on their original classification, which was derived from related families of K^+ channel genes cloned from the fruit fly, *Drosophila*. The first K^+ channel to be cloned was from fruit flies that displayed abnormal leg shaking in response to ether exposure.[42] These flies were found to lack a gene encoding a K^+ channel, the *shaker* gene, and a mammalian homolog of this channel was identified (the mammalian *shaker*-type or Kv1 subfamily of channels).[43] Three other subfamilies of K^+ channel genes were identified in *Drosophila*, and mammalian homologs of these have also been identified: *shab* (Kv2), *shaw* (Kv3), and *shal* (Kv4). Three members of the *shaker* family (Kv1.2, Kv1.4, and Kv1.5), one member of the *shab* family (Kv2.1), and one member of the *shal* family (Kv4.2) have been cloned from human heart (Fig. 7–10).[44] The Kv1.4 and Kv4.2 genes express inactivating K^+ channels (Fig. 7–10*A*), similar to the 4-aminopyridine–sensitive component of I_{TO}, whereas Kv1.2, Kv1.5, and Kv2.1 genes express (noninactivating) delayed rectifier-type K^+ channels (Fig. 7–10*B*). Kv1.5–induced K^+ currents are rapidly activating and noninactivating and have similar pharmacology to I_{Kur}, and it is possible that Kv1.5 represents the cloned isoform of the native current. Biophysical and pharmacologic considerations make Kv4.2 the more likely of the candidate genes for I_{TO}. The picture is complicated, however, by the effect of coexpression of the accessory β subunit on the function of the delayed rectifier-type K^+ channels. For example, coexpression of a β subunit with the channel encoded by Kv1.5 induces channel inactivation at positive potentials (Fig. 7–10*B, C*).[45] This intracellular subunit shares no homology with Ca^{++} or Na^+ channel subunits. It is postulated to act as an inactivation "ball" similar to the N-terminal ball of Kv1.4 and Kv4.2. A final level of complexity is the diversity of expression of K^+ channel genes in different cardiac tissues, at differing stages of development. Thus, before a candidate gene can be ascribed to an ionic current species, expression of the gene must be demonstrated and the effect of any coexpressed accessory subunits must be assessed.

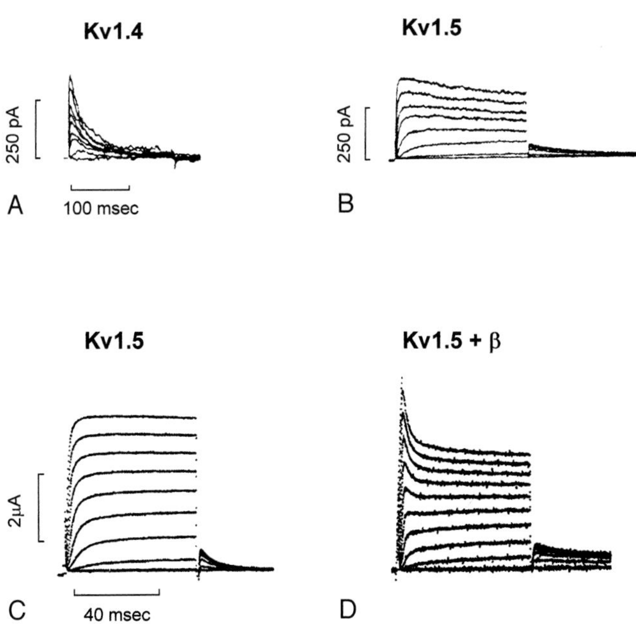

Figure 7–10 Ion currents through cloned K^+ channels. Kv1.4 *(A)* encodes an inactivating current, whereas the closely related Kv1.5 *(B)* encodes a noninactivating current. Coexpression of a β subunit (hKvβ3) with Kv1.5 induces inactivation of the macroscopic current *(C, D)*. *(A-D,* From Deal KK, England SK, Tamkun MM: Molecular physiology of cardiac potassium channels. Physiol Rev 76:49, 1996.)

The *shaker* family of genes does not express currents similar to the major components of the delayed rectifier in ventricle and Purkinje fiber, I_{Kr} and I_{Ks}. An unrelated K^+ channel gene, the *ether-a-gogo* (or *eag* gene), also originally cloned from *Drosophila*, expresses a K^+ channel structurally very similar to the *shaker* family. (The name was coined because of an atypical response of the *Drosophila* to ether.) The mammalian analog of this gene, *h-erg*, or human ether-a-gogo–related gene (see Fig. 7–8*C*), encodes an ionic current with close biophysical and pharmacologic similarity to I_{Kr} when expressed in heterologous cell lines.[46] *H-erg* channels are blocked by E4031 and dofetilide (both class III antiarrhythmic agents) and exhibit extremely rapid inactivation at positive potentials, which causes the currents to appear to inwardly rectify. The molecular basis of I_{Ks} has also been elucidated.[47] This gene (almost uniquely among human cardiac K^+ channel genes) was not originally cloned in *Drosophila*. It was identified as one of the genetic abnormalities underlying the long QT (LQT) syndrome, a rare inherited human illness that causes sudden death by ventricular arrhythmias (see later). It encodes a K^+ channel, the human LQT1 channel (or Kv LQT1), which, although unrelated to the *shaker* channel, is structurally very similar to it. In order to express fully functional channels, Kv LQT1 associates with a second, smaller molecule, I_{sK} (also known as minK), which itself was formerly thought to encode a subclass of atypical K^+ channels.

Inward Rectifying K^+ Channels

Inward rectifying K^+ channels, which are structurally and functionally distinct from other voltage-gated K^+ channels, include I_{K1}, the current primarily responsible for the resting membrane potential in atrial and ventricular myocardium, $I_{K(ACh)}$; the G protein–gated K^+ channel in atrium and nodal tissues; and $I_{K(ATP)}$, a K^+ channel activated by reduced adenosine triphosphate (ATP) levels that may be important in postischemic cardioprotection.[48] The molecular structure of inward rectifying K^+ channels is radically different from other voltage-gated K^+ channels. They contain only two transmembrane domains (see Fig. 7–8*C*), which resemble the S5/S6 pore-forming regions of other channel types. Inward rectification results from binding of intracellular divalent cations and certain polyamines to the channel molecule; removal of these agents linearizes the current-voltage relationship.[49,50] I_{K1} appears to be derived from a family of channel molecules. Two different human heart inward rectifiers have been cloned, and because, in human atrium, multiple levels of single-channel conductance have been observed, other channel subtypes may also exist. The G protein–related K^+ channel, $I_{K(ACh)}$, is formed by a heteromer of two subunits called GIRK (G protein–coupled inward rectifier) and CIR (cardiac inward rectifier), which form a tetramer.[51] Both of these clones show inward rectifier K^+ channel activity when expressed alone in some systems, but conductance is much higher when they are expressed together. Additionally, these subunits copurify during immunoaffinity purification using antibodies to GIRK.

Pacemaker Channels

The ion channel molecule underlying I_f has been identified as a member of a diverse group of cyclic nucleotide–gated channels, HCN (for *H*yperpolarization-activated *C*yclic *N*ucleotide-gated channel). HCN1 has been detected in high concentration in the sinus node, and HCN2 is found in Purkinje fibers.[52] Analogous to K^+ channels, four individual transmembrane domains, each containing six transmembrane segments, constitute the channel pore. There is a cyclic nucleotide binding site in the C-terminal peptide (Fig. 7–11*A*). Similar to Na^+, Ca^{++}, and other K^+ channels, the S4 segment of each domain is a voltage sensor, but, unique among ion channels, hyperpolarization rather than depolarization opens the pore. The cyclic nucleotide binding domain binds cAMP with much higher affinity than cGMP. In the presence of saturating concentrations of cAMP, the current in response to any hyperpolarizing clamp pulse is greatly enhanced (Fig. 7–11*B*). Diastolic depolarization is thus enhanced and heart rate increased.

Clinical Correlates

Ion Channels and Antiarrhythmic Drugs

Drug therapy of cardiac arrhythmias would ideally be targeted at an individual ionic current, with the intention of tailoring the cardiac action potential to reduce abnormal excitability, without affecting normal rhythmicity. This goal remains unrealized. The prototype antiarrhythmic agents, such as disopyramide and quinidine, have diverse effects on cardiac excitability, and these, along with agents introduced more recently, frequently exhibit significant proarrhythmia with potentially fatal consequences. In the Cardiac Arrhythmia Suppression Trial (CAST), mortality among asymptomatic post–myocardial infarction patients was approximately doubled by treatment with the potent Na^+ channel–blocking agents encainide and flecainide, an effect that is likely attributable to slowing of conduction velocity with a consequent increase in fatal reentrant arrhythmias.[53] The results of the CAST trial prompted efforts to approach antiarrhythmic drug therapy by prolonging action potential duration (e.g., with dofetilide)—a strategy with some support from animal studies but one that may also cause proarrhythmia through induction of polymorphic ventricular tachycardia (the so-called acquired LQT syndrome).[54] Drugs that prolong action potential duration share the property of blockade of I_{Kr}, and it is by no means clear that this therapeutic goal results in arrhythmia control without induction of clinically significant proarrhythmia. The only drugs currently available that definitely prolong life by reducing fatal arrhythmias are β-blockers (e.g., International Study of Infarct Survival-1, 1997), and these agents have no channel-blocking effects.

Ion Channels in Disease

Elucidation of the molecular mechanisms of the cardiac action potential is beginning to directly affect patient management, particularly in patients with inherited genetic abnormalities of ion channels leading to cardiac sudden death. Two groups of diseases serve to illustrate this point—the LQT syndrome and Brugada syndrome. An understanding of the molecular mechanism of cardiac electrical excitability is also leading to the emergence of gene therapies and stem cell therapies that may in the future allow manipulation of cardiac rhythm and function.

LONG QT SYNDROME

This excessively rare group of ion channel abnormalities causes abnormal prolongation of the cardiac action potential, resulting in early afterdepolarizations (i.e., oscillations in the action potential during the plateau phase), and death from polymorphic ventricular tachycardia (torsades de pointes type). To date, six LQT subtypes have been identified on the basis of the affected gene. They are numbered sequentially according to the date of discovery (Table 7–1), and all the loci so far identified encode ion channels except for LQT4. LQT occurs because of disruption of cardiac repolarization and in principle can occur either from enhancement of inward depolarizing current or reduction of outward current. LQT3 is a gain of function mutation of the cardiac Na^+ channel that results in failure of channel inactivation most commonly from a deletion of three amino acids from the inactivation gate. LQT1 and LQT2 result from mutations of the delayed recti-

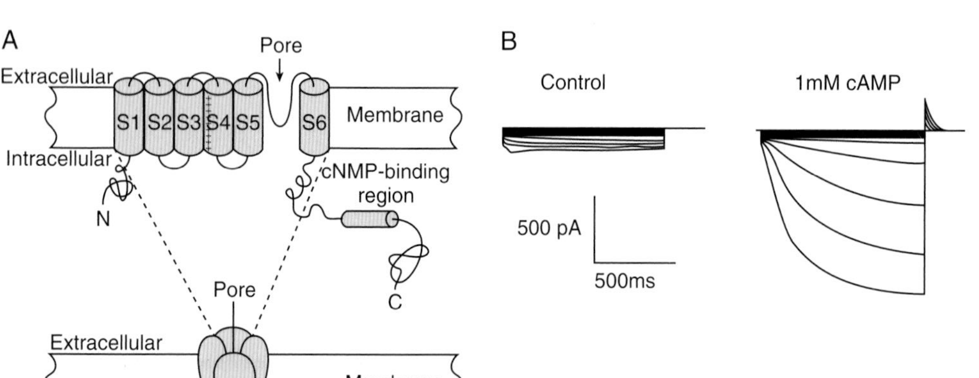

Figure 7–11 *(A)* Membrane topology of HCN channels. Note the cyclic nucleotide binding domain on the C-terminal peptide. *(B)* Dependence of HCN currents on cAMP. HCN currents are hyperpolarization-activated noninactivating currents that are enhanced in the presence of cAMP. (From Kaupp UB, Seifert R: Molecular diversity of pacemaker ion channels. Annu Rev Physiol 63:235, 2001.)

Table 7–1 Spectrum of Long QT (LQT) Syndrome

Type	Gene	Current	Chromosome	Comment
LQT1	*KCNQ1* (*Kv LQT1*)	I_{Ks}	11	Stress, exercise
LQT2	*KCNH2* (*hERG*)	I_{Kr}	7	Noise, emotional stress
LQT3	*SCN5A*	I_{Na}	3	Sleep, β-blockers less effective
LQT4	*ANKB*	—	4	Ankyrin B, transporter accessory protein
LQT5	*KCNE1* (*minK*)	I_{Ks}	21	Associated congenital deafness
LQT6	*KCNE2* (*MiRP1*)	I_{Kr}	21	Drugs, exercise

KCN = gene encoding channel underlying I_{Ks} currents and formerly known as *Kv LQT1*; *SCN5A* = gene encoding the cardiac sodium channel; *hERG* = human ether-a-gogo related, now known as *KCNH*$_2$; *MiRP1* = gene encoding an accessory protein that modulates I_{Kr} or *KCNE2*; *ANKB* = Ankyrin B, gene encoding ankyrin B transporter protein; *minK* = now known as *KCNE1* and is the gene encoding a KCNQ1 accessory protein that modulates I_{Ks}.

fier K^+ channels that underlie I_{Ks} and I_{Kr}, and LQT5 and LQT6 result in reductions of I_{Kr} and I_{Ks} through mutations in channel accessory subunits. Loss of repolarizing current prolongs the QT interval leading to the syndrome. LQT4 is unique in that it results from a mutation in ankyrin B, an adaptor protein that binds to the Na^+ pump and Na^+/Ca^{++} exchanger. The resulting effects on cellular Ca^{++} homeostasis cause ventricular arrhythmias.[55] Identification of the molecular substrate for LQT syndrome allows detection of the disease in asymptomatic carriers and may in the future allow targeted gene therapy.

BRUGADA SYNDROME

This group of ion channel abnormalities affects cardiac repolarization and results in cardiac sudden death. It is characterized by incomplete right bundle-branch block and persistent ST-segment elevation in the anterior precordial leads of the ECG.[56] Cases for which the genotype is available seem to result from reduction of depolarizing Na^+ current. A group of channel mutations have been identified that result in loss of the action potential dome, an effect that is most marked in the right ventricular epicardium where the transient outward current I_{TO1} is strongly expressed (hence the ST-segment elevation in the anterior chest ECG leads). Early repolarization of the epicardial action potential results in a transmural repolarization gradient, and this can lead to reentry and sudden cardiac death.[57] It is noteworthy that in more than two thirds of patients with Brugada syndrome, the genetic locus is unknown. Much work remains to be done to elucidate the mechanism of this condition.

CONTROLLING CARDIAC FUNCTIONING: RECEPTORS

Receptors are membrane proteins that transduce signals from the outside to the inside of the cell. When a *ligand*—a hormone carried in blood, a neurotransmitter released from a nerve ending, or a local messenger released from neighboring cells—binds to the receptor, it induces a conformational change in the receptor molecule. The configuration of the intracellular segment of the receptor changes, and results in activation of intracellular systems, with a variety of effects, ranging from enhanced phosphorylation and changes in intracellular (second) messenger concentrations to activation of ion channels.

Receptors

Receptors are grouped into several broad classes, the *protein tyrosine kinase receptors* and the *G protein–coupled receptors* (GPCRs) being the most important ones. The protein tyrosine kinase receptors are large molecular complexes. Ligand binding induces activation of a phosphorylating enzyme activity in the intracellular segment of the molecule. As phosphorylation is one of the major mechanisms of cellular regulation (e.g., the phosphorylation of the Ca^{++} channel described earlier), such receptors can have a variety of cellular effects (Box 7–4). In contrast, GPCRs are much smaller. Ligand binding results in activation of an associated protein (*G protein*) that subsequently influences cellular processes. The receptors discussed in this section all belong to the GPCR superfamily, and the properties of this class are discussed in some detail.

The number of GPCRs is large and still growing. For more than 100 receptors, the function has been defined. In addition, the olfactory epithelium expresses hundreds of GPCRs, which are thought to mediate the sense of smell, and another large

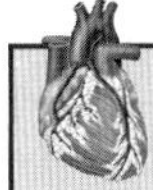

BOX 7–4 *G Protein–Coupled Receptors*

- β-Adrenergic receptors
- α-Adrenergic receptors
- Muscarinic acetylcholine receptors
- Adenosine A_1 receptors
- ATP receptors
- Histamine H_2 receptors
- Vasoactive intestinal peptide receptors
- Angiotensin II receptors

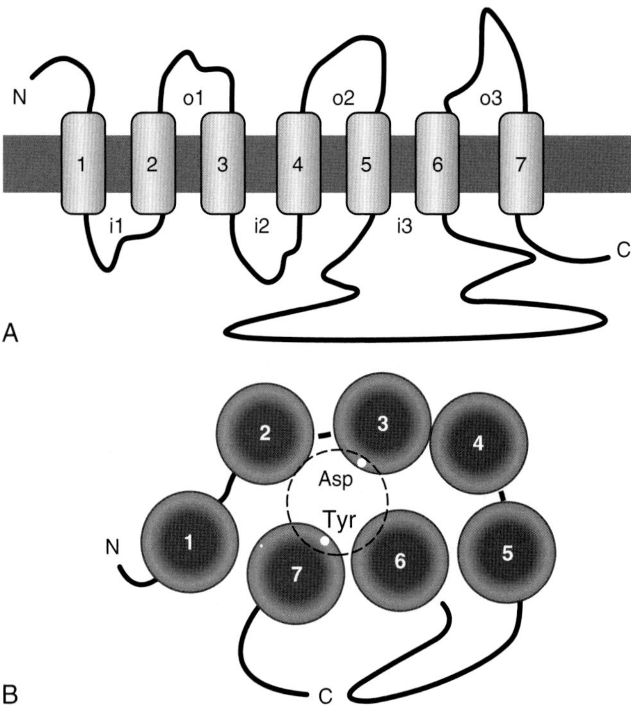

Figure 7–12 Model of G protein–coupled receptor. *(A)* Linear model. Seven hydrophobic stretches of approximately 20 amino acids are present, presumably forming α helices that pass through the cell membrane, thus forming seven-transmembrane domains (t1 through t7). Extracellularly the N terminus (N) and three outside loops (o1 through o3) are found; intracellularly there are similarly three loops (i1 through i3) and the C terminus (C). *(B)* Top-down view. Although in *(A)*, the molecule is pictured as a linear complex, the transmembrane domains are thought to be in close proximity, forming an ellipse with a central ligand-binding cavity (indicated by a *dashed circle*). Asp and Tyr refer to two amino acids important for ligand interaction. G protein binding takes place at the i3 loop and the C terminus.

group, with unknown function, is expressed on sperm cells. Taken together, the superfamily has more than 1000 members.

All of these have similar molecular characteristics. They are generally several hundred to 1000 amino acids in length and contain seven stretches of 20 to 25 hydrophobic amino acids. These hydrophobic domains are thought to form α helices and traverse the membrane, thus anchoring the receptor to the cell (Fig. 7–12). For this reason, the family is often referred to as the "seven-transmembrane" family. Although crystallographic data are not yet available for the clinically relevant GPCRs, it is thought that the seven-transmembrane domains arrange in a funnel-like structure, the inside of which forms the ligand-binding domain. The intracellular domains, particularly the third intracellular loop and the C terminus, bind to the G protein.

The heart and blood vessels express a variety of GPCRs, the most important of which are discussed below. The β-adrenergic and muscarinic acetylcholine receptors are those most important for regulation of cardiac functioning, but a number of others play relevant modulatory roles. These include the α-adrenergic, adenosine A_1, ATP, histamine H_2, vasoactive intestinal peptide (VIP), and angiotensin II receptors.

G Proteins

As do the receptors, G proteins, or GTP-binding proteins, also come in two families: the small (cytoplasmic) G proteins and the heterotrimeric (membrane) G proteins. Common to all is their mechanism of function. In their resting state, they bind a molecule of guanosine diphosphate (GDP). When activated by a GPCR (in the case of heterotrimeric G proteins) or by an intracellular messenger (in the case of cytoplasmic G proteins), this GDP is exchanged for a GTP molecule. The activated G protein can now perform functions within the cell, as discussed later, until it is inactivated when intrinsic enzyme activity hydrolyzes the GTP to GDP. The critical point about this hydrolytic activity is that it is (molecularly speaking) very slow, on the order of seconds. As a result, brief activation of a receptor (on the order of milliseconds) can lead to more prolonged activation of the intracellular signaling machinery.

GPCRs bind to *heterotrimeric* G proteins, so called because they consist of three subunits: α, β, and γ. Of these, the β and γ subunits are so tightly associated that for practical purposes they can be viewed as a single unit, often termed the ßγ unit. The α subunit contains both the GDP-GTP binding domain and the hydrolytic activity and was classically thought to be the "business end" of the molecule, with the βγ unit roaming freely and inactively, serving as an anchor and a sink of free α units. However, the βγ subunit actually has activating functions as well, as is discussed later in relation to the muscarinic K^+ channel.

Several classes of heterotrimeric G proteins exist, indicated by subscripts (Box 7–5). The classic types are G_s and G_i, which stimu-late and inhibit, respectively, the enzyme adenylate cyclase, thereby leading to changes in cytoplasmic cAMP concentrations. G_q proteins (and G_o in brain) activate phospholipase C (PLC), and thereby induce the generation of inositol-1,4,5-triphosphate (IP_3) and diacylglycerol (DAG) from phosphatidylinositol-4,5-biphosphate (PIP_2). IP_3 acts on its own receptor-channel complex on intracellular Ca^{++} storage sites and induces release of Ca^{++} from these sites, thereby raising intracellular Ca^{++} concentrations. DAG activates protein kinase C (PKC), leading to phosphorylation of a variety of targets (including the receptors that initiated the cascade). Cloning efforts have shown each of these classes of G proteins to consist of a number of members, but their functional differences are as yet incompletely defined.

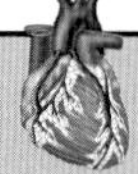

BOX 7–5 ***G Protein Classes***

- G_s: activates adenylate cyclase
- G_i: inhibits adenylate cyclase
- G_q: activates phospholipase C
- G_o: subtype of G_i, found mostly in brain, Ca^{++} also activates phospholipase C
- G_k: subtype of G_i, linked to K^+ channels

Adrenergic Receptors and Signaling Pathways

Adrenergic Receptors

Main control over cardiac contractility is provided by the β-adrenergic signaling pathways, which can be activated by circulating catecholamines (derived from the adrenal glands) or those released locally from adrenergic nerve endings on the myocardium.

The two main subtypes of β-adrenergic receptors are the β_1 and β_2 subclasses. A β_3 subtype exists as well, but its role in the cardiovascular system is unclear[58]; its most important role is in fat cells. Both β_1- and β_2-receptors are present in heart, and both contribute to the increased contractility induced by catecholamine stimulation (this is different from the situation in vascular muscle, where β-adrenergic stimulation induces relaxation). Under normal conditions, the relative ratio of β_1- to β_2-receptors in heart is approximately 70:30, but, as discussed later, this ratio can be changed dramatically by cardiac disease.

Structurally, as well as functionally, the various β-adrenergic receptors are closely related. Both couple to G_s proteins and, as described earlier, thereby activate adenylate cyclase, leading to increased intracellular levels of cAMP. There may, however, be differences in some details of their intracellular signaling. For example, it has been suggested that β_2-receptors couple more effectively than β_1-receptors and induce greater changes in cAMP levels.[59] In addition to their effect on cAMP signaling, β-receptors may couple to myocardial Ca^{++} channels.[27] However, these additional actions are species specific, and care should be taken in extrapolating animal data to humans.

The inotropic and electrophysiologic effects of β-adrenergic signaling are an indirect result of increases in intracellular cAMP levels. cAMP activates a specific protein kinase (PKA) that in turn is able to phosphorylate a number of important cardiac ion channels (including L-type Ca^{++} channels, Na^+ channels, voltage-dependent K^+ channels, and Cl^- channels). Phosphorylation alters channel functioning, and it is these changes in membrane electrophysiologic events that modify myocardial behavior.

The α-adrenergic receptors, like their β-receptor counterparts, can be divided into several molecular groups: the α_1- and α_2-receptors. Both of these groups consist of several closely related subtypes, with different tissue distributions and functions that are as yet not very well differentiated. In general, α_1-receptors couple to G_q proteins, thereby activating PLC, which increases intracellular Ca^{++} concentrations. α_2-Receptors couple to G_i, which inhibits adenylate cyclase, thereby lowering intracellular cAMP concentrations.

The primary site of importance of α-receptors is in the vasculature, where α_1-receptors on vascular smooth muscle are the main mediators of neuronally mediated vasoconstriction. α_2-Receptors on the neurons themselves function in a negative feedback loop to control α-adrenergic vasoconstriction. In the heart, the primary subtype present is α_1. Activation of these receptors leads to a modest increase in cardiac contractility.[60]

Regulation of β-Receptor Functioning

Although β-receptor stimulation allows the dramatic increases in cardiac output of which the human heart is capable, it is clearly intended to be a temporary measure. Prolonged adrenergic stimulation has highly detrimental effects on the myocardium: The pronounced increases in cAMP levels are followed by increases in intracellular Ca^{++} concentration, reductions in RNA and protein synthesis, and finally cell death. Thus, β-receptor modulation is best viewed as part of the "fight or flight" response: beneficial in the short term, but detrimental if depended on too long. Cardiac failure, in particular, has been shown to be associated with prolonged increases in adrenergic stimulation, even to the extent that norepinephrine "spillover" from cardiac nerve endings can be detected in the blood of patients in heart failure (see Chapter 10).[61]

For this reason, the regulation of β-receptor functioning has received significant attention, and it has been shown that a number of mechanisms exist to modify adrenergic responsiveness of the myocyte. Unfortunately, it appears that the reduction of adrenergic responsiveness necessary to prevent cell death in the face of adrenergic overstimulation may be in large part responsible for the decreased myocardial performance that is the hallmark of cardiac failure.

One mechanism for decreasing β-receptor functioning is the *downregulation* (i.e., decrease in density) of receptors. In cardiac failure, receptor levels are reduced up to 50%. β_1-Receptors downregulate more than do β_2-receptors, resulting in a change in the $\beta_1:\beta_2$ ratio. As mentioned earlier, the normal ratio is approximately 70:30; in the failing heart, it is approximately 3:2.[62] Various molecular mechanisms exist for this downregulation. Some of them, particularly in the longer term, are degradation and permanent removal of receptors from the cell surface. In the short term, receptors can be temporarily removed from the cell membrane and "stored" in intracellular vesicles, where they are not accessible to agonists. These receptors are, however, fully functional and can be recycled to the membrane when adrenergic overstimulation has ceased.[63]

An additional method by which β-adrenergic receptor functioning can be modified is through phosphorylation of the agonist-occupied receptor by a specific β-adrenergic receptor kinase (βARK, which can itself be activated by βγ subunits).[64] Phosphorylation by this kinase allows binding to the receptor of a protein, β-arrestin, that inhibits receptor functioning.[65] In addition, the β-receptor can be phosphorylated by PKA, which itself can be activated by several other receptors. The detrimental actions of adrenergic overstimulation can also be modified by activation of muscarinic receptors, as discussed in the next section.

Despite the existence of these various regulatory mechanisms and the known detrimental effects of adrenergic overstimulation, paradoxical increases in β-receptor functioning occur in clinical disease states. For example, under ischemic conditions, β-receptors are upregulated, so that after periods of ischemia as brief as 15 minutes, significant increases are found in expressed and functional receptor levels. Interestingly, reperfusion rapidly decreases the number of receptors back to their normal levels.

Muscarinic Receptors and Signaling Pathways

Muscarinic Acetylcholine Receptors

The second major receptor type involved in cardiac regulation is the muscarinic receptor. Although five subtypes of muscarinic receptors exist, only one of these (m2) is present in cardiac tissue. Most of these muscarinic receptors are present on the atria. Indeed, it was thought until recently that there was no vagal innervation of the ventricles, but this view turns out to be incorrect. The ventricles are innervated by the vagus, and muscarinic receptors are, in fact, present in the ventricles, albeit at lower concentrations than in the atria; the amount of muscarinic receptor protein in atrium is approximately twofold greater than in ventricle (200 to 250 versus 70 to 100 fmol/mg protein).[66] Thus, although the primary function of cardiac muscarinic signaling is heart rate control through actions at the atrial level, vagal stimulation is, in fact, able to directly influence ventricular functioning.

M2-Muscarinic receptors couple to G_i proteins, thereby inhibiting adenylate cyclase and decreasing intracellular levels of cAMP. In fact, the m2 receptors have been used as an elegant model to determine the site of G protein binding to the receptor. Exchanging approximately 20 amino acids of the third intracellular loop (i3) (see Fig. 7–12) between m2 and m3 receptors resulted in altered coupling; m2 receptors mutated in this manner were then able to release Ca^{++} from intracellular IP_3-sensitive stores by coupling to G_q.[67]

In the impulse-generating system of the heart, a more important signaling mechanism than changes in cAMP is opening of an inwardly rectifying K^+ channel (K_{ACh}) in the plasma membrane. The coupling between m2 receptor and K_{ACh} is performed by G_K, a member of the G_i class of G proteins. Interestingly, it is not the α subunit of G_K that activates K_{ACh} but rather the β subunit.[68] As seen later, cardiac adenosine receptors couple to this channel as well.

The adenylate cyclase system is ubiquitous, but differential expression of K_{ACh} determines the actions of muscarinic signaling on the heart. K_{ACh} is largely absent from ventricular tissue. Therefore, in the ventricle, muscarinic signaling primarily involves decreases in cAMP levels, and, as these are low under resting conditions, little effect is seen unless the heart has been stimulated previously by adrenergic agents. In other words, in the absence of adrenergic stimulation, acetylcholine has little effect on the ventricle; in conditions of high adrenergic tone, however, muscarinic stimulation can modify the adrenergic effects, as is discussed in the next section.

Regulation of Muscarinic Acetylcholine Receptors

The role of muscarinic receptors in atrial impulse generation and the conduction system is straightforward, but the role of ventricular muscarinic receptors is not as clear. It appears that under nonstressed conditions, muscarinic signaling has little influence on cardiac contractility. In contrast, the system might act as a brake on overstimulation by adrenergic receptors, discussed earlier. The effects of muscarinic signaling, which virtually all oppose those induced by adrenergic signaling (because muscarinic receptors couple to G_i and adrenergic receptors couple to G_s), may counteract adrenergic effects and thereby preserve cardiac functioning during prolonged stress responses.

Unfortunately, these compensatory mechanisms may not be available in the old heart. Increased age is accompanied by changes in cardiac muscarinic receptor expression that might make it more difficult for the heart to respond to adrenergic stress. In senescent rats, muscarinic receptor density was decreased by approximately 50%.[69] Adrenergic receptor levels were also decreased but to a lesser extent. As a result, the adrenergic/muscarinic receptor ratio is increased, from 0.29 in young adults to 0.42 in senescent animals. Although the physiologic implications of these changes are not well known, the data at least suggest that the muscarinic systems in the aged heart might not be as well prepared to react to prolonged adrenergic stimulation, such as observed in hypertension and cardiac failure.

With the exception of age, muscarinic receptors are little affected in settings that profoundly modify β-receptor expression. There are, for example, no consistent data supporting changes in muscarinic receptor expression in hypertension, cardiac failure, or ischemic heart disease.[70,71] Therefore, imbalances between adrenergic and muscarinic stimulation might occur in each of these situations.

Regulation of G-Protein Functioning

In view of the profound changes in GPCR expression that occur in various disease states, the expression and function of G proteins in cardiovascular disease have been studied with interest. G_s proteins appear unchanged in cardiac failure, both in expression level and in function. With G_i proteins, the situation is more interesting, as $G_{i\alpha}$ is considered to have a secondary role in addition to its inhibition of adenylate cyclase. Under normal conditions, G_i is present in greater amounts than G_s. Activation of receptors coupled to G_i would, therefore, lead to the release of a large number of free $\beta\gamma$ subunits. These could combine with any free $G_{s\alpha}$, thereby making it unavailable for activation of adenylate cyclase.[72] In addition, these $\beta\gamma$ units can enhance the phosphorylation of β-receptors by βARK.[73] In failing human cardiac tissue, the amount of G_i (as assessed by ADP-ribosylation by pertussis toxin) is increased.[74] Although this would be expected to make muscarinic signaling more efficacious (thereby helping counteract the adrenergic overstimulation), it has been difficult to correlate these changes with alterations in adenylate cyclase functioning. It is similarly unclear whether the reported increases in G_i levels are a result of increased mRNA expression or increased stability of the G protein itself.

The catalytic subunit of adenylate cyclase appears little influenced by cardiac disease. Pressure overload is the only situation in which a consistent decrease in its activity has been observed.[75,76]

Other Receptors

As stated earlier, the heart and vasculature express a large variety of GPCRs apart from the adrenergic and muscarinic receptors. A few examples are mentioned here. Angiotensin receptors mediate hormonal vasoconstriction in the vascular tree, and are also present in the heart, although their function there is not fully defined. Receptors for several purinergic compounds are expressed in the heart as well, and are the subject of intense investigation, as is discussed in the next section. In addition, histamine H_2 and VIP receptors are present, the former mediating the inotropic action of histamine.

Although less is understood about the role and regulation of these receptors, it is clear that some are affected by cardiovascular disease. For example, VIP receptors are downregulated by 70% in idiopathic dilated cardiomyopathy, whereas histamine receptors are unaffected.[77] In general, receptors coupled to G_i show little alteration in expression and function during disease states, whereas G_s-coupled receptors are affected more profoundly.

Clinical Correlate: Adenosine Signaling and Cardiac Function

Understanding of the role of adenosine in cardiac regulation has expanded significantly over the past years. Its established use as an antiarrhythmic compound (see Chapter 10) and its probable role in cardiac preconditioning (see Chapters 19 and 28) are two examples of clinical advances resulting from this increase in understanding. Adenosine acts through a GPCR, activating several intracellular signaling systems. In this section, the molecular aspects of adenosine signaling, as well as their clinical implications, are discussed. More detailed recent reviews on the topic are available.[78-80]

Adenosine Signaling

Although adenosine can be generated by several pathways, in the heart it is usually found as a dephosphorylation product of AMP.[81] As AMP accumulation is a sign of a low cellular energy charge, an increased adenosine concentration is a marker of unbalanced energy demand and supply; thus, ischemia, hypoxemia, and increased catecholamine concentrations are all associated with increased adenosine release.[82] Adenosine is rapidly degraded by various pathways, both intracellularly and extracellularly. As a result, its half-life is extremely short, on the order of 1 second.[83] Therefore, it is not only a marker of a cardiac "energy crisis," but its concentrations will fluctuate virtually instantly with the energy balance of the heart; it provides a real-time indication of the cellular energy situation.

Adenosine signals through GPCRs of the purinergic receptor family. Two subclasses of purinoceptors exist: P_1 (high affinity for adenosine and AMP) and P_2 (high affinity for ATP and ADP). The P_1-receptor class can be divided into (at least) two receptor subtypes: A_1 and A_2. A_1-receptors are present mostly in the heart, and, when activated, inhibit adenylate cyclase; A_2-receptors are present in the vasculature and, when activated, stimulate adenylate cyclase. The A_2-receptors mediate the vasodilatory actions of adenosine. The A_1-receptors mediate its complex cardiac effects.

The A_1-adenosine receptor couples to (at least) two intracellular signaling systems. Both of these actions are mediated by G proteins of the G_i class. The first intracellular system is one already encountered: the K_{ACh} channel. Presumably, through the same G_K protein, adenosine activates this channel in the same way as does m2 muscarinic stimulation, and the cardiac electrophysiologic effects of acetylcholine and adenosine are, therefore, quite similar. The specific effect of adenosine depends on the cardiac tissue studied, as K_{ACh} expression varies with location. As has been discussed, whereas the channel is present in large amounts in the atrial conduction system and atrial myocardium, it is virtually absent in ventricle. In the unstimulated heart, adenosine shortens the atrial action potential, decreases atrial refractoriness, and decreases atrial contractile force, but it is almost without effect on the ventricle.[84]

The second intracellular signaling system activated is a G_i protein that inhibits adenylate cyclase. As cAMP levels are quite low under resting conditions, this mechanism plays little role until cAMP concentrations are increased by adrenergic stimulation of the heart. cAMP-mediated cardiac actions of adenosine are observed only under conditions of adrenergic drive. Because the adenylate cyclase system is present throughout the heart, its effects are widespread: L-type Ca^{++} channel functioning is diminished (by inhibiting cAMP-induced phosphorylation of the channel) in atrium as well as ventricle, resulting in decreased inotropy and shortening of the action potential.[85,86]

Antiarrhythmic Actions of Adenosine

From these molecular actions of adenosine, its clinical effects can easily be deduced. The antiarrhythmic actions are largely a result of its activation of K_{ACh}. Remembering the tissue distribution of K_{ACh}, it could be anticipated that adenosine will be much more effective in the treatment of supraventricular arrhythmias than ventricular arrhythmias, and such is indeed the case. Because of its negative chronotropic effects on the atrial conduction system, the compound is most effective in treating supraventricular tachycardias that contain a reentrant pathway involving the atrioventricular node. The efficacy of adenosine in terminating such tachycardias has been reported as greater than 90%.[87] In contrast, it is consistently ineffective in tachycardias not involving the atrioventricular node.[88]

Most ventricular tachycardias are insensitive to adenosine. The only exception is again easily deduced from the compound's molecular mechanism of action: a rare form of exercise- or catecholamine-induced ventricular tachycardia responds promptly to adenosine.[89] Presumably, in this setting adenosine-mediated inhibition of adenylate cyclase counteracts the stimulatory effects of catecholamines.

Occasionally, adenosine may be useful because of its ability to differentiate between true ventricular tachycardia and supraventricular tachycardia with aberrant conduction. In view of concerns that the often already precarious cardiovascular status of patients in ventricular tachycardia could be temporarily worsened by vasodilatation, many clinicians have been hesitant to use adenosine for this purpose. In contrast, it has been found very useful as a diagnostic agent for supraventricular tachycardias. Care should be taken, however, in the patient with Wolff-Parkinson-White syndrome, who may respond with increases in ventricular rate and hemodynamic deterioration.

The side effects of adenosine would be significant if the half-life of the compound was not as short as it is. Many of the adverse effects result from activation of A_2-receptors in the vascular system: flushing, headache, and lightheadedness. Chest pain, anxiety, nausea, vomiting, and occasional bronchospasm are seen as well. However, these effects are usually short-lived, and if the patient has been adequately warned about their occurrence, they are rarely of significance. Profound but brief electrophysiologic responses are observed on the electrocardiogram (ECG), ranging from premature atrial and ventricular beats to short periods of asystole. Again, these are rarely of significance.

Adenosine and Myocardial Preconditioning

Myocardial preconditioning is the phenomenon in which brief exposure of the myocardium to ischemic conditions allows it to withstand a subsequent, more prolonged, exposure. The phenomenon has received much attention, as its application in the clinical setting might allow the heart to better withstand, for instance, the insults of cardiac surgery. The mechanisms of this effect were investigated in the hope that they might be activated directly, without the need for ischemia. A variety of mechanisms might account for preconditioning, as reviewed.[80,90]

A G protein–linked K^+ channel located on the mitochondrial membrane, the mitochondrial K_{ATP} channel (mito-K_{ATP}), appears to be a key mediator in myocardial preconditioning. Opening of this channel using compounds that selectively open mito-K_{ATP} without affecting other cellular K_{ATP} channels has been shown to have a protective effect, whereas inhibition of the channel (with the channel blocker glibenclamide) increases ischemic damage to the myocardium.[91] For example, abolishment by glibenclamide of preconditioning could be shown in a study measuring ST-segment changes and cardiac pain in patients undergoing balloon angioplasty.[92] Similar findings have been observed in various animal studies. K_{ATP}, like K_{ACh}, belongs to the class of G protein–coupled inward rectifier-type channels; its structure is indicated in Figure 7–12. In contrast to K_{ACh}, however, it appears to be modulated primarily by changes in intracellular ATP derivatives. For example, intracellular increases in ATP levels have a direct inhibitory effect on the channel. In addition, K_{ATP} can be modulated by PKC, which phosphorylates the channel. PKC can be activated directly by ischemic conditions or by activation of α-adrenergic and adenosine receptors. In addition, it now appears that adenosine may also be able to influence behavior of K_{ATP} in the same manner that it regulates K_{ACh}: through a G_i protein.[93] The mechanisms by which mito-K_{ATP} opening would be protective are under investigation. Potential beneficial effects involve inhibition of mitochondrial Ca^{++} uptake, regulation of mitochondrial volume, and modulation of the generation of reactive oxygen species. Of interest from the anesthesiologist's point of view are observations that volatile anesthetics induce preconditioning by similar mechanisms. For example, sevoflurane preconditions human myocardium against hypoxia through activation of K_{ATP} channels and activation of A_1-adenosine receptors.[94] Lidocaine was also shown to induce protection against inflammatory stimulation of endothelial and vascular smooth muscle cells by affecting mito-K_{ATP}.[95]

ANESTHETIC ACTIONS

Although the functioning and the physiologic role of the receptors and channels described are of obvious importance to the anesthesiologist, from a practical perspective, the interactions between anesthetic drugs and these signaling molecules are at least as relevant. As mentioned at the end of the previous section, effects of anesthetics on such proteins may be beneficial to the cardiovascular system. However, detrimental interactions may exist as well.

Volatile anesthetics are administered in extremely high doses compared with most other pharmacologic agents. Most of the commonly used pharmacologic compounds are administered in amounts that result in micromolar blood concentrations. Because current pharmacologic agents are sufficiently potent, a half-maximal effect on the site of action only requires low micromolar concentrations. Anesthetics, in contrast, require low millimolar concentrations in blood in order to be effective, almost a thousand times as much. Despite the reference to them as "potent agents," they are certainly not very potent compared with other pharmacologic compounds. As a result, it is not surprising that they have a wide range of actions in addition to their primary effect site (which, of course, is still not completely defined). In addition, volatile anesthetics are lipophilic compounds, and if, under laboratory conditions, concentrations are increased even further, they can be found to interact with almost any preparation exhibiting a certain degree of lipophilicity. As a result, data exist demonstrating interactions between volatile anesthetics and virtually every component of the cardiovascular system. The issue, then, is not with which channels and receptors the anesthetics interact but which of all these interactions are clinically important. The importance of the interactions has been difficult to determine. A first test that should be applied, of course, is that of reasonable concentrations; if effects are not observed at 1 to 2 minimal alveolar concentration (MAC) equivalents, it is very unlikely that an interaction has clinical relevance. As many experiments are performed at temperatures below 37°C, temperature correction of anesthetic solubility is an important issue. It is also important that actions are shown in several models. Effects observed in an isolated system may not necessarily be reproduced in an organ or whole-animal model; in that case, the relevance of the finding is in doubt. This issue has been reviewed in some detail.[96]

Injected anesthetics are less troublesome in this regard. Most of these act at defined sites (the γ-aminobutyric acid $[GABA]_A$ receptor-channel complex for most of them; ketamine's primary action on the *N*-methyl-D-aspartate [NMDA] receptor-channel complex is an exception). They are more potent, and they are, therefore, active at significantly lower concentrations. However, this does not necessarily mean that they are without other interactions, as their various side effect profiles show.

In this section, the focus is on some of the interactions between anesthetics and the molecular systems described in previous sections. Those interactions for which there is most support in the literature and which, in addition, help explain some of the specific side effects of anesthetic drugs are selected. Thus, rather than providing a detailed overview of all interactions reported, several well-described examples with probable clinical relevance are presented. Unfortunately, many of these interactions have not yet been described in molecular and submolecular detail. Although it may be known that an anesthetic inhibits functioning of a receptor or channel type, it is usually not known where in the molecule this interaction takes place. Most times it cannot even be ascertained that the interaction occurs with the protein itself, rather than with the lipid membrane environment surrounding the protein. Site-directed mutagenesis and the study of chimeric molecules are likely to shed light on these issues.

Interactions With Channels: Ca^{++} Channels

Of the variety of ion channels present in the heart, those most likely to be significantly affected by anesthetics in the clinical setting are the voltage-gated Ca^{++} channels. Although interactions with other cardiac channel types may also be relevant (such as those with the K_{ATP} channel, described earlier), they have not yet received as much research attention, and it is not yet possible to draw firm conclusions about the extent of these interactions. Hence, in this section the focus is only on Ca^{++} channels.

Anesthetic actions on cardiac Ca^{++} channels have been studied in a variety of models. The original observations that halothane blocked Ca^{++} flux into heart cells date back to the 1970s, and much specific information has been gained since then.[97] In particular, voltage clamp and patch clamp studies have contributed significantly to the understanding of the interactions between anesthetics and Ca^{++} channels and have elegantly described the effects of anesthetics on electrophysiologic behavior. However, it is not straightforward to assign the observed electrophysiologic effects to a molecular substrate. This issue is only beginning to be addressed with the use of recombinant technology.

Almost all volatile anesthetics inhibit L-type Ca^{++} channels.[98-100] Inhibition is modest, approximately 25% to 30% at 1 MAC anesthetic, but certainly sufficient to account for the physiologic changes induced by the anesthetics. Volatile anesthetics decrease peak current and, in addition, tend to increase the rate of inactivation.[101] Hence, maximal Ca^{++} current is depressed, and duration of Ca^{++} current is shortened. Together, these actions significantly limit the Ca^{++} influx into the cardiac myocyte. However, some specific actions may depend on the particular compound studied. In the presence of β-adrenergic stimulation, halothane, but not sevoflurane, is associated with a long-lasting enhancement of Ca^{++} channel function that may contribute to its proarrhythmic effects.[102] Xenon is without effect on cardiac Ca^{++} channels, explaining in large part its lack of effect on myocardial contractility. Other types of Ca^{++} channels have different sensitivities. Neuronal (N-type) channels have been shown to be quite resistant to volatile anesthetics. T-type channels, in general, tend to be much more sensitive than are L-type channels; at clinical concentrations of most volatile anesthetics, T currents are inhibited 50% or more.

The effects of volatile anesthetics on cardiac Ca^{++} channels can be modulated greatly by concurrent interactions of the compounds on other cardiac signaling systems. As discussed below, volatile anesthetics inhibit function of several types of muscarinic acetylcholine receptor systems. Because Ca^{++} channel function can be inhibited by muscarinic signaling, as discussed earlier, additional interactions would be anticipated when this system is exposed to volatile anesthetics, and such is indeed the case. Halothane and isoflurane further inhibit currents through these channels when either volatile anesthetic was applied following the inhibition produced by prior muscarinic stimulation. However, when muscarinic receptors were stimulated following administration of volatile anesthetic, its effect was reduced. Thus, although volatile anesthetics directly inhibit L-type channels, they also interfere with channel modulation by GPCR.[103]

Not only volatile, but also injected, anesthetics have been reported to inhibit cardiac L-type Ca^{++} channels in some models. However, the concentrations used generally exceed those used in clinical practice. Thiopental and methohexital block L-type Ca^{++} currents.[100,104] Similarly, propofol has been reported to inhibit these channels but at concentrations well beyond the clinical range.[105]

Interactions With Receptors: Muscarinic Receptors

As with cardiac channels, anesthetic interactions with a variety of GPCR may be of potential relevance to cardiovascular side effects of anesthetic compounds. However, most of these potential interactions have not been described in significant detail. The two main control systems of myocardial functioning—the muscarinic and adrenergic systems—have been studied to some extent, and a generalizing conclusion can be that muscarinic receptors are and adrenergic receptors are not sensitive to many anesthetics. Hence, the focus is on muscarinic receptors in this section.

Determination of anesthetic effects on GPCR is in some ways more complex than determination of the effects on channels. Although the receptors are molecularly smaller and only consist of a single subunit, they are only one part of very complex signaling pathways. Therefore, it is not sufficient to determine the effects on the receptor itself; actions on intracellular signaling should be investigated as well.

There is no doubt that at least some volatile anesthetics interfere with muscarinic signaling. Unfortunately, most of these investigations have not studied the heart, or even looked specifically at the m2-receptor, the only subtype expressed in cardiac tissue.

Aronstam and Dennison[106] published a series of papers reporting the effects of various anesthetics on muscarinic receptor binding. A summary of their findings has appeared in print as well. Several studies investigated the effect of halothane on agonist and antagonist binding.[107,108] The conclusions drawn from this work were that (1) the anesthetic enhanced antagonist binding by slowing the rate of ligand dissociation and (2) the anesthetic inhibited agonist binding (by 48% with 10% halothane).

The site of action of these effects was studied in more detail by investigating the interactions of anesthetics with G-protein functioning.[104,105] As discussed earlier, G proteins are activated by GDP-GTP exchange. An intrinsic, but remarkably slow, enzyme activity hydrolyzes GTP back to GDP, thereby inactivating the G protein after several seconds. While active, the G protein is no longer able to couple to the receptor, and uncoupled receptors exhibit a decreased affinity for their agonist. This decrease in activity can be induced in the experimental setting by including a nonhydrolyzable analog of GTP (such as Gpp[NH]p) in the reaction mixture, resulting in irreversibly activated G proteins. This effect is known as the GTP shift in receptor affinity. Halothane shifts the Gpp(NH)p concentration-response relationship to the right. In other words, a higher concentration of the GTP analog was necessary to induce a similar decrease in agonist binding. In the absence and presence of 5% halothane, the half-maximal inhibitory concentration (IC_{50}) values for the inhibitory effect of Gpp(NH)p were 0.7 and 83 μM, respectively, a 100-fold difference. These findings were interpreted as an ability of halothane to stabilize high-affinity G protein-receptor complexes.

Hence, it appears that halothane affects receptor binding as well as receptor–G protein interaction. In a subsequent study, the effect of the anesthetic on G-protein functioning—its ability to hydrolyze bound GTP—was investigated. Halothane was found not to inhibit binding of radiolabeled GTP analog to G proteins.[106] However, the anesthetic completely blocked the stimulation of G protein GTPase activity induced by acetylcholine, with a half-maximal effect at the clinically relevant halothane concentration of 0.3 mmol/L. The site of this effect was not determined. Largely similar findings were obtained with other anesthetics. Halothane also has been shown to interfere with G protein–mediated Ca^{++} sensitization in airway smooth muscle by inhibiting G proteins.[109] The interaction between halothane and purified, recombinant G_i was investigated. In contrast to the findings just given, no effect of the anesthetic on G_i protein function was found.[110] Hence, the earlier results may have been contaminated by interactions with other subtypes that are less relevant to muscarinic m2-receptor signaling. The conclusion to be drawn from these studies is that anesthetics may interfere with several components of the muscarinic signaling pathway. However, it should be kept in mind that (1) most often a mixture of muscarinic receptor subtypes was studied, (2) the anesthetics were administered in relatively high, and clinically unequal, concentrations, and (3) anesthetic effects on functional properties of the receptor–G protein unit were not specifically addressed.

One study has addressed this issue directly: Magyar and Szabo,[111] using the patch-clamp technique, investigated the effects of halothane (0.9 mmol/L) and isoflurane (0.8 mmol/L) on acetylcholine (10 μmol/L)-induced activation of the muscarinic K^+ channel in frog atrial myocytes. They found that if anesthetic and agonist were administered at the same time, a reduction in the peak K^+ current was observed, which was greater with halothane than with isoflurane. However, pretreatment with the anesthetic was found to have a significant, time-dependent, additional effect: 25-minute exposure to halothane restored the peak and significantly increased the steady-state current, whereas exposure to isoflurane decreased both. As equilibration of the anesthetic with the direct signaling pathway should be complete within milliseconds to seconds, the prolonged time course of these effects seems to indicate that additional intracellular pathways (such as PKC-mediated phosphorylation) are involved. Exposure of the membrane patches to the nonhydrolyzable GTP analog (GTPγS), thereby irreversibly activating G_K, prolonged the current. When single-channel measurements were performed, halothane was found to enhance the frequency of channel opening without significantly affecting the single-channel conductance. Isoflurane was without effect. Therefore, halothane affects the signaling pathway downstream of the muscarinic receptor in this model. Whether this action is on the G protein or on the channel itself cannot be conclusively determined from these studies.

When the time considerations are taken into account, it seems likely that the initial action of halothane on the system is inhibiting, whereas that of isoflurane is less so. After prolonged exposure, halothane is found to enhance signaling, whereas isoflurane inhibits it. These results are probably due to various effects of the anesthetics on intracellular systems that modify the signaling properties of the muscarinic pathway. In addition, halothane, but not isoflurane, has a direct activating effect downstream of the muscarinic receptor. The latter is consistent with findings of halothane effect on Ca^{++} channels mentioned earlier.

LOOKING AHEAD

The preceding sections have given an overview of the current understanding of the molecular biology of the cardiovascular system. There is fairly detailed insight into the basic mechanisms of cardiac regulation—that anesthetics interact significantly with at least some of these systems (although it is not always easy to correlate observed molecular effects with clinical actions of the anesthetics) and that the molecular defect is known in at least a few cardiovascular disease states. It is important to realize that virtually all these advances were made in the past 20 years, and most of them in the past decade. Therefore, even more dramatic increases in understanding can be anticipated in the next few years, and it is useful to summarize the most likely directions these developments will take. Thus, this section is a look ahead to where the clinician may expect the most from molecular biology in the next 5 to 10 years. Two areas appear to be of main importance: molecular diagnosis and molecular therapy. Both are part of the domain of medical genomics. An excellent series of reviews on this topic has appeared.[112]

Diagnosis

Now that the human genome has been cloned, researchers can expect to find the molecular substrate for an ever larger number of diseases. Genetically defined disorders, in which the defect is in a single gene, will be the most easily defined in molecular terms. This, in fact, has already been done for several cardiovascular diseases, with hemophilia and sickle cell disease as prominent examples. Undoubtedly, many more of these will be defined over the ensuing years. However, for most disorders the genetic origin is not that clearly defined. The majority of diseases have a genetically determined component (i.e., they tend to be more prevalent in certain families or genetically similar groups), but for the disease to develop more than a genetic predisposition is needed; interactions with the environment (diet, toxins, etc.) are required before the disease manifests itself. Examples of such diseases are hypertension, arteriosclerosis, and cardiac failure. For obvious reasons, it will be difficult, if not impossible, to determine a clear molecular defect for such diseases, except for a small subgroup with a very strong genetic component (an example from a different area is the relationship between the gene *BCA-1* and carcinoma of the breast—a relationship that is very strong but holds only in a small subgroup of breast cancer patients: those with strongly genetically determined cancer). However, this does not mean that there will be no place for molecular diagnosis in these diseases. In fact, the techniques can be very useful for screening. Being aware of mutations in genes known to be involved in a disorder can provide an estimate of the likelihood that a patient will develop the disease. Thus, they can help determine how aggressive a preventive regimen should be instituted. In addition, measurement of mRNA and protein expression in healthy and diseased tissues can provide valuable insight into pathophysiologic mechanisms.

How then is molecular diagnosis accomplished? Interestingly, it is possible to define the presence of a mutation, even if the gene has not been cloned, using a methodology with the rather cumbersome name of *restriction fragment length polymorphisms* (RFLP). RFLP requires the presence of a marker sequence located on the chromosome close to the gene of interest, so that the two will be co-inherited. In addition, the marker must contain a mutation that modifies a restriction site (a sequence cut by a restriction enzyme, a bacterial enzyme that cuts DNA at defined sequences), so that either the presence or absence of the mutation is inherited with the gene of interest. By cutting DNA with restriction enzymes, separating the fragments, and then determining the presence or absence of the marker restriction site, the presence or absence of the mutation in the gene of interest can be assessed. Clearly, this is a rather cumbersome technique and suitable only for a limited number of diseases. In addition, it is primarily suitable to single-gene defects.

The techniques that will be used primarily in the future employ sequence information from cloned genes, so that changes in the sequence can be directly sought. DNA or RNA hybridization with specific probes can be used. However, PCR is much more powerful and can selectively amplify certain segments of DNA for analysis. This flexible methodology is being used routinely for the diagnosis of an increasing number of disease states (for an example of the diagnosis of hemophilia A by this method, see Kogan et al[113]). Technically, PCR is relatively straightforward. The main difficulty is in interpretation. And, as with RFLP techniques, PCR is primarily useful in the setting of single-gene disorders.

Molecular diagnosis becomes much more difficult in cases in which multiple genetic changes might lead to the same clinical syndrome, such as in malignant hyperthermia,[114] and particularly in diseases in which genetic abnormalities only contribute to, rather than cause, the disorder. Diagnosis of such disorders requires that a (sometimes large) number of genes be investigated simultaneously. The technique best suited for this purpose is gene microarrays, which allow identification of sets of genes that are consistently upregulated or downregulated in a specific disease state. In microarray analysis, a large number (15,000 or such) of DNA pieces ("probes") are attached in specific spots on a chip less than 1 × 1 inch. Several approaches exist for assembling the chip, but a common one is the oligodeoxynucleotide chip, where DNA fragments are actually synthesized directly on the chip using a methodology reminiscent of the techniques used for constructing electronic integrated circuits. Each probe is able to recognize a single gene. The chip is then exposed to RNA from the patient. If a specific RNA is present in the patient sample, it will combine with the probe on the chip, in proportion to its abundance. The bound RNA can be visualized using fluorescent indicators. The chip is scanned, and the results are analyzed by computer. This technology has been used extensively in cancer research and is only beginning to be used in the setting of cardiovascular disease.[115]

Although these techniques show much promise, there are also difficult ethical issues involved. Undoubtedly, there will be an explosion of commercial tests for a variety of diseases. Determining their appropriate role in medicine, and their ethical use, will fuel debate for a number of years to come.

Therapy

Molecular diagnosis is already here, but molecular therapy appears just tantalizingly out of reach—and has seemed that way since the 1990s. The concepts are clear. The application, however, has been fraught with much more difficulty than at first appreciated.

Gene therapy attempts to modify expression of genetic material. Although myriad approaches have been suggested, those with the most promise are replacement of lacking or defective genes and selective inhibition of gene expression by antisense treatment. Another approach, further removed from clinical practice at this time, is the targeting of drug delivery to specific tissues using molecular techniques.

Replacement of genes is by now a routine technique in laboratory cell cultures, and can be performed with reasonable ease in animal models such as transgenic animals. Application in the clinical setting has been difficult, however. Obviously, most times it is not necessary to replace a gene in every cell of the body. In cystic fibrosis, for example, a disease in which gene therapy is probably closest to succeeding, the main target tissue will be the pulmonary system. The main issue then becomes the delivery of the functional gene to the target tissue in such a manner that it will be consistently expressed at adequate levels. A variety of experimental techniques exists. Cells can be removed from the patient's body, changed in culture, and then replaced. Alternatively, the gene can be incorporated in an otherwise innocuous virus that then is used to infect the patient's tissues. Both approaches show promise, but technical difficulties indicate that this is still a considerable time away from routine clinical application. Nonetheless, several clinical trials are in progress.[116,117]

Inhibition of gene expression by antisense treatment is similarly full of promise.[118-120] The technique is based on the fact that messenger RNA can no longer be translated efficiently into protein when bound to a complementary strand of nucleic acid, a so-called antisense strand. Thus, by introducing specific antisense DNA into cells, expression of a selected gene product can be inhibited. The problem here, again, is efficient targeting of the tissue of interest. Remarkably, cells are able to take up antisense material from the extracellular environment without degrading it, but the material still has to be brought in contact with the tissue of interest. A second technical problem involves the stability of the antisense DNA. As most diseases for which this technique seems suitable require constant inhibition of gene expression over long time periods, the antisense construct has to be highly stable, and this degree of stability has not yet been consistently achieved.

Thus, molecular therapy seems feasible but is not quite ready for the clinic yet. Several times over the past decade, clinicians have thought that a breakthrough would be achieved rapidly; each time they have been disappointed. It would, therefore, be dangerous to predict that these techniques will find practical clinical application in the next few years. Nonetheless, the concepts appear sound and have been proved in animal models. It seems to be only a matter of time before patients will be treated with these methods.

Somatic Gene Therapy for Cardiac Arrhythmias

Somatic gene therapy means addition of genes as either DNA or RNA to cells other than eggs or sperm with the goal of treating or preventing a disease. Early trials of somatic gene therapy were initially targeted at monogenic disorders that were easily accessible for gene transfer. Gene delivery to the cardiovascular system has complicated attempts to translate gene therapy to cardiology. Potential delivery strategies include replication-deficient viruses and physicochemical techniques such as liposomes and direct injection. The only report of in vivo utilization of gene therapy to target an arrhythmia was viral transfection of an inhibitory G protein into the AV node of pigs to control the ventricular response to atrial fibrillation.[121] The rationale for this strategy was that that overexpression of an inhibitory G protein would in effect create a localized β-receptor blockade. The success of this strategy may point to human trials in the future.

Stem Cell Therapy

Stem cells are immature tissue precursor cells that are undifferentiated and can differentiate into specialized cells including cardiomyocytes and cardiac rhythm-generating tissue. Stem cells may be isolated from the fetus, but limited supply and ethical considerations have mandated a search for a more easily accessible source. Skeletal myoblasts, endothelial progenitor cells, and adult mesenchymal stem cells have all been used. There are early reports of the use of stem cells for cellular cardiomyoplasty in patients with end-stage heart failure after myocardial infarction, but there remain concerns about incorporation of the cells into the myocardium and the possibility of arrhythmogenesis.[122] Prospective randomized trials are awaited. Human mesenchymal stem cells transfected with HCN2, a pacemaker channel, have been incorporated into canine myocardium. These cells have been shown to form gap junctions with the myocardium and to generate rhythmic activity after AV nodal blockade.[123] These experiments offer the distant prospect of a biological cardiac pacemaker.

REFERENCES

1. Watson JA, Crick FHC: Molecular structure of nucleic acids: A structure for deoxyribose nucleic acid. Nature 171:737, 1953
2. Hamill OP, Marty A, Neher E, et al: Improved patch-clamp techniques for high-resolution current recording from cells and cell-free membrane patches. Pflugers Arch Eur J Physiol 391:85, 1981
3. Sakmann B, Trube G: Voltage-dependent inactivation of inward-rectifying single-channel currents in the guinea-pig heart cell membrane. J Physiol (Lond) 347:659, 1984
4. Hume JR, Uehara A: Ionic basis of the different action potential configurations of single guinea-pig atrial and ventricular myocytes. J Physiol (Lond) 368:525, 1985
5. Moorman JR: Sodium channels. *In* Yaksh T, et al (eds): Anesthesia: Biologic Foundations. Philadelphia, Lippincott-Raven Publishers, 1997, p 145

6. Coraboeuf E, Carmeliet E: Existence of two transient outward currents in sheep cardiac Purkinje fibers. Pflugers Arch Eur J Physiol 392:352, 1982
7. Hiraoka M, Kawano S: Calcium-sensitive and insensitive transient outward current in rabbit ventricular myocytes. J Physiol (Lond) 410:187, 1989
8. Tseng GN, Hoffman BF: Two components of transient outward current in canine ventricular myocytes. Circ Res 64:633, 1989
9. Li Q, Keung EC: Effects of myocardial hypertrophy on transient outward current. Am J Physiol 266:H1738, 1994
10. Lue WM, Boyden PA: Abnormal electrical properties of myocytes from chronically infarcted canine heart. Alterations in Vmax and the transient outward current. Circulation 85:1175, 1992
11. Grant AO, Starmer CF: Mechanisms of closure of cardiac sodium channels in rabbit ventricular myocytes: Single-channel analysis. Circ Res 60:897, 1987
12. Attwell D, Cohen I, Eisner D, et al: The steady-state TTX-sensitive ("window") sodium current in cardiac Purkinje fibres. Pflugers Arch Eur J Physiol 379:137, 1979
13. Tsien RW, Bean BP, Hess P, et al: Mechanisms of calcium channel modulation by beta-adrenergic agents and dihydropyridine calcium agonists. J Mol Cell Cardiol 18:691, 1986
14. Trautwein W, Cavalie A: Cardiac calcium channels and their control by neurotransmitters and drugs. J Am Coll Cardiol 6:1409, 1985
15. Reuter H: Calcium channel modulation by neurotransmitters, enzymes and drugs. Nature 301:569, 1983
16. Bennett P, McKinney L, Begenisich T, Kass RS: Adrenergic modulation of the delayed rectifier potassium channel in calf cardiac Purkinje fibers. Biophys J 49:839, 1986
17. Sanguinetti MC, Jurkiewicz NK: Two components of cardiac delayed rectifier K+ current. Differential sensitivity to block by class III antiarrhythmic agents. J Gen Physiol 96:195, 1990
18. Wang Z, Fermini B, Nattel S: Sustained depolarization-induced outward current in human atrial myocytes. Evidence for a novel delayed rectifier K+ current similar to Kv1.5 cloned channel currents. Circ Res 73:1061, 1993
19. Trautwein W, Taniguchi J, Noma A: The effect of intracellular cyclic nucleotides and calcium on the action potential and acetylcholine response of isolated cardiac cells. Pflugers Arch Eur J Physiol 392:307, 1982
20. Giles W, Noble SJ: Changes in membrane currents in bullfrog atrium produced by acetylcholine. J Physiol (Lond) 261:103, 1976
21. Ragazzi E, Wu SN, Shryock J, Belardinelli L: Electrophysiological and receptor binding studies to assess activation of the cardiac adenosine receptor by adenine nucleotides. Circ Res 68:1035, 1991
22. Pfaffinger PJ, Martin JM, Hunter DD, et al: GTP-binding proteins couple cardiac muscarinic receptors to a K channel. Nature 317:536, 1985
23. Liu DW, Gintant GA, Antzelevitch C: Ionic bases for electrophysiological distinctions among epicardial, midmyocardial, and endocardial myocytes from the free wall of the canine left ventricle. Circ Res 72:671, 1993
24. DiFrancesco D: The onset and autonomic regulation of cardiac pacemaker activity: Relevance of the F current. Cardiovasc Res 29:449, 1995
25. DiFrancesco D, Tromba C: Acetylcholine inhibits activation of the cardiac hyperpolarizing-activated current, If. Pflugers Arch Eur J Physiol 410:139, 1987
26. DiFrancesco D, Tortora P: Direct activation of cardiac pacemaker channels by intracellular cyclic AMP. Nature 351:145, 1991
27. Yatani A, Okabe K, Codina J, et al: Heart rate regulation by G proteins acting on the cardiac pacemaker channel. Science 249:1163, 1990
28. Armstrong CM, Bezanilla F: Currents related to movement of the gating particles of the sodium channels. Nature 242:459, 1973
29. Catterall WA: Molecular properties of voltage gated ion channels in the heart. *In* Fozzard HA, Haber E, Jennings R (eds): The Heart and Cardiovascular System—Scientific Foundations. New York, Raven Press, 1992, pp 945–962
30. Lipkind GM, Fozzard HA: A structural model of the tetrodotoxin and saxitoxin binding site of the Na+ channel. Biophys J 66:1, 1994
31. Hille B: The permeability of the sodium channel to organic cations in myelinated nerve. J Gen Physiol 58:599, 1971
32. Tomaselli GF, Backx PH, Marban E: Molecular basis of permeation in voltage-gated ion channels. Circ Res 72:491, 1993
33. Terlau H, Heinemann SH, Stuhmer W, et al: Mapping the site of block by tetrodotoxin and saxitoxin of sodium channel II. FEBS Lett 293:93, 1991
34. Armstrong CM, Bezanilla F, Rojas E: Destruction of sodium conductance inactivation in squid axons perfused with pronase. J Gen Physiol 62:375, 1973
35. Miller C: Annus mirabilis of potassium channels. Science 252:1092, 1991
36. Hille B: Local anesthetics: Hydrophilic and hydrophobic pathways for the drug-receptor reaction. J Gen Physiol 69:497, 1977
37. Hondeghem LM, Katzung BG: Antiarrhythmic agents: The modulated receptor mechanism of action of sodium and calcium channel-blocking drugs. Annu Rev Pharmacol Toxicol 24:387, 1984
38. Starmer CF, Grant AO, Strauss HC: Mechanisms of use-dependent block of sodium channels in excitable membranes by local anesthetics. Biophys J 46:15, 1984
39. Ragsdale DS, McPhee JC, Scheuer T, Catterall WA: Molecular determinants of state-dependent block of Na^+ channels by local anesthetics. Science 265:1724, 1994
40. Perez-Reyes E, Schneider T: Molecular biology of calcium channels. Kidney Int 48:1111, 1995
41. Po S, Roberds S, Snyders DJ, et al: Heteromultimeric assembly of human potassium channels. Molecular basis of a transient outward current? Circ Res 72:1326, 1993
42. Salkoff L: Development of ion channels in the flight muscles of *Drosophila*. J Physiol (Paris) 80:275, 1985
43. Timpe LC, Schwarz TL, Tempel BL, et al: Expression of functional potassium channels from Shaker cDNA in Xenopus oocytes. Nature 331:143, 1988
44. Deal KK, England SK, Tamkun MM: Molecular physiology of cardiac potassium channels. Physiol Rev 76:49, 1996
45. England SK, Uebele VN, Shear H, et al: Characterization of a voltage-gated K+ channel beta subunit expressed in human heart. Proc Natl Acad Sci U S A 92:6309, 1995
46. Trudeau MC, Warmke JW, Ganetzky B, Robertson GA: HERG, a human inward rectifier in the voltage-gated potassium channel family [erratum appears in Science 272:1087, 1996; PMID:8638148]. Science 269:92, 1995
47. Barhanin J, Lesage F, Guillemare E, et al: K(V)LQT1 and lsK (minK) proteins associate to form the I(Ks) cardiac potassium current. Nature 384:78, 1996
48. Yao Z, Gross GJ: The ATP-dependent potassium channel: An endogenous cardioprotective mechanism. J Cardiovasc Pharmacol 24(suppl 4):S28, 1994
49. Vandenberg CA: Inward rectification of a potassium channel in cardiac ventricular cells depends on internal magnesium ions. Proc Natl Acad Sci U S A 84:2560, 1987
50. Kass RS, Tsien RW: Control of action potential duration by calcium ions in cardiac Purkinje fibers. J Gen Physiol 67:599, 1976
51. Krapivinsky G, Gordon EA, Wickman K, et al: The G-protein-gated atrial K+ channel IKACh is a heteromultimer of two inwardly rectifying K(+)-channel proteins. Nature 374:135, 1995
52. Kaupp UB, Seifert R: Molecular diversity of pacemaker ion channels. Annu Rev Physiol 63:235, 2001
53. Echt DS, Liebson PR, Mitchell LB, et al: Mortality and morbidity in patients receiving encainide, flecainide, or placebo. The Cardiac Arrhythmia Suppression Trial. N Engl J Med 324:781, 1991
54. Singh BN: Arrhythmia control by prolonging repolarization: The concept and its potential therapeutic impact. Eur Heart J 14(suppl H):14, 1993
55. Mohler PJ, Schott JJ, Gramolini AO, et al: Ankyrin-B mutation causes type 4 long-QT cardiac arrhythmia and sudden cardiac death. Nature 421:634, 2003
56. Brugada P, Brugada J: Right bundle-branch block, persistent ST-segment elevation and sudden cardiac death: A distinct clinical and electrocardiographic syndrome. A multicenter report. J Am Coll Cardiol 20:1391, 1992
57. Antzelevitch C, Brugada P, Brugada J, et al: Brugada syndrome: A decade of progress. Circ Res 91:1114, 2002
58. Gauthier C, Langin D, Balligand JL: Beta$_3$-adrenoceptors in the cardiovascular system. Trends Pharmacol Sci 21:426, 2000
59. Bristow MR, Hershberger RE, Port JD, et al: Beta$_1$- and beta$_2$-adrenergic receptor-mediated adenylate cyclase stimulation in nonfailing and failing human ventricular myocardium. Mol Pharmacol 35:295, 1989
60. Bristow MR, Minobe W, Rasmussen R, et al: Alpha$_1$-adrenergic receptors in the nonfailing and failing human heart. J Pharmacol Exp Ther 247:1039, 1988
61. Hasking GJ, Esler MD, Jennings GL, et al: Norepinephrine spillover to plasma in patients with congestive heart failure: Evidence of increased overall and cardiorenal sympathetic nervous activity. Circulation 73:615, 1986
62. Harding SE, Brown LA, Wynne DG, et al: Mechanisms of beta-adrenoceptor desensitisation in the failing human heart. Cardiovasc Res 28:1451, 1994

63. Maisel AS, Ziegler MG, Carter S, et al: In vivo regulation of beta-adrenergic receptors on mononuclear leukocytes and heart. Assessment of receptor compartmentation after agonist infusion and acute aortic constriction in guinea pigs. J Clin Invest 82:2038, 1988
64. Chen CY, Dion SB, Kim CM, Benovic JL: Beta-adrenergic receptor kinase. Agonist-dependent receptor binding promotes kinase activation. J Biol Chem 268:7825, 1993
65. Lohse MJ, Benovic JL, Codina J, et al: Beta-arrestin: A protein that regulates beta-adrenergic receptor function. Science 248:1547, 1990
66. Deighton NM, Motomura S, Borquez D, et al: Muscarinic cholinoceptors in the human heart: Demonstration, subclassification, and distribution. Naunyn Schmiedebergs Arch Pharmacol 341:14, 1990
67. Lechleiter J, Hellmiss R, Duerson K, et al: Distinct sequence elements control the specificity of G protein activation by muscarinic acetylcholine receptor subtypes. EMBO J 9:4381, 1990
68. Logothetis DE, Kurachi Y, Galper J, et al: The beta gamma subunits of GTP-binding proteins activate the muscarinic K+ channel in heart. Nature 325:321, 1987
69. Swynghedauw B, Besse S, Assayag P, et al: Molecular and cellular biology of the senescent hypertrophied and failing heart. Am J Cardiol 76:2D, 1995
70. Schmitz W, Boknik P, Linck B, Muller FU: Adrenergic and muscarinic receptor regulation and therapeutic implications in heart failure. Mol Cell Biochem 157:251, 1996
71. Bohm M, Gierschik P, Jakobs KH, et al: Increase of Gi alpha in human hearts with dilated but not ischemic cardiomyopathy. Circulation 82:1249, 1990
72. Fleming JW, Wisler PL, Watanabe AM: Signal transduction by G proteins in cardiac tissues [erratum appears in Circulation 86:698, 1992]. Circulation 85:420, 1992
73. Pitcher JA, Inglese J, Higgins JB, et al: Role of beta gamma subunits of G proteins in targeting the beta-adrenergic receptor kinase to membrane-bound receptors. Science 257:1264, 1992
74. Feldman AM, Jackson DG, Bristow MR, et al: Immunodetectable levels of the inhibitory guanine nucleotide-binding regulatory proteins in failing human heart: Discordance with measurements of adenylate cyclase activity and levels of pertussis toxin substrate. J Mol Cell Cardiol 23:439, 1991
75. Bristow MR, Anderson FL, Port JD, et al: Differences in beta-adrenergic neuroeffector mechanisms in ischemic versus idiopathic dilated cardiomyopathy. Circulation 84:1024, 1991
76. Bristow MR, Minobe W, Rasmussen R, et al: Beta-adrenergic neuroeffector abnormalities in the failing human heart are produced by local rather than systemic mechanisms. J Clin Invest 89:803, 1992
77. Hershberger RE, Anderson FL, Bristow MR: Vasoactive intestinal peptide receptor in failing human ventricular myocardium exhibits increased affinity and decreased density. Circ Res 65:283, 1989
78. Belardinelli L, Shryock JC, Song Y, et al: Ionic basis of the electrophysiological actions of adenosine on cardiomyocytes. FASEB J 9:359, 1995
79. Shen WK, Kurachi Y: Mechanisms of adenosine-mediated actions on cellular and clinical cardiac electrophysiology. Mayo Clin Proc 70:274, 1995
80. Murphy E: Primary and secondary signaling pathways in early preconditioning that converge on the mitochondria to produce cardioprotection. Circ Res 94:7, 2004
81. Schutz W, Schrader J, Gerlach E: Different sites of adenosine formation in the heart. Am J Physiol 240:H963, 1981
82. Schrader J: Metabolism of adenosine and sites of production in the heart. *In* Berne RM, Rall TW, Rubio R (eds): Regulatory Functions of Adenosine. The Hague, Martinus Nijhoff, 1983, p 133
83. Moser GH, Schrader J, Deussen A: Turnover of adenosine in plasma of human and dog blood. Am J Physiol 256:C799, 1989
84. Visentin S, Wu SN, Belardinelli L: Adenosine-induced changes in atrial action potential: contribution of Ca^{++} and K^{+} currents. Am J Physiol 258:H1070, 1990
85. Dobson JG Jr: Adenosine reduces catecholamine contractile responses in oxygenated and hypoxic atria. Am J Physiol 245:H468, 1983
86. Dobson JG Jr: Mechanism of adenosine inhibition of catecholamine-induced responses in heart. Circ Res 52:151, 1983
87. Rankin AC, Brooks R, Ruskin JN, McGovern BA: Adenosine and the treatment of supraventricular tachycardia. Am J Med 92:655, 1992
88. diMarco JP, Sellers TD, Lerman BB, et al: Diagnostic and therapeutic use of adenosine in patients with supraventricular tachyarrhythmias. J Am Coll Cardiol 6:417, 1985
89. Shen WK, Hamill SC: Cardiac arrhythmias. *In* Mayo Clinic Practice of Cardiology, 3rd edition. St. Louis, CV Mosby, 1996
90. Martin HB, Walter CL: Preconditioning: An endogenous defense against the insult of myocardial ischemia. Anesth Analg 83:639, 1996
91. Sato T, Sasaki N, Seharaseyon J, et al: Selective pharmacological agents implicate mitochondrial but not sarcolemmal K(ATP) channels in ischemic cardioprotection. Circulation 101:2418, 2000
92. Tomai F, Crea F, Gaspardone A, et al: Ischemic preconditioning during coronary angioplasty is prevented by glibenclamide, a selective ATP-sensitive K+ channel blocker. Circulation 90:700, 1994
93. Kirsch GE, Codina J, Birnbaumer L, Brown AM: Coupling of ATP-sensitive K+ channels to A_1-receptors by G proteins in rat ventricular myocytes. Am J Physiol 259:H820, 1990
94. Yvon A, Hanouz JL, Haelewyn B, et al: Mechanisms of sevoflurane-induced myocardial preconditioning in isolated human right atria in vitro. Anesthesiology 99:27, 2003
95. de Klaver MJ, Buckingham MG, Rich GF: Lidocaine attenuates cytokine-induced cell injury in endothelial and vascular smooth muscle cells. Anesth Analg 97:465, 2003
96. Franks NP, Lieb WR: Selective actions of volatile general anaesthetics at molecular and cellular levels [erratum appears in Br J Anaesth 71:616, 1993]. Br J Anaesth 71:65, 1993
97. Porsius AJ, van Zwieten PA: Influence of halothane on calcium movements in isolated heart muscle and in isolated plasma membranes. Arch Int Pharmacodyn Ther 218:29, 1975
98. Bosnjak ZJ, Supan FD, Rusch NJ: The effects of halothane, enflurane, and isoflurane on calcium current in isolated canine ventricular cells. Anesthesiology 74:340, 1991
99. Terrar DA, Victory JG: Effects of halothane on membrane currents associated with contraction in single myocytes isolated from guinea-pig ventricle. Br J Pharmacol 94:500, 1988
100. Yamakage M, Hirshman CA, Croxton TL: Inhibitory effects of thiopental, ketamine, and propofol on voltage-dependent Ca2+ channels in porcine tracheal smooth muscle cells. Anesthesiology 83:1274, 1995
101. Pancrazio JJ: Halothane and isoflurane preferentially depress a slowly inactivating component of Ca^{++} channel current in guinea-pig myocytes. J Physiol (Lond) 494:91, 1996
102. Fassl J, Halaszovich CR, Huneke R, et al: Effects of inhalational anesthetics on L-type Ca2+ currents in human atrial cardiomyocytes during beta-adrenergic stimulation. Anesthesiology 99:90, 2003
103. Kamatchi GL, Durieux ME, Lynch C, 3rd: Differential sensitivity of expressed L-type calcium channels and muscarinic M(1) receptors to volatile anesthetics in Xenopus oocytes. J Pharmacol Exp Ther 297:981, 2001
104. Ikemoto Y, Yatani A, Arimura H, Yoshitake J: Reduction of the slow inward current of isolated rat ventricular cells by thiamylal and halothane. Acta Anaesthesiol Scand 29:583, 1985
105. Krnjevic K, Puil E: Halothane suppresses slow inward currents in hippocampal slices. Can J Physiol Pharmacol 66:1570, 1988
106. Aronstam RS, Dennison RL Jr: Anesthetic effects on muscarinic signal transduction. Int Anesthesiol Clin 27:265, 1989
107. Aronstam RS, Anthony BL, Dennison RL Jr: Halothane effects on muscarinic acetylcholine receptor complexes in rat brain. Biochem Pharmacol 35:667, 1986
108. Dennison RL Jr, Anthony BL, Narayanan TK, Aronstam RS: Effects of halothane on high affinity agonist binding and guanine nucleotide sensitivity of muscarinic acetylcholine receptors from brainstem of rat. Neuropharmacology 26:1201, 1987
109. Kai T, Jones KA, Warner DO: Halothane attenuates calcium sensitization in airway smooth muscle by inhibiting G-proteins. 89:1543, 1998
110. Streiff J, Jones K, Perkins WJ, et al: Effect of halothane on the guanosine 5' triphosphate binding activity of G-protein alpha subunits. Anesthesiology 99:105, 2003
111. Magyar J, Szabo G: Effects of volatile anesthetics on the G protein-regulated muscarinic potassium channel. Mol Pharmacol 50:1520, 1996
112. Lorentz CP, Wieben ED, Tefferi A, et al: Primer on medical genomics, part I: History of genetics and sequencing of the human genome. Mayo Clin Proc 77:773, 2002
113. Kogan SC, Doherty M, Gitschier J: An improved method for prenatal diagnosis of genetic diseases by analysis of amplified DNA sequences. Application to hemophilia A. N Engl J Med 317:985, 1987
114. Gillard EF, Otsu K, Fujii J, et al: Polymorphisms and deduced amino acid substitutions in the coding sequence of the ryanodine receptor (RYR1) gene in individuals with malignant hyperthermia. Genomics 13:1247, 1992
115. Cook SA, Rosenzweig A: DNA microarrays: Implications for cardiovascular medicine. 91:559, 2002
116. Eisensmith RC, Woo SL: Gene therapy for phenylketonuria. 407:124, 1994
117. Alton EW, Geddes DM: Gene therapy for respiratory diseases: Potential applications and difficulties. Thorax 50:484, 1995

118. Calabretta B, Skorski T, Szczylik C, Zon G: Prospects for gene-directed therapy with antisense oligodeoxynucleotides. Cancer Treat Rev 19:169, 1993
119. Stein CA, Cheng YC: Antisense oligonucleotides as therapeutic agents—is the bullet really magical? Science 261:1004, 1993
120. Cohen JS: Selective anti-gene therapy for cancer: Principles and prospects. Tohoku J Exp Med 168:351, 1992
121. Donahue JK, Heldman AW, Fraser H, et al: Focal modification of electrical conduction in the heart by viral gene transfer. Nat Med 6:1395, 2000
122. Lee MS, Makkar RR: Stem-cell transplantation in myocardial infarction: A status report. Ann Intern Med 140:729, 2004
123. Potapova I, Plotnikov A, Lu Z, et al: Human mesenchymal stem cells as a gene delivery system to create cardiac pacemakers. Circ Res 94:952, 2004

Chapter 8
SYSTEMIC INFLAMMATION

Elliott Bennett-Guerrero, MD

KEY POINTS

1. Mortality and morbidity are relatively common after major surgery.
2. Postoperative morbidity often involves multiple organ systems, which implicates a systemic process.
3. A large body of evidence suggests that excessive systemic inflammation is a cause of postoperative organ dysfunction.
4. No interventions have been proved in large randomized clinical trials to protect patients from systemic inflammation–mediated morbidity.

Numerous advances in perioperative care have allowed increasingly high-risk patients to safely undergo cardiac surgery. Although mortality rates of 1% are quoted for "low-risk" cardiac surgery, results from large series of patients older than 65 years suggest that mortality rates are actually more substantial.[1] For example, Birkmeyer et al[2] reviewed a large number (N = 474,108) of "all-comers" undergoing coronary artery bypass graft surgery (CABG) or aortic valve surgery in the Medicare Claims Database. It is very interesting to note that 30-day all-cause mortality was in the range of 4.0% to 5.4% after CABG and 6.5% to 9.1% after aortic valve replacement. The patient population studied, although elderly (age >65 years), would not be considered to be particularly high risk by today's standards. These data do not point to the cause of death. Nevertheless, they indicate that outcome after routine cardiac surgery is poor for many patients. Outcome after these procedures is even worse if the extent of postoperative complications is considered. Postoperative morbidity is common and complications include atrial fibrillation, poor ventricular function requiring inotropic agents, and non–cardiac-related etiologies such as infection, gastrointestinal dysfunction, acute lung injury, stroke, and renal dysfunction. For example, in a large series by Rady et al[3] of patients 75 years of age undergoing cardiac surgery (N = 1157), the mortality rate was 8%. The rate of serious complications, however, exceeded 50%.

Many postoperative complications appear to be caused by an exaggerated systemic proinflammatory response to surgical trauma.[4-6] The most severe form of this inflammatory response leads to multiple organ dysfunction syndrome and death.[5,6] Milder forms of a proinflammatory response cause less severe organ dysfunction, which does not lead to admission to an intensive care unit, but nevertheless causes suffering, increased hospital length of stay, and increased cost. The etiology and clinical relevance of systemic inflammation following cardiac surgery are poorly understood. Systemic inflammation is a multifactorial process and has profound secondary effects on both injured and normal tissues. Proinflammatory mediators can have beneficial as well as deleterious effects on multiple organ systems (Box 8–1). According to most theories, tissue injury, endotoxemia, and contact of blood with the foreign surface of the cardiopulmonary bypass (CPB) circuit are some of the major factors postulated to initiate a systemic inflammatory response. Nevertheless, there is controversy surrounding the etiology as well as pathogenesis of inflammation in the perioperative period.

TERMINOLOGY

The terminology of *inflammation* is confusing and has hampered effective communication among scientists and clinicians. Despite attempts to standardize the terminology, variation in usage still exists in the scientific literature as well as the clinical setting.[7] Much of the confusion relates to the term *inflammation,* defined as "a fundamental pathologic process consisting of a dynamic complex of cytologic and chemical reactions that occur in the affected blood vessels and adjacent tissues in response to an injury or abnormal stimulation caused by a physical, chemical, or biologic agent, including (1) the local reactions and resulting morphologic changes, (2) the destruction or removal of the injurious material, and (3) the responses that lead to repair and healing."[8] This definition acknowledges the potential role of noninfectious etiologies, i.e., infection is not a prerequisite for the development of *inflammation.* The American College of Chest Physicians/Society of Critical Care Medicine Consensus Conference has developed the following definitions for terms related to inflammation (Table 8–1). Figure 8–1 demonstrates the possible interrelationships among many of these terms.

In particular, the *systemic inflammatory response syndrome* (SIRS) refers to an inflammatory process that can arise from, or in the absence of, infection. A viewpoint consistent with the recommended terminology is that systemic inflammation is a spectrum from mild systemic inflammation without organ dysfunction to a more severe form characterized by multisystem organ failure and death. There are three reasons why

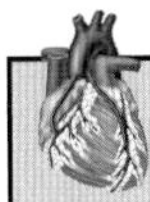

BOX 8–1 ***Organs Potentially Affected by Excessive Inflammation***

- Heart
- Lungs
- Brain
- Blood
- Blood vessels
- Gastrointestinal tract/liver
- Kidneys

Table 8–1 Definitions Related to Inflammation

Infection = microbial phenomenon characterized by an inflammatory response to the presence of microorganisms or the invasion of normally sterile host tissue by those organisms.

Bacteremia = the presence of viable bacteria in the blood.

Systemic inflammatory response syndrome (SIRS) = the systemic inflammatory response to a variety of severe clinical insults. The response is manifested by two or more of the following conditions: (1) temperature >38°C or <36°C; (2) heart rate >90 beats per minute; (3) respiratory rate >20 breaths per minute or Pa_{CO_2} <32 mm Hg; and (4) white blood cell count >12,000/mm^3, <4000/mm^3, or >10% immature (band) forms.

Sepsis = the systemic response to infection, manifested by two or more of the following conditions as a result of infection: (1) temperature >38°C or <36°C; (2) heart rate >90 beats per minute; (3) respiratory rate >20 breaths per minute or Pa_{CO_2} <32 mm Hg; and white blood cell count >12,000/mm^3, <4000/mm^3, or >10% immune (band) forms.

Severe sepsis = sepsis associated with organ dysfunction, hypoperfusion, or hypotension. Hypoperfusion and perfusion abnormalities may include, but are not limited to, lactic acidosis, oliguria, or an acute alteration in mental status.

Septic shock = sepsis-induced with hypotension despite adequate fluid resuscitation along with the presence of perfusion abnormalities that may include, but are not limited to, lactic acidosis, oliguria, or an acute alteration in mental status. Patients who are receiving inotropic or vasopressor agents may not be hypotensive at the time that perfusion abnormalities are measured.

Sepsis-induced hypotension = a systolic blood pressure <90 mm Hg or a reduction of ≥40 mm Hg from baseline in the absence of other causes of hypotension.

Multiple organ dysfunction syndrome (MODS) = presence of altered organ function in an acutely ill patient such that homeostasis cannot be maintained without intervention.

From Bone RC, Balk RA, Cerra FB, et al: Definitions for sepsis and organ failure and guidelines for the use of innovative therapies in sepsis: ACCP/SCCM consensus conference. Chest 101:1644–1655, 1992.

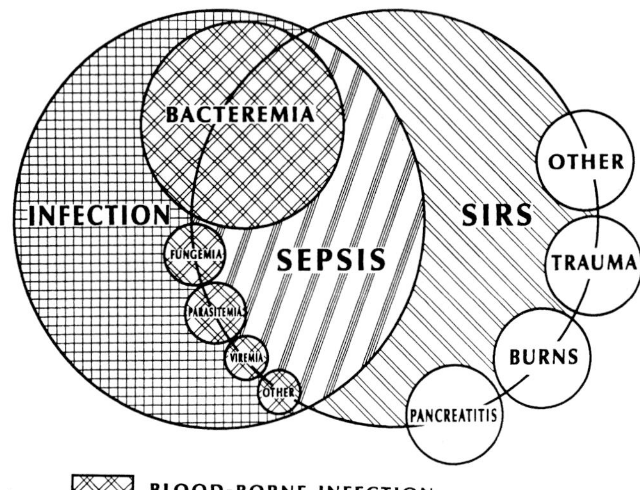

Figure 8–1 The interrelationships among systemic inflammatory response syndrome (SIRS), sepsis, and infection. (From Bone RC, Balk RA, Cerra FB, et al: Definitions for sepsis and organ failure and guidelines for the use of innovative therapies in sepsis: ACCP/SCCM Consensus Conference. Chest 101:1644, 1992.)

many clinicians do not routinely think of systemic inflammation as a clinical entity: (1) there are no universally accepted tests (i.e., physical diagnosis or laboratory assays) that can reliably and accurately measure the degree of systemic inflammation; (2) even if such a test existed and it is known that a patient has "severe" SIRS, the clinician would still not be able to predict (a) if organs will fail, (b) which organ(s) will fail, and (c) when organ(s) will fail; and (3) even if SIRS could be accurately diagnosed, currently there are no therapies in widespread clinical use for the prevention or treatment of systemic inflammation.

In the surgical population, the use of the phrase and definition for SIRS has generated some controversy.[9] This controversy relates to the fact that almost all patients following major surgery fulfill the criteria for SIRS. Most patients, however, clearly do not develop clinically significant organ dysfunction from their systemic inflammation. Critics may argue that the use of the term *SIRS* in cardiac surgery patients hence is meaningless because it does not differentiate patients who will have a benign versus a complicated postoperative course. For these reasons, the term *SIRS* is used more commonly by investigators than by practicing physicians. Use of the term *SIRS*, nevertheless, has the benefit of raising awareness regarding the many noninfectious causes of inflammation.

The distinction of systemic versus local inflammation is important. Local inflammation has several beneficial purposes. Invasion of the injured or infected tissue by inflammatory cells (i.e., neutrophils and macrophages) results in high concentrations of cells involved in host defense. Local mediator-induced edema and clotting of lymphatics by fibrinogen result in the effective "walling off" of the injured area. In contrast, systemic inflammation is not limited to the initial area of infection or injury. The systemic elaboration of inflammatory mediators may be beneficial by heightening the host's general defenses. It, however, may lead to the "autodestruction" of the host through secondary damage to tissues/organs not originally affected by the primary injury or infection.

The *acute-phase response* to tissue injury and infection is characterized by leukocytosis, fever, increased vascular permeability, a negative nitrogen balance, changes in plasma steroid and metal concentrations, and increased synthesis of hepatic acute-phase proteins. Examples of these proteins include haptoglobin, fibrinogen, C-reactive protein, complement factors (C3, factor B), serum amyloid A, α_1-acid glycoprotein, and α_1-antichymotrypsin.[10] The terms *acute-phase response* and *systemic inflammation* are often used interchangeably.

A common misconception relates to the terms *bacteremia* and *endotoxemia*. Although *bacteremia* refers to the presence of viable bacteria in the blood, *endotoxemia* refers to the presence of endotoxin in the blood. Endotoxin, also known as lipopolysaccharide (LPS), is a component of the cell membranes of gram-negative bacteria and hence its presence does not require the existence of viable organisms. In fact, it has been clearly established that cardiac surgical patients have a high incidence of intraoperative endotoxemia despite simultaneously exhibiting a low incidence of culture-proved bacteremia. This observation is consistent with the observation that "sterile" instruments and solutions, including intravenous

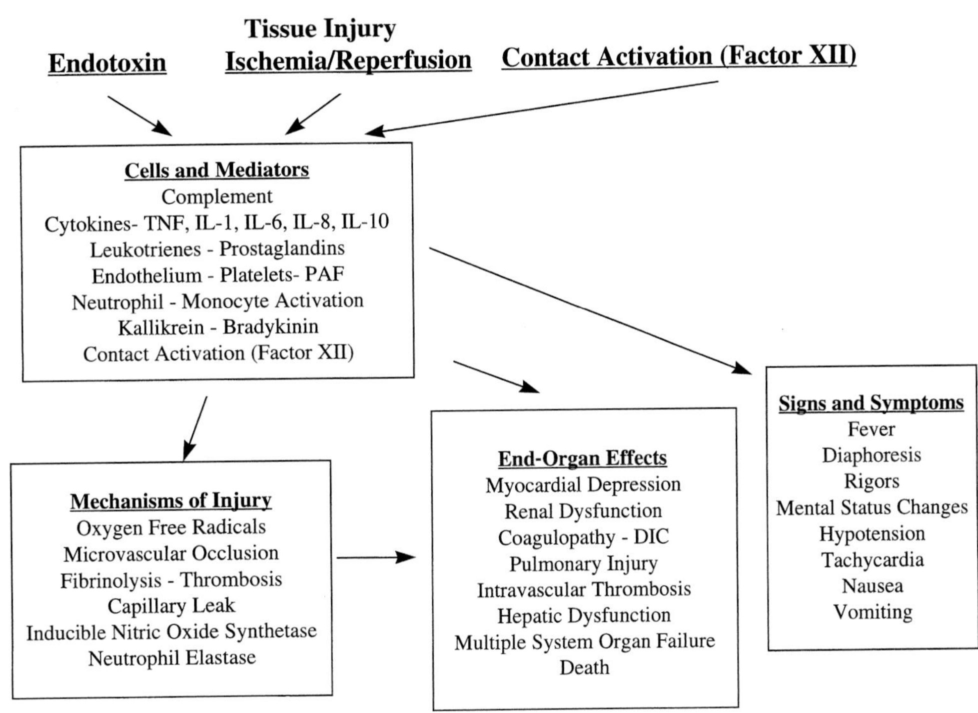

Figure 8–2 Overview of inflammation. TNF = tumor necrosis factor; IL = interleukin; PAF = platelet-activating factor; DIC = disseminated intravascular coagulation.

fluids and the CPB circuit, may be contaminated with endotoxin.[11]

SYSTEMIC INFLAMMATION AND CARDIAC SURGERY

The systemic inflammatory response following cardiac surgery is multifactorial. As described earlier, the term *SIRS* is not particularly helpful at clarifying the pathophysiology of inflammation in cardiac surgery.[9] A schematic of the inflammatory process is depicted in Figure 8–2. There does not appear to be much disagreement with the statement that all of these processes may happen and may be responsible for causing complications in cardiac surgical patients. Tissue injury, endotoxemia, and contact of blood with the foreign surface of the CPB circuit are thought to initiate a systemic inflammatory response following cardiac surgery. What is least understood and most controversial is the issue of which of these many processes is the most clinically relevant. It appears as if major surgery is an important cause of systemic inflammation and that CPB further exacerbates the elaboration of proinflammatory mediators. Various etiologies and mediators of inflammation are reviewed in the subsequent sections.

Mechanisms of Inflammation-Mediated Injury

It is not entirely clear how inflammation ultimately damages cells and organ systems. Activation of neutrophils and other leukocytes is central to most theories regarding inflammation-induced injury.[6,12-15] Neutrophil activation leads to the release of oxygen radicals, intracellular proteases, and fatty acid (e.g., arachidonic acid) metabolites. These products, as well as those from activated macrophages and platelets, can cause or exacerbate tissue injury.

In localized areas of infection, oxygen free radicals liberated by activated neutrophils aid in the destruction of pathogens.[16] Complement, in particular C5a, results in activation of leukocytes and oxygen free radical formation.[17] These activated neutrophils liberate toxic amounts of oxygen free radicals such as hydrogen peroxide, hydroxyl radicals, and superoxide anion. Oxygen free radicals are thought to cause cellular injury ultimately through damage to the lipid membrane.[18-20] Elevated levels of lipid peroxidation products (i.e., products of oxidation of membrane lipids such as malondialdehyde) are thought to reflect the severity of free radical cellular damage.[21] Consistent with this model of injury, Royston et al[22] demonstrated increased levels of peroxidation products in cardiac surgical patients. In another study, oxygen free radicals were found to be elevated in 21 patients undergoing cardiac surgery; however, the clinical relevance of these changes was not studied.[21]

A related mechanism of injury results from the degranulation of neutrophils. Activated neutrophils release granules containing myeloperoxidase, as well as other toxic digestive enzymes such as neutrophil elastase, lactoferrin, β-glucuronidase, and *N*-acetyl-β-glucosaminidase.[23-26] Release of these intracellular enzymes not only causes tissue damage but also reduces the number of cells that can participate in bacterial destruction. In one study, cardiac surgical patients who developed splanchnic hypoperfusion, a possible cause of inflammation, demonstrated increased neutrophil degranulation and increased plasma neutrophil elastase concentrations.[26]

Another mechanism of inflammation-mediated injury involves microvascular occlusion. Activation of neutrophils leads to adhesion of leukocytes to endothelium and formation of clumps of inflammatory cells as microaggregates.[14,27]

Activated leukocytes have less deformable cell membranes, which affects their ability to pass through capillaries.[28] Microaggregates can cause organ dysfunction through microvascular occlusion and a reduction in blood flow and oxygen at the local level.[22,28,29] Following the disappearance of these microaggregates and restoration of microvascular flow, reperfusion injury may occur.

Finally, activated leukocytes release leukotrienes such as leukotriene B_4. Leukotrienes are arachidonic acid metabolites generated by the lipoxygenase pathway. They markedly increase vascular permeability and are potent arteriolar vasoconstrictors. These leukotriene-mediated effects account for some of the clinical signs of systemic inflammation, in particular generalized edema as well as "third-space losses." Prostaglandins, generated from arachidonic acid via the cyclooxygenase pathway, also act as mediators of the inflammatory process.

Physiologic Mediators of Inflammation

Cytokines

Cytokines are believed to play a pivotal role in the pathophysiology of acute inflammation associated with cardiac surgery.[30,31] Cytokines are proteins released from activated macrophages, monocytes, fibroblasts, and endothelial cells that have far-reaching regulatory effects on cells.[32] They are small proteins that exert their effects by binding to specific cell surface receptors. Many of these proteins are called *interleukins* because they aid in the communication between white blood cells (leukocytes).

Cytokines are an important component of the acute-phase response to injury or infection. The acute-phase response is the host's physiologic response to tissue injury or infection and is intended to fight infection as well as contain areas of diseased or injured tissue. Cytokines mediate this attraction of immune system cells to local areas of injury or infection. They also help the host through activation of the immune system, thus providing for an improved defense against pathogens. For example, cytokines enhance the function of both B- and T-lymphocytes, thereby improving both humoral and cell-mediated immunity. Most cytokines are proinflammatory whereas others appear to exert an anti-inflammatory effect, suggesting a complex feedback system designed to limit the amount of inflammation. Excessive levels of cytokines, however, may result in an exaggerated degree of systemic inflammation, which may lead to greater secondary injury. Numerous cytokines (e.g., tumor necrosis factor [TNF], interleukin [IL]-1 to IL-16) and other protein mediators (e.g., transforming growth factors, macrophage inflammatory proteins) have been described and may play an important role in the pathogenesis of postoperative systemic inflammation. The cytokines that have received most attention related to cardiac surgery include TNF and IL-1, -1ra, -6, -8, and -10 (Box 8–2).

Tumor Necrosis Factor

TNF is one of the earliest cytokines detected in the blood following the activation of macrophages and other proinflammatory cells. One factor complicating studies of TNF relates to the fact that there are two similar forms of TNF, TNF-α and TNF-β, as well as two distinct receptors, TNFR-I and TNFR-II. TNF appears to be pivotal in initiating the complex inflammatory cascade. Endotoxin is a potent stimulus for TNF production.

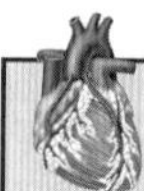

BOX 8–2 *Most Commonly Measured Biochemical Markers of Inflammation*

- Tumor necrosis factor-α
- Interleukin-6
- Interleukin-8
- C-reactive protein

Endotoxemia unequivocally results in initiation of proinflammatory pathways, most likely through stimulation of TNF.[33-36] Michie et al[33] administered endotoxin intravenously to human volunteers and detected peak levels of TNF 90 to 180 minutes later. Peak concentrations of TNF correlated with increased temperature and heart rate, as well as circulating levels of ACTH and epinephrine. In this and other studies, TNF levels soon appear following a proinflammatory stimulus and disappear quickly, which helps explain a common finding from clinical studies. TNF levels are often not elevated when measured in patients with systemic inflammation, probably because test samples are obtained long after exposure to the primary inflammatory stimulus. This issue of sampling time may partially account for the fact that some cardiac surgical studies have detected elevated TNF levels, whereas others have not.[37-53]

Interleukins

Following the appearance of TNF, levels of IL-1 increase in cardiac surgical patients.[47,50,52,54] Measured levels are low and may peak within several hours following CPB.[54] Other patients have demonstrated maximum levels 1 day following cardiac surgery, which may explain the inability of some investigators to detect IL-1 during the intraoperative period.[50] IL-1 may decrease systemic vascular resistance following CPB through induction of nitric oxide synthesis in vascular endothelial cells.[55] Although IL-1 appears to be important in the initiation and propagation of the inflammatory cascade, it is not clear whether IL-1 levels cause deleterious effects or even serve as a marker for patients who develop organ dysfunction following cardiac surgery. Some of the reported effects of IL-1 may be due instead to other cytokines, in particular TNF, which are detected at the same time.

IL-8 is also believed to be an important component of the proinflammatory cascade. It is a potent chemoattractant of neutrophils to the site of injury or infection. IL-8 is also responsible for the activation, priming, and degranulation of neutrophils.[56,57] The relevance of elevations in IL-8 levels to outcome following cardiac surgery has not been established.[42-44,46,47,51,53,58,59] Rothenburger et al observed a significant association between prolonged mechanical ventilation and postoperative IL-8 levels but not IL-6 levels.[60,61]

IL-6 levels have been shown to increase in the setting of cardiac surgery, although this is not a universal finding.[10,42,43,45-48,51-54,58,62-65] Peak levels of this cytokine appear following maximum values for TNF and IL-1. For example, Steinberg et al[54] measured plasma cytokine levels in 29 patients undergoing CPB. IL-6 levels peaked at 3 hours following separation from CPB and remained elevated 24 hours postoperatively. No association was found between IL-6 levels and hemodynamic parameters or postoperative pulmonary function.

Anti-inflammatory Cytokines

Work suggests that regulation of inflammation is complex and involves a balance between pro- and anti-inflammatory cytokines. IL-10 is a potent inhibitor of the synthesis of TNF, IL-1, IL-6, and IL-8 and increases in the perioperative period.[44,66-68] McBride et al[68] obtained blood samples perioperatively from 20 patients undergoing cardiac surgery. Prior to and during CPB, increases were observed in the proinflammatory cytokines TNF, IL-1, and IL-8. At the same time that proinflammatory cytokine levels began to decrease, increases in the anti-inflammatory cytokines IL-10 and IL-1 receptor antagonist (IL-1ra) were observed. The authors suggested that the balancing effects of these two types of cytokines may determine whether a patient has the effects of excessive systemic inflammation (e.g., postoperative organ dysfunction) or the effects of inadequate immune system enhancement (e.g., postoperative infection and poor wound healing). Use of this theory to improve outcome has not yet been translated into a clinical trial involving surgical patients. One concern related to potentially deleterious effects of inhibiting proinflammatory mediators has been borne out in sepsis trials in which mortality was increased in the group given an anti-inflammatory agent.[69] An understanding of the interaction between pro- and anti-inflammatory mediators may result in the development of an effective and safe approach to reducing complications related to excessive systemic inflammation.

Complement System

The complement system describes at least 20 plasma proteins and is involved in the chemoattraction, activation, opsonization, and lysis of cells. Complement is also involved in blood clotting, fibrinolysis, and kinin formation. These proteins are found in the plasma as well as in the interstitial spaces, mostly in the form of enzymatic precursors.

The complement cascade is illustrated in Figure 8–3. The complement cascade can be triggered by either the *classical pathway* or the *alternate pathway.* In the alternate pathway, C3 is activated by contact of complement factors B and D with complex polysaccharides, endotoxin, or exposure of blood to foreign substances such as the CPB circuit. *Contact activation* (Fig. 8–4) describes contact of blood with a foreign surface with resulting adherence of platelets and activation of factor XII (Hageman factor). Activated factor XII has numerous effects, including initiation of the coagulation cascade through factor XI and conversion of prekallikrein to kallikrein. Kallikrein leads to generation of plasmin, which is known to activate the complement as well as the fibrinolytic systems. Kallikrein generation also activates the kinin-bradykinin system.

The classical pathway involves the activation of C1 by antibody-antigen complexes. In the case of cardiac surgery, there are two likely mechanisms for the activation of the classical pathway. Endotoxin can be detected in the serum of almost all patients undergoing cardiac surgery. Endotoxin forms an antigen-antibody complex with antiendotoxin antibodies normally found in serum, which can then activate C1. The administration of protamine following separation from CPB has been reported to result in heparin/protamine complexes, which can also activate the classical pathway[70,71] (see Chapters 28 and 29). Others, however, have not observed this effect.[72] Contact activation leads to activation of factor XII, which results in the generation of plasmin. Plasmin is capable of activating complement factors C1 and C3. A summary of the physiologic effects of the complement system is presented in Table 8–2.

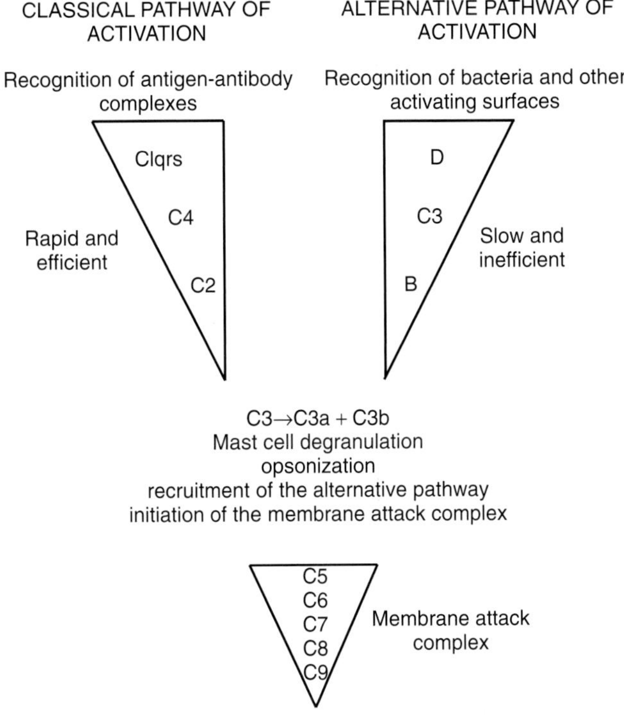

Figure 8–3 Simplified components of the complement system. (From Haynes BF, Fauci AS: Introduction to clinical immunology. *In* Braunwald E, Isselbacher KJ, Petersdorf RG, et al [eds]: Harrison's Principles of Internal Medicine, 11th edition. New York, McGraw-Hill, 1987, pp 328–337.)

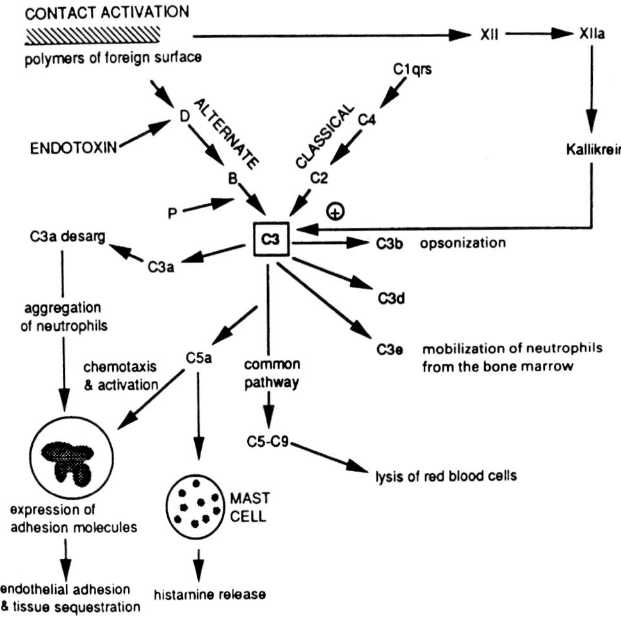

Figure 8–4 Contact activation of the complement cascade during cardiopulmonary bypass. Activation of complement occurs primarily through the alternate pathway. (From Ohri SK: The effects of cardiopulmonary bypass on the immune system. Perfusion 8:121, 1993.)

Activated C3, as well as other complement factors downstream in the cascade, has several actions. The effects of activated complement fragments on mast cells and their circulating counterparts, the basophil cells, may be relevant to

Table 8–2 Some Biologically Significant Effects of the Various Complement-Split Products

Biologic Effect	Complement-Split Products
Mast cell degranulation, contraction of smooth muscle, increased vascular permeability	C3a, C5a
Chemotaxis of neutrophils	C5a, C5a des Arg
Neutrophil aggregation	C5a, C5a des Arg
Lysosomal enzyme release	C5a, C3b
Leukocytosis	C3e
Immune adherence	C3b, C4b
Membrane lysis	C5b-9 (membrane attack complex)

From Knudsen F, Anderson LW: Immunological aspects of cardiopulmonary bypass. J Cardiothorac Anesth 4:245, 1990.

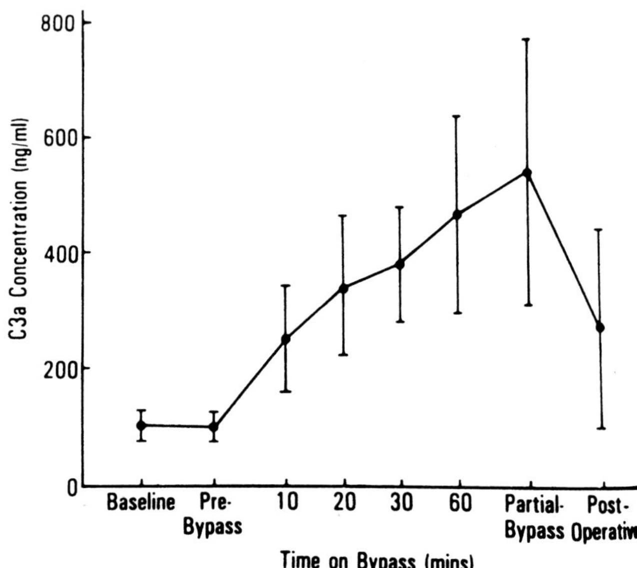

Figure 8–5 Plasma levels of C3a in patients undergoing cardiopulmonary bypass. Levels were unaffected by routine surgical procedures (prebypass) but displayed a time-dependent elevation during cardiopulmonary bypass. Postoperative levels remained elevated. Each point represents the mean (±SD) of observations in 15 patients. (From Chenowith DE, Cooper SW, Hugli TE, et al: Complement activation during cardiopulmonary bypass: Evidence for generation of C3a and C5a anaphylatoxins. N Engl J Med 304:497, 1981. Copyright 1981 Massachusetts Medical Society. All rights reserved.)

the development of postoperative complications potentially attributable to complement activation. Fragments C3a and C5a (also called "anaphylatoxins") lead to the release of numerous mediators, including histamine, leukotriene B_4, platelet-activating factor, prostaglandins, thromboxanes, and TNF. These mediators, when released from mast cells, result in endothelial leak, interstitial edema, and elevated tissue blood flow. Complement factors such as C5a and C3b complexed to microbes stimulate macrophages to secrete inflammatory mediators such as TNF. C3b activates neutrophils and macrophages and enhances their ability to phagocytose bacteria. The lytic complex or membrane attack complex, composed of complement factors C5b, C6, C7, C8, and C9, is capable of directly lysing cells. Activated complement factors make invading cells "sticky" such that they bind to one another (i.e., agglutinate). The complement-mediated processes of capillary dilation, leakage of plasma proteins and fluid, and accumulation and activation of neutrophils make up part of the acute inflammatory response.

Although some elements of complement activation have been elucidated, the clinical relevance of this process to patients undergoing cardiac surgery has only been learned recently. Several studies have reported elevated complement levels during cardiac surgery.[38,58,73-78] Chenoweth et al[73] measured plasma C3a and C5a levels at different time points in 15 adults undergoing cardiac surgery with CPB. While C3a levels were not affected by surgical stimulation, complement activation increased significantly during CPB (Fig. 8–5). This and other studies did not test the association between elevated complement levels and adverse postoperative outcome. Thus, they do not provide any evidence that complement activation causes clinically significant systemic inflammation. Kirklin et al[75] measured plasma C3a levels in 116 patients undergoing cardiac surgery with CPB and 12 patients undergoing operations without CPB. In this study, an elevation of complement activation during CPB was associated with postoperative morbidity. Patients undergoing procedures without CPB did not demonstrate elevations in complement. This result suggests that a factor unique to CPB causes activation of complement. This study, however, does not pinpoint the clinical relevance of complement activation or of the CPB circuit, in part because even patients without postoperative morbidity had elevated complement levels. Furthermore, confounding factors capable of causing SIRS, such as endotoxin, were not measured and accounted for in this study (see Chapter 28).

The results from several large randomized clinical trials in which complement activation was selectively blocked have become available.[79-81] These studies indicate that attenuation of complement activation results in less myocardial injury; however, there did not appear to be an impact on complications such as pulmonary and renal dysfunction and severe vasodilation. These results suggest that complement activation may not play as large a role in the development of systemic inflammation–mediated morbidity as previously thought. These trials are discussed in more detail later in this chapter.

Endotoxin

Endotoxin, also called lipopolysaccharide (LPS), is a component of the cell membrane of gram-negative bacteria. It is a potent activator of complement and cytokines and appears to be one of the initial triggers of systemic inflammation[12,82-84] (see Fig. 8–2). Although the LPS constituent varies from one bacterial species to another, it may be generally described with reference to Figure 8–6 as consisting of three structural regions: (1) lipid A, (2) core, and (3) *O*-polysaccharide outer region. The lipid region of lipid A is embedded in the outer leaflet of the outer membrane. The oligosaccharide core region is positioned between lipid A and the *O*-polysaccharide outer region. Lipid A has the same basic structure in practically all gram-negative bacteria and is the toxic component of endotoxin. The LPS core region shows a high degree of similarity among various bacteria. It usually consists of a limited number of sugars. For example, the inner core region is

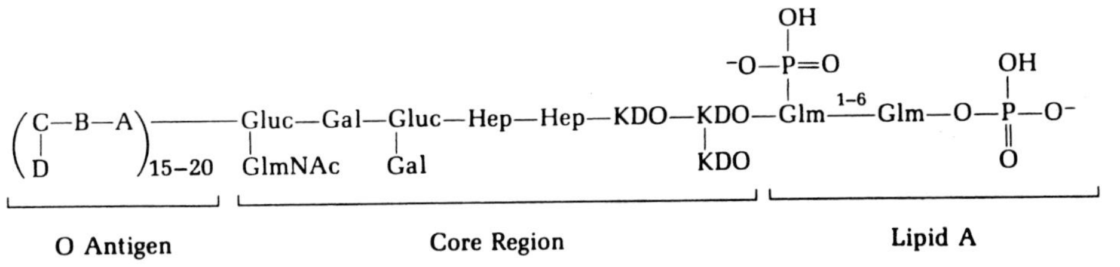

Figure 8–6 Schematic structure of one unit of *Salmonella* cell wall lipopolysaccharide (LPS) (endotoxin). The structure of the cell wall LPS may vary slightly from one genus of gram-negative organism to another, but as far as is known, all contain three general regions, as shown. Although not shown here, all free hydroxyl groups of the glucosamines in lipid A are esterified with fatty acids. The serologic differences between different strains within a genus lie in the kinds of sugars and their linkages that exist in the O-antigen region. (From Volk WA, Benjamin DC, Kadner RJ, Parsons JT [eds]: Essentials of Medical Microbiology, 3rd edition. Philadelphia, JB Lippincott, 1986, p 399.)

(C—B—A / D)15–20 —Gluc—Gal—Gluc—Hep—Hep—KDO—KDO—Glm —1–6— Glm—O—P(OH)(=O)—O⁻

(Branches: Gluc–GlmNAc; Gluc–Gal; KDO–KDO; first Glm–O–P(OH)(=O)–O⁻)

O Antigen | Core Region | Lipid A

Glm —Glucosamine
KDO —Ketodeoxyoctonic acid
Hep —Heptose
Gluc —Glucose
Gal —Galactose
GlmNAc—N-acetyl glucosamine
A,B,C,D —Monosaccharides such as mannose, galactose, rhamnose, fructose, glucose, abequose, and colitose. These sugars exist in a repeating sequence of 15 to 20 units of 3 or 4 sugars.

constituted of heptose and 3-deoxy-D-*manno*-2-octulosonate (KDO) residues; whereas the outer core region comprises galactose, glucose, or *N*-acetyl-D-glucosamine residues displayed in various manners depending upon the strain. The O-polysaccharide outer region (also called O-specific antigen or O-specific side chain) is highly variable and is composed of one or more oligosaccharide repeating units characteristic of the serotype.

ENDOTOXEMIA

Endotoxemia refers to the presence of endotoxin in the blood. Endotoxemia is common in cardiac surgical patients.[10,11,38,41,60,64,65,85-95] It is not surprising that some investigators have failed to detect endotoxemia during cardiac surgery given its transient and intermittent nature, although differences in endotoxin-assaying techniques used may also contribute to this discrepancy.[51,52,96,97] Andersen et al[11] measured circulating endotoxin levels in 10 patients undergoing cardiac surgery. All preoperative blood samples were free of endotoxin; however, substantial levels of endotoxin were detected intraoperatively. Blood endotoxin levels from eight typical patients undergoing cardiac surgery are presented[85] (Fig. 8–7). Although endotoxin can be found in sterile fluids administered to patients, it is believed that the majority of endotoxin arises through a patient's impaired gut barrier.[11] Rothenburger et al[60] studied the association of endotoxin levels with prolonged mechanical ventilation in 78 cardiac surgical patients. Endotoxin levels were three times higher in patients with a postoperative mechanical ventilation time longer than 24 hours (n = 13) than in patients with a ventilator time of less than 24 hours.

Normally, intestinal flora contain a large amount of endotoxin from gram-negative microorganisms.[98] The average human colon contains approximately 25 billion ng of endotoxin, which is an enormous quantity when 300 ng of endotoxin is considered toxic to humans.[33,34] The leakage of live bacterial cells into the bloodstream can result in infection as these viable bacteria multiply.[99] However, many of the bacteria in the intestine are dead, and thus endotoxin can also enter the bloodstream contained within cell membrane fragments of dead bacteria. In this case, infection per se does not develop.

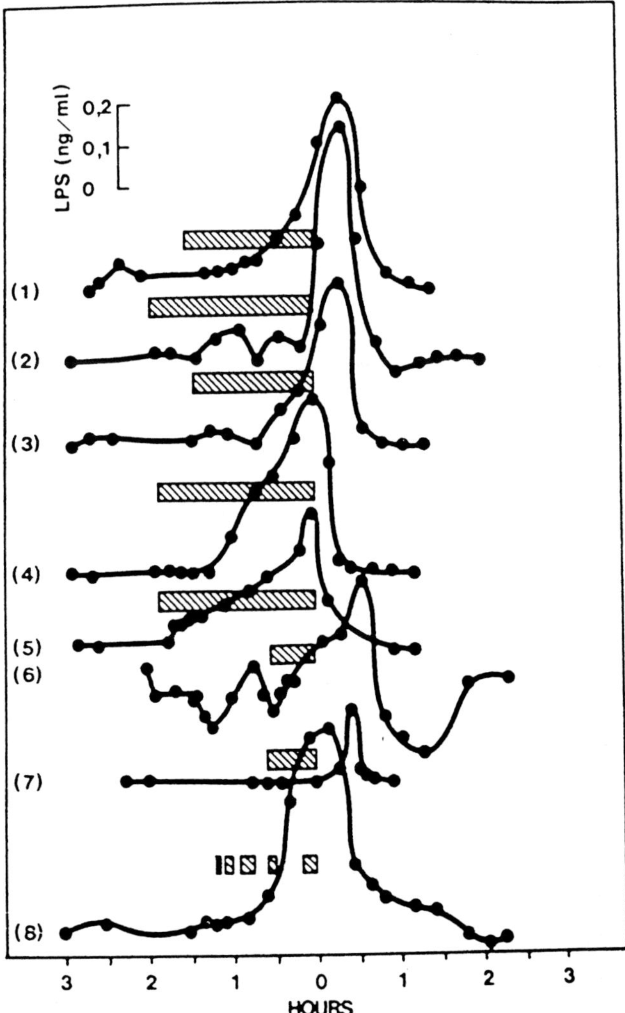

Figure 8–7 Time course of plasma lipopolysaccharide (LPS) concentrations during cardiopulmonary bypass procedures for patients 1-8. *Hatched boxes* indicate the period of aortic crossclamping. For clarity, records were offset and aligned at the time of removal of the aortic clamp. (From Rocke DA, Gaffin SL, Wells MT, et al: Endotoxemia associated with cardiopulmonary bypass. J Thorac Cardiovasc Surg 93:832, 1987.)

Instead, endotoxin may initiate a systemic inflammatory response through potent activation of macrophages and other proinflammatory cells.[100] A plasma endotoxin concentration of only 1 ng/mL has been reported to be lethal in humans.[101]

Upon entry into the bloodstream, endotoxin forms complexes with numerous intravascular compounds including high-density lipoprotein, lipopolysaccharide-binding protein, and endotoxin-specific immunoglobulins. Endotoxin has been linked to dysfunction in every organ system of the body and may be the key initiating factor in the development of systemic inflammation.[12,82-84,93]

Normal Host Defenses Against Endotoxemia

Early Tolerance

If endotoxemia is deleterious to patients, it would be logical to assume that patients have defense mechanisms against this ubiquitous toxin. Tolerance to endotoxin was studied extensively by Greisman and Hornick more than three decades ago.[102] Two distinct types of tolerance to endotoxin exist and are classified as *early tolerance* and *late tolerance.*[102] Early tolerance to endotoxin represents a reduction in the proinflammatory effects of LPS when administered several hours following a prior infusion of LPS.[103] It appears to be due to an LPS-induced refractory state of macrophages in which they release less TNF in response to endotoxin. This early refractive state shows no LPS specificity and can be overcome with increased doses of endotoxin. The degree of this tolerance is directly proportional to the dose and, hence, intensity of the initial LPS-induced inflammatory state. Early tolerance begins within hours of LPS exposure and decreases almost to baseline within 2 days. It cannot be transferred with plasma. Early tolerance may protect the host from lethal systemic inflammation following an overwhelming exposure of LPS.

Late Tolerance

Late tolerance to endotoxin is due to the synthesis of immunoglobulins, that is, antibodies, directed against the offending LPS.[102] Late tolerance begins approximately 72 hours following exposure to LPS, which correlates with the appearance of the early-appearing IgM class of antibodies. This form of tolerance persists for at least 2 weeks and correlates with the presence of serum immunoglobulins. In contrast to early tolerance, the late response is not proportional to the intensity of the initial LPS-induced inflammatory response but is related to the immunogenicity of the initial LPS. Furthermore, late tolerance does not generally protect against a subsequent challenge with a dissimilar type of LPS. In other words, late tolerance is most pronounced when the same (i.e., homologous) LPS serotype is used for both the initial and the subsequent challenge. It is not definitively understood how antiendotoxin antibodies responsible for late tolerance confer protection from LPS-induced systemic inflammation. Proposed mechanisms include increased clearance of endotoxin into the reticuloendothelial system and direct neutralization through binding.

Understanding of the host's normal humoral defense against endotoxin is further complicated owing to the numerous serotypes of endotoxin.[98] Serotype-specific antibodies, antibodies synthesized in response to a particular LPS, exhibit high-affinity binding to and protection from the specific serotype of endotoxin. These serotype, that is, O-specific, antiendotoxin antibodies, however, do not recognize the many possible variations of endotoxin *O*-polysaccharide side chains and thus are ineffective at conferring protection against the numerous serotypes of endotoxin likely to be encountered in the clinical setting. Antibodies, however, directed against the well-conserved inner core structure of endotoxin should theoretically be cross-reactive against many clinically relevant serotypes of endotoxin. Cardiac surgical patients are exposed to a wide variety of endotoxin types. For example, at least 164 O-antigens exist for *Escherichia coli,* the gram-negative bacteria most commonly isolated in high-risk surgical and intensive care unit patients.[104,105]

Antiendotoxin Antibodies

There is a growing body of evidence that suggests that antibodies to endotoxin may be an important determinant of adverse outcome following cardiac surgery. According to this theory, the presence of protective antiendotoxin antibodies *preoperatively* reduces the incidence of complications caused by LPS-induced systemic inflammation. Only antibodies that are present preoperatively can buffer the effects of perioperative endotoxemia, because a minimum of 72 hours is required for the synthesis of new antibodies following exposure to endotoxin encountered during surgery. It is also known that CPB results in denaturation of antibodies, which decreases the number of protective antibodies even further.[106,107] Moreover, there is evidence that antibody production by B-lymphocytes (plasma cells) is depressed following cardiac surgery, which reduces the effectiveness of the humoral immune response to toxins encountered during surgery.[108]

Measurement of Antiendotoxin Antibodies Before Surgery

An early study measured the preoperative presence or absence of antibodies to endotoxin in 86 cardiac surgery patients.[109] A lower incidence of fever and infections was observed in the 30 patients with the preoperative presence of antiendotoxin antibody. This study did not quantitate antiendotoxin antibodies, measure total immunoglobulins, assign risk scores to patients preoperatively, or comment on postoperative length of stay or other complications. Nevertheless, this study's results suggest that antiendotoxin-based humoral immunity is clinically relevant.

A specific type of antibody directed toward the core structure of endotoxin has been described.[110,111] These antiendotoxin-core antibodies (EndoCAb) can be measured using an enzyme-linked immunosorbent assay (ELISA), which measures antibody binding to incomplete core rough mutant LPS.[110] The serum concentration of these antibodies demonstrates marked variability. Measurement of EndoCAb in more than 1000 human volunteer blood donors demonstrated some subjects having 300-fold higher concentrations than others.[111] The reason or reasons for this variability in levels are unknown but may be due to differences in intestinal flora or to genetic differences in the ability to synthesize these antibodies. These antibodies appear to have different binding characteristics and cross-reaction against different forms of LPS from antibodies measured by other investigators.[111,112] Their binding characteristics are different from antibodies induced by vaccination with lipid A, Re chemotype LPS, as well as the extensively studied Rc-like J5 rough mutant LPS of *Escherichia coli.*[110,112-114] These other "antiendotoxin" antibodies may in fact have limited cross-reactivity, which may explain their inability to provide protection consistently in vitro or in animal and human trials.[112,114-119]

Further confirmation for the clinical relevance of EndoCAb levels comes from a study by Hamilton-Davies et al.[120] Serum levels of EndoCAb were measured preoperatively in a study of 58 European patients undergoing first-time cardiac valve replacement. In this study, low preoperative serum IgM EndoCAb levels were associated with postoperative complications. A limitation of this and other observational studies relates to the possibility that low levels of antiendotoxin antibodies may not be a cause of poor outcome but merely a marker for sicker patients with higher operative risk and poorer general immunity.

A subsequently performed study minimized this possibility by using a validated preoperative risk scoring system to quantify degree of risk in addition to measuring total immunoglobulin levels.[121] In this prospective blind cohort study, Bennett-Guerrero et al measured preoperative levels of serum EndoCAb and total immunoglobulins in 301 patients undergoing CABG, valvular heart surgery, or both. Known preoperative risk factors were collected and patients were assigned a risk score using a validated method. Major complications, defined as either in-hospital death or significantly prolonged postoperative hospital length of stay, occurred in 34 patients (11.3%). All complications were potentially attributable to the toxic effects of endotoxemia, such as pulmonary and renal dysfunction.[11,83,122] Lower IgM EndoCAb level independently predicted increased risk of major complication over and above the effects of preoperative risk score, total immunoglobulin level, and all other known preoperative risk factors (Fig. 8–8). In contrast, total IgM concentration did not predict outcome, and no association existed between risk score and level of IgM EndoCAb. This study demonstrated that there is marked preoperative variability in humoral immunity against endotoxin-core antibody, which is not accounted for by differences in known preoperative risk factors. Furthermore, low levels of antiendotoxin-core antibody were an important independent predictor of adverse postoperative outcome, which supports the theory that endotoxin-mediated systemic inflammation is an important cause of postoperative complications.

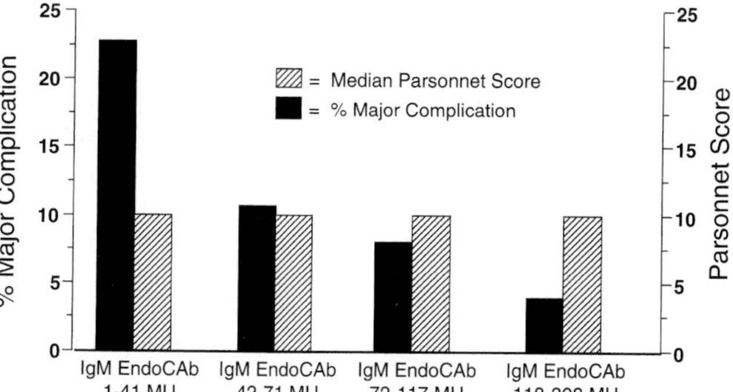

Figure 8–8 Relationship between preoperative immunoglobulin M (IgM) antiendotoxin-core antibodies (EndoCAb) levels by quartile (in median units [MU]) and Parsonnet preoperative risk score *(hatched bars)* or percentage of patients having a major complication *(solid bars)*. Median Parsonnet risk score in each of the IgM EndoCAb quartiles is the same, which illustrates the lack of correlation between IgM EndoCAb level and risk score. (From Bennett-Guerrero E, Ayuso L, Hamilton-Davies C, et al: Relationship of preoperative antiendotoxin core antibodies and adverse outcomes following cardiac surgery. JAMA 277:646, 1997.)

Mathew et al[123] reported an association between lower preoperative IgM EndoCAb levels and a greater incidence and severity of postoperative cognitive decline at 6 weeks postoperatively in 460 patients undergoing elective CABG. The mechanism underlying this association is not clear; however, there is increasing evidence that systemic inflammation plays a role in neurologic injury during surgery.

Criticisms of Endotoxin as an Etiologic Factor

There are several criticisms of the theory that endotoxemia is an important cause of postoperative morbidity. A common criticism relates to the low incidence of culture-proved bacteremia in surgical and intensive care unit patients.[124-127] Endotoxemia, however, is clearly prevalent in these patients and usually exists in the setting of negative blood cultures.[10,11,24,38,41,64,65,85-95] In fact, studies attempting to detect endotoxemia probably underestimate its incidence given its intermittent nature.

The failure of two anti–lipid A monoclonal antibodies (HA-1A, Centocor, Malvern, PA; and E5, Xoma, Berkeley, CA) to improve outcome on an "intention-to-treat" basis in intensive care unit patients with established sepsis has also been used to suggest that endotoxemia is not clinically relevant.[117,118] These monoclonal antibodies, however, were tested in patients with established sepsis and organ failure, which is an entirely different setting from elective surgical patients, who are more likely to benefit from prophylaxis with endotoxin-neutralizing drugs. There is also evidence suggesting that these anti–lipid A monoclonal antibodies may not bind to endotoxin with high affinity, which may explain, in part, their lack of demonstrable efficacy.[115] Results from controlled studies in which endotoxin is selectively neutralized are to ascertain the clinical relevance of endotoxemia in cardiac surgery.

SPLANCHNIC PERFUSION

Splanchnic hypoperfusion appears to be an important cause of systemic inflammation.[128-131] The gut is one of the most susceptible organs to hypoperfusion during conditions of trauma or stress.[131-133] In the 1960s, Price et al[132] removed 15% of the blood volume from healthy volunteers, causing a 40% reduction in splanchnic blood volume. In this study, cardiac output (CO), blood pressure (BP), and heart rate (HR) did not change from baseline. In a study conducted in the 1990s by Hamilton-Davies et al,[134] 25% of the blood volume was removed from six healthy volunteers. Gastric mucosal perfusion, as measured by saline tonometry, was the first variable to decline (in five of the six subjects). Stroke volume (SV) also decreased; however, routinely measured cardiovascular variables such as HR, BP, and CO did not change significantly from baseline values to cause suspicion of a hypovolemic state. Based on these types of studies, the advanced trauma life support (ATLS) course teaches that a 15% blood loss (class I hemorrhage) rarely results in changes in HR, BP, or urine output.[135] Significant decreases in systolic blood pressure are a late sign of shock, which typically occurs after class III hemorrhage (30% to 40% blood loss).

These studies suggest that during periods of hypovolemia, the gut vasoconstricts, thus shunting blood toward "more vital organs" such as the heart and brain.[131-133] In addition to hypovolemia, endogenously released vasoconstrictors during CPB, such as angiotensin II, thromboxane A_2, and vasopressin, may also result in decreased splanchnic perfusion.[136-139] Vasoconstrictors such as phenylephrine are routinely administered by anesthesiologists and perfusionists to increase BP and are likely to further reduce gut perfusion. Oudemans-van Straaten et al[89] measured intestinal permeability and endotoxin levels in 23 patients during cardiac surgery. Intestinal leak was measured by the amount of orally administered cellobiose present in the patients' urine. Intestinal permeability increased during surgery and correlated with circulating endotoxin levels. Administration of ephedrine, low central venous pressures, and reduced fluid balance during surgery were also associated with intestinal permeability, confirming the theory that gut perfusion is reduced by vasoconstrictors as well as hypovolemia. There is also evidence that systemic endotoxemia may worsen intestinal permeability, thus exacerbating splanchnic hypoperfusion and initiating a vicious circle.[140]

Gastric Tonometry

A Food and Drug Administration–approved monitor (the gastrointestinal tonometer) exists that can detect gut hypoperfusion.[141] The tonometer is a naso/orogastric tube that has been modified to include a silicone balloon into which air or saline is introduced (Trip Catheter; Datex-Engstrom, Tewksbury, MA) (Fig. 8–9). The gastric mucosal bed is similar to the overall splanchnic mucosa in its propensity to become hypoperfused during periods of physiologic stress. Hypoperfused areas of tissue develop regional hypercapnia (elevated P_{CO_2}), which diffuses into the tonometer balloon allowing for an indirect measurement of gastric mucosal P_{CO_2}. Hypoperfusion is manifested by a positive gap (gastric mucosal P_{CO_2} > arterial P_{CO_2}) between the gastric mucosal P_{CO_2} and the arterial P_{CO_2}. A gap greater than 8 to 10 mm Hg is considered by many investigators to reflect splanchnic hypoperfusion.[141] In theory, any gap is abnormal; however, the use of a higher cutoff value appears to improve the specificity of this monitor without significantly decreasing its sensitivity. There is no agreement yet as to exactly what magnitude of P_{CO_2} gap is "abnormal" or if this continuous measurement should be converted into a categoric outcome (i.e., abnormal versus normal).

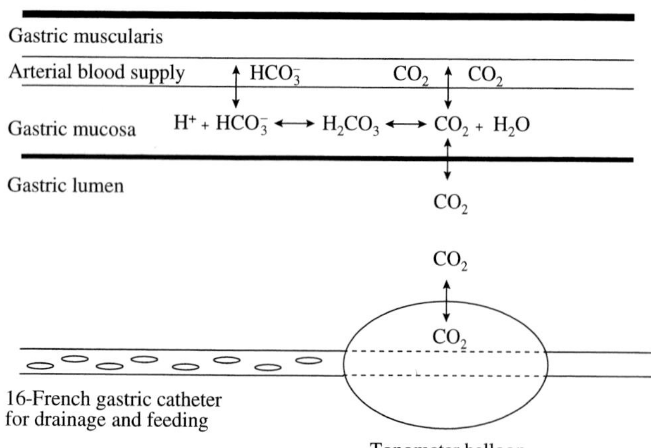

Figure 8–9 Diagram of operation of gastric tonometer in gastric lumen. Tonometer balloon is filled with either saline solution or air. Protons (H^+) are generated in the gastric mucosa from anaerobic metabolism (tissue acidosis). Protons then combine with bicarbonate (HCO_3^-) to form carbonic acid (H_2CO_3), which dissociates into carbon dioxide (CO_2) and water (H_2O). Carbon dioxide diffuses freely into the gastric lumen and tonometer balloon.

An alternative method, used exclusively in initial studies, involves the calculation of the gastric mucosal pH (pH_i). The pH_i is derived from a modified Henderson-Hasselbalch equation containing the arterial bicarbonate concentration and the gastric mucosal P_{CO_2}. Some have argued correctly that the calculation of pH_i is not specific for splanchnic pathology. An abnormal value (i.e., low pH_i) is obtained in patients with metabolic acidosis but without gut ischemia, such as in patients with diabetic ketoacidosis or bicarbonate wasting secondary to ultrafiltration during CPB.

Gastric Mucosal Hypoperfusion During Cardiac Surgery

Gut hypoperfusion can progress to ischemia, which may result in complications that take place many hours and days following an episode of hypovolemia.[99] Many of the complications seen following major surgery are consistent with a toxic exposure to endotoxemia, which presumably arises from translocation through an impaired gut mucosa.[89,128-130,142]

Several studies have observed a high incidence of splanchnic hypoperfusion during cardiac surgery, with some showing an association between abnormal gut perfusion during cardiac surgery and postoperative complications.[10,87,88,143-146] Fiddian-Green and Baker[143] used saline tonometry to measure gastric mucosal perfusion in 85 cardiac surgical patients. Half (49%) of these patients developed evidence of abnormal perfusion, and all serious postoperative complications (eight patients, including five deaths) developed in this group. Gastric tonometry was shown in this and in two other studies to be a more sensitive predictor of adverse postoperative outcome compared with more routinely used global measures such as CO, BP, HR, and urine output.[144,146]

A new version of tonometry involves the introduction of air instead of saline into the tonometer's balloon. Following a brief period of equilibration (<15 minutes), air in the balloon is assayed for P_{CO_2} by the infrared analyzer that accompanies the monitor (Tonocap; Datex-Engstrom, Tewksbury, MA). This new method allows for the determination of gastric mucosal P_{CO_2} every 5 minutes and is more likely to be used in clinical practice. A series using air tonometry demonstrated an elevated gastric mucosal P_{CO_2} in 52% of cardiac surgical patients. Thirty-five percent of these patients with abnormal perfusion developed postoperative complications, in contrast to 5% in the group without evidence of hypoperfusion.[146]

Studies that have failed to demonstrate an association between splanchnic hypoperfusion and adverse postoperative outcome are limited in part by small sample size, insensitive measures of postoperative morbidity, and deviation from validated methodology of tonometry.[87,88] Tonometric measurements of gastric mucosal perfusion during hypothermic CPB have not been validated in terms of their ability to predict postoperative morbidity.

Gastric Mucosal Hypoperfusion: Marker or Cause of Adverse Outcome?

It is unclear if splanchnic hypoperfusion is a cause of postoperative complications (possibly through translocation of endotoxin) or simply a marker for patients who have adverse outcomes through some other undetermined mechanism. There is a growing body of evidence that suggests that a causal relationship exists. Several studies have demonstrated an association between splanchnic hypoperfusion or gut permeability and systemic endotoxemia, a recognized trigger of systemic inflammation.[89,147]

A causal role is also suggested by a study involving perioperative fluid optimization.[145] Mythen and Webb hypothesized that inadequate intravascular blood volume is the most common cause of gastric mucosal hypoperfusion. The objective of their study was to avoid any hypovolemia during the intraoperative period. Patients undergoing cardiac surgery who had a left ventricular ejection fraction greater than 40% were randomized to either a control group or to a protocol group in which, in addition to routine fluid administration, 200-mL boluses of fluid were administered before and after CPB to achieve a peak stroke volume as determined by a standard esophageal Doppler technique. Gastric mucosal perfusion was measured in all patients using standard saline tonometry but was blinded and not used as a trigger for fluid therapy. Patients in the group who were fluid loaded had a lower incidence of gastric mucosal hypoperfusion (7% versus 56%). Consistent with this result, fewer patients in the protocol group had postoperative complications (0 versus 6) and mean hospital stay (days) was lower in the protocol group (6.4 versus 10.1). These results suggest that splanchnic hypoperfusion and complications can be reduced by the use of a simple low-risk strategy. Larger versions of this study are under way with the aim of confirming these encouraging findings.

POSTOPERATIVE COMPLICATIONS ATTRIBUTABLE TO INFLAMMATION

Types of Complications

Many postoperative complications appear to be caused by an exaggerated systemic proinflammatory response to surgical trauma. A common misunderstanding relates to the types of postoperative complications that may be attributable to systemic inflammation and, in particular, splanchnic hypoperfusion. Many of the complications that are thought to be linked to splanchnic hypoperfusion do not involve the gastrointestinal system. Because splanchnic hypoperfusion may cause injury through endotoxemia and resulting systemic inflammation, it would be expected that every organ system of the body would be potentially involved.[148] Endotoxin has been reported to have adverse effects on the pulmonary, renal, cardiac, and vascular systems.[41,46,83,84,122,149-151] Endotoxin affects the coagulation system and may be both antihemostatic, potentially explaining bleeding, and prothrombotic.[83,122,152] Prothrombotic effects may account for some cases of postoperative stroke, deep venous thrombosis, and pulmonary emboli. There is also circumstantial evidence that systemic inflammation may worsen neurologic injury.[153] Activation of inflammatory cascades has been shown to worsen neurologic injury in numerous animal models (see Chapter 35).

Infections are common following cardiac surgery and increase hospital length of stay and cost.[125,154,155] Infecting bacteria may arise from translocation across the patient's gastrointestinal tract.[125,128,130] Surgical wounds (sternum and lower extremity) and the respiratory tract are common sources of postoperative infection.[156] Infections of prosthetic heart valves are less common but represent a devastating complication.[157] Infections are probably not caused by the direct effects of endotoxin and inflammation but instead occur through secondary effects on host immunity.[158]

Widespread activation of the complement system results in depletion of complement factors, which are crucial to the effective opsonization of bacterial pathogens.[159,160] Systemic activation and degranulation of neutrophils render these cells less capable of destroying bacteria via phagocytosis. CPB leads to reductions in immunoglobulin levels through denaturation of these and other proteins.[106,107,160-162] Antibody production by B-lymphocytes (plasma cells) is depressed following cardiac surgery.[108] Cell-mediated immunity, revealed by decreased T-lymphocyte function, appears to be impaired following cardiac surgery.[163] Thus, reduced antibody levels and reduced B- and T-cell function in the post-CPB period may lead to increased infection rates following cardiac surgery.

Incidence of Complications

The "low" mortality rate following cardiac surgery has also been cited as evidence that splanchnic hypoperfusion, endotoxemia, and systemic inflammation only result in "rare" complications. As discussed earlier, it is clear that mortality and morbidity are still significant problems after cardiac surgery.[1,3,164] In addition, many studies only report frank organ failures or catastrophes and do not take into account less severe forms of organ dysfunction, which do not lead to admission to an intensive care unit but nevertheless cause suffering and increase hospital length of stay.

For example, a series by Huddy et al[165] of 4473 cases involving CPB demonstrated a very low incidence (0.78%) of "gastrointestinal complications." In a series of 3129 patients, Christenson et al[166] reported an incidence of 2.3% for major gastrointestinal complications following CABG. The low incidence of major gastrointestinal complications (e.g., perforation, necrotic bowel, major gastrointestinal bleed) is often used to call into question the clinical relevance of splanchnic hypoperfusion. There is growing evidence, however, that less severe forms of splanchnic dysfunction (e.g., ileus, nausea, anorexia, and abdominal distention) are clinically relevant and increase hospital length of stay.

Some series of postoperative complications have broadened their scope. In a series of 572 patients, Corwin et al[167] reported the incidence of renal failure requiring dialysis (1%) as well as the incidence of renal dysfunction not requiring dialysis (6.3%). This study demonstrates that organ dysfunction is common following surgery, despite a low incidence of organ failure.

Similarly, the incidence of acute respiratory distress syndrome (ARDS) following cardiac surgery has been reported to be very low (<2%) in several series.[168,169] The incidence, however, of less severe pulmonary dysfunction appears to be much higher, with as many as 7% of patients requiring supplemental oxygen 11 days following surgery.[170] Furthermore, a high incidence of postoperative pulmonary dysfunction, as measured by diagnostic tests, gives further support to the hypothesis that many patients have abnormal pulmonary physiology potentially attributable to systemic inflammation.[171-173]

Potential Therapies for the Prevention of Inflammation-Related Complications

Numerous strategies and pharmacologic agents have been postulated to reduce the severity and incidence of systemic inflammation. Many studies have demonstrated reductions in intermediate end-points, such as laboratory indices of

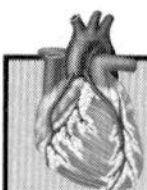

BOX 8–3 *Previously Studied Interventions*

- Steroids
- Cardiopulmonary bypass technique
- Complement inhibition
- Ultrafiltration
- Leukocyte depletion
- Aprotinin administration
- Endotoxin immune-related strategies
- E5564
- Pentoxifylline
- Anesthetic agents
- Selective digestive decontamination

complement activation and cytokinemia. Most of these studies, however, have been too small to detect improvements in clinically meaningful postoperative outcomes. On the other hand, there are studies that show an improvement in outcome using an intervention that is postulated to reduce inflammation but do not actually document that there is less systemic inflammation in the treated group. It cannot be determined whether the better outcome was attributable to reduced inflammation or some other potential mechanism. At the present time, there are no therapies in widespread clinical use for the prevention or treatment of organ dysfunction resulting from systemic inflammation, although several approaches are discussed (Box 8–3).

Steroid Administration

Several attempts have been made to prevent elevations in proinflammatory cytokines and complement activation during cardiac surgery with steroid administration.[37,86,174-182] In a randomized double-blind study of 25 cardiac surgical patients, dexamethasone administration (1 mg/kg on induction of anesthesia) prevented increases in TNF as well as reduced postoperative hyperthermia and hypotension.[175] There was a trend toward improved outcome in the treatment group, but the small sample size prevented any conclusions from being drawn regarding clinically relevant outcomes.

Inaba et al[176] randomized 17 patients undergoing cardiac surgery to placebo or methylprednisolone 30 mg/kg given immediately prior to the initiation of CPB. In this study, glucocorticoid administration minimized intraoperative elevations in both plasma endotoxin and IL-6 levels, but no improvement in postoperative outcome was reported.

Cavarocchi et al[174] randomized 91 patients undergoing CPB to bubble oxygenator without methylprednisolone (group 1), bubble oxygenator with 30 mg/kg methylprednisolone (group 2), or membrane oxygenator (group 3). C3a levels increased in all three groups during CPB but were higher in group 1 than in the other two groups. This study suggests that complement activation may be reduced by specific medical interventions (see Chapter 28). Andersen et al[86] randomized 16 patients to receive, at induction of anesthesia, either methylprednisolone (30 mg/kg) or placebo. This study demonstrated a reduction of complement activation in the protocol group.

Randomized clinical trials by Chaney et al[183,184] evaluated the effects of methylprednisolone (30 mg/kg) or placebo in cardiac surgical patients. Patients randomized to the steroid groups exhibited statistically significantly prolonged extubation times and received more vasoconstrictors. The investigators also observed significantly more hyperglycemia in the postoperative period in the methylprednisolone-treated patients. The overall data suggest that steroids are probably of limited benefit and may in fact be harmful.

Role of Cardiopulmonary Bypass Technique

Although heparin-coated circuits have many theoretic advantages, there is little evidence that their use during cardiac surgery results in fewer clinically significant adverse complications. Steinberg et al[54] found no difference in cytokine levels or markers of complement activation between patients randomized to a heparin-coated circuit and those randomized to a traditional circuit. Boroweic et al,[25] however, observed lower levels of myeloperoxidase and lactoferrin (markers of inflammation) in patients undergoing CPB with a heparin-coated circuit. Other investigators have reported reduced plasma levels of cytokines, neutrophil proteases, or both in patients subjected to CPB using heparin-coated circuits, but no improvement in outcome was observed in these small studies[23,53,185,186] (see Chapter 28).

Centrifugal vortex blood pumping has been shown to result in reduced complement and neutrophil activation as well as reduced hemolysis during cardiac surgery compared with standard roller blood pumping.[187,188] Centrifugal vortex blood pumping, however, did not significantly prevent increases in cytokines in 17 pediatric patients randomized to this bypass technique.[58]

A randomized study of 15 patients suggested that pulsatile flow CPB may result in less endotoxemia than CPB involving nonpulsatile flow.[94] Levine et al[139] randomized 20 patients to pulsatile versus nonpulsatile flow and observed a less marked increase in vasopressin levels (an endogenous vasoconstrictor) in patients perfused with pulsatile flow. Taylor et al[136] demonstrated increased levels of the endogenously produced vasoconstrictor angiotensin II in patients (total N = 24) randomized to nonpulsatile flow CPB compared with pulsatile flow. Watkins et al[138] observed fewer marked alterations in thromboxane B_2 and prostacyclin levels in patients (total N = 16) randomized to pulsatile CPB. These studies evaluating pulsatile flow suggest that splanchnic perfusion may be better preserved with pulsatile flow owing to less endogenously mediated vasoconstriction. Quigley et al,[52] however, reported a lack of endotoxemia and pathologic cytokinemia in an uncontrolled study of patients who underwent nonpulsatile CPB. They claimed that the use of "adequate flow and perfusion pressures" during CPB accounted for their findings.

The role of membrane oxygenators as a means of reducing systemic inflammation-related complications is also controversial. Less complement activation has been observed with the use of membrane oxygenators, although other studies have found no difference.[62,74,174,189-193] The use of membrane oxygenators was associated with better pulmonary function compared with the use of a bubble oxygenator, but it is unclear whether the difference observed reflected reduced systemic inflammation in the protocol group.[191] Butler et al[62] randomized 20 patients undergoing cardiac surgery to either a membrane or bubble oxygenator. IL-6 levels peaked 4 hours postoperatively, yet there were no significant differences between groups in IL-1 or IL-6 levels or in intrapulmonary shunting. This study failed to show a difference in postoperative outcome, possibly owing to short CPB durations (<1 hour) and the small sample size, which makes detecting a clinically significant difference in postoperative complications unlikely. Host defenses may be better maintained with the use of membrane oxygenators.[192]

There is also controversy as to whether hypothermia during CPB worsens systemic inflammation.[40,51,76,194-196] Hypothermia has been shown to reduce markers of complement activation.[76] Another study demonstrated reduced markers of inflammation, such as TNF and IL-6, as well as reduced neutrophil activation in the hypothermia group.[195] In contrast, another study randomized 30 cardiac surgical patients to either normothermic or hypothermic CPB.[40] No association was found between CPB temperature and plasma TNF levels at any time point in the perioperative period, suggesting a limited role for temperature as an independent cause of proinflammatory cytokine release. In one of the largest randomized trials to date, 300 elective CABG patients were randomized to either normothermic (35.5° to 36.5°C) or hypothermic (28° to 30°C) CPB.[197] No differences were seen in either short- or long-term outcome, suggesting no benefit to intraoperative hypothermia. There is evidence, however, that perioperative hyperthermia may be detrimental to the brain.[198] These investigators also observed an association between higher levels of the proinflammatory cytokine IL-6 and postoperative hyperthermia, suggesting a potential role of inflammation in the increases in temperature commonly observed after major surgery.

Finally, current data suggest that the use of CPB for cardiac surgery may not in and of itself be more deleterious than cardiac surgery without the use of CPB. Results from randomized clinical trials do not suggest that outcomes are substantially different in patients undergoing on-pump versus off-pump CABG.[199-203]

Complement Inhibition

The results from several large randomized clinical trials in which complement activation is selectively blocked have become available.[79-81] For example, in the largest randomized double-blind clinical trial conducted to date, 3099 adults undergoing CABG at 205 hospitals in North America and western Europe were enrolled.[80] Patients were randomized to placebo or to a 24-hour infusion of pexelizumab, which is a recombinant humanized single-chain antibody fragment that binds to human C5 complement and prevents its activation. The administration of pexelizumab resulted in rapid and complete inhibition of complement activation. The primary outcome variable (death or myocardial infarction within 30 days) did not achieve statistical significance ($P = 0.07$). The subset of patients undergoing CABG plus valve replacement did demonstrate a statistically significant difference ($P = 0.03$) in this outcome. This finding is somewhat contradictory to the previous phase IIb trial (N = 914) that enrolled patients undergoing CABG, valve replacement, or both and did not show a significant difference with regard to the end-point of death or myocardial infarction.[79] This previous trial did achieve significance in the subset undergoing isolated CABG, which was the apparent justification for studying isolated CABG procedures in the larger phase III trial. These studies indicate that attenuation of complement activation results in less myocardial injury; however, there did not appear to be an impact on complications such as pulmonary and renal dysfunction and severe vasodilation. These results suggest that complement activation may not play as great a role in the development of systemic inflammation–mediated morbidity as previously thought.

Ultrafiltration

Removal of excess fluid with ultrafiltration has been proposed as a method for removing proinflammatory mediators during cardiac surgery, particularly in the pediatric population.[46,204] It is unclear in studies performed thus far whether beneficial effects of ultrafiltration are due to one or some combination of the following factors: prevention of initiation of inflammation, removal of inflammatory mediators, or removal of excessive fluid alone. In one study, Journois et al[205] randomized 20 pediatric cardiac surgical patients to either a control group or high-volume, zero-fluid-balance ultrafiltration. Measured TNF, IL-1, IL-10, myeloperoxidase, and C3a levels were lower in the protocol group compared with the control group. The authors suggested that hemofiltration may have some beneficial effects that are not due to water removal alone. Patients in the ultrafiltration group had less postoperative fever, reduced perioperative blood loss, reduced time to extubation, and reduced postoperative alveolar-arterial oxygen gradient, which suggests, yet does not prove, a causal relationship between proinflammatory cytokinemia and several clinically meaningful end-points. The small sample size of this study precludes any conclusions from being made regarding other outcomes such as the incidence of multiple organ dysfunction syndrome or hospital length of stay.

Leukocyte Depletion

Removal of leukocytes during CPB with an inline leukocyte filter has been proposed as a method for reducing the concentration of activated leukocytes. This in turn may prevent inflammatory-mediated postoperative complications. Patients randomized to leukocyte depletion (n = 20) had better oxygenation following CPB; however, there were no differences in other outcomes measured.[206] A prospective randomized study of patients (total N = 50) receiving inline leukocyte filtration demonstrated decreased leukocytes, but postoperative arterial blood gases, pulmonary vascular resistance, ventilator time, and hospital length of stay were not different between groups.[207] Another study demonstrated no difference in postoperative complications or in the plasma levels of neutrophil proteases in patients undergoing leukocyte depletion with an inline filter.[208]

Davies et al[209] used another method of leukocyte depletion in which they removed platelets and leukocytes via plasmapheresis from patients prior to cardiac surgery. These patients, compared with the control group, demonstrated reduced postoperative thoracic drainage, reduced allogeneic blood product administration, and improved pulmonary function. This technique is not in widespread clinical use, owing to a lack of studies confirming its findings as well as the time and cost involved in performing plasmapheresis (see Chapter 28).

The techniques described here differ from the issue of administration of leukocyte-reduced packed red blood cells. This method of minimizing a patient's exposure to leukocytes involves the filtering of the collected blood either at the time of donation (fresh filtered) or prior to its release by the blood bank (stored filtered).[210] van de Watering and colleagues[211] reported results from a large (N = 914) randomized clinical trial in which patients undergoing cardiac surgery were randomized to receive allogeneic red cells without buffy coat, fresh-filtered allogeneic red cells, or stored filtered units. Patients randomized to either filtration group experienced a significant reduction in postoperative mortality ($P = 0.015$); this effect was most robust in patients administered more than three transfusions. It should be noted that differences between groups in the incidence of infection did not achieve statistical significance ($P = 0.13$). No differences between groups were found in intensive care unit or hospital length of stay in those patients in the overall study population or in the subset administered more than 3 units. These data are from a randomized trial and therefore should be more heavily weighted. Data from some retrospective cohort studies have shown no benefit to leukocyte reduction.[212,213]

Aprotinin Administration

Aprotinin, a 58-amino-acid serine protease inhibitor isolated from bovine lung, has been shown in numerous studies to decrease bleeding associated with cardiac surgery. It antagonizes numerous proteolytic enzymes, including plasmin and kallikrein, and may have some anti-inflammatory effects.[14,214] The blood-sparing effects of aprotinin were apparently discovered serendipitously while it was being evaluated as an anti-inflammatory agent in cardiac surgical patients. Despite more than 45 randomized clinical trials conducted to date, there are little data to support the hypothesis that aprotinin administration reduces postoperative complications attributable to excessive systemic inflammation. In these trials, numerous surrogate markers of postoperative morbidity, such as the duration of postoperative tracheal intubation, intensive care unit stay, and hospital length of stay, were not reported to be improved in aprotinin-treated patients. There is also evidence that aprotinin does not reduce cardiac surgery–induced myeloperoxidase production and complement activation[215] (see Chapter 29).

An interesting finding, however, comes from a retrospective pooling of data from U.S. clinical trials that evaluated the hemostatic effects of aprotinin. Data from randomized clinical trials suggest that aprotinin may have a protective effect.[216,217] Mechanisms to account for this potential effect include anti-inflammatory effects and inhibition of thrombus/embolus formation.[218] Administration of high-dose, but not low-dose, aprotinin resulted in improved microvascular flow, which may also account for the reduced stroke rate in aprotinin-treated patients.[28,219] This finding, however, requires confirmation in a large prospective clinical trial.

Tumor Necrosis Factor Antagonists

Soluble TNF receptor proteins antagonize the toxic effects of LPS-induced lethality in mice.[220] These agents are ineffective in the treatment of sepsis/septic shock but have not been tested in the setting of cardiac surgery.[221] Anti-TNF monoclonal antibodies have been studied in septic intensive care unit patients as well, although they have not yet been tested prophylactically in cardiac surgical patients.[69] A study involving prophylactic administration would allow for the antibody to be present prior to the TNF and thus determine if TNF has overall harmful or beneficial effects. If TNF and other cytokines are essential to the healing process, complete inhibition of their effects may result in worse rather than improved postoperative outcome. Well-designed large clinical trials could resolve these controversial issues.

Induction of Early Endotoxin Tolerance

Early endotoxin tolerance has been suggested as a way of protecting cardiac and other surgical patients from the adverse effects of endotoxemia. Astiz et al[103] administered a less toxic form of lipid A, called monophosphoryl lipid A (MPLA), to healthy volunteers. Twenty-four hours following administration of intravenous MPLA, subjects administered a challenge of *E. coli* LPS, 4 ng/kg intravenously, demonstrated less fever and fewer subjective symptoms consistent with a reduced proinflammatory response. An advantage of this technique is that it provides for nonspecific antiendotoxin tolerance. One potential drawback to this method is that early endotoxin tolerance has been shown to correlate with the intensity of the "prophylactic" LPS exposure.[102] The tachycardia and systemic proinflammatory response triggered by prophylactic LPS or MPLA may not be tolerated well by compromised patients prior to surgery. This is of particular relevance to patients with ischemic heart disease in whom increases in myocardial oxygen demand may be poorly tolerated. This technique requires hospitalization and close monitoring of the patient on the day prior to surgery, a disadvantage given the increasing percentage of patients who are admitted to the hospital on the morning of surgery.

Passive Antiendotoxin Immunization Using Antiserum

Another approach uses the principle of late endotoxin tolerance. The serum concentration of "protective" antiendotoxin antibodies can be raised by administering plasma acquired from donors with high titers of antiendotoxin antibodies.[158,222,223] This should bolster the native defenses of patients against the adverse effects of LPS, presumably by enhancing opsonization and phagocytosis of the bacterial cells or by neutralization of the biologic activity of LPS.[122] However, the effectiveness of the antisera varies greatly depending upon a large number of factors, including, for example, the composition and titer of the specific antibodies, which cannot be easily standardized.[113] To date, no "hyperimmune" plasma has been shown to confer genuine protection against forms of LPS likely to be encountered clinically in a well-controlled human clinical trial.[98,224] Other current disadvantages to this approach involve the cost and limited availability of producing hyperimmune plasma and the small but real potential risk of infectious disease transmission.

Pilz et al[225] administered intravenous immunoglobulin following cardiac surgery to 66 patients at high risk for postoperative complications or mortality. High-risk patients were identified using APACHE II scores. Mortality was lower in these treated patients than in a historical control group. This finding warrants confirmation in a prospective randomized clinical trial.

Passive Antiendotoxin Immunization Using Monoclonal Antibodies

Another possible method of passive immunization involves the use of antiendotoxin monoclonal antibodies. Two anti–lipid A monoclonal antibodies (HA-1A, Centocor; and E5; Xoma [mentioned earlier in Criticisms of Endotoxin as an Etiologic Factor]) failed to improve outcome on an "intention-to-treat" basis in intensive care unit patients with established sepsis.[117,118] This patient population is entirely different from cardiac surgical patients, who are more likely to benefit from prophylaxis with endotoxin-neutralizing drugs given prior to the initiation of a potentially deleterious systemic inflammatory response. There is also evidence suggesting that these anti–lipid A monoclonal antibodies do not bind to endotoxin with high affinity, which may explain, in part, their lack of demonstrable efficacy.[115,116] A monoclonal antibody-to-endotoxin core has been reported that appears to have favorable activity when tested in vitro and in vivo.[226] To date, a clinical trial using a monoclonal antibody with confirmed antiendotoxin properties has not been conducted in cardiac surgical patients.

Active Immunization Against Endotoxin

Another potential method of reducing endotoxin-mediated inflammatory complications involves active immunization, also referred to as vaccination. A clinically viable vaccine must fulfill two criteria, which have proved to be elusive over the past three decades. A vaccine is prophylactic by nature and must be almost devoid of toxicity. An antiendotoxin vaccine must avoid the common side effects, such as fever and malaise, which generally result when animals and humans are administered endotoxin-containing vaccines.[223,227] These side effects are particularly disadvantageous in high-risk individuals, such as cardiac surgical patients, in whom imbalances in myocardial oxygen delivery and consumption are common. The second criterion that a vaccine must meet relates to its immunogenicity. The antibodies elicited by active immunization must protect the host against forms of LPS likely to be clinically encountered. Unfortunately, no vaccine has been shown in a clinical trial to protect patients undergoing cardiac or major noncardiac surgery.

E5564

E5564 is a synthetically derived lipid A analog that is a potent Toll-like receptor 4–directed endotoxin antagonist.[228] It does not have lipid A agonist properties, and even in high doses it does not cause signs or symptoms of endotoxemia or systemic inflammation in humans and animals. Healthy volunteers were administered E5564 prior to a standard challenge dose of reference endotoxin (4 ng/kg). Single E5564 doses of 50 to 250 mg blocked or attenuated all of the effects of LPS in a dose-dependent manner. All E5564 dose groups had statistically significant reductions in elevated temperature, heart rate, C-reactive protein levels, white blood cell count, and cytokine levels (TNF-α and IL-6) compared with placebo ($P < 0.01$).[228]

Pentoxifylline

Pentoxifylline is a nonspecific phosphodiesterase inhibitor similar in chemical structure to theophylline, a common anti-inflammatory used to treat asthma. Pentoxifylline has multiple rheologic and anti-inflammatory properties, but the exact mechanism of its pharmacologic effects is poorly understood. Clinically, pentoxifylline is approved by the Food and Drug Administration to treat intermittent claudication, presumably by increasing red cell deformability, which may improve oxygen delivery to ischemic tissues. Animal studies have shown that treatment with pentoxifylline significantly attenuates endothelial damage and the formation of oxygen radicals following ischemia/reperfusion, prevents fever after the administration of LPS, and prevents leakage of bacteria from the gut during hemorrhagic shock. Clinical research studies using pentoxifylline have been performed in the setting of lung transplantation, cardiac surgery, and anemia requiring red blood cell transfusion.

In an initial study, Hoffman et al[229] randomized 40 patients with an APACHE II score of 19 or greater after cardiac surgery to placebo or pentoxifylline (1.5 mg/kg/hr for 48 hours). In this study, patients administered pentoxifylline had significantly fewer days on mechanical ventilation, less need for hemofiltration, and a shorter intensive care unit length of stay. In a historic control study, Thabut et al[230] administered pentoxifylline to 23 consecutive patients undergoing lung transplantation. Compared with historic controls, patients administered pentoxifylline experienced less allograft dysfunction, and a significant reduction in 60-day mortality was noted. These findings need to be confirmed in a prospective randomized clinical trial.

Boldt and colleagues[231,232] randomized 30 elderly (>80 years) patients undergoing cardiac surgery to placebo or pentoxifylline (300-mg bolus administered immediately after induction of general anesthesia followed by a continuous infusion of 1.5 mg/kg/hr for 48 hours). In this study, pentoxifylline administration minimized intraoperative and postoperative elevations in plasma C-reactive protein, PMN-elastase, IL-6, and IL-8 levels. Duration of mechanical ventilation was significantly lower in patients randomized to pentoxifylline. This study was not powered to detect differences in rare but serious complications.

Other Potential Antiendotoxin or Anti-Inflammatory Agents

Other potential approaches to preventing endotoxin-related complications involve the use of either synthetic or naturally occurring antiendotoxin compounds. *Bactericidal/permeability-increasing protein (BPI)* is a neutrophil granule protein and has been shown to have endotoxin-neutralizing and bactericidal activity in animal models. A human recombinant version, $rBPI_{21}$, neutralized endotoxin-mediated toxicity in humans. A recombinant version of an antiendotoxin factor, *endotoxin-neutralizing protein,* is another agent that has been shown to protect animals from endotoxin-mediated toxicity.[233] Reconstituted high-density lipoprotein (rHDL) neutralized some of endotoxin's toxic effects in an experimental model of human endotoxemia.[234] Polymyxin B neutralizes the toxic effects of endotoxin, although toxicity has prevented prophylactic intravenous use.[235] *Dextran-polymyxin B* is a variation of polymyxin B that has been reported to have antiendotoxin properties as well as minimal toxicity in animal models. *Soluble TNF receptor proteins* antagonize the toxic effects of LPS-induced lethality in mice. This agent was not effective in the treatment of sepsis/septic shock but has not been tested in the setting of cardiac surgery.[220] In addition, ethyl pyruvate is a novel anti-inflammatory agent.[236,237] It has been shown to protect the intestinal mucosa from mesenteric ischemia and reperfusion in rats and improve survival in murine models of acute endotoxemia and bacterial peritonitis. Ethyl pyruvate warrants further study in cardiac surgical patients.

ROLE OF ANESTHETIC AGENTS AND VASOACTIVE AGENTS

Anesthetic agents, defined here as drugs that induce hypnosis, amnesia, muscle relaxation, or regional anesthesia, have not been shown to result in clinically meaningful reductions in systemic inflammation after cardiac surgery. Numerous studies have evaluated the effect of these agents on the immune system with varied results, but no studies have reported a difference in outcome with one technique versus another. Ketamine is one of the more promising agents under investigation. Administration of a low dose (0.25 mg/kg) of ketamine prior to cardiac surgery prevented an increase in IL-6 for 7 days after surgery.[238] In addition, ketamine administration inhibited TNF production and leukocyte adherence in animal models and suppressed oxygen radical production in vitro. A randomized clinical trial is under way assessing the impact of low-dose ketamine on adverse outcome after cardiac surgery.

All general anesthetics can reduce splanchnic perfusion indirectly through a depression of myocardial function and a reduction in cardiac output and, hence, oxygen delivery to the splanchnic mucosa.[239,240] Isoflurane may be theoretically better than halothane, enflurane, or propofol, owing to its vasodilating properties, which may preserve splanchnic blood flow and blood volume.[239-242] A prospective randomized study of cardiac surgical patients demonstrated better splanchnic perfusion in patients maintained with isoflurane in contrast to propofol or enflurane.[243]

Although not definitively supported yet, there is evidence that splanchnic hypoperfusion and endotoxin-induced inflammation can be prevented in the operating room by strategies familiar to clinicians. Strategies involve the use of fluid loading to maximize stroke volume as well as the use of adequate levels of vasodilating volatile anesthetics.[145] Inodilating agents, such as milrinone, amrinone, dopexamine, and dobutamine, may be more protective of splanchnic perfusion than inoconstricting agents such as epinephrine, norepinephrine, and dopamine. Patients randomized to enoximone administration during cardiac surgery demonstrated lower endotoxin levels, suggesting a beneficial effect on the barrier function of the gut.[91] Endotoxemia is probably a more sensitive marker of loss of barrier function than gastric mucosal hypoperfusion, as these patients still demonstrated decreases in calculated gastric mucosal pH (pH_i). When tested in vitro, amrinone was a potent inhibitor of endotoxin-induced TNF production at clinically relevant drug concentrations, suggesting an additional advantage to the use of this phosphodiesterase inhibitor.[244] Dopamine is often touted as preserving splanchnic blood flow; however, responses to this agent are unpredictable, with vascular resistance increasing in some patients at low doses (3 to 5 μg/kg/min).

Selective Digestive Decontamination

Selective digestive decontamination represents an approach to limiting the incidence and severity of systemic inflammation. The technique attempts to reduce the total amount of endotoxin exposure by reducing the reservoir of endotoxin normally contained within the gut. Martinez-Pellús et al[65] conducted a prospective, open, randomized, controlled trial in 80 cardiac surgical patients. Patients were randomized to either a control group or up to 3 days of preoperative selective digestive decontamination accomplished with the administration of oral nonabsorbable antibiotics (polymyxin E, tobramycin, amphotericin B). Patients in the protocol group demonstrated much lower gut bacterial counts as well as lower blood levels of endotoxin and the proinflammatory cytokine IL-6 in the operating room as well as the postoperative unit. The study was not designed with sufficient power to determine whether this technique affects outcomes such as mortality and morbidity. Nevertheless, it is interesting to note that there was a trend toward improved outcome (mortality, hospital length of stay) in the protocol group.

SUMMARY

A very large body of circumstantial evidence strongly suggests that systemic inflammation is an important cause of mortality and morbidity after cardiac surgery. Although several strategies appear promising, there are little data from large randomized trials to support the widespread use of a particular intervention at the current time.

REFERENCES

1. Hammermeister KE, Burchfiel C, Johnson R, Grover FL: Identification of patients at greatest risk for developing major complications at cardiac surgery. Circulation 82:IV-380, 1990
2. Birkmeyer JD, Stukel TA, Siewers AE, et al: Surgeon volume and operative mortality in the United States. N Engl J Med 349:2117, 2003
3. Rady MY, Ryan T, Starr NJ: Perioperative determinants of morbidity and mortality in elderly patients undergoing cardiac surgery. Crit Care Med 26:225, 1998
4. Goris RJ, te Boekhorst TP, Nuytinck JK, Gimbrere JS: Multiple-organ failure. Generalized autodestructive inflammation? Arch Surg 120:1109, 1985
5. Bone RC, Balk RA, Cerra FB, et al: Definitions for sepsis and organ failure and guidelines for the use of innovative therapies in sepsis. The ACCP/SCCM Consensus Conference Committee. American College of Chest Physicians/Society of Critical Care Medicine. Chest 101:1644, 1992
6. Schlag G, Redl H, Hallstrom S: The cell in shock: The origin of multiple organ failure. Resuscitation 21:137, 1991
7. American College of Chest Physicians/Society of Critical Care Medicine Consensus Conference: Definitions for sepsis and organ failure and guidelines for the use of innovative therapies in sepsis. Crit Care Med 20:864, 1992
8. Sprayer M (ed): Stedman's Medical Dictionary, 26th ed. Baltimore, Williams & Wilkins, p 869
9. Vincent JL: Dear SIRS I'm sorry to say that I don't like you. Crit Care Med 25:372, 1997
10. Berendes E, Mollhoff T, Van Aken H, et al: Effects of dopexamine on creatinine clearance, systemic inflammation, and splanchnic oxygenation in patients undergoing coronary artery bypass grafting. Anesth Analg 84:950, 1997
11. Andersen LW, Baek L, Degn H, et al: Presence of circulating endotoxins during cardiac operations. J Thorac Cardiovasc Surg 93:115, 1987
12. Doran JE: Biological effects of endotoxin. Curr Stud Hematol Blood Transfus 59:66, 1992
13. Herskowitz A, Mangano DT: Inflammatory cascade. A final common pathway for perioperative injury? Anesthesiology 85:957, 1996
14. Royston D: Preventing the inflammatory response to open-heart surgery: The role of aprotinin and other protease inhibitors. Int J Cardiol 53(suppl):S11, 1996
15. Miller BE, Levy JH: The inflammatory response to cardiopulmonary bypass. J Cardiothorac Vasc Anesth 11:355, 1997
16. Weiss SJ: Tissue destruction by neutrophils. N Engl J Med 320:365, 1989
17. Webster RO, Hong SR, Johnston RB Jr, Henson PM: Biological effects of the human complement fragments C5a and C5ades Arg on neutrophil function. Immunopharmacology 2:201, 1980
18. Freeman BA, Crapo JD: Biology of disease: Free radicals and tissue injury. Lab Invest 47:412, 1982
19. Meerson FZ, Kagan VE, Kozlov YU, et al: The role of lipid peroxidation in pathogenesis of ischemic damage and the antioxidant protection of the heart. Basic Res Cardiol 77:465, 1982
20. Rice-Evans C, Burdon R: Free radical-lipid interactions and their pathological consequences. Prog Lipid Res 32:71–110, 1993
21. Prasad K, Kalra J, Bharadwaj B, Chaudhary AK: Increased oxygen free radical activity in patients on cardiopulmonary bypass undergoing aortocoronary bypass surgery. Am Heart J 123:37, 1992
22. Royston D, Fleming JS, Desai JB, et al: Increased production of peroxidation products associated with cardiac operations. Evidence for free radical generation. J Thorac Cardiovasc Surg 91:759, 1986
23. Fosse E, Moen O, Johnson E, et al: Reduced complement and granulocyte activation with heparin-coated cardiopulmonary bypass. Ann Thorac Surg 58:472, 1994
24. Kharazmi A, Andersen LW, Baek L, et al: Endotoxemia and enhanced generation of oxygen radicals by neutrophils from patients undergoing cardiopulmonary bypass. J Thorac Cardiovasc Surg 98:381, 1989
25. Borowiec J, Thelin S, Bagge L, et al: Heparin-coated circuits reduce activation of granulocytes during cardiopulmonary bypass. A clinical study. J Thorac Cardiovasc Surg 104:642, 1992
26. Mythen MG, Purdy G, Mackie IJ, et al: Postoperative multiple organ dysfunction syndrome associated with gut mucosal hypoperfusion, increased neutrophil degranulation and C1-esterase inhibitor depletion. Br J Anaesth 71:858, 1993

27. Bjork J, Hugli TE, Smedegard G: Microvascular effects of anaphylatoxins C3a and C5a. J Immunol 134:1115, 1985
28. Liu B, Belboul A, al-Khaja N, et al: Effect of high-dose aprotinin on blood cell filterability in association with cardiopulmonary bypass. Coron Artery Dis 3:129, 1992
29. Blauth C, Arnold J, Kohner EM, Taylor KM: Retinal microembolism during cardiopulmonary bypass demonstrated by fluorescein angiography. Lancet 2:837, 1986
30. Sheeran P, Hall GM: Cytokines in anaesthesia. Br J Anaesth 78:201, 1997
31. Tonnesen E, Christensen VB, Toft P: The role of cytokines in cardiac surgery. Int J Cardiol 53(suppl):S1, 1996
32. Baumann H, Gauldie J: The acute phase response. Immunol Today 15:74, 1994
33. Michie HR, Manogue KR, Spriggs DR, et al: Detection of circulating tumor necrosis factor after endotoxin administration. N Engl J Med 318:1481, 1988
34. Michie HR, Spriggs DR, Manogue KR, et al: Tumor necrosis factor and endotoxin induce similar metabolic responses in human beings. Surgery 104:280, 1988
35. Tracey KJ, Lowry SF, Fahey TJ 3rd, et al: Cachectin/tumor necrosis factor induces lethal shock and stress hormone responses in the dog. Surg Gynecol Obstet 164:415, 1987
36. Hesse DG, Tracey KJ, Fong Y, et al: Cytokine appearance in human endotoxemia and primate bacteremia. Surg Gynecol Obstet 166:147, 1988
37. Jansen NJ, van Oeveren W, van Vliet M, et al: The role of different types of corticosteroids on the inflammatory mediators in cardiopulmonary bypass. Eur J Cardiothorac Surg 5:211, 1991
38. Jansen NJ, van Oeveren W, Gu YJ, et al: Endotoxin release and tumor necrosis factor formation during cardiopulmonary bypass. Ann Thorac Surg 54:744, 1992; discussion 747, 1992
39. Abe K, Nishimura M, Sakakibara T: Interleukin-6 and tumour necrosis factor during cardiopulmonary bypass. Can J Anaesth 41:876, 1994
40. Tonz M, Mihaljevic T, von Segesser LK, et al: Normothermia versus hypothermia during cardiopulmonary bypass: A randomized, controlled trial. Ann Thorac Surg 59:137, 1995
41. te Velthuis H, Jansen PG, Oudemans-van Straaten HM, et al: Myocardial performance in elderly patients after cardiopulmonary bypass is suppressed by tumor necrosis factor. J Thorac Cardiovasc Surg 110:1663, 1995
42. Hennein HA, Ebba H, Rodriguez JL, et al: Relationship of the proinflammatory cytokines to myocardial ischemia and dysfunction after uncomplicated coronary revascularization. J Thorac Cardiovasc Surg 108:626, 1994
43. Wan S, Marchant A, DeSmet JM, et al: Human cytokine responses to cardiac transplantation and coronary artery bypass grafting. J Thorac Cardiovasc Surg 111:469, 1996
44. Seghaye M, Duchateau J, Bruniaux J, et al: Interleukin-10 release related to cardiopulmonary bypass in infants undergoing cardiac operations. J Thorac Cardiovasc Surg 111:545, 1996
45. Deng MC, Dasch B, Erren M, et al: Impact of left ventricular dysfunction on cytokines, hemodynamics, and outcome in bypass grafting. Ann Thorac Surg 62:184, 1996
46. Millar AB, Armstrong L, van der Linden J, et al: Cytokine production and hemofiltration in children undergoing cardiopulmonary bypass. Ann Thorac Surg 56:1499, 1993
47. Furunaga A: [Measurement of cytokines at cardiopulmonary bypass]. Nippon Kyobu Geka Gakkai Zasshi 42:2200, 1994
48. Kawamura T, Wakusawa R, Okada K, Inada S: Elevation of cytokines during open heart surgery with cardiopulmonary bypass: Participation of interleukin-8 and -6 in reperfusion injury. Can J Anaesth 40:1016, 1993
49. Markewitz A, Faist E, Lang S, et al: Regulation of acute phase response after cardiopulmonary bypass by immunomodulation. Ann Thorac Surg 55:389, 1993
50. Haeffner-Cavaillon N, Roussellier N, Ponzio O, et al: Induction of interleukin-1 production in patients undergoing cardiopulmonary bypass. J Thorac Cardiovasc Surg 98:1100, 1989
51. Frering B, Philip I, Dehoux M, et al: Circulating cytokines in patients undergoing normothermic cardiopulmonary bypass. J Thorac Cardiovasc Surg 108:636, 1994
52. Quigley RL, Caplan MS, Perkins JA, et al: Cardiopulmonary bypass with adequate flow and perfusion pressures prevents endotoxemia and pathologic cytokine production. Perfusion 10:27, 1995
53. Steinberg BM, Grossi EA, Schwartz DS, et al: Heparin bonding of bypass circuits reduces cytokine release during cardiopulmonary bypass. Ann Thorac Surg 60:525, 1995
54. Steinberg JB, Kapelanski DP, Olson JD, Weiler JM: Cytokine and complement levels in patients undergoing cardiopulmonary bypass. J Thorac Cardiovasc Surg 106:1008, 1993
55. Kilbourn RG, Belloni P: Endothelial cell production of nitrogen oxides in response to interferon gamma in combination with tumor necrosis factor, interleukin-1, or endotoxin. J Natl Cancer Inst 82:772, 1990
56. Finn A, Naik S, Klein N, et al: Interleukin-8 release and neutrophil degranulation after pediatric cardiopulmonary bypass. J Thorac Cardiovasc Surg 105:234, 1993
57. Huber AR, Kunkel SL, Todd RF 3rd, Weiss SJ: Regulation of transendothelial neutrophil migration by endogenous interleukin-8. Science 254:99, 1991
58. Ashraf SS, Tian Y, Cowan D, et al: Proinflammatory cytokine release during pediatric cardiopulmonary bypass: Influence of centrifugal and roller pumps. J Cardiothorac Vasc Anesth 11:718, 1997
59. Kawahito K, Kawakami M, Fujiwara T, et al: Proinflammatory cytokine levels in patients undergoing cardiopulmonary bypass. Does lung reperfusion influence the release of cytokines? ASAIO J 41:M775, 1995
60. Rothenburger M, Soeparwata R, Deng MC, et al: Prediction of clinical outcome after cardiac surgery: The role of cytokines, endotoxin, and antiendotoxin core antibodies. Shock 16(suppl 1):44, 2001
61. Rothenburger M, Tjan TD, Schneider M, et al: The impact of the pro- and anti-inflammatory immune response on ventilation time after cardiac surgery. Cytometry 53B:70, 2003
62. Butler J, Chong GL, Baigrie RJ, et al: Cytokine responses to cardiopulmonary bypass with membrane and bubble oxygenation. Ann Thorac Surg 53:833, 1992
63. Almdahl SM, Waage A, Ivert T, Vaage J: Release of bioactive interleukin-6 but not of tumor necrosis factor-alpha after elective cardiopulmonary bypass. Perfusion 8:233, 1993
64. Cremer J, Martin M, Redl H, et al: Systemic inflammatory response syndrome after cardiac operations. Ann Thorac Surg 61:1714, 1996
65. Martinez-Pellus AE, Merino P, Bru M, et al: Can selective digestive decontamination avoid the endotoxemia and cytokine activation promoted by cardiopulmonary bypass? Crit Care Med 21:1684, 1993
66. de Waal Malefyt R, Abrams J, Bennett B, et al: Interleukin 10 (IL-10) inhibits cytokine synthesis by human monocytes: An autoregulatory role of IL-10 produced by monocytes. J Exp Med 174:1209, 1991
67. Bogdan C, Vodovotz Y, Nathan C: Macrophage deactivation by interleukin 10. J Exp Med 174:1549, 1991
68. McBride WT, Armstrong MA, Crockard AD, et al: Cytokine balance and immunosuppressive changes at cardiac surgery: Contrasting response between patients and isolated CPB circuits. Br J Anaesth 75:724, 1995
69. Fisher CJ Jr, Agosti JM, Opal SM, et al: Treatment of septic shock with the tumor necrosis factor receptor:Fc fusion protein. The Soluble TNF Receptor Sepsis Study Group. N Engl J Med 334:1697, 1996
70. Best N, Sinosich MJ, Teisner B, et al: Complement activation during cardiopulmonary bypass by heparin-protamine interaction. Br J Anaesth 56:339, 1984
71. Kirklin JK, Chenoweth DE, Naftel DC, et al: Effects of protamine administration after cardiopulmonary bypass on complement, blood elements, and the hemodynamic state. Ann Thorac Surg 41:193, 1986
72. Chiu RC, Samson R: Complement (C3, C4) consumption in cardiopulmonary bypass, cardioplegia, and protamine administration. Ann Thorac Surg 37:229, 1984
73. Chenoweth DE, Cooper SW, Hugli TE, et al: Complement activation during cardiopulmonary bypass: Evidence for generation of C3a and C5a anaphylatoxins. N Engl J Med 304:497, 1981
74. Hammerschmidt DE, Stroncek DF, Bowers TK, et al: Complement activation and neutropenia occurring during cardiopulmonary bypass. J Thorac Cardiovasc Surg 81:370, 1981
75. Kirklin JK, Westaby S, Blackstone EH, et al: Complement and the damaging effects of cardiopulmonary bypass. J Thorac Cardiovasc Surg 86:845, 1983
76. Moore FD Jr, Warner KG, Assousa S, et al: The effects of complement activation during cardiopulmonary bypass. Attenuation by hypothermia, heparin, and hemodilution. Ann Surg 208:95, 1988
77. Riegel W, Spillner G, Schlosser V, Horl WH: Plasma levels of main granulocyte components during cardiopulmonary bypass. J Thorac Cardiovasc Surg 95:1014, 1988
78. Bonser RS, Dave JR, Davies ET, et al: Reduction of complement activation during bypass by prime manipulation. Ann Thorac Surg 49:279, 1990
79. Shernan SK, Fitch JC, Nussmeier NA, et al: Impact of pexilizumab, an anti-C5 complement antibody, on total mortality and adverse cardiovascular outcomes in cardiac surgical patients undergoing cardiopulmonary bypass. Ann Thorac Surg 77:942, 2004; discussion 949, 2004

80. Verrier ED, Shernan SK, Taylor KM, et al: Terminal complement blockade with pexilizumab during coronary artery bypass graft surgery requiring cardiopulmonary bypass: A randomized trial. JAMA 291:2319, 2004
81. Fitch JC, Rollins S, Matis L, et al: Pharmacology and biological efficacy of a recombinant, humanized, single-chain antibody C5 complement inhibitor in patients undergoing coronary artery bypass graft surgery with cardiopulmonary bypass. Circulation 100:2499, 1999
82. Morrison DC, Cochrane CG: Direct evidence for Hageman factor (factor XII) activation by bacterial lipopolysaccharides (endotoxins). J Exp Med 140:797, 1974
83. Morrison DC, Ryan JL: Endotoxins and disease mechanisms. Annu Rev Med 38:417, 1987
84. Natanson C, Eichenholz PW, Danner RL, et al: Endotoxin and tumor necrosis factor challenges in dogs simulate the cardiovascular profile of human septic shock. J Exp Med 169:823, 1989
85. Rocke DA, Gaffin SL, Wells MT, et al: Endotoxemia associated with cardiopulmonary bypass. J Thorac Cardiovasc Surg 93:832, 1987
86. Andersen LW, Baek L, Thomsen BS, Rasmussen JP: Effect of methylprednisolone on endotoxemia and complement activation during cardiac surgery. J Cardiothorac Anesth 3:544, 1989
87. Andersen LW, Landow L, Baek L, et al: Association between gastric intramucosal pH and splanchnic endotoxin, antibody to endotoxin, and tumor necrosis factor-alpha concentrations in patients undergoing cardiopulmonary bypass. Crit Care Med 21:210, 1993
88. Riddington DW, Venkatesh B, Boivin CM, et al: Intestinal permeability, gastric intramucosal pH, and systemic endotoxemia in patients undergoing cardiopulmonary bypass. JAMA 275:1007, 1996
89. Oudemans-van Straaten HM, Jansen PG, Hoek FJ, et al: Intestinal permeability, circulating endotoxin, and postoperative systemic responses in cardiac surgery patients. J Cardiothorac Vasc Anesth 10:187, 1996
90. Oudemans-van Straaten HM, Jansen PG, Velthuis H, et al: Endotoxaemia and postoperative hypermetabolism in coronary artery bypass surgery: The role of katanserin. Br J Anaesth 77:473, 1996
91. Loick HM, Mollhoff T, Berendes E, et al: Influence of enoximone on systemic and splanchnic oxygen utilization and endotoxin release following cardiopulmonary bypass. Intensive Care Med 23:267, 1997
92. te Velthuis H, Jansen PG, Oudemans-van Straaten HM, et al: Circulating endothelin in cardiac operations: Influence of blood pressure and endotoxin. Ann Thorac Surg 61:904, 1996
93. Bowles CT, Ohri SK, Klangsuk N, et al: Endotoxemia detected during cardiopulmonary bypass with a modified Limulus amebocyte lysate assay. Perfusion 10:219, 1995
94. Watarida S, Mori A, Onoe M, et al: A clinical study on the effects of pulsatile cardiopulmonary bypass on the blood endotoxin levels. J Thorac Cardiovasc Surg 108:620, 1994
95. Nilsson L, Kulander L, Nystrom SO, Eriksson O: Endotoxins in cardiopulmonary bypass. J Thorac Cardiovasc Surg 100:777, 1990
96. Myles P, Buckland M, Cannon G, et al: The association among gastric mucosal pH, endotoxemia, and low systemic vascular resistance after cardiopulmonary bypass. J Cardiothorac Vasc Anesth 10:195, 1996
97. Imai T, Shiga T, Saruki N, et al: Change in plasma endotoxin titres and endotoxin-neutralizing activity in the perioperative period. Can J Anaesth 43:812, 1996
98. Lebek G, Cottier H: Notes on the bacterial content of the gut. Curr Stud Hematol Blood Transfus 59:1, 1992
99. Fink MP: Effect of critical illness on microbial translocation and gastrointestinal mucosa permeability. Semin Respir Infect 9:256, 1994
100. Daniel M: Response of man to endotoxin. Immunobiology 187:403, 1993
101. Rubin J, Robbs JV, Gaffin SL, Wells MT: Plasma lipopolysaccharide increase after aortic aneurysm resection. S Afr Med J 74:193, 1988
102. Griesman SE, Hornick RB: Mechanism of endotoxin tolerance with special reference to man. J Infect Dis 128:265, 1973
103. Astiz ME, Rackow EC, Still JG, et al: Pretreatment of normal humans with monophosphoryl lipid A induces tolerance to endotoxin: A prospective, double-blind, randomized, controlled trial. Crit Care Med 23:9, 1995
104. Luderitz O, Staub AM, Westphal O: Immunochemistry of O and R antigens of Salmonella and related Enterobacteriaceae. Bacteriol Rev 30:192, 1966
105. Volk WA, Benjamin DC, Kadner RJ, et al: Medical Microbiology. Philadelphia, Lippincott, 1986, pp 396–398
106. van Oeveren W, Kazatchkine MD, Descamps-Latscha B, et al: Deleterious effects of cardiopulmonary bypass. A prospective study of bubble versus membrane oxygenation. J Thorac Cardiovasc Surg 89:888, 1985
107. Hairston P, Manos JP, Graber CD, Lee WH Jr: Depression of immunologic surveillance by pump-oxygenation perfusion. J Surg Res 9:587, 1969
108. Eskola J, Salo M, Viljanen MK, Ruuskanen O: Impaired B lymphocyte function during open-heart surgery. Effects of anaesthesia and surgery. Br J Anaesth 56:333, 1984
109. Freeman R, Gould FK: Prevention of fever and gram negative infection after open heart surgery by antiendotoxin. Thorax 40:846, 1985
110. Barclay GR, Scott BB: Serological relationships between Escherichia coli and Salmonella smooth- and rough-mutant lipopolysaccharides as revealed by enzyme-linked immunosorbent assay for human immunoglobulin G antiendotoxin antibodies. Infect Immun 55:2706, 1987
111. Barclay GR: Endogenous endotoxin-core antibody (EndoCAb) as a marker of endotoxin exposure and a prognostic indicator: A review. Prog Clin Biol Res 392:263, 1995
112. Poxton IR: Antibodies to lipopolysaccharide. J Immunol Methods 186:1, 1995
113. Baumgartner JD: Immunotherapy with antibodies to core lipopolysaccharide: A critical appraisal. Infect Dis Clin North Am 5:915, 1991
114. Evans ME, Pollack M, Koles NL, et al: Lipopolysaccharide heterogeneity in Escherichia coli J5 variants: Analysis by flow cytometry. J Infect Dis 166:803, 1992
115. Warren HS, Amato SF, Fitting C, et al: Assessment of ability of murine and human anti-lipid A monoclonal antibodies to bind and neutralize lipopolysaccharide. J Exp Med 177:89, 1993
116. Warren HS, Danner RL, Munford RS: Anti-endotoxin monoclonal antibodies. N Engl J Med 326:1153, 1992
117. Ziegler EJ, Fisher CJ Jr, Sprung CL, et al: Treatment of gram-negative bacteremia and septic shock with HA-1A human monoclonal antibody against endotoxin. A randomized, double-blind, placebo-controlled trial. The HA-1A Sepsis Study Group. N Engl J Med 324:429, 1991
118. Greenman RL, Schein RM, Martin MA, et al: A controlled clinical trial of E5 murine monoclonal IgM antibody to endotoxin in the treatment of gram-negative sepsis. The XOMA Sepsis Study Group. JAMA 266:1097, 1991
119. Quezado ZM, Natanson C, Alling DW, et al: A controlled trial of HA-1A in a canine model of gram-negative septic shock. JAMA 269:2221, 1993
120. Hamilton-Davies C, Barclay GR, Cardigan RA, et al: Relationship between preoperative endotoxin immune status, gut perfusion, and outcome from cardiac valve replacement surgery. Chest 112:1189, 1997
121. Bennett-Guerrero E, Ayuso L, Hamilton-Davies C, et al: Relationship of preoperative antiendotoxin core antibodies and adverse outcomes following cardiac surgery. JAMA 277:646, 1997
122. Braude AI, Douglas H, Davis CE: Treatment and prevention of intravascular coagulation with antiserum to endotoxin. J Infect Dis 128(suppl):157, 1973
123. Mathew JP, Grocott HP, Phillips-Bute B, et al: Lower endotoxin immunity predicts increased cognitive dysfunction in elderly patients after cardiac surgery. Stroke 34:508, 2003
124. DeCamp MM, Demling RH: Posttraumatic multisystem organ failure. JAMA 260:530, 1988
125. Ford EG, Baisden CE, Matteson ML, Picone AL: Sepsis after coronary bypass grafting: Evidence for loss of the gut mucosal barrier. Ann Thorac Surg 52:514, 1991
126. Moore FA, Moore EE, Poggetti R, et al: Gut bacterial translocation via the portal vein: A clinical perspective with major torso trauma. J Trauma 31:629-636; discussion 636, 1991
127. Rush BF Jr, Sori AJ, Murphy TF, et al: Endotoxemia and bacteremia during hemorrhagic shock. The link between trauma and sepsis? Ann Surg 207:549, 1988
128. Deitch EA, Berg R: Bacterial translocation from the gut: A mechanism of infection. J Burn Care Rehabil 8:475, 1987
129. Deitch EA: Bacterial translocation of the gut flora. J Trauma 30: S184, 1990
130. Deitch EA: The role of intestinal barrier failure and bacterial translocation in the development of systemic infection and multiple organ failure. Arch Surg 125:403, 1990
131. Mythen MG, Webb AR: The role of gut mucosal hypoperfusion in the pathogenesis of postoperative organ dysfunction. Intensive Care Med 20:203, 1994
132. Price HL, Deutsch S, Marshall BE, et al: Hemodynamic and metabolic effects of hemorrhage in man, with particular reference to the splanchnic circulation. Circ Res 18:469, 1966
133. Lundgren O: Physiology of the intestinal circulation. *In* Marston A Bulkley G (eds): Splanchnic Ischemia and Multiple Organ Failure. St. Louis, Mosby, 1989, pp. 29–40

134. Hamilton-Davies C, Mythen MG, Salmon JB, et al: Comparison of commonly used clinical indicators of hypovolaemia with gastrointestinal tonometry. Intensive Care Med 23:276, 1997
135. Advanced Trauma Life Support Student Manual. Chicago, American College of Surgeons, 1993, pp 81–82
136. Taylor KM, Bain WH, Russell M, et al: Peripheral vascular resistance and angiotensin II levels during pulsatile and no-pulsatile cardiopulmonary bypass. Thorax 34:594, 1979
137. Richardson PD, Withrington PG: The effects of intraportal injections of noradrenaline, adrenaline, vasopressin and angiotensin on the hepatic portal vascular bed of the dog: Marked tachyphylaxis to angiotensin. Br J Pharmacol 59:293, 1977
138. Watkins WD, Peterson MB, Kong DL, et al: Thromboxane and prostacyclin changes during cardiopulmonary bypass with and without pulsatile flow. J Thorac Cardiovasc Surg 84:250, 1982
139. Levine FH, Philbin DM, Kono K, et al: Plasma vasopressin levels and urinary sodium excretion during cardiopulmonary bypass with and without pulsatile flow. Ann Thorac Surg 32:63, 1981
140. Fink MP, Antonsson JB, Wang HL, Rothschild HR: Increased intestinal permeability in endotoxic pigs. Mesenteric hypoperfusion as an etiologic factor. Arch Surg 126:211, 1991
141. Mythen MG, Faehnrich J: Monitoring gut perfusion. *In* Rombeau JL, Takala J (eds): Gut Dysfunction in Critical Illness. Heidelberg, Springer-Verlag, 1996, pp 246–263
142. Fiddian-Green RG: Gut mucosal ischemia during cardiac surgery. Semin Thorac Cardiovasc Surg 2:389, 1990
143. Fiddian-Green RG, Baker S: Predictive value of the stomach wall pH for complications after cardiac operations: Comparison with other monitoring. Crit Care Med 15:153, 1987
144. Mythen MG, Webb AR: Intraoperative gut mucosal hypoperfusion is associated with increased postoperative complications and cost. Intensive Care Med 20:99, 1994
145. Mythen MG, Webb AR: Perioperative plasma volume expansion reduces the incidence of gut mucosal hypoperfusion during cardiac surgery. Arch Surg 130:423, 1995
146. Bennett-Guerrero E, Panah MH, Bodian CA, et al: Automated detection of gastric luminal partial pressure of carbon dioxide during cardiovascular surgery using the TONOCAP. Anesthesiology 92:38–45, 2000
147. Soong CV, Blair PH, Halliday MI, et al: Bowel ischaemia and organ impairment in elective abdominal aortic aneurysm repair. Br J Surg 81:965, 1994
148. Martich GD, Boujoukos AJ, Suffredini AF: Response of man to endotoxin. Immunobiology 187:403, 1993
149. Suffredini AF, Fromm RE, Parker MM, et al: The cardiovascular response of normal humans to the administration of endotoxin. N Engl J Med 321:280, 1989
150. Cunnion RE, Parrillo JE: Myocardial dysfunction in sepsis. Crit Care Clin 5:99, 1989
151. Hollenberg SM, Cunnion RE, Parrillo JE: The effect of tumor necrosis factor on vascular smooth muscle. In vitro studies using rat aortic rings. Chest 100:1133, 1991
152. Clauss M, Ryan J, Stern D: Modulation of endothelial cell hemostatic properties by TNF: Insights into the role of endothelium in the host response to inflammatory stimuli. *In* Beutler B (ed): Tumor Necrosis Factors: The Molecules and Their Emerging Role in Medicine. New York, Raven, 1992, pp 49–63
153. Arvin B, Neville LF, Barone FC, Feuerstein GZ: The role of inflammation and cytokines in brain injury. Neurosci Biobehav Rev 20:445, 1996
154. Loop FD, Lytle BW, Cosgrove DM, et al: J. Maxwell Chamberlain memorial paper. Sternal wound complications after isolated coronary artery bypass grafting: Early and late mortality, morbidity, and cost of care. Ann Thorac Surg 49:179, 1990; discussion 186, 1990
155. Weintraub WS, Jones EL, Craver J, et al: Determinants of prolonged length of hospital stay after coronary bypass surgery. Circulation 80:276, 1989
156. Sarr MG, Gott VL, Townsend TR: Mediastinal infection after cardiac surgery. Ann Thorac Surg 38:415, 1984
157. Miholic J, Hudec M, Domanig E, et al: Risk factors for severe bacterial infections after valve replacement and aortocoronary bypass operations: Analysis of 246 cases by logistic regression. Ann Thorac Surg 40:224, 1985
158. Kress HG, Scheidewig C, Engelhardt W, et al: Prediction and prevention, by immunological means, of septic complications after elective cardiac surgery. Prog Clin Biol Res 308:1031, 1989
159. Collett B, Alhaq A, Abdullah NB, et al: Pathways to complement activation during cardiopulmonary bypass. Br Med J (Clin Res Ed) 289:1251, 1984
160. Parker DJ, Cantrell JW, Karp RB, et al: Changes in serum complement and immunoglobulins following cardiopulmonary bypass. Surgery 71:824, 1972
161. Lee WH Jr, Krumhaar D, Fonkalsrud EW, et al: Denaturation of plasma proteins as a cause of morbidity and death after intracardiac operations. Surgery 50:29, 1961
162. van Velzen-Blad H, Dijkstra YJ, Schurink GA, et al: Cardiopulmonary bypass and host defense functions in human beings: I. Serum levels and role of immunoglobulins and complement in phagocytosis. Ann Thorac Surg 39:207, 1985
163. Markewitz A, Faist E, Lang S, et al: Successful restoration of cell-mediated immune response after cardiopulmonary bypass by immunomodulation. J Thorac Cardiovasc Surg 105:15, 1993
164. Welsby IJ, Bennett-Guerrero E, Atwell D, et al: The association of complication type with mortality and prolonged stay after cardiac surgery with cardiopulmonary bypass. Anesth Analg 94:1072, 2002
165. Huddy SP, Joyce WP, Pepper JR: Gastrointestinal complications in 4473 patients who underwent cardiopulmonary bypass surgery. Br J Surg 78:293, 1991
166. Christenson JT, Schmuziger M, Maurice J, et al: Gastrointestinal complications after coronary artery bypass grafting. J Thorac Cardiovasc Surg 108:899, 1994
167. Corwin HL, Sprague SM, DeLaria GA, Norusis MJ: Acute renal failure associated with cardiac operations. A case-control study. J Thorac Cardiovasc Surg 98:1107, 1989
168. Fowler AA, Hamman RF, Good JT, et al: Adult respiratory distress syndrome: risk with common predispositions. Ann Intern Med 98:593, 1983
169. Messent M, Sullivan K, Keogh BF, et al: Adult respiratory distress syndrome following cardiopulmonary bypass: Incidence and prediction. Anaesthesia 47:267, 1992
170. Bennett-Guerrero E: Unpublished data, January, 2000
171. Geha AS, Sessler AD, Kirklin JW: Alveolar-arterial oxygen gradients after open intracardiac surgery. J Thorac Cardiovasc Surg 51:609, 1966
172. el-Fiky MM, Taggart DP, Carter R, et al: Respiratory dysfunction following cardiopulmonary bypass: Verification of a noninvasive technique to measure shunt fraction. Respir Med 87:193, 1993
173. Turnbull KW, Miyagishima RT, Gerein AN: Pulmonary complications and cardiopulmonary bypass: A clinical study in adults. Can Anaesth Soc J 21:181, 1974
174. Cavarocchi NC, Pluth JR, Schaff HV, et al: Complement activation during cardiopulmonary bypass. Comparison of bubble and membrane oxygenators. J Thorac Cardiovasc Surg 91:252, 1986
175. Jansen NJ, van Oeveren W, van den Broek L, et al: Inhibition by dexamethasone of the reperfusion phenomena in cardiopulmonary bypass. J Thorac Cardiovasc Surg 102:515, 1991
176. Inaba H, Kochi A, Yorozu S: Suppression by methylprednisolone of augmented plasma endotoxin-like activity and interleukin-6 during cardiopulmonary bypass. Br J Anaesth 72:348, 1994
177. Niazi Z, Flodin P, Joyce L, et al: Effects of glucocorticosteroids in patients undergoing coronary artery bypass surgery. Chest 76:262, 1979
178. Miranda DR, Stoutenbeek C, Karliczek G, Rating W: Effects of dexamethasone on the early postoperative course after coronary artery bypass surgery. Thorac Cardiovasc Surg 30:21, 1982
179. Jorens PG, De Jongh R, De Backer W, et al: Interleukin-8 production in patients undergoing cardiopulmonary bypass. The influence of pretreatment with methylprednisolone. Am Rev Respir Dis 148:890, 1993
180. Tabardel Y, Duchateau J, Schmartz D, et al: Corticosteroids increase blood interleukin-10 levels during cardiopulmonary bypass in men. Surgery 119:76, 1996
181. Tennenberg SD, Bailey WW, Cotta LA, et al: The effects of methylprednisolone on complement-mediated neutrophil activation during cardiopulmonary bypass. Surgery 100:134, 1986
182. Toledo-Pereyra LH, Lin CY, Kundler H, Replogle RL: Steroids in heart surgery: A clinical double-blind and randomized study. Am Surg 46:155, 1980
183. Chaney MA, Durazo-Arvizu RA, Nikolov MP, et al: Methylprednisolone does not benefit patients undergoing coronary artery bypass grafting and early tracheal extubation. J Thorac Cardiovasc Surg 121:561, 2001
184. Chaney MA: Corticosteroids and cardiopulmonary bypass: A review of clinical investigations. Chest 121:921, 2002
185. Weerwind PW, Maessen JG, van Tits LJ, et al: Influence of Duraflo II heparin-treated extracorporeal circuits on the systemic inflammatory response in patients having coronary bypass. J Thorac Cardiovasc Surg 110:1633, 1995
186. Ovrum E, Mollnes TE, Fosse E, et al: Complement and granulocyte activation in two different types of heparinized extracorporeal circuits. J Thorac Cardiovasc Surg 110:1623, 1995

187. Jakob H, Hafner G, Iversen S, et al: Reoperation and the centrifugal pump? Eur J Cardiothorac Surg 6: S59, 1992
188. Driessen JJ, Dhaese H, Fransen G, et al: Pulsatile compared with nonpulsatile perfusion using a centrifugal pump for cardiopulmonary bypass during coronary artery bypass grafting. Effects on systemic hemodynamics, oxygenation, and inflammatory response parameters. Perfusion 10:3, 1995
189. Tamiya T, Yamasaki M, Maeo Y, et al: Complement activation in cardiopulmonary bypass, with special reference to anaphylatoxin production in membrane and bubble oxygenators. Ann Thorac Surg 46:47, 1988
190. Jones HM, Matthews N, Vaughan RS, Stark JM: Cardiopulmonary bypass and complement activation. Involvement of classical and alternative pathways. Anaesthesia 37:629, 1982
191. Byrick RJ, Noble WH: Postperfusion lung syndrome. Comparison of Travenol bubble and membrane oxygenators. J Thorac Cardiovasc Surg 76:685, 1978
192. van Oeveren W, Dankert J, Wildevuur CR: Bubble oxygenation and cardiotomy suction impair the host defense during cardiopulmonary bypass: A study in dogs. Ann Thorac Surg 44:523, 1987
193. Videm V, Fosse E, Mollnes TE, et al: Complement activation with bubble and membrane oxygenators in aortocoronary bypass grafting. Ann Thorac Surg 50:387, 1990
194. Croughwell ND, Newman MF, Lowry E, et al: Effect of temperature during cardiopulmonary bypass on gastric mucosal perfusion. Br J Anaesth 78:34, 1997
195. Menasche P, Peynet J, Lariviere J, et al: Does normothermia during cardiopulmonary bypass increase neutrophil-endothelium interactions? Circulation 90:II-275, 1994
196. Ohata T, Sawa Y, Kadoba K, et al: Normothermia has beneficial effects in cardiopulmonary bypass attenuating inflammatory reactions. ASAIO J 41:M288, 1995
197. Grigore AM, Mathew J, Grocott HP, et al: Prospective randomized trial of normothermic versus hypothermic cardiopulmonary bypass on cognitive function after coronary artery bypass graft surgery. Anesthesiology 95:1110, 2001
198. Grocott HP, Mackensen GB, Grigore AM, et al: Postoperative hyperthermia is associated with cognitive dysfunction after coronary artery bypass graft surgery. Stroke 33:537, 2002
199. van Dijk D, Nierich AP, Jansen EW, et al: Early outcome after off-pump versus on-pump coronary bypass surgery: Results from a randomized study. Circulation 104:1761, 2001
200. Puskas JD, Williams WH, Mahoney EM, et al: Off-pump vs conventional coronary artery bypass grafting: Early and 1-year graft patency, cost, and quality-of-life outcomes: A randomized trial. JAMA 291:1841, 2004
201. Nathoe HM, van Dijk D, Jansen EW, et al: A comparison of on-pump and off-pump coronary bypass surgery in low-risk patients. N Engl J Med 348:394, 2003
202. Khan NE, De Souza A, Mister R, et al: A randomized comparison of off-pump and on-pump multivessel coronary-artery bypass surgery. N Engl J Med 350:21, 2004
203. Racz MJ, Hannan EL, Isom OW, et al: A comparison of short- and long-term outcomes after off-pump and on-pump coronary artery bypass graft surgery with sternotomy. J Am Coll Cardiol 43:557, 2004
204. Andreasson S, Gothberg S, Berggren H, et al: Hemofiltration modifies complement activation after extracorporeal circulation in infants. Ann Thorac Surg 56:1515, 1993
205. Journois D, Israel-Biet D, Pouard P, et al: High-volume, zero-balanced hemofiltration to reduce delayed inflammatory response to cardiopulmonary bypass in children. Anesthesiology 85:965, 1996
206. Gu YJ, de Vries AJ, Boonstra PW, van Oeveren W: Leukocyte depletion results in improved lung function and reduced inflammatory response after cardiac surgery. J Thorac Cardiovasc Surg 112:494, 1996
207. Lust RM, Bode AP, Yang L, et al: In-line leukocyte filtration during bypass. Clinical results from a randomized prospective trial. ASAIO J 42: M819, 1996
208. Mihaljevic T, Tonz M, von Segesser LK, et al: The influence of leukocyte filtration during cardiopulmonary bypass on postoperative lung function. A clinical study. J Thorac Cardiovasc Surg 109:1138, 1995
209. Davies GG, Wells DG, Mabee TM, et al: Platelet-leukocyte plasmapheresis attenuates the deleterious effects of cardiopulmonary bypass. Ann Thorac Surg 53:274, 1992
210. Vamvakas EC: Meta-analysis of randomized controlled trials investigating the risk of postoperative infection in association with white blood cell-containing allogeneic blood transfusion: The effects of the type of transfused red blood cell product and surgical setting. Transfus Med Rev 16:304, 2002
211. van de Watering LM, Hermans J, Houbiers JG, et al: Beneficial effects of leukocyte depletion of transfused blood on postoperative complications in patients undergoing cardiac surgery: A randomized clinical trial. Circulation 97:562, 1998
212. Llewelyn CA, Taylor RS, Todd AA, et al: The effect of universal leukoreduction on postoperative infections and length of hospital stay in elective orthopedic and cardiac surgery. Transfusion 44:489, 2004
213. Dzik WH, Anderson JK, O'Neill EM, et al: A prospective, randomized clinical trial of universal WBC reduction. Transfusion 42:1114, 2002
214. Soeparwata R, Hartman AR, Frerichmann U, et al: Aprotinin diminishes inflammatory processes. Int J Cardiol 53(suppl):S55, 1996
215. Seghaye MC, Duchateau J, Grabitz RG, et al: Influence of low-dose aprotinin on the inflammatory reaction due to cardiopulmonary bypass in children. Ann Thorac Surg 61:1205, 1996
216. Levy JH, Pifarre R, Schaff HV, et al: A multicenter, double-blind, placebo-controlled trial of aprotinin for reducing blood loss and the requirement for donor-blood transfusion in patients undergoing repeat coronary artery bypass grafting. Circulation 92:2236, 1995
217. Levy JH, Murkin JM, Ramsay JG: Aprotinin reduces the incidence of strokes following cardiac surgery. Circulation 94: I, 1996
218. Murkin JM: Cardiopulmonary bypass and the inflammatory response: A role for serine protease inhibitors? J Cardiothorac Vasc Anesth 11:19, 1997; discussion 24, 1997
219. Liu B, Belboul A, Radberg G, et al: Half-dose aprotinin does not affect haemorheological properties in patients undergoing bypass surgery. Coron Artery Dis 7:609, 1996
220. Lesslauer W, Tabuchi H, Gentz R, et al: Recombinant soluble tumor necrosis factor receptor proteins protect mice from lipopolysaccharide-induced lethality. Eur J Immunol 21:2883, 1991
221. Abraham E, Glauser MP, Butler T, et al: p55 Tumor necrosis factor receptor fusion protein in the treatment of patients with severe sepsis and septic shock. A randomized controlled multicenter trial. Ro 45-2081 Study Group. JAMA 277:1531, 1997
222. Baumgartner JD, Glauser MP, McCutchan JA, et al: Prevention of gram-negative shock and death in surgical patients by antibody to endotoxin core glycolipid. Lancet 2:59, 1985
223. Ziegler EJ, McCutchan JA, Fierer J, et al: Treatment of gram-negative bacteremia and shock with human antiserum to a mutant Escherichia coli. N Engl J Med 307:1225, 1982
224. Spapen HD, Diltoer M, Huyghens LP: Passive immunotherapy of gram-negative bacteremia, sepsis and septic shock. Acta Clin Belg 48:20, 1993
225. Pilz G, Kreuzer E, Kaab S, et al: Early sepsis treatment with immunoglobulins after cardiac surgery in score-identified high-risk patients. Chest 105:76, 1994
226. Di Padova FE, Brade H, Barclay GR, et al: A broadly cross-protective monoclonal antibody binding to Escherichia coli and Salmonella lipopolysaccharides. Infect Immun 61:3863, 1993
227. DeMaria A Jr, Johns MA, Berberich H, McCabe WR: Immunization with rough mutants of Salmonella Minnesota: Initial studies in human subjects. J Infect Dis 158:301, 1988
228. Lynn M, Rossignol DP, Wheeler JL, et al: Blocking of responses to endotoxin by E5564 in healthy volunteers with experimental endotoxemia. J Infect Dis 187:631, 2003
229. Hoffmann H, Markewitz A, Kreuzer E, et al: Pentoxifylline decreases the incidence of multiple organ failure in patients after major cardiothoracic surgery. Shock 9:235, 1998
230. Thabut G, Brugiere O, Leseche G, et al: Preventive effect of inhaled nitric oxide and pentoxifylline on ischemia/reperfusion injury after lung transplantation. Transplantation 71:1295, 2001
231. Boldt J, Brosch C, Lehmann A, et al: Prophylactic use of pentoxifylline on inflammation in elderly cardiac surgery patients. Ann Thorac Surg 71:1524, 2001
232. Boldt J, Brosch C, Piper SN, et al: Influence of prophylactic use of pentoxifylline on postoperative organ function in elderly cardiac surgery patients. Crit Care Med 29:952, 2001
233. Nelson D, Kuppermann N, Fleisher GR, et al: Recombinant endotoxin neutralizing protein improves survival from Escherichia coli sepsis in rats. Crit Care Med 23:92, 1995
234. Pajkrt D, Doran JE, Koster F, et al: Antiinflammatory effects of reconstituted high-density lipoprotein during human endotoxemia. J Exp Med 184:1601, 1996
235. Palmer JD, Rifkind D: Neutralization of the hemodynamic effects of endotoxin by polymyxin B. Surg Gynecol Obstet 138:755, 1974
236. Fink MP: Ringer's ethyl pyruvate solution: A novel resuscitation fluid for the treatment of hemorrhagic shock and sepsis. J Trauma 54: S141, 2003

237. Fink MP: Ethyl pyruvate: A novel anti-inflammatory agent. Crit Care Med 31: S51, 2003
238. Roytblat L, Talmor D, Rachinsky M, et al: Ketamine attenuates the interleukin-6 response after cardiopulmonary bypass. Anesth Analg 87:266, 1998
239. Debaene B, Goldfarb G, Braillon A, et al: Effects of ketamine, halothane, enflurane, and isoflurane on systemic and splanchnic hemodynamics in normovolemic and hypovolemic cirrhotic rats. Anesthesiology 73:118, 1990
240. Stoelting RK: Pharmacology and Physiology in Anesthetic Practice. Philadelphia, JB Lippincott, 1991
241. Gelman S, Fowler KC, Smith LR: Regional blood flow during isoflurane and halothane anesthesia. Anesth Analg 63:557, 1984
242. Conzen PF, Peter K: Volatile anesthetics and organ blood flow. *In* Torri G, Damin G (eds): Update on Modern Inhalation Anesthetics. New York, Worldwide Medical Communications, 1989, pp 29–35
243. Mythen MG, Webb AR: There is no correlation between gastric mucosal perfusion (tonometer pHi) and arterial hemoglobin concentration during major surgery. Med Intens 17:S44, 1993
244. Giroir BP, Beutler B: Effect of amrinone on tumor necrosis factor production in endotoxic shock. Circ Shock 36:200, 1992

Chapter 9
PHARMACOLOGY OF ANESTHETIC DRUGS

Kelly Grogan, MD • Daniel Nyhan, MD • Dan E. Berkowitz, MD

KEY POINTS

1. In patients, the observed acute effect of any specific anesthetic agent on the cardiovascular system represents the net effect on the myocardium, coronary blood flow, electrophysiologic behavior, the vasculature, and neurohormonal reflex function. Anesthetic agents may differ from one another, either quantitatively and/or qualitatively, even within the same category, with respect to any of these variables. Moreover, the acute response to an anesthetic agent may be modulated by a patient's underlying pathology and/or pharmacologic treatment.
2. Volatile agents cause dose-dependent decreases in systemic blood pressure that for halothane and enflurane are mainly due to depression of contractile function and for isoflurane, desflurane, and sevoflurane are mainly due to decreases in systemic vascular responses. Volatile anesthetic agents cause dose-dependent depression of contractile function mediated at a cellular level by attenuating calcium currents and decreasing calcium sensitivity. Decreases in systemic vascular responses reflect variable effects on both endothelium-dependent and -independent mechanisms.
3. The net effect of volatile agents on coronary blood flow is determined by several variables, including anesthetic effects on systemic hemodynamics, myocardial metabolism, and direct effects on the coronary vasculature. When confounding variables are controlled, studies of volatile agents, including isoflurane, indicate that they exert only mild direct vasodilatory effects on the coronary vasculature.
4. In addition to causing acute coronary syndromes, myocardial ischemia can manifest itself as myocardial stunning, preconditioning, or hibernating myocardium. Volatile anesthetic agents have been demonstrated to attenuate myocardial ischemia development by mechanisms that are independent of myocardial oxygen supply and demand and to facilitate functional recovery in stunned myocardium. Volatile agents can also simulate ischemic preconditioning, a phenomenon described as anesthetic preconditioning, and the underlying mechanisms are similar to but not necessarily identical to those underlying ischemic preconditioning.
5. The intravenous induction agents/hypnotics belong to different drug classes (barbiturates, benzodiazepines, *N*-methyl-D-aspartate receptor antagonists, and α_2-adrenergic receptor agonists). Although they all induce hypnosis, their sites of action and molecular targets differ based on their class. Furthermore, their cardiovascular effects are to some degree dependent on the class to which they belong.
6. In general, studies in isolated cardiac myocytes, cardiac muscle tissue, and vascular tissue demonstrate that induction agents inhibit cardiac contractility and relax vascular tone by inhibiting mechanisms that increase intracellular Ca^{++}. This effect may be offset by mechanisms that increase myofilament Ca^{++} sensitivity in both the cardiac myocyte and vascular smooth muscle. While these effects may contribute to or modulate cardiovascular changes, the cumulative effects of the induction agents on contractility and vascular resistance and capacitance are mediated predominantly by their sympatholytic effects. It is for this reason that these agents should be used judiciously and with extreme caution in patients with shock, heart failure, or other pathophysiologic circumstances in which the sympathetic nervous system is paramount in maintaining myocardial contractility and arterial and venous tone.
7. Opioids exhibit diverse chemical structures, but all retain an essential T-shaped component necessary stereochemically for the activation of the different opioid receptors (the μ-, κ-, and δ-receptors). The latter are not confined to the nervous system and have also been identified in the myocardium and in blood vessels where endogenous opioid proteins can be synthesized.
8. Acute exogenous opioid administration modulates multiple determinants of central and peripheral cardiovascular regulation. However, the predominant clinical effect is mediated by attenuation of central sympathetic outflow.
9. Activation of the δ-opioid receptor can elicit preconditioning. The role of this mechanism in both physiologic and pathophysiologic conditions is currently an area of active investigation. In contrast to ischemia in homeotherms, hibernation is, by definition, well tolerated in certain species. This latter phenomenon may be partially dependent on mechanisms that are activated by opioids or opioid-like molecules.

An enormous body of literature has been accumulated describing the protean effects of the different anesthetic agents on the heart and the pulmonary and systemic regional vascular beds. The effects on the heart, especially, have spawned innumerable publications. More recently, this has been due to the great interest in anesthesia-induced preconditioning (APC). However, even prior to the initial description of APC, the literature detailing the influence of anesthetic agents on the myocardium was prodigious and not always consistent.[1-3] This likely reflected not only the challenges inherent in quantitating the direct effects of volatile agents on the myocyte/myocardium, but also the presence of several potential confounding variables including effects on coronary blood flow (CBF), the systemic vasculature, and the baroreceptor reflex arc. The authors divided the discussion of the effects of volatile agents, fixed agents, and narcotics on the cardiovascular system (CVS) into those that involve acute and delayed effects. Under acute effects, the influence of anesthetic agents is described on (1) myocardial function, (2) electrophysiology, (3) coronary vasoregulation, (4) systemic and pulmonary vasoregulation, and (5) the baroreceptor reflex. Within delayed effects, the focus is on APC.

VOLATILE AGENTS

Acute Effects

Myocardial Function

The influence of volatile anesthetics on contractile function has been investigated extensively in several animal species and

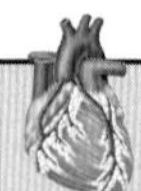

BOX 9–1 *Volatile Anesthetic Agents*

- All volatile anesthetic agents cause dose-dependent decreases in systemic blood pressure which for halothane and enflurane are predominantly due to attenuation of myocardial contractile function and which for isoflurane, desflurane, and sevoflurane are predominantly due to decreases in systemic vascular resistance. Moreover, volatile agents obtund all components of the baroreceptor reflex arc.
- The effects of volatile agents on myocardial diastolic function are not yet well characterized and await the application of "bedside" emerging technologies that have the sensitivity to quantitate indices of diastolic function.
- Volatile anesthetics lower the arrhythmogenic threshold to catecholamines. However, the underlying molecular mechanisms are not well understood.
- When confounding variables are controlled (e.g., systemic blood pressure), isoflurane does not cause "coronary steal" by a direct effect on coronary vasculature.
- The effects of volatile agents on systemic regional vascular beds and on the pulmonary vasculature are complex, and depend on variables that include, but are not confined to, the specific anesthetic under study, the specific vascular bed, the vessel size, and whether endothelial-dependent or -independent mechanisms are being investigated.

in humans using various in vitro and in vivo models.[4-12] In general, it is now widely agreed that volatile agents cause dose-dependent depression of contractile function (Box 9–1). Moreover, different volatile agents are not identical in this regard and the preponderance of information indicates that halothane and enflurane exert equal but more potent myocardial depression than do isoflurane, desflurane, or sevoflurane. This reflects in part reflex sympathetic activation with the latter agents. It is also widely accepted that in the setting of preexisting myocardial depression, volatile agents have a greater effect than in normal myocardium.[13,14] Early studies indicating that volatile agents may not have a deleterious effect on function in the setting of acute myocardial infarction (AMI) likely reflected the fact that the limited infarction did not compromise overall myocardial function.[15,16] At the cellular level, volatile anesthetics exert their negative inotropic effects mainly by modulating sarcolemmal (SL) L-type Ca^{++} channels, the sarcoplasmic reticulum (SR), and the contractile proteins. L-type Ca^{++} currents are decreased and, secondarily, SR Ca^{++} release is depressed (Figs. 9–1 and 9–2).[17] Moreover, the contractile response to lower Ca^{++} levels is further attenuated in the presence of volatile agents in that the response is decreased by volatile agents at any given Ca^{++} level, that is, volatile agents also decrease Ca^{++} sensitivity (Fig. 9–3).[17] However, the mechanisms whereby anesthetic agents modify ion channels are not completely understood. Ion channels are usually studied in ex vivo circumstances where, by definition, multiple modulating influences of the specific channel under study may be altered. Moreover, these studies are frequently undertaken in nonhuman tissue. Well-recognized species differences make extrapolation to humans difficult.[18] Nitrous oxide causes direct mild myocardial depression but also causes sympathetic activation.[19]

It is well recognized that even in the setting of normal systolic function, diastolic dysfunction occurs with increasing frequency in the elderly and is an important cause of congestive heart failure (CHF).[20-26] Diastolic dysfunction and its more

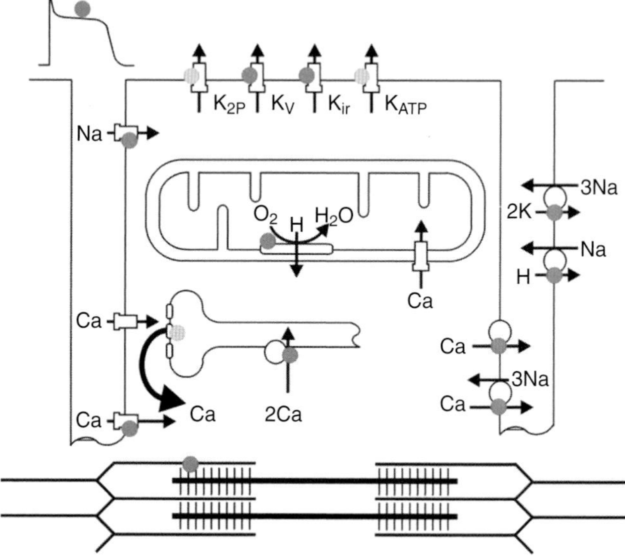

Figure 9–1 Sites of action of volatile anesthetics in a ventricular myocyte. The darker spots indicate inhibitory actions, and the lighter spots indicate stimulatory actions. (From Hanley PJ, ter Keurs HEDJ, Cannell MB: Excitation-contraction in the heart and the negative inotropic action of volatile anesthetics. Anesthesiology 101:999, 2004)

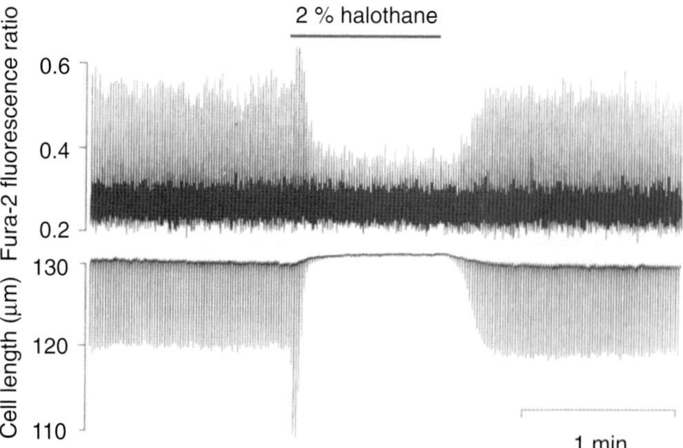

Figure 9–2 Fura-2 fluorescence (*top trace*), an index of Ca^{++}, and cell length (*bottom trace*), an index of contraction, were measured simultaneously in an electrically stimulated rat ventricular myocyte. Application of halothane initially induced a transient increase in the Ca^{++} transient and twitch force before both the Ca^{++} signals and contraction decreased. (From Harrison SM, Robinson M, Davies LA, et al: Mechanisms underlying the inotropic action of halothane on intact rat ventricular myocytes. Br J Anaesth 82:609, 1999)

severe clinical counterpart, diastolic heart failure, have protean etiologies and can be mechanistically complex[20] (Table 9–1). However, the mechanisms underlying these conditions can be categorized into those involving alterations in myocardial relaxation (e.g., SR Ca^{++} handling, phospholamdan) and those related to intrinsic properties of myocardial tissue (e.g., myocyte cytoskeletal elements), and those that are extramyocardial (e.g., loading conditions). Indices of diastolic function were not readily and reliably measured noninvasively in the past. Hence, the relatively more recent recognition and description of diastolic dysfunction and diastolic heart failure compared with perturbations in systolic function. This likely also explains the relative paucity of literature detailing the modulating effects of volatile agents on diastolic function. There is reasonable agreement in the literature that volatile agents prolong isovolumic relaxation and do so in a dose-dependent manner.[25-31] The effects of volatile agents

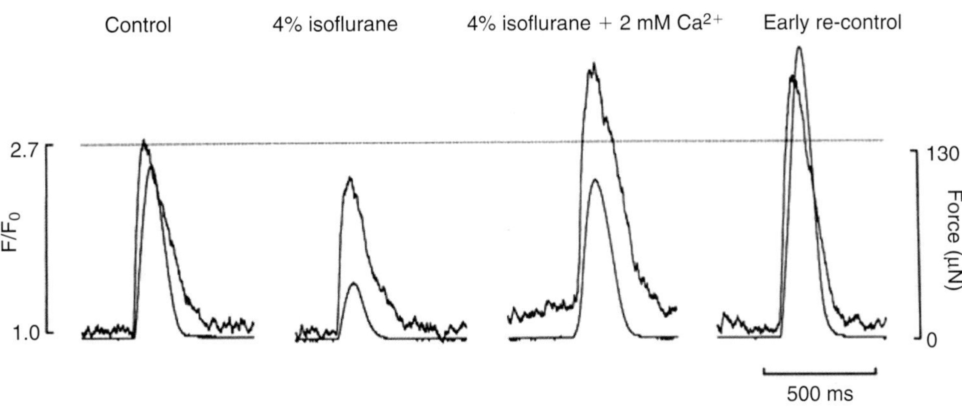

Figure 9–3 Simultaneous measurement of force and fluo-3 fluorescence, an index of Ca^{++}, in a rat cardiac trabecula. Application of isoflurane decreased force and Ca^{++}. Restoration of the Ca^{++} transient amplitude by elevation of external Ca^{++} did not recover force, indicating that, in addition to decreasing Ca^{++} availability, the anesthetic decreased Ca^{++} responsiveness of the contractile proteins. (From Hanley PJ, Loiselle DS: Mechanisms of force inhibition of halothane and isoflurane in intact rat cardiac muscle. J Physiol 506:231, 1998)

on chamber stiffness are more controversial; for example, halothane has been reported to both decrease compliance and have no effect on myocardial stiffness.[25-30,32] The effect of nitrous oxide on diastolic function has not been investigated in a manner that critically rules out confounding variables. At a molecular level, alterations in relaxation likely reflect modulation of Ca^{++} currents, including SR Ca^{++} reuptake mechanisms. Paradoxically, in the setting of reperfusion injury and Ca^{++} overload, the volatile agent sevoflurane improves indices of diastolic relaxation and attenuates myoplasmic Ca^{++} overload.[33]

Table 9–1 Diastolic Heart Failure: Mechanisms and Etiologies

Abnormalities of myocardial relaxation
Ischemia
Hypertrophy
Hypertension
Valvular heart disease
Abnormalities of myocardial compliance
Aging
Fibrosis
Hypertrophy
Diabetes mellitus
Metabolic syndrome
Infiltrative disorders—amyloidosis
Cardiomyopathies
Constrictive pericarditis

Cardiac Electrophysiology

Volatile anesthetic agents lower the arrhythmogenic threshold for epinephrine. Moreover, not all volatile agents are similar, with the order of sensitization being: halothane > enflurane > sevoflurane > isoflurane = desflurane.

The molecular mechanisms underlying this effect of volatile anesthetics are poorly understood. Anesthetic agent–induced modulation of ion channels is important mechanistically in excitation-contraction coupling (vide supra), in preconditioning (vide infra), and in modulating automaticity and arrhythmia generation[18] (Table 9–2). Although the effects of any particular volatile agent on a specific cardiac ion channel may have been characterized, this does not allow a ready extrapolation into clinical situations. This partly reflects those issues already discussed (species differences, ex vivo studies) but also the recognition that it is impossible to predict the arrhythmogenic effect that might ensue following modulation with a particular volatile agent. This should be one of the lessons garnered from the experience with the antiarrhythmic drugs such as encainide and flecainide.[34] Moreover, even in the clinical setting, not all volatile agents have the same effect.[35]

Coronary Vasoregulation

Volatile anesthetic agents modulate several determinants of both myocardial oxygen supply and demand. Moreover, it is now established that volatile agents also directly modulate the

Table 9–2 Summary of the Actions of Volatile Anesthetics on Various Ion Currents in the Heart and the Most Important Side Effects of the Drugs

Target	Effect	Anesthetic Gas	Cardiac Side Effects
L-type Ca^{++} current	Inhibition	Halothane, isoflurane, sevoflurane	**Reduced contractility,** shortened AP and refractory time
β-Adrenergic regulation of L-type Ca^{++} current	Complex interference	Halothane	Enhanced proarrhythmicity in comparison with sevoflurane?
Voltage-dependent transient outward K^+ current	Inhibition	Halothane, isoflurane, xenon	Shortened AP duration, AP duration mismatch within the heart
Voltage-dependent sustained outward K^+ current	Inhibition	Halothane, isoflurane, sevoflurane	**Delayed repolarization, mismatch of AP duration**
ATP-dependent K^+ current	Enhancement	Isoflurane, sevoflurane	Myocardial preconditioning
Fast Na^+ current	Inhibition	Halothane, isoflurane, sevoflurane	**Slowed conduction,** induction of tachyarrhythmias?

Effects of paramount importance are printed in bold.
From Huneke R, Fassl J, Rossaint R, et al: Effects of volatile anesthetics on cardiac ion channels. Acta Anaesthesiol Scand 48:547, 2004.

myocytes' response to ischemia. Thus, studies investigating the effects of volatile agents on coronary vasoregulation should be interpreted in this context.

Animal studies indicate that halothane has little direct effect on the coronary vasculature.[36-38] Likewise, clinical studies investigating the effect of halothane indicate that it has either minimal or mild coronary vasodilator effects.[39-42] The effect of isoflurane on coronary vessels was controversial and dominated much of the literature in this area in the 1980s and early 1990s. The current assessments of the effects of isoflurane have recently been succinctly detailed by Tanaka et al.[43] Several reports had indicated that it caused direct coronary arteriolar vasodilatation in vessels of 100 μm or less and that isoflurane could cause "coronary steal" in patients with "steal-prone" coronary anatomy, that is, in patients with significant coronary stenosis in a vessel subserving a region of ischemic myocardium, when presumably vessels were maximally dilated due to local metabolic autoregulation, and in whom isoflurane-induced vasodilatation in adjacent vessels resulted in diversion of coronary flow away from the ischemic region.[44,45] Several animal and human studies in which potential confounding variables were controlled indicated clearly that isoflurane did not cause coronary steal.[46-52] Studies of sevoflurane and desflurane showed similar results and are consistent with a mild direct coronary vasodilator effect of these agents.[53,54]

Ultimately, CBF (in the setting of normal systemic hemodynamics) is controlled by coronary vascular smooth muscle tone, which can be modulated directly (endothelium-independent) or indirectly via the endothelium (endothelium-dependent). Teleologically, it can be predicted that in vital organs, control of blood flow is predominantly local, acting through either endothelium-dependent or -independent mechanisms. Thus, volatile agents have the capacity to modulate mechanisms underlying vascular tone: (1) Halothane and isoflurane have been shown to attenuate endothelial-dependent tone (by receptor-dependent and receptor-dependent plus -independent mechanisms, respectively) in coronary microvessels[55]; (2) several volatile agents cause coronary vasodilation via K^+_{ATP} channel-dependent mechanisms[55-58]; and (3) sevoflurane induced K^+ and Ca^{++} channel–mediated increases in coronary collateral blood flow.[59] The effects in vivo are likely to be modest because local control mechanisms are likely to predominate.

Systemic Regional and Pulmonary Vascular Effects

Vascular tone can be modulated by volatile agents. However, the specific result can be influenced by not only the agent under study but also by the vascular bed being investigated, the vessel size/type within that vascular bed, the level of pre-existing vascular tone, age, and indirect effects of the agents, such as anesthesia-induced hypotension and reflex autonomic nervous system (ANS) activation.

All volatile anesthetic agents decrease systemic blood pressure (BP) in a dose-dependent manner. With halothane and enflurane, the decrease in systemic BP is primarily due to decreases in stroke volume (SV) and cardiac output (CO); whereas isoflurane, sevoflurane, and desflurane decrease overall systemic vascular resistance (SVR) while maintaining CO. However, these overall effects belie the multiple effects in the various regional vascular beds. Within the systemic non-coronary vasculature, aortic and mesenteric vessels have been the best studied.

Reversible inhibition of endothelium-dependent relaxation in aortic and femoral vessels was first demonstrated for halothane and has also been demonstrated for enflurane, isoflurane, and sevoflurane in both capacitance and resistance vessels.[55,60-64] However, these observations mask the differential effects of volatile agents on underlying endothelium-dependent mechanisms. Halothane and enflurane decrease agonist (bradykinin) and ATP-induced Ca^{++} increases in bovine endothelial cells, while isoflurane does not.[65] In contrast, isoflurane does attenuate histamine-induced Ca^{++} influx into human endothelial cells.[66] Alterations in endothelium-dependent mechanisms by volatile agents are not confined to attenuation of agonist-dependent and -independent activation of endothelial nitric oxide synthase (eNOS) and nitric oxide (NO) release but may also extend to other mechanisms. For example, the effects of sevoflurane on endothelial cell function may be partially due to sevoflurane-induced changes in endothelin-1 (ET-1) production and in the redox milieu of the endothelial cells (i.e., increased superoxide anion production).[67]

The effect of volatile agents on vascular smooth muscle mechanisms is equally complex and varies among agents. In endothelial cell–denuded aortic rings, halothane decreases both SL Ca^{++} influx via voltage-dependent calcium channels and SR Ca^{++} release, but sevoflurane does not.[68] Sevoflurane also inhibits angiotensin II–induced vascular smooth muscle contraction in aortic rings.[69] In mesenteric vessels, sevoflurane accentuates endothelium-dependent mechanisms and attenuates endothelium-independent mechanisms in the presence of norepinephrine.[70] Studies of the influence of volatile agents on vascular smooth muscle Ca^{++} currents indicate that both halothane and enflurane stimulate SR release and reuptake from the caffeine-sensitive pool. In contrast, halothane, enflurane, and isoflurane all increase calcium-induced calcium release (CICR) mechanisms, but sevoflurane decreases CICR mechanisms.[71] Finally, volatile agents have also been demonstrated to modulate Ca^{++} sensitivity. In mesenteric vessels, halothane relaxation is largely mediated by Ca^{++} and myosin light chain desensitizing mechanisms.[72]

The pulmonary circulation has unique features that must be taken into account when interpreting studies of this vascular bed. In addition to those issues that also apply to systemic vascular beds (vessel size, etc.), the pulmonary vasculature is a low-resistance bed (requiring preconstriction in order to access vasoactive effects), is not rectilinear (thus, changes in flow per se can change certain parameters used to calculate resistance), is contained within the chest (and thus subject to extravascular pressures, which are not atmospheric and change during the respiratory cycle), and exhibits the unique vascular phenomenon of hypoxia-induced vasoconstriction. It is clear that volatile agents modulate not only the baseline pulmonary vasculature but also multiple vasoactive mechanisms that control pulmonary vascular tone. Moreover, the effect of volatile agents is agent specific. For example, halothane causes flow-independent pulmonary vasoconstriction.[73] In contrast, the hypoxic pulmonary vasoconstrictor (HPV) response does not seem to be altered by at least two currently used volatile agents: sevoflurane and desflurane.[74] The pulmonary vascular endothelial response seems to be impaired by the volatile agents halothane and isoflurane.[75,76] Finally, pulmonary vascular smooth muscle regulatory mechanisms can also be modified by volatile agents. Halothane, enflurane, and isoflurane all attenuate pulmonary vasodilatation induced by K^+_{ATP} channel activation.[77,78] Although the

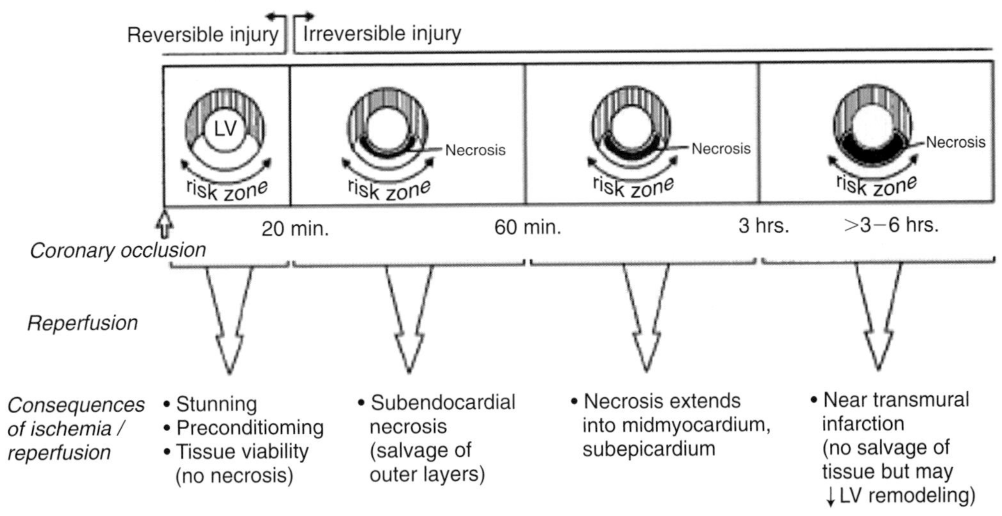

Figure 9–4 Effects of ischemia and reperfusion on the heart based on studies in anesthetized canine model of proximal coronary artery occlusion. Brief periods of ischemia of less than 20 minutes followed by reperfusion are not associated with development of necrosis (reversible injury). Brief ischemia/reperfusion results in the phenomenon of stunning and preconditioning. If duration of coronary occlusion is extended beyond 20 minutes, a wavefront of necrosis marches from subendocardium to subepicardium over time. Reperfusion before 3 hours of ischemia salvages ischemic but viable tissue. (This salvaged tissue may demonstrate stunning.) Reperfusion beyond 3 to 6 hours in this model does not reduce myocardial infarct size. Late reperfusion may still have a beneficial effect on reducing or preventing myocardial infarct expansion and left ventricular (LV) remodeling. (From Kloner RA, Jennings RB: Consequences of brief ischemia: Stunning, preconditioning, and their clinical implications. Part I. Circulation 104:2981, 2001)

effects of the different volatile agents on K^+_{ATP} channel activation are similar, β-adrenergic receptor–induced pulmonary vasodilatation is differently modulated. Halothane and isoflurane potentiate the vasodilatory response, but enflurane has no effect.[79]

Baroreceptor Reflex

All volatile agents attenuate the baroreceptor reflex. Baroreceptor reflex inhibition by halothane and enflurane is more potent than that observed with isoflurane, desflurane, or sevoflurane, each of which has a similar effect.[80,81] Each component of the baroreceptor reflex arc (afferent nerve activity, central processing, efferent nerve activity) is inhibited by volatile agents. Inhibition of afferent nerve traffic results in part from baroreceptor sensitization,[82,83] whereas attenuation of efferent activity is in part due to ganglionic inhibition as manifest by differential preganglionic and postganglionic nerve activity.[82-84]

Delayed Effects

Reversible Myocardial Ischemia

Prolonged ischemia results in irreversible myocardial damage and necrosis (Box 9–2). Shorter durations of myocardial ischemia can, depending on the duration and sequence of ischemic insults, lead to either preconditioning or myocardial stunning (Fig. 9–4).[85] Stunning, first described in 1975, occurs following brief ischemia and is characterized by myocardial dysfunction in the setting of normal restored blood flow, and by an absence of myocardial necrosis.[86] Ischemic preconditioning (IPC) was first described by Murray et al in 1986 and is characterized by an attenuation in infarct size following sustained ischemia, if this period of sustained ischemia is preceded by a period of brief ischemia (Fig. 9–5).[87] Moreover, this effect is independent of collateral flow. Thus, short periods of ischemia followed by reperfusion can lead to either stunning or preconditioning with a reduction in infarct size (Fig. 9–6).[85]

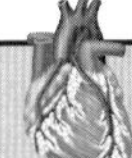

BOX 9–2 *Volatile Agents and Myocardial Ischemia*

- Volatile anesthetic agents have been demonstrated to attenuate the effects of myocardial ischemia (acute coronary syndromes).
- Nonacute manifestations of myocardial ischemia include hibernating myocardium, stunning, and preconditioning.
- Halothane and isoflurane facilitate the recovery of stunned myocardium.
- Preconditioning, a profoundly important adaptive protective mechanism in biological tissues, can be provoked by protean nonlethal stresses, including but not confined to ischemia.
- Volatile anesthetic agents can mimic preconditioning (anesthetic preconditioning), an observation that could have important clinical implications, as well as providing insight into the cellular mechanisms of action of volatile agents.

As discussed, work in the 1970s indicated that volatile anesthetic agents attenuated ST-segment elevations in the setting of short-duration ischemia,[91] and limited infarct size and lactate production following prolonged ischemia.[88,89] Moreover, these effects seemed to be independent of the main determinants of myocardial oxygen supply and demand and suggested that the volatile agents may be exerting a beneficial effect at the level of the myocyte. Upon resolution of the isoflurane "coronary steal" controversy, the first description of the salutary effects of volatile agents on the consequences of brief ischemia was made in 1988. Warltier and co-workers described the beneficial effects of halothane and isoflurane in facilitating the recovery of contractile function in stunned myocardium[90] (Fig. 9–7). However, it was almost a decade later before the effects of volatile agents on preconditioning were outlined[1,2] and the term APC was used[3] (Fig. 9–8).

The phenomenon of and the mechanisms underlying IPC are the focus of extensive investigation. IPC (1) results in two periods (termed "windows") of protection—the first (termed "early" or "classic") occurring at 1 to 3 hours and a second

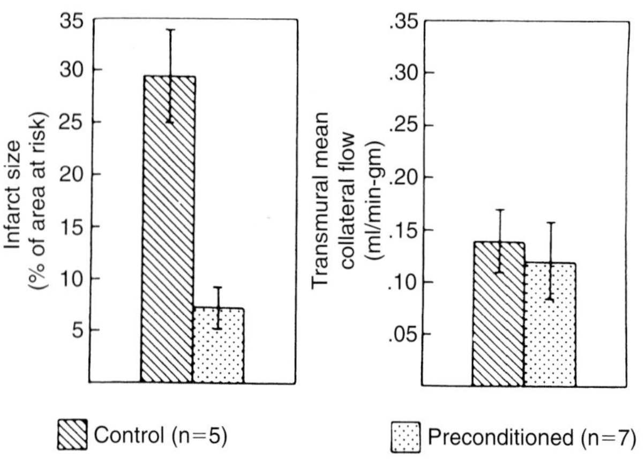

Figure 9–5 Infarct size and collateral blood flow in the 40-minute study. *Left*, Infarct size, as a percentage of the anatomic area at risk, in the control (*striped bar*) and preconditioned (*stippled bar*) hearts. Infarct size in control animals averaged 29.4% of the area at risk. Infarct size in preconditioned hearts averaged only 7.3% of the area at risk (preconditioned versus control, $P < 0.001$). Transmural mean collateral blood flow (*right*) was not significantly different in the two groups. Thus, the protective effect of preconditioning was independent of the two major baseline predictors of infarct size, area at risk and collateral blood flow. Bars represent group mean ± SEM. (From Warltier DC, al-Wathiqui MH, Kampine JP, et al: Recovery of contractile function of stunned myocardium in chronically instrumented dogs is enhanced by halothane or isoflurane. Anesthesiology 69:552, 1988)

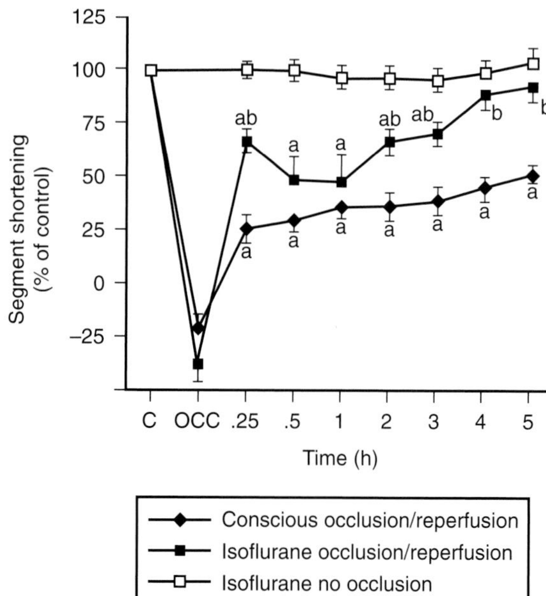

Figure 9–7 Segment shortening data (expressed as a percent of control mean ± SEM) during coronary artery occlusion (OCC) and at various times following reperfusion in conscious dogs (group 1—◆—) and in those dogs anesthetized with isoflurane (group 7—■—). Comparisons are made at various time points to those animals anesthetized with isoflurane but not undergoing coronary artery occlusion and reperfusion (group 6—□—). [a]Significant ($P < 0.05$) difference, group 6 (anesthetized without occlusion) versus 1 (conscious occlusion) or 7 (occlusion during anesthesia. [b]Significant ($P < 9.95$) difference, group 1 (conscious occlusion) versus 7 (occlusion during anesthesia). Note that the control state (C) indicates either the awake, unsedated state (group 1) or following a stable hemodynamic state after 2 hours of isoflurane anesthesia (groups 6 and 7). (From Warltier DC, al-Wathiqui MH, Kampine JP, et al: Recovery of contractile function of stunned myocardium in chronically instrumented dogs is enhanced by halothane or isoflurane. Anesthesiology 69:552, 1988)

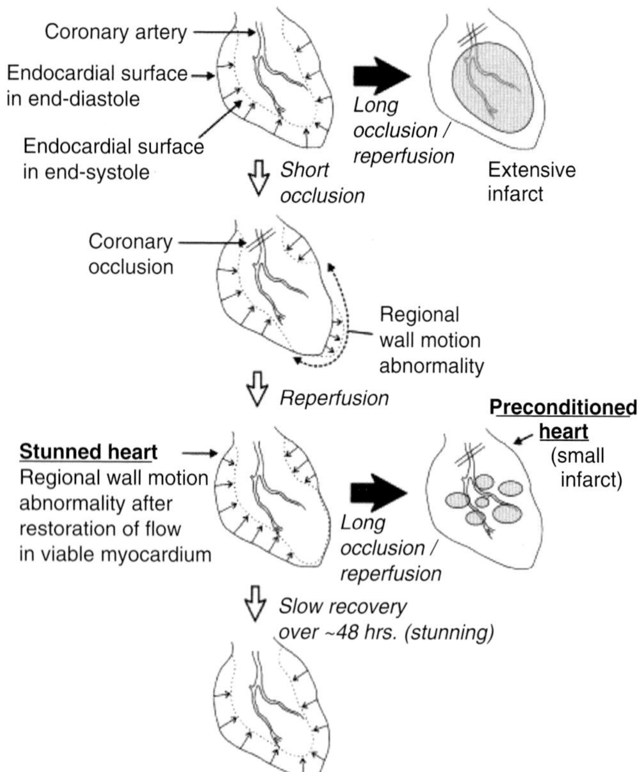

Figure 9–6 Schematic of stunning and preconditioning. Short coronary artery occlusions result in stunning, in which there is prolonged regional wall motion abnormality, despite presence of reperfusion and viable myocardial cells. Brief episodes of ischemia/reperfusion also precondition the heart. When the heart is then exposed to a longer duration of ischemia and reperfusion, myocardial infarct size is reduced. (From Kloner RA, Jennings RB: Consequences of brief ischemia: Stunning, preconditioning, and their clinical implications. Part I. Circulation 104:2981, 2001)

(termed "late" or "delayed") occurring 24 to 96 hours following the preconditioning stimulus; (2) occurs also in noncardiac tissue, such as brain and kidney; (3) is ubiquitous across species; (4) is most pronounced in larger species with lower metabolism and slower heart rates (HRs); (5) seems to be important clinically because angina within the 24-hour period preceding an AMI is associated with an improved outcome (Fig. 9–9)[91]; and (6) is mediated by multiple endogenous signaling pathways[92] (Fig. 9–10).[93] As might be predicted from the time frame of delayed IPC, it is mediated, at least in part, by transcriptional and posttranslational mechanisms[92] (Fig. 9–11). Finally, and of the utmost importance, preconditioning can be triggered by events other than ischemia (cellular stress of various forms, pharmacologic agonists, anesthetic agents) (see Fig. 9–11).[92] Moreover, the benefits of IPC are not necessarily confined to and may not include limitation of infarct size, and depend on the specific trigger for IPC, the species under study, and classic versus delayed IPC. For example, rapid pacing affords protection against arrhythmias but not against infarct evolution. In contrast, cytokine-induced IPC limits infarct size but has no effect on arrhythmias.[92] Different triggers of IPC modulating different end-points suggest that while there are fundamental mechanisms common to various triggers of IPC, there also exist mechanistic differences across triggers. Thus, APC may not be identical to IPC mechanistically.

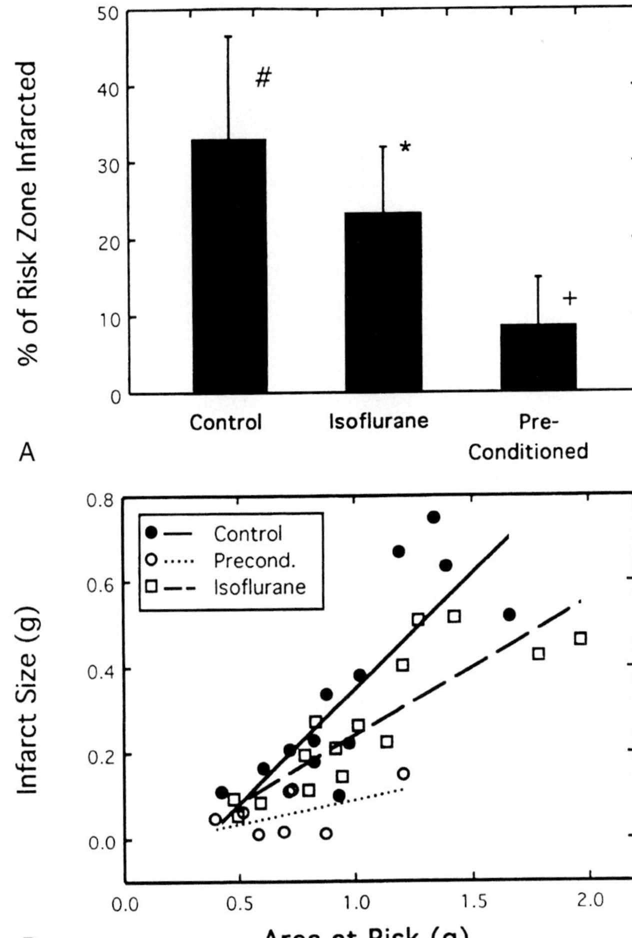

Figure 9–8 (*A*) Infarct size (mean ± SD) expressed as a percent of area at risk in rabbit hearts that were not pretreated (control, N = 13), exposed to 5 minutes of preconditioning (ischemic preconditioned, N = 8), or exposed to 15 minutes of 1.1% isoflurane (isoflurane, N = 15) before 30 minutes of anterolateral coronary occlusion. Symbols (#, *, +) indicate that statistical analysis showed that the relationship between infarct size and area at risk was different in each group ($P < 0.05$). (*B*) Relationship between infarct size and myocardium at risk for the three groups. All three regression lines were statistically different because of differences in line elevation. (From Cason BA, Gamperi AK, Slocum RE, et al: Anesthetic-induced preconditioning: Previous administration of isoflurane decreases myocardial infarct size in rabbits. Anesthesiology 87:1182, 1997)

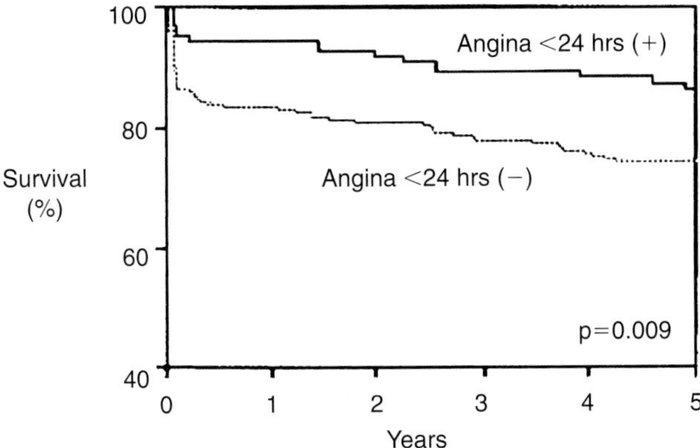

Figure 9–9 Five-year survival curves for patients with [Angina <24 hours (+)] versus those without [Angina <24 hr (–)] prodromal angina in the 24 hours before infarction. (From Ishihara M, Sato K, Tateishi H, et al: Implications of prodromal angina pectoris in anterior wall acute myocardial infarction: Acute angiographic findings and long-term prognosis. J Am Coll Cardiol 30:970, 1997)

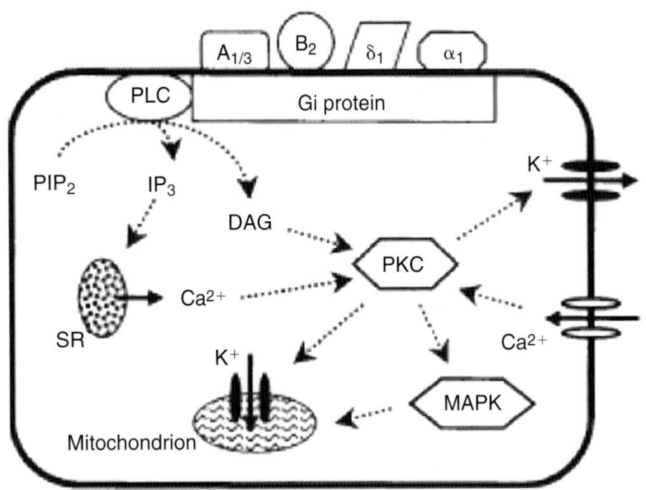

Figure 9–10 Cellular mechanism of ischemic preconditioning. Activation of adenosine A_1 and A_3 ($A_{1/3}$), bradykinin$_2$ (B_2), δ_1-opioid (δ_1), and α_1-adrenergic (α_1) receptors stimulates phospholipase C (PLC) through inhibitory guanine nucleotide-binding proteins (G_i proteins). PLC produces diacylglycerol (DAG) and inositol(1,4,5)triphosphate (IP_3). Both DAG and IP_3 activate protein kinase C (PKC). PKC enhances opening of ATP-sensitive K^+ channels (K^+_{ATP} channels), probably via mitogen-activated protein kinases (MAPK). The K^+_{ATP} channel seems to be the end-effector for inducing protection, though the downstream process is still unknown. Recently, mitochondrial K^+_{ATP} channels have been considered more important than sarcolemmal K^+_{ATP} channels. PIP_2 = phosphatidylinositol; SR = sarcoplasmic reticulum. (From Kato R, Foex P: Myocardial protection by anesthetic agents against ischemia-reperfusion injury: An update for anesthesiologists. Can J Anaesth 49:777, 2002)

Anesthetic Preconditioning

This is an area of intense investigation as reflected by two issues of *Anesthesiology* being devoted predominantly to the subject.[94,95] Following the initial description of APC,[1-3] subsequent investigations have indicated that volatile agents can elicit delayed (late), as well as classic (early) preconditioning.[96,97] Moreover, APC is dose dependent,[98-100] exhibits synergy with ischemia in affording protection,[101,102] and, perhaps not surprisingly in view of differential uptake and distribution of volatile agents, has been demonstrated to require different time intervals between exposure and the maintenance of a subsequent benefit that is agent-dependent[43](see Chapters 6 and 7).

The contributions of both SL and mitochondrial K^+_{ATP} channels in IPC have been extensively investigated, and it is now widely agreed that mitochondrial K^+_{ATP} channels play a critical role in this process. Volatile agents that exhibit APC activate mitochondrial K^+_{ATP} channels and this effect is blocked by specific mitochondrial K^+_{ATP} channel antagonists. However, the precise relative contributions of SL versus mitochondrial K^+_{ATP} channel activation to APC remain to be elucidated (Fig. 9–12)[43]. The original descriptions of APC indicated that volatile agents can trigger preconditioning without concurrent ischemia during the "triggering" period.[1-3] (see Fig. 9–8). However, studies of mitochondrial activation (via mitochondrial K^+_{ATP} channels) indicate that volatile agents on their own do not activate mitochondria but do potentiate the effects of direct mitochondrial K^+_{ATP} channel openers[100] (Fig. 9–13). These apparent inconsistencies are likely explained by the presence of multiple parallel and redundant pathways activated during APC (and IPC)[43] (Fig. 9–12). For example, it is now well established that the adenosine A-1 and δ_1-opioid G-coupled receptors can trigger IPC.

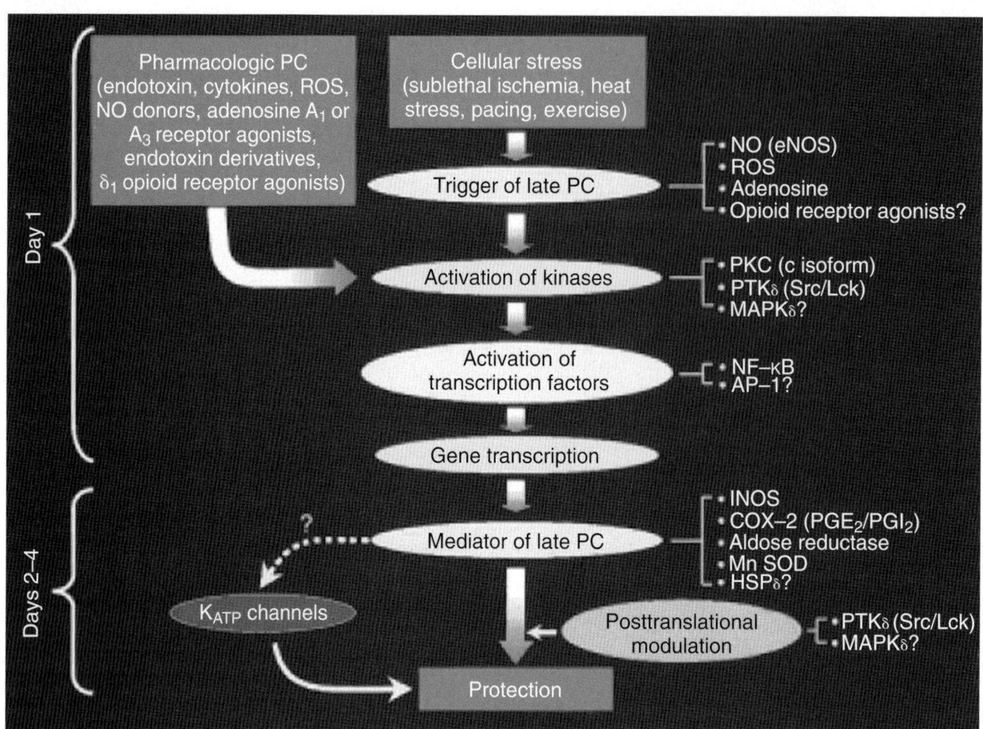

Figure 9–11 Schematic representation of the cellular mechanisms underlying late preconditioning (PC). A nonlethal cellular stress (such as reversible ischemia, heat stress, ventricular pacing, or exercise) causes release of chemical signals (NO, ROS, adenosine, and possibly opioid receptor agonists) that serve as triggers for the development of late PC. These substances activate a complex signal transduction cascade that includes PKC (specifically, the ε isoform), PTKs (specifically, Src and/or Lck), and probably other as-yet-unknown kinases. A similar activation of PKC and downstream kinases can be elicited pharmacologically by a wide variety of agents, including naturally occurring, and often noxious, substances (such as endotoxin, interleukin-1, TNFα, TNFβ, leukemia inhibitor factor, or ROS), as well as clinically applicable drugs (NO donors, adenosine A1- or A3-receptor agonists, endotoxin derivatives, or δ_1-opioid receptor agonists). The recruitment of PKC and distal kinases leads to activation of NF-κB and almost certainly other transcription factors, resulting in increased transcription of multiple cardioprotective genes and synthesis of multiple cardioprotective proteins that serve as co-mediators of protection 2 to 4 days after the PC stimulus. The mediators of late PC identified thus far include iNOS, COX-2, aldose reductase, and MnSOD. Among the products of COX-2, PGE_2 and/or PGI_2 appear to be the most likely effectors of COX-2–dependent protection. Increased synthesis of HSPs is unlikely to be a mechanism of late PC, although the role of posttranslational modification of preexisting HSPs remains to be determined. In addition, the occurrence of cardioprotection on days 2 to 4 requires the activity of PTKs and possibly p38 MAPKs, potentially because iNOS and other mediators need to undergo posttranslational modulation to confer protection against ischemia. Opening of K^+_{ATP} channels is also essential for the protection against infarction (but not against stunning) to become manifest. The exact interrelationships among iNOS, COX-2, aldose reductase, MnSOD, and K^+_{ATP} channels are unknown, although recent evidence suggests that COX-2 may be downstream of iNOS (i.e., COX-2 is activated by NO). (From Bolli R: The late phase of preconditioning. Circ Res 87:972, 2000)

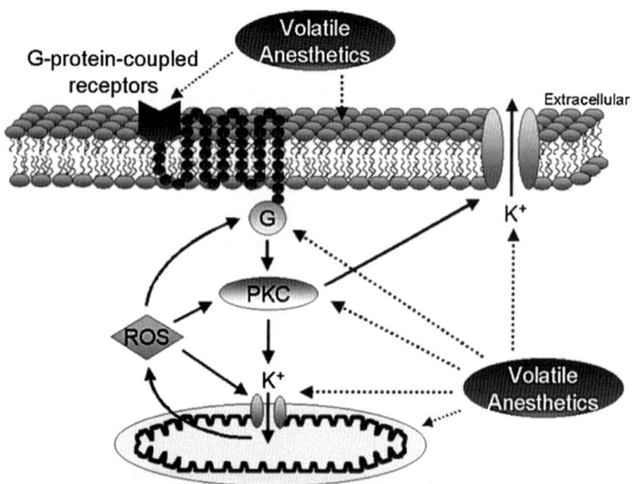

Figure 9–12 Multiple endogenous signaling pathways mediate volatile anesthetic-induced myocardial activation of an end-effector that promotes resistance against ischemic injury. Mitochondrial K^+_{ATP} channels have been implicated as the end-effector in this protective scheme, but sarcolemmal K^+_{ATP} channels may also be involved in this mechanism of protection. A trigger initiates a cascade of signal transduction events, resulting in the protection. Volatile anesthetics signal through adenosine and opioid receptors, modulate G proteins, stimulate protein kinase C (PKC) and other intracellular kinases, or have direct effects on mitochondria to generate reactive oxygen species (ROS) that ultimately enhance K^+_{ATP} channel activity. Volatile anesthetics may also directly facilitate K^+_{ATP} channel opening. *Dotted arrows* delineate the intracellular targets that may be regulated by volatile anesthetics; *solid arrows* represent potential signaling cascades. (From Tanaka K, Ludwig LM, Kersten JR, et al: Mechanisms of cardioprotection by volatile anesthetics. Anesthesiology 100:707, 2004)

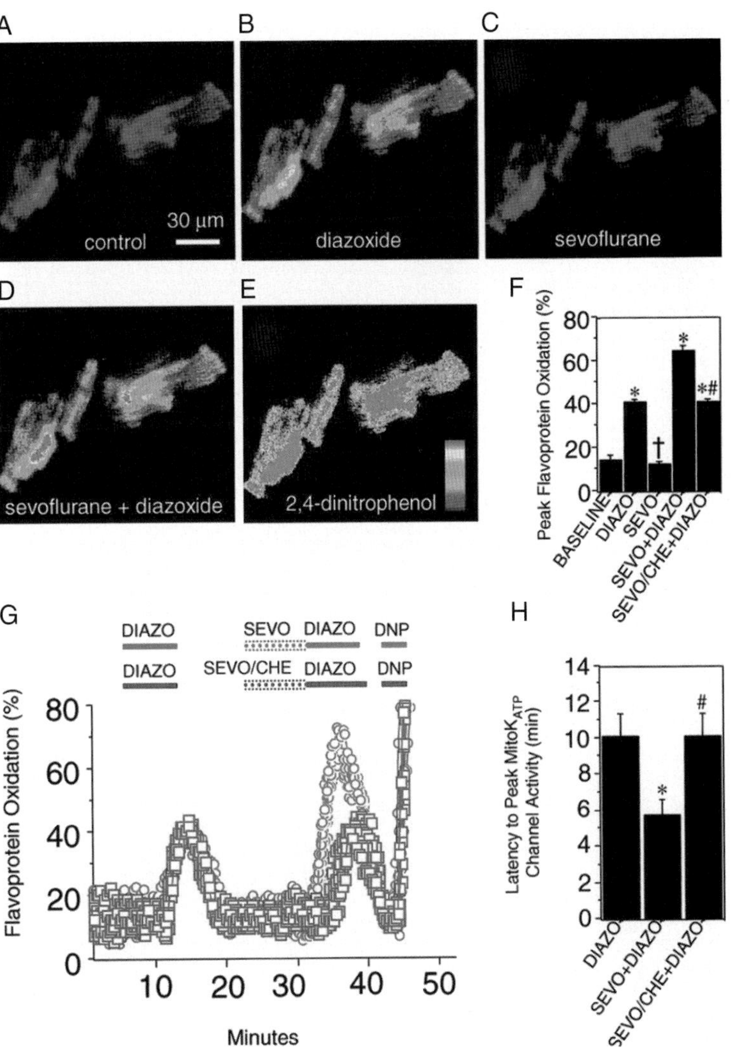

Figure 9–13 Effect of sevoflurane (SEVO) (2.8% [vol/vol]) on diazoxide (DIAZO)-induced flavoprotein oxidation in myocytes excited at 480 nm. Similar results were obtained for isoflurane. An artificial color scale (see Color Plates) was used to visualize the relative intensity of emitted fluorescence at 530 nm (dark blue indicates reduced flavoproteins, red indicates fully oxidized flavoproteins). (*A*) At baseline. (*B*) At 100 μm DIAZO (same cells). (*C*) At 2 MAC SEVO. (*D*) At 100 μm DIAZO preceded by 2 MAC SEVO. Red color indicates intense local oxidation by mitochondrial clusters. (*E*) At 100 μm 2,4-dinitrophenol (DNP). (*F*) Mean percentages of peak flavoprotein fluorescence depending on the drugs exposed to myocytes. **P* < 0.0001 versus baseline or SEVO + DIAZO versus DIAZO alone. #*P* not significantly different from DIAZO. †*P* not significantly different from baseline. SEVO/CHE indicates concomitant treatment of myocytes with SEVO and chelerythrine (CHE) at 2 μm before exposure to DIAZO. (*G*) Time-lapse analysis of alterations in fluorescence intensity in individual myocytes expressed as percentage of DNP-induced fluorescence (see text). The blue squares and red circles indicate values from eight different experiments. (*H*) Latency to peak activation of mitoK^+_{ATP} channels in response to the various treatment regimens. **P* < 0.001 versus DIAZO. #*P* not significant versus DIAZO. Data are mean ± SD. (From Zaugg M, Lucchinetti E, Spahn DR, et al: Volatile anesthetics mimic cardiac preconditioning by priming the activation of mitochondrial KATP channels via multiple signaling pathways. Anesthesiology 97:4, 2002)

Moreover, pharmacologic blockade of these receptors attenuates the positive effects of volatile agents.[98,103] Protein kinase C (PKC) and the nuclear signaling pathway, mitogen-activated protein kinase (MAPK), are important signaling pathways in preconditioning, and volatile agents have been shown to modulate at least PKC translocation.[104] Oxidant stress is a central feature of reperfusion and, depending on the specific moiety, the enzymatic source and, most importantly, the oxidant stress load, may trigger preconditioning on the one hand or mediate reperfusion injury on the other. Both indirect and direct evidence indicate that volatile agents can increase oxidant stress to levels that trigger preconditioning.[105-107]

Although the mechanisms underlying mitochondrial activation have been aggressively studied, they remain incompletely understood. For example, volatile agents cause APC but on their own do not activate mitochondrial K^+_{ATP} channels. However, it is clear that mitochondrial activation attenuates ischemia-induced oxidant stress, favorably modulates mitochondrial energetics, decreases cytochrome-*c* egress into the cytoplasm, and attenuates mitochondrial and cytoplasmic Ca^{++} overload. Mitochondrial cytochrome-*c* release is one of the important mechanisms underlying caspase activation and thus the apoptotic process[108] (Fig. 9–14). Whether by Ca^{++}-mediated or by apoptotic mechanisms, or both, volatile agents clearly attenuate cell death in models of APC[100] (Fig. 9–15). Finally, these salutary effects of volatile agents seem to have a clinical correlate[100] (Fig. 9–16).

INTRAVENOUS INDUCTION AGENTS

The drugs discussed in this section are all induction agents and hypnotics. These drugs belong to different classes (barbiturates, benzodiazepines, *N*-methyl-D-aspartate [NMDA] receptor antagonists, and α_2-adrenergic receptor agonists). Their effects on the CVS are therefore dependent on the class to which they belong. As with the inhalation anesthetic agents, the basic research that has emerged to explain the mechanisms that underlie the integrated cardiovascular effects observed in the intact organism is discussed. These effects have been studied at a cellular, tissue, organ, and whole animal level. While a detailed discussion of the molecular mechanisms underlying each agent is far beyond the scope of this chapter, a focused appraisal of well-established effects of specific drugs is given. At one level, sophisticated pharmacologic studies dissecting the signal transduction pathways may provide insights into mechanisms, but they cannot fully predict the response of the intact organisms. Because propofol is the most common

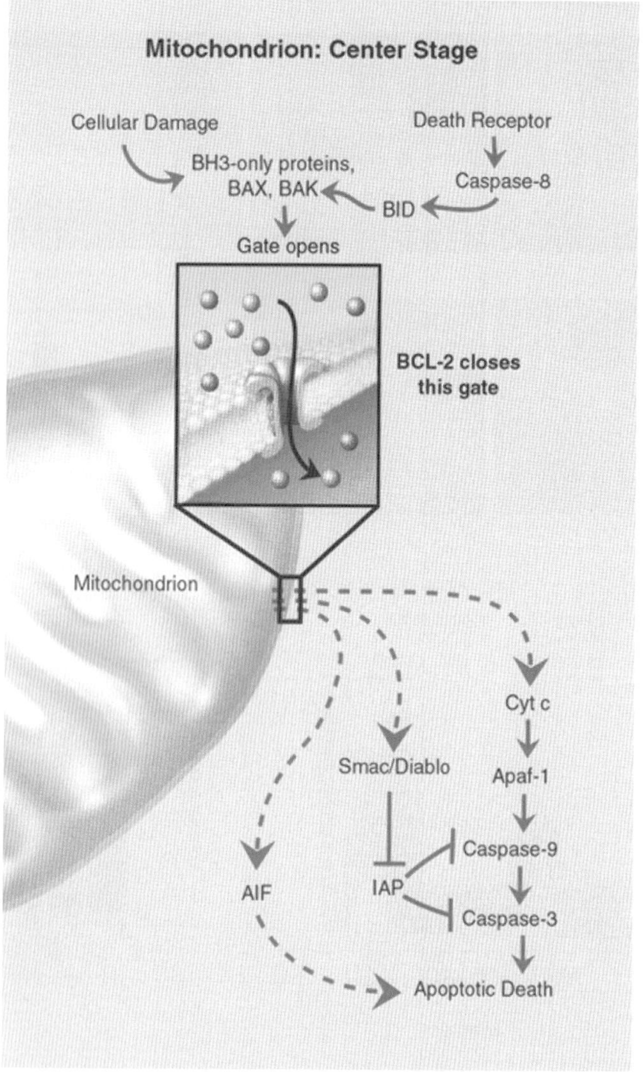

Figure 9–14 Center stage in apoptosis. In this view, numerous cell-death stimuli work through the mitochondria. They cause proapoptotic members of the BCL-2 family, such as BAX and BAK, to either open new pores or modify existing channels in the mitochondrial membrane, releasing cytochrome c and other proteins that lead to caspase activation and cell death. BCL-2 itself, which is antiapoptotic, somehow blocks the pore or channel opening. (Reprinted with permission from Science 292:624-626 (2001). Illustration: C. Slayden, Copyright 2001 AAAS)

induction agent, literature for this agent is used as the paradigm for discussing mechanisms by which cardiovascular regulation is altered by intravenous agents. A discussion summarizing the cardiovascular effects of each induction agent follows later in the chapter.

Unlike the inhalation anesthetic agents that augment IPC, there is no good evidence that the intravenous hypnotic agents demonstrate these protective effects. There is, however, emerging evidence that propofol, the mainstay of induction agents, may enhance antioxidant activity in the heart and thus may prevent lipid perioxidation following ischemia-reperfusion, offering a potential protective effect on the heart.[93]

Acute Cardiac Effects

Myocardial Contractility

To understand the effect of intravenous anesthetics on integrated cardiovascular responses is to understand the effect on the different factors that regulate the force of contraction of the heart. If the heart in isolation is considered (not coupled to the vasculature and not regulated by the autonomic system), the best methodologies for examining the effects of anesthetic agents involve using isolated myocytes and muscle tissue preparations in which the effect of the anesthetic drugs on contractile force/tension or myocyte/sarcomere shortening can be determined. With regard to propofol, the studies remain controversial as to whether there is a direct effect on myocardial contractile function at clinically relevant concentrations. However, the weight of evidence suggests that the drug has a modest negative inotropic effect, which may be mediated by inhibition of L-type Ca^{++} channels or modulation of Ca^{++} release from the SR. Thus, the effect of propofol may be mediated at multiple sites in the cardiac myocytes.

The effect of the agents may be species dependent, thus further confounding the literature regarding mechanism. For instance, van Klarenbosch et al[109] demonstrated that in contrast to rat, propofol directly depresses myocardial contractility in isolated muscle preparations from guinea pig, probably by decreasing trans-sarcolemmal Ca^{++} influx. However, there was little influence of propofol on Ca^{++} handling by the SR or on the contractile proteins in rat. In one of the few human studies using isolated atrial muscle tissue (Fig. 9–17), no inhibition of myocardial contractility was found in the clinical concentration ranges of propofol, midazolam, and etomidate. In contrast, thiopental showed strong negative inotropic properties, while ketamine showed slight negative inotropic properties (Fig. 9–18). Thus, negative inotropic effects may explain in part the cardiovascular depression on induction of anesthesia with thiopental but not with propofol, midazolam, and etomidate. Improvement of hemodynamics after induction of anesthesia with ketamine cannot therefore be explained by intrinsic cardiac stimulation but is a function of sympathoexcitation.[110]

The effect of drugs such as propofol may also be markedly affected by the underlying myocardial pathology.[111,112] For instance, Sprung et al[112] determined the direct effects of propofol on the contractility of human nonfailing atrial and failing atrial and ventricular muscles obtained from the failing human hearts of transplant patients or from nonfailing hearts of patients undergoing coronary artery bypass graft surgery (CABG). They concluded that propofol exerts a direct negative inotropic effect in nonfailing and failing human myocardium but only at concentrations larger than typical clinical concentrations. Negative inotropic effects are reversible with β-adrenergic stimulation, suggesting that propofol does not alter the contractile reserve but may shift the dose responsiveness to adrenergic stimulation. The negative inotropic effect of propofol is at least partially mediated by decreased Ca^{++} uptake into the SR; however, the net effect of propofol on contractility is insignificant at clinical concentrations because of a simultaneous increase in the sensitivity of the myofilaments to activator Ca^{++}.[112]

Molecular Mechanisms: Adrenergic Signaling, Ca^{++} Influx, and Ca^{++} Sensitivity

There are a number of suggested molecular mechanisms by which a drug such as propofol may alter cardiac contractility. Propofol may inhibit cardiac L-type calcium current by interacting with the dihydropyridine-binding site[113] (Fig. 9–19A) with resultant alteration in developed tension (Fig. 9–19B). Furthermore, as mentioned, propofol may alter adrenergic signaling in cardiac myocytes. Experiments in membranes and

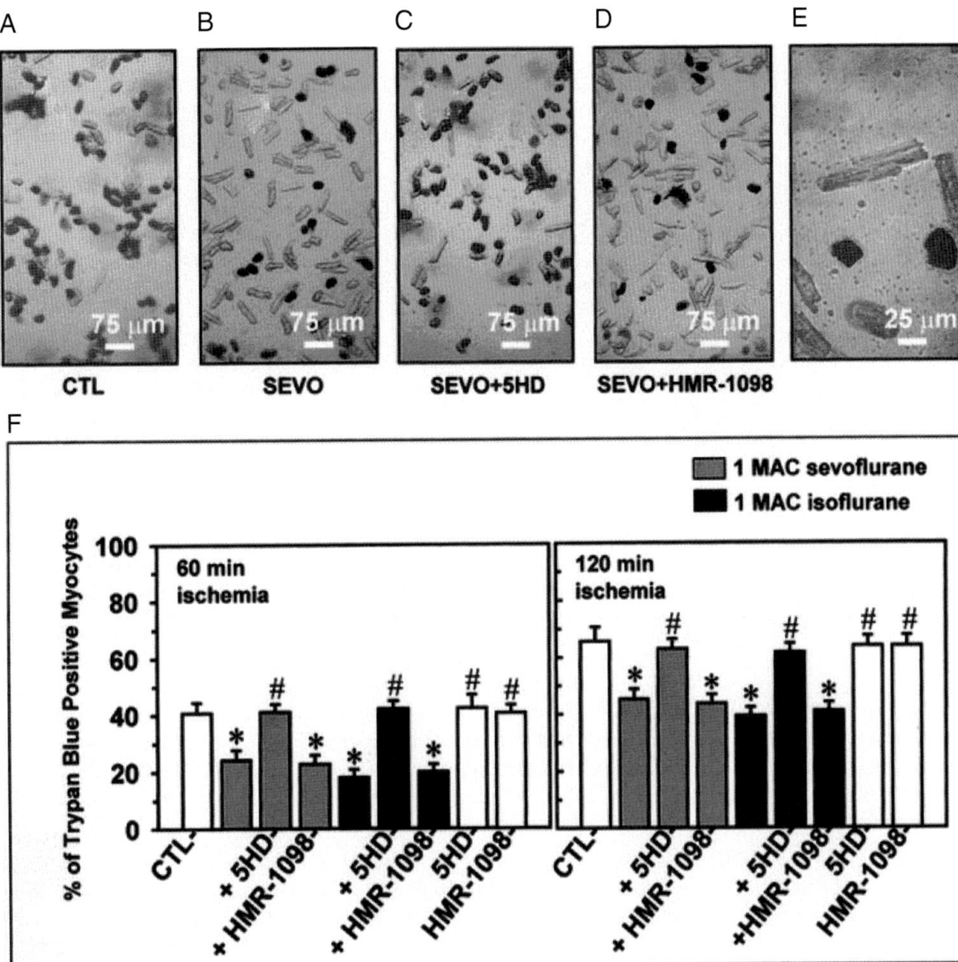

Figure 9–15 See Color Plates. Effects of the specific mitochondrial K^+_{ATP} (mitoK^+_{ATP}) channel blocker 5-hydroxy-decanoate (5HD) and the specific sarcolemmal K^+_{ATP} (sarcK^+_{ATP}) channel blocker HMR-1098 on sevoflurane (SEVO)- and isoflurane (ISO)-mediated protection at 1 MAC against 60 or 120 minutes of ischemia in myocytes as assessed by trypan blue staining. (*A*) Control myocytes after 60 min of ischemia. Myocytes staining dark blue indicate irreversible cell damage. (*B*) Myocytes exposed to SEVO before ischemia. Most myocytes retain their rod-shaped morphology. (*C*) Myocytes exposed to 5HD and SEVO before ischemia. The protective effect of SEVO is abolished. (*D*) Myocytes exposed to HMR-1098 and SEVO before ischemia. The protection by SEVO is unaffected. (*E*) Representative trypan blue–positive and –negative myocytes after exposure to ischemia seen at higher magnification. (*F*) Trypan blue–positive myocytes are indicated as percentage of total viable myocytes before ischemia. CTL indicates control group and represents myocytes exposed to 60 or 120 min of ischemia alone. Data are mean ± SD. $^*P < 0.0001$ versus respective CTL. #*P* not significant versus respective CTL. (From Zaugg M, Lucchinetti E, Spahn DR, et al: Volatile anesthetics mimic cardiac preconditioning by priming the activation of mitochondrial KATP channels via multiple signaling pathways. Anesthesiology 97:4, 2002)

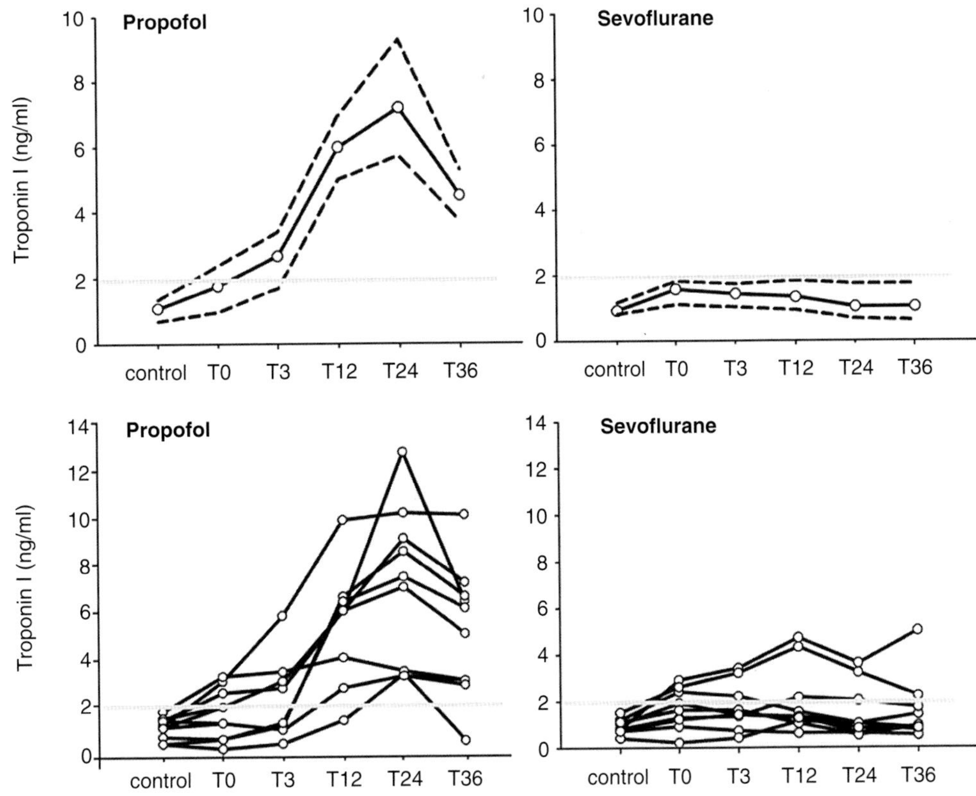

Figure 9–16 Cardiac troponin I concentrations in the propofol and sevoflurane groups before surgery (control), at arrival in the intensive care unit (T0), and after 3 (T3), 12 (T12), 24 (T24), and 36 (T36) hours. The upper panels show the median values with 95% confidence intervals. The lower panels show the evolution of the individual values. Concentrations were significantly higher with propofol. In the propofol group, all patients had troponin concentrations above the cutoff value of 2 ng/mL (gray line). (From de Hert S, ten Broecke PW, Mertens E, et al: Sevoflurane but not propofol preserves myocardial function in coronary surgery patients. Anesthesiology 97:42, 2002)

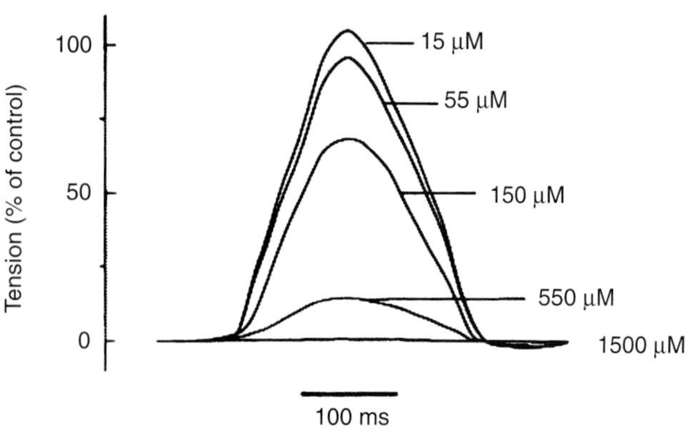

Figure 9–17 Typical experiment showing the force traces of an isometric twitch of human atrial tissue during exposure to increasing concentrations of propofol (15 to 1500 μmol/L). (From Gelissen HP, Epema AH, Henning RH, et al: Inotropic effects of propofol, thiopental, midazolam, etomidate, and ketamine on isolated human atrial muscle. Anesthesiology 84:397, 1996)

cardiac preparations isolated from rat heart demonstrate that relatively high concentrations of propofol (25 to 200 μmol/L) are required to antagonize β-adrenoceptor binding and tissue responsiveness.[114] Kurokawa et al[115] observed that clinically relevant concentrations of propofol attenuated β-adrenergic signal transduction in cardiac myocytes via inhibition of cAMP production (Fig. 9–20). The inhibitory site of action of propofol appears to be upstream of adenylyl cyclase and involves activation of PKCα.

While propofol may decrease contractile response to adrenergic stimulation, there is emerging evidence that it may enhance myofilament sensitivity to Ca^{++}. Propofol caused a leftward shift in the extracellular Ca^{++}-shortening relationship, suggesting that propofol increases the sensitivity of myofibrillar actomyosin ATPase to Ca^{++} (i.e., increases myofilament Ca^{++} sensitivity) (Fig. 9–21). This is mediated at least in part by increasing pH via protein kinase Ccdependent activation of Na^+-H^+ exchange[116] or by a PKC-dependent pathway involving the phosphorylation of MLC2.[117]

Integrated Cardiovascular Responses

The use of combined conductance-manometric catheters, which allows the simultaneous measurement of pressure and volume in the ventricle, has enabled the precise determination of the effects of anesthetic agents on integrated cardiovascular responses. These parameters include load-independent measures of contractility (slope of the end-systolic pressure-volume relationship (ESPVR), E_{es}), as well as indices of ventricular-vascular coupling (ratio of arterial elastance to ventricular elastance [E_a/E_{es}]) (see Chapters 5 and 14). In a study, the effect of propofol and pentobarbital on integrated cardiovascular function was assessed in pigs both at baseline and following an acute increase in ventricular afterload.[118] At baseline, E_{es} was lower during pentobarbital versus propofol anesthesia, suggesting a greater negative inotropic effect of barbiturates versus propofol (Fig. 9–22). On the other hand, the responses to ventricular afterload induced by aortic banding were maintained in the pentobarbital-anesthetized animals, while the responses were markedly attenuated in the propofol-anesthetized pigs, suggesting an attenuation of the baroreflex responses with propofol. Furthermore, a decrease in arterial pressure with propofol is consistent with this drug acting as a vasodilator.

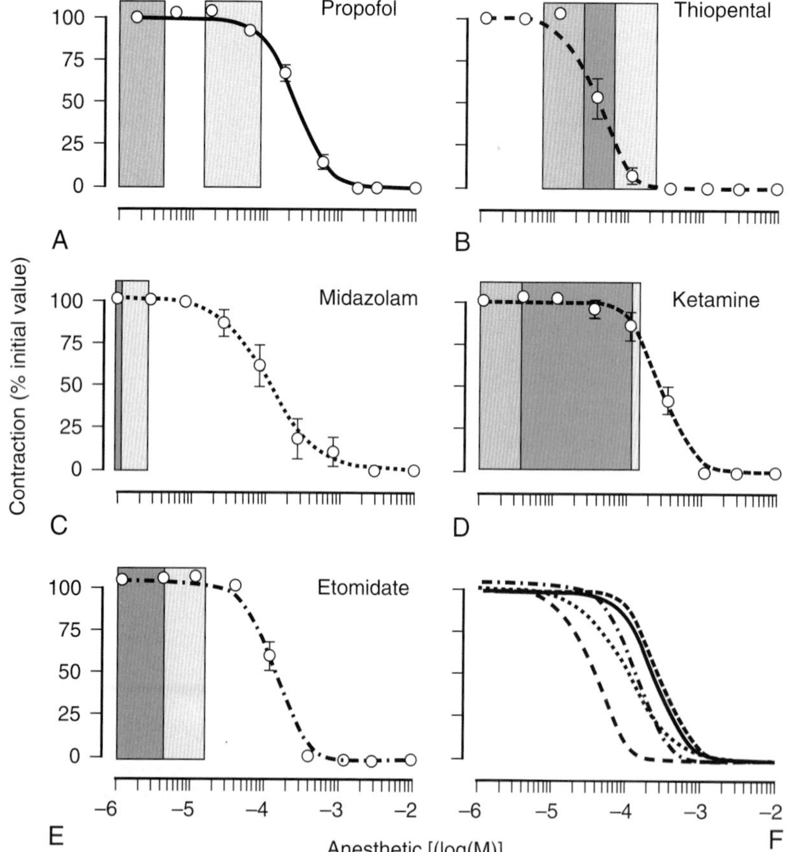

Figure 9–18 Comparative effects of increasing concentrations of anesthetic on isometric contractions of human atrial tissue induced by field stimulation. Data are mean ± SEM. Curves were plotted using logistic regression. Hatched squares indicate the clinical concentration range during anesthesia. Coarse hatching (*left*) represents the total concentration and fine hatching (*right*) shows the free fraction. (*A*) Propofol (n = 16). (*B*) Thiopental (n = 7). (*C*) Midazolam (n = 7). (*D*) Ketamine (n = 9). (*E*) Etomidate (n = 9). (*F*) Combined plot showing the concentration-response curve of the five anesthetics. (From Gelissen HP, Epema AH, Henning RH, et al: Inotropic effects of propofol, thiopental, midazolam, etomidate, and ketamine on isolated human atrial muscle. Anesthesiology 84:397, 1996)

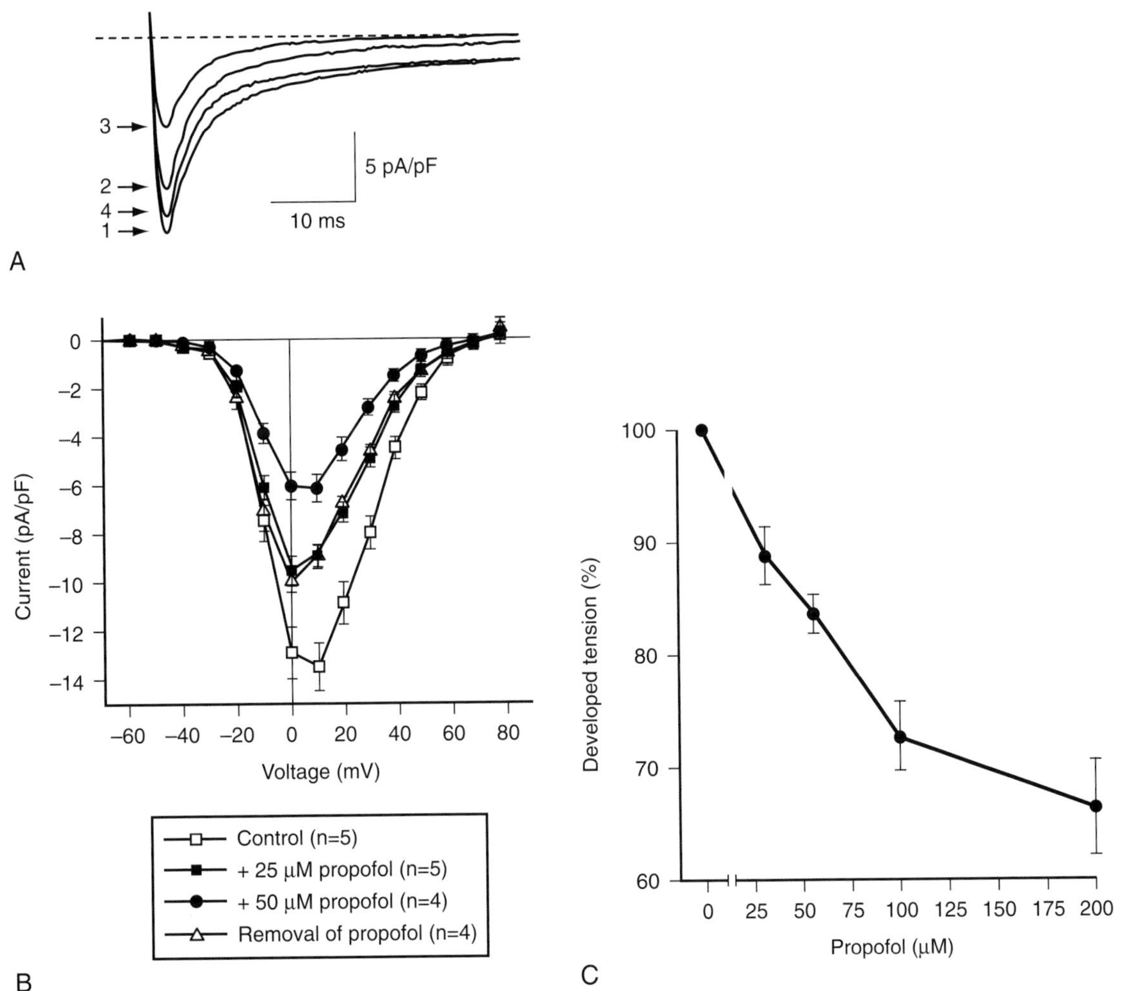

Figure 9–19 *(A)* Representative current traces of $I_{Ca,L}$ in response to depolarizing pulses to 0 μmol/L from a holding potential of −70 μV. These traces were obtained before exposure to propofol, during treatment with 25 μmol/L and 60 μmol/L of propofol, and after recovery. *(B)* The current-voltage (I-V) relation of peak $I_{Ca,L}$ as monitored before and during exposure to propofol. Cultured rat ventricular myocytes were clamped at −70 μV. $I_{Ca,L}$ was elicited by 200-ms pulses from the holding potential of −70 μV to potentials between −60 and +80 μV in 10-μV increments. Propofol dose dependently decreases calcium current. (C) Effects of propofol on developed tension in papillary muscle isolated from the rat heart. Preparations (n = 4) were bathed in an oxygenated Krebs-Henseleit solution at 37°C and paced electrically at 1 Hz. The anesthetic was added to the bathing solution cumulatively. Vertical bars represent SEM. Values on the ordinate are presented as a percentage of the developed tension recorded immediately before adding propofol (0.64 ± 0.15 g). Propofol dose dependently decreases twitch tension. (From Zhou W, Fontenot HJ, Liu S, et al: Modulation of cardiac calcium channels by propofol. Anesthesiology 86:670, 1997)

One of the questions with regard to intravenous induction agents is, What represents a clinically relevant dose? As would be predicted, with regard to the myocardial depressant effects, the coronary concentrations of propofol have been shown to be the major contributor to the cardiac depression caused by propofol but were a less significant contributor to the hypotension caused by this drug.[119]

The effects of propofol on cardiac contractility are manifest on not only ventricular but also atrial function.[120] Propofol depresses contractile function of left atrial myocardium and reduces the active left atrial contribution to left ventricular filling in vivo. Compensatory decreases in chamber stiffness, however, contribute to relative maintenance of left atrial reservoir function during the administration of propofol.

Oxidative Stress

Oxidative stress remains an important pathophysiologic mechanism for cellular injury in critically ill patients and represents an imbalance between the production of these radicals and the enzymatic defense system that removes them (Box 9–3). This has potential therapeutic implications because these agents are routinely used for sedation in the intensive care unit, in which disease processes associated with increased oxidative stress are treated.

Animal data also suggest that propofol decreases postischemic myocardial mechanical dysfunction, infarct size, and histologic evidence of injury[121-125] (Fig. 9–23). On further analysis it becomes clear that propofol has a chemical structure similar to that of phenol-based free radical scavengers, such as vitamin E, and may therefore act as a free radical scavenger.[126,127] Studies by Tsuchiya et al[128,129] demonstrated in vitro the potential for both propofol and midazolam to act as free radical scavengers at near-therapeutic doses. Propofol also impairs the activity of neutrophils by inhibiting the oxidative burst and supports a potential role for propofol in modulating injury at the critical phase of reperfusion by reducing free radicals, Ca^{++} influx, and neutrophil activity.[130] Furthermore, microsomes prepared from animals anesthetized with propofol demonstrate a significantly increased resistance to lipid peroxidation.[131] The evidence does not support propofol

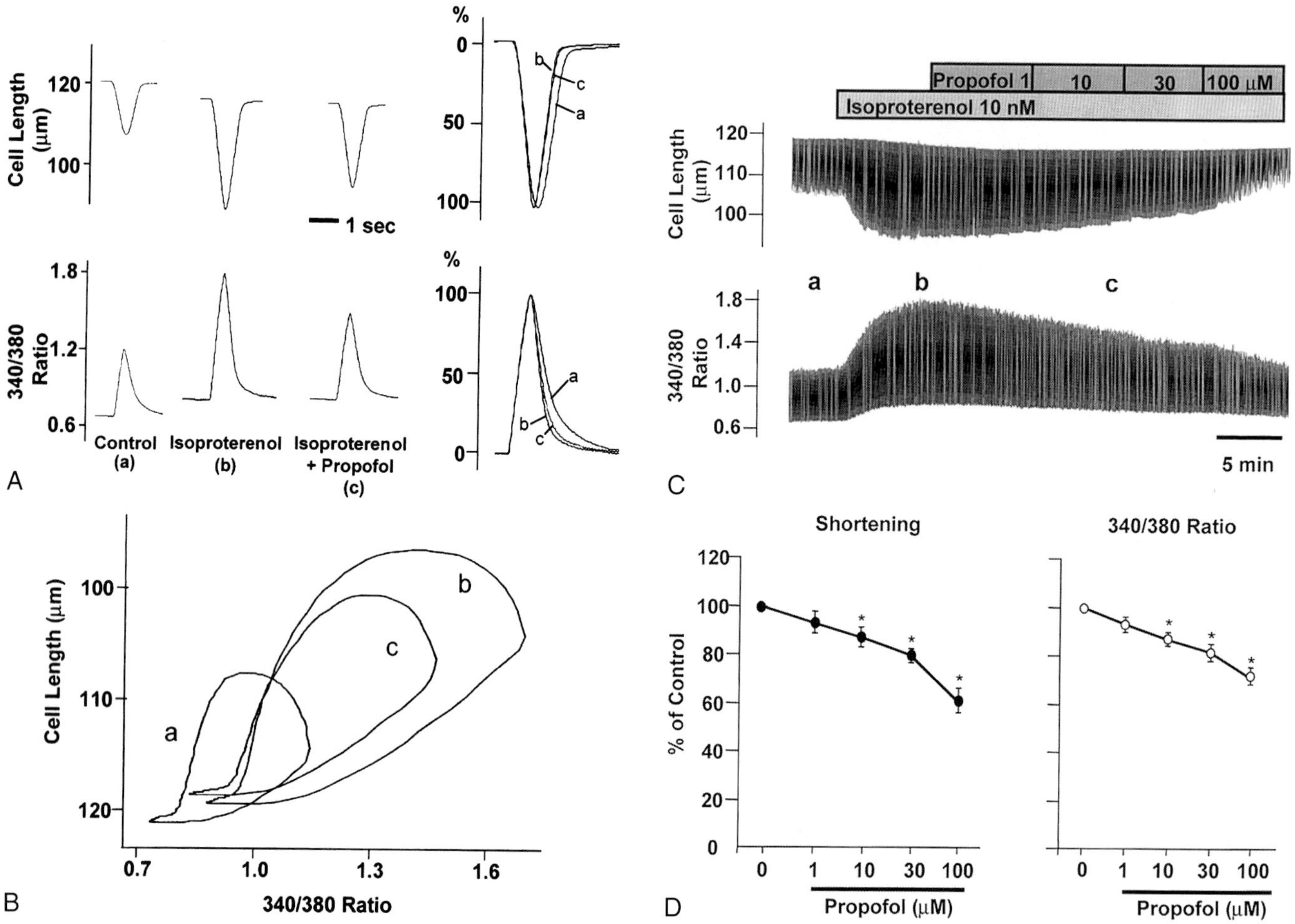

Figure 9–20 (*A and B*) Original traces depicting the dose-dependent effects of propofol on shortening and intracellular Ca^{++} concentration ($[Ca^{++}]_i$) after exposure to isoproterenol (10 nm) in a rat isolated ventricular myocyte. (*C and D*) Summarized data for the effects of propofol on isoproterenol-stimulated increases in shortening and $[Ca^{++}]_i$. Results are expressed as percent of control. Propofol inhibits β-adrenergic–mediated contractility in a dose-dependent system. (From Matsumura JS: Which formulation of propofol was used? Anesthesiology 96:1529, 2002)

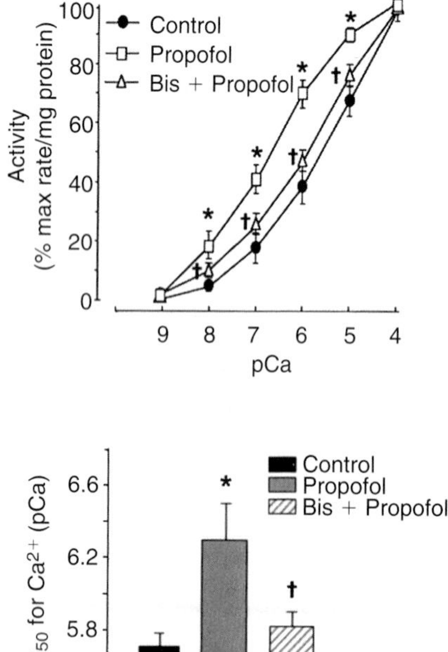

Figure 9–21 (*Top*) Summarized data depicting the effects of Bis/aprotinin kinase-C inhibition on the propofol-induced (30 μm) leftward shift in actomyosin ATPase activity in isolated myofibrils. (*Bottom*) Summarized data depicting the increase (*$P < 0.05$ versus control) in the EC_{50} value for Ca^{++} induced by propofol and inhibition of this effect (†$P < 0.05$ versus propofol) following pretreatment with Bis. Propofol increased myofilament Ca^{++} sensitivity by a protein kinase C–dependent receptor. (From Kanaya N, Gable B, Murray PA, et al: Propofol increases phosphorylation of troponin I and myosin light chain 2 via protein kinase C activation in cardiomyocytes. Anesthesiology 98:1363, 2003)

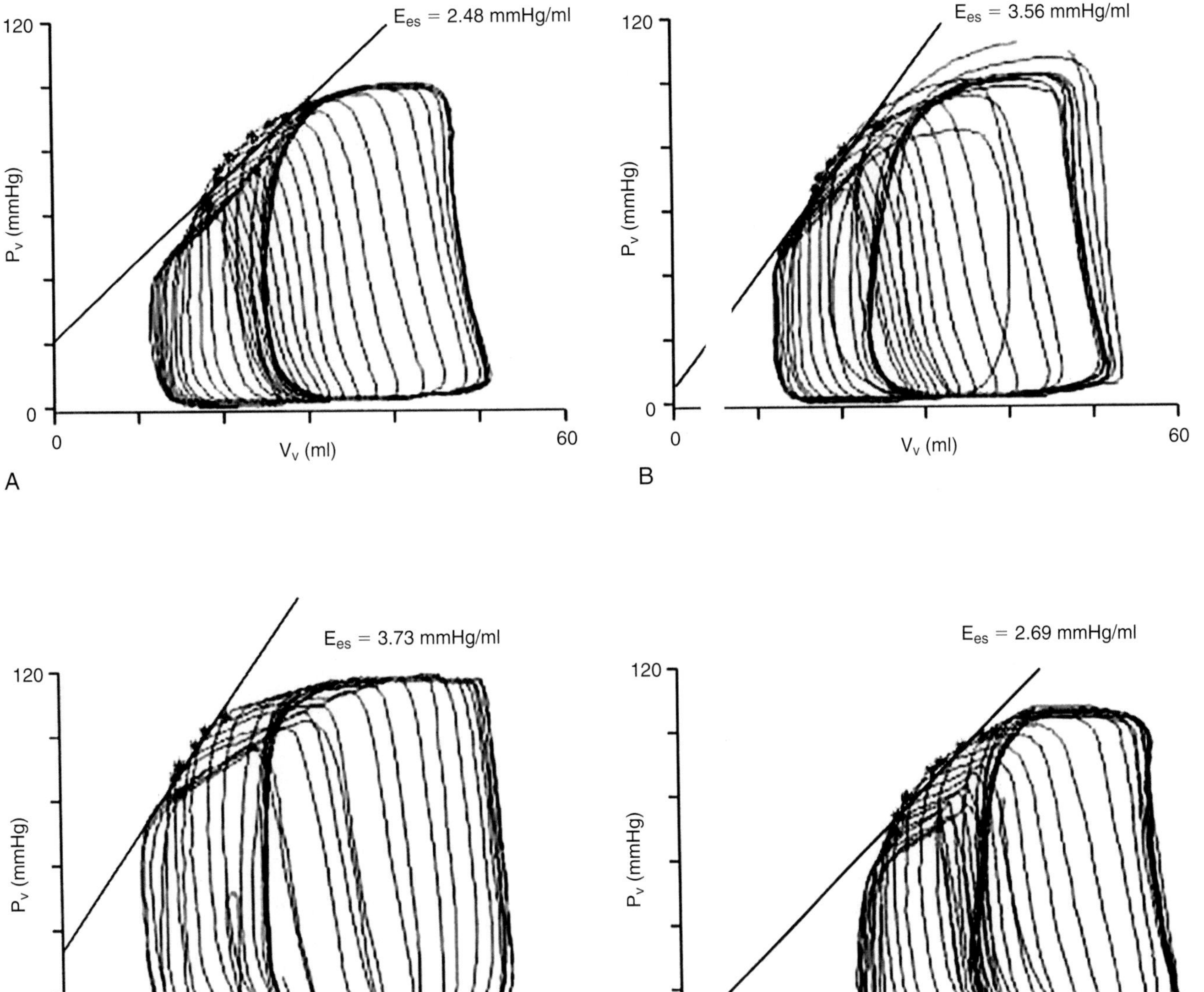

Figure 9–22 Typical pressure-volume loops recordings under pentobarbital anesthesia, at baseline (*A*) and during aortic banding (*C*); under propofol anesthesia, at baseline (*B*), and during aortic banding (*D*). (From Kolh P, Lambermont B, Ghuysen A, et al: Comparison of the effects of propofol and pentobarbital on left ventricular adaptation to an increased afterload. J Cardiovasc Pharmacol 44:294, 2004)

as an APC-inducing agent because protection was observed when the heart was treated with propofol solely during reperfusion rather than prior to or during the ischemic insult,[123] while the addition of glibenclamide, a K^+_{ATP} channel blocker, does not abolish the protection afforded by propofol.[124] There is little evidence for other intravenous induction agents having protective effects on the heart. In fact, ketamine may block IPC[132-134] by deactivating sarcolemmal K^+_{ATP} channels.[135]

Vasculature

As with the heart, the cumulative physiologic effects in the vasculature represent a summation of the effects of the agents on the central ANS, as well as the direct effects of these agents on the vascular smooth muscle, and the modulating effects on the underlying endothelium. An exhaustive review of the effects of each agent on isolated and integrated vascular function is beyond the scope of the chapter; however, a global overview of the effect of some of the most commonly used agents on vasoregulation is presented.

While there are clearly effects of anesthetic agents on vascular smooth muscle and endothelial function, controversy and diversity regarding mechanisms arise because of the species of animals studied, the vessel bed examined, and the drug dosage used. In addition, the effects may be significantly different in vessels from animals that develop disease phenotypes, such as hypertension and diabetes. Furthermore, while effects of these anesthetic agents on a variety of signal transduction pathways are invariably seen with high concentrations of agents, the clinical relevance of these effects remains unclear.

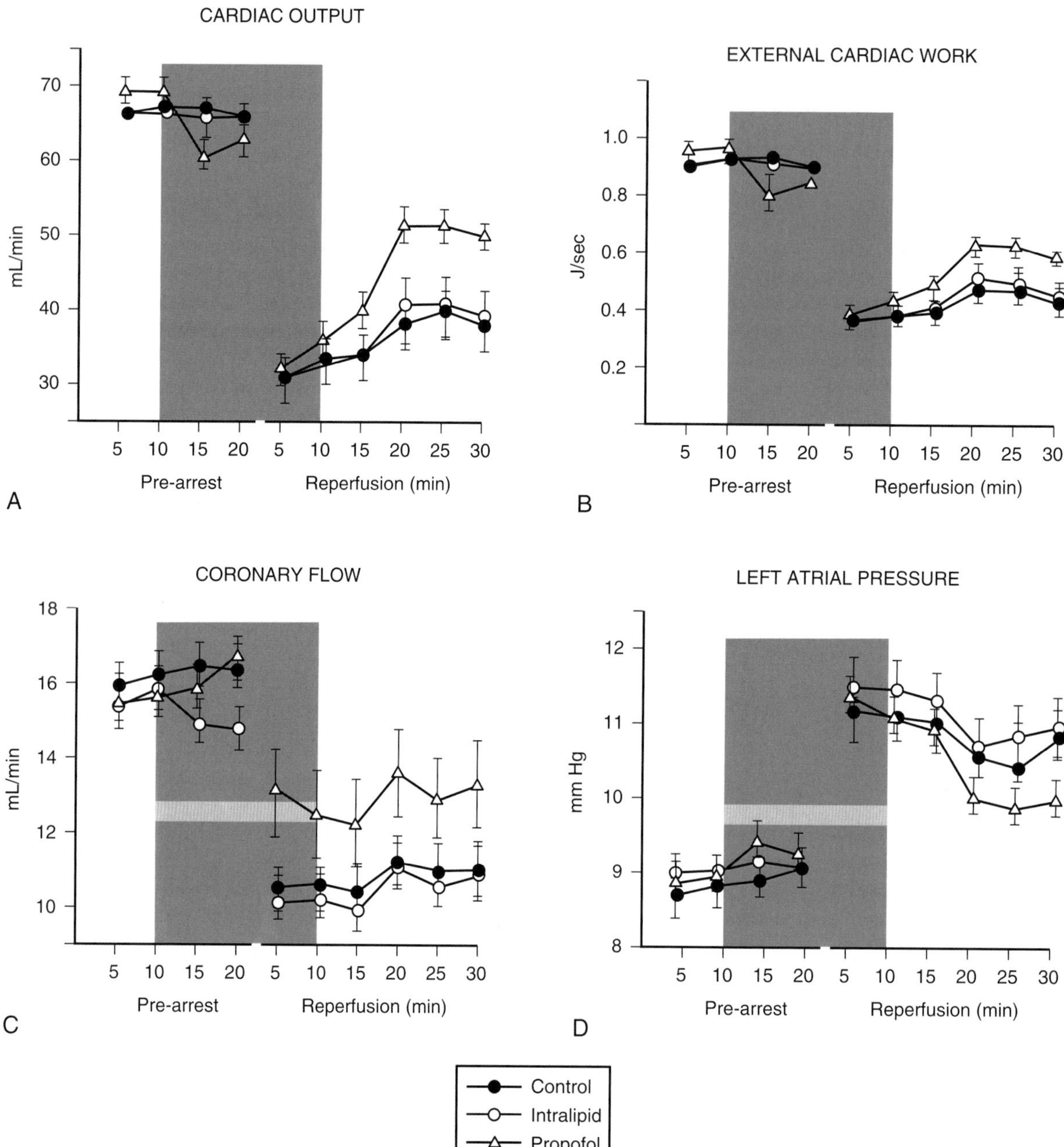

Figure 9–23 Cardiac function of the isolated working rat heart subjected to cold cardioplegic arrest and subsequent reperfusion. Propofol (4 g/mL dissolved in intralipid emulsion) or intralipid alone was added 10 minutes after initiation of the working heart mode and washed out after 10 minutes into working heart reperfusion. Data are plotted as mean ± SEM (as error bars) for the separate heart preparations: control, intralipid, and propofol (n = 12, 12, and 14, respectively). The shaded area represents the period when test agents were present. The break in the plots represents 60-minute cold cardioplegic arrest and 10 minutes of initial Langendorff reperfusion. An increase in cardiac output and a decrease in left atrial pressure in propofol-perfused hearts are apparent in the protective effect of the drug. (From Ko SH, Yu CW, Lee SK, et al: Propofol attenuates ischemia-reperfusion injury in the isolated rat heart. Anesth Analg 85:719, 1997)

Systemic Vasoregulation

It is now well established that propofol decreases SVR in humans. This was demonstrated in a patient with an artificial heart in whom the CO remained fixed.[136] As discussed later, the effect is predominantly mediated by alterations in sympathetic tone; however, in isolated arteries, propofol decreases vascular tone and agonist-induced contraction. The mechanism by which propofol mediates these effects has been attributed in part to inhibition of Ca^{++} influx through voltage or receptor-gated Ca^{++} channels, as well as inhibition of Ca^{++} release from intracellular Ca^{++} stores regulated by the ryanodine receptor.[137-140] Much of the experimental data obtained in isolated studies have focused on conduit arteries (rat aorta); however, some properties of the resistance arteries differ from the rat bioassay. Modulation of vasoconstriction by vascular smooth muscle may be mediated by (1) an alteration in endothelium-independent vasodilation[137] or (2) an alteration in the sensitivity of the myofilaments to Ca^{++}, primarily mediated by the rho activation and thereby the activation of rho kinase. In an elegant study examining the effects of propofol on resistance arteries, Imura et al[141] examined the effect of propofol on simultaneous measurements of force and in mesenteric resistance arteries.[137] They concluded that propo-

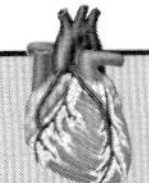

BOX 9–3 *Intravenous Induction Agents*

- Oxidative stress remains an important pathophysiologic mechanism for cellular injury in critically ill patients and represents an imbalance between the production of these radicals and the enzymatic defense system that removes them. Both propofol and midazolam act as free radical scavengers at near-therapeutic doses and support a potential role for propofol in modulating injury. This has potential therapeutic implications since these agents are routinely used for sedation in the ICU, where patients with disease processes associated with increased oxidative stress are treated.
- Evidence does not support propofol or other induction agents as preconditioning-inducing agents.
- The effect of intravenous anesthetic agents may not be solely mediated by direct acute effect on modulating vascular tone through alteration of the contractile state of the vascular smooth muscle. These agents may alter vascular smooth muscle proliferation, as well as modulate pathways that are important in angiogenesis.
- This serves to emphasize that the administration of these anesthetic agents by the anesthesiologist may have effects that last well after the drug has disappeared from the circulation.

fol attenuates norepinphrine-induced contraction through an inhibition of Ca^{++} release, as well as Ca^{++} influx through L-type Ca^{++} channels, thus partially explaining the effects of propofol on vascular adrenergic signaling (Fig. 9–24). Propofol may also modulate vascular tone by interfering with other signaling pathways involved in vasoregulation, such as endothelin-1.[141,142] Additionally, propofol may also attenuate the myogenic tone/response in pressure–flow autoregulation.[143]

Pulmonary Vasoregulation

The effects of induction agents on pulmonary vasoregulation may have important implications for the management of patients whose primary pathologies involve the pulmonary circulation when they present for cardiothoracic surgery (primary pulmonary hypertension for lung transplantation and chronic thromboembolic disease for pulmonary endarterectomy). In addition, the effects may be of importance in patients with right ventricular failure.[144] Furthermore, the effect of these agents in modulating hypoxic pulmonary vasoconstriction (HPV) may have an effect on intraoperative A-a (alveolar-arterial) gradients, particularly during one-lung ventilation. Murray and colleagues have systematically studied the effects of anesthetic agents on pulmonary vasoregulation. Specifically, they have demonstrated that propofol attenuates endothelium-dependent vasodilatation[145] via a mechanism that involves nitric oxide and endothelium-dependent hyperpolarizing factor.[146] With regard to the vascular smooth muscle, the effect appears somewhat different in the pulmonary circulation. Rather than attenuate vasoconstriction and thereby decrease tone, propofol appears to increase the sensitivity of the contractile myofilaments to Ca^{++}[147] and thereby potentiates the effect of catecholamines on pulmonary artery smooth muscle cells[148] (Fig. 9–25).

Endothelial Function

Propofol modulates the function of the endothelium, thus altering the underlying tone of the vessels. The data as to the direction and mechanism underlying this effect are widely

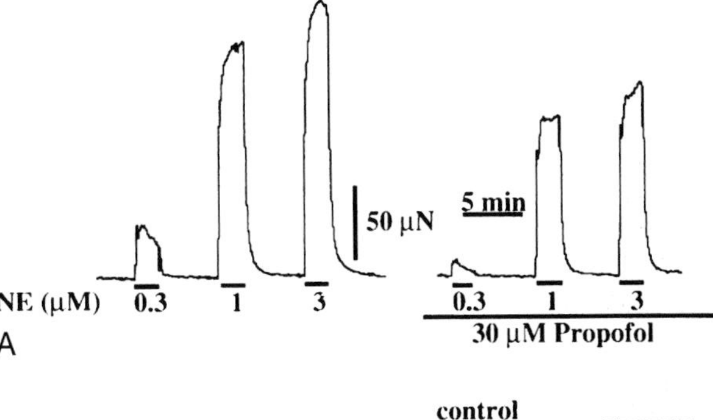

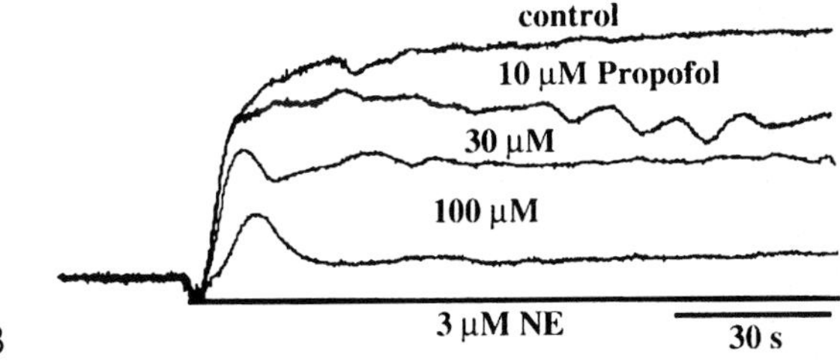

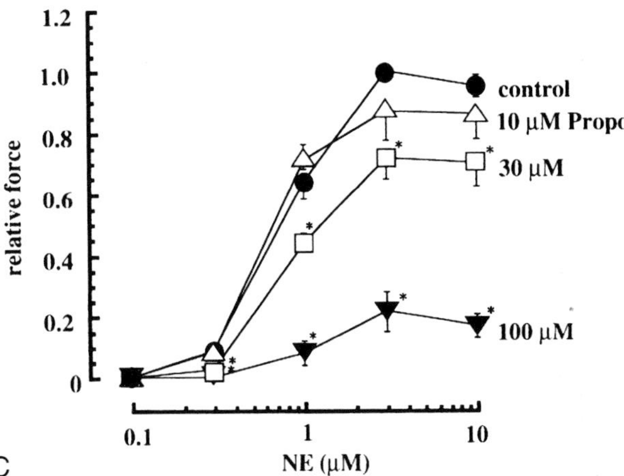

Figure 9–24 Effect of propofol on norepinephrine-induced increases in $[Ca^{++}]$I and force in smooth muscle of the rabbit mesenteric resistance artery. (From Imura N, Shiraishi Y, Katsuya H, et al: Effect of propofol on norepinephrine-induced increases in $[Ca^{++}]$ and force in smooth muscle of the rabbit mesenteric resistance artery. Anesthesiology 88:1566, 1998)

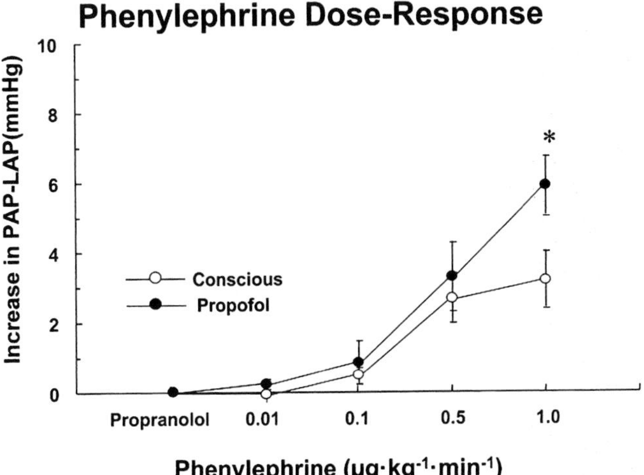

Figure 9–25 Pulmonary vascular effects of propofol at baseline, during elevated vasomotor tone, and in response to sympathetic and adrenoreceptor activation. (From Kondo U, Kim SO, Nakayama M, et al: Pulmonary vascular effects of propofol at baseline, during elevated vasomotor tone, and in response to sympathetic alpha- and beta-adrenoreceptor activation. Anesthesiology 94:815, 2001)

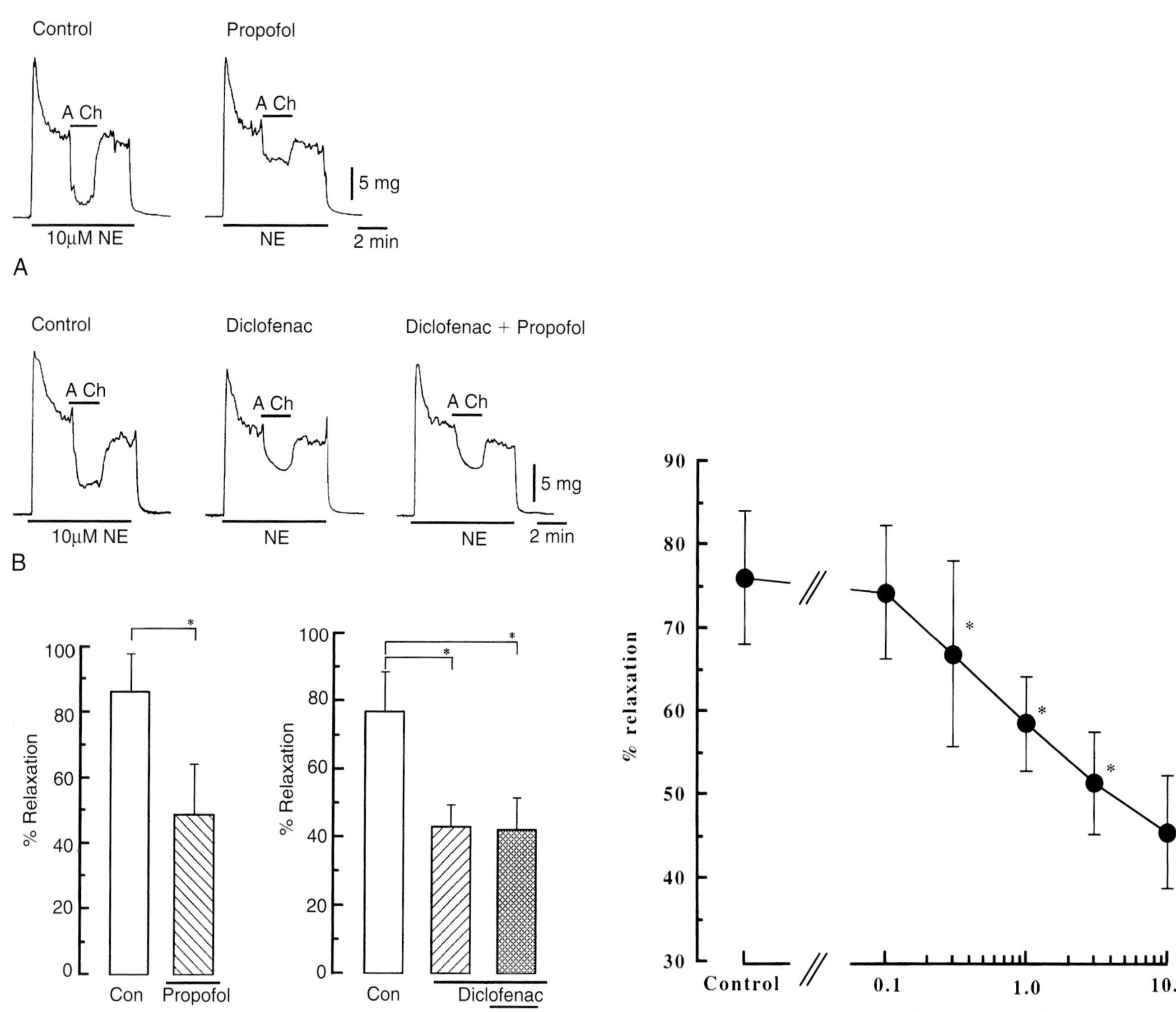

Figure 9–26 Inhibitory effects of propofol on acetylcholine-induced, endothelium-dependent relaxation and prostacyclin synthesis in rabbit mesenteric resistance arteries. (From Yamashita A, Kajikuri J, Ohashi M, et al: Inhibitory effects of propofol on acetylcholine-induced, endothelium-dependent relaxation and prostacyclin synthesis in rabbit mesenteric resistance arteries. Anesthesiology 91:1080, 1999)

divergent and are dependent on the vascular bed, species, and experimental conditions. Early studies suggested that propofol-mediated vasodilatation was a function of stimulation of nitric oxide (NO) and vasodilator prostanoids from the endothelium.[140] Other studies have demonstrated an inhibitory effect of propofol and ketamine, but not of midazolam, on endothelium-dependent relaxation.[149] Moreover, the suppressive effect of ketamine on endothelium-dependent relaxation appears to be mediated by suppression of NO formation, whereas that of propofol may be mediated at least partly by suppression of NO function. In a rabbit mesenteric resistance artery preparation, Yamashita et al[150] demonstrated that propofol inhibits prostacyclin-mediated endothelium-dependent vasodilatation by inhibition of vascular hyperpolarization (Fig. 9–26). This inhibition of hyperpolarization, and thereby inhibition of relaxation, appears to be mediated by the blockade of ATP-sensitive K^+ channels. The clinical implications of these findings are unclear; however, it may be predicted, based on the data, that the effects of propofol on the vasculature may be significantly different in patients in whom endothelial dysfunction is a significant factor, such as hypertension and atherosclerosis.

Sympathetic and Parasympathetic Nervous System

In human in vivo studies, it appears that the cumulative effects of propofol on peripheral arterial venous capacitance are mediated primarily but not solely by its effects on the sympathetic nervous system (SNS). In a well-designed study in which the effect of local infusion of propofol into the brachial artery was compared with systemic intravenous administration with induction of anesthesia, it was demonstrated that direct brachial infusion had little effect on resistance and capacitance, while the effect of intravenous administration was similar to the effect observed with sympathectomy induced by stellate ganglion block (Fig. 9–27). Thus, the peripheral vascular effects of propofol appear to be primarily mediated by reduced sympathetic vasoconstrictor nerve activity.[151] In another elegant study, Sellgren et al[152] measured the effect of propofol on the SNS using percutaneous recordings

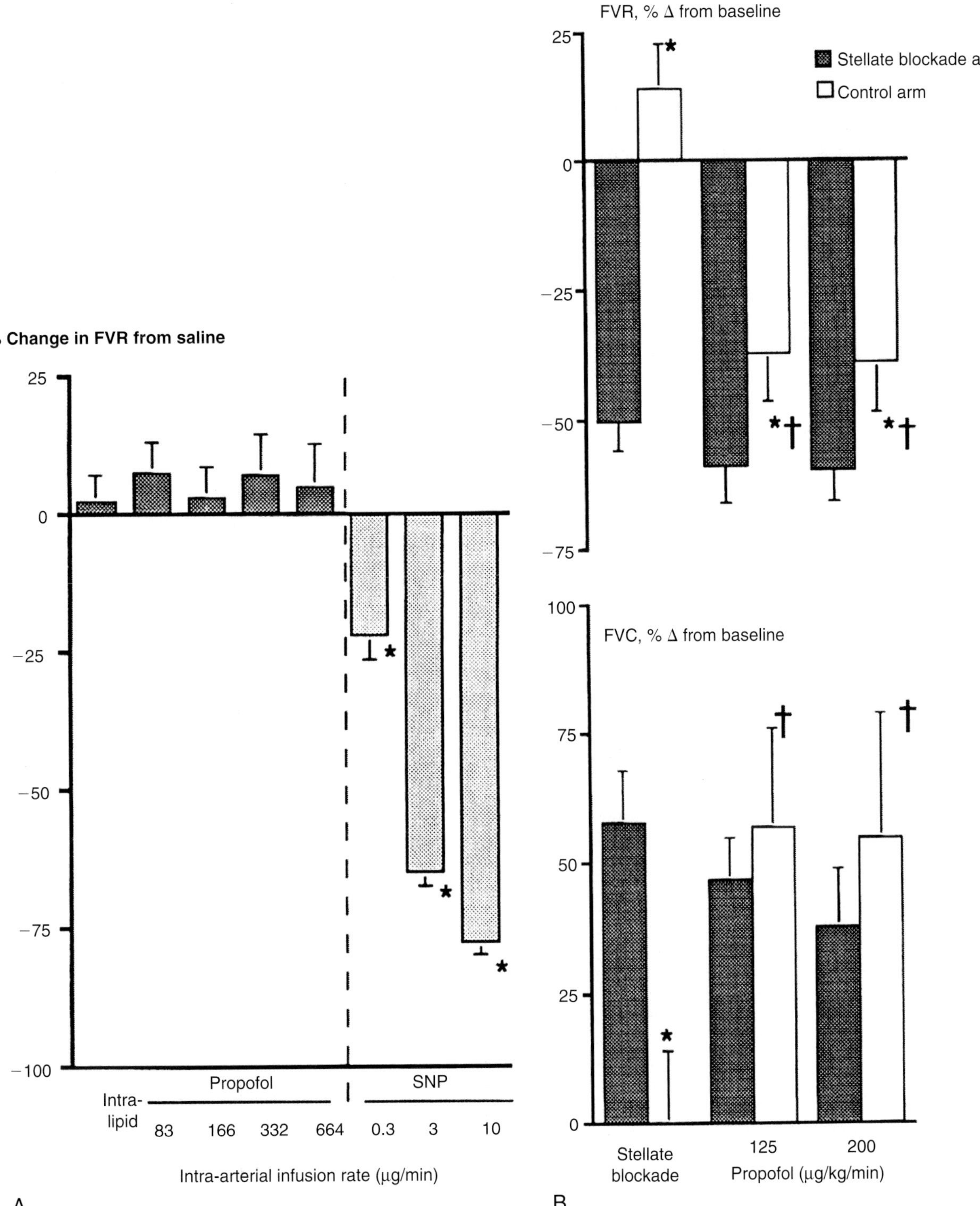

Figure 9–27 (*A*) Change in forearm vascular resistance (FVR) during brachial artery infusions of intralipid, propofol, and sodium nitroprusside (SNP). Intra-arterial infusions of propofol did not change FVR, whereas intra-arterial infusions of SNP significantly reduced FVR. Data are expressed as the percentage change from saline and are shown as mean ± SEM. *$P < 0.05$ indicates significant change from saline. (*B*) Percentage changes from awake baseline in forearm vascular resistance (FVR) and forearm venous compliance (FVC) in the left arm after stellate blockade and in the control unblocked arm before and during propofol anesthesia. Stellate blockade decreased FVR and increased FVC on the side of the blockade. During propofol anesthesia, there was no further arterial or venous dilation in the sympathectomized arm, but significant dilation occurred in the unblocked control arm. Data are mean ± SEM. *$P < 0.05$ indicates significant difference between arms. †$P < .05$ indicates significant change from prepropofol baseline. (From Robinson BJ, Ebert TJ, O'Brien TJ, et al: Mechanisms whereby propofol mediates peripheral vasodilation in humans. Sympathoinhibition or direct vascular relaxation? Anesthesiology 86:64, 1997)

of muscle sympathetic nerve activity. They demonstrated a profound decrease in SNS activity with a reciprocal increase in blood flow (measured by laser Doppler) with propofol-induced anesthesia. Furthermore, sympathetic baroreflex sensitivities were also depressed by propofol, highlighting the profound effect of this agent on central sympathetic modulation of integrated cardiovascular function. The precise locations of the central modulation by propofol have been investigated by Yang et al,[153,154] who demonstrated that propofol principally inhibits the vasomotor mechanism in the dorsomedial and ventrolateral medulla to effect its hypotensive actions. The implications of these effects are significant in that this sympathoinhibition is amplified in patients in whom SNS activity is high. Thus, caution is indicated in the administration of these agents to patients with shock, CHF, or other pathophysiologic circumstances in which the SNS is paramount in maintaining arterial and venous tone.

Remodeling and Cell Proliferation

There is emerging literature suggesting that the effects of intravenous anesthetic agents may not be solely mediated by direct modulation of vascular tone through alteration of the contractile state of the vascular smooth muscle. New studies suggest that intravenous anesthetic agents may alter vascular smooth muscle proliferation, as well as modulate pathways that are important in angiogenesis. For example, Shiga et al demonstrated the effect of ketamine (but not propofol) in inhibiting vascular smooth muscle proliferation through a PKC-dependent pathway.[155] On the other hand, midazolam, but not ketamine, was demonstrated to release vascular endothelial growth factor (VEGF), a growth factor important in angiogenesis and cellular proliferation from vascular smooth muscle cells.[156] The clinical importance of these findings remains unstudied and unclear. However, they serve to emphasize that the administration of these agents (and others) by the anesthesiologist may have effects that last well after the drug has disappeared from the core.

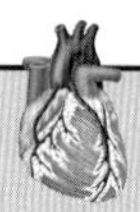

BOX 9–4 ***Intravenous Anesthetics***

- **Thiopental** decreases cardiac output by
  - A direct negative inotropic action
  - Decreased ventricular filling, resulting from increased venous capacitance
  - Transiently decreasing sympathetic outflow from the CNS
  - Because of these effects, caution should be used when thiopental is given to patients who have left or right ventricular failure, cardiac tamponade, or hypovolemia.
- **Midazolam**
  - There are only small hemodynamic changes after the intravenous administration of midazolam.
- **Etomidate**
  - Etomidate is described as the drug that changes hemodynamic variables the least. Studies in noncardiac patients and those who have heart disease document the remarkable hemodynamic stability after administration of etomidate.
  - Patients who have hypovolemia, cardiac tamponade, or low cardiac output probably represent the population for whom etomidate is better than other induction drugs, with the possible exception of ketamine.
- **Ketamine**
  - A unique feature of ketamine is stimulation of the cardiovascular system with the most prominent hemodynamic changes including significant increases in HR, CI, SVR, PAP, and systemic artery pressure. These circulatory changes cause an increase in $M\dot{V}O_2$ with an appropriate increase in coronary blood flow.
  - Studies have demonstrated the safety and efficacy of induction with ketamine in hemodynamically unstable patients and is the induction drug of choice for patients with cardiac tamponade physiology.
- **Dexmedetomidine**
  - Dexmedetomidine is a highly selective, specific and potent adrenoreceptor agonist.
  - Alpha$_2$-adrenergic agonists can safely reduce anesthetic requirements and improve hemodynamic stability. These agents may enhance sedation and analgesia without producing respiratory depression or prolonging recovery period.

INDIVIDUAL AGENTS

Thiopental

General Characteristics

Thiopental has survived the test of time as an intravenous anesthetic drug (Box 9–4). Since Lundy introduced it in 1934, thiopental has become the most widely used induction agent because of the rapid hypnotic effect (one arm-to-brain circulation time), highly predictable effect, lack of vascular irritation, and general overall safety.[157] The induction dose of thiopental is lower for older than for younger healthy patients.[158] Pharmacokinetic analyses[159-161] confirm the findings from the early classic studies of Brodie and colleagues[162] relating the awakening from thiopental to rapid redistribution. Thiopental has a distribution half-life ($t_{1/2}\alpha$) of 2.5 to 8.5 minutes, and the total body clearance varies, according to sampling times and techniques, from 0.15 to 0.26 L/kg/hr.[159-161,163,164] The elimination half-life ($t_{1/2}\beta$) varies from 5 to 12 hours.[159,160,163,164] Barbiturates[165] and drugs such as propofol[166] have increased volumes of distribution (V_d) when used during cardiopulmonary bypass (CPB). Young (less than 13 years old) patients seem to have a greater total clearance and quicker plasma thiopental clearance than do adults, which theoretically might result in earlier awakening, especially after multiple doses.[167] Because of the affinity of fat for this drug, its relatively large V_d, and its low hepatic clearance, thiopental can accumulate in tissues, especially if given in large doses over a prolonged period of time.

Cardiovascular Effects

The hemodynamic changes produced by thiopental have been studied in normal patients[158,168-174] and in patients with cardiac disease (Table 9–3).[175-180] The principal effect is a decrease in contractility,[168,169,181] which results from reduced availability of calcium to the myofibrils.[182] There is also an increase in HR.[158,168-170,173,175,177,179-181] The cardiac index (CI) is unchanged[170,175,177,179,180] or reduced,[169,172-174] and the mean aortic pressure (MAP) is maintained[170,171,177,179] or slightly reduced.[172,173,175,177,180] In the dose range studied, no relationship between plasma thiopental and hemodynamic effect has been found.[158] Early hemodynamic investigations demonstrated that thiopental (100 to 400 mg) significantly decreased CO (24%) and systemic BP (10%), presumably by reducing venous return, because of an increase in venous capacitance.[172,183]

Mechanisms for the decrease in CO include (1) direct negative inotropic action, (2) decreased ventricular filling, result-

Table 9–3 **Induction Agents and Hemodynamic Changes**

Parameter	Thiopental	Midazolam	Etomidate	Propofol	Ketamine
Heart rate	0% to +36%	−14% to +21%	0% to +22%	−6% to +12%	0% to +59%
MP^{B}	−18% to +8%	−12% to −26%	0% to −20%	0% to −47%	0% to +40%
SVR	0% to +19%	0% to −20%	0% to −17%	−9% to −25%	0% to +33%
PAP	Unchanged	Unchanged	0% to −17%	−4% to +8%	+44% to +47%
PVR	Unchanged	Unchanged	0% to +27%	—	0% to +33%
LA/PAO	Unchanged	0% to −25%	—	—	—
LVEDP/PAO	—	—	0% to −11%	+13%	Unchanged
RAP	0% to +33%	Unchanged	Unchanged	−8% to −21%	+15% to +33%
CI	0% to −24%	0% to −25%	0% to +14%	−6% to −26%	0% to +42%
SV	−12% to −35%	0% to −18%	0% to −15%	−8% to −18%	0% to −21%
LVSWI	0% to −26%	−28% to −42%	0% to −27%	−15% to −40%	0% to +27%
RVSWI	NR	−41% to −57%	—	—	—
DP/dt	−14%	0% to −12%	0% to −18%	—	Unchanged
1/PEP^{2}	−18% to −28%	—	—		
STI	—	—	Unchanged	—	NR

ing from increased venous capacitance, and (3) transiently decreased sympathetic outflow from the CNS. The increase in HR (10% to 36%) that accompanies thiopental administration probably results from the baroreceptor-mediated sympathetic reflex stimulation of the heart. Thiopental produces dose-related negative inotropic effects that appear to result from a decrease in calcium influx into the cells with a resultant diminished amount of calcium at sarcolemma sites.[184,185] Patients who had compensated heart disease and received 4 mg/kg of thiopental had a greater (18%) BP drop than did other patients. The increase in HR (11% to 36%) encountered in patients with CAD, anesthetized with thiopental (1 to 4 mg/kg), is potentially deleterious because of the obligatory increase in myocardial oxygen consumption ($M\dot{V}O_2$).

Despite the well-known potential for cardiovascular depression when thiopental is given rapidly in large doses, this drug has minimal hemodynamic effects in normal patients and in those who have heart disease when it is given slowly or by infusion. Significant reductions in cardiovascular parameters occur in patients who have impaired ventricular function. When thiopental is given to hypovolemic patients, there is a significant reduction in CO (69%), as well as a large decrease in BP, which indicate that patients without adequate compensatory mechanisms may have serious hemodynamic depression with a thiopental induction.[186] Clearly, thiopental produces greater changes in BP and HR than does midazolam when used for induction of ASA Class III and IV patients.

Uses in Cardiac Anesthesia

Thiopental can be used safely for the induction of anesthesia in normal patients and in those who have compensated cardiac disease. Because of the negative inotropic effects, increase in venous capacitance, and dose-related decrease in CO, caution should be used when thiopental is given to patients who have left or right ventricular failure, cardiac tamponade, or hypovolemia. The development of tachycardia is a potential problem in patients with ischemic heart disease.

A possible additional use for thiopental infusion is cerebral protection during CPB in patients undergoing selected cardiac operations.[187] However, the cerebral protective effect of thiopental during CPB has been challenged by Zaidan et al,[188] who demonstrated no differences in outcome between thiopental and control patients undergoing hypothermic CPB for CABG. Although the administration of a barbiturate during CPB may result in myocardial depression, necessitating additional inotropic support, a study by Ito and colleagues[189] suggested beneficial effects of a thiopental infusion during CPB in maintaining peripheral perfusion, which allowed more uniform warming, decreased base deficit, and decreased requirements for postoperative pressor support.

Midazolam

General Characteristics

Midazolam (Versed) (Fig. 9–28), a water-soluble benzodiazepine, was synthesized in the United States in 1975, in contrast to most new anesthetic drugs, which are synthesized and first tested in European countries. It is unique among benzodiazepines because of its rapid onset, short duration of action, and relatively rapid plasma clearance.[190] Although controversial, the dose for induction of general anesthesia is between 0.05 and 0.2 mg/kg and depends on the premedication and speed of injection.[191-194]

The pharmacokinetic variables of midazolam reveal that it is cleared significantly more rapidly than are diazepam and lorazepam. The rapid redistribution of midazolam, as well as high liver clearance, accounts for its relatively short hypnotic and hemodynamic effects. The $t_{1/2}\beta$ is about 2 hours, which is at least 10-fold less than for diazepam.[195-199]

Cardiovascular Effects

The hemodynamic effects of midazolam have been investigated in normal subjects,[173,200,201] in ASA Class III patients,[202] and in patients who have ischemic[203-210] and valvular[202] heart

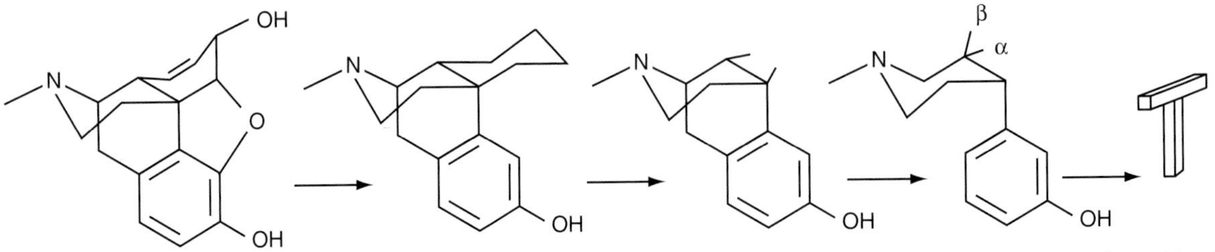

Figure 9–28 Synthetic opioids are produced by successive removal of ring structures from the five-ring phanantrene structure of morphine. However, a common core, envisaged as a T-shape, is shared by all opioids. A piperidine ring (which is believed to confer opioidlike properties to a compound) forms the crossbar, and a hydroxylated phenyl group forms the vertical axis. (With permission from Ferrante FM: Opioids. *In* Ferrante FM, VadeBoncouer TR [eds]: Postoperative Pain Management. New York, Churchill Livingstone, 1993, p 149.)

disease (VHD). Table 9–3 summarizes the hemodynamic changes after induction of anesthesia with midazolam. In general, there are only small hemodynamic changes after the intravenous administration of midazolam (0.2 mg/kg) in premedicated patients who have coronary artery disease (CAD).[203,208] Changes of potential importance include a decrease in MAP of 20% (from 102 to 81 mm Hg) and an increase in HR of 15% (from 55 to 64 beats/min).[208] The CI is maintained.[203,208] Filling pressures are either unchanged or decreased in patients who have normal ventricular function[203,208] but are significantly decreased in patients who have an elevated PCWP (18 mm Hg or higher).[209] There seems to be little effect of differences in doses on hemodynamics: 0.2 mg/kg,[203] 0.25 mg/kg,[204] and 0.3 mg/kg[207] all produce similar effects. Sedation with midazolam (0.05 mg/kg) in patients undergoing cardiac catheterization is devoid of any hemodynamic effect.[210] Marty and associates showed that induction with 0.2 mg/kg produced a 24% reduction in CBF and a 26% reduction in $M\dot{V}O_2$ in patients with CAD.[206] As in patients with ischemic heart disease, the induction of anesthesia in patients with VHD is associated with minimal changes in CI, HR, and MAP after midazolam.[210] When intubation follows anesthesia induction with midazolam, significant increases in HR and BP occur, because midazolam is not an analgesic.[173,203,205,207] Adjuvant analgesic drugs are required to block the response to noxious stimuli.

There is a suggestion that midazolam affects the capacitance vessels more than does diazepam, at least during CPB, when decreases in venous reservoir volume of the pump are greater with midazolam than with diazepam. In addition, diazepam decreases SVR more than midazolam during CPB.[211]

Midazolam (0.15 mg/kg) and ketamine (1.5 mg/kg) have proved to be a safe and useful combination for a rapid-sequence induction for emergency surgery.[171] This combination was superior to thiopental alone, because it caused less cardiovascular depression, more amnesia, and less postoperative somnolence. If midazolam is given to patients who have received fentanyl, significant hypotension may occur, as seen with diazepam and fentanyl.[212] However, midazolam is routinely combined with fentanyl for induction and maintenance of general anesthesia during cardiac surgery without adverse hemodynamic sequelae.[213,214]

Uses

Midazolam is distinctly different from the other benzodiazepines because of its rapid onset, short duration, water solubility, and failure to produce significant thrombophlebitis; it is therefore one of the mainstays of anesthesia in the cardiac operating rooms.

Etomidate

General Characteristics

Etomidate is a carboxylated imidazole derivative synthesized by Godefroi et al in 1965.[215] In animal experiments, it was found that etomidate has a safety margin four times greater than the safety margin for thiopental.[216] The recommended induction dose of 0.3 mg/kg has pronounced hypnotic effects. Etomidate is moderately lipid soluble[217] and has a rapid onset (10 to 12 seconds) and a brief duration of action.[218-220] It is hydrolyzed primarily in the liver, and in the blood as well.[221]

The administration of etomidate in a buffered solution was accompanied by a significant incidence of a burning sensation (about 40%) and myoclonic movements (about 40% to 50%).[220] The myoclonic movements were not associated with an epileptiform pattern on the electroencephalogram (EEG).[217]

Reports have shown that etomidate infusion and single injections directly suppress adrenocortical function, which in turn interferes with the normal stress response.[222-224] Blockade of 11-β-hydroxylation mediated by the imidazole radical of etomidate results in decreased biosynthesis of cortisol and aldosterone.[225] The clinical significance of etomidate-induced adrenal suppression remains undetermined.

Cardiovascular Effects

In comparative studies with other anesthetic drugs, etomidate is usually described as the drug that changes hemodynamic variables the least.[226-232] Studies in noncardiac patients[226,229-234] and those who have heart disease[177,227,228,231,235,236] document the remarkable hemodynamic stability after administration of etomidate (see Table 9–3). In normal subjects or patients who have compensated ischemic heart disease, HR, pulmonary artery pressure (PAP), pulmonary capillary wedge pressure (PCWP), left ventricular end-diastolic pressure, right atrial pressure (RAP), CI, SVR, pulmonary vascular resistance (PVR), dP/dt, and systolic time intervals (STIs) are not significantly changed after dosages of 0.15 to 0.30 mg/kg.[177,227,232,234,236] In comparison with other anesthetics, etomidate produces the least change in the balance of myocardial oxygen demand and supply. Systemic BP remains unchanged in most series[226-228,230-232] but may be decreased 10% to 19%[231,233,235] in patients who have VHD. Ammon and associates[227] found modest dose-related decreases in MAP and left ventricular stroke work index (SWI). Doses of 0.3, 0.45, and 0.6 mg/kg caused greater decreases in mean blood pressure and left ventricular SWI but had no effect on HR, PAP, PCWP, CVP, CI, SV, or SVR. Therefore, although there was a small dose-related effect on hemodynamics, the remarkable fact is that there is hemodynamic stability despite the twofold increase in dose. Dose-related changes have been demonstrated in the dog and were attributed to three possible causes: (1) decreased CNS sympathetic stimulation, (2) autoregulation secondary to decreased regional O_2 consumption, and (3) decreased SV secondary to reduced venous return.[237]

A dose-dependent direct negative inotropic effect of etomidate was demonstrated in dogs, although at equianesthetic doses it was half as pronounced as that of thiopental.[184] To determine the effects of anesthetic agents on myocardial contractility is difficult in vivo because of concomitant changes in HR, preload, and afterload. In contrast, the effects may be accurately evaluated in vitro, although this does not accurately represent what is occurring in the myocardium as a whole. Riou and associates[238] studied the effect of etomidate on intrinsic myocardial contractility, using left ventricular papillary muscle and an electromagnetic lever system. Etomidate induced a slightly positive inotropic effect, as manifested by increased maximum shortening velocity. It appears, however, that propylene glycol, the solvent in which etomidate is available, may result in sarcoplasmic reticulum dysfunction with a slight negative inotropic effect in some clinical conditions.

Etomidate (0.3 mg/kg IV), used to induce general anesthesia in patients with acute myocardial infarction under going percutaneous coronary angioplasty, did not alter HR, MAP, and rate-pressure product (RPP), demonstrating the remarkable hemodynamic stability of this agent.[239] However, the presence of VHD may influence the hemodynamic responses to etomidate. Whereas most patients can maintain their BP, patients with both aortic and mitral VHD had significant decreases of 17% to 19% in systolic and diastolic BP[231,235] and decreases of 11% and 17% in PAP and PCWP, respectively.[235] CI in patients who had VHD and received 0.3 mg/kg either remained unchanged[231,191] or decreased 13%.[235] There was no difference in response to etomidate between patients who had aortic valve disease and those who had mitral valve disease.[235]

Wauquier and colleagues[240] anticipated the widespread clinical use of etomidate in their investigation, in which they compared the effects of etomidate and thiopental in hypovolemic dogs. In a hemorrhagic shock model, dogs were bled to an MAP of 40 to 45 mm Hg and then given either etomidate (1 mg/kg) or thiopental (10 mg/kg). There was significantly more hemodynamic depression in the thiopental group and increased survival in the etomidate group. Whether this is true in humans is not known, but certainly clinical evidence suggests that etomidate is useful in hypovolemic patients.

Uses

There are certain situations in which the advantages of etomidate outweigh the disadvantages. Emergency uses include situations in which rapid induction is essential. Patients who have hypovolemia, cardiac tamponade, or low CO probably represent the population for whom etomidate is better than other drugs, with the possible exception of ketamine. The fact that the hypnotic effect is brief means that additional analgesic and/or hypnotic drugs must be administered. Etomidate offers no real advantage over most other induction drugs for patients undergoing elective surgical procedures.

Ketamine

General Characteristics

Ketamine is a phencyclidine derivative whose anesthetic actions differ so markedly from barbiturates and other CNS depressants that Corssen and Domino[241] labeled its effect *dissociative anesthesia.* The properties of ketamine and its use in anesthesia have been completely reviewed.[242] Although ketamine produces rapid hypnosis and profound analgesia, respiratory and cardiovascular functions are not depressed as much as with most other induction agents. Disturbing psychotomimetic activity (described as vivid dreams, hallucinations, or emergence phenomena) remains a problem.

Cardiovascular Effects

The hemodynamic effects of ketamine have been examined in noncardiac patients,[231,243-248] critically ill patients,[249] geriatric patients,[250] and patients who have a variety of heart diseases.[246,251-261] Table 9–3 contains the range of hemodynamic responses to ketamine. One unique feature of ketamine is stimulation of the CVS. The most prominent hemodynamic changes are significant increases in HR, CI, SVR, PAP, and systemic artery pressure. These circulatory changes cause an increase in $M\dot{V}O_2$ with an apparently appropriate increase in CBF.[254,261] Although global increases in $M\dot{V}O_2$ occur, there is some evidence that the increased work may be borne primarily by the right ventricle, because of significantly greater rises in PVR than SVR[262]; however, both ventricles certainly demonstrate increased work. The hemodynamic changes observed with ketamine are not dose related in the relatively small dose ranges examined; there is no significant difference between changes after administration of 0.5 and 1.5 mg/kg IV.[263] It is interesting that a second dose of ketamine produces hemodynamic effects opposite to those of the first.[258] Thus, the cardiovascular stimulation seen after ketamine induction of anesthesia (2 mg/kg) in a patient who has VHD is not observed with the second administration, which is accompanied instead by decreases in the BP, PCWP, and CI.

Ketamine produces similar hemodynamic changes in normal patients and in patients who have ischemic heart disease.[245] In patients who have elevated PAP (as with mitral valvular disease), ketamine seems to cause a more pronounced increase in PVR than in SVR. The presence of marked tachycardia after administration of ketamine and pancuronium can also complicate the induction of anesthesia in patients who have CAD or VHD with atrial fibrillation.[264]

The mechanism responsible for ketamine's stimulation of the circulatory system remains enigmatic. The direct effects of ketamine on the myocardium remain controversial. Riou and associates[265] demonstrated that ketamine has a dual opposing action on the myocardium: (1) a positive inotropic effect, probably secondary to increased Ca^{++} influx, and (2) an impairment of sarcoplasmic reticulum function. This impairment is significant only at supratherapeutic ketamine concentrations or in cardiomyopathic myocardium[266] and overcomes this positive inotropic effect only under these circumstances. Myocardial depression has been demonstrated in isolated rabbit hearts,[267] intact dogs, and isolated dog heart preparations.[268,269] Although the precise site of cardiovascular stimulation is still unknown, Ivankovich and colleagues[270] showed that small doses of ketamine injected directly into the CNS result in immediate hemodynamic stimulation. Ketamine also causes the sympathoneuronal release of norepinephrine, which can be measured in venous blood.[261,271,272] Blockade of this effect is possible with barbiturates, benzodiazepines,[270-273] and droperidol.[261] Animal work supports the hypothesis that the primary hemodynamic effect of ketamine is central and not peripheral.[274-281] The role of ketamine's cocaine-like neuronal inhibition of norepinephrine reuptake has yet to be defined in its overall influence on the CVS.[282,283] It is also unknown whether ketamine exerts the same effect centrally, preventing reuptake of norepinephrine in the brain.

One of the most common and successful approaches to blocking ketamine-induced hypertension and tachycardia is the prior administration of benzodiazepines. Diazepam, flunitrazepam, and midazolam all successfully attenuate the hemodynamic effects of ketamine.[171,252,257,273,284-286] For example, in a study involving 16 patients with VHD, ketamine (2 mg/kg) did not produce significant hemodynamic changes when preceded by diazepam (0.4 mg/kg).[257] Indeed, HR, MAP, and RPP were unchanged; however, there was a slight but significant decrease in CI.[257] Hatano and associates reported their experience with 200 cardiac surgical patients in whom the administration of diazepam (0.3 to 0.5 mg/kg) and then a ketamine infusion (0.7 mg/kg/hr) provided a stable hemodynamic course during induction, intubation, and incision.[284] In fact, the combination of diazepam and ketamine rivals the high-dose fentanyl technique with regard to hemodynamic stability. No patient had hallucinations, although 2% had dreams and 1% had recall of events in the operating room.[284] Levanen and colleagues[287] suggested that premedication with 2.5 μg/kg of intramuscular dexmedetomidine before ketamine-based anesthesia is as effective as midazolam in blocking the hemodynamic effects of ketamine and was more effective in reducing adverse CNS effects. Because of the propensity of dexmedetomidine to produce bradycardia, concomitant use of an anticholinergic agent was suggested.

Studies have demonstrated the safety and efficacy of induction with ketamine (2 mg/kg) in hemodynamically unstable patients who required emergency operations.[249,288,289] Most of these patients were hypovolemic because of trauma or massive hemorrhage. Ketamine induction was accompanied in the majority of patients by the maintenance of BP and, presumably, of CO as well.[249,288] In patients who have an accumulation of pericardial fluid, with or without constrictive pericarditis, induction with ketamine (2 mg/kg) maintains CI and increases BP, SVR, and RAP.[290,291] The HR in this group of patients is unchanged by ketamine, probably because cardiac tamponade already produced a compensatory tachycardia.

Uses

In adults, ketamine is probably the safest and most efficacious drug for patients who have decreased blood volume or cardiac tamponade. Undesired tachycardia, hypertension, and emergence delirium may be attenuated with benzodiazepines.

Propofol

Propofol is the most recent intravenous anesthetic to be introduced into clinical practice. It is an alkylphenol with hypnotic properties. The pharmacokinetics of propofol have been evaluated by numerous investigators and have been described by both two-compartment[292,293] and three-compartment[294,295] models.

Cardiovascular Effects

The hemodynamic effects of propofol have been investigated in healthy ASA Class I and II patients,[296] elderly patients,[297,298] patients with CAD and good left ventricular function,[299,300] and in patients with impaired left ventricular function (see Table 9–3). Numerous studies have also compared the cardiovascular effects of propofol with the most commonly used induction drugs, including the thiobarbiturates and etomidate.[301-305] Comparison of the findings between investigators is, however, difficult because of the variations in the anesthetic techniques used, doses of drugs administered, and techniques used for measuring data. It is clear that with propofol, systolic arterial pressure falls 15% to 40% after intravenous induction with 2 mg/kg and maintenance infusion with 100 μg/kg/min. Similar changes are seen in both diastolic arterial pressure and MAP.

The effect of propofol on HR is variable. The majority of studies have demonstrated significant reductions in SVR (9% to 30%), CI, SV, and left ventricular stroke work index (LVSWI) after propofol. Although controversial, the evidence points to a dose-dependent decrease in myocardial contractility.

Uses

In a study of the cerebral physiologic effects of propofol during cardiopulmonary bypass, Newman and associates[306] demonstrated that when given during nonpulsatile CPB, propofol produced statistically significant reductions in cerebral blood flow and cerebral metabolic rate in a coupled manner without adverse effects on cerebral arteriovenous oxygen content difference or jugular bulb venous saturation. The coupled reductions in cerebral blood flow and cerebral metabolic rate suggest the potential for propofol to reduce cerebral exposure to emboli during CPB.

The effect of propofol on hypoxic pulmonary vasoconstriction was minimal in thoracic surgical patients undergoing one-lung ventilation. In comparison with isoflurane, maintenance of anesthesia with propofol resulted in a lower CI and right ventricular ejection fraction, but avoided the threefold increase in shunt fraction observed with isoflurane upon commencement of one-lung ventilation.[307]

Dexmedetomidine

Dexmedetomidine, the pharmacologically active D-isomer of medetomidine, is a highly selective, specific, and potent adrenoreceptor agonist. Medetomidine has a considerably higher α_2/α_1 selectivity ratio than does the classic prototype α_2-adrenergic agonist clonidine in receptor-binding experiments. In comparison with clonidine, it is more efficacious as an α_2-adrenoreceptor agonist. It has been shown to effectively reduce volatile anesthetic requirements in experimental animals, as measured by minimal alveolar concentration, and can even be a complete anesthetic in sufficiently high doses. The exact mechanism of action and reduction of anesthetic requirement are unknown but are thought to involve an action at both presynaptic and postsynaptic α_2-adrenoreceptors in the CNS.

Cardiovascular Effects

The cardiovascular effects of dexmedetomidine are dose related. Furst and Weinger[308] demonstrated that an increase in systemic BP was associated with the pretreatment of rats with high-dose dexmedetomidine and that dexmedetomidine had little effect on arterial blood gases in spontaneously ventilating rats, consistent with minimal respiratory depression. Canine studies with medetomidine in doses of 30 μg/kg IV or 80 μg/kg IM revealed decreases in HR and CO with increased SVR after drug administration. The intravenous administration of 5 to 10 μg/kg of medetomidine to anesthetized, autonomically blocked dogs suggested that the decline in CO was not mediated by decreased contractility but rather by the effects of increased vascular resistance and decreased HR. At high doses, the increase in SVR is most likely due to the activation of peripheral postsynaptic α_2-adrenoreceptors in vascular smooth muscle.

In human studies, ASA Class I women who received low-dose premedication with 0.5 μg/kg of dexmedetomidine demonstrated modest decreases in BP and HR. Intramuscular dexmedetomidine in a dose of 2.5 μg/kg administered 45 minutes before induction of a ketamine/N_2O/oxygen anesthetic resulted in effective attenuation of the cardiostimulatory effects of ketamine but also resulted in increased intraoperative and postoperative bradycardia.[287] The use of perioperative intravenous infusions of low-dose dexmedetomidine in vascular patients at risk for CAD produced lower preoperative HR and systolic BP and less postoperative tachycardia, but also resulted in a greater intraoperative requirement for pharmacologic intervention to support BP and HR. The precise etiology of this effect is unknown, but it is possibly due to the attenuation of sympathetic outflow from the CNS.

Some controversy exists as to whether the hemodynamic effects of dexmedetomidine are influenced by the background anesthetic. In conscious animals, the hypotensive effect of the drug dominates; however, with the addition of potent inhalation anesthetics, MAP remains unchanged or increased, which implies a different mechanism of interaction of inhalation agent with this class of anesthetics. Dexmedetomidine has little effect on respiration, with minimal increase in arterial carbon dioxide tension ($PaCO_2$) after administration to spontaneously ventilating dogs; thus it has a potential advantage over other respiratory depressant anesthetics. Antinociceptive effects of medetomidine are mediated by suppression of responses of the pain-relay neurons in the dorsal horn of the spinal cord.

Uses

Clinical studies have suggested that α_2-adrenergic agonists can safely reduce anesthetic requirements and improve hemodynamic stability. These agents may enhance sedation and analgesia without producing respiratory depression or prolonging the recovery period. Levanen and colleagues[287] suggested that dexmedetomidine may be an effective alternative to benzodiazepines in attenuating the postanesthetic delirium effects of ketamine. Because α_2-adrenergic agonists potentially inhibit opiate-induced rigidity, it is clear that they may be of use as adjuvants with high-dose opioid anesthetics for cardiac surgery. In contrast to other anesthetic adjuvants, such as the benzodiazepines, the α_2-adrenoreceptor agonist dexmedetomidine does not further compromise cardiovascular or respiratory status in the presence of high-dose opioids. In summary, pharmacologic evidence suggests dexmedetomidine may be useful as an adjuvant in cardiac anesthesia.

OPIOIDS IN CARDIAC ANESTHESIA

Terminology and Classification

Various terms are commonly used to describe morphine-like drugs that are potent analgesics. The word *narcotic* is derived from the Greek word for "stupor" and refers to any drug that produces sleep. In legal terminology, it refers to any substance that produces addiction and physical dependence. Its use to describe morphine or morphine-like drugs is misleading and should be discouraged. Opiates refer to alkaloids and related synthetic and semisynthetic drugs that interact stereospecifically with one or more of the opioid receptors to produce a pharmacologic effect. The more encompassing term, *opioid*, also includes the endogenous opioids and is used in this chapter. Opioids may be agonists, partial agonists, or antagonists.

A wide diversity in chemical structure exists among the naturally occurring, semisynthetic, and synthetic opioids. Opium contains several important alkaloid constituents, which may vary markedly in their pharmacologic actions. The five major alkaloid constituents of opium can be separated into two groups based on differences in their chemical structure. The phenanthrene derivatives include morphine and codeine, as well as the convulsogenic compound thebaine, which is used as a chemical precursor in the development of many clinically useful semisynthetic opioid compounds like oxycodone. The benzylisoquinolone derivatives of opium include the phosphodiesterase inhibitor and smooth muscle relaxant papaverine and the antitussive compound noscapine.

Modification of the morphine molecule while simultaneously preserving the basic five-ring structure will result in semisynthetic compounds that also exhibit analgesic effects (e.g., hydromorphone, heroin). Progressive removal of these rings results in synthetic opioids. As long as the common core or T shape is retained stereochemically and is shared by these synthetic derivatives, opioid properties will be retained. The piperidine ring forms the crossbar and the hydroxyl phenyl group forms the vertical axis of the T shape (see Fig. 9–28).

Opioid Receptors

The postulation of opioid receptor existence was stated in the pioneering work of Beckett and Casy,[309] which in 1965 allowed Portoghese[310] to theorize the existence of separate opioid receptors by correlating analgesic activity to the chemical structure of many opioid compounds (Box 9–5). The idea of multiple opioid receptors is an accepted concept, and a number of subtypes for each class of opioid receptors have been identified. Through biochemical and pharmacologic methods, the μ-, δ-, and κ-receptors have been characterized.[311-313] Pharmacologically, it is well known that δ-opioid

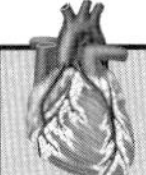

BOX 9–5 ***Opioids***

- The μ, κ, and δ-opioid receptors and endogenous opioid precursors have been identified in both cardiac and vascular tissue.
- The functional role of opioid precursors/opioid receptors in the cardiovascular system in physiologic and pathophysiologic conditions (e.g., congestive heart failure, arrhythmia development) are areas of ongoing investigation.
- The predominant cardiovascular effect of exogenously administered opioids is to attenuate central sympathetic outflow.
- Endogenous opioids and opioid receptors, especially the delta-1 receptor, are likely important contributors in effecting both early and delayed preconditioning in the heart.
- Plasma drug concentrations are profoundly altered by cardiopulmonary bypass as a result of hemodilution, altered plasma protein binding, hypothermia, exclusion of the lungs from the circulation, and altered hemodynamics that likely modulate hepatic and renal blood flow. The specific effects are drug dependent.

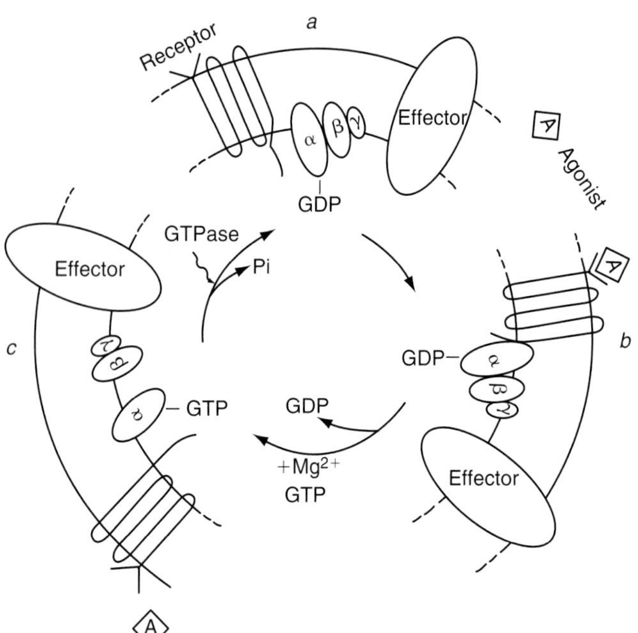

Figure 9–29 Simple scheme for G-protein signal transduction. From the unliganded state (*a*), receptor binds agonist A (for example, epinephrine/acetylcholine) which produces a change (*b*) in receptor–G protein interaction, allowing GTP in the presence of Mg^{++}, to replace GDP on the α subunit. The activated α-GTP subunit and the βγ subunits dissociate and one or both interact with effectors (for example, adenylyl cyclase, K^+ channel). Alternatively, free βγ may bind other α subunits. The intrinsic GTPase activity of the α subunit hydrolyzes GTP to GDP, releasing inorganic phosphate (P_i), and α-GDP recombines with βγ (*c*), ending the activation cycle. Nonhydrolyzable analogs of GTP such as Gpp(NH)p or GTP-γS produce persistent activation of α subunits and persistent dissociations of α from βγ because activation cannot be reversed by hydrolysis of these nucleotide analogs to GDP.

receptors consist of two subtypes: δ_1 and δ_2.[314-316] Table 9–4 lists the opioid receptors and their associated agonists and antagonists.

The μ-, κ-, and δ-opioid receptors have all been cloned, and experimental data indicate that they belong to the family of G protein–coupled receptors.[317-320] Three steps have been identified in the opioid-induced transmembrane signaling process: (1) recognition by the receptor of the extracellular opioid agonist, (2) signal transduction mediated by G protein, and (3) altered production of an intracellular second messenger (Fig. 9–29). The opioid receptors preferentially couple to a pertussis toxin–sensitive G protein (G_i/G_o) to influence one or more of three second messenger pathways: cytoplasmic free Ca^{++} $[Ca^{++}]_i$, the phosphatidylinositol-$[Ca^{++}]_i$ system, and the cyclic nucleotide cAMP. The actions of opioids are primarily inhibitory. Opioids close N-type voltage-operated Ca^{++} channels and open Ca^{++}-dependent inwardly rectifying K^+ channels. This results in hyperpolarization and a reduction in neuronal excitability.[321] κ-Receptors may only act on Ca^{++} channels.[322] There is evidence that P/Q-type Ca^{++} channels may be inhibited by μ-, but not δ-, receptor opioids.[323] These effects may be mediated via a direct coupling between G protein and the ion channels or indirectly via changes in intracellular Ca^{++}. Both Ca^{++} fluxes and the consequences of these fluxes, such as calmodulin activation, are altered by opioids. Ca^{++} ions are essential in nociception, and Ca^{++} channel blockers potentiate opioid analgesia[324,325] and reduce fentanyl requirements during cardiac surgery.[326] Opioid-induced inhibition of adenylyl cyclase, and the resultant decrease in the concentration of cAMP, may be responsible for modulation of neurotransmitter release (e.g., substance P).

Table 9–4 List of Opioid Receptor Agonist and Antagonist Drugs for the μ-, κ-, and δ-Opioid Receptors

Opioid Receptor	Agonist	Antagonist
μ	Morphine Fentanyl Levorphanol Methadone	Naloxone Naltrexone β-Funaltrexamine* Nalbuphine†
κ	U-50,488H EKC U-62,066E (spiradoline) U-69,593	Nor-BNI MR-2266 Naloxone
δ	(–)TAN-67 SIOM‡ SNC 80§	Naltrindole BNTX Naltriben

*β-FNA is an irreversible opioid receptor antagonist.
†Nalbuphine is an opioid receptor antagonist with partial agonist properties.
‡7-Spiroindinooxymorphone.
§(+)-4-[((αR)-α(2S,5R)-4-Allyl-2,5-dimethyl-1-piperazinyl)-3-methoxybenzyl]-N,N-diethylbenzamide chloride.

Opioids also have excitatory effects that involve both disinhibition of interneurons and direct excitation of neurons themselves. Nanomolar concentrations, acting via G proteins, stimulate adenylyl cyclase activity in certain neurons.[327] Another important stimulatory effect is a transient increase in cytoplasmic free Ca^{++} secondary to Ca^{++} influx via L-type Ca^{++} channel opening as well as mobilization of Ca^{++} from inositol triphosphate–sensitive intracellular stores.[328] Mu-agonists may also stimulate Ca^{++} entry into neurons via G protein–coupled activation of phospholipase-C to increase inositol(1,4,5)triphosphate formation, secondary to Ca^{++} influx via L-type Ca^{++} channel opening.[328-330]

Opioid receptors involved in regulating the CVS have been localized centrally to the cardiovascular and respiratory centers of the hypothalamus and brainstem and peripherally to cardiac myocytes, blood vessels, nerve terminals, and the adrenal medulla. It is generally accepted that opioid receptors are differentially distributed between atria and ventricles. The highest specific receptor density for binding of κ-agonists is in the right atrium and least in the left ventricle.[331,332] As with the κ-opioid receptor, the distribution of the δ-opioid receptor favors atrial tissue and the right side of the heart more than the left.[333] The data confirming the presence of the μ-opioid receptor subtype in the heart are less conclusive and most conclude that this receptor subtype is not present in cardiac tissue.[331,332,334,335] Whether these differences in receptor location are important cannot be determined, as it has not been shown whether these receptors are differentially located in cardiac muscle or cardiac nerves or are expressed on immunomodulatory cells within the heart. Based on these studies, the ability of opioid agonists to produce cardioprotection is most likely the effect of δ- and κ-receptor stimulation, and the studies performed up to the present time appear to support a role for the δ-opioid receptor as the primary receptor responsible for IPC.

Table 9–5 The Endogenous Opioid Peptide Precursors and Some of Their Active Opioid Peptide Products Involved in Cardiovascular Regulation and Function

Precursor	Opioid Peptide	Receptor*
Proenkephalin†	[Met]Enkephalin [Leu]Enkephalin	$\delta > \mu \ggg \kappa$
POMC‡	β-Endorphin	$\mu \approx \delta \gg \delta$
Prodynorphin§	Dynorphin A Dynorphin $A_{(1-8)}$ Dynorphin B	$\kappa \ggg \mu > \delta$ $\kappa \gg \mu > \delta$ $\kappa \ggg \mu > \delta$
Pronociceptin	Nociceptin	ORL_1

*The efficacy of the opioid peptide to its receptor is only qualitatively described in this table for the μ-, κ-, and δ-opioid receptor subtypes found in the central nervous system (Fowler and Fraser, 1994).

†An additional opioid peptide product from this precursor that exhibits relevant cardiovascular actions in MERF (Zhang et al, 1996).

‡An additional POMC peptide cleavage product is adrenocorticotropic hormone, which is converted to α-melanocyte-stimulating hormone-related peptides in cardiac tissue (Millington et al, 1999).

§Additional active peptides include leumorphin, α-neoendorphin, and β-neoendorphin (Fowler CV, Fraser GL: Mu-, delta-, kappa-opioid receptors and their subtypes. A critical review with emphasis on radiologand binding experiments. Neurochem Int 24:401, 1994)

Endogenous Opioids in the Heart

Myocardial cells are capable of the synthesis, storage, and release of peptides, such as opioid receptor peptides.[336] Opioid receptor peptides may be either secreted from nerves that innervate the heart or produced in myocardial tissue. Regardless of the manner of production, these peptides are devoid of activity until they undergo enzymatic proteolysis of the precursor by convertases into one (or more) active peptide products. These large stores of endogenous opioid peptide (EOP) precursors, which reside in the myocardial tissue, include proenkephalin, proendorphin, and prodynorphin.

The EOP system consists of the peptides endorphin, dynorphin, and enkephalin and their associated μ-, δ-, and κ-opioid receptors (Table 9–5). These opioid peptides and receptors are widely distributed in the body, and all have complex actions. In the heart, κ- and δ-receptor agonists have been shown to inhibit ventricular contractility, without altering atrial function.[333] A study of the actions of peptides on both electrical and mechanical properties of the isolated rat heart has shown that δ- and κ-opioid receptor agonists can directly depress cardiac function.[337] The rate of vagal firing has been shown to be regulated by opioid peptides.[338] Vagal bradycardia is inhibited by the administration of the intrinsic cardiac opioid heptapeptide MERF, presumably by the activation of D-opioid receptors on prejunctional cardiac vagal nerves or parasympathetic ganglia, reducing acetylcholine release.[339] Therefore, EOPs can mediate direct and indirect actions in various regions of the heart. Thus, in addition to complex differences in the general tissue distribution of opioid receptors, cardiac opioid peptide function is complicated by the fact that receptor expression is modulated by both physiologic states and disease.

A number of investigators have demonstrated that certain opioid peptides are released during stressful situations into the peripheral circulation.[340-343] These peptides can result in the modulation of the ANS.[344] In the heart, opioid peptides (leu- and met-enkephalins) have been shown to increase with age[345-347] as well as disease.[348-351] EOPs are involved in the modulation of hypertension and other cardiovascular conditions such as congestive heart failure and appear to be involved in arrhythmogenesis.[352] Myocardial ischemia-reperfusion has been shown to induce synthesis and release of opioid peptides.[350,353-358] In fact, several studies in humans have demonstrated that levels of circulating β-endorphins are higher in patients with acute myocardial ischemia or those undergoing angioplasty.[353-355,359] Although κ-receptor agonists have no effect on cardiovascular indices in healthy humans,[360] activation of δ- and κ-receptors during congestive heart failure decreases myocardial mechanical performance and alters regional blood flow distribution.[358] The mechanism for the negative inotropic effects is thought to be an elevation of intracellular free Ca^{++} by increasing the mobilization of calcium from intracellular stores subsequent to increased production of inositol(1,4,5)triphosphate. The increase in Ca^{++} may manifest in cardiac arrhythmias, whereas depletion of Ca^{++} from intracellular stores is responsible for a reduction in contractility.[358,361]

In patients with acute heart failure, the concentrations of EOPs are increased,[362] whereas the concentrations are decreased in patients with chronic heart failure. This has been interpreted as exhaustion of the opioid system.[363] Many studies suggest that EOPs mediate depression of myocardial function in CHF states.[341,362,364,365] Clinically, elevated levels of EOPS (β-endorphin, met-enkephalin, and dynorphin) have been found in CHF patients and these may correlate with severity. Naloxone administration to these CHF patients increased BP and HR, suggesting a homeostatic regulatory role for EOPs in CHF. However, not all clinical studies suggest that inhibition of opioid peptides is of benefit to patients with acute and chronic heart failure.[363] Oldroyd et al[366] found that plasma levels of β-endorphins were normal in patients with acute and chronic heart failure, and did not correlate with the severity of heart failure observed in their study.[366] They also found that naloxone administration did not alter cardiopulmonary exercise in these patients, and suggest that EOP inhibition is not likely to have any therapeutic potential.

Cardiac Effects of Opioids

At clinically relevant doses, the cardiovascular actions of narcotic analgesics are limited. The role that endogenously or exogenously administered opioids play in the regulation of the CVS is difficult to interpret because the physiologic effects they impart depend upon pharmacologic variables such as dose, site, and route of administration as well as receptor specificity and species. The actions opioids exhibit are mediated both by opioid receptors located centrally in specific areas of the brain and nuclei that regulate the control of cardiovascular function and peripherally by tissue-associated opioid receptors. The opioids in general exhibit a variety of complex pharmacologic actions on the CVS[341] (Fig. 9–30).

Most of the hemodynamic effects of opioids in humans can be related to their influence on the sympathetic outflow from the CNS. Current evidence shows that sympathetic overactivity favors the genesis of life-threatening ventricular tachyarrhythmias, and its control has protective effects during acute myocardial ischemia.[367] Moreover, an imbalance of the ANS, characterized by increased sympathetic activity and reduced vagal activity, results in myocardial electrical instability and promotes the occurrence of ischemic events. The pharmacologic modulation of the sympathetic activity by centrally or

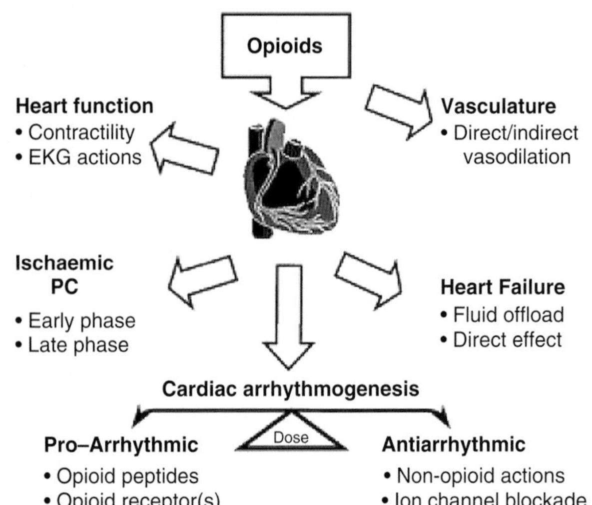

Figure 9–30 Some of the actions of opioids on the heart and cardiovascular system. Opioid actions may either involve direct opioid receptor-mediated actions, such as the involvement of the δ-opioid receptor in ischemic preconditioning (PC) or indirect, dose-dependent, non-opioid receptor–mediated actions such as ion channel blockade associated with the antiarrhythmic actions of opioids.

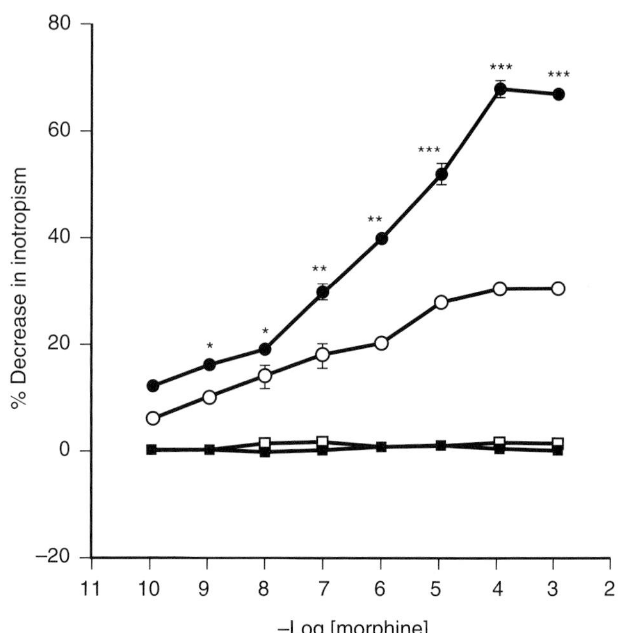

Figure 9–31 Concentration–response curves for morphine (*circles*) in isolated electrically stimulated human right atrial strips from nonfailing (*filled symbols*) and failing (*open symbols*) hearts (*squares* = control). Average auricular inotropism (mean [SEM]) for nonfailing hearts was 0.90 (0.05) g and 0.89 (0.02) g for failing hearts. **P* < 0.05, ***P* < 0.01, ****P* < 0.001 versus failing heart. Each point represents the mean (SEM) of eight experiments for each experimental group.

peripherally acting drugs elicits cardioprotective effects. Opioid receptor agonists such as fentanyl are known to exhibit significant central sympathoinhibitory effects.[368]

Fentanyl and sufentanil enhance the calcium current that occurs during the plateau phase (phase 2) of the cardiac action potential, and depress the outward potassium current responsible for terminal repolarization,[369] resulting in a significant prolongation of the duration of the action potential. Blair et al[370] suggested that the cardiac electrophysiologic effects of fentanyl and sufentanil represented a direct membrane effect resembling that produced by Class III antiarrhythmic drugs. In patients, large doses of opioids prolong the QT interval of the electrocardiogram.[369] This may explain the reported antiarrhythmic properties of opioids, particularly in the presence of myocardial ischemia.[371] Fentanyl, 60 μg/kg, and sufentanil, 10 μg/kg, significantly increased the ventricular fibrillation threshold in dogs following coronary artery occlusion.[372]

All opioids, with the exception of meperidine, produce bradycardia, although morphine given to unpremedicated normal subjects may cause tachycardia. The mechanism of opioid-induced bradycardia is central vagal stimulation. Premedication with atropine can minimize but not totally eliminate opioid-induced bradycardia, especially in patients taking β-adrenoceptor antagonists. Although severe bradycardia should be avoided, moderate slowing of the HR may be beneficial in patients with CAD by decreasing myocardial oxygen consumption.

Isolated heart or heart-muscle studies have demonstrated dose-related inotropic effects for morphine, meperidine, fentanyl, and alfentanil.[373-376] However, these effects occurred at concentrations one hundred to several thousand times those found clinically. In canine hearts, the direct intracoronary injection of fentanyl in concentrations up to 240 ng/mL produced no changes in myocardial mechanical functions.[377]

Morphine produced dose-related decreases in the contractility of atria obtained from nonfailing and failing human hearts, but the concentration-response curve was significantly shifted to the right in preparations from failing hearts[378] (Fig. 9–31). The negative inotropic effects induced by morphine in both failing and nonfailing preparations were not antagonized by naloxone, indicating that opioid receptors do not play a part in this cardiac effect of morphine. One explanation could be an interaction with β-adrenoceptors, unrelated to the binding of opioids to opioid receptors. Opioids inhibit β-adrenoceptor–sensitive adenylyl cyclase.[379]

Hypotension can occur after even small doses of morphine and is primarily related to decreases in SVR. The most important mechanism responsible for these changes is probably histamine release. The amount of histamine release is reduced by slow administration (<10 mg/min). Pretreatment with a histamine H_1 or H_2 antagonist does not block these reactions, but they are significantly attenuated by combined H_1 and H_2 antagonist pretreatment.[380] Neither morphine nor fentanyl, in clinically relevant concentrations, blocks α-adrenergic receptors in isolated vascular tissue studies.[381,382] Opioids may also have a direct action on vascular smooth muscle, independent of histamine release. In the isolated hindlimbs of dogs anesthetized with halothane, high doses of alfentanil (500 μg/kg), fentanyl (50 μg/kg), and sufentanil (6 μg/kg) caused significant decreases of 48%, 48%, and 44%, respectively, in SVR. Neither pretreatment with naloxone nor denervation changed the responses, and it was concluded that the three opioids produced vasodilation by a direct action on vascular smooth muscle.[383] Although fentanyl-induced relaxation in the rat aorta may be mediated by α-adrenergic receptors, this effect occurs only at concentrations several hundred times higher than those encountered clinically.[384]

The effects of κ-agonists on BP have been examined[385] and been shown to be dose, species, and route dependent.[385,386] U-50,488H, for example, displays a markedly different cardiovascular profile when injected intravenously as compared with injected directly into the CNS. In anesthetized dogs, κ-agonists produce dose-related decreases in BP, HR, peak sys-

Table 9–6 D_{25} Drug Doses of Arylacetamide κ-Opioid Agonists in Intact Rats: Effects on Heart Rate, Blood Pressure, and ECG Measures

Drug	Heart rate	Blood pressure	ECG Measures (msec)			
			PR	QRS	RSh	Q-T
U-50,488H	1.5	>32	20	>32	16	32
U-62,066E	4.0	8.0	15	25	2.0	10
PD117,302	5.5	0.50	3.0	7.5	1.0	6.0

The nonopioid actions of structurally related arylacetamide κ-opioid receptor agonists were examined in pentobarbital-anesthetized rats. Heart rate, blood pressure, and ECG measures were determined as D_{25}, the dose (μmol/kg/min IV) producing a 25% change in the given response. This measure allowed for a determination of the differential actions of the arylacetamides on ECG measures, an index of drug action on cardiac ion channels (n = 6). The drug dose produced a 25% change from control in intact animals for six determinations per measure. All drugs consistently reduced the heart rate but had varying D_{25} doses for blood pressure reduction. PD117,302 [(±)-*N*-methyl-*N*-[2-(1-pyrrolidinyl)cyclohexyl]benzo[**b**]thiophene-4-acetamide monohydrochloride], produced evidence of sodium channel blockade (changes in the PR, QRS, and RSh measures) and potassium channel blockade (changes in the Q-T interval) at lower D_{25} values than either of the other two drugs.

tolic pressure, and cardiac contractility when administered intravenously. The cardiovascular responses to both opioid agonists were abolished by previous administration of naloxone.[387] In addition to causing a reduction in BP, κ-opioid agonist dose dependently reduced the HR in anesthetized rats.[386] This is suggestive of an effect on either the reflex mechanisms that regulate the HR during hypotension or direct action on the electrical or mechanical properties responsible for normal cardiac contractility. Kappa agonists cause slight depressant action on the HR and BP at low doses that is not inhibited by naloxone, suggesting a lack of involvement of opioid receptors and a possible direct effect on cardiac muscle.[385] In anesthetized rats, the cardiovascular responses to κ-opioid agonists in the presence of opioid antagonists were not changed.[385,388,389] It was concluded from these studies and others[390] that because opioid receptor antagonists did not block these responses, they were not mediated by opioid receptors.

Opioid receptor agonists and antagonists have been shown to block ion channels that constitute the genesis of the action potential in neurons. Voltage-gated Na^+ channels are responsible for the initiation of membrane depolarization and the conduction of action potentials in electrically excitable cells, resulting in contraction of the heart or transmission of electrical impulses in nerves. K^+ channels are responsible for repolarization of the cell membrane and cessation of action potentials in excitable cells. Morphine and naloxone have been shown to block the propagation of action potentials in many nerve and cardiac muscle preparations by directly inhibiting voltage-dependent Na^+ and K^+ currents. In addition to the opioid receptor–independent–mediated actions of U-50,488H and related κ-agonists on BP and HR (i.e., actions not blocked by opioid receptor antagonist), these drugs produce changes in the electrocardiogram indicative of a drug interaction with cardiac ion channels.[385,391] Table 9–6 summarizes the action of several κ-opioid agonists and their actions on BP, HR, and the PR, QRS, RSh, and Q-T intervals on rat electrocardiograms. The electrocardiographic changes, including PR interval prolongation, QRS widening, and increased amplitude of the RSh, are indicative of cardiac Na^+ channel blockade. The widening of the Q-T interval, an index of cardiac repolarization, is suggestive of K^+ channel blockade.

The results of studies with opioid drugs, such as sufentanil[369] and morphine,[392] corroborate the suggestion of interaction of κ-opioids with cardiac K^+ channels. However, the opioid receptor–independent nature of the ion channel blockade may not be isolated to Na^+ and K^+ channels and may also include L-type Ca^+ channels found in cardiac muscle. The use of Ca^{++} fluorescent techniques for measurement of cardiac myocyte contractility suggested that the negative inotropic actions for κ-opioid agonists may also be due to inhibition of L-type Ca^{++} currents.[393,394] While investigating the possible cardiotoxic effects produced by opioids in human poisoning, Wu et al[395] found that opioids, like meperidine and dextropropoxyphene, exert negative inotropic actions in cardiac muscle by blockade of Ca^{++} currents in myocytes in the presence of naloxone.

Ischemic Preconditioning

Myocardial IPC is a phenomenon that occurs in cardiac muscle in which brief periods of ischemia (usually <5 minutes) render the muscle tolerant to tissue damage that occurs during a subsequent period of ischemia, following an interlude of perfusion[396] (Fig. 9–32). Such a phenomenon has been shown to occur in many species and is known to be mediated by a well-defined intracellular cascade.[397] The intercellular mediator or IPC-induction trigger appears to be diverse and has been shown to involve opioids and other substances. Thus, the nature of IPC may not be consistent between the species examined, despite a common end result.

In vivo studies show that IPC can reduce the size of an infarct resulting from prolonged ischemia.[398] There is also a reduction in damage to myocardial intracellular structure, a decrease in the dysfunction of the cardiac contractile machinery, and a direct reduction in arrhythmias associated with IPC.[398,399] The ability of IPC to limit myocardial damage occurs chronologically in two distinct phases. The first, or early phase, provides a window of protection to the heart muscle that occurs soon after IPC and declines with time during the first three hours of reperfusion. The second, late (or delayed) phase of IPC, provides a second window of protection to heart muscle that emerges after 24 hours of reper-

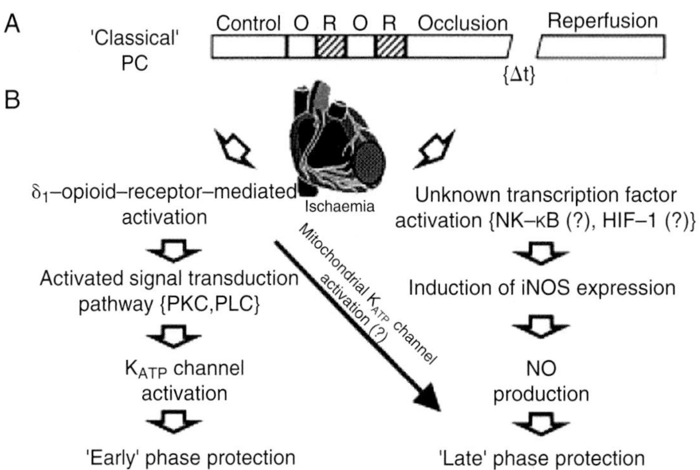

Figure 9–32 (*A*) A "typical" protocol bar that may be used in experiments that investigate the effects of agents on ischemic preconditioning (PC) in the heart. Similar protocols have been used to study opioid receptor–mediated cardioprotective mechanisms in the rat and other mammalian species. Studies may investigate the effects of ischemic PC on ischaemia and/or reperfusion arrhythmias of various durations in length (Δt). Ischemic PC usually involves a sequence of coronary artery occlusion (O), followed by reperfusion (R) cycles. In this panel, two cycles are depicted prior to coronary artery occlusion followed by reperfusion. *Note that this type of protocol may be easily amenable to modification, the protocol shown is a simplified protocol bar.* (*B*) Schematic diagram that describes the molecular pathways involved in the protective effects of ischemic PC in the heart. Brief periods of ischemia provide both an "early" and "late" phase of protection to the heart from subsequent episodes of prolonged or permanent ischaemia. The activation of G protein–coupled δ_1-opioid receptors has been shown to be involved in both protective phases. The activation of the δ_1-opioid receptor activates intracellular signal transduction pathways (including PKC, phospholipase C [PLC], and related kinase pathways). Activation of these pathways results in the phosphorylation of certain proteins such as the K^+_{ATP} channel present both on the myocyte cell surface, as well as the myocyte mitochondrial cell surface. The opening of these ion channels mediates the "early" phase of cardioprotection that lasts 2 to 3 hours after the ischaemic episode. The "late" phase of cardioprotection that results from the brief episodes of ischaemia may be mediated by the activation of oxygen-sensitive transcription factors (such as NF-κB and HIF-1). These factors subsequently induce the expression of inducible NOS (iNOS) and the production of NO, the putative mediator of the protective effect on the heart observed 24 to 48 hours after the ischaemic episode. Recently, it has been shown that δ_1-opioid receptor stimulation may also produce a "late" cardioprotective effect that may result from activation of mitochondrial K^+_{ATP} channels. (From Murry CE, Jennings RB, Reimer KA: Preconditioning with ischemia: A delay of lethal cell injury in ischemic myocardium. Circulation 74:1124, 1986)

fusion and may last up to 72 hours[400-402] (see Chapters 6, 12, and 19).

Importance of Opioid Receptors in Early Preconditioning

The involvement of opioids in IPC resulted from the recognition of their value at increasing survival time and tissue preservation prior to surgical transplantation and their possible role in enhancing tolerance to hypoxia.[403,404] The first evidence to demonstrate a role for opioids in early IPC was published by Schultz et al[404,405] in the intact blood-perfused rat heart. These investigators demonstrated that the nonselective opioid receptor antagonist naloxone completely antagonized the ability of IPC to reduce infarct size whether administered before the IPC stimulus or after the IPC stimulus just prior to the index ischemia. These results suggested that endogenous opioids serve as both a trigger and end effector of IPC in rat hearts (Fig. 9–33). Chien and Van Winkle[406] found similar results in the rabbit heart with the use of the active enantiomer, (−)-naloxone. Furthermore, Schultz et al[407] determined the role of endogenous opioids in mediating IPC and myocardial hibernation in pig hearts and observed that naloxone blocked IPC but not the effects of short-term hibernation. These data clearly suggest that an opioid receptor is mediating the effect of endogenous opioids to elicit IPC in the rat, rabbit, and pig.

Takashi et al[408] performed a study in isolated adult rabbit cardiomyocytes to determine which endogenous opioid peptides are responsible for the cardioprotective effect observed during and following IPC. They found that metenkephalin, leuenkephalin, and met-enkephalin-ang-phe (MEAP) pro-

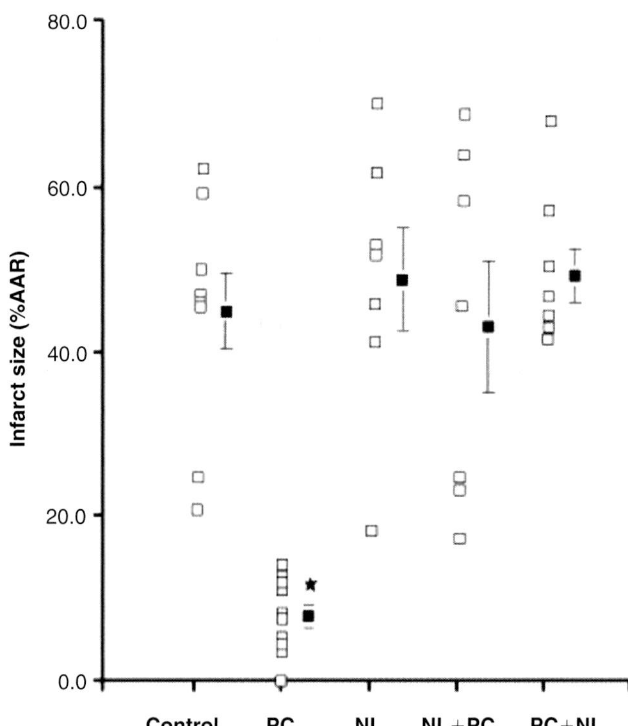

Figure 9–33 Infarct size (IS) expressed as a percentage of the area at risk (AAR) in intact rat hearts subjected to vehicle (control), ischemic preconditioning (PC), naloxone (NL) in the absence of PC, NL treatment prior to PC (NL + PC), and NL treatment after PC (PC + NL) before the index ischemic period. *Filled squares* are the mean ± SEM of each group. *$P < 0.05$ versus the control group. (From Schultz JJ, Rose E, Yao Z, et al: Evidence for involvement of opioid receptors in ischemic preconditioning in rat heart. Am J Physiol 268:157, 1995)

duced a reduction in the incidence of cell death, suggesting that the enkephalins are the most likely candidates, which serve as triggers and distal effectors of IPC in the rabbit heart.

Cardioprotective Effects of Exogenous Opioid Agonists

In 1996, Schultz and colleagues were the first to demonstrate that an opioid could attenuate ischemia-reperfusion damage in the heart. Morphine at the dose of 300 μg/kg was given before left anterior descending coronary artery occlusion for 30 minutes in rats in vivo. Infarct area/area at risk was diminished from 54% to 12% by this treatment.[409] The infarct-reducing effect of morphine has been shown in hearts in situ, isolated hearts, and cardiomyocytes.[410-412] Morphine also improved postischemic contractility.[413] It is now well accepted that morphine provides protection against ischemia-reperfusion injury. Fentanyl has been studied in a limited fashion and has had mixed results as far as its ability to protect the myocardium.[413-415] This may be due to differences in species studied and/or fentanyl concentrations. Pentazocine and buprenorphine improved postischemic contractility in rabbits in vitro.[413] Overall, the effects of opioids other than morphine have not been sufficiently investigated to allow conclusions to be drawn.

Schultz also demonstrated that the effect of IPC to reduce infarct size was mediated by the δ1-receptor but not the δ_2-, μ-, or κ-receptor, because the effects of IPC were blunted by the selective δ_1-receptor antagonist BNTX but not the δ_2-antagonist naltriben.[416] They also showed that cardioprotection was not induced by the administration of the selective μ-agonist DAMGO and that IPC was not attenuated by the μ-antagonist B-FNA.[416] In that same study, they excluded the involvement of the κ-receptor because a κ-selective antagonist could not reverse the effects of IPC to reduce infarct size. These data suggest that the δ_1-opioid receptor appears to be the primary opioid receptor involved in IPC in the intact rat heart.

While the exogenous activation of the δ-opioid receptor subtype by highly specific agonists before ischemia has been shown to reduce infarct size in a number of species, including rats,[416] rabbits,[417] and swine,[418] the role of the κ-opioid receptors in preconditioning has been a subject of much controversy. It has been reported that preischemic administration of selective κ-agonists will reduce infarct size and ischemia-induced arrhythmias in the isolated rat heart. Conversely, specific activation of the κ-opioid receptor before ischemia has also been shown to increase infarct size[404] and arrhythmias[419] and induce an "antipreconditioning"-like state in rats. It has been proposed that the κ-opioid receptor agonists exert a biphasic effect on the myocardium, producing proarrhythmic and antiarrhythmic effects in the rat.[385] Therefore, it is unclear whether selective or nonselective activation of the κ-opioid receptor subtype is beneficial during preconditioning, and although such conflicting information exists for the rat, the role of opioid receptor subtypes in IPC and pharmacologic preconditioning in other species is even more limited. Further studies are needed to address the role of the κ-receptor in arrhythmias.

Signaling Pathways Involved in Opioid-Induced Cardioprotection

Opioid-induced cardioprotection and IPC seem to share a common pathway, in that the δ-opioid receptor and the mitochondrial K^+_{ATP} channel appear to be involved in the beneficial effects observed. Additional studies show that the cardioprotective effect of IPC and δ_1-opioid receptor activation were both mediated via a G_I protein–coupled receptor.[416] To further address potential signaling pathways involved in opioid-induced protection, it was observed that morphine produced a cardioprotective effect in isolated rabbit hearts that was blocked by pretreatment with a nonselective PKC inhibitor. In summary, the beneficial effects were eliminated by a G_i protein inhibitor, a PKC inhibitor,[410,414,420,421] and a selective mitochondrial K^+_{ATP} channel blocker.[411,414,420,422-425] A schematic summary of the major pathways thought to be involved in acute opioid-induced cardioprotection is shown in Figure 9–34.

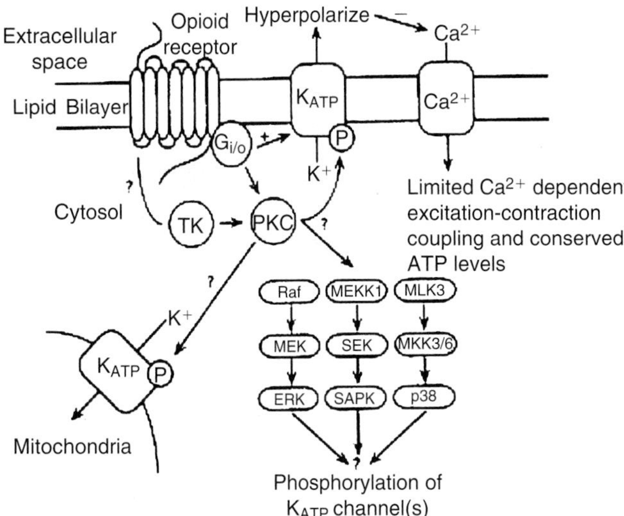

Figure 9–34 A schematic diagram of some of the major pathways thought to be involved in acute opioid-induced cardioprotection. (From Fryer RM, Hsu AK, Ells JT, et al: Opioid-induced second window of cardioprotection. Potential role of mitochondrial KATP channels. Circ Res 84:846, 1999)

Role of Opioids in Delayed Preconditioning

It appears that opioid receptors are involved in delayed cardioprotection via activation of the δ- and κ-opioid receptors. Fryer et al[424] demonstrated that TAN-67, a δ_1-opioid agonist, could also induce cardioprotection during the "second window" of IPC. They found no protective effect to reduce infarct size 12 hours after administration of the selective δ_1-opioid agonist; however, it produced a marked cardioprotective effect at 24 to 48 hours following drug administration, which disappeared at 72 hours (Fig. 9–35). The cardioprotective effects were blocked by pretreatment with a selective δ_1-antagonist, a nonselective K^+_{ATP}-channel antagonist, and a mitochondrial-selective K^+_{ATP}-channel blocker. These results suggest that δ_1-opioid receptor activation 24 to 48 hours prior to an ischemic insult results in a delayed cardioprotective effect that appears to be mediated by the mitochondrial K^+_{ATP} channel. Wu and colleagues[426] revealed that κ-opioid receptor–induced cardioprotection occurred via two phases: the first window occurred about 1 hour after receptor activation, and the second developed 16 to 20 hours following administration in isolated ventricular myocytes.

Opioids and Cardioprotection in Humans

Although the animal and cell work reviewed imply a cardioprotective effect of opioid receptor activation, it is important to demonstrate that a similar system exists in humans if these basic studies can be extrapolated to the clinical world. Tomai

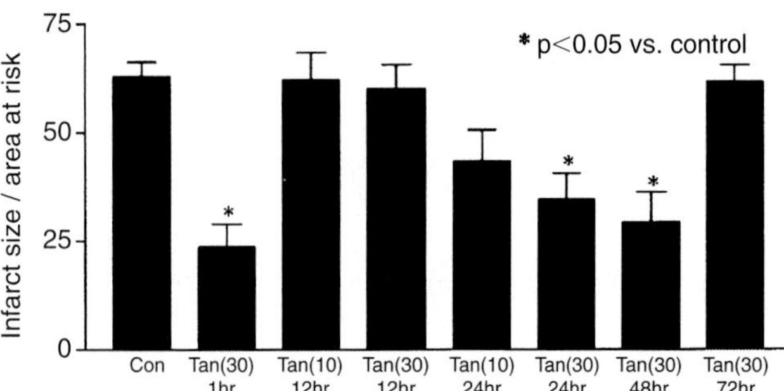

Figure 9–35 Infarct size expressed as a percent of the area at risk in rats administered 10 or 30 mg/kg of TAN-67, either 1, 12, 24, 48, or 72 hours before 30 minutes of ischemia and 2 hours of reperfusion. A 1-hour pretreatment with TAN-67 produced a significant reduction in infarct size/area at risk. Pretreatment with both doses of TAN-67 12 hours prior to ischemia/reperfusion or low-dose TAN-67 24 hours prior to ischemia/reperfusion had no significant effect on infarct size/area at risk. However, pretreatment with the large dose of TAN-67 24 to 48 hours prior to ischemia/reperfusion significantly reduced infarct size/area at risk. This cardioprotective effect was lost following 72 hours of pretreatment. All values are the mean ± SEM. *$P < 0.05$. (From Fryer RM, Hsu AK, Ells JT, et al: Opioid-induced second window of cardioprotection. Potential role of mitochondrial KATP channels. Circ Res 84:846, 1999)

et al[427] have demonstrated that naloxone could abolish the reduction in ST-segment elevation normally observed during a second balloon inflation during coronary angioplasty. Additionally, they demonstrated that in naloxone-treated patients, the severity of cardiac pain and time to onset at the end of the second balloon inflation were similar to that of the first inflation; whereas in the placebo treated patients the severity of cardiac pain during the second inflation was reduced and the time to onset of pain was lengthened versus the first inflation. This suggests a preconditioning-like effect in humans undergoing coronary angioplasty that could be attenuated by the opioid antagonist naloxone. Similarly, Xenopoulos and co-workers[428] have shown that intracoronary morphine (15 μg/kg) mimics IPC, as assessed by changes in ST segment shifts in humans undergoing percutaneous transluminal coronary angioplasty. Finally, Bell et al[423] also demonstrated that δ-opioid receptor stimulation mimics IPC in human atrial trabeculae via K^{+}_{ATP} channel activation. These results are encouraging and may suggest a possible clinical use for opioids in the therapy of acute or chronic myocardial ischemia.

Cardioplegia and hypothermia provide considerable myocardial protection against the induced ischemia of cardiac surgery. However, in certain high-risk subgroups and, to some extent in all patients, current methods of cardioprotection are still suboptimal, and there continues to be poor myocardial tolerance to ischemia. This myocardial ischemia is often evidenced by perioperative ventricular dysfunction, myocardial stunning, and poor functional recovery following an ischemic episode, which may lead to poor surgical outcome (see Chapters 28, 30, and 31). Postsurgical myocardial ischemic changes include hypothermia, intracellular acidosis, hypoxia, depletion of energy stores, and cellular volume shifts, all of which adversely affect myocardial contractility. Hibernating animals demonstrate similar cellular and molecular cardiac changes during hibernation that closely parallel those seen in hypothermic cardioplegic arrest. However, these changes are well tolerated in the myocardium of the hibernating mammals for months at a time, whereas the duration of induced ischemia tolerated surgically is limited. This process is induced by a hibernation induction trigger (HIT) molecule, which has recently been shown to have an opioid basis.[429] It has been shown that opioid peptides can induce mammalian hibernation and may provide protection against the adverse effects of hypothermic myocardial ischemia, providing potential therapeutic applications during CPB and protection of organs for heart transplantation.

In animal studies, Bolling et al[430,431] showed the δ-opioid receptor agonist DADLE protects hearts that were subjected to 18 hours of cold storage at 4°C or 2 hours of global ischemia, respectively, in the presence of a standard cardioplegic solution. Another study[432] provided evidence that pentazocine, a δ-opioid agonist, enhanced the myocardial protection of standard cardioplegia at temperatures ranging from 0° to 34°C. Subsequently, Kevelaitis and colleagues[422] have shown that stimulation of δ-opioid receptors improves recovery of cold-stored rat hearts to a state similar to IPC. These investigators showed that this opioid-induced cardioprotection is mediated through K^{+}_{ATP} channel activation.

Although the initial success of CPR is on average 39% (13% to 59%), a majority of victims die within 72 hours, primarily due to heart failure and/or recurrent ventricular fibrillation. CPR, therefore, yields a functional survival rate of only 1.4% to 5%.[433-435] Myocardial function is substantially impaired after successful resuscitation from cardiac arrest. This has led to the investigation of the use of opioid receptor agonists to improve functional outcome. Tang and colleagues[436] demonstrated that pharmacologic activation of δ-opioid receptors significantly reduced MV_{O_2} during the global myocardial ischemia of cardiac arrest. A follow-up study in rats demonstrated that the nonselective δ-opioid receptor agonist pentazocine strikingly reduced the severity of postresuscitation myocardial dysfunction and increased the duration of post-resuscitation survival.

Opioid analgesics are widely used for the treatment of pain. Although these agents are predominantly μ-opioid receptor agonists, cross-talk with δ-opioid receptors has been demonstrated. However, the Food and Drug Administration has not approved these drugs for use in patients with unstable angina or who are predisposed to myocardial infarction. This is likely due to the limited research in humans concerning the importance of opioid receptors in the myocardium and the high potential for dependence, abuse, and respiratory depression. Future avenues of research should focus on the identification of orally active compounds with high δ-opioid receptor affinity to be used as cardioprotective agents since these drugs are currently lacking.

Opioids in Cardiac Anesthesia

A technique of anesthesia for cardiac surgery involving high doses of morphine was developed in the late 1960s and early 1970s. This was based on the observation by Lowenstein et al[437] that patients requiring mechanical ventilation after surgery for end-stage VHD tolerated large doses of morphine for sedation without discernible circulatory effects. When they attempted to administer equivalent doses of morphine as the anesthetic for patients undergoing cardiac surgery, they discovered serious disadvantages including inadequate anesthesia, even at doses of 8 to 11 mg/kg, episodes of hypotension related to histamine release, and increased intraoperative and postoperative blood and fluid requirements. Attempts to overcome these problems by combining lower doses of morphine with a variety of supplements (such as N_2O, halothane, or diazepam) proved unsatisfactory, resulting in significant myocardial depression, with decreases in CO and hypotension.[438]

Because of the above problems associated with the use of morphine, several other opioids were investigated in an attempt to find a suitable alternative. The use of fentanyl in cardiac anesthesia was first reported by Stanley and Webster in 1978.[439] Since then there have been extensive investigations of fentanyl, as well as sufentanil and alfentanil, in cardiac surgery. The fentanyl group of opioids has proved to be the most reliable and effective for producing anesthesia both for patients with valvular disorders and CABG (see Chapters 19 and 20).

A major advantage of fentanyl and its analogs for patients undergoing cardiac surgery is their lack of cardiovascular depression. This is of particular importance during the induction of anesthesia, when episodes of hypotension can be critical. Cardiovascular stability may be less evident during surgery; in particular, the period of sternotomy, pericardiectomy, and aortic root dissection may be associated with significant hypertension and tachycardia. During and after sternotomy, arterial hypertension increases in SVR, and decreases in CO frequently occur.[440,441] The variability in the hemodynamic responses to surgical stimulation, even with similar doses of fentanyl, is probably a reflection of differences in the patient populations studied by different authors. One factor is the influence of β-blocking agents. In patients undergoing CABG anesthetized with fentanyl, 86% of those not taking β-blockers became hypertensive during sternal spread versus only 33% of those who were taking β-blockers.[442]

There may be differences among the opioids with regard to hemodynamic stability during surgery. One study concluded that both fentanyl and sufentanil provide similar hemodynamic stability during induction, whereas alfentanil causes hemodynamic instability and myocardial ischemia.[443] Alfentanil may also be less effective in suppressing reflex sympathetic and hemodynamic responses to stimuli than fentanyl or sufentanil.[444] In patients undergoing valvular surgery, all three opioids provided satisfactory anesthesia.[445] However, controversy still surrounds the best choice of anesthetic, at least for CABG. Two studies involving more than 2000 patients anesthetized with inhalation agents, fentanyl or sufentanil, came to the conclusion that the choice of anesthetic did not significantly influence the outcome after CABG.[446,447]

The degree of myocardial impairment will also influence the response. Critically ill patients or patients with significant myocardial dysfunction appear to require lower doses of opioid for anesthesia. This may reflect altered pharmacokinetics in those patients. A decrease in liver blood flow consequent to decreased CO and congestive heart failure reduces plasma clearance. Thus, patients with poor left ventricular function may develop higher plasma and brain concentrations for a given loading dose or infusion rate than patients with good left ventricular function. Additionally, patients with depressed myocardial function may lack the ability to respond to surgical stress by increasing CO in the face of progressive increases in SVR.[448]

An infusion of alfentanil (125 μg/kg bolus followed by 0.5 mg/kg/hr) has been compared with fentanyl, 100 μg/kg, or sufentanil, 20 μg/kg, by bolus injection, as the sole anesthetic for patients undergoing valvular surgery.[445] No differences in hemodynamic effects were found in the study and it was concluded that all three opioids can provide satisfactory anesthesia for valve replacement surgery (see Chapter 20).

Sufentanil appears to offer more stable anesthesia with less hemodynamic disturbance than fentanyl[449] and has been used successfully for cardiac transplantation.[450,451] In patients undergoing mitral or aortic valve surgery, sufentanil (total dose, 9.0 ± 0.4 μg/kg) resulted in less need for supplements and vasodilators than fentanyl, 113 ± 11 μg/kg, but sufentanil produced more hypotension during induction.[452] Howie and colleagues compared a fentanyl/isoflurane/propofol regimen with remifentanil/isoflurane/propofol for fast-track anesthesia. Significantly more patients in the fentanyl regimen experienced hypertension during skin incision and maximum sternal spread compared with patients in the remifentanil regimen. There was no difference between groups in time to extubation, discharge from the intensive care unit, electrocardiographic changes, catecholamine levels, or cardiac enzymes. The remifentanil-based anesthetic (bolus followed by continuous infusion) resulted in less need for anesthetic interventions compared with the fentanyl regimen.[453]

Samuelson et al[454] compared hemodynamic and stress responses in patients with CAD anesthetized with either sufentanil-oxygen or enflurane-nitrous oxide and oxygen. Both techniques were satisfactory and resulted in stable hemodynamics, but considerable "fine tuning" was required when enflurane was administered. The postoperative hemodynamic effects were compared in patients who received sufentanil, 25 μg/kg, or fentanyl, 100 μg/kg, for anesthesia for CABG.[455] Patients who received sufentanil had a more stable course, with higher CO, lower SVR, and a lower incidence of hypertension. The two groups had similar values for time to awakening, response to verbal commands, and extubation.

The intraoperative hemodynamic profiles and recovery characteristics of propofol-alfentanil versus a fentanyl-midazolam anesthetic in elective coronary artery surgery were compared by Collard and colleagues.[456] Cardiovascular parameters and time to extubation were recorded. Throughout surgery, hemodynamic profiles were comparable between groups except after intubation, when the MAP was significantly lower in the propofol-alfentanil group. This group also required less inotropic support and extubation was performed earlier in this group.

EFFECTS OF CARDIOPULMONARY BYPASS ON PHARMACOKINETICS AND PHARMACODYNAMICS

The pharmacokinetics of drugs in cardiac anesthesia is well covered by Wood.[457] This section focuses on the effects of CPB on pharmacokinetics as the most relevant area for the cardiac anesthesiologist.

The institution of cardiopulmonary bypass has profound effects on the plasma concentration, distribution, and elimination of administered drugs. The major factors responsible for this are hemodilution and altered plasma protein binding, hypotension, hypothermia, pulsatile versus nonpulsatile flow, isolation of the lungs from the circulation, and uptake of anesthetic drugs by the bypass circuit. These changes result in altered blood concentrations, which are also dependent on particular pharmacokinetics of the drug in question (Table 9–7).

Hemodilution

At the onset of CPB, the circuit priming fluid is mixed with the patient's blood. In adults, the priming volume is 1.5 to 2

Table 9–7 Effects of Cardiopulmonary Bypass on Drug Disposition

Pharmacokinetic Process	Pathophysiology	Pharmacokinetic Sequelae
Absorption	Hypotension and alterations in regional blood flow/perfusion	Reduced oral or intramuscular absorption
Distribution	Lung sequestration	Decreased volume of distribution
	Decreased pulmonary blood flow	Decreased pulmonary drug distribution and increase in systemic drug levels
	Hypotension, altered regional blood flow	Decreased volume of distribution
	Decreased protein binding	Increased volume of distribution
	Hemodilution	
	Dilution of binding proteins	
	Postoperative ↑ AAG	Decreased volume of distribution
	Postoperative ↑ protein binding	Interpretation of postoperative drug levels difficult
Elimination	Decreased hepatic blood flow	Decreased drug clearance
	Hypothermia	Decreased intrinsic clearance (↓ hepatic metabolism)
	Decreased renal blood flow and hypothermia	Decreased renal function

AAG = α_1 acid glycoprotein.

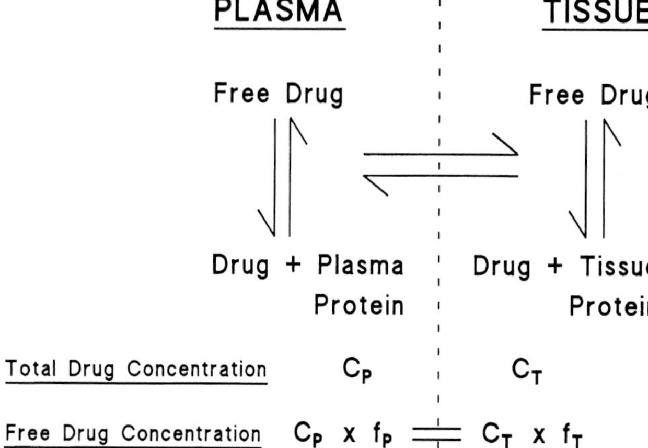

Figure 9–36 The relationship between free drug concentration in plasma and tissue. The free concentration in plasma equals the total concentration (C_p) × the free fraction in plasma (f_p). The free concentration in tissue equals the total concentration in tissue (C_T) × the free fraction in tissue (f_t).

liters and the prime may be crystalloid or may be crystalloid combined with blood or colloid. The overall result is a reduction in the patient's packed cell volume (PCV) to approximately 25% with an increase in plasma volume of 40% to 50%. This will decrease the total blood concentration of any free drug present in the blood. At the time of initiation of CPB, there is an immediate reduction in the levels of circulating proteins such as albumin and α_1-acid glycoprotein. This affects the protein binding of drugs due to alteration in the ratio of bound-to-free drug in the circulation.

In the blood, drugs exist as free (unbound) drug in equilibrium with bound (i.e., bound to plasma proteins) drug. It is the free drug that interacts with the receptor to produce the drug effect (Fig. 9–36). Drugs are primarily bound to plasma protein albumin and α_1-acid glycoprotein. Changes in protein binding are of clinical significance only for drugs that are highly protein bound. The degree of drug-protein binding depends on the total drug concentration, the affinity of the protein for the drug, and the presence of other substances that may compete with the drug or alter the drug's binding site. If the drug in question has high plasma protein binding, then hemodilution results in a potentially relatively larger increase in free fraction than for a drug with low plasma protein binding.

The effect of heparin administration on plasma protein binding is of importance. Heparin results in lipoprotein lipase and hepatic lipase release, which in turn hydrolyzes plasma triglycerides into nonesterified fatty acids. These can bind competitively to plasma proteins and result in displacement of bound drug, raising its concentration.[457]

The consequences of acute hemodilution by the pump prime on drug disposition can be summarized as follows:

1. Since plasma drug concentration is reduced without any change in the amount of drug in the body, the apparent V_d increases acutely, but by a relatively small amount.
2. After acute hemodilution, drug redistribution from tissues may occur in order to bring free drug concentrations in plasma and tissues back into equilibrium. The magnitude of this flux of drug depends on the relative amounts in tissues and plasma and on the degree of protein binding change.
3. Focus on total drug concentration of the free fraction and free concentration change may give misleading information on the expected change in the drug effect.
4. For drugs whose plasma/red cell partitioning is not equal, blood and plasma clearance will no longer bear the same relationship to each other after hemodilution and must be distinguished.
5. Heparin has an effect on measurement of drug protein binding.

There may be marked changes in acid-base balance during CPB, resulting in changes in ionized and unionized drug concentrations, again affecting drug binding. CPB may be conducted using pH-stat or alpha-stat blood gas management. The change in pH with either management scheme may affect organ blood flow.[458,459] pH management may affect the degree of ionization and protein binding of certain drugs, leading to either increased or decreased free (active) drug concentrations.

Blood Flow

Hepatic, renal, cerebral and skeletal perfusion have all been shown to be reduced during CPB, and the use of vasodilators and vasoconstrictor agents to regulate arterial pressure may further change regional blood flow. These alterations in regional blood flow distribution have implications for drug distribution and metabolism. The combination of hypotension, hypothermia, and nonpulsatile blood flow has significant impact on distribution of the circulation, with a marked reduction in peripheral flow and relative preservation of the central circulation.[460,461]

CPB may be conducted with or without pulsatile perfusion. Nonpulsatile perfusion is associated with altered tissue perfusion.[462] Nonpulsatile flow and decreased peripheral perfusion from CPB and hypothermia, as well as the administration of vasoconstrictors, may result in cellular hypoxia and probable intracellular acidosis. This may affect the tissue distribution of drugs whose tissue binding is sensitive to pH. Upon reperfusion, rewarming and the reestablishment of normal cardiac (pulsatile) function, redistribution of drugs from poorly perfused tissue is likely to add to the systemic plasma concentration, as basic drugs will have been "trapped" in acidic tissue. The degree to which pulsatile perfusion alters drug pharmacokinetics is not well studied.

Hypothermia

Hypothermia is commonly used and has been shown to reduce hepatic and possibly renal enzyme function.[463] Hypothermia depresses metabolism by inhibiting enzyme function and reduces tissue perfusion by increasing blood viscosity and activation of autonomic and endocrine reflexes to produce vasoconstriction. Hepatic enzymatic activity is decreased during hypothermia, and in addition there is marked intrahepatic redistribution of blood flow with the development of significant intrahepatic shunting. Hypothermia thus reduces metabolic drug clearance and has been shown to reduce the metabolism of propranolol and verapamil.

Altered renal drug excretion occurs as a result of decreased renal perfusion, glomerular filtration rate (GFR), and tubular secretion. In dogs, GFR is decreased by 65% at 25°C.[464]

Sequestration

When normothermia is reestablished, reperfusion of tissue might lead to washout of drug sequestered during the hypothermic CPB period. This may be one explanation for the increase in opioid plasma levels during the rewarming period.[465-467]

Many drugs bind to components of the CPB circuit and their distribution may be affected by changes in circuit design, for example, the use of membrane versus bubble oxygenators. In vitro, various oxygenators bind lipophilic agents such as volatile anesthetic agents, propofol, opioids, and barbiturates.[468-473] This phenomenon has never been demonstrated to be important in vivo, likely because any drug removed by the circuit is replaced from the much larger tissue reservoir.

During CPB, the lungs are isolated from the circulation with the pulmonary artery blood flow being interrupted. Basic drugs (lidocaine, propranolol, fentanyl) that are taken up by the lungs are therefore sequestered during CPB, and the lungs may serve as a reservoir for drug release when systemic reperfusion is established.[466] Following the onset of CPB, plasma fentanyl concentrations decrease acutely and then plateau. However, when mechanical ventilation of the lungs is instituted before separation from CPB, plasma fentanyl concentrations increase. During CPB, pulmonary artery fentanyl concentrations exceed radial artery levels, but when mechanical ventilation resumes, the pulmonary artery/radial ratio is reversed, suggesting that fentanyl is being washed out from the lungs.

Specific Agents

Opioids

All opioids show a decrease in total drug concentration on commencing CPB (Table 9–8). The degree of decrease is greater with fentanyl because a significant proportion of the drug adheres to the surface of the CPB circuit.[459,470,474] Inadequate anesthesia has been described when fentanyl was used as the major "anesthetic" agent.[475] There is high first-pass uptake of fentanyl by the lungs,[460,476] and reperfusion of the lungs at the end of CPB has been shown to result in increases in fentanyl concentrations (Figs. 9–37 and 9–38).

The decrease in total drug concentration is seen least with opioids that have a high V_d, when the addition of the prime volume is less important, and in those drugs that can equilibrate rapidly to minimize dilutional effect. In this respect sufentanil, which has the most stable total drug concentrations, may offer advantages. Studies of free alfentanil concentrations have shown that these remain relatively stable throughout CPB and therefore the pharmacologically active concentration remains unchanged. It is the bound concentration that changes, reflecting changes in both albumin and α_1-acid glycoprotein concentrations to which alfentanil is predominantly bound.[477-479] Elimination of fentanyl and alfentanil has been shown to be prolonged by CPB, whereas that of morphine was unchanged. There are inadequate data available on the elimination of sufentanil after CPB. From the pharmacokinetic information available at present,

Table 9–8 The Effect of Cardiopulmonary Bypass on the Disposition of Opioids

Opioid	Concentration: Start of CPB	Concentration: During CPB	Clearance	Half-life	Volume of Distribution
Fentanyl	Decreased	Relatively stable or increased toward end of CPB		Increased	
Alfentanil	Decrease in total alfentanil concentration; no change in free concentration	Gradual increase in total concentration toward end of CPB	Unchanged	Increased	Increased
Sufentanil	Decreased	Gradual increase			

Data from Buylaert WA, Herregods LL, Mortier EP, Bogaert MG: Cardiopulmonary bypass and the pharmacokinetics of drugs. Clin Pharmacokinet 17:10, 1989.

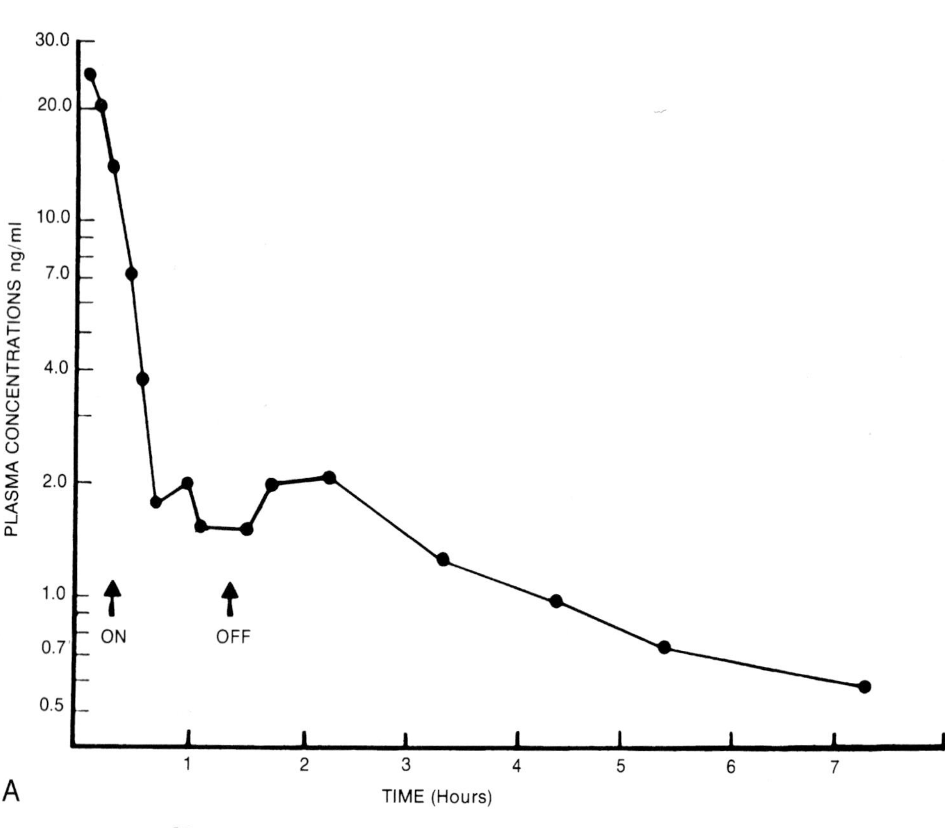

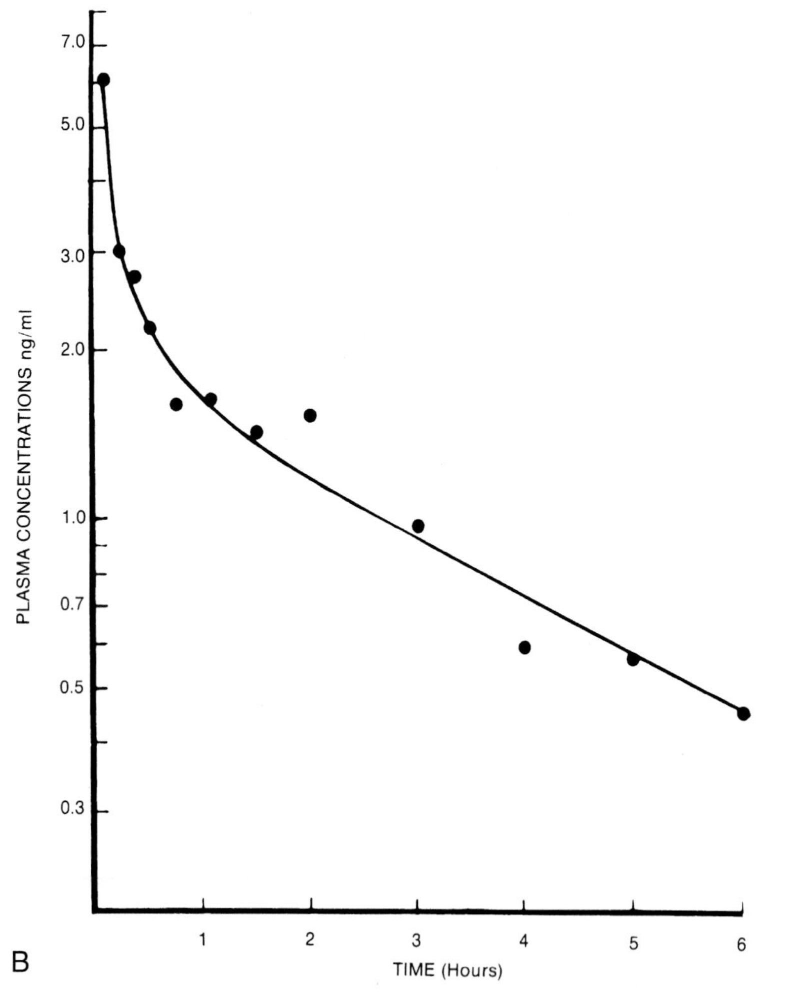

Figure 9–37 The effect of cardiopulmonary bypass (CPB) on the disposition of a single bolus injection of fentanyl. The time course of plasma fentanyl concentrations after injection of a 500 μg IV bolus at time zero. *(A)* Data from a cardiac surgery patient. Times of CPB are indicated by arrows. *(B)* Data from a vascular surgery control patient. (Reproduced from Koska AJ, Romagnole A, Karmer WG: Effect of cardiopulmonary bypass on fentanyl distribution and elimination. Clin Pharmacol Ther 29:100, 1981)

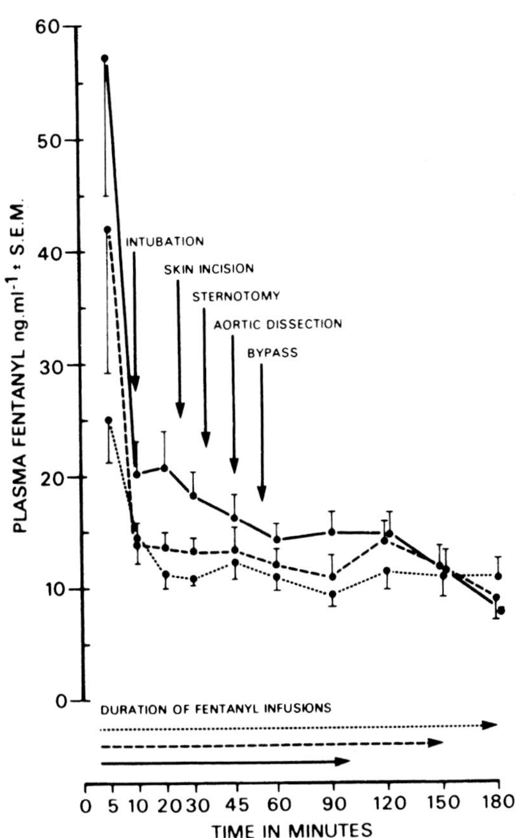

Figure 9–38 Effect of cardiopulmonary bypass (CPB) on plasma fentanyl concentrations when fentanyl is administered at various constant rate infusions for aortocoronary surgery. Plasma fentanyl concentrations and duration of fentanyl infusion for three groups of patients: those given 30 µg/kg followed by 0.3 µg/kg/min *(dotted line)*; those given 40 µg/kg followed by 0.4 µg/kg/min *(dashed line)*; and those given 50 µg/kg followed by 0.5 µg/kg/min *(solid line)*. (Reproduced from Sprigge JS, Wynands JE, Whalley DG, et al: Fentanyl infusion anesthesia for aortocoronary bypass surgery: Plasma levels and hemodynamic response. Anesth Analg 61:972, 1982)

alfentanil may be the most suitable opioid for CPB, as free concentrations have been shown to be stable during CPB and the prolongation of its half-life is much less than that of fentanyl.

Benzodiazepines

The benzodiazepines show a decrease in total concentration on commencing CPB. However, as these drugs are more than 90% protein bound, changes in free concentrations are greatly influenced by changes in protein concentrations or in factors such as acid-base balance that influence protein binding. This is particularly pertinent in the context of CPB, but no studies have commented on free versus total concentrations of benzodiazepines. Diazepam has a very long elimination half-life, even in non-CPB patients, and has been shown to be cumulative after CPB.[480] Midazolam has a shorter elimination half-life. This increases with age and is also significantly longer for CPB patients than for patients undergoing other types of major surgery (Fig. 9–39). The elimination half-life is very prolonged in a subset (6%) of patients.[481,482] However, the half-life of midazolam is shorter than that of the other benzodiazepines, and in small doses elimination was rapid in most patients. For this reason, it is the suitable benzodiazepine for use by repeated boluses of infusion. The elimination half-life of lorazepam was unchanged by CPB but was longer than that of midazolam.

Intravenous Anesthetic Agents

Thiopental and methohexital show a decrease in total drug concentration on commencing CPB, but the active free concentrations are remarkably stable.[478,483] (Fig. 9–40). Clearance of thiopental is halved during CPB, but elimination after CPB is not known. Elimination of methohexital remains unchanged. Conflicting results have been obtained for propofol.[484,485] (Fig. 9–41). The total concentration of propofol may decrease on commencing CPB with an increase in the free fraction or the total concentration may remain unchanged. A prolonged elimination half-life has been demonstrated in one study,[484] but the redistribution half-life was short, concentra-

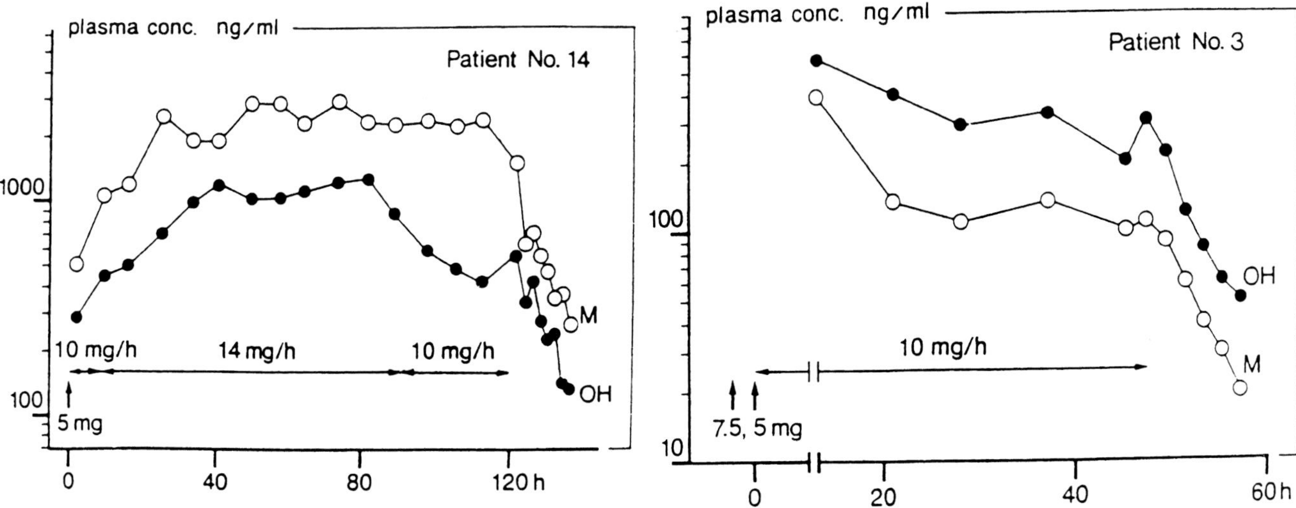

Figure 9–39 Variability of concentrations of midazolam and its metabolite in the intensive care unit. Note the difference in the two scales for concentration for the left-hand panel and right-hand panel. In the left-hand panel the concentrations of midazolam (M) are slightly higher than those of its metabolite (OH), whereas in the right-hand panel the midazolam concentrations are lower than those of the metabolite. (Reproduced from Vree TB, Shimoda M, Driessen JJ, et al: Decreased plasma albumin concentration results in increased volume of distribution and increased elimination of midazolam in intensive care patients. Clin Pharmacol Ther 46:537, 1989)

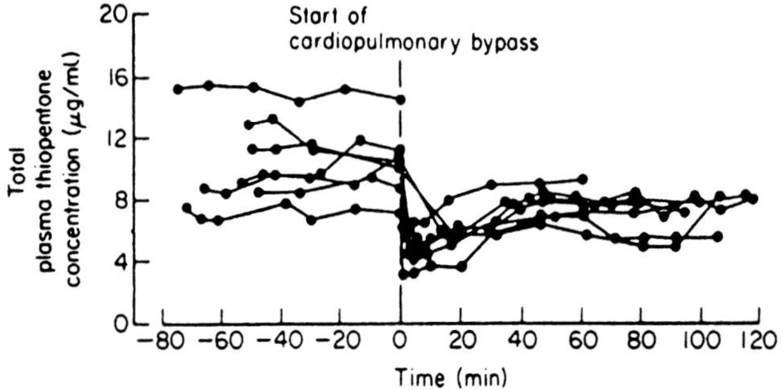

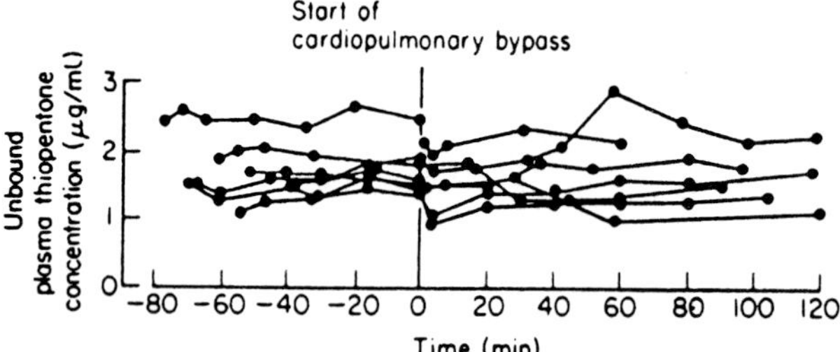

Figure 9–40 The effect of cardiopulmonary bypass on plasma thiopental concentrations during continuous infusion. *(Top)* Total plasma thiopental concentrations. *(Bottom)* Unbound (free) plasma thiopental concentrations. The point of reference (zero time) is taken as the start of bypass. (Reproduced from Morgan DJ, Crankshaw DP, Prideaux PR, et al: Thiopentone levels during cardiopulmonary bypass: Changes in plasma protein binding during continuous infusion. Anaesthesia 41:4, 1986)

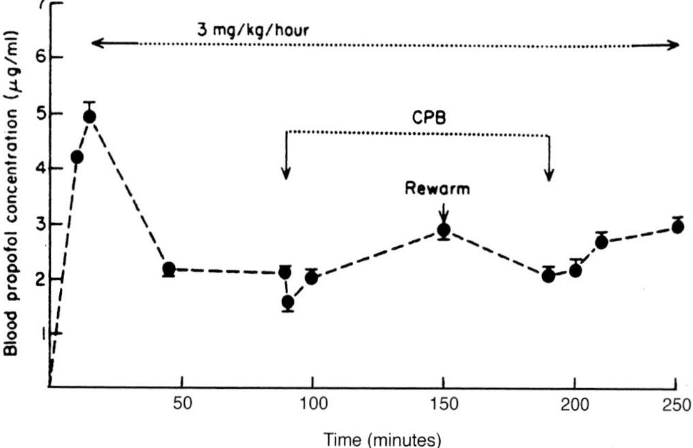

Figure 9–41 Blood propofol concentrations during coronary artery surgery and cardiopulmonary bypass. A two-stage propofol infusion (10 mg/kg/hr for 30 minutes followed by 3 mg/kg/hr thereafter) was administered. The time scale shows the mean time taken to specific events, such as the onset of cardiopulmonary bypass (CPB), induced hypothermia (25° to 27°C), and the end of bypass. (Bars represent mean concentrations ± SEM.) (Reproduced from Russell GN, Wright EL, Fox MA, et al: Propofol-fentanyl anaesthesia for coronary artery surgery and cardiopulmonary bypass. Anaesthesia 44:205, 1989)

tions decreased rapidly after stopping the drug, and patients made a rapid recovery. In general, the free active concentrations of these drugs remain unchanged, but their actions may be prolonged.

Volatile Anesthetic Agents

The effect of CPB on minimal alveolar concentration (MAC) remains uncertain. Some authors have shown that CPB reduces the MAC of enflurane by as much as 30% in animal studies, while others have failed to demonstrate any reduction.[486-488] Several groups have shown variation in MAC with temperature and with reduced volatile concentrations required at lower temperatures.[487,489-491]

The effect of CPB with cooling on the uptake of volatile anesthetics administered to the oxygenator is dependent on three factors: (1) the blood-gas solubility of the agent and the opposing effects of cooling in increasing blood-gas solubility of blood versus hemodilution, which decreases blood-gas solubility of volatile anesthetic agents[492]; (2) the increased solubility in tissue of volatile anesthetics secondary to hypothermia; and (3) uptake by the oxygenator.[493] CPB produces changes in the blood-gas partition coefficient dependent on the prime used and the temperature. Factors that alter the solubility of volatile anesthetic agents in blood and other tissues include lipid concentration, osmolarity, and packed cell volume. The changes in blood composition after the addition of a crystalloid prime tend to decrease blood solubility, favoring a more rapid attainment of steady state and a lower blood concentration of volatile agent for a given inspired concentration. However, hemodilution with a plasma prime increases solubility as volatile agents are more soluble in albumin than red cells.[494] Blood solubility is also inversely proportional to temperature. This relationship is linear, but different for individual agents, with a range of 4% to 4.9% per °C decrease in body temperature.[495] Thus, hemodilution with a crystalloid prime and hypothermia has opposite effects on the blood-gas partition coefficient. The predicted net change in solubility for isoflurane when packed cell volume (PCV) is reduced from 40% to 20% and temperature is reduced from 37° to 28°C is +2%.[496]

Volatile agents have been shown to bind to a variety of plastics,[497] and this may account for some of the decrease in concentrations on commencing bypass. A volatile agent started during hypothermic CPB takes longer to equilibrate and agents already in use need to reequilibrate, potentially changing the depth of anesthesia, until equilibration is complete. As these agents are metabolized to a small degree and washout is fast, the duration of action is not prolonged after CPB.[498,499]

Neuromuscular Blockers

It has been demonstrated that hypothermic CPB influences the concentration and the response relationships of neuromuscular blockers during hypothermia.[502] In general, the requirements for neuromuscular blockade are found to be significantly reduced as a result of a number of both pharmacokinetic and pharmacodynamic effects. Specifically, cooling influences nerve conduction in the mobilization of acetylcholine from the nerve vesicles,[503] as well as modifying cholinergic receptors. Furthermore, the effect of cooling is manifest on cholin-esterase enzyme activity, which is temperature dependent. The most important effect of cooling, however, is a decrease in the mobilization of acetylcholine that has been demonstrated both in vitro and in animal models.[504,505] Thus, during hypothermia fewer muscle relaxants are needed to obtain the same amount of muscle relaxation. In addition, cooling alters the mechanical properties of the muscle as well as having potentially significant effects on electrolytes, which modulate the contractile response.

CPB causes hemodilution, which may result in an initial decrease in the free drug concentration. However, there is also an associated decrease in the albumin concentration during CPB, so that although the total drug concentration may as a result of hemodilution be decreased, if the drug is partially bound to albumin, the free drug concentration may actually be increased. This phenomenon may occur with neuromuscular blockers such as rocuronium.[506]

Hypothermia inhibits the hepatic clearance of steroidal neuromuscular blocking agents, although it seems to promote renal clearance. This may explain why the time-course of action of steroidal neuromuscular blocking agents such as rocuronium and vecuronium, which are dependent on liver clearance, are relatively more prolonged under hypothermic conditions than those that are dependent on renal clearance, such as pancuronium and pipecuronium.[507]

Acknowledgments

We wish to thank Cheryl Dewyre for her enthusiasm and her knowledgeable administrative skills in the preparation of this chapter. We also wish to thank all of the authors of the previous chapters: Kyung W. Park, MD, J. Michael Haering, MD, Sebastian Reiz, MD, Edward Lowenstein, MD, James G. Bovill, MD, PhD, Fred Boer, MD, PhD, J. G. Reves, MD, Steven Hill, MD, Matthew R. Belmont, MD, Ralph P. F. Scott, MD, and Margaret Wood, MD, some of whose work has been reproduced into this chapter.

REFERENCES

1. Kersten JR, Lowe D, Hettrick DA, et al: Glyburide, a KATP channel antagonist, attenuates the cardioprotective effect of isoflurane in stunned myocardium. Anesth Analg 83:27, 1996
2. Kersten JR, Schmeling TJ, Pagel PS, et al: Isoflurane mimics ischemic preconditioning via activation of K(ATP) channels: Reduction of myocardial infarct size with an acute memory phase. Anesthesiology 87:361, 1997
3. Cason BA, Gamperi AK, Slocum RE, et al: Anesthetic-induced preconditioning: Previous administration of isoflurane decreases myocardial infarct size in rabbits. Anesthesiology 87:1182, 1997
4. Lynch C: Differential depression of myocardial contractility by halothane and isoflurane in vitro. Anesthesiology 64:620, 1986
5. DeTraglia MC, Komai H, Rusy BF: Differential effects of inhalational anesthetics on myocardial potentiated-state contractions in vivo. Anesthesiology 68:534, 1988
6. Housmans PR, Murat I: Comparative effects of halothane, enflurane, and isoflurane at equipotent anesthetic concentrations on isolated ventricular myocardium of the ferret. I. Contractility. Anesthesiology 69:451, 1988
7. Housmans PR, Murat I: Comparative effects of halothane, enflurane, and isoflurane at equipotent anesthetic concentrations on isolated ventricular myocardium of the ferret. II. Relaxation. Anesthesiology 69:464, 1988
8. Pagel PS, Kampine JP, Schmeling WT, et al: Evaluation of myocardial contractility in the chronically instrumented dog with intact autonomic nervous system function: Effects of desflurane and isoflurane. Acta Anaesthesiol Scand 37:203, 1993
9. Pagel PS, Kampine JP, Schmeling TJ, et al: Influence of volatile anesthetics on myocardial contractility in vivo: Desflurane versus isoflurane. Anesthesiology 74:900, 1991
10. Harkin CP, Pagel PS, Kersten JR, et al: Direct inotropic and lusitropic effects of sevoflurane. Anesthesiology 72:659, 1994
11. Kikura M, Ikeda K: Comparison of effects of sevoflurane/nitrous oxide and enflurane/nitrous oxide on myocardial contractility in humans. Anesthesiology 79:235, 1993
12. Bernard J, Wouters PF, Doursout M, et al: Effects of sevoflurane and isoflurane on cardiac and coronary dynamics in chronically instrumented dogs. Anesthesiology 72:659, 1990
13. Kemmotsu O, Hashimoto Y, Shimosato S: The effects of fluroxene and enflurane on contractile performance of isolated papillary muscles from failing hearts. Anesthesiology 30:252, 1974
14. Kemmotsu S, Hashimoto Y, Shimosato S: Inotropic effects of isoflurane on mechanics of contraction in isolated cat papillary muscles from normal and failing hearts. Anesthesiology 39:470, 1973
15. Prys-Roberts C, Roberts JG, Foex P, et al: Interaction of anesthesia, beta-receptor blockade, and blood loss in dogs with induced myocardial infarction. Anesthesiology 26:326, 1976
16. Lowenstein E, Foex P, Francis M, et al: Regional ischemic ventricular dysfunction in myocardium supplied by a narrowed coronary artery with increasing halothane concentrations in the dog. Anesthesiology 55:349, 1981
17. Hanley PJ, ter Keurs HEDJ, Cannell MB: Excitation-contraction coupling in the heart and the negative inotropic action of volatile anesthetics. Anesthesiology 101:999, 2004
18. Huneke R, Fassl J, Rossaint R, et al: Effects of volatile anesthetics on cardiac ion channels. Acta Anaesthesiol Scand 48:547, 2004
19. Pagel PS, Kampine JP, Schmeling TJ, et al: Effects of nitrous oxide on myocardial contractility as evaluated by the preload recruitable stroke work relationship in chronically instrumented dogs. Anesthesiology 73:1148, 1990
20. Zile MR, Brustsaert DL: New concepts in diastolic dysfunction and diastolic heart failure: Part II: Causal mechanisms and treatment. Circulation 105:1503, 2002
21. Aurigemma GP, Cottdiener JS, Shemanski L, et al: Predictive value of systolic and diastolic function for incidence of congestive heart failure in the elderly: The Cardiovascular Health Study. J Am Coll Cardiol 37:1042, 2001
22. Dauterman KW, Massie MB, Gheorghiade M: Heart failure associated with preserved systolic function: A common and costly clinical entity. Am Heart J 135:S310, 1998
23. Judge KW, Pawitan Y, Caldwell J, et al: Congestive heart failure in patients with preserved left ventricular systolic function: Analysis of the CASS registry. J Am Coll Cardiol 18:377, 1991
24. Brogen WC, Hillis LD, Flores ED, et al: The natural history of isolated left ventricular diastolic dysfunction. Am J Med 92:627, 1992
25. Pagel PS, Hettrick DA, Warltier DC: Amrinone enhances myocardial contractility and improves left ventricular diastolic function in conscious and anesthetized chronically instrumented dogs. Anesthesiology 79:753, 1993
26. Pagel PS, Kampine JP, Schmeling TJ, et al: Reversal of volatile anesthetic-induced depression of myocardial contractility by extracellular calcium also enhances left ventricular diastolic function. Anesthesiology 78:141, 1993
27. Pagel PS, Kampine JP, Schmeling TJ, et al: Alteration of left ventricular diastolic function by desflurane, isoflurane and halothane in the chronically instrumented dog with autonomic nervous system blockade. Anesthesiology 74:1103, 1991
28. Yamada T, Takeda J, Koyama K, et al: Effects of sevoflurane, isoflurane, enflurane, and halothane on left ventricular diastolic performance in dogs. J Cardiothorac Vasc Anesth 8:618, 1994
29. Graham MR, Thiessen DB, Mutch WAC: Isoflurane and halothane impair both systolic and diastolic function in the newborn pig. Can J Anaesth 43:495, 1996
30. Ihara T, Shannon RP, Komamura K, et al: Effects of anaesthesia and recent surgery on diastolic function. Cardiovasc Res 28:325, 1994
31. Humphrey LS, Stinson DC, Humphrey MJ, et al: Volatile anesthetic effects on left ventricular relaxation in swine. Anesthesiology 73:731, 1990
32. Shoma A, Foex P, Ryder WA: Regional distensibility, chamber stiffness, and elastic stiffness constant in halothane and propofol anesthesia. J Cardiothorac Vasc Anesth 7:188, 1993
33. Varadarajan SG, An J, Novalija E, et al: Sevoflurane before or after ischemia improves contractile and metabolic function while reducing myoplasmic Ca++ loading in intact hearts. Anesthesiology 96:125, 2002
34. Echt DS, Liebson PR, Mitchell LB, et al: Mortality and morbidity in patients receiving encainide, flecainide, or placebo. The Cardiac Arrhythmia Suppression Group Trial. N Engl J Med 324:718, 1991
35. Guler N, Kati I, Demirel CB, et al: The effects of volatile anesthetics on the Q-Tc interval. J Cardiothorac Vasc Anesth 15:188, 2001
36. Verrier ED, Edelist G, Macke C, et al: Greater coronary vascular reserve in dogs anesthetized with halothane. Anesthesiology 53:445, 1980
37. Tarnow J, Eberlein HJ, Oser G, et al: Haemodynamik, myokardkontraktilitaat, ventrikelvolumnia, and sauerstoffversorgung des herzens unter verschiedenen inhalations-anaesthetika. Anaesthetist 26:220, 1977
38. Hickey RF, Sybert PE, Verrier ED, et al: Effects of halothane, enflurane and isoflurane on coronary blood flow autoregulation and coronary vascular reserve in the canine heart. Anesthesiology 68:21, 1988
39. Wilkinson FL, Hamilton WK, Slovers JR, et al: Halothane and morphine-nitrous oxide anesthesia in patients undergoing coronary artery bypass operations: Patterns of intraoperative ischemia. J Thorac Cardiovasc Surg 82:372, 1981
40. Sonntag H, Merin RG, Donath U, et al: Myocardial metabolism and oxygenation in man awake and during halothane anesthesia. Anesthesiology 51:204, 1979
41. Reiz S, Balfors E, Gustavsson B, et al: Effects of halothane on coronary haemodynamics and myocardial metabolism in patients with ischaemic

heart disease and heart failure. Acta Anaesthesiol Scand 26:133, 1982
42. Moffitt E, Sethna D, Gray R, et al: Nitrous oxide added to halothane reduces coronary blood flow and myocardial oxygen consumption in patients with coronary artery disease. Can Anaesth Soc J 30:5, 1983
43. Tanaka K, Ludwig LM, Kersten JR, et al: Mechanisms of cardioprotection by volatile anesthetics. Anesthesiology 100:707, 2004
44. Buffington CW, Romson JL, Levine A, et al: Isoflurane induces coronary steal in a canine model of chronic coronary occlusion. Anesthesiology 66:280, 1987
45. Priebe HJ, Foex P: Isoflurane causes regional myocardial dysfunction in dogs with critical coronary artery stenoses. Anesthesiology 66:293, 1987
46. Moore PG, Kien ND, Reitan JA, et al: No evidence for blood flow redistribution with isoflurane or halothane during acute coronary artery occlusion in fentanyl-anesthetized dogs. Anesthesiology 75:854, 1991
47. Hartman JC, Kampine JP, Schmeling WT, et al: Steal-prone coronary circulation in chronically instrumented dogs: Isoflurane versus adenosine. Anesthesiology 74:744, 1991
48. Hartman JC, Kampine JP, Schmeling WT, et al: Actions of isoflurane on myocardial perfusion in chronically instrumented dogs with poor, moderate, or well-developed coronary collaterals. J Cardiothorac Anesth 4:715, 1990
49. Hartman JC, Kampine JP, Schmeling WT, et al: Alterations in collateral blood flow produced by isoflurane in chronically instrumented canine model of multivessel coronary artery disease. Anesthesiology 74:120, 1991
50. Leung JM, Goehner P, O'Kelly BF, et al: Isoflurane anesthesia and myocardial ischemia: comparative risk versus sufentanil anesthesia in patients undergoing coronary artery bypass graft surgery. The SPI (Study of Perioperative Ischemia) Research Group. Anesthesiology 74:838, 1991
51. Pulley DD, Kirvassilis GV, Kelermenos N, et al: Regional and global myocardial circulatory and metabolic effects of isoflurane and halothane in patients with steel-prone coronary anatomy. Anesthesiology 75:756, 1991
52. Diana P, Tullock WC, Gorcsan J, et al: Myocardial ischemia: A comparison between isoflurane and enflurane in coronary artery bypass patients. Anesth Analg 77:221, 1993
53. Glower DD, Spratt JA, Snow ND, et al: Linearity of the Frank-Starling relationship in the intact heart: the concept of preload recruitable stroke work. Circulation 71:994, 1985
54. Glower DD, Spratt JA, Kabas JS, et al: Quantification of regional myocardial dysfunction after acute ischemic injury. Am J Physiol 255:H85, 1988
55. Park KW, Dai HB, Lowenstein E, et al: Isoflurane and halothane attenuate endothelium-dependent vasodilation in rat coronary microvessels. Anesth Analg 84:278, 1997
56. Kersten JR, Brayer AP, Pagel PS, et al: Perfusion of ischemic myocardium during anesthesia with sevoflurane. Anesthesiology 81:995, 1994
57. Kitahata H, Kawahito S, Nozaki J, et al: Effects of sevoflurane on regional myocardial blood flow distribution: quantification with myocardial contrast echocardiography. Anesthesiology 90:1436, 1999
58. Hartman JC, Pagel PS, Kampine JP, et al: Influence of desflurane on regional distribution of coronary blood flow in a chronically instrumented canine model of multivessel coronary artery obstruction. Anesth Analg 72:829, 1991
59. Kehl F, Krolikowski JG, Tessmer JP, et al: Increases in coronary collateral blood flow produced by sevoflurane are mediated by calcium-activated potassium (BKca) channels in vivo. Anesthesiology 97:725, 2002
60. Muldoon SM, Hart JL, Bowen KA, et al: Attenuation of endothelium-mediated vasodilating by halothane. Anesthesiology 68:31, 1988
61. Yoshida K, Okabe E: Selective impairment of endothelium-dependent relaxation by sevoflurane: Oxygen free radicals participation. Anesthesiology 76:440, 1992
62. Uggeri MJ, Proctor GJ, Johns RA: Halothane, enflurane, and isoflurane attenuate both receptor- and non-receptor-mediated EDRF production in rat thoracic aorta. Anesthesiology 76:1012, 1992
63. Toda H, Nakamura K, Hatano Y, et al: Halothane and isoflurane inhibit endothelium-dependent relaxation elicited by acetylcholine. Anesth Analg 75:198, 1992
64. Akata T, Nakamura K, Kodama K, et al: Effects of volatile anesthetics on acetylcholine-induced relaxation in the rabbit mesenteric resistance artery. Anesthesiology 82:188, 1995
65. Pajewski TN, Miao N, Lynch C, et al: Volatile anesthetics affect calcium mobilization in bovine endothelial cells. Anesthesiology 85:1147, 1996
66. Tas PWL, Stossel C, Roewer N: The volatile anesthetic isoflurane inhibits the histamine-induced Ca++ influx in primary human endothelial cells. Anesth Analg 97:430, 2003
67. Arriero MM, Alameda LM, Lopez-Farre A, et al: Sevoflurane reduces endothelium-dependent vasorelaxation: Role of superoxide anion and endothelin. Can J Anaesth 49:471, 2002
68. Vinh VH, Enoki T, Hirate S, et al: Comparative contractile effects of halothane and sevoflurane in rabbit aorta. Anesthesiology 92:219, 2000
69. Yu J, Tokinaga Y, Ogawa K, et al: Sevoflurane inhibits angiotensin II-induced, protein kinase C-mediated but not Ca++-elicited contraction of rat aortic smooth muscle. Anesthesiology 100:879, 2004
70. Izumi K, Akata T, Takahashi S: The action of sevoflurane on vascular smooth muscle of isolated mesenteric resistance arteries (Part 1). Anesthesiology 92:1426, 2000
71. Akata T, Nakashima M, Izumi K: Comparison of volatile anesthetic actions on intracellular calcium stores of vascular smooth muscle. Anesthesiology 94:840, 2001
72. Tsuneyoshi I, Zhang D, Boyle W: Ca++- and myosin phosphorylation-independent relaxation by halothane in K+-depolarized rat mesenteric arteries. Anesthesiology 99:656, 2003
73. Chen BB, Nyhan D, Fehr DM, et al: Halothane anesthesia causes active flow-independent pulmonary vasoconstriction. Am J Physiol 259:H74, 1990
74. Lesitsky MA, Davis S, Murray PA: Preservation of hypoxic pulmonary vasoconstriction during sevoflurane and desflurane anesthesia compared with the conscious state in chronically instrumented dogs. Anesthesiology 89:1501, 1998
75. Gambone LM, Fujiwara Y, Murray PA: Endothelium-dependent pulmonary vasodilation is selectively attenuated during isoflurane anesthesia. Am J Physiol 272:H290, 1997
76. Oshima Y, Ishibe Y, Okazaki N, et al: Isoflurane inhibits endothelium-mediated nitric oxide relaxing pathways in the isolated perfused rabbit lung. Can J Anaesth 44:1108, 1997
77. Seki S, Sato K, Nakayama M, Murray PA: Halothane and enflurane attenuate pulmonary vasodilation mediated by adenosine triphosphate-sensitive potassium channels compared with the conscious state. Anesthesiology 86:923, 1997
78. Fujiwara Y, Murray PA: Effects of isoflurane anesthesia on pulmonary vascular response K+ ATP channel activation and circulatory hypotension in chronically instrumented dogs. Anesthesiology 90:799, 1999
79. Sato K, Seki S, Murray PA: Effects of halothane and enflurane anesthesia on sympathetic beta-adrenoreceptor-mediated pulmonary vasodilating in chronically instrumented dog. Anesthesiology 97:478, 2002
80. Ebert TJ, Harkin CP, Muzi M: Cardiovascular responses to sevoflurane: A review. Anesth Analg 81:S11, 1995
81. Muzi M, Ebert TJ: A comparison of baroreflex sensitivity during isoflurane and desflurane anesthesia in humans. Anesthesiology 82:919, 1995
82. Seagard JL, Hopp FA, Donegan JH, et al: Halothane and the carotid sinus reflex: evidence for multiple sites of action. Anesthesiology 57:191, 1982
83. Seagard JL, Elegbe EO, Hopp FA, et al: Effects of isoflurane on the baroreceptor reflex. Anesthesiology 59:511, 1983
84. Boban N, McCallum JB, Schedewie HK, et al: Direct comparative effects of isoflurane and desflurane on sympathetic ganglionic transmission. Anesth Analg 80:127, 1995
85. Kloner RA, Jennings RB: Consequences of brief ischemia: Stunning, preconditioning, and their clinical implications. Part 1. Circulation 104:2981, 2001
86. Heyndrickx GR, Millard RW, McRitchie RJ, et al: Regional myocardial functional and electrophysiological alterations after brief coronary artery occlusion in conscious dogs. J Clin Invest 56:978, 1975
87. Murry CE, Jennings RB, Reimer KA: Preconditioning with ischemia: A delay of lethal cell injury in ischemic myocardium. Circulation 74:1124, 1986
88. Bland JH, Lowenstein E: Halothane-induced decrease in experimental myocardial ischemia in the non-failing canine heart. Anesthesiology 45:287, 1976
89. Davis RF, DeBoer LW, Rude RE, et al: The effect of halothane anesthesia on myocardial necrosis, hemodynamic performance, and regional myocardial blood flow in dogs following coronary artery occlusion. Anesthesiology 59:402, 1983
90. Warltier DC, al-Wathiqui MH, Kampine JP, et al: Recovery of contractile function of stunned myocardium in chronically instrumented dogs is enhanced by halothane or isoflurane. Anesthesiology 69:552, 1988
91. Ishihara M, Sato K, Tateishi H, et al: Implications of prodromal angina pectoris in anterior wall acute myocardial infarction: Acute angiographic findings and long-term prognosis. J Am Coll Cardiol 30:970, 1997
92. Bolli R: The late phase of preconditioning. Circ Res 87:972, 2000
93. Kato R, Foex P: Myocardial protection by anesthetic agents against ischemia-reperfusion injury: An update for anesthesiologists. Can J Anaesth 49:777, 2002

94. Warltier DC, Kersten JR, Pagel PS, et al: Editorial view: Anesthetic preconditioning: Serendipity and science. Anesthesiology 97:1, 2002
95. Anesthesiology 100:469, 2004
96. Tanaka K, Ludwig LM, Krolikowski JG, et al: Isoflurane produces delayed preconditioning against myocardial ischemia and reperfusion injury: Role of cyclooxygenase. Anesthesiology 100:525, 2004
97. de Klaver MJ, Buckingham MG, Rich GF: Isoflurane pretreatment has immediate and delayed protective effects against cytokine-induced injury in endothelial and vascular smooth muscle cells. Anesthesiology 99:896, 2003
98. Ludwig LM, Patel HH, Gross GJ, et al: Morphine enhances pharmacological preconditioning by isoflurane: Role of mitochondrial KATP channels and opioid receptors. Anesthesiology 98:705, 2003
99. Kehl F, Krolikowski JG, Mraovic B, et al: Is isoflurane-induced preconditioning dose related? Anesthesiology 96:675, 2002
100. Zaugg M, Lucchinetti E, Spahn DR, et al: Volatile anesthetics mimic cardiac preconditioning by priming the activation of mitochondrial KATP channels via multiple signaling pathways. Anesthesiology 97:4, 2002
101. Toller WG, Kersten JR, Pagel PS, et al: Sevoflurane reduces myocardial infarct size and decreases the time threshold for ischemic preconditioning in dogs. Anesthesiology 91:1437, 1999
102. Mullenheim J, Ebel D, Bauer M, et al: Sevoflurane confers additional cardioprotection after ischemic late preconditioning in rabbits. Anesthesiology 99:624, 2003
103. Kersten JR, Orth KG, Pagel PS, et al: Role of adenosine in isoflurane-induced cardioprotection. Anesthesiology 86:1128, 1997
104. Hemmings HC, Adamo AI: Activation of endogenous protein kinase C by halothane in synaptosomes. Anesthesiology 84:652, 1996
105. Mullenheim J, Ebel D, Frassdorf J, et al: Isoflurane preconditions myocardium against infarction via release of free radicals. Anesthesiology 96:934, 2002
106. Tanaka K, Weihrauch D, Kehl F, et al: Mechanism of preconditioning by isoflurane in rabbits: A direct role for reactive oxygen species. Anesthesiology 97:1485, 2002
107. Novalija E, Varadarajan SG, Camara AK, et al: Anesthetic preconditioning: Triggering role of reactive oxygen and nitrogen species in isolated hearts. Am J Physiol Heart Circ Physiol 283:H44, 2002
108. Finkel E: The mitochondrion: Is it central to apoptosis? Science 292:624, 2001
109. van Klarenbosch J, Stienen GJ, de Ruijter W, et al: The differential effect of propofol on contractility of isolated myocardial trabeculae of rat and guinea pig. Br J Anaesth 132:742, 2001
110. Gelissen HP, Epema AH, Henning RH, et al: Inotropic effects of propofol, thiopental, midazolam, etomidate, and ketamine on isolated human atrial muscle. Anesthesiology 84:397, 1996
111. Hebbar L, Dorman BH, Clair MJ, et al: Negative and selective effects of propofol on isolated swine myocyte contractile function in pacing-induced congestive heart failure. Anesthesiology 86:649, 1997
112. Sprung J, Ogletree-Hughes ML, McConnell BK, et al: The effects of propofol on the contractility of failing and nonfailing human heart muscle. Anesth Analg 93:550, 2001
113. Zhou W, Fontenot HJ, Liu S, et al: Modulation of cardiac calcium channels by propofol. Anesthesiology 86:670, 1997
114. Zhou W, Fontenot HJ, Wang SN, et al: Propofol-induced alterations in myocardial beta-adrenoceptor binding and responsiveness. Anesth Analg 89:604, 1999
115. Kurokawa H, Murray PA, Damron DS: Propofol attenuates beta-adrenoreceptor-mediated signal transduction via a protein kinase C-dependent pathway in cardiomyocytes. Anesthesiology 96:688, 2002
116. Kanaya N, Murray PA, Damron DS: Propofol increases myofilament Ca++ sensitivity and intracellular pH via activation of Na+-H+ exchange in rat ventricular myocytes. Anesthesiology 94:1096, 2001
117. Kanaya N, Gable B, Murray PA, et al: Propofol increases phosphorylation of troponin I and myosin light chain 2 via protein kinase C activation in cardiomyocytes. Anesthesiology 98:1363, 2003
118. Kolh P, Lambermont B, Ghuysen A, et al: Comparison of the effects of propofol and pentobarbital on left ventricular adaptation to an increased afterload. J Cardiovasc Pharmacol 44:294, 2004
119. Zheng D, Upton RN, Martinez AM: The contribution of the coronary concentrations of propofol to its cardiovascular effects in anesthetized sheep. Anesth Analg 96:1589, 2003
120. Kehl F, Kress TT, Mraovic B, et al: Propofol alters left atrial function evaluated with pressure-volume relations in vivo. Anesth Analg 94:1421, 2002
121. Ko SH, Yu CW, Lee SK, et al: Propofol attenuates ischemia-reperfusion injury in the isolated rat heart. Anesth Analg 85:719, 1997
122. Kokita N, Hara A: Propofol attenuates hydrogen peroxide-induced mechanical and metabolic derangements in the isolated rat heart. Anesthesiology 84:117, 1996
123. Kokita N, Hara A, Arakawa J, et al: Propofol improves functional and metabolic recovery in ischemic reperfused isolated rat hearts. Anesth Analg 86:252, 1998
124. Mathur S, Farhangkhgoee P, Karmazyn M: Cardioprotective effects of propofol and sevoflurane in ischemic and reperfused rat hearts: Role of K(ATP) channels and interaction with the sodium-hydrogen exchange inhibitor HOE 642 (cariporide). Anesthesiology 91:1349, 1999
125. Javadov SA, Lim KH, Kerr PM, et al: Angelini GD, Halestrap AP. Protection of hearts from reperfusion injury by propofol is associated with inhibition of the mitochondrial permeability transition. Cardiovasc Res 45:360, 2000
126. Murphy PG, Myers DS, Davies MJ, et al: The antioxidant potential of propofol (2,6-diisopropylphenol). Br J Anaesth 68:613, 1992
127. Kahraman S, Demiryurek AT: Propofol is a peroxynitrite scavenger. Anesth Analg 84:1127, 1997
128. Tsuchiya M, Asada A, Kasahara E, et al: Antioxidant protection of propofol and its recycling in erythrocyte membranes. Am J Respir Crit Care Med 165:54, 2002
129. Tsuchiya M, Asada A, Maeda K, et al: Propofol versus midazolam regarding their antioxidant activities. Am J Respir Crit Care Med 163:26, 2001
130. Murphy PG, Ogilvy AJ, Whiteley SM: The effect of propofol on the neutrophil respiratory burst. Eur J Anesthesiol 13:471, 1996
131. Murphy PG, Bennett JR, Myers DS, et al: The effect of propofol anaesthesia on free radical-induced lipid peroxidation in rat liver microsomes. Eur J Anesthesiol 10:261, 1993
132. Mullenheim J, Rulands R, Wietschorke T, et al: Late preconditioning is blocked by racemic ketamine, but not by S(+)-ketamine. Anesth Analg 93:265, 2001
133. Mullenheim J, Frassdorf J, Preckel B, et al: Ketamine, but not S(+)-ketamine, blocks ischemic preconditioning in rabbit hearts in vivo. Anesthesiology 94:630, 2001
134. Molojavyi A, Preckel B, Comfere T, et al: Effects of ketamine and its isomers on ischemic preconditioning in the isolated rat heart. Anesthesiology 94:623, 2001
135. Ko SH, Lee SK, Han YJ, et al: Blockade of myocardial ATP-sensitive potassium channels by ketamine. Anesthesiology 87:68, 1997
136. Rouby JJ, Andreev A, Leger P, et al: Peripheral vascular effects of thiopental and propofol in humans with artificial hearts. Anesthesiology 75:32, 1991
137. Chang KS, Davis RF: Propofol produces endothelium-independent vasodilation and may act as a Ca++ channel blocker. Anesth Analg 76:24, 1993
138. Gelb AW, Zhang C, Hamilton JT: Propofol induces dilation and inhibits constriction in guinea pig basilar arteries. Anesth Analg 83:472, 1996
139. Biddle NL, Gelb AW, Hamilton JT: Propofol differentially attenuates the responses to exogenous and endogenous norepinephrine in the isolated rat femoral artery in vitro. Anesth Analg 80:793, 1995
140. Park WK, Lynch C, Johns RA: Effects of propofol and thiopental in isolated rat aorta and pulmonary artery. Anesthesiology 77:956, 1992
141. Imura N, Shiraishi Y, Katsuya H, et al: Effect of propofol on norepinephrine-induced increases in [Ca++] and force in smooth muscle of the rabbit mesenteric resistance artery. Anesthesiology 88:1566, 1998
142. Tanabe K, Kozawa O, Kaida T, et al: Inhibitory effects of propofol on intracellular signaling by endothelin-1 in aortic smooth muscle cells. Anesthesiology 88:452, 1998
143. MacPherson RD, Rasiah RL, McLeod LJ: Propofol attenuates the myogenic response of vascular smooth muscle. Anesth Analg 76:822, 1993
144. Berkowitz DE, Gaine S: Overview of the perioperative management of the patient with primary pulmonary hypertension. Probl Anesth 13:224, 2001
145. Horibe M, Ogawa K, Sohn JT, et al: Propofol attenuates acetylcholine-induced pulmonary vasorelaxation: Role of nitric oxide and endothelium-derived hyperpolarizing factors. Anesthesiology 93:447, 2000
146. Kondo U, Kim SO, Murray PA: Propofol selectively attenuates endothelium-dependent pulmonary vasodilation in chronically instrumented dogs. Anesthesiology 93:437, 2000
147. Tanaka S, Kanaya N, Homma Y, et al: Propofol increases pulmonary artery smooth muscle myofilament calcium sensitivity: Role of protein kinase C. Anesthesiology 97:1557, 2002
148. Kondo U, Kim SO, Nakayama M, et al: Pulmonary vascular effects of propofol at baseline, during elevated vasomotor tone, and in response to sympathetic alpha- and beta-adrenoreceptor activation. Anesthesiology 94:815, 2001

149. Miyawaki I, Nakamura K, Terasako K, et al: Modification of endothelium-dependent relaxation by propofol, ketamine, and midazolam. Anesth Analg 81:474, 1995
150. Yamashita A, Kajikuri J, Ohashi M, et al: Inhibitory effects of propofol on acetylcholine-induced, endothelium-dependent relaxation and prostacyclin synthesis in rabbit mesenteric resistance arteries. Anesthesiology 91:1080, 1999
151. Robinson BJ, Ebert TJ, O'Brien TJ, et al: Mechanisms whereby propofol mediates peripheral vasodilation in humans. Sympathoinhibition or direct vascular relaxation? Anesthesiology 86:64, 1997
152. Sellgren J, Ejnell H, Elam M, et al: Sympathetic muscle nerve activity, peripheral blood flows, and baroreceptor reflexes in humans during propofol anesthesia and surgery. Anesthesiology 80:534, 1994
153. Yang CY, Luk HN, Chen SY, et al: Propofol inhibits medullary pressor mechanisms in cats. Can J Anaesth 44:775, 1997
154. Yang CY, Wu WC, Chai CY, et al: Propofol inhibits neuronal firing activities in the caudal ventrolateral medulla. Chang Gung Med J 26:570, 2003
155. Shiga Y, Minami K, Segawa K, et al: The inhibition of aortic smooth muscle cell proliferation by the intravenous anesthetic ketamine. Anesth Analg 99:1408, 2004
156. Tanabe K, Dohi S, Matsuno H, et al: Midazolam stimulates vascular endothelial growth factor release in aortic smooth muscle cells: Role of the mitogen-activated protein kinase superfamily. Anesthesiology 98:1147, 2003
157. Olesen A, Huttel M, Hole P: Venous sequelae following the injection of etomidate or thiopentone IV. Br J Anaesth 56:171, 1984
158. Christensen J, Andreasen F, Jansen J: Pharmacokinetics and pharmacodynamics of thiopentone. A comparison between young and elderly patients. Anaesthesia 37:398, 1982
159. Morgan D, Blackman G, Paull J, et al: Pharmacokinetics and plasma binding of thiopental: Studies in surgical patients. Anesthesiology 54:468, 1981
160. Ghoneim M, van Hamme M: Pharmacokinetics of thiopentone: Effects of enflurane and nitrous oxide anaesthesia and surgery. Br J Anaesth 50:1237, 1978
161. Christensen J, Andreasen F, Jansen J: Pharmacokinetics of thiopentone in a group of young women and a group of young men. Br J Anaesth 52:913, 1980
162. Brodie B, Mark L, Papper E, et al: The fate of thiopental in man and a method for its estimation in biological materials. J Pharmacol Ext Ther 98:85, 1950
163. Christensen J, Andreasen F, Jansen J: Influence of age and sex on the pharmacokinetics of thiopentone. Br J Anaesth 53:1189, 1981
164. Heikkila H, Jalone J, Arola M, et al: Midazolam as adjunct to high-dose fentanyl anaesthesia for coronary artery bypass grafting operation. Acta Anaesthesiol Scand 28:683, 1984
165. Lehot J, Boulieu R, Foussadier A, et al: Comparison of the pharmacokinetics of methohexital during cardiac surgery with cardiopulmonary bypass and vascular surgery. J Cardiothorac Vasc Anesth 7:30, 1993
166. Bailey J, Mora C, Shafer S: Pharmacokinetics of propofol in adult patients undergoing coronary revascularization. The Multicenter Study of Perioperative Ischemia Research Group. Anesthesiology 84:1288, 1996
167. Sorbo S, Hudson R, Loomis J: The pharmacokinetics of thiopental in pediatric surgical patients. Anesthesiology 61:666, 1984
168. Seltzer J, Gerson J, Allen F: Comparison of the cardiovascular effects of bolus v incremental administration of thiopentone. Br J Anaesth 52:527, 1980
169. Sonntag H, Hellberg K, Schenk H, et al: Effects of thiopental (Trapanal) on coronary blood flow and myocardial metabolism in man. Acta Anaesthesiol Scand 19:69, 1975
170. Filner B, Karliner J: Alterations of normal left ventricular performance by general anesthesia. Anesthesiology 45:610, 1976
171. White P: Comparative evaluation of intravenous agents for rapid sequence induction: Thiopental, ketamine and midazolam. Anesthesiology 57:279, 1982
172. Flickinger H, Fraimow W, Cathcart R, et al: Effect of thiopental induction on cardiac output in man. Anesth Analg 40:694, 1961
173. Nauta J, Stanley T, deLange S, et al: Anaesthetic induction with alfentanil. Comparison with thiopental, midazolam, and etomidate. Can Anaesth Soc J 30:53, 1983
174. Christensen J, Andreasen F, Kristoffersen M: Comparison of the anaesthetic and haemodynamic effects of chlormethiazole and thiopentone. Br J Anaesth 55:391, 1983
175. Reiz S, Balfors E, Friedman A, et al: Effects of thiopentone on cardiac performance, coronary hemodynamics and myocardial oxygen consumption in chronic ischemic heart disease. Acta Anaesthesiol Scand 25:103, 1981
176. Lyons S, Clarke R: A comparison of different drugs for anaesthesia in cardiac surgical patients. Br J Anaesth 44:575, 1972
177. Tarabadkar S, Kopriva C, Sreenivasan N, et al: Hemodynamic impact of induction in patients with decreased cardiac reserve. Anesthesiology 53:S43, 1980
178. Fischler M, Dubois C, Brodaty D, et al: Circulatory responses to thiopentone and tracheal intubation in patients with coronary artery disease. Br J Anaesth 57:493, 1985
179. Tarnow J, Hess W, Klein W: Etomidate, althesin and thiopentone as induction agents for coronary artery surgery. Can Anaesth Soc J 27:338, 1980
180. Milocco I, Lof B, William-Olsson G, et al: Haemodynamic stability during anaesthesia induction and sternotomy in patients with ischemic heart disease. Acta Anaesthesiol Scand 29:465, 1985
181. Toner W, Howard P, McGowan W, et al: Another look at acute tolerance to thiopentone. Br J Anaesth 52:1005, 1980
182. Frankl W, Poole-Wilson P: Effects of thiopental on tension development, action potential, and exchange of calcium and potassium in rabbit ventricular myocardium. J Cardiovasc Pharmacol 3:554, 1981
183. Eckstein J, Hamilton WK, McCammond J: The effect of thiopental on peripheral venous tone. Anesthesiology 22:525, 1961
184. Kissin I, Motomura S, Aultman D, et al: Inotropic and anesthetic potencies of etomidate and thiopental in dogs. Anesth Analg 62:961, 1983
185. Komai H, Rusy B: Differences in myocardial depressant action of thiopental and halothane. Anesth Analg 63:313, 1984
186. Pedersen T, Engbaek J, Klausen N, et al: Effects of low-dose ketamine and thiopentone on cardiac performance and myocardial oxygen balance in high-risk patients. Acta Anaesthesiol Scand 26:235, 1982
187. Nussmeier N, Slogoff S: Neuropsychiatric complications after cardiopulmonary bypass. Cerebral protection by a barbiturate. Anesthesiology 64:165, 1986
188. Zaidan J, Klochany A, Martin W, et al: Effect of thiopental on neurologic outcome following coronary artery bypass grafting. Anesthesiology 74:406, 1991
189. Ito S, Tanaka A, Arakawa M, et al: Influence of thiopental administration on peripheral circulation during cardiac surgery with extracorporeal circulation. Masui 41:59, 1992
190. Reves J, Fragen R, Vinik H, et al: Midazolam: Pharmacology and uses. Anesthesiology 62:310, 1985
191. Reves J, Kissin I, Smith L: The effective dose of midazolam. Anesthesiology 55:82, 1981
192. Reves J, Samuelson P, Vinik H: Consistency of midazolam. Anesth Analg 61:545, 1982
193. Dundee J, Kwar P: Consistency of action of midazolam. Anesth Analg 61:545, 1982
194. Gross J, Caldwell C, Edwards M: Induction of dose-response curves for midazolam and ketamine in premedicated ASA class III and IV patients. Anesth Analg 64:795, 1985
195. Brown C, Sarnquist F, Canup C, et al: Clinical electroencephalographic and pharmacokinetic studies of a water-soluble benzodiazepine, midazolam maleate. Anesthesiology 50:467, 1979
196. Puglisti C, Meyer J, D'Arconte L, et al: Determination of water soluble imidazo-1,4-benzodiazepines in blood by electron-capture gas-liquid chromatography and in urine differential pulse polarography. J Chromatogr 145:81, 1978
197. Greenblatt D, Loeniskar A, Ochs H, et al: Automated gas chromatography for studies of midazolam pharmacokinetics. Anesthesiology 55:176, 1981
198. Allonen H, Ziegler G, Klotz U: Midazolam kinetics. Clin Pharmacol Ther 30:653, 1981
199. Heizmann P, Eckert M, Ziegler W: Pharmacokinetics and bioavailability of midazolam in man. Br J Clin Pharmacol 16:43S, 1983
200. Forster A, Gardaz J, Suter P, et al: IV midazolam as an induction agent for anesthesia: a study in volunteers. Br J Anaesth 52:907, 1980
201. Lebowitz P, Cote M, Daniels A, et al: Comparative cardiovascular effects of midazolam and thiopental in healthy patients. Anesth Analg 61:771, 1982
202. Lebowitz P, Cote M, Daniels A, et al: Cardiovascular effects of midazolam and thiopentone for induction of anaesthesia in ill surgical patients. Can Anaesth Soc J 30:19, 1983
203. Samuelson P, Reves J, Kouchoukos N, et al: Hemodynamic responses to anesthetic induction with midazolam or diazepam in patients with ischemic heart disease. Anesth Analg 60:802, 1981
204. Massaut J, d'Hollander A, Barvais L, et al: Haemodynamic effects of midazolam in the anaesthetized patient with coronary artery disease. Acta Anaesthsiol Scand 27:299, 1983

205. Schulte-Sasse J, Hess W, Tarnow J: Haemodynamic responses to induction of anaesthesia using midazolam in cardiac surgical patients. Br J Anaesth 54:1053, 1982
206. Marty J, Nitenberg A, Blancet F, et al: Effects of midazolam on the coronary circulation in patients with coronary artery disease. Anesthesiology 64:206, 1986
207. Kwar P, Carson I, Clarke R: Haemodynamic changes during induction of anaesthesia with midazolam and diazepam (Valium) in patients undergoing coronary artery bypass surgery. Anaesthesia 40:767, 1985
208. Reves J, Samuelson P, Lewis S: Midazolam maleate induction in patients with ischemic heart disease. Haemodynamic observations. Can Anaesth Soc J 26:402, 1979
209. Reves J, Samuelson P, Linnan M: Effects of midazolam maleate in patients with elevated pulmonary artery occluded pressure. *In* Aldrete J, Stanley T (eds): Trends in Intravenous Anesthesia. Chicago, Year Book Medical Publishers, 1980, p 253
210. Fragen R, Meyers S, Barresi V, et al: Hemodynamic effects of midazolam in cardiac patients. Anesthesiology 51:S103, 1979
211. Samuelson P, Reves J, Smith L, et al: Midazolam versus diazepam: Different effects on systemic vascular resistance. Arzneimittelforschung/Drug Res 31:2268, 1981
212. Tomichek R, Rosow C, Schneider R, et al: Cardiovascular effects of diazepam-fentanyl anesthesia in patients with coronary artery disease. Anesth Analg 61:217, 1982
213. Newman M, Reves J: Pro: Midazolam is the sedative of choice to supplement narcotic anesthesia. J Cardiothorac Vasc Anesth 7:615, 1993
214. Theil D, Stanley T, White W, et al: Midazolam and fentanyl continuous infusion anesthesia for cardiac surgery: A comparison of computer-assisted versus manual infusion systems. J Cardiothorac Vasc Anesth 7:300, 1993
215. Godefroi E, Janssen P, Van der Eycken C, et al: dl-1-(1-Arylalkyl)imadozole-5-carboxylate esters. A novel type of hypnotic agent. J Med Chem 8:220, 1965
216. Kissin I, McGee T, Smith L: The indices of potency for intravenous anesthetics. Can Anaesth Soc J 28:585, 1981
217. Ghoneim M, Yamada T: Etomidate: A clinical and electroencephalographic comparison with thiopental. Anesth Analg 56:479, 1977
218. Fragen R, Caldwell N: Comparison of a new formulation of etomidate with thiopental: Side effects and awakening times. Anesthesiology 50:242, 1979
219. Horrigan R, Moyers J, Johnson B, et al: Etomidate versus thiopental with and without fentanyl: A comparative study of awakening in man. Anesthesiology 52:362, 1980
220. Shuermans V, Dom J, Dony J, et al: Multinational evaluation of etomidate for anesthesia induction. Anaesthetist 27:52, 1978
221. Thoneim M, van Hamme M: Hydrolysis of etomidate. Anesthesiology 50:227, 1979
222. Wager R, White P: Etomidate inhibits adrenocortical function in surgical patients. Anesthesiology 61:647, 1984
223. Fragen R, Shanks C, Molteni A, et al: Effects of etomidate on hormonal responses to surgical stress. Anesthesiology 61:65, 1984
224. Wanschler M, Tonnesen E, Huttel M, et al: Effects of etomidate infusion and adrenocortical function: A study in elective surgery. Acta Anaesth Scand 29:483, 1985
225. Schrag S, Pawlik M, Mohn U, et al: The role of ascorbic acid and xylitol in etomidate-induced adrenocortical suppression in humans. Eur J Anesthesiol 13:346, 1996
226. Lamalle D: Cardiovascular effects of various anesthetics in man. Four short-acting intravenous anesthetics: Althesin, etomidate, methohexital and propanidid. Acta Anaesth Belg 27:208, 1976
227. Ammon J, Fogdall R, Garman J: Hemodynamic effects of etomidate and thiopental in patients undergoing cardiac surgery. Stanford University (unpublished manuscript).
228. Hempelmann G, Piepenbrock S, Hempelmann W, et al: Influence of althesin and etomidate on blood gases (continuous PO2 monitoring) and hemodynamics in man. Acta Anaesth Belg 25:402, 1974
229. Firestone S, Kleinman C, Jaffe C, et al: Human research and noninvasive measurement of ventricular performance. An echocardiographic evaluation of etomidate and thiopental. Anesthesiology 51:S22, 1979
230. Patschke D, Pruckner J, Eberlein J, et al: Effects of althesin, etomidate and fentanyl on haemodynamics and myocardial oxygen consumption in man. Can Anaesth Soc J 24:57, 1977
231. Kettler D, Sonntag H, Wolfram-Donath U, et al: Haemodynamics, myocardial function, oxygen requirement, and oxygen supply of the human heart after administration of etomidate. *In* Doenick A (ed): Anaesthesiology and Resuscitation. Berlin, Springer-Verlag, 1977, p 91
232. Doenicke A, Gabanyi D, Lemcke H, et al: Circulatory behaviour and myocardial function after the administration of three short-acting IV hypnotics: Etomidate, propanidid, and methohexital. Anaesthetist 23:108, 1974
233. Criado A, Maseda J, Navarro E, et al: Induction of anaesthesia with etomidate. Haemodynamic study of 36 patients. Br J Anaesth 52:803, 1980
234. Gooding J, Corssen G: Effect of etomidate on the cardiovascular system. Anesth Analg 56:717, 1977
235. Colvin M, Savege T, Newland P, et al: Cardiorespiratory changes following induction of anaesthesia with etomidate in patients with cardiac disease. Br J Anaesth 51:551, 1979
236. Gooding J, Weng J, Smith R, et al: Cardiovascular pulmonary responses following etomidate induction of anesthesia in patients with demonstrated cardiac disease. Anesth Analg 58:40, 1979
237. Prakash O, Dhasmana M, Verdouw P, et al: Cardiovascular effect of etomidate with emphasis on regional myocardial blood flow and performance. Br J Anaesth 53:591, 1981
238. Riou B, Lecarpentier Y, Chemla D, et al: In vitro effects of etomidate on intrinsic myocardial contractility in the rat. Anesthesiology 72:330, 1990
239. Kates R, Stack R, Hill R, et al: General anesthesia for patients undergoing percutaneous transluminal coronary angioplasty during acute myocardial infarction. Anesth Analg 65:815, 1986
240. Wauquier A, Hermans C, Van den Brock W, et al: Resuscitative drugs effects in hypovolemic-hypotensive animals. Part I. Comparative cardiovascular effects of an infusion of saline, etomidate, thiopental or pentobarbital in hypovolemic dogs. (Unpublished observations)
241. Corssen G, Domino E: Further pharmacologic studies and first clinical experience with the phencyclidine derivative CI. Anesth Analg 45:29, 1966
242. White P, Way W, Trevor A: Ketamine: Its pharmacology and therapeutic uses. Anesthesiology 56:119, 1982
243. Virtue R, Alanis J, Mori M, et al: An anesthetic agent: 2-Orthochlorophenyl, 2-methylamino cyclohexanone HCI (CI-581). Anesthesiology 28:823, 1967
244. Tweed W, Minuck M, Mymin D: Circulatory responses to ketamine anesthesia. Anesthesiology 37:613, 1972
245. Tweed W, Mymin D: Myocardial force-velocity relations during ketamine anesthesia at constant heart rate. Anesthesiology 41:49, 1974
246. Stanley V, Hunt J, Willis K, et al: Cardiovascular and respiratory function with CI. Anesth Analg 47:760, 1968
247. Stanley T: Blood-pressure and pulse-rate responses to ketamine during general anesthesia. Anesthesiology 39:648, 1973
248. Nishimura K, Kitamura Y, Hamai R, et al: Pharmacological studies of ketamine hydrochloride in cardiovascular system. Osaka City Med J 19:17, 1973
249. Lippman M, Appel P, Mok M, et al: Sequential cardiorespiratory patterns of anesthetic induction with ketamine in critically ill patients. Crit Care Med 11:730, 1983
250. Stefansson T, Wickstrom I, Haljamae J: Hemodynamic and metabolic effects of ketamine anesthesia in the geriatric patient. Acta Anaesth Scand 26:371, 1982
251. Lyons S, Clarke R, Dundee J: Some cardiovascular and respiratory effects of four non-barbiturate anesthetic induction agents. Eur J Clin Pharmacol 6:61, 1974
252. Jackson A, Dhadphale P, Callaghan M, et al: Haemodynamic studies during induction of anaesthesia for open-heart surgery using diazepam and ketamine. Br J Anaesth 50:375, 1978
253. Corssen G, Moustapha I, Varner E: The role of dissociative anaesthesia with ketamine in cardiac surgery: A preliminary report based on 253 patients. Presented at the Asia-Australian Congress of Anaesthesiologists, Singapore, 1974
254. Sonntag H, Heiss H, Knoll D, et al: [Coronary blood flow and myocardial oxygen consumption in patients during induction of anesthesia with droperidol/fentanyl or ketamine]. Z Kreislaufforsch 61:1092, 1972
255. Hobika G, Evers J, Mostert J, et al: Comparison of hemodynamic effects of glucagon and ketamine in patients with chronic renal failure. Anesthesiology 37:654, 1972
256. Spotoft H, Korshin J, Sorensen M, et al: The cardiovascular effects of ketamine used for induction of anaesthesia in patients with valvular heart disease. Can Anaesth Soc J 26:463, 1979
257. Dhadphale P, Jackson A, Alseri S: Comparison of anesthesia with diazepam and ketamine versus morphine in patients undergoing heart valve replacement. Anesthesiology 51:200, 1979
258. Savage T, Colvin M, Weaver E, et al: A comparison of some cardiorespiratory effects of althesin and ketamine when used for induction of anaesthesia in patients with cardiac disease. Br J Anaesth 48:1071, 1976
259. Morray J, Lynn A, Stamm S, et al: Hemodynamic effects of ketamine in children with congenital heart disease. Anesth Analg 63:895, 1984

260. Greeley W, Bushman G, Davis D, et al: Comparative effects of two induction techniques in arterial oxygen saturation during pediatric cardiovascular surgery. Society of Cardiovascular Anesthesiologists. (abstract)
261. Balfors E, Haggmark S, Nyhman H, et al: Droperidol inhibits the effects of intravenous ketamine on central hemodynamics and myocardial oxygen consumption in patients with generalized atherosclerotic disease. Anesth Analg 62:193, 1983
262. Gooding J, Dimick A, Tavakoli M, et al: A physiologic analysis of cardiopulmonary responses to ketamine anesthesia in noncardiac patients. Anesth Analg 62:193, 1977
263. Zsigmond E, Domino E: Clinical pharmacology and current uses of ketamine. *In* Aldrete J, Stanley T (eds): Trends in Intravenous Anesthesia. Chicago, Year Book Medical Publishers, 1980, p 283
264. McIntyre J, Dobson D, Aitken G: Ketamine with pancuronium for induction of anesthesia. Can Anaesth Soc J 21:475, 1974
265. Riou B, Lecarpentier Y, Viars P: Inotropic effects of ketamine on rat cardiac papillary muscle. Anesthesiology 71:116, 1989
266. Riou B, Viars P, Lecarpentier Y: Effects of ketamine on the cardiac papillary muscle of normal hamsters and those with cardiomyopathy. Anesthesiology 73:910, 1990
267. Dowdy E, Kaya K: Studies of the mechanism of cardiovascular responses to CI, Anesthesiology 29:931, 1968
268. Valicenti J, Newman W, Bagwell E, et al: Myocardial contractility during induction and steady-state ketamine anesthesia. Anesth Analg 52:190, 1973
269. Urthaler F, Walker A, James T: Comparison of the inotropic action of morphine and ketamine studied in canine cardiac muscle. J Thorac Cardiovasc Surg 72:1976, 1976
270. Ivankovich A, Miletich D, Reimann C, et al: Cardiovascular effects of centrally administered ketamine in goats. Anesth Analg 53:924, 1974
271. Zsigmond E, Kothary S, Matsuki A, et al: Diazepam for prevention of he rise of plasma catecholamines caused by ketamine. Clin Pharmacol Ther 15:223, 1974
272. Zsigmond E: Guest discussion. Anesth Analg 53:931, 1974
273. Kumar S, Kothary S, Zsigmond E: Plasma free norepinephrine and epinephrine concentrations following diazepam-ketamine induction in patients undergoing cardiac surgery. Acta Anaesth Scand 22:583, 1978
274. Slogoff S, Allen G: The role of baroreceptors in the cardiovascular response to ketamine. Anesth Analg 53:704, 1974
275. Clanachan A, McGrath J, Mackenzie J: Cardiovascular effects of ketamine in the pithed rat, rabbit, and cat. Br J Anaesth 53:704, 1976
276. Traber D, Wilson R, Priano L: Differentiation of the cardiovascular effects of CI, Anesth Analg 47:769, 1968
277. Traber D, Wilson R: Involvement of the sympathetic nervous system in the pressor response to ketamine. Anesth Analg 48:248, 1969
278. Traber D, Wilson R, Priano L: Blockade of the hypertensive response to ketamine. Anesth Analg 49:420, 1970
279. Traber D, Wilson R, Priano L: The effect of beta-adrenergic blockade on the cardiopulmonary response to ketamine. Anesth Analg 49:604, 1970
280. Traber D, Wilson R, Priano L: A detailed study of the cardiopulmonary response to ketamine and its blockade by atropine. South Med J 63:1077, 1970
281. Traber D, Wilson R, Priano L: The effect of beta-adrenergic blockade on the cardiopulmonary response to ketamine. Anesth Analg 50:737, 1971
282. Hill G, Wong K, Shaw C, et al: Interactions of ketamine with vasoactive amines at normothermia and hypothermia in the isolated rabbit heart. Anesthesiology 48:315, 1978
283. Miletich D, Ivankovich A, Albrecht R, et al: The effect of ketamine on catecholamine metabolism in the isolated perfused rat heart. Anesthesiology 39:271, 1973
284. Hatano S, Keane D, Boggs R, et al: Diazepam-ketamine anaesthesia for open heart surgery: a "micro-mini" drip administration technique. Can Anaesth Soc J 23:648, 1976
285. Freuchen I, Ostergaard J, Kuhl J, et al: Reduction of psychotomimetic side effects of Ketalar (ketamine) by Rohypnol (flunitrazepam). Acta Anaesthsiol Scand 20:97, 1976
286. Pedersen T, Engbaek J, Ording H, et al: Effect of vecuronium and pancuronium on cardiac performance and transmural myocardial perfusion during ketamine anaesthesia. Acta Anaesthesiol Scand 28:443, 1984
287. Levanen J, Makela M, Scheinin H: Dexmedetomidine premedication attenuates ketamine-induced cardiostimulatory effects and postanesthetic delirium. Anesthesiology 82:1117, 1995
288. Corssen G, Reves J, Carter J: Neurolept anesthesia, dissociative anesthesia, and hemorrhage. Int Anesthesiol Clin 12:145, 1974
289. Nettles D, Herrin T, Mullen J: Ketamine induction in poor-risk patients. Anesth Analg 52:59, 1973
290. Kingston H, Bretherton K, Halloway A, et al: A comparison between ketamine and diazepam as induction agents for pericardiectomy. Anaesth Intensive Care 6:66, 1978
291. Patel K, Gelman S, McElvein R: Ketamine in patients with pericarditis: Hemodynamic effects. VI European Congress of Anaesthesiology. Anaesthesia 427, 1982
292. Simons P, Cockshott I, Douglas E, et al: Blood concentrations, metabolism and elimination after a subanesthetic dose of 4C-propofol (Diprivan) to volunteers. Postgrad Med J 61:64, 1985
293. Adam H, Briggs L, Bahar M, et al: Pharmacokinetic evaluation of ICI 35 868 in man. Single induction doses with different rates of injection. Br J Anaesth 55:97, 1983
294. Kay N, Sear J, Upington J, et al: Disposition of propofol in patients undergoing surgery. A comparison in men and women. Br J Anaesth 58:1075, 1986
295. Kirkpatrick T, Cockshott I, Douglas E, et al: Pharmacokinetics of propofol (Diprivan) in elderly patients. Br J Anaesth 60:146, 1988
296. Coates P, Monk C, Prys-Roberts C, et al: Hemodynamic effects of infusions of the emulsion formation of propofol during nitrous oxide anesthesia in humans. Anesth Analg 66:64, 1987
297. Monk C, Coates P, Prys-Roberts C, et al: Hemodynamic effects of a prolonged infusion of propofol as a supplement to nitrous oxude anaesthesia. Br J Anaesth 59:954, 1987
298. Claeys M, Gepts E, Camu F: Hemodynamic changes during anaesthesia induced and maintained with propofol. Br J Anaesth 60:3, 1988
299. Vermeyen K, Erpels F, Janssen L, et al: Propofol-fentanyl anaesthesia for coronary bypass surgery in patients with good left ventricular function. Br J Anaesth 59:1115, 1987
300. Stephan H, Sonntag H, Schenk H, et al: Effects of propofol on cardiovascular dynamics, myocardial blood flow and myocardial metabolism in patients with coronary artery disease. Br J Anaesth 58:969, 1986
301. Profeta J, Guffin A, Mikula S, et al: The hemodynamic effects of propofol and thiamylal sodium for induction in coronary artery surgery. Anesth Analg 66:S142, 1987
302. de Hert S, Vermeyen K, Adriensen H: Influence of thiopental, etomidate and propofol on regional myocardial function in the normal and acute ischemic heart segments. Anesth Analg 70:600, 1990
303. Mulier J, Wouters P, van Aken H, et al: Cardiodynamic effects of propofol in comparison with thiopental: assessment with a transesophageal echocardiographic approach. Anesth Analg 72:28, 1991
304. Brussel T, Theissen J, Vigfusson G, et al: Hemodynamic and cardiodynamic effects of propofol and etomidate: Negative inotropic properties of propofol. Anesth Analg 69:35, 1989
305. Patrick M, Blair I, Feneck R, et al: Comparison of the hemodynamic effects of propofol (Diprivan) on thiopentone in patients with coronary artery disease. Postgrad Med J 61:23, 1985
306. Newman M, Murkin J, Roach G, et al: Cerebral physiologic effects of burst suppression doses of propofol during nonpulsatile cardiopulmonary bypass. Anesth Analg 81:452, 1995
307. Kellow N, Scott A, White S, et al: Comparison of the effects of propofol and isoflurane anaesthesia on right ventricular function and shunt fraction during thoracic surgery. Br J Anaesth 75:578, 1995
308. Furst S, Weinger M: Dexmedetomidine, a selective α2-agonist, does not potentiate the cardiorespiratory depression of alfentanil in the rat. Anesthesiology 72:882, 1990
309. Beckett AH, Casy AF: Synthetic analgesics: Stereochemical considerations. J Pharm Pharmacol 6:986, 1954
310. Portoghese PS: A new concept on the mode of interaction narcotic analgesics with receptors. J Med Chen 609, 1965
311. Martin WR: Pharmacology of opioids. Pharmacol Chem 8:283, 1983
312. Paterson SJ, Robson LE, Kosterlitz HW: Classification of opioid receptors. Br Med Bull 39:31, 1983
313. Dhawan BN, Cesselin F, Raghubir R, et al: International Union of Pharmacology, XII: Classification of opioid receptors. Pharmacol Rev 48:567, 1996
314. Jiang Q, Takemori AE, Sultana M, et al: Differential antagonism of opioid delta antinociception by [D-Ala2, Leu5, Cys6] enkephalin and naltrindole 5-isothiocyanate: Evidence for delta receptor subtypes. J Pharmacol Exp Ther 257:1069, 1991
315. Mattia A, Vanderah T, Mosberg HI, et al: Lack of antinociceptive cross-tolerance between [D-Pen2, D-Pen5] enkephalin and [D-Ala2] deltorphin II in mice: Evidence for delta receptor subtypes. J Pharmacol Exp Ther 258:583, 1991
315a. Sofouglu M, Portoghese PS, Takemori AE: Differential antagonism of delta opioid agonists by naltrindole and its benzofuran analog (NTB) in mice: Evidence for delta opioid receptor subtypes. J Pharmacol Exp Ther 257:676, 1991

316. McDonald J, Lambert D: Opioid receptors. Cont Educ Anaesth Crit Care Pain 5:1, 2005
317. Evans CJ, Keith DE Jr, Morrison H, et al: Cloning of a delta opioid receptor by functional expression. Science 258:1952, 1992
318. Kieffer BL, Befort K, Gaveriaux-Ruff C, et al: The delta opioid receptor: Isolation of a cDNA by expression cloning and pharmacological characterization. Proc Natl Acad Sci USA 89:12048, 1992
319. Chen Y, Mesick A, Liu J, et al: Molecular cloning and functional expression of a mu opioid receptor from rat brain. Mol Pharmacol 44:8, 1993
320. Minami M, Toya T, Katao Y, et al: Cloning and expression of cDNA for the rat kappa-opioid receptor. FEBS Lett 329:291, 1993
321. McFadzean I: The ionic mechanisms underlying opioid actions. Neuropeptides 11:173, 1988
322. North RA: Opioid receptor types and membranes on ion channels. Trends Neurosci 174, 1986
323. Rhim H, Miller RJ: Opioid receptors modulate diverse types of calcium channels in the nucleus tractus solitarius of the rat. J Neurosci 14:7608, 1994
324. Carta F, Bianchi M, Argenton S, et al: Effect of nifedipine on morphine-induced analgesia. Anesth Analg 70:493, 1990
325. Santillan R, Maestre JM, Hurle MA, et al: Enhancement of opiate analgesia by nimodipine in cancer patients chronically treated with morphine: A preliminary report. Pain 58:129, 1994
326. Boldt J, von Bormann B, Kling D, et al: Low-dose fentanyl analgesia modified by calcium channel blockers in cardiac surgery. Eur J Anaesthesiol 4:387, 1987
327. Crain SM, Shen KF: Opioids can evoke direct receptor-mediated excitatory effects on sensory neurons. Trends Pharmacol Sci 11:77, 1990
328. Smart D, Smith G, Lambert DG: Mu-opioids activate phospholipase C in SH-SY5Y human neuroblastoma cells via calcium-channel opening. Biochem J 305:577, 1995
329. Smart D, Smith G, Lambert DG: Mu-opioid receptor stimulation of inositol (1,4,5)triphosphate formation via a pertussis toxin-sensitive G protein. J Neurochem 62:1009, 1994
330. Wandless AL, Smart D, Lambert DG: Fentanyl increases intracellular Ca++ concentrations in SH-SY5Y cells. Br J Anaesth 76:461, 1996
331. Krumins SA, Faden AI, Feurenstein G: Opiate binding in rat hearts: Modulation of binding after hemorrhagic shock. Biochem Biophys Res Commun 127:120, 1985
332. Tai KK, Jin WQ, Wong TM: Characterization of [3H]U69,593 binding sites in the rat heart by receptor binding assays. J Mol Cell Cardiol 23:1297, 1991
333. Barron BA: Opioid peptides and heart. Cardiovasc Res 43:13, 1999
334. Ventura C, Bastagli L, Bernardi P, et al: Opioid receptors in rat cardiac sarcolemma: effect of phenylephrine and isoproterenol. Biochim Biophys Acta 987:69, 1989
335. Ela C, Barg J, Vogel Z, et al: Distinct components of morphine effects on cardiac myocytes are mediated by the kappa and delta opioid receptors. J Mol Cell Cardiol 29:711, 1997
336. Barron BA, Jones CE, Caffrey JL: Pericardial repair depresses canine cardiac catecholamines and met-enkephalin. Regul Pept 59:313, 1995
337. Vargish T, Beamer KC: Delta and mu receptor agonists correlate with greater depression of cardiac function than morphine sulfate in perfused rat hearts. Circ Shock 27:245, 1989
338. Pokrovsky VM, Osadchiy OE: Regulatory peptides as modulators of vagal influence on cardiac rhythm. Can J Physiol Pharmacol 73:1235, 1995
339. Caffrey JL: Enkephalin inhibits vagal control of heart rate, contractile force and coronary blood flow in the canine heart in vivo. J Auton Nerv Syst 76:75, 1999
340. Lewis JW, Tordoff MG, Sherman JE, et al: Adrenal medullary enkephalin-like peptides may mediate opioid stress analgesia. Science 217:557, 1982
341. Holaday JW: Cardiovascular effects of endogenous opiate systems. Annu Rev Pharmacol Toxicol 23:541, 1983
342. Akil H, Watson SJ, Young E, et al: Endogenous opioids: Biology and function. Annu Rev Neurosci 7:223, 1984
343. Howlett T, Tomlin S, Ngahfoong L: Release of beta-endorphin and met-enkephalin during exercise in normal women response to training. Br Med J 288:1950, 1984
344. Xiao RP, Pepe S, Spurgeon HA, et al: Opioid peptide receptor stimulation reverses beta-adrenergic effects in rat heart cells. Am J Physiol 272:H797, 1997
345. Boluyt MO, Younes A, Capprey JL, et al: Age-associated increase in rat cardiac opioid production. Am J Physiol 265:H212, 1993
346. Caffrey JL, Boluyt MO, Younes A, et al: Aging, cardiac proenkephalin mRNA and enkephalin peptides in the Fisher 244 rat. J Mol Cell Cardiol 26:701, 1994
347. McLaughlin PJ, Wu Y: Opioid gene expression in the developing and adult rat heart. Dev Dyn 211:153, 1998
348. Dumont M, Lemaire S: Increased content of immunoreactive Leu-enkepahlin and alteration of delta opioid receptor in hearts of spontaneously hypertensive rats. Neurosci Lett 24:114, 1988
349. Ouellette M, Brakier-Gingras L: Increase in the relative abundance of preproenkephalin messenger RNA in the ventricles of cardiomyopathic hamsters. Biochem Biophys Res Comm 155:449, 1988
350. Paradis P, Dumont M, Belicahrd P, et al: Increased preproenkephalin A gene expression in the rat heart after induction of a myocardial infarction. Biochem Cell Biol 70:593, 1992
351. Forman LJ, Hock CE, Harwell M, et al: The results of exposure to immobilization, hemorrhagic shock, and cardiac hypertrophy on beta-endorphin in rat cardiac tissue. Proc Soc Exp Biol Med 206:124, 1994
352. Lee AY: Endogenous opioid peptides and cardiac arrhythmias. Int J Cardiol 27:145, 1990
353. Falcone C, Guasti L, Ochan M, et al: Beta-endorphins during coronary angioplasty in patients with silent or symptomatic myocardial ischemia. J Am Coll Cardiol 22:1614, 1993
354. Oldroyd KG, Harvey K, Gray CE, et al: Beta endorphin release in patients after spontaneous and provoked acute myocardial ischaemia. Br Heart J 67:230, 1992
355. Miller PJ, Light KC, Bragdon EE, et al: Beta-endorphin response to exercise and mental stress in patients with ischemic heart disease. J Psychosom Res 37:455, 1993
356. Maslov LN, Lichmanov YB: Change in opioid peptide level in the heart and blood plasma during acute myocardial ischemia complicated by ventricular fibrillation. Clin Exp Pharmacol Physiol 22:812, 1995
357. Wu JP, Chen YT, Lee AY: Opioids in myocardial ischemia: Potentiating effects of dynmorphin on ischemic arrhythmia, bradycardia, and cardiogenic shock following coronary artery occlusion in the rat. Eur Heart J 14:1273, 1993
358. Imai N, Kashiki M, Woolf PD, et al: Comparison of cardiovascular effects of mu and delta opioid receptor antagonists in dogs with congestive heart failure. Am J Physiol 267:H912, 1994
359. Slepushkin VD, Pavlenko VS, Zoloyez GK, et al: The role of enkephalins in the pathogenesis of acute myocardial infarction. Exp Pathol 35:129, 1988
360. Rimoy GH, Wright DM, Bhaskar NK, et al: The cardiovascular and central nervous system effects in the human of U-62066E. A selective kappa-opioid receptor agonist. Eur J Clin Pharmacol 46:203, 1994
361. Ventura C, Spurgeon HA, Lakatta EG, et al: Kappa and delta opioid receptor stimulation affects cardiac myocyte function and Ca++ release from an intracellular pool in myocytes and neurons. Circ Res 70:66, 1992
362. Fontana F, Bernardi P, Pich EM, et al: Relationship between plasma atrial natriuretic factor and opioid peptide levels in healthy subjects and in patients with acute congestive heart failure. Eur Heart J 14:219, 1993
363. Lowe H: Role of endogenous opioids in heart failure. Z Kardiol 80:47, 1991
364. Barron BA, Gu H, Gaugl JF, et al: Screening for opioid peptides in dog hearts. J Mol Cell Cardiol 24:67, 1992
365. Llobel F, Laorden ML: Effects of mu-, delta-, and kappa-opioid antagonists in atrial preparations from nonfailing and failing human hearts. Gen Pharmacol 28:371, 1997
366. Oldroyd KG, Gray GE, Carter R, et al: Activation and inhibition of the endogenous opioid system in human heart failure. Br Heart J 73:41, 1995
367. Airaksinen KE: Autonomic mechanisms and sudden death after abrupt coronary occlusion. Ann Med 31:240, 1999
368. Flacke JW, Flacke WE, Bloor BC, et al: Effects of fentanyl, naloxone, and clonidine on hemodynamics and plasma catecholamine levels in dogs. Anesth Analg 62:305, 1983
369. Pruett JK, Blair JR, Adams RJ: Cellular and subcellular actions of opioids in the heart. *In* Estafanous FG (ed): Opioids in Anesthesia. Boston, Butterworth-Heinemann, 1991, p 61
370. Blair JR, Pruett JK, Introna RP, et al: Cardiac electrophysiologic effects of fentanyl and sufentanil in canine cardiac Purkinje fibers. Anesthesiology 71:565, 1989
371. Saini V, Carr DB, Hagestad EL, et al: Antifibrillatory action of the narcotic agonist fentanyl. Am Heart J 115:598, 1988
372. Hess L, Vrana M, Vranova Z, et al: The antifibrillatory effect of fentanyl, sufentanil, and carfentanil in the acute phase of local myocardial ischemia in the dog. Acta Cardiol 44:303, 1989
373. Goldberg AH, Padget CH: Comparative effects of morphine and fentanyl on isolated heart muscle. Anesth Analg 48:978, 1969
374. Strauer B: Contractile responses to morphine, piritramide, meperidine and fentanyl: A comparative study of effects on the isolated ventricular myocardium. Anesthesiology 37:304, 1972

375. Sullivan DC, Wong KC: The effects of morphine on the isolated heart during normothermia and hypothermia. Anesthesiology 38:550, 1973
376. Zhang CC, Su JY, Calkins D: Effects of alfentanil on isolated cardiac tissues of the rabbit. Anesth Analg 71:268, 1990
377. Kohno K, Takaki M, Ishioka K, et al: Effects of intracoronary fentanyl on left ventricular mechanoenergetics in the excised cross-circulated canine heart. Anesthesiology 86:1350, 1997
378. Llobel F, Laorden ML: Effects of morphine on atrial preparations obtained from nonfailing and failing human hearts. Br J Anaesth 76:106, 1996
379. Van Vliet BJ, Ruuls SR, Drukarch B, et al: Beta-adrenoceptor-sensitive adenylate cyclase inhibited by activation of μ-opioid receptors in rat striated neurons. Eur J Pharmacol 195:295, 1991
380. Philbin DM, Moss J, Rosow CE, et al: The use of H1 and H2 histamine antagonists with morphine anesthesia: A double blind study. Anesthesiology 55:292, 1981
381. Rorie DK, Muldoon SM, Tyce GM: Effects of fentanyl on adrenergic function in canine coronary arteries. Anesth Analg 60:21, 1981
382. Muldoon SM, Otto J, Freas W, et al: The effects of morphine, nalbuphine, and butorphanol on adrenergic function in canine saphenous veins. Anesth Analg 62:21, 1983
383. White DA, Reitan JA, Kien ND, et al: Decrease in vascular resistance in the isolated canine hindlimb after graded doses of alfentanil, fentanyl, and sufentanil. Anesth Analg 71:29, 1990
384. Karasawa F, Iwanov V, Moulds RF: Effects of fentanyl on the rat aorta are mediated by alpha-adrenoceptors rather than by the endothelium. Br J Anaesth 71:877, 1993
385. Pugsley MK, Penz WP, Walker MJ, et al: Cardiovascular actions of the kappa receptor agonist, U-50,488H, in the absence and presence of opioid receptor blockade. Br J Pharmacol 105:521, 1992
386. Pugsley MK, Penz WP, Walker MJ: Cardiovascular actions of U-50,488H and related kappa agonists. Cardiovasc Drug Rev 11:151, 1993
387. Hall ED, Wolf DL, McCall RB: Cardiovascular depressant effects of the kappa opioid receptor agonist U-50,488H and spiradoline mesylate. Circ Shock 26:409, 1988
388. Brasch H: Influence of the optical isomers (+) and (-) naloxone on beating frequency, contractile force and the action potentials of guinea-pig isolated cardiac preparations. Br J Pharmacol 88:733, 1986
389. Kaschube M, Brasch H: Negative chronotropic but no antiarrhythmic effect of (+) and (-) naloxone in rats and guinea pigs. Cardiovasc Res 25:230, 1991
390. Pugsley MK, Saint DA, Penz WP, et al: Electrophysiological and antiarrhythmic actions of the kappa agonist PD129290, and its R,R(+) enantiomer, PD 129289. Br J Pharmacol 110:1579, 1993
391. Pugsley MK, Hayes ES, Saint DA, et al: Do related kappa agonists produce similar effects on cardiac ion channels? Proc West Pharmacol Soc 38:25, 1995
392. Helgesen KG, Refsum H: Arrhythmogenic, antiarrhythmic and inotropic properties of opioids. Effects of piritramide, pethidine, and morphine compared on heart muscle isolated from rats. Pharmacology 35:121, 1987
393. Kasper E, Ventura C, Ziman BD, et al: Effect of U-50,488H on the contractile response of cardiomyopathic hamster ventricular myocytes. Life Sci 50:2029, 1992
394. Lakatta EG, Xiao RP, Ventura C, et al: Negative feedback of opioid peptide receptor stimulation of beta-adrenergic effects in heart cells. J Mol Cell Cardiol 24:S25, 1992
395. Wu C, Fry CH, Henry J: The mode of action of several opioids on cardiac muscle. Exp Physiol 82:261, 1997
396. Murry CE, Jennings RB, Reimer KA: Preconditioning with ischemia: A delay of lethal cell injury in ischemic myocardium. Circulation 74:1124, 1986
397. Dana A, Yellon DM: Angina: Who needs it? Cardioprotection in the preconditioning era. Cardiovasc Drug Ther 12:515, 1998
398. Gross GJ, Fryer RM: Sarcolemmal versus mitochondrial ATP-sensitive K+ channels and myocardial preconditioning. Circ Res 84:973, 1999
399. Light PE: Cardiac KATP channels and ischemic preconditioning: Current perspective. Can J Cardiol 15:1123, 1999
400. Bolli R, Dawn B, Tang XL, et al: The nitric oxide hypothesis of late preconditioning. Basic Res Cardiol 93:325, 1998
401. Guo Y, Wu W, Qiu Y, et al: Demonstration of an early and a late phase of ischemic preconditioning in mice. Am J Physiol 275:H1375, 1998
402. Bolli R, Marban E: Molecular and cellular mechanisms of myocardial stunning. Physiol Rev 79:609, 1999
403. Mayfield KP, D'Alecy LG: Role of endogenous opioid peptides in the acute adaptation to hypoxia. Brain Res 582:226, 1992
404. Chien CC, Brown G, Pan YX, et al: Blockade of U50,488H analgesia by antisense oligodeoxynucleotides to a kappa-opioid receptor. Eur J Pharmacol 253:R7, 1994
405. Schultz JJ, Rose E, Yao Z, et al: Evidence for involvement of opioid receptors in ischemic preconditioning in rat heart. Am J Physiol 268:157, 1995
406. Chien GL, Van Winkle DM: Naloxone blockade of myocardial ischemia preconditioning is stereoselective. J Mol Cell Cardiol 28:1895, 1996
407. Schultz R, Gres P, Heutsch G: Role of endogenous opioids in ischemic preconditioning but not in short-term hibernation in pigs. Am J Physiol 280:H2175, 2001
408. Takashi Y, Wolff RA, Chien GL, et al: Met5-enkephalin protects isolated adult rabbit cardiomyocytes via delta-opioid receptors. Am J Physiol 277:H2442, 1999
409. Schultz JJ, Hsu AK, Gross GJ: Morphine mimics the cardioprotective effect of ischemic preconditioning via a glibenclamide-sensitive mechanism in the rat heart. Circ Res 78:1100, 1996
410. Miki T, Cohen MV, Downey JM: Opioid receptor contributes to ischemic preconditioning through protein kinase C activation in rabbits. Mol Cell Biochem 186:3, 1998
411. Liang BT, Gross GJ: Direct preconditioning of cardiac myocytes via opioid receptors and KATP channels. Circ Res 84:I1396, 1999
412. Takaski Y, Wolff RA, Chien GL, et al: Met5-enkephalin protects isolated adult rabbit cardiomyocytes via delta-opioid receptors. Am J Physiol 277:H2442, 1999
413. Benedict PE, Benedict MB, Su TP, et al: Opiate drugs and delta-receptor-mediated myocardial protection. Circulation II-357, 1999
414. Kato R, Foëx P: Fentanyl reduces infarction but not stunning via delta-opioid receptors and protein kinase C in rats. Br J Anaesth 84:608, 2000
415. Kato R, Ross S, Foëx P: Fentanyl protects the heart against ischemic injury via opioid receptors, adenosine A1 receptors and KATP channel linked mechanism in rats. Br J Anaesth 84:204, 2000
416. Schultz JJ, Hsu AK, Gross GJ: Ischemic preconditioning in the intact rat heart is mediated by delta1, but not mu- or kappa-opioid receptors. Circulation 97:1282, 1998
417. Bolling SF, Badhwar V, Schwatz CF, et al: Opioids confer myocardial tolerance to ischemia: interaction of delta-opioid agonist and antagonists. J Thorac Cardiovasc Surg 122:476, 2001
418. Sigg DC, Coles JA, Oeltgen PR, et al: Role of delta-opioid receptor agonists on infarct size reduction in swine. Am J Physiol Heart Circ Physiol 282:H1953, 2002
419. Wong TM, Tai KK: Effects of drugs interacting with opioid receptors during normal perfusion of ischemia and reperfusion in the isolated rat heart: An attempt to identify cardiac opioid receptor subtype(s) involved in arrhythmogenesis. J Mol Cell Cardiol 22:1167, 1990
420. Huh J, Gross GJ, Nagase H, et al: Protection of cardiac myocytes via delta1-opioid receptors, protein kinase C, and mitochondrial KATP channels. Am J Physiol 280:H377, 2001
421. Wang GY, Wu S, Pei JM, et al: Kappa but not delta opioid receptors mediate effects of ischemic preconditioning on both infarct and arrhythmia in rats. Am J Physiol 280:H384, 2001
422. Kevelaitis E, Peynet J, Mouas C, et al: Opening of potassium channels. The common cardioprotective link between preconditioning and natural hibernation? Circulation 99:3079, 1999
423. Bell SP, Sack MN, Patel A, et al: Delta opioid receptor stimulation mimics ischemic preconditioning in human heart muscle. J Am Coll Cardiol 36:2296, 2000
424. Fryer RM, Hsu AK, Ells JT, et al: Opioid-induced second window of cardioprotection. Potential role of mitochondrial KATP channels. Circ Res 84:846, 1999
425. McPherson BC, Yao Z: Signal transduction of opioid-induced cardioprotection in ischemia-reperfusion. Anesthesiology 94:1082, 2001
426. Wu S, Li HY, Wong TM: Cardioprotection of preconditioning by metabolic inhibition in the rat ventricular myocyte: Involvement of K-opioid receptor. Circ Res 84:1388, 1999
427. Tomai F, Crea F, Gaspardone A, et al: Effects of naloxone on myocardial ischemic preconditioning in humans. J Am Coll Cardiol 33:1863, 1999
428. Xenopoulos NP, Leesar M, Bolli R: Morphine mimics ischemic preconditioning in human myocardium during PTCA. J Am Coll Cardiol 65A, 1998
429. Horton ND, et al: Isolation and partial characterization of an opioid-like 88kDa hibernation-related protein. Comp Biochem Physiol B Biochem Mol Biol 119:787, 1998
430. Bolling SF, Su TP, Childs KF, et al: The use of hibernation induction triggers for cardiac transplant preservation. Transplantation 63:326, 1997

431. Bolling SF, Tramontini NL, Kilgore KS, et al: Use of "natural" hibernation induction trigger for myocardial protection. Ann Thorac Surg 64:623, 1997
432. Schwartz CF, Georges AJ, Gallagher MA, et al: Delta opioid receptors and low temperature myocardial protection. Ann Thorac Surg 68:2089, 1999
433. Becker LB, Ostrander MP, Barrett J, et al: CPR Chicago: Outcome of cardiopulmonary resuscitation in a large metropolitan area: Where are the survivors? Ann Emerg Med 20:355, 1991
434. Brown CG, Martin DR, Pepe PE: A comparison of standard-dose and high-dose epinephrine in cardiac arrest outside the hospital. N Engl J Med 327:1051, 1992
435. Lombardi G, Gallagher J, Gennis P: Outcome of out-of-hospital cardiac arrest in New York City: the Pre-Hospital Arrest Survival Evaluation (PHASE) study. JAMA 271:678, 1994
436. Tang W, Weil MH, Yu T, et al: A delta opioid receptor agonist minimized myocardial ischemia during cardiopulmonary resuscitation. Crit Care Med A18, 2001
437. Lowenstein E, Hallowell P, Levine FH, et al: Cardiovascular response to large doses of intravenous morphine in man. N Engl J Med 281:1389, 1969
438. Lowenstein E: Morphine "anesthesia": A perspective. Anesthesiology 35:563, 1971
439. Stanley TH, Webster LR: Anesthetic requirements and cardiovascular effects of fentanyl-oxygen and fentanyl-diazepam-oxygen anesthesia in man. Anesth Analg 57:411, 1978
440. Waller JL, Hug CC, Nagle DN, et al: Hemodynamic changes during fentanyl-oxygen anesthesia for aortocoronary bypass operations. Anesthesiology 55:212, 1981
441. Sebel PS, Bovill JG, Boekhorst RA, et al. Cardiovascular effects of high-dose fentanyl anesthesia. Acta Anaesthesiol Scand 26:308, 1982
442. de Lange S, Boscoe MJ, Stanley TH: Comparison of sufentanil-O2 and fentanyl-O2 for coronary artery surgery. Anesthesiology 56:112, 1982
443. Miller DR, Wellwood M, Teasdale SJ, et al: Effects of anesthetic induction on myocardial function and metabolism: A comparison of fentanyl, sufentanil, and alfentanil. Can J Anaesth 35:219, 1988
444. Swenzen GO, Chakrabarti MK, Sapsed-Byrne S, et al: Selective depression by alfentanil of group III and IV somatosympathetic reflexes in the dog. Br J Anaesth 61:441, 1988
445. Bovill JG, Warren PJ, Schuller JL, et al: Comparison of fentanyl, sufentanil, and alfentanil anesthesia in patients undergoing valvular heart surgery. Anesth Analg 63:1081, 1984
446. Tuman KJ, McCarthy RJ, Speiss BD, et al: Does choice of anesthetic agent significantly affect outcome after coronary artery surgery? Anesthesiology 156:179, 1989
447. Slogoff S, Keats AS: Randomized trial of primary anesthetic agents on outcome of coronary artery bypass operations. Anesthesiology 70:179, 1989
448. Wynands JE, Townsend GE, Wong P, et al: Blood pressure response and plasma fentanyl concentrations during high- and very high-dose fentanyl anesthesia for coronary artery surgery. Anesth Analg 62:661, 1983
449. Butterworth JF, Bean VE, Royster RL: Sufentanil is preferable to etomidate during rapid-sequence anesthesia induction for aortocoronary bypass surgery. J Cardiothorac Anesth 3:396, 1989
450. Berberich JJ, Fabian JA: A retrospective analysis of fentanyl and sufentanil for cardiac transplantation. J Cardiothorac Anesth 1:200, 1987
451. Gutzke GE, Shah KB, Glisson SN, et al: Cardiac transplantation: A prospective comparison of ketamine and sufentanil for anesthetic induction. J Cardiothorac Anesth 3:389, 1989
452. Stanley TH, de Lange S: Comparison of sufentanil-oxygen and fentanyl-oxygen anesthesia for mitral and aortic valvular surgery. J Cardiothorac Anesth 2:6, 1988
453. Howie MB, Cheng D, Newman MF, et al: A randomized double-blinded multicenter comparison of remifentanil versus fentanyl when combined with isoflurane/propofol for early extubation in coronary artery bypass graft surgery. Anesth Analg 92:1084, 2001
454. Samuelson PN, Reves JG, Kirklin JK, et al: Comparison of sufentanil and enflurane-nitrous oxide anesthesia for myocardial revascularization. Anesth Analg 65:217, 1986
455. Howie MB, Smith DF, Reilley TE, et al: Postoperative course after sufentanil or fentanyl anesthesia for coronary artery surgery. J Cardiothorac Vasc Anesth 5:485, 1991
456. Collard E, Delire V, Mayne A, et al: Propofol-alfentanil versus fentanyl-midazolam in coronary artery surgery. J Cardiothorac Vasc Anesth 10:869, 1996
457. Wood M: Pharmacokinetics and principles of drug infusions in cardiac patients. *In* Kaplan JA (ed): Cardiac Anesthesia, 4th edition. Philadelphia, WB Saunders, 1999, pp 657–685
458. Schell RM, Kern FH, Greeley WJ, et al: Cerebral blood flow and metabolism during cardiopulmonary bypass. Anesth Analg 76:849, 1993
459. Skacel M, Knott C, Reynolds F, et al: Extracorporeal circuit sequestration of fentanyl and alfentanil. Br J Anaesth 58:947, 1986
460. Roerig DL, Kotrly KJ, Vucins EJ, et al: First pass uptake of fentanyl, meperidine, and morphine in the human lung. Anesthesiology 67:466, 1987
461. Boer F, Engbers FH, Bovill JG, et al: First-pass pulmonary retention of sufentanil at three different background concentrations of the opioid. Br J Anaesth 74:50, 1995
462. Hornick P, Taylor K: Pulsatile and nonpulsatile perfusion: The continuing controversy. J Cardiothorac Vasc Anesth 11:310, 1997
463. McAllister RG, Tan TG: Effect of hypothermia on drug metabolism. Pharmacology 20:95, 1980
464. Boylan JW, Hong SK: Regulation of renal function in hypothermia. Am J Physiol 211:1371, 1966
465. Okutanil R, Philbin DM, Rosow CE, et al: Effect of hypothermic hemodilutional cardiopulmonary bypass on plasma sufentanil and catecholamine concentrations in humans. Anesth Analg 67:667, 1988
466. Bently JB, Conahan TJ, Cork RC: Fentanyl sequestration in lungs during cardiopulmonary bypass. Clin Pharmacol Ther 34:703, 1983
467. Caspi J, Klausner JM, Safadi T, et al: Delayed respiratory depression following fentanyl anesthesia for cardiac surgery. Crit Care Med 16:238, 1988
468. Booth BP, Henderson M, Milne B, et al: Sequestration of glyceryl trinitrate (nitroglycerin) by cardiopulmonary bypass oxygenators. Anesth Analg 72:493, 1991
469. Hickey S, Goylor JD, Kenny GN: In vitro uptake and elimination of isoflurane by different membrane oxygenators. J Cardiothorac Vasc Anesth 10:352, 1996
470. Hynynen M: Binding of fentanyl and alfentanil to the extracorporeal membrane. Acta Anaesthesiol Scand 31:706, 1987
471. Hynynen M, Hammaren E, Rosenberg PH: Propofol sequestration within the extracorporeal circuit. Can J Anaesth 41:583, 1994
472. Skacel M, Knott C, Reynolds F, et al: Extracorporeal circuit sequestration of fentanyl and alfentanil. Br J Anaesth 58:947, 1986
473. Rosen DA, Rosen KR: Elimination of drugs and toxins during cardiopulmonary bypass. J Cardiothorac Vasc Anesth 11:337, 1997
474. Rosen DA, Rosen KR, Davidson B, et al: Absorption of fentanyl by the membrane oxygenator. Anesthesiology A281, 1985
475. Hug CC, Moldenhauer CC: Pharmacokinetics and dynamics of fentanyl infusions in cardiac surgical patients. Anesthesiology A45, 1982
476. Taeger K, Weninger E, Franke N, et al: Uptake of fentanyl by human lung. Anesthesiology A246, 1984
477. Hug CC, Burm AG, de Lange S: Alfentanil pharmacokinetics in cardiac surgical patients. Anesth Analg 78:231, 1994
478. Hynynen M, Hynninen M, Soini H, et al: Plasma concentration and protein binding of alfentanil during high-dose infusion for cardiac surgery. Br J Anesth 72:571, 1994
479. Kumar K, Crankshaw DP, Morgan DJ, et al: The effect of cardiopulmonary bypass on plasma protein binding of alfentanil. Eur J Clin Pharmacol 35:47, 1988
480. Lowry KG, Dundee JW, McClean E, et al: Pharmacokinetics of diazepam and midazolam when used for sedation following cardiopulmonary bypass. Br J Anesth 57:883, 1985
481. Dundee JW, Collier PS, Carlisle RJ, et al: Prolonged midazolam elimination half-life. Br J Clin Pharmacol 21:425, 1986
482. Harper KW, Collier PS, Dundee JW, et al: Age and nature of operation influence the pharmacokinetics of midazolam. Br J Anesth 57:866, 1985
483. Bjorksten AR, Crankshaw DP, Morgan DJ, et al: The effects of cardiopulmonary bypass on plasma concentrations and protein binding of methohexital and thiopental. J Cardiothorac Anesth 2:281, 1988
484. Massey NJ, Sherry KM, Oldroyd S, et al: Pharmacokinetics of an infusion of propofol during cardiac surgery. Br J Anesth 65:475, 1990
485. Russell GN, Wright EL, Fox MA, et al: Propofol-fentanyl anaesthesia for coronary artery surgery and cardiopulmonary bypass. Anesthesiology 71:205, 1989
486. Antognini JK, Kien ND: Cardiopulmonary bypass does not alter canine enflurane requirements. Anesthesiology 76:953, 1992
487. Doak GJ, Gefeng L, Hall RI, et al: Does hypothermia or hyperventilation affect enflurane MAC reduction following partial cardiopulmonary bypass in dogs? Can J Anaesth 40:176, 1993
488. Hall RI, Sullivan JA: Does cardiopulmonary bypass alter enflurane requirements for anesthesia? Anesthesiology 73:249, 1990
489. Hall RI, Hawwa R: The enflurane-sparing effect of hypothermia. Can J Anaesth S114, 1989
490. Steffey EP, Eger EI: Hyperthermia and halothane MAC in the dog. Anesthesiology 41:392, 1974

491. Vitez TA, White PF, Eger EI: Effects of hypothermia on halothane MAC and isoflurane MAC in the rat. Anesthesiology 41:80, 1974
492. Nussmeier N, Lambert M, Moskowitz G, et al: Washin and washout of three volatile anesthetics concurrently administered during cardiopulmonary bypass. Anesthesiology A84, 1988
493. Stern R, Weiss C, Steinbach J, et al: Isoflurane uptake and elimination are delayed by absorption of anesthetic by the SciMed membrane oxygenator. Anesth Analg 69:659, 1989
494. Lerman J, Gregory GA, Eger EI: Hematocrit and the solubility of volatile anesthetics in blood. Anesth Analg 63:911, 1984
495. Eger RR, Eger EI: Effect of temperature and age on the solubility of enflurane, halothane, isoflurane, and methoxyflurane in human blood. Anesth Analg 64:640, 1985
496. Feingold A: Crystalloid hemodilution, hypothermia, and halothane blood solubility during cardiopulmonary bypass. Anesth Analg 56:622, 1977
497. Targ AG, Yasuda N, Eger EI: Anesthetic plastic solubility. Anesthesiology A297, 1988
498. Nussmeier N, Lambert DG, Moskowitz G, et al: Washin and washout of isoflurane administered via bubble oxygenators during hypothermic cardiopulmonary bypass. Anesthesiology 71:519, 1989
499. Price SL, Brown DL, Carpenter RL, et al: Isoflurane elimination via a bubble oxygenator during extracorporeal circulation. J Cardiothorac Anesth 2:41, 1988
500. Finkel E: The mitochondrion: Is it central to apoptosis? Science 292:624, 2001
501. de Hert S, ten Broecke PW, Mertens E, et al: Sevoflurane but not propofol preserves myocardial function in coronary surgery patients. Anesthesiology 97:42, 2002
502. Smeulers NJ, Wierda MKH, van den Broek L, et al: Effects of hypothermic cardiopulmonary bypass on the pharmacodynamics and pharmacokinetics of rocuronium. J Cardiothorac Vasc Anesth 9:700, 1995
503. Miller RD: Factors affect the action of neuromuscular blocking drugs. *In* Agoston S, Bowman WC (eds): Muscle Relaxants. Amsterdam, Elsevier, 1990, pp 181–197
504. Boyd IA, Martin AR: Spontaneous subthreshold activity at mammalian neuromuscular junctions. J Physiol 132:61, 1956
505. Hubbard JI, Jones SF, Landau EM: The effect of temperature change upon transmitter release, facilitation and post-tetanic potentiation. J Physiol 216:591, 1971
506. Wierda JMKH, Proost JH, Muir AW, et al: Design of drugs for rapid onset. Anaesth Pharmacol Rev 1:57, 1993
507. Buzello W, Schluermann D, Schindler M, et al. Hypothermic cardiopulmonary bypass and neuromuscular blockade by pancuronium and vecuronium. Anesthesiology 62:201, 1985

Chapter 10
CARDIOVASCULAR PHARMACOLOGY

Roger L. Royster, MD • John Butterworth, MD • Leanne Groban, MD • Thomas F. Slaughter, MD • David A. Zvara, MD

KEY POINTS

Anti-Ischemic Drug Therapy

1. Ischemia during the perioperative period demands immediate attention by the anesthesiologist. The impact of ischemia may be both acute (impending infarction, hemodynamic compromise) and chronic (a marker of previously unknown cardiac disease, a prognostic indicator of poor outcome).
2. Nitroglycerin is indicated in nearly all conditions of perioperative myocardial ischemia. Mechanisms of action include coronary vasodilation and favorable alterations in preload and afterload. Nitroglycerin is contraindicated when hypotension is present.
3. Perioperative β-blockade may reduce the incidence of perioperative myocardial ischemia via a number of mechanisms. Favorable hemodynamic changes associated with β-blockade include a blunting of the stress response and reduced heart rate, blood pressure, and contractility. All of these conditions improve myocardial oxygen supply/demand ratios.
4. Calcium channel blockers reduce myocardial oxygen demand by depression of contractility, heart rate, and/or decreased arterial blood pressure. Calcium channel blockers are often administered in the perioperative period for longer term antianginal symptomatic control.

Drug Therapy for Systemic Hypertension

1. Current guidelines suggest seeking a target blood pressure of less than 140/85 mm Hg to minimize long-term risk for adverse cardiovascular morbidity and mortality.
2. For patients with diabetes, renal impairment, or established cardiovascular diseases, a lower target of less than 130/80 mm Hg is recommended.
3. Mild-to-moderate hypertension does not represent an independent risk factor for perioperative complications; however, a diagnosis of hypertension necessitates preoperative assessment for target organ damage.
4. Patients with poorly controlled preoperative hypertension experience more labile blood pressures in the perioperative setting with greater potential for hypertensive or hypotensive episodes or both.

Pharmacotherapy for Acute and Chronic Heart Failure

1. The signs, symptoms, and treatment of chronic heart failure are as related to the neurohormonal response as they are to the underlying ventricular dysfunction.
2. Current treatments for chronic heart failure are aimed at prolonging survival, not just relief of symptoms.
3. The low-cardiac-output syndrome seen after cardiac surgery has a pathophysiology, treatment, and prognosis that differ from those of chronic heart failure, with which it is sometimes compared.

Pharmacotherapy for Cardiac Arrhythmias

1. Physicians must be cautious in administering antiarrhythmic drugs because of the proarrhythmic effects that can increase mortality in certain subgroups of patients.
2. Amiodarone has become a popular intravenous antiarrhythmic drug for use in the operating room and critical care areas because it has a broad range of effects for ventricular and supraventricular arrhythmias.
3. β-Receptor antagonists are very effective but underused antiarrhythmics in the perioperative period because many arrhythmias are adrenergically mediated due to the stress of surgery and critical illness.
4. Managing electrolyte abnormalities and treating underlying disease processes such as hypervolemia and myocardial ischemia are critical treatment steps prior to the administration of any antiarrhythmic agent.

ANTI-ISCHEMIC DRUG THERAPY

Anti-ischemic drug therapy during anesthesia is indicated whenever evidence of myocardial ischemia exists. The treatment of ischemia during anesthesia is complicated by the ongoing stress of surgery, blood loss, concurrent organ ischemia, and the patient's inability to interact with the anesthesiologist. Nonetheless, the fundamental principles of treatment remain the same as in the unanesthetized state. All events of myocardial ischemia involve an alteration in the oxygen supply/demand balance (Table 10–1). The American College of Cardiology/American Heart Association (ACC/AHA) Guidelines on the Management and Treatment of Patients with Unstable Angina and Non-ST-Segment Elevation Myocardial Infarction provide an excellent framework for the treatment of patients with ongoing myocardial ischemia.[1] These guidelines detail the initial evaluation, management, hospital care, and coronary revascularization strategies in the nonanesthetized patient with an acute coronary syndrome. In the anesthetized patient with evidence of myocardial ischemia, initiation of anti-ischemic drug therapy is indicated. This section reviews the common agents used for this purpose (see Chapter 19).

Nitroglycerin

Nitroglycerin (NTG) is clinically indicated as initial therapy in nearly all types of myocardial ischemia.[2] Chronic exertional angina, de novo angina, unstable angina, Prinzmetal's angina (vasospasm), and silent ischemia respond to NTG administration.[2-6] NTG therapy decreases the incidence of anginal attacks and improves exercise tolerance before angina symp-

Table 10–1 Myocardial Ischemia: Factors Governing O_2 Supply and Demand

O_2 Supply	O_2 Demand
Heart rate*	Heart rate*
O_2 content	Contractility
Hgb, SAT%, Pa_{O_2}	Wall tension
Coronary blood flow	Afterload
CPP = DP − LVEDP*	Preload (LVEDP)*
CVR	

Hgb = hemoglobin; SAT = percent oxygen saturation; CPP = coronary perfusion pressure; DP = diastolic blood pressure; LVEDP = left ventricular end-diastolic pressure; CVR = coronary vascular resistance.
*Affects both supply and demand.
Modified from Royster RL: Intraoperative administration of inotropes in cardiac surgery patients. J Cardiothorac Anesth 6 (Suppl 5):17, 1990.

toms.[7] During therapy with intravenous (IV) NTG, if blood pressure (BP) drops and ischemia is not relieved, the addition of phenylephrine will allow coronary perfusion pressure (CPP) to be maintained while allowing higher doses of NTG to be used for ischemia relief.[8] If reflex increases in heart rate (HR) and contractility occur, combination therapy with β-adrenergic blockers may be indicated to blunt this undesired increase in HR. Combination therapy with nitrates and calcium channel blockers may be an effective anti-ischemic regimen in selected patients; however, excessive hypotension and reflex tachycardia may be a problem, especially when a dihydropyridine calcium antagonist is used.[9]

Mechanism of Action

NTG enhances myocardial oxygen delivery and reduces myocardial oxygen demand. NTG is a smooth muscle relaxant that causes vasculature dilation. Nitrate-mediated vasodilation occurs with or without intact vascular endothelium.[10] Nitrites, organic nitrites, nitroso compounds, and other nitrogen oxide–containing substances (e.g., nitroprusside) enter the smooth muscle cell and are converted to reactive nitric oxide (NO) or *S*-nitrosothiols, which stimulate guanylate cyclase metabolism to produce cGMP[10-13] (Fig. 10–1). A cGMP-dependent protein kinase is stimulated with resultant protein phosphorylation in the smooth muscle. This leads to a dephosphorylation of the myosin light chain and smooth muscle relaxation.[14,15] Vasodilation is also associated with a reduction of intracellular calcium.[16] Sulfhydryl (SH) groups are required for formation of NO and the stimulation of guanylate cyclase. When excessive amounts of SH groups are metabolized by prolonged exposure to NTG, vascular tolerance occurs.[17] The addition of *N*-acetylcysteine, an SH donor, reverses NTG tolerance.[18] The mechanism by which NTG compounds are uniquely better venodilators, especially at lower serum concentrations, is unknown but may be related to increased uptake of NTG by veins compared with arteries.[19]

Physiologic Effects

Two important physiologic effects of NTG are systemic and regional venous dilation (Fig. 10–2). Venodilation can markedly reduce venous pressure, venous return to the heart, and cardiac filling pressures. Prominent venodilation occurs at lower doses and does not increase further as the NTG dose increases.[20] Venodilation results primarily in pooling of blood in the splanchnic capacitance system.[21] Mesenteric blood volume increases as ventricular size, ventricular pressures, and intrapericardial pressure decrease.[21]

NTG increases the distensibility and conductance of large arteries without changing systemic vascular resistance (SVR) at low doses.[22] Improved compliance of the large arteries does not necessarily imply afterload reduction. At higher doses, NTG dilates smaller arterioles and resistance vessels, which reduces afterload and BP[23] (see Fig. 10–2). Reductions in cardiac dimension and pressure reduce myocardial oxygen consumption ($M\dot{V}O_2$) and improve myocardial ischemia[24] (Fig. 10–3). NTG may preferentially reduce cardiac preload while maintaining systemic perfusion pressure, an important hemodynamic effect in myocardial ischemia. However, in hypovolemic states, higher doses of NTG may markedly reduce systemic BP to dangerous levels. A reflex increase in HR may occur at arterial vasodilating doses.

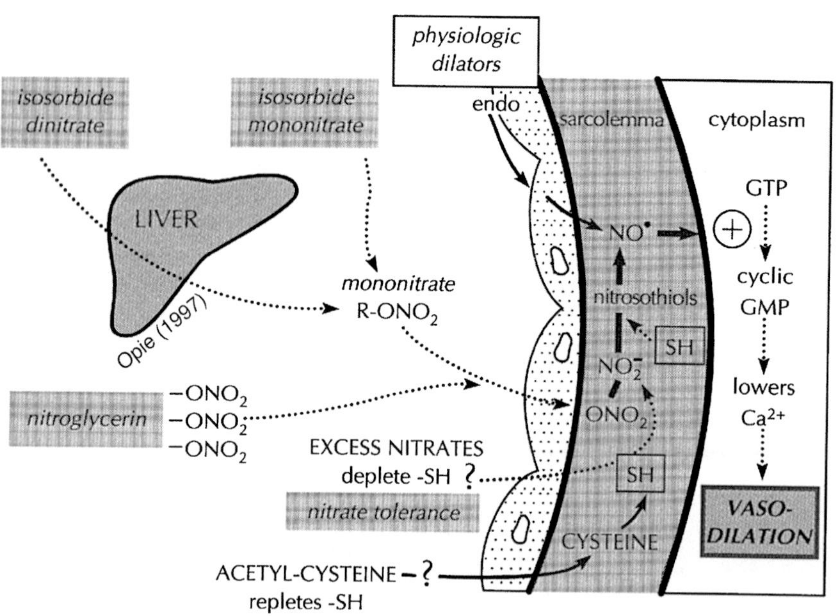

Figure 10–1 Mechanisms of the effects of nitrates in the generation of nitric oxide (NO•) and the stimulation of guanylate cyclase cyclic guanosine monophosphate (GMP), which mediates vasodilation. Sulfhydryl (SH) groups are required for the formation of NO• and the stimulation of guanylate cyclase. Isosorbide dinitrate is metabolized by the liver, whereas this route of metabolism is bypassed by the mononitrates. GTP = guanosine triphosphate. (Redrawn from Opie LH: Drugs for the Heart, 4th edition. Philadelphia, WB Saunders, 1995, p 33.)

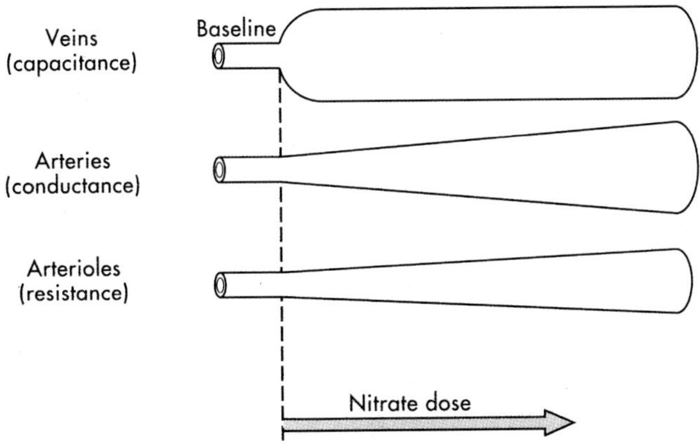

Figure 10–2 Actions of organic nitrates on the major vascular beds and relationship of vasodilation to the size of the administered dose. The venous capacitance system dilates maximally with very low doses of organic nitrates. Increasing the amount of drug does not cause appreciable additional venodilation. Arterial dilation and enhanced arterial conductance begin at low doses of nitrates, with further vasodilation as the dosage is increased. With high plasma concentrations of nitrates, the arteriolar resistance vessels dilate, resulting in decreases in systemic and regional vascular resistance. (Modified from Abrams J: Hemodynamic effects of nitroglycerin and long-acting nitrates. Am Heart J 110(part 2):216, 1985; and Abrams J: Nitrates. *In* Chatterjee K, Cheitlin MD, Karliner J, et al [eds]: Cardiology: An Illustrated Text/Reference, Vol 1. Philadelphia, JB Lippincott, 1991, pp 275–290.)

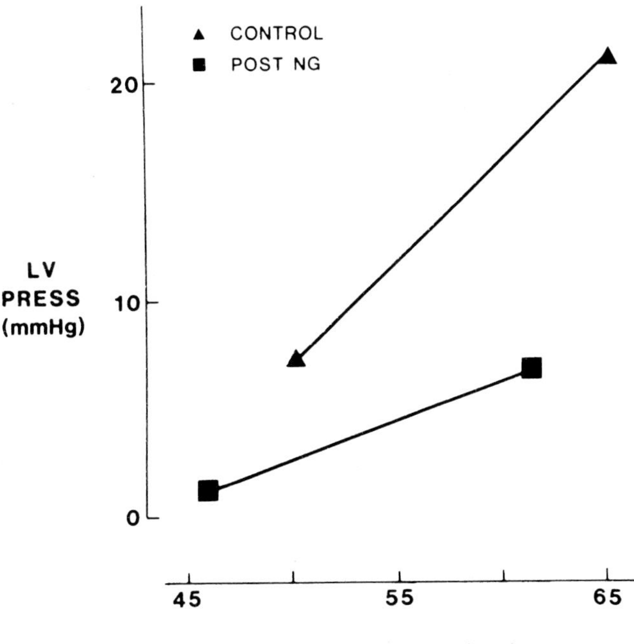

Figure 10–3 Effect of sublingual nitroglycerin (NG) on the left ventricular (LV) diastolic pressure-dimension relation in a patient with chronic aortic regurgitation. Dimensions (from an echocardiogram) and pressure data points were obtained in early diastole (minimal pressure) and at end-diastole (peak of QRS). After the administration of nitroglycerin, the pressure-dimension curve is shifted to the left. (From Smith ER, Smiseth OA, Kingma I, et al: Mechanism of action of nitrates. Role of changes in venous capacitance and in the left ventricular diastolic pressure-volume relation. Am J Med 76:14, 1984. Copyright 1984, with permission from Excerpta Medical Inc.)

NTG causes vasodilation of pulmonary arteries and veins and predictably decreases right atrial (RAP), pulmonary artery (PAP), and pulmonary capillary wedge pressures (PCWP).[23] Pulmonary artery hypertension may be reduced in various disease states and in congenital heart disease with NTG.[25,26] Renal arteries, cerebral arteries, and cutaneous

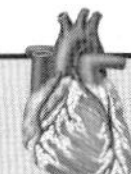

BOX 10–1 ***Effects of Nitroglycerin and Organic Nitrates on the Coronary Circulation***

- Epicardial coronary artery dilation: small arteries dilate proportionately more than larger arteries
- Increased coronary collateral vessel diameter and enhanced collateral flow
- Improved subendocardial blood flow
- Dilation of coronary atherosclerotic stenoses
- Initial short-lived increase in coronary blood flow, later reduction in coronary blood flow as $M\dot{V}O_2$ decreases
- Reversal and prevention of coronary vasospasm and vasoconstriction

Modified from Abrams J: Hemodynamic effects of nitroglycerin and long-acting nitrates. Am Heart J 110(part 2):216, 1985.

vessels also dilate with NTG.[27] Blood flow to the kidney and brain may decrease if adequate renal and cerebral perfusion pressures are not maintained.

NTG has several important effects on the coronary circulation (Box 10–1). NTG is a potent epicardial coronary artery vasodilator in both normal and diseased vessels. Stenotic lesions dilate with NTG, reducing the resistance to coronary blood flow (CBF) and improving myocardial ischemia.[28,29] Smaller coronary arteries may dilate relatively more than larger coronary vessels; however, the degree of dilation may depend on the baseline tone of the vessel.[30] NTG effectively reverses or prevents coronary artery vasospasm.[31]

Total CBF may initially increase but eventually decreases with NTG despite coronary vasodilation[32] (Fig. 10–4). Autoregulatory mechanisms probably result in decreases in total flow as a result of reductions in wall tension and myocardial oxygen consumption.[23] However, regional myocardial blood flow may improve by vasodilation of intercoronary collateral vessels or reduction of subendocardial compressive forces[33] (Fig. 10–5). Coronary arteriographic studies in humans demonstrate that coronary collateral vessels increase in size after NTG administration.[34] This effect may be especially important when epicardial vessels have subtotal or total occlusive disease.[35] Improvement in collateral flow may also be protective in situations in which coronary artery steal may occur with other potent coronary vasodilator agents. The improvement in blood flow to the subendocardium, the most vulnerable area to the development of ischemia, is secondary to both improvement in collateral flow and reductions in left ventricular end-diastolic pressure (LVEDP), which reduce subendocardial resistance to blood flow.[36] With the maintenance of an adequate CPP (e.g., with administration of phenylephrine), NTG can maximize subendocardial blood flow[8] (see Figs. 10–4 and 10–5). The ratio of endocardial to epicardial blood in transmural segments is enhanced with NTG.[36] Inhibition of platelet aggregation also occurs with NTG; however, the clinical significance of this action is unknown.[37]

Pharmacology

Organic nitrates are biotransformed by reduction hydrolysis catalyzed by the hepatic enzyme glutathione-organic nitrate reductase.[15] The rate of hepatic denitrification is characteristic of each nitrate and is further dependent on hepatic blood

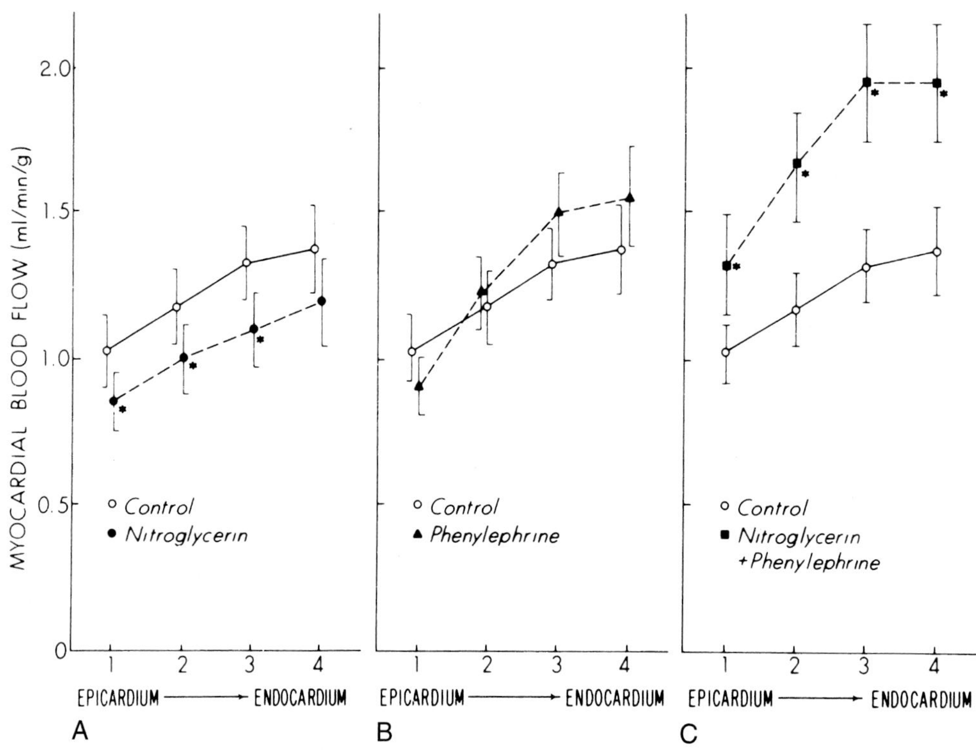

Figure 10–4 Mean blood flow (mL/min/g) ± SE to four transmural layers of anterior nonischemic myocardium during occlusion of the circumflex coronary artery in animals. Data are reported during control conditions, during infusion of nitroglycerin (0.015 mg/kg/min) *(A)*, during administration of phenylephrine to increase mean arterial pressure to 153 ± 6 mm Hg *(B)*, and during simultaneous administration of nitroglycerin and phenylephrine *(C)*. Nitroglycerin decreases blood flow, and phenylephrine generally increases blood flow in normal myocardium. The combination markedly augments flow. $^*P < 0.05$ in comparison with control measurements. *(A-C,* From Bache RJ: Effect of nitroglycerin and arterial hypertension on myocardial blood flow following acute coronary artery occlusion in the dog. Circulation 57:557, 1978. Copyright 1978, American Heart Association.)

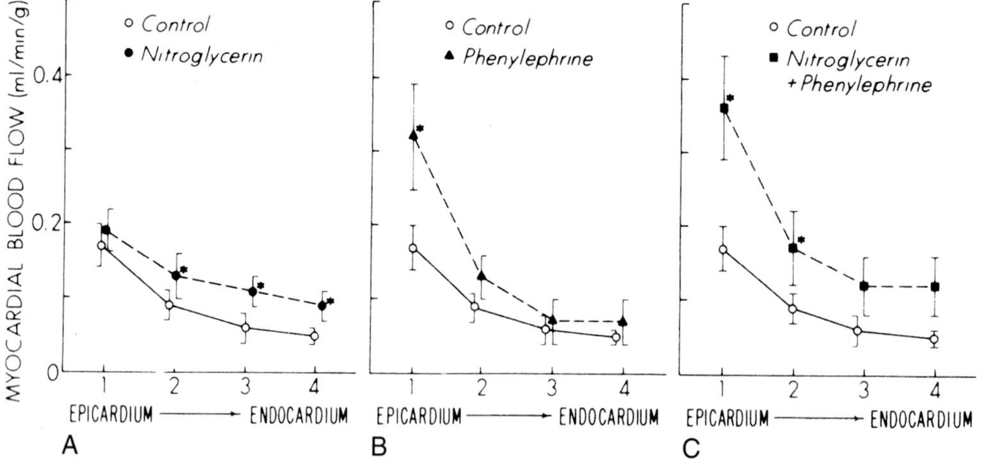

Figure 10–5 Mean blood flow (mL/min/g) ± SE to four transmural layers of the central ischemic zone during occlusion of the circumflex coronary artery in animals. Data are reported during control conditions, during infusion of nitroglycerin (0.015 mg/kg/min) *(A)*, during administration of phenylephrine to increase mean arterial pressure to 153 ± 6 mm Hg *(B)*, and during simultaneous administration of nitroglycerin and phenylephrine *(C)*. Coronary blood flow to all layers of ischemic myocardium is enhanced with the combination; $^*P < 0.05$ in comparison with control measurements. *(A-C,* From Bache RJ: Effect of nitroglycerin and arterial hypertension on myocardial blood flow following acute coronary artery occlusion in the dog. Circulation 57:557, 1978. Copyright 1978, American Heart Association.)

flow or presence of hepatic disease.[15] Common organic nitrates for clinical use are shown in Table 10–2.

Sublingual Nitroglycerin

Sublingual NTG (0.15- to 0.6-mg tablets) achieves blood levels adequate to cause hemodynamic changes within several minutes; physiologic effects last 30 to 45 minutes[38] (Table 10–3). Sublingual bioavailability is approximately 80% and bypasses the high first-pass biodegradation in the liver (90%) by nitrate reductase to glycerol dinitrate and nitrite, which are renally excreted. Plasma half-life of sublingual NTG is 4 to 7 minutes. NTG spray has pharmacokinetics and pharmacodynamics equivalent to those of a 0.4-mg sublingual tablet; however, it has a longer shelf half-life compared with the

Table 10–2 **Nitroglycerin and Nitrates in Angina**

Compound	Route	Dose/Dosage	Duration of Effect
Nitroglycerin	Sublingual tablets	0.3 to 0.6 mg up to 1.5 mg 0.4 mg as needed	1 to 7 min
	Spray	0.2 to 0.8 mg/hr every 12 hr	Similar to sublingual tablets
	Transdermal	<1 inch 2% ointment	8 to 12 hr during intermittent therapy
	Intravenous	5 to 200 μg/min	Tolerance in 7 to 8 hr
Isosorbide dinitrate	Oral Oral, slow release	5 to 80 mg, 2 or 3 times daily 40 mg once or twice daily	Up to 8 hr Up to 8 hr
Isosorbide	Oral	20 mg twice daily	12 to 24 hr
Mononitrate	Oral, slow release	60 to 240 mg once daily	
Pentaerythritol tetranitrate	Sublingual	10 to 60 mg every 6 to 8 HR	Not known
Erythritol tetranitrate	Sublingual Oral	5 to 10 mg as needed 10 to 60 mg 3 times daily	Not known Not known

Adapted from Gibbons RJ, Chatterjee K, Daley J, et al: ACC/AHA/ACP-ASIM Guidelines for the Management of Patients with Chronic Stable Angina: A report of the American College of Cardiology/American Heart Association Task Force on Practice Guidelines (Committee on the Management of Patients with Chronic Stable Angina). J Am Coll Cardiol 33:2092, 1999.

Table 10–3 **Physiologic Effects of β_1- and β_2-Receptor Stimulation**

Physiologic Effect	β_1 Response	β_2 Response
Cardiac		
Increased heart rate	++	++
Increased contractility		
Atrium	+	++
Ventricle	++	++
Increased Automaticity and Conduction Velocity		
Nodal tissue	++	++
His-Purkinje	++	++
Arterial Relaxation		
Coronary	+	++
Skeletal muscle		++
Pulmonary		+
Abdominal		+
Renal		+
Venous relaxation		++
Smooth Muscle Relaxation		
Tracheal and bronchial		+
Gastrointestinal		+
Bladder		+
Uterus		+
Splenic capsule		+
Ciliary muscle		+
Metabolic		
Renin release	++	+
Lipolysis	++	+
Insulin secretion		+
Glycogenolysis, gluconeogenesis		++
Cellular K^+ uptake		+
ADH secretion (pituitary)	+	

Modified from Lefkowitz RJ, Hoffman BB, Taylor P: Neurohumoral transmission: The autonomic and somatic motor nervous systems. *In* Gilman AG, Rall TW, Niew AS, Taylor P (eds): Goodman and Gilman's The Pharmacological Basis of Therapeutics. New York, Pergamon Press, 1990, pp 84–121. With permission of The McGraw-Hill Companies.

tablets, which decompose in air and warm temperatures.[39] A tablet that adheres to the buccal area between the upper lip and teeth has rapid onset and has the advantage of longer half-life than sublingual tablets.[40] Although NTG is readily absorbed through the gastric mucosa, the high rate of liver metabolism makes oral administration highly unpredictable.

Nitroglycerin Ointment and Patches

NTG ointment (2%) is readily absorbed through the skin, with this method of administration providing longer lasting effects.[41] Adequate NTG blood levels are reached within 20 to 30 minutes, and duration of action is 4 to 6 hours.[41] Ointment is administered in inches (15 mg/inch), but the surface area of application and not the amount administered determines the blood level achieved. NTG ointment is messy, requires application four times a day, and is most appropriate for nursing administration in special care units.[42]

NTG patches contain either liquid NTG or NTG bonded to a polymer gel and slowly released to the skin through a semipermeable membrane.[43] The pharmacokinetics approach that of a consistent intravenous infusion.[43] Blood levels are reached within 20 to 30 minutes, and a steady state is reached within 2 hours. Blood levels may be maintained up to 24 hours and are largely determined by patch size. Patches or discs contain a NTG concentration per square centimeter, and doses of 0.2 to 0.8 mg/hr are usually required for relief of myocardial ischemia. Although convenient for patients, tolerance may be a problem with these sustained-release preparations.[41] Intermittent therapy is recommended to avoid tolerance.[44]

Intravenous Nitroglycerin

NTG has been available since the early 1980s as an injectable drug with stable shelf half-life in a 400-μg/mL solution of D_5W. Blood levels are achieved instantaneously, and arterial dilating doses with resulting hypotension may quickly occur. If the volume status of the patient is unknown, initial doses of 5 to 10 μg/min are recommended. The dose necessary for relieving myocardial ischemia may vary from patient to patient, but relief is usually achieved with 75 to 150 μg/min. In a clinical study of 20 patients with rest angina, a mean dose of 72 μg/min reduced or abolished ischemic episodes in 85% of patients.[45] However, doses as high as 500 to 600 μg/min may be necessary for ischemic relief in some patients. Arterial dilation becomes clinically apparent at doses around 150 μg/min. Drug offset after discontinuation of an infusion is rapid (2 to 5 minutes). The dosage of NTG available is less when administered in plastic bags and polyvinylchloride tubing because of NTG absorption by the bag and tubing, although this is not a significant clinical problem since the drug is titrated to effect.[46]

Adverse Effects

The metabolism of NTG by liver nitrate reductase produces a nitrite that oxidizes the ferrous iron of hemoglobin to the ferric form of methemoglobin. The ferric iron does not bind or release oxygen.[47] Methemoglobin is formed normally and is reduced by enzyme systems within the red blood cell.[48] Normally, methemoglobin levels do not exceed 1%, but may increase when direct oxidants are present in the serum (nitrates, sulfonamides, aniline dye derivates). Methemoglobinemia with levels up to 20% is not a clinical problem. Documented increases in methemoglobin blood levels occur with intravenous NTG, averaging 1.5% in one study of 50 patients receiving NTG for longer than 48 hours.[49] NTG doses of 5 mg/kg/day and higher should be avoided to prevent significant methemoglobinemia.[50] However, rare instances of smaller doses causing clinically significant problems have been reported.[51] Nitrates are effective in producing methemoglobin to bind cyanide in sodium nitroprusside toxicity.

Several mechanisms of nitrate tolerance have been proposed, including a depletion of SH groups, neurohumoral activation, volume expansion, and/or downregulation of nitrate receptors.[52-57] Tolerance may occur with all forms of nitrate administration that maintain continuous blood levels of the drug.[17,58-61] Discontinuation of the drug after prolonged exposure may result in a rebound phenomenon, possibly resulting in coronary vasospasm and myocardial ischemia or infarction.[62] Tolerance to NTG apparently does not occur in all patients.[63] If tolerance develops after prolonged exposure, physiologic responsiveness may be achieved with higher doses of NTG, an important observation during NTG administration in cardiac surgery.[64] Intermittent dosing with a nitrate-free interval each day or night can maintain NTG responsiveness.[44, 65]

NTG interferes with platelet aggregation.[66] The ability of the platelet to adhere to damaged intima is reduced.[67] Primary and secondary wave aggregation of platelets is also attenuated.[68] Previously formed platelet plugs are disaggregated.[69] A clinical study of 10 patients with coronary artery disease (CAD) demonstrated that a mean dose of NTG (1.19 μg/kg/min) inhibited platelet aggregation by 50%, with a return to baseline platelet aggregation 15 minutes after the infusion was discontinued[70] (Fig. 10–6). NO production increases cGMP, which modulates intracellular platelet calcium and reduces platelet secretion of proaggregatory factors.[71] The clinical significance of these actions remains unclear. As with other potent vasodilators, NTG may increase intrapulmonary shunting of blood and reduce arterial oxygen tension.

NTG may induce resistance to the anticoagulant effects of heparin.[72] During simultaneous infusions of NTG and heparin, an increase in the NTG infusion caused the activated partial thromboplastin time to decrease.[73] Becker et al[74] reported NTG-induced heparin resistance at NTG infusion rates greater than 350 μg/min. They suggested a qualitative problem with antithrombin III (AT III), because AT III levels did not decrease. Others have suggested that NTG interferes with AT III binding to heparin by *N*-desulfation of the heparin molecule at the AT III binding sites.[75] *N*-Desulfation of heparin reduces its anticoagulant activity.[76]

NTG is contraindicated in patients who have used sildenafil (Viagra), vardenafil (Levitra), or tadalafil (Cialis) within the previous 24 to 48 hours or in patients who are hypotensive. These drugs for erectile dysfunction inhibit the phosphodiesterase (PDE5) that degrades cyclic guanosine monophosphate (cGMP), and the cGMP mediates vascular smooth muscle relaxation by nitric oxide (NO). NTG-mediated vasodilation is markedly enhanced and prolonged, resulting in cases of profound hypotension, myocardial infarction (MI), and death.[77]

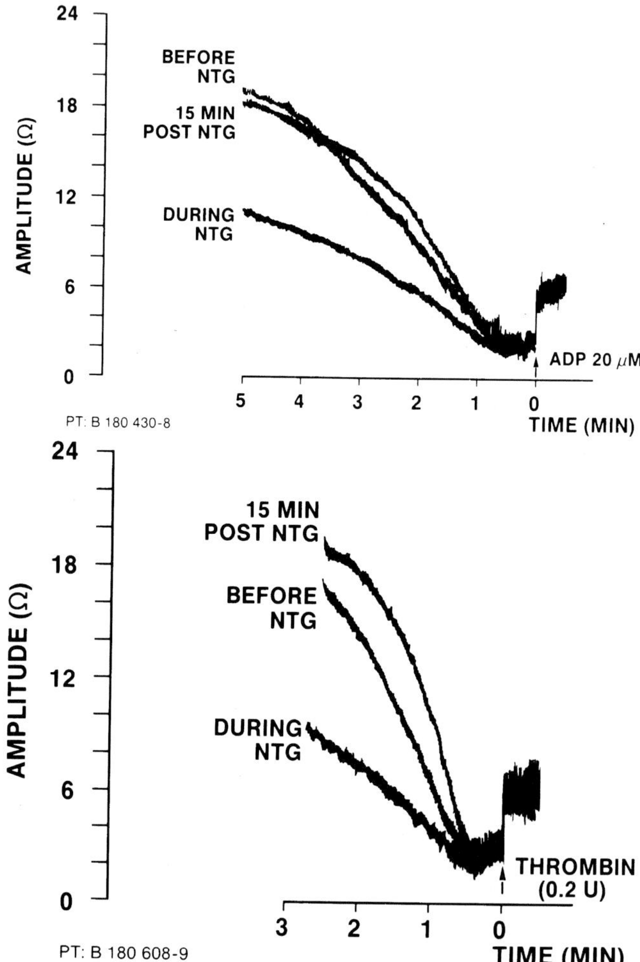

Figure 10–6 Typical examples of aggregation responses to adenosine diphosphate (ADP) *(top)* and to thrombin *(bottom)* before, during, and after infusion of nitroglycerin (NTG) in patients with coronary artery disease. The amplitude of the curve is calibrated in ohms using a dual-channel impedance aggregometer. Nitroglycerin inhibits platelet aggregation to both reagents and the effect is rapidly reversible after discontinuation of the drug. (Modified from Diodati J, Theroux P, Latour JG, et al: Effects of nitroglycerin at therapeutic doses on platelet aggregation in unstable angina pectoris and acute myocardial infarction. Am J Cardiol 66:683, 1990.)

Summary

NTG remains a first-line agent for the treatment of myocardial ischemia. Special care must be taken in patients with signs of hypovolemia or hypotension, as the vasodilating effects of the drug may worsen the clinical condition. Use of NTG in patients who have used sildenafil within the past 24 hours is contraindicated. Recommendations from the ACC/AHA on intraoperative use of NTG are given in Box 10–2.

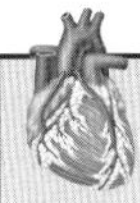

BOX 10–2 ***Recommendations for Intraoperative Nitroglycerin***

Class I*	High-risk patients previously on nitroglycerin who have active signs of myocardial ischemia without hypotension.
Class II†	As a prophylactic agent for high-risk patients to prevent myocardial ischemia and cardiac morbidity, particularly in those who have required nitrate therapy to control angina. The recommendation for prophylactic use of nitroglycerin must take into account the anesthetic plan and patient hemodynamics and must recognize that vasodilation and hypovolemia can readily occur during anesthesia and surgery.
Class III‡	Patients with signs of hypovolemia or hypotension.

*Conditions for which there is evidence for and/or general agreement that a procedure be performed or a treatment is of benefit.
†Conditions for which there is a divergence of evidence and/or opinion about the treatment.
‡Conditions for which there is evidence and/or general agreement that the procedure is not necessary.
From Eagle KA, Brundage BH, Chaitman RB, et al: Guidelines for perioperative cardiovascular evaluation of noncardiac surgery. Circulation 93:1278, 1996.

β-Adrenergic Blockers

β-Adrenergic blockers have multiple favorable effects in treating the ischemic heart during anesthesia (Box 10–3). β-Adrenergic blockers reduce oxygen consumption by decreasing HR, BP, and myocardial contractility. HR reduction increases diastolic CBF. Increased collateral blood flow and redistribution of blood to ischemic areas may occur with β-blockers. More free fatty acids may be available for substrate consumption by the myocardium. Microcirculatory oxygen delivery improves, and oxygen dissociates more easily from hemoglobin after β-adrenergic blockade. Platelet aggregation is inhibited. β-Blockers should be started early in ischemic patients in the absence of contraindications.[1] Many patients at high risk of perioperative cardiac morbidity should be started on β-blockers prior to surgery and continued for up to 30 days after surgery.[78-80] The choice of which β-blocker for any individual patient is based upon clinician familiarity and desired pharmacologic profile. There is no evidence that one specific agent is superior to another; however, β-blockers without intrinsic sympathomimetic activity are preferable when treating acute myocardial ischemia.

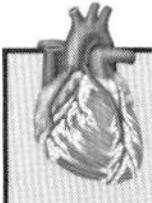

BOX 10–3 ***Effects of β-Adrenergic Blockers on Myocardial Ischemia***

- Reductions in myocardial oxygen consumption
- Improvements in coronary blood flow
- Prolonged diastolic perfusion period
- Improved collateral flow
- Increased flow to ischemic areas
- Overall improvement in supply/demand ratio
- Stabilization of cellular membranes
- Improved oxygen dissociation from hemoglobin
- Inhibition of platelet aggregation
- Reduced mortality after myocardial infarction

β-Blockers administered during MI reduce myocardial infarct size.[81] In addition, a reduction in morbidity has been shown to occur with acute intravenous metoprolol during MI.[81] Similar findings with reductions in mortality extending up to 3 years after MI have been shown in numerous trials with β-adrenergic blockers[82,83] (Fig. 10–7). The mechanisms for mortality reduction are unclear. In the absence of contraindications, β-blockers should be a routine part of care in patients with all forms of CAD, including unstable angina and recent MI.

Data confirm the important role of β-blockade in treating patients after acute MI and in reducing mortality in high-risk populations. Immediate β-blockade following thrombolytic therapy in patients with acute MI significantly decreased recurrent early myocardial ischemia and reinfarction.[84] Early β-blockade is indicated in the treatment of MI[85] (Box 10–4). In fact, β-blocker therapy after MI may be greatly underused in patients older than 65 years.[86] Atenolol has been found to reduce ischemia and adverse outcome in patients with mildly symptomatic ischemia.[87]

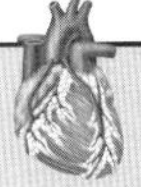

BOX 10–4 ***ACC/AHA Guidelines for Early Use of β-Adrenoceptor Blocking Agents After Myocardial Infarction***

Early Therapy

Class I*	1. Patients without a contraindication to β-adrenoceptor blocker therapy who can be treated within 12 hours of onset of infarction, irrespective of administration of concomitant thrombolytic therapy
	2. Patients with continuing or recurrent ischemic pain
	3. Patients with tachyarrhythmias, such as AF with a rapid ventricular response
Class IIb†	1. Non–Q-wave MI
Class III‡	1. Patients with moderate or severe left ventricular failure or other contraindications to β-adrenoceptor blocker therapy

*Conditions for which there is evidence for and/or general agreement that a procedure be performed or a treatment is of benefit.
†Conditions for which there is a divergence of evidence and/or opinion about the treatment.
‡Conditions for which there is evidence and/or general agreement that the procedure is not necessary.
From Ryan TJ, Anderson JL, Antman EM, et al: ACC/AHA guidelines for the management of patients with acute myocardial infarction. A report of the American College of Cardiology/American Heart Association Task Force on Practice Guidelines. J Am Coll Cardiol 28:1328, 1996.

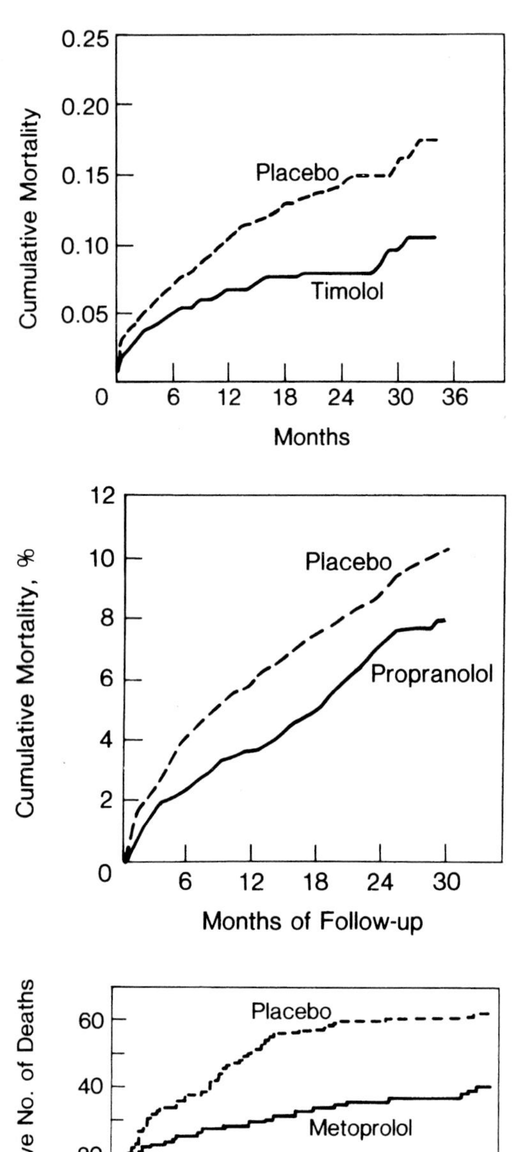

Figure 10–7 Cumulative mortality curves for timolol *(top)*, propranolol *(center)*, and metoprolol *(bottom)* post–myocardial infarction mortality reduction trials. (Modified from Turi ZG, Braunwald E: The use of β-blockers after myocardial infarction. JAMA 249:2512, 1983. Copyright 1983, American Medical Association.)

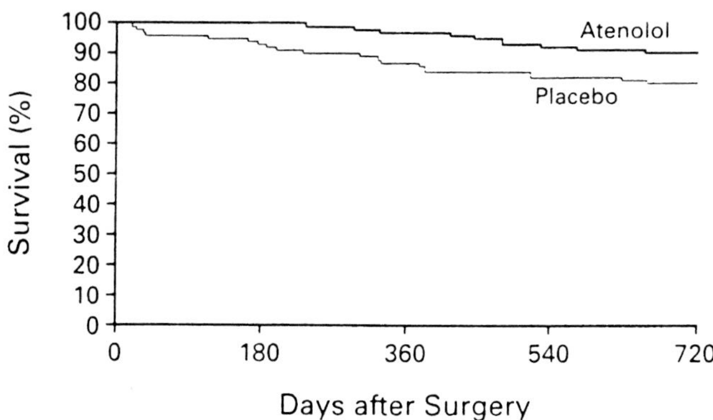

Figure 10–8 Overall survival in the 2 years after noncardiac surgery among 192 patients in the atenolol and placebo groups who survived to hospital discharge. The rate of survival at 6 months (180 days) was 100% in the atenolol group and 92% in the placebo group ($P < 0.001$); at 1 year (360 days), the rates were 97% and 86%, respectively ($P = 0.005$); and at 2 years (720 days), 90% and 79% ($P = 0.019$). (From Mangano DT, Layug EL, Wallace A, Tateo I: Effect of atenolol on mortality and cardiovascular morbidity after noncardiac surgery. N Engl J Med 335:1713, 1996.)

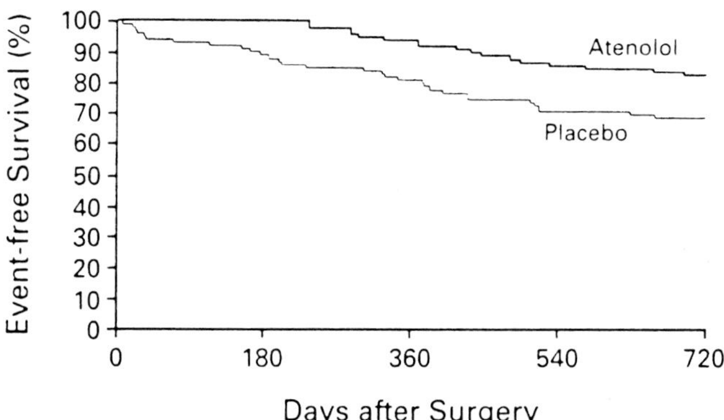

Figure 10–9 Event-free survival in the 2 years after noncardiac surgery among 192 patients in the atenolol and placebo groups who survived to hospital discharge. The outcome measure combined the following events: myocardial infarction, unstable angina, the need for coronary artery bypass surgery, and congestive heart failure. The rate of event-free survival at 6 months (180 days) was 100% in the atenolol group and 88% in the placebo group ($P < 0.001$); at 1 year (360 days), the rates were 92% and 78%, respectively ($P = 0.003$); and at 2 years (720 days), 83% and 68% ($P = 0.008$). (From Mangano DT, Layug EL, Wallace A, Tateo I: Effect of atenolol on mortality and cardiovascular morbidity after noncardiac surgery. N Engl J Med 335:1713, 1996.)

Perioperative administration of β-adrenergic blockers reduces both mortality and morbidity when given to patients at high risk for CAD who must undergo noncardiac surgery[78-80,88,89] (Figs. 10–8, 10–9, and 10–10). These data suggest that intermediate- and high-risk patients presenting for noncardiac surgery should receive perioperative β-adrenergic blockade to reduce postoperative cardiac mortality and morbidity. Recommendations on the perioperative use of β-adrenergic blockade for noncardiac surgery are given in Box 10–5.[90]

BOX 10–5 *Recommendations for Perioperative Medical Therapy*

Class I	β-Blockers required in the recent past to control symptoms of angina or symptomatic arrhythmias or hypertension
	β-Blockers: patients at high cardiac risk, owing to the finding of ischemia on preoperative testing, who are undergoing vascular surgery
Class IIa	β-Blockers: preoperative assessment identifies untreated hypertension, known coronary disease, or major risk factors for coronary disease
Class III	β-Blockers: contraindication to β-blockade

Adapted from Eagle KA, Berger PB, Calkins H, et al: ACC/AHA guideline update for perioperative cardiovascular evaluation for noncardiac surgery—executive summary: A report of the American College of Cardiology/American Heart Association Task Force on Practice Guidelines (Committee to Update the 1996 Guidelines on Perioperative Cardiovascular Evaluation for Noncardiac Surgery). J Am Coll Cardiol 39:542, 2002.

β-Receptor

The β-receptor was conceptualized by Ahlquist, who divided various physiologic effects of catecholamine stimulation into α- and β-responses.[91] The β-receptor has been identified bio-

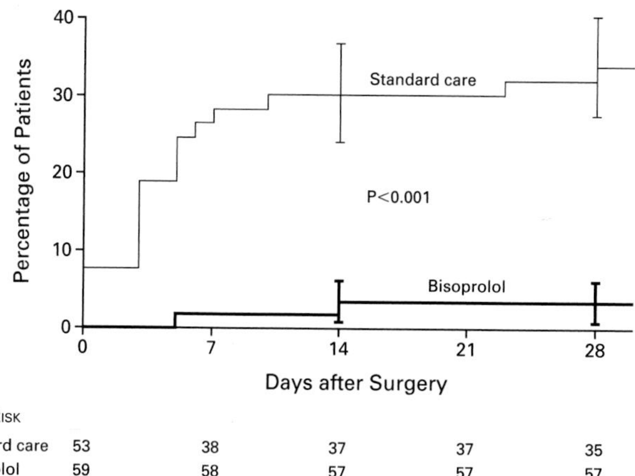

Figure 10–10 Kaplan-Meier estimates of the cumulative percentages of patients who died of cardiac causes or had a nonfatal myocardial infarction during the perioperative period and were at high risk for myocardial mortality with and without preoperative treatment of the β-adrenergic blocker bisopnolol. I bars indicate standard errors. The difference between groups was significant ($P < 0.001$ by the log-rank test). (Reprinted with permission from Poldermans D, Boersma E, Bax JJ, et al: The effect of bisoprolol on perioperative mortality and myocardial infarction in high-risk patients undergoing vascular surgery. N Engl J Med 341:1789, 1999. Copyright © 1999 Massachusetts Medical Society. All rights reserved.)

chemically as a polypeptide chain of approximately 50,000 to 60,000 kDa.[92] The receptor's structure is common to most receptor proteins that have been identified: seven transmembrane crossings with two extramembranous terminal ends[93] (Fig. 10–11). All receptors that transduce a signal through G proteins share this basic structure.[94] There are three extracellular and intracellular loops connecting the intramembranous portion of the receptor.[93] Agonist–antagonist binding occurs at the intramembranous portion, while the intracellular loops modulate interaction with the G-protein complex.[95,96] The terminal intracellular end contains amino acid residues that undergo phosphorylation, which relates to desensitization and downregulation of the receptor.[97]

Receptor stimulation activates a G protein, which stimulates adenylyl cyclase. The G-protein complex is composed of both stimulatory (G_s) and inhibitory (G_i) intermediary proteins.[94] Adenylyl cyclase converts ATP to cyclic AMP, which phosphorylates a protein kinase and produces the appropriate cellular response. A typical cascade of this sequence leading to increases in myocardial contractility from β-receptor stimulation is illustrated in Figure 10–12.

β-Receptor numbers in any tissue may decrease with chronic stimulation (downregulation) or increase with chronic blockade (upregulation). The process of desensitization of the adrenergic response in chronic stimulation (i.e., congestive heart failure [CHF]) may involve downregulation of the receptors but may involve either the G-protein complex

Figure 10–11 The human β_2-adrenergic receptor (*darkened area* represents the cell membrane). Depicted are two sites of extracellular *N*-linked glycosylation (Asn5, 16), four cysteine residues that may participate in disulfide bonds (Cys106, 184, 190, 191), an intracellular cysteine residue (Cys341) that may serve as a site of attachment for a palmitate membrane anchor, as well as multiple threonine and serine residues located in C-III and the cytoplasmic carboxyl terminus, which are potential sites of phosphorylation by protein kinase A (PKA), protein kinase C (PKC), or β-adrenergic receptor kinase (βARK). (Reproduced with permission from Raymond JR, Hnatowich M, Lefkowitz RJ, Caron MG: Adrenergic receptors. Models for regulation of signal transduction processes. Hypertension 15:119, 1990. Copyright 1990, American Heart Association.)

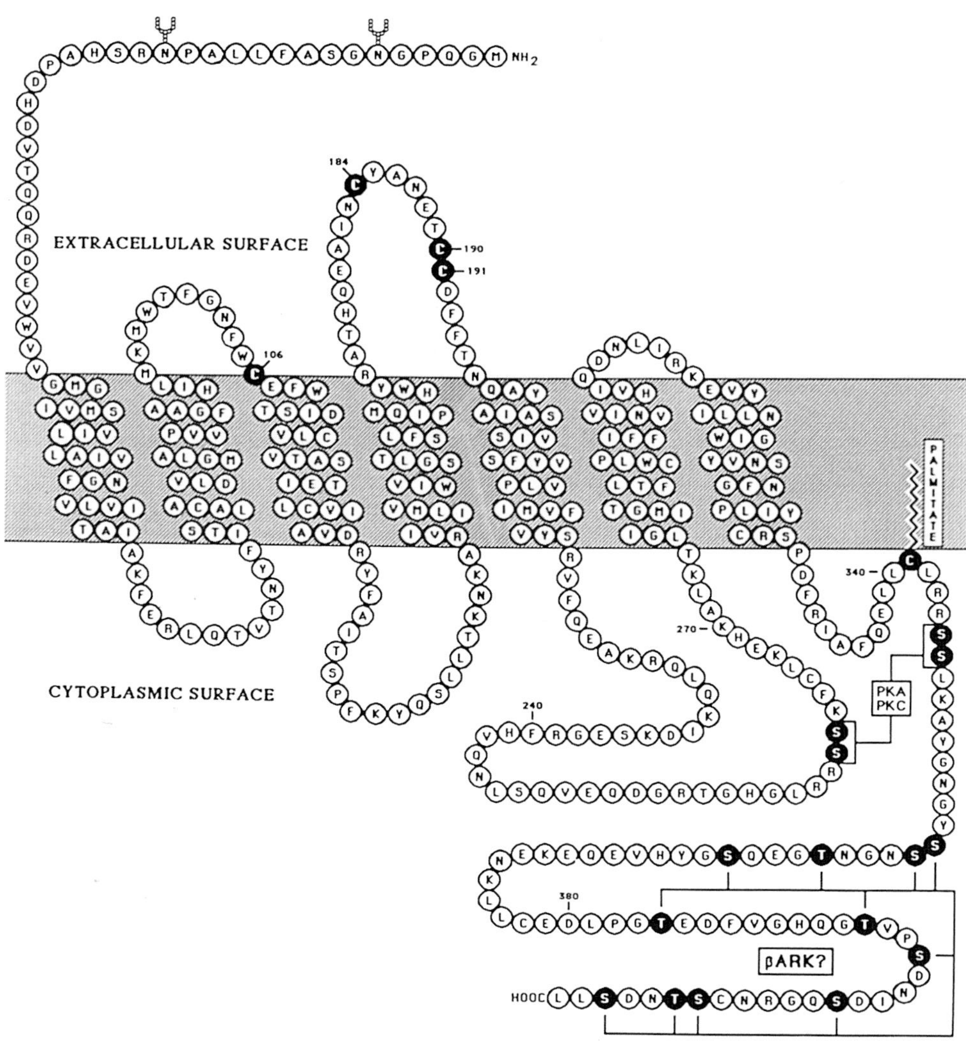

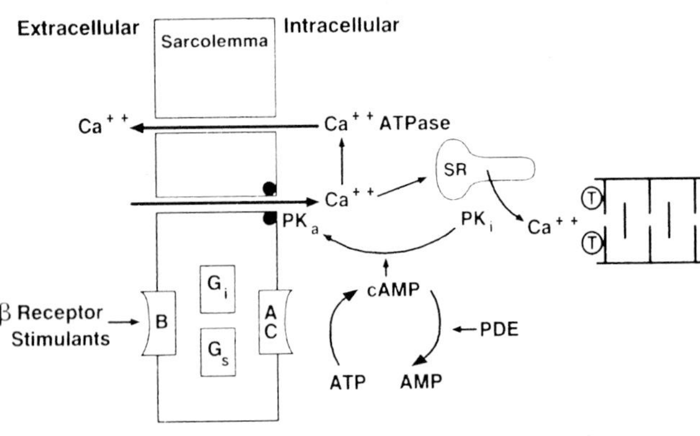

Figure 10–12 The β-receptor, G protein, adenylyl cyclase system. With β-receptor stimulation, dynamic changes occur in the G_i and G_s regulatory proteins. Ultimately, G_s stimulates adenylyl cyclase (AC) to convert adenosine triphosphate (ATP) to cyclic adenosine monophosphate (cAMP), which is metabolized by phosphodiesterase enzyme (PDE). An inactive protein kinase (PK_i) is activated (PK_a) by cAMP, which opens an energy-dependent receptor-operated calcium channel allowing calcium entry into the cell. Calcium cycling occurs with calcium actively pumped out of the cell by Ca^{++} adenosine triphosphatase (ATPase). This calcium cycling causes a release of calcium from the sarcoplasmic reticulum (SR), allowing calcium to bind to troponin C (T) with subsequent activation of the actin-myosin complex. AMP = adenosine monophosphate. (Modified from Royster RL: Intraoperative administration of inotropes in cardiac surgery patients. J Cardiothorac Anesth 4:17, 1990.)

or adenylyl cyclase. Desensitization may occur very quickly, whereas downregulation with actual internalization of the receptor within the cell may take days to weeks.[98] Myocardial ischemia increases β-receptor density, although it remains controversial whether this upregulation results in greater adrenergic response.[99] Several studies have demonstrated that high-affinity β-receptors in nonischemic tissue were shifted to a low-affinity state during ischemia.[100,101] Also, the levels of G_s and its activity are reduced during myocardial ischemia.[102] However, stimulation of these receptors with isoproterenol during ischemia does result in increases in cAMP production.[99,103]

There are two types of β-receptors with a multitude of responses[104] (see Table 10–3). Both β_1- and β_2-receptor stimulation primarily involve cardiac function (Fig. 10–13). Responses of isolated human atrial tissue demonstrated greater inotropic response to β_1- than to β_2-receptor stimulation.[105] Endogenous norepinephrine produces inotropic responses in human atrial appendages and ventricular papillary muscle by β_1-receptor stimulation, while epinephrine produces its maximal inotropic effects on the atria by β_2-receptor stimulation and up to 50% of its maximal inotropic response in the ventricle by β_2-receptor stimulation.[106,107] Sinus node, atrioventricular node, the left and right bundle branches, and the Purkinje system contain higher densities of β_2-receptors.[108] Clearly, both receptor subtypes have cardiac inotropic, chronotropic, and dromotropic properties.

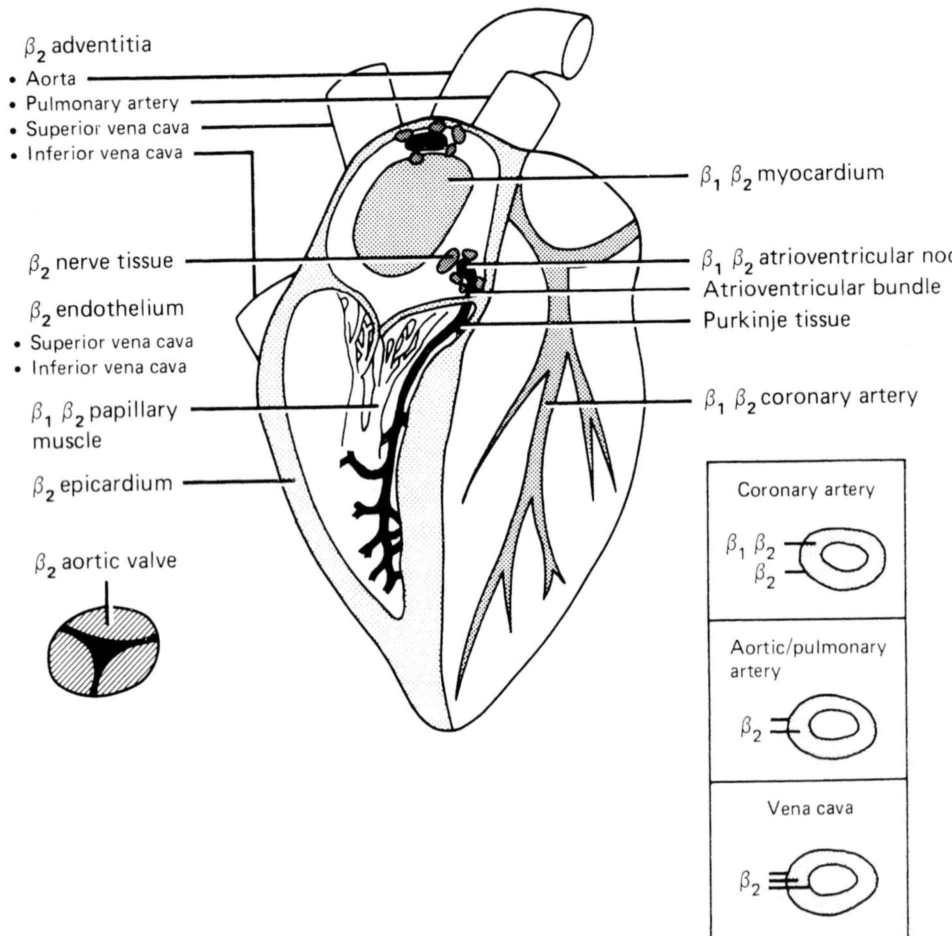

Figure 10–13 Summary of locations of β_1- and β_2-adrenoceptors in rat, guinea pig, dog, and human hearts determined by autoradiography. The β_1- and β_2-adrenoceptors are located on myocardium and specialized conducting tissue. A greater density of β_2-adrenoceptors is located on the atrioventricular node, bundle of His, and left and right bundle branches in comparison to surrounding myocardium in guinea pig. In addition, β_2-adrenoceptors are located on blood vessels, nerve tissue, epicardium and the aortic valve. In large canine coronary arteries (0.5 to 2 mm diameter), β_1-adrenoceptors account for 85% of the total population of β-adrenoceptors; in small arterioles (16 to 55 μm), β_2-adrenoceptors comprise 93% of the total population. (Modified from Summers RJ, Molena-ar P, Stephenson JA: Autoradiographic localization of receptors in the cardiovascular system. Trends Pharmacol Sci 8:272, 1987; and Jones CR: New views of human cardiac β-adrenoceptors. J Mol Cell Cardiol 21:519, 1989.)

β_2-Adrenoceptors comprise 93% of the total population of β-receptors in arterioles and 100% of receptors in epicardium, vena cava, aorta, and pulmonary artery.[107] β_2-Receptors are found on the intimal surface of human internal mammary artery, but not on the saphenous vein,[109] the two vessels most commonly used for coronary artery bypass graft surgery (CABG). β_2-Stimulation results in vascular smooth muscle relaxation and vasodilation.

β_1-Receptor stimulation increases plasma renin production and aqueous humor production. β_2-Receptor stimulation relaxes smooth muscle and produces bronchodilation and uterine relaxation. β_2-Stimulation also increases insulin secretion, glycogenolysis, and lipolysis and shifts extracellular potassium to intracellular sites.

β_3-Adrenoreceptors are found on visceral adipocytes, the gallbladder, and colon. Stimulation of β_3-receptors is thought to mediate lipolytic and thermic responses in brown and white adipose tissue.[110]

Physiologic Effects

ANTI-ISCHEMIC EFFECTS

β-Blockade on the ischemic heart may result in a favorable shift in the O_2 demand/supply ratio (see Table 10–1). The reductions in the force of contraction and HR reduce myocardial oxygen consumption and result in autoregulatory decreases in myocardial blood flow. Several studies have shown that blood flow to ischemic regions with propranolol is maintained; however, this is probably secondary to maintenance of α-vasoconstrictor tone of epicardial vessels and of a pressure gradient to the vasodilated endocardial areas of ischemia.[111,112] Reductions in blood flow in some patients with vasospastic angina may worsen with the administration of propranolol.[113] Intracoronary infusion of propranolol does not worsen stenotic lesions and actually increases the luminal size of the stenosis at rest and during exercise.[114]

ANTIHYPERTENSIVE EFFECTS

The exact mechanisms involved in BP reduction are not clear. Both β_1- and β_2-receptor blockers inhibit myocardial contractility and reduce HR; both effects should reduce BP. No acute decrease in BP occurs during acute administration of propranolol.[115] However, chronic BP reduction has been attributed to a chronic reduction in cardiac output (CO).[116] Reductions in high levels of plasma renin have been suggested as effective therapy in controlling essential hypertension.[117] However, the relationship between renin levels and hypertension is not established, and the decrease in BP in patients has no relation to the change in renin levels.[118, 119] Stimulation of prejunctional β-receptors results in norepinephrine release from postganglionic sympathetic fibers and increases in vascular tone to most major organ systems.[120] Prejunctional β-blockade reduces norepinephrine release, sympathetic nerve traffic, and vascular tone.[120]

ELECTROPHYSIOLOGIC EFFECTS

Several β-blockers have potent local anesthetic activity at higher serum levels because of sodium channel blocking activity and result in depression of phase 0 of the cardiac action potential.[121] However, this membrane-stabilizing or quinidine-like effect is of questionable clinical relevance because it is observed at concentrations far exceeding therapeutic levels.[122] Generalized slowing of cardiac depolarization results from reducing the rate of diastolic depolarization (phase 4). Action potential duration and the QT interval may shorten with β-adrenergic blockers.[121] The ventricular fibrillation threshold is increased with β-blockers.[123] These antiarrhythmic actions of β-blockers are enhanced in settings of catecholamine excess as in pheochromocytoma, acute MI, the perioperative period, and hyperthyroidism.

METABOLIC EFFECTS

Although β_2-blockers are reported to reduce insulin release, the clinical significance of this reduction is questionable.[124] Catecholamines, however, promote glycogenolysis and mobilization of glucose in response to hypoglycemia. In the diabetic patient, nonselective β-blockade may impede this process, thereby worsening recovery from a hypoglycemic episode. Also, the usual hypoglycemic symptoms of tachycardia and anxiety may be suppressed when taking β-blockers, thus delaying detection. In fact, bradycardia and hypertension have been documented as side effects of hypoglycemia in the diabetic patient receiving propranolol because of unopposed α-receptor stimulation with catecholamine release.[125]

Stimulation of β_2-receptors increases the movement of potassium into skeletal muscle cells, reduces aldosterone secretion and increases renal potassium loss, effects resulting in reduction of serum potassium. β_2-Receptor blockers aid in the maintenance of serum potassium levels by blocking the adrenergic-stimulated movement of potassium intracellularly.[126] β_2-Receptor blockers may cause mild elevations in serum potassium, which may be significant in patients with renal insufficiency.[127]

Inhibition of catecholamine-stimulated lipolysis may occur with β-blockers, which reduces the availability of free fatty acids to activate contracting muscle, such as the heart.[128] β-Adrenergic blockers produce increases in serum triglycerides, decreases in HDL cholesterol, and little change in LDL cholesterol. A proposed mechanism is an increase in the relative ratio of α- to β-activity receptors.[129] Increases in β-receptor activity result in increases in lipoprotein lipase and triglyceride levels.[130] These effects on blood lipids are concerns for patients receiving chronic therapy. However, animal studies have revealed that β-blockers actually have a retarding effect on the development of atherosclerosis.[131] β-Blockers with intrinsic sympathomimetic activity produce the smallest changes in the lipid profile.[132]

INTRINSIC SYMPATHOMIMETIC ACTIVITY

Several β-blockers (acebutolol, carteolol, penbutolol, pindolol) have agonist as well as antagonist properties and are characterized as having intrinsic sympathomimetic activity (ISA).[133] These agents are actually agonists that elicit a submaximal response and block the effects of endogenous catecholamines in a competitive fashion.[133] CO and HR are reduced less with ISA drugs.[134] Peripheral blood flow is also reduced less, making ISA agents attractive in patients with peripheral vascular disease.[135] ISA drugs also cause less bronchoconstriction and are advantageous in chronic obstructive pulmonary disease. Theoretically, differences in changes in β-receptor density should differ with ISA. The effects of ISA drugs reduce β-receptor density (similar to pure agonists), whereas non-ISA agents increase β-receptor density.[136] Although controversial, ISA drugs appear to have a role in mortality reduction after MI, similar to non-ISA β-blockers.[137]

General Pharmacology

Lipid-soluble β-blockers (propranolol, labetalol, metoprolol) are well absorbed after oral administration and attain high

Table 10–4 **Properties of β-Blockers in Clinical Use**

Drug	Selectivity	Partial Agonist Activity	Usual Dose for Angina
Propranolol	None	No	20 to 80 mg twice daily
Metoprolol	β_1	No	50 to 200 mg twice daily
Atenolol	β_1	No	50 to 200 mg/d
Nadolol	None	No	40 to 80 mg/d
Timolol	None	No	10 mg twice daily
Acebutolol	β_1	Yes	200 to 600 mg twice daily
Betaxolol	β_1	No	10 to 20 mg/d
Bisoprolol	β_1	No	10 mg/d
Esmolol (intravenous)	β_1	No	50 to 300 μg/kg/min
Labetalol*	None	Yes	200 to 600 mg twice daily
Pindolol	None	Yes	2.5 to 7.5 mg 3 times daily

*Labetalol is a combined α- and β-blocker.

Adapted from Gibbons RJ, Chatterjee K, Daley J, et al: ACC/AHA/ACP-ASIM Guidelines for the Management of Patients with Chronic Stable Angina: A report of the American College of Cardiology/American Heart Association Task Force on Practice Guidelines (Committee on the Management of Patients with Chronic Stable Angina). J Am Coll Cardiol 33:2092, 1999.

concentrations in the brain.[138] Lipid-soluble agents have a high incidence of central nervous system (CNS) side effects, such as depression, sleep disturbances, and impotence. First-pass hepatic metabolism after oral ingestion can be very high but varies from patient to patient and affects daily dosing schedules.[139] Cirrhosis, CHF, and cigarette smoking may reduce hepatic metabolism.[140] Lipophilic agents are highly protein bound. The hepatic metabolism of lipophilic agents is independent of protein binding, which is different from most drugs in which hepatic metabolism occurs only with the unbound drug.[141]

Lipid-insoluble or water-soluble agents (atenolol, nadolol, acebutolol, sotalol) are less well absorbed orally but are not hepatically metabolized. These drugs are almost entirely eliminated by renal excretion and must be used cautiously in renal insufficiency. The incidence of CNS side effects is low because of lipid insolubility.

Pindolol and timolol have intermediate lipid solubility properties and are metabolized partially by the liver (50%) and excreted through the kidneys (50%). Acebutolol, which is water soluble, has an active metabolite, diacetolol, which is water soluble and renally excreted.[142] The plasma elimination of acebutolol is more rapid than that of diacetolol. For further information on the available oral and intravenous β-adrenergic blockers for treatment of myocardial ischemia, see Table 10–4. Additional β-blockers with other indications, such as carvedilol (for CHF) and sotalol (for arrhythmias), are covered later.

Pharmacology of Intravenous β-Adrenergic Blockers

PROPRANOLOL

Propranolol has an equal affinity for β_1- and β_2-receptors, lacks ISA, and has no α-adrenergic receptor activity. It is the most lipid-soluble β-blocker and generally has the most CNS side effects. First-pass liver metabolism (90%) is very high, requiring much higher oral doses than intravenous doses for pharmacodynamic effect.[143] Although propranolol has an active metabolite (4-hydroxypropranolol), the metabolite's half-life is much shorter and does not add to the clinical effect.[144] Serum half-life of the drug after intravenous dosing is 3 to 4 hours.[145]

Because of the high hepatic extraction of propranolol, factors that affect hepatic blood flow markedly affect propranolol plasma levels. Because propranolol reduces hepatic blood flow, it can reduce its own metabolism as well as the metabolism of other drugs.[146] This must be taken into consideration during anesthetic procedures in patients with liver disease, reduced CO states, and right ventricular (RV) heart failure (HF).

Propranolol serum levels of 100 ng/mL produce a maximum β-blocking effect in relation to reducing exercise-induced tachycardia.[139] Propranolol still produces a 50% reduction of exercise-induced tachycardia at serum levels of 12 ng/mL.[147] Reductions in HR with propranolol occur at lower serum levels than depression of myocardial contractility.[148] Accordingly, as drug levels decrease after discontinuation of therapy, reductions in the chronotropic response last much longer than reductions in inotropy.[148] This is an important concept in treating tachycardias in patients with significant ventricular dysfunction and CHF.

The usual intravenous dose of propranolol initially is 0.5 to 1.0 mg titrated to effect. A titrated dose resulting in maximum pharmacologic serum levels is 0.1 mg/kg. The use of continuous infusions of propranolol has been reported after noncardiac surgery in patients with cardiac disease.[149] A continuous infusion of 1 to 3 mg/hr can prevent tachycardia and hypertension but must be used cautiously because of the potential of cumulative effects.

METOPROLOL

Metoprolol was the first clinically used cardioselective β-blocker. Its affinity for β_1-receptors is 30 times higher than its affinity for β_2-receptors as demonstrated by radioligand binding.[150] Metoprolol is lipid soluble, with 50% of the drug metabolized during first-pass hepatic metabolism, and with only 3% excreted renally.[151] Protein binding is less than 10%. Metoprolol's serum half-life is 3 to 4 hours. Because of its lipophilic properties, metoprolol has been shown in animal studies to diffuse into ischemic tissue better than atenolol, a hydrophilic β-receptor blocker.[150]

As with any cardioselective β-blocker, higher serum levels may result in greater incidence of β_2-blocking effects. Metoprolol is administered intravenously in 1- to 2-mg doses, titrated to effect. The potency of metoprolol is approximately one half that of propranolol. Maximum β-blocker effect is achieved with 0.2 mg/kg IV.

ESMOLOL

Esmolol's chemical structure is similar to that of metoprolol and propranolol, except it has a methylester group in the para position of the phenyl ring, making it susceptible to rapid hydrolysis by red blood cell esterases (9-minute half-life).[152] Esmolol is not metabolized by plasma cholinesterase. Hydrolysis results in an acid metabolite and methanol with clinically insignificant levels.[153] Ninety percent of the drug is eliminated in the form of the acid metabolite, normally within 24 hours.[153] A loading dose of 500 μg/kg given intravenously followed by a 50 to 300 μg/kg/min infusion will reach steady-state concentrations within 5 minutes. Without the loading dose, steady-state concentrations are reached in 30 minutes.[153]

Esmolol is cardioselective, blocking primarily β_1-receptors. It lacks ISA and membrane-stabilizing effects and is mildly lipid soluble. Esmolol produced significant reductions in BP, HR, and cardiac index after a loading dose of 500 μg/kg and an infusion of 300 μg/kg/min in patients with CAD, and the effects were completely reversed 30 minutes after discontinuation of the infusion.[154] Initial therapy during anesthesia may require significant reductions in both the loading and infusion doses.

Hypotension is a common side effect of intravenous esmolol. The incidence of hypotension was higher with esmolol (36%) than with propranolol (6%) at equal therapeutic end-points.[155] The cardioselective drugs may cause more hypotension because of β_1-induced myocardial depression and the failure to block β_2 peripheral vasodilation. Esmolol appears safe in patients with bronchospastic disease. In another comparative study with propranolol, esmolol and placebo did not change airway resistance, while 50% of patients treated with propranolol developed clinically significant bronchospasm.[156] Phlebitis may occur at the site of intravenous administration after prolonged infusion.[157]

Esmolol inhibits human plasma cholinesterase during in vitro studies, in which clinically insignificant prolongation of duration of succinylcholine action by esmolol was reported.[158] Digoxin levels may increase slightly with concomitant esmolol administration.[159] In addition, both esmolol and landiolol, a new short-acting β_1-receptor blocker, also suppress the bispectral index during general anesthesia.[160]

LABETALOL

Labetalol is an equal mixture of four stereoisomers with varying α- and β-blocking properties. Labetalol provides selective α_1-receptor blockade and nonselective β_1- and β_2-blockade. The potency of β-adrenergic blockade is 5- to 10-fold greater than α_1-adrenergic blockade.[15,160] Labetalol has partial β_2-agonist effects that promote vasodilation.[161] Labetalol is moderately lipid soluble and is completely absorbed after oral administration.[162] First-pass hepatic metabolism is significant with production of inactive metabolites.[162] Renal excretion of the unchanged drug is minimal. Elimination half-life is approximately 6 hours.[162]

In contrast to other β-blockers, clinically, labetalol should be considered a peripheral vasodilator that does not cause a reflex tachycardia. BP and systolic vascular resistance decrease after an intravenous dose.[163] Stroke volume (SV) and CO remain unchanged, with HR decreasing slightly.[164] The reduction in BP is dose related, and acutely hypertensive patients usually respond within 3 to 5 minutes after a bolus dose of 100 to 250 μg/kg.[165] However, the more critically ill or anesthetized patients should have their BP titrated beginning with 5- to 10-mg intravenous increments. Reduction in BP may last as long as 6 hours after intravenous dosing.

Significant Adverse Effects

CHF can be precipitated by β-adrenergic blockers, especially when other cardiac drugs with myocardial depressant properties are used, such as calcium blockers and disopyramide. β-Blockers blunt the usual reflex in sympathetic activity with these other depressant agents.[166] Similarly, these effects are additive on the conduction system, and heart block can occur. Propranolol reduces the clearance of many drugs that depend on hepatic metabolism by reducing hepatic blood flow (e.g., lidocaine).[167]

β_2-Blocker effects cause bronchospasm and peripheral vasoconstriction, which can exacerbate symptoms in patients with chronic pulmonary disease and peripheral vascular disease. Impotence is a problem in some patients. The lipophilic agents cause many CNS side effects such as depression, sleep disturbances, and fatigue. Hypoglycemia is a significant problem for diabetics.

Sudden withdrawal of β-adrenergic blockers can precipitate a state of enhanced adrenergic activity, resulting in tachycardia, hypertension, arrhythmias, myocardial ischemia, and infarction.[168] Most studies indicated that this period of hypersensitivity occurs from 2 to 6 days after withdrawal of β-blockade. This corresponds to an increase in human lymphocyte β-receptors during this period. Continuing β-receptor blockers before cardiac surgery results in a more stable anesthetic induction, intubation, and sternotomy sequence than performing anesthesia and surgery during a period of withdrawal hypersensitivity.[169,170] Furthermore, reinstitution of small doses of β-adrenergic blockade after cardiac surgery smooths the postoperative course and reduces the incidence of tachyarrhythmias.[171]

Summary

β-Adrenergic blockers are first-line agents in the treatment of myocardial ischemia. These agents effectively reduce myocardial work and oxygen demand. There is growing evidence that β-adrenergic–blocking agents may play a significant role in reducing perioperative cardiac morbidity and mortality in noncardiac surgery.[172]

Calcium Channel Blockers

Calcium channel blockers reduce myocardial oxygen demands by depression of contractility, HR, and/or decreased arterial BP.[173] Myocardial oxygen supply may be improved by dilation of coronary and collateral vessels. Calcium channel blockers are used primarily for symptom control in patients with stable angina pectoris. In an acute ischemic situation, calcium channel blockers (verapamil and diltiazem) may be used for rate control in situations when β-blockers cannot be used. The most important effects of calcium channel blockers, however, may be the treatment of variant angina. These drugs can attenuate ergonovine-induced coronary vasoconstriction in patients with variant angina, suggesting protection via coronary dilation.[174] Most episodes of silent myocardial ischemia, which may account for 70% of all transient ischemic episodes, are not related to increases in myocardial oxygen demands (HR and BP), but rather, intermittent obstruction of coronary flow likely caused by coronary vasoconstriction or spasm.[175] All calcium channel blockers are effective at reversing coronary spasm, reducing ischemic episodes, and reducing NTG consumption in patients with variant or Prinzmetal's angina.[176] Combinations of NTG and calcium channel blockers, which also effectively relieve and possibly prevent coronary spasm, are at present rational therapy for variant angina. β-Blockers may aggravate anginal episodes in some patients with vasospastic angina and should be used with caution.[177] Preservation of CBF with calcium channel blockers is a significant difference from the predominant β-blocker anti-ischemic effects of reducing myocardial oxygen consumption.

Calcium channel blockers have proven effective in controlled trials of stable angina.[178–181] However, rapid-acting dihydropyridines such as nifedipine may cause a reflex tachycardia, especially during initial therapy, and exacerbate anginal symptoms. Such proischemic effects probably explain why the short-acting dihydropyridine nifedipine in high doses produced adverse effects in patients with unstable angina. The introduction of long-acting dihydropyridines such as extended-release nifedipine, amlodipine, felodipine, isradipine, nicardipine, and nisoldipine has led to fewer adverse events. These agents should be used in combination with β-blockers. Some patients may have symptomatic relief improved more with calcium channel blockers than with β-blocker therapy, although at present it is difficult to predict which patients respond better by other than empiric observation.

The causes of unstable angina may involve coronary vasospasm, accelerated atherosclerotic process, or enhanced platelet aggregation with fibrin clot formation. Calcium channel blockers have favorable effects in all three of the processes and are effective in the relief of symptoms of unstable angina.[182] There are no significant clinical differences in the response of patients with unstable angina to β-adrenergic blockers and calcium channel blockers.[183]

Calcium Channel

Calcium channels are functional pores in membranes through which calcium flows down an electrochemical gradient when the channels are open. Calcium channels exist in cardiac muscle, smooth muscle, and probably many other cellular membranes. These channels are also present in cellular organelle membranes such as the sarcoplasmic reticulum (SR) and mitochondria. Calcium functions as a primary generator of the cardiac action potential and an intracellular second messenger to regulate various intracellular events.[184]

Calcium enters cellular membranes through voltage-dependent channels or receptor-operated channels. The voltage-dependent channels depend on a transmembrane potential for activation (opening). Receptor-operated channels either are linked to a voltage-dependent channel after receptor stimulation or directly allow calcium passage through cell or organelle membranes independent of transmembrane potentials.

There are three types of voltage-dependent channels: the T (transient), L (long-lasting), and N (neuronal) channels.[185] The T and L channels are located in cardiac and smooth muscle tissue, whereas the N channels are located only in neural tissue. The T channel is activated at low voltages (−50 mV) in cardiac tissue, plays a major role in cardiac depolarization (phase 0), and is not blocked by calcium antagonists.[186,187] The L channels are the classic "slow" channels, are activated at higher voltages (−30 mV), and are responsible for phase 2 of the cardiac action potential. These channels are blocked by calcium antagonists.[186,187]

As mentioned previously, receptor-operated channels regulate calcium entry through voltage-regulated channels or through channels regulated by the receptor system per se. The β-adrenergic receptor operates an L-type voltage-dependent channel, which is activated by phosphorylation of a protein kinase by cAMP generated by the β-adrenergic receptor.[187] α_1-Receptor stimulation activates a G protein, which causes phospholipase C to hydrolyze phosphatidylinositol diphosphate to diacylglycerol (DAG) and inositol triphosphate (IP_3).[188] DAG activates protein kinase C that likely phosphorylates an L-type channel allowing calcium entry, while IP_3 is a second messenger that interacts with the SR and directly promotes calcium release from the SR through an intracellular calcium channel.[189] A receptor-operated channel may also increase calcium entry stimulated directly by a G protein. Both α_2-receptor and β-receptor stimulation may activate G protein–regulated channels, which are not voltage dependent[190,191] (see Chapter 9).

Calcium channel blockers interact with the L-type calcium channel and are composed of drugs from four different classes: (1) the 1,4-dihydropyridine (DHP) derivatives (nifedipine, nimodipine, nicardipine, isradipine, amlodipine, and felodipine); (2) the phenylalkyl-amines, (verapamil); (3) the benzothiazepines (diltiazem); and (4) a diarylaminopropylamine ether (bepridil).[15] The L-type calcium channel has specific receptors, which bind to each of the different chemical classes of calcium channel blockers.[192] The binding to calcium blocker receptors by dihydropyridine derivatives (nifedipine) is voltage dependent.[193] Calcium channels transform from a closed resting form that can potentially open, to an activated open form, to an inactive conformation that cannot open, and finally back to the closed resting form. Nifedipine binds preferentially to the inactive receptor that has just recently undergone activation and cannot open. Nifedipine essentially acts as a plug to block the channel. Verapamil binds to the L-type channel preferentially when it is active or open.[194] The greater the period of activation of the channel, the more effective is the blockade (use dependent). Any repetitive activity, such as cardiac pacemaker activity, is sensitive to use-dependent agents.

Physiologic Effects

HEMODYNAMIC EFFECTS

Systemic hemodynamic effects of calcium channel blockers in vivo represent a complex interaction among myocardial depression, vasodilation, and reflex activation of the autonomic nervous system (Table 10–5).

Nifedipine, like all dihydropyridines, is a potent arterial dilator with few venodilating effects.[195] Reflex activation of the sympathetic nervous system may increase HR. The intrinsic

Table 10–5 Calcium Channel Blocker Vasodilator Potency and Inotropic, Chronotropic, and Dromotropic Effects on the Heart

	Amlodipine	Diltiazem	Nifedipine	Verapamil
Heart rate	↑/0	↓	↑/0	↓
Sinoatrial node conduction	0	↓↓	0	↓
Atrioventricular node conduction	0	↓	0	↓
Myocardial contractility	↓/0	↓	↓/0	↓↓
Neurohormonal activation	↑/0	↑	↑	↑
Vascular dilatation	↑↑	↑	↑↑	↑
Coronary flow	↑	↑	↑	↑

From Eisenberg MJ, Brox A, Bestawros AN. Calcium channel blockers: An update. Am J Med 116:35, 2004.

Table 10–6 Hemodynamic Effects of Intravenous Administration of Verapamil in 20 Patients With Coronary Artery Disease

	Before Verapamil*	After Verapamil*	Significance (*p*)
Heart rate (bpm)	74 ± 12	75 ± 12	NS
Mean arterial pressure (mm Hg)	94 ± 17	82 ± 13	<.0005
Right ventricular end-diastolic pressure (mm Hg)	4 ± 2	7 ± 2	<.0005
Left ventricular end-diastolic pressure (mm Hg)	12 ± 4	14 ± 4	<.25
Cardiac index (L/min/m^2)	2.8 ± 0.6	3.1 ± 0.7	<.0005
Stroke volume index (mL/m^2)	57 ± 12	63 ± 13	<.025
Systemic vascular resistance (dyne·sec·cm^{-5})	1413 ± 429	1069 ± 235	<.0005
Ejection fraction (%)	55 ± 16	61 ± 18	<.01

*Values are mean ± SD.
NS = Not significant.
Reproduced with permission from Ferlinz J, Easthope JL, Aronow WS: Effects of verapamil on myocardial performance in coronary disease. Circulation 59:313, 1979. Copyright 1979, American Heart Association.

negative inotropic effect of nifedipine is offset by potent arterial dilation, which results in lowering of BP and increase in CO in patients.[196] Dihydropyridines are excellent antihypertensive agents owing to their arterial vasodilatory effects. Antianginal effects result from reduced myocardial oxygen requirements secondary to the afterload-reducing effect and to coronary vascular dilation resulting in improved myocardial oxygen delivery.

Verapamil is a less potent arterial dilator than the dihydropyridines and results in less reflex sympathetic activation. In vivo, verapamil generally results in moderate vasodilation without significant change in HR, CO, or SV[197] (Table 10–6). Intravenous administration of verapamil in the catheterization laboratory causes increases in right ventricular pressure and LVEDP, decreases in systemic vascular resistance, improvement in ejection fraction (EF), and little change in PAPs.[198] Verapamil can significantly depress myocardial function in patients with preexisting ventricular dysfunction.[199]

Diltiazem is a less potent vasodilator and has fewer negative inotropic effects compared with verapamil. Studies in patients reveal reductions in systemic vascular resistance and BPs, with increases in CO, PAWP, and EF[200] (Fig. 10–14). Dil-

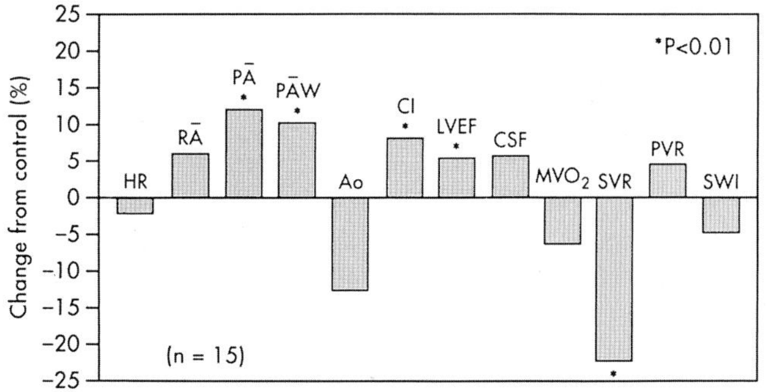

Figure 10–14 Effects of intravenous diltiazem on systemic and coronary hemodynamics and left ventricular ejection fraction in patients with coronary artery disease. (HR = heart rate; R̄A = mean right atrial pressure; P̄A = mean pulmonary artery pressure; P̄AW = mean pulmonary capillary wedge pressure; Ao = mean aortic pressure; CI = cardiac index; LVEF = left ventricular ejection fraction; CSF = coronary sinus flow; MVO_2 = myocardial oxygen consumption; SVR = systemic vascular resistance; PVR = pulmonary vascular resistance; SWI = stroke work index.) (Modified from Josephson MA, Singh BN: Use of calcium antagonists for ventricular dysfunction. Am J Cardiol 55:81B, 1985; and Abrams J: Nitrates. *In* Chatterjee K, Cheitlin MD, Karliner J, et al [eds]: Cardiology: An Illustrated Text/Reference, Vol 1. Philadelphia, JB Lippincott, 1991, pp 2.75–2.90.)

tiazem attenuates baroreflex increases in HR secondary to NTG and decreases in HR secondary to phenylephrine.[201] Regional blood flow to the brain and kidney increases, whereas skeletal muscle flow does not change.[202] In contrast to verapamil, diltiazem is not as likely to aggravate CHF, although it should be used carefully in these patients.[203]

Bepridil is a calcium channel blocker with antianginal, antihypertensive, and type 1 antiarrhythmic properties. The antianginal effects are mediated by a reduced HR and arteriolar dilation. Left ventricular performance may be improved in patients with angina.[204] Because of its effects on myocardial conduction, bepridil is contraindicated in patients with a history of serious ventricular arrhythmias, sick sinus syndrome, second- or third-degree AV block (except when a pacemaker is present), and in patients with congenital prolonged QT interval. Bepridil can cause torsades de pointes in patients with prolonged QT interval. Because of these serious side effects, bepridil should be reserved for patients refractory to other therapy.[205]

CORONARY BLOOD FLOW

Coronary artery dilation occurs with the calcium channel blockers with increases in total CBF (Fig. 10–15). Nifedipine is the most potent coronary vasodilator, especially in epicardial vessels, which are prone to coronary vasospasm. Diltiazem is effective in blocking coronary artery vasoconstriction caused by a variety of agents, including α-agonists, serotonin, prostaglandin, and acetylcholine.[174,206,207]

Calcium channel blockers may also dilate the coronary artery at the stenotic site, thus reducing the pressure gradient across the coronary lesion.[174] Diltiazem preferentially dilates coronary arteries compared with other peripheral vessels.[208] Animal studies demonstrate that nifedipine, verapamil, and diltiazem increase coronary collateral flow distal to coronary ligation in animals and improve subendocardial flow relative to subepicardial flow[209-212] (Fig. 10–16).

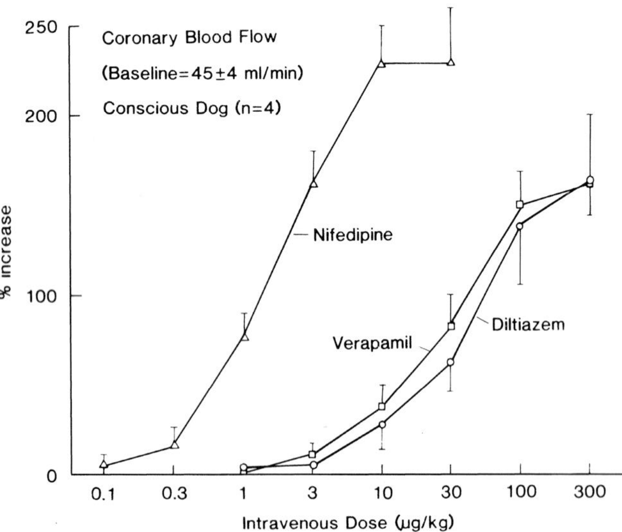

Figure 10–15 Coronary blood flow responses to intravenous diltiazem, nifedipine, and verapamil in the conscious normal dog. In contrast to nitroglycerin and β-blockers, calcium channel blockers increase total coronary flow. Data are mean values ± SE (n = 4). (Reproduced with permission from Millard RW, Grupp G, Grupp IL, et al: Chronotropic, inotropic, and vasodilator actions of diltiazem, nifedipine, and verapamil. A comparative study of physiological responses and membrane receptor activity. Circ Res 52[suppl I]:29, 1983. Copyright 1983, American Medical Association.)

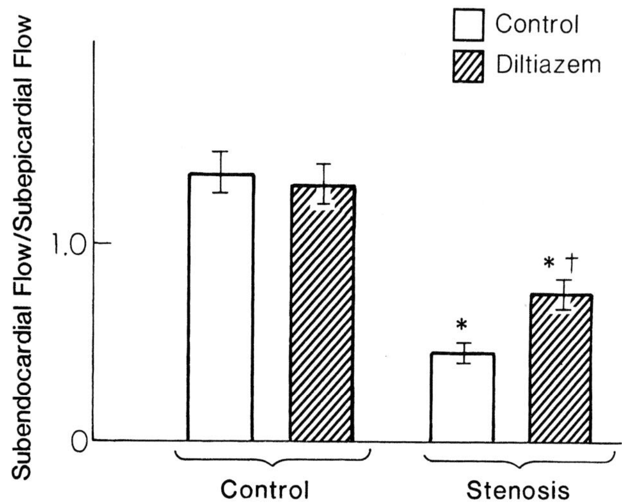

Figure 10–16 The ratio of subendocardial to subepicardial blood flow during resting control conditions and in the presence of proximal stenosis, which prevented arterial inflow from increasing above the preocclusion control after a 10-second coronary artery occlusion in animals. Diltiazem increased subendocardial to subepicardial blood flow ratio in the ischemic area. Values are mean ± SEM. *$P < .05$ compared with measurements during control conditions with unimpeded arterial inflow. †$P < .05$ compared with the control stenosis. (From Bache RJ, Dymek DJ: Effect of diltiazem on myocardial blood flow. Circulation 65[suppl I]:I, 1982. Copyright 1982, American Medical Association.)

ELECTROPHYSIOLOGIC EFFECTS

Calcium channel blockers exert their primary electrophysiologic effects on tissue of the conducting system that is dependent on calcium for generation of the action potential, primarily at the SA and AV nodes. They do not alter the effective refractory period of atrial, ventricular, or His-Purkinje tissue. Diltiazem and verapamil exert these electrophysiologic effects in vivo and in vitro, whereas the dihydropyridines' (nifedipine) electrophysiologic depression is completely attenuated by reflex sympathetic activation. Nifedipine actually can enhance SA and AV node conduction, while verapamil and diltiazem slow conduction velocity and prolong refractoriness of nodal tissue.[213-215] Bepridil is a class I antiarrhythmic, inhibiting both the slow inward Ca^{++} current and the fast inward Na^{+} current. Its use is contraindicated in many patients with electrophysiologic defects (see earlier).

ATHEROSCLEROSIS

Calcium is involved in the generation of atherosclerotic plaque and in damaged atherosclerotic tissue (calcification).[216] Verapamil and nifedipine have been found to have antiatherogenic effects.[216] Nifedipine has been shown to retard angiographic progression of CAD in humans.[217] Diltiazem may also reduce atherosclerotic progression after heart transplantation.[218] Diltiazem suppresses aortic atherosclerosis but not that of coronary arteries, inhibits spontaneous calcinosis in hypertensive rats, and prevents vitamin D–induced calcinosis in arterial elastic tissue.[219-221] Diltiazem also suppresses necrosis of aortic smooth muscle cells by hyperlipidemia serum[222] and intimal thickening in rabbit carotid arteries.[223]

PLATELET AGGREGATION

Calcium antagonists, nitrates, and β-adrenergic blockers all inhibit platelet aggregation. This could be a most important effect of all anti-ischemic drugs, especially in the treatment of

Table 10–7 Properties of Calcium Antagonists in Clinical Use

Drug	Usual Dose	Duration of Action	Side Effects
Dihydropyridines			
Nifedipine	Immediate release: 30 to 90 mg daily orally Slow release: 30 to 180 mg orally	Short Long	Hypotension, dizziness, flushing, nausea, constipation, edema
Amlodipine	5 to 10 mg once daily	Long	Headache, edema
Felodipine	5 to 10 mg once daily	Long	Headache, edema
Isradipine	2.5 to 10 mg twice daily	Medium	Headache, fatigue
Nicardipine	20 to 40 mg 3 times daily	Short	Headache, dizziness, flushing, edema
Nisoldipine	20 to 40 mg once daily	Short	Similar to nifedipine
Nitrendipine	20 mg once or twice daily	Medium	Similar to nifedipine
Miscellaneous			
Bepridil	200 to 400 mg once daily	Long	Arrhythmias, dizziness, nausea
Diltiazem	Immediate release: 30 to 80 mg 4 times daily Slow release: 120 to 320 mg once daily	Short Long	Hypotension, dizziness, flushing, bradycardia, edema
Verapamil	Immediate release: 80 to 160 mg 3 times daily Slow release: 120 to 480 mg once daily	Short Long	Hypotension, myocardial depression, heart failure, edema, bradycardia

Adapted from Gibbons RJ, Chatterjee K, Daley J, et al: ACC/AHA/ACP-ASIM Guidelines for the Management of Patients with Chronic Stable Angina: A report of the American College of Cardiology/American Heart Association Task Force on Practice Guidelines (Committee on the Management of Patients with Chronic Stable Angina). J Am Coll Cardiol 33:2092, 1999.

chronic disease. Calcium is a mediator involved in the release of platelet aggregatory factors, such as ADP, and verapamil inhibits calcium-induced release of these factors.[224] Diltiazem inhibition of platelet aggregation correlates with changes in intracellular calcium levels.[225] In vivo, diltiazem inhibits platelet aggregation after 24 hours in healthy volunteers.[226] Similar antiaggregatory effects of diltiazem were seen in patients with unstable angina, but no inhibitory effect of platelet aggregation was found with verapamil. Diltiazem metabolites are even more effective in inhibiting platelet aggregation than diltiazem.[227]

METABOLIC EFFECTS

Nifedipine may be associated with decreases in serum glucose levels in diabetics, but glucose levels in normal volunteers generally rise slightly with nifedipine and in hypertensive patients with diltiazem.[228,229] Diltiazem reportedly has no effect on insulin, glucagon, growth hormone, or cortisol levels.[230, 231] However, nifedipine apparently delays insulin release in diabetic patients.[231]

Pharmacology

Table 10–7 illustrates pharmacokinetic parameters for the Food and Drug Administration (FDA)-approved anti-ischemic calcium channel blockers.

NIFEDIPINE

Nifedipine was the first dihydropyridine derivative to be used clinically. Other dihydropyridines available for clinical use include nicardipine, isradipine, amlodipine, felodipine, and nimodipine.[232] In contrast to the other calcium channel blockers, nimodipine is highly lipid soluble and penetrates the blood-brain barrier. It is indicated for vascular spasm after intracerebral bleeding.

Nifedipine's oral bioavailability is approximately 70%, with peak plasma levels occurring within 30 to 45 minutes. Protein binding is 95%, and elimination half-life is approximately 5 hours. Nifedipine is available for oral administration in capsular form. The compound degenerates in the presence of light and moisture, preventing commercially available intravenous preparations. Puncture of the capsule and sublingual administration provide an onset of effects in 2 to 3 minutes. Nifedipine GITS (GastroIntestinal Therapeutic System, Procardia XL), a long-acting, controlled-release delivery system, is available for single daily dosing and is now the preferred preparation. It has an onset of action of 20 minutes, with steady-state plasma levels being reached in 48 hours.

NICARDIPINE

Nicardipine is a dihydropyridine agent with a longer half-life than nifedipine and with vascular selectivity for coronary and cerebrovascular beds. Nicardipine may be the most potent overall relaxant of vascular smooth muscle among the dihydropyridines.[233] Peak plasma levels are reached 1 hour after oral administration, with bioavailability of 35%.[234] Plasma half-life is approximately 8 to 9 hours. Although the drug undergoes extensive hepatic metabolism with less than 1% of the drug excreted renally, greater renal elimination occurs in some patients.[235] Plasma levels may increase in patients with renal failure; reduction of the dose is recommended in these patients.[234]

Nicardipine is a potent cerebrovascular vasodilator and may prevent ischemia-related neuronal necrosis in animal studies.[236,237] Marked improvements in CBF occur with nicardipine.[238] Although coronary vasodilation is one explanation, positive inotropic effects with either phosphodiesterase activity or calcium channel agonist (as well as antagonist) activity resulting in autoregulatory increases in blood flow may be an additional mechanism.[239]

VERAPAMIL

Verapamil's structure is similar to that of papaverine. Verapamil exhibits significant first-pass hepatic metabolism, with a bioavailability of only 10% to 20%.[240] One hepatic metabolite, norverapamil, is active and has a potency approximately 20% of that of verapamil.[240] Peak plasma levels are reached within 30 minutes. Bioavailability markedly increases in hepatic insufficiency, mandating reduced doses.[240] Intravenous verapamil achieves hemodynamic and dromotropic effects within minutes, peaking at 15 minutes and lasting up to 6 hours. Accumulation of the drug occurs with prolonged half-life during long-term oral administration.[241]

Verapamil's metabolism is dependent on hepatic blood flow and may decrease in the presence of H_2-receptor blockers. Increased metabolism may occur when hepatic enzyme–inducible agents like phenobarbital are given concomitantly. Seventy percent of verapamil's metabolites are recovered in the urine and 15% in feces.

DILTIAZEM

After oral dosing, the bioavailability of diltiazem is greater than verapamil's, varying between 25% and 50%.[242] Peak plasma concentration is achieved between 30 and 60 minutes, and elimination half-life is 2 to 6 hours.[242] Protein binding is approximately 80%. As with verapamil, hepatic clearance is flow-dependent and major hepatic metabolism occurs with metabolites having 40% of the clinical activity of diltiazem.[243,244] Hepatic disease may require decreased dosing, while renal failure does not affect dosing.[245]

BEPRIDIL

Bepridil is a diarylaminopropylamine calcium channel blocker unrelated in structure to the other calcium channel blockers. Bepridil is available for oral use, with a usual starting dose of 200 mg once daily. Peak concentrations are reached in 2 to 3 hours, and 99% of the drug is bound to plasma proteins. Metabolism is primarily hepatic, with 70% of the metabolized drug excreted in the urine.

Significant Adverse Effects

Most significant adverse hemodynamic effects can be predicted from the calcium channel blockers' primary effects of vasodilation, and negative inotropy, chronotropy, and dromotropy. Hypotension, HF, bradycardia and asystole, and AV nodal block have occurred with calcium channel blockers.[246] These side effects are more likely to occur with combination therapy with β-blockers or digoxin, in the presence of hypokalemia.[246]

Verapamil increases digoxin levels, while diltiazem has variable effects and nifedipine no effect on digoxin levels.[247-249] Cimetidine and ranitidine increase calcium blockers' serum levels either by liver enzyme induction or reductions of hepatic blood flow.[250] The physiologic effects of calcium blockers may be additive to those of anesthetic agents in animal studies, but clinically significant effects are variable.[251,252] The cautious use of intravenous verapamil with a β-adrenergic receptor antagonist is necessary because of the increased risk of AV block or severe myocardial depression.

Paradoxic aggravation of myocardial ischemia may be seen with the short-acting dihydropyridines (nifedipine).[253] This may be secondary to decreased CPP with associated hypotension, selective vasodilation in the nonischemic region (coronary steal), or increased oxygen demand as a result of reflex sympathetic stimulation and tachycardia.

Case reports of a withdrawal syndrome similar to β-blocker withdrawal have been presented. Five of 143 patients had significant ST-segment changes after diltiazem or verapamil withdrawal.[254] Myocardial infarction and coronary spasm have been reported after diltiazem withdrawal.[255,256] One study comparing propranolol to verapamil withdrawal in patients with stable angina found that 2 of 20 patients had severe exacerbation of their angina with propranolol withdrawal, and no patients had hemodynamic or symptomatic evidence of a withdrawal phenomenon with verapamil.[257] Bepridil can prolong the QT_c interval and can produce fatal cardiac arrhythmias (ventricular tachycardia, fibrillation, and torsades de pointes), especially in patients with hypokalemia. Agranulocytosis has also been reported.[205]

Summary

Calcium antagonists provide excellent symptom control in patients with unstable angina. In the absence of β-adrenergic blockade, the short-acting dihydropyridine nifedipine may increase the risk of MI or recurrent angina. When β-adrenergic blockers cannot be used, and HR slowing is indicated, verapamil and diltiazem may offer an alternative.

DRUG THERAPY FOR SYSTEMIC HYPERTENSION

Systemic hypertension, long recognized as a leading cause of cardiovascular morbidity and mortality, accounts for enormous health-related expenditures. Nearly a quarter of the U.S. population has hypertensive vascular disease; however, 30% of these individuals are unaware of their condition and another 30% to 50% are inadequately treated.[258] On a worldwide basis, nearly 1 billion individuals are hypertensive.[259] Based on data from the Framingham Heart study, normotensive patients at age 55 can expect a 90% lifetime risk for subsequent development of hypertension.[260] Furthermore, hypertension management comprises the most common reason underlying adult visits to primary care physicians, and antihypertensive drugs are the most prescribed medication class.[261]

Despite the asymptomatic nature of hypertensive disease, with symptom onset delayed 20 to 30 years after development of systemic hypertension, substantial incontrovertible evidence demonstrates a direct association between systemic hypertension and increased morbidity and mortality. The World Health Organization (WHO) estimates that hypertension underlies one in eight deaths worldwide, making elevated BP the third leading cause of mortality.[259] In fact, hypertension accounts for the single most treatable risk factor for MI, stroke, peripheral vascular disease, CHF, renal failure, and aortic dissection.[258] In prospective randomized trials, over the course of adult lifetimes, successful treatment of hypertension has been associated with 35% to 40% reductions in the incidence of stroke, 50% reductions in CHF, and 25% reductions in MIs.[258,259] Improved treatment of hypertension has been credited with the major reductions in stroke and cardiovascular mortality occurring over the past 30 years in the United States.

Pathophysiologic mechanisms underlying predisposition to hypertension remain, for the most part, unclear. Undoubtedly, both genetic and environmental factors play contributory roles.[262] Concordance for hypertension is greater between mono- or dizygotic twins, and even siblings within a single family, than that observed between unrelated individuals, supporting a genetic component. However, by some estimates genetic predeterminants account for only 30% to 40% of hypertensive disease.[262] As for environmental factors, a direct association between body mass index and hypertension has been reported, and dietary sodium intake is associated with long-term risk for development of hypertension.[263,264]

In most cases, no single reversible mechanism underlying systemic hypertensive disease can be identified—the so-called *primary or essential hypertension*. In a small subset, perhaps 5% of hypertensive patients, a distinct etiology promoting systemic hypertension is identified. The most common etiology underlying *secondary hypertension* is renal insufficiency. Other less common mechanisms include pheochromocytoma, renal artery stenosis, and hypertension resulting from adrenal cortical abnormalities such as primary aldosteronism or Cushing's syndrome. Diagnostic clues suggestive of secondary hypertension include hypertensive disease refractory to medical therapy, unusually abrupt onset with severe associated symptoms, or occurrence of hypertension at a particularly young age.

Definitions for hypertension are somewhat arbitrary, although derived from clinical trials suggesting systemic pressures at which the benefits of treatment outweigh the risk for adverse effects related to antihypertensive therapy. BP varies with normal distribution across the population at large, and aging is associated with progressive increases in systolic pressure. After 50 years of age, reductions in diastolic pressure are commonly observed, resulting in widening of pulse pressure with age. Published evidence suggests that systolic and pulse pressure are better predictors for morbidity and mortality than diastolic pressure.[261] Most recently, the Seventh Report of the Joint National Committee on Prevention, Detection, Evaluation, and Treatment of High Blood Pressure (JNC-7 Report) defined systolic BPs (Table 10–8) exceeding 140 mm Hg and diastolic BPs exceeding 90 mm Hg as stage 1 hypertension. BPs less than 120/80 mm Hg were defined as normal and those in between as consistent with "prehypertension."[258]

Although antihypertensive drug therapy is widely regarded as essential for BPs exceeding 140/90 mm Hg, recent evidence suggests benefits to more aggressive BP reduction for certain patient subsets. The association between systemic BP and cardiovascular risk has been described as a "J-curve", with progressive cardiovascular risk reductions accompanying BP reductions until a critical threshold—after which the potential for myocardial ischemia and/or other organ injury increases.[265]

Risk for cardiovascular disease appears to increase at BPs exceeding 115/75 mm Hg, with a doubling in risk associated with each 20/10-mm Hg increment in systemic pressure.[258] Thus, the most recent JNC 7 report recommends drug therapy for "prehypertensive" disease in patients with "compelling indications" such as chronic renal disease or diabetes. Antihypertensive therapy generally is targeted to achieve systemic BPs of less than 140/90 mm Hg; however, for high-risk patients such as those with diabetes, renal, or cardiovascular disease, lower BP targets are suggested, typically less than 130/80 mm Hg.[258]

Medical Treatment for Hypertension

At present, nearly 80 distinct medications are marketed for treatment of hypertension[261] (Table 10–9). Often, combined therapy with two or more classes of antihypertensive medications may be needed to achieve treatment goals[266] (Table 10–10). Although the specific drug selected for initial therapy now has been deemed less important than in the past, recognition that specific antihypertensive drug classes alleviate end-organ damage, beyond that simply associated with reductions in systemic BP, has led to targeted selection of antihypertensive drug combinations on the basis of coexisting risk factors such as recent MI, chronic renal insufficiency, or diabetes.

Diuretics

Thiazide diuretic therapy comprises the cornerstone of most antihypertensive regimens.[267,268] Three classes of diuretics have

Table 10–8 **Classification and Management of Blood Pressure for Adults Aged 18 Years or Older**

					Management* Initial Drug Therapy	
BP Classification	**Systolic BP* (mm Hg)**		**Diastolic BP* (mm Hg)**	**Lifestyle Modification**	**Without Compelling Indication**	**With Compelling Indication**
Normal	<120	and	<80	Encourage		
Prehypertension	120 to 139	or	80 to 89	Yes	No antihypertensive drug indicated	Drug(s) for the compelling indications†
Stage 1 hypertension	140 to 159	or	90 to 99	Yes	Thiazide-type diuretics for most; may consider ACE inhibitor, ARB, β-blocker, CCB, or combination	Drug(s) for the compelling indications Other antihypertensive drugs (diuretics, ACE inhibitor, ARB, β-blocker, CCB) as needed
Stage 2 hypertension	≥160	or	≥100	Yes	Two-drug combination for most (usually thiazide-type diuretic and ACE inhibitor or ARB or β-blocker or CCB)‡	Drug(s) for the compelling indications Other antihypertensive drugs (diuretics, ACE inhibitor, ARB, β-blocker, CCB) as needed

ACE = angiotensin-converting enzyme; ARB = angiotensin-receptor blocker; BP = blood pressure; CCB = calcium channel blocker.
*Treatment determined by highest BP category.
†Treat patients with chronic kidney disease or diabetes to BP goal or < 130/80 mm Hg.
‡Initial combination therapy should be used cautiously in those at risk for orthostatic hypotension.
Adapted with permission from Chobanian AV, Bakris GL, Black HR, et al. Seventh report of the Joint National Committee on Prevention, Detection, Evaluation, and Treatment of High Blood Pressure: The JNC7 Report. JAMA 289:2560, 2003.

Table 10–9 Oral Antihypertensive Drugs

Drug (Trade Name)	Usual Dose Range (mg/d)	Usual Daily Frequency
Thiazide Diuretics		
Chlorothiazide (Diuril)	125 to 500	1 to 2
Chlorthalidone (generic)	12.5 to 25	1
Hydrochlorothiazide (Microzide, Hydrodiuril†)	12.5 to 50	1
Polythiazide (Renese)	2 to 4	1
Indapamide (Lozol†)	1.25 to 2.5	1
Metolazone (Mykrox)	0.5 to 1.0	1
Metolazone (Zaroxolyn)	2.5 to 5	1
Loop Diuretics		
Bumetanide (Bumex†)	0.5 to 2	2
Furosemide (Lasix†)	20 to 80	2
Torsemide (Demadex†)	2.5 to 10	1
Potassium-Sparing Diuretics		
Amiloride (Midamor†)	5 to 10	1 to 2
Triamterene (Dyrenium)	50 to 100	1 to 2
Aldosterone Receptor Blockers		
Eplerenone (Inspra)	50 to 100	1
Spironolactone (Aldactone†)	25 to 50	1
β-Blockers		
Atenolol (Tenormin†)	25 to 100	1
Betaxolol (Kerlone†)	5 to 20	1
Bisoprolol (Zebeta†)	2.5 to 10	1
Metoprolol (Lopressor†)	50 to 100	1 to 2
Metoprolol extended release (Toprol XL)	50 to 100	1
Nadolol (Corgard†)	40 to 120	1
Propranolol (Inderal†)	40 to 160	2
Propranolol long-acting (Inderal LA†)	60 to 180	1
Timolol (Blocadren†)	20 to 40	2
β-Blockers With Intrinsic Sympathomimetic Activity		
Acebutolol (Sectral†)	200 to 800	2
Penbutolol (Levatol)	10 to 40	1
Pindolol (generic)	10 to 40	2
Combined α-Blockers and β-Blockers		
Carvedilol (Coreg)	12.5 to 50	2
Labetalol (Normodyne, Trandate†)	200 to 800	2
Angiotensin-Converting Enzyme Inhibitors		
Benazepril (Lotensin†)	10 to 40	1
Captopril (Capoten†)	25 to 100	2
Enalapril (Vasotec†)	5 to 40	1 to 2
Fosinopril (Monopril)	10 to 40	1
Lisinopril (Prinivil, Zestril†)	10 to 40	1
Moexipril (Univasc)	7.5 to 30	1
Perindopril (Aceon)	4 to 8	1
Quinapril (Accupril)	10 to 40	1
Ramipril (Altace)	2.5 to 20	1
Trandolapril (Mavik)	1 to 4	1
Angiotensin II Antagonists		
Candesartan (Atacand)	8 to 32	1
Eprosartan (Teveten)	400 to 800	1 to 2
Irbesartan (Avapro)	150 to 300	1
Losartan (Cozaar)	25 to 100	1 to 2
Olmesartan (Benicar)	20 to 40	1
Telmisartan (Micardis)	20 to 80	1
Valsartan (Diovan)	80 to 320	1 to 2
CCBs: Nondihydropyridines		
Diltiazem extended release (Cardizem CD, Dilacor XR, Tiazac†)	180 to 420	1
Diltiazem extended release (Cardizem LA)	120 to 540	1
Verapamil immediate release (Calan, Isoptin†)	80 to 320	2
Verapamil long-acting (Calan SR, Isoptin SR†)	120 to 480	1 to 2
Verapamil (Coer, Covera HS, Verelan PM)	120 to 360	1
CCB: Dihydropyridines		
Amlodipine (Norvasc)	2.5 to 10	1
Felodipine (Plendil)	2.5 to 20	1
Isradipine (Cynacirc CR)	2.5 to 10	2
Nicardipine sustained release (Cardene SR)	60 to 120	2
Nifedipine long-acting (Adalat CC, Procardia XL)	30 to 60	1
Fisoldipine (Sular)	10 to 40	1

Table 10–9 Oral Antihypertensive Drugs—(Continued)

Drug (Trade Name)	Usual Dose Range (mg/d)	Usual Daily Frequency
α_1-Blockers		
Doxazosin (Cardura)	1 to 16	1
Prazosin (Minipress†)	2 to 20	2 to 3
Terazosin (Hytrin)	1 to 20	1 to 2
Central α_2-Agonists and Other Centrally Acting Drugs		
Clonidine (Catapres†)	0.1 to 0.8	2
Clonidine patch (Catapres-TTS)	0.1 to 0.3	1 weekly
Methyldopa (Aldomet†)	250 to 1000	2
Reserpine (generic)	0.05 to 0.25	1
Guanfacine (Tenex†)	0.5 to 2	1
Direct Vasodilators		
Hydralazine (Apresoline†)	25 to 100	2
Minoxidil (Loniten†)	2.5 to 80	1 to 2

CCB = calcium channel blocker.

*In some patients treated once daily, the antihypertensive effect may diminish toward the end of the dosing interval (trough effect). BP should be measured just prior to dosing to determine if satisfactory BP control is obtained. Accordingly, an increase in dosage or frequency may need to be considered. These dosages may vary from those listed in the PDR, 51st ed.

†Available now or soon to become available in generic preparations.

Adapted with permission from Chobanian AV, Bakris GL, Black HR, et al: Seventh report of the Joint National Committee on Prevention, Detection, Evaluation, and Treatment of High Blood Pressure: The JNC7 Report. JAMA 289:2560, 2003.

Table 10–10 Combination Drugs for Hypertension

Combination Type	Fixed-Dose Combination, mg*	Trade Name
ACEIs and CCB	Amlodipine-benazepril hydrochloride (2.5/10, 5/10, 5/20, 10/20)	Lotrel
	Enalapril-felodipine (5/5)	Lexxel
	Trandolapril-verapamil (2/180, 1/240, 2/240, 4/240)	Tarka
ACEIs and Diuretics	Benazepril-hydrochlorothiazide (5/6.25, 10/12.5, 20/12.5, 20/25)	Lotensin HCT
	Captopril-hydrochlorothiazide (25/15, 25/25, 50/15, 50/25)	Capozide
	Enalapril-hydrochlorothiazide (5/12.5, 10/25)	Vaseretic
	Fosinopril-hydrochlorothiazide (10/12.5, 20/12.5)	Monopril/HCT
	Lisinopril-hydrochlorothiazide (10/12.5, 20/12.5, 20/25)	Prinzide, Zestoretic
	Moexipril-hydrochlorothiazide (7.5/12.5, 15/25)	Uniretic
	Quinapril-hydrochlorothiazide (10/12.5, 20/12.5, 20/25)	Accuretic
ARBs and Diuretics	Candesartan-hydrochlorothiazide (16/12.5, 32/12.5)	Atacand HCT
	Eprosartan-hydrochlorothiazide (600/12.5, 600/25)	Teveten-HCT
	Irbesartan-hydrochlorothiazide (150/12.5, 300/12.5)	Avalide
	Losartan-hydrochlorothiazide (50/12.5, 100/25)	Hyzaar
	Olmesartan medoxomil-hydrochlorothiazide (20/12.5, 40/12.5, 40/25)	Benicar HCT
	Telmisartan-hydrochlorothiazide (40/12.5, 80/12.5)	Micardis-HCT
	Valsartan-hydrochlorothiazide (80/12.5, 160/12.5, 160/25)	Diovan-HCT
BBs and Diuretics	Atenolol-chlorthalidone (50/25, 100/25)	Tenoretic
	Bisoprolol-hydrochlorothiazide (2.5/6.25, 5/6.25, 10/6.25)	Ziac
	Metoprolol-hydrochlorothiazide (50/25, 100/25)	Lopressor HCT
	Nadolol-bendroflumethiazide (40/5, 80/5)	Corzide
	Propranolol LA-hydrochlorothiazide (40/25, 80/25)	Inderide LA
	Timolol-hydrochlorothiazide (10/25)	Timolide
Centrally Acting Drug and Diuretic	Methyldopa-hydrochlorothiazide (250/15, 250/25, 500/30, 500/50)	Aldoril
	Reserpine-chlorthalidone (0.125/25, 0.25/50)	Demi-Regroton, Regroton
	Reserpine-chlorothiazide (0.125/250, 0.25/500)	Diupres
	Reserpine-hydrochlorothiazide (0.125/25, 0.125/50)	Hydropres
Diuretic and Diuretic	Amiloride-hydrochlorothiazide (5/50)	Moduretic
	Spironolactone-hydrochlorothiazide (25/25, 50/50)	Aldactazide
	Triamterene-hydrochlorothiazide (37.5/25, 75/50)	Dyazide, Maxzide

BB = β-blocker; ACEI = angiotensin-converting enzyme inhibitor; ARB = angiotensin-receptor blocker; CCB = calcium channel blocker.

*Some drug combinations are available in multiple fixed doses. Each drug dose is reported in milligrams.

Adapted with permission from Chobanian AV, Bakris GL, Black HR, et al. Seventh report of the Joint National Committee on Prevention, Detection, Evaluation, and Treatment of High Blood Pressure: The JNC7 Report. JAMA 289:2560, 2003.

proved efficacious in reducing systemic BP—the thiazide and related sulfonamide compounds, loop diuretics, and potassium-sparing agents. All classes of diuretics initially reduce BP by increasing urinary excretion of sodium, with resultant reductions in plasma volume and cardiac output (CO); however, over a period of 6 to 8 weeks diuretic therapy leads to reductions in SVR—hypothesized to relate to activation of vascular endothelial potassium channels.

Thiazide diuretics remain the first choice medical therapy for the majority of patients with hypertension.[269] Although the natriuretic effect achieved by blockade of sodium and chloride transport in the distal convoluted tubule is relatively weak, thiazide diuretics generally produce 10 mm Hg reductions in BP and have proved efficacious in numerous randomized trials to reduce morbidity and mortality related to hypertensive vascular disease.[261,266]

Loop diuretics, the most potent natriuretics of this class, block sodium, potassium, and chloride transport in the thick ascending loop of Henle. The loop diuretics typically are reserved for patients with renal insufficiency (serum creatinine >2 mg/dL or creatinine clearance <25 mL/min) or CHF; conditions for which thiazide diuretics are relatively ineffective. The short duration of action of loop diuretics (e.g., furosemide: 4 to 6 hours) and greater likelihood for adverse effects limit more widespread application.

Potassium-sparing and aldosterone-receptor–blocking diuretics are among the weakest natriuretics of this class. These drugs act by a variety of mechanisms to inhibit sodium reabsorption from the distal collecting duct while simultaneously reducing urinary potassium excretion. These drugs are most commonly administered in combination with a thiazide diuretic in an effort to reduce the incidence of hypokalemia or for their salutary effects in chronic HF.

Low doses of diuretic are well tolerated; however, common adverse effects related to this drug class include hypokalemia (secondary to renal potassium wasting), impaired glucose tolerance and insulin resistance, hyperuricemia, hypercalcemia, hyperlipidemia, and rarely hyponatremia. The potassium-sparing and aldosterone-receptor–blocking drugs are contraindicated in patients at risk for hyperkalemia—in particular, patients with renal insufficiency.

β-Blockers

β-Adrenergic receptor blockers, which reduce sympathetic stimulation of the heart and vasculature, comprise another common antihypertensive therapy, particularly in settings of CAD or CHF.[270-273] More specifically, β-blockers inhibit myocardial and peripheral β_1-adrenergic receptors to reduce CO. As well, β-blockers reduce renin release from renal juxtaglomerular cells and norepinephrine release by inhibition of prejunctional β_2-adrenergic receptors in the peripheral vasculature. β-Blockers traditionally are classified on the basis of cardioselectivity, lipid solubility, and intrinsic sympathetic activity—with first-generation agents such as propranolol nonselectively blocking both β_1- and β_2-adrenergic receptors. Second-generation agents (e.g., metoprolol or atenolol) exhibit a relatively cardioselective preference for β_1-adrenergic receptor blockade at low doses. Pindolol, a novel β-blocker with intrinsic sympathomimetic activity, stimulates vasodilation by activation of β_2-adrenergic receptors. Combination agents, such as labetalol, provide mixed β- and α_1-adrenergic blocking properties resulting in inhibition of sympathetic activity as well as direct vasodilatory effects.

As with the diuretics, β-blockers typically are well tolerated at low doses; however, the potential for nonselective blockade of β-adrenergic receptors may result in bronchospasm, Raynaud's phenomenon, depression, and HF or heart block. β-Blockers are relatively contraindicated in patients with asthma or reactive airways disease, heart block, or depression. Rapid withdrawal of β-blockers may be associated with rebound adrenergic stimulation and potential for exacerbating myocardial and/or peripheral vascular ischemia; therefore, β-blocker discontinuation must occur by gradual stepped reductions in dose.

Angiotensin-Converting Enzyme (ACE) Inhibitors

ACE inhibitors reduce peripheral vascular resistance by inhibiting conversion of angiotensin I (Ang I) to the highly vasoconstrictive angiotensin II (Ang II).[274] Recent evidence suggests that much of the long-term antihypertensive effect of ACE inhibitors derives from protective effects on bradykinin degradation. Bradykinin, a potent vasodilator under normal conditions, undergoes degradation by the action of angiotensin-converting enzyme. Therefore, ACE inhibition results in increased plasma and tissue concentrations of bradykinin.

Persistent dry cough accounts for the most common adverse effect associated with ACE inhibitor administration. Attributed to elevated concentrations of bradykinin, this side effect frequently leads to discontinuation of ACE inhibitor therapy. Much rarer, although substantially more serious, is the potential for angioedema, again attributable to elevated bradykinin concentrations. Angioedema may occur at any time during therapy, occurs most frequently in African Americans, and may prove fatal due to airway compromise. Increased potential for hyperkalemia occurs in patients with renal insufficiency and those receiving potassium supplements or potassium-sparing diuretics. ACE inhibitors have been reported to induce renal failure in patients with bilateral renal artery stenosis and may potentiate severe intractable hypotension in patients with particularly elevated renin activity (e.g., decompensated HF or intravascular volume depletion). Finally, ACE inhibitors pose a teratogenic risk and are therefore contraindicated in pregnancy.

Angiotensin II Antagonists

Ang II antagonists, or angiotensin-receptor blockers, are perhaps the best tolerated of all current antihypertensive therapies and rapidly are becoming a favored drug therapy for management of hypertensive vascular disease.[274] Ang II antagonists bind and competitively inhibit Ang II AT_1 receptors, thereby directly inhibiting the vasoconstrictive effects of Ang II.[275]

Similar concerns to those of ACE inhibitors exist with regard to administration of Ang II antagonists in the settings of bilateral renal artery stenosis or hypovolemia; however, Ang II antagonists typically are not associated with cough and rarely implicated in angioedema. As with the ACE inhibitors, Ang II antagonists are contraindicated in pregnancy.

Calcium Channel Blockers

Calcium channel blockers, commonly classified as either dihydropyridines or nondihydropyridines, share a common mechanism of action in that they bind various sites on the $\alpha 1$ subunit of the L-type voltage-dependent calcium channel to partially inhibit calcium entry into cells. Although all calcium channel blockers induce arterial vasodilation, the dihydropyridines more frequently induce a reflex tachycardia, whereas the nondihydropyridines (e.g., diltiazem and verapamil) may impair cardiac conduction and/or contractility.[276]

Common side effects reported with calcium channel blockers, and relating to arterial vasodilation, include ankle edema, flushing, and headaches. Nondihydropyridines are most often contraindicated in patients with preexisting HF or cardiac conduction defects due to their potential for precipitating HF and/or heart block. Controversy surrounding the safety of calcium channel blockers as antihypertensive therapy has been substantially negated by recent prospective randomized trials demonstrating the safety and efficacy of long-acting calcium channel blockers for treatment of hypertensive cardiovascular disease.[277-279] Administration of short-acting dihydropyridines (e.g., nifedipine) for rapid control of hypertension has been associated with an increased incidence of acute coronary events and is contraindicated in the acute treatment of severe hypertension.

α_1-Blockers

α_1-Adrenergic blockers competitively inhibit binding of norepinephrine to α_1-adrenergic receptors in the peripheral vasculature, thereby producing vasodilation and reducing BP. Prazosin and its congeners selectively block postsynaptic α_1-adrenergic receptors. Continued activity of the presynaptic α_1-receptors allows for down-regulation of norepinephrine release, limits occurrence of tolerance, and reduces the incidence of compensatory tachycardia. In contrast, phenoxybenzamine, commonly used in the preoperative management of pheochromocytoma, blocks both pre- and postsynaptic α_1-adrenergic receptors.

Adverse effects associated with α_1-blockers include orthostatic hypotension, fluid retention, and reflex tachycardia.[280] Although rarely administered as monotherapy, α_1-blockers continue to prove useful in combination with other antihypertensives due to their lack of metabolic side effects and propensity to dilate urethral smooth muscle, alleviating symptoms of prostatism.[261]

Central α_2-Agonists and Other Centrally Acting Drugs

Centrally acting antihypertensive agents, such as clonidine and methyldopa, stimulate α_2-adrenergic and imidazoline receptors within the central nervous system to reduce sympathetic outflow and SVR. In the case of clonidine, activation of presynaptic α-adrenergic receptors inhibits norepinephrine release and subsequent catecholamine generation.[281] Reserpine differs from the α_2-agonists in that it inhibits reuptake of norepinephrine by storage vesicles in the postganglionic adrenergic neurons depleting norepinephrine. As opposed to the α_2-agonists, reserpine's peripheral effects predominate over central activity.

More widespread use of centrally acting antihypertensives has been limited by central nervous system–mediated adverse effects including sedation, depression, and dry mouth. In addition, autoimmune hemolytic anemia has been reported with methyldopa. Despite these limitations, however, pregnancy-induced hypertension remains a common indication for this agent as long-term use has indicated no adverse effects toward the fetus. Abrupt discontinuation of clonidine frequently results in rebound hypertension, but this effect may be alleviated with transdermal clonidine patches or the longer acting oral agent guanfacine. All centrally acting antihypertensives are contraindicated in the setting of depression.

Direct Vasodilators

Both hydralazine and minoxidil produce potent direct arterial vasodilation mediated by activation of ATP-sensitive potassium channels within the arterial vasculature. The relative lack of effect by direct vasodilators on venous capacitance vessels reduces the potential for orthostatic hypotension. The potency and relatively adverse side effect profile for direct vasodilators limit applications to hypertensive disease resistant to standard pharmacologic approaches, most often in the setting of severe hypertension associated with chronic renal failure.

Both hydralazine and minoxidil cause peripheral edema formation and profound reflex sympathetic activation manifested as tachycardia, headaches, and flushing. Minoxidil, a more potent antihypertensive than hydralazine, frequently is associated with excessive growth of facial hair. Reflex sympathetic responses to direct vasodilators necessitate concomitant administration of diuretics and β-adrenergic blockers to alleviate the potential for fluid retention and myocardial ischemia.

Management of Severe Hypertension

For purposes of characterizing treatment urgency, severe hypertension is characterized as either a hypertensive *emergency* with target organ injury (e.g., myocardial ischemia, stroke, pulmonary edema) or a hypertensive *urgency* with severe elevations in BP not yet associated with target organ damage. Chronic elevations in BP, even when of a severe nature, do not necessarily require urgent intervention and often may be managed with oral antihypertensive therapy on an outpatient basis. In contrast, a hypertensive emergency necessitates immediate therapeutic intervention, most often in an intensive care setting, with intravenous antihypertensive therapy and invasive arterial BP monitoring. In the most extreme cases of *malignant hypertension*, severe elevations in BP may be associated with retinal hemorrhages, papilledema, and evidence of encephalopathy, which may include headache, vomiting, seizure, and/or coma. Progressive renal failure and cardiac decompensation are additional clinical features characteristic of the most severe hypertensive emergencies.

A common therapeutic approach to the hypertensive emergency includes a limited reduction in BP, of perhaps 10%, over the initial 1 to 2 hours of therapy followed by further reductions to a target diastolic pressure (i.e., 110 mm Hg) during the initial 12 hours of therapy. Further reductions in BP to acceptable target levels should proceed over a period of days to minimize potential for inducing ischemic injury in the setting of altered autoregulatory flow to target organ vascular beds.[261,282]

The favored parenteral drug for rapid treatment of hypertensive emergencies remains sodium nitroprusside[261] (Table 10–11). An NO donor, sodium nitroprusside, induces arterial and venous dilation, providing rapid and predictable reductions in systemic BP. Prolonged administration of large doses may be associated with cyanide or thiocyanate toxicity; however, this is rarely a concern in the setting of acute hypertensive emergencies. Although less potent and predictable than sodium nitroprusside, NTG, another NO donor, may be preferable in the setting of myocardial ischemia or after CABG. NTG preferentially dilates venous capacitance beds as opposed to arterioles; however, rapid onset of tolerance limits the efficacy of sustained infusions to maintain BP control.

Table 10–11 **Parenteral Drugs for Treatment of Hypertensive Emergencies***

Drug	Dose	Onset of Action	Duration of Action	Adverse Effects†	Special Indications
Vasodilators					
Sodium nitroprusside	0.25 to 10 µg/kg/min as IV infusion‡	Immediate	1 to 2 min	Nausea, vomiting, muscle twitching, sweating, thiocyanate and cyanide intoxication	Most hypertensive emergencies; caution with high intracranial pressure or azotemia
Nicardipine hydrochloride	5 to 15 mg/hr IV	5 to 10 min	15 to 30 min, may exceed 4 hr	Tachycardia, headache, flushing, local phlebitis	Most hypertensive emergencies except acute heart failure; caution with coronary ischemia
Fenoldopam mesylate	0.1 to 0.3 µg/kg/min IV infusion	<5 min	30 min	Tachycardia, headache, nausea, flushing	Most hypertensive emergencies; caution with glaucoma
Nitroglycerin	5 to 100 µg/min as IV infusion	2 to 5 min	5 to 10 min	Headache, vomiting, methemoglobinemia, tolerance with prolonged use	Coronary ischemia
Enalaprilat	1.25 to 5 mg every 6 hr IV	15 to 30 min	6 to 12 hr	Precipitous fall in pressure in high-renin states, variable response	Acute left ventricular failure; avoid in acute myocardial infarction
Hydralazine hydrochloride	10 to 20 mg IV 10 to 40 mg IM	10 to 20 min IV 20 to 30 min IM	1 to 4 hr IV 4 to 6 hr IM	Tachycardia, flushing, headache, vomiting, aggravation of angina	Eclampsia
Adrenergic Inhibitors					
Labetalol hydrochloride	20 to 80 mg IV bolus every 10 min 0.5 to 2.0 mg/min IV infusion	5 to 10 min	3 to 6 hr	Vomiting, scalp tingling, bronchoconstriction, dizziness, nausea, heart block, orthostatic hypotension	Most hypertensive emergencies except acute heart failure
Esmolol hydrochloride	250 to 500 µg/kg/min IV bolus, then 50 to 100 µg/kg/min by infusion; may repeat bolus after 5 min or increase infusion to 300 µg/min	1 to 2 min	10 to 30 min	Hypotension, nausea, asthma, first-degree heart block, heart failure	Aortic dissection, perioperative
Phentolamine	5 to 15 mg IV bolus	1 to 2 min	10 to 30 min	Tachycardia, flushing, headache	Catecholamine excess

*These doses may vary from those in the PDR, 51st ed.
†Hypotension may occur with all agents.
‡Requires special delivery system.
Reproduced with permission from Chobanian AV, Bakris GL, Black HR, et al. Seventh Report of the Joint National Committee on Prevention, Detection, Evaluation, and Treatment of High Blood Pressure. Hypertension 42:1206, 2003.

Nicardipine, a parenteral dihydropyridine calcium channel blocker, and fenoldopam, a selective dopamine$_1$-receptor antagonist, have been utilized increasingly in select patient populations after coronary artery bypass graft surgery and in the setting of renal insufficiency, respectively.

Several drugs remain available for intermittent parenteral administration in the setting of hypertensive emergencies or urgencies. Enalaprilat, an intravenous ACE inhibitor, has been administered in settings of severe hypertension complicated by HF. Hydralazine, labetalol, and esmolol provide additional therapeutic options for intermittent parenteral injection for hypertensive control. However, with the exception of sodium nitroprusside, the response to parenteral antihypertensive drugs remains unpredictable, posing the potential for delayed achievement of targeted BP goals, or, conversely, severe hypotensive responses. In most cases of emergent or severe hypertension, a diuretic will be required to maintain the prolonged natriuresis needed to sustain an antihypertensive response. In the setting of renal insufficiency or failure, minoxidil and even acute dialysis may be necessary to attain BP control.

Compelling Indications for Specific Antihypertensive Drug Selection

Despite compelling evidence supporting the preferential administration of thiazide diuretics as agents of choice for treatment of hypertension, most patients will require addition

TABLE 10–12 **Clinical Trial and Guideline Basis for Compelling Indications for Individual Drug Classes**

	Recommended Drugs						
Compelling Indication*	**Diuretic**	**BB**	**ACEI**	**ARB**	**CCB**	**Aldo ANT**	**Clinical Trial Basis†**
Heart failure	•	•	•	•		•	ACC/AHA Heart Failure Guideline,[270] MERIT-HF,[271] COPERNICUS,[302] CIBIS,[273] SOLVD,[661] AIRE,[662] TRACE,[663] ValHEFT,[299] RALES,[305] CHARM,[664]
Post–myocardial infarction		•	•			•	ACC/AHA Post-MI Guideline,[1] BHAT,[82] SAVE,[665] Capricorn,[272] EPHESUS,[306]
High coronary disease risk	•	•	•		•		ALLHAT,[279] HOPE,[666] ANBP2,[274] LIFE,[667] CONVINCE,[668] EUROPA,[670] INVEST,[669]
Diabetes	•	•	•	•	•		NKF-ADA Guideline,[283,671] UKPDS,[672] ALLHAT,[279]
Chronic kidney disease			•	•			NKF Guideline,[283] Captopril Trial,[285] RENAAL,[286] IDNT,[284] REIN,[673] AASK,[674]
Recurrent stroke prevention	•		•				PROGRESS,[675]

BB = β-blocker; ACEI = angiotensin-converting enzyme inhibitor; ARB = angiotensin receptor blocker; CCB = calcium channel blocker; Aldo ANT = aldosterone antagonist.

*Compelling indications for antihypertensive drugs are based on benefits from outcome studies or existing clinical guidelines. The compelling indication is managed in parallel with the blood pressure.

†Conditions for which clinical trials demonstrate benefit of specific classes of antihypertensive drugs used as part of an antihypertensive regimen to achieve blood pressure goal to test outcomes.

Reproduced with permission from Chobanian AV, Bakris GL, Black HR, et al: Seventh Report of the Joint National Committee on Prevention, Detection, Evaluation, and Treatment of High Blood Pressure. Hypertension 42:1206, 2003.

of a second nondiuretic antihypertensive drug to achieve desired target BPs.[261] Selection of a complementary antihypertensive agent necessitates a thorough understanding of the mechanisms of action so as to optimize the additive effect of combined therapy. For example, β-blockers, ACE inhibitors, and Ang II antagonists inhibit renin release. Therefore, combinations of these agents are unlikely to achieve a maximal additive antihypertensive response. Similarly, both the diuretics and dihydropyridine calcium channel blockers produce peripheral vasodilation such that combination with other antihypertensive drug classes is likely to prove more efficacious. Increasingly, data derived from ongoing outcomes-based trials of antihypertensive therapy in patients with coexisting diseases suggest that specific antihypertensive drugs reduce morbidity beyond that expected for BP reduction alone[261] (Table 10–12).

For example, in patients with ischemic heart disease, and most especially a recent MI, β-blockers have been demonstrated to reduce mortality and morbidity related to subsequent cardiac events.[82,272,283] Although precise mechanisms remain unclear, reductions in overall sympathetic stimulation and antiarrhythmic effects presumably play contributory roles. In the setting of renal insufficiency, ACE inhibitors and Ang II antagonists delay progression of both diabetic and nondiabetic-associated renal disease.[283-286] Calcium channel blockers have proved efficacious in the setting of peripheral vascular diseases, such as Raynaud syndrome, and α_1-blockers favorably influence symptoms of prostatism. In the setting of hypertension and pregnancy, methyldopa and hydralazine remain preferred antihypertensives for management of chronic hypertension and preeclampsia, respectively.[258]

Perioperative Implications of Hypertension

There is little evidence to suggest that mild-to-moderate degrees of hypertension adversely affect morbidity and mortality in the perioperative setting. In fact, ACC/AHA guidelines state that mild-to-moderate hypertension does not represent an independent risk factor for perioperative cardiovascular complications.[287] However, given the strong association between hypertension and cardiovascular diseases, a preoperative diagnosis of hypertension necessitates preoperative assessment for evidence of target organ damage (e.g., CAD, renal dysfunction, stroke, peripheral vascular disease).[288] In contrast to isolated hypertension, secondary cardiovascular diseases, in many cases, do pose increased risk for perioperative morbidity and mortality. In patients with a preoperative diagnosis of hypertension, an ECG is performed (to assess for evidence of ischemia, prior MI, or left ventricular hypertrophy) and a urinalysis and plasma creatinine determination may be obtained to assess renal function. Specific antihypertensive therapies may necessitate additional evaluations such as assessment of plasma potassium and sodium in patients taking diuretics.

In cases of mild-to-moderate hypertension, few controlled trials assessing the association between preoperative hypertension and perioperative morbidity and mortality are available. Most investigations have been observational in nature with no correction for potentially confounding risk factors. In many cases, the number of study participants has been inadequate to ensure statistical power to assess for relevant associations between outcomes and a preoperative diagnosis of hypertension. Howell and colleagues[282] published a meta-analysis summarizing 30 studies including more than 12,995 patients for whom an association between hypertension and perioperative complications could be assessed. These authors calculated an odds ratio of 1.31, suggesting a slightly increased risk for perioperative cardiovascular complications in patients with preexisting hypertension; however, given limitations of the dataset, the authors further concluded that such a small odds ratio in the setting of a "low perioperative event rate" likely represents a clinically insignificant association between preexisting hypertension and cardiac risk. Other investigators have reported similar small associations between isolated systolic hypertension preoperatively and subsequent perioperative morbidity.

As opposed to the apparently low perioperative risk posed by mild-to-moderate hypertension, cases of severe hypertension (diastolic BP >110 mm Hg) frequently lead to questions as to whether elective surgery should be postponed to allow for titration of antihypertensive therapy to acceptable systemic BPs. Again, although there are little data to support conclusive recommendations regarding acceptable preoperative BPs or the length of antihypertensive therapy necessary to achieve a new "steady state", patients with poorly controlled BP experience more labile BP responses in the perioperative setting with greater potential for hypertensive and/or hypotensive episodes.[288-290] Guidelines published by the ACC/AHA suggest that systemic BPs exceeding 180 mm Hg systolic and/or 110 mm Hg diastolic should be controlled before surgery.[287] In a review, Howell and colleagues concluded that surgery need not be canceled in the setting of severe hypertension; however, a careful preoperative assessment for target organ damage (e.g., cardiovascular, renal, cerebrovascular disease) should be performed preoperatively, and intraoperative arterial pressures should be maintained within 20% of preoperative BPs.[282] At a minimum, in patients with severe hypertension, invasive monitoring of arterial pressure with strict control of perioperative BPs, continuing into the postoperative setting, appears justified; given the predilection for CAD in these patients, perioperative therapy with β-blockers may be indicated.[88,89]

PHARMACOTHERAPY FOR ACUTE AND CHRONIC HEART FAILURE

Chronic HF is one major cardiovascular disorder that continues to increase in incidence and prevalence, both in the United States and worldwide. It affects nearly 5 million persons in the United States, and roughly 550,000 new cases are diagnosed each year.[291] Currently, 1% of those 50 to 59 years of age and 10% of individuals older than 80 have HF.[292] Because HF is primarily a disease of the elderly, its prevalence is projected to increase 2- to 3-fold over the next decade, as the median age of the U.S. population continues to increase.[293] The increasingly prolonged survival of patients with various cardiovascular disorders that culminate in ventricular dysfunction (e.g., patients with CAD are living longer rather than dying acutely with MI) further compounds the HF epidemic. Despite improvements in the understanding of the neurohormonal mechanisms underlying its pathophysiology and remarkable advances made in pharmacologic therapy, HF continues to cost the United States an estimated $38 billion annually in medical expenditures,[294] and it contributes to approximately 250,000 deaths per year.[295] Given the public health impact of the disease and the rapid pace of therapeutic advances, it is essential that the perioperative physician remain aware of contemporary clinical practice for the benefit of those patients with chronic HF presenting to the operating room or intensive care unit.

Accordingly, the pharmacologic management of HF as it relates to guidelines published by the ACC/AHA is reviewed.[270] The focus is primarily on chronic HF associated with left ventricular systolic dysfunction, although chronic HF with preserved systolic function (or diastolic HF), and acute HF are also discussed. For each drug commonly used in clinical practice, the general format of presentation includes whether it alters the progression of myocardial damage (for agents administered chronically), its mechanism(s) of action, current clinical data on trials of its use for HF, and its current place in the treatment of HF. New, nonneurohormonal, pharmacologic options in HF management are also reviewed.

Heart Failure Classification

The ACC/AHA updated guidelines for evaluating and managing HF include a new, four-stage classification system emphasizing both the evolution and progression of the disease (Box 10–6). It calls attention to patients with preclinical stages of HF to focus on halting disease progression. The staging system is meant to complement, not replace, the widely used New York Heart Association (NYHA) Classification, a semi-quantitative index of functional classification that categorizes patients with HF by the severity of their symptoms (Box 10–7). NYHA classification remains useful clinically because it reflects symptoms, which in turn correlate with quality of life and survival.[296] The new classification system for HF, recognizing its progressive course and identifying those who are at risk, reinforces the importance of determining the optimal strategy for neurohormonal antagonism in an attempt to improve the natural history of the syndrome.

Although the pathophysiology of HF has been addressed elsewhere, it is important to mention key concepts as the basis of current pharmacologic therapy. To start, HF remains the final common pathway for CAD, hypertension, valvular heart disease, and cardiomyopathy, in which the natural history results in symptomatic or asymptomatic left ventricular dysfunction (specifically, left ventricular systolic dysfunction for the purposes of this discussion). The neurohormonal responses to impaired cardiac performance (salt and water retention, vasoconstriction, sympathetic stimulation) are initially adaptive but, if sustained, become maladaptive, resulting in pulmonary congestion and excessive afterload. This, in turn, leads to a vicious cycle of increases in cardiac energy expenditure and worsening of pump function and tissue perfusion (Table 10–13). Although the cardiorenal and cardiocirculatory branches of this neurohormonal hypothesis of HF were the original foundation for the use of diuretics, vasodilators, and inotropes, respectively, seminal information in the early 1990s emerged from large, randomized clinical trials that showed ACE inhibitors[297,298] and angiotensin receptor blockers,[299,300] but not most other vasodilators,[301] prolonged survival in patients with HF. In a similar fashion, the use of β-blockers, despite their negative inotropic effects, improved morbidity and mortality in randomized controlled trials.[302-304]

The finding that low-dose aldosterone antagonists added to conventional therapy for HF reduce mortality in patients with severe HF suggests that there is more to the neurohormonal hypothesis of drug efficacy than cardiorenal and hemo-

Table 10–13 Neurohormonal Effects of Impaired Cardiac Performance on the Circulation

Response	Short-term Effects	Long-term Effects
Salt and water retention	Augments preload	Pulmonary congestion, edema
Vasoconstriction	Maintains blood pressure for perfusion of vital organs	Exacerbates pump dysfunction (excessive afterload), increases cardiac energy expenditure
Sympathetic stimulation	Increases heart rate and ejection	Increases energy expenditure

Modified from Katz AM: Heart failure. In Fozzard HA, Haber E, Jennings RB: The Heart and Cardiovascular System: Scientific Foundations. 2nd ed. New York, Raven, 1992, pp 333–353.

BOX 10–6 ***ACC/AHA Four-Stage Classification and Management Recommendations***

Stage A	High risk for developing HF. No structural or functional disorders of the heart. No symptoms of HF.
Examples	Hypertension; coronary artery disease; diabetes mellitus, history of cardiotoxic therapy or alcohol abuse; history of rheumatic heart disease; family history of cardiomyopathy
Treatment	Emphasize prevention: treat hypertension, encourage smoking cessation, treat dyslipidemia, encourage regular exercise; discourage excessive alcohol use or illicit drug use. Consider ACE inhibitor for patients with history of peripheral vascular disease, diabetes mellitus, or hypertension with associated risk factors.
Stage B	Structural heart disease strongly associated with HF. No symptoms of HF.
Examples	Patients with left ventricular hypertrophy or fibrosis, left ventricular dilatation or hypocontractility, asymptomatic valvular heart disease, or previous myocardial infarction.
Treatment	Use all preventive measures listed under stage A. ACE inhibitors and/or β-blockers are recommended for patients with recent or remote history of myocardial infarction. Consider the same for patients with reduced ejection fraction, regardless of previous myocardial infarction history.*
Stage C	Structural heart disease with prior or current symptoms of HF.
Examples	Patients with dyspnea or fatigue due to left ventricular systolic dysfunction; asymptomatic patients who are undergoing treatment for prior symptoms of HF.
Treatment	Use all measures listed in stage A. Drugs recommended for routine use include loop diuretics, ACE inhibitors, β-blockers, and digitalis.* Advise dietary salt restriction.
Stage D	Advanced structural heart disease. Marked symptoms of HF at rest despite maximal medical therapy.
Examples	Patients who are often hospitalized for HF and who cannot be safely discharged from the hospital; patients in the hospital awaiting heart transplantation; patients at home receiving continuous intravenous support for symptom relief or being supported with a mechanical circulatory assist device; patients in a hospice setting for the management of HF. Specialized interventions required.
Treatment	Use all measures listed under Stages A, B, and C. Specialized interventions include mechanical assist devices, heart transplantation, continuous intravenous inotropic infusions for palliation, hospice care.

HF = heart failure; ACE = angiotensin-converting enzyme; LV = left ventricular.
*β-Blockers are relatively contraindicated in patients with bronchospastic pulmonary disease.
Reprinted with permission from Clinical update: New guidelines for evaluating and managing heart failure. Women's Health in Primary Care 5(2):105, 2002.

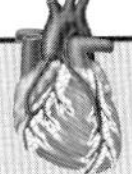

BOX 10–7 ***New York Heart Association Functional Class***

Class I:	No limitation of functional activity. Ordinary physical activity does not cause undue fatigue, palpitation, dyspnea, or anginal pain.
Class II:	Slight limitation of physical activity. Comfortable at rest, but ordinary physical activity results in fatigue, palpitation, dyspnea, or anginal pain.
Class III:	Marked limitation of physical activity. Comfortable at rest. Less than ordinary activity causes dyspnea, palpitation, fatigue, or anginal pain.
Class IV:	Severe limitation in ability to carry on any physical activity without discomfort. Symptoms of heart failure or anginal pain are present even at rest. If any physical activity is undertaken, discomfort increases.

dynamic effects alone.[305,306] Taken together with evidence from basic investigations showing that Ang II is a growth factor and a vasoconstrictor,[307] the clinical data promoted a shift in focus from cardiorenal and cardiocirculatory processes toward cardiac remodeling as the central component in the progression of this neurohormone-mediated cardiac syndrome.[308] The renin-angiotensin-aldosterone system (RAAS), excess sympathetic activity, endothelin, and various cytokines all have been implicated as stimuli of proliferative signaling that contribute to maladaptive cardiac growth. Accordingly, ventricular remodeling, or the structural alterations of the heart in the form of dilatation and hypertrophy (Boxes 10–8 and 10–9), in addition to the counterregulatory hemodynamic responses, lead to progressive ventricular dysfunction and represent the target of current therapeutic interventions (Fig. 10–17).

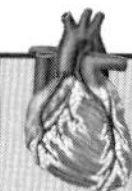

BOX 10–8 ***Pathobiology of Left Ventricular Remodeling***

Alterations in myocyte biology
- Excitation-contraction coupling
- Myosin heavy chain (fetal) gene expression
- β-Adrenergic desensitization
- Hypertrophy
- Myocytolysis
- Cytoskeletal proteins

Myocardial changes
- Myocyte loss
- Necrosis
- Apoptosis

Alterations in extracellular matrix
- Matrix degradation
- Replacement fibrosis

Alterations in left ventricular chamber geometry
- Left ventricular dilation
- Increased left ventricular sphericity
- Left ventricular wall thinning
- Mitral valve incompetence

From Mann DL: Mechanisms and models in heart failure: an approach. Circulation 100:999, 1999.

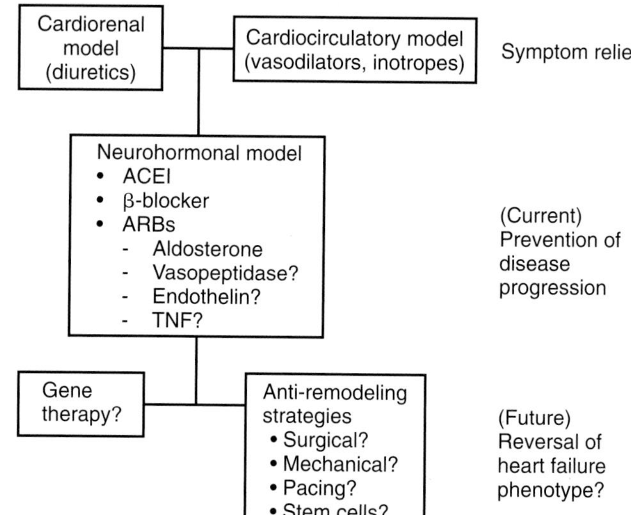

Figure 10–17 Current and future treatments of heart failure. Currently, heart failure therapies are focused on prevention of disease progression with drugs that antagonize neurohormonal systems. Future therapies may involve antagonists of other biologically active systems (e.g., endothelins, TNFα) and antiremodeling strategies that may reverse the heart failure phenotype. ACEI = angiotensin-converting enzyme inhibitor; ARB = angiotensin-receptor blocker; NEP = neutral endopeptidane blocker. (Adapted from Mann DL. Mechanisms and model in heart failure: a combinatorial approach. Circulation 100:999, 1999.)

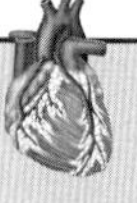

BOX 10–9 ***Mechanical Disadvantage Created by Left Ventricular Remodeling***

- Increased wall stress (afterload)
- Afterload mismatch
- Episodic subendocardial hypoperfusion
- Increased oxygen utilization
- Sustained hemodynamic overloading
- Worsening activation of compensatory mechanisms

From Mann DL: Mechanisms and models in heart failure: an approach. Circulation 100:999, 1999.

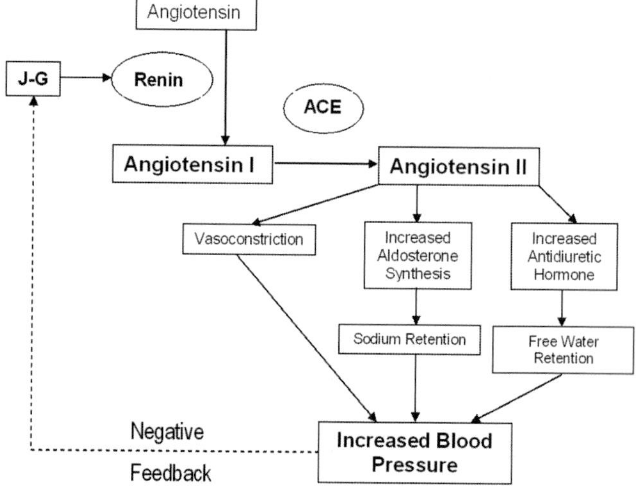

Figure 10–18 Basic pathway of the renin-angiotensin-aldosterone system (RAAS). (From Jaski BE: Basis of Heart Failure: A Problem Solving Approach. Boston, Kluwer Academic Publishers, 2000, with kind permission of Springer Science and Business Media.)

Pathophysiologic Role of the Renin-Angiotensin System in Heart Failure

The renin-angiotensin system (RAS) is one of several neuroendocrine systems that are activated in patients with HF. The RAS is also an important mediator in the progression of HF. In the short term, the juxtaglomerular cells of the kidney release the proteolytic enzyme renin in response to a decrease in BP or renal perfusion (e.g., hemorrhage) generating Ang I from circulating angiotensinogen. ACE cleavage of Ang II from Ang I in the lung produces circulating Ang II. Acutely, Ang II acts as a potent arteriolar and venous vasoconstrictor to return BP and filling pressure to baseline, respectively. Ang II also stimulates the release of aldosterone from the adrenal cortex and antidiuretic hormone from the posterior pituitary. Both contribute to increases in blood volume through their effects on the kidney to promote salt and water reabsorption, respectively. In the long term, elevations in Ang II lead to sodium and fluid retention, and increases in systemic vascular resistance, which contribute to symptoms of HF, pulmonary congestion, and hemodynamic decompensation (Fig. 10–18).

In addition to these cardiorenal and cardiocirculatory effects, most of the hormones and receptors of the RAS are expressed in the myocardium, where they contribute to maladaptive growth or remodeling, a key factor in the progression of HF. Increased expression of mRNA for angiotensinogen, ACE, and Ang II has been identified in the failing human heart.[309] Correspondingly, increased coronary sinus Ang II concentrations were measured in patients with dilated and ischemic cardiomyopathy, signifying a paracrine or autocrine action of the RAS. Moreover, progressive increases in coronary sinus Ang II production correlated with increases in NYHA functional classification of HF.[309] Taken together, these data provide evidence that intracardiac RAS is involved in the evolution of the disease process.

Table 10–14 **Cellular and Physiologic Effects of AT_1 and AT_2 Stimulation That Lead to Tissue Remodeling**

AT_1 Receptor	AT_2 Receptor
Vasoconstriction	Vasodilation
Cell growth and proliferation	Cell growth inhibition/apoptosis
Positive inotropy	Negative chronotropy
Aldosterone secretion	Natriuresis
Catecholamine release	Bradykinin release

Modified from Mann DL: Heart Failure: A Companion to Braunwald's Heart Disease. Philadelphia: Saunders, 2004.

The effects of Ang II on its receptors AT_1 and AT_2 are well appreciated. The AT_1 receptor is involved in several effects that lead to adverse cardiovascular outcomes. Activation of AT_1 receptors promotes aldosterone and vasopressin secretion with concomitant increases in salt and water reabsorption through the kidneys, vasoconstriction, catecholamine release, and cell growth and proliferation of cardiovascular tissue (Table 10–14). Stimulation of AT_2 receptors, on the other hand, results in natriuresis, vasodilation, release of bradykinin and NO, and cell growth inhibition or apoptosis. The Ang II that is formed locally in the heart acts primarily through AT_1 receptors located on myocytes and fibroblasts where it participates in the regulation of cardiac remodeling. Through complex cascades of intracellular signal transduction that activate protein transcription factors within the nucleus initiating the creation of RNA transcripts, the long-term effects of intracardiac Ang II on the AT_1 receptor result in cardiomyocyte hypertrophy, fibroblast proliferation, and extracellular matrix deposition[310] (Fig. 10–19). These processes contribute to progressive left ventricular remodeling and left ventricular dysfunction characteristic of HF.

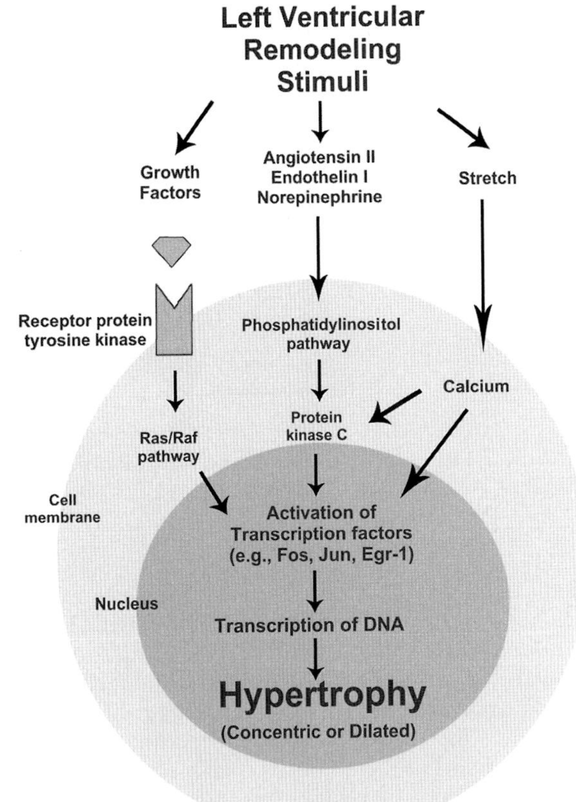

Figure 10–19 Left ventricular remodeling stimuli.

Angiotensin-Converting Enzyme Inhibitors

CLINICAL EVIDENCE

Evidence supporting the beneficial use of ACE inhibitors in HF patients comes from various randomized, placebo-controlled clinical trials (Table 10–15). Initially this class of drugs was evaluated for treatment of symptomatic HF (SOLVD, V-HeFT, CONSENSUS). Patients with NYHA class II to IV HF treated with ACE inhibitors had reductions in mortality ranging from 16% to 31%. Subsequently, ACE inhibitors were also found to improve outcome for asymptomatic patients with left ventricular systolic dysfunction in the following categories: patients with EFs less than 35% due to cardiomyopathy,[310] patients within 2 weeks following MI with EFs less than 40%,[311] and patients presenting within the first 24 hours of MI regardless of EF.[312] Recent results from the Heart Outcomes Prevention Evaluation (HOPE) study have further expanded

Table 10–15 **Selected Clinical Trials of Angiotensin-Converting Enzyme Inhibitors in Heart Failure**

Patient Subset	Heart Failure Stage	Drug	Trial
Heart Failure			
NYHA Class II-III	C	Enalapril	SOLVD (treat); V-HeFT II
NYHA Class IV	D	Enalapril	CONSENSUS I
Asymptomatic Left Ventricular Dysfunction			
Ejection fraction <35%	**B**	**Enalapril**	**SOLVD (prevent)**
Post–myocardial infarction (ejection fraction <40%)	B	Captopril	SAVE
Acute myocardial infarction	B	Captopril Lisinopril	GISSI ISIS-4
Asymptomatic High Risk (history of diabetes mellitus, pulmonary vascular disease, and coronary risk factors)	**A**	**Ramipril**	**HOPE**

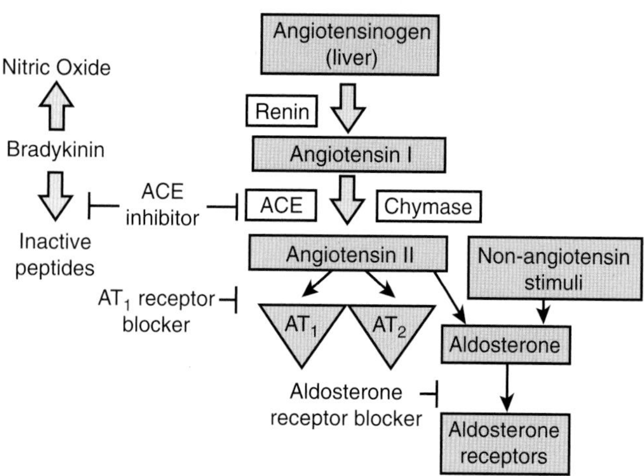

Figure 10–20 Activation of the renin-angiotensin-aldosterone system (RAAS). (Redrawn from Mann DL. Heart Therapy: A Companion to Braunwald's Heart Disease. Philadelphia: Saunders, 2004.)

the indications for this class of agents to include asymptomatic, high-risk patients to prevent new onset HF.[313] In patients with diabetes or peripheral vascular disease and an additional atherosclerotic risk factor, but without clinical HF or systolic dysfunction, ramipril (10 mg/day) reduced the HF risk by 23%. Together, these data endorse the use of ACE inhibitors as first-line therapy for a broad spectrum of patients including those with left ventricular systolic dysfunction, with or without symptoms, and in high-risk patients with vascular disease and/or diabetes, in addition to those with the traditional coronary risk factors. Since the commencement of these trials, the rationale for the use of ACE inhibitors has expanded from a reduction in the progression of clinical HF through ACE inhibitor–mediated vasodilatory action, to acknowledgment that ACE inhibitors also directly affect the cellular mechanisms responsible for progressive myocardial pathology.

MECHANISMS OF ACTION

ACE inhibitors act by inhibiting one of several proteases responsible for cleaving the decapeptide, Ang I, to form the octapeptide, Ang II. Because ACE is also the enzyme that degrades bradykinin, ACE inhibitors lead to increased circulating and tissue levels of bradykinin (Fig. 10–20). ACE inhibitors have several useful effects in chronic HF. They are potent vasodilators through decreasing Ang II and norepinephrine and increasing bradykinin, NO, and prostacyclin.[314] By reducing the secretion of aldosterone and antidiuretic hormone (ADH), ACE inhibitors also reduce salt and water reabsorption from the kidney. ACE inhibitors reduce release of norepinephrine from sympathetic nerves by acting on AT_1 receptors at the nerve terminal. Within tissue, ACE inhibitors inhibit Ang II production and thus attenuate Ang II–mediated cardiomyocyte hypertrophy and fibroblast hyperplasia.[315,316] Clinical evidence supporting an ACE inhibitor–mediated role in cardiac remodeling comes from comparative studies of enalapril versus placebo (SOLVD trial) and enalapril versus hydralazine isosorbide dinitrate (VHeft II trial).[317,318] In a subset of the SOLVD study,[317] the placebo group exhibited left ventricular dilation, whereas the enalapril group exhibited a decrease in chamber size for a given left ventricular pressure. Correspondingly, in the VHeft II trial, survival was better with enalapril versus hydralazine-isosorbide dinitrate, despite improvements in exercise capacity in the latter group, suggesting that mechanisms other than vasodilation contribute to improved survival with ACE inhibitors.[317] Chymase also catalyzes the production of Ang II from Ang I within myocardial tissue. This serine protease has nearly 20-fold greater affinity for Ang I than ACE, and it is not influenced by ACE inhibitors.[319] Accordingly, Ang II receptor blockers (ARBs) may add to the inhibition by ACE inhibitors of angiotensin-promoted progression of HF (see ARB mechanisms).

ACE inhibitors attenuate insulin resistance, a common metabolic abnormality in HF patients, independent of Ang II activity. Ang II receptor antagonists do not attenuate insulin resistance.[320] Both ACE inhibitors and ARBs have been shown to reduce proteinuria, and slow the progression to renal failure in hypertensives (and a common comorbidity in HF patients).[286,321]

DRUG SELECTION/STRATEGY FOR CLINICAL PRACTICE

Treatment guidelines for the use of ACE inhibitors including appropriate starting and target doses, and common side effects are shown in Table 10–16. Adherence to target doses of ACE inhibitors increases the likelihood of reproducing benefits demonstrated in large-scale HF trials (see Table 10–15). According to the AHA/ACC guidelines (see Table 10–13), ACE inhibitor therapy should be initiated in high-risk patients (stage A)—those with diabetes and/or peripheral vascular disease, asymptomatic patients with structural heart disease; those with previous MI and normal EFs (stage B); and all patients with EFs less than 40% (Stages C and D). The relative contraindications for the use of ACE inhibitors include (1) history of intolerance or adverse reactions, e.g., cough, angioedema, neutropenia, and rash; (2) persisting hyperkalemia greater than 5.5 mEq/L that cannot be reduced by diet or diuretic adjustment; (3) symptomatic hypotension, and (4) history of bilateral renal artery stenosis. Small doses of an agent with a short plasma half-life (e.g., captopril) are advo-

Table 10–16 ACE Inhibitors Proved Effective in Heart Failure and/or Left Ventricular Dysfunction

Drug	Half-life (hr)	Dosing Interval	Start Dose (mg)	Target Dose (mg)	Relative Tissue Binding
Captopril	3	3 Times daily	6.25	50	+
Enalapril	11	Twice daily	2.5 to 5	10	+
Lisinopril	12	Once daily	5	20	+
Ramipril	9 to 18	Twice daily	2.5	5	++
Quinapril	2(25)	Twice daily	5	20	+++
Trandolapril	6	Twice daily	1	1 to 2	NA

cated when initiating therapy in patients with marginal BP (systolic BP <90 mm Hg) or reduced renal function (baseline creatinine >2.0 mg/dL). Once it is demonstrated that a patient tolerates inhibition of RAS, dosing should be adjusted to target doses of a longer acting agent. In the ATLAS trial, lisinopril 32.5 to 35 mg/day had greater efficacy than 2.5 to 5.0 mg/day in patients with symptomatic HF and left ventricular systolic dysfunction (EF <35%).[322] Patients receiving "target doses" of ACE inhibitors are less frequently hospitalized than those receiving reduced doses.[323] The importance of differences in tissue binding among the various ACE inhibitors remains unclear.

Angiotensin II Receptor Blockers for Heart Failure

PATHOPHYSIOLOGY/MECHANISM OF ACTION

Although ACE inhibitors reduce mortality, many patients will not tolerate their side effects. ACE inhibitors incompletely antagonize Ang II. These factors have prompted the development of specific Ang II receptor blockers in the pharmacologic treatment of HF[324] (see Fig. 10–20). Non–ACE-generated Ang II within the myocardium contributes to left ventricular remodeling and HF progression through AT_1 receptor effects (see Table 10–14). Selective AT_1 blockers prevent Ang II from acting on the cell, preventing vasoconstriction, sodium retention, release of norepinephrine, and delaying or preventing left ventricular hypertrophy and fibrosis.[325] AT_2 receptors remain unaffected, and their actions, including NO release, remain intact.

CLINICAL EVIDENCE

Outcome benefits from ARBs were first shown in the ELITE I trial, which showed, as a secondary end-point, a significantly reduced risk of sudden death with losartan (4.8%) compared with captopril (8.7%),[326] despite no between-group differences in the primary end-points, renal dysfunction and hypotension. The follow-up ELITE II trial (Table 10–17), although having greater statistical power than ELITE I, failed to confirm that losartan was superior to captopril in reducing mortality in older patients with HF.[327] Moreover, in subgroup analyses, the ELITE II trial patients on preexisting β-blockers tended to have less favorable outcomes with losartan, as opposed to captopril. The two more recent trials, Valsartan in Heart Failure (Val-HeFT) and Candesartan in Heart Failure Assessment in Reduction of Mortality (CHARM), were designed to evaluate whether ARBs plus conventional therapy (including β-blockers, ACE inhibitors, and diuretics) for symptomatic HF provide additional clinical benefit. Although the findings from the Val-HeFT support the use of this ARB in patients with chronic HF who are intolerant to ACE inhibitors, those patients already on ACE inhibitors and β-blockers (93% of their patient population) showed a trend toward an increased risk of death or hospitalization when valsartan was added to their treatment regimen[299] (Fig. 10–21). This is in contrast to the CHARM-Added trial,[328] which showed safety with regard to use of candesartan in combination with ACE inhibitors and β-blockers (15% relative risk reduction in cardiovascular-related mortality or hospitalization), and in patients intolerant to ACE (alternative group), the relative risk reduction in mortality or hospitalization was 23%. On the other hand, patients with EF greater than 40% not receiving ACE inhibition (preserved group) showed no difference in cardiovascular mortality and only a small reduction in HF hospitalizations.[329,330] In the CHARM-overall trial, both cardiovascular-related death and hospitalizations were significantly reduced with candesartan use (relative risk reduction for CV death was 16%).[300]

CLINICAL PRACTICE

ARBs may be used as alternatives to ACE inhibitors for the treatment of patients with symptomatic HF if there are side effects to ACE inhibitors (e.g., persistent cough, angioedema, hyperkalemia, or worsening renal dysfunction) or persistent hypertension despite ACE inhibitors and β-blockers. Since ARBs do not affect bradykinin levels, cough and angioedema are rare side effects. Doses and dosing intervals for ARBs studied in large-scale trials are shown in Table 10–18. Similar to ACE inhibition, ARBs produce dose-dependent decreases in RAP, PCWP, and SVR. Unlike long-term ACE inhibition,[331] these hemodynamic effects and associated increases in cardiac

Table 10–17 Angiotensin Receptor Blocker Trial in Heart Failure

Trial	Agent	Population	Outcome
ELITE II	Losartan 50 mg once daily	Age ≥60 NYHA II–IV EF ≤40%	• Losartan was not better than captopril • No difference in mortality • Losartan was better tolerated • Losartan + β-blocker had worse outcome
Val-HeFT	Valsartan 160 mg twice daily or placebo plus open-label ACEI (93%)	NYHA II–IV EF <40%	• No difference in all-cause mortality • 13% Significant difference in combined morbidity/mortality • HF hospitalization decreased 27% • Most benefit observed in ACEI-intolerant patients (7% of study group) with 45% reduction in combined primary endpoints
CHARM	Candesartan 32 mg once daily versus placebo with or without open-label ACEI Added Preserved Alternative Overall	NYHA II–IV EF ≤40% EF >40% EF ≤40% ACEI intolerant	• 15% Relative risk reduction in all-cause mortality • Mild reduction in HF-related hospitalizations • 23% Relative risk reduction in HF-related mortality or hospitalization • Significant difference in all-cause mortality

ACEI = angiotensin-converting enzyme inhibitor; EF = ejection fraction; HF = heart failure.

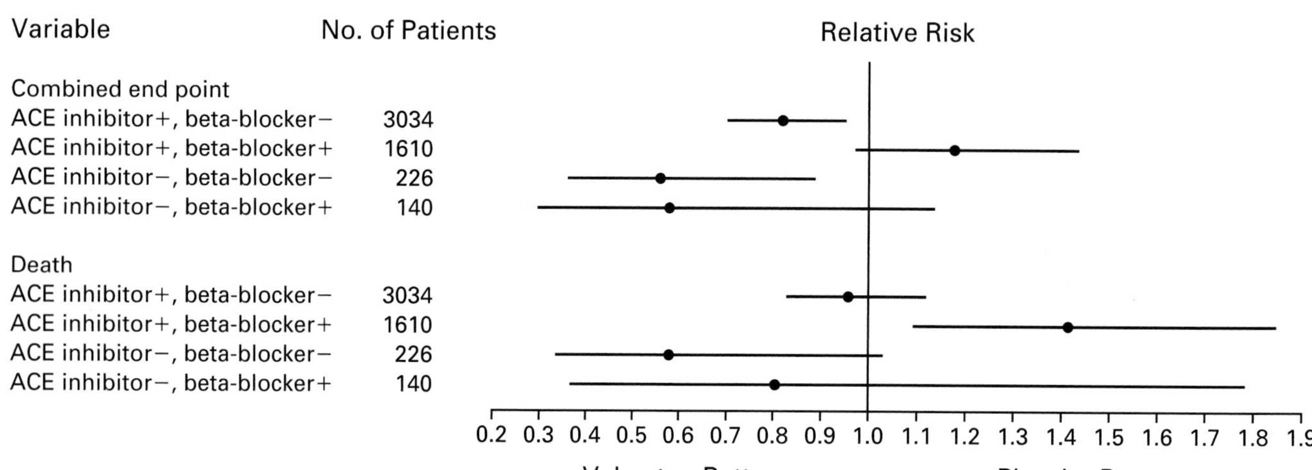

Figure 10–21 Val-HeFT subgroups. Relative risk for combined end-point (cardiovascular-related mortality and hospitalization) and death. (From Cohn JN, Tognoni G; Valsartan Heart Failure Trial Investigators: A randomized trial of the angiotensin-receptor blocker valsartan in chronic heart failure. N Engl J Med 345:1667, 2001.)

Table 10–18 **Angiotensin Receptor Blockers Evaluated in Large-Scale Trials**

Agent	Half-life (hr)	Dosing interval	Initial Dose	Target Dose
Losartan	6 to 9*	Once daily	25	50
Valsartan	9	Twice daily	40	160
Irbesartan	11 to 15	Once daily	75	150
Candesartan	3.5 to 4	Once daily	4	32

index are sustained, and the plasma levels of Ang II remain suppressed with ARB therapy. Nevertheless, there is no convincing evidence that patients with HF benefit from addition of ARBs to standard therapy with ACE I and β-blockers.

Aldosterone Receptor Antagonists

Aldosterone, a mineralocorticoid, is another important component of the neurohormonal hypothesis of HF. Although it was previously assumed that treatment with an ACE inhibitor (or ARB) would block the production of aldosterone in patients with HF, elevated levels of aldosterone have been measured despite inhibition of Ang II [332](see Fig. 10–20). Adverse effects of elevated aldosterone levels on the cardiovascular system include: sodium retention, potassium and magnesium loss, ventricular remodeling (e.g., collagen production, myocyte growth, and hypertrophy), myocardial norepinephrine release, and endothelial dysfunction[333] (Fig. 10–22). Non–Ang II–mediated aldosterone production may, in part, be due to the hypomagnesemia commonly seen in HF patients.[334] Low extracellular Mg^{++}, common in chronic illness as well as a result of loop diuretics, becomes a stimulus for adrenal aldosterone secretion.[335] Extra-adrenal production of aldosterone (e.g., in myocardial and vascular tissue) may also contribute to oxidative, proinflammatory and prothrombotic signaling pathways (NF-κB, AP-1, plasminogen activator inhibitor-1 [PAI-1]) and maladaptive processes such as left ventricular dilatation, perivascular fibrosis, and atherosclerosis.[336-338] Aldosterone produced in the brain increases sympathetic nervous system activity, a central finding in HF.[339]

Given the multiple endocrine and auto/paracrine contributions of aldosterone to the neurohormonal hypothesis of HF, the possibility that aldosterone-receptor antagonism might halt disease progression became an increasingly attractive hypothesis. Besides the traditional mechanisms of mineralocorticoidceptor blockade, including natriuresis, diuresis, and kaliuresis,[334,340] beneficial nonrenal effects of aldosterone antagonism include decreased myocardial collagen formation,[341] increased myocardial norepinephrine uptake and decreased circulating norepinephrine levels,[341] normalization of baroreceptor function, increased HR variability,[342,343] and improved endothelial vasodilator dysfunction and basal NO bioactivity at the vascular level.[344]

CLINICAL EVIDENCE

Two large-scale trials have demonstrated improved outcomes with aldosterone-receptor antagonism in chronic HF. The Randomized Aldactone Evaluation Study (RALES), conducted in more than 1600 symptomatic HF (e.g., stage C, NYHA III-IV) patients, showed the efficacy of spironolactone (26 mg/day) (in combination with standard therapy: ACE inhibitor, loop diuretic with or without digoxin and a β-blocker). Regardless of age, gender, and HF etiology, the treatment group experienced a 30% reduction in risk for all-cause mortality and in cardiovascular-related mortality compared with standard therapy[305] (Fig. 10–23). Because β-blockers were used infrequently in this study (10% to 20%), the role of spironolactone in contemporary management of HF remains unclear. Indeed, studies have reported marked increases in

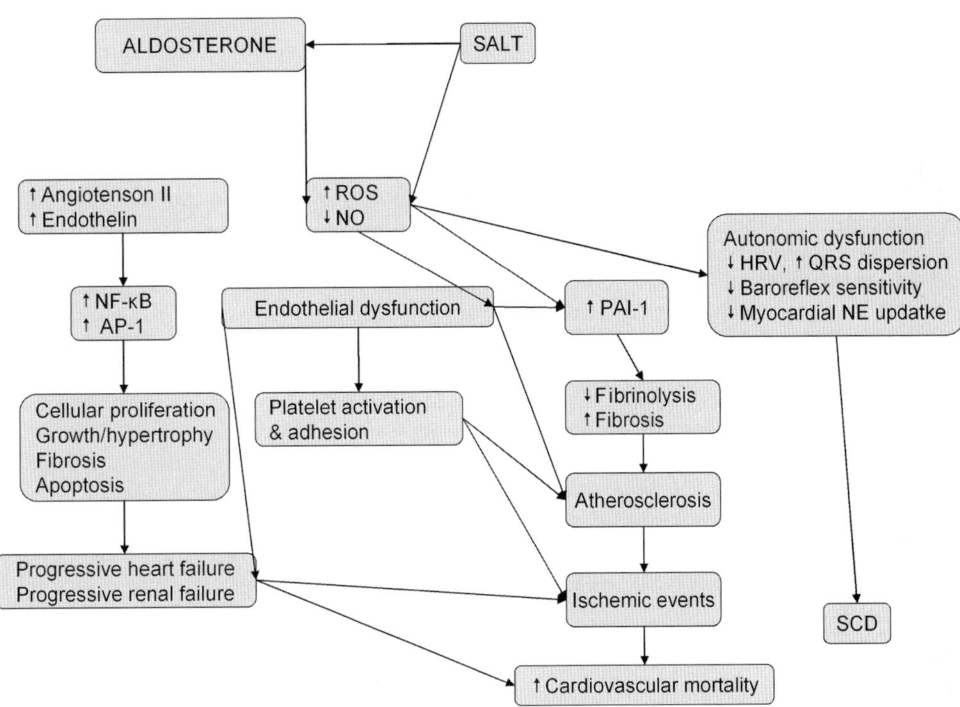

Figure 10–22 Adverse effects of aldosterone and salt on the cardiovascular system. SCD = sudden cardiac death; PAI-1 = plasminogen activator inhibitor-1; ROS = reactive oxygen species; NO = nitric oxide; HRV = heart rate variability. (From Pitt B, Rajagopalan S. In: McMurray JJV, Pfeffer MA, eds. *Heart Failure Updates*. London, England: Martin Dunitz, 2003: 129.)

hospital admission and death related to hyperkalemia subsequent to widespread use of spironolactone.[345] It has been speculated that the K^+-sparing effect of spironolactone and its ability to reduce circulating norepinephrine[346] and increase NO availability[344] may have reduced the propensity for digitalis-related arrhythmias and the subsequent risk of sudden cardiac death reported in the digitalis trial.[347] Eplerenone is a new aldosterone antagonist that lacks some of spironolactone's common side effects.[348] The Eplerenone Post-acute Myocardial Infarction Heart Failure Efficacy and Survival Study (EPHSUS), conducted in more than 6600 patients with symptomatic HF within 3 to 14 days post-MI, showed that eplerenone (25 to 50 mg/day) in combination with ACE inhibitor, loop diuretic, and β-blocker reduced all cause mortality (P = 0.008), death from cardiovascular causes (P = 0.0002), and hospitalization for cardiovascular events.[306]

While there are no large-scale trials examining the use of aldosterone receptor blockade in patients with mild-to-moderate systolic HF (NYHA II-III), there are pilot data suggesting that aldosterone inhibition may also benefit these patients through improvements in endothelial function,[350] exercise tolerance, EF,[349] and attenuation of collagen formation. As noted previously, successful use of aldosterone antagonists mandates that close attention be paid to blood [K^+].[350] Based on these data and the favorable effects of aldosterone antagonism in animal models of infarction,[336] it seems reasonable to expect that aldosterone receptor blockers may find value even in patients with *asymptomatic* systolic left ventricular dysfunction.

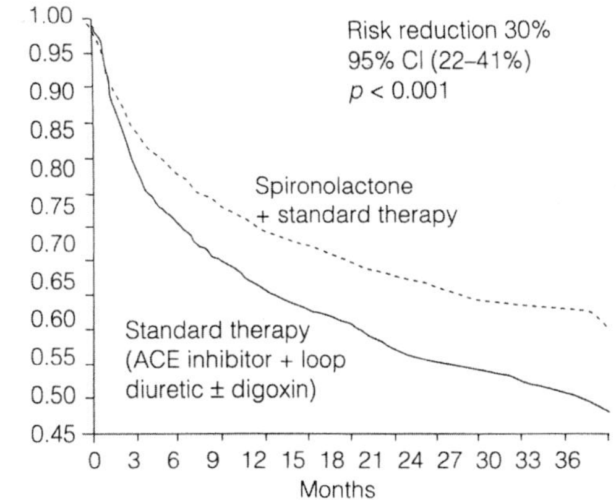

	Risk reduction (95% CI)	*p value*
Cardiac mortality	31% (18–42%)	< 0.001
Progression of heart failure	36% (20–49%)	< 0.001
Sudden cardiac death	29% (5–46%)	0.02
Total mortality	30% (18–40%)	< 0.001

Figure 10–23 The effect of spironolactone on morbidity and mortality in patients with severe heart failure. Randomized Aldactone Evaluation Study Investigators. (From Pitt B, Rajagopalan S. In: McMurray JJV, Pfeffer MA, eds. *Heart Failure Updates*. London, England: Martin Dunitz, 2003: 118.)

CLINICAL PRACTICE

Current evidence supports aldosterone antagonists only for patients with severe symptomatic HF and patients with left ventricular dysfunction after MI.[306] Aldosterone-receptor antagonists should be considered in addition to standard therapy (including ACE inhibitors) for patients with severe HF (NYHA stage IV) caused by left ventricular systolic function. Spironolactone should be initiated at 12.5 mg to 25 mg per day. Patients should have a normal serum K^+ (<5.0 mEq/L) and adequate renal function (creatinine <2.5 mg/dL and creatinine clearance >30). Regular measurement of electrolytes is mandatory to avoid hyperkalemia. In particular, dosages and/or dosing intervals should be reduced during episodes of potential dehydration (e.g., vomiting or diarrhea) and with concomitant use of pharmacologic agents that may predispose to impairments in renal function (e.g., steroidal anti-inflammatory agents). In the RALES trial, there was no significant increase in the incidence of severe hyperkalemia ($K^+ \geq$ 6.0 mEq/L), and only one death related to hyperkalemia (in the placebo arm).[305] This is in marked contrast to a recent Canadian time-series analysis that showed an abrupt increase in hyperkalemia-associated morbidity and mortality in association with the publication of the RALES data.[345] Spironolactone can occupy androgen receptors, leaving unopposed estrogen receptors and, thus, predispose to estrogen-like effects such as painful gynecomastia and menstrual disorders. Because digoxin has estrogen-like properties, its use in combination with spironolactone can also predispose to gynecomastia.[351] This usually does not pose a problem in men since they do not have biologically significant amounts of estrogen. From the EPHESUS data, it appears that the newer aldosterone receptor antagonist, eplerenone, has a lower incidence of hyperkalemia and no evidence of unopposed estrogen receptor–like properties. Unfortunately, eplerenone is *many times more expensive* than spironolactone.

With regard to patients in stage B and C HF on baseline ACE inhibitor and β-blocker therapy, clinicians look forward to findings from large-randomized trials as to whether the addition of aldosterone antagonists to standard therapy will halt progression of the disease.

β-Adrenergic Receptor Antagonists

Sympathetic Nervous System Activation and Its Role in the Pathogenesis of Heart Failure

Activation of the sympathetic nervous system (SNS) (e.g., after MI or with long-standing hypertension), much like increases in RAS activity, contributes to the pathophysiology of HF. In brief, SNS activation leads to pathological left ventricular growth and remodeling. Myocytes thicken and elongate, with eccentric hypertrophy and increases in sphericity. Wall stress is increased by this architecture, promoting subendocardial ischemia, cell death, and contractile dysfunction. Persistent SNS activation leads to altered gene expression with a shift to a fetal-like phenotype (e.g., down-regulation of cardiac a-actin and a-myosin heavy chain and upregulation of fetal forms of β-myosin heavy chain). There is down-regulation of calcium regulatory proteins, including sarcoplasmic reticulum (SR) calcium ATPase, and impairment of contractility and relaxation. The activated SNS can also be harmful to myocyctes directly through programmed cell death. As myocytes are replaced by fibroblasts, the heart function deteriorates from this "remodeling."[352] The threshold for arrhythmias may also be lowered, contributing in a vicious, deteriorating cycle.

How β-Adrenergic Receptor Blockers Influence the Pathophysiology of Heart Failure

In chronic HF, the beneficial effects of long-term β-blockade include improved systolic function and myocardial energetics, and reversal of pathologic remodeling. A shift in substrate utilization from free fatty acids to glucose, a more efficient fuel in the face of myocardial ischemia, may partly explain the improved energetics and mechanics in the failing heart treated with β-blockade.[353] HR, a major determinant of myocardial oxygen consumption, is reduced by β_1-receptor blockade. β-Blockade is also associated with a change in the molecular phenotype of the heart. Systolic dysfunction of individual myocytes is associated with upregulation in gene expression of natriuretic peptides and fetal-like β-myosin heavy chain (MHC), and increased expression of SERCA2 and α-myosin heavy chain (the more efficient, faster, adult isoform).[352] β-Blockade reverses these changes in gene expression with concurrent improvements in left ventricular function.[354] In a dog model of HF, β-blockade also reduces myocyte apoptosis.[355] Taken together, chronic β-blockade reduces the harmful effects of excessive SNS activation of the heart and can reverse left ventricular remodeling.

β-Adrenergic blockade may also limit the disturbance of excitation-contraction (E-C) coupling and predisposition to ventricular arrhythmias associated with HF. In the normal heart, the "fight or flight" response activates the SNS. This in turn stimulates a β-adrenergic receptor signaling pathway in the myocyte that increases phosphorylation of three key components of E-C coupling: the voltage-gated Ca^{2+} channel (VGCC), the SR Ca^{2+} release channel (RYR2), and the Ca^{2+} uptake pathway (phosphorylation of phospholamban reduces inhibition of the Ca^{2+}-ATPase SERCA2a), ultimately resulting in increased contractility.[356] In the low CO failing heart, the SNS is chronically activated. In this hyperadrenergically stimulated heart, ECC becomes maladaptive due to "leaky" Ca^{2+} from the sarcoplasmic reticulum. This "leaky" Ca^{2+} is due to protein kinase A (PKA)-hyperphosphorylated RyR2 channels that cause a diastolic SR Ca^{2+} leak that conspires with reduced SERCA2a-mediated SR Ca^{2+} uptake (due in part to PKA-hypophosphorylated phospholamban that inhibits SERCA2a) to deplete SR Ca^{2+} and contribute to contractile dysfunction of cardiac muscle[357,358] (Fig. 10–24). Depletion of SR Ca^{2+} stores explains, in part, the reduced contractility of failing cardiac muscle. The "leaky" Ca^{2+} may also explain the predisposition to ventricular arrhythmias thought to be initiated by delayed afterdepolarizations.[359] Briefly, the cardiac RyR has a large cytoplasmic structure that serves as a scaffold for

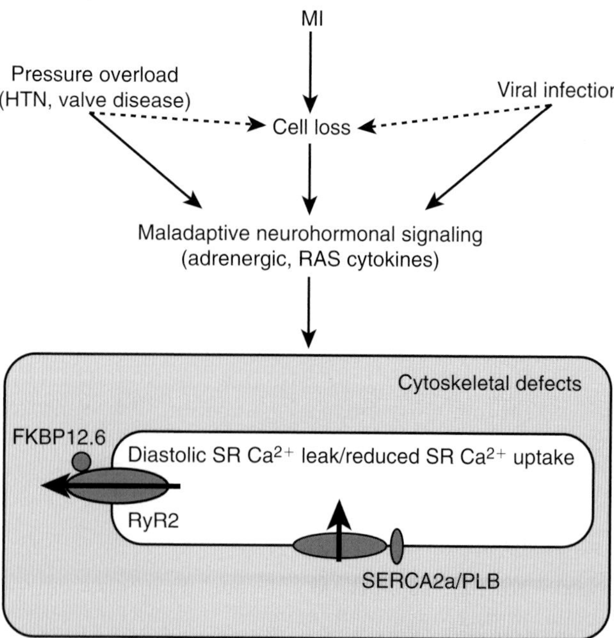

Figure 10–24 Remodeling of extracelluar matrix (MMPs and TIMPs). (Redrawn from Marks AR: A guide for the perplexed: towards an understanding of the molecular basis of heart failure. Circulation 107:1456, 2003.)

modulatory proteins that regulate the function of the channel. Protein kinase A (PKA) phosphorylation of RyR2 dissociates the regulatory protein FKBP 12.6 and regulates the open probability of the channel. In failing hearts, RyR2 is PKA-hyperphosphorylated, resulting in defective channel function due to increased sensitivity of Ca^{2+}-induced activation. Interestingly, studies in animal models of HF show that chronic β-blockade may reverse the PKA hyperphosphorylated state and restore the structure and function of the RYR2 Ca^{2+} release channel.[360,361] Thus, another potential benefit of β-adrenergic receptor blockade in the failing heart may be normalization of E-C coupling, potentially reducing the propensity for arrhythmias.

An evolving concept in the pathophysiology of HF also relates to the negative inotropic action of catecholamines and, specifically, the role of β_3-adrenoreceptors. The failing heart is resistant to exogenous inotropic stimulation compared with hearts that are not failing. This has been attributed to a down-regulation of β_1- and β_2-adrenoreceptors secondary to a hyperadrenergic state.[362,363] However, β_3-adrenoreceptors have been identified in the failing and nonfailing hearts of humans and other mammalian species.[364-366] Unlike the case for β_1- and β_2-adrenoreceptors, β_3-adrenoreceptors are upregulated in HF.[366-368] β_3-Activation decreases contractility. In contrast to the G_s protein–coupled adenylyl cyclase activation and cAMP-dependent pathway of the β_1- and β_2-adrenoreceptors, the negative inotropy that results from stimulation of β_3-adrenoreceptors appears to be due to activation of an NO pathway and an increased intracellular cGMP.[369] However, an understanding of the role of β_3-receptors in the treatment and pathophysiology of HF will await the arrival of specific β_3-adrenoceptor antagonists.

Clinical Evidence

The use of β-blockers in patients with HF was initially accepted with skepticism related to the perceived risk of decompensation from transient negative inotropic effects. However, data from both human and animal studies have shown that β-blockers improve energetics and ventricular function, and reverse pathologic chamber remodeling. Although this beneficial biologic process takes 3 months or more to manifest (Fig. 10–25), it translates into improved outcomes (reduced deaths and hospitalizations) in patients with HF. The available randomized trials show that metoprolol CR/XL, bisoprolol, and carvedilol (in conjunction with ACE inhibitors) reduce morbidity (hospitalizations) in symptomatic, stage C and D (not in cardiogenic shock) HF patients (NYHA II-IV class)[303,304,370,371] (Table 10–19). Although β-blocker therapy is recommended for asymptomatic HF patients (stages A and B), evidence from randomized trials is still lacking.[270]

β-Blockers are classified as being first-, second-, or third-generation drugs based on specific pharmacologic properties. First-generation agents, such as propranolol and timolol, block both β_1- and β_2-adrenoreceptors, are considered nonselective, and have no ancillary properties. Second-generation agents, such as metoprolol, bisoprolol, and atenolol, are specific for the β_1-adrenoreceptor subtype but lack additional mechanisms of cardiovascular activity. Third-generation agents, such as bucindolol, carvedilol, and labetalol, block both β_1- and β_2-adrenoreceptors as well as possessing vasodilatory and other ancillary properties. Specifically, labetalol and carvedilol produce vasodilation by α_1-adrenoreceptor antagonism, while bucindolol produces mild vasodilation through a cGMP-mediated mechanism. Carvedilol increases insulin sensitivity,[372] possesses antioxidant effects,[373] and has β_3-adrenoreceptor selectivity.[374,375] Although it is not entirely clear whether these ancillary properties of the third-generation β-blockers translate into better outcomes as opposed to the second-generation agents, recent findings from the Carvedilol or Metoprolol European Trial (COMET) suggest that the beneficial effect from β-blockers is not a drug "class" effect. The study compared carvedilol (25 mg twice a day) to metoprolol tartrate (50 mg twice a day) in sympto-

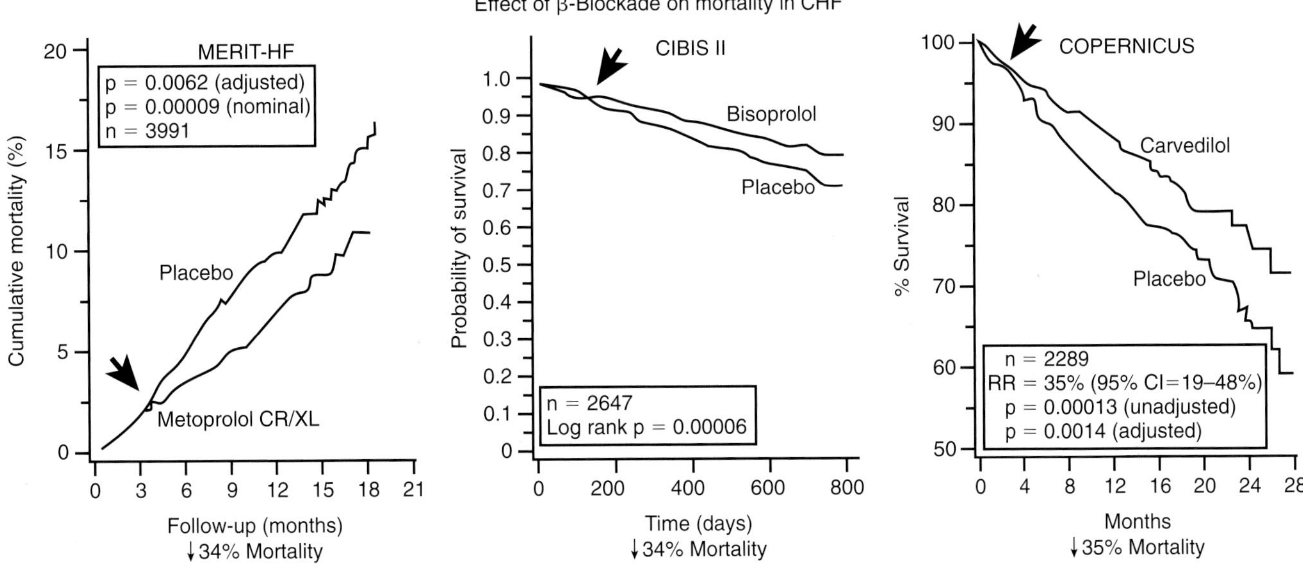

Figure 10–25 Kaplan-Meier analysis of the probability of survival among patients in the placebo and β-blocker groups in the CIBIS-2, MERIT-HF, and COPERNICUS trials. Arrows denote 3-month lag phase of beta-blocker benefit. (From Mann DL: Heart Failure: A Companion to Braunwald's Heart Disease. Philadelphia: Saunders, 2004.)

Table 10–19 Large-Scale Placebo-Controlled Mortality Trials of β-Blockade in Heart Failure

Trial	Agent	HF Severity	Patients (n)	Target Dose (mg)	Effect on All Cause	
					Mortality	Hospitalization
US Carvedilol	Carvedilol	EF ≤35%; NYHA II-III	1094	6.25 to 50 twice daily	↓ 65%	↓ 27%
CIBIS-II	Bisoprolol	EF ≤35%; NYHA III-IV	2647	10 once daily	↓ 34%	↓ 20%
MERIT-HF	Metoprolol CR/XL	EF ≤40%; NYHA II-IV	3991	200 once daily	↓ 34%	↓ 18%
BEST	Bucindolol	EF ≤35%; NYHA III-IV	2708	50 to 100 twice daily	NS	↓ 8%
COPERNICUS	Carvedilol	EF ≤25%; NYHA IV	2289	25 twice daily	↓ 35%	↓ 20%

EF = ejection fraction; NYHA = New York Heart Association.

Table 10–20 β-Blockers Proved Effective in Heart Failure

Agent	Receptor Selectivity	Start Dose (mg)	Target Dose (mg)
Metoprolol CR/XL	β_1	12.5 qd*	200 qd
Bisoprolol	β_1	1.25 qd	5 to 10 qd
Carvedilol	$\beta_1\, \beta_2 \gg \beta_3;\ \alpha_1$	3.125 qd	25 to 50 qd*

*qd = Once a day.

matic patients with EF ≤35% for 58 months and demonstrated that carvedilol reduced the risk of death significantly more than metoprolol tartrate (all-cause mortality risk reduction: 17%, $P = 0.0017$; cardiovascular death risk reduction: 20%, $P = 0.00004$).[376] Specifically, the superiority of carvedilol over metoprolol may reflect the importance of carvedilol's ancillary effects and/or pharmacodynamic (half-life) differences.[377] Findings from the BEST trial confirm that not all β-blockers improve outcome in HF and suggest that the added benefit from carvedilol might not be a β_2-antagonistic effect, as there was no improvement with bucindolol compared with placebo.[371] Whether the selective β_1-specific agents bisoprolol and metoprolol CR/XL exert similar clinical benefits to carvedilol will require additional study. Nonetheless, based on the results of COMET, carvedilol is preferred to conventional metoprolol, not metoprolol CR/XL, for HF treatment.

Clinical Practice

Current evidence suggests that β-blockers should be given to all HF patients with reduced EF (EF <0.40) who are stabilized on oral medications including ACE inhibitors and diuretics, unless there is a contraindication. This recommendation is endorsed by the ACC/AHA[270] and the European Society of Cardiology.[378] Specifically, long-term β-blockade is advocated in stage B-D HF patients in addition to ACE inhibition to limit disease progression and reduce mortality. Patients with ongoing decompensation (e.g., requiring intravenous inotropic or vasodilator therapy), overt fluid retention, or symptomatic hypotension should not receive β-blockers. There is no apparent decline in safety or efficacy when β-blockers are given to diabetics with HF. The long-term benefit of β-blocker therapy in patients with coexisting chronic obstructive pulmonary disease is uncertain, as these patients have been excluded from the major clinical trials.

The three agents with clinical trial evidence for improved morbidity and mortality in patients with HF are carvedilol, metoprolol CR/XL, and bisoprolol. Starting doses of β-blockers should be small to minimize worsening of HF symptoms, hypotension, and bradycardia. The dose should be doubled every 1 to 2 weeks, as tolerated, until target doses shown to be effective in large trials are achieved (Table 10–20). Although it is recommended that β-blocker therapy be continued indefinitely in patients with HF, if it is to be electively stopped, a slow downtitration is preferred. Acute withdrawal of β-blocker therapy in the face of high adrenergic tone may result in sudden cardiac death.[379] The adverse effects of β-blocker therapy include fatigue, dizziness, hypotension, and bradycardia. Because the absolute risk of adverse events is small compared with the overall risk reduction of cardiovascular death, few patients have been withdrawn from β-blocker therapy.[380] A practical guide to the use of β-blockers in HF patients has been published by McMurray et al.[381]

Adjunctive Drugs

In addition to ACE inhibitors and β-blockers, diuretics and digoxin are often prescribed for patients with left ventricular systolic dysfunction and symptomatic HF.

Diuretics

For most patients, volume status should be optimized prior to introduction of β-blockers and ACE inhibitors. Patients with pulmonary congestion often will require a loop diuretic in addition to standard therapy. Diuretics relieve dyspnea, decrease heart size and wall stress, and correct hyponatremia of volume overload. However, overly aggressive and especially unmonitored diuretic therapy can lead to metabolic abnormalities, intravascular depletion, hypotension, and neurohormonal activation. Loop diuretics inhibit tubular reabsorption of sodium along the ascending limb of the loop of Henle. Furosemide also reduces preload by increasing vascular capacity. Dosing recommendations and kinetic data for the commonly used loop diuretics are provided in Table 10–21. Common side effects of loop diuretics include electrolyte depletion (Na^+, K^+, Mg^+, Ca^{2+}, Cl^-), prolonged action of nondepolarizing muscle relaxants, hyperglycemia and insulin

Table 10–21 Loop Diuretics

Drug	Equivalent Doses	Initial Dose	Maximal Dose	Onset (IV)	Diuresis Peak	Duration
Furosemide	40 mg	10 to 40 mg/day	240 mg twice a day	5 min	90 min	4 to 6 hr
Bumetanide	1 mg	0.5 to 1.0 mg/day	5 mg once a day	5 min	75 to 95 min	4 to 6 hr
Torsemide	20 mg	50 mg/day	200 mg twice a day	10 min	60 min	12 hr
Ethacrynic acid*	25 mg	100 mg twice a day	100 mg twice a day	5 min	90 min	12 hr

*No longer available in the United States.

resistance. Less common side effects include skin rash, hyperuricemia, and ototoxicity.

Digoxin

Digoxin continues to be useful for patients with symptomatic HF and left ventricular systolic dysfunction despite receiving ACE inhibitor, β-blocker, and diuretic therapy. Digoxin is the only positive inotropic drug approved for the management of chronic HF. Its indirect mechanism of positive inotropy begins with inhibition of the myocardial sarcolemmal Na^+-K^+-ATPase, resulting in increased intracellular Na^+. This, in turn, prompts the Na^+/Ca^{++} exchanger to extrude Na^+ from the cell, increasing intracellular [Ca^{++}]. The increased Ca^{++} now available to the contractile proteins increases contractile function.[382] Besides its inotropic effects, digoxin has important vagotonic and sympatholytic effects. In atrial fibrillation, digoxin slows the rate of conduction at the AV node. In HF patients it reduces sympathetic efferent nerve activity to the heart and peripheral circulation through direct effects on the carotid sinus baroreceptors.[383] Digoxin increases HR variability, an additional beneficial action on autonomic function in the HF patient.[384] Although these properties are beneficial in controlling the ventricular rate in atrial fibrillation, digoxin has only a narrow therapeutic/toxicity ratio. Digoxin toxicity is dose dependent and modified by concurrent medications (non–potassium-sparing diuretics) or conditions (renal insufficiency, myocardial ischemia). Ventricular arrhythmias consequent to digoxin toxicity may be caused by calcium-dependent afterpotentials. In patients with intoxication and life-threatening arrhythmias, purified anti-digoxin FAB fragments from digoxin-specific antisera provide a specific antidote.[382]

The efficacy of digoxin for symptomatic HF was shown in randomized, controlled trials. The Digitalis Investigators Group (DIG) trial, enrolling more than 6500 patients with an average follow-up of 37 months, showed that digoxin reduced the incidence of HF exacerbations. Although the study showed no difference in survival in patients with EF less than 45% receiving either digoxin or placebo, the combined end-point of death or hospitalization for HF was significantly reduced in patients who received digoxin (27% versus 35%; relative risk, 0.72; 95% confidence interval, 0.66 to 0.79).[347] Efficacy of digoxin in patients with mildly symptomatic HF was shown in pooled results from the Prospective Randomized Study of Ventricular Function (PROVED) and the Randomized Assessment of Digoxin and Inhibitors of Angiotensin-Converting Enzyme (RADIANCE) trials. Patients randomized to digoxin withdrawal had an increased likelihood of treatment failure compared with those who continued to receive digoxin, suggesting that patients with left ventricular systolic dysfunction benefit from digoxin (or, at least, do *not* benefit from digoxin withdrawal), even when they have only mild symptoms.[385,386] Accordingly, digoxin is recommended for symptomatic HF unless contraindicated. Together with ACE inhibitors, β-blockers, and diuretics, digoxin should be added to the therapeutic armamentarium. Ideally, serum digoxin concentration should remain between 0.7 and 1.1 ng/mL. In the elderly patient with renal insufficiency, severe conduction abnormalities, or acute coronary syndromes, even a low dose of 0.125 mg/day should be used with extra caution.

Other Pharmacologic Therapies for Chronic Heart Failure Management

Anticytokines

In addition to the RAAS and the SNS, an increasing number of other vasoactive mediators and growth factors have been implicated in the progression of HF. Production of inflammatory cytokines (including tumor necrosis factor-α [TNFα] and interleukin (IL)-6) is increased in HF patients, and increased blood concentrations of these cytokines have been associated with poor short-term and long-term prognoses.[387] The value of anti-TNFα therapy with Etanercept, a TNFα receptor fusion protein, has been studied in two trials: RENAISSANCE (Randomized Etanercept North American Strategy to Study Antagonism of Cytokines) and RECOVER (Research into Etanercept: Cytokine Antagonism in Ventricular Dysfunction) and in the combined analysis, RENEWAL (Randomized Etanercept Worldwide Evaluation). However, the trials were terminated prematurely after an interim data analysis showing lack of benefit. Etanercept had no effect on clinical status and had no effect on the death or HF hospitalization end-points.[388] Accordingly, inhibition of anti-proinflammatory cytokines remains only a potential therapy for HF.

Endothelin-Receptor Antagonists

The endothelin system may also contribute to the progression of HF. Plasma levels of endothelin-1 (ET-1) are increased in patients with HF.[389] ET-1 produces vasoconstriction of the systemic, renal, pulmonary, and coronary vasculature, remodeling of the myocardium (including myocardial and vascular fibrosis), and neurohormonal activation and has proarrhythmic and negative inotropic effects. Once the central role of endothelin in pathogenesis and beneficial effect of endothelin antagonists in treating experimental HF were defined, clinical studies with endothelin antagonists began.[390,391] To date, the clinical efficacy of endothelin receptor-antagonists (e.g., Bosentan, Enrasentan, and Darusentan) have been investigated in four clinical trials, REACH-1, ENCOR, ENABLE and EARTH.[392-394] However, in none of these trials was there a significant difference between endothelin-receptor antagonists and placebo with regard to clinical status, all-cause mortality, or HF-related hospitalizations.

Vasopeptidase Inhibitors

In opposition to the endogenous vasoconstrictor systems (Ang II, the adrenergic system, ET-1, vasopressin, and aldosterone) are the endogenous vasodilator systems, including NO, endothelium-derived hyperpolarizing factor, prostaglandins, adrenomedullin, and natriuretic peptides. These vasodilating mediators not only reduce BP and improve sodium and water excretion, but they also reduce growth and fibrosis, inhibit coagulation, and reduce inflammation. However, in HF there is an imbalance that favors vasoconstriction. Accordingly, the concept of neutral endopeptidase inhibition (the major enzymatic pathway for degradation of natriuretic peptides) for the treatment of chronic HF led to two large-scale, randomized, controlled trials, OCTAVE and OVERTURE, that compared the use of omapatrilat to ACE inhibition.[395,396] Although there was no statistically significant advantage with omapatrilat regarding total mortality, the secondary end-point of cardiovascular death or HF hospitalizations was reduced in the omapatrilat group (hazard ratio 0.91; 95% confidence interval, 0.82 to 0.98; $P = 0.012$). Concerns regarding the side effect profile of omapatrilat, e.g., angioedema, however, will limit its use in the armamentarium of HF treatment.

Future Therapy

Among the promising nonpharmacologic therapies for the management of HF are the implantable defibrillators and biventricular pacemakers. In the COMPANION trial (The Comparison of Medical Therapy, Pacing, and Defibrillation in Heart Failure), cardiac-resynchronization therapy with a pacemaker combined with an implantable defibrillator significantly decreased the likelihood of death from or hospitalization for HF when compared with conventional pharmacologic therapy[397] (see Chapters 4, 13, and 25).

Stem cell therapy is another potential treatment of HF. Stem cell therapy has shown promise in the treatment for ischemic heart disease both in the laboratory and in small clinical studies.[398] Autologous bone marrow and peripheral blood stem cells transplanted in patients with acute MI improved cardiac function.[399] However, until double-blind, randomized controlled trials are performed, the true benefit of this innovative treatment remains unknown.

Management of Acute Exacerbations of Chronic Heart Failure

Patients with chronic HF, despite good medical management, may experience episodes of pulmonary edema or other signs of acute volume overload.[400] These patients may require hospitalization for intensive management if diuretics fail to relieve their symptoms. Other patients may experience exacerbations of HF associated with acute myocardial ischemia or infarction, worsening valvular dysfunction, infections (including myocarditis), or failure to maintain an established drug regimen. Fonarow et al[401] described a risk stratification system for in-hospital mortality in acutely decompensated HF using data from a national registry. Low-, intermediate-, and high-risk patients with mortality ranging from 2.1% to 21.9% were identified using BUN, creatinine, and systolic BP on admission. These patients will require all the standard medications, as outlined in previous sections, and may also require infusions of vasodilators or positive inotropic drugs.

Vasodilators

Intravenous vasodilators have long been used to treat the symptoms of low CO in patients with decompensated chronic HF. In general, vasodilators reduce ventricular filling pressures and systemic vascular resistance, while increasing SV and CO. NTG is commonly used for this purpose and has been studied in numerous clinical trials.[400] It is often initially effective at relatively small doses (20 to 40 μg/min) but frequently requires progressively increasing doses to counteract tachyphylaxis. NTG is associated with dose-dependent arterial hypotension.[402]

Nesiritide

Brain natriuretic peptide (BNP) is a 32-amino acid peptide that is mainly secreted from the cardiac ventricles.[403] In normal healthy subjects, BNP concentrations in blood increase with age and are greater in females than males. Physiologically, BNP functions as a natriuretic and diuretic. It also serves as a counterregulatory hormone to Ang II, norepinephrine, and endothelin by decreasing the synthesis of these agents and by direct vasodilation.

As the clinical severity of HF increases, the concentrations of BNP in blood also increase.[403] As a result, measurements of BNP in blood have been used to evaluate new onset of dyspnea (to distinguish between lung disease and HF). BNP concentrations in blood increase with decreasing left ventricular EF, therefore measurements of this mediator have been used to estimate prognosis. BNP concentrations decline in response to therapy with ACE inhibitors, Ang II antagonists, and aldosterone antagonists.

In addition, recombinant BNP has been released as a drug (nesiritide), indicated for patients with acute HF and dyspnea with minimal activity. Nesiritide produces arterial and venous dilatation through increasing cyclic GMP. Nesiritide does not increase HR, and has no effect on cardiac inotropy. It has a rapid onset of action and a short elimination half-life (15 minutes). In clinical studies, loading doses have ranged from 0.25 to 2 μg/kg and maintenance doses have ranged from 0.005 to 0.03 μg/kg/min. Studies have shown that nesiritide reduces symptoms of acute decompensated HF similarly to NTG, without development of acute tolerance.[404] Patients receiving nesiritide experienced fewer adverse events than those receiving NTG.[405] However, the mortality rate at 6 months was higher in the patients receiving nesiritide than in the NTG group. Compared with dobutamine, nesiritide was associated with fewer instances of ventricular tachycardia or cardiac arrest.[406]

Inotropes

Positive inotropic drugs, principally dobutamine or milrinone, have long been used to treat decompensated HF, despite the lack of data showing an outcome benefit to their use.[400] In the past, some chronic HF patients would receive intermittent infusions of positive inotropic drugs as part of their maintenance therapy. Small studies consistently demonstrate improved hemodynamic values and reduced symptoms following administration of these agents to patients with HF. Studies comparing dobutamine to milrinone for advanced decompensated HF showed large differences in drug costs, favoring dobutamine, and only small hemodynamic differences, favoring milrinone.[407]

Nevertheless, placebo-controlled studies suggest that there may be no role whatsoever for discretionary administration of positive inotropes to patients with chronic HF.[408] In this study, 951 hospitalized patients with decompensated chronic HF who did not require intravenous inotropic support were assigned to receive a 48-hour infusion of either milrinone or saline. Meanwhile, all patients received ACE inhibitors and diuretics as deemed necessary. Total hospital days did not differ between groups; however, those receiving milrinone were significantly more likely to require intervention for hypotension or to have new atrial arrhythmias. A subanalysis of these results found that patients suffering from ischemic cardiomyopathy were particularly subject to adverse events from milrinone (a 42% incidence of death or rehospitalization versus 36% for placebo).[409]

At the present, positive inotropic drug support can be recommended only when there is no alternative. Thus dobutamine and milrinone continue to be used to treat low CO in decompensated HF but only in selected patients.

Alternate Therapies

When drug treatment proves unsuccessful, HF patients may require invasive therapy, including ventricular assist devices, biventricular pacing, coronary bypass with or without surgical remodeling, or even cardiac orthotopic transplantation. These treatment options are beyond the scope of this chapter[410] (see Chapters 4, 12, 13, 19, 25, 26, and 27).

Low-Output Syndrome

Acute HF is a frequent concern of the cardiac anesthesiologist, particularly at the time of separation from cardiopulmonary bypass (CPB). The new onset of ventricular dysfunction and a low CO state after aortic clamping and reperfusion is a condition with more pathophysiologic similarity to cardiogenic shock than to chronic HF, and is typically treated with positive inotropic drugs, vasopressors (or vasodilators), if needed, and/or mechanical assistance.[411,412] The latter more commonly takes the form of intra-aortic balloon counterpulsation and less commonly includes one of the several available ventricular assist devices (see Chapters 27, 28, 31, and 33).

Causes

Most patients undergoing cardiac surgery with CPB experience a temporary decline in ventricular function, with a recovery to normal function in a period of roughly 24 hours. Thus, pathophysiologic explanations must acknowledge the (usual) temporary nature of the low-output syndrome after CPB. Most likely, this results from one of three processes, all related to inadequate oxygen delivery to the myocardium: acute ischemia, hibernation, or stunning. All three processes would be expected to improve with adequate revascularization and moderate doses of positive inotropic drugs, consistent with the typical progress of the cardiac surgery patient. All three processes would be expected to be more troublesome in patients with pre-existing chronic HF, pulmonary hypertension, or arrhythmias.

Risk Factors for the Low-Output Syndrome After Cardiopulmonary Bypass

The need for inotropic drug support after CPB can often be anticipated based on data available in the preoperative medical history, physical examination, and imaging studies. In a series of consecutive patients undergoing elective CABG, it was observed that increasing age, decreasing left ventricular EF, female sex, cardiac enlargement (on the chest radiograph), and prolonged duration of CPB were all associated with an increased likelihood that the patient would be receiving positive inotropic drugs on arrival in the intensive care unit.[413] Similarly, in a study of patients undergoing cardiac valve surgery, it was found that increasing age, reduced left ventricular EF, and the presence of CAD all increased the likelihood that a patient would receive positive inotropic drug support.[414] The lack of a between-sex difference in the likelihood of inotropic drug support after cardiac valve surgery was consistent with there being no between-sex difference in pathophysiology of valve disease, unlike the between-sex difference in pathophysiology of CAD. This latter study also illustrated another important risk factor: practitioner bias. In this study from a single cardiac surgical unit, some anesthesiologists were more likely to administer positive inotropes than others, even after a statistical adjustment for other risk factors. Such differences are even more pronounced when one cardiac surgical unit is compared with another. In a survey of 40 cardiac surgical units participating in a University Health System Consortium benchmarking project of nonemergent coronary bypass surgery, use of positive inotropic drugs ranged almost linearly and continuously from 5% to 100% of patients.

Specific Drugs for Treating the Low-Output Syndrome

While all positive inotropic drugs increase the strength of contraction in noninfarcted myocardium, mechanisms of action differ. These drugs can be divided into those that increase cyclic AMP (directly or indirectly) for their mechanisms of action and those that do not. The agents that do not depend on cyclic AMP form a diverse group, including cardiac glycosides, calcium salts, calcium sensitizers, and thyroid hormone. In contrast to chronic HF, cardiac glycosides are not used for this indication due to their limited efficacy and narrow margin of safety. Calcium salts continue to be administered for ionized hypocalcemia and hyperkalemia, common occurrences during and after cardiac surgery. Increased $[Ca^{++}]$ in buffer solutions bathing cardiac muscle in vitro unquestionably increase inotropy. However, despite long-standing contrary opinions, available studies suggest that doses of $CaCl_2$ from 5 to 10 mg/kg do not increase cardiac index (CI) in patients recovering from cardiac surgery.[415,416] Calcium sensitizers, specifically levosimendan, function by binding to troponin C in a calcium-dependent fashion. Thus, levosimendan does not impair diastolic function since its affinity for troponin C declines with $[Ca^{++}]$ during diastole. Although several reports have described the successful use of levosimendan in patients recovering from CABG, clinical experience with this agent remains limited, and there is no consensus as to how and when this agent should be used, relative to other, better established agents.[417,418]

Intravenous thyroid hormone (T_3, or liothyronine) has been studied extensively as a positive inotrope in cardiac surgery. There are multiple studies supporting the existence of euthyroid "sick" syndrome with persistent reduced concentrations of T_3 in blood after cardiac surgery in both children and adults.[415] There are also data suggesting that after ischemia and reperfusion, T_3 increases inotropy faster than and as potently as isoproterenol.[418] Nevertheless, randomized controlled clinical trials have failed to show efficacy of T_3 after CABG.[419,420]

The cyclic AMP–dependent agents form the mainstays of positive inotropic drug therapy after cardiac surgery. There are two main classes of agents: the phosphodiesterase (PDE) inhibitors and the β-adrenergic receptor agonists. There are many different phosphodiesterase inhibitors in clinical use around the world, including enoximone, inamrinone, milrinone, olprinone, and piroximone. Comparisons among the agents have failed to demonstrate important hemodynamic differences.[421] Reported differences relate to pharmacokinetics and rare side effects, typically observed with chronic oral administrations during clinical trials. All members of the class produce rapid increases in contractile function and CO, and decreases in systemic vascular resistance. The effect on BP is variable, depending on the pretreatment state of hydration and hemodynamics; nevertheless, the typical response is a small decrease in BP. There is either no effect on HR or a small increase. Inamrinone and milrinone have been shown to be effective, first-line agents in patients with reduced preoperative left ventricular function.[422,423] In one of the few studies in which outcome has been assessed after use of positive inotropic agents, it was confirmed that "prophylactic" use of milrinone in children undergoing correction of congenital heart disease improved outcomes in terms of length of stay and incidence of low-output syndrome.[424] Milrinone, the most commonly used member of the class, is most often dosed at a 50 μg/kg loading dose and 0.5 μg/kg/min maintenance infusion. It is often given in combination with a β-adrenergic receptor agonist.

Among the many β-adrenergic receptor agonists, the agents most often given to patients recovering from cardiac surgery are dopamine, dobutamine, and epinephrine. Dopamine has long been assumed to have dose-defined receptor specificity. At small doses (0.5 to 3 μg/kg/min), it is assumed to have an effect mostly on dopaminergic receptors. At intermediate doses, β-adrenergic effects are said to predominate; and at doses of 10 μg/kg/min or greater, α-adrenergic receptor effects predominate. Nevertheless, the relationship between dose and blood concentration is poorly predictable, even in normal volunteers, as was shown by MacGregor et al.[425] This makes it unlikely that the dose-response relationship is as consistent as has been described in textbooks for the past 20 years. Moreover, dopamine is a relatively weak inotrope that has a predominant effect on HR rather than on SV.[426]

Dobutamine is a selective β-adrenergic receptor agonist. Most studies suggest that it causes less tachycardia and hypotension than isoproterenol.[427,428] It has been frequently compared with dopamine, where dobutamine's greater tendency for pulmonary and systemic vasodilation is evident.[426] Dobutamine has a predominant effect on HR, compared with SV, and as the dose is increased more than 10 μg/kg/min there are further increases in HR without changes in SV.[429]

Epinephrine is a powerful adrenergic agonist, and, like dopamine, demonstrates differing effects depending on the dose. At small doses (10 to 30 ng/kg/min), despite an almost pure β-adrenergic receptor stimulus, there is almost no increase in HR.[416,430] Clinicians have long assumed that epinephrine increases HR more than dobutamine administered at comparable doses. Nevertheless, in patients recovering from cardiac surgery, the opposite is true: dobutamine increases HR more than epinephrine![430]

Other β-adrenergic agonists are used in specific circumstances. For example, isoproterenol is often used after cardiac transplantation to exploit its powerful chronotropy and after correction of congenital heart defects to exploit its pulmonary vasodilatory effects.[431] Norepinephrine is exploited to counteract profound vasodilation.[432] Outside of North America, dopexamine, a weak dopaminergic and β-agonist with a pronounced tendency for tachycardia, is sometimes used.[433]

Left Atrial Drug Administration

Based on an appeal to "common sense," clinicians faced with severe cardiac depression in a severely ill patient undergoing cardiac surgery would sometimes administer potentially "vasoconstricting" agents (for example, epinephrine or norepinephrine) into the left heart circulation (via a left atrial catheter) to avoid adverse effects on the pulmonary vascular resistance. Fullerton et al have confirmed the usefulness of this approach in showing that left atrial administration of epinephrine produces a greater CO and a more reduced pulmonary artery pressure than the same dose of epinephrine administered into the right atrium.[434]

Assist Devices

A small fraction of patients undergoing cardiac surgery develop acute HF refractory to drug treatment. For these patients, available options include intra-aortic balloon counterpulsation, extracorporeal membrane oxygenation (or extracorporeal carbon dioxide elimination), and right- or left-heart assist devices either as "destination therapy" or as a bridge to transplantation.[410] The interested reader is referred to Chapters 26 and 27 in this textbook for details.

Pharmacologic Treatment of Diastolic Heart Failure

Abnormal diastolic ventricular function is a common cause of clinical HF. As many as one in three patients presenting with clinical signs of chronic HF have a normal or near-normal EF (≥40%). The risk of diastolic HF increases with age, approaching 50% in patients over 70 years old.[435] Diastolic HF is also more common in females, and patients with hypertension or diabetes mellitus. Although the prognosis of patients with diastolic HF is better than for systolic HF, 5% to 8% versus 10% to 15% annual mortality, respectively, the complication rate is the same.[436] The one year readmission rate for patients with isolated diastolic HF approaches 50%.[435] In the chronic state, abnormal increases in systolic BP and afterload may contribute to an impaired Frank-Starling response and the resultant symptoms of exercise intolerance. Because this syndrome carries substantial morbidity (exercise intolerance, hospital admissions) and mortality, and results in substantial annual health care expenditures, pharmacotherapy of diastolic HF represents one of the current frontiers of clinical cardiovascular medicine.

In contrast to the large randomized trials that have led to the treatment guidelines for systolic HF, there are few randomized, double-blind, placebo-controlled, multicenter trials performed in patients with diastolic HF. Consequently, the guidelines are based on clinical experience, small clinical studies, and an understanding of the pathophysiologic mechanisms. The general approach to treating diastolic HF has three main components. First, treatment should reduce symptoms, primarily by lowering pulmonary venous pressure during rest and exercise by reducing left ventricular volume, maintaining atrial-ventricular synchrony, and increasing the duration of diastole by reducing HR. Second, treatment should target the underlying causes of diastolic HF. Specifically, ventricular remodeling should be reversed by controlling hypertension, replacing stenotic aortic valves, and treating ischemia. Third, treatment should target the underlying

Table 10–22 **Diastolic Heart Failure Treatments**

Goal	Management Strategy	Drugs/Recommended Doses
Reduce the Congestive State	Salt restriction Diuretics (avoid reductions in cardiac output) ACE inhibitors Angiotensin II receptor blockers	<2 g of sodium/day Furosemide, 10 to 120 mg Hydrochlorothiazide, 12.5 to 25 mg Enalapril, 2.5 to 40 mg Lisinopril, 10 to 40 mg Candesartan, 4 to 32 mg Losartan, 25 to 100 mg
Target Underlying Cause Control hypertension Restore sinus rhythm Prevent tachycardia Prevent/treat ischemia Treat aortic stenosis	Antihypertensive agents (<130/80) Cardioversion of atrial fibrillation Atrioventricular sequential pacing β-Blockers, calcium channel blockers Morphine, nitrates, oxygen, aspirin Angioplasty or revascularization? Aortic valve replacement	β-Blockers, ACE inhibitors, all receptor blockers according to published guidelines Atenolol, 12.5 to 100 mg; metoprolol, 25 to 100 mg; diltiazem, 120 to 540 mg
Target Underlying Mechanisms Promote regression of hypertrophy and prevent myocardial fibrosis	(Theoretical) Renin-angiotensin axis blockade	Enalapril, 2.5 to 40 mg Lisinopril, 10 to 40 mg Captopril, 25 to 150 mg Candesartan, 4 to 32 mg Losartan, 50 to 100 mg Spironolactone, 25 to 75 mg Eplerenone, 25 to 50 mg

ACE = angiotensin-converting enzyme.
Adapted from Aurigemma GP, Gaasch WH: Clinical practice. Diastolic heart failure. N Engl J Med 351:1097–1105, 2004.

mechanisms that are altered by the disease processes, mainly neurohormonal activation. Drug treatment of diastolic HF with respect to these three goals is shown in Table 10–22.

Many of the drugs used to treat systolic HF are also used to treat diastolic HF. However, the reason for their use and the doses used may be different for diastolic HF. For instance, in diastolic HF β-blockers are used to increase the time of diastolic filling whereas in systolic HF, β-blockers are used to reverse heart remodeling (e.g., carvedilol). In fact, metoprolol-CR/XL may be a better β-blocker choice than carvedilol for diastolic HF as too low a BP (as a consequence of carvedilol) may be detrimental for the diastolic HF patient. Similarly, diuretic and NTG doses for diastolic HF are usually much smaller than for systolic HF, as the diastolic HF patient is very sensitive to large reductions in preload. Calcium channel blockers are not a part of the armamentarium in systolic HF treatment but *may* be beneficial in diastolic HF through effects on rate control, specifically the long-acting dihydropyridine class of calcium channel blockers. With the exception of rate control in chronic atrial fibrillation, digoxin is not recommended for diastolic HF.

Ongoing clinical trials and the recently completed CHARM-Preserved trial focus on "mechanism-targeted" therapy for HF patients with preserved systolic function (Table 10–23). Two of the trials (CHARM and I-PRESERVE) examined the effects of treatment with angiotensin-receptor blockade, the PEP-CHF and Hong Kong Diastolic Heart Failure trials examined the effects of ACE-I, the SENIORS trial examined the role of β-blockers, and the MCC-135 trial examined the influence of modulation of calcium homeostasis at the sarcoplasmic reticulum and cellular membrane.

In 1999, a small trial showed that losartan, an angiotensin-receptor antagonist, improved exercise capacity in patients with diastolic HF.[437] The CHARM-Preserved Trial data indicate that treatment with the angiotensin-receptor antagonist candesartan reduces hospitalization rates but does not alter mortality in patients with diastolic HF.[330] In theory, the use of ACE inhibitors should be beneficial for patients with diastolic dysfunction by causing regression of hypertrophy, reduction of systemic BP, and prevention or modification of cardiac remodeling. Likewise, aldosterone antagonists have been proposed for use in patients with diastolic dysfunction because of their antifibrotic and antiremodeling effects.[305,306] Preliminary findings from ongoing studies suggest that aldosterone antagonists may improve exercise tolerance and quality of life in patients with diastolic HF.[438] However, until validation from adequately powered, randomized controlled trials is available, the treatment of chronic diastolic HF remains empiric.

Except in the presence of acute diastolic HF, positive inotropic and chronotropic agents should be avoided as they may worsen diastolic function by increasing contractile force and HR, or by increasing calcium concentrations in diastole. However, in the short-term management of acute diastolic dysfunction or HF (e.g., post CPB), β-adrenergic agonists (e.g., epinephrine) and phosphodiesterase inhibitors (e.g., milrinone), enhance calcium sequestration by the sarcoplasmic reticulum and thereby promote a more rapid and complete myocardial relaxation between beats.[439,440]

Current Clinical Practice

The pharmacotherapy of HF begins with primary prevention of left ventricular dysfunction. Because hypertension and CAD are leading causes of left ventricular dysfunction, adequate treatment of both hypertension and hypercholesterolemia has been endorsed following encouraging results in prevention trials.[258,440,441] Limitation of neurohormonal activation with ACE inhibitors, and possibly β-blockers, should be initiated in diabetic, hypertensive, and hypercholesterolemic patients (AHA/ACC, stage A HF) who are at increased risk for cardiovascular events, despite normal contractile function, in order to reduce the onset of new HF (HOPE trial). In patients with asymptomatic left ventricular

Table 10–23 Ongoing, Randomized Clinical Trials for Diastolic Heart Failure

	CHARM-Preserved	MCC-135	PEP-CHF	Seniors	Hong Kong	I-Preserve
Entrance Criteria						
Signs/symptoms of heart failure	Yes	Yes	Yes	Yes	Yes	Yes
NYHA functional class	II-IV	II-III	II-IV	II-IV	II-IV	II–IV
Prior hospitalization	Yes	Yes	Yes	Yes	No	Yes
Ejection fraction (%)	>40	>40	>40	>35	>45	>45
Enrollment						
Total	6500	500	1000	2000	1000	3600
Diastolic heart failure	2500	230	1000	1000	1000	3600
Drug	Candesartan	MCC-135	Perindapril	Nebivolol	Diuretic alone Diuretic + ramiprel Diuretic + Irbesartan	Irbesartan
Duration	24	6	12	18	12	24
End-points						
Death	X	X	X	X	X	X
Hospitalization	X	X	X	X	X	X
Echocardiography	X	X	X	X	X	X
Cardiac MRI		X	X	X	X	
Exercise tolerance		X				
Brain natriuretic peptide		X	X			X
Completion of study (yr)	2003 Completed	2003 Results pending	2004	2004	2004	2006

dysfunction (EF = 40%) (stage B), treatment with ACE inhibitors, and β-blockers can blunt the disease progression. In the symptomatic HF patient (stage C), diuretics are titrated to relieve symptoms of pulmonary congestion and peripheral edema and achieve a euvolemic state, while ACE inhibitors and β-blockers are recommended to blunt disease progression. Although digoxin has no effect on patient survival, it may be considered in stage C if the patient remains symptomatic despite adequate doses of ACE inhibitors and diuretics. In general, the primary treatment objectives for Stages A-C HF are to (1) improve quality of life, (2) reduce morbidity, and (3) reduce mortality. At this time, the most important factor affecting long-term outcome is blunting of neurohormonal stimulation, because this mediates disease progression. Pharmacologic therapy in stage D, or patients with severe, decompensated HF, is based on hemodynamic status to alleviate symptoms with diuretics, vasodilators, and in palliative circumstances, intravenous inotropic infusions. ACE inhibitors and β-blockers are also incorporated in the treatment regimen to retard disease progression through reductions in ventricular enlargement, vascular hypertrophy, and ventricular arrhythmias[442] (Fig. 10–26).

PHARMACOTHERAPY FOR CARDIAC ARRHYTHMIAS

Perhaps the most widely used electrophysiologic and pharmacologic classification of antiarrhythmic drugs is that proposed by Vaughan Williams[443] (Table 10–24). There is, however, substantial overlap in pharmacologic and electrophysiologic effects of specific agents among the classes and the linkage between observed electrophysiologic effects and the clinical antiarrhythmic effect is often tenuous. Likewise, especially in class I, there may be considerable diversity within a single class. Moreover, other antiarrhythmic drugs are not included in this classification such as the classic antiarrhythmic for chronic atrial fibrillation, digitalis, or adenosine, a

Table 10–24 Classification of Antiarrhythmic Drugs

	Class			
Effect	**I (Membrane Stabilizers)**	**II (β-Adrenergic Receptor Antagonists)**	**III (Drugs Prolonging Repolarization)**	**IV (Calcium Antagonists)**
Pharmacologic	Fast channel (Na^+) blockade	β-Adrenergic receptor blockade	Uncertain: possible interference with Na^+ and Ca^{++} exchange	Decreased slow-channel calcium conductance
Electrophysiologic	Decreased rate of V_{max}	Decreased V_{max}, increased APD, increased ERP, and increased ERP/APD ratio	Increased APD, increased ERP, increased ERP/APD ratio	Decreased slow-channel depolarization; decreased APD

V_{max} = maximal rate of depolarization; APD = action potential duration; ERP = effective refractory period.

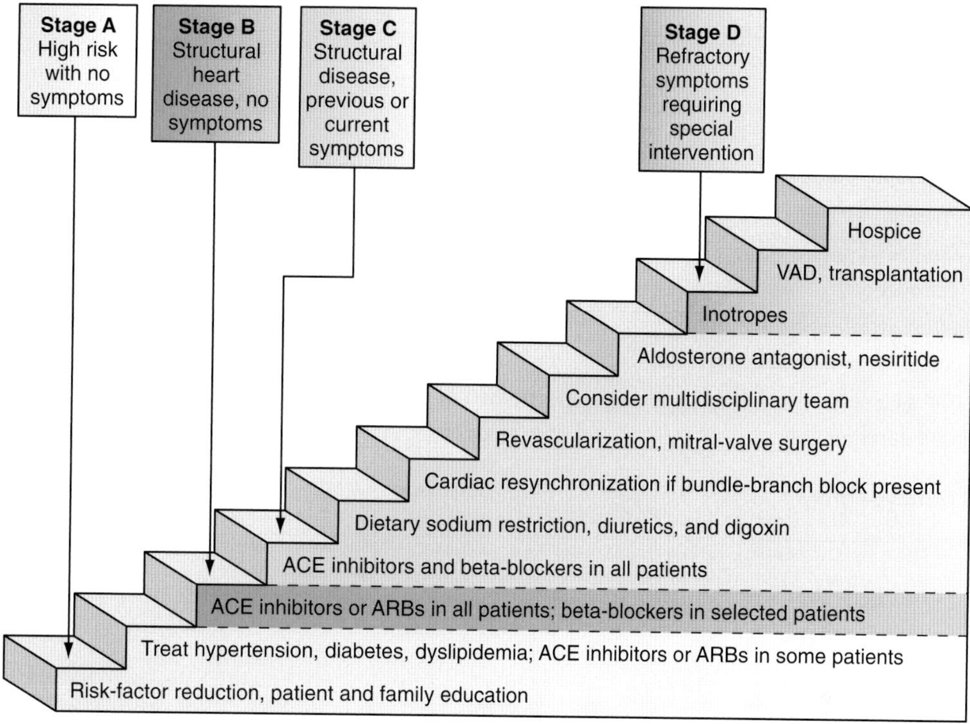

Figure 10–26 Treatment options for the stages of heart failure. (Redrawn from Jessup M, Brozena S: Heart failure. N Engl J Med 348:2007, 2003, Fig. 3, p. 2013.)

drug with potent antiarrhythmic effects mediated by a specific class of membrane receptors.[444,445]

The Cardiac Arrhythmia Suppression Trial (CAST) questions the appropriateness of treating arrhythmias with antiarrhythmic agents in certain groups of patients.[446] The CAST study was designed to test the hypothesis that suppression of ventricular ectopy seen after MI reduces the subsequent incidence of sudden death. Patients were eligible for the study if they had ventricular ectopy without sustained ventricular tachycardia (VT) following MI. The study required documented suppression of the ventricular ectopy with class IC drugs encainide and flecainide. The primary study end-points were death or cardiac arrest caused by arrhythmia. After 22 months of enrollment, of a planned 36 months, the Data and Safety Monitoring Board recommended discontinuation of the encainide and flecainide limbs of the study because of apparent excess mortality in those two treatment groups. Of the 1498 patients assigned to the encainide and flecainide groups, there were 89 deaths (63 in the active drug subgroups and 26 in the placebo subgroups; $P < 0.0001$). The mechanisms of the excess mortality were thought to be the precipitation of proarrhythmia secondary to facilitation of reentry, especially during ischemic episodes. Following this study, the use of sodium channel blocking agents was not recommended, especially in low-risk patients following MI. Encainide is now no longer available; however, flecainide is still used for supraventricular tachyarrhythmias and documented life-threatening ventricular arrhythmias.

Although the class I and especially subclass IC agents are most commonly known for their proarrhythmic effects, the other classes are not devoid of this side effect. Bretylium initially causes the release of norepinephrine, and an increased incidence of ventricular arrhythmias is often seen when therapy is initiated. In fact, in one study there was a significant arrhythmia frequency when different doses of bretylium were used.[447] Similarly, for the first week after initiation of sotalol, a nonspecific β-adrenergic blocker that is considered a class III arrhythmic agent, there is an increased incidence of torsade de pointes. The proarrhythmic effects seem increased in the presence of hypokalemia, bradycardia, CHF, and a history of sustained ventricular dysfunction (Box 10–10).[448]

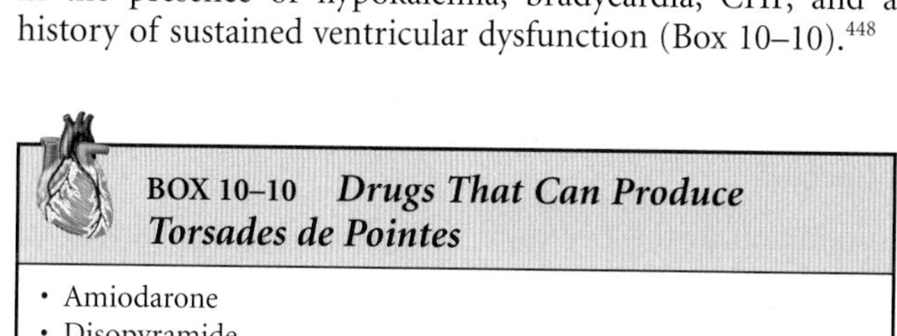

BOX 10–10 ***Drugs That Can Produce Torsades de Pointes***

- Amiodarone
- Disopyramide
- Dofetilide
- Ibutilide
- Procainamide
- Quinidine
- Sotalol

Chronic antiarrhythmic therapy should be initiated only after careful evaluation of the risks and benefits of the intervention. The appropriate use of intravenous antiarrhythmic agents with sudden-onset arrhythmias is not clear. Obviously, life-threatening ventricular arrhythmias must be treated. Patients at low risk for arrhythmic events may not benefit from therapy and indeed as learned from CAST, mortality may even increase with some of these agents. High-risk patients may be more safely treated in some cases by implantation of internal cardioverter-defibrillators (ICDs).[449]

Class I Antiarrhythmic Drugs: Sodium Channel Blockers

Class I drugs have the common property of inhibiting the fast inward depolarizing current carried by sodium ion. Because of the diversity of other effects of the class I drugs, a subgroup of the class has been proposed[450] (Table 10–25). Whether the depression of fast inward current of the sodium channel pro-

Table 10–25 **Subgrouping of Class I Antiarrhythmic Drugs**

	Subgroup		
	IA	IB	IC
Electrophysiologic Activity			
Phase 0	Decreased	Slight effect	Marked decrease
Depolarization	Prolonged	Slight effect	Slight effect
Conduction	Decreased	Slight effect	Markedly slowed
Effective refractory period (ERP)	Increased	Slight effect	Slight prolongation
Action potential duration (APD)	Increased	Decreased	Slight effect
ERP/APD ratio	Increased	Decreased	Slight effect
QRS duration	Increased	No effect during sinus rhythm	Marked increase
Prototype Drugs	Quinidine, procainamide, disopyramide	Lidocaine, mexiletine, tocainide	Propafenone, encainide, flecainide, moricizine

duces the primary antiarrhythmic effect of all class I drugs is controversial. Other proposed mechanisms involve abolishing reentry by improving conduction in the reentry pathway; however, shortening the action potential duration (APD) in ventricular pathways and improving conduction of premature impulses by shortening the refractory period of the action potential (AP) could also decrease the likelihood for reentry.[451-453]

Class IA

QUINIDINE

In addition to the electrophysiologic effects summarized in Table 10–25, quinidine decreases the slope of phase 4 diastolic depolarization at low concentrations and increases threshold potential at high concentrations.[454] Quinidine depresses cardiac contractility, which in combination with an indirect α-adrenergic blockade, can reduce arterial pressure. This hypotensive effect is the principal limitation to intravenous administration of quinidine.

Electrocardiographic effects of quinidine include an increase in sinus rate, which is perhaps a reflex response both to vasodilation and to cardiac depression. Conduction through the AV node may be enhanced or depressed or may not change, depending on the interplay of the direct slowing effect and the anticholinergic effect of quinidine. Infranodal conduction is slowed and, at high concentrations, bundle-branch block, complete AV block, or asystole may result. The QT interval possibly is prolonged by sympathetic activation.[455]

Clinically, quinidine is used primarily in oral form to treat both atrial and ventricular arrhythmias. However, quinidine may substantially accelerate the ventricular response rate in atrial fibrillation (AF) or atrial flutter. Its use in these conditions should be preceded by β-blockade or digitalization. This acceleration of ventricular response rate is a function of the direct slowing of the atrial rate produced by quinidine and its indirect anticholinergic effects. The decreased frequency of atrial depolarization allows a greater percentage of impulses to be conducted through the AV node to depolarize the His bundle.

Quinidine may be administered orally or intramuscularly. The GI absorption of quinidine is good, and plasma levels peak 1 to 2 hours after oral administration. Quinidine has an elimination half-life of 6 to 7 hours; therefore, a dose every 6 or 8 hours is appropriate, although shortening the dosage interval may more effectively maintain a stable plasma concentration than increasing the dosage. Typical maintenance doses are 300 to 600 mg, and therapeutic plasma concentrations range from 2 to 6 μg/mL.[456] Quinidine gluconate, 200 mg intramuscularly, is the preferred dose.

Quinidine is 70% to 80% protein bound in plasma, with much of that due to hemoglobin. Administration of quinidine substantially increases the plasma concentrations of digoxin, probably by releasing the glycoside from protein-binding sites.[457] Elimination of quinidine is primarily by hepatic metabolism (hydroxylation), although about 20% is excreted unchanged by the kidney. Renal excretion is by both glomerular filtration and tubular secretion and depends on urinary pH; excretion is decreased up to 50% when urine is alkaline.[458]

The most serious toxic effect of quinidine is cardiac and is largely a function of its conduction effects. Monitoring both the QRS duration and QT interval is a useful guide to therapy; a 50% increment in either should prompt a reduction in dose. Various degrees of conduction block at both the atrial and ventricular levels may occur, including asystole. "Quinidine syncope" probably relates to a proarrhythmia produced by QT interval prolongation and may not be dose related.[459] Symptoms of tinnitus, visual disturbance, and gastrointestinal irritation progressing to severe CNS symptoms (headache, diplopia, photophobia, confusion, or psychosis) are part of the spectrum of "cinchonism" produced by quinidine, by other cinchona alkaloids such as quinine, and by salicylates. Thrombocytopenia may occur with quinidine, and hypersensitivity to quinidine may appear as fever, anaphylaxis, or bronchospasm, which can be severe.

PROCAINAMIDE

Electrophysiologic effects of procainamide include decreased V_{max} and amplitude during phase 0, decreased rate of phase 4 depolarization, and prolonged effective refractory period

(ERP) and APD.[460] Clinically, procainamide prolongs conduction and increases the ERP in atrial and His-Purkinje portions of the conduction system, which may prolong PR interval and QRS complex durations; however, the QT interval is lengthened less than with quinidine. As with quinidine, AV nodal ERP may be decreased by indirect anticholinergic side effects.

Procainamide is used to treat ventricular arrhythmias and to suppress atrial premature beats to prevent the occurrence of AF and flutter. It has been very useful for chronic suppression of PVCs, but may be supplanted in this use by class IB drugs such as mexiletine. Both quinidine and procainamide are reported to reduce the frequency of short-coupling interval (<400 msec) PVCs and thereby to reduce the frequency of VT or ventricular fibrillation (VF) created by the R-on-T phenomenon.[461]

Administered intravenously, procainamide is an effective emergency treatment for ventricular arrhythmias, especially after lidocaine failure, but, recently, amiodarone has become a more popular drug for intravenous suppression of ventricular arrhythmias. Dosage is 100 mg, or approximately 1.5 mg/kg given at 5-minute intervals until the therapeutic effect is obtained or a total dose of 1 g or 15 mg/kg is given (Tables 10–26 and 10–27). Arterial pressure and ECG should be monitored continuously during loading and administration stopped if significant hypotension occurs or if the QRS complex is prolonged by 50% or more. Maintenance infusion rates are 2 to 6 mg/min to maintain therapeutic plasma concentrations of 4 to 8 μg/mL.[462]

Oral administration of procainamide has a 75% to 95% absorption rate, and plasma levels peak after 1 to 2 hours.[463] The elimination half-life of procainamide is 3 to 4 hours, and the oral dosage interval is similar; however, sustained-release preparations are available. Oral dose requirements are on the order of 50 mg/kg/24 hr or 400 to 600 mg every 3 to 4 hours.[464] Decreasing the dosage interval rather than increasing the dose may be a better method of producing a stable increase in plasma concentrations without creating peak levels that are toxic. Sustained-release forms of procainamide are available.

Table 10–26 Intravenous Supraventricular Antiarrhythmic Therapy

Class I	Procainamide (IA)—converts acute atrial fibrillation, suppresses PACs and precipitation of atrial fibrillation/flutter, converts accessory pathway SVT. 100 mg IV loading dose every 5 min until arrhythmia subsides or total dose of 15 mg/kg (rarely needed) with continuous infusion of 2 to 6 mg/min.
Class II	Esmolol—converts or maintains slow ventricular response in acute atrial fibrillation. 0.5 to 1 mg/kg loading dose with each 50 μg/kg/min increase in infusion, with infusions of 50 to 300 μg/kg/min. Hypotension and bradycardia are limiting factors.
Class III	Amiodarone—converts acute atrial fibrillation to sinus rhythm. 5 mg/kg IV over 15 min. Ibutilide (Convert)—converts acute atrial fibrillation and flutter. Adults (>60 kg): 1 mg given over 10 min IV, may repeat once Adults (<60 kg) and children: 0.01 mg/kg given over 10 min IV, may be repeated once.
Class IV	Verapamil—slow ventricular response to acute atrial fibrillation, converts AV node reentry SVT. 75 to 150 μg/kg IV bolus. Diliazem—slow ventricular response in acute atrial fibrillation, converts AV node reentry SVT. 0.25 μg/kg bolus, then 100 to 300 μg/kg/hr infusion.
Others	Adenosine—converts AV node reentry SVT and accessory pathway SVT. Aids in diagnosis of atrial fibrillation and flutter. Adults: 3 to 6 mg IV bolus, repeat with 6 to 12 mg bolus. Children: 100 μg/kg bolus, repeat with 200 μg/kg bolus. Increased dosage required with methylxanthines, decreased use required with dipyridamole. Digoxin—maintenance IV therapy for atrial fibrillation and flutter, slows ventricular response. Adults: 0.25 mg IV bolus followed by 0.125 mg each 1 to 2 hr until rate controlled, not to exceed 10 μg/kg in 24 hr. Children (<10 years of age): 10 to 30 μg/kg load given in divided doses over 24 hours. Maintenance: 25% of loading dose.

Table 10–27 Intravenous Ventricular Antiarrhythmic Therapy

Class I	Procainamide (IA)—100 mg IV loading dose every 5 min until arrhythmia subsides or total dose of 15 mg/kg (rarely needed) with continuous infusion of 2 to 6 mg/min. Lidocaine (IB)—1.5 mg in divided doses given twice over 20 min with continuous infusion of 1 to 4 mg/min.
Class II	Propranolol—0.5 to 1 mg given slowly up to a total β-blocking dose of 0.1 mg/kg. Repeat bolus as needed. Metoprolol—2.5 mg given slowly up to a total β-blocking dose of 0.2 mg/kg. Repeat bolus as needed. Esmolol—0.5 to 1.0 mg/kg loading dose with each 50 μg/kg /min increase in infusion, with infusions of 50 to 300 μg/kg/min. Hypotension and bradycardia are limiting factors.
Class III	Bretylium—5 mg/kg loading dose given slowly with a continuous infusion of 1 to 5 mg/min. Hypotension may be a limiting factor with infusion. Amiodarone—150 mg IV over 10 min, then 1 mg/min for 6 hours, then 0.5 mg/min for the next 18 hr. Repeat bolus as needed.
Others	Magnesium—2 g $MgSO_4$ over 5 min, then continuous infusion of 1 g/hr for 6 to 10 hr to restore intracellular magnesium levels.

From Royster RL: Diagnosis and Management of Cardiac Disorders. ASA Refresher Course Lectures, with permission of the American Society of Anesthesiologists, 520 N. Northwest Highway, Park Ridge, IL 60068-2573.

Procainamide has both hepatic and renal routes of elimination, with each route approximately equal in magnitude. Hepatic metabolism is by acetylation and, therefore, will be either fast or slow in individual patients as a result of genetic variation.[465] The primary metabolite, *N*-acetylprocainamide (NAPA), has antiarrhythmic effects as well as toxic side effects and is excreted almost entirely by the kidney.[466] The clinical importance is that patients with impaired hepatic or renal function, or with diminished perfusion of either organ, as in CHF, will have markedly impaired elimination of procainamide. Recommended dosages with renal impairment or CHF are a loading dose of 12 mg/kg given over 1 hour, with a maintenance dose of 1.4 mg/kg/hr.[467]

Toxic side effects of procainamide are dose related and are primarily related to plasma concentration, a function of both total dose and rate of administration during the loading technique. Serious cardiac toxicity generally requires plasma concentrations over 12 μg/mL. NAPA levels should be monitored as well. The likelihood of producing proarrhythmia as a result of QT_c prolongation is less with procainamide than with quinidine.[468] Procainamide may also produce GI disturbances, CNS symptoms (headache and sleep disturbance), rash, and agranulocytosis. Among patients receiving procainamide chronically, antinuclear antibodies develop in 50% to 70%, and approximately half will suffer fever, myalgia, rash, pleuritis, or pericarditis similar to that seen with lupus erythematosus, although renal and CNS effects are rare.[469] They are also more common among patients who are slow acetylators. After discontinuation of the drug, lupus-like symptoms resolve slowly.

Intramyocardial distribution of procainamide, especially during ischemia or infarction, is an important component of its therapeutic effect. In a canine infarction model, procainamide increased ERP more in ischemic than in nonischemic myocardium.[470] The pharmacokinetics of procainamide have been shown to differ between ischemic and nonischemic regions of myocardium; tissue concentrations of procainamide decline more rapidly in the latter.[471]

DISOPYRAMIDE

Although disopyramide is chemically different from quinidine and procainamide, electrophysiologic effects of the three drugs are similar. Conduction through the AV node may be facilitated slightly by disopyramide because of its indirect vagolytic effect.[472] Accessory pathway conduction may be slowed in patients with Wolff-Parkinson-White (WPW) syndrome.[473] Disopyramide is a potent negative inotropic drug and, after intravenous use, SVR reflexively increases.[474]

Disopyramide is therapeutically effective against supraventricular and ventricular tachyarrhythmias. However, as with quinidine and procainamide, disopyramide should not be used for ventricular tachyarrhythmias caused by prolonged QT syndrome. The marked negative inotropic and anticholinergic effects limit the usefulness of the drug.

When given orally, 80% of disopyramide is absorbed, and steady-state therapeutic plasma concentrations of 2 to 4 μg/mL can be achieved with 100 to 200 mg orally every 6 hours.[475] The elimination half-life is approximately 7 hours, and elimination occurs equally by hepatic and renal mechanisms; hepatic or renal insufficiency may necessitate smaller doses.[476] Disopyramide is approximately 30% to 50% protein bound at plasma concentrations of 3 μg/mL.[477]

Toxicity of disopyramide is most frequently anticholinergic in origin, with symptoms of gastrointestinal upset, visual disturbance, and urinary tract obstruction, which may be marked in elderly men with prostatic hypertrophy. Unless there is left ventricular failure, cardiovascular complications are infrequent; however, recurrent CHF is seen in up to 50% of patients with a history of CHF.[474] Conduction system toxicity resembles that with quinidine.

Class IB

LIDOCAINE

First introduced as an antiarrhythmic drug in the 1950s, lidocaine has become the clinical standard for the acute intravenous treatment of ventricular arrhythmias except those precipitated by an abnormally prolonged QT interval.[478-481] Lidocaine may, in fact, be one of the most useful drugs in clinical anesthesia because it has both local and general anesthetic properties, in addition to an antiarrhythmic effect.[482]

The direct electrophysiologic effects of lidocaine produce virtually all of its antiarrhythmic action. Lidocaine depresses the slope of phase 4 diastolic depolarization in Purkinje fibers and increases the VF threshold.[483] In Purkinje fibers, lidocaine increases transmembrane potassium conductance, but does not affect resting membrane potential or threshold potential.[484] At less negative (partially depolarized) initial membrane potentials, lidocaine decreases fast-channel (Na^+) responses through an increase in background outward potassium flux, an effect directly related to extracellular potassium concentration.[485,486] Lidocaine may be ineffective in hypokalemic patients.[487]

Conduction velocity is not affected by lidocaine in normal tissue, but it is significantly decreased in ischemic tissue.[488] The effects of lidocaine on APD vary by conduction system location. In atrial tissues, there is little or no effect. In contrast, in Purkinje fibers, APD is markedly decreased, and the magnitude of the decrease is directly proportional to normal APD.[452] Because lidocaine decreases APD, its antiarrhythmic effect has been attributed to improved conduction in ectopic foci, which would decrease the likelihood of reentry; however, it has been shown that lidocaine slows conduction in these areas and decreases reentrant ventricular ectopy after experimental infarction.[457,489]

The clinical pharmacokinetics of lidocaine are well described. Both distribution and elimination half-lives of lidocaine are short, approximately 60 seconds and 100 minutes, respectively.[490] Hepatic extraction of lidocaine is about 60% to 70%, and essentially all lidocaine is metabolized, because the urine contains negligible amounts of unchanged lidocaine.[456] Hepatic metabolism produces monoethylglycine-xylidide and glycine-xylidide, both of which possess antiarrhythmic effects. Metabolic products are eliminated by the kidney, and accumulation of the monoethyl metabolite is related to the toxicity of intravenous lidocaine.[491-493] In patients with impaired hepatic function or blood flow (e.g., those with CHF), the dose requirement is approximately 50% of that in the healthy person (Fig. 10–27, Table 10–28).

Therapeutic plasma levels of lidocaine range from 1.5 to 5 μg/mL; signs of toxicity are frequent with concentrations above 9 μg/mL.[492] Various intravenous dosages can be used, but the important factor is to rapidly achieve steady-state therapeutic plasma concentrations. Thus, an initial bolus dose of 1 to 1.5 mg/kg should be followed immediately by a continuous infusion of 20 to 50 μg/kg/min in order to prevent the "therapeutic hiatus" produced by the rapid redistribution half-life of lidocaine. Likewise, infusion increments should be

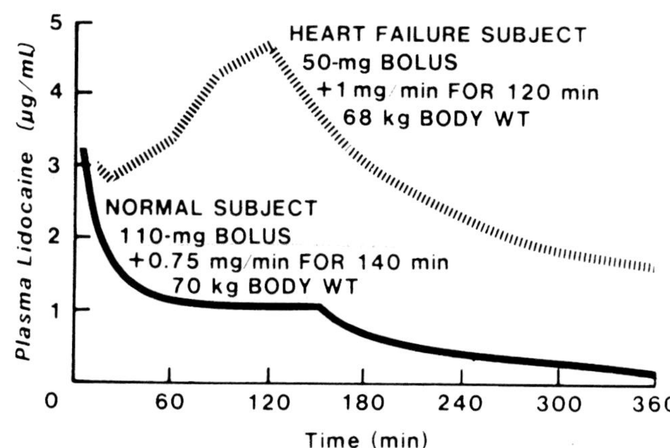

Figure 10–27 The difference between plasma level responses to infused lidocaine in a normal subject *(solid line)* and a subject with heart failure *(broken line)*. The accumulation of lidocaine in patients with depressed hepatic metabolism is dramatically illustrated. (From Textbook of Cardiac Life Support, 1987. Copyright American Heart Association.)

Table 10–28 Potential Effects of Pathophysiologic Changes in Congestive Heart Failure on Drug Disposition

Pathophysiology	Pharmacokinetic Sequelae
↓ Cardiac output and organ perfusion	↓ Hepatic and renal clearance
↑ Sympathetic activity	↓ Drug distribution
↑ Plasma norepinephrine	↓ Intramuscular absorption
Altered regional perfusion	↓ Gastrointestinal absorption
↓ Peripheral perfusion	
Changes in extracellular fluid volume and protein binding	↓ ↑ Volume of distribution
Visceral congestion	↓ Drug metabolism

accompanied by additional bolus doses to immediately increase plasma level.

The major toxic effect of lidocaine is associated with the CNS and is manifested by drowsiness and disorientation, which progress to agitation, muscle twitching, and hearing abnormalities and culminate in seizures. With regard to CNS toxicity, it is important to note that lidocaine can be an effective general anesthetic agent; cases of coma with EEG silence similar to brain death patterns, have been produced by overdose of lidocaine and have resolved completely on discontinuation of the drug. Interestingly, the direct CNS effect of lidocaine and other local anesthetics is anticonvulsant.[494-496] Local anesthetic-induced seizures do not produce permanent damage to the CNS, as long as cardiovascular and respiratory complications of the seizure are prevented. Pharmacologically, benzodiazepines are superior to barbiturates (e.g., thiopental) for stopping local anesthetic-induced seizure activity. Drug therapy alone is insufficient, however; airway control, ventilation, and especially oxygenation are paramount to prevent CNS morbidity.

MEXILETINE AND TOCAINIDE

Both drugs have electrophysiologic effects similar to those of lidocaine (decreases in APD and ERP, but little effect on conduction). Mexiletine has little effect on the QT interval. Hemodynamic effects are minor and consist primarily of small decreases of left ventricular dP/dt and increases of LVEDP.[497] Small decreases of CO, SVR, and BP have been reported; however, even in patients with CAD, acute MI, or valvular heart disease, hemodynamic effects are clinically insignificant.[498-501]

The antiarrhythmic effects decrease the frequency of acute and chronic ventricular ectopy but not supraventricular arrhythmias. Mexiletine may decrease symptomatic ventricular arrhythmias in patients not responding to other therapy and may be more effective than lidocaine when used IV to suppress PVCs and VT in acute MI.[502-505] Mexiletine, administered orally, may also be effective prophylaxis for PVCs and VT, but it may less effectively suppress closely coupled PVCs.[506-508] Mexiletine may be used in children and in patients with a long QT syndrome.

Pharmacokinetics of orally administered mexiletine reveal a bioavailability of 85% with 70% of the drug protein bound. The volume of distribution of mexiletine is 2.5 times that for other antiarrhythmics.[509] Elimination half-life is 10 hours and is suitable for twice or three times per day dosage regimens.[510] Mexiletine is eliminated by hepatic metabolism with less than 10% renally excreted unchanged in the urine. The hepatic metabolism is accelerated with microsomal enzyme induction and predictably decreased with hepatic disease, but overall metabolism is unaffected by renal failure.[511,512]

The usual dosage of mexiletine is 200 mg every 8 hours, which can be increased to 400 mg and not to exceed 1200 mg/day. Effective plasma levels of mexiletine range from 0.5 to 2 µg/mL, but there is wide individual variation of the dose required to achieve that concentration. Adverse effects of mexiletine include nausea, dysarthria, dizziness, paresthesia, tremor, vomiting, and sweating. Adverse reactions to mexiletine are dose related and may occur at serum concentrations at the high end of the therapeutic range, which requires careful titration of the drug in patients. The incidence of minor reactions is 30%, and the incidence of severe reactions (vomiting, confusion, and hypotension) is 19% when the plasma concentration is over 2 µg/mL.[513]

DIPHENYLHYDANTOIN

Diphenylhydantoin (DPH) or phenytoin is unique among class IA drugs in that it has a potent central sympatholytic effect that decreases cardiac sympathetic efferent nerve activity.[514,515] Its electrophysiologic effect in many ways bridges the IA and IB classification. In normal conduction system cells, DPH decreases V_{max} and the amplitude of phase 0, but this effect is weaker than with other class IA drugs.[516] DPH does not decrease intraventricular conduction or prolong the QT interval but shortens APD.[517] DPH can effectively abolish the delayed afterpotentials associated with digitalis intoxication.[518,519] In cells partially depolarized from cold, hypoxia, or cardiac glycoside administration, DPH increases maximal diastolic potential, V_{max} of phase 0, and the conduction velocity.[520] Thus, DPH exerts its antiarrhythmic effect by increasing the ERP/APD ratio and by decreasing automaticity, both of these effects being enhanced in partially depolarized cells.

The drug is useful to treat the atrial and ventricular arrhythmias produced by cardiac glycoside toxicity and in some patients with arrhythmias secondary to prolonged QT syndrome. It is less effective for other supraventricular arrhythmias and for suppressing chronic ventricular ectopy.

The drug is also useful in children to prevent late postoperative arrhythmias after surgical correction of congenital heart disease such as junction ectopic tachycardia.[521]

Intravenous loading of DPH is accomplished in much the same way as with procainamide. Doses of 50 to 100 mg (0.5 to 1.5 mg/kg) are given at 5-minute intervals until therapeutic effects are obtained, up to a total dose of 1 g (15 mg/kg); the usual therapeutic plasma concentration is 8 to 10 μg/mL.[522] The drug undergoes primary hepatic metabolism, with urinary excretion of unchanged DPH accounting for only 5% of the total dose.[523] Patients with impaired hepatic or renal function should be expected to have higher plasma concentrations of DPH for a given dose; therefore, the dose should be reduced to prevent toxicity.

With intravenous administration a depressor effect is seen with depressed contractile function and a moderate increase of left ventricular end-diastolic pressure (LVEDP).[524,525] These effects may, in part, be due to the solvents used for the injectable preparation, propylene glycol and ethyl alcohol.[526] Infusion rates above 50 mg/min in adults have produced cardiovascular collapse, VF, and death.[527] Other side effects include visual disturbances (nystagmus and blurring), nausea, dysarthria, and cerebellar ataxia. Chronic DPH use produces gingival hyperplasia, macrocytic anemia, and dermatologic disorders.

Class IC

FLECAINIDE

Flecainide depresses phase 0, delays repolarization in canine ventricular myocardium, and increases intracardiac monophasic APD in humans. The sodium channel depressant effects are slow onset and offset and use dependent. It can also inhibit the slow calcium channel so the drug has properties of multiple classes.[528] Minimal changes occur in ventricular or atrial refractoriness; however, the drug can markedly change accessory pathway refractoriness. The QT interval changes are also minimal.

This drug is indicated for life-threatening ventricular arrhythmias, supraventricular arrhythmias, and atrial fibrillation. It is also effective in patients with the WPW syndrome. Chronic clinical studies have shown that PVCs and VT are effectively suppressed.[529] Flecainide is probably the most effective antiarrhythmic at eliminating premature depolarizations, but as CAST showed in certain patient populations, PVC suppression may not always be in the best interest of the patient.

Flecainide decreases left ventricular dP/dt and CO experimentally.[530] Clinical studies have shown no effects of oral flecainide on BP, echocardiographic parameters, or exercise tolerance.[529,531,532] However, patients with depressed ventricular function may be more susceptible to the negative inotropic effects of flecainide.

Flecainide is well absorbed after oral administration with a plasma half-life of 20 hours. The drug is 85% excreted renally either unchanged or as an inactive metabolite. Effective plasma concentrations range from 0.2 to 1.0 ug/mL. Dosages range from 100 to 200 mg twice a day. The dose should be reduced in renal failure or HF. Flecainide increases serum digoxin and propranolol levels, while propranolol, quinidine, and amiodarone can increase flecainide levels.

Adverse effects are usually minor at doses that have a significant therapeutic effect, but the QT interval has been prolonged with induction of polymorphic VT, and the CAST study showed definite increases in mortality after MI.[533] Confusion and irritability rarely occur.

PROPAFENONE

This drug blocks the fast sodium current in a use-dependent manner. It also has a slow offset like flecainide. Propafenone also blocks β-receptors and is a weak potassium channel blocker.[534] This drug generally slows conduction and prolongs refractoriness of most cardiac conduction system tissue. Propafenone is indicated for life-threatening ventricular arrhythmias, various supraventricular arrhythmias and atrial fibrillation. In one study, a single 600-mg oral dose of propafenone converted 76% of patients in atrial fibrillation.[535]

Propafenone is well absorbed orally and is highly protein bound with an elimination half-life of 6 to 8 hours. Therapeutic serum levels are from 0.2 to 1.5 μg/mL. The metabolites of propafenone are active and demonstrate significant AP and β-blocking effects. A small percentage of patients poorly metabolize the drug and the metabolites of these patients exhibit greater β-blocking properties.

The drug has fewer proarrhythmic problems than flecainide likely due to the β-blocking effects, which tend to decrease arrhythmic traits of antiarrhythmic drugs. Worsening of bronchospastic lung disease has occurred and in a small percentage of patients dizziness, blurred vision, and taste issues, along with some gastrointestinal complaints, may develop.

MORICIZINE

Moricizine is a potent sodium-channel blocker with mild potassium-blocking effects. It prolongs AV node, HV and QRS duration. It has little effect on atrial tissue. The drug is indicated for life-threatening ventricular arrhythmias and is as effective as some of the other class I agents.

Moricizine is highly protein bound and its bioavailability is only 35%. Serum levels do not correlate with therapeutic activity. The elimination half-life is 1 to 3 hours, with the drug eliminated by both hepatic and renal routes. Dosage is 300 mg every 8 hours. Dosage may be changed to every 12 hours in patients with hepatic or renal disease or in patients with CHF.

Adverse effects include tremor, headache, vertigo, dizziness, and gastrointestinal side effects of nausea, vomiting and diarrhea. Proarrhythmic episodes can occur in up to 15% of patients. In the CAST study, the moricizine limb was continued after the encainide and flecainide limbs were stopped and analysis of the moricizine-treated patients showed an increase in mortality as well.[536]

Class II: β-Adrenergic Receptor Antagonists

β-Adrenergic receptor blockers are very effective antiarrhythmics in patients during the perioperative period or who are critically ill because many arrhythmias in these patients are adrenergically mediated.

Propranolol

Propranolol was the first major β-receptor-blocking drug to be used clinically. Propranolol is very potent, but is nonselective for $\beta_{1/2}$-receptor subtypes. It possesses essentially no intrinsic sympathomimetic activity. Because it interferes with the bronchodilating actions of epinephrine and the sympathetic stimulating effects of hypoglycemia, propranolol is less useful in patients with diabetes or bronchospasm. These difficulties with propranolol stimulated the search for β-receptor–blocking drugs with receptor subtype specificity, such as metoprolol, esmolol, and atenolol.

The electrophysiologic effects of β-receptor antagonism are decreased automaticity, increased APD, primarily in ventricular muscle, and a substantially increased ERP in the AV node. β-Blockade decreases the rate of spontaneous (phase 4) depolarization in the SA node; the magnitude of this effect depends on the background sympathetic tone. Although resting HR is decreased by β-blockade, the inhibition of the increase of HR in response to exercise or emotional stress is much more marked. Automaticity in the AV node and more distal portions of the conduction system is also depressed. β-Blockade affects the VF threshold variably, but it consistently reverses the fibrillation threshold-lowering effect of catecholamines.

In addition to β-blockade, propranolol decreases the background outward current of potassium and, at higher concentrations, also inhibits inward sodium current. Because of similarity to class I activity, these effects have been termed *membrane-stabilizing activity* (MSA) or quinidine-like effects. In very high concentrations (1000 to 3000 ng/mL), this effect increases depolarization threshold in Purkinje fibers.[121] Although effective β-blockade is achieved at propranolol concentrations of 100 to 300 ng/mL, concentrations of 1000 ng/mL may be required to control ventricular arrhythmias.[537] Propranolol decreases intramyocardial impulse conduction in acutely ischemic myocardium but does not do so in normal myocardium.[538]

Pharmacokinetics show that absorption after oral administration is virtually 100%, but bioavailability is impaired by first-pass hepatic metabolism, which accounts for approximately two thirds of the administered dose. The degree of hepatic extraction is highly variable, which probably accounts for the great variability of the plasma concentration produced by a given oral dose of propranolol. The hepatic extraction of propranolol is a saturable process, and bioavailability improves with increased oral dose or with chronic therapy.[539] Propranolol is 90% to 95% protein bound in plasma, which further confounds the use of plasma concentration as a guide to therapy.[540] Propranolol is metabolized before excretion; one product, 4-hydroxypropranolol, has a β-blocking potency similar to that of propranolol, but a short half-life prevents this metabolic product from contributing significantly to the therapeutic effect of propranolol.[541] The elimination half-life of orally administered propranolol is 3 to 4 hours, but it is increased during chronic therapy as a result of saturation of hepatic metabolic processes.[542] CPB alters the kinetics of propranolol. Heparinization doubles the free fraction of propranolol, an effect that is reversed after protamine administration. This effect is thought to be due to an increase of free fatty acid concentration produced by heparin, which decreases the protein binding of propranolol.[543]

Major toxic side effects of propranolol relate to β-blockade per se. Cardiac toxicity includes CHF (uncommon without other causes of ventricular dysfunction) and depressed AV conduction. Both complete heart block and asystole have occurred in patients with preexisting AV nodal or intraventricular conduction abnormalities. In contrast, sudden discontinuation of β-blockade therapy may precipitate a withdrawal syndrome of excessive β-adrenergic activity, as a result of the altered sensitivity associated with chronic blockade; responses to normal levels of sympathetic activity are exaggerated as the β-blockade declines, likely due to an increased receptor density or upregulation of the β-receptor.[544,545] Increased airway resistance results from β_2-receptor blockade by propranolol, and this can precipitate severe pulmonary compromise in the asthmatic patient. The hypoglycemic action of insulin is accentuated by propranolol, since the sympathomimetic effect of hypoglycemia is blocked. Side effects perhaps not related to β-receptor blockade include CNS disturbances such as insomnia, hallucinations, depression, and dizziness, and minor allergic manifestations such as rash, fever, and purpura.

An appropriate IV dose for acute control of arrhythmias is 0.5 to 1.0 mg titrated to therapeutic effect up to a total of 0.1 to 0.15 mg/kg. Stable therapeutic plasma concentrations of propranolol can be obtained with a continuous intravenous infusion. An effective level of β-blockade may be obtained with a continuous infusion approximating 3 mg/hr in adult postoperative patients previously receiving chronic treatment; however, with the availability of esmolol, the need for a propranolol infusion is no longer necessary.

Metoprolol

Metoprolol is a relatively selective β-receptor antagonist. The potency of metoprolol for β_1-receptor blockade is equal to that of propranolol, but metoprolol exhibits only 1% to 2% of the effect of propranolol at β_2-receptors.[546]

Like propranolol, metoprolol is rapidly and efficiently absorbed after oral administration; however, its first-pass extraction by the liver is lower, and 40% of the administered dose reaches the systemic circulation. Plasma half-life after oral administration is approximately 3 hours. Metoprolol is 90% metabolized, with hydroxylation and *O*-demethylation being the primary pathways. The metabolites lack β-receptor effects. As with acetylation of procainamide, the rate of hydroxylation of metoprolol is genetically determined. "Slow hydroxylators" show a markedly prolonged elimination of the parent drug and higher plasma concentrations.[547]

Toxicity of metoprolol is related primarily to its limited β_2-antagonist activity. Metoprolol increases airway resistance and decreases the FEV_1 in asthmatic patients, although to a lesser extent than does propranolol at equipotent β_1-antagonist doses. In contrast to propranolol, metoprolol does not inhibit the bronchodilation of isoproterenol. Metoprolol impairs β-receptor–mediated insulin release, and the signs of hypoglycemia will be masked as with propranolol. Other side effects of metoprolol are similar to those of propranolol.

Metoprolol is useful for treating supraventricular and ventricular arrhythmias that are adrenergically driven. The primary advantage of metoprolol is its relative lack of most of the bronchoconstrictive effects in patients with chronic obstructive pulmonary disease (COPD). Acute IV dosage is 1.0 mg titrated to therapeutic effect up to 0.1 to 0.2 mg/kg.

Esmolol

Esmolol is a cardioselective (β_1) receptor antagonist with an extremely brief duration of action.[548] In anesthetized dogs, esmolol infused at 50 μg/kg/min produced a steady-state β-blockade that was completely reversed 20 minutes after stopping the infusion.[549] Esmolol has only minimal ISA and MSA and, in conscious dogs, it has no effect on LVEDP, BP, HR, CO, or SVR; however, at 5 to 60 μg/kg/min, it does decrease left ventricular dP/dt. The decreased contractility, however, fully resolves by 20 minutes after the infusion.

Electrophysiologic effects of esmolol are those of β-adrenergic receptor antagonism. In open-chested dogs, esmolol infused at 300 μg/kg/min increased SA node recovery time and AH conduction interval, but not HV interval. Effective refractory period was increased in the AV node, but this effect does not occur in vitro at β-blocking concentrations.

Esmolol is rapidly metabolized in blood by hydrolysis of its methyl ester linkage. Its half-life in whole blood is 12.5 and 27.1 minutes in dogs and humans, respectively. The acid metabolite possesses a slight degree (1500 times less than esmolol) of β-antagonism. Esmolol is not affected by plasma cholinesterase; the esterase responsible is located in erythrocytes and is not inhibited by cholinesterase inhibitors but it is deactivated by sodium fluoride. Of importance to clinical anesthesia, no metabolic interactions between esmolol and other ester molecules are known. Specifically, esmolol doses up to 500 μg/kg/min have not modified neuromuscular effects of succinylcholine.[152]

Clinically, in asthmatic patients, esmolol (300 μg/kg/min) only slightly increases airway resistance. Also, in patients with COPD who received esmolol, no adverse pulmonary effects occurred.[550] In a multicenter trial, in a comparison with propranolol for the treatment of PSVT, esmolol was equally efficacious and had the advantage of a much faster termination of the β-blockade.[551] Esmolol has become a very useful agent in controlling sinus tachycardia in the perioperative period, a time when a titratable and brief β-blockade is highly desirable.

Dosing begins at 25 μg/kg/min and is titrated to effect up to 250 μg/kg/min. Doses higher than this may cause significant hypotension due to reduced CO in patients. Esmolol is especially effective in treating acute onset atrial fibrillation or flutter perioperatively and results in both acute control of the ventricular response and conversion of the arrhythmia back to sinus rhythm.

Class III: Agents That Block Potassium Channels and Prolong Repolarization

Amiodarone

Amiodarone is a benzofuran derivative initially introduced as an antianginal drug and was subsequently found to have antiarrhythmic effects. The drug has a wide spectrum of effectiveness including supraventricular,[552] ventricular,[553,554] and preexcitation arrhythmias[552-555] (see Tables 10–26 and 10–27). It may also be effective against VT and VF refractory to other treatment.[556] Amiodarone has been approved by the AHA as the first-line antiarrhythmic in cardiopulmonary resuscitation.[557] Amiodarone may be effective prophylactically in preventing AF postoperatively.[552] It also can decrease the number of shocks in patients who have ICDs compared with other antiarrhythmic drugs.[558]

Amiodarone used in an isolated rabbit SA node preparation increased APD and decreased the slope of diastolic (phase 4) depolarization, which depressed SA node automaticity.[559] Amiodarone prolongs repolarization and refractoriness in the SA node, in atrial and ventricular myocardium, in the AV node, and in the His-Purkinje system.[560] Resting potential and myocardial automaticity are minimally affected, but both ERP and absolute refractory period are prolonged.[561] Amiodarone blocks inactive sodium channels in Purkinje fibers, which significantly depresses phase 0.[560] In anesthetized dogs, amiodarone decreases AV junctional as well as SA nodal automaticity, and prolongs intranodal conduction.[562]

There are substantial differences in the electrophysiologic effects of acute and chronic amiodarone administration. Acutely, the drug slightly increases ERP of the His-Purkinje system and ventricular myocardium. The QTc is not prolonged by acute intravenous administration despite myocardial concentrations similar to those with chronic oral therapy.[563] However, chronic oral administration significantly increases QTc.[564] Although AV nodal ERP increases with acute IV amiodarone therapy, the increase is greater following chronic use. In other cardiac tissue, there is little or no change in ERP following intravenous administration; however, after chronic oral use, ERP is increased globally and both AH and HV conduction times are increased.[565]

The electrophysiologic effects of chronic amiodarone treatment mimic those of thyroid ablation.[566] Moreover, the repolarization effects of the drug are reversed by triiodothyronine (T_3) administration. This suggests that among the basic effects of amiodarone is the blockade of the cardiac effect of T_3; this mechanism has been proposed as an alternative to the active metabolite accumulation theory to account for the slow onset of the antiarrhythmic effect of amiodarone.[565]

Amiodarone increases the amount of electric current required to elicit VF (an increase in VF threshold). In most patients, refractory VT is suppressed by acute IV use of amiodarone. This effect has been attributed to a selectively increased activity in diseased tissue, as has been seen with lidocaine.[567] Amiodarone also has an adrenergic-receptor (α and β) antagonistic effect produced by a noncompetitive mechanism; the contribution of this effect to the antiarrhythmic action of the drug is not known.[568]

Hemodynamic effects of IV amiodarone (10 mg/kg) include decreased left ventricular dP/dt, maximal negative dP/dt, mean aortic pressure, HR, and peak left ventricular pressure after coronary artery occlusion in dogs. CO was increased despite the negative inotropic effect as a result of the more marked decrease of left ventricular afterload.[569] Clinical effects are similar; a 5 mg/kg IV dose during cardiac catheterization decreased BP, LVEDP, and SVR and increased CO, but it did not affect HR. Chronic amiodarone therapy is not associated with clinically significant depression of ventricular function in patients without left ventricular failure. Hemodynamic deterioration may occur in some patients with compensated CHF, perhaps because of the antiadrenergic effects of the drug.[570]

Pharmacokinetics of amiodarone are notable for the low bioavailability, very long elimination half-life, relatively low clearance, and large volume of distribution. Oral absorption of amiodarone is slow, with peak plasma levels occurring 3 to 7 hours after ingestion.[571] Bioavailability is variable and low, ranging from 22% to 50%. The hepatic extraction ratio, however, is only 0.13, so that the major limit to bioavailability may be incomplete absorption. Amiodarone has a large volume of distribution, variably estimated as 1.3 to 65.8 L/kg; plasma clearance rates range from 0.14 to 0.60 L/min.[572] Plasma half-life following chronic oral therapy is variably reported as from 14 to 107 days; therapeutic and steady-state plasma concentrations are slowly achieved with maintenance oral administration at 9.5 and 30 days, respectively.[573]

Because steady-state plasma levels are achieved slowly, loading techniques have been developed. Patient-specific pharmacokinetic data have been used to prescribe loading infusion rates from 0.5 to 3.9 mg/min and maintenance rates of 0.5 to 1.0 mg/min to produce plasma levels of 0.5 to 2.5 μg/mL during maintenance infusion. This dosage reduced VT by 85%, paired PVCs by 74%, and isolated PVCs by

60%.[574] A comparison of onset of antiarrhythmic effect of oral loading (800 mg/day for 7 days, then 600 mg/day for 3 days) and IV (5 mg/kg for 30 minutes) plus oral (as for oral alone) administration demonstrated that the combined IV and oral loading technique had a more rapid therapeutic effect with a lower total amiodarone dose.[575] In acute situations with stable patients, a 150-mg IV bolus is followed by a 1.0 mg/min infusion for 6 hours and then 0.5 mg/min thereafter. In CPR, a 300-mg IV bolus is given and repeated with multiple boluses as needed if defibrillation is unsuccessful.

Adverse reactions to amiodarone are numerous. Photosensitivity of the skin occurs in 57% of patients without apparent relation to dose or plasma level.[576] Other skin manifestations include abnormal pigmentation (slate gray) and an erythematous, pruritic rash. Corneal microdeposits occur in most patients taking amiodarone chronically, although visual symptoms are uncommon.

Pulmonary side effects are more severe.[577-580] Clinical features include exertional dyspnea, cough, and weight loss. Hypoxia may occur; pulmonary function studies show decreased total lung capacity and diffusion rate. Chest radiographic findings are diffuse bilateral interstitial infiltrates, which histologically may be fibrosing alveolitis. Pulmonary effects may resolve with discontinuation of treatment or with dose reduction. The pathophysiologic mechanism of these pulmonary effects is not known but may relate to abnormal production of phospholipid. The overall incidence of pulmonary toxicity is up to 6%, with a mortality rate in those affected of 20% to 25%. There are case reports of an increased risk of ARDS when amiodarone is used prior to CPB, but this association has not been proven.

Thyroid abnormalities are associated with amiodarone; the frequencies of hyperthyroidism and hypothyroidism range from 1% to 5% and 1% to 2%, respectively.[568] Amiodarone contains two iodine atoms per molecule, or 75 mg of organic iodide/200 mg of drug, and 10% of that amount may become free iodine. The iodine alone does not account for the thyroid abnormalities, because intake of an amount of inorganic iodine equivalent to that ingested with chronic amiodarone intake does not have the same effect. HR is not increased during hyperthyroidism associated with amiodarone, probably because of its antiadrenergic effects. Amiodarone therapy increases both thyroxine (T_4) and reverse T_3, but only slightly decreases T_3.[581,582]

Despite relatively widespread use of amiodarone, anesthetic complications have infrequently been reported. In two case reports, bradycardia and hypotension were prominent.[583,584] One of the reports described profound resistance to the vasoconstrictive effects of α-adrenergic agonists.[584] The slow decay of amiodarone in plasma and tissue makes such adverse reactions possible long after discontinuing its administration. Because T_3 is reported to reverse electrophysiologic effects of amiodarone, T_3 could possibly be used to reverse hemodynamic abnormalities, such as those described in these two case reports, although this theory has not been tested. Epinephrine has been shown to be more effective than dobutamine or isoproterenol in reversing amiodarone-induced cardiac depression.[585]

Bretylium

Bretylium is a quaternary ammonium compound that produces a biphasic cardiac response after acute intravenous administration. Initially, norepinephrine is displaced from adrenergic nerve endings, and there are attendant increases in BP, SVR, and cardiac automaticity. After 20 to 30 minutes, this response wanes and the adrenergic-blocking effects of bretylium predominate.[586-588] These latter effects depend on uptake of bretylium by adrenergic neurons; however, inhibition of its adrenergic-blocking effects does not impair the antiarrhythmic effect.

The direct electrophysiologic effect of bretylium is prolongation of the ventricular ERP. In this regard, the electrophysiologic effect correlates with the myocardial rather than the plasma concentrations of bretylium.[589] Bretylium delays conduction of premature impulses from normal myocardium to the border of ischemic zones and decreases the disparity between the excitation thresholds of adjoining zones of ischemic and normal myocardium. Bretylium increases the electric current required to induce VF and may spontaneously convert VF to sinus rhythm.[590] The antiarrhythmic effect of bretylium is undiminished by cardiac denervation or chronic reserpine treatment, which indicates that the antiarrhythmic effects are dissociated from the antiadrenergic effects.[591,592] Bretylium also decreases the amount of electrical current required to produce defibrillation.[593]

Results of clinical trials of bretylium in acute cardiac arrest are inconsistent. In one study in which it was compared with lidocaine, bretylium did not have a better antiarrhythmic effect, improve resuscitation, or lower mortality.[594] In contrast, in another study, bretylium (10 mg/kg) was used as a first-line treatment for out-of-hospital VF and significantly improved the outcome from resuscitation; lidocaine administered after bretylium also decreased the incidence of recurrent VF.[595] In the acute setting, bretylium is effective prophylaxis against VF.[561,596-599]

Clinical indications for bretylium include refractory VT or VF. For VF, bretylium is administered as a 5 to 10 mg/kg IV bolus, which can be repeated to a total dose of 30 mg/kg if VF persists. The antifibrillatory effect may require some time to develop, so full resuscitative efforts should continue for at least 20 to 30 minutes after bretylium has been administered. Administration for recurrent VT is similar to that for VF. Continuous infusion of 2 mg/min may be used to maintain plasma levels. As with VF, the effect of bretylium in VT may take 20 to 30 minutes to manifest.

Adverse reactions to bretylium include nausea and vomiting in conscious patients. During chronic therapy, postural hypotension may develop, but it is reduced by tricyclic drugs, which block uptake of bretylium by adrenergic neurons.

Sotalol

Sotalol is classified as a class III agent, but also has class II β-adrenergic blocking properties. Sotalol was first synthesized as a β-blocker and was initially used to treat angina and hypertension. The antiarrhythmic effect was quickly recognized and the antiarrhythmic actions were then evaluated. Sotalol prolongs refractoriness in both atrial and ventricular tissues due to blockade of the delayed rectifier potassium current. The β-blocking effects result in decreased HR and increased refractory periods at both the atrial and ventricular levels.[600] It is indicated for life-threatening ventricular arrhythmias and atrial fibrillation.

Sotalol exists as a mixture of the D and L isomers. These two isomers have different mechanisms of action. Sotalol can be administered orally or intravenously. Oral bioavailability is greater than 90%. The drug is poorly bound to plasma protein and undergoes renal excretion with an elimination half-life of 12 hours when renal function is normal. The usual starting oral dose is 80 to 160 mg every 12 hours. Peak plasma concentration is seen within 4 hours.[601]

Sotalol has been used to treat both supraventricular and ventricular tachyarrhythmias. Sotalol was found to be superior to class I agents in preventing the recurrence of ventricular arrhythmias.[602] To investigate the contribution of the β-blocking property to the efficacy of sotalol, class I agents with or without β-blocker were compared with sotalol.[603] Sotalol was more effective in preventing the recurrence of arrhythmias than class I agents with or without β-blockers. However, the mortality rates were similar when sotalol was compared with the combined class I and β-blocker regimen. Sotalol is also effective in the prevention of paroxysmal supraventricular tachyarrhythmias.[604]

Sotalol administration is not without side effects. In fact, a large prospective study of D-sotalol (not the mixture of D and L isomers) in patients with reduced left ventricular function was terminated early because of increased mortality in the treatment group.[605] D-Sotalol lacks a significant β-adrenergic receptor–blocking property, which may explain these findings. In addition, sotalol administration is also associated with increased risk of torsades de pointes and QT-interval prolongation. Females and patients with renal failure are at increased risk of the proarrhythmic side effects.

Ibutilide

Ibutilide fumarate is a methanesulfonanilide antiarrhythmic agent that is approved for the conversion of atrial flutter and atrial fibrillation to sinus rhythm. Ibutilide prolongs the cardiac refractory period at both the atrial and ventricular levels by activating a slow inward sodium current.[606] In addition, ibutilide may cause the blockade of the rapid outward delayed rectifier potassium current, which also leads to prolongation of the cardiac refractory period.[607] In vitro and at high dose, ibutilide may shorten AP, although this effect has not been observed clinically. Ibutilide may also predispose to the formation of afterdepolarizations, which may be involved in the development of torsades de pointes.

Ibutilide is administered intravenously, is 40% protein bound and undergoes hepatic metabolism. There are eight metabolites, only one with slight antiarrhythmic activity. The pharmacokinetics of ibutilide are linear. There is rapid extravascular distribution and systemic clearance is high, with the elimination half-life ranging from 2 to 6 hours.[608] The usual dose is 1 mg administered over 10 minutes. This may be followed by a second dose of 0.5 to 1 mg.

In one study, ibutilide, 0.015 mg/kg, administered intravenously over 10 minutes, resulted in conversion to sinus rhythm of about 45% of patients with atrial flutter longer than 3 hours in duration or AF 3 hours to 90 days in duration.[609] The arrhythmia was terminated in 3% of patients receiving placebo. The mean time to termination of arrhythmia was 19 minutes from the start of the infusion. In this study, termination of arrhythmias was unaffected by an enlarged left atrium, decreased EF, presence of valvular heart disease, or the use of concomitant medications such as β-blocking agents and digoxin.

In another study, the safety and efficacy of repeated intravenous doses were evaluated.[610] The investigators found a similar conversion rate to the previously mentioned study. In addition, they found that efficacy was higher in atrial flutter than fibrillation (63% versus 31%). In AF conversion rates were higher in patients with shorter arrhythmia duration or a normal left atrial size. However, the duration of arrhythmias in all patients in this study was less than 45 days.

Cardiovascular side effects occur in about 25% of patients treated with ibutilide, compared with 7% for the placebo-treated group.[611] Torsades de pointes occurred in 4.3% of these patients. Most of the proarrhythmic activity was seen within 1 hour of termination of the infusion, reflecting the short half-life and lack of metabolites with significant antiarrhythmic property. Bradycardia, low body weight, and a history of CHF were predictive of the occurrence of torsades de pointes. Electrolyte abnormalities and acquired prolong QT interval should be corrected prior to ibutilide therapy.

Dofetilide

This drug blocks the rapid component of the delayed rectifier potassium current of repolarization without slowing conduction. Similar to ibutilide, dofetilide has a profound effect on prolonging the QT interval. Atrial tissue is more affected by dofetilide's electrophysiologic effects than ventricular tissue. Thus, dofetilide is indicated for acute conversion and chronic suppression of AF.[612]

Dofetilide is only available orally and results in 90% bioavailability. About 50% of the drug is excreted in the urine with an elimination half-life of 8 to 12 hours. Several drugs have been shown to increase dofetilide serum concentrations including verapamil, cimetidine, and ketoconazole. These drugs should be avoided or cautiously used in combination with dofetilide.

Dosing is from 0.125 mg to 0.5 mg twice a day and should be performed during ECG monitoring and measuring of the QT interval. QT prolongation with polymorphic VT may occur in up to 4% of patients. Any electrolyte abnormalities should be corrected prior to administering this drug. Patients with prolonged QT intervals or history of torsades de pointes should not receive chronic therapy.

Class IV: Calcium Channel Antagonists

Although the principal direct electrophysiologic effects of the three main chemical groups of calcium antagonists (verapamil, a benzoacetonitrite; nifedipine, a dihydropyridine; and diltiazem, a benzothiazepine) are similar, verapamil and diltiazem are the primary antiarrhythmics.

As with other transmembrane ionic channels, the calcium channel is conceptualized as macromolecular protein that spans the ion-impermeable lipid bilayer of the membrane (Fig. 10–28). Such channels exhibit selectivity both for a particular ionic species and for specific transmembrane electrical potential ranges to control the permeability of the pore.[194] The decreased membrane potential produced by depolarization increases the permeability of the Ca^{++} channel for Ca^{++}, which permits Ca^{++} to pass down its concentration gradient into the cell. Conversely, the "gate" closes on repolarization. This mechanism has been termed the *voltage-dependent* or *voltage-gated* channel. In cardiac tissue, the Ca^{++} channel is also controlled by membrane β-adrenergic receptors; activation of β_1-receptors recruits additional Ca^{++} channels to the open or active state, and such channels are termed *receptor-operated* channels.[613]

Based on studies with the sodium channels in the giant axons of squid, three different activity states of the Ca^{++} channel have been distinguished: resting, open, and inactive. The resting state of the Ca^{++} channel is characterized by a

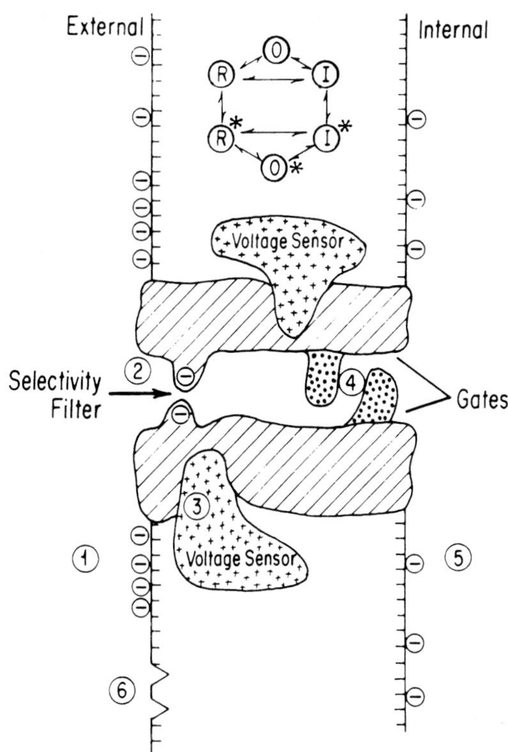

Figure 10–28 Schematic representation of a calcium channel depicted as a proteinaceous membrane pore. A selectivity filter (2) confers ion selectivity by specific molecular dimension and change density characteristics. Voltage sensor components (3) link membrane depolarization with channel opening and closing via the gating mechanism (4). Negatively charged sites on the external surface serve as calcium binding sites (1). (From Triggle DJ: Biochemical pharmacology of calcium blockers. *In* Flaim SF, Zelis R [eds]: Calcium Blockers: Mechanisms of Action and Clinical Applications. Baltimore, Urban and Schwarzenberg, 1982, pp 121–134.)

closed activation (*d*) gate on the external surface of the membrane and an opened inactivation (*f*) gate on the internal surface[614] (Fig. 10–29). Depolarization triggers the open state when the *d* gate relaxes to permit Ca^{++} influx, and also triggers the slower closure of the *f* gate, which, when complete, blocks further Ca^{++} influx; the resulting "inactive" state persists until complete repolarization resets both gates. For the Ca^{++} channel, the time constant for the transition from the resting to the open state is 520 msec, that from the open to the inactive state is 30 to 300 msec, and that from the inactive to the resting state is also 30 to 300 msec.[615]

The "use dependence" noted with Ca^{++} antagonists is the direct relation between the antagonist effect and the frequency of tissue activation. Thus, in cardiac tissue, the negative inotropic and Ca^{++} channel–blocking properties of verapamil depend on both transmembrane potential and stimulation frequency; the inhibitory activity increases with increased frequency and with partial depolarization.[616] Such findings may indicate that verapamil interacts primarily with the inactive (depolarized) state of the Ca^{++} channel. In contrast, the activation state of the membrane is less important for the inhibitory action of nifedipine.

The lipophilic nature of Ca^{++} channel antagonists is important to their effect. In skinned cardiac cells, D600, a congener of verapamil, is ineffective, which would seem to indicate a primary effect of the drug at the plasma membrane.[617] Likewise, quaternary ammonium derivatives of D600 and nifedipine, which are highly ionized and therefore less lipophilic, are also less effective Ca^{++} channel antagonists.[616] Such data indicate that perhaps the locus of activity of these Ca^{++} channel antagonists is the internal surface of the channel or within the membrane itself.

In general, the drugs commonly classified as Ca^{++} channel antagonists, typified by verapamil, diltiazem, nifedipine, and nicardipine, exhibit specificity for vascular smooth muscle and cardiac tissues; however, within the group, specificity for these tissues varies. Nifedipine and nicardipine (and other dihydropyridines) are more potent in smooth muscle than cardiac tissue, whereas verapamil and diltiazem are more potent in cardiac tissue.[618,619] Although Ca^{++} channel antagonism is the dominant effect of these agents, at sufficiently high (greater than 10^6 M) concentrations, other effects become notable. For example, verapamil and D600 at concentrations greater than 10^6 M inhibit sodium channel activity and receptor binding at muscarinic, adrenergic, and opiate receptors.[620] These latter effects do not exhibit stereoselectivity as does Ca^{++} channel–specific action.[621]

Verapamil and Diltiazem

Verapamil and diltiazem have been used extensively in the treatment of supraventricular arrhythmias, AF, and atrial flutter. They are especially effective at preventing or terminating PSVT by blocking impulse transmission through the AV node by prolonging AV nodal conduction and refractoriness.[622] They are also useful in the treatment of AF and atrial flutter by slowing AV nodal conduction and decreasing the ventricular response. The effect on ventricular response is similar to that of the cardiac glycosides, although the onset is more rapid and acutely effective for control of tachycardia in patients.[623, 624]

In the perioperative period, verapamil is a useful antiarrhythmic agent. In one study of anesthetized patients, it successfully controlled a variety of supraventricular and ventricular arrhythmias.[624] However, verapamil should be used cautiously intraoperatively because, in conjunction with inhalation anesthetics, significant cardiac depression may occur.[625,626]

A significant precaution in the use of verapamil and diltiazem to treat PSVT involves preexcitation of the AV node in WPW. If PSVT is orthodromic (anterograde conduction through the AV node and retrograde over the accessory pathway) with a narrow or normal QRS complex, verapamil has a high success rate by blocking anterograde AV nodal conduction. If the PSVT is antidromic (anterograde conduction through accessory pathway and retrograde over the AV node) with a widened QRS complex, successful blockade with verapamil is unlikely, because it has little effect on refractoriness or conduction in accessory pathways. Atrial flutter and AF may also occur in WPW. In this setting, agents that shorten the ERP of the accessory pathway or increase the ERP in the AV node (e.g., digitalis, verapamil) will often increase ventricular response and may precipitate VF.[627] Type I and III drugs, such as procainamide or amiodarone, are more effective in slowing the ventricular response in AF with an accessory pathway (see Chapter 13).

Electrophysiologic effects of verapamil and diltiazem are seen predominantly in tissues in which phase 0 or phase 4 depolarization is largely calcium dependent, namely SA and AV nodes. Discharge rate and recovery time in the SA, AV conduction time, and AV node ERP are prolonged. Clinically, the QRS complex and QT_c interval are not significantly affected,

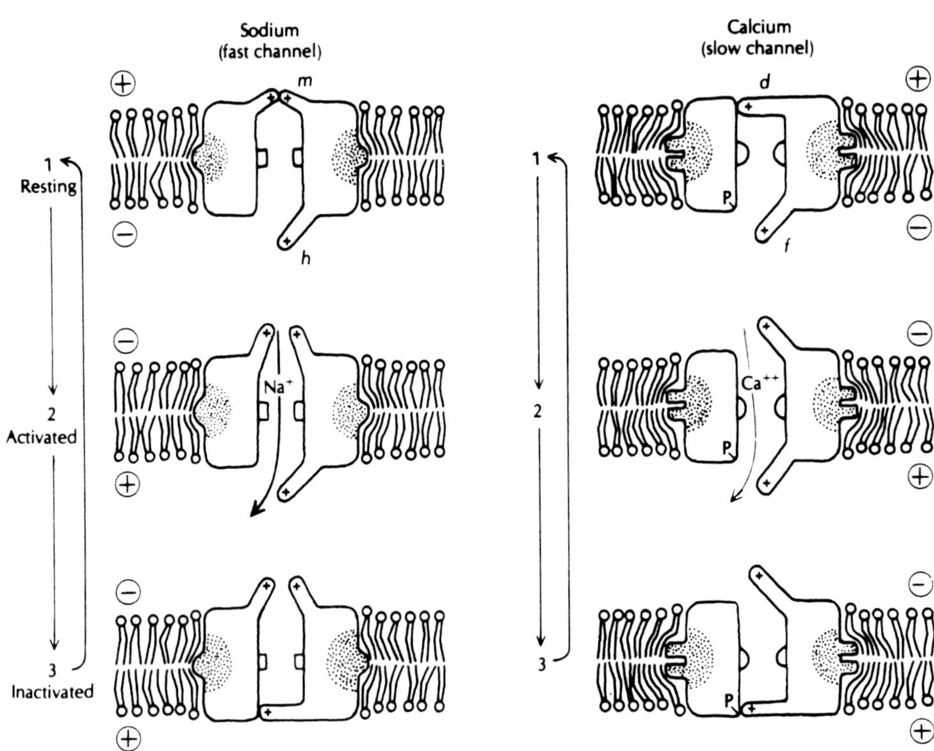

Figure 10–29 Schematic depiction of the calcium channel in the sarcolemmal membrane. The upstroke (phase 0) of the action potential, which allows rapid entry of sodium into the cell, producing the opening of the activation gates (m) in the sodium channel. The resulting change in transmembrane potential closes the inactivation gate (h), which stops sodium influx but maintains a refractory state in the cell membrane until repolarization. Similar processes occur in the calcium channel activation gate (d) and inactivation gate (f) except that at least some of the steps in slow channel activation require phosphorylation (P) by a cyclic adenosine monophosphate protein kinase. Changes in the conformation of the channel proteins provide the three functional states of the channel: (1) resting (closed and able to open); (2) activated (open); and (3) inactivated (closed and unable to open in response to depolarization). (From Katz AM, Messineo FC: Lipids and membrane function: Implications in arrhythmias. Hosp Pract 16:49, 1981.)

but AH (but not HV) conduction time is prolonged. Electrophysiologic effects of verapamil have been shown experimentally (in anesthetized dogs) to relate to plasma concentration; the AH interval was prolonged at lower concentrations than were necessary to slow the SA node or to produce AV block.[628]

As with several other antiarrhythmic drugs, the pharmacokinetics of IV and orally administered verapamil differ. The hepatic extraction of orally administered verapamil is extensive; as a result, its bioavailability, which is normally low, is increased significantly by liver disease.[240] After intravenous administration of verapamil, plasma clearance approximates splanchnic blood flow rate and, because of its lipophilic nature, the apparent volume of distribution is large. Elimination half-life of verapamil is approximately 5 hours, but it may be longer with chronic administration, perhaps because of saturation of hepatic metabolic pathways. Also, a principal metabolite, norverapamil, is biologically active, accumulates to concentrations equal to those of verapamil during chronic therapy, and has a longer half-life (8 to 13 hours).[629] Excretion of verapamil after metabolism is renal (65% to 70%), but 3% to 4% is excreted unchanged.[627] Metabolism involves *n*-dealkylation and *O*-demethylation with norverapamil (one eighth of the Ca^{++} channel–blocking potency of verapamil) as the major metabolite.[618] Verapamil and metabolites are highly protein bound (90%).

Verapamil dosage for acute intravenous treatment of PSVT is 0.07 to 0.15 mg/kg over 1 minute, with the same dose repeated after 30 minutes if the initial response is inadequate (10 mg maximum). Since the cardiovascular depressant effects of the inhalation anesthetics involve inhibition of calcium-related intracellular processes, the interaction of verapamil and these anesthetics is synergistic. In one large clinical series, verapamil given during steady-state halothane anesthesia transiently decreased BP and produced a 4% incidence of PR interval prolongation.[630] In laboratory studies, verapamil interacts similarly with halothane, enflurane, and isoflurane to mildly depress ventricular function and to slow AV conduction (PR interval).[625] AV block can occur, however, and may be refractory. In addition, AV block can occur when verapamil is combined with β-blockers.

Diltiazem in doses of 0.25 to 0.30 mg/kg administered intravenously followed by a titratable intravenous infusion of 10 to 20 mg/hr has been shown to be rapid acting and efficacious in controlling ventricular response rate in new-onset AF and atrial flutter.[631,632] In addition, the prophylactic use of intravenous diltiazem has been shown to reduce the incidence of postoperative supraventricular arrhythmias following pneumonectomy and cardiac surgery.[633] Diltiazem may also have a role in treating ventricular arrhythmias. In an experimental model, diltiazem has been shown to be protective against VF with acute cocaine toxicity.[634]

Another adverse effect of verapamil is the potentiation of neuromuscular blockade. In two laboratory studies, verapamil depressed twitch height response to indirect stimulation.[635, 636] Although the exact presynaptic versus postsynaptic site of the block was not determined, the qualitative similarity of the effect to that of pancuronium suggested an effect at the neuromuscular junction. At clinically relevant doses of verapamil, the effect is slight, but the clinical potential for synergistic interaction with residual muscle relaxants seems substantial. Cautious clinical attention to neuromuscular function is necessary to safely use verapamil in patients who are receiving or have recently received muscle relaxants.

Other Antiarrhythmic Agents

Digoxin

The primary therapeutic use of digitalis drugs is to slow the ventricular response during AF or atrial flutter, which occurs because of a complex combination of direct and indirect actions on the AV node. The primary direct pharmacologic effect of digitalis is inhibition of the membrane-bound Na^+-K^+–dependent ATPase. This enzyme provides the chemical energy necessary for the transport of sodium (out) and potassium (in) during repolarization. The glycosides bind to the enzyme in a specific saturable way that inhibits enzyme activity and impairs the active transport of sodium and potassium. The net result is a slight increase in intracellular sodium and a corresponding decrease in intracellular potassium concentration. The sodium exchanges for calcium and results in a relatively weak inotropic effect.

In Purkinje fibers, digoxin increases the slope of phase 4 depolarization and decreases resting potential or maximal diastolic potential so that the initiation of depolarization (phase 0) begins at a less negative potential; therefore, both the V_{max} and the conduction velocity of the AP are lower. The phase 4 effect is inversely related to extracellular potassium concentration. At low concentrations of potassium, the increased rate of phase 4 depolarization is augmented and automaticity increases, which may partially explain the increased risk of digoxin-related toxicity during hypokalemia or pronounced potassium fluxes, such as during cardioversion or in the period immediately surrounding CPB. At concentrations approaching toxicity, digoxin produces delayed afterpotentials, which may be sufficient to reach threshold and trigger depolarization.[637-639] The direct action of therapeutic concentrations of digoxin in Purkinje fibers, therefore, decreases conduction velocity and increases ERP.

In specialized conduction fibers in the SA and AV nodes, similar electrophysiologic effects occur; in both of these regions, however, the dominant effects are indirect and mediated by the ANS. In atrial and ventricular muscle, direct effects resemble those in Purkinje fibers. The indirect effects of digitalis, notably a decreased APD, account for the decreased QT interval in the ECG; effects of this drug during phases 2 and 3 of the AP account for the characteristic downward convexity of the ST segment.[640]

Digoxin increases vagal efferent activity, the origin of which may relate to increased sensitivity of arterial baroreceptors and an increased carotid sinus nerve activity, or to an effect on the central vagal nuclei.[641-643] In addition, SA node sensitivity to acetylcholine may be enhanced by digoxin. In high concentrations, digoxin may decrease SA and AV nodal sensitivities to catecholamines and sympathetic stimulation, although this may be due to increased sympathetic efferent activity produced by both the central nervous system (CNS, medulla) effects of digoxin and the inhibition of norepinephrine uptake at peripheral sympathetic nerve terminals.[642,643] The decreased sinus rate seen with digoxin is, therefore, due in part to both increased vagal efferent activity and decreased sympathetic tone.

The AV node is the portion of the conduction system most strongly influenced by both the direct and indirect effects of digoxin. Conduction through the AV node is slowed, and the ERP of the AV node is lengthened by digoxin. In toxic concentrations, digoxin can effectively block AV nodal transmission.

In atrial tissue, the direct and indirect (vagal) effects of digoxin are opposed. The direct effect is an increase in APD, but the indirect effect (mediated by acetylcholine release) is marked decreases in APD and ERP. At therapeutic concentrations, the indirect effect predominates, which makes the atria responsive to higher stimulation frequencies.[640] The frequency of atrial impulses arriving at the AV node is generally increased, which leads to frequent partial depolarization of the AV node (*concealed conduction*). This effect, plus the increased AV nodal ERP (produced by direct effects, vagal effects, and sympatholytic effects), result in a net decrease in the frequency of impulses that successfully traverse the AV node to depolarize the His-Purkinje system.

The main preparation of cardiac glycosides available is digoxin. Digoxin reaches peak effects in 1.5 to 2 hours, but has a significant effect within 5 to 30 minutes. For undigitalized patients, the initial dose is 0.5 to 0.75 mg of digoxin, with subsequent doses of 0.125 to 0.25 mg. The usual total digitalizing dose ranges from 0.75 to 1.0 mg by the IV route. Digoxin is approximately 25% protein bound, and the therapeutic range of plasma concentrations is 0.5 to 2.0 ng/mL.

Adenosine

Adenosine is a virtually ubiquitous endogenous nucleoside that has potent electrophysiologic effects in addition to having a major physiologic role in regulation of vasomotor tone.[644] Adenosine is unique in that it is produced as an intermediate metabolite of adenosine monophosphate (AMP). It has an extremely short half-life in plasma (on the order of 1.5 to 2 seconds) because of metabolism by adenosine deaminase to inosine, or by adenosine kinase to AMP. Both enzymes are contained within the intracellular compartment (cytosolic), indicating a rapid transmembrane transport system for adenosine. Inhibition of this transport system by dipyridamole markedly enhances the cardiac effects of adenosine.

The important cardiac electrophysiologic effects of adenosine are mediated by the A_1-receptor and consist of negative chronotropic, dromotropic, and inotropic actions. Adenosine decreases SA node activity, AV node conductivity, and ventricular automaticity. In many ways these effects mimic those of acetylcholine. The A_1-receptor is linked to the ionic channel for K^+ and Ca^{++}, and to adenylyl cyclase through guanine nucleotide-binding inhibitory protein (G_i). Activation of the A_1-receptor in the SA and AV nodes activates the outward acetylcholine-adenosine-regulated potassium current. In ventricular myocardium, adenosine antagonizes the stimulation of the inward Ca^{++} current produced by catecholamines. The primary antiarrhythmic effect of adenosine is to interrupt reentrant AV nodal tachycardia, and this effect most likely relates to the potassium current effects.

For clinical use, adenosine must be administered by a rapid IV bolus in a dose of 100 to 200 μg/kg, although continuous IV infusions of 150 to 300 μg/kg/min have been used to produce controlled hypotension. For practical purposes, in adults an IV dose of 3 to 6 mg is given by IV bolus followed by a second dose of 6 to 12 mg after 1 minute if the first dose was not effective. This therapy rapidly interrupts narrow-complex tachycardia caused by AV nodal reentry.[645] Comparison with verapamil has shown adenosine to be equally effective as an antiarrhythmic, but with the advantages of fewer adverse hemodynamic effects, a faster onset of action, and a more rapid elimination so that undesired effects are short-lived.[646] The MD_{50} of adenosine for reentrant supraventricular arrhythmias in children is 100 to 150 μg/kg.[647]

Potassium

Because of the close relationship between extracellular pH and potassium, the primary mechanism of pH-induced arrhythmias may be alteration of potassium concentration. Both hypokalemia and hyperkalemia are associated with cardiac arrhythmias; however, hypokalemia is more common perioperatively in cardiac surgical patients and is more commonly associated with arrhythmias.[648] Decreasing extracellular potassium concentration increases the peak negative diastolic potential, which would theoretically appear to decrease the likelihood of spontaneous depolarization. However, because the permeability of the myocardial cell membrane to potassium is directly related to extracellular potassium concentration, hypokalemia decreases cellular permeability to potassium. This prolongs the AP by slowing repolarization, which in turn slows conduction and increases the dispersion of recovery of excitability and, thus, predisposes to the development of arrhythmias. Electrocardiographic correlates of hypokalemia include appearance of a U wave and increased P-wave amplitude.[649] The arrhythmias most commonly associated with hypokalemia are premature atrial contractions (PACs), atrial tachycardia, and supraventricular tachycardia (SVT). Hypokalemia also accentuates the toxicity of cardiac glycosides.

Moderate hyperkalemia, in contrast, increases membrane permeability to potassium, which increases the speed of repolarization and decreases APD, thereby decreasing the tendency to arrhythmias. An increased potassium concentration also affects pacemaker activity. The increased potassium permeability caused by hyperkalemia decreases the rate of spontaneous diastolic depolarization, which slows HR and, in the extreme case, can produce asystole. The repolarization abnormalities of hyperkalemia lead to the characteristic ECG findings of T-wave peaking, prolonged PR interval, decreased QRS amplitude, and a widened QRS complex.[650] Both atrioventricular and intraventricular conduction abnormalities result from the slowed conduction and uneven repolarization.

Treatment of hyperkalemia is based on its magnitude and on the clinical presentation. For life-threatening, hyperkalemia-induced arrhythmias, the principle is rapid reduction of extracellular potassium concentration, a treatment that does not acutely decrease total body potassium content. Calcium chloride, 10 to 20 mg/kg, given by IV infusion, will directly antagonize the effects of potassium on the cardiac cell membranes. Sodium bicarbonate, 1 to 2 mEq/kg, or a dose calculated from acid-base measurements to produce moderate alkalinity (pH approximately 7.45 to 7.50), will shift potassium intracellularly. A change in pH of 0.1 unit produces a 0.5 to 1.5 mEq/L change of potassium concentration in the opposite direction. An IV infusion of glucose and insulin has a similar effect; glucose at a dose of 0.5 to 2.0 g/kg with insulin in the ratio of 1 unit to 4 g of glucose is appropriate. Sequential measurement of serum potassium is important with this treatment because marked hypokalemia can result. Loop diuretics and potassium-binding resins promote excretion of potassium, although the effects are less rapid than with the previously mentioned modalities (see Chapter 36).

With chronic potassium deficiency, the plasma level poorly reflects the total body deficit. Since only 2% of total body potassium is in plasma, and total body potassium stores may be 2000 to 3000 mEq, a 25% decline in serum potassium from 4 to 3 mEq/L indicates an equilibrium total body deficiency of 500 to 800 mEq, replacement of which should be undertaken slowly.

Acute hypokalemia frequently occurs after CPB as a result of hemodilution, urinary losses, and intracellular shifts,[651] the latter perhaps relating to abnormalities of the glucose-insulin system seen with nonpulsatile hypothermic CPB.[652] With frequent assessment of serum potassium concentrations and continuous ECG monitoring, potassium infusion at rates of up to 10 to 15 mEq/hr may be administered to treat serious hypokalemia.

Magnesium

Magnesium deficiency is also a relatively common electrolyte abnormality in critically ill patients, especially in chronic situations. Hypomagnesemia is associated with a variety of cardiovascular disturbances, including arrhythmias.[653,654] Sudden death from CAD, alcoholic cardiomyopathy, and CHF may involve magnesium deficiency.[653-655] Functionally, magnesium is required for the membrane-bound Na^+/K^+-ATPase, which is the principal enzyme that maintains normal intracellular potassium concentration. Not surprisingly, the ECG findings seen with magnesium deficiency mimic those seen with hypokalemia: prolonged PR and QT intervals, increased QRS duration, and ST-segment abnormalities. In addition, as with hypokalemia, magnesium deficiency predisposes to the development of the arrhythmias produced by cardiac glycosides.[656,657]

Arrhythmias induced by magnesium deficiency may be refractory to treatment with antiarrhythmic drugs and either electrical cardioversion or defibrillation. For this reason, adjunctive treatment of refractory arrhythmias with magnesium has been advocated even when magnesium deficiency has not been documented.[658] Magnesium deficiency is common in cardiac surgery patients due to the diuretic agents these patients are often receiving and because magnesium levels decrease with CPB because of hemodilution of the pump. Magnesium lacks a counter-regulatory hormone to increase magnesium levels during CPB in contrast with the hypocalcemia that is corrected by PTH. The results of magnesium administration trials involving CABG have been conflicting. Some studies have shown a benefit and others have not in regard to reducing the incidence of postoperative arrhythmias.

REFERENCES

1. ACC/AHA 2002 Guideline Update for the Management of Patients with Unstable Angina and NonST-Segment Elevation Myocardial Infarction. A Report of the American College of Cardiology/American Heart Association Task Force on Practice Guidelines (Committee on Management of Patients with Unstable Angina). Available: http://www.acc.org/clinical/guidelines/unstable/incorporated/UA_incorporated.pdf
2. Rutherford JR: Medical management. *In* Fuster V, Topol E, Nabel E (eds): Atherothrombosis and Coronary Artery Disease. Philadelphia, Lippincott, 2005, pp 1327–1337
3. Horowitz JD: Role of nitrates in unstable angina pectoris. Am J Cardiol 70:64B, 1992
4. Hill JA, Feldman RL, Pepine CJ, et al: Randomized double-blind comparison of nifedipine and isosorbide dinitrate in patients with coronary arterial spasm. Am J Cardiol 49:431, 1982
5. Purcell H, Mulcahy D, Fox K: Nitrates in silent ischemia. Cardiovasc Drug Ther 8:727, 1994
6. Hoekenga D, Abrams J: Rational medical therapy for stable angina pectoris. Am J Med 76:309, 1984
7. Abrams J: Usefulness of long-acting nitrates in cardiovascular disease. Am J Med 64:183, 1978
8. Miller RR, Awan NA, DeMaria AN, et al: Importance of maintaining systemic blood pressure during nitroglycerin administration for reducing ischemic injury in patients with coronary disease. Effects on CBF, myocardial energetics and left ventricular function. Am J Cardiol 40:504, 1977
9. Abrams J: Mechanisms of action of the organic nitrates in the treatment of myocardial ischemia. Am J Cardiol 70:30B, 1992
10. Murad F: Cyclic guanosine monophosphate as a mediator of vasodilation. J Clin Invest 78:1, 1986
11. Needleman P, Jakschik B, Johnson EM Jr: Sulfhydryl requirement for relaxation of vascular smooth muscle. J Pharmacol Exp Ther 187:324, 1973
12. Galvas PE, DiSalvo J: Concentration and time-dependent relationships between isosorbide dinitrate-induced relaxation and formation of cyclic GMP in coronary arterial smooth muscle. J Pharmacol Exp Ther 224:373, 1983
13. Anderson TJ, Meredith IT, Ganz P, et al: Nitric oxide and nitrovasodilators: Similarities, differences, and potential interactions. J Am Coll Cardiol 24:555, 1994
14. Waldman SA, Murad F: Cyclic GMP synthesis and function. Pharmacol Rev 39:163, 1987

15. Hardman JG, Limbird LE (eds): Goodman and Gilman's The Pharmacological Basis of Therapeutics. New York, McGraw-Hill, 1996
16. Opie LH (ed): Drugs for the Heart, 6th edition. Philadelphia, Elsevier, 2005, pp 33–49
17. Armstrong PW, Moffat JA: Tolerance to organic nitrates: Clinical and experimental perspectives. Am J Med 74;73, 1983
18. Packer M, Lee WH, Kassler PD, et al: Prevention and reversal of nitrate tolerance in patients with congestive heart failure. N Engl J Med 317:799, 1987
19. Fung H-L, Sutton SC, Kamiya A: Blood vessel uptake and metabolism of organic nitrates in the rat. J Pharmacol Exp Ther 228:334, 1984
20. Imhof PR, Ott B, Frankhauser P, et al: Difference in nitroglycerin dose-response in the venous and arterial beds. Eur J Clin Pharmacol 18:455, 1980
21. Smith ER, Smiseth OA, Kingma I, et al: Mechanism of action of nitrates. Role of changes in venous capacitance and in the left ventricular diastolic pressure-volume relation. Am J Med 76:14, 1984
22. Simon AC, Levenson JA, Levy BY, et al: Effect of nitroglycerin on peripheral large arteries in hypertension. Br J Clin Pharmacol 14:241, 1982
23. Abrams J: Hemodynamic effects of nitroglycerin and long-acting nitrates. Am Heart J 110:216, 1985
24. McGregor M: Pathogenesis of angina pectoris and role of nitrates in relief of myocardial ischemia. Am J Med 74:21, 1983
25. Pearl RG, Rosenthal MH, Schroeder JS, et al: Acute hemodynamic effects of nitroglycerin in pulmonary hypertension. Ann Intern Med 99:9, 1983
26. Ilbawi MN, Idriss FS, DeLeon SY, et al: Hemodynamic effects of intravenous nitroglycerin in pediatric patients after heart surgery. Circulation 72:II-101, 1985
27. Vatner SF, Pagani M, Rutherford JD, et al: Effects of nitroglycerin on cardiac function and regional blood flow distribution in conscious dogs. Am J Physiol 234:H244, 1978
28. Brown G, Bolson E, Peterson RB, et al: The mechanisms of nitroglycerin action. Stenosis vasodilatation as a major component of drug response. Circulation 64:1089, 1981
29. Conti CR, Feldman RL, Pepine CJ, et al: Effect of glyceryl trinitrate on coronary and systemic hemodynamics in man. Am J Med 74:28, 1983
30. Feldman RL, Pepine CJ, Conti CR: Magnitude of dilatation of large and small coronary arteries by nitroglycerin. Circulation 64:324, 1981
31. Ludmer PL, Selwyn AP, Shook TL, et al: Paradoxical vasoconstriction induced by acetylcholine in atherosclerotic coronary arteries. N Engl J Med 315:1046, 1986
32. Panzenbeck MJ, Baez A, Kaley G: Nitroglycerin and nitroprusside increase CBF in dogs by a mechanism independent of prostaglandin release. Am J Cardiol 53:936, 1984
33. Horwitz LD, Gorlin R, Taylor WJ, et al: Effects of nitroglycerin on regional myocardial blood flow in coronary artery disease. J Clin Invest 50:1578, 1971
34. Cohen MV, Downey JM, Sonnenblick EH, et al: The effects of nitroglycerin on coronary collaterals and myocardial contractility. J Clin Invest 52:2836, 1973
35. Feldman RL, Joyal M, Conti CR, et al: Effect of nitroglycerin on coronary collateral flow and pressure during acute coronary occlusion. Am J Cardiol 54:958, 1984
36. Moir TW: Subendocardial distribution of CBF and the effect of antianginal drugs. Circ Res 30:621, 1972
37. Munzel T, Mulsch A, Kleschyov A: Mechanisms underlying nitroglycerin-induced superoxide production in platelets. Circulation 106:170, 2002
38. Armstrong PW, Armstrong JA, Marks GS: Blood levels after sublingual nitroglycerin. Circulation 59:585, 1979
39. Parker JO, Vankoughnett KA, Farrell B: Nitroglycerin lingual spray: Clinical efficacy and dose-response relation. Am J Cardiol 57:1, 1986
40. Reichek N, Priest C, Kienzle M, et al: Angina prophylaxis with buccal nitroglycerin: A rapid onset long-acting nitrate. Adv Pharmacother 1:2, 1982
41. Reichek N, Goldstein RE, Redwood DR, et al: Sustained effects of nitroglycerin ointment in patients with angina pectoris. Circulation 50:348, 1974
42. Armstrong PW, Mathew MT, Boroomand K, et al: Nitroglycerin ointment in acute myocardial infarction. Am J Cardiol 38:474, 1976
43. Chien YW: Pharmaceutical considerations of transdermal nitroglycerin delivery: The various approaches. Am Heart J 108:207, 1984
44. DeMots H, Glasser SP: Intermittent transdermal nitroglycerin therapy in the treatment of chronic stable angina. J Am Coll Cardiol 13:786, 1989
45. DePace NL, Herling IM, Kotler MN, et al: Intravenous nitroglycerin for rest angina. Potential pathophysiologic mechanisms of action. Arch Intern Med 142:1806, 1982
46. Young JB, Pratt CM, Farmer JA, et al: Specialized delivery systems for intravenous nitroglycerin. Are they necessary? Am J Med 76:27, 1984
47. Darling RC, Roughton FJW: The effect of methemoglobin on the equilibrium between oxygen and hemoglobin. Am J Physiol 137:56, 1942
48. Smith RP, Olson MV: Drug-induced methemoglobinemia. Semin Hematol 10:253, 1973
49. Kaplan KJ, Taber M, Teagarden JR, et al: Association of methemoglobinemia and intravenous nitroglycerin administration. Am J Cardiol 55:181, 1985
50. Harris JC, Rumack BH, Peterson RG, et al: Methemoglobinemia resulting from absorption of nitrates. JAMA 242:2869, 1979
51. Zurick AM, Wagner RH, Starr NJ, et al: Intravenous nitroglycerin, methemoglobinemia, and respiratory distress in a postoperative cardiac surgical patient. Anesthesiology 61:464, 1984
52. Axelsson KL, Anderson RGG: Tolerance towards nitroglycerin, induced in vivo, is correlated to a reduced cGMP response and an alteration in cGMP turnover. Eur J Pharmacol 88:71, 1983
53. Thadani U: Role of nitrates in angina pectoris. Am J Cardiol 70:43B, 1992
54. Parker JD, Farrell B, Fenton T, et al: Counter-regulatory responses to continuous and intermittent therapy with nitroglycerin. Circulation 84:2336, 1991
55. Parker JD, Parker JO: Effect of therapy with an angiotensin-converting enzyme inhibitor of hemodynamic and counterregulatory responses during continuous therapy with nitroglycerin. J Am Coll Cardiol 21:1445, 1993
56. Dupuis J, Lalonde G, Lemieux R, Rouleau JL: Tolerance to intravenous nitroglycerin in patients with congestive heart failure: Role of increased intravascular volume, neurohumoral activation and lack of prevention with N-acetylcysteine. J Am Coll Cardiol 16:923, 1990
57. Watanabe H, Kakihana M, Ohtsuka S, et al: Platelet cyclic GMP. A potentially useful indicator to evaluate the effects of nitroglycerin and nitrate tolerance. Circulation 88:29, 1993
58. Bassan MM: The daylong pattern of the antianginal effect of long-term three times daily administered isosorbide dinitrate. J Am Coll Cardiol 16:936, 1990
59. Parker JO, Amies MH, Hawkinson RW, et al: Intermittent transdermal nitroglycerin therapy in angina pectoris. Clinically effective without tolerance or rebound. Circulation 91:1368, 1995
60. Munzel T, Heitzer T, Kurz S, et al: Dissociation of coronary vascular tolerance and neurohormonal adjustments during long-term nitroglycerin therapy in patients with stable coronary artery disease. J Am Coll Cardiol 27:297, 1996
61. Mangione NJ, Glasser SP: Phenomenon of nitrate tolerance. Am Heart J 128:137, 1994
62. Lange RL, Reid MS, Tresch DD, et al: Nonatheromatous ischemic heart disease following withdrawal from chronic industrial nitroglycerin exposure. Circulation 46:666, 1972
63. Elkayam V, Kulick D, McIntosh N, et al: Incidence of early tolerance to hemodynamic effects of continuous infusion of nitroglycerin in patients with coronary artery disease and heart failure. Circulation 76:577, 1987
64. Thadani U, Fung HL, Darke AC, et al: Oral isosorbide dinitrate in angina pectoris: Comparison of duration of action and dose-response relationship during acute and sustained therapy. Am J Cardiol 49:411, 1982
65. Parker JO: Eccentric dosing with isosorbide-5-mononitrate in angina pectoris. Am J Cardiol 72:871, 1993
66. Stamler JS, Loscalzo J: The antiplatelet effects of organic nitrates and related nitroso compounds in vitro and in vivo and their relevance to cardiovascular disorders. J Am Coll Cardiol 18:1529, 1991
67. Lam JYT, Chesebro JH, Fuster V: Platelets, vasoconstriction and nitroglycerin during arterial wall injury. A new antithrombotic role for an old drug. Circulation 78:712, 1988
68. Mellion BT, Ignarro LJ, Myers CB, et al: Inhibition of platelet aggregation by S-nitrosothiols. Heme-dependent activation of soluble guanylate cyclase and stimulation of cyclic GMP accumulation. Mol Pharmacol 23:653, 1983
69. Stamler JS, Vaughan DE, Loscalzo J: Synergistic disaggregation of platelets by tissue-type plasminogen activator, prostaglandin E_1, and nitroglycerin. Circ Res 65:796, 1989
70. Diodati J, Theroux P, Latour JG, et al: Effects of nitroglycerin at therapeutic doses on platelet aggregation in unstable angina pectoris and acute myocardial infarction. Am J Cardiol 66:683, 1990
71. Negrescu EV, Sazonova LN, Baldenkov GN, et al: Relationship between the inhibition of receptor-induced increase in cytosolic free calcium concentration and the vasodilator effects of nitrates in patients with congestive heart failure. Int J Cardiol 26:175, 1990
72. Pizzulli L, Nitsch J, Luderitz B: Inhibition of the heparin effect by nitroglycerin. Dtsch Med Wochenschr 113:1837, 1988

73. Habbab MA, Haft JI: Heparin resistance induced by intravenous nitroglycerin. A word of caution when both drugs are used concomitantly. Arch Intern Med 147:857, 1987
74. Becker RC, Corrao JM, Bovill EG, et al: Intravenous nitroglycerin-induced heparin resistance: A qualitative antithrombin III abnormality. Am Heart J 119:1254, 1990
75. Stanek EJ, Nair RN, Munger MA: Nitroglycerin-induced heparin resistance (letter). Am Heart J 121:1849, 1991
76. Bjornsson TD, Schneider DE, Hecht AR: Effects of *N*-deacetylation and *N*-desulfation of heparin on its anticoagulant activity and in vivo disposition. J Pharmacol Exp Ther 245:804, 1988
77. Cheitlin MD, Hutter AMJ, Brindis RG, et al: ACA/AHA expert consensus document of sildenafil in patients with cardiovascular disease: American College of Cardiology/American Heart Association. J Am Coll Cardiol 33:273, 1999
78. Auerbach AD, Goldman L: Beta-blockers and reduction of cardiac events in noncardiac surgery. JAMA 287;1435-1444, 2002
79. London MJ, Zaugg M, Schaub MC, Spahn DR: Perioperative beta-adrenergic receptor blockade. Anesthesiology 100;170, 2004
80. Stevens RD, Burri H, Tramer MR: Pharmacologic myocardial protection in patients undergoing noncardiac surgery: a quantitative systematic review. Anesth Analg 97:623, 2003
81. Peter T, Norris RM, Clarke ED, et al: Reduction of enzyme levels of propranolol after acute myocardial infarction. Circulation 57:1091, 1978
82. β-Blocker Heart Attack Trial Research Group: A randomized trial of propranolol in patients with acute myocardial infarction: I. Mortality results. JAMA 247:1707, 1982
83. Norwegian Multicenter Study Group: Timolol-induced reduction in mortality and reinfarction in patients surviving acute myocardial infarction. N Engl J Med 304:801, 1981
84. Roberts R, Rogers WJ, Mueller HS, et al: Immediate versus deferred beta-blockade following thrombolytic therapy in patients with acute myocardial infarction. Results of the Thrombolysis in Myocardial Infraction (TIMI) II-B Study. Circulation 83:422, 1991
85. Ryan TJ, Anderson JL, Antman EM, et al: ACC/AHA guidelines for the management of patients with acute myocardial infarction. A report of the American College of Cardiology/American Heart Association Task Force on Practice Guidelines. J Am Coll Cardiol 28:1328, 1996
86. Soumeral SB, Mclaughlin TJ, Spiegelman D, et al: Adverse outcomes of underuse of β-blockers in elderly survivors of acute myocardial infarction. JAMA 277:115, 1997
87. Pepine CJ, Cohn PF, Deedwania PC, et al: Effects of treatment on outcome in mildly symptomatic patients with ischemia during daily life. The Atenolol Silent Ischemia Study (ASIST). Circulation 90:762, 1994
88. Poldermans D, Boersma E, Bax JJ et al. The effect of bisoprolol on perioperative mortality and myocardial infarction in high risk patients undergoing vascular surgery. N Engl J Med 341:1789, 1999
89. Mangano DT, Layug EL, Wallace A, Tateo I: Effect of atenolol on mortality and cardiovascular morbidity after noncardiac surgery. N Engl J Med 335:1713, 1996
90. ACC/AHA Guideline Update on Perioperative Cardiovascular Evaluation for Noncardiac Surgery. A Report of the American College of Cardiology/American Heart Association Task Force on Practice Guidelines. J Am Coll Cardiol 39:542, 2002. Available at: http://www.acc.org/clinical/guidelines/perio/clean/pdf/perio_pdf.pdf
91. Ahlquist RP: A study of the adrenotropic receptors. Am J Physiol 153:586, 1948
92. Benovic JL, Shorr RGL, Caron MG, et al: The mammalian β_2-adrenergic receptor: Purification and characterization. Biochemistry 23:4510, 1984
93. Dixon RAF, Kobilka BK, Strader DJ, et al: Cloning of the gene and cDNA for mammalian β-adrenergic receptor and homology with rhodopsin. Nature 321:75, 1986
94. Gilman AG: G proteins: Transducers of receptor-generated signals. Annu Rev Biochem 56:615, 1987
95. Dohlman HG, Caron MG, Strader CD, et al: Identification and sequence of a binding site peptide of the β_2-adrenergic receptor. Biochemistry 27:1813, 1988
96. O'Dowd BF, Hnatowich M, Regan JW, et al: Site-directed mutagenesis of the cytoplasmic domains of the human β_2-adrenergic receptor. Localization of regions involved in G protein-receptor coupling. J Biol Chem 263:15985-15992, 1988
97. Bouvier M, Hausdorff WP, DeBlasi A, et al: Removal of phosphorylation sites from the β_2-adrenergic receptor delays onset of agonist-promoted desensitization. Nature 333:370, 1988
98. Benovic JL, Bouvier M, Caron MG, et al: Regulation of adenylyl cyclase-coupled β-adrenergic receptors. Annu Rev Cell Biol 4:405, 1988
99. Mukherjee A, Bush LR, McCoy KE, et al: Relationship between β-adrenergic receptor numbers and physiological responses during experimental canine myocardial ischemia. Circ Res 50:735, 1982
100. Freissmuth M, Schütz W, Weindlmayer-Göttel M, et al: Effects of ischemia on the canine myocardial β-adrenoceptor-linked adenylate cyclase system. J Cardiovasc Pharmacol 10:568, 1987
101. Vatner DE, Young MA, Knight DR, et al: β-Receptors and adenylate cyclase: Comparison of nonischemic and postmortem tissue. Am J Physiol 258:H140-H144, 1990
102. Susanni EE, Manders WT, Knight DR, et al: One hour of myocardial ischemia decreases the activity of the stimulatory guanine nucleotide regulatory protein G_s. Circ Res 65:1145, 1989
103. Maisel AS, Motulsky HJ, Insel PA: Externalization of beta-adrenergic receptors promoted by myocardial ischemia. Science 230:183, 1985
104. Lands AM, Arnold A, McAuliff JP, et al: Differentiation of receptor systems activated by sympathomimetic amines. Nature 214:597, 1967
105. Ablad B, Carlsson B, Carlsson E, et al: Cardiac effects of β-adrenergic antagonists. Adv Cardiol 12:290, 1974
106. Lemoine H, Schönell H, Kaumann AJ: Contribution of β_1- and β_2-adrenoceptors of human atrium and ventricle to the effects of noradrenaline and adrenaline as assessed with (-)-atenolol. Br J Pharmacol 95:55, 1988
107. Kaumann AJ, Lemoine H: β_2-Adrenoceptor-mediated positive inotropic effect of adrenaline in human ventricular myocardium. Quantitative discrepancies with binding and adenylate cyclase stimulation. Naunyn Schmiedebens Arch Pharmacol 335:403, 1987
108. Molena-ar P, Russell FD, Shimada T, et al: Function, characterization and autoradiographic localization and quantitation of beta-adrenoceptors in cardiac tissues. Clin Exp Physiol Pharmacol 16:529, 1989
109. Molena-ar P, Malta E, Jones CR, et al: Autoradiographic localization and function of β-adrenoceptors on the human internal mammary artery and saphenous vein. Br J Pharmacol 95:225, 1988
110. Lipworth BJ: Clinical pharmacology of β_3-adrenoreceptors. Br J Clin Pharmacol 42:291, 1996
111. Lewis CM, Brink AJ: Beta-adrenergic blockade. Hemodynamics and myocardial energy metabolism in patients with ischemic heart disease. Am J Cardiol 21:846, 1968
112. Becker LC, Fortuin NJ, Pitt B: Effect of ischemic and antianginal drugs on the distribution of radioactive microspheres in the canine left ventricle. Circ Res 28:263, 1971
113. Kern MJ, Ganz P, Horowitz JD, et al: Potentiation of coronary vasoconstriction by beta-adrenergic blockade in patients with coronary artery disease. Circulation 67:1178, 1983
114. Gaglione A, Hess OM, Corin WJ, et al: Is there coronary vasoconstriction after intracoronary beta-adrenergic blockade in patients with coronary artery disease? J Am Coll Cardiol 10:299, 1987
115. Tarazi RC, Dustan HP: Beta-adrenergic blockade in hypertension. Practical and theoretical implications of long-term hemodynamic variations. Am J Cardiol 29:633, 1972
116. Lund-Johansen P: Hemodynamic consequences of long-term beta-blocker therapy: A 5-year follow-up study of atenolol. J Cardiovasc Pharmacol 1:487, 1979
117. Bühler FR, Laragh JH, Baer L, et al: Propranolol inhibition of renin secretion. A specific approach to diagnosis and treatment of renin-dependent hypertensive diseases. N Engl J Med 287:1209, 1972
118. Hansson L: Beta-adrenergic blockade in essential hypertension. Effects of propranolol on hemodynamic parameters and plasma renin activity. Acta Med Scand 194:1, 1973
119. Man in't Veld AJ, Schalekamp MA: Effects of 10 different beta-adrenoreceptor antagonists on hemodynamics, plasma renin activity, and plasma norepinephrine in hypertension: The key role of vascular resistance changes in relation to partial agonist activity. J Cardiovasc Pharmacol 5:S30-S45, 1983
120. Yamaguchi N, de Champlain J, Nadeau RA: Regulation of norepinephrine release from cardiac sympathetic fibers in the dog by presynaptic α- and β-receptors. Circ Res 41:108, 1977
121. Davis LD, Temte JV: Effects of propranolol on the transmembrane potentials of ventricular muscle and Purkinje fibers of the dog. Circ Res 22:661, 1968
122. Henry JA, Cassidy SL: Membrane stabilizing activity: A major cause of fatal poisoning. Lancet 1:1414, 1986
123. Venditti FJ Jr, Garan H, Ruskin JN: Electrophysiologic effects of beta-blockers in ventricular arrhythmias. Am J Cardiol 60:3D-9D, 1987
124. Totterman K, Groop L, Groop P-H, et al: Effect of beta-blocking drugs on beta-cell function and insulin sensitivity in hypertensive nondiabetic patients. Eur J Clin Pharmacol 26:13, 1984
125. Ryan JR, LaCorte W, Jain A, et al: Hypertension in hypoglycemic diabetics treated with β-adrenergic antagonists. Hypertension 7:443, 1985

126. Rosa RM, Silva P, Young JB, et al: Adrenergic modulation of extrarenal potassium disposal. N Engl J Med 302:431, 1980
127. Traub YM, Rabinov M, Rosenfeld JB, et al: Elevation of serum potassium during beta-blockade: Absence of relationship to the renin-aldosterone system. Clin Pharmacol Ther 28:765, 1980
128. Juhlin-Dannfelt A: Metabolic effects of β-adrenoceptor blockade on skeletal muscle at rest and during exercise. Acta Med Scand 665:113, 1982
129. Day JL, Metcalfe J, Simpson CN: Adrenergic mechanisms in control of plasma lipid concentrations. Br Med J 284:1145, 1982
130. Rohlfing JJ, Brunzell JD: The effects of diuretics and adrenergic-blocking agents on plasma lipids. West J Med 145:210, 1986
131. Kaplan JR, Manuck SB, Adams MR, et al: The effects of beta-adrenergic blocking agents on atherosclerosis and its complications. Eur Heart J 8:928, 1987
132. van Brummelen P: The relevance of intrinsic sympathomimetic activity for beta-blocker-induced changes in plasma lipids. J Cardiovasc Pharmacol 5:S51-S55, 1983
133. Jaillon P: Relevance of intrinsic sympathomimetic activity for beta-blockers. Am J Cardiol 66:21C-23C, 1990
134. Svendsen TL, Hartling OJ, Trap-Jensen J, et al: Adrenergic beta-receptor blockade: Hemodynamic importance of intrinsic sympathomimetic activity at rest. Clin Pharmacol Ther 29:711, 1981
135. Ireland MA, Littler WA: The effects of oral acebutolol and propranolol on forearm blood flow in hypertensive patients. Br J Clin Pharmacol 12:363, 1981
136. van den Meiracker AH, Man in't Veld AJ, Boomsma F, et al: Hemodynamic and β-adrenergic receptor adaptations during long-term β-adrenoceptor blockade. Studies with acebutolol, atenolol, pindolol, and propranolol in hypertensive patients. Circulation 80:903, 1989
137. Multicentre International Study: Supplementary report. Reduction in mortality after myocardial infarction with long-term beta-adrenoceptor blockade. Br Med J 2:419, 1977
138. Myers MG, Lewis PJ, Reid JL, et al: Brain concentration of propranolol in relation to hypotensive effect in the rabbit with observations on brain propranolol levels in man. J Pharmacol Exp Ther 192:327, 1975
139. Nies AS, Shand DG: Clinical pharmacology of propranolol. Circulation 52:6, 1975
140. Branch RA, Shand DG: Propranolol disposition in chronic liver disease: A physiological approach. Clin Pharmacokinet 1:264, 1976
141. Wilkinson GR, Shand DG: Commentary: A physiological approach to hepatic drug clearance. Clin Pharmacol Ther 18:377, 1975
142. Ryan JR: Clinical pharmacology of acebutolol. Am Heart J 109:1131, 1985
143. Paterson JW, Conolly ME, Dollery CT, et al: The pharmacodynamics and metabolism of propranolol in man. Pharmacol Clin 2:127, 1970
144. Walle T, Gaffney TE: Propranolol metabolism in man and dog: Mass spectrometric identification of six new metabolites. J Pharmacol Exp Ther 182:83, 1972
145. Shand DG, Rangno RE: The disposition of propranolol. I. Elimination during oral absorption in man. Pharmacology 7:159, 1972
146. Nies AS, Evans GH, Shand DG: The hemodynamic effects of beta-adrenergic blockade on the flow-dependent hepatic clearance of propranolol. J Pharmacol Exp Ther 184:716, 1973
147. Chidsey C, Pine M, Favrot L, et al: The use of drug concentration measurements in studies of the therapeutic response to propranolol. Postgrad Med J 52:26, 1976
148. Alderman EL, Davies RO, Crowley JJ, et al: Dose-response effectiveness of propranolol for the treatment of angina pectoris. Circulation 51:964, 1975
149. Smulyan H, Weinberg SE, Howanitz PJ: Continuous propranolol infusion following abdominal surgery. JAMA 247:2539, 1982
150. Abrahamsson T, Ek B, Nerme V: The beta$_1$- and beta$_2$-adrenoceptor affinity of atenolol and metoprolol. A receptor-binding study performed with different radioligands in tissues from the rat, the guinea pig and man. Biochem Pharmacol 37:203, 1988
151. Åblad B, Borg KO, Carlsson E, et al: Animal and human pharmacological studies on metoprolol-α new selective adrenergic beta-1-receptor antagonist. Acta Pharmacol Toxicol 36:5, 1975
152. Gorczynski RJ: Basic pharmacology of esmolol. Am J Cardiol 56:3F, 1985
153. Sum CY, Yacobi A, Kartzinel R, et al: Kinetics of esmolol, an ultrashort-acting beta-blocker, and of its major metabolite. Clin Pharmacol Ther 34:427, 1983
154. Thys D, Girard D, Kaplan JA, et al: Hemodynamic effects of esmolol during CABG. Anesthesiology 65:157, 1986
155. Abrams J, Allen J, Allin D, et al: Efficacy and safety of esmolol versus propranolol in the treatment of supraventricular tachyarrhythmias: A multicenter double-blind clinical trial. Am Heart J 110:913, 1985
156. Sheppard D, DeStefano S, Byrd RC, et al: Effects of esmolol on airway function in patients with asthma. J Clin Pharmacol 26:169, 1986
157. The Esmolol Research Group: Intravenous esmolol for the treatment of supraventricular tachyarrhythmia: Results of a multicenter, baseline controlled safety and efficacy study of 160 patients. Am Heart J 112:498, 1986
158. Murthy VS, Patel KD, Elangovan RG, et al: Cardiovascular and neuromuscular effects of esmolol during induction of anesthesia. J Clin Pharmacol 26:351, 1986
159. Lowenthal DT, Porter RS, Saris SD, et al: Clinical pharmacology, pharmacodynamics and interactions with esmolol. Am J Cardiol 56:14F-18F, 1985
160. Oda Y, Nishikawa K, Hase I, Asada A: The short-acting β$_1$-adrenoreceptor antagonists esmolol and candiolol suppress the bispectral index response to tracheal intubation during sevoflurane anesthesia. Anesth Analg 100;733, 2005
161. Dage RC, Hsieh CP: Direct vasodilatation by labetalol in anaesthetized dogs. Br J Pharmacol 70:287, 1980
162. Martin LE, Hopkins R, Bland R: Metabolism of labetalol by animal and man. Br J Pharmacol 3:695, 1976
163. Kaplan JA: Treatment of hypertension: Drug therapy. *In* Kaplan JA: Clinical Hypertension, 8th edition. Philadelphia, Lippincott, 2002, pp 237–338
164. Omvik P, Lund-Johansen P: Acute hemodynamic effects of labetalol in severe hypertension. J Cardiovasc Pharmacol 4:915, 1982
165. Ronne-Rasmussen JO, Andersen GS, Bowel Jensen N, et al: Acute effect of intravenous labetalol in the treatment of systemic arterial hypertension. Br J Clin Pharmacol 3:805, 1976
166. Packer M, Meller J, Medina N, et al: Hemodynamic consequences of combined beta-adrenergic and slow calcium channel blockade in man. Circulation 65:660, 1982
167. Ochs HR, Carstens G, Greenblatt DJ: Reduction in lidocaine clearance during continuous infusion and by coadministration of propranolol. N Engl J Med 303:373, 1980
168. Egstrup K: Transient myocardial ischemia after abrupt withdrawal of antianginal therapy in chronic stable angina. Am J Cardiol 61:1219, 1988
169. Miklos D, Keertai M, Bax J, et al: Is there any reason to withhold beta-blockers from high-risk patients with coronary artery disease during surgery? Anesthesiology 100:4, 2004
170. London M, Zaugg M, Schaub M, Spahn D: Perioperative β-adrenergic receptor blockade. Anesthesiology 100:170, 2004
171. Silverman NA, Wright R, Levitsky S: Efficacy of low-dose propranolol in preventing postoperative supraventricular tachyarrhythmias: A prospective, randomized study. Ann Surg 196:194, 1982
172. Giles J, Sear J, Foex P: Effect of chronic beta-blockage on perioperative outcome in patients undergoing noncardiac surgery. Anaesthesia 59:574, 2004
173. Eisenberg MJ, Brox A, Bestawros AN. Calcium channel blockers: an update. Am J Med 116;35, 2004
174. Brown BG, Bolson EL, Dodge HT: Dynamic mechanisms in human coronary stenosis. Circulation 70:917, 1984
175. Singh BN (ed): Detection, quantification and clinical significance of silent myocardial ischemia in coronary artery disease. Am J Cardiol 58(4):1B-60B, 1986
176. Johnson SM, Mauritson DR, Willerson JT, et al: A controlled trial of verapamil in Prinzmetal's variant angina. N Engl J Med 304:862, 1981
177. Robertson RH, Wood AJJ, Vaughan WK, et al: Exacerbation of vasotonic angina pectoris by propranolol. Circulation 65:281, 1982
178. Strauss WE, McIntyre KM, Parisi AR, et al: Safety and efficacy of diltiazem hydrochloride for the treatment of stable angina pectoris: Report of a cooperative clinical trial. Am J Cardiol 49:560, 1982
179. Pine MB, Citron PD, Bailly DJ, et al: Verapamil versus placebo in relieving stable angina pectoris. Circulation 65[suppl I]:17, 1982
180. Pitt B, Byington R, Furberg C, et al: Effect of anesthesia on the progression of atherosclerosis and the occurrence of clinical events. Circulation 102:1503, 2000
181. Subramanian VB, Bowles MJ, Khurmi NS, et al: Rationale for the choice of calcium antagonists in chronic stable angina. An objective double-blind placebo-controlled comparison of nifedipine and verapamil. Am J Cardiol 50:1173, 1982
182. McCall D, Walsh RA, Frohlich ED, et al: Calcium entry blocking drugs: Mechanisms of action, experimental studies and clinical uses. Curr Probl Cardiol 10:1, 1985
183. Theroux P, Taeymans Y, Morissette D, et al: A randomized study comparing propranolol and diltiazem in the treatment of unstable angina. J Am Coll Cardiol 5:717, 1985

184. Zelis R, Moore R: Recent insights into the calcium channels. Circulation 80[suppl IV]:IV-14-IV, 1989
185. Nowycky MC, Fox AP, Tsien RW: Three types of neuronal calcium channel with different calcium agonist sensitivity. Nature 316:440, 1985
186. Mitra R, Morad M: Two types of calcium channels in guinea pig ventricular myocytes. Proc Natl Acad Sci USA 83:5340, 1986
187. Hofmann F, Nastainczyk W, Rohrkasten A, et al: Regulation of the L-type calcium channel. Trends Pharmacol Sci 8:393, 1987
188. Exton JH: Mechanisms of action of calcium-mobilizing agonists: Some variations on a young theme. FASEB J 2:2670, 1988
189. Berridge MJ, Irvine RF: Inositol triphosphate, a novel second messenger in cellular signal transduction. Nature 312:315, 1984
190. Van Meel JCA, de Jonge A, Kalkman HO, et al: Vascular smooth muscle contraction inhibited by postsynaptic a_2-adrenoceptor activation is induced by an influx of extracellular calcium. Eur J Pharmacol 69:205, 1981
191. Armstrong DL: Calcium channel regulation by calcineurin, a Ca^{2+}-activated phosphatase in mammalian brain. Trends Neurosci 12:117, 1989
192. Hosey MM, Lazdunski M: Calcium channels: Molecular pharmacology, structure and regulation. J Memb Biol 104:81, 1988
193. Schmid A, Romey G, Barhanin J, et al: SR 33557, an indolizinsultone blocker of Ca^{2+} channels. Identification of receptor sites and analysis of its mode of action. Mol Pharmacol 35:766, 1989
194. Triggle DJ, Swamy VC: Pharmacology of agents that affect calcium: Agonists and antagonists. Chest 78:174, 1980
195. Robinson BF, Dobbs RJ, Kelsey CR: Effects of nifedipine on resistant vessels, arteries and veins in man. Br J Clin Pharmacol 10:433, 1980
196. Serruys PW, Brower RW, Ten Katen JH, et al: Regional wall motion from radiopaque markers after intravenous and intracoronary injections of nifedipine. Circulation 63:584, 1981
197. Singh BN, Roche AHG: Effects of intravenous verapamil on hemodynamics in patients with heart disease. Am Heart J 94:593, 1977
198. Ferlinz J, Easthope JL, Aronow WS: Effects of verapamil on myocardial performance in coronary disease. Circulation 59:313, 1979
199. Chew CYC, Hecht HS, Collett JT, et al: Influence of severity of ventricular dysfunction on hemodynamic responses to intravenously administered verapamil in ischemic heart disease. Am J Cardiol 47:917, 1981
200. Josephson MA, Hopkins J, Singh BN: Hemodynamic and metabolic effects of diltiazem during coronary sinus pacing with particular reference to left ventricular ejection fraction. Am J Cardiol 55:286, 1985
201. Giudicelli JF, Berdeaux A, Edouard A, et al: Attenuation by diltiazem of arterial baroreflex sensitivity in man. Eur J Clin Pharmacol 26:675, 1984
202. Hof RP: Patterns of regional blood flow changes induced by five different calcium antagonists. Prog Pharmacol 5:71, 1983
203. Walsh RA, Porter CB, Starling MR, et al: Beneficial hemodynamic effects of intravenous and oral diltiazem in severe congestive heart failure. J Am Coll Cardiol 3(4):1044, 1984
204. Zusman RM, Higgins J, Christensen D, Boucher CA: Bepridil improves left ventricular performance in patients with angina pectoris. J Cardiovasc Pharmacol 22:474, 1993
205. Hollingshead LM, Faulds D, Fitton A: Bepridil. A review of its pharmacological properties and therapeutic use in stable angina pectoris. Drugs 44:835, 1992
206. Sato M, Ohashi M, Metz MZ, et al: Inhibitory effect of a calcium antagonist (diltiazem) on aortic and coronary contractions in rabbits. J Mol Cell Cardiol 14:741, 1982
207. Taira N, Satoh K, Maruyama M, et al: Sustained coronary constriction and its antagonism by calcium-blocking agents in monkeys and baboons. Circ Res 52:I-40-I, 1983
208. Nagao T, Sato M, Nakajima H, et al: Studies on a new 1,5-benzothiazepine derivative (CRD-401). II. Vasodilator actions. Jpn J Pharmacol 22:1, 1972
209. Schmier J, VanAckern K, Bruckner U: Investigations on tachyphylaxis and collateral formation after nifedipine whilst taking into consideration the direction of flow and the mortality rate due to infarction. *In* Hashimoto K, Kimura E, Kobayashi T (eds): The First Nifedipine Symposium. Tokyo, Tokyo Press, 1975, pp 45–52
210. Henry PD, Shuchleib R, Clark RE, et al: Effect of nifedipine on myocardial ischemia: Analysis of collateral flow, pulsatile heat and regional muscle shortening. Am J Cardiol 44:817, 1979
211. da Luz PL, Monteiro de Barros LF, Leite JJ, et al: Effect of verapamil on regional coronary and myocardial perfusion during acute coronary occlusion. Am J Cardiol 45:269, 1980
212. Bache RJ, Dymek DJ: Effect of diltiazem on myocardial blood flow. Circulation 65[suppl I]:I-19-I, 1982
213. Rowland E, Evans T, Krikler D: Effect of nifedipine on atrioventricular conduction as compared with verapamil. Intracardiac electrophysiological study. Br Heart J 42:124, 1979
214. Wellens HJJ, Tan SL, Bär FWH, et al: Effect of verapamil studied by programmed electrical stimulation of the heart in patients with paroxysmal re-entrant supraventricular tachycardia. Br Heart J 39:1058, 1977
215. Sugimoto T, Ishikawa T, Kaseno K, et al: Electrophysiologic effects of diltiazem, a calcium antagonist, in patients with impaired sinus or atrio-ventricular node function. Angiology 31:700, 1980
216. Henry PD: Atherosclerosis, calcium, and calcium antagonists. Circulation 72:456, 1985
217. Lichtlen PR, Hugenholtz PG, Rafflenbeul W, et al: Retardation of angiographic progression of coronary artery disease by nifedipine. Results of the International Nifedipine Trial on Antiatherosclerotic Therapy (INTACT). Lancet 335:1109, 1990
218. Schroeder JS, Gao SZ, Alderman EL, et al: A preliminary study of diltiazem in the prevention of coronary artery disease in heart transplant recipients. N Engl J Med 328:164, 1993
219. Ginsburg R, Davis K, Bristow MR, et al: Calcium antagonists suppress atherogenesis in aorta but not in the intramural coronary arteries of cholesterol-fed rabbits. Lab Invest 49:154, 1983
220. Frey M, Adelung C: Antihypertensive and anticalcinotic effects of calcium antagonists. J Mol Cell Cardiol 17stract 167], 1985
221. Zorn J, Fleckenstein A: Anticalcinotic effects of calcium antagonists in cardiac, renal, intestinal and vascular tissues (abstract). Pfluegers Arch 403:R31, 1985
222. Saito K, Birou H, Fukunaga H, et al: Diltiazem prevents the damage to cultured aortic smooth muscle cells induced by hyperlipidemic serum. Experientia 42:412, 1986
223. Naito M, Asai K, Shibata K, et al: Anti-arteriosclerotic effect of diltiazem (III) [Japanese]. Yakuri To Chiryo 13:1545, 1985
224. Chierchia S, Crea F, Bernini W, et al: Antiplatelet effects of verapamil in man [Abstract]. Am J Cardiol 47:399, 1981
225. Ware JA, Johnson PC, Smith M, et al: Inhibition of human platelet aggregation and cytoplasmic calcium response by calcium antagonists: Studies with aequorin and quin2. Circ Res 59:39, 1986
226. Alusik S, Kubis M, Hrckova Y, et al: Antiagregacni ucinek diltiazemu. Vnitr Lek 31:877, 1985
227. Kiyomoto A, Sasaki Y, Odawara A, et al: Inhibition of platelet aggregation by diltiazem. Comparison with verapamil and nifedipine and inhibitory potencies of diltiazem metabolites. Circ Res 52:I-115-I, 1983
228. Charles S, Ketelslegers JM, Buysschaert M, et al: Hyperglycaemic effects of nifedipine. Br Med J 283;19, 1981
229. Massie BM, MacCarthy EP, Ramanathan KB, et al: Diltiazem and propranolol in mild to moderate essential hypertension as monotherapy or with hydrochlorothiazide. Ann Intern Med 107:150, 1987
230. Kindermann W, Schmitt W, Wolfing A: Physical performance capacity, metabolism and hormonal behavior as affected by diltiazem. Z Kardiol 75:99, 1986
231. Ohneda A: Effect of diltiazem hydrochloride on glucose tolerance in diabetes mellitus. Jpn J Clin Exp Med 57:1, 1980
232. Allen GS, Ahn HS, Preziosi TJ, et al: Cerebral arterial spasm-α-controlled trial of nimodipine in patients with subarachnoid hemorrhage. N Engl J Med 308:619, 1983
233. Clarke B, Grant D, Patmore L: Comparative calcium entry blocking properties of nicardipine, nifedipine and Py-108068 on cardiac and vascular smooth muscle. Br J Pharmacol 79:333, 1983
234. Clair F, Bellet M, Guerret M, et al: Hypotensive effect and pharmacokinetics of nicardipine in patients with severe renal failure. Curr Ther Res 38:74, 1985
235. Dow RJ, Graham DJM: A review of the human metabolism and pharmacokinetics of nicardipine hydrochloride. Br J Clin Pharmacol 22:195S, 1986
236. Gaab MR, Czech T, Korn A: Intracranial effects of nicardipine. Br J Clin Pharmacol 20:67S-74S, 1985
237. Alps BJ, Haas WK: The potential beneficial effect of nicardipine in a rat model of transient forebrain ischemia. Neurology 37:809, 1987
238. Pepine CJ, Lambert CR: Usefulness of nicardipine for angina pectoris. Am J Cardiol 59:13J-19J, 1987
239. Thomas G, Gross R, Schramm M: Calcium channel modulation: Ability to inhibit or promote calcium influx resides in the same dihydropyridine molecule. J Cardiovasc Pharmacol 6:1170, 1984
240. Somogyi A, Albrecht M, Kliems G, et al: Pharmacokinetics, bioavailability and ECG response of verapamil in patients with liver cirrhosis. Br J Clin Pharmacol 12:51, 1981
241. McAllister RG Jr, Hamann SR, Blouin RA: Pharmacokinetics of calcium-entry blockers. Am J Cardiol 55:30B-40B, 1985
242. Hermann P, Morselli PL: Pharmacokinetics of diltiazem and other calcium-entry blockers. Acta Pharmacol Toxicol 57:10, 1985

243. Piepho RW: Comparative clinical pharmacokinetics of the calcium antagonists. *In* Hoffman BF (ed): Calcium Antagonists: The State of the Art and Role in Cardiovascular Disease. Symposia on the Frontiers of Pharmacology, Vol 2. Philadelphia, College of Physicians of Philadelphia, 1983, pp 159–174
244. Rovei V, Gomeni R, Mitchard M, et al: Pharmacokinetics and metabolism of diltiazem in man. Acta Cardiol (Brux) 35:35, 1980
245. Etoh A, Kohno K: Interactions by diltiazem (4). Relationship between first-pass metabolism of various drugs and absorption enhancement by diltiazem. Yakugaku Zasshi 103:581, 1983
246. Hedner T: Calcium channel blockers: Spectrum of side effects and drug interactions. Acta Pharmacol (Copenh) 58:119, 1986
247. Lang R, Klein HO, Weiss E, et al: Effect of verapamil on blood level and renal clearance of digoxin (abstract). Circulation 62(suppl III):83, 1980
248. Oyamar Y, Fuji S, Kana K, et al: Digoxin-diltiazem interaction. Am J Cardiol 53:1480, 1984
249. Abernathy DR, Schwartz JB: Calcium antagonist drugs. N Engl J Med 341:1447, 1999
250. Mazhar M, Popat KD, Sanders C: Effect of cimetidine on diltiazem blood levels [Abstract]. Clin Res 32:A741, 1984
251. Kapur PA, Campos JH, Buchea OC: Plasma diltiazem levels, cardiovascular function, and coronary hemodynamics during enflurane anesthesia in the dog. Anesth Analg 65:918, 1986
252. Henling CE, Slogoff S, Kodali SV, et al: Heart block after coronary artery bypass-effect of chronic administration of calcium-entry blockers and beta-blockers. Anesth Analg 63:515, 1984
253. Egstrup K, Andersen PE Jr: Transient myocardial ischemia during nifedipine therapy in stable angina pectoris, and its relation to coronary collateral flow and comparison with metoprolol. Am J Cardiol 71:177, 1993
254. Subramanian VB, Bowles MJ, Khurmi NS, et al: Calcium antagonist withdrawal syndrome: Objective demonstration with frequency-modulated ambulatory ST-segment monitoring. Br Med J 286:520, 1983
255. Kozeny GA, Ragona BP, Bansal VK, et al: Myocardial infarction with normal results of coronary angiography following diltiazem withdrawal. Am J Med 80:1184, 1986
256. Engelman RM, Hadji-Rousou I, Breyer RH, et al: Rebound vasospasm after coronary revascularization in association with calcium antagonist withdrawal. Ann Thorac Surg 37:469, 1984
257. Frishman WH, Klein N, Strom J, et al: Comparative effects of abrupt withdrawal of propranolol and verapamil in angina pectoris. Am J Cardiol 50:1191, 1982
258. Chobanian AV, Bakris GL, Black HR, et al: The Seventh Report of the Joint National Committee on Prevention, Detection, Evaluation, and Treatment of High Blood Pressure: the JNC 7 report. JAMA 289:2560, 2003
259. Whitworth JA: 2003 World Health Organization (WHO)/International Society of Hypertension (ISH) statement on management of hypertension. J Hypertens 21:1983, 2003
260. Vasan RS, Larson MG, Leip EP, et al: Assessment of frequency of progression to hypertension in nonhypertensive participants in the Framingham Heart Study: a cohort study. Lancet 358:1682, 2001
261. Chobanian AV, Bakris GL, Black HR, et al: Seventh report of the Joint National Committee on Prevention, Detection, Evaluation, and Treatment of High Blood Pressure. Hypertension 42:1206, 2003
262. Lifton RP, Gharavi AG, Geller DS: Molecular mechanisms of human hypertension. Cell 104:545, 2001
263. Whelton PK, Appel LJ, Espeland MA, et al: Sodium reduction and weight loss in the treatment of hypertension in older persons: a randomized controlled trial of nonpharmacologic interventions in the elderly (TONE). TONE Collaborative Research Group. JAMA 279:839, 1998
264. Sacks FM, Svetkey LP, Vollmer WM, et al: Effects on blood pressure of reduced dietary sodium and the Dietary Approaches to Stop Hypertension (DASH) diet. DASH-Sodium Collaborative Research Group. N Engl J Med 344:3, 2001
265. Cruickshank JM: Coronary flow reserve and the J curve relation between diastolic blood pressure and myocardial infarction. BMJ 297:1227, 1988
266. August P: Initial treatment of hypertension. N Engl J Med 348:610, 2003
267. Appel LJ: The verdict from ALLHAT—thiazide diuretics are the preferred initial therapy for hypertension. JAMA 288:3039, 2002
268. Psaty BM, Lumley T, Furberg CD, et al: Health outcomes associated with various antihypertensive therapies used as first-line agents: a network meta-analysis. JAMA 289:2534, 2003
269. Staessen JA, Gasowski J, Wang JG, et al: Risks of untreated and treated isolated systolic hypertension in the elderly: meta-analysis of outcome trials. Lancet 355:865, 2000
270. Hunt SA, Baker DW, Chin MH, et al: ACC/AHA guidelines for the evaluation and management of chronic heart failure in the adult: executive summary. A report of the American College of Cardiology/American Heart Association Task Force on Practice Guidelines (Committee to revise the 1995 Guidelines for the Evaluation and Management of Heart Failure). J Am Coll Cardiol 38:2101, 2001
271. Tepper D: Frontiers in congestive heart failure: Effect of metoprolol CR/XL in chronic heart failure: Metoprolol CR/XL Randomised Intervention Trial in Congestive Heart Failure (MERIT-HF). Congest Heart Fail 5:184, 1999
272. Dargie HJ: Effect of carvedilol on outcome after myocardial infarction in patients with left ventricular dysfunction: the CAPRICORN randomised trial. Lancet 357:1385, 2001
273. A randomized trial of beta-blockade in heart failure. The Cardiac Insufficiency Bisoprolol Study (CIBIS). CIBIS Investigators and Committees. Circulation 90:1765, 1994
274. Comfere T, Sprung J, Kumar MM, et al: Angiotensin inhibitors in a general surgical population. Anesth Analg 100:636, 2005
275. Contreras F, de la Parte MA, Cabrera J, et al: Role of angiotensin II AT_1 receptor blockers in the treatment of arterial hypertension. Am J Ther 10:401, 2003
276. Israili ZH: The use of calcium antagonists in the therapy of hypertension in the elderly. Am J Ther 10:383, 2003
277. Neal B, MacMahon S, Chapman N: Effects of ACE inhibitors, calcium antagonists, and other blood-pressure-lowering drugs: results of prospectively designed overviews of randomised trials. Blood Pressure Lowering Treatment Trialists' Collaboration. Lancet 356:1955, 2000
278. Brown MJ, Palmer CR, Castaigne A, et al: Morbidity and mortality in patients randomised to double-blind treatment with a long-acting calcium-channel blocker or diuretic in the International Nifedipine GITS study: Intervention as a Goal in Hypertension Treatment (INSIGHT). Lancet 356:366, 2000
279. Major outcomes in high-risk hypertensive patients randomized to angiotensin-converting enzyme inhibitor or calcium channel blocker vs diuretic: The Antihypertensive and Lipid-Lowering Treatment to Prevent Heart Attack Trial (ALLHAT). JAMA 288:2981, 2002
280. Major cardiovascular events in hypertensive patients randomized to doxazosin vs chlorthalidone: the antihypertensive and lipid-lowering treatment to prevent heart attack trial (ALLHAT). ALLHAT Collaborative Research Group. JAMA 283:1967, 2000
281. van Zwieten PA: Centrally acting antihypertensive drugs. Present and future. Clin Exp Hypertens 21:859, 1999
282. Howell SJ, Sear JW, Foex P: Hypertension, hypertensive heart disease and perioperative cardiac risk. Br J Anaesth 92:570, 2004
283. K/DOQI clinical practice guidelines for chronic kidney disease: evaluation, classification, and stratification. Am J Kidney Dis 39:S1-S266, 2002
284. Lewis EJ, Hunsicker LG, Clarke WR, et al: Renoprotective effect of the angiotensin-receptor antagonist irbesartan in patients with nephropathy due to type 2 diabetes. N Engl J Med 345:851, 2001
285. Lewis EJ, Hunsicker LG, Bain RP, Rohde RD: The effect of angiotensin-converting enzyme inhibition on diabetic nephropathy. The Collaborative Study Group. N Engl J Med 329:1456, 1993
286. Brenner BM, Cooper ME, de Zeeuw D, et al: Effects of losartan on renal and cardiovascular outcomes in patients with type 2 diabetes and nephropathy. N Engl J Med 345:861, 2001
287. Eagle KA, Berger PB, Calkins H, et al: ACC/AHA guideline update for perioperative cardiovascular evaluation for noncardiac surgery—executive summary: a report of the American College of Cardiology/American Heart Association Task Force on Practice Guidelines (Committee to Update the 1996 Guidelines on Perioperative Cardiovascular Evaluation for Noncardiac Surgery). Circulation 105:1257, 2002
288. Spahn DR, Priebe HJ: Editorial II: Preoperative hypertension: remain wary? "Yes"—cancel surgery? "No." Br J Anaesth 92:461, 2004
289. Howell SJ, Hemming AE, Allman KG, et al: Predictors of postoperative myocardial ischaemia. The role of intercurrent arterial hypertension and other cardiovascular risk factors. Anaesthesia 52:107, 1997
290. Williams B: Recent hypertension trials. J Am Coll Cardiol 45:813, 2005
291. American Heart Association: Heart Disease and Stroke Statistics, 2004. Dallas, TX, American Heart Association. Available at: www.americanheart.org
292. Ho KK, Pinsky JL, Kannel WB, Levy D: The epidemiology of heart failure: the Framingham Study. J Am Coll Cardiol 22(4 Suppl A):6A-13A, 1993
293. Wilhelmson L, Resengrew A, Eriksson H, et al: Heart failure in the general population on men: Morbidity, risk factors, and prognosis. J Intern Med 249:253, 2001
294. O'Connell JB, Bristow MR: Economic impact of heart failure in the United States: time for a different approach. J Heart Lung Transplant 13:S107-S112, 1994
295. Massie BM, Shah NB: Evolving trends in the epidemiologic factors of heart failure: rationale for preventive strategies and comprehensive disease management. Am Heart J 133:703, 1997

296. al-Kaade S, Hauptman PJ: Health-related quality of life measurement in heart failure: challenges for the new millennium. J Card Fail 7:194, 2001
297. Garg R, Yusuf S: Overview of randomized trials of angiotensin-converting enzyme inhibitors on morality and morbidity in patients with heart failure. JAMA 273:1450, 1995
298. Flather MD, Yusuf S, Kober L, et al: Long-term ACE inhibitor therapy in patients with heart failure or left ventricular dysfunction: a systematic overview of data from individual patients. ACE inhibitor Myocardial Infarction Collaborative Group. Lancet 355:1575, 2000
299. Cohn JN, Tognoni G: A randomized trial of the angiotensin-receptor blocker valsartan in chronic heart failure. N Engl J Med 345:1667, 2001
300. Pfeffer MA, Swedberg K, Granger CB, et al: Effects of candesartan on mortality and morbidity in patients with chronic heart failure: the CHARM-Overall programme. Lancet 362:759, 2003
301. Consensus recommendations for the management of chronic heart failure. On behalf of the membership of the advisory council to improve outcomes nationwide in heart failure. Am J Cardiol 83(Suppl 2A):1A-38A, 1999
302. Packer M, Coats AJ, Fowler MB, et al: Effect of carvedilol on survival in severe chronic heart failure. N Engl J Med 344:1651, 2001
303. The Cardiac Insufficiency Bisoprolol Study II (CIBIS-II): a randomised trial. Lancet 353:9, 1999
304. Effect of metroprolol CR/XL in chronic heart failure: Metoprolol CR/XL Randomised Intervention Trial in Congestive Heart Failure (MERIT-HF) Lancet 353:2001, 1999
305. Pitt B, Zannad F, Remme WJ, et al: The effect of spironolactone on morbidity and mortality in patients with severe heart failure. Randomized Aldactone Evaluation Study Investigators. N Engl J Med 341:709, 1999
306. Pitt B, Remme W, Zannad F, et al: Eplerenone, a selective aldosterone blocker, in patients with left ventricular dysfunction after myocardial infarction. N Engl J Med 348:1309, 2003
307. Katz AM: Angiotensin II: hemodynamic regulator or growth factor? J Mol Cell Cardiol 22:739, 1990
308. Cohn JN, Ferrari R, Sharpe N: Cardiac remodeling—concepts and clinical implications: a consensus paper from an international forum on cardiac remodeling. J Am Coll Cardiol 35:569, 2000
309. Serneri GG, Boddi M, Cecioni I, et al: Cardiac angiotensin II formation in the clinical course of heart failure and its relationship with left ventricular function. Circ Res 88:961, 2001
310. Dell'Italia LJ, A Sabri: Activation of the renin-angiotensin system in hypertrophy and heart failure. *In* Mann DL (ed): Heart Failure, a companion to Braunwald's Heart Disease. Philadelphia, W.B. Saunders, 2004, pp. 129-143.
311. Pfeffer MA, Braunwald E, Moye LA, et al: Effect of captopril on mortality and morbidity in patients with left ventricular dysfunction after myocardial infarction. Results of the survival and ventricular enlargement trial. The SAVE investigators. N Engl J Med 327:669, 1992
312. ISIS-4: A randomised factorial trial assessing early oral captorpil, oral mononitrate, and intravenous magnesium sulphate in 58,050 patients with suspected acute myocardial infarction. ISIS-4 (Fourth International Study of Infarct Survival) Collaborative Group. 1995;345:669, 1995
313. Arnold JM, Yusuf S, Young J, et al: Prevention of Heart Failure in Patients in the Heart Outcomes Prevention Evaluation (HOPE) Study. Circulation 107:1284, 2003
314. Varin R, Mulder P, Tamion F, et al: Improvement of endothelial function by chronic angiotensin-converting enzyme inhibition in heart failure: role of nitric oxide, prostanoids, oxidant stress, and bradykinin. Circulation 102:351, 2000
315. Sadoshima J, Izumo S: Molecular characterization of angiotensin II-induced hypertrophy of cardiac myocytes and hyperplasia of cardiac fibroblasts. Critical role of the AT_1 receptor subtype. Circ Res 73:413, 1993
316. Kim S, Yoshiyama M, Izumi Y, et al: Effects of combination of ACE inhibitor and angiotensin-receptor blocker on cardiac remodeling, cardiac function, and survival in rat heart failure. Circulation 103:148, 2001
317. Konstam MA, Kronenberg MW, Rousseau MF, et al: Effects of angiotensin-converting enzyme inhibitor, enalapril, on the long-term progression of left ventricular dilation in patients with asymptomatic systolic dysfunction. Circulation 88:2277, 1993
318. Cohn JN, Johnson G, Ziesche S, et al: A comparison of enalapril with hydralazine-isosorbide dinitrate in the treatment of chronic congestive heart failure. N Engl J Med 325:303, 1991
319. Dell'Italia LJ, Husain A: Dissecting the role of chymase in angiotensin II formation and heart and blood vessel diseases. Curr Opin Cardiol 17:374, 2002
320. Fogari R, Zoppi A, Corradi L, et al: Comparative effects of lisinopril and losartan on insulin sensitivity in the treatment of nondiabetic hypertensive patients. Br J Clin Pharmacol 46:467, 1998
321. Janssen JJ, Gans RO, van der Meulen J, et al: Comparison between the effects of amlodipine and lisinopril on proteinuria in nondiabetic renal failure: a double-blind, randomized prospective study. Am J Hypertens 11:1074, 1998
322. Packer M, Poole-Wilson PA, Armstrong PW, et al: Comparative effects of low and high doses of the angiotensin-converting enzyme inhibitor, lisinopril, on morbidity and mortality in chronic heart failure. ATLAS Study Group. Circulation 100:2312, 1999
323. Luzier AB, Forrest A, Feuerstein SG, et al: Containment of heart failure hospitalizations and cost by angiotensin-converting enzyme inhibitor dosage optimization. Am J Cardiol 86:519, 2000
324. Mann DL, Deswal A, Bozkurt B, Torre-Amione G: New therapeutics for chronic heart failure. Annu Rev Med 53:59, 2002
325. Burnier M, Brunner HR: Angiotensin II receptor antagonists. Lancet 355:637, 2000
326. Pitt B, Segal R, Martinez FA, et al: Randomised trial of losartan versus captopril in patients over 65 with heart failure (Evaluation of Losartan in the Elderly Study, ELITE). Lancet 349:747, 1997
327. Pitt B, Poole-Wilson PA, Segal R, et al: Effect of losartan compared with captopril on mortality in patients with symptomatic heart failure: randomised trial—the Losartan Heart Failure Survival Study ELITE II. Lancet 355:1582, 2000
328. McMurray JJ, Ostergren J, Swedberg K, et al: Effects of candesartan in patients with chronic heart failure and reduced left ventricular systolic function taking angiotensin-converting-enzyme inhibitors: the CHARM-Added trial. Lancet 362:767, 2003
329. Granger CB, McMurray JJ, Yusuf S, et al: Effects of candesartan in patients with chronic heart failure and reduced left ventricular systolic function intolerant to angiotensin-converting-enzyme inhibitors: the CHARM-Alternative trial. Lancet 362:772, 2003
330. Yusuf S, Pfeffer MA, Swedberg K, et al: Effects of candesartan in patients with chronic heart failure and preserved left ventricular ejection fraction: the CHARM-Preserved Trial. Lancet 362:777, 2003
331. Roig E, Perez-Villa F, Morales M, et al: Clinical implications of increased plasma angiotensin II despite ACE inhibitor therapy in patients with congestive heart failure. Eur Heart J 21:53, 2000
332. McKelvie RS, Yusuf S, Pericak D, et al: Comparison of candesartan, enalapril, and their combination in congestive heart failure: randomized evaluation of strategies for left ventricular dysfunction (RESOLVD) pilot study. The RESOLVD Pilot Study Investigators. Circulation 100:1056, 1999
333. Pitt B, Rajagopalan A: The role of mineralocorticoid receptor blocking agents in patients with heart failure and cardiovascular disease. In: McMurray JJ, Pfeffer MA (eds). Heart Failure Updates, 1st Ed. United Kingdom, Martin Dunitz (Taylor & Francis Group plc), 2003, pp 115–140.
334. Weber KT: Aldosterone in congestive heart failure. New Eng J Med 345:1689, 2001
335. Weber KT: Aldosteronism revisited: perspectives on less well-recognized actions of aldosterone. J Lab Clin Med 142:71, 2003
336. Delcayre C, Silvestre JS, Garnier A, et al: Cardiac aldosterone production and ventricular remodeling. Kidney Int 57:1346, 2000
337. Weber KT: Fibrosis and hypertensive heart disease. Curr Opin Cardiol 15:264, 2000
338. Rajagopalan S, Duquaine D, King S, et al: Mineralocorticoid receptor antagonism in experimental atherosclerosis. Circulation 105:2212, 2002
339. Zhang ZH, Francis J, Weiss RM, Felder RB: The renin-angiotensin-aldosterone system excites hypothalamic paraventricular nucleus neurons in heart failure. Am J Physiol 283:H423-H433, 2002
340. Stockand JD: New ideas about aldosterone signaling in epithelia. Am J Physiol 282:F559-F576, 2002
341. Zannad F, Alla F, Dousset B, et al: Limitation of excessive extracellular matrix turnover may contribute to survival benefit of spironolactone therapy in patients with congestive heart failure: insights from the randomized aldactone evaluation study (RALES). Rales Investigators. Circulation 102:2700, 2000
342. Korkmaz ME, Muderrisoglu H, Ulucam M, Ozin B: Effects of spironolactone on heart rate variability and left ventricular systolic function in severe ischemic heart failure. Am J Cardiol 86:649, 2000
343. Yee KM, Pringle SD, Struthers AD: Circadian variation in the effects of aldosterone blockade on heart rate variability and QT dispersion in congestive heart failure. J Am Coll Cardiol 37:1800, 2001
344. Farquharson CA, Struthers AD: Spironolactone increases nitric oxide bioactivity, improves endothelial vasodilator dysfunction, and suppresses vascular angiotensin I/angiotensin II conversion in patients with chronic heart failure. Circulation 101:594, 2000

345. Juurlink DN, Mamdani MM, Lee DS, et al: Rates of hyperkalemia after publication of the Randomized Aldactone Evaluation Study. N Engl J Med 351:543, 2004
346. Barr CS, Lang CC, Hanson J, et al: Effects of adding spironolactone to an angiotensin-converting enzyme inhibitor in chronic congestive heart failure secondary to coronary artery disease. Am J Cardiol 76:1259, 1995
347. The effect of digoxin on mortality and morbidity in patients with heart failure. The Digitalis Investigation Group. N Engl J Med 336:525, 1997
348. Brown NJ: Eplerenone. Cardiovascular protection. Circulation 107: 2512, 2003
349. Cicoira M, Zanolla L, Rossi A, et al: Long-term, dose-dependent effects of spironolactone on left ventricular function and exercise tolerance in patients with chronic heart failure. J Am Coll Cardiol 40:304, 2002
350. MacFadyen RJ, Barr CS, Struthers AD: Aldosterone blockade reduces vascular collagen turnover, improves heart rate variability and reduces early morning rise in heart rate in heart failure patients. Cardiovasc Res 35:30, 1997
351. Weber KT: Efficacy of aldosterone receptor antagonism in heart failure: potential mechanisms. Current Heart Failure Reports I:51, 2004
352. Eichhorn EJ, Bristow MR: Antagonism of β-adrenergic receptors in heart failure. In: Mann DL, eds. Heart Failure: A Companion to Braunwald's Heart Disease,1st ed. Philadelphia: Saunders, 2004: 619-636.
353. Wallhaus TR, Taylor M, DeGrado TR, et al: Myocardial free fatty acid and glucose use after carvedilol treatment in patients with congestive heart failure. Circulation 103:2441, 2001
354. Lowes BD, Gilbert EM, Abraham WT, et al: Myocardial gene expression in dilated cardiomyopathy treated with beta-blocking agents. N Engl J Med 346:1357, 2002
355. Sabbah HN, Sharov VG, Gupta RC, et al: Chronic therapy with metoprolol attenuates cardiomyocyte apoptosis in dogs with heart failure. J Am Coll Cardiol 36:1698, 2000
356. Marks AR: A guide for the perplexed: towards an understanding of the molecular basis of heart failure. Circulation 107:1456, 2003
357. Marx SO, Reiken S, Hisamatsu Y, et al: PKA phosphorylation dissociates FKBP12.6 from the calcium release channel (ryanodine receptor): defective regulation in failing hearts. Cell 101:365, 2000
358. Marks AR, Reiken S, Marx SO: Progression of heart failure: is protein kinase a hyperphosphorylation of the ryanodine receptor a contributing factor? Circulation 105:272, 2002
359. Schlotthauer K, Bers DM: Sarcoplasmic reticulum Ca(2+) release causes myocyte depolarization. Underlying mechanism and threshold for triggered action potentials. Circ Res 87:774, 2000
360. Reiken S, Gaburjakova M, Gaburjakova J, et al: Beta-adrenergic receptor blockers restore cardiac calcium release channel (ryanodine receptor) structure and function in heart failure. Circulation 104:2843, 2001
361. Doi M, Yano M, Kobayashi S: Propranolol prevents the development of heart failure by restoring FKBP12.6-mediated stabilization of ryanodine receptor. Circulation 105:1374, 2002
362. Bristow MR, Ginsburg R, Minobe W, et al: Decreased catecholamine sensitivity and beta-adrenergic-receptor density in failing human hearts. N Engl J Med 307:205, 1982
363. Ungerer M, Bohm M, Elce JS, et al: Altered expression of beta-adrenergic receptor kinase and beta1-adrenergic receptors in the failing human heart. Circulation 87:454, 1993
364. Gauthier C, Tavernier G, Charpentier F, et al: Functional beta3-adrenoceptor in the human heart. J Clin Invest 98:556, 1996
365. Gauthier C, Langin D, Balligand JL: Beta3-adrenoceptors in the cardiovascular system. Trends Pharmacol Sci 21:426, 2000
366. Cheng HJ, Zhang ZS, Onishi K, et al: Upregulation of functional beta(3)-adrenergic receptor in the failing canine myocardium. Circ Res 89:599, 2001
367. Morimoto A, Hasegawa H, Cheng HJ, et al: Endogenous beta3-adrenoreceptor activation contributes to left ventricular and cardiomyocyte dysfunction in heart failure. Am J Physiol Heart Circ Physiol 286:H2425-H2433, 2004
368. Moniotte S, Kobzik L, Feron O, et al: Upregulation of beta(3)-adrenoceptors and altered contractile response to inotropic amines in human failing myocardium. Circulation 103:1649, 2001
369. Gauthier C, Leblais V, Kobzik L, et al: The negative inotropic effect of beta3-adrenoceptor stimulation is mediated by activation of a nitric oxide synthase pathway in human ventricle. J Clin Invest 102:1377, 1998
370. Packer M, Bristow MR, Cohn JN, et al: The effect of carvedilol on morbidity and mortality in patients with chronic heart failure. U.S. Carvedilol Heart Failure Study Group. N Engl J Med 334:1349, 1996
371. Beta-Blocker Evaluation of Survival Trial Investigators. A trial of the beta-blocker bucindolol in patients with advanced chronic heart failure. N Engl J Med 344:1659, 2001
372. Jacob S, Rett K, Wicklmayr M, et al: Differential effect of chronic treatment with two beta-blocking agents on insulin sensitivity: the carvedilol-metoprolol study. J Hypertens 14:489, 1996
373. Dulin B, Abraham WT. Pharmacology of carvedilol. Am J Cardiol 93:3B-6B, 2004
374. Hoffmann C, Leitz MR, Oberdorf-Ma-ass S, et al: Comparative pharmacology of human beta-adrenergic receptor subtypes—characterization of stably transfected receptors in CHO cells. Naunyn Schmiedebergs Arch Pharmacol 369:151, 2004
375. Moniotte S, Balligand JL: Potential use of beta(3)-adrenoceptor antagonists in heart failure therapy. Cardiovasc Drug Rev 20:19, 2002
376. Poole-Wilson PA, Swedberg K, Cleland JG, et al: Carvedilol or Metoprolol European Trial Investigators. Comparison of carvedilol and metoprolol on clinical outcomes in patients with chronic heart failure in the Carvedilol or Metoprolol European Trial (COMET): randomised controlled trial. Lancet 362:7, 2003
377. Di Lenarda A, Sabbadini G, Sinagra G: Do pharmacological differences among beta-blockers affect their clinical efficacy in heart failure? Cardiovasc Drugs Ther 18:91, 2004
378. Remme WJ, Swedberg K: Task Force for the Diagnosis and Treatment of Chronic Heart Failure, European Society of Cardiology. Guidelines for the diagnosis and treatment of chronic heart failure. Eur Heart J 22:1527, 2001
379. Eichhorn EJ: Beta-blocker withdrawal: the song of Orpheus. Am Heart J 138:387, 1999
380. Ko DT, Hebert PR, Coffey CS, et al: Adverse effects of beta-blocker therapy for patients with heart failure: a quantitative overview of randomized trials. Arch Intern Med 164:1389, 2004
381. McMurray J, Cohen-Solal A, Dietz R, et al: Clinical Research Initiative in Heart failure. Practical recommendations for the use of ACE inhibitors, beta-blockers and spironolactone in heart failure: putting guidelines into practice. Eur J Heart Fail 3:495, 2001
382. Gheorghiade M, Adams KF Jr, Colucci WS: Digoxin in the management of cardiovascular disorders. Circulation 109:2959, 2004
383. Ferguson DW: Sympathetic mechanisms in heart failure: pathophysiological and pharmacological implications. Circulation 87(Suppl VII):68, 1993
384. Krum H, Bigger JT Jr, Goldsmith RL, et al: Effect of long-term digoxin therapy on autonomic function in patients with chronic heart failure. J Am Coll Cardiol 25:289, 1995
385. Adams KF Jr, Gheorghiade M, Uretsky BF, et al: Patients with mild heart failure worsen during withdrawal from digoxin therapy. J Am Coll Cardiol 30:42, 1997
386. Rahimtoola SH: Digitalis therapy for patients in clinical heart failure. Circulation 109:2942, 2004
387. Rauchhaus M, Doehner W, Francis DP, et al: Plasma cytokine parameters and mortality in patients with chronic heart failure. Circulation 102:3060, 2000
388. Mann DL, McMurray JJ, Packer M, et al: Targeted anticytokine therapy in patients with chronic heart failure: results of the Randomized Etanercept Worldwide Evaluation (RENEWAL). Circulation 109:1594, 2004
389. Ergul A, Grubbs AL, Zhang Y, et al: Selective upregulation of endothelin converting enzyme-1a in the human failing heart. J Card Fail 6:314, 2000
390. Sakai S, Miyauchi T, Kobayashi M, et al: Inhibition of myocardial endothelin pathway improves long-term survival in heart failure. Nature 384:353, 1996
391. Mishima T, Tanimura M, Suzuki G, et al: Effects of long-term therapy with bosentan on the progression of left ventricular dysfunction and remodeling in dogs with heart failure. J Am Coll Cardiol 35:222, 2000
392. Teerlink JR: Recent heart failure trials of neurohormonal modulation (OVERTURE and ENABLE): approaching the asymptote of efficacy? J Card Fail 8:124, 2002
393. Kalra PR, Moon JC, Coats AJ: Do results of the ENABLE (Endothelin Antagonist Bosentan for Lowering Cardiac Events in Heart Failure) study spell the end for nonselective endothelin antagonism in heart failure? Int J Cardiol 85:195, 2002
394. Neunteufl T, Berger R, Pacher R: Endothelin-receptor antagonists in cardiology clinical trials. Expert Opin Investig Drugs 11:431, 2002
395. Packer M, Califf RM, Konstam MA, et al: Comparison of omapatrilat and enalapril in patients with chronic heart failure: the Omapatrilat Versus Enalapril Randomized Trial of Utility in Reducing Events (OVERTURE). Circulation 106:920, 2002
396. Worthley MI, Corti R, Worthley SG: Vasopeptidase inhibitors: will they have a role in clinical practice? Br J Clin Pharmacol 57:27, 2004
397. Bristow MR, Saxon LA, Boehmer J, et al: Cardiac-resynchronization therapy with or without an implantable defibrillator in advanced chronic heart failure. N Engl J Med 350:2140, 2004

398. Mathur A, Martin JF: Stem cells and repair of the heart. Lancet 364:183, 2004
399. Wollert KM, Meyer GP, Lotz J, et al: Intracoronary autologous bone-marrow cell transfer after myocardial infarction: the BOOST randomised controlled clinical trial. Lancet 364:141, 2004
400. DiDomenico RJ, Park HY, Southworth MR, et al: Guidelines for acute decompensated heart failure treatment. Ann Pharmacother 38:649, 2004
401. Fonarow GC, Dams K, Abraham W, et al: Risk stratification for in-hospital mortality in acute decompensated heart failure. JAMA 293:572, 2005
402. Loh E, Elkayam U, Cody R, et al: A randomized multicenter study comparing the efficacy and safety of intravenous milrinone and intravenous nitroglycerin in patients with advanced heart failure. J Card Fail 7:114, 2001
403. de Denus S, Pharand C, Williamson DR: Brain natriuretic peptide in the management of heart failure: the versatile neurohormone. Chest 125: 652, 2004
404. Elkayam U, Akhter MW, Singh H, et al: Comparison of effects on left ventricular filling pressure of intravenous nesiritide and high-dose nitroglycerin in patients with decompensated heart failure. Am J Cardiol 93:237, 2004
405. Publication Committee for the VMAC Investigators (Vasodilatation in the Management of Acute CHF). Intravenous nesiritide vs nitroglycerin for treatment of decompensated congestive heart failure: a randomized controlled trial. JAMA 287:1531, 2002
406. Burger AJ, Horton DP, LeJemtel T, et al: Effect of nesiritide (B-type natriuretic peptide) and dobutamine on ventricular arrhythmias in the treatment of patients with acutely decompensated congestive heart failure: the PRECEDENT study. Am Heart J 144:1102, 2002
407. Yamani MH, Haji SA, Starling RC, et al: Comparison of dobutamine-based and milrinone-based therapy for advanced decompensated congestive heart failure: Hemodynamic efficacy, clinical outcome, and economic impact. Am Heart J 142:998, 2001
408. Cuffe MS, Califf RM, Adams KF Jr, et al: Short-term intravenous milrinone for acute exacerbation of chronic heart failure: a randomized controlled trial. JAMA 287:1541, 2002
409. Felker GM, Benza RL, Chandler AB, et al: Heart failure etiology and response to milrinone in decompensated heart failure: results from the OPTIME-CHF study. J Am Coll Cardiol 41:997, 2003
410. Renlund DG: Building a bridge to heart transplantation. N Engl J Med 351:849, 2004
411. Wernly JA: Ischemia, reperfusion, and the role of surgery in the treatment of cardiogenic shock secondary to acute myocardial infarction: an interpretative review. J Surg Res 117:6, 2004
412. Hochman JS: Cardiogenic shock complicating acute myocardial infarction: expanding the paradigm. Circulation 107:2998, 2003
413. Royster R, Butterworth J, Prough D, et al: Preoperative and intraoperative predictors of inotropic support and long-term outcome in patients having coronary artery bypass grafting. Anesth Analg 72:729, 1991
414. Butterworth J, Legrault C, Royster R, Hammon J: Factors that predict the use of positive inotropic drug support after cardiac valve surgery. Anesth Analg 86:461, 1998
415. Butterworth JF, Prielipp RC: Endocrine, metabolic, and electrolyte responses. In: Gravlee GP, Davis RF, Kurusz M, Utley JR, eds. Cardiopulmonary Bypass, Principles and Practice, 2nd ed. Philadelphia: Lippincott Williams & Wilkins, 2000:342-366.
416. Zaloga GP, Strickland RA, Butterworth JF IV, et al: Calcium attenuates epinephrine's beta-adrenergic effects in postoperative heart surgery patients. Circulation 81:196, 1990
417. Lekmann A, Boldt J: New pharmacologic approaches for the perioperative treatment of ischemic cardiogenic shock. J Cardiothorac Vasc Anesth 19:97, 2005
418. Siirilia-waris K, Suojaranta-Ylinen R, Harjola VP: Levosimendan in cardiac surgery. J Cardiothorac Vasc Anesth 19, 2005
419. Ririe DG, Butterworth JF IV, Royster RL, et al: Triiodothyronine increases contractility independent of beta-adrenergic receptors or stimulation of cyclic-3',5'-adenosine monophosphate. Anesthesiology 82:1004, 1995
420. Bennett-Guerrero E, Jimenez JL, White WD, et al: Cardiovascular effects of intravenous triiodothyronine in patients undergoing coronary artery bypass graft surgery. A randomized, double-blind, placebo-controlled trial. Duke T3 study group. JAMA 275:687, 1996
421. Rathmell JP, Prielipp RC, Butterworth JF, et al: A multicenter, randomized, blind comparison of amrinone with milrinone after elective cardiac surgery. Anesth Analg 86:683, 1998
422. Butterworth JF IV, Royster RL, Prielipp RC, et al: Amrinone in cardiac surgical patients with left ventricular dysfunction. A prospective, randomized placebo-controlled trial. Chest 104:1660, 1993
423. Doolan LA, Jones EF, Kalman J, et al: A placebo-controlled trial verifying the efficacy of milrinone in weaning high-risk patients from cardiopulmonary bypass. J Cardiothorac Vasc Anesth 11:37, 1997
424. Hoffman TM, Wernovsky G, Atz AM, et al: Efficacy and safety of milrinone in preventing low cardiac output syndrome in infants and children after corrective surgery for congenital heart disease. Circulation 107:996, 2003
425. MacGregor DA, Smith TE, Prielipp RC, et al: Pharmacokinetics of dopamine in healthy male subjects. Anesthesiology 92:338, 2000
426. DiSesa VJ, Gold JP, Shemin RJ, et al: Comparison of dopamine and dobutamine in patients requiring postoperative circulatory support. Clin Cardiol 9:253, 1986
427. Tinker JH, Tarhan S, White RD, et al: Dobutamine for inotropic support during emergence from cardiopulmonary bypass. Anesthesiology 44:281, 1976
428. Kersting F, Follath F, Moulds R, et al: A comparison of cardiovascular effects of dobutamine and isoprenaline after open heart surgery. Br Heart J 38:622, 1976
429. Pellikka PA, Roger VL, McCully RB, et al: Normal stroke volume and cardiac output response during dobutamine stress echocardiography in subjects without left ventricular wall motion abnormalities. Am J Cardiol 76:881, 1995
430. Butterworth JF IV, Prielipp RC, Royster RL, et al: Dobutamine increases heart rate more than epinephrine in patients recovering from aortocoronary bypass surgery. J Cardiothorac Vasc Anesth 6:535, 1992
431. Jaccard C, Berner M, Rouge JC, et al: Hemodynamic effect of isoprenaline and dobutamine immediately after correction of tetralogy of Fallot. Relative importance of inotropic and chronotropic action in supporting cardiac output. J Thorac Cardiovasc Surg 87:862, 1984
432. Leone M, Vallet B, Teboul JL, et al: Survey of the use of catecholamines by French physicians. Intensive Care Med 30:984, 2004
433. MacGregor DA, Butterworth JF IV, Zaloga CP, et al: Hemodynamic and renal effects of dopexamine and dobutamine in patients with reduced cardiac output following coronary artery bypass grafting. Chest 106:835, 1994
434. Fullerton DA, St Cyr JA, Albert JD, et al: Hemodynamic advantage of left atrial epinephrine administration after cardiac operations. Ann Thorac Surg 56:1263, 1993
435. Zile MR, Brutsaert DL: New concepts in diastolic dysfunction and diastolic heart failure: Part I: diagnosis, prognosis, and measurements of diastolic function. Circulation 105:1387, 2002
436. Aurigemma GP, Ga-asch WH: Clinical practice. Diastolic heart failure. N Engl J Med 351:1097, 2004
437. Warner JG Jr, Metzger DC, Kitzman DW, et al: Losartan improves exercise tolerance in patients with diastolic dysfunction and a hypertensive response to exercise. J Am Cardiol 33:1567, 1999
438. Daniel KR, Wells GL, Fray B, et al: The effect of spironolactone on exercise tolerance and quality of life in elderly women with diastolic heart failure. Am J Geriatr Cardiol 12:131, 2003
439. Ga-asch WH, Zile MR: Left ventricular diastolic dysfunction and diastolic heart failure Annu Rev Med 55:373, 2004
440. Lobato E, Willert J, Looke T, et al: Effects of milrinone versus epinephrine on left ventricular relaxation after cardiopulmonary bypass following myocardial revascularization. J Cardiothorac Vasc Anesth 19, 2005
441. Shephard J, Cobbe SM, Ford I, et al: Prevention of coronary artery disease with pravastatin in men with hypercholesterolemia. West of Scotland Coronary Prevention Study Group. N Engl J Med 333:1301, 1995
442. Liu P, Konstam M, Force T: Highlights of the 2004 Scientific Sessions of the Heart Failure Society of America. J Am Coll Cardiol 45:617, 2005
443. Vaughan Williams EM: Classification of antiarrhythmic drugs. J Cardiovasc Pharmacol 20:51, 1992
444. Singh S, Patrick J: Antiarrhythmic drugs. Curr Treat Options Cardiovasc Med 6:357, 2004
445. Liang BT: Adenosine receptors and cardiovascular function. Trends Cardiovasc Med 2:100, 1992
446. Echt DS, Liebson PR, Mitchell LB, et al: Mortality and morbidity in patients receiving encainide, flecainide, or placebo. N Engl J Med 324:781, 1991
447. Duff HJ, Roden DM, Yacobi A, et al: Bretylium: Relations between plasma concentrations and pharmacological actions in high-frequency ventricular arrhythmias. Am J Cardiol 55:395, 1985
448. Roden DM: Drug therapy: Drug-induced prolongation of this QT interval. N Engl J Med 350:1013, 2004
449. AVID Investigators: A comparison of antiarrhythmic drug therapy with implantable defibrillators in patients resuscitated from near-fatal ventricular arrhythmias. N Engl J Med 337:1576, 1997

450. Harrison DC, Winkle R, Sami M, et al: Encainide: a new and potent antiarrhythmic agent. Am Heart J 100:1046, 1980
451. Scheinman M, Keung E: The year in clinical electrophysiology. J Am Coll Cardiol 45:790, 2005
452. Wittig J, Harrison LA, Wallace AG: Electrophysiological effects of lidocaine on distal Purkinje fibers of canine heart. Am Heart J 86:69, 1973
453. Vaughan Williams EM: A classification of antiarrhythmic actions reassessed after a decade of new drugs. J Clin Pharmacol 24:129, 1984
454. Hoffman BF, Rosen MR, Wit AL: Electrophysiology and pharmacology of cardiac arrhythmias. VII. Cardiac effects of quinidine and procainamide. Am Heart J 90:117, 1975
455. Darbar D, Fromm MF, Dellorto S, Roden DM: Sympathetic activation enhances QT prolongation by quinidine. J Cardiovasc Electrophysiol 12:9, 2001
456. Kessler KM, Lowenthal DT, Warner H, et al: Quinidine elimination in patients with congestive heart failure or poor renal function. N Engl J Med 290:706, 1974
457. Leahey EB Jr, Reiffel JA, Drusin RE, et al: Interaction between quinidine and digoxin. JAMA 240:533, 1978
458. Gerhardt RE, Knouss RF, Thyrum PT, et al: Quinidine excretion in aciduria and alkaluria. Ann Intern Med 71:927, 1969
459. Koster RW, Wellens HJJ: Quinidine-induced ventricular flutter and fibrillation without digitalis therapy. Am J Cardiol 38:519, 1976
460. Rials SJ, Britchkow D, Marinchak RA, Kowey PR: Electropharmacologic effect of a standard dose of intravenous procainamide in patients with sustained ventricular tachycardia. Clin Cardiol 23:171, 2000
461. Krone RJ, Miller JP, Kleiger RE, et al: The effectiveness of antiarrhythmic agents on early-cycle premature ventricular complexes. Circulation 63:664, 1981
462. Rials S, Britchkow D, Marinchak R, Kowey P: Electrophysiologic effects of a standard dose of IV procainamide. Clin Cardiol 23:171, 2000
463. Graffner C, Johnsson G, Sjogren J: Pharmacokinetics of procainamide intravenously and orally as conventional slow release tablets. Clin Pharmacol Ther 17:414, 1975
464. Collste P, Karlsson E: Arrhythmia prophylaxis with procainamide: Plasma concentrations in relation to dose. Acta Med Scand 194:405, 1973
465. Reidenberg MM, Drayer DE, Levy M, et al: Polymorphic acetylation of procainamide in man. Clin Pharmacol Ther 17:722, 1975
466. Woosley RL, Roden DM: Importance of metabolites in antiarrhythmic therapy. Am J Cardiol 52:3C-7C, 1983
467. Dimarco J, Gersh B, Opie L: Antiarrhythmic drugs and strategies. In Opie L, Horsh G (eds): Drugs for the Heart. 6th ed. Philadelphia, Elsevier, 2005, pp 218–274
468. Strasberg B, Sclarovsky S, Erdberg A, et al: Procainamide-induced polymorphous ventricular tachycardia. Am J Cardiol 47:1309, 1981
469. Blomgren SE, Condemi JJ, Vaughn JH: Procainamide-induced lupus erythematosus: Clinical and laboratory observations. Am J Med 52:338, 1972
470. Michelson EL, Spear JF, Moore EN: Effects of procainamide on strength-interval relations in normal and chronically infarcted canine myocardium. Am J Cardiol 47:1223, 1981
471. Wenger TL, Browning DL, Masterton CE, et al: Procainamide delivery to ischemic canine myocardium following rapid intravenous administration. Circ Res 46:789, 1980
472. Reid DS, Williams DO, Parashar SK: Disopyramide in the sick sinus syndrome-safe or not? Br Heart J 39:348, 1977
473. Spurrell RA, Thorburn CW, Camm J, et al: Effects of disopyramide on electrophysiological properties of specialized conduction system in man and on accessory atrioventricular pathway in Wolff-Parkinson-White syndrome. Br Heart J 37:861, 1975
474. Podrid PJ, Schoeneberger A, Lown B: Congestive heart failure caused by oral disopyramide. N Engl J Med 302:614, 1980
475. Koch-Weser J: Drug therapy. Disopyramide. N Engl J Med 300:957, 1979
476. Zipes DP, Troup PJ: New antiarrhythmic agents: Amiodarone, aprinidine, disopyramide, ethmozin, mexiletine, tocainide, verapamil. Am J Cardiol 41:1005, 1979
477. Chien YW, Lambert HJ, Karim A: Comparative binding of disopyramide phosphate and quinidine sulfate to human plasma proteins. J Pharm Sci 63:1877, 1974
478. Sadowski ZP: Multicenter randomized trial and systemic overview of lidocaine in acute myocardial infarction. Am Heart J 137:792, 1999
479. Carden NL, Steinhaus JE: Lidocaine and cardiac resuscitation from ventricular fibrillation. Circ Res 4:680, 1956
480. Dorian P, Cass D, Schwartz G, et al: Amiodarone compared with lidocaine for shock-resistant ventricular fibrillation. N Engl J Med 346:884, 2002
481. Weiss WA: Intravenous use of lidocaine for ventricular arrhythmias. Anesth Analg 39:369, 1960
482. DeClive-Lowe SG, Desmond J, North J: Intravenous lignocaine anaesthesia. Anaesthesia 13:138, 1958
483. Gerstenblith G, Spear JF, Moore EN: Quantitative study of the effect of lidocaine on the threshold for ventricular fibrillation in the dog. Am J Cardiol 30:242, 1972
484. Davis LD, Temte JV: Electrophysiological actions of lidocaine on canine ventricular muscle and Purkinje fibers. Circ Res 24:639, 1969
485. Singh BN, Williams EM: Effect of altering potassium concentration on the action of lidocaine and diphenylhydantoin on rabbit atrial and ventricular muscle. Circ Res 29:286, 1971
486. Obayashi K, Hayakawa H, Mandell WJ: Interrelationships between external potassium concentration and lidocaine: Effects on canine Purkinje fiber. Am Heart J 89:221, 1975
487. Watanabe Y, Dreifus LS, Likoff W: Electrophysiological antagonism and synergism of potassium and antiarrhythmic agents. Am J Cardiol 12:702, 1963
488. Kupersmith J, Antman EM, Hoffman BF: In vivo electrophysiological effects of lidocaine in canine acute myocardial infarction. Circ Res 36:84, 1975
489. El-Sherif N, Scherlag BJ, Lazzara R, et al: Reentrant ventricular arrhythmias in the late myocardial infarction period. 4. Mechanism of action of lidocaine. Circulation 56:395, 1977
490. Covino B: Pharmacology of Local Anesthetics. Br J Anaesth 58:701, 1986
491. Blumer J, Strong JM, Atkinson AJ Jr: The convulsant potency of lidocaine and its *o*-dealkylated metabolites. J Pharmacol Exp Ther 186:31, 1973
492. Collinsworth KA, Kalman SM, Harrison DC: The clinical pharmacology of lidocaine as an antiarrhythmic drug. Circulation 50:1217, 1974
493. Smith ER, Duce BR: The acute antiarrhythmic and toxic effects in mice and dogs of 2-ethylamino-2,6-acetoxylidine (L-86), a metabolite of lidocaine. J Pharmacol Exp Ther 179:580, 1971
494. Essman WB: Xylocaine-induced protection against electrically induced convulsions in mice. Arch Int Pharmacodyn Ther 157:166, 1965
495. Bernheard CG, Bohm E: Local Anesthetics as Anticonvulsants. A Study on Experimental and Clinical Epilepsy. Stockholm, Almqvist & Wiksel, 1965
496. Hood DD, Mecca RS: Failure to initiate electroconvulsive seizures in a patient pretreated with lidocaine. Anesthesiology 58:379, 1983
497. Ikram H: Hemodynamic and electrophysiologic interactions between antiarrhythmic drugs and beta-blockers, with special reference to tocainide. Am Heart J 100:1076, 1980
498. Kuhn P, Kroiss A, Klicpera M, et al: Antiarrhythmic and haemodynamic effects of mexiletine. Postgrad Med J 53(Suppl I):81, 1977
499. Winkle RA, Anderson JL, Peters F, et al: The hemodynamic effects of intravenous tocainide in patients with heart disease. Circulation 57:787, 1978
500. Nyquist O, Forssell G, Nordlander R, et al: Hemodynamic and antiarrhythmic effects of tocainide in patients with acute myocardial infarction. Am Heart J 100:1000, 1980
501. Ryan WF, Karliner JS: Effects of tocainide on left ventricular performance at rest and during acute alterations in heart rate and systemic arterial pressure. Br Heart J 41:175, 1979
502. Abinader EG, Cooper M: Mexiletine. Use and control of chronic drug-resistant ventricular arrhythmia. JAMA 242:337, 1979
503. DiMarco JP, Garan H, Ruskin JN: Mexiletine for refractory-ventricular arrhythmias: results using serial electrophysiologic testing. Am J Cardiol 47:131, 1981
504. Podrid PJ, Lown B: Mexiletine for ventricular arrhythmias. Am J Cardiol 47:895, 1981
505. Horowitz JD, Anavekar SN, Morris PM, et al: Comparative trial of mexiletine and lignocaine in the treatment of early ventricular tachyarrhythmias after acute myocardial infarction. J Cardiovasc Pharmacol 3:409, 1981
506. Campbell RWF, Achuff SC, Pottage A, et al: Mexiletine in the prophylaxis of ventricular arrhythmias during acute myocardial infarction. J Cardiovasc Pharmacol 1:43, 1979
507. Bell JA, Thomas JM, Isaacson JR, et al: A trial of prophylactic mexiletine in home coronary care. Br Heart J 48:285, 1982
508. Chamberlain DA, Jewitt DE, Julian DG, et al: Oral mexiletine in high-risk patients after myocardial infarction. Lancet 2:1324, 1980
509. Ryden L, Arnman K, Conradson TB, et al: Prophylaxis of ventricular tachyarrhythmias with intravenous and oral tocainide. *In* Harrison DC (ed): Cardiac Arrhythmias-A Decade of Progress. Boston, GK Hall, 1981, pp 227–247

510. Pottage A: Clinical profiles of newer class I antiarrhythmic agents-tocainide, mexiletine, encainide, flecainide, and lorcainide. Am J Cardiol 52:24C-31C, 1983
511. Oltmanns D: Tocainid-pharmakokinetik bei chronischer leber-erkrankung (abstract). Z Kardiol 71:172, 1982
512. El Allaf D, Henrard L, Crochelet L, et al: Pharmacokinetics of mexiletine in renal insufficiency. Br J Pharmacol 14:431, 1982
513. Campbell NP, Kelly JG, Adgey AA, et al: The clinical pharmacology of mexiletine. Br J Clin Pharmacol 6:103, 1978
514. Gillis RA, McClellan JR, Sauer TS, et al: Depression of cardiac sympathetic nerve activity by diphenylhydantoin. J Pharmacol Exp Ther 179:599, 1971
515. Evans DE, Gillis RA: Effect of diphenylhydantoin and lidocaine on cardiac arrhythmias induced by hypothalamic stimulation. J Pharmacol Exp Ther 191:506, 1974
516. Singh BN: Explanation for the discrepancy in reported cardiac electrophysiological actions of diphenylhydantoin and lignocaine. Br J Pharmacol 41:385P, 1971
517. Bigger JT Jr, Weinberg DI, Kovalik AT, et al: Effects of diphenylhydantoin on excitability and automaticity in the canine heart. Circ Res 26:1, 1970
518. Rosen MR, Danilo P Jr, Alonso MB, et al: Effects of therapeutic concentrations of diphenylhydantoin on transmembrane potentials of normal and depressed Purkinje fibers. J Pharmacol Exp Ther 197:594, 1976
519. Peon J, Ferrier GR, Moe GK: The relationship of excitability to conduction velocity in canine Purkinje tissue. Circ Res 43:125, 1978
520. Bigger JT Jr, Bassett AL, Hollnian BF: Electrophysiological effects of diphenylhydantoin on canine Purkinje fibers. Circ Res 22:221, 1968
521. Garson A Jr, Kugler JD, Gillette PC, et al: Control of late postoperative ventricular arrhythmias with phenytoin in young patients. Am J Cardiol 46:290, 1980
522. Bigger JT Jr, Schmidt DH, Kutt H: Relationship between the plasma level of diphenylhydantoin sodium and its cardiac antiarrhythmic effects. Circulation 38:363, 1968
523. Kutt H, Winters W, Kokenge R, et al: Diphenylhydantoin metabolism, blood levels, and toxicity. Arch Neurol 11:642, 1964
524. Lieberson AD, Schumacher RR, Childress RH, et al: Effect of diphenylhydantoin on left ventricular function in patients with heart disease. Circulation 36:692, 1967
525. Conn RD, Kennedy JW, Blackmon JR: The hemodynamic effects of diphenylhydantoin. Am Heart J 73:500, 1967
526. Louis S, Kutt H, McDowell F: Cardiocirculatory changes caused by intravenous dilantin and its solvent. Am Heart J 74:523, 1967
527. Unger AH, Sklaroff HJ: Fatalities following intravenous use of sodium diphenylhydantoin for cardiac arrhythmias. JAMA 200:335, 1967
528. Olsson SB, Edvardsson N: Clinical electrophysiologic study of antiarrhythmic properties of flecainide: acute intraventricular delayed conduction and prolonged repolarization in regular paced and premature beats using intracardiac monophasic action potentials with programmed stimulation. Am Heart J 102:864, 1981
529. Duff HJ, Roden DM, Maffucci RJ, et al: Suppression of resistant ventricular arrhythmias by twice daily dosing with flecainide. Am J Cardiol 48:1133, 1981
530. Verdouw PD, Deckers JW, Conrad GJ: Antiarrhythmic and hemodynamic actions of flecainide acetate (R-818) in the ischemic porcine heart. J Cardiovasc Pharmacol 1:473, 1979
531. Hodges M, Haugland JM, Granrud G, et al: Suppression of ventricular ectopic depolarization by flecainide acetate, a new antiarrhythmic agent. Circulation 65:879, 1982
532. Anderson JL, Stewart JR, Perry BA, et al: Oral flecainide acetate for the treatment of ventricular arrhythmias. N Engl J Med 305:473, 1981
533. Lui HK, Lee G, Dietrich P, et al: Flecainide-induced QT prolongation and ventricular tachycardia. Am Heart J 103:567, 1982
534. Arias C, Gonzalez T, Moreno I, et al: Effects of propafenone and its main metabolite, 5-hydroxypropafenone, on HERG channels. Cardiovasc Res 57:660, 2003
535. Boriani G, Martignani C, Biffi M, et al: Oral loading with propafenone for conversion of recent-onset atrial fibrillation: a review on in-hospital treatment. Drugs 62:415, 2002
536. Effect of the antiarrhythmic agent moricizine on survival after myocardial infarction. The Cardiac Arrhythmia Suppression Trial II Investigators. N Engl J Med 327:227, 1992
537. Woosley RL, Shand D, Cornhauser B, et al: Relation of plasma concentration and dose of propranolol to its effect on resistant ventricular arrhythmias. Clin Res 25:262A, 1967
538. Kupersmith J, Shiang H, Litwak RS, et al: Electrophysiological and antiarrhythmic effects of propranolol in canine acute myocardial ischemia. Circ Res 38:302, 1976
539. Evans GH, Wilkinson GR, Shand DG: The disposition of propranolol. IV. A dominant role for tissue uptake in the dose-dependent extraction of propranolol by the perfused rat liver. J Pharmacol Exp Ther 186:447, 1973
540. Evans GH, Nies AS, Shand DG: The disposition of propranolol. 3. Decreased half-life and volume of distribution as a result of plasma binding in man, monkey, dog, and rat. J Pharmacol Exp Ther 186:114, 1973
541. Fitzgerald JD, O'Donnell SR: Pharmacology of 4-hydroxypropranolol, a metabolite of propranolol. Br J Pharmacol 43:222, 1971
542. Shand DG: Drug therapy: Propranolol. N Engl J Med 293:280, 1975
543. Wood M, Shand DG, Wood AJJ: Propranolol binding in plasma during cardiopulmonary bypass. Anesthesiology 51:512, 1979
544. Miller RR, Olson HG, Amsterdam EA, et al: Propranolol-withdrawal rebound phenomenon. Exacerbation of coronary events after abrupt cessation of antianginal therapy. N Engl J Med 293:416, 1975
545. Shiroff RA, Mathis J, Zelis R, et al: Propranolol rebound-a retrospective study. Am J Cardiol 41:778, 1978
546. Ablad B, Carlsson E, Ek L: Pharmacological studies of two new cardioselective adrenergic beta-receptor antagonists. Life Sci 12:107, 1973
547. Lennard MS, Silas JH, Freestone S, et al: Oxidation phenotype—a major determinant of metoprolol metabolism and response. N Engl J Med 307:1558, 1982
548. Kaplan JA: Role of ultrashort-acting beta-blockers in the perioperative period. J Cardiothorac Anesth 2:683, 1988
549. Gorczynski RJ, Shaffer JE, Lee RJ: Pharmacology of ASL, a novel beta-adrenergic receptor antagonist with an ultra short duration of action. J Cardiovasc Pharmacol 5:668, 1983
550. Steck J, Sheppard D, Byrd RC, et al: Pulmonary effects of esmolol-an ultra short-acting beta-adrenergic blocking agent. Clin Res 33:472A, 1985
551. Morganroth J, Horowitz LN, Anderson J, et al: Comparative efficacy and tolerance of esmolol to propranolol for control of supraventricular tachyarrhythmia. Am J Cardiol 56:33F-39F, 1985
552. Daoud EG, Strickberger SA, Man KC, et al: Preoperative amiodarone as prophylaxis against atrial fibrillation after heart surgery. N Engl J Med 337:1785, 1997
553. Kaski JC, Girotti LA, Messuti H, et al: Long-term management of sustained, recurrent, symptomatic ventricular tachycardia with amiodarone. Circulation 64:273, 1981
554. Nademanee K, Hendrickson JA, Cannom DS, et al: Control of refractory life-threatening ventricular tachyarrhythmias by amiodarone. Am Heart J 101:759, 1981
555. Ward DE, Camm AJ, Spurrell RA: Clinical antiarrhythmic effects of amiodarone in patients with resistant paroxysmal tachycardias. Br Heart J 44:91, 1980
556. Fogoros RN, Anderson KP, Winkle RA, et al: Amiodarone: clinical efficacy and toxicity in 96 patients with recurrent, drug-refractory arrhythmias. Circulation 68:88, 1983
557. American Heart Association. Guidelines for Cardiopulmonary Resuscitation Emergency Cardiovascular Care. Circulation 102 (suppl I): I-1-I, 2000
558. Dorian P, Mangat I: Role of amiodarone in the era of the implantable cardioverter defibrillator. J Cardiovasc Electrophysiol 14(9 Suppl):S78-S81, 2003
559. Goupil N, Lenfant J: The effects of amiodarone on the sinus node activity of the rabbit heart. Eur J Pharmacol 39:23, 1976
560. Rosen MR, Wit AL: Electropharmacology of antiarrhythmic drugs. Am Heart J 106:829, 1983
561. Dhurandhar RW, Pickron J, Goldman AM: Bretylium tosylate in the management of recurrent ventricular fibrillation complicating acute myocardial infarction. Heart Lung 9:265, 1980
562. Gloor HO, Urthaler F, James TN: Acute effects of amiodarone upon the canine sinus node and the atrioventricular junctional region. J Clin Invest 71:1457, 1983
563. Singh BN: Amiodarone: historical development and pharmacologic profile. Am Heart J 106:788, 1983
564. Heger JJ, Prystowsky EN, Jackman WM, et al: Amiodarone: Clinical efficacy and electrophysiology during long-term therapy for recurrent ventricular tachycardia or fibrillation. N Engl J Med 305:539, 1981
565. Zipes DP, Prystowsky EN, Heger JJ: Amiodarone: electrophysiologic actions, pharmacokinetics, and clinical effects. J Am Coll Cardiol 3:1059, 1984
566. Singh BN, Nadenmanee K: Amiodarone and thyroid function: clinical implications during antiarrhythmic therapy. Am Heart J 106:857, 1983
567. Hariman RJ, Gomes JAC, Kang PS, et al: Effects of intravenous amiodarone in patients with inducible repetitive ventricular responses and ventricular tachycardia. Am Heart J 107:1109, 1984

568. Marcus FI, Fontaine GH, Frank R, et al: Clinical pharmacology and therapeutic applications of the antiarrhythmic agent amiodarone. Am Heart J 101:480, 1981
569. DeBoer LWV, Nosta JJ, Kloner RA, et al: Studies of amiodarone during experimental myocardial infarction: beneficial effects on hemodynamics and infarct size. Circulation 65:508, 1982
570. Haffajee CI, Love JC, Alpert JS, et al: Efficacy and safety of long-term amiodarone in treatment of cardiac arrhythmias: dosage experience. Am Heart J 106:935, 1983
571. Canada AT, Lasko LG, Haffajee CI: Disposition of amiodarone in patients with tachyarrhythmias. Curr Ther Res 30:968, 1981
572. Latini R, Tognoni G, Kates RE: Clinical pharmacokinetics of amiodarone. Clin Pharmacokinet 9:136, 1984
573. Andreasen F, Agerbaek H, Bjerrega-ard P, et al: Pharmacokinetics of amiodarone after intravenous and oral administration. Eur J Clin Pharmacol 19:293, 1981
574. Mostow ND, Rakita L, Vrobel TR, et al: Amiodarone: intravenous loading for rapid suppression of complex ventricular arrhythmias. J Am Coll Cardiol 4:97, 1984
575. Kerin NZ, Blevins RD, Frumin H, et al: Intravenous and oral loading versus oral loading alone with amiodarone for chronic refractory ventricular arrhythmias. Am J Cardiol 55:89, 1985
576. Harris L, McKenna WJ, Rowland E, et al: Side effects and possible contraindications of amiodarone use. Am Heart J 106:916, 1983
577. Rakita L, Sobol SM, Mostow N, et al: Amiodarone pulmonary toxicity. Am Heart J 106:906, 1983
578. Marchlinski FE, Gansler TS, Waxman HL, et al: Amiodarone pulmonary toxicity. Ann Intern Med 97:839, 1982
579. Kudenchuk PJ, Pierson DJ, Greene HL, et al: Prospective evaluation of amiodarone pulmonary toxicity. Chest 86:541, 1984
580. Veltri EP, Reid PR: Amiodarone pulmonary toxicity: early changes in pulmonary function tests during amiodarone rechallenge. J Am Coll Cardiol 6:802, 1985
581. Burger A, Dinicher D, Nicod P, et al: Effect of amiodarone on serum triiodothyronine, reverse triiodothyronine, thyroxin and thyrotropin. A drug influencing peripheral metabolism of thyroid hormones. J Clin Invest 58:255, 1976
582. Kerin NZ, Blevins RD, Benaderet D, et al: Relation of serum reverse T_3 to amiodarone antiarrhythmic efficacy and toxicity. Am J Cardiol 57:128, 1986
583. Buchser E, Chiolero R, Martin P, et al: Amiodarone-induced haemodynamic complications during anaesthesia. Anaesthesia 38:1008, 1983
584. Gallagher JD, Lieberman RW, Meranze J, et al: Amiodarone-induced complications during coronary artery surgery. Anesthesiology 55:186, 1981
585. Spotnitz WD, Nolan SP, Kaiser DL, et al: The reversal of amiodarone-induced perioperative reduction in cardiac systolic reserve in dogs. J Am Coll Cardiol 12:757, 1988
586. Boura AL, Green AF: Actions of bretylium: adrenergic neuron blocking and other effects. Br Pharm Chemother 14:536, 1959
587. Chatterjee K, Mandel WJ, Vyden JK, et al: Cardiovascular effects of bretylium tosylate in acute myocardial infarction. JAMA 223:757, 1973
588. Anderson JL, Patterson E, Wagner JG, et al: Clinical pharmacokinetics of intravenous and oral bretylium tosylate in survivors of ventricular tachycardia or fibrillation: clinical application of a new assay for bretylium. J Cardiovasc Pharmacol 3:485, 1981
589. Lucchesi BR: Rationale of therapy in the patient with acute myocardial infarction and life-threatening arrhythmias: a focus on bretylium. Am J Cardiol 54:14A-19A, 1984
590. Kniffen FJ, Lomas TE, Counsell RE, et al: The antiarrhythmic and antifibrillatory actions of bretylium and its *o*-iodobenzyltrimethyl ammonium analog, UM-360. J Pharmacol Exp Ther 192:120, 1975
591. Cervoni P, Ellis CH, Maxwell RA: Anti-arrhythmic action of bretylium in normal, reserpine-pretreated and chronically denervated dog hearts. Arch Int Pharmacodyn Ther 190:91, 1971
592. Namm DH, Wang CM, El-Sayad S, et al: Effects of bretylium on rat cardiac muscle: the electrophysiological effects and its uptake and binding in normal and immunosympathectomized rat hearts. J Pharmacol Exp Ther 193:194, 1975
593. Tacker WA Jr, Niebauer MJ, Babbs CF, et al: The effect of newer antiarrhythmic drugs on defibrillation threshold. Crit Care Med 8:177, 1980
594. Haynes RE, Chinn TL, Copass MK, et al: Comparison of bretylium tosylate and lidocaine in management of out-of-hospital ventricular fibrillation: a randomized clinical trial. Am J Cardiol 48:353, 1981
595. Nowak RM, Bodnar TJ, Dronen S, et al: Bretylium tosylate as initial treatment for cardiopulmonary arrest: randomized comparison with placebo. Ann Emerg Med 10:404, 1981
596. Terry G, Vellani CW, Higgins MR, et al: Bretylium tosylate in treatment of refractory ventricular arrhythmias complicating myocardial infarction. Br Heart J 32:21, 1970
597. Bernstein JG, Koch-Weser J: Effectiveness of bretylium tosylate against refractory ventricular arrhythmias. Circulation 45:1024, 1972
598. Holder DA, Sniderman AD, Fraser G, et al: Experience with bretylium tosylate by a hospital cardiac arrest team. Circulation 55:541, 1977
599. MacAlpin RN, Zalis EG, Kivowitz CF: Prevention of recurrent ventricular tachycardia with oral bretylium tosylate. Ann Intern Med 72:909, 1970
600. Woosley RL: Antiarrhythmic drugs. *In* Hurst JW (ed): The Heart. 11th ed. New York, McGraw-Hill, 2004, pp 949–974
601. O'Callaghan PA, McGovern BA: Evolving role of sotalol in the management of ventricular tachyarrhythmias. Am J Cardiol 78:54, 1996
602. Reiter MJ: The ESVEM trial: impact on treatment of ventricular tachyarrhythmias. Electrophysiologic Study Versus Electrocardiographic Monitoring. Pacing Clin Electrophysiol 20:468, 1997
603. Reiffel JA, Hahn E, Hartz V, Reiter MJ: Sotalol for ventricular tachyarrhythmias. ESVEM Investigators: Electrophysiologic Study Versus Electrocardiographic Monitoring. Am J Cardiol 79:1048, 1997
604. Wanless RS, Anderson K, Joy M, Joseph SP: Multicenter comparative study of the efficacy and safety of sotalol in the prophylactic treatment of patients with paroxysmal supraventricular tachyarrhythmias. Am Heart J 133:441, 1997
605. Waldo AL, Camm AJ, deRuyter H, et al: Effect of D-sotalol on mortality in patients with left ventricular dysfunction after recent and remote myocardial infarction. The SWORD Investigators, Survival with Oral D-Sotalol. Lancet 348:7, 1996
606. Cropp JS, Antal EG, Talbert RL: Ibutilide: A new class III antiarrhythmic agent. Pharmacotherapy 17:1, 1997
607. Yang T, Snyders DJ, Roden DM: Ibutilide, a methanesulfonailide antiarrhythmic. Circulation 91:1799, 1995.
608. Naccarelli GV, Lee KS, Gibson JK, VanderLugt JT: Electrophysiology and pharmacology of ibutilide. Am J Cardiol 78:12, 1996
609. Ellenbogen KA, Stambler BS, Wood MA, et al: Efficacy of intravenous ibutilide for rapid termination of atrial fibrillation and atrial flutter: a dose-response study. J Am Coll Cardiol 28:130, 1996
610. Stambler BS, Wood MA, Ellenbogen KA, et al: Efficacy and safety of repeated intravenous doses of ibutilide for rapid conversion of atrial flutter or fibrillation. Circulation 94:1613, 1996
611. Kowey PR, VanderLugt JT, Luderer JR: Safety and risk/benefit analysis of ibutilide for acute conversion of atrial fibrillation/flutter. Am J Cardiol 78:46, 1996
612. Kalus JS, Mauro VF: Dofetilide: a class III-specific antiarrhythmic agent Ann Pharmaco Ther 34:44, 2000
613. Van Breemen C, Aaronson P, Loutzenhiser R: Sodium-calcium interactions in mammalian smooth muscle. Pharmacol Rev 30:167, 1978
614. Katz AM, Messineo FC: Lipids and membrane function: implications in arrhythmias. Hosp Pract 16:49, 1981
615. Gettes LS: Possible role of ionic changes in the appearance of arrhythmias. Pharmacol Ther [B] 2:787, 1976
616. Triggle DJ: Calcium antagonists: Basic chemical and pharmacological aspects. *In* Weiss GB (ed): New Perspectives on Calcium Antagonists. Bethesda, MD, American Physiological Society, 1981, pp 1–18
617. Fleckenstein A: Specific pharmacology of calcium in myocardium, cardiac pacemaker, and vascular smooth muscle. Annu Rev Pharmacol Toxicol 17:149, 1977
618. Henry PD: Comparative pharmacology of calcium antagonists: nifedipine, verapamil and diltiazem. Am J Cardiol 46:1047, 1980
619. Kazda S, Garthoff B, Meyer H, et al: Pharmacology of a new calcium antagonist compound, isobutyl methyl 1,4-dihydro-2,6-dimethyl-4-(2-nitrofentyl)-3,5-pyridinedicarb oxylate (nisoldipine, k5552). Arzneimittelforschung 30:2144, 1980
620. Triggle DJ: Biochemical pharmacology of calcium blockers. *In* Flaim SF, Xellis R (eds): Calcium Blockers: Mechanisms of Action and Clinical Applications. Baltimore, Urban and Swartzenberg, 1981
621. Satoh K, Yanagisawa T, Taira N: Coronary vasodilator and cardiac effects of optical isomers of verapamil in the dog. J Cardiovasc Pharmacol 2:309, 1980
622. Roy PR, Spurrell RA, Sowton GE: The effect of verapamil on the conduction system in man. Postgrad Med J 50:270, 1974
623. Schlepper M, Weppner HG, Merle H: Haemodynamic effects of supraventricular tachycardias and their alterations by electrically and verapamil-induced termination. Cardiovasc Res 12:28, 1978
624. Kopman EA: Intravenous verapamil to relieve pulmonary congestion in patients with mitral valve disease. Anesthesiology 58:374, 1983

625. Kapur PA, Flacke WE, Olewine SK: Comparison of effects of isoflurane versus enflurane on cardiovascular and catecholamine responses to verapamil in dogs. Anesth Analg 61:193, 1982
626. Kates RA, Kaplan JA, Guyton RA, et al: Hemodynamic interactions of verapamil and isoflurane in dogs. Anesth Analg 59:132, 1983
627. Singh BN, Nademanee K, Feld G: Calcium blockers in the treatment of cardiac arrhythmias. *In* Flaim SF, Zelis R (eds): Calcium Blockers: Mechanisms of Actions and Clinical Applications. Baltimore, Urban and Swartzenberg, 1982, p 258
628. Mangiardi LM, Hariman RJ, McAllister RG Jr, et al: Electrophysiologic and hemodynamic effects of verapamil: Correlation with plasma drug concentrations. Circulation 57:366, 1978
629. Kates RE, Keefe DLD, Schwartz J, et al: Verapamil disposition kinetics in chronic atrial fibrillation. Clin Pharmacol Ther 30:44, 1981
630. Brichard G, Zimmermann PE: Verapamil in cardiac dysrrhythmias during anaesthesia. Br J Anaesth 42:1005, 1970
631. Schreck DM, Rivera AR, Tricarico VJ: Emergency management of atrial fibrillation and flutter: intravenous diltiazem versus intravenous digoxin. Ann Emerg Med 29:135, 1997
632. Olshansky B: Management of atrial fibrillation after coronary artery bypass graft. Am J Cardiol 78:27, 1996
633. Amar D, Roistacher N, Burt ME, et al: Effects of diltiazem versus digoxin on dysrhythmias and cardiac function after pneumonectomy. Ann Thorac Surg 63:1374, 1997
634. Billman GE: Effect of calcium channel antagonists on cocaine-induced malignant arrhythmias: protection against ventricular fibrillation. J Pharmacol Exp Ther 266:407, 1993
635. Lawson NW, Kraynack BJ, Gintautas J: Neuromuscular and electrocardiographic responses to verapamil in dogs. Anesth Analg 62:50, 1983
636. Kraynack BJ, Lawson NW, Gintautas J: Neuromuscular blocking action of verapamil in cats. Can Anaesth Soc J 30:242, 1983
637. Davis LD: Effect of changes in cycle length on diastolic depolarization produced by ouabain in canine Purkinje fibers. Circ Res 32:206, 1973
638. Ferrier GR, Saunders JH, Mendez C: A cellular mechanism for the generation of ventricular arrhythmias by acetylstrophanthidan. Circ Res 32:600, 1973
639. Rosen MR, Gelband H, Merker C, et al: Mechanisms of digitalis toxicity: Effects of ouabain on phase 4 of canine Purkinje fiber transmembrane potentials. Circ Res 47:681, 1973
640. Hoffman BF, Bigger JT Jr: Digitalis and allied cardiac glycosides. *In* Gilman AG, Goodman LS, Rall TW, et al (eds): The Pharmacological Basis of Therapeutics, 7th edition. New York, Macmillan, 1985, pp 724, 725
641. Rosen MR, Wit AL, Hoffman BF: Electrophysiology and pharmacology of cardiac arrhythmias. IV. Cardiac antiarrhythmic and toxic effects of digitalis. Am Heart J 89:391, 1975
642. Mudge GH Jr, Lloyd BL, Greenblatt DJ, et al: Inotropic and toxic effects of a polar cardiac glycoside derivative in a dog. Circ Res 43:847, 1978
643. Gillis RA, Quest JA: The role of the central nervous system in the cardiovascular effects of digitalis. Pharmacol Rev 31:19, 1979
644. Lerman BB, Belardinelli L: Cardiac electrophysiology of adenosine, basic and clinical concepts. Circulation 83:1499, 1991
645. Camm AJ, Garratt CJ: Adenosine and supraventricular tachycardia. N Engl J Med 325:1621, 1991
646. Hood MA, Smith WM: Adenosine versus verapamil in the treatment of supraventricular tachycardia: A randomized double-crossover trial. Am Heart J 123:1543, 1992
647. Overholt ED, Rheuban KS, Gutgesell HP, et al: Usefulness of adenosine for arrhythmias in infants and children. Am J Cardiol 61:336, 1988
648. Mohnle P, Schwann N, Vaughn W, et al: Perturbations in laboratory values after coronary artery bypass surgery with cardiopulmonary bypass. J Cardiothorac Vasc Anesth 19:19, 2005
649. Eisenkraft J: Electrolyte disturbances and the electrocardiogram. In Thys D, Kapun JA (eds): The ECG in Anesthesia and Critical Care. New York, Churchill-Livingstone, 1987, pp 167–180
650. Chung EK: Principles of Cardiac Arrhythmias, 2nd edition. Baltimore, Williams & Wilkins, 1977, pp 25, 32, 570, 651, 668, 672
651. Pacifico AD, Digerness S, Kirklin JW: Acute alterations of body composition after open heart intracardiac operations. Circulation 41:331, 1970
652. Mandelbaum I, Morgan CR: Effect of extracorporeal circulation upon insulin. J Thorac Cardiovasc Surg 55:526, 1968
653. Burch GE, Giles TE: The importance of magnesium deficiency in cardiovascular disease. Am Heart J 94:649, 1977
654. Aglio LS, Stanford GG, Maddi R, et al: Hypomagnesemia is common following cardiac surgery. J Cardiothorac Vasc Anesth 5:201, 1991
655. Turlapaty PDMV, Altura BM: Magnesium deficiency produces spasm of coronary arteries. Relationship to etiology of sudden death and ischemic heart disease. Science 208:198, 1980
656. Seller RH, Cangiano J, Kim KE, et al: Digitalis toxicity and hypomagnesemia. Am Heart J 79:57, 1970
657. Specter MJ, Schweizer E, Goldman RH: Studies on magnesium's mechanism of action in digitalis-induced arrhythmias. Circulation 52:1001, 1975
658. Scheinman MM, Sullivan RW, Hyatt KH: Magnesium metabolism in patients undergoing cardiopulmonary bypass. Circulation 39:I235, 1969
659. Geertman H, van der Starre P, Sie H, et al: Magnesium in addition to sotalol does not influence the incidence of postoperative atrial tachyarrhythmias after coronary artery bypass surgery. J Cardiothorac Vasc Anesth 18:309, 2004
660. Toraman F, Karabulut E, Alhan H, et al: Magnesium infusion dramatically decreases the incidence of atrial fibrillation after coronary artery bypass grafting. Ann Thorac Surg 72:1256, 2001
661. The SOLVD Investigators: Effect of enalapril on survival in patients with reduced left ventricular ejection fractions and congestive heart failure. N Engl J Med 325:293, 1991
662. The Acute Infarction Ramipril Efficacy (AIRE) Study Investigators: Effect of ramipril on mortality and morbidity of survivors of acute myocardial infarction with clinical evidence of heart failure. Lancet 342:821, 1993
663. Kober L, Torp-Pedersen C, Carlsen JE, et al: A clinical trial of the angiotensin-converting-enzyme inhibitor trandolapril in patients with left ventricular dysfunction after myocardial infarction. Trandolapril Cardiac Evaluation (TRACE) Study Group. N Engl J Med 333:1670, 1995
664. McMurray J, Ostergren J, Pfeffer M, et al: Clinical features and contemporary management of patients with low and preserved ejection fraction heart failure: Baseline characteristics of patients in the Candesartan in Heart Failure-Assessment of Reduction in Mortality and morbidity (CHARM) programme. Eur J Heart Fail 5:261, 2003
665. Hager WD, Davis BR, Riba A, et al: Absence of a deleterious effect of calcium channel blockers in patients with left ventricular dysfunction after myocardial infarction: The SAVE Study Experience. SAVE Investigators. Survival and Ventricular Enlargement. Am Heart J 135:406, 1998
666. Yusuf S, Sleight P, Pogue J, et al: Effects of an angiotensin-converting-enzyme inhibitor, ramipril, on cardiovascular events in high-risk patients. The Heart Outcomes Prevention Evaluation Study Investigators. N Engl J Med 342:145, 2000
667. Dahlof B, Devereux RB, Kjeldsen SE, et al: Cardiovascular morbidity and mortality in the Losartan Intervention For Endpoint reduction in hypertension study (LIFE): a randomised trial against atenolol. Lancet 359:995, 2002
668. Black HR, Elliott WJ, Grandits G, et al: Principal results of the Controlled Onset Verapamil Investigation of Cardiovascular End Points (CONVINCE) trial. JAMA 289:2073, 2003
669. Pepine CJ, Handberg EM, Cooper-DeHoff RM, et al: A calcium antagonist vs a non-calcium antagonist hypertension treatment strategy for patients with coronary artery disease. The International Verapamil-Trandolapril Study (INVEST): A randomized controlled trial. JAMA 290:2805, 2003
670. Fox KM: Efficacy of perindopril in reduction of cardiovascular events among patients with stable coronary artery disease: Randomised, double-blind, placebo-controlled, multicentre trial (the EUROPA study). Lancet 362:782, 2003
671. Arauz-Pacheco C, Parrott MA, Raskin P: Treatment of hypertension in adults with diabetes. Diabetes Care 26 (Suppl 1): S80, 2003
672. UK Prospective Diabetes Study Group. Efficacy of atenolol and captopril in reducing risk of macrovascular and microvascular complications in type 2 diabetes: UKPDS 39. BMJ 317:713, 1998
673. Randomised placebo-controlled trial of effect of ramipril on decline in glomerular filtration rate and risk of terminal renal failure in proteinuric, non-diabetic nephropathy. The GISEN Group (Gruppo Italiano di Studi Epidemiologici in Nefrologia): Lancet 349:1857, 1997
674. Wright JT Jr, Agodoa L, Contreras G et al: Successful blood pressure control in the African American Study of Kidney Disease and Hypertension. Arch Intern Med 162:1636, 2002
675. PROGRESS Collaborative Group: Randomised trial of a perindopril-based blood-pressure-lowering regimen among 6,105 individuals with previous stroke or transient ischaemic attack. Lancet 358:1033, 2001

Part III

PREOPERATIVE EVALUATION

Chapter 11

ASSESSMENT OF CARDIAC RISK AND THE CARDIOLOGY CONSULTATION: EXAMINING, IMAGING, OPTIMIZING, AND RECOMMENDING

Jiri Horak, MD • Lee A. Fleisher, MD, FACC

KEY POINTS

1. Perioperative cardiac morbidity is multifactorial and understanding these factors helps define individual risk factors.
2. Assessment of myocardial injury is based upon the integration of information from myocardial imaging (e.g., echocardiography), electrocardiography, and serum biomarkers, with significant variability in the diagnosis based on the criteria selected.
3. Multivariate modeling has been used to develop risk indices, which focus on preoperative variables, intraoperative variables, or both.
4. Key predictors of perioperative risk are dependent on the type of cardiac operation and the outcome of interest.
5. The factors used to construct a risk index are critical in determining whether it is applicable to a given population.
6. Although coronary angiography measures anatomy, stress myocardial imaging provides a better assessment of cardiac function.
7. New risk models have become available for valvular heart surgery or combined coronary and valvular cardiac procedures.

In the early 1980s, coronary artery bypass graft surgery (CABG) was characterized by operative mortality rates in the range of 1% to 2%. Over the ensuing years, however, urgent and emergent operations and "redo" procedures became common, and higher morbidity and mortality rates were observed. Percutaneous coronary interventions absorbed low-risk patients from the surgery pool, with the net result being that the operative mortality rate rose to the range of 5% to 6%. Hospital administrators began to ask for justification of the observed increase in CABG mortality. This often prompted a time-consuming and expensive chart review to identify the differences in the patient populations that led to the higher morbidity. Even with this information, it was difficult to *objectively* determine the impact of these new and compelling factors on mortality. The impetus for the development of a risk-adjusted outcome assessment/appropriate risk adjustment scoring system was the need to compare adult cardiac surgery results in different institutions and to benchmark the observed complication rates.[1] The first risk-scoring scheme for cardiac surgery was introduced by Paiement et al at the Montreal Heart Institute in 1983.[2] Since then, multiple preoperative cardiac surgery risk indices have been developed. The patient characteristics that affected the probability of specific adverse outcomes were identified and weighted, and the resultant risk indices have been used to adjust for case-mix differences among surgeons and centers where performance profiles have been compiled. In addition to comparisons between centers, the preoperative cardiac risk indices have been used to counsel patients and their families in resource planning, in high-risk group identification for special care or research, to determine cost-effectiveness, to determine effectiveness of intervention, to improve provider practice, and to assess costs related to severity of disease.[3,4]

Anesthesiologists are interested in risk indices as a means of identifying patients who are at high risk for intraoperative cardiac injury and, along with the surgeon, to estimate perioperative risk for cardiac surgery, in order to provide objective information to patients and their families during the preoperative discussion. This chapter approaches the preoperative evaluation from this perspective.

SOURCES OF PERIOPERATIVE MYOCARDIAL INJURY IN CARDIAC SURGERY

Myocardial injury, manifested as transient cardiac contractile dysfunction ("stunning") and/or acute myocardial infarction (AMI), is the most frequent complication after cardiac surgery and is the single most important cause of hospital complications and death. Furthermore, patients who have a perioperative MI have poor long-term prognosis: only 51% of such patients remain free from adverse cardiac events after 2 years, compared with 96% of patients without MI.[5]

To understand the determinants of perioperative risk, it is important to understand the pathogenesis of this morbidity and mortality. This is particularly important with respect to cardiac outcomes, because the definition of *cardiac morbidity* represents a continuum rather than a discrete event. This understanding can help target the biologically significant risk factors, as well as interventions that may decrease irreversible myocardial necrosis.

Myocardial necrosis is the result of progressive pathologic ischemic changes that start to occur in the myocardium within minutes after the interruption of its blood flow, as seen in cardiac surgery (Box 11–1). The duration of the interruption

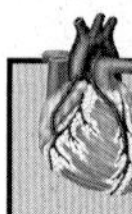

BOX 11–1 *Determinations of Perioperative Myocardial Injury*

- Disruption of blood flow
- Reperfusion of ischemic myocardium
- Adverse systemic effects of cardiopulmonary bypass

of blood flow, either partial or complete, determines the extent of myocardial necrosis. This is consistent with the finding that both the duration of the period of aortic cross-clamping (AXC) and the duration of cardiopulmonary bypass (CPB) have consistently been shown to be the main determinants of postoperative outcomes in virtually all studies. This was further supported in a study with an average follow-up of 10 years after complex cardiac surgery in which Khuri[6] observed a direct relationship between the lowest mean myocardial pH recorded both during and after the period of AXC and long-term patient survival. Patients who experienced acidosis (pH < 6.5) had decreased survival compared with those who did not. Because myocardial acidosis reflects both myocardial ischemia and poor myocardial protection during bypass, this study demonstrated the relationship of the adequacy of intraoperative myocardial protection to long-term outcome (see Chapters 6, 12, 19, and 30).

Reperfusion of an Ischemic Myocardium

Surgical interventions requiring interruption of blood flow to the heart must, out of necessity, be followed by restoration of perfusion. Numerous experimental studies have provided compelling evidence that reperfusion, although essential for tissue and/or organ survival, is not without risk, due to the extension of cell damage as a result of reperfusion itself. Myocardial ischemia of limited duration (less than 20 minutes), followed by reperfusion, is accompanied by functional recovery without evidence of structural injury or biochemical evidence of tissue injury.[7,8]

Paradoxically, reperfusion of cardiac tissue, which has been subjected to an extended period of ischemia, results in a phenomenon known as myocardial reperfusion injury.[9-11] Thus, there exists a paradox in that tissue viability can be maintained only if reperfusion is instituted within a reasonable time period but only at the risk of extending the injury beyond that due to the ischemic insult itself. This is supported by the observation that ventricular fibrillation was prominent when the regionally ischemic canine heart was subjected to reperfusion.[12] Jennings and coworkers[13] reported adverse structural and electrophysiologic changes associated with reperfusion of the ischemic canine heart, and Hearse[14] introduced the concept of an oxygen paradox in noting cardiac muscle enzyme release and alterations in ultrastructure when isolated hearts were reoxygenated after a period of hypoxic perfusion.

Myocardial reperfusion injury is defined as the death of myocytes, alive at the time of reperfusion, as a direct result of one or more events initiated by reperfusion. Myocardial cell damage results from the restoration of blood flow to the previously ischemic heart, thereby extending the region of irreversible injury beyond that due to the ischemic insult alone. The cellular damage that results from reperfusion can be reversible or irreversible, depending on the length of the ischemic insult. If reperfusion is initiated within 20 minutes after the onset of ischemia, the resulting myocardial injury is reversible and is characterized functionally by depressed myocardial contractility, which eventually recovers completely. Myocardial tissue necrosis is not detectable in the previously ischemic region, although functional impairment of contractility may persist for a variable period, a phenomenon known as myocardial stunning. Initiating reperfusion after a duration of ischemia of longer than 20 minutes, however, results in irreversible myocardial injury or cellular necrosis. The extent of tissue necrosis that develops during reperfusion is directly related to the duration of the ischemic event. Tissue necrosis originates in the subendocardial regions of the ischemic myocardium and extends to the subepicardial regions of the area at risk, often referred to as the *wavefront phenomenon*. The cell death that occurs during reperfusion can be characterized microscopically by explosive swelling, which includes disruption of the tissue lattice, contraction bands, mitochondrial swelling, and calcium phosphate deposits within mitochondria.[12]

The magnitude of reperfusion injury is directly related to the magnitude of the ischemic injury that precedes it. In its most severe form, it manifests in a "no-reflow" phenomenon. In cardiac surgery, prevention of myocardial injury after the release of the AXC, including the prevention of no reflow, is directly dependent on the adequacy of myocardial protection during the period of aortic clamping. The combination of ischemic and reperfusion injury is probably the most frequent and serious type of injury that leads to poor outcomes in cardiac surgery today (see Chapters 6, 12, 14, 15, 16, and 30).

Basic science investigations (in mouse, human, and porcine hearts) have implicated acidosis as a primary trigger of apoptosis. Acidosis, reoxygenation, and reperfusion, but not hypoxia (or ischemia) alone, are strong stimuli for programmed cell death, as well as the demonstration that cardiac apoptosis can lead to heart failure.[15,16] This suggests that apoptotic changes might be triggered in the course of a cardiac operation, thus effecting an injurious cascade of adverse clinical events that manifest late in the postoperative course.

Based on the previous discussion, it is clear that a significant portion of perioperative cardiac morbidity is related primarily to intraoperative factors. However, preoperative risk factors may influence ischemia–reperfusion injury.

Adverse Systemic Effects of Cardiopulmonary Bypass

In addition to the effects of disruption and restoration of myocardial blood flow, cardiac morbidity may result from many of the components used to perform cardiovascular operations, which lead to systemic insults that result from CPB circuit-induced contact activation. Inflammation in cardiac surgical patients is produced by complex humoral and cellular interactions, including activation, generation, or expression of thrombin, complement, cytokines, neutrophils, adhesion molecules, mast cells, and multiple inflammatory mediators.[17] Because of the redundancy of the inflammatory cascades, profound amplification occurs to produce multiorgan system dysfunction that can manifest as coagulopathy, respiratory failure, myocardial dysfunction, renal insufficiency, and neurocognitive defects. Coagulation and inflammation are also closely linked through networks of both humoral and cellular components, including proteases of the clotting and fibrinolytic cascades as well as tissue factor. Vascular endothelial cells also mediate inflammation and the cross-talk between coagulation and inflammation. Surgery alone also activates specific hemostatic responses, activation of immune mechanisms, and inflammatory responses mediated by the release of various cytokines and chemokines (see Chapters 8 and 28 through 30). This can lead to death from nonischemic causes and suggests that preoperative risk factors may not predict morbidity. The ability to risk-adjust populations is critical to study interventions that may influence these responses to CPB.

ASSESSMENT OF PERIOPERATIVE MYOCARDIAL INJURY IN CARDIAC SURGERY

Unfortunately, the current clinical armamentarium is devoid of a means by which perioperative cardiac injury can be reliably monitored in real time, leading to the use of indicators of AMI after the event occurs. Generally, there is a lack of consensus regarding how to measure myocardial injury in cardiac surgery because of the continuum of cardiac injury. Electrocardiographic changes, biomarker elevations, and measures of cardiac function have all been used, but all assessment modalities are affected by the direct myocardial trauma of surgery. The American College of Cardiology/European Society of Cardiology (ACC/ESC) published a definition of AMI in 2000, which includes a characteristic rise and fall in blood concentrations of cardiac troponins and/or creatine kinase (CK)-MB in the context of a coronary intervention, while other modalities are less sensitive and specific[18] (Fig. 11–1).

Traditionally, AMI was determined electrocardiographically (see Chapters 14 and 19). Biochemical measures have not been widely accepted because exact thresholds for myocardial injury have not been clearly defined. Cardiac biomarkers are elevated postoperatively and can be used for postoperative risk stratification, in addition to being used to diagnose acute morbidity (Box 11–2).

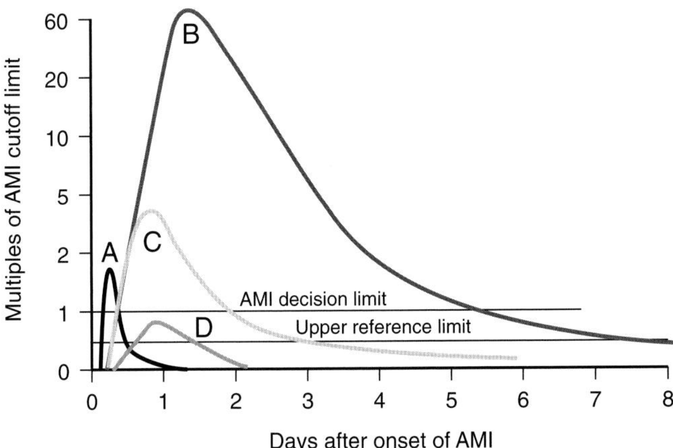

Figure 11–1 Timing of release of various biomarkers following acute, ischemic myocardial infarction. Peak A, early release of myoglobin or creatine kinase (CK)-MB isoforms after AMI (acute myocardial infarction); peak B, cardiac troponin after AMI; peak C, CK-MB after AMI; peak D, cardiac troponin after unstable angina. Data are plotted on a relative scale, where 1.0 is set at the AMI cutoff concentration. (From Apple FS, Gibler WB: National Academy of Clinical Biochemistry Standards of Laboratory Practice: Recommendations for the use of cardiac markers in coronary artery disease. Clin Chem 45:1104, 1999.)

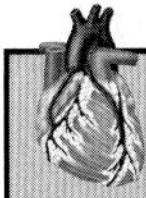

BOX 11–2 *Assessment of Perioperative Myocardial Injury*

- Assessment of cardiac function
  - Echocardiography
- Nuclear imaging
- Electrocardiography
  - Q waves
  - ST-T wave changes
- Serum biomarkers
  - Myoglobin
  - Creatine kinase
  - CK-MB
  - Troponin
  - Lactate dehydrogenase

Assessment of Cardiac Function

Cardiac contractile dysfunction is the most prominent feature of myocardial injury, despite the fact that there are virtually no perfect measures of postoperative cardiac function.

The need for inotropic support, thermodilution cardiac output (CO) measurements, and transesophageal echocardiography (TEE) may represent practical intraoperative options for cardiac contractility evaluation. The need for inotropic support and CO measurements are not reliable measures, because they depend on loading conditions and practitioner variability. Failure to wean from CPB, in the absence of systemic factors such as hyperkalemia and acidosis, is the best evidence of intraoperative myocardial injury or cardiac dysfunction but may also be multifactorial and therefore a less robust outcome measure.

Regional wall motion abnormalities (RWMAs) follow the onset of ischemia in 10 to 15 seconds. Echocardiography can therefore be a very sensitive and rapid monitor for cardiac ischemia/injury.[19] If the RWMA is irreversible, this indicates irreversible myocardial necrosis (see Chapters 14 through 16). The importance of TEE assessment of cardiac function is further enhanced by its value as a predictor of long-term survival.[20] In patients undergoing CABG, a postoperative decrease in left ventricular (LV) ejection fraction (EF) compared with preoperative baseline predicts decreased long-term survival.[21]

The use of TEE is complicated because myocardial stunning (postischemic transient ventricular dysfunction) is a common cause of new postoperative RWMAs, which are transient. However, the appearance of a new ventricular RWMA in the postoperative period, whether due to irreversible AMI or to reversible myocardial stunning, is an indication of some form of inadequate myocardial protection during the intraoperative period and therefore of interest for the assessment of new interventions. Echocardiographic and Doppler systems also have the limitation of being sensitive to alterations in loading conditions, similar to the need for inotropic support and CO determinations.[22] The interpretation of TEE images is also operator dependent.[23] In addition, there are nonischemic causes of RWMA, such as conduction abnormalities, ventricular pacing, and myocarditis, that confound the use of this outcome measure for the assessment of ischemic morbidity.

Electrocardiography Monitoring

The presence of new persistent Q waves of at least 0.03-second duration, broadening of preexisting Q waves, or new QS deflections on the postoperative ECG has been considered evidence of perioperative AMI.[24] However, new Q waves may also be due to unmasking of an old MI and therefore not indicative of a new AMI. Crescenzi and colleagues[25] demonstrated that the association of a new Q wave and high levels of biomarkers was strongly associated with postoperative cardiac events, while the isolated appearance of a new Q wave had no impact on the postoperative cardiac outcome. Additionally, new Q waves may actually disappear over time.[26] Signs of non–Q-wave MI, such as ST-T wave changes, are even less reliable signs of AMI after cardiac surgery in the absence of biochemical evidence. ST-segment changes are even less specific for perioperative MI, because they can be due to changes in body position, hypothermia, transient conduction abnormalities, and electrolyte imbalances.

Serum Biochemical Markers to Detect Myocardial Injury

Serum biomarkers have become the primary means of assessing the presence and extent of AMI after cardiac surgery. Serum biomarkers that are indicative of myocardial damage include the following (with postinsult peak time given in parentheses): myoglobin (4 hours), total CK (16 hours), CK-MB isoenzyme (24 hours), troponins I and T (24 hours), and lactate dehydrogenase (LDH) (76 hours). The CK-MB isoenzyme has been most widely used, but studies have suggested that troponin I is the most sensitive and specific in depicting myocardial ischemia and infarction.[27-32]

With respect to CK-MB, the definition of an optimal cutoff has best been defined by the correlation of multiples of the upper limit of normal for the laboratory and medium- and long-term outcomes. For example, Klatte and colleagues[33] reported on the implications of CK-MB in 2918 high-risk CABG patients enrolled in a clinical trial of an anti-ischemic agent. The unadjusted 6-month mortality rates were 3.4%, 5.8%, 7.8%, and 20.2% for patients with a postoperative peak CK-MB ratio (peak CK-MB value/upper limits of normal [ULN] for laboratory test) of less than 5, ≥5 to <10, ≥10 to < 20, and ≥20 ULN, respectively.[33] The relationship remained statistically significant after adjustment for EF, congestive heart failure (CHF), cerebrovascular disease, peripheral vascular disease, cardiac arrhythmias, and the method of cardioplegia delivery. In the Arterial Revascularization Therapies Study (ARTS), 496 patients with multivessel coronary artery disease (CAD) undergoing CABG were evaluated by CK-MB testing and followed postoperatively at 30 days and 1 year.[34] Patients with increased cardiac enzyme levels after CABG were at increased risk of both death and repeat AMI within the first 30 days. CK-MB elevation was also independently related to late adverse outcome.

Studies suggest that post–cardiac surgery monitoring of troponins can be used to assess myocardial injury and risk stratification. Increased cardiac-specific troponin I or T in patients after CABG has been associated with a cardiac cause of death and with major postoperative complications within 2 years after CABG.[35,36] The American College of Cardiology/European Society of Cardiology definition includes biomarkers but does not include specific criteria for diagnosing post-CABG AMI using cardiac biomarkers.[18]

There are a few new biomarkers of perioperative cardiac injury or ischemia under development. Brain natriuretic peptide (BNP) could be detected in the early stages of ischemia and decreases shortly after ischemic insult, allowing better detection of reinjury.[37] BNP concentrations after CABG in the patients who had cardiac events within 2 years were significantly higher than those in the patients free of cardiac events.[38] Soluble CD40 ligand (sCD40L) is another early biomarker of myocardial ischemia,[39] and CPB causes an increase in the concentration of plasma sCD40L. A corresponding decrease in platelet CD40L suggests that this prothrombotic and proinflammatory protein was derived primarily from platelets and may contribute to the thrombotic and inflammatory complications associated with CPB.[40] Future research will be required to determine how these biomarkers will be used to assess outcome after cardiac surgery.

Variability in Diagnosis of Perioperative Myocardial Infarction

The variability in diagnosing perioperative AMI has been studied by Jain and colleagues,[41] who evaluated data from 566 patients at 20 clinical sites, collected as part of a clinical trial. The occurrence of AMI by Q-wave, CK-MB, or autopsy criteria was determined. Of the 25% of patients who met the Q-wave, CK-MB, or autopsy criteria for AMI, 19% had increased CK-MB as well as electrocardiographic changes. Q-wave and CK-MB or autopsy criteria for AMI were met by 4% of patients. Multicenter data collection revealed a substantial variation in the incidence of AMI and an overall incidence of up to 25%. The definition of perioperative AMI was highly variable depending on the definitions used.

CARDIAC RISK ASSESSMENT AND CARDIAC RISK STRATIFICATION MODELS

In defining important risk factors and developing risk indices, each of the studies has used different primary outcomes. Postoperative mortality remains the most definitive outcome that is reflective of patient injury in the perioperative period. It is important to note that death can be cardiac and noncardiac and, if cardiac, may be ischemic or nonischemic in origin. Postoperative mortality is reported as either in-hospital or 30-day. The latter represents a more standardized definition, although more difficult to capture because of the cost-cutting push to discharge patients early after surgery. The value of developing risk-adjusted postoperative mortality models is the assessment of the comparative efficacy of various techniques in preventing myocardial damage, but it does not provide information that is useful in preventing the injury in real time.[42] The postoperative mortality rate has also been used as a comparative measure of quality of cardiac surgical care.[43,44]

Postoperative morbidity includes AMI and reversible events such as CHF and need for inotropic support. The problems of using AMI as an outcome of interest were described here earlier. Because resource utilization has become such an important financial consideration for hospitals, length of intensive care unit (ICU) stay has increasingly been used in the development of risk indices (see Chapter 32).

Predictors of Postoperative Morbidity and Mortality

Clinical and angiographic predictors of operative mortality were initially defined from the Coronary Artery Surgery Study (CASS).[45,46] A total of 6630 patients underwent isolated CABG between 1975 and 1978. Women had a significantly higher mortality than men; mortality increased with advancing age in men, but this was not a significant factor in women. Increasing severity of angina, manifestations of heart failure, and number and extent of coronary artery stenoses all correlated with higher mortality, while EF was not a predictor. Urgency of surgery was a very strong predictor of outcome, with those patients requiring emergency surgery in the presence of a 90% left main coronary artery stenosis sustaining a 40% mortality.

A risk-scoring scheme for cardiac surgery (CABG and valve) was introduced by Paiement et al at the Montreal Heart Institute in 1983.[2] Eight risk factors were identified: (1) poor LV function, (2) CHF, (3) unstable angina or recent (within 6 weeks) MI, (4) age greater than 65 years, (5) severe obesity (body mass index greater than 30 kg/m^2), (6) reoperation, (7) emergency surgery, and (8) other significant or uncontrolled systemic disturbances. Three classifications were identified: patients with none of these factors (normal), those presenting with one risk factor (increased risk), and those with more than one factor (high risk). In a study of 500 consecutive cardiac surgical patients, it was found that operative mortality increased with increasing risk (confirming their scoring system).

One of the most commonly used scoring systems for CABG was developed by Parsonnet and colleagues[47] (Table 11–1). Fourteen risk factors were identified for in-hospital or 30-day mortality following univariate regression analysis of 3500 consecutive operations. An additive model was constructed and prospectively evaluated in 1332 cardiac procedures. Five categories of risk were identified with increasing mortality rates, complication rates, and length of stay at the Newark Beth Israel Medical Center. The Parsonnet Index is frequently used as a benchmark for comparison between institutions. However, the Parsonnet model was created earlier than the other models and may not be representative of the current practice of CABG. During the period following publication of the Parsonnet model, numerous technical advances now in routine use have diminished CABG mortality rates.

Bernstein and Parsonnet[48] simplified the risk-adjusted scoring system in 2000 to provide a handy tool in preoperative discussions with patients and their families and for preoperative risk stratification calculation. The authors developed a logistic regression model in which 47 potential risk factors were considered, and a method requiring only simple addition and graphic interpretation was designed for relatively easily approximating the estimated risk. The final estimates provided by the simplified model correlated well with the observed mortality (Fig. 11–2).

O'Connor et al[49] used data collected from 3055 patients undergoing isolated CABG at five clinical centers between 1987 and 1989 to develop a multivariate numerical score. A regression model was developed in a training set and subsequently validated in a test set. Independent predictors of in-hospital mortality included patient age, body surface area, comorbidity score, prior CABG, EF, LV end-diastolic pressure, and priority of surgery. The validated multivariate prediction rule was very robust in predicting the in-hospital mortality for an individual patient, and the authors proposed that it could be used to contrast observed and expected mortality rates for an institution or a particular clinician.

Higgins et al[50] developed a Clinical Severity Score for CABG at The Cleveland Clinic. A multivariate logistic regression model to predict perioperative risk was developed in 5051 patients undergoing CABG between 1986 and 1988 and subsequently validated in a cohort of 4069 patients. Independent predictors of in-hospital and 30-day mortality were emergency procedure, preoperative serum creatinine level of greater than 168 μmol/L, severe LV dysfunction, preoperative hematocrit of less than 34%, increasing age, chronic pulmonary disease, prior vascular surgery, reoperation, and mitral valve insufficiency. Predictors of morbidity (AMI and

Table 11–1 Components of the Additive Model

Risk factor	Assigned weight
Female gender	1
Morbid obesity (≥1.5 × ideal weight)	3
Diabetes (unspecified type)	3
Hypertension (systolic BP > 140 mm Hg)	3
Ejection fraction (%): _______ (actual value when available)	
Good (≥50)	0
Fair (30–49)	2
Poor (<30)	4
Age (yr): _______	
70–74	7
75–79	12
≥80	20
Reoperation	
First	5
Second	10
Preoperative IABP	2
Left ventricular aneurysm	5
Emergency surgery following PTCA or catheterization complications	10
Dialysis dependency (PD or Hemo)	10
Catastrophic states (e.g., acute structural defect, cardiogenic shock, acute renal failure)*	10–50†
Other rare circumstances (e.g., paraplegia, pacemaker dependency, congenital HD in adult, severe asthma)*	2–10†
Valve surgery	
Mitral	5
PA pressure ≥ 60 mm Hg	8
Aortic	5
Pressure gradient > 120 mm Hg	7
CABG at the time of valve surgery	2

BP = blood pressure; IABP = intra-aortic balloon pump; PTCA = percutaneous transluminal coronary angioplasty; PD = peritoneal dialysis; Hemo = hemodialysis; HD = heart disease; PA = pulmonary artery; CABG = coronary artery bypass graft.

*On the actual worksheet, these risk factors require justification.

†Values were predictive of increased risk of operative mortality in univariate analysis.

From Parsonnet V, Dean D, Bernstein A: A method of uniform stratification of risk for evaluating the results of surgery in acquired adult heart disease. Circulation 79:I3, 1989.

CARDIAC SURGERY:
PREOPERATIVE RISK-ESTIMATION WORKSHEET
(not intended for retrospective risk stratification)

Newark Beth Isreal Medical Center
Division of Surgical Research

Patient's Name:
Patient Number:
Date:

INSTRUCTIONS:

Step 1. Fill in the blanks for existing risk factors, using the scores provided. (Note: Scores shown are in arbitrary units, and are not, by themselves, estimates of percent risk.)

Step 2. Add the scores to obtain a total score. (Include common risk factors on this side of the page and less common risk factors on the other side.)

Step 3. See reverse side to interpret the total score.

RISK FACTOR	SCORING (APPROXIMATE SYSTEM 97)		VALUE
Female gender		6	6
Age	70–75 76–79 80+	2.5 7 11	7
Congestive failure		2.5	
COPD, severe		6	
Diabetes		3	
Ejection fraction	30–42% <30%	6.5 8	
Hypertension	Over 140/90, or history of hypertension, or currently taking anti-hypertension medication	3	3
Left-main disease	Left-main stenosis is 50%	2.5	
Morbid obesity	Over 1.5 times ideal weight	1	1
Preoperative IABP	IABP present at time of surgery	4	
Reoperation	First reoperation Second or subsequent reoperation	10 20	
One valve, aortic	Procedure proposed	0	
One valve, mitral	Procedure proposed	4.5	
Valve + ACB	Combination valve procedure and ACB proposed	6	
Special conditions	*(see reverse side)*		
		TOTAL SCORE:	17

(See reverse side for risk estimation.)

RISK VALUES FOR SPECIAL CONDITIONS

Cardiac	
Cardiogenic shock (urinary output <10 cc/hr)	12
Endocarditis, active	5.5
Endocarditis, treated	0
LV aneurysm resected	1.5
One valve, incuspid: procedure proposed	5
Pacemaker dependency	0
Transmural acute MI within 48 hr	4
Ventricular septal defect, acute	12
Ventricular tachycardia, ventricular fibrillation, aborted sudden death	1
Pulmonary	
Asthma	1
Endotracheal tube, preoperative	4
Idiopathic thrombocytopenic purpura	12
Pulmonary hypertension (mean pressure >30)	11

Hepato-renal	
Cirrhosis	12.5
Dialysis dependency	13.5
Renal failure, acute or chronic	3.5
Vascular	
Abdominal aortic aneurysm, asymptomatic	0.5
Cartoid disease (bilateral or 100% unilateral occlusion)	2
Peripheral vascular disease, severe	3.5
Miscellaneous	
Blood products refused	11
Severe neurologic disorder (healed CVA, paraplegia, muscular dystrophy, hemiparesis)	5
PTCA or catheterization failure	5.5
Substance abuse	4.5

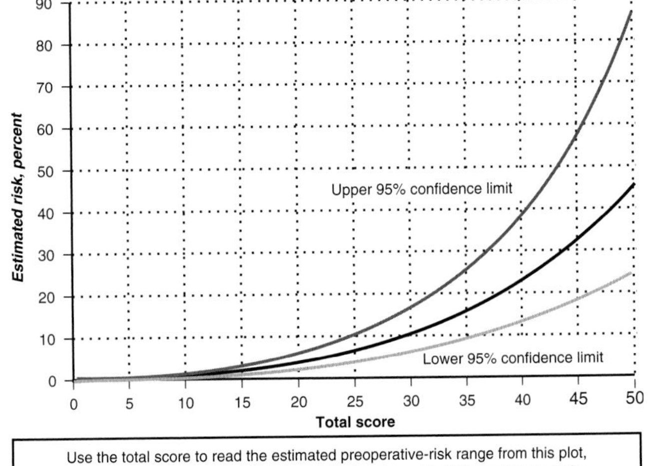

Use the total score to read the estimated preoperative-risk range from this plot, which shows the estimated risk of mortality together with 95% confidence limits.

Figure 11–2 Preoperative Risk Estimation Worksheet. (From Bernstein AD, Parsonnet V: Bedside estimation of risk as an aid for decision-making in cardiac surgery. Ann Thorac Surg 69:823, 2000, with permission from the Society of Thoracic Surgeons.)

use of intra-aortic balloon pump [IABP], mechanical ventilation for 3 or more days, neurologic deficit, oliguric or anuric renal failure, or serious infection) included diabetes mellitus, body weight of 65 kg or less, aortic stenosis, and cerebrovascular disease. Each independent predictor was assigned a weight or score, with increasing mortality and morbidity associated with an increasing total score.

The New York State model of Hannan et al[51] collected data over the years of 1989 through 1992 with 57,187 patients in a study with 14 variables. It was validated in 30 institutions. The mortality definition was "in hospital." The crude mortality rate was 3.1%; the receiver operating characteristic (ROC) curve was 0.7, with the Hosmer-Lemeshow (H-L) statistic <0.005. Observed mortality was 3.7%, and the expected mortality rate was 2.8%. They included only isolated CABG operations.

The Society of Thoracic Surgeons national database represents the most robust source of data for calculating risk-adjusted scoring systems. Established in 1989, the database has grown to include 638 participating hospitals in 2004. This provider-supported database allows participants to benchmark their risk-adjusted results against regional and national standards. New patient data are brought into the Society of Thoracic Surgeons database on an annual and, now, semiannual basis. These new data have been analyzed, modeled, and tested using a variety of statistical algorithms. Since 1990, when more complete data collection was achieved, risk stratification models were developed for both CABG and valve replacement surgery. Models developed in 1995 and 1996 were shown to have good predictive value[52,53] (Table 11–2, Fig. 11–3*A* to *C*). In 1999, the Society of Thoracic Surgeons analyzed the database for valve replacement with and without CABG to determine trends in risk stratification. Between 1986 and 1995, 86,580 patients were analyzed. The model evaluated the influence of 51 preoperative variables on operative mortality by univariate and multivariate analyses for the overall population and for each subset. After the significant risk factors were determined by univariate analysis, a standard logistic regression analysis was performed using the training-set population to develop a formal model. The test set population was then used to determine the validity of the model. The preoperative risk factors associated with highest operative mortal-

Table 11–2 Risk Model Results	
Variable	**Odds Ratio**
Age (in 10-yr increments)	1.640
Female gender	1.157
Noncaucasian	1.249
Ejection fraction	0.988
Diabetes	1.188
Renal failure	1.533
Serum creatinine (if renal failure is present)	1.080
Dialysis dependence (if renal failure is present)	1.381
Pulmonary hypertension	1.185
Cerebrovascular accident timing	1.198
Chronic obstructive pulmonary disease	1.296
Peripheral vascular disease	1.487
Cerebrovascular disease	1.244
Acute evolving, extending myocardial infarction	1.282
Myocardial infarction timing	1.117
Cardiogenic shock	2.211
Use of diuretics	1.122
Hemodynamic instability	1.747
Triple-vessel disease	1.155
Left main disease >50%	1.119
Preoperative intra-aortic balloon pump	1.480
Status	
Urgent or emergent	1.189
Emergent salvage	3.654
First reoperation	2.738
Multiple reoperations	4.282
Arrhythmias	1.099
Body surface area	0.488
Obesity	1.242
New York Heart Association Class IV	1.098
Use of steroids	1.214
Congestive heart failure	1.191
Percutaneous transluminal coronary angioplasty within 6 hr of surgery	1.332
Angiographic accident with hemodynamic instability	1.203
Use of digitalis	1.168
Use of intravenous nitrates	1.088

From Shroyer AL, Plomondon ME, Grover FL, et al: The 1996 coronary artery bypass risk model: The Society of Thoracic Surgeons Adult Cardiac National Database. Ann Thorac Surg 67:1205, 1999, with permission from Society of Thoracic Surgeons.

ity rates were salvage status, renal failure (dialysis dependent and non–dialysis dependent), emergent status, multiple reoperations, and New York Heart Association class IV. The multivariate logistic regression analysis identified 30 independent preoperative risk factors among the six valvular models, isolated or in combination with CABG. The addition of CABG increased the mortality rate significantly for all age groups and for all subset models.[54]

Tu and colleagues[55] collected data from 13,098 patients undergoing cardiac surgery between 1991 and 1993 at all nine adult cardiac surgery institutions in Ontario, Canada. Six variables (age, sex, LV function, type of surgery, urgency of surgery, and repeat operation) predicted in-hospital mortality, ICU stay, and postoperative stay in days after cardiac surgery. Subsequently, the Working Group Panel on the Collaborative CABG Database Project categorized 44 clinical variables into 7 core, 13 level 1, and 24 level 2 variables, to reflect their relative importance in determining short-term mortality after CABG. Using data from 5517 patients undergoing isolated CABG at nine institutions in Ontario in 1993, a series of models were developed. The incorporation of additional variables beyond the original six added little to the prediction of in-hospital mortality.

Spivack et al[56] collected data during the years of 1991 and 1992 and included 513 patients with 15 variables, validated only in their institution. They used only an isolated CABG population, and the outcomes measured were mortality and morbidity. The morbidity definition was ventilator time and ICU days. Both prolonged mechanical ventilation and death were rare events (8.3% and 2.0%, respectively). The combination of reduced LVEF and the presence of selected preexisting comorbid conditions (clinical CHF, angina, current smoking, diabetes) served as modest risk factors for prolonged mechanical ventilation; their absence strongly predicted an uncomplicated postoperative respiratory course.

European System for Cardiac Operative Risk Evaluation (EuroSCORE) for cardiac operative risk evaluation was constructed from an analysis of 19,030 patients undergoing a diverse group of cardiac surgical procedures from 128 centers across Europe[57,58] (Tables 11–3 and 11–4). The following risk factors were associated with increased mortality: age, female gender, serum creatinine, extracardiac arteriopathy, chronic airway disease, severe neurologic dysfunction, previous cardiac surgery, recent MI, LVEF, chronic CHF, pulmonary hypertension, active endocarditis, unstable angina, procedure urgency, critical preoperative condition, ventricular septal rupture, noncoronary surgery, and thoracic aortic surgery.

EuroSCORE provided a unique opportunity to assess the true risk of cardiac surgery in the absence of any identifiable risk factors. For the purposes of this analysis, baseline mortality figures were calculated in patients in whom no preoperative risk factors could be identified (including risk factors that were not found to have a significant impact in this study, such as diabetes and hypertension). When all such patients were excluded, it was gratifying to note the extremely low current mortality for cardiac surgery in Europe: 0% for atrial septal defect repair, 0.4% for CABG, and barely over 1% for single valve repair or replacement.

During the 2000s, this additive EuroSCORE has been widely used and validated across different centers in Europe and across the world, making it a primary tool for risk stratification in cardiac surgery.[59-70] While its accuracy has been well established for CABG and isolated valve procedures, its predictive ability in combined CABG and valve procedures has been less well studied. Karthik et al[61] showed that in patients undergoing combined procedures, the additive EuroSCORE significantly underpredicted the risk compared with the observed mortality. In this subset, they determined that the logistic EuroSCORE is a better and more accurate method of risk assessment.

Dupuis and colleagues[71] attempted to simplify the approach to risk of cardiac surgical procedures in a manner

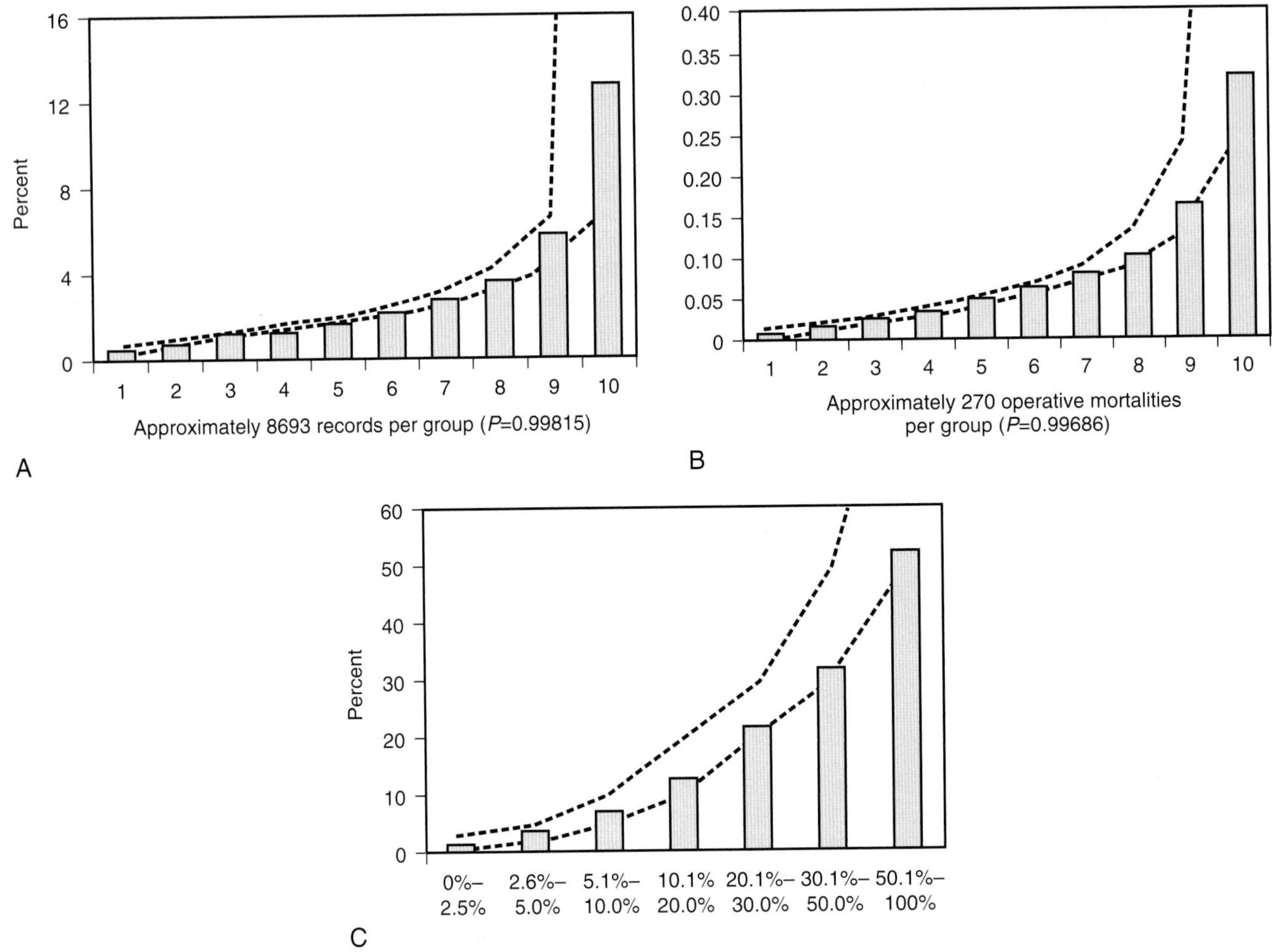

Figure 11–3 *A,* Ordered risk deciles with equal number of records per group. After the predicted risk for each patient in the test set was determined, the patient records were arranged sequentially in order of predicted risk. The population was divided into 10 groups of equal size. The predicted mortality rate was compared with the actual mortality for each of the 10 groups. Dashed lines = range of predicted mortality for a group of patients; bars = actual mortality for a group of patients. *B,* Ordered risk deciles with equal number of deaths per group. After the predicted risk for each patient in the test set was determined, the patient records were arranged sequentially in order of predicted risk. The population was divided into 10 groups with equal numbers of deaths in each group. The predicted mortality was compared with the actual mortality for each of the ten groups. Dashed lines = range of predicted mortality for a group of patients; bars = actual mortality for a group of patients. *C,* Ordered risk categories in clinically relevant groupings. After the predicted risk for each patient in the test set was determined, the patient records were arranged sequentially in order of predicted risk. The population was divided into seven clinically relevant risk categories. The predicted mortality was compared with the actual mortality for each of the seven groups. Dashed lines = range of predicted mortality for a group of patients; bars = actual mortality for a group of patients. (*A–C,* From Shroyer AL, Plomondon ME, Grover FL, et al: The 1996 coronary artery bypass risk model: The Society of Thoracic Surgeons Adult Cardiac National Database. Ann Thorac Surg 67:1205, 1999, with permission from The Society of Thoracic Surgeons.)

similar to the original ASA physical status classification. They developed a score that uses a simple continuous categorization, using five classes plus an emergency status (Table 11–5). The Cardiac Anesthesia Evaluation Score (CARE) model collected data from 1996 to 1999 and included 3548 patients to predict both in-hospital mortality and a diverse group of major morbidities. It combined clinical judgment and the recognition of three risk factors previously identified by multifactorial risk indices: comorbid conditions categorized as controlled or uncontrolled, the surgical complexity, and the urgency of the procedure. The CARE score demonstrated similar or superior predictive characteristics compared with the more complex indices.

Nowicki and colleagues[72] used data on 8943 cardiac valve surgery patients aged 30 years and older from eight northern New England medical centers from 1991 through 2001 to develop a model to predict in-hospital mortality. In the multivariable analysis, 11 variables in the aortic model (older age, lower body surface area, prior cardiac operation, elevated creatinine, prior stroke, NYHA class IV, CHF, atrial fibrillation, acuity, year of surgery, and concomitant CABG) and 10 variables in the mitral model (female sex, older age, diabetes, CAD, prior cerebrovascular accident, elevated creatinine, NYHA class IV, CHF, acuity, and valve replacement) remained independent predictors of the outcome. They developed a look-up table for mortality rate based on a simple scoring system.

Hannan and colleagues[73] also evaluated predictors of mortality after valve surgery but used data from 14,190 patients from New York State. A total of 18 independent risk factors were identified in the six models of differing combinations of valve and CABG. Shock and dialysis-dependent renal failure

Table 11–3 Risk Factors, Definitions, and Weights (Score)

	Definition	Score
Patient-Related Factors		
Age	Per 5 yr or part thereof over 60 yr	1
Sex	Female	1
Chronic pulmonary disease	Long-term use of bronchodilators or steroids for lung disease	1
Extracardiac arteriopathy	Any one or more of the following: claudication, carotid occlusion or >50% stenosis, previous or planned intervention on the abdominal aorta, limb arteries or carotids	2
Neurologic dysfunction	Disease severely affecting ambulation or day-to-day functioning	2
Previous cardiac surgery	Requiring opening of the pericardium	3
Serum creatinine	>200 μmol/L preoperatively	2
Active endocarditis	Patient still under antibiotic treatment for endocarditis at the time of surgery	3
Critical preoperative state	Any one or more of the following: ventricular tachycardia or fibrillation or aborted sudden death, preoperative cardiac massage, preoperative ventilation before arrival in the anesthetic room, preoperative inotropic support, intra-aortic balloon counterpulsation or preoperative acute renal failure (anuria or oliguria <10 mL/hr)	3
Cardiac-Related Factors		
Unstable angina	Rest angina requiring IV nitrates until arrival in the anesthetic room	2
Left ventricular dysfunction	Moderate or LVEF 30–50% Poor or LVEF >30%	1 3
Recent myocardial infarct	(<90% days)	2
Pulmonary hypertension	Systolic pulmonary artery pressure >60 mm Hg	2
Surgery-Related Factors		
Emergency	Carried out on referral before the beginning of the next working day	2
Other than isolated CABG	Major cardiac procedure other than or in addition to CABG	2
Surgery on thoracic aorta	For disorder of ascending aorta, arch or descending aorta	3
Postinfarct septal rupture		4

CABG = coronary artery bypass graft surgery; LVEF = left ventricular ejection fraction.
From Nashef SA, Roques F, Michel P, et al: European system for cardiac operative risk evaluation (EuroSCORE). Eur J Cardiothorac Surg 16:9, 1999.

Table 11–4 Application of EuroSCORE Scoring System

			95% Confidence Limits for Mortality	
EuroSCORE	**Patients (n)**	**Died (n)**	**Observed**	**Expected**
0–2 (low risk)	4529	36 (0.8%)	0.56–1.10	1.27–1.29
3–5 (medium risk)	5977	182 (3.0%)	2.62–3.51	2.90–2.94
6 plus (high risk)	4293	480 (11.2%)	10.25–12.16	10.93–11.54
Total	14,799	698 (4.7%)	4.37–5.06	4.72–4.95

From Nashef SA, Roques F, Michel P, et al: European system for cardiac operative risk evaluation (EuroSCORE). Eur J Cardiothorac Surg 16:9, 1999.

were among the most significant risk factor in all models. The risk factors and odds ratios are shown in Tables 11–6, 11–7, and 11–8. They also studied which risk factors are associated with early readmission (within 30 days) following CABG. Of 16,325 total patients, 2111 (12.9%) were readmitted within 30 days for reasons related to CABG. Eleven risk factors were found to be independently associated with higher readmission rates: older age, female sex, African American race, greater body surface area, previous AMI within 1 week, and six comorbidities. After controlling for these preoperative patient-level risk factors, two provider characteristics (annual surgeon CABG volume <100 and hospital risk-adjusted mortality rate in the highest decile) and two postoperative factors (discharge to nursing home or rehabilitation/acute care facility and length of stay during index CABG admission of ≥5 days) were also related to higher readmission rates. The devel-

Table 11–5 Cardiac Anesthesia Risk Evaluation Score

1. Patient with stable cardiac disease and no other medical problem. A noncomplex surgery is undertaken.
2. Patient with stable cardiac disease and one or more controlled medical problems.* A noncomplex surgery is undertaken.
3. Patient with any uncontrolled medical problem† or patient in whom a complex surgery is undertaken.‡
4. Patient with any uncontrolled medical problem *and* in whom a complex surgery is undertaken.
5. Patient with chronic or advanced cardiac disease for whom cardiac surgery is undertaken as a last hope to save or improve life.

E. Emergency: surgery as soon as diagnosis is made and operating room is available.

*Examples: controlled hypertension, diabetes mellitus, peripheral vascular disease, chronic obstructive pulmonary disease, controlled systemic diseases, others as judged by clinicians.

†Examples: unstable angina treated with intravenous heparin or nitroglycerin, preoperative intra-aortic balloon pump, heart failure with pulmonary or peripheral edema, uncontrolled hypertension, renal insufficiency (creatinine level >140 μmol/L, debilitating systemic diseases, others as judged by clinicians.

‡Examples: reoperation, combined valve and coronary artery surgery, multiple valve surgery, left ventricular aneurysmectomy, repair of ventricular septal detect after myocardial infarction, coronary artery bypass of diffuse or heavily calcified vessels, others as judged by clinicians.

From Dupuis JY, Wang F, Nathan H, et al: The cardiac anesthesia risk evaluation score: A clinically useful predictor of mortality and morbidity after cardiac surgery. Anesthesiology 94:194, 2001.

Table 11–6 Significant Independent Risk Factors for In-Hospital Mortality for Isolated Aortic Valve Replacement and for Aortic Valvuloplasty or Valve Replacement Plus CABG

	Isolated Aortic Valve Replacement (C = 0.809)		Aortic Valvuloplasty or Valve Replacement Plus CABG (C = 0.727)	
Risk Factor	**Odds Ratio**	**95% CI for Odds Ratio**	**Odds Ratio**	**95% CI for Odds Ratio**
Age ≥ 55 yr	1.06	1.04, 1.08	1.04	1.02, 1.06
Hemodynamic instability	3.97	1.85, 8.51	NS	. . .
Shock	8.68	2.76, 27.33	9.09	3.82, 21.62
CHF in same admission	2.26	1.54, 3.30	NS	. . .
Extensively calcified ascending aorta	1.96	1.22, 3.15	1.56	1.16, 2.08
Diabetes	2.52	1.67, 3.81	NS	. . .
Dialysis-dependent renal failure	5.51	2.58, 11.73	3.17	1.70, 5.90
Pulmonary artery systolic pressure ≥50 mm Hg	2.35	1.61, 3.41	2.28	1.75, 2.96
Body surface area	NS	. . .	0.28	0.16, 0.50
Previous cardiac operation	NS	. . .	2.13	1.54, 2.96
Renal failure, no dialysis	NS	. . .	2.36	1.32, 4.21
Aortoiliac disease	NS	. . .	1.88	1.26, 2.82

From Hannan EL, Racz MJ, Jones RH, et al: Predictors of mortality for patients undergoing cardiac valve replacements in New York State. Ann Thorac Surg 70:1212, 2000, with permission from The Society of Thoracic Surgeons.

opment of several excellent risk models for cardiac valve surgery provides a powerful new tool to improve patient care, select procedures, counsel patients, and compare outcomes[74] (see Chapter 20).

Consistency Among Risk Indices

Many different variables have been found to be associated with the increased risk at cardiac surgery, but only a few variables have consistently been found to be major risk factors across multiple and very diverse study settings. Age, female gender, LV function, body habitus, reoperation, type of surgery, and urgency of surgery were some variables consistently present in most of the models (Box 11–3).

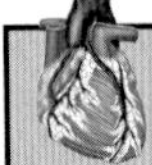

BOX 11–3 *Common Variables Associated With Increased Risk of Cardiac Surgery*

- Age
- Female gender
- Left ventricular function
- Body habitus
- Reoperation
- Type of surgery
- Urgency of surgery

Table 11–7 Significant Independent Risk Factors for In-Hospital Mortality for Isolated Mitral Valve Replacement and for Mitral Valve Replacement Plus CABG

Risk Factor	Isolated Mitral Valve Replacement (C = 0.823)		Mitral Valve Replacement Plus CABG (C = 0.718)	
	Odds Ratio	95% CI for Odds Ratio	Odds Ratio	95% CI for Odds Ratio
Age ≥55 yr	1.08	1.06, 1.11	1.07	1.05, 1.09
Carotid disease	2.98	1.65, 5.39	1.81	1.21, 2.70
Shock	9.17	4.17, 20.16	5.29	3.03, 9.22
CHF in same admission	3.03	2.01, 4.56	NS	. . .
Dialysis-dependent renal failure	5.07	1.98, 12.97	NS	. . .
Endocarditis	4.28	2.49, 7.36	NS	. . .
Ejection fraction <30%	NS	. . .	1.76	1.23, 2.51
Hemodynamic instability	NS	. . .	3.40	2.16, 5.36
Extensively calcified ascending aorta	NS	. . .	1.94	1.27, 2.96

From Hannan EL, Racz MJ, Jones RH, et al: Predictors of mortality for patients undergoing cardiac valve replacements in New York State. Ann Thorac Surg 70:1212, 2000, with permission from The Society of Thoracic Surgeons.

Table 11–8 Significant Independent Risk Factors for In-Hospital Mortality for Multiple Valvuloplasty or Valve Replacement and for Multiple Valvuloplasty or Valve Replacement Plus CABG

Risk Factor	Multiple Valvuloplasty or Valve Replacement (C = 0.764)		Multiple Valvuloplasty or Valve Replacement Plus CABG (C = 0.750)	
	Odds Ratio	95% CI for Odds Ratio	Odds Ratio	95% CI for Odds Ratio
Age ≥55 yr	1.05	1.03, 1.07	1.05	1.10, 1.08
Aortoiliac disease	3.55	1.17, 10.72	4.63	2.12, 10.10
CHF in same admission	2.18	1.44, 3.29	NS	. . .
Malignant ventricular arrhythmia	2.62	1.19, 5.78	NS	. . .
Extensively calcified ascending aorta	2.13	1.13, 4.00	NS	. . .
Diabetes	1.87	1.13, 3.10	2.49	1.46, 4.24
Renal failure without dialysis	3.55	1.88, 6.72	NS	. . .
Dialysis-dependent renal failure	9.37	4.10, 21.40	NS	. . .
Female gender	NS	. . .	1.95	1.20, 3.18
Hemodynamic instability	NS	. . .	3.65	1.50, 8.86
Shock	NS	. . .	50.19	6.08, 414.44
Hepatic failure	NS	. . .	8.21	1.84, 36.66
Endocarditis	NS	. . .	4.70	1.59, 13.87

From Hannan EL, Racz MJ, Jones RH, et al: Predictors of mortality for patients undergoing cardiac valve replacements in New York State. Ann Thorac Surg 70:1212, 2000, with permission from The Society of Thoracic Surgeons.

While a variety of investigators have found different comorbid diseases to be significant risk factors, no diseases have been shown to be consistent risk factors, with the possible exception of renal dysfunction and diabetes. These two comorbidities have been shown to be important risk factors in a majority of the studies (Box 11–4).

BOX 11–4 *Medical Conditions Associated With Increased Risk*

- Renal dysfunction
- Diabetes (inconsistent)
- Recent acute coronary syndromes

Applicability of Risk Indices to a Given Population

To understand how best to apply a given risk index to a specific patient or population, it is critical to understand how these indices were created. Specifically, the application of these risk models must be done with caution and after careful study for any specific population. One issue is that the profile of patients undergoing cardiac surgery is constantly changing, and patients who would not previously have been considered for surgery (and thus not included in the development data set) are now undergoing surgery. Therefore, the models require continuous updating and revision. Additionally, cardiac surgery itself is changing with the increasing use of off-pump and less invasive procedures, which may change the nature of the influence of preexisting conditions.

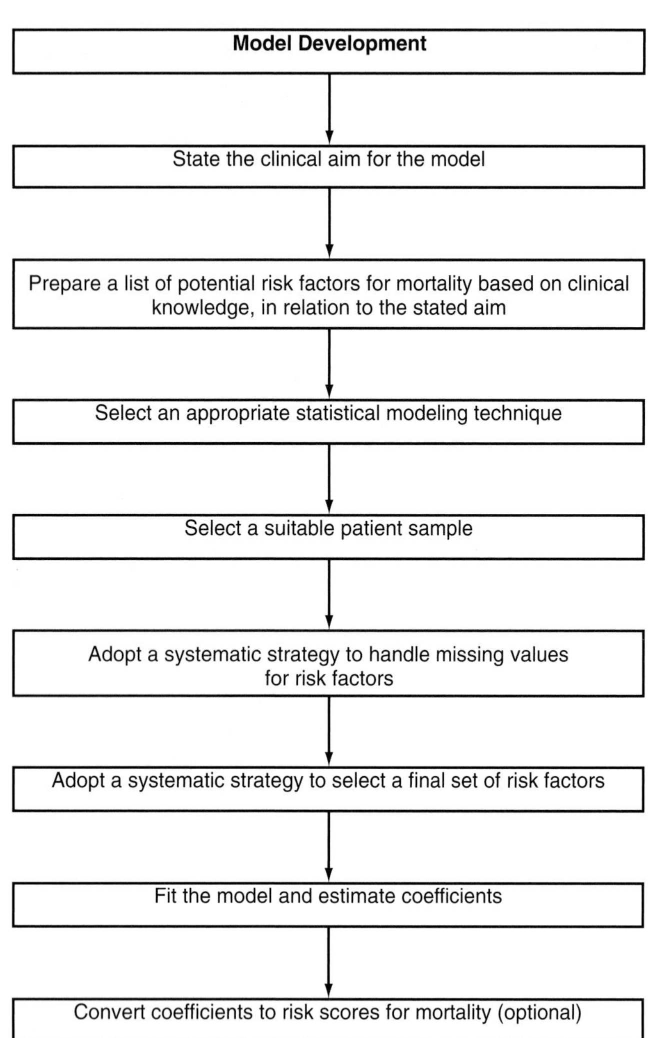

Figure 11–4 Risk model development. (From Omar RZ, Ambler G, Royston P, et al: Cardiac surgery risk modeling for mortality: A review of current practice and suggestions for improvement. Ann Thorac Surg 77:2232, 2004, with permission from The Society of Thoracic Surgeons.)

One critical factor in the choice of model to use for a given practice is to understand the clinical goals used in the original development process. Additionally, despite extensive research and widespread use of risk models in cardiac surgery, there are methodologic problems. The extent of the details in the reports varies greatly. Different conclusions can be reached depending on the risk model used. Processes critical to the development of risk models are shown in Figure 11–4.

The underlying assumption in the development of any risk index is that specific factors (disease history, physical findings, laboratory data, nature of surgery) cannot be modified with respect to their influence on outcome; that is, the perioperative period is essentially a black box. If a specific factor is left untreated, it could lead to major morbidity or mortality. For example, the urgency of the planned surgical procedure and baseline comorbidities cannot be changed. However, the models themselves depend on the appropriate selection of baseline variables or risk factors to study, and their prevalence in the population of interest is critical in order for them to affect outcome. For example, referral patterns to a given institution may result in an absence of certain patient populations and therefore the risk factor would not appear in the model. Also, the use of multivariate logistic regression may eliminate biologically important risk factors, which are not present in sufficient numbers to achieve statistical significance.

In developing a risk index, it is also important to validate the model and to benchmark it against other known means of assessing risks. It is important to determine if the index predicts morbidity, mortality, or both. Typically, a model's performance is first evaluated on the developmental data, evaluating its goodness of fit. Alternatively, the original data can be split and the model can be built on half of the data and validated on the other half. This reduces the total number of patients and outcomes available to create the model. This method is best suited to situations in which data on tens of thousands of patients are available. This internal validation does not provide the practitioner with information on the generalizability of the model. External validation on a large, completely independent test dataset is the best approach to satisfying this requirement.

In addition to validation, calibration refers to a model's ability to predict mortality accurately. There are numerous tests that can be applied, the most common being the H-L test. If the p value from an H-L test is greater than 0.05, the current practice of the developers is to claim that the model predicts mortality accurately.

Discrimination is the ability of a model to distinguish patients who die from those who survive. The area under the ROC is the common method of assessing this facet of the model. In brief, the test is determined by evaluating all possible pairs of patients, determining if the predicted probability of death should ideally be higher for the patient who died than for the one who survived. The ROC area is the percentage of pairs for which this is true. The current practice in cardiac surgery is to conclude that a model discriminates well if the ROC area is greater than 0.7. If predictions are used to identify surgical centers or surgeons with unexpectedly high or low rates, achieving a high ROC area alone is not adequate, but good calibration is also critical. A poorly calibrated model may cause large numbers of institutions or surgeons to reveal excessively high or low rates of mortality, when in fact the fault lies with the model, not the clinical performance. If predictions are used to stratify patients by disease severity in order to compare treatments or to decide on patient management, both calibration and discrimination aspects are important.

Specific Risk Conditions

Renal dysfunction has been shown to be an important risk factor for surgical mortality in patients undergoing cardiac surgery.[75-77] However, the spectrum of what constitutes renal dysfunction is broad, with some models defining it as elevated creatinine levels and others defining it as dialysis dependency. The Northern New England Cardiovascular Study Group recently reported a 12.2% in-hospital mortality following CABG in patients on chronic dialysis, versus a 3.0% mortality in patients not on dialysis.[78] However, the incidence of dialysis dependency in the cardiac surgical population is sufficiently low (e.g., 0.5% in New York State) that it may not enter into many of the models developed. The association between diabetes and mortality with cardiac surgery has been inconsistent, with some studies supporting the association while other studies do not.[79-86] Patients with a recent episode of non–ST-segment elevation acute coronary syndrome before CABG have higher rates of operative morbidity and mortality than do patients with stable coronary syndromes.[87] Investigators at the Mayo Clinic reported a postoperative mortality rate of 21% in a population of patients with severe aortic stenosis and LV dysfunction.[88]

CARDIOVASCULAR TESTING

Patients who present for cardiac surgery have extensive cardiovascular imaging prior to surgery to guide the procedure. Coronary angiography provides a static view of the coronary circulation, while exercise and pharmacologic testing provide a more dynamic view. Because both tests may be available, it is useful to review some basics of cardiovascular imaging (Box 11–5) (see Chapters 6, 12, 14, 15, 16, and 19).

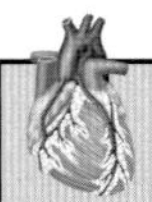

BOX 11–5 ***Preoperative Cardiovascular Testing***

- Coronary angiography
- Exercise electrocardiography
- Nonexercise (pharmacologic) stress testing
- Dipyridamole thallium scintigraphy
- Dobutamine stress echocardiography

In patients with a normal baseline electrocardiogram without a prior history of CAD, the exercise electrocardiographic response is abnormal in up to 25%, and increases up to 50% in those with a prior history of MI or an abnormal resting electrocardiogram. In the general population, the usefulness of an exercise electrocardiographic test is somewhat limited. The mean sensitivity and specificity are 68% and 77%, respectively, for detection of single-vessel disease, 81% and 66% for detection of multivessel disease, and 86% and 53% for detection of three-vessel or left main CAD.[89-91]

The level at which ischemia is evident on exercise electrocardiography can be used to estimate an "ischemic threshold" for a patient to guide perioperative medical management, particularly in the prebypass period.[92,93] This may support further intensification of perioperative medical therapy in high-risk patients, which may have an impact on perioperative cardiovascular events (see Chapters 6, 10, 12, 14, 15, 16, and 19).

Nonexercise (Pharmacologic) Stress Testing

Pharmacologic stress testing has been advocated for patients in whom exercise tolerance is limited, both by comorbid diseases and by symptomatic peripheral vascular disease. Often, these patients may not stress themselves sufficiently during daily life to provoke symptoms of myocardial ischemia or CHF. Pharmacologic stress testing techniques either increase myocardial oxygen demand (dobutamine)[94] or produce coronary vasodilatation leading to coronary flow redistribution (dipyridamole/adenosine).[95] Echocardiographic or nuclear scintigraphic imaging (SPECT) is used in conjunction with the pharmacologic therapy to perform myocardial perfusion imaging (MPI) for risk stratification and myocardial viability assessment (Box 11-6) (see Chapters 6, 12, 14, 15, 16, and 19).

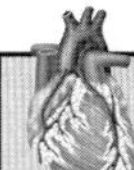

BOX 11–6 ***Indications for Myocardial Perfusion Imaging***

- Risk stratification
- Myocardial viability assessment
- Preoperative evaluation
- Evaluation following percutaneous coronary intervention or coronary artory bypass grafting
- Monitoring medical therapy in coronary artery disease

Dipyridamole-Thallium Scintigraphy

Dipyridamole works by blocking adenosine reuptake and increasing adenosine concentration in the coronary vessels. Adenosine is a direct coronary vasodilator. After infusion of the vasodilator, flow is preferentially distributed to areas distal to normal coronary arteries, with minimal flow to areas distal to a coronary stenosis.[96,97] A radioisotope, such as thallium or 99-technetium sestamibi, is then injected. Normal myocardium will show up on initial imaging, while areas of either myocardial necrosis or ischemia distal to a significant coronary stenosis will demonstrate a defect. After a delay of several hours, or after infusion of a second dose of 99-technetium sestamibi, the myocardium is again imaged. Those initial defects that remain as defects are consistent with old scar, while those defects that demonstrate normal activity on subsequent imaging are consistent with areas at risk for myocardial ischemia. In order to increase the predictive value of the test, several strategies have been suggested. The redistribution defect can be quantitated, with larger areas of defect being associated with increased risk.[97] Additionally, both increased lung uptake and LV cavity dilation have been shown to be markers of ventricular dysfunction with ischemia (Box 11-7).

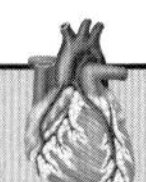

BOX 11–7 ***Scintigraphic Findings of High Risk with Coronary Artery Disease***

- Increased lung uptake
- Left ventricular dilatation
- Increased end-diastolic and end-systolic volumes
- Stress-induced ischemia
- Multiple perfusion defects

Dobutamine Stress Echocardiography

Dobutamine stress echocardiography (DSE) involves the identification of new or worsening RWMAs using two-dimensional echocardiography during infusion of intravenous dobutamine. It has been shown to have the same accuracy as dipyridamole thallium scintigraphy for the detection of CAD. There are several advantages to DSE compared with dipyridamole thallium scintigraphy: the DSE study can also assesses LV function and valvular abnormalities; the cost of the procedure is significantly lower; there is no radiation exposure; the duration of the study is significantly shorter; and results are immediately available.

CONCLUSIONS

Preoperative cardiac risk assessment and stratification in patients undergoing cardiac surgery are distinct from those in patients undergoing noncardiac surgery. In the noncardiac surgery patients, the main goal is to identify a high-risk group of patients who would benefit from either noninvasive or invasive cardiac evaluation and appropriate perioperative medical management or interventional therapy. In patients undergoing cardiac surgery, extensive cardiac evaluation is part of the routine preoperative work-up for the procedure and the patient is having corrective therapy for the underlying disease.

The main goal of cardiac risk assessment in this group of patients, from the anesthesiologist's perspective, is to provide risk-adjusted mortality rates for the preoperative patient and family counseling and identification of the high-risk group for a perioperative cardiac event. Various complex or simplified risk-adjusted morbidity and mortality models can serve as a tool for the preoperative discussion with the patient, but even a well-calibrated model with good discrimination has to be used with caution when applied to individual counseling. First, it is difficult for any model to predict morbidity/mortality, which occurs at a low incidence. Second, it has to be clear that the scoring system provides only the probability of death or major complication, but the individual patient experiences only one of the outcomes.

Clinicians are unable to reliably monitor cardiac injury intraoperatively or in real time. There is also a lack of consensus regarding the definition and quantification of AMI in the perioperative and early postoperative periods. On the other hand, postoperative mortality is easy to define. Therefore, deviation of expected mortality from observed mortality has been used as a "gold standard." However, it is important to recognize that late outcome and survival may also be reflective of intraoperative events. Preoperative cardiac risk assessment of patients undergoing cardiac surgery would ideally lead to identification of a group of patients at risk of increased morbidity and mortality due to perioperative myocardial injury. Based on individual risk factors, perioperative care would then be modified to improve the patient's outcome. To achieve this goal, a clear definition and quantification of myocardial injury in cardiac surgery patients are required. Clinicians need to be able to monitor intraoperative ischemia and intervene to prevent loss of myocardium. Anesthesiologists also need to follow both short- and long-term outcomes of cardiac surgical patients, as well as the impact of different preoperative and intraoperative strategies, on short- and long-term outcomes. Evidence-based medicine has led to an unprecedented growth in the scientific approach to decision-making in the belief that it will translate into benefits for patients to decrease their risk and improve outcomes.[100]

REFERENCES

1. Kouchoukos NT, Ebert PA, Grover FL, et al: Report of the Ad Hoc Committee on Risk Factors for Coronary Artery Bypass Surgery. Ann Thorac Surg 45:348, 1988
2. Paiement B, Pelletier C, Dyrda I, et al: A simple classification of the risk in cardiac surgery. Can Anaesth Soc J 30:61, 1983
3. Pinna-Pintor P, Bobbio M, Sandrelli L, et al: Risk stratification for open heart operations: Comparison of centers regardless of the influence of the surgical team. Ann Thorac Surg 64:410, 1997
4. Smith PK, Smith LR, Muhlbaier LH: Risk stratification for adverse economic outcomes in cardiac surgery. Ann Thorac Surg 64:S61, 1997; discussion S80, 1997
5. Guiteras Val P, Pelletier LC, Hernandez MG, et al: Diagnostic criteria and prognosis of perioperative myocardial infarction following coronary bypass. J Thorac Cardiovasc Surg 86:878, 1983
6. Khuri SF: Evidence, sources, and assessment of injury during and following cardiac surgery. Ann Thorac Surg 72:S2205, 2001
7. Heyndrickx GR, Millard RW, McRitchie RJ, et al: Regional myocardial functional and electrophysiological alterations after brief coronary artery occlusion in conscious dogs. J Clin Invest 56:978, 1975
8. Bolli R: Mechanism of myocardial "stunning." Circulation 82:723, 1990
9. Hearse DJ, Bolli R: Reperfusion-induced injury: Manifestations, mechanisms, and clinical relevance. Cardiovasc Res 26:101, 1992
10. Opie LH: Reperfusion injury and its pharmacologic modification. Circulation 80:1049, 1989
11. Braunwald E, Kloner RA: Myocardial reperfusion: A double-edged sword? J Clin Invest 76:1713, 1985
12. Park JL, Lucchesi BR: Mechanisms of myocardial reperfusion injury. Ann Thorac Surg 68:1905, 1999
13. Jennings RB, Sommers HM, Smyth GA, et al: Myocardial necrosis induced by temporary occlusion of a coronary artery in the dog. Arch Pathol 70:68, 1960
14. Hearse DJ: Ischemia, reperfusion, and the determinants of tissue injury. Cardiovasc Drugs Ther 4(suppl 4):767, 1990
15. Webster KA, Discher DJ, Kaiser S, et al: Hypoxia-activated apoptosis of cardiac myocytes requires reoxygenation or a pH shift and is independent of p53. J Clin Invest 104:239, 1999
16. Thatte HS, Rhee JH, Zagarins SE, et al: Acidosis-induced apoptosis in human and porcine heart. Ann Thorac Surg 77:1376, 2004
17. Levy JH, Tanaka KA: Inflammatory response to cardiopulmonary bypass. Ann Thorac Surg 75:S715, 2003
18. Alpert JS, Thygesen K, Antman E, et al: Myocardial infarction redefined—a consensus document of The Joint European Society of Cardiology/American College of Cardiology Committee for the redefinition of myocardial infarction. J Am Coll Cardiol 36:959, 2000
19. Comunale ME, Body SC, Ley C, et al: The concordance of intraoperative left ventricular wall-motion abnormalities and electrocardiographic S-T segment changes: Association with outcome after coronary revascularization. Multicenter Study of Perioperative Ischemia (McSPI) Research Group. Anesthesiology 88:945, 1998
20. Royster RL, Butterworth JF, Prough DS, et al: Preoperative and intraoperative predictors of inotropic support and long-term outcome in patients having coronary artery bypass grafting. Anesth Analg 72:729, 1991
21. Jacobson A, Lapsley D, Tow DE, et al: Prognostic significance of change in resting left ventricular ejection fraction early after successful coronary artery bypass surgery: a long-term follow-up study. J Am Coll Cardiol 184A, 1995
22. Fleisher LA, Tuman KJ: What can we learn from provoking ischemia? Anesth Analg 84:1177, 1997
23. Griffin M, Edwards B, Judd J, et al: Field-by-field evaluation of intraoperative transoesophageal echocardiography interpretative skills. Physiol Meas 21:165, 2000
24. Brewer DL, Bilbro RH, Bartel AG: Myocardial infarction as a complication of coronary bypass surgery. Circulation 47:58, 1973
25. Crescenzi G, Bove T, Pappalardo F, et al: Clinical significance of a new Q wave after cardiac surgery. Eur J Cardiothorac Surg 25:1001, 2004
26. Sztajzel J, Urban P: Early and late Q wave regression in the setting of acute myocardial infarction. Heart 83:708, 2000
27. Alyanakian MA, Dehoux M, Chatel D, et al: Cardiac troponin I in diagnosis of perioperative myocardial infarction after cardiac surgery. J Cardiothorac Vasc Anesth 12:288, 1998
28. Carrier M, Pellerin M, Perrault LP, et al: Troponin levels in patients with myocardial infarction after coronary artery bypass grafting. Ann Thorac Surg 69:435, 2000
29. Etievent JP, Chocron S, Toubin G, et al: Use of cardiac troponin I as a marker of perioperative myocardial ischemia. Ann Thorac Surg 59:1192, 1995
30. Greenson N, Macoviak J, Krishnaswamy P, et al: Usefulness of cardiac troponin I in patients undergoing open heart surgery. Am Heart J 141:447, 2001
31. Mair J, Larue C, Mair P, et al: Use of cardiac troponin I to diagnose perioperative myocardial infarction in coronary artery bypass grafting. Clin Chem 40:2066, 1994
32. Vermes E, Mesguich M, Houel R, et al: Cardiac troponin I release after open heart surgery: A marker of myocardial protection? Ann Thorac Surg 70:2087, 2000
33. Klatte K, Chaitman BR, Theroux P, et al: Increased mortality after coronary artery bypass graft surgery is associated with increased levels of postoperative creatine kinase-myocardial band isoenzyme release: results from the GUARDIAN trial. J Am Coll Cardiol 38:1070, 2001
34. Costa MA, Carere RG, Lichtenstein SV, et al: Incidence, predictors, and significance of abnormal cardiac enzyme rise in patients treated with bypass surgery in the Arterial Revascularization Therapies Study (ARTS). Circulation 104:2689, 2001
35. Fellahi JL, Gue X, Richomme X, et al: Short- and long-term prognostic value of postoperative cardiac troponin I concentration in patients

undergoing coronary artery bypass grafting. Anesthesiology 99:270, 2003
36. Lehrke S, Steen H, Sievers HH, et al: Cardiac troponin T for prediction of short- and long-term morbidity and mortality after elective open heart surgery. Clin Chem 50:1560, 2004
37. Baxter GF: Natriuretic peptides and myocardial ischaemia. Basic Res Cardiol 99:90, 2004
38. Watanabe M, Egi K, Hasegawa S, et al: Significance of serum atrial and brain natriuretic peptide release after coronary artery bypass grafting. Surg Today 33:671, 2003
39. Vishnevetsky D, Kiyanista VA, Gandhi PJ: CD40 ligand: A novel target in the fight against cardiovascular disease. Ann Pharmacother 38:1500, 2004
40. Nannizzi-Alaimo L, Rubenstein MH, Alves VL, et al: Cardiopulmonary bypass induces release of soluble CD40 ligand. Circulation 105:2849, 2002
41. Jain U, Laflamme CJ, Aggarwal A, et al: Electrocardiographic and hemodynamic changes and their association with myocardial infarction during coronary artery bypass surgery. A multicenter study. Multicenter Study of Perioperative Ischemia (McSPI) Research Group. Anesthesiology 86:576, 1997
42. Fleisher LA: Risk indices: What is their value to the clinician and patient? Anesthesiology 94:191, 2001
43. Hannan EL, Kilburn H Jr, Racz M, et al: Improving the outcomes of coronary artery bypass surgery in New York State. JAMA 271:761, 1994
44. Mukamel DB, Mushlin AI: Quality of care information makes a difference: An analysis of market share and price changes after publication of the New York State Cardiac Surgery Mortality Reports. Med Care 36:945, 1998
45. Coronary Artery Surgery Study (CASS): A randomized trial of coronary artery bypass surgery. Survival data. Circulation 68:939, 1983
46. Alderman EL, Fisher LD, Litwin P, et al: Results of coronary artery surgery in patients with poor left ventricular function (CASS). Circulation 68:785, 1983
47. Parsonnet V, Dean D, Bernstein A: A method of uniform stratification of risk for evaluating the results of surgery in acquired adult heart disease. Circulation 79:I-3, 1989
48. Bernstein AD, Parsonnet V: Bedside estimation of risk as an aid for decision-making in cardiac surgery. Ann Thorac Surg 69:823, 2000
49. O'Connor G, Plume S, Olmstead E, et al: Multivariate prediction of in-hospital mortality associated with coronary artery by-pass graft surgery. Circulation 85:2110, 1992
50. Higgins T, Estafanous F, Loop F, et al: Stratification of morbidity and mortality outcome by preoperative risk factors in coronary artery bypass patients. JAMA 267:2344, 1992
51. Hannan EL, Kilburn H Jr, O'Donnell JF, et al: Adult open heart surgery in New York State. An analysis of risk factors and hospital mortality rates. JAMA 264:2768, 1990
52. Shroyer AL, Grover FL, Edwards FH: 1995 Coronary artery bypass risk model: The Society of Thoracic Surgeons Adult Cardiac National Database. Ann Thorac Surg 65:879, 1998
53. Shroyer AL, Plomondon ME, Grover FL, et al: The 1996 coronary artery bypass risk model: The Society of Thoracic Surgeons Adult Cardiac National Database. Ann Thorac Surg 67:1205, 1999
54. Jamieson WR, Edwards FH, Schwartz M, et al: Risk stratification for cardiac valve replacement. National Cardiac Surgery Database. Database Committee of The Society of Thoracic Surgeons. Ann Thorac Surg 67:943, 1999
55. Tu JV, Jaglal SB, Naylor CD: Multicenter validation of a risk index for mortality, intensive care unit stay, and overall hospital length of stay after cardiac surgery. Steering Committee of the Provincial Adult Cardiac Care Network of Ontario. Circulation 91:677, 1995
56. Spivack SD, Shinozaki T, Albertini JJ, et al: Preoperative prediction of postoperative respiratory outcome. Coronary artery bypass grafting. Chest 109:1222, 1996
57. Nashef SA, Roques F, Michel P, et al: European system for cardiac operative risk evaluation (EuroSCORE). Eur J Cardiothorac Surg 16:9, 1999
58. Roques F, Nashef SA, Michel P, et al: Risk factors and outcome in European cardiac surgery: analysis of the EuroSCORE multinational database of 19030 patients. Eur J Cardiothorac Surg 15:816, 1999; discussion 822, 1999
59. Al-Ruzzeh S, Nakamura K, Athanasiou T, et al: Does off-pump coronary artery bypass (OPCAB) surgery improve the outcome in high-risk patients? A comparative study of 1398 high-risk patients. Eur J Cardiothorac Surg 23:50, 2003
60. Ghosh P, Djordjevic M, Schistek R, et al: Does gender affect outcome of cardiac surgery in octogenarians? Asian Cardiovasc Thorac Ann 11:28, 2003
61. Karthik S, Srinivasan AK, Grayson AD, et al: Limitations of additive EuroSCORE for measuring risk stratified mortality in combined coronary and valve surgery. Eur J Cardiothorac Surg 26:318, 2004
62. Kasimir MT, Bialy J, Moidl R, et al: EuroSCORE predicts mid-term outcome after combined valve and coronary bypass surgery. J Heart Valve Dis 13:439, 2004
63. Kurki TS, Jarvinen O, Kataja MJ, et al: Performance of three preoperative risk indices CABDEAL, EuroSCORE and Cleveland models in a prospective coronary bypass database. Eur J Cardiothorac Surg 21:406, 2002
64. Nakamura Y, Nakano K, Nakatani H, et al: Hospital and mid-term outcomes in elderly patients undergoing off-pump coronary artery bypass grafting—comparison with younger patients. Circ J 68:1184, 2004
65. Nilsson J, Algotsson L, Hoglund P, et al: Early mortality in coronary bypass surgery: The EuroSCORE versus The Society of Thoracic Surgeons risk algorithm. Ann Thorac Surg 77:1235, 2004; discussion 1239, 2004
66. Riha M, Danzmayr M, Nagele G, et al: Off pump coronary artery bypass grafting in EuroSCORE high and low risk patients. Eur J Cardiothorac Surg 21:193, 2002
67. Swart MJ, Joubert G: The EuroSCORE does well for a single surgeon outside Europe. Eur J Cardiothorac Surg 25:145, 2004; author reply 146
68. Toumpoulis IK, Anagnostopoulos CE, DeRose JJ, et al: European system for cardiac operative risk evaluation predicts long-term survival in patients with coronary artery bypass grafting. Eur J Cardiothorac Surg 25:51, 2004
69. Toumpoulis IK, Anagnostopoulos CE, Swistel DG, et al: Does EuroSCORE predict length of stay and specific postoperative complications after cardiac surgery? Eur J Cardiothorac Surg 27:128, 2005
70. Ugolini C, Nobilio L: Risk adjustment for coronary artery bypass graft surgery: An administrative approach versus EuroSCORE. Int J Qual Health Care 16:157, 2004
71. Dupuis JY, Wang F, Nathan H, et al: The cardiac anesthesia risk evaluation score: A clinically useful predictor of mortality and morbidity after cardiac surgery. Anesthesiology 94:194, 2001
72. Nowicki ER, Birkmeyer NJ, Weintraub RW, et al: Multivariable prediction of in-hospital mortality associated with aortic and mitral valve surgery in Northern New England. Ann Thorac Surg 77:1966, 2004
73. Hannan EL, Racz MJ, Jones RH, et al: Predictors of mortality for patients undergoing cardiac valve replacements in New York State. Ann Thorac Surg 70:1212, 2000
74. Gardner S, Grunwald G, Rumsfeld J, et al: Comparison of short-term mortality risk factors for valve replacement vs. coronary artery bypass graft surgery. Ann Thorac Surg 77:549, 2004
75. Brandrup-Wognsen G, Haglid M, Karlsson T, et al: Preoperative risk indicators of death at an early and late stage after coronary artery bypass grafting. Thorac Cardiovasc Surg 43:77, 1995
76. Conlon PJ, Little MA, Pieper K, et al: Severity of renal vascular disease predicts mortality in patients undergoing coronary angiography. Kidney Int 60:1490, 2001
77. Hayashida N, Chihara S, Tayama E, et al: Coronary artery bypass grafting in patients with mild renal insufficiency. Jpn Circ J 65:28, 2001
78. Liu JY, Birkmeyer NJ, Sanders JH, et al: Risks of morbidity and mortality in dialysis patients undergoing coronary artery bypass surgery. Northern New England Cardiovascular Disease Study Group. Circulation 102:2973, 2000
79. Yamamoto T, Hosoda Y, Takazawa K, et al: Is diabetes mellitus a major risk factor in coronary artery bypass grafting? The influence of internal thoracic artery grafting on late survival in diabetic patients. Jpn J Thorac Cardiovasc Surg 48:344, 2000
80. Clement R, Rousou JA, Engelman RM, et al: Perioperative morbidity in diabetics requiring coronary artery bypass surgery. Ann Thorac Surg 46:321, 1988
81. Devineni R, McKenzie FN: Surgery for coronary artery disease in patients with diabetes mellitus. Can J Surg 28:367, 1985
82. Engelman RM, Bhat JG, Glassman E, et al: The influence of diabetes and hypertension on the results of coronary revascularization. Am J Med Sci 271:4, 1976
83. Herlitz J, Wognsen GB, Emanuelsson H, et al: Mortality and morbidity in diabetic and nondiabetic patients during a 2-year period after coronary artery bypass grafting. Diabetes Care 19:698, 1996
84. Magee MJ, Dewey TM, Acuff T, et al: Influence of diabetes on mortality and morbidity: Off-pump coronary artery bypass grafting versus coronary artery bypass grafting with cardiopulmonary bypass. Ann Thorac Surg 72:776, 2001; discussion 780, 2001
85. Salomon NW, Page US, Okies JE, et al: Diabetes mellitus and coronary artery bypass. Short-term risk and long-term prognosis. J Thorac Cardiovasc Surg 85:264, 1983

86. Thourani VH, Weintraub WS, Stein B, et al: Influence of diabetes mellitus on early and late outcome after coronary artery bypass grafting. Ann Thorac Surg 67:1045, 1999
87. Marso SP, Bhatt DL, Roe MT, et al: Enhanced efficacy of eptifibatide administration in patients with acute coronary syndrome requiring in-hospital coronary artery bypass grafting. PURSUIT Investigators. Circulation 102:295, 2000
88. Connolly HM, Oh JK, Schaff HV, et al: Severe aortic stenosis with low transvalvular gradient and severe left ventricular dysfunction: Result of aortic valve replacement in 52 patients. Circulation 101:1940, 2000
89. Horacek BM, Wagner GS: Electrocardiographic ST-segment changes during acute myocardial ischemia. Cardiol Electrophysiol Rev 6:196, 2002
90. Schneider RM, Seaworth JF, Dohrmann ML, et al: Anatomic and prognostic implications of an early treadmill exercise test. Am J Cardiol 50:682, 1982
91. Weiner DA, McCabe CH, Ryan TJ: Prognostic assessment of patients with coronary artery disease by exercise testing. Am Heart J 105:749, 1983
92. Myers J, Prakash M, Froelicher V, et al: Exercise capacity and mortality among men referred for exercise testing. N Engl J Med 346:793, 2002
93. Balady GJ: Survival of the fittest: More evidence. N Engl J Med 346:852, 2002
94. Carstensen S: Dobutamine-atropine stress echocardiography. Heart Drug 5:101, 2005.
95. Grossman GB, Alazraki N: Myocardial perfusion imaging in coronary artery disease. Cardiology 10:1, 2004
96. Klocke FJ, Baird MG, Bateman TM, et al: ACC/AHA/ASNC guidelines for the clinical use of cardiac radionucleotide imaging: Executive summary. Circulation 108:1404, 2003
97. Beller GA: Clinical value of myocardial perfusion imaging in coronary artery disease. J Nucl Cardiol 10:529, 2003
98. Armstrong WF, Pellikka PA, Ryan T, et al: Stress echocardiography: Recommendations for performance and interpretation. J Am Soc Echocardiogr 11:97, 1998
99. Marwick TH: Quantitative techniques for stress echocardiography. Eur J Echocardiogr 3:171, 2002
100. Cheng DC, Martin JE: Raising the bar: A primer on evidence-based decision-making. Semin Cardiothoracic Vasc Anesth 9:1, 2005

Chapter 12

CARDIAC CATHETERIZATION LABORATORY: DIAGNOSTIC AND THERAPEUTIC PROCEDURES IN THE ADULT PATIENT

Mark Kozak, MD • Bryan J. Robertson, MD • Charles E. Chambers, MD

KEY POINTS

1. The cardiac catheterization laboratory has evolved from a diagnostic facility to a therapeutic one. Despite improvements in equipment, the quality of the procedure depends upon well-trained and experienced physicians with proper certification, adequate procedural volume, and personnel committed to the continuous quality improvement process.
2. Guidelines for diagnostic cardiac catheterization have established indications and contraindications, as well as criteria to identify high-risk patients. Careful evaluation of the patient before the procedure is necessary to minimize risks.
3. A general overview of hemodynamics is presented, including waveform generation and analysis, cardiac output measurement, and assessment of valvular pathology. Basic angiography is also reviewed, including ventriculography, aortography, and coronary cineangiography.
4. Interventional cardiology began in the late 1970s as balloon angioplasty with a success rate of 80% and emergent coronary artery bypass graft surgery (CABG) rates of 3% to 5%. Although current success rates exceed 95% with CABG rates less than 1%, the failed percutaneous coronary intervention (PCI) patient presents a challenge for the anesthesiologist because of hemodynamic problems, concomitant medications, and the underlying cardiac disease.
5. Thrombosis is a major cause of complications during PCI, and platelets are primary in this process. Thrombotic complications have declined with combination pharmacotherapy.
6. In the stent era, acute closure from coronary dissection has diminished significantly. Restenosis rates have fallen precipitously since the introduction of the drug-eluting stents.
7. For patients presenting with acute myocardial infarction, both primary PCI and thrombolytic therapy are effective. In multivessel disease, the advantage of CABG over PCI is narrowing, and drug-eluting stents may reverse this advantage.
8. Extensive thrombus, heavy calcification, degenerated saphenous vein grafts, and chronic total occlusions present specific challenges in PCI. Various specialty devices have been developed to address these problems with varying degrees of success.
9. The reach of the interventional cardiologist is extending beyond the coronary vessels, and now includes closure of congenital defects and percutaneous treatment of valvular disease. These long and complex procedures are more likely to require general anesthesia.

From its inception until recently, the cardiac catheterization laboratory was primarily a diagnostic unit. In the 21st century, its focus has changed to therapy. As the noninvasive modalities of echocardiography, computed tomography and magnetic resonance imaging improve in resolution, sensitivity, and specificity, the role of the diagnostic cardiac catheterization will likely decline before the end of the decade.[1,2] The diagnosis and treatment of peripheral and cerebral vascular disease are now commonly performed in catheterization laboratories previously restricted to cardiac work.[3] Newer coronary stents, as well as patent foramen ovale (PFO)/atrial septal defect (ASD)/ventricular septal defect (VSD) closure devices, are emerging as alternatives to cardiac surgery for many patients. Percutaneous valve replacement/repair is in development as well. In this arena, the need for more "routine" involvement of anesthesiologists in the catheterization laboratory will be important.

Where and how did this entity called "cardiac catheterization" begin? In 1929, Dr. Werner Forssmann was a resident in the Auguste Viktoria Hospital at Eberswald near Berlin. At that time, cardiac arrests during anesthesia and surgery were not uncommon. Treatment included heroic measures such as intracardiac injection of epinephrine, which often resulted in fatal intrapericardial hemorrhage. In an effort to identify a safer route for delivery of medicine directly into the heart, Dr. Forssmann asked a colleague to place a catheter in his arm. The catheter was successfully passed to his axilla, at which time Dr. Forssmann, under radioscopic guidance and using a mirror, advanced the catheter into his own right atrium (RA). His mentor, Professor Ferdinand Sauerbruch, a leading surgeon in Berlin at the time, was quoted as saying, "I run a clinic, not a circus!" Dr. Forssmann subsequently practiced in a small town in the Rhine Valley, but eventually shared the Nobel Prize in 1956 for this procedure.[4]

Fortunately, the remainder of the world quickly acknowledged Forssmann's accomplishments[5] with right heart catheterization; in 1930 Dewey measured cardiac output using the Fick method. In 1941 Andre Cournand published his work on right-sided heart catheterization in the *Proceedings of the Society of Experimental Biology and Medicine.* Dexter and his colleagues first reported cardiac catheterization in the pediatric population in 1947, and first documented correlation between the pulmonary capillary wedge pressure (PCWP) and the left atrial pressure (LAP). Zimmerman and Mason first performed arterial retrograde heart catheterization in 1950, and Seldinger developed his percutaneous approach in 1953. Ross and Cope developed transseptal catheterization in 1959.

This was also the same year that Mason Sones performed his first selective coronary arteriography.

Diagnostic catheterization led to interventional therapy in 1977 when Andreas Gruentzig performed his first percutaneous transluminal coronary angioplasty (PTCA). Refinements in both diagnostic and interventional equipment occurred during the decade of the 1980s, with the 1990s seeing advances in both new device technologies for coronary artery disease (CAD) and the entry of cardiologists into the diagnosis and treatment of peripheral vascular disease. The 2000s will see advances in all of these interventional areas as well as the emergence of percutaneous valve replacement/repair.

This brief historical background serves as an introduction to the discussion of diagnostic and therapeutic procedures in the adult catheterization laboratory.[6] The reader must realize the dynamic nature of this field. While failed percutaneous coronary interventions (PCIs) once occurred in up to 5% of coronary interventions, most centers now report procedural failure rates under 1%. Simultaneously, the impact on the anesthesiologist has changed. The high complication rates of years past required holding an operating room (OR) open for all PCIs, and many almost expected to see the patient in the OR. Current low complication rates lead to complacency, along with amazement and perhaps confusion when a PCI patient comes emergently to the OR. Additionally, the anesthesiologist may find the information in this chapter useful in planning the preoperative management of a patient undergoing a cardiac or a noncardiac surgical procedure based on diagnostic information obtained in the catheterization laboratory. Finally, it is the goal of these authors to provide a current overview of this field so that the collaboration between the anesthesiologist and the interventional cardiologist will be mutually gratifying.

CATHETERIZATION LABORATORY FACILITIES

Room Setup/Design/Equipment

The setup and design for the cardiac catheterization laboratory vary from a single room, as seen in a mobile catheterization laboratory or a small community hospital, to a multilaboratory facility, as is found in large tertiary care centers (Box 12–1). In these facilities with multiple laboratories, a central work area is needed to coordinate patient flow to each of the surrounding laboratories and for centralized equipment storage. Patient holding areas are used for observation and evaluation of patients before and after the procedure.

For the individual laboratory, the monitoring suite is separated from the x-ray imaging equipment by lead-lined glass as well as lead-lined walls. These areas contain the hemodynamic recorders, equipment for blood gas analysis and activated coagulation time (ACT), and x-ray controls. Voice communication from the central area is maintained with each catheterization laboratory to coordinate tasks performed in the central area (e.g., monitoring and recording data, ACT determination), thereby minimizing staff radiation exposure.[7]

A hemodynamic monitoring system with a minimum of a five-channel monitor and recorder is essential for catheterization laboratories.[8] This would include three channels for pressure monitoring and two for ECG monitoring. Pressure recordings using a common zero or baseline are displayed and recorded to allow for pressure gradient determinations.

The individual catheterization laboratory may use single-plane C-arm equipment or biplane equipment, the latter being essential for pediatric studies, placement of percutaneous closure devices, or performance of complex electrophysiologic procedures (Fig. 12–1). Standard resuscitation equipment including resuscitation drugs, a cardiac defibrillator, and external pacemaker must be readily available in each room. In addition, space for ventilators, intra-aortic balloon pumps, and equipment for cardiopulmonary resuscitation is necessary when dealing with critically ill cardiac patients. This particularly applies to acute myocardial infarction intervention.

As in the operating room, four aspects of electrical safety must be addressed in each catheterization laboratory: (1) a safe primary electrical system must be in place; (2) all equipment attached to the patient must be electrically isolated; (3) there should be an equipotential hard wire grounding system for all equipment; and (4) periodic laboratory measurement of current leakage and inspection of equipment must be performed.[9]

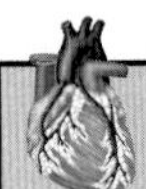

BOX 12–1 *Catheterization Laboratory Setup and Radiation Safety*

Components of a catheterization laboratory
- Imaging equipment
- Monitoring equipment
- Emergency equipment
- Radiation safety
- Shielding
- Lead aprons

Radiation Safety

Radiation safety must be considered at all times in the catheterization laboratory, from room design to everyday practice.[10] Lead-lined walls, lead-glass partitions, and mobile lead shielding are useful in limiting the daily exposure of personnel.

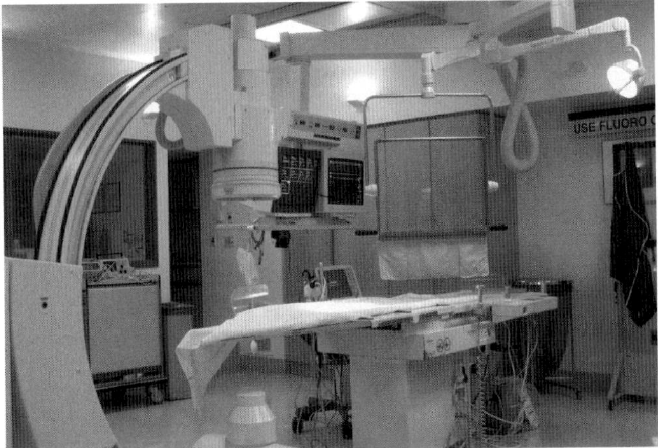

Figure 12–1 A representative cardiac catheterization laboratory with an above-table image intensifier, a below-table x-ray tube mounted on a "C" arm, table, shielding both ceiling-mounted and free-standing image monitors, emergency equipment, and the control room separated/shielded by lead glass.

A thermoluminescent film badge must be worn at all times by any personnel exposed to the x-ray equipment, with levels monitored regularly. Radiation levels should not exceed 5 rem per calendar year, and 1.25 rem per calendar quarter, or approximately 100 mrem per week.[8] Operator and staff radiation has been assessed for years. However, only recently has the issue of radiation toxicity to the patient gained attention. With long PCI and electrophysiology procedures, radiation injury to the patient has been identified, and the need for monitoring dose delivery to the patient is now appreciated.[11,12] Lead aprons are mandatory for all personnel in the procedure suite. Thyroid shielding should also be strongly considered, particularly if the clinician is working in close proximity to the x-ray source. Often cumbersome, these shields protect the gonads and about 80% of the active bone marrow.[10]

It is not in the scope of the chapter to cover all aspects of radiation. For a more complete review written for all who utilize or who are exposed to fluoroscopy, a recent consensus document was published by ACC/AHA/NASPE-HRS/SCAI.[11]

Several aspects of radiation safety require brief review. The duration of the procedure will increase exposure. Cine imaging (i.e., making a permanent recording) requires at least five times the radiation of fluoroscopy. Although newer equipment may narrow this ratio and permanently record fluoroscopic images, limiting cine imaging will decrease exposure. Proximity to the x-ray tube, situated at the bottom of the C arm, is directly related to exposure. When working in an environment where x-rays are in use, clinicians should always remember the simple rule of radiation dose: the amount of radiation exposure is related to the square of the distance from the source. No body part should ever be placed in the imaging field when fluoroscopy/cine is being performed. Finally, the cardiologist can decrease x-ray scatter by placing the imaging equipment as close to the patient as possible, thereby decreasing personnel exposure.

The anesthesiologist should recognize x-ray use in the catheterization laboratory and take appropriate precautions. This must be emphasized, particularly in emergent situations when the anesthesiologist is asked to resuscitate a critically ill patient during a catheterization procedure while the cardiologist may need fluoroscopic imaging. This may require the anesthesiologist to be within feet of, and often even straddling, the x-ray tube. With 96% of the x-ray beam scatter stopped with 0.5 mm of lead, aprons and thyroid shields are clearly needed to protect the anesthesiologist while at the head of the patient.[10] To protect personnel, the use of x-rays can almost always be interrupted; patient care may require the interruptions to be brief. A collaborative effort between the cardiologist and the anesthesiologist is necessary, and communication is essential. The goal of the anesthesiologist should be to treat the patient while protecting himself or herself from excess radiation.[12]

Filmless Imaging/Flat Panel Technology

Until the 1990s, the utilization of 35 mm film in the catheterization laboratory had been the standard for image quality as well as for both storage and information exchange in and among laboratories. The term *cine* refers to motion; although replacing 35 mm film in the catheterization laboratory is often referred to as cineless, it is best described as filmless or digital recording. Radiation is required to generate an image and recordings are made at various frequencies (frames per second) in the presence or absence of film. The best image quality for film is produced at x-ray frame rates of greater than 30 frames/sec. Digital imaging decreases radiation exposure in the laboratory by allowing for image acquisition at lower frame rates, 15 frames/sec (half the radiation dose), while still maintaining excellent image quality. Cost savings have been achieved by the elimination of the purchasing, processing, and storage of film. Film imaging was an analog technique, and a single recording was made. Copies were rarely made because of cost and degradation of image quality. If films were loaned, lost, or misplaced, the study could not be reviewed. With the current digital technology, images are archived on a central server and can be viewed on remote workstations. An infinite number of copies can be made at low cost and with no loss of image quality.

Despite its limitations, 35 mm film had the advantage of universal use, thus allowing the lending of film to another institution. In 1995 the American College of Cardiology (ACC) and the American College of Radiology (ACR), together with industry representatives from the National Electrical Manufacture Association (NEMA), working under the aegis of the Digital Imaging and Communications in Medicine (DICOM), published the industry standard for digital transfer of angiographic images.[13] By setting industry-wide standards for both coding and media (CD-ROM), this work guaranteed the ability to share images among institutions and permitted commercial development of archival systems. It also sealed the fate of film.

Data compression for storage is required to be 2:1 ("lossless") compression. Although "lossless" compression on a CD-ROM is the standard for the transfer of images between institutions, similar standards do not exist for long-term archival (no media standard) and data transfer options within a single institution (no compression standard).[14] Large amounts of memory and bandwidth are required for storage and transfer of the images in "lossless" compression. At remote viewing stations, such as those in the operating room, it is essential that the viewer be aware of the type of image compression used to transfer data. If significant image compression is used, image quality will decrease. It is essential that improper decisions not be made because of inferior image quality.

The evolution of angiographic recording has extended beyond recording formats. Charged-couple device (CCD) cameras and flat-panel detectors (FPDs) represent the next steps in this progress.[15] The image intensifier has been the standard for x-ray imaging throughout the history of the cardiac catheterization laboratory. X-rays are generated from below the patient by the x-ray tube, pass through the patient, are captured by the image intensifier, and converted into a visible light image (analog). This visible light image may then be displayed on a monitor, recorded on film, or converted to a digital image for display or recording.[16]

In 1995, flat panel technology was introduced into the catheterization laboratory. In this system, the x-rays are both acquired and digitally processed by the flat panel, eliminating a step in this process.[11] The flat panel is above the patient (analogous to the image intensifier), and the x-rays are generated below the patient, as before. This next generation of imaging in the catheterization laboratory can already deliver an improved image quality since the dynamic range of the image (number of shades of gray) is improved. It has the potential to decrease radiation exposure by providing immediate feedback to the x-ray generator.

Facility Case Load

All catheterization facilities must maintain appropriate patient volume to assure competence. ACC/AHA guidelines recommend that a minimum of 300 adult diagnostic cases and 75 pediatric cases per facility per year be performed to provide adequate care.[8,17] A case load of at least 200 percutaneous coronary interventions (PCIs) per year, with an ideal volume of 400 cases annually, is recommended.[18,19]

Facilities performing PCIs without in-house surgical backup are becoming more prevalent.[20] Despite this, national guidelines still recommend that both elective and emergent PCIs be performed in centers with surgical capabilities.[21] Although emergent CABG is infrequent in the stent era, when emergent CABG is required, the delays inherent in the transfer of patients to another hospital would compromise the outcomes of these compromised patients.[22] Primary PCI for acute myocardial infarction (AMI) is the accepted standard treatment for patients: (1) in cardiogenic shock; (2) who have contraindications to thrombolytic therapy; (3) who fail thrombolytic therapy. It is preferred therapy for those who present late in the course of an infarction, and is probably the optimal treatment for all myocardial infarctions, provided that it can be performed in a timely manner. In the situation where a patient presents with an AMI to a facility without cardiac surgical capabilities, management is controversial. Although national guidelines do not endorse the performance of PCI in this setting, they state that the operator should be qualified. In practice, this means that he or she performs elective and emergent PCIs at another facility and the total laboratory case volume should be at least 36 AMI procedures per year.[22]

Although minimal volumes are recommended, no regulatory control currently exists. In a study of volume-outcome relationships published for New York State, a clear inverse relationship between laboratory case volume and procedural mortality and coronary artery bypass graft (CABG) rates was identified.[23] In a nationwide study of Medicare patients, low-volume centers had a 4.2% 30-day mortality, whereas the high-volume centers' mortality was 2.7%.[24] The ACC clinical competence statement for PCI summarizes these studies.[25] Centers of excellence, based upon physician and facility volume as well as overall services provided, may well be the model for cardiovascular care in the future.[26]

Physician Credentialing

The more experience an operator has with a particular procedure, the more likely this procedure will have a good outcome. The American College of Cardiology Task Force has established guidelines for the volume of individual operators in addition to the facility volumes mentioned above.[8,17] The current recommendations for competence in diagnostic cardiac catheterization require a fellow perform a minimum of 300 angiographic procedures, with at least 200 catheterizations as the primary operator, during his or her training.

Prior guidelines have recommended a cardiologist perform a minimum of 150 diagnostic cases per year to maintain clinical expertise after fellowship training.[8,17] Of note, when physicians have performed more than 1000 cases independently, the individual case volume may fall for a limited period with the operator still maintaining a high level of expertise. The ideal case volume should not exceed 500 to 600 procedures per year for physicians committed to cardiac catheterization. For the physician performing pediatric procedures, annual volumes should equal or exceed 50 cases.[17] Ultimately, each hospital's quality assurance/peer review program is responsible for setting its own standards and maintaining them through performance improvement reviews.[27,28]

In 1999, the American Board of Internal Medicine established board certification for interventional cardiology. To be eligible, a physician has to complete 3 years of a cardiology fellowship, complete a (minimum) of a 1-year fellowship in interventional cardiology, and obtain board certification in general cardiology. In addition to the diagnostic catheterization experience discussed above, a trainee must perform at least 250 coronary interventional procedures. Board certification requires renewal every 10 years, and initially was offered to practicing interventionalists with or without formal training in intervention. In 2004, the "grandfather" pathway ended, and a formal interventional fellowship is required for board certification in interventional cardiology. Following board certification, the physician should perform at least 75 PCIs as a primary operator annually. Operators who perform fewer than 75 cases per year should only operate in facilities that perform more than 600 PCIs annually. In addition to case load, the physician should attend at least 30 hours every 2 years in interventional cardiology continuing education.[18,19,22] With the establishment of board certification for PCI and the correlation of outcomes to PCI volumes, it is likely that high-volume, board-certified interventional cardiologists will displace low volume PCI operators, and improved outcomes will result.[20]

The performance of peripheral interventions in the cardiac catheterization laboratory is increasing. Vascular surgeons, interventional radiologists, and interventional cardiologists all compete in this area. The claim of each subspecialty to this group of patients has merits and limitations. Renal artery interventions are the most common peripheral intervention performed by interventional cardiologists, but distal peripheral vascular interventions are performed in many laboratories. Stenting of the carotid arteries looks favorable when compared with carotid endarterectomy.[29,30] Guidelines are being developed with input from all subspecialties. These guidelines and oversight by individual hospitals will be needed to ensure that the promise of clinical trials is translated into quality patient care.

With this in mind, internal peer review is essential for the catheterization laboratory. Although separate from credentialing, the peer review process is designed to identify quality issues for the purpose of improving patient care. This involves education, clinical practice standardization, feedback and benchmarking, professional interactions, incentives, decision-support systems, and administrative interventions.[17,27,28] An internal peer review process allows the physicians to establish and maintain in-hospital practice standards essential for quality patient care.

Freestanding Diagnostic Laboratories and Non–Operating Room Interventional Laboratory Facilities

Although initially introduced in the university setting, diagnostic cardiac catheterization laboratories were established in community hospitals in the 1970s, initially with and then without the availability of cardiac surgery. Such facilities now number in excess of 2100 in the United States alone.[17] Beginning in the mid 1980s, diagnostic catheterization laboratories left the hospital as freestanding facilities and even mobile catheterization laboratories.[17,31] Advances in PCI during the

1990s reduced the need for emergent cardiac surgery to less than 1%. In response, many of these "diagnostic" catheterization laboratories began to perform PCIs without OR backup.[20]

To address the issues of the freestanding diagnostic cardiac catheterization laboratory, The Society for Cardiac Angiography and Interventions published guidelines.[32] This committee defined a freestanding cardiac catheterization laboratory as "a facility with electrocardiographic, hemodynamic, and angiographic capabilities for invasive studies of the structure and function of the heart that is neither owned nor administered by a hospital, and is geographically separate from a hospital."[32] The Society made recommendations for freestanding catheterization facilities that included appropriate local governance, formal written affiliation with a nearby hospital with cardiac surgery, and proper prescreening to avoid the high-risk patient.

PCI is currently not recommended without OR backup.[22] However, this is very controversial. Several states, such as Pennsylvania and Massachusetts, have pilot programs to address this issue. Due to the advances in PCI, particularly in coronary stenting, as well as the need for primary PCI for AMI, diagnostic catheterization laboratories have begun offering PCI without OR backup. Essential to the success of this program have been experienced interventionalists and staff with total laboratory numbers reflecting expertise in this area. In a recent publication from the Medicare PCI database, patients undergoing PCI from 178 hospitals without on-site CABG were compared with patients from 943 hospitals with on-site CABG. For patients undergoing rescue or primary PCI for AMI, no mortality difference was seen. However, for all others undergoing PCI, mortality was higher in the patients undergoing PCI without onsite CABG.[20]

PATIENT SELECTION FOR CATHETERIZATION

Indications for Cardiac Catheterization in the Adult Patient

Table 12–1 lists generally agreed on indications for cardiac catheterization. With respect to CAD, approximately 15% of the adult population studied will have normal coronary arteries.[17] This reflects limitations of the specificity of the clinical criteria and noninvasive tests used to select patients for catheterization. However, as the sensitivity and specificity of the noninvasive studies have improved, this percentage of normal studies has progressively declined.[33] Despite this, coronary angiography is, for the moment, still considered the gold standard for defining CAD. With advances in MRI and multislice CT scanning, the next decade may well see a further evolution of the catheterization laboratory to an interventional suite with fewer diagnostic responsibilities.

Table 12–1 Indications for Diagnostic Catheterization in the Adult Patient

Coronary Artery Disease
SYMPTOMS
Unstable angina
Postinfarction angina
Angina refractory to medications
Typical chest pain with negative diagnostic testing
History of sudden death
DIAGNOSTIC TESTING
Strongly positive exercise tolerance test
Early positive, ischemia in ≥5 leads, hypotension, ischemia present for ≥6 minutes of recovery
Positive exercise testing following myocardial infarction
Strongly positive nuclear myocardial perfusion test
Increased lung uptake or ventricular dilation post stress
Large single or multiple areas of ischemic myocardium
Strongly positive stress echocardiographic study
Decrease in overall ejection fraction or ventricular dilation with stress
Large single area or multiple or large areas of new wall motion abnormalities
Valvular Disease
SYMPTOMS
Aortic stenosis with syncope, chest pain, or congestive heart failure
Aortic insufficiency with progressive heart failure
Mitral insufficiency or stenosis with progressive congestive heart failure symptoms
Acute orthopnea/pulmonary edema postinfarction with suspected acute mitral insufficiency
DIAGNOSTIC TESTING
Progressive resting LV dysfunction with regurgitant lesion
↓ LV function and/or chamber dilation with exercise
Adult Congenital Heart Disease
ATRIAL SEPTAL DEFECT
Age >50 with evidence of coronary artery disease
Septum primum or sinus venosus defects
VENTRICULAR SEPTAL DEFECT
Catheterization for definition of coronary anatomy
COARCTATION OF THE AORTA
Detection of collaterals
Coronary arteriography if increased age and/or risk factors are present
Other
Acute MI therapy—consider primary PCI
Mechanical complication postinfarction
Malignant cardiac arrhythmias
Cardiac transplantation
Pretransplant donor evaluation
Posttransplant annual coronary artery graft rejection evaluation
Unexplained congestive heart failure
Research studies with institutional review board review and patient consent

LV = left ventricular.

Patient Evaluation Prior to Cardiac Catheterization

Diagnostic cardiac catheterization in the 21st century is universally considered an outpatient procedure except for the patient at high risk. Therefore, the precatheterization evaluation is essential for quality patient care. Evaluation before cardiac catheterization includes diagnostic tests that are necessary to identify the high-risk patient. An electrocardiogram (ECG) must be performed on all patients shortly before catheterization. Necessary laboratory studies before catheterization include a coagulation profile (prothrombin time [PT], partial thromboplastin time [PTT], and platelet count), hemoglobin, and hematocrit. Electrolytes are obtained along with a baseline blood urea nitrogen (BUN) and creatinine to assess renal function. Urinalysis and chest radiograph may provide useful information but are no longer routinely obtained by all operators. Prior catheterization reports should be available. If the patient had prior PCI or coronary bypass surgery, this information must also be available.

The precatheterization history is important to delineate the specifics that may place the patient at increased risk. Proper identification of prior contrast exposure with or without contrast allergic reaction must be recorded. If a true contrast reaction (rash, breathing difficulties, angioedema, and so forth) occurred with prior contrast exposure, premedication with glucocorticoids is required. Similarly, renal insufficiency will be detected if the patient is properly evaluated. The study can then be canceled or delayed. If the indication for catheterization is strong, prehydration, avoidance of certain medication (e.g., NSAIDs), and limiting the volume of contrast (i.e., assessing ventricular function by echocardiography and omitting ventriculography) will reduce the risk of worsening renal function.[17]

A review of the noninvasive cardiac evaluation prior to cardiac catheterization allows the cardiologist to formulate objectives for the procedure. In patients with hypotension on the exercise stress test, left main coronary lesions should be suspected. Knowing the location of either perfusion or wall motion abnormalities in a particular coronary distribution, the cardiologist must specifically identify or exclude coronary lesions in these areas during the procedure. Finally, in patients with echocardiographic evidence of left ventricular (LV) thrombus, left ventriculography may not be performed.

Patient medications must be addressed. On the morning of the catheterization, antianginal and antihypertensive medications are routinely continued while diuretic therapy is held. Diabetic patients are scheduled early, if possible. As breakfast is held, no short-acting insulin is given. Patients on oral anticoagulation should stop warfarin sodium (Coumadin) therapy 48 to 72 hours before catheterization (INR ≤ 1.8). In patients who are anticoagulated for mechanical prosthetic valves, the patient may best be managed with intravenous heparin before and after the procedure, when the warfarin effect is not therapeutic. Low-molecular-weight heparins (LMWH) are used in this setting, but this is controversial. LMWHs vary in their duration of action, and their effect cannot be monitored by routine tests. This effect needs to be considered, particularly with regard to hemostasis at the vascular access site. Intravenous heparin is routinely discontinued 2 to 4 hours before catheterization, except in the unstable angina patient. Aspirin therapy for angina patients or in patients with prior CABG is often continued, particularly in patients with unstable angina.[34,35]

Contraindications, High-Risk Patients, and Postcatheterization Care

Despite advances in facilities, equipment, technique, and personnel, the precatheterization evaluation must identify those patients at increased risk for complications. In a modern facility with an experienced staff, the only absolute contraindication would be the refusal by a competent patient or an incompetent patient unable to provide informed consent. Relative contraindications are listed in Box 12–2, with the primary operator responsible for this assessment.[7,17]

Box 12–3 lists criteria for identifying the high-risk patient before catheterization. Procedural alterations based on this assessment may include avoidance of crossing an aortic valve or performing ventriculography.[36,37] Regardless of the risk, determination as to whether a patient is a candidate for catheterization must be based on the risk versus benefit for each individual.

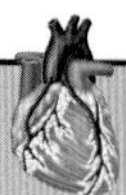

BOX 12–2 *Relative Contraindications to Diagnostic Cardiac Catheterization*

1. Uncontrolled ventricular irritability: The risk of ventricular tachycardia/fibrillation during catheterization is increased if ventricular irritability is uncontrolled.
2. Uncorrected hypokalemia or digitalis toxicity
3. Uncorrected hypertension: Predisposes to myocardial ischemia and/or heart failure during angiography.
4. Intercurrent febrile illness
5. Decompensated heart failure: especially acute pulmonary edema
6. Anticoagulation state: INR > 1.8
7. Severe allergy to radiographic contrast agent
8. Severe renal insufficiency and/or anuria: unless dialysis is planned to remove fluid and radiographic contrast load

Modified from Baim DS, Grossman W: Cardiac Catheterization, Angiography, and Intervention, 6th edition. Philadelphia, Lippincott Williams & Wilkins, 2000

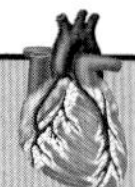

BOX 12–3 *Identification of the High-Risk Patient for Catheterization*

- Age
  - Infant <1 year
  - Elderly >70 years
- Functional class
  - Mortality ↑ 10-fold for class IV patients compared with I and II
- Severity of coronary obstruction
  - Mortality ↑ 10-fold for left main disease compared with one- or two-vessel disease
- Valvular heart disease
  - As an independent lesion
  - Greater risk when associated with coronary artery disease
- Left ventricular dysfunction
  - Mortality ↑ 10-fold in patients with low ejection fraction (≤30%)
- Severe noncardiac disease
- Renal insufficiency
- Insulin-requiring diabetes
- Advanced peripheral and cerebral vascular disease
- Severe pulmonary insufficiency

Modified from Baim DS, Grossman W: Cardiac Catheterization, Angiography, and Intervention, 6th edition. Philadelphia, Lippincott Williams & Wilkins, 2000
From Mahrer PR, Young C, Magnusson PT: Efficacy and safety of outpatient cardiac catheterization. Cathet Cardiovasc Diagn 13:304, 1987, with permission.

With the increased emphasis on outpatient procedures in medicine today, outpatient diagnostic catheterization is the standard of care for stable patients. Outpatient catheterization reduces costs, is preferred by patients, and is associated with similar outcomes.[17,38] Unstable and postinfarction patients are already hospitalized, and catheterization is usually performed before discharge. Planned PCI usually requires admission. Even when outpatient catheterization is planned, assessment of the patient following catheterization is required. Some patients, particularly those with left main disease, critical aortic stenosis, uncontrolled hypertension, significant LV dysfunction with CHF, or significant postprocedural complications such as a large groin hematoma will require admission.[17]

In addition to the high-risk cardiac patient, patients with renal insufficiency may require overnight hydration before and after catheterization. For patients on chronic anticoagulation with Coumadin, the patient requires measurement of the coagulation status and may require heparinization before and/or after the procedure. Day-of-procedure ambulation and discharge are planned for patients undergoing outpatient catheterization. Radial catheterization may expedite this discharge.[39] For patients undergoing catheterization via the percutaneous femoral approach, the cardiologist may utilize closure devices or a smaller catheter size (4 Fr) for the arterial puncture.[40] Protocols for early ambulation may permit the patient to be out of bed in 2 to 4 hours following hemostasis.[41]

CARDIAC CATHETERIZATION PROCEDURE

Whether the procedure is elective or emergent, diagnostic or interventional, coronary or peripheral, certain basic components are relatively constant in all circumstances. Variations are dependent upon the specific situation and are discussed separately in this chapter.

Patient Preparation

All patients receive a thorough explanation of the procedure, often including pamphlets and videotapes. A full explanation of technique and potential risks minimizes patient anxiety, and is similar to the preoperative anesthesia visit. It is important for the cardiologist to meet the patient before the study. This relaxes the patient while allowing the physician to be better acquainted with the patient, aiding in the decision process. Although some laboratories do allow the patient to have a clear liquid breakfast up to 2 to 3 hours prior to the procedure, outpatients are routinely asked to have no oral intake for 8 hours before the procedure, except for oral medications.

Patients with previous allergic reactions to iodinated contrast agents require adequate prophylaxis.[42] Greenberger et al[43] studied 857 patients with a prior history of an allergic reaction to contrast media. In this study, 50 mg of prednisone was administered 13, 7, and 1 hour before the procedure. Diphenhydramine, 50 mg IM, was also administered 1 hour before the procedure. Although no severe anaphylactic reactions occurred, the overall incidence of urticarial reactions in known high-risk patients was 10%. The use of nonionic contrast agents may further decrease reactions in patients with known contrast allergies.[44] The administration of H_2 blockers (cimetidine, 300 mg) is less well studied.[44] For patients undergoing emergent cardiac catheterization with known contrast allergies, 200 mg of hydrocortisone is administered intravenously immediately and repeated every 4 hours until the procedure is completed. Diphenhydramine (50 mg IV) is recommended 1 hour before the procedure.[45]

Contrast-induced nephropathy (CIN) is defined as an increase in serum Cr of more than 0.5 mg/dL or 25% above baseline level within 48 hours.[46] Although infrequent, occurring in less than 5% of PCIs, when it does occur, its impact on patient morbidity and mortality is significant.[47] Total contrast doses less than 4 mL/kg are recommended in patients with normal renal function, and lower doses are recommended for those with preexisting renal dysfunction (Cr > 2.0), particularly in diabetics (Cr > 1.5).[46] A study in more than 8000 PCI patients identified eight risk factors for CIN, and these included: hypotension, intra-aortic balloon pump, congestive heart failure, chronic kidney disease, diabetes, age greater than 75, anemia, and contrast volume.[48] It is therefore essential that the patient at high risk be identified and properly treated. Additionally, renal function should be monitored for at least 48 hours in patients at high risk for CIN, particularly if surgery or other interventions are planned.

Several methods have been employed to decrease renal toxicity from contrast agents. The two most important measures are minimizing contrast dose and adequate hydration with 0.9% saline at a rate of 1 mL/kg/hr for 12 hours before and after the procedure, if tolerated.[46] Low osmolar contrast agents are recommended.[49,50] Pre/post treatment with *N*-acetyl cysteine (Mucomyst) has had mixed results. Fenoldopam, a dopamine agonist, has been studied without benefit.[51] Ultrafiltration dialysis and sodium bicarbonate infusion have been beneficial in small studies.[46]

Patient Monitoring/Sedation

Standard limb leads with one chest lead are used for ECG monitoring during cardiac catheterization. One inferior and one anterior ECG lead are monitored during diagnostic catheterization. During an interventional procedure, two ECG leads are monitored in the same coronary artery distribution as the vessel undergoing PTCA. Radiolucent ECG leads improve monitoring without interfering with angiographic data.

Cardiac catheterization laboratories routinely monitor arterial oxygen saturation by pulse oximetry ($Sp{O_2}$) on all patients. Utilizing pulse oximetry, Dodson et al demonstrated that 38% of 26 patients undergoing catheterization had episodes of hypoxemia ($Sp{O_2} < 90\%$) with a mean duration of 53 seconds.[52] Variable amounts of premedication were administered to the patients.

Sedation in the catheterization laboratory, either from preprocedure administration or subsequent intravenous administration during the procedure, may lead to hypoventilation and hypoxemia. The administration of midazolam, 1 to 5 mg IV, with fentanyl, 25 to 100 μg, is common practice. Institutional guidelines for conscious sedation typically govern these practices. Light to moderate sedation is beneficial to the patient, particularly for angiographic imaging and interventional procedures. Deep sedation, in addition to its widely recognized potential to cause respiratory problems, poses distinct problems in the catheterization laboratory. Deep sedation often requires supplemental oxygen, and this complicates the interpretation of oximetry data and may alter hemodynamics. Furthermore, deep sedation may exacerbate respiratory variation altering hemodynamic measurements.

Sparse data exist regarding the effect of sedation on hemodynamic variables and respiratory parameters in the cardiac catheterization laboratory. One study examined the cardiorespiratory effects of diazepam sedation and flumazenil reversal of sedation in patients in the cardiac catheterization laboratory.[53] A sleep-inducing dose of diazepam was administered intravenously in the catheterization laboratory; this produced only slight decreases in mean arterial pressure (MAP), PCWP, and LV end-diastolic pressure (LVEDP), with no significant changes in intermittently sampled arterial blood gases. Flumazenil awakened the patient without significant alterations in either hemodynamic or respiratory variables.

More complex interventions have resulted in longer procedures. Although hospitals require conscious sedation policies, individual variation in the type and degree of sedation is common. While general anesthesia is rarely required for adult patients, it is needed more frequently for pediatric procedures. In the future, more complex adult interventions may well require the presence of an anesthesiologist in the catheterization laboratory, similar to the early days of adult coronary intervention.

Left-Sided Heart Catheterization

Catheterization Site and Anticoagulation

Left-sided heart catheterization has traditionally been performed by either the brachial or femoral artery approach. In the 1950s, the brachial approach was first introduced utilizing a cutdown with brachial arteriotomy. The brachial arteriotomy is often time consuming, can seldom be performed more than three times in the same patient, and has higher complication rates. This led operators to adopt the femoral approach. Introduced more than 15 years ago, the percutaneous radial artery approach is an alternative increasingly used.[39,54] The percutaneous radial approach is also more time consuming than the femoral approach but may have fewer complications.[39] This approach may be preferred in patients with significant peripheral vascular disease or recent (less than 6 months) femoral/abdominal aortic surgeries, or significant hypertension, on oral anticoagulants with PT greater than 1.8, or are morbidly obese. With increasing utilization of the radial artery as a conduit for CABG, care must be taken if this vessel has been used for radial access during catheterization.[55]

It is beyond the scope of this chapter to provide a detailed description of the brachial arteriotomy. The percutaneous radial approach is similar to a radial artery catheter access. The Allen's test, though not performed by all, is considered as part of the precatheterization evaluation. Standard access kits with needles, wires and sheaths are available to further simplify this approach. Once the sheath is in place, intravenous calcium channel blocker therapy is given to prevent spasm. Although standard catheters may be used from the radial/brachial approach, specific catheters are also available.

The percutaneous femoral artery approach is performed using catheters that allow for operator ease and speed of performance. The landmarks for the percutaneous femoral approach are illustrated in Figure 12–2. The percutaneous approach uses the Seldinger technique or modifications thereof with a Cook needle, which does not have an internal trochanter. Once the wire is successfully inserted into the vessel, standard sheaths (5 to 8 Fr) are placed in the femoral artery. Through these sheaths, separate coronary artery catheters are inserted to perform left and then right coronary cineangiography, and left ventriculography is performed using a pigtail catheter. These standard catheters and a sheath are illustrated in Figure 12–3.

In patients with synthetic grafts in the femoral area, arterial access is possible after the grafts are a few months old, and complication rates are similar to those seen with native vessels. An additional problem can be encountered with aortofemoral grafts. If the native iliac system or distal aorta is occluded, it can be a challenge to advance the catheters through the bypass conduit.

At the completion of the catheterization from the femoral approach, the patient is returned to the pre/post procedural area for sheath removal. If a right-heart catheterization is performed, arterial and venous sheaths should be removed separately to avoid the formation of an atrioventricular (AV) fistula.[56,57] Pressure is applied manually or by a compression device. The duration of bed rest depends upon the size of the sheath.[58] Closure devices have been developed to provide for more rapid hemostasis following the procedure, allowing for earlier ambulation and discharge. However, complication rates have not decreased with these devices.[40] Closure devices include collagen plugs placed within the artery that require avoidance of the site for repeat puncture for 3 months, exter-

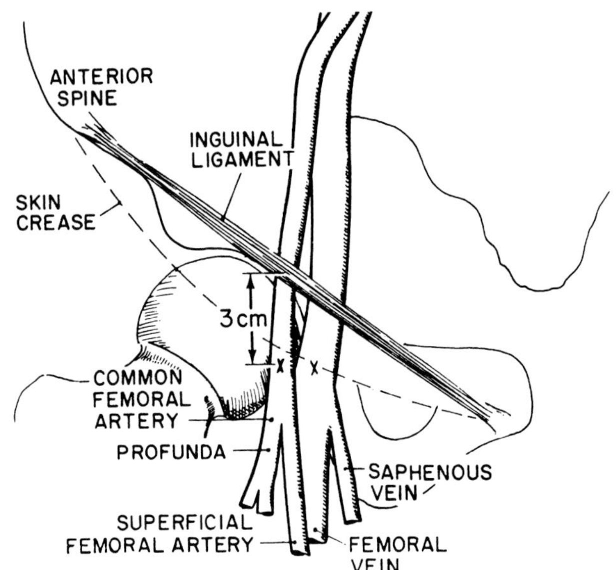

Figure 12–2 Relevant anatomy for percutaneous catheterization of femoral artery and vein. The right femoral artery and vein run underneath the inguinal ligament, which connects the anterior-superior iliac spine and pubic tubercle. The arterial puncture (indicated by X) should be made approximately 1.5 to 2 finger breadths (3 cm) below the inguinal ligament and directly over the femoral artery pulsation. The venous puncture should be made at the same level, but approximately 1 finger breadth medial. (From Baim DS, Grossman W: Percutaneous approach. *In* Grossman W [ed]: Cardiac Catheterization and Angiography, 3rd edition. Philadelphia, Lea & Febiger, 1986, p 60.)

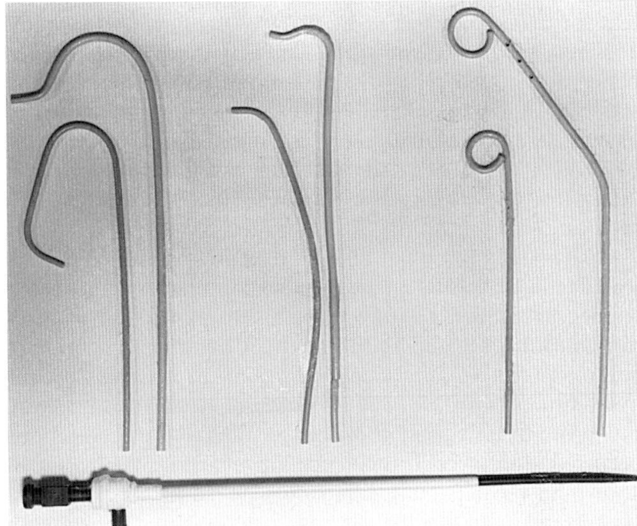

Figure 12–3 Femoral arterial catheters and sheath. (*Left*) Standard left coronary artery catheters. (*Middle*) Standard right coronary artery catheters. (*Right*) Standard ventricular pigtail catheters. (*Bottom*) Femoral artery sheath.

nal arterial/subcutaneous plugs that do not hinder repeat access, topical patches that elute coagulants to the puncture site, and suture devices that perform percutaneous arteriotomy closure. For radial closure,[57] wristbands are available to hold compression until hemostasis is achieved.

Once hemostasis has been achieved, pulse and bleeding checks should be performed on a regular basis. Sandbag placement is seldom used. In most instances, for outpatient diagnostic studies, patients are ambulatory and ready to be discharged 2 to 4 hours postprocedure.[41,58]

Theoretically, anticoagulation is necessary to prevent thrombus on catheters placed into the arterial system. Systemic heparinization with 5000 units had been the standard of care since left-sided heart catheterization was begun.[59] Heparinization during brachial and/or radial catheterization includes a bolus of about 60 units/kg. For the femoral approach, dosing regimens have employed 40 units/kg. When various doses of heparin were compared, a doubling of the PTT was achieved with a dose of 3000 units, with no embolic events reported.[59] That being stated, routine anticoagulation for diagnostic procedures from the femoral approach is often omitted due to the limited arterial access times, unproved need for anticoagulation, and risks of reversing anticoagulation and/or potential delay in sheath removal.

Contrast Agents

Adverse reactions have been the major disadvantage of the ionic contrast agents since their introduction for urinary tract visualization in 1923.[42] The two major classifications of contrast agents used today for cardiovascular imaging are based on their ability to either dissociate into ionic particles in solution (ionic media) or not dissociate (nonionic). The ionic agents were the first group developed, with sodium diatrizoate and iothalamate anions as the iodine carriers. Commercially available agents using meglumine and sodium salts of diatrizoic acid include Renografin, Hypaque, and Angiovist. In 1975, Shehadi reported on a prospective survey of 30 university hospitals in the United States, Canada, Europe, and Australia, involving 112,003 patients, using ionic contrast for cardiovascular diagnosis.[60] The overall rate of adverse reactions was 5.65%, with 0.02% having severe reactions and eight patients dying.

The next generation of contrast agents began to impact clinical practice in the 1980s. These agents, listed in Table 12–2, are predominantly monomeric, nonionic agents with the exception of the two dimers: ioxaglate (ionic) and iodixanol (nonionic). These agents, particularly the nonionic dimmer iodixnol, have lower osmolarity and, therefore, lower toxicity systemically and renally.[49]

Several areas must be discussed when comparing ionic and nonionic contrast agents. First, the ECG effects (transient heart block, QT and QRS prolongation), depression of LV contractility, and systemic hypotension from peripheral vasodilation are more pronounced with the ionic agents, but only marginally statistically different from that of the nonionic compounds.[61] The hemodynamic effects of the nonionic dimer, iodixanol, were compared with the nonionic monomer, iohexol in 48 patients. While both agents caused an increase in LV diastolic pressure (LVEDP), this was significantly less in the iodixanol group.[62] Additionally, the iodine content may vary among agents, resulting in variations in opacification. Also, for patients who have had previous anaphylactoid reactions to iodinated contrast, nonionic contrast decreases the incidence of an anaphylactoid reaction with repeat contrast exposure.[36,42,63] Finally, the nonionic agents and dimers are more expensive than the ionic agents. When first introduced, this difference was large and slowed the adoption of the newer agents. Current price differences are less dramatic, and nonionic agents are used in most laboratories.[36]

Both ionic and nonionic agents have anticoagulant and antiplatelet effects, these being pronounced with ionic agents. A comparison of the nonionic agents iohexol (monomer) and iodixanol with the ionic dimer, ioxaglate, demonstrated a clear distinction with the in vivo antiplatelet effect of the ionic agent, ioxaglate, 65% greater than the nonionic agent.[64] Regardless of the agent used, these differences are unlikely to be important for diagnostic procedures. Although minute thrombi may form when blood and nonionic contrast remain in a syringe, clinical sequelae have not been noted.[65]

Some data suggest that the nonionic contrast agents are less likely to cause contrast-induced nephropathy than the ionic agents, and that the iso-osmolar agent iodixanol (Visipaque) may be the least likely. Patients with impaired renal function, particularly if diabetic, would be most likely to benefit from the use of this agent.[50] The effects of contrast agents on the kidneys are more pronounced when large volumes are delivered near the renal vessels. Thus, arteriography of the renal

Table 12–2 Contrast Agents (Nonionic and/or Dimeric)

Product	Type of Contrast Agent	Concentration (mg/mL)	Osmolality (mOsm/kg water)
Monomers			
Iohexol (Omnipaque)	Nonionic LOCM	350	844
Iopamidol (Isovue)	Nonionic LOCM	370	796
Ioxilan (Oxilan)	Nonionic LOCM	350	695
Iopromide (Ultravist)	Nonionic LOCM	370	774
Ioversol (Optiray)	Nonionic LOCM	350	792
Dimers			
Iodixanol (Visipaque)	Nonionic IOCM	320	290
Ioxaglate (Hexabrix)	Ionic LOCM	320	600

Ultravist is a registered trademark of Berlex Laboratories.
Isovue is a registered trademark of Bracco Diagnostics.
Omnipaque and Visipaque are registered trademarks of Nycomed Inc.
Optiray is a registered trademark of Mallinckrodt Medical, Inc.
Hexabrix is a registered trademark of Guerbet, S.A.
LOCM = low osmolality contrast media; IOCM = isomolar contrast media.

arteries or abdominal aorta would be the procedures in which the choice of contrast is most important. In fact, abdominal arteriography can be done with digital subtraction techniques and the intra-arterial injection of gaseous carbon dioxide, thus avoiding the use of any iodinated contrast.

Two large, multicenter trials have compared ionic and nonionic agents in patients undergoing cardiovascular diagnostic imaging.[66,67] One performed in 109,546 patients in Australia and another, in 337,647 patients in Japan, revealed severe adverse reactions in the ionic group of 0.9 and 0.25%, respectively, whereas severe adverse reactions occurred in the nonionic group at rates of 0.02% and 0.04%, respectively. For the patient undergoing intervention, the COURT trial compared the nonionic dimer iodixanol to the ionic dimer ioxaglate in 856 PCI patients at high risk and noted a 45% reduction in major adverse cardiac events in the iodixanol group.[44] The VIP trial compared the same agents in 1411 PCI patients but failed to show a difference in cardiac events, although fewer allergic reactions were seen in the iodixanol group.[63]

Table 12–3 Indications for Diagnostic Right-Heart Catheterization During Left-Heart Catheterization

Significant valvular pathology
Suspected intracardiac shunting
Acute infarct—differentiation of free wall versus septal rupture
Evaluation of right- and/or left-heart failure
Evaluation of pulmonary hypertension
Severe pulmonary disease
Evaluation of pericardial disease
Constrictive pericarditis
Restrictive cardiomyopathy
Pericardial effusion
Pretransplant assessment of pulmonary vascular resistance and response to vasodilators

Right-Sided Heart Catheterization

Indications

The Cournand catheter was initially used to measure right-sided heart pressures, but required fluoroscopic guidance for placement. The Cournand catheter permitted the measurement of cardiac output by the Fick method. Clinical applications of right-sided heart hemodynamic monitoring changed greatly in 1970 with the flow-directed, balloon-tipped, pulmonary artery catheter (PAC) developed by Swan and Ganz. This balloon flotation catheter allowed the clinician to measure pulmonary artery (PA) and wedge pressures without fluoroscopic guidance. It also incorporated a thermistor, making the repeated measurement of cardiac output feasible. With this development, the PAC left the cardiac catheterization laboratory and entered both the operating room and intensive care unit.[68]

In the cardiac catheterization laboratory, right-sided heart catheterization is performed for diagnostic purposes. The routine use of right-sided heart catheterization during standard left-sided heart catheterization was studied by Hill et al.[69] Two hundred patients referred for only left-sided heart catheterization for suspected CAD underwent right-sided heart catheterization. This resulted in an additional 6 minutes of procedure time and 90 seconds of fluoroscopy. Abnormalities were detected in 35% of the patients. However, management was altered in only 1.5% of the patients. With this in mind, routine right-sided heart catheterization cannot be recommended. Table 12–3 outlines acceptable indications for right-sided heart catheterization during left-sided heart catheterization.

Using the thermodilution technique, cardiac output (CO) measurements during right-sided heart catheterization allow for a further assessment of ventricular function.[70] This is obviously helpful in the setting of an AMI to delineate high-risk groups and to measure the effect of cardiac medications.[71,72] Finally, measurement of CO can differentiate high-output failure states (hyperthyroidism, Paget's disease, beriberi, anemia, AV malformations, or AV fistulas) from those secondary to a low CO. In patients with congenital heart disease, right-sided heart catheterization allows for measurement of oxygen saturation in various cardiac chambers and calculation of intracardiac shunting. In patients with ASDs, the right-sided heart catheter passes through the defect into the left atrium (LA), allowing for complete saturation and pressure measurements. The thermodilution technique cannot be used to measure CO in the setting of intracardiac shunting; in such cases, the Fick method must be used. With significant tricuspid regurgitation or very low cardiac outputs, the Fick method provides a more accurate measurement of CO and is preferred.

Procedure

The brachial, femoral, and internal jugular venous approaches are most commonly used for right-sided heart catheterization in the catheterization laboratory.

The brachial approach for right-sided heart catheterization may be done percutaneously or via venotomy. The pitfalls in the brachial approach include identifying the proper vein for insertion. The basilic and brachial veins are preferable, whereas the cephalic vein on the radial aspect of the arm is tortuous in the axilla and should be avoided for catheter insertion. When the left brachial (or left internal jugular) approach is considered, the operator must be aware of the possibility of an anomalous left-sided superior vena cava (SVC). This empties into the coronary sinus, hindering catheter passage into the right ventricle (RV). Whenever the peripheral arm veins are entered, the catheter or sheath must be moist and inserted quickly to decrease venous spasm.

The femoral approach for PAC insertion is performed under fluoroscopic guidance using one of two approaches: the catheter can be advanced against the lateral wall of the atrium creating a loop in the RA, and the balloon is then inflated and advanced across the tricuspid and pulmonic valves to the PCWP position; or the catheter is passed from the RA into the RV; with clockwise rotation and balloon inflation, the catheter enters the pulmonary outflow tract and is advanced into the PA and PCWP positions.

Although it is common to obtain an oxygen saturation from the PA during right-sided heart catheterization, a complete oxygen saturation assessment is required in patients with suspected left-to-right shunts. In the adult population, an ASD or postinfarction ventricular septal defect (VSD) is the most common left-to-right shunts requiring identification. In these patients, 0.5 to 1.0 mL of blood is obtained in the following locations: high and low SVC; high and low inferior vena cava (IVC); high, mid, and low RA; RV apex and outflow tract; and main PA (rarely, right and left PA). These saturations are obtained upon entry with the PAC, with repeat sampling during pullback if the data are ambiguous. These samples must be obtained in close temporal proximity to avoid systemic factors affecting oxygen saturation (e.g., hypoventilation). A step up or step down in saturation identifies the level at which the shunt is occurring.

Pulmonic and systemic flow is calculated as modifications of the Fick equation for CO determination.[73] It is very important that measurements be made during steady state. The Q_p/Q_s ratio is calculated for patients with left-to-right shunting by the following equation:

$$Q_p/Q_s = (SAO_2 - MVO_2)/(PVO_2 - PAO_2)$$

where Q_p is pulmonary flow, Q_s is systemic flow, PVO_2 is pulmonary venous oxygen saturation,* SAO_2 is systemic arterial oxygen saturation, PAO_2 is PA oxygen saturation, and MVO_2 is mixed venous oxygen saturation.

In the presence of an RA step-up, an estimated resting MVO_2 sample is obtained by the following weighted average:

$$[3 \times (\text{SVC saturation}) + 1 \times (\text{IVC saturation})]/4$$

Saturation values are measured in high and low regions of both the SVC and IVC and are normally the same. If anomalous pulmonary venous drainage is present, regional differences in saturation in either the SVC or IVC may occur. Calculation of the Q_p/Q_s ratio does not require the measurement of oxygen consumption and can be calculated with any stable level of oxygen supplementation. Calculation of the absolute values of pulmonary and systemic flow does require this measurement, and it can be complicated to measure if supplemental oxygen is required.

Correction of the defect is required when the Q_p/Q_s ratio is greater than 2 and is unnecessary when the Q_p/Q_s ratio is less than 1.5. Ratios of 1.5 to 2.0 require additional confirmatory evidence and clinical assessment before a decision to intervene can be made.

The following example demonstrates a sample calculation of left-to-right shunting in a patient with an ASD:

Oxygen saturations: IVC = 68%; SVC = 60%; mid-RA = 77%; mid-RV = 77%; PAO_2 = 77%; and SAO_2 = 92%

$$Q_p/Q_s = 92 - 6292 - 77 = 30/15 = 2/1\text{: } Q_p/Q_s = 2/1$$

Significant bidirectional and/or right-to-left shunting are unusual in adult patients. These occur in the setting of congenital heart disease after the development of pulmonary artery disease. As more children with corrected or partially corrected congenital heart disease reach adulthood, the likelihood of encountering an adult with a complicated shunt will increase. These encounters may be further complicated by the development of adult cardiology problems, mainly CAD (see Chapter 22).

Calculation of bidirectional shunting involves determination of the effective blood flow. Effective blood flow (Q_{eff}) represents the flow if no right-to-left or left-to-right shunting exists.[74] With Q_{eff}, right-to-left shunting is equal to $Q_s - Q_{eff}$, and left-to-right shunting is equal to $Q_p - Q_{eff}$, using the following formulas derived from the Fick equation for cardiac output:

$$Q_s\ (\text{L/min}) = O_2 \text{ consumption (mL/min)}/SAO_2\ (\text{mL/L}) - MVO_2\ (\text{mL/L})$$

$$Q_p\ (\text{L/min}) = O_2 \text{ consumption (mL/min)}/PVO_2\ (\text{mL/L}) - PAO_2\ (\text{mL/L})$$

$$Q_{eff}\ (\text{L/min}) = O_2 \text{ consumption (mL/min)}/PVO_2\ (\text{mL/L}) - MVO_2\ (\text{mL/L})$$

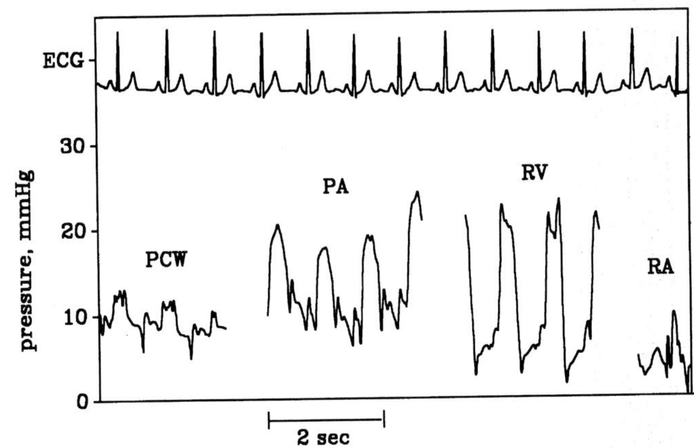

Figure 12–4 A pullback tracing obtained using a pulmonary artery catheter (PAC) from the pulmonary capillary wedge (PCW) position, to the pulmonary artery (PA), right ventricle (RV), and right atrium (RA).

Right-sided heart pressure obviously may be obtained either on entry or on pullback (Fig. 12–4). Catheter placement using the femoral approach may be time-consuming, with expedited passage necessary to prevent catheter softening. Therefore, pressure measurements are often obtained during catheter pullback to assure temporal proximity. As with all invasive procedures, complications can occur with right-heart catheterization, requiring that risks and benefits be assessed prior to undertaking this and any procedure[75] (see Chapter 14).

Diagnostic Catheterization Complications

Although adult diagnostic catheterization with coronary cineangiography had been performed from the late 1950s, complication rates were not followed until 1979 when the Society for Cardiac Angiography and Interventions established the first registry to prospectively monitor the performance of participating laboratories. In 1982 the first publication from this registry reported complication rates from a study population of more than 50,000 patients.[76] This was updated in 1989 with a report on 222,553 patients who underwent selective coronary arteriography between 1984 and 1987.[77] When compared with the earlier report, similar complication rates were noted. Complications are related to multiple factors, but severity of disease is important. Mortality rates are shown in Table 12–4. Complications are specific for both right- and left-heart catheterization (Table 12–5). The registry reported incidences of major complications as follows: death 0.1%, MI 0.06%, cerebrovascular accident (CVA) 0.07%, arrhythmia 0.47%, contrast reaction 0.23%, and vascular complications 0.46%.[77] Although advances in

*The SaO_2 value is usually used for this value.

Table 12–4 Cardiac Catheterization Mortality Data

Patient Characteristics*	Mortality Rate (%)
Overall mortality from cardiac catheterization	0.14
Age-related mortality	
<1 yr	1.75
>60 yr	0.25
Coronary artery disease	
One-vessel disease	0.03
Three-vessel disease	0.16
Left main disease	0.86
Congestive heart failure	
NYHA functional class I or II	0.02
NYHA functional class III	0.12
NYHA functional class IV	0.67
Valvular heart disease	
All valvular disease patients	0.28
Mitral valve disease	0.34
Aortic valve disease	0.19

*Other reported high-risk characteristics: unstable angina, acute myocardial infarction, renal insufficiency, ventricular arrhythmias, cyanotic congenital heart disease (including arterial desaturation and pulmonary hypertension). Detailed data from large-scale studies on these characteristics are unavailable.

From Pepine CJ, Allen HD, Bashore TM, et al: ACC/AHA guidelines for cardiac catheterization and cardiac catheterization laboratories. J Am Coll Cardiol 18:1149, 1991.

Table 12–5 Complications from Diagnostic Catheterization

Left Heart
CARDIAC
Death
Myocardial infarction
Ventricular fibrillation
Ventricular tachycardia
Cardiac perforation
NONCARDIAC
Stroke
Peripheral embolization
Air
Thrombus
Cholesterol
Vascular surgical repair
Pseudoaneurysm
AV fistula
Embolectomy
Repair of brachial arteriotomy
Evacuation of hematomas
Contrast related
Renal insufficiency
Anaphylaxis
Right Heart
CARDIAC
Conduction abnormality
RBBB
Complete heart block (RBBB superimposed on LBBB)
Arrhythmias
Valvular damage
Perforation
NONCARDIAC
Pulmonary artery rupture
Pulmonary infarction
Balloon rupture
Paradoxical (systemic) air embolus

AV = arteriovenous; RBBB = right bundle-branch block; LBBB = left bundle-branch block.

technology continue, these complication rates are still present today, most likely due to the higher risk patient undergoing catheterization.[75,76]

Vascular complications from the percutaneous femoral approach occur in less than 1% of cases, with the most common being pseudoaneurysms.[78] This risk is higher for the obese patient in whom compression is more difficult. Therapy includes either ultrasound-directed thrombin injection or surgical repair. In patients with aortic regurgitation (AR), an increased incidence of femoral arteriovenous fistulas is seen due to the widened pulse pressure.[56] Many small arteriovenous fistulas will close spontaneously. If large or if the fistula is associated with high output (rare) or edema of the affected leg, surgical correction is indicated. Thrombosis of the femoral artery occurs rarely, and underlying atherosclerotic disease is usually severe. Emergent restoration of flow is essential with a surgical approach used at some hospitals and a percutaneous one at others.

Arrhythmic complications during left-sided heart catheterization are more frequent with ionic contrast than with nonionic contrast, and they occur during coronary injection. Surprisingly, the presence of the catheter in the LV rarely causes a sustained arrhythmia. Early contrast media containing potassium produced ventricular fibrillation during coronary arteriography. However, currently, contrast materials are potassium-free, and with the addition of calcium, result in an incidence of significant ventricular arrhythmias of 0.47%.[77]

Anaphylactoid reactions occur in approximately 5% to 8% of cases when nonionic contrast is used. The definition of reaction severity as well as the differential diagnosis for severe reactions is listed in Table 12–6. If a severe anaphylactoid reaction to contrast media occurs with hypotension, refractory to rapid fluid resuscitation, and/or significant bronchospasm, immediate therapy with intravenous epinephrine, 0.1 mL of 1:10,000 solution of epinephrine (10 μg) every minute, is recommended. Subcutaneous doses, 0.3 mL of 1:1000 solution, can be administered for moderate reactions, whereas diphenhydramine is effective for mild reactions.[42]

Cholesterol embolization can occur after catheter manipulation, and has been described following cardiac catheterization.[79,80] Although the femoral approach can be used in patients with unrepaired abdominal aortic aneurysms, an increased incidence of cholesterol emboli syndrome may occur in this population.[81] Cholesterol embolization produces small vessel arterial occlusion by cholesterol crystals, resulting in a serious clinical presentation including livedo reticularis, acrocyanosis of the lower extremities, renal insufficiency, and accelerated hypertension. The clinical course is variable, does not respond to anticoagulation, and has the potential for an insidious development of progressive renal failure, accelerating hypertension, and a fatal outcome.

HEMODYNAMICS

The heart functions by converting chemical or metabolic energy into mechanical energy. The mechanical energy of the heart manifests as the development of force, or pressure, and

Table 12–6 Contrast-Induced Anaphylactoid Reactions

Severity Classification		
Minor	Moderate	Severe
Urticaria (limited)	Urticaria (diffuse)	Cardiovascular shock
Pruritus	Angioedema	Respiratory arrest
Erythema	Laryngeal edema	Cardiac arrest
	Bronchospasm	
Differential Diagnosis (Severe Reactions)		
Cardiac	Noncardiac	
Vasovagal reaction	Hypovolemia	
Cardiogenic shock	Dehydration	
Right ventricular infarction	Blood loss—gastrointestinal, vascular, external	
Cardiac tamponade	Drug related	
Cardiac rupture	Narcotic, benzodiazepine, protamine	
Bezold-Jarich reflex	Sepsis	

Adapted from Goss J, Chambers C, Heupler F, et al: Systemic anaphylactoid reactions to iodinated contrast media during cardiac catheterization procedures. Cathet Cardiovasc Diagn 34:99, 1995.

the acceleration of blood into the circulation. Myocardial work is equivalent to the product of developed pressure and the resulting blood flow; therefore, pressure and flow are important variables to be measured in the cardiac catheterization laboratory.

Pressure Measurements

Today, the usual system required to measure pressure includes a fluid-filled catheter inserted into a heart chamber or blood vessel, a coupler between the catheter and the transducer, the transducer itself, an electrical link between the transducer and output device, and an output device (typically a digital monitor and recorder). Pressure waves are measured by transduction of force per unit area into an electrical voltage, which can easily be measured and displayed as a function of time (see Chapter 14).

Harmonic Analysis of Waveforms

For a physical phenomenon displaying a cyclic repetition with time (periodicity), a means of reducing complex occurrences to their fundamental components was developed by the French mathematician and physicist Fourier. Since pressure waves in the circulation meet the criterion of being complex periodic waveforms, this type of analysis can be applied.[82] A complex wave can be separated into a series of oscillations in which each oscillation has a frequency that is an integral multiple of the same basic frequency (Fig. 12–5). The basic, or fundamental, frequency in this type of analysis is equivalent to the heart rate (HR), such that a HR of 60 beats/min (bpm), for example, would result in a fundamental frequency of 1 beat/sec, or 1 Hz. From this, an infinite number of sine and cosine functions with increasing harmonic frequencies can be added to reproduce the original pressure waveform, each adding a degree of detail. It is thought that up to the tenth

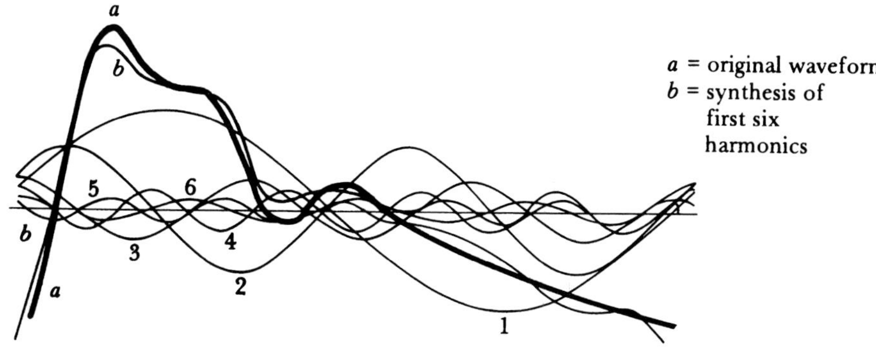

Harmonic	Amplitude (%)
1	100
2	63.2
3	29.6
4	22.2
5	14.8
6	11.8

Figure 12–5 Arterial pressure waveform *(a)*, shown with the first six harmonics (1 to 6, harmonic no. 1 being the fundamental frequency). Note that adding six harmonics *(b)* yields a close approximation of the original wave. (From Hansen AT: Pressure measurement in the human organism. Acta Physiol Scand 19:26, 1950.)

harmonic of the fundamental frequency is contained in pressure waveforms during rapid pressure changes (e.g., the dicrotic notch of the aortic pressure[74]) (see Chapter 14).

Transducer Performance

The degree of accuracy with which the transducer can convert mechanical into electrical energy is one of the main factors necessary for authentic reproduction of the pressure waveform. Transducer performance is judged in a formal manner by observing how accurately an input function is converted into an output with similar features. The output function for most transducers in clinical use is a voltage that can be displayed visually on a cathode ray screen or graphically by writing the wave on paper.

Static properties of a transducer are tested by quantifying the behavior of the transducer with inputs of incrementally varied magnitudes that do not change with time; for example, the particular voltage output of a transducer exposed to a constant pressure of 10 mm Hg from a mercury manometer should double when the pressure is increased to 20 mm Hg. The static response of a transducer should be a linear function. In most cases, the linearity of clinically used transducers is adequate.

Dynamic properties of a transducer are judged by testing its response to a sinusoidal input with constant amplitude, but varying frequency. The ideal response would be a transducer output that is not affected by an increasing input frequency. Most transducers in clinical use today are not ideal in this respect. The typical response of a transducer is to show a progressive degradation in output amplitude as the input frequency becomes greater than the resonant frequency of the transducer (Fig. 12–6).

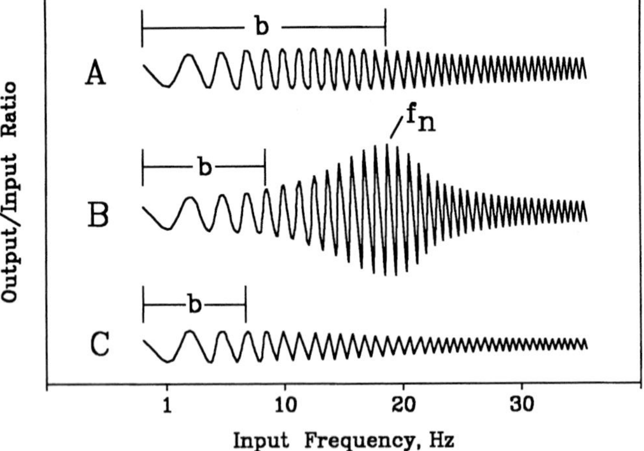

Figure 12–6 The frequency response of a transducer under three damping conditions. *Vertical axis* is the ratio of output/input signal, or amplitude. *Horizontal axis* is the input frequency in Hz. In this test system, the input magnitude is constant with increasing frequency. *(A)* Optimally damped transducer. Bandwidth (b) is "flat" (amplitude = 100 [5%]) to 19 Hz and the transducer does not display the exaggerated output near the natural frequency (f_n) of the transducer. Amplitude then decreases at frequencies greater than 20 Hz. *(B)* Underdamped transducer with an f_n of 19 Hz, indicated by the point of the maximal resonation of the transducer. Because the transducer is underdamped, the bandwidth is only about 10 Hz. This is similar to many fluid-coupled transducers in daily clinical use (see Fig. 12–2). Amplitude still drops off at input frequencies in the 20-Hz range. *(C)* Same transducer with an air bubble in system, causing significant overdamping. Bandwidth is now decreased to about 8 Hz. The amplitude drops off quickly, which indicates that f_n has also been decreased.

Ways in which the dynamic response of transducers is quantified are as follows:

Frequency-Response Curves

In this type of curve, either the transducer output or the output amplitude (output divided by input ratio) is plotted against the input frequency.

Natural (or Resonant) Frequency

All substances possess a natural frequency at which oscillations within a material or group of materials are of maximal intensity; transducers are no exception. Typically, this is in the 10- to 20-Hz range for clinical transducers. Remembering that the first 10 harmonics of the fundamental frequency (HR) are present in the pressure waveform, if the HR is 60 bpm or 1 Hz, a transducer needs to accurately reproduce the tenth harmonic with a frequency of 10 Hz in order to have an undistorted waveform. If the HR increases to 120 bpm, then the transducer's resonant frequency must be at least 20 Hz. Usually, as the input frequency approaches the natural frequency of the transducer, the output is exaggerated as the energy from the resonating transducer is added to the output amplitude (see Fig. 12–6).

Resonant frequency should be as high as possible, in order to cover the range required in clinical practice, in which HR may exceed 200 bpm. This will minimize the oscillatory contributions of the transducer itself, as well as preserving the contributions of the higher harmonic components of the pressure wave at faster heart rates.

Bandwidth

The bandwidth is defined as the useful dynamic range of input frequency in which the output closely approximates the input (output/input amplitude approaches unity). This is also described as the range of input frequency in which the output amplitude is accurate and constant, or "flat," within ±5% of the input amplitude (see Fig. 12–6).

Damping

Since most transducers resonate to some degree at frequencies in the clinical range, damping is the means by which the oscillatory energy of the transducer system is dissipated. Optimal damping maintains the frequency response flat to or past the transducer's natural frequency. An underdamped system that does not dissipate the oscillating energy will demonstrate an exaggerated output and cause an overestimation of the high and low values of a pressure wave. An overdamped system, such as that containing an air bubble, will interfere with accurate transducer response, and subsequent loss of authentic pressure displays. This is because in an overdamped system, the excessive damping also interferes with the frequency response of the transducer. This is displayed in Figures 12–7 and 12–8, in which both the natural frequency response and the LV waveform, respectively, were studied in the same transducer system under different conditions of damping.

Volume Displacement

The volume displacement of a transducer is also a measure of its elasticity. When a pressure is exerted on a transducer membrane, a small amount of displacement must take place in order for the pressure to be sensed and converted to electrical energy. The smaller the amount of volume required to be displaced to transduce the waveform, the more accurately the transducer will reproduce the pressure waveform. The volume displacement is described as:

$$\Delta\text{Pressure}/\Delta\text{Volume}$$

Transducer volume displacement is a function of the stiffness of the transducer membrane. Major advances in reproducing pressure waveforms have been made as the membrane stiffness has been improved in recent years (Table 12–7).

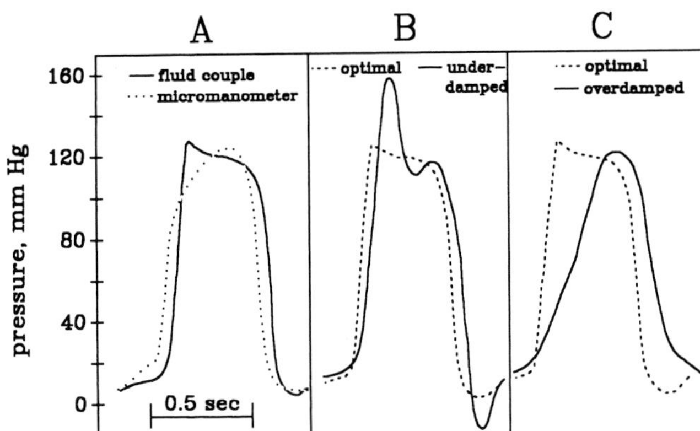

Figure 12–7 Series of ventricular pressure waves demonstrating the effects of damping and fluid coupling on a transducer connected to an 18-gauge needle in the left ventricle by 60 cm of rigid tubing filled with water. *(A)* Optimally damped fluid-coupled system (—) compared with micromanometer output (----). Inertia from fluid couple leads to a 10-msec lag in upstroke and a small systolic overshoot. *(B)* The same transducer system, underdamped (—). Oscillations of the transducer and inertial forces in the fluid couple are not properly damped, leading to a more significant overshoot and undershoot when compared with the optimally damped fluid-system (----). *(C)* The transducer system is overdamped (—), leading to loss of high-frequency contributions to the wave that are maintained with optimal damping (----).

Fluid Coupling

The most accurate transducer systems are the catheter-tipped transducers that place the transducing membrane directly in the blood stream. Due to the great expense of these catheters, it is much more common to have the transducer membrane coupled to the blood stream by a fluid column. As seen in Figure 12–7, the fluid-filled coupling introduces some char-

Table 12–7 History of Pressure Monitoring

Date	Description
1733	Stephen Hales measures height of blood in a tube inserted into the artery of a horse.
1828	Poiseuille introduces mercury U-tube for pressure measurement.
1881	Marey devises an air-filled tube with a rubber membrane on the distal end inserted into the heart chambers and a tambour controlling a writing lever on the proximal end.
1888	Hürthle replaces air with less compressible water as a coupling medium.
1903	Frank replaces the writing arm with a low-weight mirror, and increases the high-amplitude capability.
1924	Wiggers uses stiffer membranes to increase the natural frequency.
1934	Hamilton uses brass membranes to decrease transducer displacement characteristics.
1947	Lambert and Wood introduce electrical strain gauge, and increase accuracy and durability of transducers.
1973	Millar perfects catheter-tipped transducers by using unbonded semiconductor half bridges.

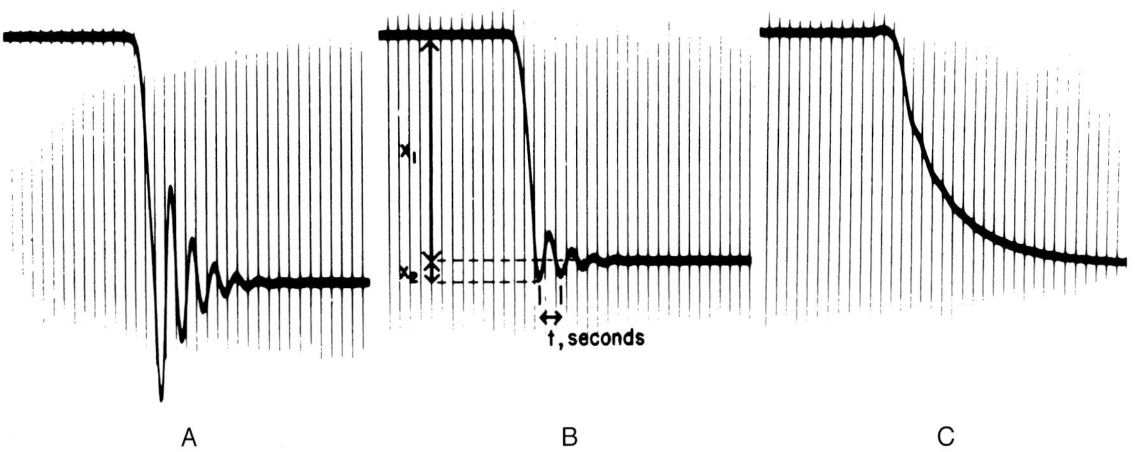

In example B, t = 40 msec, $N_D = 1/t$ = 25 cycles/second

$$D = \sqrt{\ln^2(x_2/x_1)/[\pi^2 + \ln^2(x_2/x_1)]} = .603$$

$$N = N_D/\sqrt{1-D^2} = 31.3 \text{ cycles/second}$$

Figure 12–8 Transducer output after a "shock" test (see text for explanation). The sudden withdrawal of pressure causes the transducer system to oscillate around zero pressure, which yields information about the natural frequency (N) and damping coefficient (D). Formulas for calculating N require a knowledge of the period of oscillation; the ratio of the amplitude of two successive oscillatory waves (x_2/x_1) is used to calculate D. *(A)* Underdamping leads to prolonged oscillations before the system settles (x_2x_1 is large, signifying a low D). *(B)* Optimal damping leads to minimum oscillations (low x_2x_1). *(C)* An overdamped system inaccurately produces a prolonged pressure decay to zero, which also reflects a lower natural frequency. *(A–C,* from Grossman W, Baim DS [eds]: Cardiac Catheterization, Angiography, and Intervention, 4th edition. Philadelphia, Lea & Febiger, 1991, p 131.)

acteristics that lead to inaccuracies in pressure measurement. The fluid in the tubing has inertia, which causes some distortion of the pressure waveform, especially apparent during rapid changes in the slope of the pressure wave, at the systolic peak and during early diastole. The fluid-filled systems tend to overestimate systolic pressure due to systolic overshoot, and underestimate diastolic pressure due to a similar diastolic undershoot. The fluid-filled system also adds an element of compressibility, which also tends to degrade the pressure signal by adding to the volume displacement of the transducer.

Some of the characteristics of the tubing can also impact on the pressure signal that results, such as its stiffness, length, and diameter. In summary, the impact of the components of the fluid couple can be summarized as follows:

$$f_n \text{ a } D\, L^{-}/2 \cdot (\Delta V/\Delta P)^{-}/2 \cdot \delta^{-}/2$$

where f_n is natural frequency of the entire catheter-couple-transducer system, D is tubing diameter, L is tubing length, $\Delta V/\Delta P$ is tubing compliance, and δ is density of coupling fluid.

The natural or resonant frequency of the transducer system can be maximized by using short, low-compliance tubing with as large a diameter as possible, that is filled with a low-density, noncompressible fluid, such as water, that will add little inertial energy to the system.

Measuring the Natural Frequency of the Entire Transducer-Couple System

To test the dynamic response for a catheter system, a shock wave should be applied to either end of the system (either at the tip of the catheter or at the dome of the transducer). This shock wave can be a sudden positive- or negative-pressure change. It is important to characterize catheter transducer systems, so that the clinician has some idea how much confidence to place in the resulting pressure waveforms. As the shock wave is applied to the system, this results in an oscillation of the transducer output, which then damps out. Demonstrated in Figure 12–8 is the formula by which the natural frequency and the damping coefficient of the catheter system can be calculated from the ratio of oscillation amplitudes and the period of oscillation.

Measurement Errors

Several potential errors and artifacts exist in intravascular pressure measurement. One of the most common is a low transducer frequency response. Any condition that decreases the natural frequency will result in a pressure waveform that misses many of the high-frequency waves in the original input wave. Therefore, for example, the dicrotic notch of an aortic pressure trace may be either slurred or lost altogether (see Figs. 12–5 and 12–7). Systolic pressures will tend to be underestimated, and diastolic pressures will tend to be overestimated, since the system cannot respond quickly enough to rapid changes in pressure. As was previously mentioned, an air bubble in the system is a common cause of reduction of the natural frequency of the system. In addition, any type of partial clot at the tip of the catheter will also degrade the natural frequency.

Catheter "whip" is a condition in which a catheter that is placed into a large cavity or vessel produces artifacts as it moves rapidly to and fro within the chamber. This can occur when measurements are made in the LV cavity, or in the PA. Another common error when electronic transducers are used results when the electronic balance within the transducer becomes altered. This is referred to as *transducer drift*. Since electronic transducers consist of an activating current that is sent through a variable resistor, the electronic integrity of the transducer should be checked periodically. This can be done easily by exposing the transducer to atmospheric pressure, to check to make sure the transducer reads zero.

The last type of error is a transducer position error. By convention, the electronic zero point of the transducer should be placed at the level of the RA, which is the accepted zero reference point. If the transducer height is altered from this point, significant errors can result. If the transducer is placed in a position below the RA, then the column of fluid above the transducer will result in an artificially elevated reading. Likewise, if the transducer is placed above the zero reference, the transducer will read artificially low. Therefore, correct pressure monitoring requires adherence to two types of zeroing of the transducer, both electronic and zero reference.

Definition of Pressure Waveforms—Cardiac Cycle

Right-Sided Heart Pressures

The right-sided heart pressures, as measured in the cardiac catheterization laboratory, consist of the central venous pressure (CVP) or RA pressure (RAP), RV pressure (RVP), PA pressure (PAP), and PCWP. The CVP consists of three waves and two descents (Fig. 12–9, Box 12–4). The A wave occurs synchronously with the Q wave of the ECG, and accompanies atrial contraction. Next, a smaller C wave appears, which results from tricuspid valve closure and bulging of the valve into the RA as the RV begins to contract. Following this, with the tricuspid valve in the closed position, the atrium relaxes, resulting in the X descent. This is followed by the V wave, which corresponds to RA filling that occurs during RV systole with a closed tricuspid valve. As the RV relaxes, the RVP then becomes less than the RAP, the tricuspid valve opens, and the atrial blood rapidly empties into the ventricle. This is signified by the Y descent.

Beginning in early diastole, the RV waveform reaches its minimum pressure shortly before or as the tricuspid valve opens. During the rapid filling phase of diastole, the ventricular pressure rises slowly, and usually an A wave, which signifies atrial contraction, is seen just before the onset of ventricular systole. As ventricular contraction occurs, peak

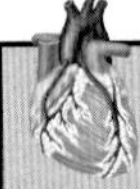

BOX 12–4 ***Hemodynamics and Valvular Pathology***

- Primary data
  - Pressures (PCW, PA, RV, RA, arterial, LV)
  - Thermodilution cardiac output
  - Oxygen saturation of blood
  - Oxygen consumption
- Calculated values
  - Valve areas
  - Vascular resistance
  - Shunt ratio
  - Fick cardiac output

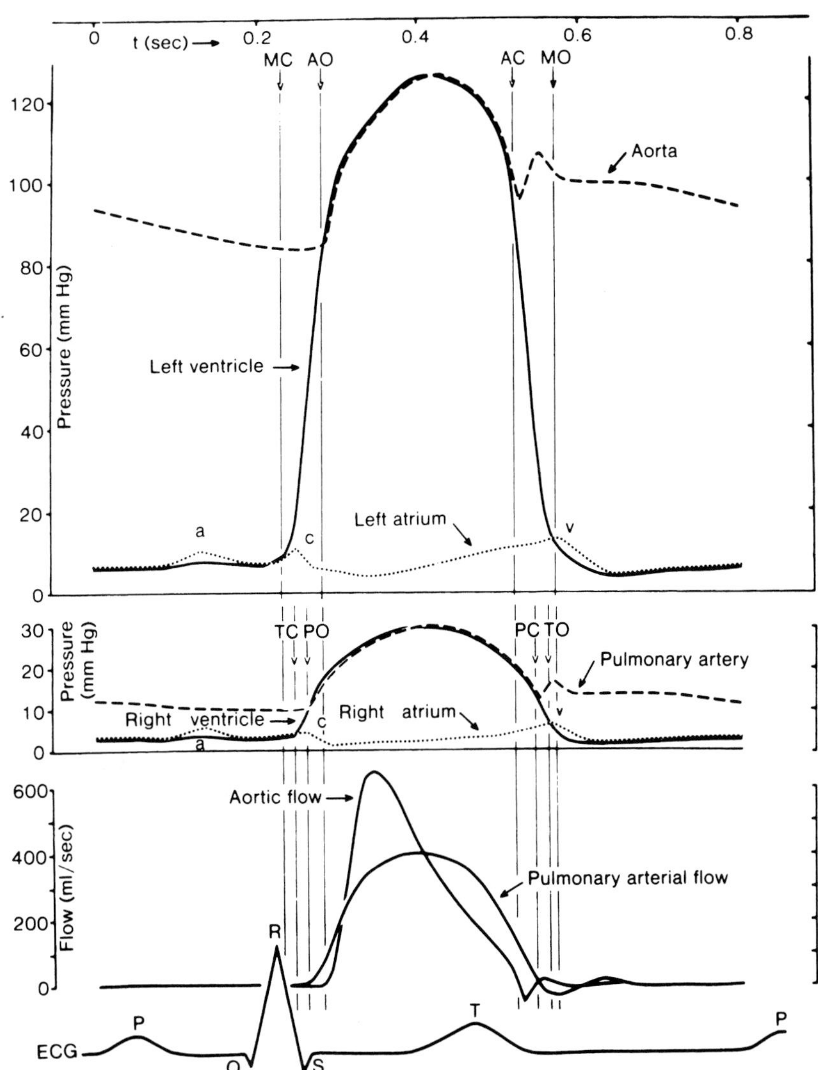

Figure 12–9 The cardiac cycle, demonstrating simultaneous left ventricular, aortic, and left atrial pressures *(top)*; right ventricular, pulmonary arterial, and right atrial pressures *(middle)*; and electrocardiogram (ECG) and aortic and pulmonary flows *(bottom)*. Also displayed are the temporal relationships of mitral valve opening (MO) and closure (MC), aortic valve opening (AO) and closure (AC), tricuspid opening (TO) and closure (TC), and pulmonic valve opening (PO) and closure (PC). (From Milnor WR: Hemodynamics, 2nd edition. Baltimore, Williams & Wilkins, 1989, p 145.)

systolic pressure is rapidly reached. Just before the onset of contraction, and after the A wave, the RV end-diastolic pressure (RVEDP) can be determined.

The PAP is usually greater than the RVP during the time the pulmonic valve is closed, during ventricular relaxation and filling. During systole, RVP crosses over PAP by a small margin, causing the pulmonic valve to open, and the ventricle ejects blood into the PA. It is not uncommon for a 5-mm gradient to exist between the RV and PA during peak systolic contraction. The minimum PA diastolic pressure can also be measured just before the onset of contraction, as an estimate of the PCWP; however, the presence of increased pulmonary vascular resistance will invalidate this correlation. With an inflated balloon, the tip of the PAC is protected from pulsatile pressures, and "looks forward" to the pressure in the pulmonary venous system and the LA. This "wedge" pressure shows many of the characteristics of the LAP. The differences between these two waves are considered in the discussion of LAP below.

Left-Sided Heart Pressures

The LA, LV, aortic, and peripheral pressures are commonly measured in the cardiac catheterization laboratory. The LAP can be measured directly if a transseptal catheter is placed.[83] Since this is not commonly done, the PCWP is used to estimate LAP. The LAP has a very similar appearance (A, C, V waves; X, Y descent) to that in the RA, although the pressures seen are about 5 mm Hg higher. The A wave in the RA tracing is normally larger than the V wave while the opposite is true in the LA (or PCWP). The PCWP provides reasonable estimations of the LAP, although the waveform is often damped and also delayed in time compared with the LAP (Fig. 12–10).

LV pressure also has many similar characteristics to the RVP, although since this is a thick-walled chamber, the generated pressures are higher than those reached in the RV (see Fig. 12–9). The central aortic pressure displays a higher diastolic pressure than that seen in the ventricle due to the properties of resistance in the arterial tree and the presence of a competent aortic valve. The dicrotic notch, which signifies the aortic valve closure, is a prominent feature of the aortic pressure wave in the central aorta. As the site of pressure measurement moves more distally in the arterial tree, there is a progressive distortion of the arterial waveform, usually demonstrated as an increase in systolic pressure. This is thought to be due to the addition of the pressure wave of reflected waves from the elastic arterial wall. Summation of reflected pressure waves has been postulated as a contributing

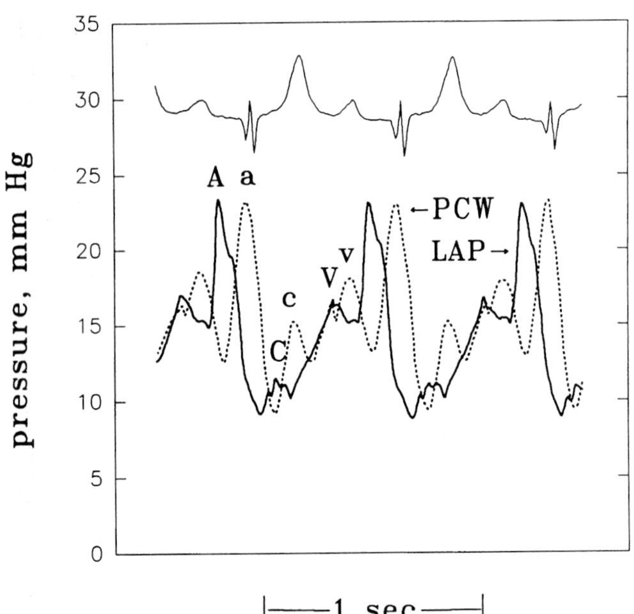

Figure 12–10 Simultaneous left atrial (LAP) and pulmonary capillary wedge (PCW) pressures, demonstrating the accuracy of the PCW in replicating the A, C, and V waves seen in the LAP (corresponding to a, c, and v waves in the PCW). Also shown is the time delay seen in the PCW trace, which results from the pressure wave traveling back through the compliant pulmonary venous system to the pulmonary artery catheter. (Modified from Grossman W, Barry WH: Cardiac catheterization. *In* Braunwald E [ed]: Heart Disease: A Textbook of Cardiovascular Medicine, 3rd edition. Philadelphia, WB Saunders Company, 1988, p 252.)

factor in aneurysm formation. Additionally, the rapid propagation of reflected waves along stiff arteries has been advanced as an explanation of the systolic hypertension seen in the elderly. Table 12–8 displays the range of normal pressures on the right and left side of the heart.

Cardiac Output Measurements

The techniques of measuring an average CO remain important means to a complete assessment of the patient in the cardiac catheterization laboratory. The measurement of CO along with other information allows the physician to estimate whether the metabolic needs of the patient are being met; that is, whether the oxygen supply or oxygen delivery is matching the oxygen demand. In addition, quantitating the CO also allows the calculation of shunt flows, regurgitant fractions, systemic vascular resistance (SVR), and pulmonary vascular resistance (PVR).

Cardiac Output Determination

Since the advent of hemodynamic monitoring, many different methods for measuring CO have been used. These can basically be divided into invasive and noninvasive techniques. Techniques such as indicator dilution and Fick CO measurements are quite invasive, involving the placement of catheters into the pulmonary and arterial circulations. Newer techniques, such as Doppler-echocardiographic and bioimpedance methods, are noninvasive. It has been difficult to judge the accuracy of any of these methods, since there is no gold standard for *in vivo* measurement of cardiac output. Correctly or incorrectly, the Fick method is usually considered to be the most accurate.[84] In studies comparing two methods, the measurements that display the greatest degree of reproducibility tend to be taken also as the most accurate, which may be misleading.[85] The literature is replete with comparisons between one method and another, but because of the pulsatile nature of flow through the systemic vasculature, as well as the second-to-second alterations in CO due to neurogenic, metabolic, and local control in the vascular beds, an exact measurement of blood flow in vivo is difficult to determine, and any method that shows a good degree of reproducibility is a reasonable choice (see Chapter 14).

Fick Method

The Fick method for CO measurement is based on a physiologic principle first described by Adolf Fick in 1870, although he never used this principle specifically for measuring cardiac output. The principle states that flow through a vascular bed is equal to the amount (A) of a substance used or produced by that bed divided by the outflow concentration (C_{out}) of the substance minus the input concentration (C_{in}) of the substance.

$$\text{Flow} = (A)/(C_{out} - C_{in})$$

It can be seen that this principle can be used to describe blood flow across any vascular bed in vivo, and can also be applied to the body as a whole. This principle is used to calculate the total CO determination, by using oxygen as the substance being measured. The inflow and outflow concentrations of oxygen can be measured across the pulmonary circulation. At steady state, oxygen is used by the systemic beds at a rate that is equal to that by which it is taken up by the lungs. Therefore, CO is equal to the minute consumption of oxygen divided by the difference between the oxygen content of the pulmonary outflow minus the pulmonary inflow. The oxygen concentration of the pulmonary outflow is equal to that found in the pulmonary veins, but this is usually estimated by taking a sample of systemic arterial blood, and the pulmonary inflow oxygen concentration is measured by sampling blood from either the RV or PA.

Measuring Oxygen Consumption

In order to accurately measure the oxygen consumption ($\dot{V}O_2$), the following must be quantified: the inspired oxygen concentration; the expired oxygen concentration; and the volume of a timed collection of expired gas. Oxygen consumption can be quantified by using one of two approaches. The first is the closed-circuit method. There are several commercially available instruments to measure the rate of oxygen usage. Usually, this entails the use of a metabolic rate computer.[86,87] A polarographic cell is used to monitor concentrations of oxygen, and a computer-controlled feedback system maintains the oxygen at a constant level in a closed rebreathing chamber by entraining additional room air into the chamber. By measuring the amount of room air entering, the $\dot{V}O_2$ can be calculated.

The open method for measuring $\dot{V}O_2$ involves making accurate timed collections of expired gas into a large reservoir such as a Douglas bag, then measuring the volume and expired oxygen concentration of the gas to calculate $\dot{V}O_2$.[84] Inspired oxygen concentration is assumed to be that of room air, or 21%. Both methods are complicated for patients receiving supplemental oxygen.

Table 12–8 Normal Values on Right and Left Side of the Heart

	a Wave	v Wave	Mean	Systolic	End-Diastolic	Mean
Pressure (mm Hg)						
Right atrium	2 to 10	2 to 10	0 to 8			
Right ventricle				20 to 30	0 to 8	
Pulmonary artery				20 to 30	10 to 15	15 to 20
Pulmonary artery "wedge"	3 to 15	3 to 12	1 to 10			
Left ventricle				100 to 140	3 to 12	
Peripheral artery or aorta			100 to 140	60 to 90	70 to 105	
Flow						
Cardiac output (L/min)	4.5 to 7.0					
Cardiac index (L/min/m^2)	2.5 to 4.2					
Oxygen consumption index (mL/min/m^2)	100 to 150					
A–VO_2 difference (mL O_2/100 mL blood)	3.0 to 5.0					
Resistance	**Wood's Unit (WU = mm Hg/min/·L)**	**Metric Units (U = dynes/sec/cm^5)**				
Systemic vascular resistance (SVR)	12 to 18 WU	900 to 1500 U				
Systemic vascular resistance index	20 to 32 WU·m^2	1700 to 2600 U·m^2				
Pulmonary vascular resistance (PVR)	0.5 to 1.5 WU	40 to 100 U				
Pulmonary vascular resistance index	0.8 to 2.3 WU·m^2	70 to 180 U·m^2				
Resistance ratio (PVR/SVR)	<0.15	<0.15				

A–VO_2 = arterial-venous oxygen difference.

Measuring Arterial-Venous Oxygen Content Difference

The measurement of the arterial-venous oxygen content difference across the pulmonary circulation is accomplished by sampling blood in the PA, or inflow to the lungs, and sampling pulmonary venous, or outflow from the lungs. As stated previously, since pulmonary venous blood is difficult to sample, arterialized blood is sampled instead. Oxygen content can be determined by the classic method of Van Slike.[88] Since this method is very time-consuming, an easier method involves measuring the hemoglobin (Hgb) concentration and the hemoglobin saturation (SaO_2), and multiplying this product times the oxygen-carrying capacity of hemoglobin, which is 1.36 mL of oxygen per gram of Hgb.

$$CaO_2 = Hgb \cdot 1.36 \cdot SaO_2$$

Generally, the dissolved portion of oxygen in blood is extremely small for the patient breathing room air. The constant, 1.36, is an adjusted one to account for this relatively small amount of oxygen.

It is important to realize the possible errors involved in sampling systemic arterial blood instead of blood from the pulmonary veins. Basically, by doing so, it is assumed that no intracardiac shunt exists. Although this is largely true, there will be a small amount of mixing of deoxygenated blood returning via the bronchial and thebesian circulations. In the normal individual, this accounts for a shunt of approximately 5%. Since the oxygen content of systemic arterial blood is usually lower than pulmonary venous blood, the estimate of CO using the Fick method will usually overestimate CO by a small degree. In terms of sampling inflow blood to the lungs, it is important that the venous blood from the IVC and SVC be adequately mixed, since blood returning via the IVC has a significantly higher saturation level than that from the SVC. Sampling from the RA could lead to significant inaccuracies due to inadequate mixing or if the sample is drawn near the ostium of the coronary sinus, a site with an extremely low oxygen saturation. The best place for sampling is from the PA, which provides for a true mixed sample. Another source of error in calculating the oxygen content of venous blood can occur if the PAC is in a wedged position, permitting arterialized blood to be withdrawn through the catheter. This too will tend to decrease the denominator of the Fick equation and overestimate CO. Normal values for CO, cardiac index (CI), oxygen consumption index, and $A\dot{V}O_2$ difference are shown in Table 12–8.

Indirect and Modified Fick Methods

The so-called indirect Fick method for measuring CO has been described.[89] In this method, the carbon dioxide rate of exchange across the lungs is used as the indicator substance. A commercially available instrument (Gould 9000N) measures carbon dioxide by absorption analysis. The equation for the indirect Fick method is similar to the standard Fick equation. In this instance, CO is equal to the minute production of carbon dioxide divided by the difference of venous carbon dioxide content minus arterial carbon dioxide content. The minute production of carbon dioxide is calculated from the minute volume and the fractional content of carbon dioxide in expired air. The arterial carbon dioxide content is also calculated from the expired carbon dioxide concentration, and the venous content of carbon dioxide is calculated using a carbon dioxide rebreathing method. This indirect Fick method displays a wide variability in its measurements, but has been described as being fairly accurate when carefully performed.

A single breath-holding method for measuring carbon dioxide has also been described.[90] In this method, the uptake of Freon-22 by the lungs is measured to derive the CO. Kendrick et al[90] have compared CO measurements and found them to be similar to those derived by the classic Fick method.

A "modified" Fick CO can also be calculated by using an estimated rather than measured oxygen consumption, since this measurement can introduce error.[91] However, others recommend that measured rather than assumed values lead to less error.[92]

Indicator Dilution Cardiac Outputs

There are two basic types of indicator dilution that are used in the cardiac catheterization laboratory. The first is an indicator dye CO method and the second is a thermodilution method. The indicator dye method uses a nontoxic dye such as indocyanine green or methylene blue that is not taken up by the lungs or tissues.[93] The dye is injected into a central venous compartment such as the RA, and becomes totally mixed in the pulmonary circulation. Following this, the dye appears in the systemic arterial system, from which blood is continually drawn and sampled to measure the concentration of the dye. The amount of dye injected is known. Integration of the concentration of the dye over time as it is sampled in the systemic circulation permits calculation of the rate of flow. A typical dye dilution curve is shown in the top of Figure 12–11.

It can be seen that the majority of the dye is contained in the first pass that appears as a large deflection, and then gives rise to an exponential decay. However, the recirculation part of the dye dilution curve, which is a normal occurrence, can also be seen. Extrapolating the exponential decay portion of the curve to the zero line, and then integrating the dye concentration-versus-time curve calculate the CO.

The presence of an intracardiac shunt, and its predominant direction, can be detected by the green dye technique, despite the fact that the actual computed number will be in error. The site of the shunt cannot be determined by this method. A fraction of the dye travels through the shunt, and causes characteristic abnormalities in the curve. These are seen in Figure 12–11. In the normal curve, dye travels through the lungs and into the periphery, reaching a high peak concentration during the first circulation time. An exponential decay follows, which is briefly interrupted by a smaller recirculation peak. In the case of a left-to-right shunt, dye injected into the RA will travel through the lungs to the LA. From here, part of the dye will travel back into the pulmonary circuit, while less will travel into the peripheral artery where it is sampled. A circular circuit is set up with some dye continuing to circulate in the lungs. This will result in a peak concentration that is less than normal, with an early recirculation peak that results from shunted dye returning early to the LA. The typical exponential decay is not present; instead, the decline is slower than normal.

For right-to-left shunts, a portion injected into the RA will be shunted directly to the LA without passing through the lungs. This will appear as an early peak that is not as tall as the normal peak. Again, both early and regular peaks are smaller than normal.

The thermodilution technique for measuring CO is probably the most commonly used method because of its ease.[70] In this instance, the indicator is a known aliquot of saline, which can either be at room temperature or iced (4°C). The indicator is injected into a central compartment such as the RA, and a thermistor in the PA measures the change in blood temperature as the cooler saline mixes with the pulmonary blood. In a manner similar to dye dilution curves, the thermistor output describes a curve, which rapidly reaches a minimum, and then shows an exponential decay. The CO can be calculated using the following formula, which is based on calculations by Hamilton for any dilution type of CO determination:

$$\text{Cardiac output} = [V_i \times (T_b - T_i) \times 60 \times 1.08]/A$$

where V_i is the volume of ejectate in mL, T_b is blood temperature, T_i is injectate temperature, 1.08 is a correction factor for

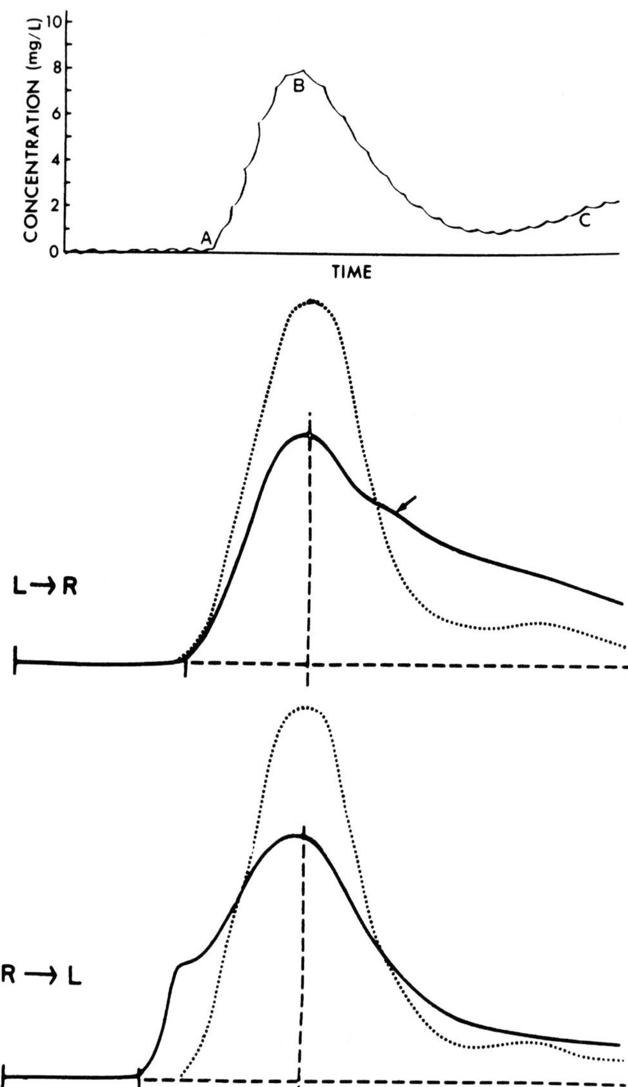

Figure 12–11 Dye dilution curve resulting from an injection of indocyanine green into the right atrium, measured by continuous spectrophotometry in blood from the radial artery. *(Top)* Normal curve, showing step rise *(A)* to a maximum *(B)*, and exponential decay, with recirculation peak *(C)*. Small scallops in curve result from individual heartbeats. The ordinate for the normal curve is plotted logarithmically in the *middle* and *bottom* traces, which show best the decay portion of the curve *(middle)*. Curve resulting from a left-to-right intracardiac shunt, showing early recirculation peak due to shunted blood reentering the pulmonary circuit *(arrow)*, nonexponential decay, and lower peak concentrations reached in the periphery *(bottom)*. Curve seen with right-to-left intracardiac shunt, demonstrating early appearance of dye in periphery that bypasses the lungs, lower peak concentrations, and normal decay (From Grossman W, Barry WH: Cardiac catheterization. *In* Braunwald E [ed]: Heart Disease: A Textbook of Cardiovascular Medicine, 3rd edition. Philadelphia, WB Saunders Company, 1988 p. 253.)

specific gravity and specific heat of the blood and the indicator, and A is the area under the dilution curve multiplied by the time required for the inscription of the curve.[94] The constant 60 is inserted to convert the CO from L/sec to L/min.

The requirements that must be satisfied in order for the thermodilution technique to accurately estimate CO are: The amount of injectate volume must be known, a rapid injection must take place (preferably within 2 seconds for a 10-mL sample), good and thorough mixing must occur, and steady-state circulatory conditions must apply[95] (see Chapter 14).

Table 12–9 outlines some sources of error for thermodilution, dye dilution, and the Fick methods for determining cardiac output.

Vascular Resistance Calculations

From the above discussions of pressure and flow measurements, it should be apparent that within a certain degree of error, hemodynamic variables can be reproducibly quantified. The flow generated by the heart, and the pressure that this flow of blood generates, will largely be determined by a third variable of the cardiovascular system: namely, the vascular resistance. Although many of the characteristics of fluid dynamics and the steady flow of fluid through a rigid tubing have been described, characterizing the vascular resistance in the body is much more complex because blood flow is pulsatile, blood is a nonhomogenous fluid (consisting of red cells, white cells, and platelets suspended in a plasma), and the vascular bed is an elastic system with many branch points. In the vascular tree, resistance continuously varies depending on the point in time of the cardiac cycle and is influenced by several factors: inertia, reflected pulse waves, and the phase angle between pulse and flow wave velocities.[96] For this reason, vascular resistance is merely estimated as the quotient of pressure divided by flow, in a manner similar to that applied in electronics:

$$R = V/I \rightarrow \text{Vascular resistance} = \text{Pressure/Flow}$$

The vascular resistance can be estimated separately across both the systemic and pulmonary beds. Thus, the SVR can help the clinician to tailor the use of vasodilator drugs. For instance, in patients with heart failure, the SVR can be greatly elevated due to increased autonomic innervations of the resistance vessels in the arterial tree. Recognition of an elevated SVR would prompt the early use of vasodilators. Likewise, the low SVR state that is common after cardiopulmonary bypass can be effectively treated with vasopressor therapy.

An elevated PVR, particularly one that does not decrease with pharmacologic therapy, predicts adverse events in several situations. For instance, the absence of pulmonary vasodilation (failure of PVR to decrease) predicts early right-heart failure after cardiac transplantation, and suggests that heart and lung transplantation may be necessary. It can also identify patients at risk for refractory right-sided heart failure after mitral valve replacement[97]; such patients may require pharmacologic or mechanical support in the postoperative period. Responsiveness to inhalation of oxygen, for example, may be helpful in identifying patients whose pulmonary reactivity is preserved.[98] In recent years, medical therapy for primary and secondary pulmonary hypertension has improved significantly with the use of calcium channel blockers, prostaglandins, and endothelin antagonists. Not all patients respond to these therapies; a decrease in PVR with pharmacologic intervention in the catheterization laboratory is evidence of preserved pulmonary arterial reactivity and predicts a response to long-term therapy.

Table 12–9 Sources of Errors in Cardiac Output Determinations

Method
Fick Method
Lack of steady state for the duration of the study
Takes at least 3 minutes to perform
Changes in mean pulmonary blood volume
Differential between oxygen taken up at mouth versus oxygen actually consumed by the body
Oxygen consumption estimate is the amount of oxygen entering the lungs, not the blood
Incomplete collection of expired air due to leak around the mouthpiece
Perforated ear drum
Assumes an RQ = 1.0
Incorrect timing of expired air collection
Abnormal hemoglobin will alter the calculation of oxygen content
Contamination of pulmonary capillary wedge blood with the mixed venous blood
Cannot check reproducibility easily because so much time is needed for one measurement
Time varying change in mixed venous PO_2
Less accurate with high outputs and narrow A–VO_2 difference (which is in the denominator of the equation)
Using assumed rather than measured values of oxygen consumption
Thermodilution
Variability in the volume of injectate
Rate of injection too slow
Differences in calculating the area under the curve
Variability of blood temperature in the lungs
Gain of heat by the indicator from the heart chambers after ejection
Overestimates cardiac outputs at low CO values due to recirculation
Variability due to respiratory effects
Errors in presence of tricuspid regurgitation
Requires invasive procedure to place a catheter into the pulmonary artery
Iced injectate can cause decrease in heart rate due to cooling of SA node
Catheter tip in peripheral pulmonary artery
Intracardiac shunt
Concomitant rapid volume infusion
Temperature of injectate may be a factor in accuracy
Dye Dilution
Errors relating to dose and rate of injection of indicator also apply
Low cardiac output states may cause inclusion of indicator recirculation and cardiac output calculation
Presence of mitral valve disease may alter cardiac output if dye is injected into the pulmonary artery
Requires invasive procedures to place central catheter or pulmonary artery catheter for injection and also systemic arterial catheter for sample withdrawal
Cannot repeat measurements often in short period of time due to build-up of dye
Inaccurate in left-sided regurgitant valve lesions

RQ = respiratory quotient; CO = cardiac output; SA = sinoatrial.

To calculate SVR, the CO divides the difference between the MAP and the RAP:

$$SVR = [MAP - RAP]/CO$$

To calculate the PVR, the difference between the mean PAP (MPAP) and the mean LAP (or PCWP) is divided by the CO:

$$PVR = [MPAP - PCWP]/CO$$

In order to normalize the SVR for body surface area (BSA), it is necessary to divide the numerator by CI rather than CO. Since the BSA is in the denominator of this term, the calculation of systemic vascular resistance index (SVRI) then equals the SVR *multiplied* by the BSA. Likewise, the pulmonary vascular resistance index (PVRI) is equal to the PVR multiplied by the BSA. The values for vascular resistance are expressed in mm Hg • min/L, which are also termed *hybrid* or *Wood units*. The Wood units can be converted to metric units by multiplying by the conversion factor of 80. The metric units are expressed in dynes/sec/cm^5 (see Table 12–8 for normal values).

Another index of pulmonary vascular disease is the ratio of pulmonary to systemic vascular resistance, also called the *resistance ratio*, calculated as R_p divided by R_s. This ratio correlates with survival, as first described by Wood.[99] More recently, studies looking at the natural history of ASDs and VSDs with pulmonary hypertension have reiterated the value of the resistance ratio in predicting outcome.[100,101] As seen in Table 12–8, the normal R_p/R_s is 0.15, but patients with an R_p/R_s of less than 0.5 have tolerated cardiac surgery.

When using either SVR or PVR calculations, it must be remembered that these are global assessments of the vascular resistance in the systemic or pulmonary arterial tree. There will certainly be differences in resistances across various vascular beds, and flow to any one bed or organ (e.g., kidneys) cannot be predicted by using the concept of total vascular resistance.

Valvular Pathology

Each type of valvular pathology has its own particular hemodynamic "fingerprint," the character of which depends on the severity of the pathology, as well as its duration (see Chapters 15, 16, and 20).

Stenotic Lesions

In order to assess the severity of stenotic lesions, the transvalvular gradient as well as the transvalvular flow must be quantified. For a given amount of stenosis, hydraulic principles state that as flow increases, so also will the pressure drop across the orifice. Both the CO and the HR determine flow; it is during the systolic ejection period that flow occurs through the semilunar valves and during the diastolic filling period for the atrioventricular (AV) valves.

Gorlin and Gorlin[102] derived a formula from fluid physics to relate valve area with blood flow and blood velocity:

$$\text{Valve area} \propto \text{Blood flow/Blood velocity}$$

In general, as a valve orifice becomes increasingly stenotic, the velocity of flow must progressively increase if total flow across the valve is to be maintained. In order to estimate valve area, flow velocity can be measured by the Doppler principle; however, in the catheterization laboratory, this is not as practical as measuring blood *pressures* on either side of the valve.

As described by Gorlin, the velocity of blood flow is related to the square root of the pressure drop across the valve:

$$P_1 - P_2 \propto (\text{Blood velocity})^2$$

Stated another way, for any given orifice size, *the transvalvular pressure gradient is a function of the square of the transvalvular flow rate.* For example, with mitral stenosis, as the valve area progressively decreases, a modest increase in the rate of flow across the valve causes progressively larger increases in the pressure gradient across the valve (Fig. 12–12).

To complete the calculation, the actual time of the cardiac cycle in which flow occurs must be known. For semilunar valves (aortic and pulmonic), flow occurs during the systolic ejection period; for AV valves (mitral and tricuspid), flow occurs during the diastolic filling period. The systolic ejection period (SEP) occurs during ventricular contraction when the aortic valve is open, and the diastolic filling period (DFP) occurs while the mitral valve is open (Fig. 12–13). The HR determines the duration of the SEP or DFP over an entire minute. Also present in the Gorlin formula is a coefficient that quantifies the conversion of potential energy (pressure energy) to kinetic energy (velocity). This term also contains an empirically derived factor, which accounts for the difference between calculated and measured valve areas at the time of surgery or postmortem.

The final Gorlin formula then becomes:

$$\text{Valve area} = \text{CO} \div [(\text{DFP or SEP})(\text{HR})] / 44.3 \cdot C \cdot (P_1 - P_2)^{1/2}$$

where CO is cardiac output (mL/min), DFP or SEP is diastolic filling period or systolic ejection period in sec/beat, HR is

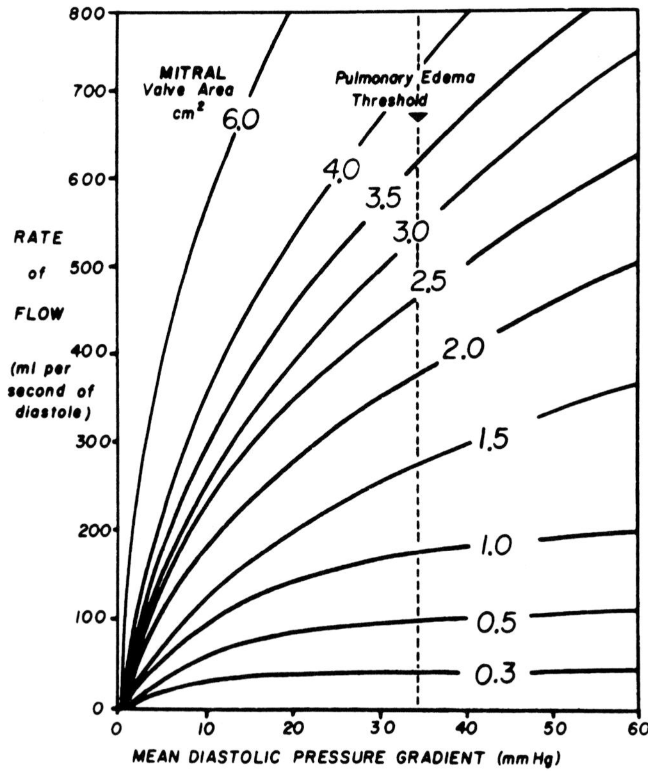

Figure 12–12 Rate of flow in diastole versus mean pressure gradient for several degrees of mitral stenosis. The pressure gradient is directly proportional to the square of the flow rate, such that as the degree of stenosis progresses, modest increases in flow (as with light exercise) will require large increases in the pressure gradient. As an example, a cardiac output (CO) of 5.2 L/min, heart rate (HR) of 60 bpm, and diastolic filling time of 0.5 second results in a 200 mL/sec flow during diastole (see text for details). For mild mitral stenosis (valve area = 2.0 cm^2), the required pressure gradient remains small (<10 mm Hg). In the case of severe stenosis (valve area < 1.0 cm^2), the resultant gradient is high enough to place the patient past the threshold for pulmonary edema. (From Wallace AG: Pathophysiology of cardiovascular disease. *In* Smith LH Jr, Thier SO [eds]: Pathophysiology: The Biological Principles of Disease. The International Textbook of Medicine, Vol 1. Philadelphia, WB Saunders Company, 1981, p 1192.)

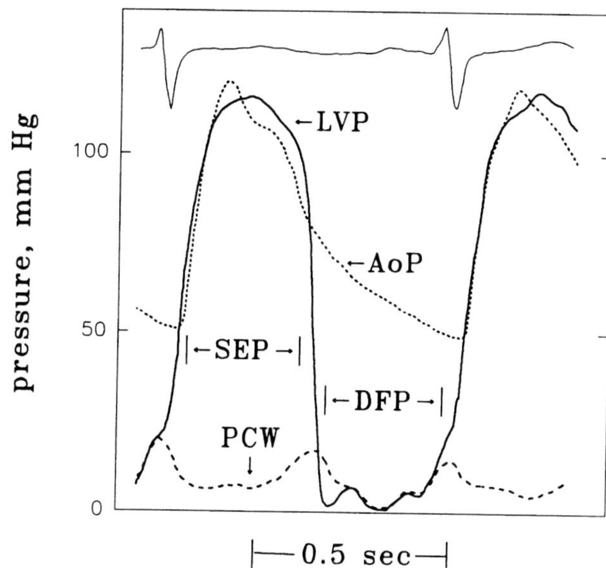

Figure 12–13 Diagram showing simultaneous left ventricular (LVP), aortic (AoP), and left atrial pressure (PCW) waveforms. The systolic ejection period (SEP) is defined as the period during which the aortic valve is open (from when LVP crosses over AoP at the beginning of systole to when AoP crosses over LVP near the end of systole) and forward blood flow is present in the aorta (see also Fig. 12–2). Diastolic filling period (DFP) is defined as that period during which the mitral valve is open (from the crossover of LVP by PCW to the crossover of PCW by LVP) and blood is flowing through the mitral valve. (Modified from Grossman W, Baim DS [eds]: Cardiac Catheterization, Angiography, and Intervention, 4th edition. Philadelphia, Lea & Febiger, 1991, p 153.)

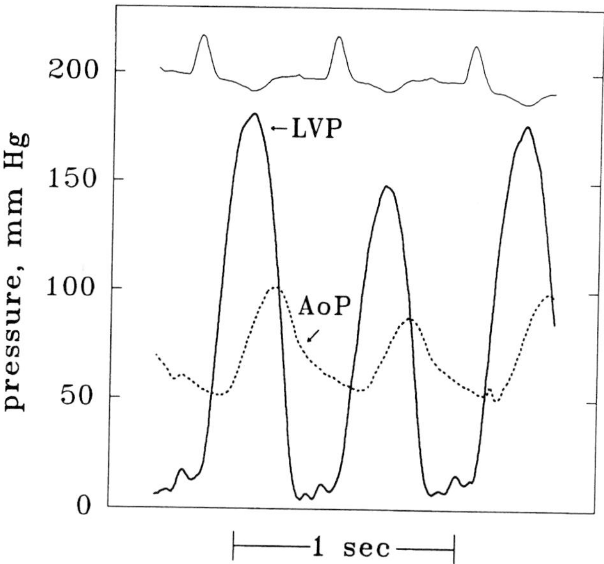

Figure 12–14 Left ventricular (LVP) and aortic (AoP) pressure waveforms in patient with aortic stenosis. Of note is the large pressure gradient from left ventricle to aorta at peak systolic pressure, the delay to the onset of aortic upstroke, and the decrease in the rate of rise of the aortic pressure. End-diastolic pressure is still normal at this stage of the disease.

heart rate in beats/min, C is orifice constant (aortic, C = 1.0; mitral, C = 0.85; tricuspid, C = 0.7), and $P_1 - P_2$ is the mean pressure difference across the orifice using computer-assisted analysis or area blanketing. The 44.3 term is derived from the energy calculation.

Aortic Stenosis

The normal adult aortic valve area is 2.6 to 3.5 cm^2, which corresponds to a normal aortic valve index of 2 cm^2/m^2. As the valve area decreases to a range of 1.5 to 2.0 cm^2 (or a valve index of 1.0 cm^2/m^2, the major hemodynamic finding is an increase in the LV systolic pressure in order to maintain a normal aortic systolic pressure. An elevation in LVEDP may also be observed, which is merely a reflection of the decrease in compliance of the hypertrophied ventricle (see Chapter 20).

As the stenosis becomes moderate and the valve area decreases to 1.0 to 1.5 cm^2, symptoms can occur. At this point, the LV exhibits a more rounded appearance at its peak systolic pressure, and a progressive increase in the LVEDP occurs. As the LV hypertrophies, its filling becomes more dependent upon the contraction of the LA; this is reflected as an augmented A wave on the ventricular tracing. At this point, the increased LA pressure makes atrial fibrillation more likely, and the decreasing compliance of the LV makes it poorly tolerated. Widening of the systolic pressure gradient from the LV to the aorta (AO), a decrease in the rate of rise of the upstroke of the aortic pressure tracing, and a delay in the time to peak aortic pressure are also seen (Fig. 12–14).

In the case of severe AS with a valve area of less than 1.0 cm^2 and a valve area index of less than 0.5 cm^2/m^2, a decrease in systolic function of the LV can occur. Increases in PAP, PCWP, and RAP, are also observed. These latter changes are often accompanied by symptoms of congestive heart failure.

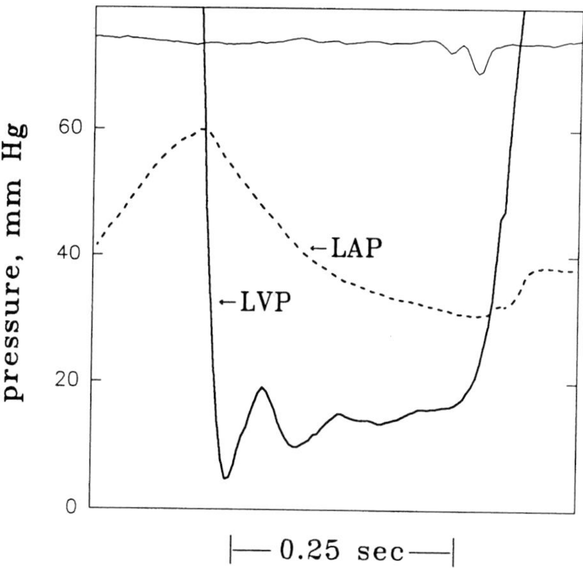

Figure 12–15 Mitral stenosis, with pressures measured at catheterization. Note the gradient during diastole between the left atrial (LAP) and the left ventricular (LVP) pressures, and the elevation in the LAP.

Mitral Stenosis

In normal adults the mitral valve orifice is 4 to 6 cm^2. Mild mitral stenosis (MS) is considered to be present when the mitral valve orifice is reduced to less than 2 cm^2. In this condition, the typical hemodynamic finding is that of an elevation in either LAP or PCWP. The increase in LAP will tend to maintain normal flow across the valve. As the mitral valve orifice becomes reduced to less than 1.0 cm^2, considered to be critical MS, a much larger LA-to-LV gradient is required to maintain reasonable flow across the valve (Fig. 12–15). An elevation in LAP during diastole leads to early opening of the mitral valve, as well as slightly delayed closure of the same valve (Fig. 12–16). It is easy to understand why a slow HR in the presence of MS is preferred, since a maximal DFP is necessary in order to maintain reasonable flow and maintain CO across the mitral valve. Another hemodynamic hallmark in patients with MS is the reduced rise in LV pressure during early diastole. Normally, a fairly rapid rise is seen during the rapid filling phase of diastole, but the slope of this pressure rise is delayed in the presence of severe MS. In the presence of severe MS, elevations in right-sided heart pressures are very common. In severe long-standing MS, the PAP can reach or exceed systemic arterial pressure. Dilation of the LA commonly leads to chronic atrial fibrillation in these patients.

Doppler echocardiography has reduced the importance of catheterization in the evaluation of valvular disease (see Chapter 15). In stenoses of borderline severity, data from the catheterization laboratory are still important for clinical decision-making. Performance of exercise or administration of inotropic agents increases the cardiac output. In addition to confirmation of inotropic reserve, this increase in output increases the flow across the valves and increases the gradient exponentially. When both the gradient across the valve and the cardiac output are low, augmentation of flow can help to distinguish severe stenosis with reversible ventricular failure from mild stenosis with irreversible ventricular failure.

Regurgitant Lesions

The severity of regurgitant lesions is quantified angiographically, and is discussed below. However, several hallmark changes occur in the presence of regurgitant lesions of either the semilunar or AV valves. As an example of semilunar valve regurgitation, the aortic valve is discussed, and the mitral valve is used as an example of AV valve regurgitation or incompetence (see Chapters 15, 16, and 20).

Aortic Regurgitation

Acute AR or insufficiency (AI) is uncommon, unless there is aortic dissection, sudden failure of a valve prosthesis, or if there is native valve destruction in the setting of bacterial endocarditis. In the presence of acute AR, there are sudden increases in systolic and end-diastolic volumes and pressures. Thus, the normal ventricle is suddenly faced with an increased load, and generates greater pressure. During relaxation, because the ventricle is filling with blood from the aorta, there is a delay in the isovolumic pressure decline, accompanied by rapid increases in ventricular diastolic pressures, both due to continued valve regurgitation. The wide pulse pressure, a characteristic of chronic AR, may not be seen in the acute setting. In addition, the dicrotic notch, which usually occurs with aortic valve closure, is absent in severe AR. A condition called *pulsus bisferiens* is a common finding in the presence of AR, and this condition is due to the "tidal-wave effect" as regurgitant blood entering the ventricle during early diastole causes a reflected pressure wave that is seen in the aorta. In the PCWP tracing, an accentuated V wave is commonly seen in the presence of AR, presumably a reflection of the decrease in compliance of the ventricles.

Chronic AR can be caused by aortic root dilation, bicuspid valves, rheumatic fever, failing prostheses, endocarditis, and other conditions. With chronic AR, the LV dilates and becomes more compliant, reflected as a lower LVEDP than in the acute phase. End-diastolic pressure may even be in the normal range until terminal failure is present. The systolic arterial pressure increases, and the diastolic pressure decreases. The former is due to the greater ventricular pressures generated, and the latter is due to continued runoff from the arterial system into the ventricle (Fig. 12–17). Aortic insuf-

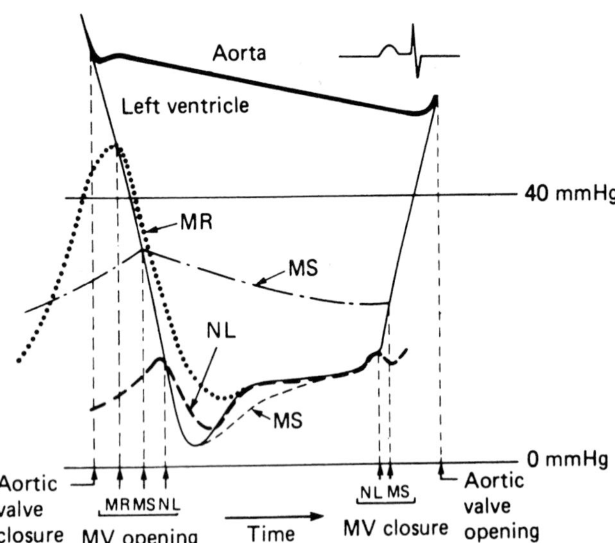

Figure 12–16 Idealized diagram summarizing mitral valve disorders, concentrating on the diastolic filling period. MR = mitral regurgitation; MS = mitral stenosis; NL = normal; MV = mitral valve. In MS, the elevation in left atrial pressure (---) versus normal atrial pressure (---) causes early MV opening and a slight delay in MV closure. Left ventricular rapid filling is delayed, which delays the rise of ventricular pressure (-----) from that seen during normal diastole (—). In MR, the left atrial pressure (. . .) has a large V wave, since not only is the atrium full of blood regurgitating through the MV, but it also receives blood from the pulmonary veins. Thus, the MV opens early. (From Braunwald E: Valvular heart disease. *In* Braunwald E [ed]: Heart Disease: A Textbook of Cardiovascular Medicine, 3rd edition. Philadelphia, WB Saunders Company, 1988, p 1024.)

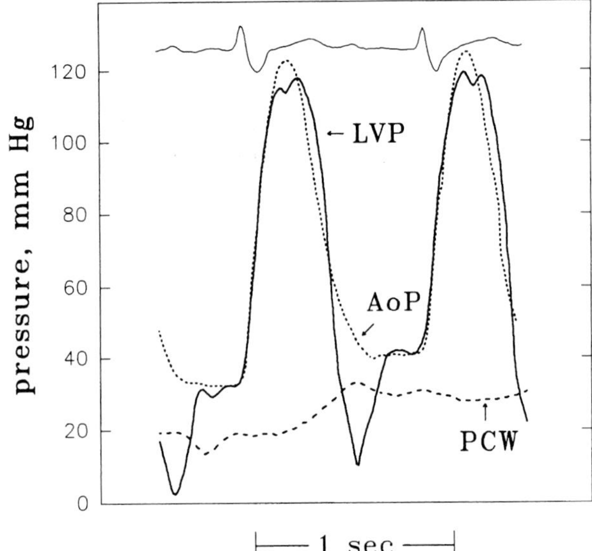

Figure 12–17 Aortic regurgitation. Simultaneous aortic (AoP), left ventricular (LVP), and pulmonary wedge (PCW) pressures demonstrate a wide aortic pulse pressure with absence of dicrotic notch, a rapid increase in LVP during early diastole due to regurgitation, and elevated PCW, reflective of elevated left ventricular end-diastolic pressure (Modified from Grossman W, Baim DS [eds]: Profiles in valvular heart disease. *In* Grossman W [ed]: Cardiac Catheterization, Angiography, and Intervention, 4th edition. Philadelphia, Lea & Febiger, 1991, p 575.)

ficiency imposes both a pressure load and a volume load on the left ventricle. Accordingly, the mass of the left ventricle can increase markedly if the condition is chronic.

Mitral Regurgitation

Mitral regurgitation (MR) can either be acute or chronic in nature. Acute MR is usually secondary to a condition such as acute ischemia leading to dysfunction of the papillary muscles of the mitral valve, or frank rupture of the structures following a significant myocardial infarction. Rupture of the chordae tendinae can occur in the setting of endocarditis or spontaneously and cause acute MR (Fig. 12–18). In this instance, it is not uncommon to see an enormously large V wave in the PCWP or LAP tracing, as ventricular blood freely flows back into a small, normal, and thus noncompliant LA. This is also accompanied by acute rises in the PAP and RAP, which can lead to significant clinical signs and symptoms.

In the setting of chronic MR, the LA can become quite large, nonfunctional, and very compliant. Thus, a significant regurgitant fraction can exist in the presence of a minimal V wave on the pressure tracing.

ANGIOGRAPHY

Ventriculography

Ejection Fraction Determination

Ventriculography is routinely performed in the single-plane 30-degree right anterior oblique (RAO) or biplane 60-degree left anterior oblique (LAO) and 30-degree RAO projections using 20 to 45 mL of contrast with injection rates of 10 to 15 mL/sec (Box 12–5). Complete opacification of the ventricle without inducing ventricular extrasystoles is necessary for accurate assessment during ventriculography. These premature contractions not only alter the interpretation of MR, but also result in a false increase in the global ejection fraction (EF).

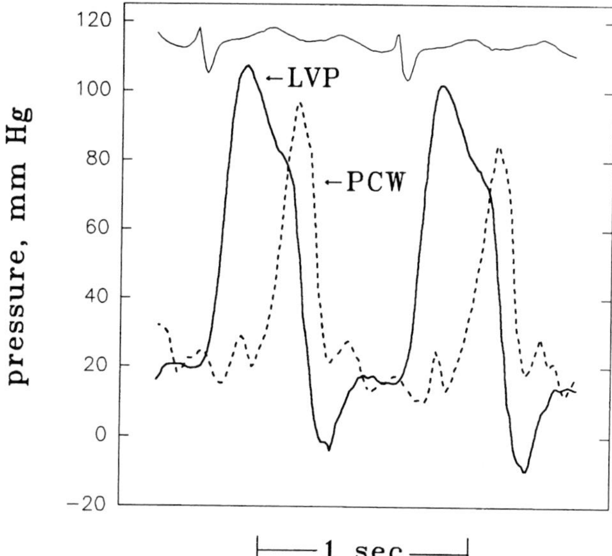

Figure 12–18 Acute mitral regurgitation due to chordae tendinae rupture. Simultaneous left ventricular (LVP) and pulmonary wedge (PCW) pressures demonstrate large V wave due to severe regurgitation into a normal-sized left atrium. Note that the V wave is delayed temporally from that shown in Figure 12–2. This delay is due to the time required for the pressure wave to travel through the compliant pulmonary venous and capillary beds to the pulmonary artery catheter (PAC). (Modified from Grossman W, Baim DS [eds]: Profiles in valvular heart disease. *In* Grossman W [ed]: Cardiac Catheterization, Angiography, and Intervention, 4th edition. Philadelphia, Lea & Febiger, 1991, p 564.)

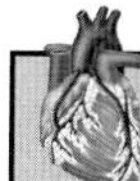

BOX 12–5 ***Angiography***

- Coronary anatomy
  - Left anterior descending coronary artery with diagonal and septal branches
  - Circumflex artery with marginal branches
  - Right coronary artery with conus, sinoatrial nodal, atrioventricular nodal, and right ventricular branches
  - Dominant circulation (posterior descending): 10% circumflex; 90% right coronary artery
- Coronary collaterals
- Coronary anomaly
- Ventriculography/aortography
- Ejection fraction calculation
- Valvular regurgitation

The EF is a global assessment of ventricular function and is calculated as follows:

$$EF = [EDV - ESV]/EDV = SV/EDV$$

where EF is ejection fraction, EDV is end-diastolic volume, ESV is end-systolic volume, and SV is stroke volume.

The primary clinical method for calculation of ventricular volumes necessary for determining the EF utilizes the area length method described by Dodge et al. in 1960.[103] Prior to calculation, visual identification is needed of the outer margin of the ventricular silhouette in both the RAO and LAO projections for both end-systole and end-diastole. To facilitate volume calculations, the ventricle is approximated as an ellipsoid (Fig. 12–19). Using biplane ventriculography to define major (L) and minor (M, N) axes, the following standard geometric formula for the area of an ellipsoid is used.[104]

$$A_{rao} = \pi[L_{rao}/2][M/2]$$
$$A_{lao} = \pi[L_{lao}/2][N/2]$$

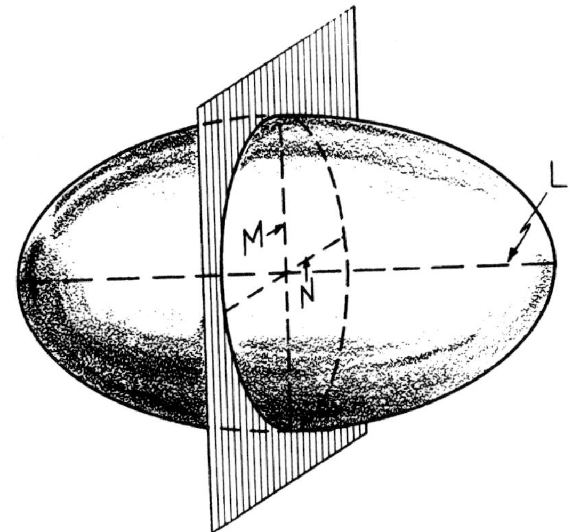

Figure 12–19 Ellipsoid used as reference figure for the left ventricle. The long axis (L) and the short axes (M and N) are shown. (From Fifer MA, Grossman W: Measurement of ventricular volumes, ejection fraction, mass, and wall stress. *In* Grossman W [ed]: Cardiac Catheterization and Angiography, 3rd edition. Philadelphia, Lea & Febiger, 1986, p 284.)

Using planimetry, the area (A) is obtained in both LAO and RAO projections with volume (V) calculated as follows:

$$V = [8/3\pi][A_{rao}(A_{lao}/L_{min})]$$

with L_{min} being the shorter of L_{rao} and L_{lao}.

Single-plane calculation in the 30-degree RAO assumes M = N and L is the true long axis. Using the ellipsoid volume calculation $V = \pi/6$ LMN, with M the planimetered area A and $M = 4A/\pi L$, the following formula is obtained:

$$V = [8A^2/3\pi L]$$

Magnification correction can be made using a calibrated grid imaged after cineangiography. More commonly, a part of the catheter that is in the ventricle is used for calibration. Catheters with precise calibration markings are available. Mathematical equations for ventricular volume overestimate true volume; therefore, regression equations are used to correct for this.[104]

There are problems with the use of EF as a measure of ventricular function. Ejection fractions calculated by various techniques (e.g., echocardiography, ventriculography, gated blood pool scanning) may not be identical because of the mathematical modeling involved. When single-plane ventriculography is used to calculate the EF, dysfunction of a nonvisualized segment (e.g., the lateral wall in an RAO ventriculogram), global function may be overestimated. Most importantly, the EF is a load-dependent measure of ventricular function. Changes in preload, afterload, and contractility can significantly alter the EF determination. Thus, the EF can vary over time without any change in the myocardium, if the loading conditions change. Identification of a load-independent measure of LV function has been the quest of many cardiologists over the years. The best approximation requires pressure-volume analysis at varying loading conditions to generate a series of curves. Although not used in routine clinical practice, pressure-volume curve analysis provides assessment of the systolic and diastolic properties of the ventricle and has been a valuable research tool (see Chapter 14). In addition to EF calculations, ventriculography allows for estimation of wall stress and LV mass.

Abnormalities in Regional Wall Motion

Segmental wall motion abnormalities (SWMAs) are defined in both the RAO and LAO projections. A 0-to-5 grading scale may be used with hypokinesis (decreased motion), akinesis (no motion), and dyskinesis (paradoxical or aneurysmal motion).

This scale is as follows:

0 = normal
1 = mild hypokinesis
2 = moderate hypokinesis
3 = severe hypokinesis
4 = akinesis
5 = dyskinesis (aneurysmal)

Each wall segment is identified as outlined in Figure 12–20 for both the LAO and RAO projections. These segments correspond roughly to vascular territories.

In addition to the information listed above, other things can occasionally be learned from the ventriculogram. Filling defects, particularly in akinetic or dyskinetic segments, can be seen and are suggestive of intracavitary thrombus. Ventricular septal defects can be detected and localized. Obliteration of the LV cavity or outflow tract during systole suggests intracavitary obstruction.

Assessment of Mitral Regurgitation

The qualitative assessment of the degree of MR can be made with LV angiography. It is dependent on proper catheter placement outside of the mitral apparatus in the setting of no ventricular ectopy. The assessment is, by convention, done on a scale of 1+ to 4+ with 1+ being mild and 4+ being severe MR. As defined by ventriculography, 1+ regurgitation is that in which the contrast clears from the LA with each beat, never causing complete opacification of the LA. Moderate or 2+ MR is present when the opacification does not clear with one beat, leading to complete opacification of the LA after several beats. In 3+ MR (moderately severe), the LA becomes completely opacified, becoming equal in opacification to the LV after several beats. In 4+ or severe regurgitation, the LA densely opacifies with one beat and the contrast refluxes into the pulmonary veins.

By combining data from left ventriculography and right-heart catheterization, a more quantitative assessment of MR can be made by calculating the regurgitant fraction. This can be effectively calculated by measuring the following: end-diastolic LV volume (EDV), end-systolic LV volume (ESV), and the difference between these two, or the total LV stroke volume (TSV). The TSV (stroke volume calculated from

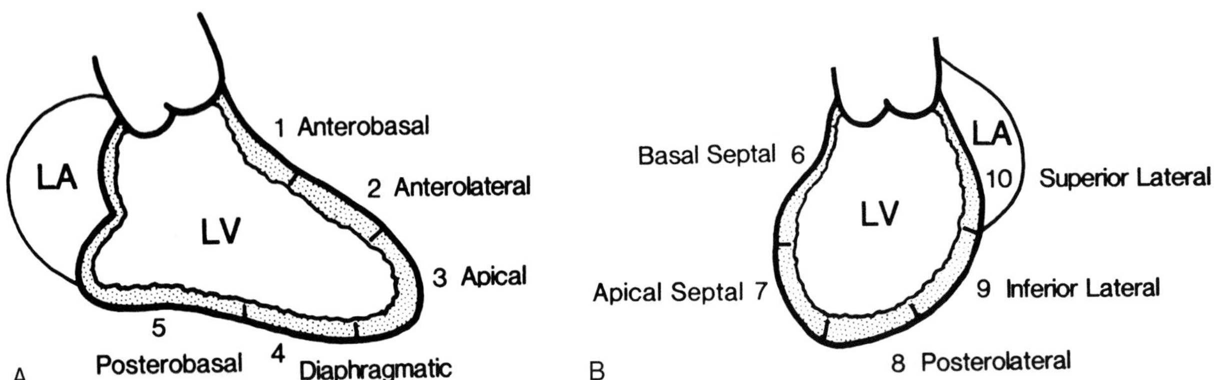

Figure 12–20 *(A)* Terminology for left ventricular segments 1 through 5 analyzed from right anterior oblique ventriculogram. LV = left ventricle; LA = left atrium. *(B)* Terminology for left ventricular segments 6 through 10 analyzed from left anterior oblique ventriculogram. LV = left ventricle; LA = left atrium. (*A, B,* from Principal Investigators of CASS and their Associates: National Heart, Lung, and Blood Institute Coronary Artery Surgery Study. Circulation 63[suppl II]:1, 1981.)

angiography) may be quite high, but it must be remembered that a significant portion of this volume will be ejected backwards into the LA. The forward stroke volume (FSV) must be calculated from a measurement of forward CO by the Fick or thermodilution method. The regurgitant stroke volume (RSV) can then be calculated by subtracting the FSV from the TSV (TSV − FSV). The regurgitant fraction (RF) is then calculated as the RSV divided by the TSV:

$$RF = (RSV)/(TSV)$$

A regurgitant fraction less than 20% is considered mild, 20% to 40% is considered moderate, 40% to 60% is considered moderately severe, and greater than 60% is considered severe MR.

Aortography

The primary indication for aortography performed in the cardiac catheterization laboratory is to delineate the extent of AR. Secondary indications include defining supravalvular lesions and determining the origins of saphenous vein grafts. Studies to differentiate proximal and distal dissections may be performed in the catheterization laboratory. However, transesophageal echocardiography (TEE), MRI, and CT scanning with contrast are more commonly utilized today to make this diagnosis.[105]

Similar to MR, AR is graded 1+ to 4+ based on the degree of contrast dye present in the LV chamber during aortography. As with MR, assessment of AR is dependent on proper catheter placement free of the valve leaflets but not too high in the ascending aorta. Mild (1+) is transient filling of the LV cavity by contrast dye clearing after each systolic beat; moderate (2+) is a small amount of contrast dye regurgitated into the LV, but present throughout the subsequent systolic beat; moderately severe AR (3+) is a significant amount of contrast dye present in the LV throughout systole, but not the intensity of that in the aorta; severe AR (4+) is contrast dye in the LV consistent with the intensity of that in the aorta with rapid ventricular opacification and delayed clearance following aortic injection.

Coronary Arteriography

Description of Coronary Anatomy

The left main coronary artery is 1 to 2.5 cm in length (Fig. 12–21). The left main bifurcates into the circumflex (CX) and left anterior descending (LAD) arteries. Occasionally, the CX and LAD arteries may arise from separate ostia, or the left main may trifurcate giving rise to a middle branch, the ramus intermedius, which supplies the high lateral ventricular wall. Both septal perforators and diagonal branch vessels arise from the LAD, which is described as proximal, mid, and distal vessel based on the location of these branch vessels. The proximal LAD artery is before the first septal and first diagonal branch; the mid LAD is between the first and second septal and diagonal branches; and the distal LAD is beyond the major septal and large diagonal vessels. The distal LAD provides the apical blood supply in two thirds of patients, with the distal right coronary artery (RCA) supplying the apex in the remaining one third (see Chapters 6 and 19).

The CX artery is located in the AV groove and is angiographically identified by its location next to the coronary sinus. The latter is seen as a large structure that opacifies

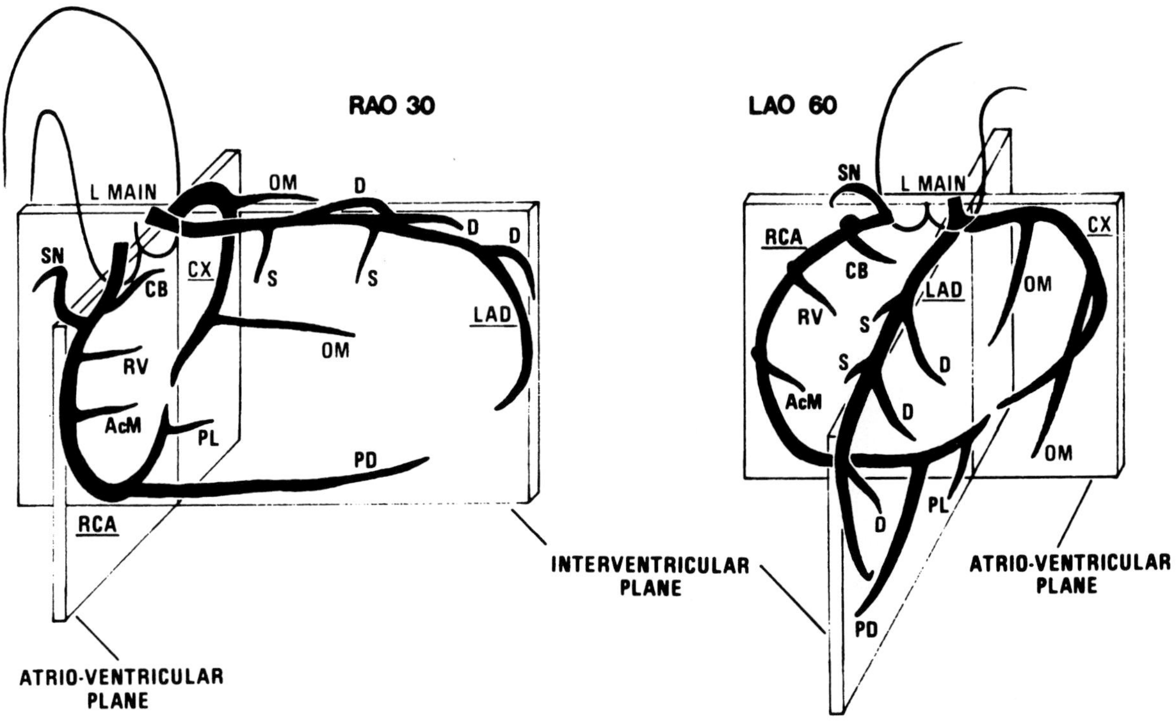

Figure 12–21 Representation of coronary anatomy relative to the interventricular and arterioventricular valve planes. RAO = right anterior oblique; LAO = left anterior oblique. Coronary branches are as indicated: L main = left main; LAD = left anterior descending; D = diagonal; S = septal; CX = circumflex; OM = obtuse marginal; RCA = right coronary; CB = conus branch; SN = sinus node; RV = right ventricle; AcM = acute marginal; PD = posterior descending; PL = posterolateral left ventricular. (From Baim DS, Grossman W: Coronary angiography. In Grossman W, Baim DS [eds]: Cardiac Catheterization, Angiography, and Intervention, 4th edition. Philadelphia, Lea & Febiger, 1991, p 200.)

during delayed venous filling after left coronary injections. Marginal branches arise from the CX artery and are the vessels in this coronary artery system usually bypassed. The CX artery in the AV groove is often not surgically approachable.

The dominance of a coronary system is defined by the origin of the posterior descending artery (PD), which through septal perforators supplies the inferior one third of the ventricular septum. The origin of the AV nodal artery is often near the origin of the PD artery. In 85% to 90% of patients, the PD originates from the RCA. In the remaining 10% to 15% of patients, the CX artery gives rise to the PD. Codominance, or a contribution from both the CX and RCA, can occur and is defined when septal perforators from both vessels arise and supply the posterior-inferior aspect of the left ventricle. Surgical bypass of this region may be difficult when this anatomy exists.

Coronary Anomalies

The coronary anomalies most frequently encountered during coronary angiography are listed in Table 12–10. Anomalous coronary origins are seldom of clinical or surgical significance, but are potentially time-consuming during coronary angiography. Rarely, anomalous coronary arteries arising from the opposite cusp and traversing between the PA and aorta may produce vessel compression and ischemia. The Bland-Garland-White syndrome occurs when the LAD arises from the PA. Although most patients present early in life, young adults with this syndrome may also present with sudden cardiac death or ischemic cardiomyopathy.[106] Coronary-cameral fistulas are not rare. Most are small and of no clinical significance.[107]

Assessing the Degree of Stenosis

By convention, the severity of a coronary stenosis is quantified as percent diameter reduction. Multiple views of each vessel are recorded, and the worst narrowing is recorded and used to make clinical decisions. This diameter reduction corresponds to cross-sectional area reduction; a 50% and 75% diameter reduction results in a 75% and 90% cross-sectional area reduction, respectively. Using the reduction in diameter as a measure of lesion severity is difficult when diffuse CAD creates difficulty in defining "normal" coronary diameter. This is particularly true in insulin-dependent diabetic patients as well as individuals with severe lipid disorders.

Table 12–10 Coronary Anomalies

Anomalous Coronary Origin
Left main coronary artery from right sinus of Valsalva separately or with right coronary artery
Circumflex artery as a separate origin off right cusp or with common origin with right coronary artery
Right coronary artery as a separate vessel from left cusp as separate ostea or as common ostea with circumflex as branch
Coronary Artery from Pulmonary Artery
Left coronary artery (Bland-Garland-White syndrome)
Right coronary artery
Fistula Formation from Normal Coronary Origin
Coronary branch vessels drain directly into right ventricle, pulmonary artery, coronary sinus, superior vena cava, pulmonary vein

Qualitative estimates of percentage of diameter reduction are highly variable among different observers, and not reflective of coronary flow. White et al,[108] using a Doppler velocity probe, demonstrated that lesion severity was underestimated in the overwhelming majority of cases. When visual interpretation is required for clinical decisions, as opposed to research purposes, there may be a systematic bias toward overestimation of lesion severity. Quantitative coronary angiography was developed to overcome the pitfalls of qualitative visual interpretation of lumen reduction. Although cumbersome in its early iterations, most contemporary imaging systems include a usable quantification program.[109] Even with quantification, the limitations of angiography remain. Intravascular ultrasound is a newer imaging modality that requires placement of a miniature transducer into the coronary artery. Thus, it entails more risk than angiography. In addition to a two-dimensional, cross-sectional view of the lumen, the vessel wall can also be seen.

Intravascular ultrasound has been a critical research tool, and is used clinically in selected situations. In a study comparing intravascular ultrasound findings with quantitative angiography, the plaque burden at maximal obstruction was frequently underestimated by quantitative angiography.[110] Tools for the physiologic assessment of coronary stenoses have been developed. Small wires (0.014 inch in diameter) containing either a pressure transducer or a Doppler probe can be passed into the artery and past the stenosis. After the intracoronary administration of a vasodilator, the pressure drop across the stenosis or the velocity response is measured. Correlation with nuclear stress testing has been good for both techniques. For instance, with the pressure wire, a ratio of the pressure distal to the stenosis to that proximal to the stenosis less than 0.75 following adenosine vasodilation predicts an abnormal nuclear perfusion scan result. This can aid in the assessment of an angiographically "borderline" stenosis. Clinical outcomes have been good for those with a higher ratio (fractional flow reserve [FFR]).[111,112]

Interpretation of coronary angiography is possible only when high-quality images are obtained. Contrast injections must be forceful to fully opacify the artery, while pressure tracings are closely observed so as to prevent coronary artery dissection. When smaller catheters are used, hand injection may require smaller syringes or power injection for adequate coronary opacification. Branch vessels must clearly be separated utilizing cranial and caudal angulations. Periodic assessment of image quality is required to assure properly functioning imaging equipment.[27]

Coronary Collaterals

Common angiographically defined coronary collaterals are described in Table 12–11. Although present at birth, these vessels become functional and enlarge only if an area of myocardium becomes hypoperfused by the primary coronary supply.[113] Angiographic identification of collateral circulation requires both the knowledge of potential collateral source as well as prolonged imaging to allow for coronary collateral opacification.

The increased flow from the collateral vessels may be sufficient to prevent ongoing ischemia. To recruit collaterals for an ischemic area, a stenosis in a main coronary or branch vessel must reduce the luminal diameter by 80% to 90%. Clinical studies suggest that collateral flow can double within 24 hours during an episode of acute ischemia.[114] However, well-developed collaterals require time to develop and only these

Table 12–11 Collateral Vessels

Left Anterior Descending Coronary Artery (LAD)
RIGHT-TO-LEFT
Conus to proximal LAD
Right ventricular branch to mid-LAD
Posterior descending septal branches at mid vessel and apex
LEFT-TO-LEFT
Septal to septal within LAD
Circumflex-OM to mid-distal LAD
Circumflex Artery (Cx)
RIGHT-TO-LEFT
Posterior descending artery to septal perforator
Posterior lateral branch to OM
LEFT-TO-LEFT
Cx to Cx in AV groove (left atrial circumflex)
OM to OM
LAD to OM via septal perforators
Right Coronary (RCA)
RIGHT-TO-RIGHT
Kugels—proximal RCA to AV nodal artery
RV branch to RV branch
RV branch to posterior descending
Conus to posterior lateral
LEFT-TO-RIGHT
Proximal mid and distal septal perforators from distal LAD
OM to posterior lateral
OM to AV nodal
AV groove Cx to posterior lateral

AV = atrioventricular; OM = obtuse marginal; RV = right ventricular.

respond to nitroglycerin (NTG). The RCA is a better collateralized vessel than the left coronary. Areas that are supplied by good collaterals are less likely to be dyskinetic or akinetic.

INTERPRETING THE CATHETERIZATION REPORT

Information obtained in the cardiac catheterization laboratory is representative of the patient's pathophysiologic process at only one point in time. Therefore, these data are static and not dynamic. In addition, alterations in fluid and medication management before catheterization can influence the results obtained. The hemodynamic information is usually obtained after the patient has fasted for 8 hours. Particularly in patients with dilated, poorly contractile hearts, the diminished filling pressures seen in the fasted state may lower the CO. In other circumstances fluid status will be altered in the opposite direction. Patients with known renal insufficiency are hydrated overnight before contrast administration. In these instances, the right- and left-sided heart hemodynamics may not reflect the patient's usual status. Additionally, medications may be held before catheterization, particularly diuretics. Acute β-blocker withdrawal can produce a rebound tachycardia, altering hemodynamics and potentially inducing ischemia.[115] These should be noted in interpreting the catheterization data.

Sedation may falsely alter blood gas and hemodynamic measurements if hypoxia occurs. Patients with chronic lung disease or Down syndrome may be particularly sensitive to sedatives, and respiratory depression may result in hypercapnia and hypoxia. Careful notations in the catheterization report must be made of medications administered as well as the patient's symptoms. Ischemic events during catheterization may dramatically affect hemodynamic data. Additionally, therapy for ischemia (e.g., NTG) may affect both angiographic and hemodynamic results.

Technical factors may influence coronary arteriography and ventriculography. The table in the catheterization laboratory may not hold very heavy patients. Patient size may limit x-ray tissue penetration and adequate visualization and may prevent proper angulations. Stenosis at vessel bifurcations may not be identified in the hypertensive patient with tortuous vessels. Catheter-induced coronary spasm, most commonly seen proximally in the RCA, must be recognized, treated with NTG, and not reported as a fixed stenosis.[116] Myocardial bridging results in a dynamic stenosis seen most commonly in the mid-LAD during systole. This is seldom of clinical significance, and should not be confused with a fixed stenosis present throughout the cardiac cycle. With ventriculography, frequent ventricular ectopy or catheter placement in the mitral apparatus may result in nonpathologic (artificial) MR. This must be recognized to avoid inappropriate therapy.

Finally, catheterization reports are often unique to institutions and are often purely computer generated, including valve area calculations. Familiarity with the catheterization report at each institution and discussions with cardiologists are essential to allow for a thorough understanding of the information and its location in the report, and the potential limitations inherent in any reporting process.

INTERVENTIONAL CARDIOLOGY: PERCUTANEOUS CORONARY INTERVENTION

This section is designed to present the current practice of interventional cardiology (Box 12–6). Although begun by Andreas Gruentzig in September 1977 as percutaneous transluminal coronary angioplasty (PTCA), catheter-based interventions have dramatically expanded beyond the balloon to include a variety of percutaneous coronary interventions (PCIs). Worldwide, this field has expanded to include approximately 900,000 PCI procedures annually.[22]

The interventional cardiology section is divided in two subsections. The first subsection consists of a general discussion of issues that relate to all catheter-based interventions. This includes a general discussion of indications, operator experience, equipment and procedures, restenosis, and complications. Anticoagulation and controversial issues in interventional cardiology are also reviewed. The second subsection is devoted to a discussion of the various catheter-based systems for PCI. Beginning with the first, PTCA, most devices

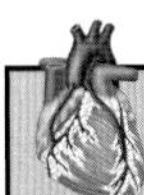

BOX 12–6 *Interventional Cardiology—Timeline*

1977 Percutaneous transluminal coronary angioplasty
1991 Directional atherectomy
1993 Rotational atherectomy
1994 Stents with extensive antithrombotic regimen
1995 Abciximab approved
1996 Simplified antiplatelet regimen after stenting
2001 Distal protection
2003 Drug-eluting stents

are presented, including current technology and devices in development. With this review, the cardiac anesthesiologist may better understand the current practice and future direction of interventional cardiology.

General Topics for All Interventional Devices

Indications

Throughout the history of PCI, both technology and operator expertise have improved continually, but this improvement has been most significant over the past decade. With the proper credentialing, experience, and current technology, the interventionalist now has the capabilities to go places in the coronary tree "where no man (or woman) has gone before." This is reflected in the expanded role for PCI. Although first restricted to patients with single-vessel disease and normal ventricular function who had a discrete, noncalcified lesion in the proximal vessel, PCI is now performed as preferred therapy in many groups of patients, including some with unprotected (no bypass grafts) left main stenosis.[117,118]

Box 12–7 provides a summary of current clinical indications for PCI. Although initially reserved only for patients who were also suitable candidates for CABG, PCI is routinely performed in patients who are not candidates for CABG.[22] In considering both the indications as well as the appropriateness of PCI, the physician must review the patient's historical presentation, including functional class, treadmill results with or without perfusion data, and wall motion assessment. Demonstrating ischemia noninvasively avoids inappropriate procedures prompted by the "ocular-dilatory reflex" (lesion seen = lesion dilated).

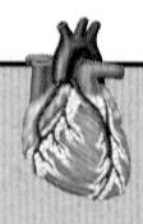

BOX 12–7 ***Clinical Indications for Percutaneous Transluminal Coronary Interventional Procedures***

Cardiac Symptoms

- Unstable angina pectoris/non–ST-segment myocardial infarction
- Angina refractory to antianginal medications
- Post–myocardial infarction angina
- Sudden cardiac death

Diagnostic Testing

- Early positive exercise tolerance testing
- Positive exercise tolerance test despite maximal antianginal therapy
- Large areas of ischemic myocardium on perfusion or wall motion studies
- Positive preoperative dipyridamole or adenosine perfusion study
- Electrophysiologic studies suggestive of arrhythmia related to ischemia

Acute Myocardial Infarction

- Cardiogenic shock
- Unsuccessful thrombolytic therapy in unstable patient with large areas of myocardium at risk
- Contraindication to thrombolytic therapy
- Cerebral vascular event
- Intracranial neoplasm
- Uncontrollable hypertension
- Major surgery <14 days
- Potential for uncontrolled hemorrhage

Absolute contraindications are few. Unprotected left main stenosis in a patient who is a surgical candidate, diffusely diseased native vessels, or a single remaining conduit for myocardial circulation is approached by PCI only after a significant discussion with patient and surgeon.[22.] Several series of unprotected left main PCIs have been published. Although the procedural risk may be low, most left main PCIs are performed in patients who are not operative candidates. By definition they are high-risk patients, and they continue to have a high rate of late events.[119,120] Multivessel PCI is frequently performed, and is a reasonable alternative to CABG in selected patients. However, CABG remains the preferred therapy for many patients, particularly diabetics. Finally, though currently performed, the role of PCI at facilities without on-site surgical capability is controversial.[20,22]

Equipment and Procedure

Significant advances have been and will continue to be made with all aspects of PCI. Although the femoral artery is still the most commonly utilized access site, the radial artery is utilized more frequently for coronary interventions. Despite numerous advances, all percutaneous coronary interventions still involve sequential placement of the following: guiding catheter in the ostium of the vessel, guiding wire across the lesion and in the distal vessel, and device(s) of choice at the lesion site.

Guiding catheters are available in multiple shapes and sizes for coronary and graft access, device support, and radial artery entry.[54,39] Guiding wires offer more flexible tips for placement in tortuous vessels as well as stiffer shafts to allow for the support of the newer devices during passage within the vessel. Separate guidewire placement within branch vessels may be required for coronary lesions at vessel bifurcations (Fig. 12–22). In selecting the appropriate device for the lesion, quantitative angiography and/or intravascular ultrasound may be used to determine the size of the vessel and composition of the lesion.[121]

While a device is in a coronary artery, blood flow is impeded to varying degrees. In vessels supplying large amounts of myocardium (e.g., proximal LAD), prolonged obstruction of flow is poorly tolerated. However, when smaller areas of myocardium are jeopardized or the distal vessel is well collateralized, longer occlusion times are possible. Distal protection devices, which involve balloon occlusion, may result in loss flow down the vessel for up to five minutes. However, with current technology, occlusion times seldom exceed one minute.

The performance of PCI immediately after a diagnostic procedure is known as ad hoc intervention. Obviously preferred in emergent situations, this strategy is increasing in popularity for elective cases as well..[22] Ad hoc PCI requires four essential components: An informed patient and family who can appreciate the risk and benefits of both the diagnostic as well as the interventional procedure. High quality imaging must be available for assessment of the extent of disease. The cardiologist must carefully assess each clinical situation and must have a collegial relationship with his or her surgical and anesthesiology colleagues if emergency backup is required. Finally, a flexible schedule must allow for the additional time required for the PCI within the catheterization laboratory.[122]

Anti-ischemic medications may permit longer periods of vessel occlusion before signs and symptoms of ischemia become limiting. This additional time could permit the com-

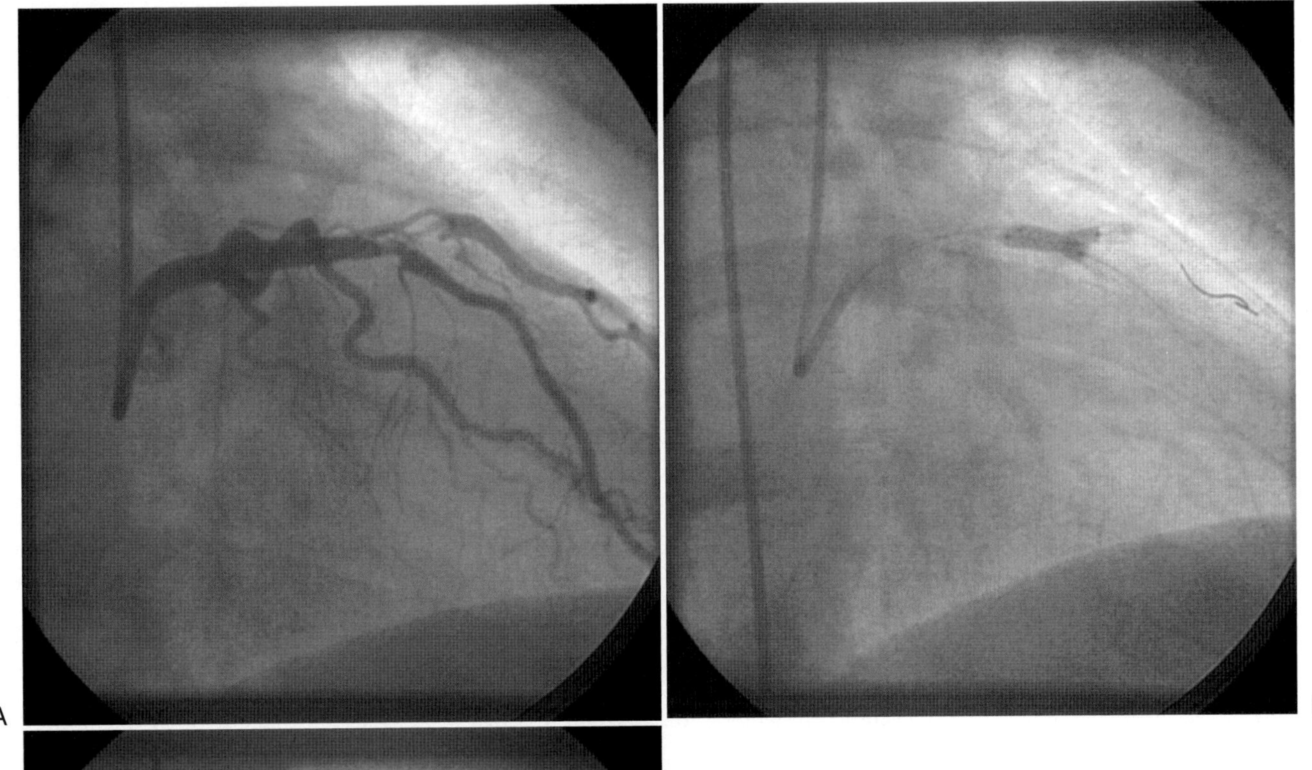

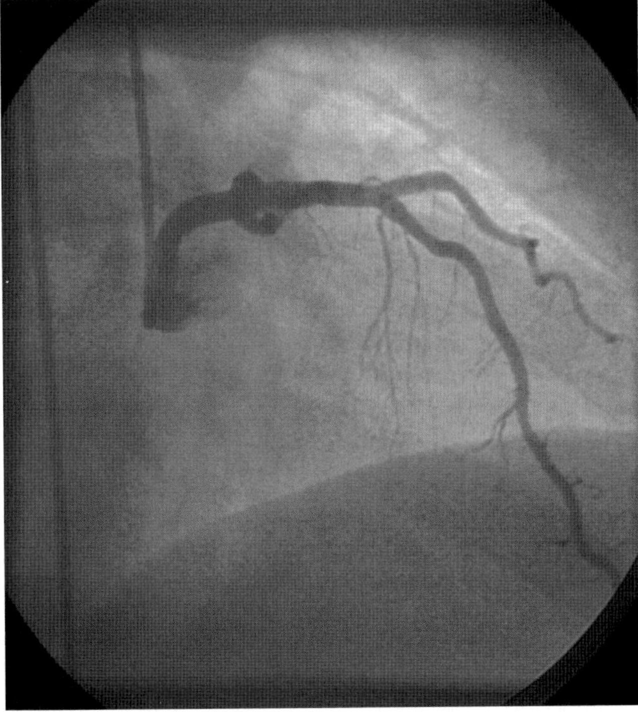

Figure 12–22 Complex coronary angioplasty. (*A*) Patient with lesion in the left anterior descending (LAD) artery at its bifurcation as well as a severe ostial diagonal stenosis. (*B*) "Kissing balloon" inflation performed simultaneously within both the deployed LAD and diagonal stents. (*C*) After dilation with patent LAD artery and diagonal branch.

pletion of a complex case or allow the use of distal protection devices. Most centers use either intracoronary or intravenous NTG at some point during the procedure to treat or prevent coronary spasm. Intracoronary calcium channel blockers are frequently used to treat vasospasm and the "no-reflow" phenomenon. The latter term describes an absence of flow in a coronary vessel when there is no epicardial obstruction. No reflow is associated with a variety of adverse outcomes; it is seen when acutely occluded vessels are opened during a myocardial infarction or when PCI is performed in old saphenous vein bypass grafts. The etiology is believed to be microvascular obstruction from embolic debris and/or microvascular spasm. Intracoronary calcium antagonists may help to restore normal flow, and nicardipine is preferred for its relative lack of hemodynamic and conduction effects.[123] NTG therapy is rarely needed after PCI unless signs of heart failure or ongoing ischemia are noted.

Restenosis

Once PTCA/PCI became an established therapeutic option for treating patients with CAD, it was soon realized that there were two major limitations: acute closure and restenosis.

Stents and antiplatelet therapy significantly decreased the incidence of acute closure. Before stents were available, restenosis occurred in 30% to 40% of PTCA procedures. With stent use, this figure decreased to about 20%. Thus, restenosis remained the Achilles heel of intracoronary intervention until the current drug-eluting stent (DES) era.

Restenosis usually occurs within the first 6 months following an intervention and has three major mechanisms: vessel recoil, negative remodeling, and neointimal hyperplasia.[124] Vessel recoil is caused by the elastic tissue in the vessel and occurs early after balloon dilation. It is no longer a significant contributor to restenosis because metal stents are nearly 100% effective in preventing any recoil.[125] Negative remodeling refers to late narrowing of the external elastic lamina and adjacent tissue. This accounted for up to 75% of lumen loss in the past.[124] This process is also prevented by metal stents, and no longer contributes to restenosis. Neointimal hyperplasia is the major component of in-stent restenosis. Neointimal hyperplasia is exuberant in the diabetic patient, and this serves to explain the increased incidence of restenosis in this population.[126]

Establishing the true rate of restenosis requires a uniform definition of restenosis. Clinical restenosis is defined as recurrence of angina or a positive stress test that results in a repeat procedure. Angiographic restenosis is defined at repeat catheterization and has higher rates than clinical restenosis. To be classified as a restenotic lesion at follow-up catheterization, at least a 50% reduction in luminal diameter must be present visually with a decrease of 0.72 mm quantitatively from the post-PTCI result.[127] Intravascular ultrasound (IVUS) can measure cross-sectional area and may also be used in assessing restenosis.[124] Since restenosis occurs within 6 months after intervention, symptoms occurring thereafter more commonly represent progression of atherosclerotic disease.[127]

Several clinical factors have been linked to restenosis. These include cigarette smoking, diabetes mellitus, male gender, absence of prior infarction, and unstable angina. Of these, only diabetes has consistently shown a statistically significant association with restenosis.[127,128] Lesion characteristics proved to predict restenosis are lesion location, baseline stenosis diameter and length, post-PTCI stenosis severity, and adjacent artery diameter.[125,128] In the stent era, baseline stenosis is no longer a predictor, while a large reference vessel diameter is associated with a lower risk of restenosis.[127,129]

Medical therapy to decrease restenosis has been unrewarding.[130-133] Aspirin decreases the risk of acute occlusion but does not significantly decrease the risk of restenosis.[130] Radiation therapy can be delivered from a source within the vessel lumen (vascular brachytherapy) and will be discussed in more detail later. Brachytherapy has been useful to treat in-stent restenosis, but results for prophylactic treatment have been disappointing.[134-136]

The major gains in combating restenosis have been in the area of stenting.[137] Intracoronary stents maximize the increase in lumen area during the PCI procedure and decrease late lumen loss by preventing recoil and negative remodeling. However, neointimal hyperplasia is enhanced due to a "foreign body-like reaction" to the stents. Different stent designs as well as varying strut thickness lead to different restenosis rates.[138,139] Systemic administration of antiproliferate drugs decreases restenosis but causes significant systemic side effects. Drug-eluting stents, with a polymer utilized to attach the antiproliferative drug to the stent, have shown the best results to date for decreasing restenosis.[140]

Anticoagulation

Thrombosis is a major component in acute coronary syndromes as well as acute complications during PCI; its management is in constant evolution[141] (Box 12–8). During interventional procedures, the guiding catheter, wire, and device in the coronary artery serve as nidi for thrombus. Additionally, most catheter interventions disrupt the vessel wall, exposing thrombogenic substances to blood. Table 12–12 summarizes the current anticoagulation agents utilized in the setting of PCI (see Chapter 29).

The primary pathway for clot formation during PCI has proved to be platelet mediated. This has prompted a focus on aggressive antiplatelet therapy. Aspirin was developed in the late 19th century and subsequently found to block platelet

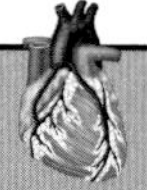

BOX 12–8 ***Anticoagulation***

- Antithrombin agents used
  - Heparin (IV during PCI)
  - Enoxaparin (SQ before, IV during PCI)
  - Bivalirudin (IV during PCI)
  - Argatroban (IV during PCI)
  - Warfarin (PO after PCI—rarely)
- Antiplatelet agents used
  - Aspirin (PO before and after PCI)
  - Ticlopidine (PO before and after PCI)
  - Clopidogrel (PO before and after PCI—preferred)
  - Abciximab (IV during PCI bolus + 12-hour infusion)
  - Eptifibatide (IV during PCI bolus + 18-hour infusion)
  - Tirofiban (IV before, during, and after PCI)

Table 12–12 Anticoagulation in Interventional Cardiology

	Dose	Mechanism of Action	Duration of Treatment	Binding
Antiplatelet Agents				
Aspirin	75 to 325 mg	Acetylates cyclooxygenase	Indefinite	Irreversible
Thienopyridines (clopidogrel)	300 to 600 mg Load 75 mg/day	Binds platelet ADP	1 to 9 mo	Irreversible
GPIIB/IIIA Inhibitors	Agent specific	Platelet IIB/IIIA Receptor	12 to 18 hr post-PTCI	Receptor
Anticoagulants				
Heparin	ACT specific	Indirect inhibition of thrombin	During PCI	60 to 90 min postinfusion
Low-molecular-weight heparin	Agent specific	Inhibition of factor Xa	During PCI	8 to 12 hr
Direct thrombin inhibitors	Agent specific	Direct inhibition of thrombin	During PCI	Slowly reversible

activation by irreversible acetylation of cyclooxygenase. It remains the foundation of antiplatelet therapy for PCI patients. When administered at least 24 and preferably up to 72 hours before the intervention in doses of 81 to 1500 mg, aspirin decreases thrombotic complications.[142]

The thienopyridines, ticlopidine (Ticlid) and clopidogrel (Plavix), block platelet activation by irreversibly binding to the ADP ($P2Y_{12}$) receptors. Ticlopidine was the initial thienopyridine used for PCI patients. However, side effects, including dyspepsia, neutropenia, and a small but clinically significant incidence of thrombotic thrombocytopenic purpura (TTP), led to its replacement by clopidogrel, which has a lower incidence of TTP.[143,144] Clopidogrel has been shown to be beneficial in patients with acute coronary syndromes for up to 9 months of therapy, both with and without PCI.[145] Clopidogrel for 1 month is standard therapy with bare metal stents, and for 3 to 6 months with drug-eluting stents.[146] As clopidogrel (and ticlopidine) is a prodrug, its onset of action is slow unless a loading dose is used. A loading dose of 300 mg of clopidogrel is ideally given at least 4 hours prior to the procedure. Recent work has shown it is possible to achieve more rapid platelet inhibition when a 600-mg bolus is administered.[147] In patients receiving either radiation therapy or drug-eluting stents, both of which have been shown to decrease endothelial overgrowth of the stent, clopidogrel has been shown to decrease stent thrombosis with prolonged therapy.[148]

Unfractionated heparin (UFH) has been used since the inception of PTCA. Traditional anticoagulant therapy for PCI was an initial heparin dose of 10,000 units. Currently, weight-adjusted heparin administration is routine. The activated coagulation time (ACT) is used to guide additional heparin therapy with the ACT in the range of 300 to 350 seconds for patients not receiving glycoprotein IIb/IIIa inhibitors and 200 to 250 seconds for patients receiving these inhibitors of platelet aggregation[149] (see Chapter 18). Protamine is not used, and the femoral sheaths are removed once the ACT is 150 seconds or less. Limitations of UFH include a variable antithrombotic effect requiring frequent ACT monitoring, inability to inhibit clot-bound thrombin, and concerns regarding heparin-induced thrombocytopenia syndrome (HITS); this has led to the search for a replacement for UFH.[150]

As an alternative to heparin, direct thrombin inhibitors have been investigated in the setting of PCI. The synthetic compound, bivalirudin (Angiomax; The Medicines Company), is the best studied of these agents. The advantage of the direct thrombin inhibitors is the direct dose response and the shorter half-life allowing for earlier sheath removal and less frequent bleeding complications. Two major PCI studies comparing UFH with bivalrudin have been performed to date. BAT (Bivalrudin Angioplasty Trial) randomized 2161 patients and supported the hypothesis that bivalirudin reduces ischemic complications and bleeding during PCI compared with UFH.[151] REPLACE-2 randomized 6010 patients and demonstrated similar clinical outcomes between bivalirudin and UFH with glycoprotein (GP) IIb/IIIa inhibition.[152] Major adverse cardiac events (MACEs) were similar between the two groups, but major bleeding was significantly less in the bivalrudin group. Argatroban is also approved for this use, although less data are available. Although easier to use than heparin, these agents are more expensive, and there is no currently known agent to reverse the effects of these new compounds (see Chapter 29).

Low-molecular-weight heparin (LMWH) is obtained by depolymerization of standard, unfractionated heparin. LMWHs were developed to overcome the limitations of UFH.[153] Enoxaparin (Lovenox) has been studied extensively in patients with acute coronary syndromes. Overall, enoxaparin use leads to a slight reduction in the occurrence of myocardial infarction when compared with UFH and has a similar side-effect profile.[154] In PCI, the NICE trials were registries of patients treated with enoxaparin instead of UFH during PCI.[155] Additionally, the SYNERGY trial was a randomized comparison of enoxaparin and UFH in patients presenting with an acute coronary syndrome in whom early catheterization was planned; about half of both groups underwent PCI.[156] Based on these and other smaller trials, enoxaparin and UFH seem to be associated with similar rates of cardiac events and bleeding complications when used during PCI. Thus, most interventionalists are comfortable with the use of enoxaparin for acute coronary syndromes and the management of patients receiving enoxaparin in the periprocedural period. However, UFH offers several advantages in the patient who arrives in the laboratory without prior antithrombin therapy: a shorter half-life, facilitating sheath removal; the ability to easily monitor its effect with the ACT; and the ability to reverse its effect with protamine.

Arterial thrombi are rich in platelets that aggregate in response to many stimuli. Aspirin inhibits only one of these pathways. The final common aggregation pathway is the IIb/IIIa glycoprotein on the platelet surface. Fibrinogen binds to this receptor to permit platelet aggregation. Several compounds target this receptor. The monoclonal antibody, abciximab (ReoPro) was the first GPIIb/IIIa inhibitor approved. Abciximab is used as a bolus followed by a 12-hour infusion. Bleeding times increase to more than 30 minutes with ex vivo platelet aggregation nearly abolished. The platelet binding of this compound is essentially irreversible, requiring more than 48 hours for normal platelet function to return. During the clinical trials of this agent, patients requiring emergency CABG experienced no significant increase in adverse events with platelet transfusions used to restore normal platelet function. In the EPIC study of high-risk PCI patients, abciximab reduced early ischemic complications by 35% and late events by 26%, with an increase in vascular complications.[157] In the EPILOG study, a similar benefit in lower risk interventional patients was seen.[158] Additionally, fewer vascular complications occurred when adjunctive heparin was used in lower doses and vascular access site management improved. Abciximab is more expensive, and its repeated use may lead to thrombocytopenia.[159]

The other GPIIb/IIIa inhibitor compounds, eptifibitide (Integrilin) and tirofiban (Aggrastat), are not antibodies but rather synthetic agents that bind reversibly to the IIb/IIIa receptor. Both have half-lives of approximately 1.5 hours in patients with normal renal function with normal hemostasis returning in under 6 hours after cessation of the medication.[160] Standard doses lead to very high plasma concentrations of these medicines; thus, platelet transfusion is less effective in correcting the hemostatic defect than with abciximab. Studies have identified the superiority of eptifibitide plus UFH to UFH alone in stable patients undergoing PCI, the superiority of abciximab plus UFH to UFH alone as well as the superiority of abciximab to tirofiban in more unstable patients undergoing PCI.[161,162] GPIs have not been proven beneficial in saphenous vein graft interventions.[163] Currently, the choice of GPIIb/IIIa inhibitor for the patient undergoing PCI is controversial. They are all expensive, but abciximab is the most expensive with a course of treatment costing about

$1500. A variety of factors, including patient acuity, presence or absence of diabetes, pretreatment with clopidogrel, use of bivalirudin, and cost enter into the decision of which, if any, GPIIb/IIIa inhibitor should be used. Adequate pretreatment with clopidogrel may provide a benefit in low-risk patients that is comparable to that from GPIs at a fraction of the cost.[164]

Thrombolytic therapy has been used for the treatment of ST-elevation acute myocardial infarction (STEMI) for more than 20 years. Although some of the early studies used intracoronary administration of thrombolytics, the need for a catheterization laboratory precluded widespread adoption, and intravenous administration of thrombolytics became standard treatment for STEMI. Several agents are available for intravenous treatment of STEMI, including streptokinase, anistreplase, alteplase, reteplase, and tenecteplase.[165] Alteplase, reteplase, and tenecteplase are recombinant variations of tissue plasminogen activator, and are all specific for fibrin (as opposed to fibrinogen). They differ primarily in their half-lives, a difference that affects the dosing regimens. Over the last 15 years, emergent PCI has evolved as an alternative to intravenous thrombolytics (vide infra). In the setting of PCI, adjunctive, intracoronary administration of thrombolytic agents may be detrimental.[166]

Outcomes: Success and Complications

In the 20 years of catheter-based interventional procedures, the marked improvement in success rates with simultaneous decrease in adverse events clearly reflects both the significant technologic advancement as well as increased operator experience. PCI was once considered successful with the luminal narrowing reduced to less than 50% residual stenosis.[167] In current practice with stent placement, seldom is a residual stenosis greater than 20% accepted, and excellent stent expansion without edge dissection is required prior to termination of the procedure.[127] The initial National Heart, Lung, and Blood Institute (NHLBI) PTCA registry from 1979 to 1983 reported a success rate of 61% and a major coronary event rate of 13.6%. The 1985 to 1986 NHLBI registry reported a success rate of 78%, with the incidence of AMI rate as 4.3% and emergency CABG rate as 3.4%.[168] In the stent era, success rates are over 90% and emergent surgery rates less than 1% in laboratories performing more than 400 PCIs.[168]

In a multicenter study of more than 8000 angioplasty patients from the 1980s, an overall cardiac mortality of 0.16% in elective cases was reported.[169] More recently, the Society for Cardiac Angiography and Interventions' registry data were published for the years 1991 to 1996. This revealed a success rate of 95%, an emergent CABG rate of 1.5%, and a mortality rate of 0.5%.[170]

The American College of Cardiology developed the National Cardiac Data Registry (NCDR) in the 1990s. Currently, approximately 400 of the more than 2100 laboratories in this country participate. Participation in ACC/NCDR requires a facility to dedicate an employee to data entry. Outcomes for both diagnostic and interventional procedures are tabulated, adjusted for baseline risk, and provided to the participating facility. Results for the most recent publication from ACC/NCDR are listed in Table 12–13.

The incidence of myocardial infarction is controversial and depends upon the definition of MI (new Q waves, total creatine kinase [CK] elevation, CK-isoform elevation, troponin).[171] Elevated CK levels occur in approximately 15% of catheter-based interventional procedures, with significant elevations (3-fold baseline) present in 8%.[171] These figures are even higher for interventions in saphenous vein grafts and with some devices. For years, routine enzymatic assessment of interventional procedural infarctions has been at the discretion of the operator. Some studies suggest that long-term outcome is adversely related to even small periprocedural elevations of CK ("infarctlets").[171] These elevations are reduced by GPIs.[158] Stone and colleagues recently published data from 7143 PCI patients.[172] In this study, CK-MB elevations of more than 8 times the upper limit of normal were predictive of death in the subsequent 2-year follow-up. However, smaller enzyme elevations, including a 17.9% 3-fold elevation of enzymes, proved to have no impact on survival.[172]

Table 12–13 Morbidity and Mortality for the PCI Patient

Complication	Outcome
Dissection	5%
Abrupt closure	1.9%
Successful reopening	41%
Angiographic success	94.5%
Post-PCI MI	0.4%
CABG	1.9%
Death	1.4%
Clinical success	92.2%
No adverse events	96.5%

From Anderson HV, Shaw R, Brindis RG, et al: A contemporary overview of percutaneous coronary interventions, the American College of Cardiology-National Cardiovascular Registry Data (ACC-NCDR). J Am Coll Cardiol 39:1096, 2002.

In 1988 and then revised in 1993, the ACC/AHA task force developed a lesion morphology classification in an attempt to correlate complexity of lesion with outcomes. This anatomic characterization of lesion complexity is outlined in Table 12–14. However, as operator experience and equipment advances have increased, complication rates have decreased across all subsets. A study in 1998 of more than 1000 consecutive lesions identified success rates for A, B1, and B2 lesions approximately equal (95% to 96%) and only C lesions having success rates of less than 90% (88%).[173] The Mayo Clinic devised a risk score for PCI and recently compared this to the ACC/AHA criteria in 5064 PCIs. They found that the ACC/AHA criteria better predicted success, while complications were better predicted with the Mayo classification.[174]

Intimal dissection was a significant issue in the pre-stent era, occurring in up to 10% of all PTCAs. *Propagation* of the intimal dissection is the leading cause of vessel occlusion during an intervention. Normally initiated by arterial disruption by the PCI device, it may also be caused by the guiding catheter or wire (Fig. 12–23). Stenting significantly reduces these events by approximating the intimal dissection flap and re-establishing flow down the true lumen.

Bifurcation lesions have become a significant area of interest in the stent era. With side-branch occlusion from displacement of plaque from the primary vessel lesion occurring in 1% to 20% of patients, bifurcation lesions often require attention to both the primary and secondary or branch vessel. Various techniques have been employed to protect the side branch, ranging from primary vessel stenting with balloon

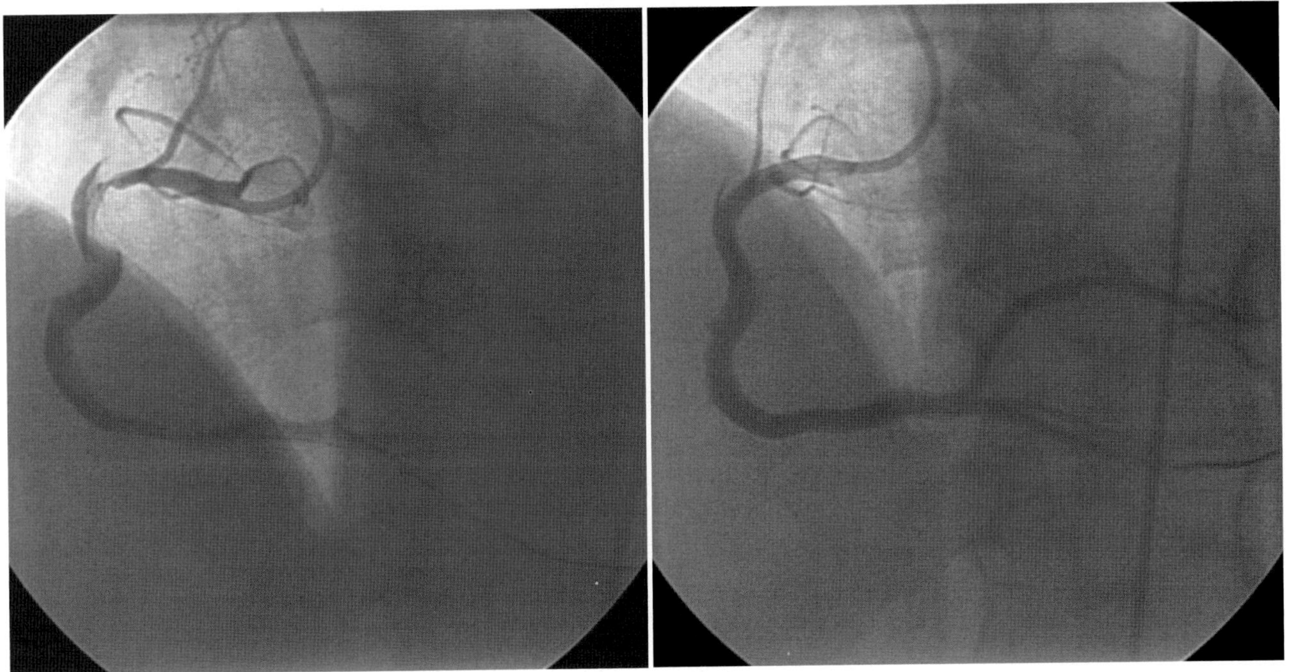

Figure 12–23 *(A)* Spiral dissection of the proximal right coronary artery (RCA) with extension of the dissection into the distal RCA severely impairing flow down the vessel. *(B)* Successful stenting of the right coronary artery dissection with flow re-established.

Table 12–14 Lesion-Specific Characteristics of Type A, B, and C Lesions*

Type A Lesions (Least Complex)	
Discrete (<10 mm length)	Little or no calcification
Concentric	Less than totally occlusive
Readily accessible	Nonostial in location
Nonangulated segment, <45 degrees	No major branch involvement
Smooth contour	Absence of thrombus
Type B Lesions (Intermediate)	
Tubular (10- to 20-mm length)	Moderate to heavy calcification
Eccentric	Total occlusions <3 mo old
Moderate tortuosity of proximal segment	Ostial in location
Moderately angulated, >45 segment degrees, <90 degrees	Bifurcation lesions requiring double guidewires
Irregular contour	Some thrombus present
Type C Lesions (Most Complex)	
Diffuse (>2 cm length)	Total occlusions >3 mo old
Excessive tortuosity of proximal segment	Inability to protect major side branches
Extremely angulated segments >90 degrees	Degenerated vein grafts with friable lesions

*American Heart Association/American College of Cardiology classification of lesion type.

From Ryan TJ, Bauman WB, Kennedy JW, et al: Guidelines for percutaneous transluminal angioplasty. J Am Coll Cardiol 22:2033, 1993, with permission.

dilation of the branch vessel through the stent struts to different types of branch vessel stenting. The "crush" technique involves stenting both the primary and branch vessels with excellent initial success rates, but side branch restenosis may be a problem[175] (see Fig. 12–29, in the Stents section). New "t"-shaped stents are under development.[176] Different debulking devices, including rotational atherectomy and the cutting balloon, have been utilized in attempts to reduce the plaque volume and prevent shifting.

The recognition of high-risk lesion and patient characteristics allows the cardiologist to better predict which patient is at increased risk for catheter-based interventional therapy. Although infrequent in current interventional practice, when the high-risk patient is identified, the cardiologist should share this information with the surgeon and anesthesiologist so that patient care is not compromised in the event of an emergency.

Operating Room Backup

When PTCA was introduced, all patients were considered candidates for CABG. The physicians' learning curve in the early 1980s was considered 25 to 50 cases; increased complications were seen during these initial cases.[18] All PCI procedures had immediate operating room (OR) availability, with the anesthesiologist often in the catheterization laboratory. In the 1990s, OR backup was needed less often. First, perfusion catheter technology developed to allow for longer inflation times with less ischemia.[177] The role for perfusion balloons and OR backup has diminished with the use of stents. With the current low incidence of emergent CABG, few institutions maintain a cardiac room on standby for routine coronary interventions.

Infrequently, high-risk interventional cases may still require a cardiac room on immediate standby. Preoperative anesthetic evaluation, which allows for preoperative assessment of the overall medical condition, past anesthetic history, current drug therapy, allergic history, and a physical examination concentrating on airway management considerations, is reserved for these high-risk cases.

As a less stringent policy for OR backup is required, PCI procedures are now performed in hospitals with no in-house cardiac surgery, though this is not standard practice and remains controversial.[178,179] Regardless of the location of the interventional procedure, when an emergency CABG is required, it is important to provide enough "lead" time to adequately prepare an OR. Additionally, since this happens infrequently, cooperation among the interventionalist, surgeon, and anesthesiologist is essential for optimal patient care in this critically ill population.

General Management for Failed Percutaneous Coronary Intervention

Several possible scenarios may result from a failed PCI (Box 12–9). First, the interventional procedure may not successfully open the vessel, but no coronary injury has occurred; the patient often remains in the hospital until a CABG can be scheduled. The second type of patient has a patent vessel with an unstable lesion. This most often occurs when a dissection cannot be contained by stents but the vessel remains open. The third patient type has an occluded coronary vessel following a failed PCI with stenting either not an option or unsuccessful. In this instance, myocardial ischemia/infarction ensues dependent upon the degree of collateralization.[180] This patient most commonly requires emergent surgical intervention.

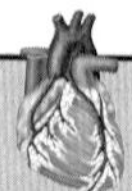

BOX 12–9 *Failed Intervention*

- Perform "usual" preoperative evaluation for emergent procedure
- Inventory of vascular access sites: pulmonary artery catheter, intra-arterial balloon pump
- Defer removal of sheaths
- Review medicines administered
  - Boluses may linger even if infusion stopped (e.g., abciximab)
  - Check medicines before catheterization laboratory (e.g., enoxparin, clopidogrel)
- Confirm availability of blood products

In preparation for the OR, a perfusion catheter, intra-aortic balloon pump, pacemaker, and/or PAC may be inserted dependent upon patient stability, OR availability, and patient assessment by the cardiologist, CT surgeon, and anesthesiologist. Although designed to better stabilize the patient, these procedures are at the expense of ischemic time. Once in the operating room, decisions on the placement of catheters for monitoring should take several details into consideration. If perfusion has been reestablished, and the degree of coronary insufficiency is mild (no ECG changes, absence of angina), time can be taken to place an arterial catheter and a PAC. *It must be remembered, however, that these patients have usually received significant anticoagulation with heparin and often glycoprotein IIb/IIIa platelet receptor inhibitors; attempts at catheter placement should not be undertaken where direct pressure cannot be applied to a vessel.* The most experienced individual should perform these procedures.

The worst scenario is the patient who arrives in the operating room either in profound circulatory shock, or full cardiopulmonary arrest. In these patients, cardiopulmonary bypass (CPB) should be established as quickly as possible. No attempt should be made to establish access for monitoring that would delay the start of surgery. The only real requirement to start a case such as this is to have good intravenous access, a five-lead ECG, airway control, a functioning blood pressure cuff, and arterial access from the PCI procedure.

In many cases of emergency surgery, the cardiologist has placed femoral artery sheaths for access during the PCI. *These should not be removed,* again because of heparin, and possibly GPIIb/IIIa inhibitor therapy during the PCI. A femoral artery sheath will provide extremely accurate pressures, which closely reflect central aortic pressure. Also, a PAC may have been placed in the catheterization laboratory, and this can be adapted for use in the operating room.

Several surgical series have looked for associations with mortality in patients who present for emergency CABG following failed PCI. The presence of complete occlusion, urgent PCI, and multivessel disease have all been associated with an increased mortality.[181]

In addition, long delays due to not having a rapid surgical alternative will lead to increases in morbidity and mortality. The paradigm shift in cardiovascular medicine toward PCIs and away from surgery will be slowed if significant numbers of serious complications occur due to prolonged delays in moving the patient to surgery.[182-185]

Support Devices for High-Risk Angioplasty

Numerous support devices for high-risk angioplasty have been used, including intraaortic balloon pumps and partial cardiopulmonary bypass via femoral cannula. National registries of elective angioplasty during partial cardiopulmonary bypass have reported that 95% of attempted vessels were successfully dilated with bypass support, but 39% of the patients incurred vascular complications.[186] In addition, 43% of the patients required transfusions. Tierstein et al compared cardiopulmonary support for high-risk angioplasty versus standby support.[187] Three hundred sixty-three patients were placed on cardiopulmonary support during angioplasty and 92 underwent standby support. The mortality in both groups was 6%.

There are several mechanical support devices under investigation in patients with cardiogenic shock that may ultimately be used in the high-risk intervention patient. The TandemHeart (CardiacAssist, Inc, Pittsburgh, PA) received CE mark approval in Europe and FDA 510(k) clearance in 2003. This device uses a cannula that is percutaneously inserted into the LA via a femoral vein and puncture of the interatrial septum. An extracorporeal pump then returns oxygenated blood to the arterial system, thereby unloading the left ventricle. The Impella Recover LP 2.5 System (Impella CardioSystems AG, Neuenhofer, Germany) is a 12.5 Fr catheter that is placed in the left ventricle. This device is inserted percutaneously and uses a transaxial flow pump to transfer up to 2.5 liters of blood per minute from the left ventricle to the ascending aorta.[188] Improved equipment and technique have made PCI safer. While this should reduce the need for mechanical support, it also permits sicker patients to be candidates for PCI (Fig. 12–24). Accordingly, the future role of mechanical support in the interventional suite remains to be determined.

Controversies in Interventional Cardiology

Therapy for Acute Myocardial Infarction: Primary Percutaneous Coronary Intervention Versus Thrombolysis

Thrombolytic therapy was introduced for AMI patients in the 1970s (Box 12–10). The decades of the 1980s and 1990s have seen extensive multicenter trials comparing the benefits of (1) thrombolytic therapy versus no thrombolytic therapy, (2) one thrombolytic agent compared with another, (3) different

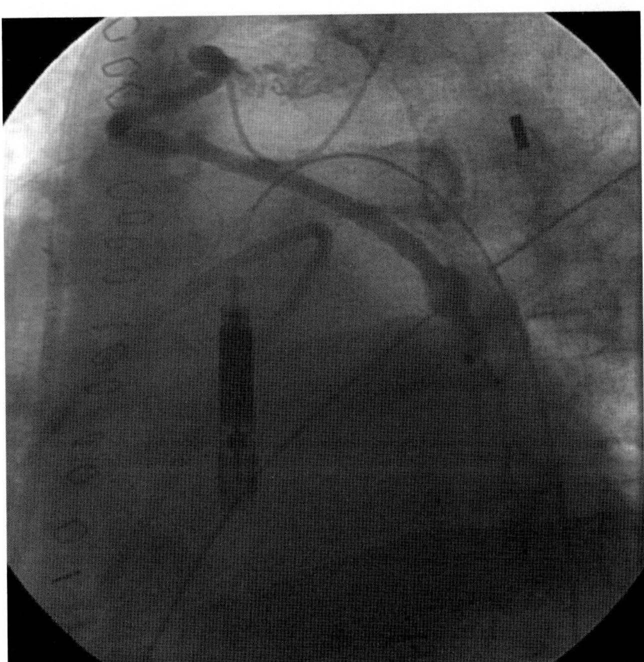

Figure 12–24 High-risk PCI with patient supported by the Impella system. A 62-year-old man, post-CABG, presented with AMI and severe hemodynamic instability refractory to maximal pressor therapy as well as an intra-aortic balloon pump. This figure illustrates Impella device in place during saphenous vein graft intervention of the LAD.

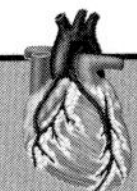

BOX 12–10 ***Coronary Intervention in Acute Myocardial Infarction (Primary Percutaneous Coronary Intervention [PCI] Versus Coronary Artery Bypass Graft [CABG] Surgery)***

- Thrombolytics preferred
  - Symptoms <3 hours
  - No contraindications
  - Would take >90 minutes until PCI (actual balloon inflation)
- Primary PCI preferred
  - Contraindications to thrombolytics (e.g., postoperatively)
  - Cardiogenic shock
  - PCI (balloon inflation) <90 minutes
  - Late presentations (probably)
  - Elderly (possibly)

adjunctive medications given with thrombolytic therapy (platelet GPIs, LMWHs, direct thrombin inhibitors), and (4) thrombolytic therapy versus primary PCI (bringing the patient directly to the catheterization laboratory).[165] Table 12–15 lists the currently available drugs used for thrombolytic therapy in AMI patients.

Before discussing thrombolytic therapy versus primary PCI for AMI, several issues must be considered. With contraindications to thrombolysis in approximately 60% of all AMI patients, PCI is often the only alternative to establish arterial patency in this group.[189] PCI has proved beneficial in patients with cardiogenic shock.[190-192] For patients who have not shown evidence of coronary reperfusion within 45 to 60 minutes following thrombolysis, cardiac catheterization and rescue PCI may be performed, particularly when large areas of myocardium are at risk (Fig. 12–25). Rescue PCI may improve outcome, particularly if done early.[193] However, other studies suggest that rescue PCI after failed thrombolysis, in the non-shock patient, may not improve 30-day survival or return of ventricular function, only decrease the need for subsequent revascularization.[194-196] Identification of reperfusion using noninvasive tests is difficult.[197] Resolution of ST-segment elevation may be the most accurate and rapid of the noninvasive markers of reperfusion, and it predicts mortality and reinfarction.[198] In patients with recurrent pain or clinical instability, cardiac catheterization following thrombolysis is often required.

Time to reperfusion is important, as long-term mortality is lowest and ventricular function improves the most when reperfusion occurs within 2 to 3 hours of symptom onset.[199] Postinfarction prognosis is also related to infarcted artery patency. Thus, strategies to promote early reperfusion are imperative, and may include prehospital protocols.[200] Transfer strategies for patients arriving in hospitals without interventional capabilities have been studied, and successful outcomes were seen when transfer times are less than 2 hours.[201]

The recently published guidelines by the ACC/AHA on management of patients with ST-elevation myocardial infarction emphasize early reperfusion and discuss the choice between thrombolytic therapy and primary PCI.[202] If a patient presents within three hours of symptom onset, the guidelines express no preference for either strategy with the following caveats: Primary PCI is preferred if (1) door-to-balloon time is less than 90 minutes and is performed by skilled personnel (operator annual volume more than 75 cases and laboratory volume more than 200 cases with 36 primary PCI); (2) thrombolytic therapy is contraindicated; and (3) the patient is in car-

Table 12–15 Current Thrombolytic Therapy

	Streptokinase	Alteplase	Reteplase	Tenecteplase
Abbreviation	SK	t-PA	r-PA	TNKase
Dose (>90 kg)	1.5 million U	100 mg	20 units	50 mg
$t_{1/2}$	23 min	<5 min	13 to 16 min	20 to 24 min
Infusion time	60 min	1.5 hr (double bolus)	30 min (double bolus)	Single bolus
Fibrin specificity	+	++	++	+++
Antigenicity	Yes	No	No	No
Concomitant heparin	No	Yes	Yes	Yes

Source: Lexi-Comp Online.

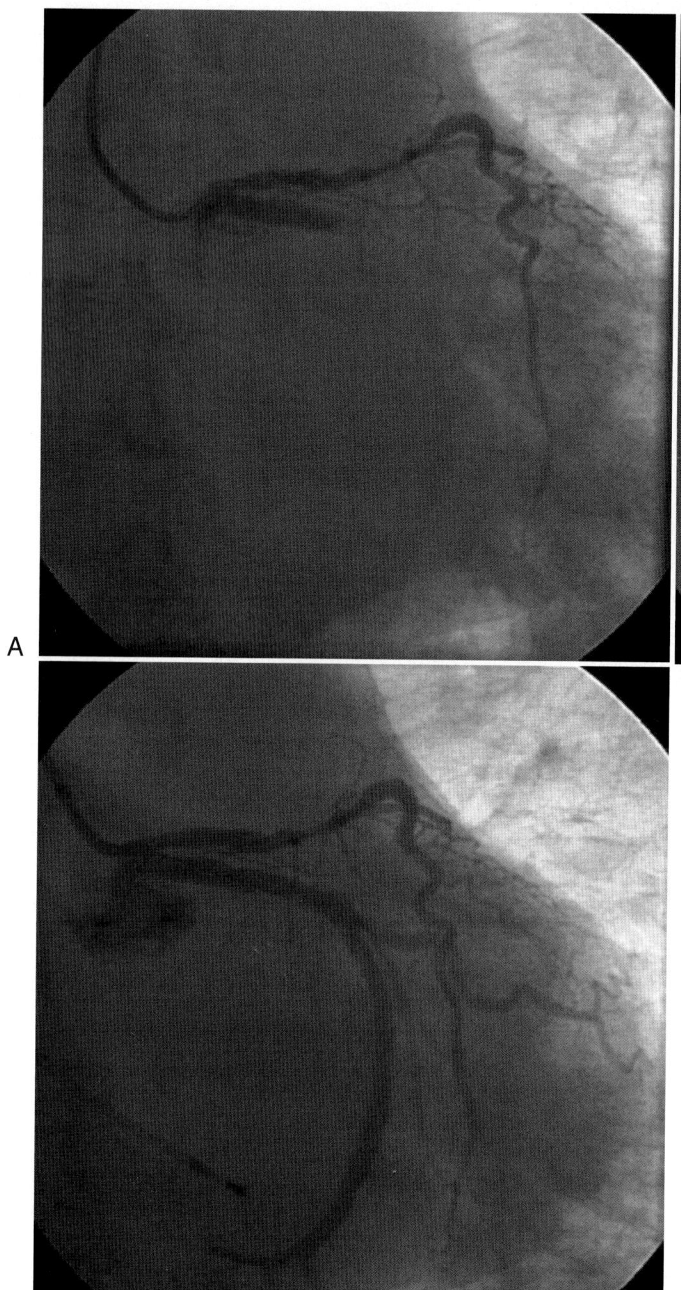

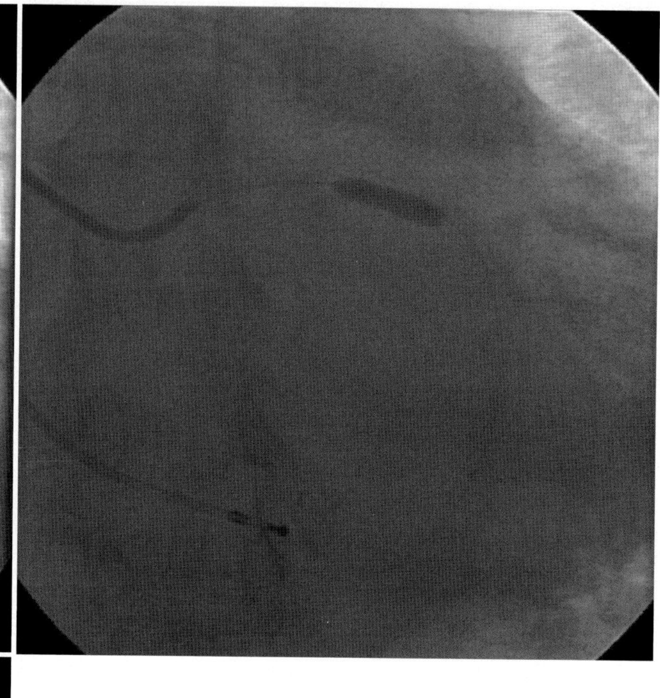

Figure 12–25 Acute myocardial infarction intervention. (*A*) Initial angiography reveals the large left circumflex artery (LCx) to be completely occluded shortly after its bifurcation with the left main. (*B*) Balloon inflation with stent deployment across the acute thrombosis. (*C*) Final angiography revealing a patent, dominant LCx artery.

diogenic shock. Thrombolytic therapy should be considered if symptom onset is less than 3 hours and door to balloon time is more than 90 minutes. Patients more than 75 years of age should be individually assessed, as they have a higher mortality from the MI but a higher risk of complications, particularly intracranial bleeding, with thrombolytic therapy.

Primary PCI is preferred when contraindications to thrombolytics exist and when patients present late. In the postoperative period, most patients will have contraindications to thrombolytic therapy. Thus, primary PCI is usually their best option. However, primary PCI requires the use of a short course of heparin and long course of aspirin. If these medicines cannot be given, primary PCI may not be possible. Ideally, primary PCI would include a GPIIb/IIIa inhibitor and stent placement, and the latter would include a course of clopidogrel. *If primary PCI is chosen, only the infarct-related artery should have the intervention in the acute case.*[202] This prevents the small potential for complications arising from other "elective lesions" compromising an already critically ill patient.

Facilitated PCI involves the administration of thrombolytic therapy, usually a reduced dose, with the intention of proceeding to PCI.[203] The PACT trial compared half-dose thrombolytic therapy to placebo in 606 patients with all patients proceeding to emergent PCI. Half-dose thrombolytic therapy was associated with improved vessel patency at catheterization, better ventricular function, and no increase in bleeding complications.[204]

All patients require risk stratification following myocardial infarction regardless of the method of reperfusion, and even, or perhaps especially, if they have not received reperfusion therapy. This includes an assessment of LV function and resid-

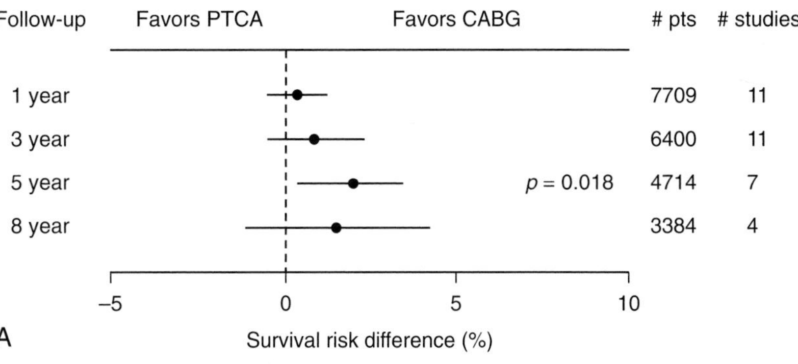

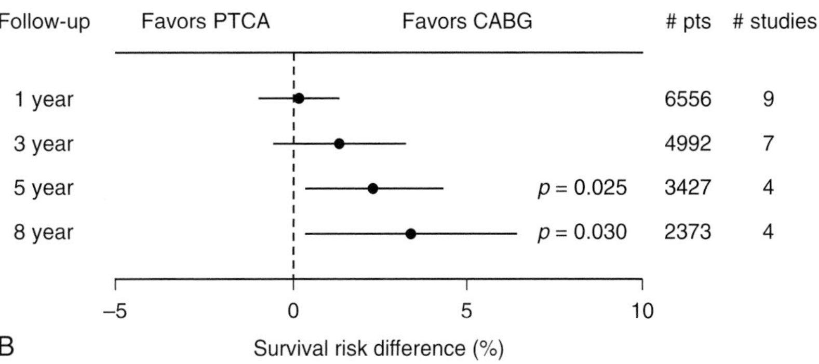

Figure 12–26 Randomized trials of coronary artery bypass graft surgery (CABG) versus coronary angioplasty (PTCA) in patients with multivessel coronary disease showing risk difference for all-cause mortality for years 1, 3, 5, and 8 post initial revascularization. (*A*) All trials. (*B*) Multivessel trials. CABG = coronary artery bypass graft surgery; PTCA = coronary angioplasty. (Redrawn from Hoffman SN, TenBrook JA, Wolf MP, et al: A meta-analysis of randomized controlled trials comparing coronary artery bypass graft with percutaneous transluminal coronary angioplasty: One- to eight-year outcomes. J Am Coll Cardiol 41:1293, 2003. Copyright 2003, with permission from The American College of Cardiology Foundation.)

ual burden of CAD. The incidence and extent of CAD in patients following thrombolysis were compiled from several large studies. In these patients, the following significant coronary lesions were present: left main in 5%, multivessel disease in 30%, single-vessel open in 35%, single-vessel closed in 15%, and minimal lesion in 15%. Obviously, the state of the other coronary arteries is assessed at the time of primary PCI. For patients treated with thrombolytic therapy or no reperfusion therapy, stress testing is an alternative method to assess the residual ischemic burden. The electrical stability of the heart must be addressed. In patients with a low ejection fraction following a myocardial infarction, prophylactic implantation of a defibrillator results in a 30% reduction in total mortality over 20 months.[205] Finally, modification of risk factors for CAD must be undertaken.

Acute MI therapy is evolving. With encouraging results from PCI in experienced hands when a facility is immediately available, more centers are considering acute primary PCI as standard of care, some in catheterization laboratories without OR backup.[206] Many patients present late or undergo thrombolytic therapy. If such patients are hemodynamically or electrically unstable, or if they have recurrent symptoms, a consensus would favor catheterization and revascularization. If such patients are stable, their management is controversial, although many cardiologists in the United States would recommend catheterization and revascularization.

PCI VERSUS CABG

The choice of therapy for multivessel CAD must be made by comparing PCI with CABG.[207] In the mid 1980s, when PCI consisted only of balloon PTCA, the first comparisons of catheter intervention to CABG were begun. By the early to mid 1990s, nine randomized clinical trials had been published comparing PTCA with CABG in patients with significant CAD. Only the BARI trial was statistically appropriate for assessing mortality.[20] These are summarized in Figure 12–26. The conclusions of these studies included similarities between the two approaches with respect to relief or angina and 5-year mortality. Costs were initially lower in the PCI group, but by 5 years had converged because of repeat PCI procedures precipitated by restenosis, occurring in 20% to 40% of the PCI group.[208]

The only clear difference between PCI and CABG for patients with multivessel disease was identified in the diabetic patient subset of the Bypass Angioplasty Revascularization Investigation (BARI) trial.[209-211] A difference in mortality was seen in a subgroup analysis of the BARI trial where both insulin-dependent and non–insulin-dependent diabetic patients with multivessel disease had a lower 5-year mortality with CABG (19.4%) than with PCI (34.5%).[211,212]

Regretfully, these trials were outdated by the time of their publication. For the patient undergoing PCI, stents had become the norm with a significant decrease in emergent CABG, due to reduced acute closure, as well as a decrease in repeat procedures, due to less restenosis.[127,129] For the patient undergoing CABG, off-pump bypass (OPCAB) became more common during this time period with its potential to decrease complications.[213,214] Additionally, the importance of arterial grafting with its favorable impact on long-term graft patency was recognized.[215,216]

To address the changes in PCI and CABG therapy, four more randomized trials were undertaken, and these are included in Figure 12–26. The results of these newer studies were similar to the results of the earlier ones. In the ARTS trial, diabetic patients had poorer outcomes with PCI. Repeat procedures, though higher in the PCI group at 20%, were significantly lower than with the earlier trials. CABG patients also had improved outcomes; for instance, cognitive impairment occurred in fewer patients in the recent studies.[208] A meta-analysis of all 13 randomized trials identified a 1.9% absolute survival advantage at 5 years in the CABG patients, but no significant difference at 1, 3, or 8 years.[217] As with the first generation of PCI versus CABG trials, the second-generation trials were outdated before publication due to the advent of the drug-eluting stents. The ARTS II and BARI II trials are now in progress and will address this issue.

Other contentious issues exist in the management of CAD. The roles of staged PCI procedures in patients with multivessel disease, ad hoc PCI, and combination procedures (LIMA to LAD and PCI of other vessels) have generated debate within the interventional and surgical communities.

In conclusion, the physician must weigh the data and explain the advantages and disadvantages of both techniques to their individual patient. CABG offers a more complete revascularization with survival advantages in selective groups and a decreased need for repeat procedures.[218] The disadvantages of a CABG are the higher early risk, longer hospitalization and recovery, initial expense, the increased difficulty of second procedures, the morbidity associated with leg incisions, and the limited durability of venous grafts. The current high cost of drug-eluting stents will negate the initial cost advantage of PCI if multiple stents are used. From the perspective of a hospital administrator in the United States, current reimbursement policies favor CABG over the placement of multiple drug-eluting stents.[182,219]

SPECIFIC INTERVENTIONAL DEVICES

Interventional Diagnostic Devices

Three intravascular diagnostic tools for the interventionalist are currently available. Angioscopy, the least applied of the three, offers the most accurate assessment of intravascular thrombus.[220] Cineangiography and intravascular ultrasound are often inadequate for visualization of thrombus. Although useful as an investigative technique, angioscopy has not entered into routine interventional practice.

Intravascular ultrasound (IVUS) is the only method by which the vessel wall of the coronary artery can be visualized in vivo. A miniature transducer mounted on the tip of a 3 Fr catheter is advanced over the standard guidewire into the coronary artery. The IVUS transducer is about 1 mm in diameter with frequencies of about 30 MHz. These high frequencies allow for excellent resolution of the vessel wall. By comparison, contrast angiography images only the lumen, with the status of the vessel wall inferred from the image of the lumen.[221] IVUS is useful in evaluating equivocal left main lesions, ostial stenoses, and vessels overlapping angiographically (Fig. 12–27).[222,223] IVUS is superior to angiography in the early detection of the diffuse, immune-mediated, arteriopathy of cardiac transplant allografts.[224]

IVUS has been used extensively in research, as it allows an excellent assessment of the post-PCI result and a precise quantitative assessment of restenosis.[225] As an adjunct to PCI, clinicians have utilized IVUS for years to assess the adequacy of stent deployment, the extent of vessel calcification, and the presence of edge dissections.[226,227] The quantitative capability of IVUS has been indispensable to researchers in preventive cardiology. It has allowed these researchers to document the benefits of aggressive lipid reduction using smaller numbers of patients and less time than would be possible with other techniques, as in the recently published PROVE-IT and REVERSAL Trials.[228,229]

Various physiologic measurements can be made in the catheterization laboratory during clinical diagnostic or interventional procedures.[230] The Doppler flow wire (Cardiometrics) was the first tool available for the interventionalist to determine the physiologic significance of an anatomic stenosis in the catheterization laboratory. Utilizing a 12-MHz

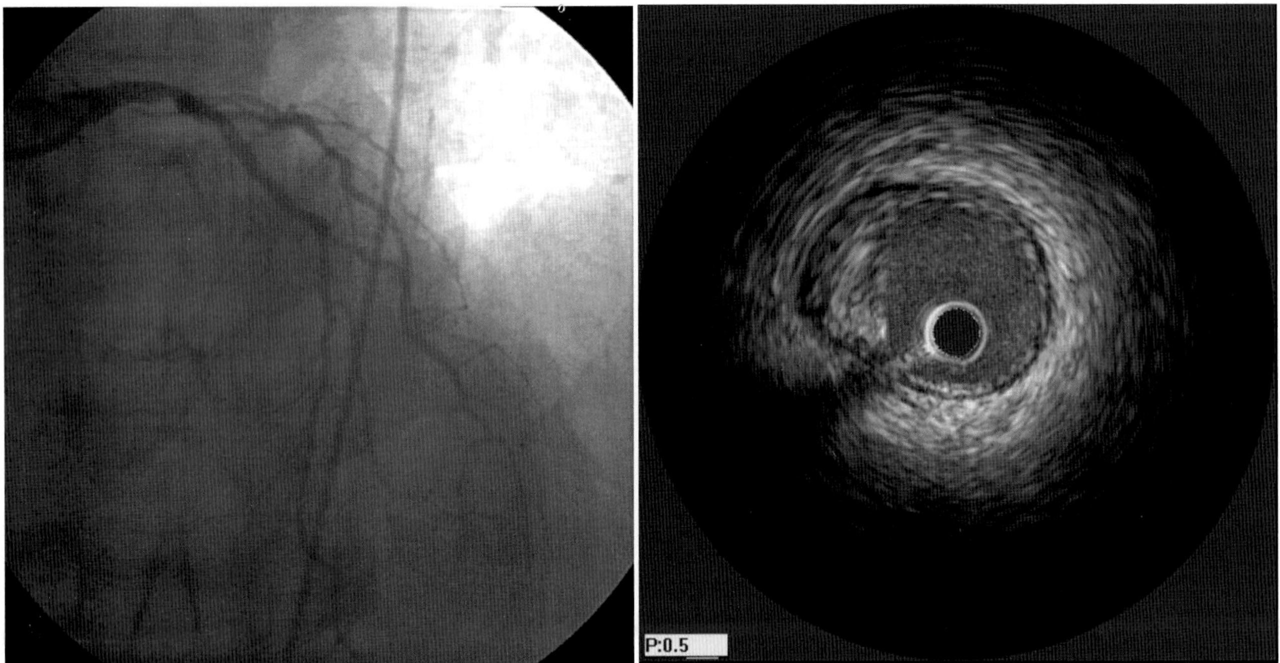

Figure 12–27 Intravascular ultrasound (IVUS). (*A*) Diagnostic angiography reveals a borderline occlusive lesion of 50% stenosis (by diameter) in the distal left main. (*B*) IVUS reveals an eccentric plaque to the left of the ultrasonographic catheter (central lucency) that is nonocclusive by both diameter and cross-sectional area.

piezoelectric ultrasound transducer on a 0.018-inch wire, it allows the measurement of coronary flow and coronary flow reserve.[231] By comparing this information to normal values, physiologic significance can be determined; these data compare favorably to stress-nuclear perfusion imaging. The interventionalist can then decide, during the diagnostic procedure, whether to proceed with PCI.[232]

In the mid 1990s, the pressure wire was introduced by Radi (Radi Medical Systems, Uppsala, Sweden). This wire has a pressure transducer near its tip, and permits measurement of a gradient across a stenosis. This gradient is measured during vasodilation after the administration of intracoronary adenosine. The ratio of pressures across a lesion during vasodilation is termed the *fractional flow reserve* (FFR). An FFR less than 0.75 signifies a significant stenosis and directs the interventionalist to proceed to PCI in a stenosis that is of borderline severity by angiography.[111] FFR has also been used to assess successful stent placement and can identify inadequate stent results predictive of restenosis.[112] Finally, a strategy of deferring PCI in patients with an FFR more than 0.75 has been tested and found to be associated with good clinical outcomes.[233]

Percutaneous Transluminal Coronary Angioplasty

When Andreas Gruentzig performed his first PTCA in 1977, the equipment was so large and bulky that he could dilate only lesions that were very proximal. Even if proximal, this equipment would not cross severe narrowings.[118] Over the last 25 years, balloon, guidewire, and guide catheter technology has advanced to allow the interventional cardiologist to place balloon catheters nearly anywhere in the arterial tree. Despite the development of new devices, "POBA" (plain old balloon angioplasty) is still an important component of the interventional procedure as it "paves the way" for stent implantation.

To better understand balloon angioplasty, the mechanism by which balloon inflation leads to vessel patency must be understood. Although four mechanisms have been described to explain the efficacy of this procedure (i.e., plaque splitting, stretching of the arterial wall, plaque compression, and plaque desquamation), the primary mechanism is *discrete* intimal dissection, which results in plaque compression into the media. Desquamation and distal embolization of superficial plaque components have been observed; however, experimental studies demonstrate this to be a minor contributor to the procedure's efficacy.[126] Propagation of the intimal dissection is the primary cause of vessel occlusion during angioplasty (see Fig. 12–23).

Although the mechanism of balloon angioplasty has not changed in 20 years, equipment and operator expertise have improved to the point that procedural success rates now exceed 90%.[170] These advances allow for the treatment of sicker patients and more complex coronary lesions while success rates continue to improve and complication rates decrease.[168]

Atherectomy Devices: Directional and Rotational

Atherectomy devices are designed to remove some amount of plaque or other material from an atherosclerotic vessel. Of these devices, directional coronary atherectomy (DCA; Guidant Corporation, Indianapolis, IN) became the first nonballoon technology to gain Food and Drug Administration (FDA) approval, in 1991. DCA removes tissue from the coronary artery, thus "debulking" the area of stenosis utilizing a low-pressure balloon located on one side of the metal housing, which when inflated, forces tissue into an elliptical opening on the opposite side of the housing. A cylindrical cutting blade shaves the tissue and stores it in the distal nose cone of the device. Although tissue removal is an attractive concept, application of DCA was limited by the need for large (9.5 to 11 Fr) guiding catheters with early devices. Trials comparing DCA with PTCA did not show improved angiographic restenosis rates, and higher rates of acute complications were seen with DCA.[234,235] Newer iterations of the device can be used with smaller (7 to 8 Fr) guiding catheters. DCA is used infrequently in most institutions because its clinical benefit is inconclusive.[236]

The FDA approved rotational coronary atherectomy in 1993. The Rotablator catheter (Boston Scientific Corp, Natick, MA) is designed to differentially remove nonelastic tissue, utilizing a diamond-studded burr rotating at 140,000 to 170,000 rpm. Designed to alter lesion compliance, particularly in heavily calcified vessels, rotational atherectomy is often used before balloon dilation to permit full expansion of the vessel.[237] The ablated material is emulsified into 5-micron particles, which pass through the distal capillary bed. Heavily calcified lesions are commonly chosen for rotational atherectomy (Fig. 12–28). Additionally, restenotic (in-stent), bifurcation, ostial, or nondilatable lesions are candidates for the Rotablator.[238] Contraindications to the Rotablator include poor ventricular function, thrombus, poor runoff, and lesions within saphenous vein grafts.[239]

The main limitation of rotational atherectomy is the "no-reflow" phenomenon. Thought secondary to particle load, this effect is associated with myocardial ischemia and occasionally infarction. Hemodynamic problems can occur, particularly in patients with depressed LV function. The frequency of "no reflow" has been reduced by shorter, slower ablation passes and variation in medications within the flush solution.[240] In heavily calcified vessels, rotational atherectomy may be the only device that can change the compliance of an artery and permit complete expansion of balloons and stents.[241,242] However, rotational atherectomy is more cumbersome and time consuming than balloon dilation. It is rarely used alone with PTCA, and stent placement is usually needed to achieve an adequate result. Therefore, though available in most interventional laboratories, rotational atherectomy is primarily relegated to vessels with significant calcification.

Cutting Balloon

Vessel wall damage during interventional procedures is generally considered the initiating factor for neointimal proliferation, which can ultimately lead to restenosis. All interventional technologies damage the vessel wall to varying degrees. In an attempt to decrease intimal injury, the cutting balloon (Boston Scientific Corp, Natick, MA) introduced the concept of microsurgical dilation. Whereas standard balloon PCI dilates haphazardly and can severely injure the arterial wall, the cutting balloon permits vessel expansion with lower pressure and less wall injury, thereby reducing the stimulus for restenosis.[243]

This device is a noncompliant balloon with three or four blades, depending on balloon size. These blades are 10 to 15 mm in length and 0.25 mm in size and attached to the

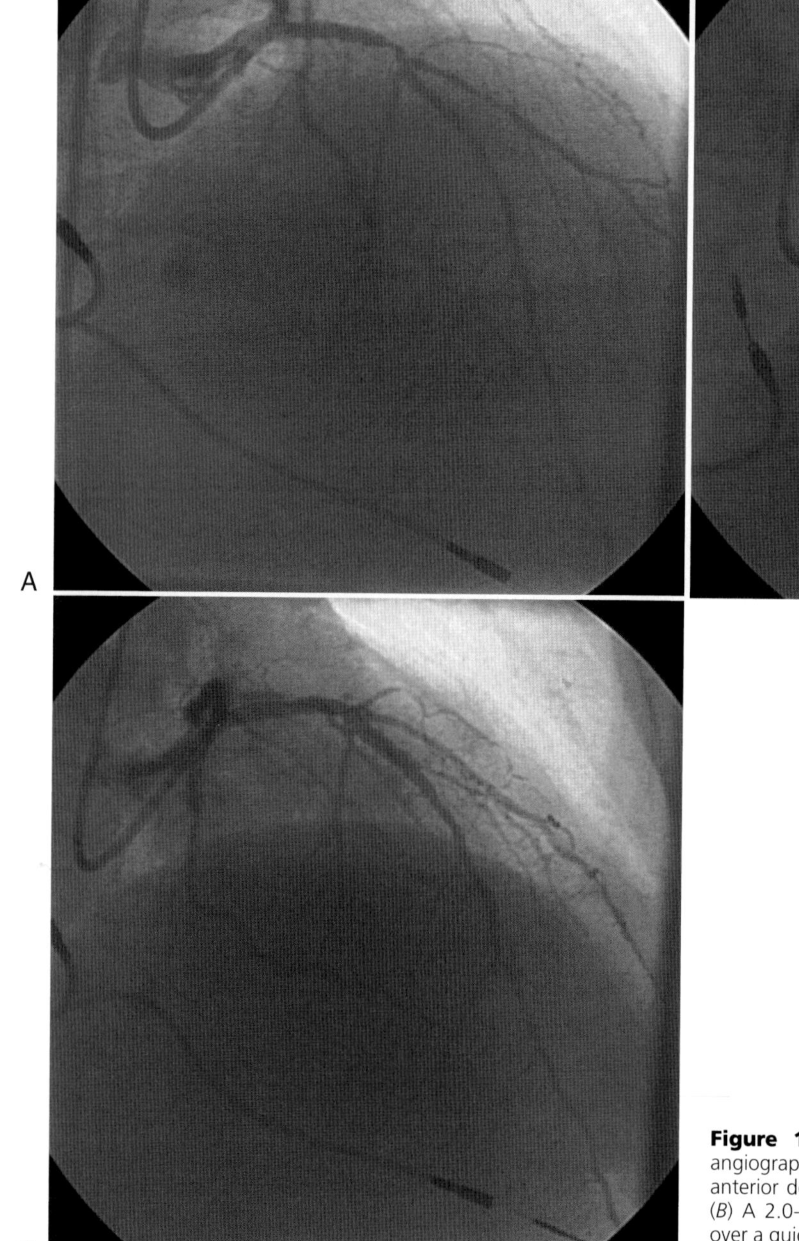

Figure 12–28 Rotational coronary atherectomy. (*A*) Diagnostic angiography reveals a complex and heavily calcified plaque in the left anterior descending artery (LAD) just proximal to the diagonal trunk. (*B*) A 2.0-mm burr rotating at 160,000 revolutions/min is advanced over a guidewire across the lesion. (*C*) Final angiography reveals a fully expanded vessel with preservation of the diagonal trunk.

balloon by a proprietary bond-to-bond manufacturing process. Once inflated, the balloon introduces these blades into the coronary intima, producing a series of tiny longitudinal incisions before balloon dilation. These microscopic cuts permit less traumatic vessel expansion. The safety and efficacy of this technique have been validated; however, there was no benefit compared with POBA when tested in a large group of patients.[244.] The cutting balloon is currently utilized for decreasing plaque shift in bifurcating lesions, changing artery compliance, and in treating in-stent restenosis.[245]

Intracoronary Laser

Excimer laser coronary angioplasty (ELCA) (Spectranetics, Colorado Springs, CO) uses xenon chloride (XeCl) and operates in the ultraviolet range (308 nm) to photochemically ablate tissue. Currently, ELCA is indicated for use in lesions that are long (>2 mm in length), ostial, in saphenous vein bypass grafts, and unresponsive to PTCA. With the development of the eccentric directional laser, treatment of eccentric or bifurcation lesions can be approached with increased success. Also, in-stent restenosis can be effectively treated with the excimer laser.[238] The Prima FX laser wire (Spectranetics, Colorado Springs, CO) is a 0.018-inch wire with the ability to deliver excimer laser energy to areas of chronic, total occlusion. With conventional equipment, failure to cross such lesions with a guidewire is frequent. The Prima FX has CE mark approval in Europe, but is investigational in the United States.[246] The optimal wavelength for the treatment of coronary atheroma has yet to be determined.

Other types of lasers have been used for various medical applications. The holmium:YAG laser (CardioGenesis, Foothill Ranch, CA) produces a wavelength in the mid-infrared spectrum.[247] The laser has been used in transmyocardial laser revascularization (TMLR), a procedure discussed later in this chapter.

Intracoronary Stent

The term *stent* was used first in reference to a dental mold developed by an English dentist, Charles Thomas Stent, in the mid nineteenth century. The word evolved to describe various supportive devices used in medicine.[248] To date, the introduction of intracoronary stents has had a larger impact on the practice of interventional cardiology than any other development.

The use of intracoronary stents exploded during the mid-1990s[249] (Box 12–11). Receiving FDA approval in April 1993, the Gianturco-Roubin (Cook Flex stent), a coiled balloon-expandable stent was approved for the treatment of acute closure after PCI. Use of the Gianturco-Roubin stent was limited by difficulties with its delivery and high rates of restenosis. The first stent to receive widespread clinical application was the Palmaz-Schatz (Johnson and Johnson, New Brunswick, NJ) tubular slotted stent approved for the treatment of de novo coronary stenosis in 1994.[250] Throughout the 1990s, multiple stents were introduced with improved support, flexibility and thinner struts, resulting in improved delivery and decreased restenosis rates (Fig. 12–29).[138,139]

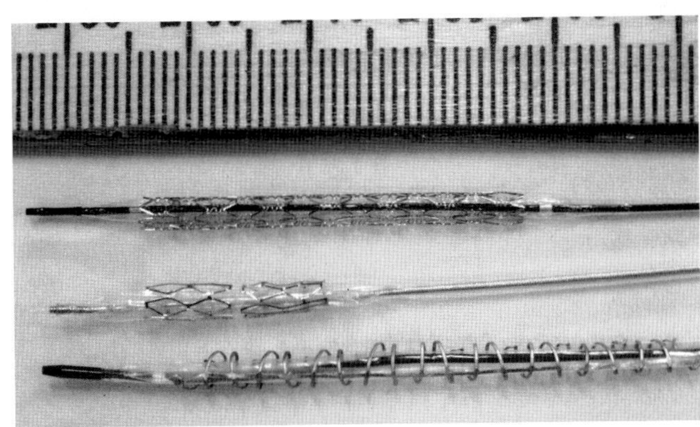

Figure 12–29 Evolution of stents: Three balloon-expandable bare metal stents are shown mounted on their delivery balloons with the above ruled marking in mms. *Bottom stent:* This is the first stent type introduced, the Gianturco-Roubin Flex-stent (Cook Cardiology, Bloomington, IN). The thick but pliable struts and low metal-to-artery ratio limited its effectiveness. *Middle stent*: The Palmaz-Schatz stent (Cordis/J&J, Warren, NJ) was the next stent type to be FDA approved for use other than acute closure. This consisted of two 8-mm relatively stiff slotted tube stents connected by a central strut. Although its introduction revolutionized PCI, its stiff structure and sheath covering limited delivery. *Top stent*: Newer stent designs produced smaller struts with increased flexibility for improved deliverability while maintaining the support structure required for long-term patency.

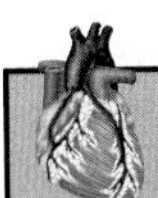

BOX 12–11 ***Stents***

- Antiplatelet therapy after stent placement
  Indefinite aspirin therapy plus.
  - Bare metal stent (BMS), clopidogrel 4 weeks
  - Cypher (sirolimus) stent, clopidogrel 3 months
  - Taxus (paclitaxel) stent, clopidogrel 6 months
- With bare metal stents, thienopyridines reduce subacute thrombosis from 3% to <1%.
- DES never tested without clopidogrel.
- Concern with DES is delay in endothelial coverage of stent, similar to brachytherapy.
- With clopidogrel, subacute thrombosis rates of DES and BMS are identical.
- Stents and elective surgery:
  - Delay until clopidogrel completed: recommended.
  - Perform during clopidogrel therapy: accept bleeding risk.
  - Discontinue clopidogrel early: not recommended.

As discussed earlier, the major limitations of catheter-based interventions had been acute vessel closure and restenosis. Stents offered an option for stabilizing intimal dissections while limiting late lumen loss, major components of acute closure and restenosis, respectively. Clinical trials have demonstrated the ability of stents not only to salvage a failed PTCA (thus avoiding emergent CABG [see Fig. 12–23]) but also to reduce restenosis.[251] Multiple studies demonstrated the benefit of stenting compared with PTCA alone in a variety of circumstances, including long lesions, vein grafts, chronic occlusions, and the thrombotic occlusions of AMI. Only in small vessels did stenting not demonstrate a restenosis benefit when compared with balloon angioplasty.[252-254] Clinical restenosis rates fell from 30% to 40% with PTCA to less than 20% with bare metal stents (BMS).[250]

Stent technology improved in incremental fashion. Modifications in coil geometry, alterations in the articulation sites, and the use of mesh-like stents offered minor advantages.[137] Different metals, such as tantalum and nitinol, were used and various coatings were applied, such as heparin, polymers, or even human cells.[138] In addition, the delivery systems that are used to implant stents have decreased in size.[139] Stent procedures, once requiring 9 Fr guiding catheters, can now be done through 5 to 6 Fr catheters. This even permits coronary stenting to be done through the radial artery.[39,54]

With the realization that restenosis involves poorly regulated cellular proliferation, researchers focused on medicines that had antiproliferative effects. Many of these medicines are toxic when given systemically, a tolerable situation in oncology, but not for a relatively benign condition like restenosis. For such medicines, local delivery was attractive, and the stent provided a vehicle.

Rapamycin, a macrolide antibiotic, is a natural fermentation product produced by *Streptomyces hygroscopicus*, which was originally isolated in a soil sample from Rapa Nui (Easter Island).[255] Rapamycin was soon discovered to have potent immunosuppressant activities, making it unacceptable as an antibiotic but attractive for prevention of transplant rejection. Rapamycin works through inhibition of a protein kinase called the mammalian target of rapamycin (mTOR), a mechanism that is distinct from other classes of immunosuppressants. Since mTOR is central to cellular proliferation as well as immune responses, this agent was an inspired choice for a stent coating. The terms *rapamycin* and *sirolimus* are often used interchangeably. A metal stent does not hold drugs well and permits little control over their release. These limitations required that polymers be developed to attach a drug to the stent and to allow the drug to slowly diffuse into the wall of the blood vessel, while eliciting no inflammatory response.[256]

The development of drug-eluting stents would not have been possible without these (proprietary) polymers. This led to the true revolution in PCI, which occurred with the approval in April, 2003 of the first drug-eluting stent (DES).[257] Johnson and Johnson/Cordis introduced their Cypher stent. This is their Velocity stent and polymer, which elutes rapamycin over 14 days; the drug is completely gone by 30 days postimplantation.[255]

The RAVEL trial randomized 238 patients to receive either a sirolimus-eluting stent (SES) or a bare metal stent (BMS). Remarkably, there was no restenosis in the group that received a sirolimus-eluting stent.[258] The SIRIUS Trial randomized 1058 patients to a sirolimus-eluting stent or a BMS. At 9 months restenosis rates were 8.9% in the SES group and 36.3% in the BMS group, with no difference in adverse events. Clinically driven repeat procedures were required in 3.9% and 16.6%,[20] respectively. This benefit was sustained, if not slightly improved at 12 months.[259] Although initially approved only for use in de novo lesions in native vessels of stable patients, subsequent publications have shown similar benefits in every clinical scenario that has been studied.[260-264] Initial concerns regarding subacute stent thrombosis (SST) have proved unjustified with the rate of SST approximately 1%, equal to that seen in BMS patients.[257]

The next DES to receive FDA approval in March of 2004 was the Taxus stent (Boston Scientific Corp). The Taxus stent uses a polymer coating to deliver paclitaxel, a drug that also has many uses in oncology. This is a lipophilic molecule, derived from the Pacific yew tree *Taxus brevifolia*. It interferes with microtubular function, affecting mitosis and extracellular secretion, thereby interrupting the restenotic process at multiple levels.[265] The Taxus IV study randomized 1314 patients to the Taxus stent or a bare metal stent. Angiographic restenosis was reduced from 26.6% in the BMS group to 7.9% in the Taxus group with no significant difference in adverse events. Clinically driven repeat procedures were required in 12.0% and 4.7% respectively.[266]

When first introduced, stents were sparingly used primarily due to the initial aggressive anticoagulation regimens recommended. These regimens included intravenous heparin and dextran along with oral aspirin, dipyridamole, and warfarin. This required long hospitalizations and led to bleeding problems at vascular access sites. These complicated combinations of medicines were used in the clinical trials that led to the approval of the stents, and were chosen based on the fear of thrombosis and limited animal data. Despite the use of these drugs, stent thrombosis still occurred in 3% to 5% of patients. The use of intracoronary ultrasound improved stent deployment by revealing incomplete expansion with conventional deployment techniques. This led to high-pressure balloon inflations, complete stent expansion, and simplified pharmacologic therapy.[267]

Initially aspirin and ticlopidine (Ticlid) were used instead of warfarin, but clopidogrel (Plavix) replaced ticlopidine because it has a better side-effect profile. The combination of a thienopyridine and aspirin has markedly reduced thrombotic events and vascular complications.[146] The timing and dosing of clopidogrel therapy are still evolving with doses of 300 to 600 mg given at least 2 to 4 hours prior to PCI.[147] Given that PCI is often performed immediately after a diagnostic study, some cardiologists begin clopidogrel before diagnostic studies. PCI can be performed immediately after the diagnostic study with a reduction in adverse events that is comparable to that seen with GPIs but at a fraction of the cost.[164] However, if the diagnostic study indicates a need for CABG, bleeding complications will be increased if clopidogrel has been given during the 5 days before CABG.[145]

Currently, stents are placed at the time of most PCI procedures, if the size and anatomy of the vessel permit (Fig. 12–30). There are several reasons not to use a DES in every procedure. First, DESs are available in fewer sizes. Second, a longer course of thienopyridine is required, and this may not be desirable if, for instance, a surgical procedure is urgently needed. Stent thromboses, myocardial infarctions, and deaths have been reported when antiplatelet therapy is interrupted.[268,269] Finally, the cost of a DES is about three times that of a BMS, and this increment is not fully reflected in reimbursement. As additional DESs reach the market, prices may decline. With the significant reduction in restenosis, DES may give PCI an advantage over CABG in multivessel disease.[266] The consequences of this may be dramatic, as hospitals (and cardiac surgeons and cardiac anesthesiologists) see reduced CABG volumes and reduced volumes of repeat PCI in restenotic vessels. If these profitable procedures are replaced by money-losing ones, as placement of multiple DESs currently is, many hospitals will suffer.[270]

Intravascular Brachytherapy

Brachytherapy was first introduced and developed for the treatment of malignant disease. In an attempt to decrease the neointimal proliferative process associated with restenosis, brachytherapy has been applied to the coronary artery. Two types of radiation are utilized in the coronary arteries: gamma and beta. Gamma-radiation, such as that from Ir-192, has no mass, only energy; therefore, there is limited tissue attenuation.[271] Beta-emitters, such as P-32 and Y-90, lose an orbiting electron or positron; the mass of this particle permits significant tissue attenuation.[271]

Radiation safety for the patient, staff, and operator is essential for intravascular brachytherapy. For the staff and the operator, radiation exposure is related to both the energy of the isotope and the type of emission. Staff exposure is much higher with gamma-emitters than with the beta-emitters, due to its insignificant tissue attenuation.[272] From the patient's perspective, brachytherapy is prescribed to provide a specific dose to the target vessel. Total body exposure is higher with gamma radiation, again because attenuation is minimal. As gamma radiation requires significant extra shielding and requires the staff to leave the room during delivery of therapy, beta radiation is used more commonly. Additionally, the long-term effects from patient exposure need to be considered.[271] Finally, significant expertise is required for intracoronary brachytherapy. In addition to the interventionalist, a radiation oncologist, medical physicist, and radiation safety officer must participate in these procedures.[272]

Brachytherapy, using either a gamma- or beta-emitter, has proved effective for the treatment of in-stent restenosis.[273,274] Following brachytherapy, clopidogrel must be continued for at least 6 to 12 months to prevent late stent thrombosis that occurs due to delayed endothelialization of the stent. The future for brachytherapy in the era of drug-eluting stents is unknown.[275] DES has significantly decreased in-stent restenosis. If restenosis does occur with DES, whether brachytherapy should be undertaken or repeat DES performed is unclear. Due to the complexity of brachytherapy, unless it is truly proved superior to other modalities, its use in the interventional suite will be limited.

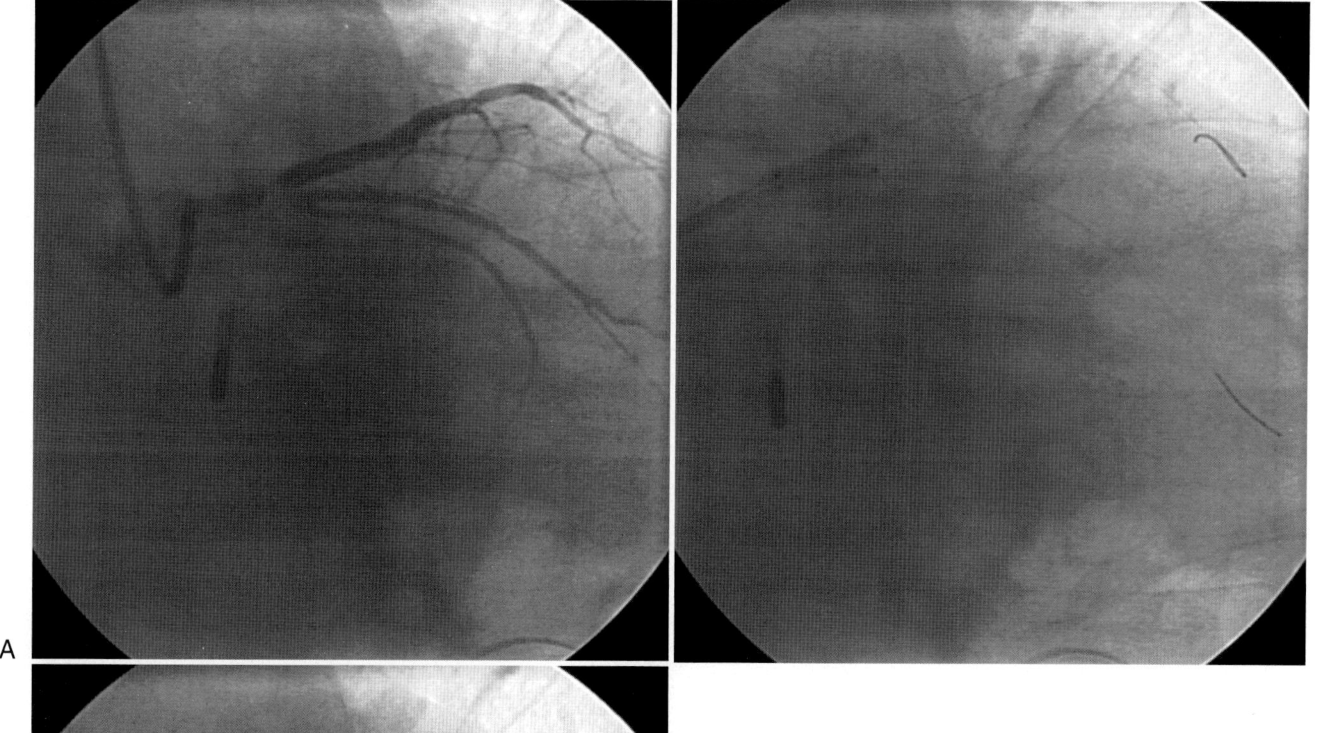

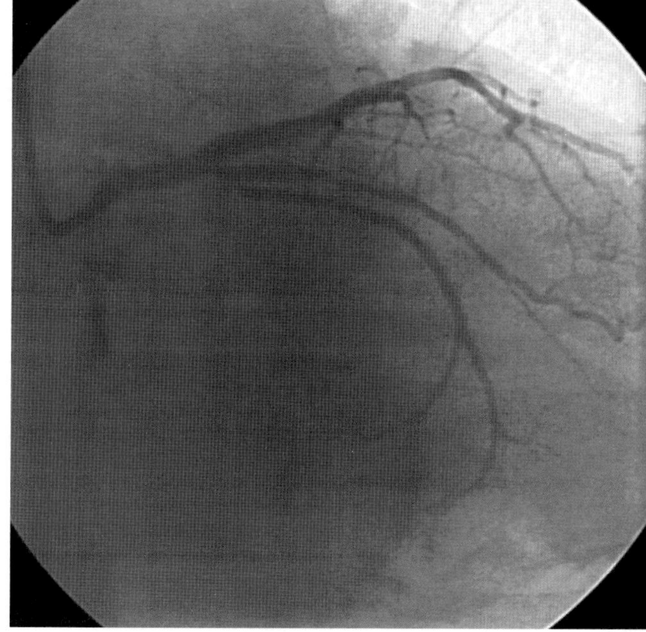

Figure 12–30 Stenting of a left main coronary artery in a nonsurgical patient with a bifurcation stenting approach, the "crush technique." (*A*) Initial angiography reveals a 90% stenosis involving the distal left main as well as the proximal left anterior descending (LAD) and left circumflex (LCx) arteries. (*B*) Simultaneously, separate stents are equally positioned from the mid left main into the LAD and LCx, respectively. First, the LCx stent is deployed and the stent delivery balloon and the LCx guidewire removed. Next, the LAD stent is deployed, "crushing" the LCx stent within the left main. Finally, the LCx guidewire is advanced through the side struts of the LCx stent and a final balloon inflation is performed simultaneously in a "kissing balloon" fashion. (*C*) Angiography reveals patent left main, LAD, and LCx arteries.

Thrombosuction/Thrombolysis

The transluminal extraction catheter (TEC) was released for use in 1993 as the first device designed to mechanically remove thrombus or other loose debris and was designed primarily for degenerated saphenous vein grafts. The TEC device was a hollow tube with a propeller-like blade on its tip that required the use of a large specially designed (10 Fr) guiding catheter. Proximal suction was applied to the rotating tube so it cut and aspirated as it was advanced into the lesion. Although an important tool when first introduced, newer thrombectomy devices have replaced this tool in the interventional suite.[276,277]

The AngioJet rheolytic thrombectomy system (Possis Medical, Minneapolis, MN) creates a Venturi effect utilizing six high-velocity saline jets distally at a pressure of 2500 psi and a flow rate of 50 mL/min to generate a low-pressure zone (less than −600 mm Hg) and cause a powerful vacuum effect. The catheter is a multilumen 4-Fr system and may be passed through a 6-Fr guiding catheter. One lumen delivers the saline, a second lumen is for guidewire passage, and a third permits thrombus evacuation utilizing a roller pump.

The system creates a recirculation pattern at the catheter tip. This emulsifies and removes thrombus without embolization. Rheolytic thrombectomy was first approved for saphenous vein grafts, utilizing a larger 6-Fr catheter. It can remove thrombus from native arteries (Fig. 12–31) and SVGs; however, some trials suggest that it may be less effective than alternative therapies for SVGs.[278-280] Although initial studies in small patient populations were encouraging for AMI patients, the recently reported but as yet unpublished AiMI

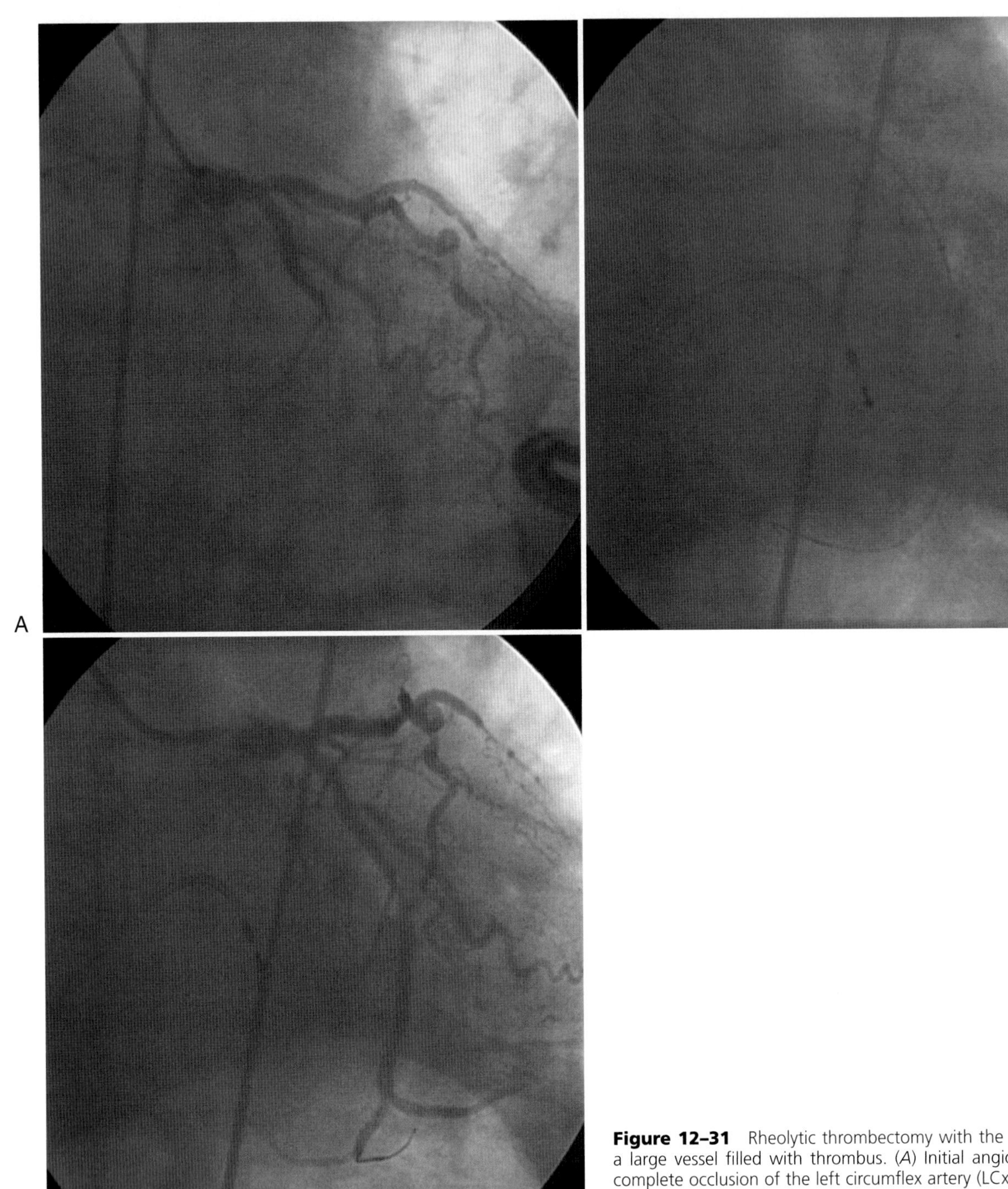

Figure 12–31 Rheolytic thrombectomy with the Possis catheter in a large vessel filled with thrombus. (*A*) Initial angiography reveals a complete occlusion of the left circumflex artery (LCx). (*B*) A guidewire is advanced across the thrombotic lesion with the Possis catheter ready for pullback. (*C*) Thrombectomy reveals the culprit LCx lesion with restoration of flow distally. The vessel was subsequently stented.

trial of 480 patients presenting within 12 hours of the onset of MI revealed higher mortality in the rheolytic thrombectomy group.[281,282] Despite these findings, this therapy remains the best option in lesions with a significant thrombus burden.[283]

Ultrasound thrombolysis is under development for the treatment of degenerated SVGs. However, the ATLAS trial in patients presenting with acute coronary syndromes and undergoing interventions in SVGs showed a higher incidence of ischemic complications with ultrasound thrombolysis.[284]

Distal Protection Devices

PCI in degenerative vein grafts is complicated by a significant incidence of myocardial infarction that is thought to result from embolization of debris. GPIIb/IIIa inhibition has not decreased myocardial infarction in this situation.[163] Although other factors, such as spasm in the distal arterial bed, may contribute to the complications during PCI in SVGs, most efforts to address this problem have focused on devices that are designed to capture potential embolic debris released as the probable cause of the "no-reflow" phenomenon during PCI. These distal protection devices come in two types: vessel occlusive and vessel nonocclusive.

Vessel-occlusive devices use a soft, compliant balloon that is incorporated into a wire. The wire is passed distal to the stenosis and inflated during the PCI. A column of blood is trapped, which includes the debris liberated during PCI. The blood and debris are aspirated before deflation of the distal balloon and restoration of flow. The GuardWire is an FDA-approved device of this type (Medtronic, Inc, Minneapolis, MN). In the SAFER Trial, 801 patients undergoing PCI in SVGs were randomized to distal protection with the GuardWire or no distal protection. The composite end-point of death, myocardial infarction, and repeat target vessel revascularization was 9.6% in the GuardWire group and 16.5% in the standard care group. Myocardial infarction was reduced by 42% in the distal protection group.[279]

A learning curve exists with this device to maximize prevention of emboli and minimize ischemic time. Patients with large areas of myocardium supplied by the SVG undergoing PCI may not be candidates due to the inability to tolerate ischemia. Also, distal lesions in an SVG may not allow for placement of the large balloon. The EMERALD trial tested the GuardWire in the setting of primary PCI of native vessels during AMI. The thrombotic AMI lesion seemed likely to benefit from aspiration of debris. However, this study showed no benefit from the device—a result attributed to the presence of side branches that are not present in SVGs.[285]

Other balloon-occlusive devices are available or in development. The Tri-Active system (Kensey-Nash) is a balloon-protected flush extraction system using distal occlusion. The recently completed but unpublished PRIDE study randomized 631 patients to either the Tri-Active device or the GuardWire. Noninferiority criteria were met, and this device is under consideration for FDA approval.

Nonocclusive devices include various forms of filters, as well as the thrombolysis or thrombectomy devices discussed above.[286] The Filter Wire (Boston Scientific) was the first filter approved. This is a 0.014-inch guidewire that incorporates a nonoccluding, polyurethane, porous membrane filter (80-micron pores). The system includes a retrieval catheter that fits over the device after PCI is completed (Fig. 12–32). Two clinical trials, the first compared with PCI alone and the second randomizing the Filter Wire EX to the GuardWire, have been completed to date.[287,288] The Filter wire was superior to PCI alone and noninferior to the GuardWire system. However, the device may not fully deploy against the vessel wall, and a new iteration of the device is currently in clinical trials.

The Rubicon Filter is an investigational device that can be placed without a delivery catheter, unlike the Filter Wire. As new devices appear, choices will be made based on ease of use, completeness of debris retrieval, amount of debris trapped before the filter is "clogged," and prevention of myocardial infarction. Filter devices are being used during interventions in the carotid arteries, a situation in which the prevention of embolization is critical and flow interruption is tolerated poorly.

Therapy for Chronic Total Occlusions

Despite steady progress in most areas of interventional cardiology, therapy for chronic total occlusions has lagged.[289] Chronic total occlusions (CTO) are defined as vessels that have been occluded for more than 3 months. They are often associated with significant collateral flow from other vessels, and are often treated conservatively (medical therapy). Guidewires with stiff tips and improved techniques have led to success rates over 70%.[289] Patients with CTO who were successfully revascularized had better long-term outcomes than those who could not be revascularized.[290,291]

Other devices for CTO are in various stages of development. The Frontrunner (LuMend, Inc. Redwood City, CA) is a bioptome-like cutting device designed to selectively remove fibrous tissue from within the lumen.[292] The Prima FX laser wire (Spectranetics, Colorado Springs, CO) has the ability to deliver excimer laser energy from the tip of the wire. The Prima FX has CE mark approval in Europe, but is investigational in the United States. As technology advances and operator experience accumulates, CTO interventions will continue to expand.

OTHER CATHETER-BASED PERCUTANEOUS THERAPIES

Percutaneous Valvular Therapy

Mitral Balloon Valvuloplasty

Percutaneous mitral valvuloplasty (PMC) was first performed in 1982 as an alternative to surgery for patients with rheumatic mitral stenosis. The procedure is usually performed via an antegrade approach and requires expertise in transseptal puncture. During the early years of PMC, the simultaneous inflation of two balloons in the mitral apparatus was required to obtain an adequate result. The development of the Inoue balloon (Toray, Inc, Houston, TX) in the 1990s simplified this procedure. This single balloon, with a central waist for placement at the valve, does not require wire placement across the aortic valve.[293]

The key to mitral valvuloplasty is patient selection. Absolute contraindications to mitral valvuloplasty include: a known LA thrombus or recent embolic event of less than 2 months and severe cardiothoracic deformity or bleeding abnormality preventing transseptal catheterization. Relative contraindications include significant MR, pregnancy, concomitant significant aortic valve disease, or significant CAD.[294]

All patients must undergo TEE to exclude LA thrombus as well as transthoracic echocardiography (TTE) to classify the patient by anatomic groups. The most widely used classification, the Wilkins score, addresses leaflet mobility, valve thickening, subvalvular thickening, and valvular calcification. These scoring systems, as well as operator experience, predict outcomes. In experienced hands, the procedure is successful in 85% to 99% of cases. Risks of PMC include a procedural mortality of 0% to 3%, hemopericardium in 0.5% to 12% and embolism in 0.5% to 5%. Severe MR occurs in 2% to 10% of procedures and often requires emergent surgery.[295] Although peripheral embolization occurs in up to 4% of patients, long-term sequelae are rare.

The procedure requires a large puncture in the interatrial septum, and this does not close completely in all patients. However, a clinically significant ASD with Q_p/Q_s of 1.5 or greater occurs in 10% or fewer of cases; surgical repair is seldom necessary. Advances in patient selection, operator experience, and equipment have significantly reduced procedural complications.[295] Restenosis rates are dependent on the degree of commissural calcium.[293] TEE or intracardiac

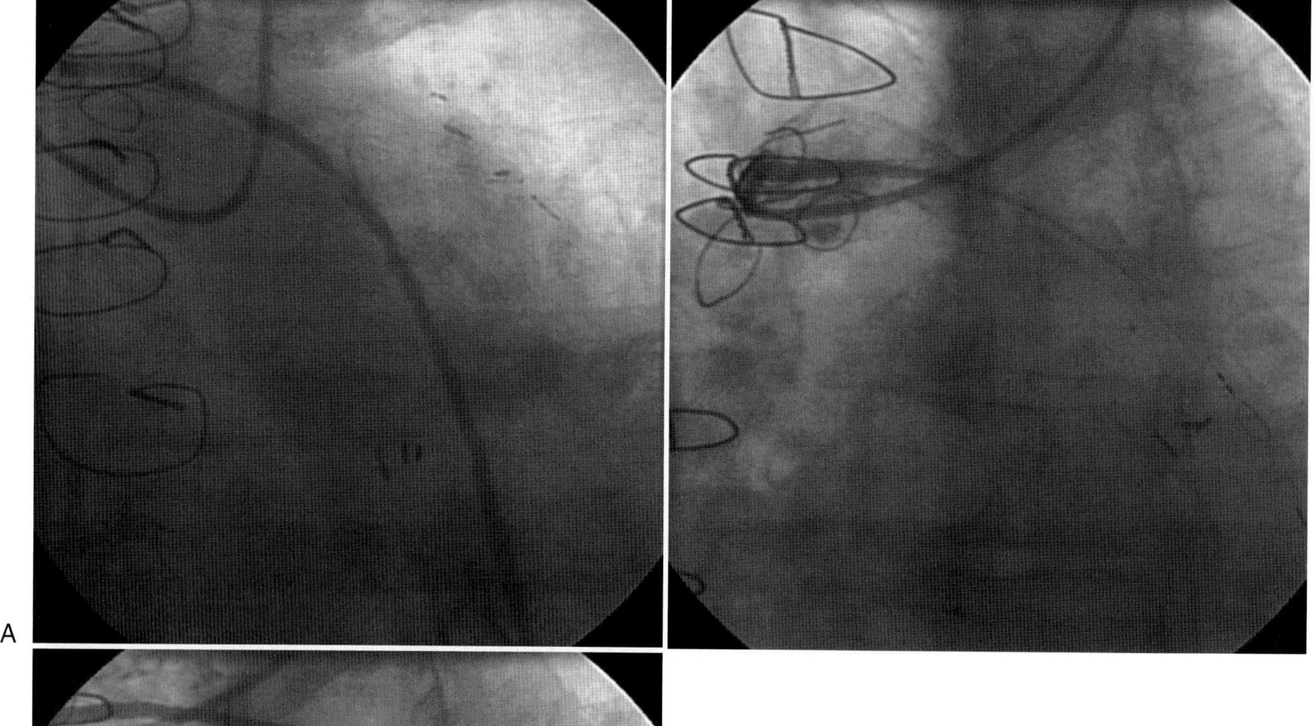

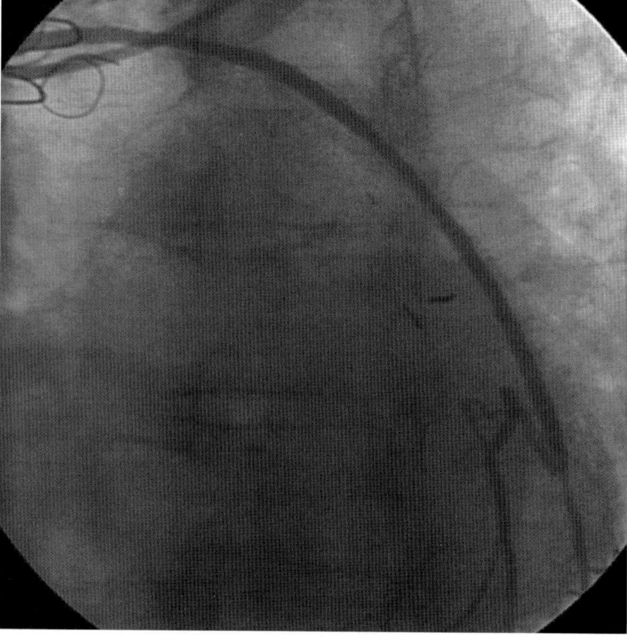

Figure 12–32 Distal protection. (*A*) Severe stenosis of a saphenous vein bypass graft to the left circumflex marginal artery. (*B*) Prior to stent placement, one of the available distal protection devices (filter wire) is seen here as a wire loop placed distal to the undeployed stent. (*C*) Final angiography reveals normal flow from the saphenous vein graft into the native coronary artery.

echocardiography (ICE) is helpful during balloon mitral valvuloplasty. These imaging modalities offer guidance with the transseptal catheter placement, verification of balloon positioning across the valve, and assessment of procedural success.[295] Long-term results have been good.[296]

Aortic Balloon Valvuloplasty

Percutaneous aortic balloon valvuloplasty was introduced in the 1980s. This procedure is usually performed via a femoral artery, using an 11-Fr sheath and 18- to 23-mm balloons. Some advocate the double-balloon technique for aortic valvuloplasty to decrease restenosis with a balloon placed through each femoral artery and inflated simultaneously.

Symptomatic improvement does occur with at least a 50% reduction in gradient in more than 80% of cases.[297] Complications include femoral artery repair in up to 10% of patients, a 1% incidence of stroke, and a less than 1% incidence of cardiac fatality.[295] Contraindications to aortic balloon valvuloplasty are significant peripheral vascular disease and moderate-to-severe aortic insufficiency. Aortic insufficiency usually increases at least one grade during valvuloplasty. The development of severe AR acutely leads to pulmonary congestion and possibly death, as the hypertrophied ventricle is unable to dilate.

Initial success rates are acceptable, but restenosis occurs as early as 6 months after the procedure and nearly all patients will have restenosis by 2 years. therefore, the use of aortic valvuloplasty has waned.[298] Current indications include the following: inoperable patient willing to accept the restenosis rate for temporary reduction in symptoms; noncardiac surgery patient hoping to decrease the surgical risk; and patient with poor LV function, in an attempt to improve ventricular function for further consideration of aortic valve replacement.

Percutaneous Valve Replacement

Surgical valve replacement is widely performed for regurgitant and stenotic valves. Although surgical morbidity and mortality continue to improve, the risks remain prohibitive for some patients. Catheter-based alternatives to surgical valve replacement have been explored since the 1960s but were not successful until recently, 2000, when percutaneous pulmonic valve replacement was performed.[299] The first procedures were performed in patients who had had prior cardiac surgery and were not considered good candidates for reoperation. The procedures are performed under general anesthesia with ICE guidance. A biologic valve is sutured onto a platinum stent and delivered on a balloon. The stent compresses the native valve against the wall of the annulus. Large 18- to 20-Fr delivery systems are used. The results in high-risk patients have been promising, and the device is now being tested in a lower risk group, that is as a true alternative to surgery. The success of percutaneous pulmonic valve replacement prompted interest in the aortic and mitral valves.

The first percutaneous aortic valve replacement in humans was performed in France in 2002. This valve is created by shaping bovine pericardium into leaflets and mounting them within a balloon-expandable stent.[300] Both retrograde and antegrade approaches have been used. Early results are encouraging, as improvements in symptoms and ventricular function are seen following percutaneous aortic valve replacement.[301]

The percutaneous approach for MR includes both attempts to replace as well as to repair the mitral valve. Preliminary work to date has included two approaches. The first approach involves placement of a device composed of a distal and proximal anchor placed within the coronary sinus. This device can then be shortened to decrease the size of the mitral annulus and decrease MR, similar to a surgically placed annuloplasty ring.[302] The second approach involves percutaneous stitching of the mitral valve, similar to the surgical Alfieri operation. Finally, both temporary and permanent mitral valve implantations have been attempted but are early in the experimental process.[295]

Although still experimental, percutaneous valve replacement and repair are exciting and offer a new dimension in catheter-based therapy. Experience to date is limited compared with the years of work and thousands of patients with surgical intervention. Although promising, enthusiasm may best be tempered at this stage.[303] However, as this field expands, the role of the cardiac anesthesiologist in the catheterization laboratory for these complex procedures will likely expand (see Chapters 16 and 20).

OTHER CATHETER-BASED INTRACARDIAC PROCEDURES

Alcohol Septal Ablation

Hypertrophic cardiomyopathy (HCM) is a genetic disorder that can present with sudden cardiac death or symptoms of heart failure. A minority of patients will have asymmetric septal hypertrophy that leads to dynamic outflow tract obstruction and produces severe symptoms. When these patients are refractory to medical therapy, a complicated surgical procedure for septal tissue removal, and often mitral valve repair or replacement, may be required. Since the mid 1990s, percutaneous methods have been studied to induce a controlled infarction and selectively ablate this overgrown septal tissue[304] (see Chapter 24).

Through a standard guiding catheter, a guidewire is placed in the large proximal septal perforator. A balloon catheter is placed over the wire, into the septal perforator, and inflated to occlude flow. The wire is removed and ethanol, 1 to 3 mL, is injected through the balloon into the septal perforator and left in place for 5 minutes. Temporary pacing is required in all patients, and a permanent pacemaker is required occasionally. When performed by experienced operators, morbidity and mortality are limited, the gradient is reduced, and symptoms are improved.[305,306]

Left Atrial Appendage Occlusion

Atrial fibrillation is responsible for up to 20% of strokes. These strokes are caused by embolization of an atrial clot, the vast majority of which arise in the LA appendage. Warfarin therapy is effective for stroke prevention but is associated with morbidity and mortality, and many patients have contraindications to warfarin. The PLAATO system (Appriva Medical, Inc, Sunnyvale, CA) is a self-expanding nitinol cage, 5 to 32 mm in diameter, covered with an occlusive polytetrafluoroethylene membrane. Placed via the transseptal approach under TEE guidance, this device is designed to occlude the atrial appendage well as become incorporated into the appendage, preventing both clot formation and embolization. Implants have been successful and safe in humans, and randomized clinical trials are in progress.[307]

Percutaneous Closure of Patent Foramen Ovale and Atrial Septal Defect

The Amplatzer device (AGA Medical Corp., Golden Valley, MN) is FDA approved and is preferred to surgical closure for isolated secundum defects. Echocardiographic guidance is required, either transesophageal or intracardiac. Accordingly, general anesthesia is used frequently to permit prolonged transesophageal imaging. Two devices (Amplatzer and CardioSEAL, NMT Medical, Inc., Boston, MA) have Humanitarian Device Exemption in the United States for use in the patient with a PFO who has a recurrent stroke while receiving warfarin. Clinical trials are in progress to determine if the devices are more effective than anticoagulation in preventing recurrent stroke after the first event (Fig. 12-33). Surgical closure has been relegated to the few patients whose anatomy precludes percutaneous closure (see Chapter 22).[308,309]

Percutaneous In Situ Coronary Venous Arterialization

Catheter-based coronary artery bypass is a novel idea for patients with diffuse coronary disease who are not candidates for surgical revascularization or PCI. A composite catheter system utilizing a phased-array ultrasound imaging system is mounted on a catheter with an extendable nitinol needle. The needle is used to exit the left anterior descending artery and enter the parallel anterior interventricular vein. The vein is then occluded proximally to permit the distal part of the vein to provide arterial blood to the capillary bed. Preliminary work has been published.[310] With the technically challenging

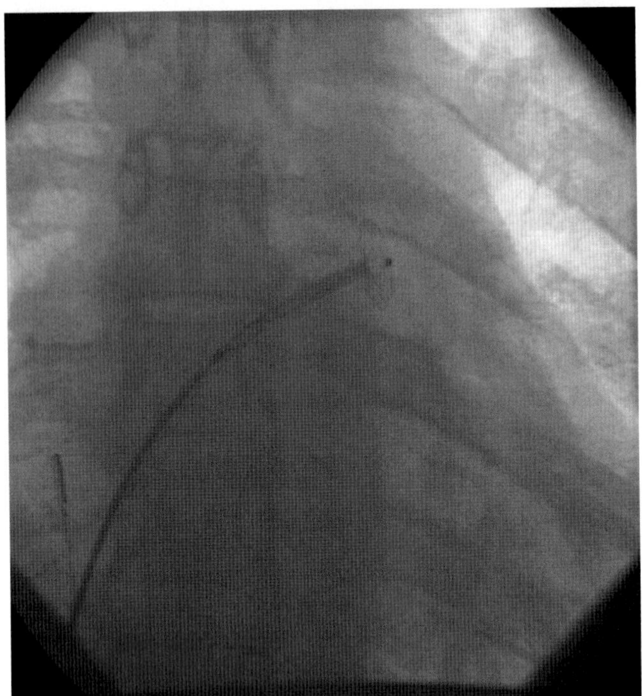

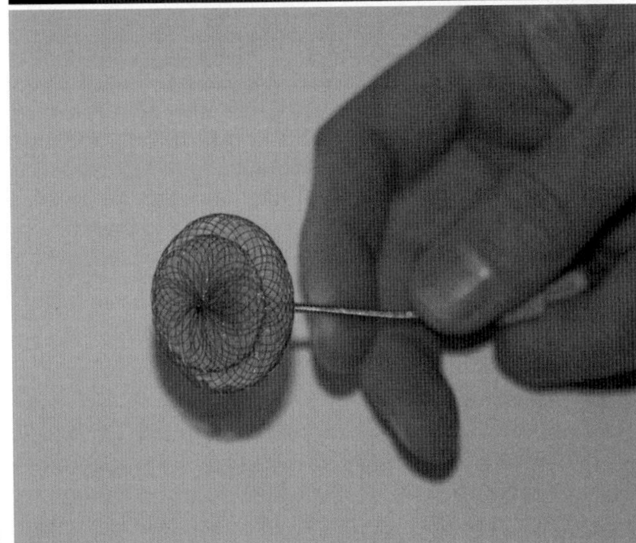

Figure 12–33 (*A*) Deployment of a PFO closure device. (*B*) PFO closure device.

components of this procedure, the limited vessel revascularization possibilities, and the advancements in other areas of PCI, the future of this technique is uncertain.

Percutaneous Transmyocardial Laser Revascularization

Surgical transmyocardial laser revascularization (TMLR) was introduced in the late 1990s. This procedure produces a series of channels from the epicardium to the endocardium, either as a primary procedure or in conjunction with CABG, in patients with refractory angina and proved ischemia who cannot be revascularized by standard techniques. TMLR can improve angina in these patients, although the mechanism is not clear.[290,311] In an attempt to avoid the risks of a thoracotomy, percutaneous transmyocardial laser revascularization (PMLR) was developed to create these channels from the endocardial surface. A randomized clinical trial in 141 patients with class III or IV angina was performed to determine if this technique was more effective in decreasing ischemia than a sham procedure. Unfortunately, this study failed to show a benefit of PMLR, and its future is uncertain.[312]

THE CATHETERIZATION LABORATORY AND THE ANESTHESIOLOGIST

The objective of this chapter has been to provide a broad overview of the catheterization laboratory for the anesthesiologist. As success rates for coronary interventions have increased and complication rates have decreased, there have been fewer opportunities for the cardiologist and the anesthesiologist to interact in the catheterization suite. However, in the 21st century, the role of the anesthesiologist in the catheterization laboratory is destined to change. In this dynamic field of interventional cardiology, more complex and prolonged procedures, such as percutaneous valvular therapy, may well require the renewed collaboration of the interventional cardiologist and the cardiac anesthesiologist.

REFERENCES

1. Kim WY, Danias PG, Stuber M, et al: Coronary magnetic resonance angiography for the detection of coronary stenoses. N Engl J Med 345:1863, 2001
2. Gibbons RJ, Aranoz PA: The year in cardiac imaging. J Am Coll Cardiol. 44:1937, 2004
3. Bittl JA, Hirsch AT: Concomitant peripheral arterial disease and coronary artery disease: Therapeutic opportunities. Circulation 109:3136, 2004
4. Verel D (ed): Cardiac Catheterization and Angiocardiography, 3rd edition. London, Churchill Livingstone, 1978
5. Forssmann-Falch R: Werner Forssman: A pioneer of cardiology. Am J Cardiol 79:651, 1997
6. Braunwald E: Cardiology: The past, the present, and the future. J Am Coll Cardiol 42:2031, 2003
7. Grossman W: Historical perspective and present practice of cardiac catheterization. *In* Baim DS, Grossman W (eds): Cardiac Catheterization, Angiography, and Intervention, 6th edition. Philadelphia, Lippincott Williams & Wilkins, 2000
8. Pepine CJ, Allen HD, Bashore TM, et al: ACC/AHA guidelines for cardiac catheterization and cardiac catheterization laboratories. J Am Coll Cardiol 18:1149, 1991
9. Judkins MP: Guidelines for electrical safety in the cardiac catheterization laboratory. Cathet Cardiovasc Diagn 10:299, 1984
10. Johnson LW, Moore RJ, Balter S: Review of radiation safety in the cardiac catheterization laboratory. Cathet Cardiovasc Diag 25:186, 1992
11. Hirshfeld JW, Balter S, Brinker JA, et al: ACCF/AHA/NASPE-HRS/SCAI Clinical Competence Statement on Physician Knowledge to Optimize Patient Safety and Image Quality in Fluoroscopically Guided invasive Cardiovascular Procedures. Am Coll Cardiol 44:2259, 2004
12. Mettler FA, Voelz GL: Major radiation exposure—what to expect and how to respond. N Engl J Med 346:1554, 2002.
13. ACC/ACR/NEMA Ad Hoc Group: American College of Cardiology, American College of Radiology and industry develop standard for digital transfer of angiographic images. J Am Coll Cardiol 25:800, 1995
14. American College of Cardiology Cardiac Catheterization Committee: Cardiac angiography without cine film: Erecting a "Tower of Babel" in the cardiac catheterization laboratory. J Am Coll Cardiol 24:834, 1994
15. Holmes DR, Laskey WK, Wondrow MA, et al: Flat-panel detectors in the cardiac catheterization laboratory: Revolution or evolution—What are the issues? Catheter Cardiovasc Interv 63:324, 2004
16. Balter S: Interventional Fluoroscopy: Physics, Technology, and Safety. Toronto, Canada, Wiley-Liss, 2001
17. Bashore TM, Bates ER, Berger PB, et al: ACC/SCA&I Expert Consensus Document on Cardiac Catheterization Laboratory Standards. J Am Coll Cardiol 37:2170, 2001

18. Ryan TJ, Klucke FJ, Reynolds WA: Clinical competence in percutaneous transluminal coronary angioplasty: A statement for physicians from the ACP/ACC/AHA Task Force on Clinical Privileges in Cardiology. Circulation 81:2041, 1990
19. American College of Cardiology Committee on Percutaneous Transluminal Coronary Angioplasty: Guidelines for percutaneous transluminal coronary angioplasty. A report of the American College of Cardiology/American Heart Association Task Force on assessment of diagnostic and therapeutic cardiovascular procedures. J Am Coll Cardiol 22:2033, 1993
20. Wennberg DE, Lucas FL, Siewers AE, et al: Outcomes of percutaneous coronary interventions performed at centers without and with onsite coronary artery bypass graft surgery. JAMA 292:1961, 2004
21. Lotfi M, Mackie K, Dzavik V, et al: Impact of delays to cardiac surgery after failed angioplasty and stenting. J Am Coll Cardiol 43:337, 2004
22. ACC/AHA Guidelines for percutaneous coronary intervention (Revision of the 1993 PTCA Guidelines)—executive summary. A report of the American College of Cardiology/American Heart Association task force on practice guidelines (Committee to revise the 1993 guidelines for percutaneous transluminal coronary angioplasty). Circulation 103:3019, 2001
23. Vakili BA, Kaplan R, Brown DL: Volume-outcome relation for physicians and hospitals performing angioplasty for acute myocardial infarction in New York state. Circulation 104:2171, 2001
24. Jollis JG, Peterson ED, DeLong ER, et al: The relation between the volume of coronary angioplasty procedures at hospitals treating Medicare beneficiaries and short-term mortality. N Engl J Med 334:1625, 1994
25. Hirshfeld JW Jr, Balter S, Brunker JA, et al: ACC Clinical Competence Statement. Recommendations for the assessment and maintenance of proficiency in coronary interventional procedures. Statement of the American College of Cardiology. J Am Coll Cardiol 31:722, 1998.
26. Epstein AJ, Rathore SS, Volpp KGM, et al: Hospital percutaneous coronary intervention volume and patient mortality, 1998 to 2000 Does the evidence support current procedure volume minimums? J Am Coll Cardiol 43:1755, 2004
27. Grossman W: Current practice standards. *In* Baim DS, Grossman W (eds): Cardiac Catheterization, Angiography, and Intervention, 5th edition. Baltimore, Williams & Wilkins, 1996, pp 9
28. Heupler FA Jr, Chambers CE, Dear WE, et al: Guidelines for internal peer review in the cardiac catheterization laboratory. Catheter Cardiovasc Diag 40:21, 1997
29. Yadav JS, Wholey MH, Kuntz RE, et al: Protected carotid-artery stenting versus endarterectomy in high-risk patients. N Engl J Med 351:1493, 2004
30. Prinssen M, Verhoeven ELG, Buth J, et al: A randomized trial comparing conventional and endovascular repair of abdominal aortic aneurysms. N Engl J Med 351:1607, 2004
31. Kahn KL: The safety and efficacy of ambulatory cardiac catheterization in the hospital and freestanding setting. Ann Intern Med 103:294, 1985
32. Society for Cardiac Angiography and Interventions, Laboratory Performance Standards Committee: Guidelines for freestanding cardiac catheterization laboratories. Soc Cardiol Angiogr 18:60, 1989
33. ACC/AHA guidelines for exercise testing. A report of the American College of Cardiology/American Heart Association task force on practice guidelines (committee on exercise testing). J Am Coll Cardiol 30:260, 1997
34. Brouwer MA, Freek VW: Oral anticoagulation for acute coronary syndromes. Circulation 105:1270, 2002
35. Hurlen M, Abdelnoor M, Smith P, et al: Warfarin, aspirin, or both after myocardial infarction. N Engl J Med 347:969, 2002
36. American College of Cardiology Cardiovascular Imaging Committee: Use of nonionic or low osmolar contrast agents in cardiovascular procedures. JACC 21:269, 1993
37. Heyder O, Schmidt H, Hackenbroch M, et al: Silent and apparent cerebral embolism after retrograde catheterization of the aortic valve in valvular stenosis: A prospective, randomized study. Lancet 361:1241, 2003
38. Block PC, Ockene I, Goldberg RJ, et al: A prospective randomized trial of outpatient versus inpatient cardiac catheterization. N Engl J Med 319:1251, 1988
39. Agostoni P, Biondi-Zoccai GL, Benedictis L, et al: Radial versus femoral approach for percutaneous coronary diagnostic and interventional procedures. J Am Coll Cardiol 44:349, 2004
40. Carey D, Martin JR, Moore CA, et al: Complications of femoral artery closure devices. Cathet Cardiovasc Intervent 52:3, 2001
41. Steffenino G, Dellavalle A, Ribichini F, et al: Ambulation three hours after elective cardiac catheterization through the femoral artery. Heart 75:477, 1996
42. Goss JE, Chambers CE, Heupler FA, et al: Systemic anaphylactoid reactions to iodinated contrast media during cardiac catheterization procedures: Guidelines for prevention, diagnosis, and treatment. Cathet Cardiovasc Diagn 34:99, 1995
43. Greenberger PA, Patterson R, Tapio CM: Anaphylaxis against repeated radiocontrast media reactions in 857 cases. Ann Intern Med 145:2197, 1985
44. Davidson CJ, Laskey WK, Hermiller JB, et al: Randomized trial of contrast media utilization in high-risk PTCA. The COURT Trial. Circulation 101:2172, 2000
45. Greenberger PA, Halwig M, Patterson R, Wallemark CB: Emergency administration of radiocontrast media in high-risk patients. J Allergy Clin Immunol 77:630, 1986
46. Maeder M, Klein M, Fehr T, et al: Contrast nephropathy: Review focusing on prevention. J Am Coll Cardiol 44:1763, 2004
47. Rihal CS, Textor SC, Grill DE, et al: Incidence and prognostic importance of acute renal failure after percutaneous coronary intervention. Circulation 105:2259, 2002
48. Mehran R, Aymong ED, Nikolsky E, et al: A simple risk score for prediction of contrast-induced nephropathy after percutaneous coronary intervention. J Am Coll Cardiol 44:1393, 2004
49. Chalmers N, Jackson RW: Comparison of iodixanol and iohexol in renal impairment. British J of Radiology 72:701, 1999
50. Aspelin P, Aubry P, Fransson S, et al: Nephrotoxic effects in high-risk patients undergoing angiography. N Engl J Med 348:491, 2003
51. Briguori C, Colombo A, Airoldi F, et al: N-Acetylcysteine versus fenoldopam mesylate to prevent contrast agent-associated nephrotoxicity. J Am Coll Cardiol 44:762, 2004
52. Dodson SR, Hensley FA Jr, Martin DE, et al: Continuous oxygen saturation monitoring during cardiac catheterization in adults. Chest 94:28, 1988
53. Geller E, Halpern P, Chernilas J, et al: Cardiorespiratory effects of antagonism of diazepam sedation with flumazenil in patients with cardiac disease. Anesth Analg 72:207, 1991
54. Kiemeneij F, Laarman GJ, Odekerken D, et al: A randomized comparison of percutaneous transluminal coronary angioplasty by the radial, brachial and femoral approaches: The access study. J Am Coll Cardiol 29:1269, 1997
55. Wakeyama T, Ogawa H, Iida H, et al: Intima-media thickening of the radial artery after transradial intervention. J Am Coll Cardiol 41:1109, 2003
56. Kron J, Sutherland D, Rosch J, et al: Arteriovenous fistula: A rare complication of arterial puncture for cardiac catheterization. Am J Cardiol 55:1445, 1985
57. Ernst SM, Tjonjoegin RM, Schreder R, et al: Immediate sealing of arterial puncture sites after cardiac catheterization and coronary angioplasty using a biodegradable collagen plug: Results of an international registry. J Am Coll Cardiol 21:851, 1993
58. Kern MJ, Cohen M, Talley JD, et al: Early ambulation after 5-French diagnostic cardiac catheterization: Results of a multicenter trial. J Am Coll Cardiol 15:1475, 1990
59. Vacek JL, Bellinger RL, Phelix J: Heparin bolus therapy during cardiac catheterization. Am J Cardiol 62:1314, 1988
60. Shehadi WH: Adverse reactions to intravascularly administered contrast media: A comprehensive study based on prospective survey. Am J Radiol 124:145, 1975
61. Salem DN, Konstam MA, Isner JM, Bonin JD: Comparison of the electrocardiographic and hemodynamic responses to ionic and nonionic radiocontrast media during left ventriculography: A randomized double-blind study. Am Heart J 111:533, 1986
62. Bergstra A, VanDijk RB, Brekke O, et al: Hemodynamic effects of iodixanol and iohexol during ventriculography in patients with compromised left ventricular function. Cathet Cardiovasc Intervent 50:314, 2000
63. Bertrand ME, Esplugas E, Piessens J, et al: Influence of a nonionic, iso-osmolar contrast medium (Iodixanol) versus an ionic, low-osmolar contrast medium (Ioxaglate) on major adverse cardiac events in patients undergoing percutaneous transluminal coronary angioplasty. A multicenter, randomized, double-blind study. Circulation 101:131, 2000
64. Markou CP, Chronos NAF, Hanson SR: Antithrombotic effects of ionic and nonionic contrast media in nonhuman primates. J Thromb Haemost 85:488, 2001
65. Grabowski EF: A hematologist's view of contrast media, clotting in angiography syringes, and thrombosis during coronary angiography. Am J Cardiol 66:23F, 1990

66. Katayama H: Report of the Japanese committee on the safety of contrast media. Presented at the Radiological Society of North America Meeting, November 1988
67. Palmer FJ: The RACR survey of intravenous contrast media reactions: A preliminary report. Australas Radiol 32:8, 1988
68. Robin ED: The cult of the Swan-Ganz catheter. Ann Intern Med 103:445, 1985
69. Hill JA, Miranda AA, Keim SG, et al: Value of right-sided cardiac catheterization in patients undergoing left-sided cardiac catheterization for evaluation of coronary artery disease. Am J Cardiol 65:590, 1990
70. Ganz W, Donoso R, Marcus HS, et al: A new technique for measurement of cardiac output by thermodilution in man. Am J Cardiol 27:392, 1971
71. Forrester JS, Diamond G, Chatterjee K, et al: Medical therapy of acute myocardial infarction by application of hemodynamic subsets (first of two parts). N Engl J Med 295:1356, 1976
72. Forrester JS, Diamond G, Chatterjee K, et al: Medical therapy of acute myocardial infarction by application of hemodynamic subsets (second of two parts). N Engl J Med 295:1404, 1976
73. Grossman W: Shunt detection and measurement. *In* Grossman W, Baim DS (eds): Cardiac Catheterization, Angiography, and Intervention, 4th edition. Philadelphia, Lea & Febiger, 1991, p 166.
74. Grossman W: Pressure measurement. *In* Grossman W, Baim DS (eds): Cardiac Catheterization, Angiography and Intervention, 4th edition. Philadelphia, Lea & Febiger, 1991, pp 123
75. Polanczyk CA, Rohde LE, Goldman L, et al: Right-heart catheterization and cardiac complications in patients undergoing noncardiac surgery. An observational study. JAMA 286:309, 2001
76. Kennedy JW, the Registry Committee of the Society for Cardiac Angiography: Complications associated with cardiac catheterization and angiography. Cathet Cardiovasc Diagn 8:5, 1982
77. Johnson W, Lozner EC, Johnson S, et al: Coronary angiography 1984: A report of the Registry of the Society for Cardiac Angiography and Interventions. I. Results and complications. Cathet Cardiovasc Diagn 17:5, 1989
78. Cohen JR, Sardari F, Glener L, et al: Complications of diagnostic cardiac catheterization requiring surgical intervention. Am J Cardiol 67:787, 1991
79. Colt HG, Begg RJ, Saporito J, et al: Cholesterol emboli after cardiac catheterization. Medicine 67:389, 1988
80. Cappiello RA, Espinoza LR, Adelman H, et al: Cholesterol embolism: A pseudovasculitic syndrome. Semin Arthritis Rheum 18:240, 1989
81. Hendel RC, Cuenoud HF, Giansiracusa DF, Alpert JS: Multiple cholesterol emboli syndrome: Bowel infarction after retrograde angiography. Arch Intern Med 149:2371, 1989
82. Attinger EO, Anne A, McDonald DA: Use of Fourier series for the analysis of biological systems. Biophys J 6:291, 1970
83. Croft CH, Lipscomb K: Modified technique of transseptal left-sided heart catheterization. J Am Coll Cardiol 5:904, 1985
84. Fagard R, Conway J: Measurement of cardiac output: Fick principle using catheterization. Eur Heart J 11(suppl I):1, 1990
85. Bland JM, Altman DG: Statistical methods for assessing agreement between two methods of clinical measurement. Lancet i:307, 1986
86. Davies GG, Jebson PJ, Glasgow BM, Hess DR: Continuous Fick cardiac output compared with thermodilution cardiac output. Crit Care Med 14:881, 1986
87. Quinn TJ, Weissman C, Kemper M: Continual trending of Fick variables in the critically ill patient. Chest 99:707, 1991
88. Van Slike DD, Neill JM: The determination of blood and other solutions by vacuum extraction and manometric measurements. J Biol Chem 61:523, 1924
89. Russell AE, Smith SA, West MJ, et al: Automated noninvasive measurement of cardiac output by the carbon dioxide rebreathing method: Comparisons with dye dilution and thermodilution. Br Heart J 63:195, 1990
90. Kendrick AH, Rozkovec A, Papouchado M, et al: Single-breath breath-holding estimate of pulmonary blood flow in man: Comparison with direct Fick cardiac output. Clin Sci 76:673, 1989
91. Dale J, Jespersen L: Determination of cardiac output with a modified Fick method using estimated instead of measured oxygen consumption. Scand J Clin Lab Invest 47:759, 1987
92. Kendrick AH, West J, Papouchado M, Rozkovec A: Direct Fick cardiac output: Are assumed values of oxygen consumption acceptable? Eur Heart J 9:337, 1988
93. Lund JP: The dye dilution method for measurement of cardiac output. Eur Heart J 11(suppl 1):6, 1990.
94. Hamilton WF, Moore JW, Kinsman JM, et al: Studies on the circulation. IV. Further analysis of the injection method, and of changes in hemodynamics under physiological and pathological conditions. Am J Physiol 99:534, 1932
95. Conway J, Lund JP: Thermodilution method for measuring cardiac output. Eur Heart J 11(suppl I):17, 1990
96. Milnor WR: Hemodynamics, 2nd edition. Baltimore, Williams & Wilkins, 1989, pp 142.
97. D'Ambra MN, LaRaia PJ, Philbin DM, et al: Prostaglandin E1. A new therapy for refractory right heart failure and pulmonary hypertension after mitral valve replacement. J Thorac Cardiovasc Surg 89:567, 1985
98. Fishman AP: Respiratory gases in the regulation of the pulmonary circulation. Physiol Rev 41:214, 1961
99. Wood P: The Eisenmenger syndrome or pulmonary hypertension with reversal of central shunt. Br Med J 2:701, 1958
100. Hashimoto A, Momma K, Hayakawa H, Hosoda S: Natural histories of atrial septal defect with pulmonary hypertension, and ventricular septal defect with pulmonary hypertension. Jpn Circ J 55:791, 1991
101. Steele PM, Fuster V, Cohen M, et al: Isolated atrial septal defect with pulmonary vascular obstructive disease: Long-term follow-up and prediction of outcome after surgical correction. Circulation 76:1037, 1987
102. Gorlin R, Gorlin G: Hydraulic formula for calculation of area of stenotic mitral valve, other cardiac values, and central circulatory shunts. Am Heart J 41:1, 1951
103. Dodge HT, Sandler H, Ballew DW, Lord JD Jr: The use of biplane angiocardiography for the measurement of left ventricular volume in man. Am Heart J 60:762, 1960
104. Fifer MA, Grossman W: Measurement of ventricular volumes, ejection fraction, mass, wall stress, and regional wall motion. *In* Grossman W, Baim DS (eds): Cardiac Catheterization, Angiography, and Intervention. Philadelphia, Lea & Febiger, 1991, p 300
105. Peterson GE, Brickner E, Reimold SC: Transesophageal echocardiography. Clinical indications and applications. Circulation 107:2398, 2003
106. Moodie DS, Fyfe D, Gill CC, et al: Anomalous origin of the left coronary artery from the pulmonary artery (Bland-White-Garland syndrome) in adult patients: Long-term follow-up after surgery. Am Heart J 106:381, 1983
107. Chaitman BR, Lesperance J, Saltiel J, Bourassa MG: Clinical, angiographic, and hemodynamic findings in patients with anomalous origin of the coronary arteries. Circulation 53:122, 1976
108. White CW, Wright CB, Doty DB, et al: Does visual interpretation of the coronary arteriogram predict the physiologic importance of a coronary stenosis? N Engl J Med 310:819, 1984
109. Mancini GBJ: Quantitative coronary arteriographic methods in the interventional catheterization laboratory: An update and perspective. J Am Coll Cardiol 17:23B, 1991.
110. Escaned J, Baptista J, DiMario C: Significance of automated stenosis detection during quantitative angiography. Insights gained from intracoronary ultrasound imaging. Circulation 94:966, 1996
111. Pijls NHJ, Bruyne B, Peels K, et al: Measurement of fractional flow reserve to assess the functional severity of coronary artery stenoses. N Engl J Med 334:1703, 1996.
112. Kern MJ, Puri S, Bach RG, et al: Abnormal coronary flow velocity reserve after coronary artery stenting in patients. Circulation 100:2491, 1999
113. Pellinen TJ, Virtanen KS, Toivonen L, et al: Coronary collateral circulation. Clin Cardiol 14:111, 1991
114. Gregg DE, Patterson RE: Functional importance of the coronary collaterals. N Engl J Med 303:1404, 1980
115. Nattel S, Rangno RE, Van Loon G: Mechanism of propranolol withdrawal phenomena. Circulation 59:1158, 1979
116. Deckelbaum LI, Isner JM, Konstam MA, Salem DN: Catheter-induced versus spontaneous spasm. Do these coronary bedfellows deserve to be estranged? Am J Med 79:1, 1985
117. Baim DS: Is it time to offer elective percutaneous treatment of the unprotected left main coronary artery? (editorial comment) J Am Coll Cardiol 35:1551, 2000
118. King SB: Percutaneous transluminal coronary angioplasty. J Am Coll Cardiol 34:615, 1999
119. Takagi T, Stankovic G, Finci L, et al: Results and long-term predictors of adverse clinical events after elective percutaneous interventions on unprotected left main coronary artery. Circulation 106:698, 2002
120. Tan WA, Tamai H, Park SJ, et al: Long-term clinical outcomes after unprotected left main trunk percutaneous revascularization in 279 patients. Circulation 104:1609, 2001
121. Hodgson J, Reddy KG, Suneja R: Intracoronary ultrasound imaging: Correlation of plaque morphology with angiography, clinical syndrome and procedural results in patients undergoing coronary angioplasty. J Am Coll Cardiol 21:35, 1993

122. Blankenship JC, Klein LW, Laskey WK, et al: SCAI statement on ad hoc versus separate performance of diagnostic cardiac catheterization and coronary intervention. Catheter Cardiovasc Inter 63; 444, 2004
123. Fugit MD, Rubal BJ, Donovan DJ: Effects of intracoronary nicardipine, diltiazem, and verapamil on coronary blood flow. J Invas Cardiol 12:80, 2000
124. Mintz GS, Popma JJ, Pichard AD: Arterial remodeling after coronary angioplasty. A serial intravascular ultrasound study. Circulation 94:35, 1996
125. Peters RJG, Kok WEM, DiMario C: Prediction of restenosis after coronary balloon angioplasty. Circulation 95:2254, 1997
126. Kornowski R, Mintz GS, Kent KM, et al: Increased restenosis in diabetes mellitus after coronary interventions is due to exaggerated intimal hyperplasia. Circulation 95:1366, 1997
127. Mercado N, Boersma E, Wijns W, et al: Clinical and quantitative coronary angiographic predictors of coronary restenosis. A comparative analysis from the balloon-to-stent era. J Am Coll Cardiol 38:645, 2001
128. Hsdai D, Garratt KN, Grill DE: Effect of smoking status on the long-term outcome after successful percutaneous coronary revascularization. N Engl J Med 336:755, 1997
129. Ruygrok PN, Webster MW, deValk V, et al: Clinical and angiographic factors associated with asymptomatic restenosis after percutaneous coronary intervention. Circulation 104:2289, 2001
130. Schwartz L, Bourassa MG, Lesperance J, et al: Aspirin and dipyridamole in the prevention of restenosis after percutaneous transluminal coronary angioplasty. N Engl J Med 318:1714, 1988
131. Powell JS, Muller RKM, Baumgartner HR: Suppression of the vascular response to injury: The role of angiotensin-converting enzyme inhibitors. J Am Coll Cardiol 17(suppl B):137B, 1991
132. Ellis SG, Bates ER, Schaible T, et al: Prospects for the use of antagonists to the platelet glycoprotein IIb/IIIa receptor to prevent post-angioplasty restenosis and thrombosis. J Am Coll Cardiol 17(suppl B):89B, 1991
133. King SB: Restenosis. The mouse that roared. Circulation 108:248, 2003
134. Lincoff AM, Topol EJ, Ellis SG: Local drug delivery for the prevention of restenosis: Fact, fancy, and future. Circulation 90:2070, 1994
135. Lowe HC, Oesterle SN, Khachigian LM, et al: Coronary in-stent restenosis: current status and future strategies. J Am Coll Cardiol 39:183, 2002
136. Williams DO: Intracoronary brachytherapy. Circulation 105:2699, 2002
137. Holmes DR, Hirshfield J, Faxon D, et al: ACC Expert consensus document on coronary artery stents. Document of the American College of Cardiology. J Am Coll Cardiol 32:1471, 1998.
138. Escaned J, Goicolea J, Alfonso F, et al: Propensity and mechanisms of restenosis in different coronary stent designs. Complementary value of the analysis of the luminal gain-loss relationship. J Am Coll Cardiol 34:1490, 1999
139. Pache J, Kastrati A, Mehilli J, et al: Intracoronary stenting and angiographic results: Strut thickness effect on restenosis outcome (ISAR-STEREO) trial. J Am Coll Cardiol 41:1283, 2003
140. Sousa JE, Serruys PW, Costa MA: New frontiers in cardiology. Drug-eluting stents: Part I. Circulation 107:2274, 2003
141. Boston DR, Malouf A, Barry WH: Management of intracoronary thrombosis complicating coronary angioplasty. Circulation 76:125, 1987
142. Awtry EH, Loscalzo J: Aspirin. Circulation 101:1206, 2000
143. Ochoa AB, Wolfe M, Lewis P, et al: Ticlopidine-induced neutropenia mimicking sepsis early after intracoronary stent placement. Clin Cardiol 21:304, 1998.
144. Bennett CL, Connors JM, Carwile JM, et al: Thrombotic thrombocytopenic purpura associated with clopidogrel. N Engl J Med 342:1773, 2000
145. Mehta SR, Yusuf S, Peters RJG, et al: Effects of pretreatment with clopidogrel and aspirin followed by long-term therapy in patients undergoing percutaneous coronary intervention: The PCI-CURE study. Lancet 358:527, 2001
146. Mishkel GJ, Aguirre FV, Ligon RW, et al: Clopidogrel as adjunctive antiplatelet therapy during coronary stenting. J Am Coll Cardiol 34:1884, 1999
147. Kastrati A, vonBeckerath N, Joost A, et al: Loading with 600 mg clopidogrel in patients with coronary artery disease with and without chronic clopidogrel therapy. Circulation 110:1916, 2004
148. Waksman R, Ajani AE, Pinnow E, et al: Twelve versus six months of clopidogrel to reduce major cardiac events in patients undergoing gamma-radiation therapy for in-stent restenosis: Washington Radiation for In-Stent restenosis Trial (WRIST) 12 versus WRIST PLUS. Circulation 106:776, 2002
149. Varga ZA, Papp L: Hemochron versus HemoTec activated coagulation time target values during percutaneous transluminal coronary angioplasty. JACC 25:803, 1995
150. Antman EM: The search for replacements for unfractionated heparin. Circulation 103:2310, 2001
151. Bird JA, Chaitman BR, Feit F, et al: Bivalirudin versus heparin during coronary angioplasty for unstable or postinfarction angina: Final report reanalysis of the bivalirudin angioplasty study. Am Heart J 142:952, 2001
152. Lincoff AM, Kleiman NS, Kereiakes DJ, et al: Long-term efficacy of bivalirudin and provisional glycoprotein IIb/IIIa blockade vs heparin and planned glycoprotein IIb/IIIa blockade during percutaneous coronary revascularization. REPLACE randomized trial. JAMA 292:696, 2004
153. Beguin S, Mardiguian J, Lindhout T, et al: The mode of action of low molecular weight heparin preparation (PK10169) and two of its major components on thrombin generation in plasma. Thromb Haemost 61:30, 1989
154. Petersen JL, Mahaffey KW, Hasselblad V, et al: Efficacy and bleeding complications among patients randomized to enoxaparin or unfractionated heparin for antithrombin therapy in nonST-Segment elevation acute coronary syndromes: A systematic overview. JAMA 292(1):89
155 Young JJ, Kereiakes DJ, Grines CL, et al: Low-molecular-weight heparin therapy in percutaneous coronary intervention: The NICE 1 and NICE 4 trials. J Invas Cardiol 12(suppl E):E14, 2000
156. Ferguson JJ, Califf RM, Antman EM, et al: Enoxaparin vs unfractionated heparin in high-risk patients with nonST-segment elevation acute coronary syndromes managed with an intended early invasive strategy: primary results of the SYNERGY randomized trial JAMA 292:45, 2004
157. The EPIC Investigators: Use of a monoclonal antibody directed against the platelet glycoprotein II_B/III_A receptor in high-risk coronary angioplasty. N Engl J Med 330:956, 1996
158. The EPILOG Investigators: Platelet glycoprotein IIb/IIIa receptor blockade and low-dose heparin during percutaneous coronary revascularization. N Engl J Med 336:1689, 1997
159. Mark DB, Talley JD, Topol EJ, et al: Economic assessment of platelet glycoprotein IIb/IIIa inhibition for prevention of ischemic complications of high-risk coronary angioplasty. Circulation 94:629, 1996
160. Kereiakes DJ, Kleiman NS, Ambrose J, et al: Randomized, double-blind, placebo-controlled dose-ranging study of tirofiban (MK) platelet IIb/IIIa blockade in high risk patients undergoing angioplasty. JACC 27:536, 1996
161. The ESPRIT Investigators: Novel dosing regimen of eptifibatide in planned coronary stent implantation (ESPRIT): A randomized, placebo-controlled trial. Lancet 356:2037, 2000
162. The EPISTENT Investigators: Randomised placebo-controlled and balloon-angioplasty-controlled trial to assess safety of coronary stenting with use of platelet glycoprotein-IIb/IIIa blockade. Lancet 352:87, 1998
163. Kereiakes DJ: Platelet glycoprotein IIb/IIIa inhibition and atheroembolism during bypass graft angioplasty. A cup half full. Circulation 106:2994, 2002
164. Kastrati A, Mehilli J, Schuhlen H, et al: Intracoronary Stenting Antithrombotic Regimen-Rapid Early Action for Coronary Treatment Study Investigators. A clinical trial of abciximab in elective percutaneous coronary intervention after pretreatment with clopidogrel. N Engl J Med 350:232, 2004
165. Armstrong PW, Collen D: Fibrinolysis for acute myocardial infarction. Current status and new horizons for pharmacological reperfusion, Part I. Circulation 103:2862, 2001
166. Ambrose JA, Almeida OD, Sharma SK, et al: Adjunctive thrombolytic therapy during angioplasty for ischemic rest angina. Results of the TAUSA Trial. TAUSA Investigators. Thrombolysis and Angioplasty in Unstable Angina trial. Circulation 90:69, 1994
167. Roubin GS, Douglas JS, King SB, et al: Influence of balloon size on initial success, acute complications, and restenosis after percutaneous transluminal coronary angioplasty. Circulation 78:557, 1988
168. Williams DO, Holubkov R, Yeh W, et al: Percutaneous coronary intervention in the current era compared with 1985. The National Heart, Lung, and Blood Institute Registries. Circulation 102:2945, 2000
169. Ellis SG, Roubin GS, King SB III, et al: In-hospital cardiac mortality after acute closure after coronary angioplasty: Analysis of risk factors from 8,207 procedures. J Am Coll Cardiol 11:211, 1988
170. Krone RJ, Laskey W, Babb J, et al: Four-year trends in coronary interventions, a report from the registry of the society for coronary angiography and interventions (abstract). Cathet Cardiovasc Diagn 41:98, 1997
171. Califf RM, Abdelmeguid AE, Kuntz RE, et al: Myonecrosis after revascularization procedures. J Am Coll Cardiol 31:241, 1998.
172. Stone GW, Mehran R, Dangas G, et al: Differential impact on survival of electrocardiographic Q-wave versus enzymatic myocardial infarction after percutaneous intervention. A device-specific analysis of 7147 patients. Circulation 104:642, 2001

173. Zaacks SM, Allen JE, Calvin JE, et al: Value of the American College of Cardiology/American Heart Association stenosis morphology classification for coronary interventions in the late 1990s. Am J Cardiol 82:43, 1998
174. Singh M, Rihal CS, Lennon RJ, et al: Comparison of Mayo Clinic risk score and American College of Cardiology/American Heart Association lesion classification in the prediction of adverse cardiovascular outcome following percutaneous coronary interventions. J Am Coll Cardiol 44:357, 2004
175. Ormiston JA, Currie E, Webster MW, et al: Drug-eluting stents for coronary bifurcations: Insights into the crush technique. Catheter Cardiovasc Interv 63:332, 2004
176. Yamashita T, Nishida T, Adamian MG, et al: Bifurcation lesions: Two stents versus one stent—immediate and follow-up results. J Am Coll Cardiol 35:1145, 2000
177. Stack RS, Quigley PJ, Collins G, Phillips HR: Perfusion balloon catheter. Am J Cardiol 61:77G, 1988
178. Vogel JHK: Changing trends for surgical standby in patients undergoing percutaneous transluminal coronary angioplasty. Am J Cardiol 69:25F, 1992
179. Weaver WD, Parsons L, Every N, et al: Primary coronary angioplasty in hospitals with and without surgery backup. J Invas Cardiol 7:34F, 1995
180. Blanke H, Cohen M, Karsch KR, et al: Prevalence and significance of residual flow to the infarct zone during the acute phase of myocardial infarction. J Am Coll Cardiol 5:827, 1985
181. Greene MA, Gray LA, Slater AD, et al: Emergency aortocoronary bypass after failed angioplasty. Ann Thorac Surg 51:194, 1991
182. Holmes DR, Firth BG, Wood DL: Paradigm shifts in cardiovascular medicine. J Am Coll Cardiol 43:507, 2004
183. O'Neill WW, Dixon SR: The year in interventional cardiology. J Am Coll Cardiol 43:875, 2004
184. Lotfi M, Mackie K, Dzavik V, Seidelin PH: Impact of delays to cardiac surgery after failed angioplasty and stenting. J Am Coll Cardiol 43:337, 2004
185. Baratke MS, Bannon PG, Hughes CF, et al: Emergency surgery after unsuccessful coronary angioplasty: A review of 15 years of experience. Ann Thorac Surg 75:1400, 2003
186. Vogel RA, Shawl FA: Report of the National Registry of Elective Supported Angioplasty: Comparison of the 1988 and 1989 results. Circulation 82(suppl II):II, 1989
187. Tierstein PS, Bogel RA, Dorros G, et al: Prophylactic vs standby cardiopulmonary support for high-risk PTCA. Circulation 82(suppl III):680, 1990
188. Satler LF: A minimally invasive, mechanical cardiovascular support system. Cath lab digest talks with Lowell F. Satler, M.D, about his experience with the Impella Recover LP 2.5 System. Cath Lab Digest, 12:1, 2004
189. International Society and Federation of Cardiology and World Health Organization Task Force on Myocardial Reperfusion: Reperfusion in acute myocardial infarction. Circulation 90:2091, 1994
190. Lee L, Erbel R, Brown TM, et al: Multicenter registry of angioplasty therapy of cardiogenic shock: Initial and long-term survival. J Am Coll Cardiol 17:599, 1991
191. Sanborn TA, Sleeper LA, Webb JG, et al: Correlates of one-year survival in patients with cardiogenic shock complicating acute myocardial infarction. Angiographic findings from the SHOCK Trial. J Am Coll Cardiol 42:1373, 2003
192. Hockman JS: Cardiogenic shock complicating acute myocardial infarction. Expanding the paradigm. Circulation 107:2998, 2003
193. Gibson CM, Cannon CP, Murphy SA, et al: Relationship of the TIMI myocardial perfusion grades, flow grades, frame count, and percutaneous coronary intervention to long-term outcomes after thrombolytic administration in acute myocardial infarction. Circulation 105:1909, 2002
194. Sutton AGC, Campbell PG, Graham R, et al: A randomized trial of rescue angioplasty versus a conservative approach for failed fibrinolysis in ST-segment elevation myocardial infarction. J Am Coll Cardiol 44:287, 2004
195. The TIMI Study Group: Comparison of invasive and conservative strategies after treatment with intravenous tissue plasminogen activator in acute myocardial infarction. Results of the thrombolysis in myocardial infarction (TIMI) Phase II Trial. N Engl J Med 320:618, 1989
196. Sutton AG, Campbell PG, Graham R, et al: A randomized trial of rescue angioplasty versus a conservative approach for failed fibrinolysis in ST-segment elevation myocardial infarction: The Middlesbrough Early Revascularization to Limit INfarction (MERLIN) trial. J Am Coll Cardiol 44:287, 2004
197. Califf RM, O'Neil W, Stack RS, et al: Failure of simple clinical measurements to predict perfusion status after intravenous thrombolysis. Ann Intern Med 108:658, 1988
198. McLaughlin MG, Stone GW, Aymong E, et al: Prognostic utility of comparative methods for assessment of ST-segment resolution after primary angioplasty for acute myocardial infarction. The controlled abiximab and device investigation to lower late angioplasty complications (CADILLAC) trial. J Am Coll Cardiol 44:1215, 2004
199. Gingliano RP, Braunwald E: Selecting the best reperfusion strategy in ST-elevation myocardial infarction. It's all a matter of time. Circulation 108:2828, 2003
200. Danchin N, Blanchard D, Steg PG, et al: Impact of prehospital thrombolysis for acute myocardial infarction on 1-year outcome. Results from the French nationwide USIC 2000 registry. Circulation 110:1909, 2004
201. Andersen HR, Nielsen TT, Rasmussen K, et al: A comparison of coronary angioplasty with fibrinolytic therapy in acute myocardial infarction. N Engl J Med 349:733, 2003
202. Antman EM, Anbe DT, Armstrong PW, et al: ACC/AHA guidelines for the management of patients with ST-elevation myocardial infarction: executive summary. Circulation 110:588, 2004
203. Gersh BJ, Stone GW, White HD, Holmes DR: Pharmacological facilitation of primary percutaneous intervention for acute myocardial infarction. JAMA 293:979, 2005
204. Ross AM, Coyne KS, Reiner JS, et al: A randomized trial comparing primary angioplasty with a strategy of short-acting thrombolysis and immediate planned rescue angioplasty in acute myocardial infarction: The PACT Trial. J Am Coll Cardiol 34:1954, 1999
205. Moss AJ, Zareba W, Hall WJ, et al: Prophylactic implantation of a defibrillator in patients with myocardial infarction and reduced ejection fraction. N Engl J Med 346:877, 2002
206. Waters RE, Singh KP, Roe MT, et al: Rationale and strategies for implementing community-based transfer protocols for primary percutaneous coronary intervention for acute ST-segment elevation myocardial infarction. J Am Coll Cardiol 43:2153, 2004
207. Chambers CE: Percutaneous transluminal coronary angioplasty versus coronary artery bypass grafting. *In* Cardiothoracic and Vascular Anesthesia Update, Vol 3, Chapter 6. Philadelphia, WB Saunders Company, 1993
208. Casey C, Faxon DP: Multi-vessel coronary disease and percutaneous coronary intervention. Heart 90:341, 2004
209. Zhao XQ, Brown G, Stewart DK, et al: Effectiveness of revascularization in the Emory angioplasty versus surgery trial. A randomized comparison of coronary angioplasty with bypass surgery. Circulation 93:1954, 1996
210. Pocock SJ, Henderson RA, Seed P, et al: Quality of life, employment status, and anginal symptoms after coronary angioplasty or bypass surgery. Three-year follow-up in the Randomized Intervention Treatment of Angina (RITA) trial. Circulation 94:135, 1996
211. Bypass Angioplasty Revascularization Investigation (BARI) Investigators: Comparison of coronary bypass surgery with angioplasty in patients with multivessel disease. N Engl J Med 335:217, 1995
212. Holmes DR: Randomized clinical trials: Do they really make a difference? BARI and diabetes mellitus. Cathet Cardiovasc Diagn 37:351, 1996
213. Khan NE, DeSouza A, Mister R, et al: A randomized comparison of off-pump and on-pump multivessel coronary-artery bypass surgery. N Engl J Med 350:21, 2004
214. Verma S, Fedak PWM, Weisel RD, et al: Off-pump coronary artery bypass surgery. Fundamentals for the clinical cardiologist. Circulation 109:1206, 2004
215. Zacharias A, Habib RH, Schwann TA, et al: Improved survival with radial artery versus vein conduits in coronary bypass surgery with left internal thoracic artery to left anterior descending artery grafting. Circulation 109:1489, 2004
216. Desai ND, Cohen EA, Naylor CD, et al: A randomized comparison of radial-artery and saphenous-vein coronary bypass grafts. N Engl J Med 351:2302, 2004
217. Hoffman SN, TenBrook JA, Wolf MP, et al: A meta-analysis of randomized controlled trials comparing coronary artery bypass graft surgery with percutaneous transluminal coronary angioplasty: One- to eight-year outcomes. J Am Coll Cardiol 41:1293, 2003
218. Leavitt BJ, O'Connor GT, Olmstead EM, et al: Use of the internal mammary artery graft and in-hospital mortality and other adverse outcomes associated with coronary artery bypass surgery. Circulation 103:507, 2001
219. Holmes DR: Stenting small coronary arteries: Works in progress. JAMA 292:2777, 2004

220. Heijer P, Foley DP, Escaned J, et al: Angioscopic versus angiographic detection of intimal dissection and intracoronary thrombus. J Am Coll Cardiol 24:649, 1994
221. vonBirgelen C, Hartmann M, Mintz GS, et al: Relationship between cardiovascular risk as predicted by established risk scores versus plaque progression as measured by serial intravascular ultrasound in left main coronary arteries. Circulation 110:1579, 2004
222. Abizaid AS, Mintz GS, Abizaid A, et al: One-year follow-up after intravascular ultrasound assessment of moderate left main coronary artery disease in patients with ambiguous angiograms. J Am Coll Cardiol 34:707, 1999
223. Nishimura RA, Higano ST, Holmes DR: Use of intracoronary ultrasound imaging for assessing left main coronary artery disease. Mayo Clin Proc 68:134, 1993
224. St Goar FG, Pinto FJ, Alderman EL, et al: Intracoronary ultrasound in cardiac transplant recipients. Circulation 85:979, 1992
225. Sousa JE, Costa MA, Sousa AGMR, et al: Two-year angiographic and intravascular ultrasound follow-up after implantation of sirolimus-eluting stents in human coronary arteries. Circulation 107:381, 2003
226. Mudra H, diMario C, deJaegere P, et al: Randomized comparison of coronary stent implantation under ultrasound or angiographic guidance to reduce stent restenosis (OPTICUS Study). Circulation 104:1343, 2001
227. Fitzgerald PJ, Oshima A, Hayase M, et al: Final results of the Can Routine Ultrasound Influence Stent Expansion (CRUISE) study. Circulation 102:523, 2000
228. Cannon CP, Braunwald E, McCabe CH, et al: Comparison of intensive and moderate lipid lowering with statins after acute coronary syndromes. N Engl J Med 350:15, 2004
229. Nissen SE, Tuzcu EM, Schoenhagen P, et al: Effect of intensive compared with moderate lipid-lowering therapy on progression of coronary atherosclerosis. A randomized controlled trial. JAMA 291:1071, 2004
230. Kern MJ: Coronary physiology revisited. Practical insights from the cardiac catheterization laboratory. Circulation 101:1344, 2000
231. Pijls NHJ, deBruyne B, Peels K, et al: Measurement of fractional flow reserve to assess the functional severity of coronary artery stenosis. N Engl J Med 334:1703, 1996
232. Miller DD, Donohue TJ, Younis LT, et al: Correlation of pharmacological (99m)Tc-sestamibi myocardial perfusion imaging with post-stenotic coronary flow reserve in patients with angiographically intermediate coronary artery stenosis. Circulation 89: 2150, 1996
233. Bech GJ, De Bruyne B, Pijls NH, et al: Fractional flow reserve to determine the appropriateness of angioplasty in moderate coronary stenosis: A randomized trial. Circulation 103:2928, 2001
234. Topol EJ, Leya F, Pinkerton CA, et al: A comparison of directional atherectomy with coronary angioplasty in patients with coronary artery disease. N Engl J Med 329:221, 1993.
235. Holmes DR, Topol EJ, Califf RM, et al: A multicenter, randomized trial of coronary angioplasty versus directional atherectomy for patients with saphenous vein bypass graft lesions. CAVEAT-II Investigators. Circulation 91:1966, 1995
236. Tsuchikane E, Sumitsuji S, Awata N, et al: Final results of the Stent versus Directional Coronary Atherectomy Randomized Trial (START). J Am Coll Cardiol 34:1050, 1999
237. Bowers TR, Stewart RE, O'Neill WW, et al: Effect of Rotablator atherectomy and adjunctive balloon angioplasty on coronary blood flow. Circulation 95:1157, 1997
238. Mehran R, Dangas G, Mintz GS, et al: Treatment of in-stent restenosis with eximer laser coronary angioplasty versus rotational atherectomy. Comparative mechanisms and results. Circulation 101:2484, 2000
239. Warth DC, Leon MB, O'Neill W, et al: Rotational atherectomy multicenter registry: Acute results, complications and 6-month angiographic follow-up in 709 patients. J Am Coll Cardiol 24:641, 1994
240. Reisman M: Technique and strategy of rotational atherectomy. Cathet Cardiovasc Diagn 3:2, 1996
241. Kaplan BM, Safian RD, Mojares JJ: Optimal burr and adjunctive balloon sizing reduces the need for target artery revascularization after coronary mechanical rotational atherectomy. Am J Cardiol 78:1224, 1996
242. Moussa I, Mario C, Moses J, et al: Coronary stenting after rotational atherectomy in calcified and complex lesions. Angiographic and clinical follow-up results. Circulation 96:128, 1997
243. Barath P: Microsurgical dilatation concept: Animal data. J Invas Cardiol 8:2A, 1996
244. Kondo T, Kawaguchi K, Awaji Y: Immediate and chronic results of cutting balloon angioplasty: A matched comparison with conventional angioplasty. Clin Cardiol 20:459, 1997
245. Albiero R, Silber S, DiMario C, et al: Cutting balloon versus conventional balloon angioplasty for the treatment of in-stent restenosis. Results of the Restenosis Cutting Balloon Evaluation Trial (RESCUT). J Am Coll Cardiol 43:943, 2004
246. Schofer J, Rau T, Schluter M, et al: Short-term results and intermediate-term follow-up of laser wire recanalization of chronic coronary artery occlusions: A single-center experience. J Am Coll Cardiol 30:1722, 1997.
247. deMarchena EJ, Mallon SM, Knoph WD, et al: Effectiveness of holmium laser-assisted coronary angioplasty. Am J Cardiol 73:117, 1994
248. Ruygrok PN, Serruys PW: Intracoronary stenting: From concept to custom. Circulation 94:882, 1996
249. Pepine CJ, Holmes DR: Coronary artery stents. J Am Coll Cardiol 28:782, 1996
250. Kiemeneij F, Serruys PW, Macaya C, et al: Continued benefit of coronary stenting versus balloon angioplasty: Five-year clinical follow-up of Benestent-I trial. J Am Coll Cardiol 37:1598, 2001
251. George B, Voorhees W, Roubin G: Multicenter investigation of coronary stenting to treat acute or threatened closure after percutaneous transluminal coronary angioplasty: Clinical and angiographic outcomes. J Am Coll Cardiol 22:135, 1993
252. Maillard L, Hamon M, Khalife K, et al: A comparison of systematic stenting and conventional balloon angioplasty during primary percutaneous transluminal coronary angioplasty for acute myocardial infarction. J Am Coll Cardiol 35:1729, 2000
253. Serruys PW, Foley DP, Suttorp MJ, et al: A randomized comparison of the value of additional stenting after optimal balloon angioplasty for long coronary lesions. Final results of the additional value of NIR stents for treatment of long coronary lesions (ADVANCE) study. J Am Coll Cardiol 39:393, 2002
254. Doucet S, Schalij MJ, Vrolix MCM, et al: Stent placement to prevent restenosis after angioplasty in small coronary arteries. Circulation 104:2029, 2001
255. Marx SO, Marks AR: Bench to bedside. The development of rapamycin and its application to stent restenosis. Circulation 104:852, 2001
256. Schwartz RS, Chronos NA, Virmani R, et al: Preclinical restenosis models and drug-eluting stents. J Am Coll Cardiol 44:1373, 2004
257. Muni NI, Gross TP: Problems with drug-eluting coronary stents—The FDA perspective. N Engl J Med 251:1593, 2004
258. Morice MC, Serruys PW, Sousa JE, et al: A randomized comparison of a sirolimus-eluting stent with a standard stent for coronary revascularization. N Engl J Med 346:1773, 2002
259. Holmes DR, Leon MB, Moses JW, et al: Analysis of 1-year clinical outcomes in the SIRUS trial. A randomized trial of a sirolimus-eluting stent versus a standard stent in patients at high risk for coronary restenosis. Circulation 109:634, 2004
260. Lemos PA, Saia F, Hofma SH, et al: Short- and long-term clinical benefit of sirolimus-eluting stents compared with conventional bare stents for patients with acute myocardial infarction. J Am Coll Cardiol 43:704, 2004
261. Schampaert E, Cohen EA, Schluter M, et al: The Canadian study of the sirolimus-eluting stent in the treatment of patients with long de nova lesions in small native coronary arteries (C-SIRIUS). J Am Coll Cardiol 43:1110, 2004
262. Colombo A, Moses JW, Morice MC, et al: Randomized study to evaluate sirolimus-eluting stents implanted at coronary bifurcation lesions. Circulation 109:1244, 2004
263. Iakovou I, Ge L, Michev I, et al: Clinical and angiographic outcome after sirolimus-eluting stent implantation in aorto-ostial lesions. J Am Coll Cardiol 44:967, 2004
264. Hoye A, Tanabe K, Lemos PA, et al: Significant reduction in restenosis after the use of sirolimus-eluting stents in the treatment of chronic total occlusions. J Am Coll Cardiol 43:1954, 2004
265. Grube E, Silber S, Hauptmann KE, et al: TAXUS I. Six- and twelve-month results from a randomized, double-blind trial on a slow-release paclitaxel-eluting stent for de nova coronary lesions. Circulation 107:38, 2003
266. Stone GW, Ellis SG, Cox DA, et al: A polymer-based, paclitaxel-eluting stent in patients with coronary artery disease. N Engl J Med 350:221, 2004
267. Colombo A, Hall P, Nakamura S, et al: Intracoronary stenting without anticoagulation accomplished with intravascular ultrasound guidance. Circulation 91:1676, 1995
268. Wilson SH, Fasseas P, Orford JL, et al: Clinical outcome of patients undergoing noncardiac surgery in the two months following coronary stenting. J Am Coll Cardiol 42:234, 2003
269. McFadden EF, Stabile E, et al: Late thrombosis in drug-eluting coronary stents after discontinuation of antiplatelet therapy. Lancet 364:1519, 2004
270. Lemos PA, Serruys PW, Sousa JE: Drug-eluting stents. Cost versus clinical benefit. Circulation 107:3003, 2003

271. Nag S: High-Dose-Rate Brachytherapy: A Textbook. Armonk, NY, Futura Publishing, 1994.
272. Teirstein P: β-Radiation to reduce restenosis, too little, too soon? Circulation 95:1095, 1997
273. Waksman R, White RL, Chan RC, et al: Intracoronary β-radiation therapy after angioplasty inhibits recurrence in patients with in-stent restenosis. Circulation 2165, 2000
274. Waksman R, Bhargava B, White L, et al: Intracoronary β-radiation therapy inhibits recurrence of in-stent restenosis. Circulation 101:1895, 2000
275. Teirstein PS, King S: Vascular radiation in a drug-eluting stent world. It's not over til it's over. Circulation 108:384, 2003
276. Parks JM: TEC before stent implantation. J Invas Cardiol 7(suppl D):10D, 1995
277. Safian RD, May MA, Lichtenberg A: Detailed clinical and angiographic analysis of transluminal extraction coronary atherectomy for complex lesions in native coronary arteries. J Am Coll Cardiol 25:848, 1995
278. Mahmud E, Pezshki B, Salami A, Keramati S: Highlights of the 2004 Transcatheter Cardiovascular Therapeutics (TCT) annual meeting: "Clinical Implications." J Am Coll Cardiol 45:798, 2005
279. Cohen DJ, Murphy SA, Baim DS, et al: Cost-effectiveness of distal embolic protection for patients undergoing percutaneous intervention of saphenous vein bypass grafts. Results from the SAFER Trial. J Am Coll Cardiol 44:1801, 2004
280. deFeyter PJ: Percutaneous treatment of saphenous vein bypass graft obstructions. A continuing obstinate problem. Circulation 107:2284, 2003
281. Antoniucci D, Valenti R, Migliorini A, et al: Comparison of rheolytic thrombectomy before direct infarct artery stenting versus direct stenting alone in patients undergoing percutaneous coronary intervention for acute myocardial infarction. Am J Cardiol 93:1033, 2004
282. Siva JA, Ramee SR, Cohen DJ, et al: Rheolytic thrombectomy during percutaneous revascularization for acute myocardial infarction: Experience with AngioJet catheter. Am Heart J 141:353, 2001
283. Gaitonde RS, Sharm N, Von Lohe E, et al: Combined distal embolization protection and rheolytic thrombectomy during percutaneous revascularization of totally occluded grafts. Cathet Cardiovasc Intervent 60:212, 2003
284. Singh M, Rosenschein U, Ho KKL, et al: Treatment of saphenous vein bypass grafts with ultrasound thrombolysis. A randomized study (ATLAS). Circulation 107:2331, 2003
285. Stone GW, Webb J, Cox DA, et al: Primary angioplasty in acute myocardial infarction with distal protection of the microcirculation: Principal results from the prospective, randomized EMERALD trial. J Am Coll Cardiol 43(suppl 2):A285, 2004
286. Li SSL, Lam CW, SoYC, et al: The use of distal occlusion balloon protection device in acute coronary syndrome. Int J Cardiol 92: 281, 2003
287. Limbruno U, Micheli A, DeCarlo M, et al: Mechanical prevention of distal embolization during primary angioplasty. Safety, feasibility, and impact on myocardial reperfusion. Circulation 108:171, 2003
288. Stone GW, Rogers C, Hermiller J, et al: Randomized comparison of distal protection with a filter-based catheter and a balloon occlusion and aspiration system during percutaneous intervention of diseased saphenous vein aorto-coronary bypass grafts. Circulation 108:548, 2003
289. Aaberge L, Rootwelt K, Blomhoff S, et al: Continued symptomatic improvement three to five years after transmyocardial revascularization with CO_2 laser. A late clinical follow-up of the Norwegian randomized trial with transmyocardial revascularization. J Am Coll Cardiol 39:1588, 2002
290. Suero JA, Marso SP, Jones PG, et al: Procedural outcomes and long-term survival among patients undergoing percutaneous coronary intervention of a chronic total occlusion in native coronary arteries: A 20-year experience. J Am Coll Cardiol 38:409, 2001
291. Olivari Z, Rubartelli P, Piscione F, et al: Immediate results and one-year clinical outcome after percutaneous coronary interventions in chronic total occlusions. Data from a multicenter, prospective, observational study (TOAST-GISE). J Am Coll Cardiol 41:1672, 2003
292. Whitlow PL, Selmon M, O'Neill W, et al: Treatment of uncrossable chronic total occlusions with the Frontrunner: Multicenter experience. J Am Coll Cardiol 39(suppl 1):29, 2002
293. Cannan CR, Nishimura RA, Reeder GS, et al: Echocardiographic assessment of commissural calcium: A simple predictor of outcome after percutaneous mitral balloon valvotomy. J Am Coll Cardiol 29:175, 1997
294. Iung B, Cormier B, Ducimetiere P, et al: Immediate results of percutaneous mitral commissurotomy: A predictive model on a series of 1514 patients. Circulation 94:2124, 1996
295. Vahanian A, Palacios IF: Percutaneous approaches to valvular disease. Circulation 109:1572, 2004
296. Hernandez R, Banuelos C, Alfonso F, et al: Long-term clinical and echocardiographic follow-up after percutaneous mitral valvuloplasty with the Inoue balloon. Circulation 99:1580, 1999
297. Kuntz RE, Tosteson ANA, Berman AD, et al: Predictors of event-free survival after balloon aortic valvuloplasty. N Engl J Med 325:17, 1991
298. Sherman W, Hershman R, Lazzam C, et al: Balloon valvuloplasty in adult aortic stenosis: Determinants of clinical outcome. Ann Intern Med 110:421, 1989
299. Bonhoeffer P, Boudjemline Y, Qureshi SA, et al: Percutaneous insertion of the pulmonary valve. J Am Coll Cardiol 39:1664, 2002
300. Cribier A, Eltchaninoff H, Bash A, et al: Percutaneous transcatheter implantation of an aortic valve prosthesis for calcific aortic stenosis. First human case description. Circulation 106:3006, 2002
301. Bauer F, Eltchaninoff H, Tron C, et al: Acute improvement in global and regional left ventricular systolic function after percutaneous heart valve implantation in patients with symptomatic aortic stenosis. Circulation 110:1473, 2004
302. Maniu CV, Patel JB, Reuter DG, et al: Acute and chronic reduction of functional mitral regurgitation in experimental heart failure by percutaneous mitral annuloplasty. J Am Coll Cardiol 44:1652, 2004
303. Fish RD: Percutaneous heart valve replacement. Circulation 110:1876, 2004
304. Hess OM, Sigwart U: New treatment strategies for hypertrophic obstructive cardiomyopathy. Alcohol ablation of the septum: The new gold standard? J Am Coll Cardiol 44:2054, 2004
305. Chang SM, Lakkis NM, Franklin J, et al: Predictors of outcome after alcohol septal ablation therapy in patients with hypertrophic obstructive cardiomyopathy. Circulation 109:824, 2004
306. Maron BJ, Dearani JA, Ommen SR, et al: The case for surgery in obstructive hypertrophic cardiomyopathy. J Am Coll Cardiol 44:2044, 2004
307. Sievert H, Lesh MD, Trepels T, et al: Percutaneous left atrial appendage transcatheter occlusion to prevent stroke in high-risk patients with atrial fibrillation. Early clinical experience. Circulation 105:1887, 2002
308. Martin F, Sanchez PL, Doherty E, et al: Percutaneous transcatheter closure of patent foramen ovale in patients with paradoxical embolism. Circulation 106:1121, 2002
309. Mullen MJ, Dias BF, Walker F, et al: Intracardiac echocardiography-guided device closure of atrial septal defects. J Am Coll Cardiol 41:285, 2003
310. Oesterle SN, Reifart N, Hauptmann E, et al: Percutaneous in situ coronary venous arterialization. Report of the first human catheter-based coronary artery bypass. Circulation 103:2539, 2001
311. Saririan M, Eisenberg MJ: Myocardial laser revascularization for the treatment of end-stage coronary artery disease. J Am Coll Cardiol 41:173, 2003
312. Stone GW, Teirstein PS, Rubenstein R, et al: A prospective, multicenter, randomized trial of percutaneous transmyocardial laser revascularization in patients with nonrecanalizable chronic total occlusions. J Am Coll Cardiol 39:1581, 2002

Chapter 13

CARDIAC ELECTROPHYSIOLOGY: DIAGNOSIS AND TREATMENT

Michael J. Andritsos, MD • Mitchell Faddis, MD, PhD • Charles W. Hogue, Jr., MD

KEY POINTS

1. Identifying the underlying mechanism(s) of an arrhythmia (e.g., either enhanced automaticity or reentry) is fundamental for either surgical or catheter ablative treatment.
2. The basic principles of surgical or catheter-based ablative therapies are (a) interposition of scar tissue along the reentrant pathway or (b) isolating an area of an ectopy.
3. Supraventricular arrhythmias can be life threatening in the presence of an accessory pathway or when occurring in the setting of structural heart disease and, if persistent, may lead to tachycardia-associated cardiomyopathy.
4. Accessory pathways are now typically interrupted using percutaneous catheter-based techniques with high success rates and complication mainly related to catheter access (hematoma and atrioventricular fistula).
5. Atrioventricular nodal reentrant tachycardia is due to altered electrophysiologic properties of the anterior fast pathway and posterior slow pathway fibers providing input to the atrioventricular node; interruption of involved pathway is curative.
6. Atrial flutter typically includes a reentrant circuit that circles the tricuspid valve crossing the myocardial isthmus between the inferior vena cava and the tricuspid valve; catheter ablation of this region can prevent the arrhythmia.
7. Intermittent or paroxysmal atrial fibrillation is often due to ectopy arising from the pulmonary veins; pulmonary vein isolation with catheter ablative energy can be curative.
8. The rapidly changing nature of the reentrant circuits associated with persistent or chronic atrial fibrillation precludes map-directed surgical or ablative strategies. Rather, surgical incisions or catheter ablative lesions are placed along cardiac structures anatomically known to support reentrant conduction.
9. Incisions for the "Maze procedure" for atrial fibrillation have been modified to avoid the sinoatrial nodal complex at the atrial–superior vena cava junction to avoid chronotropic incompetence sometimes observed in the early surgical experience.
10. In adults, most episodes of ventricular tachycardia or fibrillation are the result of coronary artery disease and the remainder are due to dilated or hypertrophic cardiomyopathy. Rarer conditions include long QT syndromes, Brugada syndrome, infiltrative cardiac conditions, and rare forms of right ventricular fatty/fibrotic infiltrative disease.
11. Substantial evidence supports implantable cardiac defibrillator placement for primary and secondary prevention of sudden cardiac death due to complications of coronary artery disease.
12. Emerging data on the effectiveness of implantable cardiac defibrillator therapy for non–coronary-related near sudden death episodes or syncope in the setting of ventricular tachycardia will lead to continued expansion of indications for implantation.

Cardiac rhythm disturbances are common and an important source of morbidity and mortality. For example, sudden cardiac death most often due to ventricular fibrillation accounts for more than 350,000 deaths annually in the United States alone.[1,2] Supraventricular tachycardias (SVTs) are more frequent, ranging in estimated incidence from 35 per 100,000 person-years for paroxysmal SVT, to 5 to 587 per 100,000 person-years for atrial flutter for individuals aged 50 years versus those older than 80 years, respectively.[3,4] By far, atrial fibrillation is the most common sustained cardiac arrhythmia in the general population, affecting more than 2.3 million Americans.[5] The prevalence of atrial fibrillation is strongly related to age, occurring in fewer than 1% of individuals less than 55 years old but in nearly 10% of those older than 80 years.[5] The occurrence of atrial fibrillation increases health resource utilization, heightens the risk for stroke, and is associated with long-term mortality.[6]

There has been a major shift in treatment paradigms of cardiac arrhythmias over the past decade, due in part to the increasing realization that pharmacologic treatments may actually increase risk for mortality rather than prevent death. This is due mostly to the negative inotropic effects and to the proarrhythmic effect of these drugs.[7,8] Data from prospective randomized trials showing improved survival for patients with implantable cardioverter-defibrillators (ICDs) compared with those given antiarrhythmic drugs have further contributed to a shift to nonpharmacologic treatments.[9] Finally, increasing successes using surgical or less invasive percutaneous catheter methods for treating patients with various arrhythmias have made these methods the treatment of choice in many instances.[10,11] Improvements in techniques and low associated morbidity will likely lead to an expansion of eligibility criteria for these interventions.

Anesthesiologists specializing in the care of patients with cardiac diseases, thus, will be increasingly challenged to provide care for patients undergoing surgical or catheter-based treatments of cardiac arrhythmias. The underlying principle for both approaches is similar: identification of the electrophysiologic mechanism of the arrhythmia followed by ablation of the involved myocardium with surgical incisions, cryothermy, or radiofrequency (RF) current. The fundamentals for the care of patients undergoing either procedure require familiarization with the anatomy of the normal cardiac conduction system, the electrophysiologic basis for common cardiac rhythm disorders, and the approaches to their ablative treatment. This chapter discusses these basic principles, along with special anesthetic considerations when unique to a particular form of treatment.

BASIC ELECTROPHYSIOLOGIC PRINCIPLES

Anatomy and Physiology of the Cardiac Pacemaker and Conduction Systems

Sinus Node

The sinoatrial (SA) node (Fig. 13–1) is a spindle-shaped structure composed of highly specialized cells located in the right atrial sulcus terminalis, lateral to the junction of the superior vena cava and the right atrium[12] (see Box 13–1 for a summary of the anatomy of the cardiac pacemaker and conduction system). Three cell types have been identified in the SA node (nodal, transitional, and atrial muscle cells), but no single cell appears to be solely responsible for initiating the pacemaker impulse. Rather, multiple cells in the SA node discharge synchronously through complex interactions.[13-15] Rather than a discrete and isolated structure, studies suggest that the SA node consists of three distinct regions, each responsive to a separate group of neural and circulatory stimuli.[16] The interrelationship of these three regions appears to determine the ultimate rate of output of the SA node. Although the SA node is the site of primary impulse formation, subsidiary atrial

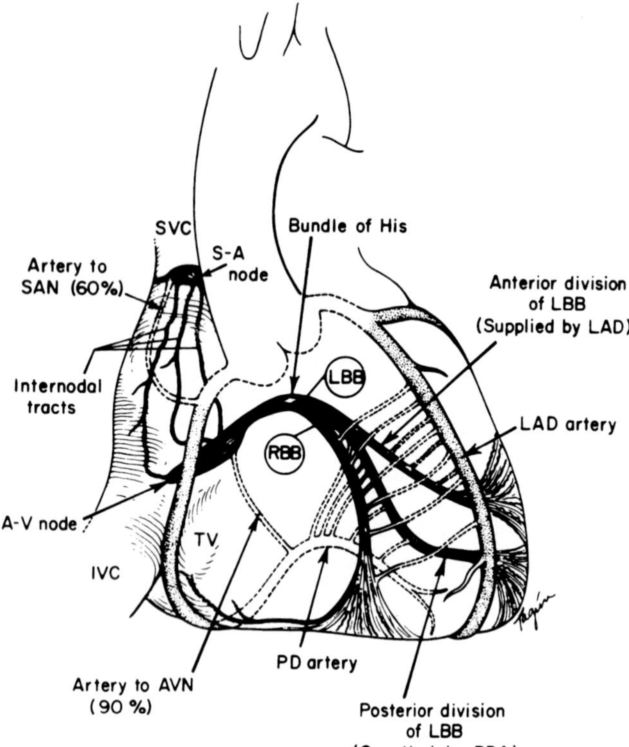

Figure 13–1 Drawing of the anatomy of the cardiac conduction system including arterial blood supply. In 60% of patients the sinoatrial (SA) nodal artery is a branch of the right coronary artery while in the remainder it arises from the circumflex artery. The atrioventricular (AV) node is supplied by a branch from the right coronary artery or posterior descending artery. SVC = superior vena cava; IVC = inferior vena cava; TV = tricuspid valve; LAD = left anterior descending coronary artery; PDA = posterior descending artery; RBB = right bundle branch; LBB = left bundle branch. (From Harthorne JW, Pohost GM: Electrical therapy of cardiac arrhythmias. *In* Levine HJ [ed]: Clinical Cardiovascular Physiology. New York, Grune & Stratton, 1976, p 854.)

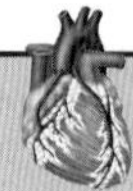

BOX 13–1 ***Anatomy of the Cardiac Pacemaker and Conduction System***

- Sinus node
- Internodal conduction
- Atrioventricular junction
- Intraventricular conduction system
  - Left bundle branch
    - Anterior fascicle
    - Posterior fascicle
  - Right bundle branch
  - Purkinje fibers

pacemakers located outside the sinus node have been demonstrated.[17-19] Subsequently, in a series of studies both in dogs and in humans, it was confirmed that there is an extensive system of atrial pacemakers widely distributed in the right and left atria, as well as in the atrial septum.[20-23] Because the atrial pacemaker system occupies a much larger area than the SA node, it can be severed during arrhythmia surgery, resulting in impaired rate responsiveness.[24]

The arterial supply to the SA node (SAN artery) is provided from either the right coronary artery (RCA) (in 60% of the population) or the left circumflex coronary artery (see Fig. 13–1). The SA node is richly innervated with postganglionic adrenergic and cholinergic nerve terminals. Vagal stimulation, by releasing acetylcholine, slows SA nodal automaticity and prolongs intranodal conduction time; whereas adrenergic stimulation increases the discharge rate of the SA node.[25,26]

Internodal Conduction

For many years, there has been much controversy concerning the existence of specialized conduction pathways connecting the SA node to the atrioventricular (AV) node. Most electrophysiologists now agree that preferential conduction is unequivocally present and that spread of activation from the SA node to the AV node follows distinct routes by necessity because of the peculiar geometry of the right atrium.[27] The orifices of the superior and inferior cava, the fossa ovalis, and the ostium of the coronary sinus divide the right atrium into muscle bands, thus limiting the number of routes available for internodal conduction (see Fig. 13–1). These routes, however, do not represent discrete bundles of histologically specialized internodal tracts comparable with the ventricular bundle branches.[27,28] It has been suggested that a parallel arrangement of myocardial cells in bundles, such as the crista terminalis and the limbus of the fossa ovalis, may account for preferential internodal conduction. Although electrical impulses travel more rapidly through these thick atrial muscle bundles, surgical transection will not block internodal conduction because alternate pathways of conduction through atrial muscle are available.[29]

Atrioventricular Junction and Intraventricular Conduction System

The AV junction (Fig. 13–2) corresponds anatomically to a group of discrete specialized cells, morphologically distinct from working myocardium and divided into a transitional cell zone, compact portion, and penetrating AV bundle (His bundle).[30] Based on animal experiments, the transitional zone appears to connect atrial myocardium with the compact AV node.[31] The compact portion of the AV node is located

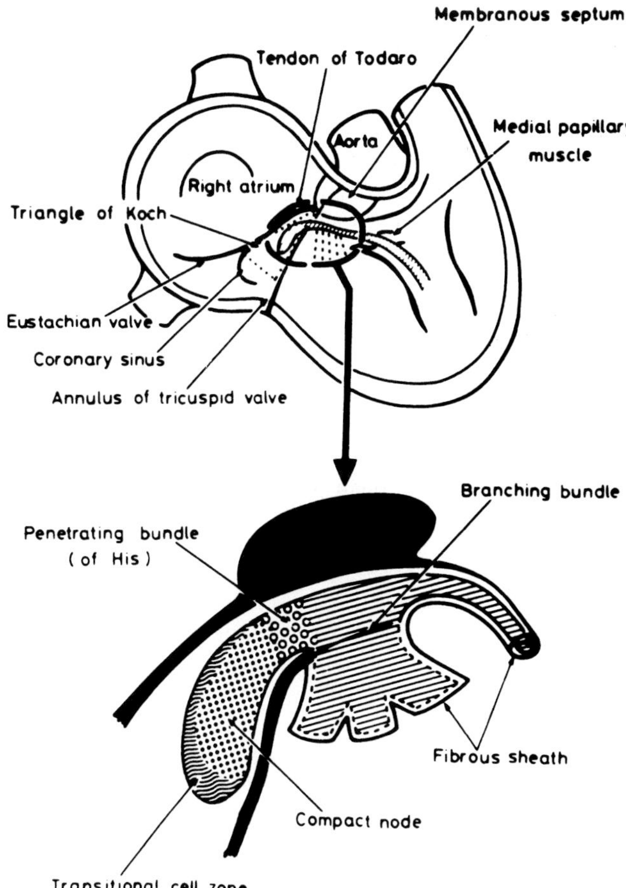

Figure 13–2 Anatomic relation of the atrioventricular junction in relation to other cardiac structures. (From Harrison DC [ed]: Cardiac Arrhythmias: A Decade of Progress. Boston, GK Hall Medical Publishers, 1981.)

superficially, anterior to the ostium of the coronary sinus above the insertion of the septal leaflet of the tricuspid valve. Based on electrophysiologic data from animals, the AV node is often classified into AN, N, and NH regions. The majority of AV nodal conduction delay occurs at the AN and N regions. The longitudinal segment of the compact AV node penetrates the central fibrous body and becomes the bundle of His. As the nodal-bundle axis descends into the ventricular musculature, it gradually becomes completely isolated by collagen and is no longer in contact with atrial fibers. The AV junction is contained within the triangle of Koch, an anatomically discrete region bounded by the tendon of Todaro, the tricuspid valve annulus, and the ostium of the coronary sinus (Fig. 13–3). This triangle is avoided in all cardiac operative procedures to prevent surgical damage to AV conduction. Individual variability in the specific anatomy of the AV nodal area is dependent on the degree of central fibrous body development.[27]

The branching of the nodal-bundle axis begins at the superior margin of the muscular interventricular septum. At this level, the bundle of His emits a broad band of fasciculi, forming the left bundle branch that extends downward as a continuous sheet into the left side of the septum beneath the noncoronary aortic cusp (see Fig. 13–1). The left bundle divides into smaller anterior and broader posterior fascicles, although this is not a consistent anatomic delineation. The right bundle branch usually originates as the final continuation of the bundle of His, traveling subendocardially on the right side of the interventricular septum toward the apex of

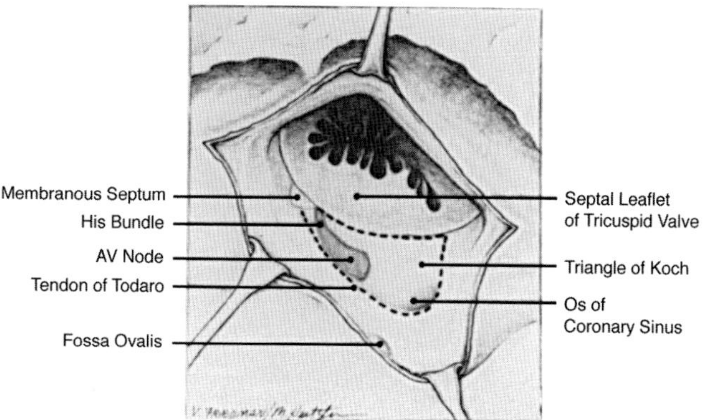

Figure 13–3 View of right atrial septum via a right atriotomy incision (superior is to the left). The triangle of Koch is an important anatomic area that includes the AV node and proximal portion of the His bundle. This anatomic region is contained in the area between the tendon of Todaro, the tricuspid valve annulus, and a line connecting the two at the level of the os of the coronary sinus. (From Cox JL, Holman WL, Cain ME: Cryosurgical treatment of atrioventricular node reentry tachycardia. Circulation 76:1331, 1987.)

the right ventricle. The distal branches of the conduction system connect with an interweaving network of Purkinje fibers expanding broadly on the endocardial surface of both ventricles. Blood supply to the AV node is mostly from the RCA (in 85% of the population) or from the left circumflex artery. The bundle of His is supplied by branches from the anterior and posterior descending coronary arteries. Innervation to the SA and AV nodes is complex because of substantial overlapping of vagal and sympathetic nerve branches. Stimulation of the right cervical vagus nerve causes sinus bradycardia, whereas stimulation of the left vagus produces prolongation of AV nodal conduction. Stimulation of the right stellate ganglion speeds SA nodal discharge rate, whereas stimulation of the left ganglion produces a shift in the pacemaker from the SA node to an ectopic site.[32]

Basic Arrhythmia Mechanisms

The mechanisms of cardiac arrhythmias are broadly classified as either focal mechanisms that include automatic or triggered arrhythmias or reentrant arrhythmias (Box 13–2). Cells that display automaticity lack a true resting membrane potential and, instead, undergo slow depolarization during diastole (Figs. 13–4 and 13–5). Diastolic depolarization results in the

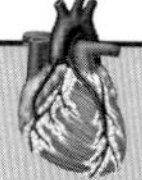

BOX 13–2 ***Arrhythmia Mechanisms***

- Focal mechanisms
  - Automatic
  - Triggered
- Reentrant arrhythmias
- Normal automaticity
  - Sinoatrial node
  - Subsidiary atrial foci
  - Atrioventricular node
  - His-Purkinje system
- Triggered mechanisms occur from repetitive afterdepolarizations
- Reentry
  - Unidirectional block is necessary
  - Slowed conduction in the alternate pathway exceeds the refractory period of cells at the site of unidirectional block

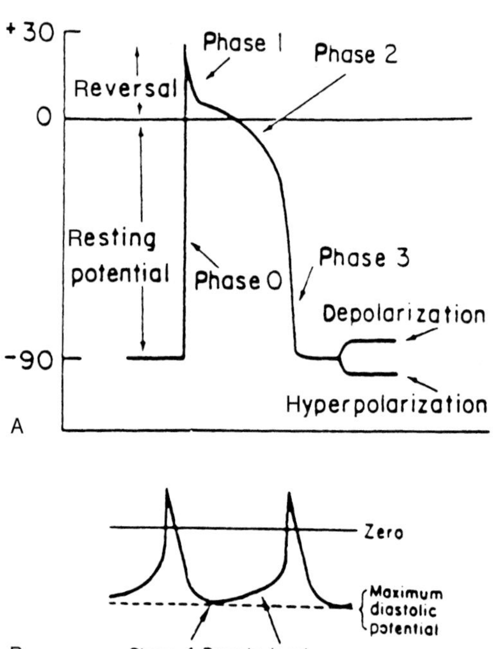

Figure 13–4 Graph depicting the cardiac cellular action potential from fast-response fiber *(A)* and slow-response fiber *(B)*. The slow-response fiber similar to that found in the SA node lacks the rapid upstroke of phase 0. (From Ferguson TB Jr: Anatomic and electrophysiologic principles in the surgical treatment of cardiac arrhythmias. Cardiac Surg 4:19, 1990.)

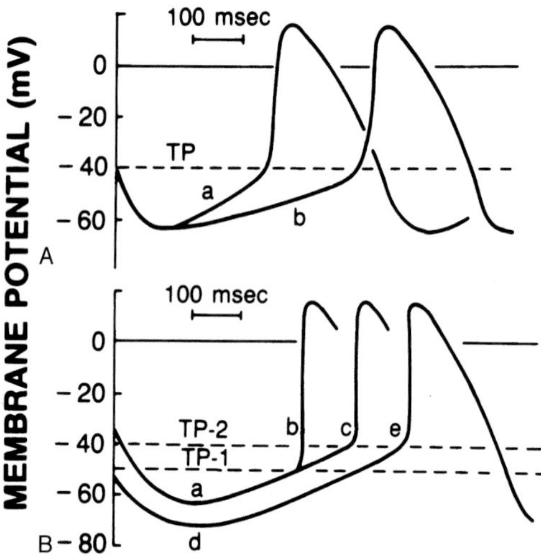

Figure 13–5 Transmembrane potential from sinus node. *(A)* A decrease in the slope of phase 4 or diastolic depolarization (from a to b) will increase the time to reach threshold potential (TP), thus slowing the heart rate. *(B)* Heart rate slowing occurs by changing from TP-1 to TP-2, such that a longer interval is needed to reach threshold potential (b to c). Increasing maximum diastolic potential (a to d) will also slow heart rate by increasing the time to reach threshold potential (b to c). (From Atlee JL III: Perioperative Cardiac Arrhythmias: Mechanisms, Recognition, Management, 2nd edition. Chicago, Year Book Medical Publishers, 1990, p 36.)

transmembrane potential becoming more positive between successive action potentials until threshold potential is reached, leading to membrane excitation. Cells possessing normal automaticity can be found in the SA node, subsidiary atrial foci, AV node, and His-Purkinje system.[14,15,33-36] The property of slow diastolic depolarization is termed "spontaneous diastolic" or phase 4 depolarization. Factors that may modify spontaneous diastolic depolarization are shown in Figure 13–5 and include alterations in the maximum diastolic potential, threshold potential, and rate or slope of diastolic depolarization. The net effect of these factors is to influence the rate (increased or decreased) at which threshold potential is achieved, resulting in either an increase or a decrease in automaticity. The ionic mechanism of diastolic depolarization may involve a decrease in net outward K^+ movement, although newer data support an inward Na^+ current, different from that causing phase 0, as the pacemaker current.[33,37-40] Pacemaker cells with the fastest rate of phase 4 depolarization become dominant in initiating the cardiac impulse, with other automatic foci subject to overdrive suppression.

When cells that normally display automaticity (e.g., SA node, AV node, Purkinje fibers) change the rate of pacemaker firing, altered normal automaticity is said to occur. While the ionic mechanisms resulting in altered normal automaticity are unchanged, other factors such as those seen in Figure 13–5 can contribute to an increase in automaticity. In contrast, automaticity resulting from abnormal ionic mechanisms, even if occurring in cells that are usually considered automatic (e.g., Purkinje fibers), is referred to as "abnormal automaticity." Abnormal automaticity may also occur in cells in which automaticity is not normally observed (e.g., ventricular myocardium).

Arrhythmias arising from a "triggered" mechanism are initiated from cells that experience repetitive afterdepolarizations. Afterdepolarizations are oscillations in the transmembrane potential that occur either before (early afterdepolarizations) or after (delayed afterdepolarizations) membrane repolarization. Different ionic mechanisms are responsible for each form of afterdepolarization, and if the oscillations in membrane potential reach threshold potential, a triggered cardiac impulse can be generated.[14] Triggered activity is often considered an abnormal form of automaticity. However, because triggered activity requires a prior cardiac impulse (in contrast to automaticity), this abnormal electrophysiologic event cannot purely be considered a form of automaticity.

Reentry is a condition in which a cardiac impulse persists to re-excite myocardium that is no longer refractory.[14] Unidirectional block of impulse conduction is a necessary condition for reentry. This unidirectional block may be in the form of differences in membrane refractoriness (dispersion of refractoriness) such that some areas of myocardium are unexcitable whereas other areas allow impulse propagation. Upon repolarization, previously refractory membranes will be available for depolarization if the initial impulse has found an alternate route of propagation and returns to the prior site of conduction block. For reentry to occur, slowed conduction in the alternate pathway must exceed the refractory period of cells at the site of unidirectional block. Partial depolarization of fast-response fibers (depressed fast response) results in reduced Na^+ channel availability with consequent reduced rate of phase 0 of the action potential. This reduced rate of action potential upstroke of phase 0 can result in slowed conduction and contribute to the above conditions conducive to reentry. Arrhythmias produced by reentrant or triggered mechanisms, but not those secondary to increased automaticity, can be induced with programmed stimulation in the setting of a diagnostic electrophysiology study (EPS). Pacemaker-induced overdrive suppression is a characteristic of arrhythmias produced by automaticity (see Chapter 25).

Diagnostic Evaluation

Most patients are asymptomatic when evaluated for cardiac arrhythmias necessitating diagnostic evaluations. The history of symptoms can often provide clues to the nature of an arrhythmia. Abrupt onset and termination of palpitations, for example, is consistent with a paroxysmal SVT most often due to atrioventricular nodal reentrant tachycardia (AVNRT) or atrioventricular reentrant tachycardia (AVRT) associated with an accessory AV bypass tract. A history of syncope should be sought and may indicate either a fast heart rate with the arrhythmia, atrial fibrillation in the presence of an accessory conduction pathway, structural heart disease (e.g., aortic stenosis or hypertrophic cardiomyopathy), or perhaps a ventricular arrhythmia. Whether palpitations are regular or irregular is useful in differentiating atrial fibrillation as a cause of the symptoms. Precipitating events, number and duration of episodes, presence of dyspnea, fatigue, or other constitutional symptoms should be sought from the history (Box 13–3).

A 12-lead electrocardiogram (ECG) should be obtained and when simultaneous with an arrhythmia can be diagnostic. Other cardiac conditions might be uncovered such as the presence of ventricular preexcitation suggesting Wolff-Parkinson-White (WPW) syndrome. Patients with a history of preexcitation presenting with an arrhythmia should be immediately evaluated, because atrial fibrillation in the presence of an accessory pathway can lead to sudden death. For all patients undergoing evaluation of an arrhythmia, an echocardiogram is essential to evaluate for cardiac structural abnormalities and ventricular function. The latter is particularly germane for patients with persistent tachycardia (weeks to months) because this can lead to tachycardia-associated cardiomyopathy.[41] Twenty-four–hour Holter monitoring might be useful in some patients with frequent but transient symptoms. Other evaluations such as exercise or pharmacologic stress testing are based on the patient's age and likelihood of coronary artery disease.

The ultimate diagnosis of the underlying mechanisms of the arrhythmia may require invasive electrophysiologic testing. These studies involve percutaneous introduction of catheters capable of electrical stimulation and recording of the electrograms from various intracardiac sites. Initial recording sites often include the high right atrium, coronary sinus, bundle of His, and apex of the right ventricle[42,43] (Figs. 13–6 and 13–7). The sequence of cardiac activation can be discerned from these recordings along with the surface ECG. This is illustrated in Figure 13–8 from a patient undergoing evaluation for an accessory AV conduction pathway. The sequence of the activation is observed by noting the timing of depolarization recorded by the respective electrodes positioned fluoroscopically at various anatomic sites. An example of a

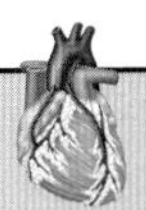

BOX 13–3 *Diagnostic Evaluation of Arrhythmias*

- History of palpitations, syncope, and constitutional symptoms; examination
- 12-Lead electrocardiogram
- Echocardiogram
- 24-Hour Holter monitoring
- Invasive electrophysiologic testing with multichannel, computerized mapping

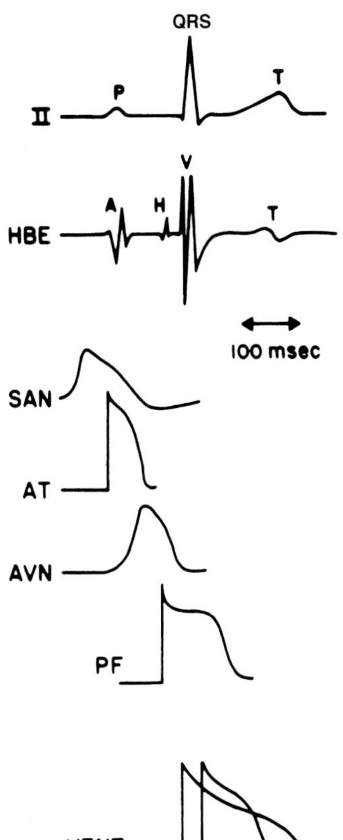

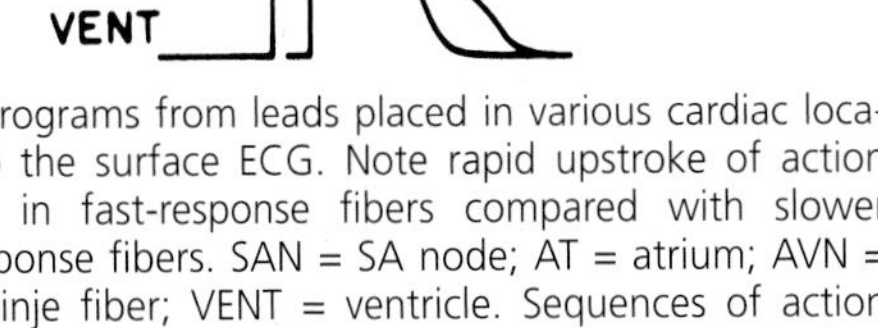

Figure 13–6 Electrograms from leads placed in various cardiac locations in reference to the surface ECG. Note rapid upstroke of action potential (phase 0) in fast-response fibers compared with slower upstroke of slow-response fibers. SAN = SA node; AT = atrium; AVN = AV node; PF = Purkinje fiber; VENT = ventricle. Sequences of action potentials from various cardiac tissues are presented in relation to surface ECG and His bundle electrogram. (From Atlee JL III: Perioperative Cardiac Arrhythmias: Mechanisms, Recognition, Management, 2nd edition. Chicago, Year Book Medical Publishers, 1990, p 27.)

recording obtained during diagnostic evaluation of a patient with a ventricular arrhythmia is shown in Figure 13–9.

The catheters are most often introduced via the femoral vessels under local anesthesia. Systemic heparinization is required, particularly when catheters are introduced into the left atrium or ventricle. The most common complications from electrophysiologic testing are those associated with vascular catheterization.[44,45] Other complications include hypotension (in 1% of patients), hemorrhage, deep venous thrombosis (in 0.4% of patients), embolic phenomena (0.4%), infection (0.2%), and cardiac perforation (0.1%).[44,45] Proper application of adhesive cardioversion electrodes prior to the procedure facilitates rapid cardioversion/defibrillation in the event of persistent tachyarrhythmia resulting from stimulation protocols.

The principles of intraoperative electrophysiologic mapping are similar to those used in the cardiac catheterization suite. These procedures have evolved from early single-point epicardial mapping systems with a hand-held electrode to sophisticated multichannel computerized systems.[10] The latter are capable of acquiring and storing multiple epicardial, intramural, and endocardial electrograms from a single depolarization. Multichannel, computerized mapping allows for rapid identification of arrhythmia pathways (e.g., accessory pathways) prior to initiation of cardiopulmonary bypass (CPB), reducing the need for excessive cardiac manipulations

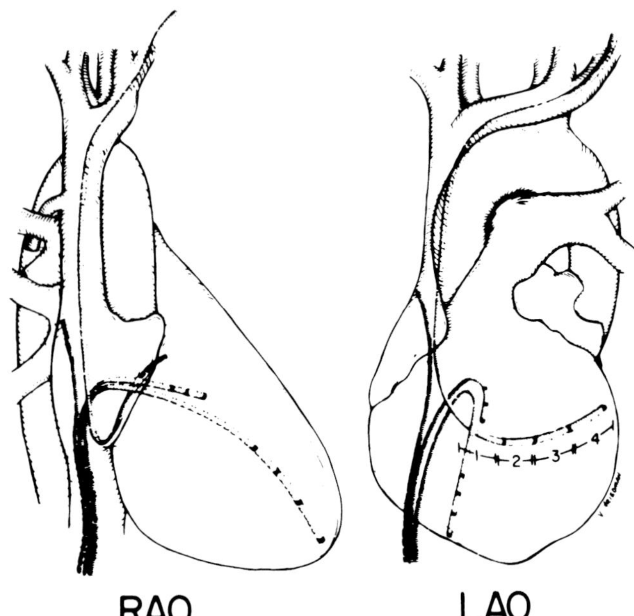

Figure 13–7 Electrophysiologic study in patient with Wolff-Parkinson-White syndrome is schematically depicted. Catheter with multiple recording/pacing electrodes is positioned in the high right atrium, coronary sinus, bundle of His region, and right ventricular apex. Right anterior oblique (RAO) projections differentiate anterior from posterior sites. Left anterior oblique (LAO) projections differentiate septal from lateral sites. Numbered zones in the LAO projection regionalize electrode positions in the coronary sinus (4, posterolateral; 3, posterior; 2, posterior; 1, posteroseptal). (From Cain ME, Cox JL: Surgical treatment of supraventricular tachyarrhythmias. *In* Platia EV [ed]: Management of Cardiac Arrhythmias: The Nonpharmacologic Approach. Philadelphia, JB Lippincott, 1987, p 307.)

necessary with a hand-held electrode, thus promoting stable conduction.

Principles of Electrophysiologic Treatment

The paradigm for ablative treatment of cardiac arrhythmias evolved from the surgical treatment of WPW syndrome and then ventricular tachycardia (VT) developed by Sealy, Boineau, and colleagues.[46-48] The fundamental paradigm for this approach is precise localization of the electrophysiologic substrate for the arrhythmia and then ablating the pathway. In the case of WPW syndrome, the accessory pathway is identified with intraoperative electrophysiologic mapping that initially used hand-held electrodes.[10,49] Development of multichannel computer-based mapping systems allowed for the identification of both the mechanisms for many arrhythmias, including VT, and their termination by interruption of the underlying substrate.[10,49] Experience and insights into arrhythmia mechanisms led to the development of catheter-based methods now routinely used for a variety of supraventricular and ventricular arrhythmias. General indications for ablative treatments include drug-resistant arrhythmias, drug intolerance, severe symptoms, and desire to avoid life-long drug treatments (Box 13–4).

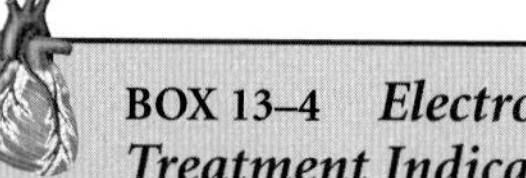

BOX 13–4 ***Electrophysiologic Ablative Treatment Indications***

- Drug-resistant arrhythmias
- Drug intolerance
- Severe symptoms
- Avoiding life-long treatments

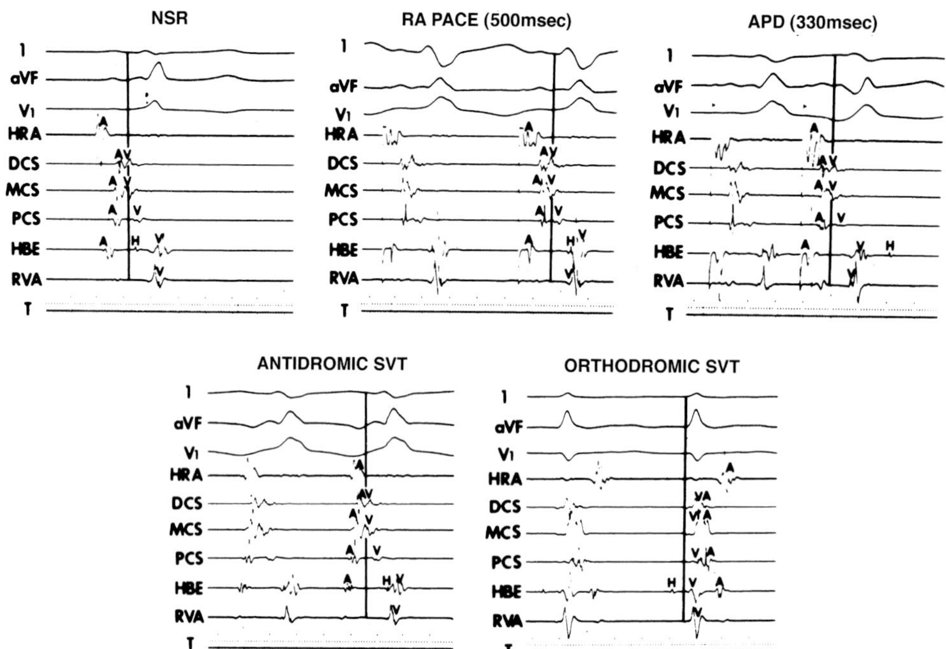

Figure 13–8 Surface ECG (leads I, aVF, and V_1) and electrograms at various intracardiac sites during sinus rhythm, pacing from the right atrium, after an atrial premature depolarization, and during antidromic and orthodromic supraventricular tachycardia. The left free wall accessory pathway is identified by noting the earliest onset of ventricular depolarization at the distal coronary sinus catheter (DCS) in relation to the delta wave on the surface ECG (solid vertical line). This is followed closely by activation in the mid- (MCS) and proximal coronary sinus (PCS) sites. Other catheter locations are the high right atrium (HRA), His-bundle region (HBE), and right ventricular apex (RVA). Conduction is followed during supraventricular tachycardia by noting the pattern of cardiac activation from the right atrium (solid vertical line) to the ventricles. (From Cain ME, Cox JL: Surgical treatment of supraventricular tachyarrhythmias. *In* Platia EV [ed]: Management of Cardiac Arrhythmias. Philadelphia, JB Lippincott, 1987, p 308.)

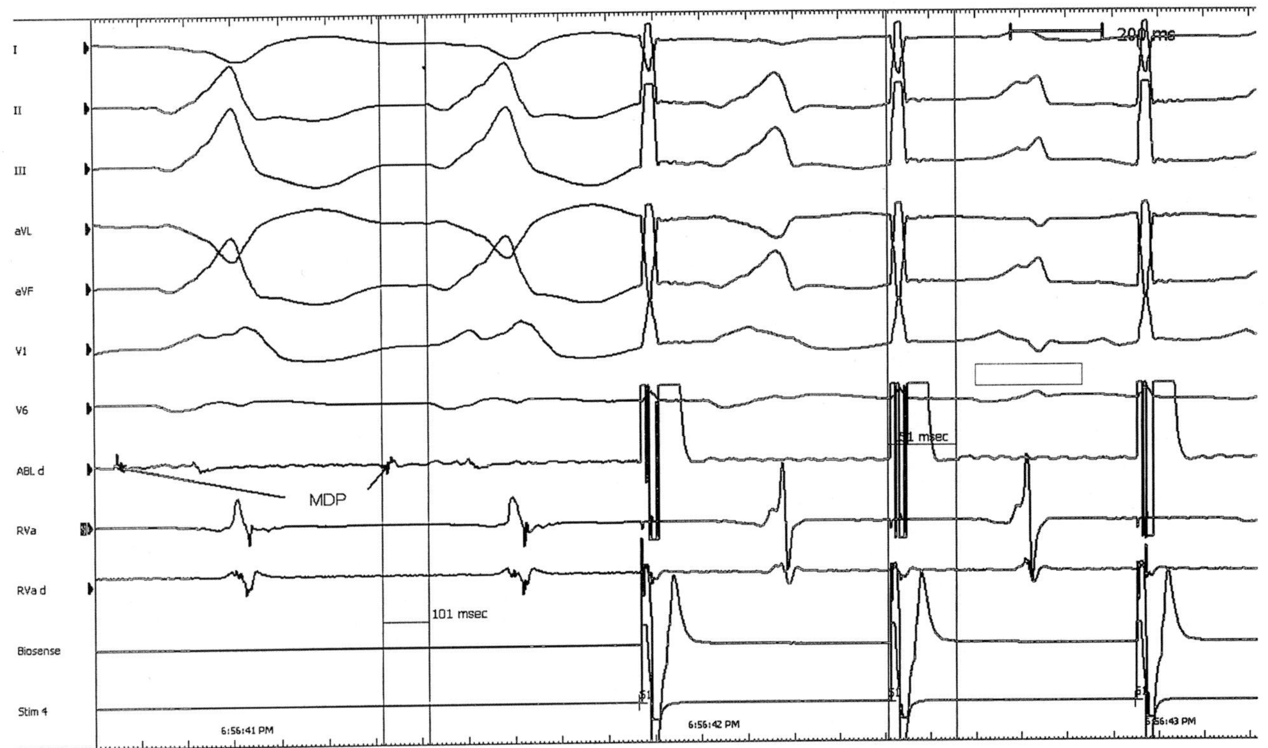

Figure 13–9 Endocardial mapping of ventricular tachycardia. Surface electrocardiograms and selected endocardial electrograms are shown during sustained ventricular tachycardia in a patient with a severe ischemic tachycardia. The mapping catheter distal electrode (ABL d) has been positioned at an endocardial site that records a mid-diastolic potential (MDP) that precedes the QRS by 101 milliseconds. Pacing at a cycle length slightly faster than the tachycardia cycle length results in ventricular capture with a QRS morphology that is slightly different from the native tachycardia. The interpretation of this maneuver is that the endocardial pacing site is not at a favorable location for catheter ablation. Pacing at an optimal site for catheter ablation produces an identical QRS morphology to the native tachycardia.

Manipulation of catheter electrodes in the heart for precise mapping and treatment of arrhythmias can be laborious and time consuming. A new stereotactic magnetic-based system can facilitate these manipulations and, it is hoped, lead to shorter ablation procedures and improved outcomes. With the system, the catheter tip is localized with three-dimensional fluoroscopy and then precisely moved to the myocardial area of interest using a magnetic field[50] (Fig. 13–10).

Surgical and catheter-based treatments of atrial fibrillation and flutter deviate from the traditional paradigm of identification and then ablation of the arrhythmogenic pathway. This is due in part to the fleeting and unpredictable nature of atrial fibrillation that precludes map-directed ablation. Further, the predictable critical anatomic substrate for atrial fibrillation and atrial flutter has allowed for the successful use of anatomic-based interventions rather than electrophysiologic map–guided ablation (see later). Regardless, the aim of electrophysiologic treatments is to interpose scar tissue within the conduction pathway of the arrhythmia. This is accomplished with a properly placed surgical incision or by inducing myocardial injury by application of an energy source from a precisely placed catheter. Various energy sources have been used including laser energy, microwave energy, and cryoablation. The most common energy source is RF energy that destroys myocardium by resistive heating. Success is determined by the volume and depth of tissue injured by RF application. Measurement of tissue impedance during application of bipolar RF energy ensures that transmural injury occurs. Because transmural scarring is not ensured with unipolar RF or microwave energy, measurement of conduction across the lesion is recommended. Failure to conduct an applied electrical stimulus indicates pathway interruption.

SPECIFIC ARRHYTHMIAS

Supraventricular Tachyarrhythmias

Supraventricular arrhythmias are defined as cardiac rhythms with a heart rate greater than 100 beats/min originating above the division of the common bundle of His. These arrhythmias are classified based on the origin (SA node, atrial myocardium, or AV junction), and they can be life threatening in the presence of an accessory pathway or when occurring in the setting of structural heart disease. Further, persistent tachycardia for weeks to months may lead to tachycardia-associated cardiomyopathy and to disabling symptoms.[41] Procedures have been developed for the treatment of supraventricular arrhythmias produced by abnormal sinus nodal function, the WPW syndrome and other forms of AV reentry, AV nodal reentry, increased atrial automaticity, and atrial fibrillation/flutter.

Atrioventricular Reentrant Tachycardia

Accessory pathways are abnormal strands of myocardium connecting the atria and ventricles across the AV groove, providing alternate routes for conduction bypassing the AV node and bundle of His (Box 13–5). Various classifications are used to describe accessory pathways based on their location by the mitral or tricuspid valves, whether conduction is decremental

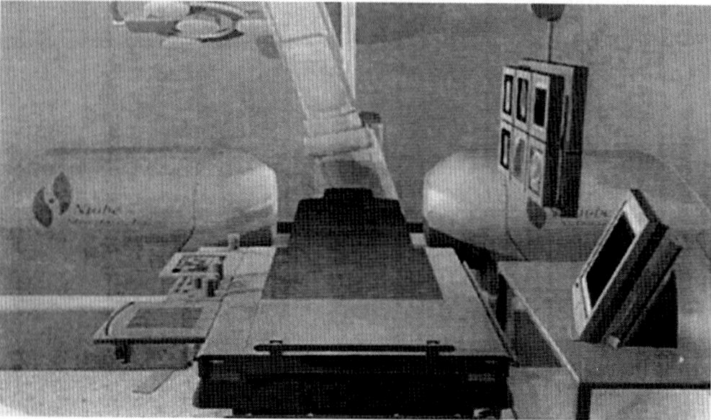

A

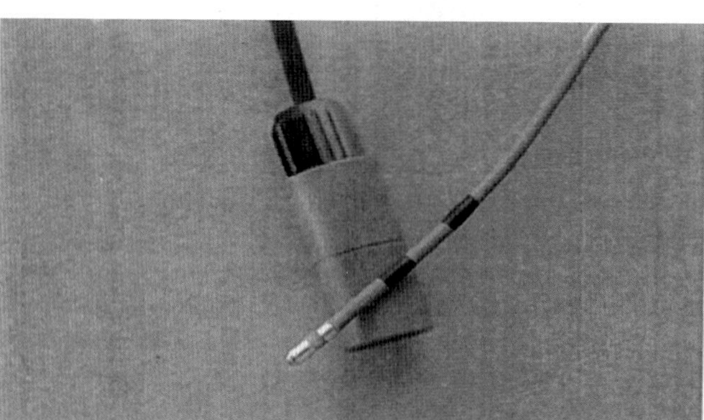

B

Figure 13–10 Stereotaxis magnetic catheter navigation system. *(A)* The Stereotaxis system consists of two permanent magnetic arrays positioned on either side of a standard fluoroscopy table and digital fluoroscopy together with a computer control system. The magnetic arrays project a composite magnetic field of 0.08 T in the region of a patient's heart to control the position of a magnetic catheter. *(B)* A 7-French magnetic catheter that is used with the Stereotaxis system is shown. The catheter has two distal electrodes for endocardial pacing, recording, and radiofrequency ablation. An internal permanent magnet allows the catheter to interact with the prevailing magnetic field for motion control.

or nondecremental with increasing pacing rates, and whether conduction is antegrade or retrograde.[51] Only a minority of accessory pathways have decremental conduction. Concealed pathways refer to the situation in which the accessory pathway only exhibits retrograde conduction. This is in contrast to manifest pathways displaying antegrade conduction on the

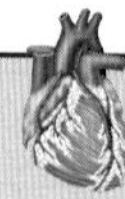

BOX 13–5 ***Atrioventricular (VA) Reentrant Tachycardia Accessory Pathways***

- Concealed: accessory pathway displays retrograde conduction
- Manifest: accessory pathway displays antegrade and retrograde conduction
- Orthodromic: antegrade conduction from atria to ventricle via the normal AV nodal conduction system and retrograde conduction via the accessory pathway
- Antidromic: antegrade conduction from atria to ventricle via the accessory pathway and retrograde conduction via the VA nodal pathway
- Treated with percutaneous radiofrequency ablation
- Treated surgically from endocardium to epicardium by transection and/or cryoablation

ECG as delta waves—the hallmark of ventricular preexcitation. Manifest pathways typically conduct in both antegrade and retrograde directions. The presence of a manifest pathway allows for the ventricle to be depolarized or "preexcited" prior to that occurring via the normal route of conduction through the AV node (Figs. 13–11 and 13–12). During preexcitation, an activation wavefront propagates simultaneously to the ventricles across the bundle of His and the accessory pathway. Because anterograde conduction is delayed at the AV node but not the accessory pathway, the impulse passing through the accessory pathway initiates ventricular depolarization prior to the impulse traveling via the normal AV conduction system. The ventricle is thus preexcited, resulting in a delta wave preceding the QRS complex (see Fig. 13–11). These ECG findings (short PR interval and delta wave) were noted by Wolff, Parkinson, and White in the 1930s in association with SVT.[52] WPW syndrome describes the condition of preexcitation when accompanied by tachyarrhythmias due to reentry via the accessory pathway. AVRT occurs in the absence of the WPW syndrome when the pathway is concealed, and not all tachyarrhythmias in patients with WPW result from the AVRT mechanism.[51]

AVRT can occur in either an orthodromic or antidromic form[53-55] (Fig. 13–13). The former refers to antegrade conduction from the atria to the ventricles via the normal AV nodal conduction system and retrograde conduction through

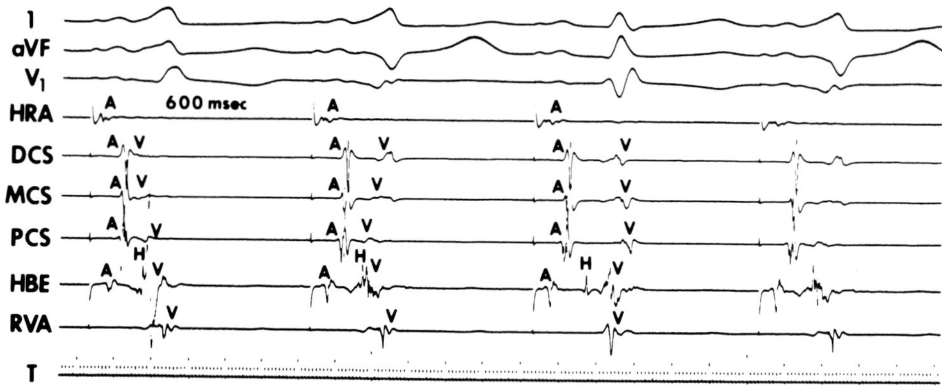

Figure 13–11 The presence of two accessory pathways is revealed during pacing. The site of earliest ventricular activation is noted with the distal coronary sinus (DCS) electrode, indicating left free-wall accessory pathway. The second paced beat shows the site of earliest ventricular activation from the proximal coronary sinus (PCS) electrode, indicating posterior septal accessory pathway. After the third paced beat neither site is activated due to anterograde conduction block. In this instance, conduction follows the normal AV-His bundle and bundle-branch pathways. Surface ECG leads and intracardiac electrograms are organized as in Figure 13-8. (From Cain ME, Cox JL: Surgical treatment of supraventricular tachyarrhythmias. *In* Platia EV [ed]: Management of Cardiac Arrhythmias. Philadelphia, JB Lippincott, 1987, p 312.)

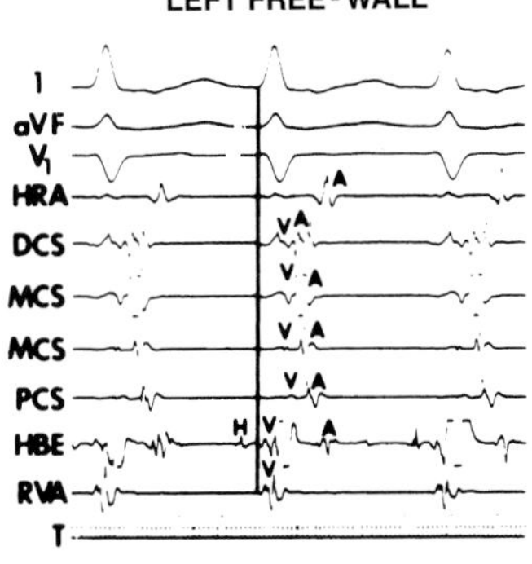

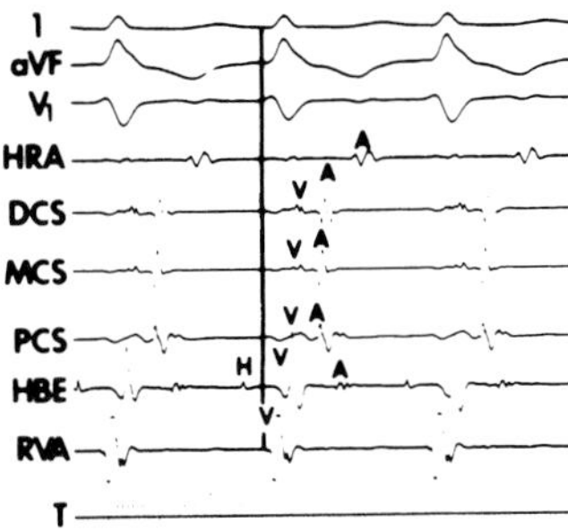

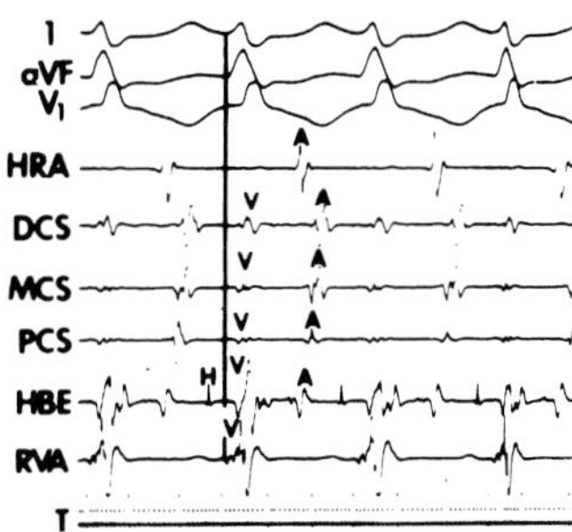

Figure 13–12 Atrial activation recordings from three different patients during orthodromic tachycardia via accessory pathways at distinct locations. Using the solid vertical line as a reference for the QRS complex from the surface ECG, the first example demonstrates the earliest atrial activation at the DCS site, indicating a left free wall accessory pathway. The posterior septal accessory pathway is indicated by earliest activation of the electrode located in the proximal coronary sinus (PCS). In the last example, atrial activation at the high right atrium (HRA) and His bundle (HBE) occurs before all the coronary sinus recording sites, indicative of a right free-wall accessory pathway. Surface ECG leads and intracardiac electrograms are organized as in Figure 13–8. (From Cain ME, Cox JL: Surgical treatment of supraventricular tachyarrhythmias. *In* Platia EV [ed]: Management of Cardiac Arrhythmias. Philadelphia, JB Lippincott, 1987, p 313.)

the accessory pathway. In contrast, antidromic tachycardia refers to antegrade conduction via the accessory pathway and retrograde conduction to the atria through the AV nodal pathway. Antidromic AVRT is much less common than the orthodromic form. Importantly, atrial fibrillation occurring in patients with WPW syndrome can rapidly progress to ventricular fibrillation and sudden death due to the lack of decremental conduction across the accessory pathway. The potential for sudden death due to atrial fibrillation in patients with WPW provides an argument for aggressive ablative treat-

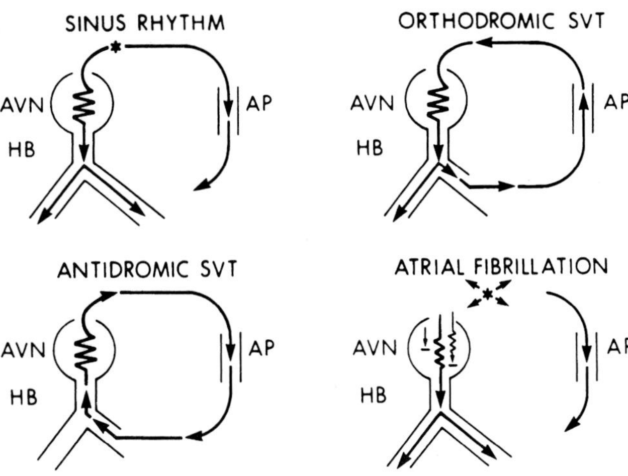

Figure 13–13 Schematic representation of conduction through an accessory pathway (AP) and the normal conduction system (AVN HB) during sinus rhythm, orthodromic supraventricular tachycardia (SVT), antidromic SVT, and atrial fibrillation. (From Lindsay BD, Branyas NA, Cain ME: The preexcitation syndrome. *In* El-Sherif N, Samet P [eds]: Cardiac Pacing and Electrophysiology, 3rd edition. Orlando, FL, Grune & Stratton, 1990.)

ment when the procedure can be performed in centers with low periprocedural morbidity.

By noting polarity of the delta wave (QRS axis) and precordial R-wave progression, the resting 12-lead ECG can provide clues about the location of the accessory pathway in either the left lateral, left posterior, posterior septal, right free wall, or anterior septal regions[56] (Table 13–1). Precise localization, though, is dependent on EPS. Additional information provided by such investigation includes documentation of the mechanism for the arrhythmia (AV versus other mechanism) and the conduction properties of the accessory pathways.[57] The atrial and ventricular insertion sites of the accessory pathway are identified by observing ventricular activation patterns during sinus rhythm and during atrial pacing (see Fig. 13–11). In the presence of an accessory pathway, the interval between the deflection denoting activation of the bundle of His and the earliest ventricular activation (delta wave) is less than the H-V interval. The area with the shortest delta-to-V interval localizes the accessory pathway's ventricular insertion. More than one accessory pathway may be present, which is suggested by observing different delta-wave morphology with increasing atrial pacing rates or with introduced atrial premature beats (see Fig. 13–12). Observing atrial activation patterns during ventricular pacing, after a ventricular premature beat, or during induced orthodromic SVT can identify the location of the atrial insertion sites.

Catheter-Based Therapy for Accessory Pathways

Percutaneous catheter ablation of accessory pathways has largely supplanted the surgical approach to treatment. RF ablation is typically performed during EPS once the accessory pathway has been localized. Transseptal or retrograde aortic catheter approaches are used to ablate left-sided accessory pathways, and right-heart catheterization via a venous approach is used to ablate right-sided pathways. Success rates of 95% have been reported using these methods.[51,58-60] Recurrence rates after successful catheter ablation of an accessory

Table 13-1 ECG Patterns Common with Different Anatomical Location of Accessory Pathways

Region	Negative Delta Wave	QRS Frontal Axis	R > S
Left lateral free-wall	I and/or aVL	Normal	V_1 to V_3
Left posterior free-wall	III and aVF	−75 to +75	V_1
Posterior septal	III and aVF	0 to −90	V_2 to V_4
Right free-wall	aVR	Normal	V_3 to V_5
Anterior septal	V_1 and V_2	Normal	V_3 to V_5

Note: R > S refers to progression of the R-wave in the precordial ECG leads. (Adapted from Lindsay BD, Crossen KL, Cain ME: Concordance of distinguishing electrocardiographic features during sinus rhythm with the location of accessory pathways in the Wolff-Parkinson-White syndrome. Am J Cardiol 59:1093, 1987.)

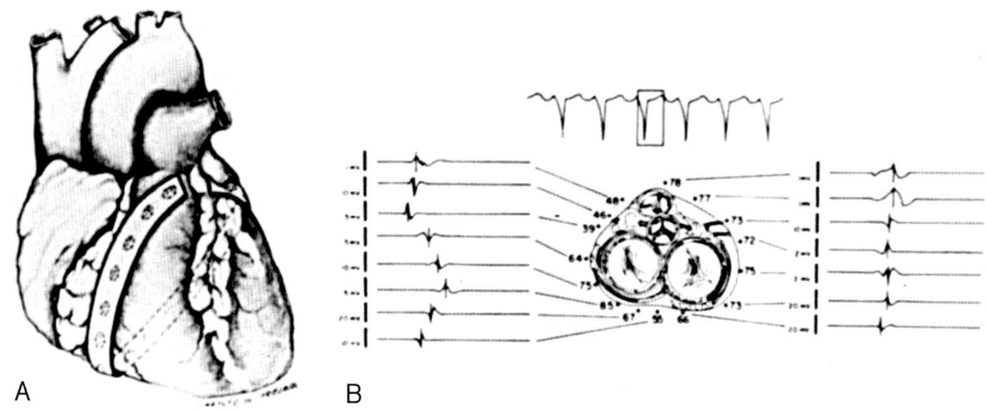

Figure 13–14 Intraoperative electrophysiologic study recorded from a band of electrodes placed on the ventricular side of the AV groove *(A)*. The single beat is analyzed *(B)* as noted by the window on the surface ECG *(top)*. The ventricular activation sequences are shown *(bottom)* noting the earliest activation on the left ventricular free wall. (From Ferguson TB Jr, Cox JL: Surgical therapy for patients with supraventricular tachycardia. Cardiol Clin 8:535, 1990.)

pathway are generally less than 5%. Overall, reported complications are low and include those related to vascular access such as hematoma and AV fistula. Other complications are related to catheter manipulations of the left- and right-sided circulation such as valvular or cardiac damage from the catheter, systemic and cerebral embolization due to catheter manipulation in the aorta, coronary sinus damage, coronary thrombosis and dissection, cardiac perforation, and cardiac tamponade. Complete AV block, cardiac perforation, and coronary spasm due to RF may also occur. A 1995 survey involving 5427 patients reported serious complications from catheter ablation of accessory pathways in 1.8% of patients and procedure-related mortality in 0.08%.[51,58] Complete AV block is more common with septal accessory pathway ablation. Procedural success with catheter ablation methods is reported to be 87% to 99%.[51,59,60] In a randomized study comparing ablation with drug treatment, quality of life, symptom scores, and exercise performance were improved with successful RF ablation.[61]

Surgical Therapy for Accessory Pathways

Due to progress with percutaneous catheter-based ablation treatments, surgical interruption of accessory pathways is limited to patients for whom RF ablation failed or those patients with concomitant cardiac disease necessitating surgery. Surgery is performed via a median sternotomy, and the patient is first prepared for CPB including cannulation of the aorta and vena cava. Electrophysiologic mapping is then performed by placing electrodes along the ventricular and atrial sides of the AV groove (Figs. 13–14 and 13–15). Overdrive atrial pacing is performed and anterograde ventricular activation assessed. Retrograde conduction is then assessed by performing ventricular pacing. The earliest site of ventricular activation in sinus rhythm or atrial pacing and the earliest atrial activation site in response to ventricular pacing indicate the sites of ventricular and atrial insertion of the accessory pathway, respectively. Because accessory pathways can originate or insert anywhere from the endocardium to the epicardium, the basic principle of surgery is to perform endocardial-to-epicardial dissection.[62-70] Accessory pathways are most often located in the left free wall followed in frequency of occurrence by the posterior septal, right free wall, and anterior septal positions (Fig. 13–16). Multiple pathways are found in 20% of patients.[63,67,70]

Accessory pathways can be approached via an endocardial or epicardial dissection. For left free wall pathways, the endocardial approach involves dissection of the entire free wall space (AV groove) to the epicardial reflection off the posterior left ventricle.[10,70,71] After the heart has been arrested with cold cardioplegia, left atriotomy is performed and a supra-annular incision is placed 2 mm above the posterior leaflet of the mitral valve extending from the left fibrous trigone to the posterior septum. A sharp nerve hook or a knife is used to transect any remaining fibers connecting the atria to the ventricle. After completion of the left-sided dissection, the supra-

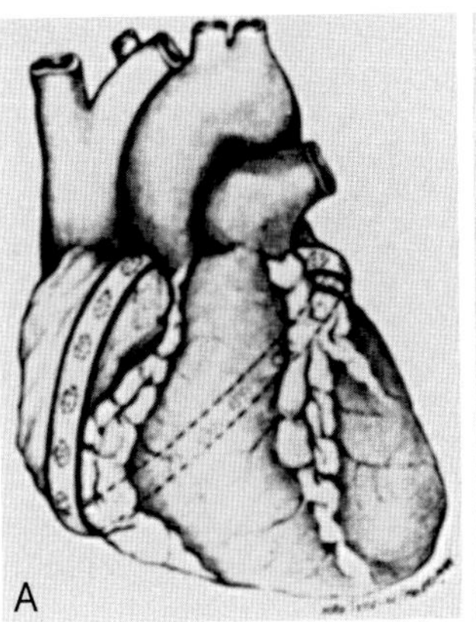

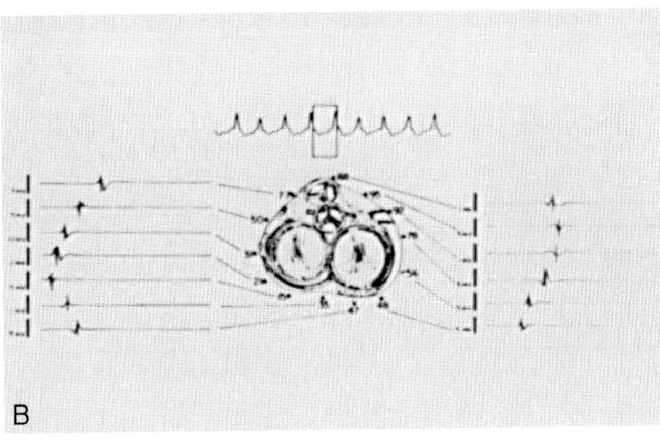

Figure 13–15 Intraoperative electrophysiologic study recorded from a band of electrodes now placed on the atrial side of the AV groove *(A)* in contrast to their location in Figure 13-9 (ventricular side of the AV groove). Atrial activation is analyzed *(B)* from a single beat isolated in the window from the surface ECG *(top)*. The site of earliest atrial activation is again noted on the left atrial free wall. (From Ferguson TB Jr, Cox JL: Surgical therapy for patients with supraventricular tachycardia. Cardiol Clin 8:535, 1990.)

annular incision is closed. The epicardial approach incorporates dissection from the left atrial side of the AV groove to the level of the posterior mitral valve annulus.[72-74] The dissection plane passes underneath the vascular structures located in the epicardial fat and divides the atrial end of the accessory pathway in this area, except for those pathways that are located immediately adjacent to the mitral valve annulus. Intraoperative mapping is then performed to evaluate the results of the dissection. If the abnormal conduction persists, cryoablation is performed (60°C for 1 to 3 minutes) at the level of the mitral valve annulus to destroy any accessory pathways that might have remained intact.

Posterior septal pathways are located in the posterior septal space between the two AV valves. Due to the proximity to the AV node and the bundle of His, heart block may occur after posterior septal accessory pathway interruption.[75] A right atriotomy is performed and the bundle of His identified with a hand-held electrode. A supra-annular incision is then made above the posterior medial tricuspid valve annulus and extended onto the free wall of the posterior right atrium. A plane of dissection is established between the fat pad occupying the posterior septal space and the posterior ventricular septum. Once this portion of the dissection is completed, the heart is arrested with cold cardioplegic solution. The dissection is then completed by following the mitral annulus over to the posterior left ventricle. Dissection in the region is via an epicardial incision placed anterior to the coronary sinus to expose the AV junction.

The epicardial approach for right free wall pathways can be performed on a beating heart. Dissection of the AV groove is carried out and cryoablation of the pathways located adjacent to the tricuspid annulus is also performed. The endocardial approach does necessitate CPB as dissection of the AV groove is performed via a right atriotomy.[76] Anterior septal pathways are approached via a right atriotomy. Typically, the pathway is located adjacent to the right fibrous trigone anterior to the bundle of His. A supra-annular incision is made above the tricuspid annulus and extended well onto the right anterior free wall. The proximal right coronary artery traverses through the AV groove in proximity to the dissection plane, necessitating extreme care with the incision to avoid injuring the vessel.[10]

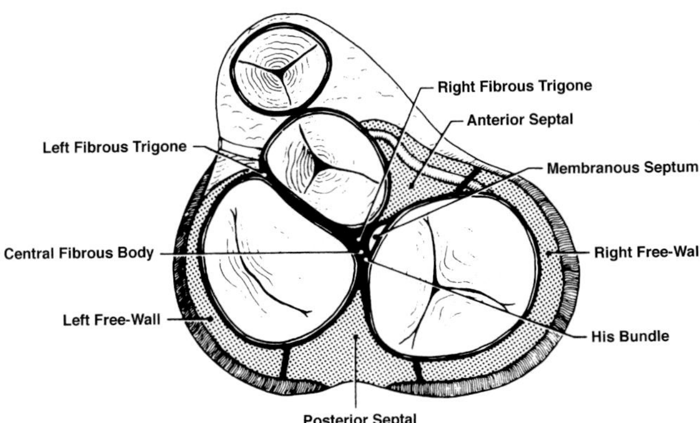

Figure 13–16 Transverse section of the heart drawn to show the four anatomic locations of accessory pathways in Wolff-Parkinson-White syndrome: left free wall, posterior septal, right free wall, and anterior septal. (From Cox JL, Ferguson TB Jr: Surgery for the Wolff-Parkinson-White syndrome: The endocardial approach. Semin Thorac Cardiovasc Surg 1:34, 1989.)

Atrioventricular Nodal Reentrant Tachycardia

AVNRT is due to altered electrophysiologic properties of the anterior fast pathway and posterior slow pathway fibers providing input to the AV node.[10,51,59,60] In the past, the only treatment for recurrent SVT due to AVNRT was total ablation of the His bundle and permanent pacemaker insertion.[10] Surgical techniques developed in the 1980s provided an alternate treatment that was associated with high procedural success, acceptable morbidity, and preservation of atrial–ventricular conduction.[77-81] Fundamentals developed with this surgical approach and increased understanding of the physiologic basis of AVNRT led to the development of percutaneous catheter-based treatments. Interruption of either the slow or fast pathway with RF ablation can eliminate AVNRT, with higher success rates reported for ablation of the slow pathway (slow-pathway ablation, 68% to 100%, versus fast-pathway ablation, 46% to 94%).[51,82-86] Complication rates are reportedly lower with slow pathway RF ablation and include AV block requiring pacemaker insertion (1%)[51] (Box 13–6).

Catheter-Based Therapy for Atrioventricular Nodal Reentrant Tachycardia

Fast pathway ablation is performed by positioning the catheter adjacent to the AV node–His bundle anterosuperior to the tricuspid valve annulus. The catheter is withdrawn until the atrial electrogram is larger than the ventricular electrogram and the His recording small or absent. The ECG is closely monitored as RF energy is applied for PR prolongation/heart

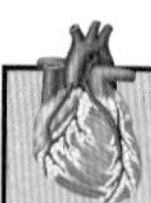

BOX 13–6 *Atrioventricular (AV) Nodal Reentrant Tachycardia (AVNRT)*

- Altered electrophysiologic properties of the anterior fast and posterior slow pathways provide input to the AV node
- Successful fast pathway ablation occurs when the PR interval is prolonged or fast-pathway conduction eliminated
- Successful slow pathway ablation occurs when induced AVNRT is eliminated
- Surgical techniques involve selective cryoablation

block. The energy is delivered until there is PR prolongation or the retrograde fast-pathway conduction is eliminated. Noninducibility of AVNRT then is confirmed. Slow pathway ablation is performed by identifying the pathway along the posteromedial tricuspid annulus near the coronary sinus. Using fluoroscopy, one approach is to divide the level of the coronary sinus os and His bundle recordings into six anatomic regions[87] (Fig. 13–17). Lesions are then placed beginning with the most posterior region moving anteriorly. Rather than the anatomic approach, the slow pathway can be mapped and then ablated by performing ventricular pacing. The end point of slow pathway ablation is elimination of induced AVNRT.[82-86] The development of junctional ectopy during RF ablation of the slow pathway is associated with successful slow-pathway ablation.[88]

Surgical Therapy for Atrioventricular Nodal Reentrant Tachycardia

Surgical techniques for treating AVNRT involve selective cryoablation of the reentrant pathway, while avoiding the normal AV conduction tract.[89] Following institution of CPB, a right atriotomy is performed and the bundle of His is identified with a hand-held electrode. Atrial pacing is performed and the AV interval is monitored. Cryolesions are then placed along the tendon of Todaro (Fig. 13–18), moving sequentially toward the apex of the triangle of Koch near the bundle of His. Cryothermia application increases the AV interval in a linear fashion, with interval prolongation of approximately 200 to 300 milliseconds, indicating impending

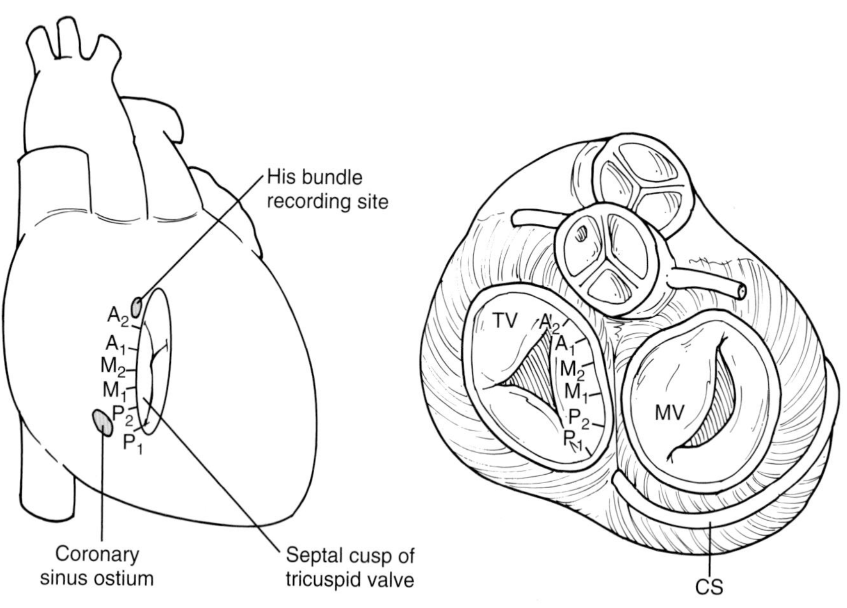

Figure 13–17 Schematic representation of sites for AV nodal modification in relation to other anatomic structures. The posterior location is usually first targeted for ablation of the slow-pathway with subsequent ablative lesions placed more anteriorly depending on the response. TV = tricuspid valve; MV = mitral valve; CS = coronary sinus. (From Akhtar M, Jazayeri MR, Sra JS, et al: Atrioventricular nodal reentry: Clinical, electrophysiologic, and therapeutic considerations. Circulation 88:282, 1993. Reprinted with permission from the American Heart Association.)

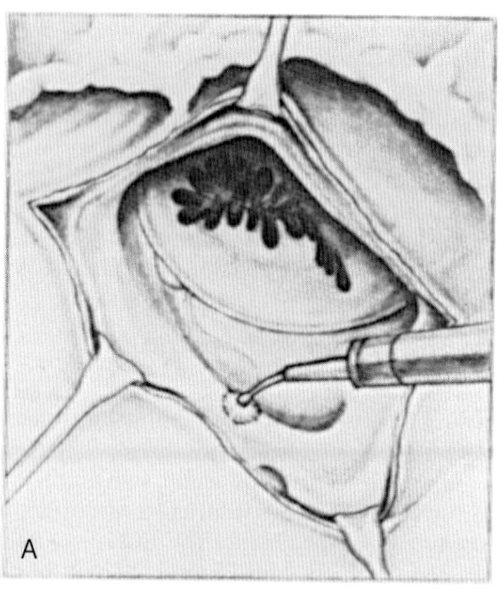

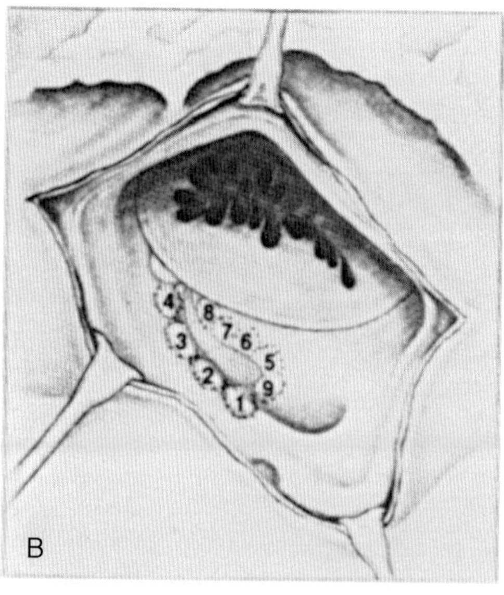

Figure 13–18 Surgical treatment of AV node reentrant tachycardia using nitrous oxide cryoprobe to place nine lesions at the atrioventricular junction starting at the coronary sinus ostia along the tendon of Todaro (sites 1, 2, 3, and 4) and the annulus of the tricuspid valve (sites 5, 6, 7, and 8). See text for detailed description. (Adapted from Cox JL, Holman WL, Cain ME: Cryosurgical treatment of atrioventricular node reentry tachycardia. Circulation 76:1329, 1987.)

complete heart block. When the AV interval reaches this level of prolongation, the cryoprobe is immediately removed to prevent permanent damage of the AV conduction system. Additional cryolesions are placed along the annulus of the tricuspid valve just beneath the os of the coronary sinus.

Focal Atrial Tachycardia

Focal atrial tachycardia is a relatively rare arrhythmia mechanism accounting for less than 15% of patients undergoing evaluation for SVT.[90] The arrhythmia is due to atrial activation from a discrete atrial area resulting in heart rates between 100 and 250 beats/min.[91] Although the 12-lead ECG might provide clues to the origin of the tachycardia based on P-wave axis, localization of the site of atrial tachycardia is made by electrophysiologic investigations and tends to "cluster" in certain anatomic zones.[51] Right-sided tachycardias typically originate along the crista terminalis from the SA node to the AV node and left-sided ones from the pulmonary veins, atrial septum, or mitral valve annulus.[91,92] The mechanisms for atrial tachycardia include abnormal automaticity, triggered activity, or micro-reentry. Characteristics of the arrhythmia might provide clues to the underlying mechanisms. Abrupt onset and offset suggest a reentrant mechanism, while a gradual onset ("warm-up") and offset ("cool-down") pattern suggests automaticity (Box 13–7).

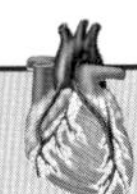

BOX 13–7 ***Focal Atrial Tachycardia***

- Mechanisms include abnormal automaticity, triggered activity, or microreentry
- Catheter-based treatment is with radiofrequency ablation
- Surgical-based treatment is with incision and cryoablation

Catheter-Based Therapy for Focal Atrial Tachycardia

Due to the discrete localized area involved in generating atrial tachycardia, the approach to catheter ablation is the same regardless of the mechanisms for the arrhythmia. The site of tachycardia onset is identified with electrophysiologic mapping and then isolated from the remaining atrium by application of RF current. Success of this approach is reported to be 86%, and recurrence rates, 8%.[51,92-96] Complications reported in these series occur in 1% to 2% of cases and include rare myocardial perforation, phrenic nerve injury, and sinus node dysfunction.[97]

Surgical Therapy for Focal Atrial Tachycardia

Due to success with catheter-based techniques, surgical ablation of atrial tachycardia is rarely performed but may be indicated for a select group of patients with concomitant cardiac disease. Surgical procedures performed in the past were successful in isolating the arrhythmogenic area of the atrium while preserving AV conduction.[10,98,99] Once the site of the tachycardia is localized based on preoperative and/or intraoperative electrophysiologic evaluation, incisions and cryoablation are used to interrupt connections of the involved atrial myocardium with the remainder of the heart. For right-sided tachycardia, care is taken to preserve the continuity of the sinoatrial node with the atrial septum and AV node while isolating the atrial myocardium responsible for the tachycardia.

Sinus Tachycardia

Sinus tachycardia is deemed inappropriate when it occurs in the absence of physiologic stressors (e.g., increased body temperature, hypovolemia, anemia, hyperthyroidism, anxiety, postural changes, drugs, etc), indicating failure of normal mechanisms controlling sinus rate. Proposed mechanisms are enhanced sinus node automaticity and/or abnormal autonomic regulation. The diagnosis is made based on nonparoxysmal, persistent resting sinus tachycardia and excessive increases in response to normal physiologic stressors and nocturnal normalization of the rate based on Holter monitoring.[51] The P-wave morphology and endocardial activation are consistent with a sinus origin and secondary causes have been excluded. Catheter-based or surgical treatments are considered for a minority of patients not responding to β-blockers and when symptoms are disabling. The aim of this treatment is RF ablative modification of the sinus node to promote dominance of slower depolarizing sinus nodal tissues. An esophageal electrode is placed and connected to the operating room ECG monitor to guide treatment. The end point of application of RF energy is change in the P-wave morphology. Reported complications include need for permanent pacemaker, superior vena cava (SVC) syndrome, phrenic nerve injury, and pericarditis.[51,100] Acute and long-term reported success rates are 76% and 66%, respectively.[51,100]

Sinus Node Reentrant Tachycardia

Reentrant pathways involving the sinus node may lead to paroxysmal tachycardia, in contrast to the nonparoxysmal inappropriate sinus tachycardia.[101] The P-wave morphology is similar to that occurring during sinus rhythm. Similar to other reentrant tachycardias, the arrhythmia is usually triggered by a premature atrial beat. Endocardial activation sequence on EPS is in the high right atrium and is similar to sinus rhythm. The arrhythmia can be initiated with a premature pace beat and is terminated by vagal maneuvers or adenosine.[51] Clinically, the arrhythmia is also responsive to β-blockers, nonhydropyridine calcium channel antagonists, and amiodarone. RF ablation of the identified reentrant pathway is an effective treatment for frequently occurring tachycardia episodes not responsive to other treatments.[102]

Atrial Flutter

Atrial flutter usually presents with acute onset of symptoms (e.g., palpitations, shortness of breath, fatigue) accompanied by a tachycardia and typical "flutter" waves on the ECG (Box 13–8). Fixed 2:1 conduction is usually present with flutter rate of 300 beats/min and ventricular rate of 150 beats/min. When AV conduction is fixed, the heart rate is regular, but varying AV conduction results in an irregular rhythm. Rapid AV conduction can occur with exercise, in patients with accessory pathways, and, paradoxically, after administration of class 1C antiarrhythmic drugs.[51] The latter results from the antiarrhythmic drugs slowing atrial

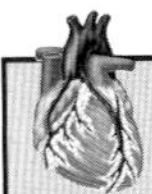

BOX 13–8 ***Atrial Flutter***

- Reentry occurs due to a large anatomic circuit
- Macroreentrant pathway is amenable to catheter ablation

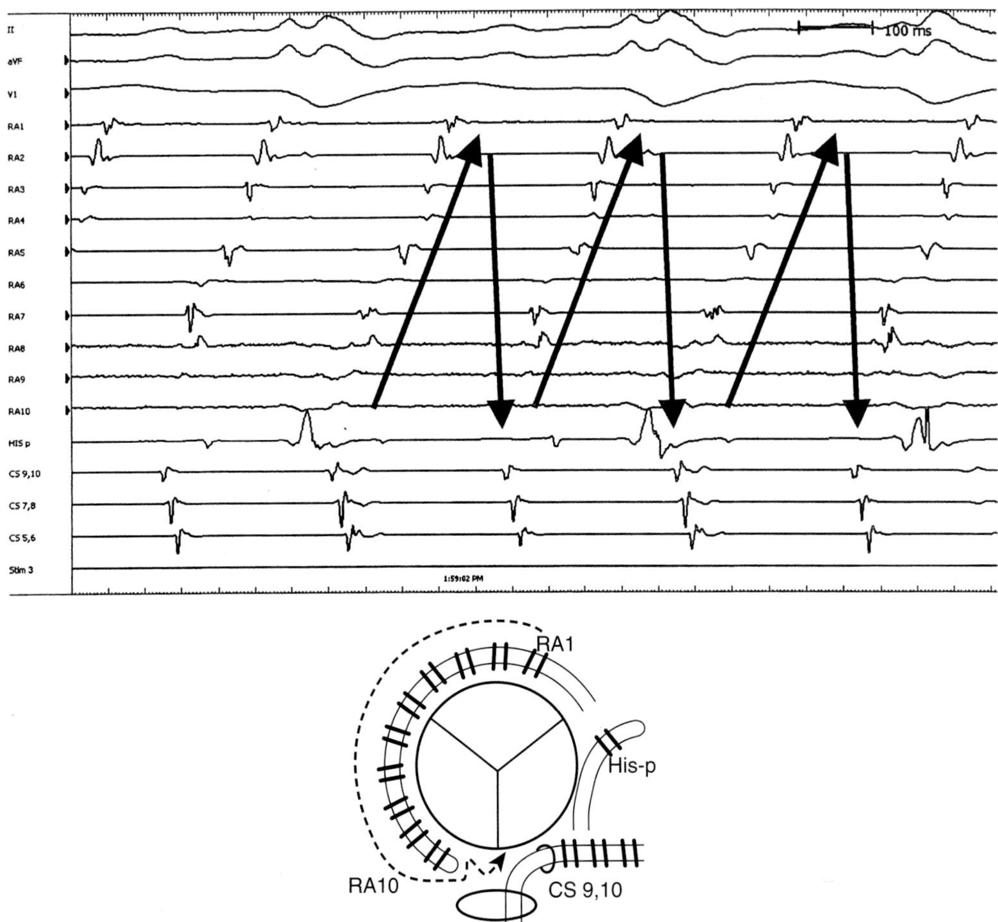

Figure 13–19 Endocardial mapping of typical atrial flutter. Endocardial signals recorded from diagnostic catheters are shown in a patient with typical atrial flutter. The anatomic basis for this circuit is an electrical wavefront circulating in a counterclockwise direction around the tricuspid valve annulus. A 20-pole catheter has been positioned around the tricuspid valve to record the passage of the activation wavefront by adjacent electrode pairs RA1 to RA10. The wavefront then proceeds across the isthmus connecting the inferior vena cava and the tricuspid valve before passing the ostium of the coronary sinus (CS), recorded by CS electrodes 9 and 10 and the His bundle recording catheter (His-p). The progress of the activation wavefront is indicated by the schematic arrows and by the diagram at the bottom of the figure.

rate, thus promoting more rapid AV conduction. This maneuver requires coadministration of drugs with AV conduction-slowing properties (e.g., β-blockers).

Atrial flutter is due to reentry that is referred to as "macroreentry" because the anatomic circuit is large. "Typical" atrial flutter occupies a circuit that circles the tricuspid valve, crossing the myocardial isthmus between the inferior vena cava (IVC) and the tricuspid valve[51,91] (Fig. 13–19). Counterclockwise rotation through the cava-tricuspid region is usually observed, although other patterns such as clockwise rotation, double-waves, and "lower loop" reentry (i.e., reentry around the inferior vena cava) might be observed.[51,103,104] Polarity of the flutter waves on the 12-lead ECG provides insight into the pattern of atrial flutter. Counterclockwise rotation is associated with negative flutter waves in the inferior leads and positive flutter waves in V_1, while the opposite is observed with clockwise rotation.[51]

The anatomic location of this macroreentrant pathway is amenable to catheter ablation and cure of atrial flutter by creating a linear conduction block across the tricuspid-IVC isthmus. Testing for bidirectional conduction block through the caval-tricuspid region after application of RF energy enhances success.[105,106]

Atrial flutter and atrial fibrillation may coexist, complicating success with catheter ablation methods. Procedural success with pure atrial flutter is reported in 80% to 100% of cases, with recurrence occurring in 16% of patients.[107-111] In a prospective, randomized trial, catheter ablation resulted in sinus rhythm in 80% of patients, compared with 36% of patients treated with antiarrhythmic drugs (mean follow-up of 21 months).[111] Fewer hospitalizations and higher scores on quality-of-life surveys are reported after catheter ablation compared with drug treatment. In the absence of atrial fibrillation, subsequent RF ablation procedures may result in successful elimination of atrial flutter. Even when not present during initial treatment, atrial fibrillation may develop after successful catheter ablation for atrial flutter in 8% to 12% of patients.[51,109]

Atrial scar tissue from prior cardiac surgery (e.g., congenital heart surgery, mitral valve surgery, Maze procedure) may provide an area for reentry leading to atrial flutter.[92,112-115] Reentrant circuits involving the caval-tricuspid area may coexist, leading to complicated, multiple reentry pathways.[51,115] Characterization of the reentry circuit with electrophysiologic mapping studies may allow for successful RF ablation in these circumstances.

Anesthetic Considerations for Supraventricular Arrhythmia Surgery/Ablation Procedures

The approach to the care of patients undergoing surgical or percutaneous therapies for supraventricular arrhythmias involves similar basic principles. Patients with WPW surgery are usually young and free of other cardiac disease. The age in larger series is reported, though, to range from 9 months to 70 years.[70] The syndrome can be accompanied by congenital cardiac abnormalities. Ebstein's anomaly, for example, is associated with WPW in up to 10% of cases.[70,116] Anesthesiologists must be familiar with preoperative EPS results and the characteristics of associated supraventricular arrhythmias (rate, associated hemodynamic disturbances, syncope, etc.), including treatments. Tachyarrhythmias might recur at any time during surgical and percutaneous treatments. Transcutaneous cardioversion/defibrillation adhesive pads are placed prior to anesthesia induction and connected to a defibrillator/cardioverter. In a series of patients undergoing WPW surgery, Irish et al[117] reported two episodes of SVT prior to induction of anesthesia and single episodes of atrial fibrillation and SVT during central venous cannulation. The development of tachyarrhythmias in this retrospective review was unrelated to any single anesthetic or adjuvant drug. In another series, tachyarrhythmias were not observed before or after induction of anesthesia in patients undergoing WPW surgery.[10,117,118] The development of atrial fibrillation may be particularly deleterious in patients with WPW syndrome. Accessory pathways lack delay in conduction as seen in the AV node such that fibrillatory impulses are rapidly conducted to the ventricle. Immediate cardioversion is required to avoid rapid degeneration to ventricular fibrillation (Box 13–9).

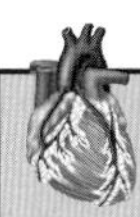

BOX 13–9 ***Anesthetic Considerations for Supraventricular Arrhythmia Surgery and Ablation Procedures***

- Familiarity with electrophysiologic study results and associated treatments
- Transcutaneous cardioversion/defibrillation pads placed prior to induction
- Hemodynamically tolerated tachyarrhythmias treated by slowing conduction across accessory pathway as opposed to atrioventricular node
- Hemodynamically significant tachyarrhythmias treated with cardioversion
- Avoid sympathetic stimulation

Treatment of hemodynamically tolerated tachyarrhythmias in this group of patients is aimed at slowing conduction across the accessory pathway as opposed to the AV node. Therapy directed at slowing conduction across the AV node (e.g., β-adrenergic–blocking drugs, verapamil, digoxin) may enhance conduction across accessory pathways and should be used only if proved safe by prior EPS. Drugs that are recommended include amiodarone and procainamide. A consideration is that antiarrhythmic drugs may interfere with intraoperative mapping. Hemodynamically significant tachyarrhythmias developing prior to intraoperative mapping are usually treated with cardioversion.

The effects of anesthetics on accessory pathway conduction have been investigated mostly to evaluate whether these agents might interfere with electrophysiologic mapping. Droperidol has been demonstrated to depress accessory pathway conduction but the clinical significance of small antiemetic doses is likely minimal.[119,120] Opioids and barbiturates have no proven electrophysiologic effect on accessory pathways and have been shown to be safe in patients with WPW syndrome.[121-124] Normal AV conduction is depressed by halothane, isoflurane, and enflurane, and preliminary evidence suggests that these volatile anesthetics may also depress accessory pathway conduction.[125-128] Although muscle relaxants with anticholinergic effects (e.g., pancuronium) have been safely used in patients with WPW, drugs lacking autonomic side effects are most often chosen.[129]

The major goal of the anesthetic management of patients undergoing supraventricular surgery or ablative procedures is to avoid sympathetic stimulation and the development of tachyarrhythmias. Clinical studies have evaluated the efficacy of various anesthetic techniques in maintaining intraoperative hemodynamic stability and in preventing arrhythmias in patients with WPW syndrome.[10,130,131] An opioid-based anesthetic technique with supplemental volatile anesthetics is typically used in patients having surgical division of accessory pathways. For surgical therapy, monitoring is based mostly on associated cardiac disorders. Care is taken with central venous cannulation or pulmonary artery catheter placement to avoid precipitating arrhythmias due to direct cardiac stimulation.[132] Intraoperative transesophageal echocardiography (TEE) during WPW surgery is also useful, especially to assist in removing air from cardiac chambers after left-sided open cardiac procedures.[10]

Atrial Fibrillation

Atrial fibrillation, the most common sustained cardiac arrhythmia in the general population, can lead to palpitations, shortness of breath, chest discomfort, or anxiety due to the irregular-irregular heart rate pattern[5] (Box 13–10). The treatment aims for atrial fibrillation include anticoagulation to decrease the risk for stroke and heart rate control to limit symptoms and reduce the risk for tachycardia-associated cardiomyopathy.[41] Restoration of sinus rhythm with either cardioversion and/or antiarrhythmic drugs is considered in some instances, but data suggest this strategy is no more effective than a strategy of anticoagulation/heart rate control for improving mortality.[133] Because antiarrhythmic drugs are associated with life-threatening proarrhythmic side effects, speculation exists that any benefits of restoring sinus rhythm might be outweighed by mortality due to drug-induced ven-

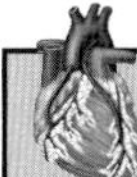

BOX 13–10 ***Atrial Fibrillation Features***

- Associated with multiple reentrant circuits
- May originate from automatic foci in pulmonary vein or vena cava
- Treatment with catheter ablation
  - Atrioventricular node ablation with pacemaker placement
  - Curative ablation to restore sinus rhythm
- Surgical therapy with the Maze procedure

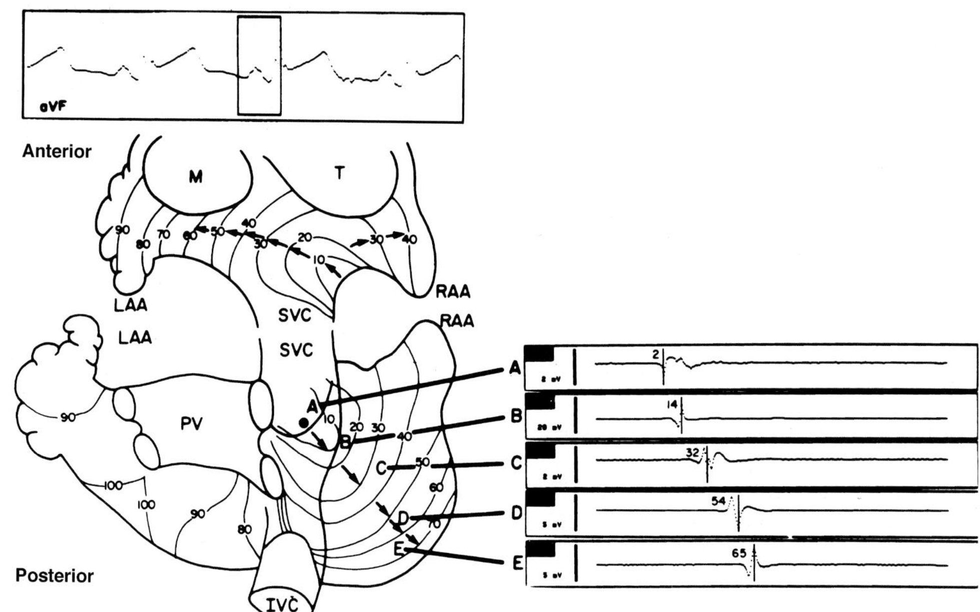

Figure 13–20 Atrial activation sequence map of a single beat during sinus rhythm in a human. Isochronous lines are in 10-millisecond increments across the anterior and posterior atrium. The upper left panel is the lead aVF from the surface ECG and the window denotes the P wave chosen to obtain atrial mapping data. The labels on each electrogram A to E correspond to the letters on the map denoting the five electrode positions shown. The time of activation from the electrodes is used to generate the isochronous representation of atrial depolarization. LAA = left atrial appendage; RAA = right atrial appendage; SVC = superior vena cava; IVC = inferior vena cava; PV = pulmonary veins; M = mitral valve; T = tricuspid valve. (From Cox JL, Canavan TE, Schuessler RB, et al: The surgical treatment of atrial fibrillation. II. Intraoperative electrophysiologic mapping and description of the electrophysiologic basis of atrial flutter and atrial fibrillation. J Thorac Cardiovasc Surg 101:406, 1991.)

tricular arrhythmias.[7] Regardless, the rising prevalence of atrial fibrillation and the limitations of pharmacologic treatments have led to much interest in nonpharmacologic treatments.

A growing understanding of the mechanisms of atrial fibrillation has led to the introduction of surgical and catheter-based procedures to restore sinus rhythm. Experimental and clinical investigations demonstrate that atrial fibrillation is associated with multiple reentrant circuits in the atrium ("multiple wavelets") that rapidly and unpredictably change their anatomic location.[134-137] Intraoperative electrophysiologic mapping of a patient in sinus rhythm (Fig. 13–20), and then after atrial fibrillation was induced by introducing atrial ectopic beats (Fig. 13–21), demonstrates the random and fleeting nature of the reentrant circuits.[137] The rapidly changing nature of the reentrant circuits preclude a map-directed surgical or ablative strategy for atrial fibrillation. Nonetheless, the realization that certain cardiac structures (e.g., pulmonary veins, valve annulus, vena cava) were necessary substrate for the fibrillatory reentrant circuits led to the development of an anatomy-based surgical procedure for atrial fibrillation (the Cox-Maze procedure) whereby macroreentrant circuits are interrupted by a series of atrial incisions and cryoablation lesions.[137-139]

Investigators have demonstrated that atrial fibrillation in some instances originates from automatic foci in the pulmonary veins or vena cava and that isolating these sites may restore sinus rhythm[140] (Fig. 13–22). Other data have demonstrated focal sources of atrial fibrillation in patients with mitral valve disease.[141,142] These findings are supported by laboratory investigations showing that atrial fibrillation can be maintained by a single atrial source of fibrillatory waves moving away from the originating circuit.[143,144] These and other findings, along with advances in computer-based electrophysiologic mapping systems, open up the possibility of map-guided strategies to eliminate the substrate for atrial fibrillation in some patients.[145-155] The latter strategy would have the benefit of perhaps higher success rates and lower complications than what occurs with current procedures.

Catheter-Based Therapy for Atrial Fibrillation

Catheter ablation approaches for atrial fibrillation include AV node ablation with permanent pacemaker placement to control ventricular rate and curative catheter ablation procedures that can restore sinus rhythm. In this latter class of procedures, two strategies are commonly practiced that are directed at the posterior left atrium in the region of the ostia of the pulmonary veins. In the first, complete electrical isolation of the pulmonary veins is achieved by sequential, segmental application of RF ablation at each pulmonary vein ostium.[140,147] Most pulmonary veins are electrically isolated by only partial circumferential ablation. An alternate strategy is to regionally isolate the posterior left atrium by encircling not only the pulmonary vein ostia but the surrounding posterior left atrial wall by a circular pattern of adjacent RF ablation lesions.[142] A randomized comparison of these two strategies has demonstrated a significantly higher success rate with the regional isolation strategy: 88% of patients were free of atrial fibrillation at 6 months compared with 67% free of atrial fibrillation at 6 months with the segmental isolation strategy.[149] The regional isolation procedure also reduces the risk of creating pulmonary venous stenosis that can be associated with the segmental isolation procedure. AV node ablation is used for medically refractory tachycardia due to atrial fibrillation or to eliminate intolerable symptoms due to irregular heart rate. The procedure requires pacemaker implantation,

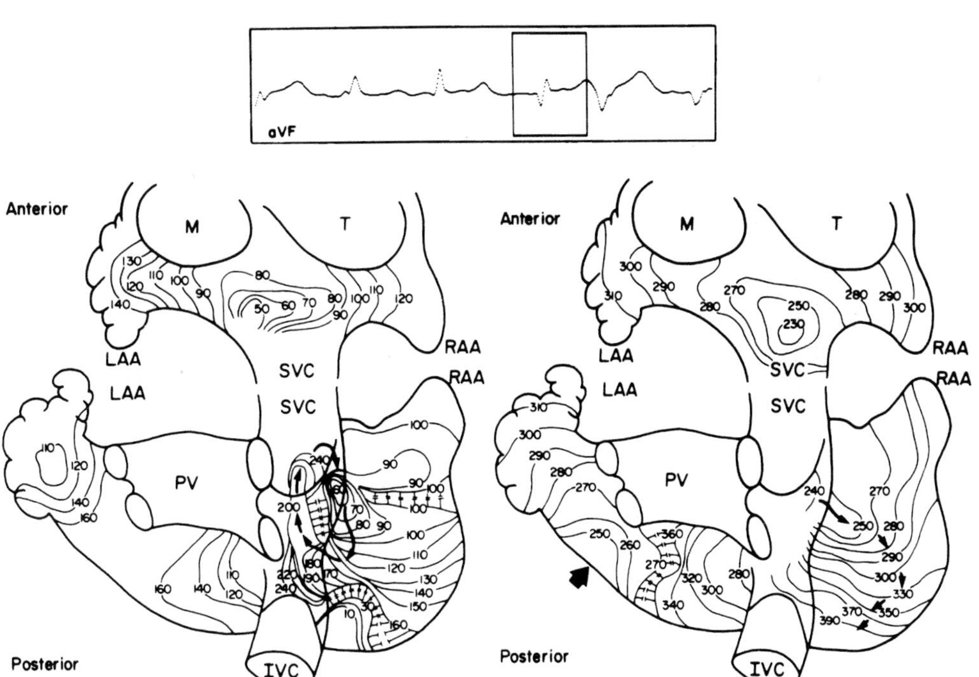

Figure 13–21 Atrial activation mapping from a human during atrial fibrillation indicating a single reentrant circuit. Recordings and isochronous mapping are the same as in Figure 13–20. The map on the left shows the first 240 milliseconds, with 230 to 400 milliseconds in the right map. The beat spreads along the anterior and posterior atria *(left)*. Posteriorly, the beat encounters several areas of conduction block, but as it spreads, it encounters myocardium now repolarized and capable of sustaining conduction. The clockwise, rotating reentrant circuit circulates around natural obstacles such as the orifices of the vena cava. SVC = superior vena cava; IVC = inferior vena cava; RAA = right atrial appendage; LAA = left atrial appendage; PV = pulmonary veins; M = mitral valve; T = tricuspid valve. (From Cox JL, Canavan TE, Schuessler RB, et al: The surgical treatment of atrial fibrillation. II. Intraoperative electrophysiologic mapping and description of the electrophysiologic basis of atrial flutter and atrial fibrillation. J Thorac Cardiovasc Surg 101:406, 1991.)

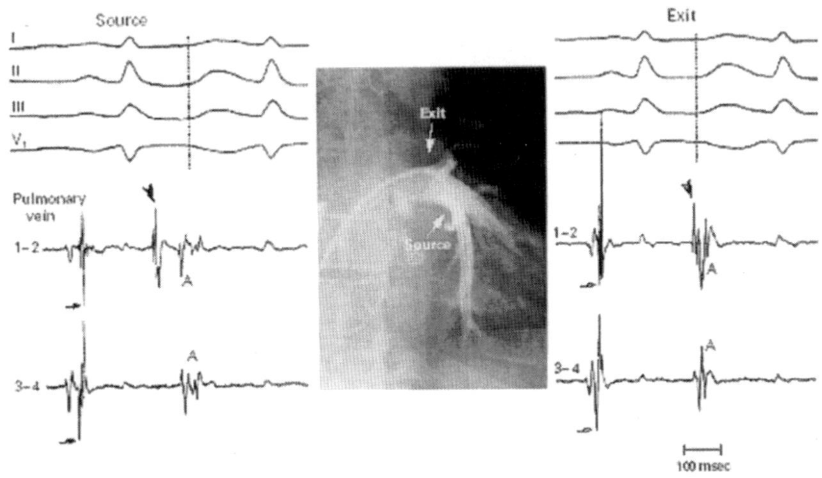

Figure 13–22 Electrophysiologic recordings and venous angiogram of the left inferior pulmonary vein from a patient with paroxysmal atrial fibrillation. Positioning of the distal catheter towards the source of ectopic beats results in progressively delayed activation in relation to the P wave during sinus rhythm *(left, arrows)*. Ectopic activity is recorded earlier *(arrowhead)*. The catheter electrode positioned at the exit of the pulmonary vein *(right)* shows the spike to be less delayed in sinus rhythm *(arrows)* and later after an ectopic beat *(arrowhead)*. The *center* panel shows a pulmonary vein angiogram demonstrating the position of the catheter. The *vertical lines* indicate the onset of an atrial ectopic beat. *A* represents near field electrical activity. Radiofrequency ablation of the ectopic source resulted in cure of atrial fibrillation. (From Haissaguerre M, Pierre J, Shah DC, et al: Spontaneous initiation of atrial fibrillation by ectopic beats originating in the pulmonary veins. N Engl J Med 339:659, 1998. Reprinted with permission for the Massachusetts Medical Society. Copyright © 1998 Massachusetts Medical Society. All rights reserved.)

does not restore atrial transport function, and does not eliminate the need for anticoagulation.

Research into methods emulating the surgical Maze procedure continues to evolve but remains investigative (see later). Linear ablation techniques involve RF energy application along critical sites for the maintenance of atrial fibrillation.[150-155] Success has been limited with this approach (28% to 57%), and the procedures are associated with long procedure duration and associated radiation exposure. Further, complication rates remain high (4% to 50%).

Surgical Therapy for Atrial Fibrillation

The growing understanding of the underlying mechanisms for atrial fibrillation led to the development of a surgical procedure developed by Cox et al termed the *Maze procedure*.[137-139,156-159] This moniker stems from the basic design of the operation to

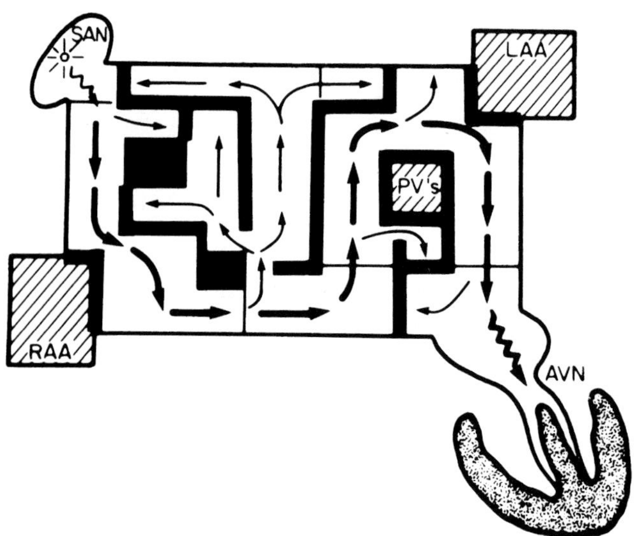

Figure 13–23 Schematic representation of the Maze I procedure for atrial fibrillation designed to allow for conduction of an impulse from the sinus nodal complex to the atria and AV node while interposing scar tissue interrupts the multiple reentrant circuits of atrial fibrillation. Atrial appendages are excised and the pulmonary veins are isolated. SAN = sinoatrial node; RAA = right atrial appendage; LAA = left atrial appendage; PVs = pulmonary veins; AVN = atrioventricular node. (From Cox JL, Schuessler RB, D'Agostino HJ Jr, et al: The surgical treatment of atrial fibrillation. III. Development of a definitive surgical procedure. J Thorac Cardiovasc Surg 101:569, 1991.)

surgically create a "Maze" of functional myocardium, allowing propagation of atrial depolarization throughout the atrium to the AV node while interposed scar tissue interrupts possible routes of reentry (Fig. 13–23). The principal goals of the Maze procedure thus are to (a) interrupt the electrophysiologic substrate for atrial fibrillation (reentrant circuits) restoring sinus rhythm, (b) maintain sinus nodal–to–AV nodal conduction thus preserving AV synchrony, and (c) preserve atrial mechanical function ("atrial kick") to improve hemodynamic function.

The Maze procedure has evolved from the original procedure (Maze I) introduced in the early 1990s. The Maze I procedure consisted of multiple atrial incisions around the SA node including an incision anterior to the atrial-SVC junction[139-141,158] (Fig. 13–24). The latter incision is through the sinus tachycardia region of the SA node resulting in the unintended consequence of blunted heart rate response to exercise and obtunded atrial mechanical function.[159-161] Subsequently, the procedure was modified (Maze II procedure) to include an incision on the anterior right atrium while allowing the sinus impulse to travel anteriorly across the left atrium but preventing it from reentering the right atrial–SVC junction (Fig. 13–25). While successfully addressing the limitations with the original procedure, the Maze II procedure was technically challenging particularly the approach to the left atrium that necessitated division and then reapproximation of the SVC. This was addressed by moving the left atrial incision to a more posterior location (Fig. 13–26). These and other modifications led to the introduction of the Maze III procedure, which reduced the frequency of chronotropic incompetence, improved atrial transport function, and shortened the procedure.[158]

Operative results from multiple centers show that greater than 90% of patients remain atrial fibrillation free after the Maze procedure.[161] Episodes of atrial flutter during the immediate perioperative period do not alter the long-term success of restoration of sinus rhythm.[161] Procedure-specific complications have included an attenuated heart rate response to exercise resulting in the need for permanent pacemaker implantation.[161] The frequency of these complications is less

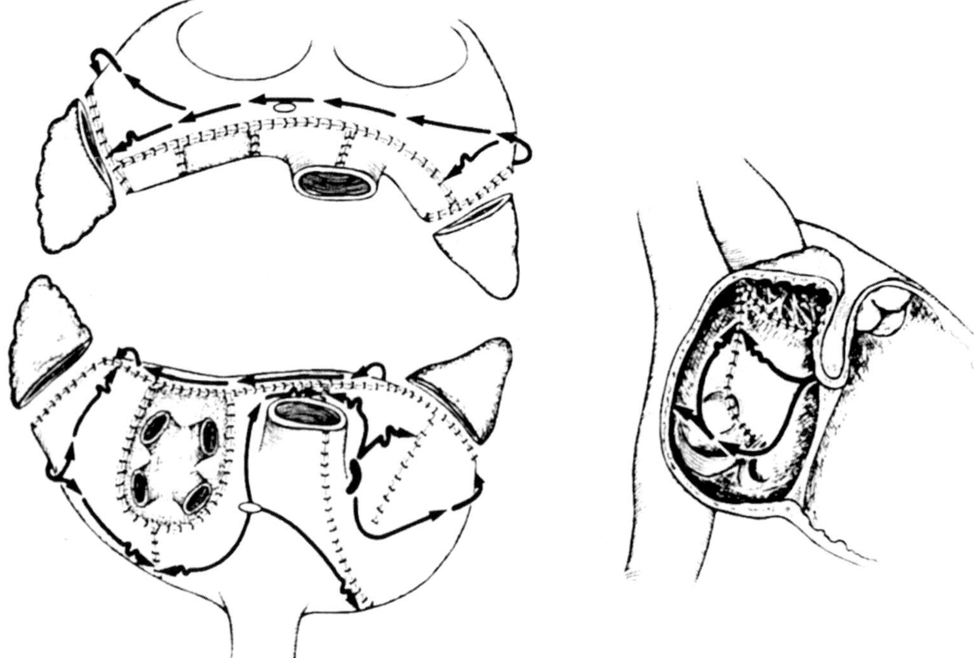

Figure 13–24 Depiction of surgical incisions and resultant conduction pathways of the Maze I procedure. The atria are shown in the *left panel* splayed open such that the anterior surface is superior and the posterior surface inferior. In the *right panel,* the atria are divided in a sagittal plane showing the right atrial septum. Incisions are placed at sites most commonly associated with reentrant circuits of atrial fibrillation to eliminate the arrhythmia. At the same time bridges of myocardium are left intact to allow the spread of conduction across the atria and to the AV node preserving atrial transport function and facilitating sinus rhythm. The pulmonary veins are isolated to eliminate potential conduction of premature beats. (From Cox JL: Evolving applications of the Maze procedure for atrial fibrillation [invited editorial]. The Annals of Thoracic Surgery 55:578–580, 1993. Reprinted with permission from the Society of Thoracic Surgeons. Copyright 1993, with permission from the Society of Thoracic Surgeons.)

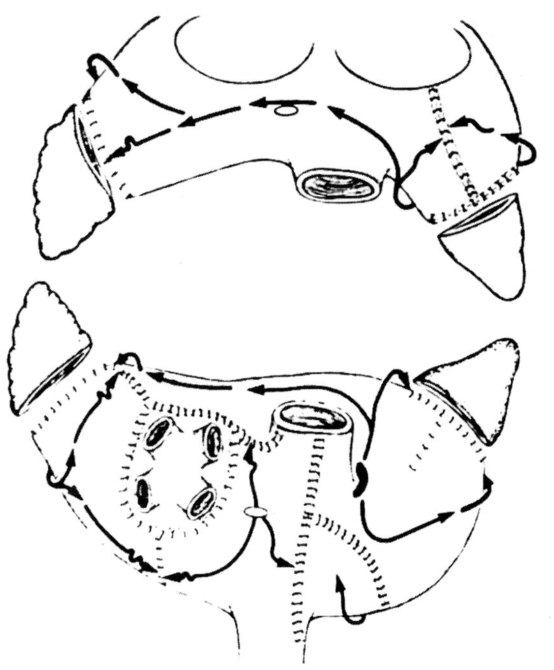

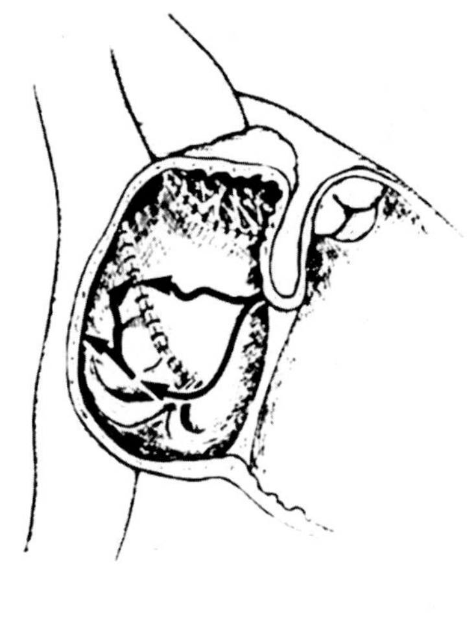

Figure 13–25 Representation of surgical incisions and conduction pathways of the Maze II procedure (similar views as in Fig. 13–24). The procedure is modified to eliminate incisions through the sinus tachycardia region of the sinus nodal complex performed in the Maze I procedure to address chronotropic incompetence. A transverse incision across the dome of the left atrium is moved posteriorly. (From Cox JL: Evolving applications of the Maze procedure for atrial fibrillation [invited editorial]. The Annals of Thoracic Surgery 55:578–580, 1993. Reprinted with permission from the Society of Thoracic Surgeons. Copyright 1993, with permission from the Society of Thoracic Surgeons.)

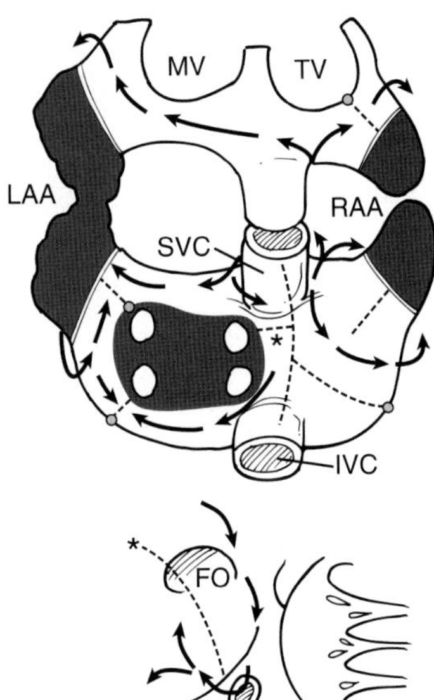

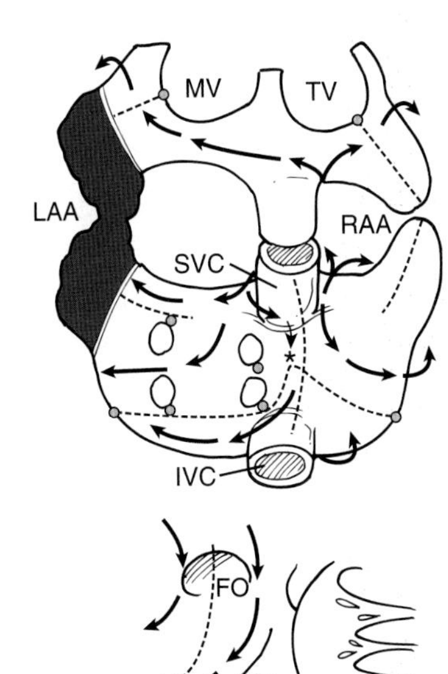

Figure 13–26 The Maze III procedure is shown using the same views. Modification of the posterior incisions to the vena cava and placement of the septal incision posterior to the orifice of the superior vena cava are noted. (From Cox JL: Evolving applications of the Maze procedure for atrial fibrillation [invited editorial]. The Annals of Thoracic Surgery 55:578–580, 1993. Reprinted with permission from the Society of Thoracic Surgeons. Copyright 1993, with permission from the Society of Thoracic Surgeons.)

with newer versions of the procedure. Fluid retention is a common problem after the Maze procedure, which is attributed to reduced secretion of atrial natriuretic peptide and elevation of antidiuretic hormone as well as aldosterone.[162,163] Furosemide, spironolactone, or both perioperatively can limit the consequences of this complication.[164]

An intended goal of the Maze procedure is preservation of atrial transport function. Follow-up of patients early in the experience at Washington University School of Medicine demonstrated that this was achieved in 98% of patients for the right atrium but in only 86% of patients for the left atrium.[165] More detailed analysis further revealed that even when left atrial contraction was present, quantitative mechanical function was lower compared with control patients.[166,167] The latter consequence was believed to be related to the incisions used to isolate the pulmonary veins that resulted in isolating nearly 30% of the left atrium myocardium from excitation.[168] To better preserve left atrial transport function, a new approach to the Maze procedure was developed whereby incisions radiate from the SA node (Fig. 13–27) along the path of coronary arteries supplying the atrium (rather than across as in the Maze III procedure).[169,170] This modification is termed the *radial procedure* and is further designed to preserve the right atrial appendage, which is an important source of atrial natriuretic peptide.[171] Compared with the standard Maze III procedure, the radial approach results in a more synchronous activation sequence of the left atrium, preserving atrial transport function, while it is equally effective in eliminating the reentrant circuits of atrial fibrillation.

Technologic advancements continue to be introduced including devices that can generate linear scars using RF energy delivered via the epicardium.[160,172,173] The availability of such devices has resulted in the modern Maze procedure becoming a hybrid operation using catheter/device-delivered RF energy and properly placed incisions. These advances shorten surgical time allowing the Maze procedure to be performed with other surgeries such as mitral valve surgery. Shortened surgical times and lower complexity further allow for expansion of eligibility criteria and foster the development of less invasive surgical approaches such as minimally invasive

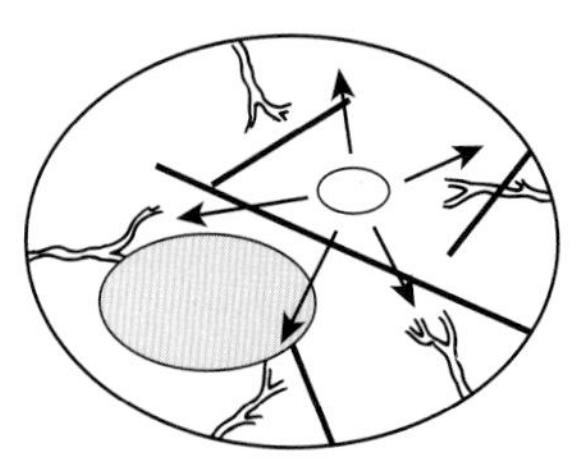

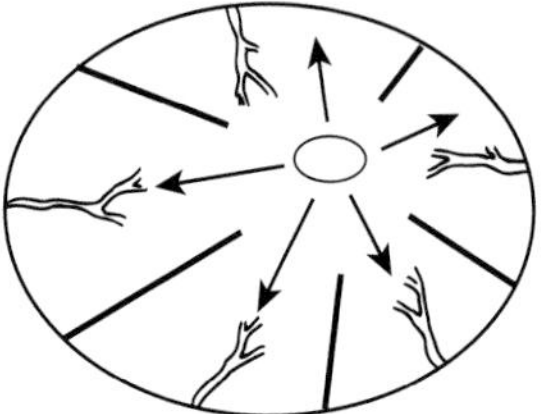

Figure 13–27 Contrasting concepts for the Maze procedure *(left)* and radial approach *(right)*. The *small circle* in the middle indicates the sinus node, the *outer circle* the atria, and the *shaded area* atrial myocardium isolated by the incisions. The atrial arterial supply is depicted. The arrows indicate propagation of the depolarizing wavefront. The radial approach preserves atrial arterial blood supply and a more physiologic activation sequence. With the Maze procedure, some arteries are divided and the atrial activation sequence disrupted. (From Nitta T, Lee R, Schuessler RB, et al: Radial approach: a new concept in surgical treatment of atrial fibrillation. I. Concept, anatomic and physiologic bases and development of a procedure. Ann Thorac Surg 67:27, 1999. Reprinted with permission from the Society of Thoracic Surgeons. Copyright 1999, with permission from the Society of Thoracic Surgeons.)

and beating-heart surgeries. A basic tenet of catheter-based energy delivery is that transmural scarring must be ensured. This can be ensured by measuring tissue impedance when using bipolar RF energy or by measuring conduction across the lesion when other energy forms are used.[161] Of concern are reports of esophageal injury following procedures using left atrial RF applications.[174] This complication appears to occur regardless of whether TEE is used during surgery.

Anesthetic Considerations

The care of the patient undergoing the Maze procedure generally includes measures taken for any patient undergoing cardiac surgery using cardiopulmonary bypass. Preoperative cardiac evaluation includes echocardiography and coronary angiography. Patients with paroxysmal atrial fibrillation further undergo electrophysiologic evaluation to exclude accessory AV pathways, AVNRT, or both.

Preparation of the patient for surgery first includes review of preoperative cardiac testing, assessment of the characteristics of the patient's arrhythmia, and review of surgical plan and whether concomitant procedures will accompany the Maze procedure (e.g., coronary artery bypass grafting, valve replacement, repair of congenital lesions).

Anesthetics chosen are based on the patient's general physical condition including comorbid conditions and ventricular dysfunction. For the most part, the anesthetic chosen is aimed at early tracheal extubation and consists of a lower dose opioid-based technique supplemented with volatile anesthetics and skeletal muscle relaxants. Patient monitoring modalities for the Maze procedure are similar to those used for other cardiac surgical procedures including TEE to evaluate for ventricular and valvular function, monitor for new wall motion abnormalities, and assist in evacuation of air from the cardiac chambers at the conclusion of surgery. Ventricular dysfunction (right more often than left ventricle), at least transiently, as well as echocardiographic and ECG ischemic changes (inferiorly more often), are common.[10] The proposed etiology includes coronary artery air embolization and/or inadequate myocardial protection. Because the Maze procedure entails placement of multiple atrial incisions, initial atrial compliance and performance of the atria appear altered. TEE evaluation of atrial activity is performed following separation from the extracorporeal circulation and decannulation.[10]

VENTRICULAR ARRHYTHMIAS

As with supraventricular arrhythmias, the treatment of ventricular fibrillation and VT is aimed at addressing underlying mechanisms (e.g., myocardial ischemia, drug induced, electrolyte or metabolic abnormalities, etc.). In most patients with life-threatening ventricular arrhythmias and structural heart disease, implantable cardioverter-defibrillator (ICD) placement is the standard of care with or without concomitant antiarrhythmic drug therapy.[175] In patients with significant structural heart disease, catheter ablation is considered as an adjuvant therapy for medically refractory monomorphic VT. Rarely, VT occurs in the setting of a structurally normal heart. This syndrome of a primary electrical disorder is typically due to a focal, triggered mechanism that occurs mostly in younger patients and originates from the right ventricular outflow tract or apical septum (Box 13–11).[176-178]

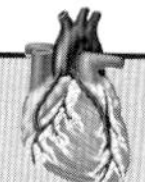

BOX 13–11 ***Ventricular Arrhythmias***

- A majority of episodes of ventricular tachycardia or fibrillation result from coronary artery disease and dilated or hypertrophic cardiomyopathy
- Implantable cardioverter-defibrillator placement is the standard of care with or without medical treatment in life-threatening ventricular arrhythmias and structural heart disease
- Catheter ablation is adjuvant therapy for medically refractory monomorphic ventricular tachycardia
- Surgical therapy includes endocardial resection with cryoablation
- Anesthetic considerations focus on preoperative catheterization, echocardiogram, and electrophysiologic testing
- Monitoring of surgical patients is dictated by the underlying cardiac disease

Catheter Ablation Therapy for Ventricular Tachycardia

The mechanism for VT can be identified in the electrophysiology suite using programmed stimulation.[179,180] Single or multiple extrastimuli are introduced during the vulnerable period of cardiac repolarization (near T wave) until sustained VT develops that is similar in morphology to that of the spontaneous arrhythmia. The diagnostic hallmark of VT due to a reentrant circuit is the ability to entrain the tachycardia by pacing slightly faster than the tachycardia cycle length.[181] Traditional catheter mapping techniques for guiding catheter ablation of VT serve to position the ablation catheter within a protected isthmus of the reentrant circuit. The pathologic characteristics of this site are thought to be viable myocardium surrounded by scar tissue that is electrically isolated from the bulk of the ventricular myocardium except at the entrance and exit sites. Important shortcomings of these techniques are that most VTs are not hemodynamically stable enough for mapping and that multiple morphologies of inducible VT are commonly present in a single patient. As a result, newer strategies that rely on three-dimensional computerized mapping techniques attempt to identify important

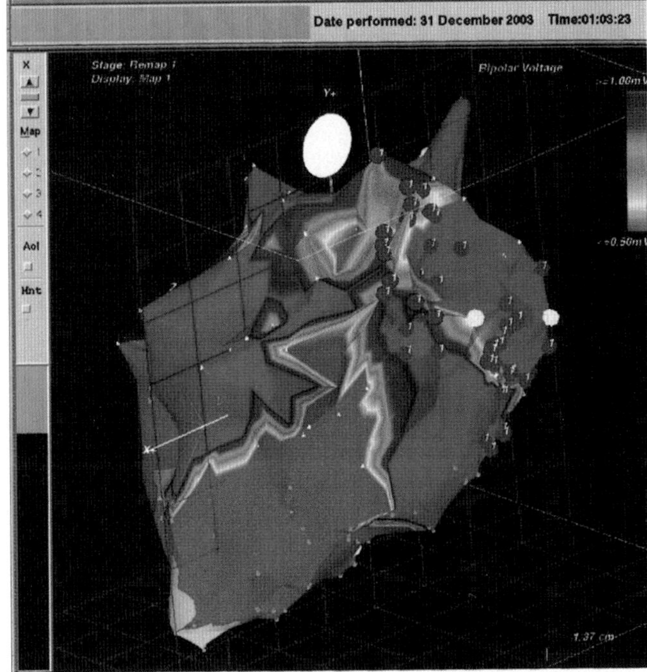

Figure 13–28 Electroanatomic mapping to guide catheter ablation of ventricular tachycardia. An electroanatomic map of the left ventricle of a patient with an ischemic cardiomyopathy complicated by ventricular tachycardia is shown. The posterolateral aspect of the left ventricle is displayed with color coding for the size of the ventricular electrograms recorded from the endocardial surface. Regions of myocardial scar are plotted in red corresponding to electrograms of less than 0.5 mV, and regions of viable myocardium corresponding to electrograms greater than 1.0 mV are plotted in purple. Border zones around myocardial scars are in between these regions. One border zone in this patient represents the location of "exit sites" for multiple forms of hemodynamically unstable ventricular tachycardia. Catheter ablation at sites plotted as red circles resulted in disruption of all forms of ventricular tachycardia. (See Color Plates.)

areas of myocardial scar, of which the perimeter may participate in reentrant circuits (Fig. 13–28). By strategic placement of areas of conduction block guided by these maps, significant cure rates have been obtained without the necessity of mapping individual reentrant circuits.[182] In rare instances, the VT circuits might involve the conduction system as in bundle-branch reentry or fascicular VT that is easily ablated with RF energy.[183]

There are no data from prospective randomized trials of VT ablation, but results from case series report success rates ranging from 37% to 86%.[183-190] The latter represent mostly patients with drug-resistant VT or multiple VT morphologies and the treatment performed as a "last-ditch effort" to control the arrhythmia. Reported success rates are higher after RF ablation for primary VT. Major complications from catheter ablation procedures for VT in the setting of structural heart disease include stroke, myocardial infarction, heart failure exacerbation, vascular injury, and death. The incidence of these complications appears to be low despite the lengthy procedure times that are commonly required.[182]

Surgical Therapy for Ventricular Tachycardia

Advances in percutaneous methods and ICD device treatments (see later) for VT have dramatically reduced the indications for surgical therapy of VT. Candidates typically have concomitant cardiac disease with drug-refractory or persistent VT despite catheter ablative therapy. In addition, these patients typically have reduced left ventricular function resulting from prior myocardial infarction associated with a left ventricular aneurysm resulting in a high risk for operative morbidity and mortality. Preoperative electrophysiologic evaluation ideally has located the arrhythmia pathway to an isolated area of the ventricle.

Based on experimental data showing that the site of VT often occurs in the endocardium at the border between viable and infarcted myocardium, endocardial resection is one approach used to surgically excise areas of the myocardium around the site of myocardial scar. This procedure is often combined with cryoablation or wide encircling endocardial ventriculotomy with endocardial resection.[10,191] Limitations of this generalized surgical approach are the extensive myocardial resection required and the risk of failure to ablate arrhythmogenic myocardium remote from the site of endocardial fibrosis. This empiric approach was largely replaced by surgical techniques based on intraoperative electrophysiologic map-guided resection.[10,191-193] Precise localization of the sites of earliest ventricular activation during induced VT allows for application of incisions or cryoablative lesions to isolate the affected myocardium. Most often, the arrhythmogenic site originates in the ventricular septum, the endocardium, or intramurally. Epicardial "sock" electrodes initially used for intraoperative mapping could identify only the site of earliest epicardial breakthrough of the induced arrhythmia.[10,194] Plunge needle electrodes were inserted at the identified epicardial sites to further locate the arrhythmogenic area. Presumed septal sites of arrhythmogenesis are approached from a right atriotomy to avoid ventricular incisions and to enhance more precise electrophysiologic mapping. Advances in multichannel computerized mapping of ventricular arrhythmias at the time of surgery provide more rapid and precise localization of the arrhythmogenic locus, which is an important determinant for limiting cardiopulmonary bypass duration in this high-risk category of patient. Once the arrhythmogenic area is localized, a ventriculotomy is performed and resection aided by cryoablation is carried out. When the arrhythmia pathway involves the papillary muscles, cryothermia is applied to their bases in an attempt to preserve mitral valvular function postoperatively.[10] Cardioplegic arrest of the heart for coronary artery bypass or other procedures is avoided until myocardial resection of the pathway is complete. This allows for subsequent attempts to reinitiate VT and electrophysiologic mapping to confirm that all arrhythmogenic pathways have been identified and interrupted.

Anesthetic Considerations

Anesthetic management of patients undergoing procedures to ameliorate ventricular arrhythmias is primarily based on the patient's underlying cardiac disease and other comorbidities. Surgical candidates often have underlying coronary artery disease, severely impaired left ventricular function, and other secondary organ dysfunction (e.g., hepatic and renal dysfunction) and are receiving multiple medications that may potentially interact with anesthetics (e.g., vasodilation from angiotensin-converting enzyme inhibitors). Consequently, a thorough review of the patient's underlying conditions and treatments is mandated. Special attention is given to cardiac catheterization results, preoperative echocardiogram findings, and the findings from preoperative electrophysiologic testing.

Information regarding characteristics of the patient's arrhythmia such as ventricular rate, hemodynamic tolerance, and method of arrhythmia termination should be sought.

Prior or current treatment with amiodarone is a particular concern. The long elimination half-life (about 60 days) of amiodarone requires that potential side effects such as hypothyroidism be considered perioperatively.[195] The α- and β-adrenergic properties of amiodarone might lead to hypotension during anesthesia, but most anesthesiologists in contemporary practice are familiar with the management of these complications. Much attention has been given to bradycardia associated with amiodarone during anesthesia that might be resistant to atropine.[196-198] Methods for temporary cardiac pacing should be readily available to care for patients receiving long-term amiodarone. Retrospective reports further suggest a higher need for inotropic support for patients receiving preoperative amiodarone therapy, because a low systemic vascular resistance has been observed in these patients.[197,198] Pulmonary complications speculated to be related to pulmonary toxicity from amiodarone have further been reported.[199,200] In a series of 67 patients receiving preoperative amiodarone, 50% developed acute respiratory distress syndrome that could not be attributed to other factors including intraoperative FIO_2 (see Chapter 10).[200]

Monitoring during surgery is dictated by the patient's underlying cardiac disease. TEE is valuable for management of these high-risk patients, especially for assessment immediately after weaning from cardiopulmonary bypass. Rapid assessment of regional and global left ventricular function and valvular function is essential in guiding pharmacologic treatments or the need for mechanical support (e.g., intra-aortic balloon pump insertion, ventricular assist device). Pulmonary artery catheters are commonly used and may be useful for guiding hemodynamic treatments after surgery when TEE monitoring is no longer used. Means for rapid cardioversion/defibrillation should be readily available when inserting any central venous catheter. Self-adhesive electrode pads are most often used and connected to a cardioverter/defibrillator prior to anesthesia induction. Premature ventricular beats induced during these procedures can easily precipitate the patient's underlying ventricular arrhythmia that might be difficult to convert to sinus rhythm.[201,202] Advancing the pulmonary artery catheter after the completion of the surgical procedure and weaning from CPB might be prudent.

Selection of anesthetics for arrhythmia ablation/surgery is dictated mostly by the patient's underlying physical state and goals of potential early tracheal extubation. Because anesthetics can influence cardiac conduction and arrhythmogenesis, there is a concern about the potential of anesthetics to alter the electrophysiologic mapping procedures.[203,204] The effects of the various volatile anesthetics on ventricular arrhythmias vary between the experimental models and, importantly, due to the mechanism of the arrhythmia. Data showing proarrhythmic, antiarrhythmic, and no effects of volatile anesthetics on experimental arrhythmias have been reported.[203-211] Opioids have been shown to have no effects on inducibility of VT.[208,212,213]

IMPLANTABLE CARDIOVERTER-DEFIBRILLATOR

Considerable progress has occurred with the ICD, including decreased device size, improved battery life, and improved treatment algorithms, all contributing to enhanced reliability (Box 13–12). Current ICDs are capable of providing tiered therapy consisting of antitachycardia pacing and shocks to terminate life-threatening ventricular arrhythmias (Fig. 13–29). Antibradycardia pacing via single-, dual-, or tri-chamber intracardiac electrodes can be used. Advances in energy delivery, including use of biphasic shock waveform, have reduced considerably defibrillation and cardioversion energy requirements.[214,215] These improvements have led to simplification of electrode implantation to now mostly consist of intravascular insertion methods rather than epicardial patch electrodes used in prior generations of devices. As a result, insertion of modern devices is nearly exclusively via percutaneous techniques rather than more invasive median sternotomy required for earlier generations of ICDs.

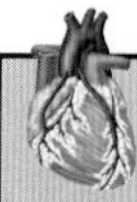

BOX 13–12 *Implantable Cardioverter-Defibrillator (ICD)*

- ICDs are capable of providing tiered therapy consisting of shocks to terminate life-threatening arrhythmias, antitachycardia pacing, and antibradycardia pacing
- Insertion of modern devices is almost exclusively via percutaneous techniques
- ICDs are indicated for the primary or secondary prevention of sudden cardiac death
- ICDs have been shown to reduce the incidence of mortality versus standard treatment alone
- Funding for ICDs is approved for those with prior myocardial infarction, left ventricular ejection fraction <0.30, and QRS duration ≥0.12 second

The ICD consists of a pulse generator and intracardiac electrodes that continuously monitor heart rate. When the heart rate exceeds a programmable limit, therapy is initiated that might include a brief burst of rapid pacing (e.g., <10 stimuli at 150 to 220 beats/min) followed by 10-J to 30-J shocks if the arrhythmia persists. Electrogram storage capabilities allow for review of appropriateness of delivered treatments as well as changes in ventricular arrhythmia characteristics. The style of ICD, either one, two, or three leads, is chosen based on a patient's requirement for antibradycardia pacing (single- or dual-lead devices) or cardiac resynchronization therapy, also known as biventricular pacing, when medically refractory heart failure and interventricular conduction delay are present.

Technologic aspects of ICDs have been reviewed and are discussed in more detail in Chapter 25.[214] Microprocessors contained in the ICD allow for filtering and processing of electrograms to minimize oversensing of T waves or electrical noise. Programmable algorithms categorize monitored sets of R-R intervals into heart rate zones of bradycardia, ventricular fibrillation, or VT. Ventricular fibrillation is detected when a set of R-R intervals falls below a programmable cycle length for a programmable duration (e.g., 10 to 24 intervals).[214] Defibrillation voltage is much higher than can be delivered with existing batteries, necessitating the use of storage capacitors. After charging, continued presence of ventricular fibrillation is confirmed prior to device discharge to reduce inappropriate defibrillation. Following delivery of energy, redetection and episode-termination algorithms assess for successful termination of the arrhythmia. VT detection algorithms can be more complex to allow discrimination of SVTs,

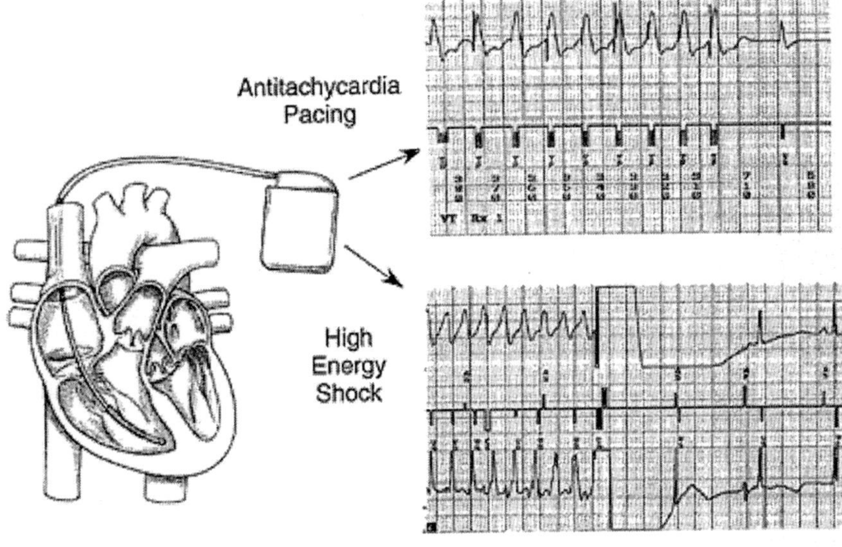

Figure 13–29 Internal cardioverter-defibrillator and attached intracardiac leads *(left panel)* and different modes of therapy for ventricular tachycardia. *Right upper panel* demonstrates antitachycardia pacing at 150 beats/min resulting in termination of ventricular tachycardia. *Right lower panel* demonstrates termination of fast ventricular tachycardia (250 beats/min) with high-energy shock. (From Exner DV, Klein GJ, Prystowsky EN: Primary prevention of sudden death with implantable defibrillator therapy in patients with cardiac disease. Circulation 104:1564, 2001. Reprinted with permission from the American Heart Association.)

especially atrial fibrillation, to avoid inappropriate device discharge. In addition to setting R-R interval definitions below which device detection pathways are activated, VT detection algorithms include criteria for suddenness of onset, QRS morphology, and rate stability (stable with VT but irregular with atrial fibrillation).[214] Presence of an atrial lead enhances the discrimination of atrial fibrillation from VT.[214]

Guidelines for implantation of antiarrhythmic devices have been issued by the American College of Cardiology, the American Heart Association, and the North American Society of Pacing and Electrophysiology[216] (Table 13–2). In general, ICDs are indicated for the primary or secondary prevention of sudden cardiac death. These recommendations are based on data from large, multicenter investigations that have compared ICD therapy with standard care including antiarrhythmic drugs. For patients with prior cardiac arrest due to VT or ventricular fibrillation (secondary prevention), the data show

Table 13-2 American College of Cardiology/American Heart Association/North American Society of Pacing and Electrophysiology Guidelines for Insertion of ICD

Class I	Spontaneous VT not amenable to other treatment in patient without structural heart disease
Class IIa	Left ventricular ejection fraction ≤0.30 at least 1 month after MI and at least 3 months after coronary revascularization surgery
Class IIb	Syncope of unexplained origin or family history of unexplained sudden cardiac death in association with typical or atypical right bundle-branch block and ST-segment elevations (Brugada syndrome)
	Syncope in patient with advanced structural heart disease in whom thorough invasive and noninvasive investigations have failed to define cause

Class I indications: evidence or general agreement that the treatment is useful and effective.
Class IIa indications: weight of the data of evidence favors benefit of the therapy.
Class IIb: conditions usefulness/efficacy of the treatment is less well established.

that ICDs lower the risk of subsequent mortality by 20% to 30% compared mostly with amiodarone or β-adrenergic receptor blockers.[216-219] Similarly, relative mortality is reduced by 49% to 54% with ICD treatment for patients with nonsustained VT or inducible ventricular arrhythmias with programmed stimulation compared with standard care or serial drug testing in patients with ischemic left ventricular dysfunction.[220,221]

The most convincing data regarding primary prevention of sudden death with ICD treatment for patients with coronary artery disease come from the MADIT II trial. In contrast to other studies, MADIT II did not require a history of inducible or spontaneous ventricular arrhythmias. Rather, enrollment criteria were simply prior myocardial infarction and left ventricular ejection fraction of 0.30 or less. Patients were continued on conventional treatments consisting mostly of β-blockers, angiotensin-converting enzyme inhibitors, and hMG-CoA reductase inhibitors ("statins"). After more than 4 years of follow-up, ICD treatment was associated with a 31% relative reduction in mortality compared with those randomized to only conventional treatment. The risk is most pronounced for patients with QRS duration greater than 0.12 second, but those with a QRS duration less than 0.12 second are not necessarily at lower risk.[221]

Benefits of ICDs have further been demonstrated for patients without coronary artery disease in the Defibrillators in Non-Ischemic Cardiomyopathy Treatment Evaluation (DEFINITE) trial.[222] In this randomized trial patients with left ventricular ejection fraction less than 36% and premature ventricular complexes or nonsustained VT had a 35% reduction in sudden death compared with standard medical care. Other conditions such as inherited long QT syndrome and hypertrophic cardiomyopathy may warrant ICD insertion for prevention of sudden cardiac death, although data from large randomized studies are lacking due to the relative rarity of the conditions. Treatment with an ICD is considered for patients with long QT syndrome when they are symptomatic or when there is a family history of sudden death.[223,224] Patients with hypertrophic cardiomyopathy and marked left ventricular hypertrophy, particularly if young, with little functional impairment and other risk factors for sudden cardiac death (e.g., family history), should receive consideration for ICD insertion.[223,225,226] In the future, genetic screening might provide valuable information about risk for sudden death for patients with both long QT syndrome and hypertrophic cardiomyopathy that might be useful for guiding treatment.[227,228]

The cost of expansion of indications for ICD therapy is a concern, particularly in light of the aging population, which portends increases in eligible patients. It is estimated that the cost of ICD therapy could double from $2 to $4 billion annually in the United States alone if MADIT II criteria are used. The Centers for Medicaid and Medicare Services have approved funding for ICD insertion for patients with prior myocardial infarction, left ventricular ejection fraction less than 0.30, and a QRS duration of 0.12 second or greater.[224] The QRS duration of 0.12 second or greater is controversial because the MADIT II did not conclusively demonstrate that shorter QRS duration indicated lower risk for sudden death.[226]

Anesthetic Considerations

Insertion of ICDs is mostly performed in the catheterization suite with only complicated cases referred to the operating room. The procedure requires defibrillation testing to ensure an acceptable margin of safety for the device. VT or ventricular fibrillation is induced by the introduction of premature beats timed to the vulnerable repolarization period. External adhesive pads are placed prior to the procedure and connected to an external cardioverter/defibrillator to provide "back-up" shocks should the device be ineffective. Monitored anesthesia care is typically chosen with a brief general anesthetic given for defibrillation testing. General anesthesia may be chosen for patients with severe concomitant diseases (e.g., chronic lung disease, sleep apnea) when control of the airway is desired. Simultaneous insertion of biventricular pacing systems with an ICD usually necessitates a general anesthetic due to the length of the procedure and the often severe impairment of left ventricular function.

In addition to standard patient monitoring, continuous arterial blood pressure monitoring is used even during monitored anesthesia care to rapidly assess for return of blood pressure after defibrillation testing. Defibrillation testing was demonstrated to be associated with ischemic electroencephalographic (EEG) changes 7.5 ± 1.8 seconds (mean ± SD) after arrest.[229] These changes were transient and not associated with persistent ischemic EEG changes or exacerbation of an existing neurologic deficit, nor was significant deterioration in neuropsychometric performance detected. Repeated defibrillation testing is usually well tolerated without deterioration of cardiac function even in patients with left ventricular ejection fractions less than 35%.[230] Nonetheless, means of pacing must be available should bradycardia develop following cardioversion/defibrillation. Often, however, restoration of circulatory function after defibrillation testing is accompanied by tachycardia and hypertension necessitating treatment with a short-acting β-blocker and/or vasoactive drugs.

Complications associated with ICD insertion include those related to insertion and those associated specifically with the device. Percutaneous insertion is typically via the subclavian vein, predisposing to pneumothorax. Cardiac injury including perforation is a remote possibility. Cerebrovascular accident and myocardial infarction have been reported, but mostly with older device insertion methods.[10] Device-related complications include those associated with multiple shocks that may lead to myocardial injury or refractory hypotension.[231,232] Device infections are particularly difficult to manage, often requiring device and lead explantation.

Acknowledgments

The authors acknowledge Demetrius Lappas, MD, Michael Cain, MD, and James Cox, MD, for their thoughtful contributions to prior editions to this book that provided the fundamental basis of this chapter.

REFERENCES

1. National Center for Health Statistics: Report of final mortality statistics, 1995. Monthly Vital Stat Rep 45:suppl 2, 1997
2. Gillum RE: Sudden coronary death in the United States: 1980-1985. Circulation 79:756, 1989
3. Orejarena LA, Vidailles H Jr, DeStefano F, et al: Paroxysmal supraventricular tachycardia in the general population. J Am Coll Cardiol 31:150, 1998
4. Granada J, Uribe W, Chyou PH, et al: Incidence and predictors of atrial flutter in the general population. J Am Coll Cardiol 36:2242, 2000
5. Sra J, Dhala A, Blanck Z, et al: Atrial fibrillation: Epidemiology, mechanisms, and management. Cur Probl Cardiol 25:405, 2000
6. Benjamin EJ, Wolf PA, D'Agostino RB, et al: Impact of atrial fibrillation on the risk of death: The Framingham Heart Study. Circulation 98:946, 1998
7. The Cardiac Arrhythmia Suppression Trial (CAST) Investigators: Preliminary report: Effect of encainide and flecainide on mortality in a randomized trial of arrhythmia suppression after myocardial infarction, N Engl J Med 321:406, 1989
8. Ben-David J, Zipes DP: Torsades de pointes and proarrhythmia, Lancet 341:1578, 1993.
9. Zipes DP: Implantable cardioverter-defibrillator: A Volkswagen or Rolls Royce? Circulation 103:1372, 2001
10. Skubas NJ, Hogue CW Jr, Cox JL, Lappas DG: Anesthesia for Electrophysiologic Procedures. *In* Kaplan J (ed): Cardiac Anesthesia, 4th Edition. Philadelphia, WB Saunders, 1999
11. Morady F: Radiofrequency ablation as treatment for cardiac arrhythmias. N Engl J Med 340:534, 1999
12. Anderson KR, Ho SY, Anderson RH: The location and vascular supply of the sinus node in the human heart. Br Heart J 41:28, 1979
13. Cranefield PF: Action potentials, afterpotentials and arrhythmias. Circ Res 41:415, 1977
14. Atlee JL: Perioperative Cardiac Arrhythmias, 2nd edition. Chicago, Year Book Medical Publishers, 1990, pp 30-35
15. Fozzard HA, Gunn RB: Membrane transport. *In* Fozzard HA, Haber E, Jennings RB, et al (eds): The Heart and Cardiovascular System. New York, Raven Press, 1986, pp 1-30
16. Boineau JP, Mooney C, Hudson R, et al: Observations on re-entrant excitation pathways and refractory period distribution in spontaneous and experimental atrial flutter in the dog. *In* Kulbertus HE (ed): Re-entrant Arrhythmias. Baltimore, University Park Press, 1977, pp 79-98
17. Goldberg JM: Intra-SA-nodal pacemaker shifts induced by autonomic nerve stimulation in the dog. Am J Physiol 229:1116, 1975
18. Randall WC, Talano J, Kaye MP, et al: Cardiac pacemakers in absence of the SA node: Responses to exercises and autonomic blockade. Am J Physiol 234:H465, 1978
19. Sealy WC, Bache RJ, Seaber AV, Bhattacharga SK: The atrial pacemaking site after surgical exclusion of the sinoatrial node. J Thorac Cardiovasc Surg 65:841, 1973
20. Boineau JP, Schuessler RB, Mooney CR, et al: Multicentric origin of the atrial depolarization wave: The pacemaker complex. Circulation 58:1036, 1978
21. Sealy WC, Seaber AV: Surgical isolation of the atrial septum from the atria: Identification of an atrial septal pacemaker. J Thorac Cardiovasc Surg 80:742, 1980
22. Boineau JP, Schuessler RB, Hackel DB, et al: Widespread distribution and rate differentiation of the atrial pacemaker complex. Am J Physiol 239:H406, 1980
23. Boineau JP, Miller CB, Schuessler RB, et al: Activation sequence and potential distribution maps demonstrating multicentre atrial impulse origin in dogs. Circ Res 54:332, 1984
24. Boineau JP, Schuessler RB: Reflections on the establishment of the electrophysiologic basis for cardiac arrhythmia surgery. Cardiac Surg 4:3, 1990

25. Levy MN, Martin PJ: Neural control of heart rate and atrioventricular conduction. *In* Abboud FM, et al (eds): Disturbances in Neurogenic Control of the Circulation. Clinical Physiology Series. Bethesda, MD, American Physiological Society, 1981, p 205
26. Randall WC, Ardell JL: Nervous control of the heart. Anatomy and pathophysiology. *In* Zipes DP, Jalife J (eds): Cardiac Electrophysiology: From Cell to Bedside. Philadelphia, WB Saunders, 1990, p 291
27. Becker AE, Bouman LN, Janse MJ, Anderson RH: Functional anatomy of the cardiac conduction system. *In* Harrison DC (ed): Cardiac Arrhythmias: A Decade of Progress. Boston, GK Hall Medical Publishers, 1981, pp 3-24
28. Hoffman BF: Fine structure of internodal pathways. Am J Cardiol 44:385, 1979
29. Cox JL: The surgical treatment of cardiac arrhythmias. *In* Sabiston DC Jr (ed): Textbook of Surgery. Philadelphia, WB Saunders, 1991, p 2058
30. Anderson RH, Davies MJ, Becker AE: Atrioventricular ring specialized tissue in the normal heart. Eur J Cardiol 2:219, 1974
31. Anderson RH, Becker AE: Anatomy of conducting tissues revisited. Br Heart J 40:2, 1979
32. Zipes DP: Genesis of cardiac arrhythmias: Electrophysiologic considerations. *In* Braunwald E (ed): Heart Disease, 3rd edition. Philadelphia, WB Saunders, 1990, pp 581-620
33. Baumgarten CM, Gozzard HA: The resting and pacemaker potentials. *In* Gozzard HA, Haber E, Jennings RB, et al (eds): The Heart and Cardiovascular System. New York, Raven Press, 1986, pp 601-626
34. Kreitner D: Electrophysiological study of the two main pacemaker mechanisms in the rabbit sinus node. Cardiovasc Res 19:304, 1985
35. Rozanski GJ, Lipsius SL: Electrophysiology of functional subsidiary pacemakers in canine right atrium. Am J Physiol 249:H504, 1985
36. Watanabe Y, Dreifus LS: Sites of impulse formation within the atrioventricular junction of the rabbit. Circ Res 22:717, 1968
37. DiFrancesco D: A new interpretation of the pacemaker current in calf Purkinje fibers. J Physiol (Lond) 314:359, 1981
38. Noble D, Tsien RW: The kinetics and rectifier properties of the slow potassium current in cardiac Purkinje fibers. J Physiol (Lond) 195:185, 1968
39. Vassalle M: Analysis of cardiac pacemaker potential using "voltage clamp" technique. Am J Physiol 210:1335, 1966
40. Vassalle M: Cardiac pacemaker potentials at different extracellular and intracellular K^+ concentrations. Am J Physiol 208:770, 1965
41. Wu EB, Chia HM, Gill JS: Reversible cardiomyopathy after radiofrequency ablation of lateral free-wall pathway-mediated incessant supraventricular tachycardia. PACE Pacing Clin Electrophysiol 23:1308, 2000
42. Platia EV: The electrophysiologic study. *In* Platia EV (ed): Management of Cardiac Arrhythmias: The Nonpharmacologic Approach. Philadelphia, JB Lippincott, 1987, pp 304-339
43. Cain ME, Lindsay BD: The preoperative electrophysiologic study. Cardiac Surg 4:53, 1990
44. DiMarco JP, Garan H, Ruskin JN: Complications in patients undergoing cardiac electrophysiologic procedures. Ann Intern Med 97:490, 1982
45. Horowitz LN, Kay HR, Kutalek SP, et al: Risks and complications of clinical cardiac electrophysiologic studies: A prospective analysis of 1,000 consecutive patients. J Am Coll Cardiol 9:1261, 1987
46. Cobb FR, Blumenschein SD, Sealy WC, et al: Successful surgical interruption of the bundle of Kent in a patient with Wolff-Parkinson-White syndrome. Circulation 38:1018, 1968
47. Sealy WC, Boineau JP, Wallace AG: The identification and division of the bundle of Kent for premature ventricular excitation and supraventricular tachycardia. Surgery 68:1009, 1970
48. Boineau JP, Moore EN, Sealy WC, Kasell JH: Epicardial mapping in Wolff-Parkinson-White syndrome. Arch Intern Med 135:422, 1975
49. Cox JL, Gallagher JJ, Cain ME: Experience with 118 consecutive patients undergoing surgery for the Wolff-Parkinson-White syndrome. J Thorac Cardiovasc Surg 90:490, 1985
50. Faddis MN, Chen J, Osborn J, et al: Magnetic guidance system for cardiac electrophysiology: A prospective trial of safety and efficacy in humans. J Am Coll Cardiol 42:1952, 2003
51. Blomström-Lundqvist C, Scheinman MM, Aliot EM, et al: ACC/AHA/ESC Guidelines for the management of patients with supraventricular arrhythmias. J Am Coll Cardiol 108:1871, 2003
52. Wolff L, Parkinson J, White PD: Bundle-branch block with short P-R interval in healthy young people prone to paroxysmal tachycardia. Am Heart J 5:685, 1930
53. Gallagher JJ, Pritchett ELC, Sealy WC, et al: The preexcitation syndromes. Prog Cardiovasc Dis 20:285, 1978
54. Bardy GH, Packer DL, German LD, et al: Pre-excited reciprocating tachycardia in patients with Wolff-Parkinson-White syndrome: Incidence and mechanisms. Circulation 70:377, 1984
55. Kuck K, Brugada P, Wellens HJ: Observations on the antidromic type of circus movement tachycardia in the Wolff-Parkinson-White syndrome. J Am Coll Cardiol 2:1003, 1983
56. Lindsay BD, Crossen KJ, Cain ME: Concordance of distinguishing electrocardiographic features during sinus rhythm with the location of accessory pathways in the Wolff-Parkinson-White syndrome. Am J Cardiol 59:1093, 1987
57. Cain ME, Lindsay BD: The preoperative electrophysiologic study. Cardiac Surg 4:53, 1990
58. Scheinman MM, Huang S: The 1998 NASPE prospective catheter ablation registry. PACE Pacing Clin Electrophysiol 23:1020, 2000
59. Calkins H, Yong P, Miller JM, et al: For the Atakr Multicenter Investigator Group: Catheter ablation of accessory pathways, atrioventricular nodal re-entrant tachycardia, and the atrioventricular junction: Final results of a prospective, multicenter clinical trial. Circulation 99:262, 1999
60. Yee R, Connolly S, Noorani H: Clinical review of radiofrequency catheter ablation for cardiac arrhythmias. Can J Cardiol 19:1273, 2003
61. Lau CP, Tai YT, Lee PW: The effects of radiofrequency ablation versus medical therapy on the quality-of-life and exercise capacity in patients with accessory pathway-mediate supraventricular tachycardia: A treatment comparison study. PACE Pacing Clin Electrophysiol 18:424, 1995
62. Gallagher JJ, Kasell JH, Sealy WC, et al: Epicardial mapping in the Wolff-Parkinson-White syndrome. Circulation 70:377, 1984
63. Cain ME, Cox JL: Surgical treatment of supraventricular tachyarrhythmias. *In* Platia EV (ed): Management of Cardiac Arrhythmias: The Nonpharmacologic Approach. Philadelphia, JB Lippincott, 1987, pp 304-339
64. Kramer JB, Cox JL, Witkowski FX, et al: Simultaneous computer mapping to facilitate localization of accessory pathways. Am J Cardiol 56:571, 1985
65. Witkowski FX, Corr PB: An automated transmural cardiac mapping system. Am J Physiol 247:H661, 1984
66. Peirick J, Pogwizd SM, Watchmaker GP, et al: The evolution of intraoperative electrophysiologic mapping procedures to guide cardiac arrhythmia surgery. Cardiac Surg 4:93, 1990
67. Cox JL: The surgical management of cardiac arrhythmias. *In* Sabiston DC, Spencer FC (eds): Gibbon's Surgery of the Chest, 5th edition. Philadelphia, WB Saunders, 1988
68. Becker AE, Anderson RH: The Wolff-Parkinson-White syndrome and its anatomical substrate. Anat Rec 201:169, 1981
69. Lunel AV: Significance of annulus fibrosis of heart in relation to A-V conduction and ventricular activation in cases of Wolff-Parkinson-White syndrome. Br Heart J 34:1263, 1972
70. Cox JL, Gallagher JJ, Cain ME: Experience with 118 consecutive patients undergoing operation for the Wolff-Parkinson-White syndrome. J Thorac Cardiovasc Surg 90:490, 1985
71. Lowe JE: The endocardial technique for left free-wall accessory pathways. Cardiac Surg 4:135, 1990
72. Cox JL, Ferguson TB Jr: Surgery for the Wolff-Parkinson-White syndrome: The endocardial approach. Semin Thorac Cardiovasc Surg 1:34, 1989
73. Guiraudon G, Klein G, Sharma A, Yee R: Left ventricular free-wall accessory pathways do not require cardiopulmonary bypass when using the "direct" epicardial approach. Circulation 80(suppl II):II, 1989
74. Klein GJ, Guiraudon GM, Perkins DG, et al: Surgical correction of the Wolff-Parkinson-White syndrome in the closed heart using cryosurgery. J Am Cardiol 3:405, 1984
75. Penn OC: The epicardial technique for left free-wall accessory pathways. Cardiac Surg 4:123, 1990
76. Hammon JW Jr: Surgery for right free-wall and anterior septal accessory pathways. Cardiac Surg 4:279, 1990
77. Holman W, Ikeshita M, Lease J, et al: Elective prolongation of atrioventricular conduction by multiple discrete cryolesions: A new technique for the treatment of paroxysmal supraventricular tachycardia. J Thorac Cardiovasc Surg 84:554, 1982
78. Holman WL, Ikeshita M, Lease JG, et al: Alteration of antegrade atrioventricular conduction by cryoablation of periatrioventricular nodal tissue. J Thorac Cardiovasc Surg 88:67, 1984
79. Holman WL, Ikeshita M, Lease JG, et al: Cryosurgical modification of retrograde atrioventricular conduction: Implications for the surgical treatment of atrioventricular node reentry tachycardia. J Thorac Cardiovasc Surg 91:826, 1986
80. Cox JL, Holman WL, Cain ME: Cryosurgical treatment of atrioventricular node reentry tachycardia. Circulation 76:1329, 1987

81. Holman WL: Paroxysmal supraventricular tachycardia due to atrioventricular nodal reentry: Electrophysiologic mechanism and surgical therapy. Cardiac Surg 4:145, 1990
82. Stein KM, Lerman BB: Evidence for functionally distinct dual atrial inputs to the human AV node. Am J Physiol 267:H2333, 1994
83. Langberg JJ, Leon A, Borganelli M, et al: A randomized, prospective comparison of anterior and posterior approaches to radiofrequency catheter ablation of atrioventricular nodal reentry tachycardia. Circulation 87:1551, 1993
84. Jazayeri MR, Akhtar M: Electrophysiological behavior of atrioventricular node after selective fast or slow pathway ablation in patients with atrioventricular nodal reentrant tachycardia. PACE Pacing Clin Electrophysiol 16:623, 1993
85. Mitrani RD, Dlien LS, Hackett FK, et al: Radiofrequency ablation for atrioventricular node reentrant tachycardia: Comparison between fast (anterior) and slow (posterior) pathway ablation. J Am Coll Cardiol 21:432, 1993
86. Chen SA, Chiang CE, Tsang WP, et al: Selective radiofrequency catheter ablation of fast and slow pathways in 100 patients with atrioventricular nodal reentrant tachycardia. Am Heart J 125:1, 1993
87. Akhtar M, Jazayeri MR, Sra JS, et al: Atrioventricular nodal reentry: Clinical, electrophysiologic and therapeutic considerations. Circulation 88:2822, 1993
88. Gentzer JH, Goyal R, Williamson BD, et al: Analysis of junctional ectopy during radiofrequency ablation of the slow pathway in patients with atrioventricular nodal reentrant tachycardia. Circulation 90:2820, 1994
89. Cox JL, Holman WL, Cain ME: Cryosurgical treatment of atrioventricular node reentry tachycardia. Circulation 76:1329, 1987
90. Steinbeck G, Hoffmann E: 'True' atrial tachycardia. Eur Heart J 19:E-10, 1998
91. Saoudi N, Cosio F, Waldo A, et al: A classification of atrial flutter and regular atrial tachycardia according to electrophysiological mechanism and anatomical bases: A statement from a joint expert group from The Working Groups of Arrhythmias of the European Society of Cardiology and the North American Society of Pacing and Electrophysiology. Eur Heart J 22:1162, 2001
92. Hoffmann E, Reithmann C, Nimmermann P, et al: Clinical experience with electroanatomic mapping of ectopic atrial tachycardia. PACE Pacing Clin Electrophysiol 25:49, 2002
93. Lai LP, Lin JL, Chen TF, et al: Clinical, electrophysiological characteristics, and radiofrequency catheter ablation of atrial tachycardia near the apex of Koch's triangle. PACE Pacing Clin Electrophysiol 21:367, 1998
94. Chen SA, Tai CT, Chiang CE, et al: Focal atrial tachycardia: Reanalysis of the clinical and electrophysiologic characteristics and prediction of successful radiofrequency ablation. J Cardiovasc Electrophysiol 9:355, 1998
95. Schmitt C, Zrenner B, Schneider M, et al: Clinical experience with a novel multielectrode basket catheter in right atrial tachycardia. Circulation 99:2414, 1999
96. Natale A, Breeding L, Tomassoni G, et al: Ablation of right and left ectopic atrial tachycardia using a three-dimensional nonfluoroscopic mapping system. Am J Cardiol 82:989, 1998
97. Anguera I, Brugada J, Roba M, et al: Outcomes after radiofrequency catheter ablation of atrial tachycardia. Am J Cardiol 87:886, 2001
98. Williams JM, Ungerleider RM, Lofland GD, et al: Left atrial isolation: New technique for the treatment of supraventricular arrhythmias. J Thorac Cardiovasc Surg 80:373, 1980
99. Harada A, D'Agostino HJ Jr, Schuessler RB, et al: Right atrial isolation: A new surgical treatment for supraventricular tachycardia. I. Surgical technique and electrophysiologic effects. J Thorac Cardiovasc Surg 95:643, 1988
100. Man KC, Knight B, Tse HF, et al: Radiofrequency catheter ablation of inappropriate sinus tachycardia guided by activation mapping. J Am Coll Cardiol 35:451, 2000
101. Cossu SF, Steinberg JS: Supraventricular tachyarrhythmias involving the sinus node: Clinical and electrophysiologic characteristics. Prog Cardiovasc Dis 41:51, 1998
102. Goya M, Iesaka Y, Takahashi A, et al: Radiofrequency catheter ablation for sinoatrial node reentrant tachycardia: electrophysiologic features of ablation sites. Jpn Circ J 63:177, 1999
103. Cheng J, Scheinman MM: Acceleration of typical atrial flutter due to double-wave reentry induced by programmed electrical stimulation. Circulation 97:1589, 1998
104. Cheng J, Cabeen WR Jr, Scheinman MM: Right atrial flutter due to lower loop reentry: Mechanism and anatomic substrates. Circulation 99:1700, 1999
105. Willems S, Weiss C, Ventura R, et al: Catheter ablation of atrial flutter guided by electroanatomic mapping (CARTO): A randomized comparison to the conventional approach. J Cardiovasc Electrophysiol 11:1223, 2000
106. Kottkamp H, Hugl B, Krauss B, et al: Electromagnetic versus fluoroscopic mapping of the inferior isthmus for ablation of typical atrial flutter: A prospective randomized study. Circulation 102:2082, 2000
107. Ward DE, Xie B, Rowland E: Ablation of atrial flutter using the anatomical method: Results and long-term follow-up. J Interv Cardiol 8:697, 1995
108. Tai CT, Chen SA, Chiang CE, et al: Long-term outcome of radiofrequency catheter ablation for typical atrial flutter: Risk prediction of recurrent arrhythmia. J Cardiovasc Electrophysiol 9:115, 1998
109. Lee SH, Tai CT, Yu WC, et al: Effects of radiofrequency catheter ablation on quality of life in patients with atrial flutter. Am J Cardiol 84:278, 1999
110. Anselmen F, Saoudi N, Poty H, et al: Radiofrequency catheter ablation of common atrial flutter: Significance of palpitations and quality-of-life evaluation in a patient with proven isthmus block. Circulation 99:534, 1999
111. Natale A, Newby KH, Pisano E, et al: Prospective randomized comparison of antiarrhythmic therapy versus first-line radiofrequency ablation in patients with atrial flutter. J Am Coll Cardiol 35:1898, 2000
112. Nakagawa H, Shah N, Matsudaira K, et al: Characterization of re-entrant circuit in macro-re-entrant right atrial tachycardia after surgical repair of congenital heart disease: Isolated channels between scars allow "focal" ablation. Circulation 103:699, 2001
113. Shah D, Jais P, Takahashi A, et al: Dual-loop intra-atrial re-entry in humans. Circulation 101:631, 2000
114. Duru F, Hindricks G, Kottkamp H: Atypical left atrial flutter after intraoperative radiofrequency ablation of chronic atrial fibrillation: Successful ablation using three-dimensional electroanatomic mapping. J Cardiovasc Electrophysil 12:602, 2001
115. Akar JG, Kok LC, Haines DE, et al: Coexistence of type I atrial flutter and intra-atrial reentrant tachycardia in patients with surgically corrected congenital heart disease. J Am Coll Cardiol 38:377, 2001
116. Lev M, Gibson S, Miller DA: Ebstein's disease with Wolff-Parkinson-White syndrome. Am Heart J 49:724, 1955
117. Irish CL, Murkin JM, Guiraudon GM: Anesthetic management for surgical cryoablation of accessory conducting pathways: A review and report of 181 cases. Can J Anaesth 35:634, 1988
118. Zamparelli R, Alessandrini F, Tavernese C, et al: L'anestesia nei pazienti affetti da sindrome da preeccitazione ventricolare soltoposti a chirurgia ablativa per via epicardica. Minerva Anestesiol 56:1007, 1990
119. Henzi I, Sonderegger J, Tramer MR: Efficacy, dose-response, and adverse effects of droperidol for prevention of postoperative nausea and vomiting. Can J Anesth 47:537-551, 2000
120. Bertolo L, Novakovic BS, Penna M: Antiarrhythmic effects of droperidol. Anesthesiology 29:529, 1972
121. Gomez-Arnau J, Mones JM, Auello F: Fentanyl and droperidol effects on the refractoriness of the accessory pathway in the Wolff-Parkinson-White syndrome. Anesthesiology 58:307, 1983
122. Sadowski AR, Moyers JR: Anesthetic management of the Wolff-Parkinson-White syndrome. Anesthesiology 51:553, 1979
123. Suppan P: Althesin in the Wolff-Parkinson-White syndrome. Br J Anaesth 51:69, 1979
124. Sharpe MD, Murkin JM, Dobkowski WB, et al: Sufentanil anesthesia has no effect on conduction of normal and accessory pathways in patients with Wolff-Parkinson-White syndrome. Anesth Analg 72:5248, 1991
125. Sharpe MD, Murkin JM, Dobkowski WB, et al: Halothane depresses conduction of normal and accessory pathways during surgery for Wolff-Parkinson-White syndrome. Anesth Analg 70:5365, 1990
126. Sharpe MD, Dobkowski WB, Murkin JM: The electrophysiologic effects of volatile anesthetics on the normal AV conduction system and accessory pathways in WPW. Anesthesiology 80:63-70, 1994
127. Dobkowski WB, Murkin JM, Sharpe MD, et al: The effect of enflurane (IMAC) on the normal AV conduction system and accessory pathways. Anesth Analg 72:550, 1991
128. Atlee JL, Yeager TS: Electrophysiologic assessment of the effects of enflurane, halothane and isoflurane on properties affecting supraventricular reentry in chronically instrumented dogs. Anesthesiology 71:941, 1989
129. Geha GD, Rozelle BC, Raessler KL, et al: Pancuronium bromide enhances atrioventricular conduction in halothane-anesthetized dogs. Anesthesiology 46:342, 1977
130. Kumazawa T: Wolff-Parkinson-White syndrome and anesthesia. Jpn J Anesthesiol 19:68, 1970
131. Van der Starr PJA: Wolff-Parkinson-White syndrome during anesthesia. Anesthesiology 48:369, 1978

132. Geha DG, Davis NJ, Lappas DG: Persistent atrial arrhythmias associated with placement of a Swan-Ganz catheter. Anesthesiology 39:651, 1973
133. Wyse DG, Waldo AL, DiMarco JP, et al: Atrial Fibrillation Follow-up Investigation of Rhythm Management (AFFIRM) Investigators. A comparison of rate control and rhythm control in patients with atrial fibrillation. N Engl J Med 347:1825, 2002
134. Moe GK: On the multiple wavelet hypothesis of atrial fibrillation. Arch Int Pharmacodyn 140:183, 1962
135. Boineau JP, Schuessler RB, Mooney CR, et al: Natural and evoked atrial flutter due to circus movement in dogs: Role of abnormal atrial pathways, slow conduction, nonuniform refractory period distribution and premature beats. Am J Cardiol 45:1167, 1980
136. Allessie MA, Bonke FIM, Schopman FG: Circus movement in rabbit atrial muscle as a mechanism of tachycardia. II. The role of nonuniform recovery of excitability in the occurrence of unidirectional block as studied with multiple microelectrodes. Circ Res 39:168, 1976
137. Cox JL, Canavan TE, Schuessler RB, et al: The surgical treatment of atrial fibrillation. II. Intraoperative electrophysiologic mapping and description of the electrophysiologic basis of atrial flutter and atrial fibrillation. J Thorac Cardiovasc Surg 101:406, 1991
138. Cox JL, Boineau JP, Schuessler RB, et al: Successful surgical treatment of atrial fibrillation. Review and clinical update. JAMA 266:1976, 1991
139. Cox JL, Boineau JP, Schuessler RB, et al: Operations for atrial fibrillation. Clin Cardiol 14:827, 1991
140. Haissaguerre M, Jais P, Shah DC, et al: Spontaneous initiation of atrial fibrillation by ectopic beats originating in the pulmonary veins. N Engl J Med 339:659, 1998
141. Yamauchi S, Tanaka S, Asano T, et al: Efficacy of combining mapping with surgery for atrial fibrillation. Rinsho Kyobu Geka 14:344-5, 1994
142. Harada A, Sasaki K, Fukushima T, et al: Atrial activation during chronic atrial fibrillation in patients with isolated mitral valve disease. Ann Thorac Surg 61:104, 1996
143. Schuessler RB, Grayson TM, Bromberg BI, et al: Cholinergically mediated tachyarrhythmias induced by a single extrastimulus in the isolated canine right atrium. Circ Res 71:1254, 1992
144. Yamauchi S, Boineau JP, Schuessler RB, Cox JL: Varying types of circus movement reentry with both normal and dissociated contralateral conduction causing different right and left atrial rhythms in canine atrial flutter. Jpn Circ J 62:201, 1998
145. Nitta T, Ishii Y, Miyagi Y, et al: Concurrent multiple left atrial focal activations with fibrillatory conduction and right atrial focal or reentrant activation as the mechanisms in atrial fibrillation. J Thorac Cardiovasc Surg 127:770, 2004
146. Schuessler RB: Do we need a map to get through the Maze? J Thorac Cardiovasc Surg 127:627, 2004
147. Haissaguerre M, Shah DC, Jais P, et al: Electrophysiological breakthroughs from the left atrium to the pulmonary veins. Circulation 102:2463, 2000
148. Pappone C, Rosario S, Oreto G, et al: Circumferential radiofrequency ablation of pulmonary vein ostia: A new anatomic approach for curing atrial fibrillation. Circulation 102:2619, 2000
149. Oral H, Scharf C, Chugh A, et al: Catheter ablation for paroxysmal atrial fibrillation: Segmental pulmonary vein ostial ablation versus left atrial ablation. Circulation 108:2355, 2003.
150. Haissaguerre M, Jais P, Shah DC, et al: Right and left atrial radiofrequency catheter therapy of paroxysmal atrial fibrillation. J Cariodvasc Electrophysiol 7:1132, 1996
151. Jais P, Shah DC, Haissaguerre M, et al: Efficacy and safety of septal and left-atrial linear ablation for atrial fibrillation. Am J Cardiol 84:R139, 1999
152. Natale A, Leonelli F, Bheiry S, et al: Catheter ablation approach on the right side only for paroxysmal atrial fibrillation therapy: Long-term results. PACE Pacing Clin Electrophysiol 23:224, 2000
153. Shah DC, Haissaguerre M, Jais P, et al: Electrophysiological endpoint for catheter ablation of atrial fibrillation initiated from multiple pulmonary venous foci. Circulation 101:1409, 2000
154. Hsieh MH, Chen SA, Tai CT, et al: Double multi-electrode mapping catheters facilitate radiofrequency catheter ablation of focal atrial fibrillation originating from pulmonary veins. J Cardiovasc Electrophysiol 10:136, 1999
155. Chen SA, Hsieh MH, Tai CT, et al: Initiation of atrial fibrillation by ectopic beats originating from the pulmonary veins: Electrophysiological characteristics, pharmacological response, and effect of radiofrequency ablation. Circulation 100:1879, 1999
156. Cox JL, Schuessler RB, D'Agostino HJ, et al: The surgical treatment of atrial fibrillation. III. Development of a definitive surgical procedure. J Thorac Cardiovasc Surg 101:569, 1991
157. Cox JL: The surgical treatment of atrial fibrillation. IV. Surgical technique. J Thorac Cardiovasc Surg 101:584, 1991
158. Cox JL, Boineau JP, Schuessler RB, et al: Modification of the Maze procedure for atrial flutter and atrial fibrillation. I. Rationale and surgical results. J Thorac Cardiovasc Surg 110:473, 1995
159. Cox JL, Jaquiss RDB, Schuessler RB, et al: Modification of the Maze procedure for atrial flutter and atrial fibrillation. II. Surgical technique of the Maze III procedure. J Thorac Cardiovasc Surg 110:485, 1995.
160. Pasic M, Musci M, Siniawski HK, et al: Transient sinus node dysfunction after the Cox-Maze III procedure in patients with organic heart disease and chronic fixed atrial fibrillation. J Am Coll Cardiol 32:1040, 1998
161. Gillinov AM, Blackstone EH, McCarthy PM: Atrial fibrillation: Current surgical options and their assessment. Ann Thorac Surg 74:2210, 2002
162. Kim KB, Lee CH, Kim CH, Cha YJ: Effect of the Cox-Maze procedure on the secretion of atrial natriuretic peptide. J Thorac Cardiovasc Surg 115:139, 1998
163. Albåge A, van der Linden J, Bengtsson L, et al: Elevations in antidiuretic hormone and aldosterone as possible causes of fluid retention in the Maze procedure. Ann Thorac Surg 72:58, 2001
164. Ad N, Suyderhoud JP, Kim YD, et al: Benefits of prophylactic continuous infusion of furosemide after the Maze procedure for atrial fibrillation. J Thorac Cardiovasc Surg 123:232, 2002
165. Cox JL, Schuessler RB, Lappas DG, Boineau JP: An 8 1/2-year clinical experience with surgery for atrial fibrillation. Ann Surg 224:267, 1996
166. Isobe F, Kawashima Y: The outcome and indications of the Cox Maze III procedure for chronic atrial fibrillation with mitral valve disease. J Thorac Cardiovasc Surg 116:220, 1998
167. Feinberg MS, Waggoner AD, Kater KM, et al: Restoration of atrial function after the Maze procedure for patients with atrial fibrillation: Assessment by Doppler echocardiography. Circulation 90(suppl II):II-285, 1994
168. Tsui SS, Grace AA, Ludman PF, et al: Maze 3 for atrial fibrillation: Two cuts too few? PACE Pacing Clin Electrophysiol 17:2163, 1994
169. Nitta T, Lee R, Schuessler RB, et al: Radial approach: A new concept in surgical treatment for atrial fibrillation. I. Concept, anatomic and physiologic bases and development of the procedure. Ann Thorac Surg 67:27, 1999
170. Nitta T, Lee R, Watanabe H, et al: Radial procedure: A new concept in surgical treatment for atrial fibrillation. II. Electrophysiologic effects and atrial contribution to ventricular filling. Ann Thorac Surg 67:36, 1999
171. Omari BO, Nelson RJ, Robertson JM: Effect of right atrial appendectomy on the release of atrial natriuretic hormone. J Thorac Cardiovasc Surg 102:272, 1991
172. Mohr FW, Fabricius AM, Falk V, et al: Curative treatment of atrial fibrillation with intraoperative radiofrequency ablation: Short-term and midterm results. J Thorac Cardiovasc Surg 123:919, 2002
173. Kottkamp H, Hindricks G, Autschblach R, et al: Specific linear left atrial lesions in atrial fibrillation. J Am Coll Cardiol 40:475, 2002
174. Doll N, Borger MA, Fabricius A, et al: Esophageal perforation during left atrial radiofrequency ablation: Is the risk too high? J Thorac Cardiovasc Surg 125:836, 2003
175. The Antiarrhythmics Versus Implantable Defibrillator (AVID) Investigators: A comparison of antiarrhythmic-drug therapy with implantable defibrillators in patients resuscitated from near-fatal ventricular arrhythmias. N Engl J Med 337:1576, 1997
176. Calkins H, Kalbfleisch SJ, el-Atassi R, et al: Relation between efficacy of radiofrequency catheter ablation and site of origin of idiopathic ventricular tachycardia. Am J Cardiol 71:827, 1993
177. Coggins DL, Lee RJ, Sweeney J, et al: Radiofrequency catheter ablation as a cure for idiopathic tachycardia of both left and right ventricular origin. J Am Coll Cardiol 23:1333, 1994
178. Thakur RK, Klein GJ, Sivaram CA, et al: Anatomic substrate for idiopathic left ventricular tachycardia. Circulation 93:497, 1996
179. Prystowsky EN, Miles WM, Evans JJ, et al: Induction of ventricular tachycardia during programmed electrical stimulation: Analysis of pacing methods. Circulation 73(suppl II):II-32, 1986
180. Bigger JT, Reiffel JA, Livelli FD Jr, et al: Sensitivity, specificity, and reproducibility of programmed ventricular stimulation. Circulation 73(suppl II):II, 1986
181. Stevenson WG, Sager PT, Friedman PL: Entrainment techniques for mapping atrial and ventricular tachycardias. J Cardiovasc Eletrophysiol 6:201, 1995
182. Marchlinski FE, Callans DJ, Gottlieb CD, et al: Linear ablation lesions for control of unmappable ventricular tachycardia in patients with ischemic and nonischemic cardiomyopathy. Circulation 101:1288, 2000
183. Mehdirad AA, Keim S, Rist K, Tchou P: Long-term clinical outcome of right bundle branch radiofrequency catheter ablation for treatment of

bundle branch reentrant ventricular tachycardia. Pacing Clin Electrophysiol 18:2135, 1995
184. Rothman SA, Hsia HH, Cossu SF, et al: Radiofrequency catheter ablation of postinfarction ventricular tachycardia: long-term success and the significance of inducible nonclinical arrhythmias. Circulation 96:3499, 1997
185. Callans DJ, Zado E, Sarter BY, et al: Efficacy of radiofrequency catheter ablation for ventricular tachycardia in healed myocardial infarction. Am J Cardiol 82:42, 1998
186. Stevenson WG, Friedman PL, Kocovic D, et al: Radiofrequency catheter ablation of ventricular tachycardia after myocardial infarction. Circulation 98:308, 1998
187. Stevenson WG, Khan H, Sage P, et al: Identification of reentry circuit sites during catheter mapping and radiofrequency ablation of ventricular tachycardia late after myocardial infarction. Circulation 88:1647, 1993
188. Gonska BD, Cao K, Schaumann A, et al: Catheter ablation of ventricular tachycardia in 136 patients with coronary artery disease: Result and long-term follow-up. J Am Coll Cardiol 24:1506, 1994
189. Kim YH, Sosa-Suarez G, Trouton TG, et al: Treatment of ventricular tachycardia by transcatheter radiofrequency ablation in patients with ischemic heart disease. Circulation 89:1094, 1994
190. Jadonath RL, Snow JS, Goldner BG, Cohen TJ: Radiofrequency catheter ablation as primary therapy for symptomatic ventricular tachycardia. J Invasive Cardiol 6:289, 1994
191. Cox JL: Patient selection criteria and results of surgery for refractory ischemic ventricular tachycardia. Circulation 79(suppl I):I163, 1989
192. Damiano R Jr: Surgical treatment of nonischemic ventricular tachycardia. Cardiac Surg 4:233, 1990
193. Cox JL: Ventricular tachycardia surgery: A review of the first decade and a suggested contemporary approach. Semin Thorac Cardiovasc Surg 1:97, 1989
194. Harrison L, Ideker RE, Smith WM, et al: The sock electrode array: A tool for determining global epicardial activation during unstable arrhythmias. PACE Pacing Clin Electrophysiol 3:531, 1980
195. Haffajje C, Lesko L, Canada A, et al: Clinical pharmacokinetics of amiodarone. Circulation 64(suppl IV):IV-263, 1981
196. Gallagher JD, Lieberman RW, Meranze J, et al: Amiodarone-induced complications during coronary artery surgery. Anesthesiology 55:186, 1981
197. Liberman BA, Teasdale SJ: Anesthesia and amiodarone. Can Anaesth Soc J 32:629, 1985
198. Feinberg BI, LaMantia KR, Levy WJ: Amiodarone and general anesthesia: A retrospective analysis. Anesth Analg 65:549, 1986
199. Schmid JP, Rosengant TK, McIntosh CL, et al: Amiodarone-induced complications after cardiac operation for obstructive hypertrophic cardiomyopathy. Ann Thorac Surg 48:359, 1989
200. Greenspon AJ, Kidwell GA, Hurley W, Mannion J: Amiodarone-related postoperative adult respiratory distress syndrome. Circulation 84(suppl III):III-407, 1991
201. Eliot GC, Zimmerman GA, Clemmen TP: Complications of pulmonary artery catheterization in the case of critically ill patients. Chest 76:647, 1979
202. Feinberg BI, LaMantia KR: Ventricular tachyarrhythmias during placement of pulmonary artery catheters in patients with recurrent ventricular tachycardia. Mt Sinai J Med 53:545, 1986
203. Kroll DA, Knight PR: Antifibrillatory effects of volatile anesthetics in acute occlusion/reperfusion arrhythmias. Anesthesiology 61:657, 1984
204. Turner LA, Bosnjak ZJ, Kampine JP: Electrophysiological effects of halothane on Purkinje fibers from normal and infarcted canine hearts. Anesthesiology 67:619, 1987
205. Atlee JL, Bosnjak ZJ: Mechanism for cardiac arrhythmias during anesthesia. Anesthesiology 72:347, 1990
206. Hunt GB, Ross DL: Comparison of effects of three anesthetic agents on induction of ventricular tachycardia in a canine model of myocardial infarction. Circulation 78:221, 1988
207. Deutsch N, Huntler CB, Tait AR, et al: Suppression of ventricular arrhythmias by volatile anesthetics in a canine model of chronic myocardial infarction. Anesthesiology 72:1012, 1990
208. MacLeod BA, Augerean P, Walker MJA: Effects of halothane anesthesia compared with fentanyl anesthesia and no anesthesia during coronary ligation in rats. Anesthesiology 58:44, 1983
209. Denniss AR, Richards DA, Taylor AT, Uther JB: Halothane anesthesia reduces inducibility of ventricular tachyarrhythmias in chronic canine myocardial infarction. Basic Res Cardiol 84:5, 1989
210. Atlee JL III: Halothane: Cause or cure for arrhythmias. Anesthesiology 67:617, 1987
211. Gallagher JD, McClernan CA: The effects of halothane on ventricular tachycardia in intact dogs. Anesthesiology 75:866, 1991
212. Saini V, Carr DB, Hagestod EL, et al: Antifibrillatory action of the narcotic agonist fentanyl. Am Heart J 115:598, 1988
213. DeSilva RA, Verrier RL, Lown B: Protective effect of the vagotonic action of morphine sulphate or ventricular vulnerability. Cardiovasc Res 12:167, 1978
214. Atlee JL, Bernstein AD: Cardiac rhythm management devices. Part I. Anesthesiology 95:1265, 2001
215. Saksena S, An H, Mehra R, et al: Prospective comparison of biphasic and monophasic shocks for implantable cardioverter-defibrillators using endocardial leads. Am J Cardiol 70:304, 1992
216. Gregoratos G, Abrams J, Epstein AE, et al: ACC/AHA/NASPE 2002 guideline update for implantation of cardiac pacemakers and antiarrhythmia devices: A report of the American College of Cardiology/American Heart Association Task Force on Practice Guidelines. Circulation 106:2145, 2002
217. The Antiarrhythmics Versus Implantable Defibrillator (AVID) Investigators: A comparison of antiarrhythmic drug therapy with implantable defibrillators in patients resuscitated for near-fatal ventricular arrhythmias. N Engl J Med 337:1576, 1997
218. Connolly SJ, Gent M, Roberts RS, et al: Canadian Implantable Defibrillator Study (CIDS): A randomized trial of the implantable cardioverter-defibrillator against amiodarone. Circulation 101:129, 2000
219. Kuck KH, Capitol R, Seibel J, et al: Randomized comparisons of antiarrhythmic drug therapy with implantable defibrillators in patients resuscitated from cardiac arrest: The Cardiac Arrest Study Hamburg (CASH). Circulation 102:748, 2000
220. Moss AJ, Hall WJ, Cannon DS, et al: Improved survival with an implanted defibrillator in patients with coronary disease at high risk for ventricular arrhythmia: Multicenter Automatic Defibrillator Implantation Trial Investigators. N Engl J Med 335:1933, 1996
221. Buxton AE, Lee KL, Fisher JD, et al: A randomized study of the prevention of sudden death in patients with coronary artery disease: Multicenter Unsustained Tachycardia Trial Investigators. N Engl J Med 341:1882, 1999
222. Kadish A, Dyer A, Daubert JP, et al: Prophylactic defibrillator implantation in patients with nonischemic dilated cardiomyopathy. N Engl J Med 350:2151, 2004
223. Exner DV, Klein GJ, Prystowsky EN: Primary prevention of sudden death with implantable defibrillator therapy in patients with cardiac disease. Circulation 104:1564, 2001
224. Epstein AE: An update on implantable cardioverter-defibrillator guidelines. Curr Opin Cardiol 19:23, 2004
225. Maron BJ, Olivotto I, Spirito P, et al: Epidemiology of hypertrophic cardiomyopathy-related death: Revisited in a large nonreferral-based patient population. Circulation 102:858, 2000
226. Elliott PM, Gimeno JR, Mahon NG, et al: Relation between severity of left-ventricular hypertrophy and prognosis in patients with hypertrophic cardiomyopathy. Lancet 357:420, 2001
227. Zareba W, Moss AJ, Schwartz PJ, et al: Influence of genotype on the clinical course of the long-QT syndrome: International Long-QT Syndrome Registry Research Group. N Engl J Med 339:960, 1998
228. Watkins H, McKenna WJ, Thierfelder L, et al: Mutations in the genes for cardiac troponin T and alpha-tropomyosin in hypertrophic cardiomyopathy. N Engl J Med 332:1058, 1995
229. Adams DC, Heyer EJ, Emerson RG, et al: Implantable cardioverter-defibrillator. Evaluation of clinical neurologic outcome and electroencephalographic changes during implantation. J Thorac Cardiovasc Surg 109:565, 1995
230. Meyer J, Mollhoff T, Seifert T, et al: Cardiac output is not affected during testing of the AICD. J Cardiovasc Electrophysiol 7:211, 1996
231. Hurst TM, Hinrichs M, Breidenbach C, et al: Detection of myocardial injury during transvenous implantation of automatic cardioverter-defibrillators. J Am Coll Cardiol 34:402, 1999
232. DiMarco JP: Implantable cardioverter-defibrillators. N Engl J Med 349:1836-1847, 2003

Part IV

MONITORING

Chapter 14

MONITORING OF THE HEART AND VASCULAR SYSTEM

David L. Reich, MD • Alexander Mittnacht, MD • Martin London, MD • Joel A. Kaplan, MD

KEY POINTS

1. Patients with severe cardiovascular disease and those undergoing surgery associated with rapid hemodynamic changes should be adequately monitored at all times.
2. Adequate monitoring is based on specific patient, surgical, and environmental factors.
3. Standard monitoring for cardiac surgery patients includes invasive blood pressure, electrocardiography, central venous pressure, urine output, temperature, capnometry, pulse oximetry, and intermittent blood gas analysis.
4. Electrocardiography remains the gold standard for myocardial ischemia monitoring. Continuous thermodilution pulmonary artery catheters and left atrial pressure catheters are invasive monitors. The risks and benefits should be considered for each patient.
5. The Society of Cardiovascular Anesthesiologists and the American Society of Echocardiography have published recommendations for intraoperative transesophageal echocardiography in various clinical settings.
6. Evidence-based data on clinical outcome and monitoring in cardiac anesthesia are difficult to obtain due to difficulties in conducting large prospective trials.

HEMODYNAMIC MONITORING

For patients with severe cardiovascular disease and those undergoing surgery associated with rapid hemodynamic changes, adequate hemodynamic monitoring should be available at all times. With the ability to measure and record almost all vital physiologic parameters, the development of acute hemodynamic changes may be observed, and corrective action may be taken in an attempt to correct adverse hemodynamics and improve outcome. Although outcome changes are difficult to prove, it is a reasonable assumption that appropriate hemodynamic monitoring should reduce the incidence of major cardiovascular complications. This is based on the presumption that the data obtained from these monitors are interpreted correctly and that therapeutic decisions are implemented in a timely fashion.

Many devices are available to monitor the cardiovascular system. These devices range from those that are completely noninvasive, such as the blood pressure (BP) cuff and electrocardiogram (ECG), to those that are extremely invasive, such as the pulmonary artery catheter (PAC). To make the best use of invasive monitors, the potential benefits to be gained from the information must outweigh the potential complications. In many critically ill patients, the benefit obtained does seem to outweigh the risks, which explains the widespread use of invasive monitoring. Transesophageal echocardiography (TEE), a minimally invasive technology, has gained in popularity as an alternative to the PAC (see Chapters 15 and 16), and is considered a standard-of-care monitoring device in the perioperative management for certain procedures such as mitral valvuloplasty or surgery for congenital heart defects.

Standard monitoring for cardiac surgical patients includes BP, ECG, central venous pressure (CVP), urine output, temperature, capnometry, pulse oximetry, and intermittent arterial blood gas analysis (Box 14–1). The next tier of monitoring includes PACs, left atrial pressure (LAP) catheters, thermodilution cardiac output (CO) measurements, TEE, and indices of tissue oxygen transport (Box 14–2). All of these measurements and their derivatives can be obtained and recorded. The interpretation of these complex data, however, requires an astute clinician who is aware of the patient's overall condition and the limitations of the monitors.

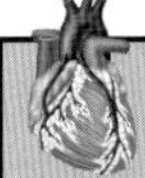

BOX 14–1 *Standard Monitoring for Cardiac Surgical Patients*

- (Invasive) blood pressure
- Electrocardiogram
- Pulse oximetry
- Capnometry
- Temperature
- Central venous pressure
- Urine output
- Intermittent arterial blood gas analysis

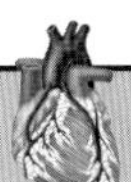

BOX 14–2 *Extended Monitoring for Patients Based on Case-Specific Factors*

- Pulmonary artery catheter
- Cardiac output measurements
- Transesophageal echocardiography
- Left atrial pressure
- Bispectral index monitoring
- Cerebral oximetry
- Jugular venous saturation or pressure
- Spinal drain (intrathecal) pressure

ARTERIAL PRESSURE MONITORING

BP monitoring is the most commonly used method of assessing the cardiovascular system. The magnitude of the BP is directly related to the CO and the systemic vascular resistance (SVR). This is analogous to Ohm's law of electricity (voltage = current × resistance), in which BP is analogous to voltage, CO to flow, and SVR to resistance. An increase in the BP may reflect an increase in CO or SVR, or both. Although BP is one of the easiest cardiovascular variables to measure, it gives only indirect information about the patient's cardiovascular status.

Mean arterial pressure (MAP) is probably the most useful parameter to measure in assessing organ perfusion, except for the heart, in which the diastolic BP is the most important. MAP is measured directly by integrating the arterial waveform tracing over time, or using the formula: MAP = (SBP + [2 × DBP])/3, in which SBP is systolic blood pressure, and DBP is diastolic blood pressure. The pulse pressure is the difference between SBP and DBP.

Anesthesia for cardiac surgery is frequently complicated by rapid and sudden lability of the BP because of several factors, including direct compression of the heart, impaired venous return due to retraction and cannulation of the vena cavae and aorta, arrhythmias from mechanical stimulation of the heart, and manipulations that may impair right ventricular (RV) outflow and pulmonary venous return. Sudden losses of significant amounts of blood may induce hypovolemia at almost any time. The cardiac surgical population also includes many patients with labile hypertension and atherosclerotic heart disease. A safe and reliable method of measuring acute changes in the BP is required during cardiac surgery with cardiopulmonary bypass (CPB).

Numerous methods of noninvasive BP measurement are clinically available.[1,2] Nevertheless, most of these require the detection of flow past an occlusive cuff, and none generate an arterial waveform suitable for cardiac surgery. Continuous BP monitoring with noninvasive devices has been introduced, but they have not proven to be suitable for cardiac surgery.[3,4] Intra-arterial monitoring provides a continuous, beat-to-beat indication of the arterial pressure and waveform, and having an indwelling arterial catheter enables frequent sampling of arterial blood for laboratory analyses. Direct intra-arterial monitoring remains the gold standard for cardiac surgical procedures.

The arterial waveform tracing can provide information beyond timely BP measurements. For example, the slope of the arterial upstroke correlates with the derivative of pressure over time, dP/dt, and gives an indirect estimate of myocardial contractility. This is not specific information, because an increase in SVR alone will also result in an increase in the slope of the upstroke. The arterial waveform can also present a visual estimate of the hemodynamic consequences of arrhythmias, and the arterial pulse contour can be used to estimate stroke volume (SV). Hypovolemia is suggested when the arterial pressure shows large SBP variation during the respiratory cycle in the mechanically ventilated patient.[5,6] Coriat et al[7] found that TEE-derived left ventricular (LV) dimensions at end-diastole correlated well with the magnitude of SBP decrease during inspiration.[7]

General Principles

The arterial pressure waveform is ideally measured in the ascending aorta. The pressure measured in the more peripheral arteries is different from the central aortic pressure, because the arterial waveform becomes progressively more distorted as the signal is transmitted down the arterial system. The high-frequency components, such as the dicrotic notch, disappear, the systolic peak increases, the diastolic trough decreases, and there is a transmission delay. These changes are caused by decreased arterial compliance in the periphery and reflection and resonance of pressure waves in the arterial tree.[8] This effect is most pronounced in the dorsalis pedis artery, in which the SBP may be 10 to 20 mm Hg higher, and the DBP 10 to 20 mm Hg lower than in the central aorta (Fig. 14–1).[9] Despite this distortion, the MAP measured in the peripheral arteries should be similar to the central aortic pressure under normal circumstances. However, this may not be the case after CPB.

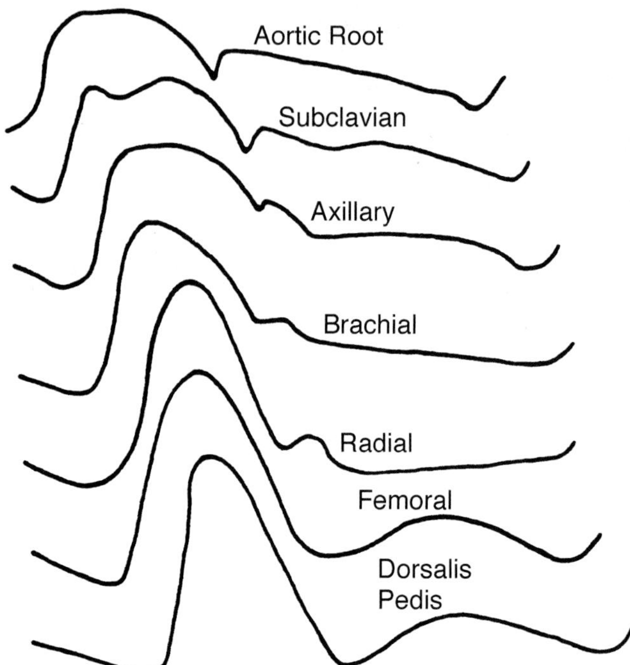

Figure 14–1 The waveform of the arterial pressure changes markedly according to the site of the intra-arterial catheter. These changes are shown as a progression from central monitoring *(top)* through peripheral monitoring *(bottom)*. These changes are thought to be caused by forward wave propagation and wave reflection. In the periphery, systolic pressure is higher, diastolic pressure is lower, and mean pressure is minimally lower. (Modified from Bedford RF: Invasive blood pressure monitoring. *In* Blitt CD [ed]: Monitoring in Anesthesia and Critical Care. New York, Churchill Livingstone, 1985, p 505.)

Pressure waves in the arterial (or venous) tree represent the transmission of forces generated in the cardiac chambers. Measurement of these forces requires their transmission to a device that converts mechanical energy into electronic signals. The components of a system for intravascular pressure measurement include an intravascular catheter, fluid-filled tubing and connections, an electromechanical transducer, an electronic analyzer, and electronic storage and display systems (see Chapter 12).

Components of a Pressure Measurement System

Intravascular Catheters

For arterial pressure measurements, short, narrow catheters are recommended (20 gauge or smaller), because they have favorable dynamic response characteristics and are less thrombogenic than larger catheters.[10] Catheters made from Teflon are most widely used because they are softer and less thrombogenic, but are prone to kinking. An artifact associated with intra-arterial catheters has been designated *end-pressure artifact.*[11] When flowing blood comes to a sudden halt at the tip of the catheter, it is estimated that an added pressure of 2 to 10 mm Hg results. Conversely, clot formation on the catheter tip will overdamp the system.

Coupling System

The coupling system usually consists of pressure tubing, stopcocks, and a continuous flushing device. This is the major source of distortion of arterial pressure tracings. Hunziker[12] studied the damping coefficients and natural frequencies of various coupling systems. All systems were severely underdamped and most led to systematic overestimation of the systolic arterial pressure.

Transducers

The function of transducers is to convert mechanical forces into electrical current or voltage. Over the years, this has been achieved by several different mechanisms, but today most transducers are of the resistance-type. Pairs of resistors are incorporated into a circuit on the arms of a Wheatstone bridge-type of electrical circuit. Most modern disposable transducers have a silicone diaphragm into which resistive elements have been etched. The manufacturers have adopted an output standard of 5 μV per volt excitation per 1 mm Hg, so that, theoretically, any transducer can be used with any monitor.[13] The dynamic response of bare transducers is usually in the 100- to 500-Hz range. Modern disposable transducers have eliminated much of the difficulties that used to require frequent recalibration due to drifting of the zero point. The major practical problem remaining with transducer systems is improper zeroing relative to the patient.

Analysis and Display Systems

Most modern equipment designed to analyze and display pressure information consists of a computerized system that handles several tasks. These include the acquisition and display of pressure signals, the derivation of numerical values for systolic, diastolic, and mean pressures, alarm functions, data storage, trend displays, and printing functions. The algorithms used to analyze the pressure information, and to provide numerical data, vary between manufacturers. When comparing displayed numerical values, and values obtained from strip chart recordings, Maloy and Gardner[14] observed frequent discrepancies between the numerical values and the pressure recordings.

Venous pressures, and arterial pressures to a lesser degree, are significantly affected by respiratory fluctuations. Several techniques have been devised to automatically recognize end-expiration because this is the preferred measurement period.[15] Most display systems average hemodynamic parameters over several cardiac cycles to minimize the effects of respiratory variability.

Flush Systems

The arterial catheter should be kept patent with a continuous infusion of normal saline solution (1 to 3 mL/hr). The infusion minimizes thrombus formation and helps prolong the usefulness of the catheter.[16] Heparin is no longer routinely recommended as an additive to flush solutions due to the risk of heparin-induced thrombocytopenia in susceptible patients. Catheters may also be flushed intermittently with small volumes (2 to 3 mL) of saline. Larger volumes, however, could potentially produce central arterial embolization and should be avoided.[17]

Characteristics of a Pressure Measurement System

The dynamic response of a pressure measurement system is characterized by its natural frequency and its damping.[18] These concepts are best understood by snapping the end of a transducer-tubing assembly with a finger. The waveform on the monitor demonstrates rapid oscillations above and below the baseline (the natural frequency), which quickly decays to a straight line due to friction in the system (damping). The peaks and troughs of an arterial pressure waveform will be amplified if the transducer-tubing-catheter assembly has a natural frequency less than 20 Hz because this is the maximal significant frequency that normally exists in the arterial BP signal.[19] This is commonly known as *ringing* or *resonance* of the system (Fig. 14–2). In practical terms, longer transducer tubing lowers the natural frequency of the system and tends to amplify the height of the SBP (peak) and the depth of the DBP (trough) values.[20,21] Boutros and Albert[22] demonstrated that by changing the length of low-compliance (rigid) tubing from 6 inches to 5 feet, the natural frequency decreased from 34 to 7 Hz. As a result of the reduced natural frequency, the SBP measured with the longer tubing exceeded reference pressures by 17.3%.

Damping is the tendency of factors such as friction, compliant (soft) tubing, and air bubbles to absorb energy and decrease the amplitude of peaks and troughs in the waveform. The optimal degree of damping is that which counterbalances the distorting effects of transducer-tubing systems with lower natural frequencies. This is very difficult to achieve. The damping of a clinical pressure measurement system can be assessed by observing the response to a rapid high-pressure flush of the transducer-tubing-catheter system (see Fig. 14–2). In a system with a low damping coefficient, a fast-flush test results in several oscillations above and below the baseline before the pressure becomes constant. In an adequately damped system, the baseline is reached after one oscillation, whereas in an overdamped system, the baseline is reached after a delay and without oscillations.[23–26]

The formulas for calculating the natural frequency and damping coefficient are as follows:

$$\text{Natural frequency: } f_n = \frac{d}{8}\sqrt{\frac{3}{\pi L \rho V_d}}$$

$$\text{Damping coefficient: } \zeta = \frac{16\eta}{d^3}\sqrt{\frac{3LV_d}{\pi\rho}}$$

In the equations, d is the tubing diameter, L is the tubing length, ρ is the density of the fluid, V_d is the transducer fluid volume displacement, and η is the viscosity of the fluid.

Arterial Cannulation Sites

Factors that influence the site of arterial cannulation include the location of surgery, the possible compromise of arterial flow due to patient positioning or surgical manipulations, and any history of ischemia of or prior surgery on the limb to be cannulated. Another factor that may influence the cannulation

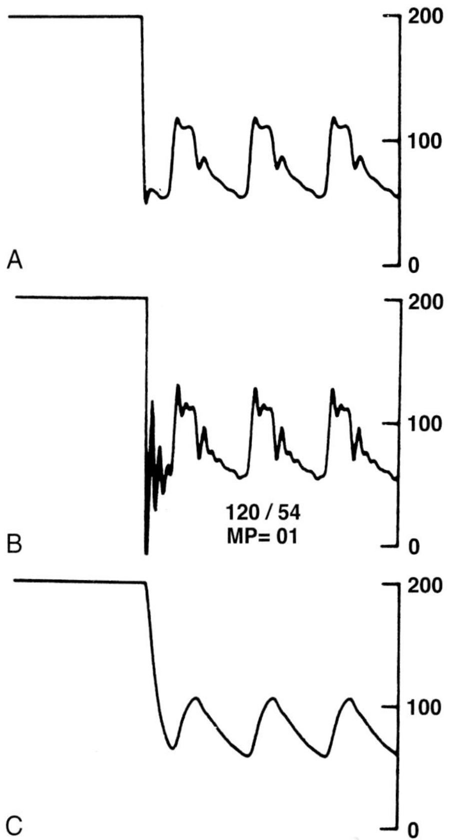

Figure 14–2 The fast-flush test demonstrates the harmonic characteristics of a pressure monitoring system (i.e., transducer, fluid-filled tubing, and intra-arterial catheter). In an optimally damped system *(A)*, the pressure waveform returns to baseline after only one oscillation. In an underdamped system *(B)*, the pressure waveform oscillates above and below the baseline several times. In an overdamped system *(C)*, the pressure waveform returns to the baseline slowly with no oscillations. *(A–C,* Adapted from Gibbs NC, Gardner RM: Dynamics of invasive pressure monitoring systems: Clinical and laboratory evaluation. Heart Lung 17:43, 1988.)

site is the presence of a proximal arterial cutdown. The proximal cutdown may cause damped waveforms or falsely low BP readings due to stenosis or vascular thrombosis.[27] Surgeons have used axillary cannulation to establish arterial access for CPB in patients with anterograde selective cerebral perfusion or a severely diseased ascending aorta.[28–30] Patients with prior axillary artery cannulation may have some degree of axillary stenosis, causing a gradient between the BP measured in the ascending aorta and the BP obtained by ipsilateral radial artery cannulation. Sites for arterial cannulation include the following:

- Radial artery
- Ulnar artery
- Brachial artery
- Axillary artery
- Femoral artery
- Dorsalis pedis or posterior tibial arteries
- Superficial temporal artery

Radial and Ulnar Arteries

The radial artery is the most commonly used artery for continuous BP monitoring because it is easy to cannulate with a short (20-gauge) catheter, readily accessible during surgery, and the collateral circulation is usually adequate and easy to check. It is advisable to assess the adequacy of the collateral circulation and the absence of proximal obstructions before cannulating the radial artery for monitoring purposes.

The ulnar artery provides most blood flow to the hand in about 90% of patients.[31] The radial and ulnar arteries are connected by a palmar arch, which provides collateral flow to the hand in the event of radial artery occlusion. Palm showed that if there is adequate ulnar collateral flow, circulatory perfusion pressure to the fingers is adequate after radial arterial catheterization.[32] Many clinicians routinely perform Allen's test before radial artery cannulation to assess the adequacy of collateral circulation to the hand.

Allen's test is performed by compressing the radial and ulnar arteries and by exercising the hand until it is pale. The ulnar artery is then released (with the hand open loosely), and the time until the hand regains its normal color is noted.[33] With a normal collateral circulation, the color returns to the hand in about 5 seconds. If, however, the hand takes longer than 15 seconds to return to its normal color, cannulation of the radial artery on that side is controversial. The hand may remain pale if the fingers are hyperextended or widely spread apart, even in the presence of a normal collateral circulation.[34] Variations on Allen's test include using a Doppler probe or pulse oximeter to document collateral flow.[35–37] If the Allen's test demonstrates that the hand depends on the radial artery for adequate filling, and other cannulation sites are not available, the ulnar artery may be selected.[38]

The predictive value of Allen's test has been challenged. In a large series of children in whom radial arterial catheterization was performed without preliminary Allen's tests, there was an absence of complications.[39] Slogoff et al[40] cannulated the radial artery in 16 adult patients with poor ulnar collateral circulation (assessed using Allen's test) without any complications. An incidence of zero in a study sample of only 16 patients, however, does not guarantee that the true incidence of the complication is negligible. In contrast, Mangano and Hickey[41] reported a case of hand ischemia requiring amputation in a patient with a normal preoperative result for Allen's test. The predictive value of Allen's test is somewhat questionable. Alternatively, pulse oximetry or plethysmography can be used to assess patency of the collateral arteries of the hand. Barbeau et al[42] compared the modified Allen's test with pulse oximetry and plethysmography in 1010 consecutive patients undergoing percutaneous radial cannulation for cardiac catheterization. Pulse oximetry and plethysmography were more sensitive than the Allen's test for detecting inadequate collateral blood supply and only 1.5% of patients were not suitable for radial artery cannulation.

Another method of radial arterial catheterization involves percutaneous insertion of a long catheter to obtain a central aortic tracing of arterial pressure.[43] There were no complications attributed to these catheters in a series of patients.[44] The advantage of a central arterial tracing is the increased accuracy compared with radial arterial pressure in patients with low-flow states or after CPB.[45,46] Although reasons for the difference between central and peripheral measurements of BP are not entirely clear—after CPB, they were transiently present in 17% to 40% of patients in several studies.[47–50] Kanazawa et al[51] suggested that a decrease in the arterial elasticity is responsible for instances in which lower radial artery pressures (compared with aortic pressures) are observed after CPB. When the palpated central aortic pressure is high despite a low radial arterial BP value, the central aortic pressure may also be temporarily monitored using a needle attached to pressure tubing placed in the aorta by the surgeon until the problem resolves. Alternatively, a femoral arterial catheter may be inserted.

Chest wall retractors, such as the Favaloro retractor, may impede radial arterial pressure monitoring in cardiothoracic procedures in some patients. The arm on the affected side may have diminished perfusion during extreme retraction of the chest wall. If the left internal mammary artery is used during myocardial revascularization, the right radial artery could be monitored to avoid this problem. Alternatively, a noninvasive BP cuff on the right side could be used to confirm the accuracy of the radial artery tracing during extreme chest wall retraction.

Monitoring of the radial artery distal to a brachial arterial cutdown site is not recommended. Acute thrombosis or residual stenosis of the brachial artery will lead to falsely low radial arterial pressure readings.[22] Other considerations related to the choice of a radial arterial monitoring site include prior surgery of the hand, selection of the nondominant hand, and the preference of the surgeon, the anesthesiologist, or both.

Brachial and Axillary Arteries

The brachial artery lies medial to the bicipital tendon in the antecubital fossa, in close proximity to the median nerve. Brachial artery pressure tracings resemble those in the femoral artery, with less systolic augmentation than radial artery tracings.[52] Brachial arterial pressures were found to more accurately reflect central aortic pressures than radial arterial pressures before and after CPB.[53] The complications from percutaneous brachial artery catheter monitoring are lower than those after brachial artery cutdown for cardiac catheterization.[54] A few series of perioperative brachial arterial monitoring have documented the relative safety of this technique.[48,49,54] Armstrong et al[55] published data on 1326 patients with peripheral vascular disease undergoing angiography with percutaneous brachial access and found an overall complication rate of 1.28% with a higher risk of thrombosis in female patients. Still, there is little or no collateral flow to the hand if brachial artery occlusion occurs. Other sites should be chosen, if possible.

The axillary artery is normally cannulated by the Seldinger technique near the junction of the deltoid and pectoral muscles. This has been recommended for long-term catheterization in the intensive care unit (ICU) and in patients with peripheral vascular disease.[56,57] Because the tip of the 15- to 20-cm catheter may lie within the aortic arch, the use of the left axillary artery is recommended to minimize the risk of cerebral embolization during flushing. Lateral decubitus positioning or adduction of the arm occasionally results in kinking of axillary catheters with damping of the pressure waveform. Arterial pressures measured in the axillary artery (by radial artery cannulation) more closely reflected central aortic BP than brachial arterial BP measurements.[49]

Femoral Artery

The femoral artery may be cannulated for monitoring purposes, but is usually reserved for situations in which other sites are unable to be cannulated or it is specifically indicated (e.g., descending thoracic aortic aneurysm surgery for distal pressure monitoring). The use of this site remains controversial because of the risk of ischemic complications and pseudoaneurysm formation after diagnostic angiographic and cardiac catheterization procedures.[58] However, these data do not pertain to the clinical situation in which the femoral artery is used for monitoring purposes because the size of the catheters for BP monitoring is considerably smaller than that of diagnostic catheters. Scheer et al[59] have reviewed the literature on peripheral artery cannulation for hemodynamic monitoring, including 3899 femoral artery cannulations. Temporary occlusion was found in 10 patients (1.45%), whereas serious ischemic complications requiring extremity amputation were reported in 3 patients (0.18%). Other complications that were summarized from the published data were pseudoaneurysm formation in 6 patients (0.3%), sepsis in 13 patients (0.44%), local infection (0.78%), bleeding (1.58%), and hematoma (6.1%). Based on the reviewed literature, they concluded that using the femoral artery for hemodynamic monitoring purposes was safer than radial artery cannulation. Older literature stated that the femoral area was intrinsically dirty, and that catheter sepsis and mortality were significantly increased compared with other monitoring sites. This could also not be confirmed by the reviewed literature.[60] Theoretically, femoral artery cannulation is less desirable in patients with peripheral vascular disease. Aortic inflow obstruction may decrease the BP in the femoral artery, or the femoral artery may have atheromatous plaques that could embolize and cause distal ischemia. Atheromatous plaque may also make it more difficult to thread catheters up this artery, necessitating the use of a J-wire.

In patients undergoing thoracic aortic surgery, distal aortic perfusion (using partial CPB, left-heart bypass, or a heparinized shunt) may be performed during aortic cross-clamping to preserve spinal cord and visceral organ blood flow. In these situations, it is useful to measure the distal aortic pressure at the femoral artery (dorsalis pedis or posterior tibial artery) to optimize the distal perfusion pressure[61] (see Chapter 23). In repairs of aortic coarctation, simultaneous femoral and radial arterial monitoring may help determine the adequacy of the surgical repair by documenting the pressure gradient after the repair. It is necessary to consult with the surgeon before cannulating the femoral vessels because these vessels may be used for extracorporeal perfusion or placement of an intra-aortic balloon pump during the surgical procedure.

Dorsalis Pedis and Posterior Tibial Arteries

The two main arteries to the foot are the dorsalis pedis artery and the posterior tibial artery, which form an arterial arch on the foot that is similar to the one formed by the radial and ulnar arteries in the hand. The dorsalis pedis or posterior tibial arteries are reasonable alternatives to radial arterial catheterization. The SBP is usually 10 to 20 mm Hg higher in the dorsalis pedis artery than in the radial or brachial arteries, whereas the diastolic pressure is 15 to 20 mm Hg lower (see Fig. 14–1).[62] The dorsalis pedis is a relatively small artery that may be cannulated when other sites are not available, but the vessel may not be palpable or present in 5% to 12% of patients.[63] The incidence of failed cannulation is up to 20%, and the incidence of thrombotic occlusion is about 8%, because of the small size of the artery.[64] A modified Allen's test may be performed by blanching the great toe during compression of the dorsalis pedis and posterior tibial arteries, and then releasing the pressure over the posterior tibial artery. These vessels should not be used in patients with severe peripheral vascular disease from diabetes mellitus or other causes.

Superficial Temporal Artery

The superficial temporal artery is a branch of the external carotid artery that passes anteriorly to the ear. It has a variable course, and this may be determined with a Doppler probe.[65] The artery may be quite tortuous and difficult to cannulate. The tip of the catheter must be positioned carefully so that embolization by the internal carotid artery to the cerebral circulation will not occur. This approach is not recommended in patients with carotid occlusive or cerebrovascular disease.

Indications

The indications for invasive arterial monitoring are provided in Box 14–3.

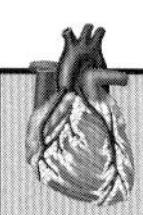

BOX 14–3 *Indications for Intra-arterial Monitoring*

- Major surgical procedures involving large fluid shifts or blood loss
- Surgery requiring cardiopulmonary bypass
- Surgery of the aorta
- Patients with pulmonary disease requiring frequent arterial blood gases
- Patients with recent myocardial infarctions, unstable angina, or severe coronary artery disease
- Patients with decreased left ventricular function (congestive heart failure) or significant valvular heart disease
- Patients in hypovolemic, cardiogenic, or septic shock, or with multiple organ failure
- Procedures involving the use of deliberate hypotension or deliberate hypothermia
- Massive trauma cases
- Patients with right heart failure, chronic obstructive pulmonary disease, pulmonary hypertension, or pulmonary embolism
- Patients requiring inotropes or intra-aortic balloon counterpulsation
- Patients with electrolyte or metabolic disturbances requiring frequent blood samples
- Inability to measure arterial pressure noninvasively (e.g., morbid obesity)

Contraindications

The contraindications to arterial cannulation include local infection, coagulopathy, proximal obstruction, vaso-occlusive disorders, and surgical considerations.

Local Infection

Placement of an arterial catheter through infected tissues is likely to result in catheter sepsis. If signs of infection develop at an existing arterial cannulation site, the catheter must be removed. A separate cannulation site should be found. Strict aseptic technique is necessary during the insertion and maintenance of arterial cannulas.

Coagulopathy

Coagulopathy is a relative contraindication because it may result in hematoma formation during arterial cannulation at peripheral sites, such as the radial and dorsalis pedis arteries. However, there is a more significant risk of exsanguination or massive hematoma formation causing vascular or neurologic compromise during axillary and femoral cannulation attempts. This is because it is more difficult to apply direct arterial pressure with failed attempts at cannulation or when the catheter is removed. In anticoagulated patients, it is recommended that more peripheral arterial cannulation sites be used when this form of monitoring is required.

Proximal Obstruction

Anatomic factors may lead to intra-arterial pressure readings that markedly underestimate the central aortic pressure. The thoracic outlet syndrome and congenital anomalies of the aortic arch vessels will obstruct flow to the upper extremities. Aortic coarctation will diminish flow to the lower extremities. Arterial pressure distal to a previous arterial cutdown site may be lower than the central aortic pressure due to arterial stenosis at the cutdown site.

Raynaud's Syndrome and Buerger's Disease

Radial and brachial arterial cannulation are contraindicated in patients with a history of Raynaud's syndrome or Buerger's disease (i.e., thromboangiitis obliterans). This is especially important in the perioperative setting, because hypothermia of the hand is the main trigger for vasospastic attacks in Raynaud's syndrome.[66] It is recommended that large arteries, such as the femoral or axillary, be used for intra-arterial monitoring if indicated in patients with either of these diseases.

Surgical Considerations

Several surgical maneuvers may interfere with intra-arterial monitoring. During mediastinoscopy, the scope intermittently compresses the innominate artery against the manubrium. In this situation, in which the arterial waveform damping is intermittent, it is advantageous to monitor radial artery pressure on the affected side, and a pulse oximeter may be placed on the opposite extremity. The surgeon can be informed whenever compression of the innominate artery occurs.

The lateral decubitus position may compromise flow to the downward arm if an axillary roll is not properly positioned. In this situation, the damping may be prolonged. Nevertheless, during descending thoracic aortic aneurysm repairs, the right radial, brachial, or axillary artery should be monitored, because the left subclavian artery may be occluded during various phases of the procedure.

Insertion Techniques

Direct Cannulation

Proper technique is helpful in obtaining a high degree of success in arterial catheterization. The wrist should be placed in a dorsiflexed position on an armboard over a pack of gauze and immobilized in a supinated position. It is helpful to draw the course of the artery for 1 inch and to be comfortably seated. Doppler devices and ultrasonic vessel finders may also be of value. Local anesthetic is injected intradermally over the artery, and a small skin nick may be made to allow passage of the catheter-over-needle assembly into the subcutaneous tissue without crimping secondary to penetration of the unit through the skin. A 20-gauge or smaller, 3- to 5-cm, nontapered Teflon catheter over needle is used, without a syringe attached, to make the puncture. If a syringe is used, the plunger should be removed to allow free flow of blood to detect when the artery has been punctured. The angle between the needle and the skin should be shallow (30 degrees or less), and the needle should be advanced parallel to the course of the artery. When the artery is entered, the angle between the

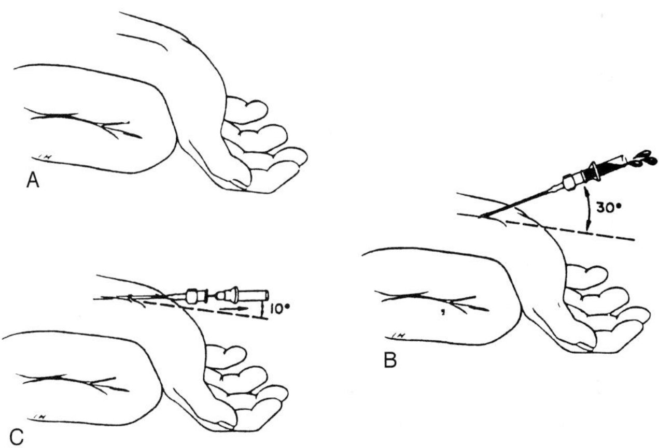

Figure 14–3 The direct-cannulation technique for the radial artery. *(A)* The wrist is dorsiflexed over a towel or a small pack of gauze and loosely taped to a stable surface such as an armboard. *(B)* The artery is directly cannulated at a 30- to 40-degree angle to the plane of the wrist. Arterial blood flows steadily into the "flashback" chamber. *(C)* The catheter-over-needle assembly is lowered until the angle is approximately 10 degrees to the plane of the wrist. The entire assembly is advanced another 1 to 2 mm, until the tip of the catheter lies within the lumen of the artery. The catheter is then advanced into the artery completely while the needle is held motionless. *(A–C,* From Lake CL: Cardiovascular Anesthesia. New York, Springer-Verlag, 1985, p 54.)

needle and skin is reduced to 10 degrees, the needle is advanced another 1 to 2 mm to ensure that the tip of the catheter also lies within the lumen of the vessel, and the outer catheter is then threaded off the needle while watching that blood continues to flow out of the needle hub (Fig. 14–3). After insertion of the catheter, the wrist should be taken out of the dorsiflexed position, because continued extreme dorsiflexion can lead to median nerve damage by stretching of the nerve over the wrist. An armboard may still be used to prevent the wrist from flexing, which causes kinking of the catheter and damping of the arterial waveform.

Transfixation

If blood ceases flowing while the needle is being advanced, the needle has penetrated the back wall of the vessel. In this technique, the artery has been transfixed by passage of the catheter-over-needle assembly "through-and-through" the artery. The needle is then completely withdrawn. As the catheter is slowly withdrawn, pulsatile blood flow emerges from the catheter when its tip is within the lumen of the artery. The catheter is then slowly advanced into the artery. A guidewire may be helpful at this point if the catheter does not advance easily into the artery. Alternatively, the catheter-over-needle assembly may be withdrawn slowly as one unit until flow of blood has returned. As soon as this occurs, the needle and catheter are most likely in the lumen of the artery and the catheter may be gently threaded off the needle into the artery.

Seldinger Technique

The artery is localized with a needle, and a guidewire is passed through the needle into the artery. A catheter is then passed over the guidewire into the artery. Alternatively, a catheter-over-needle assembly may be inserted in the artery in a through-and-through fashion, the needle withdrawn, and the wire passed through the catheter after pulsatile flow is encountered. It is very important when using this technique to avoid withdrawal of guidewires through needles to prevent shearing of the wire and embolization. Mangar et al[67] showed that when using the direct or modified Seldinger technique compared with a direct-cannulation method, the success rate of arterial catheter placement increased from 62% to 82%.

Doppler-Assisted Technique

The artery is localized using a Doppler flow probe. The direction of insertion of the percutaneous catheter is guided by the Doppler signals.[68,69] This may be especially useful in small children and infants. In adults, this may be helpful when palpation of the artery is difficult, such as in obese patients requiring femoral arterial cannulation.

Two-Dimensional Ultrasound-Assisted Method

The Doppler-assisted techniques have been largely supplanted in clinical practice by two-dimensional ultrasonic methods. In the case of arterial catheterization, especially radial artery cannulation, a high-frequency ultrasonic transducer (e.g., 9 MHz) is required to visualize small structures in the "near field." The artery is visualized in transverse section and the catheter-over-needle assembly is advanced at a 30- to 60-degree angle, starting 5 to 15 mm distal to the ultrasonic transducer. With experience, the artery and the catheter are seen to intersect within the ultrasonic imaging plane using a "triangulation" technique. Using a two-dimensional ultrasound imaging technique for radial artery cannulation has been shown to increase the success rate on the first attempt.[70] Nevertheless, there seems to be a significant learning curve involved.

Surgical Cutdown

An incision is made in the skin overlying the artery, and the surrounding tissues are dissected away from the arterial wall. Proximal and distal ligatures are passed around the artery to control blood loss, but are not tied down. Under direct vision, the artery is cannulated with a catheter-over-needle assembly. Alternatively, a small incision is made in the arterial wall to facilitate passage of the catheter.

Complications

Infection

One potential complication that is common to all forms of invasive monitoring is infection from indwelling catheters. Indwelling percutaneous catheters can become infected because of insertion through an infected skin site; poor aseptic technique during insertion or maintenance; sepsis with seeding of the catheter; and prolonged duration of cannulation with colonization by skin flora. Historically, factors that were associated with catheter infection included nondisposable transducer domes, dextrose flush solutions, contaminated blood gas syringes, and duration of insertion.[71–74] In contrast to central venous catheterization, later published data on vascular catheter infections did not find that full sterile barriers during arterial catheter placement reduced the risk of infection.[75,76] Nevertheless, these data do not exempt the practitioner from using strict aseptic technique. Guidelines for the prevention of intravascular catheter-related infections have been published by the Hospital Infection Control Practices Advisory Committee and the Centers for Disease Control and Prevention.[77]

It is still common practice to remove percutaneous catheters when vascular catheter infection is suspected. This concept has been challenged, and a watchful waiting strategy has been advocated until a catheter-related bloodstream infection has been confirmed instead of immediate removal of the catheter.[78] Whenever infection at the cannulation site or a catheter-related bloodstream infection is confirmed, the catheter should be removed. The catheter is a foreign body that cannot be sterilized with antibiotic therapy. Lymphangitic streaks or cellulitis may occur as a result of catheter infection. These problems require systemic antibiotic therapy.[79]

Hemorrhage

The use of an intra-arterial catheter carries the potential risk of exsanguination if the catheter or tubing assembly becomes disconnected. The use of Luer-Lok (instead of tapered) connections and monitors with low-pressure alarms should decrease the risk of this complication.[80] Stopcocks are an additional source of occult hemorrhage due to the potential for loose connections or inadvertent changes in the position of the control lever that would open the system to the atmosphere.

Thrombosis and Distal Ischemia

Thrombosis of the radial artery after cannulation has been extensively studied. Temporary arterial occlusion is the most commonly reported complication after radial artery cannulation.[81] Factors that correlate with an increased incidence of thrombosis include prolonged duration of cannulation,[82] larger catheters,[83] and smaller radial artery size (i.e., a greater proportion of the artery is occupied by the catheter).[84] The incidence of thrombosis is not affected by the technique of cannulation,[85] but is lowered with aspirin pretreatment.[86]

The association between radial artery thrombosis and ischemia of the hand is less certain. An abnormal result for Allen's test was not associated with hand complications after radial artery cannulation.[40] Despite the widespread use of radial artery cannulation, hand complications are rarely reported. Temporary occlusion after arterial cannulation is usually benign. Nevertheless, serious ischemic complications are reported that may require the amputation of a digit or extremity.[87–89] In the experience of Slogoff et al,[40] most ischemic complications occurred in patients who had had multiple embolic phenomena from other sources or were on high-dose vasopressor therapy with resultant ischemia in multiple extremities.

The hand should be closely examined at regular intervals in patients with axillary, brachial, radial, or ulnar arterial catheters. Because thrombosis may appear several days after the catheter has been removed, examinations should be continued through the postoperative period.[82] Although recanalization of the thrombosed artery can be expected in an average of 13 days, the collateral blood flow may be inadequate during this period.[90] Any evidence of hand ischemia should be aggressively investigated and promptly treated to prevent morbidity.[91]

The treatment plan should involve consultation with a vascular, hand, or plastic surgeon. Traditionally, treatment for arterial occlusion or thrombosis with adequate collateral flow has been conservative. However, fibrinolytic agents (e.g., streptokinase), stellate ganglion blockade, and surgical intervention are modalities that should be considered.

Skin Necrosis

Volar proximal skin necrosis has been reported in patients after radial arterial cannulation.[92,93] This has led to full-thickness skin loss over the volar aspect of the forearm. The skin necrosis is presumably due to thrombosis of the radial artery with proximal propagation of the thrombosis to involve the cutaneous branches of the radial artery.

Embolization

Particulate matter or air that is flushed forcefully into an arterial catheter can move proximally as well as distally within the artery. Cerebral embolization is most likely from axillary or temporal sites, but is also possible with brachial and radial catheters.[17,94] Emboli from the right arm are more likely to reach the cerebral circulation than those from the left arm due to the anatomy and direction of blood flow in the aortic arch. Other factors that influence the likelihood of cerebral embolization include the volume of flush solution, the rapidity of the injection, and the proximity of the intraluminal end of the catheter to the central circulation.[17]

Hematoma and Neurologic Injury

Hematoma formation may occur at any arterial puncture or cannulation site and is particularly common with a coagulopathy. Hematoma formation should be prevented by the application of direct pressure after arterial punctures and, if possible, the correction of any underlying coagulopathy. Posterior puncture/tear of the femoral or iliac arteries can produce massive bleeding into the retroperitoneal area.[95] Surgical consultation should be obtained if massive hematoma formation develops.

Nerve damage is possible if the nerve and artery lie in a fibrous sheath (e.g., the brachial plexus) or in a limited tissue compartment (e.g., the forearm).[96] Direct nerve injuries may also occur from needle trauma during attempts at arterial cannulation. The median nerve is in close proximity to the brachial artery, and the axillary artery lies within the brachial plexus sheath.

Late Vascular Complications

Incomplete disruption of the wall of an artery may eventually result in pseudoaneurysm formation.[97] The wall of the pseudoaneurysm is composed of fibrous tissue that continues to expand. If the pseudoaneurysm ruptures into a vein or if both a vein and artery are injured simultaneously, an arteriovenous fistula may result. Nonsurgical treatment options for the repair of pseudoaneurysms after arterial cannulation have been described and may replace surgery that is usually performed to treat this complication.[98]

Inaccurate Pressure Measurements

Despite the great advantages of intra-arterial monitoring, it does not always give accurate BP values. The monitoring system may be incorrectly zeroed and calibrated, or the transducers may not be at the appropriate level. The waveform will be damped if the catheter is kinked or partially thrombosed. In vasoconstricted patients, those in hypovolemic shock, and during the post-CPB period, the brachial and radial artery pressures may be significantly lower than the true central aortic pressure. Another possible cause of inaccurate measurements is unsuspected arterial stenosis proximal to the monitored artery, as occurs with thoracic outlet syndrome and subclavian stenosis. Unsuspected Raynaud's syndrome also can yield unreliable BP readings from peripheral arteries.

CENTRAL VENOUS PRESSURE MONITORING

CVP catheters are used to measure the filling pressure of the right ventricle, give an estimate of the intravascular volume status, and assess RV function. For accurate pressure measurement, the distal end of the catheter must lie within one of the large intrathoracic veins or the right atrium. Although water manometers have been used in the past, an electronic system is preferred because it allows the observation of the right atrial (RA) waveform, which provides additional information. In any pressure monitoring system, it is necessary to have a reproducible landmark (such as the midaxillary line) as a zero reference. This is especially important in monitoring venous pressures, because small changes in the height of the zero reference point produce proportionately larger errors compared with arterial pressure monitoring.

The normal CVP waveform consists of three upward deflections (A, C, and V waves) and two downward deflections (X and Y descents) (Fig. 14–4). The A wave is produced by right atrial contraction and occurs just after the P wave on the ECG. The C wave occurs because of the isovolumic ventricular contraction forcing the tricuspid valve to bulge upward into the right atrium. The pressure within the right atrium then decreases as the tricuspid valve is pulled away from the atrium during RV ejection, forming the X descent. RA filling continues during late ventricular systole, forming the V wave. The Y descent occurs when the tricuspid valve opens and blood from the right atrium empties rapidly into the right ventricle during early diastole.[99]

The CVP waveform may be useful in the diagnosis of pathologic cardiac conditions. For example, onset of an irregular rhythm and loss of the A wave suggest atrial flutter or fibrillation. Cannon A waves occur as the right atrium contracts against a closed tricuspid valve, as occurs in junctional (atrioventricular [AV] nodal) rhythm, complete heart block, and ventricular arrhythmias (Fig. 14–5). This is clinically relevant because nodal rhythms are frequently seen during anesthesia and may produce hypotension due to a decrease in SV. Cannon A waves may also be present when there is increased resistance to RA emptying, as in tricuspid stenosis, RV hypertrophy, pulmonary stenosis, or pulmonary hypertension. Early systolic or holosystolic "cannon V waves" (or C-V waves) occur if there is a significant degree of tricuspid regurgitation. Large V waves may also appear later in systole if the ventricle becomes noncompliant due to ischemia or RV failure. A comprehensive review of CVP waveform analysis in various pathophysiologic states has been published by Mark.[100]

Pericardial constriction produces characteristic waveforms in the CVP tracing (Fig. 14–6). There is a decrease in venous return because of the inability of the heart chambers to dilate due to the constriction. This causes prominent A and V waves and steep X and Y descents (creating an M configuration) resembling that seen with diseases that cause decreased RV compliance. Egress of blood from the right atrium to the right ventricle is initially rapid during early diastolic filling of the right ventricle (creating a steep Y descent), but is short lived and abruptly halted by the restrictive, noncompliant right ventricle. The RA pressure then increases rapidly and reaches a plateau until the end of the A wave, at the end of diastole. This portion of the waveform is analogous to the ventricular diastolic dip-and-plateau sign.[100] With pericardial tamponade, the X descent is steep but the Y descent is not present, because early diastolic run-off is impaired by the pericardial fluid collection.

The CVP is a useful monitor if the factors affecting it are recognized and its limitations are understood. The CVP reflects the patient's blood volume, venous tone, and RV performance. Following serial measurements (trends) is more useful than individual numbers. The response of the CVP to a volume infusion is a useful test. Thromboses of the vena cavae and alterations of intrathoracic pressure, such as those induced by positive end-expiratory pressure (PEEP), also affect measurement of the CVP.[101] Many peaks and troughs in the CVP waveform are created artifactually from the transducer-tubing monitoring system. Tachycardia produces blending of the waveforms, especially the A and C waves.

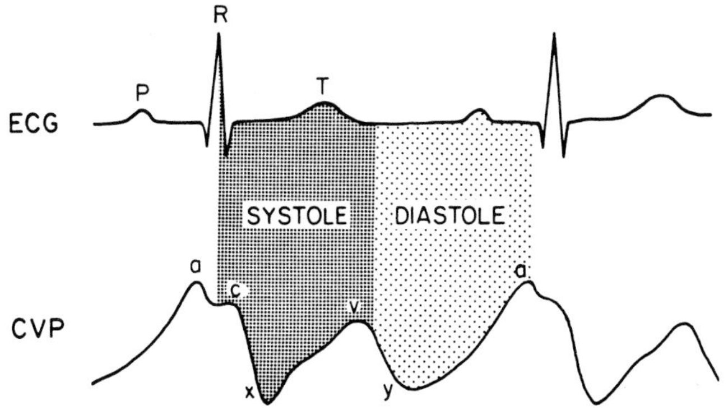

Figure 14–4 The relationship of the central venous pressure (CVP) tracing to the electrocardiogram (ECG) in normal sinus rhythm. The normal CVP waveform consists of three upward deflections (A, C, and V waves) and two downward deflections (X and Y descents). The A wave is produced by right atrial contraction and occurs just after the P wave on the ECG. The C wave occurs because of the isovolumic ventricular contraction forcing the tricuspid valve to bulge upward into the right atrium. The pressure within the right atrium (RA) then decreases as the tricuspid valve is pulled away from the atrium during right ventricular ejection, forming the X descent. The RA continues to fill during late ventricular systole, forming the V wave. The Y descent occurs when the tricuspid valve opens and blood from the RA empties rapidly into the RV during early diastole. (Adapted from Mark JB: Central venous pressure monitoring: Clinical insights beyond the numbers. J Cardiothorac Vasc Anesth 5:163, 1991.)

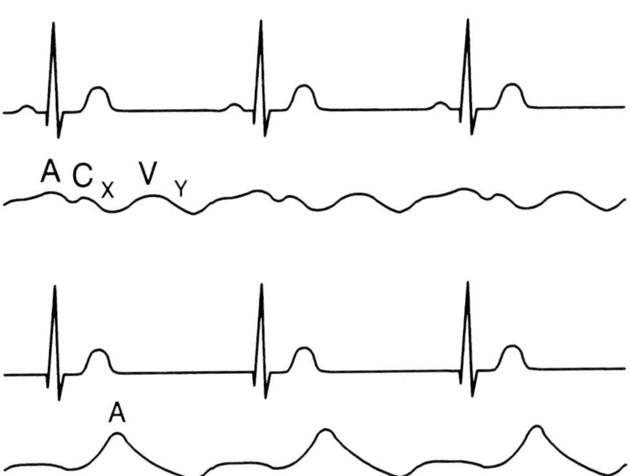

Figure 14–5 The relationship of the central venous pressure (CVP) tracing to the electrocardiogram (ECG) during junctional (atrioventricular nodal) rhythm. The contraction of the atrium against the closed tricuspid valve results in the cannon A waves; notice that the P wave is hidden within the QRS complex of the ECG.

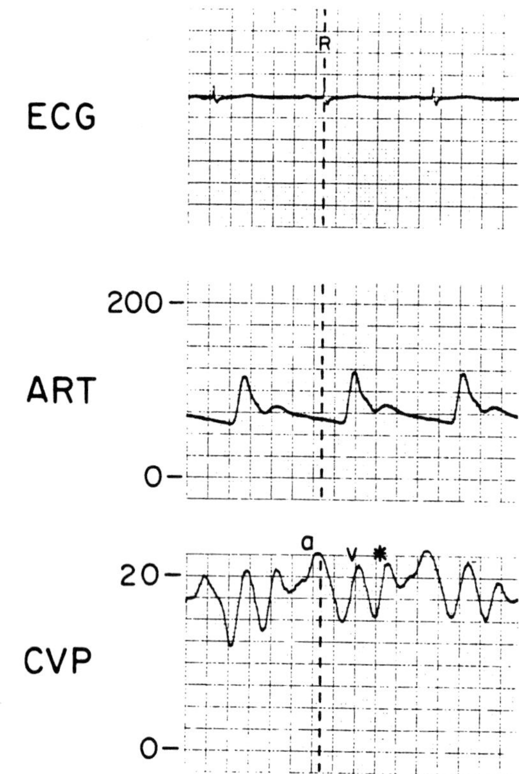

Figure 14–6 The central venous pressure (CVP) waveform during pericardial constriction. There is a characteristic M configuration with prominent A and V waves, accompanied by steep X and Y descents. An additional wave *(asterisk)* is present because of impairment of ventricular filling by the rigid pericardial shell. ART = arterial pressure; ECG = electrocardiogram. (Adapted from Mark JB: Central venous pressure monitoring: Clinical insights beyond the numbers. J Cardiothorac Vasc Anesth 5:163, 1991.)

The CVP does not give a direct indication of left-heart filling pressure, but it may be used as an estimate of left-sided pressures in patients with good LV function. Mangano showed a good correlation between the CVP and left-sided filling pressures during a change in volume status in patients with coronary artery disease and left ventricular ejection fraction (LVEF) greater than 0.4.[102] Later studies have not replicated these results, demonstrating weak relationships between the CVP and measures of LV preload.[103–106]

Techniques and Insertion Sites

Percutaneous central venous cannulation may be accomplished by catheter-through-needle, catheter-over-needle, or catheter-over-wire (Seldinger) techniques. The considerations for selecting the site of cannulation include the experience of the operator, ease of access, anatomic anomalies, and the ability of the patient to tolerate the position required for catheter insertion. The Trendelenburg position can be complicated by hypoxemia in cardiac surgical patients breathing room air, and nasal cannula oxygen may ameliorate this problem. This position is not necessary, however, when venous distention is present in the supine position as occurs in patients with high CVP or right-sided heart failure.

Internal Jugular Vein

Cannulation of the internal jugular vein (IJV) was first described by English et al in 1969.[107] Its popularity among anesthesiologists has steadily increased since that time. Advantages of this technique include the high success rate as a result of the relatively predictable relationship of the anatomic structures; a short, straight course to the right atrium that almost always assures RA or superior vena cava (SVC) localization of the catheter tip; easy access from the head of the operating room table; and fewer complications than with subclavian vein catheterization. The IJV is located under the medial border of the lateral head of the sternocleidomastoid (SCM) muscle (Fig. 14–7). The carotid artery is usually deep and medial to the IJV. The right IJV is preferred, because this vein takes the straightest course into the SVC, the right cupola of the lung may be lower than the left, and the thoracic duct is on the left side.[108]

The preferred *middle approach* to the right IJV is shown in Figure 14–8. With the patient supine or in Trendelenburg position and the head turned toward the contralateral side, the fingers of the left hand are used to palpate the two heads of the SCM muscle and the carotid pulse. These fingers then hold the skin stable over the underlying structures while local anesthetic is infiltrated into the skin and subcutaneous tissues. A 22-gauge "finder" needle is placed at the apex of the triangle formed by the two heads of the SCM muscle at a 45-degree angle to the skin, and directed toward the ipsilateral nipple. If venous blood return is not obtained, the needle is withdrawn to the subcutaneous tissue and then passed in a more lateral or medial direction until the vein is located. This needle reduces the risk of consequences related to inadvertent carotid arterial puncture and tissue trauma if localization of the vein is difficult. When venous blood is aspirated through the "finder" needle, the syringe and needle are withdrawn, leaving a small trail of blood on the drape to indicate the direction of the vein. Alternatively, the needle and syringe can be fixated and used as an identifying needle. Then, a syringe attached to an 18-gauge intravenous catheter-over-needle is inserted in an identical fashion. When venous return is present, the whole assembly is lowered to prevent the needle from going through the posterior wall of the central vein and advanced an additional 1 to 2 mm until the tip of the catheter is within the lumen of the vein. The catheter is then threaded into the vein.

Once the catheter is advanced into the vein, the needle is removed, and an empty syringe is attached to the cannula to withdraw a sample of blood. To confirm that an artery has not been inadvertently cannulated, comparison of the color of the blood sample to an arterial sample drawn simultaneously is recommended.[109] If this is inconclusive or there is no arterial catheter in place, the cannula may be attached to a transducer by sterile tubing to observe the pressure waveform.[110] Another option is to attach the cannula to sterile tubing and allow blood to flow retrograde into the tubing.[111] The tubing is then held upright as a venous manometer, and the height of the blood column is observed. If the catheter is in a vein, it will stop rising at a level consistent with the CVP and demonstrate respiratory variation. A guidewire is then passed through the 18-gauge catheter, and the catheter is exchanged over the wire for a CVP catheter. The use of more than one technique to confirm the venous location of the catheter may provide additional reassurance of correct placement before cannulation of the vein with a larger cannula.

Many other approaches to the right IJV have been described.[112] An anterior (high) approach to the IJV is performed at the level of the laryngeal cartilage. The needle enters the skin at the medial border of the SCM muscle and is directed lateral to the carotid artery pulse. The posterior

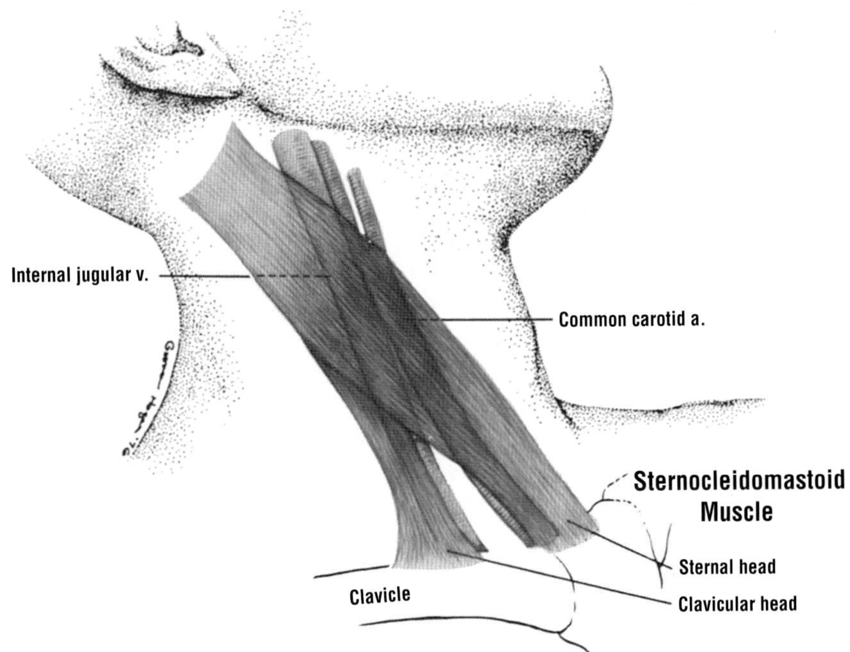

Figure 14–7 The internal jugular vein (v.) is usually located deep to the medial border of the lateral head of the sternocleidomastoid muscle, just lateral to the carotid pulse. a. = artery.

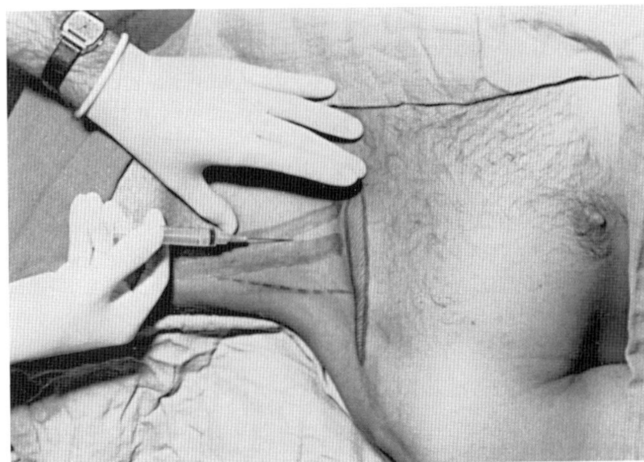

Figure 14–8 The preferred middle approach to the right internal jugular vein. The needle enters the skin at the apex of the triangle formed by the sternal and clavicular heads of the sternocleidomastoid muscle. The needle is held at a 30- to 45-degree angle to the skin and directed toward the ipsilateral nipple.

approach to the IJV is performed near the intersection of the external jugular vein (EJV) and the lateral border of the SCM muscle. The needle is directed along the posterior surface of the SCM muscle toward the sternal notch. In this technique, the needle is aimed in the direction of the carotid artery, and the incidence of carotid artery puncture therefore may be higher. These alternative approaches are less successful and produce more complications than the standard middle approach in the experience of most clinicians.

Some investigators have recommended additional techniques for cannulating the IJV to reduce the incidence of carotid artery puncture. Petty[112] recommended leaving a small identifying needle in place while advancing the larger needle. Jobes et al[110] recommended attaching a 20-gauge catheter to a transducer before passing the guidewire and observing the pressure and waveform. In a prospective study of 1284 patients, 10 episodes of arterial catheterization were diagnosed by this technique of pressure monitoring when they were not suspected by other signs. Many studies have verified the high degree of success of experienced personnel in cannulating the IJV of adult and pediatric patients.[113,114] However, Hayashi et al[115] found that age younger than 3 months or weight less than 4 kg decreased the success rate of cannulating the IJV in pediatric patients undergoing cardiovascular surgery. Experience contributed little to the success or complication rates of this technique in infants.

ULTRASONIC GUIDANCE OF INTERNAL JUGULAR VEIN CANNULATION

Ultrasound has been increasingly used to define the anatomic variations of the IJV.[116] A review and meta-analysis of randomized controlled trials looking at ultrasound-guided central venous cannulation found that real-time two-dimensional ultrasound for IJV cannulation had a significantly higher success rate overall and on the first attempt compared with the landmark method in adults.[117] In this meta-analysis, there was no significant difference between the traditional landmark method and ultrasound-guided IJV cannulation in infants. This was confirmed by a prospective study by Grebenik et al,[118] who challenged the guidelines from the National Institute for Clinical Excellence in the United Kingdom that recommended the use of ultrasound guidance for central venous catheterization in children. In this study, using ultrasound for IJV cannulation was less successful, had a higher incidence of arterial puncture, and there was no time difference compared with the landmark method. Nevertheless, there are numerous publications including prospective studies advocating the use of ultrasound for IJV cannulation in infants.[119–122] Overall, most studies have demonstrated that two-dimensional ultrasonic guidance of IJV cannulation is helpful in locating the vein, permits more rapid cannulation, and decreases the incidence of arterial puncture.[123–127] Circumstances in which ultrasonic guidance of IJV cannulation can be advantageous include patients with difficult neck anatomy (e.g., short neck, obesity), prior neck surgery, anticoagulated patients, and infants.

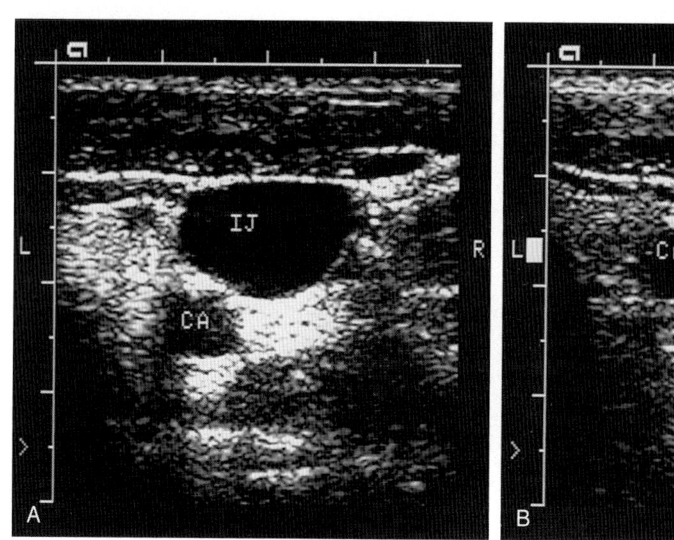

Figure 14–9 The ultrasound images depict the anatomic relationship of the right internal jugular (IJ) vein and the carotid artery (CA). *(A)* With the Valsalva maneuver or Trendelenburg position, the IJ is distended and circular. *(B)* As gentle pressure is applied with the ultrasound probe, the IJ is partially compressed and flattened anteriorly, and the CA size is unaffected. The compressibility of the IJ is its most characteristic feature during ultrasonic imaging.

Ultrasound has provided more precise data regarding the structural relationship between the IJV and the carotid artery (Fig. 14–9). Troianos et al[128] found that in more than 54% of patients, more than 75% of the IJV overlies the carotid artery. Patients who were older than 60 years were more likely to have this type of anatomy. In pediatric patients, Alderson et al[129] found that the carotid artery coursed directly posterior to the IJV in 10% of patients. Sulek et al[130] observed that there was greater overlap of the IJV and the carotid artery when the head is rotated 80 degrees compared with head rotation of only 0 to 40 degrees. The data from 2 and 4 cm above the clavicle did not differ, and the percentage overlap was larger on the left side of the neck compared with the right. Excessive rotation of the head of the patient toward the contralateral side may distort the normal anatomy in a manner that increases the risk of inadvertent carotid artery puncture. Doppler or ultrasound has also been used to demonstrate that the Valsalva maneuver increases IJV cross-sectional area by approximately 25% and that the Trendelenburg position increases it by approximately 37%.[131] Parry[132] published an ultrasound study showing that maximal right IJV diameter can be achieved by placing the patient in 15 degrees Trendelenburg position, slightly elevating the head with a small pillow, keeping the head close to midline and releasing the pressure administered to palpate the carotid artery before IJV cannulation.

Ultrasonic guidance is not the standard of care for IJV cannulation, but the accumulating evidence previously cited should be sufficient to justify the cost and effort related to acquiring this equipment and training cardiac anesthesiologists in its use. The TEE probe can be used for transpharyngeal ultrasonography at a depth of 12 to 20 cm from the teeth in patients with difficult anatomy.[133] The probe is rotated laterally 15 to 20 degrees to see the cervical vascular bundle, which appears as a mirror image with the IJV in the far field. As with most emerging techniques, the practitioner must gain experience in a number of normal IJV cannulations to gain most benefit from the technology in the more complicated patient.

External Jugular Vein

Although the EJV is another means of reaching the central circulation, the success rate with this approach is lower because of the tortuous path followed by the vein. A valve is usually present at the point where the EJV perforates the fascia to join with the subclavian vein. One study, however, reported a success rate of 90% using a J-wire to manipulate past obstructions into the central circulation.[134] The main advantage of this technique is that there is no need to advance a needle into the deeper structures of the neck.

For this approach, the patient is placed supine or in the Trendelenburg position until the EJV becomes distended. The vein is then cannulated with an intravenous catheter. A guidewire with curved tip (i.e., J-wire) is passed through the cannula and manipulated into the central circulation. The curved tip is necessary to negotiate the tortuous course between the EJV and the SVC. Manipulation of the shoulder and rotation of the guidewire between the operator's fingers may be useful maneuvers when difficulty is encountered in passing the wire into the superior vena cava.

Subclavian Vein

The subclavian vein is readily accessible from supraclavicular or infraclavicular approaches and has long been used for central venous access.[135] The success rate is higher than the EJV approach, but lower than the right IJV approach. Cannulation of the subclavian vein is associated with a higher incidence of complications than the IJV approach, especially pneumothorax.[136,137] Other complications associated with subclavian vein cannulation are arterial punctures, misplacement of the catheter tip, aortic injury, cardiac tamponade, mediastinal hematoma, and hemothorax.[138,139] This may be the cannulation site of choice, however, when CVP monitoring is indicated in patients undergoing carotid artery surgery. It is also useful for parenteral nutrition or for prolonged CVP access because the site is easier to maintain and well tolerated by patients.

The *infraclavicular approach* is performed with the patient supine or in the Trendelenburg position with a folded sheet between the scapulae and the shoulder lowered.[140] (Fig. 14–10). The head is turned to the contralateral side. A thin-walled needle or intravenous catheter is inserted 1 cm below the midpoint of the clavicle and advanced toward the suprasternal notch under the posterior surface of the clavicle. When a free flow of venous blood is obtained, the guidewire is passed into the subclavian vessel, and is exchanged for a CVP catheter.

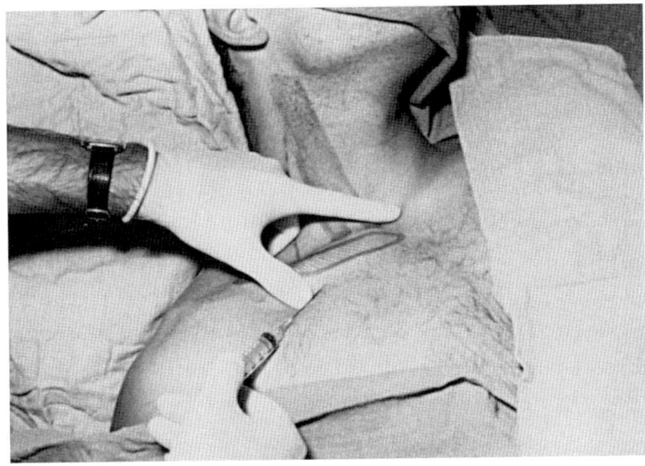

Figure 14–10 The infraclavicular approach to the right subclavian vein. The patient is positioned with a rolled towel between the scapulae to increase the distance between the clavicle and the first rib. The needle enters the skin 1 cm inferior to the midpoint of the clavicle and is directed underneath the clavicle toward the sternal notch. If the needle is directed too far posteriorly, the pleura may be punctured, resulting in a pneumothorax.

The *supraclavicular approach* is performed with the patient in the Trendelenburg position with the head turned away from the side of the insertion. This is usually not performed on the left side because of the risk of an injury to the thoracic duct. The finder needle is inserted at the lateral border of the SCM at the point of insertion into the clavicle. The needle is directed to bisect the angle between the SCM and the clavicle, and about 15 to 20 degrees posteriorly. The vessel is very superficial (about 1 to 2 cm) and lies very close to the innominate artery and the pleura.

Antecubital Veins

Another route for central venous monitoring is through the basilic or cephalic veins. The advantages of this approach are the low likelihood of complications and the ease of access intraoperatively, if the arm is exposed. The major disadvantage is that it is often difficult to assure placement of the catheter in a central vein. Studies have indicated that blind advancement will result in central venous cannulation in 59% to 75% of attempts.[141,142] Chest radiographs are usually necessary to confirm that the tip of the catheter has been appropriately placed, and this involves some time delay. Exact positioning of the catheter tip is crucial because movement of the arm will result in significant catheter migration and could cause cardiac tamponade.[143–145] Unsuccessful attempts result most frequently from failure to pass the catheter past the shoulder, or cannulation of the ipsilateral IJV. Turning the head to the ipsilateral side may help prevent IJV placement of the catheter.[146]

Artru et al[147] reported a high success rate (92%) for the placement of multiorificed catheters from the antecubital veins using intravascular electrocardiography. These catheters are positioned at the SVC-RA junction and are used for the aspiration of air emboli in neurosurgical patients. Due to problems inherent with intravascular electrocardiography, Mongan et al[148] described a method for transducing the pressure waveform and identifying the point at which the catheter tip entered the right ventricle. They then calculated the distance required to withdraw the catheters to the SVC-RA junction (for three different types of air embolism aspirating catheters). Others have used TEE to assist in the correct placement of these types of catheters.[149] Even though peripherally placed central venous catheters avoid the placement of needles into deep venous structures, there are still significant risks associated with their use.[150–153]

Femoral Vein

The femoral vein is rarely cannulated in the adult patient for intraoperative monitoring purposes. However, cannulation of this vein is technically simple, and the success rate is high. Cannulation of the vessel should be done about 1 to 2 cm below the inguinal ligament. The vein typically lies medial to the artery. Although older literature reported a high rate of catheter sepsis and thrombophlebitis with this approach, this may no longer be valid with disposable catheter kits and improved catheter technology.[154–156] Subcutaneous tunneling of femoral central venous catheters has been suggested to reduce the incidence of catheter-related infections.[157,158] In patients with SVC obstruction, the femoral vein is necessary for intravenous access and to obtain a true CVP measurement. The catheter should be long enough so that the tip lies within the mediastinal portion of the inferior vena cava.

Indications

CVP monitoring is often performed to obtain an indication of intravascular volume status. The accuracy and reliability of CVP monitoring depend on many factors, including the functional status of the right and left ventricles, the presence of pulmonary disease, and ventilatory factors, such as PEEP. The CVP may reflect left-heart filling pressures, but only in patients with good LV function. Elderly patients have a high incidence of coronary artery and pulmonary disease, and the CVP is therefore less likely to accurately reflect left-sided filling pressures in this population.[159] Perioperative indications for the insertion of a central venous catheter are listed in Box 14–4.

The CVP should be monitored in all patients during CPB. When the catheter tip is in the SVC, it indicates RA pressure and cerebral venous pressure. Significant increases in CVP can produce critical decreases in cerebral perfusion pressure. This is occasionally caused by a malpositioned SVC cannula during CPB and must be corrected immediately by the surgeon to avoid cerebral edema and poor cerebral perfusion.

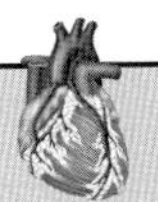

BOX 14–4 ***Indications for Central Venous Catheter Placement***

- Major operative procedures involving large fluid shifts or blood loss in patients with good heart function
- Intravascular volume assessment when urine output is not reliable or unavailable (e.g., renal failure)
- Major trauma
- Surgical procedures with a high risk of air embolism, such as sitting-position craniotomies. The central venous pressure catheter also may be used to aspirate intracardiac air.
- Frequent venous blood sampling
- Venous access for vasoactive or irritating drugs
- Chronic drug administration
- Inadequate peripheral intravenous access
- Rapid infusion of intravenous fluids (using large cannulae)
- Total parenteral nutrition

Contraindications

Absolute Contraindications

The SVC syndrome is a contraindication to placing a CVP catheter in the neck, subclavian area, or the upper extremities. Venous pressures in the head and upper extremities are elevated by the SVC obstruction, and do not reflect RA pressure. Medications that are administered in the obstructed venous circulation reach the central circulation by collateral vessels in a delayed fashion. Rapid fluid administration into the obstructed venous circulation may exacerbate the elevated venous pressures and cause more pronounced edema. The mild SVC syndrome seen with some ascending aortic aneurysms, however, does not represent a contraindication to central venous cannulation of the upper body. Infection may occur at the site of insertion.

Relative Contraindications

Coagulopathies predispose to hemorrhagic complications of CVP placement, such as airway obstruction from a neck hematoma, hemothorax, or hematoma collection with subsequent infection.

Newly inserted pacemaker wires may be dislodged during the insertion of CVP catheters. This could result in severe arrhythmia, especially if the patient is pacemaker dependent. In general, it is preferable to wait 4 to 6 weeks before placing a central catheter in a patient with newly inserted pacemaker wires.

Complications

The complications of central venous cannulation can be roughly divided into three categories: complications of vascular access, complications of catheter insertion, or complications of catheter presence. These are summarized in Box 14–5, and specific information regarding several of the complications is detailed in this section.

Inadvertent arterial puncture during central venous cannulation is not uncommon.[160] The two main reasons why this phenomenon occurs are that all veins commonly used for cannulation lie in close proximity to arteries (except the EJV and cephalic) and that the venous anatomy is quite variable. Localized hematoma formation is the usual consequence. This may be minimized if a small-gauge needle is initially used to localize the vein or ultrasonic guidance is employed.[161]

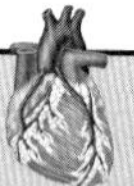

BOX 14–5 ***Complications of Central Venous Catheterization***

Complications of Central Venous Cannulation

- Arterial puncture with hematoma
- Arteriovenous fistula
- Hemothorax
- Chylothorax
- Pneumothorax
- Nerve injury
- Brachial plexus
- Stellate ganglion (Horner's syndrome)
- Air emboli
- Catheter or wire shearing
- Right atrial or right ventricular perforation

Complications of Catheter Presence

- Thrombosis, thromboembolism
- Infection, sepsis, endocarditis
- Arrhythmias
- Hydrothorax

If the arterial puncture is large, direct pressure is difficult to apply secondary to the location of the artery. If the patient has a coagulopathy, a massive hematoma may form. In the neck, this may lead to airway obstruction requiring urgent tracheal intubation. In the arm or leg, venous obstruction may occur. If the artery is cannulated with a large-bore catheter, a surgical consultation may be required before its removal. Reports about successful percutaneous repair of inadvertent arterial injuries after central venous cannulation have been published.[162,163]

Arteriovenous fistula from the carotid artery to the IJV has also been reported after central venous cannulation.[164,165] Hemothorax may occur if the subclavian artery is lacerated during cannulation attempts. Symptoms of hypovolemia may predominate because of the large capacity of the pleural cavity.[166]

Injury to the thoracic duct resulting in chylothorax has been reported after left IJV and left subclavian vein cannulation.[167,168] Fear of this complication is one of the major reasons for selecting right-sided IJV and subclavian approaches for central venous cannulation. This is a serious problem that may require surgical treatment.[169]

If the pleural cavity is entered and lung tissue is punctured during a cannulation attempt, a pneumothorax may result. Tension pneumothorax is possible if air continues to accumulate due to a "ball-valve" effect. Pneumothorax is most common with subclavian punctures and occurs only rarely with IJV cannulation.[170,171]

The brachial plexus, stellate ganglion, and phrenic nerve all lie in close proximity to the IJV. These structures may be injured during cannulation attempts. Paresthesias of the brachial plexus are not uncommon during attempts to localize the IJV. Direct needle trauma is the most likely cause of paresthesias or motor deficits, and this risk is somewhat increased by the long-beveled needles used for vascular access.[172,173] Transient deficits may result from the deposition of local anesthetic in the brachial plexus, stellate ganglion, or cervical plexus. A large hematoma or pseudoaneurysm could result in nerve injury after an inadvertent arterial puncture.[174] Horner's syndrome has also been reported after IJV cannulation.[175]

Venous air embolism is a potentially fatal complication that can occur when there is negative pressure in the venous system. Paradoxical embolization is a risk if there is a patent foramen ovale or another intracardiac defect, such as an atrial or ventricular septal defect. During central venous cannulation, air embolism can usually be prevented with positional maneuvers, such as the Trendelenburg position, which increase the venous pressure in the vessel. Once the CVP catheter has been placed, it is important to assure that the catheter is firmly attached to its connecting tubing. Air embolism may even occur after the catheter has been removed, if the subcutaneous tract persists.[176]

The diagnosis of venous air embolism is likely when there is a sudden onset of tachycardia associated with pulmonary hypertension and systemic hypotension. A new murmur may be heard due to turbulent flow in the RV outflow tract. Two-dimensional echocardiography (transesophageal or transthoracic) and precordial Doppler probe monitoring are highly sensitive methods of detecting air embolism. Venous air embolism is most effectively treated by aspirating the air by a catheter positioned at the SVC-RA junction. An older (and probably less effective) method involves turning the patient to the left lateral decubitus position to move the embolus out of the RV outflow tract.

Catheter or guidewire fragments may be sheared off by the inserting needle and embolize to the right heart and pulmonary circulation when catheter-through-needle or Seldinger-type cannulation kits are used. It is also possible to lose a guidewire within the patient by not withdrawing a sufficient length of the wire to grasp it at the external end before inserting the catheter.[177] The catheter fragment position within the right-sided circulation will determine whether surgery or percutaneous transvenous techniques are necessary for its removal.[178]

These problems can almost always be avoided using proper technique. A catheter must never be withdrawn through the inserting needle. Reinsertion of needles into standard (catheter-over-needle) intravenous cannulae cannot be recommended, but should certainly never be performed if the cannula is kinked, or resistance is encountered. Similarly, guidewires should not be inserted through cannulae if blood return is not present, or forcefully inserted if resistance is encountered. Additionally, guidewires should not be withdrawn through inserting needles. During unsuccessful catheterization, the needle and catheter or needle and guidewire must be withdrawn simultaneously.

If RA or RV perforation occurs during central venous cannulation, pericardial effusion or tamponade may result. The likelihood of this complication is increased when inflexible guidewires, long dilators, or catheters are used. This complication has also been reported with the use of an indwelling polyethylene catheter.[179] In an in vitro model, Gravenstein et al[180] evaluated the perforating aspects of central venous catheters. An angle of incidence less than 40 degrees, single-orifice catheters, polyurethane catheters, silicone rubber, and pigtail-tip catheters all significantly decreased the risk of perforation compared with conventional catheters.

Oropello et al[181] suggested that the dilators used in many of the central catheters kits may be a major cause of vessel perforation. They believe that the dilator may bend the guidewire, creating its own path, causing it to perforate a vessel wall. Several kits have dilators that are much longer than the catheters, and they constitute a further risk factor for possible perforation of the heart or vessels.

The physiology of fluid accumulation in the pericardial sac is such that sudden cardiovascular collapse occurs once a critical volume has been reached. This is explained by the compliance curve of the normal pericardium. The curve is flat until the critical volume is reached, and then rises steeply with any further increment in volume. If pericardial tamponade is imminent, immediate pericardiocentesis is indicated. A long needle attached to a syringe is directed through the skin at the junction of the xyphoid process and the sternum on the left side, and directed toward the left shoulder. The needle is advanced while suction is maintained with the syringe until free-flowing blood is obtained. An ECG electrode can show an injury current (e.g., ST-segment elevation) when the needle is in contact with the myocardium. Withdrawal of small volumes of blood results in marked hemodynamic improvement because of the nature of pericardial compliance.

If the catheter tip is placed extravascularly in the pleural cavity or erodes into this position, the fluid that is infused into the catheter will accumulate in the pleural cavity (hydrothorax). The diagnosis is made by auscultation, percussion, and radiography of the chest. A pleurocentesis or thoracostomy (chest) tube might be necessary and surgical consultation may be required.

Transient atrial and ventricular arrhythmias commonly occur as the guidewire is passed into the right atrium or right ventricle during central venous cannulation using the Seldinger technique. This most likely results from the relatively inflexible guidewire causing extrasystoles as it contacts the endocardium. Ventricular fibrillation during guidewire insertion has been reported.[182] The same investigators reported a 70% reduction in the incidence of arrhythmias when guidewire insertion was limited to 22 cm.

There are also reports of complete heart block due to guidewire insertion during central venous cannulation.[183] These cases can be successfully managed using a temporary transvenous or external pacemaker. This complication has previously been reported with pulmonary artery catheterization. The problem most likely resulted from excessive insertion of the guidewire, with impingement of the wire in the region of the right bundle branch. It is recommended that the length of guidewire insertion be limited to the length necessary to reach the SVC-RA junction to avoid these complications. It is also imperative to monitor the patient appropriately (e.g., ECG and pulse monitoring) and to have resuscitative drugs and equipment immediately available when performing central venous catheterization.

Strict aseptic technique is required to minimize catheter-related infections. Full barrier precautions during insertion of central venous catheters have been shown to decrease the incidence of catheter-related infections.[184,185] Subcutaneous tunneling of central venous catheters inserted into the internal jugular and femoral veins,[186,187] antiseptic barrier-protected hub for central venous catheters,[188] and antiseptic/antibiotic-impregnated short-term central venous catheters[189,190] have been shown to reduce catheter-related infections.[191] There is accumulating evidence that 2% chlorhexidine preparation for skin antisepsis is associated with a reduced risk of catheter-related infections, whereas other studies found that povidone-iodine solution was equally effective. [192–195] Hospital policies differ with respect to the permissible duration of catheterization at particular sites, but routine replacement of central venous catheters to prevent catheter-related infections is not recommended.[196,197]

PULMONARY ARTERIAL PRESSURE MONITORING

The introduction of the flow-directed PAC was a quantum advance in the monitoring of patients in the perioperative period. Since the 1970s, its use has increased the amount of diagnostic information that can be obtained at the bedside in critically ill patients.[198] It is impressive to observe large changes in the PAP and PCWP with almost no reflection in the CVP. Connors et al[199] prospectively analyzed 62 consecutive pulmonary artery catheterizations. They found that fewer than one half of a group of clinicians correctly predicted the PCWP or CO, and more than 50% made at least one change in therapy based on data from the pulmonary artery catheterization. Waller and Kaplan[200] demonstrated that a group of experienced cardiac anesthesiologists and surgeons who were blinded to the information from pulmonary artery catheterization during CABG surgery were unaware of any problem during 65% of severe hemodynamic abnormalities. Similarly, Iberti and Fisher[201] showed that ICU physicians were unable to accurately predict hemodynamic data on clinical grounds and that 60% made at least one change in therapy and 33% changed their diagnosis based on PAC data. The clinical significance of these changes has been questioned because the weight of evidence-based medicine on the subject does not support improvements in outcome related to PAC monitoring. Nevertheless, with increasing numbers of patients with multisystem organ dysfunction undergoing cardiac surgical procedures, PAC monitoring is prevalent in cardiac surgical settings. An understanding of the potential benefits and pitfalls of pulmonary artery catheterization is therefore essential for anesthesiologists.

Specific information that can be gathered with the PAC and the quantitative measurements of cardiovascular and pulmonary function that can be derived from this information are listed in Tables 14–1 through 14–3. Special purpose PACs for continuous CO, continuous mixed venous oximetry (SvO_2), pacing, and thermodilution right ventricular ejection fraction (RVEF) are also available.

One of the main reasons that clinicians measure PCWP and pulmonary artery diastolic pressure (PAD) is that these parameters are estimates of LAP, which is an estimate of left ventricular end-diastolic pressure (LVEDP). LVEDP is an index of left ventricular end-diastolic volume (LVEDV), which correlates well with left ventricular preload.[202] The relationship between LVEDP and LVEDV is described by the left ventricular compliance curve. This nonlinear curve is affected by many factors, such as ventricular hypertrophy and myocardial ischemia.[203–205] The PCWP and PAD do not directly measure LV preload. The relationship of these parameters is diagrammed in Figure 14–11.

The PCWP and PAD pressures will not accurately reflect LVEDP in the presence of incorrect position of the PAC catheter tip, pulmonary vascular disease, high levels of PEEP, or mitral valvular disease. The patency of vascular channels between the distal port of the PAC and the LA is necessary to ensure a close relationship between the PCWP and LAP. This condition is met only in the dependent portions of the lung (West's zone III), in which the pulmonary venous pressure exceeds the alveolar pressure.[206] Otherwise, the PCWP will reflect the alveolar pressure, not the LAP. Because PEEP decreases the size of West's zone III, it has been shown to adversely affect the correlation between the PCWP and LAP,

Table 14–1 Normal Intracardiac Pressures

Location	Mean (mm Hg)	Range (mm Hg)
Right atrium	5	1–10
Right ventricle	25/5	15–30/0–8
Pulmonary arterial systolic/diastolic	23/9	15–30/5–15
Mean pulmonary arterial	15	10–20
Pulmonary capillary wedge	10	5–15
Left atrial	8	4–12
Left ventricular end-diastolic	8	4–12
Left ventricular systolic	130	90–140

Table 14–2 Derived Hemodynamic Parameters

Formula	Normal Values
Cardiac index CI = CO/BSA	2.8–4.2 L/min/m^2
Stroke volume SV = CO × 1000/HR	50–110 mL/beat
Stroke index SI = SV/BSA	30–65 mL/beat/m^2
Left ventricular stroke work index LVSWI = 1.36 × (MAP – PCWP) × SI/100	45–60 g · m/m^2
Right ventricular stroke work index RVSWI = 1.36 × (MPAP – CVP) × SI/100	5–10 g · m/m^2
Systemic vascular resistance SVR = (MAP – CVP) × 80/CO	900–1400 dynes/sec · cm^{-5}
Systemic vascular resistance index SVRI = (MAP – CVP) × 80/CI	1500–2400 dynes/sec · cm^{-5}/m^2
Pulmonary vascular resistance PVR = (MPAP – PCWP) × 80/CO	150–250 dynes/sec · cm^{-5}
Pulmonary vascular resistance index PVRI = (MPAP – PCWP) × 80/CI	250–400 dynes/sec · cm^{-5}/m^2

BSA = body surface area; CI = cardiac index; CO = cardiac output; CVP = central venous pressure; HR = heart rate; LVSWI = left ventricular stroke work index; MAP = mean arterial pressure; PAP = pulmonary arterial pressure; PCWP = pulmonary capillary wedge pressure; PVR = pulmonary vascular resistance; PVRI = pulmonary vascular resistance index; RVSWI = right ventricular stroke work index; SI = stroke index; SV = stroke volume; SVR = systemic vascular resistance; SVRI = systemic vascular resistance index.

Table 14–3 **Oxygen Delivery Parameters**

Formula	Normal Values
Arterial oxygen content $CaO_2 = (1.39 \times Hb \times SaO_2) + (0.0031 \times PaO_2)$	18–20 mL/dL
Mixed venous oxygen content $CvO_2 = 1.39 \times Hb \times SvO_2 + 0.0031 \times PvO_2$	13–16 mL/dL
Arteriovenous oxygen content difference $avDO_2 = CaO_2 - CvO_2$	4–5.5 mL/dL
Pulmonary capillary oxygen content $CcO_2 = 1.39 \times Hb \times ScO_2 + 0.0031 \times PcO_2$	19–21 mL/dL
Pulmonary shunt fraction $Qs/Qt = 100 \times (CcO_2 - CaO_2)/(CcO_2 - CvO_2)$	2%–8%
Oxygen delivery $DO_2 = 10 \times CO \times CaO_2$	800–1100 mL/min
Oxygen consumption $VO_2 = 10 \times CO \times (CaO_2 - CvO_2)$	150–300 mL/min

a = arterial; av = arteriovenous; C = concentration; c = capillary; D = diffusing capacity; Hb = hemoglobin; PcO_2 = pulmonary capillary oxygen tension; PvO_2 = venous oxygen tension; Q = volume of blood; Qs/Qt = shunt fraction; ScO_2 = pulmonary capillary oxygen saturation; SvO_2 = venous oxygen saturation; v = venous.

From McGrath R: Invasive bedside hemodynamic monitoring. Prog Cardiovasc Dis 29:129, 1986.

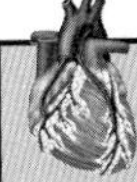

BOX 14–6 ***Conditions Resulting in Discrepancies Between Pulmonary Capillary Wedge Pressure and Left Ventricular End-Diastolic Pressure***

PCWP > LVEDP

- Positive-pressure ventilation
- PEEP
- Increased intrathoracic pressure
- Non–West lung zone III PAC placement
- Chronic obstructive pulmonary disease
- Increased pulmonary vascular resistance
- Left atrial myxoma
- Mitral valve disease (e.g., stenosis, regurgitation)

PCWP < LVEDP

- Noncompliant left ventricle (e.g., ischemia, hypertrophy)
- Aortic regurgitation (premature closure of the mitral valve)
- LVEDP > 25 mm Hg

LVEDP = left ventricular end-diastolic pressure; PAC = pulmonary artery catheter; PCWP = pulmonary capillary wedge pressure; PEEP = positive end-expiratory pressure.

Adapted from Tuman KJ, Carrol CC, Ivankovich AD: Pitfalls in interpretation of pulmonary artery catheter data. Cardiothorac Vasc Anesth Update 2:1, 1991.

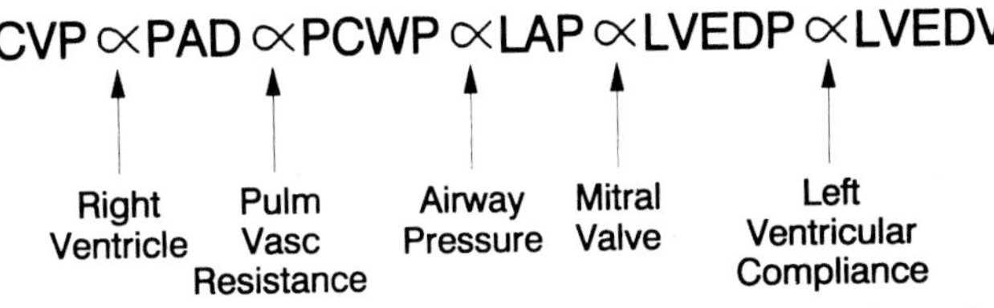

Figure 14–11 The left ventricular end-diastolic volume (LVEDV) is related to left ventricular end-diastolic pressure (LVEDP) by the left ventricular compliance. The LVEDP is related to the left atrial pressure (LAP) by the diastolic pressure gradient across the mitral valve. The pulmonary capillary wedge pressure (PCWP) is related to the LAP by the pulmonary capillary resistance. The pulmonary artery diastolic pressure (PAD) is an estimate of the PCWP. The central venous pressure (CVP) reflects the PAD if right ventricular function is normal.

especially in the hypovolemic patient.[207–209] Nevertheless, the correlation of PCWP and LAP could be maintained in the presence of PEEP by placing the catheter tip below the left atrium.[210,211] The acute respiratory distress syndrome (ARDS) seems to prevent the transmission of increased alveolar pressure to the pulmonary interstitium. This preserves the relationship between the PCWP and LAP during the application of PEEP.[212] It is not considered prudent, however, to temporarily disconnect patients from PEEP to measure preload.[213,214] The presence of large V waves in the PCWP tracing of patients with mitral regurgitation leads to an overestimation of the LVEDP.[215] In patients with mitral stenosis, using the PCWP instead of the LAP to assess the transmitral gradient has been shown to overestimate the severity of mitral stenosis.[216] However, when the PCWP was adjusted for the time delay through the pulmonary vasculature, the mean LAP and mean PCWP correlated well in another study.[217] It has been demonstrated that there is a significant positive gradient between the PCWP and the LAP in the initial hour after CPB.[218] Box 14–6 is a summary of conditions that may alter the relationship between the PCWP and the LVEDP.

The PCWP waveform is analogous to the CVP waveform described previously. The A, C, and V waves are similarly timed in the cardiac cycle. Large V waves have been described during mitral regurgitation, LV diastolic noncompliance, and episodes of myocardial ischemia.[219] They are seen as large ("giant") V waves that occur slightly later than the upstroke on the pulmonary artery tracing.[220] The V waves cause the pulmonary artery waveform to become wider and to lose the dicrotic notch (Fig. 14–12). The cause of large V waves during myocardial ischemia is probably a decrease in diastolic ventricular compliance. Alternatively, they may be caused by mitral regurgitation induced by ischemic papillary muscle dysfunction. In this instance, the V waves may occur earlier during the onset of the C wave (C-V wave). Large V waves, however, did not correlate well with other determinants of myocardial ischemia in a study of vascular surgical patients with coronary artery disease.[221] A study of patients undergoing coronary artery bypass grafting (CABG) also found that PCWP was limited as a monitoring technique for myocardial ischemia.[222]

Placement of the Pulmonary Artery Catheter

The considerations for the insertion site of a PAC are the same as for CVP catheters. The right IJV approach remains the technique of choice because of the direct path between this vessel and the right atrium. The placement of PACs through subclavian vein introducers may be complicated by kinking of the catheter when the sternum is retracted during cardiothoracic surgery. Forty-five percent of PACs (through subclavian catheters) became kinked and remained permanently nonfunctional after sternal retraction.[223]

Passage of the PAC from the vessel introducer to the PA can be accomplished by monitoring the pressure waveform from

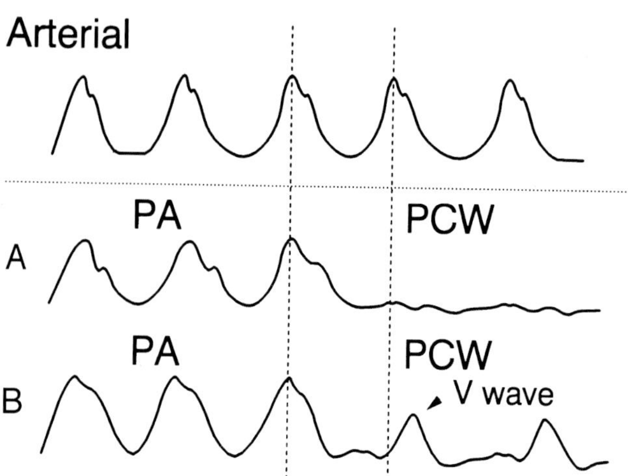

Figure 14–12 The relationship of the systemic arterial waveform, the pulmonary arterial (PA) waveform, and the pulmonary capillary wedge (PCW) waveform in the normal situation (A) and in the presence of V waves (B). Notice the widening of the PA waveform and the loss of the dicrotic notch in the presence of V waves. Also notice that the peak of the V wave occurs after the peak of the systemic arterial waveform.

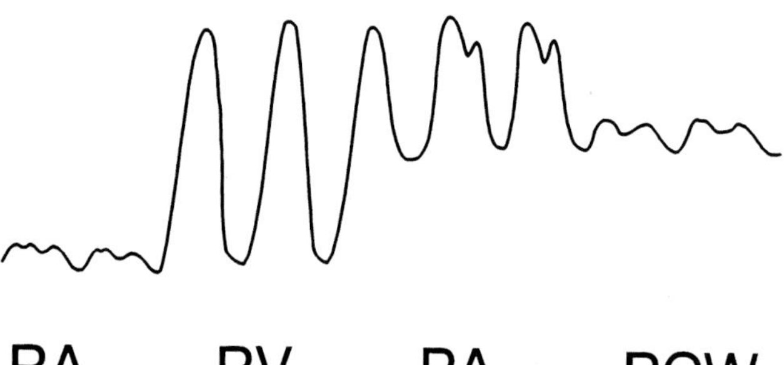

Figure 14–13 The waveforms encountered during the flotation of a pulmonary artery catheter from the venous circulation to the pulmonary capillary wedge (PCW) position. Notice the sudden increase in systolic pressure as the catheter enters the right ventricle (RV), the sudden increase in diastolic pressure as the catheter enters the pulmonary artery (PA), and the decrease in mean pressure as the catheter reaches the PCW position. RA = right atrium.

the distal port of the catheter, or under fluoroscopic guidance. Waveform monitoring is the more common technique for perioperative right-heart catheterization. First, the catheter must be advanced through the vessel introducer (15 to 20 cm) before inflating the balloon. The inflation of the balloon facilitates further advancement of the catheter through the right atrium and right ventricle into the pulmonary artery. Normal intracardiac pressures are shown in Table 14–1. The pressure waveforms seen during advancement of the PAC are illustrated in Figure 14–13. The RA waveform is seen until the catheter tip crosses the tricuspid valve and enters the right ventricle. In the right ventricle, there is a sudden increase in SBP but little change in DBP compared with the RA tracing. Arrhythmias, particularly premature ventricular complexes, usually occur at this point, but almost always resolve without treatment once the catheter tip has crossed the pulmonary valve. The catheter is rapidly advanced through the right ventricle toward the pulmonary artery. Slight reverse Trendelenburg and right lateral tilt minimize arrhythmias during passage of the catheter through the RV cavity.[224]

As the catheter crosses the pulmonary valve, a dicrotic notch appears in the pressure waveform, and there is a sudden increase in diastolic pressure. The PCWP tracing is obtained by advancing the catheter approximately 3 to 5 cm farther until there is a change in the waveform associated with a drop in the measured mean pressure. Deflation of the balloon results in reappearance of the pulmonary artery waveform and an increase in the mean pressure value. Using the right IJV approach, the right atrium is entered at 25 to 35 cm, the right ventricle at 35 to 45 cm, the pulmonary artery at 45 to 55 cm, and the PCWP at 50 to 60 cm in most patients.

If the catheter does not enter the pulmonary artery by 60 cm, the balloon should be deflated. It should be withdrawn into the right atrium, and another attempt should be made to advance the catheter into proper position. Excessive coiling of the catheter in the right ventricle should be avoided to prevent catheter knotting. The balloon should be inflated only for short periods to measure the PCWP. The pulmonary artery waveform should be continually monitored to be certain that the catheter does not float out into a constant wedge position because this may lead to pulmonary artery rupture or pulmonary infarction. The PAC is covered by a sterile sheath that must be secured at both ends to prevent contamination of the external portion of the catheter. Not infrequently, the PAC must be withdrawn a short distance because the extra catheter in the right ventricle floats out more peripherally into the pulmonary artery over time as the catheter softens.

The time for the entire PAC insertion procedure is about 10 to 15 minutes in experienced hands. Many clinicians believe that the PAC should be inserted before the induction of anesthesia. Studies by Waller et al[225] and Quintin et al[226] showed that PAC insertion in the awake patient did not result in myocardial ischemia or deleterious hemodynamic changes after preanesthetic medication and with continuation of all preoperative cardiac medications. A chest radiograph should be obtained postoperatively in all patients to check the position of the PAC. Benumof et al[227] found that most catheters pass into the right middle or lower lobes.

Indications

The indications for pulmonary artery catheterization are given in Box 14–7. The ability of PACs to positively influence patient outcome has never been conclusively proved in large-scale, prospective studies. There remains considerable controversy regarding the risk/benefit ratio of PACs.[228,229] Many studies have reported no change or even worse outcome in patients who were monitored with PACs.[230–233] Randomized trials on patients with myocardial infarction seemed to confirm these data,[234,235] whereas earlier prospective studies on surgical patients showed improved outcome.[236,237]

Major problems with PAC outcome studies include flaws in study design and insufficient statistical power. The most

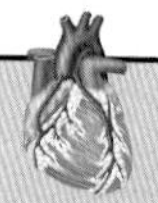

BOX 14–7 ***Indications for Pulmonary Artery Catheterization***

- Assessment of volume status
- Cardiac output measurements
- Hemodynamic measurements
- Respiratory or oxygen transport measurements

common design flaws were a lack of therapeutic protocols or treatment algorithms and inadequate randomization, which introduce observer bias.[238] Physician knowledge is another confounding variable, as demonstrated in a multicenter study that indicated competency in interpreting PAC-derived data was lacking in many individuals, and depended on such factors as the level of training and the frequency of use.[239] As many as 47% of physicians could not correctly determine the PCWP to within 5 mm Hg in that study.[240]

Another problem with PAC outcome studies is the clinical setting, specifically operating room versus ICU. Haupt et al[241] observed that patients in the ICU might have disease too far advanced to make invasive hemodynamic monitoring useful. Studies that have reported improved outcome used invasive hemodynamic monitoring to optimize oxygen delivery in the perioperative period.[242–245] In their meta-analysis, Heyland et al[246] argued similarly that "maximizing oxygen delivery" in the perioperative setting (i.e., before the onset of irreversible organ damage) is more effective in comparison with the chronic ICU setting. Based on the intention-to-treat analysis of patients with preoperative PAC placement, they reported improved survival.

Several large studies have addressed the controversies regarding the indications, risks, and benefits associated with PAC monitoring. In 1996, Connors et al[247] published the results of a large prospective cohort study. Data were collected from five U.S. teaching hospitals between 1989 and 1994. They enrolled 5735 critically ill adult patients in ICU settings and found that right-heart catheterization was associated with increased mortality in this patient population.

Adjusting for the severity of illness, Murdoch et al[248] found that the use of the PAC in ICU patients is safe, but no beneficial effect was demonstrated. Chittock et al[249] demonstrated that severity of illness may play an important role of defining subgroups of patients who may benefit from PAC monitoring. Of 7310 critically ill adult patients admitted to the ICU, those with APACHE II scores greater than 31 showed decreased mortality with PAC monitoring, whereas patients with lower APACHE II scores had increased mortality.

In 2001, Polanczyk et al[250] published the results of an observational study on 4059 patients undergoing major elective noncardiac procedures examining the relationship between pulmonary artery catheterization and postoperative cardiac complications. Right-heart catheterization was associated with an increased incidence of major postoperative cardiac events.

Sandham et al[251] reported a prospective, randomized, controlled outcome study of 1994 high-risk patients (ASA III or IV) scheduled for major surgery followed by ICU stay who were managed with or without the use of a PAC. No benefit to therapy directed by PAC compared with standard care (without the use of PAC) was found, with a higher risk of pulmonary embolism in the PAC group.

A meta-analysis by Barone et al[252] asserted that only four prospective studies were adequately randomized, and that the use of the PAC did not improve outcome in vascular surgery patients. Another meta-analysis by Ivanov et al[253] showed a significant reduction in morbidity when PAC-guided strategies were applied.

Yu et al[254] performed a prospective cohort study of the relationship between PAC use and outcome in 1010 patients with severe sepsis. PAC monitoring did not improve outcome in this patient population. A prospective randomized study by Rhodes et al[255] found no significant difference in mortality in critically ill patients treated with or without the use of a PAC. Outcomes of patients with shock and ARDS were not affected by PAC placement in a multicenter, randomized, controlled trial.[256]

Two studies looked at the use of PACs in cardiac surgery patients. Schwann et al[257] retrospectively assessed the outcome of 2685 patients undergoing CABG in whom the decision to place a PAC was based on patient characteristics and risk factors. Using a highly selective strategy, no PAC was used in 91% of cases, and the outcomes were comparable. In another retrospective trial, Ramsey et al[258] found that pulmonary artery catheterization in elective coronary artery bypass graft surgery was associated with an increased in-hospital mortality, greater length of stay, and higher total costs. This effect was more prominent in hospital settings with low PAC use.

The operative procedures and medical conditions that are cited as indications for pulmonary artery catheterization in the perioperative period remain controversial and vary by institution.[259,260] In a global sense, the indications for using a PAC are assessing volume status, measuring CO, measuring $S\text{v}O_2$, and deriving hemodynamic parameters.[261] In 2003, the American Society of Anesthesiologists (ASA) Task Force on Pulmonary Artery Catheterization published updated practice guidelines for pulmonary artery catheterization (http://www.asahq.org/publicationsAndServices/pulm_artery.pdf).[262] These guidelines emphasized that patient, surgery, and practice setting had to be considered. Generally, the routine use of PACs is indicated in high-risk patients (e.g., ASA 4 or 5) and high-risk procedures (e.g., where large fluid changes or hemodynamic disturbances are expected). The practice setting is important, because there is evidence that inadequate training or experience may increase the risk for perioperative complications associated with the use of a PAC. It is recommended that the routine use of a PAC should be confined to centers with adequate training and experience in the perioperative management of patients with PAC (Box 14–8). The authors of this chapter have composed a summary of procedural indications that is relatively aggressive (Box 14–9).

The use of the PAC has significantly contributed to the understanding and care of patients with cardiac disease. Nevertheless, further large-scale randomized controlled trials are needed to clearly define which, if any, patient populations benefit from PAC monitoring.[263] The body of evidence is inconclusive. The risks associated with perioperative PAC monitoring may outweigh the benefits in low-to-moderate risk patients, whereas high-risk patients undergoing major surgery probably benefit from right-heart catheterization. One major caveat is that the data derived from PAC monitoring must be interpreted correctly and treatment protocols should be followed to derive maximal benefit. In summary, using an evidence-based medicine approach, PAC monitoring does not improve patient outcome in most patient populations, and may actually be harmful in certain circumstances.

Contraindications

Contraindications to pulmonary artery catheterization are summarized in Box 14–10.

Absolute Contraindications

Contraindications to the use of a PAC include tricuspid or pulmonic valvular stenosis. It is unlikely that a PAC would be able to cross a stenotic valve, and it might worsen the obstruction to flow if it did.

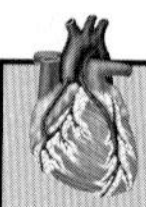

BOX 14–8 ***American Society of Anesthesiologists' Practice Guidelines for Pulmonary Catheter Use***

Opinions

- PA catheterization provides new information that may change therapy, with poor clinical evidence of its effect on clinical outcome or mortality.
- There is no evidence from large, controlled studies that preoperative PA catheterization improves outcome regarding hemodynamic optimization.
- Perioperative PAC monitoring of hemodynamic parameters leading to goal-directed therapy has produced inconsistent data in multiple studies and clinical scenarios.
- Having immediate access to PA catheter data allows important preemptive measures for selected subgroups of patients who encounter hemodynamic disturbances that require immediate and precise decisions about fluid management and drug treatment.
- Experience and understanding are the major determinants of PA catheter effectiveness.
- PA catheterization is inappropriate as routine practice in surgical patients and should be limited to cases in which the anticipated benefits of catheterization outweigh the potential risks.
- PA catheterization can be harmful.

Recommendations

- The appropriateness of routine PA catheterization depends on a combination of patient-, surgery-, and practice setting–related factors.
- Perioperative PA catheterization should be considered in patients who present with significant organ dysfunction or major comorbidity that poses an increased risk for hemodynamic disturbances or instability (e.g., ASA IV or V patients).
- Perioperative PA catheterization in surgical settings should be considered based on the hemodynamic risk of the individual case rather than generalized surgical setting-related recommendations. High-risk surgical procedures are those in which large fluid changes or hemodynamic disturbances can be anticipated and procedures that are associated with a high risk of morbidity and mortality.
- Because of the risk of complications from PA catheterization, the procedure should not be performed by clinicians or nursing staff or done in practice settings where competency in safe insertion, accurate interpretation of results, and appropriate catheter maintenance cannot be guaranteed.
- Routine PA catheterization is not recommended when the patient, procedure, or practice setting poses a low or moderate risk for hemodynamic changes.

ASA = American Society of Anesthesiologists; PA = pulmonary artery.
From American Society of Anesthesiologists: Practice guidelines for pulmonary artery catheterization: http://www.asahq.org/publicationsAndServices/pulm_artery.pdf.

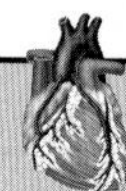

BOX 14–9 ***Clinical Indications for Pulmonary Artery Catheter Monitoring***

Major Procedures Involving Large Fluid Shifts or Blood Loss in Patients with

- Severe unstable coronary artery disease or poor left ventricular function (congestive heart failure)
- Cardiogenic or septic shock or with multiple-organ failure
- Right-heart failure, pulmonary hypertension, or pulmonary embolism
- Hemodynamic instability requiring inotropes or intra-aortic balloon counterpulsation
- Surgery of the aorta requiring cross-clamping
- Hepatic transplantation
- Massive ascites requiring major surgery

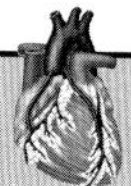

BOX 14–10 ***Contraindications for Pulmonary Artery Catheterization***

Absolute Contraindications

- Tricuspid or pulmonary stenosis
- Right atrial or right ventricular mass
- Tetralogy of Fallot

Relative Contraindications

- Severe arrhythmias
- Coagulopathy
- Newly inserted pacemaker wires

RA or RV masses (i.e., tumor or thrombus) are absolute contraindications. The catheter may dislodge a portion of the mass, causing pulmonary or paradoxical embolization.

In patients with tetralogy of Fallot, the RV outflow tract is hypersensitive. A PAC could induce a hypercyanotic episode ("tet spell") by eliciting spasm of the RV infundibulum.

Relative Contraindications

Use of a PAC may be contraindicated in patients with severe arrhythmias. Transient atrial and ventricular arrhythmias are common during PAC placement in normal patients. The risk of inducing an arrhythmia in a patient prone to malignant arrhythmias must be weighed against the potential benefits of the information gained from PAC monitoring. Appropriate preparations must be undertaken to enable the administration of antiarrhythmic drugs and cardiopulmonary resuscitation, and electrical cardioversion, defibrillation, or pacing if required.

Coagulopathy may prohibit the use of a PAC. This is related to the potential complications of obtaining central venous access in the patient with a coagulopathy. The risk of inducing endobronchial hemorrhage with inadvertent migration of the PAC or prolonged balloon inflation may be increased.

Newly inserted pacemaker wires may be a contraindication, because they may be displaced by the PAC during insertion or withdrawal. In approximately 4 to 6 weeks, the pacemaker wires become firmly embedded in the endocardium, and wire displacement becomes less likely.

Complications

The complications associated with PAC placement include almost all of those detailed in the section on CVP placement. Additional complications that are unique to the PAC are detailed here. The ASA Task Force on Pulmonary Artery Catheterization concluded that serious complications due to PAC catheterization occurs in 0.1% to 0.5% of patients monitored with a PAC.[262] Higher estimates are found in the literature and probably represent different patient populations, hospital settings, level of experience with PAC management, and other factors.[264]

Arrhythmias

The most common complications associated with PAC insertion are transient arrhythmias, especially premature ventricular contractions (PVCs).[265] However, fatal arrhythmias have rarely been reported.[266,267] Intravenous lidocaine has been used in attempts to suppress these arrhythmias, with mixed results.[268,269] However, a positional maneuver entailing 5-degree head-up and right lateral tilt was associated with a statistically significant decrease in malignant arrhythmias (compared with the Trendelenburg position) during PAC insertion.[224]

Complete Heart Block

Complete heart block may develop during pulmonary artery catheterization in patients with preexisting left bundle-branch block (LBBB).[270–272] This potentially fatal complication is most likely due to electrical irritability from the PAC tip causing transient right bundle-branch block (RBBB) as it passes through the RV outflow tract. The incidence of developing RBBB was 3% in a prospective series of patients undergoing pulmonary artery catheterization.[273] However, none of the patients with preexisting LBBB developed complete heart block in that series. In another study of 47 patients with LBBB, complete heart block occurred in 2 patients with recent-onset LBBB.[274] It is imperative to have an external pacemaker immediately available or to use a pacing PAC when placing a PAC in patients with LBBB.

Endobronchial Hemorrhage

Iatrogenic rupture of the pulmonary artery has become more common since the advent of PAC monitoring in the ICU and operating room. Numerous cases have been recorded in the medical literature.[275] The incidence of pulmonary artery–induced endobronchial hemorrhage is 0.064% to 0.20%.[265] Hannan et al[276] reported a 46% mortality rate in a review of 28 cases of pulmonary artery–induced endobronchial hemorrhage, but the mortality rate was 75% in anticoagulated patients. From these reports, several risk factors have emerged: advanced age, female sex, pulmonary hypertension, mitral stenosis, coagulopathy, distal placement of the catheter, and balloon hyperinflation. Balloon inflation in distal pulmonary arteries is probably accountable for most episodes of pulmonary artery rupture because of the high pressures generated by the balloon.[277] Hypothermic CPB may also increase risk due to distal migration of the catheter tip with movement of the heart and hardening of the PAC.[278,279] It is now common practice to pull the PAC back approximately 3 to 5 cm when CPB is instituted.

It is important to consider the cause of the hemorrhage when forming a therapeutic plan. If the hemorrhage is minimal, and a coagulopathy coexists, correction of the coagulopathy may be the only necessary therapy. Protection of the uninvolved lung is of prime importance. Tilting the patient toward the affected side, placement of a double-lumen endotracheal tube, and other lung-separation maneuvers should protect the contralateral lung.[280] Strategies proposed to stop the hemorrhage include the application of PEEP, placement of bronchial blockers, and pulmonary resection.[281] The clinician is obviously at a disadvantage unless the site of hemorrhage is known. A chest radiograph will usually indicate the general location of the lesion. Although the cause of endobronchial hemorrhage may be unclear, the bleeding site must be unequivocally located before surgical treatment is attempted. A small amount of radiographic contrast dye may help to pinpoint the lesion if active hemorrhage is present. In severe hemorrhage and with recurrent bleeding, transcatheter coil embolization has been used. This may emerge as the preferred treatment method.[282,283]

Pulmonary Infarction

Pulmonary infarction is a rare complication of PAC monitoring. An early report suggested that there was a 7.2% incidence of pulmonary infarction with PAC use.[284] However, continuously monitoring the pulmonary artery waveform and keeping the balloon deflated when not determining the PCWP (to prevent inadvertent wedging of the catheter) were not standard practice at that time. Distal migration of PACs may also occur intraoperatively due to the action of the right ventricle, uncoiling of the catheter, and softening of the catheter over time. Inadvertent catheter wedging occurs during CPB because of the diminished RV chamber size and retraction of the heart to perform the operation. Embolization of thrombus formed on a PAC could also result in pulmonary infarction.

Catheter Knotting and Entrapment

Knotting of a PAC usually occurs as a result of coiling of the catheter within the right ventricle. Insertion of an appropriately sized guidewire under fluoroscopic guidance may aid in unknotting the catheter.[285] Alternatively, the knot may be tightened and withdrawn percutaneously along with the introducer if no intracardiac structures are entangled.[286] If cardiac structures, such as the papillary muscles, are entangled in the knotted catheter, then surgical intervention may be required.[287,288] Sutures placed in the heart may inadvertently entrap the PAC. A report of such a case and the details of the percutaneous removal have been described.[289]

Valvular Damage

Withdrawal of the catheter with the balloon inflated may result in injury to the tricuspid[290] or pulmonary valves.[291] Placement of the PAC with the balloon deflated may increase the risk of passing the catheter between the chordae tendinae.[292] Septic endocarditis has also resulted from an indwelling PAC.[293,294]

Thrombocytopenia

Mild thrombocytopenia has been reported in dogs and humans with indwelling PACs.[295] This probably results from increased platelet consumption. Heparin-coated PACs can trigger the rare disease heparin-induced thrombocytopenia, which has been reported in cardiac surgical patients (see Chapter 29).[296]

Thrombus Formation

The PAC is a foreign body that may serve as a nidus for thrombus formation. The thrombogenicity of PACs seems to have been reduced up to 72 hours after the insertion by the introduction of heparin-bonded PACs.[297,298] However, the introduction of high-dose aprotinin therapy may lead to thrombus formation on PACs despite heparin bonding.[299] This phenomenon has also been reported with ε-aminocaproic acid therapy.[300] TEE can be an invaluable tool for detecting and monitoring this relatively rare complication.[301]

Incorrect Placement

The catheter may pass through an interatrial or interventricular communication into the left side of the heart. It is then possible for the catheter to enter the aorta through the LV outflow tract. A similar complication has been reported in which the catheter crossed a surgically repaired tear in the SVC into the left side of the heart.[302] This complication should be recognized by the similarity between the pulmonary artery and systemic arterial waveforms. In a case report of a patient with an ascending aortic aneurysm, compression of the SVC by the aneurysm led to traumatic placement of the PAC directly into the pulmonary vein.[303]

Hypotension secondary to balloon inflation has been reported in a patient after a pneumonectomy in whom the balloon obstructed the pulmonary circulation.[304] Venous cannula obstruction has occurred in patients during CPB.[305–307] The temporal association with the abrupt loss of venous return and the negative pressure recorded on the distal lumen tracing are important indicators that this may be occurring. This stresses the importance of monitoring the pressure waveforms during CPB. Coronary sinus obstruction has also been reported from a PAC.[308] Placement of the PAC in the liver has also been described; the wedged hepatic venous pressures may mimic the pulmonary artery pressure waveform.[309]

TEE has proved invaluable for confirming the proper placement of PACs. In many case reports, TEE detected incorrect placement and complications resulting from PACs.[301,303]

Balloon Rupture

This is not uncommon when the PAC has been left in place for several days or when the balloon is inflated with more than 1.5 mL of air. Small volumes of air injected into the PA are of little consequence, and balloon rupture is apparent if the injected air cannot be withdrawn. In patients with right-to-left shunts, carbon dioxide may be used for inflation. Great care must be taken not to rupture the balloon in these patients, with the attendant possibility of systemic gas embolization.

Ventricular Perforation

RV perforation is a rare complication with a balloon-tipped catheter, but it has been reported in the literature.[310]

Erroneous Interpretation of Data

Malfunctions of the catheter and balloon can lead to spurious numbers for the PCWP and incorrect treatment of the patient. Shin et al[311] reported the problem of eccentric inflation of the balloon, with the catheter tip impinging on the pulmonary artery wall. Several reviews have pointed out many of the problems with clinical use of the PAC.[203–205,213,312] These include errors in interpretation due to ventilation modes (Fig. 14–14), compliance changes, ventricular interdependence, and associated technical problems.

"Catheter whip" is an artifact that is associated with long catheters, such as PACs. Because the tip moves within the bloodstream of the cardiac chambers and great vessels, the fluid contained within the catheter is accelerated. This can produce superimposed pressure waves of 10 mm Hg in either direction.

Pacing Catheters

The possible indications for placement of a pacing PAC are shown in Box 14–11. The actual use in a group of 600 patients undergoing cardiac surgery is shown in Table 14–4.[313]

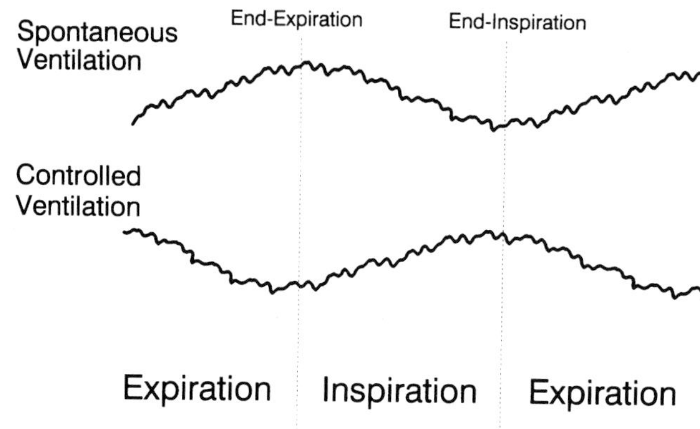

Figure 14–14 Respiratory variation of the pulmonary capillary wedge pressure waveform during spontaneous and mechanical ventilation. Inspiration is marked by negative mediastinal pressure in the spontaneously breathing patient and by positive mediastinal pressure in the mechanically ventilated patient.

Electrode Catheters

A multipurpose PAC (originally produced by Baxter Edwards) contains five electrodes for bipolar atrial, ventricular, or atrioventricular (AV) sequential pacing. With appropriate filtering, the catheter may also be used for the recording of an intracardiac ECG. The intraoperative success rates for atrial, ventricular, and AV sequential capture have been reported as 80%, 93%, and 73%, respectively.[314] Electrode detachment has been reported twice with the multipurpose catheter—with prolonged placement (60 hours)[315] and during catheter withdrawal.[316]

Pacing Wire Catheters

The Paceport and A-V Paceport catheters (Baxter Edwards, Irvine, CA) have lumina for the introduction of a ventricular wire (Paceport) or for atrial and ventricular wires (A-V Paceport) for temporary transvenous pacing. The success rate for ventricular pacing capture was 96% for the Paceport.[317] The success rates for atrial and ventricular pacing capture before CPB were 98% and 100%, respectively, in a study of the A-V Paceport.[318] The additional risk of atrial or ventricular perforation is theoretically present with these thin pacing wires, but has not yet been reported in the literature.

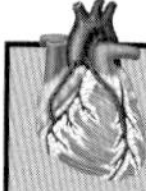

BOX 14–11 *Indications for Perioperative Placement of Pacing Pulmonary Artery Catheters*

- Sinus node dysfunction or bradycardia
- Second-degree (Mobitz II) atrioventricular block
- Complete (third-degree) atrioventricular block
- Digitalis toxicity
- Need for atrioventricular sequential pacing
- Aortic stenosis (need to maintain sinus rhythm)
- Severe left ventricular hypertrophy or noncompliant left ventricle
- Idiopathic hypertrophic subaortic stenosis/hypertrophic obstructive cardiomyopathy
- Need for an intracardiac electrogram

Table 14–4 **Use of Pacing Pulmonary Artery Catheters According to the Presence or Absence of Different Indications**

Indication	Indication Present*	Indication Present/Pacing PAC Used† (%)	Indication Absent*	Indication Absent/Pacing PAC Used† (%)	*p* Value
Sinus node dysfunction	24	6 (25.0)	576	32 (5.5)	0.002
First-degree AV block	52	1 (1.9)	548	37 (6.7)	0.24
Second-degree AV block	1	1 (100)			
Complete AV block	15	5 (33.3)	585	33 (5.6)	0.001
LBBB	41	5 (12.1)	559	33 (5.9)	0.17
RBBB	32	0 (0)	568	38 (6.6)	0.25
LAH	17	1 (5.8)	583	37 (6.3)	1.0
RBBB and LAH	5	0 (0)	595	38 (6.3)	1.0
Reoperation/with other indications present	61	14 (23.0)	539	24 (4.4)	<0.001
Reoperation/no other indications present	51	1 (1.9)	549	37 (6.7)	0.24
Aortic stenosis	88	11 (12.0)	512	27 (5.2)	0.02
Mitral stenosis	17	1 (5.8)	583	37 (6.3)	1.0
Aortic insufficiency	40	9 (22.5)	560	29 (5.1)	<0.001
Mitral regurgitation	65	7 (10.7)	535	31 (5.7)	0.17

*Total number of patients.
†Total number and percentage of patients with or without each indication.
AV = atrioventricular; LAH = Left anterior block; LBBB = left bundle-branch block; PAC = pulmonary artery catheter; RBBB = right bundle-branch block.
From Risk SC, Brandon D, D'Ambra MN, et al: Indications for the use of pacing pulmonary artery catheters in cardiac surgery. J Cardiothorac Vasc Anesth 6:275, 1992.

Right Ventricular Ejection Fraction Catheters

The rapid-response thermistor PAC (Baxter Edwards, Irvine, CA) incorporates three modifications from a standard PAC: a multihole injectate port, a rapid-response thermistor, and ECG electrodes. The catheter is positioned so that the injectate port is 2 cm cephalad to the tricuspid valve in the right atrium.[319,320] With each injection, the computer determines the RVEF from the exponential decay of the thermodilution curve. End-diastolic temperature points in the thermodilution curve are identified using the R-wave signal (Fig. 14–15). The difference in temperature between the baseline and the first end-diastolic plateau is defined as C_1, and the difference between the baseline and the second plateau is defined as C_2, etc. Residual fraction (RF), the portion of blood left in the ventricle at the end of systole, is calculated from the equations:

$$RF_1 = C_2 \div C_1$$

$$RF_2 = C_3 \div C_2$$

$$RF_{mean} = \frac{(RF_1 + RF_2)}{2}$$

in which RF_1 is the first estimate of residual fraction, and RF_2 is the second estimate of residual fraction.

The ejection fraction (EF) is calculated from the following equation:

$$EF = 1 - RF_{mean}$$

The computer also measures heart rate from the catheter ECG electrodes. From these data, SV, RV end-diastolic volume, and RV end-systolic volume are calculated. Assumptions that are essential to the accuracy of the technique include a regular RR interval, "instantaneous" mixing of the injectate with the RV blood, and absence of tricuspid regurgitation. The timing of injection with respect to the respiratory cycle also impacts the reproducibility of the measurements.[321]

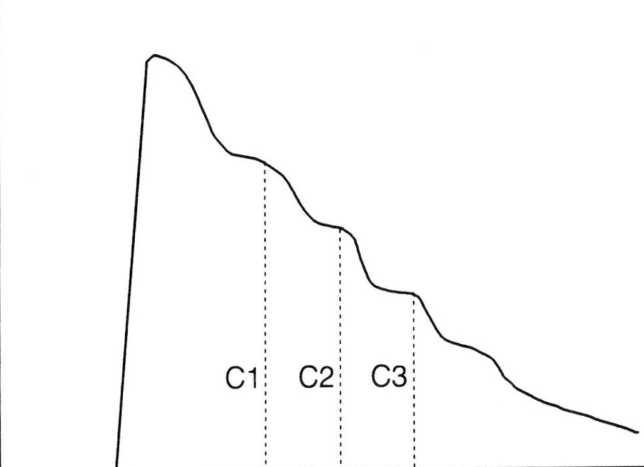

Figure 14–15 The thermodilution curve obtained from a rapid-response thermistor after the injection of a bolus of cold fluid into the right ventricle. The differences between the end-diastolic plateaus and the baseline temperature yield the constants C1, C2, and C3, which may be used to calculate right ventricular ejection fraction.

An in vitro study showed that thermodilution measurements of RVEF, CO, and SV are highly predictive of actual pulsatile flow in a pulsatile flow model ($r^2 = 0.95$, $r^2 = 0.99$, and $r^2 = 0.98$, respectively).[322] The technique has also been validated in vivo by comparison with radionuclide and angiographic determinations of RVEF.[323,324] In patients with TEE color-flow Doppler, evidence of mild tricuspid regurgitation without atrial pressure waveform abnormalities, there was no significant invalidation of RVEF data.[325] Boldt et al[326] found that RVEF was significantly more depressed in patients with right coronary artery stenosis after CPB. RVEF is extremely sensitive to alterations in afterload. Changes in RVEF may not always reflect changes in LV contractility. The use of this type of monitoring could be justified in patients with severe RV dysfunction due to myocardial infarction, right-sided coronary artery disease, pulmonary hypertension, LV failure, or intrinsic pulmonary disease.

Mixed Venous Oxygen Saturation Catheters

Monitoring the SvO_2 is a means of providing a global estimation of the adequacy of oxygen delivery relative to the needs of the various tissues. The formula for SvO_2 calculation can be derived by modifying the Fick equation and assuming that the effect of dissolved oxygen in the blood is negligible:

$$SvO_2 = SaO_2 - \frac{\dot{V}O_2}{CO \cdot 1.34 \cdot Hb}$$

A decrease in the SvO_2 can indicate one of the following situations: decreased CO; increased oxygen consumption; decreased arterial oxygen saturation; or decreased hemoglobin (Hb) concentration. To measure SvO_2, blood is aspirated from the distal port of the PAC slowly, so as not to contaminate the sample with oxygenated alveolar blood.

The addition of fiberoptic bundles to PACs has enabled the continuous monitoring of SvO_2 using reflectance spectrophotometry. The catheter is connected to a device that includes a light-emitting diode and a sensor to detect the light returning from the pulmonary artery. SvO_2 is calculated from the differential absorption of various wavelengths of light by the saturated and desaturated hemoglobin.[327]

If it is assumed that there is constant oxygen consumption and arterial oxygen content, changes in SvO_2 should reflect changes in CO. Several investigators have come to the conclusion that it provides a valuable measure of CO during surgery.[328,329] The SvO_2 has been shown to correlate with cardiac index during CABG surgery when oxygen consumption is constant,[328] but not to correlate with the cardiac index when oxygen consumption is changing, such as during shivering after anesthesia.[330] The usefulness of the catheter may primarily be its ability to continuously monitor the balance between oxygen delivery and consumption,[331–334] and SvO_2 may also help predict survival after acute myocardial infarction.[335] Severe deterioration in the condition of critically ill patients, however, was often not predicted by changes in SvO_2.[336–338] London et al[339] published a prospective, multicenter, observational study in which continuous monitoring of SvO_2 was compared with standard PAC monitoring in 3265 cardiac surgical patients. They failed to show any improved outcome associated with the use of continuous SvO_2 catheters and only a small reduction in resource use.

Continuous monitoring of SvO_2 has been complicated by artifacts due to the vessel wall and clot formation on the catheter with loss of light intensity. Varying hematocrit may also introduce error, but not with all systems.[340] The values obtained with various fiberoptic catheter systems showed good agreement with in vitro (co-oximetry) SvO_2 measurements.[341–344]

CARDIAC OUTPUT MONITORING

The CO is the amount of blood pumped to the peripheral circulation by the heart each minute. It is a measurement that reflects the status of the entire circulatory system, not just the heart, because it is governed by autoregulation from the tissues. The CO is equal to the product of the SV and the heart rate. Preload, afterload, heart rate, and contractility are the major determinants of the CO. The measurement of CO is of particular interest in patients with cardiac disease. This section will briefly describe historical methods of CO monitoring and then focus on current practices of CO measurement.

Fick Method

The Fick equation is derived from the concept that oxygen consumed by the tissues per unit time is equal to the amount of oxygen extracted per unit time from the circulation. The oxygen extracted from the circulation is the product of the arteriovenous oxygen content difference and the CO:

$$\dot{V}O_2 = (CaO_2 - CvO_2) \cdot CO$$

Rearranging the equation, CO is calculated using the following formula:

$$CO = \frac{\dot{V}O_2}{(CaO_2 - CvO_2)}$$

in which CO is the cardiac output, $\dot{V}O_2$ is the oxygen consumption, CaO_2 is the arterial oxygen content, and CvO_2 is the mixed venous oxygen content.

In the direct Fick method, oxygen consumption is measured by indirect calorimetry using algorithms based on inspired and expired oxygen concentrations and volumes. Oxygen consumption can be calculated when the rate of fresh gas flow, respiratory rate, and change of oxygen concentration are known. Arterial oxygen content is measured from an arterial blood sample, and mixed venous oxygen content can be obtained from the PAC. Due to technical difficulties, oxygen consumption in pediatric patients is commonly estimated using the formulas of LaFarge and Miettinen with the use of gender, heart rate, and age as variables.[345] Oxygen consumption and arteriovenous oxygen content differences must be measured at steady state because the Fick principle is valid only when tissue oxygen uptake equals lung oxygen uptake.

The accuracy and reproducibility of the direct Fick CO technique have been determined in a variety of animal and human experiments. They have usually been found to be high.[346] The major limitations of the direct Fick technique are related to errors in sampling and analysis, difficulty in obtaining oxygen uptake continuously in the operating room, the presence of bulky equipment surrounding the endotracheal tube, or the inability to maintain steady-state hemodynamic and respiratory conditions.[347,348]

Some of these problems have been overcome with the introduction of metabolic modules for the measurement of oxygen consumption that are incorporated into the patient monitoring system and that do not depend on collecting gases in bulky sample chambers.[349] No flow or volume transducers are incorporated into these systems. Instead, continuous measurement of expiratory carbon dioxide concentrations in a constant flow allows for the calculation of the amount of carbon dioxide eliminated by the patient. This method is referred to as the modified carbon dioxide Fick method. Inspiratory and expiratory oxygen and carbon dioxide concentrations are measured to obtain the respiratory quotient (RQ value), which is then used to derive oxygen consumption.

In the indirect Fick method of calculating CO, expired gases such as carbon dioxide (intermittent partial rebreathing of carbon dioxide) or acetylene replace oxygen consumption in the Fick equation.[350] Substituting CO_2 production for oxygen consumption, capnographic measurement of CO_2 concentrations may be used to provide a noninvasive Fick estimate of CO. The rebreathing technique is used to estimate mixed venous P_{CO_2}. In the clinical setting, patients are sedated and mechanically ventilated, and capnometry equipment is attached to a processor that calculates CO.[351] Studies comparing the CO_2 rebreathing method with standard measures of CO have yielded conflicting results.[352–356] Binder et al[357] studied postoperative cardiac surgical patients. They compared the CO_2 method with the thermodilution method and showed a good correlation. In contrast, van Heerden et al,[358] using a different device, found that CO measurements in cardiac surgery patients were overestimated using the CO_2 rebreathing technique.

Indicator Dilution

The indicator dilution method is based on the observation that, for a known amount of indicator introduced at one point in the circulation, the same amount of indicator should be detectable at a downstream point. The amount of indicator detected at the downstream point is equal to the product of CO and the change in indicator concentration over time. CO is calculated using the Stewart-Hamilton equation:

$$CO = I \times 60 \div \int C\,dt$$

in which CO is cardiac output, I is amount of indicator injected, and $\int C\,dt$ is the integral of indicator concentration over time (60 converts seconds to minutes).

Cold saline (i.e., thermodilution) or lithium ions are used as the indicator, whereas dye (e.g., indocyanine green) or radioisotopes are rarely used in current practice.[359] Blood flow is directly proportional to the amount of the indicator delivered and inversely proportional to the amount of indicator that is present at a sampling site distal to the injection site.

Thermodilution

INTERMITTENT THERMODILUTION CARDIAC OUTPUT

The thermodilution method, using the PAC, is the most commonly used method at present for invasively measuring CO in the clinical setting. With this technique, multiple COs can be obtained at frequent intervals using an inert indicator, and without blood withdrawal. A bolus of cold fluid is injected into the right atrium, and the resulting temperature change is detected by the thermistor in the pulmonary artery.[198,360] When a thermal indicator is used, the modified Stewart-Hamilton equation is used to calculate CO:

$$CO = \frac{V(T_B - T_I) \times K_1 \times K_2}{\int_0^\infty \Delta T_B(t)dt}$$

in which CO is the cardiac output (L/min), V is the volume of injectate (mL), T_B is the initial blood temperature (°C), T_I is the initial injectate temperature (°C), K_1 is the density factor, K_2 is the computation constant, and $\int_0^\infty \Delta T_B(t)dt$ is the integral of blood temperature change over time.

Solution of this equation is performed by a computer that integrates the area under the temperature versus time curve. CO is inversely proportional to the area under the curve.

Accuracy. Salgado and Galetti[361] discovered that thermodilution CO was 2.9% higher than the true flows. Bilfinger et al[362] found that the average difference between the thermodilution measurements and the reference values were 7% to 8% with room-temperature injectate and 11% to 13% with ice-cold saline injectate. Under strictly controlled in vitro conditions, the accuracy of the thermodilution CO technique varied from ±7% to ±13%.

When thermodilution measurements were compared with the direct Fick method, correlation coefficients of 0.96 were obtained in two studies.[363,364] Pelletier compared total electromagnetic flow, including coronary blood flow, with thermodilution CO in dogs.[365] He observed that, on average, thermodilution overestimated total aortic flow by ±3% compared with electromagnetic flow, whether iced or room-temperature injectate was used.

When CO measurements were compared using the thermodilution and indocyanine green method, the results varied among various studies, with some investigators finding excellent correlations over a wide range of outputs, whereas others observed that thermodilution systematically overestimated dye dilution CO.[366–368]

The temperature-versus-time curve is the crux of this technique and any circumstances that affect it have consequences for the accuracy of the CO measurement. Specifically, anything that results in less "cold" reaching the thermistor, more "cold" reaching the thermistor, or an unstable temperature baseline will adversely affect the accuracy of the technique. Less "cold" reaching the thermistor would result in overestimation of the CO. This could be caused by a smaller amount of indicator, indicator that is too warm, a thrombus on the thermistor, or partial "wedging" of the catheter. Conversely, underestimation of the CO will occur if excessive volume of injectate, or injectate that is too cold, is used to perform the measurement. Intracardiac shunts have unpredictable effects that depend on the anatomy and physiology of individual patients. Surprisingly, in one report, large left-to-right shunts were found not to adversely affect the measurement of systemic CO.[369]

Wetzel et al[370] observed variations of up to 80% in measured CO when the rate of administration of intravenous crystalloid infusions caused fluctuations in baseline blood temperature. The rapid temperature decrease seen after hypothermic CPB has been shown to result in the underestimation of CO by 0.6 to 2.0 L/min.[371] In that study, the temperature decrease after CPB was 0.14°C/min. Latson et al[372] also found that the normal changes in the pulmonary artery that occur with each respiratory cycle appear to be exaggerated in the early phase after hypothermic CPB. This may cause peak-to-peak errors in estimation of intermittent CO of up to 50% if initiated at different times during the ventilatory cycle. This effect was significantly decreased with thermal equilibration, approximately 30 minutes after CPB. This problem is less prevalent currently, because hypothermic CPB is used less commonly.

Tricuspid regurgitation has generally been considered as a source of error in thermodilution CO determinations. The scientific data, however, are contradictory. Some experimental reports indicate that tricuspid regurgitation does not impair the accuracy of thermodilution CO when compared with the Fick method[373] and electromagnetic flow probes.[374,375] In contrast, Heerdt et al[376] reported that thermodilution CO had wide variability in the direction and magnitude of error compared with Doppler and electromagnetic CO in a single patient with acute tricuspid regurgitation. The severity of tricuspid regurgitation also seems to be important in determining its effect on CO measurements by thermodilution, with underestimation of CO occurring in the presence of more severe tricuspid regurgitation.[377]

Slowing of the heart rate has been described as a side effect of rapid injection of cold injectate into the heart.[378] In a prospective study, Harris et al[379] observed that with the use of iced injectate, a decrease in heart rate of more than 10% occurred in 22% of the determinations. Nishikawa and Dohi[380] reported that heart rate slowing was more likely in patients with a low cardiac index, low mean pulmonary artery pressure, and high SVR.

Precision. In vivo reproducibility can be assessed by obtaining a large number of thermodilution COs and calculating their standard deviation. Hoel[381] postulated that a true CO could be measured by calculating the average of an infinite number of thermal injections. Using probability calculus, he found that with two injections there was only a 50% probability of being within 5% of the true CO. With three injections there was an 89% probability of being within 10% of the true CO. In an attempt to better delineate the reproducibility of the technique, Stetz et al[382] reviewed 14 publications on the use of thermodilution in clinical practice. They concluded that with the use of commercial thermodilution devices, a minimal difference of 12% to 15% (average, 13%) between determinations was required for statistical significance, provided that each determination was obtained by averaging three measurements.

A few studies have also evaluated the effects of the timing of the injection in the respiratory cycle on the reproducibility of thermodilution CO. In mechanically ventilated dogs, Snyder and Powner[383] observed that CO variations were present in each respiratory cycle and were usually greater than 10%. Stevens et al[384] studied the effects of the respiratory cycle on thermodilution CO in critically ill patients. They confirmed that injections at specific times in the respiratory cycle resulted in less variability, but possibly decreased accuracy. They nevertheless concluded that, in clinical practice, the improvement in reproducibility was more important than the decrease in accuracy.

The effects of injectate volume and temperature on the variability of thermodilution CO have also been studied in critically ill patients.[385] Six combinations of injectate volume (3, 5, and 10 mL) and temperature (iced and room temperature) were studied in 18 adult, intubated patients. The best reproducibility was obtained with 10-mL injections at 0°C or room temperature.

In summary, the precision of the thermodilution CO technique is not very good, but can be improved by ensuring that, for each determination, the rate and duration of the injection are kept as constant as possible.[386] Whenever possible, 10-mL volumes of injectate should be used, and the timing of the injection in the respiratory cycle should be the same. However, if injection is always at the same point in the respiratory cycle, some loss in accuracy is to be expected.

CONTINUOUS THERMODILUTION CARDIAC OUTPUT

Pulmonary arterial catheters with the ability to measure CO continuously were introduced into clinical practice in the 1990s. The method that has gained the most clinical use functions by mildly heating the blood in a pseudorandom stochastic fashion. In vitro as well as in vivo studies have shown that a good correlation exists between this method and other measures of CO.[387–392] Unfortunately, the correlation with CO measurements using the intermittent thermodilution method in this patient population is inconsistent.[393–395]

Bottiger et al[396] found that there was a poor correlation between intermittent and continuous thermodilution CO ($r = 0.273$) in the first 45 minutes after CPB. In contrast, there was an excellent correlation between intermittent and continuous CO measurements obtained in more physiologically stable periods. Perhaps the reason for this observation lies in the unstable thermal baseline after hypothermic CPB that was described in the previous section.

The routine use of continuous CO catheters in cardiac surgery patients has not been shown to improve outcome, and they are more expensive than standard PACs. Bolus thermodilution CO still holds its place as the gold standard of CO measurements in the clinical setting. Even though its accuracy is adversely affected by imprecise technique, it introduces extra intravenous volume, and the measurements are labor intensive. Continuous CO catheters partially alleviate these problems and provide a continuous CO trend.[397] However, there is insufficient evidence to support their routine use in cardiac surgery patients.

Dye Dilution

The indicator dilution method using indocyanine green dye had been the most popular technique of CO measurement before the introduction of the thermodilution method. Indocyanine green dye is nontoxic and is rapidly removed from the circulation by the liver. In clinical practice, it was common to inject 5 mg of indocyanine green into a central vein and to continuously sample arterial blood from an arterial catheter. The blood passed through a cuvette densitometer, and the change in indicator concentration over time was measured. A computer calculated the area under the dye concentration curve by integration of the dye concentrations over time and computed CO. After completion of the CO determination, the sampled blood was returned to the patient. Recirculation of the indicator distorts the primary time-concentration curve, and the buildup of indicator in the blood results in high background concentrations, which limits the total number of measurements that could be obtained.

Intracardiac shunting can be diagnosed by alterations of the dye dilution curve. Left-to-right shunts produce a decrease in the peak concentration of the dye, a prolonged disappearance time, and absence of the recirculation peak. In contrast, right-to-left shunts produce an early-appearing hump on the dye curve.

The introduction of lithium chloride as the indicator has led to a renaissance of the indicator dilution technique for the measurement of CO.[398] A lithium chloride solution is injected through a central venous catheter, and a lithium-selective electrode that is connected to a standard intra-arterial cannula measures plasma concentrations. Unlike thermodilution measurements of CO, no PAC needs to be inserted. Only intra-arterial and central venous catheters are required. Comparisons with standard techniques have been promising.[399,400] Peripheral venous administration of lithium chloride has shown comparable results.[401]

Cardiac Output Measurements Using Ultrasound Technology

Measurements of SV and CO can be accomplished using different echocardiographic techniques. Early attempts were made using M-mode echocardiographic dimensions and results were promising.[402,403] Two-dimensional echocardiography measurements depend on adequate imaging and calculate volume dimensions from two-dimensional data using a geometric assumption of chamber size and shape. With the introduction of three-dimensional echocardiography, it should be possible to overcome some of the problems encountered with this mathematical approach, and to determine and visualize true chamber size.[404] A different technique uses Doppler echocardiography to determine CO. Unlike two-dimensional echocardiography-derived CO measurements, Doppler echocardiography is less dependent on geometric assumptions (see Chapter 15).

Doppler Ultrasound

Ultrasound can be used for the measurement of CO based on the Doppler principle. Information on blood flow is obtained by applying Doppler frequency shift analysis to echoes reflected by the moving red blood cells. Blood flow velocity, direction, and acceleration can be instantaneously determined. From this information, SV and CO are calculated using the following formula:

$$SV = VTI \times CSA$$

in which SV is stroke volume, VTI is the Doppler velocity-time integral (i.e., area under the Doppler spectral display curve), and CSA is the cross-sectional area at the site of flow measurement. The SV is then multiplied by heart rate to calculate the CO. Blood flow in the human heart can be described by the continuity equation, which states that the flow measured at one cross-sectional area of the heart is equal to the flow measured at another cross-section (as long as there is no intracardiac shunting). Theoretically, CO may be measured at all anatomical sites in which a cross-sectional area is determined and a Doppler beam positioned. Depending on the velocity being measured, pulsed-wave Doppler or continuous-wave Doppler technology is applied. The ultrasound signals can be transmitted and detected using transthoracic, transesophageal, suprasternal, or transtracheal transducers. In clinical practice, CO measurements can be made at the aortic,[405,406] pulmonary artery,[407,408] or mitral valve positions.[409]

The degree of accuracy in comparative studies has been promising.[410–419] Technical limitations include the quality of the imaging, the accuracy of the valve or outflow tract area calculations, and the degree of alignment between the ultrasound beam and the direction of blood flow. Because the cross-sectional area is determined from two-dimensional images, converting measurements of the radius to calculate area leads to exponential increases in any errors. Calculation of the cross-sectional area at the mitral valve site gives various results because the orifice is not constant throughout the cardiac cycle.[420] The Doppler beam must be as parallel to the blood flow as possible. Angles larger than 30 degrees between the ultrasound beam and the direction of blood flow lead to increased error, despite angle-correction algorithms.

Two-Dimensional Echocardiography

Two-dimensional echocardiography allows for the calculation of CO using the following formula:

$$CO = (EDV - ESV) \times HR$$

in which CO is the cardiac output, EDV is the end-diastolic volume, ESV is the end-systolic volume, and HR is the heart rate. Two-dimensional echo-derived LV volume and CO determinations are based on geometric assumptions of chamber size and shape (i.e., Simpson's rule method). Reliable estimation of CO depends on adequate imaging that allows for exact tracing of the endocardial border. The echo-derived cardiac index shows a good correlation with the simultaneously measured value using the standard thermodilution method.[421–423]

Automated Border Detection

Automated border detection is an endocardial tracking algorithm superimposed on B-mode two-dimensional images. It is commercially available on some modern TEE machines and allows for semiautomated measurement of LV areas. The blood-endocardial interface is detected and displayed continuously. End-diastolic area, end-systolic area, and fractional area of contraction are displayed. Computer processing of the two-dimensional data (using a single-plane modification of Simpson's rule) allows for an estimation of LV volumes and EF[424,425] (see Chapter 15). Validation studies comparing automated border detection with conductance catheter volume measurement or thermodilution showed promising results.[426–430] Absolute measurements of LV dimensions tend to be systematically underestimated by automated border detection techniques; however, ABD might still be useful for detecting CO trends rather than absolute values.[431] Several difficulties must be overcome. Signal quality depends on high-quality two-dimensional echocardiographic images; a region of interest needs to be defined manually by the user; and endocardial image dropout requires repetitive readjustments by the user to optimize the image using power settings, gain adjustments, and probe manipulation.

Three-Dimensional Echocardiographic Cardiac Output

Eventually, three-dimensional echocardiography will result in a major advance in minimally invasive CO monitoring. Calculations of three-dimensional images require sequential acquisition of two-dimensional echocardiographic data from multiple imaging planes. Early results of three-dimensional evaluation of the heart were promising,[432–435] and advances in processor speed and echocardiographic technology have already helped to overcome some of the problems this technology still encounters today. Good correlation and accuracy could be demonstrated when three-dimensional echocardiographic estimates of volumetric measures were compared with established methods.[436–438] Although real-time, three-dimensional echocardiographic imaging is still limited to transthoracic imaging, advancing technology should enable real-time three-dimensional TEE in the future. Nevertheless, with economic factors being of increasing importance in current medical practice, CO monitoring using three-dimensional technology may remain too expensive for routine clinical use.

Other Techniques

Pulse Contour

Another method of CO measurement is the pulse contour analysis. The notion that SV can be quantified from the pulse pressure was derived from observations by Erlanger and Hooker in 1904. Pulse contour analysis uses the arterial pressure waveform in a mathematic model of the systemic circulation to calculate CO. Parameters used to compute CO are the resistance, compliance, and characteristic impedance of the arterial tree. These parameters are derived from specific patient information and the arterial pressure waveform. Pulse contour analysis therefore requires an arterial catheter and makes assumptions concerning the distensibility of the systemic arterial bed. The model is calibrated against a standard, recognized technique such as thermodilution or lithium chloride dilution. The system needs to be recalibrated, especially in patients who exhibit frequent changes in the parameters mentioned earlier. Accordingly, patients with poorly defined arterial waveforms, arrhythmias, or patients with abrupt changes in SVR such as cardiac surgery patients shortly after discontinuation of CPB may not be suitable candidates for this method.[439–441] Acceptable correlation with acknowledged techniques could be shown in cardiac surgical patients after admission to the ICU.[442–444] Overall, validation studies have shown various results when compared with acknowledged techniques.[445–450] Drawbacks of this technique include the need for repetitive calibrations against a standard technique, its invasive nature, and nonlinearity due to changing compliance of the arterial system.

Thoracic Electrical Bioimpedance

The first attempts at measuring CO by thoracic electrical bioimpedance began in 1966, when Kubicek et al[451] presented an empiric equation for calculation of the LV SV. To measure thoracic electrical bioimpedance, an alternating current of low amplitude and high frequency is introduced and simultaneously sensed by electrodes placed around the neck and on the chest wall or xyphoid process. Changes in thoracic impedance are induced by ventilation and pulsatile blood flow, and processing of the measured signal leads to a characteristic impedance (Z) waveform. For the measurement of SV, only the cardiac-induced pulsatile component of the total change in electrical impedance is analyzed (dZ/dt) as the respiratory component is filtered out.

Commercial systems have been introduced with improved software for advanced signal processing, but validation studies show highly inconsistent results. Although some studies trying to validate bioimpedance CO measurements found good agreement between thermodilution and bioimpedance CO,[452–456] this was not the conclusion of all investigators.[457–462]

In a prospective study, Shoemaker et al[463] compared the bioimpedance technique with standard thermodilution CO in emergency patients. The correlation was promising ($r = 0.85$), but the accuracy was not, suggesting that the bioimpedance technique may be useful for trend analysis, rather than absolute values.[464] More promising data, such as a study by Sageman et al[465] on aortocoronary bypass patients, suggest that bioimpedance can be a valid equivalent to thermodilution measurements of CO in this group of patients.

Factors that may interfere include pulmonary edema, large pleural effusions, and intracardiac shunts. Intraoperatively, lead placement may infringe on the surgical field. There may also be significant variability between different thoracic electrical impedance devices.[466] The advantage of the bioimpedance technique is the continuous on-line display of noninvasive data that may lead to prompt recognition of hemodynamic changes in patients.

The ability of bioimpedance to measure LV function remains controversial. Bioimpedance did not accurately measure LVEF compared with radionuclide imaging,[467] but dZ/dt_{max} did correlate well with LV fractional shortening as measured by echocardiography.[468]

LEFT ATRIAL PRESSURE MONITORING

In this very invasive technique, a catheter is placed by the surgeon into the right superior pulmonary vein (usually) and advanced into the left atrium. A Teflon-pledgetted purse-string stitch is placed around the catheter to provide a surface for clotting on removal of the catheter. The catheter is brought out through the skin in the subxiphoid region and is sutured in place. It is important to maintain positive airway pressure or distend the left atrium in some other way during insertion of the catheter to prevent air entry into the pulmonary vein and the left side of the heart. Another potential problem during insertion of the catheter in neonates is puncture of the right mainstem bronchus through the right superior pulmonary vein, with bronchopulmonary venous fistula formation.[469]

The LAP is an extremely informative monitor, but it also requires extreme caution. The possibility of air embolism to the coronary or cerebral circulations is always present. This problem exists on insertion and during its continued use postoperatively in the ICU. There is also the risk of clot formation on the catheter and subsequent embolization when the catheter is flushed or removed; therefore, a continuous flushing system is necessary to avoid thrombus formation on the catheter tip in the postoperative period. Postoperatively, there is also the risk of bleeding when the LAP catheter is removed. It therefore should be removed while the chest tubes are still in place to diagnose and treat this problem. Other reported complications include catheter retention and prosthetic valve entrapment.[470]

With the wider application of PAC monitoring, LAP monitoring is usually restricted to use in patients in whom PCWP determinations have been unsuccessful, are impractical, or are known to be inaccurate (e.g., in patients with pulmonary vascular disease or in small children). Continuous LAP monitoring is also useful in discontinuing CPB in some high-risk patients. The catheter may also be used to infuse inotropic agents selectively to the systemic circulation to minimize the effects on the pulmonary circulation. This was more important before therapies that selectively treat pulmonary vasoconstriction were available.

ANALYSIS AND INTERPRETATION OF HEMODYNAMIC DATA

The information provided by hemodynamic monitoring permits the calculation of various derived parameters that assist in evaluating patients clinically. The formulas, normal values, and units for the calculation of various hemodynamic parameters are presented in Table 14–2. These parameters include the SVR, pulmonary vascular resistance (PVR), SV, left ventricular stroke work (LVSW), and right ventricular stroke work (RVSW). As an example of information that may be obtained, graphs of PCWP versus SV can be constructed for individual patients; these "Starling curves" provide insight into the contractile state of the heart. Although these parameters are easily derived using the standard formulas, many modern monitors perform these calculations. To compare data among patients of different body weights and types, the various hemodynamic parameters may be normalized by indexing them to body surface area.

Systemic and Pulmonary Vascular Resistances

Systemic vascular resistance represents an estimation of the afterload of the left ventricle. Afterload is roughly defined as the force that impedes or opposes ventricular contraction. Higher SVR results in increased LV systolic wall stress. This has clinical significance because LV wall stress is one of the major determinants of myocardial oxygen consumption. Elevations in wall stress have been observed in patients with LV enlargement due to systemic hypertension, aortic stenosis, and aortic regurgitation.[471]

Clinically, calculations of SVR are used to assess the response to inotropic, vasodilatory, and vasoconstrictive agents. For example, a patient who is hypotensive despite a high normal CO has a low SVR. The SVR is calculated, and then therapy is instituted (e.g., a vasoconstrictor). A repeat calculation of the SVR enables the clinician to titrate the therapy to the appropriate end-point. Despite this common use in the operating room and ICU setting, there is good evidence that SVR is not an accurate indicator of true afterload.[472] Nevertheless, SVR remains the clinical technique for measuring afterload at the present time.

PVR remains the traditional measure of afterload of the right ventricle. This is also a flawed assumption because the recruitable nature of the pulmonary vasculature violates the assumptions of the PVR formula.[473] As the pulmonary arterial pressure (PAP) increases, the pulmonary vasculature distends (increasing the size of West's zone III of the lung).[474] The net gain in the cross-sectional area of the pulmonary vasculature results in a decrease in the measured PVR. Systolic PAP may provide a better estimation of RV afterload. PVR and PAP do provide some clinically useful information regarding the pulmonary vasculature and are readily available in patients with PACs. The PVR should be used in conjunction with other hemodynamic data to assess the response of the pulmonary vasculature to pharmacologic therapy and physiologic changes (see Chapters 10 and 33).

Frank-Starling Relationships

Myocardial function depends on the contractile state and the preload of the ventricle (sarcomere length at end-diastole). The relationship between the ventricular preload and myocardial work (ventricular stroke work) is the Frank-Starling relationship. The slope of the curve indicates the contractile state of the myocardium (Fig. 14–16). For clinical purposes, it is usually not feasible to measure actual end-diastolic volumes (can be estimated with TEE), and approximations of end-diastolic pressure, such as the PCWP or LAP, are often substituted. This introduces error, because the relationship between end-diastolic pressure and volume is usually nonlinear (as described by the diastolic ventricular compliance curve) and is dynamic. Unfortunately, the Frank-Starling relationship is extremely sensitive to changes in afterload. Patients with LV or RV dysfunction may have severe decrements in SV with increased SVR or PVR, respectively.

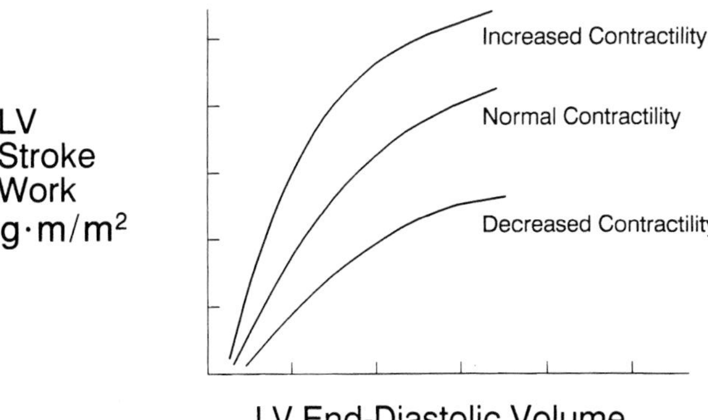

Figure 14–16 The graph of left ventricular (LV) stroke work versus LV preload (i.e., end-diastolic volume) is known as the Frank-Starling relationship. Shifting of the curve upward and to the left represents increased contractility. Shifting of the curve downward and to the right represents decreased contractility. Alterations in afterload significantly affect the curve.

End-Systolic Elastance and Pressure-Volume Loops

An important limitation of isovolumic and ejection phase indices of contractility (e.g., the Frank-Starling relationship) is their significant sensitivity to ventricular loading conditions. To overcome this shortcoming, the use of load-independent indices has been explored. One such index is the LV end-systolic pressure-volume relationship (ESPVR), also known as *end-systolic elastance.*[475] To measure this, multiple end-systolic pressures and volumes need to be measured during rapid and, preferably, pronounced alterations in LV preload (e.g., inferior vena cava occlusion). On a pressure-volume diagram, points defined by the end-systolic pressures and volumes of the several contractions will be positioned on a single line. The slope of this line is relatively independent of loading conditions and proportional to contractility; the steeper the slope, the greater the contractility (Fig. 14–17).

The intraoperative determination of contractility by this technique has been hampered by difficulties in obtaining accurate ventricular volumes and pressures. Albeit with a much more invasive approach, continuous LV pressure-volume loops may be displayed during cardiac surgery using LV conductance and micromanometry catheters that are introduced through the pulmonary veins.[476] An alternative approach using the dicrotic notch on the radial arterial tracing has been able to measure the LV end-systolic pressure with reasonable accuracy.[477] Computer software has also been described for the continuous measurement of end-systolic elastance.[478] TEE probably provides the least invasive means of measuring indices of LVEDV. However, the ESPVR is still not a practical or routine means of assessing LV contractility in the clinical setting.

PULSE OXIMETRY

Pulse oximetry is probably one of the most important advances in anesthesia monitoring technology. Pulse oxime-

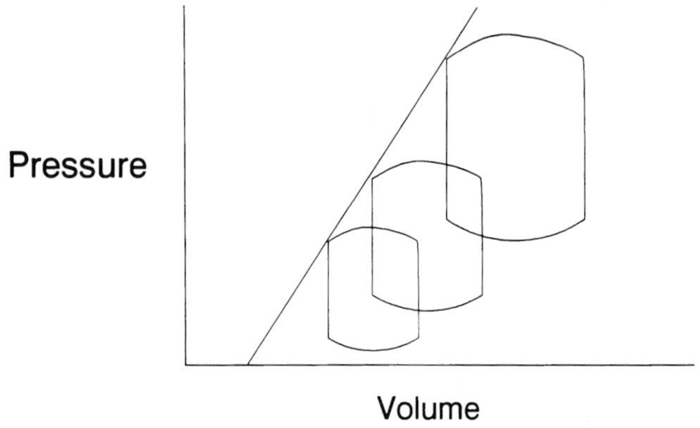

Figure 14–17 The end-systolic pressure-volume relationship, also known as end-systolic elastance, is the line connecting the end-systolic points of multiple pressure-volume loops that are obtained at various preloads. An increased slope (i.e., steeper line) represents increased contractility, and a decreased slope represents decreased contractility. This measurement is relatively insensitive to variations in afterload.

try has been accepted as an intraoperative monitoring standard, and this is reflected in current practice parameters and recommendations for perioperative anesthetic monitoring published by the American Society of Anesthesiologists.[479] This is the case despite the fact that results of outcome studies of pulse oximetry are inconsistent and that the numbers of patients who would have to be studied to answer the question are prohibitively large.[480–482] Its overwhelming acceptance as a monitoring standard has made such studies impossible.[483] The advantages and limitations of the technique merit discussion to prevent misinterpretation of data provided by pulse oximetry devices.

The absorbance spectra of oxyhemoglobin and reduced hemoglobin differ significantly. Oxyhemoglobin absorbs most infrared light (940 nm) and transmits most red light (660 nm). This may be remembered by considering that the red appearance of oxyhemoglobin would not be possible if it did not reflect (or transmit) red light. Reduced hemoglobin absorbs more red light (and appears blue) and transmits infrared light. The pulse oximeter uses this principle to determine the relative concentration of oxyhemoglobin in the blood.

Several things in addition to arterial blood also absorb red and infrared light in the tissues. These include capillary blood, venous blood, soft tissue, skin, and bone. All of these, however, absorb red and infrared light at a constant rate. The absorbance of the two waveforms of light increases as arterial blood rushes into the tissue during each cardiac cycle. It is this pulsatile component of the light absorbance that the pulse oximeter uses to calculate the arterial oxygen concentration. Many things interfere with the accuracy of pulse oximetry. Some of these include diminished tissue perfusion (e.g., limb ischemia, hypothermia, vasoconstricting drugs), ambient light, intravenous dyes, carboxyhemoglobin, and methemoglobin.[484]

There is another problem with pulse oximetry. As the signal strength of the pulse decreases in relation to the continuous absorption of the tissues, the ratio of absorbance of red to infrared light approaches unity. This would normally correlate with a saturation of 85%. It is important to regard a poor plethysmography tracing with a saturation of 85% as possibly representing artifact, and to confirm the result with an independent technique.

In the lateral decubitus position, the downward hand may give a less reliable reading due to diminished tissue perfusion. It could be argued that this might serve as a good sign of improper axillary padding. However, the information provided by pulse oximetry is probably too important to lose intermittently during the operative procedure. It has not been definitively established that a good plethysmography tracing from a pulse oximeter correlates with adequate perfusion.

Another problem in cardiac procedures is that the plethysmography tracing often decreases in amplitude over the course of the procedure until the signal-to-noise ratio is too low for accurate oximetry. This is most likely due to hypothermia of the digits, but may also be related to positioning, hypovolemia, high catecholamine levels, and extremes of age. It has been demonstrated that a digital perfusion pressure of 13 mm Hg and temperature of 24°C are the minimum requirements for accurate pulse oximetry readings before and after CPB.[485]

Reich et al[486] showed that there is a very high incidence of pulse oximetry failure in the cardiac surgery setting. The overall incidence of cases that had at least one continuous gap of 10 minutes or more in pulse oximetry data was 31%. The independent preoperative predictors of pulse oximetry data failure included American Society of Anesthesiologists (ASA) physical status 3, 4, or 5, and cardiac surgery. Intraoperative hypothermia, hypotension, and hypertension, and duration of procedure were also independent risk factors.

Electrocautery also interferes with pulse oximetry. The electromagnetic field from the cautery device induces electrical current in the wires that connect to the pulse oximetry probe. These create a very high degree of electrical noise and may disrupt the oximetry reading.

The main disadvantage of pulse oximetry is that the PaO_2 must fall below 100 mm Hg before the device will begin to detect any change, and below 60 mm Hg before rapid changes will occur. The device is not sensitive to changes in PaO_2 over wide ranges.

OXYGEN TRANSPORT CALCULATIONS

The ultimate purpose of circulation is the delivery of oxygen to the tissues. Oxygen is bound to hemoglobin and is also dissolved in the plasma (to a much smaller extent). If the hemoglobin concentration, arterial and mixed venous blood gases, and CO are available, then oxygen transport calculations may be performed. This can then allow for optimization of these parameters to improve delivery and uptake of the proper amount of oxygen to the tissues. These calculations are shown in Table 14–3.

MONITORING CORONARY PERFUSION

The coronary perfusion pressure (CPP) is usually defined as the aortic diastolic blood pressure (DAP) minus the LVEDP:

$$CPP = DAP - LVEDP$$

Elevation of the LVEDP will decrease the gradient of blood flow to the vulnerable subendocardial tissue during diastole as will a decrease in the DBP.[487] If coronary artery disease is present, significant stenosis will decrease the coronary artery DBP well below the aortic DBP, and elevation of LVEDP can seriously jeopardize the subendocardium.[488] An increase in the LVEDP is detrimental in two ways: decreased coronary blood

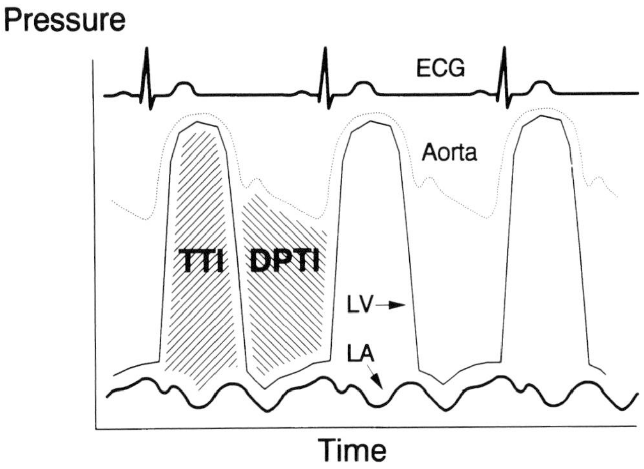

Figure 14–18 Left ventricular (LV) oxygen demand is graphically represented by the area between the LV and the left atrial (LA) waveforms during systole, which is the tension-time index (TTI). LV oxygen supply is represented by the area between the aortic and the LV waveforms during diastole, which is the diastolic pressure–time index (DPTI). Factors that decrease the DPTI (e.g., myocardial oxygen supply) include decreased aortic diastolic pressure, increased LV end-diastolic pressure, and a shortened diastolic interval. ECG = electrocardiogram.

flow and increased myocardial oxygen demand (MVO_2), which explain the severe ischemia seen with overdistention of the left ventricle. Tachycardia is also extremely detrimental because it decreases coronary filling time and increases oxygen demand. Subendocardial ischemia is commonly produced by a combination of tachycardia and elevated LVEDP.

Hoffman and Buckberg[489,490] described the endocardial viability ratio (EVR), or diastolic pressure-time index (DPTI) divided by the tension-time index (TTI), which graphically describes the ratio of myocardial oxygen supply to myocardial oxygen demand (Fig. 14–18).

$$EVR = \frac{DPTI}{TTI} = \frac{(DBP - LAP) * T_d}{SBP * T_s} = \frac{\text{Oxygen supply}}{\text{Oxygen demand}}$$

In this equation, DBP is the diastolic blood pressure, LAP is the left atrial pressure, T_d is the diastolic interval, SBP is the systolic blood pressure, and T_s is the systolic interval.

This ratio can be used to estimate subendocardial blood flow. To assess the oxygen supply, the DPTI is used, and for the oxygen demand, the TTI is used. A normal EVR is 1.0 or greater (DPTI equals or exceeds TTI). When the EVR is less than 0.7, Hoffman and Buckberg[488] found that the LV endocardial blood flow fell in proportion to the epicardial flow (decreased endocardial-to-epicardial ratio), which indicate subendocardial ischemia. The endocardial-to-epicardial ratio fell whether the decreased EVR resulted from decreased aortic DBP, increased LAP, or increased heart rate. Although the EVR is not a clinical monitoring tool, it is an elegant means of demonstrating the use of hemodynamic monitoring and treatment to assess the balance between myocardial oxygen supply and demand (e.g., the beneficial effects of the intra-aortic balloon pump).

ELECTROCARDIOGRAPHY

Interpretation of the ECG is often considered the domain of the cardiologist, but clinicians providing perioperative and critical care also derive important information from it by the standard 12-lead tracing or as a continuous "monitoring" modality. With advances in computer technology, the distinction between diagnostic ECG carts and bedside monitoring units is narrowing. Many bedside units are capable of recording diagnostic quality 12-lead ECGs for transmission over a hospital network for storage and retrieval. The diagnostic and monitoring capabilities of the ECG for the detection of arrhythmias and myocardial ischemia/infarction continue to develop and expand (Box 14–12). However, there are finite limits defined by the relationship between sensitivity and specificity (usually inversely related) for detecting coronary artery disease and its consequences. For example, during exercise testing, the 12-lead ECG has a mean sensitivity of only 68% and a specificity of 77%.[491] The resting 12-lead ECG is even less sensitive and specific. Other clinical modalities are often required (e.g., transthoracic echocardiography, TEE, pulmonary artery catheterization). Newer, more complex electrocardiographic modalities are likely to improve its utility in the future (e.g., continuous vectorcardiography, high-frequency QRS signal averaging). Routine use of digital signal processing techniques greatly facilitates continuous electrocardiographic monitoring inexpensively (Box 14–13), with minimal invasiveness.

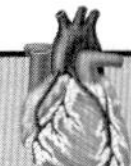

BOX 14–12 ***Basic Clinical Information Available from Electrocardiography***

Anatomy or Morphology

- Infection
- Ischemia
- Hypertrophy

Physiology

- Automaticity
- Arrhythmogenicity
- Conduction
- Ischemia
- Autonomic tone
- Electrolyte abnormalities
- Drug toxicity or effect
- Ejection fraction (?)

The practicing anesthesiologist relies on the ECG to make critical decisions at many phases of the perioperative period in patients undergoing cardiac or noncardiac (particularly vascular) surgery. In this section of the chapter, the theory and the operating characteristics of electrocardiographic hardware used in the perioperative period are presented to facilitate proper use and interpretation of monitoring data.

Historical Perspective

Willem Einthoven is universally considered the father of electrocardiography (for which he won the 1924 Nobel Prize). However, Augustus Waller actually recorded the first human ECG in 1887 using a glass capillary electrometer. This early device used changes in surface tension between mercury and sulfuric acid in a glass column induced by a varying electric potential. The level of the meniscus was magnified and recorded on moving photographic paper, describing what were initially called *A-B-C-D waves*. In 1895, Einthoven published his observations using this crude device. Frustration with its low-frequency resolution led him to develop the string

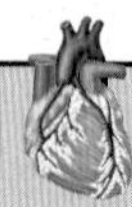

BOX 14–13 ***Data Extraction from the Electrocardiogram to Support Current and Future Clinical Uses, with or without Ancillary Correlative Modalities***

P wave
- Polarity
- Duration
- Mean amplitude
- Area
- Frequency content

PR segment
- AH interval
- HV interval

QRS complex
- Polarity
- Duration
- Area
- Mean amplitude
- Frequency content
- Late potential-power spectrum

ST-T wave
- Slope of ascending/descending limbs
- Area
- Ratio of area to peak, duration to peak
- Power spectrum of variation

Arrhythmias
- Morphology
- Coupling interval

From Garfein OB: The promise of electrocardiography in the 21st century. Ann N Y Acad Sci 601:370, 1990.

galvanometer, using a silver-coated quartz fiber suspended between the poles of a magnet. Changes induced by the electrical potentials conducted through the quartz string resulted in its movement at right angles to the magnetic field. The shadow of the string, backlit from a light source, was transmitted through a microscope (the string was only 2.1 mm in diameter) and was recorded on a moving photographic plate. He renamed the signal the P-QRS-T complex (based on standard geometric convention for describing points on curved lines).

Many of the basic clinical abnormalities in electrocardiography were first described using the string galvanometer (e.g., bundle-branch block, delta waves, ST-T changes with angina). It was used until the 1930s, when it was replaced by a system using vacuum tube amplifiers and a cathode ray oscilloscope. A portable direct-writing ECG cart was not introduced until the early 1950s (facilitated at first by transistor technology and subsequently by integrated circuits), which allowed widespread use of the ECG in clinical practice. The first analog-to-digital (A/D) conversion systems for the ECG were introduced in the early 1960s, but their clinical use was restricted until the late 1970s. In the 1980s, microcomputer technology became widely available and is now standard for all diagnostic and monitoring systems.

Technical Aspects

Power Spectrum of the Electrocardiogram

The electrocardiographic signal must be considered in terms of its amplitude (or voltage) and its frequency components

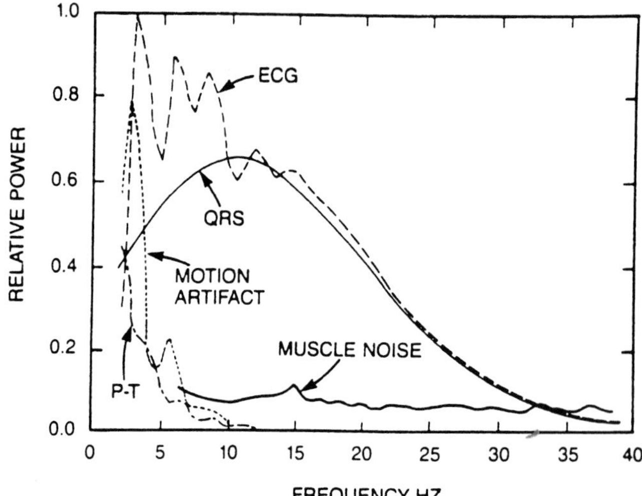

Figure 14–19 The typical power spectrum of the electrocardiogram (ECG) signal (obtained during ambulatory monitoring), including its subcomponents and common artifacts (i.e., motion and muscle noise). The power of the P and T waves (PT) is low frequency, and the QRS complex is concentrated in the mid-frequency range, although residual power extends up to 100 Hz. (From Thakor NV: From Holter monitors to automatic defibrillators: Developments in ambulatory arrhythmia monitoring. IEEE Trans Biomed Eng 31:770, 1984.)

(generally called its *phase*). Voltage considerations differ depending on the signal source. Surface recording involves amplification of smaller voltages (on the order of 1 mV) than recording sites closer to the heart beneath the electrically resistant layers of the skin (e.g., endocardial, esophageal and intratracheal leads). The "power spectrum" of the ECG (Fig. 14–19) is derived by Fourier transformation, in which a periodic waveform is mathematically decomposed to its harmonic components (sine waves of various amplitudes and frequencies). Spectra representing some of the major sources of artifact must be eliminated during the processing and amplification of the QRS complex.[492] The frequency of each of these components can be equated to the slope of the component signal.[493] The R wave with its steep slope is a high-frequency component, whereas P and T waves have lesser slopes and are lower in frequency. The ST segment has the lowest frequency, not much different from the "underlying" electrical (i.e., isoelectric) baseline of the ECG. Before the introduction of digital signal processing (DSP), accurately displaying the ST segment presented significant technical problems, particularly in operating room and ICU bedside monitoring units. Although the overall frequency spectrum of the QRS complex in Figure 14–19 does not appear to exceed 40 Hz, many components of the QRS complex, particularly the R wave, exceed 100 Hz. Very-high-frequency signals of particular clinical significance are pacemaker spikes. Their short duration and high amplitude present technical challenges for proper recognition and rejection to allow accurate determination of the heart rate (HR). The frequencies of greatest importance for optimal electrocardiographic processing are presented in Table 14–5.[494]

Intrinsic and Extrinsic Artifacts

Motion artifact and "baseline wander" result from several causes. Skin impedance has been shown to vary at different skin sites, at different times of the day as well as seasonally (likely related to humidity changes), and may be 50% higher

Processing	Frequency Range
Display	0.5 (or 0.05)–40 Hz
QRS detection	5–30 Hz
Arrhythmia detection	0.05–60 Hz
ST-segment monitoring	0.05–60 Hz
Pacemaker detection	1.5–5 kHz

Table 14–5 **Range of Signal Frequencies Included in Different Phases of Processing in an Electrocardiographic Monitor**

From Weinfurt PT: Electrocardiographic monitoring: An overview. J Clin Monit 6:132, 1990.

in females.[495] With application of a silver-silver chloride electrode, impedance decays with a time constant of 6.9 minutes as the conductive gel penetrates the skin. Deformation of the stratum granulosum generates electrical potentials of several millivolts as cells slide over each other or are stretched. Skin potentials up to 64 mV can be measured between two electrodes on the skin surface, varying with the type of electrolyte gel used. Direct current (DC) potentials are actually stored by the electrode itself (i.e., offset potentials), varying with the type of electrode used. A striking example of an offset potential is the transient obliteration of the ECG that occurs immediately after electrical defibrillation. Poor electrode contact enhances pickup of alternating current power-line interference (60-Hz signals). The second major physiologic source of artifact is electromyographic (EMG) noise produced by motor activity, either voluntary (i.e., during treadmill testing or ambulatory ST-segment monitoring) or involuntary (i.e., shivering or Parkinsonian tremor). Electromyographic noise is similar in amplitude to the ECG, but is generally of considerably higher frequency. Because it is a random signal, in contrast to the regular repetitive ECG signal, it is amenable to significant attenuation (if not outright elimination) using routine DSP techniques.[496]

There are also extrinsic or nonphysiologic causes of artifact. An important one is called *common-mode rejection.* The electrocardiographic signal is recorded as the difference in potential between two electrodes and is technically a differential signal. The body is not at absolute ground potential, which is why the right leg lead is used as a reference electrode.[497] This higher potential (over that of an absolute ground to earth) is called *common-mode potential,* because it is common to both electrode inputs to the differential amplifier used to amplify the ECG signal. Common-mode potential must be rejected or it may alter the ECG signal. The ability of the differential amplifier to reject these potentials (relative to the differential inputs) is called the *common-mode rejection ratio* (CMRR). In modern amplifiers, CMRR should be at least 100,000; in newer diagnostic digital electrocardiographic units, it is at least 1 million. Adequate CMRR is of great importance in attenuating a variety of environmental factors.

Electrical power-line interference (60 Hz) is a common environmental problem. Power lines and other electrical devices radiate energy that can enter the monitor by poor electrode contact or cracked or poorly shielded lead cables. Interference can also be induced electromagnetically as these signals radiate through the loop formed by the body, lead cables, and monitor.[498] This type of interference can be reduced by twisting the lead cables together (reducing the loop area), or by minimizing the distance between the lead cables. In newer diagnostic electrocardiographic machines, A/D signal conversion occurs in an acquisition module close to the patient, which effectively reduces the length of the lead cables and the amount of signal induction possible. A line frequency "notch" filter is often used to remove 60-Hz noise.

Electrocautery (electrosurgery) units generate radiofrequency currents at very high frequencies (800 to 2000 kHz) and high voltages (1 kV, which is 10^6 greater than the ECG signal). Older units used a modulation frequency of 60 Hz, which spread substantial electrical noise into the QRS frequency range of the ECG signal. Newer units use a modulation frequency of 20 kHz, minimizing this problem.[499] To minimize electrocautery artifact, the right leg reference electrode should be placed as close as possible to the grounding pad and the ECG monitor should be plugged into a different power outlet from the electrosurgical unit.

Technical Aspects of Electrode Placement

Monitoring electrodes should preferentially be placed directly over bony prominences of the torso (e.g., clavicular heads, iliac prominences) to minimize excursion of the electrode during respiration, which can cause baseline wander. Electrode impedance must be optimized to avoid loss and alteration of the signal. By removing a portion of the stratum corneum (e.g., gentle abrasion with a dry gauze pad resulting in a minor amount of surface erythema works well), skin impedance can be reduced by a factor of 10 to 100. Optimal impedance is 5000 ohms or less. The electrode may be covered with a watertight dressing to prevent surgical scrub solutions from undermining electrode contact.

Clinical Sources of Artifact

Devices with which the patient is in physical contact, particularly plastic tubing, may at times cause clinically significant electrocardiographic artifact.[500–504] Although the exact mechanism is uncertain, two leading explanations are a piezoelectric effect due to mechanical deformation of the plastic and a buildup of static electricity between two dissimilar materials, especially those in motion. This effect has been seen with the use of CPB and usually mimics atrial arrhythmias. A grounding lead on the CPB machine usually eliminates this. Other clinical devices associated with electrocardiographic interference, albeit rarely, include infusion pumps and blood warmers. Isolated power supply line isolation monitors (LIMs) have also been associated with 60-Hz interference. This can be diagnosed by removing the LIM fuses to see if the artifact disappears.[505]

Frequency Response of Electrocardiographic Monitors: Monitoring and Diagnostic Modes

Given the importance of the ECG in diagnosing myocardial ischemia, it is important to realize that "significant" ST-segment depression or elevation can occur solely as a result of improper signal filtering in 12-lead ECG machines and bedside or ambulatory ST-segment monitors.[506–510] This artifact was a particular problem before the introduction of DSP. The American Heart Association (AHA) Committee On Electrocardiography Standardization has addressed specific frequency requirements for monitoring in this setting.[511]

ECG signals must be amplified and filtered before display. To reproduce the component frequencies accurately, each must be amplified equally. The monitor must have a "flat amplitude response" over the wide range of frequencies present. Similarly, because the slight delay in a signal as it passes through a filter or amplifier may vary in duration with different frequencies, all frequencies must be delayed equally. This is called *linear phase response.* If the response is nonlinear, various components may appear temporally distorted (called *phase shift*).

Nonlinear frequency response in the low-frequency range (0.5 Hz) can cause artifactual ST depression, whereas phase delay in this range can cause ST-segment elevation.[493] The AHA recommends a bandwidth from 0.05 to 100 Hz (at 3 dB).[512] Although a completely linear response is desirable, with analog filters it is not generally possible. However, the response at 0.05 Hz should not be reduced by more than 30% (at 3 dB) from the response at 0.14 Hz (Fig. 14–20). Phase response is not well described, but is usually adequate when amplitude response criteria are met.[513] Because greater baseline noise is present when a 0.05-Hz cutoff is used, the 0.5 Hz cutoff is often used to display a more stable signal. This is commonly referred to as *monitoring mode,* and use of a 0.05-Hz low-frequency cutoff is known as *diagnostic mode.*[514] The difference in ST-segment morphology at various low-frequency cutoffs is illustrated in Figure 14–21. Because most newer monitors use signal averaging techniques that effectively eliminate most artifact even in the diagnostic mode, the clinician can usually (and should) avoid using the monitoring mode, whenever possible.

High-frequency response is of less importance clinically, because the ST segment and T wave reside in the low-frequency spectrum. However, at the commonly used high-frequency cutoff of 40 Hz, the amplitude of the R and S waves may diminish significantly, making it difficult to diagnose ventricular hypertrophy.[507,515] Significant reduction in QRS amplitude may occur in the following circumstances: major decreases in LV function, obesity, pericardial and pleural effusions, and infiltrative or restrictive cardiac diseases.

Newer data document significant reversible reduction of the QRS complex with whole-body fluid accumulation (e.g., anasarca). Madias et al[516] evaluated 28 patients with anasarca in whom pericardial effusions had been ruled out by serial echocardiograms. A reduction in the sum of the amplitude of QRS complexes in all 12 leads correlated well with increase in body weight and reversed direction in patients recovering from acute illness. Although a variety of potential etiologic factors may be involved (including intracavitary volume by the Brody effect), they attribute this reduction to a shunting of the cardiac potentials due to the low electrical resistance of the anasarca fluid. It may also obscure the electrocardiographic diagnosis of LV hypertrophy as well as presence of

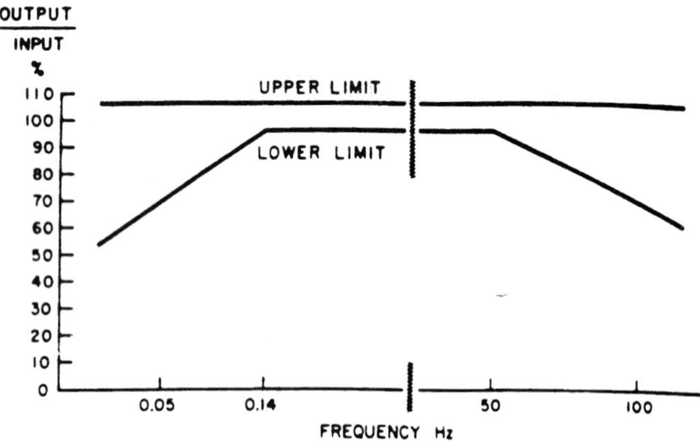

Figure 14–20 Recommended bounds to frequency response for direct-writing electrocardiograms (ECGs) recommended by the American Heart Association. The bandwidth is demarcated by the upper and lower corner frequencies (in this example, 0.05 and 100 Hz). Each of the corner frequencies is located 3 dB (roughly a 30% decrease in voltage) relative to the amplification at a frequency near the middle of the bandwidth *(vertical bar).* (From Pipberger HV, Arzbaecher RC, Berson AS, et al: Recommendations for the standardization of leads and of specifications for instruments in electrocardiography and vectorcardiography. Report of the Committee on Electrocardiography, American Heart Association. Circulation 52:11, 1975; with permission of the American Heart Association.)

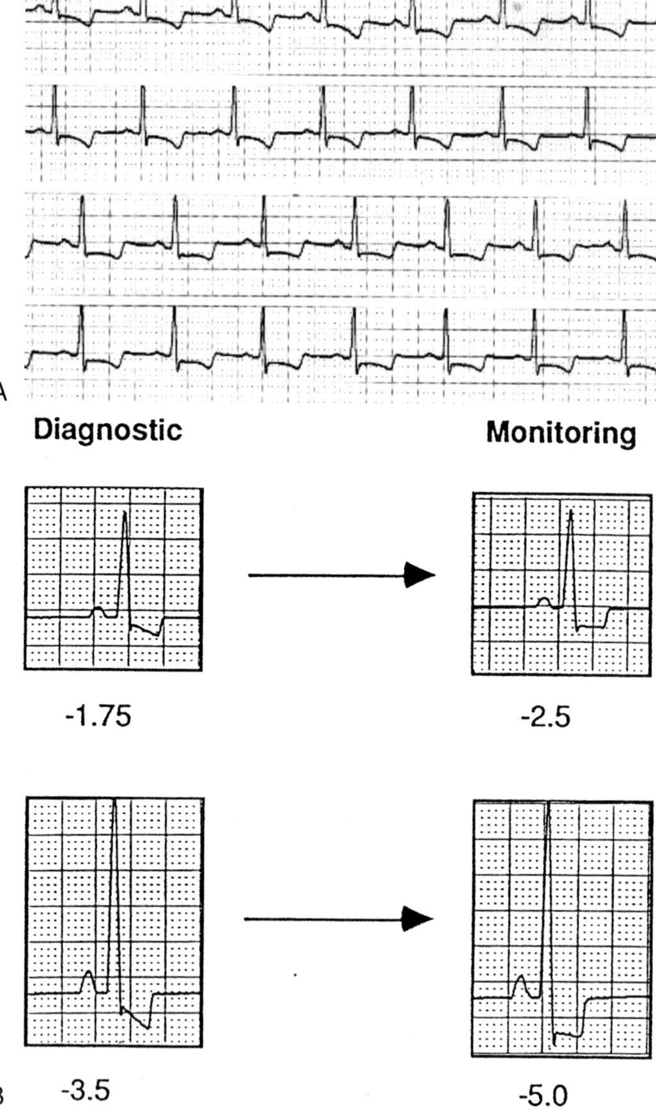

Figure 14–21 *(A)* Monitoring versus diagnostic mode in leads II *(top trace)* and V_5 *(bottom trace)* in a patient undergoing coronary artery bypass grafting. Notice the straightening of the baseline with use of the monitoring mode, which is most notable in lead II. The degree of the PR and ST segments is exaggerated in both leads. *(B)* Effects of monitoring mode on ST-segment depth and morphology are illustrated using a digital electrocardiographic simulator. A SpaceLabs PC2 monitor (Redmond, WA) was switched from monitoring (0.5 to 40 Hz) to diagnostic mode (0.05 to 70 Hz). Notice the increase in the depth of ST-segment depression and the alteration of slope in both leads. (From London MJ: Ischemia monitoring: ST segment analysis versus TEE. *In* Kaplan JA [ed]: Cardiothoracic and Vascular Anesthesia Update, Vol 3. Philadelphia, WB Saunders Company, 1993, pp 1–20.)

pacemaker spikes.[517,518] The precise clinical applications and exact sensitivity and specificity of these responses have not yet been well documented. Given the potential application of these findings for inexpensive, noninvasive monitoring of therapeutic effect (e.g., diuresis), it is likely to be a topic for further study in the ICU setting.[519]

Tsuda et al[520] studied changes in R-wave amplitude in V_5 throughout the intraoperative period in 35 patients undergoing CABG or valve replacement. Amplitude was reduced by 50% to 60% before institution of CPB. CABG patients had a slower recovery of R-wave amplitude. Marked reduction and failure of recovery of R-wave amplitudes occurred in patients dying perioperatively, a finding often observed clinically but not previously documented in the literature. Crescenzi et al[521] have extended these observations by comparing R-wave amplitude in leads V_4 and V_5 in patients undergoing CABG with (n = 35) or without CPB (n = 35). A control group of patients undergoing mitral valve repair (n = 31) without coronary artery disease were included. A lack of change of amplitude in the R wave was found in the off-pump cases in contrast to reductions of R-wave amplitude in patients undergoing CABG or mitral valve surgery with CPB (Fig. 14–22). Although biochemical markers of cardiac damage were significantly lower in the off-pump CABG group, no significant correlation was observed between alteration of R-wave amplitude and biochemical marker levels. It does not appear that fluid shifts or weight changes were considered in this analysis, factors that are more likely with the use of CPB. Larger sample sizes and more detailed analyses are required to better refine any potential clinically useful applications of QRS amplitude changes.

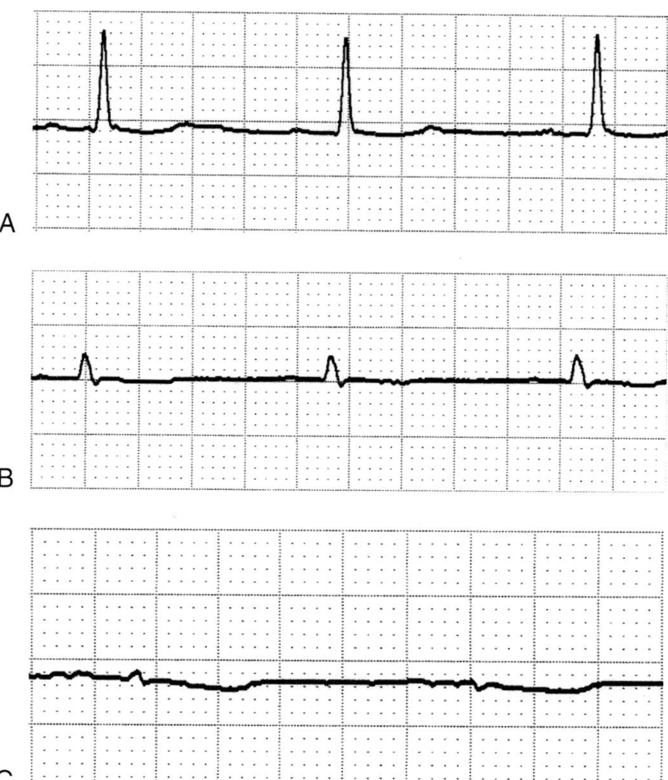

Figure 14–22 The effects of vertical suspension of the heart on electrocardiographic amplitude (Medtronic Urchin apical suction device) are depicted. *(A)* Baseline complex. *(B)*. Transition. *(C)* Complete vertical suspension.

Digital Signal Processing and Computerized Electrocardiography

The foundation of DSP is the A/D converter, which samples the incoming "continuous" analog signal (characterized by variable amplitude or voltage over time) at a very rapid rate and converts the sampled voltage into binary numbers, each of which has a precise time index or sequence. The "bit size" of the A/D converter controls the number of measurements possible within a given voltage range according to the formula $2^n - 1$, in which n is the bit size (e.g., an 8-bit converter divides the input range into 255 intervals).[522] The larger the bit size, the greater the resolution of the signal. Greater bit size and higher sampling rates, however, require more powerful microprocessors and greater computer memory. Most commercially available units use minimum sampling rates of 256 Hz (resulting in 4-msec increments) with at least 12-bit resolution. Use of lower sampling rates may result in slight differences in the times at which digitization of each QRS complex begins (i.e., phase shift); this can distort the signal as described previously. Newer diagnostic ECG units are capable of sampling at 1000 Hz (i.e., high-resolution or high-RES ECG).

After A/D conversion, the resultant data bits are inspected by a microprocessor using a mathematical model to determine where reference points (i.e., fiducial points) are located. A common method locates the point of most rapid change in amplitude (located on the downslope of the R wave). This process characterizes the baseline QRS complex (QRS recognition), providing a template on which subsequent beats are overlaid (beat alignment) and averaged (signal averaging). This allows visual display of the QRS complex and quantification of its components, as well as elimination of random electrical noise and wide complex beats that fail to meet criteria established by the fiducial points. Signal averaging is used to reduce noise by the square root of the number of beats averaged. A 10-fold reduction in noise is accomplished by averaging only 100 beats (Fig. 14–23). Because of the proprietary nature of this technology (the specific algorithms used are patented), methods may vary according to manufacturer. Consequently, processed QRS complexes may vary in the quality of representation (i.e., if noise or aberrant beats are averaged into the complex, it will vary from the raw analog complex).

The signal averaging process involves comparison of voltages at particular time points between the incoming complex and a template. The easiest method uses the mean difference between voltages to update the template, but the most accurate method uses the median difference (which is less affected by outliers, such as aberrant beats or other signals that have escaped QRS matching) (Fig. 14–24). However, median averaging is computationally more complex (i.e., memory intensive) and may have slightly higher baseline noise content. Because median averaging is impractical for continuous data acquisition, *incremental averaging* is used, a technique that minimizes the influence of outliers.[523,524] When the incoming value is above the value of the template (by any amount), a small, fixed voltage increment is added to the template (generally 10 mV/beat); when it is below the previous beat, the same value is subtracted.

Most monitors incorporate a visual trend line from which deviations in the position of the ST segment can be rapidly detected to aid on-line detection of myocardial ischemia. This can be a single summated trend of several "quasi-orthogonal" leads or multiple single leads. Most monitors also display on-

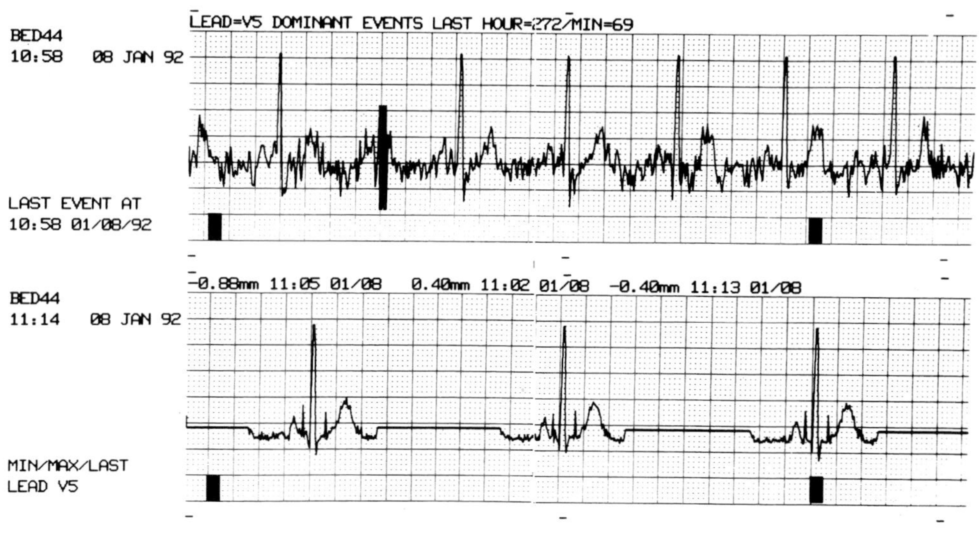

Figure 14–23 Reduction of muscle artifact (simulated) by digital signal processing using signal averaging (PC2 Bedside Monitor, SpaceLabs, Redmond, WA). *(Top)* The initial learned complex (i.e., dominant) on the left is followed by real-time complexes. *(Bottom)* Median complexes are smoothed by signal processing. Notice that the ST-segment position is isoelectric in the normal complex, but it does vary in accuracy with this degree of noise. The degree of noise reduction is proportional to the square root of the number of beats averaged.

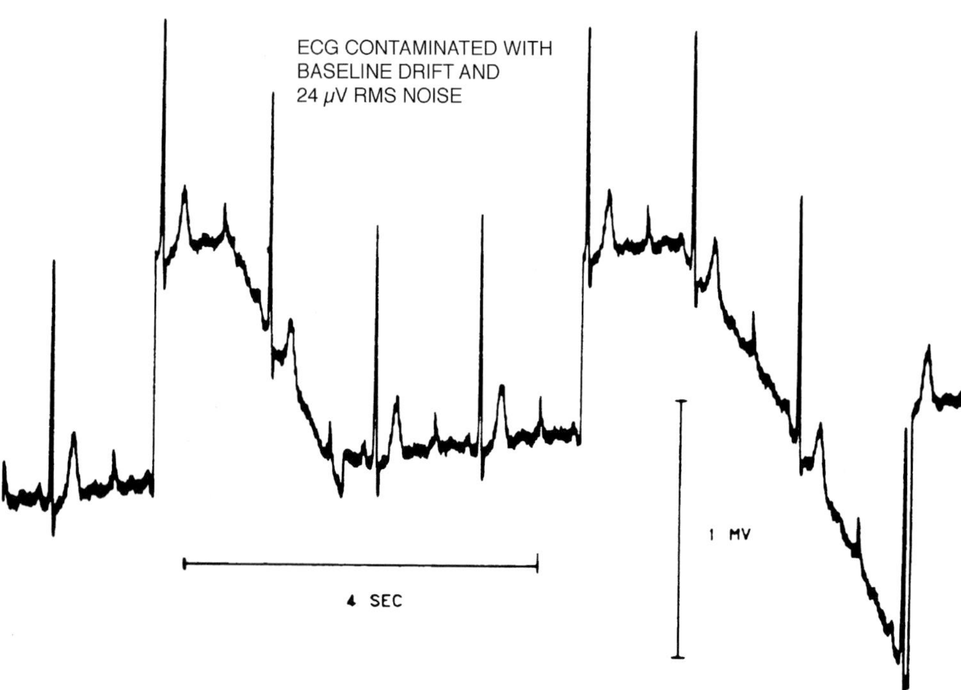

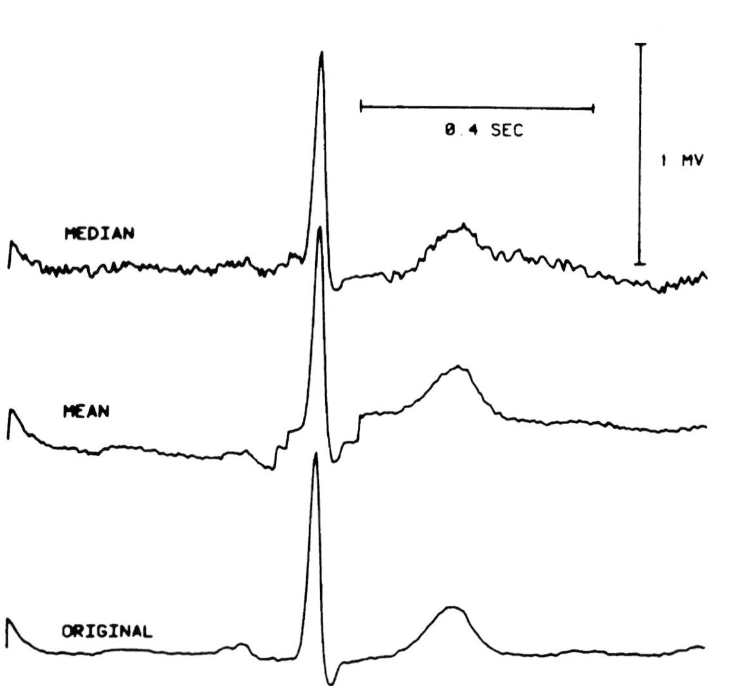

Figure 14–24 Effects of averaging techniques on resolution of an electrocardiographic signal heavily contaminated with baseline and electrical noise. Despite a greater degree of baseline and electrical noise, median averaging results in a more accurate rendition of the original signal. Notice the abnormal J-point elevation in the mean averaged complex. (From Froelicher VF: Special methods: Computerized exercise ECG analysis. *In* Exercise and the Heart. Chicago, Year Book Medical Publishers, 1987, p 36.)

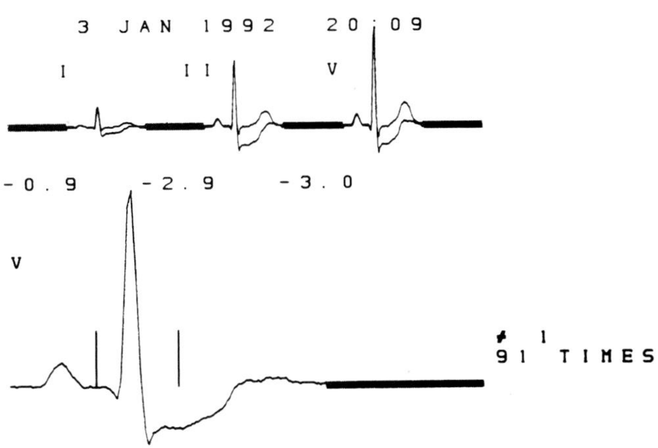

Figure 14–25 The graphic output of the ST-adjustment window from a Marquette Electronics Series 7010 monitor (Milwaukee, WI) ST-segment analyzer. This software allows trending and display of three leads (i.e., I, II, and any single V lead). In this window, the initial complex ("learned" when the program was activated) is displayed along with the current complex. Two complexes are superimposed with different intensities to facilitate comparison. ST analysis is performed automatically at 80 msec after the J point, although the user can manually adjust this. The number of QRS complexes that are input to the monitor is displayed (in this example, 91).

screen numerical values for the position of the ST segment used for ischemia detection (generally 60 to 80 msec after the J point). The specific point used is adjustable, which may be helpful with tachycardia and wide QRS complexes (Figs.14–25 and 14–26). These features enhance the diagnosis of perioperative ischemia, which is difficult to detect without some automated system.

Lead Systems

Where and how ECG electrodes are placed on the body are critical determinants of the morphology of the ECG signal. Lead systems have been developed based on theoretical considerations (e.g., orthogonal arrangement of the Frank XYZ leads) and references to anatomic landmarks that facilitate consistency between individuals (e.g., standard 12-lead system). Table 14–6 describes basic mathematical relations between the components of the 12-lead system and the Frank-Lewis orthogonal lead system.

History and Description of the 12-Lead System

Einthoven established electrocardiography using three extremities as references: the left arm (LA), right arm (RA), and left leg (LL). He recorded the difference in potential between the LA and RA (lead I), between the LL and RA (lead II), and between the LL and LA (lead III). Because the signals recorded were differences between two electrodes, these leads were called *bipolar*. The RL served only as a reference electrode. Because Kirchoff's loop equation states that the sum of the three voltage differential pairs must equal zero, the sum of leads I and III must equal lead II (which is therefore redundant).[525] The positive or negative polarity of each of the limbs was chosen by Einthoven to result in positive deflections of most of the waveforms and has no innate physiologic significance. He postulated that the three limbs defined an imaginary equilateral triangle with the heart at its center. Given the influence of Einthoven's vector analyses of frontal plane forces, others eventually incorporated the other two orthogonal planes (transverse and sagittal).

Wilson refined and introduced the unipolar precordial leads into clinical practice. To implement these leads, he postulated a mechanism whereby the absolute level of electrical potential could be measured at the site of the exploring precordial electrode (the positive electrode). A negative pole with zero potential was formed by joining the three limb electrodes in a resistive network in which equally weighted signals cancel each other out. He called this the *central terminal*, and in a fashion similar to Einthoven's vector concepts, he postulated it was located at the electrical center of the heart, representing the mean electrical potential of the body throughout the cardiac cycle. He described three additional limb leads (VL, VR, and VF). These leads measured new vectors of activation, and in this way, the hexaxial reference system for determination of electrical axis was established. He subsequently introduced the six unipolar precordial V leads in 1935 (Fig. 14–27).[526]

Clinical application of the unipolar limb leads was limited because of their significantly smaller amplitude relative to the bipolar limb leads from which they were derived. They were not clinically applied until Goldberger augmented their

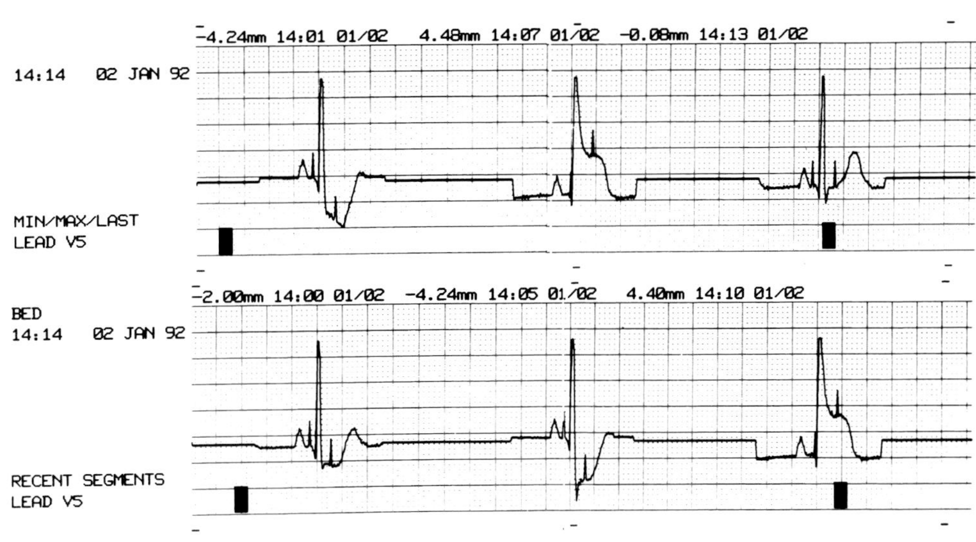

Figure 14–26 Output from ST-segment trending software from PC2 Bedside monitor (SpaceLabs, Redmond, WA). Up to nine averaged complexes can be displayed: the minimal and maximal ST change, the latest complex, and the preceding six complexes at 5-minute intervals (only three are displayed in this example). The isoelectric and ST measurement positions are indicated on each complex. An ST-segment simulator has been used to introduce episodes of ST-segment elevation and depression.

Table 14–6 Definition of Electrocardiographic Leads

Lead Type	Electrodes Used	Definition
Bipolar or limb leads (Einthoven)	LA, RA, LL, RL	I = LA − RA II = LL − RA III = LL − LA
Augmented (Goldberger)	LA, RA, LL, RL	aVR = RA − 0.5(LA + LL) aVL = LA − 0.5(LL + RA) aVF = LL − 0.5(LA + RA)
Unipolar chest leads (Wilson)*	V_1, V_2, V_3, V_4, V_5, V_6	$V_1 = v_1 - (LA + RA + LL)/3$ $V_2 = v_2 - (LA + RA + LL)/3$ $V_3 = v_3 - (LA + RA + LL)/3$ $V_4 = v_4 - (LA + RA + LL)/3$ $V_5 = v_5 - (LA + RA + LL)/3$ $V_6 = v_6 - (LA + RA + LL)/3$
Orthogonal vector leads (Frank)	I, E, C, A, M, H, F	X = 0.610A + 0.171C − 0.781I Y= 0.655F + 0.345M − 1.000H Z = 0.133A + 0.736M − 0.264I − 0.374E − 0.231C

*The lower-case v in the definitions indicates precordial voltage (i.e., before input to central terminal of Wilson).
F = foot; LA = left arm; LL = left leg; RA = right arm; RL = right leg.
From Thakor NV: Electrocardiographic monitors. *In* Webster JG (ed): Encyclopedia of Medical Devices and Instrumentation. New York, John Wiley & Sons, 1988, p 1002.

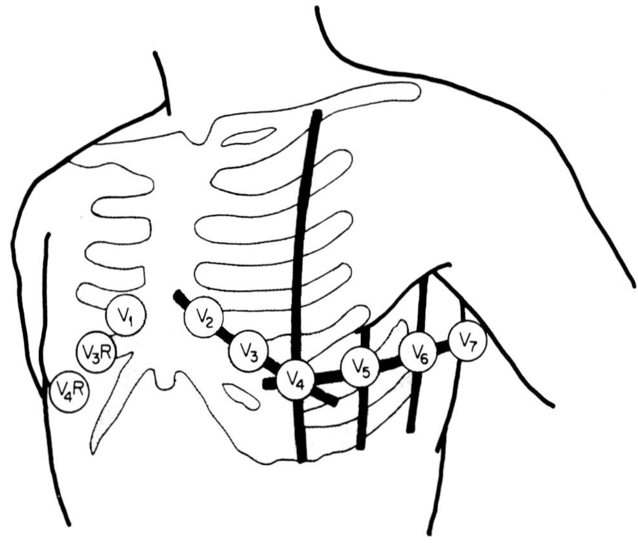

Figure 14–27 The locations of the precordial leads. *Heavy vertical lines* represent the midclavicular, anterior, axillary, and midaxillary lines (from left to right). V_1 and V_2 are referenced to the fourth intercostal space and V_4 to the fifth space. V_3 lies on a line between V_2 and V_4. V_5 and V_6 lie on a horizontal line from V_4. Additional precordial leads can be obtained on the right side (V_3R, V_4R), as well as extending farther left from V_6 (V_7). (From Friedman HH: Diagnostic Electrocardiography and Vectorcardiography. New York, McGraw-Hill, 1985, p 41; with permission of The McGraw-Hill Companies.)

amplitude (by a factor of 1.5) by severing the connection between the central terminal and the lead extremity being studied (which he called *augmented limb leads*) in 1942. These three lead groups, the bipolar limb leads, the unipolar precordial leads, and the augmented unipolar limb leads, form what was accepted by the AHA as the conventional 12-lead ECG system.[512]

Frank Leads

As early as 1920, Mann introduced the concept of vectorcardiography (VCG), which measures the time course of the mean instantaneous spatial cardiac vectors. This was represented by a loop in the frontal plane, although it was not until the invention of the cathode ray oscilloscope that it could be directly recorded. Use of the frontal plane bipolar leads has limitations. Lead I, although oriented horizontally (the x direction), is only an approximation, because current flow in the lead field is not uniform or solely in the x direction (based on the dipole theory).[525] A number of alternate lead systems allowing more accurate depiction of the vector loop in the three orthogonal axes (transverse x, vertical y, and sagittal z leads) were investigated. The most widely accepted is that of Frank, which uses seven exploring electrodes that are interconnected by a resistor network to derive approximately uniform vector fields of equal magnitude in the x, y, and z axes. It is properly called a *corrected orthogonal lead system* because it assumes that the body volume conductor is nonuniform, the heart is eccentric as a source, there are a number of dipoles, and there is variation in the vectorial expression of the magnitude of an electrical signal.[527] The Frank lead system allowed standardized recording of the VCG, although it has never been widely accepted due to its complexity. Nonetheless, the VCG may be superior to the 12-lead ECG in diagnosing myocardial infarction and in detecting RV hypertrophy or atrial enlargement.[527] Some clinical studies report increased sensitivity and earlier detection of perioperative ischemia using continuous computerized vectorcardiography, which may facilitate use of this lead system in the near future.

Detection of Myocardial Ischemia

Pathophysiology of ST-Segment Responses

The ST segment is the most important portion of the QRS complex for evaluating ischemia[528,529] (Box 14–14). The origin of this segment, at the J point, is easy to locate. Its end, which is generally accepted as the beginning of any change of slope of the T wave, is more difficult to determine. In normal individuals, there may be no discernible ST segment as the T wave starts with a steady slope from the J point, especially at rapid heart rates. The TP segment has been used as the isoelectric baseline from which changes in the ST segment are evaluated, but with tachycardia, this segment is eliminated, and during

BOX 14–14 ***Monitoring for Myocardial Ischemia***

- (Preoperative) clinical symptoms
- Electrocardiogram (leads II, $V_{3,4,5}$)
- Transesophageal echocardiography
- Pulmonary artery catheterization

exercise testing, the PR segment is used. The PR segment is used in all ST-segment analyzers.

Repolarization of the ventricle proceeds from the epicardium to the endocardium, opposite to the vector of depolarization. The ST segment reflects the midportion, or phase 2, of repolarization during which there is little change in electrical potential.[527] It is usually isoelectric. Ischemia causes a loss of intracellular potassium, resulting in a *current of injury*. The electrophysiologic mechanism accounting for ST-segment shifts (elevation or depression) remains controversial. The two major theories are based on a loss of resting potential as current flows from the uninjured to the injured area (i.e., diastolic current) and on a true change in phase 2 potential as current flows from the injured to the uninjured area (i.e., systolic current). With subendocardial injury, the ST segment is depressed in the surface leads. With epicardial or transmural injury, the ST segment is elevated. When a lead is placed directly on the endocardium, opposite patterns are recorded.

Electrocardiographic Manifestations of Ischemia

With myocardial ischemia, repolarization is affected, resulting in downsloping or horizontal ST-segment depression. Various local effects and differences in vectors during repolarization result in different ST morphologies that are recorded by the different leads. It is generally accepted that ST changes in multiple leads are associated with more severe degrees of coronary artery disease.

The classic criterion for ischemia is 0.1 mV (1 mm) of ST-segment depression measured 60 to 80 msec after the J point.[529,528] The slope of the segment must be horizontal or downsloping. Downsloping depression may be associated with a greater number of diseased vessels and a worse prognosis than horizontal depression. Slowly upsloping depression with a slope of 1 mV/sec or less is also used, but is considered less sensitive and specific (and difficult to assess clinically). The magnitude of ST-segment depression is directly related to the height of the associated R wave. Given that R waves are highest in the lateral precordium and lowest in the inferior regions, some have proposed "normalizing" ST depression for this variable.[530] However, this is controversial and not practical clinically. Nonspecific ST-segment depression can be related to drug use, particularly digoxin.[531] Interpretation of ST-segment changes in patients with LV hypertrophy is particularly controversial given the tall R-wave baseline, J-point depression, and steep slope of the ST segment. Although a number of studies have excluded such patients, others (including those using other modalities or epidemiologic studies) observed that LV hypertrophy is a highly significant predictor of adverse cardiac outcome.[532]

The criteria for ischemia with ST-segment elevation (≥0.1 mV in ≥2 contiguous leads) are used in conjunction with clinical symptoms or elevation of biochemical markers to diagnose acute coronary syndromes. It usually results from transmural ischemia, but it may potentially represent a *reciprocal change* in a lead oriented opposite to the primary vector with subendocardial ischemia (as may be seen in the reverse situation).[533,534] Perioperative ambulatory monitoring studies have also included more than 0.2 mV in any single lead as a criterion, but ST elevation is rarely reported in the setting of noncardiac surgery. It is commonly observed, however, during weaning from CPB in cardiac surgery, and during CABG surgery (on and off pump) with interruption of coronary flow in a native or graft vessel. ST elevation in a Q-wave lead should not be analyzed for acute ischemia, although it may indicate the presence of a ventricular aneurysm.

Despite the clinical focus on the ST segment for monitoring, the earliest electrocardiographic change at the onset of transmural ischemia is the almost immediate onset of tall and peaked (i.e., hyperacute) T waves, a so-called primary change. This phase is often transient. A significant increase in R-wave amplitude may also occur at this time.[535] T-wave inversions (symmetrical inversion) commonly accompany transmural ST-segment elevation changes, although most T-wave inversions or flattening observed perioperatively is nonspecific, resulting from transient alterations of repolarization due to changes in electrolytes, sympathetic tone, and other noncardiac factors.

Although repolarization changes (e.g., ST-T wave) are the focus of ischemia detection, computerized electrocardiographic analysis using signal averaging techniques has well documented changes in depolarization with ischemia manifested by reduction in high-frequency components of the QRS complex (150 to 250 Hz). Such changes are not visible on the standard ECG as they are in the range of only 10 to 20 μV and are measured quantitatively using the root mean square (RMS) value (calculated by squaring the amplitude of each sample, determining the means of the squares, and then the square root of that mean value). Absolute changes in the RMS value above 0.6 μV or relative changes of more than 20% are considered clinically significant. This effect is likely due to slowing of conduction velocity in the ischemic region.[536] One study documented higher sensitivity of this approach compared with 12-lead ST-segment analysis in the detection of acute coronary occlusion during percutaneous transluminal coronary angioplasty.[537] The overall sensitivity was 88%, compared with 71% using ST-segment elevation criteria, or 79% by combining ST-segment elevation and depression. Its greatest value was in the detection of circumflex and right coronary occlusions.

Although this technology has been applied in several studies of patients undergoing cardiac surgery, all compared preoperative data with late (>1 week) postoperative data. Matsushita et al,[538] however, described its perioperative use in 70 patients undergoing CABG or valve surgery, evaluating RMS values 1 to 2 hours after removal of the aortic cross-clamp. Dividing patients into quartiles of RMS values, they observed that decreases in cardiac index correlated significantly with progressive reductions in RMS, use of inotropes, and longer cross-clamp times. At a threshold of 35% of preoperative values, a low CO syndrome was more common. They hypothesized that the increase in intracellular calcium with ischemia is the common thread linking changes in conduction velocity with function. They recommend more common use of this technology because it is performed using an orthogonal lead set, which avoids the surgical field, is nearly real-time in nature, and extends the connection between ECG-derived parameters and cardiac function. Although intriguing, further studies from other groups are clearly required. It is unlikely this will be used commonly in the near future given the expense of replacing or upgrading existing equipment, but it remains a fertile topic for research.

Clinical Lead Systems for Detecting Ischemia

Early clinical reports of intraoperative monitoring using the V_5 lead in high-risk patients were based on observations during exercise testing, in which bipolar configurations of V_5 demonstrated high sensitivity for myocardial ischemia detection (up to 90%). Subsequent studies using 12-lead monitoring (torso mounted for stability during exercise) confirmed the sensitivity of the lateral precordial leads.[539,540] Some studies, however, reported higher sensitivity for leads V_4 or V_6 compared with V_5, followed by the inferior leads (in which most false-positive responses were reported).[541–548]

The factors responsible for precipitating ischemia during exercise testing and surgical settings may differ. For example, during exercise stress testing, most ischemia is demand related, whereas in the perioperative period, a larger proportion may be related to reduced oxygen supply. The most sensitive leads during exercise testing, however, are useful in the perioperative setting.

Given the relatively low sensitivity and specificity of the ECG, radionuclide and echocardiographic imaging are now routinely used in addition to the ECG in cardiology evaluations, but they are not practical in most perioperative settings. Other infrequently used parameters, such as R-wave amplitude and various patterns of heart rate change (e.g., heart rate recovery after exercise, heart rate change related to the slope of the ST segment) have been proposed as more sensitive means of detecting ischemia, compared with isolated ST-segment depression.

With the widespread growth of percutaneous coronary intervention for acute myocardial infraction and unstable angina in the 1990s, a number of investigators have reported on the use of continuous electrocardiographic monitoring (3 or 12 leads) in this setting. These observations have extended the classic teaching regarding localization of sites of coronary artery occlusion. Horacek and Wagner[549] reviewed the complexities and controversies regarding vessel-specific electrocardiographic responses to acute myocardial ischemia in detail. In general, ST-segment elevation in leads V_2 and V_3 is most sensitive for occlusion of the left anterior descending artery, and leads III and aVF are most sensitive for the right coronary artery. In contrast, circumflex occlusion results in variable responses, with primary elevation in the posterior precordial leads V_7 through V_9 (which are rarely monitored clinically), and reciprocal ST-segment depression in the standard precordial leads (V_2 or V_3).[550,551] For transmural ischemia, sensitivity is highest in the anterior rather than the lateral precordial leads. An international multidisciplinary working group specifically recommended continuous monitoring of leads III, V_3, and V_5 for all acute coronary syndrome patients.[552]

Intraoperative Lead Systems

Detection of perioperative myocardial ischemia has received considerable attention over the past several decades and more recently with publication of several studies of clinical monitoring and therapy (e.g., perioperative β-blockade). Many of these studies demonstrated associations of perioperative ischemia with adverse cardiac outcomes in adults undergoing

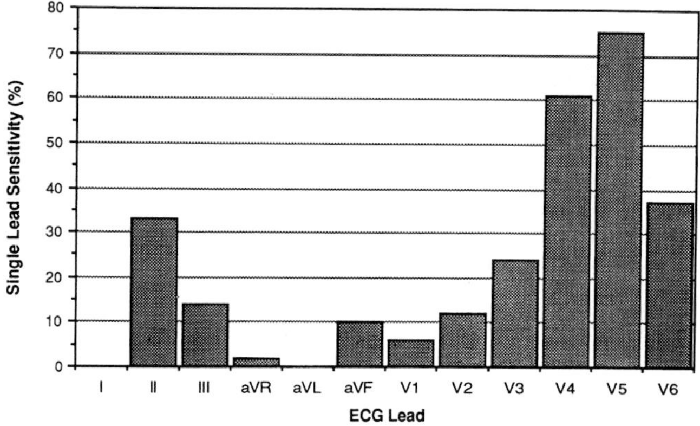

Figure 14–28 Single-lead sensitivity for the intraoperative detection of ischemia based on 51 episodes detected in 25 patients undergoing noncardiac surgery. Sensitivity was calculated by dividing the number of episodes detected in that lead by the total number of episodes. Sensitivity was greatest in lead V_5, and the lateral leads (I, aVL) were insensitive. (From London MJ, Hollenberg M, Wong MG, et al: Intraoperative myocardial ischemia: Localization by continuous 12-lead electrocardiography. Anesthesiology 69:232, 1988.)

a variety of cardiac and noncardiac surgical procedures, particularly major vascular surgery.[553–556] The ease of use of new ST-segment trending software in operating room monitors has resulted in its routine use in many low-risk surgical patients, which may result in false-positive responses (although these are uncommon). Perhaps the bigger challenge is interpreting minor ST-segment changes in the context of the overall risk profile of the patient to avoid costly diagnostic tests being performed inappropriately. Studies document that transient myocardial ischemia occurs in the absence of significant coronary artery disease in unexpected patients, such as parturients, particularly with significant hemodynamic stress or hemorrhage.[557] Although the precise cause of such changes is uncertain, significant troponin release has been documented in these patients, confirming the suspicion that these electrocardiographic changes are true ischemic responses (probably related to subendocardial ischemia due to global hypoperfusion).

The recommended leads for intraoperative monitoring, based on several clinical studies, do not differ substantially from those used during exercise testing although considerable controversy as to the optimal leads persists in both clinical settings. The coronary care unit's use of continuous electrocardiographic monitoring has received increasing attention.[558] The most widely quoted clinical study using continuous, computerized 12-lead ECG analysis in a mixed cohort (for vascular and other noncardiac procedures) by London et al[559] reported that almost 90% of responses involved ST-segment depression alone (75% in V_5 and 61% in V_4). In approximately 70% of patients, significant changes were observed in multiple leads. The sensitivity of each of the 12 leads in that study is shown in Figure 14–28. When considered in combination (as occurs clinically), the use of leads V_4 and V_5 increased sensitivity to 90%, whereas sensitivity for the standard clinical combination of leads II and V_5 was only 80%. Use of leads V_2 through V_5 and lead II captured all episodes (Table 14–7).

A larger clinical study by Landesberg et al[560] of patients undergoing vascular surgery using a longer period of monitoring (up to 72 hours) with more specific criteria for ischemia (>10 minute duration of episode) extended these observations. The reported that V_3 was most sensitive for ischemia

Table 14–7 Sensitivity for Different Electrocardiographic Lead Combinations

Number of Leads	Combination	Sensitivity (%)
1 lead	II	33
	V_4	61
	V_5	75
2 leads	II/V_5	80
	II/V_4	82
	V_4/V_5	90
3 leads	$V_3/V_4/V_5$	94
	$II/V_4/V_5$	96
4 leads	$II/V_2–V_5$	100

Data from London MJ, Hollenberg M, Wong MG, et al: Intraoperative myocardial ischemia: Localization by continuous 12-lead electrocardiography. Anesthesiology 69:232, 1988.

(87%) followed by V_4 (79%), whereas V_5 alone was only 66% sensitive.[560] In the subgroup of patients in whom prolonged ischemic episodes ultimately culminated in infarction, V_4 was most sensitive (83%). In this study, all myocardial infarctions were non-Q-wave events detected by troponin elevation. Use of two precordial leads detected 97% to 100% of changes. Based on analysis of the resting isoelectric levels of each of the 12 leads (a unique component of this study), it was recommended that V_4 was the best single choice for monitoring of a single precordial lead, as it was most likely to be isoelectric relative to the resting 12-lead preoperative ECG. In contrast, the baseline ST segment was more likely above isoelectric in V_1 through V_3 and below isoelectric in V_5 and V_6. Surprisingly, no episodes of ST elevation occurred in this study, as opposed to 12% in the earlier study of London et al,[559] in which such changes were detected in inferior and anteroseptal precordial leads.

Martinez et al[561] evaluated a cohort of vascular patients monitored in the ICU for the first postoperative day with continuous 12-lead monitoring using a threshold of 20 minutes for an ischemic episode. Eleven percent of 149 patients met criteria, with ST depression in 71% and ST elevation alone in 18% (12% had both). Most changes were detected in V_2 (53%) and V_3 (65%). Using the standard two-lead system (II and V_5), only 41% of episodes would have been detected.

Although these studies clearly support the value of precordial monitoring in patients at risk for subendocardial ischemia, clinicians must be vigilant for the rare patient with acute Q-wave infarction (most commonly in the inferior leads). The studies previously cited have all been conducted in patients undergoing noncardiac surgery, because it is not practical to conduct such studies in those with open chests or extensive surgical dressings in the precordial region. There is no reason, however, to assume that there would be any significant differences in the cardiac patient. Sudden episodes of acute transmural ischemia (associated with ST-segment elevation) are much more likely in this setting from acute ischemia/infarction (e.g., thrombotic occlusion) or surgery-induced reductions in coronary blood flow. The use of multiple precordial leads, although appealing, is not likely to become common clinical practice, due to the limitations of existing monitors (and cables). Even if such equipment were available, it is likely that considerable resistance would occur from practitioners due to the extra effort associated with this approach. Perhaps, in the future, when lower cost wireless technologies are perfected, this approach may become a clinical reality.

Arrhythmia and Pacemaker Detection

Use of inferior leads allows superior discrimination of P-wave morphology, facilitating visual diagnosis of arrhythmias and conduction disorders. Although esophageal (and even intracardiac) leads allow the greatest sensitivity in detecting P waves, these are rarely used clinically. Nevertheless, they should be kept in mind for difficult diagnoses. With the increasing use of implantable defibrillators and automatic external defibrillators to treat ventricular fibrillation and ventricular tachycardia, there is considerable interest in the refinement of arrhythmia detection algorithms and their validation.[562] As expected, the devices' accuracy for detecting ventricular arrhythmias is high, but is much lower for detecting atrial arrhythmias. In the settings of critical care and ambulatory monitoring, a variety of artifacts are common causes of false-positive responses.[563]

Detection of pacemaker spikes may be complicated by very-low-amplitude signals related to bipolar pacing leads, amplitude varying with respiration, and total-body fluid accumulation.[518,562] Most critical care and ambulatory monitors incorporate pacemaker spike enhancement for small high-frequency signals (typically 5 to 500 mV with 0.5- to 2-msec pulse duration) to facilitate recognition. However, this can lead to artifact if there is high-frequency noise within the lead system.

SUMMARY

The choice of appropriate monitoring is a difficult task. Despite many years of clinical experience, there are no convincing outcome data that demonstrate the superiority of more invasive versus less invasive monitoring techniques. The clinician therefore must make a rational decision based on the following conditions:

- The patient's underlying medical diseases
- The degree of hemodynamic compromise, myocardial ischemia risk, and fluid shift likely to result from the proposed surgery
- The effects of the anesthetic drugs and techniques on the patient's cardiovascular system
- The skills of the practitioner and his or her understanding of the risks, benefits, and alternatives to the different types of monitoring.

REFERENCES

1. O'Brien E, Waeber B, Parati G, et al: Blood pressure measuring devices: Recommendations of the European Society of Hypertension. BMJ 322:531, 2001
2. Jones DW, Appel LJ, Sheps SG, et al: Measuring blood pressure accurately: New and persistent challenges. JAMA 289:1027, 2003
3. Parati G, Ongaro G, Bilo G, Glavina F: Non-invasive beat-to-beat blood pressure monitoring: New developments. Blood Press Monit 8:31, 2003
4. Belani K, Ozaki M, Hynson J, et al: A new noninvasive method to measure blood pressure: Results of a multicenter trial. Anesthesiology 91:686, 1999
5. Dorje P, Tremper K: Systolic pressure variation: A dynamic measure of the adequacy of intravascular volume. Semin Anesth Periop Med Pain 24:147–153, 2005

6. Gunn SR, Pinsky MR: Implications of arterial pressure variation in patients in the intensive care unit. Curr Opin Crit Care 7:212, 2001
7. Coriat P, Vrillon M, Perel A, et al: A comparison of systolic blood pressure variations and echocardiographic estimates of end-diastolic left ventricular size in patients after aortic surgery. Anesth Analg 78:56, 1994
8. Remington JW: Contour changes of the aortic pulse during propagation. Am J Physiol 199:331, 1960
9. Husum B, Palm T, Eriksen J: Percutaneous cannulation of the dorsalis pedis artery. Br J Anaesth 51:1055, 1979
10. Kim JM, Arakawa K, Bliss J: Arterial cannulation: Factors in the development of occlusion. Anesth Analg 54:836, 1975
11. Grossman W, Baim DS: Cardiac Catheterization, Angiography, and Intervention. 6th edition. Baltimore, Lippincott Williams & Wilkins, 2000
12. Hunziker P: Accuracy and dynamic response of disposable pressure transducer-tubing systems. Can J Anaesth 34:409, 1987
13. Hill DW: Physics Applied to Anesthesia, 4th edition. London, Butterworth, 1980
14. Maloy L, Gardner RM: Monitoring systemic arterial blood pressure: Strip chart recording versus digital display. Heart Lung 15:627, 1986
15. Mitchell MM, Meathe EA, Jones BR, et al: Accurate, automated, continuously displayed pulmonary artery pressure measurement. Anesthesiology 67:294, 1987
16. Tuncali BE, Kuvaki B, Tuncali B, Capar E: A comparison of the efficacy of heparinized and nonheparinized solutions for maintenance of perioperative radial arterial catheter patency and subsequent occlusion. Anesth Analg 100:1117, 2005
17. Lowenstein E, Little JW, Lo HH: Prevention of cerebral embolization from flushing radial artery cannulae. N Engl J Med 285:1414, 1971
18. Kleinman B: Understanding natural frequency and damping and how they relate to the measurement of blood pressure. J Clin Monit 5:137, 1989
19. Gorback MS: Considerations in the interpretation of systemic pressure monitoring. *In* Lumb PD, Bryan-Brown CW (eds): Complications in Critical Care Medicine. Chicago, Year Book, 1988, p 296
20. Todorovic M, Jensen EW, Thogersen C: Evaluation of dynamic performance in liquid-filled catheter systems for measuring invasive blood pressure. Int J Clin Monit Comput 13:173, 1996
21. Heimann PA, Murray WB: Construction and use of catheter-manometer systems. J Clin Monit 9:45, 1993
22. Boutros A, Albert S: Effect of the dynamic response of transducer-tubing system on accuracy of direct blood pressure measurement in patients. Crit Care Med 11:124, 1983
23. Kleinman B, Frey K, Stevens R: The fast-flush test—is the clinical comparison equivalent to its in vitro simulation? J Clin Monit Comput 14:485, 1998
24. Kleinman B, Powell S, Kumar P, et al: The fast-flush test measures the dynamic response of the entire blood pressure monitoring system. Anesthesiology 77:1215, 1992
25. Schwid HA: Frequency response evaluation of radial artery catheter-manometer systems: Sinusoidal frequency analysis versus flush method. J Clin Monit 4:181, 1988
26. Gibbs NC, Gardner RM: Dynamics of invasive pressure monitoring systems: Clinical and laboratory evaluation. Heart Lung 17:43, 1988
27. Ryan JF, Raines J, Dalton BC, et al: Arterial dynamics of radial artery cannulation. Anesth Analg 52:1015, 1973
28. Shimazaki Y, Watanabe T, Takahashi T, et al: Minimized mortality and neurological complications in surgery for chronic arch aneurysm: Axillary artery cannulation, selective cerebral perfusion, and replacement of the ascending and total arch aorta. J Card Surg 19:338, 2004
29. Strauch JT, Spielvogel D, Lauten A, et al: Axillary artery cannulation: Routine use in ascending aorta and aortic arch replacement. Ann Thorac Surg 78:103, 2004
30. Sinclair MC, Singer RL, Manley NJ, et al: Cannulation of the axillary artery for cardiopulmonary bypass: Safeguards and pitfalls. Ann Thorac Surg 75:931, 2003
31. Mozersky DJ, Buckley CJ, Hagood C, et al: Ultrasonic evaluation of the palmar circulation. Am J Surg 126:810, 1973
32. Palm T: Evaluation of peripheral arterial pressure in the thumb following radial artery cannulation. Br J Anaesth 49:819, 1977
33. Allen EV: Thromboangiitis obliterans: Methods of diagnosis of chronic occlusive arterial lesions distal to the wrist with illustrated cases. Am J Med Sci 178:237, 1929
34. Greenhow DE: Incorrect performance of Allen's test: Ulnar artery flow erroneously presumed inadequate. Anesthesiology 37:356, 1972
35. Brodsky JB: A simple method to determine patency of the ulnar artery intraoperatively prior to radial artery cannulation. Anesthesiology 42:626, 1975
36. Nowak GS, Moorthy SS, McNiece WL: Use of pulse oximetry for assessment of collateral arterial flow. Anesthesiology 64:527, 1986
37. Castella X: A practical way of performing Allen's Test to assess palmar collateral circulation. Anesth Analg 77:1085, 1993
38. Kahler AC, Mirza F: Alternative arterial catheterization site using the ulnar artery in critically ill pediatric patients. Pediatr Crit Care Med 3:370, 2002
39. Marshall AG, Erwin DC, Wyse RKH, Hatch DJ: Percutaneous arterial cannulation in children. Anaesthesia 39:27, 1984
40. Slogoff S, Keats AS, Arlund C: On the safety of radial artery cannulation. Anesthesiology 59:42, 1983
41. Mangano DT, Hickey RF: Ischemic injury following uncomplicated radial artery catheterization. Anesth Analg 58:55, 1979
42. Barbeau GR, Arsenault F, Dugas L, et al: Evaluation of the ulnopalmar arterial arches with pulse oximetry and plethysmography: Comparison with the Allen's test in 1010 patients. Am Heart J 147:489, 2004
43. Gardner RM, Schwartz R, Wong HC, et al: Percutaneous indwelling radial artery catheters for monitoring cardiovascular function. N Engl J Med 290:1227, 1974
44. Rulf ENR, Mitchell MM, Prakash O: Measurement of arterial pressure after cardiopulmonary bypass with a long radial artery catheter. J Cardiothorac Anesth 4:19, 1990
45. VanBeck JO, White RD, Abenstein JP, et al: Comparison of axillary artery or brachial artery pressure with aortic pressure after cardiopulmonary bypass using a long radial artery catheter. J Cardiothorac Vasc Anesth 7:312, 1993
46. Stern DH, Gerson JL, Allen FB, et al: Can we trust the direct radial artery pressure immediately after cardiopulmonary bypass? Anesthesiology 62:557, 1985
47. Mohr R, Lavee J, Goor DA: Inaccuracy of radial artery pressure measurement after cardiac operations. J Thorac Cardiovasc Surg 94:286, 1987
48. Gravlee GP, Wong AB, Adkins TG, et al: A comparison of radial, brachial, and aortic pressures after cardiopulmonary bypass. J Cardiothorac Anesth 3:20, 1989
49. VanBeck J, White R, Abenstein J, et al: Comparison of axillary artery or brachial artery pressure with aortic pressure after cardiopulmonary bypass using a long radial artery catheter. J Cardiothorac Vasc Anesth 7:312, 1993
50. Rich G, Lubanski R, McLoughlin T: Differences between aortic and radial artery pressure associated with cardiopulmonary bypass. Anesthesiology 77:63, 1992
51. Kanazawa M, Fukuyama H, Kinefuchi Y, et al: Relationship between aortic-to-radial arterial pressure gradient after cardiopulmonary bypass and changes in arterial elasticity. Anesthesiology 99:48, 2003
52. Pascarelli EF, Bertrand CA: Comparison of blood pressures in the arms and legs. N Engl J Med 270:693, 1964
53. Bazaral MG, Welch M, Golding LAR, Badhwar K: Comparison of brachial and radial arterial pressure monitoring in patients undergoing coronary artery bypass surgery. Anesthesiology 73:38, 1990
54. Barnes RW, Foster E, Jansen GA, et al: Safety of brachial artery catheters as monitors in the intensive care unit—prospective evaluation with the Doppler ultrasonic velocity detector. Anesthesiology 44:260, 1976
55. Armstrong PJ, Han DC, Baxter JA, et al: Complication rates of percutaneous brachial artery access in peripheral vascular angiography. Ann Vasc Surg 17:107, 2003
56. Gurman GM, Kriemerman S: Cannulation of big arteries in critically ill patients. Crit Care Med 13:217, 1985
57. Yacoub OF, Bacaling JH, Kelly M: Monitoring of axillary arterial pressure in a patient with Buerger's disease requiring clipping of an intracranial aneurysm. Br J Anaesth 59:1056, 1987
58. Eriksson I, Jorulf H: Surgical complications associated with arterial catheterization. Scan J Thorac Cardiovasc Surg 4:69, 1970
59. Scheer B, Perel A, Pfeiffer UJ: Clinical review: Complications and risk factors of peripheral arterial catheters used for haemodynamic monitoring in anaesthesia and intensive care medicine. Crit Care 6:199, 2002
60. Frezza EE, Mezghebe H: Indications and complications of arterial catheter use in surgical or medical intensive care units: Analysis of 4932 patients. Am Surg 64:127, 1998
61. Kopman EA, Ferguson TB: Intraoperative monitoring of femoral artery pressure during replacement of aneurysms of the descending thoracic aorta. Anesth Analg 56:603, 1977
62. Johnstone RE, Greenhow DE: Catheterization of the dorsalis pedis artery. Anesthesiology 39:654, 1973

63. Barnhorst BA, Boener HB: Prevalence of generally absent pedal pulses. N Engl J Med 278:264, 1968
64. Youngberg JA, Miller ED: Evaluation of percutaneous cannulations of the dorsalis pedis artery. Anesthesiology 44:80, 1976
65. Prian GW: New proximal approach works well in temporal artery catheterization. JAMA 235:2693, 1976
66. Porter JM: Raynaud's syndrome. *In* Sabiston DC (ed): Textbook of Surgery. Philadelphia, WB Saunders Company, 1985, pp 1925–1932
67. Mangar D, Thrush D, Connell G, et al: Direct or modified Seldinger guidewire-directed technique for arterial catheter insertion. Anesth Analg 76:714, 1993
68. Fukutome T, Kojiro M, Tanigawa K, Sese A: Doppler-guided "percutaneous" radial artery cannulation in small children. Anesthesiology 69:434, 1988
69. Morray JP, Brandford GH, Barnes LF, et al: Doppler-assisted radial artery cannulation in infants and children. Anesth Analg 63:346, 1984
70. Levin PD, Sheinin O, Gozal Y: Use of ultrasound guidance in the insertion of radial artery catheters. Crit Care Med 31:481, 2003
71. Band JD, Maki DG: Infection caused by arterial catheters used for hemodynamic monitoring. Am J Med 67:735, 1979
72. Shinozaki T, Deane R, Mazuzan JE, et al: Bacterial contamination of arterial lines: A prospective study. JAMA 249:223, 1983
73. Weinstein RA, Stamm WE, Kramer L: Pressure monitoring devices: Overlooked sources of nosocomial infection. JAMA 236:936, 1976
74. Stamm WE, Colella JJ, Anderson RL, et al: Indwelling arterial catheters as a source of nosocomial bacteremia. N Engl J Med 292:1099, 1975
75. Rijnders BJ, Van Wijngaerden E, Wilmer A, Peetermans WE: Use of full sterile barrier precautions during insertion of arterial catheters: A randomized trial. Clin Infect Dis 36:743, 2003
76. Sherertz RJ: Update on vascular catheter infections. Curr Opin Infect Dis 17:303, 2004
77. O'Grady NP, Alexander M, Dellinger EP, et al: Guidelines for the prevention of intravascular catheter-related infections. Centers for Disease Control and Prevention. MMWR Recomm Rep 51(RR-10):1, 2002
78. Rijnders BJ, Peetermans WE, Verwaest C: Watchful waiting versus immediate catheter removal in ICU patients with suspected catheter-related infection: A randomized trial. Intensive Care Med 30:1073, 2004
79. Mermel LA, Farr BM, Sherertz RJ, et al: Guidelines for the management of intravascular catheter-related infections. Clin Infect Dis 32:1249, 2001
80. Pierson DJ, Hudson LD: Monitoring hemodynamics in the critically ill. Med Clin North Am 67:1343, 1983
81. Scheer B, Perel A, Pfeiffer UJ: Clinical review: Complications and risk factors of peripheral arterial catheters used for haemodynamic monitoring in anaesthesia and intensive care medicine. Crit Care 6:199, 2002
82. Bedford RF, Wollman H: Complications of percutaneous radial artery cannulation: An objective prospective study in man. Anesthesiology 38:228, 1973
83. Bedford RF: Radial arterial function following percutaneous cannulation with 18- and 20-gauge catheters. Anesthesiology 47:37, 1977
84. Bedford RF: Wrist circumference predicts the risk of radial arterial occlusion after cannulation. Anesthesiology 48:377, 1978
85. Jones RM, Hill AB, Nahrwold ML, Bolles RE: The effect of method of radial artery cannulation on postcannulation blood flow and thrombus formation. Anesthesiology 55:76, 1981
86. Bedford RF, Ashford TP: Aspirin pretreatment prevents post-cannulation radial artery thrombosis. Anesthesiology 51:176, 1979
87. Wong AY, O'Regan AM: Gangrene of digits associated with radial artery cannulation. Anaesthesia 58:1034, 2003
88. Green JA, Tonkin MA: Ischaemia of the hand in infants following radial or ulnar artery catheterisation. Hand Surg 4:151, 1999
89. Bright E, Baines DB, French BG, et al: Upper limb amputation following radial artery cannulation. Anaesth Intensive Care 21:351, 1993
90. Kim JM, Arakawa K, Bliss J: Arterial cannulation: Factors in the development of occlusion. Anesth Analg 54:836, 1975
91. Vender JS, Watts RD: Differential diagnosis of hand ischemia in the presence of an arterial cannula. Anesth Analg 61:465, 1982
92. Goldstein RD, Gordon MJV: Volar proximal skin necrosis after radial artery cannulation. N Y State J Med 90:375, 1990
93. Wyatt R, Glaves I, Cooper DJ: Proximal skin necrosis after radial artery cannulation. Lancet 1:1135, 1974
94. Chang C, Dughi J, Shitabata P, et al: Air embolism and the radial arterial line. Crit Care Med 16:141, 1988
95. Zavela NG, Gravlee GP, Bewckart DH, et al: Unusual cause of hypotension after cardiopulmonary bypass. J Cardiothorac Vasc Anesth 10:553, 1996
96. Qvist J, Peterfreund R, Perlmutter G: Transient compartment syndrome of the forearm after attempted radial artery cannulation. Anesth Analg 83:183, 1996
97. Edwards DP, Clarke MD, Barker P: Acute presentation of bilateral radial artery pseudoaneurysms following arterial cannulation. Eur J Vasc Endovasc Surg 17:456, 1999
98. Knight CG, Healy DA, Thomas RL: Femoral artery pseudoaneurysms: Risk factors, prevalence, and treatment options. Ann Vasc Surg 17:503, 2003
99. O'Rourke RA, Silverman ME, Shaver J: The history, physical examination, and cardiac auscultation. *In* Fuster V, Alexander RW, O'Rourke RA, et al (eds): The Heart, 11th edition. New York, McGraw-Hill, 2004, pp 217–294
100. Mark JB: Central venous pressure monitoring: Clinical insights beyond the numbers. J Cardiothorac Anesth 5:163, 1991
101. Luecke T, Roth H, Herrmann P, et al: Assessment of cardiac preload and left ventricular function under increasing levels of positive end-expiratory pressure. Intensive Care Med 30:119, 2004
102. Mangano DT: Monitoring pulmonary arterial pressure in coronary artery disease. Anesthesiology 53:364, 1980
103. Kumar A, Anel R, Bunnell E, et al: Pulmonary artery occlusion pressure and central venous pressure fail to predict ventricular filling volume, cardiac performance, or the response to volume infusion in normal subjects. Crit Care Med 32:691, 2004
104. Buhre W, Weyland A, Schorn B, et al: Changes in central venous pressure and pulmonary capillary wedge pressure do not indicate changes in right and left heart volume in patients undergoing coronary artery bypass surgery. Eur J Anaesthesiol 16:11, 1999
105. Godje O, Peyerl M, Seebauer T, et al: Central venous pressure, pulmonary capillary wedge pressure and intrathoracic blood volumes as preload indicators in cardiac surgery patients. Eur J Cardiothorac Surg 13:533, 1998
106. Lichtwarck-Aschoff M, Beale R, Pfeiffer UJ: Central venous pressure, pulmonary artery occlusion pressure, intrathoracic blood volume, and right ventricular end-diastolic volume as indicators of cardiac preload. J Crit Care 11:180, 1996
107. English IC, Frew RM, Pigott JF, et al: Percutaneous catheterization of the internal jugular vein. Anesthesia 24:521, 1969
108. Muralidhar K: Left internal versus right internal jugular vein access to central venous circulation using the Seldinger technique. J Cardiothorac Anesth 9:115, 1995
109. Neustein S, Narang J, Bronheim D: Use of the color test for safer internal jugular vein cannulation. Anesthesiology 76:1062, 1992
110. Jobes DR, Schwartz AJ, Greenhow DE, et al: Safer jugular vein cannulation: Recognition of arterial puncture. Anesthesiology 59:353, 1983
111. Fabian JA, Jesudian MC: A simple method for improving the safety of percutaneous cannulation of the internal jugular vein. Anesth Analg 64:1032, 1985
112. Petty C: Alternate methods of internal jugular venipuncture for monitoring central venous pressure. Anesth Analg 54:157, 1975
113. Kuramoto T, Sakav T: Comparison of success in jugular versus basilic vein techniques for central venous pressure catheter positioning. Anesth Analg 54:696, 1975
114. Prince SR, Sullivan RL, Hackel A: Percutaneous catheterization of the internal jugular vein of infants and children. Anesthesiology 44:170, 1976
115. Hayashi Y, Uchida O, Takaki O, et al: Internal jugular vein catheterization in infants undergoing cardiovascular surgery: An analysis of the factors influencing successful catheterization. Anesth Analg 74:688, 1992
116. Denys BG, Uretsky BF: Anatomical variations of internal jugular vein location: Impact on central venous access. Crit Care Med 19:1516, 1991
117. Hind D, Calvert N, McWilliams R, et al: Ultrasonic locating devices for central venous cannulation: Meta-analysis. BMJ 327:361, 2003
118. Grebenik CR, Boyce A, Sinclair ME, et al: NICE guidelines for central venous catheterization in children. Is the evidence base sufficient? Br J Anaesth 92:827, 2004
119. Asheim P, Mostad U, Aadahl P: Ultrasound-guided central venous cannulation in infants and children. Acta Anaesthesiol Scand 46:390, 2002
120. Liberman L, Hordof AJ, Hsu DT, et al: Ultrasound-assisted cannulation of the right internal jugular vein during electrophysiologic studies in children. J Interv Card Electrophysiol 5:177, 2001
121. Verghese ST, McGill WA, Patel RI, et al: Ultrasound-guided internal jugular venous cannulation in infants: A prospective comparison with the traditional palpation method. Anesthesiology 91:71, 1999
122. Verghese ST, McGill WA, Patel RI, et al: Comparison of three techniques for internal jugular vein cannulation in infants. Paediatr Anaesth 10:505, 2000

123. Randolph AG, Cook DJ, Gonzales CA, Pribble CG: Ultrasound guidance for placement of central venous catheters: A meta-analysis of the literature. Crit Care Med 24:2053, 1996
124. Gratz I, Ashar M, Kidwell P, et al: Doppler-guided cannulation of the internal jugular vein: A prospective, randomized trial. J Clin Monit 10:185, 1994
125. Troianos CA, Jobes DR, Ellison N: Ultrasound-guided cannulation of the internal jugular vein: A prospective, randomized study. Anesth Analg 72:823, 1991
126. Riopelle J, Ruiz D, Hunt J, et al: Circumferential adjustment of ultrasound probe position to determine the optimal approach to the internal jugular vein: A noninvasive geometric study in adults [Erratum in Anesth Analg 101:924, 2005]. Anesth Analg 100:512, 2005
127. Denys BG, Uretsky BF, Reddy PS: Ultrasound assisted cannulation of the internal jugular vein. A prospective comparison to the external landmark-guided technique. Circulation 87:1557, 1993
128. Troianos CA, Kuwik R, Pasqual J, et al: Internal jugular vein and carotid artery anatomic relation as determined by ultrasonography. Anesthesiology 85:43, 1996
129. Alderson PJ, Burrows FA, Stemp LI, et al: Use of ultrasound to evaluate internal jugular vein anatomy and to facilitate central venous cannulation of paediatric patients. Br J Anaesth 70:145, 1993
130. Sulek CA, Gravenstein N, Blackshear RH, Weiss L: Head rotation during internal jugular vein cannulation and the risk of carotid artery puncture. Anesth Analg 82:125, 1996
131. Mallory DL, Showker T, Evans G, et al: Effects of clinical maneuvers on sonographically determined internal jugular vein size during venous cannulation. Crit Care Med 18:1269, 1990
132. Parry G: Trendelenburg position, head elevation and a midline position optimize right internal jugular vein diameter. Can J Anaesth 51:379, 2004
133. Bevilacqua S, Romagnoli S, Ciappi F, et al: Transpharyngeal ultrasonography for cannulation of the internal jugular vein. Anesthesiology 102:873, 2005
134. Blitt CD, Wright WA, Petty WC, et al: Cardiovascular catheterization via the external jugular vein: A technique employing the J-wire. JAMA 229:817, 1974
135. Defalque RJ: Subclavian venipuncture: A review. Anesth Analg 47:677, 1968
136. Wistbacka JO, Nuutinen LS: Catheter-related complications of total parenteral nutrition (TPN): A review. Acta Anaesthesiol Scand 29:S84, 1985
137. Kaufman B: Pitfalls of central hemodynamic monitoring. Resident Staff Physician 30:27, 1992
138. Lefrant JY, Muller L, De La Coussaye JE, et al: Risk factors of failure and immediate complication of subclavian vein catheterization in critically ill patients. Intensive Care Med 28:1036, 2002
139. Fangio P, Mourgeon E, Romelaer A, et al: Aortic injury and cardiac tamponade as a complication of subclavian venous catheterization. Anesthesiology 96:1520, 2002
140. Kitagawa N, Oda M, Totoki T, et al: Proper shoulder position for subclavian venipuncture. Anesthesiology 101:1306–1312, 2004
141. Kellner GA, Smart JF: Percutaneous placement of catheters to monitor "central venous pressure." Anesthesiology 36:515, 1972
142. Webre DR, Arens JF: Use of cephalic and basilic veins for introduction of cardiovascular catheters. Anesthesiology 38:389, 1973
143. Nadroo AM, Lin J, Green RS, et al: Death as a complication of peripherally inserted central catheters in neonates. J Pediatr 138:599, 2001
144. Nadroo AM, Glass RB, Lin J, et al: Changes in upper extremity position cause migration of peripherally inserted central catheters in neonates. Pediatrics 110:131, 2002
145. Loewenthal MR, Dobson PM, Starkey RE, et al: The peripherally inserted central catheter (PICC): A prospective study of its natural history after cubital fossa insertion. Anaesth Intensive Care 30:21, 2002
146. Burgess GE, Marino RJ, Peuler MJ: Effect of head position on the location of venous catheters inserted via the basilic vein. Anesthesiology 46:212, 1977
147. Artru AA, Colley PS: Placement of multiorificed CVP catheters via antecubital veins using intravascular electrocardiography. Anesthesiology 69:132, 1988
148. Mongan P, Peterson R, Culling R: Pressure monitoring can accurately position catheters for air embolism aspiration. J Clin Monit 8:121, 1992
149. Roth S, Aronson S: Placement of a right atrial air aspiration catheter guided by transesophageal echocardiography. Anesthesiology 83:1359, 1995
150. Kumar M, Amin M: The peripherally inserted central venous catheter: friend or foe? Int J Oral Maxillofac Surg 33:201, 2004
151. Parikh S, Narayanan V: Misplaced peripherally inserted central catheter: An unusual cause of stroke. Pediatr Neurol 30:210, 2004
152. Pettit J: Assessment of infants with peripherally inserted central catheters. Part 1. Detecting the most frequently occurring complications. Adv Neonatal Care 2:304, 2002
153. Smith JR, Friedell ML, Cheatham ML, et al: Peripherally inserted central catheters revisited. Am J Surg 176:208, 1998
154. Bansmer G, Keith D, Tesluk H: Complications following the use of indwelling catheters of the inferior vena cava. JAMA 167:1606, 1958
155. Durbec O, Viviand X, Potie F, et al: A prospective evaluation of the use of femoral venous catheters in critically ill adults. Crit Care Med 25:1986, 1997
156. Pawar M, Mehta Y, Kapoor P, et al: Central venous catheter-related bloodstream infections: Incidence, risk factors, outcome, and associated pathogens. J Cardiothorac Vasc Anesth 18:304, 2004
157. Timsit JF, Bruneel F, Cheval C, et al: Use of tunneled femoral catheters to prevent catheter-related infection. A randomized, controlled trial. Ann Intern Med 130:729, 1999
158. Nahum E, Levy I, Katz J, et al: Efficacy of subcutaneous tunneling for prevention of bacterial colonization of femoral central venous catheters in critically ill children. Pediatr Infect Dis J 21:1000, 2002
159. Del Guercio LR, Cohn JD: Monitoring operative risk in the elderly. JAMA 243:1350, 1980
160. Applebaum RM, Adelman MA, Kanschuger MS, et al: Transesophageal echocardiographic identification of a retrograde dissection of the ascending aorta caused by inadvertent cannulation of the common carotid artery. J Am Soc Echocardiogr 10:749, 1997
161. Eckhardt W, Iaconetti D, Kwon J, et al: Inadvertent carotid artery cannulation during pulmonary artery catheter insertion. J Cardiothorac Vasc Anesth 10:283, 1996
162. Fraizer MC, Chu WW, Gudjonsson T, Wolff MR: Use of a percutaneous vascular suture device for closure of an inadvertent subclavian artery puncture. Catheter Cardiovasc Interv 59:369, 2003
163. Berlet MH, Steffen D, Shaughness G, Hanner J: Closure using a surgical closure device of inadvertent subclavian artery punctures during central venous catheter placement. Cardiovasc Intervent Radiol 24:122, 2001
164. Gobiel F, Couture P, Girard D, et al: Carotid artery-internal jugular fistula: Another complication following pulmonary artery catheterization via the internal jugular venous route. Anesthesiology 80:230, 1994
165. Robinson R, Errett L: Arteriovenous fistula following percutaneous internal jugular vein cannulation: A report of carotid artery-to-internal jugular vein fistula. J Cardiothorac Anesth 2:488, 1988
166. Kim J, Ahn W, Bahk JH: Hemomediastinum resulting from subclavian artery laceration during internal jugular catheterization. Anesth Analg 97:1257, 2003
167. Kwon SS, Falk A, Mitty HA: Thoracic duct injury associated with left internal jugular vein catheterization: Anatomic considerations. J Vasc Interv Radiol 13:337, 2002
168. Khalil DG, Parker FB, Mukherjee N, Webb WR: Thoracic duct injury: A complication of jugular vein catheterization. JAMA 221:908, 1972
169. Teba L, Dedhia HV, Bowen R, Alexander JC: Chylothorax review. Crit Care Med 13:49, 1985
170. Cook TL, Deuker CW: Tension pneumothorax following internal jugular cannulation and general anesthesia. Anesthesiology 45:554, 1976
171. Plewa MC, Ledrick D, Sferra JJ: Delayed tension pneumothorax complicating central venous catheterization and positive-pressure ventilation. Am J Emerg Med 13:532, 1995
172. Porzionato A, Montisci M, Manani G: Brachial plexus injury following subclavian vein catheterization: A case report. J Clin Anesth 15:582, 2003
173. Selander D, Dhuner K-G, Lundborg G: Peripheral nerve injury due to injection needles used for regional anesthesia. An experimental study of the acute effects of needlepoint trauma. Acta Anaesth Scand 21:182, 1977
174. Nakayama M, Fulita S, Kawamata M, et al: Traumatic aneurysm of the internal jugular vein causing vagal nerve palsy: A rare complication of percutaneous catheterization. Anesth Analg 78:598, 1994
175. Parikh RD: Horner's syndrome: A complication of percutaneous catheterization of the internal jugular vein. Anaesthesia 27:327, 1972
176. Turnage WS, Harper JV: Venous air embolism occurring after removal of a central venous catheter. Anesth Analg 72:559, 1991
177. Akazawa S, Nakaigawa Y, Hotta K: Unrecognized migration of an entire guidewire on insertion of a central venous catheter into the cardiovascular system. Anesthesiology 84:241, 1996
178. Smyth NPD, Rogers JB: Transvenous removal of catheter emboli from the heart and great veins by endoscopic forceps. Ann Thorac Surg 11:403, 1971
179. Friedman BA, Jergeleit HC: Perforation of atrium by polyethylene central venous catheter. JAMA 203:1141, 1968
180. Gravenstein N, Blackshear R: In vitro evaluation of relative perforating potential of central venous catheters: Comparison of materials, selected

models, number of lumens, and angles of incidence to simulated membrane. J Clin Monit 7:2, 1991

181. Oropello J, Leibowitz A, Manasia A, et al: Dilator-associated complications of central venous catheter insertion: Possible mechanisms of injury and suggestions. J Cardiothorac Vasc Anesth 10:634, 1996
182. Royster RL, Johnston WE, Gravlee GP, et al: Arrhythmias during venous cannulation prior to pulmonary artery catheter insertion. Anesth Analg 64:1214, 1985
183. Eissa NT, Kvetan V: Guidewire as a cause of complete heart block in patients with preexisting left bundle-branch block. Anesthesiology 73:772, 1990
184. O'Grady NP, Alexander M, Dellinger EP, et al: Guidelines for the prevention of intravascular catheter-related infections. Infect Control Hosp Epidemiol 23:759, 2002
185. Hu KK, Lipsky BA, Veenstra DL, Saint S: Using maximal sterile barriers to prevent central venous catheter-related infection: A systematic evidence-based review. Am J Infect Control 32:142, 2004
186. Timsit JF, Sebille V, Farkas JC, et al: Effect of subcutaneous tunneling on internal jugular catheter-related sepsis in critically ill patients: A prospective randomized multicenter study. JAMA 276:1416, 1996
187. Timsit JF, Bruneel F, Cheval C, et al: Use of tunneled femoral catheters to prevent catheter-related infection. A randomized, controlled trial. Ann Intern Med 130:729, 1999
188. Leon C, Alvarez-Lerma F, Ruiz-Santana S, et al: Antiseptic chamber-containing hub reduces central venous catheter-related infection: A prospective, randomized study. Crit Care Med 31:1318, 2003
189. Veenstra DL, Saint S, Saha S, et al: Efficacy of antiseptic-impregnated central venous catheters in preventing catheter-related bloodstream infection: A meta-analysis. JAMA 281:261, 1999
190. McGee D, Gould M: Preventing complications of central venous catheterization. N Engl J Med 348:1123, 2003
191. Cicalini S, Palmieri F, Petrosillo N: Clinical review: New technologies for prevention of intravascular catheter-related infections. Crit Care 8:157, 2004
192. Maki DG, Ringer M, Alvarado CJ: Prospective randomised trial of povidone-iodine, alcohol, and chlorhexidine for prevention of infection associated with central venous and arterial catheters. Lancet 338:339, 1991
193. Mimoz O, Pieroni L, Lawrence C, et al: Prospective, randomized trial of two antiseptic solutions for prevention of central venous or arterial catheter colonization and infection in intensive care unit patients. Crit Care Med 24:1818, 1996
194. Chaiyakunapruk N, Veenstra DL, Lipsky BA, Saint S: Chlorhexidine compared with povidone-iodine solution for vascular catheter-site care: A meta-analysis. Ann Intern Med 136:792, 2002
195. Humar A, Ostromecki A, Direnfeld J, et al: Prospective randomized trial of 10% povidone-iodine versus 0.5% tincture of chlorhexidine as cutaneous antisepsis for prevention of central venous catheter infection. Clin Infect Dis 31:1001, 2000
196. Mermel LA: Prevention of intravascular catheter-related infections. Ann Intern Med 132:391, 2000
197. Polderman KH, Girbes AR: Central venous catheter use. Part 2. Infectious complications. Intensive Care Med 28:18, 2002
198. Swan HJC, Ganz W, Forrester JS, et al: Catheterization of the heart in man with the use of a flow-directed balloon-tipped catheter. N Engl J Med 283:447, 1970
199. Connors AF, McCaffree DR, Gray BA: Evaluation of right-heart catheterization in the critically ill patient. N Engl J Med 308:263, 1983
200. Waller JL, Johnson SP, Kaplan JA: Usefulness of pulmonary artery catheters during aortocoronary bypass surgery. Anesth Analg 61:221, 1982
201. Iberti T, Fisher CJ: A prospective study on the use of the pulmonary artery catheter in a medical intensive care unit-Its effect on diagnosis and therapy. Crit Care Med 11:238, 1983
202. Lappas D, Lell WA, Gabel JC, et al: Indirect measurement of left atrial pressure in surgical patients—pulmonary capillary wedge and pulmonary artery diastolic pressures compared with left atrial pressure. Anesthesiology 38:394, 1973
203. Raper R, Sibbald WJ: Misled by the wedge? Chest 89:427, 1986
204. Nadeau S, Noble WH: Misinterpretation of pressure measurements from the pulmonary artery catheter. Can Anaesth Soc J 33:352, 1986
205. Tuman KJ, Carroll G, Ivankovich AD: Pitfalls in interpretation of pulmonary artery catheter data. J Cardiothorac Anesth 3:625, 1989
206. West JB: Ventilation/blood flow and gas exchange, 4th edition. Oxford, Blackwell Scientific Publications, 1970
207. Shasby DM, Dauber IM, Pfister S, et al: Swan-Ganz catheter location and left atrial pressure determine the accuracy of the wedge pressure when positive end-expiratory pressure is used. Chest 80:666, 1980
208. Lorzman J, Powers SR, Older T, et al: Correlation of pulmonary wedge and left atrial pressure: A study in the patient receiving positive end-expiratory pressure ventilation. Arch Surg 109:270, 1974
209. Kane PB, Askanazi J, Neville JF Jr, et al: Artifacts in the measurement of pulmonary artery wedge pressure. Crit Care Med 6:36, 1978
210. Rajacich N, Burchard KW, Hasan FM, Singh AK: Central venous pressure and pulmonary capillary wedge pressure as estimates of left atrial pressure: Effects of positive end-expiratory pressure and catheter tip malposition. Crit Care Med 17:7, 1989
211. Shasby DM, Dauber IM, Pfister S, et al: Swan-Ganz catheter location and left atrial pressure determine the accuracy of the wedge pressure when positive end-expiratory pressure is used. Chest 80:666, 1981
212. Teboul J-L, Zapol WM, Brun-Buisson C, et al: A comparison of pulmonary artery occlusion pressure and left ventricular end-diastolic pressure during mechanical ventilation with PEEP in patients with severe ARDS. Anesthesiology 70:261, 1989
213. Kaufman B: Pitfalls of central hemodynamic monitoring. Resident Staff Physician 30:27, 1992
214. Pinsky M, Vincent JL, DeSmet JM: Estimating the left ventricular filling pressure during positive end-expiratory pressure. Am Rev Respir Dis 25:143, 1991
215. Haskell RJ, French WJ: Accuracy of left atrial and pulmonary artery wedge pressure in pure mitral regurgitation in predicting left ventricular end-diastolic pressure. Am J Cardiol 61:136, 1988
216. Hildick-Smith DJ, Walsh JT, Shapiro LM: Pulmonary capillary wedge pressure in mitral stenosis accurately reflects mean left atrial pressure but overestimates transmitral gradient. Am J Cardiol 85:512, 2000
217. Lange RA, Moore DM, Cigarroa RG, Hillis LD: Use of pulmonary capillary wedge pressure to assess severity of mitral stenosis: Is true left atrial pressure needed in this condition? J Am Coll Cardiol 13:825, 1989
218. Entress JJ, Dhamee S, Olund T, et al: Pulmonary artery occlusion pressure is not accurate immediately after CPB. J Cardiothorac Anesth 4:558, 1990
219. Schmitt EA, Brantigan CO: Common artifacts of pulmonary artery pressures: Recognition and interpretation. J Clin Monit 2:44, 1986
220. Moore RA, Neary MJ, Gallagher HD, Clark DL: Determination of the pulmonary capillary wedge position in patients with giant left atrial V waves. J Cardiothorac Anesth 1:108, 1987
221. Haggmark S, Hohner P, Ostman M, et al: Comparison of hemodynamic, electrocardiographic, mechanical, and metabolic indicators of intraoperative myocardial ischemia in vascular surgical patients with coronary artery disease. Anesthesiology 70:19, 1989
222. van Daele ME, Sutherland GR, Mitchell MM, et al: Do changes in pulmonary capillary wedge pressure adequately reflect myocardial ischemia during anesthesia? Circulation 81:865, 1990
223. Mantia AM, Robinson JN, Lolley DM, et al: Sternal retraction and pulmonary artery catheter compromise. J Cardiothorac Anesth 2:430, 1988
224. Keusch DJ, Winters S, Thys DM: The patient's position influences the incidence of dysrhythmias during pulmonary artery catheterization. Anesthesiology 70:582, 1989
225. Waller JL, Zaidan JR, Kaplan JA, et al: Hemodynamic response to preoperative vascular cannulation in patients with coronary artery disease. Anesthesiology 56:219, 1982
226. Quintin L, Whalley DG, Wynands JE, et al: The effects of vascular catheterization upon heart rate and blood pressure before aortocoronary bypass surgery. Can Anaesth Soc J 28:244, 1981
227. Benumof JL, Saidman IJ, Arkin DB, et al: Where pulmonary artery catheters go: Intrathoracic distribution. Anesthesiology 46:336, 1977
228. Robin ED: Defenders of the pulmonary artery catheter. Chest 93:1059, 1988
229. Dalen JE, Bone RC: Is it time to pull the pulmonary artery catheter? JAMA 276:916, 1996
230. Afessa B, Spencer S, Khan W, et al: Association of pulmonary artery catheter use with in-hospital mortality. Crit Care Med 29:1145, 2001
231. Gattinoni L, Brazzi L, Pelosi P, et al: A trial of goal-oriented hemodynamic therapy in critically ill patients. N Engl J Med 333:1025, 1995
232. Tuman KJ, McCarthy RJ, Spiess BD, et al: Effect of pulmonary artery catheterization on outcome in patients undergoing coronary artery surgery. Anesthesiology 70:199, 1989
233. Taylor RW: Controversies in pulmonary artery catheterization. New Horizons 5:173, 1997
234. Guyatt G, Ontario Intensive Care Group: A randomised control trial of right heart catheterization in critically ill patients. J Intensive Care Med 6:91, 1991
235. Gore JM, Goldberg RJ, Spodick DH, et al: A community-wide assessment of the use of pulmonary artery catheters in patients with acute myocardial infarctions. Chest 92:721, 1987

236. Shoemaker WC, Appel PL, Kram HB, et al: Prospective trial of supranormal values of survivors as therapeutic goals in high-risk surgical patients. Chest 94:1176, 1988
237. Boyd O, Grounds RM, Bennett ED: A randomised clinical trial of the effect of deliberate perioperative increase of oxygen delivery on mortality in high-risk surgical patients. JAMA 270:2699, 1993
238. Sandham JD: Pulmonary artery catheter use—refining the question. Crit Care Med 32:1070, 2004
239. Gnaegi A, Feihl F, Perret C: Intensive care physicians' insufficient knowledge of right-heart catheterization at the bedside: Time to act? Crit Care Med 25:213, 1997
240. Iberti TJ, Fischer EP, Leibowitz AB, et al: A multicenter study of physicians' knowledge of the pulmonary artery catheter. JAMA 264:2928, 1990
241. Haupt M, Shoemaker W, Haddy F, et al: Correspondence: Goal-oriented hemodynamic therapy. N Engl J Med 334:799, 1996
242. Shoemaker WC, Appel PL, Kram HB, et al: Prospective trial of supranormal values of survivors as therapeutic goals in high-risk surgical patients. Chest 94:1176, 1988
243. Boyd O, Grounds RM, Bennett ED: The beneficial effect of supranormalization of oxygen delivery with dopexamine hydrochloride on perioperative mortality. JAMA 270:2699, 1993
244. Rao TLK, Jacobs KH, El-Etr AA: Reinfarction following anesthesia in patients with myocardial infarction. Anesthesiology 59:499, 1983
245. Moore CH, Lombardo TR, Allums JA, Gordon FT: Left main coronary artery stenosis: Hemodynamic monitoring to reduce mortality. Ann Thorac Surg 26:445, 1978
246. Heyland DK, Cook DL, King D, et al: Maximizing oxygen delivery in critically ill patients: A methodologic appraisal of the evidence. Crit Care Med 24:517, 1996
247. Connors AF, Speroff T, Dawson NV, et al: The effectiveness of right-heart catheterization in the initial care of critically ill patients. JAMA 276:889, 1996
248. Murdoch SD, Cohen AT, Bellamy MC: Pulmonary artery catheterization and mortality in critically ill patients. Br J Anaesth 85:611, 2000
249. Chittock DR, Dhingra VK, Ronco JJ, et al: Severity of illness and risk of death associated with pulmonary artery catheter use. Crit Care Med 32:911, 2004
250. Polanczyk CA, Rohde LE, Goldman L, et al: Right-heart catheterization and cardiac complications in patients undergoing noncardiac surgery: An observational study. JAMA 286:309, 2001
251. Sandham JD, Hull RD, Brant RF, et al: A randomized, controlled trial of the use of pulmonary artery catheters in high-risk surgical patients. N Engl J Med 348:5, 2003
252. Barone JE, Tucker JB, Rassias D, Corvo PR: Routine perioperative pulmonary artery catheterization has no effect on rate of complications in vascular surgery: A meta-analysis. Am Surg 67: 674, 2001
253. Ivanov R, Allen J, Calvin JE: The incidence of major morbidity in critically ill patients managed with pulmonary artery catheters: A meta-analysis. Crit Care Med 28:615, 2000
254. Yu DT, Platt R, Lanken PN, Black E, et al: Relationship of pulmonary artery catheter use to mortality and resource utilization in patients with severe sepsis. Crit Care Med 31:2734, 2003
255. Rhodes A, Cusack RJ, Newman PJ, et al: A randomised, controlled trial of the pulmonary artery catheter in critically ill patients. Intensive Care Med 28:256, 2002
256. Richard C, Warszawski J, Anguel N, et al: Early use of the pulmonary artery catheter and outcomes in patients with shock and acute respiratory distress syndrome: A randomized controlled trial. JAMA 290:2713, 2003
257. Schwann TA, Zacharias A, Riordan CJ, et al: Safe, highly selective use of pulmonary artery catheters in coronary artery bypass grafting: An objective patient selection method. Ann Thorac Surg 73:1394, 2002
258. Ramsey SD, Saint S, Sullivan SD, et al: Clinical and economic effects of pulmonary artery catheterization in nonemergent coronary artery bypass graft surgery. J Cardiothorac Vasc Anesth 14:113, 2000
259. Weintraub AC, Barash PG: A pulmonary artery catheter is indicated in all patients for coronary artery surgery. Pro: A pulmonary artery catheter is indicated in all patients for coronary artery surgery. J Cardiothorac Anesth 1:358, 1987
260. Bashein G, Ivey TD: A pulmonary artery catheter is indicated in all patients for coronary artery surgery. Con: A pulmonary artery catheter is not indicated for all coronary artery surgery. J Cardiothorac Anesth 1:362, 1987
261. Vender JS: Pulmonary artery and mixed venous monitoring: Appropriate use. Annu Refresher Course Lect 144:1, 1995
262. American Society of Anesthesiologists Task Force on Pulmonary Artery Catheterization: Practice guidelines for pulmonary artery catheterization: An updated report by the American Society of Anesthesiologists Task Force on Pulmonary Artery Catheterization. Anesthesiology 99:988, 2003
263. Bernard GR, Sopko G, Cerra F, et al: Pulmonary artery catheterization and clinical outcomes: National Heart, Lung, and Blood Institute and Food and Drug Administration Workshop Report. Consensus Statement. JAMA 283:2568, 2000
264. Poses RM, McClish DK, Smith WR, et al: Physicians' judgments of the risks of cardiac procedures. Differences between cardiologists and other internists. Med Care 35:603, 1997
265. Shah KB, Rao TLK, Laughlin S, El-Etr AA: A review of pulmonary artery catheterization in 6245 patients. Anesthesiology 61:271, 1984
266. Lopez-Sendon J, Lopez de Sa E, Gonzalez Maqueda I, et al: Right ventricular infarction as a risk factor for ventricular fibrillation during pulmonary artery catheterization using Swan-Ganz catheters. Am Heart J 119:207, 1990
267. Spring CL, Pozen RG, Rozanski JJ, et al: Advanced ventricular arrhythmias during bedside pulmonary artery catheterization. Am J Med 72:203, 1982
268. Salmenperä M, Peltola K, Rosenberg P: Does prophylactic lidocaine control cardiac arrhythmias associated with pulmonary artery catheterization? Anesthesiology 56:210, 1982
269. Shaw TJI: The Swan-Ganz pulmonary artery catheter. Incidence of complications with particular reference to ventricular dysrhythmias and their prevention. Anaesthesia 34:651, 1979
270. Patil AR: Risk of right bundle-branch block and complete heart block during pulmonary artery catheterization. Crit Care Med 18:122, 1990
271. Abernathy WS: Complete heart block caused by a Swan-Ganz catheter. Chest 65:349, 1974
272. Thomson IR, Dalton BC, Lappas DG, et al: Right bundle-branch block and complete heart block caused by the Swan-Ganz catheter. Anesthesiology 51:359, 1979
273. Sprung CL, Elser B, Schein RMH, et al: Risk of right bundle-branch block and complete heart block during pulmonary artery catheterization. Crit Care Med 17:1, 1989
274. Morris D, Mulvihill D, Lew WYW: Risk of developing complete heart block during bedside pulmonary artery catheterization in patients with left bundle-branch block. Arch Intern Med 147:2005, 1987
275. McDaniel DD, Stone JG, Faltas AN, et al: Catheter-induced pulmonary artery hemorrhage. J Thoracic Cardiovasc Surg 82:1, 1981
276. Hannan AT, Brown M, Bigman O: Pulmonary artery catheter-induced hemorrhage. Chest 85:128, 1984
277. Durbin CG: The range of pulmonary artery catheter balloon inflation pressures. J Cardiothorac Anesth 4:39, 1990
278. Dhamee MS, Pattison CZ: Pulmonary artery rupture during cardiopulmonary bypass. J Cardiothorac Anesth 1:51, 1987
279. Cohen JA, Blackshear RH, Gravenstein N, Woeste J: Increased pulmonary artery perforating potential of pulmonary artery catheters during hypothermia. J Cardiothorac Vasc Anesth 5:234, 1991
280. Stein JM, Lisbon A: Pulmonary hemorrhage from pulmonary artery catheterization treated with endobronchial intubation. Anesthesiology 55:698, 1981
281. Purut CM, Scott SM, Parham JV, Smith PK: Intraoperative management of severe endobronchial hemorrhage. Ann Thorac Surg 51:304, 1991
282. Laureys M, Golzarian J, Antoine M, Desmet JM: Coil embolization treatment for perioperative pulmonary artery rupture related to Swan-Ganz catheter placement. Cardiovasc Intervent Radiol 27:407, 2004
283. Abreu AR, Campos MA, Krieger BP: Pulmonary artery rupture induced by a pulmonary artery catheter: A case report and review of the literature. J Intensive Care Med 19:291, 2004
284. Foote GA, Schabel SI, Hodges M: Pulmonary complications of the flow-directed balloon-tipped catheter. N Engl J Med 290:927, 1974
285. Mond HG, Clark DW, Nesbitt SJ, Schlant RC: A technique for unknotting an intracardiac flow-directed balloon catheter. Chest 67:731, 1975
286. England MR, Murphy MC: A knotty problem. J Cardiothorac Vasc Anesth 11:682, 1997
287. Georghiou GP, Vidne BA, Raanani E: Knotting of a pulmonary artery catheter in the superior vena cava: Surgical removal and a word of caution. Heart 90:e28, 2004
288. Arnaout S, Diab K, Al-Kutoubi A, Jamaleddine G: Rupture of the chordae of the tricuspid valve after knotting of the pulmonary artery catheter. Chest 120:1742, 2001
289. Lazzam C, Sanborn TA, Christian F: Ventricular entrapment of a Swan-Ganz catheter: A technique for nonsurgical removal. J Am Coll Cardiol 13:1422, 1989
290. Boscoe MJ, deLange S: Damage to the tricuspid valve with a Swan-Ganz catheter. BMJ 283:346, 1981

291. O'Toole JD, Wurtzbacher JJ, Wearner NE, Jain AC: Pulmonary valve injury and insufficiency during pulmonary artery catheterization. N Engl J Med 301:1167, 1979
292. Kainuma M, Yamada M, Miyake T: Pulmonary artery catheter passing between the chordae tendineae of the tricuspid valve (correspondence). Anesthesiology 83:1130, 1995
293. Rowley KM, Clubb KS, Smith GJ, Cabin HS: Right-sided infective endocarditis as a consequence of flow-directed pulmonary artery catheterization. A clinicopathological study of 55 autopsied patients. N Engl J Med 311:1152, 1984
294. Greene JF Jr, Fitzwater JE, Clemmer TP: Septic endocarditis and indwelling pulmonary artery catheters. JAMA 233:891, 1975
295. Kim YL, Richman KA, Marshall BE: Thrombocytopenia associated with Swan-Ganz catheterization in patients. Anesthesiology 53:261, 1980
296. Moberg PQ, Geary VM, Sheikh FM: Heparin-induced thrombocytopenia: A possible complication of heparin-coated pulmonary artery catheters. J Cardiothorac Anesth 4:226, 1990
297. Hofbauer R, Moser D, Kaye AD, et al: Thrombus formation on the balloon of heparin-bonded pulmonary artery catheters: An ultrastructural scanning electron microscope study. Crit Care Med 28:727, 2000
298. Mangano DT: Heparin bonding and long-term protection against thrombogenesis. N Engl J Med 307:894, 1982
299. Böhrer H, Fleischer F, Lang J, Vahl C: Early formation of thrombi on pulmonary artery catheters in cardiac surgical patients receiving high-dose aprotinin. J Cardiothorac Anesth 4:222, 1990
300. Dentz M, Slaughter T, Mark JB: Early thrombus formation on heparin-bonded pulmonary artery catheters in patients receiving epsilon aminocaproic acid (case reports). Anesthesiology 82:583, 1995
301. Martins P, Driessen J, Vandekerckhove Y, et al: Transesophageal echocardiography detection of a right atrial thrombus around a pulmonary artery catheter. Anesth Analg 75:847, 1992
302. Allyn J, Lichtenstein A, Koski G, et al: Inadvertent passage of a pulmonary artery catheter from the superior vena cava through the left atrium and left ventricle into the aorta. Anesthesiology 70:1019, 1989
303. Saad R, Loubser P, Rokey R: Intraoperative transesophageal and contrast echocardiographic detection of an unusual complication associated with a misplaced pulmonary artery catheter. J Cardiothorac Vasc Anesth 10:247, 1996
304. Willis C, Wight D, Zidulka A: Hypotension secondary to balloon inflation of a pulmonary artery catheter. Crit Care Med 12:915, 1984
305. Gilbert T, Scherlis M, Fiocco M, et al: Pulmonary artery catheter migration causing venous cannula obstruction during cardiopulmonary bypass. Anesthesiology 82:596, 1995
306. Meluch A, Karis JH: Obstruction of venous return by a pulmonary artery catheter during cardiopulmonary bypass. Anesth Analg 70:121, 1990
307. Oyarzun JR, Donahoo JS, McCormick JR, Herman S: Venous cannula obstruction by Swan-Ganz catheter during cardiopulmonary bypass. Ann Thorac Surg 62:266, 1996
308. Kozlowski JH: Inadvertent coronary sinus occlusion by a pulmonary artery catheter. Crit Care Med 14:649, 1986
309. Tewari P, Kumar M, Kaushik S: Pulmonary artery catheter misplaced in liver. J Cardiothorac Vasc Anesth 9:482, 1995
310. Karakaya D, Baris S, Tur A: Pulmonary artery catheter-induced right ventricular perforation during coronary artery bypass surgery. Br J Anaesth 82:953, 1999
311. Shin B, McAslan TC, Ayella RJ: Problems with measurements using the Swan-Ganz catheter. Anesthesiology 43:474, 1975
312. Schmitt EA, Brantigan CO: Common artifacts of pulmonary artery pressures: Recognition and interpretation. J Clin Monit 2:44, 1986
313. Risk SC, Brandon D, D'Ambra MN, et al: Indications for the use of pacing pulmonary artery catheters in cardiac surgery. J Cardiothorac Vasc Anesth 6:275, 1992
314. Zaidan J, Freniere S: Use of a pacing pulmonary artery catheter during cardiac surgery. Ann Thorac Surg 35:633, 1983
315. Macander PJ, Kuhnlein JL, Buiteweg J, et al: Electrode detachment: A complication of the indwelling pacing Swan-Ganz catheter. N Engl J Med 314:1711, 1986
316. Heiselman DE, Maxwell JS, Petro V: Electrode displacement from a multipurpose Swan-Ganz catheter. PACE 9:134, 1986
317. Mora CT, Seltzer JL, McNulty SE: Evaluation of a new design pulmonary artery catheter for intraoperative ventricular pacing. J Cardiothorac Anesth 2:303, 1988
318. Trankina MF, White RD: Perioperative cardiac pacing using an atrioventricular pacing pulmonary artery catheter. J Cardiothorac Anesth 3:154, 1989
319. Kay HR, Afshari M, Barash P, et al: Measurement of ejection fraction by thermal dilution techniques. J Surg Res 34:337, 1983
320. Spinale FG, Zellner JL, Mukherjee R, Crawford FA: Placement considerations for measuring thermodilution right ventricular ejection fraction. Crit Care Med 19:417, 1991
321. Assmann R, Heidelmeyer CF, Trampisch HJ, et al: Right ventricular function assessed by thermodilution technique during apnea and mechanical ventilation. Crit Care Med 19:810, 1991
322. Ferris S, Konno M: In vitro validation of a thermodilution right ventricular ejection fraction method. J Clin Monit 8:74, 1992
323. Dhainaut JF, Brunet F, Monsallin J, et al: Bedside evaluation of right ventricular performance using a rapid computerized thermodilution method. Crit Care Med 15:148, 1987
324. Urban P, Scheidegger D, Gabathuler J, Rutishauser W: Thermodilution determination of right ventricular ejection fraction: A comparison with biplane angiography. Crit Care Med 15:652, 1987
325. Donahue PJ, Hansen DD, Mayer JE: A new complication of left atrial catheters. J Cardiothorac Vasc Anesth 3:757, 1991
326. Boldt J, Kling D, Thiel A, et al: Revascularization of the right coronary artery: Influence on thermodilution right ventricular ejection fraction. J Cardiothorac Anesth 2:140, 1988
327. Krouskop RW, Cabatu EE, Chelliah BP, et al: Accuracy and clinical utility of an oxygen saturation catheter. Crit Care Med 11:744, 1983
328. Waller JL, Kaplan JA, Bauman DI, Craver JM: Clinical evaluation of a new fiberoptic catheter oximeter during cardiac surgery. Anesth Analg 61:676, 1982
329. Norwood SH, Nelson LD: Continuous monitoring of mixed venous oxygen saturation during aortofemoral bypass grafting. Am Surg 52:114, 1986
330. Guffin A, Girard D, Kaplan JA: Shivering following cardiac surgery: Hemodynamic changes and reversal. J Cardiothorac Anesth 1:24, 1987
331. Heiselman D, Jones J, Cannon L: Continuous monitoring of mixed venous oxygen saturation in septic shock. J Clin Monit 2:237, 1986
332. Nelson LD: Continuous venous oximetry in surgical patients. Ann Surg 203:329, 1986
333. Thys DM, Cohen E, Eisenkraft JB: Mixed venous oxygen saturation during thoracic anesthesia. Anesthesiology 69:1005, 1988
334. Linton D, Gilon D: Advances in noninvasive cardiac output monitoring. Ann Card Anaesth 5:141, 2002.
335. Vaughn S, Puri VK: Cardiac output changes and continuous mixed venous oxygen saturation measurement in the critically ill. Crit Care Med 16:495, 1988
336. Boutrous AR, Lee C: Value of continuous monitoring of mixed venous blood oxygen saturation in the management of critically ill patients. Crit Care Med 14:132, 1986
337. Jastremski MS, Chelluri L, Beney K, et al: Analysis of the effects of continuous on-line monitoring of mixed venous oxygen saturation on patient outcome and cost-effectiveness. Crit Care Med 17:148, 1989
338. Pearson KS, Gomez MN, Moyers JR, et al: A cost/benefit analysis of randomized invasive monitoring for patients undergoing cardiac surgery. Anesth Analg 69:336, 1989
339. London MJ, Moritz TE, Henderson WG, et al: Standard versus fiberoptic pulmonary artery catheterization for cardiac surgery in the Department of Veterans Affairs: A prospective, observational, multicenter analysis. Anesthesiology 96:860, 2002
340. Woerkens EC, Trouwborst A, Tenbrinck R: Accuracy of a mixed venous saturation catheter during acutely induced changes in hematocrit in humans. Crit Care Med 19:1025, 1991
341. Reinhart K, Kuhn HJ, Hartog C, Bredle DL: Continuous central venous and pulmonary artery oxygen saturation monitoring in the critically ill. Intensive Care Med 30:1572, 2004
342. Scuderi P, MacGregor D, Bowton D, et al: A laboratory comparison of three pulmonary artery oximetry catheters. Anesthesiology 81:245, 1994
343. Pond CG, Blessios G, Bowlin J, et al: Perioperative evaluation of a new mixed venous oxygen saturation catheter in cardiac surgical patients. J Cardiothorac Vasc 6:280, 1992
344. Armaganidis A, Dhainaut JF, Billard JL, et al: Accuracy assessment for three fiberoptic pulmonary artery catheters for SvO_2 monitoring. Intensive Care Med 20:484, 1994
345. LaFarge CG, Miettinen OS. The estimation of oxygen consumption. Cardiovasc Res 4:23, 1970
346. Wood EH, Bowers D, Shepherd JT, et al: O_2 content of mixed venous blood in man during various phases of the respiratory and cardiac output cycles in relation to possible errors in measurement of cardiac output by conventional applications of the Fick method. J Appl Physiol 215:605, 1968

347. Grossman W: Fick oxygen method. *In* Cardiac Catheterization and Angiography, 3rd edition. Philadelphia, Lea & Febiger, 1986, p 105
348. Guyton AC: The Fick principle. *In* Guyton AC, Jones CE, Coleman TG (eds): Circulatory Physiology: Cardiac Output and Its Regulation, 2nd edition. Philadelphia, WB Saunders Company, 1973, p 21
349. Tissot S, Delafosse B, Bertrand O, et al: Clinical validation of the Deltatrac monitoring system in mechanically ventilated patients. Intensive Care Med 21:149, 1995
350. Johnson BD, Beck KC, Proctor DN, et al: Cardiac output during exercise by the open circuit acetylene washing method: Comparison with direct Fick. J Appl Physiol 88:1650, 2000
351. Jaffe MB: Partial CO_2 rebreathing cardiac output: Operating principles of the NICOTM system. J Clin Monit 15:387, 1999
352. Rocco M, Spadetta G, Morelli A, et al: A comparative evaluation of thermodilution and partial CO_2 rebreathing techniques for cardiac output assessment in critically ill patients during assisted ventilation. Intensive Care Med 30:82, 2004
353. Nilsson LB, Eldrup N, Berthelsen PG: Lack of agreement between thermodilution and carbon dioxide-rebreathing cardiac output. Acta Anaesthesiol Scand 45:680, 2001
354. Arnold JH, Stenz RI, Grenier B, et al: Noninvasive determination of cardiac output in a model of acute lung injury. Crit Care Med 25:864, 1997
355. Russell AE, Smith SA, West MJ, et al: Automated non-invasive measurements of cardiac output by the carbon dioxide rebreathing method: Comparisons with dye dilution and thermodilution. Br Heart J 63:195, 1990
356. Arnold JH, Stenz RI, Thompson JE, Arnold LW: Noninvasive determination of cardiac output using single-breath CO_2 analysis. Crit Care Med 24:1701, 1996
357. Binder JC, Parkin WG: Non-invasive cardiac output determination: Comparison of a new partial-rebreathing technique with thermodilution. Anaesth Intensive Care 29:19, 2001
358. van Heerden PV, Baker S, Lim SI, et al: Clinical evaluation of the non-invasive cardiac output (NICO) monitor in the intensive care unit. Anaesth Intensive Care 28:427, 2000
359. Kurita T, Morita K, Kato S, et al: Comparison of the accuracy of the lithium dilution technique with the thermodilution technique for measurement of cardiac output. Br J Anaesth 79:770, 1997
360. Forrester JS, Ganz W, Diamond G, et al: Thermodilution cardiac output determination with a single flow-directed catheter. Am Heart J 83:306, 1972
361. Salgado CR, Galletti PM: In vitro evaluation of the thermodilution technique for the measurement of ventricular stroke volume and end-diastolic volume. Cardiologia 49:65, 1966
362. Bilfinger TV, Lin CY, Anagnostopoulos CE: In vitro determinations of accuracy of cardiac output measurements by thermal dilution. J Surg Res 33:409, 1982
363. Goodyer AVN, Huvos A, Eckhardt WF, et al: Thermal dilution curves in the intact animal. Circ Res 7:432, 1959
364. Pavek K, Lindquist O, Arfors KE: Validity of thermodilution method for measurement of cardiac output in pulmonary oedema. Cardiovasc Res 7:419, 1973
365. Pelletier C: Cardiac output measurement by thermodilution. Can J Surg 22:347, 1979
366. Runciman WB, Ilsley AH, Roberts JG: Thermodilution cardiac output—a systematic error. Anaesth Intensive Care 9:135, 1981
367. Sorensen MB, Bille-Brahe NE, Engell HC: Cardiac output measurement by thermodilution. Ann Surg 183:67, 1976
368. Weisel RD, Berger RL, Hechtman HB, et al: Measurement of cardiac output by thermodilution. N Engl J Med 292:682, 1975
369. Pearl RG, Siegel LC: Thermodilution cardiac output measurement with a large left-to-right shunt. J Clin Monit 7:146, 1991
370. Wetzel RC, Latson TW: Major errors in thermodilution cardiac output measurement during rapid volume infusion. Anesthesiology 62:684, 1985
371. Bazaral M, Petre J, Novoa R: Errors in thermodilution cardiac output measurements caused by rapid pulmonary artery temperature decreases after cardiopulmonary bypass. Anesthesiology 77:31, 1992
372. Latson TW, Whitten CW, O'Flaherty D, et al: Ventilation, thermal noise, and errors in cardiac output measurements after cardiopulmonary bypass. Anesthesiology 79:1233, 1993
373. Hamilton MA, Stevenson LW, Woo M, et al: Effect of tricuspid regurgitation on the reliability of the thermodilution cardiac output in congestive heart failure. Am J Cardiol 64:945, 1989
374. Buffington CW, Nystrom EUM: Neither the accuracy nor the precision of thermal dilution cardiac output measurements is altered by acute tricuspid regurgitation in pigs. Anesth Analg 98:884, 2004
375. Kashtan HI, Maitland A, Salerno TA, et al: Effects of tricuspid regurgitation on thermodilution cardiac output: Studies in an animal model. Can J Anaesth 34:246, 1987
376. Heerdt PM, Pond CB, Blessios GA, Rosenbloom M: Inaccuracy of cardiac output by thermodilution during acute tricuspid regurgitation. Ann Thorac Surg 53:706, 1992
377. Balik M, Pachl J, Hendl J, et al: Effect of the degree of tricuspid regurgitation on cardiac output measurements by thermodilution. Intensive Care Med 28:1117, 2002
378. Nishikawa T, Dohi S: Slowing of heart rate during cardiac output measurement by thermodilution. Anesthesiology 57:538, 1982
379. Harris AP, Miller CF, Beattie C, et al: The slowing of sinus rhythm during thermodilution cardiac output determination and the effect of altering injectate temperature. Anesthesiology 63:540, 1985
380. Nishikawa T, Dohi S: Hemodynamic status susceptible to slowing of heart rate during thermodilution cardiac output determination in anesthetized patients. Crit Care Med 18:841, 1990
381. Hoel BL: Some aspects of the clinical use of thermodilution in measuring cardiac output. Scand J Clin Lab Invest 38:383, 1978
382. Stetz CW, Miller RG, Kelly GE, et al: Reliability of the thermodilution method in the determination of cardiac output in clinical practice. Am Rev Respir Dis 126:1001, 1982
383. Snyder JV, Powner DJ: Effects of mechanical ventilation on the measurement of the cardiac output by thermodilution. Crit Care Med 10:677, 1982
384. Stevens JH, Raffin TA, Mihm FG, et al: Thermodilution cardiac output measurement: Effects of the respiratory cycle on its reproducibility. JAMA 253:2240, 1985
385. Pearl RG, Rosenthal MH, Nieson L, et al: Effect of injectate volume and temperature on thermodilution cardiac output determination. Anesthesiology 64:798, 1986
386. Nelson LD, Houtchens BA: Automatic versus manual injections for thermodilution cardiac output determinations. Crit Care Med 10:190, 1982
387. Neto EP, Piriou V, Durand PG et al: Comparison of the two semicontinuous cardiac output pulmonary artery catheters after valvular surgery. Crit Care Med 27:2694, 1999
388. Jacquet L, Hanique G, Glorieux D, et al: Analysis of the accuracy of continuous thermodilution cardiac output measurement. Comparison with intermittent thermodilution and Fick cardiac output measurements. Intensive Care Med 22:1125, 1996
389. Jakobsen CJ, Melsen NC, Andresen EB: Continuous cardiac output measurements in the perioperative period. Acta Anaesthesiol Scand 39:485, 1995
390. Mihaljevic T, von Segesser LK, Tonz M, et al: Continuous thermodilution measurements of cardiac output: In-vitro and in-vivo evaluation. Thorac Cardiovasc Surg 42:32, 1994
391. Hogue CW, Rosenbloom M, McCawley C, Lappas DG: Comparison of cardiac output measurements by continuous thermodilution with electromagnetometry in adult cardiac surgical patients. J Cardiothorac Vasc Anesth 8:631, 1994
392. Zollner C, Polasek J, Kilger E, et al: Evaluation of a new continuous thermodilution cardiac output monitor in cardiac surgical patients: A prospective criterion standard study. Crit Care Med 27:293, 1999
393. Zollner C, Goetz AE, Weis M, et al: Continuous cardiac output measurements do not agree with conventional bolus thermodilution cardiac output determination. Can J Anaesth 48:1143, 2001
394. Zollner C, Polasek J, Kilger E, et al: Evaluation of a new continuous thermodilution cardiac output monitor in cardiac surgical patients: A prospective criterion standard study. Crit Care Med 27:293, 1999
395. Leather HA, Vuylsteke A, Bert C, et al: Evaluation of a new continuous cardiac output monitor in off-pump coronary artery surgery. Anaesthesia 59:385, 2004
396. Bottiger BW, Rauch H, Bohrer H, et al: Continuous versus intermittent cardiac output measurement in cardiac surgical patients undergoing hypothermic cardiopulmonary bypass. J Cardiothorac Vasc Anesth 9:405, 1995
397. Medin DL, Brown DT, Wesley R: Validation of continuous thermodilution cardiac output in critically ill patients with analysis of systematic errors. J Crit Care13:184, 1998
398. Linton RA, Band DM, Haire KM. A new method of measuring cardiac output in man using lithium dilution. Br J Anaesth 71:262, 1993
399. Kurita T, Morita K, Kato S, et al: Comparison of the accuracy of the lithium dilution technique with the thermodilution technique for measurement of cardiac output. Br J Anaesth 79:770, 1997
400. Linton R, Band D, O'Brian T, et al: Lithium dilution cardiac output measurement: A comparison with thermodilution. Crit Care Med 25:1767, 1997

401. Garcia-Rodriguez C, Pittman J, Cassell CH, et al: Lithium dilution cardiac output measurement: A clinical assessment of central venous and peripheral venous indicator injection. Crit Care Med 30:2199, 2002
402. Feigenbaum H, Popp RL, Wolfe SB, et al: Ultrasound measurements of the left ventricle: A correlative study with angiocardiography. Ann Intern Med 129:461, 1972
403. Kronik G, Slany J, Moslacher H: Comparative value of eight M-mode echocardiographic formulas for determining left ventricular stroke volume. Circulation 60:1308, 1979
404. Nosir YF, Fioretti PM, Vletter WB, et al: Accurate measurement of left ventricular ejection fraction by three-dimensional echocardiography. A comparison with radionuclide angiography. Circulation 94:460, 1996
405. Katz WE, Gasior TA, Quinland JJ, Gorscan J III. Transgastric continuous wave Doppler to determine cardiac output. Am J Cardiol 71:853, 1993
406. Darmon PL, Hillel Z, Mogtabar A, et al: Cardiac output by transesophageal echocardiography using continuous wave Doppler across the aortic valve. Anesthesiology 80:796, 1994
407. Roewer N, Bednarz F, Schulte am Esch J: Continuous measurement of intracardiac and pulmonary blood flow velocities with transesophageal pulsed Doppler echocardiography: Technique and initial clinical experience. J Cardiothorac Anesth 1:418, 1987
408. Muhiudeen IA, Kuecherer HF, Lee E, et al: Intraoperative estimation of cardiac output by transesophageal pulsed Doppler echocardiography. Anesthesiology 74:9, 1991
409. Pu M, Griffin BP, Vandervoort PM, et al: Intraoperative validation of mitral inflow determination by transesophageal echocardiography: Comparison of single-plane, biplane and thermodilution techniques. J Am Coll Cardiol 26:1047, 1995
410. Estagnasie P, Djedaini K, Mier L, et al: Measurement of cardiac output by transesophageal echocardiography in mechanically ventilated patients. Comparison with thermodilution. Intensive Care Med 23:753, 1997
411. Perrino AC Jr, Harris SN, Luther MA: Intraoperative determination of cardiac output using multiplane transesophageal echocardiography: A comparison to thermodilution. Anesthesiology 89:350, 1998
412. Dabaghi SF, Rokey R, Rivera J, et al: Comparison of echocardiographic assessment of cardiac hemodynamics in the intensive care unit with right-sided cardiac catheterization. Am J Cardiol 76:392, 1995
413. Roewer N, Bednarz F, Dziadka A, et al: Intraoperative cardiac output determination from transmitral and pulmonary blood flow measurements using transesophageal pulsed Doppler. J Cardiothorac Anesth 1:418, 1987
414. Savino JS, Trolanos CA, Aukburg S, et al: Measurement of pulmonary blood flow with two-dimensional echocardiography and Doppler echocardiography. Anesthesiology 75:445, 1991
415. Miller WE, Richards KL, Crawford MH: Accuracy of mitral Doppler echocardiographic cardiac output determinations in adults. Am Heart J 119:905, 1990
416. Maslow A, Communale M, Haering M, et al: Pulsed-wave Doppler measurements of cardiac output from the right ventricular outflow tract. Anesth Analg 83:466, 1996
417. Darmon P, Hillel Z, Mogtader A, et al: Cardiac output by transesophageal echocardiography using continuous-wave Doppler across the aortic valve. Anesthesiology 80:796, 1994
418. Hillel Z, Thys DM, Keene D, et al: A method to improve the accuracy of esophageal Doppler cardiac output determinations. Anesthesiology 71: A386, 1989
419. Siegel LC, Shafer SL, Martinez GM, et al: Simultaneous measurements of cardiac output by thermodilution, esophageal Doppler, and electrical impedance on anesthetized patients. J Cardiothorac Anesth 2:590, 1989
420. Muhiudeen IA, Kuecherer HF, Lee E, et al: Intraoperative estimation of cardiac output by transesophageal pulsed Doppler echocardiography. Anesthesiology 79:9, 1991
421. Ryan T, Burwash I, Lu J, et al: The agreement between ventricular volumes and ejection fraction by transesophageal echocardiography or a combined radionuclear and thermodilution technique in patients after coronary artery surgery. J Cardiothorac Vasc Anesth 10:323, 1996
422. Urbanowicz JH, Shaaban MJ, Cohen NH, et al: Comparison of transesophageal echocardiographic and scintigraphic estimates of left ventricular end-diastolic volume index and ejection fraction in patients following coronary artery bypass grafting. Anesthesiology 72:607, 1990
423. Liu N, Darmon PL, Saada M, et al: Comparison between radionuclide ejection fraction and fractional area changes derived from transesophageal echocardiography using automated border detection. Anesthesiology 85:468, 1996
424. Goens MB, Martin GR: Acoustic quantification: A new tool for diagnostic echocardiography. Curr Opin Cardiol 11:52, 1996
425. Perez JE, Miller JG, Holland MR, et al: Ultrasonic tissue characterization: Integrated backscatter imaging for detecting myocardial structural properties and on-line quantitation of cardiac function. Am J Card Imaging 8:106, 1994
426. Gorcsan J III, Morita S, Mandarino WA, et al: Two-dimensional echocardiographic automated border detection accurately reflects changes in left ventricular volume. J Am Soc Echocardiogr 6:482, 1993
427. Gorcsan J III, Denault A, Mandarino WA, Pinsky MR: Left ventricular pressure-volume relations with transesophageal echocardiographic automated border detection: Comparison with conductance-catheter technique. Am Heart J 131:544, 1996
428. Pinto FJ, Siegel LC, Chenzbraun A, Schnittger I: On-line estimation of cardiac output with a new automated border detection system using transesophageal echocardiography: A preliminary comparison with thermodilution. J Cardiothorac Vasc Anesth 8:625, 1994
429. Tardif JC, Cao QL, Pandian NG, et al: Determination of cardiac output using acoustic quantification in critically ill patients. Am J Cardiol 74:810, 1994
430. Morrissey RL, Siu SC, Guerrero JL, et al: Automated assessment of ventricular volume and function by echocardiography: Validation of automated border detection. J Am Soc Echocardiogr 7:107, 1994
431. Katz WE, Gasior TA, Reddy SCR, Gorscan J III: Utility and limitations of biplane transesophageal echocardiographic automated border detection for estimation of left ventricular stroke volume and cardiac output. Am Heart J 128:389, 1994
432. Kuhl HP, Franke A, Janssens U, et al: Three-dimensional echocardiographic determination of left ventricular volumes and function by multiplane transesophageal transducer: Dynamic in vitro validation and in vivo comparison with angiography and thermodilution. J Am Soc Echocardiogr 11:1113, 1998
433. Lee D, Fuisz AR, Fan PH, et al: Real-time 3-dimensional echocardiographic evaluation of left ventricular volume: Correlation with magnetic resonance imaging-a validation study. J Am Soc Echocardiogr 14:1001, 2001
434. Panza JA: Real-time three-dimensional echocardiography: An overview. Int J Card Imaging 17:227, 2001
435. Pandian NG, Roelandt J, Nanda NC, et al: Dynamic three-dimensional echocardiography: Methods and clinical potential. Echocardiography 11:237, 1994
436. Arai K, Hozumi T, Matsumura Y, et al: Accuracy of measurement of left ventricular volume and ejection fraction by new real-time three-dimensional echocardiography in patients with wall motion abnormalities secondary to myocardial infarction. Am J Cardiol 94:552, 2004
437. Kawai J, Tanabe K, Morioka S, Shiotani H: Rapid freehand scanning three-dimensional echocardiography: Accurate measurement of left ventricular volumes and ejection fraction compared with quantitative gated scintigraphy. J Am Soc Echocardiogr 16:110, 2003
438. Jenkins C, Bricknell K, Hanekom L, Marwick TH: Reproducibility and accuracy of echocardiographic measurements of left ventricular parameters using real-time three-dimensional echocardiography. J Am Coll Cardiol 44:878, 2004
439. Rauch H, Muller M, Fleischer F, et al: Pulse contour analysis versus thermodilution in cardiac surgery patients. Acta Anaesthesiol Scand 46:424, 2002
440. Zollner C, Haller M, Weis M, et al: Beat-to-beat measurement of cardiac output by intravascular pulse contour analysis: A prospective criterion standard study in patients after cardiac surgery. J Cardiothorac Vasc Anesth 14:125, 2000
441. Rodig G, Prasser C, Keyl C, et al: Continuous cardiac output measurement: Pulse contour analysis vs thermodilution technique in cardiac surgical patients. Br J Anaesth 82:525, 1999
442. Goedje O, Hoeke K, Lichtwarck-Aschoff M, et al: Continuous cardiac output by femoral arterial thermodilution calibrated pulse contour analysis: Comparison with pulmonary arterial thermodilution. Crit Care Med 27:2407, 1999
443. Godje O, Hoke K, Lamm P, et al: Continuous, less invasive, hemodynamic monitoring in intensive care after cardiac surgery. Thorac Cardiovasc Surg 46:242, 1998
444. Zollner C, Haller M, Weis M, et al: Beat-to-beat measurement of cardiac output by intravascular pulse contour analysis: A prospective criterion standard study in patients after cardiac surgery. J Cardiothorac Vasc Anesth 14:125, 2000
445. Jansen JR, Schreuder JJ, Mulier JP, et al: A comparison of cardiac output derived from the arterial pressure wave against thermodilution in cardiac surgery patients. Br J Anaesth 87:212, 2001

446. Godje O, Friedl R, Hannekum A: Accuracy of beat-to-beat cardiac output monitoring by pulse contour analysis in hemodynamically unstable patients. Med Sci Monit 7:1344, 2001
447. Linton NWF, Linton RAF: Estimation of changes in cardiac output from the arterial blood pressure waveform in the upper limb. Br J Anaesth 86:486, 2001
448. Rodig G, Prasser C, Keyl C: Continuous cardiac output measurement: Pulse contour analysis vs thermodilution technique in cardiac surgical patients. Br J Anaesth 82:525, 1999
449. Buhre W, Weyland A, Kazmaier S, et al: Comparison of cardiac output assessed by pulse-contour analysis and thermodilution in patients undergoing minimally invasive direct coronary artery bypass grafting. J Cardiothorac Vasc Anesth 13:437, 1999
450. Godje O, Friedl R, Hannekum A: Accuracy of beat-to-beat cardiac output monitoring by pulse contour analysis in hemodynamically unstable patients. Med Sci Monit 7:1344, 2001
451. Kubicek WG, Karegis JN, Patterson RP, et al: Development and evaluation of an impedance cardiac output system. Aerosp Med 37:1208, 1966
452. Cohen AJ, Arnaudov D, Zabeeda D, et al: Non-invasive measurement of cardiac output during coronary artery bypass grafting. Eur J Cardiothorac Surg 14:64, 1998
453. Shoemaker WC, Wo CC, Bishop MH, et al: Multicenter trial of a new thoracic electrical bioimpedance device for cardiac output estimation. Crit Care Med 22:1907, 1994
454. Belardinelli R, Ciampani N, Costanini C: Comparison of impedance cardiography with thermodilution and direct Fick methods for noninvasive measurements of stroke volume and cardiac output during incremental exercise in patients with ischemic cardiomyopathy. Am J Cardiol 77:1293, 1996
455. Spiess BD, Patel MA, Soltow LO, Wright IH: Comparison of bioimpedance versus thermodilution cardiac output during cardiac surgery: Evaluation of a second-generation bioimpedance device. J Cardiothorac Vasc Anesth 15:567, 2001
456. Spinale FG, Reines HD, Crawford FA Jr: Comparison of bioimpedance and thermodilution methods for determining cardiac output: Experimental and clinical studies. Ann Thorac Surg 45:421, 1988
457. Fuller HD: The validity of cardiac output measurements by thoracic impedance: A meta-analysis. Clin Invest Med 15:103, 1992
458. van der Meer BJ, de Vries JP, Schreuder WO, et al: Impedance cardiography in cardiac surgery patients: Abnormal body weight gives unreliable cardiac output measurements. Acta Anaesthesiol Scand 41:708, 1997
459. Barry BN, Mallick A, Bodenham AR, et al: Lack of agreement between bioimpedance and continuous thermodilution measurement of cardiac output in intensive care unit patients. Crit Care 1:71, 1997
460. Young JD, McQuillan P: Comparison of thoracic electrical bioimpedance and thermodilution for the measurement of cardiac index in patients with severe sepsis. Br J Anaesth 70:58, 1993
461. Sagemann WS, Amundsen DE: Thoracic electrical bioimpedance measurements of cardiac output in postaortocoronary bypass patients. Crit Care Med 21:1139, 1993
462. Siegel LC, Shafer SL, Martinez GM, et al: Simultaneous measurements of cardiac output by thermodilution, esophageal Doppler, and electrical impedance in anesthetized patients. J Cardiothorac Anesth 2:590, 1988
463. Shoemaker WC, Belzberg H, Wo C, et al: Multicenter study of noninvasive monitoring systems as alternatives to invasive monitoring of acutely ill emergency patients. Chest 114:1643, 1998
464. Perrino AC Jr, Lippman A, Ariyan C, et al: Intraoperative cardiac output monitoring: Comparison of impedance cardiography and thermodilution. J Cardiothorac Vasc Anesth 8:24, 1994
465. Sageman WS, Riffenburgh RH, Spiess BD: Equivalence of bioimpedance and thermodilution in measuring cardiac index after cardiac surgery. J Cardiothorac Vasc Anesth 16:8, 2002
466. Gotshall RW, Wood VC, Miles DS: Comparison of two impedance cardiographic techniques for measuring cardiac output in critically ill patients. Crit Care Med 17:806, 1989
467. Miles DS, Gotshall RW, Quinones JD, et al: Impedance cardiography fails to measure accurately left ventricular ejection fraction. Crit Care Med 18:221, 1990
468. Spinale FG, Smith AC, Crawford FA: Relationship of bioimpedance to thermodilution and echocardiographic measurements of cardiac function. Crit Care Med 18:414, 1990
469. Donahue PJ, Hansen DD, Mayer JE: A new complication of left atrial catheters. J Cardiothorac Vasc Anesth 3:757, 1991
470. Carvalho R, Loures D, Brofman P, et al: Left atrial catheter complications. J Thorac Cardiovasc Surg 92:162, 1986
471. Bashore T: Afterload reduction in chronic aortic regurgitation: It sure seems like a good idea. J Am Coll Cardiol 45:1031, 2005
472. Lang RM, Borow KM, Neumann A, et al: Systemic vascular resistance: An unreliable index of left ventricular afterload. Circulation 74:1114, 1986
473. Gorback MS: Problems associated with the determination of pulmonary vascular resistance. J Clin Monit 6:118, 1990
474. West JB: Recruitment in networks of pulmonary capillaries. J Appl Physiol 39:976, 1975
475. Suga H, Sagawa K: Instantaneous pressure-volume relationships and their ratio in the excised, supported canine left ventricle. Circ Res 35:117, 1974
476. Schreuder JJ, Biervliet JD, van der Velde ET, et al: Systolic and diastolic pressure-volume relationships during cardiac surgery. J Cardiothorac Vasc Anesth 5:539, 1991
477. Dahlgren G, Veintemilla F, Settergren G, Liska J: Left ventricular end-systolic pressure estimated from measurements in a peripheral artery. J Cardiothorac Vasc Anesth 5:551, 1991
478. Ward JA, Kingsley CP, Silverman SM: Computer software for the on-line measurement of the left ventricular end-systolic pressure-dimension relationship. J Cardiothorac Vasc Anesth 5:554, 1991
479. American Society of Anesthesiologists: Standards for basic anesthetic monitoring. Available at: http://www.asahq.org/publicationsAndServices/standards/02.pdf. Accessed September 23, 2005
480. Pedersen T, Petersen P, Moller AM: Pulse oximetry for perioperative monitoring. Cochrane Database Syst Rev 2:CD002013, 2001
481. Moller JT, Pedersen T, Rasmussen LS, et al: Randomized evaluation of pulse oximetry in 20,802 patients. I. Design, demography, pulse oximetry failure rate, and overall complication rate. Anesthesiology 78:436, 1993
482. Moller JT, Johannessen NW, Espersen K, et al: Randomized evaluation of pulse oximetry in 20,802 patients. II. Perioperative events and postoperative complications. Anesthesiology 78:445, 1993
483. Keats AS: Anesthesia mortality in perspective. Anesth Analg 71:113, 1990
484. Tremper KK, Barker SJ: Pulse oximetry. Anesthesiology 70:98, 1989
485. Pälve H, Vuori A: Minimum pulse pressure and peripheral temperature needed for pulse oximetry during cardiac surgery with cardiopulmonary bypass. J Cardiothorac Vasc Anesth 5:327, 1991
486. Reich DL, Timcenko A, Bodian CA, et al: Predictors of pulse oximetry failure. Anesthesiology 84:859, 1996
487. Gamble WJ, LaFarge CG, Fyler DC, et al: Regional coronary venous oxygen saturation and myocardial oxygen tension following abrupt changes in ventricular pressure in the isolated dog heart. Circ Res 34:672, 1974
488. Hoffman JIE, Buckberg GD: Regional myocardial ischemia: Causes, prediction and prevention. Vasc Surg 8:115, 1974
489. Hoffman JIE, Buckberg GD: Transmural variations in myocardial perfusion. *In* Yu PN, Goodwin JF (eds): Progress in Cardiology. Philadelphia, Lea & Febiger, 1976, p 37
490. Hoffman JIE, Buckberg GD: Pathophysiology of subendocardial ischemia. BMJ 1:76, 1975
491. Stern S: Angina pectoris without chest pain: Clinical implications of silent ischemia. Circulation 106:1906, 2002
492. Thakor NV: Electrocardiographic monitors. *In* Webster JG (ed): Encyclopedia of Medical Devices and Instrumentation. New York, John Wiley & Sons, 1988, pp 1002–1017
493. Tayler D, Vincent R: Artefactual ST segment abnormalities due to electrocardiograph design. Br Heart J 54:121, 1985
494. Weinfurt PT: Electrocardiographic monitoring: An overview. J Clin Monit 6:132, 1990
495. Carim HM: Bioelectrodes. *In* Webster JG (ed): Encyclopedia of Medical Devices and Instrumentation. New York, John Wiley & Sons, 1988, pp 195–224
496. de Pinto V: Filters for the reduction of baseline wander and muscle artifact in the ECG. J Electrocardiol 25(suppl):40, 1992
497. Thakor NV: Electrocardiographic monitors. *In* Webster JG (ed): Encyclopedia of Medical Devices and Instrumentation. New York, John Wiley & Sons, 1988, pp 1002–1017
498. Gardner RM, Hollingsworth KW: Optimizing the electrocardiogram and pressure monitoring. Crit Care Med 14:651, 1986
499. Weinfurt PT: Electrocardiographic monitoring: An overview. J Clin Monit 6:132, 1990
500. Lampert BA, Sundstrom FD: ECG artifact simulating supraventricular tachycardia during automated percutaneous lumbar discectomy. Anesth Analg 67:1096, 1988
501. Paulsen AW, Pritchard DG: ECG artifact produced by crystalloid administration through blood/fluid warming sets (letter). Anesthesiology 69:803, 1988

502. Khambatta HJ, Stone JG, Wald A, et al: Electrocardiographic artifacts during cardiopulmonary bypass. Anesth Analg 71:88, 1990
503. Kleinman B, Shah K, Belusko R, et al: Electrocardiographic artifact caused by extracorporeal roller pump (letter). J Clin Monit 6:258, 1990
504. Metz S: ECG artifacts during cardiopulmonary bypass—an alternative method (letter). Anesth Analg 72:715, 1991
505. Marsh R: ECG artifact in the OR. Health Devices 20:140, 1991
506. Berson AS, Pipberger HV: The low-frequency response of electrocardiographs, a frequent source of recording errors. Am Heart J 71:779, 1966
507. Meyer JL: Some instrument-induced errors in the electrocardiogram. JAMA 201:351, 1967
508. Bragg-Remschel DA, Anderson CM, Winkle RA: Frequency response characteristics of ambulatory ECG monitoring systems and their implications for ST segment analysis. Am Heart J 103:20, 1982
509. Bragg-Remschel DA: Problems with ST-segment analysis in ambulatory ECG monitoring systems. *In* Rutishauser W, Roskamm H (ed): Silent myocardial ischemia. Berlin, Springer-Verlag, 1984, pp 90–99
510. Bailey JJ, Berson AS, Garson A Jr, et al: Recommendations for standardization and specifications in automated electrocardiography: Bandwidth and digital signal processing. A report for health professionals by an ad hoc writing group of the Committee on Electrocardiography and Cardiac Electrophysiology of the Council on Clinical Cardiology, American Heart Association. Circulation 81:730, 1990
511. Mirvis DM, Berson AS, Goldberger AL, et al: Instrumentation and practice standards for electrocardiographic monitoring in special care units. A report for health professionals by a Task Force of the Council on Clinical Cardiology, American Heart Association. Circulation 79:464, 1989
512. Pipberger HV, Arzbaecher RC, Berson AS, et al: Recommendations for standardization of leads and of specifications for instruments in electrocardiography and vectorcardiography. Report of the Committee on Electrocardiography, American Heart Association. Circulation 52:11, 1975
513. Mirvis DM, Berson AS, Goldberger AL, et al: Instrumentation and practice standards for electrocardiographic monitoring in special care units. A report for health professionals by a Task Force of the Council on Clinical Cardiology, American Heart Association. Circulation 79:464, 1989
514. London MJ: Ischemia monitoring: ST segment analysis versus TEE. *In* Kaplan JA (ed): Cardiothoracic and Vascular Anesthesia Update. Philadelphia, WB Saunders Company, 1993, pp 1–18
515. Garson JA: Clinically significant differences between the "old" analog and the "new" digital electrocardiograms. Am Heart J 114:194, 1987
516. Madias JE, Bazaz R, Agarwal H, et al: Anasarca-mediated attenuation of the amplitude of electrocardiogram complexes: A description of a heretofore unrecognized phenomenon. J Am Coll Cardiol 38:756, 2001
517. Madias JE: Concealment of electrocardiographically based diagnosis of left ventricular hypertrophy by anasarca. Am J Hypertens 17:897, 2004
518. Madias JE: Decrease/disappearance of pacemaker stimulus "spikes" due to anasarca: Further proof that the mechanism of attenuation of ECG voltage with anasarca is extracardiac in origin. Ann Noninvasive Electrocardiol 9:243, 2004
519. Madias JE: Recognizing the link between peripheral edema and voltage attenuation of QRS complexes: Implications for the critical care patient. Chest 124:2041, 2003
520. Tsuda H, Tobata H, Watanabe S, et al: QRS complex changes in the V_5 ECG lead during cardiac surgery. J Cardiothorac Vasc Anesth 6:658, 1992
521. Crescenzi G, Scandroglio AM, Pappalardo F, et al: ECG changes after CABG: The role of the surgical technique. J Cardiothorac Vasc Anesth 18:38, 2004
522. Bhargava V, Watanabe K, Froelicher VF: Progress in computer analysis of the exercise electrocardiogram. Am J Cardiol 47:1143, 1981
523. Watanabe K, Bhargava V, Froelicher V: Computer analysis of the exercise ECG: A review. Prog Cardiovasc Dis 22:423, 1980
524. Rowlandson I: Computerized electrocardiography. A historical perspective. Ann N Y Acad Sci 601:343, 1990
525. Plonsey R: Electrocardiography. *In* Webster JG (ed): Encyclopedia of Medical Devices and Instrumentation. New York, John Wiley & Sons, 1988, pp 1017–1040
526. Kossman CE: Unipolar electrocardiography of Wilson: A half century later. Am Heart J 110:901, 1985
527. Castellanos A, Interian A, Myerburg R: The resting electrocardiogram. In Fuster V, Alexander R, O'Rourke R (eds): The Heart, 11th ed. New York, McGraw-Hill, 2004, pp 295–324
528. Fletcher GF, Froelicher VF, Hartley LH, et al: Exercise standards: A statement for health professionals from the American Heart Association. Circulation 82:2286
529. Froelicher VF: Interpretation of specific exercise test responses. *In* Exercise and the Heart. Chicago, Year Book Medical Publishers, 1987, pp 81–145
530. Hollenberg M, Mateo G, Massie BM, et al: Influence of R-wave amplitude on exercise-induced ST depression: Need for a "gain factor" correction when interpreting stress electrocardiograms. Am J Cardiol 56:13, 1985
531. Goldberger AL: Electrocardiogram in coronary artery disease: Limitations in sensitivity. *In* Myocardial Infarction: Electrocardiographic Differential Diagnosis. St Louis, CV Mosby, 1984, pp 303–308
532. Hollenberg M, Mangano DT, Browner WS, et al: Predictors of postoperative myocardial ischemia in patients undergoing noncardiac surgery. The Study of Perioperative Ischemia Research Group. JAMA 268:205, 1992
533. Croft CH, Woodward W, Nicod P, et al: Clinical implications of anterior ST segment depression in patients with acute myocardial infarction. Am J Cardiol 50:428, 1982
534. Mirvis DM: Physiologic bases for anterior ST segment depression in patients with acute inferior wall myocardial infarction. Am Heart J 116:1308, 1988
535. Brody DA: A theoretical analysis of intracavitary blood mass influence on the heart-lead relationship. Circ Res 4:731, 1956
536. Abboud S, Berenfeld O, Sadeh D: Simulation of high-resolution QRS complex using a ventricular model with a fractal conduction system. Effects of ischemia on high-frequency QRS potentials. Circ Res 68:1751, 1991
537. Pettersson J, Pahlm O, Carro E, et al: Changes in high-frequency QRS components are more sensitive than ST-segment deviation for detecting acute coronary artery occlusion. J Am Coll Cardiol 36:1827, 2000
538. Matsushita S, Sakakibara Y, Imazuru T, et al: High-frequency QRS potentials as a marker of myocardial dysfunction after cardiac surgery. Ann Thorac Surg 77:1293, 2004
539. Blackburn H, Katigbak R: What electrocardiographic leads to take after exercise? Am Heart J 67:184, 1964
540. Mason RE, Likar I: A new system of multiple-lead exercise electrocardiography. Am Heart J 71:196, 1966
541. Mason RE, Likar I, Biern RO, et al: Multiple-lead exercise electrocardiography: Experience in 107 normal subjects and 67 patients with angina pectoris, and comparison with coronary cinearteriography in 84 patients. Circulation 36:517, 1967
542. Tubau JF, Chaitman BR, Bourassa MG, et al: Detection of multivessel coronary disease after myocardial infarction using exercise stress testing and multiple ECG lead systems. Circulation 61:44, 1980
543. Koppes G, McKiernan T, Bassan M, et al: Treadmill exercise testing. Part I. Curr Probl Cardiol 7:1, 1977
544. Chaitman BR, Bourassa MG, Wagniart P, et al: Improved efficiency of treadmill exercise testing using a multiple lead ECG system and basic hemodynamic exercise response. Circulation 57:71, 1978
545. Miller TD, Desser KB, Lawson M: How many electrocardiographic leads are required for exercise treadmill tests? J Electrocardiol 20:131, 1987
546. Lam J, Chaitman BR: Exercise lead systems and newer electrocardiographic parameters. J Card Rehabil 4:507, 1984
547. Chaitman BR: The changing role of the exercise electrocardiogram as a diagnostic and prognostic test for chronic ischemic heart disease. J Am Coll Cardiol 8:1195, 1986
548. Chaitman BR, Hanson JS: Comparative sensitivity and specificity of exercise electrocardiographic lead systems. Am J Cardiol 47:1335, 1981
549. Horacek BM, Wagner GS: Electrocardiographic ST-segment changes during acute myocardial ischemia. Card Electrophysiol Rev 6:196, 2002
550. Carley SD: Beyond the 12 lead: Review of the use of additional leads for the early electrocardiographic diagnosis of acute myocardial infarction. Emerg Med (Fremantle) 15:143, 2003
551. Zimetbaum PJ, Josephson ME: Use of the electrocardiogram in acute myocardial infarction. N Engl J Med 348:933–940, 2003
552. Drew BJ, Krucoff MW: Multilead ST-segment monitoring in patients with acute coronary syndromes: A consensus statement for healthcare professionals. ST-Segment Monitoring Practice Guideline International Working Group. Am J Crit Care 8:372, 1999
553. Mangano DT, Browner WS, Hollenberg M, et al: Association of perioperative myocardial ischemia with cardiac morbidity and mortality in men undergoing noncardiac surgery. The Study of Perioperative Ischemia Research Group. N Engl J Med 323:1781, 1990
554. London MJ: The significance of perioperative ischemia in vascular surgery. *In* Kaplan JA (ed): Cardiothoracic and Vascular Anesthesia Update. Philadelphia, WB Saunders Company, 1993, pp 1–18

555. Slogoff S, Keats AS: Randomized trial of primary anesthetic agents on outcome of coronary artery bypass operations. Anesthesiology 70:179, 1989
556. London MJ: Perioperative myocardial ischemia in patients undergoing myocardial revascularization. Curr Opin Anesthesiol 6:98, 1993
557. Karpati PC, Rossignol M, Pirot M, et al: High incidence of myocardial ischemia during postpartum hemorrhage. Anesthesiology 100:30, 2004
558. London MJ: Multilead precordial ST-segment monitoring: "The next generation?" Anesthesiology 96:259, 2002
559. London MJ, Hollenberg M, Wong MG, et al: Intraoperative myocardial ischemia: Localization by continuous 12 lead electrocardiography. Anesthesiology 69:232, 1988
560. Landesberg G, Mosseri M, Wolf Y, et al: Perioperative myocardial ischemia and infarction: Identification by continuous 12-lead electrocardiogram with online ST-segment monitoring. Anesthesiology 96:264, 2002
561. Martinez EA, Kim LJ, Faraday N, et al: Sensitivity of routine intensive care unit surveillance for detecting myocardial ischemia. Crit Care Med 31:2302, 2003
562. Balaji S, Ellenby M, McNames J, et al: Update on intensive care ECG and cardiac event monitoring. Card Electrophysiol Rev 6:190, 2002
563. Marquez MF, Colin L, Guevara M, et al: Common electrocardiographic artifacts mimicking arrhythmias in ambulatory monitoring. Am Heart J 144:187, 2002

Chapter 15

INTRAOPERATIVE ECHOCARDIOGRAPHY

Ronald A. Kahn, MD • Stanton K. Shernan, MD •
Steven N. Konstadt, MD, FACC

KEY POINTS

1. An ultrasound beam is a continuous or intermittent train of sound waves emitted by a transducer or wave generator that is composed of density or pressure. Ultrasound waves are characterized by their wavelength, frequency, and velocity.
2. Waves interact with the medium in which they travel and with one another, and the manner in which waves interact with a medium is determined by its density and homogeneity. When a wave is propagated through an inhomogenous medium, it is partly absorbed, partly reflected, and partly scattered.
3. Doppler frequency shift analysis can be used to obtain blood flow velocity, direction, and acceleration of red blood cells, where the magnitude and direction of the frequency shift are related to the velocity and direction of the moving target.
4. Doppler shifts above the Nyquist limit will create artifacts described as "aliasing" or "wraparound," and blood flow velocities will appear in a direction opposite to the conventional one. To optimize Nyquist limits, the ultrasound frequency should be low and the sampling frequency should be high.
5. Normally, red blood cells scatter ultrasound waves weakly, resulting in a black appearance on ultrasonic examination. Contrast echocardiography uses gas microbubbles to present additional gas–liquid interfaces, which substantially increase the strength of the returning signal. This augmentation in signal strength may be used to better define endocardial borders, optimize Doppler envelope signals, and estimate myocardial perfusion.
6. *Axial resolution* is the minimum separation between two interfaces located in a direction parallel to the ultrasound beam so that they can be imaged as two different interfaces. *Lateral resolution* is the minimum separation of two interfaces aligned along a direction perpendicular to the beam. *Elevational resolution* refers to the ability to determine differences in the thickness of the imaging plane.
7. Absolute contraindications to transesophageal echocardiography in intubated patients include esophageal stricture, diverticula, tumor, recent suture lines, and known esophageal interruption. Relative contraindications include symptomatic hiatal hernia, esophagitis, coagulopathy, esophageal varices, and unexplained upper gastrointestinal bleeding.
8. Horizontal imaging planes are obtained by moving the transesophageal echocardiography probe up and down (upper esophageal: 20 to 25 cm; mid-esophageal: 30 to 40 cm; transgastric: 40 to 45 cm; deep transgastric: 45 to 50 cm). Multiplane probes may further facilitate interrogation of complex anatomic structures by allowing up to 180° of axial rotation of the imaging plane without manual probe manipulation.
9. The dynamic assessment of ventricular function with echocardiography is based on derived indices of muscle contraction and relaxation. Echocardiography indices of left ventricular function that incorporate endocardial border outlines and Doppler techniques can be used to estimate cardiac output, stroke volume, ejection fraction, and parameters of ventricular relaxation and filling.
10. There are three primary stages of diastolic dysfunction: impaired relaxation, pseudonormalization, and restrictive cardiomyopathy. The evaluation of diastolic function may be performed using Doppler analysis of mitral valve inflow and pulmonary vein flow, color M-mode propagation velocities, and tissue Doppler analysis of the mitral valve annulus.
11. The summation of flow velocities in a given period of time is called the *velocity-time integral*. Flow across the orifice is equal to the product of the cross-sectional area of the orifice and the velocity-time integral.

Few areas in cardiac anesthesia have developed as rapidly as the field of intraoperative echocardiography. In the early 1980s, when transesophageal echocardiography (TEE) was first used in the operating room, its main application was the assessment of global and regional left ventricular (LV) function. Since that time, there have been numerous technical advances: biplane and multiplane probes; multifrequency probes; enhanced scanning resolution; color-flow, pulsed-wave, and continuous-wave Doppler; automatic edge detection, Doppler tissue imaging, three-dimensional (3D) reconstruction, and digital image processing. With these advances, the number of clinical applications of TEE has markedly increased. The common applications of TEE include (1) assessment of valvular anatomy and function, (2) evaluation of the thoracic aorta, (3) detection of intracardiac defects, (4) detection of intracardiac masses, (5) evaluation of pericardial effusions, (6) detection of intracardiac air and clots, and (7) assessment of biventricular systolic and diastolic function. In many of these evaluations, TEE is able to provide unique and critical information that was not previously available in the operating room (Box 15–1).

The future will certainly bring new technology—such as 3D imaging, improved contrast agents, higher-resolution images, and more automated computer processing—into the operating room. Future research will attempt to define new applications of TEE, outcome determinants, and cost-benefit

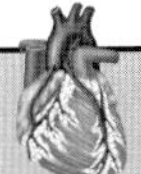

BOX 15–1 ***Common Applications of Transesophageal Echocardiography***

- Assessment of valvular anatomy and function
- Evaluation of the thoracic aorta
- Detection of intracardiac defects
- Detection of intracardiac masses
- Evaluation of pericardial effusions
- Detection of intracardiac air and clots
- Assessment of biventricular systolic and diastolic function

issues. This chapter covers the important topics needed to begin the study of intraoperative echocardiography.

BASIC CONCEPTS

Properties of Ultrasound

In echocardiography, the heart and great vessels are insonated with ultrasound, which is sound above the human audible range. The ultrasound is sent into the thoracic cavity and is partially reflected by the cardiac structures. From these reflections, distance, velocity, and density of objects within the chest are derived.[1]

Wavelength, Frequency, and Velocity

An ultrasound beam is a continuous or intermittent train of sound waves emitted by a transducer or wave generator. It is composed of density or pressure waves and can exist in any medium with the exception of a vacuum (Fig. 15–1). Ultrasound waves are characterized by their wavelength, frequency, and velocity. *Wavelength* is the distance between the two nearest points of equal pressure or density in an ultrasound beam, and *velocity* is the speed at which the waves propagate through a medium. As the waves travel past any fixed point in an ultrasound beam, the pressure cycles regularly and continuously between a high and a low value. The number of cycles per second (Hertz) is called the *frequency* of the wave. Ultrasound is sound with frequencies above 20,000 Hz, which is the upper limit of the human audible range. The relationship among the frequency (f), wavelength (λ), and velocity (v) of a sound wave is defined by the formula:

$$v = f \times \lambda \qquad (15\text{–}1)$$

The velocity of sound varies with the properties of the medium through which it travels. For soft tissues, this velocity approximates 1540 m/sec. Because the frequency of an ultrasound beam is determined by the properties of the emitting transducer and the velocity is a function of the tissues through which the sound travels, wavelengths vary according to the relationship expressed in Equation 15–1.

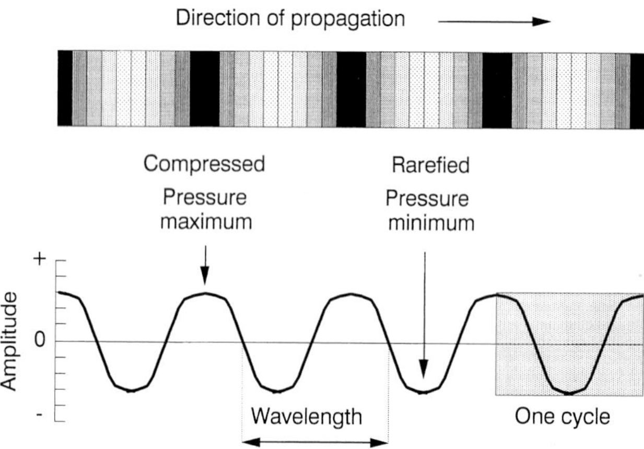

Figure 15–1 A sound wave is a series of compressions and rarefactions. The combination of one compression and one rarefaction represents one cycle. The distance between the onset (peak compression) of one cycle and the onset of the next is the wavelength. (From Thys DM, Hillel Z: How it works: Basic concepts in echocardiography. *In* Bruijn NP, Clements F [eds]: Intraoperative Use of Echocardiography. Philadelphia, JB Lippincott, 1991.)

Piezoelectric crystals convert the energy between ultrasound and electrical signals. When presented with a high-frequency electrical signal, these crystals produce ultrasound energy, which is directed toward the areas to be imaged. Commonly, a short ultrasound signal is emitted from the piezoelectric crystal. After ultrasound wave formation, the crystal "listens" for the returning echoes for a given period of time and then pauses prior to repeating this cycle. This cycle length is known as the *pulse repetition frequency* (PRF). This cycle length must be long enough to provide enough time for a signal to travel to and return from a given object of interest. Typically, PRFs vary from 1 to 10 kHz, which results in 0.1- to 1-msec intervals between pulses. When reflected ultrasound waves return to these piezoelectric crystals, they are converted into electrical signals, which may be appropriately processed and displayed. Electronic circuits measure the time delay between the emitted and received echo. Because the speed of ultrasound through tissue is a constant, this time delay can be converted into the precise distance between the transducer and tissue.

The 3D shape of the ultrasound beam is dependent on both physical aspects of the ultrasound signal and the design of the transducer. An unfocused ultrasound beam may be thought of as an inverted funnel, where the initial straight columnar area is known as the "near field" (also known as Fresnel zone) followed by conical divergent area known as the "far field" (also known as Fraunhofer zone). The length of the near field is directly proportional to the square of the transducer diameter and inversely proportional to the wavelength, specifically,

$$F_n = D^2/4\lambda \qquad (15\text{–}2)$$

where F_n is the near-field length, D is the diameter of the transducer, and λ is the ultrasound wavelength. Increasing the frequency of the ultrasound increases the length of the near field. The angle of the far-field convergence (θ) is directly proportional to the wavelength and inversely proportional to the diameter of the transducer and is expressed by the equation:

$$\sin\theta = 1.22\lambda/D \qquad (15\text{–}3)$$

Further shaping of the beam geometry may be adjusted using acoustical lenses or the shaping of the piezoelectric crystal. Ideally, imaging should be performed within the near field or focused aspect of the ultrasound beam, because the ultrasound beam is most parallel and the tissue interfaces are most perpendicular to these ultrasound beams.

Attenuation, Reflection, and Scatter

Waves interact with the medium in which they travel and with one another. Interaction among waves is called *interference*. The manner in which waves interact with a medium is determined by its density and homogeneity. When a wave is propagated through an inhomogenous medium (and all living tissue is essentially inhomogenous), it is partly absorbed, partly reflected, and partly scattered. *Attenuation* refers to the loss of ultrasound power as it transverses tissue. Tissue attenuation is dependent on ultrasound reflection, scattering, and absorption. The absorption occurs as a result of the conversion of ultrasound energy into heat. The greater the ultrasound reflection and scattering, the less ultrasound energy is available for penetration and resolution of deeper structures; this effect is especially important during scanning with higher frequencies. While water, blood, and muscle have low tissue impedance with resultant low ultrasound attenuation, air and

Table 15–1 Half-Power Distances for Tissues and Substances Important in Echocardiography

Material	Half-Power Distance (cm)
Water	380
Blood	15
Soft tissue (except muscle)	1 to 5
Muscle	0.6 to 1
Bone	0.2 to 0.7
Air	0.08
Lung	0.05

bone have very high tissue ultrasound impedance, limiting the ability of ultrasound to transverse these structures. Table 15–1 gives the distance in various tissues at which the intensity or amplitude of an ultrasound wave of 2 MHz is halved (the half-power distance). Echo studies across lung or other gas-containing tissues are not feasible, nor are those across dense structures such as bone or strongly scattering tissues such as thick muscle. Reflected echoes, also called specular echoes, are usually much stronger than scattered echoes. A grossly inhomogenous medium, such as a stone in a water bucket or a cardiac valve in a blood-filled heart chamber, produces strong specular reflections at the water–stone or blood–valve interface. Conversely, media that are inhomogenous at the microscopic level, such as muscle, produce more scatter than specular reflection. Specular reflections are obtained when the width of the reflecting object is larger than one fourth of the wavelength of the ultrasound. To visualize smaller objects, ultrasound of shorter wavelengths must be used. Because the velocity of sound in soft tissue is approximately constant, shorter wavelengths are obtained by increasing the frequency of the ultrasound beam (see Eq. 15–1). While smaller objects can be visualized with higher frequencies, more scatter is produced by insignificant inhomogeneities in the medium, confusing signals are generated, ultrasound beams are attenuated, and the depth of ultrasound penetration is limited.

Imaging Techniques

M Mode

The most basic form of ultrasound imaging is M-mode echocardiography. In this mode, the density and position of all tissues in the path of a narrow ultrasound beam (i.e., *along a single line*) are displayed as a scroll on a video screen. The scrolling produces an updated, continuously changing time plot of the studied tissue section, several seconds in duration. Because this is a timed *motion display* (normal cardiac tissue is always in motion), it is called M mode. Because only a very limited part of the heart is being observed at any one time and because the image requires considerable interpretation, M mode is not currently used as a primary imaging technique. This mode is, however, useful for the precise timing of events within the cardiac cycle and is often used in combination with color-flow Doppler for the timing of abnormal flows (see later). Quantitative measurements of size, distance, and velocity are also easily performed in the M mode without the need for sophisticated analysis stations. Because M-mode images are updated 1000 times per second, they provide greater temporal resolution than 2D echocardiography; thus, more subtle changes in motion or dimension can be appreciated.

Two-dimensional Mode

By rapid, repetitive scanning along *many different radii* within an area in the shape of a fan (sector), echocardiography generates a 2D image of a section of the heart. This image, which resembles an anatomic section and, thus, can be more easily interpreted, is called a *two-dimensional scan.* Information on structures and motion in the plane of a 2D scan is updated 30 to 60 times per second. This repetitive update produces a "live" (real-time) image of the heart. Scanning 2D echo devices image the heart by using either a mechanically steered transducer or, as is common in many of the modern devices, an electronically steered ultrasound beam (phased-array transducer).

Doppler Techniques

Most modern echo scanners combine Doppler capabilities with their 2D imaging capabilities. After the desired view of the heart has been obtained by 2D echocardiography, the Doppler beam, represented by a cursor, is superimposed on the 2D image. The operator positions the cursor as parallel as possible to the assumed direction of blood flow and then empirically adjusts the direction of the beam to optimize the audio and visual representations of the reflected Doppler signal. At the present time, Doppler technology can be used in at least four different ways to measure blood velocities: pulsed wave, high repetition frequency, continuous wave, and color flow. Each of these methods has specific applications; they may be concurrently available on some echocardiographic devices.

Doppler Effect

Information on blood flow dynamics can be obtained by applying Doppler frequency shift analysis to echoes reflected by the moving red blood cells.[2,3] Blood flow velocity, direction, and acceleration can be instantaneously determined. This information is different from that obtained in 2D imaging and, hence, complements it.

The Doppler principle as applied in echocardiography states that the frequency of ultrasound reflected by a moving target (red blood cells) is different from the frequency of the reflected ultrasound. The magnitude and direction of the frequency shift are related to the velocity and direction of the moving target. The velocity of the target is calculated with the Doppler equation:

$$v = (cf_d)/(2f_0 \cos\theta) \qquad (15\text{–}4)$$

where v is the target velocity (blood flow velocity), c is the speed of sound in tissue, f_d is the frequency shift, f_0 is the frequency of the emitted ultrasound, θ is the angle between the ultrasound beam and the direction of the target velocity (blood flow).

The only ambiguity in the equation is that theoretically the direction of the ultrasonic signal could refer to either the transmitted or the received beam; however, by convention, Doppler displays are made with reference to the received beam, and thus if the blood flow and the reflected beam travel in the same direction, the angle of incidence is zero degrees and the cosine is +1. As a result, the frequency of the reflected signal will be higher than the frequency of the emitted signal.

Equipment currently used in clinical practice displays Doppler blood flow velocities as waveforms. The waveforms consist of a spectral analysis of velocities on the ordinate and time on the abscissa. By convention, blood flow toward the transducer is represented above the baseline. If the blood flows away from the transducer, the angle of incidence will be 180 degrees, the cosine will equal −1; the waveform will be displayed below the baseline. When the blood flow is perpendicular to the ultrasonic beam, the angle of incidence will be 90 or 270 degrees, the cosine of either angle will be zero, and no blood flow will be detected. Because the cosine of the angle of incidence is a variable in the Doppler equation, blood flow velocity is measured most accurately when the ultrasound beam is parallel or antiparallel to the direction of blood flow. In clinical practice, a deviation from parallel of up to 20 degrees can be tolerated, because this only results in an error of 6% or less.

Pulsed-Wave Doppler

In pulsed-wave (PW) Doppler, blood flow parameters can be determined at precise locations within the heart by emitting repetitive short bursts of ultrasound at a specific frequency (pulse repetition frequency [PRF]) and analyzing the frequency shift of the reflected echoes at an identical sampling frequency (f_s). A time delay between the emission of the ultrasound signal burst and the sampling of the reflected signal determines the depth at which the velocities are sampled. The delay is proportional to the distance between the transducer and the location of the velocity measurements. To sample at a given depth (D), sufficient time must be allowed for the signal to travel a distance of 2 × D (from the transducer to the sample volume and back). The time delay, T_d, between the emission of the signal and the reception of the reflected signal, is related to D, and to the speed of sound in tissues (c), by the following formula:

$$D = cT_d/2 \qquad (15\text{–}5)$$

The operator varies the depth of sampling by varying the time delay between the emission of the ultrasonic signal and the sampling of the reflected wave. In practice, the sampling location or *sample volume* is represented by a small marker, which can be positioned at any point along the Doppler beam by moving it up or down the Doppler cursor. On some devices, it is also possible to vary the width and height of the sample volume.

The trade-off for the ability to measure flow *at precise locations* is that *ambiguous information* is obtained when flow velocity is very high. A simple reference to Western movies will clearly illustrate this point. When a stagecoach gets under way, its wheel spokes are observed as rotating in the correct direction. As soon as a certain speed is attained, rotation in the reverse direction is noted because the camera frame rate is too slow to correctly observe the motion of the wheel spokes. In PW Doppler, the ambiguity exists because the measured Doppler frequency shift (f_D) and the sampling frequency (f_s) are in the same frequency (kilohertz) range. Ambiguity will be avoided only if the f_D is less than half the sampling frequency:

$$f_D < f_s/2 \qquad (15\text{–}6)$$

The expression $f_s/2$ is also known as the Nyquist limit. Doppler shifts above the Nyquist limit will create artifacts described as *aliasing* or *wraparound,* and blood flow velocities will appear in a direction opposite to the conventional one. Blood flowing with high velocity toward the transducer will result in a display of velocities above and below the baseline. This artifact can be avoided by increasing the PRF, but this then limits the time available for a pulse to travel to the sample volume and back, thus limiting the range. The relationship between the maximum detectable velocity and the range at which it can be detected is known as the range-velocity product, or V_mR:

$$V_m R = c^2/8f_0 \qquad (15\text{–}7)$$

where V_m is the maximal velocity that can be unambiguously measured, R is the range or distance from the transducer at which the measurement is to be made, c is the speed of sound in tissue, and f_0 is the frequency of emitted ultrasound.

PW Doppler measurements are performed with the same transducer as the one used for imaging.

High Pulse Repetition Frequency Doppler

On some instruments, PW Doppler can be modified to a high-PRF mode. Whereas in conventional PW Doppler only a single burst of ultrasound is considered to be in the body at any given time, in high-PRF Doppler two to five sample volumes are simultaneously present in the tissues. Information coming back to the transducer may be coming back from depths of either two, three, or four times the initial sample volume depth. The returning signals can be a mix of signals that have previously been emitted and have traveled to distant gates and other signals that were just sent and returned from the first range gate.

The high-PRF mode allows increasing the sampling frequency because the scanner does not wait for the return of the information from distant gates; nonetheless, it receives information back within the specified time-gate period. Higher velocities can be measured with this method than with PW Doppler; however, the exact gate from which the ultrasound signals are reflected is unknown (range ambiguity).

Continuous-Wave Doppler

The continuous-wave (CW) Doppler technique uses continuous, rather than discrete, pulses of ultrasound waves. As a result, the region where flow dynamics are measured cannot be precisely localized. Blood flow velocity is, however, measured with great accuracy even at high flows. CW Doppler is particularly useful for the evaluation of patients with valvular lesions or congenital heart disease. It is also the preferred technique when attempting to derive hemodynamic information from Doppler signals (Box 15–2).

Color-Flow Mapping

Advances in electronics and computer technology have allowed the development of color-flow Doppler ultrasound scanners capable of displaying real-time blood flow within the heart as colors, while also showing 2D images in black and

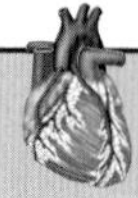

BOX 15–2 *Pulsed-Wave Versus Continuous-Wave Doppler Analysis*

- Pulsed-wave Doppler
  - Spatial specificity
  - Ambiguity in the measurement of high velocities
- Continuous-wave Doppler
  - Able to measure high velocities accurately
  - Spatial ambiguity

white. In addition to showing the location, direction, and velocity of cardiac blood flow, the images produced by these devices allow estimation of flow acceleration and differentiation of laminar and turbulent blood flow. Color-flow Doppler echocardiography is based on the principle of multigated, PW Doppler in which blood flow velocities are sampled at many locations along many lines covering the entire imaging sector.[4] At the same time, the sector is also scanned to generate a 2D image.

A location in the heart where the scanner has detected flow toward the transducer (the top of the image sector) is assigned the color red. Flow away from the direction of the top is assigned the color blue. This color assignment is arbitrary and determined by the equipment manufacturer and the user's color mapping. In the most common color-flow coding scheme, the faster the velocity (up to a limit), the more intense is the color. Flow velocities that change by more than a preset value within a brief time interval (flow variance) have the color green added to either the red or the blue. Both rapidly accelerating laminar flow (change in flow speed) and turbulent flow (change in flow direction) satisfy the criteria for rapid changes in velocity. In summary, the brightness of the red or blue colors at any location and time is usually proportional to the corresponding flow velocity, while the hue is proportional to the temporal rate of change of the velocity.

Contrast Echocardiography

Normally, red blood cells scatter ultrasound waves weakly, resulting in their black appearance on ultrasonic examination. Contrast echocardiography is performed by injecting nontoxic solutions containing gaseous microbubbles. These microbubbles present additional gas–liquid interfaces, which substantially increase the strength of the returning signal. This augmentation in signal strength may be used to better define endocardial borders, optimize Doppler envelope signals, and estimate myocardial perfusion.

Gramiak et al[5] originally reported the use of contrast echocardiography in 1968. They described visualization of aortic valve (AV) incompetence during left-heart catheterization (Box 15–3). Subsequently, contrast echocardiography has been used to image intracardiac shunts,[6] valvular incompetence,[7] and pericardial effusions.[8] In addition, LV injections of hand-agitated microbubble solutions have been used to identify semiquantitative LV endocardial edges,[9] cardiac output,[10] and valvular regurgitation.[11]

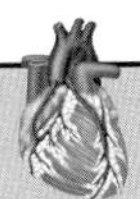

BOX 15–3 *Diagnostic Applications for Contrast Echocardiography*

- Assessment of congenital heart disease
- Enhancement of endocardial borders for qualitative assessment of wall-motion abnormalities
- Measurement of left ventricular function
- Quantification of valvular regurgitation
- Enhancement of color-flow Doppler signals
- Assessment of myocardial perfusion
- Measurements of perfusion area after coronary artery bypass graft surgery
- Assessment of quality of coronary bypass grafts and cardioplegia distribution
- Correct assessment of the results of surgery for ventricular septal defect

Contrast agents are microbubbles, consisting of a shell surrounding a gas. Initial contrast agents were agitated free air in either a saline or blood/saline solution. These microbubbles were large and unstable, so they were unable to cross the pulmonary circulation; they were effective only for right-sided heart contrast. Because of their thin shell, the gas quickly leaked into the blood with resultant dissolution of the microbubble. Agents with a longer persistence were subsequently developed.

More modern contrast agents have improved both the shell surrounding the microbubble and modification of the gas. The shell must inhibit the diffusion of gas into the blood and must enhance the pressure that a microbubble can tolerate before dissolving.[12] Gases with low shell diffusivity and blood saturation concentration result in a microbubble of increased survival, because the gas would rapidly equilibrate with blood and tend to stay within the shell. Improvements in the shell both increase the tolerance of the microbubble to ultrasound energies and decrease the diffusion of the gas into the blood; both changes further increase the persistence of the microbubbles. At the same time, there must be an element of fragility; the microbubbles must be disrupted by ultrasound signals producing appropriate imaging effects. The use of high-molecular-weight and less-soluble gases further increases the persistence of the contrast agents. Presently the perfluorocarbons are the most common gases used in contrast agents. The microbubbles need to be small enough to transverse the pulmonary circulation with a predominant size particle that approaches the size of an erythrocyte. The number of larger particles needs to be minimized to reduce the risk of obstruction of pulmonary capillary flow. Because the reflected energy of contrast agents is high, attenuation of the ultrasound signal is common. This signal attenuation interferes with visualization of distal structures.

An ultrasound signal produces compression and rarefaction (expansion) of the medium through which it travels. When this compression and rarefaction have impact with a microbubble, the bubble is compressed and expanded, respectively.[13] These changes result in alterations in the bubble volume, causing bubble vibrations with subsequent effects on the returning ultrasound signal to allow it to be "seen." These bubble pulsations may result in changes in the bubble radius by a factor of 20 or more.[14]

The acoustical properties of these microbubbles depend on the amplitude of the ultrasound signal. The amplitude of an ultrasound signal is usually defined by its mechanical index (MI), which is the peak negative pressure divided by the square root of the ultrasound frequency. Normally, when bubbles are insonated by ultrasound at their intrinsic resonate frequency, they vibrate; during the peak of the signal, they are compressed, and at the nadir of the signal, they expand. An ideal bubble will oscillate at the insonated ultrasound frequency.[15] At low ultrasound amplitudes (MI <0.1), the microbubbles oscillate at the frequency of the insonated signal with the degree of compression being equal to the degree of expansion. This is called *linear oscillation.* With fundamental imaging, no special contrast echo signals are produced.[16] With increasing signal amplitudes (MI = 0.2 to 0.7), the degree of expansion exceeds the degree of compression, which results in nonlinear oscillations. These nonlinear oscillations result in the creation of ultrasound waves at harmonic frequencies of the delivered ultrasound waves. While some bubble destruction will occur at all amplitudes, further increases in ultrasound amplitude (0.8 to 1.9) results in more compression and expansion with subsequent extensive bubble destruction. This bubble destruction, called *scintillation*, results in a brief but high output signal. Because of the extensive bubble destruction, intermittent imaging must be performed to allow contrast replenishment.

Further improvements in image acquisition can be achieved using harmonic imaging.[14] As explained previously, nonlinear oscillations result in the creation of harmonics. It was theorized that if the receiver were tuned to receive the first harmonic of the transmitted ultrasound signal, the signal-to-noise ratio could be improved by predominantly imaging signals from the microbubbles producing these harmonics. Because tissues also produce harmonics, tissue gray-scale imaging was also enhanced. Further improvements may include subharmonic and ultraharmonic imaging, which may provide more specific contrast enhancement. Harmonic imaging with TEE improves endocardial visualization and allows partial assessment of myocardial perfusion.[17] Harmonic power Doppler is more sensitive for detecting basilar perfusion in the far field compared with harmonic gray-scale imaging.[18]

The safety of contrast echocardiography must be considered. The contrast agents themselves must have a high therapeutic index. Multiple large bubbles may obstruct pulmonary microcirculation. The disruption of microbubbles by high-amplitude ultrasound may cause rupture of capillaries and injury to surrounding tissue.[19] Premature ventricular contractions have been described during high-intensity triggered imaging.[20] Other investigators were not able to demonstrate an increase in premature ventricular complex occurrence during or after imaging with triggered ultrasound at an MI of 1.[21] If current recommendations are followed, contrast echocardiography rarely results in significant side effects.[12]

The first-generation agents were Albunex and Levovist. Optison (Mallinckrodt Inc., St. Louis, MO), Imagent (Alliance Pharmaceuticals, San Diego, CA), and Definity (DuPont Pharmaceuticals, Waltham, MA) are presently available in the United States for use; Levovist and SonoVue (Bracco Diagnostics Inc., Princeton, NJ) are approved in Europe. Albunex is no longer available. Albunex utilized albumin encapsulation to stabilize a 4-μm air bubble that could opacify the LV but did not result in good microvascular perfusion. Levovist uses an air microbubble within a fatty acid shell.

Optison is a refinement of Albunex, with the substitution of perfluoropropane within an albumin shell. Definity uses perfluoropropane within a liposome shell, and Imagent encases a perfluorohexane/air combination in a phospholipid surfactant shell. SonoVue consists of hexafluoride with a phospholipid shell. New agents under development may use polymer shells whose flexibility and size can be more precisely controlled. These agents may be targeted to specific organs or vectors.

CLINICAL APPLICATIONS

Diagnostic applications for contrast echocardiography include enhancement of endocardial borders from qualitative assessment of wall motion abnormalities, measurement of LV function, assessment of congenital heart disease, quantification of valvular regurgitation, enhancement of color-flow Doppler signals, and assessment of myocardial perfusion. During cardiac surgery, the special and unique applications of myocardial contrast echocardiography (MCE) include measurements of perfusion area after coronary artery bypass graft surgery (CABG), assessment of quality of coronary bypass grafts and cardioplegia distribution, and visualization of the results of surgery for ventricular septal defect (VSD). Noncardiac intraoperative applications include assessment of perfusion in the kidney and in skeletal muscle. Work is ongoing to investigate the potential for analyzing cerebral blood flow with contrast-echo techniques.

Hand-agitated saline solutions are still useful to enhance right-sided structures. These saline solutions can be easily prepared by hand agitation of saline between two 10-mL Luer-Lok syringes connected by a three-way stopcock; small amounts of blood or air may be added to improve right-sided opacification. This technique is most commonly used to opacify the right atrium (RA) and ventricle (RV), assisting in the diagnosis of intra-atrial and ventricular shunts and to enhance pulmonary artery (PA) Doppler signals. The most common indication is the detection of a patent foramen ovale (PFO). After obtaining a bicaval view, a Valsalva maneuver is induced, and hand-agitated saline is injected into a large vein. After the RA is opacified, the Valsalva is released, and the left atrium (LA) is examined for contrast.

The commercially available contrast agents allow for opacification of the LV as well. This LV opacification leads to enhancement of LV endocardial borders as well as enhancement of color-flow Doppler mapping of the LA during evaluation of mitral regurgitation and enhancement of CW Doppler signals during evaluation of aortic stenosis. The second-generation agents allow for perfusion of the myocardial microcirculation. This perfusion permits assessment of perfusion patterns, coronary artery stenosis, and myocardium at risk during acute coronary syndromes.[16]

MYOCARDIAL CONTRAST ECHOCARDIOGRAPHY

Coronary artery stenosis and flow reserve may be estimated by contrast echocardiography. Lindner et al[22] described a method for the quantification of myocardial blood flow. If a contrast agent is administered at a steady rate, the blood concentration and myocardial concentration of the contrast agent equilibrate. If a single high-amplitude (i.e., high MI) ultrasound pulse is delivered to a myocardial region of interest, the microbubbles will be destroyed, but will be replenished as the contrast-filled blood perfuses the myocardium. The rate of contrast replenishment in the myocardium is directly related to myocardial blood flow. Repeated ultrasound pulses are delivered at shorter frequencies until a maximum myocardial contrast-enhanced ultrasound signal is obtained. A time–myocardial contrast intensity curve is constructed. MCE-derived indications of myocardial perfusion rate have relatively good between-study and between-reading reproducibility.[23]

If contrast echocardiography is used in conjunction with traditional echocardiography, different flow patterns can be described as outlined in Table 15–2. A fixed myocardial deficit may be diagnosed with a perfusion deficit during rest and stress with akinetic segments during both of these periods. An ischemic segment may be defined as a segment with normal perfusion and wall motion with rest and a perfusion deficit during stress that is accompanied by a regional wall motion abnormality (RWMA). Myocardial stunning may be diagnosed if normal perfusion is observed during rest in the presence of a hypokinetic rest wall motion, and hibernation may be diagnosed with rest hypoperfusion and a hypokinetic RWMA. The addition of MCE may increase the sensitivity, but not specificity, of dipyridamole-exercise echocardiography. Moir et al[24] combined MCE with dipyridamole-exercise echocardiography in 85 patients. They detected significant

Table 15–2 Diagnosis of Fixed Myocardial Deficits, Ischemia, Stunning, and Hibernation Based on Perfusion and Wall Motion Findings

	Rest Perfusion	Stress Perfusion	Rest Wall Motion	Stress Wall Motion
Fixed deficit	Deficit	Deficit	Akinetic	Akinetic
Ischemia	Normal	Deficit	Normal	Regional wall motion abnormality
Stunning	Normal		Regional wall motion abnormality	
Hibernation	Hypoperfusion		Hypokinetic	

coronary artery stenosis in 43 patients involving 69 coronary areas. The addition of MCE improved sensitivity for the detection of coronary artery disease (CAD) (91% versus 74%, $p = 0.02$) and accurate recognition of disease extent (87% versus 65% of territories, $p = 0.003$).

Measurements of myocardial blood flow by MCE are comparable to other techniques. Senior et al[25] compared MCE and single-photon emission computed tomography (SPECT) for the detection of CAD in 55 patients with a medium probability of disease. The sensitivity of MCE was significantly greater than that of SPECT for the detection of CAD (86% versus 43%, $p < 0.0001$); however, the specificities were not significantly different (88% and 93%, $p = 0.52$). In another investigation, quantitative real-time MCE with dipyridamole defined the presence and severity of CAD in a manner that compares favorably with quantitative SPECT.[26]

Microvascular perfusion is a prerequisite for ensuring viability early after acute myocardial infarction (AMI). For adequate assessment of myocardial perfusion, both myocardial blood volume and velocity need to be evaluated. Due to its high frame rate, low-power continuous MCE can assess both myocardial blood volume and velocity, allowing for assessment of microvascular perfusion.[27] In order to differentiate necrotic from viable myocardium after reperfusion therapy, Janardhanan et al[27] examined 50 patients with low-power continuous MCE 7 to 10 days after acute myocardial perfusion. Myocardial perfusion (contrast opacification) was assessed over 15 cardiac cycles after the destruction of microbubbles, and wall thickening was assessed at baseline. Regional and global LV function was reassessed after 12 weeks. Of the segments without contrast enhancements, 93% showed no recovery of function; in the segments with contrast opacification, 84% showed functional recovery. The greater the extent and intensity of contrast opacification, the better was the LV function at 3 months ($p < 0.001$, $r = -0.91$). Almost all patients (94%) with less than 20% perfusion in dysfunctional myocardium (assessing various cutoffs) failed to demonstrate an improvement in LV function.

Janardhanan et al[28] performed MCE in 70 patients with AMI after thrombolysis. Myocardial perfusion was examined in the akinetic areas in 20 patients with an occluded infarct-related artery that was subsequently revascularized. Contractile reserve was evaluated in these segments 12 weeks after revascularization with dobutamine stress echocardiography (DSE). Of the 102 akinetic segments, 37 (36%) showed contractile reserve. Contractile reserve was present in 24 of the 29 segments (83%) with homogenous contrast opacification and absent in 60 of the 73 segments (82%) with reduced opacification. Quantitative measurements of myocardial blood flow were significantly higher ($p < 0.0001$) in the segments with contractile reserve than in those without contractile reserve. MCE may thus be used as a reliable bedside technique for the accurate evaluation of collateral blood flow in the presence of an occluded infarct-related artery after AMI. MCE performed early after percutaneous coronary interventions provides information on the extent of infarction, and hence the likelihood for recovery of contractile reserve. The presence of perfusion before this intervention predicts the maintenance of perfusion and recovery of systolic function.[29]

MCE may be a useful tool in the detection of myocardial viability prior to coronary revascularization. In a study by Korosoglou et al,[30] contrast echocardiography was compared with low-dose dobutamine stress echocardiography (DSE) and combined technetium-99 sestamibi SPECT and fluorodeoxyglucose-18 positron emission tomography. Myocardial recovery was predicted by contrast echocardiography with a sensitivity of 86% and a specificity of 43%, and by nuclear imaging with a sensitivity of 90% and specificity of 44%, whereas DSE was similarly sensitive (83%) but more specific (76%). A combination of quantitative MCE and DSE provided the best diagnostic characteristics, with a sensitivity of 96%, a specificity of 63%, and an accuracy of 83%. Fukuda et al[31] performed MCE on 28 patients with chronic stable CAD and LV dysfunction before and after coronary revascularization. Of the 101 revascularized dysfunctional segments, MCE was adequately visualized in 91 (90%) segments, and wall motion was recovered in 45 (49%) segments. Quantitative measurements of myocardial blood flow in the recovery segments were significantly higher than those in nonrecovery segments. The investigators concluded that quantitative intravenous MCE can predict functional recovery after coronary revascularization.

Echo Scanners

Basic Principles

The conversion of reflected ultrasound echoes into 2D video images is a complicated process involving numerous electronic and digital manipulations. A 2D echo image is generated by scanning the heart every 17 msec, or 60 times each second. The image generated from a single 1/60th-second scan is called a "field." A process called "interlacing" combines two scans or fields into a frame of 1/30th of a second. Because the eye cannot capture an image lasting 1/30th of a second, microprocessors further process the frame electronically in real time. The intrinsic persistence of the television screen enhances image quality, and the end result is a fairly smooth picture.

Resolution

An ultrasound image may be described by its axial, lateral, or elevational resolution (Box 15–4). *Axial resolution* is the minimum separation between two interfaces located in a

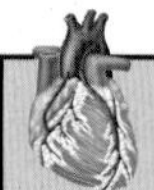

BOX 15–4 *Optimization of Resolution*

- Axial
  - High ultrasound frequency
  - Short duration of ultrasound pulse
  - High-frequency bandwidth
- Lateral
  - Narrow beam width
- Elevational
  - Thickness of the ultrasound beam

direction parallel to the beam so that they can be imaged as two different interfaces. The most precise image resolution is along this axial plane. The higher the frequency of the ultrasound signal, the greater is the axial resolution, because ultrasound waves of shorter wavelengths may be used. The shorter the burst of the emitted ultrasound wave (i.e., the shorter the pulse length), the greater is the axial resolution, because of the increased ability to differentiate adjacent interfaces. Pulse length should be no more than two or three cycles. The range of frequencies contained within a given ultrasound transmission is referred to as the *frequency bandwidth.* Generally, the shorter the pulse of the ultrasound produced, the greater is the frequency bandwidth. Because of the relationship between short pulse lengths and high bandwidths, high bandwidths are associated with better axial resolution. High transducer bandwidths also allow for better resolution of deeper structures.

Lateral resolution is the minimum separation of two interfaces aligned along a direction perpendicular to the ultrasound beam. The most important determinant of lateral resolution is the ultrasound beam width or ultrasound beam focusing; the narrower the beam, the better is the lateral resolution. If a small object appears within the "near field," it can be resolved laterally accurately; however, if it appears within the "far field," the size of this small object will appear to increase with the increase in the width of the ultrasound beam. This increase in size associated with object resolution in the far field results in blurring of deeper structures. *Elevational resolution* refers to the ability to determine differences in the thickness of the imaging plane. The thickness of the ultrasound beam is a major determinant of elevational resolution.

Preprocessing

Ultrasound echoes are received and converted to electronic signals by the transducer. On most modern echo scanners, the analog electronic signals undergo several modifications before being digitized and eventually displayed as an image. Preprocessing describes the modifications performed on the analog and digital signal prior to storage in the computer memory.

DYNAMIC RANGE MANIPULATION

The intensity of echo signals spans a wide range from very weak to very strong. Very strong signals falling beyond the saturation level of the electronic circuitry and very weak signals below the sensitivity of the instrument are automatically eliminated. The dynamic range (DR) of the instrument is defined by the limits at which extremely strong or weak signals are eliminated; DR is under operator control (Fig. 15–2). In this manner, signals of low intensity that contain little useful information, and mostly noise, can be selectively rejected.

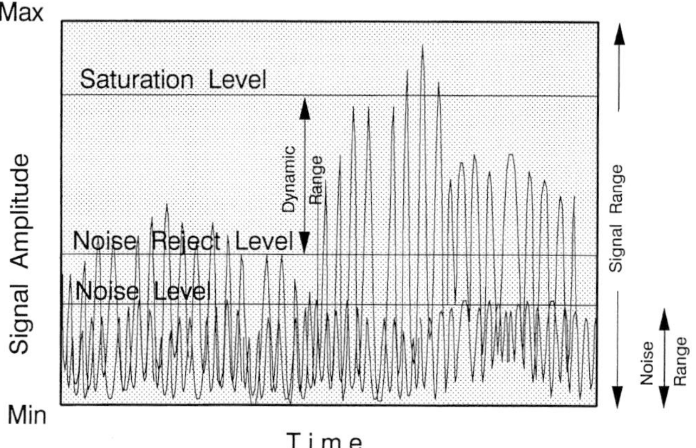

Figure 15–2 Dynamic range of a representative echocardiographic display system. All ultrasound signals begin at zero signal level and can increase in amplitude until they reach the signal "saturation" level. Many of the low-intensity signals fall within the range of the background noise and are, therefore, obscured. All systems have a built-in system reject, which eliminates both the system noise and the low-intensity echoes that lie just above the noise level. The dynamic range of the system is between the noise reject level and the saturation level. Signals within the dynamic range appear on the image display. (From Thys DM, Hillel Z: How it works: Basic concepts in echocardiography. *In* Bruijn NP, Clements F [eds]: Intraoperative Use of Echocardiography. Philadelphia, JB Lippincott, 1991.)

A wide DR is needed for high resolution, whereas a narrow range facilitates the discrimination between true image signals and noise. In clinical echocardiography, strong signals that arise from dense tissues (e.g., cardiac valves) and weaker signals arising from soft tissues (e.g., myocardium) are of interest. To give the weaker signals a greater representation in the DR, an amplifier converts the linear signal intensity scale into a logarithmic scale. While this increases the number of weaker signals detected, it also, unfortunately, tends to amplify noise.

GAIN, ATTENUATION, AND DAMPING

The gain and attenuation controls of a scanner increase and decrease the intensity of all signals in a proportional manner. As a result, they change the number of detected echo signals by bringing them above or below the rejection threshold of the DR. To deal with the potential loss of image quality caused by the display of the larger number of insignificant echoes obtained at high settings, a "damping" adjustment exists. Damping does not modify the received signal directly, but it decreases the strength of the emitted ultrasound beam by limiting the duration of the pulses that form the beam. Because less power is sent toward the target, fewer noise signals are generated. Damping also enhances the image, since it improves resolution by decreasing the number of cycles in each ultrasound pulse.

LATERAL GAIN CONTROL

An innovation allows the application of gain control to selected sectors of the ultrasound image. This feature appears particularly useful for the enhancement of image strength of structures that are nearly parallel to the ultrasound beam (e.g., the septum and lateral wall on a short-axis view at the level of the papillary muscles) (Fig. 15–3).

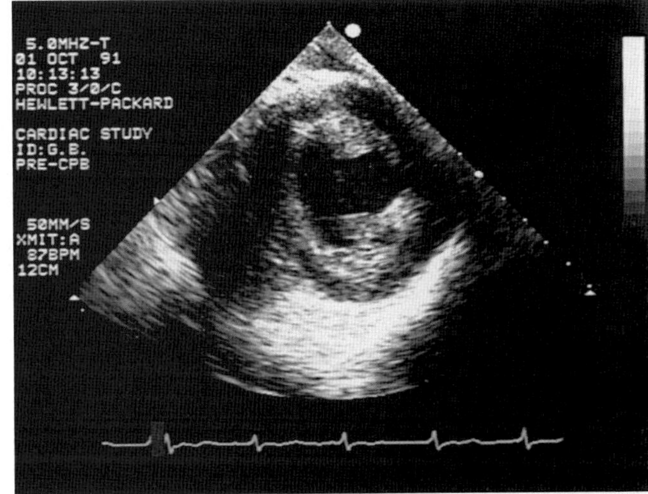

A

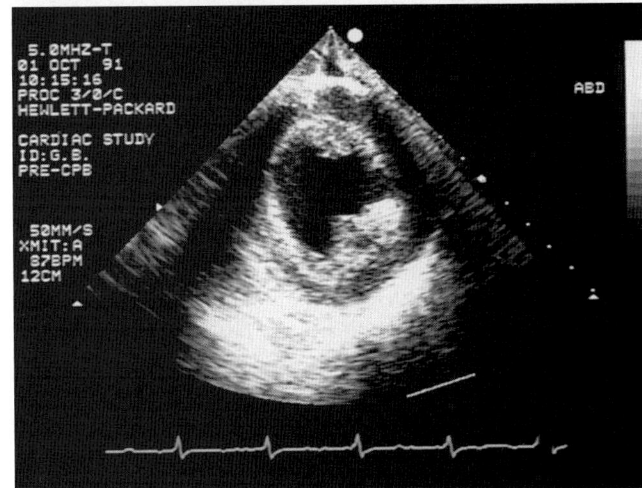

B

Figure 15–3 (*A*) Standard two-dimensional short-axis view of the left ventricle at the level of the papillary muscles. Note that the image drops out in the septal and lateral walls (vertical portions of the wall). (*B*) Identical view after application of lateral gain adjustments. The septal and lateral walls appear brighter, and less dropout is seen.

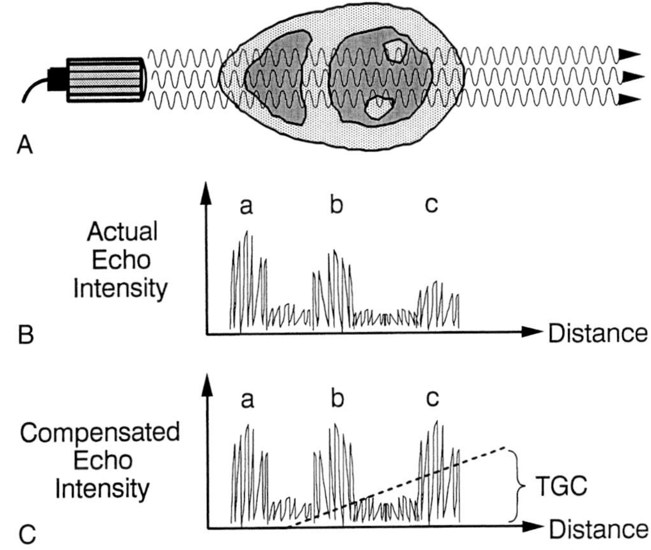

Figure 15–4 (*A*) As an ultrasound beam is aimed across the heart, specular echoes are reflected at the right ventricular wall (*a*), the septum (*b*), and the left ventricular wall (*c*). (*B*) The normal loss of echo strength is due to the decreasing intensity of the beam as it propagates through the heart. (*C*) Time-gain compensation (TGC) allows the intensity of the far-field signals to be increased selectively. (*A–C*, From Thys DM, Hillel Z: How it works: Basic concepts in echocardiography. *In* Bruijn NP, Clements F [eds]: Intraoperative Use of Echocardiography. Philadelphia, JB Lippincott, 1991.)

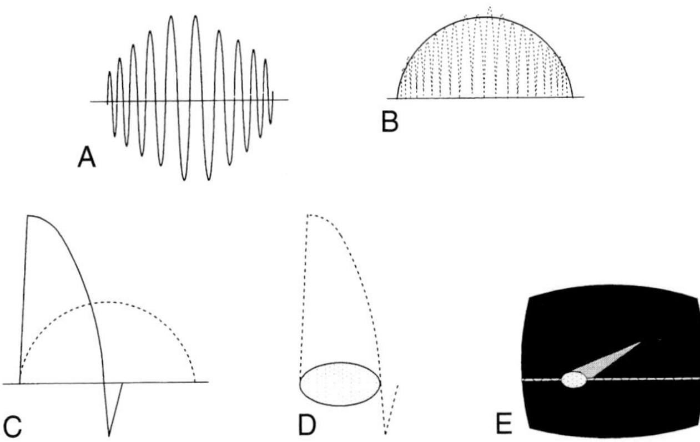

Figure 15–5 Leading-edge enhancement techniques. (*A*) Radiofrequency (RF) type of echo display. (*B*) This video represents the average height of the upper half of the RF signal. (*C*) Differentiation is obtained by taking the first derivative of the video display. (*D, E*), Intensity modulation represents the conversion of signal amplitude to intensity, changing the signal from a spike to a dot. (*A–E*, From Thys DM, Hillel Z: How it works: Basic concepts in echocardiography. *In* Bruijn NP, Clements F [eds]: Intraoperative Use of Echocardiography. Philadelphia, JB Lippincott, 1991.)

TIME-GAIN COMPENSATION

Because any wave traveling through tissues is attenuated proportional to the traveled distance, it is necessary to compensate for the fact that echoes returning from more distant objects will be weaker than those from equally dense objects closer to the transducer. A mechanism called "depth compensation" or "time-gain compensation" (TGC) is used to achieve this. The manner in which TGC is obtained is illustrated in Figure 15–4. TGC can be manually or automatically controlled.

LEADING-EDGE ENHANCEMENT

Leading-edge enhancement, or differentiation, is another type of preprocessing used to sharpen the video image. The reflected echo signal undergoes half-wave rectification and is smoothed into a signal envelope (Fig. 15–5*A*, *B*). An amplifier then differentiates the leading edge of the smoothed signal envelope to its first mathematical derivative (Fig. 15–5*C*), and a narrower and brighter image spot is formed (Fig. 15–5*D*). Because a 2D-echo image is composed of multiple radially juxtaposed scan lines, excessive edge enhancement narrows bright spots in the direction of travel of the echo beam (i.e., axially but not laterally). For this reason, leading-edge enhancement is primarily performed on M-mode scans, whereas instruments with 2D-mode capability use little or no edge enhancement in the 2D mode. Therefore, M-mode images often have better resolution than 2D images and are better suited for quantitative measurements.

Postprocessing

DIGITAL SCAN CONVERSION

After completing analog preprocessing, ultrasound devices digitize the image data with an analog-to-digital (A-D) converter (Fig. 15–6). Further processing is done while data are

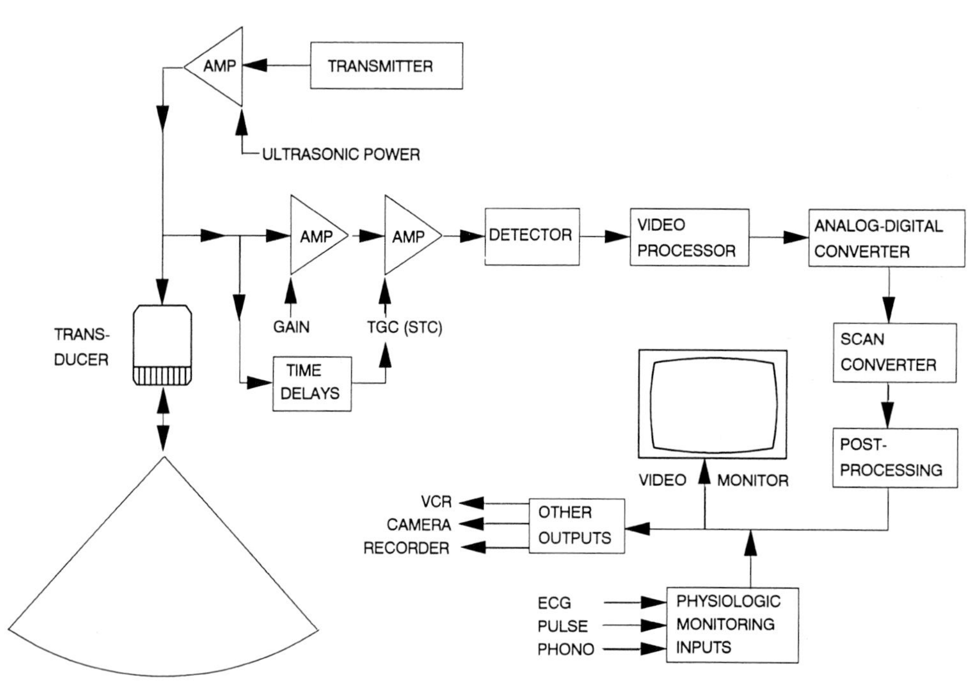

Figure 15–6 Schematic of a modern ultrasound scanner. The *arrows* indicate the directions for the flow of information or electronic power. AMP = electronic amplifier; TGC (STC) = time-gain compensation; VCR = videocassette recorder. (From Thys DM, Hillel Z: How it works: Basic concepts in echocardiography. *In* Bruijn NP, Clements F [eds]: Intraoperative Use of Echocardiography. Philadelphia, JB Lippincott, 1991.)

stored in the digital memory (input processing) or as they are received from the memory (output processing). An early step in digital processing uses a scan converter to transform the information obtained as radial sector scan lines into a rectangular (Cartesian) format for television screen display.

The memory stores the information of two adjacent scan fields consisting of a total of 128 scan lines. Each scan line is assigned to one column of memory. There is also one row of memory for each of the 512 horizontal television image lines (raster lines). Therefore, a typical television display of an echo image consists of 128 columns by 512 rows for a total of 65,536 picture elements, or *pixels.* While the monitor only displays 64 shades of gray for each pixel, the memory unit assigned to each pixel has the capacity to store 1024 degrees of brightness. Each pixel is assigned 10 binary bits of memory for a total of 2^{10} (1024) possible storage combinations.

TEMPORAL PROCESSING

As digital data are entered into memory, they can undergo temporal averaging in one of two modes. In the variable persistence mode, information from previous images is combined with current image data. A weighted average of the old and new data is then entered in memory as the new current data. A mechanism is built in to allow variable representation of old data into the new image. A different input-processing option calculates the arithmetic mean of the new data and up to nine frames of existing data.

Input processing is mainly used to improve the signal-to-noise ratio. In a 2D-echo image, a lower signal-to-noise ratio means a less granular appearance (the result of microscopic scatter) and less echo dropout (the result of very weak signals that are difficult to detect on the screen). Time averaging is most useful for enhancing slowly varying images.

HISTOGRAM EQUALIZATION

The video image is generated from data retrieved from memory via the scan converter. During retrieval, data can be subjected to histogram equalization. This process redistributes the gray-level assignment of each pixel according to the relative frequency of occurrence of the gray level in the entire image in an equalitarian manner. All levels of gray receive some representation even though the original image may have been formed from only a limited range of grays.

GRAY-SCALE PROCESSING

Each unit of memory assigned to a pixel can store 1 to 24 values of echo intensity, whereas the pixel itself can only display 64 shades of gray; thus, each gray level represents multiple echo intensities. The gray level reassignment is done by transfer functions of variable shapes, slopes, and end-points. An inverting transfer function allows the M-mode display to exist as a dark background with white lines or as a light background with dark lines. Gray-scale processing greatly affects image quality.

SPATIAL PROCESSING OR CONVOLUTION OPERATIONS

Spatial processing is a very sophisticated type of averaging that involves modifications in the content of a pixel based on the content of its neighbors. In Figure 15–7*A*, the gray level at pixel A_{11} is replaced by the average gray level of all pixels within the "kernel" $W_1 \ldots W_9$ or, simply stated, by the average of itself and the eight surrounding gray levels ($A_{11} = 1/9\ [A_2 + A_3 + A_4 + A_{10} + A_{11} + A_{12} + A_{18} + A_{19} + A_{20}]$). This operation is done for all pixels, and the new pixels are stored in a new image memory area. This produces spatial smoothing of the image and is particularly useful for parts of the image in which no abrupt changes in the echo density occur. It also eliminates "noise." When the detection of subtle changes in density is desired, such as in endocardial border detection, an edge-enhancing, convolution process is used. Applying the kernels shown in Figure 15–7*B,* the new A_{11} value would be $A_{11} = 1/9\ (A_2 + A_3 + A_4 + A_{18} + A_{19} + A_{20})$. To enhance vertical edges, a similar transformation can be used with the values of the kernel mask rotated 90 degrees. Edge enhancement has limited success because most ultrasound image edges are rel-

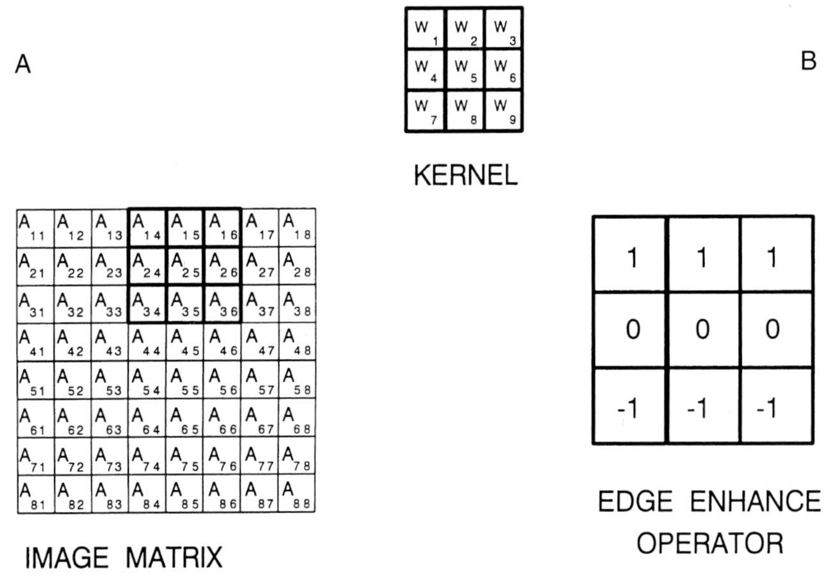

Figure 15–7 (*A, B*) Digital spatial processing by convolution operators. (*A, B*, From Thys DM, Hillel Z: How it works: Basic concepts in echocardiography. *In* Bruijn NP, Clements F [eds]: Intraoperative Use of Echocardiography. Philadelphia, JB Lippincott, 1991.)

atively smooth and the enhancement operator works best with images in which light and dark regions abruptly change.

Image Storage

All modern echo scanners allow the operator to store or "freeze" a single echo image on the display screen. This allows the scrutiny of any unusual transient anatomic or physiologic observations. Once frozen, an image can also be subjected to some simple quantitative measurements. With the continuous motion of the cardiac structures, it is often difficult, however, to capture the exact frame that is to be analyzed. For this reason, techniques to acquire several consecutive frames have been developed.

Cine Memory

One of the widely used techniques for information storage is cine memory. When activated, this mode captures a sequence of several echo images in digital memory. Because of the digital storage technique, the quality of the stored images is high. They can be displayed again in several different ways. In one method, the frames are displayed one by one as the operator manually controls the transition from one frame to the next, using a trackball. Any amount of time can be spent on a single frame. The images can also be replayed continuously in repeated endless-loop fashion, at the same speed as the original recording speed or at a different speed.

Videotape

The video recorder is the most common long-term, mass storage medium used in echocardiography. Most echo scanners are equipped with $^{3}/_{4}$-inch VHS, "super" VHS, or $^{1}/_{2}$-inch videocassette recorders (VCRs). Their advantages include low cost and their ability to record multiple cardiac cycles, facilitating the creation of a 3D image in the reviewer's mind.[32] Because VCRs store images in analog format, the quality of videotaped images is currently inferior to the real-time display, the digital cine memory replay, or digital storage. In the United States, videotape records images using NTSC (National Television Standards Committee) format. When videotape is used, resolution is limited by this NTSC format; resolution is not lost with digital storage.[32] Other disadvantages are the inability to randomly access parts of the current examination or previous examinations, difficulty sharing examinations with colleagues, as well as the degradation of videotape quality over time.[32]

Digital Storage Media

Digital paper chart recorders are available for most devices and are used to record the continuously scrolled information of M-mode and PW Doppler. The scrolls can subsequently be used for quantitative analysis of these types of data. These devices can also provide prints of single-frame 2D images. Most equipment contains a color video printer as well.

Digital image storage is rapidly becoming an alternative to videotape storage. The advantages of digital image storage include easy review, comparison with previous examinations, and postprocessing and quantitative analysis. Because of the vendor-independent communications protocols, storage and sharing examinations are simplified, allowing for easy transmission over high-bandwidth communication lines.

The DICOM (digital imaging and communications in medicine) standard for echocardiography was established in 1993 and 1994.[33] The main purpose of this protocol is to allow for independence of vendor-specific solutions.[34] It is a set of rules that govern the sharing of information between devices. The DICOM standard is a communications protocol that allows transmission and exchange of images among ultrasound machines, archives, and reviewing stations.

In order to efficiently store echocardiographic images, the digital image must be compressed. A single digital frame requires approximately 1 megabyte of storage. If 30 frames per second is assumed, a 15-minute study would use 25 to 30 gigabytes of space.[35] Because of the electronic size of the examination, the digital files are typically compressed using lossless run length encoding (RLE) or JPEG (Joint Photographic Expert Group) compression. This compression algorithm is designed primarily for still-frame images and provides compression ratio of at least 20:1. JPEG compression of this magnitude is similar in quality to S-VHS images.[35] Higher compression ratios (200:1) afforded by MPEG-1 (Moving Pictures Export Group) use redundant frame-to-frame information and do not decrease visualization scores of myocardial wall segments.[36] MPEG-1 is, however, presently not supported by DICOM. With standard DICOM compression, adult echocardiographic examinations may be up to 100 megabytes in size.

During the performance of an echocardiographic examination, 1 to 10 cardiac cycle loops of each of the standard ASE recommended views (see later) should be obtained and stored on the local hard drive of the echocardiography machine. Alternatively, 1 to 10 seconds may be recorded. Generally, a single cardiac cycle suffices for adults and is accurate (or superior) to videotape images.[37] After the examination is completed, the entire examination may be sent over a high-speed Ethernet connection through a network switch to a server. Alternatively, the examination may be stored on optical disks either for long-term storage or as a way of transfer to the server. Current examinations are stored on a RAID array (redundant array of inexpensive hard disks) with longer-term storage being provided with either a jukebox of optical disks or digital tapes. Random access to different parts of the examination, as well as comparison to previous examinations, is also facilitated. Postprocessing measurements are facilitated by DICOM calibration information.[33] Workstations can be connected to the local server for image analysis and review.

EQUIPMENT

Because fat, bone, and air-containing lung interfere with sound wave penetration, clear transthoracic echocardiogram (TTE) views are particularly difficult to obtain in patients with obesity, emphysema, or abnormal chest wall anatomy. To avoid these problems, TEE transducers were developed. Sound waves emitted from an esophageal transducer only have to pass through the esophageal wall and the pericardium to reach the heart, improving image quality and increasing the number of echocardiographic windows. Other advantages of TEE include the stability of the transducer position and the possibility of obtaining continuous recordings of cardiac activity for extended periods of time.

The first TEE examination was performed in 1975. The probe used allowed only M-mode imaging and had limited control of direction. Two-dimensional TEE was first performed with a mechanical system.[38,39] The system consisted of a vertical and a horizontal mechanical scanner connected to a 3.5-MHz ultrasonic transducer contained in a 12 × 20 × 6-mm oil bag. The transducers were rotated by a single-phase commutator motor via flexible shafts.

Subsequently, phased-array transducers were mounted into gastroscope housings.[40,41] With their greater flexibility and control, these probes allowed 2D scanning of the heart through many planes, and the probes became the prototypes of the currently used models. Annular array probes have also been introduced. These two types of systems offer a multitude of imaging capabilities: (1) M mode; (2) 2D (gray scale and B color, in which the typical gray scale is replaced by a range of colors); (3) high-resolution modes; (4) PW Doppler; (5) CW Doppler; (6) color-flow mapping; and (7) computerized data processing for measurements and cine loop display.

All TEE probes share several common features. All of the currently available probes employ a multifrequency transducer that is mounted on the tip of a gastroscope housing. The majority of the echocardiographic examination is performed using ultrasound between 3.5 and 7 MHz. The tip can be directed by the adjustment of knobs placed at the proximal handle. In most adult probes there are two knobs; one allows anterior and posterior movement, and the other permits side-to-side motion. Multiplane probes also include a control to rotate the echocardiographic array from 0 to 180 degrees. Thus, in combination with the ability to advance and withdraw the probe and to rotate it, many echocardiographic windows are possible. Another feature common to most probes is the inclusion of a temperature sensor to warn of possible heat injury from the transducer to the esophagus.

Currently, most adult echocardiographic probes are multiplane (variable orientation of the scanning plane), whereas pediatric probes are either multiplane or biplane (transverse and longitudinal orientation, parallel to the shaft). The adult probes usually have a shaft length of 100 cm and are between 9 and 12 mm in diameter. The tips of the probes vary slightly in shape and size but are generally 1 to 2 mm wider than the shaft. The size of these probes requires the patient to weigh at least 20 kg. Depending on the manufacturer, the adult probes contain between 32 and 64 elements per scanning orientation. In general, the image quality is directly related to the number of elements used. The pediatric probes are mounted on a narrower, shorter shaft with smaller transducers. These probes may be used in patients as small as 1 kg. Because of size limitations, these probes may not possess a lateral control knob. The question has been asked, Why not use the pediatric probe on all patients to decrease the risk of esophageal injury? The answer is that the smaller probes provide less diagnostic information. The number of elements is reduced, the aperture is smaller, there is less control of the tip, and the smaller transducer tip does not usually make good contact in the adult esophagus. These factors combine to significantly reduce image quality.

An important feature that is often available is the ability to alter the scanning frequency. A lower frequency, such as 3.5 MHz, has greater penetration and is more suited for the transgastric view. It also increases the Doppler velocity limits. Conversely, the higher frequencies yield better resolution for detailed imaging. One of the limitations of TEE is that structures very close to the probe are seen only in a very narrow sector. Newer probes may also allow a broader near-field view. Finally, newer probes may possess the ability to scan simultaneously in more than one plane.

COMPLICATIONS

Complications resulting from intraoperative TEE can be separated into two groups: injury from direct trauma to the airway and esophagus, and indirect effects of TEE (Box 15–5). In the first group, potential complications include esophageal bleeding, burning, tearing, dysphagia, and laryngeal discomfort. Many of these complications could result from pressure exerted by the tip of the probe on the esophagus and the airway. Although in most patients even maximal flexion of the probe will not result in pressure above 17 mm Hg, occasionally, even in the absence of esophageal disease, pressures greater than 60 mm Hg will result.[42] To look more closely at the effects on the esophagus, animal autopsy studies have been performed. In dogs as small as 5 kg on cardiopulmonary bypass (CPB) with full heparinization, no evidence of macroscopic or microscopic injury to the esophageal mucosa was noted following 6 hours of maximally flexed probe positioning.[43]

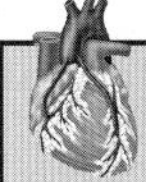

BOX 15–5 ***Complications from Intraoperative Transesophageal Echocardiography***

- Injury from direct trauma to the airway and esophagus
  - Esophageal bleeding, burning, tearing
  - Dysphagia
  - Laryngeal discomfort
  - Bacteremia
  - Vocal cord paralysis
- Indirect effects
  - Hemodynamic and pulmonary effects of airway manipulation
  - Distraction from patient

Further confirmation of the low incidence of esophageal injury from TEE is apparent in the few case reports of complications. In the world's literature, there are only a few reports of a fatal esophageal perforation[44,45] and one report of a benign Mallory-Weiss tear following intraoperative TEE.[46]

Another possible complication of esophageal trauma is bacteremia. Studies have shown that the incidence of positive blood cultures in patients undergoing upper gastrointestinal endoscopy is 4% to 13%,[47,48] and that in patients undergoing TEE is 0% to 17%.[49-51] Even though bacteremia may occur, it does not always cause endocarditis. Antibiotic prophylaxis in accordance with the American Heart Association guidelines is not routinely recommended but is optional in patients with prosthetic or abnormal valves or who are otherwise at high risk for endocarditis.[52]

In one of the earliest studies using TEE, transient vocal cord paralysis was reported in two patients undergoing neurosurgery in the sitting position with the head maximally flexed and the presence of an armored endotracheal tube.[53] This complication was believed to be due to the pressure the TEE probe exerted against the larynx. Since this initial report, no further problems of this kind have been reported with the use of the newer equipment.

The second group of complications that result from TEE includes hemodynamic and pulmonary effects of airway manipulation and, particularly for new TEE operators, distraction from patient care. Fortunately, in the anesthetized patient there are rarely hemodynamic consequences to esophageal placement of the probe, and there are no studies that specifically address this question. One potential hemodynamic effect of TEE, even in the well-anesthetized patient, is direct cardiac irritation from the probe with resultant atrial and ventricular arrhythmias. More important for the anesthesiologist are the problems of distraction from patient care. Although these reports have not appeared in the literature, the authors have heard of several endotracheal tube disconnections that went unnoticed to the point of desaturation during TEE. Additionally, there have been instances in which severe hemodynamic abnormalities have been missed because of fascination with the images or the controls of the echocardiograph machine. Clearly, new echo operators should enlist the assistance of an associate to watch the patient during the echo examination. This second anesthesiologist will become unnecessary after sufficient experience is gained. It is also important to be sure that all of the respiratory and hemodynamic alarms are activated during the echo examination. One report that did appear in the literature showed that, during TEE, an esophageal stethoscope was inadvertently pushed into the patient's stomach and was noticed to be missing only when the patient developed a small bowel obstruction.[54]

SAFETY GUIDELINES AND CONTRAINDICATIONS

To ensure the continued safety of TEE, the following recommendations are made. The probe should be inspected prior to each insertion for cleanliness and structural integrity. If possible, the electrical isolation should also be checked. The probe should be inserted gently and, if resistance is met, the procedure aborted. Minimal transducer energy should be used and the image frozen when not in use. Finally, when not imaging, the probe should be left in the neutral, unlocked position to avoid prolonged pressure on the esophageal mucosa.

Absolute contraindications to TEE in intubated patients include esophageal stricture, diverticula, tumor, recent suture lines, and known esophageal interruption. Relative contraindications include symptomatic hiatal hernia, esophagitis, coagulopathy, esophageal varices, and unexplained upper gastrointestinal bleeding. It should be noted that, despite these relative contraindications, TEE has been used in patients undergoing hepatic transplantation without reported sequelae.[55,56]

TRAINING/QUALITY ASSURANCE

This is an era in medicine in which the observance of guidelines for training, credentialing, certifying, and recertifying medical professionals has become increasingly common. Although there have been warnings and objections to anesthesiologists making diagnoses and aiding in surgical decision-making, there is no inherent reason that an anesthesiologist cannot provide this valuable service to the patient.[57] The key factors are proper training, extensive experience with TEE, and available backup by a recognized echocardiographer.

In cardiovascular medicine, formal policy standards for performing diagnostic and therapeutic techniques have been recommended by a number of societies. Although general guidelines for echocardiography have existed since 1990, no absolute minimum training criteria for intraoperative TEE have been established, nor is there any organization that grants certification in intraoperative TEE. Because the focus of recommendations for training, performance, and application of echocardiography has principally been directed at non–operating room environments, there remains a need for guidelines, training direction, and competence evaluation in the use of intraoperative and perioperative echocardiography.

In 1990, a task force from the American College of Physicians, the American College of Cardiology (ACC), and the American Heart Association (AHA) created initial general guidelines for echocardiography.[58] The American Society of Echocardiography (ASE) also provided recommendations for general training in echocardiography and has introduced a self-assessment test for measuring proficiency. These organizations recommended the establishment of three levels of performance with a minimum number of cases for each level: level 1, introduction and an understanding of the indications

(120 2D and 60 Doppler cases); level 2, independent performance and interpretation (240 2D and 180 Doppler cases); and level 3, laboratory direction and training (590 2D and 530 Doppler cases).[59,60] However, these guidelines are limited because they are not based on objective data or achievement. Furthermore, because different individuals learn at different rates, meeting these guidelines does not ensure competence, nor does failure to meet these guidelines preclude competence. In addition, these guidelines did not focus on intraoperative applications of echocardiography. In 1997, a revision of these same guidelines by the ACC and AHA also did not include specific recommendations for intraoperative applications.[61]

Proficiency in echocardiography can be more efficiently achieved in a limited setting (i.e., the perioperative period) with fewer clinical applications (e.g., interpreting wall motion, global function, and mitral regurgitation severity) than in a setting that introduces every aspect of echocardiography. The American Society of Anesthesiologists (ASA) and the Society of Cardiovascular Anesthesiologists (SCA) have worked together to create a document on practice parameters for perioperative TEE.[62] The SCA then created a Task Force on Certification for Perioperative TEE to develop a process that acknowledged basic competence and offered the opportunity to demonstrate advanced competence as outlined by the SCA/ASA practice parameters. This process resulted in the development of the PTEeXAM. Previous work has shown that an examination focused on intraoperative problems can serve as a test of TEE competence.[63]

TEE training should begin with a dedicated training period. This is most easily accomplished during a cardiac anesthesia fellowship but can be done by postgraduate physicians as well (see Chapter 41). The subject can be approached through a combination of tutorials, scientific review courses, self-instruction with teaching tapes, interactive learning programs, and participation in echo reading sessions.[64,65] Frequently, a symbiotic relationship with the cardiology division can be established in which anesthesiologists can teach the fundamentals of airway management, operating room physiology, and the use of local anesthetics while learning the principles of echocardiography from the cardiologists.

The ASE and the SCA combined to create guidelines for training in perioperative echocardiography. These guidelines have two levels: basic and advanced. In the basic level, at least 50 examinations must be performed and at least 150 observed. Competence at this level involves safe insertion, a complete examination, and the ability to perform a wide variety of applications. The advanced level requires performing at least 150 examinations with observation of at least 300 examinations. Competence at this level involves the full spectrum of perioperative applications. The National Board of Echocardiography (NBE) has also created Certification in Perioperative TEE. Certification is offered only for those with advanced level training. Certification requires successful completion of the PTEeXAM, a current medical license, board certification, and documented specific training in the care of patients with cardiovascular disease or 24 months of dedicated experience. This NBE certification is not board certification in TEE and only certifies that the PTEeXAM was passed.[66]

Quality assurance is another area for which no specific guidelines currently exist for TEE. One model for quality assurance was proposed by Rafferty et al.[67] At the very least, each echocardiogram should be recorded in a standardized fashion and accompanied by a written report for inclusion in the patient's chart. Images may also be copied and included in the chart. Careful records of any complications should be kept. To ensure that the proper images are being obtained and that the interpretations are correct, the studies should be periodically reviewed. This is another area in which the relationship between cardiology and anesthesiology can be productive.

It is important to recognize that practice guidelines are systematically developed *recommendations* that assist the practitioner and patient in making decisions about health care. These recommendations may be adopted, modified, or rejected according to clinical needs and constraints. Practice guidelines are not intended as standards or absolute requirements, and their use cannot guarantee any specific outcome. Practice guidelines are subject to revisions from time to time as medical knowledge, technology, and technique evolve. Guidelines are supported by analysis of the current literature and by synthesis of expert opinion, open forum commentary, and clinical feasibility data.

TECHNIQUE OF PROBE PASSAGE

Anesthesiologists may need to insert TEE probes in awake or anesthetized patients. Awake insertions are identical in technique to awake upper gastrointestinal endoscopy and should be performed when the patient has an empty stomach. It is also important to use a bite block. Probe insertion usually requires topical oral and pharyngeal anesthesia, as well as moderate sedation. The probe is well lubricated, and the function of the directional controls is tested prior to insertion. The vast majority of patients are able to assist the probe's passage through the pharynx with a swallowing action. The presence of a TEE probe, however, would complicate airway management during anesthetic induction. Thus, most anesthesiologists introduce TEE probes in anesthetized patients after tracheal intubation. To improve image quality, it is also useful to evacuate the stomach via suction prior to probe insertion.

The passage of a TEE probe through the oral and pharyngeal cavities in anesthetized patients may be challenging at times. The usual technique is to place the well-lubricated probe in the posterior portion of the oropharynx with the transducer element pointing inferiorly and anteriorly. The remainder of the probe may be stabilized by looping the controls and the proximal portion of the probe over the operator's neck and shoulder. The operator's left hand then elevates the mandible by inserting the thumb behind the teeth, grasping the submandibular region with the fingers, and then gently lifting. The probe is then advanced against a slight but even resistance, until a loss of resistance is detected as the tip of the probe passes the inferior constrictor muscle of the pharynx. This usually occurs 10 cm past the lips in neonates to 20 cm past the lips in adults. Further manipulation of the probe is performed under echocardiographic guidance.

Difficult TEE probe insertion may be caused by the probe tip abutting the pyriform sinuses, vallecula, posterior tongue, or an esophageal diverticulum. Overinflation of the endotracheal tube cuff could also obstruct passage of the probe. Maneuvers that might aid the passage of the probe include changing the neck position, realigning the TEE probe, and applying additional jaw thrust by elevating the angles of the mandible. The probe may also be passed with the assistance of laryngoscopy. The probe should never be forced past an obstruction. This could result in airway trauma or esophageal perforation.

ANATOMY AND TRANSESOPHAGEAL ECHOCARDIOGRAPHY VIEWS

Over the past two decades, perioperative TEE has become recognized as a valuable hemodynamic monitor and diagnostic tool. In 1993, the ASE established the Council for Intraoperative Echocardiography (IOC) to address issues related to the rapidly increasing utility of TEE in the perioperative period and its important impact on anesthesia and surgical decision-making. In 1997, the board members of the IOC decided to create the ASE/SCA Guidelines for Performing a Comprehensive Intraoperative Multiplane Examination,[68,69] which included the collective endorsement of a standard recommended set of anatomically directed cross-sectional views and the corresponding nomenclature. As implied in the original manuscript,[68,69] these guidelines were established to

1. Facilitate training in intraoperative TEE by providing a framework in which to develop the necessary knowledge and skills.
2. Enhance and improve the technical quality and completeness of individual studies.
3. Facilitate the communication of intraoperative echocardiographic data between centers to provide a basis for multicenter investigations.
4. Standardize the description of intraoperative echocardiographic data to encourage industrial development of efficient and rapidly acquiring labeling, storage, and analysis systems.

The guidelines for the intraoperative TEE examination were not intended to be all encompassing but rather to serve as a framework for a systematic and complete examination of cardiac and great vessel anatomy of the "normal patient and to serve as a baseline for later comparison."[68,69] This examination may require 20 minutes to complete by the beginner who must balance both comprehension and expedience in obtaining each 2D image and sequentially view one structure at a time. The experienced and competent echocardiographer, however, should be able to complete this examination in less than 10 minutes in order to provide timely and relevant diagnostic information. A more thorough intraoperative TEE examination, including the delineation of detailed intracardiac and extracardiac anatomy, description of congenital heart defects, and qualitative/quantitative Doppler analysis, is certainly recommended and warranted in appropriate patients. Ideally, a complete intraoperative TEE examination not only provides information that is relevant to the particular diagnosis in question but also identifies unanticipated findings that may have a significant impact on perioperative management (e.g., PFO, atrial thrombus, severe aortic atherosclerosis).

Multiplane Transesophageal Echocardiography Probe Manipulation: Descriptive Terms and Technique

The process of obtaining a comprehensive intraoperative multiplane TEE examination begins with a fundamental understanding of the terminology and technique for probe manipulation (Fig. 15–8). Efficient probe manipulation minimizes esophageal injury and facilitates the process of acquiring and sweeping through 2D image planes. Horizontal imaging planes are obtained by moving the TEE probe up and down (proximal and distal) in the esophagus at various depths relative to the incisors (upper esophageal: 20 to 25 cm; mid-esophageal: 30 to 40 cm; transgastric: 40 to 45 cm; deep transgastric: 45 to 50 cm) (Table 15–3). Vertical planes are obtained by manually turning the probe to the patient's left or right.

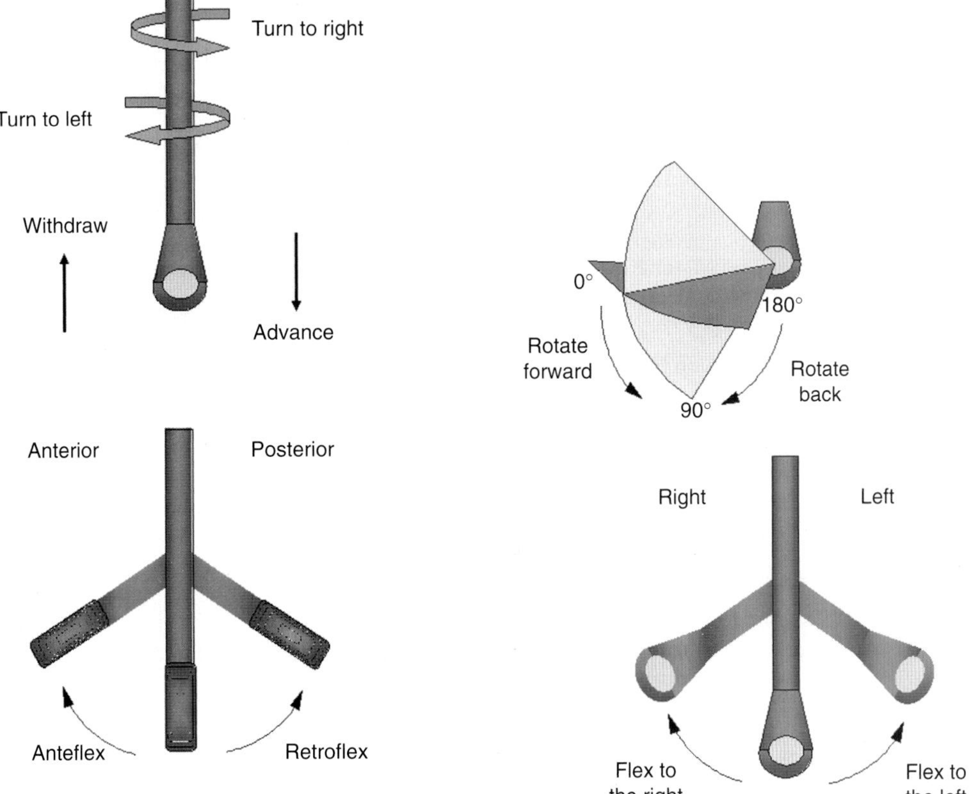

Figure 15–8 Ways to adjust the probe. *Top left*, Probe movement in the esophagus. *Top right*, Scanning angles obtained by crystal rotation. *Bottom left*, Movement of the tip forward and back. *Bottom right*, Movement of the tip from side to side.

Table 15–3 The Comprehensive Intraoperative Multiplane Transesophageal Echocardiographic Examination

Probe Tip Depth (from lips)	**Upper Esophageal (20 to 25 cm)**
VIEW	AORTIC ARCH: LONG AXIS
Multiplane angle range	0°
Anatomy imaged	Aortic arch; left brachiocephalic vein; left subclavian and carotid arteries; right brachiocephalic artery
Clinical utility	Ascending aorta and arch pathology: atherosclerosis, aneurysms, and dissections Aortic CPB cannulation site evaluation
VIEW	AORTIC ARCH: SHORT AXIS
Multiplane angle range	90°
Anatomy imaged	Aortic arch; left brachiocephalic vein; left subclavian and carotid arteries; right brachiocephalic artery; main pulmonary artery and pulmonic valve
Clinical utility	Ascending aorta and arch pathology: atherosclerosis, aneurysms and dissections; pulmonary embolus; pulmonary valve evaluation (insufficiency, stenosis, Ross procedure) Pulmonary artery catheter placement
Probe Tip Depth	**Mid Esophageal (30 to 40 cm)**
VIEW	FOUR CHAMBER
Multiplane angle range	0° to 20°
Anatomy imaged	Left ventricle and atrium Right ventricle and atrium Mitral and tricuspid valves Interatrial and interventricular septa Left pulmonary veins: slight probe withdrawal and turning to left Right pulmonary veins: slight probe withdrawal and turning to right Coronary sinus: slight probe advancement and turning to right
Clinical utility	Ventricular function: global and regional Intracardiac chamber masses: thrombus, tumor, air; foreign bodies Mitral and tricuspid valve evaluation: pathology, pathophysiology Congenital or acquired interatrial and ventricular septal defects evaluation Hypertrophic obstructive cardiomyopathy evaluation Ventricular diastolic evaluation via transmitral and pulmonary vein Doppler flow profile analysis Pericardial evaluation: pericarditis; pericardial effusion Coronary sinus evaluation: coronary sinus catheter placement; dilation secondary to persistent left superior vena cava
VIEW	MITRAL COMMISSURAL
Multiplane angle range	60° to 70°
Anatomy imaged	Left ventricle and atrium Mitral valve
Clinical utility	Left ventricular function: global and regional Left ventricular and atrial masses: thrombus, tumor, air; foreign bodies Mitral valve evaluation: pathology, pathophysiology Ventricular diastolic evaluation via transmitral Doppler flow profile analysis
VIEW	TWO CHAMBER
Multiplane angle range	80° to 100°
Anatomy imaged	Left ventricle, atrium and atrial appendage Mitral valve Left pulmonary veins: turning probe to left Coronary sinus (short axis or long axis by turning probe tip to left)
Clinical utility	Left ventricular function: global and regional Left ventricular and atrial masses: thrombus, tumor, air; foreign bodies Mitral valve evaluation: pathology, pathophysiology Ventricular diastolic evaluation via transmitral and pulmonary vein Doppler flow profile analysis Coronary sinus evaluation: coronary sinus catheter placement; dilation secondary to persistent left superior vena cava
VIEW	LONG AXIS
Multiplane angle range	120° to 160°
Anatomy imaged	Left ventricle and atrium Left ventricular outflow tract Aortic valve Mitral valve Ascending aorta
Clinical utility	Left ventricular function: global and regional Left ventricular and atrial masses: thrombus, tumor, air; foreign bodies Mitral valve evaluation: pathology, pathophysiology Ventricular diastolic evaluation via transmitral Doppler flow profile analysis Aortic valve evaluation: pathology, pathophysiology Ascending aorta pathology: atherosclerosis, aneurysms, dissections Hypertrophic obstructive cardiomyopathy evaluation
VIEW	RIGHT VENTRICULAR INFLOW-OUTFLOW ("WRAP-AROUND")
Multiplane angle range	60° to 90°
Anatomy imaged	Right ventricle and atrium Left atrium

Table 15–3 The Comprehensive Intraoperative Multiplane Transesophageal Echocardiographic Examination—(Continued)

Clinical utility	Tricuspid valve Aortic valve Right ventricular outflow tract Pulmonic valve and main pulmonary artery Right ventricular and right and left atrial masses: thrombus, embolus, tumor, foreign bodies Pulmonic valve and subpulmonic valve: pathology; pathophysiology Pulmonary artery catheter placement Tricuspid valve: pathology; pathophysiology Aortic valve: pathology; pathophysiology
VIEW	AORTIC VALVE SHORT AXIS
Multiplane angle range	30° to 60°
Anatomy imaged	Aortic valve Interatrial septum Coronary ostia and arteries Right ventricular outflow tract Pulmonary valve
Clinical utility	Aortic valve: pathology; pathophysiology Ascending aorta pathology: atherosclerosis, aneurysms and dissections Left and right atrial masses: thrombus, embolus, air, tumor, Foreign bodies Congenital or acquired interatrial septal defects evaluation
VIEW	AORTIC VALVE LONG AXIS
Multiplane angle range	120° to 160°
Anatomy imaged	Aortic valve Proximal ascending aorta Left ventricular outflow tract Mitral valve Right pulmonary artery
Clinical utility	Aortic valve: pathology; pathophysiology Ascending aorta pathology: atherosclerosis, aneurysms and dissections Mitral valve evaluation: pathology, pathophysiology
VIEW	BICAVAL
Multiplane angle range	80° to 110°
Anatomy imaged	Right and left atrium Superior vena cava (long axis) Inferior vena cava orifice: advance probe and turn to right to visualize inferior vena cava in the long axis, liver, hepatic and portal veins Interatrial septum Right pulmonary veins: turn probe to right Coronary sinus and thebesian valve Eustachian valve
Clinical utility	Right and left atrial masses: thrombus, embolus, air, tumor, foreign bodies Superior vena cava pathology: thrombus, sinus venosus atrial septal defect Inferior vena cava pathology (thrombus, tumor) Femoral venous catheter placement Coronary sinus catheter placement Right pulmonary vein evaluation: anomalous return, Doppler evaluation for left ventricular diastolic function Congenital or acquired interatrial septal defects evaluation Pericardial effusion evaluation
VIEW	ASCENDING AORTIC SHORT AXIS
Multiplane angle range	0° to 60°
Anatomy imaged	Ascending aorta Superior vena cava (short axis) Main pulmonary artery Right pulmonary artery Left pulmonary artery (turn probe tip to left) Pulmonic valve
Clinical utility	Ascending aorta pathology: atherosclerosis, aneurysms and dissections Pulmonic valve: pathology; pathophysiology Pulmonary embolus/thrombus evaluation Superior vena cava pathology: thrombus, sinus venosus atrial septal defect Pulmonary artery catheter placement
VIEW	ASCENDING AORTA LONG AXIS
Multiplane angle range	100° to 150°
Anatomy imaged	Ascending aorta Right pulmonary artery
Clinical utility	Ascending aorta pathology: atherosclerosis, aneurysms and dissections Anterograde cardioplegia delivery evaluation Pulmonary embolus/thrombus

Table continued on following page

Table 15–3 The Comprehensive Intraoperative Multiplane Transesophageal Echocardiographic Examination—(Continued)

VIEW	DESCENDING AORTA SHORT AXIS
Multiplane angle range	0°
Anatomy imaged	Descending thoracic aorta Left pleural space
Clinical utility	Descending aorta pathology: atherosclerosis, aneurysms and dissections Intra-aortic balloon placement evaluation Left pleural effusion
VIEW	DESCENDING AORTA LONG AXIS
Multiplane angle range:	90° to 110°
Anatomy imaged	Descending thoracic aorta Left pleural space
Clinical utility	Descending aorta pathology: atherosclerosis, aneurysms and dissections Intra-aortic balloon placement evaluation Left pleural effusion
Probe Tip Depth	**Transgastric (40 to 45 cm)**
VIEW	BASAL SHORT AXIS
Multiplane angle range	0° to 20°
Anatomy imaged	Left and right ventricle Mitral valve Tricuspid valve
Clinical utility	Mitral valve evaluation ("fish-mouth view"): pathology, pathophysiology Tricuspid valve evaluation: pathology, pathophysiology Basal left ventricular regional function Basal right ventricular regional function
VIEW	MID SHORT AXIS
Multiplane angle range	0° to 20°
Anatomy imaged	Left and right ventricle Papillary muscles
Clinical utility	Mid left and right ventricular regional and global function Intracardiac volume status
VIEW	TWO CHAMBER
Multiplane angle range	80° to 100°
Anatomy imaged	Left ventricle and atrium Mitral valve: chordae and papillary muscles Coronary sinus
Clinical utility	Left ventricular regional and global function (including apex) Left ventricular and atrium masses: thrombus, embolus, air, tumor, foreign bodies Mitral valve: pathology and pathophysiology
VIEW	LONG AXIS
Multiplane angle range	90° to 120°
Anatomy imaged	Left ventricle and outflow tract Aortic valve Mitral valve
Clinical utility	Left ventricular regional and global function Mitral valve: pathology and pathophysiology Aortic valve: pathology and pathophysiology
VIEW	RIGHT VENTRICULAR INFLOW
Multiplane angle range	100° to 120°
Anatomy imaged	Right ventricle and atrium Tricuspid valve: chordae and papillary muscles
Clinical utility	Right ventricular regional and global function Right ventricular and atrium masses: thrombus, embolus, tumor, foreign bodies Tricuspid valve: pathology and pathophysiology
Probe Tip Depth	**Deep Transgastric (45 to 50 cm)**
VIEW	LONG AXIS
Multiplane angle range	0° to 20° (anteflexion)
Anatomy imaged	Left ventricle and outflow tract Interventricular septum Aortic valve and ascending aorta Left atrium Mitral valve Right ventricle Pulmonic valve
Clinical utility	Aortic valve and subaortic pathology and pathophysiology Mitral valve pathology and pathophysiology Left and right ventricular global function Left and right ventricular masses: thrombus, embolus, tumor, Foreign bodies Congenital or acquired interventricular septal defect evaluation

Further alignment of the imaging plane can be obtained by manually rotating one of the two control wheels on the probe handle, which flexes the probe tip to the left or right direction or in the anterior or posterior plane. Multiplane probes may further facilitate interrogation of complex anatomic structures, such as the mitral valve (MV), by allowing up to 180 degrees of axial rotation of the imaging plane without manual probe manipulation.

The Comprehensive Intraoperative Transesophageal Echocardiography Examination: Imaging Planes and Structural Analysis

Left and Right Ventricles

The LV should be carefully examined for global and regional function using multiple transducer planes, depths, and rotational and angular orientations (Fig. 15–9). Although a 17-segment model for assessing regional ventricular function has been developed[70] (Fig. 15–10*A*), the original comprehensive intraoperative TEE examination[68,69] proposes a regional assessment scheme that requires a systematic approach to evaluate each of the 16 individual LV segments: 6 basal, 6 mid, and 4 apical (Fig. 15–10*B*). Analysis of segmental function is based upon a qualitative visual assessment that includes the following grading system of both LV wall thickness and motion (endocardial border excursion) during systole: 1 = normal (>30% thickening); 2 = mild hypokinesis (10% to 30% thickening); 3 = severe hypokinesis (<10% thickening); 4 = akinesis (no thickening); 5 = dyskinesis (paradoxical motion). The *mid-esophageal (ME) four-chamber* view at 0 to 20 degrees (see Fig. 15–9*A*) and *two-chamber* view at approximately 80 to 100 degrees (Fig. 15–9*B*) enable visualization of the septal and lateral as well as the inferior and anterior segments at the basal, mid, and apical level segments, respectively. The *ME long-axis (LAX) view* at 120 to 160 degrees (Fig. 15–9*C*) allows evaluation of the remaining anteroseptal and posterior LV segments. Because the LV is usually oriented inferiorly to the true horizontal plane, slight retroflexion of the probe tip may be required to minimize LV foreshortening. The *transgastric mid short-axis view (TG mid SAX)* at 0 to 20 degrees (Fig. 15–9*D*) is the most commonly used view for monitoring LV function because it allows a mid-papillary assessment of the LV segments supplied by the corresponding coronary arteries (right [RCA], left circumflex [CX], and left anterior descending [LAD]). This view also enables qualitative and quantitative evaluation of pericardial effusions. Advancing or withdrawing the probe at the transgastric depth enables LV evaluation at the respective apical and basal levels (*TG basal SAX*—Fig. 15–9*F*). Further evaluation of the LV can be obtained at the mid-papillary transgastric depth by rotating the probe forward to the *TG two-chamber* (80 to 100 degrees) (Fig. 15–9*E*) and *TG LAX* (90 to 120 degrees) (Fig. 15–9*J*).

Text continued on p. 460

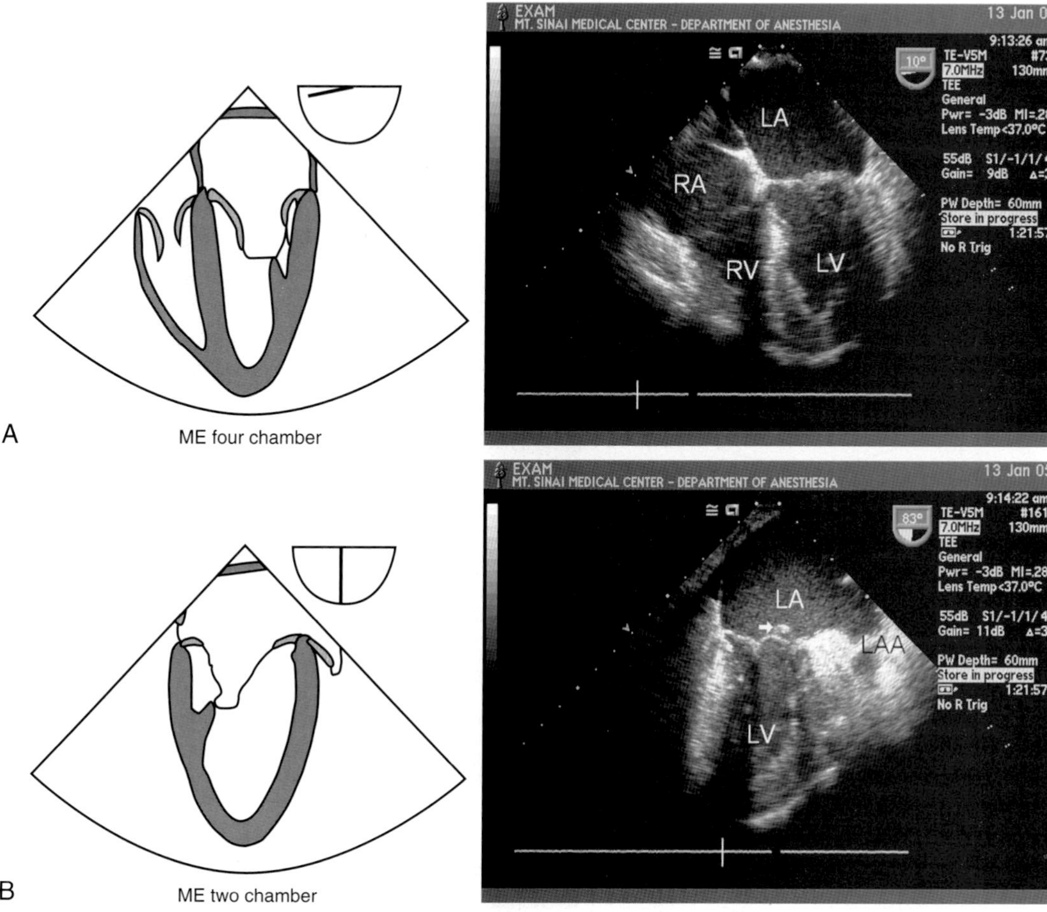

Figure 15–9 Schematic drawings and corresponding echo images of the comprehensive TEE exam. (*A*) ME four-chamber view. (*B*) ME two-chamber view; the *arrow* points to a prolapsing posterior mitral leaflet.

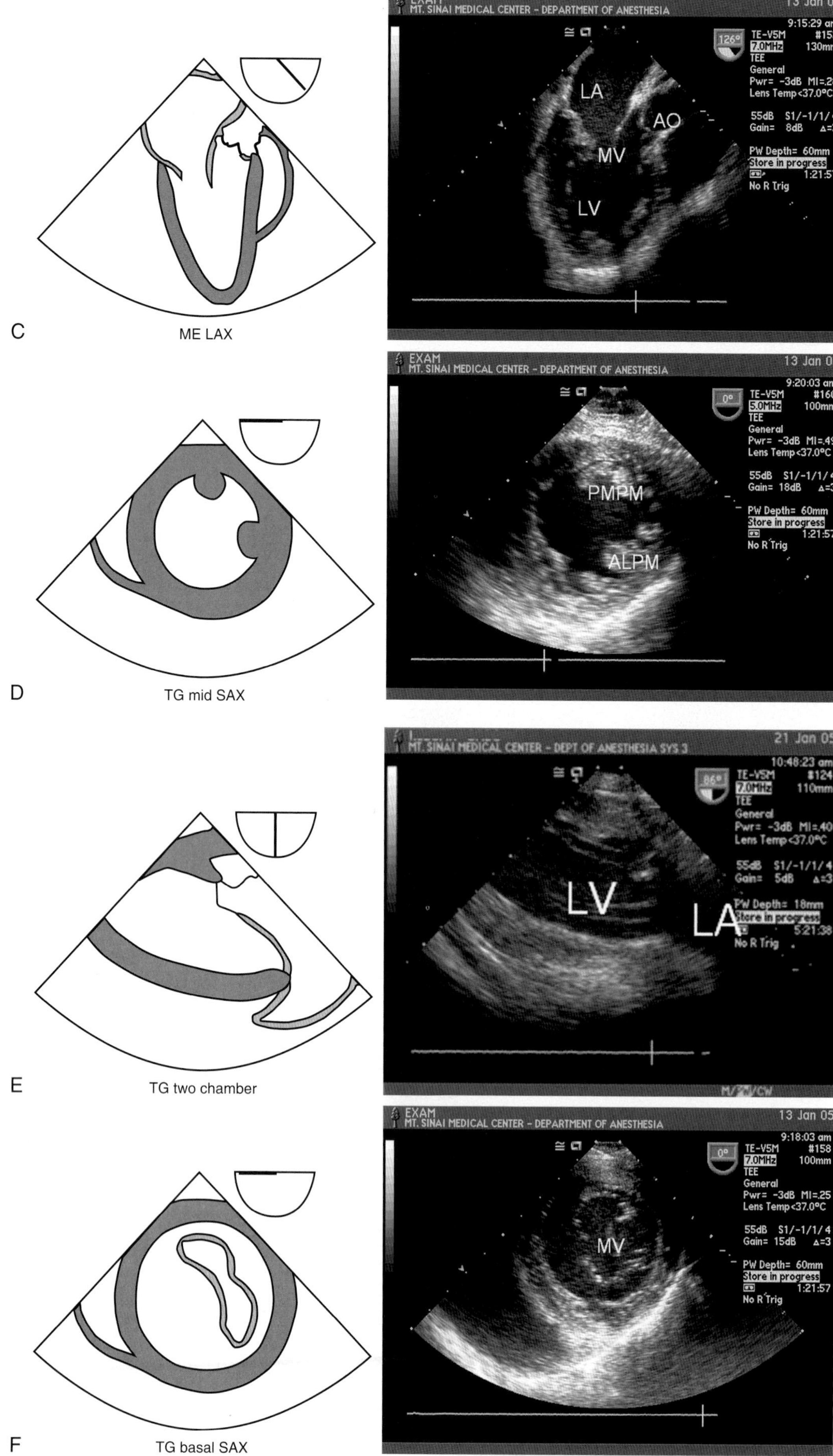

Figure 15–9, cont'd (*C*) ME LAX view. (*D*) TG mid SAX view. (*E*) TG two-chamber view. (*F*) TG basal SAX view.

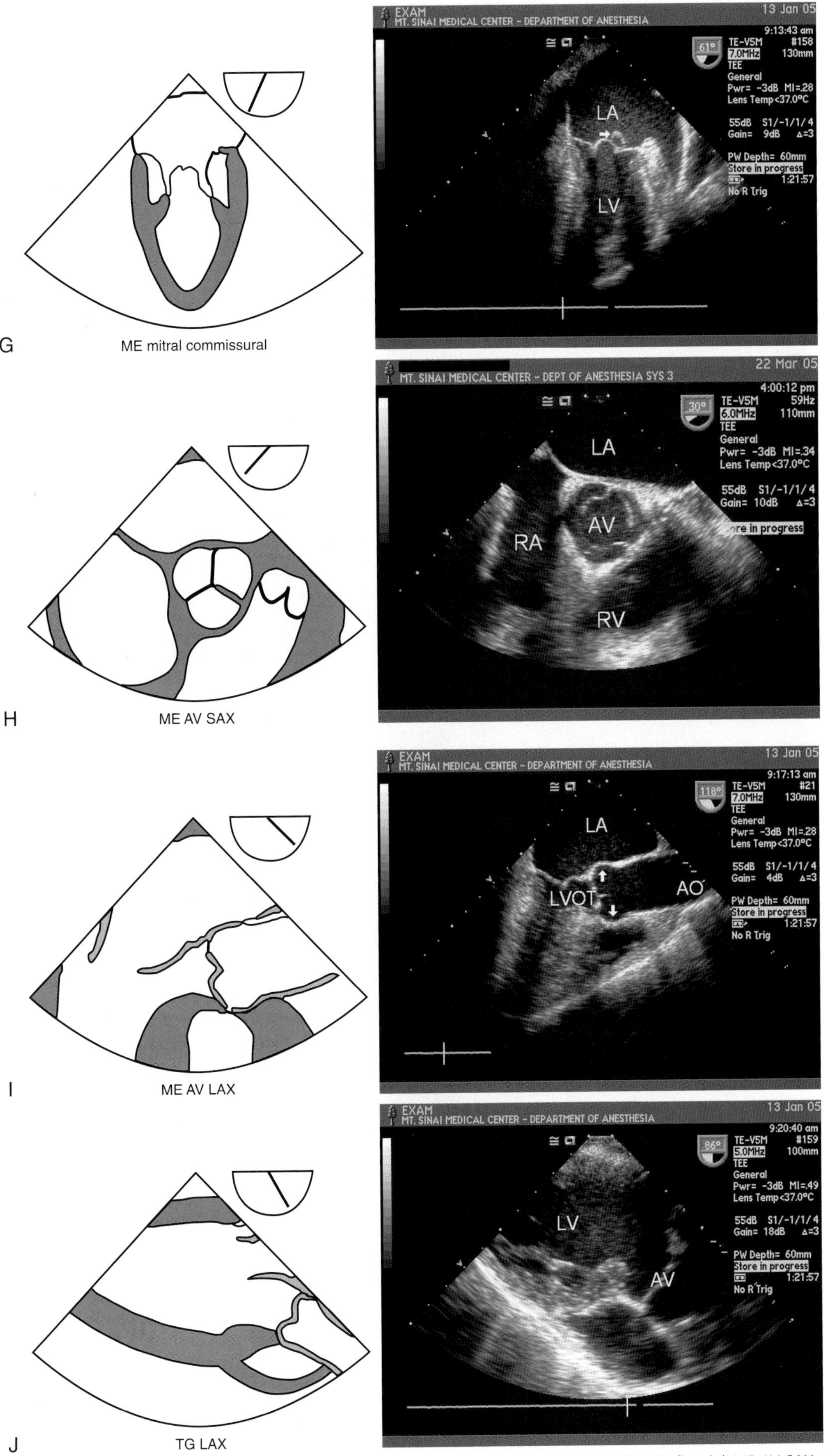

Figure 15–9, cont'd (*G*) ME mitral commissural view; the *arrow* points to a prolapsing posterior mitral leaflet. (*H*) ME AV SAX view. (*I*) ME AV LAX view; the *arrows* point to the aortic sinuses. (*J*) TG LAX view.

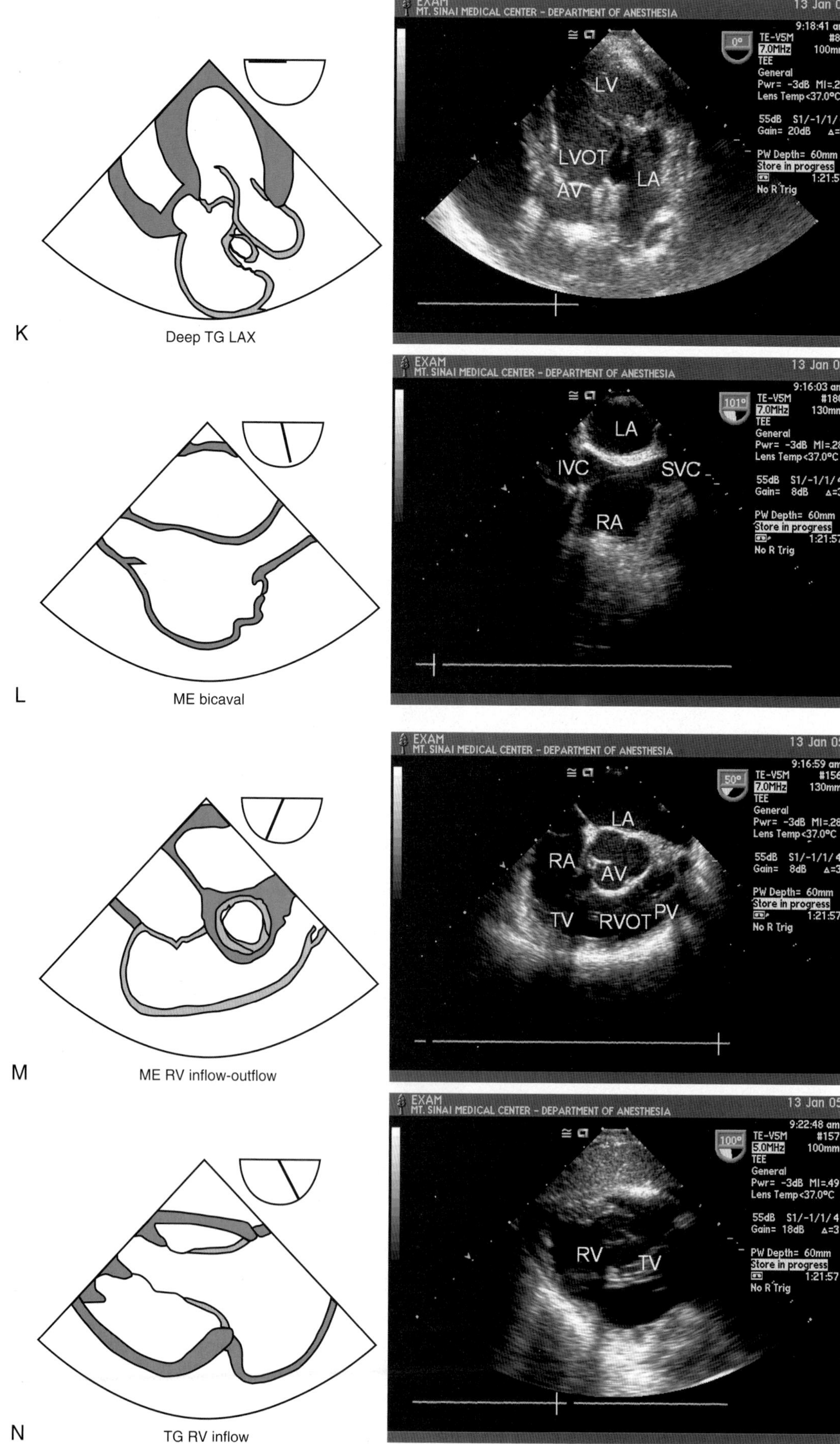

Figure 15–9, cont'd (*K*) Deep TG LAX view. (*L*) ME bicaval view. (*M*) ME RV inflow-outflow view. (*N*) TG RV inflow view.

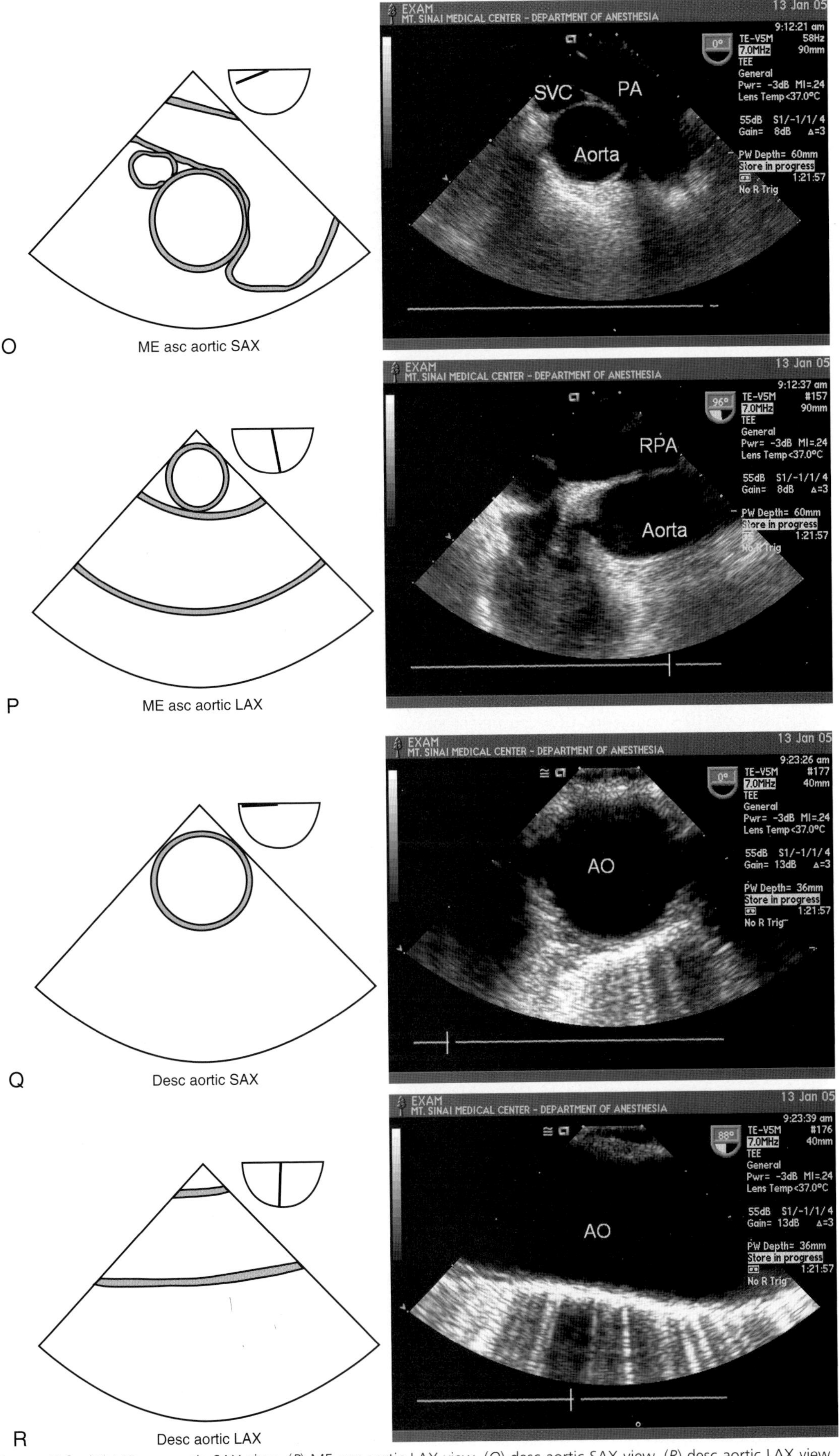

Figure 15–9, cont'd (*O*) ME asc aortic SAX view. (*P*) ME asc aortic LAX view. (*Q*) desc aortic SAX view. (*R*) desc aortic LAX view.

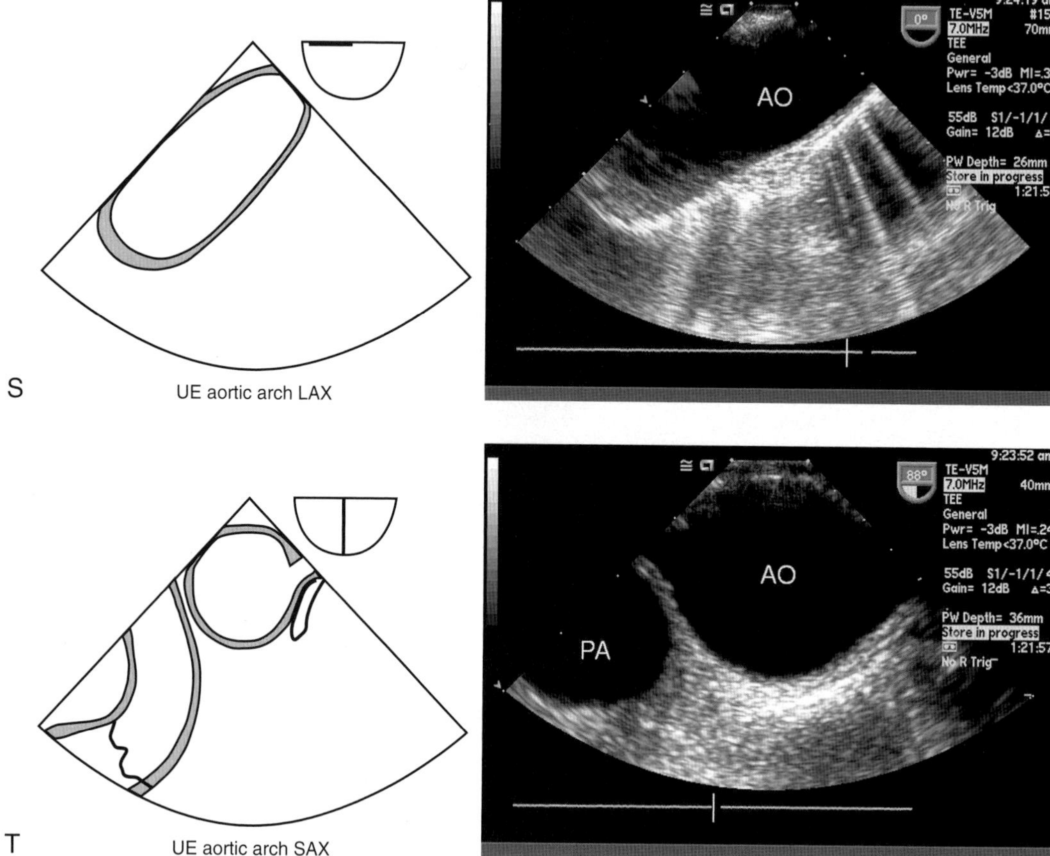

Figure 15–9, cont'd (*S*) UE aortic arch LAX view. (*T*) UE aortic arch SAX view. ME = mid-esophageal; SAX = short axis; LAX = long axis; AV = aortic valve; RV = right ventricle; TG = transgastric; UE = upper esophageal; asc = ascending aorta; desc = descending aorta; LA = left atrium; MV = mitral valve; LVOT = left ventricular outflow tract; RA = right atrium; LV = left ventricle; TV = tricuspid valve; PV = pulmonic valve; RVOT = right ventricular outflow tract; ALPM = anterior lateral papillary muscle; PMPM = posterior medial papillary muscle; IVC = inferior vena cava; SVC = superior vena cava.

Global LV function requires assessment of dilatation (>6 cm at end diastole), hypertrophy (>1.2 cm at end diastole), and contractility. A more extensive quantitative evaluation of ventricular performance can be acquired by planimetry measurements of end-diastolic and end-systolic areas from which ejection fractions (EFs), ventricular volumes, cardiac output (CO), and mean circumferential shortening can be calculated.

Right ventricular (RV) regional and global function can be assessed from the ME four-chamber view (Fig. 15–9*A*), which allows visualization of the septal and free walls. Although a formal segmental scheme has not been developed for the RV free wall, regional assessment of the septum can be performed. Turning the probe to the right and advancing slightly from the mid-esophageal depth allows visualization of the tricuspid valve (TV), coronary sinus (CS), and RV apex. Rotating the probe between 60 and 90 degrees reveals the *ME RV inflow-outflow* view (Fig. 15–9*M*), in which the RA, TV, inferior RV free wall, right ventricular outflow tract (RVOT), pulmonic valve (PV), and main PA can be viewed "wrapping around" the centrally oriented AV. This view often allows optimal Doppler beam alignment to evaluate the TV and can also be helpful for directing PA catheter floating and positioning. The TG mid SAX view (Fig. 15–9*D*) displays the crescent-shaped, thinner-walled RV to the left of the LV (i.e., to the right side of the LV). The *TG RV inflow* view (Fig. 15–9*N*) is developed by turning the probe to the right to center the RV at this depth and rotating the multiplane angle forward to 100 to 120 degrees, thereby revealing the inferior RV free wall. Slight anteflexion, advancement, and rotation of the probe back toward 0 degrees can often reveal the RVOT and PV. Despite the asymmetric shape of the RV, global function can still be assessed from the ME four-chamber, TG mid SAX, ME RV inflow-outflow, and TG RV inflow views (Fig. 15–9*A, D, M, N*) using a quantitative evaluation scheme similar to that previously delineated for the LV. Qualitative echocardiographic findings consistent with a diagnosis of global RV dysfunction include dilatation and hypertrophy, flattened or leftward shift of the atrial and ventricular septum, tricuspid regurgitation, and a dilated CS.

Mitral Valve

The echocardiographic evaluation of the MV requires a thorough assessment of its leaflets (anterior and posterior), annulus, and the subvalvular apparatus (chordae tendineae, papillary muscles, and adjacent LV walls) in order to locate lesions and define the etiology and severity of the pathophysiology. The mitral leaflets can be further divided into posterior leaflet scallops, lateral (P1), middle (P2), and medial (P3), that correspond with respective anterior leaflet sections, lateral third (A1), middle third (A2), and medial third (A3). The leaflets are united at the anterolateral and posteromedial

Left Ventricular Regional Nomenclature

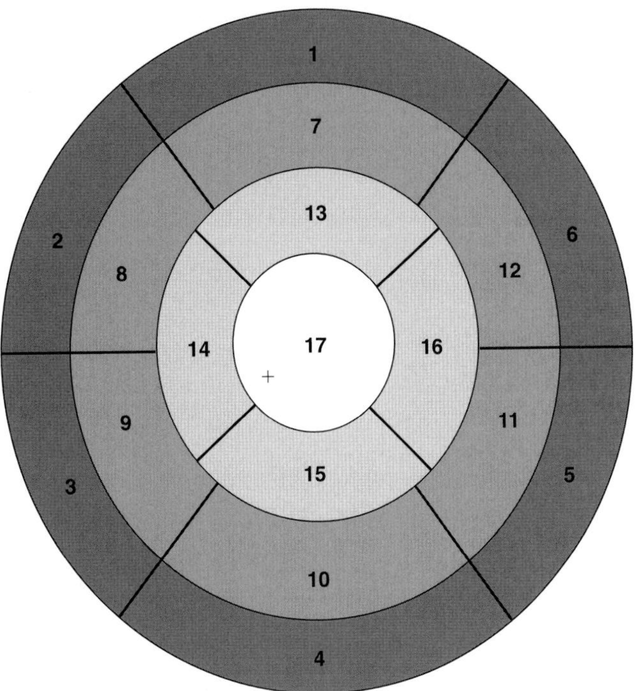

A
1. Basal anterior
2. Basal anteroseptal
3. Basal inferoseptal
4. Basal inferior
5. Basal inferolateral
6. Basal anterolateral
7. Mid anterior
8. Mid anteroseptal
9. Mid inferoseptal
10. Mid inferior
11. Mid inferolateral
12. Mid anterolateral
13. Apical anterior
14. Apical septal
15. Apical inferior
16. Apical lateral
17. Apex

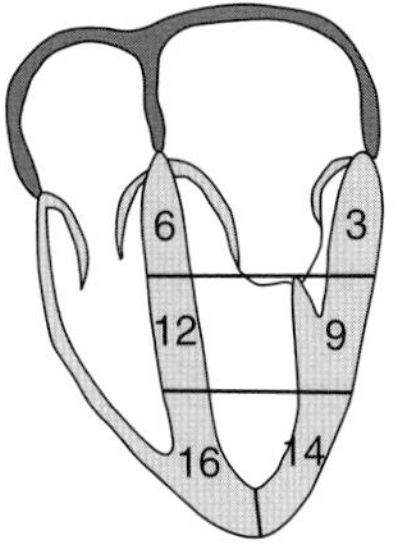

four chamber view

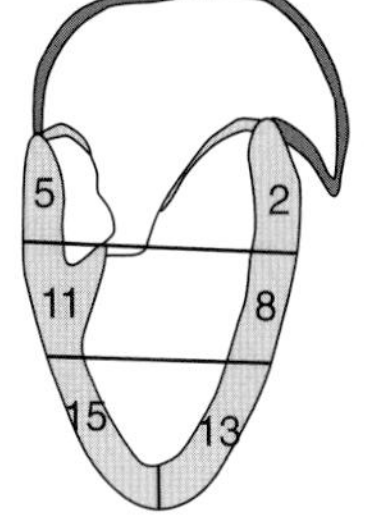

two chamber view

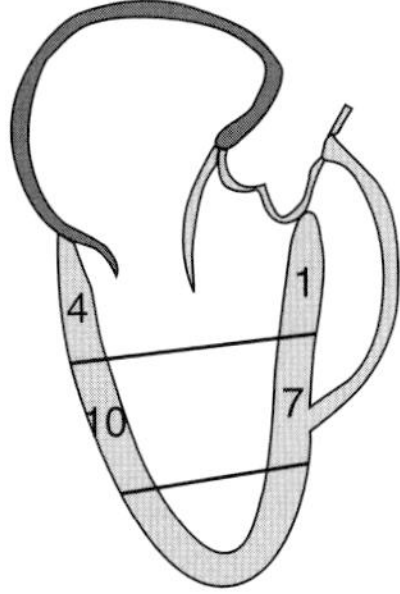

long axis view

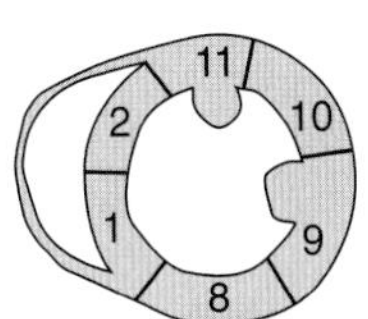

mid short axis view

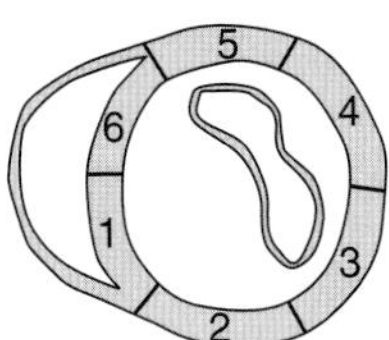

basal short axis view

B

Basal segments
1= Basal anteroseptal
2= Basal anterior
3= Basal lateral
4= Basal posterior
5= Basal inferior
6= Basal septal

Mid segments
7= Mid anteroseptal
8= Mid anterior
9= Mid lateral
10= Mid posterior
11= Mid inferior
12= Mid septal

Apical segments
13= Apical anterior
14= Apical lateral
15= Apical inferior
16= Apical septal

Figure 15–10 Left ventricular segmental nomenclature. (*A*) 17 segments; (*B*) 16 segments.

commissures. The ME four-chamber view (Fig. 15–9*A*) displays the larger appearing anterior leaflet (A3) to the left of the posterior leaflet (P1). Anteflexing the probe provides imaging of the anterior aspect of the MV, while gradual advancement of the probe and retroflexion shifts the image plane to the posterior aspect of MV. Maintaining the probe at the ME depth and rotating the multiplane angle forward to 60 to 70 degrees develops the *ME mitral commissural* view (Fig. 15–9*G*) in which A2 is flanked by P1 on the right and P3 on the left, giving A2 the appearance of a "trap-door" as it moves in and out of the imaging plane throughout the cardiac cycle. Further forward rotation of the probe to 80 to 100 degrees develops the ME two-chamber view (Fig. 15–9*B*), revealing P3 to the left and A1 on the right. Final forward probe rotation to 120 to 160 degrees reveals the ME LAX view (Fig. 15–9*C*), which images P2 on the left and A2 on the right. The TG basal SAX view (Fig. 15–9*F*) enables visualization of both MV leaflets ("fish-mouth view") if the probe is anteflexed and withdrawn slightly from the mid-papillary level of the LV. In this view, the posteromedial commissure is in the upper left, the anterolateral commissure to the lower right, the posterior leaflet is to the right, and the anterior leaflet to the left of the displayed image. Rotation of the probe to 80 to 100 degrees develops the TG two-chamber view (Fig. 15–9*E*), which is especially useful for evaluating the chordae tendineae and corresponding papillary muscles. Further functional evaluation of the MV requires a quantitative Doppler evaluation (pulsed-wave [PWD], continuous-wave [CWD], and color-flow [CFD]) of transmitral and pulmonary venous flow (PVF) for assessing MV regurgitation, stenotic lesions, and LV diastolic function.

Aortic Valve, Aortic Root, and Left Ventricular Outflow

The three cusps of the semilunar AV are best visualized simultaneously in the *ME AV SAX* view (Fig. 15–9*H*), which is obtained by rotating the probe forward to 30 to 60 degrees. The noncoronary cusp is superior, lying adjacent to the atrial septum, the right cusp is inferiorly imaged, and the left cusp lies to the right pointing in the direction of the LA appendage (LAA). This view permits planimetry of the AV orifice, evaluation of congenital anomalies of the AV (e.g., bicuspid AV), and qualitative assessment of aortic regurgitation (AR) when CFD is used. Withdrawing the probe slightly through the sinuses of Valsalva allows for imaging the RCA inferiorly and the left main coronary artery branching into the LAD and CX. The *ME AV LAX* (Fig. 15–9*I*) view can be obtained at the same depth while rotating the probe to 120 to 160 degrees, allowing for visualization of the LVOT, AV annulus and leaflets (right and either noncoronary or left), sinuses of Valsalva, sinotubular junction, and proximal ascending aorta. This view is particularly useful for evaluating AR with CFD, systolic anterior motion of the MV, and proximal aortic pathology (dissections, aneurysms). Rotating the probe back to 90 to 120 degrees and advancing into the stomach to the transgastric level develops the TG LAX view (Fig. 15–9*J*). In this view, the LVOT and AV are oriented to the right and inferiorly in the displayed image, thereby providing an optimal window for parallel Doppler beam alignment for the assessment of flows and pressure gradients (aortic stenosis, hypertrophic obstructive cardiomyopathy). Rotating the probe back further to 0 to 20 degrees, advancing deep into the stomach and anteflexing the tip so that it lies adjacent to the LV apex allows for the development of the *deep TG LAX* view (Fig. 15–9*K*), which also provides optimal Doppler beam alignment for measuring transaortic valve and LVOT flow velocities and may also provide an additional window for assessing flows through muscular VSDs and LV apical pathology (thrombus, aneurysms).

Tricuspid Valve

The echocardiographic evaluation of the TV requires a thorough assessment of its three leaflets (anterior, posterior, and septal), annulus, chordae tendineae, papillary muscles, and the corresponding RV walls. In the ME four-chamber view (Fig. 15–9*A*), the septal TV leaflet is displayed on the right side and the posterior TV leaflet on the left side of the annulus. Rotating the multiplane angle to 60 to 90 degrees develops the ME RV inflow-outflow view (Fig. 15–9*M*), which displays the posterior TV leaflet on the left side of the image and the anterior TV leaflet on the right side of the image adjacent to the AV. The *TG RV inflow* view (Fig. 15–9*N*) is obtained by advancing the probe into the stomach and rotating to 100 to 120 degrees. This view is ideal for visualizing the chordae tendineae and papillary muscles in the RV. Rotating back to the TG mid SAX at 0 to 20 degrees and slightly withdrawing the probe provides a cross-sectional view of the TV, displaying the anterior leaflet in the far field, the posterior leaflet to the left in the near field, and the septal leaflet on the right side of the image. A more extensive quantitative analysis of TV pathophysiology requires the use of Doppler echocardiography (PWD, CWD, and CFD) by aligning the beam parallel to transtricuspid flow in either the ME RV inflow-outflow or ME four-chamber view.

Pulmonic Valve and Pulmonary Artery

The pulmonic valve (PV) is a trileaflet, semilunar valve. The ME AV SAX view (Fig. 15–9*H*) displays the transition between the RVOT and PV. Rotating the probe back toward 0 degrees and withdrawing slightly develops the *ME ascending aortic SAX* view (Fig. 15–9*O*), displaying the transition between the RV and main PA and its bifurcation. Although the right PA is usually easy to visualize by turning the probe to the right, the left PA is often obscured by the interposing, air-filled, left main-stem bronchus. This view can be used in the Doppler echocardiographic assessment of PV pathophysiology because of the parallel alignment of the beam relative to the flow and can also be used to locate pulmonary emboli. The ME RV inflow-outflow (Fig. 15–9*M*) view can also be used to assess RV, PV, and main PA, which lie on the right side of the image adjacent to the AV, although the *upper esophageal aortic arch SAX* view (Fig. 15–9*T*), which displays the PV oriented to the left of the cross-sectional view of the aortic arch, usually provides a more parallel Doppler beam orientation for the evaluation of pulmonic regurgitation or stenosis. Withdrawing the probe slightly in the *deep TG LAX* view (Fig. 15–9*K*) in combination with slight anteflexion and turning to the right can often allow visualization of the RVOT and PV to the left in the far field and provide an alternative imaging plane for Doppler echocardiographic evaluation in patients with subpulmonic and pulmonary valve pathology.

Left Atrium, Left Atrial Appendage, Pulmonary Veins, and Atrial Septum

The LA is the closest cardiac structure to the TEE probe when positioned in the esophagus. Consequently, the LA is usually easily displayed in the superior aspect of the 2D image sector.

The ME four-chamber view (Fig. 15–9*A*) displays the LA almost in its entirety with the LAA oriented to its superior and lateral aspect when the probe is slightly withdrawn. The muscular ridges of the pectinate muscles within the LAA should not be confused with thrombi. Slight further withdrawal of the probe and turning it to the left allows the left upper pulmonary vein (LUPV) to be imaged as it enters the LA from the anterior to posterior direction separated from the lateral border of the LAA by the "warfarin ridge." In contrast to the LUPV, which is usually optimally aligned for parallel Doppler beam alignment, the left lower pulmonary vein (LLPV) enters the LA just below the LUPV in a lateral-to-medial direction and is more perpendicularly aligned. Pulmonary venous Doppler flow-velocity profiles are useful for the qualitative and quantitative assessment of LV diastolic function. Turning the probe to the right at this depth reveals the right upper pulmonary vein (RUPV) entering the LA in an anterior-to-posterior direction. The right lower pulmonary vein (RLPV) can sometimes be visualized as it enters perpendicular to the long axis of the LA, by slightly advancing the probe.

The interatrial septum (IAS), consisting of thicker limbus regions flanking the thin fossa ovalis, can also be imaged in the ME four-chamber view. Benign lipomatous hypertrophy of the IAS must be distinguished from pathologic lesions such as atrial myxomas. The patency of the IAS and presence of PFO or congenital atrial septal defects (ASDs) should be assessed with Doppler echocardiography and intravenous injections of agitated saline or other contrast agents. Advancing and rotating the probe to 80 to 100 degrees develops the ME two-chamber view (Fig. 15–9*B*), which allows for further imaging of the LA from left to right. The LAA and LUPV can be seen by turning the probe slightly to the left. Rotating the probe to the right at this level and adjusting the multiplane angle to 80 to 110 degrees develops the *ME bicaval view* (Fig. 15–9*L*), which delineates the superior vena cava (SVC) entering the RA to the right of the image and the inferior vena cava (IVC) entering from the left. The IAS can be seen in the middle of the image separating the LA and RA. The RUPV and RLPV can usually be seen if the probe is turned farther to the right just beyond the point at which the long axis of the SVC can no longer be visualized. This transition of images can also be used in conjunction with Doppler echocardiography to identify sinus venosus ASDs and anomalous pulmonary venous return.

Right Atrium and Coronary Sinus

The RA can be most easily visualized in the ME four-chamber view (Fig. 15–9*A*) by turning the probe to the patient's right side. In this view, the entire RA can be visualized for size, overall function, and the presence of masses (thrombi, tumors). Rotating the multiplane angle to 80 to 110 degrees develops the *ME bicaval* view (Fig. 15–9*L*), which displays the RA and its internal structures (Eustachian valve, Chiari network, crista terminalis). The SVC can be imaged entering the RA on the right, superior to the right atrial appendage (RAA), and the IVC enters the RA on the left of the display. Advancing and turning the probe to the right allows for a qualitative evaluation of the intrahepatic segment of the IVC and hepatic veins. Pacemaker electrodes and central venous catheters for hemodynamic monitoring or CPB can be easily imaged in this view.

The coronary sinus (CS) lies posteriorly in the atrioventricular groove, emptying into the RA at the inferior extent of the atrial septum. The CS can be viewed in long axis entering the RA just superior to the tricuspid annulus by advancing and slightly retroflexing the probe from ME four-chamber view (Fig. 15–9*A*). The CS can be imaged cross-sectionally in short axis in the ME two-chamber (Fig. 15–9*B*) view in the upper left of the display. Turning the probe to the left in this view often allows visualization of the CS in long axis as it traverses the atrioventricular groove. The CS and thebesian valve can also be visualized in the *ME bicaval* view (Fig. 15–9*L*) on the upper right of the image as the CS enters the RA at an obtuse angle, by turning the probe to leftward simultaneously with retro- and leftward flexion. Echocardiographic visualization of the CS can be useful for directing the placement of CS catheters used for CPB with retrograde cardioplegia.

Thoracic Aorta

The proximal and mid-ascending thoracic aorta can be visualized in short axis in the ME ascending aortic SAX view (Fig. 15–9*O*). Advancing and withdrawing the probe should enable visualization of the thoracic aorta from the sinotubular junction to a point 4 to 6 cm superior to the AV and allow inspection for aneurysms and dissections. Rotating the multiplane angle to 100 to 150 degrees develops the ME ascending aortic LAX view (Fig. 15–9*P*), which optimally displays the parallel anterior and posterior walls for measuring proximal and mid-ascending aortic diameters. This view can also be obtained from the ME AV LAX view (Fig. 15–9*I*) by slightly withdrawing and turning the probe to the left.

TEE imaging of the aortic arch is often obscured by the interposing, air-filled trachea. The most optimal views of the aortic arch are obtained by withdrawing the probe from the ME ascending aortic SAX view at 0 degrees (Fig. 15–9*O*) and rotating to the left to obtain the *upper esophageal aortic arch LAX* view (Fig. 15–9*S*), which displays the proximal arch followed by the mid-arch, the great vessels (brachiocephalic, left carotid and left subclavian artery) and distal arch before it joins the proximal descending thoracic aorta imaged in cross section. Alternatively, rotating the probe to 90 degrees develops the *upper esophageal aortic arch SAX* view (Fig. 15–9*T*). Turning the probe to the left, this view delineates the transition of the distal arch with the proximal descending thoracic aorta. Turning the probe to the right and slightly withdrawing allows for the mid-arch and great vessels to be imaged on the right side of the screen, followed by the distal ascending aorta when the probe is subsequently advanced and rotated forward to 120 degrees (ME ascending aortic LAX view (Fig. 15–9*P*). Epiaortic scanning may be particularly useful for assessing the extent of ascending aortic and arch pathology (e.g., aneurysms, dissection, atherosclerosis) in order to determine cross-clamping and cannulation sites for CPB.

A short-axis image of the descending thoracic aorta is obtained by turning the probe leftward from the ME four-chamber view (Fig. 15–9*A*) to produce the *descending aortic SAX* view (Fig. 15–9Q). Rotating the multiplane angle of the probe from 0 degrees to 90 to 110 degrees produces a long-axis image, the *descending aortic LAX* view (Fig. 15–9*R*). The descending thoracic aorta should be interrogated in its entirety, beginning at the distal aortic arch by continually advancing the probe and turning slightly to the left until the celiac and superior mesenteric arteries are visualized branching tangentially from the anterior surface of the abdominal aorta when the probe is in the stomach. Thorough examination of the descending thoracic aorta may be necessary to evaluate the distal extent of an aneurysm or dissection. In addition, the descending aortic SAX and LAX views can be useful for confirming appropriate intra-aortic balloon positioning.

CLINICAL APPLICATIONS

Ventricular Function

Cardiovascular function, such as the global indices of muscle contraction or regional indices described by segmental wall motion, is assessed by analyzing moving echocardiographic images. Assessment of global and regional ventricular function has become the cornerstone for evaluating patients with ischemic heart disease (IHD). The dynamic assessment of ventricular function with echocardiography is based on derived indices of muscle contraction and relaxation. Echocardiographic indices of LV function that incorporate endocardial border outlines and Doppler techniques can be used to estimate CO, stroke volume (SV), EF, and parameters of ventricular relaxation and filling.

Global LV performance is directly related to preload, contractility, and afterload. Cardiac output reflects systolic function and is an important factor in oxygen delivery. Alteration in LV diastolic function may result from systolic dysfunction or, in as many as 40% of patients, may be the primary and main etiology of cardiac failure.[71]

The development of quantitative analytical techniques for TEE applications has been fairly rapid because many of its mathematical models had already been used for transthoracic or epicardial echocardiography. The practical applications of quantitative TEE analysis have been limited by the necessity for time-consuming tracings and the meticulous attention to detail that is essential to avoiding errors. Thus, the best quantitative TEE analyses are performed some time after the images have been acquired, i.e., "off-line." In addition, the well-trained echocardiographer may be capable of qualitatively grading myocardial performance in a clinically useful way during the actual examination, i.e., "on-line." The development of accurate, reliable, on-line, automated endocardial border detection is the factor that is bringing quantitative analysis to the forefront of TEE techniques.

Visual Estimation of Function

In routine clinical work, the anesthesiologist-echocardiographer must make visual estimates of ventricular wall motion and overall function. These depend on the ability of the individual to interpret the images and correctly "quantify" subjective assessments of ventricular function. The clinician may be aided by video recordings of prior function or video images stored on split screens. These estimations of global ventricular function are usually performed in the short-axis view of the LV, but additional information can also be gained by assessing the long-axis views of the LV. In this assessment, the observer examines the end-diastolic image and compares it with the end-systolic frame to determine the degree of ejection. The rate of ejection is also estimated.

Clements et al[72] demonstrated that regional wall motion abnormalities (RWMAs) may be identified on visual inspection of echo images by anesthesiologists. However, later work by Hillel et al[73] and Saada et al[74] has shown that EF and RWMAs may not be adequately detected by visual inspection alone. The preliminary data in these two studies are further supported by Lazar et al,[75] who found that qualitative scoring did not detect improvements in regional LV function detected by off-line quantitative wall thickening analysis. In contrast, several studies have documented that an educated visual analysis of echocardiographic images provides a better estimation of LVEF than more sophisticated and time-consuming computer techniques.[76,77]

Echocardiographic Tracing

Consistency in the acquisition and analysis of 2D TEE images is required if meaningful data are to be obtained from a 2D view of a 3D heart. For the purposes of LV wall motion analysis, the TG midpapillary SAX view of the LV (Fig. 15–9*D*) has become the standard view because maximal ventricular excursion is seen in this view. However, the short-axis view is somewhat difficult to maintain, because slight anteroflexion or retroflexion of the probe leads to multiple oblique views that are similar in appearance but yield widely varying information. Thus, the papillary muscle morphology must be continually observed to maintain a consistent short-axis view.

Other issues that are essential to the consistency of quantitative analysis are stability of cardiac rhythm, surgical manipulations, and the respiratory cycle. Ectopic and postextrasystolic beats yield abnormal values when compared with normal sinus rhythm. Irregular cardiac rhythms, such as atrial fibrillation, are problematic because the derived parameters vary from beat to beat. Averaging of information from several beats may be necessary. Surgical manipulations may alter loading conditions (e.g., vena caval obstruction, aortic retraction), temporarily alter cardiac function (e.g., pericardial irritation with hot solutions), or change the echocardiographic image (retraction or lifting of the heart). The respiratory cycle also results in cyclical changes in loading conditions and the anatomic relationship of the heart to the esophagus.

Once the echocardiographic image has been acquired, the methods of tracing the endocardial and/or epicardial borders are important. Echocardiographic images may be traced using software that is included in most echocardiography machines or by using a separate workstation. The ability to identify borders is aided by viewing the moving echocardiographic image just prior to tracing. Cine loops and videotape playback help the operator to determine what represents the actual border and to "fill in" missing or unclear regions using the operator's knowledge of the shape of the border.

Trabeculation of the ventricular wall and the observed "thickness" of the endocardial border complicate the tracing of endocardial borders. As diagrammed in Figure 15–11, the endocardial border appears thicker at the anterior and posterior walls where the border runs perpendicular to the ultrasound transmission. This perceived thickness has a leading edge and a trailing edge. The accepted method of tracing endocardial borders uses the "leading edge–leading edge" outline. Wyatt et al[78] found that this technique led to acceptable correlations with in vitro measurements. For all quantitative echocardiographic measurements, it is recommended that the average of at least four consecutive contractions be used because of the considerable beat-to-beat variation.

Preload/Diastolic Function

End-Diastolic Dimensions

While in conventional hemodynamics preload is often estimated by measuring left-sided heart filling pressures (pulmonary capillary wedge pressure [PCWP], left atrial pressure

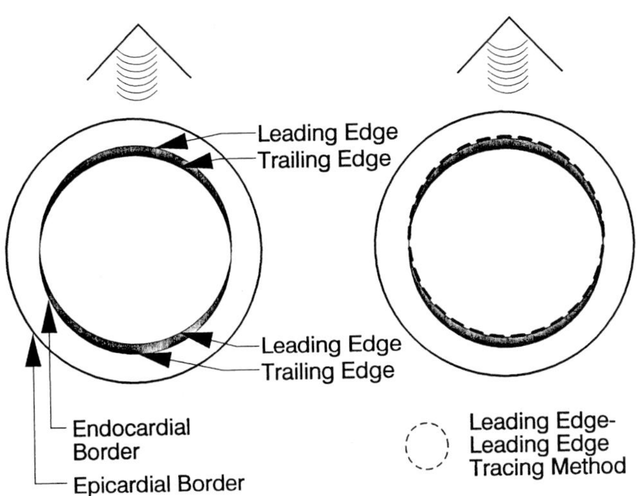

Figure 15–11 Endocardial border analysis.

[LAP], or LV end-diastolic pressure [LVEDP]), in echocardiography it can be determined by measuring LV end-diastolic dimensions or calculating LV end-diastolic pressures. In M-mode echocardiography a single ventricular diameter is obtained, whereas in 2D echocardiography one or multiple tomographic cuts are recorded. It has been proposed that end-diastolic dimensions provide a better index of preload than the PCWP. When PCWP and end-diastolic volume (EDV), derived from short-axis areas at the level of the papillary muscles, were compared as predictors of cardiac index (CI) in patients undergoing CABG, a strong correlation was observed between end-diastolic area (EDA), or EDV, and CI, whereas no significant correlation was found between PCWP and CI.[79] Konstadt et al[80] compared TEE short-axis images with images generated directly from the cardiac surface during cardiac surgery. There was a close correlation between end-diastolic and end-systolic areas and area EFs derived from the two methods ($r = 0.88$ and 0.94).

In a study of 32 patients during cardiovascular surgery, Beaupre et al[81] provided evidence for the clinical value of intraoperative TEE for monitoring LV short-axis dimension (preload) changes. They compared short-axis area changes with simultaneous PCWP changes obtained from PA catheters. Their results showed that estimates of SV derived from short-axis area changes were consistent with thermodilution data in 91% of patients. In contrast, EDA changes correlated with PCWP changes in only 23% of patients. Because LV compliance changes dramatically during cardiovascular surgery, PCWP may be an inadequate guide to LV preload.

Clements et al[82] studied 14 patients during resection of abdominal aortic aneurysm. At multiple times during surgery, echocardiograms and first-pass radionuclide studies were recorded simultaneously. The correlation between echocardiographic and radionuclide estimates was excellent; however, virtually no correlation was seen between estimates from either of these techniques and PA pressures. Thus, TEE provides the anesthesiologist with a direct, quantitative method to assess LV preload and ejection. However, if severe RWMAs are present, information from a single cross-section may not be adequate for estimating these parameters.

TEE is often, for practical reasons, limited to a single short-axis view at the level of the papillary muscles. Some evidence suggests that short-axis EDAs measured at this level correlate reasonably well with measurements obtained by on-heart echocardiography and with EDVs measured simultaneously using radionuclides. However, findings by Urbanowicz et al[83] were in disagreement with these conclusions. Using a combined radionuclide and thermodilution technique, these investigators found that the correlation coefficient between the LVEDA by TEE and the LVEDV was only 0.74. In addition, they noted discordant changes in four of nine patients. Overall, it has been shown that despite variable loading conditions, changes in LV short-axis area reflect changes in LV pressure or compliance factors. There are two main echocardiographic signs of decreased preload: (1) decrease in EDA ($<5.5\ cm^2/m^2$) invariably reflects hypovolemia. It is, however, difficult to set an upper limit of EDA below which hypovolemia can be confirmed. This is particularly true in patients with impaired contractility in whom a compensatory baseline increase in preload makes the echocardiographic diagnosis of hypovolemia difficult. (2) Obliteration of the end-systolic area (ESA) ("the kissing ventricle sign") accompanies the decrease in EDA in severe hypovolemia.

Transmitral Blood Flow

Another approach to the evaluation of LV filling is to examine the flow across the MV. This approach adds information during the entire diastolic period, not just end-diastole. After valvular dysfunction has been excluded, the sample volume of the PW Doppler system is placed in the mitral inflow. The best location for the sample volume is in the center of the mitral flow, just slightly to the ventricular side of the MV. Flow velocity measured with the sample volume in this location results in a typical flow-velocity pattern (Fig. 15–12). After opening of the MV, the early inflow into the LV will be recognized as a large velocity peak (E peak). It is followed by a period of diastasis and a second, smaller velocity peak (A peak) representing flow produced by atrial contraction. Analysis of the diastolic inflow includes the measurements of E-peak and A-peak velocities and their ratio (E/A), the derivation of acceleration and deceleration for each peak, calculation of various time intervals, and integration of total area (velocity–time integral [VTI]) under the velocity display.

Deviations from the normal diastolic velocity pattern have been described under various circumstances. Fusion of the E and A peaks occurs with tachycardia, while the A-peak and the E-peak velocity exceed values observed in normal subjects. The diastolic inflow of the patient with mitral stenosis is marked by high E-peak velocity, prolonged deceleration from the peak velocity, and continuous flow throughout diastole. The most commonly observed abnormality is early LV filling. This has been noted with advanced age, IHD, hypertrophic cardiomyopathy, secondary LV hypertrophy, dilated cardiomyopathy, and RV pressure overload.

The determinants of E-peak velocity have been investigated in recent animal and human studies. Variables that have been clearly recognized as determinants of E-peak velocity include the LA "V" wave pressure, the LV relaxation rate, and the systemic arterial pressure. The E-peak velocity varies directly with increasing LAP and inversely with increases in the time constant of relaxation or systemic arterial pressure.[84]

PVF, as measured by PWD echocardiography, can also be used to assess LAP. In using this technique, the flow recording is compared with a simultaneous ECG tracing so that the systolic and diastolic peaks can be identified and their respective VTI measurements can be performed. When LAP is below 15 mm Hg, the PVF velocities are greatest in systole. Increases in

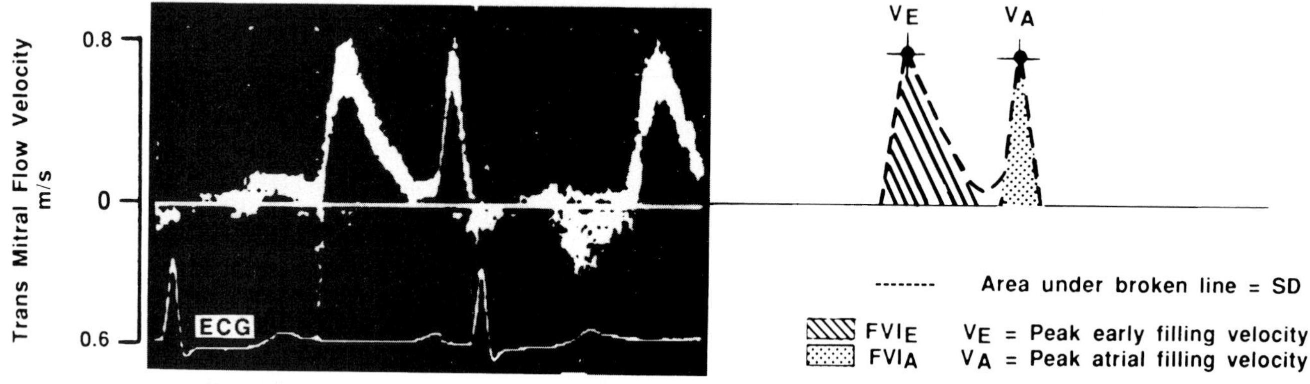

Figure 15–12 Transmitral flow-velocity profile and diagrammatic representation of its quantification.

LAP (>15 mm Hg) have been shown to result in a shift of higher flow velocities toward earlier diastole.[85]

Other factors that have not been directly associated with the E-peak velocity, but are nonetheless important for the onset of diastolic flow, include the ventricular suction effect and mitral ring recoil. Interpretation of diastolic peak velocity is further confounded by changes in heart rate and loading conditions. In one study, Nishimura et al[86] observed that, with fluid infusion leading to an increased PCWP, E-peak velocity increased, whereas phenylephrine infusion had the opposite effect.

ACCELERATION AND DECELERATION

Acceleration of flow in early diastole is the result of the pressure gradient between the LA and LV, and deceleration coincides with the reversal of the pressure gradient between these chambers.[87] Under normal circumstances, the average forward gradient associated with acceleration is significantly greater than the reverse gradient associated with deceleration. The determinants of E-wave deceleration are similar to those of E-peak velocity.

AREA INTEGRATION

Integration of *partial* areas under the flow–velocity curve has been suggested for the assessment of the ventricular filling and diastolic function.[88] Some of the areas that have been studied include the areas for the first 33% of diastole, the first 50% of diastole, the area under the E peak (E*i*), and the area under the A peak (A*i*). Using the ratio E*i*/A*i*, Pearson et al[89] observed an inverse linear relationship between age and early diastolic filling. This observation suggests that, with increasing age, the filling of the LV becomes more dependent on atrial contraction. In children, Snider et al[90] found that the ratio of the area under the first 33% of diastole over the total area was larger in normal than in hypertensive children. Conversely, the ratio of A*i* to total area was larger in hypertensive patients.

INTRAOPERATIVE APPLICATIONS

Diastolic function has been assessed intraoperatively by PW Doppler echocardiography in only a few studies. In cardiac surgical patients, it was observed that some patients with normal mitral inflow patterns before CPB had signs of impaired ventricle filling after bypass.[91] Rinder et al[92] reported that diastolic filling was significantly impaired 2 hours after CPB. They noted a trend toward recovery by 4 hours and a return to baseline by 18 hours. Other potential intraoperative applications of the determination of diastolic mitral flow by PW Doppler echocardiography include the following topics.

ASSESSMENT OF ATRIAL CONTRIBUTION TO STROKE VOLUME

The contribution of the atrial contraction to ventricular filling is ideally studied by the measurement of mitral flow velocity. The area under the A peak is directly proportional to the fraction of the SV contributed by the atrial contraction. In cardiac surgical patients, it has been demonstrated that the decrease in CI occurring as a result of the loss of the atrial contraction is greater in patients with lower E/A ratios. Others have used PW Doppler echocardiography to document increased CI with atrioventricular versus ventricular pacing or to optimize atrioventricular delay intervals during atrioventricular sequential pacing.[93-95]

DETECTION OF ISCHEMIA

Because the rate of LV relaxation is an important determinant of early ventricular filling, it would be expected that impaired relaxation would result in impaired early ventricular filling. Ventricular relaxation is an energy-requiring process, and one of the early consequences of myocardial ischemia is an impairment in ventricular relaxation. When myocardial ischemia is produced by transient occlusion of a coronary artery, as occurs during angioplasty, the observation of a rapid reduction in E-peak velocity is suggestive of impaired relaxation. Diastolic LV dysfunction was the earliest change noted after coronary occlusion, and it often preceded the development of abnormal systolic function. In another study, it was further observed that acute ischemia not only altered early ventricular filling, but also produced marked abnormalities in late ventricular filling.[96]

Diastolic Function

Evaluation of diastolic function implies that it is possible to assess the pressure-volume relationship of LV diastolic filling. This relationship can only be measured hemodynamically. Doppler echocardiography attempts to evaluate diastolic filling by evaluating patterns and time of flow, such as from the LA into the LV or pulmonary veins into the LA. The main determination of flow is the pressure differences in the two chambers. The early diastolic pressure difference between the LA and the LV mainly reflects the rate of LV relaxation. Thus, if filling is delayed, impaired relaxation is usually present. It is

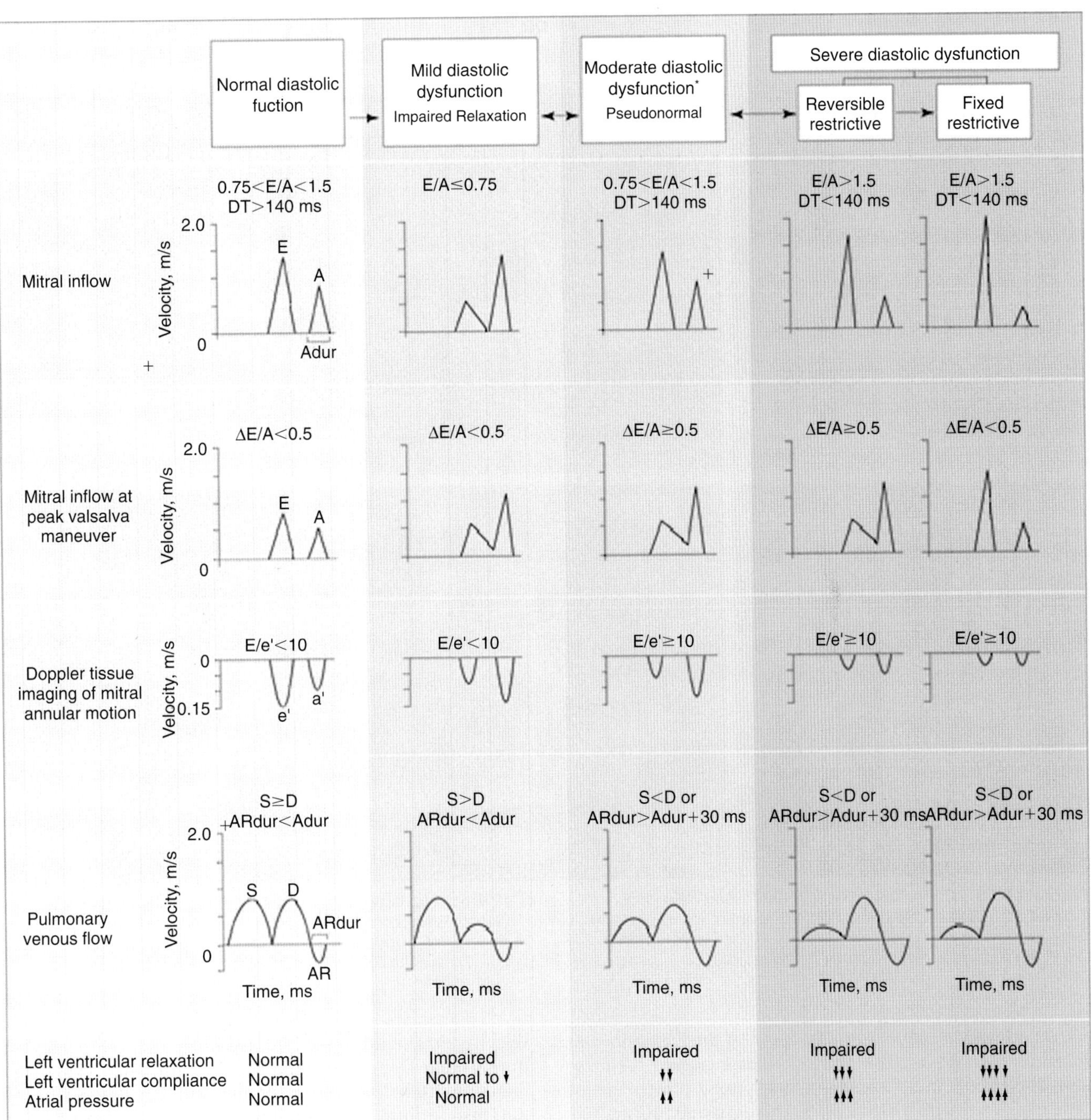

Figure 15–13 Doppler criteria for classification of diastolic function. (Reproduced with permission from Redfield MM, Jacobsen SJ, Burnett JC Jr, et al: Burden of systolic and diastolic ventricular dysfunction in the community: Appreciating the scope of the heart failure epidemic. JAMA 289:194, 2003.)

important to remember that other factors, such as chamber and myocardial compliance, LV loading conditions, ventricular interaction, and pericardial constraint, can also influence rates of LV filling.

There are three primary stages of diastolic dysfunction: impaired relaxation, pseudonormalization, and restrictive cardiomyopathy. The evaluation of diastolic function may be evaluated using Doppler analysis of MV inflow and PVF, color M-mode propagation velocities, and tissue Doppler analysis of the MV annulus[97,98] (Fig. 15–13). Diastolic function can be assessed by PWD interrogation of MV inflow velocity in the long-axis view of the LV (see Fig. 15–9C). To assess diastolic function, the velocities are recorded at the tips of the open MV leaflets. With normal diastolic function, the E/A ratio of mitral valve inflow is between 0.75 and 1.5 with an E-wave deceleration time of greater than 140 msec. The atrial systolic component of the PVF (i.e., atrial reversal) velocity is usually less than 35 cm/sec, and its duration is usually less than the transmitral E-wave duration. With impaired relaxation, there is an increase in the A-wave velocity with respect to the E wave, such that the E/A ratio is less than 0.75. E-wave deceleration time is usually greater than 220 msec. Further worsening in diastolic function results in increases in LA pressure. This increased LA pressure both increases the E-wave veloc-

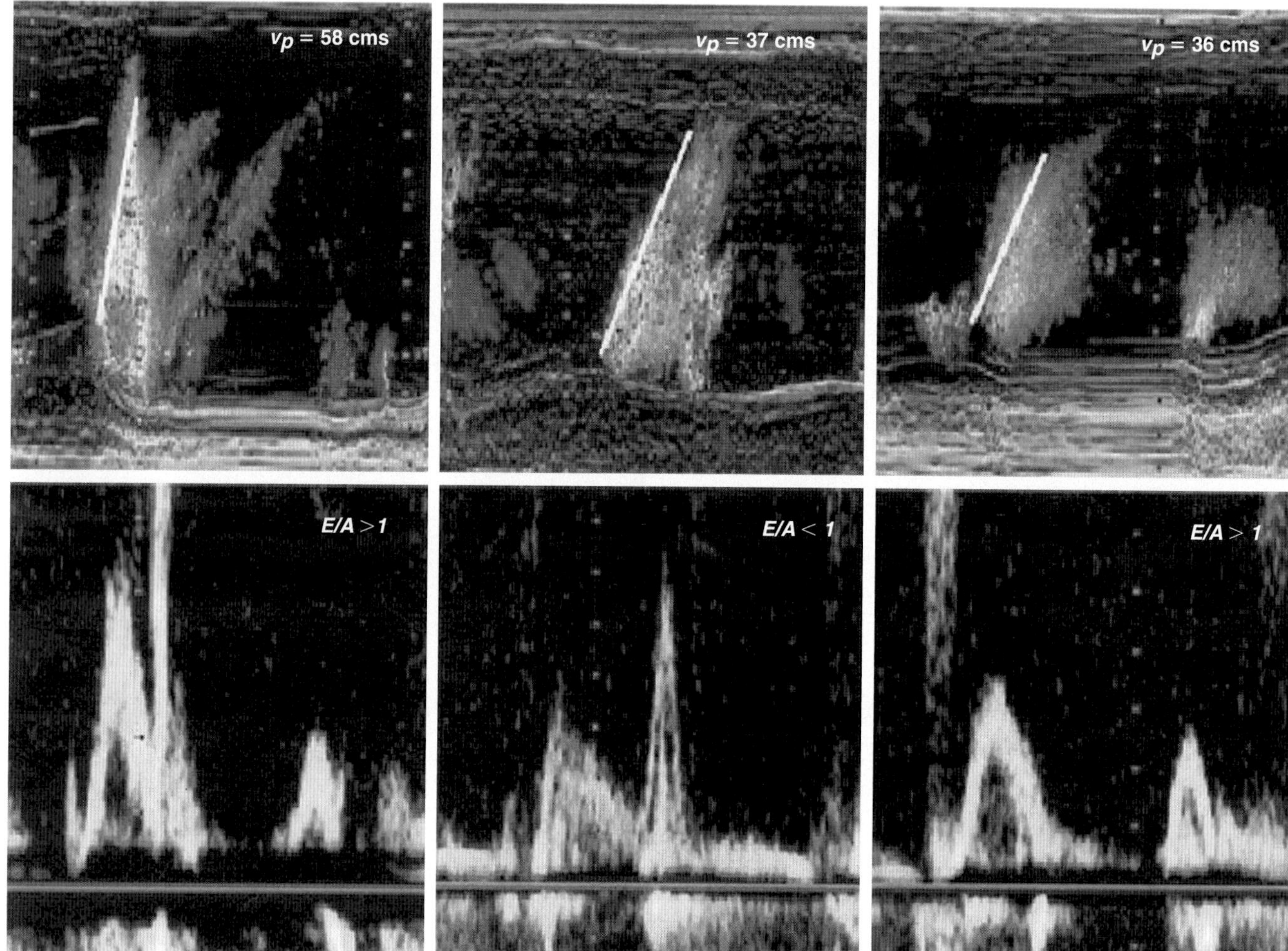

Figure 15–14 Color M-mode Doppler and pulsed-wave Doppler images of left ventricular filling. *Left*, Normal filling pattern (vp = 58 cm/sec, E/A > 1). *Middle*, Delayed relaxation (DR) filling pattern (vp = 37 cm/sec, E/A < 1). *Right*, Pseudonormal (PN) filling pattern (vp = 36 cm/sec, E/A > 1). (Reproduced with permission from De Meya S, De Sutterb J, Vierendeelsa J, Verdoncka P: Diastolic filling and pressure imaging: Taking advantage of the information in a colour M-mode Doppler image. Eur J Echocardiogr 2:219, 2001, copyright 2001, with permission from the European Society of Cardiology.)

ity, resulting in a "pseudonormalization" of the E/A ratio, and increases E-wave deceleration time. This increased LA pressure also results in a blunting of the systolic component of PVF compared with diastolic PVF. During pseudonormalization, there are also changes in the atrial systole component of the PVF; the velocity is greater than 35 cm/sec and the duration is at least 30 msec greater than transmitral E-wave duration. Further progression to restrictive cardiomyopathy is marked by an E/A wave ratio greater than 1.5 and an E-wave deceleration time less than 140 msec.

During determination of color M-mode propagation velocity, the M-mode scan line is displayed extending through the MV leaflet opening to the LV apex.[99] If CFD is superimposed on this path, the velocity of flow progression can be determined (Fig. 15–14). With normal diastolic function and impaired relaxation, the M-mode propagation velocity is greater than 45 cm/sec. During progression to "pseudonormalization" and restrictive disease, the M-mode propagation velocity is less than 45 cm/sec.

Spectral Doppler can be used to determine blood flow velocities. Because these velocities are relatively high and the amplitude of the Doppler signal is low, high-amplitude/low-velocity ultrasound signals are usually ignored. Alternatively, during tissue Doppler examination, primary interest lies in the high-amplitude/low-velocity ultrasound signals created by the myocardium; low-amplitude/high-velocity signals are ignored. Doppler tissue imaging (DTI) of the MV annulus may also be used to judge diastolic function.[100] Normally, this DTI wave consists of two diastolic components: one in early diastole (E_a) and one in late diastole (Fig. 15–15). These two signals are in the opposite direction of MV inflow. In normal cases, E_a velocity is greater than 8 cm/sec; with diastolic dysfunction, Ea velocity is less than 8 cm/sec.[97] E/E_a ratios greater than 10 are also consistent with diastolic dysfunction.

Afterload

Although afterload cannot be determined by echocardiography alone, the combination of ventricular dimensions with ventricular wall thickness and systolic arterial pressure yields end-systolic wall stress. Ventricular wall thickness is derived by calculating the difference between the epicardial and endocardial areas, whereas the ventricular dimension corresponds to the endocardial area[101] (see Chapters 5 and 14).

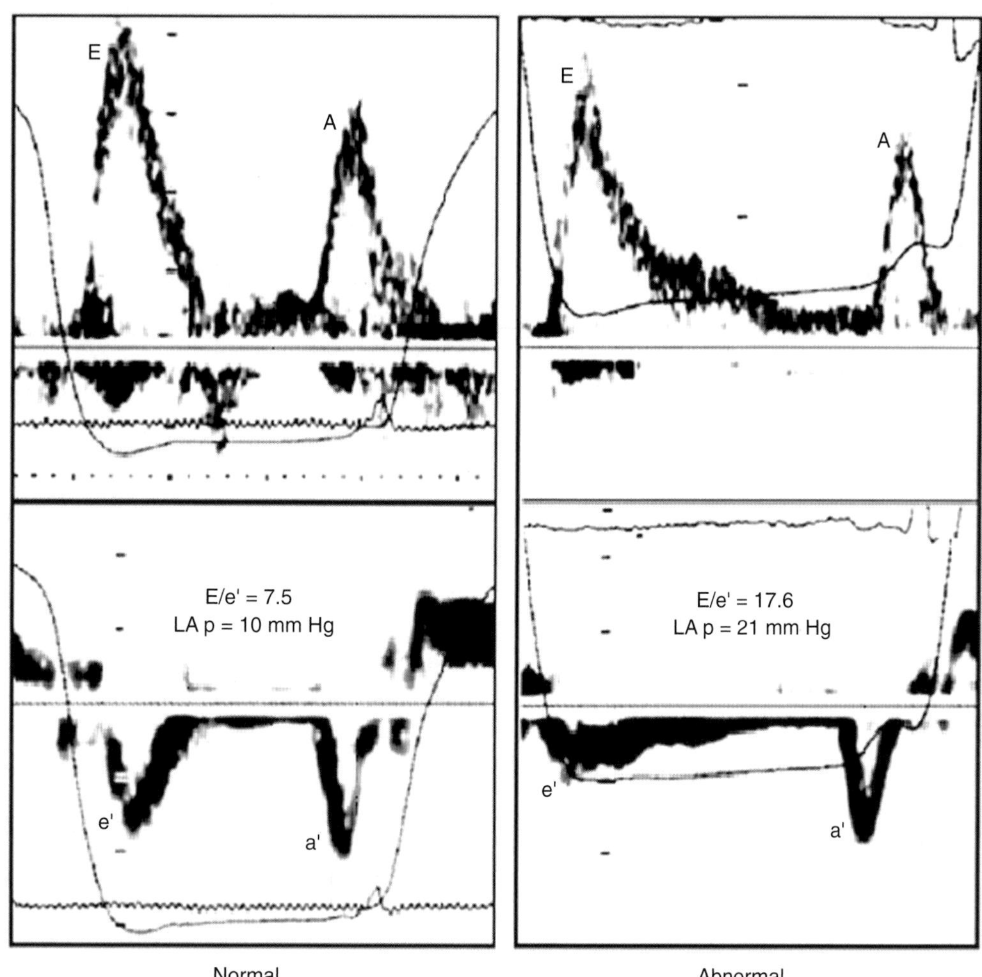

Figure 15–15 The tissue Doppler velocity of the mitral annulus can help distinguish between normal and abnormal filling. On the *left*, a normal mitral annular velocity and E/e′ ratio indicate normal filling pressures. On the *right*, the mitral annular e′ velocity is reduced and the E/e′ ratio elevated in a patient with high left atrial pressure. A = mitral filling at atrial contraction; a′ = late mitral annulus diastolic velocity; E = mitral early filling wave; e′ = early mitral annulus diastolic velocity; E/e′ = ratio of mitral early filling wave to early mitral annulus velocity; LA p = left atrial pressure. (Reproduced from Ommen SR, Nishimura RA: A clinical approach to the assessment of left ventricular diastolic function by Doppler echocardiography: Update 2003. Heart 89[suppl III]:III-18, 2003, with permission from the BMJ Publishing Group.)

The formula to calculate wall stress was derived by Sandler and Dodge from the basic Laplace equation:

$$\text{Wall stress} = 1.33 \times P \times LVEDD/4WT \; (1 + WT/LVEDD) \qquad (15\text{–}8)$$

where P is the systolic blood pressure, WT is wall thickness, LVEDD is end-diastolic cavity dimension, and 1.33 is the conversion factor for mm Hg to dynes/cm^2.

A simplified version of the wall stress equation states that

$$\text{Wall stress} = P \times LVEDD/WT \qquad (15\text{–}9)$$

where P is systolic arterial pressure, LVEDD is LV end-diastolic dimension, and WT is LV wall thickness.

Diastolic dimensions are selected because it is assumed that peak-systolic wall stress occurs during isovolumic ventricular contractions, while the ventricle still possesses its diastolic anatomic configuration.

Reichek et al[101] demonstrated that the arterial systolic pressure, obtained noninvasively with a blood pressure cuff, can be substituted for the LV end-systolic pressure, if a correcting factor is used (LVESP = 0.89 SAP ± 8.1) in the absence of significant mitral regurgitation. In healthy subjects, the end-systolic wall stress is equal to approximately 65 × 10^3 dynes/cm^2.

Elevations in wall stress have been observed in patients with LV enlargement caused by systemic hypertension.[102] Wall stress provides a better index of afterload than systemic vascular resistance (SVR) when forward SV is not equal to the total ventricular ejection, such as in mitral regurgitation or in the presence of a VSD. Whether the same is true in patients without lesions is unclear. In one animal study, it was observed that, during pharmacologic interventions, SVR and wall stress did not correlate well and occasionally varied in opposite directions.[103]

In cardiac surgical patients, similarly poor correlations between SVR and end-systolic wall stress were observed.[101] In patients undergoing carotid artery surgery, Smith et al[104] studied wall stress under various anesthetic regimens. They noted that, during carotid artery cross-clamping, patients receiving high concentrations of volatile agents, with phenylephrine to maintain blood pressure, had significantly higher wall stress values than those receiving low concentrations of volatile agents without phenylephrine.

Contractility

Echocardiography has been used to estimate contractility in a variety of ways. It is best suited for evaluating contractility during the ejection phase of contraction, but the use of other approaches has been explored.

Ejection Phase Indices

Using echocardiography, contractility has most frequently been estimated with ejection phase indices. A wide array of ejection phase indices have been described, but all require that end-diastolic and end-systolic dimensions be measured. In M-mode echocardiography, these dimensions are often simple, linear, internal dimensions of the LV cavity. The following ratio yields fractional shortening (FS), a basic ejection phase index of contractility:

$$FS = (LVIDD - LVISD)/LVIDD \qquad (15\text{–}10)$$

where LVIDD is LV internal diastolic dimension and LVISD is LV internal systolic dimension.

With 2D echocardiography, multiple tomographic cuts can be obtained and used to calculate ventricular volumes using a variety of formulas such as Simpson's rules.[113] Using the ventricular volumes, EF can be calculated using the standard formula:

$$EF = (LVEDV - LVESV)/LVEDV \qquad (15\text{–}11)$$

where LVEDV is LV end-diastolic volume and LVESV is LV end-systolic volume.

During intraoperative TEE, it is most convenient to monitor a single, short-axis view at the level of the midpapillary muscles. Once the end-diastolic and end-systolic endocardial areas have been delineated with the help of tracing software, contractility may be estimated using the fractional area of contraction (FAC) or the ejection fraction area (EFA):

$$EFA = (LVEDA - LVESA)/LVEDA \qquad (15\text{–}12)$$

where LVEDA is LV end-diastolic area and LVESA is LV end-systolic area.

Isovolumic Phase Indices

The standard isovolumic phase index, dP/dt, cannot be obtained using TEE. Some information on the isovolumic phase can, however, be gathered by measuring the length of the preejection period (PEP). The PEP is the time between the onset of the Q wave on the electrocardiogram (ECG) and the opening of the AV on M-mode echocardiography. The usefulness and limitations of PEP, as well as of the other systolic time intervals, have been extensively reviewed elsewhere.[105,106]

The maximal acceleration of blood flow in the aorta is another measurement related to the isovolumic phase of contraction.[107] Maximal blood flow acceleration occurs in the early part of LV ejection and can be measured by Doppler echocardiography. It is determined by placing a Doppler transducer in the suprasternal notch and aiming the ultrasound beam at the AV. A variety of studies have demonstrated that maximum blood flow acceleration, sampled in this manner, provides information on LV contractility.[108-110] However, the currently available TEE imaging planes are not suitable for this type of measurement.

The circumferential fiber shortening rate (V_{cf}) is an index of contractility that incorporates a time-related element and seems to be less preload dependent than EF:

$$V_{cf} = EDC - ESC/EDC \times LVET \qquad (15\text{–}13)$$

where EDC and ESC are the end-diastolic and end-systolic circumferences of the LV, respectively, measured at the transgastric short-axis view, and LVET is the LV ejection time obtained from a Doppler analysis of the LVOT. Its value in normal individuals is 1.2 ± 0.1 cm/sec.

End-Systolic Pressure-Volume Relationship

An important limitation of isovolumic and ejection phase indices of contractility is their significant sensitivity to ventricular loading conditions. The use of load-independent indices has been explored in order to circumvent this problem. One such index is the LV end-systolic pressure-volume relationship (ESPVR), or end-systolic elasticity.[111] Multiple end-systolic pressures and volumes must be measured during rapid alterations in LV preload (e.g., vena caval occlusion) in order to calculate ESPVR (see Chapters 5 and 14).

On a pressure-volume diagram, points defined by the end-systolic pressures and volumes of several cardiac cycles are positioned on a single line. The slope of this line is relatively independent of loading conditions and proportional to contractility. The intraoperative determination of contractility by this technique has been hampered by difficulties in obtaining accurate ventricular volumes and pressures and the ability to sufficiently vary preload. Nonetheless, using single short-axis views of the LV and radial arterial pressures, the linearity of ESPVR was confirmed.[112] In addition, predicted changes in the direction of the slope were demonstrated after the administration of known positive and negative inotropic agents.

An echocardiography-based system, which uses ultrasonic backscatter technology to characterize tissue properties, incorporates a border detection algorithm for delineating the endocardial–blood interface. The system enables automatic tracking of endocardial boundary and volume (area) determination in real time.[113] These measurements of on-line, beat-to-beat values for LV cavity area and volume can be used to estimate load-dependent parameters of systolic performance (EF and SV) in real time. In addition, it is possible to generate load-independent parameters of systolic performance, such as ESPVRs. With automated border detection, volume-versus-time relationships during systole and diastole can be compared. In addition, LV ESPVRs have been proposed as load-independent indices of contractile function. The combination of continuous volume-dimension assessment with automatic border detection, together with pressure data acquisition, has enabled the generation of end-systolic pressure-volume loops.[112]

Other Techniques

Because of the difficulties in measuring ESPVR, alternative approaches have been attempted. One such alternative is the use of the end-systolic stress/end-systolic area (ESS/ESA) relationship.[114] Initial work with this relationship has shown that it is linear over a wide range of systolic pressures and that it shifted in an appropriate fashion during postextrasystolic potentiation. Further work to define the effects of positive and negative inotropes on the ESS/ESA is needed to determine the applicability of this relationship. Simonson and Schiller[115] proposed an interesting alternative approach to the determination of LV function. They studied the systolic excursion of the mitral LVEF. They found that in normal subjects the excursion of the ventricular base was always at least 8 mm, whereas it was less in patients with decreased ventricular function. They also observed that the relationship between this variable and LVEF was linear.

Cardiac Output

M-Mode Echocardiographic Measurement

Early in the development of echocardiography, Feigenbaum et al[116] compared echocardiographic and angiographic volumes in an attempt to show that M-mode echo measurements were related to actual ventricular size. They cubed single M-mode echocardiographic dimensions and correlated them with their angiographic equivalents. Although reasonably good correlations were obtained, they never intended to use M-mode ventricular diameters for the actual, clinical measurements of ventricular volumes.

Nevertheless, the good correlations between echocardiographic and angiographic volumes prompted other investigators to develop several methods for deriving ventricular volumes from single M-mode dimensions. Kronik et al[117] calculated SV from M-mode echocardiography using a number of these methods and compared their findings with SV measured by thermodilution in patients with and without symmetric ventricular contractions. They concluded that clinically useful SV could be obtained using the Teicholz equation, provided the ventricular contraction was symmetric or nearly symmetric. The other formulas were found unsatisfactory in patients with a similar contraction pattern, while all formulas failed in patients with asymmetric contractions.

Using the Teicholz equation, ventricular volumes are calculated as:

$$\text{Volume} = 7D3/(2.4 + D) \qquad (15\text{–}14)$$

where D is the ventricular internal dimension.

SV is calculated as the difference between EDV and ESV. The ASE has recommended that the diastolic dimension coincide with the Q wave on the ECG. The end-systolic dimension is best measured at the time of the peak downward motion of the posterior endocardium. When TEE was used to obtain ventricular dimensions, correlations between echo and indicator dilution varied from $r = 0.72$ in patients undergoing cardiac surgery to $r = 0.97$ in critically ill patients.[118]

Two-Dimensional Echocardiographic Measurement

In patients undergoing CABG, SV was derived from 2D short-axis views using echocardiography.[79] Comparisons of echo-derived CI with simultaneous thermodilution-derived CI yielded a correlation coefficient of 0.80 (see Chapter 14).

Doppler Measurements

Integration of the *total* area under the transmitral Doppler flow-velocity display has been used for the measurement of SV. The FVI is multiplied by CSA of the MV to determine SV. However, there are different models for the calculations of MV CSA.[119,120] Using TEE, Roewer et al[121] calculated SV in 27 surgical patients. A comparison of Doppler-determined CO values with those obtained by thermodilution yielded an excellent correlation ($r = 0.95$). LaMantia et al,[122] who performed a similar study in 13 cardiac surgical patients, found only a modest correlation ($r = 0.68$).

Flow across the orifice is equal to the product of the CSA of the orifice and the flow velocity. Because flow velocity is not constant throughout a flow cycle, the sum of all of the flow velocities during the entire ejection period is integrated to measure total flow. This summation of flow velocities in a given period of time is called the VTI. The VTI is represented by the area enclosed within the baseline and spectral Doppler signal. In essence, the VTI is the planimetry of the Doppler signal over time.

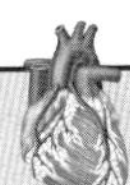

BOX 15–6 ***Assumptions of Flow Calculations***

- Laminar blood flow in the area interrogated
- A flat or blunt flow-velocity profile, such that the flow across the entire cross-sectional area interrogated is relatively uniform
- Doppler angle of incidence between the Doppler beam and the main direction of blood flow is less than 20 degrees

Once VTI is determined, then SV and CO can be calculated:

$$\text{SV} = \text{CSA} \times \text{VTI and CO} = \text{SV} \times \text{HR} \qquad (15\text{–}15)$$

In using these equations, there are a number of assumptions, including (1) laminar blood flow in the area interrogated; (2) a flat or blunt flow-velocity profile, such that the flow across the entire CSA interrogated is relatively uniform; and (3) Doppler angle of incidence between the Doppler beam and the main direction of blood flow is less than 20 degrees, so that the underestimation of the flow velocity is less than 60% (Box 15–6).

A number of Doppler methods have been attempted. Probably the most popular and accepted utilize aortic flow. Other methods using the mitral, tricuspid, and pulmonic orifice have been attempted with variable results. Their respective accuracy is dependent on the angle of insonation. The major determinant of variability in estimating SV by the use of any technique is the accurate measurements of the CSA. The CSA for a circular orifice, such as the AV (also the aortic root and for the LV outflow tract orifice), is:

$$\pi(D/2)^2 \qquad (15\text{–}16)$$

where D represents the diameter obtained by 2D imaging. Therefore, any error in diameter measurement would be squared in the final results. There have been a number of methods suggested for measuring the diameter of the AV orifice. In the absence of AV disease, the diameter at the level of the aortic root either at the level of the sinuses of Valsalva or immediately above them has been used to define the aortic orifice area. However, in the presence of aortic stenosis, the aortic orifice area should be measured at the level of the LVOT, immediately underneath the AV insertion. If the LVOT diameter is used as the aortic CSA to obtain determinations of CO, changes in the diameter of the aortic root will be minimized throughout the cardiac cycle (systole versus diastole).

A second source of variability in measuring aortic flow involves the proper recording of reproducible Doppler signals. If the LVOT is chosen as the CSA, the VTI should be obtained from the Doppler signal at this level. For this purpose, the systolic forward flow must be obtained from an apical five- or two-chamber view. The sample volume of the pulsed Doppler should be placed in the high portion of the LVOT *exactly* at the same level where the diameter was measured. If the aortic root is chosen as the CSA, the VTI can be derived from the systolic aortic flow velocities obtained by continuous-wave Doppler from the apex, suprasternal, or right parasternal areas, wherever the most representative Doppler signal is obtained. Occasionally, the Doppler signal is difficult to obtain and the morphology of the spectrum may be similar to a triangle with a spike at the peak velocity rather than a round "bell-shaped" flow signal. Under such circumstances, it is inappropriate to estimate the VTI, because underestimations or overestimations are likely to result. If attention is given to proper recording techniques, the interobserver variability in measuring the aortic VTI in normal subjects should be less than 5%.

When the results of various studies are compared, it is important to know the method of calculating the VTI and the CSA, as well as where the Doppler sampling volume was located. Because PW Doppler provides a spectral display of instantaneous velocities, mean velocities or velocity modes are used for the integration of flow velocity. The measurement of the mitral orifice diameter should probably be repeated at various cosines. It has been well established that the size of the mitral orifice varies with varying flows. Sample volume location is very important. The SV is underestimated when the sampling volume is placed at the mitral leaflet tips and overestimated when placed at the mitral annulus.

Some investigations have used PA Doppler FVIs and estimations of the vessel area to perform off-line calculations of SV and CO.[123] Muhiudeen et al[124] found that transmitral Doppler CO did not correlate with that obtained by thermodilution and that PA Doppler CO correlated only weakly ($r = 0.65$) with that obtained by thermodilution. They concluded that transesophogeal Doppler has significant limitations as an off-line monitor of CO. In contrast, Savino et al[123] found good agreement and correlation ($r = 0.93$) between transesophageal PA Doppler and thermodilution CO. They were, however, unable to visualize the main PA in 24% of patients. In addition, the method was tedious and not suitable for on-line analysis.

Other Applications

Determination of Intravascular Pressures

In an interesting application of echocardiography, various echocardiographic techniques have been used to gauge intracardiac or intravascular pressures. Based on the Doppler shift principle, blood flow velocity can be used to determine pressure gradients. The modified Bernoulli equation describes the relationship between pressure gradients and blood flow velocities. When flow acceleration and viscous friction variables of blood are ignored and flow velocity proximal to a fixed obstruction (V1) is significantly less than flow velocity after the obstruction (V2), the following formula applies:

$$P1 - P2 = 4(V2)^2 \qquad (15\text{–}17)$$

With this formula, the pressure gradient across a fixed orifice can be calculated.

Application of Pressure Gradient Calculation

The velocity of a regurgitant valve is a direct application of pressure gradient calculations, as it represents the pressure drop across that valve, and, therefore, can be used to calculate intracardiac pressure. For example, tricuspid regurgitation (TR) velocity reflects systolic pressure differences between the RV and RA. RV systolic pressure can be obtained by adding RA pressure (estimated or measured) to $(\text{TR velocity})^2 \times 4$. In the absence of RVOT obstruction, PA systolic pressure will be the same as RVESP. For example,

$$\text{TR velocity} = 3.8\ \text{m/sec};\ \text{RAP} = 10\,\text{mm Hg}$$

then

$$\text{RVESP} = (\text{TR velocity})^2 \times 4 + \text{RAP}$$
$$4(3.8)^2 = 58\,\text{mm Hg} + 10\,\text{mm Hg}$$
$$\text{RVESP} = \text{PA systolic} = 68\,\text{mm Hg}$$

Similarly, pulmonary regurgitation (PR) velocity represents the diastolic pressure difference between the PA and the RV. Therefore, PAEDP = RVEDP + 4 (PR end-diastolic velocity)^2. Note that RVEDP is equal to RAP (estimated or measured). Mitral regurgitation (MR) velocity represents the systolic pressure difference between the LV and the LA. In patients without LVOT obstruction, systolic blood pressure is essentially equal to LV systolic pressure; therefore, LAP is equal to SBP – 4(MR)^2. Finally, aortic regurgitation (AR) velocity reflects the diastolic pressure gradient between the aorta and the LV. Note also that LVEDP can be estimated by various diastolic filling patterns from mitral and pulmonary venous flow velocity patterns. In summary,

$$\text{PAP systolic} = \text{RVESP} = 4\ (\text{TR})^2 + \text{RAP}$$
$$\text{PAP diastolic} = 4(\text{PR})^2 + \text{RAP}$$
$$\text{LAP} = \text{SBP} - 4(\text{MR})^2 \times 4$$
$$\text{LVEDP} = \text{DBP} - (\text{AR})^2 \times 4$$

Regarding inspection of spectral signal and application of the Bernoulli equation for measuring pressure gradients, some useful concepts to remember include the following: (1) The preejection period is the time from Q-wave onset of flow. (2) Peak acceleration time is the most rapid portion at the onset of early systolic flow. (3) Time to peak velocity is the time from onset of flow to peak flow. (4) Systolic ejection time is the time from onset to end of flow (i.e., the period of blood flow across the AV). (5) The peak (or maximal pressure difference) is measured easily in the echo laboratory and in the catheterization laboratory, but is of little clinical use in gauging severity of most valve lesions. It is always higher than the peak-to-peak pressure difference at cardiac catheterization. (6) Mean pressure differences are measured in both the echo and catheterization laboratories, and are the most clinically useful parameters. (7) Peak-to-peak pressure differences between nonsimultaneous events are measured in the catheterization laboratory, but not in the echo laboratory.

Stevenson compared six different echocardiographic techniques to measure PA pressure.[125] When compared with direct measurements, some of these techniques yielded highly accurate correlations ($r = 0.97$), but they were not always applicable in all patients. Using TEE, several investigators have attempted to derive PCWP or LAP from pulmonary venous Doppler velocity signals. In one study the LAP correlated best with the systolic forward flow in the LUPV, while in others it correlated best with flow-velocity reversal in that vein during atrial contraction.[126]

Myocardial Ischemia Monitoring

Regional Wall Motion and Systolic Wall Thickness

The relationship of echocardiographic indices of regional myocardial function to ischemia has been compared with changes that occur with the surface ECG, PCWP, and the onset of chest pain. As early as 1935, it was recognized that acute myocardial ischemia results in abnormal inward motion and thickening of the affected myocardial region.[127] Since then, RWMAs have been shown to occur within seconds of inadequate blood flow or oxygen supply.[128] These abnormal contraction patterns typically occur at the same time as regional lactate production.[129,130]

Diagnosis of Ischemia

The precise sequence of functional changes that occur in the myocardium after interruption of flow has been studied in models of acute ischemia, including PTCA.[131-133] Abnormalities in diastolic function usually precede abnormal changes in systolic function. Normal function is critical for LV filling and is dependent on ventricular relaxation, compliance, and atrial contraction. Diastolic ventricular function can be assessed by monitoring the rate of filling associated with changes in the chamber dimensions (see above). Regional systolic function can be estimated by echocardiographic determination of wall thickening and wall motion during systole in both long- and short-axis views of the ventricle. The short-axis view of the LV at the papillary muscle level displays myocardium perfused by the three main coronary arteries and is, therefore, very useful (Fig. 15–9D). However, because the short-axis view does not image the ventricular apex and this is a very common location of ischemia, the long-axis and longitudinal ventricle views are also clinically important.[134]

In the clinical assessment of regional function with the short-axis view, the ventricle is usually subdivided into four quadrants: inferior, anterior, septal, and lateral. Regional function can be evaluated by wall motion and/or wall thickening. Wall thickening can be assessed qualitatively or it can be quantitatively evaluated by calculating systolic wall thickening from the following equation:

$$\text{PSWT} = \text{SWT} - \text{DWT}/\text{SWT} \times 100 \qquad (15\text{–}18)$$

where PSWT is percentage of systolic wall thickening, SWT is end-systolic wall thickening, and DWT is end-diastolic wall thickening.

Although wall thickening is probably a more specific marker of ischemia than wall motion, its measurement requires visualization of the epicardium, which is not always possible. Alternatively, by observing the movement of the endocardium toward the center of the cavity during systole, RWMAs can almost always be assessed. As the myocardial oxygen supply/demand balance worsens, graded RWMAs progress from mild hypokinesia to severe hypokinesia, akinesia, and finally dyskinesia.[135] *Normal contraction* is defined as greater than 30% shortening of the radius from the center to the endocardial border. *Mild hypokinesia* refers to inward contraction that is slower and less vigorous than normal during systole, with radial shortening of 10% to 30%. *Severe hypokinesia* is defined as less than 10% radial shortening. The precise distinction between varying degrees of hypokinesia can be difficult. *Akinesia* refers to the absence of wall motion or no inward movement of the endocardium during systole. *Dyskinesia* refers to paradoxical wall motion or movement outward during ventricular systole. These measurements of regional wall motion are obviously based on the determination of the center of the ventricular cavity. Unfortunately, because of cardiac translation, this center may move during the cardiac cycle. Two reference systems have been used: fixed reference and floating reference. Because of its relative simplicity and the fact that in most situations the impact of translation is minimal, the fixed reference system is generally used. In conditions of significant translation, such as after CPB, the more cumbersome floating system may be more appropriate[136] (Fig. 15–16).

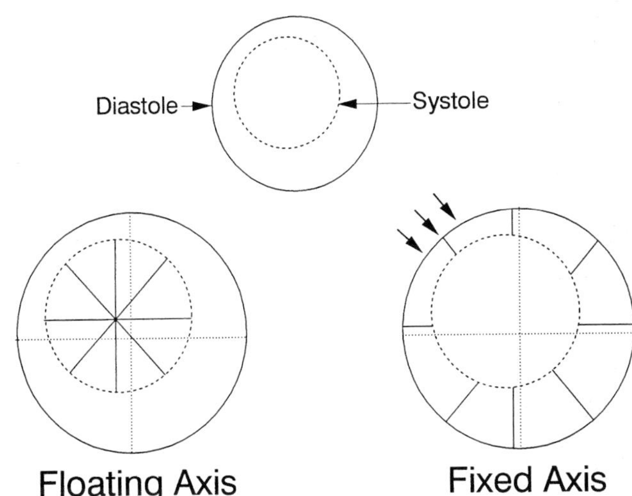

Figure 15–16 Comparison of fixed and floating axis systems. In the fixed-axis system, there is an apparent motion abnormality (delineated by the *arrows*). Conversely, in the floating-axis system, the effects of translation are negated and no abnormality is observed.

Stress Echocardiography

Dynamic imaging with *stress echocardiography* was first introduced in the late 1970s and has been rigorously evaluated as a method to better distinguish viable from nonviable myocardium. Stress echocardiography uses mechanical, pharmacologic, or other stresses to the heart to achieve predetermined peak stress levels. Over the past decade, stress echocardiography has emerged as a safe and sensitive method for the detection of CAD and a cost-efficient alternative to scintigraphy. Reversible RWMAs due to transient myocardial ischemia are the hallmark of atherosclerotic CAD. Among the means for initiating the stress response are exercise, atrial pacing, intravenous dipyridamole, adenosine, and dobutamine. Exercise and dobutamine cause myocardial ischemia through marked increases in heart rate, systolic blood pressure, and contractility. Dipyridamole-induced ischemia, on the other hand, is mainly due to blood flow maldistribution, with a reduction in subendocardial flow in the regions of myocardium supplied by a stenotic coronary artery. Because dipyridamole predominantly affects the supply part of the supply-demand ratio, flow maldistribution may not be severe enough to always induce endocardial ischemia. It is not surprising that sensitivity is greater for detecting IHD with exercise followed by dobutamine, whereas specificity is greater with dipyridamole echocardiography. The application of stress echocardiography for assessment of perioperative cardiac risk in patients undergoing major vascular surgery has been investigated and shown to be a safe and cost-efficient method for identifying patients at high and low risk of perioperative cardiac events. A meta-analysis by Srinivas et al[137] determined that its positive predictive value compares favorably with dipyridamole-thallium, Holter ECG, and radionuclide ventriculography for perioperative risk stratification (see Chapters 11 and 12).

Relation to Other Monitors

Clinical studies have indicated that RWMAs occur earlier and are a more sensitive indicator of myocardial ischemia than the abnormal changes detected with an ECG or PAC.[138-144] In one study, 30 patients undergoing PTCA were simultaneously monitored with 12-lead ECGs and echocardiography.[141] All the patients had isolated obstructive lesions in their LADs, stable angina, normal baseline ECGs, normal baseline myocardial function with no prior history of infarction, and no angiographic evidence of collateralization. In the study, all patients developed RWMAs approximately 10 seconds after coronary artery occlusion. ECG changes occurred in 27 of 30 patients approximately 22 seconds after coronary occlusion.

Smith et al[140] evaluated 50 patients at high risk for myocardial ischemia during peripheral vascular or cardiac surgery with TEE and a multilead ECG. In their study, 6 patients had repolarization changes diagnostic of ischemia and 24 had new evidence of RWMAs. ECG repolarization changes were always accompanied by a corresponding RWMA. In 50% of the patients who experienced ST-segment changes, the RWMA had occurred minutes before. Three patients with evidence of new RWMAs developed perioperative MIs; however, only one patient of the three had evidence of ST-segment changes.

The value of PCWP monitoring for ischemia has also been compared with changes in regional LV function assessed with TEE. In one study, PCWP, 12-lead ECG, and LV wall motion were evaluated in 98 patients before CABG at predetermined intervals.[142] Myocardial ischemia was diagnosed by TEE in 14 patients. In 10 of the 14 patients, ischemia was associated with repolarization changes on the ECG. An increase of at least 3 mm Hg in PCWP was tested as an indicator for ischemia and was sensitive only 33% of the time, with a positive predictive value of only 16%. Overall, most studies indicate that the sensitivity of wall motion analysis for detection of myocardial ischemia is generally superior to that of the ECG or PCWP (see Chapter 14).

Limitations

Although TEE appears to have many advantages over traditional intraoperative monitors of myocardial ischemia, there remain potential limitations as well (Table 15–4). The most obvious limitation of TEE monitoring is the fact that ischemia cannot be detected during critical periods, such as induction, laryngoscopy, intubation, emergence, and extubation. In addition, the adequacy of RWMA analysis may be influenced by artifact.[145] The ultrasound system itself or the particular tangential section being imaged can produce artifacts.

The septum in particular must be given special consideration with respect to wall motion and wall thickness assessment.[145,146] The septum is composed of two parts: the lower muscular portion and the basal membranous portion. The basal septum does not exhibit the same degree of contraction as the lower muscular part. At the most superior basal portion, the septum is attached to the aortic outflow track. Its movement at this level is normally paradoxical during ventricular systole. The septum is also a unique region of the LV, because it is a region of the RV as well, and is therefore influenced by forces from both ventricles. In addition, sternotomy, pericardiotomy, and CPB have been found to alter the translational and rotational motion of the heart within the chest, which may cause changes in ventricular septal motion.[146]

For these reasons, use of a floating reference system in the intraoperative period is recommended. Consequently, the exact imaging plane for wall motion assessment is critical. The short-axis view of the LV at the level of the midpapillary muscles is used to ensure constant internal landmarks as reference (anterior and posterior papillary muscles) and to ensure monitoring of the muscular septal region. It must be recognized that, although myocardial blood flow from the coronary arteries is best represented at the short-axis midpapillary muscle level, there may be other myocardial regions that are underperfused and not adequately represented in one echocardiographic imaging plane.[147] One solution to this problem is to frequently reposition the probe to view other cross sections of the heart.

Another potential problem of RWMA assessment is evaluation of the dys-synchronous contraction that occurs as a result of a bundle-branch block or ventricular pacing. In these situations, the system used to assess RWMAs must compensate for global motion of the heart (usually done with a floating frame of reference) and evaluate not only regional endocardial wall motion but also myocardial thickening.

Not all RWMAs are indicative of myocardial ischemia or infarction. Clearly, under normal conditions, all hearts do not contract in a homogenous and consistent manner.[148] It is reasonable to assume, however, that most of the time an acute change in the regional contraction pattern of the heart during surgery is likely attributable to myocardial ischemia. An important exception to this rule may apply in models of acute coronary artery occlusion. In these models, it has been established that myocardial function becomes abnormal in the center of an ischemic zone, but it is also true that the myocardial regions adjacent to the ischemic zones become dysfunctional as well. Several studies have reported that the total area of dysfunctional myocardium commonly exceeds the area of ischemic or infarcted myocardium.[149,150] The impairment of function in nonischemic tissue has been thought to be caused by a "tethering effect" (Fig. 15–17). Tethering, or the attachment of noncontracting tissue that is normally perfused, probably accounts for the consistent overestimation of infarct size by echocardiography when compared with postmortem studies.[151]

Another limitation of RWMA analysis during surgery is that it does not differentiate stunned or hibernating myocardium from acute ischemia, nor does it differentiate the cause of ischemia between increased oxygen demand and decreased oxygen supply.[152] Finally, it should be noted that areas of previous ischemia or scarring may become unmasked by changes in afterload and appear as new RWMAs.[153] This is particularly important in vascular surgery, in which major abrupt changes in afterload occur.

Table 15–4 Limitations of Transesophageal Echocardiography

Incompatibility: induction, laryngoscopy intubation, emergence, extubation
Artifact interference: electronic, septum, bundle-branch block
Lack of specificity: tethering effect, scar, afterload changes, stunned myocardium

Outcome Significance

Data regarding the significance of intraoperative detection of RWMAs suggest that transient abnormalities unaccompanied by hemodynamic or ECG evidence of ischemia may not represent significant myocardial ischemia and are usually not associated with postoperative morbidity.[154] Hypokinetic myocardial segments appear to be associated with minimal perfusion defects compared with the significant perfusion defects that accompany akinetic or dyskinetic segments.

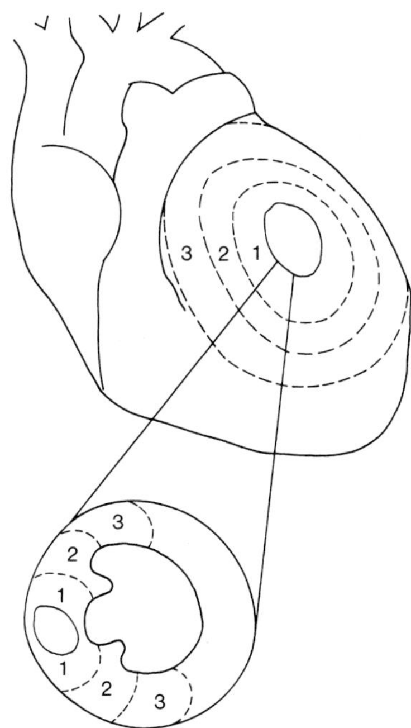

Figure 15–17 Tethering effect. Myocardial function becomes abnormal in the center of an ischemic zone as well as in regions adjacent to the ischemic zone. Attachment of noncontracting tissue (the central zone) mechanically impairs contraction in normally perfused adjacent tissue (zones 1 through 3).

Hence, hypokinesia may be a less predictive marker for postoperative morbidity.[104,140,155,156]

Intraoperative detection of new or worsened and persistent RWMAs during peripheral vascular surgery has been reported to be associated with postoperative cardiac morbidity by several investigators. The occurrence of new RWMAs during vascular surgery appears to be common; however, most of the time they are transient and clinically insignificant.[104,154-156] New RWMAs that are recognized to persist until the conclusion of surgery, in contrast, imply perioperative AMI. Intraoperative RWMAs, therefore, may be spurious, reversible with or without treatment, or irreversible. The former may be associated with clinically insignificant short periods of ischemia, whereas the latter are associated with significant ischemia or infarction.[104,140,155,156]

Intraoperative TEE has helped predict the results of CABG. Following CABG of previously dysfunctional segments, immediate improvement of regional myocardial function (which is sustained) has been demonstrated.[157-160] In addition, prebypass compensatory hypercontracting segments have been reported to revert toward normal immediately following successful CABG.[161] Persistent RWMAs following CABG appear to be related to adverse clinical outcomes, and lack of evidence of RWMAs following CABG has been shown to be associated with a postoperative course without cardiac morbidity.[152]

Ischemia-Related Diagnoses

Echocardiography is widely used in patients with IHD for characterization of cardiac anatomy as well as for analysis of intracardiac flow velocities by Doppler echocardiographic modalities. Two-dimensional TEE has been shown to greatly enhance the diagnostic potential for detecting life-threatening sequelae of MI, such as a ruptured ventricular septum or ruptured papillary muscles.[162,163] It has also been recognized that TEE may enable the identification of subtle, but potentially significant, problems that complicate the management of IHD, such as anomalous coronary artery origins and atrial infarction.[164] In addition, it is important to note that the assessment of right- as well as left-sided heart function can be accomplished with intraoperative echocardiography. The assessment of right- as well as left-sided heart damage during intraoperative ischemia monitoring is essential because the presence of RV dysfunction may be a limiting factor and, thus, influence perioperative treatment strategies[165,166] (see Chapters 31 and 33). An echocardiographic examination for IHD should routinely include a functional assessment of valvular competency, with emphasis on the MV because of the high incidence of MV insufficiency that accompanies IHD.[167]

The potential to evaluate coronary blood flow reserve following administration of coronary artery vasoactive drugs may prove to be another application of transesophageal Doppler echocardiography. Several investigators have reported that, because 2D TEE enables imaging of the proximal coronary artery anatomy, it can be used together with PW Doppler to evaluate coronary blood flow velocity.[168,169]

FUTURE TECHNOLOGY

While much intraoperative echocardiographic research has been directed toward estimating pressures (e.g., PCWP) and flow (e.g., CO) to replace catheter-based techniques, new innovative technologies are exploring means of providing information distinct from and complementary to the traditional measurement of global cardiac hemodynamics and performance. Novel information can be extracted from the complex image analysis of the Doppler and echocardiographic signals to provide quantitative measures of endocardial position and excursion, intramyocardial velocity of shortening, and 3D reconstruction of cardiac anatomy. These techniques are currently in evolution and will need to undergo technical refinement before they become routine during intraoperative evaluation. There is the opportunity for clinical investigation to define the physiologic significance of the data derived by these techniques in the complex and dynamic intraoperative environment. These techniques can analyze common pathophysiologic problems encountered in the operating room in novel ways to shed new insights on clinical decision making. Although it is unlikely that these echocardiographic techniques will supplant traditional monitoring techniques, when used in concert with a comprehensive hemodynamic assessment of cardiac loading conditions and intracardiac blood flow, important information about global cardiac performance, regional diastolic and systolic function, and complex 3D relationships is likely to emerge. For instance, while existing techniques permit reasonable assessment of overall LV systolic function by EF and SV calculations, there may be ways of evaluating LV myocardial shortening in relation to systolic wall stress for specific layers of the myocardium, which may define the mechanisms of impaired systolic contraction; specific spatial or temporal contraction patterns may distinguish myocardial stunning, hibernating myocardium, myocardial edema, myocardial inflammation, or postcardioplegic myocardial dysfunction. These are unrealized potential applications that will provide the stimulus for future investigation and development of new echocardiographic technologies.

Automated Endocardial Border Detection and Tissue Characterization Using Integrated Backscattered Ultrasound

Online detection of the endocardium has been a subject of intense research interest in the field of echocardiographic image processing. Reliable automated detection of endocardial and epicardial interfaces would potentially permit online rapid calculation of ventricular mass, ventricular volume, endocardial excursion, and transmural wall thickening. Theoretically, derived indices of global systolic and diastolic function could be obtained with such measurements. Hemodynamic data measured simultaneously by catheter techniques might permit the assessment of myocardial contractility by the afterload-scaled, end-systolic wall stress versus end-systolic cavity area method of analysis.[170] Similarly, online analysis of instantaneous LV volumes and intraventricular pressure (measured by catheter techniques) would provide the means to measure diastolic parameters such as LV chamber compliance.

An approach to automated endocardial border detection has been developed utilizing backscattered ultrasound energy rather than reflected energy from myocardial tissue. Clinical echocardiographic imaging devices image from reflected ultrasound, representing the returning signal from specular reflectors such as the blood–endocardium interface. These specular reflectors have intrinsic dimensions, which are larger than the wavelength of the ultrasound beam. Much smaller objects such as the structural inhomogeneities within the myocardium have physical dimensions less than the wavelength of the ultrasound beam and are referred to as "Raleigh scatterers."[171,172] Rather than reflecting the incident ultrasound beam (as a function of angle of incidence and relative change in acoustic impedance at a specular reflecting interface), these Raleigh scatterers distribute ultrasound scatter in all directions. The portion of the scattered energy that returns to the transducer (path of travel 180 degrees to the incident beam) is called "backscatter."

The unprocessed backscattered radiofrequency signal derived from each radial line of the imaging sector is processed in the time domain by squaring and integrating the signal over a finite interval. This integrated backscattered signal is typically collected from 100 range gates along each radial line. The integrated backscattered signal represents the average power returning along a radial line of ultrasound interrogation and is expressed in decibels relative to a system reference power standard.[172] This integrated backscattered signal is a function of the overall transmitted power settings as well as receiver gain controls, but independent of operator-defined post-processing curves and choice of signal compression (steps in the normal image processing train occurring after the radiofrequency signal is sampled for quantitative analysis).

The integrated backscattered signal from intramyocardial scatterers varies during the cardiac cycle, having higher intensity in late diastole and lower intensity in systole.[172] The backscatter may arise from interaction of ultrasound energy with small structures such as individual myofilaments, and the magnitude of the backscatter and its cyclic variation are influenced by myofiber orientation.[172,173] If the ultrasound beam is parallel to the myofibers responsible for the scattering interaction, integrated backscatter is reduced and cyclic variation in integrated backscatter is attenuated. Initial investigations have demonstrated that analysis of the magnitude of cyclic variation of integrated backscattered ultrasound may be utilized to differentiate normal, stunned, and infarcted myocardium.[174,175] Even though conventional echocardiographic imaging (based on images derived from specular reflectors) may show stunned and infarcted segments of the myocardium to be akinetic, differences in cyclic variation in integrated backscatter permit differentiation among these conditions. There are also data to suggest that analysis of cyclic variations in integrated backscatter may be useful in identifying immunologic rejection in patients who have undergone orthotopic heart transplantation.[176]

The processing of integrated backscattered signals has been applied to the task of distinguishing the LV blood pool from myocardium during online acquisition of echocardiographic images.[171,172,177] In a commercially available implementation of this automated endocardial tracking algorithm, conventional B-mode images of the LV are obtained as transmitted power settings and receiver gain are optimized to display endocardial borders throughout the cardiac cycle with minimal endocardial dropout (Fig. 15–18). A region of interest is traced on the screen to identify the portion of the image where endocardial-to-blood pool interface tracking is desired. Upon selection of automated endocardial tracking, the echocardiograph analyzes the relative power of the integrated backscattered signal and employs a proprietary thresholding technique to discriminate blood pool from myocardial tissue. The boundary between pixels assigned to blood pool and pixels assigned to myocardium is demonstrated by a closed loop superimposed on the conventional B-mode image. Fine tuning of the image to ensure that the automated endocardial tracking agrees with the echocardiographer's perception of where the endocardium lies is required to optimize the measurement. The computer can compute the time-varying endocardial cavity area for the short axis of the LV. After defining the region of interest for the blood pool myocardial interface in a four-chamber image of the LV, the computer identifies the mitral annular plane and the LV long axis. From automated endocardial tracking and application of a single-plane modified Simpson rule, an approximation of LV volume can be computed online and displayed as a time-varying waveform along with its first derivative (Fig. 15–19). Average LVEDV, ESV, EF, peak diastolic filling rate, peak systolic ejection rate, and time to peak diastolic filling rate are also displayed.

A novel reconfiguration of these data to a color-encoded display format permits a depiction of regional LV endocardial motion.[178,179] The automated endocardial tracking algorithm can sequentially identify the endocardial borders at specified time intervals following the QRS of the ECG. In one implementation of this process, 12 sequential endocardial contours at 33-msec intervals following the QRS can be displayed superimposed upon the conventional B-mode echocardiographic image. These sequential "isochronal" maps of endocardial position are color encoded to provide a temporal map of sequential regional wall motion during early systole. For instance, in Figure 15–19, orange encodes the earliest centripetal endocardial motion (first 33 msec following the QRS), whereas yellow, green, and blue encode successive endocardial positions in systole. The timing of endocardial motion and the magnitude of endocardial motion (area of the color contour within a specified segment) for any given isochronal interval are inherently quantifiable entities that can be used to assess regional wall motion. The isochronal maps could be extracted for diastole, in order to assess regional LV cavity expansion during ventricular filling.

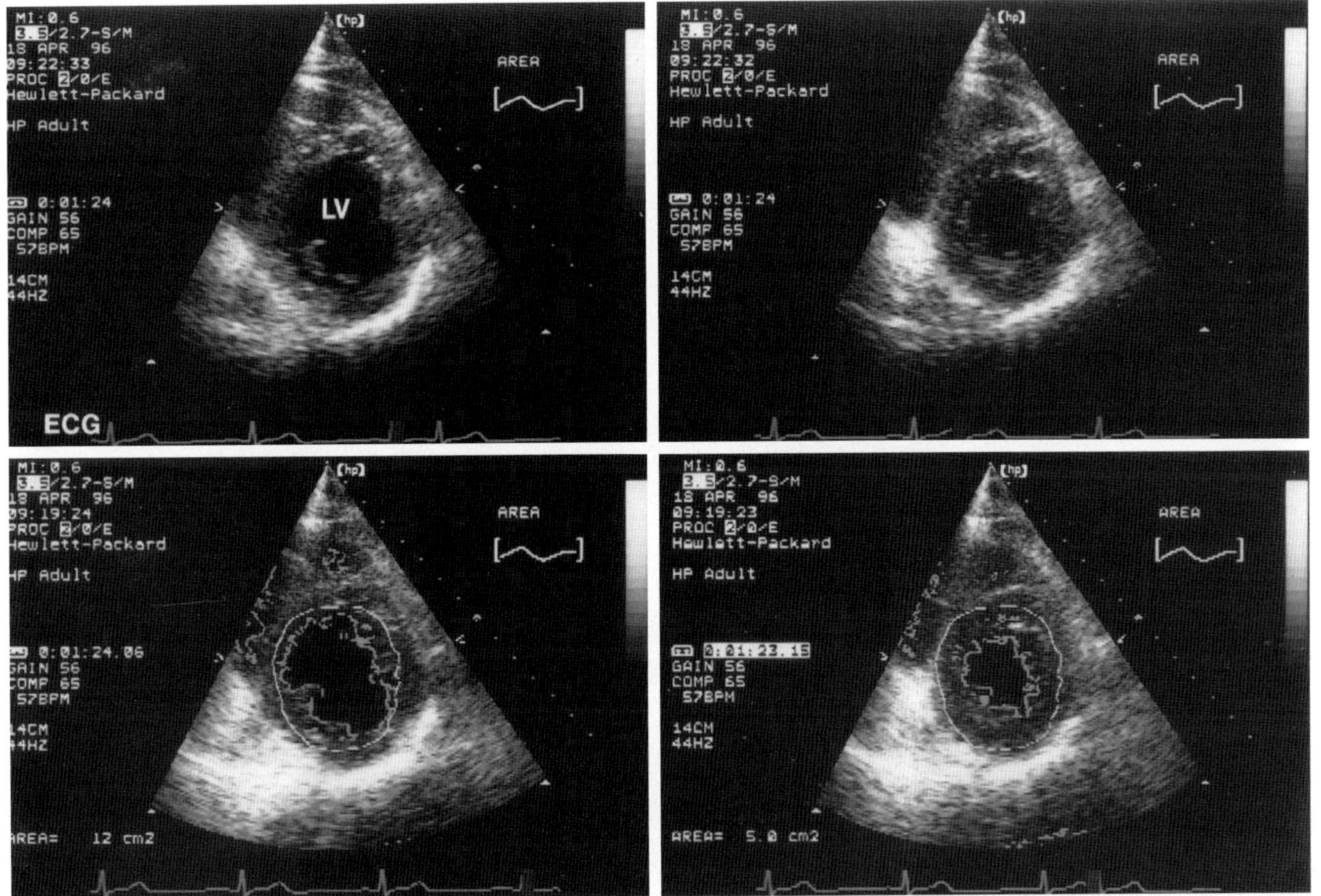

Figure 15–18 Automated endocardial tracking derived from the analysis of integrated backscattered ultrasound signals from the interface between blood pool and myocardium. All four stop-frame transthoracic echocardiographic images display the short-axis profile of the left ventricle (LV) at the level of the papillary muscles with anterior structures near the apex of the sector and the patient's left positioned on the right side of the image. An electrocardiographic (ECG) trace is depicted in green and interrupted at the point of acquisition of the stop-frame image. Depth calibrations are at 1.0-cm intervals. *Upper left panel:* Diastolic stop-frame image of the short-axis image of the LV cavity demonstrates distinct endocardial margins. *Lower left panel:* Diastolic stop frame image of the LV (corresponding to *upper left panel*) with superimposed user-defined region of interest (blue closed loop). Automated endocardial tracking is depicted by light brown-colored contours and closely follows the endocardial contours depicted in the *upper left panel. Upper right panel:* Systolic stop-frame image of the short-axis image of the LV cavity demonstrates clear delineation of the endocardium. *Lower right panel:* Systolic stop-frame image of the LV (corresponding to *upper right panel* with superimposed user-defined region of interest (blue closed loop). Automated endocardial tracking is depicted by light brown-colored contours of the blood pool myocardial interface, which closely follows the endocardium depicted in the upper right panel. (See Color Plate VI.) (From Louie EK, Louie DS: New echocardiographic technology: Does it add to clinical decision making? Semin Cardiothorac Vasc Anesth 1:16, 1997.)

Validation of automated endocardial tracking derived from integrated backscattered ultrasound signals has provided evidence that LV systolic function can be estimated by this technique. Acceptable correlations with SV and CO measured by thermal dilution techniques or aortic electromagnetic flow probes have been obtained.[180,181] Absolute measurements of SV and CO tend to be systematically underestimated by these automated endocardial tracking techniques, suggesting that the technique might be useful for tracking directional changes in a given patient but not for providing absolute measurement of SV.[180-182] Estimates of LVEF obtained from single-plane modified Simpson's rule measurements of LV volume with application of automated endocardial tracking of the integrated backscattered signal have been compared with EF estimates obtained by gated radionuclide ventriculography.[183-185] These correlations are generally good (r = 0.81 to 0.91), but absolute measurements of LVEF are systematically underestimated by the automated endocardial tracking derived from the integrated backscattered signal.[185] Because the automated endocardial tracking techniques derive volume estimates from only a single plane, Simpson's rule estimations of LV volume are likely to provide a good estimate of true ventricular volume if the ventricle contracts uniformly. When there are RWMAs outside the imaging plane,[185] and when asymmetry of LV shape is inadequately represented in a single four-chamber view of the heart, estimates of ventricular volume will be inaccurate.[186,187] Thus, the correlation coefficient between LVEF measured by automated endocardial tracking and radionuclide angiography for all patients was 0.81 but fell to 0.69 when analysis was confined to patients with regional asynergy. These techniques have been successfully applied to TEE imaging[183,185] and have been used to monitor LV systolic function of patients during cardiac surgery.[188]

As illustrated in Figure 15–20, LV diastolic filling can be characterized by quantitation of the derived LV volume curve. As with the assessment of systolic function, it would be predicted that automated endocardial tracking of diastolic volume changes from a single tomographic plane would be

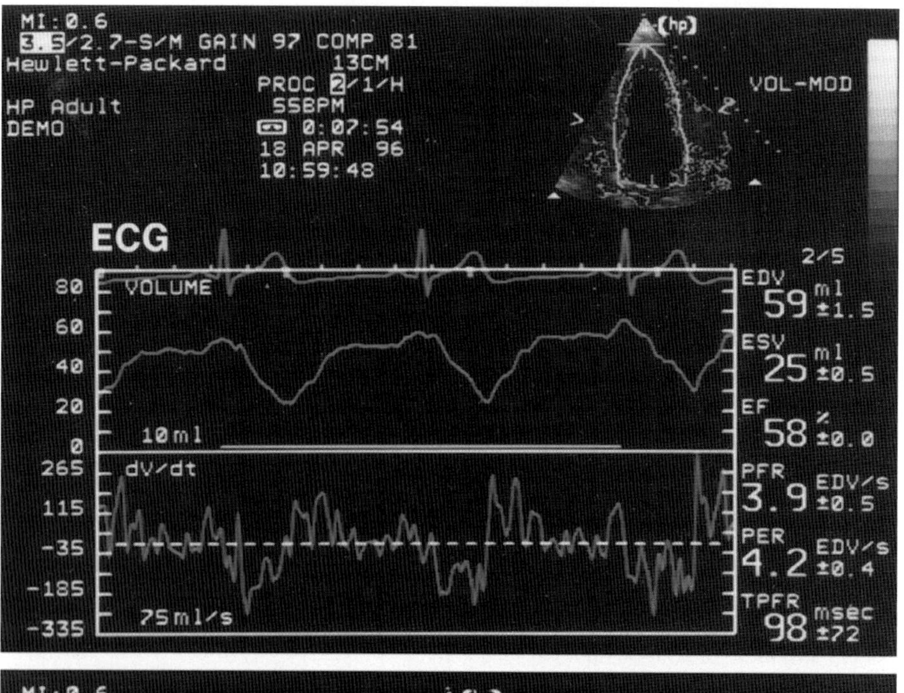

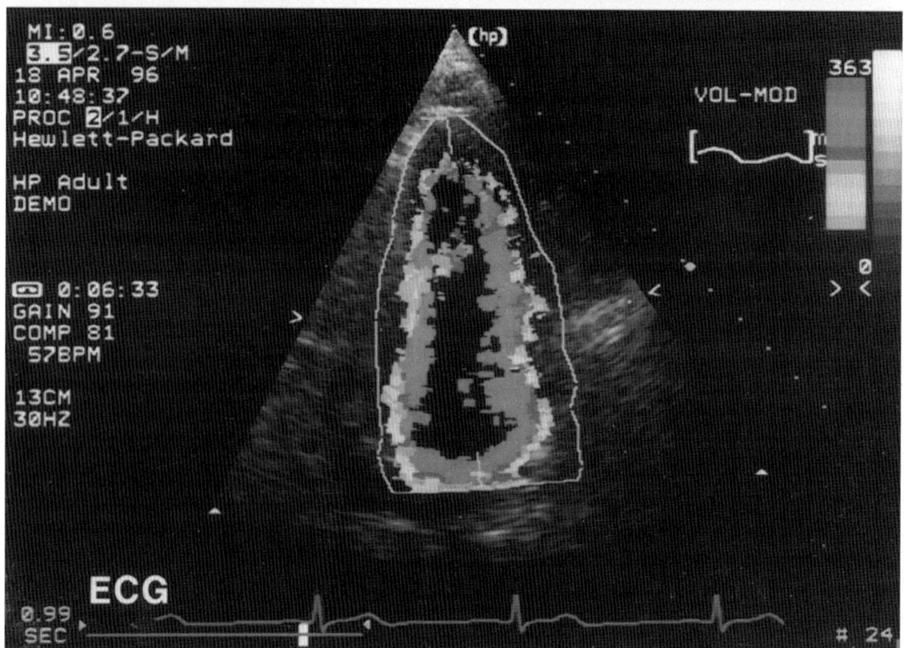

Figure 15–19 Derived indices of global and regional systolic left ventricular function from automated endocardial tracking of integrated backscattered ultrasound signals. The miniature B-mode image in the *upper right hand corner of the upper panel* (transthoracic echocardiographic apical four-chamber view) displays the image of the left ventricle along with the user-defined region of interest (blue closed loop that includes a semiautomated determination of the mitral annular plane and the left ventricular long axis). The light brown trace indicates the tracking of the left ventricular endocardium and the mitral annular plane. The apical four-chamber image permits derivation of left ventricular volumes by a single-plane modified Simpson formula. Depth calibrations are at 1.0-cm intervals. Derived parameters are presented as time varying graphics (green traces) below the electrocardiogram (ECG). The instantaneous time varying volume curve for the left ventricle is represented by the *upper trace* and permits derivation of the average left ventricular end-diastolic volume (59 + 1.5 mL), end-systolic volume (25 + 0.5 mL), and ejection fraction (58 + 0.0 percent). The *lower trace* represents the first derivative (dV/dt) of the volume curve and permits measurement of the peak left ventricular diastolic filling rate (3.9 + 0.5 end-diastolic volumes/sec), peak systolic ejection rate (4.2 + 0.4 end-diastolic volumes/sec), and the time from the QRS to the peak filling rate (98 + 72 msec). *Lower panel:* Color-encoded isochronal maps of systolic endocardial excursion are mapped onto the B-mode echocardiographic image of the transthoracic apical four-chamber view of the left ventricle. The blue closed loop represents the user-defined region of interest. The color scale (*upper right corner*) represents isochronal intervals beginning with the initial 33-msec interval following the QRS (orange) and successively progressing at 33-msec intervals through shades of yellow, green, and blue. The concentric rings of color superimposed on the B-mode echocardiographic image of this normal left ventricle represent successive isochronal maps of the inward excursion of the endocardium during systole. The width of any given color zone represents the magnitude of endocardial excursion at that particular segment of the left ventricle for the specified isochronal interval. Qualitative and quantitative assessment of regional systolic function is possible from such images. Equivalent isochronal maps of diastolic endocardial motion could also be constructed to assess global and regional left ventricular filling patterns. (See Color Plate 15–19.)

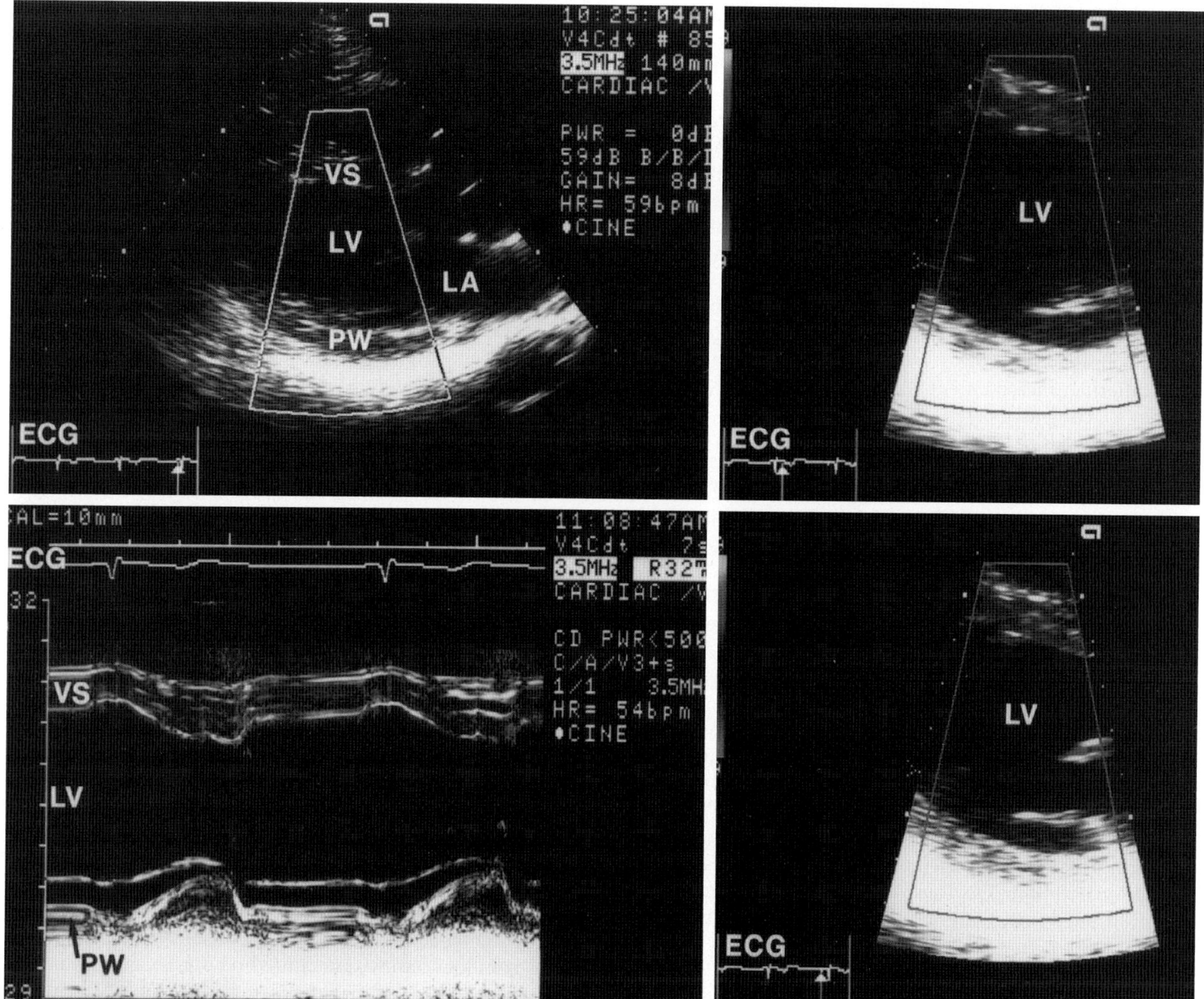

Figure 15–20 Color Doppler myocardial velocity mapping. *Upper left panel:* Stop-frame diastolic image from a cine loop of the transthoracic parasternal long-axis image of the left ventricle (LV) and left atrium (LA). The ventricular septum (VS) and left ventricular posterior walls (PW) are clearly imaged. Timing of the stop frame is indicated by the *arrow* referenced to the electrocardiogram (ECG) in the *lower left corner of the panel.* The quadrilateral region of interest superimposed on the B-mode image is redisplayed in the upper and lower right panels. Depth calibrations are at 5-cm intervals (bright dots) and 1-cm intervals (subdued dots). *Upper right panel:* Early systolic stop-frame image from the transthoracic parasternal long-axis image of the LV with superimposed color Doppler myocardial velocity mapping. Myocardial velocities relative to the transducer (located at the apex of the sector) range from shades of blue (9 cm/sec directed away from the transducer) to shades of red (9 cm/sec directed toward the transducer) as depicted by the color bar on the *left side of the panel.* Note the ventricular septum is encoded blue as it contracts toward the center of the LV (away from the transducer) and the posterior wall is encoded red as it contracts toward the center of the LV (toward the transducer). *Lower right panel*: The display format is the same as in the upper right panel except a late diastolic stop-frame image is shown. Now the left ventricular septum is moving outward (encoded red for motion towards the transducer) and the posterior wall is also moving away from the center of the left ventricle (encoded blue for motion away from the transducer). *Lower left panel*: M-mode echocardiogram at the level of the chordae tendineae targeted from a transthoracic parasternal long-axis view of the LV (such as that portrayed in the *upper left panel*). The superimposed color Doppler map of myocardial velocities is derived from a transducer located at the top of the M-mode image. The VS and PW are clearly delineated and the simultaneous ECG is provided for timing purposes. Depth calibrations are at 1.0-cm intervals and time calibrations are at 200-msec intervals (minor divisions). The VS is encoded blue during systole, because it is moving toward the center of the LV and away from the transducer and red during diastole when it is moving away from the center of the LV and toward the transducer. The PW shows a reciprocal pattern of color Doppler myocardial velocity mapping, which is less well demonstrated in this image. The inherently high sampling rate of the dedicated single M-mode Doppler sampling beam permits high temporal resolution of the myocardial velocity map. (See Color Plate VIII.)

more accurate for uniformly contracting LVs than for ventricles with marked RWMAs.[189] Correlations have been demonstrated for a number of diastolic filling parameters (e.g., peak filling rate, time to peak filling rate) derived by automated endocardial tracking when compared with related parameters measured by transmitral Doppler echocardiography and gated radionuclide angiography.[184-192]

There are several limitations to the use of integrated backscatter measurements for the quantitative assessment of ultrasound data. First, the power of the signal is expressed in decibels relative to a proprietary reference standard. The relevant reference standard should be a signal of known initial power emanating from the patient and, hence, appropriately corrected for depth-dependent attenuation and potential variations with the cardiac and respiratory cycles. Since such a true reference standard is not available and attenuation effects are not easily estimated, the significance of the absolute value of integrated backscatter measurement is uncertain. Second, the previously noted cyclic variations in intramyocardial integrated backscatter intensity have not been taken into account in this analysis. Presumably, the differences in integrated backscatter between blood pool and myocardium are so great that the threshold selection for "blood-tissue discrimination" is unambiguous and, hence, these considerations can be neglected.

A practical technical concern in the optimization of images for automated endocardial tracking is the angle dependence of the technique. The angle between the line of sight for the backscattering measurements and the orientation of the myofibers acting as Raleigh scatterers influence the intensity of the integrated backscattered signal. This may account for the difficulties in endocardial tracking of the anterolateral wall and the posterior septum on short-axis views of the LV. In the four-chamber view, the majority of the LV myocardium (ventricular septum and lateral wall) may be suboptimally positioned for automated endocardial tracking. One solution to this problem is to enhance the receiver gain of signals returning from the lateral portions of the sector ("lateral gain control") to improve tracking of these portions of the myocardium.

Two considerations relevant to image analysis in general and its use in the assessment of cardiac physiology are the impact of frame rate upon temporal resolution of physiologic events and the influence of cardiac translation and rotation upon measurement of intrinsic cardiac motion. High-fidelity volumetric analysis by cine ventriculography is performed at 60 frames per second in patients with basal heart rates ranging from 60 to 100 bpm. Obviously, the higher the frame rate at any given heart rate, the greater the temporal resolution for differentiating events within the cardiac cycle. To distinguish subtle differences in the regional timing of systolic contraction patterns or diastolic expansion, frame rates significantly greater than 30 frames per second achieved with conventional echocardiographic techniques may be required. For example, to distinguish the site of systolic preexcitation in the Wolff-Parkinson-White syndrome to permit intraoperative ablation of a bypass tract may require distinguishing earliest systolic endocardial motion to within 15 msec. This would require that endocardial tracking techniques be performed at 60 frames/sec. Because the ultrasound probe is fixed in position with respect to the human body and not with respect to the center of contraction of the LV, endocardial tracking describes the motion of the endocardium as a vector sum of intrinsic endocardial excursion relative to a floating frame of reference (the center of contraction of the LV) and extrinsic motion of the heart relative to the ultrasound probe. Thus, when the automated endocardial tracking algorithm identifies a given pixel as changing from blood pool to tissue, it cannot distinguish between true endocardial motion and swinging of the heart. Consequently, an infarcted akinetic segment may still show motion tracked by the system, which may be explained by the motion of the entire heart within the thoracic cavity. One solution to this problem might be to track epicardium and endocardium simultaneously and compute instantaneous LV wall thickening. Though translation and rotation would create small errors in the measurement of wall thickening (through misregistration of corresponding systolic and diastolic targets), a large component of the error encountered with translational effects would be eliminated. While simple thresholding techniques for endocardial tracking have been implemented, there are substantial challenges to devising algorithms for epicardial tracking because the difference in integrated backscattered signals between myocardium and extracardiac soft tissues is not as great as the difference in signals between myocardium and blood pool.

Current clinical implementation of automated endocardial tracking requires an excellent echocardiographic image and a significant degree of operator experience. "Fine tuning" the standard B-mode image by trimming the time-gain compensation, adjusting lateral gain, and optimizing transmit power and overall receiver gain is necessary to achieve images in which the entire endocardium is reliably tracked. Between 59% and 78% of patients have technically adequate transthoracic echocardiograms for automated endocardial tracking.[183,184] Although the images afforded by TEE offer a greater opportunity for successful automated endocardial tracking, experienced investigators have reported acceptable tracking in only 72% to 84% of patients undergoing TEE studies.[188] In addition, suboptimal LV apical imaging by TEE in a small but significant number of patients can result in significant underestimation of LV volume from four- or two-chamber views.[182]

Automated endocardial tracking by integrated backscatter analysis has not solved the problem of inherently "noisy" echocardiographic images. The technique cannot "extract" endocardial contours from suboptimal images. The technique should not be thought of as a low-level algorithm for improving signal-to-noise ratio. Rather, the application of the technique requires very high-resolution images with distinct endocardial contours from which visual recognition and manual tracing of the endocardium can be performed with ease. What is unique about the technique is that it automates this process and provides online quantitative data, which would be impractical to obtain by manual, labor-intensive, off-line digital analysis. Because the absolute radiofrequency signal is influenced by transmitted power, receiver gain, and attenuation effects, a "higher order" of "oversight" (currently the operator's intuition as to what constitutes the appropriate estimate of systolic function, but perhaps supplanted by "artificial intelligence" in the future) is required to adjust instrument settings to an appropriate level before automatic tracking can be initiated.

Myocardial Velocity Mapping

Pulsed-Doppler spectral analysis has been adapted to measure endocardial motion and to characterize instantaneous endocardial velocity. Pulsed-Doppler analysis of mitral annular motion relative to the LV apex can characterize LV diastolic long-axis expansion velocities in patients with pericardial constriction and restrictive cardiomyopathy.[193] A related technique involves the direct mapping of Doppler-determined myocardial velocities onto the 2D echocardiographic image of the heart.[194]

Color-flow Doppler technology, which maps average regional velocities of intracardiac flow to the 2D echocardiographic image by an autocorrelation algorithm, has been adapted to map myocardial tissue velocities to the image.[194] Whereas normal forward intracardiac flow velocities are in the range of 100 to 150 cm/sec, typical myocardial velocities of systolic contraction are on the order of less than 20 cm/sec. The amplitude of the Doppler-shifted signal returning from intracardiac flow is relatively low (<20 dB), whereas the amplitude of Doppler-shifted signals returning from the LV wall may be in excess of 40 dB.[194,195] Color-flow Doppler measurements from intracardiac blood flow are optimized for low-amplitude high Doppler frequency-shifted signals by high-pass filtering, which eliminates "wall-motion artefacts." In contrast, color Doppler measurement of myocardial tissue velocities uses the lowest possible "wall or clutter filter" settings or eliminates high-pass filtering altogether to detect the velocity of wall motion.[195] As illustrated in Figure 15–20, these high-amplitude, low Doppler frequency-shifted signals from tissue motion are assigned a color scale with low Nyquist limits (in this example, +9 cm/sec), allowing for the measurement of small changes in myocardial velocity anticipated for myocardial motion. An area of interest is selected on the conventional B-mode echocardiographic image, and a color overlay is superimposed on the echocardiographic image. A variety of displays are possible, but the fundamental display encodes varying shades of red (brighter shades for higher velocities) for myocardium moving toward the transducer and varying shades of blue for myocardium moving away from the transducer. The spatial mapping of Doppler-derived myocardial velocities affords the opportunity for regional assessment of myocardial velocity contraction patterns. In addition, discrimination of endocardial, midmyocardial, and epicardial velocities is potentially possible.[196,197] Such data may shed light on ischemic myocardial dysfunction, since the earliest metabolic and contractile abnormalities occur in the subendocardium and spread to the epicardium in a wavefront of ischemic injury. In addition to providing spatial maps of myocardial velocity, there is the potential for extraction of quantitative data from pixels within the region of interest as small as 3 × 3 mm.[197] The first derivative of myocardial tissue velocities and an index of the power or energy of the color Doppler signal can also be derived. Clinical application has demonstrated the feasibility of characterizing RWMAs with the color Doppler mapping of myocardial velocities.[197]

There are theoretic advantages and limitations of color Doppler velocity mapping, which are common to intracardiac blood flow analysis and myocardial velocity mapping. One advantage of the technique is that the absolute value of the Doppler frequency shift is not affected by tissue attenuation and can be interpreted without reference to a patient-specific standardization procedure and without correction for signal attenuation.[196] This stands in contrast to conventional B-mode imaging of signals from specular reflectors and integrated backscattered data from Raleigh scatterers, which are subject to attenuation effects. An important theoretic limitation of the Doppler technique, however, is that the technique can only measure the component of velocity parallel to the Doppler beam. Off-axis myocardial targets, whose motion is not aligned with the interrogating Doppler beam, will be subject to significant underestimation of myocardial velocity by this technique.[195,198] One solution to this problem involves the calculation of the systolic myocardial velocity gradient across the LV wall in the direction parallel to endocardial motion.[198] The myocardial velocity gradient at any given point in time is equal to the instantaneous fractional change in wall thickening per unit time and thus is equivalent to the instantaneous fractional rate of systolic wall thickening, providing a quantitative index of regional systolic function.[199]

Computation of the myocardial velocity gradient from the short-axis image of the LV requires some operator-dependent "higher order" assumptions about the pattern of LV contraction.[198] The theoretic center of contraction for the short-axis profile of the LV must be selected by the operator so that the color-encoded myocardial velocities can be corrected for the angle of incidence of the interrogating Doppler beam. The angle-corrected velocity profile along each radial line from the center of contraction across the myocardial wall can then be obtained. The myocardial velocity gradient is computed as the slope of the least squares linear regression of the transmural velocity profile. The derived myocardial velocity gradients are then reencoded as shades of red for positive transmural gradients (absolute value of endocardial velocity > absolute value of epicardial velocity) and shades of blue for negative transmural gradients. The short-axis polar map of myocardial velocity gradients in a normal individual might show a uniform red ring indicating uniform fractional rate of wall thickening around the circumference of the LV. In contrast, the raw color Doppler myocardial velocity map would encode the anterior septum as blue in systole (moving toward the center of the LV away from the transducer) and the posterior wall as red (moving toward the center of the LV and toward the transducer). Qualitative assessment of the color patterns on the myocardial velocity gradient polar map can identify RWMAs that are not apparent from a qualitative assessment of the raw color Doppler myocardial velocity map.[198] While the myocardial velocity gradient technique corrects velocity of myocardial motion for Doppler angle of incidence, those portions of the myocardium that move almost perpendicular to the Doppler beam and have a negligible component of velocity parallel to the Doppler beam cannot be accurately corrected for angle of incidence. This novel method of analyzing the dynamics of wall thickening as an index of systolic function can potentially be refined to minimize operator-dependent "higher order" manipulations of the data and automated for eventual online analysis during image acquisition. Additional imaging from orthogonal planes may be required to circumvent the problem of angle-correcting velocities from targets moving perpendicular to the initial direction of Doppler interrogation.[198]

As in all physiologic analysis of cardiac motion, the impact of cardiac translation and rotation as well as acquisition frame rate must be considered. The myocardial velocity gradient potentially corrects for the angle dependence of Doppler measurements and partially corrects for the effects of cardiac translation and rotation. To the extent that LV wall thickness is small relative to LV short-axis cavity radius, the myocardial velocity gradient technique is independent of translation and rotational effects that act on the heart. This occurs because the myocardial velocity gradient is calculated as the difference in velocity from endocardium to epicardium and the translational and rotational vectors for the equivalent endocardial and epicardial targets cancel each other out.[198] High frame rates are particularly critical to the assessment of myocardial tissue velocities, where the assessment of regional wall motion and earliest endocardial motion are important diagnostic considerations. One approach to this problem is to employ color M-mode Doppler myocardial imaging, which capitalizes on the intrinsically high sampling rate achieved, when Doppler information is collected along a single interrogating ray (see Fig. 15–20). This approach sacrifices 2D spatial orientation and limits the potential segments of the LV wall, which are accessible for analysis. Miyatake et al[195] and Uematsu et al[198] report the achievement of frame rates up to 57 frames/sec in the clinical application of 2D color Doppler myocardial velocity mapping. Such increases in frame rate are achieved by a 50% reduction in data sampling along each interrogating ray, an increase in pitch (1.5×) of each ray, and the use of parallel processing technology.

Color Doppler mapping of myocardial velocities can take advantage of the high-resolution images obtained by TEE; however, operator experience is required to achieve interpretable color Doppler myocardial velocity maps. As refinements in processing speed, frame rate, and potential automation of the myocardial velocity gradient technique become possible, there will probably be expanded applications for this new diagnostic technique. While equivalent approaches for measuring intramyocardial shortening and shortening velocities have been developed by magnetic resonance myocardial tagging techniques, the Doppler echocardiographic approach has obvious practical advantages in the operating room and the critical care environment.

Three-Dimensional Reconstruction

Although the concept of 3D echocardiography was first introduced in the early 1970s, its utility in the perioperative environment has only recently acquired appropriate recognition.[200,201] Advantages of both conventional 3D reconstruction and real-time 3D imaging (RT3DE) techniques for enhancing the diagnostic confidence of conventional echocardiography in the perioperative period have begun to emerge in the literature. Primary areas of interest have included the utility of 3D echocardiography in *preoperative* surgical planning, *intraoperative* assessment of the surgical procedure, and *postoperative* early and long-term follow-up to determine the need for further intervention.[202]

Three-dimensional reconstruction of echocardiographic data requires sequential acquisitions of 2D echocardiographic data from multiple imaging planes, digitization of echocardiographic data points in appropriate 3D spatial registration, and off-line reconstruction of the 3D data set into a comprehensible display format. These computationally intensive and time-consuming manipulations of the data are not feasible for rapid, online analysis and are therefore not currently applicable as an intraoperative echocardiographic technique.[203] It can be anticipated, however, that innovative means for expediting the acquisition of multiple imaging planes may bring 3D imaging closer to being a clinically applicable tool in the operating room.

Three-dimensional cardiac imaging may be used to explicitly portray 3D spatial relationships that are normally inferred in the mind of the echocardiographer from the interrelationships between multiple 2D images, to quantitate anatomic blood flow data that do not conform to simple geometric models, to provide a surface or volume rendering of a cardiac structure that facilitates understanding of a pathologic condition, or to dissect a complex structure by displaying a synthetic 2D tomographic image (derived from the 3D data set) from a perspective that cannot be achieved with conventional transducer positioning. Three-dimensional reconstruction of echocardiographic data requires acquisition of the image data, digital formatting of the data, and generation of a display that exploits the advantages of 3D presentation of the data. Data are acquired with appropriate registration of time in the cardiac cycle (ECG gating), time in the respiratory cycle (thoracic impedance gating), and spatial registration of the various imaging planes. Spatial registration may occur by external determination of the physical coordinates of each randomly acquired imaging plane.[203] Acoustic spark gap locators (not appropriate in an environment with explosive gases such as the operating room) or mechanical articulating arms attached to the transducer are two approaches employed in transthoracic imaging. Predetermined and calibrated incremental motion of the probe represents an approach that has been readily adapted to TEE and may eventually become applicable to studies conducted in the operating room.[203] A TEE probe rigidly aligned to obtain sequential parallel transverse plane images by withdrawing the probe along the length of the esophagus (via a stepper motor) represents one approach. Sequential rotation of the transesophageal longitudinal plane imaging crystal using the esophagus as the axis of rotation creates imaging planes of the heart that resemble the "pages" of a book radiating from the esophagus, which serves as the "spine of the book."[204] Finally, sequential rotations of a multiplane transesophageal crystal fixed at one acoustic window provide a family of imaging planes intersecting along the axis of rotation of the crystal.[205,206]

Subsequent digitization and formatting of the acquired data involve the detection of borders (endocardium and epicardium), segmentation of the data to confine attention to regions of particular interest, and interpolation between points of acquisition to fill in the gaps. Finally, the data must be presented in a display format that captures the unique information inherent to the 3D format. This may involve surface rendering, volume rendering, or the generation of synthetic tomographic imaging planes. To these static 3D renditions of the data set, the element of time to show the motion of structures in 3D during the cardiac cycle may be added. Clearly, 3D echocardiography will have to undergo revolutionary technical advances before these processing steps can reasonably be applied in the operating room or the critical care environment. The exciting new structural and functional relationships revealed by such data transformations, however, will address important questions for surgeons and anesthesiologists.

The utility of 3D echocardiographic techniques in providing preoperative, noninvasive imaging of intracardiac lesions from the surgeon's visual perspective, has been demonstrated in patients with congenital heart and valvular lesions. Lange et al[207] compared preoperative 2D and 3D TTE evaluations with intraoperative findings in 15 patients with atrioventricular septal defect morphology. In comparison with preoperative 2D echocardiography, 3D TTE reconstruction provided superior imaging of the MV and TV function. In addition, 3D TTE provided a more precise description of primum ASD size, secundum ASD fenestrations, and VSD size. Thus, preoperative 3D TTE enhanced the diagnostic capability of standard 2D TTE in patients with common atrioventricular junction congenital heart disease. Acar et al also performed preprocedural 3D TTE in 62 consecutive patients aged 2 to 18 years with ASDs scheduled for either transcatheter (n = 42) or surgical (n = 20) closure.[208] Preprocedural 3D TTE measurement of ASD size correlated well with findings obtained intraoperatively and during transcatheter closure. A similar degree of accuracy for 3D TTE evaluation of VSD size prior to closure has also been demonstrated.[209] Additional reported applications for preoperative 3D echocardiography have included a complementary role to conventional echocardiographic techniques in facilitating surgical planning for defining the shape, dimensions, location, origin, mobility, and valve involvement of cardiac tumors.[210] Furthermore, preoperative 3D echocardiographic reconstruction was shown to enhance accurate imaging of the spatial relationship among mobile LV thrombi, the myocardial wall and the valvular apparatus, which subsequently influenced the selection of the most appropriate surgical approach for urgent thrombectomy.[211] Thus, preoperative 3D echocardiography may facilitate surgical planning by providing superior imaging of intracardiac structures.

The accuracy, feasibility, and value of 3D echocardiography have also been demonstrated in the intraoperative environment. Abraham et al[212] performed intraoperative 2D and 3D reconstruction TEE examinations on 60 patients undergoing valve surgery. In this study, 3D acquisitions were completed in 87% of the patients within a mean acquisition time of 2.8 ± 0.2 minutes and reconstruction time within 8.6 ± 0.7 minutes. Three-dimensional echocardiography detected all salient valve morphologic pathology (leaflet perforations, fenestrations, and masses), which was subsequently confirmed on pathologic examination in 84% of the patients. In addition, intraoperative 3D TEE provided new additional information not obtained by 2D TEE in 15 patients (25%), and in one case influenced the surgeon's decision to perform a valve repair rather than a replacement. Furthermore, intraoperative 3D reconstruction TEE provided worthwhile and complementary anatomic information that explained the mechanism of valve dysfunction demonstrated by 2D imaging and CF Doppler. Ahmed et al evaluated the potential utility of 3D TEE in identifying individual MV scallop prolapse in 36 adult patients undergoing surgical correction.[213] Perfect correlation between 3D TEE and surgical findings was noted in 78% of the patients. Similarly, De Castro et al[214] demonstrated superior concordance between intraoperative 3D TEE surgical identification of prolapsing anterior and posterior MV scallops compared to 2D TEE. Intraoperative 3D TEE has also been used to identify distortion and folding of the mitral annulus as a cause of functional mitral stenosis or worsening mitral regurgitation during beating heart surgery while positioning to access the back of the heart.[215] Furthermore, in studies comparing 2D versus 3D TEE for measuring MV area and volume in patients with stenosis undergoing percutaneous MV balloon valvuloplasty, 3D TEE enabled a better description of valve anatomy including the identification of commissural splitting and leaflet tears following valvuloplasty.[216,217] Finally, intraoperative 3D TEE has been shown to be valuable in patients undergoing surgery for congenital heart lesions.[218,219] For example, the superiority of intraoperative 3D TEE compared to 2D has been demonstrated in providing en face and oblique views of left atrioventricular valve septal malformations in patients undergoing reoperation for persistent regurgitant lesions after previous repair of partial atrioventricular septal defects[218] (see Chapters 4, 12, 20, and 21).

The recent development and availability of RT3DE has introduced additional opportunities for noninvasive diagnostic imaging to influence perioperative decision-making. Compared with conventional 3D reconstruction, RT3DE permits faster acquisition without a dependency on the ECG or respiratory gating and allows simultaneous visualization of orthogonal planes with 2D resolution.[220] Disadvantages compared with conventional 2D imaging include decreased line density in the acquired volume and slower frame rates.[220] In addition, compared to conventional TEE probes, the larger dimensions of RT3DE transducers currently available for clinical utilization limit their utilization to TTE or intraoperative epicardial viewing planes. Nonetheless, comprehensive RT3DE epicardial examinations can be efficiently performed, and permit rapid acquisition of immediately available data to assist intraoperative surgical decision-making.[221] The utility of intraoperative epicardial RT3DE has been reported in a patient with hypertrophic cardiomyopathy undergoing septal myectomy, for enhancing the spatial assessment, extent of septal thickening, MV systolic anterior motion and postsurgical LV outflow tract patency.[222] In addition, Suematsu et al[223] used RT3DE in a beating heart animal model to monitor off-pump ASD closure. Finally, Qin et al[224] performed intraoperative epicardial and postoperative transthoracic RT3DE to evaluate changes in LV volume and function in cardiac surgical patients undergoing infarct exclusion surgery for ischemic cardiomyopathy. In contrast to 3D echocardiographic imaging, conventional 2D methods may not accurately quantify LV volumes in patients with severe ischemic cardiomyopathy, especially in the presence of significant geometric changes due to an LV aneurysm. Thus, assuming inevitable growth in the technological development of more sophisticated ultrasound transducers in the near future, the introduction of improvements in image acquisition, processing speed, real-time volume rendering and transducer miniaturization may promote RT3DE into becoming the technique of choice for noninvasive intraoperative cardiac imaging.[220]

REFERENCES

1. Thys DM, Hillel Z: How it works: Basic concepts in echocardiography. *In* Bruijn NP, Clements F (eds): Intraoperative Use of Echocardiography. Philadelphia, JB Lippincott Company, 1991, pp 13–44
2. Hatle L, Angelsen B: Doppler Ultrasound in Cardiology, 2nd edition. Philadelphia, Lea & Febiger, 1984
3. Kisslo J, Adams D, Mark DB: Basic Doppler Echocardiography. New York, Churchill Livingstone, 1986
4. Kisslo J, Adams DB, Belkin RN: Doppler Color-Flow Imaging. New York, Churchill Livingstone, 1988
5. Gramiak R, Shah PM, Kramer DH: Ultrasound cardiography: Contrast studies in anatomy and function. Radiology 92:939, 1969
6. Serwer GA, Armstrong BE, Anderson PA, et al: Use of contrast in ventricular septal defects. Circulation 58:327, 1978
7. Melzer RS, Hoogenhuyze DV, Serruys PW: Diagnosis of tricuspid regurgitation by contrast echocardiography. Circulation 63:1093, 1981
8. Roelandt J: Contrast echocardiography. Ultrasound Med Biol 8:471, 1982
9. Armstrong WF, West SR, Mueller TM, et al: Assessment of location and size of myocardial infarction abnormalities with contrast-enhanced echocardiography. J Am Coll Cardiol 2:63, 1983
10. DeMaria A, Bommer W, Kuan OL, et al: In vivo correlation of thermodilution cardiac output and videodensitometry indicator-dilution curves obtained from contrast two-dimensional echocardiograms. J Am Coll Cardiol 3:999, 1984
11. Goldman ME, Mindich BP, Teicholz LE, et al: Intraoperative contrast echocardiography to evaluate mitral valve operations. J Am Coll Cardiol 4:1035, 1984
12. Raisinghani A, DeMaria AN: Physical principles of microbubble ultrasound contrast agents. Am J Cardiol 90:3J, 2002
13. Frinkin PJA, Bouakaz A, Kirkhorn J, et al: Ultrasound contrast imaging: Current and new potential methods. Ultrasound Med Biol 26:965, 2000
14. Stewart MJ: Contrast echocardiography. Heart 89:342, 2003
15. Kaul S: Instrumentation for contrast echocardiography: Technology and techniques. Am J Cardiol 18:8J, 2002
16. Miller AP, Nanda NC: Contrast echocardiography: New agents. Ultrasound Med Biol 30:425, 2004
17. Ward RP, Collins KA, Balasia B, et al: Harmonic imaging for endocardial visualization and myocardial contrast echocardiography during transesophageal echocardiography. J Am Soc Echocardiogr 17:10, 2004
18. Masugata H, Yukiiri K, Takagi Y, et al: Potential pitfalls of visualization of myocardial perfusion by myocardial contrast echocardiography with harmonic gray scale B-mode and power Doppler imaging. Int J Cardiovasc Imaging 20:117, 2004
19. Skyba DM, Price RJ, Linka AZ, et al: Direct in vivo visualization of intravascular destruction of microbubbles by ultrasound and its local effects on tissue. Circulation 98:290, 1998
20. van Der Wouw PA, Brauns AC, Bailey SE, et al: Premature ventricular contractions during triggered imaging with ultrasound contrast. J Am Soc Echocardiogr 13:288, 2000

21. Raisinghani A, Wei KS, Crouse L, et al: Myocardial contrast echocardiography (MCE) with triggered ultrasound does not cause premature ventricular complexes: Evidence from PB127 MCE studies. J Am Soc Echocardiogr 16:1037, 2003
22. Lindner JR, Wei K, Kaul S: Imaging of myocardial perfusion with SonoVue(r) in patients with a prior myocardial infarction. Echocardiography 16:753, 1999
23. Palmieri V, Arezzi E, Pezzullo S, et al: Inter- and intra-study reproducibility of contrast echocardiography for assessment of interventricular septal wall perfusion rate in humans. Eur J Echocardiogr 5:367, 2004
24. Moir S, Haluska BA, Jenkins C, et al: Incremental benefit of myocardial contrast to combined dipyridamole-exercise stress echocardiography for the assessment of coronary artery disease. Circulation 110:1108, 2004
25. Senior R, Lepper W, Pasquet A, et al: Myocardial perfusion assessment in patients with medium probability of coronary artery disease and no prior myocardial infarction: Comparison of myocardial contrast echocardiography with 99mTc single-photon emission computed tomography. Am Heart J 147:1100, 2004
26. Peltier M, Vancraeynest D, Pasquet A, et al: Assessment of the physiologic significance of coronary disease with dipyridamole real-time myocardial contrast echocardiography. Comparison with technetium-99m sestamibi single-photon emission computed tomography and quantitative coronary angiography. J Am Coll Cardiol 43:257, 2004
27. Janardhanan R, Swinburn JM, Greaves K, et al: Usefulness of myocardial contrast echocardiography using low-power continuous imaging early after acute myocardial infarction to predict late functional left ventricular recovery. Am J Cardiol 92:493, 2003
28. Janardhanan R, Burden L, Senior R: Usefulness of myocardial contrast echocardiography in predicting collateral blood flow in the presence of a persistently occluded acute myocardial infarction-related coronary artery. Am J Cardiol 93:1207, 2004
29. Balcells E, Powers ER, Lepper W, et al: Detection of myocardial viability by contrast echocardiography in acute infarction predicts recovery of resting function and contractile reserve. J Am Coll Cardiol 41:827, 2003
30. Korosoglou G, Hansen A, Hoffend J, et al: Comparison of real-time myocardial contrast echocardiography for the assessment of myocardial viability with fluorodeoxyglucose-18 positron emission tomography and dobutamine stress echocardiography. Am J Cardiol 94:570, 2004
31. Fukuda S, Hozumi T, Muro T, et al: Quantitative intravenous myocardial contrast echocardiography predicts recovery of left ventricular function after revascularization in chronic coronary artery disease. Echocardiography 21:119, 2004
32. Sable C: Digital echocardiography and telemedicine applications in pediatric cardiology. Pediatr Cardiol 23:358, 2002
33. Thomas JD, Greenberg NL, Garcia MJ: Digital echocardiography 2002: Now is the time. J Am Soc Echocardiogr 15:831, 2002
34. Mildenberger P, Eichelberg M, Martin E: Introduction to the DICOM standard. Eur Radiol 12:920, 2002
35. Karson TH, Zepp RC, Chandra S, et al: Digital storage of echocardiograms offers superior image quality to analog storage, even with 20:1 digital compression: Results of the Digital Echo Record Access Study. J Am Soc Echocardiogr 9:769, 1996
36. Spencer K, Weinert L, Mor-Avi V, et al: Electronic transmission of digital echocardiographic studies: Effects of MPEG compression. Int J Cardiol 75:141, 2000
37. Segar DS, Skolnick D, Sawada SG, et al: Comparison of the interpretation of digitized and videotape recorded echocardiograms. J Am Soc Echocardiogr 12:714, 1999
38. Hisanaga K, Hisanaga A, Nagata K, et al: A new transesophageal real-time two-dimensional echocardiographic system using a flexible tube and its clinical application. Proc Jpn J Med Ultrasonogr 32:43, 1977
39. Matsomoto M, Oka Y, Lin Y, et al: Transesophageal echocardiography for assessing ventricular performance. N Y State J Med 79:19, 1979
40. Matsumoto M, Oka Y, Strom J, et al: Application of transesophageal echocardiography to continuous intraoperative monitoring of left ventricular performance. Am J Cardiol 46:95, 1980
41. Schluter M, Langenstein B, Polster J, et al: Transesophageal cross-sectional echocardiography with a phased array transducer system. Technique and initial clinical results. Br Heart Jr 48:68, 1982
42. Urbanowicz JH, Kernoff RS, Oppenheim G, et al: Transesophageal echocardiography and its potential for esophageal damage. Anesthesiology 72:40, 1990
43. O'Shea JP, Southern JF, D'Ambra MN, et al: Effects of prolonged transesophageal echocardiographic imaging and probe manipulation on the esophagus: An echocardiographic-pathologic study. J Am Coll Cardiol 17:1426, 1991
44. Daniel WG, Erbel R, Kasper W, et al: Safety of transesophageal echocardiography: A multicenter survey of 10,419 examinations. Circulation 83:817, 1991
45. Kharasch ED, Sivarajan M: Gastroesophageal perforation after intraoperative transesophageal echocardiography. Anesthesiology 85:426, 1996
46. Dewhurst WE, Stragand JJ, Fleming BM: Mallory-Weiss tear complicating intraoperative transesophageal echocardiography in a patient undergoing aortic valve replacement. Anesthesiology 73:777, 1990
47. Everett ED, Hirschman JV: Transient bacteremia and endocarditis prophylaxis. Medicine 56:61, 1977
48. Botoman VA, Surawicz CM: Bacteremia with gastrointestinal endoscopic procedures. Gastrointest Endosc 32:342, 1986
49. Nikutta P, Mantey-Stiers F, Becht I, et al: Risk of bacteremia induced by transesophageal echocardiography: Analysis of 100 consecutive procedures. J Am Soc Echocardiogr 5:168, 1992
50. Melendez LJ, Kwan-Leung Chan, Cheung PK, et al: Incidence of bacteremia in transesophageal echocardiography: A prospective study of 140 consecutive patients. J Am Coll Cardiol 18:1650, 1991
51. Steckelberg JM, Khandheria BK, Anhalt JP, et al: Prospective evaluation of the risk of bacteremia associated with transesophageal echocardiography. Circulation 84:177, 1991
52. Dajani AS, Bisno AAL, Chung KJ, et al: Prevention of bacterial endocarditis. JAMA 264:2919, 1990
53. Cucchiara RF, Nugent M, Seward JB, et al: Air embolism in upright neurosurgical patients: Detection and localization by two-dimensional transesophageal echocardiography. Anesthesiology 60:353, 1984
54. Humphrey LS: Esophageal stethoscope loss complicating transesophageal echocardiography. J Cardiothorac Anesth 3:356, 1988
55. Ellis JE, Lichtor JL, Feinstein SB, et al: Right heart dysfunction, pulmonary embolism, and paradoxical embolization during liver transplantation. Anesth Analg 68:777, 1989
56. Suriani RJ, Cutrone A, Feierman D, et al: Intraoperative transesophageal echocardiography during liver transplantation. J Cardiothorac Vasc Anesth 10:699, 1996
57. Kaplan JA: Monitoring technology: Advances and restraints. J Cardiothorac Anesth 3:257, 1989
58. Popp RL, Williams SV, et al: ACP/ACC/AHA Task Force on Clinical Privileges in Cardiology: Clinical competence in adult echocardiography. J Am Coll Cardiol 15:1465, 1990
59. Pearlman AS, Gardin JM, Martin RP, et al: Guidelines for physician training in transesophageal echocardiography: Recommendations of the American Society of Echocardiography Committee for Physician Training in Echocardiography. Am Soc Echocardiogr 5:187, 1992
60. Pearlman AS, Gardin JM, Martin RP, et al: Guidelines for optimal physician training in echocardiography. Recommendations of the American Society of Echocardiography Committee for Physician Training in Echocardiography. Am J Cardiol 60:158, 1987
61. Cheitlin MD, Alpert JS, Armstrong WF, et al: Committee on Clinical Application of Echocardiography: ACC/AHA Guidelines for the clinical application of echocardiography: Executive summary. J Am Coll Cardiol 29:862, 1997
62. Practice guidelines for perioperative transesophageal echocardiography. A report by the American Society of Anesthesiologists and the Society of Cardiovascular Anesthesiologists Task Force on Transesophageal Echocardiography. Anesthesiology 84:986, 1996
63. Konstadt SN, Reich DL, Rafferty T: Validation of a test of competence in transesophageal echocardiography. J Cardiothorac Vasc Anesth 10:311, 1996
64. Calahan MK, Foster E: Training in transesophageal echocardiography: In the lab or on the job? Anesth Analg 81:217, 1995
65. Savage RM, Licina MG, Koch CG, et al: Educational program for intraoperative transesophageal echocardiography. Anesth Analg 81:399, 1995
66. Quinones M, Doulgas P, Foster E, et al: American College of Cardiology/American Heart Association clinical competence statement of echocardiography. Circulation 107:1068, 2003
67. Rafferty T, LaMantia KR, Davis E, et al: Quality assurance for intraoperative transesophageal echocardiography monitoring: A report of 836 procedures. Anesth Analg 76:228, 1993
68. Shanewise J, Cheung A, Aronson S, et al: ASE/SCA Guidelines for Performing a Comprehensive Intraoperative Multiplane Transesophageal Echocardiography Examination: Recommendations of the American Society of Echocardiography Council for Intraoperative Echocardiography and the Society of Cardiovascular Anesthesiologists Task Force for Certification in Perioperative Transesophageal Echocardiography. Anesth Analg 89:870, 1999

69. Shanewise J, Cheung A, Aronson S, et al: ASE/SCA Guidelines for Performing a Comprehensive Intraoperative Multiplane Transesophageal Echocardiography Examination: Recommendations of the American Society of Echocardiography Council for Intraoperative Echocardiography and the Society of Cardiovascular Anesthesiologists Task Force for Certification in Perioperative Transesophageal Echocardiography. J Am Soc Echocardiogr 12:884, 1999
70. Cerqueira M, Weissman NJ, Dilsizian V, et al: Standardized myocardial segmentation and nomenclature for tomographic imaging of the heart: A statement for healthcare professionals from the Cardiac Imaging Committee of the Council on Clinical Cardiology of the American Heart Association. Circulation 105:539, 2002
71. Rakowski H, Appleton C, Kwan-Leung C, et al: Canadian consensus recommendations for the measurement and reporting of diastolic dysfunction by echocardiography. J Am Soc Echocardiogr 9:736, 1996
72. Clements FM, Hill R, Kisslo J, et al: How easily can we learn to recognize regional wall motion abnormalities with two-dimensional-transesophageal echocardiographic images? Presented at the 11th Annual Meeting of the Society of Cardiovascular Anesthesiologists, Seattle, WA, 1989
73. Hillel Z, Thys D, Ali J: Can left ventricular ejection fraction be estimated by visual inspection of two-dimensional echocardiographic images? Presented at the 11th Annual Meeting of the Society of Cardiovascular Anesthesiologists, Seattle, WA, 1989
74. Saada M, Cahalan MK, Lee E, et al: Real-time evaluation of segmental wall motion abnormalities. Anesth Analg 68:S242, 1989
75. Lazar HL, Plehn J, Schick EM, et al: Effects of coronary revascularization on regional wall motion. J Thorac Cardiovasc Surg 98:498, 1989
76. Amico AF, Lichtenberg GS, Reisner SA, et al: Superiority of visual versus computerized echocardiographic estimation of radionuclide left ventricular ejection fraction. Am Heart J 118:1259, 1989
77. Stauffer JC, Mueller X, Homsi L, et al: Echocardiographic determination of ejection fraction with various methods: Comparison with contrast angiography. J Am Soc Echocardiogr 3:7-I, 1990
78. Wyatt HL, Haendchen RV, Meerbaum S, et al: Assessment of quantitative methods for 2-dimensional echocardiography. Am J Cardiol 52:396, 1983
79. Thys DM, Hillel Z, Goldman ME, et al: A comparison of hemodynamic indices by invasive monitoring and two-dimensional echocardiography. Anesthesiology 67:630, 1987
80. Konstadt SN, Thys D, Mindich BP, et al: Validation of quantitative intraoperative transesophageal echocardiography. Anesthesiology 65:418, 1986
81. Beaupre PN, Kremer PF, Cahalan MK, et al: Intraoperative changes in left ventricular segmental wall motion by transesophageal two-dimensional echocardiography. Am Heart J 107:1021, 1984
82. Clements FM, Harpole D, Quill T, et al: Simultaneous measurements of cardiac volumes, areas and ejection fractions by transesophageal echocardiography and first-pass radionuclide angiography. Anesthesiology 69:A4, 1988
83. Urbanowicz JH, Shaaban MJ, Cohen NH, et al: Comparison of transesophageal echocardiographic and scintigraphic estimates of left ventricular end-diastolic volume index and ejection fraction in patients following coronary artery bypass grafting. Anesthesiology 72:607, 1990
84. Choong CY, Abascal V, Thomas JD, et al: Combined influence of ventricular loading and relaxation on the transmitral flow velocity profile in dogs measured by Doppler echocardiography. Circulation 78:672, 1988
85. Kuecherer HF, Muhiudeen IA, Lee E, et al: Estimation of left atrial pressure by Doppler interrogation of phasic pulmonary venous flow: An intraoperative transesophageal study. Circulation 80(suppl II), 1989
86. Nishimura RA, Abel MD, Housmans PR, et al: Mitral flow velocity curves as a function of different loading conditions: Evaluation by intraoperative transesophageal Doppler echocardiography. J Am Soc Echocardiogr 2:79, 1989
87. Courtois M, Kovacs SJ, Ludbrook PA: Transmitral pressure-flow velocity relation. Circulation 78:661, 1988
88. Kuo LC, Quinones MA, Rokey R, et al: Quantification of atrial contribution to left ventricular filling by pulsed Doppler echocardiography and the effects of age in the normal and diseased heart. Am J Cardiol 59:1174, 1987
89. Pearson AC, Labovitz AJ, Mrosek D, et al: Assessment of diastolic function in normal and hypertrophied hearts: Comparison of Doppler echocardiography and M-mode echocardiography. Am Heart J 113:1417, 1987
90. Snider AR, Gidding SS, Rocchini AP, et al: Doppler evaluation of left ventricular diastolic filling in children with systemic hypertension. Am J Cardiol 56:921, 1985
91. Thys DM, Hillel Z, Konstadt S, et al: The intraoperative evaluation of left ventricular filling by esophageal Doppler echocardiography. Abstracts of the Eighth Annual Meeting of the Society of Cardiovascular Anesthesiologists, Montreal, Canada, 1986, p 80
92. Rinder CS, Wheeler LR, Alpern WD: Pulsed Doppler assessment of diastolic function before and after cardiopulmonary bypass. Anesthesiology 69:A2, 1988
93. Stewart WJ, Dicola VC, Harthorne W, et al: Doppler ultrasound measurement of cardiac output in patients with physiologic pacemakers. Am J Cardiol 54:308, 1984
94. Haskell RJ, French WJ: Optimum AV interval in dual chamber pacemakers. PACE 9:670, 1986
95. Pearson AC, Janosik DL, Redd RM, et al: Prediction of hemodynamic benefit of physiologic pacing from baseline Doppler-echocardiographic parameters. PACE 10:127A, 1987
96. Bowman LK, Cleman MW, Cabin HS, et al: Dynamics of early and late left ventricular filling determined by Doppler two-dimensional echocardiography during percutaneous transluminal coronary angioplasty. Am J Cardiol 61:541, 1988
97. Khouri SJ, Maly GT, Suh DD, Walsh TE: A practical approach to the echocardiographic evaluation of diastolic function. J Am Soc Echocardiogr 17:290, 2004
98. Redfield MM, Jacobsen SJ, Burnett JC Jr, et al:. Burden of systolic and diastolic ventricular dysfunction in the community: Appreciating the scope of the heart failure epidemic. JAMA 289:194, 2003
99. De Meya S, De Sutterb J, Vierendeelsa J, Verdoncka P: Diastolic filling and pressure imaging: Taking advantage of the information in a colour M-mode Doppler image. Eur J Echocardiogr 2:219, 2001
100. Ommen SR, Nishimura RA: A clinical approach to the assessment of left ventricular diastolic function by Doppler echocardiography: Update 2003. Heart 89(suppl III):III-18, 2003
101. Reichek N, Wilson J, St John Sutton M, et al: Noninvasive determination of left ventricular end-systolic stress: Validation of the method and initial application. Circulation 65:99, 1982
102. Hartford M, Wilstand JCM, Wallentin I, et al: Left ventricular wall stress and systolic function in untreated primary hypertension. Hypertension 7:97, 1985
103. Lang RL, Borow KM, Newman A, et al: Systemic vascular resistance: An unreliable index of afterload. Circulation 74:1114, 1986
104. Smith JS, Roizen MF, Cahalan MK, et al: Does anesthetic technique make a difference? Augmentation of systolic blood pressure during carotid endarterectomy: Effects of phenylephrine versus light anesthesia and of isoflurane versus halothane on the incidence of myocardial ischemia. Anesthesiology 69:846, 1988
105. Weissler AM: Systolic time intervals. N Engl J Med 296:321, 1977
106. Lewis RP, Rittgers SE, Forester WF, et al: A critical review of the systolic time intervals. Circulation 56:146, 1977
107. Noble MIM, Trenchard D, Guz A: Left ventricular ejection in conscious dogs: 1. Measurement and significance of the maximum acceleration of blood from the left ventricle. Circ Res 19:139, 1966
108. Bennett ED, Else W, Miller GAH, et al: Maximum acceleration of blood from the left ventricle in patients with ischaemic heart disease. Clin Sci Mol Med 46:49, 1974
109. Mehta N, Bennett DE: Impaired left ventricular function in acute myocardial infarction assessed by Doppler measurement of ascending aortic blood velocity and maximum acceleration. Am J Cardiol 57:1052, 1986
110. Sabbah HN, Khaja F, Brymer JF, et al: Noninvasive evaluation of left ventricular performance based on peak aortic blood acceleration measured with a continuous-wave Doppler velocity meter. Circulation 74:323, 1986
111. Suga H, Sagawa K: Instantaneous pressure-volume relationships and their ratio in the excised, supported canine left ventricle. Circ Res 35:117, 1974
112. Hillel Z, Thys DM, Mindich BP, et al: A new method for the intraoperative determination of contractility. Anesth Analg 65:S72, 1986
113. Gorscan J, Morita S, Mandareno WA, et al: Two dimensional echocardiographic automated border detection accurately reflects changes in left ventricular volume. J Am Soc Echocardiogr 5:482, 1992
114. Marwick TH: Techniques for comprehensive 2D echocardiographic assessment of left ventricular systolic function. Heart 89:(Suppl 3)2, 2003
115. Simonson JS, Schiller NB: Descent of the base of the left ventricle: An echocardiographic index of left ventricular function. J Am Soc Echocardiogr 2:25, 1989
116. Feigenbaum H, Popp RL, Wolfe SB, et al: Ultrasound measurements of the left ventricle: A correlative study with angiocardiography. Arch Intern Med 129:461, 1972

117. Kronik G, Slany J, Mosslacher H: Comparative value of eight M-mode echocardiographic formulas for determining left ventricular stroke volume. Circulation 60:1308, 1979
118. Terai C, Venishi M, Sugimoto H, et al: Transesophageal echocardiographic dimensional analysis of four cardiac chambers during positive end-expiratory pressure. Anesthesiology 63:640, 1985
119. Fisher DC, Sahn DJ, Allen HD, et al: The mitral valve orifice method for noninvasive two-dimensional echo Doppler determinations of cardiac output. Circulation 67:872, 1983
120. Lewis JF, Kuo LC, Nelson JG, et al: Pulsed Doppler echocardiographic determination of stroke volume and cardiac output: Clinical validation of two new methods using the apical window. Circulation 70:425, 1984
121. Roewer N, Bednarz F, Dziadka A, et al: Intraoperative cardiac output determination from transmitral and pulmonary blood flow measurements using transesophageal pulsed Doppler. J Cardiothorac Anesth 1:418, 1987
122. LaMantia K, Harris S, Mortimore K, et al: Transesophageal pulse-wave Doppler assessment of cardiac output. Anesthesiology 69:A1, 1988
123. Savino JS, Troianos CA, Aukburg S, et al: Measurement of pulmonary blood flow with two-dimensional echocardiography and Doppler echocardiography. Anesthesiology 75:445, 1991
124. Muhiudeen IA, Kuecherer HF, Lee E, et al: Intraoperative estimation of cardiac output by transesophageal pulsed Doppler echocardiography. Anesthesiology 74:9, 1991
125. Stevenson JG: Comparison of several noninvasive methods for estimation of pulmonary artery pressure. J Am Soc Echocardiogr 2:157, 1989
126. Weyman AF: The year in echocardiography. J Am Coll Cardiol 45:48, 2005
127. Tennant R, Wiggers CJ: The effect of coronary occlusion on myocardial infarction. Am J Physiol 112:351, 1935
128. Vatner SF: Correlation between acute reductions in myocardial blood flow and function in conscious dogs. Circ Res 47:201, 1980
129. Waters DD, Luz PD, Wyatt HL, et al: Early changes in regional and global left ventricular function induced by graded reductions in regional coronary perfusion. Am J Cardiol 39:537, 1977
130. Hauser AM, Gangadharan V, Ramos R, et al: Sequence of mechanical, electrocardiographic and clinical effects of repeated coronary artery occlusion in human beings: Echocardiographic observations during coronary angioplasty. J Am Coll Cardiol 5:193, 1985
131. Massre BM, Botvinick EH, Brundage BH, et al: Relationship of regional myocardial perfusion to segmental wall motion: A physiological basis for understanding the presence of reversibility of asynergy. Circulation 58:1154, 1978
132. Alam M, Khaja F, Brymer J, et al: Echocardiographic evaluation of left ventricular function during coronary angioplasty. Am J Cardiol 57:20, 1986
133. Labovitz AJ, Lewen MK, Kern M, et al: Evaluation of left ventricular systolic and diastolic dysfunction during transient myocardial ischemia by angioplasty. J Am Coll Cardiol 10:748, 1988
134. Shah PM, Shunei K, Matsumura M, et al: Utility of biplane transesophageal echocardiography in left ventricular wall motion analysis. J Cardiothorac Anesth 5:316, 1991
135. Pandian NG, Kerber RE: Two-dimensional echocardiography in experimental coronary stenosis. I. Sensitivity and specificity in detecting transient myocardial dyskinesis: Comparison with sonomicrometers. Circulation 66:597, 1982
136. Thys DM: The intraoperative assessment of regional myocardial performance: Is the cart before the horse? J Cardiothorac Anesth 1:273, 1987
137. Srinivas M, Roizen MF, Barnard J, et al: Relative effectiveness of four preoperative tests to predict adverse cardiac outcomes following vascular surgery: A metaanalysis. Anesth Analg 79:422, 1994
138. Battler A, Forelicher VF, Gallagher KT, et al: Dissociation between regional myocardial dysfunction and ECG changes during ischemia in the conscious dog. Circulation 62:735, 1980
139. Tomoike H, Franklin D, Ross J Jr: Detection of myocardial ischemia by regional dysfunction during and after rapid pacing in conscious dogs. Circulation 58:48, 1978
140. Smith JS, Cahalan MK, Benefiel DJ, et al: Intraoperative detection of myocardial ischemia in high-risk patients: Electrocardiography versus two-dimensional transesophageal echocardiography. Circulation 72:1015, 1985
141. Wohlgelernter D, Jaffe CC, Cabin HS, et al: Silent ischemia during coronary occlusion produced by balloon inflation: Relation to regional myocardial dysfunction. J Am Coll Cardiol 10:491, 1987
142. VanDaele ME, Sutherland GR, Mitchell MM, et al: Do changes in pulmonary capillary wedge pressure adequately reflect myocardial ischemia during anesthesia? Circulation 81:865, 1990
143. Leung JM, O'Kelley B, Browner WS, et al: Prognostic importance of postbypass regional wall motion abnormalities in patients undergoing coronary artery bypass graft surgery. Anesthesiology 71:16, 1989
144. Leung JM, O'Kelley BF, Mangano DT: Relationship of regional wall motion abnormalities to hemodynamic indices of myocardial supply and demand in patients undergoing CABG surgery. Anesthesiology 73:802, 1990
145. Clements FM, de Bruijn NP: Perioperative evaluation of regional wall motion by transesophageal two-dimensional echocardiography. Anesth Analg 66:249, 1987
146. Lehman KG, Korrester AL, MacKenzie WB, et al: Onset of altered intraventricular septal motion during cardiac surgery. Circulation 82:1325, 1990
147. Chung F, Seyone C, Rakowski H: Transesophageal echocardiography may fail to diagnose perioperative myocardial infarction. Can J Anaesth 38:98, 1991
148. Pandian NG, Skorton DJ, Collins SM, et al: Heterogeneity of left ventricular segmental wall motion thickening and excursion in 2-dimensional echocardiograms of normal human subjects. Am J Cardiol 51:1667, 1983
149. Liberman AN, Weiss JL, Judutt BD, et al: Two-dimensional echocardiography and infarct size: Relationship of regional wall motion and thickening to the extent of myocardial infarction in the dog. Circulation 63:739, 1981
150. Luma JAC, Becker LA, Melin JA, et al: Impaired thickening of nonischemic myocardium during acute regional ischemia in the dog. Circulation 71:1048, 1985
151. Force T, Kemper A, Perkins L, et al: Overestimation of infarct size by quantitative two-dimensional echocardiography: The role of tethering and of analytic procedures. Circulation 73:1360, 1986
152. Braunwald E, Kloner RA: The stunned myocardium: Prolonged, postischemic ventricular dysfunction. Circulation 66:1146, 1982
153. Buffington CW, Coyle RJ: Altered load dependence of postischemic myocardium. Anesthesiology 75:464, 1991
154. London MJ, Tubau JF, Wong MG, et al: The "natural history" of segmental wall motion abnormalities in patients undergoing noncardiac surgery. Anesthesiology 73:644, 1990
155. Roizen MF, Beaupre PN, Alpert RA, et al: Monitoring with two-dimensional transesophageal echocardiography. Comparison of myocardial function in patients undergoing supraceliac, suprarenal-infraceliac, or infrarenal aortic occlusion. J Vasc Surg 2:300, 1984
156. Gewertz BL, Kremser PC, Zarins CK, et al: Transesophageal echocardiographic monitoring of myocardial ischemia during vascular surgery. J Vasc Surg 5:607, 1987
157. Comunale M, Body S, Ley C, et al: The concordance of intraoperative LVWMA and ECG ST segment changes: Association with outcome after CABG. Anesthesiology 88:945, 1998
158. Fleisher L, Welskopf R: Real-time intraoperative monitoring of myocardial ischemia in noncardial surgery. Anesthesiology 92:1183, 2000
159. Topol EJ, Weiss JL, Guzman PA, et al: Immediate improvement of dysfunctional myocardial segments after coronary revascularization: Detection by intraoperative transesophageal echocardiography. J Am Coll Cardiol 4:1123, 1984
160. Koolen JJ, Visser CA, Van Wezel HB, et al: Influence of coronary artery bypass surgery on regional left ventricular wall motion: An intraoperative two-dimensional transesophageal echocardiography study. J Cardiovasc Anesth 1:276, 1987
161. Voci P, Billotta F, Aronson S, et al: Changes in myocardial segmental wall motion, systolic wall thickening, and ejection fraction immediately following CABG: An echocardiographic analysis comparing dysfunctional and normal myocardium. J Am Soc Echocardiogr 4:289, 1991
162. Koenig K, Kasper W, Hofman T, et al: Transesophageal echocardiography for diagnosis of rupture of the ventricular septum or left ventricular papillary muscle during acute myocardial infarction. Am J Cardiol 59:362, 1987
163. Patel AM, Miller FA, Khandheria BK, et al: Role of TEE in the diagnosis of papillary muscle rupture secondary to myocardial function. Am Heart J 118:1330, 1989
164. Garther NS, Rogan KM, Stajduhar K, et al: Anomalous origin and course of coronary arteries in adults: Identification and improved imaging utilizing transesophageal echocardiography. Am Heart J 122:69, 75, 1991
165. Dell Italia LJ, Starling MR, Blumhardt R, et al: Comparative effects of volume loading, dobutamine, and nitroprusside in patients with predominant right ventricular function. Circulation 72:1327, 1985

166. Vitanen A, Salmenpera M, Heinonen S: Right ventricular response to hypercarbia after cardiac surgery. Anesthesiology 73:393, 1990
167. Balu V, Heshowitz S, Zaki Masud AR, et al: Mitral regurgitation in coronary artery disease. Chest 5:550, 1982
168. Iliceto S, Marangelli V, Memmola C, Rizzou P: Transesophageal Doppler echocardiography evaluation of coronary blood flow velocity in baseline conditions and during dipyridamole-induced coronary vasodilation. Circulation 83:61, 1991
169. Biagini A, Maffei S, Baroni M, et al: Early assessment of coronary reserve after bypass surgery by dipyridamole transesophageal echocardiographic stress test. Am Heart J 120:1097, 1990
170. O'Kelly BF, Tubau JF, Knight AA, et al: Measurement of left ventricular contractility using transesophageal echocardiography in patients undergoing coronary artery bypass grafting. Am Heart J 122:1041, 1991
171. Goens MB, Martin GR: Acoustic quantification: A new tool for diagnostic echocardiography. Curr Opin Cardiol 11:52, 1996
172. Perez JE, Miller JG, Holland MR, et al: Ultrasonic tissue characterization: Integrated backscatter imaging for detecting myocardial structural properties and on-line quantitation of cardiac function. Am J Cardiac Imaging 8:106, 1994
173. O'Brien PD, O'Brien WD Jr, Rhyne TL, et al: Relation of ultrasonic backscatter and acoustic propagation properties to myofibrillar length and myocardial thickness. Circulation 91:171, 1995
174. Milunski MR, Mohr GA, Perez JE, et al: Ultrasonic tissue characterization with integrated backscatter. Acute myocardial ischemia, reperfusion, and stunned myocardium in patients. Circulation 80:491, 1989
175. O'Brien WD, Sagar KB, Warltier DC, Rhyne TL: Acoustic propagation properties of normal, stunned and infarcted myocardium. Morphological and biochemical determinants. Circulation 9:154, 1995
176. Masuyama T, Valantine HA, Gibbons R, et al: Serial measurement of integrated ultrasonic backscatter in human cardiac allografts for the recognition of acute rejection. Circulation 81:829, 1990
177. Perez JE, Waggoner AD, Barzilai B, et al: On-line assessment of ventricular function by automated boundary detection and ultrasonic backscatter imaging. J Am Coll Cardiol 19:313, 1992
178. Lang RM, Vignon P, Weinert L, et al: Echocardiographic quantification of regional left ventricular wall motion with color kinesis. Circulation 93:1877, 1996
179. Vignon P, Mor-Avi V, Bednarz J, et al: Automated diagnosis of regional wall motion abnormalities using segmental analysis of end-systolic color kinesis images (abstract). J Am Coll Cardiol 27(suppl A):48A, 1996
180. Gorscan J, Gasior TA, Mandarino WA, et al: On-line estimation of changes in left ventricular stroke volume by transesophageal echocardiographic automated border detection in patients undergoing coronary artery bypass grafting. Am J Cardiol 72:721, 1993
181. Tardif JC, Cao QL, Pandian NG, et al: Determination of cardiac output using acoustic quantification in critically ill patients. Am J Cardiol 74:810, 1994
182. Katz WE, Gasior TA, Reddy SCR, Gorscan J III: Utility and limitations of biplane transesophageal echocardiographic automated border detection for estimation of left ventricular stroke volume and cardiac output. Am Heart J 128:389, 1994
183. Gorscan J, Lazar JM, Schulman DS, Follansbee WP: Comparison of left ventricular function by echocardiographic automated border detection and by radionuclide ejection fraction. Am J Cardiol 72:810, 1993
184. Lindower PD, Rath L, Preslar J, et al: Quantification of left ventricular function with an automated border detection system and comparison with radionuclide ventriculography. Am J Cardiol 73:195, 1994
185. Yvorchuk KJ, Davies RA, Chan KL: Measurement of left ventricular ejection fraction by acoustic quantification and comparison with radionuclide angiography. Am J Cardiol 74:1052, 1994
186. Lin SS, Reynertson SI, Louie EK, Levitsky S: Right ventricular volume overload results in depression of left ventricular ejection fraction: Implications for the surgical management of tricuspid valve disease. Circulation 90(suppl II), 1994
187. Louie EK, Lin SS, Reynertson SI, et al: Pressure and volume loading of the right ventricle have opposing effects on left ventricular ejection fraction. Circulation 92:819, 1995
188. Cahalan MK, Ionescu P, Melton HEJ, et al: Automated real time analysis of intraoperative transesophageal echocardiograms. Anesthesiology 78:477, 1993
189. Stoddard MF, Keedy DL, Longaker RA: Two dimensional transesophageal echocardiographic characterization of ventricular filling in real time by acoustic quantification: Comparison with pulsed Doppler echocardiography. J Am Soc Echocardiogr 7:116, 1994
190. Chenzbraun A, Pinto FJ, Popylisen S, et al: Filling patterns in left ventricular hypertrophy: A combined acoustic quantification and Doppler study. J Am Coll Cardiol 23:1179, 1994
191. Kimball TR, Witt SA, Daniels SR, et al: The role of automatic endocardial edge detection in the evaluation of left ventricular diastolic function in children. J Am Soc Echocardiogr 9:18, 1996
192. Vitarelli A, Penco M, Ferro-Luzzi M, et al: Assessment of diastolic left ventricular filling by echocardiographic automated border detection and comparison with radionuclide ventriculography. J Am Soc Echocardiogr 9:135, 1996
193. Garcia MJ, Rodriguez L, Ares M, et al: Differentiation of constrictive pericarditis from restrictive cardiomyopathy: Assessment of left ventricular diastolic velocities in longitudinal axis by Doppler tissue imaging. J Am Coll Cardiol 27:108, 1996
194. Flachskampf F: Recent progress in quantitative echocardiography. Curr Opin Cardiol 10:634, 1995
195. Miyatake K, Yamagishi M, Tanaka N, et al: New method for evaluating left ventricular wall motion by color-coded tissue Doppler imaging: In vitro and in vivo studies. J Am Coll Cardiol 25:717, 1995
196. McDicken WN, Sutherland GR, Moran CM, et al: Colour Doppler velocity imaging of the myocardium. Ultrasound Med Biol 18:651, 1992
197. Sutherland GR, Stewart MJ, Groundstroem KWE, et al: Color Doppler myocardial imaging: A new technique for the assessment of myocardial function. J Am Soc Echocardiogr 7:441, 1994
198. Uematsu M, Miyatake K, Tanaka N: Myocardial velocity gradient as a new indicator of regional left ventricular contraction: Detection by a two-dimensional tissue Doppler imaging technique. J Am Coll Cardiol 26:217, 1995
199. Louie EK, Louie DS: New echocardiographic technology: Does it add to clinical decision making? Semin Cardiothorac Vasc Anesth 1:16, 1997
200. Dekker DL, Piziaii RL, Dong E Jr: A system for ultrasonically imaging the human heart in three dimensions. Comput Biomed Res 7:544, 1974
201. Matsumoto M, Matsuo H, Kitabatake A, et al: Three-dimensional echocardiograms and two-dimensional echocardiographic images at desired planes by a computerized system. Ultrasound Med Biol 3:163, 1977
202. Gunasegaran K, Yao J, De Castro S, et al: Three-dimensional transesophageal echocardiography (TEE) and other future directions. Cardiol Clin 18: 893, 2000
203. Pandian NG, Roelandt J, Nanda NC, et al: Dynamic three-dimensional echocardiography: Methods and clinical potential. Echocardiography 11:237, 1994
204. Belohlavek M, Foley DA, Gerber TC, et al: Three dimensional reconstruction of color Doppler jets in the human heart. J Am Soc Echocardiogr 7:553, 1994
205. Roelandt TRC, ten Cate FJ, Vletter WB, et al: Ultrasonic dynamic three dimensional visualization of the heart with a multiplane transesophageal imaging transducer. J Am Soc Echocardiogr 7:217, 1994
206. Salustri A, Becker AE, van Herwerden L, et al: Three dimensional echocardiography of normal and pathologic mitral valve: A comparison with two-dimensional transesophageal echocardiography. J Am Coll Cardiol 27:1502, 1996
207. Lange A, Mankad P, Walayat M, et al: Transthoracic 3D echocardiography in the preoperative assessment of atrioventricular defect morphology. Am J Cardiol 85:630, 2000
208. Acar P. Roux D, Dulac Y, et al: Transthoracic 3D echocardiography prior to closure of atrial septal defects in children. Cardiol Young 13:58, 2003
209. Acar P, Abdel-Massih T, Douste-Blazy M, et al: Assessment of muscular VSD closure by transcatheter or surgical approach: A 3D echocardiographic study. Eur J Echocardiogr 3:185, 2002
210. Borges AC, Witt C, Bartel T, et al: Preoperative two-dimensional and three-dimensional echocardiographic assessment of heart tumors. Ann Thorac Surg 61:1163, 1996
211. Muller S, Bartel T, Laube H: Left ventricular thrombus after pregnancy: Choice of surgical access using dynamic three-dimensional echocardiography. Echocardiography 13:293, 1996
212. Abraham T, Warner J, Kon N, et al: Feasibility, accuracy, and incremental value of intraoperative three-dimensional transesophageal echocardiography in valve surgery. Am J Cardiol 80:1577, 1997
213. Ahmed S, Nanda N, Miller A, et al: Usefulness of transesophageal three-dimensional echocardiography in the identification of individual segment/scallop prolapse of the mitral valve. Echocardiography 20:203, 2003
214. De Castro S, Salandin V, Cartoni D, et al: Qualitative and quantitative evaluation of mitral valve morphology by intraoperative volume-rendered three-dimensional echocardiography. J Heart Valve Dis 11:173, 2002
215. George S, Al-Russeh S, Amrani M: Mitral annulus distortion during beating heart surgery: A potential cause for hemodynamic distur-

bance—a three-dimensional echocardiographic reconstruction study. Ann Thorac Surg 73:1424, 2002

216. Langerveld J, Valocik G, Plokker T, et al: Additional value of three-dimensional transesophageal echocardiography for patients with mitral valve stenosis undergoing balloon valvuloplasty. J Am Soc Echocardiogr 16:841, 2003
217. Applebaum RM, Kasliwal RR, Kanojia A, et al: Utility of three-dimensional echocardiography during balloon mitral valvuloplasty. J Am Coll Cardiol 32:1405, 1998
218. Miller A, Nanda N, Aaluri S, et al: Three-dimensional transesophageal echocardiographic demonstration of anatomical defects in AV septal defect patients presenting for reoperation. Echocardiography 20:105, 2003
219. Acar P, Laskari C, Rhodes J, et al: Three-dimensional echocardiographic analysis of valve anatomy as a determinant of mitral regurgitation after surgery for atrioventricular septal defects. Am J Cardiol 83:745, 1999
220. Weyman A: The year in echocardiography. J Am Coll Cardiol 43:140, 2004
221. Eltzschig H, Kallmeyer I, Alapati S, et al: A practical approach to epicardial echocardiography. J Thorac Cardiovasc Anesth 422, 2003
222. Nash P, Agler D, Shin J, et al: Epicardial real-time 3-dimensional echocardiography during septal myectomy for obstructive hypertrophic cardiomyopathy. Circulation 108:e54, 2003
223. Suematsu Y, Takamoto S, Kaneko Y, et al: Beating atrial septal defect closure monitored by epicardial real-time three-dimensional echocardiography without cardiopulmonary bypass. Circulation 107:785, 2003
224. Qin J, Shiota T, McCarthy P, et al: Real-time three-dimensional echocardiographic study of left ventricular function after infarct exclusion surgery for ischemic cardiomyopathy. Circulation 102:III, 2000

Chapter 16

DECISION-MAKING AND PERIOPERATIVE TRANSESOPHAGEAL ECHOCARDIOGRAPHY

Stuart J. Weiss, MD, PhD • Joseph S. Savino, MD

KEY POINTS

1. The first step in decision-making is to "frame" the problem by defining the parameters, priorities, and pertinent criteria.
2. The second step is the directed acquisition of data, "data collection," that includes all pertinent information, regardless whether it is confirmatory or contradictory. The supplemental information from the preoperative evaluation should always be taken into consideration.
3. A comprehensive systematic transesophageal echocardiography examination permits the acquisition and interpretation of both qualitative and quantitative echocardiographic data for most cardiovascular diseases. The greatest risk and source of error is that of omission or misinterpretation leading to mismanagement and poor outcome.
4. The decision regarding patient management of a specific anatomic abnormality should be an evidence-based approach reflecting the severity of the lesion, coexisting factors, patient's wishes, and the current literature.
5. Intraoperative findings should be objectively and effectively characterized and discussed with the pertinent clinicians, surgeon, or cardiologist.
6. The decision and recommendations should be formally communicated through a reporting document that is accessible to other health care providers.
7. A systematic process for learning from the results of past decisions (quality improvement program) and continued education are critical for the future success of any intraoperative transesophageal echocardiography program.

In the affair of so much importance, wherein you ask my advice, I cannot make for want of sufficient premises advise you what to determine, but if it please I will tell you how.

Benjamin Franklin

All too often in medicine, critical decisions are made without the benefit of a thorough consideration of data, evidence, and framework. The paucity of clinical outcomes research in echocardiography, especially in the perioperative period, dampens the prospects for evidence-based decision-making. In the absence of evidence-directed practice, decision-making is typically based on anecdote, clinical impression, and tradition, with little effort devoted to the process of reaching an intelligent conclusion. The quantity of information is increasingly abundant in medicine, and in the operating room is no exception. Its acquisition, interpretation, and application for decision-making can be cumbersome, distracting, and misguided. In the era of increasing information, there is an imperative to develop a systematic process of handling data streams, organizing ideas and thoughts, defining and prioritizing problems, and effecting care through a well-thought-out decision. A formalized approach to the acquisition of data and decision-making (Fig. 16–1) enhances the quality of the intraoperative echocardiogram, its interpretation, and the confidence with which the findings are communicated to other members of the operative and nonoperative teams. The poor decision is not made by the physician with bad intentions. Poor decisions are commonly the result of individuals relying on limited medical knowledge (a database typically defined by the narrow bounds of their profession), narrow framing, and false or tenuous anchors. The echocardiographer who is overly confident in the abilities of his or her surgical counterpart may be falsely anchored to the prior performances of the surgeon, with little or no reliance on a formalized decision-making process. The lack of a structured paradigm for decision-making is most worrisome when clinicians with lesser ability or experience are making the decisions. The least-accomplished clinicians often have the most inflated estimate of their own abilities, thus lending themselves to the vulnerabilities of limited skills plus lack of a decision-making process.[1]

The intraoperative consultant in echocardiography is confronted with multiple channels of information (Boxes 16–1, 16–2, and 16–3). The broad database that is required to formulate an intelligent decision includes provider- and patient-specific data. Patient-specific data include history and demographics, preoperative diagnostic examinations, admitting diagnosis and comorbidities, the patient's wishes, recommendations of referring physicians, and intraoperative data. Intraoperative data include hemodynamic data, visual inspec-

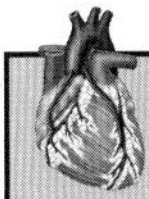

BOX 16–1 ***Patient History and Physical Signs***

Symptoms
- Shortness of breath
- New York Heart Association classification for heart failure
- Level of activity
- Functional disability
- Age

- Signs: Vital signs, rales, peripheral edema, peripheral circulation
- Cardiac and noncardiac comorbidities, including esophageal disease
- Patient preferences (e.g., Jehovah's Witness)

Define the purpose for the intraoperative TEE examination

Confirm preoperative diagnosis Diagnose new abnormalities Influence the conduct of cardiopulmonary bypass Titrate pharmacologic therapy Placement of cannulas, intra-aortic balloon pump	Evaluate: Global and regional function Myocardial ischemia Intracardiac masses Endocarditis Congenital pathology Intracardiac air Aortic pathology/trauma Surgical intervention

↓

Approach to initial operative TEE examination

Review preoperative studies/reports
Perform a standard, organized comprehensive echo exam
Complete a focused and quantitative evaluation
Assess severity by use of 2D/Doppler/secondary findings

↓

Write preCPB echo report

↓

Decision process

1. Framing of clinical problem
2. Data collection/integration of data
   TEE, patient factors, acuity,
   operative factors,
   current knowledge base
3. Decision and reassessment

↓

Communication: Discussion with stakeholders (surgeon/cardiologist/family/colleague)

↓

Learning (feedback, case conferences, specialty meetings, published literature)

Figure 16–1 An algorithm for the decision-making process.

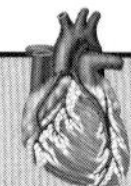

BOX 16–2 ***Patient Data***

- Intraoperative transesophageal echocardiography
- Left ventricle: systolic/diastolic function, ejection fraction, chamber size, wall thickness, regional wall motion
- Valvular function: pathology, severity, positron, vena contracta, annular size, size of donor chamber, pressure gradient, flow-velocity profiles
- Cardiac catheterization
- Chest radiographs, electrocardiogram, blood tests, radionucleotide studies, positron-emission tomography scans, stress test, transthoracic echocardiography
- Hemodynamics
- Surgical inspection of the pathology

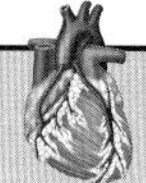

BOX 16–3 ***Operative Factors***

- Complexity of planned surgery
- Alternatives to the planned surgery
- Anticipated risk of a failed intervention
- Alternatives if original procedure is unsuccessful
- Equipment availability (VAD back-up, special retractors, specific valves, homografts, etc.)
- Expertise and experience of the operating team

tion, surgical input, and the transesophageal echocardiographic (TEE) examination. A systematic TEE examination of the heart and great vessels permits the acquisition and interpretation of qualitative and quantitative echocardiographic data applied to intraoperative decision-making. The provider-specific data are composed of an accumulated database of knowledge acquired from training, experience, and continuous medical education. Expertise is gained from experience and enhances the repertoire of experiences from which a practitioner can draw but does not alter the cognitive engine and does not immunize the practitioner from errors in decision-making. Intuition and experience are not reliable predictors of success. Learning through methods of trial and error and self-education by exploratory problem-solving have little role in the arena of cardiac surgery. Heuristic methods of decision-making often create a systematic and predictable bias. It is acceptable to be wrong. It is unacceptable to be consistently wrong in the same direction. A structured process of assessing all the data and weighing various alternatives (cognitive engine) will enable the physician to formulate a concise, organized approach to problem-solving, communicating the findings and management alternatives.

Decision-making can be encumbered by cognitive and emotional attachments that limit clinicians' intellectual flexibility. Poor problem-solving and poor outcome can follow a single poor decision of great magnitude. However, the "creep effect" of a series of small poor decisions can insidiously lead to a poor outcome. The adherence to a poor course of action because of an attachment to the original decision is common in medicine. "The escalating commitment to a losing course of action often begins with small steps" (Roch Parayre, MBA, personal communication). In the perioperative setting, this process is most vivid in the care of critically ill patients with little or no hope for survival. Continued commitment of resources and intervention often contribute to patient discomfort and cost without benefit in quality of life or longevity. The prior commitment of resources often encourages further commitment and investment in a losing cause. The echocardiographic decisions during surgery may become part of an intraoperative sequence of diagnostic and therapeutic interventions in which the best course of action is a complete reversal in direction. Repeated attempts at repairing a mitral valve (MV) may follow an initial unsuccessful repair. The decision to replace the valve instead of repairing it is often not considered until late in the course. Repeated intervals of cardiopulmonary bypass (CPB) and aortic cross-clamping are not without their complications and associated morbidity. It is often difficult to retain an open mind and to consider alternative diagnoses or therapeutic alternatives. Effective decision-makers are able, if necessary, to abandon the original decision to repair an MV and move toward valve replacement.

An intraoperative TEE examination can correct preoperative inaccuracies in diagnosis or detect occult disease. With increasing emphasis on decreasing preoperative testing, avoiding redundant testing, and decreasing costs, accurate diagnoses of disease may not occur until the time of surgery. The increased reliance on the intraoperative TEE is fiscally wise but places greater responsibility and impact on the intraoperative echocardiographer. The detection of occult disease not appreciated during the preoperative evaluation often impacts operative management. It is necessary to reframe a problem when the data acquired reveal new insights. The detection of mobile atheroma in the ascending aorta may dissuade the juxtaposition of an aortic infusion cannula, hence changing circulatory management and the operation.[2-4] The rationale for changing management in respect to otherwise asymptomatic and clinically silent findings is often not obvious and typically invokes controversy. The change in the operation has typically not been discussed with the patient, as the findings were unanticipated. The intraoperative diagnosis of moderate aortic valve regurgitation (AR) that was not detected preoperatively will create a clinical challenge for the surgical team with the decision of whether to replace the aortic valve (AV). Hence, the decision to proceed with an unplanned AV replacement (AVR) relies on the ability of the echocardiographer to establish the diagnosis and mechanism of valvular pathology, define the pertinent factors that sway the decision (preoperative symptoms of congestive heart failure [CHF], ventricular size and function, pulmonary hypertension), and communicate with the surgeon and the other pertinent stakeholders. The finding of moderate AR with normal ventricular systolic function and chamber size, normal left atrial (LA) pressure, and no preoperative history of CHF may sway the operative team to proceed with the originally planned surgery and to treat the occult finding medically with postoperative afterload reduction and follow-up serial echocardiograms. In contrast, in a patient with otherwise unexplained shortness of breath, pulmonary hypertension, and a dilated left ventricle (LV), the presence of moderate AR typically leads to AVR. The introduction of new findings to the operative team often warrants a "time out" approach to determine the impact of the findings on the operative care.

CASE STUDY

A patient was scheduled for an AVR for the presumptive diagnosis of aortic stenosis (AS) based on a transthoracic echocardiogram (TTE) showing a sclerotic AV, an LV-to-aorta pressure gradient of 100 mm Hg, and severe LV hypertrophy. The intraoperative TEE confirmed the preoperative findings but added new information. Inspection of the valve revealed a mobile sclerotic three-cusp AV with a valve area consistent with only mild AS. The LV outflow tract (LVOT), however, contained an obstructing membrane that contributed to the "apparent" transvalvular pressure gradient. The surgeon, confronted with information that significantly altered the operative plan, called for an intraoperative "time out" and contacted the referring cardiologist who performed the original echocardiogram. After discussion among the referring cardiologist, the intraoperative echocardiographer, and the cardiac surgeon, the patient underwent an AVR and surgical excision of the obstructing membrane in the outflow tract.

If a suggestion by the echocardiographer for a proposed course of action is rejected or modified, it is counterproductive to interpret the disagreement as a personal rejection. The echocardiographer is a consultant who performs, analyzes, and interprets findings in an objective manner. The final decision and ultimate responsibility of the operative plan typically belong to the attending cardiac surgeon, although this may be institution-dependent. A shared responsibility held by the surgeon and the intraoperative echocardiographer seems to be gaining momentum as diagnostic abilities in the operating room continue to advance.

DECISION-MAKING PROCESS

The process of decision-making is in essence "deciding how to decide."[5] What is the primary issue that needs to be addressed? What are the pitfalls in the decision? What are the consequences of the decision? What tools and resources does the decision-maker require? What information is needed to make an informed decision? Is there evidence to support one decision over another? How much time does the decision-maker need to make the decision? Rarely is there a valid reason for not taking enough time to make a well-thought-out decision, even in the high productivity, high throughput environment of the operating room. Does the decision-maker need help? We have applied the methods of Russo and Schoemaker[5] to decision-making in medicine:

1. *Framing:* Framing defines the question that is being asked of the decision-maker, sets the vantage point of the decision-maker, and defines the boundaries, parameters, and priorities. Framing defines the criteria that may sway the decision-maker. By performing this process, in the early stages of problem-solving, it permits focus and bounded rationality. However, the price of focusing on a specific issue may be loss of peripheral vision. Adopting a narrowed vantage point can inadvertently impose significant bias and limitation. The decision should be addressed from a variety of vantage points, so that all aspects of the decision can be considered.

   Failure to work beyond an individual conceptual frame can lead to difficulties in communication among the different participants of the care team. In the setting of a complex MV repair, the intraoperative echocardiographer is often focused on performance of the TEE, successful remedy of hemodynamic disturbances, surgical intervention, and documentation. If the echocardiographer is also the anesthesiologist, his or her frame is broadened to include patient safety and comfort, vigilance, and maintaining body homeostasis. The surgeon's frame includes his or her ability and limitations in achieving a competent surgical repair, alternatives in surgical management, and covenant with the patient and family regarding surgical management (e.g., repair versus replacement, bioprosthesis versus mechanical prosthesis), patient overall outcome, and his or her reputation as a surgeon. The patient's vantage point may differ from those of the operative team. The patient wants the mitral regurgitation (MR) to be fixed, for the symptoms to be resolved, to return to a "normal routine," for the remedy to be long lasting, and to be able to ride a Harley Davidson, which he or she would otherwise have to forfeit if he was taking life-long Coumadin. Hence, as a decision-maker, broadening the understanding of the issues and consideration of multiple frames will account for the interests of multiple parties.

2. *Data Collection:* Data collection is aimed at reducing uncertainty. Uncertainty is never eliminated and hence needs to be managed. The perioperative echocardiographer manages uncertainty not through pinpoint predictions but by uncertainty estimates. It is imperative in the decision-making process to systematically identify the causes that could lead to decision failure and to quantify the likelihood of such causes occurring. A dilated mitral annulus with a flailed middle scallop of the posterior leaflet and two ruptured chordae are associated with a high rate of successful surgical repair. However, factors that are likely to affect this outcome include the technical ability of the surgeon, a parameter that is difficult to estimate and creates uncertainty in the expected outcome.

   The data should include echocardiographic and nonechocardiographic data (see Boxes 16–1 through 16–3). The importance and impact of TEE decisions have been generally recognized and accepted. The ability to make an appropriate decision is predicated on a comprehensive examination. Confirmatory information is useful, as is contradictory information. The process of decision-making also includes defining what information "not to collect." Collecting as much data as possible typically leads to confusion and loss of direction in the reasoning process. A common hazard for the echocardiographer is the performance of an abridged examination, due to either increased clinical demands or reliance on a preoperative examination. The conclusions drawn from an intraoperative examination and associated decisions should not be hurried and should be based on all aspects of the examination. Although physical injury from the TEE examination is a serious matter, the greater risk is that of errors of omission or misinterpretation, leading to mismanagement and poor outcome.[6-11]

3. *Decision and Implementation:* A clinical decision is made based on the integration of knowledge, framing, and information (Box 16–4). Primary knowledge is "knowing what you know" and "knowing what you do not know," with the latter prompting a practitioner to seek assistance. Second-order knowledge is "not knowing what you do not know"; hence, diagnoses are missed rather than misinterpreted. The broader the repertoire of primary knowledge, the more informed is the decision-maker, and the more reliable is the decision.

   The echocardiographer is an intraoperative consultant who generates vital information that has a direct impact on intraoperative care and decision-making. As consultants, suggestions and recommendations are offered, but rarely does the echocardiographer dictate the management to the operative team. The decision/recommendation is shared with the stakeholders (surgeons, perfusionists, nurses, referring cardiologists, postoperative intensivists, and family and patient) and is communicated verbally and by written report. Decisions often are accompanied by discussion and sometimes persuasion. Making a sound decision concerning the surgical approach to an anatomic problem can benefit the patient only if it is effectively communicated to the operating surgeon. However, clinical judgment must take into account the skills set of the operative team and the pitfalls associated with each intervention. Persuading a surgeon to proceed with a complex reconstruction may appear to be the appropriate course of action according to an echocardiographer, but it may be the wrong thing to do if the surgeon is unfamiliar with the recommended repair (i.e., poor framing).

4. *Learning:* A systematic process for learning from the results of past decisions is designed to increase the decision-maker's primary knowledge base and defines an effective clinical quality improvement program. The ability to achieve success or failure may depend on the ability of the decision-maker to learn from past decisions and the decisions of others.[5] A fund of knowledge gained through training, continuous medical education, readings, and the performance of echocardiograms on a regular basis maintains the skills of the echocardiographer. Although it is often difficult to obtain feedback regarding the impact of decisions on long-term outcome, the increment in effort to seek such insight always renders the echocardiographer more prepared for the next clinical scenario that shares common cardiovascular themes. Feedback can be sought from a variety of sources: surgeon, cardiologist, outpatient echocardiography data files, etc. Participation in quality improvement forums with cardiologists and cardiac surgeons who tend to follow the patients longitudinally is a useful learning tool.

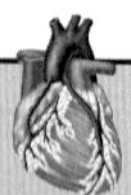

BOX 16–4 ***Decision Process***

Projecting the impact of:
- Progression of disease
- Risk of redo surgery
- Short- and long-term outcome
- Associated risks (e.g., anticoagulation)
- Size mismatch of prosthesis
- Effect of prolonged cardiopulmonary bypass on immediate postoperative outcome

Does the decision account for:
- Inconsistencies (among two-dimensional/Doppler/patient symptoms/preoperative evaluation)
- Plausibility of alternate explanation
- Alternate therapy
- Current literature
- Preoperative evaluations
- Patient factors (age, cardiac status, ability to tolerate anticoagulation, etc.)

Although all four processes above are important, the initial framing of the problem prompts the subsequent steps of data collection, conclusion, and learning. Framing begins by articulating a question. By addressing the problem in terms of a specific question, a clinical situation is framed in a more manageable context. A framing strategy can be an effective method to rationally limit decision options and form the basis of communication.

Performance of the decision-maker is judged based on final outcome. However, decision-making should be based on the information the decision-maker had at the time of the decision. A significant limitation of measuring performance during uncertainty is that it is often judged, not by the decision-making process but by single case results. If the decision is followed by a good outcome, the decision-maker is often applauded with little regard to the ability to reach an intelligent conclusion. A poor outcome does not necessarily imply a poor process or poor decision. High-risk surgery leads to poor outcomes in many cases despite robust decisions. In medicine, this often leads to individuals being reluctant to make any decision at all, knowing that a poor outcome is likely and that it will be linked to their decision-making. The reality of performance assessment is that even if the decision to proceed with therapy is substantiated, a poor outcome will often reflect negatively on the abilities of the echocardiographer, anesthesiologist, surgeon, and the operative team. Conversely, a good outcome does not imply a good process or a good decision.[5] The surgeon's decision to perform a posterior sliding mitral valvuloplasty and quadrilateral resection of the posterior leaflet based on a dilated mitral annulus with normal leaflet motion as defined by TEE may result in a technically competent MV repair and good long-term results. The decision to perform a posterior sliding valvuloplasty may or may not have been a wise decision. Equally good results may have occurred with the insertion of an annular ring without leaflet resection. The measure of an outcome by recording a metric is only a valid assessment of quality if the metric is a function of the actions of the provider.[12] The outcome cannot be random; otherwise, there is no basis for estimating quality.

CASE STUDY

A 48-year-old asymptomatic woman presented for elective MV repair secondary to MR. She was otherwise healthy, except for mild pulmonary hypertension and rapidly increasing LV dimensions. The woman was a union carpenter and absolutely refused to be subjected to lifelong anticoagulation. Physical examination was notable for a loud holosystolic murmur from the apex to the axilla. The lungs were clear. Baseline ECG was normal, as were all laboratory blood tests. Preoperative chest wall echocardiogram demonstrated severe MR, no regional wall motion abnormalities (RWMAs), and a flail MV. Intraoperatively, after induction of general anesthesia and tracheal intubation, the TEE was performed and demonstrated a severely dilated LA, dilated LV, flail and thickened middle scallop of the posterior leaflet with multiple ruptured primary and secondary chordae to all scallops of the posterior leaflet, prolapse of the anterior leaflet, and a small perforation. The short-axis view of the MV suggested three regurgitant orifices. The surgeon was experienced in complex mitral repairs with extensive experience in repairing myxomatous valves and chordal transfer. Consultation between the surgeon and the echocardiographer resulted in the surgeon proceeding with an MV repair, resection of excessive leaflet tissue of the posterior leaflet, chordal transfer from the anterior leaflet, and patch closure of the perforation, plus a mitral annular ring. Separation from CPB was facilitated with epinephrine, but the postrepair TEE demonstrated residual moderate central MR and residual anterior leaflet prolapse. No systolic anterior motion of the MV was evident. No gradient existed between the LV and the aorta. CPB was reinstituted, and the MV was exposed again through a left atriotomy. The surgeon elected to replace the MV with a pericardial bioprosthesis, despite the patient's young age. The patient returned to the operating room on the evening of surgery due to mediastinal bleeding, requiring the transfusion of blood, plasma, and platelets. The patient emerged from the anesthetic and surgery on postoperative day 1 edematous and confused. Heart function showed a cardiac index of 2.4 L/min/m^2, mild pulmonary hypertension, and bounding peripheral pulses. Neurologic function recovered fully before discharge on postoperative day 7. Was the initial decision to repair the MV a sound decision? Do the poor initial results of the operation suggest the decision was a poor one? Was the better decision to proceed directly to an MV replacement, decreasing the cardiopulmonary and aortic cross-clamp times?

INTRAOPERATIVE TRANSESOPHAGEAL ECHOCARDIOGRAPHY: INDICATIONS

The first decision by the echocardiographer is whether TEE is indicated. Application of intraoperative TEE in the care of the patient with mitral disease is widely accepted. Even in this area, however, there is a paucity of data supporting an improved outcome for intraoperative patients cared for with TEE compared with no TEE. The decision to perform TEE during cardiac surgery is substantiated by practice expectations and consensus opinion. In an attempt to develop an evidence-based approach to this expanding technology, the American Society of Anesthesiologists (ASA) and the Society of Cardiovascular Anesthesiologists (SCA) cosponsored a task force to develop guidelines for defining the indications for perioperative TEE. Despite the scarcity of outcome data to support the application of TEE in the perioperative period, TEE had rapidly been adopted by cardiac surgeons and cardiac anesthesiologists as a routine monitoring and diagnostic modality during cardiac surgery. In 1996, the task force published their guidelines designed to establish the scientific merit of TEE and justification of its use in defined patient cohorts.[13] The indications were grouped into three categories based on the strength of the supporting evidence/expert opinion that TEE improves outcome (Box 16–5). Category I indications suggested strong evidence/expert opinion that TEE was useful in improving clinical outcome. Category II indications suggested there was weak evidence/expert opinion that TEE improves outcome in these settings. Category III indications suggested there was little or no scientific merit or expert support for the application of TEE in these settings (see Chapter 15).

TEE is not without its serious complications. The risks of intraoperative TEE include physical injury to the mouth, dentition, and esophagus, plus the misinterpretation of a finding leading to mismanagement and poor outcome. When making the decision of whether to perform an intraoperative TEE, the physician should consider the cumulative effects of the indications and the cumulative effects of the risks. A TEE should not be performed if the appropriate equipment, safety precautions, and skilled examiners are not available.

Population-based management decisions are driven by clinical trials, cost-effectiveness analysis, and resource allocation. However, few physicians take care of populations. Most physicians care for individuals. Evidence-based practice paradigms based on "population medicine" define the most effective management scheme for groups of patient cohorts but not every patient. Individual patient decisions by physicians are not consistently based on evidence but are often made in the context of "What would I do if it was my mother?" with the premise that more information is better. Should every patient undergoing repair of an abdominal aortic aneurysm undergo

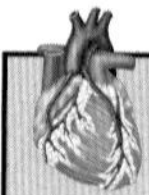

BOX 16–5 ***Indications for the Use of Transesophageal Echocardiography***

Category I

- Heart valve repair
- Congenital heart surgery
- Hypertrophic obstructive cardiomyopathy
- Endocarditis
- Acute aortic dissection
- Acute, unstable aortic aneurysm
- Aortic valve function in the setting of aortic dissection
- Traumatic thoracic aortic disruption
- Pericardial tamponade

Category II

- Myocardial ischemia and coronary artery disease
- Increased risk of hemodynamic disturbances
- Heart valve replacement
- Aneurysms of the heart
- Intracardiac masses
- Intracardiac foreign bodies
- Air emboli
- Intracardiac thrombi
- Massive pulmonary emboli
- Traumatic cardiac injury
- Chronic aortic dissection
- Chronic aortic aneurysm
- Detection of aortic atheromatous disease as a source of emboli
- Evaluating the effectiveness of pericardiectomies
- Heart-lung transplantation
- Mechanical circulatory support

Category III

- Other cardiomyopathy
- Emboli during orthopedic procedures
- Uncomplicated pericarditis
- Pleuropulmonary disease
- Placement of intra-aortic balloon pump, pulmonary artery catheter
- Monitoring the administration of cardioplegia

Modified from published guidelines of the American Society of Anesthesiologists and the Society of Cardiovascular Anesthesiologists.[13]

dipyridamole or dobutamine stress testing? The evidence does not support their use. Nonetheless, the practice in many centers is to obtain a dipyridamole or adenosine thallium stress test, even if the patient is asymptomatic. Should every patient undergoing heart surgery have a TEE? The answer is unknown. Despite the reassurances provided by large clinical trials, practitioners do not consistently adhere to their recommendations and often rely on tradition, anecdote, and impression in their decision-making. The anchor to a "last case" experience creates bias and is all too prevalent in medicine where the experience from the previous case dictates the decision-making on the subsequent one. If physicians are to remain the dispensers of medical care and resources, then they need to be cognizant of the effects of their decisions on all patients, not just the one lying on the operating room table. It is inappropriate to accrue health care costs without evidence that such financial investment provides any health care benefit. Unfortunately, the risk of uncertainty and medicolegal liability results in more testing than is often indicated.[14]

INTRAOPERATIVE TRANSESOPHAGEAL ECHOCARDIOGRAPHY: PERFORMANCE OF THE INTRAOPERATIVE ECHO EXAMINATION

The careful consideration of TEE data precedes decision-making. It takes time to consider all variables and make a decision in the operative environment. Hasty decisions because of perceived time pressures may unduly introduce misconceptions or surgical bias. It is more detrimental to retract a preliminary diagnosis or recommendation than it is to take a few extra minutes to assemble the facts and present a concise coherent assessment.

The ability to render a sound conclusion is often predicated on the performance of a complete and quantitative echocardiographic examination. Incomplete and qualitative assessments may be subject to missed or inaccurate diagnoses. The complete TEE examination has been described through a consensus opinion.[15] The sequence of the comprehensive examination is less important than is adherence to it. A common practice is to perform a targeted examination, followed by the complete examination. This method allows for capture of the most important information should the patient become unstable and necessitate rapid initiation of CPB prior to completion of the TEE. The "soft" interpretation of "mild to moderate" is not always avoidable. The ability to "nail down" a diagnosis and establish a quantifiable measure of dysfunction allows for serial follow-up and comparison before and after treatment. The imperative for quantitative measures is directed at producing reproducible conclusions and trackable results.

Aliasing of color-flow Doppler in the LVOT is highly sensitive for detection of outflow obstruction but lacks specificity. Altered loading conditions, contractility, obstructive myopathy, and systolic anterior mitral motion may produce similar color Doppler findings. Spectral Doppler offers distinct advantages to color Doppler by measuring gradients and analysis of blood flow velocity profiles, rendering the interpretation of abnormal flow patterns and pressure gradients more reliable and quantifiable. A similar approach is applied to assess abnormal blood flow velocities across the MV (see Chapter 15).

Time permitting, the echocardiographer is encouraged to document in writing the prebypass TEE findings at the time they are discovered. It is acceptable to document a finding only to discover later that there is poor agreement with the surgical findings. This practice fosters learning and a systematic process. The process of writing a report ensures a formalized approach to evaluating the TEE.

Cardiac Function and Regional Wall Motion Abnormalities

Framing

Ventricular function is a predictor of outcome after heart surgery and a predictor of long-term outcome in patients with cardiovascular disease. Patients with compensated CHF may have severely decreased ejection fraction (EF) with minimal symptoms. Regional ventricular dysfunction is most commonly caused by myocardial ischemia or infarction. Hence, there is an imperative to detect ventricular dysfunction and institute treatment in an attempt to prevent acute or long-term consequences.

Is ventricular function normal or abnormal? Is the abnormal function global or regional? What is the coronary distribution that relates to an RWMA? Is the ventricle big or small? Is the myocardium thinned or hypertrophied? Is the abnormal function new or old? Does the medical or surgical intervention improve or deteriorate ventricular function?

Data Collection

LV systolic function is assessed echocardiographically based on regional and global wall motion. Methods of assessment include changes in regional wall thickness, radial shortening with endocardial excursion, fractional area change (FAC), and systolic displacement of the mitral annulus. Off-line measurements of EF can be calculated using Simpson's rule. FAC is the most common metric used to assess global LV function. Other measures include end-diastolic area (EDA), end-systolic area (ESA), and meridional wall stress.[16]

Regional assessment provides an index of myocardial well-being that can be linked to coronary anatomy and blood flow. Although the measurement of coronary blood flow is not achieved by TEE, the perfusion beds and corresponding myocardium for the left anterior descending (LAD), left circumflex (LCx), and right coronary (RCA) arteries are relatively distinct and can be scrutinized by TEE using multiplane imaging. The transgastric and long-axis imaging views of the LV are the most widely used for evaluating wall motion abnormalities. Digital archival systems have gained popularity for their ability to capture a single cardiac cycle that can then be examined more closely as a continuous cine loop. Cine loops can also permit side-by-side display of images obtained under varying conditions (e.g., prebypass and postbypass). Regional myocardial ischemia produces focal changes in the corresponding ventricular walls before changes occur on the ECG.[17] Changes progress from normal wall motion to hypokinesis or akinesis. Dyskinesis, thinning, and calcification of the myocardium suggest a nonacute process, likely a prior infarction.

Assessment of right ventricular (RV) systolic function is more problematic because it is less quantifiable. The crescent-shaped RV is not amenable to quantitative measures of differences in chamber size during the cardiac cycle. Characterization of the RV is accomplished by comparing the size of the RV chamber to that of the LV and assessing the relative contractile function of the RV free wall and that of the interventricular septum (IVS).

Ventricular failure can be caused by diastolic dysfunction: the compromised ability of the ventricle to accommodate diastolic filling. Diastolic dysfunction is assessed echocardiographically by examining volumetric filling of the ventricle at the mitral or tricuspid valves. Normal diastolic filling is biphasic with an early (passive) component that exceeds the late (active) inflow velocities. Abnormalities of ventricular filling (e.g., impaired ventricular relaxation, restriction, constriction) produce characteristic changes in the spectral recordings of Doppler inflow velocities. Abnormalities of diastolic function can lend insight into the mechanisms of circulatory instability (see Chapter 15).

Discussion

Preexisting ventricular dysfunction suggests increased risk for surgery and poorer long-term outcome. The presence of such ventricular dysfunction may deteriorate intraoperatively, requiring the need for marked pharmacologic or mechanical support. A patient with a preoperative EF of 10% scheduled for coronary artery bypass grafting (CABG) and MV repair is at increased risk of intraoperative ischemia, acute heart failure, and difficulty maintaining hemodynamic stability during the immediate postbypass period. Anticipating such problems, placement of an intra-aortic balloon pump or femoral arterial catheter is considered during the prebypass period (Fig. 16–2). The same patient is likely to benefit from the administration of inotropic agents.

A marked decrement or unexpected decrease in global cardiac function after release of the aortic cross-clamp can be caused by poor myocardial preservation during cross-clamping or distention of the heart during bypass. The risk of such incidents can be reduced by the monitoring of the electrical activity of the heart and pulmonary artery pressures and for distention of the RV and LV. Effective venting of the heart is often difficult to discern by visual inspection alone, especially with the use of minimally invasive surgery through small incisions. TEE imaging can diagnose ventricular distention produced by AV insufficiency.

Not all preexisting regional wall motion abnormalities benefit from coronary revascularization. Regions of akinesia and dyskinesia are usually the result of a myocardial infarction and may reflect nonviable myocardium, although "hibernating" myocardium is possible. Hypokinetic segments are generally viable and may represent active ischemia.[18] Preoperative positron emission tomography (PET) scanning can detect hibernating myocardium and may be cost-effective to guide CABG.[19-21] The detection of hibernating myocardium in an area of chronic ischemia and regional hypokinesis will direct the surgeon to revascularize the corresponding stenosed coronary artery. In contrast, an occluded coronary artery with downstream infarction may not benefit from revascularization, as contractile function may be irreversibly lost. However, in this latter scenario, revascularization postinfarction may provide some benefit in decreasing the risk of ventricular aneurysm formation.[22]

Diastolic dysfunction is associated with significant increases in mortality during long-term follow-up.[23] Characterization of abnormalities of diastolic function lends insight into the mechanisms of circulatory instability and hypotension. Severe LV hypertrophy with a noncompliant LV and hyperdynamic systolic function may produce severe heart failure if adequate loading is not achieved. Hemodynamic indices obtained from a pulmonary artery catheter may be misleading. The findings of a small LV chamber size, blunted transmitral filling velocities, and an increased FAC reveal the cause of the hypotension. The decision to administer volume may be appropriate despite the increased pulmonary artery pressures.

If the intraoperative examination reveals new ventricular dysfunction, the intraoperative team must determine the etiology and severity and plan a treatment. Other etiologies of RWMAs such as conduction abnormalities (left bundle-branch block or ventricular pacing) can be difficult to distinguish. Treatment of myocardial ischemia may include optimizing hemodynamics; administering anticoagulants, nitrates, calcium channel blockers, or β-blockers; inserting an intra-aortic balloon pump; or instituting CPB and coronary revascularization. The presence of a new-onset RWMA after separation from bypass is worrisome for myocardial ischemia. Even the patient without coronary artery disease remains at risk because of hypotension, shower of air or debris into the coronary circulation, or coronary spasm. The patient with coronary artery disease undergoing coronary

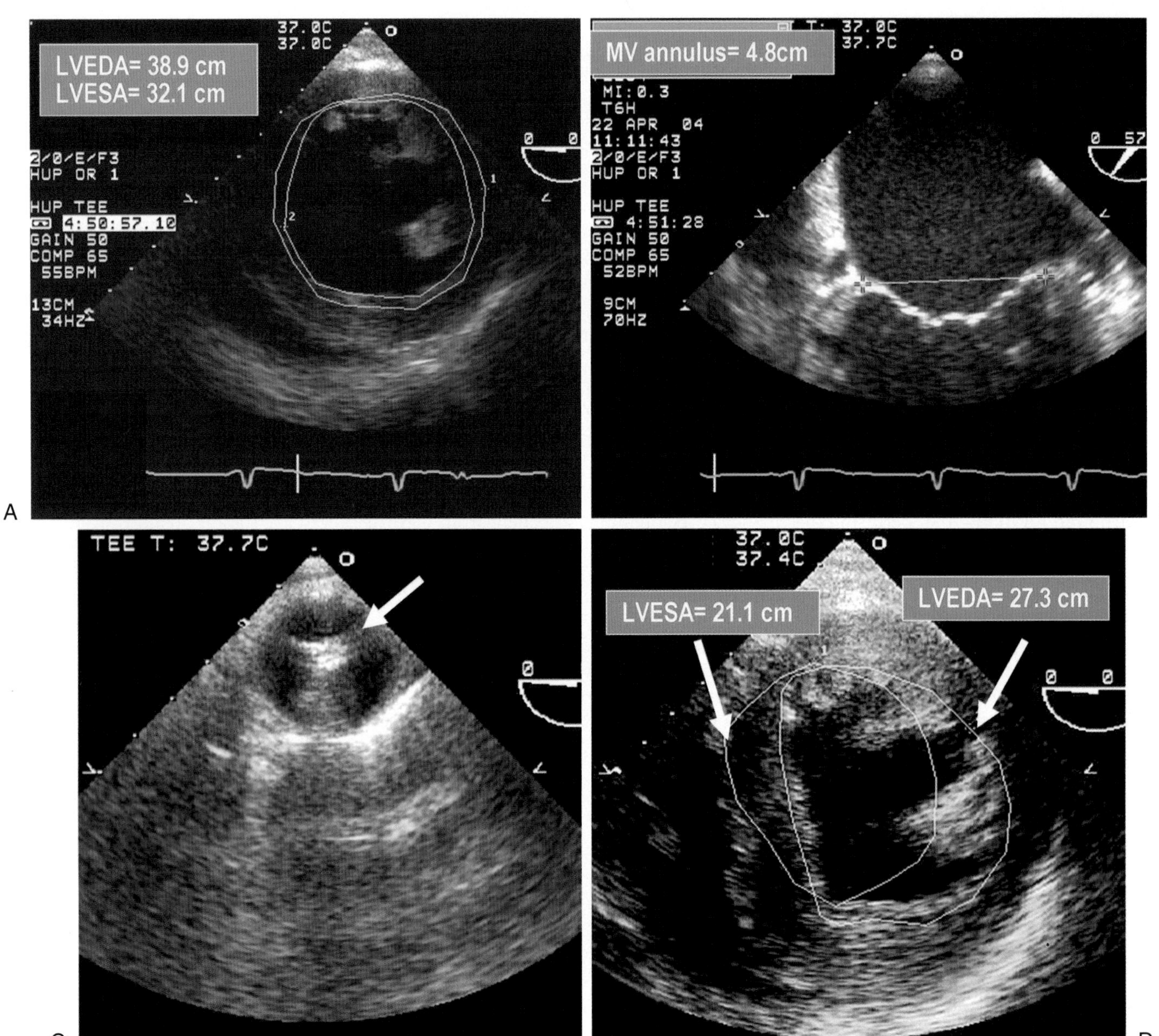

Figure 16–2 The prebypass transesophageal echocardiography (TEE) examination may have predictive value for postbypass circulatory management. A 63-year-old woman with a past medical history of hypertension, congestive heart failure, pulmonary edema, dilated cardiomyopathy, diabetes, and obesity was scheduled for coronary artery bypass grafting (CABG) and mitral valve (MV) repair. The preoperative evaluation documented moderate to severe mitral regurgitation (MR) with reversal of systolic pulmonary vein blood flow velocity. The prebypass TEE mid-esophageal four-chamber view showed a markedly dilated left ventricle (LV) and mildly dilated right ventricle (RV) with mildly decreased global dysfunction (*A*). The transgastric view was characterized by severe global dysfunction and a LV end-diastolic diameter of 6.6 cm (*A*). The fractional area change (FAC) was 17% [FAC = (LV end-diastolic area – LV end-systolic area)/LV end-diastolic area × 100]. Revascularization alone was unlikely to significantly improve MV function. The mid-esophageal bicommissural view of the MV (*B*) demonstrated marked dilation of the MV annulus (major axis = 4.8 cm) and tethering of the leaflets below the valve plane that was caused by LV chamber dilation. A femoral arterial line was inserted for monitoring of central aortic pressure and/or possibly placing an intra-aortic balloon pump. The patient underwent a CABG × 3 and MV annuloplasty for moderate MR. The separation from bypass was difficult, requiring milrinone, epinephrine, vasopressin, and placement of an intra-aortic balloon pump. TEE, which was used to initially confirm the location of the femoral guidewire (*C*), was later used to position the balloon pump just downstream to the left subclavian artery. Worsening of RV function that was characterized by increased central venous pressure, new-onset tricuspid regurgitation, and a hypokinetic RV can be appreciated by ventricular septal flattening and dilation of the RV (*D*). The LV ejection fraction did not decrease as might be expected; after correcting MR, the FAC improved slightly from 17% to 22% postbypass. Cardiac function continued to improve, and the counterpulsation device was removed without complication on the first day after surgery. The infusions of milrinone and epinephrine were continued for several days.

Table 16–1 Management Strategies for New-Onset Myocardial Ischemia Postbypass	
Diagnosis	**Plausible Treatment**
Coronary graft occlusion	Revise coronary graft
Coronary air emboli	Increase coronary perfusion pressure, administer coronary dilators
Coronary calcium/atheroma emboli	Support circulation
Dissection of the aortic root	Repair dissection
Coronary spasm	Administer coronary dilators

revascularization may have all the above risks, technical difficulties at the anastomotic site, injury to the native coronary (e.g., stitch caught the back wall), or occlusion of the coronary graft by thrombosis or aortic dissection. The coronary arteries, grafts, and anastomoses should be carefully inspected for patency and flow. Graft patency in the operating room is difficult to determine. Techniques include manual stripping and refill, measuring coronary flow by hand-held Doppler, or administration of echo contrast agents (see Chapter 15). In the future, miniaturization and enhanced fluoroscopy systems may prompt imaging of the coronary circulation angiographically during surgery. A new RWMA in the distribution of a new coronary graft can prompt the decision-making strategies listed in Table 16–1 (see Chapters 19, 31, and 33).

Transesophageal Echocardiography as a Rescue Device: Management of Marked Hemodynamic Instability

Framing

There are many instances during the perioperative period when the patient may exhibit progressive, unremitting hemodynamic deterioration, or acute cardiovascular collapse. Echocardiography offers a versatile modality to quickly and accurately diagnose the etiology of hypotension and develop management strategies.

The echocardiographer may be summoned to evaluate an unstable patient in the operating room, intensive care unit, or emergency department with little or no preceding knowledge of the patient. Typically, there will be no consent for the TEE procedure; occasionally, a family member may be available to provide consent on the patient's behalf. TEE may need to be postponed in the trauma patient with suspected cervical spine injury or esophageal injury. The trauma patient with an unstable cervical spine is at increased risk of spinal cord injury with passive movement of the head and neck. Until the cervical spine has been documented to be stable, TTE is the alternative. The risk of further esophageal injury in patients with a penetrating trauma poses an additional challenge. Esophagoscopy prior to TEE probe insertion is performed in patients with suspected esophageal injury. However, delay in diagnosis is not without cost. Time must be used efficiently, as permanent vital organ injury relates to the magnitude and duration of hypotension and malperfusion. To guide the discussion and development of rational management strategies, a number of issues should be considered.

What is the cause of the hypotension? Does the cardiac or vascular pathology detected by TEE explain the decrease in blood pressure? Is the heart big or small? Is it full or empty? What is the global function of both ventricles? Are there RWMAs? Is there fluid in the pericardium? Is the observed decrease in cardiac function the primary cause, or is it a consequence of the decreased blood pressure? Is this event related to the patient's past medical history or current operative procedure? What specific parameters of the ventricle may help explain the current episode of hypotension? What interventions or therapy can be performed to improve hemodynamics? Once therapy is initiated, what index or parameter should be monitored to guide management?

Data Collection

Clinicians must not underestimate the importance of past medical history, chief complaint, and operative course when attempting to discern the causes of hemodynamic instability in the acute setting. Important hemodynamic indices include heart rhythm, rate, and blood pressure, concentration of exhaled carbon dioxide, and central venous or pulmonary artery pressure, if available. Echocardiography can be used to develop a rational approach based on the critical factors of cardiac performance. The determinants of cardiac performance include SV and heart rate (HR), as elucidated by the following equation: $CO = SV \times HR$. The three components of SV that can be affected are preload, afterload, and myocardial contractility. Although quantitative analysis is possible, qualitative online analysis will generally yield sufficient information to form the basis of initial therapeutic intervention. Preload of the ventricle can be determined by assessing end-diastolic area (EDA), afterload can be estimated by assessing the end systolic area (ESA), and contractility can be estimated by the velocity of circumferential shortening, FAC, or EF.

Discussion

Initial inspection determines heart size and overall contractile function of both ventricles. Estimates of EDA and EF of the LV provide an index of ventricular load and global function. Attention to both RV and LV size and function helps distinguish between different inciting events. The common causes of intraoperative or perioperative hypotension include intravascular hypovolemia, myocardial ischemia, myocardial infarction, and systemic vasodilatation, either pathologic from infection or inflammation or iatrogenic from drug administration (e.g., vancomycin). The MV is inspected for incompetence. Acute MR is rare in the absence of myocardial ischemia or infarction. A diagnosis of dynamic LV outflow tract obstruction, an uncommon cause during the perioperative period, is difficult to manage in the absence of more invasive monitoring such as TEE (Fig. 16–3).

Mechanical causes of hypotension are typically related to compressive forces impairing the heart's ability to fill or eject (e.g., pericardial fluid, tension pneumothorax). Systemic hypotension with a dilated RV and a small, underfilled LV implies either primary RV failure (e.g., myocardial ischemia or infarction in the distribution of the RCA) or secondary RV failure from acute increases in pulmonary vascular resistance (e.g., pulmonary embolus [Fig. 16–4], pneumothorax).

The distribution of the right coronary system of most patients (right dominant system) includes the RV and the posterior descending coronary artery, which provides blood supply to the inferior and inferoseptal walls of the LV. Acute

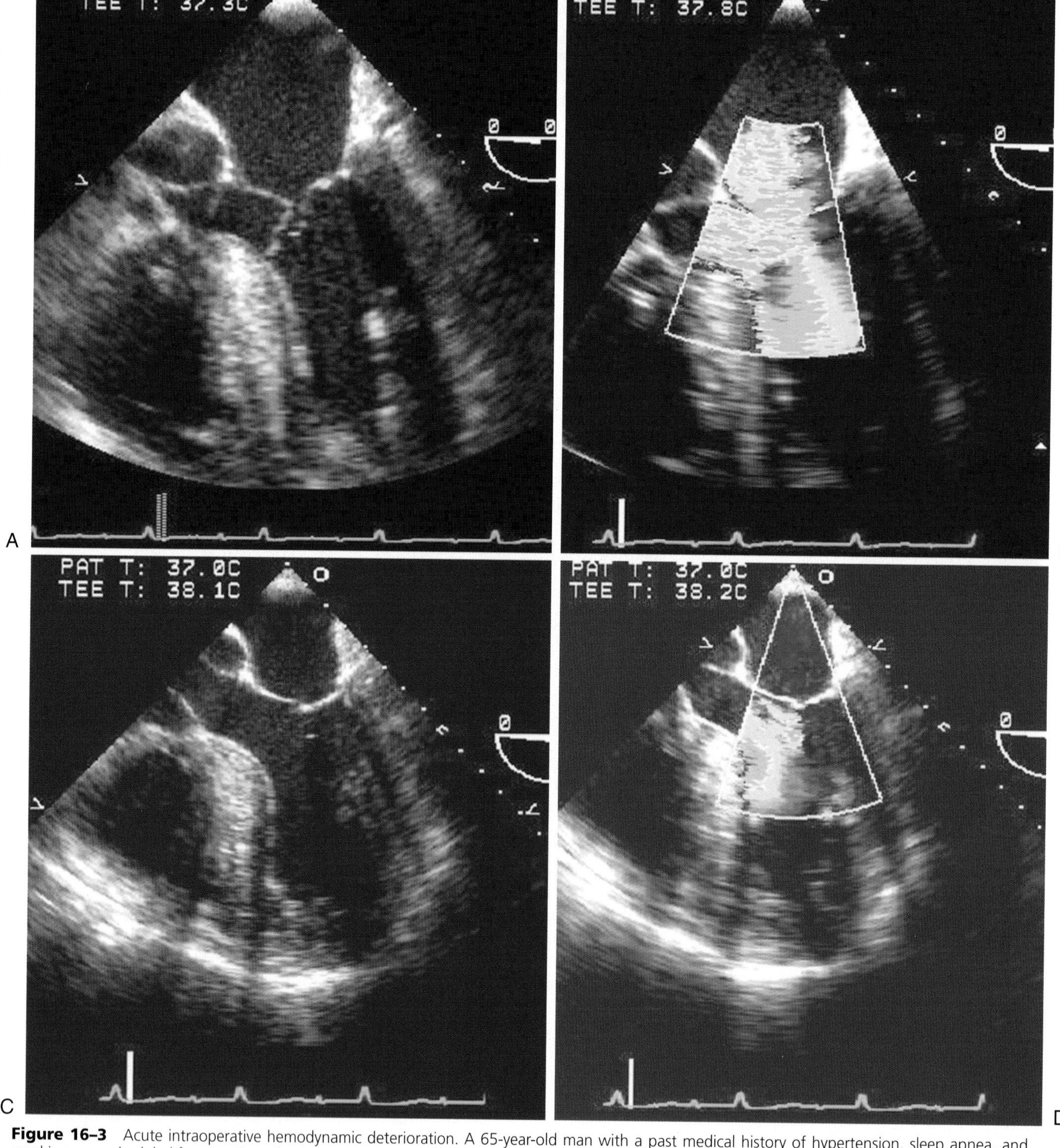

Figure 16–3 Acute intraoperative hemodynamic deterioration. A 65-year-old man with a past medical history of hypertension, sleep apnea, and smoking was scheduled for resection of colon cancer. During the bowel resection, the patient had a profound episode of hypotension and new-onset hypoxia. Although the patient's hemodynamic condition initially improved after administration of phenylephrine and ephedrine, the patient became more hypotensive and hypoxic with evidence of pulmonary edema. Transesophageal echocardiography (TEE) was requested and was emergently placed to diagnose the etiology of cardiovascular collapse and guide management. The mid-esophageal four-chamber view showed a moderately hypertrophied left ventricle (LV) (*A*). LV systole was associated with displacement of the mitral leaflet and chordae down into the outflow tract. The resulting defect in leaflet coaptation of the mitral valve (MV) and abnormal chordal position that was noted in *A* were associated with overwhelming mitral regurgitation (MR) and LV outflow tract obstruction. (*B*) Administration of inotropes (epinephrine and ephedrine) was discontinued; the management strategy was changed to volume resuscitation and pressor administration. The hemodynamics normalized and the examination was repeated 10 minutes later (*C, D*). Displacement of the mitral leaflet and chordae had resolved along with the findings of MR and outflow tract obstruction. The patient was believed to have experienced a profound acute drop in the systemic vascular resistance in response to the release of vasoactive substances during bowel manipulation. The initial exacerbation of the hemodynamics was created by the relative hypovolemia and use of inotrope, leading to dynamic LV outflow tract obstruction. The concomitant episodes of hypoxia and pulmonary edema, which were attributed to the severe MR and increased left atrial pressures, resolved with the decrease in MR. The application of TEE was critical in making the correct diagnosis, altering management strategies, and initiating the appropriate therapy.

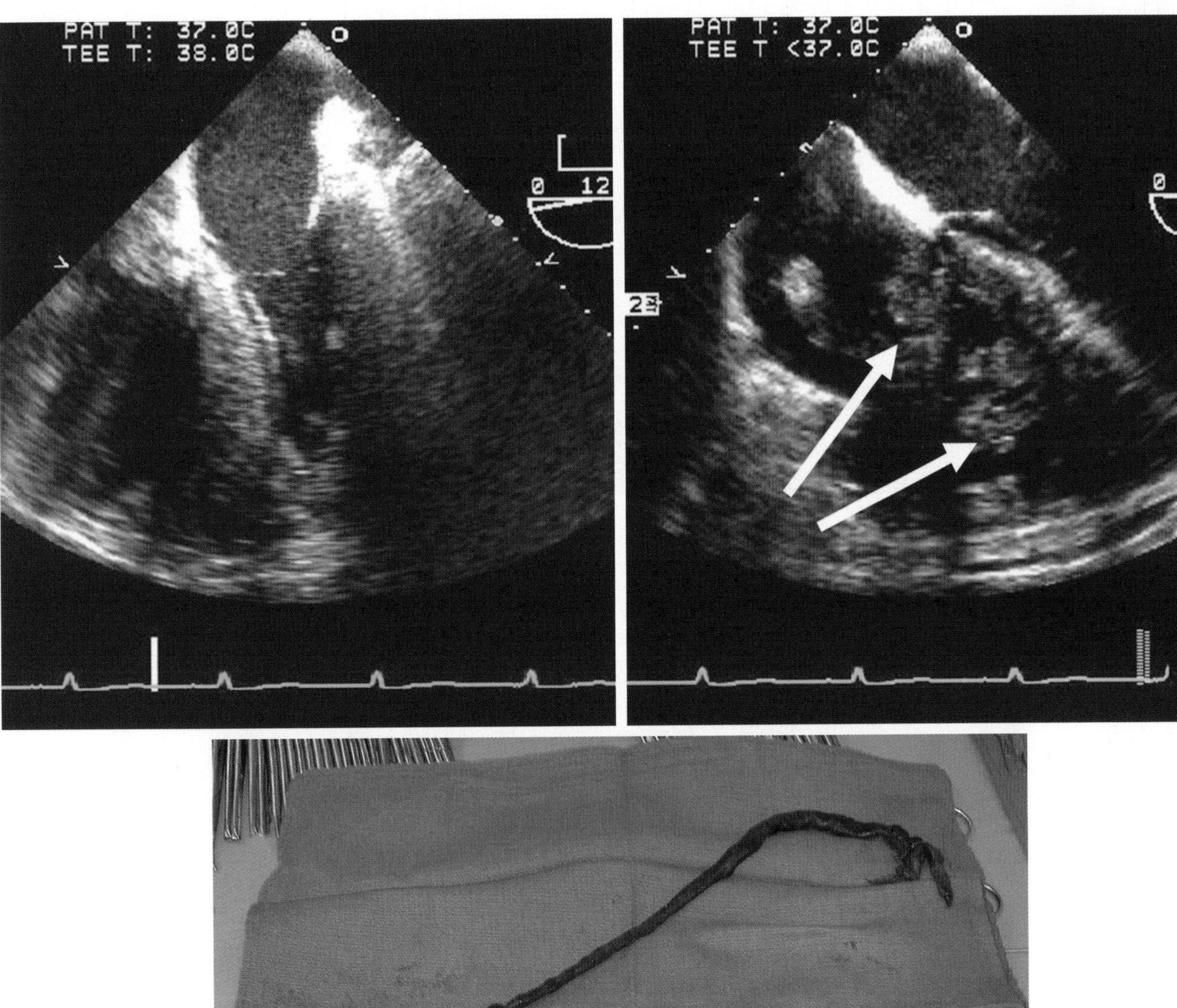

Figure 16–4 Progressive hypoxia and hypotension after cardiac surgery. A 58-year-old morbidly obese patient with a past medical history of hypertension, diabetes, and smoking had recently undergone coronary artery bypass grafting × 3. Five days after surgery, the patient developed new-onset atrial fibrillation along with progressive hypoxia and hypotension requiring readmission to the intensive care unit. The patient's condition continued to deteriorate and required tracheal intubation, ventilator support, and infusions of vasoactive agents. Transesophageal echocardiography (TEE) was performed to evaluate cardiac function and rule out a pericardial effusion. The mid-esophageal four-chamber view (*A*) revealed a dilated right ventricle (RV) coincident with a relatively underfilled left ventricle (LV) and abnormal positioning of the ventricular septum. The displacement of the septum into the LV was consistent with RV dysfunction and RV volume overload. Inspection of the right heart revealed a dilated hypokinetic RV and a serpiginous density that extended from the right atrium into the RV (*B*). The thrombus appeared to be entangled in the chordal structure of the tricuspid valve. Although no thrombus was noted in the pulmonary arteries, the diagnosis of pulmonary embolism was made and the patient underwent an emergent embolectomy. A right atriotomy was performed and a 64-cm thrombus was extracted from the RV along with additional clots from both the right and left pulmonary arteries (*C*). The postbypass TEE documented improved RV function and filling of the LV. TEE was critical in making the diagnosis and the decisions to institute and guide therapy.

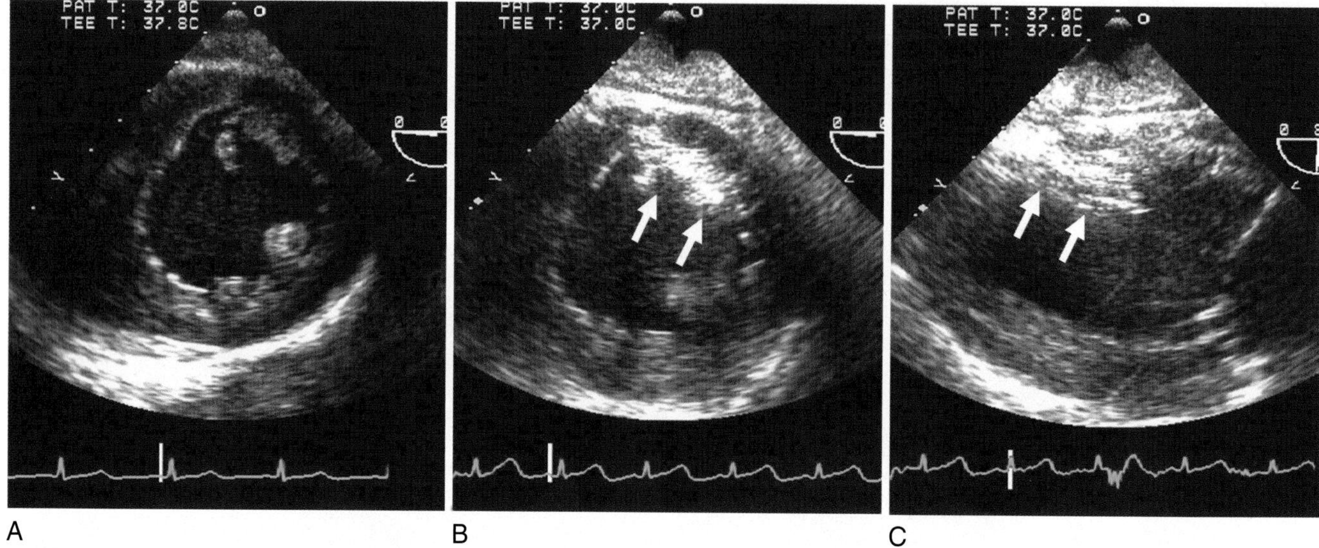

Figure 16–5 Air embolism after open-chamber procedure. A 57-year-old patient underwent surgical intervention to treat severe mitral regurgitation (MR) and two-vessel coronary artery disease. After performing the mitral valve (MV) repair, the right superior pulmonary vein vent catheter was advanced through the mitral valve to facilitate deairing. The patient was positioned in Trendelenburg and the aortic cross-clamp removed. After ventricular ejection, the left atrium and ventricle (LV) were relatively clear of air and the left atrial vent was removed. An aortic vent that had previously served as the cardioplegia cannula was used to vent the residual air from the ascending aorta. The patient was separated from bypass in normal sinus rhythm and maintained good hemodynamics. The initial postbypass transesophageal echocardiogram (TEE) showed normal ventricular function and filling (*A*). Shortly after starting administration of protamine, the blood pressure decreased and the electrocardiogram demonstrated ST-segment changes consistent with ischemia. The protamine administration was stopped, and vasopressors and inotropes were quickly administered. The TEE documented reduced cardiac function in the right ventricle and hypokinesis in the inferior and inferoseptal walls of the LV. The transgastric short- and long-axis views of the LV (*B* and *C*) showed that the myocardium in the distribution of the right coronary artery, as designated by the *arrows,* was characterized by increased echogenicity. Note the significantly elevated ST segments observed in *B* and *C* compared with the baseline (*A*). The absence of pulmonary hypertension and adequate diastolic filling of the LV supported a diagnosis other than acute anaphylactic protamine response or pulmonary embolism. The most likely culprit was air embolization causing transient myocardial ischemia. Air bubbles that migrated from the LV chamber embolized into the ostium of the right coronary artery, which lies at the most anterior aspect of the sinus of Valsalva. TEE served a crucial role in quickly evaluating and diagnosing the etiology of hypotension. The hemodynamics, which were temporarily supported by boluses of vasopressors and inotropes, stabilized, and the protamine dose was completed. The patient was transferred to the intensive care unit without any further incident.

RV dysfunction is not uncommon after the release of the aortic cross-clamp. Preservation of the RV is less reliable compared with the LV because of its exposure to ambient room temperature and variability in its coronary circulation. Open-chamber procedures increase the risk of RV dysfunction because of retained intracardiac air. In the supine patient, the right coronary ostium is located in the least-dependent portion of the aortic root, predisposing for the embolization of air bubbles into it. Air embolization to the RCA produces acute ST-segment changes, marked global RV dysfunction, and RWMAs of the inferior wall of the LV (Fig. 16–5). Conservative treatment includes increasing the blood pressure to promote coronary perfusion while continuing CPB.

As a consequence of decreased systemic vascular resistance (SVR) during sepsis or a systemic inflammatory reaction, the RV and LV often have decreased end-systolic area (ESA) and increased ventricular contractility (increased velocity of circumferential shortening), with concomitant increases in the EF and FAC. The increase in cardiac performance can be quantified by measuring the cardiac output (CO). In cases of hypotension associated with a markedly increased CO, the treatment of choice would be the administration of a vasopressor, such as phenylephrine or vasopressin. If decreased SVR and CO are present, administration of a positive inotrope having vasopressor actions, such as epinephrine or norepinephrine, might be more appropriate.

Pericardial Effusion and Tamponade

Framing

Small effusions are common after heart surgery, especially after removal of chest tubes. In isolation, pericardial effusion may not require surgical intervention. Cardiac tamponade occurs when the pressure exerted by the presence of a pericardial effusion (or any structure adjacent to the heart) compresses the heart, limits diastolic filling of any of the chambers of the heart, and impairs CO. Cardiac tamponade is an emergency, necessitating immediate diagnosis and intervention.

Is a pericardial effusion present? If so, does it contribute to cardiac dysfunction? What is the etiology of the effusion? Is the pericardial effusion the sequela of another cardiovascular event or process? Are there invaginations of the free walls of the RA, RV, or LA? Are the effusions loculated? Where is it located? Is there tamponade?

Data Collection

Echocardiography is the standard diagnostic modality for diagnosis of pericardial fluid. However, the diagnosis of cardiac tamponade is a clinical diagnosis based on hemodynamics and the patient's condition. Low CO, hypotension, equalization of pressures, and high venous pressure are all signs of cardiac tamponade. Echo findings consistent with tamponade include presence of pericardial fluid, compression of the atria, compression of the RV, and loss of normal respiratory variability of ventricular inflow velocities.

The TEE examination quickly determines whether pericardial effusion is present, the location of the effusion (loculated, free flowing), and invagination of select chambers. Location of the effusion is paramount should pericardiocentesis be deemed necessary for acute decompression. RA and RV collapse are the most sensitive signs of increased pericardial pressure. The effusion need not be a large circumferential effusion to significantly impact heart function. Postcardiotomy pericardial clot may be smaller and more compartmentalized than a chronic circumferential effusion that may be free flowing. Interpreting the clinical significance on cardiac hemodynamics may be complicated by factors such as lability of hemodynamics, decreased intravascular volume, depressed cardiac function, mechanical ventilation and pulmonary dysfunction, soft tissue changes, and chest tubes that obstruct some of the echocardiographic windows. Doppler is used as a complementary method of demonstrating the hemodynamic derangements of tamponade and to determine the clinical significance of an effusion. The echocardiographer should interrogate the phasic respiratory variation of blood flow through the tricuspid valve and MV. Although not specific for tamponade, the changes in respiratory variation of inflow velocity are the hallmark of increased pericardial pressure. Significant respiratory variation of blood inflow velocities may also be seen in constrictive pericarditis or conditions associated with changes in intrathoracic pressure, such as increased work of breathing, asthma, or positive-pressure ventilation, and may be exacerbated in patients on positive end-expiratory pressure (PEEP).

Discussion

The American College of Cardiology/American Heart Association/American Society of Echocardiography (ACC/AHA/ASE) task force assigned a class I recommendation to the use of echocardiography in patients with suspected bleeding in the pericardial space. Echocardiography is portable, quick, and noninvasive, yet it is a sensitive and specific modality for the detection and impact of a pericardial effusion. Pericardial effusions can be diagnosed and cardiovascular effects determined by TTE or TEE. However, during the post–cardiac surgery period, the presence of positive-pressure ventilation, chest tubes, and bandages may severely limit the capability of TTE to assess fluid in the pericardium.

The effusion need not be a large circumferential effusion to significantly affect heart function. Loculated effusion may impinge only on the LA and may not be discernible by the traditional acoustic windows used by TTE. A hemodynamically significant localized hematoma compressing only the LA may not produce RA and RV collapse, or the constellation of equalization of pressures. Small effusions are common after heart surgery, especially after removal of chest tubes, and in heart transplant recipients in whom there is a mismatch between heart size and pericardial cradle. The presence of a pericardial effusion in the nonpostcardiotomy patient must lead to a search for the etiology of the effusion. Pericardial effusion mandates close scrutiny of the aortic root for possible aortic dissection. Pericardial effusion in a trauma patient is worrisome for cardiac rupture, ventricular contusion, or foreign body injury.

Not all pericardial effusions require immediate intervention. Development of cardiac tamponade is related to the rate of accumulation of pericardial fluid and the capacity for the pericardium to stretch and accommodate fluid. Chronic pericardial effusions, which occur in cases of malignancy, uremia, connective tissue disease, Dressler's syndrome, and postinfection pericarditis, uncommonly require emergent intervention. Acute pericardial effusions that occur postcardiotomy are usually more ominous and often result in hemodynamic compromise, requiring treatment (see Chapter 24).

Acute cardiac tamponade in the nonpostcardiotomy patient can develop after introduction of as little as 60 to 100 mL of blood. The cause may include type A aortic dissection, myocardial infarction with rupture, acute pericarditis, bleeding from malignancy, myocardial contusion, or myocardial perforation from penetrating trauma. These life-threatening conditions may present with hypotension, tachycardia, plethora, and jugular venous distention. Other classic findings include narrowed pulse pressure, pulsus paradoxus, widening of the mediastinum on chest radiography, and electrical alternans on the ECG. Treatment is immediate decrease in pericardial pressure that could be accomplished through the removal of a relatively small volume of fluid. This temporizing measure can be life saving until more definitive therapy is instituted.

Hemodynamics may temporarily improve with the administration of volume, altering intrathoracic pressure (decreasing peak inflation pressure), but may still require drainage of the effusion. Chronic malignant effusions will temporarily improve following pericardiocentesis but often require a pericardial window for more definitive therapy. Effusions resulting from acute aortic syndromes or cardiac trauma require timely surgical intervention. Post–cardiac surgery patients may require urgent reexploration for evacuation of pericardial hematoma and to address the cause of continued bleeding. If hemodynamics improve following sternotomy but minimal clot is found, the physiologic tamponade may be related to generalized tissue edema and pulmonary dysfunction. In cases of poor cardiac function, the sternal incision may need to remain open and covered with a sterile dressing until edema recedes and cardiac function improves.

Management of Ischemic Mitral Regurgitation

Framing

Ischemic heart disease is the most common cause of mitral insufficiency in the United States. Mechanisms of valve incompetence are varied and include annular dilatation, papillary muscle dysfunction from active ischemia or infarction, papillary muscle rupture, or ventricular remodeling from scar, often leading to a tethering effect of the subvalvular apparatus. Mitral regurgitation leads to pulmonary hypertension, pulmonary vascular congestion, and pulmonary edema with functional disability. Ventricular function deteriorates as the LV becomes volume overloaded with corresponding chamber dilatation. Left untreated, severe MR from ischemic heart disease has a poor prognosis, hence the imperative for diagnosis and treatment.[24-27] Less certain is the impact of lesser degrees of mitral insufficiency on functional status and long-term morbidity and mortality. Patients presenting for surgical coronary revascularization often have concomitant MR of a mild or moderate degree. The intraoperative team is confronted with the decision of whether to surgically address the MV during the coronary operation.

Does MR warrant mitral surgery? What is the mechanism of the regurgitation? What is the grade of the MR? Is the MR likely to improve by coronary revascularization alone?

Data Collection

Pertinent data, including preoperative functional status and evaluation, need to be considered to appropriately interpret and place the intraoperative data in context. The preoperative echocardiogram and ventriculogram need to be reviewed. The intraoperative hemodynamic data are coupled with TEE information to complete the dataset needed to move forward with the decision-making process. The severity of MR on TEE is measured by the vena contracta, maximum area of the regurgitant jet, regurgitant orifice area, and pulmonary vein blood flow velocities. Wall motion assessment and the ECG are used for detecting reversible myocardial dysfunction that may benefit from revascularization. The hemodynamic and TEE data are coupled with provocative testing of the MV in an attempt to emulate the working conditions of the MV in an awake, unanesthetized state. It is not uncommon that preoperative mild to moderate MR with a structurally normal valve totally resolves under the unloading conditions of general anesthesia.[28-30]

Discussion

Most cases of ischemic MR are categorized as "functional" rather than structural. In a study of 482 patients with ischemic MR, 76% had functional ischemic MR, compared with 24% having significant papillary muscle dysfunction.[31] The mechanism of ischemic MR is attributed to annular dilatation, secondary to LV enlargement and regional LV remodeling with papillary muscle displacement, causing apical tethering and restricted systolic leaflet motion.[32] The importance of local LV remodeling with papillary muscle displacement as a mechanism for ischemic MR has been reproduced in an animal model.[33]

The MR is prioritized in accordance with principal diagnosis (e.g., coronary artery disease), comorbidities, functional disability, and short- and long-term outcome. Ischemic MR is quantitated and the mechanism of valve dysfunction is defined. Intraoperative MR is compared with preoperative findings. Discrepancies between the preoperative and intraoperative assessment of the valve may reflect the pressure and volume unloading effects of general anesthesia. In patients with functional ischemic MR who have 1 to 2+ MR, the MV is often not repaired or replaced. However, the need for surgical intervention in patients with 2+ MR under anesthesia remains a point of debate and has not been definitively answered by prospective studies. MV surgery is typically recommended to improve functional status and long-term outcome for patients with 3+ ischemic MR or greater.[31] Ignoring significant ischemic MR at the time of CABG can limit the functional benefit derived from surgery.

The risks to the patient of not surgically altering the MV and anticipated residual regurgitation is weighted against the risk of atriotomy, mitral surgery, extending cardiopulmonary and aortic cross-clamp times, and the likelihood that the coronary surgery will be successful at decreasing the severity of MR. Added risk includes commitment to a mechanical prosthesis should a reparative procedure prove unsuccessful. MR due to acute ischemia may resolve after restoration of coronary blood flow (Fig. 16–6). The reversibility of the regurgitation is difficult to predict: factors supporting reversibility (and hence no immediate need to surgically address the valve) include a structurally normal MV, normal LA and LV dimension, including the mitral annulus, and RWMAs associated with transient regurgitation and pulmonary edema. Revascularization of the culprit myocardium with improvement in regional function may be all that is necessary to restore normal mitral coaptation.[34,35] Myocardial infarction with a fixed wall motion defect or aneurysm, chronically dilated left-sided heart, dilated annulus, or other structural abnormalities that are not reversible (ruptured papillary muscle or chordae, leaflet prolapse, leaflet perforation) suggest myocardial revascularization is unlikely to correct the valvular incompetence.

The decision to proceed or not to proceed with mitral surgery in the setting of ischemic heart disease is institution and surgeon dependent. Centers may elect to surgically address any degree of MR detected during the preoperative or intraoperative work-up of a patient scheduled for coronary surgery. Less aggressive sites elect to proceed with coronary revascularization, followed by repeat scrutiny of the ventricular wall motion and MV. If revascularization has not corrected the MR, the surgeon proceeds with CPB and mitral surgery. With the advent of off-pump coronary artery bypass (OPCAB) surgery, this process has gained another level of complexity, as decisions to proceed with mitral repair will commit the patient to CPB. Off-pump mitral surgical procedures may be possible in the near future. A device that decreases the minor annular axis by adjusting the length of an artificial subvalvular chord that spans the ventricle between anterior and posterior epicardial pads has been used to treat functional MR.[36,37] Likewise, percutaneous endovascular procedures to "clip" the free edges of the anterior and posterior mitral leaflets akin to the Alfierri surgical technique are aimed at noninvasively improving leaflet coaptation.[38,39] Short- and long-term outcome data regarding such investigational techniques remain forthcoming (see Chapters 4, 12, 19, 20, and 21).

Myxomatous Degeneration of the Mitral Valve and Mitral Regurgitation

Framing

Myxomatous degeneration of the MV is a common cause of MR. Patients are often young and otherwise quite healthy. The diagnosis is commonly established preoperatively, and patients are scheduled for elective surgery unless acute leaflet or chordal rupture leads to acute pulmonary edema and emergency surgery. The decisions to be addressed in this setting include the following: Can the surgeon perform an MV repair to address the MR, or is valve replacement necessary? What does the surgeon need to know to assess the possibility of repair and how to accomplish it? What are the possible complications of MV repair? Is the MV repair acceptable?

Data Collection

The surgeon cannot rely on visual inspection of the native MV in the flaccid arrested heart to discern the mechanism of MR. Unless the patient had a preoperative TEE as part of the preoperative evaluation, the intraoperative study is often critical in assisting the surgeon to plan the appropriate surgical correction.

The intraoperative TEE examination targets the MR, LA, LV, and RV. Myxomatous MR is typically amenable to valve repair. Typical findings of myxomatous valves include excessive leaflet motion, redundant leaflet tissue, and a dilated mitral annulus. Leaflets commonly prolapse into a dilated LA, the degree of which is based on the chronicity of the illness. Chordal rupture is common and leads to flail leaflets and

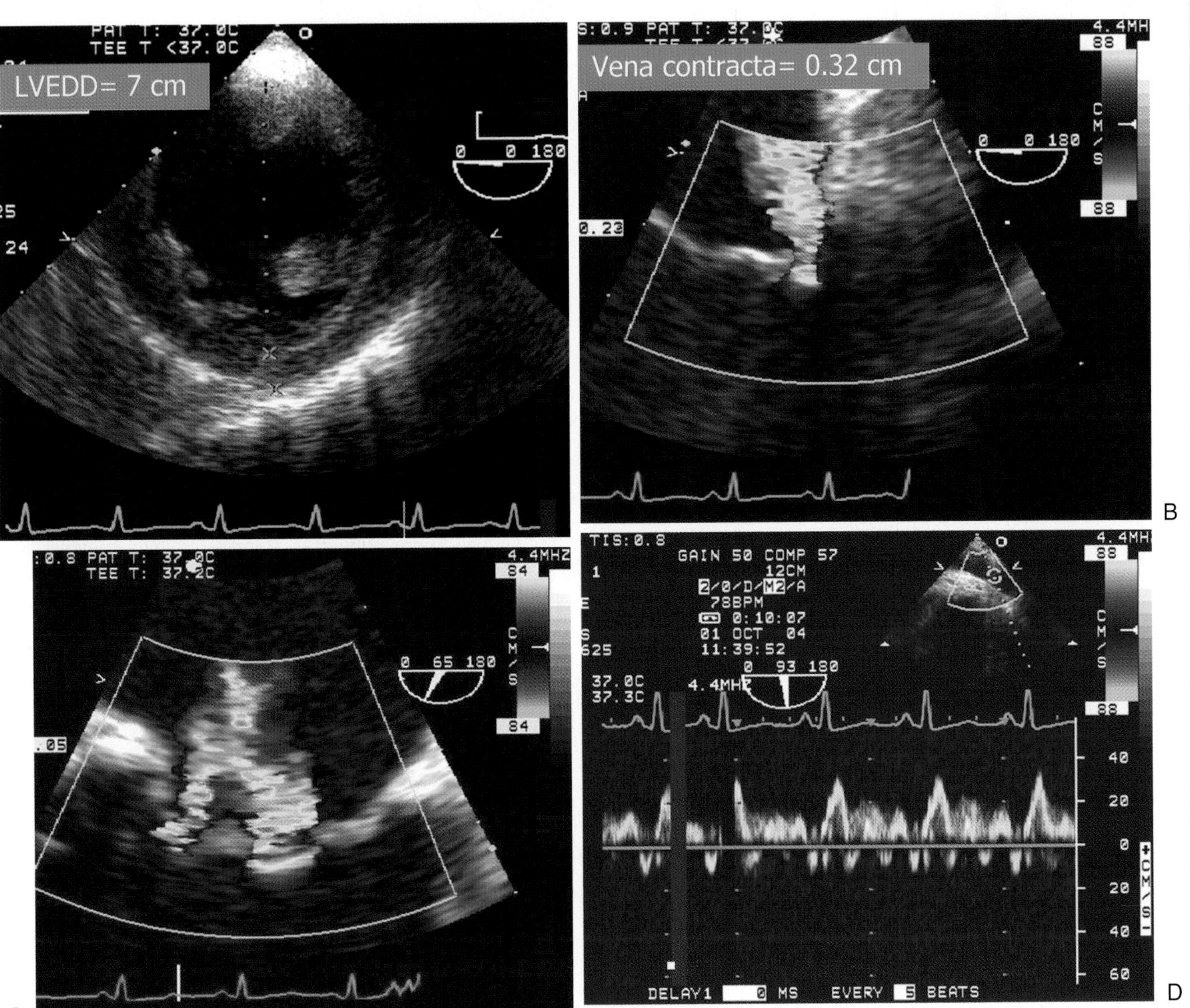

Figure 16–6 Evaluation of mitral regurgitation (MR) in a patient undergoing coronary artery bypass grafting. A 63-year-old man was scheduled to undergo off-pump coronary artery revascularization. The patient had a history of progressive congestive heart failure without evidence of acute pulmonary edema. The physical examination was significant for diffuse laterally displaced point of maximum impulse (PMI) and a systolic murmur at the apex that radiated to the axilla. The patient received an intraoperative transesophageal echocardiography (TEE) examination to evaluate the severity of MR. The left ventricle (LV) was significantly dilated with an LV end-diastolic dimension of 7 cm (*A*) and had depressed systolic function with an estimated ejection fraction of 40%. The MR was characterized by color-flow Doppler imaging to be a central jet of mild to moderate severity. The grading of MR was based on the area of the regurgitant jet and the vena contracta (*B*) viewed in a bicommissural view. The pathogenesis of MR was believed to be functional and resulted from restricted leaflet mobility caused by the dilated LV. The coaptation of the anterior and posterior leaflets was below the valve plane (*C*). The absence of reversal of pulmonary vein blood flow measured in the left lower pulmonary vein (*C*) supported the assessment of moderate MR. Because the annulus was not significantly dilated (the minor axis measured 2.97 cm) and the MR graded as only mild to moderate, the surgeon proceeded with his initial plan of off-pump coronary artery bypass grafting. The MR decreased immediately after revascularization, and the patient's symptoms were expected to further improve with afterload reduction.

severe MR. The imperative is to be exact in the descriptive anatomy of the MV. The accepted nomenclature of the anatomy of the MV is stated in a consensus guideline.[15] The locus of flail scallops or leaflets and regurgitant orifice, the width of the anterior and posterior leaflets, the bisecting widths of the mitral annulus (minor and major axes), the locus of a perforation, severity of annular calcification (less common in isolated ischemic or myxomatous disease), and the size of the LA all contribute significantly to the planned repair. The findings of long and redundant anterior and posterior leaflets increase the risk of postoperative systolic anterior motion (SAM) of the MV. Maslow et al[40] examined the predictors of outflow tract obstruction after MV repair. In this study of patients who were undergoing repair for myxomatous valve disease, 11 of 33 patients developed SAM and outflow tract obstruction. The major predictive factors were smaller anteroposterior length ratio (annulus to coaptation) (0.99 versus 1.95) and short distance from septum to MV coaptation point (2.53 versus 3.00 cm). The surgeon may elect to perform a posterior sliding valvuloplasty to move the point of coaptation laterally, thereby decreasing the risk of outflow obstruction and mitral incompetence associated with SAM.

Although assessment of valvular incompetence is made and the need for repair/replacement is generally decided prior to surgery, the severity and pathogenesis of MR should again be determined intraoperatively. The severity of MR can be quite variable and depend on the hemodynamic loading conditions and its pathogenesis. Discrepancies between preoperative and intraoperative assessment of MR are less likely in patients with structural abnormalities (e.g., ruptured chordae or leaflet perforation) of their MVs, in contrast to patients with functional MR (e.g., ischemic MR)

The repaired MV is closely scrutinized, with the ventricular vent removed at the discontinuation of bypass under typical loading conditions. The systolic and diastolic functions of the valve are examined for residual regurgitation, stenosis, and the presence of outflow tract obstruction. The postbypass examination is critical for determining the acceptability of the repair or guiding the subsequent revision, should the initial repair be unacceptable. Systolic valve dysfunction after repair typically produces residual MR. Residual MR after mitral repair is not uncommon and may not necessitate revision if the grade is trace or mild. Diastolic mitral function is ascertained by Doppler flow measurements across the mitral orifice to provide assurance that the repaired valve has not been rendered stenotic. Peak transvalvular blood flow velocities and pressure half-times are measured to calculate valve gradients and valve areas.

Discussion

There is a growing imperative to repair instead of replace myxomatous MVs. The intraoperative echocardiographer soon becomes familiar with the abilities and limitations of his or her surgical counterparts. Outcomes may be quite dependent on the ability of the individual surgeon, more so than in valve replacement surgery. Hence, it may be prudent to track short-term (intraoperative) results of these operations, as outcomes may be less defined by national databases and more so by individual provider. In general, the likelihood of a successful repair is based on the severity and extent of involvement of the mitral leaflets. Isolated prolapse of the middle scallop of the posterior mitral leaflet associated with eccentric MR that overrides an otherwise normal anterior leaflet is associated with a high success rate. However, cases of extensive leaflet degeneration with bileaflet prolapse, multiple chordal ruptures from both leaflets, leaflet destruction from preceding endocarditis, two or more regurgitant orifices, and extensive calcification are associated with a significantly lower success rate for repair.[41] Many patients leave the operating room with a prosthetic MV replacement with preservation of the subchordal apparatus with excellent long-term results. Retention of the subvalvular apparatus preserves longitudinal shortening of the LV and decreases the incidence of heart failure in the long term.[42,43] In a comparative study, the EF of patients without chordal transfer decreased 24% postoperatively compared with patients having chordal transfer who maintained preoperative function.[43]

Some degree of residual MR after repair is common. Most surgeons will not accept residual MR of 2+ or greater and will readdress the valve surgically. Assessment of valve function postbypass under unloaded conditions (decreased afterload with relative hypovolemia) may erroneously predict MR in the long term or under provoked conditions of exercise. Hypotension with decreased LV contractility and chamber dilatation often responds to inotropic agents with improved coronary perfusion and decreased MR.

The mechanism of the failed repair is paramount to the decision process and treatment. Residual mild regurgitation associated with persistent leaflet prolapse may warrant further leaflet resection. Mild residual regurgitation in the setting of a "normal" MV may sway the surgeon to accept it. The presence of a central jet of MR may require resizing (smaller) or repositioning of the annular ring. The decision of re-repair or valve replacement is often a difficult one, weighing the balance between the risks of reoperation versus the risk of residual MR. The final decision of what is acceptable residual valvular regurgitation is patient specific (e.g., age, anticipated level of activity, ability to tolerate a return to bypass).

The finding of LV outflow tract obstruction caused by SAM after valve repair is usually repairable (Fig. 16–7). The locus of leaflet coaptation that is now displaced anteriorly causes the anterior leaflet to paradoxically move into the LV, rather than toward the LA late in systole.[44] Displacing the anterior leaflet into the LV outflow tract during ventricular ejection (Venturi effect) produces outflow tract obstruction, early closure of the AV, and MR. SAM may be intermittent, depending on loading conditions, typically exacerbated by hypovolemia, vasodilatation, and increased inotropy. If possible, patients should be examined in sinus rhythm as compared with pacing. Acutely, RV pacing may cause decreased inward movement of the ventricular septum, thereby increasing systolic LV outflow tract dimensions and reducing the velocity of LV outflow.[45] This in turn tends to reduce SAM, further diminishing LV outflow obstruction and MR. Persistent SAM should be treated surgically. The management of intermittent SAM, based on loading conditions, is controversial and depends on several patient factors and the surgeon. Aggressive treatment would include return to CPB and revising the mitral repair (e.g., posterior sliding mitral valvuloplasty to shift the locus of coaptation laterally) or possibly MV replacement. Resolution of SAM with volume loading and treatment with a vasoconstrictor may not predict resolution of the problem in the long term. Patients who transiently demonstrate SAM or turbulence in the outflow tract may be at increased risk after surgery (see Fig. 16–3). An important role of the clinical echocardiographer is to recognize potentially important findings that may have an impact on subsequent patient care (see Chapters 15 and 24).

Occult Congenital Abnormalities: Persistent Left-Sided Superior Vena Cava

Framing

The finding of a persistent left-sided superior vena cava (SVC) is not a common incidental finding, but its diagnosis has important implications for the conduct of circulatory management during CPB.

What echocardiographic findings suggest persistent left-sided SVC? What confirmatory test can be performed? Does the finding of an anomalous left-sided SVC have implications for the conduct of bypass?

Data Collection

The echocardiographer should suspect a persistent left-sided SVC if the coronary sinus is significantly dilated or if significant difficulty was encountered while attempting to place a pulmonary artery catheter. Because the differential diagnosis of a dilated coronary sinus includes pathology associated with increased right-sided pressures, confirmation should be

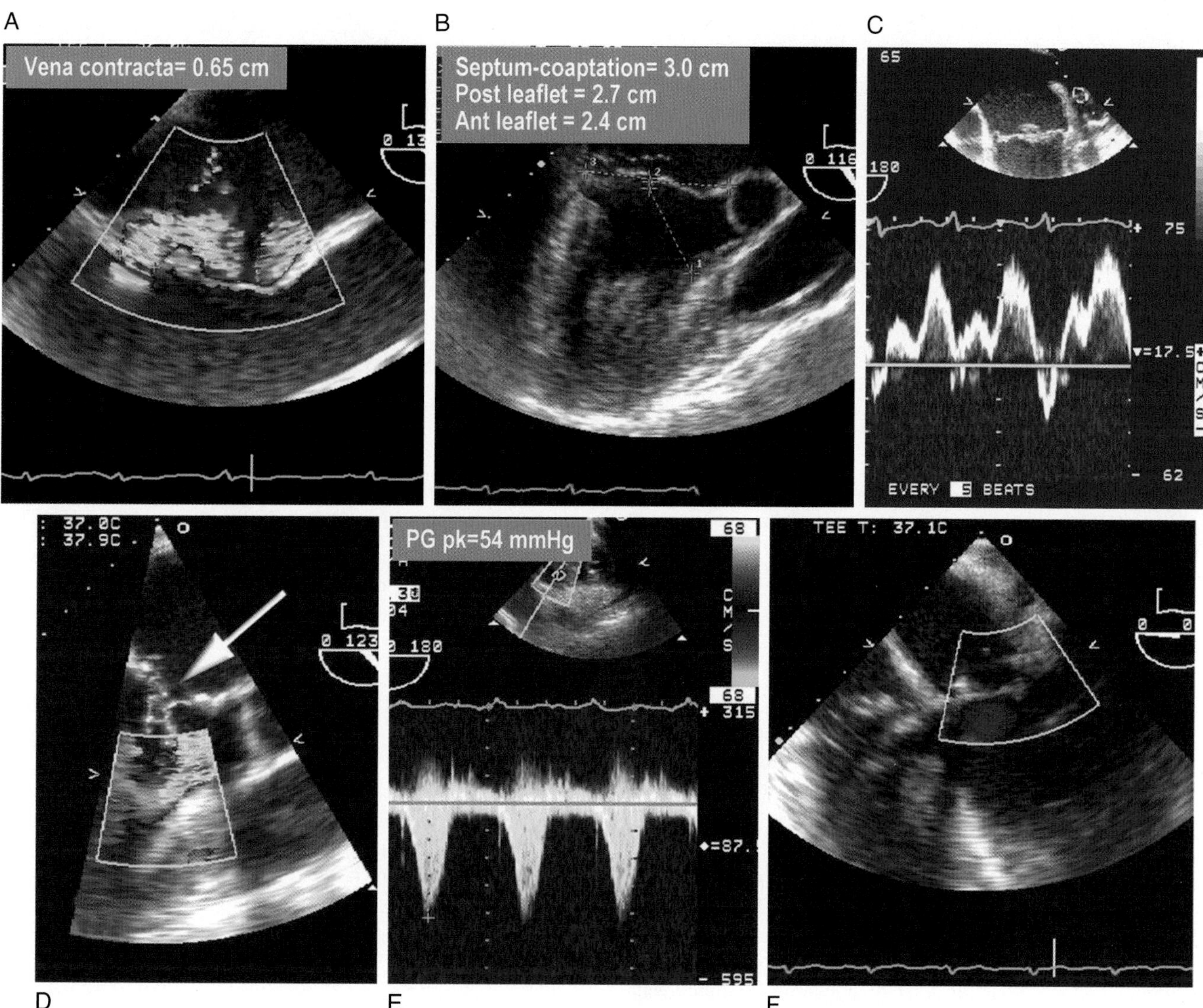

Figure 16–7 Complex mitral valve (MV) replacement/repair revision. A 58-year-old woman with severe MR and a history of congestive heart failure, pulmonary edema, and hypertension was scheduled for surgical repair of mitral insufficiency. The prebypass transesophageal echocardiogram (TEE) characterized the MV as having severe mitral regurgitation (MR) with mildly thickened, myxomatous leaflets and several ruptured chordae. The markedly dilated annulus was consistent with the chronic disease process. Prolapse of the posterior leaflet resulted in the MR jet overriding the anterior leaflet (*A*). Although the distance from the septum to the coaptation point of the MV was greater than the value cited by Maslow as predictive of postbypass SAM, the ratio of the length of the anterior and posterior leaflets (0.89) suggested a risk for LV outflow obstruction (*B*).[40] The mid-esophageal long-axis view demonstrates several ruptured chordae (*B*) that resulted in MR having a vena contracta of 0.65 cm. Blunting of the systolic component of pulmonary vein blood flow velocity corroborated the diagnosis of significant MR (*C*). The surgeon performed a quadrangular resection of the posterior leaflet and secured the annulus with a No. 30 Physio ring. The postbypass imaging of the mid-esophageal long-axis view demonstrated a coaptation defect, designated by the *arrow*, and nonlaminar flow in the LV outflow tract (*D*). Shift of the coaptation point medially created laxity of the redundant chordae that were drawn into the outflow tract by systolic LV ejection (*D*). The outflow tract obstruction was characterized by a pressure gradient of 54 mm Hg as determined by continuous-wave Doppler through the outflow tract using the transgastric long-axis view (*E*). Neither the MR nor the outflow tract obstruction was effectively addressed by volume loading and decreasing the inotropic support. Circulatory bypass was reinstituted, and the surgeon revised the previous repair by further resecting the posterior leaflet and enlarging the annular ring to a No. 34. The patient was successfully separated from bypass using minimal support and had resolution of LV outflow tract obstruction, return of normal hemodynamics, and reduction of MR to trace severity (*F*).

obtained by injecting agitated saline contrast into an intravenous catheter in the left arm. In the case of a persistent left-sided SVC, opacification of the coronary sinus occurs before that of the RA or RV (Fig. 16–8). Once the diagnosis is confirmed, the echocardiographer should look for other associated congenital anomalies, including atrial septal defects (ASDs) or an unroofed coronary sinus with communication between the coronary sinus and the floor of the LA.

Discussion

Left-sided SVC is the consequence of arrested embryologic development that results in the left brachiocephalic vein emptying into the coronary sinus with subsequent flow into the RA return of blood. As a consequence, cannulation of the coronary sinus with administration of retrograde cardioplegia will be ineffective at providing cardiac protection during

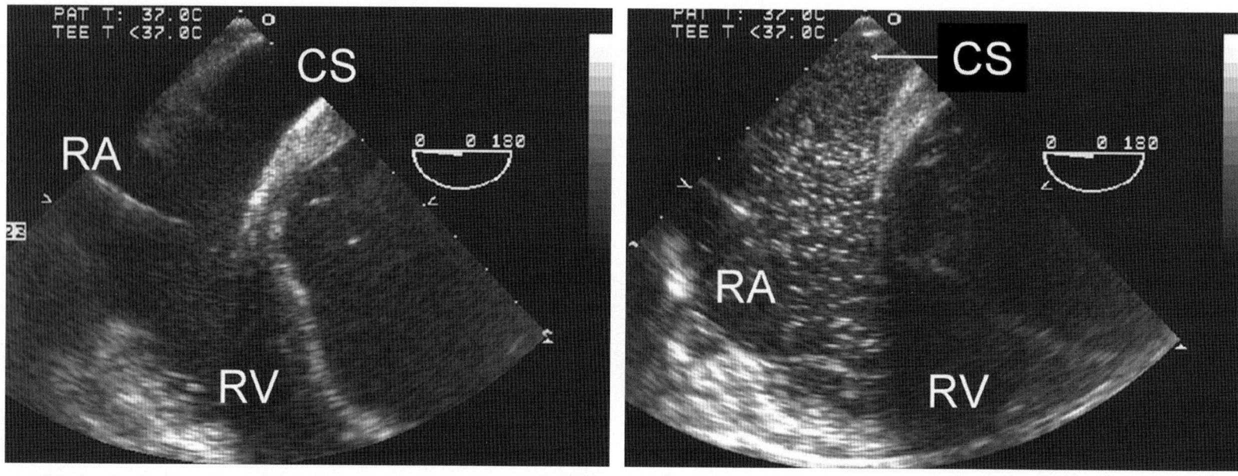

Figure 16–8 Detection of occult persistent left superior vena cava alters circulatory management. A 57-year-old patient was scheduled to undergo an aortic valve replacement for severe aortic stenosis. The intraoperative transesophageal echocardiography examination documented a bicuspid aortic valve (AV) with a dilated aortic root and ascending aorta, preserved left ventricular (LV) systolic function, moderate LV hypertrophy, and dilated coronary sinus (CS) (*A*). The diagnosis of persistent left superior vena cava was considered. An agitated mixture of saline, blood, and air was injected into the intravenous access in the left arm, and the diagnosis was confirmed when the coronary sinus was opacified before the right atrium (RA) and ventricle (RV). The diagnosis of a persistent left superior vena cava altered conduct of bypass by negating the standard use of retrograde cardioplegia and by relying solely on antegrade cardioplegia.

cardiac arrest. Once the diagnosis is confirmed, the surgeon is informed to modify the conduct of cardiac protection during bypass. If TEE is unable to confirm the diagnosis (absence of venous access in the left arm to inject contrast), the surgeon can confirm its presence by direct inspection.

Occult Congenital Abnormalities: Atrial Septal Defects and Patent Foramen Ovale

Framing

Incidental detection of an ASD or a patent foramen ovale (PFO) is a common occurrence. The clinical implications of an intracardiac defect are shunting, stroke, headaches, pulmonary hypertension, RV dysfunction, and paradoxical embolization. If transseptal flow is present, it is generally from left to right, because LA pressure is generally greater throughout the cardiac cycle. Bidirectional flow is possible with transient increases of right atrial (RA) pressure that can be observed during normal respiratory maneuvers (i.e., Valsalva, coughing, and physical straining).[46] Routine physical activities associated with a Valsalva maneuver include heavy physical activity, *lifting heavy objects*, defecation, or vigorous coughing.[47] Although uncommon, right-to-left shunting can produce episodes of relative hypoxia and paradoxical embolization. TEE is an extremely sensitive technique to detect an ASD or a PFO.[48] ASD or PFO is generally well tolerated and often remains asymptomatic into adulthood; hence, their detection is often incidental during a routine intraoperative TEE examination.

What type of ASD is present: primum, secundum, sinus venosus, or PFO? What is the size of the defect? Does the defect produce transseptal blood flow? What is the shunt fraction: Q_s/Q_t? Does the patient have any symptoms such as CHF, increased shortness of breath, history of stroke or transient ischemic attack, or refractory hypoxia? What is the pulmonary artery pressure and RV function? Does the patient have any associated congenital abnormalities, such as a cleft MV with a primum ASD? Does the surgery as initially planned require the use of bypass? If so, was single or bicaval cannulation planned? Does the interatrial defect need to be closed?

Data Collection

The application of two-dimensional echocardiography, color-flow Doppler imaging, and contrast administration in the mid-esophageal four-chamber and mid-esophageal bicaval views provides for high sensitivity of detection and diagnosis of ASD and PFOs. The clinical implication of these findings is determined by the type of pathology. The PFO may be detected in about 30% of adults; it occurs when the secundum septum fails to close or is stretched open because of elevated pressures in the LA (Fig. 16–9). Ostium secundums, which account for 70% of ASDs, are located in the area of the foramen ovale. The etiology of this lesion is attributed to poor growth of the secundum septum or excessive absorption of the primum septum. MV prolapse is present in up to 70% of patients with this abnormality and may be related to a change in the LV geometry resulting from RV volume overload. The primum ASD develops when the septum fails to fuse with the endocardial cushion at the base of the interatrial septum (IAS). A primum ASD is commonly associated with cleft anterior leaflet of the MV and MR. The tricuspid valves may also be abnormal. The final type of ASD is a sinus venosus defect, which comprises only 10% of ASDs. It is commonly associated with abnormal insertion of the pulmonary veins into the RA or SVC.

Discussion

In general, patients benefit from ASD closure. ASDs and PFOs are the most common congenital cardiac anomalies. ASDs are often asymptomatic but may present with atrial arrhythmias, heart murmur, abnormal ECG, dyspnea, cerebrovascular injury or stroke, or migraine headaches. Medical management and surgical closure of secundum ASDs were compared in randomized trials; surgical closure was associated with significantly decreased morbidity and mortality.[49] However, there are little data concerning treatment strategies and outcomes

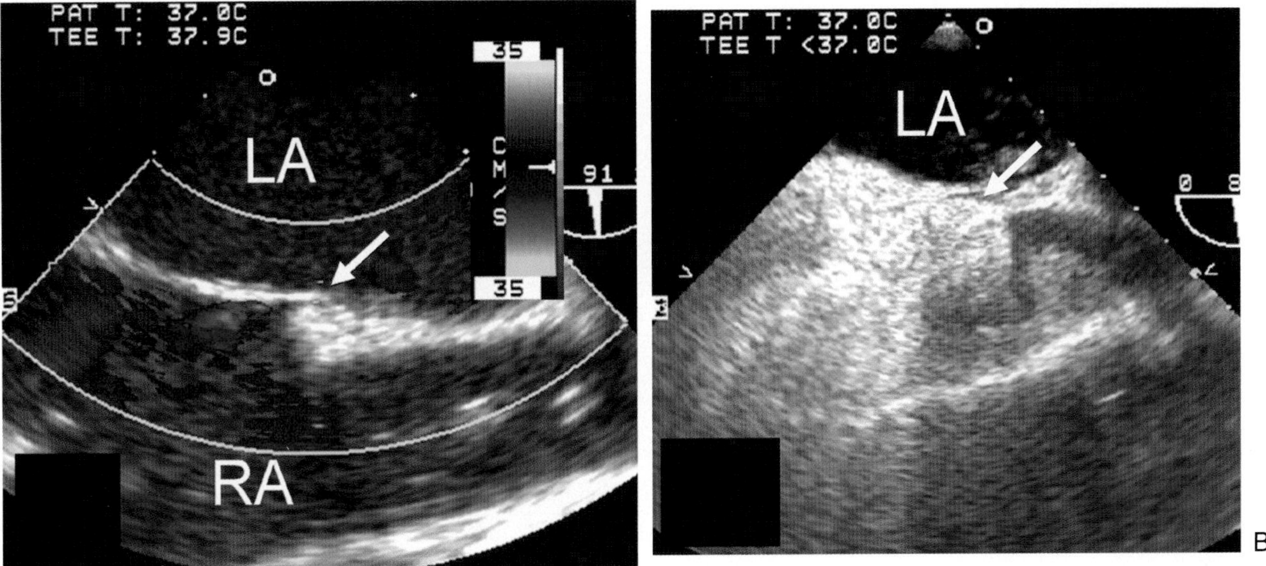

Figure 16–9 Detection of a patent foramen ovale in a patient undergoing cardiac surgery. A 68-year-old patient was undergoing two-vessel off-pump coronary artery bypass grafting (OPCAB). In addition to coronary artery disease, the patient had a past medical history of hypertension, non–insulin-dependent diabetes, and a stroke of unknown etiology. The intraoperative transesophageal echocardiography (TEE) examination that included an inspection of the interatrial septum in the mid-esophageal four-chamber and bicaval imaging planes revealed a new finding of an aneurysmal interatrial septum with a patent foramen ovale (PFO, *arrow*). Color-flow Doppler showed minimal shunt flow from the left atrium (LA) to the right atrium (RA). The presence of the PFO, which was initially diagnosed by color-flow Doppler imaging (*A*), was confirmed by the transient flow of injected contrast (*arrow*) into the LA (*B*), after it was injected into the venous circulation. A provocative maneuver such as Valsalva transiently increases RA pressure more than that of the LA, increasing the sensitivity of PFO detection.[48] Because of the patient's history of a cryptogenic stroke, the surgical plan and circulatory management were altered. The patient was fully heparinized and circulation supported by an extracorporeal pump, while the CABG was performed and the PFO was closed.

for the occult ASD or PFO detected intraoperatively. When PFO detection occurs during OPCAB, surgical correction of the PFO necessitates marked change in the conduct of both the operation and circulatory management. In the absence of recognized consensus guidelines, the decision to proceed with definitive closure should be based on the following factors: history of neurologic event without a definite etiology, recurrent stroke while receiving anticoagulation, significant shunting through the defect, previous episode of hypoxia that may be related to intracardiac shunting, RV dysfunction, or previous paradoxical embolism.

Pulmonary hypertension may increase risk. Detection of a primum or sinus venosus defect requires a more involved surgical procedure, and associated anomalies must be addressed. Undiagnosed complex congenital abnormalities are uncommon in the patient presenting for cardiac surgery. Alternatives to operative closure are increasing as transvenous percutaneous closure devices become increasingly applicable.

Transvenous catheter–based closure of an ASD by interventional cardiologists can be performed only on a secundum ASD or PFO (Fig. 16–10). Approximately 30% of secundum ASDs are amenable to percutaneous closure.[50] The technique optimally requires a defect with limited size and a rim of tissue surrounding the defect of at least 5 mm to prevent obstruction of the coronary sinus or impingement of the AV (see Chapters 12 and 22).

A number of studies have found an increased prevalence of PFO and atrial septal aneurysms in patients having cryptogenic stroke (i.e., no identified cardioembolic or large vessel source).[51-58] Atrial septal aneurysm is a congenital outpouching of the IAS at the fossa ovalis and is strongly associated with PFOs.[51,52,54] The occurrence of atrial septal aneurysms detected by echocardiography is about 10% in the general population and up to 28% in patients with a history of stroke or transient ischemic episode.[53-55,59] A meta-analysis of these case-control studies found that PFO, atrial septal aneurysms, or both were significantly associated with ischemic stroke in patients younger than 55 years.[60] However, the relationship between septal pathology and neurologic events in patients older than 55 is less clear. The data on treating patients with atrial septal abnormalities for either primary or secondary prevention of stroke are limited. The Patent Foramen Ovale in Cryptogenic Stroke Study and a meta-analysis by Oregera found that warfarin treatment was superior to other antiplatelet therapy and comparable to surgical PFO closure for the prevention of recurrent cerebral events.[60] Chronic anticoagulation is associated with complications. The decision regarding closure of an incidental PFO considers the presence of RV dysfunction that may increase the risk of right-to-left transatrial blood flow and cryptogenic stroke. For patients already undergoing cardiac surgery, the incremental risk associated with atriotomy and closure of the PFO is unknown. There are no data, and practices are typically based on individual surgical preferences. However, there are several case reports that describe postoperative complications related to hypoxia and neurologic events in patients with persistent PFOs.[61-64]

The benefit of aggressive management of a PFO in the absence of other interatrial septal abnormalities is less clear and is more controversial. Sometimes surgical intervention requires a significant alteration of the surgical plan and therefore may significantly increase operative risk. In cases in which PFO detection occurs during OPCAB, surgical intervention necessitates marked changes in the conduct of both the operation and circulatory management. The OPCAB patient with a small PFO will typically remain untreated. In the absence of recognized consensus guidelines, the decision to proceed with

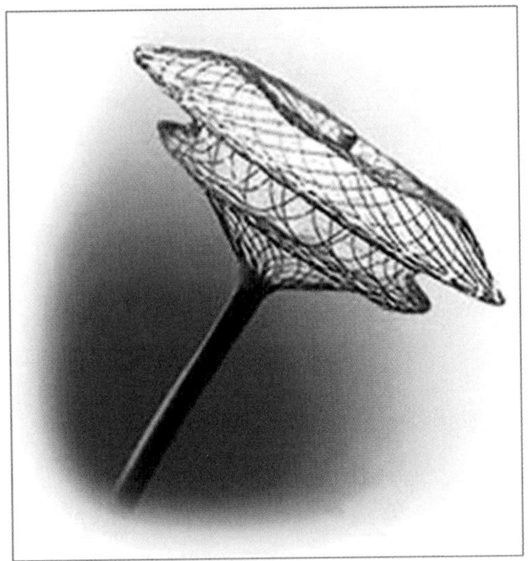

A

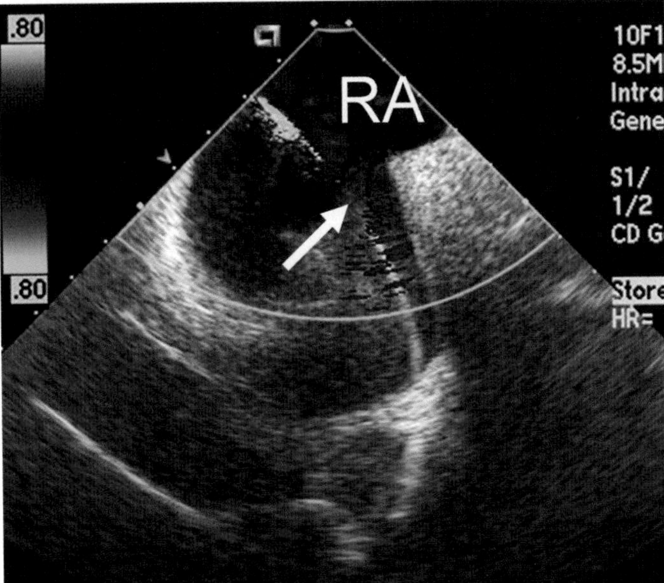

B

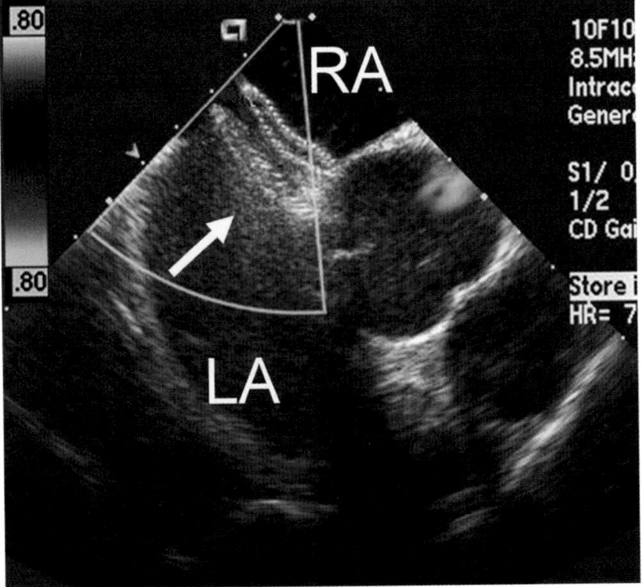

C

Figure 16–10 Transvenous approach to closure of atrial septal defects (ASDs). Patent foreman ovale and secundum ASDs can be closed by deploying a transvenous closure device as an alternative to surgical intervention. (*A*) Self-expanding Amplatzer occlusion device (AGA Medical Corporation, MN) that is made from wires tightly woven into two interconnected disks. The device is deployed from the femoral vein and positioned using transesophageal echocardiography (TEE) or intravascular ultrasound. (*B*) Color-flow Doppler image from an intravascular ultrasound that shows the deployment catheter as it enters through the right atrium (RA) and spans the secundum ASD. (*C*) Color-flow Doppler ultrasound image showing the Amplatzer (arrowhead) in position across the interatrial septum, preventing shunt flow across the ASD.

definitive closure should be based on the following factors: history of neurologic event without a definite etiology, recurrent stroke while receiving anticoagulation, significant shunting through the defect, previous episode of hypoxia that may be related to intracardiac shunting, RV dysfunction, or previous paradoxical embolism.

Management of Previously Undiagnosed Aortic Valve Disease

Framing

A relatively common clinical scenario for the echocardiographer is to assess the significance of previously unrecognized AV pathology. This discussion has pertinence for the echocardiographer faced with the new diagnosis of a bicuspid valve, AS, or insufficiency.

What are the symptoms that brought the patient to medical attention? What is the patient's baseline function? What is the anatomy of the AV? What is the severity of AR, of AS? How do the intraoperative findings of AV disease differ from the preoperative assessment? Would surgical repair or replacement of the AV benefit the patient's short- or long-term outcome? What is the planned procedure, and how would the risks be changed if the procedure was altered to address the new finding? Does another health care provider need to be involved in the decision of whether to surgically address the valve? Is the pathology of the AV significant enough to require surgical intervention at this time?

Data Collection and Characterization of the Aortic Valve

Multiplane TEE permits an accurate assessment of AV area, valvular pathology, severity of regurgitation and stenosis, and detection of secondary cardiac changes. In the case of AS, the severity of valvular dysfunction is determined by measuring the transvalvular pressure gradient, calculating the AV area using the continuity equation, and by planimetry of the AV

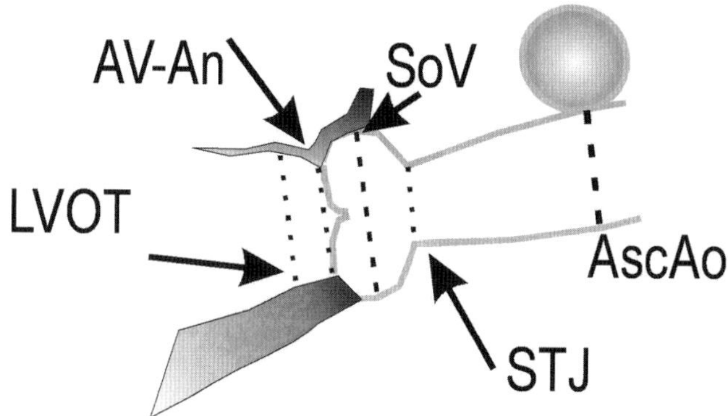

Figure 16–11 Anatomy of the aortic root. This schematic figure of the aortic valve in long axis shows the components of the aortic root, which include sinotubular junction (STJ), sinus of Valsalva (SoV), and the annulus of the aortic valve (AV-An). LVOT = left ventricular outflow tract; AscAo = ascending aorta.

systolic orifice. Planimetry of the AV orifice with TEE is more closely correlated with the catheterization-determined valve area (using the Gorlin formula) than the value derived from TTE ($r = 0.91$ versus 0.84).[65] The severity of AR by TEE is generally graded with color-flow Doppler imaging with measurement of the width of the regurgitant jet relative to the width of the LV outflow tract. TEE is sensitive to even the most trivial amount of AR. Jet areas measured by TEE tend to be larger, and their severity is graded as greater compared with AR assessed by TTE.[66] Determining the clinical significance of AR typically requires assessment of more than just regurgitant grade although severe 4+ AR is never left unaddressed. A more challenging decision is whether to surgically address lesser degrees of AR in patients requiring heart surgery for another reason (see Chapters 12, 20, and 23).

The etiology and extent of AV disease can be best delineated by TEE, as shown in Figure 16–11. The relatively high resolution of the AV and associated structures in the near field of the mid-esophageal short and longitudinal axis views permits an accurate assessment of the severity and mechanism of valvular disease. The aortic leaflets should be inspected in the mid-esophageal long-axis view for the presence of vegetations, perforation, restriction, thickening/calcification, malcoaptation, and leaflet prolapse. The presence of subvalvular disease, such as a discrete fibrous subaortic membrane, can also be reliably excluded. The ascending aorta from the valve to the right pulmonary artery also should be viewed in long axis. This view is usually optimal for examining associated pathology of the aortic root and ascending aorta (e.g., aortoannular ectasia, bicuspid valve, type A aortic dissection).

AS is caused by calcification of the AV and rheumatic heart disease. Bicuspid AVs are at greater risk compared with the general population. AS produces a systolic pressure gradient between the LV and aorta. Secondary findings are dependent on where the patient's condition is along the natural course of the disease. Secondary findings often contribute to the decision-making process, as they infer the effects or consequences of the disease. AS is commonly associated with LV hypertrophy and abnormal filling of the LV. The diastolic function is often impaired due to a thickened, noncompliant LV. Hence, MV and pulmonary vein blood flow velocities would demonstrate a blunted passive filling phase of the ventricle. Systolic function is often normal or hyperdynamic. The LV chamber size is normal or small. However, longstanding AS results in progressive ventricular systolic dysfunction and heart failure. The LV becomes dilated with compromised contractile function. As the ventricle fails, CO decreases with a resultant decrease in trans-AV pressure gradient. Hence, the pressure gradient across an AV may be misleading as a measure for severity of AS.

Bicuspid Aortic Valve

A bicuspid AV is at increased risk of degeneration and calcification, leading to AR and calcific AS. Bicuspid AVs predispose for ascending aortic and arch aneurysm formation, and are associated with an increased incidence of aortic coarctation and ASD. The diagnosis of bicuspid AV prompts the echocardiographer to search for other commonly associated findings. The presence of isolated asymptomatic bicuspid AV without AS or AR does not mandate corrective surgery.

Bicuspid AVs are common in the general population, with an estimated incidence between 0.9% and 2.25%. The natural history of bicuspid valves is variable. Patients can go late into adulthood without AV or aortic disease. Bicuspid AVs can function without major hemodynamic abnormality well into the seventh decade of life.[67] In contrast, a significant percentage of patients experience progressive dilatation of the aortic root, producing AR, or premature calcification of the valve; producing AS.[68-72] For patients in their fourth decade of life, the predominant lesion at surgery is AR. With increasing age, the predominant lesion associated with bicuspid AVs becomes AS.[73] The architectural makeup of the wall of the aorta is abnormal in patients with a bicuspid AV, predisposing for aneurysm formation.[74-77] The decision-making process in regard to surgical correction of a bicuspid AV must account for the size of the aortic root and the likelihood the patient will return for aortic root surgery in the not too distant future. The rate of ascending aortic dilatation in patients with a bicuspid AV may be as high as 0.9 mm/year.[78] Even though patients with a bicuspid AV are at increased risk for cardiac surgery at a later time in life, surgical intervention is not recommended for a bicuspid AV in the absence of aortic root aneurysm, AS, or AR. A normally functioning bicuspid AV may have a longer duration than a bioprosthetic artificial valve. Some centers in North America have adopted a more aggressive stance toward repairing a mildly dilated ascending aorta (≥4-cm diameter) because of the increased risk of acute aortic dissection and ruptures.[79]

The majority of young patients with a bicuspid AV have a regurgitant lesion. If found as an incidental finding, valvular dysfunction is usually minimal, and patients do not have a significantly increased risk of heart failure and death. Although AVR is associated with a low risk of mortality, the lifelong cumulative risk of valve replacement is not insignificant. Mechanical heart valves are associated with low but significant rates of valve thrombosis, thromboembolism, and hemorrhagic complications from lifelong anticoagulation. Biologic prosthetic valves are limited by degeneration of the bioprosthetic material. The use of a homograft or pulmonary autograft provides alternatives for patients who do not want to be or are at high risk for anticoagulation. Bicuspid AVs that can be rendered competent and nonstenotic may be "repaired" in the setting of surgery for aortic dissection or aneurysm. Reconstruction of an isolated, severely regurgitant bicuspid AV has been attempted and described[80-83] but is not in the mainstream of cardiac surgery in the United States due to the risk of recurrent AR. Surgical advances of AV repair have raised the hope of increased valve longevity that rivals or exceeds that of a biologic prosthesis (see Chapter 20).

Natural Course of Aortic Stenosis

The natural course of AS in the adult begins with a prolonged asymptomatic period associated with minimal mortality. Progression of the disease is manifested by a reduction in the valve area and an increase in the transvalvular systolic pressure gradient. The progression is quite variable, exhibiting a decrease in effective valve area ranging from approximately 0.1 to 0.3 cm^2/year. AV calcification, as depicted by echocardiography, has been suggested to be an independent predictor of outcome. Patients with no or mild valvular calcification, compared with those with moderate or severe calcification, had significantly increased rates of event-free survival at 1 and 4 years (92% versus 60% and 75% versus 20%, respectively).[84] Decisions regarding valve replacement for mild or moderate AV disease in the setting of cardiac surgery for another cause are complicated by the variability in the natural progression of the disease. The pathogenesis of AS is an active process having many similarities to the progression of atherosclerosis.[85] AV calcification is not a random degenerative process but an actively regulated disease associated with hypercholesterolemia, inflammation, and osteoblast activity. More aggressive medical control of these processes might be expected to have a positive impact on outcome by retarding the degenerative process. Statin therapy prescribed to older patients with AS was associated with a significantly slower (smaller annualized decrease) decrease in AV area and a slower increase in mean pressure gradient across the AV.[86] The definitive role of such therapies attenuating the progress of AV disease remains unclear but should be forthcoming. If the progression of AV stenosis can be attenuated, the need for AVRs would decrease significantly (see Chapter 20).

Assessment of Mild and Moderate Aortic Stenosis

The intraoperative management of mild to moderate AS at the time of cardiac surgery remains controversial. A patient arrives in the operating room scheduled for a CABG but is discovered to also have mild or moderate AS that was unappreciated preoperatively. The operative team must decide whether to surgically address the AV. The ACC/AHA task force recommends valve replacement at the time of coronary surgery if the asymptomatic patient has severe AS but acknowledges there are very limited data to support intervention in the case of mild or moderate AS. It is in this exact scenario that the rate of progression of AS is of value but it is rarely obtainable. A rapidly calcifying valve in a young patient that is becoming rapidly stenotic would sway the operative team to perform an AVR. A combined double cardiac procedure (CABG/AVR) increases the initial perioperative risk, as well as those risks associated with long-term prosthetic valve implantation. A delay in AVR and commitment to a second heart operation in the future subjects the patient to the risk of a redo sternotomy in the setting of patent coronary grafts and its associated morbidities. If the AV is not operated on during the initial presentation for CABG, the development of symptomatic AS may be quite delayed or may not happen.

A review of 1,344,100 patients in the national database of the Society of Thoracic Surgeons having CABG, CABG/AVR, or AVR alone culminated in a decision paradigm recommendation.[87] The study assumed rates of AV disease progression (pressure gradient of 5 mm Hg/yr), valve-related morbidity, and age-adjusted mortality rates that were obtained from published reports. The authors proposed three factors in the consideration of CABG or AVR/CABG: age (life expectancy), peak pressure gradient, and rate of progression of the AS (if known). Since the latter is difficult to discern, the analysis assumed an average rate of disease progression and recommended patients should undergo AVR/CABG when the pressure gradient exceeds 30 mm Hg. The threshold (AS pressure gradient) to perform both procedures is increased for patients greater than 70 years of age because the reduced life expectancy diminishes the likelihood that they will become symptomatic from the AV disease. Whether to perform a concomitant AVR at the time of revascularization was also addressed by Rahimtoola, who advocated a less aggressive approach.[88] One problem with both studies is that they analyzed the transvalvular pressure gradient, which may be a misleading measure of the degree of stenosis of the AV, as its value is dependent on CO. A low CO and flow rate will produce a low transvalvular pressure gradient, even in the setting of a severely stenotic AV. However, in the setting of preserved ventricular systolic function and mild or moderate AS, a pressure gradient is a useful metric. The variable rate of disease progression and the controversy regarding the indications for "prophylactic" AVR preclude a simple algorithm for dealing with this patient cohort. Increased age, lack of symptoms, minimal LV hypertrophy, with a valve area suggesting milder disease, and a pressure gradient less than 30 mm Hg would sway the decision to not replace the AV. In an asymptomatic young patient, a severely calcified valve, bicuspid valve, and LV hypertrophy in the setting of moderate stenosis, and a pressure gradient greater than 30 mm Hg would suggest that an AVR might be beneficial in the long term. It is often useful to include the patient's primary cardiologist and family in the decision-making process.

Assessment of Low Pressure Gradient Aortic Stenosis

Patients with LV dysfunction and decreased CO in the setting of AS often present with only modest transvalvular pressure gradients (less than 30 mm Hg). Distinguishing patients with a low CO and severe AS from patients with mild to moderate AS can be challenging (Fig. 16–12). The standard for assessing severity of AS is AV area, typically calculated using either a continuity method or by planimetry. Patients with low-gradient AS with severe LV dysfunction who received an AVR had improved survival and functional status compared with patients who did not have a valve replacement.[89-91]

A low pressure gradient related to LV dysfunction may not open the AV to its maximum capacity. Dobutamine challenge in a patient with low pressure gradient AS can be useful in establishing true AV area. The ability to distinguish between true AV stenosis and a state of "pseudostenosis" relies upon characteristic changes in hemodynamic and structural measurements in response to the augmented CO. The test is not typically performed in the operative setting, but rather as a preoperative evaluation. The increase in calculated AV area is related to the increase in the CO, and is attributed to partial reversal of primary cardiac dysfunction.[92-95] If dobutamine improves CO and increases AV area, it is likely the baseline calculations overestimated the severity of the AS. The dobutamine challenge is conducted as follows: patients with low-gradient AS receive intravenous dobutamine at 5 μg/kg/min with stepwise increases in dose.[93] Patients may exhibit a significant increase in AV area (0.8 cm^2 to 1.1 cm^2)

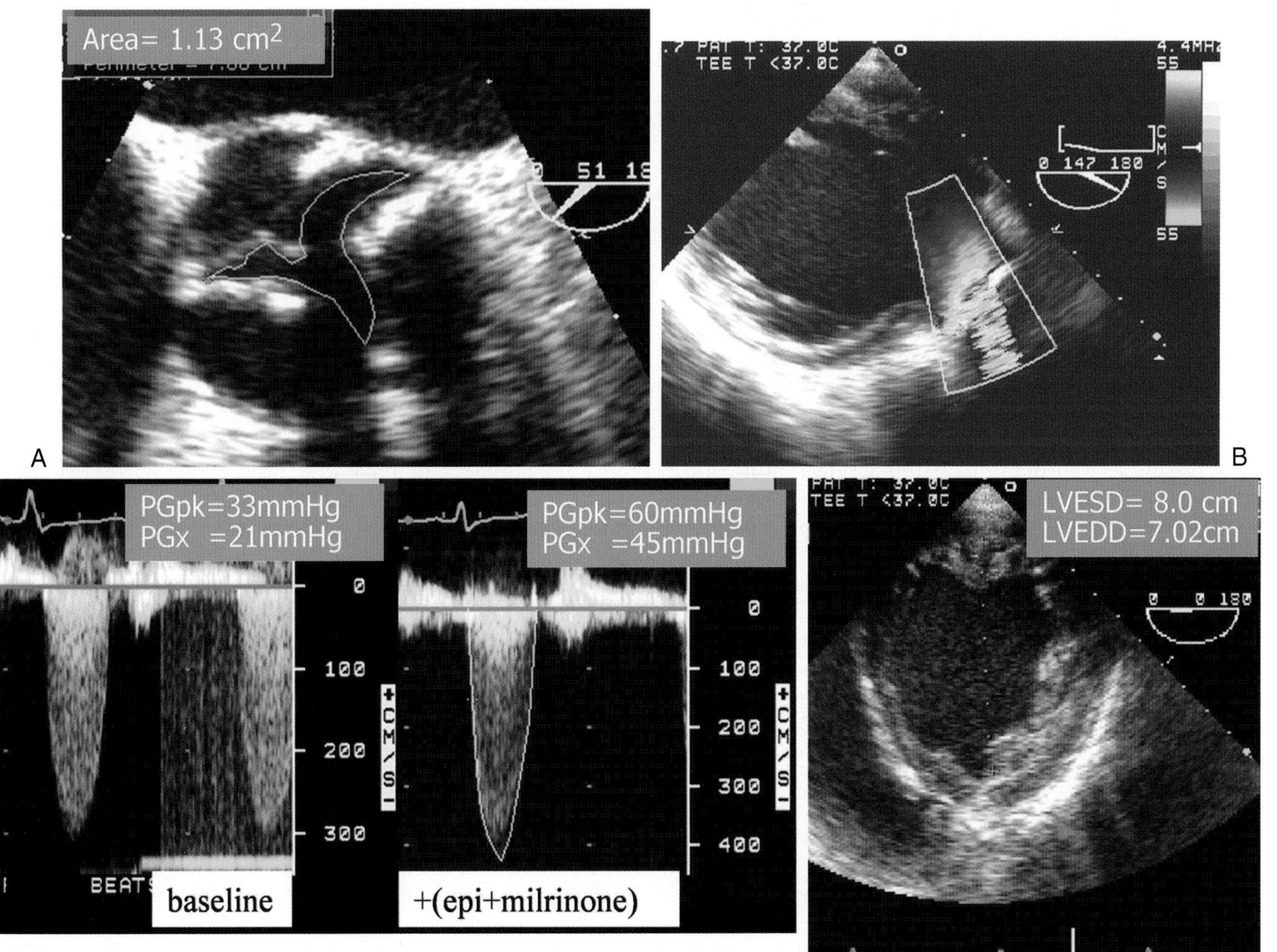

Figure 16–12 Low pressure gradient severe aortic stenosis. A 76-year-old cachetic man was scheduled to undergo corrective surgery for severe mitral regurgitation (MR) and possibly clinically significant aortic stenosis (AS). The mid-esophageal short-axis view of the aortic valve (AV) showed a highly calcified trileaflet valve with restricted mobility (*A*). The measurement of AV area, 1.13 cm^2, which was obtained by planimetry, was believed to underestimate the severity of AS because of the shadowing artifacts related to the severity of calcification. The transgastric long axis of the left ventricle (LV) was obtained (*B*), and the velocity profiles of blood flow within the LV outflow tract and the AV were measured. Although the patient had a diagnosis of severe AS, the maximal and mean pressure gradients were 33 mm Hg and 21 mm Hg, respectively (*C*). The area of the AV was calculated to be 0.83 cm^2 using the continuity equation. The LV function was characterized by a severe dilated cardiomyopathy with an ejection fraction of 8%, LVESD of 7 cm, and LVEDD of 8 cm (*D*). The diagnosis of low pressure gradient AS was considered, and infusions of epinephrine and milrinone were started. Cardiac performance improved from 2.4 L/min to 4.5 L/min, and the pressured gradients increased to 60 mm Hg, peak, and 41 mm Hg, mean (*C*). Although the calculated valve area that was recorded under conditions of inotrope support slightly increased to 0.9 cm^2, transesophageal echocardiography (TEE) clarified that the marked increase in the pressure gradient was consistent with a diagnosis of low-gradient AS and confirmed the presence of cardiac reserve.

and a decline in valve resistance after dobutamine challenge. Patients with fixed, high-grade AS would demonstrate no change in valve area and an increase in valve resistance. The 2003 ACC/AHA/ASE Task Force gave a class IIb recommendation (usefulness/efficacy is less well established by evidence/opinion) for the use of dobutamine echocardiography in the evaluation of patients with low-gradient AS and ventricular dysfunction.[96] In addition to its role in distinguishing between true stenosis and pseudostenosis, low-dose dobutamine echocardiography is helpful in risk stratifying of patients with severe true AS. Patients with augmented contractile function after dobutamine administration have an improved outcome after surgery.[97,98]

Aortic Regurgitation: Natural Course and Management

Many elderly patients undergoing cardiac surgery will have some degree of AR. In most cases, the patients are asymptomatic and the severity is graded as trace to mild. The presence of AR has implications regarding the conduct of circulatory management, administration of cardioplegia, management of hemodynamics, and possible alteration of the surgical plan. The presence of AR obligates the echocardiographer to monitor for distention of the LV during CPB and cardiac arrest, and during the administration of antegrade cardioplegia. Upon release of the aortic cross-clamp, the heart may not instantaneously revert to an organized rhythm, precluding ejection of LV blood and predisposing for ventricular distention. The latter is particularly problematic in the setting of AR. The decision of whether to surgically address the valvular dysfunction should not be based on LV distention during CPB but should be considered in the context of the data set that includes the natural history of AR in adults, established guidelines and published outcomes, in addition to individual patient variables as previously described.

Chronic AR generally evolves in a slow and insidious manner with a very low morbidity during a long asymptomatic phase. Some patients with mild AR may remain asymptomatic for decades. Others exhibit progressive worsening of the regurgitant lesion and develop LV systolic dysfunction, leading eventually to heart failure. Evaluation of LV size and function is important because of the poor correlation between symptoms and severity of cardiac pathology. The nature of the transition between the compensated and uncompensated periods is poorly understood. Clinicians should be reluctant to consider valve replacement in an asymptomatic patient with preserved LV function (Fig. 16–13). Early surgery exposes the patient to perioperative mortality and morbidity, and to the long-term complications of a prosthetic valve. Guidelines for AV surgery in patients with AR were published in 1998 by the ACC/AHA Task Force, and in 2002 by the Working Group on Valvular Heart Disease of the European Society of Cardiology.[99,100] AVR is clearly indicated for symptomatic patients with chronic AR and LV dysfunction. However, the decision to perform valve replacement is less apparent for asymptomatic patients. The published recommendations suggest serial examinations to detect the progression of LV dysfunction. In a strategy similar to that applied for patients with low-gradient AS, the induction of stress exercise testing may be helpful for assessing functional capacity and timing of surgery. However, intraoperative detection of occult AR does not provide for the luxury of serial examinations.

The intraoperative decision for asymptomatic patients should be based on the severity of AR and the presence of LV dysfunction. Patients with an LV end-systolic dimension less than 50 mm would be expected to remain asymptomatic for the next few years; the risk of developing symptoms or LV dysfunction would range from 1% to 2% per year to as high as 6% per year.[101,102] However, the yearly rate of becoming symptomatic or developing significant LV dysfunction increases to greater than 20% when the LV end-systolic dimension exceeds 50 mm.[101,103]

Choice of Surgical Intervention

Framing

Once the decision to surgically intervene has been established, the echocardiographer can have a valuable role in assisting the surgeon in formulating and implementing the intended change of plans for surgical management.

What information would be required for the surgeon to determine whether surgical valve repair or valve replacement is more appropriate? Is the choice of surgical intervention limited by surgical experience or prosthesis availability? What type of valve prosthesis is most appropriate for this patient in these circumstances? What size of valve prosthesis can be inserted? Could valve replacement have unintended consequences that could be prevented or detected and treated?

Data Collection

The choice of specific intervention, whether to repair or to replace the valve, will depend on pathology of the diseased valve, experience of the surgical team, and discussion between the surgeon and the cardiologist, in addition to patient variables. The echocardiographer can best contribute to the surgeon's understanding of the pathogenesis of AV disease by assessing function and structure in the short- and long-axis imaging planes. The surgeon is provided with a complete anatomic echocardiographic assessment of the AV and root, including dimensions of the annulus, sinus of Valsalva and sinotubular junction, leaflet anatomy, primary mechanism of regurgitation, and severity of thickening/calcification.

Discussion

The development of reparative procedures for the AV has lagged behind those implemented for the MV or for the development of prosthetic devices. Some of the major factors are the apparently irreversible changes produced by calcification of the cusps, the retraction of cusp tissue in AR, and the lack of durable biological material suitable for supplementing the valvular apparatus. It is unlikely that surgical repair of stenotic and highly calcified valves will achieve much success within the near future. However, aortic valvular repair has been successfully applied for the resuspension of the AV to correct acute AR resulting from an aortic dissection. Yacoub, Cohn, and others report improved short- and long-term results for minimizing residual AR and freedom from reoperation.[104-106]

A diseased valve characterized by thickened, calcified leaflets and having restricted mobility is not a candidate for valve repair, and would require valve replacement. Alternatively, remodeling of the aortic root and AV to improve the geometry of the tricuspid AV has been successfully used in cases of acute type A aortic dissection. In addition, a select cohort of patients having AR as the primary valvular diagnosis may be candidates for surgical repair. In the case of bicuspid AVs or isolated AR, successful repair of the AV was more likely when the anatomy demonstrated left coronary/right coronary cusp fusion and when the primary mechanism of AR was leaflet prolapse or commissural separation, compared with poor leaflet coaptation of a "central defect."[104] Although a complete review of the technical aspects and controversy of AV-sparing surgeries are beyond the scope of this chapter, it should be noted that aortic dilatation has a negative prognostic implication for successful long-term outcome. A more detailed discussion of surgical repair of the AV can be found in Chapter 20 and in literature reviews.[105,106]

Valve repair and replacement surgery for patients having symptomatic valve disease have been heralded as significant successes. Advances in surgical technique and perioperative care have enabled the morbidity and mortality of valve replacement to decrease despite the increasing proportion of high-risk patients. The choice of prosthetic heart valve replacement is generally based on patient age, size, and wishes[107] (Fig. 16–14). A joint decision with the patient, the cardiologist, and the cardiac surgeon is indicated before surgery.

Compared with nature's own heart valves, prosthetic valves are relatively stenotic. Prosthetic valves are sized based on their external diameter even though their transvalvular gradient reflects the internal diameter and orifice size. Each valve has an "effective orifice area" (EOA) that is based on in vitro studies performed by the manufacturer. The clinical impor-

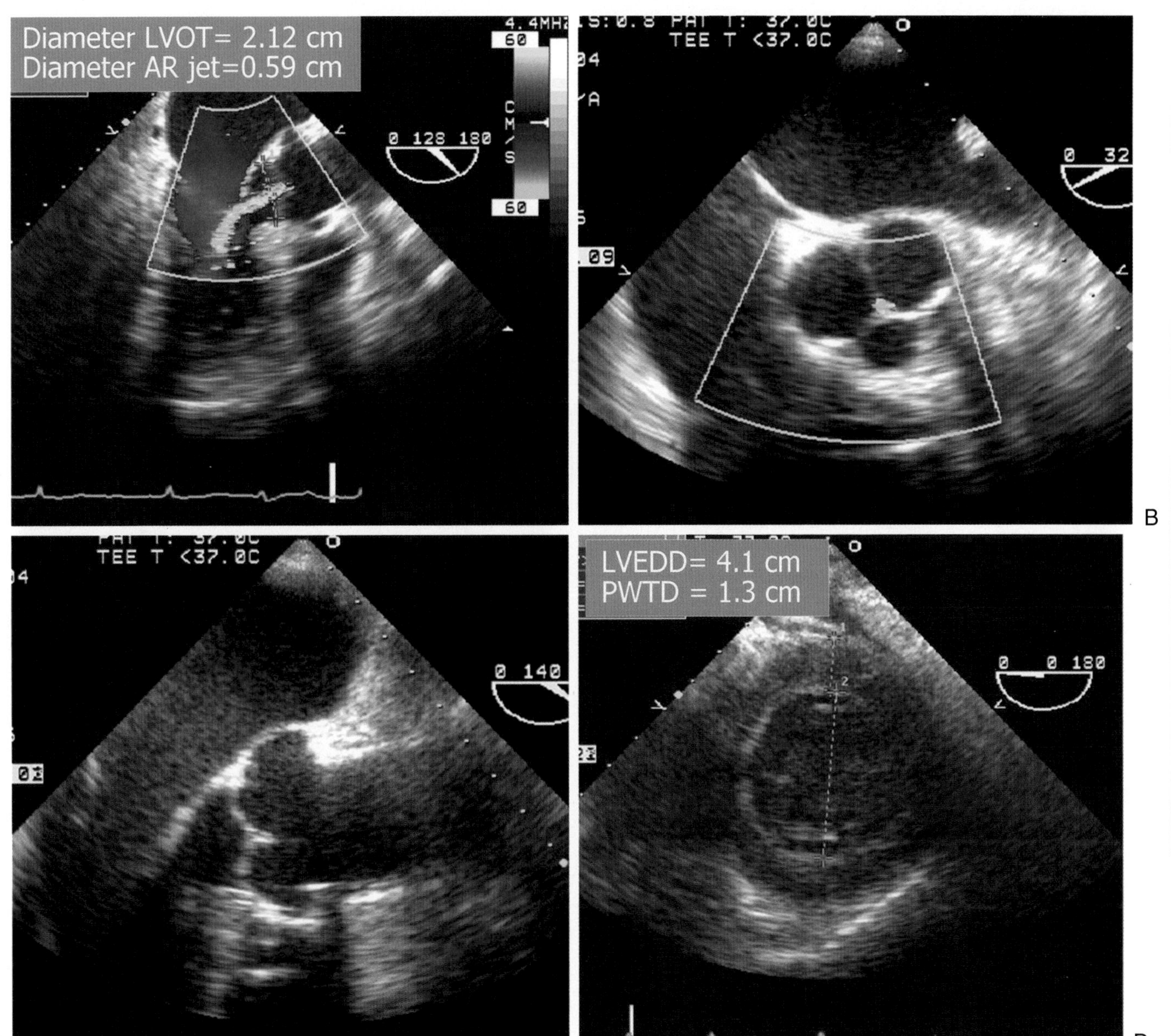

Figure 16–13 Detection of occult aortic regurgitation (AR) during nonvalvular cardiac surgery. A 66-year-old woman was scheduled to undergo coronary artery bypass grafting using extracorporeal circulatory support. An intraoperative transesophageal echocardiography (TEE) examination diagnosed presence of a central AR jet that extended halfway into the left ventricle (LV). The severity of AR, which was graded as mild, was based on assessing the retrograde flow in the LV outflow tract using color-flow Doppler imaging in mid-esophageal long-axis plane. The severity of AR is determined by comparing the width of the AR jet, 0.59 cm, to the diameter of the LV outflow tract, 2.12 cm; the ratio of 0.28 is graded as mild (*A*). The anatomy of the valve was that of a normal trileaflet structure with mildly thickened leaflets (*A, B*). No leaflet prolapse, vegetations, or annular/root dilation was present. In addition, no significant aortic stenosis was detected by Doppler or calcification of the leaflets. LV chamber size was normal, LVEDD was 4.14 cm, and presence of LV hypertrophy was consistent with hypertension (*C*). Because the severity of AR was not clinically significant and it was not expected to markedly increase, surgical intervention to the aortic valve was deferred. However, the diagnosis of AR altered circulatory management by increasing the vigilance of the echocardiographer to monitor LV chamber size during antegrade cardioplegia and initiating supplemental retrograde cardioplegia.

tance of the disparity between prosthesis annular size and EOA becomes evident when relatively small prosthetic valves are inserted into comparatively large patients. Prosthetic valve/patient mismatch results when transvalvular flow through a prosthetic valve is limited and produces clinically significant stenosis (Fig. 16–15). The increase in transvalvular blood flow velocity necessary to accommodate and sustain an acceptable SV in a large patient with a prosthetic AV can produce surprisingly high transvalvular pressure gradients.

An objective of valve replacement surgery is to provide the patient with the largest effective orifice area. Prosthetic valve mismatch is more likely to occur in older patients, those with increased body surface area (BSA), smaller prosthetic valve size, and preoperative diagnosis of valvular stenosis.[108] The incidence of AV mismatch increases with prosthetic annular size less than 21 mm. In larger patients, mismatch can occur in patients receiving prosthetic AVs greater than 21 mm because dominant factors in determining the pressure gradi-

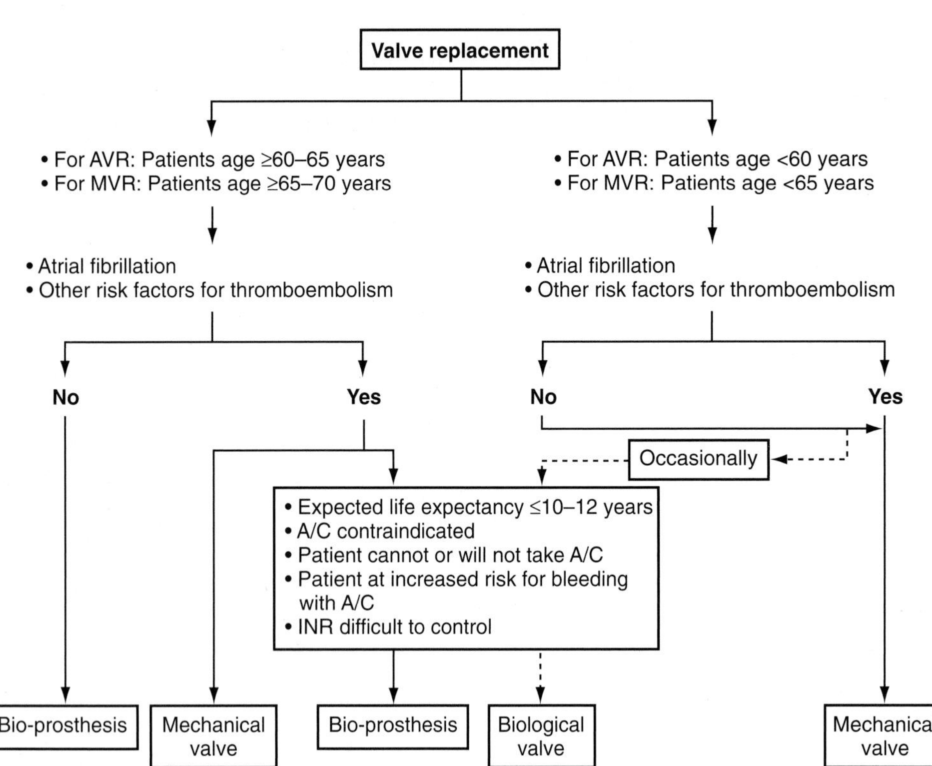

Figure 16–14 An algorithm for choice of prosthetic heart valve. A/C = anticoagulation; AVR = aortic valve replacement; INR = international normalized ratio; MVR = mitral valve replacement. (Redrawn from Figure 8 from Rahimtoola, 2003.[107])

ent are the SV and CO which are related to body size and level of activity. The association of mismatch with stenotic native AVs is a result of calcified native valves, a calcified annulus, and a smaller annular size. The treatment of AS through AVR in the setting of preserved ventricular systolic function may result in dramatic increases in SV and CO. The resultant increase in transvalvular flow produces a large transprosthetic pressure gradient. In contrast, valvular insufficiency is usually associated with annular dilatation and decreased systolic function. Hence, patients with annuloectasia often receive larger prosthetic valves implanted and functional AS post-AVR is rarely a problem.

Increased postoperative transvalvular gradients have been implicated in increasing long-term morbidity and mortality.[109-111] The short-term clinical significance of prosthetic valve size mismatch is controversial and may be associated with immediate postoperative risk of cardiovascular complications and mortality. Controversy stems in part from studies with limited sample populations and the failure to normalize specific valvular EOA to a metric of patient size. Nonetheless, the concept of prosthetic valve mismatch adversely affecting outcome is generally accepted. The long-term risk of prosthetic valve mismatch is inability to restore or improve functional capacity. A consequence of an increased residual transvalvular pressure gradient is to prevent or attenuate regression of LV hypertrophy.[112] LV hypertrophy is associated with diastolic dysfunction, decreased exercise capacity, and a predictor of increased mortality. Significant differences in regression of LV hypertrophy occur in patients who received prosthetic AVs larger than 21 mm (−21%) compared with patients with prosthetic valves that were less than 21 mm (−8%).[112,113] Hence, it would be expected that a corresponding difference in functional capacity would parallel these differences in hypertrophy regression. A decreased indexed EOA (EOA/BSA = cm^2/m^2) was an independent predictor of long-term morbidity following aortic and MV replacement.[114]

In general, an indexed effective orifice area for a prosthetic AV should be greater than 0.85 cm^2/m^2.[114] For a similar external rim size, the EOA can vary considerably between mechanical and bioprosthetic AVs and by manufacturer. Bioprosthetic valves tend to have a significantly larger EOA compared with mechanical valves. Biologic aortic roots have even larger effective orifice areas. If the anatomy of the aortic root precludes implantation of a suitably sized prosthesis, the surgeon may perform a supra-annular implantation, allowing the placement of a larger valve. Alternatively, creation of a larger effective orifice area may require enlargement of the aortic root, a biologic aortic root, a pulmonic valve autograft (Ross procedure), or implantation of a stentless valve (see Chapters 20 and 23).

Aortic Valve: Concomitant Mitral Regurgitation

Framing

Valvular diseases do not often occur in isolation. Other anatomic structures may be influenced, either by the same pathophysiology or as a secondary consequence of the primary valvular lesion. Mitral insufficiency is a common finding, occurring in about two-thirds of the patients having significant AS.[115] Patients presenting for AVR commonly have MR and pose the question of whether to repair or replace the MV in addition to the AV (Fig. 16–16). Such an undertaking is not without risk. Patients undergoing double-valve replacement have increased mortality compared with isolated AVR.

Should moderate MR be surgically addressed in patients undergoing AVR for AS? Does the severity of MR regress after AVR? Does the presence of AR in patients with severe AS alter the expected prognosis of the regression of MR after AVR? Can it be predicted which cohort of patients with AS would benefit from concomitant MV repair? In which patient cohort

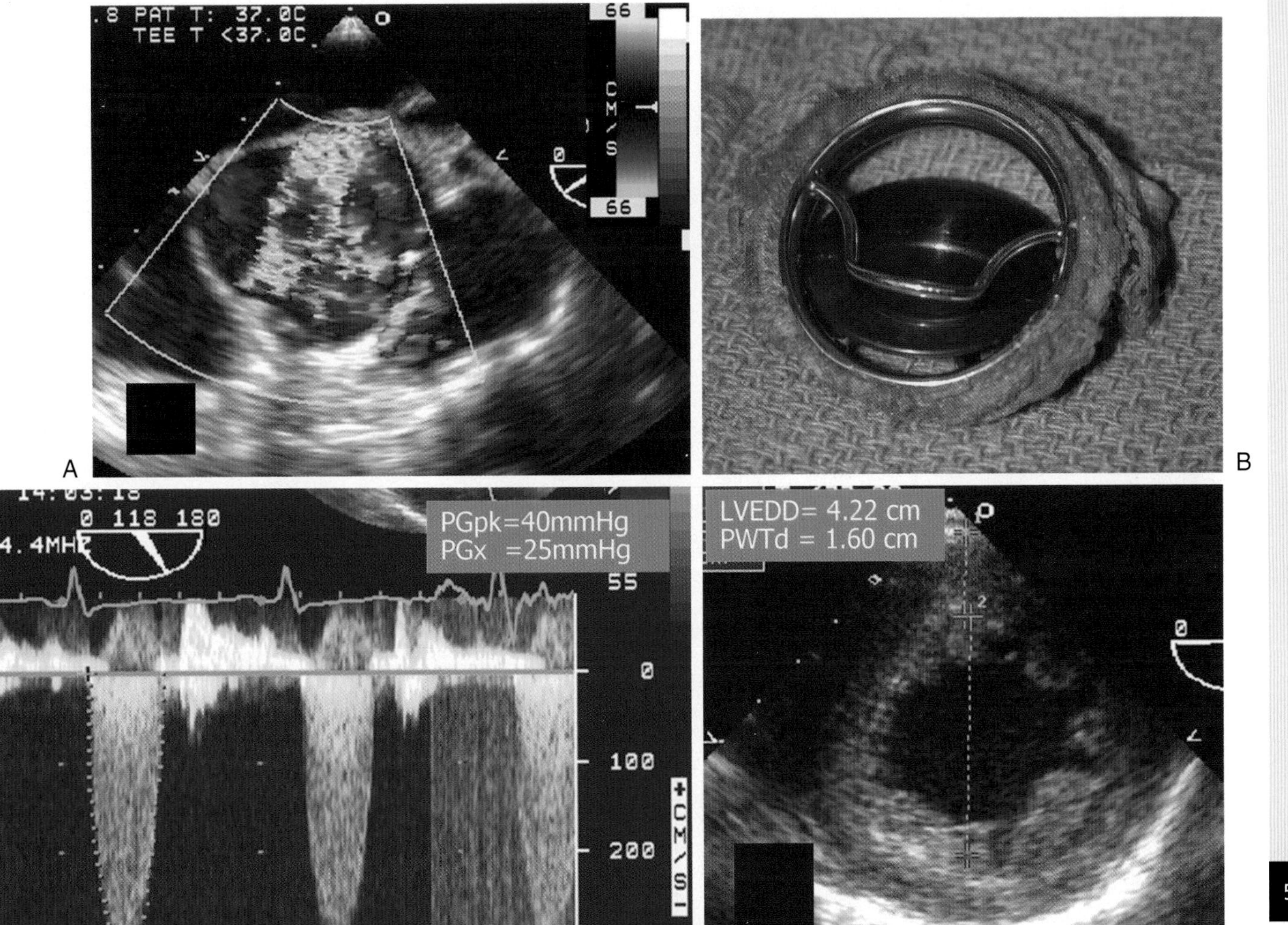

Figure 16–15 Detection of a significant transvalvular pressure gradient across a previously implanted prosthetic aortic valve (AV). Patient who underwent a previous AV replacement (AVR) was now scheduled for coronary artery bypass grafting and possible AVR for aortic stenosis. The preoperative evaluation included an echocardiogram that demonstrated a small paravalvular leak and blood cultures that were negative. (*A*) Color-flow Doppler image of the AV in mid-esophageal short-axis imaging plane that shows turbid flow from the orifice of the 19-mm Bjork-Shiley mechanical valve. The aortic annulus and other valves were inspected for evidence of active infection or abscess, but none was found. The clinical decision was to replace the AV or repair the paravalvular leak. The prosthetic valve appeared to be functioning normally aside from a small paravalvular leak. The intraoperative transesophageal echocardiography (TEE) examination documented preserved left ventricular (LV) systolic function and significant LV hypertrophy with a posterior wall thickness of 1.6 cm. Examination of the mechanical prosthetic valve showed a well-seated valve with a small paravalvular leak at the fibromuscular continuity and the absence of any abscess or vegetations (*B*). Although the valve appeared to be functioning normally, the transvalvular pressure gradient was 40 mm Hg in the absence of any outflow tract obstruction (*C, D*). The presence of a significant gradient in a normally functioning valve and presence of significant LV hypertrophy raised the possibility of valve mismatch; the small paravalvular leak was determined not to significantly contribute to the transvalvular gradient. The patient was an active 64-year-old man who weighed 98 kg and had a body surface area of 2.2 mm^2. The presence of a significant transvalvular gradient across an apparently normally functioning valve in a large patient supported the diagnosis of prosthetic valve mismatch. The patient underwent a root replacement (No. 23) and had a transvalvular pressure gradient of 14 mm Hg.

would the MR be expected to regress with the unloading effects of replacing a stenotic AV?

Data Collection

The most important data for these decisions are the grade of MR, AV area, and anatomy of the MV. Patients are likely to have the signs and symptoms of AS and MR and pulmonary hypertension. The grade of MR is often not evident until a TEE is performed and may be underestimated by a preoperative transthoracic examination. An enlarged LA suggests the MR is not acute.

Discussion

MR is a maladaptive consequence of increasing AS. More significant MR is associated with greater trans-AV pressure gradients as well as more progressive dilation and worsening systolic function.[116,117] If MV anatomy is markedly abnormal and the severity of regurgitation is severe, the decision is relatively obvious: MV repair or replacement at the time of AVR. If the MV is anatomically normal (no leaflet prolapse, no perforation, no rheumatic changes) and the regurgitation is trace or mild, the decision is also relatively obvious: correct the AS and do not surgically address the MV. In the setting of

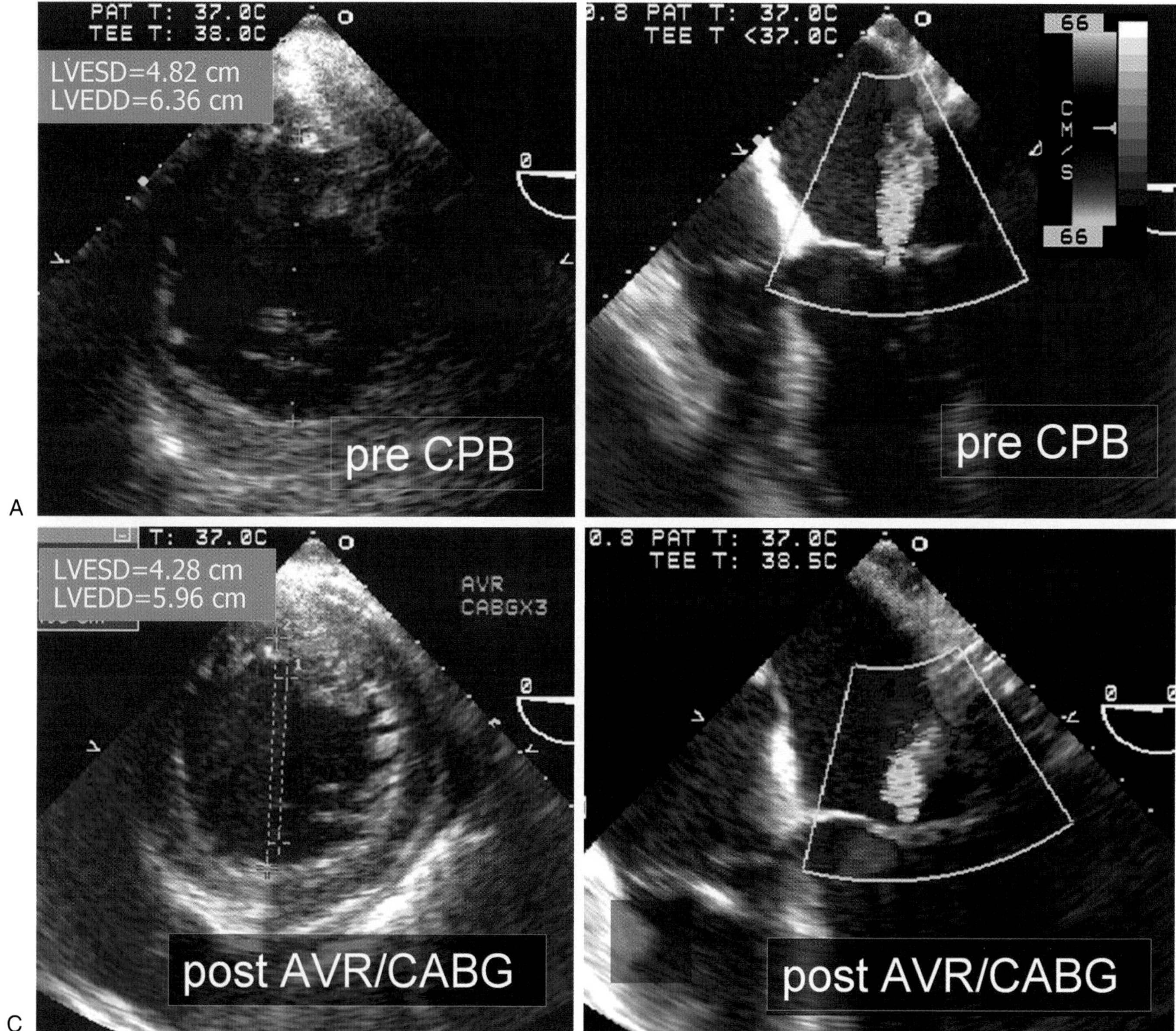

Figure 16–16 Management of concurrent mitral regurgitation (MR) in a patient undergoing aortic valve replacement (AVR) for aortic stenosis (AS). The patient is a 70-year-old who underwent an AVR for critical AS. The patient had history of hypertension, moderate MR, congestive failure, and episodes of shortness of breath. Left ventricular function was moderately depressed and the chamber size was dilated (LVEDD = 6.36 cm) (*A*). (*B*) The patient had a central jet of MR that was graded as mild; the annulus was mildly dilated; and the pathology of the leaflets and apparatus was only mildly thickened. The pulmonary vein blood flow showed minimal blunting of the systolic component, consistent with increased left atrial pressures but not clinically significant MR. The discrepancy in the severity of MR between the preoperative study and intraoperative transesophageal echocardiogram (TEE) reflects the effect of general anesthesia upon loading conditions. After reviewing the prebypass TEE examination and the patient's history, it was decided to perform only an AVR. A bioprosthetic valve was chosen by the surgeon because of the patient's age, thus eliminating the requirement for anticoagulation. Because the MR was believed to be more functional, the replacement of the severely stenotic AV, the major pathologic lesion, was anticipated to decrease MR over time. The choice of implanting a No. 23 pericardial prosthetic valve was based on the annular size that was measured before initiation of bypass. The postbypass TEE examination documented that the gradient across the AV decreased from 74 mm Hg to 18 mm Hg and that cardiac function (*C*) and MR (*D*) improved after AVR.

rheumatic AS, it is common to have other valves involved in the disease process. Hence, mitral calcification, thickening, and leaflet fusion are common in patients with rheumatic AS. The MV is rarely replaced based on anatomic abnormality alone in the absence of significant stenosis or regurgitation.

The more controversial decision is whether to surgically address the MV that has mild to moderate regurgitation when a patient presents for AVR for AS. There is neither an absolute answer nor consensus. The uncertainty of the decision is based on the unpredictability of the residual MR after the AV is replaced. If the grade of MR of moderate or severe were expected to be reduced to mild, the operative team might elect not to operate on the MV. A confounding factor is the grade of MR during general anesthesia may be underestimated and not reflect the grade during the awake or exercising state. Furthermore, the lasting effects of replacing an AV in the setting of MR are not established immediately after CPB. The heart undergoes significant change after AVR for AS, including changes in pressure-volume relationships of the LV, transmitral pressure gradients, and LV remodeling.

MR with an anatomically normal MV is referred to as "functional MR." Increased LV afterload, driving pressure, and LV remodeling have been implicated in the development of functional MR in patients with severe AS. The natural history and clinical impact of mild to moderate MR in patients undergoing AVR for AS suggest that concurrent MV surgery may not be warranted in all cases. In the cohort of patients with functional MR and severe AS, the decrease in MR after AVR alone was variable; between 39% and 90% of patients having moderate MR experienced a regression in its severity following AVR.[118-123] In general, patients with functional MR of moderate grade had significant improvement (decrease) in the MR after AVR, suggesting leaving the MV alone in this setting is not unreasonable. Conversely, a significant number of patients, between 8% and 64%, had either no change or an increase in MR severity. In a study of 196 patients who had concomitant MR, Moazami[122] noted a decrease in 3-year survival for those patients whose moderate to severe MR persisted after AVR and recommended surgical intervention for this cohort of patients.

In general, functional MR of moderate severity will usually regress at least one grade after AVR for severe AS (see Fig. 16–16). Mild to moderate MR that improves after AVR for AS seems to be a lasting phenomenon.[118] Unfortunately, there has been little control for the severity of concurrent AR, which is a common finding associated with AS. Although the physiologic load of patients with combined AS and AR is different, the particular pathology of the AV did not affect regression of MR after AVR.[122] Harris et al[121] ascribed the decrease in the severity of MR after AVR to several anatomic changes: decreases in mitral annular area, LA size, and LV length. Along with the decrease in driving pressure that occurs with resolution of AS, all three of these anatomic changes alter the architecture of the MV and ventricle and contribute to decreasing functional MR. The greater the decrease in systolic area and increase in fractional area change of the LV post-AVR, the greater is the reduction in postoperative MR.[121]

It is difficult to define the negative predictors for the regression of MR after AVR. The presence of valvular abnormalities, such as leaflet thickening, calcification or prolapse, and chordal pathology that could contribute to a "nonfunctional" cause of MR would most likely persist. Mitral annular calcification is a potential complicating factor and its impact is unclear. Annular calcification would be expected to impede the reduction in MV area that normally occurs during systole. This reduction appears to be important in the mechanism of MR reduction after AVR for AS. Likewise, mitral annular calcification renders mitral surgery more difficult and the implantation of a mitral prosthesis more problematic, likely increasing the risk of paravalvular leak and AV groove disruption. Many patients with severe AS have a calcified AV with concomitant MV annular calcification. Mitral annular calcifications may be predictive of fixed MR post-AVR.[124] Ischemic MR may improve after revascularization as a more favorable balance of myocardial oxygen supply/demand is produced after AVR.[119,125] "Functional" MR of moderate to severe grade that is not operated on during AVR may remain unchanged after AVR and require reinstitution of CPB for MV surgery. In the absence of more predictable criteria to define this group, patients with moderate to severe MR caused by intrinsic valvular pathology should be considered for surgical intervention. Reports suggest that AVR combined with MV repair can be accomplished with excellent long-term results and minimal effect on mortality.[119]

Ascending Aorta, a Source of Embolization

Framing

The most disabling complication following cardiac surgery is stroke. Major focal and nonfocal neurologic deficits, cognitive decline, and coma following surgery are common. The pathogenesis of cerebral damage is multifactorial with embolism considered a major contributor. Other factors include hypotension, low flow, reperfusion injury, and inflammation. Embolic events are strongly associated with the severity of atherosclerotic disease characterized by plaque thickness of greater than 4 mm, ulcerated plaques, and mobile protruding plaques in the aorta.[126,127] The severity of atherosclerosis of the descending aorta, as determined by TEE, is a significant risk factor and an independent predictor of adverse cardiac and neurologic outcome in patients undergoing CABG.[128] Surgical manipulation of the thoracic aorta may liberate debris from diseased aortic tissue. The process of microembolization has been detected by transcranial Doppler during aortic cannulation, application and removal of the aortic cross-clamp, commencement of bypass, and initiation of ventricular ejection. The clinical consequence of distal embolization is dependent on the number, composition (e.g., air bubbles, fat particles, platelet aggregates, and calcium deposits), size, and location of the emboli (see Chapters 15, 17, 19, 20, 23, 28, 30, and 35).

Is the patient at increased risk of postoperative neurologic dysfunction? Would epiaortic ultrasound or TEE improve detection of significant atheromatous disease? What modifications to the conduct of the general anesthesia, monitoring, CPB or cardiac surgery could be implemented in a risk reduction effort? Is epiaortic scanning necessary?

Data Collection

TEE imaging of the anterior wall of the ascending aorta is limited by far field imaging resolution and its juxtaposition to air in the open chest. Imaging of the mid and distal ascending aorta by TEE is limited by the interposition of the airway with the esophagus and aorta. Epiaortic ultrasound can provide high-definition imaging of these otherwise hidden portions of the aorta. Epiaortic scanning offers higher sensitivity for detection of atheroma of the ascending aorta, as compared with TEE, especially in the mid and distal segments.[3,129] The descending aorta is immediately adjacent to the esophagus and easily imaged using conventional TEE. A common practice is the interrogation of the descending thoracic aorta for high-grade atheroma. In the absence of atheromatous disease in the descending aorta, the ascending aorta and locus of aortic cannulation are significantly less likely to have high-grade disease. If the descending aorta contains high-grade or mobile atheroma, it may be prudent to examine the ascending aorta with epiaortic scanning for potential sites for aortic cannulation and clamping (Fig. 16–17).

Discussion

Historically, surgeons palpate the ascending aorta to determine the extent of intraluminal atherosclerotic disease in an effort to choose an appropriate location for cannulation, cross-clamping, and proximal graft anastomosis. However, palpation is a notoriously poor predictor of atheromatous disease.[130-132] The occurrence of atheroma in the ascending aorta of cardiac surgery patients may be as high as 60% to 90%.[131,133] Advanced age, hypertension, and diabetes are risk

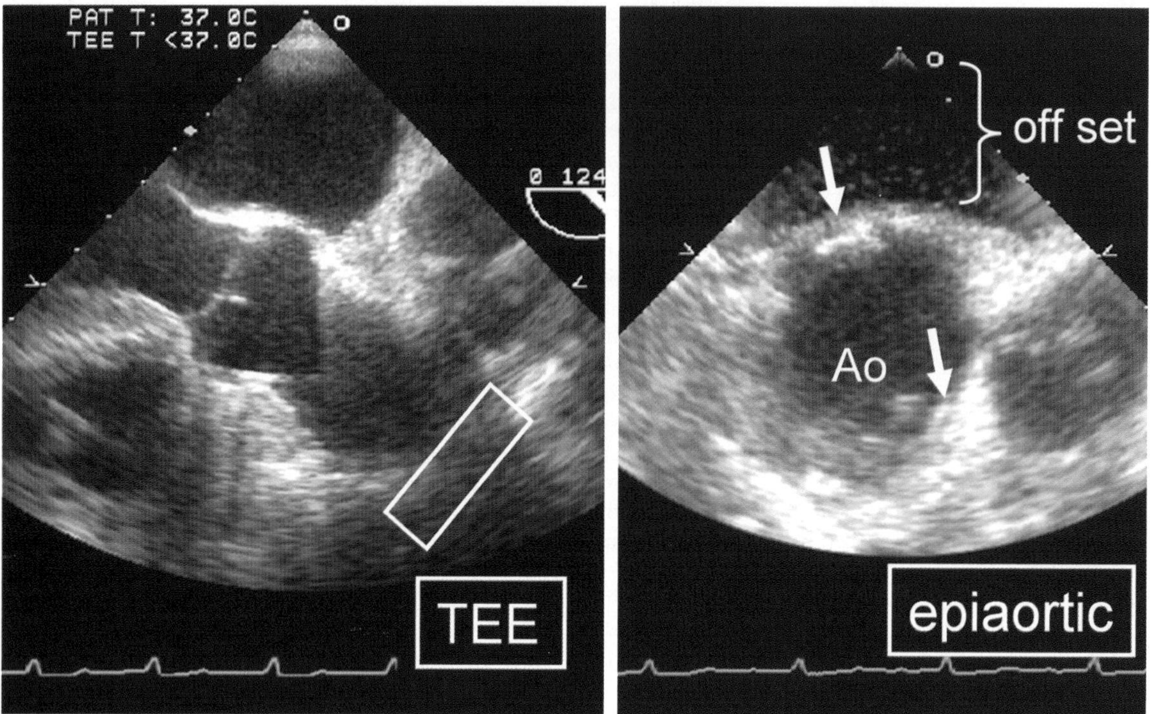

Figure 16–17 Detection of atheromatous plaque by epiaortic ultrasound. A 67-year-old patient was scheduled to undergo coronary artery bypass grafting × 3. The transesophageal echocardiography (TEE) examination was performed to evaluate the mitral valve for mitral regurgitation that might necessitate surgical intervention. Routine examination of the descending thoracic aorta detected severe atherosclerotic disease characterized by several ulcerated areas and plaques with a thickness of 4 mm. Because the severity of atherosclerotic disease in the descending aorta predicts significant disease in the ascending aorta,[128] examination of the ascending aorta was attempted. TEE examination of the ascending aorta at the site of aortic cross-clamp and cannulation (designated by the *white rectangle*) was limited by poor resolution in the far field and interposition of the trachea (*A*). A handheld probe that was placed in a sterile sleeve was used to examine the aorta (*B*). The bottom of the sleeve was filled with saline as an offset to better image the anterior surface of the aorta (Ao). Several calcified plaques, as designated by the *arrows*, were detected. Based on findings of the epiaortic scanning, the surgeon modified the site of cannulation and used a single cross-clamp technique to avoid a second clamping of the aorta during the proximal anastomosis.

factors for atheromatous disease of the aorta and stroke after heart surgery.[3,134] The information provided by ultrasound imaging of the aorta defines the location and severity of atheromatous disease, which can guide the surgeon to more strategically choose the cannulation, cross-clamp, and anastomotic sites.

Possible modifications to the conduct of cardiac surgery and bypass include (1) altering the site of cannulation, (2) aborting CPB altogether and performing the CABG surgery as an off-bypass procedure, (3) performing the surgery on a fibrillating heart without aortic cross-clamping, (4) performing aortic atherectomy or replacement of the ascending aorta, or (5) attempting a "no touch" technique using deep hypothermic circulatory arrest. Epiaortic scanning combined with modification of surgery techniques in patients undergoing CABG decreased the number of emboli as detected by transcranial Doppler and significantly reduced neurologic behavioral changes at 1 week and 1 month after surgery.[135] Modifications in the methods used in CABG revascularization, including the avoidance of proximal aortic graft anastomoses after detection of atheroma by echocardiography, resulted in a lower incidence of late neurologic complications.[2] Although somewhat counterintuitive, late neurologic dysfunction appears to also be related to increased number of microemboli that were detected by transcranial Doppler imaging during the operative period and aortic manipulation.

The application of epiaortic scanning for all patients undergoing cardiac surgery is controversial. Epiaortic scanning takes time and expertise in its interpretation and poses the potential risk of wound contamination. There are insufficient data to support its use in all cardiac patients, although high-risk patients (advanced age, diabetes, hypertension) are the most likely to benefit.[136,137] As the profile of patients undergoing cardiac surgery ages, they have a higher incidence of atherosclerosis of the aorta and the presence of concomitant risk factors for postoperative complications. Echocardiographers working in the operating room need the skills set to interrogate the aorta by hand-held ultrasound and the ability to guide the surgeon in performing the examination. It could be potentially life saving in high-risk patients. A diagnostic scan of the ascending aorta and arch to evaluate the location of possible cannulation and clamp sites can be performed in several minutes. Standardized approaches to a comprehensive organized intraoperative epiaortic and epicardial examination are useful guides.[138]

Intracardiac Clot, Calcium, and Air

Framing

The incidence of postoperative neurologic dysfunction is greater in patients undergoing open cardiac procedures. The sources of microemboli include atheroma, calcified debris, tissue, and entrapped air. The particulate matter can embolize to the coronary circulation (see Fig. 16–5), causing acute RV or LV dysfunction; to the cerebral circulation, producing postoperative neurologic deficits; and/or to distal vital organs.[139-141]

Which patients are at risk of embolization from an intracardiac or aortic source? What are the echocardiographic characteristics that define this high-risk population? What techniques can be applied to detect intracardiac or aortic sources of emboli? Are any anesthetic or surgical interventions useful in decreasing the risk of embolic stroke during heart surgery?

Data Collection

TEE data collection is focused on intracardiac air, thrombus, calcium, or other particulate matter that is at high risk for embolization (e.g., endocarditis). Cardiac ultrasound is highly sensitive in the detection of intracardiac air. The ASA/SCA task force suggested the detection of air emboli during cardiotomy, heart transplant operations, and upright neurosurgical procedures to be classified as IIa indication for perioperative TEE. Classification IIa suggests a condition in which the existing evidence/opinion was in favor of the application of the technology. Entrapped air appears as bright, highly reflective particles that produce a shadowing artifact when the air coalesces. When performing deairing maneuvers prior to release of the aortic cross-clamp and separation from bypass, the patients are placed in Trendelenburg. In addition, an ascending aortic vent can be placed to aspirate the debris/air that was not removed by the LV vent.

Discussion

The surgical team can perform several maneuvers to reduce sources of embolization that originate with open-chamber cardiac procedures. Placement of a drainage cannula in the LV via the right superior pulmonary vein can aspirate much of the debris that is suspended in solution. A small vent cannula in the anterior portion of the proximal ascending aorta is often inserted to aspirate gas bubbles or debris as they are ejected by LV contraction. The heart is often agitated by the surgeon in an attempt to eject the LV debris or air while the "protective" aortic root vent continues to aspirate. The agitation often results in the release of pockets of air that may reside at the LA appendage, IAS, apex of the LV, or entrapped in the chordal structures or ventricular muscles of the heart. There is no consensus regarding when to terminate the de-airing process and separate from CPB. Not until some degree of pulmonary blood flow is restored is it possible to eliminate most of the retained intracardiac air. The aortic root vent is often left on continual aspiration even after CPB with judicious volume replenishment through other sources. The aortic root vent should be discontinued before the administration of protamine. Although there is a paucity of evidence to support improved outcome, TEE is commonly used in the detection of retained air and the monitoring of the de-airing procedures. The effectiveness of de-airing can be tracked qualitatively. The relationship between degree of "echo contrast" and actual quantity of air is unknown.

Aortic Pathology and Transesophageal Echocardiography

Framing

The utility of TEE has expanded beyond simply examining cardiac performance and pathology. TEE is well suited as a quick, highly sensitive, and specific tool to detect the presence of aortic pathology and some of its life-threatening sequelae. The detection and differentiation of true aneurysms and pseudoaneurysms, aortic dissections and transections, intraluminal atherosclerotic disease, and abnormalities of the aortic root are often the challenge of the intraoperative team (see Chapter 23).

What are the limitations of TEE for evaluation of the thoracic aorta? Is TEE the most appropriate diagnostic test to evaluate aortic pathology in the elective and emergency patient? Does the acuity of the patient preclude other imaging modalities, such as magnetic resonance imaging (MRI) or computed tomography (CT) scanning? What are the quantitative measures that impact surgical management of aortic dissection, aortic aneurysms, aortic root disease, and aortic transection? What information can the echocardiographer provide the surgeon to assist in formulating a management strategy? What degree of aortic dilatation is sufficient to necessitate replacement? What is the risk of not replacing an aneurysmal aorta?

Data Collection

Data acquired in the assessment of the patient with aortic disease include a targeted history for evidence of malperfusion or vital organ injury (e.g., stroke) and examination of blood pressure and pulse in each of the extremities, carotid arteries, and abdominal aorta. A history of chest or back pain is common with aortic dissection or aneurysm with tearing of the aorta and its adventitia. Increasing shortness of breath may occur with AR heart failure or a left pleural effusion. Patients may present with hoarseness related to recurrent laryngeal nerve damage causing vocal cord dysfunction. The preoperative blood work may detect renal insufficiency with an elevated blood creatinine concentration. The chest radiograph often shows a widened mediastinum or calcification of the thoracic aorta. The TEE data are aimed at dimensional and anatomic assessment of the aortic root, ascending arch, and descending aorta. The echocardiographer measures and reports the size of the aortic annulus, sinus of Valsalva, sinotubular junction, and ascending aorta (see Fig. 16–11). LV hypertrophy may suggest long-lasting hypertension. A dilated LV may accompany chronic AR. Dilatation of the aortic root is common in the setting of AV stenosis and AR. Patients with a congenital predisposition for aortic aneurysm, such as Marfan's syndrome or bicuspid AV, often develop a dilated and aneurysmal ascending aorta. Epiaortic scanning increases the sensitivity of detecting abnormalities of the ascending aorta as it is in the far field from a transesophageal window and may be hidden by the interposition of the trachea and left mainstem bronchus, which obstructs the distal half of the ascending aorta.[129]

Discussion

The echocardiographer may determine the definitive diagnosis and the extent of the disease. The information contributes to the decision of surgical management.

Aneurysm rupture occurs at a stunningly high frequency of 32% to 68% in patients with thoracic aortic aneurysms managed by conservative medical treatment and accounted for 32% to 47% of deaths. The 1-, 3-, and 5-year survival of unoperated thoracic aneurysms was 65%, 36%, and 20%, respectively.[142-144] The risk of aortic rupture is a function of the size and rate of growth of the aneurysm. The risk of rupture for aneurysms less than 40 mm, 40 to 59 mm, and greater than 60 mm was 0%, 16%, and 31%, respectively.[145] The diameter of aneurysms tends to grow at a rate of approximately 5 mm/year. However, the rate of aneurysm expansion is variable. In general, the change in diameter of thoracic aortic aneurysms is a function of the initial diameter and increases more quickly in larger aneurysms.

Surgical intervention is a consideration for patients having an aneurysm of the aorta that is greater than 5 cm, accelerated rate of growth of the aneurysm, or the patient has a collagen vascular disease, such as Marfan's syndrome. The incidence and progression of disease in the ascending aorta and arch after previous sternotomy have not been reported. The scarring and connective tissue growth around the mediastinal structures (aortic root, ascending aorta, and arch) after previous heart surgery would not be expected to alter the rate of aneurysm enlargement. However, it may change the pattern of rupture, likely decreasing the risk of frank rupture into a risk of a contained rupture. No consensus exists regarding management of cardiac patients having an incidental finding of an ascending aorta greater than 4 cm in diameter. The decision to pursue surgical intervention at the time of surgery depends on the pathogenesis of the disease, presence of symptoms, age of the patient, progression, and other operative and patient factors. A young patient with a 4.5-cm ascending aorta that is thinned and is associated with a bicuspid AV is more likely to undergo a root replacement and ascending aorta graft compared with an elderly patient with a similar aortic diameter who is undergoing CABG and whose aortic size has remained stable over the previous decade. Surgical replacement of the ascending aorta and arch is complex, requiring specialized surgical training. Significant modification of the initial surgical procedure may increase the risk of perioperative complications and potentially jeopardize the success of the originally planned operation. Extensive ascending aortic surgery involving the arch vessels requires hypothermic circulatory arrest followed by controlled exsanguination to allow for visualization of the operative field.

Disease of the AV is often accompanied by abnormalities of the thoracic aorta. Aortic root dilatation may require ascending aortic replacement. The decision is based on size of the aortic root diameter, and presence of abnormalities of the aortic wall, such as thrombus, dissection, or focal aneurysm. There are no strict guidelines that dictate practice. The surgeon might choose to replace the entire root or just the AV and ascending aorta, sparing the sinuses of Valsalva. The Wheat procedure is a replacement of the AV and ascending aorta while preserving the native sinuses of Valsalva and coronary ostia. Alternatively, in the setting of a dilated or aneurysmal sinus, the surgeon may elect to replace the entire aortic root. Choice of implanting a biologic root or composite AVR is a surgical decision based on many of the factors presented in Table 16–1. Implantation of a root or composite graft necessitates reattachment of the coronary arteries, increasing the risk of postoperative bleeding and coronary ischemia.[146] Despite a history of normal coronary arteries, the close scrutiny of regional wall motion postbypass is aimed at detecting newly created abnormalities of coronary blood flow. Air into the coronary circulation or compromise of coronary blood flow through the newly constructed coronary buttons may produce severe myocardial dysfunction. Kinking of the coronaries or stenosis at the ostia often produces transmural ischemia that is not subtle. Enlargement of the sinus segment may facilitate coronary anastomoses. A prosthetic graft with an enlarged area to mimic the sinus of Valsalva has been developed. Enlargement of the sinus segment may facilitate coronary anastomoses, and thus may decrease the risk of such complications, but this remains to be proven.

No consensus guidelines exist on the specific dimensions of the aortic root beyond which a root replacement is deemed necessary. However, distortion of the root producing severe AR or disruption in its integrity requires surgical attention. The echocardiographer reports the size of the aortic annulus, sinus of Valsalva, sinotubular junction, and ascending aorta (see Fig. 16–11). These measurements are obtained using the AV long-axis view. The short- and longitudinal-axis views from TEE can define the severity and mechanism of AR, and the success of AV repair. Patients scheduled for aorta surgery with an intrinsically normal AV with AR due to a correctable aortic lesion (incomplete leaflet closure, leaflet prolapse, or dissection flap prolapse) can undergo AV repair.[105,147] In contrast, valvular pathology that includes connective tissue degeneration (Marfan or bicuspid valve), aortitis, or severe calcification would most likely require valve replacement.

Acute Aortic Syndromes

Framing

The unstable patient with suspected acute aortic disease or injury is often the most challenging of TEE cases. There are few more crucially important decisions that are posed to the intraoperative echocardiographer than to quickly and accurately diagnose the nature and extent of acute aortic injury. Hypotension and respiratory distress may prevent a complete and comprehensive evaluation before surgery (Fig. 16–18). History is often unobtainable. The echocardiographer becomes a detective. Clues are quickly gathered from the available clinical presentation, past history, and associated physical findings. The TEE is often the only modality used to establish the diagnosis and define the surgical plan.

CASE STUDY

It is midnight on a gloomy rainy night. The hospital helicopter calls in ". . . young women, unrestrained driver, deceleration injury, steering wheel impact, chest contusion, unconscious, hypotensive. She is intubated with bilateral breath sounds. Her blood pressure is 70/40 mm Hg with a HR = 125 sinus tachycardia. She is being fluid resuscitated and being transported directly to the cardiac operating room." The patient is too unstable for MRI or CAT scanning. The patient arrives with a portable chest radiograph obtained as she traveled through the emergency department, showing a widened mediastinum. The vital signs have not changed except that she is receiving dopamine at 10 μg/kg/min. Pulses are palpable in the groins and the neck. The attending surgeon turns to the echocardiographer-anesthesiologist and asks, "I need to know whether this is an anterior injury with heart contusion, injury to the ascending aorta, tamponade with blood in the pericardium or is this a transected aorta or does the patient have a non-operable injury? The former will require a sternotomy. The transections will require a left thoracotomy. If we make the incorrect decision, the patient will surely die." The patient is stabilized in the operating room and the TEE probe is inserted. After the diagnosis is made, the patient is positioned and prepped accordingly for the definitive surgery.

The sensitivity and specificity of TEE to detect and diagnose injury or disease of the thoracic aorta are significantly

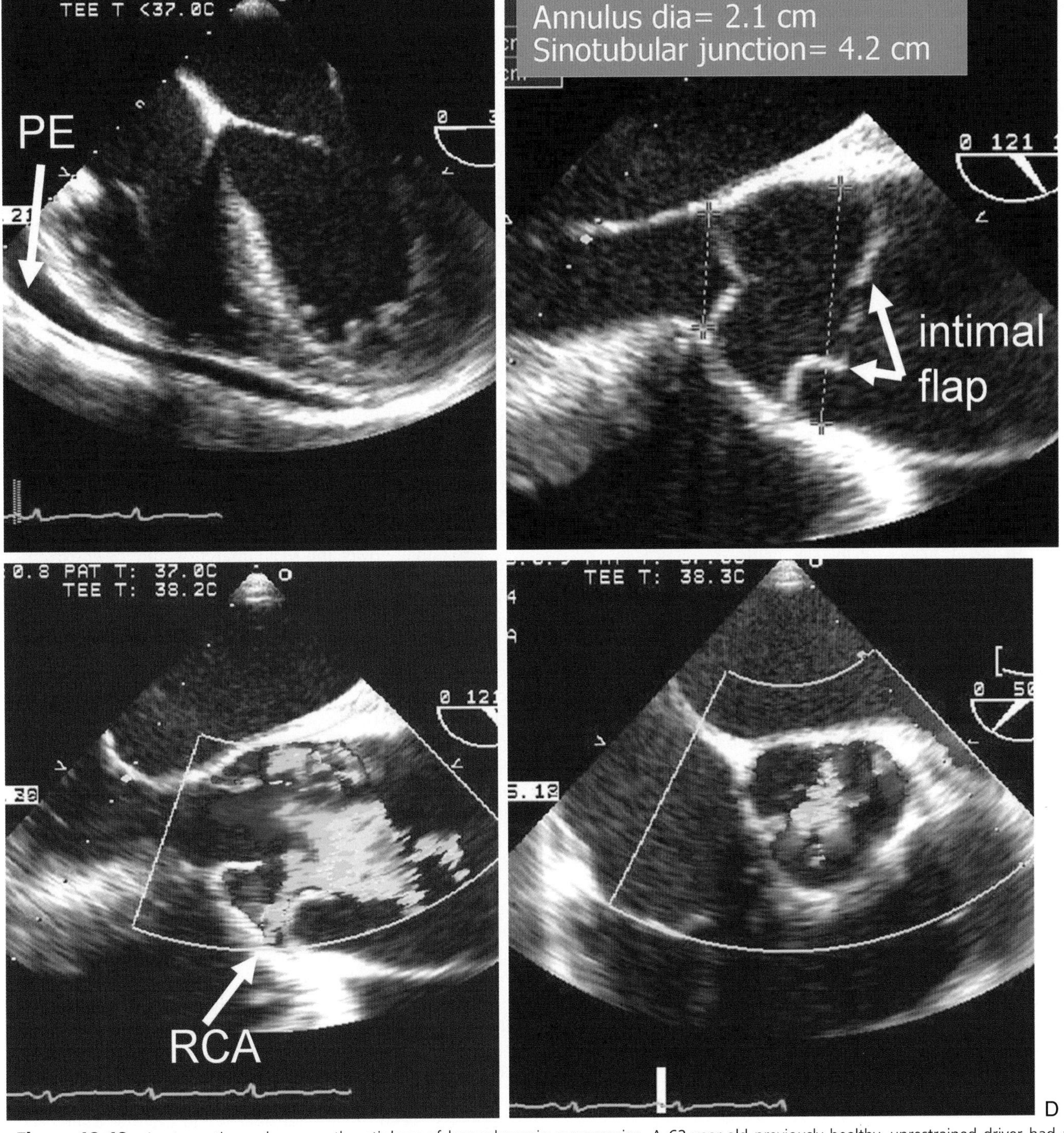

Figure 16–18 Acute aortic syndrome as the etiology of hemodynamic compromise. A 62-year-old previously healthy, unrestrained driver had a motor vehicle accident. On arrival to the emergency department, the patient was hypotensive (BP = 90/45) and tachycardic (HR = 120). He described an episode of loss of consciousness that was associated with severe chest pain but could not recall if the syncopal episode preceded the accident. The chest radiograph was significant for several fractured ribs, widened mediastinum, and a pleural effusion. The patient became progressively more unstable and was transferred to the operating room to perform diagnostic transesophageal echocardiography (TEE) and definitive surgical procedure if necessary. The echocardiographer performed a quick transthoracic echocardiographic examination that confirmed the presence of pericardial effusion with findings that were consistent for tamponade. After fluid resuscitation and induction of anesthesia, a TEE examination was performed. The mid-esophageal four-chamber view showed presence of a pericardial effusion (PE) that compromised right atrial filling (*A*). The mid-esophageal long-axis view of the aortic valve revealed a type A dissection that was characterized by intimal flaps within the aortic root and that extended distally into the descending thoracic aorta. (*B*) The annulus of the aortic valve was of normal size, but the sinus and root were markedly enlarged (diameter of sinotubular junction = 4.22 cm). The dissection extended into the noncoronary and right coronary sinus segments, narrowing blood flow at the coronary ostia (*C, arrow*). Although the electrocardiogram did not show acute ischemia, the right ventricular function and inferior wall of the left ventricle were mildly hypokinetic. Although an effaced aortic root, ascending aortic aneurysm, and acute dissection in this age group are suggestive of congenital bicuspid valve, the short-axis view of the aortic valve (*D*) showed a trileaflet valve with a coaptation defect with aortic insufficiency at the noncoronary cusp. The surgeon resuspended the aortic valve and replaced the ascending aorta and hemiarch with a tube graft. The valve repair was successful with only +1 aortic insufficiency and cardiac return to normal after surgery.

better than the sensitivity and specificity of TTE and are comparable to CAT scan and MRI.[148,149] TEE provides information regarding cardiac performance and the presence of other critically important sequelae that may be important in determining the approach and timing for surgical intervention. Hence, TEE is indicated even if MRI or CT scanning has confirmed the diagnosis.

Can consent be obtained from the patient or family members? In these emergency circumstances, it may be more prudent to proceed with the TEE examination rather than delaying diagnosis and treatment in an attempt to find family members. What is the differential diagnosis of a widened mediastinum? How does TEE discriminate the different causes of a widened mediastinum? Is the TEE performed in the awake distressed patient, or is the TEE done under more controlled conditions of an anesthetized, intubated patient? Is there a risk of cervical spine injury? Is there a risk of esophageal injury? Can insertion of the TEE probe further compromise the patency of mediastinal structures? Is there fluid in the pericardium? What is the biventricular function? Is there myocardial rupture? Is there aortic rupture? Is the thoracic aorta intact? Is there an intimal flap and a dissection? Is there a transection? Is there a pleural or periaortic effusion/hematoma? What factors determine the urgency of intervention and strategies for management?

Data Collection

Because the diagnosis and cause for instability are not established, the entire mediastinum, including the left pleural space, is interrogated before definitive therapy is initiated. Rarely is there not enough time to do a complete TEE examination. The operative team can often proceed with confidence in the management of these critically ill patients with only TEE to guide the treatment. The primary event in aortic dissection is a tear and separation of the aortic intima. It is uncertain whether the inciting event is a primary rupture of the intima with secondary dissection of the media, or hemorrhage within the media and subsequent rupture of the overlying intima. Systolic ejection forces blood into the aortic media through a tear that leads to the separation of the intima from the surrounding media, creating a false lumen. Blood flow may exist in both the false and true lumens through communicating fenestrations. Aortic dissections are classified by one of two anatomic schemes (the DeBakey and Stanford classifications). Transection is diagnosed through the detection of para-aortic hematoma near the isthmus and a "step-up" in the internal media wall (see Chapter 23).

Discussion

Acute dissections (Stanford type A or DeBakey type I or type II) involving the ascending aorta or arch are considered acute surgical emergencies. In contrast, dissections confined to the descending aorta (distal to the left subclavian artery; Stanford type B or DeBakey type III) are treated medically unless the patient demonstrates proximal extension, hemorrhage, or malperfusion. From the International Registry of Acute Aortic Dissection (IRAD), 73% of the 384 patients with type B dissections were managed medically; in-hospital mortality was 10%.[150] The long-term survival rate after applying medical therapy is approximately 60% to 80% at 4 to 5 years[150-153] and approximately 40% to 45% at 10 years.[152,153] Survival is best in patients with noncommunicating and retrograde dissections.[154] From the IRAD registry, in-hospital mortality for surgical patients was significantly higher (32%).[150] The increased rate of mortality for surgically treated patients is likely influenced by selecting a cohort of patients with more advanced disease and complicated course (malperfusion, leakage, extension). The overall reported short- and long-term outcomes are similar for medically treated patients with type B dissections.[153] Of 142 patients with type B aortic dissections, there was a trend toward lower mortality with medical therapy compared with surgical treatment at 1 year (15% versus 33%). Both groups had similar survival at 5 and 10 years (60% and 35%).[153]

Endovascular stent grafting for descending thoracic aortic dissections is gaining momentum as a less invasive alternative to surgery in stable patients with type B dissections.[155,156] The stent graft is positioned to cover the intimal flap and seal the entry site of the dissection, resulting in thrombosis of the false lumen. In one nonrandomized evaluation of 24 consecutive patients with a subacute or chronic thoracic type B dissection, there was no morbidity (paraplegia, stroke, embolization, malperfusion syndrome, or infection) or mortality with stent grafting.[155] In contrast, surgical intervention was associated with a 33% mortality and a 42% incidence of adverse events within a 12-month interval. Other studies are promising but less positive.[157] In a series of 19 patients with acute dissections (15 type B and 4 type A dissections), the major morbidity rate was 21% (small bowel and renal infarction and lower extremity ischemia) and 30-day mortality was 16%. However, there were no additional deaths or instances of aneurysm/aortic rupture during the subsequent 13-month follow-up period.

Ascending aortic dissections (involving the aortic root, ascending aorta, or arch) are acute surgical emergencies, because of the high risk for a life-threatening complication such as AR, cardiac tamponade, myocardial infarction, rupture, and stroke. The mortality rate is as high as 1% to 2%/hour early after symptom onset.[158] Neither acute myocardial ischemia nor cerebral infarction should contraindicate urgent intervention. Although patients with stroke in progress may be at increased risk for hemorrhagic cerebral infarction due to intraoperative anticoagulation, leading to hemorrhagic stroke, the authors have seen several patients who experienced dramatic neurologic recovery. Operative mortality for ascending aortic dissections at experienced centers varies from 7% to 36%, well below the greater than 50% mortality with medical therapy.[151,158-165]

Traumatic aortic rupture is a life-threatening vascular injury that often results in lethal hemorrhage. In a multicenter trial of 274 patients, the overall mortality rate reached 31%, with 63% of deaths attributable to aortic rupture.[166] Aortic transection and rupture usually occur at the aortic isthmus (between the left subclavian and the first intercostal arteries) and result from shear forces generated by unrestrained frontal collisions.[167] Although aortography had been considered the gold standard for the diagnosis of transection, TEE and contrast-enhanced spiral CT and MRI are currently favored, especially for patients with renal insufficiency.[168-172] Intravascular ultrasonography has been proposed as a potential diagnostic tool for the identification of limited aortic injuries.[173] Traumatic aortic rupture needs to be distinguished from an aortic dissection. Imaging of a dissected aorta typically reveals true and false lumens at multiple levels. The focal aortic injury of aortic transection is quite localized and may be overlooked when performing a cursory examination. A second potential diagnostic problem is that protuberant atherosclerotic changes of the aorta may be difficult to differentiate from partial aortic tears. The thick and irregular intraluminal flap, which corresponds to disruption of both intimal and medial aortic layers, can be imaged in both the short- and long-axis planes in the vicinity of the isthmus. In the longitudinal view, the medial flap is nearly perpendicular to the aortic wall because traumatic lesions are usually confined within a few centimeters distal to the left subclavian. The formation of a localized contained rupture of the false aneurysm is common.[169,174] Color-flow Doppler imaging and spectral Doppler can be used to detect turbulence associated with nonlaminar flow at the aortic defect and the presence of a pressure gradient. Traditional treatment includes immediate surgical invention using a right lateral decubitus approach and resection of the aorta with insertion of a tube graft. Deployment of endovascular stent grafts has been successful. Two series that included a total of 16 patients having aortic transection reported successful repair with no mortality or serious morbidity.[175,176] However, the application of this device under such conditions poses a high risk for left subclavian malperfusion and paraplegia.[177] The decision regarding appropriate management and time course of therapy will depend on the technical availability and expertise within the institution and the forthcoming results of clinical trials that use newer, less invasive technologies.

Intramural Hematoma

Framing

The presence of an intramural hematoma is a subtle finding that may be missed when evaluating the thoracic aorta for a dissection or rupture. Intramural hematoma is distinct from a classic aortic dissection but has been considered by some as being a variant.[178]

What are the characteristics of an intramural hematoma? What are the common findings and symptoms at presentation? What, if any, is the clinical significance of this pathologic finding? Does location influence the choice of medical or surgical approach? What are the prognostic indicators of progression?

Data Collection

Aortic intramural hematoma is often considered a variant of an aortic dissection.[178] Although many of the patients may present with chest or back pain, many of the associated sequelae, such as pericardial or pleural effusions, stroke, and myocardial infarction, are absent.[179-181] It is characterized by the absence of a detectable intimal tear. The hematoma is probably produced by a hemorrhage of the vaso vasorum into the aortic wall. In a meta-analysis, acute aortic intramural hematoma was most often associated with long-standing hypertension; traumatic etiology was also a significant factor for 6% of cases.[179] In the meta-analysis of 143 cases, 81% were diagnosed by CT and the remaining patients by MRI and/or TEE.[179] The sensitivity and specificity of TEE to detect an intramural hematoma were reported to be 100% and 91%, respectively.[181] The diagnosis is characterized by the absence of a dissecting flap or intimal disruption with specific regional thickening of the aortic wall of greater than 7 mm in a crescent or circular shape. On MRI or CT, this crescent-shaped or circular area in the aortic wall demonstrates high attenuation that does not enhance with contrast.[182] Although intramural hematomas can be detected in any portion of the aorta, the location appears to be a factor in its etiology and prognosis. The ascending aorta, which was involved in 33% to 57% of cases, appeared to represent the early stage of a classic dissection,[179,180,182-184] whereas traumatic intramural hematomas typically involved the descending thoracic aorta.[183]

Discussion

Acute management is similar to that of a classic aortic dissection. In the meta-analysis of 143 patients with aortic intramural hematoma, lesions of the ascending aorta were associated with a lower early mortality with surgical intervention than medical treatment (14% versus 36%); lesions of the descending aorta had a similar mortality with medical or surgical therapy (14% versus 20%).[179] Although surgery may be preferred, it may not be performed in some patients because of old age and comorbid conditions. Progression of disease in patients who are medically managed is attenuated by the use of β-blockers.[185] The force of LV systolic blood pressure, the driving force for disease progression, is reduced by the administration of β-blockers. Medically treated patients with aortic intramural hematoma appear to do better than patients having a classic ascending aortic dissection.[184] In contrast, several Korean studies have reported success in initially using a medical approach and reserving surgery for patients who developed sequelae or frank aortic dissection.[184] Their results may reflect the lower incidence and severity of atherosclerotic and hypertensive disease in this select patient cohort. Until more definitive data are available, surgery should be considered the first choice for proximal aortic intramural hematomas.

Patients with an intramural hematoma in the descending thoracic aorta should be medically treated using β-blockers. Attempts have been made to identify predictors of progression. In two studies with 88 patients, independent predictors of progression included maximum aortic diameter of 40 mm, maximum aortic thickness of 10 mm,[186] and age greater than 70 years.[187] Another predictor of progression with medical therapy is the presence of an ulcer-like projection into the hematoma.[187,188] This subpopulation seems to be at significantly greater risk of rupture, dissection, and hematoma expansion and may require more aggressive management and follow-up. Future management approaches may include the use of intravascular aortic stents.

In conclusion, the intraoperative echocardiographer is confronted with a broad array of diseases that require on-site decision-making in the perioperative setting. The key ingredients to sound decision-making are a broad fund of knowledge (database), a systematic approach with attention to all vantage points and frames, and identifying, addressing, and prioritizing the pertinent questions.

Plans are nothing, ... Planning is everything.

Dwight Eisenhower

REFERENCES

1. Kruger J, Dunning D: Unskilled and unaware of it: How difficulties in recognizing one's own incompetence lead to inflated self-assessments. J Person Soc Psychol 77:1121, 1999
2. Royse AG, Royse CF, Ajani AE, et al: Reduced neuropsychological dysfunction using epiaortic echocardiography and the exclusive Y graft. Ann Thorac Surg 69:1431, 2000
3. Sylivris S, Calafiore P, Matalanis G, et al: The intraoperative assessment of ascending aortic atheroma: Epiaortic imaging is superior to both transesophageal echocardiography and direct palpation. J Cardiothorac Vasc Anesth 11:704, 1997
4. Ura M, Sakata R, Nakayama Y, et al: Extracorporeal circulation before and after ultrasonographic evaluation of the ascending aorta. Ann Thorac Surg 67:478, 1999

5. Russo JE, Schoemaker PJH: The Power of Frames, Winning Decisions. New York, New York, Doubleday, 2002, p 34
6. Kallmeyer IJ, Collard CD, Fox JA, et al: The safety of intraoperative transesophageal echocardiography: A case series of 7200 cardiac surgical patients. Anesth Analg 92:1126, 2001
7. MacGregor DA, Zvara DA, Treadway RM Jr, et al: Late presentation of esophageal injury after transesophageal echocardiography. Anesth Analg 99:41, 2004
8. Olenchock SA Jr, Lukaszczyk JJ, Reed J III, Theman TE: Splenic injury after intraoperative transesophageal echocardiography. Ann Thorac Surg 72:2141, 2001
9. Pong MW, Lin SM, Kao SC, et al: Unusual cause of esophageal perforation during intraoperative transesophageal echocardiography monitoring for cardiac surgery—a case report. Acta Anaesthesiol 41:155, 2003
10. Savino JS, Hanson CW III, Bigelow DC, et al: Oropharyngeal injury after transesophageal echocardiography. J Cardiothorac Vasc Anesth 8:76, 1994
11. Venticinque SG, Kashyap VS, O'Connell RJ: Chemical burn injury secondary to intraoperative transesophageal echocardiography. Anesth Analg 97:1260, 2003
12. Silber JH: Using outcomes analysis to assess quality of care: Applications for cardiovascular surgery, outcome measurements. *In* Tuman KJ (ed): Cardiovascular Medicine. Philadelphia, Lippincott, Williams and Wilkins, 1999, p 1
13. Practice guidelines for perioperative transesophageal echocardiography. A report by the American Society of Anesthesiologists and the Society of Cardiovascular Anesthesiologists Task Force on Transesophageal Echocardiography. Anesthesiology 84:986, 1996
14. Savino JS, Fleisher LA: Assessment of the patient with heart disease undergoing non-cardiac surgery. *In* Rosendorff C (ed): Essential Cardiology, Principles and Practice, 2nd edition. Totowa, NY, Humana Press, 2004
15. Shanewise JS, Cheung AT, Aronson S, et al: ASE/SCA guidelines for performing a comprehensive intraoperative multiplane transesophageal echocardiography examination: recommendations of the American Society of Echocardiography Council for Intraoperative Echocardiography and the Society of Cardiovascular Anesthesiologists Task Force for Certification in Perioperative Transesophageal Echocardiography. Anesth Analg 89:870, 1999
16. Gorcsan J III, Gasior TA, Mandarino WA, et al: Assessment of the immediate effects of cardiopulmonary bypass on left ventricular performance by on-line pressure-area relations. Circulation 89:180, 1994
17. Battler A, Froelicher VF, Gallagher KP, et al: Dissociation between regional myocardial dysfunction and ECG changes during ischemia in the conscious dog. Circulation 62:735, 1980
18. Foster E, O'Kelly B, LaPidus A, et al: Segmental analysis of resting echocardiographic function and stress scintigraphic perfusion: Implications for myocardial viability. Am Heart J 129:7, 1995
19. Jacklin PB, Barrington SF, Roxburgh JC, et al: Cost-effectiveness of preoperative positron emission tomography in ischemic heart disease. Ann Thorac Surg 73:1403, 2002
20. Landoni C, Lucignani G, Paolini G, et al: Assessment of CABG-related risk in patients with CAD and LVD. Contribution of PET with [18F]FDG to the assessment of myocardial viability. J Cardiovasc Surg (Torino) 40:363, 1999
21. Kozman H, Cook JR, Wiseman AH, et al: Presence of angiographic coronary collaterals predicts myocardial recovery after coronary bypass surgery in patients with severe left ventricular dysfunction. Circulation 98:II-57, 1998
22. Premaratne S, Razzuk A, Koduru S, et al: Incidence of postinfarction aneurysm within one month of infarct: Experience with 16 patients in Hawaii. J Cardiovasc Surg 40:473, 1999
23. Redfield MM, Jacobsen SJ, Burnett JC J, et al: Burden of systolic and diastolic ventricular dysfunction in the community: Appreciating the scope of the heart failure epidemic. JAMA 289:194, 2003
24. Tischler MD, Cooper KA, Rowen M, LeWinter MM: Mitral valve replacement versus mitral valve repair. A Doppler and quantitative stress echocardiographic study. Circulation 89:132, 1994
25. Grigioni F, Enriquez-Sarano M, Zehr KJ, et al: Ischemic mitral regurgitation: Long-term outcome and prognostic implications with quantitative Doppler assessment. Circulation 103:1759, 2001
26. Feinberg MS, Schwammenthal E, Shlizerman L, et al: Prognostic significance of mild mitral regurgitation by color Doppler echocardiography in acute myocardial infarction. Am J Cardiol 86:903, 2000
27. Grossi EA, Goldberg JD, LaPietra A, et al: Ischemic mitral valve reconstruction and replacement: Comparison of long-term survival and complications. J Thorac Cardiovasc Surg 122:1107, 2001
28. Bach DS, Deeb GM, Bolling SF: Accuracy of intraoperative transesophageal echocardiography for estimating the severity of functional mitral regurgitation. Am J Cardiol 76:508, 1995
29. Choi H, Lee K, Lee H, et al: Quantification of mitral regurgitation using proximal isovelocity surface area method in dogs. J Vet Sci 5:163, 2004
30. Grewal KS, Malkowski MJ, Piracha AR, et al: Effect of general anesthesia on the severity of mitral regurgitation by transesophageal echocardiography. Am J Cardiol 85:199, 2000
31. Gillinov AM, Wierup PN, Blackstone EH, et al: Is repair preferable to replacement for ischemic mitral regurgitation? J Thorac Cardiovasc Surg 122:1125, 2001
32. Yiu SF, Enriquez-Sarano M, Tribouilloy C, et al: Determinants of the degree of functional mitral regurgitation in patients with systolic left ventricular dysfunction: A quantitative clinical study. Circulation 102:1400, 2000
33. Gorman JH III, Gorman RC, Jackson BM, et al: Annuloplasty ring selection for chronic ischemic mitral regurgitation: Lessons from the ovine model. Ann Thorac Surg 76:1556, 2003
34. Guy TS, Moainie SL, Gorman JH III, et al: Prevention of ischemic mitral regurgitation does not influence the outcome of remodeling after posterolateral myocardial infarction. J Am Coll Cardiol 43:377, 2004
35. Miller DC: Ischemic mitral regurgitation redux—To repair or to replace? J Thorac Cardiovasc Surg 122:1059, 2001
36. Inoue M, McCarthy PM, Popovic ZB, et al: Mitral valve repair without cardiopulmonary bypass or atriotomy using the Coapsys device: Device design and implantation procedure in canine functional mitral regurgitation model. Heart Surg Forum 7: E117, 2004
37. Fukamachi K, Popovic ZB, Inoue M, et al: Changes in mitral annular and left ventricular dimensions and left ventricular pressure-volume relations after off-pump treatment of mitral regurgitation with the Coapsys device. Eur J Cardiothorac Surg 25:352, 2004
38. Fann JI, St Goar FG, Komtebedde J, et al: Beating heart catheter-based edge-to-edge mitral valve procedure in a porcine model: efficacy and healing response. Circulation 110:988, 2004
39. Condado JA, Velez-Gimon M: Catheter-based approach to mitral regurgitation. J Interv Cardiol 16:523, 2003
40. Maslow AD, Regan MM, Haering JM, et al: Echocardiographic predictors of left ventricular outflow tract obstruction and systolic anterior motion of the mitral valve after mitral valve reconstruction for myxomatous valve disease. J Am Coll Cardiol 34:2096, 1999
41. Hellemans IM, Pieper EG, Ravelli AC, et al: Prediction of surgical strategy in mitral valve regurgitation based on echocardiography. Interuniversity Cardiology Institute of the Netherlands. Am J Cardiol 79:334, 1997
42. Lee EM, Shapiro LM, Wells FC: Superiority of mitral valve repair in surgery for degenerative mitral regurgitation. Eur Heart J 18:655, 1997
43. Rozich JD, Carabello BA, Usher BW, et al: Mitral valve replacement with and without chordal preservation in patients with chronic mitral regurgitation. Mechanisms for differences in postoperative ejection performance. Circulation 86:1718, 1992
44. Charls LM: SAM—Systolic anterior motion of the anterior mitral valve leaflet postsurgical mitral valve repair. Heart Lung 32:402, 2003
45. Fananapazir L, Epstein ND, Curiel RV, et al: Long-term results of dual-chamber (DDD) pacing in obstructive hypertrophic cardiomyopathy. Evidence for progressive symptomatic and hemodynamic improvement and reduction of left ventricular hypertrophy. Circulation 90:2731, 1994
46. Movsowitz C, Podolsky LA, Meyerowitz CB, et al: Patent foramen ovale: A nonfunctional embryological remnant or a potential cause of significant pathology? J Am Soc Echocardiogr 5:259, 1992
47. Langholz D, Louie EK, Konstadt SN, et al: Transesophageal echocardiographic demonstration of distinct mechanisms for right to left shunting across a patent foramen ovale in the absence of pulmonary hypertension. J Am Coll Cardiol 18:1112, 1991
48. Augoustides JG, Weiss SJ, Weiner J, et al: Diagnosis of patent foramen ovale with multiplane transesophageal echocardiography in adult cardiac surgical patients. J Cardiothorac Vasc Anesth 18:725, 2004
49. Attie F, Rosas M, Granados N, et al: Surgical treatment for secundum atrial septal defects in patients >40 years old. A randomized clinical trial. J Am Coll Cardiol 38:2035, 2001
50. Ferreira SM, Ho SY, Anderson RH: Morphological study of defects of the atrial septum within the oval fossa: Implications for transcatheter closure of left-to-right shunt. Br Heart J 67:316, 1992
51. Mugge A, Daniel WG, Angermann C, et al: Atrial septal aneurysm in adult patients. A multicenter study using transthoracic and transesophageal echocardiography. Circulation 91:2785, 1995
52. Belkin RN, Kisslo J: Atrial septal aneurysm: Recognition and clinical relevance. Am Heart J 120:948, 1990

53. Cabanes L, Mas JL, Cohen A, et al: Atrial septal aneurysm and patent foramen ovale as risk factors for cryptogenic stroke in patients less than 55 years of age. A study using transesophageal echocardiography. Stroke 24:1865, 1993
54. Mattioli AV, Aquilina M, Oldani A, et al: Atrial septal aneurysm as a cardioembolic source in adult patients with stroke and normal carotid arteries. A multicentre study. Eur Heart J 22:261, 2001
55. Agmon Y, Khandheria BK, Meissner I, et al: Frequency of atrial septal aneurysms in patients with cerebral ischemic events. Circulation 99:1942, 1999
56. Pearson AC, Nagelhout D, Castello R, et al: Atrial septal aneurysm and stroke: A transesophageal echocardiographic study. J Am Coll Cardiol 18:1223, 1991
57. Webster MW, Chancellor AM, Smith HJ, et al: Patent foramen ovale in young stroke patients. Lancet 2:11, 1988
58. Lechat P, Mas JL, Lascault G, et al: Prevalence of patent foramen ovale in patients with stroke. N Engl J Med 318:1148, 1988
59. Burger AJ, Sherman HB, Charlamb MJ: Low incidence of embolic strokes with atrial septal aneurysms: A prospective, long-term study. Am Heart J 139:149, 2000
60. Overell JR, Bone I, Lees KR: Interatrial septal abnormalities and stroke: A meta-analysis of case-control studies. Neurology 55:1172, 2000
61. Rose GC, Armstrong WF, Mahomed Y, Feigenbaum H: Atrial level right to left intracardiac shunt associated with postoperative hypoxemia: Demonstration with contrast two-dimensional echocardiography. J Am Coll Cardiol 6:920, 1985
62. Kollar A, Reames MK, Coyle JP: Patent foramen ovale and pulmonary embolism. An underestimated co-morbidity following cardiac surgery. J Cardiovasc Surg (Torino) 39:355, 1998
63. Yasu T, Fujii M, Saito M: Long-term follow-up of an interatrial right-to-left shunt that appeared after cardiac surgery—Evaluation by transesophageal Doppler echocardiography. Jpn Circ J 60:70, 1996
64. Akhter M, Lajos TZ: Pitfalls of undetected patent foramen ovale in off-pump cases. Ann Thorac Surg 67:546, 1999
65. Stoddard MF, Arce J, Liddell NE, et al: Two-dimensional transesophageal echocardiographic determination of aortic valve area in adults with aortic stenosis. Am Heart J 122:1415, 1991
66. Smith MD, Harrison MR, Pinton R, et al: Regurgitant jet size by transesophageal compared with transthoracic Doppler color flow imaging. Circulation 83:79, 1991
67. Fenoglio JJ Jr, McAllister HA Jr, DeCastro CM, et al: Congenital bicuspid aortic valve after age 20. Am J Cardiol 39:164, 1977
68. Osler W: The bicuspid condition of the aortic valves. Trans Assoc Am Physicians 1:185, 1886
69. Grant RT, Wood JE Jr, Jones TD: Heart valve irregularities in relation to subacute bacterial endocarditis. Heart 14:247, 1928
70. Keith JD: Bicuspid aortic valve. *In* Keith JD, Rowe RD, Vlad P (eds): Heart Disease in Infancy and Childhood. London, MacMillan, 1978, p 728
71. Roberts WC: The congenitally bicuspid aortic valve. A study of 85 autopsy cases. Am J Cardiol 26:72, 1970
72. Larson EW, Edwards WD: Risk factors for aortic dissection: A necropsy study of 161 cases. Am J Cardiol 53:849, 1984
73. Novaro GM, Tiong IY, Pearce GL, et al: Features and predictors of ascending aortic dilatation in association with a congenital bicuspid aortic valve. Am J Cardiol 92:99, 2003
74. Borger MA, Preston M, Ivanov J, et al: Should the ascending aorta be replaced more frequently in patients with bicuspid aortic valve disease? J Thorac Cardiovasc Surg 128:677, 2004
75. Olearchyk AS: Congenital bicuspid aortic valve and an aneurysm of the ascending aorta. J Card Surg 19:462, 2004
76. Olearchyk AS: Congenital bicuspid aortic valve disease with an aneurysm of the ascending aorta in adults: Vertical reduction aortoplasty with distal external synthetic wrapping. J Card Surg 19:144, 2004
77. Fedak PW, de Sa MP, Verma S, et al: Vascular matrix remodeling in patients with bicuspid aortic valve malformations: Implications for aortic dilatation. J Thorac Cardiovasc Surg 126:797, 2003
78. Ferencik M, Pape LA: Changes in size of ascending aorta and aortic valve function with time in patients with congenitally bicuspid aortic valves. Am J Cardiol 92:43, 2003
79. Borger MA, Preston M, Ivanov J, et al: Should the ascending aorta be replaced more frequently in patients with bicuspid aortic valve disease? J Thorac Cardiovasc Surg 128:677, 2004
80. Cosgrove DM, Rosenkranz ER, Hendren WG, et al: Valvuloplasty for aortic insufficiency. J Thorac Cardiovasc Surg 102:571, 1991
81. Haydar HS, He GW, Hovaguimian H, et al: Valve repair for aortic insufficiency: Surgical classification and techniques. Eur J Cardiothorac Surg 11:258, 1997
82. Moidl R, Moritz A, Simon P, et al: Echocardiographic results after repair of incompetent bicuspid aortic valves. Ann Thorac Surg 60:669, 1995
83. Casselman FP, Gillinov AM, Akhrass R, et al: Intermediate-term durability of bicuspid aortic valve repair for prolapsing leaflet. Eur J Cardiothorac Surg 15:302, 1999
84. Rosenhek R, Binder T, Porenta G, et al: Predictors of outcome in severe, asymptomatic aortic stenosis. N Engl J Med 343:611, 2000
85. Rajamannan NM, Subramaniam M, Springett M, et al: Atorvastatin inhibits hypercholesterolemia-induced cellular proliferation and bone matrix production in the rabbit aortic valve. Circulation 105:2660, 2002
86. Bellamy MF, Pellikka PA, Klarich KW, et al: Association of cholesterol levels, hydroxymethylglutaryl coenzyme-A reductase inhibitor treatment, and progression of aortic stenosis in the community. J Am Coll Cardiol 40:1723, 2002
87. Smith WT, Ferguson TB Jr, Ryan T, et al: Should coronary artery bypass graft surgery patients with mild or moderate aortic stenosis undergo concomitant aortic valve replacement? A decision analysis approach to the surgical dilemma. J Am Coll Cardiol 44:1241, 2004
88. Rahimtoola SH: "Prophylactic" valve replacement for mild aortic valve disease at time of surgery for other cardiovascular disease? No. J Am Coll Cardiol 33:2009, 1999
89. Pereira JJ, Lauer MS, Bashir M, et al: Survival after aortic valve replacement for severe aortic stenosis with low transvalvular gradients and severe left ventricular dysfunction. J Am Coll Cardiol 39:1356, 2002
90. Brogan WC III, Grayburn PA, Lange RA, Hillis LD: Prognosis after valve replacement in patients with severe aortic stenosis and a low transvalvular pressure gradient. J Am Coll Cardiol 21:1657, 1993
91. Connolly HM, Oh JK, Schaff HV, et al: Severe aortic stenosis with low transvalvular gradient and severe left ventricular dysfunction: Result of aortic valve replacement in 52 patients. Circulation 101:1940, 2000
92. Ford LE, Feldman T, Chiu YC, Carroll JD: Hemodynamic resistance as a measure of functional impairment in aortic valvular stenosis. Circ Res 66:1, 1990
93. deFilippi CR, Willett DL, Brickner ME, et al: Usefulness of dobutamine echocardiography in distinguishing severe from nonsevere valvular aortic stenosis in patients with depressed left ventricular function and low transvalvular gradients. Am J Cardiol 75:191, 1995
94. Bermejo J, Garcia-Fernandez MA, Torrecilla EG, et al: Effects of dobutamine on Doppler echocardiographic indexes of aortic stenosis. J Am Coll Cardiol 28:1206, 1996
95. Lin SS, Roger VL, Pascoe R, et al: Dobutamine stress Doppler hemodynamics in patients with aortic stenosis: feasibility, safety, and surgical correlations. Am Heart J 136:1010, 1998
96. Cheitlin MD, Armstrong WF, Aurigemma GP, et al: ACC/AHA/ASE 2003 guideline update for the clinical application of echocardiography—summary article: A report of the American College of Cardiology/American Heart Association Task Force on Practice Guidelines (ACC/AHA/ASE Committee to Update the 1997 Guidelines for the Clinical Application of Echocardiography). J Am Coll Cardiol 42:954, 2003
97. Nishimura RA, Grantham JA, Connolly HM, et al: Low-output, low-gradient aortic stenosis in patients with depressed left ventricular systolic function: The clinical utility of the dobutamine challenge in the catheterization laboratory. Circulation 106:809, 2002
98. Monin JL, Quere JP, Monchi M, et al: Low-gradient aortic stenosis: operative risk stratification and predictors for long-term outcome: A multicenter study using dobutamine stress hemodynamics. Circulation 108:319, 2003
99. ACC/AHA guidelines for the management of patients with valvular heart disease. A report of the American College of Cardiology/American Heart Association. Task Force on Practice Guidelines (Committee on Management of Patients with Valvular Heart Disease). J Am Coll Cardiol 32:1486, 1998
100. Lung B, Gohlke-Barwolf C, Tornos P, et al: Recommendations on the management of the asymptomatic patient with valvular heart disease. Eur Heart J 23:1252, 2002
101. Bonow RO, Rosing DR, McIntosh CL, et al: The natural history of asymptomatic patients with aortic regurgitation and normal left ventricular function. Circulation 68:509, 1983
102. Bonow RO, Lakatos E, Maron BJ, Epstein SE: Serial long-term assessment of the natural history of asymptomatic patients with chronic aortic regurgitation and normal left ventricular systolic function. Circulation 84:1625, 1991
103. Henry WL, Bonow RO, Rosing DR, Epstein SE: Observations on the optimum time for operative intervention for aortic regurgitation. II. Serial echocardiographic evaluation of asymptomatic patients. Circulation 61:484, 1980

104. Nash PJ, Vitvitsky E, Cosgrove DM, et al: Echocardiographic predictors of aortic valve repair in patients with bicuspid valves and aortic regurgitation. J Am Coll Cardiol 41:516, 2003
105. Yacoub MH, Cohn LH: Novel approaches to cardiac valve repair: From structure to function: Part II. Circulation 109:1064, 2004
106. Carr JA, Savage EB: Aortic valve repair for aortic insufficiency in adults: A contemporary review and comparison with replacement techniques. Eur J Cardiothorac Surg 25:6, 2004
107. Rahimtoola SH: Choice of prosthetic heart valve for adult patients. J Am Coll Cardiol 41:893, 2003
108. Girard SE, Miller FA Jr, Orszulak TA, et al: Reoperation for prosthetic aortic valve obstruction in the era of echocardiography: Trends in diagnostic testing and comparison with surgical findings. J Am Coll Cardiol 37:579, 2001
109. Rao V, Jamieson WR, Ivanov J, et al: Prosthesis-patient mismatch affects survival after aortic valve replacement. Circulation 102:III-5, 2000
110. He GW, Grunkemeier GL, Gately HL, et al: Up to thirty-year survival after aortic valve replacement in the small aortic root. Ann Thorac Surg 59:1056, 1995
111. Yazdanbakhsh AP, van den Brink RB, Dekker E, de Mol BA: Small valve area index: Its influence on early mortality after mitral valve replacement. Eur J Cardiothorac Surg 17:222, 2000
112. Barner HB, Labovitz AJ, Fiore AC: Prosthetic valves for the small aortic root. J Card Surg 9:154, 1994
113. Gonzalez-Juanatey JR, Garcia-Acuna JM, Vega FM, et al: Influence of the size of aortic valve prostheses on hemodynamics and change in left ventricular mass: Implications for the surgical management of aortic stenosis. J Thorac Cardiovasc Surg 112:273, 1996
114. Pibarot P, Dumesnil JG: Hemodynamic and clinical impact of prosthesis-patient mismatch in the aortic valve position and its prevention. J Am Coll Cardiol 36:1131, 2000
115. Come PC, Riley MF, Ferguson JF, et al: Prediction of severity of aortic stenosis: Accuracy of multiple noninvasive parameters. Am J Med 85:29, 1988
116. Palta S, Gill KS, Pai RG: Role of inadequate adaptive left ventricular hypertrophy in the genesis of mitral regurgitation in patients with severe aortic stenosis: Implications for its prevention. J Heart Valve Dis 12:601, 2003
117. Brener SJ, Duffy CI, Thomas JD, Stewart WJ: Progression of aortic stenosis in 394 patients: Relation to changes in myocardial and mitral valve dysfunction. J Am Coll Cardiol 25:305, 1995
118. Absil B, Dagenais F, Mathieu P, et al: Does moderate mitral regurgitation impact early or mid-term clinical outcome in patients undergoing isolated aortic valve replacement for aortic stenosis? Eur J Cardiothorac Surg 24:217, 2003
119. Christenson JT, Jordan B, Bloch A, Schmuziger M: Should a regurgitant mitral valve be replaced simultaneously with a stenotic aortic valve? Tex Heart Inst J 27:350, 2000
120. Goland S, Loutaty G, Arditi A, et al: Improvement in mitral regurgitation after aortic valve replacement. Isr Med Assoc J 5:12, 2003
121. Harris KM, Malenka DJ, Haney MF, et al: Improvement in mitral regurgitation after aortic valve replacement. Am J Cardiol 80:741, 1997
122. Moazami N, Diodato MD, Moon MR, et al: Does functional mitral regurgitation improve with isolated aortic valve replacement? J Card Surg 19:444, 2004
123. Tunick PA, Gindea A, Kronzon I: Effect of aortic valve replacement for aortic stenosis on severity of mitral regurgitation. Am J Cardiol 65:1219, 1990
124. Tassan-Mangina S, Metz D, Nazeyllas P, et al: Factors determining early improvement in mitral regurgitation after aortic valve replacement for aortic valve stenosis: A transthoracic and transesophageal prospective study. Clin Cardiol 26:127, 2003
125. Akins CW, Buckley MJ, Daggett WM, et al: Myocardial revascularization with combined aortic and mitral valve replacements. J Thorac Cardiovasc Surg 90:272, 1985
126. Amarenco P, Cohen A, Tzourio C, et al: Atherosclerotic disease of the aortic arch and the risk of ischemic stroke. N Engl J Med 331:1474, 1994
127. Davila-Roman VG, Barzilai B, Wareing TH, et al: Atherosclerosis of the ascending aorta. Prevalence and role as an independent predictor of cerebrovascular events in cardiac patients. Stroke 25:2010, 1994
128. Hartman GS, Yao FS, Bruefach M III, et al: Severity of aortic atheromatous disease diagnosed by transesophageal echocardiography predicts stroke and other outcomes associated with coronary artery surgery: A prospective study. Anesth Analg 83:701, 1996
129. Konstadt SN, Reich DL, Quintana C, Levy M: The ascending aorta: How much does transesophageal echocardiography see? Anesth Analg 78:240, 1994
130. Katz ES, Tunick PA, Rusinek H, et al: Protruding aortic atheromas predict stroke in elderly patients undergoing cardiopulmonary bypass: Experience with intraoperative transesophageal echocardiography. J Am Coll Cardiol 20:70, 1992
131. Marshall WG Jr, Barzilai B, Kouchoukos NT, Saffitz J: Intraoperative ultrasonic imaging of the ascending aorta. Ann Thorac Surg 48:339, 1989
132. Hosoda Y, Watanabe M, Hirooka Y, et al: Significance of atherosclerotic changes of the ascending aorta during coronary bypass surgery with intraoperative detection by echography. J Cardiovasc Surg (Torino) 32:301, 1991
133. Ohteki H, Itoh T, Natsuaki M, et al: Intraoperative ultrasonic imaging of the ascending aorta in ischemic heart disease. Ann Thorac Surg 50:539, 1990
134. Davila-Roman VG, Barzilai B, Wareing TH, et al: Intraoperative ultrasonographic evaluation of the ascending aorta in 100 consecutive patients undergoing cardiac surgery. Circulation 84:III-47, 1991
135. Hammon JW Jr, Stump DA, Kon ND, et al: Risk factors and solutions for the development of neurobehavioral changes after coronary artery bypass grafting. Ann Thorac Surg 63:1613, 1997
136. Wilson MJ, Boyd SY, Lisagor PG, et al: Ascending aortic atheroma assessed intraoperatively by epiaortic and transesophageal echocardiography. Ann Thorac Surg 70:25, 2000
137. Konstadt SN, Reich DL, Kahn R, Viggiani RF: Transesophageal echocardiography can be used to screen for ascending aortic atherosclerosis. Anesth Analg 81:225, 1995
138. Eltzschig HK, Kallmeyer IJ, Mihaljevic T, et al: A practical approach to a comprehensive epicardial and epiaortic echocardiographic examination. J Cardiothorac Vasc Anesth 17:422, 2003
139. Chandraratna A, Ashmeg A, Pasha HC: Detection of intracoronary air embolism by echocardiography. J Am Soc Echocardiogr 15:1015, 2002
140. Baker RC, Graham AN, Phillips AS, Campalani G: An unusual iatrogenic cause of right coronary air embolism. Ann Thorac Surg 68:575, 1999
141. Ohnishi Y, Uchida O, Hayashi Y, et al: [Relationship between retained microbubbles and neuropsychologic alterations after cardiac operation]. Masui 44:1327, 1995
142. Bickerstaff LK, Pairolero PC, Hollier LH, et al: Thoracic aortic aneurysms: A population-based study. Surgery 92:1103, 1982
143. Pressler V, McNamara JJ: Thoracic aortic aneurysm: natural history and treatment. J Thorac Cardiovasc Surg 79:489, 1980
144. Crawford ES, DeNatale RW: Thoracoabdominal aortic aneurysm: observations regarding the natural course of the disease. J Vasc Surg 3:578, 1986
145. Clouse WD, Hallett JW Jr, Schaff HV, et al: Improved prognosis of thoracic aortic aneurysms: A population-based study. JAMA 280:1926, 1998
146. Sioris T, David TE, Ivanov J, et al: Clinical outcomes after separate and composite replacement of the aortic valve and ascending aorta. J Thorac Cardiovasc Surg 128:260, 2004
147. Feindel CM, David TE: Aortic valve sparing operations: Basic concepts. Int J Cardiol 97:61, 2004
148. Nienaber CA, von Kodolitsch Y, Nicolas V, et al: The diagnosis of thoracic aortic dissection by noninvasive imaging procedures. N Engl J Med 328:1, 1993
149. Roudaut RP, Billes MA, Gosse P, et al: Accuracy of M-mode and two-dimensional echocardiography in the diagnosis of aortic dissection: An experience with 128 cases. Clin Cardiol 11:553, 1988
150. Suzuki T, Mehta RH, Ince H, et al: Clinical profiles and outcomes of acute type B aortic dissection in the current era: Lessons from the International Registry of Aortic Dissection (IRAD). Circulation 108(suppl II):II-312, 2003
151. Doroghazi RM, Slater EE, DeSanctis RW, et al: Long-term survival of patients with treated aortic dissection. J Am Coll Cardiol 3:1026, 1984
152. Bernard Y, Zimmermann H, Chocron S, et al: False lumen patency as a predictor of late outcome in aortic dissection. Am J Cardiol 87:1378, 2001
153. Umana JP, Lai DT, Mitchell RS, et al: Is medical therapy still the optimal treatment strategy for patients with acute type B aortic dissections? J Thorac Cardiovasc Surg 124:896, 2002
154. Erbel R, Oelert H, Meyer J, et al: Effect of medical and surgical therapy on aortic dissection evaluated by transesophageal echocardiography. Implications for prognosis and therapy. The European Cooperative Study Group on Echocardiography. Circulation 87:1604, 1993
155. Nienaber CA, Fattori R, Lund G, et al: Nonsurgical reconstruction of thoracic aortic dissection by stent-graft placement. N Engl J Med 340:1539, 1999
156. Nienaber CA, Eagle KA: Aortic dissection: New frontiers in diagnosis and management: Part II: Therapeutic management and follow-up. Circulation 108:772, 2003

157. Dake MD, Kato N, Mitchell RS, et al: Endovascular stent-graft placement for the treatment of acute aortic dissection. N Engl J Med 340:1546, 1999
158. Nienaber CA, Eagle KA: Aortic dissection: New frontiers in diagnosis and management: Part I: From etiology to diagnostic strategies. Circulation 108:628, 2003
159. Mehta RH, Suzuki T, Hagan PG, et al: Predicting death in patients with acute type A aortic dissection. Circulation 105:200, 2002
160. Miller DC, Mitchell RS, Oyer PE, et al: Independent determinants of operative mortality for patients with aortic dissections. Circulation 70:I-153, 1984
161. Haverich A, Miller DC, Scott WC, et al: Acute and chronic aortic dissections—Determinants of long-term outcome for operative survivors. Circulation 72:II-22, 1985
162. Pansini S, Gagliardotto PV, Pompei E, et al: Early and late risk factors in surgical treatment of acute type A aortic dissection. Ann Thorac Surg 66:779, 1998
163. Sabik JF, Lytle BW, Blackstone EH, et al: Long-term effectiveness of operations for ascending aortic dissections. J Thorac Cardiovasc Surg 119:946, 2000
164. Kawahito K, Adachi H, Yamaguchi A, Ino T: Preoperative risk factors for hospital mortality in acute type A aortic dissection. Ann Thorac Surg 71:1239, 2001
165. Lai DT, Robbins RC, Mitchell RS, et al: Does profound hypothermic circulatory arrest improve survival in patients with acute type A aortic dissection? Circulation 106:I-218, 2002
166. Fabian TC, Richardson JD, Croce MA, et al: Prospective study of blunt aortic injury: Multicenter Trial of the American Association for the Surgery of Trauma. J Trauma 42:374, 1997
167. Fisher RG, Hadlock F: Laceration of the thoracic aorta and brachiocephalic arteries by blunt trauma. Report of 54 cases and review of the literature. Radiol Clin North Am 19:91, 1981
168. Ben Menachem Y: Assessment of blunt aortic-brachiocephalic trauma: Should angiography be supplanted by transesophageal echocardiography? J Trauma 42:969, 1997
169. Vignon P, Lang RM: Use of transesophageal echocardiography for the assessment of traumatic aortic injuries. Echocardiography 16:207, 1999
170. Goarin JP, Cluzel P, Gosgnach M, et al: Evaluation of transesophageal echocardiography for diagnosis of traumatic aortic injury. Anesthesiology 93:1373, 2000
171. Vignon P, Boncoeur MP, Francois B, et al: Comparison of multiplane transesophageal echocardiography and contrast-enhanced helical CT in the diagnosis of blunt traumatic cardiovascular injuries. Anesthesiology 94:615, 2001
172. Patel NH, Stephens KE Jr, Mirvis SE, et al: Imaging of acute thoracic aortic injury due to blunt trauma: A review. Radiology 209:335, 1998
173. Malhotra AK, Fabian TC, Croce MA, et al: Minimal aortic injury: A lesion associated with advancing diagnostic techniques. J Trauma 51:1042, 2001
174. Goarin JP, Catoire P, Jacquens Y, et al: Use of transesophageal echocardiography for diagnosis of traumatic aortic injury. Chest 112:71, 1997
175. Ott MC, Stewart TC, Lawlor DK, et al: Management of blunt thoracic aortic injuries: Endovascular stents versus open repair. J Trauma 56:565, 2004
176. Scheinert D, Krankenberg H, Schmidt A, et al: Endoluminal stent-graft placement for acute rupture of the descending thoracic aorta. Eur Heart J 25:694, 2004
177. Lorenzen HP, Geist V, Hartmann F, et al: Endovascular stent-graft implantation in acute traumatic aortic dissection with contained rupture and hemorrhagic shock. Z Kardiol 93:317, 2004
178. Svensson LG, Labib SB, Eisenhauer AC, Butterly JR: Intimal tear without hematoma: an important variant of aortic dissection that can elude current imaging techniques. Circulation 99:1331, 1999
179. Maraj R, Rerkpattanapipat P, Jacobs LE, et al: Meta-analysis of 143 reported cases of aortic intramural hematoma. Am J Cardiol 86:664, 2000
180. Moizumi Y, Komatsu T, Motoyoshi N, Tabayashi K: Clinical features and long-term outcome of type A and type B intramural hematoma of the aorta. J Thorac Cardiovasc Surg 127:421, 2004
181. Kang DH, Song JK, Song MG, et al: Clinical and echocardiographic outcomes of aortic intramural hemorrhage compared with acute aortic dissection. Am J Cardiol 81:202, 1998
182. Song JK, Kim HS, Song JM, et al: Outcomes of medically treated patients with aortic intramural hematoma. Am J Med 113:181, 2002
183. Vilacosta I, San Roman JA, Ferreiros J, et al: Natural history and serial morphology of aortic intramural hematoma: A novel variant of aortic dissection. Am Heart J 134:495, 1997
184. Song JK, Kim HS, Kang DH, et al: Different clinical features of aortic intramural hematoma versus dissection involving the ascending aorta. J Am Coll Cardiol 37:1604, 2001
185. von Kodolitsch Y, Csosz SK, Koschyk DH, et al: Intramural hematoma of the aorta: predictors of progression to dissection and rupture. Circulation 107:1158, 2003
186. Sueyoshi E, Imada T, Sakamoto I, et al: Analysis of predictive factors for progression of type B aortic intramural hematoma with computed tomography. J Vasc Surg 35:1179, 2002
187. Kaji S, Akasaka T, Katayama M, et al: Long-term prognosis of patients with type B aortic intramural hematoma. Circulation 108(suppl II):II-307, 2003
188. Ganaha F, Miller DC, Sugimoto K, et al: Prognosis of aortic intramural hematoma with and without penetrating atherosclerotic ulcer: A clinical and radiological analysis. Circulation 106:342, 2002

Chapter 17

CENTRAL NERVOUS SYSTEM MONITORING

Harvey L. Edmonds, Jr., PhD

KEY POINTS

1. Cardiac surgery–associated brain injury is common, multifactorial, and often preventable.
2. Electroencephalography can detect cerebral ischemia/hypoxia and seizures and measure hypnotic effect.
3. Middle-latency auditory evoked potentials objectively document inadequate hypnosis.
4. Brainstem auditory evoked potentials measure the effects of cooling and rewarming on deep brain structures.
5. Transcranial Doppler ultrasound assesses the direction and character of blood flow through large intracranial arteries and identifies microemboli.
6. Cerebral oximetry, using spatially resolved transcranial near-infrared spectroscopy, provides a continuous measure of change in the balance of cerebral oxygen supply and demand.
7. Used in concert, these technologies can reduce the incidence of brain injury and ensure the adequacy of hypnosis.

Nearly half of the 1 million patients undergoing cardiac surgery each year worldwide will likely experience persistent cognitive decline.[1] The direct annual cost to U.S. insurers for brain injury from just one type of cardiac surgery, myocardial revascularization, is estimated at $4 billion.[2] Furthermore, the same processes that injure the central nervous system (CNS) also appear to cause dysfunction of other vital organs. Thus, there are enormous clinical and economic incentives to improve CNS protection during cardiac surgery.

Historically, there has been little enthusiasm for neurophysiologic monitoring during cardiac surgery because of the presumed key role of macroembolization. It is widely assumed that most brain injuries during adult cardiac surgery result from cerebral embolization of atheromatous or calcified material dislodged from sclerotic blood vessels during their manipulation. Until the introduction of myocardial revascularization without cardiopulmonary bypass (CPB) or aortic clamp application, these injuries often have been viewed as unavoidable and untreatable.

Technical developments have begun to alter this perception. First, CNS injuries still occur despite reductions in aortic manipulation with the new approaches to coronary artery bypass and aortic surgery.[3] Second, neurophysiologic studies have implicated hypoperfusion and dysoxygenation as major causative factors in CNS injury[4,5] (Box 17–1). Because these functional disturbances are often detectable and correctable, there is an impetus to examine the role of neurophysiologic monitoring in CNS protection (see Chapter 35).

Cardiac anesthesia provider familiarity with neuromonitoring is becoming increasingly important. The introduction of compact and simplified monitors of brain electrical activity, blood flow velocity, and oxygenation promises to integrate these devices and their information into cardiac anesthetic management. The goal of this chapter is to highlight the practical issues involved with these emerging neuromonitoring technologies. This emphasis on practicality limits discussion to Food and Drug Administration–approved devices.

ELECTROENCEPHALOGRAPHY

Electroencephalographic (EEG) monitoring for ischemia detection has been performed since the first CPB procedures, but this long experience is not broad.[6] In contrast to its widespread use during carotid endarterectomy, EEG monitoring for cardiac surgery is performed primarily in academic centers or those specializing in pediatric surgery. Limited use appears to have several causes.

First, small, practical, and affordable EEG monitors have only recently become available. For example, using a book-sized box of electronics and a notebook computer, it is now possible to concurrently display multichannel conventional and processed EEG, as well as bilateral transcranial Doppler (TCD) ultrasonic spectra and cerebral oxygen saturation. All of the resulting data can be easily transmitted over high-speed data lines for Web-based consultation or archival or post hoc analysis.

Second, the traditional diagnostic approach to EEG analysis depended on complex pattern recognition of 16-channel analog waveforms to identify focal ischemic changes.[7] Because this analytic format necessitated extensive training and constant vigilance, cardiac surgery EEG monitoring directly by anesthesia providers has often been viewed as impractical. However, Craft et al[8] and Edmonds et al[9] have shown that a four-channel recording, which included bilateral activity from both the anterior and posterior circulation, was effective in identifying focal ischemia. In addition, computerized processing of EEG signals provides simplified trend displays that have helped to overcome many of the earlier complexities.

Third, EEG analysis during cardiac surgery was often confounded by anesthetics, hypothermia, and roller-pump artifacts.[10] Fortunately, the troublesome roller pumps have been replaced with centrifugal pumps or eliminated entirely; moderate-to-deep hypothermia is now usually applied only in aortic arch reconstruction; and fast-track anesthesia protocols avoid marked EEG suppression.

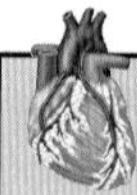

BOX 17–1 *Factors Contributing to Brain Injury During Cardiac Surgery*

- Atheromatous emboli from aorta manipulation
- Lipid microemboli from recirculation of unwashed cardiotomy suction
- Gaseous microemboli from air leakage and cavitation
- Cerebral hypoperfusion from dysautoregulation
- Cerebral hyperperfusion
- Cerebral hyperthermia

BOX 17–2 *EEG Frequency Bands*

Delta	0.5 to 2 Hz
Theta	3 to 7 Hz
Alpha	8 to 12 Hz
Beta	13 to 24 Hz
Gamma	25 to 55 Hz

Physiologic Basis of Electroencephalography

EEG-directed interventions designed to correct cerebral hypoperfusion during cardiac surgery require an appreciation of the underlying neurophysiologic substrate. Scalp-recorded EEG signals reflect the temporal and spatial summation of long-lasting (10 to 100 milliseconds) postsynaptic potentials, which arise from columnar cortical pyramidal neurons (Fig. 17–1). These potentials are produced by dipoles distributed over soma-dendritic surfaces. Pyramidal neurons have a long vertically oriented apical dendrite and shorter basal dendrites radiating from the soma base. Near-synchronous excitation (or inhibition) of neighboring dendritic membranes produces large-amplitude spatially summating vertical dipoles, whereas radial current layers are generated in the somatic region. Simultaneous current generation in the two regions may appear to be self-canceling at distant surface electrodes. In addition, traditional EEG depicts only voltage change, not absolute voltage. Thus, sustained high-frequency neuronal activity may result in a large but nonvarying surface voltage deviation, which would be invisible to the conventional EEG. These important EEG characteristics should be appreciated when interpreting low-amplitude signals; they do not necessarily indicate synaptic quiescence.

EEG rhythms represent regularly recurring waveforms of similar shape and duration. These signal oscillations depend on the synchronous excitation of a neuronal population. The descriptive nature of conventional EEG characterizes the oscillations (measured in cycles per second [cps] or Hertz [Hz]) as sinusoids that were classified according to their amplitude and frequency. The terminology used to describe the frequency bands of the most common oscillatory patterns is illustrated (Fig. 17–2). In addition, a high-frequency (25 to 55 Hz) gamma band is recognized (Box 17–2).

EEG oscillatory patterns are functional manifestations of specific intraneuronal networks. The extent of cortical processing among neighboring neuronal columns influences the extent of scalp-recorded EEG waveform synchronization and is not necessarily dependent on the subcortically mediated arousal level. At a high level of cortical processing, each neu-

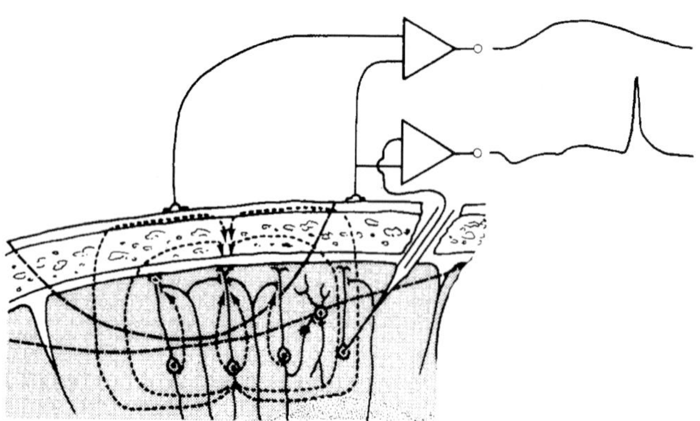

Figure 17–1 The production of EEG waves. Scalp electrodes record potential differences that are caused by postsynaptic potentials in the cell membrane of cortical neurons. The closed loops of the lighter dashed lines represent the summation of extracellular currents produced by the postsynaptic potentials. Open segments of the heavier dashed lines connect all points having the same voltage level. The two scalp electrodes record changes in the voltage difference over time (*top trace at upper right*). The *lower trace* from a microelectrode inserted in a single cortical neuron has little direct relationship to the summated EEG wave. (Modified from Fisch BJ: EEG Primer, 3rd edition, 1999, p. 6 with the permission of the publisher, Elsevier, New York, NY.)

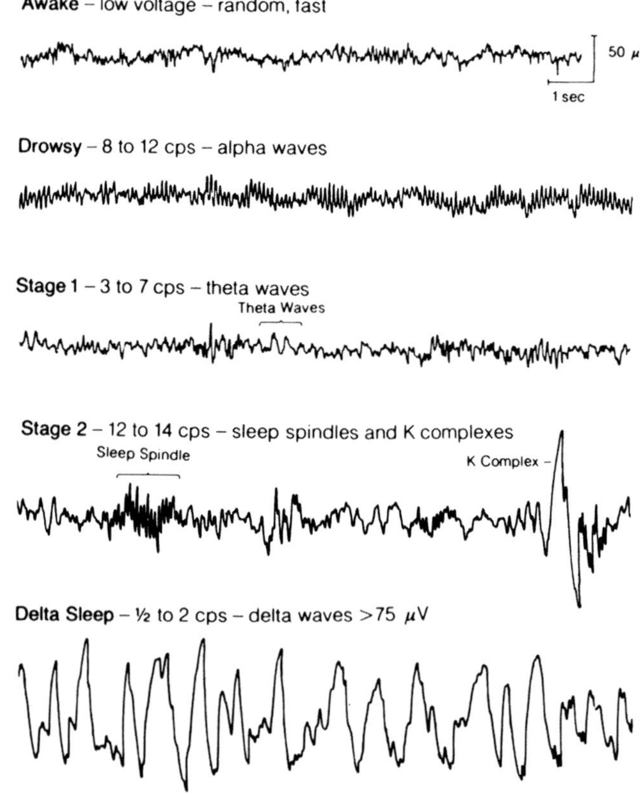

Figure 17–2 The specific EEG characteristics of the different stages of the human sleep-wakefulness cycle are shown. Note the appearance of the four most common frequency bands from the lowest frequency delta, through theta and alpha to high-frequency beta. An even higher gamma frequency band (25 to 55 cps) is also described. (Modified from Yli-Hankala A [ed]: Handbook of Four-Channel EEG in Anesthesia and Critical Care, 2004, p 5, with permission of the publisher, GE Medical, Datex-Ohmeda Division, Helsinki, Finland.)

ronal palisade may function in relative independence. The resultant EEG signal will be of low amplitude, representing the distance-weighted average of many desynchronized micropotentials. The large number of small potentials is reflected in an EEG pattern characterized by a high dominant frequency (13- to 24-Hz beta waves). Such a pattern may be seen during very different vigilance states, such as awake, mentally alert (see Fig. 17–2, top trace) versus rapid-eye-movement (i.e., dream) sleep (see Fig. 17–2, bottom trace). Partial cortical columnar synchronization develops with a reduction in information processing, resulting in higher amplitude and lower frequency EEG oscillations associated with a relaxed, drowsy state (see Fig. 17–2; 8- to 12-Hz alpha rhythm). Progressive suppression is associated with lower frequency 3- to 7-Hz theta waves. Minimal processing leads to the very high-amplitude, low-frequency hypersynchronous 0.5- to 2-Hz delta waves seen during the low vigilance states of deep coma, deepest sleep, hypoxia, ischemia, and some forms of surgical anesthesia.

Synchronization of cortical columns is influenced by subcortical structures, including the thalamus (Fig. 17–3) and reticular activating system (Fig. 17–4). Reticular inhibition can block the passage of sensory information to the cortex that is routed through thalamic relays. This state of functional deafferentation results in unconsciousness, an essential component of both natural sleep and surgical anesthesia.[11] However, the individual components of a modern balanced anesthetic technique may differentially affect the separate control mechanisms for sensory processing and vigilance. Thus, an EEG pattern suggestive of a low vigilance state (i.e., surgical hypnosis) does not necessarily guarantee the absence of subcortical (i.e., unconscious) sensory perception (i.e., reflexive response to painful stimuli).[12] Furthermore, because the neuronal basis for the EEG is primarily of cortical origin, it is not surprising that many univariate (i.e., single variable) EEG amplitude or frequency descriptors are only weakly correlated with clinical measures of anesthetic effect or developing pathology involving primarily or exclusively subcortical structures.

Practical Considerations of Electroencephalographic Recording and Signal Processing

This section describes practical issues involved in the conversion of these tiny potentials into interpretable EEG displays. The process begins with choice of scalp electrodes (subdermal needle, metallic disc, or silver chloride gel self-adhesive patch) and their location. All three electrode types provide high-quality signals. Single-use sterile needle electrodes are easy to apply but are invasive, relatively expensive, and not well tolerated by conscious patients. Reusable disk electrodes, held in place with conductive paste or built into a nylon mesh cap, may be used on conscious patients and are the least costly option. Adhesive patch electrodes can only be used on glabrous skin and have a cost midway between the other options.

Standardized electrode placement is based on the International 10-20 System (Fig. 17–5). It permits uniform spacing of electrodes, independent of head circumference, in scalp regions known to correlate with specific areas of cerebral cortex. Four anatomic landmarks are used—the nasion, inion,

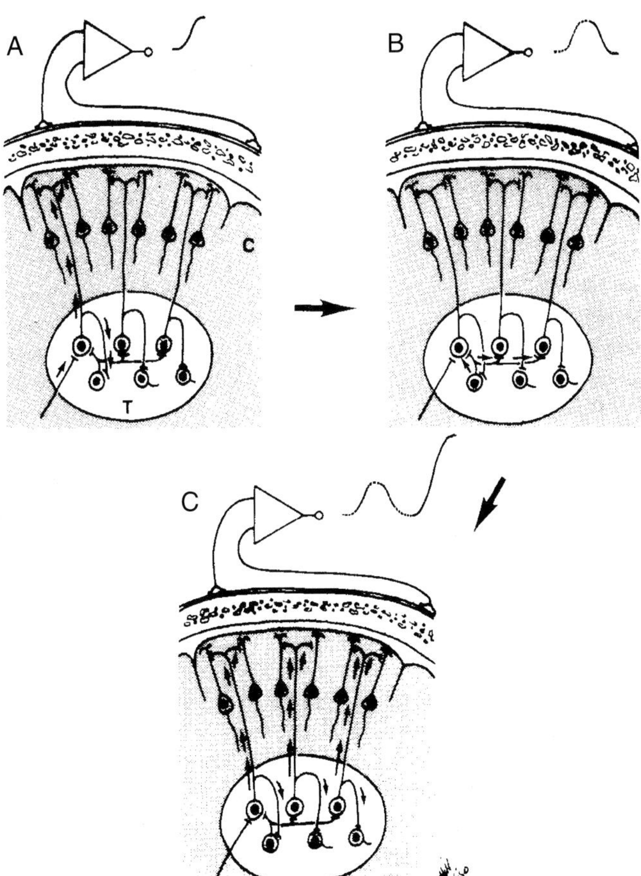

Figure 17–3 The steps involved in the production of rhythmic EEG activity. *(A)* Initiation of an EEG wave results from afferent excitation of a thalamocortical relay neuron (TCR) in the thalamus (T) and subsequent simultaneous transmission to a cortical and inhibitory thalamic interneuron. *(B)* Output from the thalamic inhibitory interneuron suppresses neighboring TCR neurons, leading to the termination of the first EEG wave. *(C)* Following the inhibitory phase, additional TCR depolarization produces another EEG wave. (Modified from Fisch BJ: EEG Primer, 3rd edition, 1999, p 10 with the permission of the publisher, Elsevier, New York, NY.)

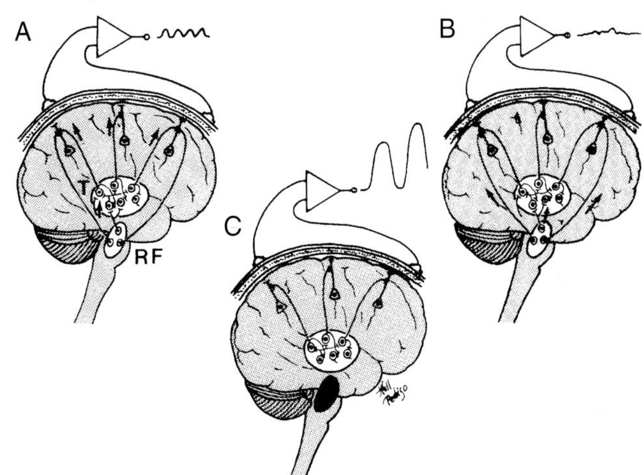

Figure 17–4 These diagrams depict the role of the mesencephalic reticular formation (RF) in the generation of rhythmical EEG activity. *(A)* In the absence of strong RF input, the thalamic pacemaker cells produce rhythmical EEG activity. *(B)* RF activation sends inhibitory signals to the thalamus, suppressing rhythmic EEG and leading to a desynchronized pattern. *(C)* In contrast, anesthetic or hypnotic RF suppression augments cortical EEG rhythms. (Modified from Fisch BJ: EEG Primer, 3rd edition, 1999, p 12 with the permission of the publisher, Elsevier, New York, NY.)

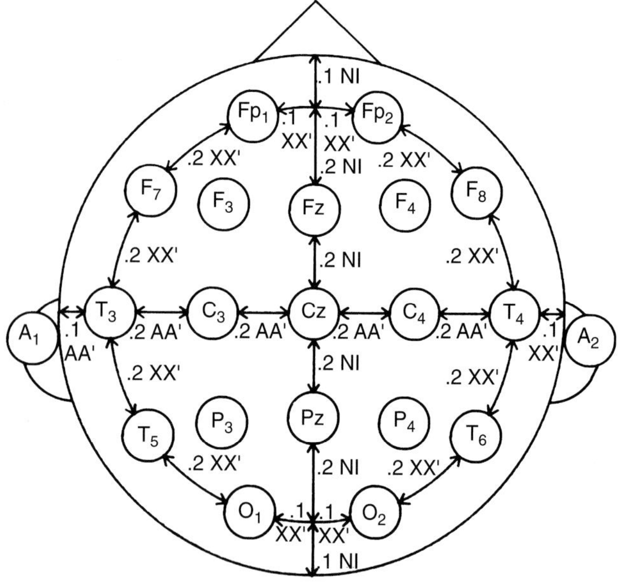

Figure 17–5 The position of the electrodes in the International 10-20 system according to scalp measurements. The sagittal hemicircumference (labeled AA′) is measured from the root of one zygoma (just anterior to the ear) to the other, across the vertex. The third measurement is the ipsilateral hemicircumference (XX′) measured from a point 10% of the coronal hemicircumference above the zygoma. Through these intersecting lines all of the scalp electrodes may be located, except frontal (F3, F4) and parietal (P3, P4). The frontal and parietal electrodes are placed along the frontal or parietal coronal line midway between the middle electrode and the electrode marked in the circumferential ring.

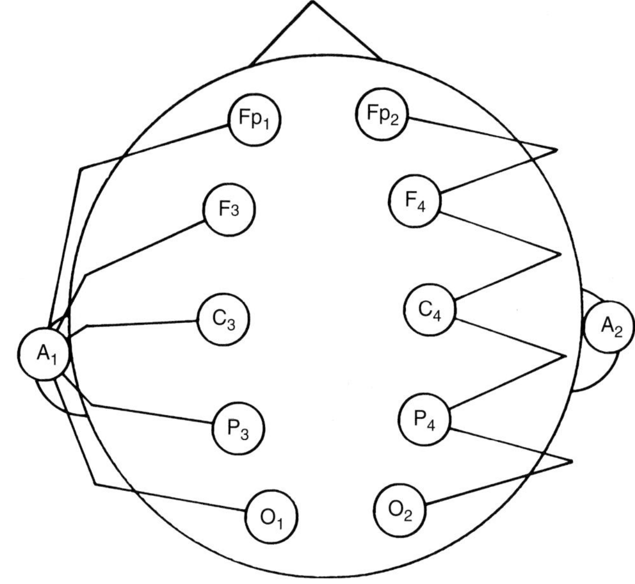

Figure 17–6 Bipolar and common reference montages are shown. The left parasagittal electrodes are connected in a common reference montage using the left earlobe (A1) as the common reference electrode. Five channels are recorded, each of them between the parasagittal electrode and the ear electrode. Differences among these channels represent differences in cerebral activity among the various parasagittal electrodes because each channel is recorded as the difference between the activity at the parasagittal electrode and the activity at the ear electrode. For comparison, the right parasagittal electrodes are connected in a bipolar chain. In this configuration, only four channels of EEG data are recorded. Each channel of data represents the electrical difference between the two electrodes.

and preauricular points. Electrodes are located at 10% or 20% segments of the distance between two of these landmarks. The alphanumeric label for each site uses an initial upper case letter to signify the skull region (i.e., frontal, central, temporal, parietal, occipital, auricular, mastoid). Second and sometimes third letters, in lowercase, further delineate position (e.g., "p" represents frontal pole, while "z" indicates zero or midline). Subscripted numbers represent left (odd) or right (even) and specific hemispheric location, with the lowest numbers closest to midline. The prime notation (′) is used to signify specialized locations designed for certain evoked potential applications (e.g., C_3' and C_4' represent 2 cm posterior to C_3 and C_4, directly over upper limb sensory cortex).

The differential amplifiers used in EEG recording measure the voltage difference between two inputs. By convention, a negative voltage at input 1 relative to input 2 results in an upward deflection of the tracing. With a referential arrangement (montage) of recording channel selections (Fig. 17–6, left), the input 2 connections from a series of channels are connected to a single electrode, while input 1 electrode connections all differ. Alternatively, in bipolar recordings, a common reference is not used (Fig. 17–6, right).

Although an array of scalp electrodes theoretically permits many possible montages to be used, the capability to quickly change montage varies greatly among different EEG monitors. This ability to quickly change recording montage may be important in the detection and characterization of both focal and diffuse abnormalities. With a referential montage (Fig. 17–7), the transient will be distorted if the reference lies within the transient electric field. Alternatively, with a bipolar montage, the potential may actually disappear due to in-phase cancellation.

Montage choice also influences susceptibility to artifact. For example, millivolt ECG potentials may contaminate the thousand-fold smaller EEG signal. Contamination is often problematic with an ear or mastoid reference montage, but may be invisible with an anterior-to-posterior bipolar montage (Fig. 17–8). The extreme lateral placement of ear or mastoid references maximizes contamination by the perpendicularly oriented high-voltage dipole generated by the heart.

The frequency range involved in production of the EEG waveform is termed its *bandwidth*. The upper and lower bandwidth boundaries are controlled by filters that reject frequencies above and below the EEG bandwidth. Both the appearance of the unprocessed EEG waveform and the value of univariate numeric EEG descriptors such as the mean frequency may be heavily influenced by signal bandwidth. The same cerebral biopotential recorded by different EEG devices may result in dissimilar waveforms and numeric values.

Modern EEG monitors use digital microprocessors to analyze the amplified analog biopotentials. Yet, analog-to-digital conversion imposes limitations on signal processing. Digitization converts a continuously varying biopotential into a series (i.e., sample) of discrete quantal values. To minimize conversion inaccuracies, at least two samples per period are required. Sampling (Nyquist) frequency must be greater than twice the highest frequency of interest. For example, with an EEG bandwidth of 50 Hz, the minimum acceptable sampling frequency is 100 Hz (e.g., 10-millisecond sampling interval). Aliasing, the counting of high-frequency signals as low-frequency input, may occur if the complex biopotential contains frequencies above the Nyquist frequency. Therefore, most EEG monitors contain antialiasing filters that sharply

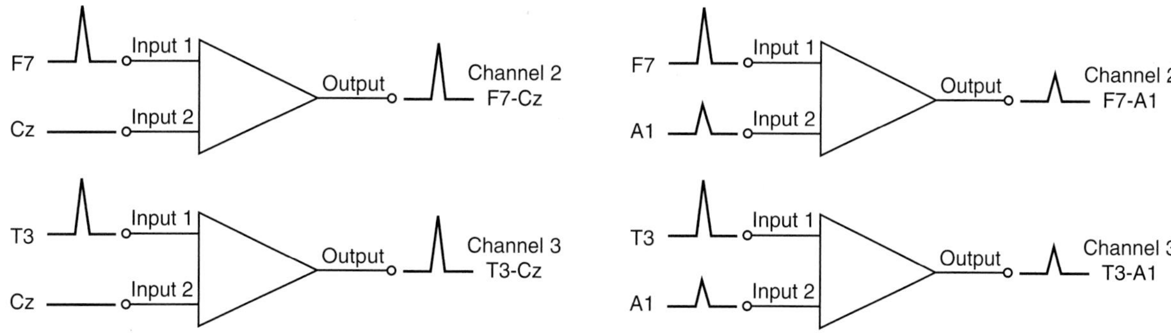

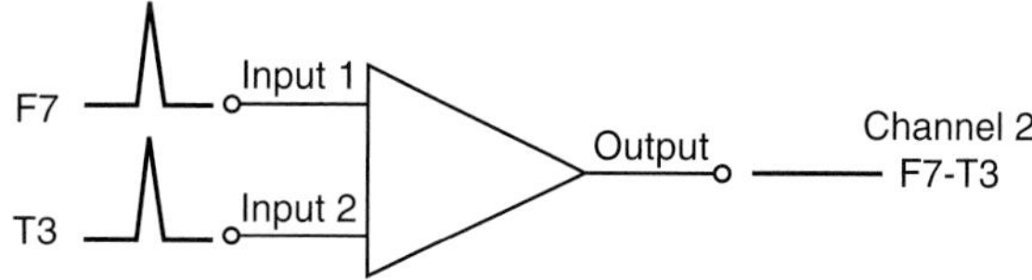

Figure 17–7 Accurate characterization of focal abnormalities requires that one of the amplifier's inputs be outside the field distribution of the transient. If both inputs lie within the transient field, the signal may become invisible due to in-phase cancellation. (Modified from Goldenshohn ES, Legatt AD, Koszer S, et al [eds]: Goldensohn's EEG Interpretation, 2nd edition, 1999, p 16 with permission of the publisher, Futura Publishing, Armonk, NY.)

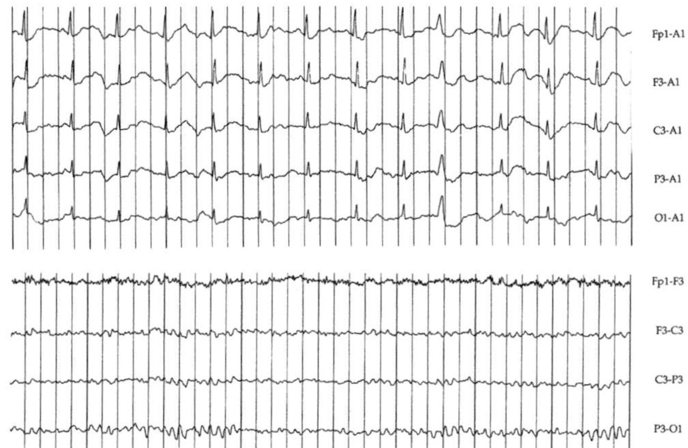

Figure 17–8 Ear-reference montages are particularly susceptible to ECG artifact since their dipoles are oriented transversely to the prominent electrocardiac vector. In contrast, the anterior-posterior orientation of bipolar temporal chain scalp dipoles is oriented in parallel with the powerful cardiac vector. As a result, such montages are relatively immune from ECG artifact. (Modified from Goldenshohn ES, Legatt AD, Koszer S, et al [eds]: Goldensohn's EEG Interpretation, 2nd edition, 1999, p 72 with permission of the publisher, Futura Publishing, Armonk, NY.)

attenuate waveform components above the Nyquist frequency. The details of filtering further add to the manufacturer-specific characteristics of processed EEG.

The continuous analog signal is also simplified into a (usually) discontinuous set of segments of a fixed duration (i.e., epoch). Window functions can minimize, but not totally eliminate, digital distortion produced by the abrupt truncation of a continuously varying waveform. These window functions are numerical series containing the same number of elements as the epoch. Their purpose is to reduce the value of epoch terminal elements. In addition to windowing, commercial EEG analyzers often use another form of signal conditioning called *whitening*. The energy content of the EEG is not uniform at all frequencies but instead is heavily skewed to the lower range. Whitening mathematically alters the momentary frequency-amplitude relationships to achieve nearly equal energy per octave and may improve pattern recognition in processed waveforms. Antialiasing, windowing, and whitening may vary not only among different devices but also among software versions used with a single device. The user should be aware that a standard unprocessed analog EEG signal may generate digitally processed displays and numeric descriptors that are unique for each monitor design and software version.

Display of Electroencephalographic Information

Time-Domain Analysis

Traditional display of the EEG is a graph of biopotential voltage (*y*-axis) as a function of time and, consequently, is described as a time-domain process. The objective of a diagnostic EEG is to identify the most likely cause of a detected abnormality at one moment in time. Typically, a diagnostic EEG is obtained under controlled conditions, using precisely defined protocols. Recorded EEG appearance is visually compared with reference patterns. Interpretation is based on recognition of unique waveform patterns that are pathognomonic for specific clinical conditions.[13] In contrast, the goal of EEG monitoring is to identify clinically important change from an individualized baseline. Unlike diagnostic EEG interpretation, monitoring requires immediate assessment of continuously fluctuating signals in an electronically hostile, complex, and poorly controlled recording environment. Therefore, of necessity, interpretation relies less on pattern recognition and more on statistical characterization of change. Simple numerical descriptors thus may appropriately form an integral part of EEG monitoring.

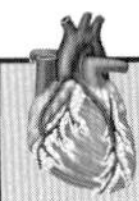

BOX 17–3 ***Law of the EEG***

- In the absence of pathology, EEG amplitude and frequency are inversely related.
- Simultaneous decrease may indicate ischemia, anoxia, or excessive hypnosis.
- Simultaneous increase may indicate seizure or artifact.

Both EEG diagnostic and monitoring interpretations are based, in part, on the "Law of the EEG" (Box 17–3). It states that amplitude and dominant frequency are inversely related. As described earlier, synchronously generated postsynaptic potentials may produce large-amplitude biopotentials. However, long membrane time constants limit the number of changes that may occur per second (e.g., high amplitude, low frequency). Conversely, summation of spatially distributed asynchronous potentials results in EEG signals of low amplitude but relatively high frequency. Thus, the inverse relationship between amplitude and frequency generally is maintained during unchanging cerebral metabolic states. Parallel increases in both may occur in some hypermetabolic states such as seizure activity, while decreases may be seen in hypometabolic states such as hypothermia. In the absence of these influences, simultaneous decreases in both amplitude and frequency may indicate ischemia or anoxia (Fig. 17–9), while a parallel increase may be artifact (Fig. 17–10).

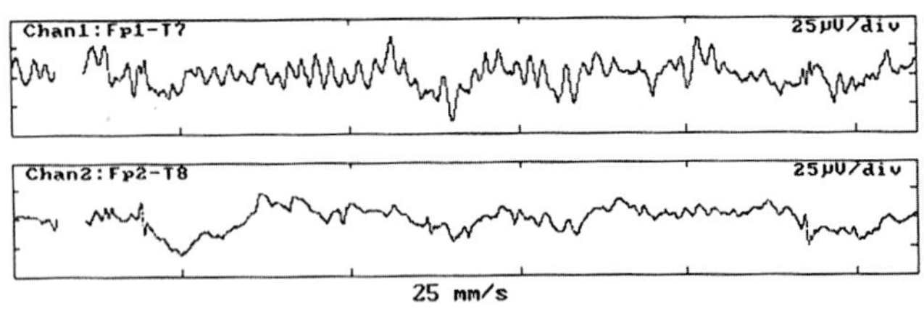

Figure 17–9 This two-channel EEG recording was made immediately after induction of anesthesia, prior to head repositioning for insertion of a central venous catheter. Anesthetic induction apparently uncovered a preexisting asymmetry that was not evident in the waking EEG. Although the patient had a history of an earlier mild cerebrovascular accident and transient ischemic attacks, he appeared neurologically normal at preoperative assessment. (Modified from Yli-Hankala A [ed]: Handbook of Four-Channel EEG in Anesthesia and Critical Care, 2004, p 31, with permission of the publisher, GE Medical, Datex-Ohmeda Division, Helsinki, Finland.)

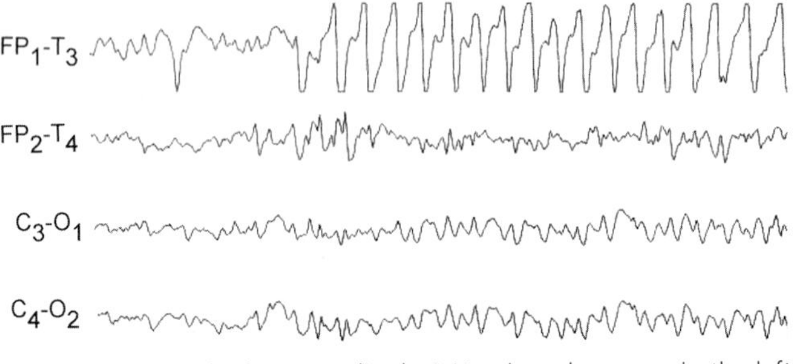

Figure 17–10 The large-amplitude 2-Hz triangular waves in the left frontotemporal derivation *(top trace)* are the result of temporalis muscle activation with a nerve stimulator. Current spread from the stimulating to the EEG recording electrodes may be minimized with use of the appropriate facial nerve stimulation site at the jaw angle. (Modified from Yli-Hankala A [ed]: Handbook of Four-Channel EEG in Anesthesia and Critical Care, 2004, p 18, with permission of the publisher, GE Medical, Datex-Ohmeda Division, Helsinki, Finland.)

Time domain analysis of traditional electroencephalography uses linear amplitude voltage and time scales. The amplitude range of EEG signals is quite large (several hundred microvolts) and univariate statistical measures of its central tendency and dispersion may contain clinically useful information.[14] Furthermore, amplitude variation may present clinically significant changes in reactivity that can be obscured by frequency-domain analysis.[15] Advances in the technology of EEG amplitude integration have prompted a resurgent interest in this attractively simple approach, particularly in pediatrics.[16]

Frequency Domain Analysis

An alternative method, frequency domain analysis, is exemplified by the prismatic decomposition of white light into its component frequencies (i.e., color spectrum). As the basis of spectral analysis, the Fourier theorem states that a periodic function can be represented, in part, by a sinusoid at the fundamental frequency and an infinite series of integer multiples (i.e., harmonics). The Fourier function at a specific frequency equals the amplitude and phase angle of the associated sinusoid. Graphs of amplitude and phase angle as functions of frequency are called Fourier spectra (i.e., spectral analysis). The EEG amplitude spectral scale (Fig. 17–11) squares voltage values to eliminate troublesome negative values. Squaring changes the unit of amplitude measure from microvolts to either picowatts (pW) or nanowatts (nW). However, a power amplitude scale tends to overemphasize large-amplitude changes. Clinically important changes in lower amplitude components that are readily discernible in the linearly scaled unprocessed EEG waveform may become invisible in power spectral displays.

Simplification of the large amount of spectral information generally has been achieved through the use of univariate numeric descriptors. Most commonly, the power contained in a specified traditional EEG frequency band (delta, theta, alpha, or beta) is calculated in absolute, relative, or normalized terms. Relative amplitude represents the fraction of total power contained in a specified frequency band (relative delta power = delta [–0.5 to 2 Hz] power/total [0.5 to 55 Hz]

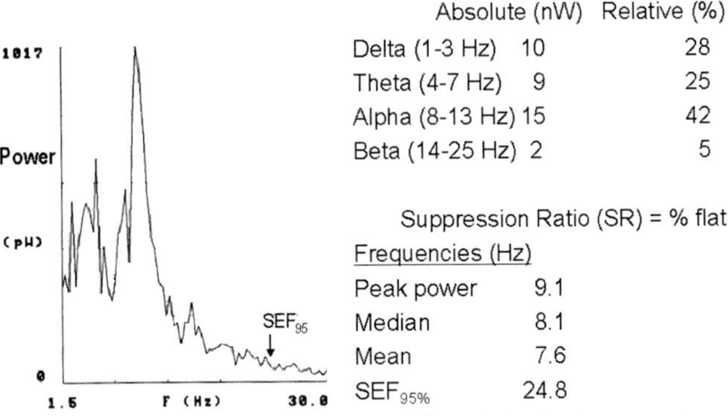

Figure 17–11 EEG frequency spectral pattern obtained from a patient anesthetized with 1 MAC isoflurane. It illustrates some of the many univariate numeric EEG descriptors.

power). Normalization equalizes the total power of successive epochs to that of some arbitrary reference before the calculation of relative power (the delta power is described as z-score change from a previous individualized baseline). The latter two derived measures are particularly useful in minimizing misinterpretation of spectral changes. For example, during the production of hypothermia, absolute delta power declines in parallel with cerebral metabolism, while the fraction of the total power in the delta band remains unchanged. In this circumstance, exclusive focus on absolute delta would lead to the erroneous conclusion that the hypnotic state is decreasing.

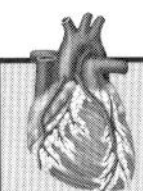

BOX 17–4 *Common Univariate EEG Descriptors Detecting Ischemia*

- Total power
- Peak power frequency
- Mean frequency
- Median frequency
- 95% Spectral edge frequency (SEF)
- Suppression ratio (SR)

The most widely used univariate frequency descriptors are (1) peak power frequency (the single frequency of the spectrum that contains the highest amplitude), (2) median power frequency (frequency below which 50% of the spectral power occurs), (3) mean spectral frequency (sum of power contained at each frequency of the spectrum times its frequency divided by the total power), (4) spectral edge frequency (SEF; frequency below which a predetermined fraction, usually 95%, of the spectral power occurs), and (5) suppression ratio (SR; percent of flat-line EEG contained within sampled epochs). The performance of two descriptors in characterizing clinically important EEG changes is compared (Fig. 17–12). Note, at anesthetic induction, the large transient decrease in SEF and reciprocal SR increase. However, later transient SR increases signifying marked EEG suppression were not detected by SEF, apparently due to low-level radio frequency contamination (Box 17–4).

Pronk[17] evaluated computer-processed univariate descriptors of EEG changes occurring before, during, and after CPB. Mean spectral frequency alone was sufficient to adequately

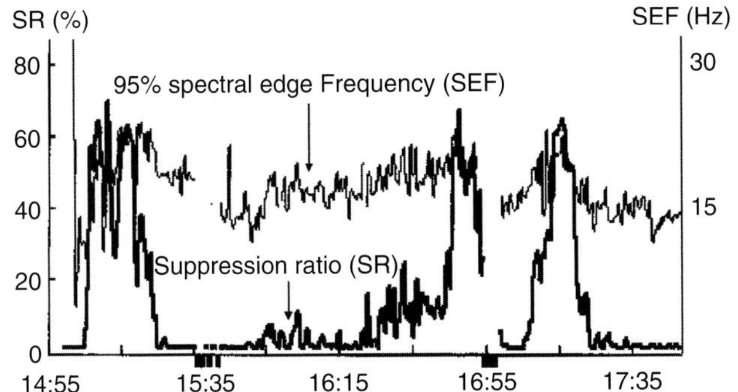

Figure 17–12 Certain univariate EEG descriptors are particularly susceptible to the confounding influence of electronic interference. Note the peak in the suppression ratio (SR) trend at 17:00, correctly identifying marked EEG suppression. In contrast, the spectral edge frequency remains unchanged because of the presence of low-intensity electronic noise.

describe all EEG changes except those occurring at very low amplitudes. Addition of a single-amplitude factor improved agreement with visual interpretation to 90%. Further factor addition did not improve agreement.

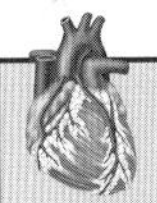

BOX 17–5 *Multivariate EEG Descriptors Primarily Measuring Hypnotic Effect*

- Bispectral index (BIS)
- Patient state index (PSI)
- Spectral entropy

Multivariate (i.e., composed of several variables) descriptors have been developed to improve simple numeric characterization of clinically important EEG changes. With this approach, algorithms are used to generate a single number that represents the pattern of amplitude-frequency-phase relationships occurring in a single epoch. Several commercially available monitors provide unitless numbers that have been transformed to an arbitrary 0-to-100 scale. Each monitor provides a different probability estimate of patient response to verbal instruction. Current examples of these descriptors include the bispectral index (BIS; Aspect Medical, Newton, MA), the patient state index (PSI; Physiometrix, North Billerica, MA), and spectral entropy (Entropy; Datex-Ohmeda division of GE Medical, Helsinki, Finland).[18-20] BIS and PSI are empirically derived proprietary indices developed from proprietary patient databases. In contrast, spectral entropy is neither empirical nor proprietary but rather represents the novel application of long-established physical sciences entropy equations to the analysis of cranial biopotentials. Each product is designed to require the use of proprietary self-adhesive forehead sensors. Collectively, these products are now in widespread use as objective measures of hypnotic effect (Box 17–5).

These three hypnotic indices appear to provide clinically useful information. However, their fundamental differences may result in distinctly unique performances. Close agreement among these measures should not be expected. For example, Figure 17–13 illustrates a BIS–versus–spectral entropy difference during emergence from anesthesia.

The proprietary BIS algorithm is a multivariate discriminant function that incorporates three EEG time and frequency domain features with empirically derived weighting coefficients.[21] Features include (1) a rule-based SR, (2) relative power in the high-frequency EEG/upper facial electromyographic (EMG) band, and (3) a bispectral measure of phase coupling.[22] The bispectral component is thought to correct for nonlinearities, which may confound rule-based algorithms.[21] The weighting coefficients are not constant but adaptive following a rule-based approach. For example, with low SR values, the variable is relatively underweighted, whereas overweighting occurs with SR greater than 50. As a consequence, high SR very heavily influences BIS.[20]

Like BIS, the PSI is also an empirically derived proprietary quantitative multivariate forehead EEG measure designed to measure the sedation–hypnosis continuum.[23-25] Rule-based algorithms remove artifact, detect EEG suppression, and combine spectral descriptors with weighting coefficients into a proprietary discriminant function. The recommended PSI

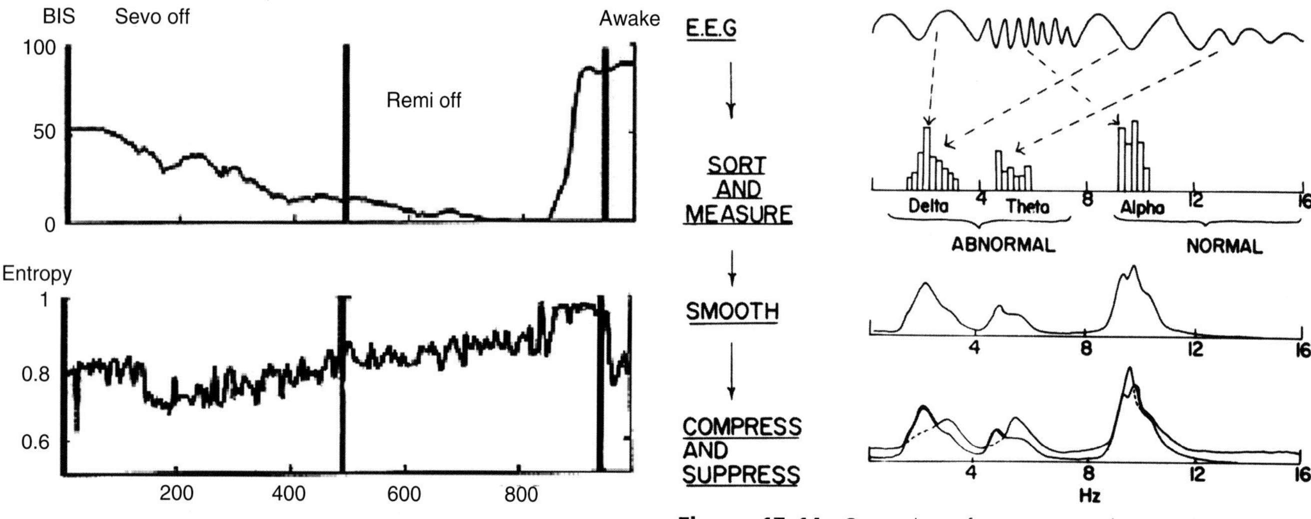

Figure 17–13 BIS and spectral entropy (response entropy) are compared during emergence from anesthesia. The sevoflurane vaporizer was turned off at time zero and the remifentanil infusion stopped at 500 seconds. Entropy successfully characterized the diminishing hypnotic effect, but BIS did not. (Modified from Muncaster AG, Sleigh JW, Williams M: Anesth Analg 96:722, 2003 with permission of the publisher, Lippincott Williams & Wilkins, Baltimore, MD.)

Figure 17–14 Generation of a compressed spectral array (CSA) display. *Top panel* represents the unprocessed EEG time domain waveform. *Panel 2* depicts Fourier transformation of the signal into the frequency domain. Smoothing of spectral data contained in individual frequency bins occurs in *panel 3*, while compressed sequencing of successive spectra with hidden-line suppression occurs in the *bottom panel*. (Modified from Myers RR, Stockard JJ, Fleming NI, et al: Br J Anaesth 45:664, 1973 with permission of the publisher, Oxford University Press, Oxford, England.)

range for adequate hypnosis of 25 to 50 is lower than the 40 to 60 BIS range. In contrast to BIS, the PSI weighting coefficients are modified by two observer functions representing SR and abrupt changes relative to a conscious baseline. Incorporation of the conscious comparison is claimed to produce a measure that is relatively agent independent.[24]

Most hypnotics decrease EEG complexity (i.e., variability) in a dose-related fashion. This long-established observation provides the rationale for the use of nonproprietary spectral entropy analysis as an objective measure of hypnotic effect.[26] The absence of an empirical rule–based approach avoids the need for arbitrary weighting coefficients and minimizes the potentially distorting influences of very low– and very high–amplitude EEG signals.

In addition, the Datex-Ohmeda version of spectral entropy views upper facial electromyographic (fEMG) activity as a useful signal, rather than noise to be eliminated. During consciousness and light sedation, gamma power (i.e., 25 to 55 Hz) is a mixture of cortically mediated EEG and subcortically influenced fEMG. Muscle activity makes a larger contribution because of closer proximity to the recording electrodes. Hypnotics and analgesics typically suppress both cerebral and muscle activities, resulting in reduced gamma power. Because the upper facial muscles are relatively insensitive to moderate neuromuscular blockade, they may remain reactive to noxious stimuli.[22] Nociception results in sudden gamma power increase, independent of activity in the lower frequency classical EEG bands.

Analysis in the Datex-Ohmeda Entropy Module incorporates two distinct spectral entropy indices: Response Entropy and State Entropy. Response Entropy describes the broad band (0.8 to 47 Hz) complexity of composite EEG and fEMG signals. The frequency range between 32 and 47 Hz is analyzed with successive brief 2-second epochs. Response Entropy provides an immediate indication of fEMG activation and changes readily with nociception or arousal. In contrast, State Entropy measures a narrower band (0.8 to 32 Hz) complexity of longer 15- to 60-second epochs, which excludes most fEMG activity. The two indices are claimed by the manufacturer to facilitate distinction between changes in hypnosis and analgesia, although supporting evidence for this proposition awaits carefully designed prospective studies. EEG suppression decreases both entropy indices, because noise-free flat-line EEG segments are generally thought to have near-zero entropy. However, during cardiac surgery, EEG signals that appear to be totally suppressed may be associated with paradoxically very high entropy values. The Datex-Ohmeda version of spectral entropy uses a special algorithm that assigns zero entropy to totally suppressed EEG epochs.

The use of pseudo-three-dimensional plots to display successive power spectra as a function of time was originated by Joy[27] and popularized by Bickford, who coined the term "compressed spectral array," or CSA.[28] This technique now represents one of the most common displays of computer-processed EEG in the frequency domain. Popularity stems from enormous data compression. For example, the essential information contained in a 4-hour EEG recording consuming more than 1000 pages of unprocessed waveforms can be displayed in CSA format on a single page.

With CSA (Fig. 17–14), successive power spectra of brief (2- to 60-second) EEG epochs are displayed as smoothed histograms of amplitude as a function of frequency. Spectral compression is achieved by partially overlaying successive spectra, with time represented on the *z*-axis. Hidden-line suppression improves clarity by avoiding overlap of successive traces. Although the display is esthetically attractive, it has limitations. The extent of data loss due to spectral overlapping depends on the nonstandard axial rotation that varies among EEG monitors. More important, epoch duration and the frequency with which each is measured (i.e., update rate) may critically affect the presentation of clinically important change. For example, there are three distinctly different burst-suppression CSA patterns: high-amplitude bursts, flat line, or a combination of the two.[29]

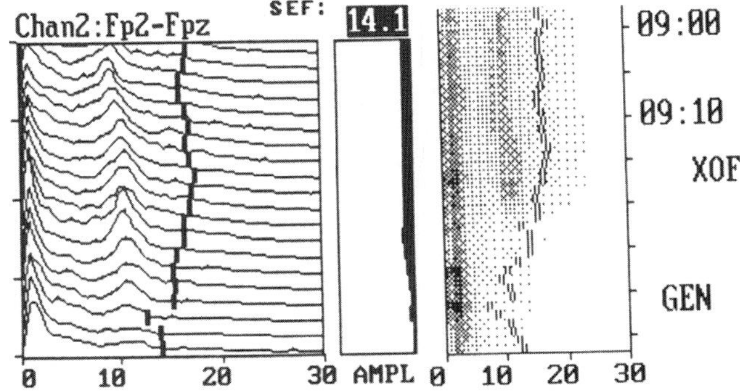

Figure 17–15 The same EEG segments are shown in the compressed spectral array (CSA, *left*), total power trend *(middle)*, and density-modulated spectral array (DSA, *right*). Note the improved amplitude resolution of the CSA display, although some information is obscured by foreground peaks. (Modified from Yli-Hankala A [ed]: Handbook of Four-Channel EEG in Anesthesia and Critical Care, 2004, p 14, with permission of the publisher, GE Medical, Datex-Ohmeda Division, Helsinki, Finland.)

Fleming and Smith[30] designed an alternative to the CSA display to reduce data loss. Density-modulated spectral array (DSA) uses a two-dimensional dot matrix plot of time as a function of frequency (Fig. 17–15). The density of dots indicates the amplitude at a particular time-frequency intersection (e.g., an intense large spot indicates high amplitude). Clinically significant shifts in frequency may be detected earlier and more easily than with CSA. However, the resolution of amplitude changes is reduced. Therefore, some DSA analyzers use color-modulated amplitude displays, provide a separate indication for mean or total power, or both. Neither the CSA nor DSA display is well suited for the detection of nonstationarity or transient phenomena like burst suppression.

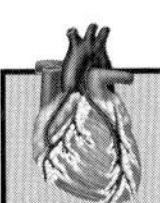

BOX 17–6 *Measures That Define EEG Changes*

- Maximum peak-to-peak amplitude (or total power)
- Relation of maximum amplitude to dominant frequency
- Amplitude and frequency variability
- Right-left symmetry

In summary, a quick assessment of EEG change in either the time or frequency domain focuses on (1) maximal peak-to-peak amplitude, (2) relation of maximal amplitude to dominant frequency, (3) amplitude and frequency variability, and (4) new or growing asymmetry between homotopic (i.e., same position on each cerebral hemisphere) EEG derivations. These objectives are generally best achieved through the viewing of both unprocessed and processed displays with a clear understanding of the characteristics and limitations of each (Box 17–6).

Electroencephalography for Injury Prevention During Cardiac Surgery

There is normally a tight coupling among cerebral cortical synaptic activity, metabolism, and blood flow. Such coupling is necessary because of the large energy requirements of interneuronal communication. Indeed, at least 60% of neuronal oxygen and glucose is consumed in the processes of synaptic and axonal transmission, while the remainder is used to maintain cellular integrity. Neurons rapidly adjust their signaling capabilities to conserve vital energy stores. Even a slight new imbalance between supply and consumption of energy substrates is manifested by altered synaptic activity. The EEG provides a sensitive measure of this synaptic change and represents an early warning of developing injury. Identification and correction of the physiologic imbalance may then avert serious injury. It must be emphasized that EEG alterations signify imbalance, not necessarily injury. For example, using functional brain imaging with fluorodeoxyglucose, Alkire[31] demonstrated EEG relative alpha power to be linearly related to cerebral metabolism during propofol and isoflurane anesthesia. In this case, the synaptic depression manifested by the reduction in high-frequency activity signified anesthetic effect, not ischemia.

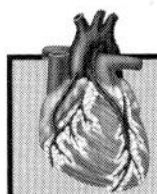

BOX 17–7 *Important Considerations During EEG Interpretation*

- EEG change signifies imbalance, not necessarily injury.
- The EEG is sensitive to imbalance but not specific for its cause.
- EEG prediction of neurologic outcome is good but not perfect.

Furthermore, because clinically apparent neurologic injury often involves subcortical circuits and structures invisible to the EEG, an expectation of perfect agreement between specific EEG change and neurologic outcome is unjustified. Imbalance in neuronal homeostasis may lead to either enhanced or diminished excitability. The majority of cortical neurons are small interneurons involved with maintenance of inhibitory tone. Their limited capacity for ionic buffering and energy storage makes them especially susceptible to imbalance. Early signs of energy deficiency may paradoxically result in EEG signs of excitation due to disinhibition.[32] Conversely, with inadequate analgesia, intense sensory stimuli occasionally result in a paradoxically depressed EEG activity resembling ischemia[33] (Box 17–7).

Although the EEG is a very sensitive indicator of cerebrocortical synaptic depression, possibly signifying cerebral ischemia or hypoxia, it is not specific. EEG suppression may also be the result of cooling or hypnotic agents. Fortunately, the time course of EEG suppression and information available from other monitors usually permit distinction between potentially harmful (e.g., ischemia) and harmless (e.g., hypothermia) causes. The following clinical situations provide the rationale for routine EEG monitoring during cardiac surgery: documentation of preexisting abnormalities, hypnotic adequacy, perfusion, cooling, rewarming, seizure detection, and other conditions.

Documentation of Preexisting Electroencephalographic Abnormalities

Because there is a high likelihood of latent cerebrovascular disease in many older cardiac surgery patients, it is essential to examine the waking EEG for signs of marked asymmetry prior to the induction of anesthesia. This serves both to alert the anesthesia provider to the patient's increased vulnerability and to document the previously unappreciated risk.

Objective Measurement of Hypnotic Effect

Recording the transition from wakefulness to unresponsiveness permits detection of unusual sensitivity or resistance to general anesthetics (Fig. 17–16). Such information is vital

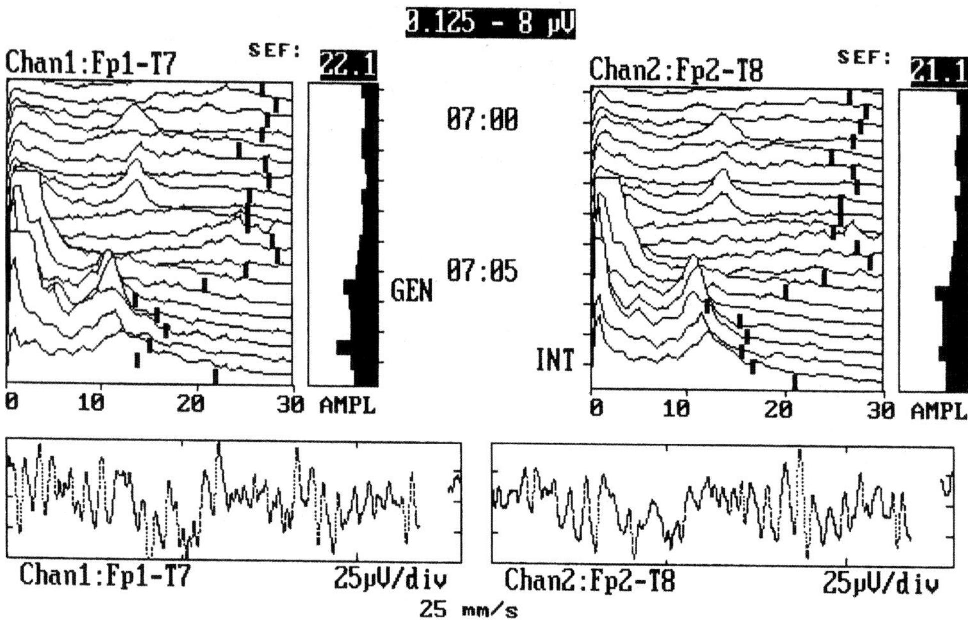

Figure 17–16 This two-channel EEG recording begins before induction of anesthesia at 07:03 and ends shortly after endotracheal intubation (INT). Note the loss of high-frequency activity with unconsciousness and the relative symmetry of the postinduction 12-Hz anesthesia peak. (Modified from Yli-Hankala A [ed]: Handbook of Four-Channel EEG in Anesthesia and Critical Care, 2004, p 30, with permission of the publisher, GE Medical, Datex-Ohmeda Division, Helsinki, Finland.)

during fast-track anesthesia protocols to avoid excessive or inadequate anesthesia. Although no available neurophysiologic monitoring modality is an infallible predictor of anesthetic inadequacy, characteristic changes in the EEG frequency pattern provide an easily recognized warning of potential patient awareness. EEG detection of excessive or inadequate hypnosis may be aided by the multivariate EEG descriptors—BIS, PSI, and spectral entropy.

Head Position

Because of the diffuse nature of atherosclerotic vascular disease, many elderly patients are at increased risk for positional focal or regional cerebral ischemia that may occur prior to incision. Head rotation for surgical positioning or insertion of a pulmonary artery catheter may compress a vital carotid or vertebral artery. Such ischemia is generally identified by marked depression in the affected frontotemporal EEG derivation (Fig. 17–17).

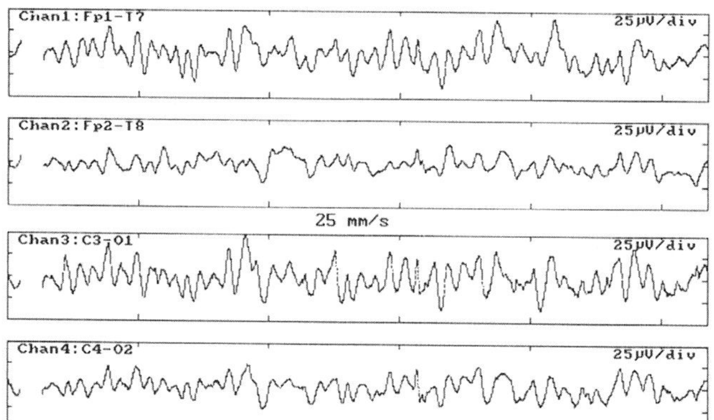

Figure 17–17 This four-channel unprocessed EEG display indicates developing cerebrocortical suppression in the right hemisphere (channel 2: Fp2-T8; channel 4: C4-O2) associated with head turning for pulmonary artery catheter placement. Symmetrical traces were restored with return of the head to a neutral position (not shown). This transient EEG change prior to surgical incision emphasizes the importance of obtaining a baseline EEG record prior to anesthetic induction to document any preexisting asymmetry or other abnormalities. (Modified from Yli-Hankala A [ed]: Handbook of Four-Channel EEG in Anesthesia and Critical Care, 2004, p 30, with permission of the publisher, GE Medical, Datex-Ohmeda Division, Helsinki, Finland.)

Vascular Obstruction and Flow Misdirection

Manipulation or torsion of the aorta or vena cava may result in regional or global cerebral ischemia. During CPB, the aortic cannula can misdirect either cardiac or pump flow away from one or more head vessels while leaving the radial artery pressure unaltered. Alternatively, a malpositioned venous cannula may impair return from the head without noticeable change in central venous pressure or return flow to the venous reservoir.[34] Resulting intracranial hypertension leads to ischemic depression of the EEG (Fig. 17–18).

Nonpulsatile Perfusion

Nonpulsatile perfusion used with CPB and some new left ventricular assist devices may result in microcirculatory collapse in susceptible regions of the cerebral cortex, despite "acceptable" radial artery pressures. EEG-guided increases in arterial pressure, circulating volume, or both may be needed to restore perfusion in the microvasculature.

Hemodilution

Hemodilution is used to improve vital organ perfusion by reducing viscosity. However, it may cause inadequate delivery of oxygenated hemoglobin to a high-demand brain, even though hematocrit and systemic venous oxygen saturation are within normal limits.[35] EEG deterioration may thus serve as an objective indicator for transfusion.

Hypocarbia and Hypercarbia

Cerebral arteries normally constrict in response to decreased carbon dioxide tension or hydrogen ion concentration. With reactive arteries, hypocarbia may lead to cerebral ischemia, because flow is reduced 4%/mm Hg [CO_2]. In this circumstance, return to normocarbia can markedly improve cerebral perfusion.[36] Conversely, hypercarbia may steal blood from the dilated vessels of an already underperfused region, resulting in focal EEG slowing. This circumstance may be exacerbated by the use of volatile anesthetics causing cerebral vasodilation.

Cooling

During cardiac surgery requiring deep hypothermic circulatory arrest, the EEG provides an effective method for

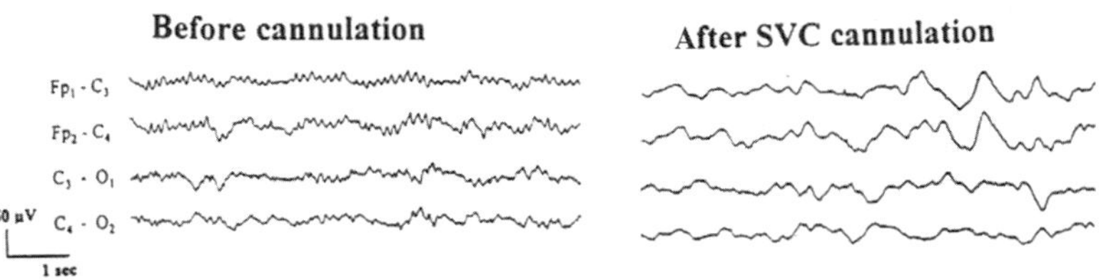

Figure 17–18 Insertion of a 14-French venous cannula in this pediatric patient during repair of an atrial septal defect caused a sudden diffuse EEG slowing. The heart rate and blood pressure remained unchanged, although the central venous pressure rose from 6 to 45 mm Hg. Cannula repositioning restored both the former EEG pattern and central venous pressure. (Modified from Rodriguez RA, Cornel G, Semelhago L, et al: Ann Thorac Surg 64:1820, 1997. Copyright 1997, with permission of the Society of Thoracic Surgeons.)

Figure 17–19 *(A)* This two-channel combined unprocessed EEG and CSA recording illustrates the loss of EEG activity during cooling. Note the flat-line waveform signifying that optimal cooling was achieved. *(B)* This recording, obtained from the same patient, shows gradual recovery of EEG activity with rewarming. (Both *A* and *B* are modified from Yli-Hankala A [ed]: Handbook of Four-Channel EEG in Anesthesia and Critical Care, 2004, p 32, with permission of the publisher, GE Medical, Datex-Ohmeda Division, Helsinki, Finland.)

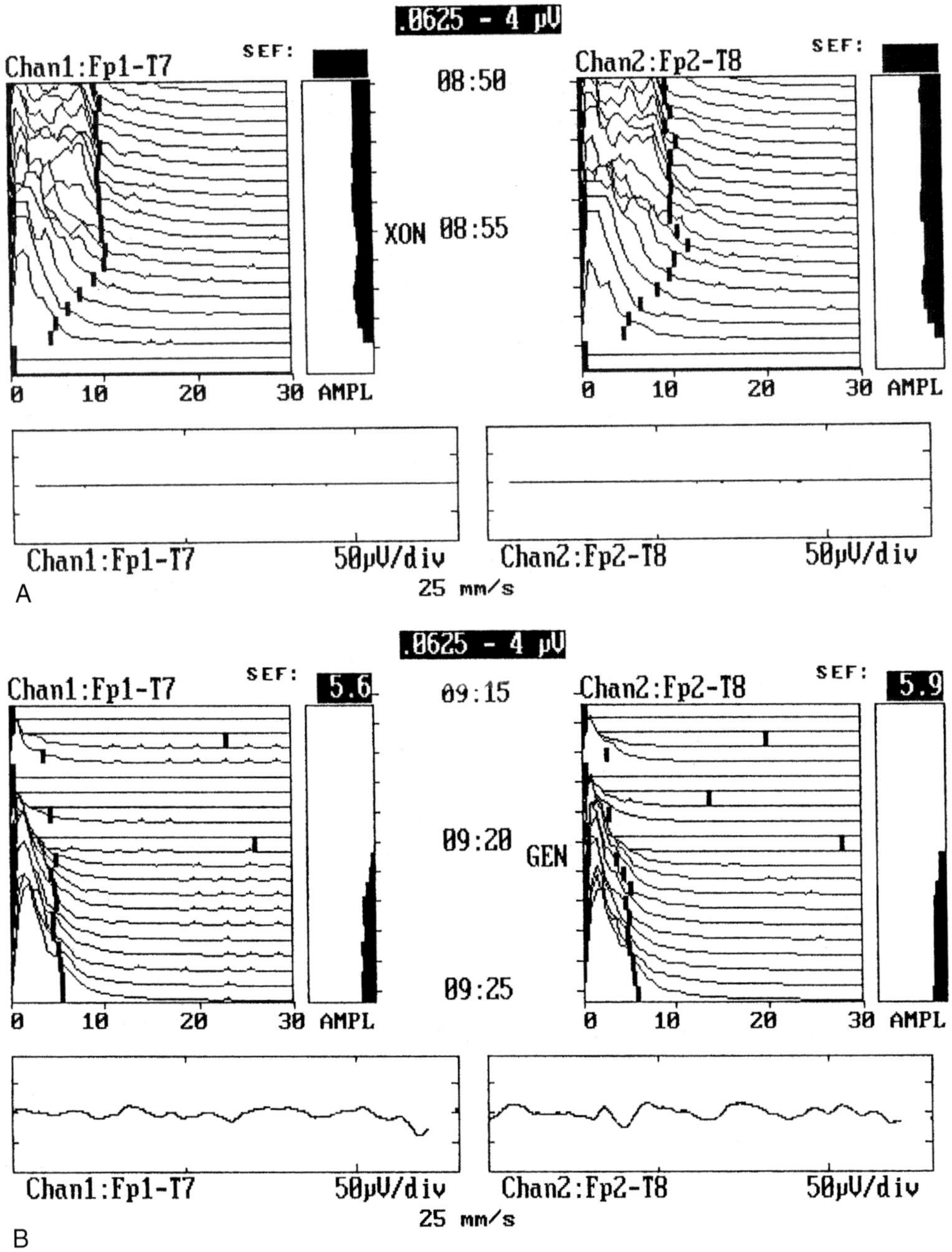

assessing the effects of cooling. Optimal brain temperature may be viewed as a balance between decreased cerebral oxygen consumption and increased risk of coagulopathy. Actual brain temperature cannot be measured directly and appears to be influenced by many variables including the rate of cooling as well as acid-base and anesthetic management. The EEG is often used to assess the functional consequences of brain cooling, because a flat-line pattern signifies cortical synaptic quiescence. The wide interpatient variation in flat-line temperature is the rationale for EEG guidance of the cooling process.[37] Alternative use of a fixed temperature criterion increases the risks of both excessive and inadequate brain cooling.

As nasopharyngeal or tympanic temperature decreases to 28°C (Fig. 17–19), there is a gradual loss of absolute spectral power across all frequency bands.[38,39] Although the reversible decreases in absolute spectral band power are quite large, computing these changes as relative spectral band power minimizes these changes, suggesting that initial brain cooling exerts a similar decrease in spectral power across all frequency bands and cortical regions.[39] Cooling below 28°C leads to progressive slowing of the residual EEG until the EEG waveform becomes a flat line.

Rewarming

After circulatory arrest, the EEG documents the recovery of synaptic function during rewarming. However, rapid rewarming may result in cerebral ischemia due to cold-triggered vasoparesis, which uncouples cerebral blood flow and metabolism. In this case, rewarming-induced increase in metabolic demand increase may outpace the lagging delivery of essential nutrients.[40] This situation is indicated by a loss of EEG high-frequency activity accompanying the increase in cranial temperature (Fig. 17–20). Although the practice is controversial, administration of a metabolic suppressant drug such as propofol, dosed to EEG burst suppression, may facilitate balancing cerebral perfusion with metabolic demand.[41]

Myocardial Revascularization Without Extracorporeal Support

The most recent significant advance in cardiac surgery has been myocardial revascularization on a beating heart. Avoidance of CPB may protect patients from the many potential hazards of this nonphysiologic insult.[42] In addition, its potential economic advantages promise widespread application. Figure 17–21 illustrates the typical remarkable stability of the EEG during a beating heart coronary revascularization despite transient hypotension and bradycardia. However, some surgeons believe that neuromonitoring is mandatory because the combination of controlled hypotension and vascular torsion can suddenly disrupt cerebral perfusion. In the absence of the neuroprotective effects of mild hypothermia, even relatively brief episodes of cerebral ischemia may result in injury.

Seizure Detection

Certain anesthetics and adjuvants such as etomidate, sevoflurane, and the opioid analgesics may produce seizure-like EEG activity, although the clinical manifestations may be obscured by neuromuscular blockade (Fig. 17–22).[43-45] The consequences of this anesthetic-induced seizure-like activity have not been established in adults. However, they are clearly deleterious in the developing brain. Bellinger et al[46] showed that perioperative EEG seizure activity in infant cardiac surgery patients was associated with a 10-point decline in expected IQ when subsequently measured in the patients' fifth year after surgery (Box 17–8).

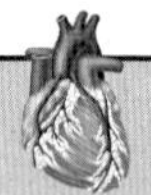

BOX 17–8 *Important Imbalances Identified With EEG*

- Preexisting EEG abnormality
- Hypnotic effect
- Head malposition
- Hypocarbia-induced cerebral ischemia
- Malperfusion syndrome
- Need for blood replacement
- Optimal cooling and rewarming technique
- Seizures

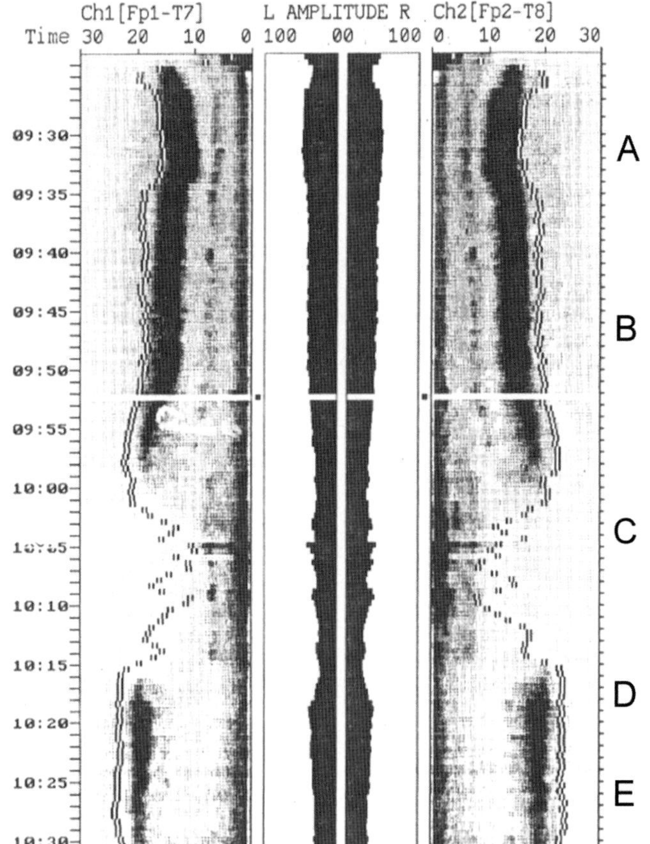

Figure 17–20 Left and mirror image right frontal density spectral array (DSA) displays of EEG changes occurring from the onset of cardiopulmonary bypass (9:26) until its termination at marker E (*left* and *right*, respectively). *Middle*, left and mirror image right frontal cortex trend plots of EEG total power. Loss of high-frequency activity began shortly after marker B. The loss was indicated by a gradual disappearance of the dark 10- to 16-Hz band. Note that there was only a small decrease in total power *(middle)*. This EEG "slowing" was associated with an increase in nasopharyngeal temperature. Further suppression was manifested by a profound decrease in spectral edge frequency *(parallel horizontal bars)*. It occurred following release of the aortic cross-clamp at marker C and was associated with transient hypotension. Note again the modest total power change. High-frequency activity returned at marker D with blood pressure increase, restoration of pulsatile perfusion, and discontinuation of rewarming. (Modified from Yli-Hankala A [ed]: Handbook of Four-Channel EEG in Anesthesia and Critical Care, 2004, p 38, with permission of the publisher, GE Medical, Datex-Ohmeda Division, Helsinki, Finland.)

AUDITORY EVOKED POTENTIALS

Auditory evoked potentials (AEPs) assess specific areas of the brainstem, midbrain, and auditory cortices. Because of their simplicity, objectivity, and reproducibility, AEPs are suitable for monitoring patients during cardiovascular surgery. Specific applications of AEP monitoring in this environment are the assessment of temperature effects on brainstem function and evaluation of hypnotic effect. Direct involvement of cardiac anesthesia providers with AEP monitoring is likely to increase following the introduction of EEG/AEP modules designed for use with available operating room physiologic monitors.

Acoustic stimuli trigger a neural response integrated by a synchronized neuronal depolarization that travels from the auditory nerve to the cerebral cortex. Scalp-recorded signals,

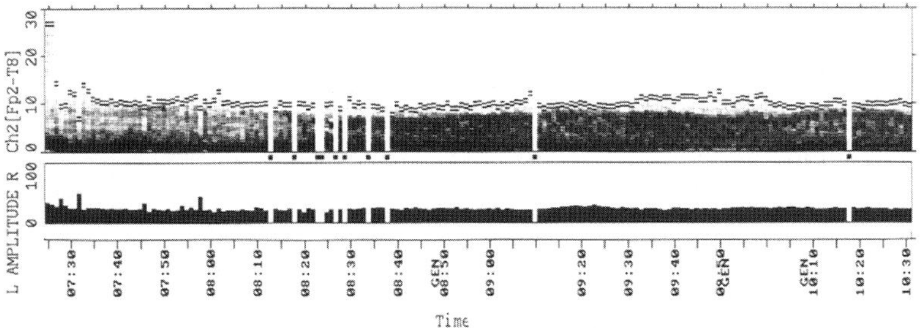

Figure 17–21 Note the stability of the EEG during this myocardial revascularization without cardiopulmonary bypass. (Modified from Yli-Hankala A [ed]: Handbook of Four-Channel EEG in Anesthesia and Critical Care, 2004, p 39, with permission of the publisher, GE Medical, Datex-Ohmeda Division, Helsinki, Finland.)

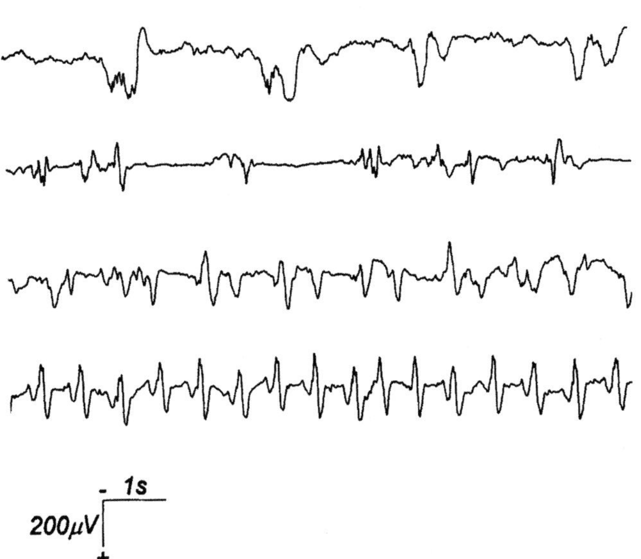

Figure 17–22 These epileptiform EEG patterns are associated with mask induction of sevoflurane in adults. The patterns include (1) slow delta monophasic activity with spikes, (2) burst suppression with spikes, (3) polyspikes, and (4) rhythmic polyspikes. (Modified from Yli-Hankala A, Vakkuri A, Sarkela M, et al: Anesthesiology 91:1596, 1999, with permission of the publisher, Lippincott Williams & Wilkins, Baltimore, MD.).

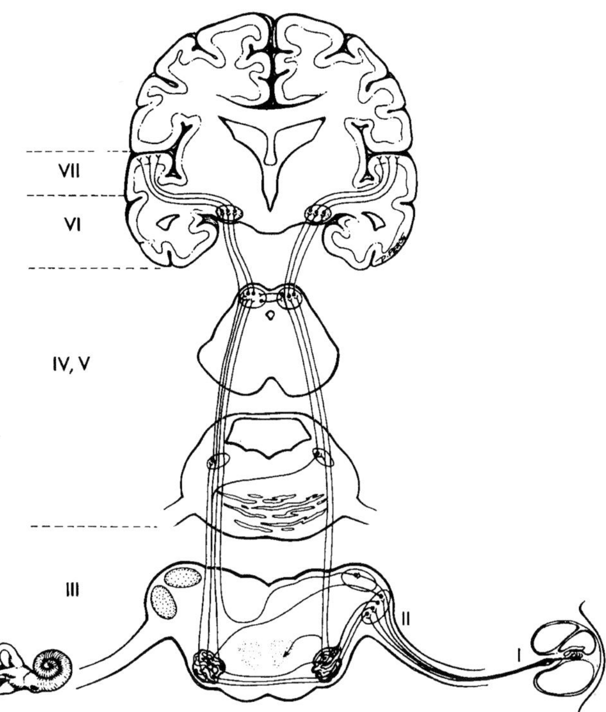

Figure 17–23 Putative sites at which the brainstem auditory evoked potential is generated include the cochlear nerve, cochlear nucleus, trapezoid complex, lateral lemniscus, inferior colliculus, medial geniculate nucleus, and auditory radiations. Wave I is generated in the distal cochlear nerve near the spiral ganglion, and wave II is generated in the proximal cochlear nerve near the brainstem. All other waveforms are generated in multiple brainstem sites and do not bear a one-to-one relationship to any particular structures, although the later waveforms do tend to be generated in more rostral sites. (Modified from Friedman WA, et al: Advances in Anesthesia 6:244, 1989 with permission of the publisher, Yearbook Medical Publishers, Chicago, IL.)

obtained from electrodes located at the vertex and ear lobe, contain both the AEPs and other unrelated EEG and EMG activity. Extraction of the relatively low-amplitude AEPs from the larger amplitude background activity requires signal-averaging techniques.[47] Because the AEP character remains constant for each stimulus repetition, averaging of many repetitions suppresses the inconstant background. For the AEP sensory stimulus, acoustic clicks are the most commonly used.[48] These broad-band signals are generated by unidirectional rectangular short pulses (40 to 500 microseconds) with frequency spectra below 10 KHz.

The AEPs comprise a series of biopotentials generated at all levels of the auditory system in response to an acoustic stimulus (Fig. 17–23). Using scalp electrodes, a dozen peaks have been identified within the first 100 milliseconds after stimulus onset.[47] Each peak is described by its poststimulus latency and peak-to-peak amplitude. AEPs are commonly classified as early or middle-latency potentials.[48] Figure 17–24 is a schematic representation of the AEPs most commonly used for surgical monitoring. Early AEPs are generated from the auditory nerve and the brainstem and include a series of wavelets recorded within the first 10 milliseconds poststimulus. These evoked responses have been designated brainstem auditory evoked potentials (BAEPs). Seven waves (I to VII) characterize the adult BAEPs. Peaks I and II are generally thought to originate from the distal and proximal parts of the eighth nerve, and peak III arises from the cochlear nucleus. Peak IV sources include the superior olivary complex, cochlear nucleus, and nucleus of the lateral lemniscus. Peak V contributors seem to include both the lateral lemniscus and inferior colliculus. Peak VI and VII origins are not well defined but may arise from the medial geniculate body and the acoustic radiations. BAEPs are useful in assessing brainstem and subcortical function during surgery, in part because of their relative resistance to the suppressant effects of most anesthetics.[49]

The middle-latency auditory evoked potentials (MLAEPs), with poststimulus latencies between 10 and 100 milliseconds, are generated in the midbrain and primary auditory cortex.[50] In an awake adult subject, the MLAEPs usually consist of three main peaks: Na, Pa, and Nb with respective latencies near 15, 28, and 40 milliseconds (Fig. 17–24). During physiologic sleep, the Pa amplitude and latency appear to be related to the depth of sleep.[50] Children under general anesthesia commonly display the trimodal configuration of the adult MLAEP waveform (Na, Pa, Nb waves), although neonates may exhibit only a small Pa wave.[51] Many agents with hypnotic effects prolong the latency and suppress the amplitude of Pa and Nb in a concentration-dependent manner.[52] It appears that the latency and amplitude changes allow reliable detection of consciousness during general anesthesia.[52]

The specific benefit of AEPs to cardiac surgery derives from their temperature sensitivity, because cooling slows both axonal conduction and synaptic transmission. During cooling, the BAEP wave V Q_{10} (ratio of two values separated by 10°C) is 2.2.[53] A decrease of tympanic or nasopharyngeal temperature from 35° to 25°C doubles wave V latency. Further cooling will eventually suppress waves III to V completely, signifying the virtual elimination of synaptic transmission within the brainstem auditory circuits. BAEPs document complete deep hypothermic electrocerebral silence prior to temporary circulatory arrest.[53]

The critical protective action of hypothermia on the brain cannot be accurately assessed by thermometry because of marked individual differences in thermal compartmentation throughout the body.[54] Even within the brain, cooling technique (e.g., rapid versus slow, alpha-stat versus pH-stat acid-base balance, α-adrenergic blockade versus none) may result in substantial thermal inhomogeneity within the cerebrum.[53-55] Therefore, hypothermia-induced electrocortical silence (i.e., flat EEG) does not necessarily indicate cessation of synaptic activity within deep brain structures. The high metabolic rates of some of these structures (e.g., basal ganglia and inferior colliculus) render them particularly vulnerable to ischemic injury.[55] EEG quiescence plus a loss of BAEP waves III to V (Fig. 17–25) ensure thorough cooling of the brain core. This approach appears to offer an optimal neuroprotective environment during temporary cessation of cerebral perfusion (Box 17–9).

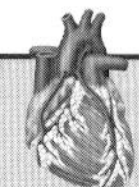

BOX 17–9 *Auditory Evoked Potentials*

- Brainstem auditory evoked potentials measure temperature effects on brain core.
- Middle latency auditory evoked potentials document inadequate hypnotic levels.

TRANSCRANIAL DOPPLER (TCD) ULTRASOUND

Ultrasound Technology

Ultrasonic probes of a clinical TCD sonograph contain an electrically activated piezoelectric crystal that transmits low power 1- to 2-MHz acoustic vibrations (i.e., insonation) through the thinnest portion of temporal bone (i.e., acoustic window) into brain tissue. Blood constituents (predominantly erythrocytes), contained in large arteries and veins, reflect these ultrasonic waves back to the probe, which also serves as a receiver. Because of laminar blood flow, erythrocytes traveling in the central region of a large blood vessel move with higher velocity than those near the vessel wall. Thus, within each vascular segment (i.e., sample volume), a series of echoes associated with varying velocities is created. The frequency differences between the insonation signal and each echo in the series are proportional to the associated velocity, and this velocity is determined from the Doppler equation. Although several large intracranial arteries may be insonated through the temporal window, the middle cerebral artery (MCA) is generally monitored during cardiac surgery because it carries approximately 40% of the hemispheric blood flow.

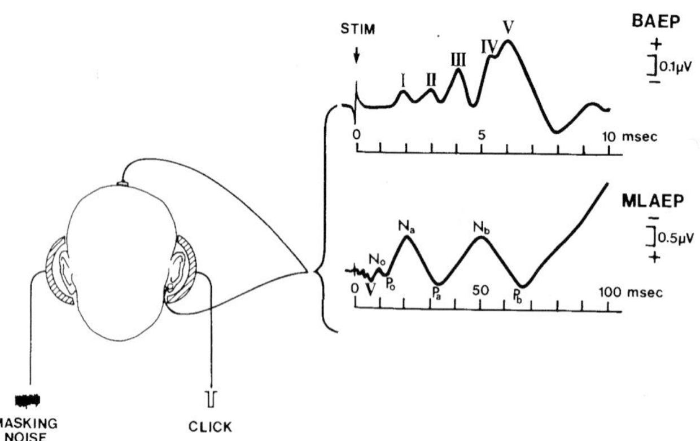

Figure 17–24 Schematic diagram of brainstem (BAEP) and middle-latency (MLAEP) auditory evoked potential production. Stimulation of one ear and recording between the ipsilateral earlobe and vertex produce sequences of peaks that can be displayed at two different recording speeds and gain settings. Recording with a short 10-millisecond time base at a high gain reveals the first five peaks that comprise the BAEP. With a longer 100-millisecond time base and lower gain, the MLAEP peaks become evident. By a rather confusing convention, BAEP peaks represent positive deflections, whereas MLAEP peaks indicate negative deflections. (Modified from Spehlmann R: Evoked Potential Primer, 1985, p 196, with permission of the publisher, Butterworth, Boston, MA.)

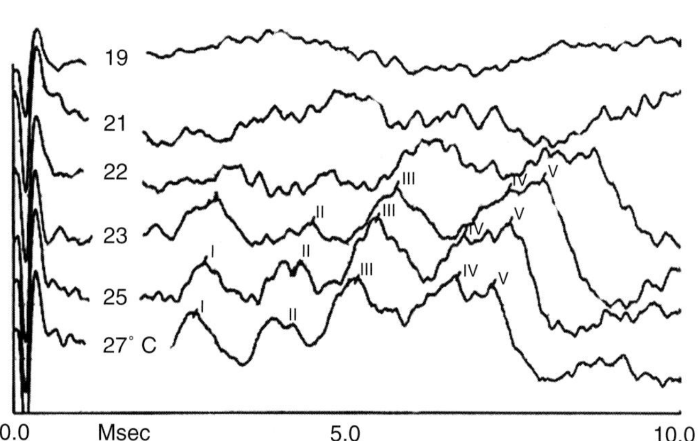

Figure 17–25 During repair of an aortic arch aneurysm, slow cooling resulted in a gradual loss of brainstem auditory evoked potentials (EPs), progressing cephalad to caudad. Loss of wave III and later components ensured a cold-induced cessation of synaptic activity within the entire cerebrum. The global cessation indicated maximal neuroprotection during circulatory arrest. (Modified from Yli-Hankala A [ed]: Handbook of Four-Channel EEG in Anesthesia and Critical Care, 2004, p 45, with permission of the publisher, GE Medical, Datex-Ohmeda Division, Helsinki, Finland.)

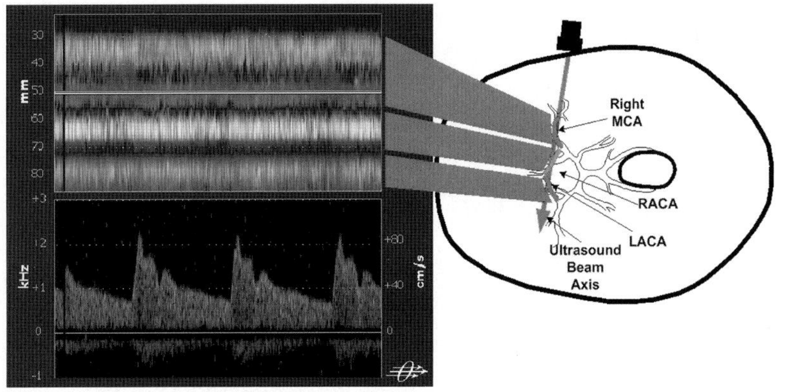

Figure 17–26 Comparison of the appearance of the transcranial Doppler continuous wave M-mode *(top)* and pulsed-wave spectral *(bottom)* displays. The horizontal bands of the M-mode display represent ultrasonic reflections from erythrocytes traveling through several vessels intersected by the path of the ultrasonic beam. Signals in the 30- to 50-mm depth range represent flow in an ipsilateral M2 segment of the middle cerebral artery that is directed towards the ultrasonic probe. Signals in the 55- to 70-mm depth range emanate from the ipsilateral anterior cerebral artery with flow directed away from the probe. Signals in the 72- to 85-mm range arise from the contralateral anterior cerebral artery with flow directed toward the probe. The *solid white horizontal line* at a depth of 50 mm below the skull surface indicates the measurement site for the lower spectral display. The waveform represents changes in the distribution of erythrocyte velocities associated with each cardiac cycle. Variation is the greatest during peak systole and least during end-diastole. (The M-mode display figure is courtesy of Dr. Mark Moehring, Spencer Technologies, Seattle, WA).

Pulsed-Wave Spectral Display

Pulsed-wave Doppler samples the ultrasonic echoes at a user-selected distance (i.e., single gate) below the scalp. The frequency composition of these Doppler-shifted echoes is analyzed by Fourier analysis, the same technique used to quantify EEG frequency patterns. The analysis produces a momentary amplitude spectrum displayed as a function of blood flow velocity (e.g., Doppler-shift frequency). This relationship is mapped as one vertical strip in the spectrogram display (Fig. 17–26, bottom). Amplitude at each frequency is expressed as log change (i.e., dB) from the background composed of random echoes. The momentary analysis is repeated 100 times a second to produce a scrolling spectrogram of time-related changes in flow velocity. Sampling echoes at multiple loci (multigating) produces spectrograms for each of the different probe-to-sample site distances (Fig. 17–27).

Signal amplitude at each frequency shift–time intersection is indicated by monochromatic dot density or color coding. The maximum velocity, the upper edge (envelope) of the velocity spectrum (analogous to the EEG spectral edge frequency), represents the maximum Doppler shift (erythrocyte velocity) in the vessel center. Peak systolic and end-diastolic velocities are derived from this spectral edge. Intensity-weighted mean velocity is calculated by weighted averaging of the intensity of all Doppler spectral signals in a vessel cross-section.

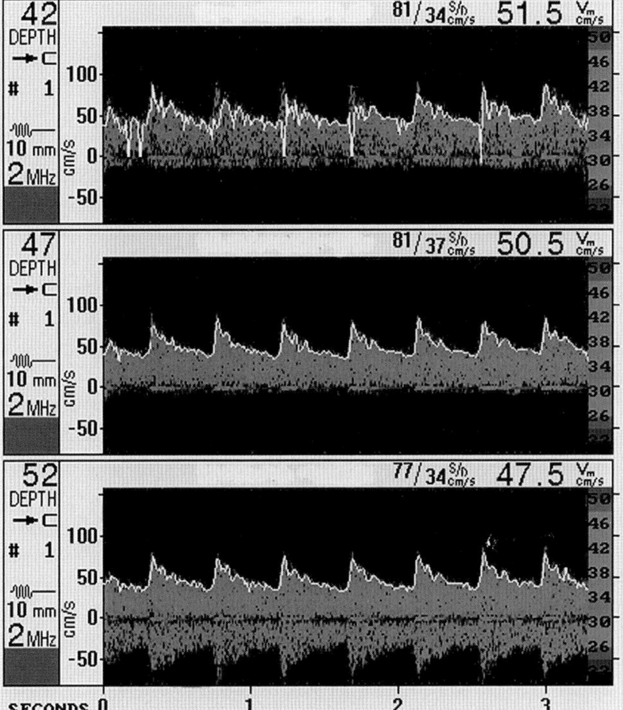

Figure 17–27 Multigating of a pulsed-wave spectral display is shown. This technique permits simultaneous insonation at several intracranial loci.

Power M-Mode Doppler Display

An alternative method for processing pulsed-wave Doppler echoes is nonspectral power M-mode Doppler (PMD). Unlike the series of spectra generated with multigating, PMD creates one image with each depth represented by a plot of signal amplitude (i.e., power) and depth as functions of time. A color scale signifies flow direction (red is flow directed toward the probe; blue is flow reversal), while color intensity is directly related to signal power.

Embolus Detection

Erythrocytes (approximately 5 million/mL) are the most acoustically reflective nonpathologic elements (i.e., high acoustic impedance) in plasma. However, emboli, gaseous more than particulate, are better reflectors of sound than erythrocytes. The presence of high-intensity transient signals (HITS) within either the PMD or spectral TCD display may signify the presence of an embolus. Because a true embolus, particle or bubble, cannot simultaneously appear at all distances from the probe, either PMD or a multigated spectral display may be used to distinguish them from acoustic artifact (tapping on the ultrasonic probe produces a high-intensity transient acoustic artifact at all distances). Figure

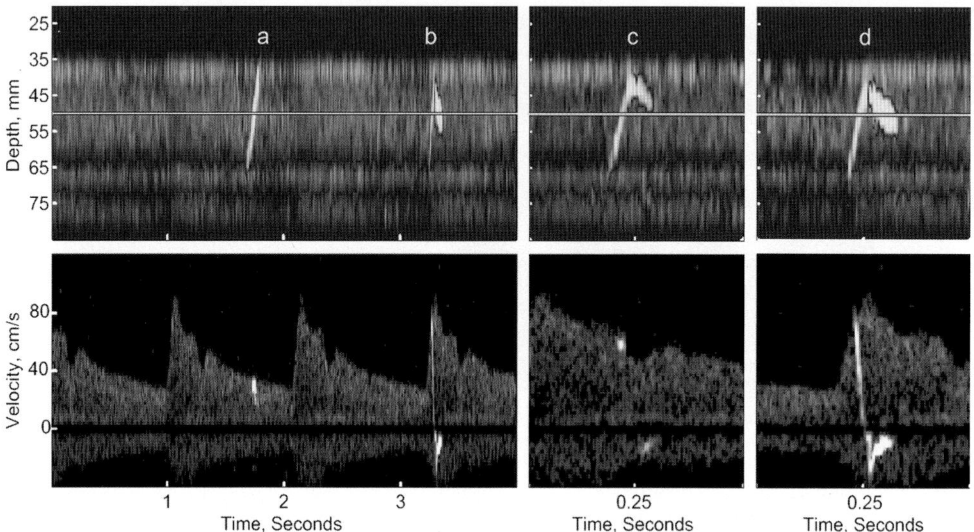

Figure 17–28 Comparison of the appearance of emboliform high-intensity transient signals (HITS) using the M-mode and spectral displays. The *white horizontal line* at a depth of 50 mm depicts the site of the spectral measurement along the axis of the vessel. HIT_a represents linear migration of an embolus in the M2 segment of the ipsilateral middle cerebral artery. A single HIT is noted on the spectral display as the embolus passes through the 50-mm measurement site. In contrast, emboli in the remaining panels suddenly change direction as they pass into a smaller branch vessel. HIT_b and HIT_d direction changes are noted on the spectral displays as the characteristic "lambda" sign. However, the HIT_c behavior is misidentified as two emboli because the direction change occurs outside the spectral sample volume. (The M-mode display courtesy of Dr. Mark Moehring, Spencer Technologies, Seattle, WA.)

17–28 illustrates the appearance of HITS in the two TCD display formats. The bottom spectral displays are generated from a small vascular segment at a distance of 50 ± 3 mm (6-mm sample volume) from the probe surface. The midpoint of the spectral sample is indicated on the top PMD displays as a light horizontal line at a 50-mm depth. An embolic track labeled "a" is a single embolus that is shown in the top PMD display moving toward the probe (i.e., decreasing distance from the probe face over time). Embolic tracks "b" and "d" display the characteristic "lambda" acoustic signature in the spectral display. The PMD shows that this pattern is due to embolus direction reversal within the spectral sample volume. The true behavior of the spectrally paradoxical track "c" (start and end-points of the single acoustic signature are not connected) becomes clear in the PMD view. Track "c" direction reversal is invisible on the spectral display because it occurs outside the sampling region. Currently available spectral or PMD TCD monitors can determine neither the size nor composition of emboliform material responsible for HITS. TCD devices designed for surgical monitoring typically provide a semiquantitative estimate of aggregate HITS, irrespective of their origin (Box 17–10).

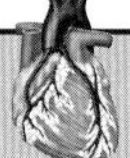

BOX 17–10 *Transcranial Doppler Ultrasonography*

- Detects change in intracranial blood flow
- Detects emboli—particulate or gaseous

Intervention Threshold

Because erythrocyte velocity and flow may be differentially influenced by vessel diameter, blood viscosity, and pH, as well as temperature, TCD does not provide a reliable measure of cerebral blood flow.[56] However, in the absence of hemodilution, *change* in TCD velocity does correlate closely with *change* in blood flow.[57] Sudden large changes in velocity or direction are readily detected by continuous TCD monitoring. A large multicenter retrospective study found that severe ischemia (high probability of new neurologic deficit) was associated with a greater than 85% reduction in flow velocity, while moderate ischemia occurred with a 60% to 85% decrease.[58] The clinical significance of velocity changes also has been assessed during implantable cardioverter/defibrillator and tilt-table testing in conscious patients.[59,60] In both circumstances, syncope resulting from systemic hypotension was accompanied by a mean velocity decline of greater than 60% and absent diastolic velocity.

In general, reduction of flow velocity indicating severe ischemia is associated with profound depression of EEG activity.[61] However, with adequate leptomeningeal collateral flow, EEG activity occasionally remains unchanged in the presence of a severely decreased or absent MCA flow velocity. Together, these findings form the rationale for a TCD-based intervention threshold. Mean velocity reductions of greater than 60% or velocity loss during diastole suggest clinically significant cerebral hypoperfusion.

Clinical Basis for Intervention

Before Cardiopulmonary Bypass

TCD provides cerebral hemodynamic information for the timely detection and correction of perfusion abnormalities that may occur *prior* to the onset of CPB. Vascular torsion during neck extension or axial head rotation may result in regional cerebral hypoperfusion detectable by TCD.[61] Excessive hyperventilation may result in inadvertent cerebral ischemia, because blood flow falls by 4%/mm Hg Pa_{CO_2} in normally reactive cerebral arteries.[62] Cerebral dysautoregulation is often seen in hypertensive and diabetic patients.[63] This abnormality may result in pressure-dependent brain perfusion and place the patient at risk for ischemic brain injury during even moderate hypotension. TCD may be used to identify pressure dependency and facilitate appropriate individualization of acceptable perfusion pressure.[63] In addition, TCD has been used to identify the optimal aortic cannulation site.[64] For example, Mullges et al[65] observed that the mean aggregate MCA embolic load was significantly lower with a distal arch cannulation compared with the traditional ascending aorta site. These results are consistent with the studies using epiaortic ultrasound. Detection of malpositioned aortic or superior vena caval perfusion cannula is rapidly achieved with TCD monitoring.[66] In the former case, the malposition results in a sudden profound decrease in the peak systolic velocity (Fig. 17–29), whereas in the latter, diastolic velocity is compromised (Fig. 17–30).

During Cardiopulmonary Bypass

TCD is the only available method to continuously assess changes in cerebral hemodynamics associated with CPB. Despite the confounding influences of hemodilution, altered acid-base management, and cooling on absolute flow velocity, TCD nevertheless indicates the presence and direction of cerebral blood flow. A sudden large decrease, increase, or asymmetry indicates, respectively, inadvertent occlusion of a great vessel, hyperperfusion of a single cranial artery, or misdirection of aortic cannula flow[67] (Fig. 17–31). During surgical repair of the aortic arch, TCD documents cerebral artery flow direction during attempts at supplemental retrograde (Fig. 17–32) or antegrade (Fig. 17–33) cerebral perfusion during systemic circulatory arrest.[67,68] Because peak velocity changes in large basal cerebral arteries are directly related to peak flow changes, TCD may aid in the determination of safe upper and lower limits for pump flow and perfusion pressure.[68] Deep cooling and circulatory arrest may produce a transient cerebral vasoparesis and result in uncoupling of cerebral blood flow and metabolism.[68] TCD identifies this phenomenon as an unchanging flow velocity during rewarming. Emboli detection by TCD can improve surgical and perfusion technique and facilitate correction of technical problems such as an air leak[69-71] (Fig. 17–33, Box 17–11).

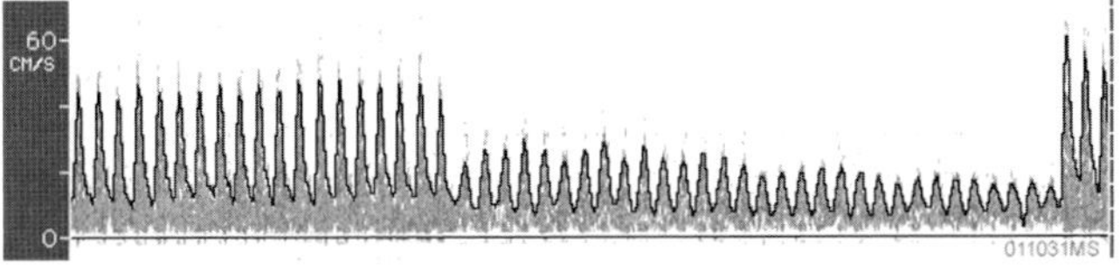

Figure 17–29 Malposition of an aortic perfusion cannula was identified upon its insertion by the sudden large decrease in peak systolic velocity. Repositioning led to a prompt recovery of cerebral perfusion.

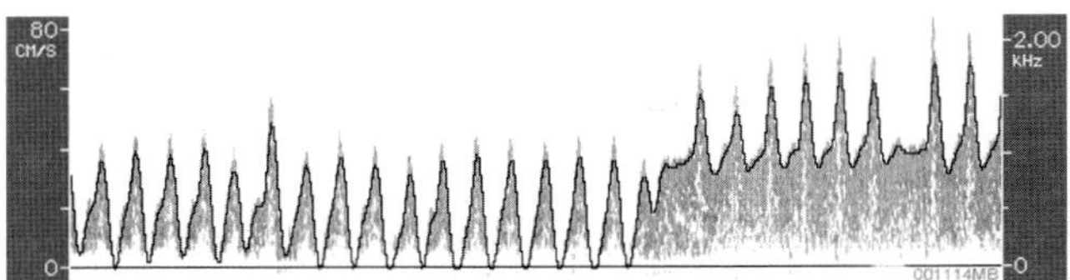

Figure 17–30 Malposition of a superior vena cava perfusion cannula was identified shortly after its insertion by the loss of end-diastolic velocity. Repositioning led to a prompt recovery of cerebral perfusion.

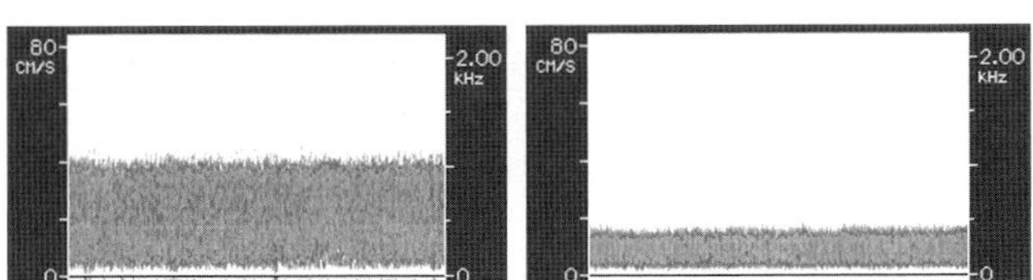

Figure 17–31 Misdirection of cerebral perfusion was identified by asymmetric peak flow velocity. A slight change in the position of the aortic perfusion cannula corrected the problem.

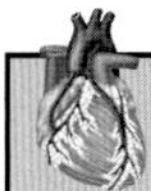

BOX 17–11 *Important Imbalances Identified by TCD Ultrasonography*

- Preexisting cerebral hemodynamic abnormalities
- Head malposition
- Hypocarbia-induced ischemia
- Appropriate aortic cannulation site
- Perfusion cannula malposition
- Malperfusion syndrome
- Successful supplementary cerebral perfusion during circulatory arrest
- Flow–metabolism uncoupling

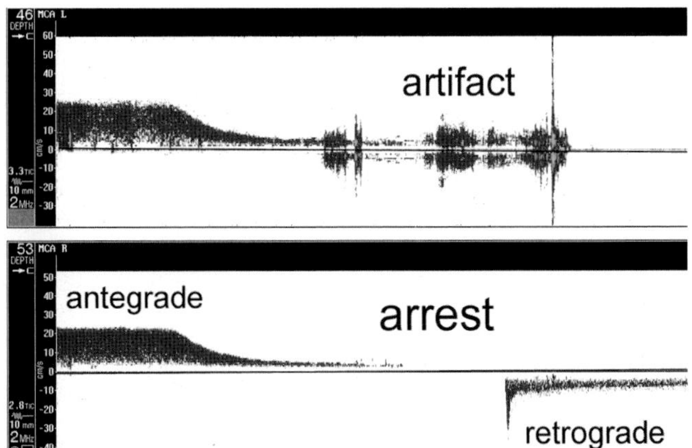

Figure 17–32 These two TCD spectral displays show changes in left *(top)* and right *(bottom)* middle cerebral artery flow velocity during circulatory arrest and attempted supplemental retrograde cerebral perfusion via the superior vena cava with carotid drainage. Spectral patterns above the zero baseline (i.e., positive values on the vertical velocity scale) indicate antegrade blood flow directed toward the ultrasound probe. Retrograde flow directed away from the probe is shown by spectral patterns below zero baseline (i.e., negative velocity scale). The perfusion pump is turned off at the 15-second time marker, and all measurable flow ceases within 20 seconds. Retrograde flow only in the right middle cerebral artery is successfully initiated within 10 seconds (at the 50-second time marker). Note the appearance of acoustic artifact in the upper spectral display, indicated by perfectly symmetrical mirror image spectral patterns above and below the zero baseline.

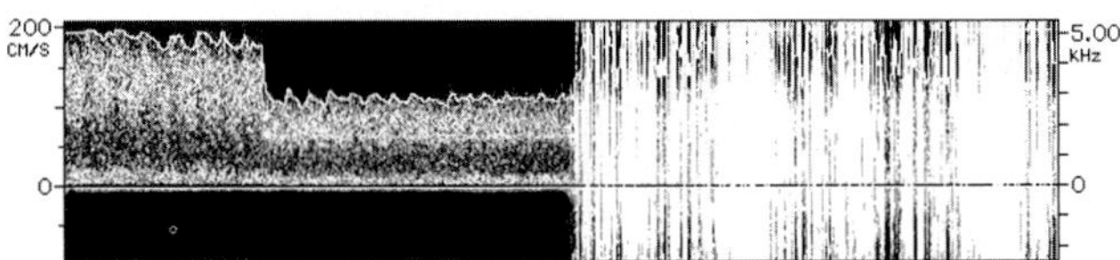

Figure 17–33 Overperfusion of the right middle cerebral artery was identified by TCD during attempted supplemental antegrade cerebral perfusion during total circulatory arrest. Repositioning of the right axillary perfusion cannula led to a reduction in velocity followed shortly thereafter by the accidental introduction of a small amount of air. The leak was quickly identified and corrected.

Reasons for Limited Transcranial Doppler Utilization

To date, TCD monitoring during cardiac surgery has not enjoyed wide popularity. The limited utilization results from a set of methodologic constraints. First, the quality of the information provided by TCD is very user-dependent; reliability is heavily influenced by the skill, experience, and practice of the sonographer.[72] In this respect, its use appears to be analogous to pulmonary artery pressure monitoring. Both techniques require specialized knowledge and practiced manual skills.

Second, continuous MCA insonation requires precise and stable probe fixation. The peak velocity is influenced by the orientation of the ultrasonic beam with respect to the reference blood vessel. Even small changes in this insonation angle may result in spurious large changes in velocity measurement. Available probe fixation appliances vary widely in their ease of use and performance characteristics. An unfortunate product selection could easily discourage use of this valuable technology.

Third, the ease of obtaining a useful TCD signal is affected by patient demographics. Effective transtemporal insonation of intracranial arteries and veins is most likely in young white males and least likely in elderly African American or Asian females. As a result, it is not currently possible to monitor intracranial hemodynamics in all patients. However, valuable information may still be obtained through submandibular insonation of the common carotid artery. Such monitoring readily permits detection of flow disruption to the brain and the presence of microemboli in all patients. Some manufacturers offer probe fixation devices for this essential objective, whereas others do not.

Fourth, TCD devices promoted for surgical monitoring vary widely in their sensitivity to radiofrequency interference. Such interference is problematic because harmonics of the electrocautery and ambient FM radio signals are in the same frequency range as that used to measure TCD shift. With ineffective noise-reduction circuitry, TCD spectral signals may be severely contaminated, making monitoring and/or trending impossible.

Fifth, success in signal acquisition is heavily dependent on probe design. For patient safety, the maximum power and frequency range available for brain insonation are established by the U.S. Food and Drug Administration. Nevertheless, TCD monitor-specific performance is far from uniform. Thus, user dissatisfaction with TCD performance is often due to an unfortunate choice of probe design rather than a fundamental limitation of the underlying technology.

JUGULAR BULB OXIMETRY

Oximeter catheters transmitting three wavelengths of light are inserted into the cerebral venous circulation to directly and continuously measure cerebral venous oxygen saturation ($SjvO_2$). Commercially available devices are modifications of the catheter oximeter originally developed for the pulmonary circulation. External preinsertion calibration of the catheter and documentation of catheter position in the jugular bulb are required for accurate measurements. In vivo calibrations against co-oximeter samples can also be performed. Reflected light signals are averaged, filtered, and displayed. Conditions affecting the accuracy of these measurements include catheter kinking, blood flow around the catheter, changes in hematocrit, fibrin deposition on the catheter, and changes in temperature.

There are two major limitations of the technology. First, $SjvO_2$ represents a global measure of venous drainage from unspecified cranial compartments. Because cerebral and extracranial venous anatomy is notoriously varied, clinical interpretation of measured change is a major challenge. The difficulty is exemplified by the study of Mutch et al,[73] who used both $SjvO_2$ and T2*-weighted magnetic resonance imaging to measure oxyhemoglobin and deoxyhemoglobin in a porcine model of CPB. Imaging demonstrated substantial hypoxic regions within the cerebral parenchyma that were invisible to the global jugular oxygen saturation measurement. Second, accurate measurement using jugular oximetry requires continuous adequate flow past the catheter. Low- or no-flow states such as profound hypoperfusion or complete ischemia render $SjvO_2$ unreliable.[74]

CEREBRAL OXIMETRY

Near-Infrared Technology

Intravascular regional hemoglobin oxygen saturation (rSO_2) may be measured noninvasively with transcranial near-infrared spectroscopy (NIRS) because the human skull is translucent to infrared light. An infrared light source contained in a self-adhesive patch affixed to glabrous skin of the scalp transmits photons through underlying tissues to the outer layers of the cerebral cortex. Adjacent sensors separate photons reflected from the skin, muscle, skull, and dura from those of the brain tissue (Fig. 17–34). Transcranial NIRS measures all hemoglobin, not just the pulsatile arterial component contained in a mixed vascular bed primarily composed of gas-exchanging vessels, venules in particular.[75] The measurement is thought to reflect 16% arterial and 84% venous

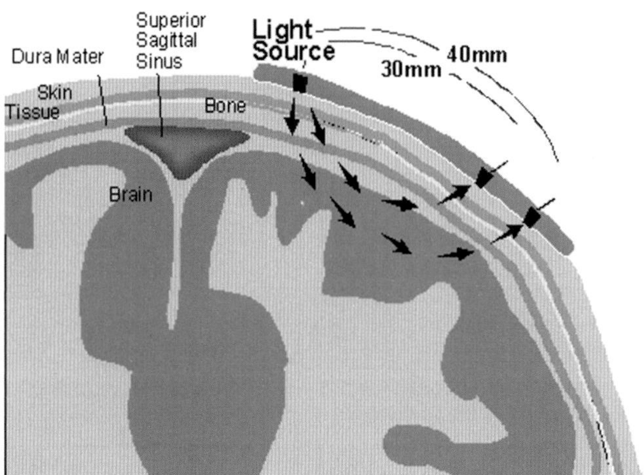

Figure 17–34 The mean photon path traveling through the cranium from the infrared source to sensors on neighboring scalp is banana shaped. Subtraction of the near (30 mm) from the distant (40 mm) signal effectively removes most extracranial "contamination" of the rSO_2 value. (Modified from Gugino LD, et al: Neurophysiological monitoring in vascular surgery. *In* Thomson DA, Gelman S [eds]: Clin Anaesthesiol 14:50, 2000, with permission of the publisher, Baillière Tindall, London, England.)

contributions.[75] This ratio remains nearly constant in normoxia, hypoxia, and hypocapnia.[75] Cerebral oximetry appears to both reliably quantify change from an individualized baseline and offer an objective measure of regional hypoperfusion.[76,77] Unlike pulse and jugular bulb oximetry, respectively, cerebral oximetry may be used during nonpulsatile CPB and circulatory arrest.

Similar to TCD monitoring, cerebral oximetry is primarily used to quantify change. An adverse shift in oxygen supply-demand balance is indicated by a decreasing oxyhemoglobin fraction. The clinical significance of the decline has been determined in conscious patients during G-force studies with high-speed centrifugation, implantable cardioverter/defibrillator testing, tilt-table testing, carotid artery occlusion, and intracranial artery balloon occlusion.[59,60,78-80] In each setting, a decline of greater than 20% was associated with syncope or signs of focal cerebral ischemia. The magnitude and duration of cerebral dysoxygenation are associated with both the severity of postoperative neurocognitive dysfunction and hospital cost-driver increase.[81-83]

Technologic Limitations

The technical limitations of cerebral oximetry primarily involve factors influencing photon migration. Sensor placement is currently limited to glabrous skin (e.g., forehead) lateral to the midline. Such placement prevents monitoring the critical posterior watershed at the juncture of the anterior, middle, and posterior cerebral arteries (Fig. 17–35). Dark hair and the follicles of dark hair absorb near-infrared light and can substantially reduce the signal-to-noise ratio. Thus, de Letter et al,[84] using a parietotemporal placement in head-shaved neurosurgical patients, failed to obtain saturation values in 18% of their patients. Weak signals may also result from hematoma or sensor placement over a venous sinus.[85] In either case, the large hemoglobin volume acts as a photon sink. Conversely, recording failures may arise from excessively large signals, such as those produced by a skull defect.[86]

Validation

The rSO_2 value has been validated from arterial and jugular bulb oxygen saturation measurements in pediatric and adult subjects.[87,88] In these studies, hypoxemia involving cerebral tissue proximate to the sensors was consistently detected by this technology. Except during ischemia and CPB, $SjvO_2$ and rSO_2 generally correlate in the midrange saturation, although discrepancies may appear at the extremes.[89] The validity of rSO_2 also has been assessed by comparison with direct microprobe measurement of brain tissue oxygen partial pressure (tPO_2). Reasonable agreement between these two measures has been found in neurosurgical patients.[90,91]

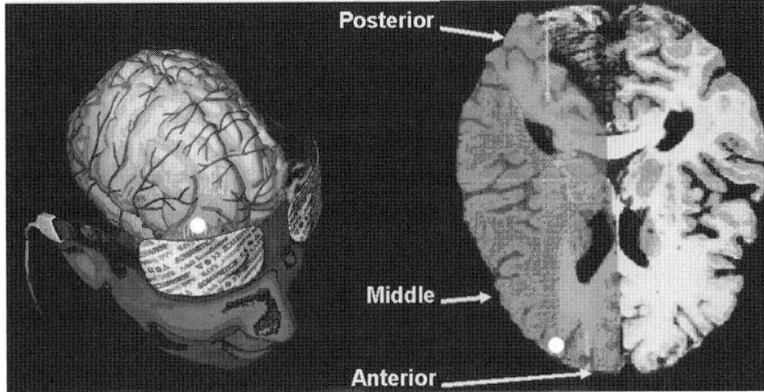

Figure 17–35 The regions of the frontal cortex sampled by the cerebral oximeter. When the infrared sensor-containing patches are properly positioned on the forehead above each eye, the sample volume (P5 mL) typically lies in the ischemia-sensitive border zone between the anterior and middle cerebral artery. (Courtesy of Ron Widman, Somanetics Corp, Troy, MI.)

Controversies

As with many new technologies, the emergence of cerebral oximetry has spawned criticism, some of it based on misunderstanding. Criticisms include the lack of absolute oxyhemoglobin quantification; inadequacy of intravascular oxygenation as an index of intracellular oxygenation; inaccuracy arising from the use of a fixed arterial/venous ratio in the rSO_2 computational algorithm; confounding influences of large shifts in hematocrit, temperature, and hydrogen ion concentration[92]; and inconsistencies with alternative estimates of brain oxygenation or blood flow.[75,76,92-95]

There appear to be two primary sources of misunderstanding. One source involves an observed oximeter "failure" to meet an unjustified investigator expectation. This phenomenon is typified by Schwartz et al,[96] who examined rSO_2 in cadavers and found that some values exceeded those obtained from healthy subjects. As a result, the authors questioned the validity of rSO_2 measurement. In fact, such an overlap in rSO_2 values from live and dead brain is to be expected. Tissue oxygen saturation may be nearly normal in dead or nonmetabolizing brain because of sequestered cerebral venous blood in capillaries and venous capacitance vessels.[97] In contrast, desaturation occurs in ischemic metabolizing brain due to an oxygen supply insufficient to meet cerebral metabolic demand. In support of this view, Maeda et al[98] examined cerebral venous oxygen saturation during 214 autopsies and found values ranging from 1% to 95%. Variation appeared to depend on the total hemoglobin content, cause of death, and cadaver storage conditions.

The other major source of misunderstanding is an apparent lack of appreciation for recent advances in NIRS technology. As a result, early negative findings continue to be referenced in discussions critical of the current technology. This inappropriate comparison may be misleading, because the performance of the current Food and Drug Administration–approved spectrometers (INVOS 4100 and 5100; Somanetics Corporation, Troy, MI) has improved substantially from previous models. Most notably, there has been a 10-fold increase in the infrared source output with a narrower bandwidth and center wavelength deviation that approaches the performance of laser diodes. As a result, the signal-to-noise ratio has been increased by a factor of 10 and the averaging interval shortened from 20 to 4 seconds or less.[88]

Perhaps as a result of this recent progress in NIRS technology, there is expanding use of rSO_2 monitoring during cardiovascular surgery. According to the manufacturer's website (www.Somanetics.com), cerebral oximetry is currently used in half of the U.S. institutions performing pediatric cardiac surgery and 10% of those performing adult cardiovascular procedures.

Normative Values

Kishi et al[99] examined surgical patient demographic influences on rSO_2. The measure appeared to be independent of weight, height, head size, or gender, although it was negatively correlated with age and positively correlated with hemoglobin concentration. Values were also affected as the sensor was moved laterally from the recommended position above the eye. In contrast, Misra et al[100] found no association between rSO_2 and age, gender, skin color, height, weight, tobacco use, or caffeine intake in 94 adult healthy subjects. This suggests that the apparent age influence on rSO_2 actually may reflect advancing pathology in older patients.

Development of local physiologic norms is a common practice in neurophysiology units. Following this practice, in 1000 elective adult cardiac surgery patients (age range, 21 to 91; females, 32%), this author has determined a preprocedure rSO_2 value of 67 ± 10 scale units.[101] This value is significantly less than the 71 ± 6 previously reported for healthy volunteers (age range, 20 to 36).[88] The mean and median left-right difference was zero, and only 5% of the differences were greater than 10. Only 5% of the rSO_2 baseline values were less than 50 or above 80. Thus, from a statistical perspective, an awake rSO_2 value in adult elective cardiac surgery patients is abnormal if it is either outside the range of 50 to 80 or there is a right-left difference of greater than 10.

Intervention Threshold

Absence of an accepted intervention threshold is often used as an excuse to avoid this new technology. However, there is substantial agreement among investigators attempting to define a rSO_2 ischemic/hypoxic threshold. Cho et al[102] found that desaturation of greater than 10 scale units below baseline or an absolute value below 50 was associated with decreased somatosensory evoked potential (SSEP) amplitude following carotid occlusion during carotid endarterectomy performed under general anesthesia. With regional anesthesia and cerebral oximeter monitoring, Roberts et al[103] observed four patients with clamp-related transient neurologic deficits. The decreases in rSO_2 ranged from 27% to 31% below preclamp values. Symptoms and desaturation resolved with shunt insertion or blood pressure increase.

Samra et al[104] confirmed this observation in 10 symptomatic and 90 asymptomatic patients. Carotid occlusion associated with neurologic symptoms of regional ischemia resulted in an average 20% decline in rSO_2 below the preocclusion baseline, whereas only a 9% decline was seen in asymptomatic patients. Using the criterion of a 20% rSO_2 decline to predict clinical signs of ischemia, there was a 2.6% false-negative rate, with a sensitivity of 80% and specificity of 82%. The use of a 20% rSO_2 decrease as an ischemic threshold for carotid endarterectomy compares favorably with that observed during syncope induced in conscious patients or subjects by implantable cardioverter/defibrillator testing, tilt-table testing, balloon occlusion of the internal carotid artery, and negative gravitational force testing.[80,105-107]

An alternative basis for an ischemic threshold is a fixed rSO_2 value. The increased simplicity must be weighed against the likelihood of decreased sensitivity and specificity. Nevertheless, decreases of rSO_2 below 50, even for brief intervals, are associated with significant increases in cognitive or neurologic injury, length of critical care or total hospital stay, and hospital charges.[108-111] In practice, either approach may be suitable because a 20% decline from the normative mean rSO_2 of 66 would be 53, close to the fixed threshold of 50. Using either criterion, patient management could be adjusted to prevent further desaturation (Box 17–12).

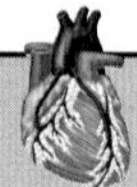

BOX 17–12 ***Cerebral Regional Oxygen Saturation (rSO_2)***

- It detects imbalance in oxygen supply and demand.
- Normative range for adult cardiac surgery patient is 67 ± 10.
- Clinically important decrease is 20% below baseline.

Intervention Rationale

Baseline rSO_2

Surgical cerebral oximetric monitoring should be initiated immediately after patient entry to the operating room. Self-adhesive patches containing the infrared light source with shallow (proximate) and deep (distant) sensors are fixed on the forehead on both sides of the midline. The initial objective is the establishment of a reference baseline prior to preoxygenation and anesthetic induction (Fig. 17–36).

A high cerebral metabolic demand for oxygen may result in abnormally low rSO_2 values despite normal pulse oximetry readings. For example, the cerebral oximeter detected oxygen imbalance during high-altitude trekking that was unrecognized by pulse oximetry.[112] Similarly, patients in heart failure often have preoperative baseline values far below the normative range.[113] Abnormally high rSO_2 values may signify a silent infarction, because injured or dead neurons consume little oxygen. Abnormal (>10 scale units) right-left rSO_2 may be caused by unrecognized carotid or intracranial arterial stenosis, intracranial space-occupying lesion, old infarction, skull defect, or extracranial sources such as a hemangioma, sinusitis, or artifactual interference from an infrared-emitting device.[114-117] An asymmetry or abnormal rSO_2 baseline, high or low, alerts the operative team to the increased potential for cerebral oxygen imbalance during surgical challenge and may alter the plan of anesthetic management.

Developing rSO_2 Asymmetry

A new asymmetry, signifying cerebral dysoxygenation, may develop quickly during anesthetic induction, pulmonary artery catheter insertion, or final patient positioning. During head rotation, rSO_2 (see Fig. 17–36) may decrease contralateral

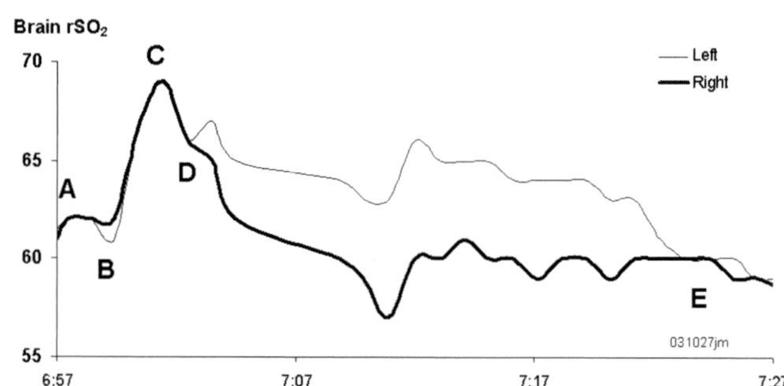

Figure 17–36 Clinically important changes in the intraoperative rSO_2 trend prior to skin incision are shown. The *thick line* represents the right frontal cortex and, *thin line,* the left. Values at marker A were obtained in the awake patient before preoxygenation. General anesthetic induction began at marker B, and tracheal intubation was successfully completed at marker C. Note the symmetrical rSO_2 increase associated with CO_2 accumulation and hypnotic suppression of cerebral oxygen demand. A left-right asymmetry appeared at marker D coincident with axial head rotation to the left for insertion of a pulmonary artery catheter. The asymmetry disappeared at marker E as the head was returned to a neutral position.

to a stenotic carotid artery.[117] Axial head rotation displaces the lateral mass of the contralateral atlas forward behind the internal carotid artery, just below its entrance into the carotid canal at the skull base. If this process is prolonged or if the artery is adherent to adjacent tissue, it can be compressed from behind, resulting in decreased flow.[118,119] Furthermore, volatile anesthetics may interfere with the regulatory mechanisms that normally maintain effective cerebral perfusion bilaterally during head rotation in conscious patients.[120]

The cerebral oximeter has detected potentially catastrophic cerebral desaturation due to great vessel torsion during cardiac manipulation.[121] Desaturation often appears to be the result of compromised venous return. Particularly in pediatric cardiac operations and in myocardial revascularization without CPB, cardiac manipulation may produce sudden large rso_2 decreases without any appreciable change in mean arterial pressure or arterial oxygen saturation.

Fukada et al[122] reported cerebral oximetric detection and successful correction of a malperfusion syndrome during acute type A aortic dissection repair. Although parallel recording of radial and femoral arterial pressures is widely used to detect malperfusion, no pressure difference was seen in this case due to maintenance of perfusion in the leftmost arch branch. Malperfusion-related cerebral ischemia may often be identified by EEG or SSEP, but these signals are susceptible to compromise by electrocautery, deep anesthesia, and hypothermia.[123] Cerebral oximetry is also used during extracorporeal membrane oxygenation to detect regional deficiencies in brain perfusion associated with carotid cannulation.[124]

rso_2 Responsiveness to CO_2

Induction of anesthesia and its attendant apnea during tracheal intubation often transiently alters the brain oxygen supply-demand relationship. Hypnotic agents may transiently suppress cerebral metabolism more than blood flow, resulting in an rso_2 increase.[125] With normally reactive cerebral arterioles, ventilation disruption and CO_2 accumulation during tracheal intubation further increase rso_2 as a result of the increased delivery of hyperoxygenated blood to a metabolically suppressed brain. Under these circumstances, even mild hypercapnia augments cerebral perfusion and oxygenation through local vasodilation.[126] Several investigators have demonstrated an rso_2 increase (see Fig. 17–36) associated with hypercapnia.[127]

Holzschuh et al[90] found significant correlation between changes in xenon-measured cerebral blood flow and rso_2 in response to acetazolamide. The authors concluded that "NIRS can be used as a noninvasive screening method to test the cerebrovascular reserve capacity." Absence of the hyperoxic response suggests impairment of both CO_2 reactivity and cerebral autoregulation. Asymmetry warns of a potential vasculopathy (e.g., intracranial stenosis or silent infarction) and may prompt alterations in anesthetic and perfusion management to maintain cerebral perfusion in both hemispheres.

Acid-base management during CPB remains controversial, particularly during deep cooling. Some propose that the higher CO_2 tension afforded by pH-stat acid-base management results in fewer neurologic complications.[128] Vijay et al[129] observed that during adult near-normothermic myocardial revascularization, vasopressor-induced perfusion pressure increases alone were sometimes inadequate to correct decreased rso_2 occurring during CPB. In this situation, judiciously applied permissive hypercapnia often was effective in restoring rso_2 to baseline.

Despite these seeming benefits, hypercapnia has potentially deleterious effects. Hypercapnia-induced cardiac output and heart rate also increase myocardial oxygen demand, while cerebral vasodilation may exacerbate preexisting intracranial hypertension. Cerebral oximetry provides a convenient method to document appropriate bihemispheric CO_2 reactivity. In addition, continuous measurement of brain oxygen saturation permits CO_2 titration to achieve optimal tissue perfusion at the lowest risk.[102,104] Individualized management of carbon dioxide tension facilitated by cerebral oximetry enhances the opportunity for anesthesia providers and perfusionists to positively affect cardiovascular surgery outcome.

rso_2 as a Transfusion Trigger

Two important determinants of tissue oxygenation are hemoglobin availability and plasma volume.[130,131] Madl et al[132] examined the relationship between hemoglobin and rso_2 in patients with septic shock. If a low hemoglobin (<8.5 mg/dL) was associated with an rso_2 below the normative range (i.e., <60%), transfusion consistently increased both variables. However, transfusion had no effect on rso_2 values above 65%. Blas et al[133] described profound desaturation accompanying hemodilution (hematocrit of 16%), despite the absence of low perfusion pressure and hypocapnia, as well as high arterial oxygen tension and mixed venous oxygen saturation. Brain saturation responded immediately to 2 units of packed red cells in this patient with bilateral carotid artery occlusions.

Because of the apparent association between rso_2 and hemoglobin, transient brain oxygen desaturation is to be expected at the onset of CPB, as the pump prime solution briefly displaces hemoglobin in the cerebral circulation. Vijay et al[134] demonstrated that the magnitude of this transient desaturation was related directly to the volume of crystalloid prime. The hemoglobin influence on rso_2 is the basis for use of cerebral oximetry as a transfusion trigger.[135]

rso_2 and Blood Volume

Tissue oximetry has been used to visualize the effect of volume expansion on cerebral perfusion during tilt-table diagnostic testing for syncope.[136] An rso_2 sensor was placed on the gastrocnemius muscle to measure upright tilt-induced desaturation resulting from lower limb venous pooling. In susceptible patients, extensive pooling resulted in cerebral dysoxygenation and syncope. Crystalloid volume expansion reduced lower limb hemoglobin sequestration and prevented syncope. This same concept may be applied to cardiac surgery. Vasopressor ineffectiveness in the correction of an rso_2 decline may indicate compromised microcirculatory gas exchange due to hypovolemia. In this circumstance, low rso_2 values often respond to volume augmentation.

rso_2 and Autoregulation

Numerous studies have concluded that cerebral autoregulation remains intact during cardiac operations, both before and during CPB. Although this conclusion may be correct for large groups of patients, it does not necessarily apply to each individual. Cerebral oximetry can identify the lower limit of autoregulation, the point at which brain blood flow and tissue oxygenation become pressure dependent. The independence of mean arterial pressure (MAP) and rso_2 establishes intact cerebral autoregulation.[137]

Figure 17–37 illustrates the use of rso_2 measurement in the determination of the lower autoregulatory limit. The rso_2-versus-MAP relationship in the top graph depicts intact

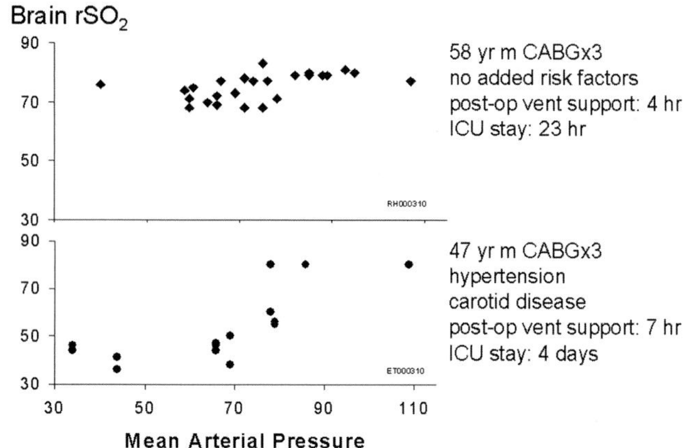

Figure 17–37 The relationship between rso_2 and mean arterial pressure during cardiopulmonary bypass is depicted. Each symbol represents a single point paired measurement obtained at 5-minute intervals. *Top,* intact cerebral autoregulation with clear independence of rso_2 and mean arterial pressure (MAP) over a wide range. The patient's outcome was uneventful. In contrast, the *bottom* depicts dysautoregulation with the classic appearance of a vascular waterfall. Each time the MAP fell below 80 mm Hg, a marked rso_2 decrease occurred, indicating that the cerebral perfusion pressure had fallen below the lower limit of autoregulation. Presumably, as a result of suboptimal cerebral perfusion the patient experienced a prolonged recovery complicated by delirium.

autoregulation. The rso_2 values remain independent of MAP over a wide pressure range. The bottom graph, generated later the same day in the same operating room by the same surgical team, depicts dysautoregulation, because rso_2 declines each time MAP falls below 80 mm Hg. Examination of MAP-rso_2 relationships from a large series of cardiac operations resulted in two findings.[138] First, the lower limit of autoregulation varies widely among patients, from a mean arterial pressure of less than 40 to more than 100 mm Hg. Second, a substantial proportion of cardiac patients do not, in fact, maintain autoregulation throughout the entirety of the operation. These observations illustrate the potential benefit of continuously monitoring the adequacy of cerebral perfusion during cardiovascular surgery.

The driving force for hemoglobin through the gas-exchanging microvasculature is not arterial pressure per se, but the arterial-venous pressure difference. Factors that increase cerebral venous pressure will compromise oxygen delivery, even if the arterial pressure remains in the normally acceptable range. It is most useful to examine a trend of the relationship between rso_2 and cerebral perfusion pressure (MAP − [the higher of central venous or intracranial pressure]).

rso_2 and Brain Temperature

Temperature has important effects on tissue oxygenation.[139] Because standard temperature monitoring during CPB does not accurately characterize the efficacy of brain cooling, cerebral oximetry may facilitate management of hypothermic neuroprotection.[140,141] In theory, temperature with CPB and alpha-stat acid-base management results in a linear decrease in cerebral blood flow and an exponential decline in metabolic rate.[142] Consequently, predicted "luxury" flow should ensure adequate cerebral oxygenation during cooling. However, Daubeney et al[121] demonstrated that other variables were also involved in the maintenance of adequate tissue oxygenation during deep hypothermia in pediatric patients. The rso_2 at a 20°C target cooling temperature varied inversely with the cooling rate by the equation: $rso_2 = -20.5$ (cooling rate, °C/min) + 97.4. In addition, they found that the rate of desaturation during total circulatory arrest was a function of the nasopharyngeal temperature at arrest onset, described by the equation: desaturation rate = 0.19 (nasopharyngeal temp, °C) − 2.5. At 20°C, the mean desaturation rate was 0.25% min, although decay was not linear. At temperatures slightly above 20°C (21° to 26°C), desaturation rate increased nearly 10-fold (2.0% min). In normothermic infants, transient disruption of cerebral perfusion resulted in another 10-fold increase (i.e., ≈20% min) in the rate of desaturation.[143] The desaturation rates in hypothermic pediatric patients are somewhat less than those reported in adults.[144] The differences may reflect the relative ease of homogenous cooling of the pediatric brain or intrinsic differences in neonatal cerebral oxygen utilization.[145]

Deep hypothermia may also produce transient cerebral vasoparesis.[121,146] Consequently, rewarming may result in desaturation as the temperature-induced increase in cerebral metabolism is unsupported by adequate flow increase. Daubeney et al[121] described an inverse relationship between rso_2 and nasopharyngeal temperature during rewarming in pediatric patients, given by the equation: $rso_2 = -2.9$ (nasopharyngeal temp) + 148. Liu et al[125] observed similar cerebral desaturation during rewarming in adult cardiac surgery patients. Small perfusion deficits decreased rso_2 as oxygen extraction is increased to meet rising demand. When the oxygen extractive capacity is exceeded, functional compromise will be manifested by EEG or evoked potential abnormalities.[147]

rso_2 Guides Supplemental Cerebral Perfusion

Deeb et al[148] demonstrated that rso_2-guided retrograde cerebral perfusion extended the "safe time" for hypothermic circulatory arrest during adult aortic arch reconstruction. Blas et al[133] reported on the use of cerebral oximetry for detection of a superior vena cava cannula malposition during retrograde cerebral perfusion. Higami et al[149] found rapid desaturation with total circulatory arrest, slow continual desaturation with retrograde cerebral perfusion, and no desaturation with supplemental antegrade cerebral perfusion (Fig. 17–38). There was a high incidence of neurologic deficit in patients whose saturation declined more than 30% below the conscious baseline.

Cerebral oximetry also appears to be a useful guide for the management of regional low-flow perfusion (RLFP) during neonatal aortic arch reconstruction.[150] RLFP (≈20 mL/kg/min) via the innominate artery maintained brain rso_2. In contrast, profound desaturation occurred with total circulatory arrest. Monitoring of rso_2 helped to prevent both cerebral hypoperfusion and hyperperfusion. In agreement with these observations, Hofer et al[151] found a linear relationship between rso_2 and antegrade supplemental cerebral perfusion pump flow in neonates undergoing aortic arch reconstruction.

rso_2 and Anesthetic Adequacy

Another important determinant of tissue oxygenation is pain-induced stress.[152] With inadequate hypnosis or analgesia, pain-induced stress may result in cerebral oxygen consumption exceeding delivery and decreasing rso_2. Concomitant use of quantitative EEG and upper facial muscle EMG measures of hypnotic and analgesic adequacy can facilitate the prompt

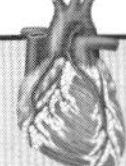

BOX 17–13 ***Important Imbalances Identified by Cerebral Oximetry***

- Preexisting cerebral oxygen imbalance
- Position-related asymmetry
- Cerebral arterial CO_2 reactivity and autoregulation
- Need for blood replacement
- Volume status
- Perfusion cannula malposition
- Malperfusion syndrome
- Optimal brain cooling and rewarming
- Successful supplementary cerebral perfusion during circulatory arrest

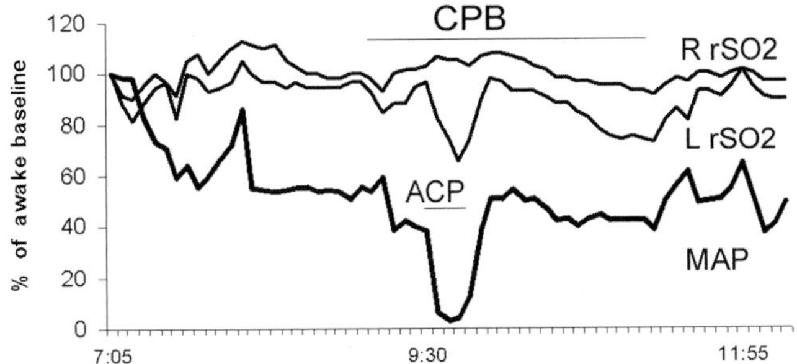

Figure 17–38 Cerebral oximetry provides continuous objective assessment of supplemental antegrade cerebral perfusion (ACP) during deep hypothermic systemic circulatory arrest. In this case a single perfusion cannula for ACP was located in the right axillary artery. The stable rSO_2 value in the right hemisphere and falling rSO_2 in the left hemisphere document that ACP was only partially successful. Had a longer arrest period been anticipated, this information would have prompted the surgeon to cannulate the left carotid as well.

identification and correction of this source of cerebral dysoxygenation (Box 17–13).

NEUROMONITORING AND OUTCOME

Outcome studies of EEG monitoring primarily have concentrated on process variables, describing occurrences of ischemic EEG changes and their possible association with neurologic complications. To date, the results of only one adequately powered prospective randomized study on EEG clinical and economic benefit have been published. Myles et al[153] demonstrated a significant 82% decrease in awareness with BIS monitoring. This finding replicated the results of a large nonrandomized study, which showed that BIS monitoring was associated with a 78% decrease in awareness.[154] Both these results are consistent with a number of smaller, nonrandomized studies.

Outcome studies on TCD efficacy for surgical monitoring have thus far been limited to carotid endarterectomy. Spencer[155] used a retrospective control group to demonstrate a significant reduction in stroke incidence with TCD monitoring. The contemporaneous study of Lennard et al[156] lacked an unmonitored comparison group but achieved an impressive 0% stroke incidence in a cohort of 100 TCD-monitored patients. Subsequently, the Washington State Blue Shield carrier endorsed TCD as medically necessary for "assessing initial collateral blood flow and embolization during carotid endartectomy."[157]

Outcome studies for AEPs and jugular bulb oximetry are not available. However, the author has conducted four nonrandomized controlled cardiac surgery outcome studies for cerebral oximetry as the sole approach to neuromonitoring.[82,83,101,111] Because all findings were similar, their collective

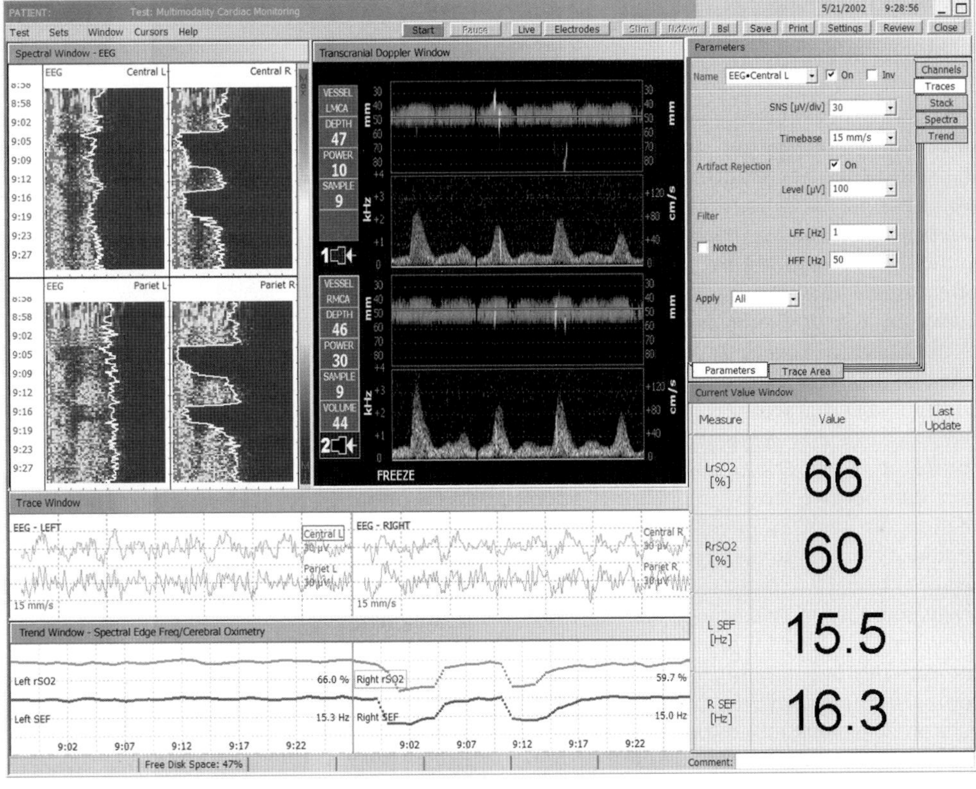

Figure 17–39 Multimodality neuromonitoring (EEG, TCD, and cerebral oximetry) now may be viewed on a single computer screen. Note the loss in right hemisphere EEG high-frequency activity with associated declines in both SEF and rSO_2 and the presence of emboliform HITS in the power M-mode and spectral TCD displays. (Courtesy of Howard Bailin, Axon Instruments, Hauppauge, NY.)

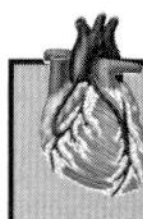

BOX 17–14 *Multimodality Neuromonitoring for Cardiac Surgery*

Modality	**Function**
Electroencephalography	Cortical synaptic activity
Middle latency auditory evoked potentials	Subcortical-cortical activity
Brainstem auditory evoked potentials	Brainstem synaptic activity
Transcranial Doppler	Blood flow change and emboli
Cerebral oximetry	Cortical oxygen balance

result may be most informative. In the combined study population of 3742 patients, cerebral oximetric monitoring was associated with an average 1.7-day decline in length of hospital stay. All of these studies suggest that improved oxygenation benefits not only the brain but also all vital organs.

There are two outcome studies that have examined the impact of multimodality neuromonitoring using a combination of EEG, TCD, and cerebral oximetry[158,159] (Fig. 17–39). Both found a 2.7-day reduction in length of stay associated with multimodality neuromonitoring. The study of Edmonds[158] also noted an 11% reduction in hospital expenses. In addition to the substantial reductions in hospital stay, charges, and neurologic complications, the results suggested possible benefit to other vital organ systems. This finding is not unexpected because the same processes that injure the brain may also injure other organs.[71] Future studies of neuromonitoring efficacy should not overlook these important accessory benefits. In addition, Lozano and Mossad[160] reviewed studies of neuromonitoring during pediatric cardiac surgery and showed that the monitoring was associated with enhanced outcomes (Box 17–14).

SUMMARY

The EEG is an exquisitely sensitive measure of synaptic function. Modern display and numeric trending techniques make it practical for the cardiac anesthesia provider to monitor multichannel EEG and AEPs. The EEG aids rapid detection of cerebral ischemia/hypoxia and seizure activity. Both EEG and MLAEPs quantify hypnotic adequacy. EEG and BAEPs offer simple functional measures of effective brain cooling. However, despite their sensitivity, EEG and AEP information is not specific. The cause of detected synaptic suppression must be determined by other techniques such as TCD, which continuously characterizes brain blood flow changes. In addition, TCD detects cerebral microemboli, regardless of their source or composition. Vital cerebral hemodynamic imbalance can be detected by TCD, but it offers no direct information on neuronal metabolism. This essential element is provided by cerebral oximetry, which describes changes in the regional balance of oxygen supply and demand. Thus, collectively, these monitoring modalities function "hand-in-glove." Together, they identify physiologic imbalance, its causes, and the patient's response to corrective action. The risks of neuromonitoring are nil, the costs modest, and the clinical and economic benefits substantial; cardiac surgery neuromonitoring has come of age.

Acknowledgments

The author has no personal financial relationship with any manufacturer or distributor of neuromonitoring devices, but he has at some time received research support from each of the following sources: Aspect Medical Systems, Axon Systems, Baxter Healthcare, Cadwell Laboratories, Datex-Ohmeda, DWL, ElectroCap International, Nicolet Vascular, Physiometrix, Spencer Technologies, Somanetics Corporation, and Terumo. The author is grateful for financial support provided by Norton HealthCare, Jewish HealthCare Services, and Baptist Hospital East, all of Louisville, KY, and the editorial assistance of his wife, Jeanne.

REFERENCES

1. Newman MF, Kirchner JL, Phillips-Bute B, et al: Longitudinal assessment of neurocognitive function after coronary artery bypass surgery. N Engl J Med 344:395, 2001
2. Roach GW, Kanchuger M, Mangano CM, et al: Adverse cerebral outcomes after coronary bypass surgery. N Engl J Med 335:1857, 1996
3. Kilo J, Dzerny M, Gorlitzer M et al: Cardiopulmonary bypass affects cognitive brain function after coronary artery bypass grafting. Ann Thorac Surg 72:1926, 2001
4. Edmonds HL Jr, Rodriguez RA, Audenaert SM, et al: The role of neuromonitoring in cardiovascular surgery. J Cardiothorac Vasc Anesth 10:15, 1996
5. Edmonds HL Jr: Detection and treatment of cerebral hypoxia is key to avoiding intraoperative brain injuries. J Clin Monit Comput 16:69, 2000
6. Theye RA, Patrick RT, Kirklin JW: The electroencephalogram in patients undergoing open intracardiac operations with the aid of extracorporeal circulation. J Thorac Surg 34:709, 1957
7. Blume WT, Sharbrough FW: EEG monitoring during carotid endarterectomy and open heart surgery. *In* Niedermeyer E, Lopes Da Silva F (eds): Electroencephalography, 4th edition. Philadelphia, Lippincott Williams & Wilkins, 1999, p 797
8. Craft RM, Losasso TJ, Perkins WJ, et al: EEG monitoring or cerebral ischemia during carotid endarterectomy: How much is enough? Anesthesiology 81(3A):A214, 1994 (abstract)
9. Edmonds HL Jr, Sehic A, Gruenthal M: Comparison of 2-, 4- and 16-channel EEG for detection of cerebral ischemia. Anesthesiology 97(3A):A-305, 2002 (abstract)
10. Levy WJ: Monitoring of the electroencephalogram during cardiopulmonary bypass. Know when to say when. Anesthesiology 76:876, 1992
11. Timofeev I, Contreras D, Steriade M: Synaptic responsiveness of cortical and thalamic neurons during various phases of slow sleep oscillation in cat. J Neurophysiol (Lond) 494:265, 1996
12. Stockard J, Bickford RG: The neurophysiology of anaesthesia. *In* Gordon E (ed): A Basis and Practice of Neuroanaesthesia. Amsterdam, Excerpta Medica, 1975, p 3
13. Sharbrough FW: Nonspecific abnormal EEG patterns. *In* Niedermeyer E, Lopes da Silva F (eds): Electroencephalography, 4th edition. Philadelphia, Lippincott Williams & Wilkins, 1999, p 215
14. Goldstein L: Psychotropic drug-induced EEG changes as revealed by the amplitude integration method. Mod Probl Pharmacopsychiatr 8:131, 1974
15. Prior PM, Maynard DE, Sheaff PC, et al: Monitoring cerebral function: Clinical experience with a new device for continuous recording of electrical activity of the brain. Br Med J 2:215, 1971
16. Hellström-Westas L, de Vries LD, Rosén I: An Atlas of Amplitude-Integrated EEGs in the Newborn. Boca Raton, Parthenon, 2003
17. Pronk RAF: EEG Processing in Cardiac Surgery. Utrecht, Inst Med Physics TNO, 1982
18. Rampil I: EEG processing and the bispectral index. Anesthesiology 89:815, 1998
19. Gugino LD, Chabot RJ, Prichep LSD, et al: Quantitative EEG changes associated with loss and return of consciousness in healthy adult volunteers anaesthetized with propofol or sevoflurane. Br J Anaesth 87:421, 2001
20. Vakkuri A, Yli-Hankala A, Talja P, et al: Time-frequency balanced spectral entropy as a measure of anesthetic effect in central nervous system during sevoflurane, propofol, and thiopental anesthesia. Acta Anaesthesiol Scand 48:145, 2004
21. Rampil IJ: A primer for EEG signal processing in anesthesia. Anesthesiology 89:980, 1998
22. Paloheimo M: Quantitative surface electromyography (qEMG): Applications in anaesthesiology and critical care. Acta Anaesthesiol Scand Suppl 93:1, 1990

23. John ER, Prichep LS, Kox W, et al: Invariant reversible QEEG effects of anesthetics. Conscious Cognit 10:165, 2001
24. Prichep LS, Gugino LD, John ER, et al: The patient state index as an indicator of the level of hypnosis under general anesthesia. Br J Anaesth 92:1, 2004
25. Drover D, Lemmons H, Loyd G, et al: Patient state index (PSI) sensitivity to changes in anesthetic state and optimization of delivery and recovery from anesthesia. Anesthesiology 97:82, 2002
26. Viertiö-Oja H, Maja V, Särkelä M, et al: Description of the Entropy™ algorithm as applied in the Datex-Omeda S/5™ Entropy Module. Acta Anaesthesiol Scand 48:154, 2004
27. Joy RM: Spectral analysis of long EEG samples for comparative purposes. Neuropharmacology 10:471, 1971
28. Myers RR, Stockard JJ, Fleming NI, et al: The use of on-line telephonic computer analysis of the EEG in anaesthesia. Br J Anaesth 45:664, 1973
29. Pichylmayr I, Lips U: EEG monitoring in anesthesiology and intensive care. Neuropsychobiology 10:239, 1983
30. Fleming RA, Smith NT: An inexpensive device for analyzing and monitoring the electroencephalogram. Anesthesiology 50:456,1979
31. Alkire MT: Quantitative EEG correlation with brain glucose metabolic rate during anesthesia in volunteers. Anesthesiology 89:323, 1998
32. Gusev EI, Fedin Al, Erokhin OY, et al: Compressed spectral analysis of the EEG in patients with acute cerebrovascular disturbance. Neurosci Behav Physiol 15:144, 1985
33. Bischoff P, Kochs E, Droese D, et al: Topographic quantitative EEG analysis of the paradoxical arousal reaction. EEG changes during urologic surgery using isoflurane/N_2O anesthesia. Anesthesist 42:142, 1993 [In German]
34. Rodriguez RA, Cornel G, Semelhago L, et al: Cerebral effects in superior vena caval obstruction: The role of brain monitoring. Ann Thorac Surg 64:1820, 1997
35. Orth VH, Rehm M, Thiel M, et al: First clinical implications of perioperative red cell volume measurement with a nonradioactive marker. Anesth Analg 87:1234, 1998
36. Hanel F, von Knobelsdorff G, Werner C, et al: Hypercapnia prevents jugular bulb desaturation during rewarming from hypothermic cardiopulmonary bypass. Anesthesiology 89:19, 1998
37. Edmonds HL Jr, Rodriguez RA, Audenaert S, et al: The role of neuromonitoring in cardiovascular surgery. J Cardiothorac Vasc Anesth 10:15, 1996
38. Edmonds HL Jr, Griffiths L, Van der Laken J, et al: Quantitative electroencephalographic monitoring during myocardial revascularization predicts postoperative disorientation and improves outcome. J Thorac Cardiovasc Surg 103:555, 1992
39. Gugino LD, Chabot RJ, Aglio LS, et al: QEEG changes during cardiopulmonary bypass: Relationship to postoperative neuropsychological function. Clin Electroencephalogr 30:53, 1999
40. Croughwell ND, Newman MF, Blumenthal JA, et al: Jugular bulb saturation and cognitive dysfunction after cardiopulmonary bypass. Ann Thorac Surg 58:1702, 1994
41. Ederberg S, Westerlind A, Houltz E, et al: The effects of propofol on cerebral blood flow velocity and cerebral oxygen extraction during cardiopulmonary bypass. Anesth Analg 86:1201, 1998
42. BhaskerRao B, VanHimbergen D, Edmonds HL Jr, et al: Evidence for improved cerebral function after minimally invasive bypass surgery. J Card Surg 13:27, 1998
43. Reddy RV, Moorthy SS, Dierdorf SF, et al: Excitatory effects and electroencephalographic correlation of etomidate, thiopental, methohexital and propofol. Anesth Analg 77:1008, 1993
44. Yli-Hankala A, Vakkuri A, Sarkela M, et al: Epileptiform EEG during induction of anesthesia with sevoflurane mask. Anesthesiology 91:1596, 1999
45. Kearse LA Jr, Koski G, Husain MV, et al: Epileptiform activity during opioid anesthesia. Electroencephalogr Clin Neurophysiol 87:374, 1993
46. Bellinger DC, Wypij D, Kuban KC, et al: Developmental and neurological status of children at 4 years of age after heart surgery with hypothermic circulatory arrest or low-flow cardiopulmonary bypass. Circulation 100:526, 1999
47. Picton TW, Hillyard SA, Krausz HI: Human auditory evoked potentials. I. Evaluation of components. Electroencephalogr Clin Neurophysiol 36:179, 1974
48. Picton TW, Rodriguez RA, Linden RD: The neurophysiology of human hearing. Human Communication, Canada 9:127, 1985
49. Thornton C: Evoked potentials in anaesthesia. Eur J Anaesth 8:89, 1991
50. Kraus N, McGee T: The middle latency response generating system. Electroencephalogr Clin Neurophysiology Suppl 44:93, 1995
51. Kraus N, Smith DI, Reed NL: Auditory middle latency responses in children: Effects of age and diagnostic category. Electroencephalogr Clin Neurophysiol 62:343, 1985
52. Kumar A, Bhattacharya A: Evoked potential monitoring in anaesthesia and analgesia. Anaesthesia 55:225, 2000
53. Rodriguez RA, Audenaert SM, Austin EH: Auditory evoked responses in children during hypothermic cardiopulmonary bypass. J Clin Neurophysiol 12:168-176, 1995.
54. Stone JG, Young WL, Smith CR et al: Do standard monitoring sites reflect true brain temperature when profound hypothermia is rapidly induced and reversed? Anesthesiology 82:344, 1995
55. Duebener LF, Hagino I, Sakamoto T, et al: Effects of pH management during deep hypothermic bypass on cerebral microcirculation: Alpha-stat versus pH-stat. Circulation 106(12 suppl I):I-103, 2002
56. Kontos HA: Validity of cerebral arterial blood flow calculations from velocity measurements. Stroke 20:1, 1989
57. Burrows FA, Bissonnette B: Monitoring the adequacy of cerebral perfusion during cardiopulmonary bypass in children using transcranial Doppler technology. J Neurosurg Anesthesiol 5:209, 1993
58. Halsey J: Risks and benefits of shunting in carotid endarterectomy. The International Transcranial Doppler Collaborators. Stroke 23:1583, 1992
59. Singer I, Edmonds HL Jr: Changes in cerebral perfusion during third-generation implantable cardioverter-defibrillator testing. Am Heart J 127:1052, 1994
60. Edmonds HL Jr, Singer I, Sehic A, et al: Multimodality neuromonitoring for neurocardiology. J Interven Cardiol 11:197, 1998
61. Steiger HJ: Monitoring for carotid surgery. *In* Newell DW, Aaslid R (eds): Transcranial Doppler. New York, Raven Press, 1992, p 197
62. Gundamraj RN, Lauer KK: Diagnosis of intracranial arterial stenosis using transcranial Doppler flowmetry. Anesth Analg 98:1776, 2004
63. Blaber A, Bondar RL, Stein F, et al: Transfer function analysis of cerebral autoregulation dynamics in autonomic failure patients. Stroke 28:1686, 1997
64. Borger MA, Taylor RL, Weisel RD, et al: Decreased cerebral emboli during distal aortic arch cannulation: A randomized clinical trial. J Thorac Cardiovasc Surg 118:740, 1999
65. Mullges W, Franke D, Reents W, et al: Brain microembolic counts during extracorporeal circulation depend on aortic cannula position. Ultrasound Med Biol 27:933, 2001
66. Rodriguez RA, Cornel G, Semelhago L, et al: Cerebral effects in superior vena caval cannula obstruction: The role of brain monitoring. Ann Thorac Surg 64:1820, 1997
67. Ganzel BL, Edmonds HL Jr, Pank JR, et al: Neurophysiological monitoring to assure delivery of retrograde cerebral perfusion. J Thorac Cardiovasc Surg 113:748, 1997
68. Gugino LD, Aglio LS, Edmonds HL Jr: Neurophysiological monitoring in vascular surgery. Bailliere's Clin Anaesth 2000;14:17–62
69. Jones TJ, Deal DD, Vernon JC, et al: How effective are cardiopulmonary bypass circuits at removing gaseous microemboli? J Extra Corpor Technol 34:151, 2002
70. Yeh TJ Jr, Austin EH III, Sehic A, et al: Role of neuromonitoring in the detection and correction of cerebral air embolism. J Thorac Cardiovasc Surg 126:589, 2003
71. Edmonds HL Jr: Emboli and renal dysfunction in CABG patients (editorial). J Cardiothorac Vasc Anesth 18: 545-547, 2004.
72. Shen Q, Stuart J, Venkatesh B, et al: Interobserver variability of the transcranial Doppler ultrasound technique. Impact of lack of practice on the accuracy of measurement. J Clin Monit Comput 15:179, 1999
73. Mutch WAC, Ryner LN, Kozlowski P, et al: Cerebral hypoxia during cardiopulmonary bypass: A magnetic resonance imaging study. Ann Thorac Surg 64:695, 1997
74. de Vries JW, Visser GH, Bakker PFA: Neuromonitoring in defibrillation threshold testing. A comparison between near-infrared spectroscopy and jugular bulb oximetry. J Clin Monit 13:303, 1997
75. Watzman HM, Kurth CD, Montenegro LM, et al: Arterial and venous contributions to near-infrared cerebral oximetry. Anesthesiology 93:947, 2000
76. Kurth CD, Steven JM, Benaron D, et al: Near-infrared monitoring of the cerebral circulation. J Clin Monit 9:163, 1993
77. Stingele R, Schnippering H, Keller E, et al: Transcranial oximetry using fast near-infrared spectroscopy can detect failure of collateral blood supply in humans. Comp Biochem Physiol (Part A) 134:534, 2003
78. Chelette TL, Albery WB, Esken RL, et al: Female exposure to high G: Performance of simulated flight after 24 hours of sleep deprivation. Aviat Space Environ Med 69:862, 1998
79. Roberts KW, Crnkowic AP, Linneman LJ: Near-infrared spectroscopy detects critical cerebral hypoxia during carotid endarterectomy in awake patients. Anesthesiology 89(3A):A934, 1998

80. Hernandez-Avila G, Dujovny M, Slavin KV, et al: Use of transcranial cerebral oximetry to monitor regional cerebral oxygen saturation during neuroendovascular procedures. Amer J Neuroradiol 16:1618, 1995
81. Edmonds HL Jr, Sehic A, Pollock SB Jr, et al: Low cerebrovenous oxygen saturation predicts disorientation. Anesthesiology 89(3A):A941, 1998
82. Edmonds HL Jr, Yu Q-J, Ganzel BL: Cost of cerebral macroembolization and oxygen desaturation during myocardial revascularization. Stroke 29:2238, 1998
83. Edmonds HL Jr, Toney KA, Thomas MH, et al: Neuromonitoring cost-benefit for adult cardiac surgery. Anesthesiology 87(3A):A426, 1997
84. de Letter J, Sie HT, Moll F, et al: Transcranial cerebral oximetry during carotid endarterectomy: Agreement between frontal and lateral probe measurements as compared with an electroencephalogram. Cardiovasc Surg 6:373, 1998
85. Gopinath SP, Robertson CS, Grossman RG, et al: Near-infrared spectroscopic localization of intracranial hematomas. J Neurosurg 79:43, 1993
86. Sehic A, Thomas MH: Cerebral oximetry during carotid endarterectomy: Signal failure resulting from large frontal sinus defect. J Cardiothorac Vasc Anesth 13:444, 2000
87. Pigula FA, Siewers RD, Nemoto E: Hypothermic cardiopulmonary bypass alters oxygen/glucose uptake in the pediatric brain. J Thorac Cardiovasc Surg 121:366, 2001
88. Kim MB, Ward DS, Cartwright CR: Estimation of jugular venous O_2 saturation from cerebral oximetry or arterial O_2 saturation during isocapnic hypoxia. J Clin Monit 16:191, 2000
89. Daubeney PE, Pilkington SN, Janke E: Cerebral oxygenation measured by near-infrared spectroscopy: Comparison with jugular bulb oximetry. Ann Thorac Surg 61:930, 1996
90. Holzschuh M, Woertgen C, Metz C: Dynamic changes of cerebral oxygenation measured by brain tissue oxygen pressure and near-infrared spectroscopy. Neurol Res 19:246, 1997
91. Brawanski A, Faltermeier R, Rothoerl RD: Comparison of near-infrared spectroscopy and tissue PO_2 time series in patients after head injury and aneurysmal subarachnoid hemorrhage. J Cereb Blood Flow Metab 22:605, 2002
92. Kurth CD, Steven JM, Nicolson SC: Cerebral oxygenation during pediatric cardiac surgery using deep hypothermic circulatory arrest. Anesthesiology 82:74, 1995
93. Büchner K, Meixensberger J, Dings J: Near-infrared spectroscopy—not useful to monitor cerebral oxygenation after severe brain injury. Zentralbl Neurochir 61:69, 2000
94. Gagnon RE, Macnab AJ, Gagnon FA: Comparison of two spatially resolved NIRS oxygen indices. J Clin Monit 17:385, 2002
95. Dullenkopf A, Frey B, Baenziger O: Measurement of cerebral oxygenation in anaesthetized children using the INVOS 5100 cerebral oximeter. Pediatr Anaesth 13:384, 2003
96. Schwartz G, Litscher G, Kleinert R: Cerebral oximetry in dead subjects. J Neurosurg Anesthesiol 8:189, 1996
97. Dunham C, Sosnowski C, Porter J: Correlation of noninvasive cerebral oximetry with cerebral perfusion in the severe head injured patients: A pilot study. J Trauma 52:40, 2002
98. Maeda H, Fukita K, Oritani S: Evaluation of postmortem oximetry with references to the causes of death. Forens Sci Int 87:201, 1997
99. Kishi K, Kawaguchi M, Yoshitani K: Influence of patient variables and sensor location on regional cerebral oxygen saturation measured by INVOS 4100 near-infrared spectrometer. J Neurosurg Anesth 15:302, 2003
100. Misra M, Stark J, Dujovny M: Transcranial cerebral oximetry in random normal subjects. Neurol Res 20:137, 1998
101. Edmonds HL Jr, Ganzel BL, Austin EH 3rd: Cerebral oximetry for cardiac and vascular surgery. Semin Cardiothorac Vasc Anesth 8: 147-66, 2004.
102. Cho H, Nemoto E, Yonas H: Cerebral monitoring by means of oximetry and somatosensory evoked potentials during carotid endarterectomy. J Neurosurg 89:533, 1998
103. Roberts KW, Crnkowic AP, Linneman LJ: Near-infrared spectroscopy detects critical cerebral hypoxia during carotid endarterectomy in awake patients. Anesthesiology 89(3A):A934, 1998
104. Samra SK, Dy EA, Welch K: Evaluation of a cerebral oximeter as a monitor of cerebral ischemia during carotid endarterectomy. Anesthesiology 93:964, 2000
105. Singer I, Dawn B, Edmonds HL Jr: Syncope is predicted by neuromonitoring in patients with ICDs. PACE Pacing Clin Electrocardiol 21(pt II):216, 1998
106. Rodriguez-Nuñez A, Couceiro J, Alonso C: Cerebral oxygenation in children with syncope during head-upright tilt test. Pediatr Cardiol 18:406, 1997
107. Tripp LD, Chelette T, Savul S: Female exposure to high G: Effects of simulated combat sorties on cerebral and arterial O_2 saturation. Aviat Space Environ Med 69:869, 1998
108. Monk TG, Reno KA, Olsen BS, et al: Postoperative cognitive dysfunction is associated with cerebral oxygen desaturations. Anesthesiology 93:A167, 2000
109. BhaskerRao B, VanHimbergen D, Jaber S, et al: Evidence for improved cerebral function after minimally invasive bypass surgery. J Cardiac Surg 13:27, 1998
110. Yao FSF, Tseng CC, Trifiletti RR, et al: Low preoperative cerebral oxygen saturation is associated with postoperative frontal lobe and cognitive dysfunction and prolonged ICU and hospital stays. Anesth Analg 90:SCA30, 2000
111. Edmonds HL Jr, Austin EH III, Seremet V, et al: Cost-benefit analysis of neuromonitoring for pediatric cardiac surgery. Anesth Analg 84:SCA22, 1997
112. Hadolt I, Litscher G: Noninvasive assessment of cerebral oxygenation during high altitude trekking in the Nepal Himalayas (2850-5600 m). Neurol Res 25:183, 2003
113. Madsen PL, Nielsen HB, Christiansen P: Well-being and cerebral oxygen saturation during acute heart failure in humans. Clin Physiol 20:158, 2000
114. Konishi A, Kikuchi K: Significance of regional cerebral oxygen saturation (rSO_2) during open heart surgery. J Clin Anesth Jpn 19:1759, 1995
115. Nemoto E, Yonas H, Kassam A: Clinical experience with cerebral oximetry in stroke and cardiac arrest. Crit Care Med 28:1052, 2000
116. Sehic A, Thomas MH: Cerebral oximetry during carotid endarterectomy: Signal failure resulting from large frontal sinus defect. J Cardiothorac Vasc Anesth 13:244, 2000
117. Bar-Yosef S, Sanders EG, Grocott HP: Asymmetric cerebral near-infrared oximetric measurements during cardiac surgery. J Cardiothorac Vasc Anesth 17:773, 2003
118. Boldrey E, Maass L, Miller ER: Role of atlantoid compression in etiology of internal carotid thrombosis. J Neurosurg 13:127, 1956
119. Hardesty WH, Roberts S, Toole JF: Studies of carotid artery blood flow in man. N Engl J Med 263:944, 1960
120. Fuchs G, Schwarz G, Kulier A: The influence of positioning on spectroscopic measurements of brain oxygenation. J Neurosurg Anesthesiol 12:75, 2000
121. Daubeney PEF, Smith DC, Pilkington SN: Cerebral oxygenation during paediatric cardiac surgery: Identification of vulnerable periods using near-infrared spectroscopy. Eur J Cardiothorac Surg 13:370, 1998
122. Fukada J, Morishita K, Kawaharada N: Isolated cerebral perfusion for intraoperative cerebral malperfusion in type A aortic dissection. Ann Thorac Surg 75:266, 2003
123. Borst HC, Laas J, Heinemann M: Type A aortic dissection: Diagnosis and management of malperfusion phenomena. Semin Thorac Cardiovasc Surg 3:238, 1991
124. DuPlessis AJ: Near-infrared spectroscopy for the in vivo study of cerebral hemodynamics and oxygenation. Curr Opin Pediatr 7:632-639, 1995
125. Liu R, Sun D, Hang Y, et al: Evaluation of cerebral oxygen balance by cerebral oximeter and transcranial Doppler during hypothermic cardiopulmonary bypass. Anesthesiology 89:A309, 1998
126. Kontos H: Regulation of cerebral circulation. Annu Rev Physiol 43: 397, 1989
127. Akça O, Liem E, Suleman M-I: Effect of intraoperative end-tidal carbon dioxide partial pressure on tissue oxygenation. Anaesthesia 58:536, 2003
128. Du Plessis AJ, Jonas RA, Wypij D: Perioperative effects of alpha-stat versus pH-stat strategies for deep hypothermic cardiopulmonary bypass in infants. J Thorac Cardiovasc Surg 114:991, 1997
129. Vijay V, McCusker K, Stasko A, et al: Cerebral oximetry-directed permissive hypercapnia enhances cerebral perfusion during CPB for heart failure surgery. Heart Surg Forum 6:205, 2003
130. Gosain A, Rabin J, Reymond JP: Tissue oxygen tension and other indicators of blood loss or organ perfusion during graded hemorrhage. Surgery 109:523, 1991
131. Arkilic CF, Akça O, Taguchi M: Temperature monitoring and management during neuraxial anesthesia: An observational study. Anesth Analg 91:662, 2000
132. Madl C, Eisenhuber E, Kramer L, et al: Impact of different hemoglobin levels on regional cerebral oxygen saturation, cerebral extraction of oxygen and sensory evoked potentials in septic shock. Crit Care Med 25(suppl):4, 1997
133. Blas M, Sulek C, Martin T: Use of near-infrared spectroscopy to monitor cerebral oxygenation during coronary artery bypass surgery in a patient with bilateral internal carotid artery occlusion. J Cardiothorac Vasc Anesth 6:732, 1999

134. Vijay V, McCusker K, Stasko A, et al: Cerebral oximetry-based comparison of cerebral perfusion with standard versus condensed extracorporeal circuits in adult cardiac surgery. Heart Surg Forum 6:201, 2003
135. Torella F, Haynes SL, McCollum CN: Cerebral and peripheral oxygen saturation during red cell transfusion. J Surg Res 110:217, 2003
136. Villafane J, Edmonds HL Jr: Volume expansion prevents tilt-induced syncope. Cardiol Young 11(suppl 1):1168, 2001
137. Jalowiecki P, Plóro A, Dzlurdzlk P: Regional cerebral oxygenation monitoring in children undergoing elective scoliosis surgery with controlled urapidil-induced hypotension. Med Sci Monit 4:987, 1998
138. Edmonds HL Jr, Thomas MH, Ganzel BL, et al: Effect of volatile anesthetics on cerebral autoregulation during cardiopulmonary bypass (abstract). Anesthesiology 95:A306, 2001
139. Plattner O, Semsroth M, Sessler DI: Lack of nonshivering thermogenesis in infants anesthetized with fentanyl and propofol. Anesthesiology 86:772, 1997
140. Kern FH, Jonas RA, Mayer JE: Temperature monitoring during CPB in infants: Does it predict efficient brain cooling? Ann Thorac Surg 54:749, 1992
141. Wardle SP, Yoxall CW, Weindling AM: Cerebral oxygenation during cardiopulmonary bypass. Arch Dis Child 78:26, 1998
142. Greeley WJ, Kern FH, Mault JR: Mechanisms of injury and methods of protection of the brain during cardiac surgery in neonates and infants. Cardiol Young 3:317, 1993
143. de Vries JW, Hoorntje T, Bakker PFA: Cerebral oxygen saturation monitoring in an infant undergoing ICD implantation. J Cardiothorac Vasc Anesth 12:442, 1998
144. Ausman JI, McCormick PW, Stewart M: Cerebral oxygen metabolism during hypothermic arrest in humans. J Neurosurg 77:656, 1993
145. Dullenkopf A, Frey B, Baenziger O: Measurement of cerebral oxygenation in anaesthetized children using the INVOS 5100 cerebral oximeter. Pediatr Anaesth 13:384, 2003
146. Manecke GR, Nieman JD, Phillips P: Deep hypothermia alters the vascular response to thiopental (abstract). Anesthesiology 96(3A):A169, 2002
147. Jones TH, Morawetz RB, Crowell RM: Threshold of focal cerebral ischemia in awake monkeys. J Neurosurg 54:773, 1981
148. Deeb GM, Jenkins E, Bolling SF: Retrograde cerebral perfusion during hypothermic circulatory arrest reduces neurologic morbidity. J Thorac Cardiovasc Surg 109:259, 1995
149. Higami T, Kozawa S, Asada T: Retrograde cerebral perfusion versus selective cerebral perfusion as evaluated by cerebral oxygen saturation during aortic arch reconstruction. Ann Thorac Surg 67:1091, 1999
150. Pigula FA, Nemoto EM, Griffith BP: Regional low-flow perfusion provides cerebral circulatory support during neonatal aortic arch reconstruction. J Thorac Cardiovasc Surg 199:331, 2000
151. Hofer AA, Haizinger B, Geiselseder G: Near-infrared spectroscopy to monitor cerebral oxygenation during antegrade cerebral perfusion in neonates undergoing cardiosurgical repair (abstract). Anesthesiology 96:A1284, 2002
152. Akça O, Melischek M, Scheck T: Postoperative pain and subcutaneous oxygen tension. Lancet 354:41, 1999
153. Myles PS, Leslie K, McNeil J, et al: Bispectral index monitoring to prevent awareness during anesthesia: The B-Aware randomized controlled trial. Lancet 363:1757, 2004
154. Ekman A, Lindholm M-L, Lenmarken C, et al: Reduction in the incidence of awareness using BIS monitoring. Acta Anaesthesiol Scand 48:20, 2004
155. Spencer MP: Transcranial Doppler monitoring and causes of stroke from carotid endarterectomy. Stroke 28:685, 1997
156. Lennard N, Smith J, Dumville J, et al: Prevention of postoperative thrombotic stroke after carotid endarterectomy: The role of transcranial Doppler ultrasound. J Vasc Surg 26:579, 1997
157. Blue Shield of Washington State. Provisions 3:13, 1999
158. Edmonds HL Jr: Multi-modality neurophysiologic monitoring for cardiac surgery. Heart Surg Forum 5:225, 2002
159. Laschinger J, Razumovsky AY, Stierer KA, et al: Cardiac surgery: Value of neuromonitoring. Heart Surg Forum 6:204, 2003
160. Lozano S, Mossad E: Cerebral function monitors during pediatric cardiac surgery: Can they make a difference? J Cardiothorac Vasc Anesth 18:645, 2004

Chapter 18
COAGULATION MONITORING

Linda Shore-Lesserson, MD

KEY POINTS

1. Monitoring the effect of heparin is done using an activated coagulation time (ACT), a functional test of heparin anticoagulation. The ACT is susceptible to elevation due to hypothermia, hemodilution, and the use of aprotinin (celite ACT).
2. Heparin resistance can be congenital or acquired. Pretreatment heparin exposure predisposes a patient to altered heparin responsiveness due to either antithrombin III (ATIII) depletion, platelet activation, or activation of extrinsic coagulation.
3. Heparin-induced thrombocytopenia type I is benign and is a normal aggregation response of platelets to heparin. Heparin-induced thrombocytopenia type II is an abnormal immunologic response to the heparin/platelet factor 4 complex and is sometimes associated with overt thrombosis.
4. Protamine neutralization of heparin can be associated with "protamine reactions," which include vasodilatory hypotension, anaphylactoid reactions, and pulmonary hypertensive crises (types 1, 2, and 3).
5. Before considering a transfusion of plasma, it is important to document that the effect of heparin has been neutralized. This can be done using a heparinase-neutralized test or a protamine-neutralized test.
6. Point-of-care tests are available for use in transfusion algorithms that can measure coagulation factor activity (international normalized ratio, activated partial thromboplastin time) and platelet function.
7. Fibrinolysis is common after cardiopulmonary bypass when antifibrinolytic therapy is not used.
8. New thrombin inhibitor drugs are available for anticoagulation in patients who cannot receive heparin. These can be monitored using the ecarin clotting time or a modified ACT. Bivalirudin and hirudin are the two new drugs that have been used most often in cardiac surgery.
9. Platelet dysfunction is the most common reason for bleeding after cardiopulmonary bypass. There are point-of-care tests that can be used to measure specific aspects of platelet function.
10. The degree of platelet inhibition as measured by standard or point-of-care instruments has been shown to correlate with decreased ischemic outcomes after coronary intervention. However, cardiac surgical patients who are receiving antiplatelet medication are at increased risk for postoperative bleeding.

Cardiac surgery is an area in which coagulation monitoring has vital applications. Cardiopulmonary bypass (CPB) procedures could not be performed without an effective method of preventing blood from clotting in the extracorporeal circuit. In the early part of the twentieth century, heparin was discovered to have anticoagulant properties; it remains the anticoagulant most commonly used during CPB. Reversal of heparin effect is most frequently performed using protamine, although a number of different pharmacologic agents and reversal techniques can be used.

CPB itself induces a "whole-body inflammatory response" due to contact of blood and cellular elements with the extracorporeal circuit. The resultant alterations include leukocyte activation, release of inflammatory mediators, free radical formation, complement activation, kallikrein release, platelet activation, and stimulation of the coagulation and fibrinolytic cascades. This complex interplay of systems induces a coagulopathy characterized by microvascular coagulation, platelet dysfunction, and enhanced fibrinolysis.[1,2] The homeostatic perturbations incurred during CPB are a major etiology for the postbypass coagulopathy that is seen even after the effects of heparin are reversed with protamine.

The need to monitor anticoagulation during and after surgery is the reason that the cardiac surgical arena has evolved into a major site for the evaluation and use of hemostasis monitors. The rapid and accurate identification of abnormal hemostasis has been the major impetus toward the development of point-of-care tests that can be performed at the bedside or in the operating room. The detection and treatment of specific coagulation disorders in a timely and cost-efficient manner are major goals in hemostasis monitoring for the cardiac surgical patient. This chapter discusses the mechanisms of normal coagulation and how they are affected by CPB. The latter portion discusses the laboratory and point-of-care tests available for monitoring the coagulation system. A comprehensive overview of hemostasis, transfusion medicine, and the management of coagulopathy and bleeding disorders after CPB is provided in Chapter 29.

HEMOSTASIS

Hemostasis is the body's normal response to vascular injury and involves a complex interplay of systems within the body that helps to seal the endovascular defect and prevent exsanguination. The three major components of hemostasis include the vascular endothelium; the platelets, which constitute primary hemostasis; and the coagulation cascade glycoproteins, which constitute secondary hemostasis. Fibrinolysis is the normal physiologic response to clot formation, which ensures that coagulation remains localized to the area of vascular injury.

Anticoagulation for Cardiopulmonary Bypass

The safe conduct of CPB could not be accomplished without anticoagulation of blood in preparation for its contact with the extracorporeal circuit. An ideal anticoagulant should be easy to administer, rapid in onset, titratable, predictable, measurable in a timely fashion, and reversible. Heparin use during CPB has continued until the present time, most likely due to its rapid onset, ease of measurement, and ease of reversibility. Decades of the use of heparin are either a testimonial to its effectiveness or demonstrative of the inability to find a more suitable alternative.

Heparin acts as an antithrombin III (ATIII) agonist and accelerates ATIII binding to thrombin.[3-5] In the absence of ATIII, heparin is clinically ineffective as an anticoagulant; adequate ATIII activity is necessary in patients about to undergo heparinization for cardiac surgical procedures.[6-9]

MONITORING HEPARIN EFFECT

Cardiac surgery had been performed for decades using empiric heparin dosing in the form of a bolus and subsequent interval dosing. Empiric dosing continued due to the lack of an easily applicable bedside test to monitor the anticoagulant effects of heparin. Many assays are available to measure the response to the heparin dose given to institute extracorporeal circulation. These tests are in the form of functional tests of anticoagulation or quantitative measures of the level of circulating heparin. The anticoagulant effect of heparin can be monitored using a variety of different techniques.

The first clotting time to be used to measure heparin's effect was the whole-blood clotting time (WBCT), or the Lee-White WBCT. This simply requires whole blood to be placed in a glass tube, maintained at 37°C, and manually tilted until blood fluidity is no longer detected. This test fell out of favor for monitoring the cardiac surgical patient because it was so labor intensive and required the undivided attention of the person performing the test for periods up to 30 minutes. Although the glass surface of the test tube acts as an activator of factor XII, the heparin doses used for cardiac surgery prolong the WBCT to such a profound degree that the test is impractical as a monitor of the effect of heparin during cardiac surgery.[10] To speed the clotting time so that the test was appropriate for clinical use, activators were added to the test tubes, and the activated coagulation time (ACT) was introduced into practice.[11]

Activated Coagulation Time

The ACT was first introduced by Hattersley in 1966 and is still the most widely used monitor of heparin effect during cardiac surgery. Whole blood is added to a test tube containing an activator—diatomaceous earth (celite) or kaolin. The presence of activator augments the contact activation phase of coagulation, which stimulates the intrinsic coagulation pathway. ACT can be performed manually, whereby the operator measures the time interval from when blood is injected into the test tube to when clot is seen along the sides of the tube. More commonly, the ACT is automated as it is in the Hemochron and Hemotec systems. In the automated system, the test tube is placed in a device that warms the sample to 37°C. The Hemochron device (International Technidyne Corp., Edison, NJ) rotates the test tube, which contains celite activator and a small iron cylinder, to which 2 mL of whole blood is added. Before clot forms, the cylinder rolls along the bottom of the rotating test tube. When clot forms, the cylinder is pulled away from a magnetic detector, interrupts a magnetic field, and signals the end of the clotting time. Normal ACT values range from 80 to 120 seconds. The Hemochron

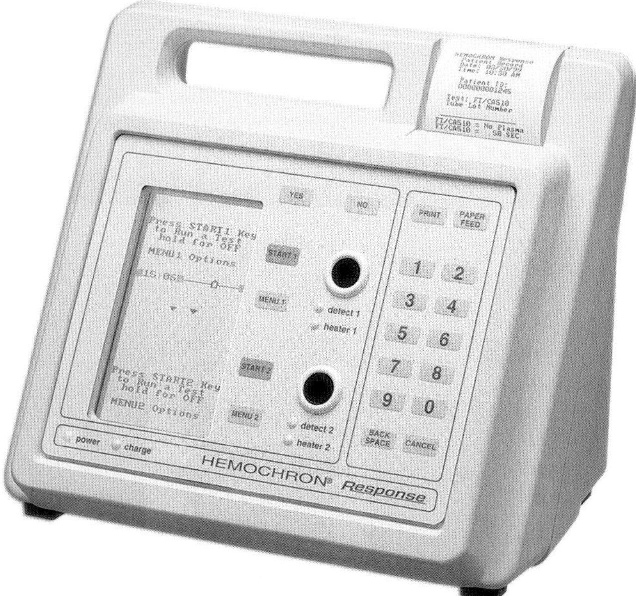

Figure 18–1 The Hemochron Response is a dual chamber point-of-care coagulation monitor that is capable of measuring clotting times that are compatible with Hemochron technology. This system has software capability for calculation, data management, and storage of results. (Courtesy of International Technidyne Corp., Edison, NJ, http://www.itcmed.com)

ACT can also be performed using kaolin as the activator in a similar manner (Fig. 18–1).

The Hemotec ACT device (Medtronic Hemotec, Parker, CO) is a cartridge with two chambers that contain kaolin activator and is housed in a heat block. Blood (0.4 mL) is placed into each chamber and a daisy-shaped plunger is raised and passively falls into the chamber. The formation of clot will slow the rate of descent of the plunger, and this decrease in velocity of the plunger is detected by a photo-optical system that signals the end of the ACT test. The Hemochron and Hemotec ACTs have been compared in a number of investigations and have been found to differ significantly at low heparin concentrations.[12] However, differences in heparin concentration, activator concentration, and the measurement technique make comparison of these tests difficult and have led to the realization that the Hemochron ACT result and the Hemotec ACT result are not interchangeable. In adult patients given 300 U/kg of heparin for CPB, the Hemochron and Hemotec (Hepcon) ACTs were both therapeutic at all time points; however, at two points, the Hemochron ACT was statistically longer[13] (Fig. 18–2). This difference was even more pronounced in pediatric patients, who have higher heparin consumption rates (Fig. 18–3). The apparent "overestimation" of ACT by the Hemochron device during hypothermic CPB may be due to the different volumes of blood that each assay warms to 37°C.

The ACT test can be modified by the addition of heparinase. Using this modification, the coagulation status of the patient can be monitored during CPB while the anticoagulant effects of heparin are eliminated. Because this test is a side-by-side comparison of the untreated ACT to the heparinase ACT, it also has the advantage of being a rapid test for the assessment of a circulating heparin-like substance or for residual heparinization after CPB.[14]

With the introduction of ACT monitoring into the cardiac surgical arena, clinicians have been able to more accurately titrate heparin and protamine dosages.[11,15] As a result, many investigators report reductions in blood loss and transfusion

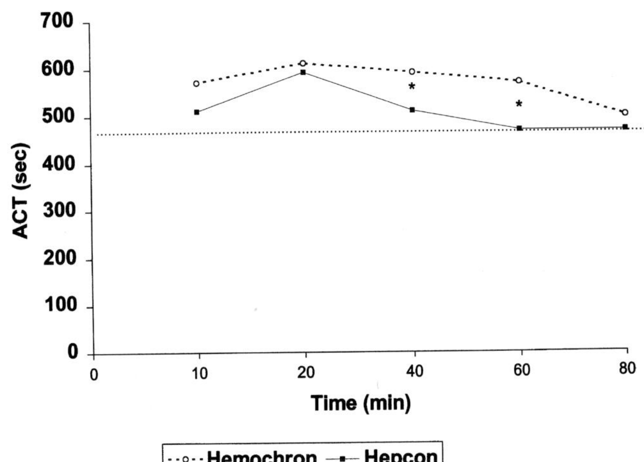

Figure 18–2 The Hemochron and Hemotec (Hepcon) activated coagulation time (ACT) values in 20 adults at five time points during cardiopulmonary bypass (CPB). At 40 and 80 minutes on CPB, the Hemochron ACT was significantly higher. *$P < 0.01$. (Copyright 1992, with permission from the Society of Thoracic Surgeons [The Annals of Thoracic Surgery 53:822–826, 1992].)

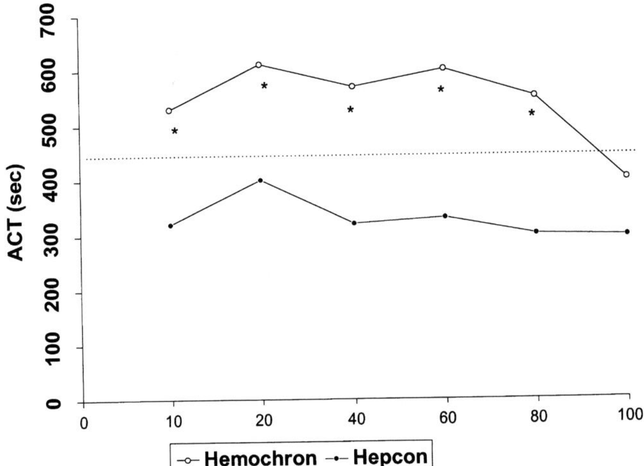

Figure 18–3 The Hemochron and Hemotec (Hepcon) activated coagulation time (ACT) values in 22 pediatric patients at six time points during cardiopulmonary bypass (CPB). Hemochron ACT was significantly higher than Hemotec ACT at five time points. *$P < 0.01$. (Copyright 1992, with permission from the Society of Thoracic Surgeons [The Annals of Thoracic Surgery 53:822–826, 1992].)

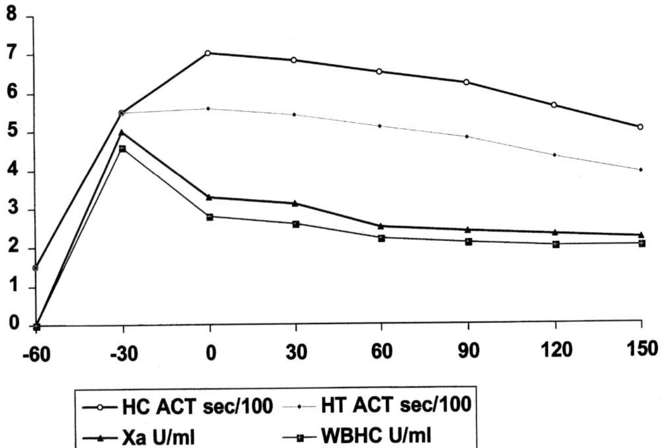

Figure 18–4 Anticoagulation measured at baseline (–60 minutes), heparinization (–30 minutes), and six time points after institution of cardiopulmonary bypass (CPB). Note the close correlation between the anti–factor Xa (Xa) activity and whole blood heparin concentration (WBHC), which does not parallel the change in Hemochron (HC ACT) or Hemotec activated coagulation time (HT ACT). (Modified from Despotis GJ, Summerfield AL, Joist JH: Comparison of activated coagulation time and whole blood heparin measurements with laboratory plasma anti-Xa heparin concentration in patients having cardiac operations. J Thorac Cardiovasc Surg 108:1076–1082, 1994.)

requirements, though many of these studies used retrospective analyses.[16] The improvements in postoperative hemostasis documented with ACT monitoring are potentially attributed to better intraoperative suppression of microvascular coagulation and improved monitoring of heparin reversal with protamine.[17]

ACT monitoring of heparinization is not without pitfalls, and its use has been criticized because of the extreme variability of the ACT and the absence of a correlation with plasma heparin levels (Fig. 18–4). Many factors have been suggested to alter the ACT, and these factors are prevalent during cardiac surgical procedures. When the extracorporeal circuit prime is added to the patient's blood volume, hemodilution occurs and may theoretically increase ACT. Evidence suggests that this degree of hemodilution alone is not enough to actually alter ACT. Hypothermia increases ACT in a "dose-related" fashion. It has been shown by Culliford et al[18] that although hemodilution and hypothermia significantly increase the ACT of a heparinized blood sample, similar increases do not occur in the absence of added heparin. The effects of platelet alterations are a bit more problematic. At mild-to-moderate degrees of thrombocytopenia, the baseline and heparinized ACT are not affected. It is not until platelet counts are reduced to below 30,000 to 50,000/μL that ACT may be prolonged.[19] Patients treated with platelet inhibitors such as prostacyclin, aspirin, or platelet membrane receptor antagonists have a prolonged heparinized ACT compared with patients not treated with platelet inhibitors.[20] This ACT prolongation is not exclusively related to decreased levels of platelet factor 4 (PF4) (PF4 is a heparin-neutralizing substance), because it also occurs when blood is anticoagulated with substances that are not neutralized by PF4. Platelet lysis, however, significantly shortens the ACT due to the release of PF4, and other platelet membrane components, which may have heparin-neutralizing activities.[21] Gravlee et al[22] showed that anesthesia and surgery decrease the ACT and create a hypercoagulable state, possibly by creating a thromboplastic response or through activation of platelets.

During CPB, heparin decay varies substantially and its measurement is problematic because hemodilution and hypothermia alter the metabolism of heparin. In a CPB study, Mabry et al[23] found that the consumption of heparin varied from 0.01 to 3.86 U/kg/min and that there was no correlation between the initial sensitivity to heparin and the rate of heparin decay.[23] In the pediatric population, the consumption of heparin is increased above that of adult levels. The heparin administration protocol for pediatric patients undergoing CPB should account for a large volume of distribution, increased consumption, and a shorter elimination half-life. In monitoring the effects of heparin in pediatric patients, the minimum acceptable ACT value should be increased or an additional monitor should be used. The discrepancy between the Hemochron ACT and the Hemotec ACT that is demonstrated in Figure 18–2 is even more pronounced in pediatric patients (see Fig. 18–3). Some investigators recommend the maintenance of heparin concentrations in addition to ACT during pediatric congenital heart surgery to ensure that optimal anticoagulation is being achieved.[24,25]

Heparin Resistance

Heparin resistance is documented by an inability to raise the ACT of blood to expected levels despite an adequate dose and plasma concentration of heparin. In many clinical situations, especially when heparin desensitization or a heparin inhibitor is suspected, heparin resistance can be treated by administering increased doses of heparin in a competitive fashion. If an adequately prolonged clotting time is ultimately achieved using higher-than-expected doses of heparin, a better term than *heparin resistance* would be *heparin tachyphylaxis* of "altered heparin responsiveness." During cardiac surgical procedures, the belief that a safe minimum ACT value of 300 to 400 seconds is required for CPB is based on a few clinical studies and a relative paucity of scientific data. However, inability to attain this degree of anticoagulation in the heparin-resistant patient engenders the fear among cardiac surgical providers that the patient will experience a microvascular consumptive coagulopathy or that clots will form in the extracorporeal circuit. This potential for fibrin formation in the extracorporeal circuit was reported by Young et al,[26] who found increased production of fibrin monomer and consumption of fibrinogen and platelets in six of nine rhesus monkeys when the ACT fell below 400 seconds. However, Metz and Keats[27] reported no adverse effects of thrombosis or excessive bleeding in 51 patients undergoing CPB whose ACT was less than 400 seconds. In a porcine model, the group whose ACT was maintained between 250 and 300 seconds did not have excessive consumption of coagulation factors, increases in fibrin monomer formation, or changes in oxygenator performance compared with the group whose ACT was maintained at greater than 450 seconds.[28]

Many clinical conditions are associated with heparin resistance.[29] Sepsis, liver disease, and pharmacologic agents represent just a few[30,31] (Table 18–1). Many investigators have documented decreased levels of ATIII secondary to heparin pretreatment,[32] whereas others have not found decreased ATIII levels.[33] Esposito et al[34] measured coagulation factor levels in patients receiving preoperative heparin infusions and found that a lower baseline ACT was the only risk factor for predicting heparin resistance compared with patients not receiving preoperative heparin.

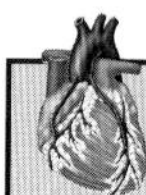

BOX 18–1 *Heparin Resistance*

- It is primarily due to ATIII deficiency in pediatric patients.
- It is multifactorial in adult cardiac surgical patients.
- The critical ACT value necessary in patients who demonstrate acquired heparin resistance is not yet determined.
- Heparin resistance can also be a sign of heparin-induced thrombocytopenia.

Patients receiving preoperative heparin therapy traditionally require larger heparin doses to achieve a given level of anticoagulation when that anticoagulation is measured by the ACT. Presumably, this "heparin resistance" is due to deficiencies in the level or activity of ATIII.[31,34-37] Other possible etiologies include enhanced factor VIII activity and platelet dysfunction causing a decrease in ACT response to heparin. Levy et al[37] have shown that the in vitro addition of ATIII enhances the ACT response to heparin. Lemmer and Despotis[36] demonstrated that this heparin resistance, as measured by the ACT, does not correlate with preoperative ATIII levels. It is unclear that these patients have increased heparin requirements during CPB because the ideal ACT and monitoring techniques have yet to be elucidated. Nicolson et al[38] demonstrated that the temporal courses of ACT and ATIII concentration do not parallel each other, further suggesting that ATIII depletion is not the sole cause of heparin resistance during CPB. Lower ACTs were tolerated in this study with no adverse outcome. ATIII concentrate is now available and represents a reasonable method of treating patients with documented ATIII deficiency (Box 18–1).

Heparin-Induced Thrombocytopenia

The syndrome known as heparin-induced thrombocytopenia (HIT) develops in anywhere from 5% to 28% of patients

Table 18-1 Disease States Associated With Heparin Resistance

Disease State	Comment
Newborn	Decreased ATIII levels until 6 months of age
Venous thromboembolism	May have increased factor VIII level Accelerated clearance of heparin
Pulmonary embolism	Accelerated clearance of heparin
Congenital ATIII deficiency	
Type I	40% to 60% of normal ATIII concentration Reduced synthesis of normal/abnormal ATIII
Type II	Molecular defect within the ATIII molecule
Acquired ATIII deficiency:	<25% of normal ATIII concentration
Preeclampsia	Levels unchanged in normal pregnancy
Cirrhosis	Decreased protein synthesis
Nephrotic syndrome	Increased urinary excretion of ATIII
DIC	Increased consumption of ATIII
Heparin pretreatment	85% of normal ATIII concentration due to accelerated clearance
Estrogen therapy	
Cytotoxic drug therapy (L-asparaginase)	Decreased protein synthesis

ATIII = antithrombin III; DIC = disseminated intravascular coagulation.

receiving heparin. HIT is commonly categorized into two subtypes. HIT type I is characterized by a mild decrease in platelet count and is the result of the proaggregatory effects of heparin on platelets. HIT type II is considerably more severe, most often occurs after more than 5 days of heparin administration (average onset time, 9 days), and is mediated by antibody binding to the complex formed between heparin and PF4. Associated immune-mediated endothelial injury and complement activation cause platelets to adhere, aggregate, and form platelet clots, or "white clots." Among patients developing HIT II, the incidence of thrombotic complications approximates 20%, which in turn may carry a mortality rate as high as 40%. Demonstration of heparin-induced proaggregation of platelets confirms the diagnosis of HIT type II. This can be accomplished with a heparin-induced serotonin release assay or a specific heparin-induced platelet activation assay. A highly specific enzyme-linked immunosorbent assay for the heparin/PF4 complex has been developed and has been used to delineate the course of IgG and IgM antibody responses in patients exposed to unfractionated heparin during cardiac surgery. Bedside antibody tests are being developed that may speed the diagnosis of this condition.

The risks and appropriate courses of action in patients with HIT II are unclear because the antibodies associated with HIT often become undetectable several weeks after discontinuing heparin. Also, the clinical syndrome does not always recur upon reexposure to the drug and sometimes resolves despite continued drug therapy. Many patients never develop thrombosis and disseminated intravascular coagulation despite positive laboratory testing. HIT should possibly be considered in the differential diagnosis of intraoperative heparin resistance in patients receiving preoperative heparin therapy.

The options for treating these patients are few. If the clinician has the luxury of being able to discontinue the heparin for a few weeks, often the antibody disappears and allows a brief period of heparinization for CPB without complication.[39,40] Changing the tissue source of heparin was an option when bovine heparin was predominantly in use. Some types of low-molecular-weight heparin (LMWH) have been administered to patients with HIT, but reactivity of the particular LMWH with the patient's platelets should be confirmed in vitro. Supplementing heparin administration with pharmacologic platelet inhibition using prostacyclin, iloprost, aspirin, or aspirin and dipyridamole has been reported, all with favorable outcomes. The use of tirofiban with unfractionated heparin has been used in this clinical circumstance. Plasmapheresis may be used to reduce antibody levels. The use of heparin could be avoided altogether through anticoagulation with direct thrombin inhibitors such as argatroban, hirudin, or bivalirudin. These thrombin inhibitors have become standard of care in the management of the patient with HIT II (Box 18–2). Monitoring their effects during CPB is more complex and is discussed later in this chapter.

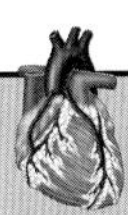

BOX 18–2 *Heparin-Induced Thrombocytopenia*

- The immunologic form is mediated by an antibody to the heparin-platelet factor 4 complex.
- This disease has variable penetrance even in the same individual.
- There is an associated 30% risk of thrombosis.
- Thrombosis carries a 50% mortality rate.

Measurement of Heparin Sensitivity

Even in the absence of heparin resistance, patient response to an intravenous bolus of heparin is extremely variable.[41] The variability stems from different concentrations of various endogenous heparin-binding proteins such as vitronectin and PF4. This variability exists whether measuring heparin concentration or the ACT; however, variability seems to be greater when measuring the ACT. Because of the large interpatient variation in heparin responsiveness and the potential for heparin resistance, it is critical that a functional monitor of heparin anticoagulation (with or without a measure of heparin concentration) be used in the cardiac surgical patient. Bull et al[42] documented a threefold range of ACT response to a 200-U/kg heparin dose and similar discrepancy in heparin decay rates and thus recommended the use of individual patient dose-response curves to determine the optimal heparin dose. This is the concept on which point-of-care individual heparin dose-response (HDR) tests are based.

An HDR curve can be generated manually using the baseline ACT and the ACT response to an in vivo or in vitro dose of heparin. Extrapolation to the desired ACT provides the additional heparin dose required for that ACT. Once the actual ACT response to the heparin dose is plotted, further dose-response calculations are made based on the average of the target ACT and the actual ACT (Fig. 18–5). This methodology was first described by Bull et al[42] and forms the scientific basis for the automated dose-response systems manufactured by Hemochron and Hemotec. The Hemochron RxDx system uses the heparin-response test (HRT), which is an ACT with a known quantity of in vitro heparin (3 IU/mL). Using an algorithm that incorporates the patient's baseline ACT, estimated blood volume, and HRT, a dose-response curve is generated that enables calculation of the heparin dose required to attain the target ACT. The patient's heparin sensitivity can be calculated in seconds/IU/mL by dividing the HRT by 3 IU/mL.

The RxDx system also provides an individualized protamine dose using the PRT (protamine response test). This is an ACT with one of two specific quantities of protamine, depending on the amount of circulating heparin suspected (2 IU/mL or 3 IU/mL). Using the patient's heparinized ACT, the PRT, and an estimate of the patient's blood volume, the protamine dose needed to return the ACT to baseline can be calculated based on a protamine-response curve. Jobes et al[43] reported that the heparin dose directed by the RxDx system resulted in ACT values well above the target ACT. In their patients, in vivo heparin sensitivity was higher than in vitro sensitivity. RxDx also resulted in lower protamine doses, lower postoperative mediastinal tube losses, and reduced transfusion requirements compared with a ratio-based system of heparin/protamine administration. In a larger study that standardized the treatment of heparin rebound, the reduced protamine dose was confirmed; however, the reductions in bleeding were not substantiated.[44] The use of a protamine dose-response curve has been shown to successfully reduce the protamine dose in vascular surgery compared with standard weight-based protamine dosing.[45]

The Hepcon HMS system uses the HDR cartridge in the Hepcon instrument (Fig. 18–6). Each cartridge houses six chambers. Chambers 1 and 2 contain heparin at a concentration of 2.5 U/mL, chambers 3 and 4 contain heparin at a concentration of 1.5 U/mL, and chambers 5 and 6 do not contain heparin. Once information regarding patient weight, height, and CPB prime volume is entered, the information that can

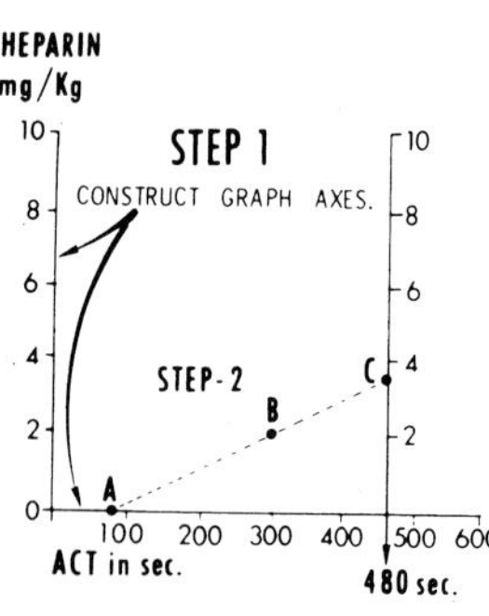

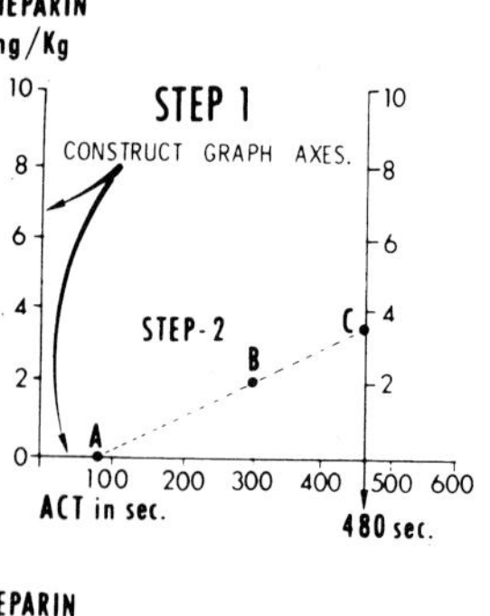

STEP 2

DETERMINE INITIAL ACT (A) AND ADMINISTER 2 mg/kg HEPARIN, THEN

MEASURE ACT (B) AND PLOT BOTH VALUES.

EXTRAPOLATE AN IMAGINARY LINE THROUGH "A" AND "B" TO INTERSECT WITH 480 second LINE TO FIND POINT "C".

EXAMPLE: 3.5 mg/kg HEPARIN IS NEEDED TO PRODUCE 480 sec. ACT OR 1.5 mg/kg IN ADDITION TO THE 2 mg/kg HEPARIN ALREADY GIVEN.

STEP 3

AFTER REQUIRED HEPARIN HAS BEEN GIVEN, MEASURE ACT. PLOT POINT "D".

IF POINT "D" DOES NOT SUPERIMPOSE ON POINT "C", THEN A DOSE RESPONSE CURVE IS DRAWN FROM "A" TO A POINT MIDWAY BETWEEN "C" AND "D".

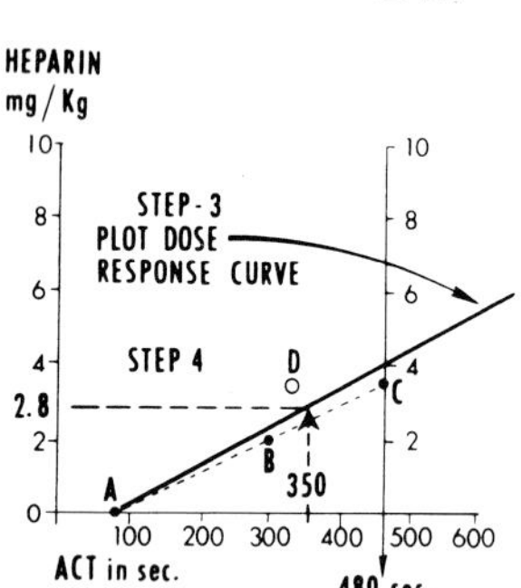

STEP 4

AFTER 60 minutes, MEASURE THE ACT. DETERMINE AMOUNT OF HEPARIN IN PATIENT'S CIRCULATION FROM THE DOSE RESPONSE CURVE.

EXAMPLE: ASSUME AN ACT OF 350 sec.; THE HEPARIN LEVEL WOULD BE 2.8 mg/kg. TO RETURN TO 480 sec., 1.2 mg/kg OF HEPARIN IS NEEDED.

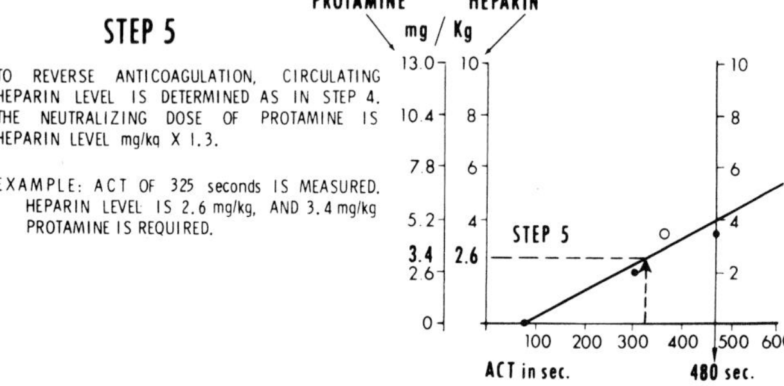

Figure 18–5 Construction of a dose-response curve for heparin. ACT = activated coagulation time. (From Bull BS, Huse WM, Brauer FS, et al: Heparin therapy during extracorporeal circulation: II. The use of a dose-response curve to individualize heparin and protamine dosage. J Thorac Cardiovasc Surg 69:685–689, 1975.)

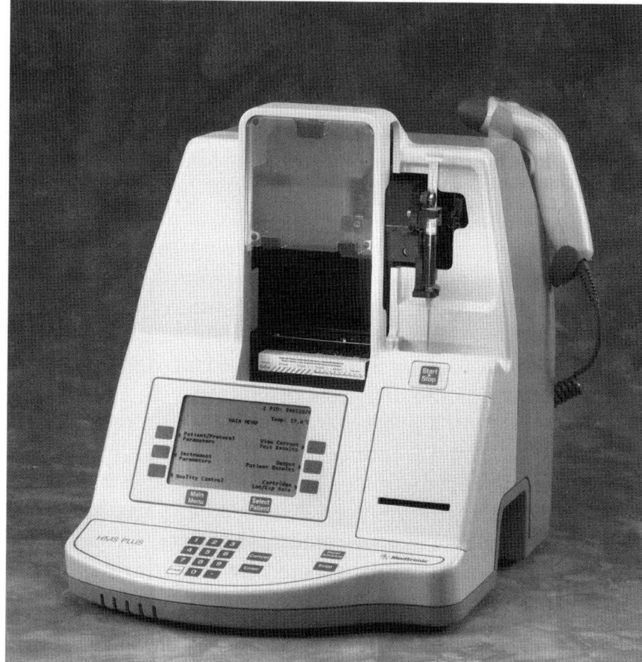

Figure 18–6 The HMS heparin management system has an automated dispenser that places the appropriate volume of whole blood into each chamber of the test cartridge. A variety of assays can be performed in this instrument, depending on the cartridge used. (Courtesy of Medtronic Inc., Parker, CO, http://www.medtronic.com/cardsurgery/bloodmgmt/hmsplus.html)

be obtained from this test includes the baseline ACT (chambers 5 and 6) and an HDR slope. The dose-response slope, which is the increase in ACT from 1.5 U/mL to 2.5 U/mL heparin, is extrapolated to the desired target ACT or target heparin concentration and the heparin dose is calculated.[29,46]

Heparin Concentration

Proponents of ACT measurement to guide anticoagulation for CPB argue that a functional assessment of the anticoagulant effect of heparin is mandatory and that the variability in ACT represents a true variability in the coagulation status of the patient. Opponents argue that during CPB the sensitivity of the ACT to heparin is altered and ACT does not correlate with heparin concentration or with anti–factor Xa activity measurement. Heparin concentration can be measured using the Hepcon HMS system (Medtronic Hemotec), which uses an automated protamine titration technique. With a cartridge with four or six chambers containing tissue thromboplastin and a series of known protamine concentrations, 0.2 mL of whole blood is automatically dispensed into the chambers. The first channel to clot is the channel whose protamine concentration most accurately neutralizes the heparin without a heparin or a protamine excess. Because protamine neutralizes heparin in the ratio of 1 mg of protamine per 100 U of heparin, the concentration of heparin in the blood sample can be calculated. A cartridge that monitors heparin concentration over a wide range can be used first, followed by another cartridge that can measure heparin concentrations within a more narrow range. The maintenance of a stable heparin concentration rather than a specific ACT level usually results in higher doses of heparin being administered because the hemodilution and hypothermia on CPB increase the sensitivity of the ACT to heparin. The measure of heparin concentration has been shown to more closely correlate with anti–factor Xa activity measurements than the ACT during CPB[47] (Fig. 18–7), although the precision and bias of the test may not prove to be acceptable for exclusive use clinically (Fig. 18–8).

In a small prospective randomized study comparing ACT and heparin concentration monitoring, Gravlee et al[48] demonstrated increased mediastinal tube drainage postoperatively in the heparin concentration group, a finding that was initially attributed to higher total heparin doses. However, heparin rebound was not systematically assessed. In a follow-up study, the authors found a higher incidence of heparin rebound in the heparin concentration group, which, when treated, resulted in no difference in bleeding between the ACT and heparin concentration groups.[49] In a prospective randomized trial, Despotis et al[50] demonstrated that by using a transfusion algorithm in association with Hepcon-based heparin management, chest tube drainage was minimally reduced and transfusion of non–red blood cell products could be significantly reduced relative to a group of patients who had ACT-based heparin management. They attributed their results to better preservation of the coagulation system by high heparin doses because the doses of heparin administered in the Hepcon group were nearly twice the doses used in the ACT management group. However, Gravlee et al[48] were unable to

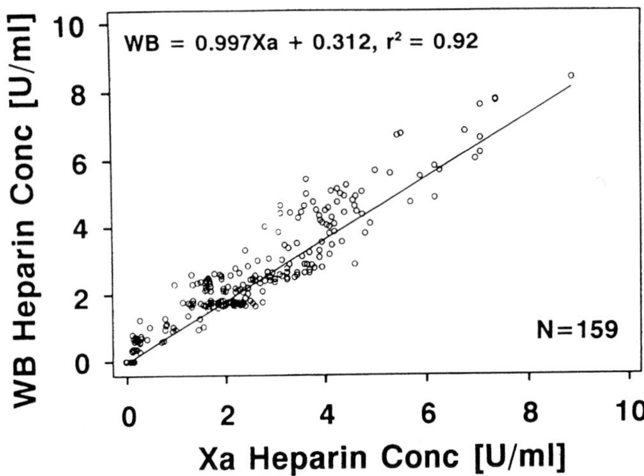

Figure 18–7 There is a strong linear relationship between whole blood heparin concentration (WB Heparin Conc) and the anti-Xa plasma heparin concentration (Xa Heparin Conc). WB Heparin Conc was measured using the Hepcon protamine titration assay and was corrected for hematocrit value. The Xa Heparin Conc was measured in plasma using a substrate assay. (From Despotis GJ, Summerfield AL, Joist JH: Comparison of activated coagulation time and whole blood heparin measurements with laboratory plasma anti-Xa heparin concentration in patients having cardiac operations. J Thorac Cardiovasc Surg 108:1076–1082, 1994.)

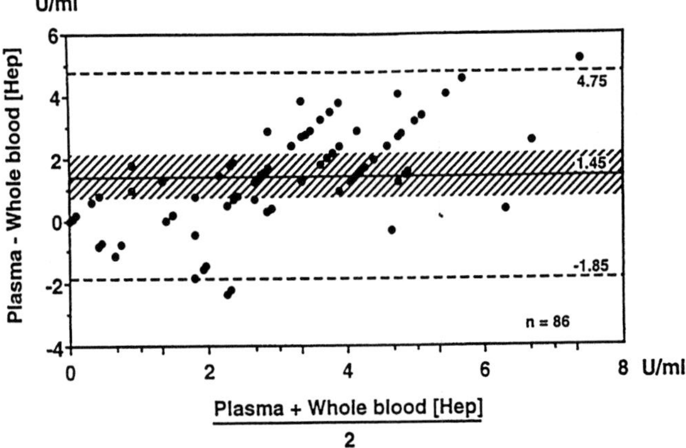

Figure 18–8 A Bland-Altman plot analyzing the limits of agreement between the whole blood heparin concentration and the plasma anti-Xa heparin concentration. The bias (1.45) and 2 standard deviations are determined to be the limits of agreement. Note that the limits of agreement do not lie within the predetermined acceptable difference between the tests. (From Hardy J-F, Belisle S, Robitaille D, et al: Measurement of heparin concentration in whole blood with the Hepcon/HMS device does not agree with laboratory determination of plasma heparin concentration using a chromogenic substrate for activated factor X. J Thorac Cardiovasc Surg 112:154–161, 1996.)

confirm suppression of ongoing coagulation using Hepcon CPB management. With the exception of during cold CPB, fibrinopeptide A (FPA) levels in patients who had heparin concentration monitoring were virtually indistinguishable from those in patients who had ACT monitoring (Fig. 18–9). The Hepcon, however, remains one of the more sensitive tests for detecting residual heparinization after protamine reversal because the heparin concentration can be measured by protamine titration to levels as low as 0.4 IU/mL (see Monitoring for Heparin Rebound).

Other tests that have been used to measure the heparin concentration include polybrene titration (functions similarly to protamine titration) and factor Xa inhibition. The latter

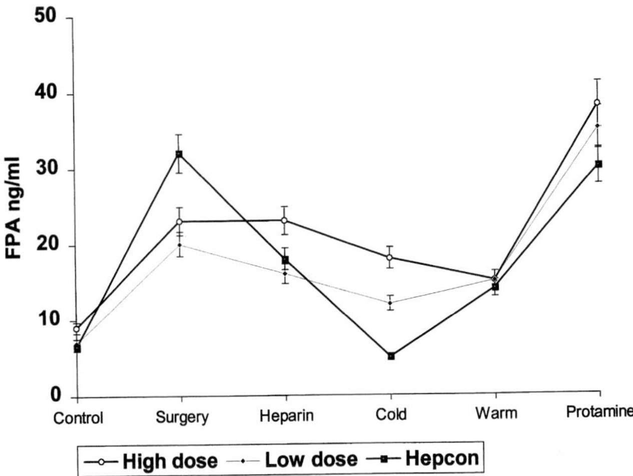

Figure 18–9 Fibrinopeptide A (FPA) levels during cardiopulmonary bypass (CPB) were measured in three groups of patients at: Control = before anesthetic induction; Heparin = after heparin administration; Cold = lowest temperature on CPB; Warm = esophageal temperature >36°C; Protamine = 5 minutes after completion of the protamine dose. Group 1 = patients receiving heparin 300 IU/kg with activated coagulation time (ACT) heparin management. Group 2 = patients receiving heparin 250 IU/kg with ACT management. Group 3 = patients receiving 350 to 400 IU/kg with Hepcon heparin management. There were no differences in FPA levels among groups except during cold CPB group 3 versus group 1, $P < 0.05$. (From Gravlee GP, Haddon WS, Rothberger HK, et al: Heparin dosing and monitoring for cardiopulmonary bypass. A comparison of techniques with measurement of subclinical plasma coagulation. J Thorac Cardiovasc Surg 99:518–527, 1990.)

requires plasma separation and is not practical for intraoperative monitoring. A modification of the thrombin time (TT) can be useful in monitoring heparin levels. One application would be an assay in which a known quantity of thrombin is added to patient blood or plasma. When mixed with a fibrin product, cleavage of the fibrin product can be measured fluorimetrically. Only thrombin not bound by the heparin–ATIII complex is available to cleave fibrin, thus yielding an indirect measure of heparin concentration.

High-Dose Thrombin Time

A functional test of heparin-induced anticoagulation that correlates well with heparin levels is the high-dose thrombin time (HiTT; International Technidyne Inc, Edison, NJ). The TT is a clotting time that measures the conversion of fibrinogen to fibrin by thrombin. The TT is prolonged by the presence of heparin and by hypofibrinogenemias or dysfibrinogenemias. Because the TT is sensitive to very low levels of heparin, a high dose of thrombin is necessary in the TT to accurately assay the high doses of heparin used for CPB. The HiTT is performed by adding whole blood to a prewarmed, prehydrated test tube that contains a lyophilized thrombin preparation. After the addition of 1.5 mL of blood, the tube is inserted into a Hemochron well and the time to clot formation is measured. In vitro assays indicate that HiTT is equivalent to the ACT in evaluation of the anticoagulant effects of heparin at heparin concentrations in the range of 0 to 4.8 IU/mL (Fig. 18–10). Unlike ACT, HiTT is not altered by hemodilution and hypothermia and has been shown to correlate better with heparin concentration than the ACT during CPB.[51] While on CPB, heparin concentration and HiTT decrease while the Hemochron and the Hepcon ACT increase (Fig. 18–11). Another potential advantage of HiTT monitoring occurs

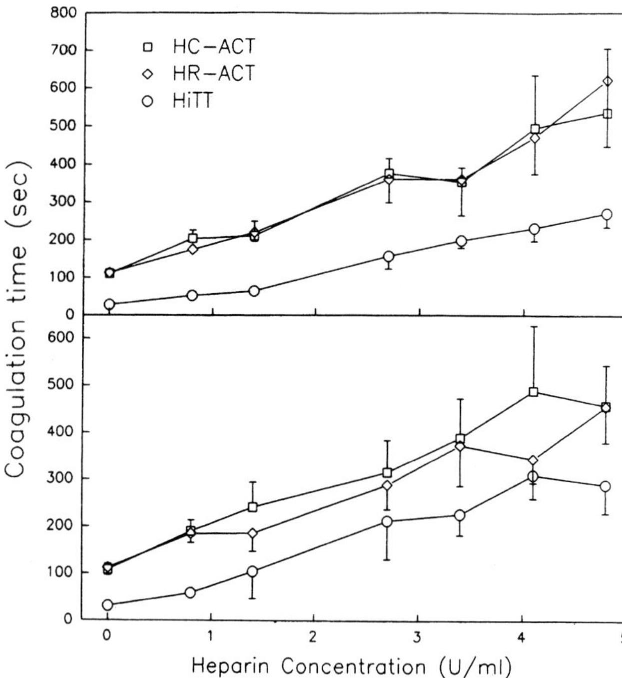

Figure 18–10 Hemochron ACT (HC-ACT), Hepcon ACT (HR-ACT), and high-dose thrombin time (HiTT) at different in vitro heparin concentrations. The relationship is linear in each group. (From Wang J-S, Lin C-Y, Karp RB: Comparison of high-dose thrombin time with activated clotting time for monitoring of anticoagulant effects of heparin in cardiac surgical patients. Anesth Analg 79:9–13, 1994.)

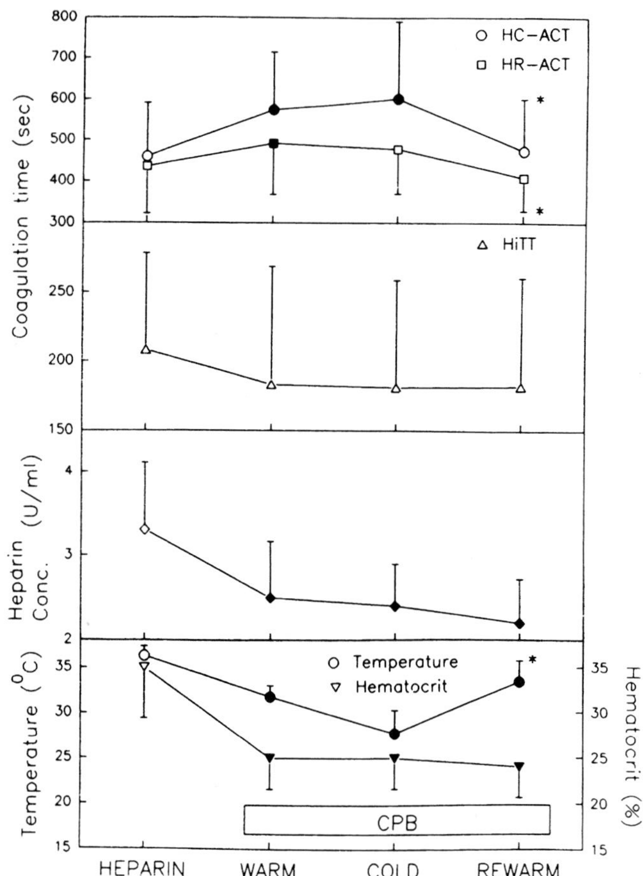

Figure 18–11 Changes over time in the Hemochron ACT (HC-ACT), Hepcon ACT (HR-ACT), and high-dose thrombin time (HiTT) in cardiac surgical patients. HiTT is unaffected by the changes in temperature and hematocrit during cardiopulmonary bypass (CPB). The HC-ACT and HR-ACT increase with the initiation of CPB and the heparin concentration and HiTT decrease. *Significant difference from previous time point ($P <$ 0.05). (From Wang J-S, Lin C-Y, Karp RB: Comparison of high-dose thrombin time with activated clotting time for monitoring of anticoagulant effects of heparin in cardiac surgical patients. Anesth Analg 79:9–13, 1994.)

for patients receiving aprotinin therapy. In the presence of heparin, aprotinin augments the celite ACT,[52] possibly because its kallikrein-inhibiting capacity prolongs activation of the intrinsic coagulation pathway by XIIa. This should not be interpreted to represent enhanced anticoagulation. The kaolin ACT is less affected by aprotinin therapy than the celite ACT, perhaps because kaolin, unlike celite, *activates* the intrinsic pathway by stimulation of factor XI directly.[53] Others have suggested that kaolin binds to aprotinin and reduces the anticoagulant effect of aprotinin in vitro. However, the heparinized kaolin ACT is still somewhat prolonged in the presence of aprotinin. HiTT is not affected by aprotinin therapy and can be used as a measure of heparinization for CPB patients receiving aprotinin therapy.[52] The high-dose thromboplastin time is another measure of anticoagulation that is not affected by aprotinin therapy.[54] The high-dose thromboplastin time is a whole blood clotting time in which celite is replaced by 0.3 mL of rabbit brain thromboplastin to which 1.2 mL of blood is added. This test measures the time to coagulation via activation of the extrinsic pathway. This pathway of coagulation is also stimulated during pericardiotomy due to the rich thromboplastin environment of the pericardial cavity.

HEPARIN NEUTRALIZATION

Protamine Effects on Coagulation Monitoring

Reversal of heparin-induced anticoagulation is most frequently performed with protamine. Biologically, protamine binds to positively charged groups such as phosphate groups and may have important properties in angiogenesis and immune function. Different successful dosing plans have been proposed.[55,56] The recommended dose of protamine for heparin reversal is 1 to 1.3 mg protamine per 100 U heparin; however, this dose often results in a protamine excess.

Protamine injection causes adverse hemodynamic effects.[57] Protamine reactions have been classified into three types.[58] The most common of these reactions is the type I reaction characterized by hypotension. Type II (immunologic) reactions are categorized as IIA (anaphylaxis), IIB (anaphylactoid), and IIC (noncardiogenic pulmonary edema). Type III reactions are heralded by hypotension and catastrophic pulmonary hypertension leading to right heart failure.[30,45,59]

In addition to hemodynamic sequelae, protamine has adverse effects on coagulation.[60] Large doses prolong the WBCT and the ACT, possibly via thrombin inhibition.[61] In animals and in humans, protamine has been associated with thrombocytopenia, likely due to activation of the complement cascade.[57] The anticoagulant effect of protamine may also be due to inhibition of platelet aggregation, alteration in the platelet surface membrane, or depression of the platelet response to various agonists.[61-63] These alterations in platelet function result from the presence of the heparin–protamine complex, not protamine alone. Protamine–heparin complexes activate ATIII in vitro and result in complement activation.

The anticoagulant effects of free protamine occur when protamine is given in doses in excess of those used clinically; however, the risk of free protamine being the cause of a hemostatic defect is small, given the rapid clearance of protamine relative to heparin.

Monitoring for Heparin Rebound

The phenomenon referred to as heparin rebound describes the reestablishment of a heparinized state after heparin has been neutralized with protamine. Various explanations for heparin rebound have been proposed.[9,49,64,65] The most commonly postulated is that rapid distribution and clearance of protamine occur shortly after protamine administration, leaving unbound heparin remaining after protamine clearance. Furthermore, endogenous heparin antagonists have an even shorter life span than protamine and are eliminated rapidly, resulting in free heparin concentrations. Also possible is the release of heparin from tissues considered heparin storage sites (endothelium, connective tissues). Endothelial cells bind and depolymerize heparin via PF4. Uptake into the cells of the reticuloendothelial system, vascular smooth muscle, and extracellular fluid may account for the storage of heparin that contributes to reactivation of heparin anticoagulation, referred to as *heparin rebound*.[9]

Residual low levels of heparin can be detected by sensitive heparin concentration monitoring in the first hour after protamine reversal and can be present for up to 6 hours postoperatively. A study by Gravlee et al[49] suggests that without careful monitoring for heparin rebound in the postoperative period, increased bleeding as a result of heparin rebound may occur, specifically when higher doses of heparin have been administered. Monitoring for heparin rebound can be accomplished using tests that are sensitive to low levels of circulating heparin.[45,50,66,67] These tests are also useful monitors for confirmation of heparin neutralization at the conclusion of CPB (see later).

HEPARIN NEUTRALIZATION MONITORS

To administer the appropriate dose of protamine at the conclusion of CPB, it would be ideal to measure the concentration of heparin present and give the dose of protamine necessary to neutralize only the circulating heparin. As a result of heparin metabolism and elimination, which vary considerably among individuals, the dose of protamine required to reverse a given dose of heparin decreases over time. Furthermore, protamine antagonizes the anti-IIa effects of heparin more effectively than the anti-Xa effects and thus varies in its potency depending on the source of heparin and its anti-IIa properties. Administration of a large fixed dose of protamine or a dose based upon the total heparin dose given is no longer the standard of care and may result in an increased incidence of protamine-related adverse effects. An optimal dose of protamine is desired because unneutralized heparin results in clinical bleeding and an excess of protamine may produce an undesired coagulopathy. The use of individualized protamine dose-response curves uniformly results in a reduced protamine dose and has been shown to reduce postoperative bleeding.[42,66] One such dose-response test, the Hemochron PRT test, is an ACT performed on a heparinized blood sample that contains a known quantity of protamine. With knowledge of the ACT, PRT, and the estimated blood volume of the patient, the protamine dose needed to neutralize the existing heparin level

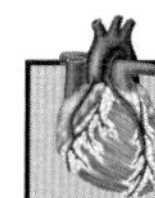

BOX 18–3 ***Heparin Neutralization***

- The most benign form of bleeding after cardiac surgery is due to residual heparinization.
- Treatment is either protamine or another heparin-neutralizing product.
- Transfusion of allogeneic blood products is rarely indicated.
- Residual heparin can be measured by using
  - A protamine titration assay
  - A heparin neutralized thrombin time assay
  - A heparinase ACT compared with ACT or
  - Any other heparinase test that compares itself with the test without heparinase added

can be extrapolated. The Hepcon instrument also has a protamine dose-response test, which is the protamine titration assay. The chamber that clots first contains the dose of protamine that most closely approximates the circulating dose of heparin. By measuring the circulating heparin level, the protamine dose required for its neutralization is calculated based on a specified heparin/protamine dose ratio.

At the levels of heparinization needed for cardiac surgery, tests that are sensitive to heparin become not clottable. ACT is relatively insensitive to heparin and is ideal for monitoring anticoagulation at high heparin levels but is too insensitive to accurately diagnose incomplete heparin neutralization. Reiner et al[68] showed that ACT had a high predictive value for adequate anticoagulation (confirmed by laboratory activated partial thromboplastin time [aPTT]) when greater than 225 seconds but was poorly predictive for inadequate anticoagulation when less than 225 seconds. The low levels of heparin present when heparin is incompletely neutralized are best measured by other more sensitive tests of heparin-induced anticoagulation, such as heparin concentration, aPTT, and TT. Thus, after CPB, confirmation of return to the unanticoagulated state should be performed with a sensitive test for heparin anticoagulation[69-72] (Box 18–3).

Thrombin Time

TT is the time it takes for the conversion of fibrinogen to fibrin clot when blood or plasma is exposed to thrombin. Fibrin strands form in seconds. Detection of fibrin formation using standard laboratory equipment involves incubation of the blood or plasma sample within the chamber in which an optical or electrical probe sits. A detector senses either movement of the probe or the creation of an electrical field (electrical detection) due to fibrin formation and hence signals the end of the test. Hemochron manufactures a point-of-care TT test that uses a lyophilized preparation of thrombin in a Hemochron test tube to which 1 mL of blood is added. Identification of fibrin formation in a Hemochron machine uses the standard Hemochron technology described previously with the ACT. The manufacturer suggests that the normal TT is 39 to 53 seconds for whole blood and 43 to 68 seconds for citrated blood. Because the TT specifically measures the activity of thrombin, it is very sensitive to heparin-induced enhancement of ATIII activity. It is a useful test in the post-CPB period for differentiating the cause of bleeding when both prothrombin time (PT) and aPTT are prolonged, because it excludes the intrinsic and extrinsic coagulation pathway limbs and evaluates the conversion of factor I to Ia.

The TT is elevated in the presence of heparin, hypofibrinogenemia, dysfibrinogenemia, amyloidosis, or antibodies to thrombin.[73] The TT is also elevated in the presence of fibrin degradation products if the systemic fibrinogen concentration is low.

The TT is an appropriate laboratory test for monitoring the degree of fibrinolytic activity in patients receiving thrombolytic therapy. Measurements of the quantity of fibrinogen, plasminogen, or plasma proteins generated during fibrinolysis are difficult to interpret and yield no prognostic information for dose adjustments. Thrombolytic agents activate the fibrinolytic system to generate plasmin, which then causes clot dissolution and decreases the quantities of fibrinogen and fibrin. This effect can be monitored using the TT. The TT should be measured at baseline (prior to institution of fibrinolytic therapy) and 3 to 4 hours after therapy is initiated. If it is prolonged by 1.5 to 5 times the baseline value, therapy should be considered effective. If the TT is prolonged by greater than 7 times the baseline value, an increased risk of bleeding is incurred; if the TT is not prolonged at all, therapy has failed to activate fibrinolysis.

Bedside Tests of Heparin Neutralization

Hepcon measures heparin concentration via a protamine titration assay. Cartridges with varying ranges of protamine concentration are available for use. The cartridge with the lower concentration of protamine in the titration is useful for the detection of residual circulating heparin and is sensitive to levels of heparin as low as 0.2 U/mL. Whole blood PT and aPTT assays are sensitive to deficiencies in coagulation factors and overly sensitive to low levels of heparin (aPTT); they lack specificity in assessing residual heparinization. The heparin-neutralized thrombin time (HNTT) is a TT assay with a small dose of protamine sufficient to neutralize 1.5 U/mL of heparin. Because the TT is elevated in the presence of heparin, hypofibrinogenemia, or dysfibrinogenemia, to discriminate among these three causes, HNTT and TT should be performed together. A normal HNTT in the presence of an elevated TT virtually confirms residual heparin effect and would indicate the need for protamine administration. If HNTT is prolonged as well as the TT, the cause of bleeding may be attributed either to a fibrinogen problem or to a concentration of heparin higher than that which could be neutralized by the HNTT. In one study comparing bedside monitors of anticoagulation, the TT-HNTT difference bore a significant correlation with the aPTT elevation. Using the line of best fit, aPTT elevation of 1.5 times the control corresponded to a 31-second difference in the TT and HNTT, indicating a convenient threshold value of TT-HNTT for the administration of protamine.[73]

Platelet Factor 4 (PF4)

This component of the alpha granule of platelets binds to and inactivates heparin. The physiologic role of PF4 is that at the site of vascular injury, PF4 is released from platelets, binds heparin (or heparin-like compounds), and promotes thrombin and clot formation. PF4 adequately neutralizes heparin inhibition of factors Xa and IIa and may be superior to protamine in neutralizing anti-Xa effects. Animal data suggest that PF4 is devoid of the adverse hemodynamic effects seen with protamine and that it may be able to be infused more rapidly.[74,75] Heparin reversal has been documented by WBCT, ACT, and heparin concentration at a PF4 concentration of 40 μ/mL, approximately twice the reversal dose of protamine.[74] Levy et al[76] subsequently found the reversal dose of PF4 to be approximately 60 μ/mL and documented similar ACT and viscoelastic measurements of clot formation compared with protamine.

Heparinase

Heparinase (Neutralase I) is an enzyme that specifically degrades heparin by catalyzing cleavage of the saccharide bonds found in the heparin molecule. As demonstrated by the ACT, heparinase in a dose of 5 μg/kg has been shown to successfully neutralize heparin effects in healthy volunteers and in patients who have undergone CPB. A dose of 7 μg/kg has been demonstrated to be even more efficacious in returning ACT to baseline values. Doses sufficient to neutralize a dose of 300 U/kg had no significant hemodynamic effects in a canine model.[77] Investigators have not found any platelet-depressive effects of heparinase in contrast with the well-documented platelet dysfunction associated with protamine therapy.[62] Return to the unanticoagulated state after the use of heparinase has been confirmed using ACT monitoring or heparin concentration monitoring.

TESTS OF COAGULATION

Standard tests of coagulation, the PT and the aPTT, are performed on plasma to which the anticoagulant citrate has been added. Because these tests are performed on plasma, they require centrifugation of blood and are generally not feasible for use at the bedside. The aPTT tests the integrity of the intrinsic and the final coagulation pathways and is more sensitive to low levels of heparin than the ACT. Factors IX and X are most sensitive to heparin effects, and thus the aPTT will be prolonged even at very low heparin levels. The test uses a phospholipid substance to simulate the interaction of the platelet membrane in activating factor XII. (Thromboplastin is a tissue extract containing tissue factor and phospholipid. The term *partial thromboplastin* refers to the use of the phospholipid portion only.) The aPTT is prolonged in the presence of deficiencies of factors XII, XI, IX, and VIII, HMWK, and kallikrein. The aPTT reaction is considerably slower than the PT, and in order to speed activation of factor XII, an activator such as celite or kaolin is added to the assay. After incubation of citrated plasma with phospholipid and activator, calcium is added and the time to clot formation is measured. Normal aPTT is 28 to 32 seconds, which is often expressed as a ratio with a control plasma sample from the same laboratory. This is important because partial thromboplastin reagents have different sensitivities to heparin and many have nonlinear responses to heparin in various concentration ranges.

PT measures the integrity of the extrinsic and common coagulation pathways. PT will be prolonged in the presence of factor VII deficiency, Coumadin (warfarin sodium) therapy, or vitamin K deficiency. Large doses of heparin also prolong the PT because of inactivation of factor II. The addition of thromboplastin to citrated plasma results in activation of extrinsic coagulation. After a 3-minute incubation and recalcification, the time to clot formation is measured and is recorded as the PT. Normal PT is 12 to 14 seconds; however, due to differences in the quality and lot of the thromboplastin used, absolute

PT values are not standardized and are difficult to compare across different testing centers. The international normalized ratio (INR) has been adopted as the standard for coagulation monitoring. The INR is an internationally standardized laboratory value that is the ratio of the patient's PT to the result that would have been obtained if the International Reference Preparation (IRP) had been used instead of the laboratory reagents. Each laboratory uses reagents with a specific sensitivity (International Sensitivity Index [ISI]) relative to the IRP. The ISI of a particular set of reagents is provided by each manufacturer so that the INR can be reported.

Bedside Tests of Coagulation

PT and aPTT tests performed on whole blood are available for use in the operating room or at the bedside. The Hemochron PT test tube contains acetone-dried rabbit brain thromboplastin to which 2 mL of whole blood is added and the tube is inserted into a standard Hemochron machine. Normal values range from 50 to 72 seconds and are automatically converted by a computer to the plasma equivalent PT and INR. Hemochron aPTT contains kaolin activator and a platelet factor substitute and is performed similarly to the PT. The aPTT is sensitive to heparin concentrations as low as 0.2 U/mL and displays a linear relationship with heparin concentration up to 1.5 U/mL.

The Ciba Corning Biotrack 512 coagulation monitor for evaluating bedside PT and aPTT uses 0.1 mL of whole blood placed into a disposable plastic cartridge for either PT or aPTT. The sample is drawn by capillary action into a heated chamber where exposure to reagents occurs. The PT uses rabbit brain thromboplastin. The aPTT uses soybean phosphatide as the platelet substitute and bovine brain sulfatide as the activator. From the reaction chamber, blood traverses a reaction path where clot formation is detected by a laser optical system. The resulting time to clot formation is converted to a ratio of the control value by a microprocessor that has control values encoded.

Many investigators have studied the Ciba Corning Biotrack system for monitoring anticoagulation in different clinical scenarios. For patients receiving oral anticoagulant therapy, the Biotrack 512 monitor has been found to be suitable for monitoring PT and INR. Reiner et al[68] compared the bedside Biotrack aPTT with the laboratory aPTT and heparin level in patients receiving therapeutic heparinization after interventional cardiac catheterization. The authors found a strong correlation ($r = 0.89$) between the Biotrack aPTT and the aPTT from the hospital laboratory. The correlation between Biotrack aPTT and heparin level was not strong, probably due to the many other factors such as heparin neutralization and clearance that affect the heparin concentration in vivo.[78] Another study in patients receiving heparin compared the Ciba Corning Biotrack aPTT assay with standard laboratory aPTT and documented that Biotrack was less sensitive to heparin than the laboratory aPTT; however, the correlation coefficient of these two tests was $r = 0.82$.[79] In patients on warfarin therapy, the Biotrack aPTT was more sensitive than the laboratory aPTT and yielded consistently higher results for aPTT value. In another study in patients being anticoagulated for nonsurgical applications, the bedside aPTT was similar to the standard aPTT in its prediction of treatment in simple therapeutic algorithms. However, in more complex clinical situations, there was less agreement between the bedside aPTT and laboratory aPTT.[80]

In a comparison of bedside coagulation monitors after cardiac surgical procedures, Reich et al[73] documented acceptable accuracy and precision levels for Hemochron and Ciba Corning Biotrack PT in comparison with standard laboratory plasma PT, making them potentially valuable for use in the perioperative period. Neither Hemochron nor Ciba Corning aPTT reached this level of clinical competence compared with standard laboratory tests. Others have documented that this monitor seems to be more precise for PT than for aPTT.[81] Because of rapid turn-around times, these point-of-care coagulation monitors may be useful in predicting patients who will bleed after cardiac surgery[82] and have also been successfully used in transfusion algorithms to decrease the number of allogeneic blood products given to cardiac surgical patients.[83,84]

Measures of Fibrin Formation

The "Tenase complex" is the group of factors and cofactors that includes Xa, platelet-bound factor Va, platelet factor 3, and Ca^{++}. All adhere on the platelet surface and catalyze the cleavage of prothrombin (factor II) to thrombin (factor IIa). Thrombin then catalyzes the cleavage of fibrinogen to form fibrin monomer and fibrinopeptide A and fibrinopeptide B. These end-products of fibrinogen cleavage are commonly measured serum markers that help to quantify the degree of coagulation that occurs in certain experimental or clinical situations.

One such experimental situation is the use of heparin-bonded extracorporeal circuits during CPB with the expectation that thrombin activation and fibrin formation will be minimized. Coating of the extracorporeal circuit with the heparin ligand makes the circuit more biocompatible such that the inflammatory response elicited is diminished or nonexistent. Heparin-bonded circuits have been extensively studied and considered advantageous due to their ability to reduce the inflammatory response to CPB. Human studies reveal decreases in enzymes that mark leukocyte activation, thus showing a reduction in the whole-body inflammatory response similar to that seen with leukocyte depletion techniques.[85-87]

Further enhancements in biocompatibility include less leukocyte activation and preserved platelet function. Reductions in thrombin generation have been difficult to document.[88] The increases in the fibrinogen fragment F1.2 and in D-dimer levels when heparin-coated circuits are used are similar to those seen when uncoated circuits are used.[89,90] Human studies have documented less bleeding and reduced transfusion requirements with the use of a heparin-coated extracorporeal circulation when these circuits are used in conjunction with a reduced systemic heparin dose.[91,92] In this circumstance, markers of thrombin generation are increased even above those in patients in whom full-dose heparin and uncoated circuits are used. In fact, increases are seen in fibrinopeptide A, prothrombin fragment F1.2, thrombin–antithrombin III complexes, D-dimers, and plasminogen activators during CPB and after protamine administration regardless of whether heparin-coated circuits are used and regardless of heparin dose.[93] Despite this, the use of reduced heparin doses and coated circuitry has resulted in diminished transfusion requirements and reduced chest tube drainage volumes without evidence of complications.[90,94] Because microvascular coagulation is not fully inhibited, the use of a reduced dose of heparin cannot be systematically advocated and should be implemented with caution.

Fibrinogen Level

Fibrinogen concentration is traditionally measured using either clottable protein methods, end-point detection techniques, or immunochemical tests. Of the former, the most commonly used fibrinogen assay relies on the method of Clauss. This method involves a 10-fold dilution of plasma, which ensures that fibrinogen is the rate-limiting step in clot formation. Subsequently, an excess of thrombin is added to the sample and the time to clot formation is measured. The clotting time is inversely related to the fibrinogen concentration. Because this assay relies on detection of actual clot, it can be affected by fibrin degradation products, polymerization inhibitors, or other inhibitors of fibrin formation. Because of the thrombin excess, small clinical concentrations of heparin do not affect fibrinogen determination according to the Clauss technique.

A whole blood point-of-care fibrinogen assay is available using the Hemochron system. The specific test tube contains a lyophilized preparation of human thrombin, snake venom extract, protamine, buffers, and calcium stabilizers. The test tube is incubated with 1.5 mL of distilled water and heated in the Hemochron instrument for 3 minutes. Whole blood is placed into a diluent vial, where it is 50% diluted, and from this vial, 0.5 mL of diluted whole blood is placed into the specific fibrinogen test tube. The clotting time is measured using standard Hemochron technology as described previously. The fibrinogen concentration is determined by comparison with a standard curve for this test. Normal fibrinogen concentration of 180 to 220 mg/dL correlates with a clotting time of 54 ± 2.5 seconds. Fibrinogen deficiency of 50 to 75 mg/dL correlates with a clotting time of 150 ± 9.0 seconds.

Unlike the method of Clauss, the end-point detection assays rely on the detection of changes in turbidity of plasma when clot is formed. This technique does not require the maintenance of a stable cross-linked fibrin product and therefore does not report underestimated fibrinogen measurements due to the presence of inhibitors. Immunochemical measures of fibrinogen concentration are a direct and accurate measurement technique; however, they are expensive and time consuming and require specialized laboratory facilities.

MONITORING FIBRINOLYSIS

Fibrinolysis, the dissolution of fibrin, is the normal modifier of hemostasis that ensures that coagulation does not proceed unchecked. It occurs in the vicinity of a clot and dissolves clot when local endothelial healing occurs. Fibrinolysis is mediated by the serine protease plasmin, which is the product of the cleavage of plasminogen by tissue plasminogen activator (tPA). Fibrinolysis is a normal phenomenon in response to clot formation; when it occurs systemically, it represents a pathologic condition.

Fibrinolysis can be primary or secondary. Primary fibrinolysis occurs when fibrinolytic activators are released or produced in excess and do not represent a response to the coagulation process. Examples of primary fibrinolysis include the release of plasminogen activators during liver transplantation surgery and the exogenous administration of fibrinolytic agents such as streptokinase. During primary fibrinolysis, plasmin cleaves fibrinogen, yielding fibrinogen degradation products. These end-products can be measured using immunologic techniques.

When fibrinolysis is a result of enhanced activation of the coagulation system, secondary fibrinolysis ensues. A well-known extreme form of secondary fibrinolysis is seen during disseminated intravascular coagulation, when both systemic coagulation and fibrinolysis are occurring in excess. During CPB, fibrinolysis is most likely secondary to the microvascular coagulation that is occurring despite attempts at suppression using high doses of heparin.[95,96]

The identification of fibrinolysis can be accomplished through either direct measurement of the clot lysis time (manual or viscoelastic tests) or measurement of the end-products of fibrin degradation. The manual clot lysis time simply involves the placement of whole blood into a test tube. This blood clots in a matter of minutes. Visual inspection determines the end-point for observation of clot lysis, and this time period is the clot lysis time. This technique is considerably time consuming and requires constant observation by the person performing the test.

Viscoelastic Tests

Viscoelastic tests measure the unique properties of the clot as it is forming, organizing, strengthening, and lysing. As a result, fibrinolysis determination by this methodology requires that time elapse during which clot formation is occurring. It is subsequent to clot formation and platelet-fibrin linkages that clot lysis parameters can be measured. For this reason, viscoelastic tests often require longer than 1 hour to detect the initiation of fibrinolysis; however, if fibrinolysis is enhanced, results can often be obtained in 30 minutes.

End-Products of Fibrin Degradation

Other methods for quantifying fibrinolysis include measurement of the end-products of fibrin degradation. Fibrin degradation products are the result of the cleavage of fibrin monomers and polymers and can be measured using a latex agglutination assay. When plasmin cleaves cross-linked fibrin, dimeric units are formed that comprise one D-domain from each of two adjacent fibrin units. These "D-dimers" are frequently measured by researchers in clinical and laboratory investigations. They are measured by either enzyme-linked immunosorbent assays or latex agglutination techniques and thus are not available for on-site use. Controversy still exists regarding whether D-dimer level or fibrin degradation products are the most sensitive test for detecting fibrinolysis, but most agree that the presence of D-dimers is the most specific for cross-linked fibrin degradation.[97]

Monitoring the Thrombin Inhibitors

A new class of drugs, the selective thrombin inhibitors, is a viable alternative to heparin anticoagulation for CPB. These agents include hirudin, argatroban, and other experimental agents. A major advantage of these agents over heparin is that they are able to effectively inhibit clot-bound thrombin in an ATIII-independent fashion.[98] The platelet thrombin receptor is believed to be the focus of thrombin's procoagulant effects in states of thrombosis such as after coronary artery angioplasty. Because surface-bound thrombin is more effectively suppressed, thrombin generation can be reduced at lower levels of systemic anticoagulation than are achieved during anticoagulation by the heparin–ATIII complex. This translates into less bleeding despite the lack of a clinically useful antidote for the thrombin antagonists.[99,100] Thrombin antagonists are also not susceptible to neutralization by PF4 and thus are not neutralized at endothelial sites where activated platelets reside. They are also useful in patients with HIT in whom the administration of heparin and subsequent antibody-induced platelet aggregation would be dangerous.[101] The lack of a potent antidote (such as protamine) and a prolonged duration of action are the major reasons that hirudin and other thrombin inhibitors have not found widespread clinical acceptance for use in CPB procedures (see Chapter 29).

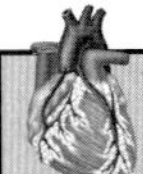

BOX 18–4 *Thrombin Inhibitors*

- These anticoagulant drugs are superior to heparin.
- They inhibit both clot-bound and soluble thrombin.
- They do not require a cofactor, activate platelets, or cause immunogenicity.
- Heparin remains an attractive drug due to its long history of safe use and the fact that it has a specific drug antidote, protamine.
- These drugs include hirudin, argatroban, and bivalirudin.

Hirudin

Hirudin, a coagulation inhibitor isolated from the salivary glands of the medicinal leech (*Hirudo medicinalis*), is a potent inhibitor of thrombin that, unlike heparin, acts independently of ATIII and inhibits clot-bound thrombin as well as fluid-phase thrombin. Hirudin does not require a cofactor and is not susceptible to neutralization by PF4. This would seem to be beneficial in patients in whom platelet activation and thrombosis are potential problems. Recombinant hirudin (r-hirudin) was administered as a 0.25-mg/kg bolus and an infusion to maintain the hirudin concentration at 2.5 μg/mL as determined by the ecarin clotting time in studies by Koster et al.[102-110] The ecarin clotting time, modified for use in the TAS analyzer, has been used in large series of patients with HIT.[102-107] Compared with standard treatment with heparin or LMWHs, r-hirudin–treated patients maintained platelet counts and hemoglobin levels and had few bleeding complications, if renal function was normal.[108,109] Hirudin is a small molecule (molecular weight 7 kDa) that is eliminated by the kidney and is easily hemofiltered at the end of CPB.[110]

Bivalirudin

Bivalirudin is a small 20–amino acid molecule with a plasma half-life of 24 minutes. It is a synthetic derivative of hirudin and thus acts as a direct thrombin inhibitor. Bivalirudin binds to both the catalytic binding site and the anion-binding exosite on fluid phase and clot-bound thrombin. The part of the molecule that binds to thrombin is actually cleaved by thrombin itself, so the elimination of bivalirudin activity is independent of specific organ metabolism. Bivalirudin has been used successfully as an anticoagulant in interventional cardiology procedures as a replacement for heparin therapy. In fact, in interventional cardiology, bivalirudin has been associated with less bleeding and equivalent ischemic outcomes compared with heparin plus a platelet inhibitor.[111] This may be the result of bivalirudin being both an antithrombin anticoagulant and an antithrombin at the level of the platelet. Merry et al[112] showed equivalence with regard to bleeding outcomes and an improvement in graft flow after off-pump cardiac surgery when bivalirudin was used (0.75-mg/kg bolus, 1.75-mg/kg/hr infusion). Case reports confirm the safety of bivalirudin use during CPB, although current trials are under way.[113-115] Monitoring of anticoagulant activity is performed using the ecarin clotting time with similar prolongation to that seen with hirudin anticoagulation.[116] The ecarin clotting time has a closer correlation with anti-IIa activity and plasma drug levels than does the ACT. For this reason, standard ACT monitoring during antithrombin therapy is not preferred if ecarin clotting time can be measured.

The anticoagulant effects of the thrombin antagonists can be monitored using the ACT, aPTT, or the TT. The bleeding time may also be prolonged. In a canine CPB model, dogs receiving a synthetic thrombin inhibitor had less postoperative blood loss and higher platelet counts than those receiving heparin; however, those who received a large dose of the thrombin inhibitor still had ACT elevations at 2 hours after CPB.[117] There were no differences in hemodynamics noted in the groups.

Bivalirudin has been favorably compared with heparin in patients undergoing coronary angioplasty for unstable angina.[118] The half-life of aPTT prolongation is approximately 40 minutes, and reductions in formation of fibrinopeptide A are evidence of thrombin inhibition and fibrinogen preservation. Careful monitoring should be used because there may be a rebound prothrombotic state after cessation of therapy, which could lead to recurrence of anginal symptoms (Box 18–4).

Evaluation of a Prolonged aPTT

The first step in evaluation of a prolonged aPTT is the elimination of heparin contamination as a cause of the elevation. Other potential causes of an elevated aPTT are the presence of factor deficiencies or inhibitors of coagulation. Factor deficiencies can be ruled out by mixing studies in which patient plasma is mixed with an equal volume of plasma derived from normal volunteers. The test results should return to normal if a deficiency is present, because mixing with normal plasma yields higher than the required concentrations of coagulation proteins for adequate clotting. If an inhibitor is present, mixing studies will not return the aPTT to normal values.

Inhibitors of factors VIII and IX and the "lupus anticoagulants" are the most common inhibitors encountered. The lupus anticoagulants are antiphospholipid antibodies that react with the phospholipid surfaces required for coagulation, thus the prolongation of the clotting time. In patients who do not have systemic lupus, this syndrome is referred to as *primary antiphospholipid syndrome*. Testing for this inhibitor has been performed using the aPTT or a dilute viper venom time. The latter consists of activation of factor X by venom and measurement of the clotting time, which will be prolonged if an inhibitor is present. Immunologic assays for anticardiolipin antibodies are available. Patient serum is incubated with solid-phase cardiolipin and bound immunoglobulin is measured.

MONITORING PLATELET FUNCTION

Circulating platelets adhere to the endothelium via platelet surface receptors that bind exposed collagen and become activated. This initiates platelet activation, because collagen is a potent platelet activator. The unstimulated platelet, which is discoid in shape, undergoes a conformational change when activated. The activated platelet is spherical, extrudes pseudopodia, and expresses an increased number of activated surface receptors that can be measured to quantify the degree of platelet reactivity. The intensity of this platelet activation occurs in proportion to the quantity and nature of the platelet stimulus and increases in a graded fashion with increasing concentrations of agonists. The glycoprotein (GP) IIb/IIIa receptor is the primary receptor responsible for fibrinogen binding and the formation of the platelet plug.

Platelet Count

Numerous events occur during cardiac surgical procedures that predispose patients to platelet-related hemostasis defects. The two major categories are thrombocytopenia and qualitative platelet defects. Thrombocytopenia commonly occurs during cardiac surgery as a result of hemodilution, sequestration, and destruction by nonendothelial surfaces. Platelet counts commonly fall to 100,000/μL or slightly below; however, the final platelet count is greatly dependent on the starting value and the duration of platelet destructive interventions (i.e., CPB).[119] Between 10,000/μL and 100,000/μL, bleeding time decreases directly; however, at platelet counts greater than 50,000/μL, neither the bleeding time nor platelet count has any correlation with postoperative bleeding in cardiac surgical patients. On the other hand, platelet size or mean platelet volume does have some correlation with hemostatic function. Larger, younger platelets are more hemostatically active than smaller ones.[120,121] Mean platelet volume multiplied by the platelet count gives an estimation of overall platelet mass and is referred to as the *plateletcrit*. It is important to appreciate the inverse relationship between platelet volume and platelet count when using a measure such as the plateletcrit to assess the viability of the existing platelet population. Because the mean platelet volume is dependent on the method of specimen collection, the anticoagulant used, and temperature of the storage conditions, its reproducibility is dependent on standardized laboratory procedures.

Qualitative platelet defects occur more commonly than thrombocytopenia during CPB procedures. The range of possible etiologies of platelet dysfunction includes traumatic extracorporeal techniques, pharmacologic therapy, hypothermia, and fibrinolysis; the hemostatic insult increases with the duration of time spent on CPB.[122] The use of bubble oxygenators, noncoated extracorporeal circulation, and cardiotomy suctioning may cause platelets to become activated, initiate the release reaction, and partly deplete platelets of the contents of their alpha granules. Many of these changes are only transiently associated with CPB. Khuri et al[123] characterized the hematologic changes associated with CPB in a group of 85 patients. While the platelet count falls and reaches a plateau at 2 hours after CPB, mean platelet volume reaches its nadir at 2 hours after CPB and then begins to rise during the ensuing 72 hours[121,123] (Figs. 18–12 and 18–13). The relative thrombocytopenia seen up to 72 hours after cardiac surgery is not consistently associated with a bleeding diathesis. Similarly, the clotting proteins fibrinogen, factor VIII–von Willebrand factor (vWF), and factor VIII-C also rise to levels above baseline in the 2 to 72 hours after CPB (Fig. 18–14).

Large doses of heparin have been shown to reduce the ability of the platelets to aggregate and to reduce clot strength.[61] This effect is not reversed when protamine is administered; however, it may be mitigated by the prophylac-

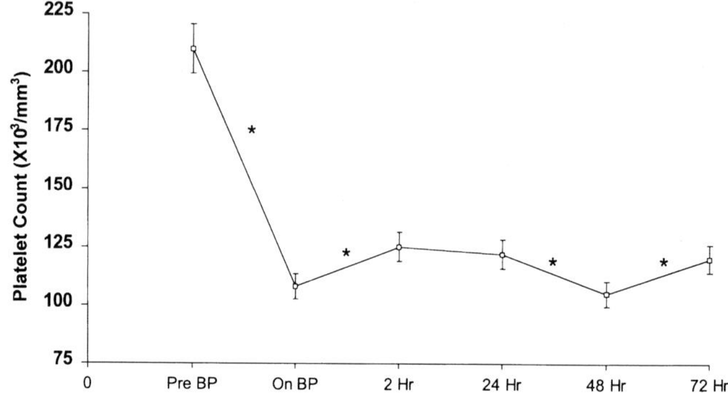

Figure 18–12 Platelet count changes in patients undergoing cardiopulmonary bypass (CPB). Significant decrease in platelet count occurs upon initiation of CPB and remains until at least 72 hours postoperatively. *$P < 0.05$ change from previous value. (From Khuri SF, Wolfe JA, Josa M, et al: Hematologic changes during and after cardiopulmonary bypass and their relationship to the bleeding time and nonsurgical blood loss. J Thorac Cardiovasc Surg 104:94–107, 1992.)

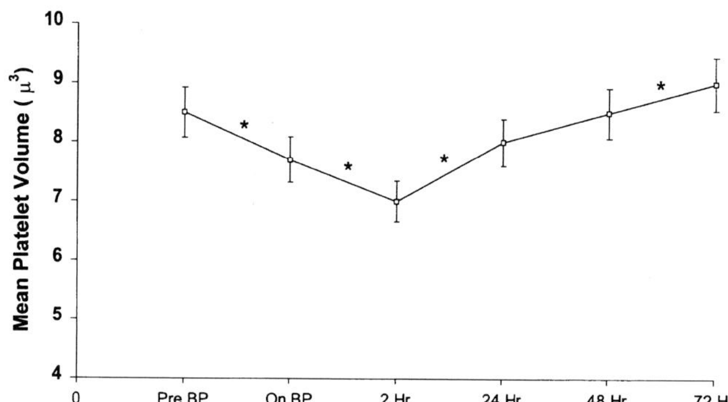

Figure 18–13 Changes in mean platelet volume (MPV) in patients undergoing cardiopulmonary bypass (CPB). Note that the decrease in MPV that occurs during CPB returns to and exceeds baseline values at 24 hours postoperatively. *$P < 0.05$ change from previous value. (From Khuri SF, Wolfe JA, Josa M, et al: Hematologic changes during and after cardiopulmonary bypass and their relationship to the bleeding time and nonsurgical blood loss. J Thorac Cardiovasc Surg 104:94–107, 1992.)

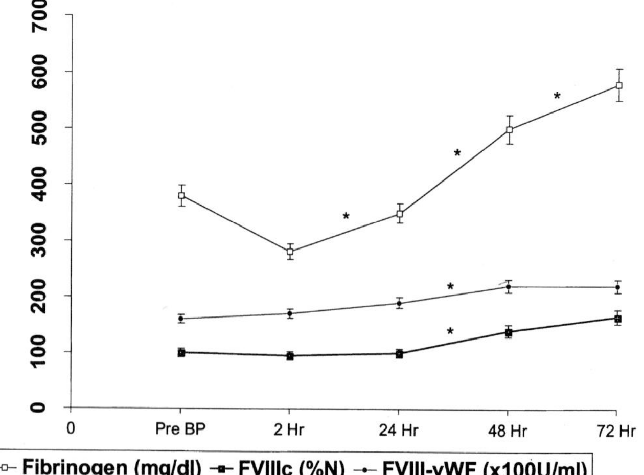

Figure 18–14 Fibrinogen values decrease during cardiopulmonary bypass (CPB). All three clotting proteins increase above baseline levels in the 24 to 72 hours after CPB. *$P < 0.05$ change from previous value. Pre BP = pre-bypass; FVIIIc = factor VIIIc; FVIII-vWF = factor VIII–von Willebrand factor. (From Khuri SF, Wolfe JA, Josa M, et al: Hematologic changes during and after cardiopulmonary bypass and their relationship to the bleeding time and nonsurgical blood loss. J Thorac Cardiovasc Surg 104:94–107, 1992.)

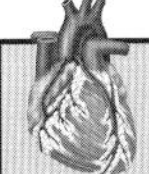

BOX 18–5 *Platelet Function*

- The measure of platelet count does not correlate with bleeding after cardiac surgery.
- Patients frequently have extreme degrees of thrombocytopenia but do not bleed because they have adequate platelet function.
- It is the measure of platelet function that correlates temporally with the bleeding course seen after cardiac surgery.
- The thromboelastogram maximal amplitude, mean platelet volume, and other functional platelet tests are very useful in transfusion algorithms.

tic administration of aprotinin.[124,125] The adverse effects of heparin on platelet function may be due to its ability to inhibit the formation of thrombin, the most potent in vivo platelet activator.[126] However, heparin also activates the fibrinolytic system, a system that, through plasmin and other activators, has the ability to depress platelet function through other mechanisms. In an extracorporeal baboon model, intravenous heparin administration resulted in increases in plasmin activity, in the quantity of immunoreactive plasmin light chain, and in immunoreactive fibrinogen fragment E.[1,127] Additionally, various degrees of fibrinolysis occur after CPB. Circulating plasmin causes dissolution of the GP Ib platelet receptor and decreases the adhesiveness of platelets. Because fibrinolysis is partly responsible for the platelet dysfunction seen after heparin administration and CPB, the efficacy of antifibrinolytic agents as hemostatic drugs can be better appreciated. In addition to reducing platelet adhesiveness to vWF, the fibrin degradation products formed depress platelet responsiveness to agonists.[128,129]

Protamine–heparin complexes and protamine alone also contribute to platelet depression after CPB. Mild-to-moderate degrees of hypothermia are associated with reversible degrees of platelet activation and platelet dysfunction,[130] which may be partly mitigated by the use of aprotinin therapy.[131] Overall, the potential coagulation benefits of normothermic CPB compared with hypothermic CPB require further study in well-conducted randomized trials (Box 18–5).

Bleeding Time

The bleeding time is performed by creating a skin incision and measuring the time to clot formation via the platelet plug. The Ivy bleeding time is performed on the volar surface of the forearm above which a cuff is inflated to 40 mm Hg (above venous pressure). Using a template, two parallel incisions are made and the incisions blotted with filter paper every 30 seconds until no further bleeding occurs. The time from incision to cessation of blood seepage is the template bleeding time. The Duke bleeding time is performed on the earlobe and has advantages for cardiac surgery because the earlobe is more accessible and less likely to be subjected to the peripheral vasoconstriction seen after hypothermia. However, because neither the width/depth of the incision nor the venous pressure can be controlled in the Duke bleeding time, the Ivy bleeding time is considered the superior test. Normal bleeding time is 4 to 10 minutes.

Numerous prospective blinded investigations have confirmed that bleeding time has little or no value in predicting excessive hemorrhage after cardiac surgery.[132,133] Even in

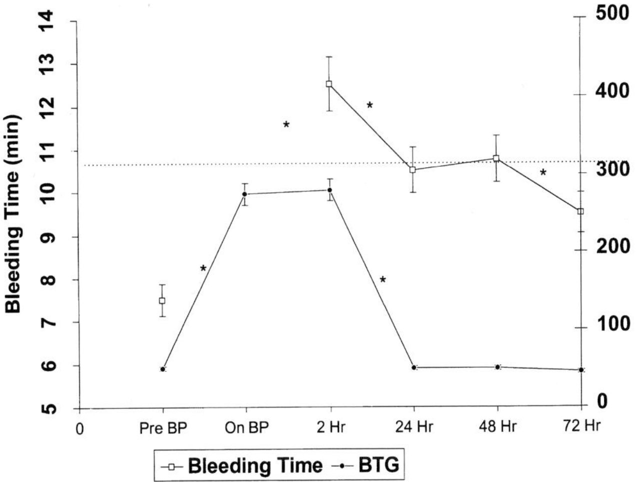

Figure 18–15 Bleeding time increases on cardiopulmonary bypass (CPB) and remains elevated until at least 72 hours postoperatively. However, platelet activation is maximal during CPB. The increase in β-thromboglobulin (BTG), indicating platelet activation, occurs upon initiation of CPB and returns to baseline by 24 hours afterward. *$P < 0.05$ change from previous value. (From Khuri SF, Wolfe JA, Josa M, et al: Hematologic changes during and after cardiopulmonary bypass and their relationship to the bleeding time and nonsurgical blood loss. J Thorac Cardiovasc Surg 104:94–107, 1992.)

patients receiving therapeutic doses of aspirin, an increase in bleeding time does not necessarily translate into an increase in mediastinal tube drainage or transfusions if reinfusion and blood conservation techniques are used aggressively. There is substantial evidence that platelet-directed therapy in the form of platelet transfusions or desmopressin acetate shortens a prolonged bleeding time in patients with clinical hemorrhage.[134,135] In a study of 85 patients undergoing CPB, Khuri et al[123] demonstrated that bleeding time becomes abnormally elevated during CPB and does not return to baseline even by 72 hours postoperatively, whereas markers of platelet activation return to baseline by 24 hours postoperatively (Fig. 18–15). Because the bleeding time does not follow the temporal course of postoperative coagulopathy, the bleeding time may be a nonspecific and impractical test for detecting an existing platelet defect but may be suitable for following patient response to platelet-directed therapies.

Aggregometry

Activated platelets undergo aggregation, which is initially a reversible process. Activation also induces the release of substances from alpha and dense platelet granules and platelet lysosomes. Because platelet granules contain many platelet agonists, the release of granular contents further stimulates platelet activation and is responsible for the secondary phase of platelet aggregation. This secondary phase of platelet aggregation is dependent on the release of thromboxane and other substances from the platelet granules, is an energy-consuming process, and is irreversible (Table 18–2).

Aggregometry is a useful research tool for measuring platelet responsiveness to a variety of different agonists. The end result, platelet aggregation, is an objective measure of platelet activation. Platelet aggregometry uses a photo-optical instrument to measure light transmittance through a sample of whole blood or platelet-rich plasma. Platelet-rich plasma undergoes a decrease in light transmittance on the early phase of platelet activation due to the change in platelet shape from

Table 18–2 Platelet Adhesion and Aggregation

Ligand	Receptor	Properties
Collagen	GP Ia/IIa, GP IIb/IIIa, GP IV	Adhesion, aggregation, secretion
Thrombospondin	GP IV, $\alpha_v\beta_3$	Adhesion, antiadhesion
vWF	GP Ib/IX, GP IIb/IIIa	Adhesion
Fibrinogen	GP IIb/IIIa	Aggregation
Laminin	GP Ic/IIa	Attachment
Vitronectin	$\alpha_v\beta_3$, GP IIb/IIIa	$\alpha_v\beta_3$ = vitronectin receptor
Fibronectin	GP Ic/IIa, GP IIb/IIIa	Attachment, spreading

GP = glycoprotein; vWF = von Willebrand factor.

discoid to spherical. When exposed to a platelet agonist such as thrombin, adenosine diphosphate (ADP), epinephrine, collagen, or ristocetin, the initial reversible aggregation phase results in increased light transmittance due to the platelet aggregates that decrease the turbidity of the sample. The larger the platelet aggregates, the greater is the transmittance of light. In the absence of further activation, disaggregation occurs and the plasma sample becomes turbid. However, when the platelet release reaction occurs, thromboxane and other activators are released from the platelet alpha granules and the phase of secondary, or irreversible, aggregation occurs. This results in a further increase in light transmittance.

Defects in platelet aggregation can be seen in patients with storage pool deficiency, Bernard-Soulier syndrome, or Glanzmann's thrombasthenia and in patients taking salicylates. Impaired platelet aggregation has been demonstrated to occur after extracorporeal circulation, but investigators have had difficulty showing a correlation between impaired aggregation and clinical bleeding.[136,137] One ex vivo study demonstrated a significant correlation between platelet aggregation and 3-hour postoperative bleeding; however, correlations were highest when preoperative aggregometry was performed using whole blood samples and when postoperative measurements were performed using platelet-rich plasma.[137] The assessment of the platelet defect induced by aspirin consumption is more sensitive when whole blood aggregometry is performed. The extreme sensitivity of this assay to minor defects in platelet function has resulted in a high negative predictive value but a rather low positive predictive value for bleeding. Its inability to be easily performed in the clinical arena has designated platelet aggregometry as strictly a research tool with occasional clinical applications.

Platelet-Mediated Force Transduction

An instrument that measures the force developed by platelets during clot retraction has been shown to be directly related to platelet concentration and function[138] (Hemodyne). The apparatus consists of a cup and a parallel upper plate. The cup is filled with blood or the platelet-containing solution, and the upper plate is lowered onto the clotting solution. Clot forms and adheres to the outer edges of the cup and to the plate above. A thin layer of oil is deposited onto the surfaces that are exposed to air. The upper plate is coupled to a displacement transducer that translates displacement due to platelet retraction into a force. Normal values for platelet force development have been suggested by the investigators.[63] The antiplatelet effects of heparin have been evaluated using this force retractometer. Using this instrument, investigators have shown that high heparin concentrations completely abolish platelet force generation.[61] Furthermore, the concentration of protamine required to reverse the anticoagulant effects of heparin is not sufficient to reverse these antiplatelet effects. The antiplatelet effects of protamine alone have also been evaluated using this monitor.

Fluorescence Flow Cytometry

The introduction of fluorescence flow cytometry into the clinical laboratory has provided a sensitive and specific means for assessing etiologies of platelet dysfunction. Disadvantages of the in vitro assays, such as shear-induced stress and clot retraction measurements, are that they represent nonspecific markers of platelet defects. The measure of specific serum markers of platelet activation, such as β-thromboglobulin and PF4, can be performed; however, plasma collection techniques for these tests are very cumbersome and the assays are often affected by other metabolic functions. Aggregometry is only a semiquantitative process and requires a high concentration of platelets for its optimal performance.

Flow cytometry is ideal for the detection of low concentrations of specific proteins within a large population of cells. These proteins may either be static portions of the platelet surface or dynamic products of platelet activation. The platelet release reaction enables specific integrin proteins, which are a part of the platelet alpha granule membrane, to incorporate themselves into the platelet surface membrane through a mechanism analogous to exocytosis. A portion of the GP IIb/IIIa receptor is also a protein of the alpha granule membrane that becomes exposed on the surface membrane of the platelet in response to platelet activation. Flow cytometry allows for the detection and quantification of many of these surface membrane constituents as a result of immunofluorescent innovations.[139]

Flow cytometry techniques have been enhanced by the development of specific monoclonal antibodies, which recognize antigens on the platelet (or white blood cell) surface. Antibodies developed are so specific that different ligand binding sites can be measured on the same GP IIb/IIIa molecule that characterizes different phases of receptor activation. Some of the epitopes for which monoclonal antibodies have been developed include PADGEM and GMP-140 (markers of platelet activation), the activated GP IIb/IIIa complex, and the GP Ib receptor.[140-142] A large number of monoclonal antibodies are available for identification of specific platelet ligand-binding sites (Table 18–3). Antibodies that bind specifically to

Table 18–3 **Monoclonal Antibodies to Platelet Antigens**

Antibody Binding Site (Other Name)	Antibodies Available	Requirement for Binding/Functional Activity
GP Ib (CD42b)	AP-1; 6D1	von Willebrand receptor; platelet adhesion
GP IX	FMC25	Platelet adhesion to endothelium
GP IIb/IIIa complex (αIIBβ3, CD41)	7E3; 10E5; 4F10; A2A9	Fibrinogen receptor; platelet aggregation
GP IIb/IIIa (αIIBβ3, CD41a)	PAC1	Active conformation of GPIIb/IIIa only
Fibrinogen	2G5; 9F9	Receptor-induced changes due to bound fibrinogen
GP IIb heavy chain of GP IIb/IIIa	P2; PMI-1	Ligand-induced changes in GP IIb
IIIa portion of GP IIb/IIIa		
(CD61)	AP6; Ab15; Y2/51	Receptor bound by fibrinogen
GMP140 (CD62P, PADGEM, P-selectin)	S12; KC4; VH10	Alpha granule membrane protein, mediates platelet-leukocyte interactions
LAMP-1 (CD63)	CLB-gran/12; H5G11	Lysosome membrane protein, expressed after platelet secretion
40-kDa protein	D495	Dense granule membrane protein
Thrombospondin	P8	Bound thrombospondin
Factor VIIIa light chain	1B3	Present on a procoagulant surface
Factor Va light chain	V237	Present on a procoagulant surface

GP = glycoprotein.

activated platelets but minimally to unstimulated platelets are referred to as *activation dependent*. In utilizing activation-dependent monoclonal antibodies, flow cytometry measures the platelet reactivity or response to the addition of platelet agonists. The technique of flow cytometry can be performed using whole blood or platelet-rich plasma. The fluorescent-labeled monoclonal antibody directed against a specific platelet membrane protein is quantified by the flow cytometer, which is an instrument equipped with a laser or a light source of a specific excitation wavelength. Light scatter data are collected that help to differentiate platelets from other cellular particles. Fluorescent antibody detection is expressed as percent of the total number of particles or as fluorescence intensity.

The ability to specifically identify platelet defects by fluorescence flow cytometry has greatly aided in the characterization of hematologic disease states such as the Bernard-Soulier syndrome and Glanzmann's thrombasthenia.[143,144] In the cardiac surgical arena, flow cytometry has aided in diagnosing the disorders of platelet function induced by CPB and protamine administration.[62,130,145,146] Kestin et al[126] used flow cytometric techniques to study the effects of CPB on the in vivo time-dependent upregulation of P-selectin in blood emerging from a bleeding wound. They showed that P-selectin expression is depressed after heparinization and during CPB and recovers at approximately 2 hours after the conclusion of CPB. In contrast, in vitro activation of CPB blood with the platelet agonist phorbol myristate acetate did not reveal this depression of P-selectin expression at any time point. Using another platelet activator (thrombin receptor agonist peptide) and flow cytometry, others did not demonstrate depression of P-selectin expression early in CPB but did so after 90 minutes of CPB and after protamine administration.[147]

Much uncertainty still exists regarding GP Ib receptor modulation in response to CPB. Using flow cytometry, George et al[139] found a modest reduction in platelet surface GP Ib during CPB. However, a subsequent study by van Oeveren et al[2] confirming a reduction in GP Ib subjected the platelets to centrifugation and processing techniques that may have induced in vitro artifactual platelet activation. Kestin et al[126] used monoclonal antibodies to many epitopes expressed on GP Ib and concluded that expression of this receptor is not reduced during CPB.

As a result of the many monoclonal antibodies directed at specific epitopes on the GP IIb/IIIa receptor, investigations into the dynamics of this receptor during CPB have yielded variable results. Some studies have confirmed modest reductions in the expression of GP IIb/IIIa, although not all have used whole blood techniques. Rinder et al,[145] using a whole blood technique, demonstrated a small decrease in GP IIb/IIIa expression. Monoclonal antibodies are available that bind to the GP IIb/IIIa fibrinogen binding site, and others are available that recognize receptor-bound fibrinogen. Flow cytometric techniques have also helped to characterize the mechanisms of action of several pharmacologic agents that have shown hemostatic potential in the perioperative period.[62]

BEDSIDE PLATELET FUNCTION TESTING

Viscoelastic Tests: Thromboelastography and Sonoclot

It was the late nineteenth century when investigators first began to explore the possibility that viscoelastic tests of blood might yield information regarding coagulation status. The changes that occur in the viscosity of blood as it clots could be studied and measured, and this information would certainly reflect certain aspects of coagulation function. During the early part of the twentieth century, many primitive viscometers were developed that use the basic mechanisms and principles upon which modern viscoelastic tests are based.

Thromboelastography

The coaguloviscometers that were developed in the 1920s formed the basis of viscoelastic coagulation testing that is now

Table 18–4 **Mechanisms of Point-of-Care Platelet Function Monitors**

Instrument	Mechanism	Agonist	Clinical Utility
Thromboelastograph[150]	Viscoelastic	Thrombin (native), ADP, arachidonic acid	Post-CPB, liver transplant, pediatric, obstetrics, drug efficacy
Sonoclot[167]	Viscoelastic	Thrombin (native)	Post-CPB, liver transplant
Hemostatus[134]	ACT reduction	PAF	Post-CPB, DDAVP, transfusion algorithm
PlateletWorks[183]	Platelet count ratio	ADP, collagen	Post-CPB, ?drug therapy
PFA-100[184]	In vitro bleeding time	ADP, epinephrine	vWD, congenital disorder, aspirin therapy, ?post-CPB
Ultegra[185]	Agglutination	TRAP, ADP	GP IIb/IIIa receptor blockade therapy, drug therapy, ?post-CPB
Clot Signature Analyzer[186]	Shear-induced in vitro bleeding time	Collagen (one channel only)	Post-CPB, drug effects
Whole blood aggregometry[137]	Electrical impedance	Multiple	Post-CPB

CPB = cardiopulmonary bypass; ACT = activated clotting time; PAF = platelet-activating factor; DDAVP = desmopressin; VWD = von Willebrand's disease; TRAP = thrombin receptor agonist peptide; GP = glycoprotein.

known as thromboelastography. Thromboelastography in its current form was developed by Hartert in 1948 and has been used in many different clinical scenarios to diagnose coagulation abnormalities.[148-150] Although not yet truly portable, the thromboelastograph (TEG; Haemoscope, Skokie, IL) can be performed "on site" either in the operating room or in a laboratory and provides a rapid whole blood analysis that yields information about clot formation and clot dissolution (Table 18–4). Within minutes, information is obtained regarding the integrity of the coagulation cascade, platelet function, platelet-fibrin interactions, and fibrinolysis. The principle is as follows: Whole blood (0.36 mL) is placed into a plastic cuvette into which a plastic pin is suspended; this plastic pin is attached to a torsion wire that is coupled to an amplifier and recorded; a thin layer of oil is added to the surface of the blood to prevent drying of the specimen; and the cuvette oscillates through an arc of 4 degrees, 45 minutes at 37°C. When the blood is liquid, movement of the cuvette does not affect the pin. However, as clot begins to form, the pin becomes coupled to the motion of the cuvette and the torsion wire generates a signal that is recorded. The recorded tracing can be stored by computer, and the parameters of interest are calculated using a simple software package. Alternatively, the tracing can be generated on line with a recording speed of 2 mm/min. The tracing generated has a characteristic conformation that is the signature of the TEG (Fig. 18–16).

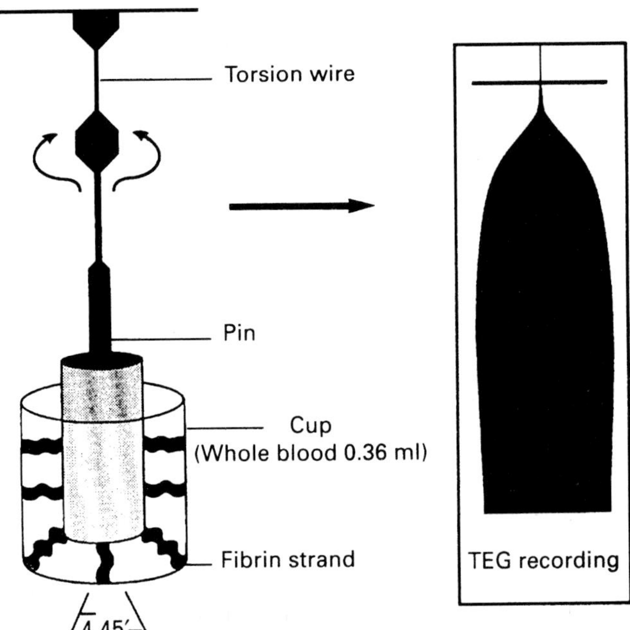

Figure 18–16 Schematic diagram of the thromboelastograph instrumentation *(left)* and a sample tracing *(right)*. A whole blood sample is placed into the cup into which a plastic pin is suspended. This plastic pin is attached to a torsion wire that is coupled to an amplifier and recorder. See text for details. (From Mallett SV, Cox DJA: Thromboelastography. Br J Anaesth 69:307–313, 1992.)

The specific parameters measured by the TEG include the reaction time (R value), coagulation time (K value), a angle, maximal amplitude (MA), amplitude 60 minutes after the maximal amplitude (A60), and clot lysis indices at 30 and 60 minutes after MA (LY30 and LY60, respectively). The reaction time, R, represents the time for initial fibrin formation and is a measure of the intrinsic coagulation pathway, the extrinsic coagulation pathway, and the final common pathway. R is measured from the start of the bioassay until fibrin begins to form and the amplitude of the tracing is 2 mm. Normal values vary depending on the type of activator used and range from 7 to 14 minutes using celite activator and are as short as 1 to 3 minutes using tissue factor activator. The K value is a measure of the speed of clot formation and is measured from the end of the R time to the time that the amplitude reaches 20 mm. Normal values (3 to 6 minutes) also vary with the type of activators used. The a angle, another index of speed of clot formation, is the angle formed between the horizontal axis of the tracing and the tangent to the tracing at 20-mm amplitude. Alpha values normally range from 45 to 55 degrees. Because both the K value and the a angle are measures of the speed of clot strengthening, each is improved by high levels of functional fibrinogen. MA (normal is 50 to 60 mm) is an index of clot strength as determined by platelet function, the cross-linkage of fibrin, and the interactions of platelets with polymerizing fibrin. The peak strength of the clot, or the shear elastic modulus "G," has a curvilinear relation with MA and is defined as G = (5000 • MA)/(96 – MA). The percent reduc-

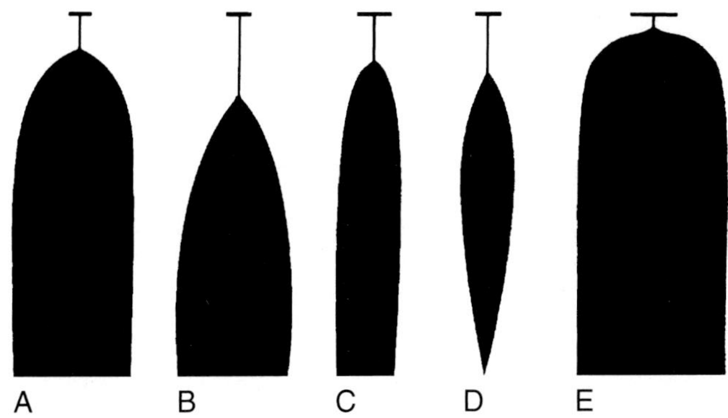

Figure 18–17 Signature thromboelastograph tracings. Tracing identification from left to right. A = normal; B = coagulation factor deficiency; C = platelet dysfunction or deficiency; D = fibrinolysis; E = hypercoagulability. (From Mallett SV, Cox DJA: Thromboelastography. Br J Anaesth 69:307–313, 1992.)

tion in MA after 30 minutes reflects the fibrinolytic activity present and is normally not more than 7.5%.

Characteristic TEG tracings can be recognized to be indicative of particular coagulation defects. A prolonged R value indicates a deficiency in coagulation factor activity or level and is seen typically in patients with liver disease and in patients on anticoagulants such as Coumadin or heparin. MA and a angle are reduced in states associated with platelet dysfunction or thrombocytopenia and are even further reduced in the presence of a fibrinogen defect. LY 30, or the lysis index at 30 minutes after MA, is increased in conjunction with fibrinolysis. These particular signature tracings are depicted in Figure 18–17.

TEG is a useful tool for diagnosing and treating perioperative coagulopathy in patients undergoing cardiac surgical procedures due to a variety of potential coagulation defects that may exist.[149] Within 15 to 30 minutes, on-site information is available regarding the integrity of the coagulation system, the platelet function, fibrinogen function, and fibrinolysis.[150] With the addition of heparinase, TEG can be performed during CPB and can provide valuable and timely information regarding coagulation status.[151] Because TEG is a viscoelastic test and evaluates whole blood hemostasis interactions, it is suggested that TEG is a more accurate predictor of postoperative hemorrhage than routine coagulation tests that analyze individual components of the hemostasis system. A number of clinical trials have confirmed that in cardiac surgical patients TEG has a greater predictive value and greater specificity than routine coagulation tests for diagnosing patients known as "bleeders."[152] Tuman et al[150] studied 42 patients, of whom 9 were classified as bleeders. A routine coagulation screen consisting of ACT, PT, aPTT, and platelet count had only a 33% accuracy for predicting bleeding, whereas TEG and Sonoclot (Sienco Inc, Morrison, CO) (another viscoelastic test) had 88% and 74% accuracy, respectively. Mongan and Hosking[153] also found that TEG abnormalities predict postoperative bleeding and, using TEG parameters, they were also able to identify a population of patients who respond to therapy with desmopressin acetate. In a prospective study of 16-hour postoperative blood loss, Gravlee et al[154] reported on 897 cardiac surgical patients in whom routine coagulation tests were measured immediately upon heparin reversal in the operating room. The weak correlations and poor predictive values of these tests confirm that these tests perform poorly as predictors of bleeding. TEG was not studied in this trial.

In a large retrospective evaluation in more than 1000 patients, Spiess et al[155] found that the institution of a transfusion algorithm using TEG resulted in a significant reduction in the incidence of mediastinal exploration and in the rate of transfusion of allogeneic blood products. Because of its ease of use and application at the bedside, TEG has been used in many research settings to assess drug effects on platelet function and clot strength.[156,157] Information from the TEG has also been used to guide clinical decision making during orthotopic liver transplantation, obstetric procedures, and vascular surgical procedures.[157-160]

Thromboelastography Modifications

TEG was originally performed using recalcified citrated whole blood or celite activator. The addition of recombinant human tissue factor as an activator can be used to accelerate the rate of thrombin formation and thus the formation of fibrin.[161] This serves to shorten the time required for development of the MA. Because the MA is primarily reflective of clot strength and platelet function, this information can be obtained more quickly with tissue factor enhancement. The recombinant tissue factor is a thromboplastin agent and is available from a number of manufacturers.

An application of thromboelastography in the clinical arena is its use in monitoring GP IIb/IIIa receptor blockade and ADP receptor blockade in patients treated with specific antiplatelet agents. TEG with tissue factor acceleration speeds the appearance of MA and is accurate for monitoring the platelet inhibition by large concentrations of GP IIb/IIIa receptor blockers. Using this technique with platelet-rich plasma, the reduction of the MA has been used as an index of platelet inhibition by GP IIb/IIIa receptor blockers in the catheterization laboratory.[160] Comparison with the baseline MA yields a relative measure of the degree of platelet inhibition. Thrombin receptor agonist peptide (TRAP)–induced aggregation correlates strongly with the TEG values measured in this fashion.[160]

Because the MA is a function of the platelet–fibrinogen interaction, a reduction in the MA can be accomplished by the addition of potent GP IIb/IIIa receptor blockade to the assay. The resultant MA, in the presence of excessively high GP IIb/IIIa receptor blockade, is primarily due to the fibrinogen concentration and the strength of fibrin alone. This value (called Ma_f) correlates strongly with plasma fibrinogen concentration.[162,163]

The thienopyridine ADP-receptor blockers, clopidogrel and ticlopidine, are widely used in cardiovascular medicine. The ability to measure the platelet defect induced by these drugs is very difficult unless sophisticated laboratory techniques such as ADP-aggregometry are used. Aggregometry yields accurate results; however, it is not readily available in the perioperative period as a point-of-care test. Native TEG analysis does not measure the thienopyridine-induced platelet defect because the formation of thrombin in the assay has an overwhelming effect on the development of the TEG MA. A modification of the TEG removes thrombin from the assay and studies a nonthrombin clot, strengthened by the addition of ADP. Figure 18–18 depicts the different signature TEG tracings that are used to calculate the platelet contribution to MA when a platelet inhibitor is present. This assay was specifically created to measure the platelet inhibition by ADP antagonists

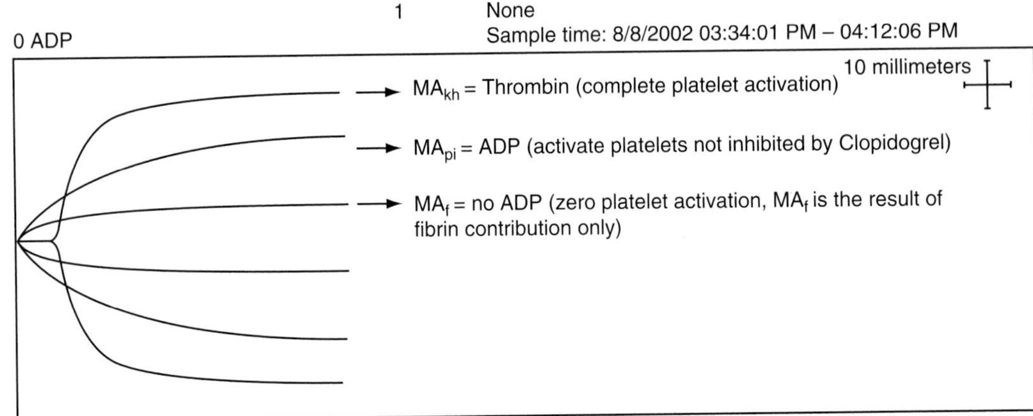

Figure 18–18 Thromboelastograph tracings using the modification to measure platelet inhibition by the thienopyridine drugs clopidogrel or ticlopidine. The measurements made are the maximal amplitude allowing thrombin activation of platelets (MA_{kh}). This is the standard kaolin-activated MA. Also measured is the maximal amplitude measuring only the fibrinogen component of MA (MA_f) using a fibrinogen activator, and the maximal amplitude measuring the platelet contribution to MA by platelets able to be activated by ADP (MA_{pi}). This is using a fibrinogen activator plus ADP. Only platelets that are responsive to ADP will contribute to the MA_{pi}.

such as clopidogrel and is referred to as the platelet mapping assay. The MA_{kh} is the maximal activation of platelets and fibrin and is the largest amplitude that can be achieved. The MA_f is the maximal amplitude that is obtained when a thrombin-depleted fibrin clot is formed without a platelet contribution. The MA_{pi} is the MA_f contribution plus the platelet contribution. MA_{pi} is created by adding an activator such as ADP to the MA_f assay (for clopidogrel testing). Only platelets that can be activated by ADP contribute to the MA_{pi}. The following formula calculates the percent reduction in platelet activity using this assay.

$$100 - [(MA_{pi} - MA_f)/(MA_{kh} - MA_f)] \times 100$$

Clopidogrel, ticlopidine, and even aspirin inhibition can now be studied at the point-of-care using this modification.[164,165]

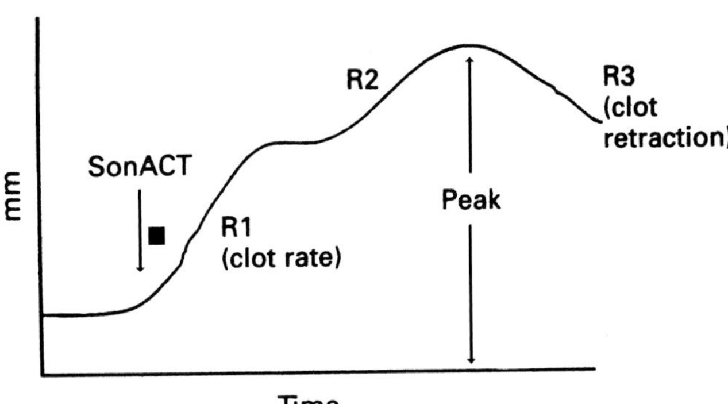

Figure 18–19 The normal Sonoclot tracing. See text for details. (From Hett DA, Walker D, Pilkington SN, Smith DC: Sonoclot analysis. Br J Anaesth 75:771–776, 1995. BMJ Publishing Group.)

Sonoclot

Another test of viscoelastic properties of blood is the Sonoclot. In 1975, von Kaulla introduced the Sonoclot, which is a coagulation analyzer that measures the changing impedance on an ultrasonic probe that is immersed in a coagulating blood sample.[166] The machine consists of a plastic disposable probe mounted on an ultrasonic transducer that vibrates vertically at 200 Hz. The probe is immersed to a standard depth into 0.4 mL of whole blood or plasma. The fluid exerts a force, or resistance, on the probe, which does not allow it to vibrate freely, and when the sample begins to clot, fibrin strands form on the tip of the probe and further increase the resistance. The electronic mechanism that drives the probe's vibration also acts as a transducer and measures the impedance to vibration and subsequently converts it to a signal on paper. This signature of the Sonoclot reflects coagulation in real time, from the start of fibrin formation, to fibrin cross-linkage, platelet-mediated clot strengthening, and eventually to clot retraction and fibrinolysis.

Immersion of the probe into the blood sample causes an initial increase in the signal due to the increased impedance to vibration by fluid relative to air. The onset time is the time for initial fibrin formation and is defined as the time taken to reach an amplitude of 1 mm. This time has also been referred to as the SonACT (Fig. 18–19). Further increase in the signal occurs due to an increased rate of fibrinogen conversion to fibrin. The rate of rise of this first peak (R1) is expressed as the percentage of the peak amplitude per unit time (normal values 18% to 45%). After R1, there is a shoulder or a dip before the rise in amplitude that characterizes R2. This shoulder is a result of the action of platelets and fibrin in producing clot retraction. As the clot retracts from the walls of the cuvette, the impedance to vibration briefly decreases. As fibrinogen converts to fibrin, and fibrin polymerizes, the speed of clot formation and the platelet–fibrin interactions are reflected by the slope R2, the second wave. In the presence of higher concentrations of fibrinogen, a larger clot mass is represented by a greater amplitude of the R2 wave due to a greater impedance to vibration. The amplitude of the peak of R2 is therefore related to the concentration of normal functional fibrinogen. The subsequent downward slope, R3, occurs as a result of platelet-mediated clot retraction that causes plasma expulsion and clot size diminution, thus a lower impedance. The magnitude of the R3 drop is reflective of platelet number and function. Figure 18–19 demonstrates the normal Sonoclot tracing. Figure 18–20 depicts a tracing in a patient with dysfunctional or deficient fibrinogen levels. When fibrinolysis occurs, the signal decreases even further to baseline values. The time for fibrinolysis to occur varies with each sample and

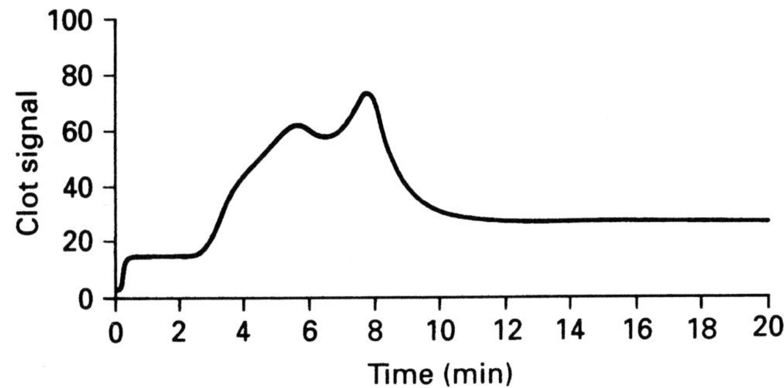

Figure 18–20 Sonoclot tracing in a patient with fibrinogen deficiency. In the presence of lower concentrations of fibrinogen, a smaller clot mass is represented by a smaller amplitude of the R2 wave due to less impedance to vibration. The amplitude of the peak of R2 is therefore directly related to the concentration of normal functional fibrinogen. (From Hett DA, Walker D, Pilkington SN, Smith DC: Sonoclot analysis. Br J Anaesth 75:771–776, 1995. BMJ Publishing Group.)

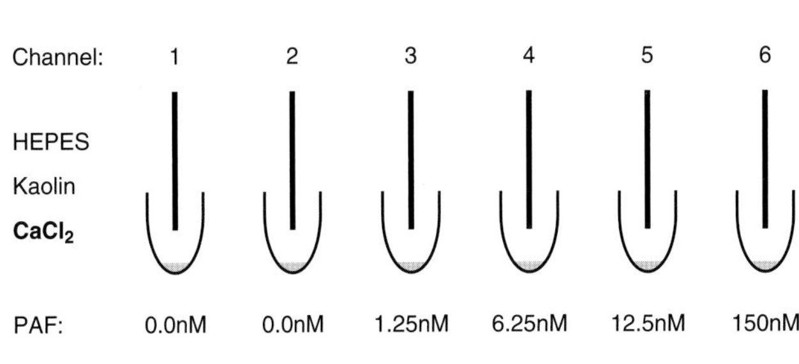

$$\text{clot ratio}(\%) = \frac{1 - \dfrac{ACT_n}{ACT_{\overline{1+2}}}}{0.51}$$

Figure 18–21 Schematic diagram of the HemoSTATUS measurement of platelet function. A specific cartridge placed into a Hepcon machine measures the reduction in the activated clotting time as a result of the addition of increasing amounts of platelet-activating factor. See text for further details. ACT = activated coagulation time; ACT_n = ACT of selected channel number; ACT_{1+2} = ACT average of channels 1 and 2.

is usually seen on Sonoclot analysis only if a patient has accelerated fibrinolysis.

Sonoclot and TEG have been studied in the surgical arena because of their ability to measure viscoelastic properties of coagulation and their on-site applications. Tuman et al[150] found an accuracy of 74% using Sonoclot and an accuracy of 88% using TEG to predict bleeding after cardiac surgery. The reason that viscoelastic tests have been able to predict bleeding so successfully probably relates to their ability to measure platelet function, a major determinant of postoperative hemostasis.[167] Significant correlations have been documented between specific Sonoclot parameters and platelet count and coagulation factor assays. This reproducibility has allowed the use of Sonoclot to also predict and successfully treat coagulation abnormalities in patients undergoing liver transplantation.[168] Like the TEG, Sonoclot is also useful in the diagnosis of hypercoagulable states.[169]

A direct comparison of TEG with Sonoclot is not likely to reveal a significant advantage of one test over the other because both tests measure the dynamic process of hemostasis by transducing the impedance changes that occur as blood clots. Both tests are easy to perform, can be performed on whole blood, and can be conveniently located in the operating room. Tuman et al[150] did not document a statistical difference between these two tests in clinical accuracy; however, they did show the viscoelastic tests to be superior to routine plasma coagulation testing. Sonoclot may provide coagulation information earlier since the initial deflection occurs when the first fibrin strands are forming. However, both TEG and Sonoclot accurately reflect the platelet-fibrin interactions required for clot formation.

Tests of Platelet Response to Agonist

HemoSTATUS

Despite the introduction of numerous point-of-care coagulation analyzers that allow for rapid determination of a patient's coagulation status, the qualitative measure of platelet function, at the bedside, remains an elusive challenge. HemoSTATUS (Medtronic Inc, Parker, CO) is a point-of-care platelet function assay that uses the Hepcon monitoring system to measure platelet reactivity. A six-channel cartridge measures the heparinized kaolin-activated ACT without platelet activator (channels 1 and 2), and with incrementally increasing doses of platelet-activating factor [PAF] (channels 3 to 6). The ACT of the PAF-activated channels will be shortened due to the ability of activated platelets to speed coagulation. The respective doses of PAF in channels 3 through 6 are 1.25, 6.25, 12.5, and 150 nmol/L. For each of channels 3 through 6, the degree of shortening of the ACT as a ratio to the ACT without PAF is the "clot ratio" and is calculated as $1 - (ACT_{activated}/ACT_{control})$. The "maximal" clot ratio is the clot ratio for channel 6 that was derived using blood from normal volunteers (Fig. 18–21). A comparison of the patient clot ratio to the maximal clot ratio (derived from normal volunteers) yields a comparative measure of platelet function, termed the *percent of maximal platelet function*.

The potential ability to measure the qualitative function of platelets using a point-of-care assay provides innumerable advantages for clinicians caring for cardiac surgical patients. Platelet dysfunction is one of the more common hemostasis defects incurred during CPB, yet it is difficult to specifically measure platelet function rapidly and at the bedside. Viscoelastic tests conveniently measure platelet function, but their use in transfusion algorithms is limited by a lack of specificity to the measure of platelet dysfunction. Transfusion algorithms like the one published by Despotis et al,[84] which have been suggested to result in reduced transfusions in cardiac surgical patients, have incorporated only the measure of platelet number, because the on-site ability to measure platelet function has been so elusive. Inclusion of a measure of platelet function into a transfusion algorithm would potentially reduce allogeneic transfusions even further.

An initial investigation of HemoSTATUS in cardiac surgical patients was performed by Despotis et al.[134] The authors studied 150 patients and conducted multivariate analyses to evaluate the relationship between postoperative blood loss and multiple demographic, operative, and hemostatic measurements. They demonstrated a significant correlation between HemoSTATUS measurements upon arrival in the intensive care unit (ICU) and 4-hour postoperative mediastinal tube drainage ($r = -0.85$, channel 5; $r = -0.82$, channel 6). Using receiver operating characteristic (ROC) curves for the detection of excessive mediastinal tube drainage, the accuracy of a number of hemostasis assays was measured. The highest predictability for bleeding was found in both the channel 5 clot ratio and the bleeding time. The PT, aPTT, and platelet count had much lower predictive value. HemoSTATUS-derived clot ratios also had the capability to detect enhanced platelet function after the administration of pharmacologic platelet therapy (desmopressin acetate) and after the transfusion of platelet concentrates. Subsequent investigations in cardiac surgical patients have confirmed a significant yet weak correlation of HemoSTATUS with postoperative bleeding but have not found this test to be superior to TEG or routine coagulation tests in its predictive value.[152]

Validation studies have been performed to compare the assessment of platelet reactivity using HemoSTATUS to that measured by fluorescence flow cytometry. Using each patient's baseline platelet function as the control, the percent reduction in platelet function at multiple time points during cardiac surgery was compared using the two methodologies. Both tests reflected a similar degree of platelet dysfunction at the time points 90 minutes into CPB, after protamine, and at ICU arrival. Differences in the type of assay and the type of platelet activators used (thrombin peptide versus PAF) may have accounted for the inability of the tests to correlate with each other at all of the time points studied.[147]

Other Platelet Function Tests

Ultegra (Accumetrics, San Diego, CA), or "rapid platelet function assay," is a point-of-care monitor designed specifically to measure the platelet response to a thrombin-receptor-agonist peptide (TRAP). This technology was approved by the U.S. Food and Drug administration for use as a platelet function assay. In whole blood, it measures TRAP activation-induced platelet agglutination of fibrinogen-coated beads using an optical detection system. Because of the importance of the GP IIb/IIIa receptor in mediating fibrinogen–platelet interactions, the Ultegra has been especially useful in accurately measuring receptor inhibition in the invasive cardiology patients receiving GP IIb/IIIa–inhibiting drugs.[170-172]

The Hemostatometer has been more recently renamed the Clot Signature Analyzer (CSA; Xylum, Scarsdale, NY). Whole blood is maintained under a constant driving pressure of 60 mm Hg as it is forced out into a synthetic vessel. The pressure distally in the vessel is monitored. The tubing of this synthetic vessel is perforated and the distal pressure drop is measured. The time to restoration of this distal pressure will be a function of development of a platelet plug. Thus the time for initial closure is a measure of platelet function. A subsequent time is measured and that is the time to complete pressure loss due to complete vessel occlusion. This clot is the result of coagulation and clot formation, and the time to the second pressure drop is reflective of coagulation function. Another chamber of this device contains a collagen-coated fibril upon which platelets adhere and form a plug. A similar pressure measurement technique indicates the formation of a platelet thrombus. This point-of-care assay has been used to measure platelet reactivity in high-risk patients with atherosclerotic coronary artery disease.[173-175] However, in cardiac surgical patients, preoperative platelet reactivity did not have predictive accuracy for bleeding.[176] Data evaluating the CSA in the postoperative period to predict bleeding are lacking.

The Platelet Function Analyzer (PFA-100) (Dade Behring, Miami, FL) is a monitor of platelet adhesive capacity that is currently approved by the Food and Drug Administration and is valuable in its diagnostic abilities to identify drug-induced platelet abnormalities, platelet dysfunction of von Willebrand's disease, and other acquired and congenital platelet defects.[177,178] The test is conducted as a modified in vitro bleeding time. Whole blood is drawn through a chamber by vacuum and is perfused across an aperture in a collagen membrane coated with an agonist (epinephrine or ADP). Platelet adhesion and formation of aggregates seal the aperture, thus indicating the "closure time" measured by the PFA-100.[179,180] In cardiac surgical patients, the preoperative PFA-100 closure time significantly correlated with postoperative blood loss ($r = 0.41$, $P = 0.022$).[181] However, preliminary evidence with post-CPB sampling and with in vitro addition of GP IIb/IIIa–inhibiting drugs suggests that these closure times may exceed those measurable using standard testing with the PFA-100.[182]

"Platelet Works" Ichor (Array Medical, Somerville, NJ) is a test that uses the principle of the platelet count ratio to assess platelet reactivity. The instrument is a Coulter counter that measures the platelet count in a standard EDTA-containing tube. Platelet count is also measured in tubes containing the platelet agonist ristocetin, ADP, epinephrine, collagen, or thrombin. Addition of blood to these agonist tubes causes platelets to activate, adhere to the tube, and be effectively eliminated from the platelet count. The ratio of the activated platelet count to the nonactivated platelet count is a function of the reactivity of the platelets. Early investigation in cardiac surgical patients indicates that this assay is useful in providing a platelet count and that it is capable of measuring the platelet dysfunction that accompanies CPB[183] (Box 18–6).

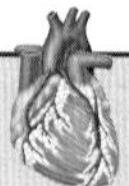

BOX 18–6 ***Platelet Function Tests***

- The appropriate test to measure platelet function depends on the suspected platelet defect.
- The TEG and the Hemostatus are useful to measure the post-CPB platelet defect. Ultegra is useful to measure the effects of GP IIb/IIIa receptor-blocker therapy.
- The PFA-100 is useful to measure the effects of aspirin on platelet adhesion.
- It is very important to understand the platelet defect being sought to accurately use the proper test.

SUMMARY

It is essential to understand the complex array of hemostatic insults that occur as a result of extracorporeal circulation before selecting an appropriate coagulation or hemostasis monitor during cardiac surgery. Preoperative, intraoperative, and postoperative testing may be mandated for patients in whom a coagulation defect may predispose to serious degrees of postoperative coagulopathy. Even in hemostatically normal individuals, CPB induces a heparin effect, platelet dysfunction, fibrinolysis, and coagulation factor defects for which there are many clinical laboratory tests available for accurate diagnoses. With the increase in prescriptions of antithrombotic platelet inhibitors, the hemostatic defect after CPB is even more pronounced.[184-186] This chapter has introduced the basic principles of hemostasis and the utility of many commonly used monitors for detecting disorders of the coagulation cascade, platelet function, and fibrinolysis. Additionally, an increased emphasis on health care economics has created a milieu in which patients have a rapid transit time through the cardiac operating room with minimal exposure to allogeneic blood products. Prophylactic measures such as heparin-bonded circuitry and antifibrinolytics have reduced the actual incidence of microvascular bleeding in this population. However, when microvascular bleeding does occur, rapid diagnosis and therapeutic intervention are made possible by point-of-care hemostasis testing, which can take place directly in the operating room. If on-site testing is not available or does not provide sufficient timely information regarding the patient's coagulation defect, transfusion therapy for cardiac surgical patients will remain indiscriminate and empiric, at best.

REFERENCES

1. Khuri SF, Valeri CR, Loscalzo J, et al: Heparin causes platelet dysfunction and induces fibrinolysis before cardiopulmonary bypass. Ann Thorac Surg 60:1008, 1995
2. van Oeveren W, Harder MP, Roozendaal KJ, et al: Aprotinin protects platelets against the initial effect of cardiopulmonary bypass. J Thorac Cardiovasc Surg 99:788, 1990; discussion 796, 1990
3. Marciniak E: Physiology of antithrombin III. Ric Clin Lab 14:475, 1984
4. Marciniak E, Gora-Maslak G: Enhancement by heparin of thrombin-induced antithrombin III proteolysis: Its relation to the molecular weight and anticoagulant activity of heparin. Thromb Res 28:411, 1982
5. Marciniak E, Romond EH: Catabolism and distribution of functionally heterogeneous human antithrombin III. J Lab Clin Med 109:89, 1987
6. Marciniak E: Thrombin-induced proteolysis of human antithrombin III: an outstanding contribution of heparin. Br J Haematol 48:325, 1981
7. Hashimoto K, Yamagishi M, Sasaki T, et al: Heparin and antithrombin III levels during cardiopulmonary bypass: Correlation with subclinical plasma coagulation. Ann Thorac Surg 58:799, 1994; discussion 804, 1994
8. Heller EL, Paul L: Anticoagulation management in a patient with an acquired antithrombin III deficiency. J Extra Corpor Technol 33:245, 2001
9. Teoh KH, Young E, Bradley CA, Hirsh J: Heparin binding proteins. Contribution to heparin rebound after cardiopulmonary bypass. Circulation 88:II-420, 1993
10. Jaberi M, Bell WR, Benson DW: Control of heparin therapy in open-heart surgery. J Thorac Cardiovasc Surg 67:133, 1974
11. Roth JA, Cukingnan RA, Scott CR: Use of activated coagulation time to monitor heparin during cardiac surgery. Ann Thorac Surg 28:69, 1979
12. Reich DL, Zahl K, Perucho MH, Thys DM: An evaluation of two activated clotting time monitors during cardiac surgery. J Clin Monit 8:33, 1992
13. Horkay F, Martin P, Rajah SM, Walker DR: Response to heparinization in adults and children undergoing cardiac operations. Ann Thorac Surg 53:822, 1992
14. Despotis GJ, Summerfield AL, Joist JH, et al: In vitro reversal of heparin effect with heparinase: Evaluation with whole blood prothrombin time and activated partial thromboplastin time in cardiac surgical patients. Anesth Analg 79:670, 1994
15. Jobes DR, Schwartz AJ, Ellison N, et al: Monitoring heparin anticoagulation and its neutralization. Ann Thorac Surg 31:161, 1981
16. Niinikoski J, Laato M, Laaksonen V, et al: Use of activated clotting time to monitor anticoagulation during cardiac surgery. Scand J Thorac Cardiovasc Surg 18:57, 1984
17. Babka R, Colby C, El-Etr A, Pifarre R: Monitoring of intraoperative heparinization and blood loss following cardiopulmonary bypass surgery. J Thorac Cardiovasc Surg 73:780, 1977
18. Culliford AT, Gitel SN, Starr N, et al: Lack of correlation between activated clotting time and plasma heparin during cardiopulmonary bypass. Ann Surg 193:105, 1981
19. Ammar T, Fisher CF, Sarier K, Coller BS: The effects of thrombocytopenia on the activated coagulation time. Anesth Analg 83:1185, 1996
20. Ammar T, Scudder LE, Coller BS: In vitro effects of the platelet glycoprotein IIb/IIIa receptor antagonist c7E3 Fab on the activated clotting time. Circulation 95:614, 1997
21. Bode AP, Lust RM: Masking of heparin activity in the activated coagulation time (ACT) by platelet procoagulant activity. Thromb Res 73:285, 1994
22. Gravlee GP, Whitaker CL, Mark LJ, et al: Baseline activated coagulation time should be measured after surgical incision. Anesth Analg 71:549, 1990
23. Mabry CD, Read RC, Thompson BW, et al: Identification of heparin resistance during cardiac and vascular surgery. Arch Surg 114:129, 1979
24. Andrew M, Ofosu F, Schmidt B, et al: Heparin clearance and ex vivo recovery in newborn piglets and adult pigs. Thromb Res 52:517, 1988
25. Andrew M, MacIntyre B, MacMillan J, et al: Heparin therapy during cardiopulmonary bypass in children requires ongoing quality control. Thromb Haemost 70:937, 1993
26. Young JA, Kisker CT, Doty DB: Adequate anticoagulation during cardiopulmonary bypass determined by activated clotting time and the appearance of fibrin monomer. Ann Thorac Surg 26:231, 1978
27. Metz S, Keats AS: Low activated coagulation time during cardiopulmonary bypass does not increase postoperative bleeding. Ann Thorac Surg 49:440, 1990
28. Cardoso PF, Yamazaki F, Keshavjee S, et al: A reevaluation of heparin requirements for cardiopulmonary bypass. J Thorac Cardiovasc Surg 101:153, 1991
29. Gravlee GP, Brauer SD, Roy RC, et al: Predicting the pharmacodynamics of heparin: A clinical evaluation of the Hepcon System 4. J Cardiothorac Anesth 1:379, 1987
30. Utley JR: Pathophysiology of cardiopulmonary bypass: current issues. J Card Surg 5:177, 1990
31. Young E, Prins M, Levine MN, Hirsh J: Heparin binding to plasma proteins, an important mechanism for heparin resistance. Thromb Haemost 67:639, 1992
32. Marciniak E, Gockerman JP: Heparin-induced decrease in circulating antithrombin-III. Lancet 2:581, 1977
33. Linden MD, Schneider M, Baker S, et al: Decreased concentration of antithrombin after preoperative therapeutic heparin does not cause heparin resistance during cardiopulmonary bypass. J Cardiothorac Vasc Anesth 18:131, 2004
34. Esposito RA, Culliford AT, Colvin SB, et al: Heparin resistance during cardiopulmonary bypass. The role of heparin pretreatment. J Thorac Cardiovasc Surg 85:346, 1983
35. Kanbak M: The treatment of heparin resistance with antithrombin III in cardiac surgery. Can J Anaesth 46:581, 1999
36. Lemmer JH Jr, Despotis GJ: Antithrombin III concentrate to treat heparin resistance in patients undergoing cardiac surgery. J Thorac Cardiovasc Surg 123:213, 2002
37. Levy JH, Montes F, Szlam F, Hillyer CD: The in vitro effects of antithrombin III on the activated coagulation time in patients on heparin therapy. Anesth Analg 90:1076, 2000
38. Nicholson SC, Keeling DM, Sinclair ME, Evans RD: Heparin pretreatment does not alter heparin requirements during cardiopulmonary bypass. Br J Anaesth 87:844, 2001
39. Warkentin TE, Kelton JG: Temporal aspects of heparin-induced thrombocytopenia. N Engl J Med 344, 2001
40. Warkentin TE, Greinacher A: Heparin-induced thrombocytopenia and cardiac surgery. Ann Thorac Surg 76:638, 2003
41. Mabry CD, Thompson BW, Read RC: Activated clotting time (ACT) monitoring of intraoperative heparinization in peripheral vascular surgery. Am J Surg 138:894, 1979
42. Bull BS, Huse WM, Brauer FS, Korpman RA: Heparin therapy during extracorporeal circulation. II. The use of a dose-response curve to individualize heparin and protamine dosage. J Thorac Cardiovasc Surg 69:685, 1975
43. Jobes DR, Aitken GL, Shaffer GW: Increased accuracy and precision of heparin and protamine dosing reduces blood loss and transfusion in patients undergoing primary cardiac operations. J Thorac Cardiovasc Surg 110:36, 1995
44. Shore-Lesserson L, Reich DL, DePerio M: Heparin and protamine titration do not improve haemostasis in cardiac surgical patients. Can J Anaesth 45:10, 1998
45. Szalados JE, Ouriel K, Shapiro JR: Use of the activated coagulation time and heparin dose-response curve for the determination of protamine dosage in vascular surgery. J Cardiothorac Vasc Anesth 8:515, 1994
46. Despotis GJ, Levine V, Joiner-Maier D, Joist JH: A comparison between continuous infusion versus standard bolus administration of heparin based on monitoring in cardiac surgery. Blood Coagul Fibrinolysis 8:419, 1997
47. Despotis GJ, Summerfield AL, Joist JH, et al: Comparison of activated coagulation time and whole blood heparin measurements with laboratory plasma anti-Xa heparin concentration in patients having cardiac operations. J Thorac Cardiovasc Surg 108:1076, 1994
48. Gravlee GP, Haddon WS, Rothberger HK, et al: Heparin dosing and monitoring for cardiopulmonary bypass. A comparison of techniques with measurement of subclinical plasma coagulation. J Thorac Cardiovasc Surg 99:518, 1990
49. Gravlee GP, Rogers AT, Dudas LM, et al: Heparin management protocol for cardiopulmonary bypass influences postoperative heparin rebound but not bleeding. Anesthesiology 76:393, 1992

50. Despotis GJ, Joist JH, Hogue CW Jr, et al: The impact of heparin concentration and activated clotting time monitoring on blood conservation. A prospective, randomized evaluation in patients undergoing cardiac operation. J Thorac Cardiovasc Surg 110:46, 1995
51. Wang JS, Lin CY, Karp RB: Comparison of high-dose thrombin time with activated clotting time for monitoring of anticoagulant effects of heparin in cardiac surgical patients. Anesth Analg 79:9, 1994
52. Wang JS, Lin CY, Hung WT, Karp RB: Monitoring of heparin-induced anticoagulation with kaolin-activated clotting time in cardiac surgical patients treated with aprotinin. Anesthesiology 77:1080, 1992
53. Dietrich W, Dilthey G, Spannagl M, et al: Influence of high-dose aprotinin on anticoagulation, heparin requirement, and celite- and kaolin-activated clotting time in heparin-pretreated patients undergoing open-heart surgery. A double-blind, placebo-controlled study. Anesthesiology 83:679, 1995; discussion 29A, 1995
54. Tabuchi N, Njo TL, Tigchelaar I, et al: Monitoring of anticoagulation in aprotinin-treated patients during heart operation. Ann Thorac Surg 58:774, 1994
55. Dercksen SJ, Linssen GH: Monitoring of blood coagulation in open heart surgery. II. Use of individualized dosages of heparin and protamine controlled by activated coagulation times. Acta Anaesthesiol Belg 31:121, 1980
56. Dercksen SJ, Linssen GH: Monitoring of blood coagulation in open heart surgery. I. Effects of conventional dosages of heparin and protamine. Acta Anaesthesiol Belg 31:113, 1980
57. Ellison N, Jobes DR, Schwartz AJ: Implications of anticoagulant therapy. Int Anesthesiol Clin 20:121, 1982
58. Jobes DR: Safety issues in heparin and protamine administration for extracorporeal circulation. J Cardiothorac Vasc Anesth 12:17, 1998
59. Habazettl H, Conzen PF, Vollmar B, et al: Effect of leukopenia on pulmonary hypertension after heparin-protamine in pigs. J Appl Physiol 73:44, 1992
60. Warkentin TE, Crowther MA: Reversing anticoagulants both old and new. Can J Anaesth 49:S11, 2002
61. Carr ME Jr, Carr SL: At high heparin concentrations, protamine concentrations which reverse heparin anticoagulant effects are insufficient to reverse heparin anti-platelet effects. Thromb Res 75:617, 1994
62. Ammar T, Fisher CF: The effects of heparinase 1 and protamine on platelet reactivity. Anesthesiology 86:1382, 1997
63. Carr ME Jr: Measurement of platelet force: The Hemodyne hemostasis analyzer. Clin Lab Manage Rev 9:312, 1995
64. Martin P, Horkay F, Gupta NK, et al: Heparin rebound phenomenon—much ado about nothing? Blood Coagul Fibrinolysis 3:187, 1992
65. Jobes DR, Schwartz AJ, Ellison N: Heparin rebound (letter). J Thorac Cardiovasc Surg 82:940, 1981
66. LaDuca FM, Zucker ML, Walker CE: Assessing heparin neutralization following cardiac surgery: Sensitivity of thrombin time-based assays versus protamine titration methods. Perfusion 14:181, 1999
67. Ohata T, Sawa Y, Ohtake S, et al: Clinical role of blood heparin level monitoring during open heart surgery. Jpn J Thorac Cardiovasc Surg 47:600, 1999
68. Reiner JS, Coyne KS, Lundergan CF, Ross AM: Bedside monitoring of heparin therapy: Comparison of activated clotting time to activated partial thromboplastin time. Cathet Cardiovasc Diagn 32:49, 1994
69. D'Ambra M: Restoration of the normal coagulation process: Advances in therapies to antagonize heparin. J Cardiovasc Pharmacol 27:S58, 1996
70. Martindale SJ, Shayevitz JR, D'Errico C: The activated coagulation time: suitability for monitoring heparin effect and neutralization during pediatric cardiac surgery. J Cardiothorac Vasc Anesth 10:458, 1996
71. Moriau M, Masure R, Hurlet A, et al: Haemostasis disorders in open heart surgery with extracorporeal circulation. Importance of the platelet function and the heparin neutralization. Vox Sang 32:41, 1977
72. Shigeta O, Kojima H, Hiramatsu Y, et al: Low-dose protamine based on heparin-protamine titration method reduces platelet dysfunction after cardiopulmonary bypass. J Thorac Cardiovasc Surg 118:354, 1999
73. Reich DL, Yanakakis MJ, Vela-Cantos FP, et al: Comparison of bedside coagulation monitoring tests with standard laboratory tests in patients after cardiac surgery. Anesth Analg 77:673, 1993
74. Williams RD, D'Ambra MN, Maione TE, et al: Recombinant platelet factor 4 reversal of heparin in human cardiopulmonary bypass blood. J Thorac Cardiovasc Surg 108:975, 1994
75. Cook JJ, Niewiarowski S, Yan Z, et al: Platelet factor 4 efficiently reverses heparin anticoagulation in the rat without adverse effects of heparin-protamine complexes. Circulation 85:1102, 1992
76. Levy JH, Cormack JG, Morales A: Heparin neutralization by recombinant platelet factor 4 and protamine. Anesth Analg 81:35, 1995
77. Michelsen LG, Kikura M, Levy JH, et al: Heparinase I (Neutralase) reversal of systemic anticoagulation. Anesthesiology 85:339, 1996
78. Bain B, Forster T, Sleigh B: Heparin and the activated partial thromboplastin time—a difference between the in-vitro and in-vivo effects and implications for the therapeutic range. Am J Clin Pathol 74:668, 1980
79. Ray MJ, Carroll PA, Just SJ, et al: The effect of oral anticoagulant therapy on APTT results from a bedside coagulation monitor. J Clin Monit 10:97, 1994
80. Werner M, Gallagher JV, Ballo MS, Karcher DS: Effect of analytic uncertainty of conventional and point-of-care assays of activated partial thromboplastin time on clinical decisions in heparin therapy. Am J Clin Pathol 102:237, 1994
81. Samama CM, Quezada R, Riou B, et al: Intraoperative measurement of activated partial thromboplastin time and prothrombin time with a new compact monitor. Acta Anaesthesiol Scand 38:232, 1994
82. Nuttall GA, Oliver WC, Beynen FM, et al: Determination of normal versus abnormal activated partial thromboplastin time and prothrombin time after cardiopulmonary bypass. J Cardiothorac Vasc Anesth 9:355, 1995
83. Despotis GJ, Santoro SA, Spitznagel E, et al: Prospective evaluation and clinical utility of on-site monitoring of coagulation in patients undergoing cardiac operation. J Thorac Cardiovasc Surg 107:271, 1994
84. Despotis GJ, Grishaber JE, Goodnough LT: The effect of an intraoperative treatment algorithm on physicians' transfusion practice in cardiac surgery. Transfusion 34:290, 1994
85. Borowiec J, Bagge L, Saldeen T, Thelin S: Biocompatibility reflected by haemostasis variables during cardiopulmonary bypass using heparin-coated circuits. Thorac Cardiovasc Surg 45:163, 1997
86. Jansen PG, te Velthuis H, Huybregts RA, et al: Reduced complement activation and improved postoperative performance after cardiopulmonary bypass with heparin-coated circuits. J Thorac Cardiovasc Surg 110:829, 1995
87. Gu YJ, Boonstra PW, Rijnsburger AA, et al: Cardiopulmonary bypass circuit treated with surface-modifying additives: A clinical evaluation of blood compatibility. Ann Thorac Surg 65:1342, 1998
88. Gorman RC, Ziats N, Rao AK, et al: Surface-bound heparin fails to reduce thrombin formation during clinical cardiopulmonary bypass. J Thorac Cardiovasc Surg 111:1, 1996; discussion 11, 1996
89. Baufreton C, Jansen PG, Le Besnerais P, et al: Heparin coating with aprotinin reduces blood activation during coronary artery operations. Ann Thorac Surg 63:50, 1997
90. Ovrum E, Holen EA, Tangen G, et al: Completely heparinized cardiopulmonary bypass and reduced systemic heparin: Clinical and hemostatic effects. Ann Thorac Surg 60:365, 1995
91. Aldea GS, Doursounian M, O'Gara P, et al: Heparin-bonded circuits with a reduced anticoagulation protocol in primary CABG: A prospective, randomized study. Ann Thorac Surg 62:410, 1996
92. Weiss BM, von Segesser LK, Turina MI, et al: Perioperative course and recovery after heparin-coated cardiopulmonary bypass: Low-dose versus high-dose heparin management. J Cardiothorac Vasc Anesth 10:464, 1996
93. Kuitunen AH, Heikkila LJ, Salmenpera MT: Cardiopulmonary bypass with heparin-coated circuits and reduced systemic anticoagulation. Ann Thorac Surg 63:438, 1997
94. Ovrum E, Brosstad F, Am Holen E, et al: Effects on coagulation and fibrinolysis with reduced versus full systemic heparinization and heparin-coated cardiopulmonary bypass. Circulation 92:2579, 1995
95. Muller N, Popov-Cenic S, Buttner W, et al: Studies of fibrinolytic and coagulation factors during open heart surgery. II. Postoperative bleeding tendency and changes in the coagulation system. Thromb Res 7:589, 1975
96. Umlas J: Fibrinolysis and disseminated intravascular coagulation in open heart surgery. Transfusion 16:460, 1976
97. Whitten CW, Greilich PE, Ivy R, et al: D-dimer formation during cardiac and noncardiac thoracic surgery. Anesth Analg 88:1226, 1999
98. Weitz J, Klement P: Bivalirudin as an alternative anticoagulant to heparin in cardiopulmonary bypass: Data from a porcine model (abstract). Anesthesiology 99:A, 2003
99. Lincoff AM, Bittl JA, Kleiman NS, et al: Comparison of bivalirudin versus heparin during percutaneous coronary intervention (the Randomized Evaluation of PCI Linking Angiomax to Reduced Clinical Events [REPLACE] trial). Am J Cardiol 93:1092, 2004
100. Merry AF: Bivalirudin, blood loss, and graft patency in coronary artery bypass surgery. Semin Thromb Hemost 30:337, 2004
101. Greinacher A: The use of direct thrombin inhibitors in cardiovascular surgery in patients with heparin-induced thrombocytopenia. Semin Thromb Hemost 30:315, 2004
102. Koster A, Kuppe H, Hetzer R, et al: Emergent cardiopulmonary bypass in five patients with heparin-induced thrombocytopenia type II employing recombinant hirudin. Anesthesiology 89:777, 1998

103. Koster A, Crystal GJ, Kuppe H, Mertzlufft F: Acute heparin-induced thrombocytopenia type II during cardiopulmonary bypass. J Cardiothorac Vasc Anesth 14:300, 2000
104. Koster A, Hansen R, Kuppe H, et al: Recombinant hirudin as an alternative for anticoagulation during cardiopulmonary bypass in patients with heparin-induced thrombocytopenia type II: A 1-year experience in 57 patients. J Cardiothorac Vasc Anesth 14:243, 2000
105. Koster A, Loebe M, Hansen R, et al: A quick assay for monitoring recombinant hirudin during cardiopulmonary bypass in patients with heparin-induced thrombocytopenia type II: Adaptation of the ecarin clotting time to the act II device. J Thorac Cardiovasc Surg 119:1278, 2000
106. Koster A, Kuppe H, Crystal GJ, Mertzlufft F: Cardiovascular surgery without cardiopulmonary bypass in patients with heparin-induced thrombocytopenia type II using anticoagulation with recombinant hirudin. Anesth Analg 90:292, 2000
107. Koster A, Hansen R, Grauhan O, et al: Hirudin monitoring using the TAS ecarin clotting time in patients with heparin-induced thrombocytopenia type II. J Cardiothorac Vasc Anesth 14:249, 2000
108. Koster A, Pasic M, Bauer M, et al: Hirudin as anticoagulant for cardiopulmonary bypass: Importance of preoperative renal function. Ann Thorac Surg 69:37, 2000
109. Koster A, Loebe M, Mertzlufft F, et al: Cardiopulmonary bypass in a patient with heparin-induced thrombocytopenia II and impaired renal function using heparin and the platelet GP IIb/IIIa inhibitor tirofiban as anticoagulant. Ann Thorac Surg 70:2160, 2000
110. Koster A, Merkle F, Hansen R, et al: Elimination of recombinant hirudin by modified ultrafiltration during simulated cardiopulmonary bypass: Assessment of different filter systems. Anesth Analg 91:265, 2000
111. Maroo A, Lincoff AM: Bivalirudin in PCI: An overview of the REPLACE Trial. Semin Thromb Hemost 30:329, 2004
112. Merry AF, Raudkivi PJ, Middleton NG, et al: Bivalirudin versus heparin and protamine in off-pump coronary artery bypass surgery. Ann Thorac Surg 77:925, 2004
113. Davis Z, Anderson R, Short D, et al: Favorable outcome with bivalirudin anticoagulation during cardiopulmonary bypass. Ann Thorac Surg 75:264, 2003
114. Gordon G, Rastegar H, Schumann R, et al: Successful use of bivalirudin for cardiopulmonary bypass in a patient with heparin-induced thrombocytopenia. J Cardiothorac Vasc Anesth 17:632, 2003
115. Vasquez JC, Vichiendilokkul A, Mahmood S, Baciewicz FA Jr: Anticoagulation with bivalirudin during cardiopulmonary bypass in cardiac surgery. Ann Thorac Surg 74:2177, 2002
116. Koster A, Spiess B, Chew DP, et al: Effectiveness of bivalirudin as a replacement for heparin during cardiopulmonary bypass in patients undergoing coronary artery bypass grafting. Am J Cardiol 93:356, 2004
117. Chomiak PN, Walenga JM, Koza MJ, et al: Investigation of a thrombin inhibitor peptide as an alternative to heparin in cardiopulmonary bypass surgery. Circulation 88:II-407, 1993
118. Bittl JA, Strony J, Brinker JA, et al: Treatment with bivalirudin (Hirulog) as compared with heparin during coronary angioplasty for unstable or postinfarction angina. Hirulog Angioplasty Study Investigators. N Engl J Med 333:764, 1995
119. Zilla P, Fasol R, Deutsch M, et al: Whole blood aggregometry and platelet adenine nucleotides during cardiac surgery. Scand J Thorac Cardiovasc Surg 22:165, 1988
120. Halbmayer WM, Haushofer A, Radek J, et al: Platelet size, fibrinogen and lipoprotein(a) in coronary heart disease. Coron Artery Dis 6:397, 1995
121. Boldt J, Zickmann B, Benson M, et al: Does platelet size correlate with function in patients undergoing cardiac surgery? Intensive Care Med 19:44, 1993
122. Despotis GJ, Filos KS, Zoys TN, et al: Factors associated with excessive postoperative blood loss and hemostatic transfusion requirements: A multivariate analysis in cardiac surgical patients. Anesth Analg 82:13, 1996
123. Khuri SF, Wolfe JA, Josa M, et al: Hematologic changes during and after cardiopulmonary bypass and their relationship to the bleeding time and nonsurgical blood loss. J Thorac Cardiovasc Surg 104:94, 1992
124. Bertolino G, Locatelli A, Noris P, et al: Platelet composition and function in patients undergoing cardiopulmonary bypass for heart surgery. Haematologica 81:116, 1996
125. Boldt J, Schindler E, Knothe C, et al: Does aprotinin influence endothelial-associated coagulation in cardiac surgery? J Cardiothorac Vasc Anesth 8:527, 1994
126. Kestin AS, Valeri CR, Khuri SF, et al: The platelet function defect of cardiopulmonary bypass. Blood 82:107, 1993
127. Upchurch GR, Valeri CR, Khuri SF, et al: Effect of heparin on fibrinolytic activity and platelet function in vivo. Am J Physiol 271:H528, 1996
128. Adelman B, Michelson AD, Loscalzo J, et al: Plasmin effect on platelet glycoprotein Ib-von Willebrand factor interactions. Blood 65:32, 1985
129. Adelman B, Michelson AD, Greenberg J, Handin RI: Proteolysis of platelet glycoprotein Ib by plasmin is facilitated by plasmin lysine-binding regions. Blood 68:1280, 1986
130. Michelson AD, MacGregor H, Barnard MR, et al: Reversible inhibition of human platelet activation by hypothermia in vivo and in vitro. Thromb Haemost 71:633, 1994
131. Boldt J, Zickmann B, Czeke A, et al: Blood conservation techniques and platelet function in cardiac surgery. Anesthesiology 75:426, 1991
132. Burns ER, Billett HH, Frater RW, Sisto DA: The preoperative bleeding time as a predictor of postoperative hemorrhage after cardiopulmonary bypass. J Thorac Cardiovasc Surg 92:310, 1986
133. Burns ER, Lawrence C: Bleeding time. A guide to its diagnostic and clinical utility. Arch Pathol Lab Med 113:1219, 1989
134. Despotis GJ, Levine V, Filos KS, et al: Evaluation of a new point-of-care test that measures PAF-mediated acceleration of coagulation in cardiac surgical patients. Anesthesiology 85:1311, 1996
135. Despotis GJ, Levine V, Saleem R, et al: Use of point-of-care test in identification of patients who can benefit from desmopressin during cardiac surgery: A randomised controlled trial. Lancet 354:106, 1999
136. Mohr R, Martinowitz U, Lavee J, et al: The hemostatic effect of transfusing fresh whole blood versus platelet concentrates after cardiac operations. J Thorac Cardiovasc Surg 96:530, 1988
137. Ray MJ, Hawson GA, Just SJ, et al: Relationship of platelet aggregation to bleeding after cardiopulmonary bypass. Ann Thorac Surg 57:981, 1994
138. Carr ME, Jr.: In vitro assessment of platelet function. Transfus Med Rev 11:106, 1997
139. George JN, Pickett EB, Saucerman S, et al: Platelet surface glycoproteins. Studies on resting and activated platelets and platelet membrane microparticles in normal subjects, and observations in patients during adult respiratory distress syndrome and cardiac surgery. J Clin Invest 78:340, 1986
140. Adelman B, Michelson AD, Handin RI, Ault KA: Evaluation of platelet glycoprotein Ib by fluorescence flow cytometry. Blood 66:423, 1985
141. Michelson AD, Barnard MR: Thrombin-induced changes in platelet membrane glycoproteins Ib, IX, and IIb-IIIa complex. Blood 70:1673, 1987
142. Nieuwenhuis HK, van Oosterhout JJ, Rozemuller E, et al: Studies with a monoclonal antibody against activated platelets: Evidence that a secreted 53,000-molecular weight lysosome-like granule protein is exposed on the surface of activated platelets in the circulation. Blood 70:838, 1987
143. Michelson AD: Flow cytometric analysis of platelet surface glycoproteins: phenotypically distinct subpopulations of platelets in children with chronic myeloid leukemia. J Lab Clin Med 110:346, 1987
144. LaRosa CA, Rohrer MJ, Benoit SE, et al: Neutrophil cathepsin G modulates the platelet surface expression of the glycoprotein (GP) Ib-IX complex by proteolysis of the von Willebrand factor binding site on GPIb alpha and by a cytoskeletal-mediated redistribution of the remainder of the complex. Blood 84:158, 1994
145. Rinder CS, Mathew JP, Rinder HM, et al: Modulation of platelet surface adhesion receptors during cardiopulmonary bypass. Anesthesiology 75:563, 1991
146. Sloand JA, Sloand EM: Studies on platelet membrane glycoproteins and platelet function during hemodialysis. J Am Soc Nephrol 8:799, 1997
147. Shore-Lesserson L, Ammar T, DePerio M, et al: Platelet-activated clotting time does not measure platelet reactivity during cardiac surgery. Anesthesiology 91:362, 1999
148. Miller BE, Mochizuki T, Levy JH, et al: Predicting and treating coagulopathies after cardiopulmonary bypass in children. Anesth Analg 85:1196, 1997
149. Spiess BD: Thromboelastography and cardiopulmonary bypass. Semin Thromb Hemost 21:27, 1995
150. Tuman KJ, Spiess BD, McCarthy RJ, Ivankovich AD: Comparison of viscoelastic measures of coagulation after cardiopulmonary bypass. Anesth Analg 69:69, 1989
151. Tuman KJ, McCarthy RJ, Djuric M, et al: Evaluation of coagulation during cardiopulmonary bypass with a heparinase-modified thromboelastographic assay. J Cardiothorac Vasc Anesth 8:144, 1994
152. Ereth MH, Nuttall GA, Klindworth JT, et al: Does the platelet-activated clotting test (HemoSTATUS) predict blood loss and platelet dysfunction associated with cardiopulmonary bypass? Anesth Analg 85:259, 1997
153. Mongan PD, Hosking MP: The role of desmopressin acetate in patients undergoing coronary artery bypass surgery. A controlled clinical trial with thromboelastographic risk stratification. Anesthesiology 77:38, 1992

154. Gravlee GP, Arora S, Lavender SW, et al: Predictive value of blood clotting tests in cardiac surgical patients. Ann Thorac Surg 58:216, 1994
155. Spiess BD, Gillies BS, Chandler W, Verrier E: Changes in transfusion therapy and reexploration rate after institution of a blood management program in cardiac surgical patients. J Cardiothorac Vasc Anesth 9:168, 1995
156. Whitten CW, Allison PM, Latson TW, et al: Evaluation of laboratory coagulation and lytic parameters resulting from autologous whole blood transfusion during primary aortocoronary artery bypass grafting. J Clin Anesth 8:229, 1996
157. Greilich PE, Alving BM, O'Neill KL, et al: A modified thromboelastographic method for monitoring c7E3 Fab in heparinized patients. Anesth Analg 84:31, 1997
158. Kang YG, Martin DJ, Marquez J, et al: Intraoperative changes in blood coagulation and thromboelastographic monitoring in liver transplantation. Anesth Analg 64:888, 1985
159. Martin LK, Kang Y, De Wolf AM: Coagulation changes immediately following liver graft reperfusion. Transplant Proc 23:19461991
160. Khurana S, Mattson JC, Westley S, et al: Monitoring platelet glycoprotein IIb/IIIa-fibrin interaction with tissue factor-activated thromboelastography. J Lab Clin Med 130:401, 1997
161. Shore-Lesserson L, Manspeizer HE, DePerio M, et al: Thromboelastography-guided transfusion algorithm reduces transfusions in complex cardiac surgery. Anesth Analg 88:312, 1999
162. Gottumukkala VN, Sharma SK, Philip J: Assessing platelet and fibrinogen contribution to clot strength using modified thromboelastography in pregnant women. Anesth Analg 89:1453, 1999
163. Greilich PE, Alving BM, Longnecker D, et al: Near-site monitoring of the antiplatelet drug abciximab using the Hemodyne analyzer and modified thromboelastograph. J Cardiothorac Vasc Anesth 13:58, 1999
164. Craft RM, Chavez JJ, Bresee SJ, et al: A novel modification of the Thromboelastograph assay, isolating platelet function, correlates with optical platelet aggregation. J Lab Clin Med 143:301, 2004
165. Shore-Lesserson L, Fischer G, Sanders J, et al: Clopidogrel induces a platelet aggregation defect that is partially mitigated by ex-vivo addition of aprotinin. Anesthesiology 101:A, 2004
166. Hett DA, Walker D, Pilkington SN, Smith DC: Sonoclot analysis. Br J Anaesth 75:771, 1995
167. Stern MP, DeVos-Doyle K, Viguera MG, Lajos TZ: Evaluation of post-cardiopulmonary bypass Sonoclot signatures in patients taking non-steroidal anti-inflammatory drugs. J Cardiothorac Anesth 3:730, 1989
168. Chapin JW, Becker GL, Hulbert BJ, et al: Comparison of Thromboelastograph and Sonoclot coagulation analyzers for assessing coagulation status during orthotopic liver transplantation. Transplant Proc 21:3539, 1989
169. Peck SD: Evaluation of the in vitro detection of the hypercoagulable state using the thrombin generation test and plasma clot impedance test. Thromb Haemost 42:764, 1979
170. Smith JW, Steinhubl SR, Lincoff AM, et al: Rapid platelet-function assay: An automated and quantitative cartridge-based method. Circulation 99:620, 1999
171. Coller BS, Lang D, Scudder LE: Rapid and simple platelet function assay to assess glycoprotein IIb/IIIa receptor blockade. Circulation 95:860, 1997
172. Coller BS, Folts JD, Scudder LE, Smith SR: Antithrombotic effect of a monoclonal antibody to the platelet glycoprotein IIb/IIIa receptor in an experimental animal model. Blood 68:783, 1986
173. Ikarugi H, Taka T, Nakajima S, et al: Norepinephrine, but not epinephrine, enhances platelet reactivity and coagulation after exercise in humans. J Appl Physiol 86:133, 1999
174. John LC, Rees GM, Kovacs IB: Inhibition of platelet function by heparin. An etiologic factor in postbypass hemorrhage. J Thorac Cardiovasc Surg 105:816, 1993
175. Kovacs IB, Mayou SC, Kirby JD: Infusion of a stable prostacyclin analogue, iloprost, to patients with peripheral vascular disease: Lack of antiplatelet effect but risk of thromboembolism. Am J Med 90:41, 1991
176. Ratnatunga CP, Rees GM, Kovacs IB: Preoperative hemostatic activity and excessive bleeding after cardiopulmonary bypass. Ann Thorac Surg 52:250, 1991
177. Bock M, De Haan J, Beck KH, et al: Standardization of the PFA-100 (R) platelet function test in 105 mmol/L buffered citrate: Effect of gender, smoking, and oral contraceptives. Br J Haematol 106:898, 1999
178. Escolar G, Cases A, Vinas M, et al: Evaluation of acquired platelet dysfunctions in uremic and cirrhotic patients using the platelet function analyzer (PFA-100): Influence of hematocrit elevation. Haematologica 84:614, 1999
179. Kundu SK, Heilmann EJ, Sio R, et al: Description of an in vitro platelet function analyzer—PFA-100. Semin Thromb Hemost 21:106, 1995
180. Mammen EF, Comp PC, Gosselin R, et al: PFA-100 system: A new method for assessment of platelet dysfunction. Semin Thromb Hemost 24:195, 1998
181. Wahba A, Sander S, Birnbaum DE: Are in-vitro platelet function tests useful in predicting blood loss following open heart surgery? Thorac Cardiovasc Surg 46:228, 1998
182. Nuttall G, Oliver WC Jr, Ereth MH, et al: The PFA 100, correlation with platelet aggregometry with GP IIB/IIIA receptor antagonists (abstract). Anesthesiology 91:A518, 1999
183. Carville DG, Schleckser PA, Guyer KE, et al: Whole blood platelet function assay on the ICHOR point-of-care hematology analyzer. J Extra Corpor Technol 30:171, 1998
184. Slaughter TF, Sreeram G, Sharma AD, et al: Reversible shear-mediated platelet dysfunction during cardiac surgery as assessed by the PFA-100 platelet function analyzer. Blood Coagul Fibrinolysis 12:85, 2001
185. Steinhubl SR, Talley JD, Braden GA, et al: Point-of-care measured platelet inhibition correlates with a reduced risk of an adverse cardiac event after percutaneous coronary intervention: Results of the GOLD (AU-Assessing Ultegra) multicenter study. Circulation 103:2572, 2001
186. Faraday N, Guallar E, Sera VA, et al: Utility of whole blood hemostatometry using the clot signature analyzer for assessment of hemostasis in cardiac surgery. Anesthesiology 96:1115, 2002

Part V

ANESTHESIA TECHNIQUES FOR CARDIAC SURGICAL PROCEDURES

Chapter 19

ANESTHESIA FOR MYOCARDIAL REVASCULARIZATION

Martin London, MD • Alexander Mittnacht, MD • Joel A. Kaplan, MD

KEY POINTS

1. The risk profile of the average patient presenting for CABG has increased with greater numbers of patients with triple vessel disease, poor targets, reduced ventricular function, and reoperations.
2. The pathophysiology of a myocardial infarction has been clarified, with an understanding that it is an acute obstruction of a coronary artery caused by an acute thrombosis in the lumen that often results from the rupture of a vulnerable arterial plaque. Inflammation plays a crucial role in development of the plaque, along with the deposits of lipoproteins.
3. Preoperative ordering of premedication should include careful consideration of all of the patient's relevant antihypertensive, antianginal, and other medications.
4. Preexisting abnormalities of ventricular function, wall motion, and ischemic mitral regurgitation, along with long ischemic time during CPB, are predictors of difficulty in weaning and postoperative low cardiac output states.
5. PAC may still be of particular benefit in patients with impaired ventricular function and major comorbidities who require postoperative cardiac output monitoring.
6. The days of high-dose opioid anesthesia for CABG are over with nearly universal adoption of fast-tracking programs aimed at early extubation with reduced ICU and hospital stay.
7. All contemporary inhalation agents have been shown to have potent ischemic preconditioning effects, and newer randomized trials have demonstrated reductions in postoperative troponin release and improved ventricular function relative to exclusively intravenous techniques.
8. Intraoperative recall is a risk in all cardiac surgical procedures, although its incidence appears to have declined substantially with the increased continuous use of inhalation anesthetics associated with fast-tracking.
9. Off-pump CABG is the greatest change in surgical revascularization technique in the past 2 decades.
10. The hemodynamic changes associated with off-pump CAB include reduction in cardiac output, stroke volume, and mean arterial pressure.
11. Intravenous nitroglycerin and short-acting beta-blockers, such as esmolol, remain the mainstay of treatment for perioperative myocardial ischemia.

Providing anesthesia care for patients undergoing coronary artery bypass grafting (CABG) continues to be a challenging yet rewarding endeavor. Surgical, anesthetic, and technologic advances continue to drive changes in clinical routines at a rapid pace, even at a time when the numbers of cases have declined because of the growth of percutaneous coronary interventions (PCIs). Administrative, social, and economic forces mandate that clinicians be as efficient as possible in how they practice to keep the substantial costs of CABG in balance with increasing health care costs.

Cardiac anesthesiologists who have been in practice for the past several decades have seen a variety of anesthetic and surgical practices come into vogue and fall out of favor based on new research and economic pressures. Perhaps the most striking example is the rise and fall of high-dose opioid anesthesia, which was initially driven by concern about excessive cardiovascular depression by volatile anesthetics in the 1970s and further accelerated in the mid-1980s by concerns about potential coronary steal with isoflurane.[1,2] The prolonged postoperative mechanical ventilation resulting from the shift to high-dose opioids was also thought important to reduce stress on the recently revascularized myocardium.[3] However, during the following decade, this approach was completely reversed by new basic and clinical research, such as lack of evidence for adverse effects of volatile agents, particularly as related to potential effects of coronary vasodilation on coronary steal, and by strong evidence of their benefits via rapid preconditioning)[4]; by social and economic factors (i.e., safety and efficacy of fast-tracking for most patients and recognition that time on the ventilator for many patients is an uncomfortable experience)[5]; and by the rapid rise in off-pump coronary artery bypass grafting (OPCAB), which by avoiding adverse physiologic effects of cardiopulmonary bypass (CPB) facilitates more rapid emergence and recovery in many patients.[6] In the past decade, newer surgical approaches (e.g., robotic surgery) were introduced that are likely to change current practices (see Chapter 21). In some cases, these new procedures have not proved as effective or efficient as initially expected and have (at least for now) fallen out of favor (e.g., minimally invasive port-access CABG).[7] Given the increasing emphasis on pain control in all surgical patients and its reported association with enhanced postoperative outcome in a variety of surgical subgroups, there has been a resurgence in the use of neuraxial techniques in cardiac surgery, particularly in European countries.[8,9] Although not commonly used in the United States due to logistical issues and perhaps liability concerns, the rapidly growing literature base mandates that clinicians familiarize themselves with their potential benefits and risks.

The cardiac anesthesiologist must also be familiar with a wider variety of monitoring practices than ever before and must be nimble in adapting to substantial variation in local practices ranging from "low tech" to "high tech" based on their availability, surgeon preferences, sophistication of ICU services, and other factors. Among the major monitors, use of

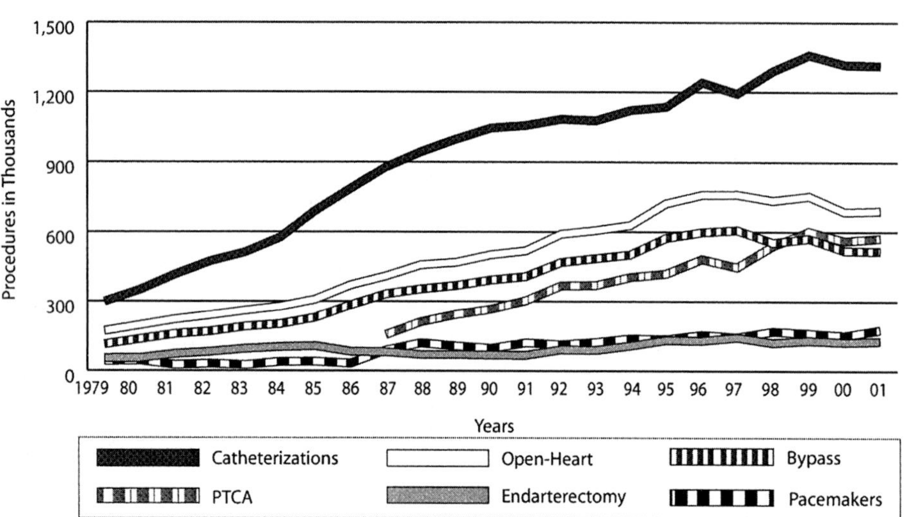

Figure 19–1 Trends in cardiovascular operations and procedures from 1979 to 2001. (From American Heart Association: Heart Disease and Stroke Statistics—2004 Update. Dallas, TX, American Heart Association, 2004, p 41.)

transesophageal echocardiography (TEE) continues to increase, and use of the pulmonary artery catheter (PAC) appears to be declining.

This chapter provides a sequential approach to the major management issues faced by the practitioner providing anesthesia for CABG from the preoperative period through the operative and early postoperative periods. Based on several unique challenges necessitating minor or major differences in anesthetic management, redo-CABG and OPCAB procedures are also considered (see Chapter 21 for other minimally invasive and robotic procedures).

EPIDEMIOLOGY AND RISK ASSESSMENT

In 2001, coronary artery disease (CAD) was estimated to occur in 13,200,000 individuals in the United States (6.4%), resulting in approximately 500,000 deaths, 2 million hospital discharges, and a societal cost of $133 billion.[10] CABG surgery is clearly the established cornerstone of treatment of advanced degrees of CAD. Although its absolute frequency has recently declined, there is no doubt that it will remain a common procedure, and that its complexity will continue to increase for many decades to come. An understanding of the basic epidemiology of CABG surgery and of risk assessment for patients undergoing it is important for the anesthesiologist for a variety of reasons, including interactions with surgeons and cardiologists; enhancing clinical management of patients by recognizing high-risk characteristics and situations where preoperative management may not be adequate (such that delay of a planned elective procedure or additional perioperative interventions are required); developing a better sense of long-term trends in surgical practice that may impact on future practice volume (e.g., growth or decline of CABG techniques); and changes in complexity of such procedures which may influence reimbursement or additional training requirements.

It is important to realize how complex it is to accurately analyze what is happening in this rapidly evolving field. Health care analysts now spend entire careers studying use and risk assessment data for cardiac surgical procedures. Dozens of publications appear monthly in many journals. Developing an efficient means to stay informed on an ongoing basis is an important strategy for the active practitioner, including an appreciation of the major subspecialty societies (e.g., Society of Thoracic Surgeons [STS], Society of Cardiovascular Anesthesiologists, American Heart Association Scientific Council on Cardiovascular Surgery and Anesthesia), their respective journals (e.g., *Annals of Thoracic Surgery*, *Anesthesia & Analgesia*, *Circulation*), and their web sites (e.g., www.sts.org, www.ctsnet.org, www.scahq.org, www.americanheart.org). A variety of other societies (e.g., European Society of Cardiothoracic Surgery) and subspecialty journals (e.g., *Journal of Cardiothoracic and Vascular Anesthesia*) are important resources for the busy clinician.

Although precise data on the annual number of CABG and PCI procedures performed are not available, numerical estimates based on sampling of large administrative and clinical databases, along with publications from discrete health care systems, have been used to derive strong estimates.[10-13] The most widely cited data for nonfederal institutions in the United States are obtained from the U.S. Department of Health and Human Services National Hospital Discharge Survey (NHDS).[13] The latest data available (reported in May 2004) from 2002 estimated 515,000 hospital discharges in 306,000 patients with an ICD-9 code for CABG at time of discharge. In contrast, there were 1,204,000 discharges for patients undergoing PCI procedures. The rapid growth of both procedures from 1979 through 2001 (Fig. 19–1) is seen clearly from these NHDS estimates. The crossover and decline in the volume of CABG versus PCI is apparent starting in 1998. Mack et al[12] reported detailed epidemiologic, use, and outcome data on 148,396 patients undergoing PCI or CABG in a large, for-profit healthcare system (HCA, Inc.) at 69 of the 200 hospitals performing these procedures in 23 states (primarily in the south, southeast, and southwestern states) from 1999 to 2002. In this private, predominantly low-volume caseload per hospital system (approximately 220 CABGs per hospital annually), 65% of all revascularizations were done by PCI, increasing 6.8% annually, and CABG declined 1.9% annually, with the greatest changes observed from 1999 to 2000. As expected, CABG was predominantly reserved for those with triple-vessel disease, and PCI was limited to a single vessel in 83% of interventions.

Operative mortality (usually defined as death within 30 days of surgery) as expected varies widely with patient risk, acuity, and previous cardiac surgery (Fig. 19–2). However, on

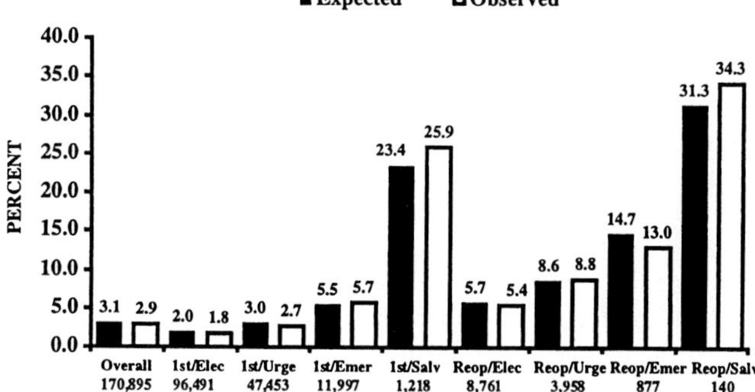

Figure 19–2 Distribution of risk of mortality for various groups of patients in the Society of Thoracic Surgeons database in 1996. The risk is highest for patients undergoing salvage procedures or reoperation. (From Grover FL: The Society of Thoracic Surgeons National Database: Current status and future directions. Ann Thorac Surg 68:367, 1999. Copyright 1999, with permission from the Society of Thoracic Surgeons.)

average, it appears that mortality has progressively declined over the past decade or more despite increases in patient risk (Fig. 19–3).[14]

The rapid growth of PCI has led to the perception of a shunting of healthier patients away from CABG leaving a greater percentage of older and sicker patients not studied in the original CABG efficacy trials (e.g., the seminal CASS trial excluded patients with ejection fractions [EFs] less than 35%). Publications over the past decade addressing the question of whether patients presenting for CABG are sicker or at higher risk than they were previously have uniformly answered this affirmatively noting older patients, worse ventricular function, and more emergent cases.[15] Despite these findings, operative mortality continues to decline. Davierwala et al[16] observed that left ventricular dysfunction and reoperative status have decreased in significance as predictors of mortality in a large cohort of Canadian patients, whereas emergency surgery has increased in importance in predicting adverse outcome.

Based on the NHDS estimates, the ACC/AHA CABG Surgery Practice Guidelines group estimated that approximately $10 billion are spent annually on this operation in the United States alone ($30,000 by 300,000 patients).[17,18] Mack et al[12] reported an increase in CABG cost from 1999 to 2002 of 30% from $23,880 to $31,184. In that report, OPCAB was reported to incur a differential cost savings of approximately $2500. Despite these substantial costs, CABG, particularly for patients with left main and three-vessel disease, is considered a very cost-effective procedure at $9000 and $18,000 spent per quality-adjusted life-year gained ($/QALY), respectively. In patients with one- or two-vessel disease, cost-effectiveness is closely related to the presence of left anterior descending (LAD) coronary artery disease and the presence of severe angina.[19]

Preoperative risk assessment for patients undergoing CABG has evolved dramatically over the past 2 decades driven by a variety of diverse factors. Institution of a federally mandated accounting of surgical outcomes for cardiac surgery in the Department of Veterans Affairs in the 1970s led to the establishment of what is considered the first large-scale, multicenter surgical outcomes database applying rigorous statistical methodology for comparing outcomes between centers.[20,21] This group and others have pioneered methodology for adjusting for different severity of illness between patients (i.e., risk adjustment) using multiple preoperative and perioperative variables thought to be of intrinsic value (usually by expert consensus) that could be easily captured and have high consistency of definition. Entering these variables into logistic regression models of mortality (considering all of the patients operated on in the particular time frame in which the variables were collected) allows determination of an

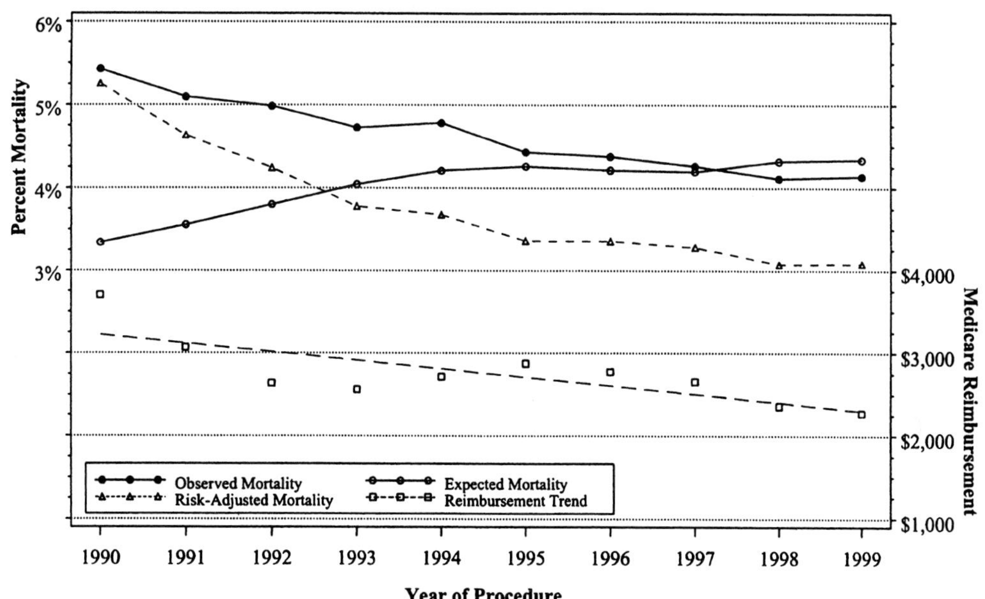

Figure 19–3 Composite figure demonstrating increase in risk profile with declining mortality and part B Medicare reimbursement for patients undergoing CABG between 1990 and 1999. (From Ferguson TB Jr, Hammill BG, Peterson ED, et al: A decade of change—risk profiles and outcomes for isolated coronary artery bypass grafting procedures, 1990–1999: A report from the STS National Database Committee and the Duke Clinical Research Institute. Society of Thoracic Surgeons. Ann Thorac Surg 73:480, 2002. Copyright 2002, with permission from the Society of Thoracic Surgeons.)

"expected" mortality based on coefficients of the regression equation most correlated with outcome. By simple comparison of the "observed" to "expected" (i.e., the value calculated by entering a unique patient's coefficients into the general population mortality model) mortality ratio (O/E ratio), hospitals in a particular system can be ranked from best (low O/E ratio) to worst (high O/E ratio).[22] However, as observed by a variety of experts, caution is advised in use of such adjectives given inherent assumptions and controversies in the statistical approaches for determining thresholds for "quality" and problems in "gaming" of the system by exploiting variables with imprecise definitions[23] (see Chapters 11 and 39).

Nonetheless, this methodology and its variants have been widely adopted by many organizations as a measure of quality of care.[24] The Society of Thoracic Surgeons (STS) instituted a voluntary clinical database system with this approach in the early 1990s which has continued to grow rapidly (containing data on more than 1.5 million isolated CABG cases as of 2003) as cardiac surgical groups are increasingly interested in benchmarking their practices against others.[25,26] Many tertiary centers (e.g., Cleveland Clinic, Duke, Texas Heart Institute) and regional consortiums of hospitals (e.g., Northern New England Cardiovascular Disease Study Group, Alabama CABG Project) maintain databases and some publish statistical models.[27-30] Many states have established and maintain risk-adjusted mandatory reporting systems for hospital and individual surgeon performance (with New York State being an early and influential pioneer).[31] A natural offshoot of this approach has been the exploration of surgeon and hospital volumes as predictors of outcome, a topic which has generated substantial controversy in the literature given conflicting findings (i.e., low-volume centers in which "high-volume" surgeons operate appear to do as well as high-volume centers, and low-risk patients do better relative to high-risk patients at high-volume centers).[32,33] This is a hotly contested topic given the high stakes involved in federal and private sector initiatives to regionalize cardiac surgery care into "centers of excellence"[34] (see Chapter 39). A new scoring system (EuroSCORE) based on outcomes in 128 centers in eight European countries has received increasing attention. It appears to compare favorably with the STS model in North American patients.[35,36] It is freely accessible by means of an interactive web-based calculator (www.euroscore.org) and is decidedly simpler and faster to use than the STS's scoring system, which is now also freely accessible to the public at http://www.sts.org/sections/stsnationaldatabase/riskcalculator/index.html.

Given the mass of literature on this topic and the large number of risk models available, some of which are easily calculated (e.g., a simple additive score), whereas others require manipulation of a logistic regression equation on an advanced calculator or microcomputer, there is considerable debate about how they are best applied. The ACC/AHA CABG guidelines group accords a IIa recommendation (level of evidence C) to their use for predicting hospital mortality. However, they caution that risk scores should be individually calibrated for regional mortality rates (a difficult task), and updated periodically to maintain accuracy (many have not been, with the exception of the Department of Veterans Affairs program and the STS).[17]

Nonetheless, consideration of risk models allows the clinician to better appreciate major variables related to mortality, because many of the important variables are relatively constant between different models.[37] In the mid-1990s a group of experts rigorously evaluated 7 databases available at the time, grouping variables by level of perceived importance and retesting them in different data sets. Seven "core" and 13 "level 1" variables were found to account for between 45% and 83% of the predictive information.[38] Those related to acuteness of surgery, age, and prior CABG were most important, whereas those describing coronary anatomy were least predictive. However, this approach has never been updated, and the conclusions must be viewed cautiously. The accuracy and availability of several key variables of interest to the surgeon and anesthesiologist, particularly EF, is problematic in many databases given different methods for its determination or lack of measurement in many patients. Table 19–1 presents an evaluation of the importance of risk factors in several major risk models and large-scale outcome analyses grouped by the classification advocated by Jones et al.[12,21,26,28,38-40]

The major database models only predict perioperative mortality (usually defined as death within 30 days of surgery although some use any death directly related to a perioperative complication regardless of the time interval, a factor further complicating comparison of models). As such, these models are often of less practical importance to the cardiac anesthesiologist. Predicting which patients are most likely to be difficult to wean from CPB due to development of a low cardiac output syndrome (LCOS) (in the operating room or early postoperative period), or who may develop postoperative complications, is of greater interest to the anesthesiologist. Despite publication of several studies, difficulty in standardization of what constitutes difficult weaning or LCOS has limited generalization of findings. However, given that most CABG mortality is related to difficulty in revascularization and/or myocardial protection, the risk factors are quite similar to those reported for overall mortality.[41,42] An analysis of 1009 patients undergoing CABG at Duke University, all of whom were monitored with TEE, found six independent predictors of inotrope support, which was required in 39% of the cohort during weaning from CPB (Table 19–2 and Figure 19–4).[43]

The introduction and rapid growth of OPCAB has complicated matters because large-scale, well-calibrated outcome models are not yet available for this procedure. Initial publications have addressed this topic.[44,45] Further extensions of this approach are the modeling of lengths of stay, time to

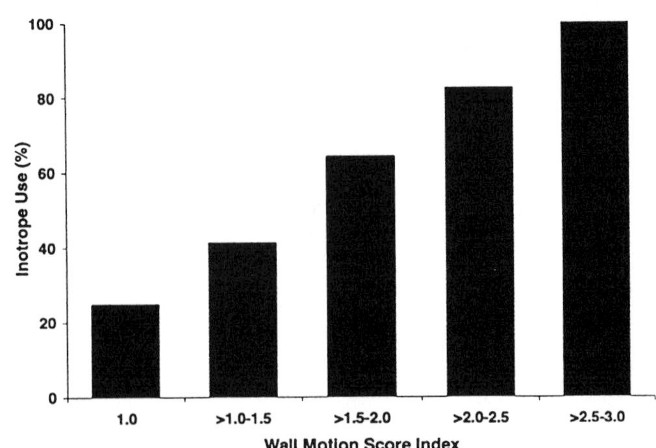

Figure 19–4 Correlation of degree of wall motion abnormalities before cardiopulmonary bypass (CPB) as reflected by an increasing wall motion score index associated with a greater use of inotropes during weaning from CPB. (From McKinlay KH, Schinderle DB, Swaminathan M, et al: Predictors of inotrope use during separation from cardiopulmonary bypass. J Cardiothorac Vasc Anesth 18:404, 2004.)

Table 19–1 **Preoperative Risk Stratification Based on Clinical Databases**

Variables	Society of Thoracic Surgeons*	Dept. of Veterans Affairs†	EuroSCORE‡	New York State§	Cleveland Clinic‖	HCA, Inc.¶
Risk equation units	OR (95% CI)	OR	Additive score	OR (95% CI)	Additive score	OR (95% CI)
Core variables						
Acuity (stability)	Status: urgent or emergent = 1.96 (1.88–2.05); shock = 2.04 (1.90–2.19); IABP = 1.46 (1.37–1.55)	IABP = 1.7	Score 3 for critical preop state = V. tach, V. fib, CPR, IABP, inotropes, or acute renal failure; score 2 for emergency	IABP = 1.39 (1.15–1.69); disaster = 3.98 (31.2–5.08)	Score 6 for emergency	Cardiogenic shock = 8.35 (6.79–10.27); acute MI = 1.80 (1.38–1.84); IABP = 5.26 (4.57–6.05)
Prior cardiac surgery	First = 2.76 (2.62–2.91); multiple = 4.19 (3.61–4.86)	2.1	Score 3	3.73 (3.29–4.24)	Score 3	1.8 (1.34–2.43)
Age	1.05 (1.05–1.05)	1.5 (per 10 yr)	Score 1 per 5 yr over 60	1.05 (1.03–1.07) for >70 yr	Score 2 for age < 75 yr; score 1 for age 65–74 yr	1.04 (1.04–1.05)
Ejection fraction	EF < 50% = 0.98 (0.98–0.98)	Cardiomegaly = 1.5	Score 1 for EF = 30%–50%; score 3 for <30%	<20% = 4.06 (3.16–5.21); 20% to 29% = 2.12 (1.89–2.58); 30% to 39% = 1.63 (1.43–1.86)	Score 3 for severe left ventricular dysfunction	NA
Sex	Male = 0.84 (0.80–0.98)	Female = 2.6	Score 1 for female	Female = 1.52 (1.36–1.69)	NA	Male = 0.71 (0.63–0.80)
Diseased vessels	Triple vessel = 1.21 (1.17–1.26)	NA	NA	NA	NA	Multivessel intervention = 0.64 (0.50–0.82)
Diseased left main	1.18 (1.14–1.24)	NA	NA	1.43 (1.23–1.67)	NA	NA
Level 1 variables						
Creatinine	Renal failure/dialysis = 1.88 (1.80–1.96)	1.5–3.0 mg/dL = 1.6; >3.0 = 2.6	Score 2 for >100 μmol/L	Dialysis = 2.80 (2.26–3.46)	Score 4 for >1.9 mg/dL; score 1 for 1.6–1.8 mg/dL	Hemodialysis = 1.05 (10.56–16.13, chronic renal failure = NS
Cardiovascular disease	1.10 (1.04–1.17)	1.3			Score 1	
Myocardial infarction	1.18 (1.16–1.21)	>7 days preop = 1.2; <7 days preop = 2.1	Score 2 for <90 days preop	<7 days preop = 1.69 (1.45–1.97)	NA	0.80 (0.65–0.97)
Congestive heart failure	NS; NYHA class IV = 1.15 (1.10–1.20)	NYHA class II = 1.5; III = 1.5; IV = 2.3		1.77 (1.53–2.04)	NA	NA
Peripheral vascular disease	PVD/CVD = 1.29 (1.25–1.34)	1.4	Score 2 for carotid, aortic, or lower extremity disease	NA	Score 2 for prior vascular surgery	1.21 (1.03–1.43); AAA = 2.47 (1.79–3.40)
PTCA current admission	<6 hr preop = 1.32 (1.18–1.48)	NA	NA	NA	NA	Thrombolytics = 0.42 (0.18–0.96; use of GPIIB/IIIa = 0.47 (0.30–0.71)
Arrhythmia	NA	1.3	Score 3 for critical preop state = V. tach, V. fib, CPR, IABP, inotropes, or acute renal failure; score 2 for emergency	NA	NA	NA

Table continued on following page

Table 19–1 Preoperative Risk Stratification Based on Clinical Databases—(Continued)

Variables	Society of Thoracic Surgeons[*]	Dept. of Veterans Affairs[†]	EuroSCORE[‡]	New York State[§]	Cleveland Clinic[‖]	HCA, Inc.[¶]
COPD	1.41 (1.36–1.48)	Resting ST depression = 1.4; CSS grade II = 1.0; III = 1.0; IV = 1.4	Score 1 for long-term use of bronchodilator or steroids	1.36 (1.20–1.54)	Score 2 on medication	1.41 (1.23–1.61)
Angina	NA	NA	Score 3 for unstable angina	Unstable angina = 1.42 (1.27–1.60)	NA	NA
Mitral regurgitation	MR = 1.22 (1.17–1.28); aortic stenosis = 1.40 (1.21–1.61)	NA	NA	NA	Score 3	Valve disease = 1.03 (1.08–1.56)
Diabetes	IDDM = 1.50 (1.42–1.58); oral therapy = 1.15 (1.09–1.21)	NA	NA	1.50 (1.34–1.67)	Score 1 on any medication	IDDM, NIDDM = NS
Weight/height	BSA = 0.91 (0.89–0.93)	NA	NA	Morbid obesity = 1.49 (1.20–1.84)	Score 1 for <65 kg	NA
Level 2 variables						
Smoking	NS	NA	NA	NA	NA	NA
Hypertension	1.12 (1.08–1.17)	NA	NA	NA	NA	0.82 (0.72–0.93)
Liver disease	NA	NA	NA	NA	NA	10.00 (6.83–14.63)
Malignancy	NA	NA	NA	NA	NA	NA
Immunosuppression	1.75 (1.57–1.95)	NA	NA	NA	NA	NA
Prior PTCA	NA	NA	NA	NA	NA	NS
Race	Black = 1.34 (1.23–1.45)	NA	NA	NA	NA	NA
Miscellaneous features						
Hypercholesterolemia	0.82 (0.79–0.86)					
Neurologic dysfunction			Score 2			
Active endocarditis			Score 3			
Other procedure			Score 2 for other procedure; score 3 for surgery on thoracic aorta			
Postinfarct septal rupture			Score 4			
Pulmonary hypertension			Score 2 for syst. PA > 60 mm Hg			
Anemia					Score 2 for hematocrit <34%	

*Data from Shroyer AL, Coombs LP, Peterson ED, et al: The Society of Thoracic Surgeons: 30-day operative mortality and morbidity risk models. Ann Thorac Surg 75:1856–1864, 2003.

†Data from Grover FL, Cleveland JC Jr, Shroyer LW: Quality improvement in cardiac care. Arch Surg 137:28–36, 2002.

‡Data from Nashef SA, Roques F, Michel P, et al: European system for cardiac operative risk evaluation (EuroSCORE). Eur J Cardiothorac Surg 16:9–13, 1999.

§Data from Hannan EL, Kilburn H Jr, Racz M, et al: Improving the outcomes of coronary artery bypass surgery in New York State. JAMA 271:761–766, 1994.

‖Higgins TL, Estafanous FG, Loop FD, et al: Stratification of morbidity and mortality outcome by preoperative risk factors in coronary artery bypass patients. A clinical severity score [published erratum appears in JAMA 268:1860, 1992]. JAMA 267:2344–2348, 1992.

¶Mack MJ, Brown PP, Kugelmass AD, et al: Current status and outcomes of coronary revascularization 1999 to 2002: 148,396 surgical and percutaneous procedures. Ann Thorac Surg 77:761–766, 2004.

AAA = abdominal aortic aneurysm; BSA = body surface area; CCS = Canadian Cardiovascular Society grade scale for angina; CI = confidence interval; COPD = chronic obstructive pulmonary disease; CPR = cardiopulmonary resuscitation; CVA, cerebrovascular accident; CVD = cardiovascular disease; EF = ejection fraction; GP = glycoprotein; IDDM = insulin-dependent diabetes mellitus; MI = myocardial infarction; MR = mitral regurgitation; NA = not available; NS = not significant; IABP = intra-aortic balloon pump; NIDDM = non–insulin-dependent diabetes mellitus; NYHA = New York Heart Association; OR = odds ratio; PTCA = percutaneous transluminal coronary angioplasty; PVD = peripheral vascular disease; V. fib = ventricular fibrillation; V. tach = ventricular tachycardia.

Adapted from Jones RH, Hannan EL, Hammermeister KE, et al: Identification of preoperative variables needed for risk adjustment of short-term mortality after coronary artery bypass graft surgery. The Working Group Panel on the Cooperative CABG Database Project. J Am Coll Cardiol 28:1478, 1996.

Table 19–2 Multivariable Predictors of Inotrope Use

Variable	Parameter Estimate	Odds Ratio (95% CI)	*p* Value
Intercept	−3.2827		
Cross-clamp time (min)	0.0133	1.013 (1.008–1.019)	<0.001
WMSI	1.4389	4.216 (2.438–7.292)	<0.001
Reoperation	0.8562	2.375 (1.083–5.212)	<0.001
CABG + MVRR	1.2829	3.607 (1.376–9.456)	0.009
Moderate/severe MR	0.4144	2.277 (1.169–4.435)	0.016
LVEF <35%	0.8654	2.376 (1.303–4.332)	0.005

CABG = coronary artery bypass grafting; CI = confidence interval; LVEF = left ventricular ejection fraction; MR = mitral regurgitation; MVRR = mitral valve repair or replacement; WMSI = wall motion score index.

From McKinlay KH, Schinderle DB, Swaminathan M, et al: Predictors of inotrope use during separation from cardiopulmonary bypass. J Cardiothorac Vasc Anesth 18:404, 2004.

extubation, and other measures of resource use. Modeling of *process variables* (i.e., patient level variables specific to how care is delivered such as the specific type of anesthetic administered) and *structure variables* (i.e., variables specific to the environment in which the care is delivered such as a specific piece of equipment or a healthcare provider) have been reported.[46-48] However, this approach suffers from substantial statistical complexity and at the present time remains more theoretical than practical, especially for prediction of infrequent outcome events such as mortality which require large sample sizes for adequate statistical power.

Although surgeons are closely scrutinized, the role of the anesthesiologist in perioperative morbidity and mortality is poorly defined and likely to remain so given the multiplicity of variables involved and low event rates associated with contemporary cardiac surgery. Despite availability of large databases, anesthesia provider information is in most instances not recorded. Detecting trends in mortality on a practitioner level (and untangling the stronger role of the surgeon) requires complex statistical modeling which even if feasible, would likely result in high levels of uncertainty. Only one analysis using this approach has specifically identified the anesthesiologist as a risk factor with no further work reported in more than a decade[49] (see Chapters 39 and 40).

Over the past 2 decades there has been considerable data reported on the potential impact of various anesthetic techniques on outcomes, particularly effects on pre-CPB myocardial ischemia and postoperative myocardial infarction. However, much of this data suffers from inadequate statistical power, use of single centers, and difficulties in standardization of definitions or reporting of *surrogate* (otherwise called *soft*) outcomes. Earlier reports supported a lack of effect of the anesthetic technique suggesting that hemodynamic control was more important (e.g., "it's not what you use, but how you use it"), particularly for prevention of ischemia.[50,51] However, newer data support various degrees of efficacy with different approaches for preserving ventricular function with volatile anesthetics on weaning from CPB,[52,53] or high sympathetic blockade relative to intravenous techniques.[54] Some of these have been linked to improved recovery or shorter lengths of stay. However, the advantages appear to be modest and demonstration of an overt reduction in serious morbidity or mortality in large-scale, multicenter cohorts has not yet been reported. Similar data suggest that although use of a specific anesthetic agent (e.g., opioid or neuromuscular agent) may facilitate earlier extubation, the small magnitude of effect in most instances does not appear to reduce overall length of hospital stay, have significant effects on recovery, or substantially reduce cost.[55,56] Nonetheless, nearly all anesthesiologists continue to strive for the "perfect technique."

Several publications have attempted to more precisely delineate the association of perioperative hemodynamics with outcomes in larger cohorts of patients than have been previously reported in the older randomized trials of anesthetic techniques. Reich et al[57] merged computerized anesthesia record data from 2149 CABG patients (with CPB) at two New York Hospitals from 1993 to 1995 with outcome data from the state's mandatory reporting database. Four independent predictors of mortality were identified: Very high mean pulmonary arterial pressure pre-CPB (>30 mm Hg; OR = 2.1), low mean arterial pressure (MAP) during CPB (40 to 49 mm Hg; OR = 1.3), very high heart rate (HR > 120 bpm; OR = 3.1), and very high diastolic pulmonary arterial pressure (>20 mm Hg; OR = 1.2) post-CPB. The investigators observed that three of the four are markers of severe left ventricular (LV) dysfunction. Although low MAP on CPB can be associated with inadequate perfusion, the value also can be artifactual during weaning given the known problem with exaggerated aortic to radial artery pressure gradients. Curiously, with regard to postoperative myocardial infarction, high HR (101 to 120 bpm; OR = 2.0), and low HR (30 to 39 bpm; OR = 2.9) were independent predictors, although both had wide 95% confidence intervals.

Fillinger et al[58] reported data on a larger cohort of 5934 CABG patients studied at six northern New England hospitals between 1995 and 2000, although their analysis was limited to preinduction HR only. Data were correlated with a large battery of preoperative risk variables. Only 15% of patients had a HR greater than 80 bpm, and only 5% had a HR of more than 90 bpm, most likely reflecting increased β-blocker use (although this variable was not captured and is therefore a major confounder in interpretation of these data). Patients with high HRs were more likely to be female, younger, have chronic obstructive pulmonary disease, diabetes, congestive heart failure, and urgent or emergent status. They observed a significant trend of increasing mortality ($p < 0.001$) and intraoperative need for an intra-aortic balloon pump (IABP) ($p < 0.002$) with HR after adjustment for preoperative risk.

Although the C-index (reported later in a letter to the editor) for the Reich et al[57] mortality model is quite high (0.87), these types of observational analyses are usually limited to "hypotheses generation," although they clearly delineate known correlations of hemodynamics with underlying pathophysiologic conditions on a population basis.

Investigators from Duke University have reported a similar approach focusing specifically on a small subset of physiologic variables (i.e., mean arterial pressure, lowest hematocrit, maximum glucose concentration, and total duration) obtained from continuous data collection during CPB in 2862 CABG patients (1993 to 1996).[59,60] Surprisingly, they found no correlation of these variables with in-hospital mortality; paradoxically, low MAP (<50 mm Hg) was associated with a lower incidence of stroke or coma. This contrasts with a much smaller, but randomized, trial of blood pressure management on CPB by Gold et al,[61] in which an opposite effect was observed.

Although there are no reports specifically examining deaths due to anesthesia in the CABG population, various nonselected studies of anesthesia-related mortality report a wide range of 0.05 to 10 deaths per 10,000 anesthetics.[62] In some of these studies, only deaths due to intraoperative cardiac arrest are reported, and in most cases, such deaths result from anesthetic mishap, such as failure to ventilate or inadvertent drug overdose. Although it could be argued that the array of monitoring techniques commonly used during cardiac surgery might reduce the risk of mishaps, there are no data to suggest that this is the case. As demonstrated by Arbous et al,[62] a variety of "good" and "bad" anesthetic practices continue to influence adverse events (e.g., machine check, lack of turnover of case, reversal of blockade). In a large cohort, Newland et al[63] reported 15 of 144 cardiac arrests (from 72,959 anesthetics between 1989 and 1999) were most commonly associated with medication administration, airway management, and central venous access. It is likely that the rates are higher for cardiac cases given greater challenges with at least two of the three identified factors.

Morbidity and mortality are also influenced by events in the operating room, including time on CPB and aortic cross-clamping, adequacy of revascularization, and complications such as cardiovascular decompensation or bleeding. Reevaluation of the patient's risk can be performed on arrival in the intensive care unit (ICU) at the start of the postoperative period. The APACHE III system has been modified for CABG patients, and Becker et al[64] found that predictors of outcome included the risk score, age, reoperative status, and number of grafts. Higgins et al[65] devised the Cleveland Clinic ICU admission score, which includes preoperative and physiologic factors present on admission to the ICU. Morbidity was 3% with scores of 5 or less, and the rate rose to 83% with scores higher than 20.

PATHOPHYSIOLOGY OF CORONARY ARTERY DISEASE

Anatomy

The anesthesiologist should be familiar with coronary anatomy if only to interpret the significance of angiographic findings. An extensive review of cardiac anatomy can be found in reference cardiology or cardiac surgery texts and in studies using newer technology, such as myocardial contrast perfusion echocardiography and positron emission tomography.[66,67] The following is an abbreviated description of the epicardial coronary anatomy. The coronary circulation and common sites for placement of distal anastomoses during CABG are shown in Figures 19–5 to 19–7. The aortic root contains three cusps: right, left, and noncoronary.

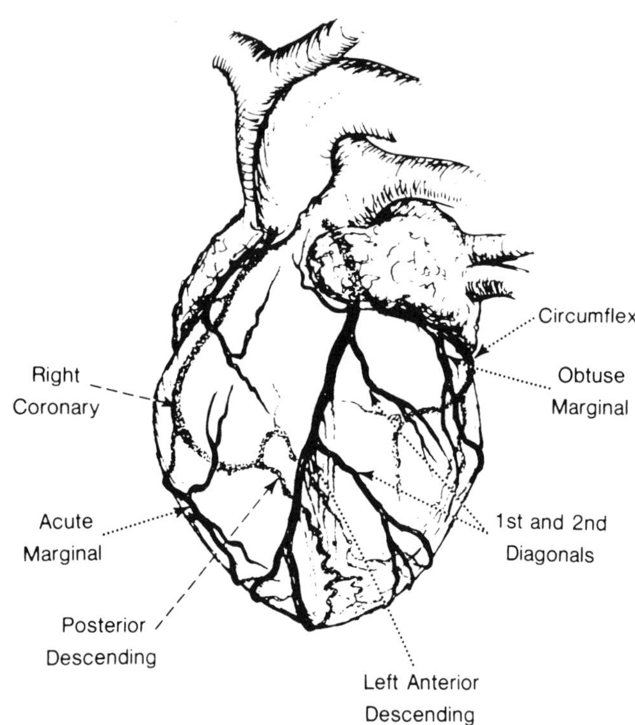

Figure 19–5 Thirty-degree left anterior oblique angiographic view of the heart, which best shows the right coronary artery. *Arrows* indicate common sites of distal vein graft anastomoses. (From Stiles QR, Tucker BL, Lindesmith GG, et al: Myocardial Revascularization: A Surgical Atlas. Boston, Little, Brown, 1976.)

The right coronary artery (RCA) arises from the right sinus of Valsalva and is best seen in the left anterior oblique view on coronary cineangiography (see Fig. 19–5). It passes anteriorly for the first few millimeters, then follows the right atrioventricular (AV) groove, and curves posteriorly within the groove to reach the crux of the heart, the area where the interventricular septum (IVS) meets the AV groove. In 84% of cases, it terminates as the posterior descending artery (PDA), which is its most important branch, being the sole supply to the posterior-superior IVS. Other important branches are those to the sinus node in 60% of patients and the AV node in approximately 85% of patients. Anatomists consider the RCA to be dominant when it crosses the crux of the heart and continues in the AV groove regardless of the origin of the PDA. Angiographers, however, ascribe dominance to the artery, right coronary or left coronary (circumflex), that gives rise to the PDA.

The vertical and superior orientation of the RCA ostium allows easy passage of air bubbles during aortic cannulation, CPB, or during open valve surgery. In sufficient concentration (e.g., coronary air embolus), myocardial ischemia involving the inferior LV wall segments and the right ventricle may occur (Fig. 19–8). In contrast, the near perpendicular orientation of the left main coronary ostium makes air embolization much less common.

The left coronary artery arises from the left sinus of Valsalva as the left main coronary artery. This is best seen in a

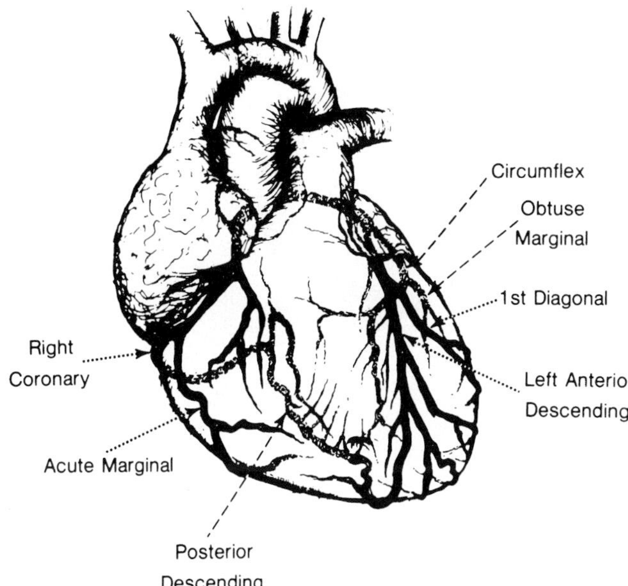

Figure 19–6 Ten-degree right anterior oblique angiographic view of the heart, which best shows the left main coronary artery dividing into the circumflex and left anterior descending arteries. *Arrows* indicate common sites of distal vein graft anastomoses. (Adapted from Stiles QR, Tucker BL, Lindesmith GG, et al: Myocardial Revascularization: A Surgical Atlas. Boston, Little, Brown, 1976.)

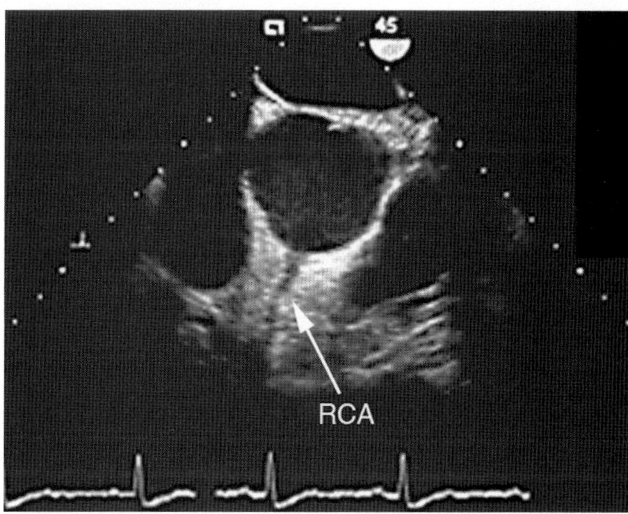

Figure 19–8 The vertical and superior orientation of the right coronary artery arising from the aortic root is identified by transesophageal echocardiography (TEE). The TEE transducer in the esophagus is on the top of the screen, and the patient's chest wall is on the bottom. Retained air preferentially enters the right coronary artery (RCA), which may cause inferior ischemia, depending on the amount of air and the coronary perfusion pressure. Elevation of perfusion pressure using phenylephrine is often used to treat coronary air embolus. The left main artery (not visible) arises at approximately 3 o'clock on this image. (Image courtesy of Martin J. London, MD, University of California, San Francisco, CA [www.ucsf.edu/teeecho].)

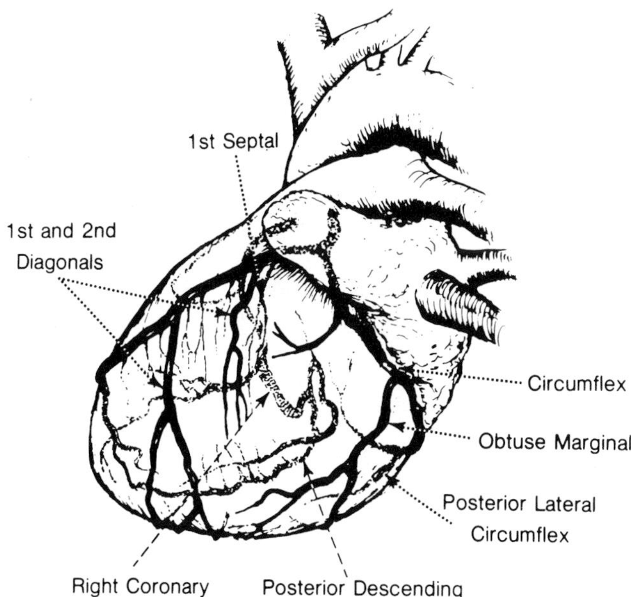

Figure 19–7 Seventy-five degree left anterior oblique angiographic view of the heart, which best shows branches of the left anterior descending and circumflex coronary arteries. (Adapted from Stiles QR, Tucker BL, Lindesmith GG, et al: Myocardial Revascularization: A Surgical Atlas. Boston, Little, Brown, 1976.)

shallow right anterior oblique projection (see Fig. 19–6). The left main coronary artery courses anteriorly and to the left, where it divides in a space between the aorta and pulmonary artery. Its branches are the left anterior descending (LAD) and circumflex arteries. The LAD passes along the anterior intraventricular groove. It may reach only two thirds of the distance to the apex or extend around the apex to the diaphragmatic portion of the left ventricle. Major branches of the LAD are the diagonal branches, which supply the free wall of the left ventricle, and septal branches, which course posteriorly to supply the major portion of the IVS. Although there may be many diagonal and septal branches, the first diagonal and first septal branches serve as important landmarks in the descriptions of lesions of the LAD (see Fig. 19–7).

The circumflex arises at a sharp angle from the left main coronary artery and courses toward the crux of the heart in the AV groove. When the circumflex gives rise to the PDA, the circulation is said to be left dominant, and the left coronary circulation supplies the entire IVS and the AV node. In approximately 40% of patients, the circumflex supplies the branch to the SA node. Up to four obtuse marginal (OM) arteries arise from the circumflex and supply the lateral wall of the left ventricle (see Fig. 19–7). All of the previously described epicardial branches give rise to small vessels that supply the outer third of the myocardium and penetrating vessels that anastomose with the subendocardial plexus. This capillary plexus is unique in that it functions as an end-arterial system. Each epicardial arteriole supplies a capillary plexus that forms an end loop rather than anastomosing with an adjacent capillary from another epicardial artery.[68] Significant collateral circulation does not exist at the microcirculatory level. This capillary anatomy explains the very distinct areas of myocardial ischemia or infarction that can be related to disease in a discrete epicardial artery (see Chapters 6 and 12).

CAD most commonly affects the epicardial muscular arteries with rare intramyocardial lesions. However, severe disorders of the microcirculation and primary impairment of coronary vascular reserve in normal coronary arteries have been described, especially in diabetics, female patients, and those with variant angina.[69-71] Atherosclerosis in all organs is most common at the outer edges of vessel bifurcations, because in these regions blood flow is slower and changes direction during the cardiac cycle resulting in less net shear stress (i.e., frictional force per unit area) than in other regions

O_2 Supply:

- O_2 content of arterial blood
- Coronary blood flow

O_2 Demands:

- Contractile state
- Afterload
- Preload
- Heart rate

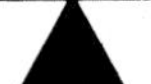

MYOCARDIAL O_2 BALANCE

Figure 19–9 Factors determining myocardial oxygen supply and demand.

with more steady blood flow and higher shear stress.[72] Low shear stress has been shown to stimulate an atherogenic phenotype in the endothelium. Epicardial lesions can be single but are more often multiple. A combined lesion of the RCA and both branches of the left coronary artery is referred to as triple-vessel disease. The left coronary artery supplies the thickest portions of the left ventricle, at least the exterior two thirds of the IVS, and the greater part of the atria. Most bypass grafts are done on the left coronary system.

Venous drainage of the myocardium is primarily to the coronary sinus, which drains 96% of the LV free wall and septum, and the remainder of the venous return goes directly into the right atrium.[67] A small fraction may enter other cardiac chambers directly through the anterior-sinusoidal, anterior-luminal, and thebesian veins.[73]

Myocardial Ischemia and Infarction

In patients with CAD, myocardial ischemia usually results from increases in myocardial oxygen demand (Fig. 19–9) that exceed the capacity of the stenosed coronary arteries to increase their oxygen supply. However, the determinants of myocardial oxygen balance are complex, and alterations may have several effects. For example, an increase in blood pressure (i.e., increased afterload) increases wall tension and oxygen demand while also increasing coronary blood flow (CBF). It is now appreciated that myocardial ischemia may occur without changes in systemic hemodynamics and in awake patients may occur in the absence of chest pain (i.e., silent ischemia), particularly in diabetic patients.

In atherosclerotic heart disease, the fundamental lesion is an intimal lipid plaque that causes chronic stenosis and episodic thrombosis, occurring most often in an epicardial coronary artery (Fig. 19–10), thereby reducing myocardial blood supply. Characteristics of the vulnerable plaque include high lipid content, a thin fibrous cap, a reduced number of smooth muscle cells, and increased macrophage activity.[74-76] The lipid core is the most thrombogenic component of the plaque. Fuster[77] described five phases in the progression of CAD by plaque morphology. Phase 1 is a small plaque present in many people younger than 30 years and usually progresses very slowly depending on the presence of risk factors associated with CAD (i.e., elevated low-density lipoprotein cholesterol). Phase 2 is a plaque with a high lipid content that has the potential to rupture. If it ruptures, it will lead to thrombosis and increased stenosis (phase 5), possibly producing unstable angina or an acute coronary syndrome. The phase 2 plaque usually does not rupture; it instead progresses onto phases 3 and 4, with enlargement and fibrous tissue organization, which may ultimately produce an occlusive plaque at phase 5.

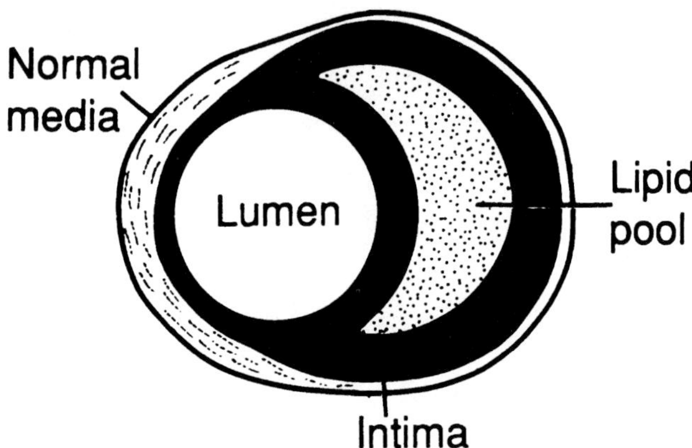

Figure 19–10 Lipoid plaque lesion of a coronary artery. (From Davies MJ: A macro and micro view of coronary vascular insult in ischemic heart disease. Circulation 82(suppl II):II-38, 1990, with permission of American Heart Association.)

Acute coronary syndromes (ACSs) are produced by sudden decreases in CBF. In unstable angina, a relatively small fissure in a plaque may produce a temporary thrombotic occlusion of a vessel lasting 10 to 20 minutes.[74] Release of vasoactive substances from platelets and white blood cells, as well as dysfunction of the endothelium, may lead to vasoconstriction and reduction of CBF.[75,76] If the occlusion lasts up to 1 hour, it may produce a small non-Q-wave MI. The duration of myocardial ischemia may be limited by reduced vasoconstriction, spontaneous thrombolysis, or the opening of collateral channels. A larger plaque disruption and prolonged thrombosis will produce a Q-wave infarction with transmural myocardial necrosis. The potential lesions seen with plaque fissure are shown in Figure 19–11. Several studies have found that the coronary artery responsible for an acute infarction is often only moderately obstructed.[78,79] It is the extent of plaque rupture and thrombosis that determines the size and extent of an infarction, rather than the degree of stenosis. Patients with severely obstructed coronary arteries often have extensive collateral circulations that protect them from infarction. Similar

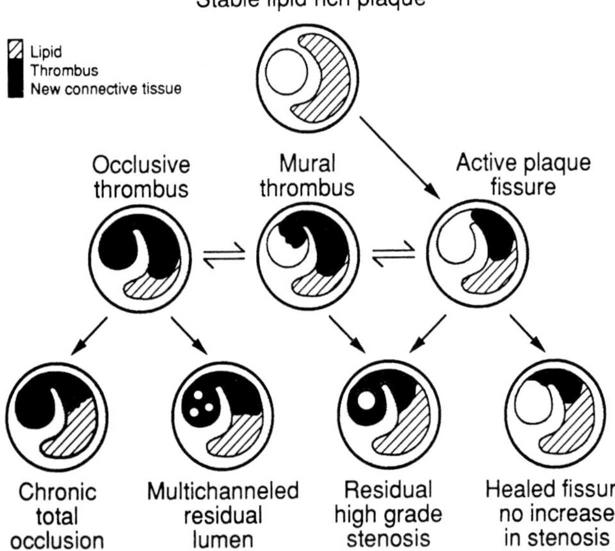

Figure 19–11 Possible outcomes of intimal plaque rupture. (From Davies MJ: A macro and micro view of coronary vascular insult in ischemic heart disease. Circulation 82(suppl II):II-38, 1990, with permission of American Heart Association.)

findings have been reported in patients developing postoperative myocardial infarction after noncardiac surgery.[80-82]

The physiology of the coronary circulation is reviewed in Chapter 6. CBF is in the normal individual independent of perfusion pressure, but it is related to tissue oxygen demand, perhaps through a metabolite such as adenosine.[67,83] This phenomenon is referred to as *autoregulation*. Autoregulation affects all layers of the ventricular wall, maintaining essentially equal flows from the epicardium to endocardium.[84,85] The difference between autoregulated flow and maximal flow constitutes the coronary vascular reserve. As an obstruction of a coronary artery increases in size, dilation of the capillary bed occurs, with maintenance of adequate blood supply as the result. Coronary flow reserve, however, is diminished and eventually is exhausted and autoregulation begins to fail. Autoregulatory failure is loss of metabolic control of CBF and the sole dependence on pressure gradients to determine flow. Autoregulation fails first in the subendocardium, where blood flow fails to match demand, resulting in subendocardial ischemia and dysfunction.[71,83]

Autoregulation is pressure-dependent, in that as perfusion pressure falls below a critical value, autoregulation begins to fail. In conscious animals, the pressure at which autoregulation begins to fail is very low (map of 38 to 40 mm Hg).[86] Because CBF reserve is diminished in CAD, the pressure at which subendocardial autoregulation fails is raised.[83] HR also appears to have an effect on autoregulation. In an unanesthetized animal model, when the HR was doubled, the perfusion pressure that produced failure of subendocardial autoregulation was raised from a mean of 38 mm Hg at the normal HR to a mean of 61 mm Hg at the doubled rate.[87] This pressure is not that much below normal perfusion pressures. This effect of HR on subendocardial autoregulation is related to the increased myocardial oxygen consumption and flow caused by tachycardia and to the reduction in diastolic time and therefore perfusion. The net effect is a reduction in coronary vascular reserve and earlier failure of autoregulation, with resultant subendocardial ischemia. Tachycardia, because of its effects on demand and supply (reduction in diastolic perfusion time), is especially deleterious in the presence of CAD, in which perfusion pressures beyond an epicardial arterial obstruction are unknown.[88] Avoidance of hypotension and tachycardia has been the basic tenet of anesthetic practice in patients with CAD for many years.

A coronary arterial stenosis may be rigid or, more commonly (70%), compliant in nature.[89] When the pressure in the coronary circulation distal to a fixed stenosis is decreased, flow across the stenotic area decreases. On the other hand, when the pressure distal to a compliant obstruction is increased, flow across the lesion is increased.[90] The clinical implication is that decreased blood pressure to an area of myocardium supplied by a vessel with a variable stenosis will decrease blood supply to the myocardium by two mechanisms: loss of collateral flow and decreased flow across the compliant stenosis. Collateral vessels exist in normal hearts, but in the presence of CAD they are increased in size and number.[91] When a coronary vessel has a high-grade stenosis, the microvasculature distal to it may be maximally dilated even at rest and subject to ischemia. Collaterals may develop between this ischemic zone and an adjacent nonischemic area supplied by a different vessel. When vasodilation of the microcirculation is induced by exercise or drugs, perfusion of the ischemic bed by the collateral circulation may be decreased or cut off, particularly when the collateral vessels are poorly developed, because these present a higher degree of resistance than collaterals that are well developed. When vasodilation occurs in the nonischemic bed, pressure within it is decreased, and flow across collateral vessels with high resistance is reduced. An increase in myocardial blood flow in one region that reduces flow in another is referred to as a coronary steal.[92,93] In experimental models, a partial lesion of the epicardial artery supplying the collateral vessel is required to produce a coronary steal.[92] This anatomic configuration, called *steal-prone anatomy*, occurs in 23% of patients with symptomatic CAD in one large registry of coronary angiograms.[94] Some observers believe it is unlikely that a steal mechanism precipitates myocardial ischemia by itself, but it may intensify ischemia in areas supplied by collateral vessels.

The hallmark symptom of myocardial ischemia is pain. It has been shown, however, that significant ischemia may occur without pain.[95,96] Early research with ambulatory electrocardiographic (ECG) monitoring reported that these episodes were frequent and occur at lower HRs and activity levels when compared with exercise stress test data for the same individuals.[97] These researchers also demonstrated that the "silent" ischemic episodes were not an electrical anomaly, but were the result of myocardial perfusion impairment and resulted in impaired regional function.[98] A study of patients presenting for elective CABG has confirmed these findings in the perioperative period: 42% of 50 patients studied had ischemic episodes preoperatively, 87% of these episodes were clinically silent, and few were precipitated by adverse hemodynamics.[99] However, in the cardiology community there exists considerable controversy regarding "hemodynamically silent" ischemia. Deedwania and Nelson subsequently reported that most silent episodes were associated with elevations of HR or blood pressure and were often closely linked to circadian sleep-wake cycles, with the highest incidence occurring in the morning.[100,101] Although interest in ambulatory silent ischemia using ambulatory monitoring has been limited given cardiologists' preferences for easier, more sensitive, and more specific monitoring techniques (e.g., stress testing methods), Deedwania's findings are commonly cited. However, there is no doubt that primary reductions in myocardial oxygen supply due to hypotension, anemia, or coronary vasoconstriction are important mechanisms in development of ischemia, particularly in the perioperative period.

ANESTHESIA FOR CORONARY ARTERY BYPASS GRAFTING

Conventional CABG with CPB is still the most commonly performed cardiac surgical procedure (Box 19–1). Fast-track management with early extubation (4 to 8 hours postoperatively) has become the standard of care in nearly all centers. OPCAB is increasing steadily, although its use tends to be very frequent in some centers or infrequent in others as various surgeons have become "early adopters" or are waiting for firm evidence-based recommendations from future randomized, controlled trials. However, anesthetic management of the sickest patients undergoing multivessel operations combined with valve repair or replacement, repeat operations, and other complex procedures (e.g., ventricular septal defect repairs along with CABG after acute myocardial infarction) has changed relatively little over the past decade as the long duration of surgery usually mandates greater cumulative doses of fixed anesthetic agents with overnight or even prolonged post-

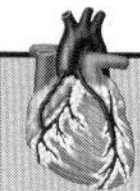

BOX 19–1 *Management Strategies for Anesthesia for Myocardial Revascularization*

Preoperative Evaluation and Management

Assessment of Cardiac Characteristics

1. Cardiac history and presenting symptoms
   Acute unstable angina, acute myocardial infarction, congestive heart failure, cardiogenic shock highest risk (possible intra-aortic balloon pump, left ventricular assist device)
2. Coronary artery anatomy
   Left main high-grade lesion, triple-vessel disease, proximal left anterior descending artery lesions: highest risk
   Status of collateral circulation and microcirculation, diffuse distal disease
3. Ventricular function
   Ejection fraction: >50%, low risk; <50%, intermediate risk; <25% to 30%, high risk
4. Valvular and structural anatomy and function
   Best assessed by echocardiogram and/or cardiac catheterization
   Concurrent aortic stenosis (potential for subendocardial ischemia), mitral regurgitation (may be related to acute or chronic ischemia, papillary rupture), aortic insufficiency (dilated ventricle, increased wall tension, problems with administration of anterograde cardioplegia, ventricular dilation during surgery), ventricular septal defect (acute), ventricular aneurysm or pseudoaneurysm
5. Electrocardiogram
   Q waves (ischemic potential, reduced function), ST-T depression or elevation (ischemic potential)
   Left bundle-branch block (advanced coronary artery disease, depressed function, potential complete heart block with passage of pulmonary artery catheter)
   PR interval (prolongation with β-blockers and calcium channel blockers, progression to more advanced block)
   Rhythm: atrial fibrillation, flutter, supraventricular tachycardia (instability during case, increased risk of perioperative cerebrovascular accident)
6. Chest radiograph
   Cardiomegaly (depressed function, pericardial effusion or tamponade, persistent left-sided superior vena cava with potentially difficult central venous pressure or pulmonary artery catheter placement)
   Aortic calcification (inability to cross-clamp aorta, "porcelain aorta")
   Lung fields (acute or chronic heart failure, pleural effusions)

Assessment of Major Comorbidities

1. Carotid and cerebrovascular disease
   Assess for presence of high-grade occlusive disease (unusual in absence of symptoms or previous cerebrovascular accident); carotid duplex ultrasound examination of all high-risk patients
2. Peripheral vascular disease
   Usually obvious, aortic disease associated with inability to pass an intra-aortic balloon pump (IABP) in normal manner, difficult radial artery catheterization possible
3. Diabetes
   Hyperglycemia associated with impaired endothelial function and attenuation of preconditioning
   Serum potassium abnormalities with glucose or acid-base management, type II renal tubular acidosis
4. Renal disease
   For dialysis patients, ensure recent dialysis and verify serum potassium level
   Careful fluid and medication management
   Systemic acidosis and hyperkalemia more likely
   More frequent blood gas and electrolyte sampling required
5. Pulmonary disease
   Bronchospasm, air trapping, high dead space with slower inhalational agent uptake, transpulmonary passage of air or embolic debris more likely, atelectasis, segmental and lobar collapse possible

Preoperative Medication Management

1. β-Adrenergic blockers
   Recommended for all patients unless contraindicated (clonidine or nondihydropyridine calcium entry blockers such as diltiazem are alternatives) to reduce risk of ischemia
   Clinical data dispute efficacy in prevention of acute cardiopulmonary bypass induced adrenoreceptor desensitization
2. Calcium channel blockers
   Higher incidence of heart block or need for pacing with concurrent β-blocker therapy
   Efficacy in ischemia prevention controversial, recent meta-analysis suggests efficacy
3. Angiotensin-converting enzyme inhibitor
   Clinical studies controversial regarding increased propensity for hypotension during induction
4. Diuretics
   No firm recommendations; ensure adequate serum potassium levels
5. Statins
   Observational data suggest beneficial anti-inflammatory effects and improved outcome independent of lipid lowering effects; no data available from randomized, controlled trials
   No data to suggest they should not be continued for patients already receiving them, despite known risks of rhabdomyolysis and hepatic injury with chronic use
6. Aspirin
   Strong data to suggest they should be continued despite increased bleeding, especially for early and late graft patency and mortality[145]
7. Other antiplatelet agents or glycoprotein IIa/IIIb inhibitors
   Associated with increased bleeding, hold as appropriate, treat with factor, platelets, or recombinant factor VII as necessary
8. Heparin
   Regimen often surgeon specific, usually discontinued 4 hours preoperatively for stable patients, continued up to and through pre-cardiopulmonary bypass period for critical left main disease or acutely unstable angina patients
9. Insulin
   Continuous infusion for poorly controlled hyperglycemia, insulin resistance may be encountered during hypothermic cardiopulmonary bypass
10. Oral hypoglycemic agents, such as metformin, glipizide, or glyburide
   Metformin associated with lactic acidosis in patients developing perioperative low cardiac output, optimal to hold administration several half-lives preoperatively
   Glyburide experimentally blocks preconditioning by closure of ATP-mediated potassium channels, no clinical evidence for adverse effects documented
11. Antibiotic prophylaxis
   Cephazolin (1 g IV) or cefuroxime (1.5 g IV) less than 60 minutes before incision; vancomycin (1 g by slow infusion to avoid hypotension and flushing) or clindamycin (600 to 900 mg IV) for penicillin or cephalosporin allergy; adjust as appropriate for renal failure
   Repeat: cefazolin every 2 to 5 hours, cefuroxime every 3 to 4 hours, vancomycin every 6 to 12 hours, clindamycin every 3 to 6 hours; adjust as appropriate for renal failure

12. Anxiolytic or analgesic premedication
    Oral diazepam (5 to 10 mg) at least 1 hour before induction, supplement with intravenous fentanyl or midazolam after insertion of intravenous line as needed
    Intramuscular lorazepam (1 to 2 mg) or morphine (approximately 0.15 mg/kg) at least 1 hour before induction, depending on age, comorbidities, anxiety level
    Supplemental nasal prong or facemask oxygen to avoid desaturation and ischemia
13. Preoperative epidural insertion
    Uncommon in United States, but it may reduce stress response, preserve adrenoreceptor function, and decrease time to extubation, pulmonary complications and pain scores.[483]
    Use for conscious off-pump coronary artery bypass has been increasingly reported from European centers (limited to one- or two-vessel procedures).
    Optimal to place at least 6 to 8 hours preoperatively to ensure adequate hemostasis

Intraoperative Management

1. Intravenous access
   One or two large-bore peripheral intravenous lines; fluid warmer for blood administration
2. Electrocardiographic monitoring
   V_3 to V_5 precordial lead monitoring most sensitive for ischemia, recommended for all patients with the exception of those with left bundle-branch block
   Inferior lead for rhythm monitoring
3. Blood pressure monitoring
   Radial artery catheter: right arm may be preferable because of potential effects of retraction for left internal mammary artery dissection (with newer surgical retractors, this is likely less problematic).
   Backup cuff for arterial monitoring failure and correlation of pressures
4. Intrathecal medication
   Low-dose intrathecal morphine (0.005 to 0.01 mg/kg) may reduce postoperative pain; efficacy data inconclusive, especially with fast track techniques; use 25-gauge needle to minimize vascular trauma.
5. Anesthetic induction
   Ensure surgeon and perfusionist are available in the rare event of cardiac arrest during induction, which may require emergency femoral-femoral CPB if the patient is unresponsive to conventional therapy.
   Fast-tracking routines using reduced doses of opioids and or benzodiazepines are standard in most centers. Various combinations of opioid boluses with or without continuous infusion (fentanyl, 10 to 20 μg/kg; sufentanil, 2.5 to 5 μg/kg; remifentanil infusion) and volatile agents (isoflurane, sevoflurane, or desflurane) with or without supplemental intravenous drugs (midazolam, 0.05 to 1 mg/g; propofol or dexmedetomidine bolus or infusions) are used. Given the increasing evidence for preconditioning effects, liberal volatile agent use is encouraged. Avoid nitrous oxide because of the adverse impact of possible hypoxemia on myocardial oxygen delivery and the possible expanding effects on cerebral or coronary gaseous emboli.
   Muscle relaxation with nondepolarizing neuromuscular blockers is almost always used, although this appears not to be absolutely necessary (e.g., movement may precede recall).
   Maintain heart rate as low as allowed based on adequate blood pressure and cardiac output to maximize coronary blood flow, which in the left ventricle occurs exclusively during diastole. The heart rate can be influenced by β-blocker or calcium channel blocker use, valvular disease, ejection fraction, or opioid dosing.
   Maintain adequate perfusion pressure based on coronary, cerebrovascular, renal, and other involved organ systems, based on examination of preoperative values and reduction in demand during stable anesthetic.
   Baseline arterial blood gas determination is recommended after intubation, along with routine clinical examination for proper endotracheal tube placement.
   Baseline activated coagulation time is required before heparin administration; heparin dose response system is used in many centers, particularly when aprotinin is administered.
   Foley placement for all patients
   Temperature monitoring: bladder or esophageal (core temperature) and nasopharyngeal or tympanic (brain temperature) are recommended for all cardiopulmonary bypass cases to minimize temperature gradients during rewarming and to minimize risk of cerebral hyperthermia with potential cerebral venous desaturation (implicated in neurocognitive dysfunction). For off-pump coronary artery bypass grafting, bladder only is sufficient. Use care when inserting nasopharyngeal probe because of the later use of heparin.
   Cerebral monitoring: use of bispectral or similar monitors (e.g., entropy, PSArray) are increasingly used in cardiac patients because of the increased risk of recall and for better titration of anesthetics, particularly with fast-track techniques. Efficacy remains controversial. Regardless of their use, care should be taken at all times to monitor for evidence of lightness, especially during periods of hemodynamic instability in which the anesthetic level is reduced.
6. Pulmonary artery catheter or central venous pressure catheter placement
   Central venous pressure catheter is considered standard of care; pulmonary artery catheter use is very center specific and appears to be declining for routine on-pump coronary artery bypass grafting but is common for off-pump coronary artery bypass grafting (including common unsubstantiated recommendations in the literature for the use of continuous SvO_2 catheters).
   Need for placement of pulmonary artery catheter before induction is controversial, but severe concurrent valve disease and a low ejection fraction are strong indications.
   When using pulmonary artery catheter, ensure the catheter does not wedge inadvertently during surgical manipulation of the heart (closes the loop, advancing it outward). Transesophageal echocardiography (TEE) can easily verify positioning; otherwise, withdrawing the catheter several centimeters before institution of cardiopulmonary bypass is usually effective.
   Avoid pulmonary artery catheter balloon inflation, particularly when the patient is heparinized or hypothermic.
7. Pharmacologic adjuncts
   Antifibrinolytic therapy
      Used primarily for cardiopulmonary bypass cases, although practices vary in European countries; strong evidence for efficacy with aprotinin (also most expensive)
      ε-Aminocaproic acid (Amicar): continuous infusion from skin incision and bolus dosing (5 g) after heparin administration and after cardiopulmonary bypass weaning are used with variable efficacy. Although there are concerns regarding renal vasoconstriction and thrombosis, both appear to lack clinical significance. Do not use concurrently with aprotinin.
      Aprotinin: strong evidence in the literature for efficacy and safety in redo cases. Several regimens have been investigated, although the high-dose Hammersmith protocol (7 to 8 million units cumulative dose) is most common. Highest risk from anaphylaxis associated with reexposure during first 6 to 8 weeks after initial therapy.
      Tranexamic acid: strong evidence in the literature for efficacy; not available in the United States
   Steroid administration
      High dose before cardiopulmonary bypass; methylprednisolone (2 to 3 g) is used in some centers to block some components

Box continued on following page

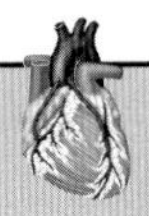

BOX 19–1 ***Management Strategies for Anesthesia for Myocardial Revascularization—(Continued)***

of inflammatory response, but results of clinical studies do not support efficacy and suggest potentially adverse effects on pulmonary function.

8. Insertion for TEE
   - Use can be heavily influenced by surgeon's preference, center's resources, anesthesia or cardiology expertise, and availability; routine use common in many centers for all patients
   - Can be of particular value in guiding anesthetic (fluid administration, detection of new ischemia, verification of pulmonary artery catheter placement in proximal pulmonary artery) and surgery (verification of retrograde cardioplegia cannula, IABP tip relative to arch vessels, presence of aortic root and arch calcification and of ulceration or mobile components, placement of left ventricular vent, ischemic changes, and other determinations)
   - Stomach decompression before and after placement of probe is recommended to decrease risk of postoperative passive aspiration.
   - Esophageal perforation is a rare but increasingly recognized as a complication that must be considered, especially with development of septic changes with new bilateral pleural effusions postoperatively.
9. Sternotomy
   - It is a very stimulating stress; ensure adequate anesthesia, especially if preparation and drape period is prolonged.
   - "Let down the lungs" to avoid potential pleural tear from sternal saw.
   - Redo sternotomy
     - Uses different technique: oscillating saw on outer sternal table, wires removed manually, and blunt dissection with scissor used on the inner table of the sternum.
     - Risks include right ventricular perforation, damage to existing vein grafts, and ventricular fibrillation from electrocautery energy transmitted by a sternal wire.
     - Use external defibrillation pads on all redo cases.
     - Ensure that blood (preferably 2 units checked) is close at hand during opening.
     - Usual presenting sign of right ventricular perforation is ventricular fibrillation, often with little obvious bleeding; emergent femoral-femoral cardiopulmonary bypass usually required

Management before Revascularization

1. Maintain "favorable hemodynamics," with low heart rate and maintenance of systemic blood pressure depending on the preoperative baseline, age, coronary anatomy, and presence of other compromised organs (e.g., brain, kidney). Hypotension with surgical manipulation of the heart and aorta is unavoidable but is usually treated with phenylephrine, volume supplementation, and Trendelenburg position. Close communication with the surgeon is essential.
2. Left internal mammary artery dissection: elevate table, rotate to left, and reduce tidal volumes (increase rate) to facilitate surgeon's exposure. Similar maneuvers for the less commonly performed right internal mammary artery dissection. Heparin is usually administered before clamping of the left internal mammary artery pedicle to avoid thrombosis. Papaverine is often injected retrograde by the surgeon, which occasionally causes hypotension.
3. Conventional coronary artery bypass grafting (CABG)
   - Passive hypothermia is likely protective, given the reduction in myocardial oxygen demands and cerebral protective effects.
   - Pre-bypass phlebotomy is popular in certain centers, although evidence of its efficacy is controversial. Blood may be sequestered before heparinization into storage bags, usually by central venous pressure catheter access, which may require additional fluid administration or by the right atrial cannula just before institution of bypass, usually with the assistance of phenylephrine. The latter technique is also a component of retrograde autologous priming, whose efficacy is controversial.
   - Retrograde cardioplegia may be used alone or, more commonly, in combination with anterograde techniques. Perfusion of the right ventricle is limited by this technique. TEE can assist in placement and confirmation of the catheter in the coronary sinus.
4. Redo cases
   - Atheroma in prior vein grafts is sandy and often loose. Sudden, profound ischemia may occur with surgical manipulation of grafts due to distal embolization. This may require emergent institution of cardiopulmonary bypass.
   - Adequate conduits are essential for performing anastomoses. This can be problematic in redo patients.
   - Exposure for cannulation and exposure of the left ventricle is often more complex because of adhesions and accounts for increased blood loss.
5. Off-pump coronary artery bypass grafting
   - Maintenance of normothermia is desirable to reduce bleeding and in case of severe hypothermia, propensity toward ventricular fibrillation, and for facilitating intraoperative extubation if planned. This can be challenging, although forced air and water blankets can be helpful.
6. Heparin administration
   - Administer 300 to 400 IU/kg. Higher dose required with aprotinin or with heparin resistance (most commonly associated with prolonged preop administration). Resistance is usually easily treated with 1 unit of fresh frozen plasma or recombinant antithrombin III. Activated coagulation time between 450 and 500 seconds is required for institution of cardiopulmonary bypass.
   - Dosing of heparin for off-pump coronary artery bypass cases is controversial, with centers using full- or low-dose regimens (e.g., 150 U/kg).
   - Only use kaolin activated coagulation time tubes with concurrent aprotinin administration.
   - Mild hypotension due to vasodilation is common with heparin administration.
   - For patients with heparin-induced thrombocytopenia, direct thrombin inhibitors have been used with success (although usually with significantly greater blood loss).
7. Cannulation
   - Aortic cannula
     - Examination of cannulation site by epicardial imaging may be used particularly if surgical palpation is suspicious for calcium or TEE examination reveals prominent distal arch or proximal aortic root disease. Surgical response to severe disease ranges from no change to "no touch" techniques to potential circulatory arrest.
     - Ensure that systemic pressure is lowered to lowest safe level (90 to 110 mm Hg systolic) during cannulation to minimize risk of dissection.
     - Adequate eye protection is required at all times and particularly during this period due to splash hazard.
     - Surgeon inspects lines for air bubbles before hooking up circuit.
     - Hypotension can be effectively treated by perfusionist infusing fluid ("give 100") into the aortic cannula given the resistance (versus venous capacitance) effects on compliance of the aorta.
   - Retrograde cannula
     - Inserted in the coronary sinus with insertion site near the right atrial appendage. TEE can guide approximately but is limited

by its two-dimensional imaging. Proper placement can be verified by TEE, surgical palpation in great cardiac vein, and dark color of the coronary sinus blood. Pressure monitoring is used to ensure adequate infusion (if low, it is likely in the right ventricle; if excessively high, rupture could occur).

Insertion can be difficult and cause major hemodynamic compromise and arrhythmias. For sick redo or low ejection fraction, insertion after institution of CPB or preparation for rapid institution of CPB may occasionally be required as arrest may occur.

Venous cannula

For isolated CABG, a single large-bore venous cannula is inserted through the right atrium into the inferior vena cava. It can be partially imaged by TEE in the bicaval view.

Left ventricular vent

Inserted after institution of CPB via the left superior pulmonary vein in many but not all cases. Can be visualized on TEE short-axis view. Verification of absence of thrombus in the LV is essential in patient with a recent anterior wall MI or aneurysm.

Revascularization Management

1. Conventional CABG

   On institution of cardiopulmonary bypass with full flow, discontinue mechanical ventilation. Passive insufflation of oxygen (200 mL/min) is usually continued. Discontinue all maintenance intravenous fluid. Turn off power to the TEE transducer if present. Verify pulmonary artery catheter tip position to avoid inadvertent wedging. Drain urine bag or mark value before cardiopulmonary bypass.

   Myocardial preservation by surgeon and perfusionist involves anterograde or retrograde cardioplegia (or both), arrest with high-potassium cardioplegia, and in most centers, hypothermia (systemic, topical, and by cardioplegia).

2. Off-pump coronary artery bypass grafting

   Left anterior descending and diagonal vessels

   Only mild left ventricular displacement is required (packs under left ventricle with mild rotation of the left ventricle upward and to the left); hemodynamic effects are usually minimal in the absence of ischemia or a very low ejection fraction. Diagonal visualization requires additional rotation. Stabilizer placement is usually well tolerated. Hemodynamic changes (hypotension) are usually easily treated with fluids, Trendelenburg position, or phenylephrine.

   Posterior descending and circumflex vessels

   Moderate to severe left ventricular displacement (verticalization), most pronounced for circumflex anastomoses, is required. Application of an apical suction device is common, although other, simpler methods are used. With proper placement, hypotension is usually mild but more common than with left anterior descending or diagonal grafts. With improper placement or a large left ventricle or right ventricle, compressive effects on the right ventricle can be severe, leading to a major reduction in cardiac output. Opening of the right pleural space may accommodate the right ventricle, relieving the compression with hemodynamic improvement. Trendelenburg positioning is helpful for maintaining hemodynamics and for the surgeon's visualization.

   Mechanical ischemic preconditioning (5-minute occlusion followed by 5-minute reperfusion) is used by some surgeons. However, evidence for efficacy, especially with concurrent volatile agent use, is weak.

   Some clinicians use "reperfusion prophylaxis," similar to the cardiac catheter lab setting during acute MI with lidocaine, thrombolytics, and magnesium sulfate. With routine off-pump coronary artery bypass, there is little evidence for this because most patients have native and collateral flow.

   Ischemia during anastomosis can be treated with insertion of an intracoronary shunt. Some surgeons use these routinely, although there is concern regarding endothelial damage with their use, and many surgeons avoid them unless absolutely necessary.

   TEE can be helpful. However, with verticalization and application of a stabilizer, visualization of all walls and interpretation of wall motion can be difficult. Electrocardiographic amplitude is often markedly diminished with verticalization for posterior descending artery and circumflex anastomoses. Detection of new mitral regurgitation strongly suggests new ischemia.

Management after Revascularization

1. Cardiopulmonary bypass weaning

   Plan ahead for potential inotrope and other vasoactive drug use based on presence of known predictors of difficult weaning, particularly low ejection fraction before cardiopulmonary bypass.

   Epicardial leads (atrial and ventricular) should be placed. Atrioventricular block and bradycardia are common in patients with severe ischemia, those on β-blockers and calcium channel antagonists. Impaired diastolic relaxation is common, reducing the effectiveness of the Frank-Starling mechanism for augmentation of cardiac output. Heart rate plays a larger role, and maintaining heart rate at 80 to 90 beats per minute for several hours avoids ventricular distention. Frequent evaluation for return of the patient's underlying sinus rhythm is optimal because it may be associated with the best cardiac output.

   Augmentation of cardiac index with catecholamines (epinephrine, dopamine, dobutamine) and/or phosphodiesterase inhibitors (amrinone, milrinone) may be required for low cardiac index (generally <2.0 L/min/m^2) or elevation of pulmonary artery occlusion pressure (generally >18 to 20 mm Hg).

   Intra-aortic balloon counterpulsation is used when inotrope therapy alone is insufficient. IABP augments diastolic coronary perfusion and forward flow ("suction effect"). Aortic insufficiency is a relative contraindication to IABP. Evaluate with TEE to avoid ventricular distention, and check placement below the level of the left subclavian and carotid vessels.

2. Off-pump coronary artery bypass grafting

   Assuming adequate anastomoses have been performed, cardiac index returns to normal levels immediately. Function may deteriorate if significant ischemia has occurred, although this is unusual.

3. Reversal of heparin and hemostasis

   Protamine is usually administered empirically in a 1 to 1 ratio in the absence of use of automated systems such as the Heparin Dose Response System (Medtronic, Inc., Minneapolis, MN).

   Avoid a rapid bolus. Exact infusion rates remain controversial.

4. Chest closure and transport

   Remove TEE, and decompress stomach with orogastric tube.

   Monitor blood pressure, electrocardiogram, and SaO_2 for transport.

   Ensure chest tubes (if present) are on water seal because tension pneumothorax is a known hazard during transport.

   Ensure patency of mediastinal drainage because tamponade is a known hazard.

operative mechanical ventilation. However, many clinicians have adopted use of infusions of shorter acting agents (e.g., sufentanil, propofol, remifentanil), avoided large cumulative dosing of fixed agents with potentially long half lives (e.g., midazolam), and rely on a volatile anesthesia "base," taking a "wait and see" attitude toward early extubation if surgery is "smooth" and physiologic parameters remain within acceptable limits (e.g., good urine output, normothermic, adequate hematocrit). Often the results are quite impressive relative to older management routines.

Premedication

The concept of "premedication" has been evolving with new knowledge and the increasing role of the cardiac anesthesiologist as a "perioperative physician." Simply discussing the rationale for ordering of sedative-hypnotics or related agents to reduce patient anxiety and promote amnesia is no longer adequate. The cardiac anesthesiologist must be familiar with the potential benefits of administering (or hazards of not administering) a variety of cardiovascular medications, particularly anti-anginal medications, and ensure that appropriate medications are ordered for morning administration with sips of water. The anesthesiologist, in concert with the surgeon and other consultants, may directly impact on patient outcome, as well as provide anxiolysis, amnesia, and analgesia in the early intraoperative period.

Anxiolysis, Amnesia, and Analgesia

The purposes of premedication are to pharmacologically reduce apprehension and fear, to provide analgesia for potentially painful events before induction (e.g., vascular cannulation), and to produce some degree of amnesia. In patients with CAD, premedication may help prevent preoperative anginal episodes that are relatively commonly observed on continuous ambulatory ECG monitoring but are often silent clinically.[99,102] Regardless of the drugs used, the clinician should be prepared to give intravenous drugs (e.g., benzodiazepines, opiates) when the patient arrives in the preoperative area to supplement inadequate sedation. All patients receive supplemental oxygen after premedication and are monitored with at least pulse oximetry during vascular cannulation (if performed before entry into the operating room suite).

A variety of drugs and regimens are used for sedation depending on the practice setting (e.g., same-day admission), the patient's condition (e.g., age, comorbidities, preoperative heparin infusion), and the clinician's preferences. Use of oral, intramuscular, or intravenous benzodiazepines is very common and provides effective anxiolysis and some degree of amnesia. Diazepam remains popular as an oral premedicant (0.1 to 0.15 mg/kg), and midazolam is most popular intravenously (1 to 2 mg), followed by lorazepam, which is commonly administered intramuscularly (1 to 2 mg). Oral diazepam is a very popular premedication for cardiac catheterization, as beneficial hemodynamic effects (vasodilation, increased venous capacitance, and decreased ventricular wall tension) have been demonstrated in this setting.[103] Unfortunately, there is a very wide interpatient variability in sedative effect with this class of drugs, with some patients having virtually no sedation and others heavily sedated after similar dosages. Opioids, most commonly morphine (0.1 to 0.15 mg/kg) given by the intramuscular route, and fentanyl (50 to 75 μg), administered intravenously, are recommended to provide analgesia, particularly during radial artery cannulation. Scopolamine, usually given intramuscularly (0.2 to 0.4 mg) but occasionally intravenously, has been commonly used for its potent amnestic effects. Given its potential to induce delirium and disorientation, particularly in the elderly, it is less frequently used today. Acute toxicity associated with overdosage can be effectively reversed with physostigmine.

Addition of opioids to a benzodiazepine premedication is more likely to cause greater sedation, more frequent arterial desaturation, increase in arterial pCO2, and hemodynamic instability compared with sublingual lorazepam alone, as demonstrated in a randomized study of 68 CABG patients by Saccomanno et al.[104] Thomson et al[105] examined the interaction of premedicant drugs with a high-dose opioid induction and different muscle relaxants. Their findings suggest that clinically indistinguishable sedation may be achieved with lorazepam alone or morphine plus scopolamine, but that the HR and BP response during anesthetic induction are quite different and influenced by the muscle relaxant chosen. Patients receiving morphine and scopolamine premedication with pancuronium were more likely to become tachycardic and hypertensive with fentanyl or sufentanil than if they received lorazepam alone. Tomicheck et al[106] reported that intravenous diazepam given just before induction with fentanyl plus pancuronium significantly reduced the BP and HR response. These studies indicate that more profound sympatholysis may be expected at the time of anesthetic induction, after the use of a benzodiazepine taken orally or administered intravenously for premedication.

Concurrent use of antianginal and antihypertensive medications will likely further influence these responses. Despite these reports, the hemodynamic changes encountered are usually easily treated with small doses of phenylephrine or ephedrine, supplemental fluids, and use of the Trendelenburg position. Newer techniques using gradual titration of opioids with primarily inhaled inductions are likely to encounter fewer overt hemodynamic episodes than those with older "fixed-dose" opioid-benzodiazepine inductions.

The sedative and anesthetic sparing actions of α_2-adrenergic agonists (clonidine, 5 mg/kg orally) have been evaluated for their efficacy in several studies of CABG patients alone[107] or in combination with a benzodiazepine.[108] Both studies report favorable sedation relative to conventional regimens with reduction in the stress response and anesthetic requirements. However, clonidine is infrequently or never used in most centers. Increasing familiarity with dexmedetomidine may increase interest in clonidine. A meta-analysis reported a reduction in mortality and postoperative myocardial infarction with their use in cardiac surgery (started preoperatively and often continuing until CPB).[109] Nevertheless, some of the hemodynamic side effects of α_2-agonists warrant caution in certain patient populations. Decreased HR, MAP, CO, contractility, transiently increased systemic vascular resistance (SVR), and hypotension during anesthesia induction have been reported in general and cardiac surgery patients premedicated with α_2-agonists.[110,111] Consequently, α_2-agonists should be used cautiously in patients with preexistent severe bradycardia, conduction problems such as second- or third-degree heart block, hypovolemia, or hypotension (see Chapter 9).

Management of Antianginal and Antihypertensive Medications

β-ADRENERGIC RECEPTOR ANTAGONISTS

For the newly trained anesthesiologist who is told to provide "perioperative β-blockade" to all patients with known CAD, or those with multiple risk factors undergoing major noncardiac (particularly vascular) surgery, it may come as a surprise that in 1972, a case series from the prestigious Cleveland Clinic admonished clinicians to withdraw such medication at least 2 weeks before CABG surgery reporting that 5 such patients died within 24 hours of surgery.[112] Several years later, Kaplan et al[113,114] reported that it was safe to continue β-blockade and that operative mortality was similar in patients in whom propranolol had been continued within 24 to 48 hours of surgery. Slogoff et al[115] performed a randomized trial evaluating the safety of administration of propranolol within 12 hours of surgery. Based on a significantly greater increase in the incidence of pre-CPB ischemia in patients withdrawn from propranolol (within 24 to 72 hours), they also recommended continuation of therapy up until the time of surgery. Further work by these and other investigators in the 1980s documented the efficacy of continuation of β-blockers through surgery with regard to reducing pre-CPB ischemia and their superior efficacy over the increasingly popular calcium channel blockers.[116,117] These studies were instrumental in laying the groundwork for the subsequent noncardiac surgery studies in the late 1980s.[118-120] These led to the contemporary randomized perioperative β-blocker trials of Polderman et al[121] and Mangano et al,[122] which despite ongoing controversy regarding the exact efficacy of this therapy resulted in it becoming a clinical routine.[123-125] Several contemporary observational studies have documented associations of β-blocker therapy with reduction in perioperative mortality in CABG patients.[126-128] The largest of these by Ferguson et al[128] considered 629,877 patients in the STS database (1996 to 1999) in which a modest, but statistically significant reduction in 30-day risk adjusted mortality was reported (OR = 0.94, 95% CI = 0.91 to 0.97). This treatment effect was observed in many high-risk subgroups, although a trend toward increased mortality was seen in patients with EF less than 30% (OR = 1.13; 95% CI, 0.96 to 1.33). Considerable efforts are being expended by major organizations (STS, ACC) in increasing compliance with existing guidelines for use of β-blockers at the time of hospital discharge (along with use of aspirin, statins, and ACE inhibitors)[129,130] (see Chapter 10).

There is little doubt that β-blockers are beneficial for most CABG patients. When acutely administered in adequate dosage, they significantly reduce myocardial oxygen demand and the incidence of atrial and ventricular arrhythmias. However, since the 1980s, there has been ongoing controversy over their precise pharmacokinetic and dynamic effects (particularly in chronically treated patients, and in those treated with β_1-selective versus nonselective agents) as well as the relationship of resting HR to the supposed level of β-blockade.[88,131-136] The β-selective blockers may also limit the activation of inflammatory responses involved in CAD progression.[137]

The newest area of investigation with regard to β-blockade in this setting is the issue of desensitization of the myocardial β-adrenergic receptor induced by sudden high levels of catecholamines induced by institution of CPB.[138,139] This desensitization is associated with a reduced response to inotropic stimulation that would be potentially detrimental during weaning from CPB. Investigators at Duke University have reported a series of studies incorporating human and canine models documenting this desensitization,[138] and the lack of efficacy of chronic oral β-blockade in CABG patients in attenuating it. They documented a similar lack of efficacy of acutely administered pre-CPB intravenous metoprolol, which contrasts with earlier canine data on the effects of intravenous esmolol.[140,141] However, they observed a significant reduction in postoperative supraventricular arrhythmias with high-dose metoprolol. In contrast, later data from this same group suggests that high spinal anesthesia (37.5 mg of bupivicaine, administered just before induction of general anesthesia) is effective in attenuating CPB-induced receptor desensitization.[139]

OTHER MEDICATIONS

Aspirin (and other platelet inhibitors such as dipyridamole) have long been recognized to have strong efficacy in the prevention of early graft thrombosis after CABG,[142] and are a well-recognized component of primary and secondary prevention strategies for all patients with ischemic heart disease.[129] Mangano,[143] in a large observational analysis, reported substantial reduction in overall mortality (1.3% versus 4.0%) and ischemic complications of the heart, brain, kidneys, and gastrointestinal tract in 5065 patients at 70 hospitals when aspirin was administered within 48 hours after surgery. However, patients receiving aspirin immediately before surgery have more mediastinal bleeding and may receive more blood products. A consensus conference of the American College of Chest Physicians on antithrombotic and thrombolytic therapies recommends institution of aspirin within 6 hours after CABG surgery over continuation of preoperative therapy (level of evidence Ia).[144] In those with ongoing bleeding, it should be administered "as soon as possible thereafter." In those allergic to aspirin, clopidogrel should be used instead. For those undergoing internal mammary artery (IMA) grafting, low-dose aspirin should be continued indefinitely. The STS has released formal practice guidelines on this topic. In high-risk patients (those with unstable angina or recent myocardial infarction) requiring urgent or emergent CABG, aspirin should be continued until the time of surgery (class IIa recommendation) unless they are in an "aspirin-sensitive high-risk subgroup" (i.e., those on other antiplatelet or anticoagulants or those who have platelet abnormalities). For elective patients in whom active platelet aggregation is less likely to be a critical factor in precipitating ischemia, they recommend discontinuation of aspirin for 3 to 5 days preoperatively to reduce transfusion requirements (class IIa) with reinstitution in the early postoperative period (class I).[145]

The efficacy of calcium channel antagonists with regard to their anti-ischemic properties in patients undergoing CABG is a controversial topic. Early observational studies suggest they were ineffective, particularly relative to β-blockers.[116,117] Subsequently, there was even less enthusiasm for their use given concerns in the mid-1990s of excess mortality with shorter-acting preparations (in particular nifedipine which was thought to cause reflex adrenergic activation due to abrupt vasodilation with each dose).[146] Two meta-analyses evaluating their efficacy in noncardiac surgery produced conflicting information.[147,148] However, one meta-analysis and a large observational cohort study with propensity matching adjustment suggest they are effective in reducing mortality in CABG patients.[149,150] Despite these reports (both from the same research group), there appears to be little enthusiasm to prove their efficacy in large randomized trials (as observed in an accompanying editorial by a prominent cardiac surgeon).[151] For patients taking them chronically, it appears prudent to continue them perioperatively. Caution is advised with concurrent administration of nondihydropyridine drugs (diltiazem) and β-blockers, although the risk (purported to be possible precipitation of advanced degrees of AV block) appears to be minor, based on a lack of problems in a reported large cohort of thoracotomy patients in which this was frequently done.[152]

Angiotensin-converting enzyme (ACE) inhibitors and statins are receiving attention as agents given a variety of important "pleiotropic" effects (e.g., effects independent of their primary actions of antihypertensive effects or lipid-lowering effects, respectively).[153-155] Potent anti-inflammatory effects and beneficial effects on endothelial function have been reported for both agents, as well as less clear effects on angiogenesis.[156] Both agents are commonly administered acutely during PCI for their purported benefits.[157,158] ACE inhibitors are widely considered to be vasculoprotective, particularly with regard to ventricular remodeling after acute myocardial infarction, and they appear to reduce damage after ischemic reperfusion (likely related to reduction in ischemic-induced vasoconstriction and reduction in leukocyte adhesion). Statins have been reported by one group of investigators to reduce circulating levels of adhesion molecules, which have been implicated in endothelial dysfunction after CPB (Fig. 19–12).[159,160] Both agents appear to have direct effects on platelet aggregation and plasminogen activator inhibitors.[161] Of the two classes of drugs, the greatest interest appears to be on the statins because of the greater number of publications and intense concurrent interest with regard to cardioprotection for noncardiac (particularly vascular) surgery.[162-164] Several investigators have published similar reports of efficacy in observational cohorts of CABG patients.[165,166] Only one small and underpowered randomized, controlled trial of statin use (for vascular surgery) has been reported, and none has been reported for ACE inhibitors. However, a high percentage of CABG patients are taking these medications chronically. There are no evidence-based recommendations to start these agents in patients not already taking them for their primary actions.

With regard to risks, statins have been rarely associated with perioperative rhabdomyolysis, and a current ACC/AHA advisory advises against their continuation (based solely on anecdotal data).[167] However, most clinicians continue them routinely (albeit orally only). ACE inhibitors have been controversial with conflicting data as to whether their vasodilatory effects are associated with greater degrees of hypotension during induction or even profound degrees of vasodilation during CPB and weaning.[168-174] A greater concern observed by Lazar[154] is in relation to potential antagonism between ACE inhibitors and aspirin, because ACE inhibitors increase prostaglandin levels, whereas aspirin inhibits them. Despite strongly promoting their perioperative use, he advises they be held for 24 to 48 hours before surgery if possible and restarted postoperatively after reinstitution of β-blockade (assuming SBP > 100 mm Hg). They are otherwise contraindicated with renal insufficiency, and their rare side effect of cough can be detrimental to sternal stability in the early postoperative period (see Chapter 10).

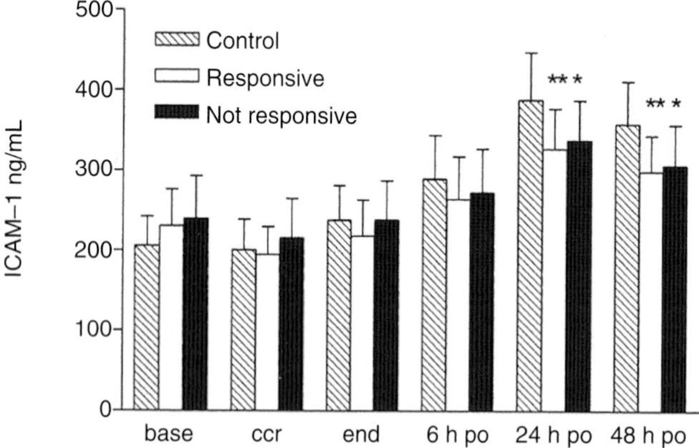

Figure 19–12 Bar graph of the mean values of circulating intercellular adhesion molecule-1 (ICAM-1), a glycoprotein circulating adhesion molecule expressed by endothelial cells in response to inflammation. Levels in response to cardiopulmonary bypass are shown for 15 controls, 15 patients on simvastatin with good control of cholesterol (i.e., responsive), and 15 patients on the drug but with poor control (i.e., not responsive) of cholesterol. Statin patients had lower ICAM-1 levels at 24 and 48 hours postoperatively, suggesting possible anti-inflammatory properties. Base = baseline; ccr = cross-clamp release; end = end of cardiopulmonary bypass; 6 h po, 24 h po, and 48 h po = postoperative periods. (From Chello M, Carassiti M, Agro F, et al: Simvastatin blunts the increase of circulating adhesion molecules after coronary artery bypass surgery with cardiopulmonary bypass. J Cardiothorac Vasc Anesth 18:605, 2004.)

Monitoring

Electrocardiogram

On arrival in the operating room, the patient undergoing CABG should have routine monitors placed, including pulse oximetry, noninvasive BP, and the electrocardiogram. A multilead ECG system and recorder is extremely useful in managing patients with ischemic heart disease. Observing the oscilloscope screen alone results in failure to detect 50% to 80% of episodes of myocardial ischemia detected by continuous recording techniques. Although a continuous paper write-out is useful, online ST-segment trending systems may be more beneficial in the early diagnosis of myocardial ischemia. Recording capability is necessary to provide visual analysis and is invaluable in diagnosing arrhythmias. Transmural myocardial ischemia is a regional disorder; therefore, placement of leads in areas known angiographically to be at risk may increase ECG sensitivity for ischemia detection, whereas subendocardial ischemia is localized nearly exclusively to ST-segment depression in the lateral precordial leads.[175] The ECG detection of myocardial ischemia is reviewed in Chapter 14.

Arterial Pressure Monitoring

The radial artery is usually cannulated for BP monitoring during CABG. Dissection of the IMA with forceful retraction of the sternum may result in tenting of the subclavian artery, with a resultant reduction in flow and inaccuracies in the displayed pressure. Some centers routinely monitor the side opposite the proposed IMA dissection to avoid this problem, whereas others use this side to detect the problem. The use of newer retractors make this substantially less problematic. Others prefer to use the nondominant hand to avoid serious quality of life issues should the rare ischemic complication occur.[176] With increasing use of radial artery grafts, the placement of the arterial catheter will be determined by the results of an ultrasound evaluation of palmar arch flow. Accurate measurement of the BP is important, because it is relied on to help determine anesthetic depth and to gauge vasoactive drug requirements. The noninvasive BP should be used as an accuracy check when there is any doubt. Radial arterial pressures are quite distal to the central circulation and have been shown to be inaccurate immediately after hypothermic CPB. Substantial reductions in radial arterial versus aortic pressure have been reported in several clinical investigations (10 to 30 mm Hg), often requiring 20 to 60 minutes after CPB to resolve.[177-181] Alterations in forearm vascular resistance (decrease) are felt to be responsible for this common phenomenon. This problem can be overcome by temporarily transducing pressure directly from the aorta (by a needle or a cardioplegia cannula) or by insertion of a femoral arterial catheter (see Chapter 14).

Central Venous Cannulation

The placement of a central venous pressure (CVP) catheter is a standard of practice in cardiac anesthesia both for pressure measurement and for infusing vasoactive drugs. Some centers routinely place two catheters (a large introducer and a smaller CVP catheter) in the central circulation to facilitate volume infusion and vasoactive or inotropic drug administration. Increasingly, ultrasound guidance is used for placement, although there remains controversy in the literature regarding whether it is a standard of care[182] (see Chapter 14).

Pulmonary Artery Catheterization

The efficacy of PAC in medical and surgical settings has evolved over the past 20 years from steadily increasing use in the 1980s and 1990s to distinctly lower use now. Increasing literature evidence from a variety of experimental designs has strongly suggested that despite the substantial amount of physiologic information obtained, major clinical outcomes (particularly mortality) are little influenced and may be increased (possibly due to the potential arrhythmogenic effects of the catheter or thrombus formation on it) with its use. Earlier studies suggested that clinicians were unable to accurately judge filling pressures based on clinical signs and that therapy could be influenced by this data in the surgical and medical settings.[183] Intraoperatively, PAC was also shown to detect decreased LV compliance associated with myocardial ischemia.[184] It also appeared better suited for monitoring high-risk patients as found by Mangano who evaluated the correlation between CVP and pulmonary capillary wedge pressure (PCWP) in a study of 30 patients having CABG. He demonstrated that CVP and PCWP correlated well preoperatively and postoperatively only in patients with an EF greater than 0.4, and in patients without significant dyssynergy, defined as two or more LV segments with less than 20% normal contraction.[185]

It was recommended that patients with a lower EF or segmental wall motion abnormalities (SWMAs) would be more appropriately managed with a PAC. With the increasing sophistication of CABG surgery performed on sicker patients with a greater disease burden in the 1980s, PAC use increased dramatically in many centers despite early retrospective data by Bashein et al[186] in 1275 patients (with a 45% PAC rate) documenting no major differences in outcome. Although not formally reported, PAC was almost never used at the prestigious, high volume Texas Heart Institute. In the late 1980s, questions regarding the sensitivity of PAC in detecting ischemia and in accurately estimating the more important end-diastolic left ventricular volume (most closely related to stroke volume by the Frank-Starling mechanism), particularly in relation to the increasingly popular and less invasive TEE, led to increased skepticism.[187-191] Tuman et al,[192] in a prospective observational study, examined the effect of the PAC on outcome in 1094 patients. Although no direct data on LV function were provided, there was no difference in the incidence of LV dysfunction between the group treated with a CVP versus the group treated with a PAC. In this study, the investigators could not demonstrate that a PAC had any effect on outcome; however, 7% of the patients initially assigned to CVP monitoring subsequently required a PAC for management. In 1993, the first ASA-sanctioned Practice Guidelines for PACs were published. These were updated in 2003.[193] Unfortunately, they were completed just before publication of the Sandham et al[194] randomized, controlled trial (which the group declined to comment on). The ASA Guidelines provide no distinct criteria for PAC use, focusing more on the inconclusive state of the literature, and a complex discussion of methodologic aspects of developing the guidelines. As with the earlier guidelines, there is no objective evidence of how it has impacted anesthesiologists' practice.

PAC use in the ICU setting also appears to be steadily decreasing. With the publication in the *New England Journal of Medicine* of the first widely respected, large-scale randomized, controlled trial, it is likely to be relegated to only the most critically ill patients with known cardiac disease (e.g., cardiogenic shock or severe valvular disease). In their study, Sandham et al[194] randomized 1994 high-risk surgical patients (i.e., age > 60 years; ASA III or IV; abdominal, thoracic, vascular, and orthopedic surgery) to PAC or no PAC. Perioperative, 6-month, and 12-month mortality were not different, whereas a higher incidence of pulmonary embolism was observed in the PAC group. These data confirm the results of several similar large observational analyses reported previously.[195,196]

Several reports have focused exclusively on PAC use in CABG surgery. Stewart et al[197] reported a retrospective analysis of 312 patients undergoing CABG (in 1996) who were felt to be low risk and suitable for CVP monitoring alone. Of these, 32% had a PAC placed and received greater volumes of fluid, gained more weight, and had longer times to extubation.[197] Ramsey et al[198] retrospectively analyzed a commercial health care outcomes benchmarking database (i.e., 13,907 patients undergoing nonemergent CABG in 1997 in 56 hospitals) (Fig. 19–13); 58% of patients had PAC and were found to have a higher risk of mortality after risk adjustment (relative risk = 2.1), longer lengths of stay, and higher total costs particularly in the hospitals with low rates of PAC use. Schwann et al[199] retrospectively analyzed 2685 consecutive CABG patients at a single private center (1994 to 1998) in which PAC use was "highly selective" (i.e., used in only 9% based on consideration of multiple cardiac risk factors). Of these PACs, 6.6% were planned with the remainder placed postoperatively in response to adverse intraoperative events. Multivariate analysis revealed EF, STS risk score, use of IABP, congestive heart failure, redo operation, and New York Heart Association (NYHA) class IV to be independent predictors of PAC use. Based on their reported overall mortality (2.3%), it appears as if this highly selective approach was safe, although the data are not necessarily generalizable outside this particular center given multiple other process variables involved in providing care for these patients.[199] London et al[200] documented the high rate of use of PAC based on analysis of 3256 CABG patients included in a larger multicenter observational study of cardiac surgery in the Department of Veterans Affairs (1994 to 1996). More than 95% of all cases were monitored with PAC, and 49% of these used the more expensive mixed venous oxygen saturation catheter. Use of this catheter was clearly center specific, and with the exception of a small reduction in number of postoperative arterial blood gas and thermodilution cardiac output measurements, it was unassociated with improvement in outcome over the routine PAC.

Based on the existing literature it is not possible to give precise criteria for PAC use in CABG surgery (see Chapter 14). The higher the patient risk (based primarily on established

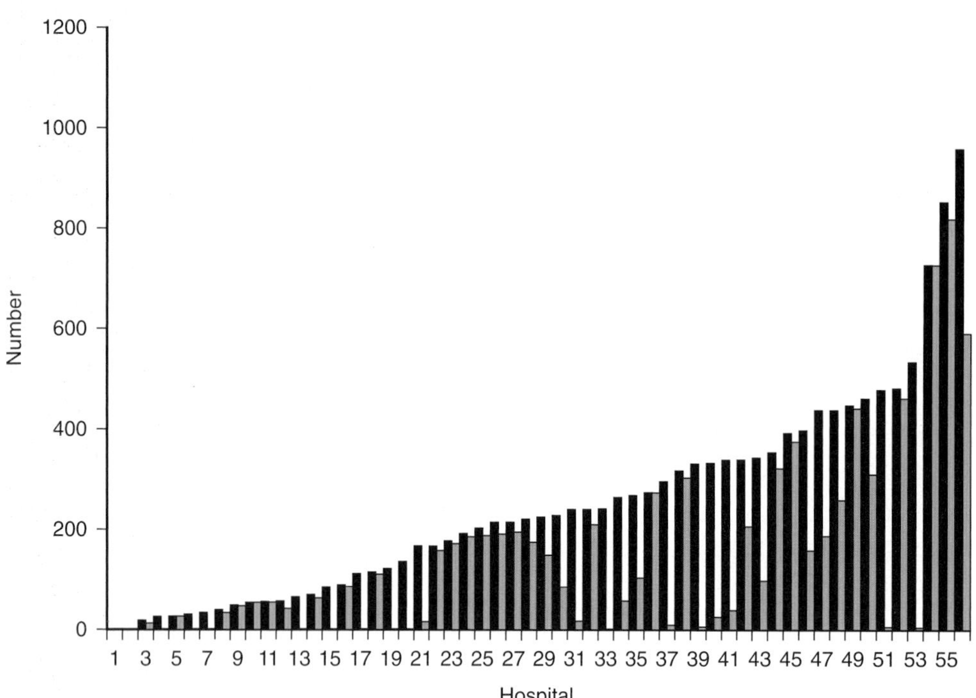

Figure 19–13 Variation in the use of pulmonary artery catheter (PAC) for elective coronary artery bypass grafting (CABG) in 13,907 patients at 56 community-based hospitals in 26 states in 1997, with data obtained from an administrative health outcomes benchmarking database. PAC was used in 58% and was associated with greater risk of in-hospital mortality, particularly in hospitals with the lowest use of PAC, hospital length of stay, and costs. *Solid bars* indicate the total number of CABG cases; *shaded bars* indicate the number of patients with PAC. (From Ramsay SD, Saint S, Sullivan SD, et al: Clinical and economic effects of pulmonary artery catheterization in nonemergent coronary artery bypass graft surgery. J Cardiothorac Vasc Anesth 14:113, 2000.)

preoperative clinical predictors), the more favorable the risk-benefit ratio is. Risk factors include the following:

1. Significant impairment of ventricular function (EF < 40%, evidence of acute or chronic congestive heart failure, known elevation of LVEDP on preoperative cath, need for preoperative IABP, acute or chronic severe mitral regurgitation due to ischemia, VSD after myocardial infarction, or other mechanical complications).
2. High risk for intraoperative ischemia or difficult revascularization (i.e., recent, large myocardial infarction or severe unstable angina, known poor revascularization targets or severe microcirculatory disease, reoperation, catheterization laboratory PCI "crash").
3. Severe co-morbidities (e.g., renal failure, on or approaching need for dialysis; severe chronic obstructive pulmonary disease).
4. Combined procedures which significantly lengthen duration of surgery or add significant blood loss (e.g., CABG-carotid, other vascular procedures).

Although most of the recent clinical reports of patients undergoing OPCAB have used, and many recommend use of, PAC, it is not possible to give firm recommendations on this due to the lack of evidence-based data. Although a PAC is commonly used for all of these patients, it is highly likely that similar findings will emerge once OPCAB becomes more popular as have been reported with conventional CABG (especially given the high concurrent use of TEE).

For patients in whom PAC is used, there is ongoing controversy regarding the optimal timing for its insertion before or after induction. Clinicians have argued a variety of points, including patient safety (e.g., how stable is the patient during induction?) and logistics of starting the case (e.g., can it be inserted while the patient is being prepared and draped?). The former is often a greater concern in teaching institutions, whereas the latter is more likely to be a concern in a busy nonteaching setting. Wall et al[201] reported a randomized, controlled trial of 200 patients at a single teaching hospital involving 32 anesthesia residents and attendings where PAC was placed before or after induction. They studied elective cases although specific exclusion criteria are not reported nor are details of use of ultrasound guidance. They found faster placement (17%) with fewer punctures and no differences in ST-segment changes, fluid or vasopressor use, or hemodynamic changes in the postinduction group. This study suggests, but is underpowered statistically to conclusively prove, that for most patients, PAC itself adds little to the safety of anesthetic induction (this group also observed that insertion postinduction has become the norm for their valve cases). However, in patients with marked impairment of ventricular function or poorly compensated valve disease, PAC can provide valuable information, guide acute management, and is strongly encouraged. It can also reveal abnormalities that were not revealed during the preoperative workup, particularly when a right-heart catheterization was not performed (e.g., unsuspected severe pulmonary hypertension). Szabo has recently reported uncontrolled data on a "simple" technique to facilitate sometimes difficult passage of a PAC in the anesthetized patient by placing the head up and right side down to position the pulmonic valve in a superior position.[202] An inspiratory pause when the catheter is in the RV outflow tract is thought to facilitate passage into the pulmonary artery.

Transesophageal Echocardiography

It is appreciated that the earliest signs of myocardial ischemia include diastolic dysfunction followed by systolic SWMAs that occur within seconds of acute coronary occlusion. Comparison of TEE with continuous (Holter) electrocardiograms have shown a greater incidence of SWMAs than ECG changes in patients with CAD. However, it is thought that new SWMAs detected in the intraoperative period may frequently occur due to nonischemic causes, particularly changes in loading conditions, and alteration in electrical conduction in the heart. The use of inotropic agents or elevations of catecholamine levels can aggravate (by increased oxygen demand) or improve wall motion (due to improvement in "hibernating" myocardium). Changes in preload and afterload are likely the most important factors in the CABG setting; transient reversible SWMAs are commonly related to acute myocardial stunning due to ischemia before or during weaning from CPB. TEE is highly sensitive but not specific for myocardial ischemia.[203,204] The short-axis midpapillary muscle view, commonly used because of its inclusion of myocardium supplied by the three major coronary arteries, may entirely miss SWMAs occurring in the basal or apical portions of the heart. These changes necessitate interrogation of additional components of the comprehensive TEE examination recommended by the ASE/SCA Task Force before and after CPB or after completion of revascularization in OPCAB.[205] The ASA Practice Guidelines for TEE (which have not been revised since their initial publication in 1996) list the perioperative uses in patients with increased risk of myocardial ischemia or infarction as a category II indication (supported by weaker evidence and expert consensus).[206] The indication is strengthened when ECG monitoring cannot be used to diagnose ischemia (e.g., in patients with left bundle-branch block, extensive Q waves, or ST-T abnormalities on the baseline electrocardiogram), and it is weakened when baseline SWMAs are present (particularly akinesis or dyskinesis due to fibrotic, calcified, or aneurysmal myocardium). Use of perioperative TEE to evaluate myocardial perfusion, coronary anatomy, or graft patency is listed as a category III indication, but newer technology will upgrade this indication.

With increasing sophistication of TEE probes and systems, strong educational emphasis on residency and fellowship training and on subspecialty society levels, TEE use continues to increase for CABG surgery. A wide variety of uses aside from detection of ischemia are well documented for TEE (e.g., verification of PAC location; placement of retrograde cardioplegia cannula, LV vent, or IABP tip; detection of atheromatous disease in the ascending aorta; intracardiac air; fluid status; and valve function). Morewood et al[207] obtained more than 1800 survey responses from members of the Society of Cardiovascular Anesthesiologists in 2000. Of approximately 1500 clinicians involved in CABG, only 11% reported never using TEE, but more than 30% used it frequently or always. This number is probably higher today because of the growth of OPCAB and ongoing popularity of the technology. A variety of observational studies over the past decade have supported the efficacy of this technique, although in the absence of a true randomized, controlled trial, it is impossible to conclusively prove efficacy or the impact of other key factors (e.g., surgeon and anesthesiologist).[208-210] The finding of a large-scale observational analysis of nearly 5000 patients undergoing cardiac surgery in the Department of Veterans Affairs in which TEE appeared to be an independent risk factor for mortality seems to suggest that the providers are key factors (although further analysis to identify provider level linkage has not been reported from this data set).[46] Proper education and certification is critical.[211] The clinician must realize that there are serious complications that can and do occur (albeit rarely) with TEE, and that an association between esophageal dysmotility and aspiration, particularly in elderly patients, has been strongly suggested in several observational reports[212-217] (see Chapters 15, 16, and 41).

Induction and Maintenance

Induction of anesthesia should take place in a calm and relaxed manner, preferably in a quiet operating room. Attention should be paid to the ambient room temperature because entry into an excessively cold operating room can elicit a sympathetic response increasing blood pressure and sometimes HR, particularly in the elderly and thin patients. Allaying the patient's anxiety with premedication and calm, reassuring verbal interaction is also critical. Preoxygenation should be used and monitoring should be in place, including the PAC in patients at very high risk, who may be unstable during or after induction.

There are two main considerations in choosing an induction technique for patients undergoing CABG. The first is LV function. Patients with good LV function (and particularly those with left ventricular hypertrophy) often have a strong sympathetic response to surgical stimulation and may require supranormal doses of anesthetics, plus the addition of β-blockers with or without vasodilators (which alone may induce further reflex tachycardia), to control these responses. Patients with poor LV function often do not tolerate normal doses of anesthetics and are unable to produce a significant hemodynamic response to sympathetic stimulation or the response may precipitate major reductions in cardiac output (e.g., tachycardia leading to ischemia in a patient with a low EF or concurrent aortic stenosis).

The second consideration is the desirability of early extubation. Time spent in the ICU is one of the most expensive aspects of hospital care for CABG and is heavily influenced by postoperative ventilator management. The patient with normal preoperative LV function, assuming an uneventful intraoperative course, will have recovered 90% of baseline LV function by 4 hours postoperatively, and can usually be extubated within 4 to 6 hours postoperatively if attention is paid to adequate rewarming and postoperative analgesia, and if high doses of respiratory depressant anesthetics (particularly opioids and benzodiazepines) have been avoided. With the routine application of fast-track techniques, some centers have adopted immediate extubation in the operating room. However, this remains relatively uncommon and requires the close cooperation of a highly coordinated team. Because this is not always the case (particularly in teaching institutions in which residents and fellows rotate for short intervals or in some private institutions in which staffing at night is relatively low), many centers take a more measured less aggressive approach.

After the induction of anesthesia, the pre-bypass period (for conventional CABG) may last less than an hour (e.g., only one or two saphenous vein grafts harvested) or several hours (e.g., for dissection of the left IMA, right IMA, or radial or gastroepiploic arteries after a repeat sternotomy). Surgical stimulus may be severe, such as during sternotomy or dissection around the ascending aorta. Between 50% and 70% of patients in most series presenting for CABG have normal LV function (when not ischemic) and are capable of mounting significant BP and HR responses to noxious stimuli, whereas others with poor LV function may require pharmacologic support of the BP for such stimuli. It is evident that no single approach to anesthesia for CABG procedures is suitable for all patients. Most hypnotics, opioids, and volatile agents have been used in different combinations for the induction and maintenance of anesthesia with good results in the hands of experienced clinicians.

Primary Induction Agents

Considerations for choice of induction agent in the patient undergoing CABG are based on theoretical and practical clinical considerations. Avoidance of hypertension and tachycardia, most likely to occur in the patient with normal ventricular function, hypertension, and left ventricular hypertrophy; avoidance of hypotension and excessive myocardial depression in a patient with depressed ventricular function or with severe flow dependent stenoses (particularly coronary and cerebral); and provision of smooth intubating conditions with a lack of effect on airway resistance are desirable goals. The cardiac effects of each of the commonly used induction agents have been investigated over many years, sometimes with conflicting results. Increasing sophistication of experimental preparations and measurements is providing new information. Unraveling the direct versus indirect effects of a particular drug on the heart and circulation is complex as overall effects are based on contractility, vascular tone, and response of the autonomic nervous system and baroreceptors. Closely related to this are the details of the animal preparation (e.g., species, acute versus chronic preparation, open versus closed chest) or the clinical setting (e.g., type and speed of induction, use of concurrent β-blockers or other antihypertensives, sophistication of cardiac monitoring) in which the drug is investigated. Rarely is one drug used exclusively (particularly in this setting where opioids, volatile agents, and benzodiazepines are often used simultaneously). All of the drugs are usually titrated to effect (see Chapter 9).

Thiopental has been used for decades for induction in this setting. Its predominant hemodynamic effects include reduction in mean arterial pressure (MAP) and cardiac output (CO) accompanied by a modest increase in HR. These are felt to result from a combination of direct myocardial depression, venodilation, and a decrease in central sympathetic outflow. In isolated muscle, whole animal,[218] and clinical studies (including use of load independent measures of contractility),[218-220] it is generally reported to have greater negative inotropic effects than propofol. A greater degree of vasodilation with propofol may also account for less depression of cardiac output.[221,222] A study of isolated human atrial muscle from CABG patients reported no effect of propofol, midazolam, and etomidate on contractility in contrast to strong effects for thiopental and, paradoxically, slight negative effects for ketamine.[223] However, a recent conscious sheep preparation, in which "site directed" coronary arterial injection was used to isolate direct cardiac effects using doses small enough to preclude indirect effects from recirculated drug in the central nervous system, reported similar direct cardiac depressant effects for thiopental and propofol (including the thiopental enantiomer and racemate).[224] Despite these findings and its use in epidemiologic studies of anesthetic techniques for CABG,[51] the use of thiopental in most centers has declined substantially in favor of propofol. Adverse effects on airway resistance, a greater propensity to elicit bronchospasm, and a greater association with postoperative nausea and vomiting are other potential factors.

Administration of ketamine is generally associated with increases in HR and MAP through indirect central and peripheral sympathetic stimulation (e.g., inhibition of neuronal reuptake of catecholamines). In states associated with depletion of catecholamines and in isolated preparations, ketamine appears to have direct negative inotropic and vasodilating effects,[223,225] and it may have a negative lusitropic effect decreasing diastolic compliance.[226] In a double-blind, randomized, controlled trial, Zilberstein et al[227] documented a potent anti-inflammatory effect (i.e., suppression of increases in superoxide anion production after CPB) with a very small dose of ketamine (0.25 mg/kg) that persisted for several days postoperatively. Its lack of effect on respiration and its adjuvant properties in modulating acute pain are desirable properties.[228,229] Although its use is relatively infrequent in CABG patients (reserved primarily for induction in those with severe reduction of EF), it has been a routine part of an intravenous technique in numerous clinical reports as a bolus (1 to 3 mg/kg) with or without continuous infusion (1 mg/kg/hr).[51,230,231]

Etomidate appears to have minimal or no direct negative inotropic effects or sympathomimetic effects.[218,222,223] In an isolated rabbit heart preparation, Komai et al[232] demonstrated that at very high concentrations etomidate inhibited the influx of extracellular calcium but had no effect on availability of intracellular calcium required for excitation-contraction coupling. It is known to inhibit adrenal mitochondrial hydroxylase activity resulting in reduced steroidogenesis even after a single bolus dose, although the studies are conflicting.[233] Although this has not been considered a significant clinical problem, controversy remains (particularly in unstable ICU patients with sepsis) even after 20 years.[234] Its use for induction in the cardiac patients with impaired ventricular function is common and increasing. It is also used commonly for cardioversion in these patients. Myoclonic jerking can be observed in the absence of muscle relaxation. The investigators caution against routine use in patients with normal ventricular function because blunting of the adrenergic response to intubation is poor and may result in hypertension and tachycardia, particularly with the low-dose opioid techniques used today.

The clinical effects of propofol are in general similar to those of thiopental. However, it has numerous advantages over thiopental based on its predictable pharmacokinetics and dynamics.[235,236] Based on these, it has been widely adopted in the operating room for anesthesia delivery by computer-controlled devices and for postoperative ICU sedation. It is often used for sedation after CABG surgery,[237] although with the recent approval of dexmedetomidine for this indication,[238] its use may decline. Its isolated effects on contractility are controversial with conflicting findings depending on the model used. A sophisticated analysis of its effects in CABG patients using TEE assessment of preload-adjusted maximal power, a load-independent measure of contractility, at four different plasma concentrations (0.6 to 2.6 mg/mL) found no effect on contractility although it lowered preload and afterload.[239] It was previously evaluated in numerous clinical studies for induction and maintenance with an opioid (most commonly sufentanil) compared with a volatile-opioid combination for CABG in patients with normal and depressed EF. These studies report minimal differences in hemodynamics or in the incidence of myocardial ischemia.[240-245] However, more sophisticated and larger contemporary studies closely evaluating ventricular function on weaning from CPB and perioperative release of markers of ischemia consistently report better myocardial protective properties with the use of volatile agents over a total intravenous anesthetic (TIVA) technique with propofol. This is apparently related to preconditioning effects of volatile agents which are absent with propofol.[4,52,53,236-249] Propofol has been reported to have strong free radical scavenging properties that in one CABG study appear to have attenuated myocardial lipid peroxidation in atrial tissue biopsies.[250] Clinically, in the period before CPB it can be a very effective and short-acting means to treat acute episodes of hypertension due to light anesthesia or surgical manipulation of the aorta just before cannulation.

Research into newer formulations of propofol, including those with reduced lipid emulsion concentrations[251] (similar properties but with more pain on injection) and a nonlipid-based prodrug formulation[252] (lower peak but significantly prolonged serum levels), has been reported. There are no reports of either formulation used in cardiac surgery.

Benzodiazepines

Benzodiazepines are commonly used in combination with a narcotic to induce anesthesia for CABG. In most settings, midazolam has replaced diazepam given its numerous advantages (particularly water solubility, a shorter half-life and absence of metabolites capable of accumulation prolonging sedative effects).[253] Stanley et al[254,255] and Liu et al[256] were among the first to report on the addition of diazepam to high-dose morphine and, shortly thereafter, fentanyl anesthesia for CABG. They reported a mild-to-moderate reduction in CO (approximately 20% relative to opioid alone with the greatest decrease in the fentanyl group). These studies suggested that diazepam should not be used, particularly in patients with impaired ventricular function. However, with the realization that breakthrough adrenergic responses, as well as a substantial incidence of anesthetic recall with fentanyl alone can occur, supplementation with diazepam or midazolam quickly grew in popularity along with high-dose opioids in the early to middle 1980s.

Numerous clinical series of widely different sizes and designs, reporting on the efficacy of diazepam or, more commonly, midazolam (with isolated reports on lorazepam)[257] used with high-dose opioids, were subsequently published.[50,230,231,258-266] Moderate degrees of hypotension were reported in most studies primarily attributed to a reduction in systemic vascular resistance (or from the effects of the high-dose opioid itself given the very potent bradycardic effects of high-dose sufentanil). With rare exception, most investigators considered it safe and effective.[260]

There has been relatively little research on midazolam's direct cardiac effects (see section on Thiopental). Messina et al[267] reported a clinical study of 40 CABG patients in which 0.1 mg/kg of midazolam was administered after induction and intubation with thiopental, fentanyl, and pancuronium. Using the short-axis TEE view, end-systolic meridional wall stress (ESS) was estimated using the relation of LV systolic shortening and ESS as an index of contractility. Contractility was depressed by midazolam although afterload was reduced simultaneously resulting in no net change in cardiac index. Patients with depressed baseline EF had lower indices of contractility at baseline, but a similar magnitude of change. This study provides clinical confirmation of the safety of midazolam in clinical practice, particularly given its experimental design. Most clinicians have reduced dosing of midazolam to the range used in the latter study. Midazolam is widely used given clinicians concerns regarding recall. However, with the use of continuous volatile anesthesia and availability of convenient neuromonitoring techniques, it should no longer be considered a necessity, particularly with use of small amounts as a component of the premedication. Midazolam has been investigated for ICU sedation by continuous infusion, although its use today is mostly limited to patients undergoing alcohol withdrawal given the more favorable kinetics of propofol and dexmedetomidine.[268-273]

Opioids

High-dose opioid anesthesia was introduced into cardiac surgery by Lowenstein et al[1] in 1969, in an attempt to provide safe anesthesia without myocardial depression in patients with severe valvular heart disease and compromised cardiac function. Although this revolutionized anesthesia for patients with cardiac dysfunction, it was apparent that morphine had several disadvantages: vasodilation from histamine release, increased requirements for fluids and vasoconstrictors, and prolonged respiratory depression. When morphine was given to patients with normal LV function, with most patients undergoing CABG particularly in the previous decades, dramatic hemodynamic responses occurred with surgical stress, and amnesia could not be guaranteed; the anesthesia was often inadequate.

In the late 1970s, Stanley and collaborators first reported on the use of high-doses of the synthetic opioid fentanyl for CABG, with and without supplemental benzodiazepines.[255,256,274] It was rapidly adopted by clinicians worldwide who perceived the lack of histamine release to be a very favorable property.[106,275-280] However, it was recognized early on that recall could still be a problem.[281] Reports on the use of the more potent sufentanil appeared at the same time as fentanyl, although most studies were not reported until the late 1980s.[230,263,264,282-288] It too was widely adopted although there was concern over its very potent bradycardic effects at high dosages, particularly when administered with nonvagolytic muscle relaxants.[289,290] Alfentanil was released later in the 1980s, and although reports of its use in CABG were published (primarily by European investigators) it was never widely adopted in the United States.[283,291-296] In the mid-1990s, remifentanil was introduced. Fueled by intense interest in fast-tracking (being promoted in the same time frame), it has been intensively investigated.[297-305] However, despite reports of efficacy, it does not appear to be commonly used, most likely due to its duration of action being too short. This ultrashort action necessitates careful planning with regard to when it is terminated, lest patients wake up too quickly (e.g., in the operating room if the infusion is inadvertently interrupted or early in the ICU with inadequate supplementary analgesia). There have been reports of greater degrees of hypotension than with fentanyl or sufentanil.[306,307] Based on computer modeling and clinical data, sufentanil appears to have the most favorable characteristics for continuous infusion with very predictable termination of effect.[308,309] This characteristic was felt to be particularly important in the early 1990s when early postoperative suppression of ischemia by "intensive analgesia" was proposed as an important treatment goal just before widespread interest in fast-tracking.[3] However, a lack of subsequent evidence and the overwhelming interest in early extubation have negated this hypothesis. Sufentanil's substantially higher costs (than fentanyl) and the apparent aversion of many cardiac anesthesiologists to use continuous anesthetic infusions have limited its use. Most evidence suggests that despite documented associations of sufentanil use with shorter times to extubation, overall costs and hospital lengths of stay are unaffected relative to fentanyl.[55,310,311] Nonetheless, it remains popular with many clinicians, many of whom infuse it continuously during surgery.

These drugs are pure opioid agonists and none provide complete anesthesia as defined by predictable dose response relations for suppression of the stress response and release of endogenous catecholamines (particularly norepinephrine)

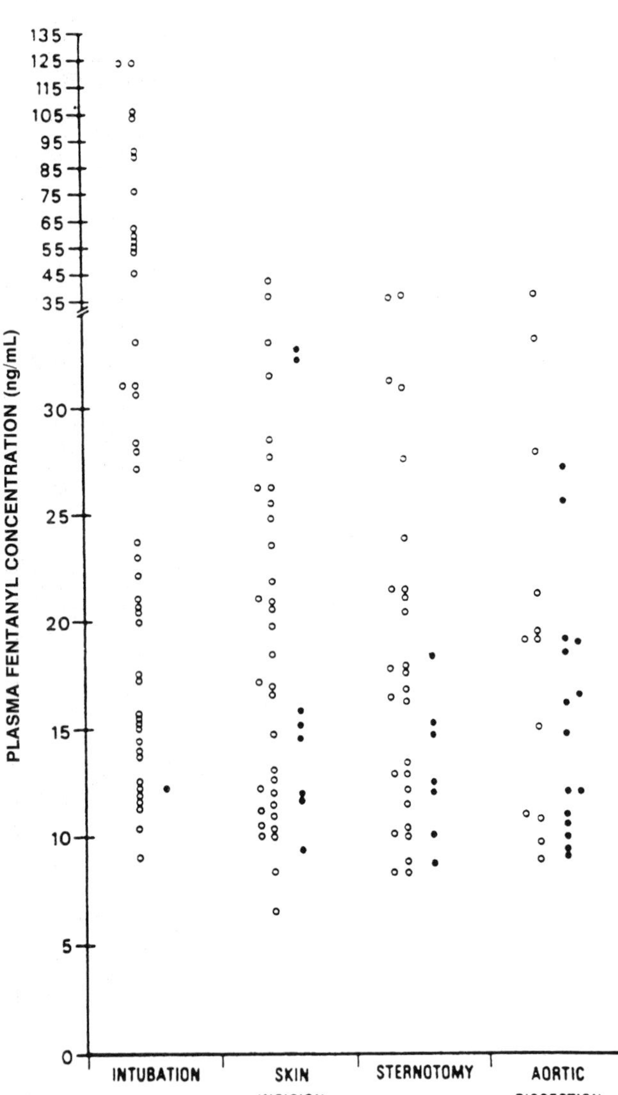

Figure 19–14 The plasma fentanyl concentration and number of patients with a hypertensive response at each event studied. *Filled circles* indicate hypertensive status; *open circles* indicate normotensive status. (From Wynands JE, Townsend GE, Wong P, et al: Blood pressure response and plasma fentanyl concentrations during high and very high-dose fentanyl anesthesia for coronary artery surgery. Anesth Analg 62:661, 1983.)

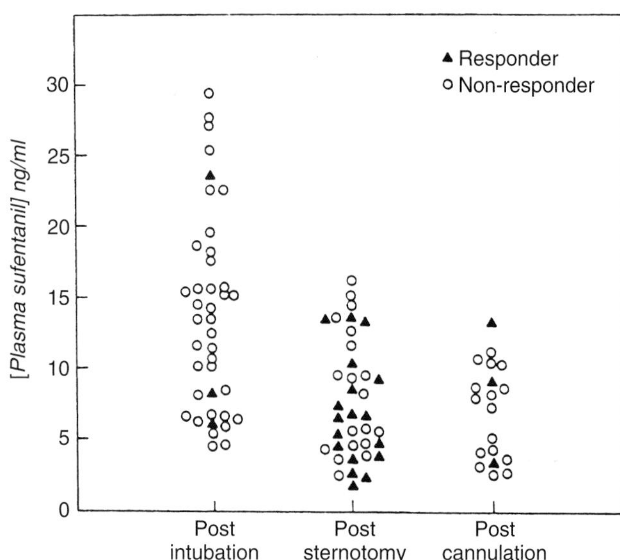

Figure 19–15 The graph plots patients with a hemodynamic response and the plasma sufentanil concentration at that time, as well as the sufentanil concentrations for the nonresponders. Therapy was initiated at the time of the initial response, and no further data points were included for those patients. (From Philbin DM, Rosow CE, Schneider RC, et al: Fentanyl and sufentanil anesthesia revisited: How much is enough? Anesthesiology 73:5, 1990.)

even with high serum concentrations.[312-314] Hypertension and tachycardia have been commonly reported in response to induction/intubation and surgical stimuli (particularly with sternotomy) in older studies of high-dose opioid anesthesia with fentanyl or sufentanil.[280,315] Figures 19–14 and 19–15 demonstrate this lack of association of serum levels with hemodynamic responses.

The seminal study of Philbin et al[316] (see Fig. 19–15) investigated the relationship between opioid dose and hemodynamic effect with fentanyl or sufentanil in a randomized study of CABG patients. Forty premedicated patients were allocated to receive fentanyl (50 or 100 μg/kg) or sufentanil (10 or 20 μg/kg) in bolus dosing with 100% oxygen and the relaxant metocurine with an additional 40 patients randomized to sufentanil bolus dosing (10, 20, or 40 μg/kg, followed by continuous infusions). Plasma opioid (only for sufentanil in the bolus/continuous infusion groups) and catecholamine concentrations were obtained after intubation and after sternotomy. A hemodynamic response was defined as a 15% or greater increase in systolic blood pressure (HRs were not reported), and a hormonal response was a 50% or greater increase from control. For both opioids, the frequency of hemodynamic responders (33% to 60%) was similar between all fentanyl and sufentanil bolus groups. In the sufentanil infusion groups, the plasma concentrations were consistent and dose-related with wide spreads between the groups. Twenty-four of the 40 patients were hemodynamic responders (with 18 occurring with sternotomy), and the frequency of response was unrelated to plasma sufentanil levels. Although this study has design flaws (e.g., small sample sizes and lack of power analyses, lack of reporting of actual hemodynamics), it is widely quoted to support the contention that even high-dose opioids alone provide incomplete anesthesia. Despite this, "narcotic anesthesia" was for many years considered synonymous with a "cardiac anesthetic" that should be used in all patients with CAD. It is only recently that this erroneous association is being laid to rest as volatile-based fast-tracking techniques gain popularity.

To provide complete anesthesia if high-dose opioids are used, the usual practice is to supplement with inhaled or other intravenous agents (e.g., midazolam). This permits a reduction in the total dose of opioid and particularly with volatile agents, more rapid return of respiratory drive facilitating early extubation. Thomson et al[317] have incorporated this approach and extended the concepts investigated by Philbin et al[316] in a small but sophisticated study of CABG patients whereby specific effect site concentrations of fentanyl or sufentanil were targeted by using a computer-assisted infusion (STANPUMP). Three targeted concentrations for each opioid were evaluated: sufentanil 0.4, 0.8, and 1.2 ng/mL and fentanyl 5, 10, and 15 ng/mL and the end-tidal concentration of isoflurane required to control MAP and HR in the pre-bypass period by predetermined criteria was monitored. The sufentanil subgroups required approximately 1.9, 3.1, and 4.9 μg/kg, and fentanyl subgroups received 18.8, 33.9, and 50.4 μg/kg in this period. The average end-tidal concentration of isoflurane was significantly greater between the low and medium/high groups with no difference between medium and high groups. Most of the responses were increases in MAP (incidentally the prime focus of the Philbin et al[316] study). Regression analysis revealed significant correlations between serum opioid concentrations and isoflurane concentrations at most of the time points sampled in the pre-CPB period. By inspecting plots of the data pairs, they were able to ascertain the inflection point at which the isoflurane concentration began to rise rapidly, indicating poor control of hemodynamics by the respective opioid. For sufentanil, this was 0.71 ± 0.13 ng/mL, and for fentanyl, it was 7.3 ± 1.1 ng/mL. Given the use of fast-tracking with approximate ranges of 20 μg/kg for fentanyl and 3 μg/kg for sufentanil for the entire case, it is unlikely these concentrations will be obtained. However, reliance on volatile anesthesia, benzodiazepines, propofol, or dexmedetomidine infusion can provide hemodynamic control. The level of preexisting β- and or calcium channel blockade and the type of muscle relaxant used influence each patient's response.

Inhalation Anesthetics and Myocardial Protection

There is steadily increasing evidence from laboratory and clinical studies that inhalation anesthetic agents have favorable properties in patients undergoing CABG surgery, particularly in comparison to TIVA approaches. Along with the now routine use of fast-track anesthesia techniques, there has been a major resurgence in their use as the primary anesthetic for cardioprotection, with opioids and benzodiazepines increasingly relegated to a "supplemental" status (see Chapter 9).

MYOCARDIAL PROTECTION

Inhalation anesthetics are thought to protect the myocardium against ischemia by their ability to mimic ischemic preconditioning. The latter has been shown to reduce myocardial infarction size after periods of ischemia,[318] protect the heart against postischemic LV dysfunction,[4] and reduce the incidence of arrhythmias after cardiac surgery.[319] Intravenous anesthetics such as propofol do not appear to have the same cardioprotective properties. In an animal model, recovery from myocardial stunning was faster in dogs anesthetized with desflurane compared with propofol.[320] In a prospective, randomized, nonblinded study, DeHert et al[53] compared the inhalation anesthetics desflurane and sevoflurane to an intravenous anesthetic technique with a continuous propofol infusion in high-risk patients undergoing CABG surgery. Myocardial function was better preserved and troponin I levels were lower with the volatile anesthetics. They also reported shorter ICU and hospital length of stay (LOS) compared with propofol or midazolam-based anesthetic regimens in this setting.[52] There is some evidence that inhalation anesthetics are associated with a reduced incidence of postoperative arrhythmias although this remains controversial and has not been conclusively demonstrated.[319-321] Inhalational anesthetics may be effective in blunting the deleterious effects of postischemic reperfusion injury, and the inflammatory response syndrome after cardiac surgery.[322] Inhalation anesthetics also preserve cardiac function after reperfusion and decrease ischemia-induced intracoronary adhesion of polymorphonuclear neutrophils and platelets.[323-327] Most available data has been derived from animal and in vitro studies. Nevertheless, there is increasing evidence from prospective randomized clinical studies in patients undergoing CABG surgery that volatile anesthetic agents should be part of the anesthetic regimen, particularly in patients at high risk for ischemic events.[328]

MYOCARDIAL PRECONDITIONING

Murry et al[329] first described that brief periods of ischemia before 40 minutes of coronary artery occlusion significantly reduced infarction size after myocardial reperfusion. Exposing the myocardium to short periods of ischemia followed by reperfusion is called *ischemic preconditioning* (IPC). These brief periods of ischemia initiate signaling pathways that render the myocardium resistant to subsequent prolonged periods of ischemia (i.e., memory effect).[330] After a short ischemic period (i.e., preconditioning signal), the myocardium is rendered more resistant to prolonged ischemia when the subsequent ischemic event occurs within a certain time window. This may occur in two distinct phases as early preconditioning (about 2 hours) and delayed preconditioning (24 to 72 hours), although not all stimuli elicit both responses. Even though multiple approaches are used to protect the heart during CPB (e.g., blood cardioplegia, topical hypothermia, pharmacologic additives), aortic cross-clamping defines a period of myocardial ischemia that often results in transient or prolonged dysfunction after reperfusion.[331,332] Brief periods of aortic cross-clamping with consequent reperfusion intervals before a period of ventricular fibrillation has been shown to preserve ATP content, decrease markers of ischemia such as troponin I, and improve cardiac function in patients undergoing CABG.[333-336] However, this approach is controversial and cumbersome. Pharmacologic interventions have been sought that mimic IPC. There is increasing evidence that volatile anesthetics and opioids trigger preconditioning. Pharmacologic preconditioning and IPC initiate similar pathways that protect the myocardial cell against ischemic damage. The pathways associated with myocardial preconditioning involve a variety of triggering stimuli, mediators, receptors, and effectors.[337] It is thought that activation of sarcolemmal and mitochondrial K_{ATP} channels play a pivotal role in the preconditioning process.[338] Opening of these channels protects the myocardium by preventing cytosolic and mitochondrial Ca^{++} overload.

The exact mechanisms of preconditioning are still actively under investigation. After the administration of a preconditioning signal such as ischemia, inhalation anesthetics, opioids, bradykinin, or nitroglycerin, membrane-bound receptors (adenosine A_1, adrenergic, bradykinin, muscarinic, delta-1 opioid) coupled to inhibitory G-proteins are activated.[339-343] Consequently, products of intracellular transduction pathways (e.g., protein kinase C [PKC], tyrosine kinases, MAP kinases) mediate the opening and stabilization of ATP-sensitive mitochondrial K_{ATP} channels, the effectors thought to be mainly responsible for the preconditioning phenomenon.[344,345] Increased formation of nitric oxide,[346,347] free oxygen radicals,[337] and enzymes such as cyclooxygenase-2[348] are also involved in the preconditioning process. The delayed phase of myocardial protection, which may last well beyond the documented 24 to 72 hours, is probably based on transcriptional changes of protective proteins.[349]

Until recently, most data was based on in vitro studies or from data obtained during percutaneous coronary interventions. Whether these results can be generalized to cardiac surgery remains questionable. Several studies have investigated the clinical relevance of anesthetic preconditioning and its impact on patient outcome. Belhomme et al[350] exposed patients to 5 minutes of preconditioning with a 2.5 minimum alveolar concentration (MAC) of isoflurane after the onset of CPB but before aortic cross-clamping. Troponin I and CK-MB levels were not significantly different from those of the control group. Nevertheless, patients who were exposed to isoflurane had an increased activity of 5-nucleotidase, a marker for PKC activation, early evidence of preconditioning pathway activation similar to the in vitro findings. Penta de Peppo et al[351] reported on myocardial function and the preconditioning effect of enflurane in patients undergoing CABG surgery. Myocardial function was assessed using the end-systolic pressure-area relationship, a relatively load independent index of myocardial contractility. Although the number of patients studied was small, myocardial function was better preserved in patients who were exposed to enflurane before cardioplegic arrest.

Julier et al,[248] in a double-blinded, placebo controlled, multicenter study, reported on the effect of sevoflurane preconditioning on biochemical markers for myocardial and renal dysfunction in patients undergoing CABG surgery. Patients who had sevoflurane preconditioning during the first 10 minutes of CPB had lower levels of biochemical markers of myocardial and renal impairment. Brain natriuretic peptide level as an indicator of myocardial dysfunction was significantly decreased in the sevoflurane group. The same group of investigators has reported on the results of a prospective, randomized study of the effect of sevoflurane preconditioning (10 minutes before aortic cross-clamping) on late cardiac events.[249] Coronary artery reocclusion, congestive heart failure, and cardiac death were assessed at 6 and 12 months postoperatively. Preconditioning with sevoflurane significantly reduced the incidence of late cardiac events. Whereas some of the studies use brief periods of anesthetic preconditioning before aortic cross-clamping, others have reported on use of volatile anesthetics throughout the operative period. The older studies using brief periods of preconditioning showed improved cardiac function, although markers of myocardial injury such as CK-MB or troponin I often were not significantly different from the control group's. DeHert et al[246] showed that the best results for myocardial protection were achieved when sevoflurane was administered throughout the intraoperative period. Most similarly designed studies have shown similar results. Conzen et al[247] studied randomized patients undergoing OPCAB surgery with a propofol infusion versus a continuous inhalation-based anesthetic technique with sevoflurane. Patients in the sevoflurane group had significantly lower troponin I levels, as well as better LV function. Nader et al[352] added vaporized sevoflurane (2%) versus oxygen alone to a cold blood cardioplegia solution in a small randomized trial of patients undergoing CABG surgery. Markers of the inflammatory response (i.e., neutrophil β-integrins, tumor necrosis factor-α, and interleukin-6) were lower and cardiac function (i.e., stroke work index and wall motion analysis) was better preserved in the sevoflurane group (Fig. 19–16). Table 19–3 summarizes the results of the randomized, prospective clinical studies.[4,52,53,246-249,350-354]

Research on pharmacologic preconditioning is not only restricted to inhalation anesthetics. There is increasing evidence that a variety of drugs that are administered perioperatively have cardioprotective properties involving preconditioning pathways. Besides inhalation anesthetics, opioids (delta-opioid receptor), adenosine (adenosine A_1

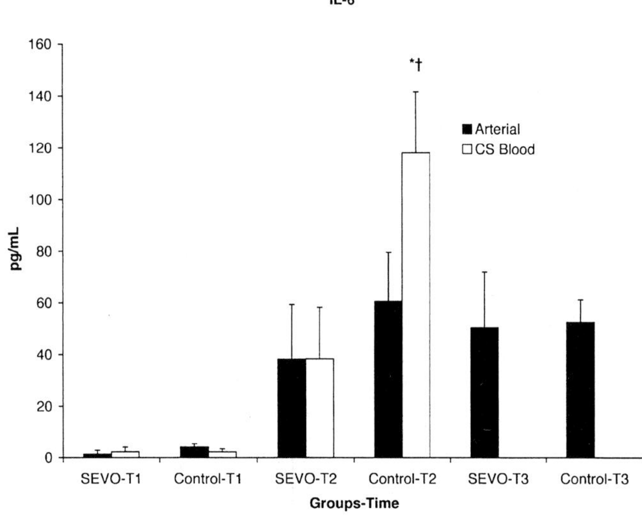

Figure 19–16 Blunting of elevation of interleukin-6 (IL-6) levels in response to cardiopulmonary bypass (CPB) in patients receiving 2% sevoflurane (SEVO) added to the cardioplegia solution (1.4 ± 1.2 to 38.2 ± 21.6 pg/mL versus 4.1 ± 1.4 to 118.2 ± 23.5 pg/mL, $p < 0.05$). Levels were similar by 6 hours after CPB. CS = coronary sinus; T1 = baseline; T2 = after separation from CPB; T3 = 6 hours after separation from CPB. (From Nader ND, Li CM, Khadra WZ, et al: Anesthetic myocardial protection with sevoflurane. J Cardiothorac Vasc Anesth 18:269, 2004.)

receptor), and bradykinin have been investigated for their preconditioning effects with variable results[355-358] (see Chapter 9).

During cardiac surgery, several of the known preconditioning triggering agents may be used and appear to be additive or synergistic in effect. Toller et al[359] reported that the administration of sevoflurane and mechanical IPC reduced infarction size significantly compared with either stimulus alone. Ludwig et al[355] demonstrated the additive effect of isoflurane and morphine on the reduction of infarction size. Some data indicate that the preconditioning effects of inhalation anesthetics are related to timing, dose, and total duration of administration.[360,361] When sevoflurane was added to the anesthesia regimen after the coronary anastomoses were completed, myocardial recovery was faster compared with a propofol-based anesthetic technique. Nevertheless, patients who received sevoflurane during the entire procedure had the lowest troponin I levels, and the stroke volume changed the least compared with baseline levels.[246] Patients undergoing OPCAB surgery may benefit more from anesthetic preconditioning when compared with CABG surgery with CPB and cardioplegic arrest although this is controversial.[362]

Several clinical factors appear to impair the protective effects of preconditioning. Two groups of patients, diabetics and females, appear to have attenuated responses to mechanical preconditioning signals (during PCI).[363] Intraoperative hyperglycemia blocks the preconditioning effect, although this effect may be reversed by *N*-acetylcysteine, an oxygen radical scavenger.[364-367] Other anesthetic agents such as etomidate, propofol, and midazolam have not been shown to affect mitochondrial K_{ATP} channels. In an in vitro model, ketamine, *S*-ketamine, and thiopental inhibited diazoxide-induced mitochondrial K_{ATP} channel opening, whereas fentanyl facilitated it.[368]

In summary, there is increasing evidence that the choice of anesthetic in patients at risk for cardiac events may have a significant effect on myocardial protection. Inhalation

Table 19–3 Clinical Studies of Volatile Agent Preconditioning for Coronary Artery Bypass Grafting

Study	Drugs, Route	*N*	End Points	Results	Comments
Belhomme, 1999[350]	ISO (2.5 MAC on CPB) for 5 min before AoX vs. case-matched controls; TIVA propofol-opioid base anesthetic	18	A. CK-MB/Trop I B. ecto-5′-nucleotidase	0 1 (increase activity)	 Marker of protein kinase C activation
Penta de Peppo, 1999[351]	ENF (0.5%–2.0%) to reduce SPB by 25% 5 min before AoX vs. control; TIVA propofol-opioid base anesthetic	16	A. CK-MB/Trop I B. CI C. LV contractility	0 0 1 (preserved)	 Pressure-area loops measured by TEE
Tomai, 1999[353]	ISO before AoX	40	A. CK-MB/Trop I	0	Significant only with preop EF <50%
Haroun-Birzi, 2001[354]	ISO (approx 1 MAC) before CPB vs. control; TIVA propofol-opioid base anesthetic	49	A. CI B. ST-segment changes	1 (higher in ISO) 1 (less in ISO)	
De Hert, 2002[4]	SEVO continuous (0.5%–2%) vs. PROP; remifentanil in both	20	A. Trop I B. LV systolic/diastolic function (LVP parameters pre/post leg elevation)	1 (lower in SEVO) 1 (preserved in SEVO)	
Julier, 2003[248]	SEVO (2 MAC) vaporized on CPB for 10 min before AoX vs. control; TIVA propofol-opioid base anesthetic	72	A. CK-MB/Trop T/Holter ST segments B. Brain natruretic peptide C. Protein kinase C translocation D. Plasma cystatin C	0 1 (lower in SEVO) 1 (greater in SEVO) 1 (lower in SEVO)	 Marker of contractile dysfunction Immunohistologic analysis from atrial tissue Marker of renal dysfunction
Conzen, 2003[247]	SEVO (approx 1 MAC) continuous vs. PROP (OPCAB); sufentanil base in both	20	A. CK-MB B. Trop I C. CI	0 1 (lower in SEVO) 1 (higher in SEVO)	

Table continued on following page

Table 19–3 Clinical Studies of Volatile Agent Preconditioning for Coronary Artery Bypass Grafting—(Continued)

Study	Drugs, Route	*N*	End Points	Results	Comments
De Hert, 2003[53]	SEVO (0.5%–2%), DES (1%–4%), PROP (2–4 μg/mL target concentration); high-risk elderly patients	45	A. Trop I B. LV systolic/diastolic function (LVP parameters pre/post leg elevation)	1 (high in PROP) 1 (preserved in SEVO, DES)	Cohort: age >70 yr, EF <50% with impaired length–dependent regulation of myocardial function
De Hert, 2004[52]	SEVO (0.5%–2%), DES (1%–4%), MIDAZ (0.5–1.5 μg/kg/min), PROP (2 μg/mL target concentration); remifentanil base anesthetic	320	A. Trop I B. LOS in ICU or hospital C. Inotrope use D. LV function	1 (lower in SEVO, DES) 1 (less in SEVO, DES) 1 (less in SEVO, DES) 1 (preserved in SEVO, DES)	
De Hert, 2004[246]	SEVO pre-CPB vs. SEVO post-CPB vs. SEVO-continuous vs. PROP alone; TIVA propofol-opioid base anesthetic	200	A. Trop I B. LOS in ICU C. Inotrope use D. LV systolic/diastolic function (LVP parameters pre/post leg elevation)	1 (lower in SEVO continuous) 1 (less in SEVO continuous) 1 (less in SEVO continuous) 1 (better preserved in SEVO esp. continuous)	
Nader, 2004[352]	SEVO, placebo (2% SEVO vaporized in cardioplegia); TIVA propofol-opioid base anesthetic	21	A. LV function (TEE, LVSWI) B. Inflammatory response (neutrophil β-integrins, tumor necrosis factor, interleukin-6)	1 (better preserved in SEVO) 1 (lower in SEVO)	
Garcia, 2004[249]	12-mo follow-up of Julier et al cohort	72	A. Endothelial function (transcript levels of PECAM-1, catalase, heat shock protein) B. Late cardiac events (6 to 12 months)	1 (better with SEVO) 1 (lower with SEVO)	PECAM-1 levels lower in SEVO, may have role in transition of coronary plaques to unstable state 3% vs. 17% for composite outcome ($p = 0.04$); peak periop BNP and Trop I higher in patients with events; no deaths

AoX = aortic cross-clamping; BNP = brain natriuretic peptide; CI, confidence interval; CK-MB = isoenzyme of creatine kinase with muscle and brain subunits; CPB = cardiopulmonary bypass; DES = desflurane; EF = ejection fraction; ENF = enflurane; ICU = intensive care unit; ISO = isoflurane; LOS = length of stay; LV = left ventricular; LVP = left ventricular pressure; LVSWI = left ventricular stroke work index; MAC = minimum alveolar concentration; MIDAZ = midazolam; OPCAB = off-pump coronary artery bypass grafting; PECAM-1 = platelet–endothelial cell adhesion molecule-1; PROP = propofol; SEVO = sevoflurane; SPB = systolic blood pressure; TEE = transesophageal echocardiography; TIVA = total intravenous anesthetic; Trop I = troponin I.

anesthetics have multiple cardioprotective effects, including triggering the preconditioning cascade and blunting of reperfusion injury. The mode of administration, dose, timing, differences between various inhalation agents, patient selection, and the impact on cardiac morbidity and mortality remain to be more precisely elucidated by larger randomized clinical trials.

SEVOFLURANE

Sevoflurane has been increasingly used during cardiac surgery due to its favorable hemodynamic effects and cardioprotective properties. When sevoflurane was compared with desflurane in healthy volunteers, the sympathetic activation seen with rapid increases in desflurane could not be documented with sevoflurane.[369] Although both agents decreased SVR, arterial BP, and CO in a dose-dependent fashion, administration of sevoflurane showed a tendency to lower HRs, which is advantageous in most patients with ischemic heart disease.[370,371]

Sevoflurane is a potent trigger of the preconditioning cascade.[372,373] It has beneficial effects on intraoperative myocardial function after CPB, and it may also favorably influence long-term morbidity and mortality after CABG.[4,52,53,246-249]

In animal studies, sevoflurane caused no maldistribution of coronary blood flow or signs of coronary steal.[374,375] The frequency of myocardial ischemia with its use has been shown to be no different from isoflurane in noncardiac and CABG surgery.[376-378] Although prolongation of the QT interval (including QTc) has been reported with sevoflurane, there is no evidence that this has adverse clinical effects.[379,380]

Potential adverse effects on renal function by sevoflurane were originally a concern on its clinical introduction due to production of plasma fluoride and compound A particularly with low-flow techniques (<2 L/min of fresh gas flow). However, a variety of clinical studies have not shown demonstrable adverse effects on renal function in normal clinical use of sevoflurane (particularly because most gas flows exceed 2 L/min).[381] In a randomized trial of patients undergoing CABG surgery, sevoflurane administration was not associated with increased plasma creatinine concentrations when compared with propofol or isoflurane based anesthetic techniques.[382] Despite package insert warnings to avoid prolonged low-flow administration, one report described no adverse effects in a small clinical cohort.[383] Other studies report no adverse effects in patients with preexisting renal insufficiency or chronic hypertension.[377,384,385] Other concerns have been raised regarding the rare occurrence of exothermic reactions with use of low-flow sevoflurane and desiccated CO_2 absorbent.[386,387] Sevoflurane's predictable and salutary hemodynamic and cardioprotective properties and favorable safety profile would appear to make it an ideal inhalation agent for patients undergoing CABG.

DESFLURANE

Desflurane has unique hemodynamic effects particularly in relation to sevoflurane. These have resulted in controversy regarding its use in patients with coronary artery disease. Desflurane, similar to isoflurane, decreases SVR, BP, and LV systolic and diastolic function in a dose-dependent fashion.[388] Desflurane and isoflurane maintain the cardiac index; however, desflurane causes a significant increase in HR, pulmonary artery pressure, and pulmonary capillary wedge pressure.[389,390] This increased sympathetic activity is most pronounced when desflurane concentrations are increased rapidly and with higher absolute concentrations.[391-393] However, activation appears greatest with the initial increase in concentration.[394] The resulting increase in HR could possibly lead to myocardial ischemia in patients presenting with ischemic heart disease, particularly in the setting of a less than optimal anesthetic regimen (e.g., absence of opioid supplement or with excessive myocardial depression from a negative inotrope induction agent).[288]

Unlike isoflurane, desflurane administration is associated with increased plasma norepinephrine concentrations during anesthesia induction despite a concomitant decrease in arterial blood pressure.[395] Grundmann et al[390] compared the cardiovascular effects of desflurane and isoflurane in patients with coronary artery disease. When desflurane concentrations were increased rapidly, a transient increase in arterial blood flow, followed by a decreased arterial blood flow, could be demonstrated. Direct airway mucosa irritation and sites within the lung that respond to desflurane administration were postulated as possible causes of the increased sympathetic activation seen with desflurane.[396] Rodig et al[397] compared desflurane and sevoflurane administered by the oxygenator's gas supply line during CPB to eliminate the effects of pulmonary irritation. Plasma norepinephrine and epinephrine concentrations remained unchanged compared with baseline levels in the desflurane group and decreased when sevoflurane was added on CPB. There is evidence for a systemic response and localized airway irritation or pulmonary stimulation as possible causes of the increased plasma catecholamine levels seen with desflurane.[398,399] However, inhalation anesthetics are usually not given as the sole anesthetic and supplemental agents are nearly always used. The administration of fentanyl, β-blockade, and clonidine have been demonstrated to partially blunt this sympathetic activation.[400,401]

Desflurane has been shown to have preconditioning-like cardioprotective effects in vitro and in vivo.[402,403] It preconditions human myocardium by activation of K_{ATP} channels, stimulation of adenosine A_1 receptors, and nitric oxide release.[404] Because of its sympathetic stimulation, desflurane, unlike other inhalation agents, also activates α- and β-adrenoceptor–mediated preconditioning of the human myocardium.[405]

Desflurane has been used safely and effectively in CABG surgery worldwide. However, the clinician must remain aware of its sympathetic stimulating properties, particularly with rapid increases in concentration. Its use in certain subgroups of patients may be deleterious (e.g., chronic hypertensive patient with severe left ventricular hypertrophy and CAD in whom increases in HR are likely poorly tolerated), whereas in others, it may be advantageous (e.g., patients with depressed EF and poor ventricular compliance in which CO may rely more on HR than on the Frank Starling mechanism).

ISOFLURANE

Preconditioning with isoflurane has been documented in multiple studies. Its hemodynamic properties and its effect on the preconditioning cascade are similar to sevoflurane. When isoflurane was compared with sevoflurane in patients with cardiac disease undergoing noncardiac surgery, there was no significant difference in perioperative ischemic events, adverse cardiac outcomes, intraoperative hemodynamic stability, and inotropic support between the two groups.[378] Isoflurane mimics IPC through activation of mitochondrial K_{ATP} channels and the generation of free radicals.[406-410] Unlike IPC, its effect on the late phase of preconditioning is less clear.[411,412] Its preconditioning effect appears to be potentiated by concurrent opioid administration.[355]

HALOTHANE AND ENFLURANE

There is limited data on the ability of halothane to trigger preconditioning pathways or its cardioprotective properties. In an isolated heart model, halothane administration before ischemia preserved adenosine triphosphate levels and postischemic cardiac function.[413] Its efficacy for preconditioning in whole animal models is controversial with positive[414] and negative[415] results. In an in vitro study of human myocardial tissue, halothane did not exhibit preconditioning effects. The effect of halothane on the cardiac K_{ATP} channel seems to differ from other volatile anesthetics such as isoflurane.[415,416] Halothane has been shown to have protective effects with regard to ischemia in canine models, perhaps by a reduction in calcium-induced cell injury. Neither halothane nor enflurane is a potent coronary vasodilator nor have they been implicated in causing coronary steal.

α_2-Agonists: Dexmedetomidine

Centrally acting α_2-adrenergic receptor agonists such as clonidine or dexmedetomidine have unique properties (Box 19–2) that explain their increasing use in cardiac surgery patients. Although the FDA approved clonidine in 1974, availability in only an oral formulation greatly limited its widespread use. In 1999, the FDA approved dexmedetomidine for continuous (up to 24 hours) intravenous sedation in the ICU setting. It is seeing increasing use in the operating room and ICU settings.

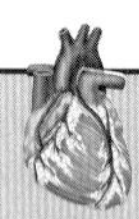

BOX 19–2 *α_2-Agonist Properties*

- Sedation
- Anxiolysis
- Analgesia
- Hemodynamic stability
- Central sympatholytic effect
- Decreased blood pressure and heart rate
- Decreased perioperative oxygen consumption
- Decreased plasma catecholamine levels
- Decreased incidence of tachyarrhythmias
- Facilitation of diuresis
- Prevention of histamine-induced bronchoconstriction
- Treatment and prevention of postoperative shivering
- Treatment and prevention of postoperative delirium
- Blunting of withdrawal symptoms in drug and alcohol addicts
- Possible inhibition of inflammatory response

PHARMACODYNAMICS AND PHARMACOKINETICS

Dexmedetomidine is a more selective α_2-adrenoceptor agonist than clonidine (approximately 8 times greater). It exhibits both central sympatholytic and peripheral vasoconstrictive effects. Intravenous infusion of dexmedetomidine (0.2 to 0.7 µg/kg/hr) causes transient increases of MAP and SVR due to stimulation of α- and β_2-adrenergic receptors in vascular smooth muscle. This is followed by a decrease in MAP, HR, SV, CO, and plasma catecholamine levels.[417,418] Higher doses of dexmedetomidine result in more profound sedation and analgesia with a persistent increase in MAP, SVR, and mean pulmonary artery pressure.[419]

There is limited data from animal studies demonstrating potential coronary vasoconstrictive and cardiodepressant effects.[420-423] However, coronary vasoconstriction was mainly seen with bolus doses of 10 µg/kg and higher. At the recommended loading doses (0.5 to 2 µg/kg) and maintenance (0.2 to 0.7 µg/kg/h), dexmedetomidine most likely has a favorable effect on myocardial perfusion.[424] Roekaerts et al[425,426] showed an increase in endocardial-to-epicardial blood flow ratio in the postischemic myocardium, with an overall reduction of myocardial oxygen demand after experimentally induced myocardial ischemia in dogs. As expected, the greatest reduction in oxygen demand is seen when baseline HR and arterial BP are increased.[424] Intravenous dexmedetomidine exhibits a rapid distribution phase with a distribution half-life of about 6 minutes. Dexmedetomidine shows high protein binding (94%) and undergoes extensive biotransformation in the liver with direct glucuronidation and cytochrome P450 mediated metabolism. Although dexmedetomidine is mainly excreted renally (95%), no dose adjustments are necessary in patients with renal insufficiency, although, slightly prolonged sedation should be expected.[427] Severe hepatic impairment may necessitate a dose reduction (see Chapter 9).

INTRAOPERATIVE USE

Intraoperatively, α_2-agonists can be useful adjuncts given their sedative, analgesic, and hemodynamic stabilizing properties. α_2-Agonists prevent hypertension and tachycardia during intubation, surgical stimulation, and emergence from anesthesia, and decrease plasma catecholamine levels.[428-430] Jalonen et al, in a randomized double-blind study, administered dexmedetomidine or placebo to CABG patients starting before induction (50 ng/kg/min for 30 min) and continued until the end of surgery (7 ng/kg/min).[423] Patients receiving dexmedetomidine had significantly lower plasma norepinephrine levels and more stable hemodynamics (less increase in MAP and HR during induction, less intraoperative variability of systolic arterial pressure). Dexmedetomidine administration was associated with a decreased incidence of intraoperative (5% versus 32%) and postoperative (4% versus 40%) tachycardia when compared with placebo. Patients who received dexmedetomidine were less likely to receive β-blocker therapy for tachycardia. Despite the findings before and after bypass, a higher incidence of hypotension (MAP < 30 mm Hg) was seen during CPB (22% versus 0% patients, dexmedetomidine versus placebo). These data demonstrate that dexmedetomidine is effective in attenuating sympathetic responses although this effect may predispose patients toward hypotension.

Because of the decreased oxygen demand and HR seen with dexmedetomidine administration, it may be beneficial during OPCAB.[431] Nevertheless, in a small series of OPCAB patients, hypotension (12 mm Hg below baseline) occurred shortly after its administration during rewarming in the ICU prompting the study authors to recommend volume loading and normothermia before its use.[431] Experimental data demonstrates a decrease in the inflammatory response to endotoxin-induced shock in a rat model.[432] Its effects on CPB-induced inflammatory responses have yet to be reported.

EARLY POSTOPERATIVE USE

Dexmedetomidine may be a very useful agent in the early postoperative period as its sedative properties are associated with minimal respiratory depression, and, in this regard, appear to mimic natural sleep patterns.[433] When administered continuously in postsurgical patients it caused no statistical differences in respiratory rate, oxygen saturation, arterial pH, and arterial carbon dioxide tension when compared with placebo.[434] These patients were usually effectively sedated but still arousable and cooperative to verbal stimulation.[435] Due to its analgesic properties, it significantly reduces additional opioid analgesia requirements in mechanically ventilated patients in the ICU.[436-438] In a multicenter randomized study, Herr et al[238] compared a dexmedetomidine-based sedation regimen to propofol sedation after CABG in the ICU. Although there were no differences in time to extubation, the investigators found a significantly reduced need for additional analgesics (i.e., propofol-sedated patients required four times the mean dose of morphine), antiemetics, diuretics, and had fewer episodes of tachyarrhythmias requiring β-blockade (ventricular tachycardia in 5% of the propofol-sedated group versus none in the dexmedetomidine group). However, hypotension was more common in the dexmedetomidine group compared with the propofol-sedated patients (24% versus 16%) (Fig. 19–17). Approximately 25% of the dexmedetomidine-associated hypotension occurred in the first hour of the study (starting at sternal closure), particularly during or within 10 minutes after the loading infusion of 1 μg/kg. The combination of reduction of preload during sternal closure and the loading dose would seem to indicate this was not the optimal manner in which to use this agent.

The α_2-agonists have been used successfully in patients with postoperative delirium, withdrawal symptoms in alcohol or drug addicts, and are associated with a low rate of shivering.[439,440] Overall, cardiac surgical patients who are sedated with dexmedetomidine should benefit from more stable hemodynamic control in the postoperative period, with a decrease in oxygen demand and a lower incidence of tachyarrhythmias.

Neuromuscular Blocking Agents

All of the available neuromuscular blocking agents have been used to produce adequate intubating conditions and relaxation during CABG surgery (Table 19–4). Murphy et al[441] conducted a national survey of more than 400 active members of the Society of Cardiovascular Anesthesiologists evaluating their neuromuscular blocking drug of choice in the cardiac surgical setting. Despite availability of newer short-acting neuromuscular blocking agents, pancuronium was still used in most patients undergoing on-pump and off-pump cardiac surgical procedures. Traditionally, pancuronium had been advocated for use with high-dose narcotic techniques, as it offsets opioid-induced bradycardia. However, it has long been recognized that clinically significant tachycardia resulting in myocardial ischemia could occur during induction of anesthesia with high-dose fentanyl and pancuronium.[442] With the increasing popularity of fast-track cardiac surgery, early extubation is now most desirable and the longer duration of action of pancuronium is a potential disadvantage. Several studies have compared the duration of action of pancuronium and rocuronium in patients undergoing cardiac surgery. Irrespective of a single intubating dose or a continuous infusion, patients receiving rocuronium had significantly less residual neuromuscular blockade[443] and shorter time to extubation.[444,445] When continuous infusions of rocuronium and cisatracurium were compared in prolonged surgical procedures, recovery to 75% of the train of four (TOF) was faster in patients receiving cisatracurium.[446] Reich et al[447] compared neuromuscular transmission recovery times in pediatric

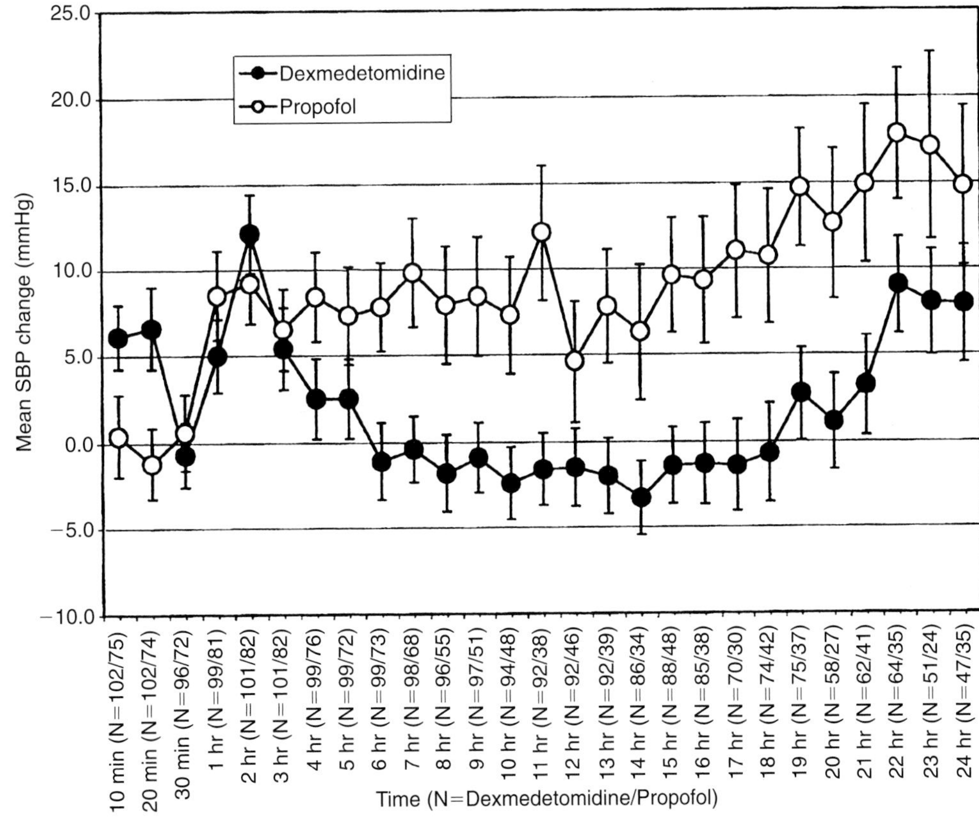

Figure 19–17 Changes from baseline in systolic blood pressure (SPB) between coronary artery bypass grafting (CABG) patients sedated with dexmedetomidine *(filled circles)* or propofol *(open circles)*. The baseline is mean systolic pressure for each treatment group just before sternal closure. Numbers of patients receiving each drug (x-axis) declines progressively as they are extubated postoperatively. (From Herr DL, Sum-Ping ST, England M: ICU sedation after coronary artery bypass graft surgery: Dexmedetomidine-based versus propofol-based sedation regimens. J Cardiothorac Vasc Anesth 17:576, 2003.)

Table 19–4 Nondepolarizing Neuromuscular Blocking Agents Commonly Used in Cardiac Anesthesia

Relaxant	Intubating Dose (mg/kg)	Maintenance	Clinical Duration (min)	Hemodynamic Effects	Special Considerations
Pancuronium	0.08–0.12	0.01 mg/kg q20–60 min	60–120	Vagolytic ++ at clinical dosages, releases Norepinephrine	Reduce dose or avoid completely in renal insufficiency
Vecuronium	0.08–0.2	0.8–2 μg/kg/hr	45–90	Insignificant	Accumulation of active metabolite with long-term use
Cisatracurium	0.15–0.2	1–2 μg/kg/min	40–75	Insignificant	Hoffman elimination
Rocuronium	0.4–1.0	0.01 mg/kg/min	35–75	Mildly vagolytic (high dosage)	No active metabolites

cardiac patients receiving cisatracurium or vecuronium infusions in the ICU setting. Cisatracurium was associated with significantly faster spontaneous recovery of the neuromuscular function. Especially in fast-track cardiac surgery, shorter-acting neuromuscular blocking agents such as cisatracurium or rocuronium are recommended to avoid residual paralysis and to allow for early extubation and ICU discharge. Neuromuscular transmission monitoring to assess for residual blockade and use of pharmacologic reversal is advisable especially if a fast-track anesthesia technique is used.[448,449] In patients with a potentially difficult airway or emergency patients who are not NPO, succinylcholine is still the agent of choice.

Additional considerations are warranted in patients with underlying comorbidities such as chronic renal failure that may alter pharmacokinetics. When magnesium is administered to cardiac surgical patients for prophylaxis of perioperative arrhythmias, blockade from nondepolarizing neuromuscular blocking agents may be significantly prolonged.[450] There remains the question as to whether continuous neuromuscular blockade for cardiac surgery is really necessary. Gueret et al[451] showed that a single intubating dose of atracurium or cisatracurium provided adequate paralysis and surgical conditions leading to quicker neuromuscular blockade recovery in cardiac surgical patients. Advocates of this technique also point to potential advantages with regard to prevention of recall (as indicated by patient movement). However, potential disadvantages include the possibility of greater oxygen demand and consumption, or movement during surgery.

Intraoperative Awareness and Recall

Intraoperative awareness (i.e., recall), usually defined as postoperative memory for intraoperative events, is an infrequent but well-recognized phenomenon during general anesthesia. Awareness, a conscious subjective experience (i.e., implicit memory) may be much more frequent than conscious recall (i.e., explicit memory) of intraoperative events.[452] In a prospective, nonrandomized, descriptive cohort study of more than 19,000 patients undergoing surgery with general anesthesia at seven academic medical centers in the United States, awareness with explicit recall occurred in 0.13% of the cases.[453] Patients undergoing cardiac surgery have always been considered to be at increased risk due to anesthetic regimens intentionally devoid of cardiodepressant inhalation anesthetics (before the era of improved myocardial preservation and fast-tracking), and due to frequent periods of light anesthesia in the presence of hemodynamic instability resulting from surgical manipulation of the heart and great vessels, depressed contractility after CPB, or bleeding. The published incidence of awareness in patients undergoing cardiac surgery is significantly higher than that reported for general surgery with older reports of up to 23%.[454] However, the introduction of fast-track anesthesia techniques and the recognition that inhalation agents are useful in intraoperative preconditioning before CPB have changed anesthetic regimens for cardiac surgery. It is now recognized that use of inhalation agents during cardiac surgery (including during CPB) reduces the risk of awareness. Ranta et al[455] found definite intraoperative awareness with recall in 0.5% of patients undergoing cardiac surgery under general anesthesia with various anesthesia regimes using inhalation or TIVA techniques. Higher doses of benzodiazepines, such as midazolam, resulted in a lower incidence of awareness. Phillips et al[456] interviewed 700 patients after cardiac surgery with CPB and found that 8 patients (1.8%) reported intraoperative recall regardless of whether benzodiazepines or inhalation agents were used. Fast-track anesthesia techniques typically combine low-dose narcotics with short-acting anesthetics such as inhalation agents or propofol infusions. Dowd et al[457] reported a low incidence (0.3%) of intraoperative awareness with this technique attributing it to the continuous administration of volatile anesthetics or propofol.

Measures to prevent intraoperative awareness are typically based on anesthetic regimens that interfere with memory processing, such as the use of inhalation anesthetics and benzodiazepines. However, the anesthesia technique does not always correlate with the incidence of intraoperative awareness. In a large series of more than 11,000 patients undergoing general anesthesia, 18 cases of recall occurred (0.18%), but the analysis suggested that this number could not have been reduced with monitoring of end-tidal anesthetic gas concentrations or more frequent use of preoperatively administered benzodiazepines.[458] Efforts to determine time periods that are prone to awareness or recall are usually based on physiologic or hemodynamic parameters that indicate light anesthesia, such as tachycardia, arterial hypertension, or patient movement. Nevertheless, Kerssens et al[459] showed that hemodynamic variables were poor predictors of intraoperative awareness, although these parameters were able to differentiate between patients with or without *conscious* recall. In contrast, electroencephalogram (EEG)–derived parameters were highly significant predictors of intraoperative awareness but were not able to detect patients with conscious recall.

Consequently, if hemodynamic parameters or measures of anesthetic concentrations are insufficient in preventing intraoperative awareness, the question arises if monitoring neurophysiologic parameters such as processed EEG data decreases the incidence of intraoperative awareness or recall. Neurophysiologic monitoring is usually based on fast Fourier transformation and bispectral analysis of one-channel EEG data obtained from electrodes on the patient's forehead. Several devices have been approved by the U.S. Food and Drug Administration (FDA).[460-464] Two large studies showed a significant reduction in awareness under general anesthesia when the Bispectral Index (BIS) was monitored. Myles et al[465] studied 2463 patients considered to be at high risk for awareness in a prospective, randomized, double-blinded, multicenter trial with 45% undergoing high-risk cardiac surgery or OPCAB. Patients were randomized to BIS-guided or routine anesthesia care. BIS monitoring reduced the risk of awareness by 82% although the absolute number of confirmed events was small (2 versus 11). In patients undergoing cardiac surgery, three events occurred (2 routine, 1 BIS). "Possible" awareness events (not confirmed by the endpoint committee) occurred irrespective of the use of BIS monitoring. Ekman et al, in a large nonrandomized, historically controlled study also showed a significantly reduced incidence of intraoperative awareness (0.04% versus 0.18%) in the BIS monitored patients.[466] However, in a small series of patients Barr et al[467] found no correlation between bispectral EEG analysis of anesthesia depth and conscious recall in patients undergoing cardiac surgery. This was attributed to exclusive use of midazolam and fentanyl. Besides monitoring anesthetic depth, neurophysiologic monitoring may also help to decrease the incidence of hemodynamic disturbances,[468,469] may guide titration of anesthetic agents to their effective dose,[461,470] and may be associated with improved patient satisfaction.[471] In clinical experience, the use of BIS monitoring has been helpful in more accurately gauging the need for reinstitution of volatile anesthesia after weaning from CPB (Fig. 19–18). In this potentially unstable period with a depressed myocardium or untoward responses to protamine, this can be an important factor. Often the BIS remains in the low range for the first 15 to 30 minutes after weaning, especially in older patients with longer pump times. It is also helpful to ensure adequacy of burst suppression for hypothermic circulatory arrest.

In summary, published data seem to indicate that despite a substantial reduction in awareness resulting from a shift to greater use of volatile anesthetics, patients undergoing cardiac surgery are still at risk for intraoperative awareness or recall. Neurophysiologic monitoring decreases the incidence of these events, but given the low incidence, a large number of patients have to be monitored to prevent one case of intraoperative awareness. The implications of intraoperative awareness or conscious recall are not yet fully understood. These events may be unrecognized or not necessarily experienced as unpleasant,[472] but they also may lead to severe posttraumatic stress disorders with chronic health impairment.[473]

Choice of Technique

A wide variety of techniques have been used for anesthetic induction and maintenance for CABG. Hemodynamic alterations such as hypotension after induction, or hypertension and tachycardia at intubation, are not infrequent. They can be readily treated with small doses of vasopressors, such as phenylephrine or ephedrine for hypotension, or deepening anesthesia or adding β-blockade to treat hyperdynamic

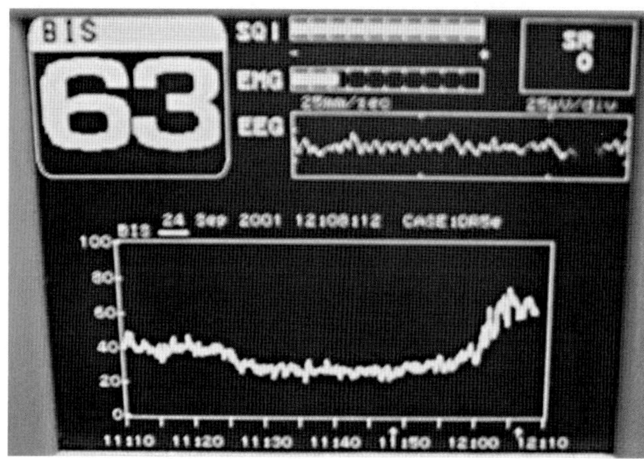

Figure 19–18 Portion of a Bispectral Index (BIS) tracing from a patient undergoing coronary artery bypass grafting with sufentanil infusion and sevoflurane-oxygen anesthesia. Isoflurane was administered during hypothermic cardiopulmonary bypass (CPB) (approximately 11:15 to 12:00), and a modest reduction in BIS was observed. Shortly after weaning from CPB, the patient developed bronchospasm with difficulty in maintaining adequate level of anesthesia due to inability to attain an adequate end-tidal concentration of volatile agent. Propofol infusion was instituted with reduction of BIS level below 60 (considered safest with regard to risk of recall) until the bronchospasm resolved. (Images courtesy of Martin J. London, MD, University of California, San Francisco, CA [www.ucsf.edu/teeecho].)

responses. In two large outcome studies,[50,51] no single technique was demonstrated to be superior in terms of reduced intraoperative ischemia, postoperative myocardial infarction, or death. These studies have been critically appraised and found wanting in terms of outcome measures and design. However, both represent large study groups and suggest that other variables such as severity of CAD, particularly the presence of significant ongoing ischemia, whether silent or clinically apparent, adequacy of myocardial revascularization, and ischemic (cross-clamp) time are much more predictive of outcome than the anesthetic regimen (see Chapter 39). It has been suggested that the anesthesiologist's primary responsibility is to *control the heart rate,* because it is the hemodynamic change most likely to result in myocardial ischemia.[50] Others would modify that statement to say that the anesthesiologist's job is to assess the patient, surgeon, and anesthetic technique and to provide an anesthetic with minimal hemodynamic disturbance plus active, continuous ischemia monitoring and aggressive treatment of hemodynamic abnormalities and myocardial ischemia. If this is done poorly, the anesthesiologist can become a major risk factor.

Interest in the use of thoracic epidural anesthesia (TEA) for cardiac surgery has steadily increased over the past 15 years. It has been long appreciated that thoracic sympathectomy has favorable effects on the heart and coronary circulation.[9] Its coronary vasodilating effects have been well documented and it has been used to treat unstable angina for many years albeit very infrequently due to logistics and the contemporary standard of use of potent antiplatelet agents. There has been a resurgence in interest, including reports of using chronically implanted patient controlled catheters.[474-478] It is frequently used as a supplement to general anesthesia for cardiac surgery, particularly in Europe and Asia (Fig. 19–19).[479-481] However, in the United States, medicolegal concerns about the rare but present danger of a devastating neurologic injury and the substantial logistical issues regarding placement the night before

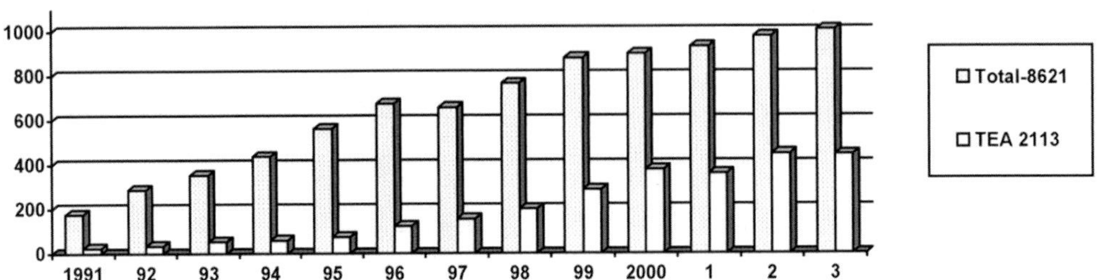

Figure 19–19 Frequency of use of thoracic epidural anesthesia (TEA) at a single center over the past 31 years (total of 2013 patients). All catheters were placed the day before surgery between C7 and T3. Dural puncture occurred in 0.9%, and temporary neurologic deficits occurred in 0.2%. No permanent deficits occurred. (From Chakravarthy M, Thimmangowda P, Krishnamurthy J, et al: Thoracic epidural anesthesia in cardiac surgical patients: A prospective audit of 2,113 cases. J Cardiothorac Vasc Anesth 19:44, 2005.)

surgery, increased time to place relative to inducing general anesthesia, and the potential for cancellation of a case in event of bloody return are major limiting factors. The advent of fast-tracking could be considered a potential driving force (e.g., ability to extubate faster and have a more comfortable patient with TEA) although most evidence suggests that a wide variety of techniques can be effectively used to facilitate early extubation and that the cardioprotective effects of volatile agents may be as effective as the beneficial effects of thoracic sympathectomy.

Liu et al[483] reported a meta-analysis of 15 randomized trials of TEA in 1178 patients. In contrast to an earlier mixed meta-analysis (i.e., cardiac and noncardiac surgery, observational and randomized),[482] there were no effects on postoperative myocardial infarction or mortality.[483] However, significant favorable effects were observed for arrhythmias (OR = 0.5), pulmonary complications (OR = 0.4), time to extubation (by 4.5 hours), and reduction in visual analog pain scales (8 to 11 at rest and with activity, respectively). In contrast, 17 trials of intrathecal morphine alone in 668 patients demonstrated only a modest reduction in systemic morphine use and decreased pain scores (by 16). However, this advantage was associated with an increase in pruritus (10% versus 25%).

The potential advantages of TEA on cardiac function were investigated specifically in several studies. Berendes et al[54] reported improved regional LV function (by wall motion score index) with lower troponin I and atrial and brain natruretic peptide levels. However, the control for this study was a TIVA technique, and it is unclear whether a volatile anesthetic can have similar effects, as demonstrated by several investigators. Lee et al[484] addressed a slightly different question, using total spinal sympathectomy (bupivacaine, 37.5 mg) before induction of general anesthesia. Patients randomized to bupivacaine had less β-receptor dysfunction in response to CPB of more than 1 hour, with lower catecholamine levels, a higher cardiac index, and a lower pulmonary vascular resistance index in the post-CPB period.

TEA in conscious patients (with supplemental intravenous sedation) appears to be increasingly used for off-pump CABG (OPCAB or MIDCAB approaches) with recent reports from diverse settings (e.g., Germany, Turkey, India) and has been designated conscious off-pump coronary artery bypass (COPCAB) (Fig. 19–20).[485-490] Although most reports are of relatively small patient cohorts (15 to 30), Karagoz et al[488] described 137 patients, of whom 97% were successfully managed. In the reported series, most grafts are single-vessel left IMA to LAD grafts, although two-vessel and even a small group of three-vessel procedures were performed successfully.

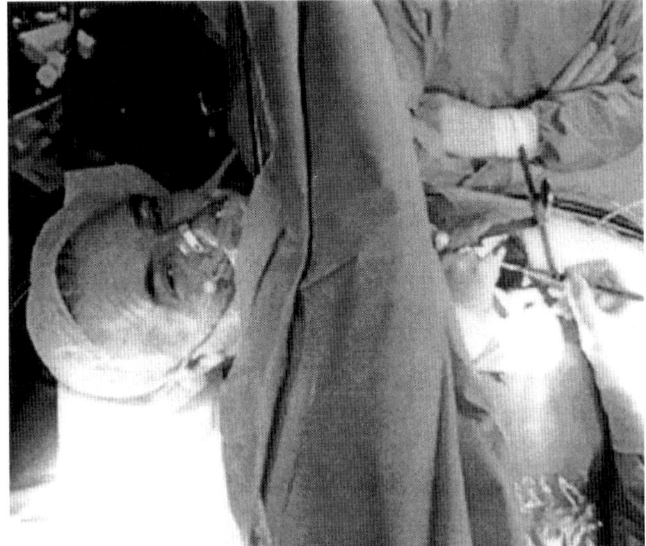

Figure 19–20 Photograph of a patient undergoing off-pump coronary artery bypass under thoracic epidural anesthesia. (From Aybek T, Kessler P, Dogan S, et al: Awake coronary artery bypass grafting: Utopia or reality? Ann Thorac Surg 75:1165, 2003. Copyright 2003, with permission from the Society of Thoracic Surgeons.)

In most series, 2% to 3% of catheters are unable to be placed in potential candidates, and 2% to 3% of patients are converted to general anesthesia because of a large pneumothorax or incomplete analgesia. Patients were fast-tracked, an ICU stay was not used, and some were discharged from the hospital the day of surgery. Patient acceptance appeared to be quite high. No complications related to TEA were observed. This is clearly an area of growing interest and one that has potential advantages, particularly for countries with different health care systems, resource constraints, and sociocultural differences. Given the fact that most are performed for single-vessel LAD lesions, the sophistication and aggressiveness of the interventional cardiologists at a particular institution are obviously major variables.

Safety concerns are a major consideration in use of TEA in this setting given chronic use of antiplatelet agents, use of systemic anticoagulation and platelet inhibition for acute therapy of unstable angina, and systemic anticoagulation and potential coagulopathy induced by CPB. The true incidence of serious complications (particularly epidural hematoma) is unknown. A widely quoted and detailed opinion piece estimates 1 in 1528 for TEA with 95% confidence and 1 in 1000 with 99% confidence. Intrathecal risks are quoted as 1 in 3610 and 1 in 2400, respectively. These estimates were based on consideration of more than 4000 reported cases (cardiac surgery) up to 1999 in which no complications were reported.[491] Chakravarthy et al[492] recently presented an audit of 2113 cardiac surgery TEA cases over a 13-year period with no permanent neurologic deficits, a 0.9% dural puncture rate, and 0.2% transient neurologic deficits. Pastor et al[493] reported 714 uneventful cases over a 7-year period, emphasizing their use of safety guidelines in which antiplatelet drugs were discontinued 7 days before surgery and routine coagulation tests and neurologic examinations were performed postoperatively.

FAST-TRACK MANAGEMENT FOR CORONARY ARTERY BYPASS GRAFTING

Efforts to reduce resource consumption for patients undergoing CABG have received considerable attention by a variety of interested payors over the last decade. With the changing pattern of reimbursement based on the ever-escalating costs of health care, payors have drastically reduced incentives to expend unnecessary resources with hospitals and clinicians attempting to minimize consumption yet maintain patient safety. The financial pressures are illustrated by the observation that Medicare costs for CABG increased from $2.8 billion in 1990 to $7.3 billion in 1997, whereas case volume increased only 40% (see Chapter 38). In 1990, Krohn et al[494] reported a study of 240 patients undergoing CABG at a private southern California hospital between 1984 and 1986 describing a clinical pathway emphasizing early extubation, rapid mobilization, intraoperative fluid restriction, and steroid administration. This program was associated with a median postoperative LOS of 4 days and in-hospital mortality of only 2%. This program itself was forged out of intense economic competition with the first major incursion of managed care into this area's competitive market. This particular pathway is widely recognized as the first formal report of what is now called *fast-tracking* for cardiac surgery. In a similar time frame, reports from the financially constrained U.K. health care system, in which formal ICU care was "bypassed" based primarily on rapid early extubation (with apparent success) appeared.[495,496] The publicity associated with these reports contributed to Medicare's interest in cost reduction leading to the Medicare Participating Heart Bypass Center Demonstration conducted between 1991 and 1996 in which seven participating hospitals agreed to a single sharply discounted rate for CABG (in return for preferential market share, a concept that ultimately has not materialized).[497] Over the 5-year period, it is estimated that $50.3 million dollars were saved. In their summary report, reduction of cost and LOS by retooling processes of care is emphasized (and reducing time to extubation was considered a key factor). In the participating centers, LOS along with mortality all declined annually despite increased severity of case mix. Observational data by Engleman et al[498,499] from the Baystate Medical Center of a large case series of fast-track patients generated additional widespread publicity in the surgical community (particularly among members of the influential Society of Thoracic Surgery).

Although the fast-track clinical pathway encompasses a variety of perioperative (and after hospital discharge) management strategies, early extubation is the one that has received perhaps the greatest attention (Box 19–3). Because it is a simple, continuous variable (e.g., hours to extubation), it is one that many observational reports and a smaller number

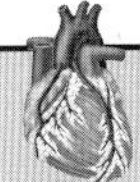

BOX 19–3 ***Perioperative Goals of Fast-Track Management***

- Preoperative education
- Same-day admission whenever possible
- Anesthetic technique tailored to early extubation and effective early postoperative analgesia
- Flexibility in the use of recovery areas (e.g., use of postanesthesia care unit instead of an intensive care unit)
- Early extubation incorporating nurse- or respiratory therapist–driven protocols for stable patients
- Early mobilization and removal of catheters, tubes, and similar devices
- Early intensive care unit and hospital discharge for patients meeting criteria
- Early follow-up (e.g., telephone, office visits) after hospital discharge
- Formalized clinical pathway and interdisciplinary continuous quality improvement strategies

of randomized, controlled trials have reported. It also appears to be the only one that has resulted in meta-analyses showing the practice is safe and effective.[5,500] Early extubation is acknowledged as a key component of the fast-track clinical pathway and one that was considered perhaps the most radical change in practice during the peak of scrutiny of the fast-track pathway (middle to late 1990s) (Box 19–4). Reports of prolonged ventilatory management after cardiac surgery first appeared in the late 1950s (for valve surgery as CABG was not yet performed) and those from the 1960s (including the first reports of CABG patients) strongly advocated its routine use.[501] This was further emphasized with the adoption of high-dose morphine (and subsequently fentanyl and sufentanil) at the end of that decade.[1,255]

As early as 1974, the first reports advocating early extubation (primarily by greater reliance on volatile anesthesia) appeared.[502] In 1980, Quasha et al[503] reported the first small, randomized, controlled trial enrolling CABG patients (n = 38), in which 89% were extubated in less than 8 hours. Ramsay et al[504] reported a small, randomized, controlled trial ($n = 20$) in which opioid reversal with nalbuphine was used. However, this resulted in an unacceptable increase in postoperative pain. The larger and more rigorous randomized, controlled trial reported by Cheng et al[505] in 1996 ($n = 100$), in which mean time to extubation was 4.1 hours, is generally recognized as the most influential of the contemporary studies of early extubation. During the past decade, reports of successful use of fast-tracking in a variety of patient populations have been reported, including academic,[55,506] private,[301,507-510] elderly,[511-513] and rural settings and Veterans Affairs patients[56,514] from the United States and many other countries. It is now used as a quality improvement marker in many health care systems.[30,55,506] In some of these, alterations of the traditional models of ICU care have been adopted, although many use routine ICU models, just with shorter stays. It has been clearly pointed out that the ability to maximize the potential of early extubation with regard to saving money and reducing LOS involves close coordination of a particular center's staffing (particularly nursing), which often is not (and in many centers remains) not very efficient.[515,516] Despite these issues, average LOS for CABG has declined substantially over the past decade in the United States.

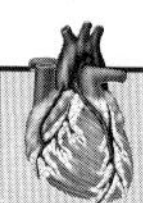

BOX 19–4 ***Suggested Criteria for Early Extubation***

Systemic
1. Body temperature stable and >36°C or <38°C
2. Arterial pH >7.30

Cardiovascular
1. Stable hemodynamics on minimal or decreasing doses of inotrope or vasodilator therapy; cardiac index >2.0 L/min/m^2, stable SvO_2, minimal base deficit
2. Stable cardiac rhythm or good response to pacing

Respiratory
1. Spontaneous respiratory rate >10 to 12 and <25 to 30, vital capacity >10 mL/kg, maximal negative inspiratory force >−20 cm H_2O with minimal respiratory support (e.g., low levels of continuous positive airways pressure, pressure support)
2. Adequate arterial blood gases: PaO_2 > 70 to 80 mm Hg (FIO_2 = 0.4 to 0.5), $PaCO_2$ < 40 to 45 mm Hg
3. Chest radiograph without major abnormalities (e.g., minimal atelectasis)

Renal
1. Adequate urine output (non–dialysis-dependent patients), stable electrolytes, and input/output values for patients on preoperative dialysis

Neurologic
1. Awake, alert, cooperative, moving all extremities
2. Adequate motor strength (e.g., hand grip); if not, consider relaxant reversal, especially for patients receiving pancuronium

Surgical
1. Adequate hemostasis with decreasing or stable mediastinal drainage

Based on accumulated data from randomized, controlled trials, the first meta-analyses of early extubation were reported. Myles et al[5] reviewed studies in which fast-tracking was defined as use of reduced opioid dosing (fentanyl ≤ 20 μg/kg) with stated intention to attempt extubation in less than 10 hours postoperatively. They identified 10 trials (n = 1800), with most involving CABG patients, from 1989 to 2002. As expected, fast-track groups had shorter times to extubation (by 8.1 hours), with no significant differences in major morbidity or mortality and only one instance of reintubation. ICU LOS was reduced by 5.4 hours, although hospital LOS was not shortened.

Hawkes et al[500] reported a meta-analysis from the United Kingdom–based Cochrane Collaboration. These investigators considered only randomized, controlled trials in which time to extubation was defined as within 8 hours and which specifically evaluated mortality (in ICU, 30 days and up to 1 year), incidence of postoperative myocardial ischemia (e.g., biomarkers, electrocardiogram), and pulmonary outcomes (e.g., reintubation, respiratory dysfunction). Secondary outcomes of ICU and hospital LOS were analyzed. Given their more stringent requirements and predetermined hypotheses for testing, they found only six studies (n = 871) meeting criteria and almost one half of the patients were from a single study (Reyes et al).[503,505,517-520] That study is unusual because both treatment groups received high-dose fentanyl, in contrast to all other studies of fast-tracking in which opioid doses are deliberately lower. However, exclusion of this study did not alter the findings. Three of the studies excluded patients older than 70 to 75 years, and 144 patients did not undergo CABG (i.e., had valve-only or other cardiac surgery). Most cases were elective (24 urgent or emergent), and all studies excluded patients "at high risk," although the criteria varied among the studies. This analysis also included the "old" study of Quasha et al,[503] which is clearly from a different generation with regard to contemporary processes of care (but is numerically small). Because not all of the studies reported on the specific outcomes of interest, the number of studies for each analysis varied from one to six. With regard to mortality, ICU (4 studies) and 30-day mortality (two studies) were no different. One-year mortality was only assessed in one study (no difference). The incidence of postoperative myocardial ischemia (six studies) was not different (although methods for detection of this diagnosis varied). The incidence of early reintubation (1.6%) within 24 hours (four studies) was no different, with two studies having none. Late reintubation after 24 hours (three studies) was no different, with two studies having none and one study having a rate of 1.5%. Consideration of respiratory outcomes was not possible due to variable methodology. Atelectasis did not appear to vary between groups. With regard to secondary outcomes, ICU LOS (four studies) was significantly reduced by 7 hours, and hospital LOS (two studies) was significantly reduced by 1.1 days. The study authors described several important issues. No studies have been properly statistically powered to determine whether outcome rates are equivalent, only whether there was no difference. This is a subtle point, but statistical methodology for this requires much larger sample sizes. They also observed that early extubation has become routine clinical practice and that further research is needed to evaluate the impact of very early extubation on pain control, stress modification, and long-term outcome (Table 19–5).

It can be seen that the fast-track knowledge base is incomplete with regard to defining all patient subgroups (e.g., who is at high risk for early extubation?) despite meta-analyses because these studies cannot always accurately risk adjust the patient groups. For the anesthesiologist, reintubation is of particular interest. London et al[311] summarized the data and observed that although the rate of early reintubation is very low with fast-track management, the frequency of later reintubation is substantial in many series (up to 6.6%). In a series of Veterans Affairs patients, a group that most clinicians consider to be at high risk for adverse respiratory outcomes due to the high prevalence of chronic obstructive pulmonary disease and smoking, only 1 of 304 fast-track patients was reintubated emergently, but 5% went on to later reintubation.[514] More research is needed to clearly define who is at risk although female gender and longer periods of initial ventilation (no fast-tracking) have been reported as risk factors.[506,521]

Despite gaps in knowledge, it is clear that various centers (most often related to a single surgeon with a large volume practice) have adopted very aggressive fast-track programs. Walji et al[510] coined the term *ultra-fast-tracking* to describe their practice, reporting a 56% hospital discharge rate by postoperative day 4 (of 258 patients) and 23% discharge by postoperative day 2 (although the readmission rate was 3.9%, albeit with no early mortality). Perhaps most impressive is the report of Ovrum et al[522] from Norway on a cohort of 5658 CABG patients in whom 99% were extubated by 5 hours (median, 1.5 hours), with a 1.1% reintubation rate. More than 99% of patients were able to be transferred to the ward the next morning, and a similar percentage were walking outdoors by postoperative day 7. An impressive in-hospital mortality rate of only 0.4% was reported. Precise time of discharge was

Table 19–5 Contemporary Randomized, Controlled Trials of Fast-Tracking in Cardiac Surgery

Study	Inclusion Criteria	Anesthesia	*N*	Time to Extubation (hr)	Extubated (%)	Reintubation (%)	SICU LOS	Mortality (%)	Comments
Cheng, 1996[505]	Elective CABG, age <75 yr, first case								
	Early	Fent, Prop, Iso	60	4.1 ± 1.1*	85	1.6	42 ± 12*	0	ICU stats "by criteria"
	Conventional	Fent, Midaz, Iso	60	18.9 ± 1.4	85	0	57 ± 29	5	
Myles, 1997[537]	Elective CABG; low/med risk patients								
	Early	Fent (15 μg/kg), Prop	58	9.1 median*	100	NR	22 median	NR	
	Conventional	Enf, Fent (31 μg/kg), Midaz	66	12.3 median	100	NR	22 median	NR	
Reyes, 1997[519]	Low or intermed risk patients; all CABG or valve	All with "high-dose fentanyl," Benzo induction							
	Early	Fent (65 μg/kg)	201	10 median*	60	6.5‡	27 median*	9.0	
	Conventional	Fent (67 μg/kg)	203	21 median	74	3.5	44 median	7.4	
Berry, 1998[517]	Elective CABG, low/med risk patients								No intent to treat, primary study of ischemia
	Early	Fent (15 μg/kg), Iso	50 (43 analyzed)	1.8 median†	94	NR	NR	0	No differences in indices of ischemia, including Holter ST
	Conventional	Fent (50 μg/kg), Iso	48 (42 analyzed)	12.6 median	100	NR	NR	2%	
Michalopoulos, 1998[518]	Elective CABG; age <70 yr, low/med risk patients								
	Early	Fent (15–20 μg/kg), Iso or halo or prop, Midaz	72	6.3 ± 0.7*	100	0	17 ± 1.3*	0	
	Conventional	Fent (50 μg/kg), Iso or Halo, Midaz	72	11.6 ± 1.3	100	0	22 ± 1.2	0	
Silbert, 1998[520]	Elective CABG; low-risk patients								No intent to treat
	Early	Fent (15 μg/kg), Prop	50 (38 analyzed)	4.0 median*	100	0	NR	2% (of 50)	
	Conventional	Fent (50 μg/kg), Midaz, Prop	50 (42 analyzed)	7.0 median	100	0	NR	2% (of 50)	

Benzo = benzodiazepine; CABG = coronary artery bypass grafting; Enf = enflurane; Fent = fentanyl; Halo = halothane; ICU, intensive care unit; Iso = isoflurane; Midaz = midazolam; NR = not reported; Prop = propofol.

*$p < 0.05$ or smaller between early and conventional groups.

†Statistic not reported.

‡$p < 0.04$, worse in early group.

not reported, and the study authors observed that readmission (with the exception of deep sternal infections) was not tracked (as it occurred at other hospitals). With the exception of a low incidence of redo patients (1.8%, who are said to have similar times to extubation), the cohort appears similar in risk to U.S. centers (with IMA grafting in 99% and a median of four distal anastomoses). As expected, CPB time was short (median, 55 minutes). With regard to anesthetic management, low-dose diazepam or midazolam (0 to 0.2 mg/kg), fentanyl (4 to 8 μg/kg), pancuronium, isoflurane, or nitrous oxide were used. A PAC was only used in cases of severe cardiac decompensation (precise figure not given but only 2% received prolonged inotropes or IABP therapy) and TEE was never used. Given these impressive results and Spartan clinical practices, perhaps the term *uber fast-tracking* might be appropriate. Both reports make the point that their on-pump results are equal to, or even better than, results of many off-pump studies. It will be interesting to see whether with ongoing adoption of OPCAB that these results can be further improved on. The lack of advanced monitoring in the Ovrum series would appear to put pressure on academic anesthesia to continue to rigorously explore the efficacy of advanced monitoring for CABG.

CORONARY ARTERY BYPASS GRAFTING WITHOUT CARDIOPULMONARY BYPASS

OPCAB is the single greatest change in CABG techniques in the past 2 decades[523,524] (see Chapters 2, 4, and 21). Although this term encompasses a range of surgical approaches (based on the degree of invasiveness encompassing full, limited, or no sternotomy), the technique that is most commonly performed is OPCAB with a full sternotomy (see Chapter 21 for information on minimally invasive cardiac revascularization). The precise number of such procedures performed remains largely speculative; however, it is likely in the 15% to 20% range at the present time. Surgeons appear to adopt it enthusiastically or not at all, an unsurprising finding given the unsettled state of the literature. Although the literature base (incorporating a large number of observational series and a smaller number of true randomized, controlled trials) is increasing rapidly, the final word is still years away (given several large ongoing randomized, controlled trials). However, it appears that OPCAB is as effective as routine CABG, is safer for certain patient subsets, and may be associated with improvement in several outcomes at slightly lower resource use.[6,524,525] Its use is likely to increase, especially for high-risk patients with serious comorbidities associated with higher morbidity/mortality from CPB (e.g., severe cerebrovascular and renal disease). The clinician will immediately notice that the pace and tempo of anesthetic management differs substantially from that of conventional CABG. The focused involvement of the anesthesiologist is perhaps more important in OPCAB than during on-pump CABG (including use of TEE and at least for now nearly routine use of PAC). Many anesthesiologists perceive OPCAB to be a unique opportunity to enhance the visibility and importance of the specialty.

Although OPCAB is perceived as a contemporary development, surgery on the beating heart was first performed in the 1950s and early 1960s, preceding the widespread use of CPB-based CABG because of the slower development and application of CPB techniques in the late 1960s[524] (see Chapters 1 to 4). In the late 1980s and early 1990s, introduction of the short-acting β-blocker esmolol led some surgeons to "experiment" with OPCAB (on the LAD) by lowering of the HR. However, it was not until the mid-to-late 1990s when surgical researchers developed efficient mechanical stabilizer devices that minimized motion around the anastomosis site (independent of HR) that this technique became widespread. The ability to expose the posterior surface of the heart to access the posterior descending and the circumflex vessels using suction devices usually placed on the apex of the heart, pericardial retraction sutures, slings, or other techniques, without producing major hemodynamic compromise was critical for multivessel application of this technique. This is commonly referred to as *verticalization*, in contrast to *displacement* for the LAD and diagonal anastomoses (Fig. 19–21).

OPCAB extends the range of surgeon-induced hemodynamic changes the anesthesiologist encounters relative to routine CABG. The skilled cardiac anesthesiologist must be able to anticipate, and communicate with the surgeon to minimize the adverse impact of these changes on the heart and other important organs. The surgical manipulations involve a variety of geometric distortions of cardiac anatomy (most notably compression of the right ventricle[526] and, to a lesser degree, some distortion of the mitral valve annulus[527]). The magnitude of distortion varies with the patient's individual anatomy (most notably the size and shape of their right and left ventricles), the skill of the surgeon in placement of stabilizer devices, use of "deep" pericardial stay sutures (which facilitate forward superior apical displacement for LAD anastomosis), and manipulation of the pleural space (e.g., right pleural incision to create space for the compressed right ventricle). With a skilled surgeon, the changes are usually modest or easily treated with the Trendelenburg position, use of vasoconstrictors or inotropes, and judicious volume expansion. However, severe changes due to acute ischemia, mitral regurgitation, or unrecognized right ventricular compression may occur, necessitating emergent conversion to CPB. Knowledge is currently strongest on the hemodynamic effects of OPCAB in contrast to more subtle alterations of blood flow to the brain, kidneys, and other organs.

Cardiovascular Effects of Off-Pump Coronary Artery Bypass Grafting

Evaluation of the hemodynamic consequences of OPCAB involves the two independent variables of distortion of the right or left atria and ventricles by stabilizer and suspension devices, and the effects of myocardial ischemia induced by vessel occlusion during anastomosis.

Effect of Cardiac Displacement and Stabilization

Grundeman et al[526] have investigated hemodynamics, coronary blood flow (CBF), and echocardiographic changes with use of the suction cup Octopus stabilizer systems (Medtronic, Inc, Minneapolis, MN) during verticalization to 90 degrees anterior displacement of the posterior wall (as would be used to access circumflex vessels during OPCAB) in an anesthetized and β-blocked pig model. With the stabilizer alone, they found significant reductions in SV (44% reduction), CO (32%), MAP (26%), and HR (26%) that were corrected with 20% head-down tilt. They also evaluated CBF in the three major coronary distributions using flow probes.[528] With a 42% decrease in CO, coronary flow was reduced in all three distri-

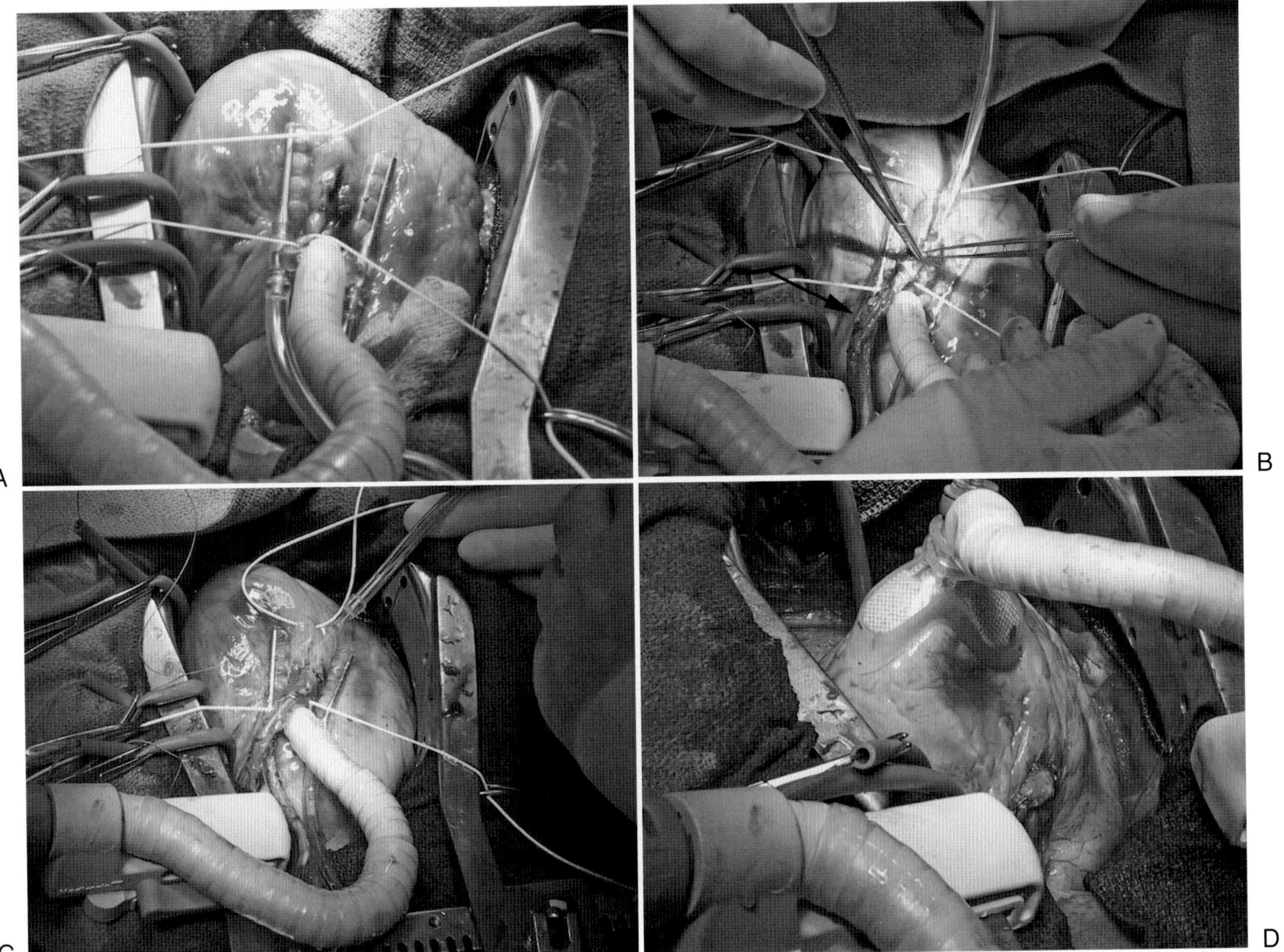

Figure 19–21 Series of images depicting the left anterior descending (LAD) artery and posterior descending artery (PDA) anastomoses during off-pump coronary artery bypass grafting using a left internal mammary artery (LIMA) and saphenous vein (SV) graft, respectively. *(A)* Packing has been placed under the heart, rotating it toward the midline and elevating it for surgical access to the LAD (partially dissected here). The Medtronic Octopus suction stabilizer is in place along with elastic stay sutures used to transiently occlude the artery. *(B)* The LIMA *(arrow)* is being anastomosed to the LAD, assisted by use of pressurized and heavily humidified carbon dioxide ("mister blower" metal cannula) to facilitate visualization of the vessel lumen. *(C)* Completed LAD-LIMA anastomosis. *(D)* Application of the Medtronic Starfish apical suction device to verticalize the heart. This view is from the anesthesiologist's vantage point, with the recently completed LAD-LIMA graft visible at the base. *Continued*

butions, with the greatest decline in the circumflex distribution (50%). However, with Trendelenburg position, the changes were largely ameliorated. Placement of an omniplane TEE probe between the two arms of the Octopus stabilizer demonstrated substantial compression of the right ventricle with a decrease in diastolic cross-sectional area of 62%, but the LV area only declined by 20% (Fig. 19–22). No valvular incompetence was observed, and institution of right-heart CPB restored all hemodynamic parameters; LV bypass had only marginal effects. This documents the importance of compression of the thin-walled, low-pressure right ventricle in hemodynamic compromise during OPCAB. They also reported on use of the Starfish apical suction device (Medtronic, Inc. Minneapolis, MN) using this pig model.[529,530] They observed substantially fewer hemodynamic changes, with only a 6% reduction in SV and 5% reduction in MAP; no reduction in coronary flows; and, approximately 30% increases in right ventricular (RV) and LV end-diastolic pressures. With institution of Trendelenburg position, mild overshoot in SV and MAP occurred with greater increases in RVEDP and LVEDP, suggesting that this maneuver is not required. Using a sheep model, Porat et al[531] demonstrated significant hemodynamic benefits using a right-heart internal cannula system that expels blood from the right atrium into the pulmonary artery, bypassing the compressed right ventricle (increasing CO and MAP with reduction in CVP by 49%).

Human Clinical Data

Hemodynamic effects in human clinical series have been reported primarily using routine monitoring (e.g., PAC, TEE, SvO_2) although several have used more sophisticated methods (right ventricular EF, pressure-volume loops).[532,533] Most of the data have been obtained from patients with normal or only mildly depressed ventricular function without significant valvular disease. Mathison et al[534] measured RV and LV end-diastolic pressures in 44 patients (i.e., using catheters inserted through the pulmonary veins, as is done for LV venting, and by pulling back the PAC during measurements for the right ventricle). They evaluated the effects of displacement with the Octopus stabilizer in Trendelenburg position.

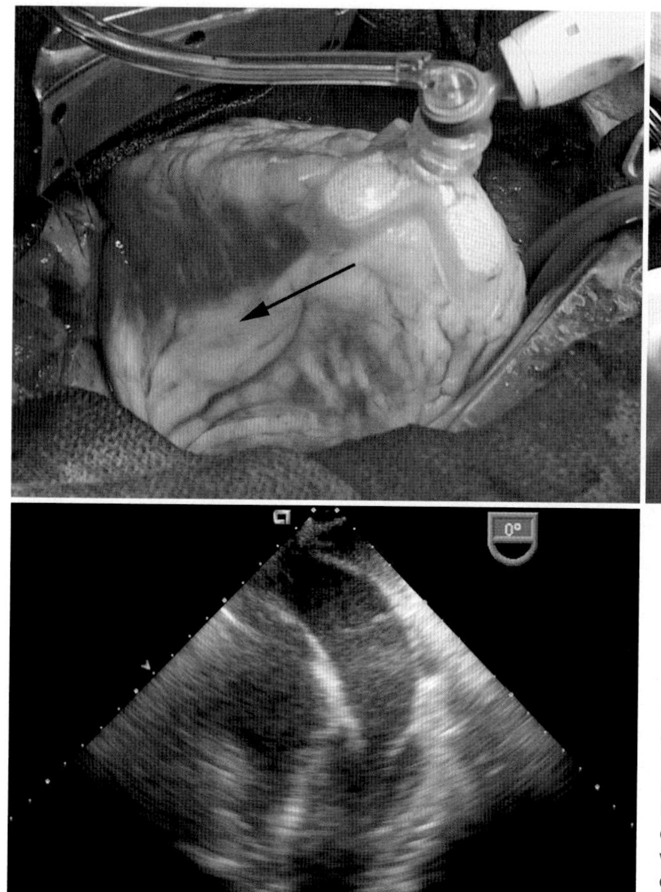

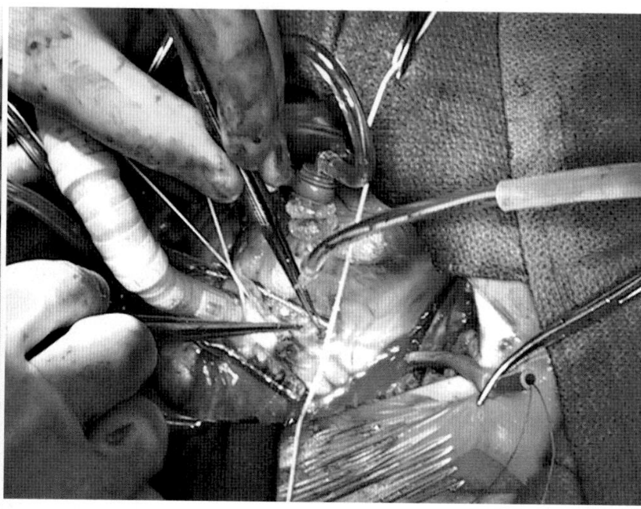

Figure 19–21 (*Continued*) *(E)* The inferior surface of the left ventricle is well visualized with the PDA *(arrow)* easily accessible. The patient is placed in a steep Trendelenburg position to facilitate exposure and maintain adequate preload. *(F)* The Octopus stabilizer is placed, and the PDA-SV anastomosis is being performed. *(G)* Characteristic appearance on transesophageal echocardiography of the four-chamber view in the verticalized heart using an apical suction device. Notice the elongation of the left atrium and compression of the right atrium and ventricle. (*A–G*, Images courtesy of Martin J. London, MD, University of California, San Francisco, CA [www.ucsf.edu/teeecho].)

RVEDP increased in each position, with the greatest increase with exposure of the circumflex vessels (Fig. 19–23). This position was associated with the greatest deterioration of SV (approximately 29% versus 22% for PDA and 18% for LAD). When comparing patients with EFs of more than or less than 40%, there were nonsignificant trends toward greater reduction in MAP and CO with lower EF. TEE, used in 31 patients, revealed moderate to severe biventricular compression with CX and PDA positioning. Nierich et al[535] reported on use of the Octopus stabilizer in a larger cohort (n = 150 patients, including 54 patients with anterolateral thoracotomy exposure undergoing LAD or diagonal anastomosis only). Although only routine hemodynamics were presented, this study also evaluated hemodynamic effects during the actual surgical anastomotic period (in contrast to Mathison et al[534]). Stroke volume decreased 6% with LAD, 14% with RCA, and 21% with OM anastomoses. Trendelenburg position was required in only 50% of LAD anastomoses, increasing to 100% with OM anastomosis. Dopamine was used in only 5% of LAD anastomoses, increasing to 30% with OM anastomoses (Fig. 19–24).

Mishra et al[536] have reported large-scale, prospective observational data on patients undergoing OPCAB at a tertiary center in New Delhi. TEE and PAC were used in all patients and approximately 40% were considered high-risk. In contrast to some of the smaller studies mentioned earlier, the degree of hemodynamic compromise was greater. In their first report of 500 patients, verticalization for exposure of the posterior wall was associated with a reduction in MAP by 18%, increase in CVP by 66%, reduction in SV by 36%, and cardiac index by 45%. New wall motion abnormalities were common (60%) and global function decreased in a similar proportion. Their practice involved use of inotropes during this period (79% versus 22% for the anterior wall). However, only 11% required IABP, and 0.7% required CPB; in-hospital mortality was 1.2%. They reported on predictors of need for IABP or conversion to CPB in an additional 500 patients (4.8% of patients). On multivariate analysis, an EF less than 25%, myocardial infarction within the prior month, congestive heart failure, and preoperative hemodynamic instability (the latter was only marginally significant) were identified. The in-hospital mortality for the latter 500 patients was only 0.8%.

Although these are excellent outcome statistics, our clinical experience differs with regard to the use of inotropes. Vasoconstrictor and volume therapy are preferred with inotrope use only with severe hemodynamic compromise, because the greater increase in oxygen demand with inotropes in the setting of ongoing ischemia may place the patient at substantial risk for myocardial injury. This difference in approach may be one factor involved in the various amounts of intraoperative fluids that have been reported with OPCAB. Staton et al[537] reported the pulmonary outcomes from a randomized, controlled trial of 200 patients at Emory in which intraoperative fluid balance was substantially greater with OPCAB (3.9 versus 1.7 L) than CABG. A greater reduction in postoperative pulmonary compliance occurred, although the OPCAB group had better gas exchange and earlier extubation. There were no differences in chest radiograph abnormalities,

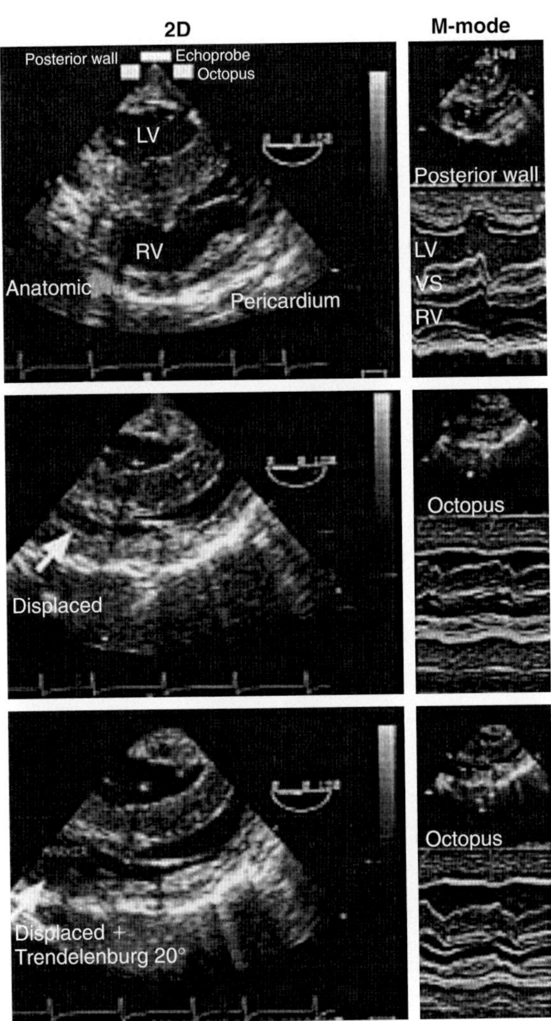

Figure 19–22 Alteration in right ventricular (RV) and left ventricular (LV) chamber sizes with verticalization of the heart and subsequent Trendelenburg positioning in a porcine open chest model obtained from a transesophageal echocardiographic probe placed between the two arms of a stabilizer device on the posterior wall. Two-dimensional *(left)* and M-mode images *(right)* are displayed. (From Grunderman PF, Borst C, Verlaan CW, et al: Exposure of circumflex branches in the tilted, beating porcine heart: Echocardiographic evidence of right ventricular deformation and the effect of right or left heart bypass. J Thorac Cardiovasc Surg 118:316,1999.)

spirometry, or adverse outcomes. This cohort is unique in its very aggressive extubation strategy, with 32% of on-pump and 45% of OPCAB patients extubated in the operating room.

Monitoring for Off-Pump Coronary Artery Bypass Grafting

Hemodynamic changes with OPCAB vary with location of the anastomosis and type of stabilizer or verticalizer system used, although most of the available hemodynamic data was obtained from low-risk patients. At present, there is no clear consensus or guidelines with regard to the type of monitoring recommended for OPCAB. Most observational studies have used fairly extensive monitoring with PAC at a minimum and often with SvO_2 and PAC. TEE appears to be widely used, despite problems with imaging during the anastomotic period, particularly when the heart is verticalized (see Fig. 19–21G). As with on-pump CABG, it is likely that as this procedure is more widely adopted and clinicians gain increasing familiarity, that monitoring recommendations, particularly for low risk patients, will become less sophisticated.

Outcomes in Off-Pump Coronary Artery Bypass Grafting

Several investigators and working groups have comprehensively reviewed outcomes in patients undergoing OPCAB.[6,524,525] Raja and Dreyfus have reviewed observational and randomized trials scoring efficacy of OPCAB by levels of literature evidence on outcomes related to various organ systems and processes of care.[524] Although this grading must be considered informal (given lack of a formal consensus panel of experts), it mirrors results obtained from a meta-analysis of randomized trials by Cheng et al.[6]

These investigators analyzed 37 randomized trials of 3369 patients with comparable treatment groups with the exception of a marginal difference in number of grafts performed (2.6 OPCAB versus 2.8 CABG). All but one of the studies specifically excluded "high-risk" patients. Although various definitions were used, most excluded patients with low EF, redo procedures, renal failure, and several studies excluded patients with diseased circumflex vessels. As expected, not all studies reported on all outcomes. The investigators found no significant differences in 30-day or 1- to 2-year mortality, myocardial infarction, stroke (30 day and 1 to 2 years), renal dysfunction, need for IABP, wound infection, or reoperation for bleeding or reintervention (for ischemia). OPCAB was associated with a significant reduction in atrial fibrillation (OR = 0.58), numbers of patients transfused (OR = 0.43), respiratory infections (OR = 0.41), need for inotropes (OR = 0.48), duration of ventilation (weighted mean difference [WMD] of 3.4 hours), ICU LOS (WMD of 0.3 day), and hospital LOS (WMD of 1.0 days). Changes in neurocognitive dysfunction were not different in the immediate postoperative period; they were significantly improved at 2 to 6 months (OR = 0.57); but there were no differences seen at 12 months. The critical issue of graft patency was addressed in only four studies and these varied substantially with regard to when this was assessed (3 months in two and 12 months in two). Only one study reported a difference (reduction in circumflex patency with OPCAB). Because of the small numbers of patients, the overall data for this category were considered inadequate for meta-analysis. A large-scale, randomized, controlled trial is being conducted by the Department of Veterans Affairs with evaluation of graft patency at 1 year postoperatively. Four randomized, controlled trials have analyzed quality of life. Various methods precluded inclusion in the meta-analysis, but it generally appears there is little difference between operations. Of the 20 trials reporting conversion rates, 8% of OPCAB patients required conversion to CABG, whereas only 1.7% were converted from CABG to OPCAB. The conversion rate for OPCAB in these low- to medium-risk patients is substantial and would be expected to be even higher in higher-risk patients with greater disease burdens, more complex lesions, or impaired ventricular function in whom tolerance of stabilization and verticalization may be less. The anesthesiologist must be prepared for rapid institution of CPB at all times.

This comprehensive analysis suggests that for every 1000 patients undergoing OPCAB, 91 fewer patients would develop atrial fibrillation, 143 fewer would require transfusion, 83 fewer would require inotropes, 53 fewer would develop

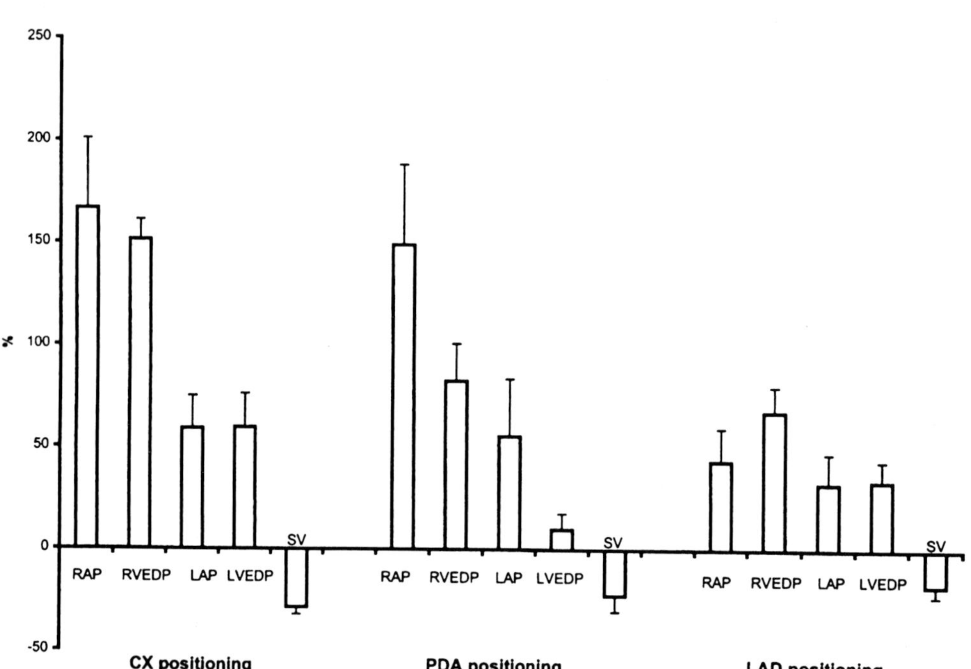

Figure 19–23 Hemodynamic changes (mean ± standard error) with off-pump coronary artery bypass (OPCAB) grafting cardiac positioning with application of the stabilizer in 44 patients. CX = circumflex artery; LAD = left anterior descending artery; LAP = left atrial pressure; LVEDP = left ventricular end-diastolic pressure; PDA = posterior descending artery; RAP = right atrial pressure; RVEDP = right ventricular end-diastolic pressure; SV = stroke volume. (From Mathison M, Edgerton JR, Horswell JL, et al: Analysis of hemodynamic changes during beating heart surgical procedures. Ann Thorac Surg 70:1355, 2000. Copyright 2000, with permission from the Society of Thoracic Surgeons.)

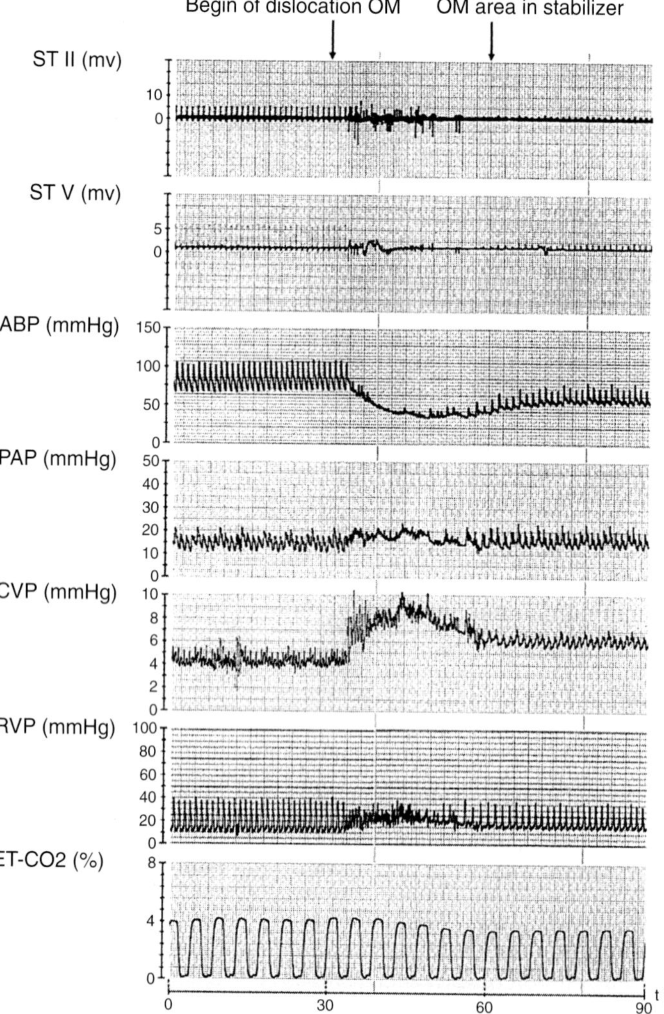

Figure 19–24 Acute hemodynamic alterations during verticalization and placement of a stabilizer in an actual patient demonstrating reduction in electrocardiographic voltage, wedging of the pulmonary artery catheter, decrease of end-tidal carbon dioxide (ET-CO2), and increase in central venous pressure (CVP). Changes partially resolve after stabilizer placement. ABP = arterial blood pressure; OM = obtuse marginal arteries; RVP = right ventricular pressure. (From Nierich AP, Diephuis J, Jansen EW, et al: Heart displacement during off-pump CABG: How well is it tolerated? Ann Thorac Surg 70:466, 2000. Copyright 2000, with permission from the Society of Thoracic Surgeons.)

respiratory infections, 100 fewer would have cognitive dysfunction at 2 to 6 months postoperatively, and there would be 300 fewer ICU days and 1000 fewer hospital days. The neutral findings regarding stroke, renal failure, myocardial infarction, and mortality are surprising, but may be found to be different in higher-risk patients once additional data is accumulated in high-risk trials.

A working group of the American Heart Association's Council on Cardiovascular Surgery and Anesthesia analyzed the current literature and several small meta-analyses, but not that of Cheng et al.[6] In an informal manner, they concluded that OPCAB is probably associated with less bleeding, less renal dysfunction, less short-term neurocognitive dysfunction (especially in patients with calcified aortas), and shorter hospital LOS. However, they also observed that it is more technically demanding, has a greater "learning curve," and may be associated with lower rates of long-term graft patency. Perhaps related to the greater technical demands, surgeons appear to place fewer grafts relative to on-pump CABG, a factor that could influence long-term outcomes. They emphasize the ongoing need for large-scale, randomized study data.

The ultimate adoption of OPCAB resides in demonstration of similar rates of long-term graft patency. Given the longevity of most grafts, particularly the IMA (>15 years),[17] this will take some time to be conclusively established. With ongoing technologic advances, it is likely this approach will continue to expand in numbers of patients and surgical complexity.

MYOCARDIAL ISCHEMIA DURING REVASCULARIZATION

Incidence of Myocardial Ischemia in Patients Undergoing Revascularization Surgery

In addition to providing anesthesia, a major concern of the anesthesiologist is the prevention and treatment of myocardial ischemia. Numerous laboratory and clinical studies have examined the incidence of myocardial ischemia in the perioperative period, as it relates to the administration of anesthetic drugs. Although the incidence of pre-bypass ischemia in patients appears to be between 10% and 50%, it is not at all clear that the anesthetic drug combination per se is a determinant of this incidence. Several studies have addressed whether the anesthetic technique (e.g., fast-track or early extubation, high thoracic epidural) is related to perioperative morbidity and myocardial ischemic events. An extensive meta-analysis of more than 30 randomized, controlled trials of patients undergoing cardiac surgery showed no difference in the relative risk of postoperative myocardial ischemia when early extubation protocols were compared with conventional extubation management.[500]

Hemodynamic Changes Related to Myocardial Ischemia

Besides ECG abnormalities, some hemodynamic changes should alert the anesthesiologist to the possibility of intraoperative myocardial ischemia. The association of tachycardia with hypotension or increased LV filling pressure (both of which reduce coronary perfusion pressure [CPP] is a particularly undesirable combination jeopardizing the oxygen supply-demand relationship. Figure 19–25 demonstrates how hypertension in the absence of tachycardia, in response to surgical stress (skin incision), can be associated with pulmonary hypertension, elevated PCWP, and prominent A and V waves on the PCWP waveform.[184] Although ECG changes occurred later, the early hemodynamic abnormalities almost certainly were the result of ischemic LV dysfunction. Treatment included deepening anesthesia and administering a nitroglycerin infusion.

LV diastolic dysfunction detected with TEE is the earliest change identified after coronary artery occlusion, and it often precedes the development of abnormal systolic function. Regional wall motion abnormalities also have been described as early signs of ischemia. They occur within seconds of inadequate blood flow or oxygen supply. Regional wall motion abnormalities detected by TEE have been shown to be a more sensitive method of detecting myocardial ischemia in patients undergoing CABG, compared with ST-segment changes.[203] Myocardial ischemia or repositioning the heart during

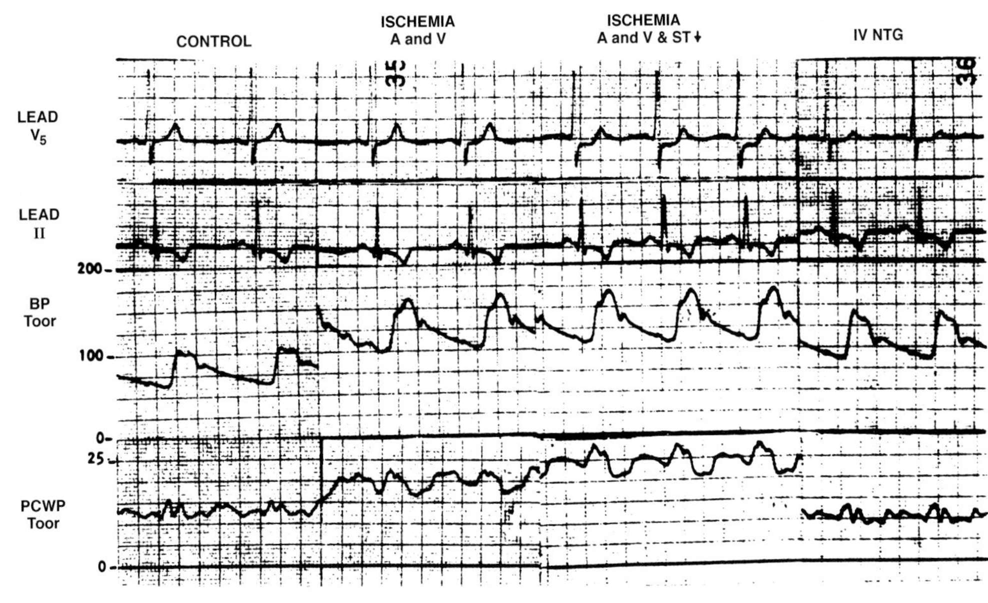

Figure 19–25 Nitroglycerin (NTG) relieved postintubation intraoperative myocardial ischemia, as evidenced by large V waves in the pulmonary capillary wedge pressure (PCWP) tracing and then by ST-segment depression. BP = blood pressure. (From Kaplan JA, Wells PH: Early diagnosis of myocardial ischemia using the pulmonary arterial catheter. Anesth Analg 60:789, 1981.)

OPCAB can be the cause of a sudden onset of mitral regurgitation (MR) or worsening of preexisting MR, both of which can be detected with TEE monitoring (see Chapters 6, 15, 16, and 20).

Intraoperative Treatment of Myocardial Ischemia

Close attention to hemodynamic control and rapid treatment of abnormalities are fundamental principles of the intraoperative management of the patient with CAD. If there is a hemodynamic abnormality that is temporally related to the onset of ischemia, it should be treated accordingly. Hemodynamic treatment to ensure an adequate CPP (diastolic blood pressure minus left ventricular end-diastolic pressure) should be a priority, as should control of HR, the single most important treatable determinant of myocardial oxygen consumption. Table 19–6 summarizes the treatment of acute perioperative myocardial ischemia. The earliest objective evidence of successful treatment of ischemia may be the return to normal of the PAP and the PCWP waveforms. In the following paragraphs, some of the routinely used pharmacologic interventions for intraoperative myocardial ischemia will be discussed.

Intravenous Nitroglycerin

Since the introduction in 1976 by Kaplan et al of the V_5 lead to diagnose myocardial ischemia[538] and intravenous nitroglycerin to treat it,[539] nitroglycerin has been one of the mainstays in the treatment for perioperative myocardial ischemia. Intravenous nitroglycerin acts immediately to reduce LV preload and wall tension, primarily by decreasing venous tone in lower doses, whereas in larger doses, it may also decrease arterial resistance and epicardial coronary arterial resistance.[540,541] Nitroglycerin has been shown to consistently decrease LV filling pressure, systemic BP, and myocardial oxygen consumption and to improve LV performance in patients with severe dysfunction.[542] It is most effective in treating acute myocardial ischemia with induced ventricular dysfunction accompanied by sudden elevations in LVEDV, LVEDP, and PAP. These elevations in LV preload and wall tension further exacerbate perfusion deficits to the ischemic subendocardium and usually respond immediately to nitroglycerin (Fig. 19–26).

Preoperatively, it is often used to treat patients with unstable angina or ischemic mitral regurgitation, and to limit the size of an evolving myocardial infarction, reduce associated complications, and reverse SWMAs.[543,544] In the pre-CPB period and during OPCAB, nitroglycerin is used to treat signs of ischemia such as ST-segment depression, hypertension uncontrolled by the anesthetic technique, ventricular dysfunction, or coronary artery spasm (Box 19–5). During CPB, nitroglycerin can be used to control the MAP with a time to onset of effect ranging from 4.1 ± 0.8 to 7.8 ± 2.8 minutes at doses of 1.7 ± 0.3 to 2.9 ± 0.7 μg/kg/min.[545] However, nitroglycerin is not always effective in controlling MAP during CPB (approximately 60% of patients respond) because of alterations of the pharmacokinetics and pharmacodynamics of the drug with CPB. Factors contributing to the reduction of its

Table 19–6 Acute Treatments for Suspected Intraoperative Myocardial Ischemia*

Associated Hemodynamic Finding	Therapy	Dosage
Hypertension, tachycardia†	Deepen anesthesia Intravenous (IV) β-blockade IV nitroglycerin	 Esmolol, 20–100 mg, +50–200 μg/kg/min PRN Metoprolol, 0.5–2.5 mg Labetalol, 2.5–10 mg Nitroglycerin, 33–330 μg/min‡
Normotension, tachycardia†	Ensure adequate anesthesia, change anesthetic regimen IV β-blockade	β-blockade, as above
Hypertension, normal heart rate	Deepen anesthesia IV nitroglycerin or nicardipine	Nicardipine, 1–5 mg, +1–10 μg/kg/min Nitroglycerin, as above
Hypotension, tachycardia†	IV α-agonist Alter anesthetic regimen (e.g., lighten) IV nitroglycerin when normotensive	Phenylephrine, 25–100 μg Norepinephrine, 2–4 μg Nitroglycerin, as above
Hypotension, bradycardia	Lighten anesthesia IV ephedrine IV epinephrine IV atropine IV nitroglycerin when normotensive	 Ephedrine, 5–10 mg Epinephrine, 4–8 μg Atropine, 0.3–0.6 mg Nitroglycerin, as above
Hypotension, normal heart rate	IV α-agonist/ephedrine IV epinephrine Alter anesthesia (e.g., lighten) IV nitroglycerin when normotensive	α-Agonist, as above Epinephrine, as above Nitroglycerin, as above
No abnormality	IV nitroglycerin IV nicardipine	Nitroglycerin, as above Nicardipine, as above

*Ensure adequacy of oxygenation, ventilation, and intravascular volume status and consider surgical factors, such as manipulation of heart of coronary grafts.
†Tachyarrhythmias (e.g., PAT, atrial fibrillation) should be treated directly with synchronized cardioversion or specific pharmacologic agents.
‡Bolus doses (25–50 μg) and high infusion rate may be required initially.

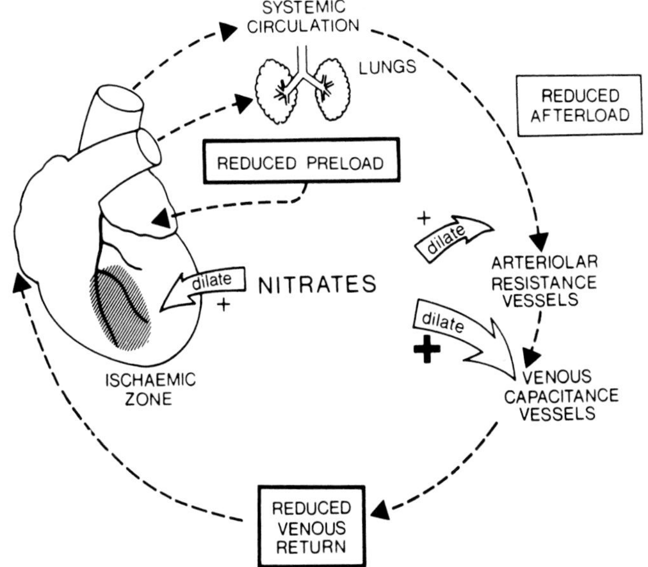

Figure 19–26 The effects of nitrates on the circulation include prominent venodilation and reduction of preload. Afterload is decreased because of mild arteriolar dilatation. Coronary dilation also occurs to benefit the ischemic myocardium. (From Opie LH: Drugs and the heart. II. Nitrates. Lancet 1:750, 1980.)

effectiveness include adsorption to the plastic in the CPB system, alterations in regional blood flow, hemodilution, and hypothermia. Booth et al[546] have shown that different oxygenators and filters sequester up to 90% of circulating nitroglycerin during CPB. After revascularization, nitroglycerin is used to treat residual ischemia or coronary artery spasm, reduce preload and afterload, and may be combined with vasopressors (e.g., phenylephrine) to increase the CPP when treating coronary air embolism (Box 19–6).

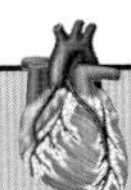

BOX 19–5 ***Profile for Intraoperative Use of Intravenous Nitroglycerin***

Hypertension >20% above control values
Pulmonary capillary wedge pressure >18 to 20 mm Hg
AC and V waves >20 mm Hg
ST changes >1 mm
New segmental wall motion abnormalities on transesophageal echocardiography
Acute right ventricular or left ventricular dysfunction
Coronary artery spasm

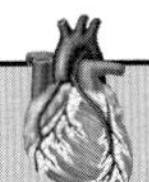

BOX 19–6 ***Uses of Intravenous Nitroglycerin on Termination of Cardiopulmonary Bypass***

- Elevated pulmonary capillary wedge pressure
- Elevated systemic vascular resistance or pulmonary vascular resistance
- Infusion of oxygenator reservoir volume
- Incomplete revascularization
- Ischemia
- Intraoperative myocardial infarction
- Coronary artery spasm

However, studies on the prophylactic role of nitroglycerin in preventing perioperative myocardial ischemia have shown mixed results, with most studies showing no effects of nitroglycerin infusions on the incidence of perioperative myocardial ischemic events.[547-549] In a prospective, double-blinded, placebo-controlled study, Zvara et al[550] randomized patients undergoing CABG surgery using a fast-track anesthesia technique to 2 μg/kg/min of nitroglycerin or placebo starting before induction and continuing until 6 hours after extubation in the ICU. They found a similar incidence, severity of symptoms, and duration of myocardial ischemia, regardless if the patients received nitroglycerin or placebo (37% versus 35%, respectively). Even though there were more patients in the placebo group with positive enzymes and ECG signs of myocardial infarction, these findings were statistically not significant. Similarly, in a prospective, randomized, controlled study, 0.5 to 1 μg/kg/min of nitroglycerin administered after aortic cross-clamp release in patients undergoing CABG surgery did not decrease the incidence of postoperative myocardial ischemia[551] (see Chapter 10).

Intravenous nitroglycerin has been compared with other vasodilators such as nitroprusside and the calcium channel blockers during CABG and in other clinical situations. Kaplan and Jones[552] demonstrated that nitroglycerin was preferable to nitroprusside during CABG. Both drugs were shown to control intraoperative hypertension and to decrease myocardial oxygen consumption; however, nitroglycerin improved ischemic changes on the electrocardiogram, but nitroprusside did not. The lack of improvement in the ischemic ST segments with nitroprusside was thought to result from a decrease in CPP or the production of an intracoronary steal. When nitroglycerin was compared with calcium channel blockers in patients undergoing CABG surgery, the results depended on the class of calcium channel blocker, the usage of arterial conduits, and the administered doses.

Calcium Channel Antagonists

The calcium antagonists are a structurally diverse group of drugs that inhibit the passage of calcium through the slow channels of the cell membrane (see Chapters 7 and 10). These agents collectively relax arterial smooth muscle, with little effect on most venous beds. Despite areas of commonality, however, the calcium antagonists differ in their actions and hemodynamic effects. For example, nifedipine acts primarily on vascular smooth muscle, with little effect on the AV node. In contrast, verapamil acts mainly on the cardiac conduction system and has less effect on vascular smooth muscle and the myocardium. Neither diltiazem nor verapamil has been found to significantly increase CBF or to consistently decrease coronary vascular resistance. Verapamil and diltiazem have been shown to produce significant hemodynamic changes with myocardial depression and conduction disturbances during anesthesia.[553,554] This limits their use in the treatment of perioperative myocardial ischemia. Nevertheless, the perioperative use of nicardipine and recent studies showing a reduced incidence of cardiac events in patients who received calcium antagonists during cardiac surgery have led to an increased interest in this diverse group of drugs in patients presenting for CABG or OPCAB surgery.[555,556]

Calcium antagonists have been found to be cardioprotective against reperfusion injury. This is due to their energy-saving actions of negative inotropy and chronotropy. These antagonists have also been shown to reduce reperfusion arrythmias and attenuate myocardial stunnine. In a review of methods to reduce ischemia during OPCAB, Kwak included the calcium antagonists along with newer drugs such as nitric oxide-releasing agents, free radical scavengers, and Na^+/H^+ exchange inhibitors in the management of ischemia-reperfusion injury.[557]

Nicardipine is a short-acting dihydropyridine calcium antagonist similar to nifedipine, but possessing a tertiary amine structure in the ester side chain. Unlike other available dihydropyridines, nicardipine is stable as a parenteral solution and therefore can be administered intravenously.[558] It has highly specific modes of action, which include coronary antispasmodic and vasodilatory effects and systemic vasodilation. Among the calcium antagonists, nicardipine is unique in its consistent augmentation of CBF and its ability to induce potent and more selective vasodilator responses in the coronary bed than in the systemic vascular bed. Other important hemodynamic effects include reductions in BP and SVR and increases in myocardial contractility and CO.[559,560] Nicardipine also produces minimal myocardial depression and significant improvement in diastolic function in patients with ischemic heart disease.[561,562] Intravenous doses of 5 to 10 mg of nicardipine administered to patients with CAD produce therapeutic plasma levels. Plasma concentrations decline in a biphasic manner, with an initial half-life of 14 minutes and a terminal half-life of 4.75 hours.[558] Clearance of nicardipine results mainly from its metabolism by the liver, and excretion is primarily through bile and the feces. It undergoes rapid and extensive first-pass hepatic metabolism with the production of inactive metabolites.

Nicardipine's rapid onset and cessation of action make it an attractive drug for the perioperative management of hypertension or myocardial ischemia.[563] It has been administered to control hemodynamics during and after noncardiac vascular surgery and CABG. Begon et al[564] demonstrated that 5 mg of nicardipine was effective in treating intraoperative hypertension. The MAP decreased by 35%, with the peak onset of action in 6 minutes and duration of action of 45 minutes. Van Wezel et al[565] used a 3 to 12 μg/kg/min infusion of nicardipine and compared it with a 1 to 3 μg/kg/min infusion of nitroprusside. Both drugs were found to be equally effective in controlling BP; however, there was a 24% incidence of ST-segment depression in the nitroprusside group versus 9% in the nicardipine group. Van Wezel et al[566] also compared intravenous nitroglycerin with the intravenous administration of verapamil or nifedipine in patients undergoing CABG. Nitroglycerin was found to be the drug of choice, because it controlled BP while not producing as much tachycardia (as nifedipine) or myocardial depression and conduction blockade (seen with verapamil). Apostolidou et al[551] randomized patients undergoing CABG surgery with CPB to nicardipine (0.7 to 1.4 μg/kg/min), nitroglycerin (0.5 to 1 μg/kg/min), or placebo. Immediately after coronary revascularization (after aortic cross-clamp release until end of surgery), there were significantly less episodes of myocardial ischemia in the nicardipine group (0% versus 10% versus 24%, respectively). During the following postoperative period, there was no difference regarding myocardial ischemia between the drug groups. Apart from preventing myocardial ischemia, nicardipine effectively controls arterial hypertension in the postoperative period.[567,568] From these studies, nicardipine appears to offer significant advantages over other drugs such as nitroprusside in the intraoperative and postoperative management of hypertension and myocardial ischemia after CABG surgery (see Chapters 10, 31, and 33).

Esmolol

Hypertension, tachycardia, arrhythmias, and myocardial ischemia from sympathetic stimulation are common occurrences in the perioperative period. Despite the benefits of early use of β-blockers in the treatment of myocardial ischemia, the relatively long half-life and prolonged duration of action of previously available β-blockers have limited their usefulness during surgery and the immediate postoperative period.[569] The introduction of esmolol, an ultra-short-acting cardioselective β_1-blocker with a half-life of 9 minutes because of rapid esterase metabolism, provides a β-blocker that is extremely useful in the perioperative period. Esmolol has been shown to be effective in treating patients with acute unstable angina or during acute coronary occlusion. A mean esmolol dose of 17 ± 16 mg/min, with a range of 8 to 24 mg/min, was found to be effective in alleviating chest pain while increasing CO in patients with unstable angina.[570] LV diastolic function was shown to improve with β-blockade. Kirshenbaum et al[571] showed that esmolol was effective in treating acute myocardial ischemia even in patients with poor LV function (increased PCWP of 15 to 25 mm Hg). Esmolol was infused in these patients in doses up to 300 μg/kg/min and produced decreases in HR, BP, and CI. However, the PCWP was not significantly altered by the drug infusion. These results suggested that even in the presence of moderate LV dysfunction, esmolol can safely reduce BP and HR in patients with acute myocardial ischemia. During percutaneous transluminal coronary angioplasty, esmolol was also found to reduce the amount of ST-segment elevation and the onset of SWMAs.[572] Esmolol has been used during CABG in a prophylactic manner to prevent hypertension, tachycardia, and myocardial ischemia.[573,574] Before the introduction of newer stabilizing mechanical devices, it had been used frequently during OPCAB procedures to slow the HR during the surgical procedure. Esmolol has also been used to treat intraoperative hypertension, tachycardia, and myocardial ischemia. Bolus doses of 1.5 mg/kg have been found to be effective in treating ST-segment changes in patients with CAD.[574] More commonly, a smaller bolus dose is used and is combined with an infusion of esmolol. Bolus doses ranging from 0.5 to 1.0 mg/kg have been used, followed by infusions of 50 to 300 μg/kg/min.[575] These doses have been found to effectively treat increases in HR that occur during surgery and to block the β-adrenergic effects of catecholamines associated with surgical stress.

Coronary Artery and Arterial Conduit Spasm

Since 1981, when Buxton et al[576] first reported coronary artery spasm immediately after CABG, there have been numerous descriptions of this problem. Spasm has usually been associated with profound ST-segment elevation on the electrocardiogram, hypotension, severe dysfunction of the ventricles, and myocardial irritability. Many hypotheses have been put forward to explain the origin of coronary artery spasm; some of the mechanisms that may play a role are demonstrated in Figure 19–27.[577] The mechanism of postoperative spasm may or may not be the same as that underlying Prinzmetal's variant angina, but the same stimuli seem to be present and therapy is usually effective with a wide range of vasodilators such as nitroglycerin, calcium channel blockers, milrinone, or combinations of nitroglycerin and calcium channel blockers in both

Figure 19–27 Schematic representation of the pathogenesis of coronary artery spasm.

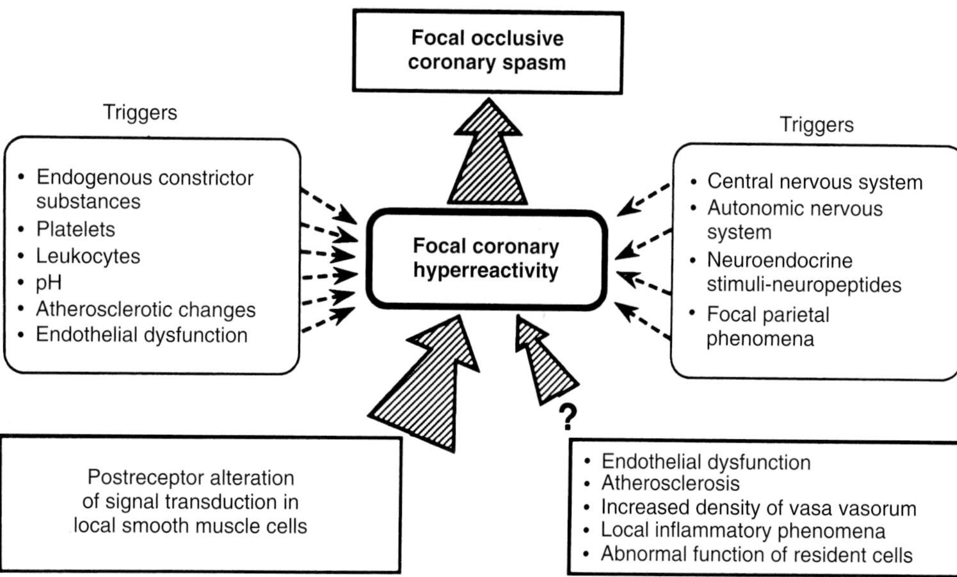

situations. Arterial grafts such as the IMA, and particularly radial artery grafts, are prone to spasm after revascularization and its prevention and recognition are crucial to prevent serious complications.[578] He et al[579] tested the reactivity of ring segments of human IMAs in organ baths to various constrictor and dilator agents. It was found that thromboxane was the most potent IMA constrictor, followed by norepinephrine, serotonin, phenylephrine, and potassium chloride. Nitroglycerin, nitric oxide, papaverine, and the calcium channel blockers nifedipine, verapamil, and diltiazem, as well as milrinone, all produced relaxation. In a similar study, Mussa et al[580] observed the vasodilating properties of topically applied phenoxybenzamine. It prevented vasoconstriction in response to various vasoconstrictors with a long-lasting effect (>5 hours), followed by verapamil/nitroglycerin (5 hours), and papaverine (1 hour). In vivo, for prophylaxis of IMA spasm, the calcium antagonists, especially diltiazem, were thought to be as useful as nitroglycerin.[581-583]

Nevertheless, prevention and treatment of arterial conduit spasm with diltiazem may cause serious side effects such as low cardiac output or conduction abnormalities. Diltiazem is a more expensive drug compared with nitroglycerin. Shapira et al[584] showed in vitro (radial artery, IMA, saphenous vein) and in vivo (radial artery) that nitroglycerin was a superior vasodilator compared with diltiazem. The same investigators monitored patients undergoing CABG surgery using radial artery grafts who were randomized to receive nitroglycerin or diltiazem intravenously after induction of anesthesia followed by a nitroglycerin patch or oral diltiazem postoperatively for 6 months. There was no significant difference in outcome (morbidity, myocardial infarction, CK-MB) between the two groups. Nevertheless, a 6-month diltiazem treatment was associated with 16-fold higher costs and significantly more patients requiring cardiac pacing compared with nitroglycerin (28% versus 13%, respectively).[585] In a double-blind, randomized study, Mollhoff et al[586] compared milrinone (0.375 μg/kg/min) to nifedipine (0.2 μg/kg/min) in patients with impaired left ventricular function undergoing CABG surgery. ST changes after revascularization (including the use of the IMA graft) indicative of myocardial ischemia occurred in 33.3% of the milrinone group compared with 86.6% in the nifedipine group. Biochemical markers of myocardial damage (CK-MB and troponin-I) after 24 hours were significantly higher in the nifedipine group.

CONCLUSIONS

Anesthesia for myocardial revascularization continues to evolve rapidly with advances in anesthetic pharmacology, monitoring technologies, as well as basic science, clinical and epidemiologic research. Considerable health care resources are consumed by revascularization procedures relative to other medical therapies. Yet, there is an urgent need to better control hospital costs and LOS. Over the past decade, major changes in practice have occurred with high-dose opioid-benzodiazepine anesthesia being replaced by fast-tracking with volatile anesthesia and early extubation. This has been closely followed by the spectacular rise in OPCAB and minimally invasive revascularization procedures in a variety of forms with which fast-track anesthesia appears well suited. The once routinely used PAC is now used less commonly, but TEE use continues to increase with its strong emphasis in training programs and by organizations such as the Society of Cardiovascular Anesthesiologists. Regional anesthesia for CABG and OPCAB has enjoyed resurgence in interest, although its use in the United States remains low. Anesthesiologists are increasingly involved in perioperative medical issues preoperatively and postoperatively with active, ongoing research.

CABG volume has been decreasing due to major advances in PCI therapies. However, data from the New York State Cardiac Registries (see Chapter 39) may produce a resurgence in volume for both CABG and OPCAB procedures. Hannan et al[587] showed improved long-term outcomes for patients with two or more diseased coronary arteries who had CABG surgery rather than PCI with stenting. This risk adjusted outcome data was better for CABG with all of the anatomic variants of double- and triple-vessel CAD. The number of additional revascularization procedures was reduced by CABG surgery. Cardiac anesthesiologists will continue to see sicker and more interesting cases, and the well-prepared and engaged anesthesiologist will be a strong component of successful surgical interventions for many years to come.

REFERENCES

1. Lowenstein E, Hallowell P, Levine FH, et al: Cardiovascular response to large doses of intravenous morphine in man. N Engl J Med 281:1389, 1969
2. Reiz S, Balfors E, Sorensen MB, et al: Isoflurane—a powerful coronary vasodilator in patients with coronary artery disease. Anesthesiology 59:91, 1983
3. Mangano DT, Siliciano D, Hollenberg M, et al: Postoperative myocardial ischemia. Therapeutic trials using intensive analgesia following surgery. Anesthesiology 76:342, 1992
4. De Hert SG, ten Broecke PW, Mertens E, et al: Sevoflurane but not propofol preserves myocardial function in coronary surgery patients. Anesthesiology 97:42, 2002
5. Myles PS, Daly DJ, Djaiani G, et al: A systematic review of the safety and effectiveness of fast-track cardiac anesthesia. Anesthesiology 99:982, 2003
6. Cheng DC, Bainbridge D, Martin JE, et al: Does off-pump coronary artery bypass reduce mortality, morbidity, and resource utilization when compared with conventional coronary artery bypass? A meta-analysis of randomized trials. Anesthesiology 102:188, 2005
7. Chaney MA, Durazo-Arvizu RA, Fluder EM, et al: Port-access minimally invasive cardiac surgery increases surgical complexity, increases operating room time, and facilitates early postoperative hospital discharge. Anesthesiology 92:1637, 2000
8. Chakravarthy M, Thimmangowda P, Krishnamurthy J, et al: Thoracic epidural anesthesia in cardiac surgical patients: A prospective audit of 2,113 cases. J Cardiothorac Vasc Anesth 19:44, 2005
9. Meissner A, Rolf N, Van Aken H: Thoracic epidural anesthesia and the patient with heart disease: Benefits, risks, and controversies. Anesth Analg 85:517, 1997
10. American Heart Association: Heart Disease and Stroke Statistics—2004 Update. Dallas, TX, American Heart Association, 2004.
11. Maynard C, Sales AE: Changes in the use of coronary artery revascularization procedures in the Department of Veterans Affairs, the National Hospital Discharge Survey, and the Nationwide Inpatient Sample, 1991–1999. BMC Health Serv Res 3:12, 2003
12. Mack MJ, Brown PP, Kugelmass AD, et al: Current status and outcomes of coronary revascularization 1999 to 2002: 148,396 surgical and percutaneous procedures. Ann Thorac Surg 77:761, 2004
13. DeFrances C, Hall M: National Hospital Discharge Survey. Advance Data from Vital and Health Statistics, no 342. Hyattsville, MD, National Center for Health Statistics, 2004
14. Ferguson TB Jr, Hammill BG, Peterson ED, et al: A decade of change—risk profiles and outcomes for isolated coronary artery bypass grafting procedures, 1990–1999: A report from the STS National Database Committee and the Duke Clinical Research Institute. Society of Thoracic Surgeons. Ann Thorac Surg 73:480; discussion 489, 2002
15. Warner CD, Weintraub WS, Craver JM, et al: Effect of cardiac surgery patient characteristics on patient outcomes from 1981 through 1995. Circulation 96:1575, 1997
16. Davierwala PM, Maganti M, Yau TM: Decreasing significance of left ventricular dysfunction and reoperative surgery in predicting coronary artery bypass grafting-associated mortality: A twelve-year study. J Thorac Cardiovasc Surg 126:1335, 2003
17. Eagle KA, Guyton RA, Davidoff R, et al: ACC/AHA 2004 guideline update for coronary artery bypass graft surgery: Summary article: A report of the American College of Cardiology/American Heart Association Task Force on Practice Guidelines (Committee to Update the 1999 Guidelines for Coronary Artery Bypass Graft Surgery). Circulation 110:1168, 2004
18. Eagle KA, Guyton RA, Davidoff R, et al: ACC/AHA 2004 guideline update for coronary artery bypass graft surgery: A report of the American College of Cardiology/American Heart Association Task Force on Practice Guidelines (Committee to Update the 1999 Guidelines for Coronary Artery Bypass Graft Surgery). American College of Cardiology Web Site. Available at: http://www.acc.org/clinical/guidelines/cabg/cabg.pdf, 2004
19. Kupersmith J, Holmes-Rovner M, Hogan A, et al: Cost-effectiveness analysis in heart disease, Part III: Ischemia, congestive heart failure, and arrhythmias. Prog Cardiovasc Dis 37:307, 1995
20. Grover FL, Shroyer AL, Hammermeister KE: Calculating risk and outcome: The Veterans Affairs database. Ann Thorac Surg 62:S6, 1996
21. Grover FL, Cleveland JC Jr, Shroyer LW: Quality improvement in cardiac care. Arch Surg 137:28, 2002
22. Daley J, Henderson WG, Khuri SF: Risk-Adjusted Surgical Outcomes. Annu Rev Med 52:275, 2001
23. Shahian DM, Normand SL, Torchiana DF, et al: Cardiac surgery report cards: Comprehensive review and statistical critique. Ann Thorac Surg 72:2155, 2001
24. Shahian DM, Blackstone EH, Edwards FH, et al: Cardiac surgery risk models: A position article. Ann Thorac Surg 78:1868, 2004
25. Grover FL: The Society of Thoracic Surgeons National Database: Current status and future directions. Ann Thorac Surg 68:367, 1999
26. Shroyer AL, Coombs LP, Peterson ED, et al: The Society of Thoracic Surgeons: 30-day operative mortality and morbidity risk models. Ann Thorac Surg 75:1856, 2003
27. O'Connor GT, Plume SK, Olmstead EM, et al: A regional prospective study of in-hospital mortality associated with coronary artery bypass grafting. The Northern New England Cardiovascular Disease Study Group. JAMA 266:803, 1991
28. Hannan EL, Kilburn H Jr, Racz M, et al: Improving the outcomes of coronary artery bypass surgery in New York State. JAMA 271:761, 1994
29. O'Connor GT, Plume SK, Olmstead EM, et al: A regional intervention to improve the hospital mortality associated with coronary artery bypass graft surgery. The Northern New England Cardiovascular Disease Study Group JAMA 275:841, 1996
30. Holman WL, Sansom M, Kiefe CI, et al: Alabama coronary artery bypass grafting project: Results from phase II of a statewide quality improvement initiative. Ann Surg 239:99, 2004
31. Hannan EL, Kilburn H Jr, O'Donnell JF, et al: Adult open heart surgery in New York State. An analysis of risk factors and hospital mortality rates JAMA 264:2768, 1990
32. Peterson ED, Coombs LP, DeLong ER, et al: Procedural volume as a marker of quality for CABG surgery. JAMA 291:195, 2004
33. Glance LG, Dick AW, Mukamel DB, et al: Is the hospital volume-mortality relationship in coronary artery bypass surgery the same for low-risk versus high-risk patients? Ann Thorac Surg 76:1155, 2003
34. Vaughan-Sarrazin MS, Hannan EL, Gormley CJ, et al: Mortality in Medicare beneficiaries following coronary artery bypass graft surgery in states with and without certificate of need regulation. JAMA 288:1859, 2002
35. Roques F, Nashef SA, Michel P, et al: Risk factors and outcome in European cardiac surgery: Analysis of the EuroSCORE multinational database of 19030 patients. Eur J Cardiothorac Surg 15:816, 1999
36. Nashef SA, Roques F, Hammill BG, et al: Validation of European System for Cardiac Operative Risk Evaluation (EuroSCORE) in North American cardiac surgery. Eur J Cardiothorac Surg 22:101, 2002
37. Higgins TL: Quantifying risk and assessing outcome in cardiac surgery. J Cardiothorac Vasc Anesth 12:330, 1998
38. Jones RH, Hannan EL, Hammermeister KE, et al: Identification of preoperative variables needed for risk adjustment of short-term mortality after coronary artery bypass graft surgery. The Working Group Panel on the Cooperative CABG Database Project. J Am Coll Cardiol 28:1478, 1996
39. Higgins TL, Estafanous FG, Loop FD, et al: Stratification of morbidity and mortality outcome by preoperative risk factors in coronary artery bypass patients. A clinical severity score [published erratum appears in JAMA 268:1860, 1992]. JAMA 267:2344, 1992
40. Nashef SA, Roques F, Michel P, et al: European system for cardiac operative risk evaluation (EuroSCORE). Eur J Cardiothorac Surg 16:9, 1999
41. Rao V, Ivanov J, Weisel RD, et al: Predictors of low cardiac output syndrome after coronary artery bypass. J Thorac Cardiovasc Surg 112:38, 1996
42. Ferraris VA, Ferraris SP: Risk factors for postoperative morbidity. J Thorac Cardiovasc Surg 111:731, 1996
43. McKinlay KH, Schinderle DB, Swaminathan M, et al: Predictors of inotrope use during separation from cardiopulmonary bypass. J Cardiothorac Vasc Anesth 18:404, 2004
44. Plomondon ME, Cleveland JC, Ludwig ST, et al: Off-pump coronary artery bypass is associated with improved risk-adjusted outcomes. Ann Thorac Surg 72:114, 2001
45. Wu Y, Grunkemeier GL, Handy JR Jr: Coronary artery bypass grafting: Are risk models developed from on-pump surgery valid for off-pump surgery? J Thorac Cardiovasc Surg 127:174, 2004
46. O'Brien MM, Shroyer AL, Moritz TE, et al: Relationship between processes of care and coronary bypass operative mortality and morbidity. Med Care 42:59, 2004
47. London MJ, Shroyer AL, Grover FL, et al: Evaluating anesthesia health care delivery for cardiac surgery. The role of process and structure variables. Med Care 33:OS66, 1995

48. Shroyer AL, London MJ, Sethi GK, et al: Relationships between patient-related risk factors, processes, structures, and outcomes of cardiac surgical care. Conceptual models. Med Care 33:OS26, 1995
49. Merry AF, Ramage MC, Whitlock RM, et al: First-time coronary artery bypass grafting: The anaesthetist as a risk factor. Br J Anaesth 68:6, 1992
50. Slogoff S, Keats AS: Randomized trial of primary anesthetic agents on outcome of coronary artery bypass operations. Anesthesiology 70:179, 1989
51. Tuman KJ, McCarthy RJ, Spiess BD, et al: Does choice of anesthetic agent significantly affect outcome after coronary artery surgery? Anesthesiology 70:189, 1989
52. De Hert SG, Van der Linden PJ, Cromheecke S, et al: Choice of primary anesthetic regimen can influence intensive care unit length of stay after coronary surgery with cardiopulmonary bypass. Anesthesiology 101:9, 2004
53. De Hert SG, Cromheecke S, ten Broecke PW, et al: Effects of propofol, desflurane, and sevoflurane on recovery of myocardial function after coronary surgery in elderly high-risk patients. Anesthesiology 99:314, 2003
54. Berendes E, Schmidt C, Van Aken H, et al: Reversible cardiac sympathectomy by high thoracic epidural anesthesia improves regional left ventricular function in patients undergoing coronary artery bypass grafting: A randomized trial. Arch Surg 138:1283, 2003
55. Butterworth J, James R, Prielipp RC, et al: Do shorter-acting neuromuscular blocking drugs or opioids associate with reduced intensive care unit or hospital lengths of stay after coronary artery bypass grafting? CABG Clinical Benchmarking Data Base Participants. Anesthesiology 88:1437, 1998
56. London MJ, Shroyer AL, Coll JR, et al: Early extubation following cardiac surgery in a veterans population. Anesthesiology 88:1447, 1998
57. Reich DL, Bodian CA, Krol M, et al: Intraoperative hemodynamic predictors of mortality, stroke, and myocardial infarction after coronary artery bypass surgery. Anesth Analg 89:814, 1999
58. Fillinger MP, Surgenor SD, Hartman GS, et al: The association between heart rate and in-hospital mortality after coronary artery bypass graft surgery. Anesth Analg 95:1483, 2002
59. Hill SE, van Wermeskerken GK, Lardenoye JW, et al: Intraoperative physiologic variables and outcome in cardiac surgery. Part I. In-hospital mortality. Ann Thorac Surg 69:1070, 2000
60. van Wermeskerken GK, Lardenoye JW, Hill SE, et al: Intraoperative physiologic variables and outcome in cardiac surgery. Part II. Neurologic outcome. Ann Thorac Surg 69:1077, 2000
61. Gold JP, Charlson ME, Williams-Russo P, et al: Improvement of outcomes after coronary artery bypass. A randomized trial comparing intraoperative high versus low mean arterial pressure. J Thorac Cardiovasc Surg 110:1302, 1995
62. Arbous MS, Meursing AE, van Kleef JW, et al: Impact of anesthesia management characteristics on severe morbidity and mortality. Anesthesiology 102:257, 2005
63. Newland MC, Ellis SJ, Lydiatt CA, et al: Anesthetic-related cardiac arrest and its mortality: A report covering 72,959 anesthetics over 10 years from a US teaching hospital. Anesthesiology 97:108, 2002
64. Becker RB, Zimmerman JE, Knaus WA, et al: The use of APACHE III to evaluate ICU length of stay, resource use, and mortality after coronary artery by-pass surgery. J Cardiovasc Surg (Torino) 36:1, 1995
65. Higgins TL, Estafanous FG, Loop FD, et al: ICU admission score for predicting morbidity and mortality risk after coronary artery bypass grafting. A Thorac Surg 64:1050, 1997
66. Nakagawa Y, Nakagawa K, Sdringola S, et al: A precise, three-dimensional atlas of myocardial perfusion correlated with coronary arteriographic anatomy. J Nucl Cardiol 8:580, 2001
67. Wei K, Kaul S: The coronary microcirculation in health and disease. Cardiol Clin 22:221, 2004
68. Factor SM, Okun EM, Minase T, et al: The microcirculation of the human heart: End-capillary loops with discrete perfusion fields. Circulation 66:1241, 1982
69. Panting JR, Gatehouse PD, Yang GZ, et al: Abnormal subendocardial perfusion in cardiac syndrome X detected by cardiovascular magnetic resonance imaging. N Engl J Med 346:1948, 2002
70. Egashira K, Inou T, Hirooka Y, et al: Evidence of impaired endothelium-dependent coronary vasodilatation in patients with angina pectoris and normal coronary angiograms. N Engl J Med 328:1659, 1993
71. Rajappan K, Rimoldi OE, Dutka DP, et al: Mechanisms of coronary microcirculatory dysfunction in patients with aortic stenosis and angiographically normal coronary arteries. Circulation 105:470, 2002
72. Malek AM, Alper SL, Izumo S: Hemodynamic shear stress and its role in atherosclerosis. JAMA 282:2035, 1999
73. Tian G, Dai G, Xiang B, et al: Effect on myocardial perfusion of simultaneous delivery of cardioplegic solution through a single coronary artery and the coronary sinus. J Thorac Cardiovasc Surg 122:1004, 2001
74. Yeghiazarians Y, Braunstein JB, Askari A, et al: Unstable angina pectoris. N Engl J Med 342:101, 2000
75. Virmani R, Burke AP, Farb A, et al: Pathology of the unstable plaque. Prog Cardiovasc Dis 44:349, 2002
76. Shah PK: Pathophysiology of coronary thrombosis: Role of plaque rupture and plaque erosion. Prog Cardiovasc Dis 44:357, 2002
77. Fuster V, Moreno PR, Fayad ZA, et al: Atherothrombosis and high-risk plaque. J Am Coll Cardiol 46:937, 2005
78. Naghavi M, Libby P, Falk E, et al: From vulnerable plaque to vulnerable patient: A call for new definitions and risk assessment strategies. Part II. Circulation 108:1772, 2003
79. Naghavi M, Libby P, Falk E, et al: From vulnerable plaque to vulnerable patient: A call for new definitions and risk assessment strategies. Part I. Circulation 108:1664, 2003
80. Dawood MM, Gutpa DK, Southern J, et al: Pathology of fatal perioperative myocardial infarction: Implications regarding pathophysiology and prevention. Int J Cardiol 57:37, 1996
81. Cohen MC, Aretz TH: Histological analysis of coronary artery lesions in fatal postoperative myocardial infarction. Cardiovasc Pathol 8:133, 1999
82. Ellis SG, Hertzer NR, Young JR, et al: Angiographic correlates of cardiac death and myocardial infarction complicating major nonthoracic vascular surgery. Am J Cardiol 77:1126, 1996
83. Hoffman JIE: Transmural myocardial perfusion. Prog Cardiovasc Dis 29:429, 1987
84. Hoffman JI: Maximal coronary flow and the concept of coronary vascular reserve. Circulation 70:153, 1984
85. DeFily DV, Chilian WM: Coronary microcirculation: Autoregulation and metabolic control. Basic Res Cardiol 90:112, 1995
86. Canty JM Jr: Coronary pressure-function and steady-state pressure-flow relations during autoregulation in the unanesthetized dog. Circ Res 63:821, 1988
87. Hoffman JI: Autoregulation and heart rate. Circulation 82:1880, 1990
88. Boudoulas H, Lewis RP, Rittgers SE, et al: Increased diastolic time: A possible important factor in the beneficial effect of propranolol in patients with coronary artery disease. J Cardiovasc Pharmacol 1:503, 1979
89. Schwartz JS: Effect of distal coronary pressure on rigid and compliant coronary stenoses. Am J Physiol 245:H1054, 1983
90. Brown BG, Bolson EL, Dodge HT: Dynamic mechanisms in human coronary stenosis. Circulation 70:917, 1984
91. Gregg DE, Patterson RE: Functional importance of the coronary collaterals. N Engl J Med 303:1404, 1980
92. Becker LC: Conditions for vasodilator-induced coronary steal in experimental myocardial ischemia. Circulation 57:1103, 1978
93. Bache RJ, Dymek DJ: Local and regional regulation of coronary vascular tone. Prog Cardiovasc Dis 24:191, 1981
94. Buffington CW, Davis KB, Gillispie S, et al: The prevalence of steal-prone coronary anatomy in patients with coronary artery disease: An analysis of the Coronary Artery Surgery Study Registry. Anesthesiology 69:721, 1988
95. Cohn PF: Prognosis in exercise-induced silent myocardial ischemia and implications for screening asymptomatic populations. Prog Cardiovasc Dis 34:399, 1992
96. Deanfield JE, Maseri A, Selwyn AP, et al: Myocardial ischaemia during daily life in patients with stable angina: Its relation to symptoms and heart rate changes. Lancet 2:753, 1983
97. Chierchia S, Gallino A, Smith G, et al: Role of heart rate in pathophysiology of chronic stable angina. Lancet 2:1353, 1984
98. Chierchia S, Lazzari M, Freedman B, et al: Impairment of myocardial perfusion and function during painless myocardial ischemia. J Am Coll Cardiol 1:924, 1983
99. Knight AA, Hollenberg M, London MJ, et al: Perioperative myocardial ischemia: Importance of the preoperative ischemic pattern. Anesthesiology 68:681, 1988
100. Deedwania PC, Nelson JR: Pathophysiology of silent myocardial ischemia during daily life. Hemodynamic evaluation by simultaneous electrocardiographic and blood pressure monitoring. Circulation 82:1296, 1990
101. Deedwania PC, Stone PH: Ambulatory electrocardiographic monitoring for myocardial ischemia. Curr Probl Cardiol 26:680, 2001
102. Slogoff S, Keats AS: Further observations on perioperative myocardial ischemia. Anesthesiology 65:539, 1986

103. Cote P, Gueret P, Bourassa MG: Systemic and coronary hemodynamic effects of diazepam in patients with normal and diseased coronary arteries. Circulation 50:1210, 1974
104. Saccomanno PM, Kavanagh BP, Cheng DC, et al: Comparison of lorazepam alone vs lorazepam, morphine, and perphenazine for cardiac premedication. Can J Anaesth 44:146, 1997
105. Thomson IR, Bergstrom RG, Rosenbloom M, et al: Premedication and high-dose fentanyl anesthesia for myocardial revascularization: A comparison of lorazepam versus morphine-scopolamine. Anesthesiology 68:194, 1988
106. Tomicheck RC, Rosow CE, Philbin DM, et al: Diazepam-fentanyl interaction—hemodynamic and hormonal effects in coronary artery surgery. Anesth Analg 62:881, 1983
107. Thomson IR, Peterson MD, Hudson RJ: A comparison of clonidine with conventional preanesthetic medication in patients undergoing coronary artery bypass grafting. Anesth Analg 87:292, 1998
108. Howie MB, Hiestand DC, Jopling MW, et al: Effect of oral clonidine premedication on anesthetic requirement, hormonal response, hemodynamics, and recovery in coronary artery bypass graft surgery patients. J Clin Anesth 8:263, 1996
109. Wijeysundera DN, Naik JS, Beattie WS: Alpha-2 adrenergic agonists to prevent perioperative cardiovascular complications: A meta-analysis. Am J Med 114:742, 2003
110. Dorman BH, Zucker JR, Verrier ED, et al: Clonidine improves perioperative myocardial ischemia, reduces anesthetic requirement, and alters hemodynamic parameters in patients undergoing coronary artery bypass surgery. J Cardiothorac Vasc Anesth 7:386, 1993
111. Scheinin H, Jaakola ML, Sjovall S, et al: Intramuscular dexmedetomidine as premedication for general anesthesia. A comparative multicenter study. Anesthesiology 78:1065, 1993
112. Viljoen J, Estafanous F, Kellner G: Propranolol and cardiac surgery. J Thorac Cardiovasc Surg 64:826, 1972
113. Kaplan JA, Dunbar RW, Bland JW, et al: Propranolol and cardiac surgery: A problem for the anesthesiologist? Anesth Analg 54:571, 1975
114. Kaplan JA, Dunbar RW: Propranolol and surgical anesthesia. Anesth Analg 55:1, 1976
115. Slogoff S, Keats AS, Ott E: Preoperative propranolol therapy and aortocoronary bypass operation. JAMA 240:1487, 1978
116. Slogoff S, Keats AS: Does chronic treatment with calcium entry blocking drugs reduce perioperative myocardial ischemia? Anesthesiology 68:676, 1988
117. Chung F, Houston PL, Cheng DC, et al: Calcium channel blockade does not offer adequate protection from perioperative myocardial ischemia. Anesthesiology 69:343, 1988
118. Pasternack PF, Imparato AM, Baumann FG, et al: The hemodynamics of beta-blockade in patients undergoing abdominal aortic aneurysm repair. Circulation 76:III1, 1987
119. Stone JG, Foëx P, Sear JW, et al: Myocardial ischemia in untreated hypertensive patients: Effect of a single small oral dose of a beta-adrenergic blocking agent. Anesthesiology 68:495, 1988
120. Stone JG, Foëx P, Sear JW, et al: Risk of myocardial ischaemia during anaesthesia in treated and untreated hypertensive patients. Br J Anaesth 61:675, 1988
121. Poldermans D, Boersma E, Bax JJ, et al: The effect of bisoprolol on perioperative mortality and myocardial infarction in high-risk patients undergoing vascular surgery. N Engl J Med 341:1789, 1999
122. Mangano DT, Layug EL, Wallace A, et al: Effect of atenolol on mortality and cardiovascular morbidity after noncardiac surgery. N Engl J Med 335:1713, 1996
123. London MJ: Perioperative beta blockade: Facts and controversies. Ann Cardiac Anaesth 6:117, 2003
124. London MJ, Zaugg M, Schaub MC, et al: Perioperative beta-adrenergic receptor blockade: physiologic foundations and clinical controversies. Anesthesiology 100:170, 2004
125. London MJ, Itani KM, Perrino AC Jr, et al: Perioperative beta-blockade: A survey of physician attitudes in the Department of Veterans Affairs. J Cardiothorac Vasc Anesth 18:14, 2004
126. Weightman WM, Gibbs NM, Sheminant MR, et al: Drug therapy before coronary artery surgery: Nitrates are independent predictors of mortality and beta-adrenergic blockers predict survival. Anesth Analg 88:286, 1999
127. ten Broecke PW, De Hert SG, Mertens E, et al: Effect of preoperative beta-blockade on perioperative mortality in coronary surgery. Br J Anaesth 90:27, 2003
128. Ferguson TB Jr, Coombs LP, Peterson ED: Preoperative beta-blocker use and mortality and morbidity following CABG surgery in North America. JAMA 287:2221, 2002
129. Denton TA, Fonarow GC, LaBresh KA, et al: Secondary prevention after coronary bypass: The American Heart Association "Get with the Guidelines" program. Ann Thorac Surg 75:758, 2003
130. Ferguson TB Jr, Peterson ED, Coombs LP, et al: Use of continuous quality improvement to increase use of process measures in patients undergoing coronary artery bypass graft surgery: A randomized controlled trial. JAMA 290:49, 2003
131. Salmenpera M, Yrjola H, Heikkila J: Hemodynamic responses to beta-adrenergic blockade with metoprolol and pindolol after coronary artery bypass surgery. Chest 83:739, 1983
132. Hammon JW Jr, Wood AJ, Prager RL, et al: Perioperative beta blockade with propranolol: Reduction in myocardial oxygen demands and incidence of atrial and ventricular arrhythmias. Ann Thorac Surg 38:363, 1984
133. Heikkila H, Jalonen J, Laaksonen V, et al: Metoprolol medication and coronary artery bypass grafting operation. Acta Anaesthesiol Scand 28:677, 1984
134. Sill JC, Nugent M, Moyer TP, et al: Influence of propranolol plasma levels on hemodynamics during coronary artery bypass surgery. Anesthesiology 60:455, 1984
135. Sill JC, Nugent M, Moyer TP, et al: Plasma levels of beta-blocking drugs prior to coronary artery bypass surgery. Anesthesiology 62:67, 1985
136. Yndgaard S, Lippert FK, Bigler D, et al: Monitoring of beta-receptor sensitivity in cardiac surgery. J Cardiothorac Vasc Anesth 13:454, 1999
137. Yeager MP, Fillinger MP, Hettleman BD, Hartman GS: Perioperative beta-blockade and late cardiac outcomes: A complementary hypothesis. J Cardiothorac Vasc Anesth 19:237, 2005
138. Booth JV, Landolfo KP, Chesnut LC, et al: Acute depression of myocardial beta-adrenergic receptor signaling during cardiopulmonary bypass: Impairment of the adenylyl cyclase moiety. Duke Heart Center Perioperative Desensitization Group. Anesthesiology 89:602, 1998
139. Gerhardt MA, Booth JV, Chesnut LC, et al: Acute myocardial beta-adrenergic receptor dysfunction after cardiopulmonary bypass in patients with cardiac valve disease. Duke Heart Center Perioperative Desensitization Group. Circulation 98:II275, 1998
140. Booth JV, Spahn DR, McRae RL, et al: Esmolol improves left ventricular function via enhanced beta-adrenergic receptor signaling in a canine model of coronary revascularization. Anesthesiology 97:162, 2002
141. Booth JV, Ward EE, Colgan KC, et al: Metoprolol and coronary artery bypass grafting surgery: Does intraoperative metoprolol attenuate acute beta-adrenergic receptor desensitization during cardiac surgery? Anesth Analg 98:1224, 2004
142. Chesebro JH, Clements IP, Fuster V, et al: A platelet-inhibitor-drug trial in coronary-artery bypass operations: Benefit of perioperative dipyridamole and aspirin therapy on early postoperative vein-graft patency. N Engl J Med 307:73, 1982
143. Mangano DT: Aspirin and mortality from coronary bypass surgery. N Engl J Med 347:1309, 2002
144. Stein PD, Schunemann HJ, Dalen JE, et al: Antithrombotic therapy in patients with saphenous vein and internal mammary artery bypass grafts: The Seventh ACCP Conference on Antithrombotic and Thrombolytic Therapy. Chest 126:600S, 2004
145. Ferraris VA, Ferraris SP, Moliterno DJ, et al: The Society of Thoracic Surgeons practice guideline series: Aspirin and other antiplatelet agents during operative coronary revascularization (executive summary). Ann Thorac Surg 79:1454, 2005
146. Opie LH, Yusuf S, Kubler W: Current status of safety and efficacy of calcium channel blockers in cardiovascular diseases: A critical analysis based on 100 studies. Prog Cardiovasc Dis 43:171, 2000
147. Stevens RD, Burri H, Tramer MR: Pharmacologic myocardial protection in patients undergoing noncardiac surgery: A quantitative systematic review. Anesth Analg 97:623, 2003
148. Wijeysundera DN, Beattie WS: Calcium channel blockers for reducing cardiac morbidity after noncardiac surgery: A meta-analysis. Anesth Analg 97:634, 2003
149. Wijeysundera DN, Beattie WS, Rao V, et al: Calcium antagonists are associated with reduced mortality after cardiac surgery: A propensity analysis. J Thorac Cardiovasc Surg 127:755, 2004
150. Wijeysundera DN, Beattie WS, Rao V, et al: Calcium antagonists reduce cardiovascular complications after cardiac surgery: A meta-analysis. J Am Coll Cardiol 41:1496, 2003
151. Ferguson TB Jr: Preoperative calcium-channel blockade in cardiac surgery: The good, the bad, the issues. J Thorac Cardiovasc Surg 127:622, 2004
152. Amar D, Roistacher N, Rusch VW, et al: Effects of diltiazem prophylaxis on the incidence and clinical outcome of atrial arrhythmias after thoracic surgery. J Thorac Cardiovasc Surg 120:790, 2000

153. Halcox JP, Deanfield JE: Beyond the laboratory: Clinical implications for statin pleiotropy. Circulation 109:II42, 2004
154. Lazar HL: Role of angiotensin-converting enzyme inhibitors in the coronary artery bypass patient. Ann Thorac Surg 79:1081, 2005
155. Vaughan CJ, Gotto AM Jr: Update on statins: 2003. Circulation 110:886, 2004
156. Ray KK, Cannon CP: The potential relevance of the multiple lipid-independent (pleiotropic) effects of statins in the management of acute coronary syndromes. J Am Cell Cardiol 46:1425, 2005
157. Chan AW, Bhatt DL, Chew DP, et al: Early and sustained survival benefit associated with statin therapy at the time of percutaneous coronary intervention. Circulation 105:691, 2002
158. Chan AW, Bhatt DL, Chew DP, et al: Relation of inflammation and benefit of statins after percutaneous coronary interventions. Circulation 107:1750, 2003
159. Chello M, Mastroroberto P, Patti G, et al: Simvastatin attenuates leucocyte-endothelial interactions after coronary revascularisation with cardiopulmonary bypass. Heart 89:538, 2003
160. Chello M, Carassiti M, Agro F, et al: Simvastatin blunts the increase of circulating adhesion molecules after coronary artery bypass surgery with cardiopulmonary bypass. J Cardiothorac Vasc Anesth 18:605, 2004
161. Pretorius M, Murphey LJ, McFarlane JA, et al: Angiotensin-converting enzyme inhibition alters the fibrinolytic response to cardiopulmonary bypass. Circulation 108:3079, 2003
162. Poldermans D, Bax JJ, Kertai MD, et al: Statins are associated with a reduced incidence of perioperative mortality in patients undergoing major noncardiac vascular surgery. Circulation 107:1848, 2003
163. Lindenauer PK, Pekow P, Wang K, et al: Lipid-lowering therapy and in-hospital mortality following major noncardiac surgery. JAMA 291:2092, 2004
164. O'Neil-Callahan K, Katsimaglis G, Tepper MR, et al: Statins decrease perioperative cardiac complications in patients undergoing noncardiac vascular surgery the Statins for Risk Reduction in Surgery (StaRRS) study. J Am Coll Cardiol 45:336, 2005
165. Dotani MI, Morise AP, Haque R, et al: Association between short-term simvastatin therapy before coronary artery bypass grafting and postoperative myocardial blood flow as assessed by positron emission tomography. Am J Cardiol 91:1107, 2003
166. Pan W, Pintar T, Anton J, et al: Statins are associated with a reduced incidence of perioperative mortality after coronary artery bypass graft surgery. Circulation 110:II45, 2004
167. Pasternak RC, Smith SC Jr, Bairey-Merz CN, et al: ACC/AHA/NHLBI clinical advisory on the use and safety of statins. Circulation 106:1024, 2002
168. Coriat P, Richer C, Douraki T, et al: Influence of chronic angiotensin-converting enzyme inhibition on anesthetic induction. Anesthesiology 81:299, 1994
169. Tuman KJ, McCarthy RJ, O'Connor CJ, et al: Angiotensin-converting enzyme inhibitors increase vasoconstrictor requirements after cardiopulmonary bypass. Anesth Analg 80:473, 1995
170. Deakin CD, Dalrymple-Hay MJ, Jones P, et al: Effects of angiotensin converting enzyme inhibition on systemic vascular resistance and vasoconstrictor requirements during hypothermic cardiopulmonary bypass. Eur J Cardiothorac Surg 13:546, 1998
171. Brabant SM, Bertrand M, Eyraud D, et al: The hemodynamic effects of anesthetic induction in vascular surgical patients chronically treated with angiotensin II receptor antagonists. Anesth Analg 89:1388, 1999
172. Pigott DW, Nagle C, Allman K, et al: Effect of omitting regular ACE inhibitor medication before cardiac surgery on haemodynamic variables and vasoactive drug requirements. Br J Anaesth 83:715, 1999
173. Bertrand M, Godet G, Meersschaert K, et al: Should the angiotensin II antagonists be discontinued before surgery? Anesth Analg 92:26, 2001
174. Meersschaert K, Brun L, Gourdin M, et al: Terlipressin-ephedrine versus ephedrine to treat hypotension at the induction of anesthesia in patients chronically treated with angiotensin converting-enzyme inhibitors: A prospective, randomized, double-blinded, crossover study. Anesth Analg 94:835, 2002
175. London MJ: Multilead precordial ST-segment monitoring: "the next generation"? Anesthesiology 96:259, 2002
176. Mangar D, Laborde RS, Vu DN: Delayed ischaemia of the hand necessitating amputation after radial artery cannulation. Can J Anaesth 40:247, 1993
177. Rich GF, Lubanski RE Jr, McLoughlin TM: Differences between aortic and radial artery pressure associated with cardiopulmonary bypass. Anesthesiology 77:63, 1992
178. Thrush DN, Steighner ML, Rasanen J, et al: Blood pressure after cardiopulmonary bypass: Which technique is accurate? J Cardiothorac Vasc Anesth 8:269, 1994
179. Dorman T, Breslow MJ, Lipsett PA, et al: Radial artery pressure monitoring underestimates central arterial pressure during vasopressor therapy in critically ill surgical patients. Crit Care Med 26:1646, 1998
180. Chauhan S, Saxena N, Mehrotra S, et al: Femoral artery pressures are more reliable than radial artery pressures on initiation of cardiopulmonary bypass. J Cardiothorac Vasc Anesth 14:274, 2000
181. Kanazawa M, Fukuyama H, Kinefuchi Y, et al: Relationship between aortic-to-radial arterial pressure gradient after cardiopulmonary bypass and changes in arterial elasticity. Anesthesiology 99:48, 2003
182. McGee DC, Gould MK: Preventing complications of central venous catheterization. N Engl J Med 348:1123, 2003
183. Eisenberg PR, Jaffe AS, Schuster DP: Clinical evaluation compared to pulmonary artery catheterization in the hemodynamic assessment of critically ill patients. Crit Care Med 12:549, 1984
184. Kaplan JA, Wells PH: Early diagnosis of myocardial ischemia using the pulmonary arterial catheter. Anesth Analg 60:789, 1981
185. Mangano DT: Monitoring pulmonary arterial pressure in coronary-artery disease. Anesthesiology 53:364, 1980
186. Bashein G, Johnson PW, Davis KB, et al: Elective coronary bypass surgery without pulmonary artery catheter monitoring. Anesthesiology 63:451, 1985
187. van Daele ME, Sutherland GR, Mitchell MM, et al: Do changes in pulmonary capillary wedge pressure adequately reflect myocardial ischemia during anesthesia? A correlative preoperative hemodynamic, electrocardiographic, and transesophageal echocardiographic study. Circulation 81:865, 1990
188. Haggmark S, Hohner P, Ostman M, et al: Comparison of hemodynamic, electrocardiographic, mechanical, and metabolic indicators of intraoperative myocardial ischemia in vascular surgical patients with coronary artery disease. Anesthesiology 70:19, 1989
189. Hansen RM, Viquerat CE, Matthay MA, et al: Poor correlation between pulmonary arterial wedge pressure and left ventricular end-diastolic volume after coronary artery bypass graft surgery. Anesthesiology 64:764, 1986
190. Fontes ML, Bellows W, Ngo L, et al: Assessment of ventricular function in critically ill patients: Limitations of pulmonary artery catheterization. J Cardiothorac Vasc Anesth 13:521, 1999
191. Kumar A, Anel R, Bunnell E, et al: Pulmonary artery occlusion pressure and central venous pressure fail to predict ventricular filling volume, cardiac performance, or the response to volume infusion in normal subjects. Crit Care Med 32:691, 2004
192. Tuman KJ, McCarthy RJ, Spiess BD, et al: Effect of pulmonary artery catheterization on outcome in patients undergoing coronary artery surgery. Anesthesiology 70:199, 1989
193. Anonymous: Practice guidelines for pulmonary artery catheterization: An updated report by the American Society of Anesthesiologists Task Force on Pulmonary Artery Catheterization. Anesthesiology 99:988, 2003
194. Sandham JD, Hull RD, Brant RF, et al: A randomized, controlled trial of the use of pulmonary-artery catheters in high-risk surgical patients. N Engl J Med 348:5, 2003
195. Connors AF Jr, Speroff T, Dawson NV, et al: The effectiveness of right heart catheterization in the initial care of critically ill patients. SUPPORT Investigators. JAMA 276:889, 1996
196. Polanczyk CA, Rohde LE, Goldman L, et al: Right heart catheterization and cardiac complications in patients undergoing noncardiac surgery: An observational study. JAMA 286:309, 2001
197. Stewart RD, Psyhojos T, Lahey SJ, et al: Central venous catheter use in low-risk coronary artery bypass grafting. Ann Thorac Surg 66:1306, 1998
198. Ramsey SD, Saint S, Sullivan SD, et al: Clinical and economic effects of pulmonary artery catheterization in nonemergent coronary artery bypass graft surgery. J Cardiothorac Vasc Anesth 14:113, 2000
199. Schwann TA, Zacharias A, Riordan CJ, et al: Safe, highly selective use of pulmonary artery catheters in coronary artery bypass grafting: An objective patient selection method. Ann Thorac Surg 73:1394, 2002
200. London MJ, Moritz TE, Henderson WG, et al: Standard versus fiberoptic pulmonary artery catheterization for cardiac surgery in the Department of Veterans Affairs: A prospective, observational, multicenter analysis. Anesthesiology 96:860, 2002
201. Wall MH, MacGregor DA, Kennedy DJ, et al: Pulmonary artery catheter placement for elective coronary artery bypass grafting: Before or after anesthetic induction? Anesth Analg 94:1409, 2002
202. Szabo Z: A simple method to pass a pulmonary artery flotation catheter rapidly into the pulmonary artery in anaesthetized patients. Br J Anaesth 90:794, 2003
203. Comunale ME, Body SC, Ley C, et al: The concordance of intraoperative left ventricular wall-motion abnormalities and electrocardiographic

S-T segment changes: Association with outcome after coronary revascularization. Multicenter Study of Perioperative Ischemia (McSPI) Research Group. Anesthesiology 88:945, 1998
204. Skidmore KL, London MJ: Myocardial ischemia. Monitoring to diagnose ischemia: How do I monitor therapy? Anesthesiol Clin North Am 19:651, 2001
205. Shanewise JS, Cheung AT, Aronson S, et al: ASE/SCA guidelines for performing a comprehensive intraoperative multiplane transesophageal echocardiography examination: Recommendations of the American Society of Echocardiography Council for Intraoperative Echocardiography and the Society of Cardiovascular Anesthesiologists Task Force for Certification in Perioperative Transesophageal Echocardiography. Anesth Analg 89:870, 1999
206. Anonymous: Practice guidelines for perioperative transesophageal echocardiography. A report by the American Society of Anesthesiologists and the Society of Cardiovascular Anesthesiologists Task Force on Transesophageal Echocardiography. Anesthesiology 84:986, 1996
207. Morewood GH, Gallagher ME, Gaughan JP, et al: Current practice patterns for adult perioperative transesophageal echocardiography in the United States. Anesthesiology 95:1507, 2001
208. Kato M, Nakashima Y, Levine J, et al: Does transesophageal echocardiography improve postoperative outcome in patients undergoing coronary artery bypass surgery? J Cardiothorac Vasc Anesth 7:285, 1993
209. Bergquist BD, Leung JM, Bellows WH: Transesophageal echocardiography in myocardial revascularization: I. Accuracy of intraoperative realtime interpretation. Anesth Analg 82:1132, 1996
210. Bergquist BD, Bellows WH, Leung JM: Transesophageal echocardiography in myocardial revascularization. II. Influence on intraoperative decision making. Anesth Analg 82:1139, 1996
211. Jacka MJ, Cohen MM, To T, et al: The use of and preferences for the transesophageal echocardiogram and pulmonary artery catheter among cardiovascular anesthesiologists. Anesth Analg 94:1065, 2002
212. Hogue CWJ, Lappas GD, Creswell LL, et al: Swallowing dysfunction after cardiac operations. Associated adverse outcomes and risk factors including intraoperative transesophageal echocardiography. J Thorac Cardiovasc Surg 110:517, 1995
213. Brinkman WT, Shanewise JS, Clements SD, et al: Transesophageal echocardiography: Not an innocuous procedure. Ann Thorac Surg 72:1725, 2001
214. Han YY, Cheng YJ, Liao WW, et al: Delayed diagnosis of esophageal perforation following intraoperative transesophageal echocardiography during valvular replacement—a case report. Acta Anaesthesiol Sin 41:81, 2003
215. Lecharny JB, Philip I, Depoix JP: Oesophagotracheal perforation after intraoperative transoesphageal echocardiography in cardiac surgery. Br J Anaesth 88:592, 2002
216. Massey SR, Pitsis A, Mehta D, et al: Oesophageal perforation following perioperative transoesophageal echocardiography. Br J Anaesth 84:643, 2000
217. Zalunardo MP, Bimmler D, Grob UC, et al: Late oesophageal perforation after intraoperative transoesophageal echocardiography. Br J Anaesth 88:595, 2002
218. De Hert SG, Vermeyen KM, Adriaensen HF: Influence of thiopental, etomidate, and propofol on regional myocardial function in the normal and acute ischemic heart segment in dogs. Anesth Analg 70:600, 1990
219. Mulier JP: Cardiodynamic effects of propofol in comparison to thiopental. Use of the end-systolic pressure-volume relationship and arterial elastance. Anesth Analg 76:677, 1993
220. Mulier JP, Wouters PF, Van Aken H, et al: Cardiodynamic effects of propofol in comparison with thiopental: Assessment with a transesophageal echocardiographic approach. Anesth Analg 72:28, 1991
221. Rouby JJ, Andreev A, Leger P, et al: Peripheral vascular effects of thiopental and propofol in humans with artificial hearts. Anesthesiology 75:32, 1991
222. Gauss A, Heinrich H, Wilder-Smith OH: Echocardiographic assessment of the haemodynamic effects of propofol: A comparison with etomidate and thiopentone. Anaesthesia 46:99, 1991
223. Gelissen HP, Epema AH, Henning RH, et al: Inotropic effects of propofol, thiopental, midazolam, etomidate, and ketamine on isolated human atrial muscle. Anesthesiology 84:397, 1996
224. Mather LE, Duke CC, Ladd LA, et al: Direct cardiac effects of coronary site-directed thiopental and its enantiomers: A comparison to propofol in conscious sheep. Anesthesiology 101:354, 2004
225. Pagel PS, Kampine JP, Schmeling WT, et al: Ketamine depresses myocardial contractility as evaluated by the preload recruitable stroke work relationship in chronically instrumented dogs with autonomic nervous system blockade. Anesthesiology 76:564, 1992
226. Pagel PS, Schmeling WT, Kampine JP, et al: Alteration of canine left ventricular diastolic function by intravenous anesthetics in vivo. Ketamine and propofol. Anesthesiology 76:419, 1992
227. Zilberstein G, Levy R, Rachinsky M, et al: Ketamine attenuates neutrophil activation after cardiopulmonary bypass. Anesth Analg 95:531, 2002
228. Kissin I, Bright CA, Bradley EL Jr: The effect of ketamine on opioid-induced acute tolerance: Can it explain reduction of opioid consumption with ketamine-opioid analgesic combinations? Anesth Analg 91:1483, 2000
229. Luginbuhl M, Gerber A, Schnider TW, et al: Modulation of remifentanil-induced analgesia, hyperalgesia, and tolerance by small-dose ketamine in humans. Anesth Analg 96:726, 2003
230. Raza SM, Masters RW, Zsigmond EK: Haemodynamic stability with midazolam-ketamine-sufentanil analgesia in cardiac surgical patients. Can J Anaesth 36:617, 1989
231. Gordon AR, O'Connor JP, Ralley FE, et al: Midazolam-ketamine vs sufentanil for rapid sequence induction of anaesthesia for CABG surgery. Can J Anaesth 37:S43, 1990
232. Komai H, DeWitt DE, Rusy BF: Negative inotropic effect of etomidate in rabbit papillary muscle. Anesth Analg 64:400, 1985
233. Donmez A, Kaya H, Haberal A, et al: The effect of etomidate induction on plasma cortisol levels in children undergoing cardiac surgery. J Cardiothorac Vasc Anesth 12:182, 1998
234. Jackson WL Jr: Should we use etomidate as an induction agent for endotracheal intubation in patients with septic shock? A critical appraisal. Chest 127:1031, 2005
235. Shafer SL: Advances in propofol pharmacokinetics and pharmacodynamics. J Clin Anesth 5:14S, 1993
236. Barr J, Egan TD, Sandoval NF, et al: Propofol dosing regimens for ICU sedation based upon an integrated pharmacokinetic-pharmacodynamic model. Anesthesiology 95:324, 2001
237. Hall RI, MacLaren C, Smith MS, et al: Light versus heavy sedation after cardiac surgery: Myocardial ischemia and the stress response. Anesth Analg 85:971, 1997
238. Herr DL, Sum-Ping ST, England M: ICU sedation after coronary artery bypass graft surgery: Dexmedetomidine-based versus propofol-based sedation regimens. J Cardiothorac Vasc Anesth 17:576, 2003
239. Schmidt C, Roosens C, Struys M, et al: Contractility in humans after coronary artery surgery. Anesthesiology 91:58, 1999
240. Bell J, Sartain J, Wilkinson GA, et al: Propofol and fentanyl anaesthesia for patients with low cardiac output state undergoing cardiac surgery: Comparison with high-dose fentanyl anaesthesia. Br J Anaesth 73:162, 1994
241. Hall RI, Murphy JT, Moffitt EA, et al: A comparison of the myocardial metabolic and haemodynamic changes produced by propofol-sufentanil and enflurane-sufentanil anaesthesia for patients having coronary artery bypass graft surgery. Can J Anaesth 38:996, 1991
242. Hall RI, Murphy JT, Landymore R, et al: Myocardial metabolic and hemodynamic changes during propofol anesthesia for cardiac surgery in patients with reduced ventricular function. Anesth Analg 77:680, 1993
243. Jain U, Body SC, Bellows W, et al: Multicenter study of target-controlled infusion of propofol-sufentanil or sufentanil-midazolam for coronary artery bypass graft surgery. Multicenter Study of Perioperative Ischemia (McSPI) Research Group. Anesthesiology 85:522, 1996
244. Engoren MC, Kraras C, Garzia F: Propofol-based versus fentanyl-isoflurane-based anesthesia for cardiac surgery. J Cardiothorac Vasc Anesth 12:177, 1998
245. Sorbara C, Pittarello D, Rizzoli G, et al: Propofol-fentanyl versus isoflurane-fentanyl anesthesia for coronary artery bypass grafting: Effect on myocardial contractility and peripheral hemodynamics J Cardiothorac Vasc Anesth 9:18, 1995
246. De Hert SG, Van der Linden PJ, Cromheecke S, et al: Cardioprotective properties of sevoflurane in patients undergoing coronary surgery with cardiopulmonary bypass are related to the modalities of its administration. Anesthesiology 101:299, 2004
247. Conzen PF, Fischer S, Detter C, et al: Sevoflurane provides greater protection of the myocardium than propofol in patients undergoing off-pump coronary artery bypass surgery. Anesthesiology 99:826, 2003
248. Julier K, da Silva R, Garcia C, et al: Preconditioning by sevoflurane decreases biochemical markers for myocardial and renal dysfunction in coronary artery bypass graft surgery: A double-blinded, placebo-controlled, multicenter study. Anesthesiology 98:1315, 2003
249. Garcia C, Julier K, Bestmann L, et al: Preconditioning with sevoflurane decreases PECAM-1 expression and improves one-year cardiovascular outcome in coronary artery bypass graft surgery. Br J Anaesth 2004

250. Sayin MM, Ozatamer O, Tasoz R, et al: Propofol attenuates myocardial lipid peroxidation during coronary artery bypass grafting surgery. Br J Anaesth 89:242, 2002
251. Song D, Hamza M, White PF, et al: The pharmacodynamic effects of a lower-lipid emulsion of propofol: A comparison with the standard propofol emulsion. Anesth Analg 98:687, 2004
252. Fechner J, Ihmsen H, Hatterscheid D, et al: Pharmacokinetics and clinical pharmacodynamics of the new propofol prodrug GPI 15715 in volunteers. Anesthesiology 99:303, 2003
253. Brown CR, Sarnquist FH, Canup CA, et al: Clinical, electroencephalographic, and pharmacokinetic studies of a water-soluble benzodiazepine, midazolam maleate. Anesthesiology 50:467, 1979
254. Stanley TH, Bennett GM, Loeser EA, et al: Cardiovascular effects of diazepam and droperidol during morphine anesthesia. Anesthesiology 44:255, 1976
255. Stanley TH, Webster LR: Anesthetic requirements and cardiovascular effects of fentanyl-oxygen and fentanyl-diazepam-oxygen anesthesia in man. Anesth Analg 57:411, 1978
256. Liu WS, Bidwai AV, Stanley TH, et al: The cardiovascular effects of diazepam and of diazepam and pancuronium during fentanyl and oxygen anaesthesia. Can Anaesth Soc J 23:395, 1976
257. Benson KT, Tomlinson DL, Goto H, et al: Cardiovascular effects of lorazepam during sufentanil anesthesia. Anesth Analg 67:996, 1988
258. Samuelson PN, Reves JG, Kouchoukos NT, et al: Hemodynamic responses to anesthetic induction with midazolam or diazepam in patients with ischemic heart disease. Anesth Analg 60:802, 1981
259. Schulte-Sasse U, Hess W, Tarnow J: Haemodynamic responses to induction of anaesthesia using midazolam in cardiac surgical patients. Br J Anaesth 54:1053, 1982
260. Heikkila H, Jalonen J, Arola M, et al: Midazolam as adjunct to high-dose fentanyl anaesthesia for coronary artery bypass grafting operation. Acta Anaesthesiol Scand 28:683, 1984
261. Kawar P, Carson IW, Clarke RS, et al: Haemodynamic changes during induction of anaesthesia with midazolam and diazepam (Valium) in patients undergoing coronary artery bypass surgery. Anaesthesia 40:767, 1985
262. Raza SM, Zsigmond EK, Barabas E: Midazolam causes no adverse hemodynamic effects in cardiac patients. Clin Ther 10:40, 1987
263. Raza SM, Masters RW, Vasireddy AR, et al: Haemodynamic stability with midazolam-sufentanil analgesia in cardiac surgical patients. Can J Anaesth 35:518, 1988
264. Tuman KJ, McCarthy RJ, el-Ganzouri AR, et al: Sufentanil-midazolam anesthesia for coronary artery surgery. J Cardiothorac Anesth 4:308, 1990
265. van der Maaten JM, Epema AH, Huet RC, et al: The effect of midazolam at two plasma concentrations of hemodynamics and sufentanil requirement in coronary artery surgery. J Cardiothorac Vasc Anesth 10:356, 1996
266. Driessen JJ, Giart M: Comparison of isoflurane and midazolam as hypnotic supplementation to moderately high-dose fentanyl during coronary artery bypass grafting: Effects on systemic hemodynamics and early postoperative recovery profile. J Cardiothorac Vasc Anesth 11:740, 1997
267. Messina AG, Paranicas M, Yao FS, et al: The effect of midazolam on left ventricular pump performance and contractility in anesthetized patients with coronary artery disease: Effect of preoperative ejection fraction. Anesth Analg 81:793, 1995
268. Barvais L, Dejonckheere M, Dernovoi B, et al: Continuous infusion of midazolam or bolus of diazepam for postoperative sedation in cardiac surgical patients. Acta Anaesthesiol Belg 39:239, 1988
269. Somma J, Donner A, Zomorodi K, et al: Population pharmacodynamics of midazolam administered by target controlled infusion in SICU patients after CABG surgery. Anesthesiology 89:1430, 1998
270. Higgins TL, Yared JP, Estafanous FG, et al: Propofol versus midazolam for intensive care unit sedation after coronary artery bypass grafting. Crit Care Med 22:1415, 1994
271. Roekaerts PM, Huygen FJ, de Lange S: Infusion of propofol versus midazolam for sedation in the intensive care unit following coronary artery surgery. J Cardiothorac Vasc Anesth 7:142, 1993
272. Chaudhri S, Kenny GN: Sedation after cardiac bypass surgery: Comparison of propofol and midazolam in the presence of a computerized closed loop arterial pressure controller. Br J Anaesth 68:98, 1992
273. Carrasco G, Molina R, Costa J, et al: Propofol vs midazolam in short-, medium-, and long-term sedation of critically ill patients. A cost-benefit analysis. Chest 103:557, 1993
274. Lunn JK, Stanley TH, Eisele J, et al: High dose fentanyl anesthesia for coronary artery surgery: Plasma fentanyl concentrations and influence of nitrous oxide on cardiovascular responses. Anesth Analg 58:390, 1979
275. Bovill JG, Sebel PS: Pharmacokinetics of high-dose fentanyl. A study in patients undergoing cardiac surgery. Br J Anaesth 52:795, 1980
276. Prakash O, Verdouw PD, de Jong JW, et al: Haemodynamic and biochemical variables after induction of anaesthesia with fentanyl and nitrous oxide in patients undergoing coronary artery by-pass surgery. Can Anaesth Soc J 27:223, 1980
277. Sebel PS, Bovill JG, Schellekens AP, et al: Hormonal responses to high-dose fentanyl anaesthesia. A study in patients undergoing cardiac surgery. Br J Anaesth 53:941, 1981
278. Waller JL, Hug CC Jr, Nagle DM, et al: Hemodynamic changes during fentanyl—oxygen anesthesia for aortocoronary bypass operation. Anesthesiology 55:212, 1981
279. Walsh ES, Paterson JL, O'Riordan JB, et al: Effect of high-dose fentanyl anaesthesia on the metabolic and endocrine response to cardiac surgery. Br J Anaesth 53:1155, 1981
280. Sonntag H, Larsen R, Hilfiker O, et al: Myocardial blood flow and oxygen consumption during high-dose fentanyl anesthesia in patients with coronary artery disease. Anesthesiology 56:417, 1982
281. Hilgenberg JC: Intraoperative awareness during high-dose fentanyl—oxygen anesthesia. Anesthesiology 54:341, 1981
282. Dubois-Primo J, Dewachter B, Massaut J: Analgesic anesthesia with fentanyl (F) and sufentanil (SF) in coronary surgery. A double blind study. Acta Anaesthesiol Belg 30:113, 1979
283. de Lange S, Boscoe MJ, Stanley TH, et al: Antidiuretic and growth hormone responses during coronary artery surgery with sufentanil-oxygen and alfentanil-oxygen anesthesia in man. Anesth Analg 61:434, 1982
284. de Lange S, Boscoe MJ, Stanley TH, et al: Comparison of sufentanil—O_2 and fentanyl—O_2 for coronary artery surgery. Anesthesiology 56:112, 1982
285. Bovill JG, Sebel PS, Fiolet JW, et al: The influence of sufentanil on endocrine and metabolic responses to cardiac surgery. Anesth Analg 62:391, 1983
286. O'Young J, Mastrocostopoulos G, Hilgenberg A, et al: Myocardial circulatory and metabolic effects of isoflurane and sufentanil during coronary artery surgery. Anesthesiology 66:653, 1987
287. Thomson IR, Hudson RJ, Rosenbloom M, et al: A randomized double-blind comparison of fentanyl and sufentanil anaesthesia for coronary artery surgery. Can J Anaesth 34:227, 1987
288. Helman JD, Leung JM, Bellows WH, et al: The risk of myocardial ischemia in patients receiving desflurane versus sufentanil anesthesia for coronary artery bypass graft surgery. The S.P.I. Research Group. Anesthesiology 77:47, 1992
289. Spiess BD, Sathoff RH, El-Ganzouri ARS, et al: High-dose sufentanil: Four cases of sudden hypotension on induction. Anesth Analg 65:703, 1986
290. Starr NJ, Sethna DH, Estafanous FG: Bradycardia and asystole following the administration of sufentanil with vecuronium. Anesthesiology 64:521, 1986
291. de Lange S, Stanley TH, Boscoe MJ, et al: Catecholamine and cortisol responses to sufentanil-O_2 and alfentanil-O_2 anaesthesia during coronary artery surgery. Can Anaesth Soc J 30:248, 1983
292. Hynynen M, Takkunen O, Salmenpera M, et al: Continuous infusion of fentanyl or alfentanil for coronary artery surgery. Plasma opiate concentrations, haemodynamics and postoperative course. Br J Anaesth 58:1252, 1986
293. Robbins GR, Wynands JE, Whalley DG, et al: Pharmacokinetics of alfentanil and clinical responses during cardiac surgery. Can J Anaesth 37:52, 1990
294. Manara AR, Monk CR, Bolsin SN, et al: Total I.V. anaesthesia with propofol and alfentanil for coronary artery bypass grafting. Br J Anaesth 66:716, 1991
295. Tritapepe L, Voci P, Di Giovanni C, et al: Alfentanil and sufentanil in fast-track anesthesia for coronary artery bypass graft surgery. J Cardiothorac Vasc Anesth 16:157, 2002
296. Roekaerts PM, Gerrits HJ, Timmerman BE, et al: Continuous infusions of alfentanil and propofol for coronary artery surgery. J Cardiothorac Vasc Anesth 9:362, 1995
297. Egan TD, Lemmens HJ, Fiset P, et al: The pharmacokinetics of the new short-acting opioid remifentanil (GI87084B) in healthy adult male volunteers. Anesthesiology 79:881, 1993
298. Latham P, Zarate E, White PF, et al: Fast-track cardiac anesthesia: A comparison of remifentanil plus intrathecal morphine with sufentanil in a desflurane-based anesthetic. J Cardiothorac Vasc Anesth 14:645, 2000
299. Olivier P, Sirieix D, Dassier P, et al: Continuous infusion of remifentanil and target-controlled infusion of propofol for patients undergoing cardiac surgery: A new approach for scheduled early extubation. J Cardiothorac Vasc Anesth 14:29, 2000

300. Cheng DC, Newman MF, Duke P, et al: The efficacy and resource utilization of remifentanil and fentanyl in fast-track coronary artery bypass graft surgery: A prospective randomized, double-blinded controlled, multi-center trial. Anesth Analg 92:1094, 2001
301. Engoren M, Luther G, Fenn-Buderer N: A comparison of fentanyl, sufentanil, and remifentanil for fast-track cardiac anesthesia. Anesth Analg 93:859, 2001
302. Howie MB, Cheng D, Newman MF, et al: A randomized double-blinded multicenter comparison of remifentanil versus fentanyl when combined with isoflurane/propofol for early extubation in coronary artery bypass graft surgery. Anesth Analg 92:1084, 2001
303. Mollhoff T, Herregods L, Moerman A, et al: Comparative efficacy and safety of remifentanil and fentanyl in 'fast track' coronary artery bypass graft surgery: A randomized, double-blind study. Br J Anaesth 87:718, 2001
304. Myles PS, Hunt JO, Fletcher H, et al: Remifentanil, fentanyl, and cardiac surgery: A double-blinded, randomized, controlled trial of costs and outcomes. Anesth Analg 95:805, 2002
305. Reddy P, Feret BM, Kulicki L, et al: Cost analysis of fentanyl and remifentanil in coronary artery bypass graft surgery without cardiopulmonary bypass. J Clin Pharm Ther 27:127, 2002
306. Elliott P, O'Hare R, Bill KM, et al: Severe cardiovascular depression with remifentanil. Anesth Analg 91:58, 2000
307. Pleym H, Stenseth R, Wiseth R, et al: Supplemental remifentanil during coronary artery bypass grafting is followed by a transient postoperative cardiac depression. Acta Anaesthesiol Scand 48:1155, 2004
308. Shafer SL, Varvel JR: Pharmacokinetics, pharmacodynamics, and rational opioid selection. Anesthesiology 74:53, 1991
309. Ethuin F, Boudaoud S, Leblanc I, et al: Pharmacokinetics of long-term sufentanil infusion for sedation in ICU patients. Intensive Care Med 29:1916, 2003
310. Sanford TJ, Smith NT, Dec-Silver H, et al: A comparison of morphine, fentanyl, and sufentanil anesthesia for cardiac surgery: Induction, emergence, and extubation. Anesth Analg 65:259, 1986
311. London MJ, Shroyer ALW, Grover FL: Fast tracking into the new millennium: An evolving paradigm. Anesthesiology 91:936, 1999
312. Wynands JE, Townsend GE, Wong P, et al: Blood pressure response and plasma fentanyl concentrations during high- and very-high-dose fentanyl anesthesia for coronary artery surgery. Anesth Analg 62:661, 1983
313. Lacoumenta S, Yeo TH, Paterson JL, et al: Hormonal and metabolic responses to cardiac surgery with sufentanil-oxygen anaesthesia. Acta Anaesthesiol Scand 31:258, 1987
314. Thomson IR, Hudson RJ, Rosenbloom M, et al: Catecholamine responses to anesthetic induction with fentanyl and sufentanil. J Cardiothorac Anesth 2:18, 1988
315. Sonntag H, Stephan H, Lange H, et al: Sufentanil does not block sympathetic responses to surgical stimuli in patients having coronary artery revascularization surgery. Anesth Analg 68:584, 1989
316. Philbin DM, Rosow CE, Schneider RC, et al: Fentanyl and sufentanil anesthesia revisited: How much is enough? Anesthesiology 73:5, 1990
317. Thomson IR, Henderson BT, Singh K, et al: Concentration-response relationships for fentanyl and sufentanil in patients undergoing coronary artery bypass grafting. Anesthesiology 89:852, 1998
318. Cope DK, Impastato WK, Cohen MV, et al: Volatile anesthetics protect the ischemic rabbit myocardium from infarction. Anesthesiology 86:699, 1997
319. Wu ZK, Iivainen T, Pehkonen E, et al: Arrhythmias in off-pump coronary artery bypass grafting and the antiarrhythmic effect of regional ischemic preconditioning. J Cardiothorac Vasc Anesth 17:459, 2003
320. Meissner A, Weber TP, Van Aken H, et al: Recovery from myocardial stunning is faster with desflurane compared with propofol in chronically instrumented dogs. Anesth Analg 91:1333, 2000
321. Novalija E, Hogan QH, Kulier AH, et al: Effects of desflurane, sevoflurane and halothane on postinfarction spontaneous dysrhythmias in dogs. Acta Anaesthesiol Scand 42:353, 1998
322. El Azab SR, Rosseel PM, De Lange JJ, et al: Effect of sevoflurane on the ex vivo secretion of TNF-alpha during and after coronary artery bypass surgery. Eur J Anaesthesiol 20:380, 2003
323. Kowalski C, Zahler S, Becker BF, et al: Halothane, isoflurane, and sevoflurane reduce postischemic adhesion of neutrophils in the coronary system. Anesthesiology 86:188, 1997
324. Heindl B, Becker BF, Zahler S, et al: Volatile anaesthetics reduce adhesion of blood platelets under low-flow conditions in the coronary system of isolated guinea pig hearts. Acta Anaesthesiol Scand 42:995, 1998
325. Heindl B, Reichle FM, Zahler S, et al: Sevoflurane and isoflurane protect the reperfused guinea pig heart by reducing postischemic adhesion of polymorphonuclear neutrophils. Anesthesiology 91:521, 1999
326. Heindl B, Conzen PF, Becker BF: The volatile anesthetic sevoflurane mitigates cardiodepressive effects of platelets in reperfused hearts. Basic Res Cardiol 94:102, 1999
327. Hu G, Salem MR, Crystal GJ: Isoflurane and sevoflurane precondition against neutrophil-induced contractile dysfunction in isolated rat hearts. Anesthesiology 100:489, 2004
328. Zaugg M, Lucchinetti E, Garcia C, et al: Anaesthetics and cardiac preconditioning. Part II. Clinical implications. Br J Anaesth 91:566, 2003
329. Murry CE, Jennings RB, Reimer KA: Preconditioning with ischemia: A delay of lethal cell injury in ischemic myocardium. Circulation 74:1124, 1986
330. Zaugg M, Lucchinetti E, Uecker M, et al: Anaesthetics and cardiac preconditioning. Part I. Signalling and cytoprotective mechanisms. Br J Anaesth 91:551, 2003
331. Stein KL, Breisblatt W, Wolfe C, et al: Depression and recovery of right ventricular function after cardiopulmonary bypass. Crit Care Med 18:1197, 1990
332. Breisblatt WM, Stein KL, Wolfe CJ, et al: Acute myocardial dysfunction and recovery: A common occurrence after coronary bypass surgery. J Am Coll Cardiol 15:1261, 1990
333. Illes RW, Swoyer KD: Prospective, randomized clinical study of ischemic preconditioning as an adjunct to intermittent cold blood cardioplegia. Ann Thorac Surg 65:748, 1998
334. Laurikka J, Wu ZK, Iisalo P, et al: Regional ischemic preconditioning enhances myocardial performance in off-pump coronary artery bypass grafting. Chest 121:1183, 2002
335. Jenkins DP, Pugsley WB, Alkhulaifi AM, et al: Ischaemic preconditioning reduces troponin T release in patients undergoing coronary artery bypass surgery. Heart 77:314, 1997
336. Baldwin D, Chandrashekhar Y, McFalls E, et al: Ischemic preconditioning prior to aortic cross-clamping protects high-energy phosphate levels, glucose uptake, and myocyte contractility. J Surg Res 105:153, 2002
337. Tanaka K, Ludwig LM, Kersten JR, et al: Mechanisms of cardioprotection by volatile anesthetics. Anesthesiology 100:707, 2004
338. Riess ML, Stowe DF, Warltier DC: Cardiac pharmacological preconditioning with volatile anesthetics: From bench to bedside? Am J Physiol Heart Circ Physiol 286:H1603, 2004
339. Kudo M, Wang Y, Xu M, et al: Adenosine A(1) receptor mediates late preconditioning via activation of PKC-delta signaling pathway. Am J Physiol Heart Circ Physiol 283:H296, 2002
340. Zhao TC, Hines DS, Kukreja RC: Adenosine-induced late preconditioning in mouse hearts: Role of p38 MAP kinase and mitochondrial K(ATP) channels. Am J Physiol Heart Circ Physiol 280:H1278, 2001
341. Leesar MA, Stoddard MF, Dawn B, et al: Delayed preconditioning-mimetic action of nitroglycerin in patients undergoing coronary angioplasty. Circulation 103:2935, 2001
342. Leesar MA, Stoddard MF, Manchikalapudi S, et al: Bradykinin-induced preconditioning in patients undergoing coronary angioplasty. J Am Coll Cardiol 34:639, 1999
343. Cohen MV, Yang XM, Liu GS, et al: Acetylcholine, bradykinin, opioids, and phenylephrine, but not adenosine, trigger preconditioning by generating free radicals and opening mitochondrial K(ATP) channels. Circ Res 89:273, 2001
344. Wolfrum S, Schneider K, Heidbreder M, et al: Remote preconditioning protects the heart by activating myocardial PKCepsilon-isoform. Cardiovasc Res 55:583, 2002
345. da Silva R, Grampp T, Pasch T, et al: Differential activation of mitogen-activated protein kinases in ischemic and anesthetic preconditioning. Anesthesiology 100:59, 2004
346. Laude K, Favre J, Thuillez C, et al: NO produced by endothelial NO synthase is a mediator of delayed preconditioning-induced endothelial protection. Am J Physiol Heart Circ Physiol 284:H2053, 2003
347. Bell RM, Yellon DM: The contribution of endothelial nitric oxide synthase to early ischaemic preconditioning: The lowering of the preconditioning threshold. An investigation in eNOS knockout mice. Cardiovasc Res 52:274, 2001
348. Alcindor D, Krolikowski JG, Pagel PS, et al: Cyclooxygenase-2 mediates ischemic, anesthetic, and pharmacologic preconditioning in vivo. Anesthesiology 100:547, 2004
349. Zaugg M, Schaub MC: Signaling and cellular mechanisms in cardiac protection by ischemic and pharmacological preconditioning. J Muscle Res Cell Motil 24:219, 2003
350. Belhomme D, Peynet J, Louzy M, et al: Evidence for preconditioning by isoflurane in coronary artery bypass graft surgery. Circulation 100:II340, 1999

351. Penta de Peppo A, Polisca P, Tomai F, et al: Recovery of LV contractility in man is enhanced by preischemic administration of enflurane. Ann Thorac Surg 68:112, 1999
352. Nader ND, Li CM, Khadra WZ, et al: Anesthetic myocardial protection with sevoflurane. J Cardiothorac Vasc Anesth 18:269, 2004
353. Tomai F, De Paulis R, Penta de Peppo A, et al: Beneficial impact of isoflurane during coronary bypass surgery on troponin I release. G Ital Cardiol 29:1007, 1999
354. Haroun-Bizri S, Khoury SS, Chehab IR, et al: Does isoflurane optimize myocardial protection during cardiopulmonary bypass? J Cardiothorac Vasc Anesth 15:418, 2001
355. Ludwig LM, Patel HH, Gross GJ, et al: Morphine enhances pharmacological preconditioning by isoflurane: Role of mitochondrial K(ATP) channels and opioid receptors. Anesthesiology 98:705, 2003
356. Bolling SF, Badhwar V, Schwartz CF, et al: Opioids confer myocardial tolerance to ischemia: Interaction of delta opioid agonists and antagonists. J Thorac Cardiovasc Surg 122:476, 2001
357. Wei M, Wang X, Kuukasjarvi P, et al: Bradykinin preconditioning in coronary artery bypass grafting. Ann Thorac Surg 78:492, 2004
358. Muraki S, Morris CD, Budde JM, et al: Experimental off-pump coronary artery revascularization with adenosine-enhanced reperfusion. J Thorac Cardiovasc Surg 121:570, 2001
359. Toller WG, Kersten JR, Pagel PS, et al: Sevoflurane reduces myocardial infarct size and decreases the time threshold for ischemic preconditioning in dogs. Anesthesiology 91:1437, 1999
360. Kehl F, Krolikowski JG, Mraovic B, et al: Is isoflurane-induced preconditioning dose related? Anesthesiology 96:675, 2002
361. Riess ML, Kevin LG, Camara AK, et al: Dual exposure to sevoflurane improves anesthetic preconditioning in intact hearts. Anesthesiology 100:569, 2004
362. Ghosh S, Galinanes M: Protection of the human heart with ischemic preconditioning during cardiac surgery: Role of cardiopulmonary bypass. J Thorac Cardiovasc Surg 126:133, 2003
363. Laskey WK, Beach D: Frequency and clinical significance of ischemic preconditioning during percutaneous coronary intervention. J Am Coll Cardiol 42:998, 2003
364. Kersten JR, Schmeling TJ, Orth KG, et al: Acute hyperglycemia abolishes ischemic preconditioning in vivo. Am J Physiol 275:H721, 1998
365. Kehl F, Krolikowski JG, Mraovic B, et al: Hyperglycemia prevents isoflurane-induced preconditioning against myocardial infarction. Anesthesiology 96:183, 2002
366. Kehl F, Krolikowski JG, Weihrauch D, et al: *N*-acetylcysteine restores isoflurane-induced preconditioning against myocardial infarction during hyperglycemia. Anesthesiology 98:1384, 2003
367. Kersten JR, Toller WG, Gross ER, et al: Diabetes abolishes ischemic preconditioning: Role of glucose, insulin, and osmolality. Am J Physiol Heart Circ Physiol 278:H1218, 2000
368. Zaugg M, Lucchinetti E, Spahn DR, et al: Differential effects of anesthetics on mitochondrial K(ATP) channel activity and cardiomyocyte protection. Anesthesiology 97:15, 2002
369. Ebert TJ, Muzi M, Lopatka CW: Neurocirculatory responses to sevoflurane in humans. A comparison to desflurane. Anesthesiology 83:88, 1995
370. Ebert TJ, Harkin CP, Muzi M: Cardiovascular responses to sevoflurane: A review. Anesth Analg 81:S11, 1995
371. Bennett SR, Griffin SC: Sevoflurane versus isoflurane in patients undergoing coronary artery bypass grafting: A hemodynamic and recovery study. J Cardiothorac Vasc Anesth 13:666, 1999
372. Hara T, Tomiyasu S, Sungsam C, et al: Sevoflurane protects stunned myocardium through activation of mitochondrial ATP-sensitive potassium channels. Anesth Analg 92:1139, 2001
373. Chen Q, Camara AK, An J, et al: Sevoflurane preconditioning before moderate hypothermic ischemia protects against cytosolic [Ca(2+)] loading and myocardial damage in part via mitochondrial K(ATP) channels. Anesthesiology 97:912, 2002
374. Kersten JR, Brayer AP, Pagel PS, et al: Perfusion of ischemic myocardium during anesthesia with sevoflurane. Anesthesiology 81:995, 1994
375. Kitahata H, Kawahito S, Nozaki J, et al: Effects of sevoflurane on regional myocardial blood flow distribution: quantification with myocardial contrast echocardiography. Anesthesiology 90:1436, 1999
376. Searle NR, Martineau RJ, Conzen P, et al: Comparison of sevoflurane/fentanyl and isoflurane/fentanyl during elective coronary artery bypass surgery. Sevoflurane Venture Group. Can J Anaesth 43:890, 1996
377. Rooke GA, Ebert T, Muzi M, et al: The hemodynamic and renal effects of sevoflurane and isoflurane in patients with coronary artery disease and chronic hypertension. Sevoflurane Ischemia Study Group. Anesth Analg 82:1159, 1996
378. Ebert TJ, Kharasch ED, Rooke GA, et al: Myocardial ischemia and adverse cardiac outcomes in cardiac patients undergoing noncardiac surgery with sevoflurane and isoflurane. Sevoflurane Ischemia Study Group. Anesth Analg 85:993, 1997
379. Kleinsasser A, Kuenszberg E, Loeckinger A, et al: Sevoflurane, but not propofol, significantly prolongs the Q-T interval. Anesth Analg 90:25, 2000
380. Kuenszberg E, Loeckinger A, Kleinsasser A, et al: Sevoflurane progressively prolongs the QT interval in unpremedicated female adults. Eur J Anaesthesiol 17:662, 2000
381. Sakamoto H, Mayumi T, Morimoto Y, et al: Sevoflurane metabolite production in a small cohort of coronary artery bypass graft surgery patients. J Cardiothorac Vasc Anesth 16:463, 2002
382. Story DA, Poustie S, Liu G, et al: Changes in plasma creatinine concentration after cardiac anesthesia with isoflurane, propofol, or sevoflurane: A randomized clinical trial. Anesthesiology 95:842, 2001
383. Kharasch ED, Frink EJ Jr, Artru A, et al: Long-duration low-flow sevoflurane and isoflurane effects on postoperative renal and hepatic function. Anesth Analg 93:1511, 2001
384. Litz RJ, Hubler M, Lorenz W, et al: Renal responses to desflurane and isoflurane in patients with renal insufficiency. Anesthesiology 97:1133, 2002
385. Higuchi H, Adachi Y, Wada H, et al: The effects of low-flow sevoflurane and isoflurane anesthesia on renal function in patients with stable moderate renal insufficiency. Anesth Analg 92:650, 2001
386. Woehlck HJ: Sleeping with uncertainty: Anesthetics and desiccated absorbent. Anesthesiology 101:276, 2004
387. Laster M, Roth P, Eger EI 2nd: Fires from the interaction of anesthetics with desiccated absorbent. Anesth Analg 99:769, 2004
388. Lowe D, Hettrick DA, Pagel PS, et al: Influence of volatile anesthetics on left ventricular afterload in vivo. Differences between desflurane and sevoflurane. Anesthesiology 85:112, 1996
389. Weiskopf RB: Cardiovascular effects of desflurane in experimental animals and volunteers. Anaesthesia 50(suppl):14, 1995
390. Grundmann U, Muller M, Kleinschmidt S, et al: Cardiovascular effects of desflurane and isoflurane in patients with coronary artery disease. Acta Anaesthesiol Scand 40:1101, 1996
391. Weiskopf RB, Moore MA, Eger EI 2nd, et al: Rapid increase in desflurane concentration is associated with greater transient cardiovascular stimulation than with rapid increase in isoflurane concentration in humans. Anesthesiology 80:1035, 1994
392. Moore MA, Weiskopf RB, Eger EI 2nd, et al: Rapid 1% increases of end-tidal desflurane concentration to greater than 5% transiently increase heart rate and blood pressure in humans. Anesthesiology 81:94, 1994
393. Muzi M, Lopatka CW, Ebert TJ: Desflurane-mediated neurocirculatory activation in humans. Effects of concentration and rate of change on responses. Anesthesiology 84:1035, 1996
394. Weiskopf RB, Eger EI 2nd, Noorani M, et al: Repetitive rapid increases in desflurane concentration blunt transient cardiovascular stimulation in humans. Anesthesiology 81:843, 1994
395. Leung JM, Pastor DA: Dissociation between haemodynamics and sympathetic activation during anaesthetic induction with desflurane. Can J Anaesth 45:533, 1998
396. Muzi M, Ebert TJ, Hope WG, et al: Site(s) mediating sympathetic activation with desflurane. Anesthesiology 85:737, 1996
397. Rodig G, Keyl C, Kaluza M, et al: Effects of rapid increases of desflurane and sevoflurane to concentrations of 1.5 MAC on systemic vascular resistance and catecholamine response during cardiopulmonary bypass. Anesthesiology 87:801, 1997
398. Weiskopf RB, Eger EI, Daniel M, et al: Cardiovascular stimulation induced by rapid increases in desflurane concentration in humans results from activation of tracheopulmonary and systemic receptors. Anesthesiology 83:1173, 1995
399. Gormley WP, Murray JM, Trinick TR: Intravenous lidocaine does not attenuate the cardiovascular and catecholamine response to a rapid increase in desflurane concentration. Anesth Analg 82:358, 1996
400. Pacentine GG, Muzi M, Ebert TJ: Effects of fentanyl on sympathetic activation associated with the administration of desflurane. Anesthesiology 82:823, 1995
401. Weiskopf RB, Eger EI 2nd, Noorani M, et al: Fentanyl, esmolol, and clonidine blunt the transient cardiovascular stimulation induced by desflurane in humans. Anesthesiology 81:1350, 1994
402. Toller WG, Gross ER, Kersten JR, et al: Sarcolemmal and mitochondrial adenosine triphosphate-dependent potassium channels: Mechanism of desflurane-induced cardioprotection. Anesthesiology 92:1731, 2000
403. Piriou V, Chiari P, Gateau-Roesch O, et al: Desflurane-induced preconditioning alters calcium-induced mitochondrial permeability transition. Anesthesiology 100:581, 2004

404. Tsai SK, Lin SM, Huang CH, et al: Effect of desflurane-induced preconditioning following ischemia-reperfusion on nitric oxide release in rabbits. Life Sci 76:651, 2004
405. Hanouz JL, Yvon A, Massetti M, et al: Mechanisms of desflurane-induced preconditioning in isolated human right atria in vitro. Anesthesiology 97:33, 2002
406. Kersten JR, Schmeling TJ, Pagel PS, et al: Isoflurane mimics ischemic preconditioning via activation of K(ATP) channels: Reduction of myocardial infarct size with an acute memory phase. Anesthesiology 87:361, 1997
407. Cason BA, Gamperl AK, Slocum RE, et al: Anesthetic-induced preconditioning: Previous administration of isoflurane decreases myocardial infarct size in rabbits. Anesthesiology 87:1182, 1997
408. Tanaka K, Weihrauch D, Kehl F, et al: Mechanism of preconditioning by isoflurane in rabbits: A direct role for reactive oxygen species. Anesthesiology 97:1485, 2002
409. Ludwig LM, Tanaka K, Eells JT, et al: Preconditioning by isoflurane is mediated by reactive oxygen species generated from mitochondrial electron transport chain complex III. Anesth Analg 99:1308, 2004
410. Mullenheim J, Ebel D, Frassdorf J, et al: Isoflurane preconditions myocardium against infarction via release of free radicals. Anesthesiology 96:934, 2002
411. Kehl F, Pagel PS, Krolikowski JG, et al: Isoflurane does not produce a second window of preconditioning against myocardial infarction in vivo. Anesth Analg 95:1162, 2002
412. Tanaka K, Ludwig LM, Krolikowski JG, et al: Isoflurane produces delayed preconditioning against myocardial ischemia and reperfusion injury: Role of cyclooxygenase-2. Anesthesiology 100:525, 2004
413. Boutros A, Wang J, Capuano C: Isoflurane and halothane increase adenosine triphosphate preservation, but do not provide additive recovery of function after ischemia, in preconditioned rat hearts. Anesthesiology 86:109, 1997
414. Piriou V, Chiari P, Lhuillier F, et al: Pharmacological preconditioning: Comparison of desflurane, sevoflurane, isoflurane and halothane in rabbit myocardium. Br J Anaesth 89:486, 2002
415. Roscoe AK, Christensen JD, Lynch C 3rd: Isoflurane, but not halothane, induces protection of human myocardium via adenosine A1 receptors and adenosine triphosphate-sensitive potassium channels. Anesthesiology 92:1692, 2000
416. Kwok WM, Martinelli AT, Fujimoto K, et al: Differential modulation of the cardiac adenosine triphosphate-sensitive potassium channel by isoflurane and halothane. Anesthesiology 97:50, 2002
417. Bloor BC, Ward DS, Belleville JP, et al: Effects of intravenous dexmedetomidine in humans. II. Hemodynamic changes. Anesthesiology 77:1134, 1992
418. Talke P, Richardson CA, Scheinin M, et al: Postoperative pharmacokinetics and sympatholytic effects of dexmedetomidine. Anesth Analg 85:1136, 1997
419. Ebert TJ, Hall JE, Barney JA, et al: The effects of increasing plasma concentrations of dexmedetomidine in humans. Anesthesiology 93:382, 2000
420. Flacke WE, Flacke JW, Bloor BC, et al: Effects of dexmedetomidine on systemic and coronary hemodynamics in the anesthetized dog. J Cardiothorac Vasc Anesth 7:41, 1993
421. Coughlan MG, Lee JG, Bosnjak ZJ, et al: Direct coronary and cerebral vascular responses to dexmedetomidine. Significance of endogenous nitric oxide synthesis. Anesthesiology 77:998, 1992
422. Talke P, Lobo E, Brown R: Systemically administered alpha2-agonist-induced peripheral vasoconstriction in humans. Anesthesiology 99:65, 2003
423. Jalonen J, Hynynen M, Kuitunen A, et al: Dexmedetomidine as an anesthetic adjunct in coronary artery bypass grafting. Anesthesiology 86:331, 1997
424. Lawrence CJ, Prinzen FW, de Lange S: The effect of dexmedetomidine on the balance of myocardial energy requirement and oxygen supply and demand. Anesth Analg 82:544, 1996
425. Roekaerts PM, Prinzen FW, de Lange S: Coronary vascular effects of dexmedetomidine during reactive hyperemia in the anesthetized dog. J Cardiothorac Vasc Anesth 10:619, 1996
426. Roekaerts PM, Prinzen FW, De Lange S: Beneficial effects of dexmedetomidine on ischaemic myocardium of anaesthetized dogs. Br J Anaesth 77:427, 1996
427. De Wolf AM, Fragen RJ, Avram MJ, et al: The pharmacokinetics of dexmedetomidine in volunteers with severe renal impairment. Anesth Analg 93:1205, 2001
428. Talke P, Chen R, Thomas B, et al: The hemodynamic and adrenergic effects of perioperative dexmedetomidine infusion after vascular surgery. Anesth Analg 90:834, 2000
429. Hogue CW Jr, Talke P, Stein PK, et al: Autonomic nervous system responses during sedative infusions of dexmedetomidine. Anesthesiology 97:592, 2002
430. Lawrence CJ, De Lange S: Effects of a single pre-operative dexmedetomidine dose on isoflurane requirements and peri-operative haemodynamic stability. Anaesthesia 52:736, 1997
431. Ruesch S, Levy JH: Treatment of persistent tachycardia with dexmedetomidine during off-pump cardiac surgery. Anesth Analg 95:316, 2002
432. Taniguchi T, Kidani Y, Kanakura H, et al: Effects of dexmedetomidine on mortality rate and inflammatory responses to endotoxin-induced shock in rats. Crit Care Med 32:1322, 2004
433. Hsu YW, Cortinez LI, Robertson KM, et al: Dexmedetomidine pharmacodynamics. Part I. Crossover comparison of the respiratory effects of dexmedetomidine and remifentanil in healthy volunteers. Anesthesiology 101:1066, 2004
434. Venn RM, Hell J, Grounds RM: Respiratory effects of dexmedetomidine in the surgical patient requiring intensive care. Crit Care 4:302, 2000
435. Venn RM, Grounds RM: Comparison between dexmedetomidine and propofol for sedation in the intensive care unit: Patient and clinician perceptions. Br J Anaesth 87:684, 2001
436. Martin E, Ramsay G, Mantz J, et al: The role of the alpha2-adrenoceptor agonist dexmedetomidine in postsurgical sedation in the intensive care unit. J Intensive Care Med 18:29, 2003
437. Triltsch AE, Welte M, von Homeyer P, et al: Bispectral index-guided sedation with dexmedetomidine in intensive care: A prospective, randomized, double blind, placebo-controlled phase II study. Crit Care Med 30:1007, 2002
438. Arain SR, Ruehlow RM, Uhrich TD, et al: The efficacy of dexmedetomidine versus morphine for postoperative analgesia after major inpatient surgery. Anesth Analg 98:153, 2004
439. Dobrydnjov I, Axelsson K, Berggren L, et al: Intrathecal and oral clonidine as prophylaxis for postoperative alcohol withdrawal syndrome: A randomized double-blinded study. Anesth Analg 98:738, 2004
440. Kranke P, Eberhart LH, Roewer N, et al: Single-dose parenteral pharmacological interventions for the prevention of postoperative shivering: A quantitative systematic review of randomized controlled trials. Anesth Analg 99:718, 2004
441. Murphy GS, Szokol JW, Vender JS, et al: The use of neuromuscular blocking drugs in adult cardiac surgery: Results of a national postal survey. Anesth Analg 95:1534, 2002
442. O'Connor JP, Ramsay JG, Wynands JE, et al: The incidence of myocardial ischemia during anesthesia for coronary artery bypass surgery in patients receiving pancuronium or vecuronium. Anesthesiology 70:230, 1989
443. McEwin L, Merrick PM, Bevan DR: Residual neuromuscular blockade after cardiac surgery: Pancuronium vs rocuronium. Can J Anaesth 44:891, 1997
444. Murphy GS, Szokol JW, Marymont JH, et al: Impact of shorter-acting neuromuscular blocking agents on fast-track recovery of the cardiac surgical patient. Anesthesiology 96:600, 2002
445. Thomas R, Smith D, Strike P: Prospective randomised double-blind comparative study of rocuronium and pancuronium in adult patients scheduled for elective 'fast-track' cardiac surgery involving hypothermic cardiopulmonary bypass. Anaesthesia 58:265, 2003
446. Jellish WS, Brody M, Sawicki K, et al: Recovery from neuromuscular blockade after either bolus and prolonged infusions of cisatracurium or rocuronium using either isoflurane or propofol-based anesthetics. Anesth Analg 91:1250, 2000
447. Reich DL, Hollinger I, Harrington DJ, et al: Comparison of cisatracurium and vecuronium by infusion in neonates and small infants after congenital heart surgery. Anesthesiology 101:1122, 2004
448. Murphy GS, Szokol JW, Marymont JH, et al: Recovery of neuromuscular function after cardiac surgery: Pancuronium versus rocuronium. Anesth Analg 96:1301, 2003
449. Cammu G, De Keersmaecker K, Casselman F, et al: Implications of the use of neuromuscular transmission monitoring on immediate postoperative extubation in off-pump coronary artery bypass surgery. Eur J Anaesthesiol 20:884, 2003
450. Pinard AM, Donati F, Martineau R, et al: Magnesium potentiates neuromuscular blockade with cisatracurium during cardiac surgery. Can J Anaesth 50:172, 2003
451. Gueret G, Rossignol B, Kiss G, et al: Is muscle relaxant necessary for cardiac surgery? Anesth Analg 99:1330; 2004
452. Adams DC, Hilton HJ, Madigan JD, et al: Evidence for unconscious memory processing during elective cardiac surgery. Circulation 98:II289, 1998

453. Sebel PS, Bowdle TA, Ghoneim MM, et al: The incidence of awareness during anesthesia: A multicenter United States study. Anesth Analg 99:833, 2004
454. Goldmann L, Shah MV, Hebden MW: Memory of cardiac anaesthesia. Psychological sequelae in cardiac patients of intra-operative suggestion and operating room conversation. Anaesthesia 42:596, 1987
455. Ranta SO, Herranen P, Hynynen M: Patients' conscious recollections from cardiac anesthesia. J Cardiothorac Vasc Anesth 16:426, 2002
456. Phillips AA, McLean RF, Devitt JH, et al: Recall of intraoperative events after general anaesthesia and cardiopulmonary bypass. Can J Anaesth 40:922, 1993
457. Dowd NP, Cheng DC, Karski JM, et al: Intraoperative awareness in fast-track cardiac anesthesia. Anesthesiology 89:1068, 1998
458. Sandin RH, Enlund G, Samuelsson P, et al: Awareness during anaesthesia: A prospective case study. Lancet 355:707, 2000
459. Kerssens C, Klein J, Bonke B: Awareness: Monitoring versus remembering what happened. Anesthesiology 99:570, 2003
460. White PF, Tang J, Ma H, et al: Is the patient state analyzer with the PSArray2 a cost-effective alternative to the Bispectral Index monitor during the perioperative period? Anesth Analg 99:1429, 2004
461. Bauer M, Wilhelm W, Kraemer T, et al: Impact of Bispectral Index monitoring on stress response and propofol consumption in patients undergoing coronary artery bypass surgery. Anesthesiology 101:1096, 2004
462. Schmidt GN, Bischoff P, Standl T, et al: SNAP index and Bispectral Index during different states of propofol/remifentanil anaesthesia. Anaesthesia 60:228, 2005
463. Schmidt GN, Bischoff P, Standl T, et al: Comparative evaluation of Narcotrend, Bispectral Index, and classical electroencephalographic variables during induction, maintenance, and emergence of a propofol/remifentanil anesthesia. Anesth Analg 98:1346, 2004
464. Ellerkmann RK, Liermann VM, Alves TM, et al: Spectral entropy and Bispectral Index as measures of the electroencephalographic effects of sevoflurane. Anesthesiology 101:1275, 2004
465. Myles PS, Leslie K, McNeil J, et al: Bispectral Index monitoring to prevent awareness during anaesthesia: The B-Aware randomised controlled trial. Lancet 363:1757, 2004
466. Ekman A, Lindholm ML, Lennmarken C, et al: Reduction in the incidence of awareness using BIS monitoring. Acta Anaesthesiol Scand 48:20, 2004
467. Barr G, Anderson RE, Samuelsson S, et al: Fentanyl and midazolam anaesthesia for coronary bypass surgery: A clinical study of bispectral electroencephalogram analysis, drug concentrations and recall. Br J Anaesth 84:749, 2000
468. Puri GD, Murthy SS: Bispectral Index monitoring in patients undergoing cardiac surgery under cardiopulmonary bypass. Eur J Anaesthesiol 20:451, 2003
469. Heck M, Kumle B, Boldt J, et al: Electroencephalogram Bispectral Index predicts hemodynamic and arousal reactions during induction of anesthesia in patients undergoing cardiac surgery. J Cardiothorac Vasc Anesth 14:693, 2000
470. Forestier F, Hirschi M, Rouget P, et al: Propofol and sufentanil titration with the Bispectral Index to provide anesthesia for coronary artery surgery. Anesthesiology 99:334, 2003
471. Lehmann A, Karzau J, Boldt J, et al: Bispectral Index-guided anesthesia in patients undergoing aortocoronary bypass grafting. Anesth Analg 96:336, 2003
472. Ranta SO, Laurila R, Saario J, et al: Awareness with recall during general anesthesia: Incidence and risk factors. Anesth Analg 86:1084, 1998
473. Lennmarken C, Bildfors K, Enlund G, et al: Victims of awareness. Acta Anaesthesiol Scand 46:229, 2002
474. Blomberg S, Curelaru I, Emanuelsson H, et al: Thoracic epidural anaesthesia in patients with unstable angina pectoris. Eur Heart J 10:437, 1989
475. Gramling-Babb P, Miller MJ, Reeves ST, et al: Treatment of medically and surgically refractory angina pectoris with high thoracic epidural analgesia: Initial clinical experience. Am Heart J 133:648, 1997
476. Olausson K, Magnusdottir H, Lurje L, et al: Anti-ischemic and anti-anginal effects of thoracic epidural anesthesia versus those of conventional medical therapy in the treatment of severe refractory unstable angina pectoris. Circulation 96:2178, 1997
477. Overdyk FJ, Gramling-Babb PM, Handy JR Jr, et al: Thoracic epidural anesthesia as the last option for treating angina in a patient before coronary artery bypass surgery. Anesth Analg 84:213, 1997
478. Gramling-Babb PM, Zile MR, Reeves ST: Preliminary report on high thoracic epidural analgesia: Relationship between its therapeutic effects and myocardial blood flow as assessed by stress thallium distribution. J Cardiothorac Vasc Anesth 14:657, 2000
479. Liem TH, Booij LH, Hasenbos MA, et al: Coronary artery bypass grafting using two different anesthetic techniques. Part I. Hemodynamic results. J Cardiothorac Vasc Anesth 6:148, 1992
480. Liem TH, Hasenbos MA, Booij LH, et al: Coronary artery bypass grafting using two different anesthetic techniques. Part 2. Postoperative outcome. J Cardiothorac Vasc Anesth 6:156, 1992
481. Liem TH, Booij LH, Gielen MJ, et al: Coronary artery bypass grafting using two different anesthetic techniques. Part 3. Adrenergic responses. J Cardiothorac Vasc Anesth 6:162, 1992
482. Beattie WS, Badner NH, Choi P: Epidural analgesia reduces postoperative myocardial infarction: A meta-analysis. Anesth Analg 93:853, 2001
483. Liu SS, Block BM, Wu CL: Effects of perioperative central neuraxial analgesia on outcome after coronary artery bypass surgery: A meta-analysis. Anesthesiology 101:153, 2004
484. Lee TW, Grocott HP, Schwinn D, et al: High spinal anesthesia for cardiac surgery: Effects on beta-adrenergic receptor function, stress response, and hemodynamics. Anesthesiology 98:499, 2003
485. Aybek T, Kessler P, Khan MF, et al: Operative techniques in awake coronary artery bypass grafting. J Thorac Cardiovasc Surg 125:1394, 2003
486. Aybek T, Kessler P, Dogan S, et al: Awake coronary artery bypass grafting: Utopia or reality? Ann Thorac Surg 75:1165, 2003
487. Chakravarthy M, Jawali V, Patil TA, et al: High thoracic epidural anesthesia as the sole anesthetic for performing multiple grafts in off-pump coronary artery bypass surgery. J Cardiothorac Vasc Anesth 17:160, 2003
488. Karagoz HY, Kurtoglu M, Bakkaloglu B, et al: Coronary artery bypass grafting in the awake patient: Three years' experience in 137 patients. J Thorac Cardiovasc Surg 125:1401, 2003
489. Kessler P, Neidhart G, Bremerich DH, et al: High thoracic epidural anesthesia for coronary artery bypass grafting using two different surgical approaches in conscious patients. Anesth Analg 95:791, 2002
490. Meininger D, Neidhart G, Bremerich DH, et al: Coronary artery bypass grafting via sternotomy in conscious patients. World J Surg 27:534, 2003
491. Ho AM, Chung DC, Joynt GM: Neuraxial blockade and hematoma in cardiac surgery: Estimating the risk of a rare adverse event that has not (yet) occurred. Chest 117:551, 2000
492. Chakravarthy M, Thimmangowda P, Krishnamurthy J, et al: Thoracic epidural anesthesia in cardiac surgical patients: A prospective audit of 2,113 cases. J Cardiothorac Vasc Anesth 19:44, 2005
493. Pastor MC, Sanchez MJ, Casas MA, et al: Thoracic epidural analgesia in coronary artery bypass graft surgery: Seven years' experience. J Cardiothorac Vasc Anesth 17:154, 2003
494. Krohn BG, Kay JH, Mendez MA, et al: Rapid sustained recovery after cardiac operations. J Thorac Cardiovasc Surg 100:194, 1990
495. Chong JL, Pillai R, Fisher A, et al: Cardiac surgery: Moving away from intensive care. Br Heart J 68:430, 1992
496. Chong JL, Grebenik C, Sinclair M, et al: The effect of a cardiac surgical recovery area on the timing of extubation. J Cardiothorac Vasc Anesth 7:137, 1993
497. Cromwell J, Dayhoff DA, McCall NT, et al: Medicare participating heart bypass center demonstration (extramural research report), Health Care Financing Administration, 1998
498. Engelman RM, Rousou JA, Flack JE 3rd, et al: Fast-track recovery of the coronary bypass patient. Ann Thorac Surg 58:1742, 1994
499. Engelman RM: Fast-track recovery in the elderly patient. Ann Thorac Surg 63:606, 1997
500. Hawkes CA, Dhileepan S, Foxcroft D: Early extubation for adult cardiac surgical patients. Cochrane Database Syst Rev 4:CD003587, 2003
501. Lefemine AA, Harken DE: Postoperative care following open-heart operations: Routine use of controlled ventilation. J Thorac Cardiovasc Surg 52:207, 1966
502. Midell AI, Skinner DB, DeBoer A, et al: A review of pulmonary problems following valve replacement in 100 consecutive patients. Ann Thorac Surg 18:219, 1974
503. Quasha AL, Loeber N, Feeley TW, et al: Postoperative respiratory care: A controlled trial of early and late extubation following coronary-artery bypass grafting. Anesthesiology 52:135, 1980
504. Ramsay JG, Higgs BD, Wynands JE, et al: Early extubation after high-dose fentanyl anaesthesia for aortocoronary bypass surgery: Reversal of respiratory depression with low-dose nalbuphine. Can Anaesth Soc J 32:597, 1985
505. Cheng DC, Karski J, Peniston C, et al: Morbidity outcome in early versus conventional tracheal extubation after coronary artery bypass grafting: A prospective randomized controlled trial. J Thorac Cardiovasc Surg 112:755, 1996
506. Butterworth J, James R, Prielipp R, et al: Female gender associates with increased duration of intubation and length of stay after coronary artery surgery. CABG Clinical Benchmarking Database Participants. Anesthesiology 92:414, 2000

507. Arom KV, Emery RW, Petersen RJ, et al: Cost-effectiveness and predictors of early extubation. Ann Thorac Surg 60:127, 1995
508. Arom KV, Emery RW, Petersen RJ, et al: Patient characteristics, safety, and benefits of same-day admission for coronary artery bypass grafting. Ann Thorac Surg 61:1136, 1996
509. Habib RH, Zacharias A, Engoren M: Determinants of prolonged mechanical ventilation after coronary artery bypass grafting. Ann Thorac Surg 62:1164, 1996
510. Walji S, Peterson RJ, Neis P, et al: Ultra-fast track hospital discharge using conventional cardiac surgical techniques. Ann Thorac Surg 67:363, 1999
511. Ott RA, Gutfinger DE, Miller MP, et al: Rapid recovery after coronary artery bypass grafting: Is the elderly patient eligible? Ann Thorac Surg 63:634, 1997
512. Ott RA, Gutfinger DE, Miller M, et al: Rapid recovery of octogenarians following coronary artery bypass grafting. J Card Surg 12:309, 1997
513. Lee JH, Graber R, Popple CG, et al: Safety and efficacy of early extubation of elderly coronary artery bypass surgery patients. J Cardiothorac Vasc Anesth 12:381, 1998
514. London MJ, Shroyer AL, Jernigan V, et al: Fast-track cardiac surgery in a Department of Veterans Affairs patient population. Ann Thorac Surg 64:134, 1997
515. Dexter F, Macario A, Dexter EU: Computer simulation of changes in nursing productivity from early tracheal extubation of coronary artery bypass graft patients. J Clin Anesth 10:593, 1998
516. Cheng DC: Fast track cardiac surgery pathways: Early extubation, process of care, and cost containment. Anesthesiology 88:1429, 1998
517. Berry PD, Thomas SD, Mahon SP, et al: Myocardial ischaemia after coronary artery bypass grafting: Early vs late extubation. Br J Anaesth 80:20, 1998
518. Michalopoulos A, Nikolaides A, Antzaka C, et al: Change in anaesthesia practice and postoperative sedation shortens ICU and hospital length of stay following coronary artery bypass surgery. Respir Med 92:1066, 1998
519. Reyes A, Vega G, Blancas R, et al: Early vs conventional extubation after cardiac surgery with cardiopulmonary bypass. Chest 112:193, 1997
520. Silbert BS, Santamaria JD, O'Brien JL, et al: Early extubation following coronary artery bypass surgery: A prospective randomized controlled trial. The Fast Track Cardiac Care Team. Chest 113:1481, 1998
521. Engoren M, Buderer NF, Zacharias A, et al: Variables predicting reintubation after cardiac surgical procedures. Ann Thorac Surg 67:661, 1999
522. Ovrum E, Tangen G, Schiott C, et al: Rapid recovery protocol applied to 5,658 consecutive "on-pump" coronary bypass patients. Ann Thorac Surg 70:2008, 2000
523. Chassot PG, van der Linden P, Zaugg M, et al: Off-pump coronary artery bypass surgery: Physiology and anaesthetic management. Br J Anaesth 92:400, 2004
524. Raja SG, Dreyfus GD: Off-pump coronary artery bypass surgery: To do or not to do? Current best available evidence. J Cardiothorac Vasc Anesth 18:486, 2004
525. Sellke FW, DiMaio JM, Caplan LR, et al: Comparing on-pump and off-pump coronary artery bypass grafting: Numerous studies but few conclusions: A scientific statement from the American Heart Association council on cardiovascular surgery and anesthesia in collaboration with the interdisciplinary working group on quality of care and outcomes research. Circulation 111:2858, 2005
526. Grundeman PF, Borst C, Verlaan CW, et al: Exposure of circumflex branches in the tilted, beating porcine heart: Echocardiographic evidence of right ventricular deformation and the effect of right or left heart bypass. J Thorac Cardiovasc Surg 118:316, 1999
527. George SJ, Al-Ruzzeh S, Amrani M: Mitral annulus distortion during beating heart surgery: A potential cause for hemodynamic disturbance—a three-dimensional echocardiography reconstruction study. Ann Thorac Surg 73:1424, 2002
528. Grundeman PF, Borst C, van Herwaarden JA, et al: Vertical displacement of the beating heart by the octopus tissue stabilizer: Influence on coronary flow. Ann Thorac Surg 65:1348, 1998
529. Grundeman PF, Budde R, Beck HM, et al: Endoscopic exposure and stabilization of posterior and inferior branches using the endo-starfish cardiac positioner and the endo-octopus stabilizer for closed-chest beating heart multivessel CABG: Hemodynamic changes in the pig. Circulation 108(suppl 1):II34, 2003
530. Grundeman PF, Verlaan CW, van Boven WJ, et al: Ninety-degree anterior cardiac displacement in off-pump coronary artery bypass grafting: The Starfish cardiac positioner preserves stroke volume and arterial pressure. Ann Thorac Surg 78:679, 2004
531. Porat E, Sharony R, Ivry S, et al: Hemodynamic changes and right heart support during vertical displacement of the beating heart. Ann Thorac Surg 69:1188, 2000
532. Biswas S, Clements F, Diodato L, et al: Changes in systolic and diastolic function during multivessel off-pump coronary bypass grafting. Eur J Cardiothorac Surg 20:913, 2001
533. Kwak YL, Oh YJ, Jung SM, et al: Change in right ventricular function during off-pump coronary artery bypass graft surgery. Eur J Cardiothorac Surg 25:572, 2004
534. Mathison M, Edgerton JR, Horswell JL, et al: Analysis of hemodynamic changes during beating heart surgical procedures. Ann Thorac Surg 70:1355, 2000
535. Nierich AP, Diephuis J, Jansen EW, et al: Heart displacement during off-pump CABG: How well is it tolerated? Ann Thorac Surg 70:466, 2000
536. Mishra M, Shrivastava S, Dhar A, et al: A prospective evaluation of hemodynamic instability during off-pump coronary artery bypass surgery. J Cardiothorac Vasc Anesth 17:452, 2003
537. Staton GW, Williams WH, Mahoney EM, et al: Pulmonary outcomes of off-pump vs on-pump coronary artery bypass surgery in a randomized trial. Chest 127:892, 2005
538. Kaplan JA, King SB 3rd: The precordial electrocardiographic lead (V5) in patients who have coronary-artery disease. Anesthesiology 45:570, 1976
539. Kaplan JA, Dunbar RW, Jones EL: Nitroglycerin infusion during coronary-artery surgery. Anesthesiology 45:14, 1976
540. Kaplan JA, Jones EL: Vasodilator therapy during coronary artery surgery. Comparison of nitroglycerin and nitroprusside. J Thorac Cardiovasc Surg 77:301, 1979
541. Parker JD, Parker JO: Nitrate therapy for stable angina pectoris. N Engl J Med 338:520, 1998
542. Kelly RA, Han X: Nitrovasodilators have (small) direct effects on cardiac contractility: is this important? Circulation 96:2493, 1997
543. Jugdutt BI, Warnica JW: Intravenous nitroglycerin therapy to limit myocardial infarct size, expansion, and complications. Effect of timing, dosage, and infarct location [Erratum in Circulation 79:1151, 1989]. Circulation 78:906, 1988
544. Fujita M, Yamanishi K, Hirai T, et al: Significance of collateral circulation in reversible left ventricular asynergy by nitroglycerin in patients with relatively recent myocardial infarction. Am Heart J 120:521, 1990
545. Townsend GE, Wynands JE, Whalley DG, et al: A profile of intravenous nitroglycerin use in cardiopulmonary bypass surgery. Can Anaesth Soc J 30:142, 1983
546. Booth BP, Henderson M, Milne B, et al: Sequestration of glyceryl trinitrate (nitroglycerin) by cardiopulmonary bypass oxygenators. Anesth Analg 72:493, 1991
547. Gallagher JD, Moore RA, Jose AB, et al: Prophylactic nitroglycerin infusions during coronary artery bypass surgery. Anesthesiology 64:785, 1986
548. Lell W, Johnson P, Plagenhoef J, et al: The effect of prophylactic nitroglycerin infusion on the incidence of regional wall-motion abnormalities and ST segment changes in patients undergoing coronary artery bypass surgery. J Card Surg 8(suppl):228, 1993
549. Thomson IR, Mutch WA, Culligan JD: Failure of intravenous nitroglycerin to prevent intraoperative myocardial ischemia during fentanyl-pancuronium anesthesia. Anesthesiology 61:385, 1984
550. Zvara DA, Groban L, Rogers AT, et al: Prophylactic nitroglycerin did not reduce myocardial ischemia during accelerated recovery management of coronary artery bypass graft surgery patients. J Cardiothorac Vasc Anesth 14:571, 2000
551. Apostolidou IA, Despotis GJ, Hogue CW Jr, et al: Antiischemic effects of nicardipine and nitroglycerin after coronary artery bypass grafting. Ann Thorac Surg 67:417, 1999
552. Kaplan JA, Jones EL: Vasodilator therapy during coronary artery surgery. Comparison of nitroglycerin and nitroprusside. J Thorac Cardiovasc Surg 77:301, 1979
553. Kates RA, Kaplan JA: Cardiovascular responses to verapamil during coronary artery bypass graft surgery. Anesth Analg 62:821, 1983
554. Griffin RM, Dimich I, Jurado R, Kaplan JA: Haemodynamic effects of diltiazem during fentanyl-nitrous oxide anaesthesia. An in vivo study in the dog. Br J Anaesth 60:655, 1988
555. Wijeysundera DN, Beattie WS, Rao V, Karski J: Calcium antagonists reduce cardiovascular complications after cardiac surgery: A meta-analysis. J Am Coll Cardiol 41:1496, 2003
556. Wijeysundera DN, Beattie WS, Rao V, et al: Calcium antagonists are associated with reduced mortality after cardiac surgery: A propensity analysis. J Thorac Cardiovasc Surg 127:755, 2004
557. Kwak YL: Reduction of ischemia during off-pump coronary artery bypass graft surgery. J Cardiothorac Vasc Anesth 19:667, 2005
558. Turlapaty P, Vary R, Kaplan JA: Nicardipine, a new intravenous calcium antagonist: A review of its pharmacology, pharmacokinetics, and perioperative applications. J Cardiothorac Anesth 3:344, 1989

559. Parmley W: New calcium antagonists: Relevance of vasoselectivity. Am Heart J 120(Pt 1):1408, 1990
560. Pepine CJ, Lambert CR: Effects of nicardipine on coronary blood flow. Am Heart J 116(Pt 1):248, 1988
561. Ogawa T, Sekiguchi T, Ishii M, et al: Acute effects of intravenous nicardipine on hemodynamics and cardiac function in patients with a healed myocardial infarction and no evidence of congestive heart failure. Am J Cardiol 68:301, 1991
562. Aroney CN, Semigran MJ, Dec GW: Left ventricular diastolic function in patients with left ventricular systolic dysfunction due to coronary artery disease and effect of nicardipine. Am J Cardiol 67:823, 1991
563. Kaplan JA: Clinical considerations for the use of intravenous nicardipine in the treatment of postoperative hypertension. Am Heart J 119:443, 1990
564. Begon C, Dartayet B, Edouard A, et al: Intravenous nicardipine for treatment of intraoperative hypertension during abdominal surgery. J Cardiothorac Anesth 3:706, 1984
565. Van Wezel HB, Koolen JJ, Visser CA, et al: The efficacy of nicardipine and nitroprusside in preventing poststernotomy hypertension. J Cardiothorac Anesth 3:700, 1989
566. Van Wezel HB, Bovill JG, Schuller J, et al: Comparison of nitroglycerin, verapamil and nifedipine in the management of arterial pressure during coronary artery surgery. Br J Anaesth 58:267, 1986
567. Kwak YL, Oh YJ, Bang SO: Comparison of the effects of nicardipine and sodium nitroprusside for control of increased blood pressure after coronary artery bypass graft surgery. J Int Med Res 32:342, 2004
568. Halpern NA, Goldberg M, Neely C, et al: Postoperative hypertension: A multicenter, prospective, randomized comparison between intravenous nicardipine and sodium nitroprusside. Crit Care Med 20:1637, 1992
569. Kaplan JA: Role of ultrashort-acting beta-blockers in the perioperative period. J Cardiothorac Anesth 2:683, 1988
570. Barth C, Ojile M, Pearson AC, Labovitz AJ: Ultra short-acting intravenous beta-adrenergic blockade as add-on therapy in acute unstable angina. Am Heart J 121(Pt 1):782, 1991
571. Kirshenbaum JM, Kloner RF, McGowan N, Antman EM: Use of an ultrashort-acting beta-receptor blocker (esmolol) in patients with acute myocardial ischemia and relative contraindications to beta-blockade therapy. J Am Coll Cardiol 12:773, 1988
572. Labovitz AJ, Barth C, Castello R, et al: Attenuation of myocardial ischemia during coronary occlusion by ultrashort-acting beta-adrenergic blockade. Am Heart J 121:1347, 1991
573. Nicolson SC, Jobes DR, Quinlan JJ: Cardiovascular effects of esmolol in patients anesthetized with sufentanil-pancuronium for myocardial revascularization. J Cardiothorac Anesth 4(suppl 2):55, 1990
574. Girard D, Shulman BJ, Thys DM, et al: The safety and efficacy of esmolol during myocardial revascularization. Anesthesiology 65:157, 1986
575. Reves JG, Croughwell NC, Hawkins E, et al: Esmolol for treatment of intraoperative tachycardia and/or hypertension in patients having cardiac operations. Bolus loading technique. J Thorac Cardiovasc Surg 100:221, 1990
576. Buxton AE, Goldberg S, Harken A, et al: Coronary-artery spasm immediately after myocardial revascularization: Recognition and management. N Engl J Med 304:1249, 1981
577. Kaski JC: Mechanisms of coronary artery spasm. Trends Cardiovasc Med 1:289, 1991
578. Apostolidou IA, Skubas NJ, Despotis GJ, et al: Occurrence of myocardial ischemia immediately after coronary revascularization using radial arterial conduits. J Cardiothorac Vasc Anesth 15:433, 2001
579. He GW, Rosenfeldt FL, Buxton BF, Angus JA: Reactivity of human isolated internal mammary artery to constrictor and dilator agents. Implications for treatment of internal mammary artery spasm. Circulation 80(suppl I):I141, 1989
580. Mussa S, Guzik TJ, Black E, et al: Comparative efficacies and durations of action of phenoxybenzamine, verapamil/nitroglycerin solution, and papaverine as topical antispasmodics for radial artery coronary bypass grafting. J Thorac Cardiovasc Surg 126:1798, 2003
581. He GW, Buxton BF, Rosenfeldt FL, et al: Pharmacologic dilatation of the internal mammary artery during coronary bypass grafting. J Thorac Cardiovasc Surg 107:1440, 1994
582. Jett GK, Guyton RA, Hatcher CR, Abel PW: Inhibition of human internal mammary artery contractions. An in vitro study of vasodilators. J Thorac Cardiovasc Surg 104:977, 1992
583. Du ZY, Buxton BF, Woodman OL: Tolerance to glyceryl trinitrate in isolated human internal mammary arteries. J Thorac Cardiovasc Surg 104:1280, 1992
584. Shapira OM, Xu A, Vita JA, et al: Nitroglycerin is superior to diltiazem as a coronary bypass conduit vasodilator. J Thorac Cardiovasc Surg 117:906, 1999
585. Shapira OM, Alkon JD, Macron DS, et al: Nitroglycerin is preferable to diltiazem for prevention of coronary bypass conduit spasm. Ann Thorac Surg 70:883, discussion 888, 2000
586. Mollhoff T, Schmidt C, Van Aken H, et al: Myocardial ischaemia in patients with impaired left ventricular function undergoing coronary artery bypass grafting—milrinone versus nifedipine. Eur J Anaesthesiol 19:796, 2002
587. Hannan EL, Racz MJ, Walford G, et al: Long-term outcomes of coronary-artery bypass grafting versus stent implantation. N Engl J Med 352:2174, 2005

Chapter 20

VALVULAR HEART DISEASE: REPLACEMENT AND REPAIR

David J. Cook, MD • Philippe R. Housmans, MD, PhD • Kent H. Rehfeldt, MD

KEY POINTS

1. Although various valvular lesions generate different physiologic changes, all valvular heart disease is characterized by abnormalities of ventricular loading.
2. The left ventricle normally compensates for increases in afterload by increases in preload. This increase in end-diastolic fiber stretch or radius further elevates wall tension in accordance with Laplace's law, resulting in a reciprocal decline in myocardial fiber shortening. The stroke volume is maintained because the contractile force is augmented at the higher preload level.
3. Factors that influence heart function include afterload stress, preload reserve, ventricular compliance, contractility, and the existence of pathology such as valve lesions, aortic stenosis, and hypertrophy.
4. Treatment modalities for hypertrophic obstructive cardiomyopathy, a relatively common genetic malformation of the heart, include β-adrenoceptor antagonists, calcium channel blockers, and myectomy of the septum. Newer approaches include dual-chamber pacing and septal reduction (ablation) therapy with ethanol.
5. The severity and duration of symptoms of aortic regurgitation may correlate poorly with the degree of hemodynamic and contractile impairment, delaying surgical treatment while patients are undergoing progressive deterioration.
6. Mitral regurgitation causes left ventricular volume overload. Treatment depends on the underlying mechanism and includes early reperfusion therapy, angiotensin-converting enzyme inhibitors, and surgical repair or replacement of the mitral valve.
7. Rheumatic disease and congenital abnormalities of the mitral valve are the main causes of mitral stenosis, a slowly progressive disease. Surgical treatment options include closed and open commissurotomy and percutaneous mitral commissurotomy.
8. Most tricuspid surgery occurs in the context of significant aortic or mitral disease, and anesthetic management is primarily determined by the left-sided valve lesion.
9. Innovations in surgical valve repair include aortic valve repair and closed- and open-chamber procedures for mitral regurgitation.

In many ways, surgery for coronary artery disease (CAD) has matured. Although there will continue to be incremental advances such as off-pump surgery, anastomotic connectors, and endoscopic vein harvest, coronary artery surgery may have seen its best days, in no small part because of advances in interventional cardiology. The same has not been true of valve surgery. At surgical institutions where valve surgery is well represented, surgical volumes are stable or increasing. This fact reflects the aging of the population and the lesser impact of cardiologic interventions on the valvular heart disease (VHD) process.

From the standpoint of anesthetic care, valve surgery is also usually very different from coronary artery bypass grafting (CABG). Over the natural history of VHD, the physiologic characteristics change markedly, and in the operating room, physiologic and hemodynamic conditions are quite variable and are readily influenced by anesthetic interventions. For some types of valve lesions, it can be relatively difficult to predict preoperatively how the heart will respond to the altered loading conditions associated with valve repair or replacement.

It is essential to understand the natural history of each of the major adult-acquired valve defects and how the pathophysiologic conditions evolve. Surgical decision making regarding valve repair or replacement must also be understood, because a valve operated on at the appropriate stage of its natural history will have a good and more predictable outcome than one operated on at a late stage, when the perioperative result can be quite poor. Because pathophysiologic conditions are dynamic and differ significantly among valve lesions, understanding the physiology and natural history of individual valve defects is the foundation of developing an anesthetic plan that includes various requirements for pacing rate and rhythm, use of inotropes (or negative inotropes), and use of vasodilators or vasoconstrictors to alter loading conditions.

Although valvular lesions impose various physiologic changes, all VHD is characterized by abnormalities of ventricular loading. The status of the ventricle changes over time as ventricular function and the valvular defect are influenced by the progression of volume or pressure overload. The clinical status of patients with VHD therefore can be complex and dynamic. It is possible to have clinical decompensation in the context of normal ventricular contractility or ventricular decompensation with normal ejection indices. The altered loading conditions characteristic of VHD may result in a divergence between the function of the heart as a systolic pump and the intrinsic inotropic state of the myocardium. This divergence between cardiac performance and inotropy occurs as a result of compensatory physiologic mechanisms specific to each of the ventricular loading abnormalities.

In analyzing the physiologic response of the left ventricle to a variety of abnormal loading conditions, it is useful to consider the concepts of afterload mismatch and preload reserve.[1] These concepts frame discussions of the pathophysiology of the individual valvular lesions. Other physiologic concepts

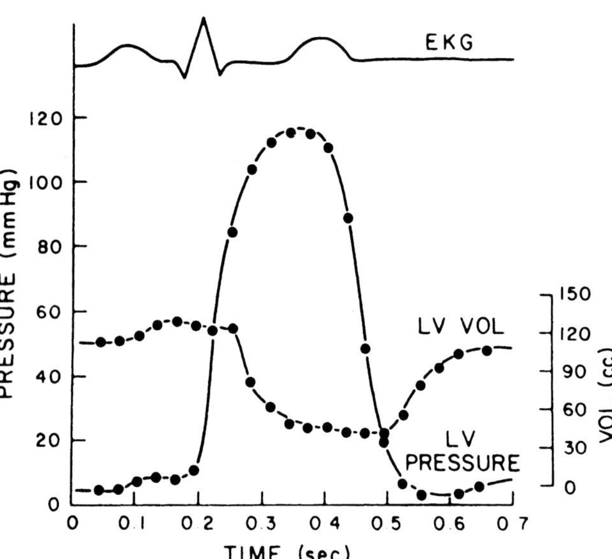

Figure 20–1 Simultaneous left ventricular volume and pressure during one cardiac cycle. (From Barash PG, Kopriva DJ: Cardiac pump function and how to monitor it. *In* Thomas SJ [ed]: Manual of Cardiac Anesthesia. New York, Churchill Livingstone, 1984, p 1.)

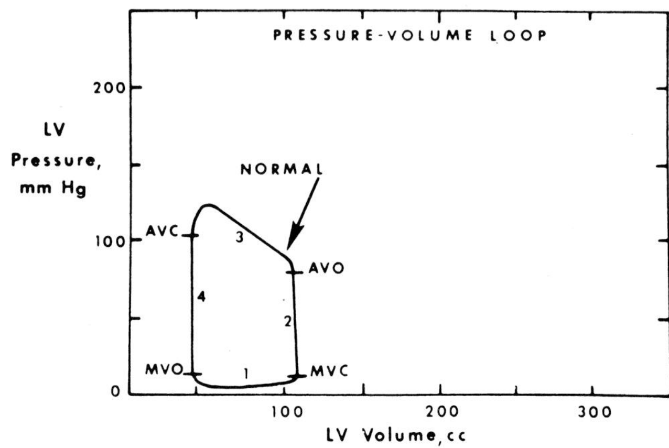

Figure 20–2 An idealized pressure-volume loop for a single cardiac cycle. (From Jackson JM, Thomas SJ, Lowenstein E: Anesthetic management of patients with valvular heart disease. Semin Anesth 1:239, 1982.)

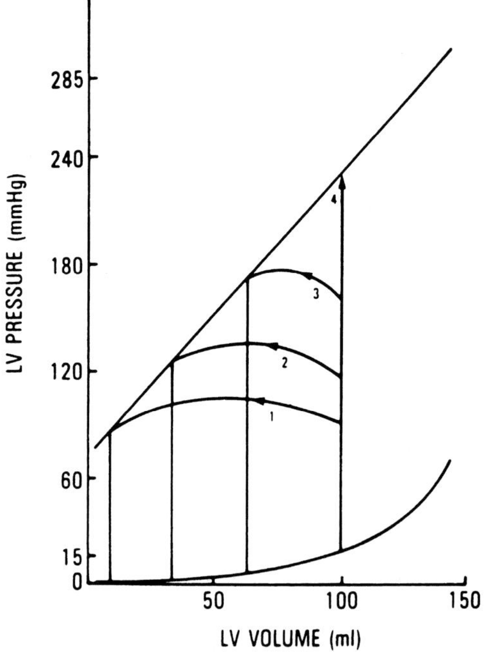

Figure 20–3 Pressure-volume loops illustrating the response of the left ventricle to progressive increases in afterload when the preload is artificially held constant. (From Ross J Jr: Afterload mismatch in aortic and mitral valve disease: Implications for surgical therapy. J Am Coll Cardiol 5:811, 1985.)

essential to understanding VHD and its evolution are pressure-volume loops and the linear end-systolic pressure-volume relationship (ESPVR). The former provides a graphic analysis of ventricular pressure-volume relationships in a single beat, whereas the latter is a method of quantifying the intrinsic contractility of the myocardium over multiple contractions and is relatively independent of changes in loading conditions (see Chapters 5, 14, and 15).

PATHOPHYSIOLOGY

Pressure-Volume Loops

The pressure and volume changes occurring during a normal cardiac cycle are depicted in Figure 20–1. A pressure-volume loop is generated when ventricular volumes are plotted against simultaneously occurring ventricular pressures for a single contraction (Fig. 20–2). Familiarity with this graphic analysis of cardiac function, the normal pressure-volume loop of the left ventricle, provides a basis for appreciating a load-insensitive index of contractility, the ESPVR. Phase 1 in Figure 20–2 shows ventricular filling and represents the loading of the heart before contraction (i.e., preload). During early and middle diastole, filling of the ventricle is rapid, depending on the pressure gradient between the left atrium and the left ventricle. In late diastole, the left atrium contracts (*a* wave), which results in the final left ventricular end-diastolic volume (LVEDV) and pressure (LVEDP). Atrial contraction in the normal heart accounts for 15% to 20% of ventricular filling. The normal ventricle accommodates large changes in ventricular volume with only a small change in ventricular diastolic pressure.

Ventricular systole occurs in two stages: the isovolumic and ejection phases. During isovolumic, or isometric, systole (phase 2 of the cardiac cycle), intraventricular pressure rises dramatically. However, there is little or no concurrent decrease in ventricular volume, because the aortic valve is still closed. Phase 3 is the systolic ejection period. When intraventricular pressure exceeds aortic pressure, the aortic valve opens, and ejection begins. At the end of phase 3, the aortic valve closes. This point is the end-systolic pressure-volume coordinate, which may uniquely reflect the cardiac inotropic state.

Afterload Stress and Preload Reserve

Figure 20–3 shows the response of the LV to changes in afterload, with preload held constant, in the context of the pressure-volume loops from single contractions. These curves are constructed experimentally by infusing a pure α-adrenergic agonist while simultaneously measuring the corresponding end-systolic volumes. The resultant curves describe the diastolic pressure-volume relationship (ventricular compliance) and the linear ESPVR at a given level of myocardial contrac-

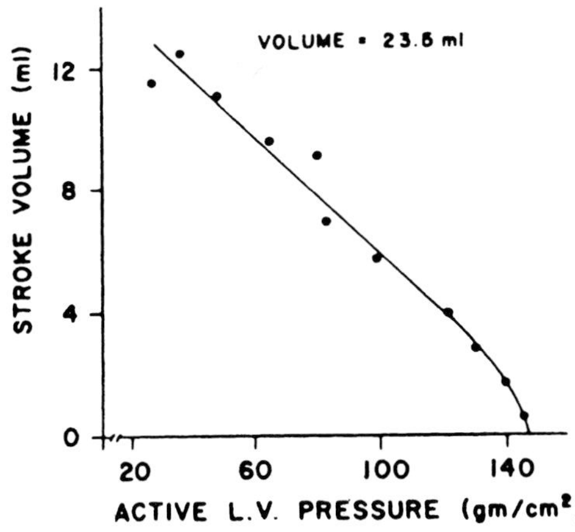

Figure 20–4 Plot of left ventricular stroke volume versus left ventricular systolic pressure when the ventricle's end-diastolic volume is held constant (the inverse force-velocity relationship). (From Burns JW, Covell JW, Ross J Jr: Mechanics of isotonic left ventricular contractions. Am J Physiol 224:725, 1973.)

tility. Each counterclockwise loop represents a cardiac cycle. The stroke volume (SV) progressively decreases as the impedance to ejection increases from beats 1 to 3. This pattern continues until beat 4, when the peak ventricular systolic pressure fails to open the aortic valve and only isovolumic contraction ensues.[1] This inverse relationship between afterload and SV (inverse force-velocity relationship) was also documented experimentally in a canine preparation in which the LVEDV was held constant (Fig. 20–4).[2] In the intact heart, afterload is a function of ventricular size and arterial pressure.[3] Its pivotal role in cardiovascular regulation is summarized in Figure 20–5. Afterload is defined as the tension, or force per unit of cross-sectional area, in the ventricular wall during ejection.[4] Laplace's law provides a mathematical expression for the wall tension[5] (in which P is the intraventricular pressure) developed in a spherical chamber of radius R and wall thickness h:

$$\text{Wall tension} = \frac{P \times R}{2h}$$

This means that ventricular afterload, a function of the constantly changing intraventricular pressure and radius, varies continuously during systole. It is extremely difficult to precisely quantify afterload in the clinical setting, and commonly used approximations such as blood pressure or systemic vascular resistance (SVR) are inherently misleading, because they fail to reflect instantaneous pressure-volume variations. LV size or preload is a determinant of the SV and afterload.[6] Normally, the left ventricle compensates for increases in afterload by increases in preload. This increase in end-diastolic fiber stretch or radius further elevates wall tension in accordance with Laplace's law, resulting in a reciprocal decline in myocardial fiber shortening (i.e., inverse force-velocity relationship). Despite this relative decline in fiber shortening, the SV is maintained because contractile force is augmented at the higher preload (i.e., Starling or length-active tension effect). This increased contractility at higher LVEDVs may be mediated by an increased sensitivity to the inotropic effects of extracellular calcium at longer muscle lengths.[7-9]

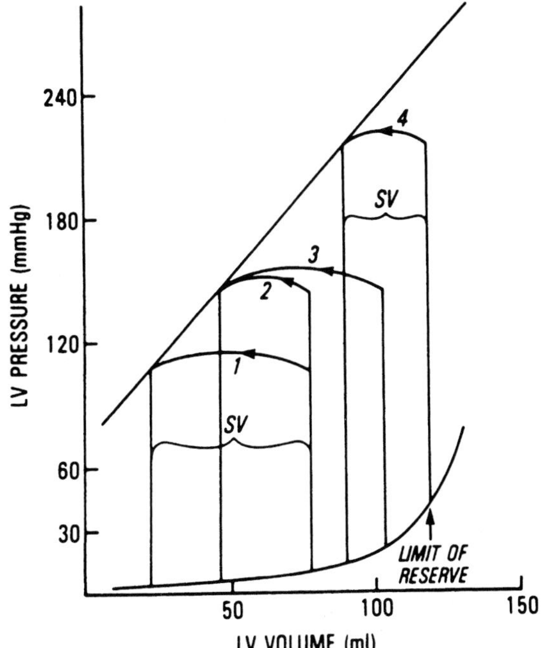

Figure 20–6 Pressure-volume loops illustrating the concept of preload reserve. An increase in afterload elicits a compensatory increase in left ventricular end-diastolic volume (LVEDV) such that stroke volume (SV) is maintained at the higher afterload. (From Ross J Jr: Afterload mismatch in aortic and mitral valve disease: Implications for surgical therapy. J Am Coll Cardiol 5:811, 1985.)

Use of this "preload reserve" allows the left ventricle to maintain its SV in the face of an afterload stress,[1] as shown in Figure 20–6.[1] The increase in afterload (beat 2) elicits a compensatory increase in end-diastolic volume (EDV; beat 3), preserving SV at the higher afterload. However, when the ventricle reaches the limit of its preload reserve, it overdistends, and preload behaves as if it were fixed. SV then decreases with further increases in the systolic pressure (afterload mismatch; beat 4), a clinical corollary of the inverse force-velocity relationship.

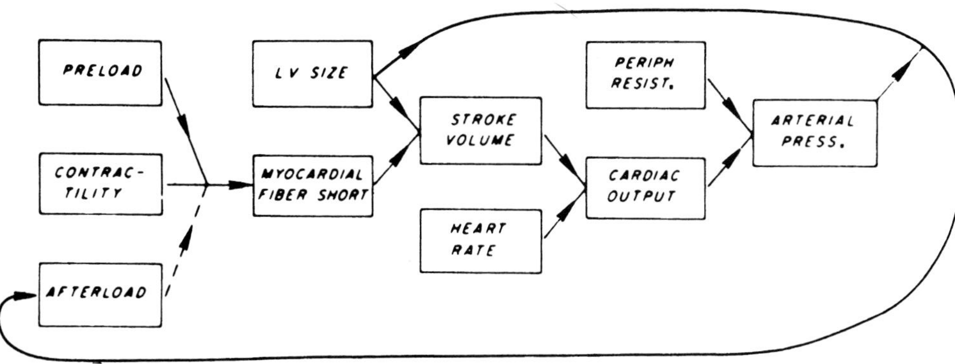

Figure 20–5 Role of afterload in cardiac regulation. (From Braunwald E: Regulation of the circulation. N Engl J Med 290:1124, 1974.)

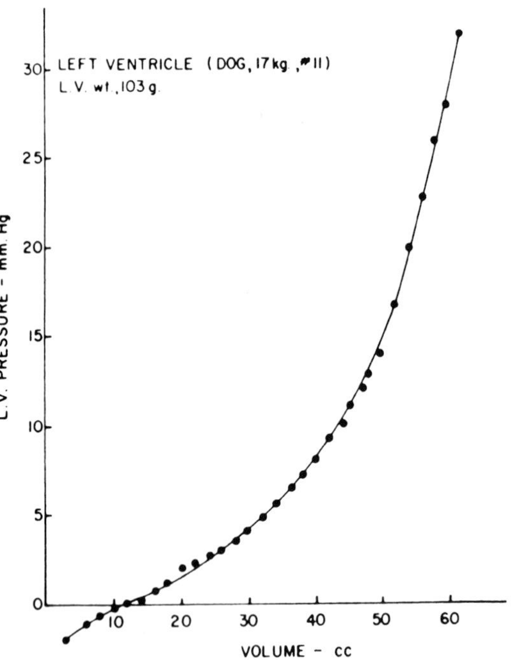

Figure 20–7 The normal diastolic pressure-volume relationship. (From Spotnitz HM, Sonnenblick EH, Spiro D: Relation of ultrastructure to function in the intact heart: Sarcomere structure relative to pressure-volume curves of the intact left ventricles of dog and cat. Circ Res 18:49, 1966.)

Ventricular Compliance

Translating this physiologic analysis to the clinical setting is complicated by a number of practical constraints. One of the most important is the inconstant relationship between LVEDV and LVEDP. The diastolic pressure-volume relationship for the normal mammalian left ventricle is a curvilinear function (Fig. 20–7).[3,10] The slope of this curve (i.e., ratio of change in volume to change in pressure during diastole) is the ventricular compliance (dV/dP). Although the normal ventricle is extremely compliant in the physiologic range, the instantaneous compliance decreases with increments in diastolic filling. This progressively increasing slope of the pressure-volume curve becomes evident at the extremes of ventricular volume, in which succeeding increments in volume result in exponentially greater rises in end-diastolic pressure. Patients with acute aortic regurgitation experience the hemodynamic consequences of this phenomenon. The catastrophic increases in ventricular filling pressure reflect the absolute magnitude of the volume overload and are a corollary of a precipitously declining compliance relationship.

These hemodynamic manifestations of acute shifts up and down a single compliance curve must be distinguished from chronic, pathologic alterations in ventricular compliance, which produce actual shifts of the entire curve relating diastolic pressure and volume. For example, in animal models of chronic volume overload, the entire pressure-volume curve is shifted to the right, such that substantial increases in ventricular volume are tolerated with relatively little change in end-diastolic pressure (Fig. 20–8).[11] In this example, the slope of the new pressure-volume curve (i.e., compliance) is decreased. Similarly, time-dependent, rightward shifts of the entire pressure-volume relationship have been shown to occur in patients with severe ventricular volume overload resulting from chronic aortic regurgitation.[12] In these examples, the development of a new relationship between pressure and volume may reflect the physiologic process of *creep*, the time-dependent change in size or the dimension of tissue maintained at a constant level of stress.[4]

Myocardial wall thickness is an important determinant of diastolic compliance. In clinical settings of chronic pressure overload (e.g., aortic stenosis, chronic hypertension), diastolic compliance and ventricular wall thickness have been shown to be linearly and inversely related (Fig. 20–9).[13] This may explain why the normal, thinner-walled right ventricle is more compliant than the normal left ventricle, even though the ventricles share similar qualities of intrinsic myocardial stiffness.[3,14] This association between pathologic hypertrophy of the ventricle and deterioration in its diastolic compliance is a well-documented but poorly understood phenomenon.

It has become customary to characterize diastolic function in certain disease states as normal or abnormal, such as diastolic dysfunction or diastolic failure.[15,16] The latter condition is a distinct pathophysiologic entity that results from an increased resistance to ventricular filling and leads to an inappropriate upward shift of the diastolic pressure-volume relationship.[17] For example, diastolic dysfunction is seen in ischemic cardiomyopathy, particularly when combined with pressure overload hypertrophy.[18]

In certain diseases, these primary derangements of diastolic function may predominate over abnormalities of diastolic function associated with ventricular hypertrophy. For example, in hypertrophic cardiomyopathy, the impaired ventricular relaxation inherent in the myopathic process appears to play the greater role in the observed abnormalities of diastolic filling, because the diastolic dysfunction is often dispro-

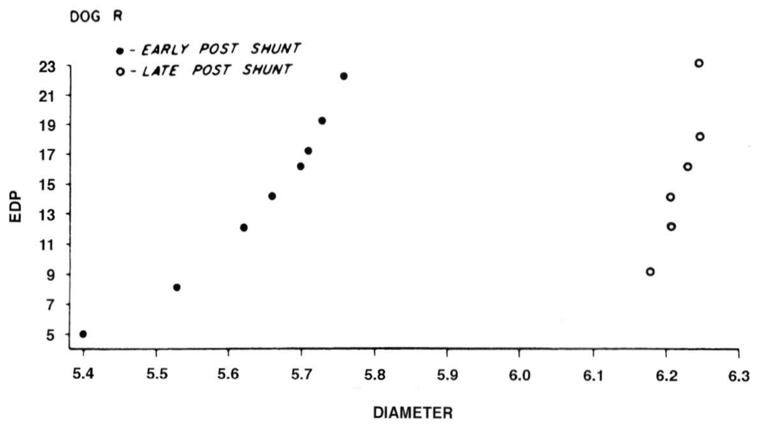

Figure 20–8 The relations between left ventricular end-diastolic pressure (EDP) and volume (diameter) in an animal studied early and late after the production of chronic volume overloading (arteriovenous fistula). (From McCullagh WH, Covell JW, Ross J Jr: Left ventricular dilation and diastolic compliance changes during chronic volume overloading. Circulation 45:943, 1972.)

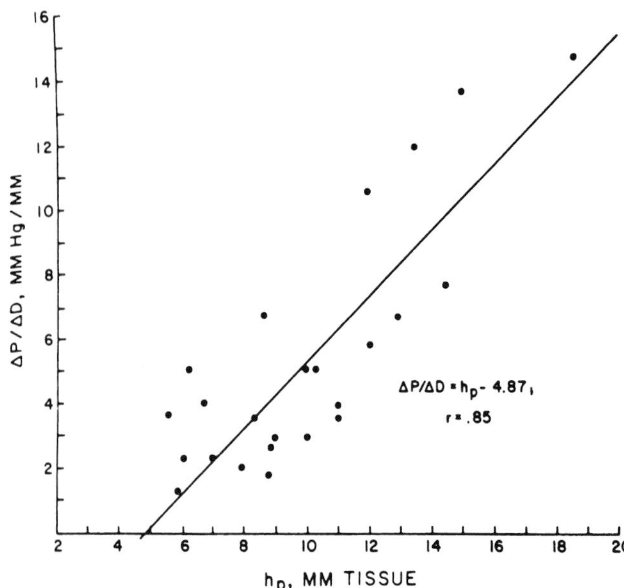

Figure 20–9 The relation between chamber stiffness (DP/DD, the inverse of compliance) and ventricular wall thickness. (From Grossman W, McLaurin P, Moos SP, et al: Wall thickness and diastolic properties of the left ventricle. Circulation 49:129, 1974.)

portionate to the degree of ventricular hypertrophy.[19,20] The effects of pathologic hypertrophy on diastolic compliance and ventricular relaxation are complex and are considered in more detail in the sections on "Aortic Stenosis" and "Hypertrophic Cardiomyopathy."

Filling of one ventricle or changes in its configuration or compliance properties can significantly alter the diastolic pressure-volume characteristics of the other ventricle.[21,22] Progressive increases in right ventricular (RV) filling shift the LV compliance curve up and to the left. This effect is greatest at high RV filling pressures and is accentuated by the presence of the pericardium.[23] With severe RV distention, the interventricular septum encroaches on the left ventricle. This encroachment reduces the size of the left ventricle and alters its geometric configuration such that its compliance declines.[21] As a result, LV filling pressures may fail to reflect even directional changes in LV size.[24]

Contractility

Myocardial contractility can be defined as the ability of the heart to generate force at a given preload.[25] Although most clinicians and researchers seem to be comfortable with their intuitive notions of the cardiac inotropic state, the search for a consensus on a quantitative yardstick of ventricular inotropy has proved to be elusive. Its accurate and reproducible measurement is of more than theoretical interest because the contractile function of the heart is a key determinant of prognosis for most cardiac diseases, and it is especially important in critical decisions regarding the timing of surgical correction in patients with VHD.

Historically, methods of assessing myocardial contractility have been divided into two groups, based on analysis of the isovolumetric or the ejection phase of cardiac contraction.[4] Details of their clinical determination and relative reproducibility are beyond the scope of this discussion, but more information can be found in several excellent reviews[4,26,27] and Chapters 5 and 14. The isovolumetric indices include measurements such as maximal velocity of myocardial fiber shortening (V_{max}), peak pressure development (dP/dt), and peak dP/dt measured at an instantaneous pressure (dP/dt/P). Although relatively insensitive to loading conditions, these tests poorly reflect basal levels of contractility and are unreliable for comparing contractility among patients or assessing directional changes in contractility in an individual patient over time.[26]

Ejection phase indices, such as the ejection fraction (EF), are determined in part by the intrinsic inotropic state and can be used to define basal levels of contractility.[26] Such measurements are extremely useful in evaluating ventricular function in patients with CAD or other conditions that do not significantly alter ventricular loading conditions.[28] Ejection phase indices are understandably popular because they are readily available, and they are the most widely used clinical measures of LV function. However, these indices are directly proportional to preload, vary inversely with ventricular afterload, and are accordingly unreliable for assessing contractile performance in patients with most forms of VHD.

The use of the pressure-volume diagram and analysis of the ESPVR allow a more precise appreciation of LV contractility, which is independent of preload.[29] The extent of myocardial shortening, and therefore of end-systolic fiber length, is a direct function of afterload (i.e., inverse force-velocity relationship), and myocardial contractility can be evaluated by making use of this fundamental property. In most instances, end-systolic pressure (ESP) can be substituted for afterload. Only with pathologic degrees of ventricular hypertrophy is there a major divergence between ESP and afterload. This means that for any level of contractility, the end-systolic volume (ESV) to which a ventricle contracts is a linearly increasing function of ESP. A stronger ventricle contracts to a smaller ESV (i.e., empties more completely) at any given level of ventricular afterload. Changes in the inotropic state can also be viewed in the context of the idealized pressure-volume loop. Positive inotropic interventions shift the curve up and to the left, increasing the work that can be performed at any given EDV (preload). Conversely, negative inotropic interventions shift the curve down and to the right[30] (Fig. 20–10) (see Chapters 5 and 14). These load-independent indices of contractility are largely research tools, but in the future, it may be possible to construct pressure-volume loops and quantify ESPVRs in real time with echocardiographic equipment featuring automated border detection[31] (see Chapter 15).

Clinical studies of patients with relatively normal loading conditions have shown that variations in the ESV reliably correlate with changes in ejection phase indices (Fig. 20–11).[32] The ESPVR represents an index of contractility that depends on systolic ventricular pressure (i.e., afterload) but is independent of end-diastolic length (i.e., preload).[28,33,34] Pressure-volume loops also provide a framework for considering the interactions between systolic (inotropic) and diastolic (lusitropic) function. Although the preload (i.e., EDV) is an independent determinant of SV, because of the circular nature of blood flow, the SV ultimately determines venous return and the resultant preload for the next cardiac cycle.[30] The "inotropically determined" ESV is the other element besides the venous return that contributes to the EDV. Just as the ESPVR uniquely describes systolic function, the end-diastolic pressure-volume relationship (EDPVR) is a manifestation of the intrinsic relaxation (lusitropic) properties of the ventricle. Positive lusitropic interventions facilitate ventricular filling and shift

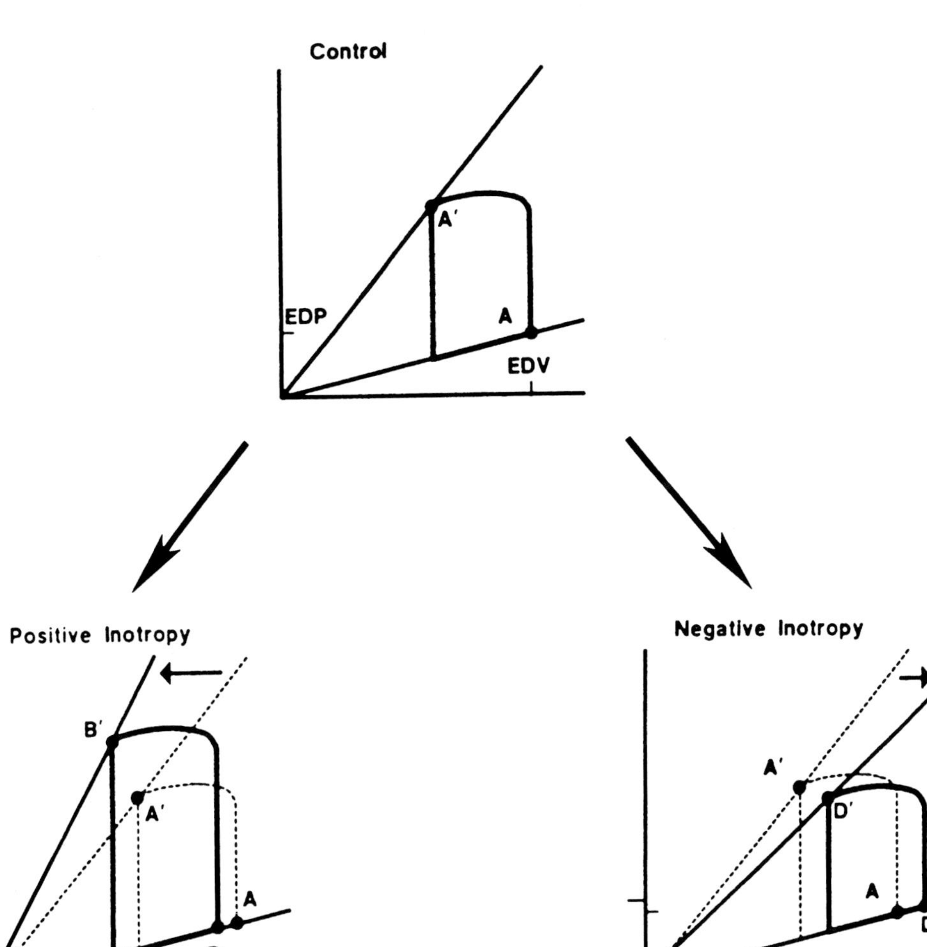

Figure 20–10 A positive inotropic intervention increases the heart's ability to do work at a given end-diastolic volume and pressure. As shown in this example, increased inotropy need not imply an increased stroke volume (SV); however, the latter is maintained despite a higher peak systolic pressure, producing the upward and leftward shift of the end-systolic pressure-volume point. Negative inotropy shifts the end-systolic pressure-volume point down and to the right. The SV is unchanged, but the end-diastolic and end-systolic volumes are increased, and the peak systolic pressure achieved is reduced. (From Katz AM: Influence of altered inotropy and lusitropy on ventricular pressure-volume loops. J Am Coll Cardiol 11:438, 1988.)

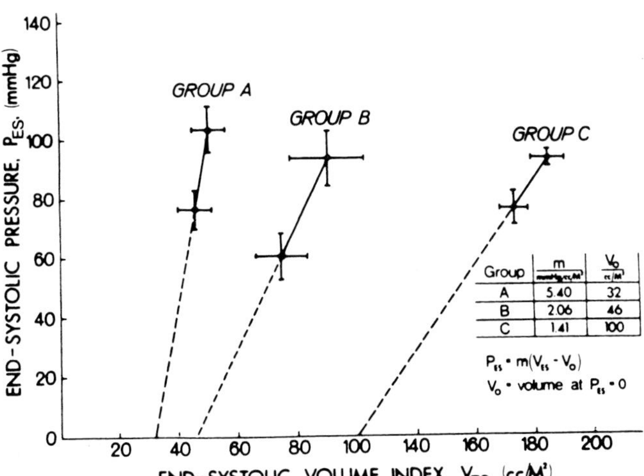

Figure 20–11 Average values of end-systolic pressure versus end-systolic volume (at two levels of afterload) plotted for groups (A, B, and C) with different contractile performance as evaluated by ejection fraction (A > 0.6; B = 0.41 to 0.59; C < 0.4). The end-systolic volume point correlates inversely with contractility. (From Grossman W, Braunwald E, Mann T, et al: Contractile state of the left ventricle in man as evaluated from end-systolic pressure-volume relations. Circulation 56:845, 1977.)

the EDPVR down and to the right, and a negative lusitropic intervention shifts it up and to the left (Fig. 20–12).

AORTIC STENOSIS

Clinical Features and Natural History

Aortic stenosis is the most common cardiac valve lesion in the United States. Approximately 1% to 2% of the population is born with a bicuspid aortic valve, which is prone to stenosis with aging, and the population is aging. Calcific aortic stenosis has several features in common with CAD. Both conditions are more common in men, older people, and patients with hypercholesterolemia, and both result in part from an active inflammatory process. There is clinical evidence of an atherosclerotic hypothesis for the cellular mechanism of aortic valve stenosis. There is a clear association between clinical risk factors for atherosclerosis and the development of aortic stenosis: elevated lipoprotein levels, increased low-density lipoprotein (LDL) cholesterol, cigarette smoking, hypertension, diabetes mellitus, increased serum calcium and creatinine levels, and male gender.[35] Homozygous familial hypercholesterolemia produces a severe form of aortic stenosis in children.[36] The early lesion of aortic valve sclerosis may be associated with CAD and vascular atherosclerosis. The extent of aortic valve calcification was observed as an important predictor of poor outcome in patients with aortic

Figure 20–12 Positive lusitropic interventions enhance diastolic filling, shifting the end-diastolic pressure-volume point down and to the right. A negative lusitropic intervention shifts the end-diastolic pressure-volume point up and to the left. (From Katz AM: Influence of altered inotropy and lusitropy on ventricular pressure-volume loops. J Am Coll Cardiol 11:438, 1988.)

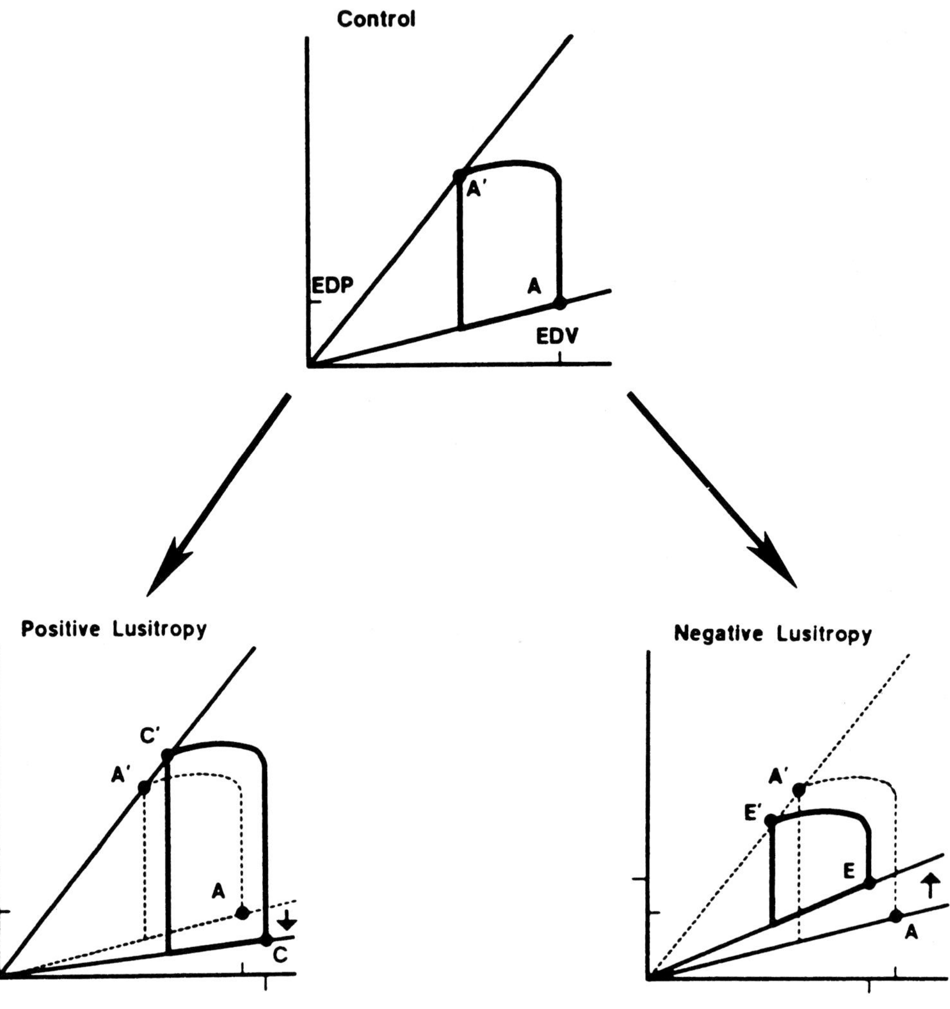

stenosis.[37] These and other studies suggest that aortic valve calcification is an inflammatory process promoted by atherosclerotic risk factors.

The early lesion of aortic stenosis resembles that of the initial plaque of CAD, and there is a close correlation between calcification found in coronary arteries and the amount of calcification found in the aortic valve. Pathologic studies of aortic valves revealed the presence of LDL , suggesting a common cellular mechanism for the genesis of valvular and vascular atherosclerotic disease.[35] Degenerative lesions on aortic valves contain an inflammatory infiltrate of nonfoam cells and foam cell macrophages, T lymphocytes, and other inflammatory cells. Lipid is accumulated in the fibrosa immediately below the endothelium layer on the aortic side of the valve. LDL- and apoE-containing lipoproteins are present as well. Little is known about the synthesis of bone matrix proteins in calcific aortic valve stenosis. The calcifications are composed of hydroxyapatite on a matrix of collagen, osteopontin, and other bone matrix proteins.

A potential mechanism for this cellular inflammation process involves the combination of macrophages, LDL, and the secretion by macrophages of transforming growth factor-β (TGF-β) and platelet-derived growth factor (PDGF) to stimulate the conversion of valvular fibroblast cells into osteoblasts that produce bone proteins.[35] Most surprising are the findings that 3-hydroxy-3-methylglutaryl coenzyme A (HMG CoA) reductase inhibitors (e.g., statins) retard the progression of CAD and of aortic stenosis.[38,39] The odds ratio of aortic stenosis progression was 0.46 in 38 treated patients compared with 118 untreated patients.[40] Other studies have shown similar results, and it is possible that therapy with statins or other drugs may be used to block or slow the progression of valve lesions in the future.[35,41]

The rate of progression is on average a decrease in aortic valve area (AVA) of 0.1 cm^2/year, and the peak instantaneous gradient increases by 10 mm Hg/year.[42] The rate of progression of aortic stenosis in men older than 60 years is faster than in women, and it is faster in women older than 75 years than in women 60 to 74 years old.[43] Treatment with hemodialysis, the use of calcium supplements, and elevated serum creatinine levels correlated with rapid progression of aortic stenosis.[44] Plasma brain natriuretic peptide (BNP), produced to a large extent by the ventricles, and the N-terminal part of the propeptide (NT-proBNP) may serve as early markers of left ventricular hypertrophy (LVH), whereas atrial natriuretic peptide (ANP) and NT-proANP reflect atrial pressure increase.[45] Repeated measurements of this marker may reflect information on the stage of aortic stenosis and its hemodynamic impact.[46]

Angina, syncope, and congestive heart failure (CHF) are the classic symptoms of the disease, and their appearance is of serious prognostic significance, because postmortem studies

indicate that symptomatic aortic stenosis is associated with a life expectancy of only 2 to 5 years.[47-49] These early natural history studies were completed before the availability of cardiac catheterization studies, and some patients, although symptomatic, may have had objectively less severe degrees of stenosis. The "hemodynamically insignificant murmur of aortic stenosis" seen so often in cardiologic consultations does not portend such dire consequences, although it is sometimes difficult to correlate aortic stenosis severity with clinical symptoms. There is evidence that patients with moderate aortic stenosis (i.e., valve areas of 0.7 to 1.2 cm^2) are also at increased risk for the development of complications, with the appearance of symptoms further increasing their risk.[50]

An interesting question is whether the natural history of aortic stenosis has changed significantly in recent years.[51] The question is prompted by two trends. The first, at least in North America, is related to the steadily diminishing number of patients with rheumatic disease. Today, aortic stenosis is essentially the bicuspid, the calcific, or what has been traditionally referred to as the senile variety. The second trend is related to the senile attribution. People are living longer, particularly those with heart disease. The typical patient with aortic stenosis is older and much more likely to have other significant medical problems, including major coexisting cardiac disease, most often CAD.

Angina is a frequent and classic symptom of the disease, occurring in approximately two thirds of patients with critical aortic stenosis, and about one half of symptomatic patients are found to have anatomically significant CAD.[52-54] However, a controversy persists about the incidence of CAD in patients with aortic stenosis who do not have angina, and the controversy probably reflects this underlying sense of a change in the natural history of the disease. Some studies report that the absence of angina virtually excludes the possibility of atherosclerotic heart disease.[55,56] In contrast, a 25% incidence of angiographically significant (>70% obstruction) coronary occlusions was described in angina-free patients, most of whom had single-vessel disease.[57] However, a much larger study found that 14% of patients with triple-vessel or left main CAD and aortic stenosis presented without angina.[58] Underscoring the continued lack of a consensus on this topic is the finding of a review that the reported incidences of significant CAD in asymptomatic patients range from 0% to 33%.[59] Identification of asymptomatic patients is important because although coexistent, untreated (i.e., unbypassed) CAD has a detrimental effect on early and late survival after aortic valve replacement (AVR), concomitant CABG with AVR does not increase perioperative mortality.[60-63] It appears that a substantial number of patients with coexisting coronary disease may have symptoms other than chest pain.[64] However, there do not appear to be other significant differences in the clinical or hemodynamic findings between patients with normal coronary arteries and those with coexistent coronary stenoses.

If the traditional natural history of aortic stenosis is perhaps more ominous in the elderly patient with likely coexistent coronary disease, is there any rationale for prophylactic AVR? With steady improvement in surgical results, this question has been raised, although rigorous studies still suggest that asymptomatic patients with hemodynamically significant disease face a very low risk of sudden death before the onset of symptoms.[65-67] As if by way of settling this particular question, an editorial by Braunwald stated that there was no role for prophylactic AVR and that "operative treatment is the most common cause of sudden death in asymptomatic patients with aortic stenosis."[68] These patients warrant very careful follow-up, and the case against prophylactic surgical intervention is further supported by studies showing that ventricular function is preserved and myocardial hypertrophy regresses after successful valve replacement.[69-71]

It is probably never too late to operate on patients with symptomatic aortic stenosis.[72,73] First, unlike aortic regurgitation, most symptomatic patients undergo valve replacement when LV function is still normal. Second, even when impaired LV function develops in aortic stenosis, the relief of pressure overload almost always restores normal function or at least produces considerable improvement. Morbidity rates, mortality rates, and clinical results are very favorable even in the oldest surgical candidates.[74,75]

The preoperative assessment of aortic stenosis with Doppler echocardiography includes measurement of the AVA and the transvalvular pressure gradient.[76,77] The latter is calculated from the Doppler-quantified transvalvular velocity of blood flow, which is increased in the presence of aortic stenosis. This maximal velocity (v) is then inserted in the modified Bernoulli equation to determine the pressure gradient (PG) between the left ventricle and the aorta (see Fig. 20–2):

$$PG = P\ (\text{left ventricle}) - P\ (\text{aorta}) = 4\ (v^2)$$

The *pressure gradient* is the maximal difference between the left ventricle and aortic pressures that occurs during ventricular systole.[78,79] This maximal instantaneous gradient is not the same as the peak-to-peak gradient determined by cardiac catheterization. The peak-to-peak gradient is determined by separate measurements of events that are not synchronous in real time. Of more practical interest is the fact that the best estimate of obstruction severity, as determined from pressure data alone, is the mean systolic gradient, which is calculated online by Doppler equipment[80] (see Chapters 12 and 15).

The Doppler-calculated gradient is subject to the same flow limitation as invasively calculated gradients. Best understood by considering the extreme, this means that a patient with true end-stage aortic stenosis would exhibit a relatively low calculated gradient because of minimal flow across a critically narrowed valve. In part because of this flow dependency, pressure gradients determined invasively or by Doppler echocardiography correctly classify aortic stenosis severity in less than 50% of cases compared with estimates of AVA.[81] However, the latter can also be determined by Doppler echocardiographic techniques. The preferred method requires only two Doppler-generated velocities: those proximal and those distal to the stenotic valve. These values are inserted in the continuity equation, which relates the respective velocities and cross-sectional areas proximal and distal to a stenotic area (see Fig. 20–3). Specifically, the equation states:

$$V_{max} \times AVA = \text{area (LVOT)} \times V\ (\text{LVOT})$$

in which AVA is the aortic valve area, V is the volume, and LVOT is the left ventricular outflow tract. Several studies have demonstrated the reliability of these Doppler-determined valve areas.[78-81]

Although advances in Doppler technology allow completely noninvasive evaluation of a large number of patients, coronary angiography is probably indicated in all patients older than 50 years who are demonstrated to have significant aortic stenosis. Angiography and, if indicated, CABG may improve the long-term outlook for patients with CAD who

undergo AVR.[58] Angiography also can identify a smaller number of patients whose CAD alone would warrant CABG.

Pathophysiology

The normal AVA is 2.6 to 3.5 cm^2, with hemodynamically significant obstruction usually occurring at cross-sectional valve areas of 1 cm^2 or less. Generally accepted criteria for critical outflow obstruction include a systolic pressure gradient greater than 50 mm Hg, with a normal cardiac output and an AVA of less than 0.4 cm^2. In view of the ominous natural history of severe aortic stenosis (AVA < 0.7 cm^2),[82,83] symptomatic patients with this degree of aortic stenosis are generally referred for immediate AVR.[84] The Hakki equation is a simplification of the gorlin equation to calculate the AVA based on the cardiac output (CO) and the peak pressure gradient (PG) across the valve.

$$\text{Valve area} \approx \frac{\text{CO}}{\sqrt{(\text{PG})}}$$

An obvious corollary of the previously described relationship is that "minimal" pressure gradients may actually reflect critical degrees of outflow obstruction when the cardiac output is significantly reduced (i.e., the generation of a pressure gradient requires some finite amount of flow). Clinicians have long recognized this phenomenon as a "paradoxical" decline in the intensity of the murmur (i.e., minimal transvalvular flow) as the aortic stenosis worsens.

Stenosis at the level of the aortic valve results in a pressure gradient from the left ventricle to the aorta. The intracavitary systolic pressure generated to overcome this stenosis directly increases myocardial wall tension in accordance with Laplace's law:

$$\text{Wall tension} = \frac{P \times R}{2h}$$

in which P is the intraventricular pressure, R is the inner radius, and h is the wall thickness.

This elevation of wall tension is believed to be the direct stimulus for the further parallel replication of sarcomeres, which produces the concentrically hypertrophied ventricle characteristic of chronic pressure overload.[85,86] The consequences of this LV hypertrophy include alterations in diastolic compliance, potential imbalances in the myocardial oxygen supply and demand relationship, and possible deterioration of the intrinsic contractile performance of the myocardium.

Figure 20–13 shows a typical pressure-volume loop for a patient with aortic stenosis. Two differences from the normal curve are immediately apparent. First, the peak pressure generated during systole is much higher because of the high transvalvular pressure gradient. Second, the slope of the diastolic limb is steeper, reflecting the reduced LV diastolic compliance that is associated with the increase in chamber thickness.[13] Clinically, this means that small changes in diastolic volume produce relatively large increases in ventricular filling pressure.

This increased chamber stiffness places a premium on the contribution of atrial systole to ventricular filling, which in patients with aortic stenosis may account for up to 40% of the LVEDV, rather than the 15% to 20% characteristic of the normal left ventricle. Echocardiographic and radionuclide studies have documented that diastolic filling and ventricular relaxation are abnormal in patients with hypertrophy from a

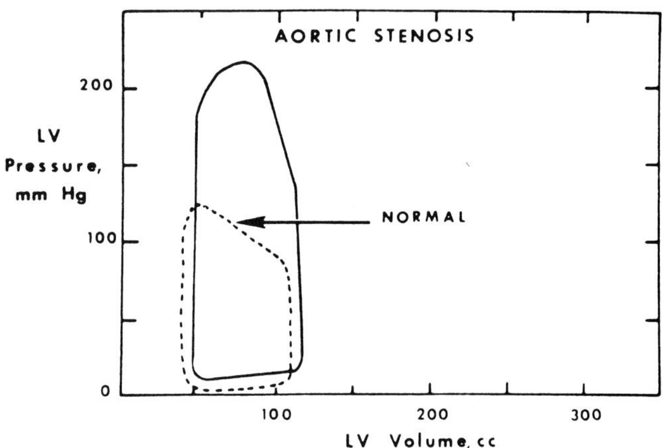

Figure 20–13 Pressure-volume loop in aortic stenosis. (From Jackson JM, Thomas SJ, Lowenstein E: Anesthetic management of patients with valvular heart disease. Semin Anesth 1:239, 1982.)

variety of causes, with significant prolongation of the isovolumic relaxation period being the most characteristic finding.[87-90] This necessarily compromises the duration and amount of filling achieved during the early rapid diastolic filling phase and increases the relative contribution of atrial contraction to overall diastolic filling (Fig. 20–14). A much higher mean left atrial (LA) pressure is necessary to distend the left ventricle in the absence of the sinus mechanism. One treatment of junctional rhythm is volume infusion.

The systolic limb of the pressure-volume loop shows preservation of pump function, as evidenced by maintenance of the SV and EF (see Fig. 20–13). It is likely that use of preload reserve and adequate LV hypertrophy are the principal compensatory mechanisms that maintain forward flow. Clinical studies have confirmed that ejection performance is preserved at the expense of myocardial hypertrophy, and the adequacy of the hypertrophic response has been related to the degree to which it achieves normalization of wall stress, in accordance with the Laplace relationship.[91-93] LV hypertrophy can be viewed as a compensatory physiologic response that completes a negative feedback loop (Fig. 20–15). It is possible, however, that severe afterload stress and proportionately massive LV hypertrophy could decrease subendocardial perfusion and superimpose a component of ischemic contractile dysfunction.

In patients with aortic stenosis, LVH develops as a result of the increase in pressure load. The development of LVH and its regression after therapeutic interventions are accompanied by changes in the cardiac extracellular matrix guided by an increase in *ECM1* gene expression during LVH and complete regression after complete correction.[94]

Systemic hypertension and aortic stenosis represent an increase in afterload to the left ventricle, and each contributes to LV remodeling and LVH. In a large series of 193 patients with aortic stenosis, 62 of whom were hypertensive, symptoms manifested with larger AVAs and lower stroke work loss.[95] Patterns of LV remodeling (i.e., concentric versus eccentric remodeling and hypertrophy) were not different between hypertensive and normotensive patients. LV mass decreased by 23% 1 year after AVR, back into the normal range, in patients with normal preoperative ventricular function; diastolic function improved concomitantly. Improvements in myocardial blood flow and coronary vasodilator reserve after

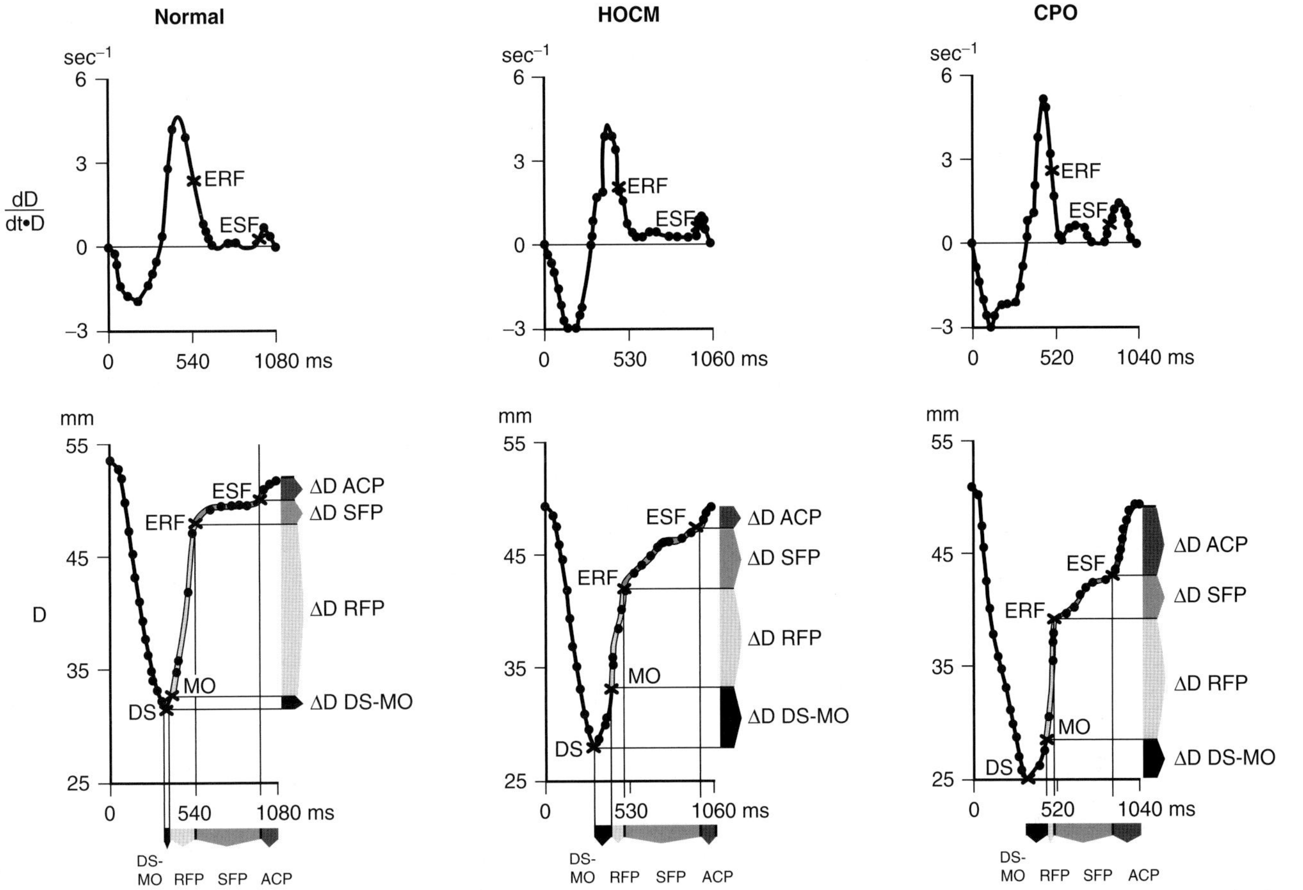

Figure 20–14 Computer-generated echograms of left venticular (LV) cavity size in normal subjects and patients with ventricular hypertrophy (i.e., hypertrophic obstructive cardiomyopathy [HOCM] or chronic pressure overload [CPO]). Upper panels show the rate of ventricular dimensional change. In the lower panels, for patients with both forms of hypertrophy, the mitral valve opening (MO) with regard to end-systolic LV dimension (DS) is delayed, and the dimensional change during this interval (ΔD DS-MO) is abnormally large. The duration of the rapid-filling phase (RFP) and the volume change during this interval (ΔD RFP) are correspondingly reduced. This is followed by a large dimensional increase during the atrial contraction phase (ΔD ACP) in the patient with chronic pressure overload. (From Hanrath P, Mathey DG, Siegert R, et al: Left ventricular relaxation and filling pattern in different forms of left ventricular hypertrophy: An echocardiographic study. Am J Cardiol 45:15, 1980.)

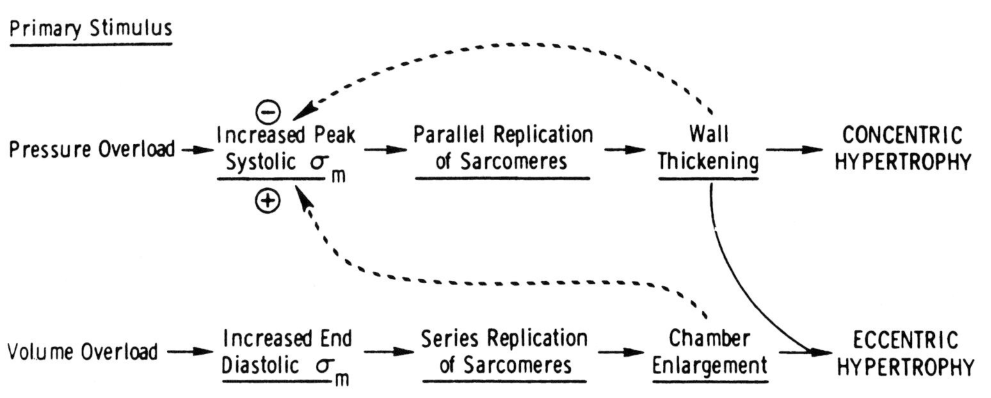

Figure 20–15 The increased peak systolic wall stress resulting from chronic pressure overload directly stimulates concentric ventricular hypertrophy, which tends to counteract or "normalize" the elevated ventricular wall stress. (From Grossman W, Jones D, McLaurin LP: Wall stress and patterns of hypertrophy in the human left ventricle. J Clin Invest 56:56, 1975.)

AVRs result from reduced extravascular compression and increased diastolic perfusion time.[96-98]

Ejection phase indices of contractile function are abnormal in many patients with aortic stenosis.[100,101] However, indices of contractile function, which are exquisitely sensitive to afterload, are inherently unreliable for quantitating the inotropic state in a disease such as aortic stenosis, in which the essence of the hemodynamic insult is the severely elevated ventricular afterload. This in no way excludes the possibility that a subset of patients may also experience some intrinsic depression of myocardial contractility. For example, patients with aortic stenosis may be particularly at risk for superimposed, ischemic ventricular dysfunction, but this possibility can be assessed only by the application of load-insensitive measurements of contractile function.

In most patients, however, load-insensitive indices of contractility (i.e., end-systolic stress-diameter determinations) are virtually identical before and after the development of hypertrophy, suggesting that the increase in chamber thickness compensates for the afterload stress, and myocardial con-

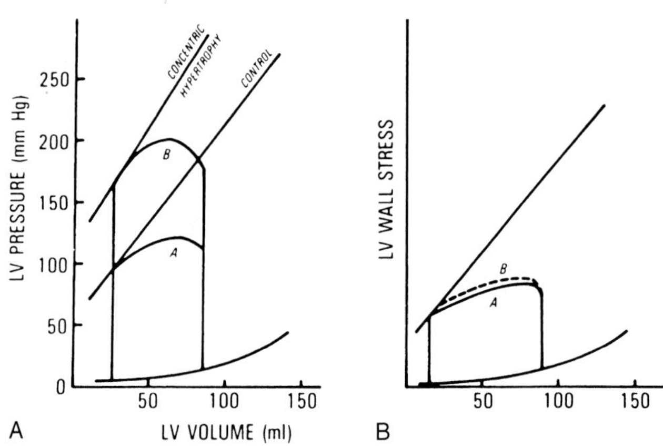

Figure 20–16 Adaptation to pressure overload. *(A)* Pressure-volume curves and the linear end-systolic pressure-volume relationship before and after the development of concentric hypertrophy. After hypertrophy, the end-systolic pressure-volume relationship is shifted upward and to the left (i.e., apparent supranormal contractility). *(B)* The same relationships are plotted as wall stress-volume loops. The loops before and after concentric hypertrophy are essentially the same, reaching the identical end-systolic wall stress-volume point (i.e., contractility unchanged). (From Ross J Jr: Afterload mismatch in aortic and mitral valve disease: Implications for surgical therapy. J Am Coll Cardiol 5:811, 1985.)

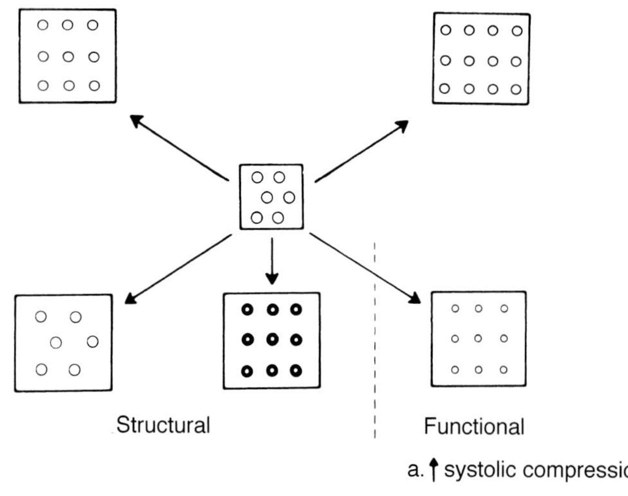

Figure 20–17 Possible coronary circulatory changes accompanying ventricular hypertrophy. The size of the box indicates myocardial mass, and the area of circles indicates the cross-sectional area of coronary vasculature. The relationship may be normal, as illustrated by top left box, when growth of the coronary bed has kept pace with ventricular hypertrophy. Experimental data support two possible anatomic derangements: inadequate growth of structurally normal vessels (bottom left) or appropriate growth of abnormally thickened resistance vessels whose luminal area is accordingly compromised. (From Marcus ML: Effects of cardiac hypertrophy on the coronary circulation. *In* Marcus ML [ed]: The Coronary Circulation in Health and Disease. New York, McGraw-Hill, 1983.)

tractility is therefore normal, albeit appropriate for the higher afterload. Figure 20–16 illustrates the adaptation of the left ventricle to chronic pressure overload. Figure 20–16*A* shows the pressure-volume relationship before (loop A) and after (loop B) the development of concentric hypertrophy. The linear ESPVR is shifted up and to the left after concentric hypertrophy occurs. However, the ESPVR may not be as accurate or load insensitive in assessing contractility at the extremes of afterload. Figure 20–16*B* shows normalization of this apparently supranormal contractility, when wall stress (rather than pressure) is used as a more exact measure of ventricular afterload. Concentric hypertrophy normalizes wall stress and contractility remains unchanged. A decline in any index of myocardial contractility in patients with aortic stenosis may represent relatively inadequate hypertrophy for the degree of wall stress, some intrinsic depression of contractility, or a combination of these two factors.[52,102,103] The fact that most patients have normal contractility is the reason for the usually favorable response to AVR.

In aortic stenosis, signs and symptoms of CHF usually develop when preload reserve is exhausted, not because contractility is intrinsically or permanently impaired. This contrasts with mitral and aortic regurgitation, in which irreversible myocardial dysfunction may develop before the onset of significant symptoms. An important exception is the patient with aortic stenosis whose symptoms of CHF occur in the setting of associated mitral regurgitation. The latter may accompany hypertrophy-induced LV chamber or mitral annular enlargement. Mitral regurgitation in patients with aortic stenosis is often referred to as *functional* as opposed to anatomic mitral insufficiency. The implication is that with relief of the high intracavitary systolic pressure, the mitral regurgitation will largely resolve, given an anatomically normal mitral valve. It is not uncommon for grade 2 or 3 mitral regurgitation to be significantly reduced after AVR.

More commonly, intrinsic contractility is preserved, and the major threat to the hypertrophied ventricle is its exquisite sensitivity to ischemia. Ventricular hypertrophy directly elevates basal myocardial oxygen demand ($M\dot{V}O_2$). The other major determinants of overall $M\dot{V}O_2$ are heart rate, contractility, and most important, wall tension. Increases in the latter occur as a direct consequence of Laplace's law in patients with relatively inadequate hypertrophy. The possibility of ischemic contractile dysfunction in the inadequately hypertrophied ventricle arises from increases in wall tension, which directly parallels the imbalance between the elevated peak systolic pressure and the degree of mural hypertrophy. Although there is considerable evidence for "supply-side" abnormalities in the myocardial supply and demand relationship in patients with aortic stenosis, clinical data also support increased $M\dot{V}O_2$ as important in the genesis of myocardial ischemia.

On the supply side, the higher LVEDP of the poorly compliant ventricle inevitably narrows the diastolic coronary perfusion pressure (CPP) gradient. With severe outflow obstruction, decreases in SV and resultant systemic hypotension may critically compromise coronary perfusion. A vicious cycle may develop because ischemia-induced abnormalities of diastolic relaxation can aggravate the compliance problem and further narrow the CPP gradient.[104] This sets the stage for ischemic contractile dysfunction, additional decreases in SV, and worsening hypotension.

Cardiac hypertrophy is also associated with structural abnormalities of the coronary circulation (Fig. 20–17).[105,106] Animal models have documented that epicardial coronary vessels do not enlarge proportionately when the left ventricle is subjected to a chronic pressure load.[107,108] LV hypertrophy accompanying chronic hypertension is associated with an increased wall lumen ratio of the coronary arterioles, a change that limits vessel dilation and augments active constriction.[109,110] Animal models of pressure-induced myocardial hypertrophy have also shown a decrease in the capillary density of about 20% to 30%.[105,107,109-113] There is considerable

evidence that in LV hypertrophy due to pressure overload, a reduction in the coronary vascular reserve may underlie episodes of myocardial ischemia[114,115] (see Chapter 6).

Echocardiographic and hemodynamic assessments of the myocardial oxygen supply and demand ratio are not significantly different in the presence or absence of angina in patients with aortic stenosis.[116] However, considerable data indicate that dynamic factors relative to oxygen supply may be crucial to the pathogenesis of angina in these patients.[117] Several clinical studies have documented a decrease in coronary vascular reserve in adult and pediatric patients with significant LV or RV hypertrophy.[118-120] It is further postulated that repeated episodes of subendocardial ischemia may contribute to the development of subendocardial fibrosis, a component of ischemic contractile dysfunction.[105]

It is possible that myocardial ischemia underlies the impaired ventricular relaxation that has been documented in patients with myocardial hypertrophy due to a variety of causes.[87,89,90] Prolongation of ventricular relaxation and resultant diastolic dysfunction (i.e., poor compliance) are probably universal features of myocardial ischemia in a variety of clinical settings.[121-125] Experimental data suggest that ischemia-induced impairment of calcium sequestration by the sarcoplasmic reticulum may underlie the increased diastolic chamber stiffness.[126] Prevention of ischemia-induced myoplasmic calcium overload may be the mechanism by which the calcium channel blockers are able to improve diastolic dysfunction in patients with CAD.[127] These drugs also ameliorate ventricular relaxation and diastolic filling in patients with hypertrophic cardiomyopathy, although the mechanism of action is controversial.[87,128-130] The absence of diastolic filling abnormalities in patients with physiologic, as opposed to pathologic, hypertrophy may also reflect the relative likelihood of ischemia in the two conditions.[131-133]

In summary, the pathophysiologic response to chronic pressure overload is a complex one characterized by unique interaction among the divergent effects of hypertrophy on systolic and diastolic function. Mural thickening enhances systolic performance, maximizing the mechanical work performed while minimizing its metabolic cost. The price of this systolic efficiency is relatively inadequate growth of the coronary microcirculation, which contributes to relaxation abnormalities, diastolic dysfunction, and the potential for superimposition of ischemia-induced abnormalities of systolic dysfunction (Table 20–1).[134] The potentially deleterious effects of LV hypertrophy cannot be overemphasized. Even in the absence of aortic stenosis, in which LV hypertrophy can be viewed as a compensatory and potentially beneficial pathophysiologic response, LV hypertrophy has been found to have an independent adverse effect on survival.[135,136]

Table 20–1 Pressure-Overload Hypertrophy

Beneficial Aspects	Detrimental Aspects
Increases ventricular work	Decreases ventricular diastolic distensibility
Normalizes wall stress	Impairs ventricular relaxation
Normalizes systolic shortening	Impairs coronary vasodilator reserve, leading to subendocardial ischemia

From Lorell BH, Grossman W: Cardiac hypertrophy: The consequences for diastole. J Am Coll Cardiol 9:1189, 1987.

Difficulty of Low-Gradient, Low-Output Aortic Stenosis

A subset of patients with severe aortic stenosis, LV dysfunction, and low transvalvular gradient suffers a high operative mortality rate and poor prognosis.[137] It is difficult to accurately assess the AVA in this low-flow, low-gradient aortic stenosis because the calculated valve area is proportional to forward SV and because the Gorlin constant varies in low-flow states. Some patients with low-flow, low-gradient aortic stenosis have a decreased AVA as a result of inadequate forward SV rather than anatomic stenosis. Surgical therapy is unlikely to benefit these patients because the underlying pathology is a weakly contractile myocardium. However, patients with severe anatomic aortic stenosis may benefit from valve replacement despite the increased operative risk associated with the low-flow, low-gradient hemodynamic state.[137] Guidelines from the American College of Cardiology (ACC) and American Heart Association (AHA) call for a dobutamine echocardiography evaluation to distinguish patients with fixed anatomic aortic stenosis from those with flow-dependent aortic stenosis with LV dysfunction.[138] Low-flow, low-gradient aortic stenosis is defined for a mean gradient of less than 30 mm Hg and a calculated AVA less than 1.0 cm^2.

Dobutamine echocardiography revealed three basic response patterns—fixed aortic stenosis, relative aortic stenosis, and absence of contractile reserve—in an initial study by DeFilippi et al.[139] In a series of 45 patients with low-flow, low-gradient aortic stenosis, the 30-day operative mortality rate was 8% for patients with contractile reserve and 50% for those without contractile reserve.[140] Dobutamine challenges during cardiac catheterization provided unique insights into low-flow, low-gradient aortic stenosis, and the details are summarized in Figure 20–18.[141] In panel A, the transvalvular gradient and cardiac output increased, and the valve area did not change. Patients represented in panel B increased their cardiac output with little or no change in gradient, and the calculated valve area increased slightly. This group still benefited from surgery. The third group of patients had no contractile reserve because cardiac output did not increase with dobutamine, and the transvalvular gradient decreased (Fig. 20–18, Panel C). Dobutamine infusion in the cardiac catheterization laboratory appears to be helpful in identifying patients with low-flow, low-gradient aortic stenosis who have a truly fixed anatomical stenosis that may benefit from valve replacement. The findings of these studies also emphasize that contractile reserve is an important prognostic indicator in these patients and dobutamine challenge may help select patients for valve replacement. It appears that patients with contractile reserve and fixed aortic stenosis have a relatively good prognosis with valve replacement. LV contractile reserve appears to be a critical variable for prognosis.

Developments in the Hemodynamic Management of Critical Aortic Stenosis Patients

The use of vasodilators is traditionally contraindicated in patients with severe aortic stenosis because cardiac output is relatively fixed across a narrowed orifice. Vasodilation reduces SVR without any possibility for a compensatory increase in cardiac output and severe hypotension would typically result. This traditional paradigm was recently reexamined in patients

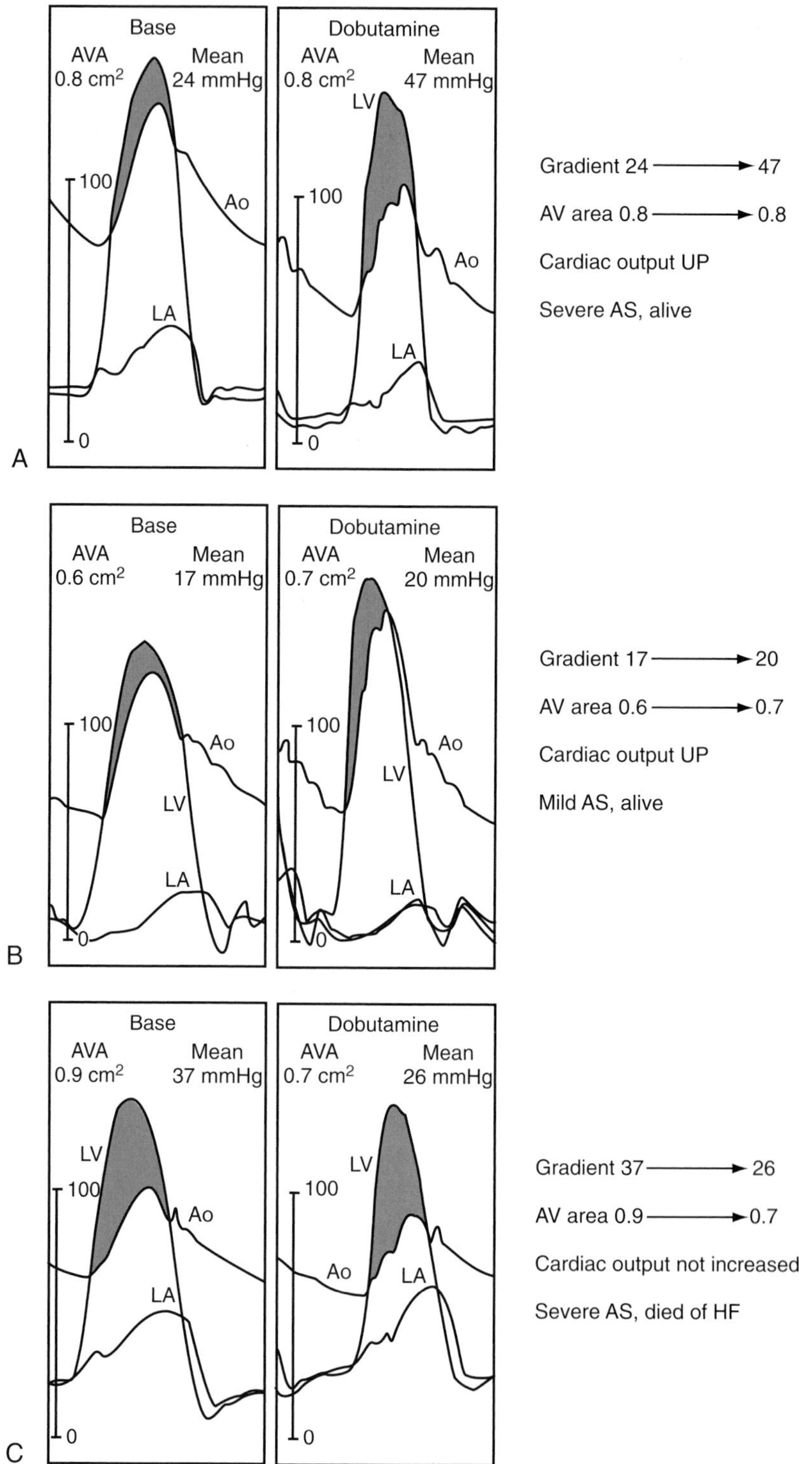

Figure 20–18 Hemodynamic tracings from three patients representing three different responses to dobutamine. (Adapted from Nishimura RA, Grantham JA, Connolly HM, et al: Low-output, low-gradient aortic stenosis in patients with depressed left ventricular systolic function: the clinical utility of the dobutamine challenge in the catheterization laboratory. Circulation 106:809, 2002.)

with fixed, severe aortic stenosis (area < 1.0 cm²) and LV dysfunction (EF < 0.35).[142] Nitroprusside was carefully titrated to maintain a mean arterial pressure (MAP) of more than 60 mm Hg with concomitant hemodynamic monitoring. The cardiac index increased over 24 hours from a mean of 1.60 to 2.52 L/min/m² with no changes in heart rate and MAP (Fig. 20–19). The pulmonary capillary wedge pressure (PCWP) and SVR decreased while SV increased.

It appears that this treatment is effective to alleviate to some extent the LV dysfunction component of the complete syndrome. LV dysfunction benefits derived from unloading and careful titration of the nitroprusside most likely allowed SVR to decrease without changes in MAP. This titrated unloading may benefit patients with severe aortic stenosis and LV dysfunction, and it may serve as a temporary bridge to AVR or oral vasodilator therapy.[142] It is unclear whether treatment with positive inotropic agents would produce similar effects with fewer risks. Adequate treatment of patients with aortic stenosis, a depressed EF, and a low transvalvular gradient continues to pose a diagnostic and therapeutic challenge.[143] The use of nitroprusside in aortic stenosis in the absence of ventricular dysfunction may not be as effective and even be deleterious because of the prompt decrease in preload by nitroprusside.

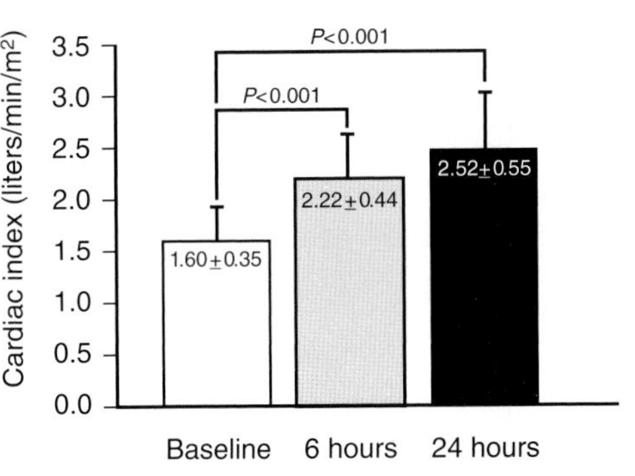

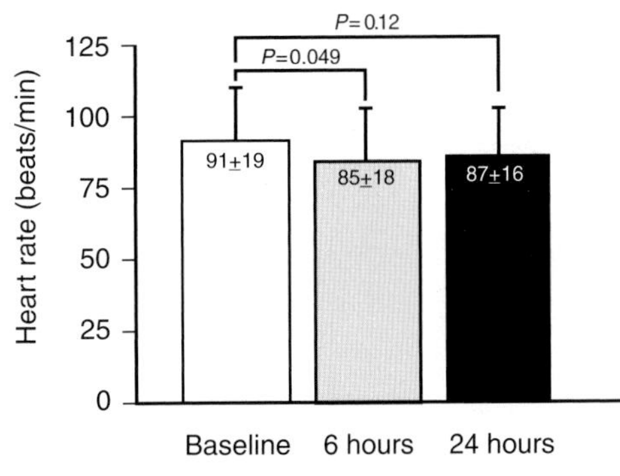

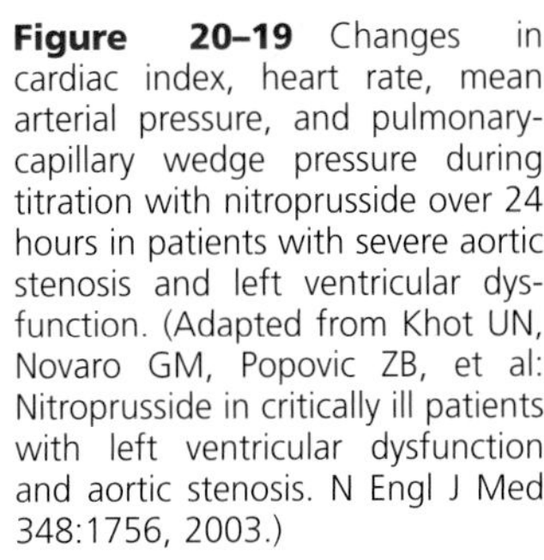
Figure 20–19 Changes in cardiac index, heart rate, mean arterial pressure, and pulmonary-capillary wedge pressure during titration with nitroprusside over 24 hours in patients with severe aortic stenosis and left ventricular dysfunction. (Adapted from Khot UN, Novaro GM, Popovic ZB, et al: Nitroprusside in critically ill patients with left ventricular dysfunction and aortic stenosis. N Engl J Med 348:1756, 2003.)

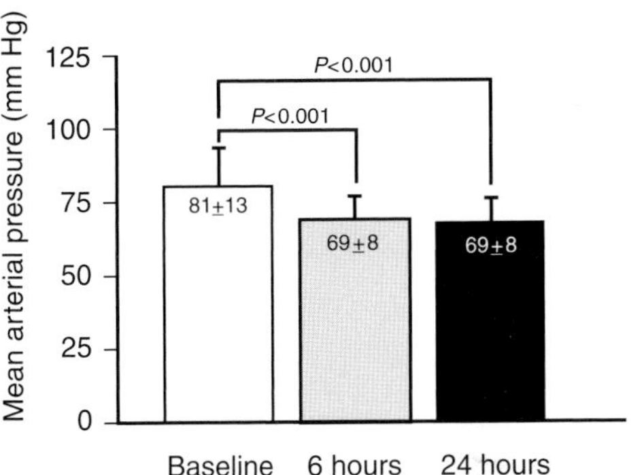

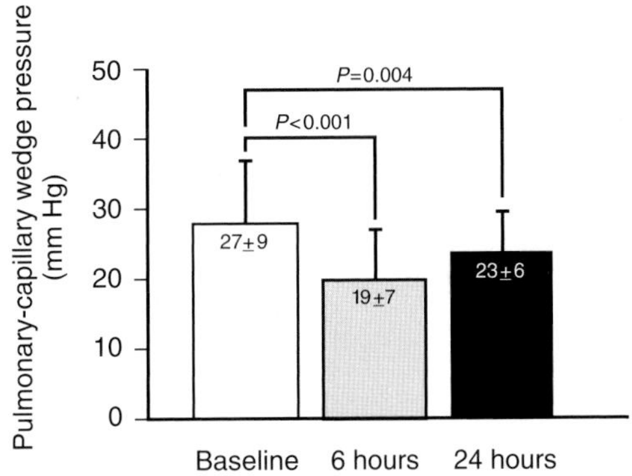

Timing of Intervention

In asymptomatic patients with aortic stenosis, it appears to be relatively safe to delay surgery until symptoms develop, but outcomes vary widely. The presence of moderate or severe valvular calcification along with a rapid increase in aortic-jet velocity identifies patients with a very poor prognosis. These patients should be considered for early valve replacement rather than delaying until symptoms develop.[37]

Echocardiography and exercise testing may identify asymptomatic patients who are likely to benefit from surgery.[144] In a study of 58 asymptomatic patients, 21 had symptoms for the first time during exercise testing.[145] Guidelines for AVR in patients with aortic stenosis are shown in Table 20–2.

Functional outcome after AVR in patients older than 80 years is excellent, operative risk is limited, and late survival rates are good.[146] In patients with severe LV dysfunction and low transvalvular mean gradient, operative mortality is increased, but AVR was associated with improved functional status.[147] Postoperative survival was best in younger patients and with larger prosthetic valves, whereas medium-term survival was related to improved postoperative functional class.[147]

Anesthetic Considerations

The foregoing pathophysiologic principles dictate that anesthetic management be based on the avoidance of systemic hypotension, maintenance of sinus rhythm and an adequate intravascular volume, and awareness of the potential for myocardial ischemia (Box 20–1). In the absence of CHF, adequate premedication may reduce the likelihood of undue preoperative excitement, tachycardia, and the resultant potential for exacerbating myocardial ischemia and the transvalvular pressure gradient. In patients with truly critical outflow tract obstruction, however, heavy premedication with an exaggerated venodilatory response can reduce the appropriately elevated LVEDV (and LVEDP) needed to overcome the systolic

Table 20–2 Recommendations for the Use of Aortic Valve Replacement in Patients with Aortic Stenosis

Replacement Indicated	Replacement Possibly Indicated
Patients with severe aortic stenosis and any of its classic symptoms (e.g., angina, syncope, dyspnea)	Patients with moderate aortic stenosis who require coronary artery bypass surgery or surgery on the aorta or heart valves
Patients with severe aortic stenosis who are undergoing coronary artery bypass surgery	Asymptomatic patients with severe aortic stenosis and at least one of the following: ejection fraction of no more than 0.50, hemodynamic instability during exercise (e.g., hypotension), ventricular tachycardia; not indicated to prevent sudden death in asymptomatic patients who have none of the findings listed
Patients with severe aortic stenosis who are undergoing surgery on the aorta or other heart valves	

Adapted from the American Heart Association web site (www.americanheart.org).

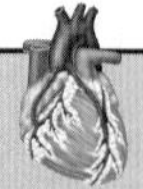

BOX 20–1 *Aortic Stenosis*

Preload:	Increased
Afterload:	Increased
Goal:	Sinus rhythm
Avoid:	Hypotension, tachycardia, bradycardia

pressure gradient. In these patients in particular, the additional precaution of administering supplementary oxygen may provide worthwhile insurance against the possibility of a similarly pronounced response to the sedative effects of the premedicant.

Intraoperative monitoring should include a standard five-lead electrocardiographic (ECG) system, including a V_5 lead, because of the left ventricle's vulnerability to ischemia. A practical constraint in terms of interpretation is that these patients usually exhibit ECG changes because of preoperative LV hypertrophy. The associated ST-segment abnormalities (i.e., strain pattern) may be indistinguishable from or at least very similar to those of myocardial ischemia, making the intraoperative interpretation difficult. Lead II and possibly an esophageal electrocardiogram should be readily obtainable, because they may be useful for assessing the P-wave changes in the event of supraventricular arrhythmias (see Chapter 14).

Hemodynamic monitoring is controversial, and few prospective data are available on which to base an enlightened clinical decision. The central venous pressure (CVP) is a particularly poor estimate of LV filling when LV compliance is reduced. A normal CVP can significantly underestimate the LVEDP or PCWP. The principal risks, although minimal, of using a pulmonary artery catheter (PAC) in the patient with aortic stenosis are arrhythmia-induced hypotension and ischemia. Loss of synchronous atrial contraction or a supraventricular tachyarrhythmia can compromise diastolic filling of the poorly compliant left ventricle, resulting in hypotension and the potential for rapid hemodynamic deterioration. The threat of catheter-induced arrhythmias is significant for the patient with aortic stenosis. However, accepting a low-normal CVP as evidence of good ventricular function can lead to similarly catastrophic underfilling of the left ventricle on the basis of insufficient replenishment of surgical blood loss. To some extent, even the PCWP can underestimate the LVEDP (and LVEDV) when ventricular compliance is markedly reduced. Placement of a PAC also allows for measurement of cardiac output, derived hemodynamic parameters, mixed venous oxygen saturation (SvO_2), and possible transvenous pacing (see Chapter 14).

Intraoperative fluid management should be aimed at maintaining appropriately elevated left-sided filling pressures. This is one reason why many clinicians believe that the PAC is worth its small arrhythmogenic risk. Keeping up with intravascular volume losses is particularly important in noncardiovascular surgery, in which the shorter duration of the operation may make an inhalation or potentially vasodilating regional anesthetic preferable to a narcotic technique.

Patients with symptomatic aortic stenosis are usually encountered only in the setting of cardiovascular surgery because of their ominous prognosis without AVR. Few studies have specifically addressed the response of these patients to the standard intravenous and inhalation induction agents; however, the responses to narcotic[148,149] and nonnarcotic[150,151] intravenous agents are apparently not dissimilar from those of patients with other forms of VHD. The principal benefit of a narcotic induction is the assurance of an adequate depth of anesthesia during intubation, which reliably blunts potentially deleterious reflex sympathetic responses capable of precipitating tachycardia and ischemia.

Many clinicians also prefer a pure narcotic technique for maintenance. The negative inotropy of the inhalation anesthetics is a theoretical disadvantage for a myocardium faced with the challenge of overcoming outflow tract obstruction. A more clinically relevant drawback may be the increased risk of arrhythmia-induced hypotension, particularly that associated with nodal rhythm and resultant loss of the atrium's critical contribution to filling of the hypertrophied ventricle[152,153] (see Chapter 9).

Occasionally, surgical stimulation elicits a hypertensive response despite the impedance posed by the stenotic valve and a seemingly adequate depth of narcotic anesthesia. In such patients, a judicious trial of low concentrations of an inhalation agent, used purely for control of hypertension, may prove efficacious. The ability to concurrently monitor cardiac output is useful in this situation. The temptation to control intraoperative hypertension with vasodilators should be resisted in most cases. Given the risk of ischemia, nitroglycerin seems to be a particularly attractive drug. Its effectiveness in relieving subendocardial ischemia in patients with aortic stenosis is controversial[154,155]; however, there is always the risk of even transient episodes of "overshoot." The hypertrophied ventricle's critical dependence on an adequate CPP may be very unforgiving of even a momentary dip in the systemic arterial pressure.

Intraoperative hypotension, regardless of the primary cause, should be treated immediately and aggressively with a direct α-adrenergic agonist such as phenylephrine.[156] The goal should be to immediately restore the CPP and then to address the underlying problem (e.g., hypovolemia, arrhythmia). After the arterial pressure responds, treatment of the precipitating event should be equally aggressive, but rapid transfusion or cardioversion should not delay the administration of a direct-acting vasoconstrictor. Patients with severe aortic stenosis in whom objective signs of myocardial ischemia persist despite restoration of the blood pressure should be treated extremely aggressively. This may mean the immediate use of an inotropic agent or simply accelerating the institution of cardiopulmonary bypass (CPB).

Intraoperative myocardial ischemic injury in the patient with aortic stenosis has been appreciated for some time, and there are several theories regarding its pathogenesis. The potential vulnerability of the hypertrophied myocardium to ischemic damage was initially speculated on by cardiac surgeons who described the phenomenon of irreversible ischemic contracture—what they called the *stone heart*—occurring after AVR in a group of patients with severe LV hypertrophy.[157] The anatomic and hemodynamic bases for an unfavorable myocardial oxygen supply and demand relationship have already been considered, but the possibility that these patients might be experiencing pre-bypass ischemic injury remains a plausible, although unproven, hypothesis.

Most attention has been focused on the potential for irreversible cellular damage occurring during the period of ischemic cardiac arrest. Although there is a consensus that improved myocardial preservation has been crucial in reduc-

ing the mortality rate after CABG, there is evidence that current cardioplegic techniques may provide suboptimal protection for patients with VHD.[158,159] Specifically, there is ultrastructural evidence (e.g., intracellular or mitochondrial edema) suggesting that the hypertrophied myocardium is uniquely susceptible to ischemic damage during the aortic cross-clamp interval, despite the presumed protection. Although these changes are observed in patients whose clinical course is seemingly unremarkable, such ischemic cellular damage also may underlie the frequent occurrence of postoperative low-output syndromes and the higher mortality rates associated with valvular operations.[160]

Although a detailed consideration of myocardial preservation is beyond the scope of this chapter (see Chapters 28 and 30), certain aspects are peculiar to the operative management of patients with aortic stenosis, and it is likely that improved cardioplegic techniques will play an important role in reducing operative morbidity and mortality rates. Because the operation requires an ascending aortotomy, many surgeons routinely use direct coronary ostial cannulation for the delivery of the cardioplegic solution. Problems associated with this approach are uncommon but include the inherent hazard of injury to the coronary ostia; cannula-induced late stenosis of the left main coronary artery has also been described.[161] Coronary ostial delivery required interrupting the surgical procedure for subsequent reinfusions of the cardioplegic solution. These problems are obviated by the use of cardioplegia delivery by the coronary sinus. The retrograde technique is commonly used in conjunction with an initial dose of antegrade cardioplegia; the latter provides for a more immediate electromechanical arrest.[162-164]

Noncardiac Surgery in the Patient with Aortic Stenosis

Patients with aortic stenosis who undergo noncardiac surgery were identified by Goldman et al[145] as being at increased risk for cardiac complications, including myocardial infarction, CHF, and supraventricular tachyarrhythmias. Likewise, the ACC Task Force on perioperative evaluation of the cardiac patient identified patients with severe or symptomatic aortic stenosis as being at increased risk for serious perioperative cardiac morbidity.[165] It states that symptomatic stenotic lesions are associated with the risk of perioperative severe CHF or shock and often require percutaneous valvotomy or valve replacement before noncardiac surgery to lower cardiac risk. With the overall aging of the surgical population and given a peak incidence of significant aortic stenosis in the fifth and sixth decades, it is likely that these patients will be encountered with increasing frequency in the setting of noncardiac surgery. Given the natural history of the disease and following the conservative ACC guidelines cited previously, one approach is to recommend immediate but elective AVR to all aortic stenosis patients, before any noncardiac procedures. Although there is a rationale for this "shotgun" solution, a variety of ethical, practical, and economic constraints argue for a more selective approach.

A common clinical problem is the elderly, asymptomatic patient, with a harsh systolic ejection murmur, who is scheduled for noncardiac surgery. Risk assessment for the asymptomatic patient is challenging because the prognosis in the absence of AVR may be quite benign. However, symptoms correlate poorly with aortic stenosis severity, which may by itself portend a more ominous natural history. In these patients, the use of a two-dimensional Doppler echocardiographic examination allows for the noninvasive assessment of the severity of stenosis[53] and for some quantification of contractile function (see Chapter 15). Patients with moderate aortic stenosis have a higher, short-term incidence of cardiovascular complications, and this risk is further increased by the presence of symptoms or objective evidence of contractile impairment.[50] Armed with the echocardiographic evaluation (e.g., stenosis severity, contractile state), the clinician can make an initial assessment of relative risk. Depending on the overall clinical picture, some of these patients may warrant immediate elective AVR, whereas in others, it may be more appropriate to proceed with the noncardiac operation, with hemodynamic monitoring as dictated by the echocardiographic data and the nature of the surgery. A reality of the clinical setting is that the overall picture often seems to dictate that the anesthesiologist should proceed with the originally planned operation, albeit at increased risk of perioperative cardiac morbidity.

HYPERTROPHIC CARDIOMYOPATHY

Hypertrophic Obstructive Cardiomyopathy

Hypertrophic obstructive cardiomyopathy (HOCM) is a relatively common genetic malformation of the heart with a prevalence of approximately 1 in 500 (see Chapter 24). The hypertrophy initially develops in the septum and extends to the free walls, often giving a picture of concentric hypertrophy. Asymmetric septal hypertrophy leads to a variable pressure gradient between the apical LV chamber and the LVOT. The LVOT obstruction leads to increases in LV pressure, which fuels a vicious cycle of further hypertrophy and increased LVOT obstruction.[166] Various treatment modalities include β-adrenoceptor antagonists, calcium channel blockers, and surgical myectomy of the septum. For more than 40 years, the traditional standard treatment has been the ventricular septal myotomy-myomectomy of Morrow, in which a small amount of muscle from the subaortic septum is resected.[167] Two new treatment modalities have gained popularity in recent years, dual-chamber pacing and septal reduction (ablation) therapy with ethanol.

Dual-chamber DDD pacing is based on the observation that excitation of the septum of the left ventricle contracts it away from the apposing wall, which may reduce the LVOT gradient. The precise mechanism by which dual-chamber pacing decreases LVOT gradient or improves symptoms is uncertain. Possible mechanisms are asynchronous ventricular activation, paradoxical septal wall motion, a negative inotropic effect, an increase in end-systolic volume, decreased systolic anterior leaflet motion, altered myocardial perfusion, and regression of LVH.[168] The AV interval must be sufficiently short to guarantee early RV apical activation without conduction through the His-Purkinje system. Although some studies have shown a decrease in the LVOT gradient of 25%, there are still variable results with respect to improvements in exercise capacity and symptoms.[168-171]

Patients with severe, drug-resistant symptoms of CHF, angina, or syncope are considered for nonsurgical septal reduction therapy. In one series, patients with a resting gradient of more than 40 mm Hg or a dobutamine-induced gradient of more than 60 mm Hg were included.[172] After coronary angiography to exclude significant CAD and after placement of temporary pacing wires, the LVOT gradient was measured

at rest and during various interventions (e.g., Valsalva, postextrasystolic, isoproterenol, amyl nitrite). The coronary septal branches were cannulated with a small balloon-equipped catheter. The balloon was inflated to prevent overflow or spillage into the left anterior descending coronary artery. Depending on the septal branch size and area of septal hypertrophy, a dose of 2 to 5 mL of ethanol was slowly injected through the balloon catheter lumen. The LVOT gradient decreased immediately in 85% to 90% of patients. Further decreases in gradient were reported after 6 months.[168] The septal muscle mass was not decreased adequately through alcohol injections at the time of the intervention, but ventricular remodeling continued and led to sustained symptomatic improvement most dramatically over the first 3 to 6 months.[166] Exercise tolerance increased as well, but atrioventricular block, right bundle-branch block, and left bundle-branch block were frequent adverse consequences. Permanent heart blocks still occur in 5% to 10% of cases.[173]

Clinical Features and Natural History

Hypertrophic cardiomyopathy (HCM) is an uncommon familial disorder in which there is pronounced hypertrophy of histologically abnormal sarcomeres with characteristically disproportionate involvement of the interventricular septum.[174-176] This disease has numerous pathologic and pathophysiologic features, which vary in their relative predominance in individual patients. A variety of other names have been applied to the disorder, including asymmetric septal hypertrophy, muscular subaortic stenosis, and idiopathic hypertrophic subaortic stenosis, with each emphasizing some aspect of the disease that may or may not be a prominent feature of its presentation in an individual patient. The cause and exact pattern of inheritance of the disease remain unknown, although it appears to be an autosomal dominant trait expressed with a high degree of penetrance[176-178] (see Chapter 24).

Patients vary widely in their clinical presentation. The contribution of echocardiography to the diagnosis has unquestionably increased the number of asymptomatic patients who carry the diagnosis. Most patients with HCM are asymptomatic and have been seen by the echocardiographer because of relatives having clinical disease. Follow-up remains an important problem for cardiologists because sudden death or cardiac arrest may occur as the presenting symptom in slightly more than one half of previously asymptomatic patients.[179]

Less dramatic frequently presenting complaints include dyspnea, angina, and syncope.[176] The clinical picture is often similar to valvular aortic stenosis. The symptoms may share a similar pathophysiologic basis (e.g., poor diastolic compliance) in the two conditions. The prognostic implications of clinical disease, however, are less certain for patients with HCM. Although cardiac arrest may be an unheralded event, other patients may have a stable pattern of angina or intermittent syncopal episodes for many years.[180] Palpitations are also frequently described and may be related to a variety of underlying arrhythmias. Of patients studied with continuous ambulatory monitoring, ventricular arrhythmias occur in more than 75%, supraventricular tachycardias in 25%, and atrial fibrillation in 5% to 10%.[181-183] The latter often precipitates clinical deterioration because of the dependence of the noncompliant left ventricle on atrial systole for its filling.[184]

The natural history of patients with HCM is also extremely variable. These patients are all at risk for sudden death, although those with a family history of this problem form an especially high-risk group.[185] Unfortunately, younger and previously asymptomatic patients with minimal subaortic gradients may also be at greater risk for sudden death due to their more frequent and vigorous physical activity.[179,186] It is unknown whether vigorous physical activity in patients with HCM is an independent risk factor for sudden death, but this disease is the most frequent autopsy finding in previously healthy competitive athletes who die suddenly.[187]

Although patients referred to diagnostic centers for evaluation of HCM are usually young to middle-aged persons, a syndrome with similar clinical and echocardiographic findings has been identified in the elderly.[89] Echocardiographically, these patients exhibit a similarly thickened and hypercontractile left ventricle. Their most common symptoms are those of CHF and are thought to reflect severe reductions in the ventricular diastolic compliance. As in younger patients with classic HCM, there is marked systolic anterior motion (SAM) of the mitral apparatus. However, in HCM of the elderly, the SAM is seemingly caused or at least accentuated by a severe degree of mitral annular calcification, which results in a particularly small LVOT.[188] Previously asymptomatic, these patients often experience the onset of progressively severe symptoms in the sixth decade of life, and the response to medical therapy, usually calcium channel blocking drugs, has been poor.[188] This lack of improvement with medical therapy may reflect the fact that mitral annular calcification plays a key role in producing a truly physical (i.e., less dynamic) subaortic obstruction. This would also explain the female predominance of the disease, because mitral annular calcification is more common in elderly women. It is unclear whether this represents a true variant of classic HCM with late onset or it is perhaps etiologically linked to long-standing systemic hypertension, with secondary, unexplained, disproportionate involvement of the interventricular septum.[89]

Pathophysiology

In HCM, the principal pathophysiologic abnormality is myocardial hypertrophy. The hypertrophy is a primary event in these patients and occurs independently of outflow tract obstruction. Unlike aortic stenosis, the hypertrophy begets the pressure gradient, not the other way around. Histologically, the hypertrophy consists of myocardial fiber disarray, and anatomically, there is usually disproportionate enlargement of the interventricular septum.[189]

There is controversy concerning the intrinsic contractile strength of the myocardium in patients with HCM. Several studies have demonstrated normal or supranormal indices of systolic function in patients with this disease.[190-192] LV ejection is rapid, with 80% of the SV being ejected very early during systole.[190,193] This is true regardless of the presence, temporal location during systole, or magnitude of outflow tract obstruction. However, studies have shown that end-systolic stress is significantly reduced in relation to end-systolic volume (Fig. 20–20).[194,195] Reinspection of the Laplace formula for wall stress, $P \times R/2h$, shows that in HCM, the degree of primary hypertrophy (i.e., with increased wall thickness [h]) should minimize instantaneous LV afterload. As a result, there is preservation, perhaps even elevation, of afterload-sensitive indices of systolic function, such as the EF.[196] Myocardial hypertrophy, particularly to the extent that it accentuates subaortic obstruction, increases the ESPVR, widening the divergence between it and the more accurate (load-

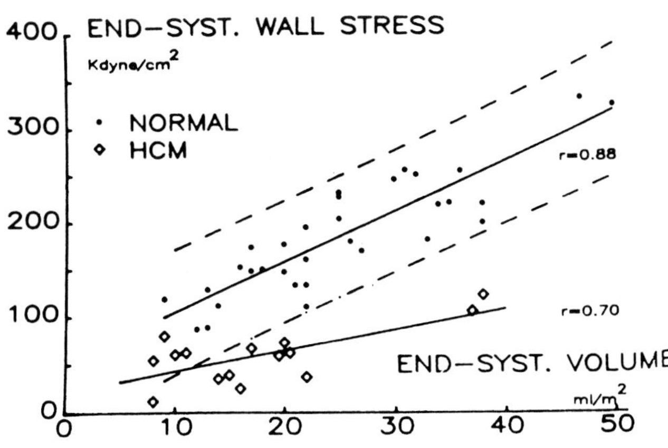

Figure 20–20 End-systolic stress versus end-systolic volume in normal subjects and in patients with hypertrophic cardiomyopathy (HCM), with *dashed lines* indicating the 95% confidence limit. Stress-volume data for most patients with HCM are located downward and to the right of the confidence band (i.e., decreased end-systolic stress related to volume), which is indicative of intrinsically depressed myocardial contractility. (From Pouleur H, Rousseau MF, van Eyll C, et al: Force-velocity-length relations in hypertrophic cardiomyopathy: Evidence of normal or depressed myocardial contractility. Am J Cardiol 52:813, 1983.)

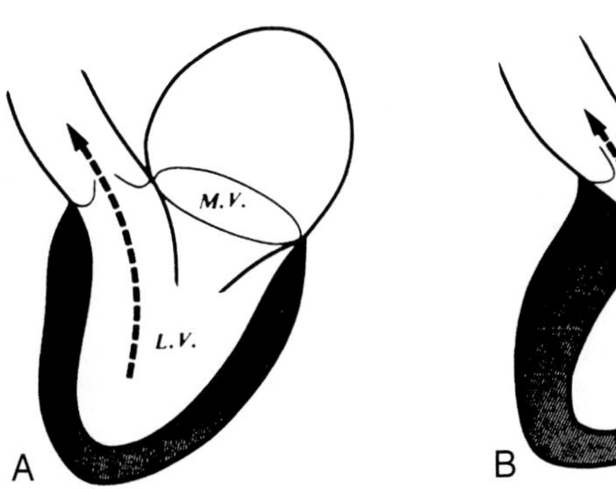

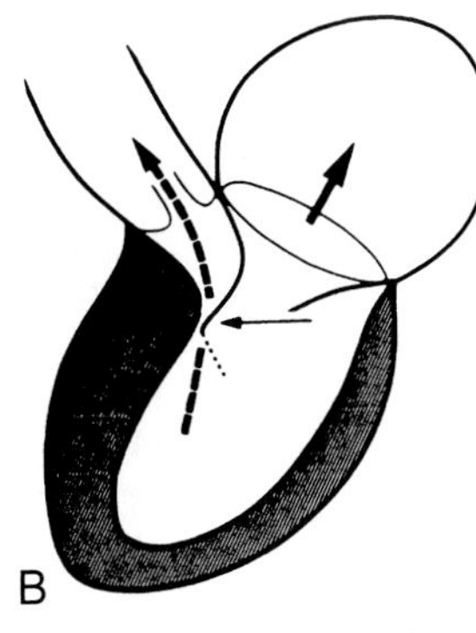

Figure 20–21 Proposed mechanism of systolic anterior motion (SAM) in hypertrophic cardiomyopathy (HCM). *(A)* Normally, blood is ejected from the left ventricle through an unimpeded outflow tract. *(B)* Thickening of the ventricular septum results in a restricted outflow tract, and this obstruction causes the blood to be ejected at a higher velocity, closer to the area of the anterior mitral valve leaflet. As a result of its proximity to this high-velocity fluid path, the anterior mitral valve leaflet is drawn toward the hypertrophied septum by a Venturi effect *(arrow)*. (From Wigle ED, Sasson Z, Henderson MA, et al: Hypertrophic cardiomyopathy: The importance of the site and the extent of hypertrophy. A review. Prog Cardiovasc Dis 28:1, 1985.)

insensitive) ratio of end-systolic wall stress to ESV. High peak systolic pressures (i.e., subaortic obstruction), elevation of ejection phase indices, and low ESV (i.e., minimal afterload) may reflect uncontrolled hypertrophy of an abnormal and perhaps intrinsically depressed myocardium. Whether overall contractility is normal, supranormal, or impaired in a given patient, it is likely that there will be regional differences in a ventricle's contractile function, which correlate with the histologic heterogeneity so characteristic of this disease.[197]

A consensus exists that the disease is characterized by a wide spectrum of the severity of obstruction. It is totally absent in some patients, may be variable in others, or may be critically severe. Its most distinctive qualities are its dynamic nature (depending on contractile state and loading conditions), its timing (begins early, peaks variably), and its subaortic location.[190,198] Those accepting the phenomenon of physical subaortic obstruction believe that it arises from the hypertrophied septum's encroachment on the systolic outflow tract, which is bounded anteriorly by the interventricular septum and posteriorly by the anterior leaflet of the mitral valve. In most patients with obstruction, exaggerated anterior (i.e., toward the septum) motion of the anterior mitral valve leaflet during systole accentuates the obstruction.[199] The cause of this SAM is unclear. One possibility is that the mitral valve is pulled toward the septum by contraction of the papillary muscles, whose orientation is abnormal because of the hypertrophic process.[200] Another theory is that vigorous contraction of the hypertrophied septum results in rapid acceleration of the blood through a simultaneously narrowed outflow tract. This could generate hydraulic forces consistent with a Venturi effect whereby the anterior leaflet of the mitral valve would be drawn close to or within actual contact with the interventricular septum[201] (Fig. 20–21). This means that after the obstruction is triggered, the mitral valve leaflet is forced against the septum by the pressure difference across the orifice. However, the pressure difference further decreases orifice size and further increases the pressure difference in a time-dependent amplifying feedback loop.[202] This analysis is also consistent with observations that the measured gradient is directly correlated with the duration of mitral-septal contact. Although still controversial,[203-205] there appears to be good correlation between the degree of SAM and the magnitude of the pressure gradient.[206,207] The SAM-septal contact also underlies the severe subaortic obstruction characteristic of HCM of the elderly, although the narrowing is usually more severe, and the contribution of septal movement toward the mitral valve is usually greater.[188]

The timing of SAM-septal contact is also important, because the magnitude of the subaortic gradient is proportional to the fraction of forward flow ejected in the presence of anatomic obstruction.[208] In general, large gradients occur as a result of early and prolonged SAM-septal contact, and small gradients arise from delayed and brief SAM-septal contact.[201,206] In studies of patients with various degrees of subaortic obstruction, the proportion of flow ejected in the presence of a gradient has varied between 30% and 70%.[206,209,210] Patients with evidence of systolic obstruction at rest have the longest intervals of systolic contact between the anterior leaflet of the mitral valve and the septum.[211] However, if SAM-septal contact is restricted to late systole, a pressure gradient may occur on the basis of "cavity obliteration" in the absence of any functional obstruction to blood flow.[212,2133] In such patients, 95% of the SV may be ejected by the halfway point in systole, when SAM-septal contact is just beginning.[190,206] Despite its seemingly critical role in producing outflow tract obstruction, SAM of the mitral valve is not a specific finding for HCM, and it may occur in patients with HCM who do not have obstruction.[203,204,211]

In addition to SAM, approximately two thirds of patients exhibit a constellation of structural malformations of the mitral valve.[214] These malformations include increased leaflet area and elongation of the leaflets or anomalous papillary muscle insertion directly into the anterior mitral valve leaflet. HCM is not a disease process confined to cardiac muscle alone, as these anatomic abnormalities of the mitral valve are unlikely to be acquired or secondary to mechanical factors.

Three basic mechanisms—increased contractility, decreased afterload, and decreased preload—exacerbate the

degree of SAM-septal contact and produce the dynamic obstruction characteristic of patients with HCM. The common pathway is a reduction in ventricular volume (actively by increased contractility, directly or reflexly in response to vasodilation, or passively by reduced preload), which increases the proximity of the anterior mitral valve leaflet to the hypertrophied septum.[176,180,215] Factors that usually impair contractile performance, such as myocardial depression, systemic vasoconstriction, and ventricular overdistention, characteristically improve systolic function in patients with HCM and outflow tract obstruction. Diagnostically, these paradoxes are exploited by quantifying the degree of subaortic obstruction after isoproterenol (e.g., increased inotropy, tachycardia, and decreased volume) and the Valsalva maneuver (e.g., decreased venous return and ventricular volume), both of which reliably elicit increases in the pressure gradient. In the operating room, catheter-induced ectopy or premature ventricular contractions resulting from cardiac manipulation may also transiently exacerbate the gradient by increased inotropy from postextrasystolic potentiation. Therapeutically, volume loading, myocardial depression, and vasoconstriction should minimize obstruction and augment forward flow.

Patients with HCM demonstrate critical derangements in diastolic function which, although in some ways more subtle than the unique phenomenon of subaortic obstruction, may contribute equally to the challenge posed.[216-219] These abnormalities include prolongation of the isovolumic relaxation time (i.e., aortic valve closure to mitral valve opening) and reduction in the peak velocity of LV filling.[87,192] Diastolic dysfunction exhibits the same heterogeneity characteristic of its systolic function, probably because its underlying cause is intrinsic to the primary myopathic process and not merely secondary to the associated chamber hypertrophy.[220] Accordingly, diastolic filling abnormalities in HCM are largely independent of the magnitude of LVH and are seen even in patients with only mild, localized hypertrophy.[20]

Poor diastolic compliance is the most clinically apparent manifestation of the relaxation abnormalities. LV filling pressures are markedly elevated despite enhanced systolic ejection and the normal or subnormal EDV. This reduced ventricular volume reemphasizes the pivotal role played by the hypertrophied but intrinsically depressed myocardium. Reductions in afterload, mediated by hypertrophy, support the ventricle's systolic performance, resulting in increased emptying and a small diastolic volume. However, hypertrophy also impairs relaxation, resulting in poor diastolic compliance and an elevated ventricular filling pressure. The key point is that the high filling pressure does not reflect distention of a failing ventricle, even though stress-volume relationships suggest that its contractility is intrinsically depressed (Fig. 20–22 and Table 20–3). This disease is characterized by systolic and diastolic dysfunction.

As in patients with valvular aortic stenosis, relatively high filling pressures reflect the LVEDV (i.e., degree of preload reserve) needed to overcome the outflow obstruction. Intervention with vasodilators is therefore inappropriate. The poor ventricular compliance also means that patients with HCM depend on a large intravascular volume and the maintenance of sinus rhythm for adequate diastolic filling. The atrial contribution to ventricular filling is even more important in HCM than in valvular aortic stenosis, and it may approach 75% of total SV.[129]

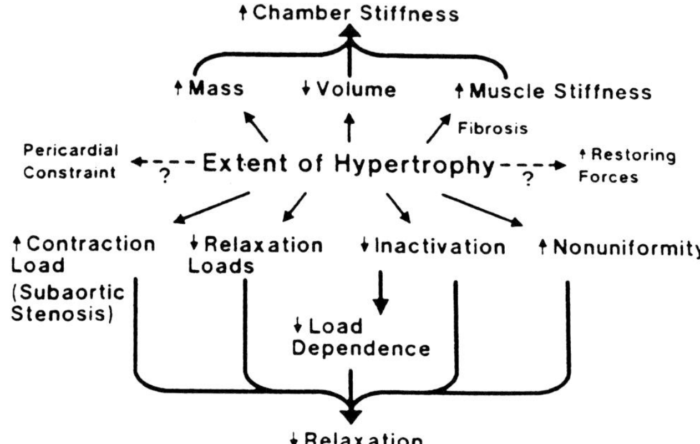

Figure 20–22 Proposed interactions between myocardial hypertrophy and other related properties of ventricular function. (From Wigle ED, Sasson Z, Henderson MA, et al: Hypertrophic cardiomyopathy: The importance of the site and the extent of hypertrophy. A review. Prog Cardiovasc Dis 28:1, 1985.)

Table 20–3 Factors Affecting Left Ventricular Diastolic Filling in Hypertrophic Cardiomyopathy

Chamber stiffness*
Relaxation
Loads
Contraction load
Subaortic stenosis
Relaxation loads
Late-systolic loading
End-systolic deformation (restoring forces)
Coronary filling
Ventricular filling
Inactivation
Myoplasmic calcium overload
Primary
Ischemic
Nonuniformity of load and inactivation in space and time†
Pericardial constraints and ventricular interaction
Effect of extent of hypertrophy on the preceding factors

*Chamber stiffness = Myocardial mass × Myocardial stiffness / Ventricular volume.
†Nonuniformity of contraction and relaxation.
From Wigel ED, Wilansky S: Diastolic dysfunction in hypertrophic cardiomyopathy. Heart Failure 3:85, 1987.

Another similarity between HCM and valvular aortic stenosis is that the combination of myocardial hypertrophy, with or without LVOT obstruction, may precipitate imbalances in the myocardial oxygen supply and demand relationship. Angina-like discomfort is one of the classic symptoms of patients with HCM, and its pathogenesis has been attributed to increases in $M\dot{V}O_2$, specifically the increased overall muscle mass and the high systolic wall tension generated by the ventricle's ejection against the dynamic subaortic obstruction. However, as in patients with aortic stenosis, there is also evidence of a compromise in myocardial oxygen supply.[221,222] Patients with HCM suffer from several types of hypertrophy-related abnormalities of the coronary circulation; some are common to other conditions associated with pathologic hypertrophy (e.g., aortic stenosis), and others are apparently unique to this distinctive form of hypertrophy.[223] A reduced capillary density in the hypertrophied myocardium prevents flow from increasing in proportion to the increase in myocar-

dial mass.[224] It is also possible that there are primary HCM-associated abnormalities of the coronary circulation that are unrelated to myocardial hypertrophy.[225] In addition to these coronary circulatory abnormalities, there is evidence of a metabolic derangement in the hypertrophied interventricular septum, whereby there is a decreased use of adequately delivered metabolic substrates.[222]

The reduction in coronary vascular reserve is similar to that observed in patients with valvular aortic stenosis, in whom $M\dot{V}O_2$ may be presumed to be uniformly elevated.[115] However, angina also occurs in patients with HCM in the absence of subaortic obstruction. Although basal $M\dot{V}O_2$ is elevated in proportion to the increased muscle mass, it is particularly interesting that clinical studies support a greater pathogenetic role for coronary circulatory abnormalities in producing ischemia in patients with nonobstructive hypertrophy.[226]

Hemodynamic derangements peculiar to the disease may aggravate the ventricle's anatomic vulnerability to ischemia. The increased LVEDP for any LVEDV (i.e., poor compliance) inevitably narrows the diastolic CPP gradient. This may precipitate subendocardial ischemia in some patients with HCM, particularly those faced with the increased oxygen demand of overcoming late-systolic obstruction.[216] There is evidence that hypertrophy-induced myocardial ischemia may underlie the diastolic dysfunction characteristic of HCM.[227] As in patients with valvular aortic stenosis, ischemia-induced abnormalities of diastolic calcium sequestration may further exacerbate relaxation abnormalities, initiating a vicious cycle (Fig. 20–23).[104,119,134,157,158,228]

β-Blockers and calcium channel blockers form the basis of medical therapy for HCM. β-Blockade is most useful for preventing sympathetically mediated increases in the subaortic gradient and for the prevention of tachyarrhythmias, which can also exacerbate outflow obstruction. Disopyramide has also been used to reduce contractility and for its antiarrhythmic properties.[229] Calcium channel blockers often prove clinically effective in patients with HCM regardless of the presence or absence of systolic obstruction.[230] The mechanism of action involves improvement in diastolic relaxation, allowing an increase in LVEDV at a relatively lower LVEDP. The negative inotropy may attenuate the subaortic pressure gradient, although in selected patients, the gradient may worsen because of pronounced and unpredictable degrees of vasodilation.[231,232]

Surgery—a septal myotomy or partial myomectomy by the aortic approach—is reserved for those patients who remain symptomatic despite maximal pharmacologic therapy. In a long-term retrospective study, the cumulative survival rate was significantly better in surgically than in pharmacologically treated patients.[233] However, it is quite likely that pharmacologic therapy may be more appropriate for the patient with a dynamic component to their degree of subaortic obstruction.[234] Further improvement in the clinical outcome of surgically treated patients may be achieved with the addition of verapamil, presumably reflecting a two-pronged attack on the systolic (myomectomy) and diastolic (verapamil) components of the disease. Enthusiasm continues for the therapeutic use of dual-chamber pacing in this disease, with some patients demonstrating reductions in their subaortic gradients.[168-171,235,236] It was not an option for patients in atrial fibrillation.

Myomectomy usually results in significant symptomatic improvement along with a reduction in the subaortic gradient.[237] The intraoperative guidance and evaluation of the surgical result by an experienced echocardiographer are essential for the success of this procedure.[238-240] In successful cases, the postmyomectomy study will show dramatic septal thinning, widening of the LVOT, and resolution of SAM and the LVOT color mosaic (see Chapter 15).

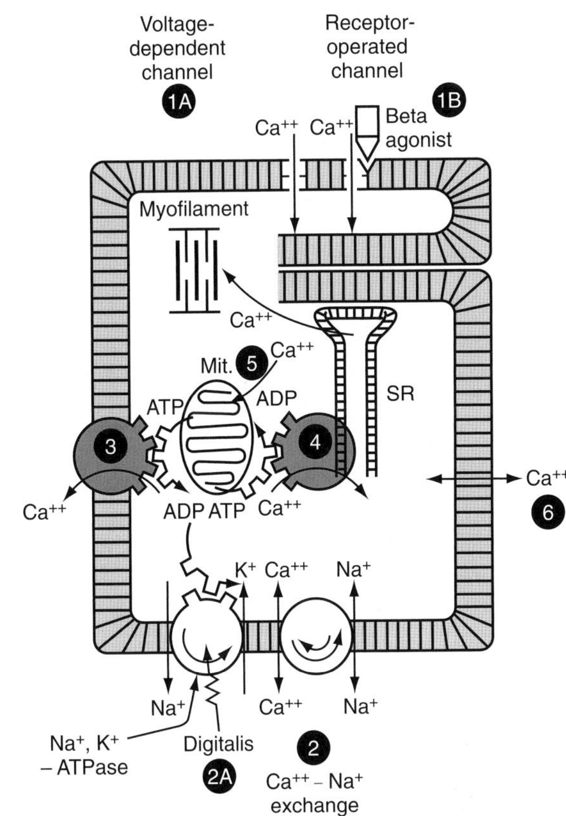

Figure 20–23 Regulation of cytoplasmic calcium. The diastolic extrusion of calcium from the myofilaments occurs at several sites. At two of the most important sites, energy (ATP) is required for the active reuptake of calcium by the sarcolemma (3) and the sarcoplasmic reticulum (4). (From Braunwald E: Mechanisms of action of calcium channel blocking agents. N Engl J Med 307:1618, 1982.)

As in any disease with diverse diagnostic criteria, it is difficult to compare mortality rates among various series, but perioperative mortality rates for isolated septal myomectomy are below 2%, although operative risks are higher when combined with other procedures.[241,242] However, clinical studies of predominantly elderly patients report mortality rates in excess of 15%. Complications other than heart block are infrequent, although more than one third of patients will experience new, clinically insignificant aortic regurgitation.[243] It is unclear whether this new aortic regurgitation poses a long-term risk for these patients from the standpoint of CHF, but it probably warrants the continued use of endocarditis prophylaxis.

Anesthetic Considerations

Priorities in anesthetic management are to avoid aggravating the subaortic obstruction while remaining aware of the derangements in diastolic function that may be somewhat less amenable to direct pharmacologic manipulation (Box 20–2). It is therefore necessary to maintain an appropriate intravascular volume while avoiding direct or reflex increases in con-

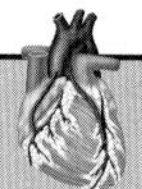

BOX 20–2 ***Hypertrophic Cardiomyopathy***

Preload:	Increased
Afterload:	Increased
Goal:	Myocardial depression
Avoid:	Tachycardia, inotropes, vasodilators

tractility or heart rate. The latter goals can be achieved with a deep level of general anesthesia and the associated direct myocardial depression. Regardless of the specific technique, the preservation of an adequate CPP, using vasoconstrictors rather than inotropes, is necessary to avoid myocardial ischemia. Heavy premedication is advisable with a view to avoiding anxiety-induced tachycardia or a reduction in ventricular filling. Chronic β-blockade or calcium channel blockade, or both, should be continued up to and including the day of surgery. These medications should be restarted immediately after surgery, particularly in those patients undergoing noncardiac surgery.

Intraoperative monitoring should include an ECG system with the capability of monitoring a V_5 lead and each of the six limb leads. Inspection of lead II may be helpful in the accurate diagnosis of supraventricular and junctional tachyarrhythmias, which may precipitate catastrophic hemodynamic deterioration due to the potential for inadequate ventricular filling resulting from the reduction in diastolic time or loss of the atrial contribution to ventricular filling. The latter may be crucial in patients with significantly reduced diastolic compliance.[129] Abnormal Q waves have been described on the electrocardiograms in 20% to 50% of patients with HCM.[176] These waves should not raise concern about a previous myocardial infarction; instead, they probably represent accentuation of normal septal depolarization or delay in depolarization of electrophysiologically abnormal cells.[244] Some patients exhibit a short PR interval with initial slurring of the QRS complex, and they may be at increased risk for supraventricular tachyarrhythmias on the basis of preexcitation.[245] Although the specific predisposing factors are unknown, patients with HCM are at increased risk for any type of arrhythmia in the operative setting.[246]

Given the pronounced abnormalities in LV diastolic compliance, the CVP is likely to be an inaccurate guide to changes in LV volume. However, a CVP catheter is extremely useful for the prompt administration of vasoactive drugs if they become necessary. As in valvular aortic stenosis, the information provided by insertion of a PAC is worth the small arrhythmogenic risk. The potential for hypovolemia-induced exacerbation of outflow tract obstruction makes it crucial that the clinician have an accurate gauge of intravascular filling. The reduced diastolic compliance means that the PCWP will overestimate the patient's true volume status, and a reasonable clinical objective is to maintain the PCWP in the high-normal to elevated range. A PAC with pacing capability is ideal because atrial overdrive pacing can effect immediate hemodynamic improvement in the event of episodes of junctional rhythm (see Chapters 14, 24, and 25). The absolute requirement of these patients for an adequate preload cannot be overemphasized, because even abrupt positioning changes have resulted in acute hemodynamic deterioration, including acute pulmonary edema.[247]

Intraoperative arrhythmias require aggressive therapy. During cardiac surgery, insertion of the venous cannulae may precipitate atrial arrhythmias. Because the resultant hypotension may be severe, the surgeon should cannulate the aorta before any atrial manipulations. Supraventricular or junctional tachyarrhythmias may require immediate cardioversion if they precipitate catastrophic degrees of hypotension. Although verapamil is one drug of choice for paroxysmal atrial and junctional tachycardia, it has the potential of disastrously worsening the LVOT obstruction if it elicits excessive vasodilation or if it is used in the setting of severe hypotension.[232] Cardioversion is preferable when the MAP is already very low; the concurrent administration of phenylephrine is also advisable. This drug is almost always a low-risk, high-yield choice for the hypotensive patient with HCM. It augments perfusion, may ameliorate the pressure gradient, and often elicits a potentially beneficial vagal reflex when used to treat tachyarrhythmia-induced hypotension.

The inhalation anesthetics are commonly used for patients with HCM. Their dose-dependent myocardial depression is ideal because negative inotropy reduces the degree of SAM-septal contact, which results in LVOT obstruction. Hypotension is almost always the result of underlying hypovolemia, which is potentially exacerbated by anesthetic-induced vasodilation. Inotropes, β-adrenergic agonists, and calcium are all contraindicated because they worsen the systolic obstruction and perpetuate the hypotension. In most cases, a beneficial response can be obtained with aggressive replenishment of intravascular volume and concurrent infusion of phenylephrine.

Several investigators have suggested that regional anesthesia, with its potential for accentuating peripheral vasodilation, may be relatively contraindicated in the management of patients with HCM.[248,249] The theoretical constraints are similar to those for patients with valvular aortic stenosis, and the same clinical caveats apply. If the vascular system is kept appropriately full and "tight" with vasopressors, it is reasonable to consider these techniques in the light of other clinical advantages they might offer the patient. Catheter techniques (e.g., continuous spinals, epidurals) may be preferable to the bolus administration of local anesthetics to achieve a finer degree of control of the anesthetic level.[250] There is unquestionably the potential for a cascade of iatrogenic complications if sympatholytic hypotension is treated in a knee-jerk fashion with ephedrine, epinephrine, or a variety of other equally contraindicated β-adrenergic agonists.

Although echocardiography has undoubtedly contributed to an increased frequency of diagnosis of this disease, an occasional patient escapes detection by ultrasound examination in the course of the preoperative work-up. When other objective data, including the physical examination, ECG results, and chest radiograph, show only nonspecific abnormalities, it is easy to disregard vague or atypical complaints of chest pain, presyncope, and dyspnea. This is particularly true when the symptoms might reasonably be attributed to the primary condition that brought the patient to surgery (e.g., CABG).[251] Other identifiable populations are said to be at high risk for occult HCM. HCM of the elderly has already been discussed, and probably only a fraction of such patients arrive in the operating room with such a formal diagnosis. However, it is not uncommon for the anesthesiologist to encounter an elderly patient with long-standing systemic hypertension and unexplained episodes of pulmonary congestion for whom the

primary physician has prescribed a digitalis preparation. Anesthesiologists may occasionally be presented with the opportunity to diagnose unsuspected HCM or one of its variants. Intraoperative events that could conceivably provoke or accentuate physiologic manifestations of the disease include hypovolemia, tachycardia, spontaneous or "manipulative" ectopy, and paradoxic responses to vasoactive drugs (e.g., inotropes, vasodilators, and vasoconstrictors) or anesthetic agents.[251,252] Clues such as these allow the experienced and astute clinician to recognize the phenomenon of dynamic subaortic obstruction when it occurs in less obvious clinical settings.

AORTIC REGURGITATION

Clinical Features and Natural History

Aortic regurgitation may result from an abnormality of the valve itself, from bicuspid anatomy, have a rheumatic or infectious origin, or occur in association with any condition producing dilation of the aortic root and leaflet separation. Nonrheumatic valvular diseases commonly resulting in aortic regurgitation include infective endocarditis, trauma, and connective tissue disorders such as Marfan's syndrome or cystic medionecrosis of the aortic valve.[52] Aortic dissection from trauma, hypertension, or chronic degenerative processes can also result in dilatation of the root and functional incompetence (see Chapter 23).

The natural history of chronic aortic regurgitation is that of a long asymptomatic interval during which the valvular incompetence and secondary ventricular enlargement become progressively more severe.[3,138] When symptoms do appear, they are usually those of CHF, and chest pain, if it occurs, is often nonexertional in origin. The life expectancy for patients with significant disease has historically been about 9 years, and in contrast to aortic stenosis, the onset of symptoms due to aortic regurgitation does not portend an immediately ominous prognosis.[253,254] In the absence of surgery, early recognition of aortic regurgitation and chronic use of vasodilators appear to be prolonging life span in this patient population.[138,255]

A relatively unique and problematic feature of chronic aortic regurgitation is that the severity of symptoms and their duration may correlate poorly with the degree of hemodynamic and contractile impairment.[138,256] The issue in surgical decision making is that many patients can remain asymptomatic, during which time they are undergoing progressive deterioration in their myocardial contractility. Noninvasive diagnostic studies (e.g., radionuclide cineangiography and two-dimensional and Doppler echocardiographic assessment of response to pharmacologic afterload stress) may facilitate the detection of early derangements in contractile function in relatively asymptomatic patients.[257-259] This finding is important to the cardiologist when considering surgical referral, because patients with depressed preoperative LV function have a higher perioperative mortality rate and are at increased risk for persistent postoperative heart failure.[260-262]

As in acute mitral regurgitation, the physiology of acute aortic regurgitation is quite different from chronic aortic regurgitation. Common causes include endocarditis, trauma, and acute aortic dissection. Because of a lack of chronic compensation, these patients usually present with pulmonary edema and heart failure refractory to optimal medical therapy. These patients are often hypotensive and clinically appear to be on the verge of cardiovascular collapse.

Pathophysiology

LV volume overload is the pathognomonic feature of chronic aortic regurgitation. The degree of volume overload is determined by the magnitude of the regurgitant flow, which is related to the size of the regurgitant orifice, the aorta-ventricular pressure gradient, and the diastolic time. It has been suggested that the size of the regurgitant aortic orifice is constant and independent of changes in loading conditions.[263] However, in other valvular lesions (e.g., aortic stenosis, mitral regurgitation), the orifice size is not constant and is dependent on the hemodynamic state. There is some evidence, in an experimental model of acute aortic regurgitation, that the regurgitant orifice area can change with increases or decreases in the transvalvular pressure gradient.[264] When aortic regurgitation occurs in the absence of valvular fibrosis or calcification (valve elasticity is preserved), reduction of regurgitant area may be one of the mechanisms of the beneficial effect of afterload reduction.

The hemodynamic effects of changes in heart rate are also less straightforward than might be assumed.[265] Theoretically, tachycardia should maximize net forward flow by shortening the regurgitant diastolic time interval. This hypothesis, first offered by Corrigan in 1832, may be the pathophysiologic basis for the seemingly paradoxic observation that patients with aortic regurgitation may tolerate exercise despite having symptoms of pulmonary congestion at rest. Sympathetically mediated vasodilation, increased inotropy, and tachycardia may contribute to the increased cardiac output achieved during isometric exercise in patients with aortic regurgitation.[266] Chronically, similar, reflex-induced hemodynamic changes may contribute to the beneficial effects of arteriolar dilators.[267] The peripheral vasculature directly affects regurgitant volume through reflex changes in heart rate; it also can alter volume loading by effects on the diastolic time. It plays a key role in the overall pathophysiology of aortic regurgitation[268,269] (Fig. 20–24).

Despite these observations, the beneficial effects of shortened diastolic time alone may be less clear-cut. Angiographic study of subjects with chronic aortic regurgitation has shown that pacing-induced tachycardia can decrease the SV, LVEDV, and LVEDP and can increase cardiac output,[270] but that the ratio of the regurgitant volume to the total SV may remain unchanged. This occurs because tachycardia shortens diastolic period per stroke but increases the number of strokes per minute, leaving the net diastolic time per minute relatively unchanged. Similar observation has been made with radionuclide studies that demonstrated that tachycardia can increase cardiac output and decrease LVEDV; however, pulmonary arterial pressure and PCWP may not change with increasing heart rate.[271] This divergence between the effects of tachycardia on LV volume (decreased) and filling pressures (unchanged) may reflect the pronounced rightward shift of the LV pressure-volume loop that is characteristic of long-standing aortic regurgitation.

Chronically, aortic regurgitation results in a state of LV volume and pressure overload. Progressive volume overloading from aortic regurgitation increases end-diastolic wall tension (i.e., ventricular afterload) and stimulates the serial replication of sarcomeres, producing a pattern of eccentric ventricular hypertrophy.[93,262] This dilation of the ventricle, in

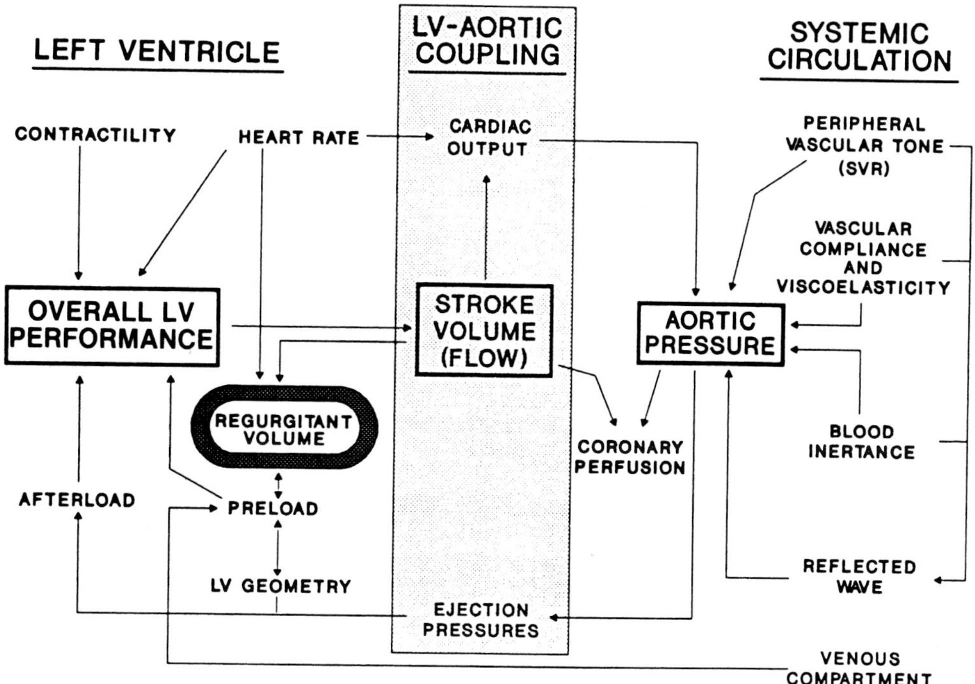

Figure 20–24 The peripheral circulation plays a pivotal role in supporting left ventricular performance in the face of chronic volume overloading. (From Borow KM, Marcus RH: Aortic regurgitation: The need for an integrated physiologic approach. J Am Coll Cardiol 17:898, 1991.)

accordance with Laplace's law, also elevates the systolic wall tension, stimulating some concentric hypertrophy. The result is normalization of the ratio of ventricular wall thickness to cavitary radius.[93] This process of eccentric hypertrophy results in the greatest absolute degrees of cardiomegaly seen in valve disease. End-diastolic volume may be three to four times normal, and very high cardiac outputs can be sustained.[272]

Figure 20–25 shows the pressure-volume loops for acute and chronic aortic regurgitation. In the chronic form, the diastolic pressure-volume curve is shifted far to the right. This permits a tremendous increase in LVEDV with minimal change in filling pressure, a property frequently described as high diastolic compliance.[273] However, animal models of chronic LV volume overloading instead suggest that the entire diastolic pressure-volume curve is shifted to the right (see Fig. 20–8).[11] This accounts for the apparent paradox of high ventricular volumes at relatively low filling pressures.

The parallel shifts of the entire curve relating diastolic pressure and volume are a manifestation of the physiologic process known as "creep."[4] This refers to the time-dependent increase in dimension that occurs as a result of an applied stress—in this case, volume overload. Because of this chronic adaptation, LV filling pressures are in the low-to-normal range and are relatively insensitive to changes in intravascular volume. This is not true of higher filling pressures, for which elevations are a reliable guide to volume overload and ventricular distention.

Because the increase in preload is compensated for by ventricular hypertrophy, cardiac output is maintained by the Frank-Starling mechanism, and cardiac failure is not seen. This is true despite probable decreases in contractility.[255] There is virtually no isovolumic diastolic phase, because the ventricle is filling throughout diastole. The isovolumic phase of systole is also brief because of the low aortic diastolic pressure. This minimal impedance to the forward ejection of a large SV allows for the performance of maximal myocardial work at a minimum of oxygen consumption. Eventually however, progressive volume overload increases ventricular

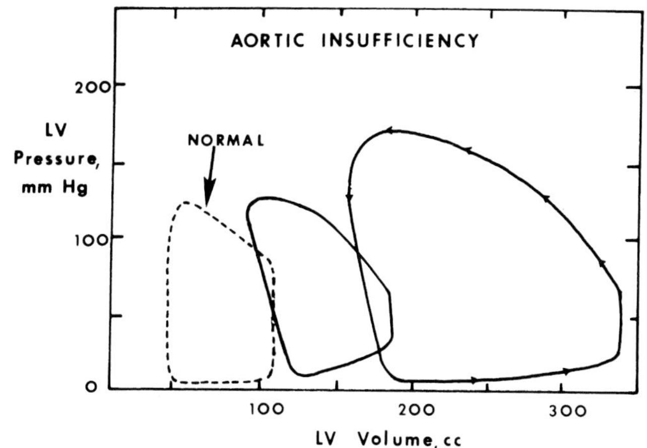

Figure 20–25 Pressure-volume loop in aortic regurgitation (AR). Acute AR (middle loop); chronic AR (right loop). (Adapted from Jackson JM, Thomas SJ, Lowenstein E: Anesthetic management of patients with valvular heart disease. Semin Anesth 1:239, 1982.)

end-diastolic volume to the point that compensatory hypertrophy is no longer sufficient to compensate, and a decline in systolic function occurs. As systolic function declines, end-systolic dimension increases further, LV wall stress increases, and LV function is further compromised by the excessive ventricular afterload. At this point, the decline of ventricular function is progressive and can be quite rapid. As is shown in Figure 20–26*A* in the patient with compensated aortic regurgitation, the eccentrically dilated ventricle maintains its SV and EF by using preload reserve; wall stress is only slightly elevated. In Figure 20–26*B*, the limit of preload reserve has been reached and ventricular dysfunction has shifted the end-systolic wall stress relation to the right. As a result of the higher wall stress, the SV and EF inevitably decline. In patients in whom the EF has become less than 25% or the end-systolic

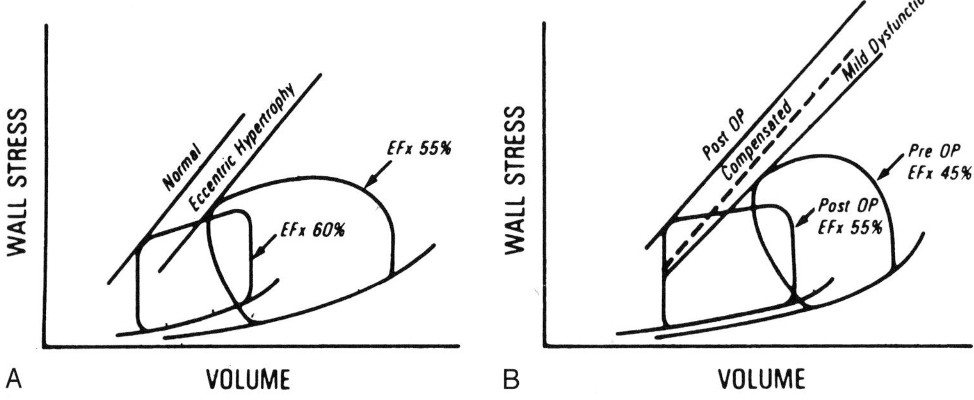

Figure 20–26 Adaptation to volume overload. *(A)* Stress-volume curves and the linear end-systolic stress-volume relationship are shifted to the right in compensated aortic regurgitation compared with normal. The stroke volume and ejection fraction are maintained despite slightly elevated systolic wall stress. *(B)* The same associations in a hypothetical patient with mild left ventricular dysfunction as evidenced by rightward shift of the end-systolic wall stress-volume relationship. Exhaustion of preload reserve causes wall stress to increase, resulting in reciprocal declines in the stroke volume and the ejection fraction. Valve replacement corrects afterload mismatch, allowing the end-diastolic and end-systolic volume relations to shift to the left. Lower wall stress allows the ejection fraction to return to normal. (From Ross J Jr: Afterload mismatch in aortic and mitral valve disease: Implications for surgical therapy. J Am Coll Cardiol 5:811, 1985.)

diameter larger than 60 mm, irreversible myocardial changes are likely to have occurred.[138]

The primary determinants of $M\dot{V}O_2$—contractility and wall tension—are usually not significantly elevated with chronic aortic regurgitation, although calculated myocardial work may be twice normal. Actual $M\dot{V}O_2$ may be only minimally elevated because the greater proportion of myocardial work is spent in the energy-efficient process of fiber shortening, with little increase occurring in oxygen-consuming tension development[274] (see Fig. 20–26).

Despite the relatively normal $M\dot{V}O_2$, angina can occur in one third of patients with severe aortic regurgitation, even in the absence of CAD.[275] Patients with chronic aortic regurgitation may be at risk for myocardial ischemia caused by hypertrophy-induced abnormalities of the coronary circulation. The increase in total myocardial mass can increase baseline $M\dot{V}O_2$, and there is evidence that total coronary blood flow (CBF), although increased, fails to keep pace with the increase in myocardial mass. Evidence suggests that the insidious development of contractile dysfunction may in part have an ischemic basis.[276]

Despite these rather favorable considerations in terms of myocardial energetics, an increase in $M\dot{V}O_2$ may pose a threat to the patient with chronic aortic regurgitation because of decreased coronary vascular reserve.[277] Although this phenomenon has been more thoroughly documented in patients with chronic pressure-induced hypertrophy, some studies indicate that the coronary vascular reserve is similarly compromised in patients with LV volume overload.[278,279] The process of hypertrophy may be a double-edged sword from the standpoint of the myocardial oxygen balance. Hypertrophy minimizes oxygen consumption as measured by wall stress, but elevates basal $M\dot{V}O_2$ and may elicit derangements in the quality or quantity of the coronary vasculature.

Intraoperatively, patients with chronic aortic regurgitation may be at risk for acute ischemia with episodes of significant bradycardia. Because bradycardia prolongs diastolic time, it increases regurgitant flow, and LV diastolic pressure and wall tension rise rapidly. Simultaneously, the CPP is decreased as aortic runoff occurs during diastole and diastolic ventricular pressure is increased.[52] Under these conditions, myocardial perfusion pressure may be insufficient. Clinically, very rapid decompensation can occur. The ischemic ventricle can rapidly dilate such that progressively increased end-systolic dimensions are seen, and ischemia and ventricular failure become a positive feedback loop.

Surgical Decision Making

From the discussion of the pathophysiology of chronic aortic regurgitation, it is evident that an accurate assessment of contractility is crucial to surgical decision making, because the clinical history may be an unreliable index of ventricular function. It is not uncommon for asymptomatic patients to have ventricular dysfunction, whereas symptomatic patients may be free of even modest myocardial depression. A variety of prognostic indicators have been used to identify early ventricular dysfunction as a trigger for surgical intervention. Clinical status, such as exercise capacity and New York Heart Association (NYHA) class, and noninvasive and invasive laboratory tests have been used. Hemodynamic parameters such as the end-systolic stress-volume relationship and estimates of the LV contractile state have been evaluated as predictors of worsening LV function.

Although ejection phase indices (e.g., EF) are most familiar to anesthesiologists, they are inherently unreliable for quantifying ventricular function in the setting of chronic volume overloading, because the Starling mechanism continues to support increases in the SV long after the onset of intrinsic myocardial depression. LV dilation, compensatory hypertrophy, and minimal afterload may normalize the EF, even though contractility is significantly depressed.[255] Preload can be exquisitely sensitive to changes in heart rate and systemic vascular tone. Ventricular performance therefore may not be adequately reflected by the EF.[280,281] The often-reported regurgitant volume or regurgitant fraction are similarly rate and load dependent, and they may correlate poorly with the underlying inotropic state.[282]

A variety of end-systolic indices have been examined in chronic aortic regurgitation, and these provide a more load-independent assessment of the inotropic state. Although the left ventricular end-systolic volume (LVESV) is preload independent, it does vary with myocardial contractility and afterload. An increased end-systolic volume may reflect a depressed inotropic state, or it may increase because of an increased LV afterload resulting from increased chamber size or pressure.[280] There is also evidence that the relative load independence of the LVESV is limited when ventricular hypertrophy is primarily eccentric.[25] However, with long-standing volume overload, virtually all studies have found that an increased end-systolic dimension correlates with a poor prognosis and a significantly depressed contractile state.[258,283]

When valve surgery is performed after ventricular decompensation has occurred, the immediate and long-term results are marginal. Much of the increased mortality is a function of postoperative deaths from heart failure.[262,284] When valve surgery occurs before significant ventricular decompensation, ventricular recovery is remarkable, with remodeling and a reduction in LV size beginning as early as 2 weeks postoperatively.[138,262] Because delays in surgical intervention can be catastrophic and because the response to surgery is so good, there is evidence of a shift toward earlier valve replacement and surgery in relatively asymptomatic patients has been advocated.[262] Based on review of the published literature, the ACC and the AHA have provided practice guidelines for surgical intervention in chronic aortic regurgitation.[138] Valve surgery is recommended for asymptomatic patients with LV systolic dysfunction. Surgery should also be considered if ventricular dilation has occurred in the asymptomatic patient, even if the EF is normal. In patients who are symptomatic but have normal ventricular function, the ACC and AHA recommend further evaluation for an unrelated cause and observation. In these cases, serial echocardiographic assessment is appropriate. Symptomatic patients with LV dysfunction should undergo surgery.[138]

Acute Aortic Regurgitation

In acute aortic regurgitation, sudden diastolic volume overload of a nonadapted left ventricle results in a precipitous rise in the end-diastolic pressure because the ventricle is operating on the steepest portion of the diastolic pressure-volume curve (see Fig. 20–25).[285] In severe acute aortic regurgitation, the LVEDP can equilibrate with aortic diastolic pressure and exceed the LA pressure in late diastole. This may be sufficient to cause closure of the mitral valve before atrial systole.[286] This is an important echocardiographic finding indicative of severe aortic regurgitation.[287] Although this phenomenon initially shields the pulmonary capillaries from the full force of the dramatically elevated LVEDP, the protection may be short-lived.[288] Severe LV distention often follows and produces mitral annular enlargement and functional mitral regurgitation.

The inevitable fall in SV in acute decompensating aortic regurgitation elicits a reflex sympathetic response so that tachycardia and a high SVR (SVR) are common. Moderate tachycardia beneficially shortens the regurgitant time without reducing the transmitral filling volume.[289] Vasoconstriction, however, preserves CPP at the expense of increasing the aorta-ventricular gradient and regurgitation.

As may be expected, patients with acute aortic regurgitation may be at greater risk for myocardial ischemia. As with chronic aortic regurgitation and bradycardia, coronary perfusion may be compromised by the combination of a low diastolic arterial pressure and the precipitously increased LVEDP. This narrowing of CPP may be so severe that the phasic epicardial blood flow may change to a predominantly systolic pattern with very severe acute aortic regurgitation.[290] Dissection of the coronary ostia is rare but frequently causes fatality in patients with acute aortic regurgitation. In addition to the structural impediment to myocardial oxygen delivery, catastrophic hypotension and high LVEDP combine to cause accentuated ischemia and ventricular dilation. Immediate surgical correction is the only hope for salvaging these patients, who often prove refractory to inotropes and vasodilators. Attempts at stabilizing the ischemic component of their injury with the intra-aortic balloon are usually contraindicated, because augmenting the diastolic pressure worsens regurgitation.

Acute aortic regurgitation is most commonly caused by infective endocarditis or aortic dissection, and intraoperative transesophageal echocardiography (TEE) has assumed increasing importance in diagnosis of acute aortic regurgitation and in decisions regarding its surgical management.[291] TEE studies are highly sensitive and specific for the diagnosis of infective endocarditis, and they are significantly more sensitive than transthoracic echocardiography (TTE).[292] TEE has been particularly useful in the diagnosis of abscesses associated with endocarditis[293] and may detect previously unsuspected abnormalities.[293] Although an area of active investigation, there is no completely satisfactory noninvasive method for quantifying the severity of aortic regurgitation. Premature closure of the mitral valve, determination of the pressure half-time of aortic regurgitation, and color-flow estimation of the regurgitant jet's width and its size in relation to the LVOT are commonly described techniques[294-296] (see Chapters 15 and 16).

Anesthetic Considerations

Intraoperative monitoring should include an ECG system with the capability of monitoring a lateral precordial lead, because ischemia is a potential hazard (Box 20–3). For most valvular procedures, a PAC provides very useful information. A PAC allows determination of basal filling pressures and cardiac output, which is particularly useful in chronic aortic regurgitation given the potential unreliability of the clinical history and EF. Equally important is the ability to accurately monitor ventricular preload and cardiac output response to pharmacologic interventions. The aggressive use of vasodilators is often appropriate therapy perioperatively for the failing ventricle, but their use can compromise the preload to which the ventricle has chronically adjusted. Concurrent preload augmentation, guided by the pulmonary artery diastolic pressure or PCWP, may be crucial to optimize cardiac output when afterload is pharmacologically manipulated[297-299] (see Chapters 10, 14, 16, 31, and 33). The other requirement for a PAC is to allow for pacing when it is anticipated. The deleterious effects of significant bradycardia in aortic regurgitation

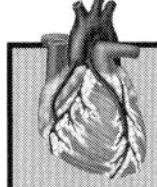

BOX 20–3 ***Aortic Regurgitation***

Preload:	Increased
Afterload:	Decreased
Goal:	Augmentation of forward flow
Avoid:	Bradycardia

have been described. In patients who arrive in the operating room with heart rates less than 70 or in patients for whom rapid epicardial pacing may be difficult to establish (e.g., redo operations), placement of a pacing wire is probably indicated. Typically, only a ventricular wire would be appropriate; it is more reliable than atrial pacing, and in aortic regurgitation, the atrial contribution to ventricular diastolic volume usually is not essential. Capturing the ventricle with a pulmonary artery–based, transvenous wire can be difficult because of the very large ventricular cavity size in patients with chronic aortic regurgitation.

Because patients with aortic regurgitation may differ widely in their degree of myocardial dysfunction, anesthetic management must be appropriately individualized. For cardiac or noncardiac surgery, the hemodynamic goals are a mild tachycardia, a positive inotropic state, and a controlled reduction in SVR. For cardiac surgery, dopamine or dobutamine, pancuronium, ketamine, and nitroprusside infusions are excellent choices. For the patient with acute aortic regurgitation, the goals are the same, but urgency must be stressed. It is essential to try to rapidly reduce end-diastolic and end-systolic ventricular volumes with the very aggressive use of inotropes (e.g., epinephrine) and vasodilators. (There is sometimes concern that inotropes may exacerbate the root dissection in acute aortic regurgitation by increasing the shear force on the aortic wall. Despite this theoretical concern, positive inotropes should not be withheld from the patient who deteriorates in the operating room because they may provide the precious additional minutes of hemodynamic stability needed to get on CPB.) In acute and chronic forms of aortic regurgitation, serial measurements of cardiac output can indicate that ventricular size and cardiac output have been optimized, regardless of the systemic pressure. TEE is also useful to look at ventricular size, but probably maximizing cardiac output under these conditions gets closer to the therapeutic goal than looking at ventricular size alone. With acute aortic regurgitation and premature closure of the mitral valve, the pulmonary artery pressures may grossly underestimate the LVEDP, which continues to rise under the influence of the diastolic regurgitant jet from the aorta. For noncardiac surgery in the patient with aortic regurgitation, there are advantages to epidural or other regional techniques when appropriate. Epidural anesthesia is usually preferable to spinal techniques where more precipitous drops in SVR can occur.

Predicting the response of the patient with aortic regurgitation to anesthetic interventions can be difficult if the contractile state of the ventricle is unknown. Although reductions in functional status or EF are broadly indicators of poorer outcomes, examining the medical history for *serial* measurements of EF or ventricular end-systolic volumes may be most useful. Because patients with chronic aortic regurgitation are subject to a rapid, self-perpetuating decline in ventricular performance, demonstration of recent decreases in EF or increases in ventricular size may be the best indicators of a challenging intraoperative course.

A few other practical points bear comment in surgery for aortic regurgitation. The early and late phases of CPB can be a real problem in aortic regurgitation, particularly in redo operations. Before cross-clamp placement, the ventricle is at risk for distention if it is not ejecting or being vented. If the ventricle dilates with aortic regurgitation during bypass, the intraventricular pressures may equilibrate with the aortic root pressures. Under these conditions, there is no coronary perfusion, and the ventricle may rapidly dilate and become profoundly ischemic. This can occur before cross-clamp placement with bradycardia, ventricular fibrillation, tachycardia, or even with a rapid supraventricular rhythm that compromises organized mechanical activity. Correcting the rhythm, pacing, cross-clamping the aorta, or venting the ventricle addresses this problem. This can also occur in cardiac surgery for conditions other than aortic regurgitation. In patients with unknown or uncorrected aortic regurgitation, removal of the cross-clamp causes the same ventricular dilation and ischemia if a rhythm and ejection are not rapidly established. Ventricular venting or pacing may be essential until an organized, mechanically efficient rhythm is established. This problem must be considered in patients referred for coronary surgery alone, in those with mild or moderate aortic regurgitation not having AVR, and in patients in whom intraoperative TEE is not used.

MITRAL REGURGITATION

Clinical Features and Natural History

Unlike mitral stenosis, which is almost always the result of rheumatic valve disease, mitral regurgitation may result from a variety of disease processes that affect the valve leaflets, the chordae tendineae, the papillary muscles, the valve annulus, or the left ventricle. Mitral regurgitation can be classified as organic or functional. Organic mitral regurgitation describes diseases that result in distortion, disruption, or destruction of the mitral leaflets or chordal structures. In Western countries, degenerative processes that lead to leaflet prolapse with or without chordal rupture represent the most common cause of mitral regurgitation.[300] Other causes of organic mitral regurgitation include infective endocarditis, mitral annular calcification, rheumatic valve disease, and connective tissue disorders such as Marfan or Ehlers-Danlos syndrome. Much less common causes of organic mitral regurgitation include congenital mitral valve clefts, diet-drug or ergotamine toxicity, and carcinoid valve disease with metabolically active pulmonary tumors or right-to-left intracardiac shunting.[301]

Functional mitral regurgitation describes cases in which mitral regurgitation occurs despite structurally normal leaflets and chordae tendineae. Resulting from altered function or geometry of the left ventricle or mitral annulus, functional mitral regurgitation often occurs in the setting of ischemic heart disease, and the term *ischemic mitral regurgitation* is sometimes used interchangeably with *functional mitral regurgitation*. However, the functional form can occur in patients without demonstrable CAD, such as those with idiopathic dilated cardiomyopathy and mitral annular dilatation. The term *ischemic mitral regurgitation* probably best applies to functional cases with a known ischemic cause. Rupture of a papillary muscle with acute, severe mitral regurgitation is somewhat more difficult to classify. Although usually a sequela of acute myocardial infarction (AMI) with normal leaflets and chordae, there is an obvious anatomic disruption of the mitral apparatus.

Because it can be caused by a wide variety of disease processes, the natural history of mitral regurgitation is quite variable.[301] Even among patients with acute-onset disease, the clinical course depends on the mechanism of regurgitation and the response to treatment. For instance, patients presenting with acute, severe mitral regurgitation due to a ruptured papillary muscle have a dismal outcome without surgery.[301]

However, the clinical course of acute mitral regurgitation due to endocarditis could be favorable if the patient responds well to antibiotic therapy.[301] Although those with chronic mitral regurgitation usually enter an initial, often asymptomatic, compensated phase, the time course for progression to LV dysfunction and symptomatic heart failure is unpredictable.[301] The literature reflects the wide variability in the natural history of mitral regurgitation, with published 5-year survival rates for patients with mitral regurgitation of 27% to 97%.[302] Selection bias, small study populations, and poorly defined degrees of mitral regurgitation likely explain these discrepancies.[303] Later studies better define the clinical course of certain subgroups of patients with mitral regurgitation. For instance, Ling et al[304] examined the natural history of patients with mitral regurgitation due to flail leaflets. Among this select group, the investigators observed an excess annual mortality of 6.3% with a combined rate of death or surgery of 90% within a 10-year period.[304] Patients with flail mitral valve leaflets also experience an increased risk of sudden death.[305] Grigioni et al[305] reported a 1.8% per year rate of sudden death among patients with flail mitral leaflets who were being medically managed. The rate of sudden death diminished after surgical intervention in this population.[305]

The application of quantitative Doppler echocardiography to the prospective study of mitral regurgitation has allowed researchers to document the progressive nature of this condition. Enriquez-Sarano et al[306] found that, on average, the regurgitant volume increases 7.5 mL and the effective regurgitant orifice increases 5.9 mm^2 each year. However, as with the natural history of mitral regurgitation in general, there was significant variability in the rate of progression among patients. Rapid progression of its severity occurred among patients who developed flail leaflets, but mitral regurgitation regressed in 11% of those studied.[306]

Pathophysiology

Mitral regurgitation causes LV volume overload. The regurgitant volume combines with the normal LA volume and returns to the left ventricle during each diastolic period. This elevated preload leads to increased sarcomere stretch and, in the initial phases of the disease process, augmentation of LV ejection performance by the Frank-Starling mechanism. Systolic ejection into the relatively low-pressure left atrium further enhances the contractile appearance of the left ventricle.

The presentation of patients with mitral regurgitation varies depending on the pathophysiology of the specific condition, which is affected by the mechanism, severity, and acuity of the mitral regurgitation. In cases of acute, severe mitral regurgitation, such as patients with a ruptured papillary muscle after AMI, the sudden increase in preload enhances LV contractility by the Frank-Starling mechanism. Despite the increased preload, LV size is initially normal. Normal LV size combined with the ability to eject into a low-pressure circuit (i.e., the left atrium) results in decreased afterload in the acute setting. The measured LV EF in cases of sudden, severe mitral regurgitation may approach 75%, although forward SV is reduced.[301] However, because the left atrium has not yet dilated in response to the large regurgitant volume, LA pressure rises acutely and may lead to pulmonary vascular congestion, pulmonary edema, and dyspnea.[301]

Many patients with mitral regurgitation, particularly those whose valvular incompetence develops more slowly, may enter a chronic, compensated phase. In this phase, chronic volume overload triggers LV cavity enlargement by promoting eccentric hypertrophy (see Fig. 20–15). Elevated preload continues to augment LV systolic performance. At the same time, the left atrium dilates in response to the ongoing regurgitant volume. Although LA dilatation maintains a low-pressure circuit that facilitates LV systolic ejection, the increased radius of the LV cavity leads to increased wall tension according to the law of Laplace, which was given earlier.

Unlike the case of sudden, acute mitral regurgitation, which is characterized by normal LV size and reduced afterload, afterload remains in the normal range in the chronic, compensated phase of mitral regurgitation.[307] The changes seen in chronic, compensated mitral regurgitation are represented graphically in Figure 20–27. The isovolumic contraction phase is shortened as the blood is ejected into the low-pressure left atrium early in the cycle of ventricular systole. Because the dilated, compliant left ventricle accepts increased diastolic volumes at low or normal filling pressures, some physicians believe that LV diastolic function is enhanced in patients with chronic mitral regurgitation.[307] Whereas dilatation of the left heart chambers permits LV filling at low or normal pressures, chamber enlargement progressively dilates the mitral annulus, potentially increasing the effective regurgitant orifice and regurgitant volume over time. Patients may tolerate the phase of chronic, compensated mitral regurgitation for many years because elevated preload maintains LV ejection performance. If symptoms develop during this time, they are often related to diminished forward cardiac output because the regurgitant fraction may exceed 50%. Rather than dyspnea or signs of pulmonary congestion, fatigue and weakness predominate.

With the eventual decline in LV systolic function, patients enter a decompensated phase. Progressive LV dilatation increases wall stress and afterload, causing further deterioration in LV performance,[301] mitral annular dilatation, and worsening of the mitral regurgitation. LV end-systolic pressure increases. The increased LV filling pressures result in elevation of LA pressures and, given time, pulmonary vascular congestion, pulmonary hypertension, and RV dysfunction. In addition to fatigue and weakness, patients with decompensated, chronic mitral regurgitation may also report dyspnea

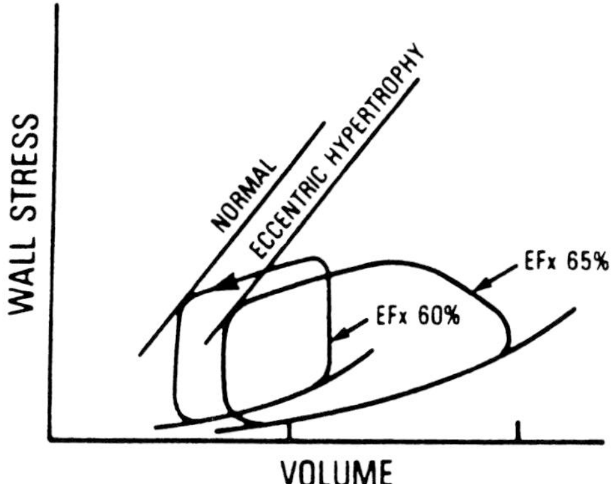

Figure 20–27 Volume overload with mitral regurgitation (MR). As in volume overloading from aortic regurgitation, wall stress-volume loops of the eccentrically hypertrophied left ventricle are shifted to the right. However, in chronic MR, retrograde ejection into the low-pressure left atrium minimizes ventricular wall stress, supporting the ejection fraction. (From Ross J Jr: Afterload mismatch in aortic and mitral valve disease: Implications for surgical therapy. J Am Coll Cardiol 5:811, 1985.)

and orthopnea. It is difficult to predict when a patient with mitral regurgitation is likely to decompensate clinically. The progression of disease in any given patient depends on the underlying cause of mitral regurgitation, its severity, the response of the left ventricle to volume overload, and possibly the effect of medical management.[301,308]

Assessment of LV function in patients with mitral regurgitation is controversial but critically important for clinical decision making.[302] As in aortic regurgitation, the altered loading conditions that characterize mitral regurgitation confound traditional, load-dependent measures of LV systolic function such as EF. Although numerous methods of assessing LV function have been proposed, no consensus exists.[302] Despite its limitations, EF remains the most studied variable of LV function in patients with mitral regurgitation and the most predictive of clinical outcome. For instance, preoperative EF is the most important prognostic factor for long-term survival after surgery for mitral regurgitation.[309] Preoperative EF also predicts postoperative EF and the occurrence of CHF after the surgical correction of mitral regurgitation.[310,311] Because of the combination of increased preload and the ability to eject into the low-pressure left atrium, a normally functioning left ventricle should display an elevated EF in presence of significant mitral regurgitation. Conversely, an EF considered normal in a patient with competent valves may represent diminished LV function in the setting of mitral regurgitation. In patients with severe mitral regurgitation, an EF in the range of 50% to 60% likely represents significant LV dysfunction and is itself an indication for surgery.[138] Enriquez-Sarano et al[309] reported that the postoperative survival after mitral repair or replacement declines after the preoperative EF falls below 60%.

A number of studies provide insight into the origin of LV dysfunction in the setting of mitral regurgitation. In animal models of the disease, myocardial mass accumulates mainly through a decrease in the natural degradation of cellular elements, rather than by an increased rate of protein synthesis.[312-314] In contrast, myocardial protein synthesis increases within hours of the creation of simulated aortic stenosis and LV pressure overload.[315] Histologic preparations from animals with experimental mitral regurgitation and LV dysfunction also show a 35% reduction in contractile elements within individual myocytes.[316] Examination of pressure-volume loops from patients with aortic stenosis and mitral regurgitation is also insightful (see Figs. 20–13 and 20–27). If the area contained within each loop is examined, it can be seen that this area, or stroke work, is similar for the two disease states. However, patients with aortic stenosis generally display a greater degree of myocardial hypertrophy when compared with patients suffering from mitral regurgitation. Stroke work per gram of myocardium is greater in patients with mitral regurgitation, a finding that may also explain LV dysfunction in this patient population.[307]

Ischemic Mitral Regurgitation

Ischemic mitral regurgitation (IMR) represents mitral regurgitation occurring in the setting of ischemic heart disease in patients without significant abnormalities of the valve leaflets or chordal structures. Some clinicians use the terms IMR and functional mitral regurgitation interchangeably. However, IMR more accurately describes those cases of functional mitral regurgitation that occur in the setting of CAD. Papillary muscle rupture, which is almost always a sequela of AMI, may also be classified as IMR, although a clear organic defect of the mitral apparatus exists.

Clinicians are increasingly recognizing the importance of IMR, because it is quite common. The incidence of mitral regurgitation after AMI as detected by echocardiography ranges from 39% to 73%.[308] Echocardiographic studies also demonstrate that in 13% to 29% of cases, the IMR is at least moderate in severity.[308] The presence of IMR also portends a worse clinical outcome. For instance, patients with IMR after AMI experience a twofold to sixfold increase in cardiovascular mortality in the first year after the ischemic event.[317] Patients with severe IMR have a 1-year mortality rate that approaches 50%.[318] However, in evaluating patients with mitral regurgitation presumed to be of ischemic origin, clinicians should attempt to identify the severity of the regurgitation, the time of onset, and the likely mechanism of valvular incompetence because these factors influence prognosis and treatment. For instance, patients with mild IMR in the early phase of an AMI rarely experience hemodynamic sequelae from this mitral leakage, whereas those with ischemic rupture of a papillary muscle often present with acute CHF and have a poor prognosis without surgical intervention.

Investigators have identified certain patient characteristics associated with an increased incidence of IMR. For instance, patients with advanced age, inferior or posterior AMI, spherical LV geometry, and multiple-vessel CAD tend to display higher rates of IMR.[308,319] Other factors associated with increased rates of IMR include LA enlargement, mitral annular dilatation, and decreased EF.[308] Frank rupture of a papillary muscle, which occurs in 1% of AMI cases, usually involves the posteromedial papillary muscle as its blood supply is derived from a single coronary artery.

The understanding of the pathophysiologic basis of IMR continues to evolve. Early investigators proposed ischemic papillary muscle dysfunction as a primary cause of IMR.[320-322] Later studies indicate that isolated ischemia of one or both papillary muscles does not cause significant mitral regurgitation.[323-326] Instead, ischemia of the papillary muscle and the adjacent myocardium is necessary to produce IMR.[308,323,325,326] Myocardial ischemia may result in focal or global LV bulging and, with time, ventricular remodeling to a more spherical shape. Such geometric changes cause outward migration of the papillary muscles. The finding most strongly correlated with chronic IMR is outward papillary muscle displacement.[308,327] When the papillary muscles are displaced outward, the point of mitral leaflet coaptation moves apically and away from the mitral annulus resulting in the appearance of valve tenting. Besides outward bulging of the left ventricle, scarring and retraction of the papillary muscles may also produce mitral leaflet tethering with the net effect of incomplete leaflet coaptation and valvular incompetence. Some investigators believe that papillary muscle dysfunction may reduce the degree of IMR in certain patients.[328,329] Komeda et al[329] suggested that reduced contractility of the papillary muscles may counteract the tethering effect of ischemic myocardium, thereby allowing leaflet coaptation to occur closer to the mitral annulus. An additional potential mechanism of IMR is decreased contractility of the posterior mitral annulus. During systole, annular contraction reduces the mitral orifice area by 25%.[330-332] Because the anterior portion of the mitral annulus is more fibrous, posterior annular contraction plays a greater role in reducing the size of the mitral orifice. Loss of posterior annular contraction may contribute to mitral regurgitation in the setting of myocardial ischemia.

The clinical approach to IMR depends on its underlying mechanism. Timely surgical intervention is often warranted in cases of papillary muscle rupture. For patients with an intact mitral apparatus who present with IMR in the setting of AMI, early reperfusion therapy improves regional and global LV function, reduces ventricular dilatation, and decreases the likelihood of adverse remodeling and associated papillary muscle displacement.[328,333-336] The resultant improvements in ventricular function and geometry combine to reduce the incidence of IMR. Clinicians often prescribe angiotensin-converting enzyme (ACE) inhibitors to patients with ischemic heart disease. Chronic ACE inhibitor therapy may decrease the incidence and severity of IMR by preventing LV remodeling, although data to support this theory are lacking.[328]

Assessment of Mitral Regurgitation

Clinicians may suspect mitral regurgitation on the basis of current symptoms, past medical history, or findings on physical examination. Echocardiography with the capability of two-dimensional and Doppler (including color-flow) imaging represents the diagnostic modality of choice for the assessment of mitral regurgitation. TTE is readily available in most areas, is noninvasive, and provides detailed information about the mechanism of mitral regurgitation, its severity, and its impact on cardiac chamber size and function. Additional information available from TTE includes calculation of RV systolic pressure based on the peak velocity of the tricuspid regurgitant signal and an estimate of right atrial pressure. Whenever possible, echocardiographers should attempt to provide a quantitative assessment of mitral regurgitation severity. Techniques that allow the determination of effective regurgitant orifice, regurgitant volume, or regurgitant fraction include the proximal isovelocity surface area (PISA) method and the continuity equation. Other echocardiographic findings such as pulmonary vein systolic flow reversals suggest severe mitral regurgitation, and they should be reported if present. Assessment of the size of the regurgitant jet in the left atrium may provide a gross estimation of mitral regurgitation severity but is limited by factors such as LA size and pressure, machine settings such as color-flow gain and aliasing velocity, and the orientation of the regurgitant jet itself. Eccentric regurgitant jets propagating along the wall of the left atrium often appear smaller than a centrally directed jet of equivalent severity. When transthoracic echocardiography is suboptimal, patients may be referred for TEE. Because of the proximity of the transducer to the mitral valve, TEE often produces superior images of the mitral valve. When performing intraoperative TEE examinations, anesthesiologists should recall that altered loading conditions, such as anesthetic-induced decreases in SVR, might favor forward cardiac output and diminish the observed amount of mitral regurgitation. A more detailed discussion of the echocardiographic evaluation of the mitral valve is presented in Chapters 15 and 16.

Cardiac catheterization with left ventriculography may also be used to evaluate mitral regurgitation. This invasive procedure is often reserved for cases in which the echocardiographic data are suboptimal, conflicting, or discordant with the clinical findings.[301] Assessment of severity by ventriculography requires analysis of the amount of contrast material that enters the left atrium after injection into the left ventricle. However, the amount of contrast material appearing in the left atrium depends on the severity of mitral regurgitation and on the volume of the left atrium, the catheter position, and the rate of contrast injection.[301] Right-heart catheterization may or may not demonstrate the presence of v waves in patients with significant mitral regurgitation. A high degree of LA compliance makes the appearance of prominent v waves less likely.

Other diagnostic tests commonly obtained in patients with mitral regurgitation include an electrocardiogram and chest radiograph. ECG findings such as atrial fibrillation, LA enlargement, and ST-segment abnormalities may be observed in patients with mitral regurgitation, but they are not specific.[301] Similarly, chest radiographs may identify enlargement of the left heart chambers and pulmonary vascular congestion, but such findings are not specific for mitral regurgitation.

Surgical Decision Making

Just as progress in the understanding of the pathophysiology of mitral regurgitation has evolved, so too has the surgical approach to this disease process. A high operative mortality associated with the surgical correction of mitral regurgitation in the 1980s led many clinicians to manage patients conservatively.[302,303,337] Because favorable loading conditions and high LA compliance allow even patients with significant mitral regurgitation to remain asymptomatic for long periods, it is likely that many patients did not undergo surgery until the onset of disabling symptoms. Studies show that more severe preoperative symptoms are associated with a lower EF and a higher incidence of postoperative CHF.[303,310,311] Historically poor outcomes after surgery for mitral regurgitation might have occurred because clinicians did not appreciate the true degree of LV dysfunction at the time of surgery in symptomatic patients. An EF of less than 60% in the setting of severe mitral regurgitation represents significant LV dysfunction and predicts a worse outcome with surgery or medical management.[304,309] Surgical techniques common in the 1980s probably also contributed to unfavorable postoperative outcomes. For instance, although the mechanisms are incompletely understood, resection of the subvalvular apparatus contributes to decreased LV systolic performance after mitral replacement.[338]

In part because of improved surgical techniques, the operative mortality rate for patients with organic mitral regurgitation who are younger than 75 years is about 1% in some centers.[309] Besides preservation of the subvalvular apparatus, valve repair represents another surgical technique associated with improved postoperative outcome.[303,339] Although not applicable to all patients, such as those with advanced rheumatic disease, the popularity of valve repairs continues to grow. Studies indicate numerous benefits associated with mitral repair. For instance, after accounting for baseline characteristics, patients who undergo mitral repair instead of replacement experience lower operative mortality and better long-term survival largely because of improved postoperative LV function.[303,339] The survival benefit that accompanies valve repair is also observed among patients undergoing combined valve and coronary artery surgery.[339] Valve repair does not increase the likelihood of reoperation when compared with replacement.[339] Although originally used most often for posterior leaflet disease, surgeons now routinely repair anterior mitral leaflets with good success.[340] When repairing anterior leaflet prolapse, surgeons may insert artificial chordae.[341,342] The approach to flail or prolapsing posterior mitral leaflet segments often involves resection of a portion of the leaflet.[342] In addition to resecting a portion of the leaflet and plicating the redundant tissue, an annuloplasty ring is often placed to reduce mitral orifice size and return the annulus to a more anatomic shape.[342] Some surgeons favor a flexible, partial, posterior annuloplasty band, which may allow improved systolic contraction of the posterior annulus and better postoperative LV function.[331,342,343]

Timely and appropriate surgical referral helps improve the perioperative outcome of patients with mitral regurgitation. To appropriately refer patients for surgery, clinicians should have an understanding of the factors that influence surgical risk in this population.[302] The factors that correlated best with increased operative risk in patients with significant mitral regurgitation include age older than 75 years, severe preoperative symptoms of CHF, and concomitant CAD.[309,344,345] Even though they represent a high-risk group, patients with severe mitral regurgitation and symptoms of heart failure should still be referred for surgery, because valve repair or replacement offers a survival advantage compared with medical management.[302,304] Similarly, although perioperative risk remains elevated, patients with evidence of LV dysfunction, such as an EF less than 60% or an end-systolic LV diameter greater than 45 mm, should be referred for surgery to prevent further, possibly irreversible deterioration in ventricular performance.[138,302] Asymptomatic patients without evidence of LV dysfunction should also be considered for surgery if conditions such as atrial fibrillation, ventricular tachycardia, or pulmonary hypertension are identified or the effective regurgitant orifice is greater than 40 mm.[2,138,302] Institutional experience, particularly with techniques such as valve repair, is an important consideration for clinicians contemplating early surgical referral[302] (see Chapters 12, 16, 21, and 27).

Anesthetic Considerations

Patients who present to the operating room with mitral regurgitation may differ significantly with respect to duration of disease, symptoms, hemodynamic stability, ventricular function, and involvement of the right heart and pulmonary circulation (Box 20–4). For instance, a patient presenting with severe mitral regurgitation due to acute papillary muscle rupture may enter the operating room in cardiogenic shock with pulmonary congestion requiring intra-aortic balloon pump (IABP) augmentation. Another patient with a newly diagnosed flail posterior mitral leaflet may enter the surgical suite with relatively preserved LV function and no symptoms whatsoever. In the latter patient, the compliance of the left atrium may have prevented pulmonary vascular congestion, pulmonary hypertension, and RV dysfunction. Despite the differences in presentation, the general management goals remain similar and include maintenance of forward cardiac output and reduction in the mitral regurgitant fraction. The anesthesiologist must also seek to optimize RV function, in part by avoiding increases in pulmonary vascular congestion and pulmonary hypertension. Various degrees of intervention are needed to achieve these hemodynamic management goals depending on the patient's presentation.

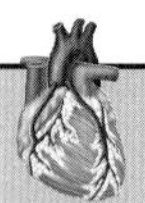

BOX 20–4 ***Mitral Regurgitation***

Preload:	Increased
Afterload:	Decreased
Goal:	Mild tachycardia, vasodilation
Avoid:	Myocardial depression

Information obtained during the preoperative interview and examination provides the anesthesiologist with important insight into the patient's degree of hemodynamic compromise. For example, a patient who reports dyspnea at rest or with minimal activity may have significant pulmonary vascular congestion and possibly compromised RV function. This information combined with the estimated pulmonary artery systolic pressure derived from the preoperative TTE report helps the anesthesiologist prepare for potential right-heart dysfunction intraoperatively. In such a patient, the anesthesiologist avoids heavy premedication with its attendant risk of obtundation, hypoventilation, and further elevation of pulmonary artery pressures. Auscultation of the heart may reveal rhythm disturbances such as atrial fibrillation and the systolic murmur of mitral regurgitation. Clinicians should recall, however, that in cases of acute, severe mitral regurgitation, a significant elevation in LA pressure decreases the systolic pressure gradient between the left heart chambers, and the murmur of mitral regurgitation may be diminished or even absent.[301]

Invasive hemodynamic monitoring provides the anesthesiologist with a wealth of important information. Arterial catheters are essential for monitoring beat-to-beat changes in blood pressure that occur in response to a variety of surgical and anesthetic manipulations. PACs facilitate many aspects of intraoperative patient management. Intraoperative use of a PAC allows the anesthesiologist to more carefully optimize left-sided filling pressures. Although the PCWP and pulmonary artery diastolic pressure depend on LA and LV compliance and filling, examination of intraoperative trends in these variables enhances the ability of the anesthesiologist to provide appropriate levels of preload while avoiding volume overload. Periodic determination of cardiac output allows a more objective assessment of the patient's response to interventions such as fluid administration or inotropic infusion. The presence or size of a v wave on a PCWP tracing does not reliably correlate with the severity of mitral regurgitation, because this finding depends on LA compliance. Just as in the management of patients with aortic valvular regurgitation, another benefit of PAC insertion is the ability to introduce a ventricular pacing wire to rapidly counteract hemodynamically significant bradycardia. In patients with RV compromise, monitoring trends in the CVP recording may also be helpful. Tricuspid regurgitation detected through analysis of the CVP tracing may suggest RV dilatation, which may be caused by pulmonary hypertension.[346]

Intraoperative TEE provides invaluable information during the surgical correction of mitral regurgitation. It reliably identifies the mechanism of mitral regurgitation, thereby guiding the surgical approach,[347] and it objectively demonstrates the size and function of the cardiac chambers. TEE can readily identify the cause of hemodynamic derangements, facilitating proper intervention. For instance, the appearance of SAM of the mitral apparatus immediately after valve repair allows the anesthesiologist to intervene with volume infusion and medications such as esmolol or phenylephrine as appropriate. In rare circumstances when hemodynamically significant SAM persists despite these interventions, the surgeon may elect to further repair or even replace the mitral valve.

TEE also identifies concomitant pathology that may warrant surgical attention, such as atrial level shunts and additional valve disease (see Chapters 15 and 16).

The intraoperative management of patients with mitral regurgitation before the institution of CPB focuses on optimizing forward cardiac output, minimizing the mitral regurgitant volume, and preventing deleterious increases in pulmonary artery pressures. Maintaining adequate LV preload is essential. An enlarged left ventricle that operates on a higher portion of the Frank-Starling curve requires adequate filling. At the same time, excessive volume administration is to be avoided because it may cause unwanted dilatation of the mitral annulus and worsening of the mitral regurgitation. Excessive fluid administration may precipitate RV failure in patients with pulmonary vascular congestion and pulmonary hypertension. Optimization of preload is aided by analysis of data obtained from PAC measurements and TEE images. Because significant LV dysfunction is present in many patients with mitral regurgitation, anesthesiologists often select specific induction and maintenance regimens to avoid further depressing LV function. For this reason, large doses of narcotics have been popular in the past.[148,149] Other researchers have shown that smaller doses of narcotics combined with vasodilating inhalation anesthetics also produce acceptable intraoperative hemodynamics.[348,349] By reducing the amount of narcotics administered, the addition of a vasodilating inhalation agent to the anesthetic regimen may allow for faster extubation of the trachea postoperatively. With the current trend toward early referral of asymptomatic patients for mitral repair, anesthetic regimens that reduce the duration of postoperative mechanical ventilation may be advantageous.

In patients with severe LV dysfunction, infusions of inotropic medications such as dopamine, dobutamine, or even epinephrine may be required to maintain an adequate cardiac output. Phosphodiesterase inhibitors such as milrinone may also augment systolic ventricular performance and reduce pulmonary and peripheral vascular resistances. By reducing pulmonary and peripheral vascular resistance, forward cardiac output is facilitated. Nitroglycerin and sodium nitroprusside represent two additional options for reducing the impedance to ventricular ejection. If patients prove refractory to inotropic and vasodilator therapy, insertion of an IABP should be strongly considered (see Chapters 10, 16, 27, 31, and 33).

Manipulation of the heart rate may be necessary in some patients to optimize hemodynamics. Bradycardia should generally be avoided as slower heart rates allow for larger filling volumes, potentially resulting in LV distention and mitral annular dilatation. Regurgitant volumes may increase at slower heart rates. Slightly increased heart rates, especially when combined with increased LV contractility, favor a smaller mitral annular area and may decrease the regurgitant fraction. Sinus rhythm and preserved atrial contraction are less important in patients with mitral regurgitation compared with patients with stenotic valves. Mitral annular dilatation accompanies most cases of long-standing mitral regurgitation. Patients with pure mitral regurgitation generally have no impedance to LV filling and atrial fibrillation is usually better tolerated than in patients with stenotic lesions.

Because severe mitral regurgitation may result in pulmonary hypertension and RV dysfunction, anesthesiologists should tailor their intraoperative management strategies accordingly. Hypercapnia, hypoxia, and acidosis elevate pulmonary artery pressures and should be avoided. Mild hyperventilation may be beneficial in some patients. The effect of nitrous oxide on pulmonary vascular resistance (PVR) and pulmonary hypertension is controversial. Some studies show no change in PVR when administered to anesthetized patients with CAD or VHD.[350-352] Other studies in patients with mitral stenosis demonstrate an elevation in PVR after nitrous oxide administration and in vitro evidence suggests that nitrous oxide increases norepinephrine release from the pulmonary artery.[353-355]

Patients with severe RV dysfunction after CPB can prove exceptionally difficult to manage. Besides avoiding the factors known to increase PVR, only a few options exist for these patients. Inotropic agents with vasodilating properties such as dobutamine, isoproterenol, and milrinone augment RV systolic performance and decrease PVR, but their use is often confounded by systemic hypotension. Prostaglandin E_1 (PGE_1) reliably reduces PVR and undergoes extensive first-pass metabolism in the pulmonary circulation.[356,357] Although PGE_1 reduces pulmonary artery pressures after CPB, systemic hypotension requiring infusions of vasoconstrictors through an LA catheter has also occurred.[358-361] Inhaled nitric oxide represents another alternative available for the treatment of RV failure in the setting of pulmonary hypertension. Nitric oxide reliably relaxes the pulmonary vasculature and is then immediately bound to hemoglobin and inactivated. Studies indicate that systemic hypotension during nitric oxide therapy is unlikely.[362,363]

LV dysfunction may also contribute to post-CPB hemodynamic instability. With mitral competence restored, the low-pressure outlet for LV ejection is removed. The enlarged left ventricle must then eject entirely into the aorta. Because LV enlargement leads to increased wall stress, a condition of elevated afterload often exists after CPB. At the same time, the preload augmentation inherent to mitral regurgitation is removed. It is therefore not surprising that the systolic performance of the left ventricle often declines after surgical correction of mitral regurgitation. Treatment options in the immediate post-CPB period include inotropic and vasodilator therapy and, if necessary, IABP augmentation.

MITRAL STENOSIS

Clinical Features and Natural History

Clinically significant mitral stenosis in adult patients usually is a result of rheumatic disease. Congenital abnormalities of the mitral valve represent a rare cause of mitral stenosis in younger patients. Other uncommon conditions that do not directly involve the mitral valve apparatus but may limit LV inflow and simulate the clinical findings of mitral stenosis include cor triatriatum, large LA neoplasms, and pulmonary vein obstruction.[364]

A decades-long asymptomatic period characterizes the initial phase of rheumatic mitral stenosis. Symptoms rarely appear until the normal mitral valve area of 4 to 6 cm^2 (Fig. 20–28) has been reduced to 2.5 cm^2 or less.[365] When the mitral valve area reaches 1.5 to 2.5 cm^2, symptoms usually occur only in association with exercise or other conditions, such as fever, pregnancy, or atrial fibrillation, that lead to an increase in heart rate or cardiac output.[366,367] After the mitral valve area falls below 1.5 cm^2, symptoms may develop at rest. Some patients are able to remain asymptomatic for long periods by gradually reducing their level of activity.[364] Patients with

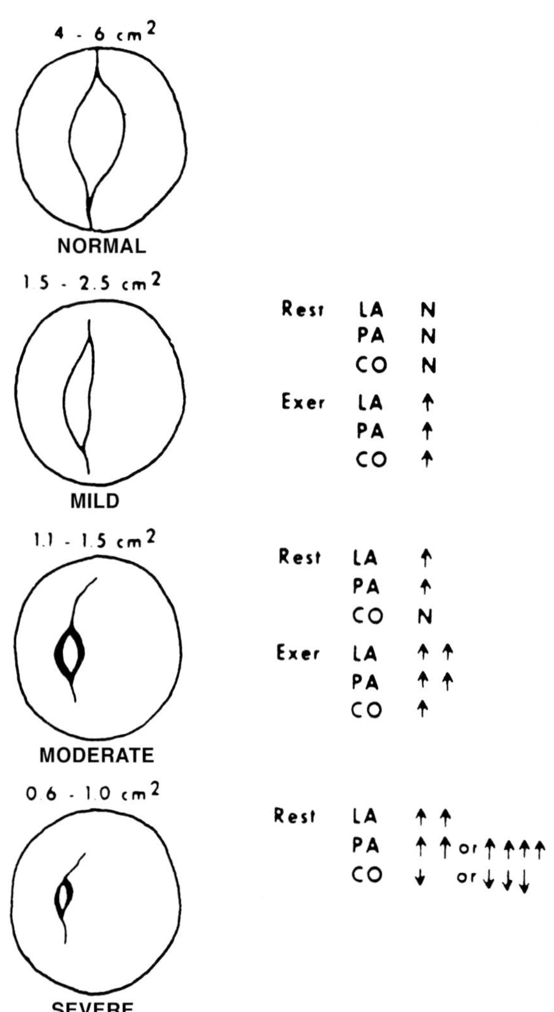

Figure 20–28 Hemodynamic changes with progressive narrowing of the mitral valve. (From Rapaport E: Natural history of aortic and mitral valve disease. Am J Cardiol 35:221, 1971.)

mitral stenosis commonly report dyspnea as their initial symptom, a finding reflective of elevated LA pressure and pulmonary congestion. In addition to dyspnea, patients may report palpitations that signal the onset of atrial fibrillation. Systemic thromboembolization occurs in 10% to 20% of patients with mitral stenosis and does not appear to be correlated with the mitral valve area or LA size.[366] Chest pain that simulates angina is present in a small number of patients with mitral stenosis and may result from RV hypertrophy rather than CAD.[366]

There has been a change in the typical age of presentation of patients with mitral stenosis.[366] Previously, patients, often women, presented with mitral stenosis while in their 20s and 30s.[366,368,369] In the past 15 years, perhaps because of more slowly progressive disease in the United States, patients have been presenting in their 40s and 50s.[366,370,371] After symptoms develop, mitral stenosis remains a slow, progressive disease. Often, patients live 10 to 20 years with mild symptoms, such as dyspnea with exercise, before disabling NYHA class III and IV symptoms develop. The symptomatic state of the patient predicts the clinical outcome. For instance, the 10-year survival rate of patients with mild symptoms approaches 80%, but the 10-year survival rate of patients with disabling symptoms is only 15% without surgery.[366,371-373]

Pathophysiology

Rheumatic mitral stenosis results in valve leaflet thickening and fusion of the commissures. Later in the disease process, leaflet calcification and subvalvular chordal fusion may occur.[366] These changes combine to reduce the effective mitral valve area and limit diastolic flow into the left ventricle. As a result of the fixed obstruction to LV inflow, LA pressures rise. Elevated LA pressures limit pulmonary venous drainage and result in elevated pulmonary artery pressures.[309] Over time, pulmonary arteriolar hypertrophy develops in response to chronically elevated pulmonary vascular pressures.[310] Pulmonary hypertension may trigger increases in RV end-diastolic volume and pressure, and in some patients, signs of RV failure such as ascites or peripheral edema may appear.[368,369] LA enlargement is an almost universal finding in patients with established mitral stenosis and is a risk factor for the development of atrial fibrillation.

Patients with mitral stenosis tolerate tachycardia particularly poorly. LV inflow, already limited by a mechanically abnormal valve, is further compromised by the disproportionate decline in the diastolic period that accompanies tachycardia. To maintain LV filling in a shorter diastolic period, the flow rate across the stenotic valve must increase. Because the valve area remains constant, the pressure gradient between the left atrium and left ventricle increases by the square of the increase in the flow rate, according to the Gorlin formula, in which PG is the transvalvular pressure gradient:

$$\text{Valve area} = \frac{\text{Transvalvular flow rate}}{\text{Constant} \times \sqrt{\text{PG}}}$$

Tachycardia necessitates a significant increase in the transvalvular pressure gradient and may precipitate feelings of breathlessness in awake patients. In patients with atrial fibrillation, it is the elevated ventricular rate that is most deleterious, rather than the loss of atrial contraction.[311] Although coordinated atrial activity is always preferable, the primary goal in treating patients with mitral stenosis and atrial fibrillation should be control of the ventricular rate.

Mitral stenosis results in diminished LV preload reserve. As seen in the pressure-volume loop in Figure 20–29, LVEDV and LVEDP are reduced with an accompanying decline in SV. Controversy exists, however, regarding the contractile state of the left ventricle in these patients. Gash et al[374] reported that almost one third of their study population of patients with mitral stenosis had an EF less than 50%. Limited preload may contribute to a reduced EF in some of these patients. However, the observation that LV contractile impairment persists postoperatively in some patients suggests that other causes of LV dysfunction may exist. Rheumatic myocarditis has been reported, although its role in producing LV contractile dysfunction is uncertain.[374] Other investigators have described posterobasal regional wall motion abnormalities, perhaps a consequence of thickening and calcification of the mitral apparatus.[313,314] Vasoconstriction occurring in response to diminished cardiac output may also impair LV ejection.[375] Afterload may also be increased due to inadequate myocardial wall thickness.[374] The lack of adequate wall thickness leads to elevations in wall stress in accordance with the law of Laplace.

In addition to abnormalities in systolic function, patients with mitral stenosis may have impaired diastolic function. Mitral stenosis creates an obvious impairment of LV diastolic filling. However, the intrinsic compliance of the left ventricle may also be reduced by the rheumatic disease process. Using

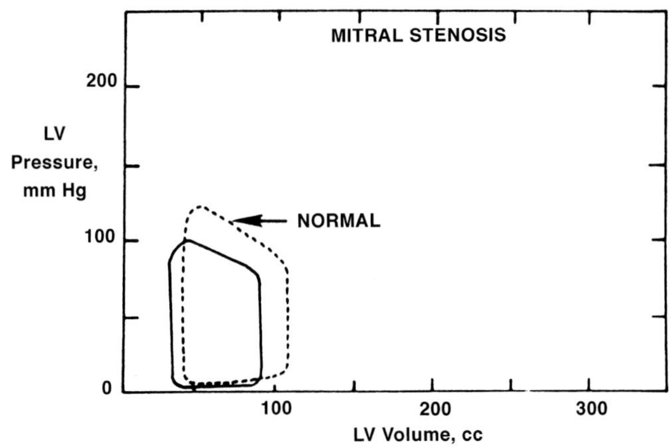

Figure 20–29 Pressure-volume loop in mitral stenosis. (From Jackson JM, Thomas SJ, Lowenstein E: Anesthetic management of patients with valvular heart disease. Semin Anesth 1:239, 1982.)

conductance catheter and micromanometer techniques, Liu et al[376] discovered decreased LV compliance in a group of patients with mitral stenosis scheduled for mitral balloon valvuloplasty. On repeat measurements taken immediately after valvuloplasty, the investigators observed a significant increase in LV compliance. Because the increase in compliance occurred immediately after valvuloplasty, the physicians hypothesized that the changes associated with rheumatic mitral stenosis create an internal constraint that limits LV compliance.

Assessment of Mitral Stenosis

As for patients with mitral regurgitation, echocardiography represents the diagnostic modality of choice for patients with suspected mitral stenosis.[364,377,378] Two-dimensional and Doppler echocardiographic techniques are able to accurately and noninvasively measure the transvalvular pressure gradient and mitral valve area. Because the pressure gradient varies with the flow rate and diastolic period, the assessment of mitral stenosis severity ideally should be based on the measured or calculated mitral valve area.[364] Echocardiographic methods used to obtain mitral valve area include the pressure half-time technique, the continuity equation, planimetry of the valve orifice, and PISA analysis. Other invaluable information obtained during an echocardiographic study includes the size and function of the ventricles and an estimation of the pulmonary artery pressure.

Exercise echocardiography can be employed when the patient's symptoms and the resting echocardiographic data are discordant.[377] In such cases, echocardiography may be performed while the patient exercises on a supine bicycle. If during exercise the transmitral gradient or pulmonary artery pressure increases significantly, mitral stenosis is the likely cause of the patient's symptoms.[377]

With the accuracy and widespread use of echocardiography, cardiac catheterization and invasive measurements of hemodynamics are almost never necessary.[366,378] Even patients referred for preoperative coronary angiography need not undergo invasive hemodynamic studies at the time of catheterization if adequate echocardiographic data have already been obtained.[378] Catheter-based hemodynamic assessments are reserved for situations in which echocardiographic studies are suboptimal or conflict with the clinical picture, because invasive mitral valve hemodynamic studies are complex and limited.[366] For instance, to measure the LA-to-LV pressure gradient directly, a transseptal puncture is required and entails risks such as tamponade, aortic injury, and heart block.[366] If the PCWP is used in place of direct LA pressure measurements, the gradient derived is less accurate than that obtained with Doppler echocardiography.[318]

Similar to patients with mitral regurgitation, nonspecific findings are commonly seen on electrocardiograms and chest radiographs in patients with mitral stenosis. Potential ECG findings include atrial fibrillation and LA enlargement. Radiographs may also reveal LA enlargement and pulmonary vascular congestion.

Surgical Decision Making

Appropriate referral of patients for surgical intervention requires integration of clinical and echocardiographic data. Patients presenting with severe symptoms (i.e., NYHA class III and IV) should be immediately referred for surgery because their outcome is poor if treated medically.[312,366] Patients with only mild mitral stenosis and few or no symptoms may be managed conservatively with periodic evaluation. Patients who are asymptomatic but have moderate mitral stenosis (i.e., mitral valve area between 1.0 and 1.5 cm^2) require careful assessment. If significant pulmonary hypertension (i.e., pulmonary artery systolic pressure >50 mm Hg) is present, surgical intervention should be considered.[312] Intervention may also be indicated if a patient becomes symptomatic or pulmonary artery pressures increase significantly during exercise testing.[366]

The surgical options for treating mitral stenosis continue to evolve. Closed commissurotomy, in which the surgeon fractures fused mitral commissures, was first performed in the 1920s. It became popular in the 1940s and is still used to treat mitral stenosis in developing countries.[377] With the advent of CPB in the 1950s, techniques of open commissurotomy developed, allowing the surgeon to directly inspect the valve before splitting the commissures.[377] The common goals of closed and open mitral commissurotomy include increasing the effective mitral valve area and decreasing the LA-to-LV pressure gradient with a resultant relief in the patient's symptoms (see Chapters 1 to 3).

Percutaneous mitral commissurotomy (PMC) allows a less invasive, catheter-based approach to mitral stenosis (see Chapters 4 and 12). First reported by Inoue in 1984,[379] clinicians worldwide perform PMC more than 10,000 times each year.[380] The technique of PMC involves directing a balloon-tipped catheter across the stenotic mitral valve. Specifically designed balloons allow sequential inflation of the distal and proximal portions of the balloon, ensuring correct positioning across the mitral valve before the middle portion of the device is inflated to split the fused commissures.[381] Patient selection for PMC requires careful echocardiographic evaluation. Echocardiographic grading scales have been developed to evaluate mitral leaflet mobility, thickness, calcification, and subvalvular fusion.[382] Patients who score favorably on such echocardiographic assessments (i.e., adequate leaflet mobility with little calcification) may be referred for PMC. Success rates for PMC are similar to those achieved with surgical commissurotomy, and most patients experience a doubling in the effective mitral valve area.[377] An increase in the amount of mitral regurgitation represents the most common complication associated with PMC.[377]

Not all patients are candidates for surgical commissurotomy or PMC. For instance, those with heavily calcified valves or significant mitral regurgitation are likely to experience suboptimal results after commissurotomy. Mitral valve anatomy unsuitable for PMC is more commonly encountered in Western countries, where patients with mitral stenosis typically present at an older average age.[380] Mitral valve replacement is commonly recommended for these patients. The risk of mitral valve replacement depends on patient characteristics such as age, functional status, and other co-morbid conditions.[377] Surgical risk in younger patients with few coexisting medical problems generally is less than 5%. Conversely, surgical risk in elderly patients with severe symptoms related to mitral stenosis and multiple co-morbidities may be 10% to 20%.[377]

Anesthetic Considerations

Several important goals should guide the anesthetic management of patients with significant mitral stenosis. First, the anesthesiologist should seek to prevent tachycardia and treat it promptly if it develops in the perioperative period (Box 20–5). Maintenance of LV preload without exacerbation of pulmonary vascular congestion represents a second management goal. Third, anesthesiologists should avoid factors that aggravate pulmonary hypertension and impair RV function.

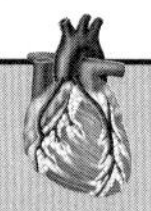

BOX 20–5 *Mitral Stenosis*

Preload:	Normal or increased
Afterload:	Normal
Goal:	Controlled ventricular response
Avoid:	Tachycardia, pulmonary vasoconstriction

Prevention and treatment of tachycardia are central to the perioperative management of these patients. Tachycardia shortens the diastolic filling period. To maintain LV preload with a shortened diastolic period, an elevation in transvalvular flow rate is required with a resultant increase in the LA-to-LV pressure gradient. Avoidance of tachycardia begins in the preoperative period. Anxiety-induced tachycardia may be treated with small doses of narcotics or benzodiazepines. However, excessive sedation is counterproductive because sedative-induced hypoventilation can result in hypoxemia or hypercarbia, potentially aggravating a patient's underlying pulmonary hypertension, and because large doses of premedication can jeopardize the patient's already limited LV preload. Appropriate monitoring and supplemental oxygen therapy should be considered for patients receiving preoperative narcotics or benzodiazepines. Medications taken by the patient preoperatively to control heart rate, such as digitalis, β-blockers, calcium receptor antagonists, or amiodarone, should be continued in the perioperative period. Additional doses of β-blockers and calcium-receptor antagonists may be required intraoperatively, particularly to control the ventricular rate in patients with atrial fibrillation. Control of the ventricular rate remains the primary goal in managing patients with atrial fibrillation, although cardioversion should not be withheld from patients with atrial tachyarrhythmias who become hemodynamically unstable. Narcotic-based anesthetics are often helpful in avoiding intraoperative tachycardia. However, clinicians should realize these patients may be receiving other vagotonic drugs and that profound bradycardia is possible in response to large doses of narcotics.[325,326] The selection of a muscle relaxant such as pancuronium may help prevent the unwanted bradycardia associated with high-dose narcotics.

Maintenance of preload is another important goal for managing patients who have a fixed obstruction to LV filling. Appropriate replacement of blood loss and prevention of excessive anesthetic-induced venodilation help preserve hemodynamic stability intraoperatively. Invasive hemodynamic monitoring allows the anesthesiologist to maintain adequate preload while avoiding excessive fluid administration that could aggravate pulmonary vascular congestion. Placement of an arterial catheter facilitates timely recognition of hemodynamic derangements. PACs can be invaluable in the management of patients with significant mitral stenosis. Even though the PCWP overestimates LV filling and the pulmonary artery diastolic pressure may not accurately reflect left heart volume in patients with pulmonary hypertension, examination of trends and responses to intervention can be more readily assessed. Tachycardia increases the pressure gradient between the left atrium and left ventricle. Elevated heart rates widen the discrepancy between the PCWP and the true LVEDP. Despite these limitations, the PAC remains a useful monitoring tool, providing information on cardiac output and pulmonary artery pressures. As anesthesiologists gain an increasing appreciation for the role of intraoperative TEE, this powerful imaging modality will no doubt be used more frequently to assess ventricular filling and function.

Many patients with mitral stenosis present with pulmonary hypertension. Anesthetic techniques that avoid increases in PVR are likely to benefit these patients and prevent additional RV embarrassment. Meticulous attention to arterial blood gas results allows appropriate adjustment of ventilatory parameters. Vasodilator therapy in patients with pulmonary hypertension generally is ineffective as the venodilation produced further limits LV filling and does not improve cardiac output. The only mitral stenosis patients who may benefit from vasodilator therapy are those with concomitant mitral regurgitation or those with severe pulmonary hypertension and RV dysfunction in whom pulmonary vasodilation can facilitate transpulmonary blood flow and improve LV filling.[324] The treatment of RV dysfunction has been discussed in preceding sections.

TRICUSPID REGURGITATION

Clinical Features and Natural History

Surgical tricuspid disease is caused by a structural defect in the valve apparatus or is a functional lesion. Functional tricuspid regurgitation is far more common and usually results from RV overload and tricuspid annular dilation. Left-sided valvular disease, usually mitral regurgitation, is most commonly responsible. Functional tricuspid incompetence can also result from mitral stenosis, aortic regurgitation, or stenosis or from isolated pulmonary hypertension. When mitral regurgitation is severe enough to warrant valve repair or replacement, tricuspid regurgitation may be present in 30% to 50% of patients.[383-385]

Tricuspid regurgitation may also be caused by structural defects as in rheumatic valve disease, carcinoid syndrome, endocarditis, Epstein's anomaly, or trauma.[386,387] In rheumatic disease, histologic involvement of the tricuspid valve may occur in 46% of patients, but it is rarely clinically severe, and in these cases, the valve is usually also stenotic.[52,388] Tricuspid regurgitation has also been described in association with CAD as a result of ischemia, infarction, or rupture of the RV papillary muscles.[389]

Another cause of structural tricuspid valve defects may be occurring with increasing frequency. Although this has not been reported in the literature, at some institutions such as that of the authors, there appears to be an increasing incidence of isolated tricuspid insufficiency related to long-standing transvenous pacemaker wires. Given the rapid escalation of the use of pacemakers and the aging of the population, this result is expected. This is occurring in the absence of endocarditis. The presence of the pacemaker wire tends to scar and tether one of the tricuspid leaflets. Historically, isolated tricuspid repair or replacement has been uncommon, but physicians may see more of this procedure for this reason.

Symptoms of isolated tricuspid insufficiency are usually minor in the absence of concurrent pulmonary hypertension. Intravenous drug abusers who develop tricuspid endocarditis are the classic example. In these patients, structural damage to the valve may be quite severe, but because they are free of other cardiac disease, they can tolerate complete excision of the tricuspid valve with few adverse effects.[390] Excision of the tricuspid valve in endocarditis has been common because of the undesirability of placing a valve prosthesis in a region of infection.[387] Surgical annuloplasty may be a better long-term option if the valve is structurally salvageable. Another factor that broadly favors tricuspid repair rather than replacement is the high incidence of thrombotic complications with a valve in this position. The lower pressure and flow state on the right side of the heart are responsible for this phenomenon. Increasingly, valve replacement in the tricuspid area is relegated to those patients who truly have unreconstructable rheumatic valve disease, totally destroyed tricuspid valves from endocarditis, or rare congenital lesions.[391-397] This is true because the literature shows improved longer-term outcomes with valve repair over replacement.[398]

In chronic tricuspid regurgitation due to RV dilation, the clinical scenario is often much different from that of isolated tricuspid disease. The major hemodynamic derangements are usually those of the associated mitral or aortic valve disease. The right ventricle dilates in the face of the afterload stress from long-standing pulmonary hypertension, and the resultant increase in end-diastolic fiber stretch (i.e., preload reserve) promotes increases in SV mediated by the Starling mechanism. These increases are negated by a concurrently rising RV afterload, however, because of relatively inadequate RV hypertrophy.[399] Regurgitation through the tricuspid valve reduces RV wall tension at the price of a decrease in effective forward SV.

An important corollary of RV chamber enlargement is the possibility of a leftward shift of the interventricular septum and encroachment on the LV cavity.[400] This phenomenon can reduce the LV chamber size and the slope of the LV diastolic pressure-volume curve, rendering the left ventricle less compliant.[401-403] Septal encroachment may mask LV underfilling by decreasing LV compliance, thereby artificially elevating LVEDP. A failing right ventricle underloads the left side by reduced effective SV and anatomic (septal shift) mechanisms.

RV failure may be relatively mild early in the course of functional tricuspid regurgitation, but over time, the regurgitation will worsen, with further dilation leading to further RV volume overload and chamber enlargement, which may worsen the tricuspid incompetence.[386] As in mitral regurgitation, the incompetent tricuspid valve serves as a pop-off circulation during RV systole, and over time, the capacitance of the right atrium and vena cavae can increase dramatically. Untreated, this eventually leads to systemic venous congestion, hepatic congestion, severe peripheral edema, and ascites. Because tricuspid insufficiency in the absence of pulmonary hypertension is rare, it has been difficult to demonstrate that chronic volume overload and ventricular dilation result in RV cardiomyopathy. However, when RV volume overload occurs in the context of pulmonic valve insufficiency, RV failure results from volume overload.[404] Clinical experience supports the presumption of RV cardiomyopathy in severe tricuspid regurgitation as well. In late tricuspid insufficiency, RV function can decline when tricuspid valve repair renders the valve competent.

Surgical Decision Making

In structural tricuspid insufficiency, the decision to repair or replace the valve is straightforward. The same cannot be said of functional tricuspid regurgitation. Because most functional cases are the consequence of left-sided valve lesions with RV overload, the tricuspid regurgitation usually improves significantly after the aortic or mitral valve is repaired or replaced, typically at least one grade. It can be unclear in the operating room whether addition of a tricuspid procedure to the left-sided valve surgery is indicated. In this situation, intraoperative TEE plays an essential role. If the tricuspid regurgitation is severe in the pre-CPB assessment, tricuspid valve surgery is almost always performed.[383] However, the evidence is less clear when the regurgitation is graded as moderate. Some surgeons choose to repair the tricuspid with moderate regurgitation, but others advocate observation.[383,385,405] It is common with moderate or moderate-to-severe tricuspid regurgitation, in the context of left-sided valve surgery, to complete the left-sided procedure and then reassess the tricuspid valve with TEE when the heart is full and ejecting.[406,407] If the regurgitation remains more than moderate after the left-sided valve is fixed, many surgeons then do the tricuspid procedure. If the regurgitation is moderate or less, the appropriate surgical course may remain unclear. Some patients having left-sided valve procedures must return to the operating room in the future for tricuspid surgery, and data from the Mayo Clinic suggest that this problem may be increasing.[408] When this occurs, the morbidity and mortality rates are probably significantly increased over what would have been experienced were the tricuspid valve fixed at the time of the aortic or mitral valve procedure. Decision making in functional tricuspid regurgitation is made more complicated by the inability to rigorously quantify the severity of the regurgitation and RV dysfunction.[408] When regurgitation is severe or mild, the assessment of the severity of tricuspid regurgitation is not critical to surgical decision making, but determinations from mild to moderate and moderate to severe are essential.

As with mitral regurgitation and the left ventricle, the presence of significant tricuspid regurgitation makes RV function difficult to assess, because the regurgitant fraction leads to a falsely elevated EF. In the absence of sophisticated echocardiographic assessments, such as determination of rate of RV pressure rise with pulsed Doppler, it is common to look at enlarged RV chamber size and any decrease in RV EF as indicators of decompensation.[408,409] Clinical experience suggests that pulmonary hypertension is also likely to be a marker for RV failure after tricuspid surgery, but studies of sufficient size are still lacking. Like assessment of RV function, grading of severity of tricuspid regurgitation is at best semiquantitative. Color-flow mapping of the volume of the regurgitant jet within the right atrium is standard,[398] and this can be supplemented by looking for systolic flow reversal in the portal veins using pulsed-wave Doppler.[410] Even though the assessment of residual tricuspid regurgitation after left-sided valve surgery is very important, the tricuspid valve is sometimes difficult to examine with TEE, and the presence of an aortic or particularly a mitral mechanical prosthesis makes this assessment more difficult.

Anesthetic Considerations

Because most tricuspid surgery occurs in the context of significant aortic or mitral disease, anesthetic management is primarily determined by the left-sided valve lesion. The exception to this is when significant pulmonary hypertension and RV failure are present. Under these conditions, the primary impediment to hemodynamic stability after surgery will be RV failure rather than the left-sided process.

If RV dysfunction is predicted, it is useful to place a PAC, even if the tricuspid valve will be replaced. Even if the PAC has to be removed because of tricuspid valve replacement, it still can be helpful to obtain cardiac outputs and pulmonary artery pressures before CPB to get insight into RV function and anticipate the hemodynamic support that may be required. A PAC is also of greater use than a central venous catheter alone because the CVP is a poor index of intravascular filling and the degree of tricuspid regurgitation. This is true because the atrium and vena cavae are highly compliant and will accept large regurgitant volumes with relatively little change in pressure. A PAC is also useful even if intraoperative TEE is used. As in aortic insufficiency with the left ventricle, the right ventricle in chronic tricuspid regurgitation is volume overloaded and dilated and requires a large end-diastolic volume to maintain forward flow. At the same time, because of the unreliability of the CVP as an indicator of filling, it is possible to volume overload patients with tricuspid regurgitation and RV failure. Cardiac output in RV failure can often be augmented with the use of vasodilators, and even though RV dimensions can be followed intraoperatively with TEE, maximizing cardiac output (sometimes at the cost of systemic arterial pressure) is best done with serial cardiac output measurements (as in aortic regurgitation). Whenever there is significant RV distention, the possibility of septal shift and secondary deterioration of LV diastolic compliance should be carefully considered. Echocardiography is uniquely helpful for this assessment.

The post-CPB management of the patient undergoing an isolated tricuspid valve procedure is usually straightforward. These patients usually do not have significant RV failure or pulmonary hypertension and typically require only a brief period of CPB without aortic cross-clamping. A larger group of patients, particularly those with tricuspid regurgitation related to aortic stenosis, typically come off CPB with little need for support of the right ventricle. These patients often do well because the improvement in LV function after AVR for aortic stenosis is usually sufficient to reduce pulmonary artery pressures significantly and offload the right heart. When the left-sided valve surgery is for mitral disease, the improvement is usually not as marked, and greater degrees of inotropic support of the right ventricle are often indicated. The combination of a phosphodiesterase inhibitor with a vasodilator and a catecholamine infusion is useful. Serial cardiac output measurements to balance systemic pressure and RV output and filling are critical.

A few other practical points on tricuspid valve repair and replacement should be made. First, because right-sided pressures can be chronically elevated with tricuspid regurgitation, it is important to look for a patent foramen ovale and the potential for right-to-left shunting before initiation of CPB. Second, intravascular volume may be quite high in this patient population, and it is often practical to avoid red blood cell transfusion by hemofiltration during bypass. Third, if significant RV dysfunction is present or there is peripheral edema or ascites, there is the potential for a coagulopathy related to liver congestion, and the patient should be managed accordingly. Fourth, it is important to ensure that central venous catheters, particularly PACs, are not entrapped in right atrial suture lines.

INNOVATIONS IN VALVE REPAIR

Interventional cardiology has had a significant impact on the volume of CABG surgery, and it can be predicted that interventional cardiology will alter surgery for VHD over time. Multiple, less invasive approaches to mitral valve repair are being examined in animal or early clinical trials, and significant inroads have been made in percutaneous replacement of the aortic and pulmonic valves. Innovations in surgical valve repair are also being made. These include aortic valve repair and closed- and open-chamber procedures for mitral regurgitation.

Aortic Valve Repair

Over the past several years, there has been a major shift from valve replacement to valve repair in degenerative mitral valve disease. The same has not been true of the aortic valve, in part because the valve disease is different in most patients, but also because the high flow and pressure conditions across the aortic valve might make repair more prone to failure. That said, aortic valve repair is being increasingly done as an appropriate patient population is being defined. Valve repair for aortic regurgitation has found broader use when regurgitation is associated with dissection or dilation of the aortic root, but isolated valve repair has been less common.[411,412] A growing body of data suggests that aortic valve repair may offer advantages over valve replacement in younger individuals with atrial insufficiency caused by bicuspid valves.[411,413] In contrast to AVR, this eliminates the need for anticoagulation for a mechanical valve and may delay the need for reoperation if a tissue valve has been placed. When regurgitation occurs with a bicuspid valve, the insufficiency is usually caused by retraction or prolapse of the conjoined cusp and repair consists of a triangular incision to shorten and elevate that cusp to improve apposition (Fig. 20–30). Although very long-term follow-up has not been reported, in a large series from the Mayo Clinic with a mean follow-up of 4.2 years, late failure of the repair requiring reoperation occurred in 14 of 160 con-

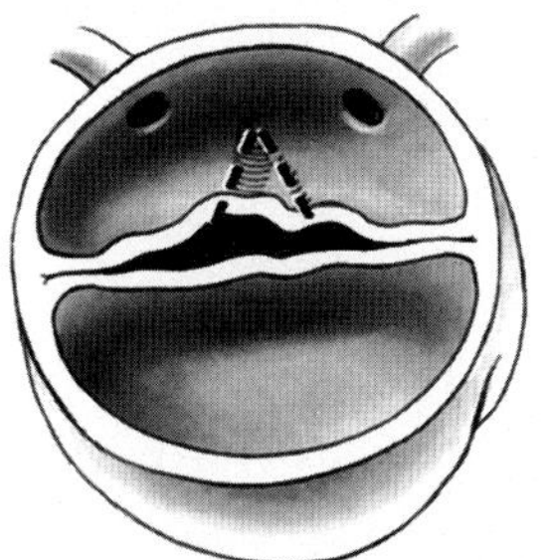

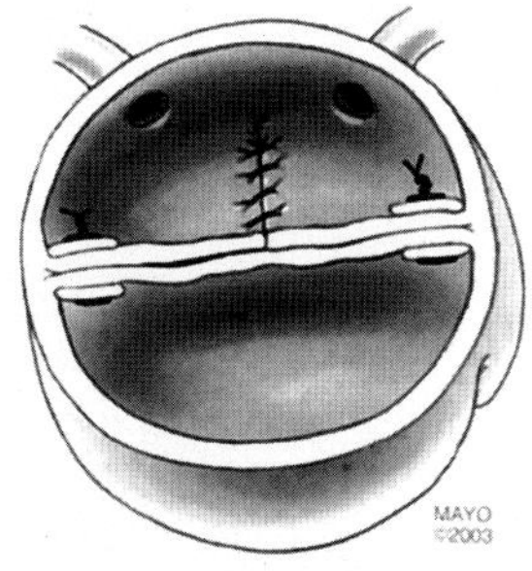

Figure 20–30 Bicuspid aortic valve with prolapse of the conjoint cusp. Triangular resection is made in the midportion of the conjoint cusp and then repaired. Commissural plication stitches also are inserted. (From Minakata K, Schaff HV, Zehr KJ, et al: Is repair of aortic valve regurgitation a safe alternative to valve replacement? J Thorac Cardiovasc Surg 127:647, 2004.)

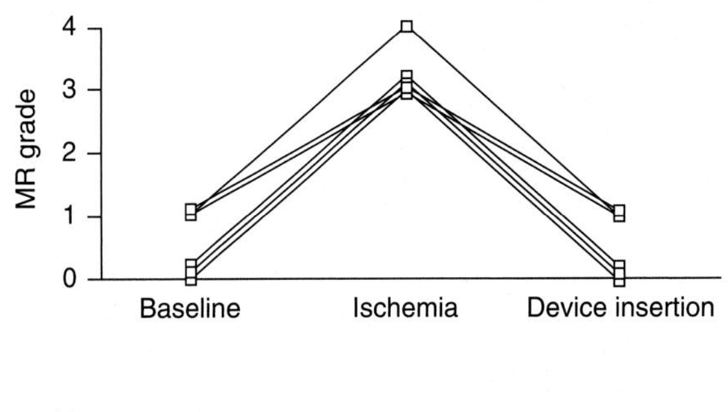

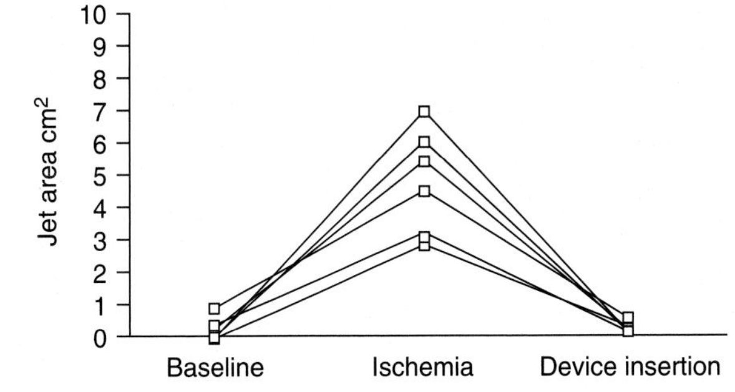

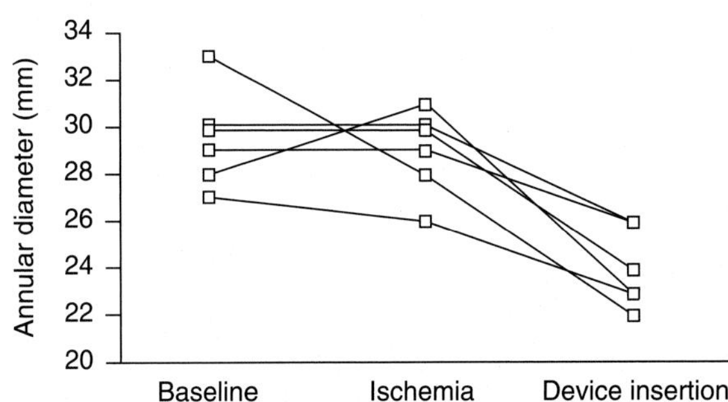

Figure 20–31 Effect of annuloplasty device on acute ischemic mitral regurgitation. *(A)* Mitral regurgitation grade. *(B)* Mitral regurgitant jet area. *(C)* Mitral annular diameter in the septal-lateral dimension. (From Liddicoat JR, Mac Niell BD, Gillinov AM, et al: Percutaneous mitral valve repair: A feasibility study in a bovine model of acute ischemic mitral regurgitation. Catheter Cardiovasc Interv 60:413, 2003.)

secutive patients, with most of that failure occurring from repairs done in the first decade of the 15-year experience.[411]

As a result of this experience, aortic valve repair is likely to find increasing application in this patient population. For this group anesthetic management is usually straightforward although the clinical indications for valve repair in aortic insufficiency are the same as those for AVR. The compelling issue for the anesthesiologist in these cases is TEE assessment of the valve for suitability of repair and the adequacy of the repair after the procedure.

Techniques for Mitral Valve Repair

Mitral regurgitation is frequently associated with CHF. In dilated and ischemic cardiomyopathy, enlargement of the mitral annulus results in a failure of coaptation of the mitral leaflets and valve incompetence. Although cardiac surgery is an effective treatment, morbidity can be high. Three different approaches have been developed to address mitral regurgitation occurring in the absence of structural mitral pathology. These approaches address the failure of leaflet coaptation at the level of the valve leaflets or the valve annulus or by altering the anatomic relationship of the septal and lateral walls of the left ventricle.

Mitral Leaflet Repair

Alfieri et al[414] showed that mitral regurgitation could be improved using an edge-to-edge technique by which mitral valve leaflets are brought together by a central suture. This surgical approach led to a catheter-based technology, which results in edge-to-edge repair by apposing the edges of a regurgitant mitral valve. The Evalve device consists of a catheter-mounted clip that is threaded using a femoral and trans-septal approach.[415] Under general anesthesia with echocardiographic and fluoroscopic guidance, the clip is placed to achieve apposition of the central portion of the anterior and posterior leaflets. If the severity of mitral regurgitation is not reduced, the device can be opened and repositioned. Animal studies show incorporation of the device into the leaflets at 6 to 10 weeks with persistent coaptation, and clinical trials are beginning.[415]

Percutaneous Mitral Annuloplasty

The second type of approach to functional mitral regurgitation is alteration of the mitral annulus, as might occur with a traditional open mitral repair, but with the percutaneous approach, the annulus is downsized by an extracardiac restraint (Figs. 20–31 and 20–32).[416,417] With this technique, interventional cardiologists percutaneously thread a wire from the venous system into the right atrium and the coronary sinus. The relationship between the coronary sinus and posterior leaflet allows downsizing of the septal-lateral diameter from this position. Under echocardiographic guidance, tension is applied to cinch the mitral annulus smaller, and an anchor is deployed to maintain position. In trials using a sheep model, a significant reduction in mitral annular dimension was achieved, and mitral regurgitation was eliminated in 7 of 9 animals.[416] Only trivial mitral regurgitation was present in the remaining two animals. Pulmonary artery pressures were significantly reduced, and cardiac output increased.

Altering Ventricular Anatomy to Reduce Mitral Regurgitation

The third approach to closed mitral valve repair consists of altering the geometry of the lateral and septal LV walls to bring the valve leaflets together. The commercial Coapsys device has entered clinical trials. This device consists of anterior and posterior epicardial pads connected by a cord. With an open chest,

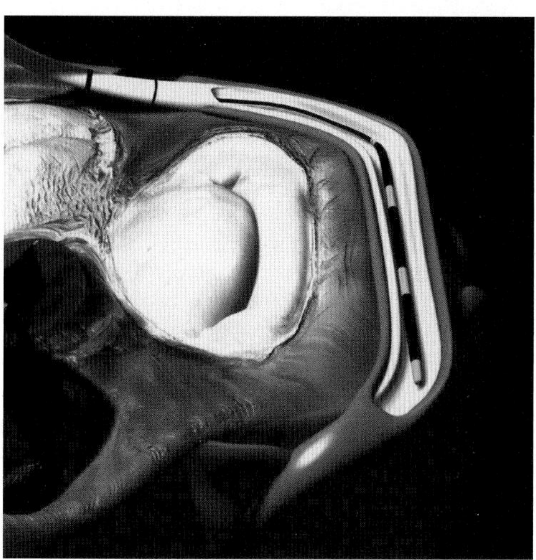

Figure 20–32 Effect of annuloplasty device on mitral annular geometry. The annuloplasty device decreases the distance between the anterior and posterior annulus, increasing leaflet coaptation. (From Liddicoat JR, Mac Niell BD, Gillinov AM, et al: Percutaneous mitral valve repair: A feasibility study in a bovine model of acute ischemic mitral regurgitation. Catheter Cardiovasc Interv 60:411, 2003.) (See Color Plates.)

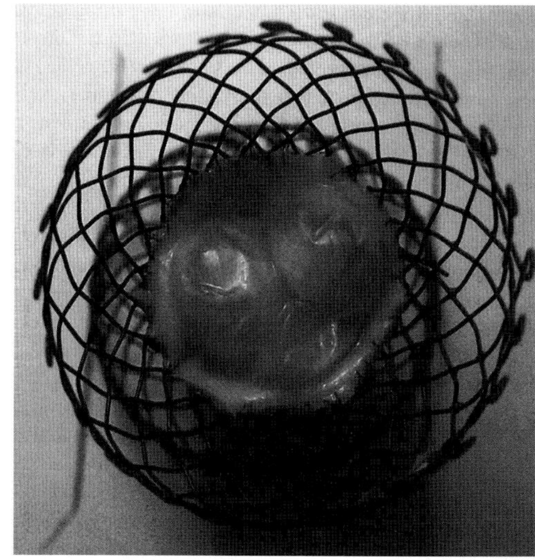

Figure 20–33 A front view of the stent, showing the pulmonary valve in the closed position, as seen from the ventricular side. (From Boudjemline Y, Agnoletti G, Bonnet D, et al: Percutaneous pulmonary valve replacement in a large right ventricular outflow tract. J Am Coll Cardiol 43:1082, 2004. Copyright 2004, with permission from The American College of Cardiology Foundation.) (See Color Plates.)

the cord is placed transventricularly in a subvalvular position and the tension on the cord is adjusted before the opposing epicardial pad is fixed in place.[418] This effectively brings the ventricular walls together and in doing so improves leaflet coaptation. TEE is used to optimize cord length and pad positioning. In contrast to the leaflet-based and annular-based approaches, the Coapsys approach is surgical, requiring an open chest but not CPB. The position of the epicardial vessels and the relationship of the submitral apparatus could pose significant risk, but the device has been used successfully in animal models and preliminary clinical trials.

Percutaneous Valve Replacement

Although surgery, particularly for aortic valve disease, has expanded to include a much older population in recent years, there remains a subset of patients for whom cardiac surgery may entail unacceptable risks. For this population, less invasive techniques such as percutaneous AVR replacement are being developed. The initial clinical experience with percutaneous AVR has been reported.[419]

The study population was six patients with severe aortic stenosis and class IV heart failure who had been denied surgery because of excessive risk. The mean AVA was 0.49 cm^2, with a low transvalvular gradient reflecting ventricular decompensation. Patients had a mean EF of 24%. Under local anesthesia with sedation, the femoral vein was catheterized, and using a transseptal approach, a balloon-tipped catheter was placed across the stenotic aortic valve. After valvuloplasty, the aortic valve stent (with incorporated leaflets) was seated at the native valve over a second balloon. In one patient, the valve was ejected into the ascending aorta on placement, and the patient died shortly thereafter. In two patients, hemodynamic collapse occurred during the initial valvuloplasty, but both patients were resuscitated.

In this small clinical trial, the mean AVA improved significantly, as did EF. Although two of six patients had aortic regurgitation before the procedure, all six had it afterward. In all the subjects, regurgitation was perivalvular, reflecting an undersized valve or fit to an irregular contour within the native valve. Of the six patients in the study, four died within 18 weeks.[419]

Although pulmonic valve disease is much less common than aortic, progress in percutaneous pulmonic valve replacement is also undergoing investigation.[420] In a sheep model, Boudjemline et al[420] implanted a pulmonary artery stent and valve using a percutaneous approach from the internal jugular vein (Fig. 20–33). This has been done in single- and two-stage approaches. One subgroup of animals underwent stent and valve insertion simultaneously, and in another group, the stent was placed in the first step and the valve was inserted into the stent 6 to 10 weeks later.

In 8 of 10 animals, the stent and graft were successfully implanted, and there was no early or late stent migration. The two failures resulted from anatomic problems related to the anatomic relationship between the tricuspid valve and the RV outlet. The valves placed into the stent percutaneously were competent angiographically and hemodynamically at follow-up.

It is likely that many of these technologies will come to clinical trial and will demonstrate various degrees of efficacy. However, it is unclear what the long-term benefits of these less invasive interventions will be or how they will compare with each other or with traditional surgical approaches. Some may find use in high-risk patients as temporizing procedures, in place of reoperations, or in conjunction with percutaneous approaches for coronary disease.[421] These technologies will get better, and there will be pressure for clinical application. The most important factors will be case selection and long-term follow-up of outcomes; otherwise, these innovations and others like them will add markedly to the burden of health care costs without clear social benefit.[422,423] For any of the percutaneous valves to succeed, they must demonstrate long-term successful clinical outcomes similar to the excellent results seen with mechanical or tissue valves for more than 10 to 15 years.[424]

Acknowledgments

The authors of this chapter thank Dr. John Jackson and Dr. Stephen Thomas for their contributions from the fourth edition.

REFERENCES

1. Ross J Jr: Afterload mismatch in aortic and mitral valve disease: Implications for surgical therapy. J Am Coll Cardiol 5:811, 1985
2. Burns JW, Covell JW, Ross J Jr: Mechanics of isotonic left ventricular contractions. Am J Physiol 224:725, 1973
3. Braunwald ER: Contraction of the normal heart. *In* Braunwald E (ed): Heart Disease. Philadelphia, WB Saunders Company, 1992
4. Braunwald E, Ross J Jr, Sonnenblick EHR: Mechanisms of contraction of the normal and failing heart. Boston, Little, Brown, 1976
5. Baudeer HSR: Contractile tension in the myocardium. Am Heart J 66:432, 1963
6. Braunwald ER: Regulation of the circulation. I. N Engl J Med 290:1124, 1974
7. Jewell BRR: Activation of contraction in cardiac muscle. Mayo Clin Proc 57(suppl):6, 1982
8. Fabiato A, Fabiato FR: Dependence of calcium release, tension generation and restoring forces on sarcomere length in skinned cardiac cells. Eur J Cardiol 4(suppl):13, 1976
9. Gordon AM, Pollack GHR: Effects of calcium on the sarcomere length-tension relation in rat cardiac muscle. Implications for the Frank-Starling mechanism. Circ Res 47:610, 1980
10. Grossman W, McLaurin LPR: Diastolic properties of the LV. Ann Intern Med 84:316, 1976
11. McCullagh WH, Covell JW, Ross J Jr: Left ventricular performance following correction of free aortic regurgitation. Circulation 45:943, 1972
12. Gault JH, Covell JW, Braunwald E, et al: Left ventricular performance following correction of free aortic regurgitation. Circulation 42:773, 1970
13. Grossman W, McLaurin LP, Moos SP, et al: Wall thickness and diastolic properties of the LV. Circulation 49:129, 1974
14. Leyton RA, Spotnitz HM, Sonnenblick EHR: Cardiac ultrastructure and function: Sarcomeres in the right ventricle. Am J Physiol 221:902, 1971
15. Gaasch WHR: Diagnosis and treatment of heart failure based on left ventricular systolic or diastolic dysfunction (see comment). JAMA 271:1276, 1994
16. Little WC, Applegate RJR: Congestive heart failure: Systolic and diastolic function. J Cardiothorac Vasc Anesth 7(suppl 2):2, 1993
17. Brutsaert DL, Sys SU, Gillebert TCR: Diastolic failure: Pathophysiology and therapeutic implications [erratum appears in J Am Coll Cardiol 22:1272, 1993]. J Am Coll Cardiol 22:318, 1993
18. Eberli FR, Apstein CS, Ngoy S, et al: Exacerbation of left ventricular ischemic diastolic dysfunction by pressure-overload hypertrophy. Modification by specific inhibition of cardiac angiotensin converting enzyme. Circ Res 70:931, 1992
19. Spirito P, Maron BJR: Relation between extent of left ventricular hypertrophy and diastolic filling abnormalities in hypertrophic cardiomyopathy (see comment). J Am Coll Cardiol 15:808, 1990
20. Wigle EDR: Impaired left ventricular relaxation in hypertrophic cardiomyopathy: Relation to extent of hypertrophy (see comment). J Am Coll Cardiol 15:814, 1990
21. Bemis CE, Serur JR, Borkenhagen D, et al: Influence of right ventricular filling pressure on left ventricular pressure and dimension. Circ Res 34:498, 1974
22. Glantz SA, Parmley WWR: Factors which affect the diastolic pressure-volume curve. Circ Res 42:171, 1978
23. Spadaro J, Bing OH, Gaasch WH, et al: Pericardial modulation of right and left ventricular diastolic interaction. Circ Res 48:233, 1981
24. Santamore WP, Lynch PR, Meier G, et al: Myocardial interaction between the ventricles. Journal of Applied Physiology 41:362, 1976
25. Carabello BA: Ratio of end-systolic stress to end-systolic volume: Is it a useful clinical tool? J Am Coll Cardiol 14:496, 1989
26. Braunwald ER: Assessment of cardiac function. *In* Braunwald E (ed): Heart Disease. Philadelphia, WB Saunders Company, 1992
27. Ross J Jr: Cardiac function and myocardial contractility: A perspective. J Am Coll Cardiol 1:52, 1983
28. Carabello BA, Spann JF: The uses and limitations of end-systolic indexes of left ventricular function. Circulation 69:1058, 1984
29. Carabello BA: Clinical practice: Aortic stenosis. N En J Med 346:677, 2002
30. Katz AMR: Influence of altered inotropy and lusitropy on ventricular pressure-volume loops. J Am Coll Cardiol 11:438, 1988
31. Gorcsan J 3rd, Romand JA, Mandarino WA, et al: Assessment of left ventricular performance by on-line pressure-area relations using echocardiographic automated border detection. J Am Coll Cardiol 23:242, 1994
32. Grossman W, Braunwald E, Mann T, et al: Contractile state of the LV in man as evaluated from end-systolic pressure-volume relations. Circulation 56:845, 1977
33. Sagawa KR: The end-systolic pressure-volume relation of the ventricle: Definition, modifications and clinical use. Am J Cardiol 40:748, 1977
34. Sagawa KR: End-systolic pressure/volume ratio: A new index of ventricular contractility. Circulation 63:1223, 1981
35. Rajamannan NM, Gersh B, Bonow RO: Calcific aortic stenosis: From bench to the bedside—emerging clinical and cellular concepts. Heart 89:801, 2003
36. Sprecher DL, Schaefer EJ, Kent KM, et al: Cardiovascular features of homozygous familial hypercholesterolemia: Analysis of 16 patients. Am J Cardiol 54:20, 1984
37. Rosenhek R, Binder T, Porenta G, et al: Predictors of outcome in severe, asymptomatic aortic stenosis. N Engl J Med 343:611, 2000
38. Carabello BA: Evaluation and management of patients with aortic stenosis. Circulation 105:1746, 2002
39. Novaro GM, Tiong IY, Pearce GL, et al: Effect of hydroxymethylglutaryl coenzyme-a reductase inhibitors on the progression of calcific aortic stenosis. Circulation 104:2205, 2001
40. Bellamy MF, Pellikka PA, Klarich KW, et al: Association of cholesterol levels, hydroxymethylglutaryl coenzyme-a reductase inhibitor treatment, and progression of aortic stenosis in the community. J Am Coll Cardiol 40:1723, 2002
41. Mitka M: Researchers probe aortic stenosis: An active, potentially treatable disease process? JAMA 289:2197, 2003
42. Otto CM, Burwash IG, Legget ME, et al: Prospective study of asymptomatic valvular aortic stenosis. Clinical, echocardiographic, and exercise predictors of outcome. Circulation 95:2262, 1997
43. Nassimiha D, Aronow WS, Ahn C, et al: Rate of progression of valvular aortic stenosis in patients > or = 60 years of age. Am J Cardiol 87:807, A809, 2001
44. Wongpraparut N, Apiyasawat S, Crespo G, et al: Determinants of progression of aortic stenosis in patients aged > or = 40 years. Am J Cardiol 89:350, 2002
45. Qi W, Mathisen P, Kjekshus J, et al: Natriuretic peptides in patients with aortic stenosis. Am Heart J 142:725, 2001
46. Gerber IL, Stewart RA, Legget ME, et al: Increased plasma natriuretic peptide levels reflect symptom onset in aortic stenosis. Circulation 107:1884, 2003
47. Ross Jr J, Braunwald ER: The influence of corrective operations on the natural history of aortic stenosis. Circulation 37(suppl 5):61, 1968
48. Rotman M, Morris JJ Jr, Behar VS, et al: Aortic valvular disease. Comparison of types and their medical and surgical management. Am J Med 51:241, 1971
49. Frank S, Johnson A, Ross J Jr: Natural history of valvular aortic stenosis. Br Heart J 35:41, 1973
50. Kennedy KD, Nishimura RA, Holmes DR Jr, et al: Natural history of moderate aortic stenosis. J Am Coll Cardiol 17:313, 1991
51. Selzer AR: Changing aspects of the natural history of valvular aortic stenosis. N Engl J Med 317:91, 1993
52. Bonow RO, Braunwald E: Valvular heart disease. *In* Zipes DP, Libby P, Bonow RO, Braunwald E (eds): Braunwald's Heart Disease. Philadelphia, Elsevier, 2005, pp 1553–1632
53. Berger M, Berdoff RL, Gallerstein PE, et al: Evaluation of aortic stenosis by continuous wave doppler ultrasound. J Am Coll Cardiol 3:150, 1984
54. Hakki AH, Kimbiris D, Iskandrian AS, et al: Angina pectoris and CAD in patients with severe aortic valvular disease. Am Heart J 100:441, 1980
55. Graboys TB, Cohn PFR: The prevalence of angina pectoris and abnormal coronary arteriograms in severe aortic valvular disease. Am Heart J 93:683, 1977
56. Bonchek LI, Anderson RP, Rosch JR: Should coronary arteriography be performed routinely before valve replacement? Am J Cardiol 31:462, 1973
57. Green SJ, Pizzarello RA, Padmanabhan VT, et al: Relation of angina pectoris to CAD in aortic valve stenosis. Am J Cardiol 55:1063, 1985
58. Mullany CJ, Elveback LR, Frye RL, et al: Coronary artery disease and its management: Influence on survival in patients undergoing aortic valve replacement. J Am Coll Cardiol 10:66, 1987
59. Exadactylos N, Sugrue DD, Oakley CMR: Prevalence of CAD in patients with isolated aortic valve stenosis. Br Heart J 51:121, 1984

60. Lytle BW, Cosgrove DM, Loop FD, et al: Replacement of aortic valve combined with myocardial revascularization: Determinants of early and late risk for 500 patients, 1967–1981. Circulation 68:1149, 1983
61. Magovern JA, Pennock JL, Campbell DB, et al: Aortic valve replacement and combined aortic valve replacement and coronary artery bypass grafting: Predicting high risk groups. J Am Coll Cardiol 9:38, 1987
62. Czer LS, Gray RJ, Stewart ME, et al: Reduction in sudden late death by concomitant revascularization with aortic valve replacement. J Thorac Cardiovasc Surg 95:390, 1988
63. Lytle BW, Cosgrove DM, Gill CC, et al: Aortic valve replacement combined with myocardial revascularization. Late results and determinants of risk for 471 in-hospital survivors. J Thorac Cardiovasc Surg 95:402, 1988
64. Lombard JT, Selzer AR: Valvular aortic stenosis. A clinical and hemodynamic profile of patients. Ann Intern Med 106:292, 1987
65. Lund OR: Preoperative risk evaluation and stratification of long-term survival after valve replacement for aortic stenosis. Reasons for earlier operative intervention (see comment). Circulation 82:124, 1990
66. Cheitlin MDR: Should an asymptomatic patient with hemodynamically severe aortic stenosis ever have aortic valve surgery? Cardiol Rev 1:344, 1993
67. Pallikka PA, Nishimura RA, Bailey KR, et al: The natural history of adults with asymptomatic hemodynamically significant aortic stenosis. J Am Coll Cardiol 15:1012, 1990
68. Braunwald ER: On the natural history of severe aortic stenosis (see comment). J Am Coll Cardiol 15:1018, 1990
69. Pantely G, Morton M, Rahimtoola SHR: Effects of successful, uncomplicated valve replacement on ventricular hypertrophy, volume, and performance in aortic stenosis and in aortic incompetence. J Thorac Cardiovasc Surg 75:383, 1978
70. Kennedy JW, Doces J, Stewart DKR: Left ventricular function before and following aortic valve replacement. Circulation 56:944, 1977
71. Schwarz F, Flameng W, Schaper J, et al: Myocardial structure and function in patients with aortic valve disease and their relation to postoperative results. Am J Cardiol 41:661, 1978
72. Croke RP, Pifarre R, Sullivan H, et al: Reversal of advanced left ventricular dysfunction following aortic valve replacement for aortic stenosis. Ann Thorac Surg 24:38, 1977
73. Smith N, McAnulty JH, Rahimtoola SHR: Severe aortic stenosis with impaired left ventricular function and clinical heart failure: Results of valve replacement. Circulation 58:255, 1978
74. Peter M, Hoffmann A, Parker C, et al: Progression of aortic stenosis. Role of age and concomitant CAD (see comment). Chest 103:1715, 1993
75. Culliford AT, Galloway AC, Colvin SB, et al: Aortic valve replacement for aortic stenosis in persons aged 80 years and over. Am J Cardiol 67:1256, 1991
76. Yeager M, Yock PG, Popp RLR: Comparison of Doppler-derived pressure gradient to that determined at cardiac catheterization in adults with aortic valve stenosis: Implications for management. Am J Cardiol 57:644, 1986
77. Tribouilloy C, Shen WF, Peltier M, et al: Quantitation of AVA in aortic stenosis with multiplane transesophageal echocardiography: Comparison with monoplane transesophageal approach. Am Heart J 128:526, 1994
78. Hegrenaes L, Hatle LR: Aortic stenosis in adults. Noninvasive estimation of pressure differences by continuous wave Doppler echocardiography. Br Heart J 54:396, 1985
79. Hatle L, Angelsen BA, Tromsdal AR: Noninvasive assessment of aortic stenosis by Doppler ultrasound. Br Heart J 43:284, 1980
80. Miller FA Jr: Aortic stenosis: Most cases no longer require invasive hemodynamic study. J Am Coll Cardiol 13:551, 1989
81. Oh JK, Taliercio CP, Holmes DR Jr, et al: Prediction of the severity of aortic stenosis by Doppler AVA determination: Prospective Doppler-catheterization correlation in 100 patients. J Am Coll Cardiol 11:1227, 1988
82. Chizner MA, Pearle DL, deLeon AC Jr: The natural history of aortic stenosis in adults. Am Heart J 99:419, 1980
83. Selzer AR: Changing aspects of the natural history of valvular aortic stenosis. N Engl J Med 317:91, 1987
84. Schwarz F, Baumann P, Manthey J, et al: The effect of aortic valve replacement on survival. Circulation 66:1105, 1982
85. Hood WP Jr, Rackley CE, Rolett ELR: Wall stress in the normal and hypertrophied human LV. Am J Cardiol 22:550, 1968
86. Peterson MB, Lesch MR: Protein synthesis and amino acid transport in the isolated rabbit right ventricular papillary muscle. Effect of isometric tension development. Circ Res 31:317, 1972
87. Hanrath P, Mathey DG, Siegert R, et al: Left ventricular relaxation and filling pattern in different forms of left ventricular hypertrophy: An echocardiographic study. Am J Cardiol 45:15, 1980
88. Betocchi S, Bonow RO, Bacharach SL, et al: Isovolumic relaxation period in hypertrophic cardiomyopathy: Assessment by radionuclide angiography. J Am Coll Cardiol 7:74, 1986
89. Topol EJ, Traill TA, Fortuin NJR: Hypertensive hypertrophic cardiomyopathy of the elderly. N Engl JMed 312:277, 1985
90. Sanderson JE, Traill TA, Sutton MG, et al: Left ventricular relaxation and filling in hypertrophic cardiomyopathy. An echocardiographic study. Br Heart J 40:596, 1978
91. Huber D, Grimm J, Koch R, et al: Determinants of ejection performance in aortic stenosis. Circulation 64:126, 1981
92. Henry WL, Bonow RO, Borer JS, et al: Evaluation of aortic valve replacement in patients with valvular aortic stenosis. Circulation 61:814, 1980
93. Grossman W, Jones D, McLaurin LP: Wall stress and patterns of hypertrophy in the human LV. J Clin Invest 56:56, 1975
94. Walther T, Schubert A, Falk V, et al: Regression of left ventricular hypertrophy after surgical therapy for aortic stenosis is associated with changes in extracellular matrix gene expression. Circulation 104(suppl I):I-54, 2001
95. Antonini-Canterin F, Huang G, Cervesato E, et al: Symptomatic aortic stenosis: Does systemic hypertension play an additional role? Hypertension 41:1268, 2003
96. Kuhl HP, Franke A, Puschmann D, et al: Regression of left ventricular mass one year after aortic valve replacement for pure severe aortic stenosis. Am J Cardiol 89:408, 2002
97. Ikonomidis I, Tsoukas A, Parthenakis F, et al: Four year follow-up of aortic valve replacement for isolated aortic stenosis: A link between reduction in pressure overload, regression of left ventricular hypertrophy, and diastolic function. Heart 86:309, 2001
98. Beyerbacht HP, Lamb HJ, van Der Laarse A, et al: Aortic valve replacement in patients with aortic valve stenosis improves myocardial metabolism and diastolic function. Radiology 219:637, 2001
99. Rajappan K, Rimoldi OE, Dutka DP, et al: Mechanisms of coronary microcirculatory dysfunction in patients with aortic stenosis and angiographically normal coronary arteries. Circulation 105:470, 2002
100. Liedtke AJ, Gentzler RD 2nd, Babb JD, et al: Determinants of cardiac performance in severe aortic stenosis. Chest 69:192, 1976
101. Thompson R, Yacoub M, Ahmed M, et al: Influence of preoperative left ventricular function on results of homograft replacement of the aortic valve for aortic stenosis. Am J Cardiol 43:929, 1979
102. Sasayama S, Franklin D, Ross JJR: Hyperfunction with normal inotropic state of the hypertrophied LV. Am J Physiol 232:H418, 1977
103. Gunther S, Grossman WR: Determinants of ventricular function in pressure overload hypertrophy in man. Circulation 59:679, 1977
104. Brutsaert DL, Rademakers FE, Sys SU: Triple control of relaxation: Implications in cardiac disease. Circulation 69:190, 1984
105. Marcus MLR: Effects of cardiac hypertrophy on the coronary circulation. *In* Marcus ML (ed): The Coronary Circulation in Health and Disease. New York, McGraw-Hill, 1983
106. Tomanek RJR: Response of the coronary vasculature to myocardial hypertrophy. J Am Coll Cardiol 15:528, 1990
107. Stack RS, Schirmer B, Greenfield JCR: Coronary artery luminal diameters in normal and hypertrophied canine ventricles (abstract). Circulation 62(suppl III): III-64, 1980
108. Alyono D, Anderson RW, Parrish DG, et al: Alterations of myocardial blood flow associated with experimental canine left ventricular hypertrophy secondary to valvular aortic stenosis. Circ Res 58:47, 1986
109. Yamori Y, Mori C, Nishio T, et al: Cardiac hypertrophy in early hypertension. Am J Cardiol 44:964, 1979
110. Hallback-Nordlander M, Noresson E, Thoren PR: Hemodynamic consequences of left ventricular hypertrophy in spontaneously hypertensive rats. Am J Cardiol 44:986, 1979
111. Hinquell L, Odoroff CL, Honig CRR: Intercapillary distance and capillary reserve in hypertrophied rat hearts beating in situ. Circ Res 41:400, 1979
112. Murray PA, Baig H, Fishbein MC, et al: Effects of experimental right ventricular hypertrophy on myocardial blood flow in conscious dogs. J Clin Invest 64:421, 1979
113. Rakusan KR: Quantitative morphology of capillaries of the heart. Number of capillaries in animal and human hearts under normal and pathological conditions. Methods Achievements Exp Pathol 5:272, 1971
114. Opherk D, Mall G, Zebe H, et al: Reduction of coronary reserve: A mechanism for angina pectoris in patients with arterial hypertension and normal coronary arteries. Circulation 69:1, 1984

115. Marcus ML, Doty DB, Hiratzka LF, et al: Decreased coronary reserve: A mechanism for angina pectoris in patients with aortic stenosis and normal coronary arteries. N Engl JMed 307:1362, 1982
116. Nadell R, DePace NL, Ren JF, et al: Myocardial oxygen supply/demand ratio in aortic stenosis: Hemodynamic and echocardiographic evaluation of patients with and without angina pectoris. J Am Coll Cardiol 2:258, 1983
117. Marcus ML, White CWR: Coronary flow reserve in patients with normal coronary angiograms. J Am Coll Cardiol 6:1254, 1985
118. Marcus ML, Doty DB, Hiratzka LFR: Impaired coronary reserve in children with cyanotic congenital heart disease. Circulation 64:32, 1981
119. Brutsaert DL, Housmans PR, Goethals MAR: Dual control of relaxation. Its role in the ventricular function in the mammalian heart. Circ Res 47:637, 1980
120. Brutsaert DL, Rademakers FE, Sys SU, et al: Analysis of relaxation in the evaluation of ventricular function of the heart. Prog Cardiovasc Dis 28:143, 1985
121. Grossman WR: Why is left ventricular diastolic pressure increased during angina pectoris? J Am Coll Cardiol 5:607, 1985
122. McLaurin LP, Rolett EL, Grossman WR: Impaired left ventricular relaxation during pacing-induced ischemia. Am J Cardiol 32:751, 1973
123. Bourdillon PD, Lorell BH, Mirsky I, et al: Increased regional myocardial stiffness of the LV during pacing-induced angina in man. Circulation 67:316, 1983
124. Carroll JD, Hess OM, Hirzel HO, et al: Exercise-induced ischemia: The influence of altered relaxation on early diastolic pressures. Circulation 67:521, 1983
125. Serruys PW, Wijns W, van den Brand M, et al: Left ventricular performance, regional blood flow, wall motion, and lactate metabolism during transluminal angioplasty. Circulation 70:25, 1984
126. Paulus WJ, Serizawa T, Grossman WR: Altered left ventricular diastolic properties during pacing-induced ischemia in dogs with coronary stenoses. Potentiation by caffeine. Circ Res 50:218, 1982
127. Lorell BH, Turi Z, Grossman WR: Modification of left ventricular response to pacing tachycardia and nifedipine in patients with CAD. Am J Med 71:667, 1981
128. Bonow RO, Rosing DR, Bacharach SL, et al: Effects of verapamil on left ventricular systolic function and diastolic filling in patients with hypertrophic cardiomyopathy. Circulation 64:787, 1981
129. Hanrath P, Mathey DG, Kremer P, et al: Effect of verapamil on left ventricular isovolumic relaxation time and regional left ventricular filling in hypertrophic cardiomyopathy. Am J Cardiol 45:1258, 1980
130. Brown RO, Rosing DR, Bacharach SLR: Left ventricular systolic function and diastolic filling in patients with hypertrophic cardiomyopathy. Circulation 62(suppl III):III-317, 1980
131. Colan SD, Sanders SP, MacPherson D, et al: Left ventricular diastolic function in elite athletes with physiologic cardiac hypertrophy. J Am Coll Cardiol 6:545, 1985
132. Granger CB, Karimeddini MK, Smith VE, et al: Rapid ventricular filling in left ventricular hypertrophy. I. Physiologic hypertrophy. J Am Coll Cardiol 5:862, 1985
133. Smith VE, Schulman P, Karimeddini MK, et al: Rapid ventricular filling in left ventricular hypertrophy. II. Pathologic hypertrophy. J Am Coll Cardiol 5:869, 1985
134. Lorell BH, Grossman WR: Cardiac hypertrophy: The consequences for diastole. J Am Coll Cardiol 9:1189, 1987
135. Ghali JK, Liao Y, Simmons B, et al: The prognostic role of left ventricular hypertrophy in patients with or without CAD. Ann Intern Med 117:831, 1992
136. Sullivan JM, Vander Zwaag RV, el-Zeky F, et al: Left ventricular hypertrophy: Effect on survival. J Am Coll Cardiol 22:508, 1993
137. Grayburn PA, Eichhorn EJ: Dobutamine challenge for low-gradient aortic stenosis. Circulation 106:763, 2002
138. Bonow RO, Carabello B, de Leon AC, et al: ACC/AHA guidelines for the management of patients with valvular heart disease. Executive summary. A report of the American College of Cardiology/American Heart Association Task Force on Practice Guidelines (Committee on Management of Patients with Valvular Heart Disease). J Heart Valve Dis 7:672, 1998
139. deFilippi CR, Willett DL, Brickner ME, et al: Usefulness of dobutamine echocardiography in distinguishing severe from nonsevere valvular aortic stenosis in patients with depressed left ventricular function and low transvalvular gradients. Am J Cardiol 75:191, 1995
140. Monin JL, Monchi M, Gest V, et al: Aortic stenosis with severe left ventricular dysfunction and low transvalvular pressure gradients: Risk stratification by low-dose dobutamine echocardiography. J Am Coll Cardiol 37:2101, 2001
141. Nishimura RA, Grantham JA, Connolly HM, et al: Low-output, low-gradient aortic stenosis in patients with depressed left ventricular systolic function: The clinical utility of the dobutamine challenge in the catheterization laboratory. Circulation 106:809, 2002
142. Khot UN, Novaro GM, Popovic ZB, et al: Nitroprusside in critically ill patients with left ventricular dysfunction and aortic stenosis. N Engl J Med 348:1756, 2003
143. Zile MR, Gaasch WH: Heart failure in aortic stenosis—improving diagnosis and treatment. N Engl J Med 348:1735, 2003
144. Carabello BA: Clinical practice. Aortic stenosis. N Engl J Med 346:677, 2002
145. Goldman L, Caldera DL, Nussbaum SR, et al: Multifactorial index of cardiac risk in noncardiac surgical procedures. N Engl JMed 297:845, 1977
146. Sundt TM, Bailey MS, Moon MR, et al: Quality of life after aortic valve replacement at the age of >80 years. Circulation 102(suppl 3):III-70, 2000
147. Connolly HM, Oh JK, Schaff HV, et al: Severe aortic stenosis with low transvalvular gradient and severe left ventricular dysfunction: Result of aortic valve replacement in 52 patients. Circulation 101:1940, 2000
148. Stanley TH, Webster LR: Anesthetic requirements and cardiovascular effects of fentanyl-oxygen and fentanyl-diazepam-oxygen anesthesia in man. Anesth Analg 57:411, 1978
149. Bovill JG, Warren PJ, Schuller JL, et al: Comparison of fentanyl, sufentanil, and alfentanil anesthesia in patients undergoing valvular heart surgery. Anesth Analg 63:1081, 1984
150. Dhadphale PR, Jackson AP, Alseri SR: Comparison of anesthesia with diazepam and ketamine vs. morphine in patients undergoing heart-valve replacement. Anesthesiology 51:200, 1979
151. Lindeburg T, Spotoft H, Bredgaard Sorensen M, et al: Cardiovascular effects of etomidate used for induction and in combination with fentanyl-pancuronium for maintenance of anaesthesia in patients with valvular heart disease. Acta Anaesthesiol Scand 26:205, 1982
152. Atlee JL 3rd, Alexander SC: Halothane effects on conductivity of the AV node and His-Purkinje system in the dog. Anesth Analg 56:378, 1977
153. Atlee JL 3rd, Rusy BF, Kreul JF, et al: Supraventricular excitability in dogs during anesthesia with halothane and enflurane. Anesthesiology 49:407, 1978
154. Perloff JG, Ronan JA, deLeon AC Jr: The effect of nitroglycerin on left ventricular wall tension in fixed orifice aortic stenosis. Circulation 32:204, 1965
155. Grose R, Nivapumin TR: Mechanisms of nitroglycerin action in valvular aortic stenosis. Am J Cardiol 44:1371, 1965
156. Goertz AW, Lindner KH, Seefelder C, et al: Effect of phenylephrine bolus administration on global left ventricular function in patients with CAD and patients with valvular aortic stenosis. Anesthesiology 78:834, 1993
157. Cooley DA, Reul GJ, Wukasch DCR: Ischemic contracture of the heart: "Stone heart." Am J Cardiol 29:575, 1972
158. Buckberg GDR: Antegrade cardioplegia, retrograde cardioplegia, or both? Ann Thorac Surg 45:589, 1988
159. Kirklin JW, Conti VR, Blackstone EHR: Prevention of myocardial damage during cardiac operations. N Engl JMed 301:135, 1979
160. Warner KG, Khuri SF, Kloner RA, et al: Structural and metabolic correlates of cell injury in the hypertrophied myocardium during valve replacement. J Thorac Cardiovasc Surg 93:741, 1987
161. Menasche P, Piwnica AR: Cardioplegia by way of the coronary sinus for valvular and coronary surgery. J Am Coll Cardiol 18:628, 1991
162. Partington MT, Acar C, Buckberg GD, et al: Studies of retrograde cardioplegia. II. Advantages of antegrade/retrograde cardioplegia to optimize distribution in jeopardized myocardium. J Thorac Cardiovasc Surg 97:613, 1989
163. Buckberg GD, Beyersdorf F, Allen BSR: Integrated myocardial management in valvular heart disease. J Heart Valve Dis 4(suppl 2):S198; discussion S212, 1995
164. Menasche P, Tronc F, Nguyen A, et al: Retrograde warm blood cardioplegia preserves hypertrophied myocardium: A clinical study. Ann Thorac Surg 57:1429; discussion 1434, 1994
165. American College of Cardiology: Report of the American College of Cardiology/AHA Task Force on Practice Guidelines (Committee on Perioperative Cardiovascular Evaluation for Noncardiac Surgery). Anesth Analg 82:854, 1996
166. Roberts R, Sigwart U: New concepts in hypertrophic cardiomyopathies, part II. Circulation 104:2249, 2001
167. Spencer WH 3rd, Roberts R: Alcohol septal ablation in hypertrophic obstructive cardiomyopathy: The need for a registry. Circulation 102:600, 2000
168. Lakkis N: New treatment methods for patients with hypertrophic obstructive cardiomyopathy. Curr Opin Cardiol 15:172, 2000

169. Nishimura RA, Trusty JM, Hayes DL, et al: Dual-chamber pacing for hypertrophic cardiomyopathy: A randomized, double-blind, crossover trial. J Am Coll Cardiol 29:435, 1997
170. Maron BJ, Nishimura RA, McKenna WJ, et al: Assessment of permanent dual-chamber pacing as a treatment for drug-refractory symptomatic patients with obstructive hypertrophic cardiomyopathy. A randomized, double-blind, crossover study. Circulation 99:2927, 1999
171. Erwin JP 3rd, Nishimura RA, Lloyd MA, et al: Dual chamber pacing for patients with hypertrophic obstructive cardiomyopathy: A clinical perspective in 2000. Mayo Clin Proc 75:173, 2000
172. Lakkis NM, Nagueh SF, Kleiman NS, et al: Echocardiography-guided ethanol septal reduction for hypertrophic obstructive cardiomyopathy. Circulation 98:1750, 1998
173. Talreja DR, Nishimura RA, Edwards WD, et al: Alcohol septal ablation versus surgical septal myectomy: Comparison of effects on atrioventricular conduction tissue. J Am Coll Cardiol 44:2329, 2004
174. Louie EK, Edwards LC 3rd: Hypertrophic cardiomyopathy. Prog Cardiovasc Dis 36:275, 1994
175. Nishimura RA, Holmes DR: Hypertrophic obstructive cardiomyopathy. N Engl J Med 350:1320, 2004
176. Wynne J, Braunwald ER: The cardiomyopathies and myocarditides. *In* Zipes DP, Libby P, Bonow RO, Braunwald E (eds): Braunwald's Heart Disease. Philadelphia, Elsevier, 2005, pp 1659–1696
177. Ciro E, Nichols PF 3rd, Maron BJR: Heterogeneous morphologic expression of genetically transmitted hypertrophic cardiomyopathy. Two-dimensional echocardiographic analysis. Circulation 67:1227, 1983
178. Clark CE, Henry WL, Epstein SER: Familial prevalence and genetic transmission of idiopathic hypertrophic subaortic stenosis. N Engl JMed 289:709, 1973
179. Maron BJ, Roberts WC, Edwards JE, et al: Sudden death in patients with hypertrophic cardiomyopathy: Characterization of 26 patients with functional limitation. Am J Cardiol 41:803, 1978
180. Braunwald E, Lambrew CT, Rockoff SDR: Idiopathic hypertrophic subaortic stenosis. Circulation 29/30:IV-1, 1964
181. McKenna WJ, Chetty S, Oakley CM, et al: Arrhythmia in hypertrophic cardiomyopathy: Exercise and 48 hour ambulatory electrocardiographic assessment with and without beta adrenergic blocking therapy. Am J Cardiol 45:1, 1980
182. Savage DD, Seides SF, Maron BJ, et al: Prevalence of arrhythmias during 24-hour electrocardiographic monitoring and exercise testing in patients with obstructive and nonobstructive hypertrophic cardiomyopathy. Circulation 59:866, 1979
183. McKenna WJ, England D, Doi YL, et al: Arrhythmia in hypertrophic cardiomyopathy. I. Influence on prognosis. Br Heart J 46:168, 1981
184. Bonow RO, Frederick TM, Bacharach SL, et al: Atrial systole and left ventricular filling in hypertrophic cardiomyopathy: Effect of verapamil. Am J Cardiol 51:1386, 1983
185. Maron BJ, Lipson LC, Roberts WC, et al: "Malignant" hypertrophic cardiomyopathy: Identification of a subgroup of families with unusually frequent premature death. Am J Cardiol 41:1133, 1978
186. Maron BJ, Roberts WC, Epstein SE: Sudden death in hypertrophic cardiomyopathy: A profile of 78 patients. Circulation 65:1388, 1982
187. Maron BJ: Sudden death in young athletes. Circulation 62:218, 1980
188. Lewis JF, Maron BJR: Elderly patients with hypertrophic cardiomyopathy: A subset with distinctive left ventricular morphology and progressive clinical course late in life. J Am Coll Cardiol 13:36, 1989
189. Wigle ED, Silver MDR: Myocardial fiber disarray and ventricular septal hypertrophy in asymmetrical hypertrophy of the heart. Circulation 58:398, 1978
190. Murgo JP, Alter BR, Dorethy JF, et al: Dynamics of left ventricular ejection in obstructive and nonobstructive hypertrophic cardiomyopathy. J Clin Invest 66:1369, 1980
191. Pohost GM, Vignola PA, McKusick KE, et al: Hypertrophic cardiomyopathy. Evaluation by gated cardiac blood pool scanning. Circulation 55:92, 1977
192. Sutton MG, Tajik AJ, Gibson DG, et al: Echocardiographic assessment of left ventricular filling and septal and posterior wall dynamics in idiopathic hypertrophic subaortic stenosis. Circulation 57:512, 1978
193. Wilson WS, Criley JM, Ross RSR: Dynamics of left ventricular emptying in hypertrophic subaortic stenosis. A cineangiographic and hemodynamic study. Am Heart J 73:4, 1967
194. Pouleur H, Rousseau MF, van Eyll C, et al: Force-velocity-length relations in hypertrophic cardiomyopathy: Evidence of normal or depressed myocardial contractility. Am J Cardiol 52:813, 1983
195. Hirota Y, Furubayashi K, Kaku K, et al: Hypertrophic nonobstructive cardiomyopathy: A precise assessment of hemodynamic characteristics and clinical implications. Am J Cardiol 50:990, 1982
196. Cannon RO 3rd, Schenke WH, Bonow RO, et al: Left ventricular pulsus alternans in patients with hypertrophic cardiomyopathy and severe obstruction to left ventricular outflow. Circulation 73:276, 1986
197. Kramer CM, Reichek N, Ferrari VA, et al: Regional heterogeneity of function in hypertrophic cardiomyopathy. Circulation 90:186, 1994
198. Morrow AG, Braunwald ER: Functional aortic stenosis: A malformation characterized by resistance to left ventricular outflow without anatomic obstruction. Circulation 20:181, 1959
199. Henry WL, Clark CE, Glancy DL, et al: Echocardiographic measurement of the left ventricular outflow gradient in idiopathic hypertrophic subaortic stenosis. N Engl JMed 288:989, 1973
200. Cape EG, Simons D, Jimoh A, et al: Chordal geometry determines the shape and extent of systolic anterior mitral motion: In vitro studies. J Am Coll Cardiol 13:1438, 1989
201. Wigle ED, Sasson Z, Henderson MA, et al: Hypertrophic cardiomyopathy. The importance of the site and the extent of hypertrophy. A review. Prog Cardiovasc Dis 28:1, 1985
202. Sherrid MV, Chu CK, Delia E, et al: An echocardiographic study of the fluid mechanics of obstruction in hypertrophic cardiomyopathy. J Am Coll Cardiol 22:816, 1993
203. King JF, DeMaria AN, Miller RRR: Markedly abnormal mitral valve motion without simultaneous intraventricular pressure gradient due to uneven mitral-septal contact in idiopathic hypertrophic subaortic stenosis. Am J Cardiol 50:360, 1982
204. Rossen RM, Goodman DJ, Ingham RE, et al: Echocardiographic criteria in the diagnosis of idiopathic hypertrophic subaortic stenosis. Circulation 50:747, 1974
205. Feizi O, Emanuel RR: Echocardiographic spectrum of hypertrophic cardiomyopathy. Br Heart J 37:1286, 1975
206. Pollick C, Rakowski H, Wigle EDR: Muscular subaortic stenosis: The quantitative relationship between systolic anterior motion and the pressure gradient. Circulation 69:43, 1984
207. Lin CS, Chen KS, Lin MC, et al: The relationship between systolic anterior motion of the mitral valve and the left ventricular outflow tract doppler in hypertrophic cardiomyopathy. Am Heart J 122:1671, 1991
208. Levine RH, Weyman AER: Dynamic subaortic obstruction in hypertrophic cardiomyopathy: Criteria and controversy. J Am Coll Cardiol 6:15, 1985
209. Ross J Jr, Braunwald E, Gault JH, et al: The mechanism of the intraventricular pressure gradient in idiopathic hypertrophic subaortic stenosis. Circulation 34:558, 1966
210. Maron BJ, Gottdiener JS, Arce J, et al: Dynamic subaortic obstruction in hypertrophic cardiomyopathy: Analysis by pulsed doppler echocardiography. J Am Coll Cardiol 6:1, 1985
211. Gilbert BW, Pollick C, Adelman AG, et al: Hypertrophic cardiomyopathy: Subclassification by M mode echocardiography. Am J Cardiol 45:861, 1980
212. Criley JM, Lewis KB, White RI Jr, et al: Pressure gradients without obstruction. A new concept of "hypertrophic subaortic stenosis." Circulation 32:881, 1965
213. Criley JM, Siegel RJR: Has "obstruction" hindered our understanding of hypertrophic cardiomyopathy? Circulation 72:1148, 1985
214. Klues HG, Maron BJ, Dollar AL, et al: Diversity of structural mitral valve alterations in hypertrophic cardiomyopathy. Circulation 85:1651, 1992
215. Glancy DL, Shepherd RL, Beiser D, et al: The dynamic nature of left ventricular outflow obstruction in idiopathic hypertrophic subaortic stenosis. Ann Intern Med 75:589, 1971
216. Lorell BH, Paulus WJ, Grossman W, et al: Modification of abnormal left ventricular diastolic properties by nifedipine in patients with hypertrophic cardiomyopathy. Circulation 65:499, 1982
217. Rosing DR, Epstein SER: Verapamil in the treatment of hypertrophic cardiomyopathy. Ann Intern Med 96:670, 1982
218. Rosing DR, Kent KM, Borer JS, et al: Verapamil therapy: A new approach to the pharmacologic treatment of hypertrophic cardiomyopathy. I. Hemodynamic effects. Circulation 60:1201, 1979
219. TenCate FJ, Serruys PW, Mey S, et al: Effects of short-term administration of verapamil on left ventricular relaxation and filling dynamics measured by a combined hemodynamic-ultrasonic technique in patients with hypertrophic cardiomyopathy. Circulation 68:1274, 1983
220. Losi MA, Betocchi S, Grimaldi M, et al: Heterogeneity of left ventricular filling dynamics in hypertrophic cardiomyopathy. Am J Cardiol 73:987, 1994
221. O'Gara PT, Bonow RO, Maron BJ, et al: Myocardial perfusion abnormalities in patients with hypertrophic cardiomyopathy: Assessment with thallium-201 emission computed tomography. Circulation 76:1214, 1987
222. Grover-McKay M, Schwaiger M, Krivokapich J, et al: Regional myocardial blood flow and metabolism at rest in mildly symptomatic patients

with hypertrophic cardiomyopathy (see comment). J Am Coll Cardiol 13:317, 1989
223. Maron BJ, Wolfson JK, Epstein SE, et al: Intramural ("small vessel") CAD in hypertrophic cardiomyopathy. J Am Coll Cardiol 8:545, 1986
224. Pasternac A, Noble J, Streulens Y, et al: Pathophysiology of chest pain in patients with cardiomyopathies and normal coronary arteries. Circulation 65:778, 1982
225. Camici P, Chiriatti G, Lorenzoni R, et al: Coronary vasodilation is impaired in both hypertrophied and nonhypertrophied myocardium of patients with hypertrophic cardiomyopathy: A study with nitrogen-13 ammonia and positron emission tomography. J Am Coll Cardiol 17:879, 1991
226. Cannon RO 3rd, Schenke WH, Maron BJ, et al: Differences in coronary flow and myocardial metabolism at rest and during pacing between patients with obstructive and patients with nonobstructive hypertrophic cardiomyopathy. J Am Coll Cardiol 10:53, 1987
227. Hayashida W, Kumada T, Kohno F, et al: Left ventricular regional relaxation and its nonuniformity in hypertrophic nonobstructive cardiomyopathy. Circulation 84:1496, 1991
228. Miyamoto MI, Rockman HA, Guth BD, et al: Effect of alpha-adrenergic stimulation on regional contractile function and myocardial blood flow with and without ischemia. Circulation 84:1715, 1991
229. Pollick CR: Muscular subaortic stenosis: Hemodynamic and clinical improvement after disopyramide. N Engl J Med 307:997, 1982
230. Chatterjee K, Raff G, Anderson D, et al: Hypertrophic cardiomyopathy—therapy with slow channel inhibiting agents. Progress in Cardiovascular Diseases 25:193, 1982
231. Bonow RO, Ostrow HG, Rosing DR, et al: Effects of verapamil on left ventricular systolic and diastolic function in patients with hypertrophic cardiomyopathy: Pressure-volume analysis with a nonimaging scintillation probe. Circulation 68:1062, 1983
232. Epstein SE, Rosing DRR: Verapamil: Its potential for causing serious complications in patients with hypertrophic cardiomyopathy. Circulation 64:437, 1981
233. Seiler C, Hess OM, Schoenbeck M, et al: Long-term follow-up of medical versus surgical therapy for hypertrophic cardiomyopathy: A retrospective study (see comment). J Am Coll Cardiol 17:634, 1991
234. Chahine RAR: Surgical versus medical therapy of hypertrophic cardiomyopathy: Is the perspective changing? (see comment). J Am Coll Cardiol 17:643, 1991
235. Fananapazir L, Cannon RO 3rd, Tripodi D, et al: Impact of dual-chamber permanent pacing in patients with obstructive hypertrophic cardiomyopathy with symptoms refractory to verapamil and beta-adrenergic blocker therapy. Circulation 85:2149, 1992
236. Maron BJR: Appraisal of dual-chamber pacing therapy in hypertrophic cardiomyopathy: Too soon for a rush to judgment? (see comment). J Am Coll Cardiol 27:431, 1996
237. Williams WG, Wigle ED, Rakowski H, et al: Results of surgery for hypertrophic obstructive cardiomyopathy. Circulation 76(Pt 2):V104, 1987
238. Grigg LE, Wigle ED, Williams WG, et al: Transesophageal Doppler echocardiography in obstructive hypertrophic cardiomyopathy: Clarification of pathophysiology and importance in intraoperative decision making (see comment). J Am Coll Cardiol 20:42, 1992
239. Joyce FS, Lever HM, Cosgrove DM 3rd: Treatment of hypertrophic cardiomyopathy by mitral valve repair and septal myectomy. Ann Thorac Surg 57:1025, 1994
240. Gilligan DM, Chan WL, Stewart R, et al: Cardiac responses assessed by echocardiography to changes in preload in hypertrophic cardiomyopathy. Am J Cardiol 73:312, 1994
241. Cohn LH, Trehan H, Collins JJ Jr: Long-term follow-up of patients undergoing myotomy/myectomy for obstructive hypertrophic cardiomyopathy. Am J Cardiol 70:657, 1992
242. ten Berg JM, Suttorp MJ, Knaepen PJ, et al: Hypertrophic obstructive cardiomyopathy. Initial results and long-term follow-up after morrow septal myectomy (see comment). Circulation 90:1781, 1994
243. Sasson Z, Prieur T, Skrobik Y, et al: Aortic regurgitation: A common complication after surgery for hypertrophic obstructive cardiomyopathy. J Am Coll Cardiol 13:63, 1989
244. Cosio FG, Moro C, Alonso M, et al: The Q wave hypertrophic cardiomyopathy: An electrophysiologic study. N Engl JMed 302:96, 1980
245. Krikler DM, Davies MJ, Rowland E, et al: Sudden death in hypertrophic cardiomyopathy: Associated accessory atrioventricular pathways. Br Heart J 43:245, 1980
246. Anderson KP, Stinson EB, Derby GC, et al: Vulnerability of patients with obstructive hypertrophic cardiomyopathy to ventricular arrhythmia induction in the operating room. Analysis of 17 patients. Am J Cardiol 51:811, 1983
247. Wulfson HD, LaPorta RFR: Pulmonary oedema after lithotripsy in a patient with hypertrophic subaortic stenosis. Can J Anaesth 40(Pt 1):465, 1993
248. Thompson RC, Liberthson RR, Lowenstein ER: Perioperative anesthetic risk of noncardiac surgery in hypertrophic obstructive cardiomyopathy. JAMA 254:2419, 1985
249. Loubser P, Suh K, Cohen SR: Adverse effects of spinal anesthesia in a patient with idiopathic hypertrophic subaortic stenosis. Anesthesiology 60:228, 1984
250. Larson CP Jr: Use of spinal anesthesia in patients with idiopathic hypertrophic subaortic stenosis. Anesthesiology 61:229, 1984
251. Pearson J, Reves JGR: Unusual cause of hypotension after coronary artery bypass grafting: Idiopathic hypertrophic subaortic stenosis. Anesthesiology 60:592, 1984
252. Lanier W, Prough DSR: Intraoperative diagnosis of hypertrophic obstructive cardiomyopathy. Anesthesiology 60:61, 1984
253. Smith HJ, Neutze JM, Roche AH, et al: The natural history of rheumatic aortic regurgitation and the indications for surgery. Br Heart J 38:147, 1976
254. Goldschlager N, Pfeifer J, Cohn K, et al: The natural history of aortic regurgitation. A clinical and hemodynamic study. Am J Med 54:577, 1973
255. Ishii K, Hirota Y, Suwa M, et al: Natural history and left ventricular response in chronic aortic regurgitation. Am J Cardiol 78:357, 1996
256. Schwarz F, Flameng W, Langebartels F, et al: Impaired left ventricular function in chronic aortic valve disease: Survival and function after replacement by Bjork-Shiley prosthesis. Circulation 60:48, 1979
257. Tam JW, Antecol D, Kim HH, et al: Low dose dobutamine echocardiography in the assessment of contractile reserve to predict the outcome of valve replacement for chronic aortic regurgitation. Can J Cardiol 15:73, 1999
258. Padial LR, Oliver A, Vivaldi M, et al: Doppler echocardiographic assessment of progression of aortic regurgitation (see comment). Am J Cardiol 80:306, 1997
259. Levine HJ, Gaasch WHR: Ratio of regurgitant volume to end-diastolic volume: A major determinant of ventricular response to surgical correction of chronic volume overload. Am J Cardiol 52:406, 1983
260. Henry WL, Bonow RO, Borer JS, et al: Observations on the optimum time for operative intervention for aortic regurgitation. I. Evaluation of the results of aortic valve replacement in symptomatic patients. Circulation 61:471, 1980
261. Bonow RO, Rosing DR, Kent KM, et al: Timing of operation for chronic aortic regurgitation. Am J Cardiol 50:325, 1982
262. Green GR, Miller DC: Continuing dilemmas concerning aortic valve replacement in patients with advanced left ventricular systolic dysfunction. J Heart Valve Dis 6:562, 1997
263. Eichorn EJ, Konstam MAR: Quantitation of aortic regurgitation. *In* Gaasch WH, Levine JH (eds): Chronic Aortic Regurgitation. Boston, Kluwer Academic, 1988, p 108
264. Reimold SC, Byrne JG, Caguioa ES, et al: Load dependence of the effective regurgitant orifice area in a sheep model of aortic regurgitation. J Am Coll Cardiol 18:1085, 1991
265. Enriquez-Sarano M, Tajik AT: Clinical practice. Aortic regurgitation. N Engl J Med 351:1539, 2004
266. Elkayam U, McKay CR, Weber L, et al: Favorable effects of hydralazine on the hemodynamic response to isometric exercise in chronic severe aortic regurgitation. Am J Cardiol 53:1603, 1984
267. Greenberg BH, DeMots H, Murphy E, et al: Mechanism for improved cardiac performance with arteriolar dilators in aortic insufficiency. Circulation 63:263, 1981
268. Devlin WH, Petrusha J, Briesmiester K, et al: Impact of vascular adaptation to chronic aortic regurgitation on left ventricular performance. Circulation 99:1027, 1999
269. Borow KM, Marcus RH: Aortic regurgitation: The need for an integrated physiologic approach (see comment). J Am Coll Cardiol 17:898, 1991
270. Judge TP, Kennedy JW, Bennett LJ, et al: Quantitative hemodynamic effects of heart rate in aortic regurgitation. Circulation 44:355, 1971
271. Firth BG, Dehmer GJ, Nicod P, et al: Effect of increasing heart rate in patients with aortic regurgitation. Effect of incremental atrial pacing on scintigraphic, hemodynamic and thermodilution measurements. Am J Cardiol 49:1860, 1982
272. Dodge HT, Kennedy JW, Petersen JLR: Quantitative angiocardiographic methods in the evaluation of valvular heart disease. Prog Cardiovasc Dis 16:1, 1973
273. Dodge HT, Hay RE, Sandler HR: Pressure-volume characteristics of diastolic LV of man with heart disease. Am Heart J 64:503, 1962

274. Segal J, Harvey WP, Hufnagel C: A clinical study of one hundred cases of severe aortic insufficiency. Am J Med 21:200, 1956
275. Johnson AE, Engler RL, LeWinger M: The medical and surgical management of patients with aortic valve disease. A symposium. West J Med 126:460, 1977
276. Kawachi K, Kitamura S, Oyama C, et al: Relations of preoperative hemodynamics and coronary blood flow to improved left ventricular function after valve replacement for aortic regurgitation. J Am Coll Cardiol 11:925, 1988
277. Eastham CL, Doty DB, Hiratzka LF: Volume-overload left ventricular hypertrophy impairs coronary reserve in humans. Circulation 64(suppl IV): IV-26, 1981
278. Strauer BE: Ventricular function and coronary hemodynamics in hypertensive heart disease. Am J Cardiol 44:999, 1979
279. Tauchert M, Hilger HH: Application of the coronary reserve concept to the study of myocardial perfusion. *In* Schaper W (ed): The Pathophysiology of Myocardial Perfusion. Amsterdam, Elsevier/North-Holland, 1979, pp 141–167
280. Borow KM: Surgical outcome in chronic aortic regurgitation: A physiologic framework for assessing preoperative predictors. J Am Coll Cardiol 10:1165, 1987
281. Gerson MC, Engel PJ, Mantil JC, et al: Effects of dynamic and isometric exercise on the radionuclide-determined regurgitant fraction in aortic insufficiency. J Am Coll Cardiol 3:98, 1984
282. Huxley RL, Gaffney FA, Corbett JR, et al: Early detection of left ventricular dysfunction in chronic aortic regurgitation as assessed by contrast angiography, echocardiography, and rest and exercise scintigraphy. Am J Cardiol 51:1542, 1983
283. Tarasoutchi F, Grinberg M, Spina GS, et al: Ten-year clinical laboratory follow-up after application of a symptom-based therapeutic strategy to patients with severe chronic aortic regurgitation of predominant rheumatic etiology (see comment). J Am Coll Cardiol 41:1316, 2003
284. Verheul HA, van den Brink RB, Bouma BJ, et al: Analysis of risk factors for excess mortality after aortic valve replacement. J Am Coll Cardiol 26:1280, 1995
285. Welch GH Jr, Braunwald E, Sarnoff SJ: Hemodynamic effects of quantitatively varied experimental aortic regurgitation. Circ Res 5:546, 1957
286. Mann T, McLaurin L, Grossman W, et al: Assessing the hemodynamic severity of acute aortic regurgitation due to infective endocarditis. N Engl J Med 293:108, 1975
287. Botvinick EH, Schiller NB, Wickramasekaran R, et al: Echocardiographic demonstration of early mitral valve closure in severe aortic insufficiency. Its clinical implications. Circulation 51:836, 1975
288. Wigle ED, Labrosse CJ: Sudden, severe aortic insufficiency. Circulation 32:708, 1965
289. Laniado S, Yellin EL, Yoran C, et al: Physiologic mechanisms in aortic insufficiency. I. The effect of changing heart rate on flow dynamics. II. Determinants of Austin Flint murmur. Circulation 66:226, 1982
290. Ardehali A, Segal J, Cheitlin MD: Coronary blood flow reserve in acute aortic regurgitation. J Am Coll Cardiol 25:1387, 1995
291. van Herwerden LA, Gussenhoven EJ, Roelandt JR, et al: Intraoperative two-dimensional echocardiography in complicated infective endocarditis of the aortic valve. J Thorac Cardiovasc Surg 93:587, 1987
292. Shapiro SM, Bayer AS: Transesophageal and Doppler echocardiography in the diagnosis and management of infective endocarditis. Chest 100:1125, 1991
293. Daniel WG, Mugge A, Martin RP, et al: Improvement in the diagnosis of abscesses associated with endocarditis by transesophageal echocardiography (see comment). N Engl J Med 324:795, 1991
294. Teague SM, Heinsimer JA, Anderson JL, et al: Quantification of aortic regurgitation utilizing continuous wave doppler ultrasound. J Am Coll Cardiol 8:592, 1986
295. Perry GJ, Helmcke F, Nanda NC, et al: Evaluation of aortic insufficiency by Doppler color flow mapping. J Am Coll Cardiol 9:952, 1987
296. Oh JK, Hatle LK, Sinak LJ, et al: Characteristic doppler echocardiographic pattern of mitral inflow velocity in severe aortic regurgitation. J Am Coll Cardiol 14:1712, 1989
297. Stone JG, Hoar PF, Khambatta HJ: Influence of volume loading on intraoperative hemodynamics and perioperative fluid retention in patients with valvular regurgitation undergoing prosthetic replacement. Am J Cardiol 52:530, 1983
298. Stone JG, Hoar PF, Calabro JR, et al: Afterload reduction and preload augmentation improve the anesthetic management of patients with cardiac failure and valvular regurgitation. Anesth Analg 59:737, 1980
299. Cohn JN, Franciosa JA: Vasodilator therapy of cardiac failure. Parts 1 and 2. N Engl J Med 297:27, 254, 1977
300. Olson LJ, Subramanian R, Ackermann DM, et al: Surgical pathology of the mitral valve: A study of 712 cases spanning 21 years. Mayo Clin Proc 62:22, 1987
301. Karon BL, Enriquez-Sarano M: Valvular regurgitation. *In* Murphy JG (ed): Mayo Clinic Cardiology Review. Philadelphia, Lippincott Williams & Wilkins, 2000, pp 303–330
302. Enriquez-Sarano M, Avierinos JF, Messika-Zeitoun D, et al: Quantitative determinants of the outcome of asymptomatic mitral regurgitation. N Engl J Med 352:875, 2005
303. Enriquez-Sarano M, Orszulak TA, Schaff HV, et al: Mitral regurgitation: A new clinical perspective. Mayo Clin Proc 72:1034, 1997
304. Ling LH, Enriquez-Sarano M, Seward JB, et al: Clinical outcome of mitral regurgitation due to flail leaflet. N Engl J Med 335:1417, 1996
305. Grigioni F, Enriquez-Sarano M, Ling LH, et al: Sudden death in mitral regurgitation due to flail leaflet. J Am Coll Cardiol 34:2078, 1999
306. Enriquez-Sarano M, Basmadjian AJ, Rossi A, et al: Progression of mitral regurgitation: A prospective doppler echocardiographic study. J Am Coll Cardiol 34:1137, 1999
307. Carabello BA: The pathophysiology of mitral regurgitation. J Heart Valve Dis 9:600, 2000
308. Otsuji Y, Handschumacher MD, Kisanuki A, et al: Functional mitral regurgitation. Cardiologia 43:1011, 1998
309. Enriquez-Sarano M, Tajik AJ, Schaff HV, et al: Echocardiographic prediction of survival after surgical correction of organic mitral regurgitation. Circulation 90:830, 1994
310. Enriquez-Sarano M, Tajik AJ, Schaff HV, et al: Echocardiographic prediction of left ventricular function after correction of mitral regurgitation: Results and clinical implications. J Am Coll Cardiol 24:1536, 1994
311. Enriquez-Sarano M, Schaff HV, Orszulak TA, et al: Congestive heart failure after surgical correction of mitral regurgitation. A long-term study. Circulation 92:2496, 1995
312. Matsuo T, Carabello BA, Nagatomo Y, et al: Mechanisms of cardiac hypertrophy in canine volume overload. Am J Physiol 275(Pt 2):H65, 1998
313. Carabello BA, Nakano K, Corin W, et al: Left ventricular function in experimental volume overload hypertrophy. Am J Physiol 256(Pt 2):H974, 1989
314. Kleaveland JP, Kussmaul WG, Vinciguerra T, et al: Volume overload hypertrophy in a closed-chest model of mitral regurgitation. Am J Physiol 254(Pt 2):H1034, 1988
315. Imamura T, McDermott PJ, Kent RL, et al: Acute changes in myosin heavy chain synthesis rate in pressure versus volume overload. Circ Res 75:418, 1994
316. Urabe Y, Mann DL, Kent RL, et al: Cellular and ventricular contractile dysfunction in experimental canine mitral regurgitation. Circ Res 70:131, 1992
317. Lehmann KG, Francis CK, Dodge HT: Mitral regurgitation in early myocardial infarction. Incidence, clinical detection, and prognostic implications. Ann Intern Med 117:10, 1992
318. Tcheng JE, Jackman JD Jr, Nelson CL, et al: Outcome of patients sustaining acute ischemic mitral regurgitation during myocardial infarction. Ann Intern Med 117:18, 1992
319. Lamas GA, Mitchell GF, Flaker GC, et al: Clinical significance of mitral regurgitation after acute myocardial infarction. Survival and ventricular enlargement investigators. Circulation 96:827, 1997
320. Phillips JH, Burch GE, Depasquale NP: The syndrome of papillary muscle dysfunction. Its clinical recognition. Ann Intern Med 59:508, 1963
321. Burch GE, DePasquale NP, Phillips JH: The syndrome of papillary muscle dysfunction. Am Heart J 75:399, 1968
322. Burch GE, De Pasquale NP, Phillips JH: Clinical manifestations of papillary muscle dysfunction. Arch Intern Med 112:112, 1963
323. Levine RA: Dynamic mitral regurgitation—more than meets the eye. N Engl J Med 351:1681, 2004
324. Kaul S, Spotnitz WD, Glasheen WP, et al: Mechanism of ischemic mitral regurgitation. An experimental evaluation. Circulation 84:2167, 1991
325. Mittal AK, Langston M Jr, Cohn KE, et al: Combined papillary muscle and left ventricular wall dysfunction as a cause of mitral regurgitation. An experimental study. Circulation 44:174, 1971
326. Tsakiris AG, Rastelli GC, Amorim S, et al: Effect of experimental papillary muscle damage on mitral valve closure in intact anesthetized dogs. Mayo Clin Proc 45:275, 1970
327. Otsuji Y, Handschumacher MD, Schwammenthal E, et al: Insights from three-dimensional echocardiography into the mechanism of functional mitral regurgitation: Direct in vivo demonstration of altered leaflet tethering geometry. Circulation 96:1999, 1997
328. Birnbaum Y, Chamoun AJ, Conti VR, et al: Mitral regurgitation following acute myocardial infarction. Coron Artery Dis 13:337, 2002

329. Komeda M, Glasson JR, MacIsaac A, et al: Systolic "dysfunction" of ischemic papillary muscle may serve as a compensatory mechanism for left ventricular wall motion abnormality (abst). Circulation 92(suppl I):I357, 1995
330. Dent JM, Spotnitz WD, Kaul S: Echocardiographic evaluation of the mechanisms of ischemic mitral regurgitation. Coron Artery Dis 7:188, 1996
331. Ormiston JA, Shah PM, Tei C, et al: Size and motion of the mitral valve annulus in man. I. A two-dimensional echocardiographic method and findings in normal subjects. Circulation 64:113, 1981
332. Tsakiris AG, Von Bernuth G, Rastelli GC, et al: Size and motion of the mitral valve annulus in anesthetized intact dogs. J Appl Physiol 30:611, 1971
333. Ma HH, Honma H, Munakata K, et al: Mitral insufficiency as a complication of acute myocardial infarction and left ventricular remodeling. Jpn Circ J 61:912, 1997
334. Tenenbaum A, Leor J, Motro M, et al: Improved posterobasal segment function after thrombolysis is associated with decreased incidence of significant mitral regurgitation in a first inferior myocardial infarction. J Am Coll Cardiol 25:1558, 1995
335. Leor J, Feinberg MS, Vered Z, et al: Effect of thrombolytic therapy on the evolution of significant mitral regurgitation in patients with a first inferior myocardial infarction. J Am Coll Cardiol 21:1661, 1993
336. Kinn JW, O'Neill WW, Benzuly KH, et al: Primary angioplasty reduces risk of myocardial rupture compared to thrombolysis for acute myocardial infarction. Cathet Cardiovasc Diagn 42:151, 1997
337. Scott WC, Miller DC, Haverich A, et al: Operative risk of mitral valve replacement: Discriminant analysis of 1329 procedures. Circulation 72(Pt 2): II108, 1985
338. Rozich JD, Carabello BA, Usher BW, et al: Mitral valve replacement with and without chordal preservation in patients with chronic mitral regurgitation. Mechanisms for differences in postoperative ejection performance. Circulation 86:1718, 1992
339. Enriquez-Sarano M, Schaff HV, Orszulak TA, et al: Valve repair improves the outcome of surgery for mitral regurgitation. A multivariate analysis. Circulation 91:1022, 1995
340. Mohty D, Orszulak TA, Schaff HV, et al: Very long-term survival and durability of mitral valve repair for mitral valve prolapse. Circulation 104(suppl 1):I1-I7, 2001
341. David TE, Armstrong S, Sun Z: Replacement of chordae tendineae with Gore-Tex sutures: A ten-year experience. J Heart Valve Dis 5:352, 1996
342. Pearson PJ, Schaff HV: Valve repair and choice of valves. *In* Yusuf S, Cairns JA, Camm AJ, et al (eds): Evidence-Based Cardiology. London, BMJ Books, 2003, pp 809–816
343. David TE, Komeda M, Pollick C, et al: Mitral valve annuloplasty: The effect of the type on left ventricular function. Ann Thorac Surg 47:524; discussion 527, 1989
344. Tribouilloy CM, Enriquez-Sarano M, Schaff HV, et al: Impact of preoperative symptoms on survival after surgical correction of organic mitral regurgitation: Rationale for optimizing surgical indications. Circulation 99:400, 1999
345. Tribouilloy CM, Enriquez-Sarano M, Schaff HV, et al: Excess mortality due to CAD after valve surgery. Secular trends in valvular regurgitation and effect of internal mammary artery bypass. Circulation 98(suppl II):II-108, 1998
346. Grose R, Strain J, Yipintosoi T: Right ventricular function in valvular heart disease: Relation to pulmonary artery pressure. J Am Coll Cardiol 2:225, 1983
347. Enriquez-Sarano M, Freeman WK, Tribouilloy CM, et al: Functional anatomy of mitral regurgitation: Accuracy and outcome implications of transesophageal echocardiography. J Am Coll Cardiol 34:1129, 1999
348. Bastard OG, Carter JG, Moyers JR, et al: Circulatory effects of isoflurane in patients with ischemic heart disease: A comparison with halothane. Anesth Analg 63:635, 1984
349. Smith JS, Cahalan MK, Benefiel DJ: Fentanyl versus fentanyl and isoflurane in patients with impaired left ventricular function. Anesthesiology 63: A18, 1985
350. McCammon RL, Hilgenberg JC, Stoelting RK: Hemodynamic effects of diazepam and diazepam-nitrous oxide in patients with CAD. Anesth Analg 59:438, 1982
351. Price HL, Cooperman LH, Warden JC, et al: Pulmonary hemodynamics during general anesthesia in man. Anesthesiology 30:629, 1969
352. Stoelting RK, Reis RR, Longnecker DE: Hemodynamic responses to nitrous oxide-halothane and halothane in patients with valvular heart disease. Anesthesiology 37:430, 1972
353. Schulte-Sasse U, Hess W, Tarnow J: Pulmonary vascular responses to nitrous oxide in patients with normal and high pulmonary vascular resistance. Anesthesiology 57:9, 1982
354. Hilgenberg JC, McCammon RL, Stoelting RK: Pulmonary and systemic vascular responses to nitrous oxide in patients with mitral stenosis and pulmonary hypertension. Anesth Analg 59:323, 1980
355. Rorie DK, Tyce GM, Sill JC: Nitrous oxide increases norepinephrine release from pulmonary artery. Anesthesiology 63:A89, 1985
356. Hammond GL, Cronau LH, Whittaker D, et al: Fate of prostaglandins E(1) and A(1) in the human pulmonary circulation. Surgery 81:716, 1977
357. Said SI: Pulmonary metabolism of prostaglandins and vasoactive peptides. Annu Rev Physiol 44:257, 1982
358. Mikawa K, Maekawa N, Goto R, et al: Use of prostaglandin E1 to treat peri-anaesthetic pulmonary hypertension associated with mitral valve disease. J Intern Med Res 21:161, 1993
359. Kunimoto F, Arai K, Isa Y, et al: A comparative study of the vasodilator effects of prostaglandin E1 in patients with pulmonary hypertension after mitral valve replacement and with adult respiratory distress syndrome (see comment). Anesth Analg 85:507, 1997
360. D'Ambra MN, LaRaia PJ, Philbin DM, et al: Prostaglandin E1. A new therapy for refractory right heart failure and pulmonary hypertension after mitral valve replacement. J Thorac Cardiovasc Surg 89:567, 1985
361. Vincent JL, Carlier E, Pinsky MR, et al: Prostaglandin E1 infusion for right ventricular failure after cardiac transplantation (see comment). J Thorac Cardiovasc Surg 103:33, 1992
362. Fullerton DA, Jones SD, Jaggers J, et al: Effective control of pulmonary vascular resistance with inhaled nitric oxide after cardiac operation. J Thorac Cardiovasc Surg 111:753; discussion 762, 1996
363. Fullerton DA, McIntyre RC Jr: Inhaled nitric oxide: Therapeutic applications in cardiothoracic surgery (see comment). Ann Thorac Surg 61:1856, 1996
364. Nishimura RA: Valvular stenosis. *In* Yusuf S (ed): Evidence-Based Cardiology, 2nd edition. London, BMJ Books, 2003, pp 285–301
365. Gorlin R, Gorlin SG: Hydraulic formula for calculation of the area of stenotic mitral valve, other cardiac valves and central circulatory shunts. I. Am Heart J 41:1, 1951
366. Bruce CJ, Nishimura RA: Clinical assessment and management of mitral stenosis. Cardiol Clin 16:375, 1998
367. Hugenholtz PG, Ryan TJ, Stein SW, et al: The spectrum of pure mitral stenosis. Hemodynamic studies in relation to clinical disability. Am J Cardiol 10:773, 1962
368. Wood P: An appreciation of mitral stenosis. I. Clinical features. Br Med J 4870:1051, 1954
369. Wood P: An appreciation of mitral stenosis: Ii. Investigations and results. Br Med J 4871:1113, 1954
370. Carroll JD, Feldman T: Percutaneous mitral balloon valvotomy and the new demographics of mitral stenosis. JAMA 270:1731, 1993
371. Selzer A, Cohn KE: Natural history of mitral stenosis: A review. Circulation 45:878, 1972
372. Rowe JC, Bland EF, Sprague HB, et al: The course of mitral stenosis without surgery: Ten- and twenty-year perspectives. Ann Intern Med 52:741, 1960
373. Olesen KH: The natural history of 271 patients with mitral stenosis under medical treatment. Br Heart J 24:349, 1962
374. Gash AK, Carabello BA, Cepin D, et al: Left ventricular ejection performance and systolic muscle function in patients with mitral stenosis. Circulation 67:148, 1983
375. Carabello BA: Mitral valve disease: Indications for surgery. *In* Yusuf S Evidence-Based Cardiology, 2nd edition. London, BMJ Books, 2003, pp 758–766
376. Liu CP, Ting CT, Yang TM, et al: Reduced left ventricular compliance in human mitral stenosis. Role of reversible internal constraint. Circulation 85:1447, 1992
377. Bruce CJ, Nishimura RA: Newer advances in the diagnosis and treatment of mitral stenosis. Curr Probl Cardiol 23:125, 1998
378. Popovic AD, Stewart WJ: Echocardiographic evaluation of valvular stenosis: The gold standard for the next millennium? Echocardiography 18:59, 2001
379. Inoue K, Owaki T, Nakamura T, et al: Clinical application of transvenous mitral commissurotomy by a new balloon catheter. J Thorac Cardiovasc Surg 87:394, 1984
380. Iung B, Vahanian A: The long-term outcome of balloon valvuloplasty for mitral stenosis. Curr Cardiol Rep 4:118, 2002
381. Nishimura RA, Holmes DR Jr, Reeder GS: Efficacy of percutaneous mitral balloon valvuloplasty with the Inoue balloon. Mayo Clin Proc 66:276, 1991
382. Abascal VM, Wilkins GT, Choong CY, et al: Mitral regurgitation after percutaneous balloon mitral valvuloplasty in adults: Evaluation by pulsed Doppler echocardiography. J Am Coll Cardiol 11:257, 1988

383. Mueller XM, Tevaearai HT, Stumpe F, et al: Tricuspid valve involvement in combined mitral and aortic valve surgery. J Cardiovasc Surg 42:443, 2001
384. Cohen SR, Sell JE, McIntosh CL, et al: Tricuspid regurgitation in patients with acquired, chronic, pure mitral regurgitation. I. Prevalence, diagnosis, and comparison of preoperative clinical and hemodynamic features in patients with and without tricuspid regurgitation. J Thorac Cardiovasc Surg 94:481, 1987
385. Katircioglu SF, Yamak B, Ulus AT, et al: Treatment of functional tricuspid regurgitation by bicuspidalization annuloplasty during mitral valve surgery. J Heart Valve Dis 6:631, 1997
386. Messika-Zeitoun D, Thomson H, Bellamy M, et al: Medical and surgical outcome of tricuspid regurgitation caused by flail leaflets. J Thorac Cardiovasc Surg 128:296, 2004
387. Sons H, Dausch W, Kuh JH: Tricuspid valve repair in right-sided endocarditis. J Heart Valve Dis 6:636, 1997
388. Chopra P, Tandon HD: Pathology of chronic rheumatic heart disease with particular reference to tricuspid value involvement. Acta Cardiol 32:423, 1977
389. Vatterott PJ, Nishimura RA, Gersh BJ, et al: Severe isolated tricuspid insufficiency in CAD. Int J Cardiol 14:295, 1987
390. Arbulu A, Holmes RJ, Asfaw I: Tricuspid valvulectomy without replacement. Twenty years' experience. J Thorac Cardiovasc Surg 102:917, 1991
391. Arbulu A, Asfaw I: Tricuspid valvulectomy without prosthetic replacement. Ten years of clinical experience. J Thorac Cardiovasc Surg 82:684, 1981
392. Farid L, Dayem MK, Guindy R, et al: The importance of tricuspid valve structure and function in the surgical treatment of rheumatic mitral and aortic disease. Eur Heart J 13:366, 1992
393. Gayet C, Pierre B, Delahaye JP, et al: Traumatic tricuspid insufficiency. An underdiagnosed disease. Chest 92:429, 1987
394. Kaul TK, Ramsdale DR, Mercer JL: Functional tricuspid regurgitation following replacement of the mitral valve. Int J Cardiol 33:305, 1991
395. McGrath LB, Gonzalez-Lavin L, Bailey BM, et al: Tricuspid valve operations in 530 patients. Twenty-five-year assessment of early and late phase events. J Thorac Cardiovasc Surg 99:124, 1990
396. Morrison DA, Ovitt T, Hammermeister KE: Functional tricuspid regurgitation and right ventricular dysfunction in pulmonary hypertension. Am J Cardiol 62:108, 1988
397. Mullany CJ, Gersh BJ, Orszulak TA, et al: Repair of tricuspid valve insufficiency in patients undergoing double (aortic and mitral) valve replacement. Perioperative mortality and long-term (1 to 20 years) follow-up in 109 patients. J Thorac Cardiovasc Surg 94:740, 1987
398. Bajzer CT, Stewart WJ, Cosgrove DM, et al: Tricuspid valve surgery and intraoperative echocardiography: Factors affecting survival, clinical outcome, and echocardiographic success. J Am Coll Cardiol 32:1023, 1998
399. Iskandrian AS, Hakki AH, Ren JF, et al: Correlation among right ventricular preload, afterload and ejection fraction in mitral valve disease: Radionuclide, echocardiographic and hemodynamic evaluation. J Am Coll Cardiol 3:1403, 1984
400. Kerber RE, Dippel WF, Abboud FM: Abnormal motion of the interventricular septum in right ventricular volume overload. Experimental and clinical echocardiographic studies. Circulation 48:86, 1973
401. Laver MB, Strauss HW, Pohost GM: Herbert Shubin memorial lecture. Right and left ventricular geometry: Adjustments during acute respiratory failure. Crit Care Med 7:509, 1979
402. Ross J Jr: Acute displacement of the diastolic pressure-volume curve of the LV: Role of the pericardium and the right ventricle. Circulation 59:32, 1979
403. Taylor RR, Covell JW, Sonnenblick EH, et al: Dependence of ventricular distensibility on filling of the opposite ventricle. Am J Physiol 213:711, 1967
404. Discigil B, Dearani JA, Puga FJ, et al: Late pulmonary valve replacement after repair of tetralogy of Fallot. J Thorac Cardiovasc Surg 121:344, 2001
405. Shatapathy P, Aggarwal BK, Kamath SG: Tricuspid valve repair: A rational alternative. J Heart Valve Dis 9:276, 2000
406. Wong M, Matsumura M, Kutsuzawa S, et al: The value of Doppler echocardiography in the treatment of tricuspid regurgitation in patients with mitral valve replacement. Perioperative and two-year postoperative findings. J Thorac Cardiovasc Surg 99:1003, 1990
407. Lambertz H, Minale C, Flachskampf FA, et al: Long-term follow-up after Carpentier tricuspid valvuloplasty. Am Heart J 117:615, 1989
408. Staab ME, Nishimura RA, Dearani JA: Isolated tricuspid valve surgery for severe tricuspid regurgitation following prior left heart valve surgery: Analysis of outcome in 34 patients. J Heart Valve Dis 8:567, 1999
409. Pai RG, Bansal RC, Shah PM: Determinants of the rate of right ventricular pressure rise by doppler echocardiography: Potential value in the assessment of right ventricular function. J Heart Valve Dis 3:179, 1994
410. Loperfido F, Lombardo A, Amico CM, et al: Doppler analysis of portal vein flow in tricuspid regurgitation. J Heart Valve Dis 2:174, 1993
411. Minakata K, Schaff HV, Zehr KJ, et al: Is repair of aortic valve regurgitation a safe alternative to valve replacement? J Thorac Cardiovasc Surg 127:645, 2004
412. Fraser CD Jr, Wang N, Mee RB, et al: Repair of insufficient bicuspid aortic valves. Ann Thorac Surg 58:386, 1994
413. Casselman FP, Gillinov AM, Akhrass R, et al: Intermediate-term durability of bicuspid aortic valve repair for prolapsing leaflet. Eur J Cardiothorac Surg 15:302, 1999
414. Fucci C, Sandrelli L, Pardini A, et al: Improved results with mitral valve repair using new surgical techniques. Eur J Cardiothorac Surg 9:621; discussion 626, 1995
415. Block PC: Percutaneous mitral valve repair for mitral regurgitation. J Int Cardiol 16:93, 2003
416. Kaye DM, Byrne M, Alferness C, et al: Feasibility and short-term efficacy of percutaneous mitral annular reduction for the therapy of heart failure-induced mitral regurgitation. Circulation 108:1795, 2003
417. Liddicoat JR, Mac Neill BD, Gillinov AM, et al: Percutaneous mitral valve repair: A feasibility study in an ovine model of acute ischemic mitral regurgitation. Cathet Cardiovasc Interven 60:410, 2003
418. Inoue M, McCarthy PM, Popovic ZB, et al: The Coapsys device to treat functional mitral regurgitation: In vivo long-term canine study. J Thorac Cardiovasc Surg 127:1068; discussion 1076, 2004
419. Cribier A, Eltchaninoff H, Tron C, et al: Early experience with percutaneous transcatheter implantation of heart valve prosthesis for the treatment of end-stage inoperable patients with calcific aortic stenosis. J Am Coll Cardiol 43:698, 2004
420. Boudjemline Y, Agnoletti G, Bonnet D, et al: Percutaneous pulmonary valve replacement in a large right ventricular outflow tract: An experimental study (see comment). J Am Coll Cardiol 43:1082, 2004
421. Byrne JG, Leacche M, Unic D, et al: Staged initial percutaneous coronary intervention followed by valve surgery ("hybrid approach") for patients with complex coronary and valve disease. J Am Coll Cardiol 45:14, 2005
422. Rahimtoola SH: The year in valvular heart disease. J Am Coll Cardiol 43:491, 2004
423. Rahimtoola SH: The year in valvular heart disease. J Am Coll Cardiol 45:111, 2005
424. Rahimtoola SH: Choice of prosthetic heart valve for adult patients. J Am Coll Cardiol 41:893, 2003

Chapter 21
MINIMALLY INVASIVE CARDIAC SURGERY

Marianne Coutu, MD • Lishan Aklog, MD

KEY POINTS

1. The goals of minimally invasive cardiac surgery are decreased pain, shorter hospital stays, accelerated recuperation, and improved cosmetics.
2. These "less invasive" surgical procedures span a wide spectrum from full sternotomy off-pump surgery to totally endoscopic procedures done through small ports.
3. Anesthetic management for minimally invasive cardiac surgery ranges from fast-track general anesthesia through awake patients under thoracic epidural anesthesia.
4. Cardiopulmonary bypass may or may not be used in minimally invasive surgery. One approach for cardiopulmonary bypass is to use the "Port-Access" system developed by Heartport, Inc.
5. Minimally invasive direct coronary artery bypass is a coronary revascularization procedure performed through a small anterolateral thoracotomy.
6. The development of computer-enhanced telemanipulators has enabled the development of robotically assisted cardiac surgery and totally endoscopic coronary artery revascularization.
7. Totally endoscopic coronary artery revascularization procedures can be performed on the arrested heart or on the beating heart.
8. Valvular procedures such as aortic valve replacement and mitral valve replacement or repair can now be performed using minimally invasive procedures.
9. Other minimally invasive cardiac procedures include congenital heart surgery, arrhythmia surgery, and ventricular resynchronization procedures.

Since its early days, cardiac surgery has typically involved large incisions with complete access to the heart and great vessels. Following the popularization of minimally invasive techniques in general surgery, cardiac surgeons began to experiment with less invasive procedures in the early 1990s. Although the goals of minimally invasive cardiac surgery (MICS) are fairly well established as decreased pain, shorter hospital stay, accelerated recuperation, and improved cosmesis, a strict definition of *minimally invasive cardiac surgery* has been more elusive. "Less invasive" is probably a more appropriate term, because these procedures span a wide spectrum from full sternotomy off-pump procedures to totally endoscopic procedures. There has been an ongoing debate within the specialty whether eliminating sternotomy or cardiopulmonary bypass (CPB) is a more fundamental component of MICS. Some have even argued that cardiac surgery will not be truly minimally invasive until general anesthesia itself is eliminated and a handful of centers have reported on various off-pump coronary artery bypass (OPCAB) procedures performed with high thoracic epidural anesthesia alone.

This chapter focuses on the anesthetic implications of operations performed through an incision other than a full sternotomy or thoracotomy and does not address the various endovascular procedures under development. The common incisions used for these procedures are shown in Figure 21–1 and include partial sternotomies (upper versus lower, unilateral versus bilateral) and minithoracotomies (anterior versus anterolateral versus posterolateral, nonspreading versus spreading) in addition to totally endoscopic procedures done exclusively through thoracoscopic ports (defined as <15 mm). This chapter focuses primarily on minimally invasive coronary and valve surgery while briefly summarizing its role in congenital, pericardial, and electrophysiologic surgery.

GENERAL ANESTHETIC CONSIDERATIONS*

Patient Setup

Position, Prepping, and Draping

Conventional cardiac surgery is almost always performed with the patient flat and supine, prepped, and draped with the sterile field extending from mid neck to the ankles (Box 21–1). Many MICS procedures, however, require different positions and sterile field setups. For example, most procedures performed through anterior minithoracotomies or exclusively thoracoscopically are done with the patient's left or right side elevated approximately 30 degrees. Some thoracoscopic procedures are performed in the left or right lateral decubitus position, typically with the hips rotated to expose one or both groins for possible femoral vascular cannulation. Unlike conventional sternotomy procedures, surgical access to remote areas (neck, lateral chest wall, groin) may be necessary for peripheral cannulation, placement of camera/instrument ports, or transcutaneous retraction sutures. This should be taken into consideration when placing electrocardiographic leads or other items on the skin during setup.

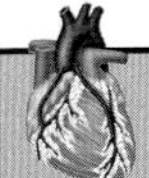

BOX 21–1 ***Anesthetic Considerations***

- Position, prepping, and draping
- Temperature management
- Hemodynamic monitoring
- Airway management
- Anesthetic regimen
- Pain management

*David Reich, MD, consulted on this anesthetic section.

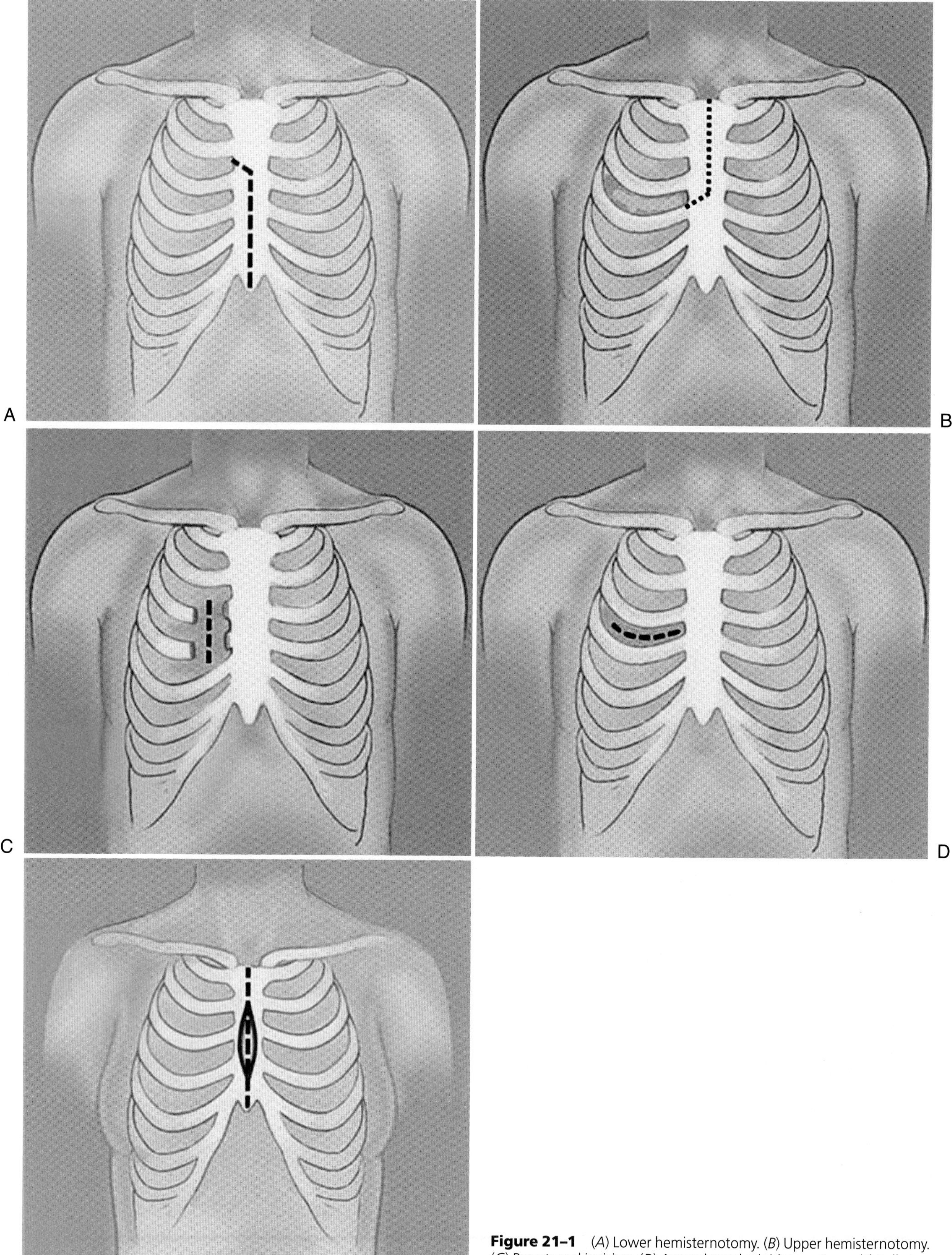

Figure 21–1 (*A*) Lower hemisternotomy. (*B*) Upper hemisternotomy. (*C*) Parasternal incision. (*D*) Anterolateral minithoracotomy. (*E*) Full sternotomy with small skin incision.

Because, by definition, access to the heart is limited in most MICS, *external defibrillator pads* should be considered mandatory. Again, care should be taken with placement and draping to ensure the current passes through the heart and that burns associated with seepage of prep solution or other liquids under the pads are avoided.

Temperature Management

Because nearly all MICS and all off-pump procedures are performed under normothermic conditions, careful temperature management is critical to avoid hypothermia, which not only can lead to ventricular fibrillation and bleeding but also can negate some of the potential benefits of MICS by prolonging the time to extubation. In addition to maintaining room temperature, one of a variety of *warming blankets* is usually required. Although conventional water or forced warm air blankets can suffice, more innovative solutions such as the Kimberly-Clark Patient Warming System (formerly the Arctic Sun) may be particularly advantageous in MICS.[1] The primary advantage of this circulating water system is that the adhesive gel pads are highly efficient at transferring heat, minimizing the required area of coverage and maximizing surgical access.

Hemodynamic Monitoring

Hemodynamic monitoring requirements for MICS are typically not different from conventional cardiac surgery. Most patients have radial arterial and pulmonary arterial catheters (PACs) placed. Some centers limit themselves to a central venous pressure catheter, especially in patients with normal ventricular function undergoing MICS. Intraoperative *transesophageal echocardiography (TEE)* is the standard of care for all valvular surgery, and it can be critical in MICS cases to assess ventricular preload and pick up early changes in regional or global ventricular function, because visualization of the heart may be limited. In addition, TEE is helpful and often necessary to guide placement of various catheters, cannulae, and balloons. Because access to a ventricular wall for temporary pacing wire placement can be limited in some MICS approaches, a PAC with a pacing port can be helpful in valve procedures or other cases in which the need for temporary cardiac pacing may arise (see Chapters 14 through 16).

Anesthetic Technique

Airway

Many MICS procedures, including all minithoracotomy and thoracoscopic approaches, require at least some period of *one-lung ventilation*. Double-lumen endotracheal tubes are generally preferred because they are less likely to be dislodged during repositioning. It is critical to take the time to confirm proper placement and lung isolation prior to and just after positioning, because loss of lung isolation during an anastomosis or during some other critical stage of the procedure can be extremely dangerous.

Carbon dioxide insufflation of the hemithorax is frequently used during thoracoscopic MICS procedures, especially during robotic procedures.[2] Insufflation to a pressure of 8 to 15 cm H_2O can dramatically increase the working space in the chest by shifting the mediastinal structures posteriorly and to the contralateral chest. Because there is always some obligatory leak around ports and incisions, the constant flow of CO_2 also clears smoke generated during electrocauterization of tissues. The intrathoracic pressure should be set to the minimal value necessary to achieve adequate exposure, and very careful monitoring of hemodynamics and gas exchange is essential, because the physiology is effectively that of a controlled tension pneumothorax. Although generally well tolerated, significant hypotension, hypercapnia, or hypoxia can occur if the pressure is set too high, particularly in patients with ventricular dysfunction or lung disease.[3]

Anesthetic Regimen

For a detailed discussion of anesthetic regimens, see Chapters 9 and 19. Because accelerated recovery and discharge are major goals of MICS, it is important to note that careful selection of the anesthetic agents is necessary to ensure that the patient obtains the full benefit from the minimally invasive approach. Most centers will use some sort of *"fast-track" anesthesia* regimen—typically very short-acting narcotics and muscle relaxants in conjunction with an inhalation agent.[4] Some have advocated precise pharmacokinetically *controlled total intravenous anesthesia* (TIVA) regimens.[5,6] Routine intraoperative extubation of MICS patients is controversial. Although some centers have established protocols whereby nearly all patients are extubated at the completion of the procedure,[7-9] others have argued that a clinical or economic benefit is difficult to document unless the patient recovers in a postoperative acute care unit setting without an overnight intensive care unit stay.[10,11]

A few centers have been exploring the radical notion that cardiac surgery, especially MICS coronary artery surgery, can be routinely performed in "awake" patients *without general anesthesia*.[12-14] Special challenges with these techniques include precise titration of sedatives, chest wall stiffness and movement, as well as managing inadvertent small pneumothoraces during the procedure. The specific benefits relative to "ultra-fast-track" general anesthetic techniques remain to be determined.

Pain Management

Aggressive pain management is another critical component of the care of patients undergoing MICS, without which it is difficult to obtain the full benefit of this approach. Successful pain management permits intraoperative or early postoperative extubation, early ambulation, and discharge. There is some evidence that the amount of pain in the early postoperative period may not be significantly less in many types of MICS and that it may actually be higher in some, particularly those involving rib-spreading thoracotomies.[15,16] The pain, however, seems to dissipate more rapidly than with full sternotomy; most patients are off narcotic pain medicines within a week or two of surgery.[17-19]

Spinal/Epidural

Spinal and epidural anesthetics have been used as an adjunct to general anesthesia at many institutions practicing MICS. A single intrathecal dose of a long-acting narcotic can be beneficial in reducing intraoperative and postoperative parenteral or enteral narcotic requirements.[20-22] A thoracic epidural catheter with narcotic or local anesthetics can be administered continuously or with patient-controlled dosing.[23,24] The excellent pain control and potential cardioprotective benefits from this approach, however, are mitigated by the additional operative time, the small but finite additional risk from the epidural, and its potential to delay the typically rapid mobilization and discharge of MICS patients (see Chapters 19 and 37).

Local

Every effort should be made to supplement the pain management of MICS with local measures at the surgical site. This can include conventional methods such as direct infiltration of the wound with a long-acting local anesthetic such as bupivacaine or *intercostal rib blocks* extending a couple of interspaces above and below the incision. Two innovations in local pain control in patients with thoracotomy incisions include continuous infusion *intercostal analgesia catheters* and *intercostal nerve cryotherapy.*[25-28] The latter involves applying a cryoablation probe directly to the intercostal nerves, causing axonal degeneration but preservation of the endoneurium, which allows axonal regeneration in 1 to 2 months.

GENERAL CARDIOPULMONARY BYPASS CONSIDERATIONS

Although nearly all minimally invasive coronary artery bypass (MICAB) surgery is performed on a beating heart, without the use of CPB, minimally invasive surgery of the cardiac valves and other intracardiac structures requires creative and innovative techniques to safely establish CPB (Box 21–2). There are a variety of approaches depending on the incision and access to cardiovascular structures. Some minimally invasive approaches permit direct, central cannulation similar to conventional cardiac surgery but typically with relatively small cannulae and vacuum-assisted venous drainage. On the other end of the spectrum, "Port-Access" techniques, pioneered by Heartport, Inc. (now a part of Johnson & Johnson) in the early 1990s, sought to have all elements of the CPB circuit enter peripherally, preferably percutaneously, to allow procedures to be performed through very small incisions or totally endoscopically. The anesthesiologist plays a central role in all "Port-Access" procedures from insertion of certain cannulae to monitoring cannula position and function by TEE.[29]

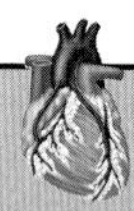

BOX 21–2 *Cardiopulmonary Bypass Considerations*

- Arterial cannulation
- Venous cannulation
- Aortic occlusion and cardioplegia
- Cardiac decompression and deairing

Cannulation

Arterial

Some MICS approaches, including most partial-sternotomy incisions, permit direct cannulation of the ascending aorta in a fashion similar, if not identical, to conventional approaches. Some surgeons use aortic cannulae with tapered dilators designed to be inserted over a guidewire to facilitate direct cannulation through a limited incision. Through many MICS approaches, however, the ascending aorta cannot be safely cannulated and peripheral cannulation is necessary. The femoral approach is most commonly used. The axillary artery is a viable alternative but is not usually used in MICS since accessing it usually requires a cosmetically prominent 3- to 6-cm incision. TEE assessment of the descending aorta is important prior to considering femoral artery cannulation to rule out extensive atherosclerotic disease, which can lead to retrograde embolization and neurologic injury.

Femoral arterial cannulation can be achieved percutaneously but is usually performed through a very small transverse incision guided by the pulse or a Doppler signal. The cannulae can be short, with the tip sitting in the pelvis, or long, extending into the thoracic aorta with multiple side ports. Contraindications include significant peripheral vascular disease. Potential complications include retrograde dissection, embolization, and perforation with retroperitoneal hemorrhage.[30,31]

Venous

Even though the right atrium (RA) is accessible in many MICS approaches, percutaneous femoral venous cannulation has become popular since it removes the venous cannulae from the operative field, enhancing exposure. The right femoral vein is usually used because the right common iliac vein joins the inferior vena cava (IVC) at a much straighter angle, facilitating advancement into the RA. Modern, highly efficient long venous cannulae as small as 20 to 21 French, coupled with vacuum-assisted venous drainage, can support full CPB flows even in large individuals. TEE is used to confirm guidewire and cannula position during percutaneous insertion.

A single cannula with the tip near the RA–superior vena cava (SVC) junction and side ports spanning the RA usually suffices for aortic valve operations. Situations in which surgical manipulation can interfere with SVC drainage must be considered to avoid complications due to upper body venous hypertension. In mitral valve operations, for example, retraction of the RA and septum can interfere with drainage. The Chitwood transthoracic aortic clamp, used commonly in videoscopic and robotic mitral valve surgery, passes over the SVC and can compress it. RA procedures (atrial septal defects [ASDs], tricuspid surgery) usually require separate IVC and SVC drainage. In these situations, improved drainage can be assured by using a two-stage long venous cannula that can be advanced into the SVC itself. Another approach is to cannulate the right internal jugular vein percutaneously with a small cannula advanced into the SVC.

As previously mentioned, routine use of vacuum-assisted venous drainage is typical in MICS and is more often than not necessary to maintain adequate flows through long, small-caliber venous cannulae. Although there are several large series that have documented the safety and efficacy of this technique,[32-34] some have cautioned that there may be an increased risk of gas emboli and hemolysis.[35-38]

Aortic Occlusion and Cardioplegia

Intracardiac procedures usually require aortic occlusion and cardioplegic arrest. In direct-access MICS procedures, direct clamping of the aorta can be achieved with conventional, slightly streamlined, or articulating aortic clamps. Videoscopic and robotic procedures, however, require some type of remote aortic occlusion. The two most common options are the Chitwood transthoracic clamp and balloon occlusion. The Chitwood clamp has conventional jaws, but a long shaft, and is passed through a separate port in the right chest with the posterior jaw in the transverse sinus.

Balloon aortic occlusion is the centerpiece of most Port-Access approaches. A catheter with a large, low-pressure balloon is passed via the femoral artery and positioned with the balloon in the ascending aorta under echocardiographic guidance. The balloon is inflated until the pressure in the port distal to the balloon falls, confirming occlusion of the ascending aorta. The right and left radial artery pressures are monitored simultaneously to ensure the balloon is not impinging on the orifice of the innominate artery. Balloon migration can be an irritating problem early in the learning curve, but experienced centers report good results with routine use of this technique. However, all centers emphasize careful collaboration among the surgery, anesthesia, and perfusion teams. Continuous TEE monitoring of balloon position is important to prevent complications.[39] The most dreaded complication of this technique is aortic dissection, and some reports indicate that the incidence may be higher than in conventional surgery.[40]

Myocardial protection during MICS can be achieved via an anterograde, retrograde, or combined approach. In direct-access and videoscopic approaches, the anterograde cardioplegia catheter is usually directly inserted into the ascending aorta. In the Port-Access approach, the cardioplegic solution is infused through the distal port of the balloon catheter into the aortic root. In direct-access approaches, a retrograde catheter can be advanced into the coronary sinus, with or without echocardiographic guidance. The Port-Access system includes a percutaneous retrograde coronary sinus catheter that is inserted by the anesthesia team through the right internal jugular vein and advanced under echocardiographic guidance.

Cardiac Decompression/Dealring

Limited visibility of and access to the cardiac chambers during MICS can make the critical steps of cardiac decompression and deairing more difficult and requires special attention to avoid the potentially devastating complications arising from unsuspected sustained myocardial distention or air embolism.

The most vulnerable period for distention is during administration of antegrade cardioplegia and immediately after removing the cross-clamp prior to restoration of ventricular ejection. The ventricular dimensions on TEE and the pulmonary artery pressures should be monitored closely to ensure adequate ventricular decompression. Patients with thick, small-cavity ventricles may be particularly difficult to monitor since the ventricle may not appear particularly dilated on TEE despite an elevated cavitary pressure and because they are more susceptible to subendocardial ischemia. A left ventricular (LV) vent can be inserted through the right superior pulmonary vein in some patients undergoing direct-access MICS. The Port-Access system includes a percutaneous pulmonary artery vent that is advanced through the jugular vein and can maintain decompression. A terminal dose of warm blood in the aortic root can rouse the heart and initiate ventricular ejection prior to removing the cross-clamp, avoiding distention.

Since manual manipulation of the cardiac chambers is usually impossible with MICS, the best way to deal with intracardiac air is to prevent it from accumulating in the first place. Flooding the surgical field with CO_2 while the chambers are open can dramatically decrease the amount of air.[41,42] Some deairing is usually necessary and manipulation of the table while ventilating and filling the heart usually facilitates this.

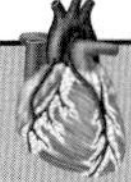

BOX 21–3 *Minimally Invasive Coronary Artery Surgery*

- Off-pump coronary artery bypass (OPCAB) (see Chapter 19)
- Minimally invasive direct coronary artery bypass (MIDCAB)
  - Enhanced (robotic-assisted) MIDCAB
- Total endoscopic coronary artery revascularization (TECAB)
  - TECAB on the arrested heart
  - TECAB on the beating heart
- Multivessel small thoracotomy revascularization

MINIMALLY INVASIVE CORONARY ARTERY BYPASS GRAFTING

The goals of minimally invasive coronary artery bypass grafting are to reduce the surgical trauma by minimizing access and to obviate the need for extracorporeal circulation (Box 21–3). These procedures encompass minimally invasive direct coronary artery bypass, totally endoscopic coronary artery bypass on an arrested or beating heart, and multivessel small thoracotomy revascularization and are discussed in this section (see Chapter 19 for OPCAB procedures).

Minimally Invasive Direct Coronary Artery Bypass

Minimally invasive direct coronary artery bypass (MIDCAB) is a coronary revascularization procedure through an anterolateral thoracotomy. Patients who should be considered for a MIDCAB are those with isolated left anterior descending (LAD) or right coronary artery (RCA) stenosis, patients with multivessel disease in which the lesion in the other vessels can be addressed percutaneously (hybrid procedure), and patients with multiple comorbidities (elderly, cerebral and peripheral vascular disease, chronic renal insufficiency, or chronic obstructive pulmonary disease) who have a higher risk of complications.[43]

The patient is positioned supine on the operating table. External defibrillator pads are placed allowing space for sternotomy access in the event of a conversion. A double-lumen endotracheal tube or a bronchial blocker is used to collapse the left lung. Standard monitoring for cardiac surgery is used, plus TEE to monitor cardiac filling and myocardial segmental abnormalities.

This procedure is performed through a small anterolateral thoracotomy (Fig. 21–1*D*). A 6- to 10-cm incision is made over the fourth intercostal space, the pleural space is opened, and the ribs are spread with a specialized left internal mammary artery (LIMA) retractor. The LIMA is harvested as a pedicle (length of about 15 cm) and prepared after systemic heparinization. The LAD is then identified, dissected, and opened after the heart has been stabilized (Fig. 21–2). Finally, the LIMA is anastomosed to the LAD on a beating heart through the thoracic incision. This procedure can also be performed for a proximal high-grade RCA stenosis through a right anterolateral thoracotomy using the right internal mammary artery (RIMA).

The main advantages of the MIDCAB procedure are the avoidance of CPB and median sternotomy, potentially less postoperative pain, and faster recovery to normal activities. Calafiore et al[44] reported their experience of more than 500

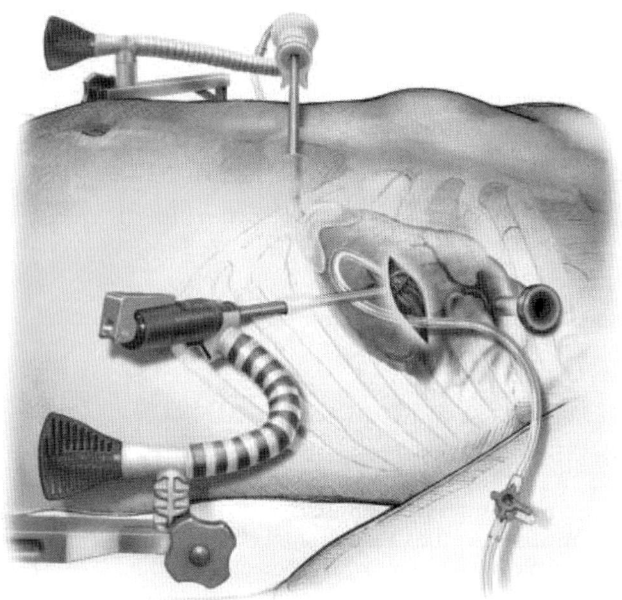

Figure 21–2 Stabilization of the LAD with a commercialized retractor during multivessel small thoracotomy revascularization (MVST). (Nonsternotomy surgical solutions: Octopus NS Tissue Stabilizer and Starfish NS Heart Positioner Medtronic, Inc., Minneapolis, MN.)

patients with low mortality and morbidity rates. Studies showed good short-term patency rates of the LIMA-to-LAD anastomosis.[45]

Totally Endoscopic Coronary Artery Revascularization

It is the development of computer-enhanced telemanipulators that has enabled robotically assisted surgery and totally endoscopic coronary artery revascularization. The currently available system, the DaVinci Telemanipulation System (Intuitive Surgical, Inc., Sunnyvale, CA), provides a high-resolution three-dimensional videoscopic image and allows remote, tremor-free, and scaled control of endoscopic surgical instruments with 6 degrees of freedom. It consists of a master console for remote control of microinstruments mounted on a surgical cart with three arms (one stereoendoscope and two endothoracic end-effectors) (Fig. 21–3). This procedure can be done on the arrested heart and on the beating heart and is most often performed for single- or double-vessel coronary artery disease.

Totally Endoscopic Coronary Artery Bypass on the Arrested Heart

The most frequently performed procedure using this technique to date is revascularization of the LAD with the LIMA via a left-sided approach.[46-48] The RCA can also be grafted with the RIMA via a right-sided approach.

For robotically assisted IMA harvest, patients are placed in a supine position with the left side of the chest elevated 30 to 40 degrees. Ventilation of the right lung is performed. A 30° scope angled up is inserted at the fourth intercostal space (ICS) in the left anterior axillary line. Continuous CO_2 insufflation (<10 mm Hg) of the thoracic cavity is used to enhance exposure by increasing the available space between the heart and the sternum. Two endoscopic instruments used for IMA

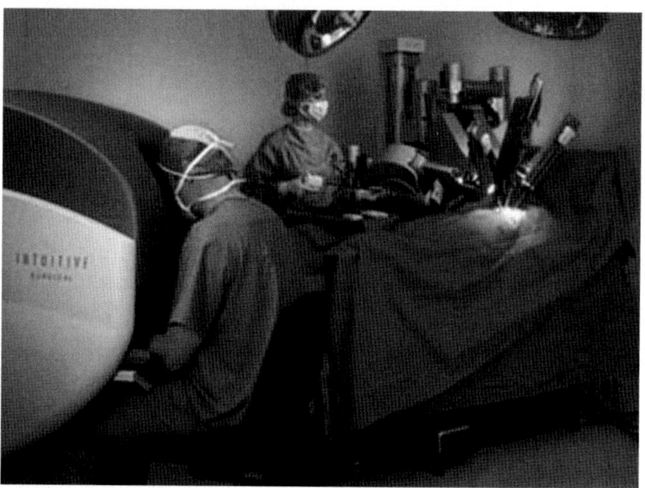

A

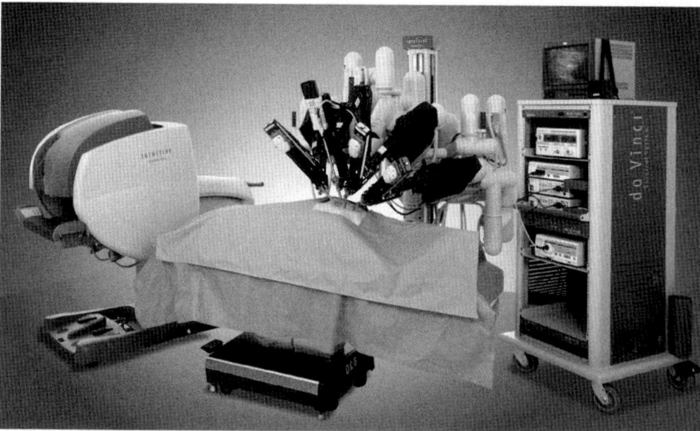

B

Figure 21–3 (*A*) DaVinci surgeon's console. (*B*) Cart-mounted manipulator.

harvesting are then placed under direct vision through ports in the third and seventh ICS in the midaxillary line. The LIMA is dissected as a pedicle from the subclavian artery to the bifurcation. After systemic heparinization, the LIMA is transected at its distal end. Femoral-femoral CPB is initiated by using the Port-Access system for closed-chest and antegrade cardioplegic cardiac arrest. The femoral venous cannula is positioned in the RA under echocardiographic guidance. After institution of CPB, the pericardium is opened, the target vessel is identified on the beating heart, and the epicardium over the anastomotic region is dissected. The heart is arrested using the endoaortic occlusion catheter and cardioplegia administration. The coronary anastomosis is performed end-to-side with a running suture (7-0 or 8-0 Prolene) or interrupted sutures (U-clips). After completion of the anastomosis, the endoaortic occlusion catheter is deflated and the patient is weaned from CPB.

Totally Endoscopic Coronary Artery Bypass on the Beating Heart

The development of endoscopic CABG on the beating heart required the development of endoscopic stabilizers and methods for temporary coronary occlusion. Vascular occlusion can be achieved by using vascular clamps or Silastic bands. For this procedure, the patient is prepared as described earlier. In addition to the three left-sided ports, an endoscopic epicardial stabilizer is inserted through a subxyphoid port

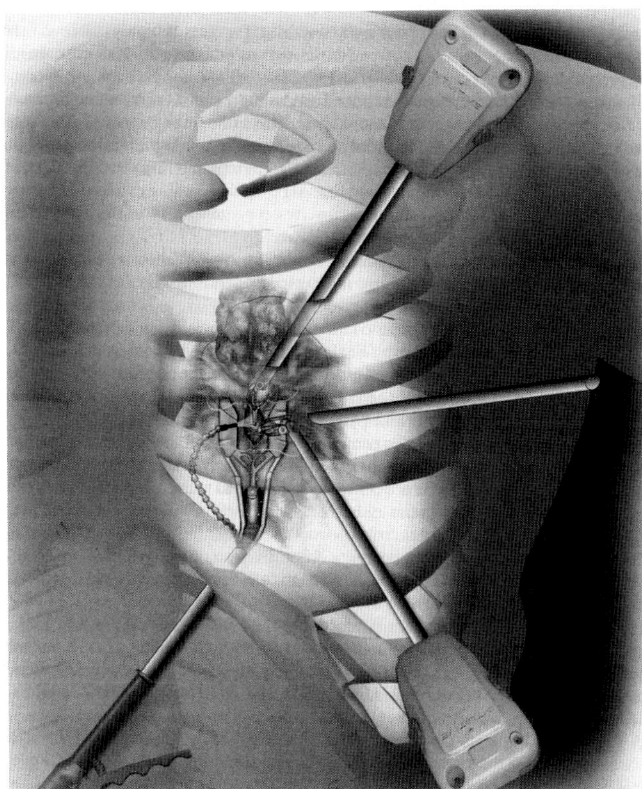

Figure 21–4 Totally endoscopic coronary artery revascularization on the beating heart: The stabilizer is inserted through a subxiphoid incision.

after harvest and preparation of the LIMA (Fig. 21–4). Endoscopic stabilizers use combined pressure and suction stabilization to facilitate the performance of the anastomosis. Because the heart is not decompressed with this technique, the space in the thoracic cavity is limited despite CO_2 insufflation. In this particular situation, CO_2 pressure may be increased above 12 mm Hg if the heart is sufficiently filled and myocardial contractility is adequate.[49] Compared with full-sternotomy beating heart surgery, the myocardial tolerance to ischemia in beating heart totally endoscopic coronary artery bypass (TECAB) is reduced. After occlusion of the target vessel, if severe ST-segment elevation or multiple extrasystoles appear on the ECG, the conversion threshold to MIDCAB should be low.[50] The anastomosis is performed with a running suture (7-0 or 8-0 Prolene), interrupted sutures (U-clips), or distal anastomotic devices.

The first successful TECAB procedure on the arrested heart was reported by Loulmet et al in 1999.[51] Most recent reported CPB and cross-clamp times are in the range of 80 to 120 and 40 to 60 minutes, respectively. The conversion rate to a sternotomy is now less than 10%, and the reported patency rate at 3-month follow-up angiography is 96%.[52] Complete TECAB procedures on the beating heart were first reported by groups in Leipzig and Dresden.[53] Approximately 80 closed-chest procedures have been reported in the literature. Based on an intention-to-treat, the conversion rate is currently between 30% and 50%. LAD occlusion times are in the range of 25 to 40 minutes.[54,55]

Even as progress has been made, as with all new technologies, a learning curve has to be overcome. Operating times are still long and conversions to open surgery are frequently necessary. A lot of steps occurring between IMA takedown and performance of the anastomosis are hampered by the lack of assistance, limited space, the lack of fine tactile feedback, and a limited number of instruments.

Enhanced Minimally Invasive Direct Coronary Artery Bypass and Multivessel Small Thoracotomy Revascularization

Enhanced MIDCAB and multivessel small thoracotomy (MVST) revascularization are procedures performed on the beating heart with robotically assisted IMA harvest and where coronary anastomoses are performed under direct vision through either a mini (MIDCAB) or a small anterolateral thoracotomy (MVST) (see Fig. 21–2). Indications for these procedures are single-vessel and multivessel disease. Anesthesiology considerations and surgical technique are similar to those described in the beating heart TECAB section. The main advantages of these procedures in comparison to the conventional MIDCAB are that the length if the IMA robotically harvested is longer and the skin incision can be kept down to 4 to 5 cm, leading to a better cosmetic result and less postoperative pain.

MINIMALLY INVASIVE VALVULAR SURGERY

Valvular procedures such as aortic valve replacement (AVR) and mitral valve replacement and repair are now performed using different types of minimally invasive procedures (Box 21–4). This section describes these techniques using smaller incisions, avoidance of sternotomy, Port-Access CPB, endoscopic instruments, and/or robotic technology (see Chapters 16 and 20).

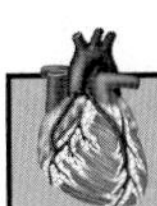

BOX 21–4 ***Minimally Invasive Valvular Surgery***

- Minimally invasive aortic valve surgery
- Minimally invasive mitral valve surgery (MIMVS)
- Direct-vision MIMVS
- Video-assisted and directed MIMVS
- Robot-directed MIMVS telemanipulation and computer-enhanced MIMVS

Minimally Invasive Aortic Valve Surgery

The goals of minimally invasive aortic valve surgery are to reduce the incision size and decrease the surgical trauma and pain, in addition to improving cosmetics, patient satisfaction, and recovery times. This must be realized without compromising the efficacy and the safety of the conventional aortic valve surgery.[56]

Minimally invasive aortic valve surgery has been performed via several approaches such as a right parasternal incision, right anterolateral thoracotomy, and transverse sternotomy, but the most frequently performed approach is the partial upper sternotomy or "ministernotomy" (Fig. 21–5). This latter approach allows excellent exposure for aortic root procedures and aortic valve replacement or repair. It is particularly useful for reoperative valve surgery and has been

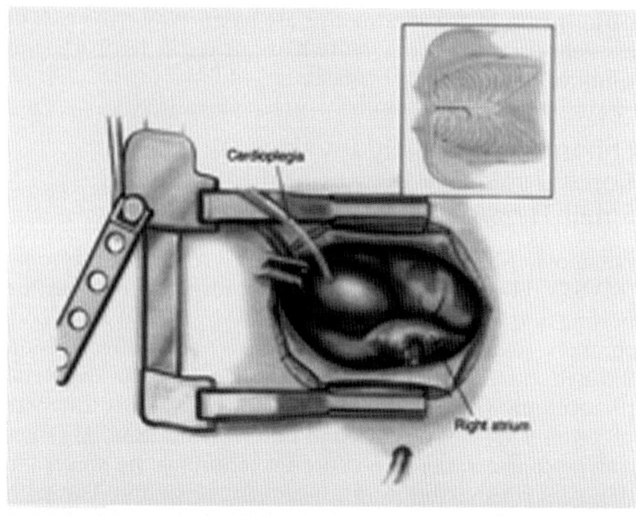

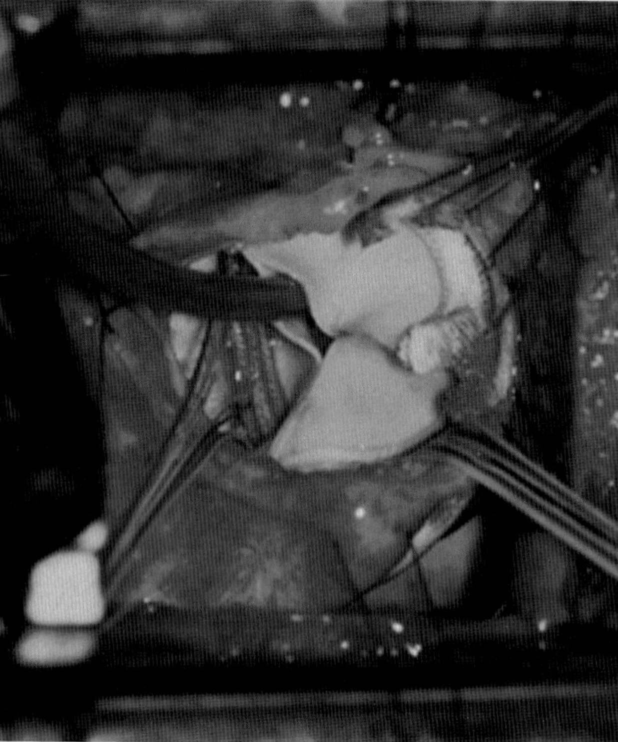

Figure 21–5 Aortic valve exposure through an upper ministernotomy. (From Edmunds LH Jr, Cohn LH [eds]: Cardiac Surgery in the Adult. New York, McGraw-Hill, 2003, p 1078, Fig 44-2A.)

reported to decrease blood loss, transfusion requirements, wound complications, and total operative times compared with a full sternotomy technique.[57] Contraindications to this technique are high-risk and elderly patients, significant coronary artery disease that needs to be corrected, chest wall deformities, cardiac malposition, and morbid obesity.[56]

For the ministernotomy, transcutaneous defibrillator pads, a PAC, and TEE are used, and the patient is prepped in a supine position. Following a 6- to 10-cm skin incision, a longitudinal midsternal cut is made from the notch to the third or fifth ICS, deviating to the right (see Fig. 21–1*B*). Care is taken not to injure the internal thoracic vessels. Right femoral venous cannulation is performed, and with echocardiographic guidance, the cannula is advanced into the RA. Direct venous cannulation in the RA can also be done but reduces the surgeon's exposure. Arterial cannulation is performed in the ascending aorta or in the femoral artery, and CPB is initiated. Both antegrade and retrograde cardioplegia are used for myocardial protection. After cross-clamping, antegrade cardioplegia is given either in the aortic root or directly into the coronary ostia, and retrograde cardioplegia is delivered via a transjugular catheter directed into the coronary sinus (Heartport, Inc., Redwood City, CA). The aortic valve procedure is then performed as usual. After cross-clamp removal, intracardiac air is carefully monitored with TEE, the patient is weaned from CPB, and sternal closure is performed as usual.

The Brigham and Women's Hospital surgeons reported their series of more than 500 mini-invasive AVR with an operative mortality of 2% and a freedom from reoperation at 6 years of 99%.[58]

Minimally Invasive Mitral Valve Surgery

Developments in minimally invasive mitral valve surgery (MIMVS) started in the mid 1990s with the work of Cohn et al[59] and Cosgrove et al.[60] Within a few years, with technological advancements in instrumentation, assisted vision, and CPB support, conventional mitral valve surgery through a full sternotomy evolved to a totally endoscopic operation. This surgical evolution led to four levels of surgical invasiveness that are discussed in this section: (1) mini-incision and direct vision; (2) video-assisted and directed; (3) robot-directed; and (4) telemanipulation and robotically enhanced operations.[61,62] These procedures are currently performed in several centers in the United States and Europe. Most suitable candidates are patients with primary valve disease, reoperative mitral valve disease, and obesity. Contraindications to these techniques are highly calcified mitral annulus, prior right chest surgery, or significant coronary artery disease and peripheral vascular disease. In addition to improved cosmetics, these procedures are associated with less perioperative blood loss, fewer blood transfusions, shorter intubation time and length of stay, and faster recovery.[61-63]

Level 1: Direct-Vision Minimally Invasive Mitral Valve Surgery

Direct-vision MIMVS can be performed through a ministernotomy, a parasternal incision, or through a limited anterolateral thoracotomy. CPB is instituted in a standard fashion or using the Port-Access system. The right parasternal approach is performed through a 6- to 10-cm incision overlying the second and the third costal cartilage (see Fig. 21–1*C*). Both cartilages are removed.[60] The limited anterolateral thoracotomy is accomplished through the right fourth intercostal space (see Fig. 21–1*D*). The "ministernotomy" or lower partial sternotomy is performed through a small 6- to 8-cm incision overlying distal aspect of the sternum (see Fig. 21–1*A*). The sternotomy is extended from the sternoxiphoid junction upward to the second intercostal space and extended into the right intercostal space. After the incision, a longitudinal pericardial incision is performed above the phrenic nerve. The pericardium is suspended to the skin to raise the right side of the heart. Arterial cannulation is done through the femoral artery in the parasternal and in the limited thoracotomy approaches, but it can sometimes be accomplished directly in the ascending aorta in the lower partial sternotomy approach. Venous cannulation is accomplished by direct cannulation of the SVC (with a right-angled cannula) through the incision. The IVC is cannulated with a small percutaneous transfemoral cannula advanced over a guidewire and under guidance of TEE. The aorta is usually clamped through the incision. Finally, the mitral valve is approached either directly (standard left atriotomy) or transseptally via the RA.[59]

The first MIMVS was done by the Stanford group in 1996 using the Port-Access technology.[62] Subsequently, surgeons of the University of Leipzig reported their experience of 24 mitral valve repairs done through a minithoracotomy.[39] Later, they reported a high incidence of retrograde acute aortic dissection and neurologic complications related to the Port-Access system (intra-aortic balloon occlusion).[40] The Brigham group published their experience of 1000 minimally invasive valve operations.[58] They performed 474 mitral procedures through a lower sternotomy, a right parasternal, or a right thoracotomy incision. They reported excellent results with operative and late mortality rates of 0.2% and 3.0%, respectively, and freedom from reoperation at 6 years was 95%. Compared with patients who had a full sternotomy incision, those who had a minimally invasive approach had shorter CPB and cross-clamp times, fewer myocardial infarctions, fewer pacemaker insertions, and a shorter length of stay (2 days).

Level 2: Video-Assisted and -Directed Minimally Invasive Mitral Valve Surgery

Video-assisted mitral valve surgery was developed to allow smaller incisions without compromising the results of the procedure and the patient's safety. A telescope and a thoracoscopic camera are used to perform the surgery. The camera is manipulated by an assistant under the guidance of the surgeon. Mitral valve repair and replacement are performed using assisted vision through the thoracoscope.

Carpentier was the pioneer of video-assisted MIMVS. He and his group performed the first video-assisted mitral valve repair through a minithoracotomy using hypothermic ventricular fibrillation.[64] Chitwood and his team modified the original technique, using a minithoracotomy, percutaneous transthoracic aortic occlusion, video assistance, and peripheral CPB.[65]

The patient is positioned with the right side of the chest elevated 30 to 45 degrees. External defibrillator pads are applied. The surgery starts with a 6-cm right anterolateral, inframammary incision, and a segment of the fifth rib is excised. The space obtained obviates the need for rib spreading (Fig. 21–6). CPB is accomplished with peripheral arterial perfusion and centrifugal pump venous return. Cardiac arrest is induced by means of a transthoracic aortic clamp inserted through a 4-mm incision in the third ICS, in front of the SVC, and through the transverse sinus (Fig. 21–7). Antegrade cardioplegia and aortic venting are provided by a videoscopically placed needle in the ascending aorta. Retrograde cardioplegia can also be used through the RA. A thoracoscopic camera is inserted through a port placed through the fourth or fifth ICS, and a 5-mm telescope is passed into the heart through a 4-cm left atriotomy, anterior to the superior pulmonary vein. Cross-clamp placement, valve inspection, annular suture placement, chord replacement, and knot tying are directed by thoracoscopic vision. Posterior leaflet repairs and atriotomy closure are done by direct vision.

There are benefits to the transthoracic aortic clamping over intraluminal aortic balloon occlusion (Port-Access). First, it reduces the risk of aortic dissection and of neurologic complications caused by migration of the balloon. Second, it can be used in patients with small peripheral arteries and aortoil-

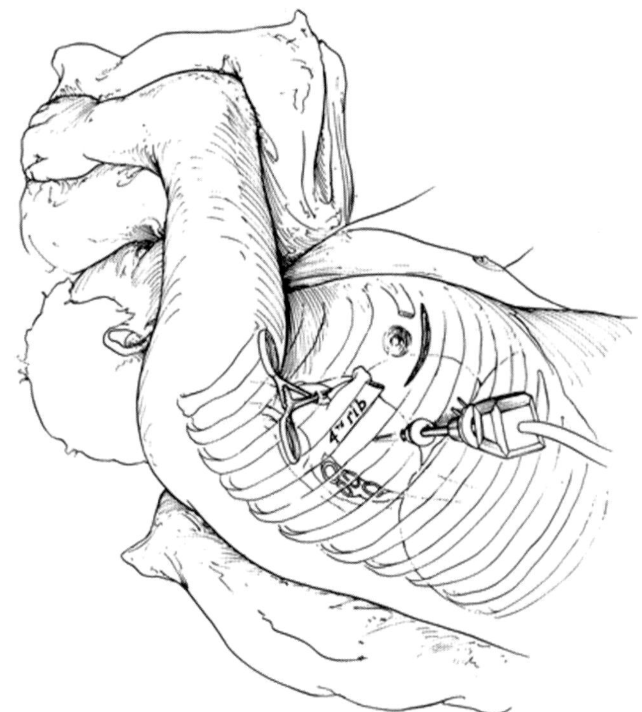

Figure 21–6 The patient positioned with the right chest elevated 30 to 45 degrees. The incision is placed in the inframammary fold over the fifth rib. The rib is excised. The 5-mm telescope and thoracoscopic camera are shown through the port in the fourth intercostal space. (From Chitwood WR Jr, Wixon CL, Elbeery JR, et al: Video-assisted minimally invasive mitral valve surgery. J Thorac Cardiovasc Surg 114:773, 1997, Fig. 2b. Copyright 1997, with permission from the American Association for Thoracic Surgery.)

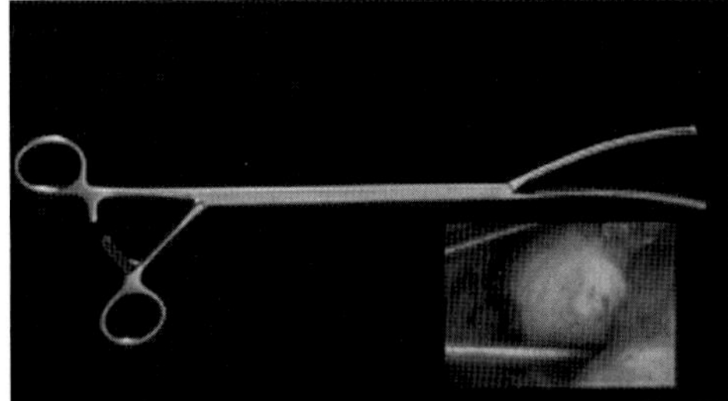

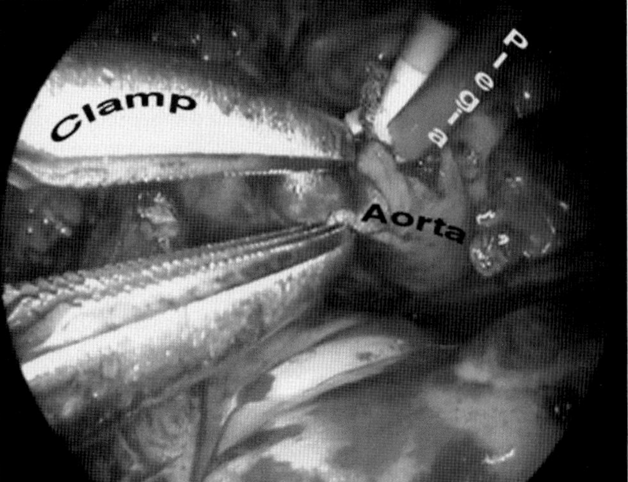

Figure 21–7 The Chitwood transthoracic aortic cross-clamp. (From Edmunds LH Jr, Cohn LH [eds]: Cardiac Surgery in the Adult. New York, McGraw-Hill, 2003, Fig. 44-13A, p 1083.)

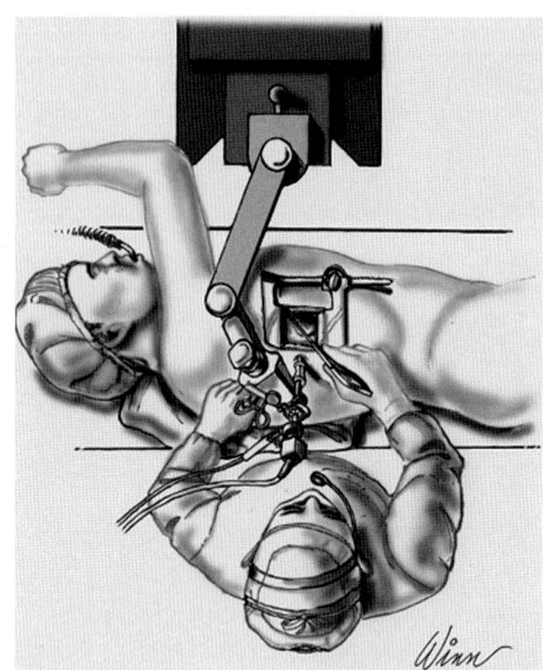

Figure 21–8 AESOP 3000 voice-activated system. Operative maneuvers are made through the 5-cm incision using long instruments and secondary instruments. (From Edmunds LH Jr, Cohn LH [eds]: Cardiac Surgery in the Adult. New York, McGraw-Hill, 2003, Fig. 44-15A, p 1085.)

iac occlusive disease. Finally, it reduces the cost associated with the Port-Access technology.

Chitwood et al[65] reported their experience with 31 consecutive patients (20 mitral repairs and 11 replacements) with excellent results. Thirty-day mortality was 3.2%. No stroke or aortic dissection was reported. Compared with patients who had conventional mitral valve surgery, these patients had significantly shorter hospitalization times, less perioperative pain, and faster recovery. In addition, hospital charges were reduced.

Level 3: Robot-Directed Minimally Invasive Mitral Valve Surgery

In robotically directed MIMVS, a voice-activated system (AESOP 3000; Computer Motion, Inc., Santa Barbara, CA) is attached to the thoracoscope. The motion of the robot is controlled by the surgeon with voice activation and one- or two-word commands (Fig. 21–8). The surgical technique is similar to the one described above for the video-assisted and -directed MIMVS. Compared with manually guided videoscopic assistance, this system provides smoother and more precise movements and zooming maneuvers and thus results in superior exposure of all valvular and subvalvular structures. It also eliminates the need for a human assistant to guide the scope.

Falk et al reported the first series of patients in 1998.[47,66] They showed that the system increased the overall performance of the procedure by allowing a full range of motion and a steady operative field and by decreasing the number of lens cleanings and, hence, operating times. Chitwood's group published their experience of robotically directed MIMVS with low mortality and morbidity. Seventy percent of the cases were repairs. They reported that the robotically directed technique showed significant decreases in blood loss, ventilator time, and hospitalization compared with the sternotomy-based technique.[67]

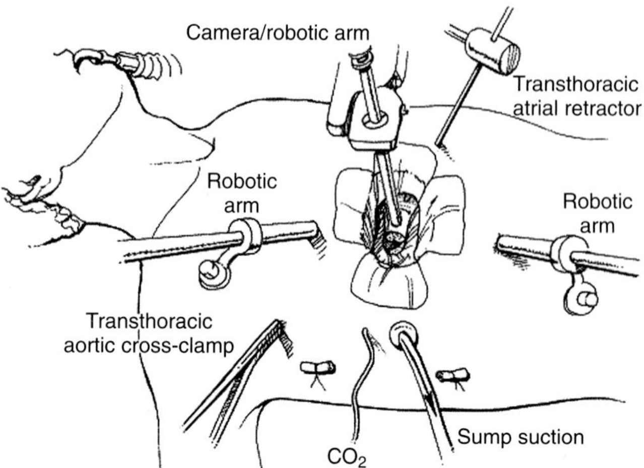

Figure 21–9 Typical setup for a robotic mitral valve repair. (From Kypson AP, Chitwood WR Jr: Robotic mitral valve surgery. Am J Surg 188[4A suppl]:83S, 2004, Fig. 1. Copyright 2004, with permission from Excerpta Medica Inc.)

Level 4: Telemanipulation and Computer-Enhanced Minimally Invasive Mitral Valve Surgery

Mitral valve surgery can now be done completely endoscopically using the DaVinci system (Intuitive Surgical, Inc., Sunnyvale, CA). This system is comprised of three components: (1) a surgeon console, (2) an instrument cart, and (3) a vision platform. The operative console is removed physically from the patient and allows the surgeon to sit comfortably. The surgeon's fingers and wrist movements are registered through sensors in computer motor banks, and then these actions are transferred to the instrument cart, which operates synchronous end-effector instruments. A three-dimensional digital visioning system enables natural depth perception with high-power magnification.

The operative approach is similar to the videoscopic mitral valve procedure using a right minithoracotomy, as previously described.[68] All patients have a preoperative TEE that guides the operative planning. Patients are anesthetized and positioned, with the right chest elevated to 30 degrees and the right arm tucked by the side. One-lung ventilation is performed to improve pericardial, aortic, and cardiac exposure. CPB is accomplished at 26°C using femoral arterial inflow. If the femoral artery is too small or diseased, a transthoracic cannula can be placed through a second right anterior ICS port. Kinetic venous drainage is provided using both a 21- to 23-F femoral view cannula to the RA and a right jugular vein (17-F) cannula. A 4- to 5-cm incision is performed and the chest is entered through the fourth intercostal space. Under direct vision, the pericardium is incised 2 cm anterior and parallel to the phrenic nerve and pulled laterally using transthoracic sutures. Antegrade cardioplegia is given by an aortic root needle/vent placed under direct vision or videoscopically. For aortic occlusion, a transthoracic cross-clamp (Scanlan International Inc., Minneapolis, MN) is passed through a 4-mm incision in the midaxillary third ICS (Fig. 21–9). Intermittent antegrade cold-blood cardioplegia is administered every 20 minutes to maintain cardiac arrest and myocardial protection. After cardioplegic arrest, a transthoracic left atrial roof retractor is used to expose the mitral valve through a 3- to 4-cm left atriotomy made medial to the right superior pulmonary vein. A right trocar is placed in the fifth ICS posterolaterally to the incision and parallel to the right inferior pulmonary vein. A left trocar is placed 6 cm cephalad and medial to the right trocar. A high-magnification (×10) camera is used with a 30-degree (looking upward), three-dimensional endoscope placed through the medial portion of the minithoracotomy. An assistant can use the remainder of the incision as a working port for needle and suture retrieval. Operative procedures are performed from the surgeon's console. Valve repairs, such as ring annuloplasty, posterior leaflet resection, sliding annuloplasty, cleft repair, chordal transfer and replacement, edge-to-edge repair (Alfieri), and valve replacements, have been reported with this technique.

Patients who are good candidates for this kind of procedure are those with isolated degenerative mitral valve disease. Exclusion criteria for robotic mitral valve surgery were described by Kypson and Chitwood[68] and are as follows: previous right thoracotomy, renal failure, liver dysfunction, bleeding disorders, severe pulmonary hypertension (PAS >60 mm Hg), significant aortic or tricuspid valve disease, coronary artery disease requiring surgery, recent myocardial infarction (<30 days), recent stroke (<30 days), and severely calcified mitral valve annulus. Patients with poor lung function undergo pulmonary testing to make sure that they can tolerate one-lung ventilation. Should they not be able to tolerate it, CPB is instituted earlier for intrathoracic preparation.

In 1998, Carpentier et al[69] in Paris and Mohr et al[40] in Leipzig performed the first truly endoscopic mitral valve repair using the early prototype of the DaVinci Surgical System. In North America, the first case was done by Chitwood and colleagues in 2000.[70] This latter team has completed more than 150 robotic mitral valve repairs with the DaVinci system. They had 1 operative death (0.67%) and 2 (1.3%) late deaths, and reoperations had to be performed on 4 patients (2.7%) for midterm valve failure.[68,71]

OTHER MINIMALLY INVASIVE CARDIAC PROCEDURES

In addition to coronary revascularization and valve repair or replacement, advances in robotic technology and imaging systems have enabled the application of minimally invasive techniques in congenital (pediatric and adult) heart surgery, arrhythmia surgery, and ventricular resynchronization procedures.

Congenital Heart Surgery

In pediatric cardiac surgery, current robotic systems have been used primarily to facilitate thoracoscopic pediatric procedures on extracardiac lesions, such as ligation of patent ductus arteriosus (PDA) and division of vascular rings.[72] With the present technology, patients weighing less than 15 kg cannot undergo a robotically assisted surgery because the instruments are too big and occupy the entire ICS of most small infants. To date, only one clinical report of a robotically assisted procedure for PDA ligation in children by Le Bret and colleagues[73] and a report on a robotically assisted division of vascular rings by Mihaljevic et al[74] have been published.

Le Bret and associates[73] compared a robotically assisted technique for PDA closure with the standard video-assisted thoracoscopic surgery (VATS) (n = 28 in each group). The procedure was performed through the left chest and with the Zeus system (Intuitive Surgical Inc., Sunnyvale, CA) with a voice-activated arm for scope holding and two additional arms for instrument control for the robotically assisted technique. The operative time was significantly longer in the robotically assisted group and the mean hospital stay was the same (3 days). The authors concluded that a robotic approach for PDA interruption in children offers no particular advantage over the VATS technique.

Mihaljevic and colleagues[74] reported the successful use of the DaVinci Surgical System for the division of a vascular ring in two patients (8 and 10 years old). Both patients' recovery was excellent, and the length of their postoperative hospital stay was short compared with that required for a conventional thoracotomy approach. The surgeons experienced enhanced intracorporeal dexterity, optimized hand-eye alignment, and tremor filtering, making tissue handling and dissection easy and accurate. For these reasons, they concluded that robotic surgical systems offer significant advantages in terms of safety.

Intracardiac lesion repair had been performed by robotically assisted surgery in the adult population (see Chapter 22). Argenziano et al[75] reported a series of 17 patients (12 secundum-type ASDs and 5 patent foramen ovales [PFOs]). Patients included were aged between 18 and 80 years old, had a Q_p:Q_s greater than 1.5, or a PFO with a documented neurologic event. Patients excluded were those who could not tolerate one-lung ventilation, those with severe peripheral vascular disease, and those with dense right pleural adhesions. After induction, left-sided single ventilation was performed, a TEE probe was inserted, and bilateral arterial monitoring catheters were inserted to facilitate monitoring of the endoaortic balloon positioning. The patients were placed in a modified left lateral decubitus position, with the right arm either suspended above the head or tucked at the side. The pelvis was placed flat to facilitate femoral cannulation. After systemic heparinization, the femoral vessels were cannulated, with the tip of the venous cannula advanced to the junction of the IVC and the RA. A percutaneous right internal jugular vein cannula was inserted and echocardiographically guided to the junction of the SVC and the RA. After establishment of selective left-lung ventilation, a port incision was made in the fourth ICS in the midclavicular line and a 12-mm trocar inserted. Two more 8-mm incisions were made in the third and sixth ICS, in the anterior axillary line. A fourth port was made (15 mm) in the fifth ICS in the posterior axillary line, for use as a service entrance. A pericardiotomy was performed and pericardial stay sutures placed. Caval snares were placed to avoid flooding of blood into the RA. CPB was initiated and the patient was cooled to 32°C. The endoaortic balloon was inflated and antegrade cardioplegia was administered through the distal cannula port. After cardiac arrest, a right atriotomy was created, the ASD or the PFO presence was confirmed, and the entire fossa was closed with a double-layer primary suture technique. Before tying the atrial suture, the left atrium was deaired by inflating the left lung. After the suture was tied, the endoaortic balloon was deflated, the patient was rewarmed, the right atriotomy was closed, and the patient was weaned from CPB. Argenziano et al reported no mortality, median aortic cross-clamp and CPB times of 32 and 122 minutes, respectively, and a successful repair rate of 94% (16 of 17). They also reported that this technique hastened postoperative recovery and improved quality of life.[76] Finally, Bacha and colleagues[77] reported the first robotically assisted sinus venosus defect repair in a 40-year-old man. The sinus venosus defect was closed with a glutaraldehyde-treated pericardial patch sutured over the inferior portion with figure-of-eight sutures of 4-0 polypropylene and then over the superior-anterior aspect (limbus) with nitinol U-clips.

Surgery for Atrial Fibrillation

Robotic telemanipulation systems have also been used to perform surgery for atrial fibrillation (AF) and ventricular resynchronization (see Chapters 13 and 25). Surgical treatment of AF allows elimination of the arrhythmia in two ways: first, creation of a contiguous encircling lesion around the pulmonary veins that prohibits the propagation of current and future foci of automaticity from the pulmonary veins and, second, creation of linear lesions in other parts of the atrium designed to interrupt potential macroreentrant circuits.[78] Pulmonary vein isolation with a mitral valve annulus connecting lesion can be performed during concomitant open procedures utilizing CPB and direct access to the left atrial endocardium. On a beating heart, pulmonary vein isolation is achieved by the application of a chosen ablative energy source on the epicardium of the closed left atrium. Two sets of lesions are currently described. The first lesion set comprises one contiguous encircling lesion around all pulmonary veins that traverses along the interatrial groove, posterior to the SVC, along the transverse and the oblique sinuses, posterior to the IVC, and returning in the interatrial groove. The second lesion set isolates the left and the right pulmonary veins, separately forming two ovals with an additional lesion that connects the ovals at the point of their closest proximity. The mitral annulus lesion repair is performed less often in beating heart surgery due to the immediate proximity of the circumflex artery. The ablative procedure is completed by amputation or suture exclusion of the left atrial appendage to decrease the risks of thromboembolism. It can be accomplished by ligation from within during open procedures and by resection or stapling techniques during epicardial procedures.

Minimally invasive techniques for the surgical treatment of AF are described as procedures that eliminate large chest incisions and CPB. Pulmonary vein isolation can be accomplished through a minithoracotomy in patients undergoing mitral valve procedures or ASD repair. The endocardial ablation can be performed using different energy sources. The ablation can also be done epicardially through the same incision with microwave energy with a special probe (Flex-10; Fig. 21–10) that can be easily manipulated and placed on the atrium in the intended lesion pattern. The Flex-10 probe can also be positioned epicardially around the four pulmonary veins, via a right minithoracotomy, with left thoracoscopy to confirm probe position, and to carry out left atrial appendage resection. The next lower level of invasiveness is epicardial pulmonary vein isolation completed endoscopically with robotic assistance (DaVinci system) and through three right thoracoscopic ports. Garrido and colleagues recently performed their first totally endoscopic, off-pump human AF epicardial ablation, using robotic assistance. The patient, who has been in AF for 20 years, remained in normal sinus rhythm after 3 months.

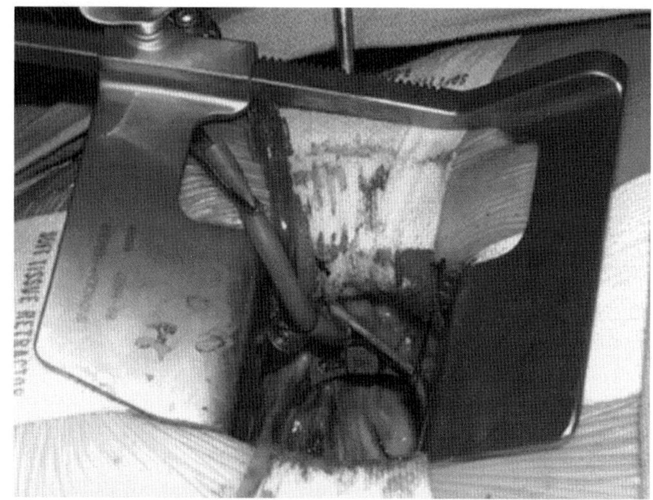

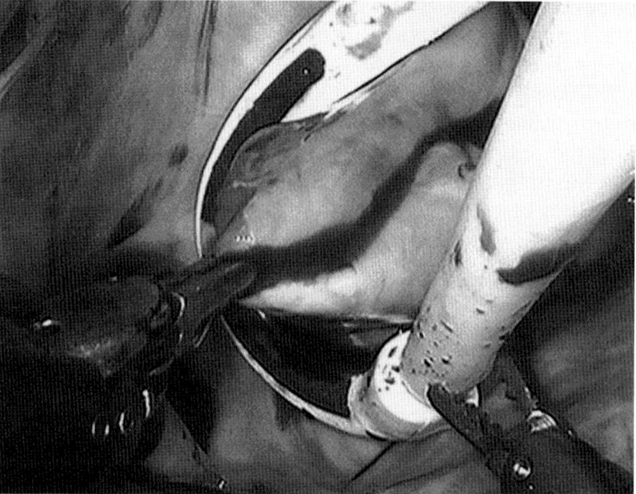

Figure 21–10 Robotically assisted atrial fibrillation ablation. (From DeRose JJ Jr, Kypson AP: Robotic arrhythmia surgery and resynchronization. Am J Surg 188[suppl]:104S, 2004. Copyright 2004, with permission from Excerpta Medica Inc.)

Cardiac Resynchronization

Close to 30% of patients diagnosed with congestive heart failure exhibit significant ventricular dyssynchrony secondary to alterations in intraventricular conduction. Also, alterations in the timing between LV and right ventricle (RV) contraction may exacerbate heart failure symptoms. Prospective randomized trials have demonstrated improvements in ventricular function, exercise capacity, and quality of life among patients undergoing ventricular resynchronization therapy via LV and RV pacing. Usually, transvenous biventricular pacing is performed by placing standard endocardial RA and RV leads. The LV lead is positioned through the coronary sinus, in one of the venous tributaries. However, technical limitations secondary to individual variations in coronary sinus anatomy result in a 10% to 15% failure rate of LV lead positioning. When percutaneous lead placement was unsuccessful, LV lead placement used to be done through a limited anterior thoracotomy. However, DeRose and Kypson[79] developed the robotic, totally endoscopic approach for posterolateral lead placement in patients with failure of coronary sinus cannulation.

Robotic approaches to resynchronization are typically best performed in the full posterolateral thoracotomy position. This procedure is performed under general anesthesia with selective right-lung ventilation. A camera port is placed in the seventh ICS in the posterior axillary line. The left and right arms of the robot are positioned in the ninth and the fifth ICS, respectively (Fig. 21–11). A 10-mm working port is inserted posterior to the camera port and is used for the introduction of the leads and sutures. The pericardium is opened posterior to the phrenic nerve, retracted posteriorly with sutures, and

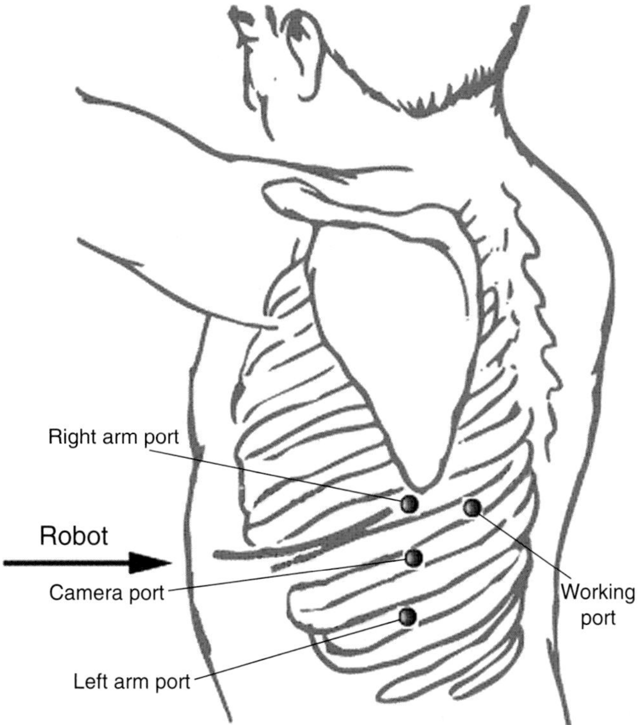

Figure 21–11 Port location and patient position for robotic left ventricular epicardial lead placement via the posterior approach. (From DeRose JJ Jr, Kypson AP: Robotic arrhythmia surgery and resynchronization. Am J Surg 188[suppl]:104S, 2004, Fig. 4. Copyright 2004, with permission from Excerpta Medica Inc.)

the first and the second obtuse marginal vessels are identified. A pacing lead is then introduced into the chest through the working port. The LV surface is mapped for threshold resistance and lateness within the native QRS. The robotic arms are used to fix a lead to the LV surface via either screw-in fixation or suture technique. This lead is capped and delivered into the chest. The second lead is positioned the same way. The pericardium is then closed over the leads to aid in permanent fixation. The first lead is retrieved from the chest through the right arm port. Both leads are then tunneled to an incision in the axilla. A chest tube is placed through the left arm port for evacuation of air and is removed before leaving the operating room. The port sites are closed, and the lead thresholds are determined. The one with the best threshold is used as a pacing lead and is connected to the device, and the second lead is secured to the fascia as a backup lead for the future. DeRose and Kypson[79] reported a series of 35 patients, including 19 patients who had undergone at least one previous heart operation, with no mortality and no conversion to thoracotomy.

CONCLUSIONS

Minimally invasive cardiac surgery spans a wide spectrum of procedures on nearly any cardiothoracic structure. The anesthetic management of patients undergoing these procedures requires detailed knowledge of the technical aspects of the surgery along with expertise in a variety of procedures and techniques that are not typically required in conventional cardiac surgery.

REFERENCES

1. Grocott HP, Mathew JP, Carver EH, et al: A randomized controlled trial of the Arctic Sun Temperature Management System versus conventional methods for preventing hypothermia during off-pump cardiac surgery. Anesth Analg 98:298, 2004
2. Ohtsuka T, Imanaka K, Endoh M, et al: Hemodynamic effects of carbon dioxide insufflation under single-lung ventilation during thoracoscopy. Ann Thorac Surg 68:29; discussion 32, 1999
3. Vassiliades TA Jr: The cardiopulmonary effects of single-lung ventilation and carbon dioxide insufflation during thoracoscopic internal mammary artery harvesting. Heart Surg Forum 5:22, 2002
4. Myles PS, Daly DJ, Djaiani G, et al: A systematic review of the safety and effectiveness of fast-track cardiac anesthesia. Anesthesiology 99:982, 2003
5. Myles PS, McIlroy D: Fast-track cardiac anesthesia: Choice of anesthetic agents and techniques. Semin Cardiothorac Vasc Anesth 9:5, 2005
6. Ahonen J, Olkkola KT, Verkkala K, et al: A comparison of remifentanil and alfentanil for use with propofol in patients undergoing minimally invasive coronary artery bypass surgery. Anesth Analg 90:1269, 2000
7. Royse CF, Royse AG, Soeding PF: Routine immediate extubation after cardiac operation: A review of our first 100 patients. Ann Thorac Surg 68:1326, 1999
8. Straka Z, Brucek P, Vanek T, et al: Routine immediate extubation for off-pump coronary artery bypass grafting without thoracic epidural analgesia. Ann Thorac Surg 74:1544, 2002
9. Lee TW, Jacobsohn E: Pro: Tracheal extubation should occur routinely in the operating room after cardiac surgery. J Cardiothorac Vasc Anesth 14:603, 2000
10. Montes FR, Sanchez SI, Giraldo JC, et al: The lack of benefit of tracheal extubation in the operating room after coronary artery bypass surgery. Anesth Analg 91:776, 2000
11. Peragallo RA, Cheng DC: Con: tracheal extubation should not occur routinely in the operating room after cardiac surgery. J Cardiothorac Vasc Anesth 14:611, 2000
12. Stritesky M, Semrad M, Kunstyr J, et al: On-pump cardiac surgery in a conscious patient using a thoracic epidural anesthesia—an ultra fast track method. Bratisl Lek Listy 105:51, 2004
13. Meininger D, Neidhart G, Bremerich DH, et al: Coronary artery bypass grafting via sternotomy in conscious patients. World J Surg 27:534, 2003
14. Aybek T, Dogan S, Neidhart G, et al: Coronary artery bypass grafting through complete sternotomy in conscious patients. Heart Surg Forum 5:17; discussion 20, 2002
15. Trehan N, Malhotra R, Mishra Y, et al: Comparison of ministernotomy with minithoracotomy regarding postoperative pain and internal mammary artery characteristics. Heart Surg Forum 3:300, 2000
16. Niinami H, Ogasawara H, Suda Y, et al: Single-vessel revascularization with minimally invasive direct coronary artery bypass: Minithoracotomy or ministernotomy? Chest 127:47, 2005
17. Bucerius J, Metz S, Walther T, et al: Endoscopic internal thoracic artery dissection leads to significant reduction of pain after minimally invasive direct coronary artery bypass graft surgery. Ann Thorac Surg 73:1180, 2002
18. Grossi EA, Zakow PK, Ribakove G, et al: Comparison of postoperative pain, stress response, and quality of life in port access vs. standard sternotomy coronary bypass patients. Eur J Cardiothorac Surg 16(suppl 2):S39, 1999
19. Walther T, Falk V, Metz S, et al: Pain and quality of life after minimally invasive versus conventional cardiac surgery. Ann Thorac Surg 67:1643, 1999
20. Parlow JL, Steele RG, O'Reilly D: Low dose intrathecal morphine facilitates early extubation after cardiac surgery: Results of a retrospective continuous quality improvement audit. Can J Anaesth 52:94, 2005
21. Bowler I, Djaiani G, Abel R, et al: A combination of intrathecal morphine and remifentanil anesthesia for fast-track cardiac anesthesia and surgery. J Cardiothorac Vasc Anesth 16:709, 2002
22. Boulanger A, Perreault S, Choiniere M, et al: Intrathecal morphine after cardiac surgery. Ann Pharmacother 36:1337, 2002
23. Kessler P, Aybek T, Neidhart G, et al: Comparison of three anesthetic techniques for off-pump coronary artery bypass grafting: general anesthesia, combined general and high thoracic epidural anesthesia, or high thoracic epidural anesthesia alone. J Cardiothorac Vasc Anesth 19:32, 2005
24. Pastor MC, Sanchez MJ, Casas MA, et al: Thoracic epidural analgesia in coronary artery bypass graft surgery: Seven years' experience. J Cardiothorac Vasc Anesth 17:154, 2003
25. Debreceni G, Molnar Z, Szelig L, et al: Continuous epidural or intercostal analgesia following thoracotomy: A prospective randomized double-blind clinical trial. Acta Anaesthesiol Scand 47:1091, 2003

26. Bucerius J, Metz S, Walther T, et al: Pain is significantly reduced by cryoablation therapy in patients with lateral minithoracotomy. Ann Thorac Surg 70:1100, 2000
27. Dowling R, Thielmeier K, Ghaly A, et al: Improved pain control after cardiac surgery. J Thor Cardiovasc Surg 126:1271, 2003
28. Moorjani N, Zhao F, Tian Y, et al: Effects of cryoanalgesia on post-thoracotomy pain and on the structure of intercostal nerves: A human prospective randomized trial and a histological study. Eur J Cardiothorac Surg 20:502, 2001
29. Ceriana P, Pagnin A, Locatelli A, et al: Monitoring aspects during Port-Access cardiac surgery. J Cardiovasc Surg (Torino) 41:579, 2000
30. Muhs BE, Galloway AC, Lombino M, et al: Arterial injuries from femoral artery cannulation with port access cardiac surgery. Vasc Endovasc Surg 39:153, 2005
31. Coddens J, Callebaut F, Hendrickx J, et al: Case 5, Port-access cardiac surgery and aortic dissection: The role of transesophageal echocardiography. J Cardiothorac Vasc Anesth 15:251, 2001
32. Banbury MK, White JA, Blackstone EH, et al: Vacuum-assisted venous return reduces blood usage. J Thorac Cardiovasc Surg 126:680, 2003
33. Carrier M, Cyr A, Voisine P, et al: Vacuum-assisted venous drainage does not increase the neurological risk. Heart Surg Forum 5:285, 2002
34. Mueller XM, Tevaearai HT, Horisberger J, et al: Vacuum assisted venous drainage does not increase trauma to blood cells. ASAIO J 47:651, 2001
35. Kurusz M, Butler BD: Bubbles and bypass: An update. Perfusion 19(suppl 1):S49, 2004
36. Jones TJ, Deal DD, Vernon JC, et al: Does vacuum-assisted venous drainage increase gaseous microemboli during cardiopulmonary bypass? Ann Thorac Surg 74:2132, 2002
37. Willcox TW: Vacuum-assisted venous drainage: To air or not to air, that is the question. Has the bubble burst? J Extra Corpor Technol 34:24, 2002
38. Cirri S, Negri L, Babbini M, et al: Haemolysis due to active venous drainage during cardiopulmonary bypass: Comparison of two different techniques. Perfusion 16:313, 2001
39. Falk V, Walther T, Diegeler A, et al: Echocardiographic monitoring of minimally invasive mitral valve surgery using an endoaortic clamp. J Heart Valve Dis 5:630, 1996
40. Mohr FW, Falk V, Diegeler A, et al: Minimally invasive Port-Access mitral valve surgery. J Thorac Cardiovasc Surg 115:567; discussion 574, 1998
41. Kalpokas MV, Nixon IK, Kluger R, et al: Carbon dioxide field flooding versus mechanical de-airing during open-heart surgery: A prospective randomized controlled trial. Perfusion 18:291, 2003
42. Webb WR, Harrison LH Jr, Helmcke FR, et al: Carbon dioxide field flooding minimizes residual intracardiac air after open heart operations. Ann Thorac Surg 64:1489, 1997
43. Dullum MKC, Pfister AJ: The MIDCAB operation. *In* Goldstein DJ, Oz MC (eds): Minimally Invasive Cardiac Surgery. Totowa, NJ, Humana Press, 2003, p 113
44. Calafiore AM, Contini M: Minimally invasive cardiac surgery on the beating heart: The European experience. *In* Goldstein DJ, Oz MC (eds): Minimally Invasive Cardiac Surgery. Totowa, NJ, Humana Press, 2003, p 129
45. Mack MJ, Magovern JA, Acuff TA, et al: Results of graft patency by immediate angiography in minimally invasive coronary artery surgery. Ann Thorac Surg 68:383; discussion 389, 1999
46. Wimmer-Greinecker G, Deschka H, Aybek T, et al: Current status of robotically assisted coronary revascularization. Am J Surg 188(4A suppl):76S, 2004
47. Mohr FW, Falk V, Diegeler A, et al: Computer-enhanced "robotic" cardiac surgery: Experience in 148 patients. J Thorac Cardiovasc Surg 121:842, 2001
48. Dogan S, Aybek T, Andressen E, et al: Totally endoscopic coronary artery bypass grafting on cardiopulmonary bypass with robotically enhanced telemanipulation: Report of forty-five cases. J Thorac Cardiovasc Surg 123:1125, 2002
49. Byhahn C, Mierdl S, Meininger D, et al: Hemodynamics and gas exchange during carbon dioxide insufflation for totally endoscopic coronary artery bypass grafting. Ann Thorac Surg 71:1496; discussion 1501, 2001
50. Mierdl S, Byhahn C, Lischke V, et al: Segmental wall motion abnormalities during minimally invasive and endoscopic coronary artery bypass grafting. Anesth Analg 100:306, 2005
51. Loulmet D, Carpentier A, d'Attellis N, et al: Endoscopic coronary artery bypass grafting with the aid of robotic assisted instruments. J Thorac Cardiovasc Surg 118:4, 1999
52. Falk V, Diegeler A, Walther T, et al: Total endoscopic computer enhanced coronary artery bypass grafting. Eur J Cardiothorac Surg 17:38, 2000
53. Falk V, Diegeler A, Walther T, et al: Total endoscopic off-pump coronary artery bypass grafting. Heart Surg Forum 3:29, 2000
54. Kappert U, Cichon R, Schneider J, et al: Technique of closed chest coronary artery surgery on the beating heart. Eur J Cardiothorac Surg 20:765, 2001
55. Kappert U, Cichon R, Schneider J, et al: Closed-chest coronary artery surgery on the beating heart with the use of a robotic system. J Thorac Cardiovasc Surg 120:809, 2000
56. Sepic J, Cohn L: Minimally invasive aortic valve surgery. *In* Goldstein DJ, Oz MC (eds): Minimally Invasive Cardiac Surgery. Totowa, NJ, Humana Press, 2003, p 293
57. Byrne JG, Aranki SF, Couper GS, et al: Reoperative aortic valve replacement: Partial upper hemisternotomy versus conventional full sternotomy. J Thorac Cardiovasc Surg 118:991, 1999
58. Mihaljevic T, Cohn LH, Unic D, et al: One thousand minimally invasive valve operations: Early and late results. Ann Surg 240:529; discussion 534, 2004
59. Cohn LH, Adams DH, Couper GS, et al: Minimally invasive cardiac valve surgery improves patient satisfaction while reducing costs of cardiac valve replacement and repair. Ann Surg 226:421; discussion 427, 1997
60. Cosgrove DM 3rd, Sabik JF, Navia JL: Minimally invasive valve operations. Ann Thorac Surg 65:1535; discussion 1538, 1998
61. Chitwood WR Jr, Nifong LW: Minimially invasive and robotic valve surgery. *In* Edmunds LH Jr, Cohn LH (eds): Cardiac Surgery in the Adult. New York, McGraw-Hill, 2003, p 1075
62. Fann JI, Pompili MF, Burdon TA, et al: Minimally invasive mitral valve surgery. Semin Thorac Cardiovasc Surg 9:320, 1997
63. Chu VF, Nifong LW, Chitwood WR Jr: Minimally invasive mitral valve surgery. *In* Goldstein DJ, Oz MC (eds): Minimally Invasive Cardiac Surgery. Totowa, NJ, Humana Press, 2003, p 255
64. Carpentier A, Loulmet D, Carpentier A, et al: [Open heart operation under videosurgery and minithoracotomy. First case (mitral valvuloplasty) operated with success]. C R Acad Sci III 319:219, 1996
65. Chitwood WR Jr, Wixon CL, Elbeery JR, et al: Video-assisted minimally invasive mitral valve surgery. J Thorac Cardiovasc Surg 114:773; discussion 780, 1997
66. Falk V, Walther T, Autschbach R, et al: Robot-assisted minimally invasive solo mitral valve operation. J Thorac Cardiovasc Surg 115:470, 1998
67. Felger JE, Chitwood WR Jr, Nifong LW, et al: Evolution of mitral valve surgery: Toward a totally endoscopic approach. Ann Thorac Surg 72:1203; discussion 1208, 2001
68. Kypson AP, Chitwood WR Jr: Robotic mitral valve surgery. Am J Surg 188(4A suppl):83S, 2004
69. Carpentier A, Loulmet D, Aupecle B, et al: [Computer assisted open heart surgery. First case operated on with success]. C R Acad Sci III 321:437, 1998
70. Chitwood WR Jr, Nifong LW, Elbeery JE, et al: Robotic mitral valve repair: Trapezoidal resection and prosthetic annuloplasty with the DaVinci Surgical System. J Thorac Cardiovasc Surg 120:1171, 2000
71. Nifong LW, Chu VF, Bailey BM, et al: Robotic mitral valve repair: Experience with the DaVinci system. Ann Thorac Surg 75:438; discussion 443, 2003
72. Suematsu Y, del Nido PJ: Robotic pediatric cardiac surgery: Present and future perspectives. Am J Surg 188(4A suppl):98S, 2004
73. Le Bret E, Papadatos S, Folliguet T, et al: Interruption of patent ductus arteriosus in children: Robotically assisted versus videothoracoscopic surgery. J Thorac Cardiovasc Surg 123:973, 2002
74. Mihaljevic T, Cannon JW, del Nido PJ: Robotically assisted division of a vascular ring in children. J Thorac Cardiovasc Surg 125:1163, 2003
75. Argenziano M, Oz MC, Kohmoto T, et al: Totally endoscopic atrial septal defect repair with robotic assistance. Circulation 108(suppl II):II-191, 2003
76. Morgan JA, Peacock JC, Kohmoto T, et al: Robotic techniques improve quality of life in patients undergoing atrial septal defect repair. Ann Thorac Surg 77:1328, 2004
77. Bacha EA, Bolotin G, Consilio K, et al: Robotically assisted repair of sinus venosus defect. J Thorac Cardiovasc Surg 129:442, 2005
78. Garrido MJ, Williams M, Argenziano M: Minimally invasive surgery for atrial fibrillation: Toward a totally endoscopic, beating heart approach. J Card Surg 19:216, 2004
79. DeRose JJ Jr, Kypson AP: Robotic arrhythmia surgery and resynchronization. Am J Surg 188(suppl):104S, 2004

Chapter 22
CONGENITAL HEART DISEASE IN ADULTS

Victor C. Baum, MD

KEY POINTS

1. Due to surgical successes in treating congenital cardiac lesions, there are currently as many or more adults than children with congenital heart disease (CHD).
2. These patients may require cardiac surgical intervention for primary cardiac repair, repair following prior palliation, revision of repair due to failure or lack of growth of prosthetic material, or conversion of a suboptimal repair to a more modern operation.
3. These patients will be encountered by noncardiac anesthesiologists for a vast array of ailments and injuries requiring surgery.
4. If at all possible, noncardiac surgery on adult patients with moderate-to-complex CHD should be done at an adult congenital heart center with the consultation of an anesthesiologist experienced with adult CHD.
5. Delegation of one anesthesiologist as the liaison with the cardiology service for preoperative evaluation and triage of adult CHD patients will be helpful.
6. All relevant cardiac tests and evaluations should be reviewed in advance.
7. Sketching out the anatomy and path(s) of blood flow is often an easy and enlightening aid in simplifying apparently very complex lesions.

Advances in perioperative care for children with congenital heart disease (CHD) over the past several decades has resulted in an ever-increasing number of these children reaching adulthood with their cardiac lesions palliated or repaired. The first paper on adult CHD was published in 1973; the field has grown such that there is now a text devoted to it, and even a specialty society dedicated to it, the International Society for Adult Congenital Cardiac Disease (http://www.isaccd.org).[1,2] There are estimated to be about 32,000 new cases of CHD each year in the United States and 1.5 million worldwide.[3] More than 85% of infants born with CHD are expected to grow to adulthood. It is estimated that there are more than 500,000 adults in the United States with CHD; 55% of these adults remain at moderate-to-high risk, and more than 115,000 have complex disease.[4] Put another way, there are as many adults with CHD as there are children, and the number of adults will only continue to increase.[5] These patients can be seen by anesthesiologists for primary cardiac repair, repair following a prior palliation, revision of repair due to failure or lack of growth of prosthetic material, or conversion of a suboptimal repair to a more modern operation (Box 22–1). In addition, these adults with CHD will be seen for all the other ailments of aging and trauma that require surgical intervention. Although it has been suggested that teenagers and adults can have repair of congenital cardiac defects with morbidity and mortality approaching that of surgery done during childhood, these data are limited and may reflect only a relatively young and acyanotic sampling.[6] Other data suggest that, in general, adults over 50 years of age represent an excessive proportion of the early postoperative mortality encountered, and the number of previous operations and cyanosis are both risk factors.[7] Risk factors for noncardiac surgery include heart failure, pulmonary hypertension, and cyanosis.[8]

These patients bring with them anatomic and physiologic complexities of which physicians accustomed to caring for adults may be unaware, and medical problems associated with aging or pregnancy that might not be familiar to physicians used to caring for children. This problem has led to the establishment of the growing subspecialty of adult CHD. There have been two Bethesda conferences devoted to the issue, most recently in 2001.[5] An informed anesthesiologist is a critical member of the team required to care optimally for these patients. A specific recommendation of that conference was that noncardiac surgery on adult patients with moderate-to-complex CHD be done at an adult congenital heart center (regional centers) with the consultation of an anesthesiologist experienced with adult CHD.[5,9] In fact, one of the founding fathers of the subspecialty wrote: "A cardiac anesthesiologist with experience in CHD is pivotal.... The cardiac anesthesiologist and the attending cardiologist are more important than the noncardiac surgeon."[3] Centers may find it helpful to delegate one attending anesthesiologist to be the liaison with the cardiology service to centralize preoperative evaluations and triage of patients to an anesthesiologist with specific expertise in managing patients with CHD, rather than random consultations with generalist anesthesiologists.

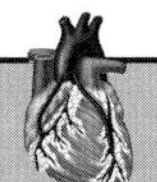

BOX 22–1 ***Indications for Cardiac Surgery in Adults With CHD***

- Primary repair
- Total correction following palliation
- Revision of total correction
- Conversion of suboptimal obsolescent operation into more modern repair

GENERAL NONCARDIAC ISSUES WITH LONGSTANDING CONGENITAL HEART DISEASE

A variety of organ systems can be affected by longstanding CHD; these are summarized in Table 22–1 and Box 22–2. Because congenital cardiac disease can be one manifestation of a multiorgan genetic or dysmorphic syndrome, all patients require a full review of systems and examination.

Table 22–1 Potential Noncardiac Organ Involvement in Patients With Congenital Heart Disease

Potential Respiratory Implications
Decreased compliance (with increased pulmonary blood flow or impediment to pulmonary venous drainage)
Compression of airways by large, hypertensive pulmonary arteries
Compression of bronchioles
Scoliosis
Hemoptysis (with end-stage Eisenmenger syndrome)
Phrenic nerve injury (prior thoracic surgery)
Recurrent laryngeal nerve injury (prior thoracic surgery; very rarely from encroachment of cardiac structures)
Blunted ventilatory response to hypoxemia (with cyanosis)
Underestimation of Pa_{CO_2} by capnometry in cyanotic patients
Potential Hematologic Implications
Symptomatic hyperviscosity
Bleeding diathesis
Abnormal von Willebrand factor
Artifactually elevated prothrombin/partial thromboplastin times with erythrocytic blood
Artifactual thrombocytopenia with erythrocytic blood
Gallstones
Potential Renal Implication
Hyperuricemia and arthralgias (with cyanosis)
Potential Neurologic Implications
Paradoxic emboli
Brain abscess (with right-to-left shunts)
Seizure (from old brain abscess focus)
Intrathoracic nerve injury (iatrogenic phrenic, recurrent laryngeal, or sympathetic trunk injury)

Pulmonary

Any lesion that results in either increased pulmonary blood flow or pulmonary venous obstruction can cause increased pulmonary interstitial fluid with decreased pulmonary compliance and increased work of breathing.[10] Patients with cyanotic heart disease have increased minute ventilation and maintain normocarbia.[11] These patients have a normal ventilatory response to hypercapnea but a blunted response to hypoxemia that normalizes after corrective surgery and the establishment of normoxia.[12-14] End-tidal CO_2 underestimates arterial Pa_{CO_2} in cyanotic patients with decreased, normal, or even increased pulmonary blood flow.[15]

Although enlarged hypertensive pulmonary arteries or an enlarged left atrium can impinge on bronchi in children, this is rare in adults. Late-stage Eisenmenger syndrome can result in hemoptysis, and patients with Eisenmenger physiology and erythrocytosis can develop thrombosis of upper lobe pulmonary arteries.[16] Prior thoracic surgery could have injured the phrenic nerve with resultant diaphragmatic paresis or paralysis.

Scoliosis can occur in up to 19% of CHD patients, most commonly in cyanotic patients. It can also develop in adolescence, years after surgical resolution of cyanosis.[17] The relative contributions of cyanosis and early lateral thoracotomy remain unclear. Scoliosis is rarely severe enough to impact respiratory function.

In an attempt to increase pulmonary blood flow, large collateral vessels originating from the aorta may have developed. These are sometimes embolized in the catheterization laboratory prior to thoracic surgery to prevent excessive intraoperative blood loss.

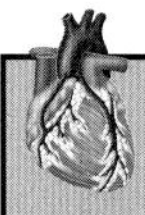

BOX 22–2 *Noncardiac Organ Systems With Potential Involvement by Longstanding CHD*

- Pulmonary
- Hematologic
- Renal
- Neurologic
- Vasculature
- Genitourinary (pregnancy)
- Psychosocial

Hematologic

Hematologic manifestations of chronic CHD are primarily a consequence of longstanding cyanosis and incorporate abnormalities of both hemostasis and red cell regulation. Longstanding hypoxemia causes increased erythropoietin production in the kidney and resultant increased red cell mass. Because solely red cell production is affected, these patients are correctly referred to as erythrocytotic rather than polycythemic. There is, however, a fairly poor relationship among oxygen saturation, red cell mass, and 2,3-diphosphoglycerate.[18] The oxygen–hemoglobin dissociation curve is normal or minimally shifted to the right. Most patients have established an equilibrium state at which they have a stable hematocrit and are iron replete. Some patients, however, develop excessive hematocrits and are iron deficient, causing a hyperviscous state. Iron-deficient red cells are less deformable and cause increased viscosity for the same hematocrit.[19] Symptoms of hyperviscosity typically develop only at hematocrits exceeding 65% providing the patient is iron replete. Iron deficiency also shifts the oxygen–hemoglobin dissociation curve to the right, decreasing oxygen affinity in the lungs.[20] Symptoms of hyperviscosity are listed in Box 22–3. Iron deficiency can be the

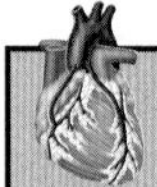

BOX 22–3 *Symptoms of Hyperviscosity*

- Headache
- Faintness, dizziness, light-headedness
- Blurred or double vision
- Fatigue
- Myalgias, muscle weakness
- Paresthesias of fingers, toes, or lips
- Depressed or dissociative mentation

result of misguided attempts to lower the hematocrit by means of repeated phlebotomies. The red cells in these patients will be hypochromic and microcytic despite the high hematocrit. Treatment with oral iron needs to be undertaken with care, as rapid increases in hematocrit can result.

Symptomatic hyperviscosity is the indication for treatment to temporarily relieve symptoms. It is not indicated to treat otherwise asymptomatic elevated hematocrits. Treatment is by means of a partial isovolumic exchange transfusion, and it is assumed that the increased hematocrit is not related to dehydration. Partial isovolumic exchange transfusion usually results in regression of symptoms within 24 hours. It is rare to require exchange of more than 1 unit of blood. Preoperatively, phlebotomized blood can be banked for autologous perioperative retransfusion if required. Elective preoperative isovolumic exchange transfusion has decreased the incidence of hemorrhagic complications of surgery.[21,22]

Hyperviscosity and erythrocytosis can cause cerebral venous thrombosis in younger children, but it is not a problem in adults, regardless of the hematocrit.[16] Protracted preoperative fasts need to be avoided in erythrocytotic patients, as they can be accompanied by rapid elevations in the hematocrit.

A variety of clotting abnormalities have been described in association with cyanotic CHD, although none uniformly.[23] Bleeding dyscrasias are uncommon until the hematocrit exceeds 65%, although excessive surgical bleeding can occur at lower hematocrits. Generally, higher hematocrits are associated with a greater bleeding diathesis. Abnormalities of a variety of factors in both the intrinsic and extrinsic coagulation pathways have been described inconsistently. Both cyanotic and acyanotic patients have been reported with deficiencies of the largest von Willebrand factor multimers, which have normalized following reparative surgery.[24] Fibrinolytic pathways are normal.[25]

The decreased plasma volume in erythrocytic blood can result in spuriously elevated measures of the prothrombin and partial thromboplastin times, and the fixed amount of anticoagulant will be excessive, as it presumes a normal plasma volume in the blood sample. Erythrocytic blood has more red cells and less plasma in the same volume. If informed in advance of a patient's hematocrit, the clinical laboratory can provide an appropriate sample tube. Normalizing to a hematocrit of 45%, the amount of citrate added to the tube can be calculated:

$$\text{mL citrate} = (0.1 \times \text{blood volume collected}) \times [(100 - \text{patient's hematocrit})/55]$$

Platelet counts are typically normal or occasionally low, but bleeding is not due to thrombocytopenia. Platelets are reported per milliliter of blood, not milliliter of plasma. When corrected for the decreased plasma fraction in erythrocytic blood, the total plasma platelet count is closer to normal. That said, abnormalities in platelet function and life span have on occasion been reported.[26,27] Patients with low-pressure conduits or synthetic vascular anastomoses are often maintained on antiplatelet drugs.

Cyanotic erythrocytotic patients have excessive hemoglobin turnover, and adults have an increased incidence of calcium bilirubinate gallstones. Biliary colic can develop years after cyanosis has been resolved by cardiac surgery.[16]

A variety of mechanical factors can also affect excessive surgical bleeding in cyanotic CHD patients. These factors include increased tissue capillary density, elevated systemic venous pressure, aortopulmonary and transpleural collaterals that have developed to increase pulmonary blood flow, and prior thoracic surgery. Aprotinin and ε-aminocaproic acid improve postoperative hemostasis in patients with cyanotic CHD.[28] The results with tranexamic acid have been mixed.[29]

Renal

Adult patients with cyanotic CHD can develop abnormal renal histology with hypercellular glomeruli and basement membrane thickening, focal interstitial fibrosis, tubular atrophy, and hyalinized afferent and efferent arterioles.[30] Cyanotic CHD is often accompanied by elevations in plasma uric acid levels that are due to inappropriately low fractional uric acid excretion.[31] Decreased urate reabsorption is thought to result from renal hypoperfusion with a high filtration fraction. Despite the elevated uric acid levels, urate stones and urate nephropathy are rare.[32] Although arthralgias are common, true gouty arthritis is less frequent than would be expected from the degree of hyperuricemia.[31] There appears to be an increased incidence of post–cardiopulmonary bypass renal dysfunction in adults with longstanding cyanosis.[33]

Neurologic

Adults with persistent or potential intracardiac shunts remain at risk for paradoxic embolism. Paradoxic emboli can occur even through shunts that are predominantly left-to-right, because during the cardiac cycle there can be small transient reversals of the shunt direction. It has been said that, unlike in children, adults with cyanotic CHD are not at risk for the development of cerebral thrombosis despite the hematocrit.[16,34] However, this assertion has been challenged by Ammash and Warnes,[35] who suggested an association of stroke not with red cell mass, but with iron deficiency and repeated venesection. Adults do, however, remain at risk for the development of brain abscess. A healed childhood brain abscess can provide the nidus for the development of seizures throughout life.

Prior thoracic surgery can result in permanent peripheral nerve damage. Surgery at the apices of the lungs is particularly associated with the risk of nerve damage. These operations would include Blalock-Taussig shunts, ligation of patent ductus arteriosus (PDA), banding of the pulmonary artery, and repair of aortic coarctation. Nerves that are susceptible to injury include the recurrent laryngeal nerve, the phrenic nerve, and the sympathetic chain.

Vasculature

Vessel abnormalities can be congenital or iatrogenic. They can affect the suitability of vessels for cannulation by the anesthesiologist or measurement of correct pressures. These abnormalities are described in Table 22–2.

Pregnancy

The physiologic changes of pregnancy, labor, and delivery can significantly alter the physiologic status of women with CHD. There are several texts available that specifically discuss issues of the pregnant woman with CHD in more detail than is possible here.[2,36,37] Management and clinical outcomes during pregnancy and delivery for several cardiac lesions are included under the discussions of those lesions later.

Successful pregnancy to term with vaginal delivery is possible for most patients with congenital defects. High-risk factors for mother and fetus include pulmonary arterial

Table 22–2 Potential Vascular Access Issues

Vessel	Possible Problem
Femoral vein(s)	May have been ligated if cardiac catheterization was done by cutdown. Large therapeutic catheters in infants often thrombose femoral veins.
Inferior vena cava	Some lesions, particularly when associated with heterotaxy (polysplenia), have discontinuity of the inferior vena cava. Will not be able to pass a catheter from the groin to the right atrium.
Left subclavian and pedal arteries	Distal blood pressure will be low in the presence of coarctation of the aorta or following subclavian flap repair (subclavian artery only), and variably so if postoperative recoarctation. Pulses can be absent or palpable with abnormal blood pressure.
Subclavian artery	Blood pressure low with classic Blalock-Taussig shunt on that side, and variably so with modified Blalock-Taussig shunt.
Right subclavian artery	Blood pressure artifactually high with supravalvular aortic stenosis (Coanda effect).
Superior vena cava	Risk of catheter-related thrombosis with Glenn operation.

hypertension, poor ventricular function, and cyanosis. Eisenmenger physiology is a particular risk factor. Up to 47% of cyanotic women have worsening of functional capacity during pregnancy.[38] The increases in stroke volume and cardiac output during pregnancy can stress an already pressure-overloaded ventricle. The decrease in systemic vascular resistance that accompanies pregnancy is better tolerated by women with regurgitant lesions and typically offsets the added insult of pregnancy-related hypervolemia. The decrease in systemic vascular resistance can, however, increase right-to-left shunting. Hypervolemia can be problematic in patients with poor ventricular function. Maternal cyanosis is associated with an increased incidence of prematurity and intrauterine growth retardation. Profound cyanosis is associated with a high rate of spontaneous abortion.[39] Endocarditis prophylaxis is not currently recommended for uncomplicated deliveries; however, an episiotomy would be an indication for prophylaxis.[40] The recurrence risk of any congenital cardiac defect in a newborn is 2.3% with one affected older sibling (any defect), 7.3% with two, 6.7% if the mother has a congenital cardiac defect, but only 2.1% if the father is affected.[3] If possible, pregnancies in mothers with CHD should be managed in a high-risk obstetric center with experienced cardiologists.

Psychosocial

Teenagers with CHD are certainly no different from other teenagers in that issues of denial, a sense of immortality, and risk-taking behavior can affect optimal care for these youngsters. Bodies that carry scars from prior surgery and physical limitations can complicate the body-conscious teenage years. Although most adolescents and adults with CHD function well, adults with CHD are less likely to be married or cohabitating and are more likely to be living with their parents.[41] There are several series of adolescent and adult patients and psychosocial outcome, but there are no well-done controlled studies.[42-48] It has been suggested that depression is common and can exacerbate the clinical consequences of the cardiac defect.

Adult CHD patients have higher medical care expenses than the general population, and they can have difficulty in obtaining life and health insurance after they can no longer be covered under their parents' policies.[49-51] Life insurance is somewhat more available to adult CHD patients than in the past; however, policies vary widely among insurers.[52]

CARDIAC ISSUES

The basic hemodynamic effects of an anatomic cardiac lesion can be modified by time and by the superimposed effects of chronic cyanosis, pulmonary disease, or the effects of aging. Although surgical cure is the goal, true universal cure, without residua, sequelae, or complications, is uncommon on a population-wide basis. Exceptions include closure of a non–pulmonary hypertensive PDA or atrial septal defect (ASD), probably in childhood. Although there have been reports of series of surgeries on adults with CHD, the wide variety of defects and sequelae from prior surgery make generalizations difficult, if not impossible. Poor myocardial function can be inherent in the CHD but can also be affected by longstanding cyanosis or superimposed surgical injury, including inadequate intraoperative myocardial protection.[52,53] This is particularly true of adults who had their cardiac repair several decades ago when myocardial protection may not have been as good and when repair was undertaken at an older age. Postoperative arrhythmias are common, particularly when surgery entailed long atrial suture lines. Thrombi can be found in these atria precluding immediate cardioversion.[54] Bradyarrhythmias can be secondary to surgical injury to the sinus node or conducting tissue or can be a component of the cardiac defect.

The number of cardiac lesions and subtypes, together with the large number of contemporary and obsolescent palliative and corrective surgical procedures, make a complete discussion of all CHD impossible. The reader is referred to one of the current texts on pediatric cardiac anesthesia for more detailed descriptions of these lesions, the available surgical repairs, and the anesthetic implications during primary repair.[55,56] Some general perioperative guidelines to caring for these patients are offered in Table 22–3. This chapter provides a discussion of the more common and physiologically important defects that will be encountered in an adult CHD population. Defining outcome after CHD surgery is like trying to hit a continuously moving target. Both short-term and long-term results from older series can differ significantly from contemporary results.

Aortic Stenosis

Most aortic stenosis in adults is due to a congenitally bicuspid valve that does not become problematic until late middle

Table 22–3 **General Approaches to Anesthesia for Congenital Heart Disease (CHD) Patients**

General
The best care for both cardiac and noncardiac surgery in adult patients with CHD is afforded in a center with a multidisciplinary team experienced in the care of adults with CHD and knowledgeable about both the anatomy and physiology of CHD and also the manifestations and considerations specific to adults with CHD.
Preoperative
Review most recent laboratory data, catheterization, and echocardiogram, and other imaging data. The most recent office letter from the cardiologist is often most helpful. Obtain and review these in advance.
Drawing a diagram of the heart with saturations, pressures, and direction of blood flow often clarifies complex and superficially unfamiliar anatomy and physiology
Avoid prolonged fast if patient is erythrocytotic to avoid hemoconcentration.
No generalized contraindication to preoperative sedation
Intraoperative
Large-bore intravenous access for redo sternotomy and cyanotic patients. (See Table 22–2 for vascular access considerations)
Avoid air bubbles in all intravenous catheters. There can be transient right-to-left shunting even in lesions with predominant left-to-right shunting (filters are available but will severely restrict ability to give volume and blood).
Apply external defibrillator pads for redo sternotomies and patients with poor cardiac function.
Appropriate endocarditis prophylaxis (orally or intravenously prior to skin incision)[40]
Consider antifibrinolytic therapy, especially for patients with prior sternotomy.
Transesophageal echocardiography for cardiac operations
Modulate pulmonary and systemic vascular resistances as appropriate pharmacologically and by modifications in ventilation.
Postoperative
Appropriate pain control (cyanotic patients have normal ventilatory response to hypercarbia and narcotics)
Maintain hematocrit appropriate for arterial saturation.
Maintain central venous and left atrial pressures appropriate for altered ventricular diastolic compliance or presence of beneficial atrial level shunting.
Pa_{O_2} may not increase significantly with the application of supplemental oxygen in the face of right-to-left shunting. Similarly, neither will decrease much with the withdrawal of oxygen (in the absence of lung pathology).

age or later, although endocarditis risk is lifelong. Once symptoms (angina, syncope, near-syncope, heart failure) develop, survival is markedly shortened. Median survival is 5 years after the development of angina, 3 years after syncope, and 2 years after heart failure.[57] Anesthetic management of aortic stenosis does not vary whether the stenosis is congenital (most common) or acquired (see Chapter 20).

Most mothers with aortic stenosis can successfully carry pregnancies to term and have vaginal deliveries. Severe stenosis (valve area <1.0 cm^2) can result in clinical deterioration and maternal and fetal mortality. Hemodynamic monitoring during delivery with maintenance of adequate preload and avoidance of hypotension is critical. When surgical intervention is required during pregnancy, percutaneous balloon valvuloplasty appears to carry lower risk than open valvotomy.

Aortopulmonary Shunts

Depending on their age, adult patients may have had one or more of several aortopulmonary shunts to palliate cyanosis during childhood. These are shown in Figure 22–1. Although life saving, there were considerable shortcomings of these shunts in the long term. All were inherently inefficient, as some of the oxygenated blood returning through the pulmonary veins to the left atrium and ventricle would then return to the lungs through the shunt, thus volume loading the ventricle. It was difficult to quantify the size of the earlier shunts such as the Waterston (side-to-side ascending aorta to right pulmonary artery) and Potts (side-to-side descending aorta to left pulmonary artery). If too small, the patient was left excessively cyanotic; if too large, there was pulmonary overcirculation with the risk of developing pulmonary vascular disease. The Waterston, in fact, could on occasion result in a hyperperfused, hypertensive ipsilateral pulmonary artery and a hypoperfused contralateral pulmonary artery as it could direct flow to the ipsilateral side. There were also surgical issues when complete repair became possible. Takedown of Waterston shunts often required a pulmonary arterioplasty to correct deformity of the pulmonary artery at the site of the anastomosis, and the posteriorly located Potts anastomoses could not be taken down from a median sternotomy. Patients with a classic Blalock-Taussig shunt almost always lack palpable pulses on the side of the shunt. Even if there is a palpable pulse (from collateral flow around the shoulder), blood pressure obtained from that arm will be artifactually low. Even after a modified Blalock-Taussig shunt (using a piece of Gore-Tex tubing instead of an end-to-side anastomosis of the subclavian and pulmonary arteries), there can be a blood pressure disparity between the arms. To ensure a valid measurement, preoperative blood pressure should be measured in both arms (Box 22–4).

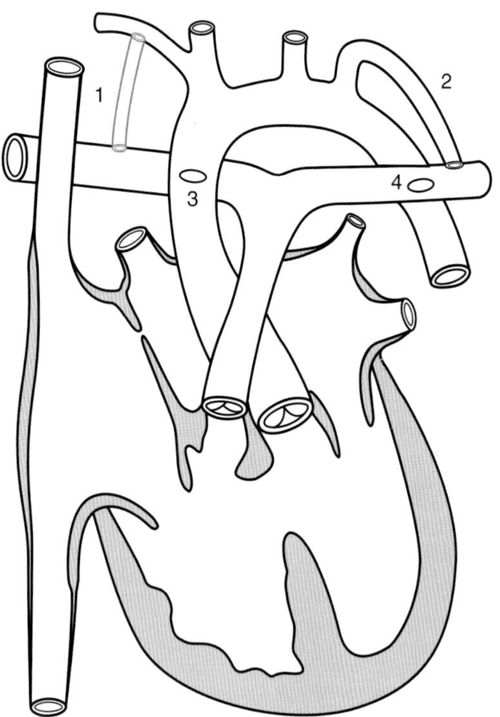

Figure 22–1 The various aortopulmonary anastomoses. The illustrated heart is one with tetralogy of Fallot. The anastomoses are 1, modified Blalock-Taussig; 2, classic Blalock Taussig; 3, Waterston (Waterston-Cooley); and 4, Potts. (Reprinted with permission from Baum VC: The adult with congenital heart disease. J Cardiothorac Vasc Anesth 10:261, 1996.)

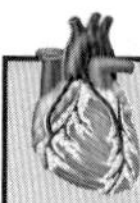

BOX 22–5 ***Complications of Atrial Septal Defect in Adulthood***

- Paradoxic emboli
- Effort dyspnea
- Atrial tachyarrhythmias
- Right-sided failure with pregnancy
- Pulmonary hypertension
- ↑ Right-sided failure with ↓ left ventricular compliance with aging
- Mitral insufficiency

Atrial Septal Defect and Partial Anomalous Pulmonary Venous Return

There are several anatomic types of ASD. The most common type, and if otherwise undefined the presumptive type, is the secundum type located in the midseptum. The primum type at the lower end of the atrial septum is a component of the endocardial cushion defects, the most primitive of which is the common atrioventricular canal (see later). The sinus venosus type, high in the septum near the entry of the superior vena cava, is almost always associated with partial anomalous pulmonary venous return, most frequently drainage of the right upper pulmonary vein to the low superior vena cava. An uncommon atrial septal–type defect is when blood passes from the left atrium to the right via an unroofed coronary sinus. For purposes of this section, only secundum defects are considered, although the natural histories of all of the defects are similar (Box 22–5).

Both the natural history and the postoperative outcome of ASDs and the physiologically related partial anomalous venous return are similar.[58-60] Because the symptoms and clinical findings of an ASD can be quite subtle and patients often remain asymptomatic until adulthood, ASDs represent approximately one third of all CHD discovered in adults. Although asymptomatic survival to adulthood is common, significant shunts ($\dot{Q}_p/\dot{Q}_s$ >1.5:1) will probably cause symptoms over time, and paradoxic emboli can occur through defects with smaller shunts. Effort dyspnea occurs in 30% by the third decade, and atrial flutter or fibrillation in about 10% by age 40.[59] The avoidance of complications developing in adulthood provides the rationale for surgical repair of asymptomatic children. The mortality for a patient with an uncorrected ASD is 6% per year over 40 years of age, and essentially all patients over 60 years of age are symptomatic.[58-60] Large nonrepaired defects can cause death from atrial tachyarrhythmias or right ventricular failure in 30- to 40-year-old patients.[61] With the decreased left ventricular diastolic compliance accompanying the systemic hypertension or coronary artery disease that is common with aging, left-to-right shunting increases with age. Pulmonary vascular disease typically does not develop until after the age of 40, unlike ventricular or ductal level shunts, which can lead to it in early childhood. Mitral insufficiency can be found in adult patients and is significant in about 15% of adult patients.[62] Paradoxic emboli remain a lifelong risk.

Late closure of the defect, after 5 years of age, has been associated with incomplete resolution of right ventricular dilation.[63] Left ventricular dysfunction has been reported in some patients having defect closure in adulthood, and closure particularly in middle age may not prevent the development of atrial tachyarrhythmias or stroke.[64-67] Survival of patients without pulmonary vascular disease has been reported to be best if operated on before 24 years of age, intermediate if operated on between 25 and 41 years of age, and worst if operated on thereafter.[65] However, more recent series have shown that even at ages over 40, surgical repair provides an overall survival and complication-free benefit compared with medical management.[68] Surgical morbidity in these patients is pri-

BOX 22–4 ***Aortopulmonary Shunts***

• Waterston	Ascending aorta→right pulmonary artery	No longer done
• Potts	Descending aorta→left pulmonary artery	No longer done
• Classic Blalock-Taussig	Subclavian artery→ipsilateral pulmonary artery	No longer done
• Modified Blalock-Taussig	Gore-Tex tube subclavian artery→ipsilateral pulmonary artery	Current
• Central shunt	Gore-Tex tube ascending aorta→main pulmonary artery	Current

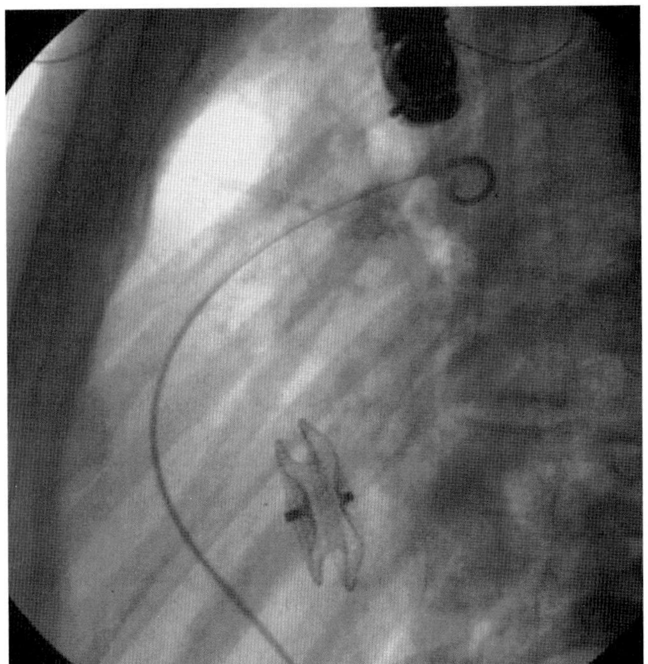

A

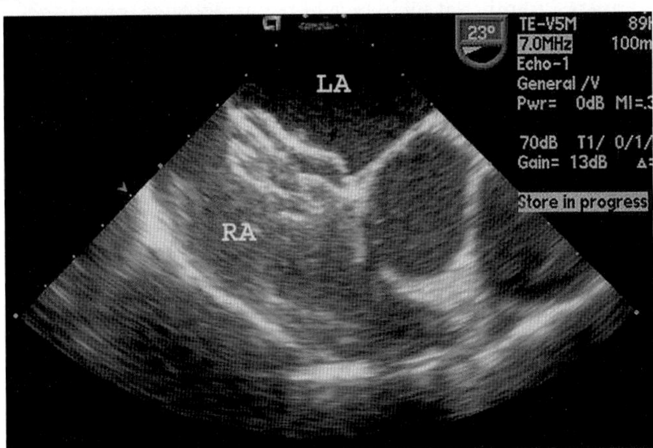

B

Figure 22–2 Closure of an atrial septal defect in an adult with use of a transvascular device (the Amplatzer septal occluder). (*A*) Radiograph. (*B*) Transesophageal echocardiogram. The device is clearly visualized spanning and occluding the atrial septal defect. RA = right atrium, LA = left atrium. (Courtesy of Dr. Scott Lim.)

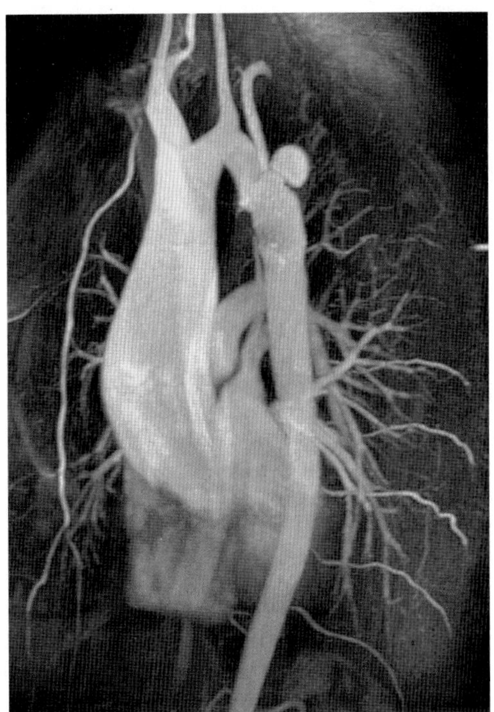

Figure 22–3 Magnetic resonance image of a 37-year-old man showing descending thoracic aortic pseudoaneurysm at the site of a coarctation that had been repaired years earlier. This patient also has a bicuspid aortic valve and an aneurysm of the ascending aorta that was later repaired. (Courtesy of Dr. Christopher Kramer.)

marily atrial fibrillation, atrial flutter, or junctional rhythm.[67] Current practice is to close these defects in adults in the catheterization laboratory via transvascular devices if anatomically practical (Fig. 22–2). For example, there needs to be an adequate rim of septum around the defect to which the device can attach. Device closure is inappropriate if the defect is associated with anomalous pulmonary venous drainage. The indications for closure are the same as for surgical closure.[69]

An otherwise uncomplicated secundum ASD, unlike most congenital cardiac defects, is not associated with an increased endocarditis risk.[40] Presumably this is because the shunt, although potentially large, is low pressure and unassociated with jet lesions of the endocardium.

Although some discussion is given to onset times with intravenous or inhalation induction agents, clinical differences are hard to notice with modern low-solubility volatile agents. Thermodilution cardiac output reflects pulmonary blood flow, which will be in excess of systemic blood flow. Pulmonary arterial catheters are not routinely indicated. Patients generally do tolerate any appropriate anesthetic; however, particular care should be taken in patients with pulmonary arterial hypertension or right-sided failure.

The vast majority of women with an ASD tolerate pregnancy well. However, the normal hypervolemia associated with pregnancy can result in heart failure in women with large defects.

Coarctation of the Aorta

Nonrepaired coarctation of the aorta in the adult brings with it significant morbidity and mortality. Mortality is 25% by age 20, 50% by age 30, 75% by age 50, and 90% by age 60.[61,70-72] Left ventricular aneurysm, rupture of cerebral aneurysms, and dissection of a postcoarctation aneurysm all contribute to the excessive mortality. Left ventricular failure can occur in patients over 40 with nonrepaired lesions. If repair is not undertaken early, there is incremental risk for the development of premature coronary atherosclerosis. Even with surgery, coronary artery disease remains the leading cause of death 11 to 25 years after surgery.[73] Coarctation is accompanied by a bicuspid aortic valve in the majority of patients. Although endocarditis of this abnormal valve is a lifelong risk, these valves often do not become stenotic until middle age or later. Coarctation can also be associated with mitral valve abnormalities (Box 22–6).

Aneurysms at the site of coarctation repair can develop years later (Fig. 22–3), and restenosis as well can develop in adolescence or adulthood. Repair includes resection of the coarctation and end-to-end reanastomosis. Because this

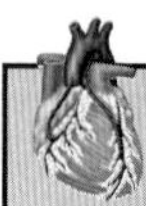

BOX 22–6 *Complications of Aortic Coarctation in Adulthood*

- Left ventricular failure
- Premature coronary atherosclerosis
- Rupture of cerebral aneurysm
- Aneurysm at site of coarctation repair
- Complications of associated bicuspid aortic valve
- Exacerbation of hypertension during pregnancy

sometimes resulted in recoarctation when done in infancy, for many years a common repair was the Waldhausen or subclavian flap operation, in which the left subclavian artery is ligated and the proximal segment opened and rotated as a flap to open the area of the coarctation. Aneurysms in the area of repair are a particular concern in adolescents and adults following coarctectomy. Persistent systemic hypertension is common following coarctation repair.[74] Adult patients require continued periodic follow-up for hypertension. A pressure gradient of 20 mm Hg or more (less in the presence of extensive collaterals) is an indication for treatment.[75] Recoarctation can be treated surgically or by balloon angioplasty with stenting.[76] Surgical repair of recoarctation or aneurysm in adults is associated with increased mortality and can be associated with significant intraoperative bleeding. It requires lung isolation for optimal surgical exposure and placement of an arterial catheter in the right arm.

Half of patients operated on after age 40 have persistent hypertension, and many of the remainder have an abnormal hypertensive response to surgery. Long-term survival is worse for patients having repair later in life. Patients over 40 having repair have a 15-year survival of only 50%.[73]

Blood pressure should be obtained in the right arm unless pressures in the left arm or legs are known to be unaffected by residual or recurrent coarctation. Postoperative hypertension is common after repair of coarctation and often requires treatment for some months. Postoperative ileus is also common, and patients should be maintained NPO for about 2 days.

Pregnancy can exacerbate preexisting hypertension in women with nonrepaired lesions, increasing the risk of aortic dissection or rupture, heart failure, angina, and rupture of a circle of Willis aneurysm. Adequate blood pressure control during pregnancy is paramount in these women. Most aortic ruptures during pregnancy occur during labor and delivery. Presumably, epidural analgesia would moderate hypertension during delivery.

Congenitally Corrected Transposition of the Great Vessels (L-Transposition, Ventricular Inversion)

"Transposition" in this context refers solely to the fact that the aorta arises anterior to the pulmonary artery. It bears no reference to the origin of blood in the aorta or pulmonary artery or to the ventricle of origin of those vessels. In L-transposition, as a consequence of the embryonic heart tube rotating to the left rather than to the right, the flow of blood is through normal vena cavae to the right atrium, through a mitral valve to a right-sided anatomic left ventricle, to the pulmonary artery, through the pulmonary circulation, to the left atrium, through a tricuspid valve to a left-sided anatomic right ventricle, and thence to the aorta. Because of the abnormal anatomic relationships, the aortic valve is located anterior and to the left of the pulmonic valve. Although anatomically altered, the physiologic flow of blood is appropriate and there are no associated shunts. L-Transposition of the great vessels (L-TGV) is frequently associated with other cardiac defects, most commonly a ventricular septal defect (VSD) and subpulmonic stenosis.

When L-transposition is an isolated lesion, most patients maintain normal biventricular function through early adulthood. However, failure of the systemic right ventricle can develop with aging, and asymptomatic aging is relatively uncommon.[77] By age 45, heart failure will be present in 67% of those patients with associated lesions and 25% of those without.[78] These patients can be born with congenital heart block, which can progress in degree. Second- or third-degree heart block occurs at a rate of about 2% per year. More than 75% of patients develop some degree of heart block, although the intrinsic pacemaker remains above the His bundle with a narrow QRS complex. L-transposition can be associated with an Ebstein's-like deformity of the (left-sided) tricuspid valve, and there can be a bundle of Kent causing the Wolff-Parkinson-White syndrome associated with that abnormal valve. There is a significant incidence of tricuspid valve insufficiency in the systemic ventricle, and this is higher still in patients with an Ebstein's deformity of the valve.[79] Anesthetic management depends on the presence of any associated lesions and the adequacy of right (systemic) ventricular function.

Ebstein's Anomaly of the Tricuspid Valve

This defect, one of arrested or incomplete exfoliation of the embryonic tricuspid valve from the right ventricular myocardium, resulting in apically displaced valve tissue, is the most common cause of congenital tricuspid insufficiency. The septal leaflet tends to be the most dysplastic. The anterior leaflet tends to be large and redundant. The defect is associated with a patent foramen ovale or a secundum ASD. Apicalization of the tricuspid valve results in a portion of the heart above the valve having a ventricular intracardiac electrogram but atrial pressures. The right atrium can be massively enlarged (Fig. 22–4), and the right ventricle, lacking the inflow portion that is now part of the right atrium, is smaller than usual with varying degrees of pulmonic stenosis. Patients with L-transposition (see earlier) can have Ebstein's anomaly of a left-sided tricuspid valve.

Symptoms will vary based on the amount of displacement of the valve and the size of the smaller-than-normal right ventricle. Cyanosis from atrial-level right-to-left shunting can be a neonatal phenomenon, resolving with the normal postnatal decrease in pulmonary vascular resistance, only to recur in adolescence or adulthood. Very mild disease is quite compatible with asymptomatic survival into adulthood, although overall earlier reports suggested a mean age at death of about 20 years with about one third dying before 10 years of age and only 15% survival by 60 years.[80-82] About one half develop arrhythmias, typically supraventricular tachyarrhythmias. Once symptoms develop, disability rapidly progresses.

Valve repair is currently the approach of choice, and only uncommonly will tricuspid valve replacement be required. Additional intervention may be required for progressive insufficiency, stenosis, prosthetic valve failure, or valve replacement with growth. Following valve replacement, up to 25% of

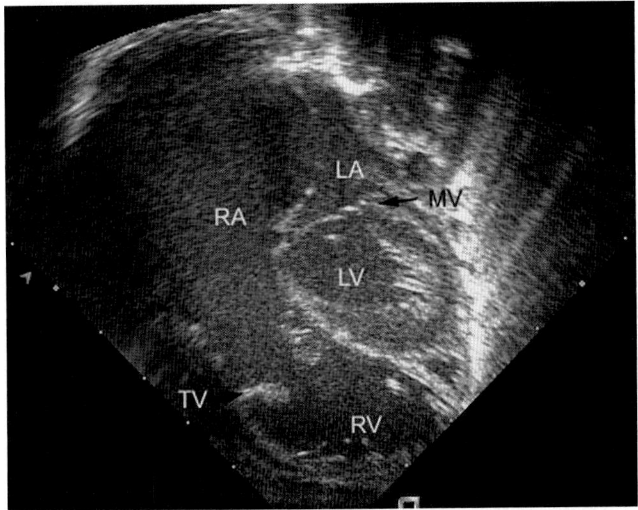

Figure 22–4 Ebstein's anomaly of the tricuspid valve. This echocardiogram shows the apically displaced redundant tricuspid valve tissue and a massively enlarged right atrium with bowing of the atrial septum to the left. RA = right atrium, LA = left atrium, TV = tricuspid valve, MV = mitral valve, RV = right ventricle, LV = left ventricle. (Reprinted with permission from Baum VC: Abnormalities of the atrioventricular valves. *In* Lake CL, Booker P [eds]: Pediatric Cardiac Anesthesia, 4th edition. 2004, with permission of Lippincott Williams and Wilkins.)

Table 22–4 Findings in Eisenmenger Syndrome

- Physical examination: Loud pulmonic component of the second heart sound, single or narrowly split second heart sound, Graham-Steell murmur of pulmonary insufficiency, pulmonic ejection sound ("click")
- Chest radiography: Decreased peripheral pulmonary arterial markings with prominent central pulmonary vessels ("pruning")
- Electrocardiogram: Right ventricular hypertrophy
- Impaired exercise tolerance
- Exertional dyspnea
- Palpitations (often due to atrial fibrillation or flutter)
- Complications from erythrocytosis/hyperviscosity
- Hemoptysis from pulmonary infarction, rupture of pulmonary vessels or aortopulmonary collateral vessels
- Complications from paradoxic embolization
- Syncope from inadequate cardiac output or arrhythmias
- Heart failure (usually end stage)

patients develop high-grade atrioventricular block. Ebstein's valves are often associated with a right-sided bypass tract causing Wolff-Parkinson-White syndrome. This is of concern, as 25% to 30% of patients develop supraventricular tachyarrhythmias. This is in addition to the subset that develop atrial fibrillation as they age, and the bypass tract allows for rapid ventricular rates and possibly ventricular fibrillation.

The major concerns when anesthetizing patients who have Ebstein's anomaly include decreased cardiac output, right-to-left atrial-level shunting with cyanosis, and the propensity for atrial tachyarrhythmias. The right atria of these patients are very sensitive and arrhythmias are easily induced by catheters or guidewires passed into the right atrium or during surgical manipulation; arrhythmias remain a concern into the postoperative period. Supraventricular arrhythmias should be treated aggressively. If associated with significant hypotension, the arrhythmia needs to be electrically cardioverted.

In the absence of marked cyanosis, pregnancy and delivery are generally well tolerated. There is, however, an increased incidence of prematurity and fetal loss and birth weights are lower in infants of cyanotic mothers.[83]

Eisenmenger Syndrome

Eisenmenger described a particular type of large VSD with dextroposition of the aorta.[84] In a general way, the term "Eisenmenger syndrome" has come to describe the clinical setting in which a large left-to-right cardiac shunt results in the development of pulmonary vascular disease. Although early on the pulmonary vasculature remains reactive, with continued insult pulmonary hypertension becomes fixed and does not respond to pulmonary vasodilators. Ultimately, the level of pulmonary vascular resistance is so high that the shunt reverses and becomes right-to-left. The development of pulmonary vascular disease is dependent on shear rate. Lesions with high shear rates, such as a large VSD or a large PDA, can result in pulmonary hypertension in early childhood. Lesions such as an ASD with high pulmonary blood flow but low pressure may not result in pulmonary vascular disease until late middle age. Pulmonary vascular disease progression is also accelerated in patients living at altitude.

Eisenmenger physiology is compatible with survival into adulthood.[85] However, reported rates of survival after diagnosis vary, probably based on the relatively long life expectancy and variability in the time of diagnosis. Cantor et al[86] reported median survival to 53 years but with wide variation. Saha et al[87] reported survival of 80% at 10 years after diagnosis and 42% at 25 years. Oya et al,[88] however, reported survival of 77% at 5 years and 58% at 10 years. Syncope, increased central venous pressure, and arterial desaturation to less than 85% are all associated with poor short-term outcome.[85] Most deaths are sudden cardiac deaths. Other causes of death include heart failure, hemoptysis, brain abscess, thromboembolism, and complications of pregnancy and noncardiac surgery.[89] These patients face potentially significant perioperative risks. Findings of Eisenmenger syndrome are summarized in Table 22–4.

Surgical closure of cardiac defects with fixed pulmonary vascular hypertension is associated with very high mortality. Lung or heart-lung transplantation is a surgical alternative.[90] Although there are several surgical series reporting survival after heart-lung or single- or double-lung transplantation performed for primary pulmonary hypertension, it is unclear if this cohort of patients is similar to patients with Eisenmenger physiology.

Fixed pulmonary vascular resistance precludes rapid adaptation to perioperative hemodynamic changes. Changes in systemic vascular resistance are mirrored by changes in intracardiac shunting. A decrease in systemic vascular resistance is accompanied by increased right-to-left shunting and a decrease in systemic oxygen saturation. Systemic vasodilators, including regional anesthesia, need to be used with caution, and close assessment of intravascular volume is important. Epidural analgesia has been used successfully in patients with Eisenmenger physiology, but the local anesthetic needs to be delivered slowly and incrementally with close observation of blood pressure and oxygen saturation.[91] Postoperative postural hypotension can also increase the degree of right-to-left shunting, and these patients should change position slowly.

Placement of pulmonary artery catheters in these patients is problematic for a variety of reasons and of less utility than might be expected. Pulmonary arterial hypertension is a risk factor for pulmonary artery rupture from a pulmonary artery catheter. Rupture is particularly worrisome in these cyanotic patients who can also have hemostatic deficits associated with erythrocytosis.[92] Abnormal intracardiac anatomy and right-to-left shunting can make successful passage into the pulmonary artery difficult without fluoroscopy. Relative resistances of the pulmonary and systemic beds are reflected in the systemic oxygen saturation, readily measured by pulse oximetry, so measures of pulmonary artery pressure are not required. In addition, in the presence of right-to-left shunting, thermodilution cardiac outputs do not accurately reflect systemic output. Thus, the value of pulmonary artery catheters in these patients is minimal at best, and they essentially are never indicated. The one potential exception is the patient with an ASD who is at risk to develop right ventricular failure if suprasystemic right ventricular pressure develops.[93]

Fixed pulmonary vascular resistance is by definition unresponsive to pharmacologic manipulation. That said, it would seem prudent to avoid factors known to increase pulmonary vascular resistance, including cold, hypercarbia, acidosis, hypoxia, and α-adrenergic agonists. Although the last of these is commonly listed to be avoided, it seems that in the face of pulmonary vascular disease due to intracardiac shunting, the systemic vasoconstrictive effects predominate and systemic oxygen saturation increases.

Nerve blocks offer an attractive alternative to general anesthesia if otherwise appropriate. If patients have general anesthesia, consideration should be given to postoperative observation in an intensive or intermediate care unit. Because of the increased perioperative risk, patients should be observed overnight, particularly if they have not had recent surgery or anesthesia, because their responses will be unknown. Ambulatory surgery is possible for patients having uncomplicated minor surgery with sedation or nerve block.

Pregnancy carries a very high mortality risk and risk of premature delivery. From 20% to 30% of pregnancies result in spontaneous abortions, and premature delivery occurs in about half.[94] At least half of newborns have intrauterine growth retardation. From 30% to 45% of all pregnancies end in maternal death intrapartum or during the first postpartum week, and successful first pregnancy does not preclude maternal death during a subsequent pregnancy.[95] The hemodynamic changes of both pregnancy and delivery increase maternal risk. Pulmonary microembolism and macroembolism have caused peripartum maternal deaths, even days after delivery. Factors influencing mortality include thromboembolism (44%), hypovolemia (26%), and preeclampsia (18%).[94,95] Mortality is similar with cesarean section or vaginal delivery, and both are significantly higher than the mortality rate for spontaneous abortions. Women should be closely monitored with arterial catheters during delivery. Epidural analgesia, delivered slowly and incrementally, can moderate many of the deleterious hemodynamic changes of active labor. Pulmonary arterial catheters are of little to no use during delivery. Prompt treatment of blood loss and hypotension during delivery is absolutely required. Postpartum observation should be in an intensive care setting. Pulmonary hypertension in pregnancy was reviewed in detail.[96,97]

Endocardial Cushion Defects (Atrioventricular Canal Defects)

The endocardial cushions are embryonic cardiac tissue that form the crux of the heart—the primum (lower) atrial septum, the posterior basal part of the ventricular septum, the septal leaflet of the tricuspid valve, and the anterior leaflet of the mitral valve. The endocardial cushion defects then consist of one or more of a primum ASD, VSD, cleft septal leaflet of the tricuspid valve, and/or cleft anterior leaflet of the mitral valve. The most primitive form is the complete atrioventricular canal. In this defect, there is a single large atrioventricular valve with mitral and tricuspid components with large ASDs and VSDs. This valve is usually "balanced." In the more complex, unbalanced defects, one component of the valve can be predominant, and this large valve is not centered over the ventricular septum, leading to underfilling of one of the ventricles. These defects can occur alone or can be part of more complex cardiac defects such as tetralogy of Fallot or single ventricle. Half of all children with Down syndrome have CHD; one half of these have an endocardial cushion defect. These lesions are marked by a typical electrocardiogram with first-degree block and a superior QRS axis with a counterclockwise QRS loop.

There is much subtlety required to construct two separate functional atrioventricular valves without residual stenosis or insufficiency of either component. Postoperative or residual mitral insufficiency is not uncommon, and 10% to 30% require repeat surgery.[98] Anesthesia for these patients depends on the degree of shunt, valve insufficiency, and pulmonary vascular disease.

Fontan Physiology

Originally proposed as a curative operation for tricuspid atresia and subsequently used to repair a variety of lesions associated with only one functional ventricle, the Fontan operation has undergone many iterations and modifications since its original description in 1971 (Fig. 22–5). The original operation used a homograft valve at the inferior vena cava–right atrial junction and a homograft valve between the right atrium and the pulmonary artery. The right atrium delivered systemic venous blood from both vena cavae to the pulmonary arteries. With time, it was appreciated that the valve at the inferior vena cava was not needed, and in fact the valve at the pulmonary artery was unnecessary. For a time the right atrium was directly anastomosed to the pulmonary artery. However, the incidence of atrial complications led to the desire to decrease the portion of the right atrium exposed to high venous pressure and produced the lateral tunnel modification (see Fig. 22–5). In this operation, the superior vena cava is transected and two end-to-side anastomoses are made with the right pulmonary artery. The atrial septum is excised, and a sheet of polytetrafluoroethylene (Gore-Tex) is used as a baffle to direct inferior vena cava blood through the right atrium to the superior vena cava. Thus, only the lateral free wall of the right atrium is exposed to high pressures. In addition, this Gore-Tex sheet allows use when there is only a single large common atrioventricular valve.

It is recognized that the upper limb of this anastomosis represents a bidirectional Glenn shunt. Glenn shunts, when done alone in adults, have poor results.[99] A further modification is to have this baffle external to the right atrium, the extracardiac Fontan. However, patients who have had this operation have not yet reached adulthood. If right-sided pressure is excessive, forward flow in the absence of a subpulmonary ventricle will be inadequate. As a safety measure, a fenestration is often left in the Fontan baffle. In the face of increased pressures, blood shunts to the left atrium. The cost is some arterial desaturation; however, forward systemic flow is maintained. If the surgical results are good, these fenestrations can be closed with devices in the catheterization laboratory. These would, of course, also serve as a potential site for passage of a paradoxic embolus.

Originally hoped to be curative, it became apparent that there is significant long-term morbidity and mortality, as alluded to earlier.[100-102] Atrial arrhythmias are commonly encountered and are present in 15% to 20% of patients at 5 years.[103] These arrhythmias are presumably related to long right atrial suture lines and high right atrial pressure. New-onset atrial fibrillation suggests possible obstruction to the Fontan baffle. Right atrial thrombus and ventricular dysfunction can also be encountered. Chylothorax and protein-losing enteropathy from increased venous pressure can be devastating postoperative complications in the short and medium term. Protein-losing enteropathy is found in 2% to 3% of patients and can cause generalized edema, ascites, pleural effusion, and chronic diarrhea.[104] The Fontan procedure is being done in younger children and can be accomplished toward the end of the first year of life. Teenagers are likely to have already developed decreased ventricular function and valve dysfunction from years of cyanosis and ventricular volume loading.[105-107] This is important as most late deaths are due to ventricular failure. Postoperative atrial arrhythmias and late postoperative arrhythmic deaths are more common in children who have surgery at older ages[108] (Box 22–7).

Fontan patients are often receiving aspirin, due to the low-pressure conduit. Uncommonly, they are on an additional antiplatelet drug, and they may be receiving Coumadin (warfarin) if they are in atrial flutter or fibrillation. Because there is no subpulmonary ventricle, it is important to minimize pulmonary vascular resistance perioperatively. Routine measures such as avoiding cold, hypoxia, hypercarbia, and acidosis are important. In addition, in an effort to minimize pulmonary vascular resistance, functional residual capacity should be maintained by the application of small amounts of positive end-expiratory pressure (PEEP) or continuous positive airway pressure (CPAP), and excessive lung volumes should be avoided. PEEP or CPAP will not significantly impede cardiac output if less than 6 cm H_2O. Spontaneous ventilation has been assumed to be optimal for these patients to minimize intrathoracic pressure and encourage forward flow into the pulmonary circulation; but as discussed by Steven and McGowan,[109] hard evidence for this approach is mostly lacking. Pressure in the inferior vena cava reliably reflects pressure in the Fontan lateral tunnel and pulmonary arteries in the supine patient in the absence of an anatomic obstruction.[110] Following Fontan surgery, there appears to be an increased risk for miscarriage but no additional risk for term delivery.[111]

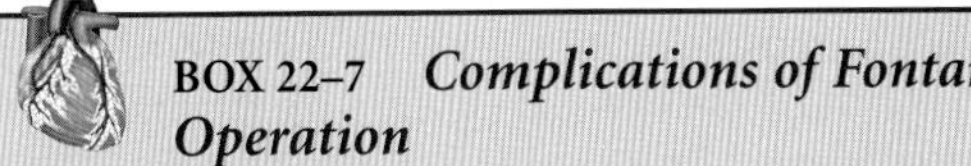

BOX 22–7 *Complications of Fontan Operation*

- Atrial thrombus
- Atrial arrhythmia
- Ventricular dysfunction
- Chylothorax
- Protein-losing enteropathy

Patent Ductus Arteriosus

Beyond the neonatal period, spontaneous closure of a PDA is uncommon. The risk of a longstanding moderate-to-large PDA is volume overloading of the left atrium and left ventricle with the risk of development of pulmonary vascular disease. With time, the ductus can become calcified or aneurysmally dilated with a risk of rupture. Ductal calcification or aneurysm increases the risk of surgery, which rarely requires cardiopulmonary bypass.[112] Nonrepaired, the natural history is for one third of patients to die of heart failure, pulmonary hypertension, or endocarditis by 40 years of age and two thirds by age 60.[113] Although small PDAs are of no hemo-

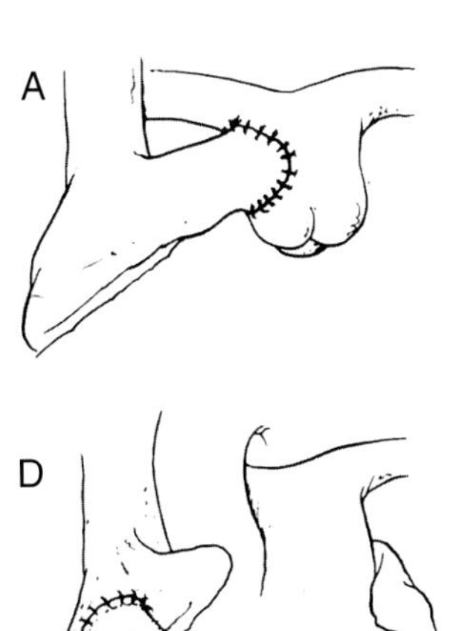

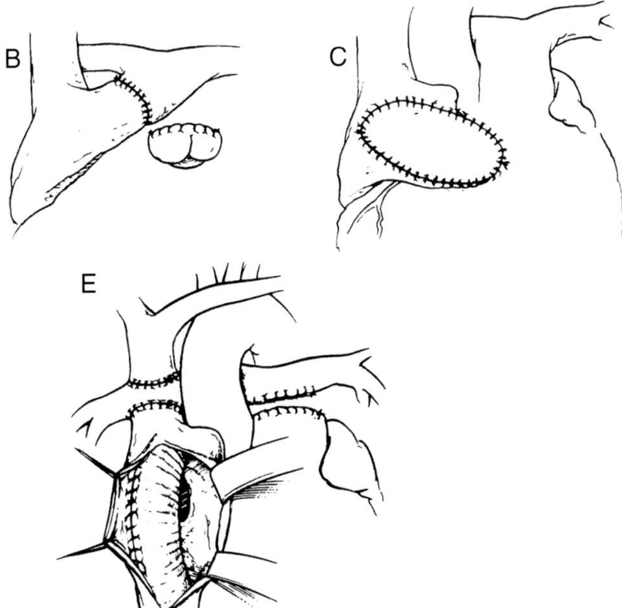

Figure 22–5 Historic modifications of the Fontan operation. (*A*) Direct connection of the right atrial appendage and main pulmonary artery. (*B*) Connection of the right atrial appendage to the distal end of a transected pulmonary artery. (*C*) Pericardial patch connection of right atrium to right ventricle. (*D*) Right atrium to right ventricle connection by a valved conduit. (*E*) Total cavopulmonary connection using a lateral tunnel within the right atrium. (Reprinted from Lowe DA, Stayer SA, Rehman MA: Abnormalities of the atrioventricular valves. *In* Lake CL [ed]: Pediatric Cardiac Anesthesia, 3rd edition. 1998, with permission of The McGraw-Hill Companies.)

dynamic consequence, even small PDAs carry relatively high endocarditis risk. Surgical closure should be considered for all adults with PDA, and transvascular closure by means of one of several devices is possible.[112]

Small PDAs do not carry a hemodynamic risk for pregnancy. The decrease in systemic vascular resistance accompanying pregnancy could lead to right-to-left shunting in a woman with a large PDA.

Pulmonary Valve Stenosis

Long-term asymptomatic survival is typical of patients, with the exception of neonates with critical stenosis.[114] There is a 94% survival rate 20 years after diagnosis, and adults generally do not require surgical intervention.[115] With aging, however, right ventricular fibrosis and failure can develop, and this is the most common cause of death, usually in the fourth decade. Almost all patients who have relief of stenosis either surgically or by balloon valvuloplasty have normal right ventricular function postoperatively. However, abnormal ventricular function may not resolve after late surgical correction. Isolated pulmonary valvular stenosis, even of a severe degree, is usually well tolerated during pregnancy, even in the face of the volume overload that accompanies it.

In patients with significant right ventricular hypertension, right ventricular ischemia can occur if systemic hypotension and decreased coronary perfusion occur. This is manifest on the electrocardiogram. Coronary ischemia resolves if coronary perfusion pressure is increased, as with use of phenylephrine.

Single-Ventricle Anatomy

This large rubric includes a variety of lesions resulting in a single functional ventricle. Long-term survival and function, then, depend on the type and degree of coexisting defects. Both pulmonic stenosis (protecting the pulmonary vascular bed from excessive flow) and a competent atrioventricular valve improve long-term survival. A single ventricle with left ventricular morphology allows better long-term function than one of right ventricular morphology.[116] Palliation with an aortopulmonary shunt (such as a Blalock-Taussig) volume loads the ventricle and function decreases with age. Cavopulmonary shunts such as a Glenn shunt or a Fontan operation decrease ventricular volume loading.

In the past, there was much consideration about possible biventricular repair in some of these patients. Many patients were thought to be inoperable and received only palliation. Currently, most are repaired with some modification of the Fontan operation. Anesthetic management depends on the specific physiology.

There is a high incidence of fetal loss, prematurity, and small-for-dates infants in pregnancies of women with single ventricle. The risk of pregnancy increases with increasing degrees of cyanosis.

Tetralogy of Fallot

As with many things in medicine, tetralogy of Fallot was first described by someone else—probably in 1673 by Steno. The classic description of tetralogy of Fallot includes (1) a large, nonrestrictive malaligned VSD, with (2) an overriding aorta, (3) infundibular pulmonic stenosis, and (4) consequent right ventricular hypertrophy, all derived from an embryonic anterocephalad deviation of the outlet septum. However, there is a spectrum of disease, with more severe defects including stenosis of the pulmonary valve, stenosis of the pulmonary valve annulus, or stenosis and hypoplasia of the pulmonary arteries in the most severe cases. Pentalogy of Fallot refers to the addition of an ASD. With advances in genetics, up to one third or more of cases of tetralogy have been ascribed to one of several genetic abnormalities, including trisomy 21, the 22q11 microdeletion, the genes *NKX 2.5* and *FOG 2.4*, and others. Tetralogy of Fallot is the most common cyanotic lesion encountered in the adult population. Nonrepaired or nonpalliated, approximately 25% of patients survive to adolescence, after which the mortality is 6.6% per year. Only 3% survive to age 40.[117] Unlike children, teenagers and adults with tetralogy do not develop "tet spells." Long-term survival with a good quality of life is expected after repair. The 32- to 36-year survival has been reported to be 85% to 86%, although symptoms, primarily arrhythmias and decreased exercise tolerance, occur in 10% to 15% at 20 years after the primary repair[118-121] (Box 22–8).

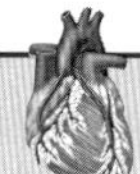

BOX 22–8 ***Risk Factors for Sudden Death After Repair of Tetralogy of Fallot***

- Repair requiring ventriculotomy
- Older age at repair
- Severe left ventricular dysfunction
- Postoperative right ventricular hypertension (residual outflow tract obstruction)
- Wide-open pulmonary insufficiency
- Prolongation of the QRS

It is uncommon to encounter an adolescent or adult with nonrepaired tetralogy. However, it can be encountered in immigrants or in patients whose anatomic variation was considered to be inoperable when they were children. In tetralogy, the right ventricle "sees" the obstruction from the pulmonic stenosis. Pulmonary vascular resistance is typically normal to low. Right-to-left shunting is unaffected by attempts at modulating pulmonary vascular resistance. Shunting is minimized, however, by pharmacologically increasing systemic vascular resistance. Increases in the inotropic state of the heart increase the dynamic obstruction at the right ventricular infundibulum and worsen right-to-left shunting. β-Blockers are often used to decrease inotropy. Although halothane was the historic anesthetic of choice in children with tetralogy due to its myocardial depressant effects and ability to maintain systemic vascular resistance, current practice is to use sevoflurane, without undue consequence from a reduction in systemic vascular resistance.[122] Anesthetic induction in adults can easily be achieved with narcotics.

Patients require closure of the VSD and resolution of the pulmonic stenosis. Although current practice is to repair the VSD through the right atrium in an effort to maintain competence of the pulmonary valve and limit any ventriculotomy, older patients will likely have had repair via a right ventriculotomy. A large right ventriculotomy increases the risks of arrhythmias and sudden death.[123] Patients who have had a right ventriculotomy will have an obligate right bundle-branch block pattern on the electrocardiogram. However, unlike the more usual bundle-branch block in adults, this represents disruption of the His-Purkinje system only in the right ventricular outflow, in the area of the right ventricular incision. Because the vast majority of His-Purkinje conduction is intact, it does not carry increased risk for the development of complete heart block. These patients can have an abnormal response to exercise.

Some patients require repair of pulmonic stenosis by placement of a transannular patch, with obligate residual pulmonary insufficiency. Isolated mild-to-moderate pulmonary insufficiency is generally well tolerated, but in the long term, it can contribute to right ventricular dysfunction with a risk of ventricular tachycardia and sudden death. Atrial tachyarrhythmias occur in about one third of adults late after repair and can contribute to late morbidity.[124,125] The development of atrial flutter or atrial reentrant tachycardia is often a harbinger of hemodynamic compromise. The substrate is usually an atrial surgical scar and the trigger is atrial dilation, such as from tricuspid insufficiency with right ventricular dysfunction. The mechanism for the development of ventricular arrhythmias is presumably the same, namely dilation superimposed on surgical scar.

In some cases, the right ventricular outflow tract patch needs to be extended onto the branch pulmonary arteries to relieve obstruction. Patients with abnormal coronary arteries may have required repair using a right ventricle–to–pulmonary artery conduit to avoid doing a right ventriculotomy in the area of the coronary artery. Repair at a younger age (<12 years) results in better postoperative right ventricular function.[126] Because there is an unrestrictive VSD, in the nonrepaired adult systemic hypertension developing in adult life imposes an additional load on both ventricles, not just the left. The increase in systemic vascular resistance decreases right-to-left shunting and diminishes cyanosis but at the expense of right ventricular or biventricular failure.

Sudden death or ventricular tachycardia requiring treatment can occur in up to 5.5% of postoperative patients over 30 years, often years postoperatively.[118,119,127] The foci for these arrhythmias are typically in the right ventricular outflow tract in the area that has had surgery, and they can be ablated in the catheterization laboratory. Older age at repair, severe left ventricular dysfunction, postoperative right ventricular hypertension from residual or recurrent outflow tract obstruction, wide-open pulmonary insufficiency, and prolongation of the QRS are all predictors of sudden death.[123,128] Premature ventricular contractions and even nonsustained ventricular tachycardia are not rare but do not seem to be associated with sudden death, making appropriate treatment options difficult.[129] It has been suggested that QRS prolongation to longer than 180 milliseconds is a risk factor. This marker, although highly sensitive, has a low positive predictive value.[130] The impact of this risk factor in the current group of younger patients who have not had ventriculotomies is unclear, as their initial postoperative QRS durations are shorter than in patients who had a right ventriculotomy.

Although for many years it was thought that moderate-to-severe pulmonary insufficiency in these patients was well tolerated, it has become apparent from a number of series that right ventricular dysfunction and both atrial and ventricular arrhythmias can be common long-term sequelae. For this reason, patients with symptomatic pulmonary insufficiency from a transannular patch or aneurysm formation at the site of a right ventricular outflow tract patch can require reoperation to replace a widely incompetent pulmonary valve with a bioprosthetic valve with or without a tricuspid annuloplasty.[131] Interestingly, the incidence of atrial arrhythmias may not be diminished when adult patients have a pulmonary valve placed, although the incidence of ventricular arrhythmias is decreased. Right ventricular dysfunction improves in a variable number of adults, suggesting that pulmonary valve placement be done sooner rather than later. There is very early experience with a pulmonary valve that can be inserted transvenously in the catheterization laboratory, although currently it is appropriate only for a limited range of pulmonary artery sizes.

Additional possible late-term complications include residual VSD, patch dehiscence, progressive aortic insufficiency, left ventricular dysfunction from surgical injury to an anomalous coronary artery or longstanding preoperative cyanosis, and heart block from VSD closure (uncommon today). Because patients who have had repairs using a conduit require multiple sternotomies and the valved conduit tends to lie immediately behind and in close proximity to the sternum, sternotomy carries with it significant potential risk for laceration of the conduit. On occasion, the femoral vessels are cannulated for bypass prior to sternotomy.

Most adult patients require reoperation to repair the right ventricular outflow tract or to insert or replace a valve in the pulmonic position. Other reasons for reoperation include repair of an outflow tract aneurysm at the site of a patch, repair of a residual VSD, or repair of an incompetent tricuspid valve.[121] These patients often have diminished right ventricular diastolic compliance and require higher-than-normal central venous pressure. Postoperative management includes minimizing pulmonary vascular resistance and maintaining central venous pressure. Patients often require treatment post-bypass with an inotrope and afterload reduction.[132]

Women with good surgical results without residual defects should tolerate pregnancy and delivery well with outcomes approximating those of the general population. Women with uncorrected tetralogy, particularly those with significant cyanosis, have a high incidence of fetal loss (80% with hematocrit >65%). The fall in systemic vascular resistance that accompanies pregnancy and delivery can worsen cyanosis, and the physiologic volume loading of pregnancy can exaggerate failure of both ventricles.

Transposition of the Great Arteries (D-Transposition)

In D-transposition of the great arteries, there is a discordant connection of the ventricles and the great arteries. The aorta (with the coronary arteries) arises from the right ventricle, and the pulmonary artery arises from the left ventricle. Thus, the two circulations are separate. Postnatal survival requires interchange of blood between the two circulations, typically via a patent foramen ovale and/or a PDA. With a 1-year mortality approximating 100%, all adults with D-transposition have had some type of surgical intervention. Adults will have had atrial-type repairs (Mustard or Senning), whereas children born after the mid-1980s will have had repair by arterial switch (the Jatene operation). Some will also have had repair of D-transposition with a moderate-to-large VSD by means of a Rastelli operation (see later).

Atrial repairs function by redirecting systemic venous blood to the left ventricle (and thence to the transposed pulmonary artery) and pulmonary venous blood to the right ventricle (and thence to the aorta). The Mustard operation uses an intra-atrial conduit of native pericardium (Fig. 22–6), whereas the Senning operation uses native atrial tissue to fashion the

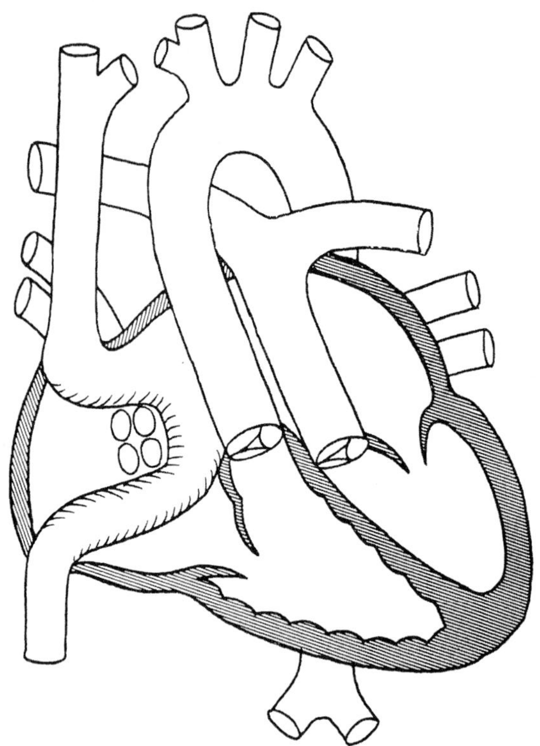

Figure 22–6 The Mustard operation. An intra-atrial baffle has directed vena caval blood across the excised atrial septum to the mitral valve and pulmonary venous blood to the tricuspid valve. The right ventricle remains as the systemic ventricle and the left ventricle as the subpulmonary ventricle. (Reprinted from Mullins C, Mayer D: Congenital Heart Disease. A Diagrammatic Atlas. 1988 with permission of Wiley-Liss, Inc., a subsidiary of John Wiley & Sons, Inc.)

conduit. The arterial switch operation transposes transected aorta and pulmonary artery such that they now arise above the appropriate ventricle. This operation also requires transposing the coronary arteries from the aorta to the pulmonary root, which, following the procedure, becomes the aortic root. The Rastelli procedure closes the VSD on a bias such that the left ventricle empties into the aorta and connects the right ventricle to the pulmonary artery by means of a valved conduit.

Atrial repairs result in a systemic right ventricle, and these patients consistently have abnormal right ventricular function that can be progressive with a right ventricular ejection fraction of about 40%.[133] Mild tricuspid insufficiency is common, but severe tricuspid insufficiency suggests the development of severe right ventricular dysfunction. There is an 85% to 90% 10-year survival with these operations, but by 20 years, survival is less than 80%.[134,135] Over 25 years, about half develop moderate right ventricular dysfunction and one third develop severe tricuspid insufficiency.[135-138] Although it always remains abnormal, it has been suggested that earlier surgery minimizes right ventricular dysfunction.[139] Because of the incidence of right ventricular dysfunction, some patients with atrial repairs have been converted to an arterial switch, following preparation of the left ventricle by a pulmonary artery band to prepare it to tolerate systemic arterial pressure.[140]

Atrial repairs bring an incidence of late electrophysiologic sequelae including sinus node dysfunction (bradycardia), junctional escape rhythms, atrioventricular block, and supraventricular arrhythmias. Atrial flutter occurs in 20% of patients by age 20 with half having progressive sinus node dysfunction by that time.[134,138] On occasion these tachyarrhythmias can result in sudden death, presumably from 1:1 conduction producing ventricular fibrillation.[134,141] The loss of sinus rhythm in the face of right ventricular (the systemic ventricle) dysfunction can also contribute to late sudden death. The risk of late death after an atrial repair is almost three times higher if there is an associated VSD. The incidence of tachyarrhythmias does decrease, however, after the tenth postoperative year.

An arterial switch operation can be done after a failed atrial repair in adults, but the outcome is generally poor. It is suggested that younger patients do better.[142]

Very-long-term outcome after the arterial switch procedure is still not known. It does appear that there is essentially no mortality after 5 years postoperatively, and late surgical reintervention is mostly due to supravalvular pulmonic stenosis.[143] Although many of these children have abnormal resting myocardial perfusion, up to 9% can have evidence of exercise-induced myocardial ischemia.[144] The implication for the development of premature coronary artery disease in adulthood is not known, and there is also some concern about the ultimate function of the neoaortic valve.

Following an atrial or a Rastelli repair, pregnancy and delivery are generally well tolerated, although right ventricular failure and deterioration in functional capacity can occur. There is an increased incidence of prematurity and small-for-date infants in these women.

Truncus Arteriosus

Truncus arteriosus derives from lack of septation of the embryonic truncus arteriosus into aortic and pulmonary artery components, resulting in a single semilunar valve with variable numbers of cusps and a single great vessel, the aorta, arising from the heart. A large malalignment-type VSD allows filling from both ventricles. The pulmonary arteries arise from the ascending aorta. Although various types have been ascribed depending on the exact anatomy of the pulmonary artery origin, there is really a spectrum of types I through III. Type IV, or pseudotruncus, describes the situation of pulmonary atresia with VSD and supply of the pulmonary arteries from large collaterals originating from the descending aorta. Repair is by closure of the VSD and connection of the right ventricle to the pulmonary artery (or pulmonary arteries) by a conduit containing a homograft valve.

Because of the very high risk of congestive heart failure followed by pulmonary vascular disease in childhood from high pulmonary blood flow from the aorta, essentially all patients who survive to adolescence have had surgical repair or will have inoperable pulmonary vascular disease. The rare exception is the patient with stenosis near the origin of the pulmonary arteries from the aorta. Patients with valved conduits placed in infancy and early childhood have requisite reoperations to replace the conduit with patient growth, even in the face of adequate valve function. Conduits placed in later childhood can suffice until adulthood. There can be ongoing problems with incompetence and stenosis of the truncal valve (postoperatively functioning as the aortic valve), and eventual dysfunction from stenosis and/or incompetence of the homograft conduit is routinely encountered, requiring replacement.[145,146] Because these patients require multiple sternotomies and the valved conduit tends to lie immediately behind and in close proximity to the sternum, sternotomy carries with it significant potential risk for laceration of the conduit. On occasion the femoral vessels are cannulated for bypass prior to sternotomy.

Ventricular Septal Defects

The natural history of VSDs has been reviewed in detail.[114] More than 75% of small and moderate VSDs close spontaneously during childhood by a gradual ingrowth of surrounding septum. Of those that close spontaneously, almost all have closed by 10 years of age. Other mechanisms for natural closure include closure by tricuspid valve tissue, closure by prolapsed aortic leaflet, and closure by endocarditis. Some VSDs result in the development of aortic insufficiency in adults from prolapse of the aortic valve into the defect.[147] Although the risk of endocarditis is ongoing, there is no hemodynamic risk of a small VSD in the adult. If pulmonary vascular disease is present, it can progress if closure of a large VSD is delayed.

Although some studies have reported possible ventricular dysfunction years after surgical repair, these are older reports and patients were operated on later than by current standards.[148-150] It does appear, though, that the ventricle successfully remodels from chronic volume overload if surgical correction is done by 5 years of age and perhaps up to 10 to 12 years of age.

Although some discussion is given to onset times with intravenous or inhalation induction agents, clinical differences are hard to notice with modern low-solubility volatile agents. Thermodilution cardiac output reflects pulmonary blood flow, which will be in excess of systemic blood flow. Pulmonary arterial catheters are not routinely indicated. In the patient with a moderate or large left-to-right shunt, low inspired oxygen and moderate hypercarbia avoid intraoperative decreases in pulmonary vascular resistance with pulmonary overcirculation and left ventricular dilation. However, unlike children, it would be rare to encounter adults with large left-to-right shunts. Adults with nonrepaired lesions would have either small shunts or would have had large shunts that caused Eisenmenger physiology.

Pregnancy is well tolerated in the absence of preexisting heart failure or pulmonary hypertension. Pregnancy with a naturally or surgically closed defect carries with it no additional risk, in the absence of additional cardiac problems.

REFERENCES

1. Perloff JK: Pediatric congenital cardiac becomes a postoperative adult. The changing population of congenital heart disease. Circulation 47:606, 1973
2. Gatzoulis M, Webb GD, Daubeney PEF: Diagnosis and Management of Adult Congenital Heart Disease, Philadelphia, Churchill Livingstone, 2003
3. Perloff JK, Warnes CA: Challenges posed by adults with repaired congenital heart disease. Circulation 103:2637, 2001
4. Warnes CA, Liberthson R, Danielson GK, et al: Task force 1: The changing profile of congenital heart disease in adult life. J Am Coll Cardiol 37:1170, 2001
5. Webb GD, Williams RG: Care of the adult with congenital heart disease: introduction. J Am Coll Cardiol 37:1166, 2001
6. Andropoulos DB, Stayer SA, Skjonsby BS, et al: Anesthetic and perioperative outcome of teenagers and adults with congenital heart disease. J Cardiothorac Vasc Anesth 16:731, 2002
7. Dore A, Glancy DL, Stone S, et al: Cardiac surgery for grown-up congenital heart patients: Survey of 307 consecutive operations from 1991 to 1994. Am J Cardiol 80:906, 1997
8. Warnes CA: The adult with congenital heart disease: Born to be bad? J Am Coll Cardiol 46:1–8, 2005
9. Landzberg MJ, Murphy DJ Jr, Davidson WR Jr, et al: Task force 4: Organization of delivery systems for adults with congenital heart disease. J Am Coll Cardiol 37:1187, 2001
10. Bancalari E, Jesse MJ, Gelband H, Garcia O: Lung mechanics in congenital heart disease with increased and decreased pulmonary blood flow. J Pediatr 90:192, 1977
11. Sietsema KE, Perloff JK: Cyanotic congenital heart disease: Dynamics of oxygen uptake and control of ventilation during exercise. *In* Perloff JK, Child JS (eds): Congenital Heart Disease in Adults. Philadelphia, WB Saunders, 1991, pp 104–110
12. Sorensen SC, Severinghaus JW: Respiratory insensitivity to acute hypoxia persisting after correction of tetralogy of Fallot. J Appl Physiol 25:221, 1968
13. Edelmann NH, Lahiri S, Braudo L, et al: The ventilatory response to hypoxia in cyanotic congenital heart disease. N Engl J Med 282:405, 1970
14. Blesa MI, Lahiri S, Rashkind WJ, Fishman AP: Normalization of the blunted ventilatory response to acute hypoxia in congenital cyanotic heart disease. N Engl J Med 296:237, 1977
15. Burrows FA: Physiologic dead space, venous admixture, and the arterial to end-tidal carbon dioxide difference in infants and children undergoing cardiac surgery. Anesthesiology 70:219, 1989
16. Perloff JK, Rosove MH, Child JS, Wright GB: Adults with cyanotic congenital heart disease: hematologic management. Ann Intern Med 109:406, 1988
17. Kawakami N, Mimatsu K, Deguchi M, et al: Scoliosis and congenital heart disease. Spine 20:1252, 1995
18. Berman WJ, Wood SC, Yabek SM, et al: Systemic oxygen transport in patients with congenital heart disease. Circulation 75:360, 1987
19. Linderkamp O, Klose HJ, Betke K, et al: Increased blood viscosity in patients with cyanotic congenital heart disease and iron deficiency. J Pediatr 95:567, 1979
20. Gidding SS, Stockman JA 3rd: Effect of iron deficiency on tissue oxygen delivery in cyanotic congenital heart disease. Am J Cardiol 61:605, 1988
21. Wedemeyer AL, Lewis JH: Improvement in hemostasis following phlebotomy in cyanotic patients with heart disease. J Pediatr 83:46, 1973
22. Maurer HM, McCue CM, Robertson LW, Haggins JC: Correction of platelet dysfunction and bleeding in cyanotic congenital heart disease by simple red cell volume reduction. Am J Cardiol 35:831, 1975
23. Tempe DK, Virmani S: Coagulation abnormalities in patients with cyanotic congenital heart disease. J Cardiothorac Vasc Anesth 16:752, 2002
24. Weinstein M, Ware JA, Troll J, Salzman E: Changes in von Willebrand factor during cardiac surgery: Effect of desmopressin acetate. Blood 71:1648, 1988
25. Rosove MH, Hocking WG, Harwig SS, Perloff JK: Studies of beta-thromboglobulin, platelet factor 4, and fibrinopeptide A in erythrocytosis due to cyanotic congenital heart disease. Thromb Res 29:225, 1983
26. Ware JA, Reaves WH, Horak JK, Solis RT: Defective platelet aggregation in patients undergoing surgical repair of cyanotic congenital heart disease. Ann Thorac Surg 36:289, 1983
27. Waldman JD, Czapek EE, Paul MH, et al: Shortened platelet survival in cyanotic heart disease. J Pediatr 87:77, 1975
28. Chauhan S, Kumar BA, Rao BH, et al: Efficacy of aprotinin, epsilon aminocaproic acid, or combination in cyanotic heart disease. Ann Thorac Surg 70:1308, 2000
29. Levin E, Wu J, Devine DV, et al: Hemostatic parameters and platelet activation marker expression in cyanotic and acyanotic pediatric patients undergoing cardiac surgery in the presence of tranexamic acid. Thromb Haemost 83:54, 2000
30. Spear GS: The glomerular lesion of cyanotic congenital heart disease. Johns Hopkins Med J 140:185, 1977
31. Ross EA, Perloff JK, Danovitch GM, et al: Renal function and urate metabolism in late survivors with cyanotic congenital heart disease. Circulation 73:396, 1986
32. Young D: Hyperuricemia in cyanotic congenital heart disease. Am J Dis Child 134:902, 1980
33. Dittrich S, Kurschat K, Dahnert I, et al: Renal function after cardiopulmonary bypass surgery in cyanotic congenital heart disease. Int J Cardiol 73:173, 2000
34. Perloff JK, Marelli AJ, Miner PD: Risk of stroke in adults with cyanotic congenital heart disease. Circulation 87:1954, 1993
35. Ammash N, Warnes CA: Cerebrovascular events in adult patients with cyanotic congenital heart disease. J Am Coll Cardiol 28:768, 1996
36. Warnes CA, Elkayam U: Congenital heart disease and pregnancy. *In* Elkayam U, Gleicher N (eds): Cardiac Problems in Pregnancy, 3rd edition. New York, Wiley-Liss, 1998, pp 39–53
37. Colman JM, Sermer M, Seaward G, Siu SC: Congenital heart disease: Pathophysiology, clinical recognition, diagnosis, and management. *In* Wilansky S, Willerson JT (eds): Heart Disease in Women. New York, Churchill Livingstone, 2002, pp 443–455
38. Shime J, Mocarski EJ, Hastings D, et al: Congenital heart disease in pregnancy: Short- and long-term implications. Am J Obstet Gynecol 156:313, 1987

39. Presbitero P, Somerville J, Stone S, et al: Pregnancy in cyanotic congenital heart disease. Outcome of mother and fetus. Circulation 89:2673, 1994
40. Dajani AS, Taubert KA, Wilson W, et al: Prevention of bacterial endocarditis. Recommendations by the American Heart Association. JAMA 277:1794, 1997
41. Foster E, Graham TP Jr, Driscoll DJ, et al: Task force 2: Special health care needs of adults with congenital heart disease. J Am Coll Cardiol 37:1176, 2001
42. Bromberg JI, Beasley PJ, D'Angelo EJ, et al: Depression and anxiety in adults with congenital heart disease: A pilot study. Heart Lung 32:105, 2003
43. van Rijen EH, Utens EM, Roos-Hesselink JW, et al: Psychosocial functioning of the adult with congenital heart disease: A 20-33 year follow-up. Eur Heart J 24:673, 2003
44. Lane DA, Lip GY, Millane TA: Quality of life in adults with congenital heart disease. Heart 88:71, 2002
45. Kamphuis M, Ottenkamp J, Vliegen HW, et al: Health-related quality of life and health status in adult survivors with previously operated complex congenital heart disease. Heart 87:356, 2002
46. Kamphuis M, Vogels T, Ottenkamp J, et al: Employment in adults with congenital heart disease. Arch Pediatr Adolesc Med 156:1143, 2002
47. Cox D, Lewis G, Stuart G, Murphy K: A cross-sectional study of the prevalence of psychopathology in adults with congenital heart disease. J Psychosom Res 52:65, 2002
48. Lip GY, Lane DA, Millane TA, Tayebjee MH: Psychological interventions for depression in adolescent and adult congenital heart disease. Cochrane Database Syst Rev CD004394, 2003
49. Moons P, Siebens K, De Geest S, et al: A pilot study of expenditures on, and utilization of resources in, health care in adults with congenital heart disease. Cardiol Young 11:301, 2001
50. Skorton DJ, Garson A Jr, Allen HD, et al: Task Force 5: Adults with congenital heart disease: Access to care. J Am Coll Cardiol 37:1193, 2001
51. Vonder Muhll I, Cumming G, Gatzoulis MA: Risky business: Insuring adults with congenital heart disease. Eur Heart J 24:1595, 2003
52. Truesdell SC, Clark EB: Health insurance status in a cohort of children and young adults with congenital cardiac diagnoses. Circulation 84(suppl II), 1991
53. Graham TP Jr, Cordell GD, Bender HW: Ventricular function following surgery. *In* Kidd BS, Rowe RD (eds): The Child With Congenital Heart Disease After Surgery. Mt. Kisco, NY, Futura, 1995
54. Feltes TF, Friedman RA: Transesophageal echocardiographic detection of atrial thrombi in patients with nonfibrillation atrial tachyarrhythmias and congenital heart disease. J Am Coll Cardiol 24:1365, 1994
55. Lake CL, Booker PD: Pediatric Cardiac Anesthesia, 4th edition. Philadelphia, Lippincott-Williams and Wilkins, 2004
56. Andropoulos DB, Stayer SA, Russell IA: Anesthesia for Congenital Heart Disease. Armonk, NY, Futura, 2004
57. Carabello BA, Crawford FA Jr: Valvular heart disease. N Engl J Med 337:32, 1997
58. Markman P, Howitt G, Wade EG: Atrial septal defect in the middle-aged and elderly. Q J Med 34:409, 1965
59. Craig RJ, Selzer A: Natural history and prognosis of atrial septal defect. Circulation 37:805, 1968
60. Mattila S, Merikallio E, Tala P: ASD in patients over 40 years of age. Scand J Thorac Cardiovasc Surg 13:21, 1979
61. Campbell M: Natural history of coarctation of the aorta. Br Heart J 32:633, 1970
62. Boucher CA, Liberthson RR, Buckley MJ: Secundum atrial septal defect and significant mitral regurgitation: Incidence, management and morphologic basis. Chest 75:697, 1979
63. Liberthson RR, Boucher CA, Strauss HW, et al: Right ventricular function in adult atrial septal defect. Preoperative and postoperative assessment and clinical implications. Am J Cardiol 47:56, 1981
64. Davies H, Oliver GC, Rappoport WJ, Gazetopoulos N: Abnormal left heart function after operation for atrial septal defect. Br Heart J 32:747, 1970
65. Murphy JG, Gersh BJ, McGoon MD, et al: Long-term outcome after surgical repair of isolated atrial septal defect. Follow-up at 27 to 32 years. N Engl J Med 323:1645, 1990
66. Konstantinides S, Geibel A, Olschewski M, et al: A comparison of surgical and medical therapy for atrial septal defect in adults. N Engl J Med 333:469, 1995
67. Gatzoulis MA, Freeman MA, Siu SC, et al: Atrial arrhythmia after surgical closure of atrial septal defects in adults. N Engl J Med 340:839, 1999
68. Attie F, Rosas M, Granados N, et al: Surgical treatment for secundum atrial septal defects in patients >40 years old. A randomized clinical trial. J Am Coll Cardiol 38:2035, 2001
69. Du ZD, Hijazi ZM, Kleinman CS, et al: Comparison between transcatheter and surgical closure of secundum atrial septal defect in children and adults: Results of a multicenter nonrandomized trial. J Am Coll Cardiol 39:1836, 2002
70. Abbott ME: Coarctation of the aorta of adult type: II. A statistical study and historical retrospect of 200 recorded cases with autopsy, of stenosis or obliteration of the descending arch in subjects above the age of two years. Am Heart J 3:392, 1928
71. Reifenstein GH, Levine SA, Gross RE: Coarctation of the aorta: A review of 104 autopsied cases of the "adult type," 2 years of age or older. Am Heart J 33:146, 1947
72. Mitchell SC, Korones SB, Berendes HW: Congenital heart disease in 56,109 births. Incidence and natural history. Circulation 43:323, 1971
73. Maron BJ, Humphries JO, Rowe RD, Mellits ED: Prognosis of surgically corrected coarctation of the aorta. A 20-year postoperative appraisal. Circulation 47:119, 1973
74. Clarkson PM, Nicholson MR, Barratt-Boyes BG, et al: Results after repair of coarctation of the aorta beyond infancy: A 10-to-28 year follow-up with particular reference to late systemic hypertension. Am J Cardiol 51:1481, 1983
75. Therrien J, Gatzoulis M, Graham T, et al: Canadian Cardiovascular Society Consensus Conference 2001 update: Recommendations for the Management of Adults with Congenital Heart Disease—Part II. Can J Cardiol 17:1029, 2001
76. Hamdan MA, Maheshwari S, Fahey JT, Hellenbrand WE: Endovascular stents for coarctation of the aorta: Initial results and intermediate-term follow-up. J Am Coll Cardiol 38:1518, 2001
77. Graham TP Jr, Parrish MD, Boucek RJJ, et al: Assessment of ventricular size and function in congenitally corrected transposition of the great arteries. Am J Cardiol 51:244, 1983
78. Graham TP Jr, Bernard YD, Mellen BG, et al: Long-term outcome in congenitally corrected transposition of the great arteries: A multi-institutional study. J Am Coll Cardiol 36:255, 2000
79. Connelly MS, Robertson P, Liu P, et al: Congenitally corrected transposition of the great arteries in adults: Natural history. Circulation 90:I, 1994
80. Kumar AE, Fyler DC, Miettinen OS, Nadas AS: Ebstein's anomaly. Clinical profile and natural history. Am J Cardiol 28:84, 1971
81. Celermajer DS, Cullen S, Sullivan ID, et al: Outcome in neonates with Ebstein's anomaly. J Am Coll Cardiol 19:1041, 1992
82. Spitaels SE: Ebstein's anomaly of the tricuspid valve complexities and strategies. Cardiol Clin 20:431, 2002
83. Connolly HM, Warnes CA: Ebstein's anomaly: Outcome of pregnancy. J Am Coll Cardiol 23:1194, 1994
84. Eisenmenger V: Die angeborenen Defects des Kammerscheidewand des Herzen. Z Klin Med 32(suppl):1, 1897
85. Vongpatanasin W, Brickner ME, Hillis LD, Lange RA: The Eisenmenger syndrome in adults. Ann Intern Med 128:745, 1998
86. Cantor WJ, Harrison DA, Moussadji JS, et al: Determinants of survival and length of survival in adults with Eisenmenger syndrome. Am J Cardiol 84:677, 1999
87. Saha A, Balakrishnan KG, Jaiswal PK, et al: Prognosis for patients with Eisenmenger syndrome of various aetiology. Int J Cardiol 45:199, 1994
88. Oya H, Nagaya N, Uematsu M, et al: Poor prognosis and related factors in adults with Eisenmenger syndrome. Am Heart J 143:739, 2002
89. Daliento L, Somerville J, Presbitero P, et al: Eisenmenger syndrome. Factors relating to deterioration and death. Eur Heart J 19:1845, 1998
90. Bando K, Armitage JM, Paradis IL, et al: Indications for and results of single, bilateral, and heart-lung transplantation for pulmonary hypertension. J Thorac Cardiovasc Surg 108:1056, 1994
91. Holzman RS, Nargozian CD, Marnach R, McMillan CO: Epidural anesthesia in patients with palliated cyanotic congenital heart disease. J Cardiothorac Vasc Anesth 6:340, 1992
92. Devitt JH, Noble WH, Byrick RJ: A Swan-Ganz catheter-related complication in a patient with Eisenmenger's syndrome. Anesthesiology 57:335, 1982
93. Perloff JK: The Clinical Recognition of Congenital Heart Disease, 3rd edition. Philadelphia, WB Saunders, 1987
94. Avila WS, Grinberg M, Snitcowsky R, et al: Maternal and fetal outcome in pregnant women with Eisenmenger's syndrome. Eur Heart J 16:460, 1995
95. Gleicher N, Midwall J, Hochberger D, Jaffin H: Eisenmenger's syndrome and pregnancy. Obstet Gynecol Surv 34:721, 1979
96. Weiss BM, Zemp L, Seifert B, Hess OM: Outcome of pulmonary vascular disease in pregnancy: A systematic overview from 1978 through 1996. J Am Coll Cardiol 31:1650, 1998

97. Weiss BM, Hess OM: Pulmonary vascular disease and pregnancy: Current controversies, management strategies, and perspectives. Eur Heart J 21:104, 2000
98. Masuda M, Kado H, Kajihara N, et al: Early and late results of total correction of congenital cardiac anomalies in infancy. Jpn J Thorac Cardiovasc Surg 49:497, 2001
99. Elizari A, Somerville J: Experience with the Glenn anastomosis in the adult with cyanotic congenital heart disease. Cardiol Young 9:257, 1999
100. Fontan F, Kirklin JW, Fernandez G, et al: Outcome after a "perfect" Fontan operation. Circulation 81:1520, 1990
101. Driscoll DJ, Offord KP, Feldt RH, et al: Five- to fifteen-year follow-up after Fontan operation. Circulation 85:469, 1992
102. Veldtman GR, Nishimoto A, Siu S, et al: The Fontan procedure in adults. Heart 86:330, 2001
103. Durongpisitkul K, Porter CJ, Cetta F, et al: Predictors of early- and late-onset supraventricular tachyarrhythmias after Fontan operation. Circulation 98:1099, 1998
104. Mertens L, Hagler DJ, Sauer U, et al: Protein-losing enteropathy after the Fontan operation: An international multicenter study. PLE study group. J Thorac Cardiovasc Surg 115:1063, 1998
105. Pasque MK: Fontan hemodynamics. J Card Surg 3:45, 1988
106. Kirklin JK, Blackstone EH, Kirklin JW, et al: The Fontan operation. Ventricular hypertrophy, age, and date of operation as risk factors. J Thorac Cardiovasc Surg 92:1049, 1986
107. Mayer JE Jr, Helgason H, Jonas RA, et al: Extending the limits for modified Fontan procedures. J Thorac Cardiovasc Surg 92:1021, 1986
108. Cromme-Dijkhuis AH, Hess J, Hahlen K, et al: Specific sequelae after Fontan operation at mid- and long-term follow-up. Arrhythmia, liver dysfunction, and coagulation disorders. J Thorac Cardiovasc Surg 106:1126, 1993
109. Steven JM, McGowan FX: Neuraxial blockade for pediatric cardiac surgery: Lessons yet to be learned. Anesth Analg 90:1011, 2000
110. Chait HI, Kuhn MA, Baum VC: Inferior vena caval pressure reliably predicts right atrial pressure in pediatric cardiac surgical patients. Crit Care Med 22:219, 1994
111. Canobbio MM, Mair DD, van der Velde M, Koos BJ: Pregnancy outcomes after the Fontan repair. J Am Coll Cardiol 28:763, 1996
112. Fisher RG, Moodie DS, Sterba R, Gill CC: Patent ductus arteriosus in adults—long-term follow-up: Nonsurgical versus surgical treatment. J Am Coll Cardiol 8:280, 1986
113. Campbell M: Natural history of patent ductus arteriosus. Br Heart J 30:4, 1968
114. O'Fallon WM, Weidman WH: Long-term follow-up of congenital aortic stenosis, pulmonary stenosis and VSD. Circulation 87(suppl I), 1993
115. Hayes CJ, Gersony WM, Driscoll DJ, et al: Second natural history study of congenital heart defects. Results of treatment of patients with pulmonary valvular stenosis. Circulation 87:I-28, 1993
116. Sano T, Ogawa M, Taniguchi K, et al: Assessment of ventricular contractile state and function in patients with univentricular heart. Circulation 79:1247, 1989
117. Bertranou EG, Blackstone EH, Hazelrig JB, et al: Life expectancy without surgery in tetralogy of Fallot. Am J Cardiol 42:458, 1978
118. Murphy JG, Gersh BJ, Mair DD, et al: Long-term outcome in patients undergoing surgical repair of tetralogy of Fallot. N Engl J Med 329:593, 1993
119. Nollert G, Fischlein T, Bouterwek S, et al: Long-term survival in patients with repair of tetralogy of Fallot: 36-Year follow-up of 490 survivors of the first year after surgical repair. J Am Coll Cardiol 30:1374, 1997
120. Harrison DA, Harris L, Siu SC, et al: Sustained ventricular tachycardia in adult patients late after repair of tetralogy of Fallot. J Am Coll Cardiol 30:1368, 1997
121. Oechslin EN, Harrison DA, Harris L, et al: Reoperation in adults with repair of tetralogy of Fallot: Indications and outcomes. J Thorac Cardiovasc Surg 118:245, 1999
122. Russell IA, Miller Hance WC, Gregory G, et al: The safety and efficacy of sevoflurane anesthesia in infants and children with congenital heart disease. Anesth Analg 92:1152, 2001
123. Gatzoulis MA, Balaji S, Webber SA, et al: Risk factors for arrhythmia and sudden cardiac death late after repair of tetralogy of Fallot: A multicentre study. Lancet 356:975, 2000
124. Roos-Hesselink J, Perlroth MG, McGhie J, Spitaels S: Atrial arrhythmias in adults after repair of tetralogy of Fallot. Correlations with clinical, exercise, and echocardiographic findings. Circulation 91:2214, 1995
125. Harrison DA, Siu SC, Hussain F, et al: Sustained atrial arrhythmias in adults late after repair of tetralogy of Fallot. Am J Cardiol 87:584, 2001
126. Rammohan M, Airan B, Bhan A, et al: Total correction of tetralogy of Fallot in adults—surgical experience. Int J Cardiol 63:121, 1998
127. Kavey RE, Blackman MS, Sondheimer HM: Incidence and severity of chronic ventricular dysrhythmias after repair of tetralogy of Fallot. Am Heart J 103:342, 1982
128. Abd El Rahman MY, Abdul-Khaliq H, Vogel M, et al: Relation between right ventricular enlargement, QRS duration, and right ventricular function in patients with tetralogy of Fallot and pulmonary regurgitation after surgical repair. Heart 84:416, 2000
129. Cullen S, Celermajer DS, Franklin RC, et al: Prognostic significance of ventricular arrhythmia after repair of tetralogy of Fallot: A 12-year prospective study. J Am Coll Cardiol 23:1151, 1994
130. Gatzoulis MA, Till JA, Somerville J, Redington AN: Mechanoelectrical interaction in tetralogy of Fallot. QRS prolongation relates to right ventricular size and predicts malignant ventricular arrhythmias and sudden death. Circulation 92:231, 1995
131. Discigil B, Dearani JA, Puga FJ, et al: Late pulmonary valve replacement after repair of tetralogy of Fallot. J Thorac Cardiovasc Surg 121: 344, 2001
132. Heggie J, Poirer N, Williams RG, Karski J: Anesthetic considerations for adult cardiac surgery patients with congenital heart disease. Semin Cardiothorac Vasc Anesth 7:141, 2003
133. Graham TP Jr: Ventricular performance in congenital heart disease. Circulation 84:2259, 1991
134. Gelatt M, Hamilton RM, McCrindle BW, et al: Arrhythmia and mortality after the Mustard procedure: A 30-year single-center experience. J Am Coll Cardiol 29:194, 1997
135. Wilson NJ, Clarkson PM, Barratt-Boyes BG, et al: Long-term outcome after the Mustard repair for simple transposition of the great arteries. 28-Year follow-up. J Am Coll Cardiol 32:758, 1998
136. Warnes CA, Somerville J: Transposition of the great arteries: Late results in adolescents and adults after the Mustard procedure. Br Heart J 58:148, 1987
137. Myridakis DJ, Ehlers KH, Engle MA: Late follow-up after venous switch operation (Mustard procedure) for simple and complex transposition of the great arteries. Am J Cardiol 74:1030, 1994
138. Puley G, Siu S, Connelly M, et al: Arrhythmia and survival in patients >18 years of age after the Mustard procedure for complete transposition of the great arteries. Am J Cardiol 83:1080, 1999
139. Graham TP Jr, Burger J, Bender HW, et al: Improved right ventricular function after intra-atrial repair of transposition of the great arteries. Circulation 72(suppl II):II-45, 1985
140. Cochrane AD, Karl TR, Mee RB: Staged conversion to arterial switch for late failure of the systemic right ventricle. Ann Thorac Surg 56:854, 1993
141. Garson AJ: The emerging adult with arrhythmias after congenital heart disease: Management and financial health care policy. PACE 13:951, 1990
142. Mavroudis C, Backer CL: Arterial switch after failed atrial baffle procedures for transposition of the great arteries. Ann Thorac Surg 69:851, 2000
143. Losay J, Touchot A, Serraf A, et al: Late outcome after arterial switch operation for transposition of the great arteries. Circulation 104:I-121, 2001
144. Mahle WT, McBride MG, Paridon SM: Exercise performance after the arterial switch operation for D-transposition of the great arteries. Am J Cardiol 87:753, 2001
145. Rajasinghe HA, McElhinney DB, Reddy VM, et al: Long-term follow-up of truncus arteriosus repaired in infancy: A twenty-year experience. J Thorac Cardiovasc Surg 113:869, 1997
146. Schreiber C, Eicken A, Balling G, et al: Single centre experience on primary correction of common arterial trunk: Overall survival and freedom from reoperation after more than 15 years. Eur J Cardiothorac Surg 18:68, 2000
147. Wilson NJ, Neutze JM: Adult congenital heart disease: Principles and management guidelines: Part II. Aust N Z J Med 23:697, 1993
148. Jarmakani JM, Graham TP Jr, Canent RV Jr, Capp MP: The effect of corrective surgery on left heart volume and mass in children with VSD. Am J Cardiol 27:254, 1971
149. Jarmakani JM, Graham TPJ, Canent RVJ: Left ventricular contractile state in children with successfully corrected VSD. Circulation 45(suppl 1):102, 1972
150. Maron BJ, Redwood DR, Hirshfeld JWJ, et al: Postoperative assessment of patients with VSD and pulmonary hypertension. Response to intense upright exercise. Circulation 48:864, 1973

Chapter 23

THORACIC AORTA

Enrique J. Pantin, MD • Albert T. Cheung, MD

KEY POINTS

1. Deliberate hypothermia is the most important therapeutic intervention to prevent cerebral ischemia during temporary interruption of cerebral perfusion during aortic arch reconstruction.
2. Selective antegrade cerebral perfusion should be considered if the anticpiated duration of deep hypothermic circulatory arrest is greater than 30 to 45 minutes.
3. Early detection and interventions to increase spinal cord perfusion pressure are effective for the treatment of delayed-onset spinal cord ischemia after thoracic or thoracoabdominal aortic aneurysm repair.
4. Stanford type A aortic dissection involving the ascending aorta and aortic arch is a surgical emergency.
5. Stanford type B aortic dissection confined to the descending thoracic or abdominal aorta should be managed medically when possible.
6. Thoracic aortic aneurysms can cause compression of the trachea, left main stem bronchus, right ventricular outflow tract, right pulmonary artery, or esophagus.
7. Intraoperative transesophageal echocardiography can be used to diagnose type A aortic dissection or traumatic aortic injuries that require emergency operation.
8. Intraoperative transesophageal echocardiography and ultrasound imaging of the carotid arteries are useful for the diagnosis of aortic regurgitation, cardiac tamponade, myocardial ischemia, or cerebral malperfusion complicationg type A aortic dissection.
9. Severe atheromatous disease or thrombus in the thoracic or descending aorta is a risk factor for stroke.
10. Distal aortic perfusion pressure should be maintained to prevent spinal cord ischemia in patients with aortic coarctation.

Thoracic aortic diseases are generally surgical problems and require surgical treatment (Table 23–1). Acute aortic dissections, rupturing aortic aneurysms, and traumatic aortic injuries are surgical emergencies. Subacute aortic dissection and expanding aortic aneurysms require urgent surgical intervention. Stable thoracic or thoracoabdominal aortic aneurysms (TAAAs), aortic coarctation, or atheromatous disease causing embolization may be considered for elective surgical repair. Increased public awareness of thoracic aortic disease, early recognition of acute aortic syndromes by emergency medical personnel, improved diagnostic imaging technology for the diagnosis of thoracic aortic disease, and an aging population all contribute to the increased number of patients requiring aortic surgery. Furthermore, improvements in the surgical treatment of thoracic aortic diseases combined with increased treatment options such as endovascular stent repair have led to an increased number of patient referrals to centers specializing in the management of patients with thoracic aortic diseases. Improved treatment and survival after aortic surgical procedures often provide a cure for the original disease but have created new and unique problems. An increasing number of patients who have had prior aortic surgical procedures require reoperation for long-term complications of aortic surgery such as bioprosthetic valve or graft failure, aortic pseudoaneurysm at old vascular graft anastomosis, endocarditis, or progression of the original disease process into native segments of the thoracic aorta.

The anesthetic management of surgical patients requiring aortic surgery presents some distinctive medical problems in addition to the usual considerations associated with major thoracic or thoracoabdominal operations. The process of repairing or replacing a portion of the thoracic aorta usually requires the temporary interruption of blood flow, creating the potential for ischemia or infarction of almost any major organ system in the body. Strategies to provide organ perfusion, to protect organs from the consequences of hypoperfusion, and to monitor and treat end-organ ischemia during aortic operations are critical aspects of the anesthetic management for thoracic aortic diseases and contribute importantly to the overall success of operations. Some of the procedures performed and managed by surgeons and anesthesiologists for organ protection during thoracic aortic operations, such as partial left heart bypass for distal aortic perfusion, deep hypothermic circulatory arrest (DHCA), selective antegrade or retrograde cerebral perfusion, and lumbar cerebrospinal fluid (CSF) drainage, are practiced routinely in no other area of medicine.

ANATOMY OF THE AORTA

The aorta is the large conducting vessel that starts at the aortic valve and ends at the iliac bifurcation. The aorta serves both as a conducting vessel and as a secondary passive pump as a consequence of its elastic recoil. During ventricular systole, the aortic lumen distends as it receives the cardiac stroke volume. In diastole, after aortic valve closure, blood is propelled forward in response to the elastic recoil of the vessel. The pulse wave is transmitted distally into the aorta at approximately 5 m/sec, exceeding the actual aortic blood flow velocity of 40 to 50 cm/sec. Systolic blood pressure within the aorta is generated by the combined effects of stroke volume, aortic compliance, and peripheral vascular resistance. With aging, isolated systolic hypertension develops when the aorta loses elasticity and is unable to dampen the stroke volume.

During fetal development, the ductus arteriosus diverts blood entering the pulmonary artery away from the lungs and into the distal aortic arch. After birth, expansion of the lungs and constriction of the ductus arteriosus in response to an increase in the oxygen content of the blood direct blood flow

Table 23–1 Diseases of the Thoracic Aorta That Are Amenable to Surgical Treatment

Aneurysm
Congenital or developmental
Marfan's syndrome, Ehlers-Danlos syndrome
Degenerative
Cystic medial degeneration
Annuloaortic ectasia
Atherosclerotic
Traumatic
Blunt and penetrating trauma
Inflammatory
Takayasu's arteritis, Bechet's syndrome, Kawasaki's disease
Microvascular diseases (polyarteritis)
Infectious (mycotic)
Bacterial, fungal, spirochetal, viral
Mechanical
Post-stenotic, associated with an arteriovenous fistula
Anastomotic (postarteriotomy)
Pseudoaneurysm
Aortic dissection
Stanford type A
Stanford type B
Intramural hematoma
Penetrating atherosclerotic ulcer
Atherosclerotic disease
Traumatic aortic injury
Aortic coarctation

Adapted from Kouchoukos NT, Dougenis D: Surgery of the aorta. N Engl J Med 336:1876, 1997.

from the pulmonary artery into the pulmonary circulation. The ductus arteriosus is functionally closed in most newborns by 48 hours of life and permanently closed by 3 weeks after birth.[1] After closure, the ductus arteriosus fibroses and becomes the "ligament arteriosum." Occasionally the ductus arteriosus does not close and it persists as a patent ductus arteriosus. Sometimes, distal closure of the ductus, but incomplete proximal closure, leaves a ductal diverticulum that can be confused with an aortic injury by angiographic studies. Aortic coarctation may be caused by ductal tissue remaining in the aortic wall that causes narrowing of the aortic lumen as it constricts.

Similar to other arteries in the body, the aorta is composed of three layers: a thin intima or inner layer lined by endothelium, a thick media or middle layer, and a thin adventitia or outermost layer. The endothelium is in direct contact with blood, is easily traumatized, and is the site for atherosclerosis. The media comprises 80% of the aortic wall thickness and is composed of multiple spirally arranged intertwining layers of elastic tissue that provide tensile strength and elasticity to the vessel. The adventitia is composed mainly of collagen and houses the vasa vasorum. The vasa vasorum nourishes the outer half of the aortic wall but is absent in the infrarenal segment of the aorta, a possible explanation for the frequency of infrarenal aortic aneurysms. The layers of the aorta are normally indistinguishable by current clinical imaging techniques, including transesophageal echocardiography (TEE). Diseases or traumatic injury to the aortic wall can disrupt individual layers or cause the layers to separate, making them visible on computed tomography (CT), magnetic resonance imaging (MRI), angiography, or TEE.

The thoracic aorta is anatomically divided into three major segments: the ascending aorta, the arch, and the descending aorta. The ascending aorta is approximately 9 cm long and is subdivided further into the aortic root and ascending aorta. The aorta originates at the aortic valve just to the right of midline at the base of the left ventricle. The aortic root and proximal ascending aorta lie within the pericardial sac. The aorta travels superiorly, anteriorly, and to the left and then turns posteriorly and towards the left up to the level of the body of the fourth thoracic vertebrae. From there it continues inferiorly, initially somewhat anterior and to the left side of the spine, crossing the diaphragm until it ends in front of the fourth lumbar vertebra. The aortic root begins at the aortic valve annulus, includes the sinuses of Valsalva, and ends at the sinotubular junction. The origin of the innominate artery marks the end of the ascending aorta and the beginning of the aortic arch. The aortic arch lies within the superior mediastinum between the ascending and descending thoracic aorta. The aortic arch ends after the origin of the left subclavian artery. The aortic isthmus is the segment of aorta where the distal aortic arch becomes the descending thoracic aorta. At the aortic isthmus, the somewhat mobile ascending aorta and arch joins the descending thoracic aorta that is fixed to the posterior thoracic cage by pleural reflections, the intercostal arteries, the ligamentum arteriosum, and the left subclavian artery. For this reason, the aortic isthmus is subjected to high shear forces in response to blunt trauma or rapid deceleration making this area especially vulnerable to traumatic injury. The aortic isthmus is also the most common site for aortic coarctation.

The left and right coronary arteries are the first branches of the aorta. The aortic arch gives origin to the innominate, left carotid, and left subclavian arteries that supply blood to the arms, head, and neck. The innominate artery or brachiocephalic trunk is the first branch arising from the summit of the aortic arch, followed by the left common carotid artery, and then the left subclavian artery. The isolated left vertebral artery is a left vertebral artery that originates directly from the aortic arch, is one of the most common aortic arch branch anomalies, and occurs in about 4% of the general population.[2] There are multiple aortic arch anatomic variations, including vascular rings, right-sided aortic arch, and one or more branching anomalies. A right-sided aortic arch is found in 0.1% of autopsies and radiographic series. Anatomic variations can also exist in the number, origin, and branching of the aortic arch branch vessels.

The aortic arch functions also to modulate blood pressure and contains baroreceptors within its outer wall. The aortic bodies are located inferior to the aortic arch and signal changes in the oxygen content of the blood. Compared with the carotid sinus, aortic baroreceptors respond to a higher threshold pressure and are less sensitive than the carotid sinus receptors. The aortic baroreceptors are derived from the aortic nerve, via the vagus nerve, and send impulses to the brainstem that act on the cardiovascular center in the medulla to modulate autonomic nervous system activity.[3]

GENERAL CONSIDERATIONS FOR THE PERIOPERATIVE CARE OF AORTIC SURGICAL PATIENTS

Patients undergoing thoracic aortic operations of any type share common considerations for the safe conduct of anesthesia and perioperative care (Table 23–2). The common elements in the perioperative care of thoracic surgical patients are addressed in this section. Unique considerations and specialized care that apply for specific pathologic conditions or operative procedures are addressed individually in the sections devoted to the management of each disease class.

Preanesthetic Assessment

The preanesthetic assessment and management of the thoracic aortic surgical patient begin ideally before the patient even enters the operating room. The first step is to determine if the planned operative procedure is emergent, urgent, or elective. For urgent or emergent operations, it is useful to assign individual members of the team specific tasks to prepare the patient and the operating room in the most efficient manner. For example, one individual can be assigned to gather patient information, review diagnostic studies, and formulate an anesthetic plan. Another individual can be assigned to interview the patient and obtain informed consent. Others can simultaneously secure intravascular access, obtain laboratory specimens including a blood sample for type and crossmatch, apply physiologic monitors, and prepare the operating room.

Second, it is important to determine the operative diagnosis because both the anesthetic management and surgical approach are dictated by the anatomic extent of the lesion and the physiologic consequences of the disease. Diseases involving the aortic root, ascending aorta, and proximal aortic arch are generally approached through a median sternotomy, whereas diseases of the distal aortic arch or descending thoracic aorta are approached through a left thoracotomy or thoracoabdominal incision. Sometimes, the operative diagnosis can be established in advance. Other times, a presumptive diagnosis has been made based on patient symptoms or available reports, and the definitive diagnosis needs to be verified after patient arrival into the operating room by direct review of the diagnostic studies or by intraoperative transesophageal echocardiography. In either case, it is important to discuss the anesthetic and operative plan with the surgical team to be properly prepared for all possible contingencies. Direct review of the actual diagnostic imaging studies such as the angiogram, CT scan, MRI, or echocardiogram not only verifies the operative diagnosis but also provides important information that determines the surgical options. Knowing the size and anatomic extent of aortic pathology provides information about the physiologic impact and consequences of the lesion, permitting the anesthesiologist to anticipate potential difficulties associated with anesthetic procedures, problems related to the surgical repair, and postoperative complications.

Assessing the medical condition of the aortic surgical patient should be approached methodically to evaluate each body system in terms of how it will affect the conduct of anesthesia and surgery. The baseline functional reserve of each body system also determines the spectrum of complications that can be anticipated during and after surgery, and priority can be assigned to strategies directed toward the protection of specific organ systems. For example, baseline renal insufficiency affects fluid management, alters the choice of drugs that have the potential to cause nephrotoxicity, and changes the dosing of drugs that are excreted through the kidneys. The presence of cerebrovascular disease dictates, among other considerations, blood pressure management to ensure adequate cerebral perfusion. Hepatic and hematologic dysfunction may be associated with coagulopathy, increased risk of bleeding and hemorrhagic complications, and increased need for transfusion. The presence of lung disease may indicate an increased risk of postoperative respiratory failure or pneumonia. Severe atherosclerosis or peripheral vascular disease increases the risk of stroke, embolic complications, and limb ischemia. Coronary artery disease, valvular heart disease, or cardiomyopathy increases the risk of heart failure, myocardial ischemia or infarction, arrhythmias, and pulmonary edema.

Table 23–2 General Considerations for the Anesthetic Care of Thoracic Aortic Surgical Patients

Preanesthetic assessment
Urgency of the operation (emergent, urgent, or elective)
Pathology and anatomic extent of the disease
Median sternotomy vs. thoracotomy vs. endovascular approach
Mediastinal mass effect
Airway compression or deviation
Preexisting or associated medical conditions
Aortic valve disease
Cardiac tamponade
Coronary artery stenosis
Cardiomyopathy
Cerebrovascular disease
Pulmonary disease
Renal insufficiency
Esophageal disease (contraindications to TEE)
Coagulopathy
Prior aortic operations
Preoperative medications
Coumadin
Antiplatelet therapy
Antihypertensive therapy
Anesthetic management
Hemodynamic monitoring
Proximal aortic pressure
Distal aortic pressure
Central venous pressure
Pulmonary artery pressure and cardiac output
TEE
Neurophysiologic monitoring
Electroencephalography (EEG)
Somatosensory evoked potentials (SSEPs)
Motor evoked potentials (MEPs)
Jugular venous oxygen saturation
Lumbar CSF pressure
Body temperature
Single-lung ventilation for thoracotomy
Double-lumen endobronchial tube
Endobronchial blocker
Potential for bleeding
Large-bore intravenous access
Blood product availability
Antifibrinolytic therapy
Antibiotic prophylaxis
Postoperative care considerations and complications
Hypothermia
Hypotension
Hypertension
Bleeding
Spinal cord ischemia
Stroke
Renal insufficiency
Respiratory insufficiency
Phrenic nerve injury
Diaphragmatic dysfunction
Recurrent laryngeal nerve injury
Pain management

Preoperative Medications

Preoperative medications and the dose of medication should be noted and often provide information about the nature and severity of preexisting medical conditions. As a general rule, all cardiac, pulmonary, and antiseizure medications should be continued up until the morning of surgery. All oral antihyperglycemic agents should be discontinued the night before surgery to avoid hypoglycemia. Metformin should be discontinued at least 24 hours prior to surgery to avoid the potential risk of severe lactic acidosis in response to the administration of iodinated contrast agents or perioperative hypovolemia. If a patient is receiving insulin, one third or one half the usual dose should be given the morning of surgery and glucose concentrations closely monitored. Warfarin or Coumadin should be discontinued 3 to 7 days before the surgery to allow full recovery of the coagulation function verified by a normalized INR. If a patient requires anticoagulation until the time of surgery, the patient should be admitted and placed on a heparin infusion that can then be discontinued shortly before surgery. Patients who are on low-molecular-weight heparin, aspirin, or adenosine diphosphate platelet receptor inhibitors (clopidogrel and ticlopidine) or who received platelet glycoprotein IIb/IIIa inhibitors (abciximab, eptifibatide, tirofiban) are at increased risk of perioperative bleeding. Optimally, aspirin and clopidogrel should be discontinued at least 1 week prior to surgery and ticlopidine discontinued at least 14 days before surgery because their antiplatelet actions cannot be immediately reversed even with platelet transfusions.[4]

Finally, the need, risks, and conduct of anesthetic procedures need to be considered. For example, preexisting coagulopathy or use of antiplatelet therapy may increase the risk of hemorrhagic complications as a consequence of lumbar CSF drainage or epidural analgesia. Cervical spine or esophageal disease may prohibit the use of intraoperative TEE. Aortic pathology distorting the trachea or bronchus may increase the difficulty of tracheal intubation or techniques to provide one-lung ventilation. Large aneurysms or a contained rupture of the aorta may produce a mass effect in the mediastinum or thorax, causing airway or vascular compromise after the induction of general anesthesia.

Anesthetic Management

Considered as a group, any operative procedure involving the aorta from endovascular stent repairs to open repair of TAAAs is associated with the potential for catastrophic bleeding and cardiovascular collapse. For this reason, continuous diagnostic electrocardiographic monitoring, intra-arterial blood pressure monitoring, large-bore vascular access for rapid volume expansion, and ensuring the immediate availability or packed red blood cells can be justified in virtually every patient. Central venous access for monitoring the right atrial pressure and the administration of vasoactive drug therapy to control the circulation can also be justified in almost all cases. Pulmonary artery catheterization to measure pulmonary artery pressures, cardiac output, and mixed venous oxygen saturation is useful for operations involving cardiopulmonary bypass (CPB), DHCA, partial left-sided heart bypass, or cross-clamping of the thoracic aorta. Routine availability and use of intraoperative TEE provide both diagnostic information and the ability to assess ventricular function.

Arguments can be made for using either the left or right radial artery for intra-arterial blood pressure monitoring. A right radial arterial catheter can detect partial occlusion or obstruction of flow into the innominate artery caused by inadvertent placement of the aortic cross-clamp too near to the origin of the innominate artery during the course of operations involving the ascending aorta or aortic arch. A right radial arterial catheter also permits monitoring of blood pressure during repair of the proximal thoracic aorta or distal aortic arch if the left subclavian artery has to be clamped. A left radial arterial catheter must be used for selective antegrade cerebral perfusion (ACP) via the right axillary artery. Sometimes bilateral radial arterial catheters are necessary. A femoral arterial catheter is necessary to monitor distal aortic pressure when partial left heart bypass is used to provide distal aortic perfusion.

Large-bore peripheral intravenous catheters that are 16 gauge or larger provide satisfactory sites for rapid intravascular volume expansion. An intravenous administration set integrated with a fluid warming unit is desirable particularly for the rapid administration of blood products. Often, patients coming to the operating room from other areas of the hospital already have established intravascular access with small-bore intravenous catheters at the site of large veins. One approach in this scenario is to exchange the small-bore catheter with a commercially available 7.5 Fr to 8.5 Fr large-bore rapid infusion catheter over a sterile guide wire. The only precaution in the use of these catheters is to ensure that the vein is large enough to accept the larger diameter catheter. Alternatively, a large-bore central venous catheter, usually an 8.5 Fr introducer sheath, 9 Fr introducer–multiple-access catheter, or hemodialysis catheter, placed in the internal jugular, subclavian, or femoral vein can be used for volume expansion. When a pulmonary artery catheter is necessary, a second introducer sheath for volume expansion can be placed also into the right internal jugular vein. For this procedure, both guide wires should be placed with at least 2 cm of separation between them. Central venous cannulation can be achieved by either anatomic landmark guidance or ultrasound guidance. Ultrasound guidance may increase both the speed and safety of venous cannulation, which is particularly advantageous in emergency operations or when the patient is hemodynamically unstable. A urinary catheter with a temperature probe to measure core temperature, together with a nasopharyngeal temperature probe, is necessary to monitor both the absolute temperature and rate of change of body temperature during deliberate hypothermia and subsequent rewarming. The temperature probe of the pulmonary artery catheter can provide core temperature monitoring, and a rectal temperature probe can be used to monitor shell temperature.

The hemodynamic condition of the patient should be reassessed immediately prior to the induction of general anesthesia. The decrease in arterial pressure in response to anesthetic drugs and subsequent increase in response to tracheal intubation should be anticipated. Both vasopressor drugs and vasodilator drugs should be immediately available to provide precise control of the blood pressure. Intravenous vasodilator drugs being infused to treat preoperative hypertension often need to be reduced in dose or discontinued upon induction of general anesthesia. Etomidate is a useful induction agent for patients in cardiogenic shock because it does not attenuate sympathetic nervous system responses and has no direct actions on myocardial contractility or vascular tone. In hemodynamically unstable patients, a narcotic such as fentanyl in combination with a benzodiazepine such as midazolam can be subsequently titrated incrementally to maintain general anesthesia after induction with etomidate. In elective cases, general anesthesia can be induced with routine intravenous hypnotic drugs followed by a narcotic to attenuate the hypertensive responses to tracheal intubation and skin incision. Antibiotic prophylaxis administration should optimally be completed at least 30 minutes before skin incision to achieve adequate bactericidal levels in tissue. Antifibrinolytic therapy, if used, should be administered prior to full anticoagulation for extracorporeal circulation.

The maintenance of general anesthesia can usually be accomplished with a combination of narcotic analgesics, benzodiazepine sedative hypnotics, an inhaled general anesthetic, and a nondepolarizing muscle relaxant. Anesthetics can be reduced in response to moderate hypothermia in the range of 30°C and then discontinued during deep hypothermia at 18°C and resumed upon rewarming. When electroencephalographic (EEG) or somatosensory evoked potential (SSEP) monitoring is required during surgery, barbiturates or bolus doses of propofol are avoided and the dose of the inhaled anesthetic is reduced to 0.5 MAC and kept constant to prevent anesthetic-induced changes in the monitored signals. Propofol, narcotics, and neuromuscular blocking drugs can be used during SSEP monitoring. When intraoperative motor evoked potential (MEP) monitoring is required, total intravenous anesthesia with propofol in combination with remifentanil or similar narcotic without neuromuscular blockade is necessary to ensure consistent reproducible recordings and a good-quality signal. In the majority of cases, the duration of general anesthesia is designed to persist for approximately 1 to 2 hours after patient transfer to the intensive care unit (ICU) to permit a gradual and controlled emergence from general anesthesia. If epidural analgesia is used intraoperatively, a dilute solution of local anesthetic and narcotic is preferred to prevent hypotension caused by sympathetic nervous system blockade and to prevent complete motor or sensory blockade to permit neurologic assessment of lower extremity function.

The potential for blood loss and bleeding is always a consideration in operations on the thoracic aorta. The presence of intrinsic disease of the vessel wall, construction of numerous vascular anastomosis in large conducting vessels, need for extracorporeal circulation, and application of deliberate hypothermia all combine to create a situation where blood loss and transfusion therapy are commonplace.[5] Because blood loss can occur rapidly and unpredictably and be difficult to control, it is often prudent to have fresh frozen plasma and platelets available to provide ongoing replacement of coagulation factors during transfusion of packed red blood cells. The time delay required for laboratory testing to verify the depletion of platelets and clotting factors in the setting of ongoing blood loss is often too long to be useful as a guide for transfusion therapy. Strategies to decrease the risk of bleeding and to conserve blood include discontinuation of anticoagulation and antiplatelet therapy prior to surgery, antifibrinolytic therapy, the routine use of intraoperative cell salvage, biologic glue, and precise control of arterial pressure and prevention of hypertensive episodes in the perioperative period. The antifibrinolytic agents, ε-aminocaproic acid or tranexamic acid, have been safely used in the setting of thoracic aortic surgery with DHCA. Early experience with the use of aprotinin in cases requiring DHCA raised concerns about its safety,[6,7] but subsequent experience suggested that it was safe when the dose of heparin was adjusted accordingly and the activated coagulation time (ACT) was measured properly using kaolin assay and maintained during the period of extracorporeal circulation.[8-10] The infusion of antifibrinolytic should be discontinued during the period of DHCA and resumed upon reperfusion. Aprotinin should not be combined or administered together with ε-amiocaproic acid to avoid the risk of intravascular thrombosis. Recombinant activated factor VIIa is a synthetic hemostatic agent that promotes hemostasis by binding with tissue factor at the site of tissue injury to promote clot formation.[11] Although experience with this agent has been limited, dramatic responses to this drug have been observed in response to coagulopathic bleeding refractory to conventional therapy in the setting of trauma, cardiac, and aortic surgery.[12-14] In the surgical setting, recombinant activated factor VIIa is administered at dose of 90 μg/kg IV and repeated once after 2 hours. Recombinant activated factor VIIa has an estimated plasma half-life of 2.6 hours and causes a rapid decrease in the prothrombin time.

Postoperative Care

After completion of the operation, the patient should be transported directly from the operating room into the intensive care unit or postanesthetic care unit for recovery. Transfer of information to the critical care team in advance to receiving the patient is necessary to ensure an uninterrupted transition of care. Immediate application of forced-air warming prevents further temperature drift and restores normothermia even in the moderately hypothermic patient.[15] In the absence of complications and when the medical condition of the patient is stable, the patient can be allowed to emerge from the effects of general anesthesia. Early emergence from general anesthesia is preferable because it permits early postoperative assessment of neurologic function. If the physiologic condition of the patient does not permit safe emergence from general anesthesia, sedation and analgesia can be provided in combination with mechanical ventilatory or circulatory support until the condition of the patient improves.

Common early complications include hypothermia, bleeding, hypertension, hypotension, ischemia, embolism, stroke, agitation and confusion, respiratory failure, and renal failure. Hyperglycemia, anemia, coagulopathy, electrolyte disturbances, and acid-base abnormalities are also common. Frequent hemodynamic assessment is important to control the circulation with short-acting vasoactive drug therapy and to detect cardiac arrhythmias. Arterial blood gas analysis and respiratory assessment are necessary to adjust the level of mechanical ventilatory support and determine the optimal time for safe extubation of the trachea. Laboratory testing to measure electrolyte concentration, hematologic parameters, and coagulation profile is necessary to institute immediate corrective measures. Maintaining glucose concentrations within the normal physiologic range is considered important because hyperglycemia has been associated with increased risk of infection, increased ICU mortality, and adverse neurologic outcome.[16] The chest roentgenogram is obtained to verify the proper position of the endotracheal tube and the position of intravascular catheters and to diagnose pneumothorax, atelectasis, pleural effusions, or pulmonary edema. Perioperative antibiotic prophylaxis is typically continued for 48 hours after surgery to decrease the risk of wound and endovascular infections.

THORACIC AORTIC ANEURYSM

An aortic aneurysm is a dilatation of the aorta containing all three layers of the vessel wall that has a diameter of at least 1.5 times that of the expected normal diameter of that given aortic segment.[17] Thoracic aortic aneurysms are common, detected in 10% of autopsies, have an incidence of 5.9 per 100,000 person-years, and are the most common reason for thoracic aortic surgery. The median age at the time of diagnosis is 65 years, and it occurs 2 to 4 times more frequently in males. Common risk factors for thoracic aortic aneurysms include hypertension, hypercholesterolemia, prior tobacco use, collagen vascular disease, and family history of aortic disease. Thoracic aortic aneurysms are classified by their location, size, shape, and etiology. Among thoracic aortic aneurysms, descending thoracic aortic aneurysms are most common, followed by ascending aortic aneurysms, and less often by aortic arch aneurysms.[18]

The anatomic location of the aneurysm and its extent determine its pathophysiologic consequences, operative approaches, and postoperative complications. Aneurysms involving the aortic root and ascending aorta are commonly associated with bicuspid aortic valve or aortic regurgitation (AR). Aneurysms extending into or involving the aortic arch require temporary interruption of cerebral blood flow to accomplish the operative repair. Endovascular stent repair is an option for aneurysms isolated to the descending thoracic aorta ending above the diaphragm. Repair of descending TAAAs requires the sacrifice of some or all of the segmental intercostal arteries branches and is associated with a risk of postoperative paraplegia from spinal cord ischemia or infarction. Aneurysmal disease of the thoracic aorta is often a diffuse process affecting multiple segments of the aorta and producing vessel tortuosity and often coexists in combination with isolated aneurysms of the abdominal aorta.

The shape of thoracic aortic aneurysms can be described as either fusiform or saccular. Fusiform aneurysms are more common, associated with atherosclerotic or collagen vascular disease, and usually affect a longer segment of the aorta, producing a dilation of the entire circumference of the vessel wall. Saccular aneurysms are more localized, confined to an isolated segment of the aorta, and produce a localized outpouching of the vessel wall. Pseudoaneurysm or a false aneurysm is a localized dilation of the aorta that does not contain all three layers of the vessel wall and instead consists of connective tissue, clot, or other surrounding tissues making up parts of the wall. Pseudoaneurysms are caused by a contained rupture of the aorta or arise from intimal disruptions, penetrating atheromas, or partial dehiscence of the suture line at the site of a previous aortic prosthetic vascular graft. Aortic aneurysms can also be associated with dissection of the vessel wall.

Atherosclerosis is the most common cause or contributing cause of aortic aneurysm. The disease process is associated with the breakdown of collagen and elastin matrix within the medial layer of the aorta leading to cystic medial necrosis, structural weakness, a predisposition to dissection, and an increase in the vessel diameter. *Annuloaortic ectasia* is a term used to describe isolated dilatation of the ascending aorta, aortic root, and aortic valve annulus. Dilation of the aortic valve annulus, aortic root, and ascending aorta pulls the aortic leaflets apart and causes central AR. Cystic medial necrosis is also an underlying pathology. Annuloaortic ectasia is a relatively common cause of pure AR, commonly seen in younger men in their fourth to sixth decades of life, associated with bicuspid aortic valve, and is a predisposition to aortic dissection.[19] Before antibiotics, tertiary syphilis was also a common cause of aortic aneurysm. Other inflammatory causes for aneurysm include giant cell arteritis, mycotic aneurysm from endocarditis, or Takayasu arteritis. Genetic defects in collagen synthesis cause thoracic aortic aneurysms in patients with Marfan syndrome or Ehlers-Danlos syndrome and possibly contribute to other familial forms of aortic aneurysms. Atherosclerotic disease of the thoracic aorta causing aneurysm is a systemic process and often associated with thromboembolic disease, intimal damage resulting in dissection, or occlusive peripheral vascular disease. Patients who survive aortic dissection often progress to develop aortic aneurysm as a consequence of the chronic dissection, weakened vessel wall, and expansion of the false lumen.

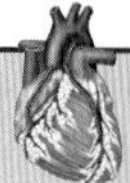

BOX 23–1 *Potential Complications of Thoracic Aortic Aneurysms*

- Rupture
- Aortic regurgitation
- Trachea or left main stem bronchial compression
- Right pulmonary artery or right ventricular outflow tract obstruction
- Esophageal compression

Most thoracic aortic aneurysms are asymptomatic and discovered incidentally through screening or as a consequence of medical workup for other cardiovascular diseases[18] (Box 23–1). The most common initial symptoms of thoracic aortic aneurysm are chest or back pain caused by aneurysmal expansion, rupture, or bony erosion. The mass effect of the aneurysm can cause hoarseness from stretching or compression of the recurrent laryngeal nerve, atelectasis from compression of the left lung, superior vena cava syndrome from compression of the superior vena cava or innominate vein, dysphagia from compression of the esophagus, or dyspnea from compression of the trachea, mainstem bronchus, or pulmonary artery. Other symptoms include wheezing, cough, hemoptysis, or hematemesis.[20] Aneurysm of the aortic root causing AR may present with dyspnea on exertion, heart failure, or pulmonary edema. Atherosclerotic aneurysms with mural thrombus may present with embolism, stroke, mesenteric ischemia, renal insufficiency, or limb ischemia.[21]

Leakage or rupture of thoracic aortic aneurysms should be treated as a surgical emergency. Expansion and impending rupture are often heralded by the development of new or worsening pain, often of sudden onset. Rupture is accompanied by the dramatic onset of excruciating pain and hypotension. Rupture of an ascending aortic aneurysm into the pericardial sac causes cardiac tamponade. Rupture of a descending aortic aneurysm may cause hemothorax, aortobronchial fistula, or aortoesophageal fistula. If surrounding tissue does not contain a ruptured aortic aneurysm, the patient will exsanguinate and die.

Diagnostic Imaging for Thoracic Aortic Aneurysms

An abnormal chest roentgenogram is common in patients with thoracic aortic aneurysms, but the routine chest radiograph provides limited diagnostic information for characterizing the location, size, and extent of aneurysms. A widened mediastinum, enlarged aortic knob, dilated descending thoracic aorta, calcifications within the aortic shadow, leftward deviation of the trachea, upward deviation of the left main stem bronchus, or a new left pleural effusion observed on the chest radiograph may suggest the presence of thoracic aortic disease and warrants additional imaging studies. Abdominal duplex ultrasound examination is useful for screening, detecting, and quantifying the size of abdominal aortic aneurysms or for detecting abdominal extension of a thoracic aortic aneurysm.[22-23] The lungs and sternum in the chest limit the acoustic windows for transthoracic ultrasound examination of the thoracic aorta, but in general a fair examination of the thoracic aorta can be obtained. Aortic angiography and digital subtraction angiography were traditionally the standard for diagnosis and evaluation of thoracic aortic aneurysm, but CT, MRI, and TEE imaging techniques have largely replaced the catheter-based technique. Angiography remains an important imaging technique for the evaluation and mapping of aortic branch vessels, obtaining physiologic information such as pressure measurements, and for interventional procedures such as endovascular stent repair. The risk of radiocontrast-induced nephropathy should always be considered in patients undergoing angiography prior to surgery.

Computed tomographic angiography (CTA) images the vasculature by rapid acquisition of images during the arterial phase of an intravenous radiocontrast agent injection. In addition to defining vascular anatomy, CTA provides high-resolution visualization of surrounding soft tissue and adjacent nonvascular structures. Extravasation of contrast out of the vessel lumen indicates aneurysm rupture or leak. The advantages of CTA include high spatial resolution, wide availability, rapid acquisition, and the ability to image calcifications and metallic implants such as stents. Postproccessing of the CTA data can also be used to generate volumetrically rendered images of the aorta that can be useful for characterizing complex anatomic features or for designing and sizing intravascular stent grafts. As with angiography, use of iodinated contrast agents in doses averaging 2 mg of iodine/kg has the potential to cause nephrotoxicity. If feasible, the administration of acetylcysteine or sodium bicarbonate may help to reduce the risk of nephrotoxicity.[24,25]

Contrast-enhanced three-dimensional magnetic resonance angiography (MRA) with gadolinium-based contrast injection agents also provides excellent detail of the aortic vascular anatomy. The spatial resolution of MRA is slightly inferior to CTA, but the variety of imaging sequences available with MRA allows some degree of tissue or fluid characterization. The disadvantages of MRA include limited availability of scanners and radiographers for interpretation of studies, the inability to study patients with metallic implants or artificial pacemakers, difficulty performing studies on patients requiring continuous hemodynamic monitoring being managed on continuous intravenous infusions, and the time required for image acquisition. Advantages of MRA and MRI are the avoidance of ionizing radiation and the lack of renal toxicity.[24]

TEE can also be used to diagnose and characterize aneurysms of the thoracic aorta. TEE can image the thoracic aorta from the aortic valve to the distal ascending aorta and from the distal aortic arch to the proximal abdominal aorta. The distal ascending aorta and aortic arch cannot be reliably imaged by TEE because the intervening trachea and left main stem bronchus obstructs the acoustic window from the esophagus in those regions. TEE has the advantages of portability and findings can be interpreted in real-time. TEE can also be performed at the bedside as well as during surgery without interfering with the conduct of surgery. The ability to image motion and combine information from Doppler color flow imaging enables TEE to detect AR, dissection, characterize blood flow within the aorta, and assess cardiac function. Disadvantages of TEE include the requirement for topical anesthesia of the airway and sedation or anesthesia, inability to provide volumetric renditions of vascular anatomy, and risk of injury to patients with large or inflammatory thoracic aortic aneurysms impinging upon the esophagus.

General Surgical Considerations for Thoracic Aortic Aneurysms

The objective of surgical repair is to replace the aneurysmal segment of aorta with a tube graft to prevent morbidity and mortality as a consequence of aneurysm rupture. The indications for aneurysm repair and optimal timing of the repair remain controversial and are often based on clinical judgment. In general, indications for operative repair include the presence of symptoms refractory to medical management, evidence of rupture, an aneurysm diameter of 5.0 to 5.5 cm for an ascending aortic aneurysm, an aneurysm diameter of 6.0 to 7.0 cm for a descending thoracic aneurysm, or an increase in aneurysm diameter greater than or equal to 10 mm/yr[26,27] (Table 23–3). Earlier surgical intervention may be justified in patients with Marfan's disease, a family history of aortic disease, or dissection.[27] In several series, 1-, 3-, and 5-year survival was as high as 65%, 36%, and 20% for medically treated patients with thoracic aortic aneurysms, respectively.[28,29] Aneurysm rupture may account for up to 32% to 47% of deaths.

An important factor that dictates how the surgical repair is performed is the location and extent of the thoracic aortic aneurysm. Thoracic aortic aneurysms of the ascending aorta and aortic arch are approached from a median sternotomy incision. Standard CPB can be used for the repair of aneurysms limited to the aortic root and ascending aorta that do not extend into the aortic arch by cannulating the distal ascending aorta or proximal aortic arch and applying an aortic cross-clamp between the aortic cannula and the aneurysm. Aneurysms that involve the aortic arch require CPB with

Table 23–3 Indications for Surgical Repair of Thoracic Aortic Aneurysms

Atherosclerotic aneurysm diameter	
Ascending aorta	≥5.5 cm
Descending aorta	≥6.5 cm
Marfan's or familial thoracic aneurysm diameter	
Ascending aorta	≥5.0 cm
Descending aorta	≥6.0 cm
Severe aortic regurgitation	
Aortoannular ectasia with dilated aortic root	
Congenital bicuspid aortic valve	
Contained or impending rupture	
Refractory pain	

temporary interruption of cerebral perfusion.[30] Neuroprotection strategies that involve a combination of deliberate hypothermia, selective ACP, and retrograde cerebral perfusion are important to protect the brain from ischemic injury during reconstruction of the aortic arch. Aortic aneurysms that involve the descending thoracic aorta are approached from a lateral thoracotomy or thoracoabdominal incision. Reconstruction of the descending thoracic aorta can be accomplished without extracorporeal circulation by cross-clamping the thoracic aorta or with extracorporeal circulation using partial left heart bypass to provide distal aortic perfusion. Partial left heart bypass is accomplished through cannulation of the left atrium via a left pulmonary vein and cannulation of the distal aorta, internal iliac artery, or femoral artery. If the descending thoracic aortic aneurysm extends into the distal aortic arch, DHCA may be necessary to construct the proximal aortic anastomosis. Operations for descending thoracic aortic aneurysms require consideration of strategies to protect the mesenteric organs, spinal cord, and lower extremities from ischemia as a consequence of temporary interruption of organ blood flow or the sacrifice of collateral vessels to accomplish the repair.

The surgical repair of thoracic aortic aneurysms generally involves partial resection of the aneurysm, reconstruction or replacement of the aortic lumen with a prosthetic tube graft, and re-anastomosis or bypass grafting of the major aortic branch vessels. Endovascular stent graft repair is an option for aneurysms confined to the descending thoracic aorta. An important advance in aortic surgery has been the development of biological adhesives.[31-33] Biological glue applied to augment the vessel wall, reinforce the suture line, or even seal the intima to the adventitia in the presence of a dissection reinforces the strength of major vascular anastomosis and decreases the risk of bleeding. Biological glues containing glutaraldehyde can cause nerve injury, and it is important to avoid applying glue in the vicinity of the sinus node, cardiac conduction system, phrenic nerve, or recurrent laryngeal nerves.

A

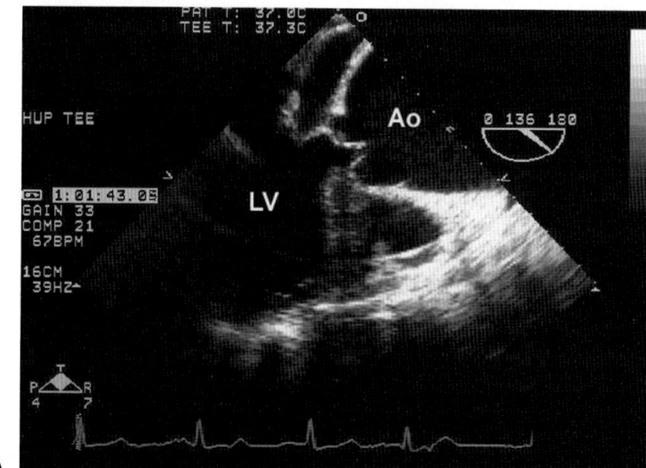

B

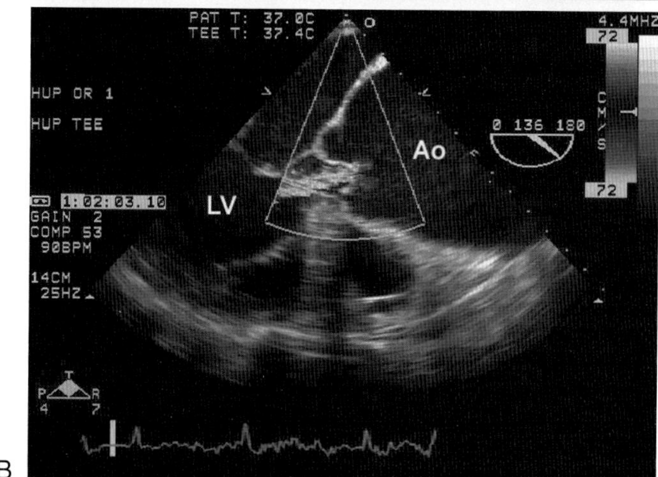

Figure 23–1 TEE mid-esophageal long-axis images of the aortic valve demonstrating aneurysmal dilation of the aortic root and ascending aorta *(A)*. Doppler color flow imaging *(B)* demonstrating severe aortic regurgitation caused by outward tethering of the aortic valve cusps by the aortic aneurysm. LV = left ventricle; Ao = aorta. (See Color Plates.)

Surgical Repair of Ascending Aortic and Arch Aneurysms

The surgical options for repair of ascending aortic aneurysms depend upon the presence of aortic valve disease, aneurysm of the sinuses of Valsalva, and distal extension of the aneurysm into the aortic arch. Intraoperative TEE is useful for evaluating the aortic valve to determine if a valve-sparing surgery is feasible, to determine the aortic valve annular diameter in relation to the diameter of the sinotubular junction to assess aneurysmal dilation of the aortic root, and to detect and quantify the presence of AR after valve repair. The most common aortic valve diseases associated with ascending aortic aneurysm are bicuspid aortic valve or AR caused by dilation of the aortic root (Fig. 23–1). If the aortic valve and aortic root are normal, a simple tube graft can be used to replace the ascending aorta. If the aortic valve is diseased but the sinuses of Valsalva are normal, an aortic valve replacement combined with a tube graft for the ascending aorta without need for reimplantation of the coronary arteries can be performed (Wheat procedure) (Fig. 23–2). If disease involves the aortic valve, aortic root, and ascending aorta, the options include tube graft of the ascending aorta in combination with aortic valve repair, reconstruction of the aortic root with sparing or repair of the aortic valve, bioprosthetic aortic root replacement, composite valve–graft conduit aortic root replacement (Bentall procedure) (Fig. 23–3), or replacement of the aortic root with a pulmonary autograft (Ross procedure). Replacement of the aortic root requires re-implantation of the coronary arteries or aortocoronary bypass grafting (Cabrol technique) (Fig. 23–4). Aortic valve repair or valve-sparing procedures may be considered for AR caused by outward tethering of the aortic valve cusps by the aneurysm and corrected by resuspending the aortic valve within a remodeled aortic root. It is important to assess the coronary anatomy before aneurysm repair. If there is evidence of significant coronary artery disease, a combined ascending aortic aneurysm repair and coronary artery bypass grafting (CABG) may be necessary.

Repairing aortic aneurysms that extend into or involve the aortic arch require temporary interruption of blood flow to the aortic arch branch vessels. For ascending aortic aneurysms that involve only the proximal aortic arch, a tube graft can be interposed between the ascending aorta or aortic root and the underside of the aortic arch. Ascending aorta and hemiarch reconstruction is often performed using DHCA or selective cerebral perfusion to enable construction of the distal anastomosis using an "open technique" when cross-clamping the distal ascending aorta or aortic arch cannot be performed

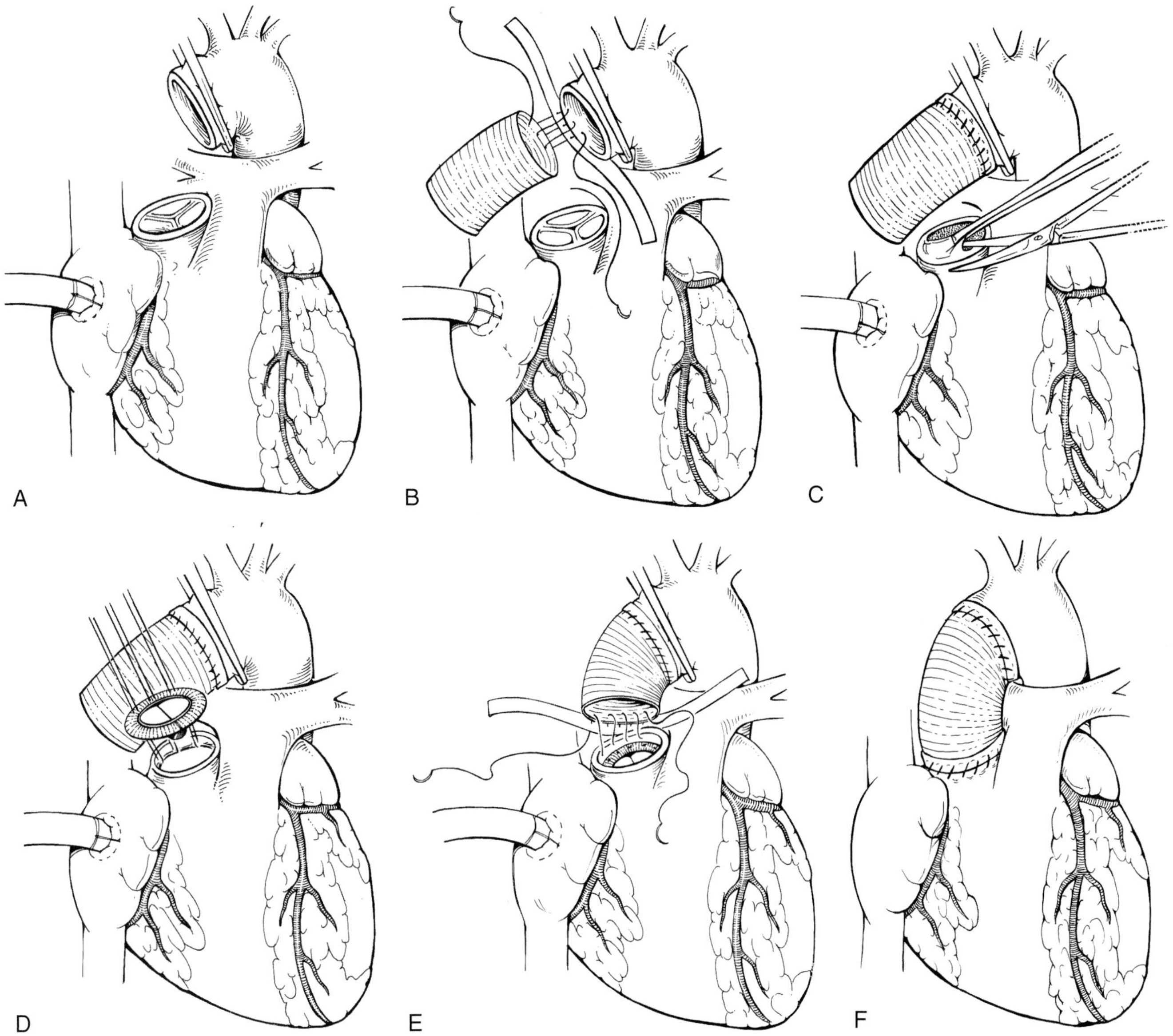

A B C D E F

Figure 23–2 Replacement of the ascending aorta with a prosthetic tube graft for ascending aortic aneurysm or type A aortic dissection. In the presence of aortic valvular disease, the aortic valve can be replaced *(C, D,* and *E)* or repaired (not shown). Extension of the aneurysm or dissection into the aortic arch may require replacement of part or all of the aortic arch with a prosthetic tube graft (not shown). A small rim of the native aortic root containing the right and left coronary ostia was left behind in this repair. (Adapted with permission from Downing SW, Kouchoukos NT: Ascending aortic aneurysm. *In* Edmunds LH [ed]: Cardiac Surgery in the Adult. New York, McGraw-Hill, 1997, p 1176.)

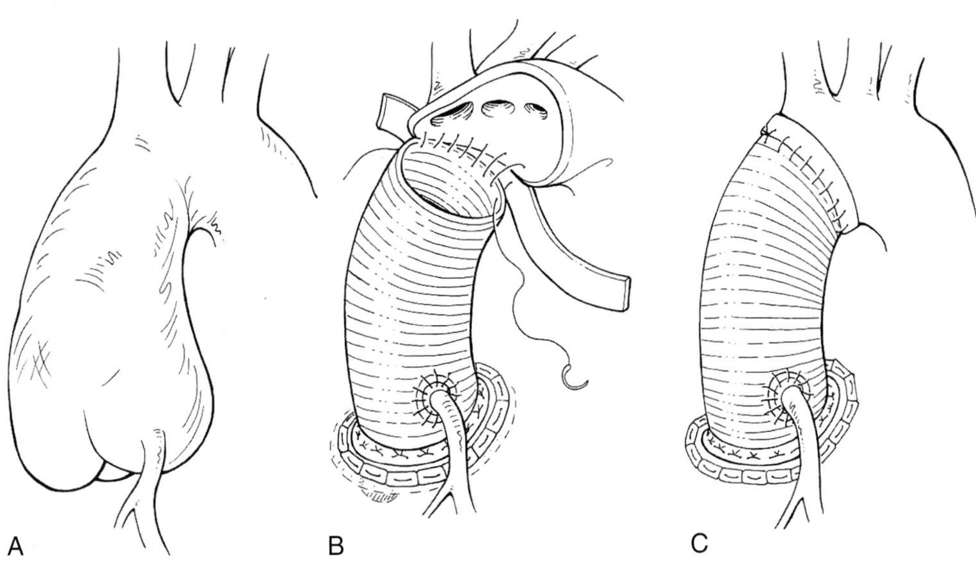

Figure 23–3 Replacement of the entire aortic root with a composite valved conduit for ascending aortic aneurysm. The underside of the aortic arch was also incorporated into the prosthetic graft. The right and left coronary arteries were re-implanted into the graft. Alternatively, the aortic root can be replaced with a cryopreserved homograft or porcine bioprosthesis (not shown). (Adapted with permission from Griepp RB, Ergin A: Aneurysms of the aortic arch. *In* Edmunds LH [ed]: Cardiac Surgery in the Adult. New York, McGraw-Hill, 1997, p 1209.)

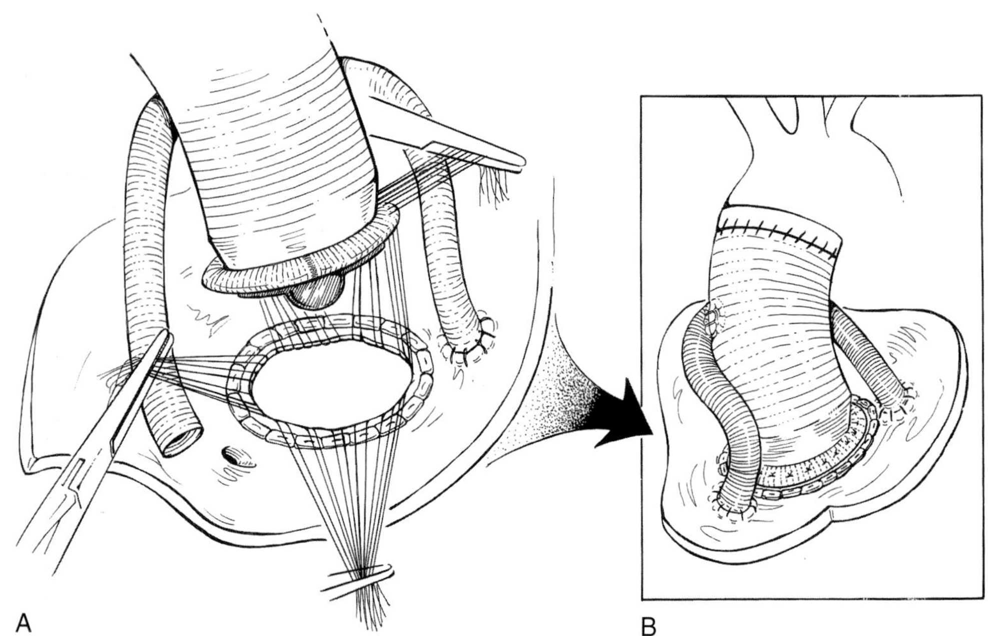

Figure 23–4 Replacement of the entire aortic root with a composite valved conduit for ascending aortic aneurysm combined with end-to-end anastomosis of the right and left coronary arteries to an 8-mm or 10-mm prosthetic tube graft that was then anastomosed to the aortic root. (Adapted with permission from Downing SW, Kouchoukos NT: Ascending aortic aneurysm. *In* Edmunds LH [ed]: Cardiac Surgery in the Adult. New York, McGraw-Hill, 1997, p 1181).

safely. Ascending aortic aneurysms that extend through the aortic arch into the descending aorta can be repaired using an "elephant trunk" technique[34] (Fig. 23–5). Aortic arch aneurysms that extend into the aortic branch vessels may require repair with branched or trifurcated tube grafts to permit separate anastomosis to the innominate, left carotid, and left subclavian arteries.

Anesthetic Management for Ascending Aorta and Arch Aneurysms

The conduct of general anesthesia for repair of ascending aortic aneurysms requires attention to a number of specific concerns. A large ascending aortic aneurysm can cause a mediastinal mass effect (Fig. 23–6). The CT or MRI studies should be reviewed to assess for aneurysm compression of the right pulmonary artery, right ventricular outflow track, trachea, or left mainstem bronchus. A right radial arterial catheter is preferred for most cases. If arterial cannulation of the right axillary, subclavian, or innominate artery is planned for CPB or selective cerebral perfusion, bilateral radial arterial catheters are often necessary to measure cerebral and systemic perfusion pressures. Nasopharyngeal, tympanic, and bladder temperatures are important for estimating brain and core temperatures for monitoring the conduct of deliberate hypothermia and DHCA. EEG, SEP, or oximetric jugular bulb venous oxygen saturation monitoring is sometimes useful for assessing cerebral metabolic activity for the conduct of DHCA. Control of the arterial pressure and prevention of hypertension are important to decrease left ventricular afterload in patients with AR and to decrease the risk of aneurysm rupture or expansion during induction of general anesthesia and surgical exposure. In patients with AR, antihypertensive drugs that decrease heart rate or myocardial contractility should be used cautiously to avoid heart failure. Intraoperative TEE is useful for evaluating the aortic valve and aortic root to determine the need for aortic root replacement or the feasibility of aortic valve repair (see Fig. 23–1). In patients with AR, a left ventricular vent is necessary to prevent ventricular distention during CPB. Patients with AR also require direct coronary cannulation for delivery of antegrade cardioplegic solution or a coronary sinus catheter to provide retrograde cardioplegia.

Neuroprotection Strategies for Temporary Interruption of Cerebral Blood Flow

Thoracic aortic surgery requiring temporary interruption of cerebral perfusion has been associated with the highest incidence of brain injury in comparison to other cardiac operations.[35] Many reports assessing the incidence of neurologic injury were based on retrospective data collection or clinically diagnosed stroke. These reports suggest an incidence of stroke in the range of 7% to 9%.[36,37] Studies that included a more detailed neurologic assessment and neuropsychological testing have found that neurologic deficits were more frequent in older patients and those subjected to DHCA for 25 minutes[38,39] (see Chapter 35).

Two major mechanisms are believed to explain high incidence of stroke and neurocognitive dysfunction related to thoracic aortic operations. The first is cerebral ischemia or infarction caused by hypoperfusion or the need for temporary circulatory arrest during reconstruction of the aortic arch. The second is cerebral ischemia or infarction caused by cerebral embolization as a consequence of extracorporeal circulation or intrinsic vascular disease. Arterial emboli causing stroke can originate from multiple sources during thoracic aortic operations and include air introduced into the circulation from open cardiac chambers, vascular cannulation sites, or arterial anastomosis. Atherosclerotic or particulate debris may be released during clamping and unclamping of the aorta, the creation of anastomoses in the ascending aorta and aortic arch, or the excision of severely calcified and diseased cardiac valves. CPB may result in the generation of platelet aggregates, fat particles, and other microparticulate debris. The turbulent high-velocity blood flow out of the aortic cannula employed for CPB may also dislodge atherosclerotic debris within the aorta. Retrograde blood flow through a diseased descending thoracic aorta as a consequence of CPB conducted with femoral artery cannulation may cause retrograde cerebral

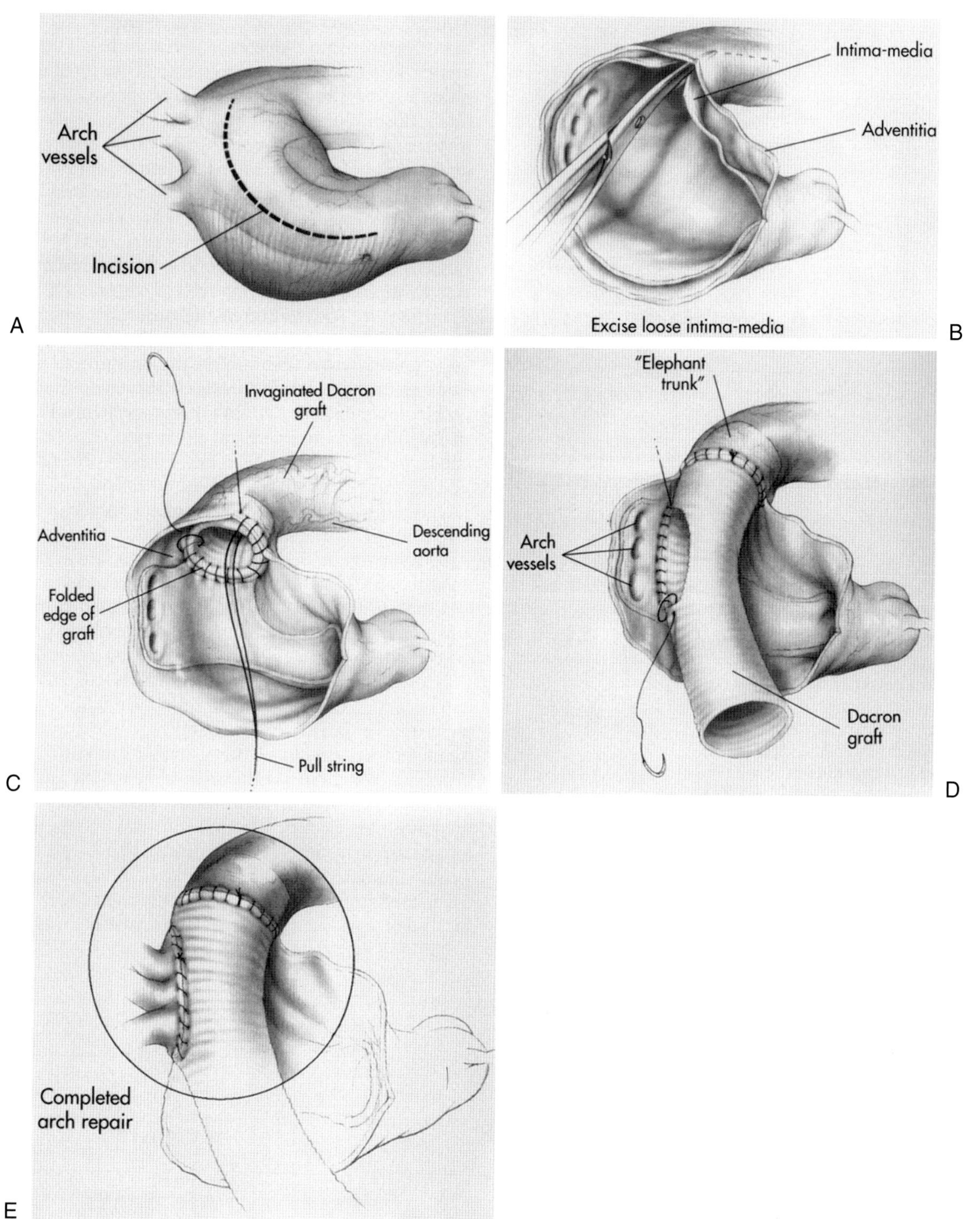

Figure 23–5 Elephant trunk procedure for prosthetic graft replacement of the ascending aorta, aortic arch, and descending thoracic aorta. The aortic aneurysm or dissection is opened its entire length and extended through the aortic arch *(A* and *B)*. The prosthetic tube graft is implanted with its distal end extending into the descending thoracic aorta, "elephant trunk" *(C* and *D)*. The graft is pulled back into the arch for implantation of the arch branch vessels and construction of the proximal anastomosis *(D* and *E)*. In the second stage of the procedure, the descending thoracic aorta is replaced by constructing a proximal graft-to-graft anastomosis (not shown). (From Doty DB: Aortic aneurysm. *In* Brown M, Baxter S [eds]: Cardiac Surgery: Operative Technique. St. Louis, Mosby-Year Book, 1997, p 324.)

embolization. For all these reasons, strategies to provide neurologic protection are important in the conduct of thoracic aortic operations (Box 23–2).

Deep Hypothermic Circulatory Arrest

The brain is exquisitely susceptible to ischemic injury within minutes after the onset of circulatory arrest because it has a high metabolic rate, continuous requirement for metabolic substrate, and limited reserves of high-energy phosphates. In the 1970s, deep hypothermia and circulatory arrest were introduced to protect the brain from ischemic injury for operations on the aortic arch requiring temporary interruption of cerebral blood flow.[40,41] The physiologic basis for deep hypothermia as a neuroprotection strategy is to decrease

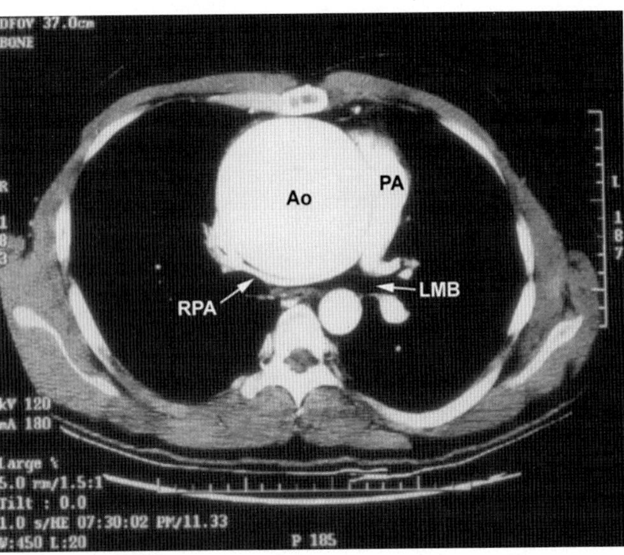

Figure 23–6 CT angiogram of the chest demonstrating a large ascending aortic aneurysm (Ao) causing compression of the right pulmonary artery (RPA), distal trachea, and left main stem bronchus (LMB).

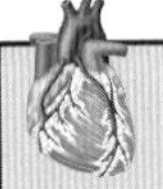

BOX 23–2 ***Brain Protection for Aortic Arch Reconstruction***

- Deep systemic hypothermia
- Topical cerebral cooling
- Retrograde cerebral perfusion
- Selective antegrade cerebral perfusion
- Prevent cerebral hyperthermia during rewarming

cerebral metabolic rate and oxygen demands to increase the period of time that the brain can tolerate circulatory arrest. Existing evidence indicates that autoregulation of cerebral blood flow is maintained during deliberate hypothermia with alpha-stat blood gas management. In adults, a 10°C decrease in body temperature decreases cerebral metabolic rate by an average factor of 2.6, a factor commonly referred to as the Q_{10} ratio.[42,43] Assuming an ischemic tolerance of 3 to 5 minutes under normothermic conditions, a Q_{10} ratio of 2.6 predicts an ischemic tolerance in the range of 20 to 34 minutes at a brain temperature of 17°C or 53 to 88 minutes at a brain temperature of 7°C. More recent estimations of cerebral metabolism in adults undergoing DHCA suggest an ischemic tolerance of 30 minutes at 15°C and 40 minutes at 10°C.[44] Direct measurement of cerebral metabolites and brainstem electrical activity in adults undergoing DHCA with retrograde cerebral perfusion at 14°C indicated the onset of cerebral ischemia after only 18 to 20 minutes[45] (Fig. 23–7). It is also possible that hypothermia provides brain protection through mechanisms other than the reduction in cerebral metabolic rate. Despite an incomplete understanding of the mechanism and efficacy of hypothermia for cerebral protection, the large body of experimental evidence and clinical experience with the deliberate hypothermia suggest that it is the single most important intervention for preventing neurologic injury in response to circulatory arrest.

Despite the proven efficacy of hypothermia for operations that require circulatory arrest, no consensus exists on an optimal protocol for the conduct of deliberate hypothermia for circulatory arrest. The average nasopharyngeal temperature used for DHCA in several reported clinical series was 18°C, but the optimal temperature for DHCA has not been established. One problem with establishing the optimal temperature for DHCA is the inability to measure directly the brain temperature. In a study using EEG monitoring to establish physiologic criteria for cerebral metabolic suppression in response to hypothermia, the median nasopharyngeal temperature that electrocortical silence was achieved was 18°C, but a nasopharyngeal temperature of 12.5°C was necessary to ensure that 99.5% of patients achieved electrocortical silence[46] (Fig. 23–8). Another criterion that correlated with electrocortical silence on the EEG in 99.5% of patients was cooling on

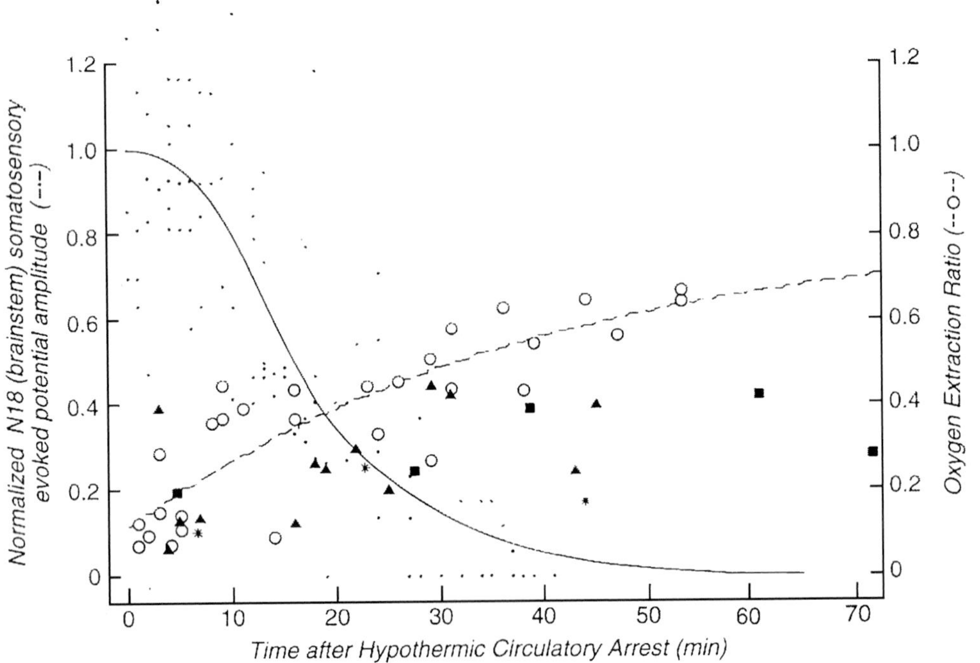

Figure 23–7 Changes in brainstem (N18) somatosensory evoked potential amplitudes (dots) after initiation of deep hypothermic circulatory arrest with retrograde cerebral perfusion superimposed on the change in brain oxygen extraction ratio (OER) in patients without strokes (circles; n = 19), preoperative strokes (triangles; n = 4), intraoperative strokes (squares; n = 3), and both preoperative and intraoperative strokes (asterisks; n = 1). The N18 somatosensory evoked potential decayed to half its original amplitude at 16 minutes after interruption of antegrade cerebral perfusion. The OER decreased to half its maximal value of 0.66 also at 16 minutes after interruption of antegrade cerebral perfusion. (Adapted from Cheung AT, et al: Oxygen delivery during retrograde cerebral perfusion in humans. Anesth Analg 88:14, 1999.)

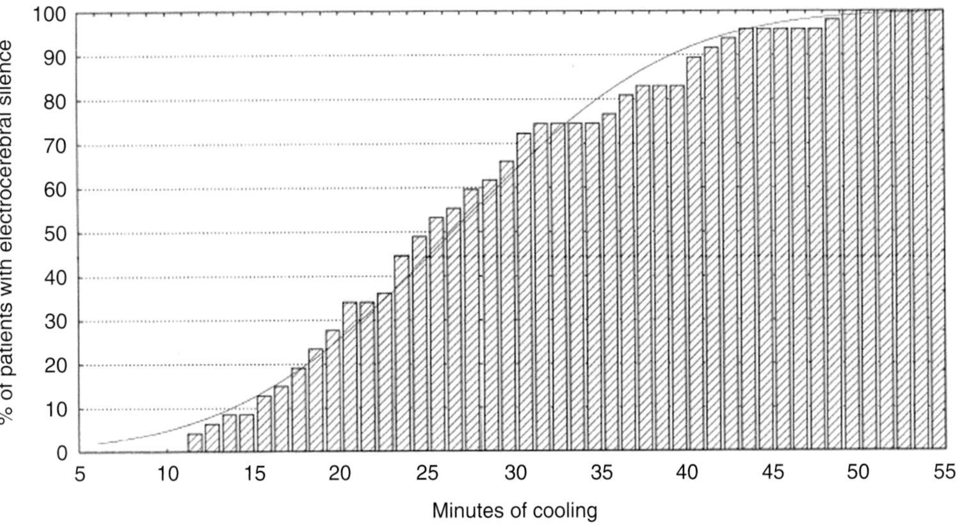

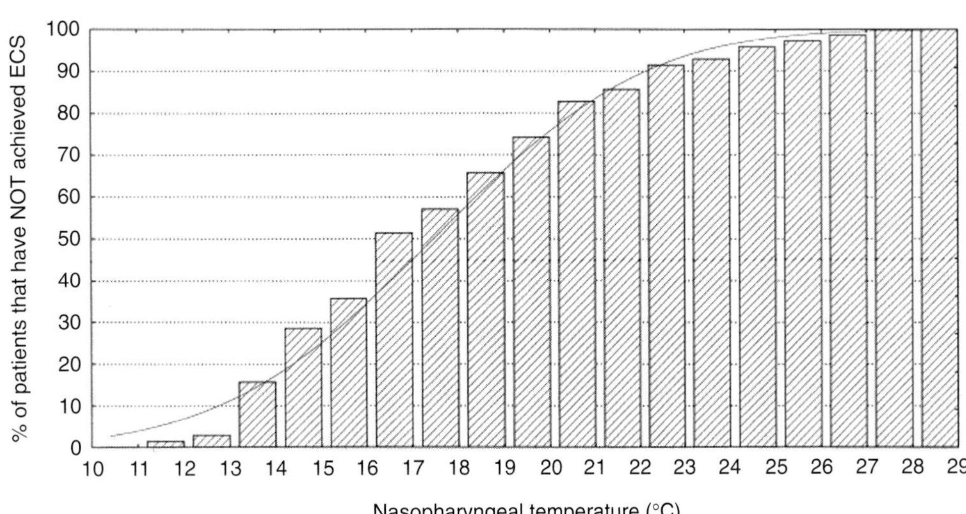

Figure 23–8 The relation between EEG activity to minutes of cooling *(top)* and nasopharyngeal temperature *(bottom)* prior to deep hypothermic circulatory arrest in 109 patients undergoing thoracic aortic operations requiring circulatory arrest. Electrocortical silence was achieved by EEG in all patients after 50 minutes of cooling or at a nasopharyngeal temperature of 12.5°C, At a nasopharyngeal temperature of 18°C, only 50% of patients had electrocortical silence by EEG. (Adapted from Stecker MM, et al: Deep hypothermic circulatory arrest: I, Effects of cooling on electroencephalogram and evoked potentials. Ann Thorac Surg 71:19, 2001. Copyright 2001, with permission from the Society of Thoracic Surgeons.)

CPB for at least 50 minutes[46] (see Fig. 23–8). Although EEG can be used as a physiologic end point for cerebral metabolic suppression during cooling, its outcome benefit remains to be demonstrated.[46-48] A jugular bulb venous oxygen saturation greater than 95% measured using an oximetric catheter has also been advocated as a means to detect maximum cerebral metabolic suppression for DHCA.[38] Based on physiologic measurements and clinical outcome studies, recent trends favor nasopharyngeal temperatures in the range of 11°C to 14°C for DHCA and a maximum safe duration of DHCA of 30 minutes.[38,49,50] Several clinical series have suggested that DHCA duration greater than 25 to 33 minutes was associated with neurocognitive dysfunction.[38,51] In addition to systemic hypothermia produced by extracorporeal circulation, topical hypothermia by packing the head in ice has been advocated to prevent passive warming of the head during circulatory arrest.[38] When providing topical hypothermia, care should be exercised to protect the eyes, nose, and ears from frostbite by protecting vulnerable areas with a thick gauze pad or avoiding direct contact with ice. Others do not believe that topical hypothermia provides any added protection to systemic hypothermia because the net effect of topical hypothermia on brain temperature is negligible during CPB and circulatory arrest.

The conduct of DHCA has several potential adverse sequelae. Lowering the target brain temperature extends the duration of CPB necessary for cooling and rewarming and all the problems inherent with prolongation of CPB such as injury to blood elements and the potential for cerebral embolization. Rewarming increases cerebral metabolic rate and has the potential to make the brain more vulnerable to ischemic injury, particularly during reperfusion after circulatory arrest. For these reasons, strategies to decrease the risk of brain injury during rewarming include delaying the start of rewarming by a period of hypothermic reperfusion, maintaining a temperature gradient of no more than 10°C in the heat exchanger, preventing the nasopharyngeal temperature from exceeding 37.5°C, or incomplete rewarming. Systemic hypothermia has commonly been associated with coagulopathy and increased risk of bleeding, but it has not been firmly established whether hypothermia is the underlying etiology of coagulopathy and bleeding. It is possible that systemic hypothermia is a consequence of prolonged surgery, blood transfusion therapy, and intravascular volume expansion.

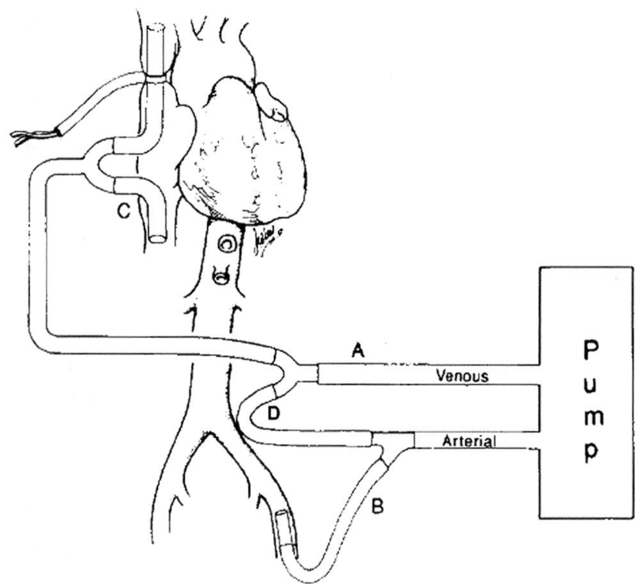

Figure 23–9 Extracorporeal perfusion circuit used to deliver retrograde cerebral perfusion. The bridge *(D)* is clamped during CPB. After initiation of deep hypothermic circulatory arrest, clamps are placed on the venous return line *(A)*, the proximal arterial cannula *(B)*, and inferior vena caval cannula *(C)*; and, the bridge *(D)* is unclamped to permit retrograde perfusion into the superior vena cava. (Adapted from Bavaria JE, et al: Retrograde cerebral and distal aortic perfusion during ascending and thoracoabdominal aortic operations. Ann Thorac Surg 60:347, 1995. Copyright 1995, with permission from the Society of Thoracic Surgeons.)

Retrograde Cerebral Perfusion

Retrograde cerebral perfusion (RCP) was first described for the treatment of massive cerebral air embolism.[50] In 1990, RCP was reported as a means to deliver metabolic substrate to the brain during operations involving the aortic arch that required the interruption of ACP.[52] RCP is performed by infusing cold oxygenated blood into the superior vena cava cannula at a temperature of 8°C to 14°C via the CBP machine (Fig. 23–9). The internal jugular venous pressure is maintained at less than or equal to 25 mm Hg to prevent cerebral edema. Internal jugular venous pressure is measured from the introducer port of the internal jugular venous cannula at a site proximal to the superior vena cava perfusion cannula and zeroed at the level of the ear. The patient is positioned in 10 degrees of Trendelenburg to decrease the risk of cerebral air embolism and prevent trapping of air within the cerebral circulation in the presence of an open aortic arch. RCP flow rates of 200 to 600 mL/min can usually be achieved. The potential benefits of RCP for neuroprotection include prolonging the safe period of DHCA by providing some metabolic substrate delivery to the brain, flushing embolic material from the cerebral arterial vasculature to decrease the risk of cerebral embolization upon resuming ACP, and providing a means to maintain cerebral hypothermia during DHCA.[53-57]

The clinical benefit of RCP is based on several uncontrolled clinical series that indicated lower stroke rates and in-hospital mortality compared with historical controls.[34,48,52,53,58-63] Subsequent studies have questioned the benefits of RCP and suggested that neurologic outcomes depend primarily on the duration of DHCA independent of whether RCP is used.[64] Direct imaging of cerebral blood flow during RCP in human patients demonstrates perfusion of the cerebral cortex, but some experimental models suggest that venovenous shunting during RCP provides limited brain perfusion.[65] In a well-controlled human study where the mean DHCA time was 32 ± 9 minutes, RCP failed to attenuate the metabolic changes associated with DHCA.[66] A small prospective trial showed that DHCA with or without RCP was associated with a high incidence of neuropsychometric change, and RCP did not improve outcome.[35] Patients in the study who had RCP had worse total test scores at 6 weeks, but scores at 12 weeks were not different. The greatest neuropsychometric change occurred in the domain of higher cortical function. However, the study was underpowered to exclude a beneficial effect of RCP in certain population subgroups. Other clinical experiences with RCP have been disappointing as well.[67] RCP also has the potential to increase the risk of cerebral edema as a consequence of excessive venous and intracranial pressures.[68] The risk of cerebral edema as a consequence of RCP may also be greater in patients with occlusive cerebrovascular disease. An early clinical study suggested that metabolic substrate delivery by RCP delayed the decay in brain electrical activity during DHCA,[54] but a subsequent clinical study demonstrated that substrate delivery by RCP was insufficient to fully support metabolic demands despite deep hypothermia.[45]

Existing evidence suggests that RCP should not be considered a substitute for hypothermia, and RCP might not prolong the safety of DHCA beyond 30 minutes.

A porcine study found that none of the animals that underwent 90 minutes ACP had neurohistopathologic evidence of injury compared with injury in 27% of those treated with RCP, and 47% of those treated with DHCA alone.[68] In another model of DHCA, brain protection was better with lower RCP infusate temperatures of 9° to 14°C supporting the concept that sustained brain hypothermia was the primary protective effect of RCP.[56] The absence of a protective effect of RCP in a well-controlled human study may also be explained by insufficient hypothermia or the presence of competent jugular vein valves that would impede retrograde flow even at relatively high pressures.[66] In baboons under DHCA, RCP did not perfuse the brain due to massive venovenous shunting, despite perfusion cannulas placed in both internal jugular veins.[65] In another porcine study, the benefit of RCP was primarily due to the maintenance of a consistent level of brain hypothermia.[57] Another potential benefit of RCP is to flush air, atheromatous debris, and toxic metabolites out of the arterial vessels to decrease the risk of emboli upon antegrade reperfusion.[48,55,63] In a porcine model of cerebral embolization, RCP decreased the overall brain embolic count compared with controls but the neurologic outcome was worse.[68] In summary, the potential benefits of RCP have not been proven and long durations of RCP greater than 30 to 40 minutes were associated with higher rates of neurologic complications.[64] Nevertheless, RCP remains a safe, simple, and easily implemented technique that can be considered as an adjunct to maintain cerebral hypothermia, provide partial metabolic substrate delivery, and decrease the risk of cerebral embolization for operations requiring DHCA.[50,54,58]

Selective Antegrade Cerebral Perfusion

Selective ACP was developed out of necessity to protect the brain from cerebral ischemia during complex operations of the aortic arch. ACP should be considered for all operations in which the duration of the repair is anticipated to exceed 30 to 45 minutes. ACP is initiated after achieving deep hypothermia by CPB and typically used in combination with brief periods of DHCA. ACP can be delivered by selective cannula-

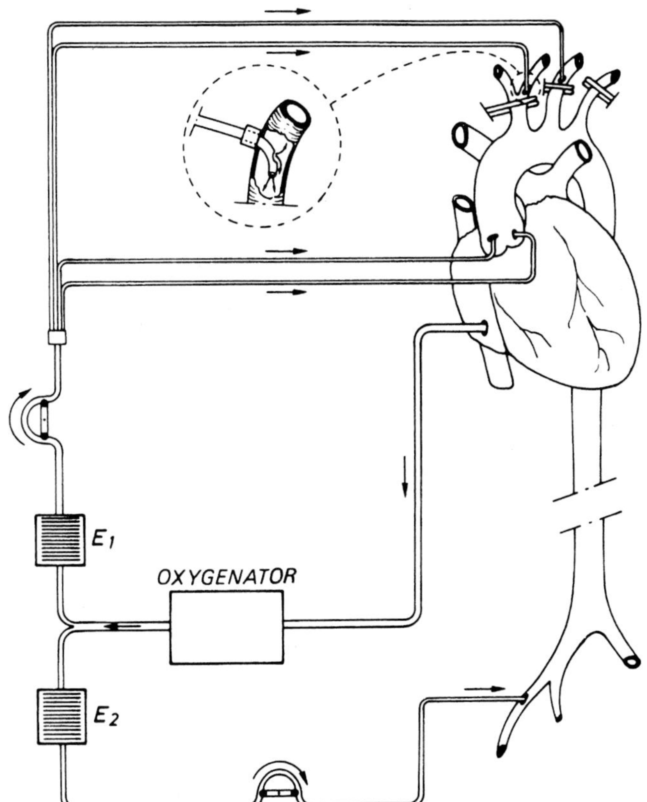

Figure 23–10 Extracorporeal perfusion circuit used for selective antegrade cerebral perfusion. After achieving deep hypothermia on CPB, individual cannulas are inserted into the coronary, innominate, and left carotid arteries for selective antegrade perfusion of the heart and brain. (From Bachet J, Teodori G, Goudot B, et al: Replacement of the transverse aortic arch during emergency operations for type A acute aortic dissection. J Thorac Cardiovasc Surg 96:878, 1988.)

tion of the right axillary artery, right subclavian artery, innominate artery, or left common carotid artery (Fig. 23–10). In transverse aortic arch reconstruction procedures, ACP can be accomplished by inserting individual perfusion cannulas into the open end of the aortic branch vessels after opening the aortic arch. After reattachment of the aortic arch branch vessels to the vascular graft, ACP can then be provided through a separate arm of the vascular graft or by direct cannulation of the graft. A functional circle of Willis may provide contralateral brain perfusion during interruption of antegrade perfusion in the innominate, left carotid, or left subclavian arteries during construction of the vascular anastomoses. ACP with oxygenated blood at 10°C to 14°C at flow rates in the range of 250 to 1000 mL/min typically achieves a cerebral perfusion pressure in the range of 50 to 80 mm Hg.

The effectiveness of selective ACP is supported by case series that described the successful application of this technique with acceptable morbidity rates for aortic arch reconstruction.[69-71] In one clinical series, the duration of ACP ranged from 75 to 235 minutes and the duration of ACP was not found to correlate with neurologic injury.[72] Experimental models also support the efficacy of ACP. In one study, low flow cerebral perfusion was found to be more effective for brain protection than no flow.[73] A porcine study found that animals that underwent 90 minutes ACP had no histopathologic evidence of neurologic injury compared with the detection of injury in 27% of those that had RCP, and 47% of those that had DHCA alone.[55] Concerns pertaining to the use of ACP include increased complexity of the procedure, the risk of cerebral embolization, vessel injury, nonuniform perfusion as a consequence of limited ability to control individual flow rates in different perfusion cannulas, or malperfusion caused by cannula obstruction or malpositioning.[63] The use of intraoperative transcranial Doppler monitoring of middle cerebral artery blood flow may detect flow disturbances and embolic events in the cerebral circulation and may decrease the incidence of these potential complications, but the experience is too small to provide general recommendations for its routine use.[74-76] The use of intraoperative cerebral oximetry is another potentially useful early indicator of brain hypoperfusion. Although initial reports using cerebral oximetry in the pediatric patients undergoing aortic arch reconstruction were promising, more experience is required to test the usefulness of these devices in adults[77] (see Chapter 17).

Pharmacologic Neuroprotection Strategies for Deep Hypothermic Circulatory Arrest

There are no proven pharmacologic regimens that have demonstrated effectiveness for decreasing the risk or severity of neurologic injury in the setting of thoracic aortic operations. Barbiturates or other central nervous system depressants decrease cerebral oxygen consumption and in theory offer the potential for cerebral protection in the setting of incomplete ischemia. There have been two randomized clinical studies evaluating the use of barbiturates to achieve EEG burst suppression throughout the period of CPB. One study demonstrated a reduced incidence of neurologic injury in the setting of open cardiac operations and the other study did not show any effect of barbiturate administration.[78,79] The additive benefit of barbiturates or other central nervous system depressant drugs in combination with deliberate hypothermia has not been proved. Experimental studies have also demonstrated that inhaled anesthetic agents can protect against cerebral ischemia through ischemic preconditioning, but clinical studies have yet to quantify this potential benefit.[80] Experimental studies and several clinical series support the administration of high dose glucocorticoid to protect against cerebral and end-organ injury in the setting of DHCA leading to the routine administration of methylprednisolone 1 g IV or dexamethasone 100 mg IV to patients undergoing thoracic aortic operations that require DHCA at many centers.[64,66,81-83] Other unproved pharmacologic adjuncts that are routinely administered in an effort to provide organ protection in the setting of thoracic aortic operations requiring DHCA include magnesium sulfate 1 to 2 g IV, lidocaine 200 mg IV, or mannitol 25 g IV. In general, the existing evidence suggests that pharmacologic neuroprotection is unreliable and should not be considered a substitute for hypothermia to protect against cerebral ischemia in the setting of hypoperfusion.

DESCENDING THORACIC AND THORACOABDOMINAL AORTIC ANEURYSMS

The objective of surgical repair for descending thoracic aortic aneurysms or TAAAs is to replace the diseased portion of the aorta with a prosthetic tube graft. The surgical approach to repair is through a lateral thoracotomy or thoracoabdominal incision. Despite technological improvements, major challenges remain in the surgical management patients with TAAA. The major etiology of this disease is atherosclerosis and the typical patient requiring surgery often is elderly with coexisting peripheral vascular disease, cerebral vascular disease, renal vascular disease, coronary artery disease, and frequently chronic obstructive pulmonary disease from a history of tobacco use (Table 23–4). Patients are particularly susceptible to renal, mesenteric, and lower extremity ischemia as a consequence of thromboembolic disease, the temporary interruption of blood flow to these organs, reperfusion injury, and difficulties encountered in the reconstruction of branch vessel anastomosis during the course of surgical repair. The need for a thoracoabdominal incision, division of the diaphragm, and surgical dissection in the proximity of the phrenic nerve, recurrent laryngeal nerve, and the esophagus represents major physiologic trespasses that increase the risk of postoperative wound dehiscence, respiratory failure, and dysphagia and is associated with a prolonged convalescence in many patients. Finally, the inability to identify or reattach all intercostal arteries to accomplish the repair decreases the vascular collateral supply to the spinal cord, making postoperative paraplegia a recognized complication of these operations. As a consequence of these medical, physiologic, and surgical challenges, repair of TAAA is considered a high-risk procedure and associated with high morbidity and mortality that vary depending on the hospital volume and surgical experience. In a nationwide sample of 1542 patients, the overall average mortality rate associated with TAAA repair was 22.3% with a cardiac complication rate of 14.8%, pulmonary complication rate of 19%, and acute renal failure rate of 14.2%[84] (Table 23–5). Because outcomes and mortality rates differ among centers, operative technique, reported surgical case series, and use of various perioperative organ protection strategies, it is difficult or impossible to compare the advantages and disadvantages of any specific methodology.

Thoracic aortic aneurysms and TAAAs are classified according to the anatomic extent of the aneurysmal segment. The most commonly used classification scheme is that described by Crawford that categorizes aneurysm extent into four major groups (Fig. 23–11). Extent I TAAA involves the entire descending thoracic aorta from the origin of the left subclavian artery down to the level of the diaphragm ending above the renal arteries. Extent II TAAA involves the entire descending thoracic aorta with extension across the

Table 23–4 Preoperative Characteristics of 1220 Patients Undergoing Thoracoabdominal Aortic Aneurysm Repair

Characteristic	No. of Patients (%)
Crawford extent	
Extent I	423 (34.7)
Extent II	371 (30.4)
Extent III	201 (16.5)
Extent IV	225 (18.4)
Acute dissection	46 (3.8)
Chronic dissection	272 (22.3)
Marfan's syndrome	72 (5.9)
Symptomatic aneurysms	855 (70.1)
Acute presentation	112 (9.2)
Rupture	76 (6.2)
Preoperative paraplegia or paraparesis	16 (1.3)
Concurrent aneurysm	224 (18.4)
Prior aneurysm repair	502 (41.2)
Prior thoracic aortic aneurysm repair	281 (23.0)
Diabetes	69 (5.7)
Hypertension	940 (77.1)
Coronary artery disease	435 (35.7)
Prior coronary artery bypass or angioplasty	202 (16.6)
Cerebrovascular disease	135 (11.1)
Renal arterial occlusive disease	312 (25.6)
Renal insufficiency	151 (12.4)
Chronic obstructive lung disease	491 (40.3)
Peptic ulcer disease	83 (6.8)

From Coselli JS, et al: Mortality and paraplegia after thoracoabdominal aortic aneurysm repair: A risk factor analysis. Ann Thorac Surg 69:409, 2000.

Table 23–5 Postoperative Complications and Mortality After Thoracoabdominal Aortic Aneurysm (TAAA) Repair in the United States From 1988 to 1998

Complication	Intact TAAA (n = 1542)	Ruptured TAAA (n = 321)
Cardiac	14.8%	18.1%
Pulmonary	19.0%	12.7%
Hemorrhage	12.4%	10.9%
Acute renal failure	14.2%	28.0%
Paraplegia	—*	3.4%
Any complication	55.2%	51.7%
In-hospital mortality	22.3%	53.8%

*Incidence of paraplegia not reported.

Data from Cowan JA, et al: Surgical treatment of intact thoracoabdominal aortic aneurysms in the United States: Hospital and surgeon volume-related outcomes. J Vasc Surg 37:1169, 2003; and Cowan JA, et al: Ruptured thoracoabdominal aortic aneurysm treatment in the United States: 1988 to 1998. J Vasc Surg 38:312, 2003.

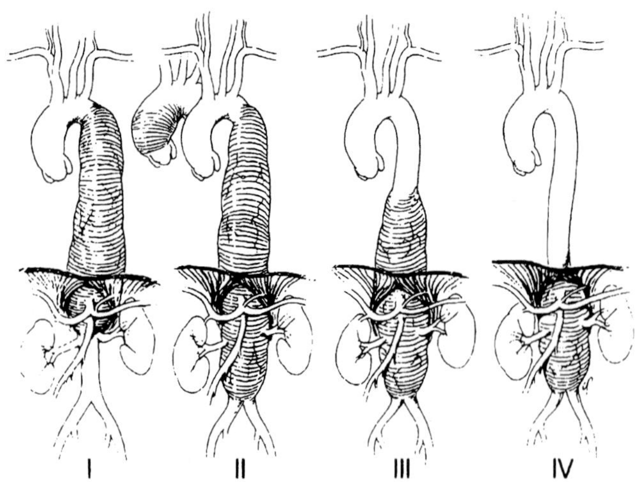

Figure 23–11 Crawford classification of thoracoabdominal aortic aneurysm extent. (From Coselli JS, Descending thoracoabdominal aortic aneurysms. *In* Edmunds LH [ed]: Cardiac Surgery in the Adult. New York, McGraw-Hill, 1997, p 1232.)

Table 23–6 **Mortality and Paraplegia After Thoracoabdominal Aortic Aneurysm (TAAA) Repair in 1220 Consecutive Patients**

TAAA Extent	No. of Patients	30-Day Mortality	Hospital Mortality	Paraplegia/Paraparesis
I	400 (35.1%)	20 (5.0%)	30 (7.5%)	16 (4.1%)
II	343 (30.1%)	18 (5.2%)	29 (8.5%)	28 (8.2%)
III	184 (16.1%)	9 (4.9%)	9 (4.9%)	7 (3.8%)
IV	213 (18.7%)	7 (3.3%)	12 (5.6%)	3 (1.4%)

From Coselli JS, et al: Mortality and paraplegia after thoracoabdominal aortic aneurysm repair: A risk factor analysis. Ann Thorac Surg 69:409, 2000.

diaphragm into and through the abdominal aorta all the way to the aortic bifurcation. Extent III TAAA involves the distal half of the descending thoracic aorta, crosses the diaphragm, and involves most of the abdominal aorta. Extent IV TAAA is confined to the upper abdominal aorta. Extent I and extent II TAAA can be further classified into those that involve the distal aortic arch and those that do not involve the distal aortic arch. Surgical repair of extent I and extent II TAAA that involve the distal aortic arch may require a two-stage "elephant trunk" procedure or DHCA to construct the proximal anastomosis. Isolated thoracic aortic aneurysms can be used to describe aneurysms confined to the descending thoracic aorta between the origin of the left subclavian artery and the diaphragm. TAAA can be further subdivided into those with dissection and those without dissection. Classification of TAAA provides a useful guide to the surgical approach, anesthetic management, and rough estimation of perioperative mortality and postoperative paraplegia (Table 23–6).

Surgical repair of TAAA with an interposition tube graft can be accomplished by three major techniques that are used in varying degrees at different centers (Fig. 23–12). The original technique for repair was accomplished by cross-clamping the thoracic aorta proximal to the aneurysm. The simple cross-clamp technique was subsequently refined by the application of arterial shunting (Gott shunt) or partial left heart bypass using extracorporeal circulation to provide distal aortic perfusion while the proximal descending thoracic aorta was cross-clamped. The third technique is to perform the repair using DHCA alone or in combination with retrograde perfusion or selective antegrade perfusion of the brain or mesen-

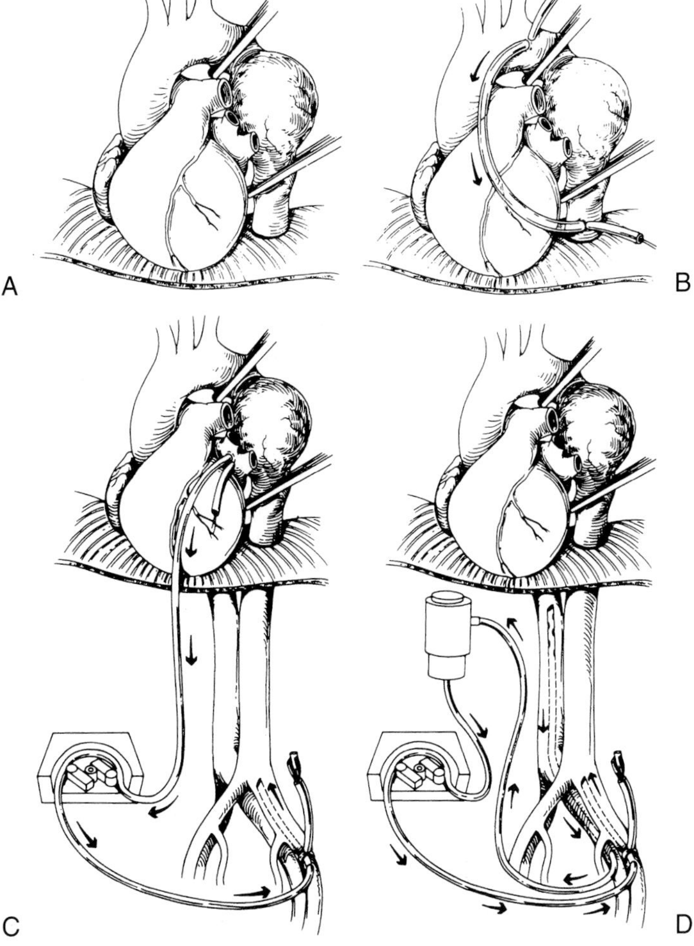

Figure 23–12 Operative techniques for repair of thoracic or thoracoabdominal aortic aneurysms. In the clamp-and-sew technique, the distal aorta is not perfused *(A)*. Alternatively, distal aortic perfusion during repair can be provided by a passive Gott shunt *(B)*, partial left heart bypass *(C)*, or partial cardiopulmonary bypass *(D)*. Deep hypothermic circulatory arrest may be necessary if the proximal cross-clamp cannot be safely applied in aneurysms extending into the distal aortic arch (not shown). (From O'Connor CJ, Rothenberg DM: Anesthetic considerations for descending thoracic aortic surgery: Part II. J Cardiothorac Vasc Anesth 9:734, 1995.)

teric organs. With all of the techniques, an attempt is usually made to reattach intercostal, lumbar, and sacral arteries to the graft to decrease the risk of spinal cord ischemia.[85,86] Endovascular stent repair is becoming a fourth option, and clinical trials to assess its safety and efficacy are well under way.

Simple Aortic Cross-Clamp Technique

In 1965, Crawford developed the technique of aortic cross-clamping for TAAA repair and subsequently reported a mortality rate of 8.9% in more than 600 TAAA cases repaired with the simple cross-clamp technique.[29,87] Mortality and paraplegia were related to the position and length of the resected aorta, the condition of the patient at the time of presentation, and the duration of time that the aorta was cross-clamped. A major disadvantage of the simple cross-clamp technique is the obligatory ischemic period to the body and organs distal to the aortic cross-clamp. For this reason, when the simple-cross-clamp technique is used, the surgeon must clamp and sew as quickly as possible to limit ischemia time to the spinal cord and distal aortic territory. The incidence of paraplegia and renal failure has been observed to correlate with the duration of the aortic cross-clamp time and was increased significantly for aortic cross-clamp times greater than 30 minutes.[88] Other disadvantages associated with cross-clamping the descending thoracic aorta include proximal aortic hypertension, bleeding from arterial collaterals, and hemodynamic instability upon reperfusion. Proximal aortic hypertension during the period that the aorta is cross-clamped may be poorly tolerated in patients with abnormal left ventricular function, regurgitant cardiac valve disease, or ischemic coronary artery disease.[89] Blood loss as a result of bleeding from arterial collaterals can be minimized by the use of intraoperative red blood cell salvaging. Hemodynamic instability during release of the aortic cross-clamp and reperfusion often has to be managed with correction of metabolic acidosis, rapid intravascular volume expansion, vasopressor therapy, or the intermittent reapplication and gradual release of the aortic cross-clamp. Adjuncts to protect end-organ function from ischemia during aortic cross-clamping include mild deliberate hypothermia and selective cooling of the spinal cord. Despite the physiologic consequences, the aortic cross-clamp technique remains a relatively simple technique with proven clinical outcomes and is still favored by many surgeons (Table 23–7).

Gott Shunt

Passive shunting of blood from the proximal to distal aorta has been used to provide distal aortic perfusion during aortic cross-clamping for TAAA repair. A Gott shunt is a tapered heparin-coated tube designed so that both ends can serve as arterial cannulas[90] (see Fig. 23–12B). The ascending aorta or aortic arch can serve as the proximal cannulation site for the Gott shunt. The distal descending thoracic aorta, iliac artery, or femoral artery can serve as the distal cannulation site for the Gott shunt. Blood flow from the proximal to distal aorta through the Gott shunt is variable and governed by the proximal aortic pressure, diameter and length of the shunt, and distal aortic pressure. Monitoring the distal aortic pressure through a femoral arterial catheter can be used to assess distal aortic perfusion and shunt flow. Advantages of the Gott shunt are that it is simple, inexpensive, requires only partial anticoagulation, and does not require perfusion personnel. Disadvantages of the Gott shunt include technical difficulty with cannulation in some patients, vessel injury, dislodgment, bleeding from the cannulation site, embolic stroke, and unproven efficacy for the prevention of paraplegia and end-organ dysfunction.[91] An alternative technique to provide passive distal aortic perfusion is to perform an axillofemoral bypass prior to aortic cross-clamping.[92]

Table 23–7 Advantages and Disadvantages of Distal Perfusion Techniques for Thoracic or Thoracoabdominal Aortic Reconstruction

Potential advantages
Control of proximal hypertension
Decrease left ventricular afterload
Less hemodynamic perturbations with aortic clamping and unclamping
Decrease duration of mesenteric ischemia
Decrease risk of paraplegia from spinal cord ischemia
Ability to control systemic temperature with heat exchanger
Vascular access for rapid volume expansion
Ability to oxygenate blood with extracorporeal oxygenator
Capability to selectively perfuse mesenteric organs or aortic branch vessels
Maintain lower extremity SSEPs and MEPs for neurophysiologic monitoring
Potential disadvantages
Require greater level of systemic anticoagulation
Increase risk of vascular injury at cannulation sites
Increase risk of thromboembolic events.
Require perfusion team
Need to monitor and control upper and lower body arterial pressure and flow
Increase technical complexity of operation

Partial Left Heart Bypass

Partial left-heart bypass with extracorporeal circulation is a method of controlling both proximal aortic and distal aortic perfusion during aortic cross-clamping for TAAA repair. The technique of partial left heart bypass involves cannulation of the left atrium from a left thoracotomy incision usually via a left pulmonary vein (see Fig. 23–12). Oxygenated blood from the left atrium is directed through the extracorporeal circuit with a centrifugal pump and into an arterial cannula placed in either the distal aorta, iliac artery, or femoral artery.[94-95] The extracorporeal circuit used to provide partial left heart bypass can be modified in a number of ways to include or not include a heat exchanger, membrane oxygenator, or venous reservoir. Heparin requirements for partial left heart bypass range from minimal to no heparin when heparin-coated circuits without oxygenators are used to full systemic anticoagulation with ACT >400 seconds when circuits with membrane oxygenators and heat exchangers are used.[95-96] During partial left heart bypass, the mean arterial pressure in the proximal aorta monitored by a radial arterial catheter is generally maintained in the range of 90 mm Hg. Bypass flow rates in the range of 1.5 to 2.5 L/min are usually necessary to maintain a distal aortic mean arterial pressure in the range of 60 to 70 mm Hg measured through a femoral arterial catheter.[94-95] Sequential advancement of the distal aortic cross-clamp during partial left heart bypass after successive reattachment of intercostal arteries, mesenteric artery, and the renal arteries to the graft permits segmental reconstruction of the thoracoabdominal aorta to decrease end-organ ischemia. Advantages of partial left heart bypass include the ability to control proximal aortic and distal aortic perfusion pressures, control systemic

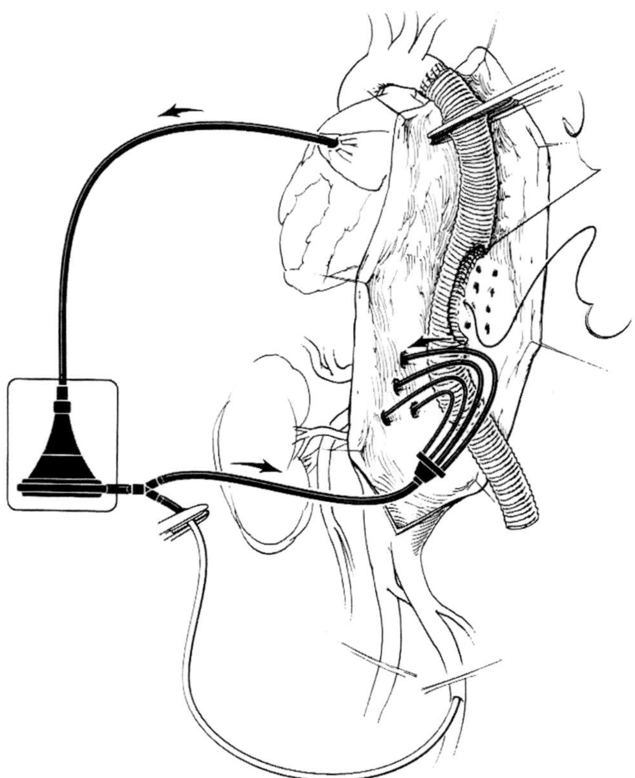

Figure 23–13 Extracorporeal perfusion circuit for repair of an extensive thoracoabdominal aortic aneurysm. Cannulation of the left atrium and femoral artery provides distal aortic perfusion by partial left heart bypass. Visceral perfusion can be provided by selective cannulation of the celiac, superior mesenteric, and renal arteries. (Adapted from Coselli JS, Descending thoracoabdominal aortic aneurysms. *In* Edmunds LH [ed]: Cardiac Surgery in the Adult. New York, McGraw-Hill, 1997, p 1237.)

temperature with a heat exchanger, provide reliable perfusion to the lower body and mesenteric organs, permit selective cannulation and antegrade perfusion of mesenteric branch vessels, and preserve lower extremity somatosensory and motor nerve function for intraoperative neurophysiologic monitoring[58,97,99-102] (Fig. 23–13). Two contemporary clinical series have suggested that use of partial left heart bypass was protective against postoperative paraplegia.[94,103] Disadvantages to partial left heart bypass include increased expense, increased complexity, and requirement for systemic anticoagulation (see Table 23–7).

Cardiopulmonary Bypass and Deep Hypothermic Circulatory Arrest

Extracorporeal circulatory support for TAAA repair can also be accomplished with partial CPB. Venous return for partial CPB can be established by cannulating the right atrium directly or with a venous cannula inserted in the femoral vein. Intraoperative TEE is often useful to assist and verify proper placement of the venous cannula emerging from the inferior vena cava, entering the right atrium, and positioned with its tip in the superior vena cava. Assisted venous drainage is sometimes necessary to generate flow rates to support full CPB. The aorta, iliac artery, or femoral artery can be cannulated for arterial inflow. CPB is useful for cardiopulmonary support in patients with lung disease who cannot tolerate single-lung ventilation for left thoracotomy. Full CPB is necessary for TAAA repair performed with DHCA and requires complete systemic anticoagulation.

Full CPB and DHCA has been described for TAAA repair with acceptable morbidity.[96,104,105] DHCA is necessary for construction of the proximal graft anastomosis if the aneurysm extends into the distal aortic arch or if the proximal descending aorta cannot be cross-clamped because the aorta is heavily calcified or cross-clamping compromises flow in the left common carotid artery. DHCA has also been advocated as an alternative method to protect the spinal cord and mesenteric organs from ischemia prior to the reattachment of branch vessels. If full CPB and DHCA is planned for TAAA repair through a left thoracotomy incision, preoperative echocardiography or intraoperative TEE is necessary to evaluate for the presence of AR so that a left ventricular vent can be inserted during surgery to prevent overdistention of the left ventricle with the onset of asystole during deliberate hypothermia. DHCA has the advantage of providing a bloodless surgical field for open anastomosis. Potential disadvantages of CPB and DHCA is the limited safe period for circulatory arrest, risk of stroke from cerebral embolization caused by retrograde perfusion of the aortic arch through a diseased descending thoracic aorta, increased duration of CPB for deliberate hypothermia and rewarming, and possibly increased risk of bleeding from hypothermia. For TAAA with extension into the distal aortic arch, a two-stage elephant trunk procedure can be performed instead of using CPB with DHCA. In the two-stage elephant trunk procedure, the transverse aortic arch graft is performed first through a median sternotomy leaving a short segment of graft extending into the descending aorta. The second stage of the repair is performed through a left thoracotomy incision to access and anastomose the distal end of the transverse arch graft to the proximal end of the descending thoracic aortic graft. This two-stage repair avoids the need for retrograde CPB perfusion through the diseased descending thoracic aorta and decreases the risk of injury to the recurrent laryngeal nerve, esophagus, and pulmonary artery located in the proximity of the distal aortic arch.

Endovascular Stent Graft Repair of Thoracic Aortic Aneurysms

Endovascular stent grafts are fabric or synthetic tube grafts reinforced by a wire frame that can be collapsed within a catheter for delivery and deployment within the aortic lumen. The endovascular stent graft is designed to be deployed within the aorta to span the length of the aneurysm and exclude blood flow into the aneurysm cavity. Endovascular stent graft repair for thoracic aortic aneurysms remains investigational but has been reported for the repair of isolated descending thoracic aortic aneurysms, repair of distal aortic arch aneurysms with partial arch reconstruction, and a few cases of transverse aortic arch aneurysms with dissection.[106-108] Endovascular stent repair requires the existence of a 1-cm-long nontapered region of aorta on either end of the aneurysm, often called the aneurysm neck, to provide a landing zone for each end of the graft. Furthermore, aneurysms that span essential aortic branch vessels require extra-anatomic bypass of those vessels before endovascular stent grafting.

Endovascular stent graft repair for isolated descending thoracic aortic aneurysms with a proximal neck that involves the origin of the left subclavian artery can be accomplished using a two-stage procedure (Fig. 23–14). In the first stage, the left subclavian artery can be divided and anastomosed onto the left common carotid artery. This first stage of the procedure

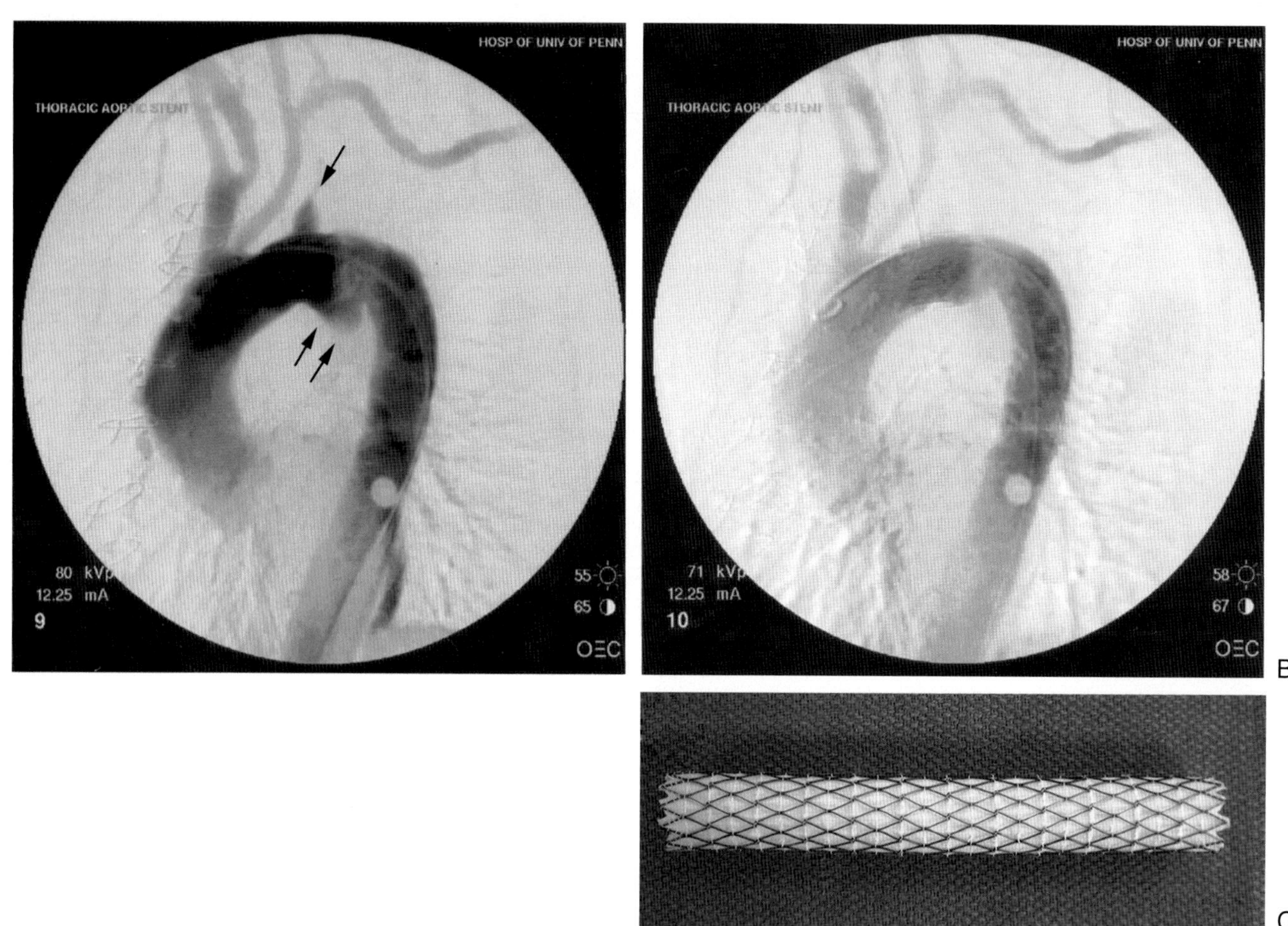

Figure 23–14 Intraoperative angiogram demonstrating an isolated saccular aneurysm *(double arrows)* of the thoracic aorta *(A)*. The left subclavian artery *(single arrow)* was previously divided and transposed onto the left carotid artery to create a proximal landing site for endovascular stent repair *(A)*. Intraoperative angiogram *(B)* after deployment of the endovascular stent graft *(C)* demonstrated exclusion of the aneurysm.

provides a proximal landing zone allowing the deployment of the endovascular stent graft over the left subclavian artery branch in the distal aortic arch in the second stage of the procedure without compromising flow through the vessel. Endovascular stent graft repair of aortic arch aneurysms in two patients with previous ascending aortic grafts have been accomplished without CPB. The stent graft procedure required re-implantation of the innominate and left common carotid arteries to the ascending aortic graft using a partial aortic occlusion clamp and ligation of the left subclavian artery prior to deployment of an endovascular stent graft spanning the entire aortic arch via the femoral artery.[107] Other new technical approaches for the treatment of aneurysms and pseudoaneurysm of the aortic arch using combined endovascular and surgical approaches have also been described.[109-114] Intraoperative angiography is the main imaging modality for aortic endovascular procedures, although intraoperative TEE can sometimes be useful.

Long-term results and efficacy of endovascular stent repair of thoracic aortic aneurysms remain to be determined. Problems that have been encountered with endovascular stent graft repair include vessel injury caused by the delivery catheter, intravascular migration of the graft, strut fracture of the stent frame, postoperative paraplegia, and endovascular leak at the graft ends, between graft segments, or from segmental arteries within the aneurysm cavity.

Anesthetic Management for Thoracoabdominal Aortic Aneurysm Repair

The anesthetic management of patients undergoing TAAA repair requires several special considerations. Selective one-lung ventilation is required for left thoracotomy or thoracoabdominal incision. Paraplegia is a major complication of the procedure, and an important aspect of the anesthetic management is directed toward strategies to decrease the risk of postoperative paraplegia from spinal cord ischemia in high-risk patients. A right radial arterial catheter is preferred to monitor proximal aortic pressure if the aortic cross-clamp has to be applied across the left subclavian artery or if the left brachial artery has to be accessed for endovascular stent graft deployment. A femoral artery or distal aortic cannula is necessary to measure distal aortic perfusion pressure for partial left heart bypass or when a Gott shunt is used. Hemodynamic monitoring of the central venous pressure, pulmonary artery pressure, and cardiac output is useful for managing the circulation during proximal aortic cross-clamping, distal aortic reperfusion, partial left heart bypass, or partial CPB. Intraoperative neurophysiologic monitoring with SSEPs or MEPs for the detection of spinal cord ischemia requires specific attention to the type and dose of anesthetic agents used for the operation. Perioperative renal insufficiency from mesenteric ischemia may complicate intravascular fluid and electrolyte management and require adjustment in the dose of drugs cleared by renal excretion. Left thoracotomy, thoracoabdominal incision, division of the diaphragm, and dissection near the recurrent laryngeal and phrenic nerve increase the risk of postoperative respiratory failure and aspiration pneumonia. Postoperative pain is also an important concern, and effective postoperative pain management by intravenous analgesics or epidural analgesia may improve pulmonary function (see Chapter 37).

Lung Isolation Techniques

Selective right lung ventilation is required for left thoracotomy or left thoracoabdominal approach to TAAA repair. Selective ventilation of the right lung and collapsing the left lung during TAAA repair improves surgical exposure and decreases the risk of pulmonary contusion or torsion of the left lung. One-lung ventilation also serves to protect the right lung in the event of hemoptysis or bleeding from the left lung. Although it is possible to accomplish TAAA repair with a single-lumen endotracheal tube and lung retraction, anesthetic techniques to provide one-lung ventilation are always preferable.

Two major techniques are available to provide one-lung ventilation (Fig. 23–15). The first is selective endobronchial intubation with a double-lumen endobronchial tube. The second is the use of a bronchial blocker. The routine use of fiberoptic bronchoscopic guidance has increased the reliability of achieving satisfactory lung isolation with either of the techniques. Although a right or left endobronchial double lumen endotracheal tube can be used for lung isolation, a left-sided endobronchial tube is used most commonly. The increased length of the left mainstem bronchus makes it easier to properly position the endobronchial lumen of a left-sided double-lumen tube and makes it less prone to dislodgement or malposition during surgery. Commercially available integrated airway devices (Arndt blocker, Cohen blocker, or Univent tube) to accomplish endobronchial blockade has also improved the ease and reliability of this technique compared with improvisation using a Fogarty balloon-tipped catheter.[115] Wire-guided endobronchial blocking catheters permit the balloon-tipped catheter to be guided and positioned precisely in the left mainstem bronchus with a fiberoptic bronchoscope.

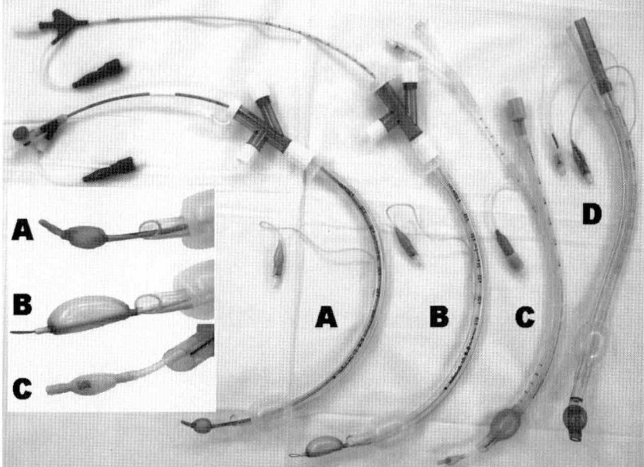

Figure 23–15 Single-lung ventilation for thoracic or thoracoabdominal aortic aneurysm repair requiring a left thoracotomy can be accomplished using a Cohen bronchial blocker inserted through a standard endotracheal tube *(A)*, an Arndt wire-guided bronchial blocker inserted through a standard endotracheal tube *(B)*, a Univent endotracheal tube with an integrated bronchial blocker *(C)*, or a left-sided double lumen endobronchial tube *(D)*.

Decisions regarding the choice of a particular technique for lung isolation in an individual patient should be based upon familiarity with the technique, the equipment or devices that are available, and the upper airway anatomy. The advantages of the double-lumen endotracheal tube are the ability to reliably isolate the left lung, intermittently ventilate and collapse the left lung, apply selectively continuous positive airway pressure to the left lung, and suction airway secretions from either the left or right mainstem bronchus. The disadvantages of using a double-lumen endobronchial tube include increased difficulty inserting the tube in patients with a difficult airway or under emergency circumstances, risk of endobronchial injury in cases where the aortic aneurysm has distorted the endobronchial anatomy or compressed the left mainstem bronchus, and need to exchange the single-lumen endotracheal tube in patients with an existing endotracheal tube. The major advantage of the endobronchial blocker is the ability to insert and position the endobronchial blocker through an existing standard 8.0-mm endotracheal tube and remove the device at the end of the operation without need for exchanging the endotracheal tube. The ease of insertion and removal of the endobronchial blocker through a standard endotracheal tube is particularly useful for emergency operations, in patients with difficult airways, or if re-exploration of the left chest is required for bleeding in the early postoperative period. Disadvantages of the bronchial blocker include increased time to collapse the left lung, inability to selectively suction the left main stem bronchus, and occasional dislodgement of the bronchial blocker during surgical manipulation of the left lung.

The majority of patients will require temporary mechanical ventilatory support in the postoperative period. If a double-lumen endobronchial tube was used to accomplish lung isolation during the operation, it will need to be exchanged for a standard single-lumen endotracheal tube at the end of the procedure. Intensive care unit personnel are usually not routinely accustomed to manage patients with double-lumen or Univent tubes, because these tubes are not ideal for long-term ventilatory support due to risk of tube malposition, airway obstruction, and difficulty removing airway secretions. Exchanging the endotracheal tube at the end of the procedure can be difficult because the airway may be edematous. For this reason, it is recommended that experienced assistance and equipment for emergency airway management be immediately available when performing the procedure. The use of an endotracheal tube exchange catheter inserted through the tracheal lumen of the double-lumen tube in combination with direct laryngoscopy may increase the safety of the tube exchange. A specially designed endotracheal tube exchange catheter (Cook Critical Care, Bloomington, IN) provides adequate length (100 cm) and stiffness for removal of the double lumen tube and guidance of the single-lumen tube into the trachea. Sometimes, airway edema permits only a smaller-diameter endotracheal tube to be placed. A central lumen through the airway exchange catheter can also be used to provide jet ventilation or oxygen insufflation in the event that an endotracheal tube cannot be advanced into the trachea.

Paraplegia After Thoracoabdominal Aortic Aneurysm Repair

The most devastating complication of TAAA repair is postoperative paraplegia caused by spinal cord ischemia and infarction. Although the exact pathophysiology and clinical events that lead to paraplegia after TAAA repair are incompletely understood, temporary interruption of distal aortic perfusion and sacrifice of intercostal and segmental arteries to accomplish TAAA repair are central events that predispose the spinal cord to ischemia and subsequent infarction. The incidence of paraplegia or paraparesis after TAAA repair based on clinical series reported in the literature varies widely and ranges from 2.9% to 32%.[86,116] Factors believed to contribute or influence the risk of postoperative paraplegia include the extent of the TAAA, acute presentation, aneurysm rupture, the duration of ischemia as a consequence of aortic cross-clamping, the loss of critical intercostal arteries, the presence of dissection, the surgical technique used to accomplish the repair, and the use of techniques to protect the spinal cord[117] (Table 23–8). The extent of the neurologic deficit in paraplegia or paraparesis varies from patient to patient but typically extends from the lumbosacral cord to the mid to high thoracic level. Postoperative paraplegia is particularly poorly tolerated in elderly patients, associated with respiratory insufficiency, and has a mortality rate that ranges from 63% to 100% depending on the length of follow-up. Although controversial, it is likely that perioperative management strategies directed at the detection and treatment of spinal cord ischemia have the potential to decrease the risk of paraplegia after TAAA repair (Table 23–9).

The anatomic distribution of arteries that supply the spinal cord provides a partial explanation of the risk and clinical features of postoperative paraplegia after TAAA repair (Fig. 23–16). The anterior spinal artery supplies the anterior two thirds of the spinal cord, and a pair of posterior spinal arteries supplies the posterior third of the spinal cord. Branches from each vertebral artery join to form the anterior spinal artery that descends along the mid-line of the anterior surface of the spinal cord. As it descends, the anterior spinal artery is sometimes discontinuous and fed in a variable extent by radicular arteries derived from ascending cervical, deep cervical, intercostal, lumbar, and sacral segmental arteries. The paired posterior spinal arteries also branch off the vertebral arteries and receive flow to a varying extent from posterior radicular arteries. The terminal region of the spinal cord and the caudal extent of the anterior and posterior spinal arteries are supplied by radicular arteries that arise from the internal iliac, lateral sacral, iliolumbar, and middle sacral arteries.[118,119] The thoracic and lumbosacral regions of the spinal cord often receive blood supplied from more than one arterial source and are particularly vulnerable to ischemia if suddenly deprived of blood from one of the sources. In these watershed regions, blood supply from one or several large radicular arteries may be crucial. In some patients, a particularly large radicular artery arising from an intercostal artery between T9-T12 in 75% of patients, T8-L3 in 15%, and L1-L2 in 10%, often called the arteria magna or artery of Adamkiewicz, can be identified.[101,120] Based upon the anatomic distribution of vessels supplying the spinal cord, temporary or permanent disruption of flow to the segmental arteries arising from the descending thoracic aorta can make the spinal cord vulnerable to ischemia and subsequent infarction.

Postoperative paraplegia can be subdivided into those with immediate-onset paraplegia and those with delayed-onset paraplegia. Delayed-onset paraplegia accounts for approximately 30% to 70% of patients with postoperative paraplegia or paraparesis.[94,116] The extent of the neurologic deficit often varies among patients. In patients with postoperative neurologic deficits, the incidence of paraplegia and paraparesis is equally divided.[116,121] Infarction in the territory of the anterior spinal artery classically causes motor paralysis with preservation of proprioception or some sensory function, but clinical experience has demonstrated that the pattern of paraplegia

Table 23–8 Potential Factors That Contribute to Postoperative Paraplegia From Spinal Cord Ischemia After Thoracic or Thoracoabdominal Aortic Procedures

Factor
Thoracoabdominal aortic aneurysm extent
Hypotension or cardiogenic shock
Emergency operation
Aortic rupture
Presence of aortic dissection
Duration of aortic cross clamp
Sacrifice of intercostal or segmental artery branches
Prior thoracic or abdominal aortic aneurysm repair
Prior repair of type A aortic dissection
Occlusive peripheral vascular disease
Anemia

Table 23–9 Strategies to Decrease the Risk of Paraplegia From Spinal Cord Ischemia After Thoracic or Thoracoabdominal Aortic Procedures

Minimize aortic cross-clamp time
Distal aortic perfusion
Passive shunt (Gott)
Partial left heart bypass
Partial cardiopulmonary bypass
Deliberate hypothermia
Mild to moderate systemic hypothermia (32°C to 35°C)
Deep hypothermic circulatory arrest (14°C to 18°C)
Selective spinal cord hypothermia (epidural cooling, 25°C)
Increase spinal cord perfusion pressure
Re-implantation of critical intercostal and segmental arterial branches
Lumbar cerebrospinal fluid drainage (CSF pressure ≤10 mm Hg)
Arterial pressure augmentation (MAP ≥85 mm Hg)
Intraoperative monitoring of lower extremity neurophysiologic function
Somatosensory evoked potentials (SSEPs)
Motor evoked potentials (MEPs)
Postoperative neurologic assessment for early detection of delayed-onset paraplegia
Serial neurologic examinations
Pharmacologic neuroprotection
Glucocorticoid
Barbiturate or CNS depressants
Magnesium sulfate
Mannitol
Naloxone
Lidocaine
Intrathecal papaverine

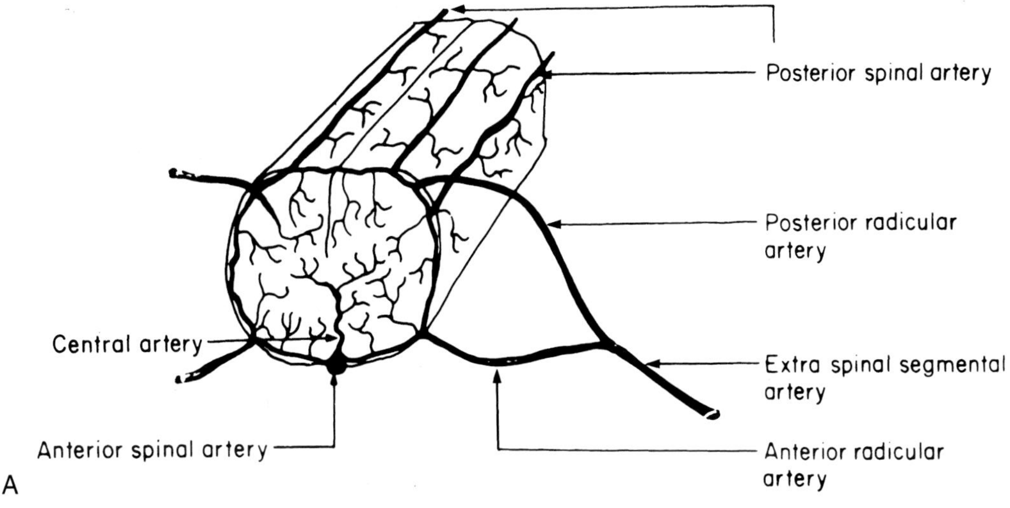

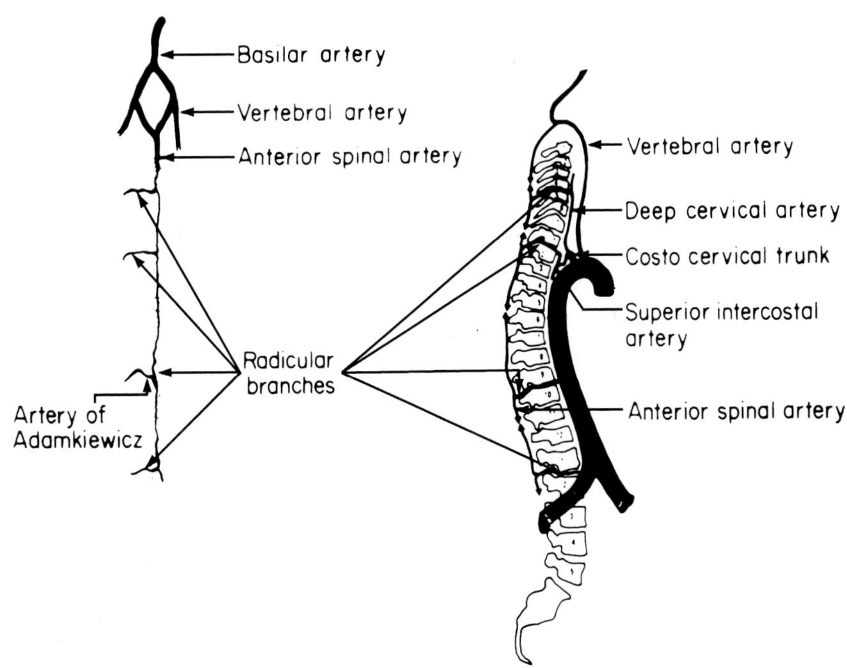

Figure 23–16 The arterial supply to the spinal cord is provided by the anterior spinal artery and paired posterior spinal arteries that branch off the vertebral arteries. Radicular arterial branches off the descending thoracic aorta provide collateral arterial supply to the anterior and posterior spinal arteries. The arteria magna or artery of Adamkiewicz refers to a large radicular branch located between the T9 to L2 vertebral levels that supplies the anterior spinal artery.

and paraparesis after TAAA is variable and often asymmetric and can affect either or both motor and sensory function.[94,120]

In immediate-onset paraplegia, the patient is paraplegic upon emergence from general anesthesia after TAAA repair. Immediate-onset paraplegia is likely a consequence of spinal cord ischemia leading to infarction that occurred at some time during surgery while the patient was under general anesthesia. In contrast to delayed-onset paraplegia, recovery or response to treatment in immediate-onset paraplegia has not been consistently demonstrated. The lack of improvement in response to measures to improve spinal cord perfusion in immediate-onset paraplegia indicate that irreversible injury had already occurred by the time paraplegia was diagnosed. For this reason, strategies to prevent immediate-onset paraplegia are directed toward protection of the spinal cord from ischemia and infarction during surgery (Box 23–3). Intraoperative efforts to protect the spinal cord from ischemia include augmentation of the arterial pressure, lumbar CSF drainage, providing distal aortic perfusion with partial left heart bypass, minimizing the ischemic time, deliberate hypothermia, segmental reconstruction of the aorta, re-implantation of intercostal arteries, or pharmacologic neuroprotection. The objective of using intraoperative neurophysiologic monitoring during general anesthesia is to detect spinal cord ischemia to permit immediate interventions to improve spinal cord perfusion during general anesthesia. Distal aortic perfusion maintains spinal cord function during aortic cross-clamping and improves the ability to monitor spinal cord integrity

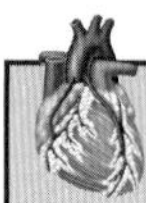

BOX 23–3 *Techniques to Decrease the Risk of Intraoperative Spinal Cord Ischemia*

- Mild systemic hypothermia
- Lumbar cerebrospinal fluid drainage
- Selective spinal cord cooling
- Distal aortic perfusion
- Intraoperative motor or somatosensory evoked potential monitoring
- Arterial pressure augmentation

during surgery with somatosensory or motor evoked potentials.

Delayed-onset paraplegia or paraparesis is the onset of spinal cord ischemia several hours or days after TAAA repair in a patient who awakes after surgery without evidence of neurologic dysfunction.[94,122] The syndrome of delayed-onset paraplegia indicates that the spinal cord was successfully protected during TAAA repair but remains vulnerable to ischemia and infarction in the early postoperative period. The abrupt onset of paraplegia or paraparesis in a patient with an initially intact neurologic examination after surgery suggests that immediate interventions to improve spinal cord perfusion may be effective for reversing spinal cord ischemia and preventing or limiting the extent of subsequent infarction. The clinical presentation of delayed onset paraplegia or paraparesis can be variable and include progressive loss of lower extremity motor strength or sensation. Findings are sometimes asymmetric, affecting one side more than the other. The cause or events provoking delayed-onset paraplegia are not fully understood, but a number of reports suggest that it is often preceded by hypotension. Strategies to prevent and treat delayed-onset paraplegia are directed at preventing hypotension after TAAA repair, early recovery from general anesthesia to permit neurologic assessment and detection of delayed-onset paraplegia, serial monitoring of lower extremity motor and sensory function, and lumbar CSF drainage for the initial 24 to 72 hours after surgery if a lumbar CSF catheter was placed during surgery (Box 23–4). Success in the treatment of delayed-onset paraplegia or paraparesis has been reported in response to immediate interventions directed at increasing the spinal cord perfusion pressure. Full or partial recovery of neurologic function after delayed-onset paraplegia has been reported in response to lumbar CSF drainage, arterial pressure augmentation, and intravenous naloxone used alone or in combination. Two reports suggested that early or immediate implementation of treatment at the onset of symptoms was more effective.[94,123] Considering the morbidity and mortality associated with permanent paraplegia after TAAA repair, all reasonable attempts to treat delayed-onset paraplegia can be justified.

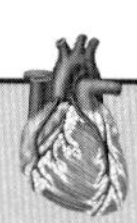

BOX 23–4 *Prevention and Treatment of Delayed-Onset Spinal Cord Ischemia*

- Maintain mean arterial pressure ≥85 mm Hg
- Serial neurologic assessment for lower extremity weakness or sensory loss
- Immediate treatment to augment spinal cord perfusion pressure
- Arterial pressure augmentation with vasopressor therapy
- Lumbar cerebrospinal fluid drainage
- Prevent hypotension

Lumbar Cerebrospinal Fluid Drainage

Lumbar CSF drainage is a recognized adjunct for the prevention and treatment of paraplegia caused by spinal cord ischemia after TAAA repair. The physiologic rationale for lumbar CSF drainage is that reduction of lumbar CSF pressure improves spinal cord perfusion pressure. It is also believed that CSF drainage counters an abnormal increase in lumbar CSF pressure in response to aortic cross-clamping, reperfusion, increased central venous pressure, or spinal cord edema.[124] A number of case reports attest to the efficacy of lumbar CSF drainage for the treatment of postoperative paraplegia,[125-130] but a meta-analysis published in 2000 failed to substantiate the benefit of lumbar CSF drainage for preventing paraplegia.[131] Interpreting the contribution of CSF drainage for the prevention and treatment of postoperative paraplegia has been difficult because any incremental benefit of lumbar CSF drainage must be considered in the context of heterogeneous patient populations, differences in the surgical technique, and lack of control of the arterial pressure. A randomized, controlled trial of 150 patients undergoing extent I and extent II TAAA repair using a uniform surgical technique employing distal aortic perfusion with partial left heart bypass demonstrated that lumbar CSF drainage was associated with an 80% risk reduction of postoperative paraplegia.[93] Two clinical series suggest that lumbar CSF drainage used in combination with arterial pressure augmentation to increase spinal cord perfusion pressure was effective for the treatment of delayed-onset paraplegia when the intervention was employed immediately after the onset of symptoms.[94,123]

Lumbar CSF drainage is performed by the insertion of a silicon elastomer ventriculostomy catheter via a 14-gauge Tuohy needle at the L3-L4 vertebral interspace. The catheter is usually advanced 10 cm to 15 cm into the subarachnoid space and securely fastened to the skin to prevent catheter movement while the patient is anticoagulated. The open end of the catheter is attached to a sterile reservoir, and CSF is allowed to drain when the lumbar CSF pressure exceeds 10 mm Hg. The lumbar CSF pressure is measured with a pressure transducer zero-referenced to the midline of the brain. At present, the best strategy to manage a traumatic lumbar puncture or the drainage of blood-tinged CSF has not been determined. For surgery, the lumbar CSF drainage catheter is inserted before or at the time of surgery and CSF drainage is continued typically for the first 24 hours after surgery. The lumbar drainage catheter can then be capped and left in place for the next 24 hours and then removed if the patient demonstrates a normal neurologic examination and coagulation function is satisfactory. Some clinicians use the catheter up to 72 hours after surgery.

The potential complications of lumbar CSF drainage include epidural hematoma, intradural hematoma, catheter fracture, meningitis, intracranial hypotension, and post lumbar puncture headache.[96] The potential for hemorrhagic complications as a consequence of dural puncture with a large-bore needle for insertion of the lumbar CSF drainage catheter in patients subjected to subsequent systemic anticoagulation during surgery remains an important concern. Despite the perceived risks of hemorrhagic complications of lumbar CSF drainage in aortic surgical patients, there are few reports in the literature to support this concern.[132] Precautions to minimize the risk of hemorrhagic complications include avoiding the procedure in the presence of coagulopathy, allowing a delay of several hours after placement of the lumbar drainage catheter before administration of systemic anticoagulation, and ensuring adequate coagulation function upon removal of the CSF drainage catheter. Intracranial hypotension as a consequence of excessive CSF drainage may cause brain herniation or subdural hematoma from stretching and rupture of the bridging dural veins. In one reported clinical series, the incidence of subdural hematoma was 3.5% when the lumbar CSF pressure was maintained at a pressure of 5 cm H_2O (3.7 mm Hg) associated with the drainage of 690 mL of CSF.[133] The risk of intracranial hypotension may be reduced by monitoring the lumbar CSF pressure during and after surgery with a pressure transducer not attached to a pressurized flush apparatus. For routine use, CSF should only be drained, using a closed circuit reservoir, when the lumbar CSF pressure exceeds 10 mm Hg. The risk of meningitis increases with the duration of lumbar CSF drainage and has been reported as high as 4.2% in a neurosurgical patient population.[134] Meningitis should be suspected in patients with high fever and altered mentation. Lumbar puncture demonstrating CSF pleocytosis or bacteria is diagnostic for meningitis. The risk of catheter fracture can be reduced by attention to patient position during catheter removal to prevent the catheter from being trapped between the posterior spinal processes.

Arterial Pressure Augmentation

The importance of arterial pressure augmentation for the prevention and treatment of spinal cord ischemia after TAAA repair has been recognized.[94,119,123] The basis for arterial pressure augmentation to prevent and treat postoperative paraplegia is loss of segmental arteries as a consequence of TAAA repair makes the spinal cord vulnerable to hypotensive infarction. Further, hypotension has been observed to precede or possibly trigger the onset of postoperative paraplegia and controlling the arterial pressure is an important component in combination with CSF drainage to support spinal cord perfusion pressure[122,135] (Fig. 23–17). Spinal cord perfusion pressure can be estimated as the mean arterial pressure minus the lumbar CSF pressure. In general, the spinal cord perfusion pressure should be maintained above 70 mm Hg after TAAA repair. Neurogenic shock or sympathetic nervous system dysfunction may be a contributing factor for hypotension that is associated with postoperative paraplegia. Spinal cord ischemia as a consequence of TAAA repair typically involves the lumbar to mid or high thoracic segments, and ischemia in these cord segments is likely to cause sympathetic nervous system dysfunction and hypotension that contribute further to spinal cord hypoperfusion. Early intervention to treat hypotension with vasopressor therapy may counter the autonomic nervous system dysfunction accompanying spinal cord ischemia and also augment spinal cord perfusion pressure. As in the treatment of neurogenic shock, high-dose vasopressor therapy with norepinephrine, phenylephrine, epinephrine, or vasopressin is often necessary to maintain mean arterial pressure in the range of 80 to 100 mm Hg.[94,119,123] Maintenance of the arterial pressure is also important in combination with lumbar CSF drainage to improve spinal cord perfusion pressure because decreasing lumbar CSF pressure alone may only have a negligible effect on spinal cord perfusion if the arterial pressure is insufficient. Recovery from spinal cord ischemia is often accompanied by an increase in the arterial pressure that may also reflect the recovery of sympathetic nervous system function.[94,119] When treating hypertension in patients during and after TAAA repair, the risks of hypotension and spinal cord ischemia must be weighed against the risk of hypertension and arterial bleeding.

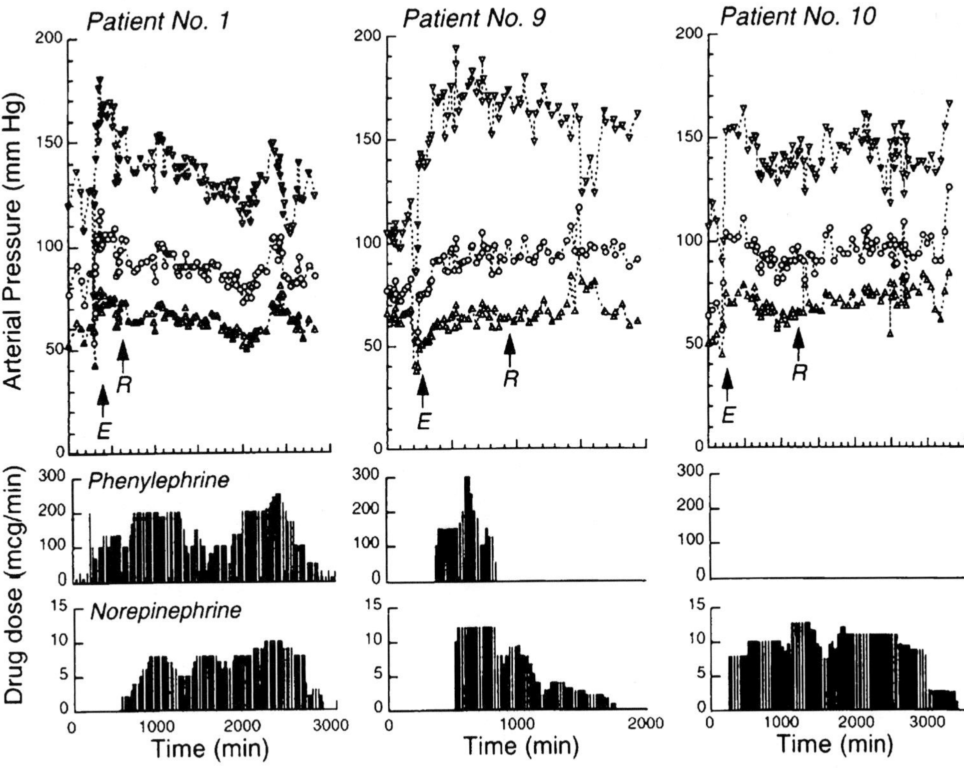

Figure 23–17 Systolic, mean, and diastolic blood pressures in the period surrounding the onset (E) and recovery (R) from delayed-onset paraplegia in three patients after thoracoabdominal aortic aneurysm repair. Autonomic nervous system dysfunction caused by spinal cord ischemia may have contributed to the decrease in arterial pressure during the events. Arterial pressures were augmented with vasopressor therapy *(bottom)*. Vasopressor requirements decreased after recovery from spinal cord ischemia. (From Cheung AT, et al: Interventions for reversing delayed-onset postoperative paraplegia after thoracic aortic reconstruction. Ann Thorac Surg 74:417, 2002. Copyright 2002, with permission from the Society of Thoracic Surgeons.)

Intraoperative Neurophysiologic Monitoring

The objective of intraoperative neurophysiologic monitoring is to permit the detection of spinal cord ischemia during surgery while the patient is under general anesthesia. The ability to detect intraoperative spinal cord ischemia may permit immediate interventions to improve spinal cord perfusion and prevent immediate onset postoperative paraplegia. Two neurophysiologic monitoring techniques have been used to detect intraoperative spinal cord ischemia during TAAA repair (see Chapter 17). SSEP monitoring is performed by applying electrical stimuli to peripheral nerves and recording the evoked potential that is generated at the level of the peripheral nerves, spinal cord, brainstem, thalamus, and cerebral cortex.[97,136-138] MEP monitoring is performed by applying paired stimuli to the scalp and recording the evoked potential that is generated in the anterior tibialis muscle.[139] Paraplegia caused by spinal cord ischemia causes a decrease in amplitude or disappearance of lower extremity evoked potentials compared with the upper extremity evoked potentials (Fig. 23–18). Comparing the lower to the upper extremity evoked potentials during surgery is useful to distinguish changes caused by spinal cord ischemia from changes caused by the systemic effects of anesthetic agents, hypothermia, or electrical interference. SSEP monitoring can usually be accomplished using a balanced anesthetic technique with narcotic, muscle relaxant, benzodiazepine and/or propofol, and keeping the inhaled anesthetic concentration less than 0.5 MAC. MEP monitoring requires total intravenous anesthesia without neuromuscular blockade.

The efficacy of intraoperative neurophysiologic monitoring for the detection and prevention of postoperative paraplegia remains controversial. A criticism of SSEP monitoring is that it only measures the integrity of the posterior columns of the spinal cord and fails to detect isolated motor defects associated with the spinal cord ischemia in the distribution of the anterior spinal artery. In addition, disappearance of SSEP during aorta cross-clamping did not always predict postoperative paraplegia.[140] However, studies have indicated that SSEP were preserved during TAAA repair with partial left heart bypass and distal aortic perfusion and that sensory defects were present in 90% of patients with postoperative paraplegia.[94] Another controversy surrounding the use of intraoperative neurophysiologic monitoring is that it is difficult to determine whether interventions prompted by abnormalities in the intraoperative SSEP or MEP can be attributed to improvements in clinical outcome. Clinical interventions in response to abnormalities in lower extremity SSEP or MEP that have been described in an attempt to decrease the risk of paraplegia include increasing the proximal aortic perfusion pressure, increasing the distal aortic perfusion pressure, increasing the distal aortic flow rate, modifying the

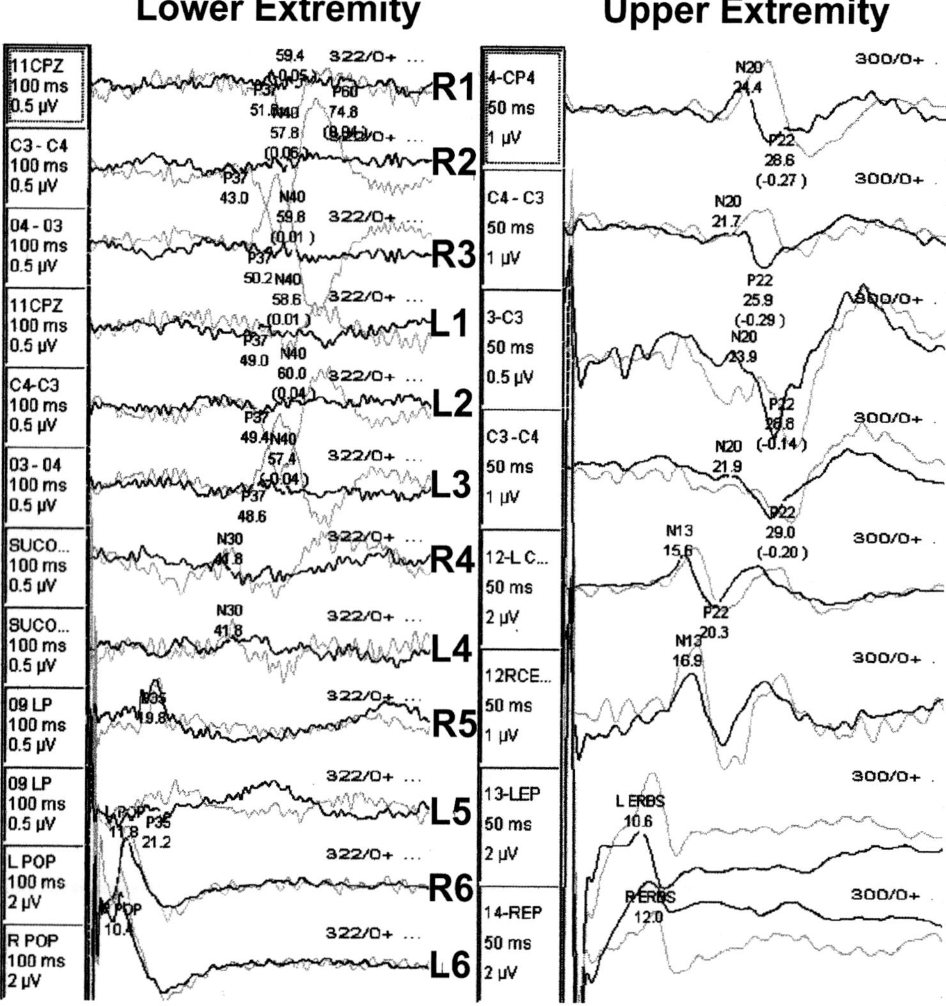

Figure 23–18 Intraoperative somatosensory evoked potential (SSEP) recordings from the lower *(left)* and upper *(right)* extremities that demonstrated spinal cord ischemia during thoracoabdominal aortic aneurysm repair. Disappearance of SSEP signals from the right (R) and left (L) lower extremities recorded at the cortex (R1, R2, R3, L1, L2, L3) and spine (R4, L4) with preservation of SSEP signals from the lumbar plexus (R5, L5) and popliteal nerves (R6, L6) indicated the acute onset of spinal cord ischemia. Upper extremity SSEP signals were maintained during the episode. The light gray tracings were the baseline SSEP signals used for comparison.

position of the proximal or distal aortic cross-clamp, and reattachment of additional intercostal, lumbar, or sacral arteries.[136,137,139,142,143]

Selective Spinal Cord Cooling

In addition to deep hypothermia and moderate systemic hypothermia,[97,144] selective cooling of the spinal cord by the infusion of cold saline into the epidural space has been described as a technique to protect the spinal cord from ischemia during TAAA repair. The original technique for selective spinal cord cooling described the infusion of 4°C saline at flow rates up to 33 mL/min through a standard 4 Fr epidural catheter inserted at the T11-T12 vertebral interspace.[86,122] A second 4 Fr thermister-tipped catheter inserted 4 cm into the subarachnoid space at the L3-L4 vertebral interspace was used to measure CSF temperature, measure CSF pressure, and act as a conduit for CSF drainage. A CSF temperature of around 26°C was achieved after the infusion of an average of 489 mL of iced saline into the epidural space over 50 minutes. CSF hypothermia was maintained by the additional infusion of 347 mL of iced saline into the epidural space while the aorta was cross-clamped. CSF was intermittently drained from the subarachnoid catheter to maintain a mean arterial to CSF pressure gradient of 30 mm Hg to 50 mm Hg to ensure spinal cord perfusion. The technique of selective spinal cord cooling is predominantly used in combination with the clamp-and-sew technique, but has also been described for use in cases performed with CPB.[145] The clinical experience with selective spinal cord cooling has been limited to only a few institutions. A case series of 170 patients undergoing TAAA repair with this technique reported a postoperative paraparesis or paraplegia rate of 7%.[86,122,146] A potential problem with the technique was excessive CSF pressures in response to epidural infusion that may have contributed to the development of a proximal cord compression syndrome in two individual patients.[122]

Pharmacologic Protection of the Spinal Cord

Various pharmacologic adjuncts have been described in an attempt to prevent and treat spinal cord ischemia as a consequence of TAAA repair. Glucocorticoids such as methylprednisolone, 1 gr to 30 mg/kg IV, thiopental, 0.5 to 1.5 g IV, mannitol, 12.5 to 25 g IV, magnesium, 1.0 to 2.0 g IV, or calcium channel antagonists are commonly administered alone or together as part of a multimodal clinical intervention strategy in an effort to protect the spinal cord from ischemia, but it is difficult to determine the individual contribution of each agent to overall clinical outcomes.[147] A small randomized trial demonstrated a lower incidence of postoperative paraplegia after TAAA repair in patients managed with lumbar CSF drainage and intrathecal administration of preservative-free papaverine, 30 mg, but again the independent contribution of papaverine to the improved outcome in the test group cannot be determined.[148] Several reports have also suggested that naloxone administered systemically at a dosage of 1 µg/kg/hr was associated with improved neurologic outcomes and even reversed the neurologic deficit in selected patients.[149,150]

Postoperative Analgesia After Thoracoabdominal Aortic Aneurysm Repair

It is well recognized that thoracotomy and thoracoabdominal incision is very painful and may cause respiratory splinting and retention of airway secretions that may contribute to the development of postoperative respiratory failure (see Chapter 37). Epidural analgesia is a proven method of providing postoperative pain relief for thoracotomy, laparotomy, and other surgical incisions that span the regions innervated by the spinal nerves.[151] Although the clinical efficacy of epidural analgesia for postoperative pain relief has not been specifically tested in patients undergoing TAAA repair, an effort is usually made to supplement systemic opioid analgesia with epidural analgesia to achieve patient comfort during convalescence. Further, providing effective postoperative analgesia may permit patients to awake earlier after surgery for assessment and monitoring of neurologic function.

The usual management of epidural anesthesia and analgesia may need to be modified when applied to the patient undergoing TAAA repair because the complications of epidural analgesia are difficult to distinguish from postoperative paraplegia caused by spinal cord ischemia.[152] The epidural analgesia regimen should be formulated to minimize interference with the ability to monitor lower extremity neurologic function and not cause sympathetic blockade that may contribute to postoperative hypotension. For example, bupivacaine 0.05% combined with fentanyl, 2 µg/mL, can be administered via a patient controlled epidural analgesia infusion pump at a basal rate of 4 to 8 mL/hr initiated after surgery and after the patient exhibits normal neurologic function.[94,119] Bolus administration of concentrated local anesthetic through the epidural catheter should be discouraged to avoid sympathetic blockade and associated hypotension. The epidural catheter can be inserted prior to, at the time of surgery, or in the postoperative period. Hemorrhagic complications attributed to epidural catheter insertion or removal have been rare, but care should be exercised to verify that the patient is not being treated with antiplatelet or anticoagulant drugs and that coagulation parameters are satisfactory prior to insertion and during removal of the epidural catheter.[153,154]

AORTIC DISSECTION

Aortic dissection is caused by a tear in the intima of the aorta, exposing the underlying diseased medial layer to the pulsatile pressure of the blood within the aortic lumen (Fig. 23–19). Blood exiting the true lumen of the aorta into the medial layer of the vessel through the intimal tear causes the intima to separate or dissect circumferentially and longitudinally within the aorta creating a true and false lumen contained by the adventitia.[26,155] The aortic dissection may remain localized to an isolated segment of the aorta at the primary entry site at the original intimal tear. Often, the aortic dissection extends distally along the length of the aorta starting at the primary entry site, but it can also propagate proximally or in a retrograde direction. As the dissection propagates along the length of the vessel, the dissection can extend into the aortic branch vessels, cause occlusion of branch vessels, or the intima may shear at the site of branch vessels creating multiple fenestrations. Propagation of the dissection into the aortic root can cause AR. The development of a false lumen and weakening of the aortic wall caused by the dissection is often accompanied by dilation and expansion in the diameter of the aorta.

Thoracic aortic dissections can be classified according to the location and extent of the aortic dissection. There are two generally accepted classification schemes for thoracic aortic dissections[156] (Table 23–10). The DeBakey scheme classifies aortic dissections into three groups[157] (Fig. 23–20). DeBakey

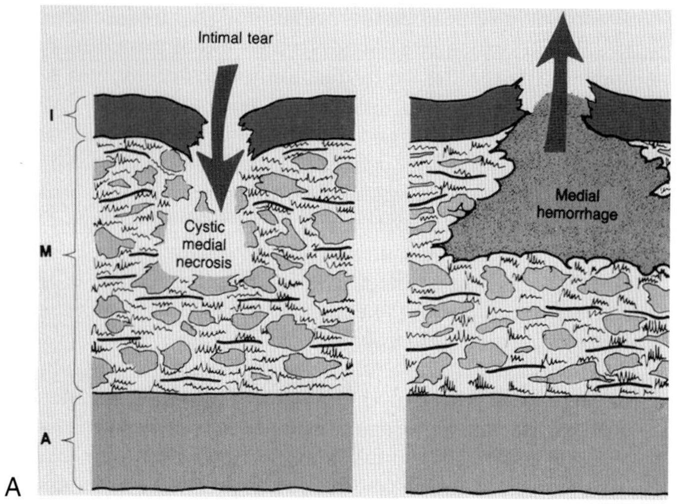

Figure 23–19 A potential mechanism for aortic dissection is cystic medial necrosis with an intimal tear allowing blood from the aortic lumen to enter the medial layer of the aorta (M) leading to separation of the intima (I) from the adventitia (A). (From Eagle KA, De Sanctis RW: Diseases of the aorta. *In* Braunwald E [ed]: Heart Disease, 4th edition. Philadelphia, WB Saunders, 1992, p 1528.)

type I dissections originate from a primary entry site in the ascending aorta and extend to involve the entire aorta. DeBakey type II dissections originate from a primary entry site in the ascending aorta and are confined to the ascending aorta. DeBakey type III dissections originate from a primary entry site in the descending thoracic aorta and are confined to the descending thoracic aorta distal to the origin of the left subclavian artery. DeBakey type III dissections can also be subdivided into subtype IIIA that is confined to the descending thoracic aorta above the diaphragm and subtype IIIB that extends below the diaphragm into the abdominal aorta. The Stanford scheme described by Daily classifies aortic dissections into two groups[158] (Fig. 23–21). Stanford type A dissections are aortic dissections that involve the ascending aorta regardless of extent, origin, or the entry sites. Stanford type B dissections are confined to the descending thoracic aorta distal to the origin of the left subclavian artery regardless of the extent or entry sites.

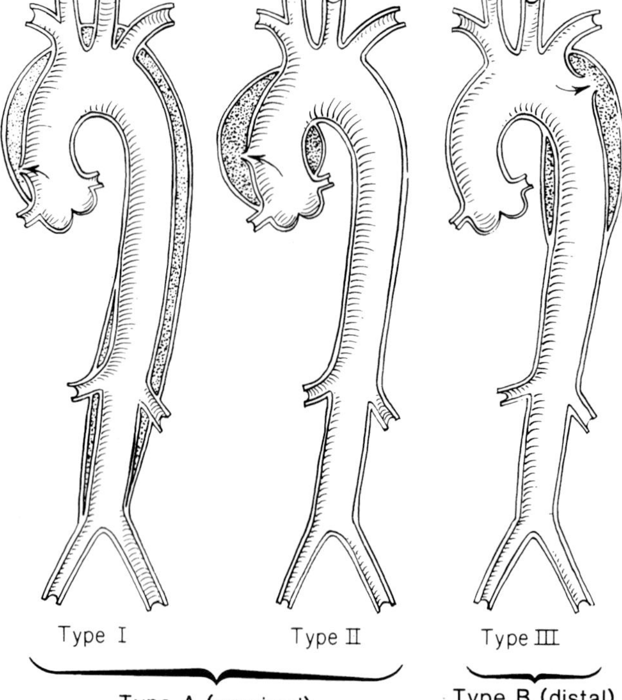

Figure 23–20 DeBakey classification of aortic dissections. Type I: intimal tear in the ascending aorta with extension of the dissection to the descending aorta. Type II: ascending intimal tear with dissection limited to the ascending aorta. Type III: intimal tear in the descending aorta with proximal extension of the dissection to involve the ascending aorta. Type IIIB: intimal tear in the descending aorta with dissection limited to the descending aorta. (Reprinted by permission of the publisher from Larson EW, Edwards WD: Risk factors for aortic dissection: A necropsy study of 161 cases. Am J Cardiol 53:849. Copyright 1984 by Excerpta Medica, Inc.)

Type A Aortic Dissection

Aortic dissections that involve the ascending aorta (Stanford type A) are considered surgical emergencies (Box 23–5). From 60% to 70% of patients presenting with aortic dissection will have a Stanford type A dissection.[159-160] According to an international registry for acute aortic dissection, mortality rates for patients with Stanford type A aortic dissection managed without surgery were estimated to be approximately 1% to 2% per hour following the initial symptom onset, and 1% per hour thereafter for the first 48 hours, 60% by day 6, 74% by 2

Table 23–10 Classification of Acute Aortic Dissection

DeBakey Classification
Type I: The entire aorta is involved (ascending, arch, and descending).
Type II: Confined to the ascending aorta.
Type III: Intimal tear originating in the descending aorta with either distal or retrograde extension.
Type IIIA: Intimal tear originating in the descending aorta with extension distally to the diaphragm or proximally into the aortic arch.
Type IIIB: Intimal tear originating in the descending aorta with extension below the diaphragm or proximally into the aortic arch.

Stanford Classification
Type A: Involvement of the ascending aorta or aortic arch regardless of the site of origin or distal extent.
Type B: Confined to the descending aorta distal to the origin of the left subclavian artery.

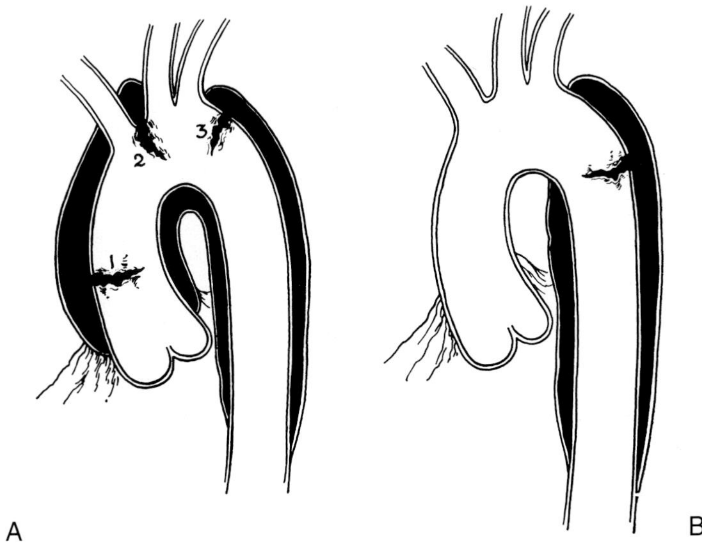

Figure 23–21 Stanford classification of aortic dissection. In type A aortic dissection, the ascending aorta is dissected regardless of the location or number of intimal tears *(A)*. In type B aortic dissection, the dissection is limited to the descending aorta *(B)* distal to the origin of the left subclavian artery. (Reprinted with permission from the Society of Thoracic Surgeons [The Annals of Thoracic Surgery, 10:237, 1970].)

weeks, and 91% by 6 months[159,161] (Fig. 23–22). When managed with surgery, the mortality rate for type A aortic dissection was 26%[159] (Table 23–11). The causes of death and morbidity attributed to type A aortic dissection included rupture of the ascending aorta causing cardiac tamponade, myocardial ischemia or infarction when the dissection involves the coronary ostia, heart failure caused by acute AR, stroke caused by malperfusion of the aortic arch branch vessels, mesenteric malperfusion causing renal failure or ischemic bowel, or limb ischemia[155,159,161,162] (Table 23–12). Aortic dissection can also rupture into the right atrium, the right ventricle, or the left atrium causing intracardiac shunting with congestive heart failure. An aortic dissection can be considered chronic after 2 weeks, as mortality tends to level off at that time.[159] Late complications of type A aortic dissection include worsening AR, aneurysm formation, or aortic rupture.

Type B Aortic Dissection

Aortic dissections that are confined to the descending thoracic aorta (Stanford type B) are considered surgical emergencies only if there is evidence of a life-threatening complication such as malperfusion or aortic rupture. Patients with type B aortic dissection are generally older, with an average age of 66 years.[159] Mortality in patients with acute type B aortic dissec-

Table 23–11 Mortality in Acute Aortic Dissection According to Dissection Type and Management

Dissection Type	N	Hospital Mortality (%)
Stanford Type A	289	101 (34.9)
Medical management	81	47 (58.0)
Surgical management	208	54 (26.0)
Stanford Type B	175	26 (14.9)
Medical management	140	15 (10.7)
Surgical management	35	11 (31.4)

Adapted from Hagan PG, et al: The International Registry of Acute Aortic Dissection (IRAD). New insights into an old disease. JAMA 283:897, 2000.

BOX 23–5 ***Potential Complications of Acute Type A Aortic Dissection***

- Cardiac tamponade
- Aortic regurgitation
- Myocardial infarction
- Stroke
- Limb ischemia
- Mesenteric ischemia

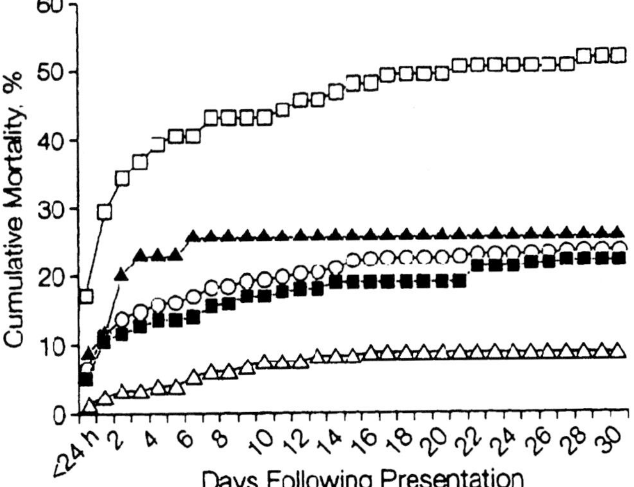

Figure 23–22 Thirty-day mortality in 464 patients from the International Registry of Aortic Dissection (IRAD) stratified by medical and surgical treatment in both type A and type B aortic dissection. (From Nienaber CA, Eagle KA: Aortic dissection: New frontiers in diagnosis and management. Part I: From etiology to diagnostic strategies. Circulation 108:631, 2003.)

Table 23–12 Complications of Acute Stanford Type A Aortic Dissection (n = 513)

Complications	Percent
All neurologic defects	18.0%
Coma/altered consciousness	14.0%
Myocardial ischemia/infarction	10.0%
Limb ischemia	10.0%
Mesenteric ischemia/infarction	4.0%
Acute renal failure	6.2%
Hypotension	26.0%
Cardiac tamponade	17.0%
Mortality	30.0%

Adapted from Bossone E, et al: Usefulness of pulse deficit to predict in-hospital complications and mortality in patients with acute type A aortic dissection. Am J Cardiol 89:851, 2002.

Table 23–13 Aortic Intramural Hematoma

Diagnostic criteria
Crescent-shaped or circumferential thickening of aortic wall
Hematoma thickness >7 mm
No dissection flap
No intimal tear
No blood flow within hematoma
Risk factors for mortality or progression
Ascending aorta or arch involvement (type A)
Aortic diameter >45 mm
Hematoma thickness >11 mm

tion managed surgically was 31.4% at 30 days compared with a mortality rate of 10.7% at 30 days in the medically managed patients[159] (see Table 23–11). The high surgical mortality in type B aortic dissection may be attributed to the presence of complications such as aortic rupture or visceral ischemia that required emergent surgery in addition to the severity of the operation. Other clinical series have also reported high surgical mortality rates that range from 21% to 45% for patients with acute type B aortic dissection.[163-165] Late complications of type B aortic dissection include aneurysm formation, aortic rupture, extension of the original dissection, or new dissection at a secondary site.[166]

Aortic Intramural Hematoma

Aortic intramural hematoma is a variant of the classic aortic dissection and is believed to account for 10% to 20% of acute aortic syndromes.[167] In a series of 464 patients with the clinical diagnosis of acute aortic dissection, 10% had aortic intramural hematoma with two-thirds of those cases classified as type B or involving only the descending thoracic aorta.[159] In aortic intramural hematoma, the intima is separated from the adventitia circumferentially and longitudinally by a greater than 7-mm-thick hematoma in the medial layer of the vessel wall[167,168] (Table 23–13). Aortic intramural hematoma differs from classic aortic dissection in that there is no intimal flap, and the intimal tear or primary entry site cannot always be identified. AR or malperfusion syndromes attributed to aortic intramural hematoma are also less common than in classic aortic dissection.[169] Although the experience is limited, the natural history of acute aortic intramural hematoma appears to be similar to classic aortic dissection. In a recent multicenter study, early mortality was 8% in patients with type A aortic intramural hematoma managed with surgery compared with a mortality rate of 55% in those managed medically.[169] Causes of mortality with aortic intramural hematoma were rupture, cardiac tamponade, and progression to classic aortic dissection, or progression to aneurysm.[169-171] The etiology of aortic intramural hematoma may include infarction of the vasa vasorum of the adventitia, intimal disruption from trauma, or penetrating atherosclerotic ulcers.[167,168,172] A rare variant of aortic dissection occurs as a consequence of a 360-degree circumferential tear in the intima causing catastrophic intimal-intimal intussusception, and distal ischemia.[173,174]

Clinical Diagnosis and Imaging Studies for Aortic Dissection

Aortic dissection is a disease that can affect a wide demographic population. Aortic dissection occurs in patients aged between 35 and 85 years with a peak incidence in the sixth and seventh decades of life.[159,161] Aortic dissection is more common in men than in women with a gender ratio of 2:1 to 3:1.[159,161] Patients with hereditary collagen vascular diseases such as Marfan's syndrome, Ehlers-Danlos syndrome, annuloaortic ectasia, bicuspid aortic valve, aortic coarctation, or familial aortic dissection may develop aortic dissection at an earlier age. The most common acquired conditions associated with aortic dissection are hypertension, cystic medial degeneration, and atherosclerosis. Other predisposing factors or conditions associated with aortic dissection include pregnancy, crack cocaine abuse, arteritis, and aortic trauma.[161,175-189] Iatrogenic aortic dissection as a consequence of cardiac surgery, valve replacement, or catheter interventions have been associated with a higher complication and mortality rate.[190,191]

The most common initial symptom in acute dissection is sudden and severe pain localized to the chest, back, or abdomen where the aorta is dissecting. The pain has been described as an acute "tearing," "ripping," "sharp," "stabbing," or "dull, pressure-like sensation" and is present in 80% to 90% of the patients.[159,192] Most patients who are diagnosed with chronic dissection do not have pain at the time of diagnosis. Patients with suspected aortic dissection should be managed as a medical emergency. The detection of pulse deficits suggests the presence of malperfusion and limb ischemia. Hypotension or jugular venous distention indicates cardiac tamponade or heart failure. Dyspnea, rales, and a diastolic murmur are signs of AR. Syncope, altered consciousness, weakness, or paresis may indicate stroke from cerebral malperfusion. Abdominal pain or oliguria indicate mesenteric ischemia. Other less common signs of dissection include hoarseness, dysphagia, dyspnea from upper airway obstruction, hemoptysis from rupture into the tracheobronchial tree, hematemesis from rupture into the esophagus, superior vena cava syndrome, pulsating neck masses, paraplegia from spinal cord malperfusion, or Horner's syndrome.

Diagnostic imaging studies are essential for establishing the diagnosis of aortic dissection and useful for detecting complications related to the dissection. Diagnostic imaging studies are also necessary to identify patients with Stanford type A aortic dissections who require emergent surgery. The specific diagnostic tests used to evaluate patients with suspected aortic dissection often depend on test availability at the admitting hospital or the sequence of the diagnostic evaluation. In the international registry for acute aortic dissection, the first diagnostic test was CT scan in 61%, transthoracic echocardiography or TEE in 33%, angiography in 4%, and MRI in 2%.[155,159] There are advantages and disadvantages to each imaging modality for the initial evaluation. Factors that should be considered when choosing an imaging modality include whether the condition of the patient is stable enough to tolerate transport to the study location for the duration of the study, the impact of radiographic contrast agents on renal function, the presence of implanted metallic devices prohibiting the use of MRI, or existing esophageal disease that would increase the risk of TEE.

Abnormalities are often present on the chest radiograph that is performed as part of the initial workup, but the findings are nonspecific and not usually diagnostic for aortic dissection. Mediastinal widening can be detected in 81% to 90% of patients. Other findings include the double aortic knob sign, loss of the aortic knob contour, poor definition or irregularity of the aortic contour, diffuse enlargement of the aorta, medial displacement of aortic intimal calcifications, tracheal displacement to the right, left pleural effusion indicating hemothorax, enlargement of the cardiac silhouette, or pulmonary edema.[175,192-195]

The most common imaging study used to diagnose aortic dissection is contrast-enhanced spiral CT or CT angiography. Equipment for performing a CT scan is widely available, and the test can be performed quickly to distinguish type A from type B aortic dissections. CT findings in acute aortic dissection include the detection of an intimal flap within the lumen of the ascending or descending thoracic aorta, inward displacement of intimal calcifications within the lumen of the vessel, and dilation of the aorta[193,196] (Fig. 23–23). Aortic intramural hematoma appears as a crescent-shaped high attenuation thickening of the aortic wall in noncontrast CT or a low attenuation thickening that does not enhance on the contrast-enhanced CT scan[172,197,198] (Fig. 23–24). CT demonstrating the presence of a pericardial effusion and extravasation of radiographic contrast outside of the aorta indicates rupture. CT angiography can determine whether there is obstruction of the mesenteric vessels and whether the aortic branch vessels are perfused from the true or false lumen of the aorta. The CT scan also provides adequate resolution of the aortic arch branch vessels to detect dissection extending into the innominate, carotid, or subclavian arteries. MRI and MRA studies have also been demonstrated to diagnose aortic dissection with a comparable sensitivity of 94% to 100% and a specificity of 95% to 100%, but facilities to perform MRI or MRA are less widely available and the test takes longer to perform[196] (Fig. 23–25).

Echocardiography is useful for the diagnosis of aortic dissection and for detecting the physiologic consequences of aortic dissection. Transthoracic echocardiography is portable, can be performed rapidly, and is a useful initial screening tool for the assessment of patients with suspected aortic dissection, but has limited ability to exclude type A aortic dissection.[193,196,199] TEE provides high-resolution images of the ascending and descending thoracic aorta and comparable sensitivity and specificity for diagnosis of type A or type B aortic dissection at experienced centers.[192,196,199] TEE has an added advantage over CT and MRA in that it is possible to evaluate the aortic valve for AR and identify the mechanism of AR, assess ventricular function and detect segmental wall motion abnormalities that may indicate myocardial ischemia, diagnose cardiac tamponade in the presence of a pericardial effusion, identify the location of intimal tears, and provide real-time information during surgery. Aortic dissection appears on TEE examination as an undulating intimal flap within the aorta separating a true and false lumen (Fig. 23–26). It is sometimes difficult to distinguish the true lumen from the false lumen, but the true lumen tends to be smaller with pulsatile high-velocity flow in systole. Doppler color flow imaging can be used to detect flow communication between the true and false lumens at intimal tear sites. Aortic intramural hematoma appears as an echo-dense crescent-shaped thickening (>7 mm) of the aortic wall on short-axis images that sometimes contains echolucent pockets of noncommunicating blood (see Fig. 23–24).

Conventional aortic angiography sometimes provides the diagnosis of aortic dissection but has been replaced based on the advantages of CT, MRI, and TEE. Diagnosis of aortic dis-

A

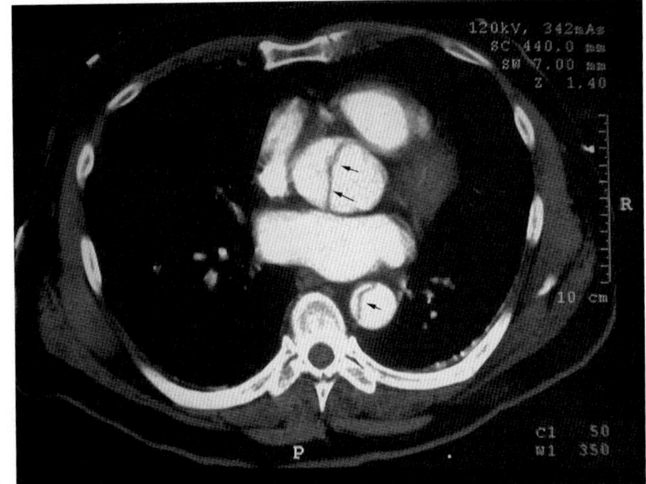

B

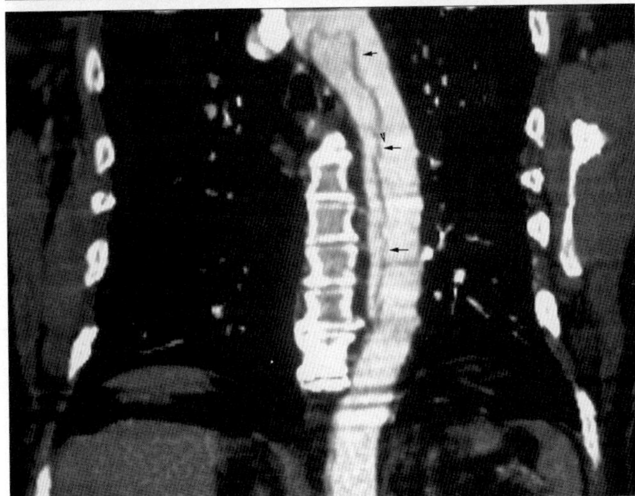

Figure 23–23 CT angiogram in a patient with a type A aortic dissection. Axial images of the chest *(A)* demonstrated an intimal flap that extended from the ascending aorta *(double arrows)* into the descending thoracic aorta *(single arrow)*. Sagittal reconstruction *(B)* demonstrated the presence of an intimal flap in the descending thoracic aorta *(single arrows)*.

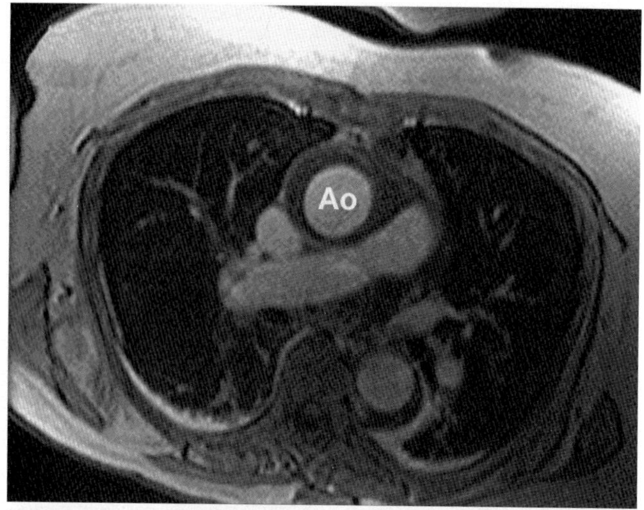

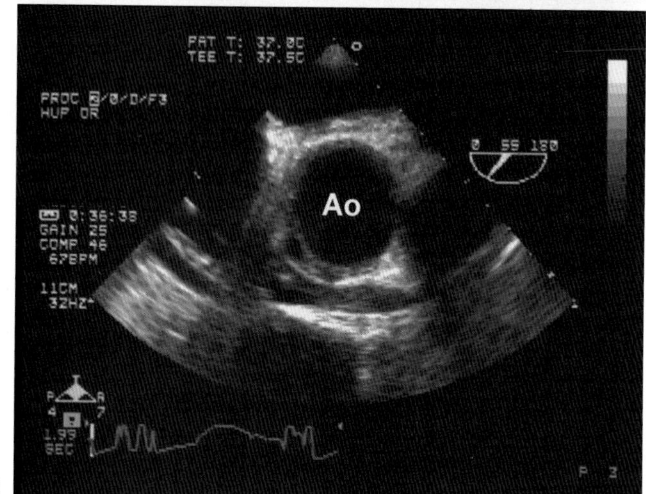

Figure 23–24 CT angiogram of the chest *(A)* and TEE upper esophageal short-axis images of the aorta *(B)* demonstrating an aortic intramural hematoma that extended from the ascending aorta into the descending thoracic aorta. A crescent-shaped or circumferential thickening of the aortic wall is diagnostic for aortic intramural hematoma.

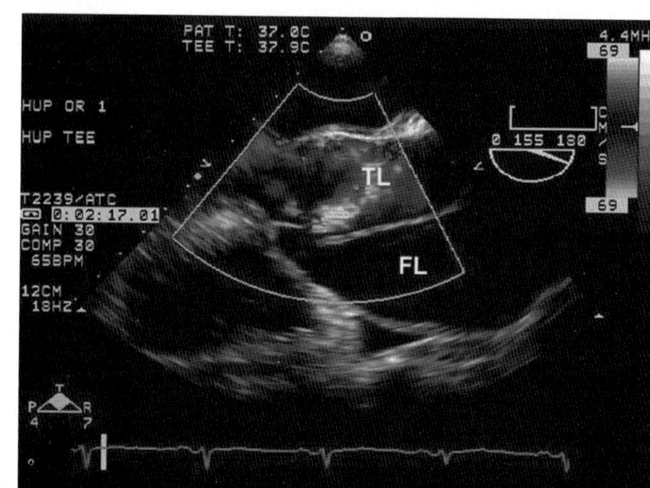

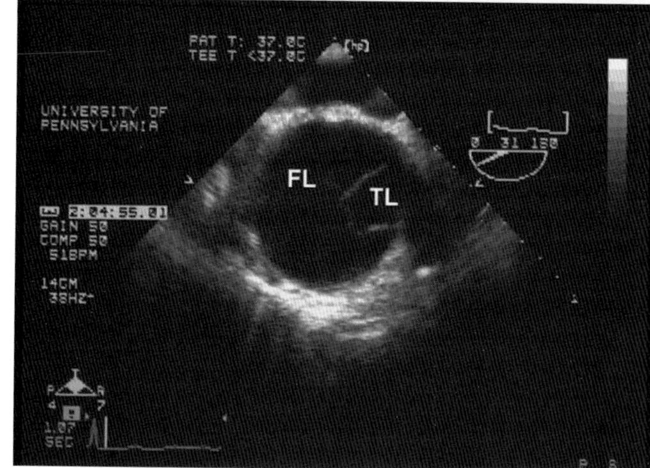

Figure 23–26 TEE mid-esophageal long-axis image of the aortic valve *(A)* and short-axis image of the ascending aorta *(B)* in a patient with a type A aortic dissection. An intimal flap separating the true lumen (TL) of the aorta with the false lumen (FL) was demonstrated in the aortic root and ascending aorta. Extension of the dissection into the aortic root may cause aortic regurgitation or coronary insufficiency. (See Color Plates.)

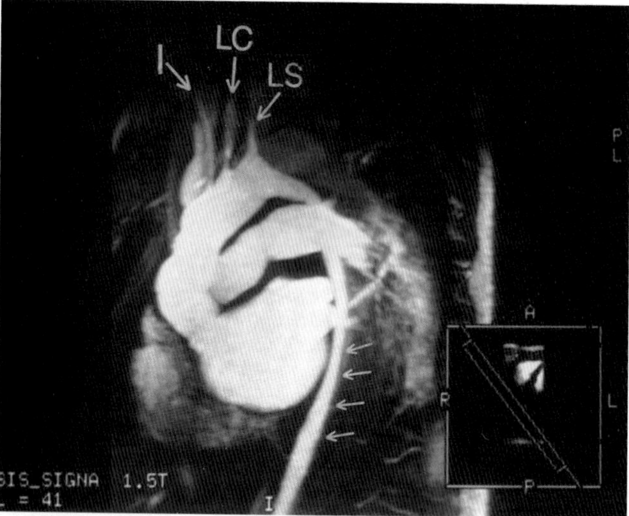

Figure 23–25 Magnetic resonance imaging of the chest with gadolinium contrast injection in a patient with a type A aortic dissection. The dissection extended into the innominate artery (I), left carotid artery (LC), left subclavian artery (LS), and into the descending aorta *(arrows)*.

section by aortic angiography is usually made during the course of cardiac catheterization for the evaluation of patients who present with chest pain. Opacification of a false lumen with compression of the true lumen and a line of demarcation indicating the intimal flap that separates the two channels within the aorta are diagnostic features of aortic dissection by aortography. Aortic angiography has a low sensitivity (19%) for detecting aortic intramural hematoma because there is no compression of the aortic lumen, and cannot be used to exclude the presence of aortic intramural hematoma.[200] Aortic intramural hematoma is almost impossible to diagnose with aortography. Although involvement of one or more of the coronary ostia occurs in 5% to 35% of type A aortic dissections, coronary angiography prior to emergency repair of the aortic dissection is not routinely warranted because of the associated risks and obligatory delay in surgery.

Anesthetic Management for Aortic Dissection

Acute aortic dissection is a medical emergency, and the medical management and diagnostic evaluation of a patient with suspected aortic dissection should proceed simultaneously. Time is of the essence because an initial mortality of 3% when surgery is expedited increases to as high as 20% when preoperative preparation is prolonged and diagnostic testing delays the start of surgery.[201] Diagnostic studies are directed to verify the diagnosis of aortic dissection, identify patients with type A aortic dissections that require emergent surgery, and detect complications associated with aortic dissection. Patients who are unstable with a high likelihood of aortic dissection based on clinical evaluation and existing diagnostic studies should be transported immediately to the operating room where TEE can be performed to verify the diagnosis and surgery can proceed immediately thereafter. Acute medical management is directed at treatment of pain and decreasing the arterial pressure with antihypertensive agents to prevent aortic rupture or extension of the aortic dissection. In general, the anesthetic preparation and management of patients with type A aortic dissection is similar to the requirements for the management of patients with ascending aortic aneurysm that require DHCA. The anesthetic preparation and management of patients with type B aortic dissections who require emergent surgery are similar to the requirements for the management of patients undergoing TAAA repair.

Large-bore intravenous catheters should be inserted for intravenous medications and intravascular volume expansion. An arterial catheter is necessary for continuous arterial pressure monitoring. A radial arterial catheter is preferred over a femoral artery catheter to allow for cannulation of the femoral artery for CPB. If a pulse deficit is detected, the site for arterial pressure monitoring should be chosen to best represent the central aortic pressure. A central venous line or pulmonary artery line to monitor central venous pressure, pulmonary artery pressure, and cardiac output is useful and can usually be inserted at the time of surgery before or after the induction of general anesthesia. Preparations should also be made to perform intraoperative TEE usually after the induction of general anesthesia.

Patients with aortic dissection who require surgery typically present with hypertension or are being treated with antihypertensive therapy. An optimal range for blood pressure in acute aortic dissection has not been established but general consensus recommends that the systolic pressure should be decreased to a range of 100 to 110 mm Hg. The objective is to maintain the lowest level of blood pressure that allows adequate vital organ perfusion to minimize the hydrostatic pressure within the aorta and reduce dP/dT or the shear forces acting on the aortic wall. Vasodilator drugs such a nitroprusside at a dosage of 0.5 to 2.0 μg/kg/min IV or nicardipine at a dose of 1 to 15 mg/hr IV are usually administered in combination with a β-blocker to decrease both the arterial pressure and dP/dT. Esmolol is a particularly useful β-blocker because it has a short pharmacologic half-life and can be rapidly titrated. Esmolol can be administered as an initial bolus of 5 to 25 mg IV, followed by a continuous infusion at a rate of 25 to 300 μg/kg/min titrated to keep the heart rate between 60 and 80 beats per minute. Alternatively, labetolol, a drug that has a 1:7 ratio of β-blocker to α-blocker activity, can be administered as a 20 to 80 mg IV bolus followed by an infusion at 0.5 to 2.0 mg/min IV. Metoprolol, a cardioselective β-blocker, may be advantageous in patients with reactive airway disease who are sensitive to β-adrenergic antagonists. Metoprolol is administered at a dose of 5 to 15 mg IV every 4 to 6 hours. A nondihydropyridine calcium channel antagonist such as verapamil or diltiazem may be necessary to control heart rate and blood pressure for patients with severe reactive airway disease. The choice of antihypertensive drug must be adjusted in patients with severe AR or cardiac tamponade associated with aortic dissection because excessive slowing of the heart rate or myocardial depression as a consequence of β-blockade can cause cardiogenic shock in this condition. Vasodilator therapy alone provides left ventricular afterload reduction and serves to maintain or improve the cardiac output in patients with acute AR. Pain caused by the aortic dissection should be treated with a narcotic analgesic.

Critically unstable patients or patients in shock should be treated like any other patient requiring cardiopulmonary resuscitation and life support by securing the airway, providing mechanical ventilation, and administering vasopressor and inotropic drugs to support the circulation. Emergent bedside or intraoperative TEE should be performed to verify the diagnosis of type A aortic dissection and detect the presence of cardiac tamponade, hypovolemia from aortic rupture, AR, or heart failure from coronary insufficiency. If TEE detects a pericardial effusion with cardiac tamponade, immediate sternotomy with preparations to institute CPB via femoral artery cannulation should be performed. Opening the pericardium and relief of cardiac tamponade can be followed by hypertension causing aortic rupture. Percutaneous pericardiocentesis for hemopericardium has been attempted as a temporizing measure, but is associated with a very high mortality and is not recommended.[202]

The induction of general anesthesia in hemodynamically stable patients with aortic dissection should proceed in a cautious manner. The dose of intravenous antihypertensive drugs may need to be reduced at the time of anesthetic induction to prevent severe hypotension when combined with anesthetic drugs. Hypotension may also occur upon anesthetic induction in response to the attenuation of sympathetic nervous system tone or decreased cardiac preload caused by venodilation and positive pressure ventilation in patients with preexisting concentric left ventricular hypertrophy. The hypertensive response to endotracheal intubation, TEE probe insertion, and sternotomy should be anticipated and attenuated with narcotic analgesics.

Surgical Treatment of Stanford Type A Aortic Dissection

Surgical therapy for type A aortic dissection is superior to medical management.[26,155,156,203,204] The objective of surgical repair for type A aortic dissection is to prevent death caused by AR, cardiac tamponade caused by rupture of the ascending aorta, myocardial infarction caused by dissection into the coronary ostia, and stroke caused by dissection into the aortic arch branch vessels.[26,156] Intraoperative TEE is useful for detecting AR, identifying the mechanism of AR to assess the feasibility of aortic valve repair, and assess the function of the aortic valve after completion of a valve-sparing aortic root replacement. Intraoperative TEE is also useful for evaluating right and left ventricular function to assess the need for coronary artery bypass grafting.

CPB is accomplished by cannulating the femoral artery and inserting a venous cannula into the right atrium. Selective cannulation of the inferior vena cava and superior vena cava is necessary for retrograde cerebral perfusion. Upon institution of CPB, retrograde perfusion through the true lumen of the aorta can be verified with intraoperative TEE. Acute cerebral malperfusion upon institution of CPB via the femoral artery is rare but can be detected by the acute decrease in EEG frequency and amplitude if EEG monitoring is used. Alternatively, duplex vascular ultrasound imaging of the carotid arteries in the neck can also be used to detect extension of the dissection into the carotid arteries or an acute decrease in carotid artery blood flow. Acute malperfusion can be treated by immediately discontinuing CPB if there is a perfusing cardiac rhythm and cannulating the contralateral femoral artery. In the absence of a cardiac rhythm, fenestrating the intimal flap within the aorta through a transverse incision in the vessel may be necessary.

Operations that are performed to treat type A aortic dissection include composite aortic root replacement with reimplantation of the coronary arteries (see Fig. 23–3), bioprosthetic aortic root replacement with reimplantation of the coronary arteries, aortic valve-sparing aortic root replacement, ascending aortic interposition tube graft, or aortic valve replacement and ascending aortic graft (see Fig. 23–2). Repair or replacement of the aortic root is typically performed in combination with graft repair of the ascending aorta and aortic arch. Partial or transverse aortic arch reconstruction requires temporary interruption of ACP (see Neuroprotection Strategies for Repair of Ascending Aorta and Aortic Arch Aneurysms) (see Figs. 23–9 and 23–10). Coronary artery bypass grafting is sometimes necessary for aortic dissections that involve the coronary ostia. Electing not to replace diseased segments of the aorta may increase the risk of aneurysm or pseudoaneurysm formation requiring reoperation at a later date.

Medical and Surgical Management of Stanford Type B Aortic Dissection

Because operative mortality in acute type B dissection is greater than 30%, operations are performed only in response to life-threatening complications such as intractable pain, rapidly expanding aortic diameter, imminent aortic rupture, bowel ischemia, or limb ischemia (see Fig. 23–22). Surgical repair by construction of an interposition graft in the descending thoracic or thoracoabdominal aorta is performed through a thoracotomy or thoracoabdominal incision in a manner similar to that used for TAAA repair (see section on descending thoracic and thoracoabdominal aortic aneurysms). Malperfusion syndromes can be treated with surgical fenestration of the intimal flap or by extra-anatomic bypass with a vascular graft, but survival is usually poor.[205] Aortic fenestration by endovascular intervention with the intent to redirect blood into the true lumen and restore branch vessel blood flow is an alternative approach for treating ischemic complications of type B aortic dissections.[206] Aortic fenestration with or without stenting of an underperfused vessel may be another option for the treatment of the obstructed aortic branches.[207,208] Endovascular stenting of the dissected aortic wall has also been reported to restore renal, visceral, and lower extremity flow in selected patients.[209-211] Percutaneous endovascular stent graft repair for the management of aortic dissection appears to be safer and to produce better results than surgery for type B dissection as suggested by reports but remains investigational.[26,212-215]

All other patients with type B aortic dissection should be treated conservatively with medical therapy because patients with acute distal aortic dissection have a lower risk of early death from complications of the dissection compared with those with proximal dissection.[26,155,216] Medical therapy for type B aortic dissection is directed at control of systemic hypertension to prevent aortic aneurysm formation, aortic rupture, and extension of the aortic aneurysm. Combination therapy with a diuretic, β-blocker, angiotensin-converting enzyme inhibitor, or other antihypertensive agents is usually necessary to achieve and maintain blood pressure less than 130/80 mm Hg. All patients after repair of type A aortic dissection should also be managed aggressively with antihypertensive therapy because many are left with a residual distal aortic dissection after repair. Serial imaging of the aorta is necessary to detect expansion of the aortic lumen and aneurysm development that may warrant surgical repair.

PENETRATING ATHEROSCLEROTIC ULCER

Penetrating atherosclerotic ulcer is the term used to describe an isolated disruption of the intimal layer of the aortic wall at the site of atheromatous disease (Fig. 23–27). A penetrating atherosclerotic ulcer can occur anywhere within the aorta, but most commonly affects the descending thoracic aorta. Disruption of the intima caused by the penetrating atherosclerotic ulcer can cause a localized rupture of the aorta or aortic intramural hematoma as a consequence of hemorrhage into the medial layer of the aorta.[217] Over time, a penetrating atherosclerotic ulcer can also rupture, become a pseudoaneurysm, evolve into a saccular or fusiform aneurysm, but rarely progress into a classic aortic dissection.[190,198,218,219] Penetrating atherosclerotic ulcers typically occur in elderly patients with systemic manifestations of atherosclerotic cardiovascular disease and a medical history of hypertension. Initial symptoms attributed to the acute onset of a penetrating atherosclerotic ulcer include chest and back pain similar to that of aortic dissection, and the majority of patients are hypertensive at initial evaluation.[197,198] Diagnosis is typically made with contrast-enhanced CT or MRI. Penetrating atherosclerotic ulcers tend to be localized to a relatively small segment of the aorta, and unlikely to cause vascular compromise.[220] Most patients with penetrating atherosclerotic ulcer are managed medically unless there is evidence of thoracic pain, acute expansion, aneurysm, pseudoaneurysm, rupture,

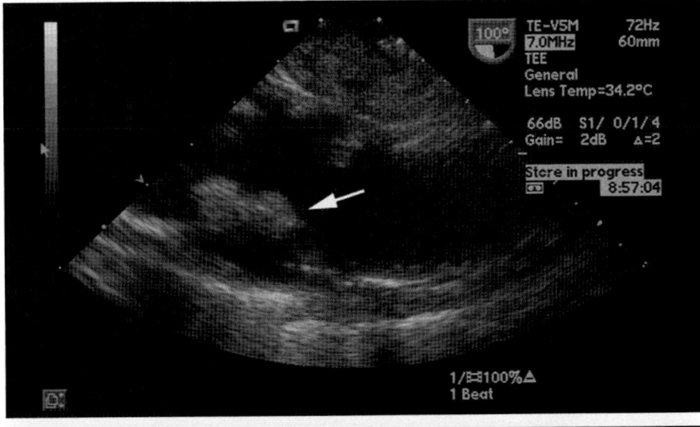

A

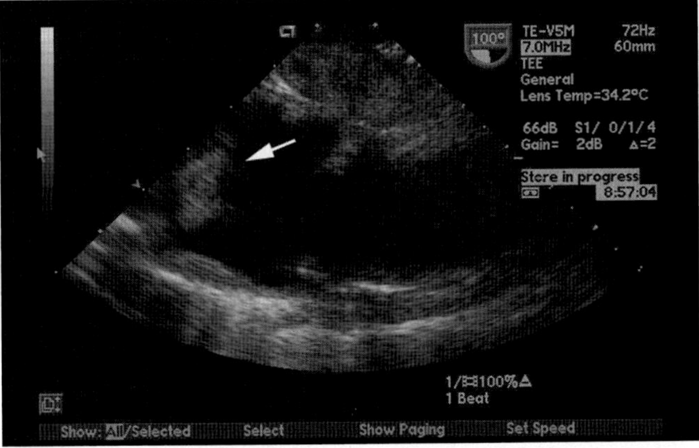

B

Figure 23–27 TEE long-axis images of the descending thoracic aorta demonstrating severe atherosclerotic disease with atheroma protruding into the vessel lumen. Images obtained in diastole (*A*) and in systole (*B*) demonstrated a large mobile atheroma (*arrow*) that may represent an atheromatous plaque that has ruptured and detached from the aortic wall.

or severe embolic disease. Some reports suggest that patients with penetrating atherosclerotic ulcers in the ascending aorta and arch are at high risk of rupture and should be treated surgically.[198] Endovascular stent graft repair may be an option for the treatment of penetrating atherosclerotic ulcer.

TRAUMATIC AORTIC INJURY

The most common cause of traumatic aortic injury is blunt trauma to the chest or rapid deceleration injuries as a consequence of motor vehicle accidents or falls. Approximately 4% to 17% of patients with chest trauma will also have an injury to the aorta.[221] Traumatic aortic rupture is lethal in 75% to 90% of patients and only 15% to 20% of patients arrive at the hospital alive. Ninety percent of patients with aortic injury who arrive alive at the hospital have an injury in the region of the aortic isthmus, followed by injuries to the ascending aorta, at the origin of the innominate artery, the descending thoracic aorta, and the arch vessels in decreasing order of frequency.[222,223] Injury at the site of the aortic isthmus may be the result of traction tears caused by cranial or caudal displacement of the aorta whereas injuries to the ascending aorta may be the result of traction or shear forces caused by displacement of the ascending aorta. The estimated mortality among patients who survive the initial injury is 30% within the first 24 hours and 50% within the first week. Nonpenetrating traumatic injury to the heart may be associated with severe chest trauma in 10% and 75% of patients, although these lesions are usually not lethal or may manifest only at a later time.[224] Patients with traumatic aortic injury commonly will have other associated injuries to the lung, brain, liver, spleen, pelvis, long bones, and spine.

TEE is considered by many as the diagnostic technique of choice for traumatic aortic injury. TEE is portable, can be performed in the operating room, does not require instrumentation of the aorta or radiographic contrast injection, and provides a rapid diagnosis.[225,226] TEE can also detect cardiac tamponade, left pleural effusion, hypovolemia, ventricular dysfunction from myocardial contusion, or vascular injuries from penetrating chest wounds. A potential disadvantage of TEE is that it cannot always be performed safely in patients with facial injuries or suspected cervical spine injuries. Further, the distal ascending aorta and transverse arch cannot reliably be imaged by TEE potentially limiting its sensitivity. In one reported series, TEE had a sensitivity of 57% and specificity of 91% for the detection of traumatic aortic injury compared with a sensitivity of 89% and a specificity of 100% for aortic angiography.[227]

The characteristic features of traumatic aortic injury detected by TEE are a mural flap at the site of intimal disruption and regional deformities of the aortic wall caused by the contained rupture (Fig. 23–28). The mural flap is commonly limited to a 1- or 2-cm segment of the aorta located at the aortic isthmus just distal to the origin of the left subclavian artery. This mural flap is usually thick compared with the intimal flap seen in aortic dissection and is less mobile because it usually contains several layers of the vessel wall. Sometimes a small defect or intramural hematoma is detected in the aortic wall instead of a mural flap.[225-228] Traumatic hemomediastinum is another sign of aortic injury and is defined by a greater than 3-mm separation between the TEE probe within the esophagus and the anteromedial wall of the aortic isthmus or the presence of blood detected between the posterolateral aortic wall and the left visceral pleura.[228] Contrast-enhanced CT, MRI, and aortic angiography can also be used to diagnose traumatic aortic injury and permit evaluation of the distal ascending aorta and aortic arch vessels when TEE is nondiagnostic or cannot be performed safely.[228]

An important consideration when evaluating a patient for repair of a traumatic aortic injury is to assess the risk of bleeding from other sites of injury. A CT scan of the head and cervical spine is especially important for assessing the presence of head or cervical spine injuries. The risks associated with systemic anticoagulation or extracorporeal circulation need to be addressed with the surgical team. Injuries to the ascending aorta or aortic arch require CPB and possibly DHCA for repair. Injuries to the aortic isthmus can be repaired through a left thoracotomy incision applying one-lung ventilation. The aorta can be repaired with an interposition graft using the clamp-and-sew technique, but clamping the proximal descending thoracic aorta causes proximal aortic hypertension and lower body ischemia. Distal aortic perfusion can be provided during the repair with partial left heart bypass, right atrial–to–femoral artery partial CPB, or a passive shunt. The risk of postoperative paraplegia is rare when distal aortic perfusion is provided (Table 23–14), because only a short segment of the thoracic aorta is replaced.[223,229-231] Endovascular stent graft repair for the treatment of traumatic aortic injury has also been reported.[215,232]

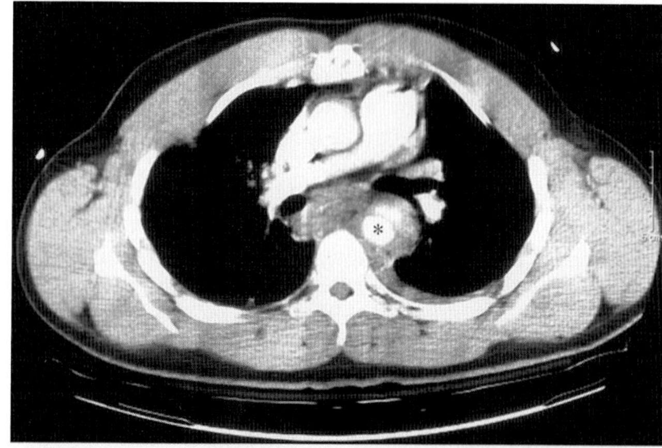

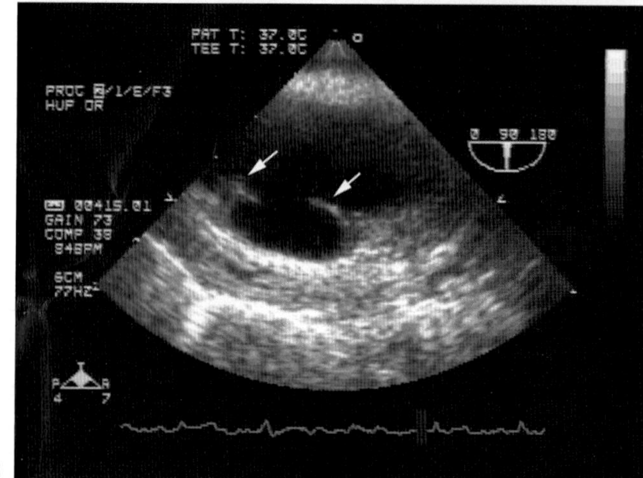

Figure 23–28 CT angiogram of the chest *(A)* in a trauma patient who presented with a widened mediastinum on the chest roentgenogram demonstrating traumatic intimal disruption of the aorta in the region of the aortic isthmus (*). Perivascular hematoma and extravasation of contrast agent into the mediastinum and left pleural cavity indicated a rupture of the descending aorta. Intraoperative TEE long-axis image of the proximal descending thoracic aorta *(B)* demonstrated a thick mural flap *(arrows)* and surrounding hematoma at the site of the intimal disruption.

AORTIC ATHEROMATOUS DISEASE

Atherosclerotic disease of the thoracic aorta has been recognized as an important cause of stroke and peripheral embolic events.[233-242] The risk of stroke and thromboembolism increases in relation to the severity of the atheromatous disease.[235,243,244] Surgical treatment with graft reconstruction of the thoracic aorta specifically for atherosclerotic disease is performed rarely and only for patients with mobile atheroma associated with recurrent life-threatening thromboembolic events (see Fig. 23–27). Sometimes, thoracic aortic reconstruction for severe atheromatous disease of the thoracic aorta is performed in combination with another reason for cardiac surgery such as aortic valve replacement or coronary artery bypass grafting. The anesthetic management of patients undergoing thoracic aortic reconstruction for atheromatous disease is similar to that described for the management of patients with thoracic aortic aneurysms involving corresponding segments of the thoracic aorta. Intraoperative epiaortic ultrasound imaging has been demonstrated to be superior to manual palpation or TEE for evaluating the location and extent of atherosclerosis in the thoracic aorta.[245,246]

Table 23–14 Incidence of Postoperative Paraplegia After Surgical Repair of Traumatic Aortic Injury in Relation to Operative Technique

Operative Technique	No. of Patients	Paraplegia (%)
Clamp and sew	73	16.4*†
Distal aortic perfusion	134	4.5
Gott shunt	4	0
Full CPB	22	4.5
Partial CPB	39	7.7
Centrifugal pump	69	2.9*

*$p < 0.004$, distal aortic perfusion vs. clamp and sew.
†$p < 0.01$, centrifugal pump vs. clamp and sew.
Adapted from Fabian TC, et al: Prospective study of blunt aortic injury: Multicenter trial of the American Association for the Surgery of Trauma. J Trauma 42:374, 1997.

Identifying the location of atheroma in the thoracic aorta is important for selecting the optimal site for aortic cannulation for CPB or placement of the aortic cross-clamp to minimize the risk of thromboembolic events.

TAKAYASU ARTERITIS

Takayasu arteritis is a chronic vasculitis that affects primarily the thoracic aorta, its branches, and even the pulmonary artery (Fig. 23–29). Takayasu arteritis occurs most frequently in young Asian women, although it has been observed worldwide. The disease is more common in women than men (10:1). The onset of Takayasu arteritis is insidious, and the early systemic manifestations are often vague or pass unrecognized. Vascular thickening and narrowing of the aortic arch branch vessels eventually cause signs and symptoms of vascular insufficiency. Dilation and aneurysm formation may also occur in diseased segments of the aorta. Diagnostic criteria are onset of disease at age less than or equal to 40 years, claudication of the extremities, decreased brachial pulses, systolic blood pressure difference of at least 10 mm Hg in each arm, bruit over the subclavian arteries or abdominal aorta, and angiographic narrowing of the aorta, its primary branches, or large arteries in the proximal upper or lower extremities.[247] Arterial angiography, CTA, MRA, or ultrasound imaging can all be used to characterize the location and extent of disease.

The initial treatment objective in Takayasu arteritis is to arrest disease progression with glucocorticoids. Methotrexate, azathioprine, mycophenolate, leflunomide, or cyclophosphamide can be tried for disease refractory to glucocorticoid therapy.[248] Percutaneous transluminal angioplasty is considered for arterial stenosis with ischemic symptoms. Surgical revascularization or bypass grafting is reserved for severe cases or cases with aneurysmal dilation of the aorta or its major branch vessels.[249] The anesthetic management of patients with Takayasu arteritis is complicated because sites for arterial blood pressure measurement are often limited. The femoral artery may be the only site for accurate measurement of central aortic pressure in patients with stenosis of both subclavian arteries. Patients with Takayasu arteritis requiring anesthesia should be assessed for cerebrovascular disease, renovascular disease, and coronary artery disease to decrease the risk of perioperative ischemic events.

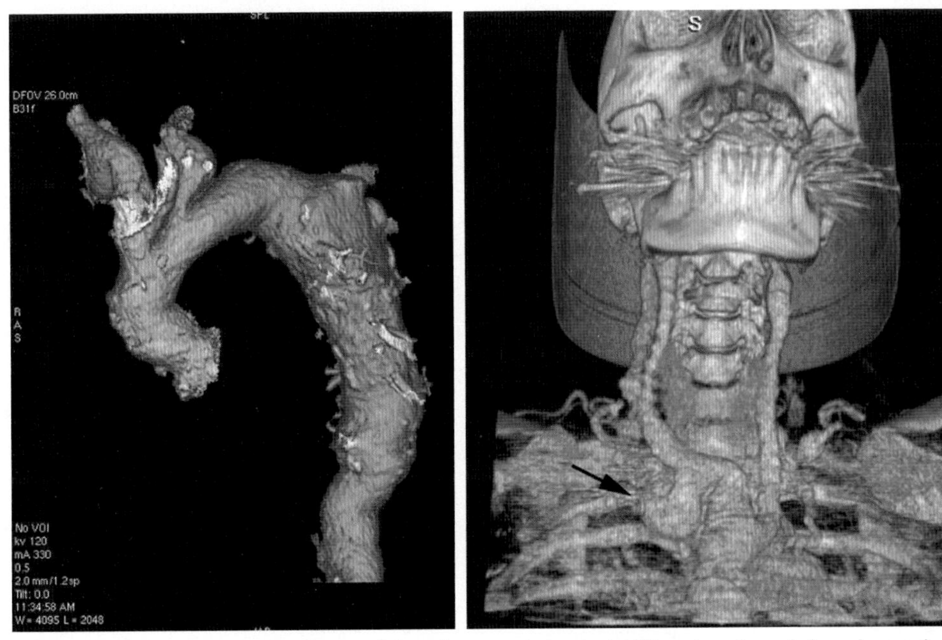

Figure 23–29 Three-dimensional reconstruction from a CT angiogram of the aorta *(A)* and aortic arch branch vessels *(B)* from a patient with Takayasu's arteritis. The reconstructions demonstrated aneurysmal dilation of the descending thoracic aorta, proximal innominate artery, and both subclavian arteries. The left and right *(arrow)* subclavian arteries were occluded distal to the aneurysm. (See Color Plates.)

AORTIC COARCTATION

Aortic coarctation is a common malformation and accounts for 6% to 8% of congenital heart defects. The anatomic defect ranges from a discrete narrowing of the aorta to a long hypoplastic segment of the vessel to complete discontinuity of the aorta (Fig. 23–30). The site of coarctation can be variable but is typically juxtaductal in location affecting the proximal descending thoracic aorta just distal to the origin of the left subclavian artery. The distal descending aorta is often hypoplastic in severe cases. Conditions associated with aortic coarctation include Turner's syndrome, bicuspid aortic valve, ventricular septal defect, patent ductus arteriosus, and intracerebral aneurysm (see Chapter 22).

The characteristic manifestation of aortic coarctation is hypertension measured in the upper extremities and hypotension with diminished pulses in the lower extremities. If the origin to the left or both subclavian arteries is distal to the coarctation, blood pressure in the arms may also be diminished. Adults with coarctation may present with headache, epistaxis, heart failure, or lower extremity claudication. Cardiac catheterization, MRI, CT scan, or echocardiography confirms the diagnosis of coarctation. Cardiac catheterization, MRI, and echocardiography are useful also to detect associated cardiac abnormalities. The chest roentgenogram often shows notching of the posterior one third of the ribs caused by the enlarged intercostal arteries that serve as collateral vessels to supply the lower body. The electrocardiogram often shows left ventricular hypertrophy.

Balloon angioplasty with or without stenting is the preferred treatment when coarctation is limited to a discrete segment of the aorta.[250,251] Balloon angioplasty and stent implantation can be performed using local anesthesia with sedation. General anesthesia is sometimes necessary because dilation of the coarctation can be quite painful or when it is necessary to keep the patient immobile for the procedure.

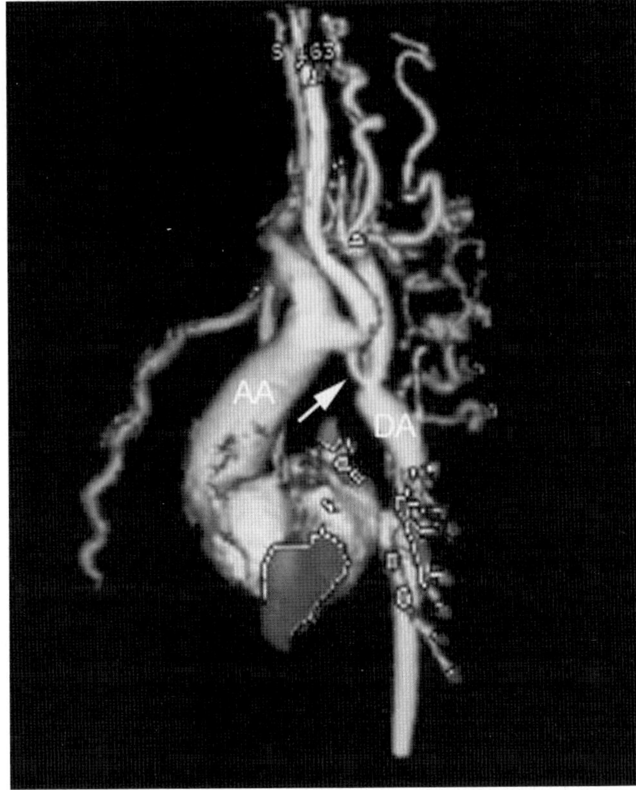

Figure 23–30 Three-dimensional reconstruction from a CT angiogram of a patient with aortic coarctation. In this patient, the site of coarctation was located between the left carotid and left subclavian arteries *(arrow)*. Repair was performed by construction of an extra-anatomic bypass graft between the ascending and descending thoracic aorta.

Reported complications of balloon angioplasty have included residual stenosis, recoarctation, paracoarctation aortic dissection or rupture, aortic aneurysm, and injury to the femoral artery. Aortic dissection or aneurysm at or near the angioplasty site may be a consequence of mechanical damage to the aortic wall or congenital defects of the aortic wall.

Techniques for operative repair of aortic coarctation include resection with end-to-end anastomosis, subclavian flap aortoplasty, interposition graft repair, extra-anatomic bypass grafting from the proximal aorta or left subclavian artery to the descending aorta, or prosthetic patch aortoplasty.[252,253] Prosthetic patch aortoplasty is rarely performed because of the high incidence of pseudoaneurysm after this procedure. Extra-anatomic bypass is advantageous for reoperations or in adults when the distal aortic arch cannot be mobilized to perform an end-to-end anastomosis. Avoiding surgical dissection in the region of the distal aortic arch also decreases the risk of injury to the recurrent laryngeal or phrenic nerves. Surgical mortality for repair of aortic coarctation is low, but patients are at risk for spinal cord or even mesenteric ischemia during repair if collateral circulation to the lower body is inadequate or if distal aortic perfusion pressure becomes too low. Intraoperative monitoring of distal aortic perfusion pressure using a femoral arterial catheter, monitoring lower extremity SSEPs or MEPs, mild deliberate hypothermia, and distal aortic perfusion using partial left heart bypass or partial right atrial to femoral artery bypass are techniques to decrease the risk of postoperative paraplegia.[101] Postoperative hypertension after repair can be severe, especially in older patients, and requires close monitoring and treatment.

REFERENCES

1. Corbet AJ: Medical manipulation of the ductus arteriosus. *In* Garson A, Bricker T, Fisher D, Neish S (eds): The science and practice of pediatric cardiology, 2nd edition. Baltimore, Williams & Wilkins, 1997, p 2489
2. Kern MJ, Serota H, Callicoat P, et al: Use of coronary arteriography in the preoperative management of patients undergoing urgent repair of the thoracic aorta. Am Heart J 119:143, 1990
3. Sanders JS, Ferguson DW, Mark AL: Arterial baroreflex control of sympathetic nerve activity during elevation of blood pressure in normal man: Dominance of aortic baroreflexes. Circulation 77:279, 1988
4. Horlocker, TT, Wedel DJ, Benzon H, et al: Regional anesthesia in the anticoagulated patient: defining the risk. Reg Anesth Pain Med 29(suppl 1):1, 2004
5. Svensson LG, Sun J, Nadolny E, et al: Prospective evaluation of minimal blood use for ascending aorta and aortic arch operations. Ann Thorac Surg 59:1501, 1995
6. Sundt TM, et al: Renal dysfunction and intravascular coagulation with aprotinin and hypothermic circulatory arrest. Ann Thorac Surg 55:1418, 1993
7. Westaby S, et al: Aprotinin and bleeding in profoundly hypothermic perfusion. Eur J Cardiothorac Surg 8:82, 1994
8. Parolari A, et al: Aprotinin and deep hypothermic circulatory arrest: There are no benefits even when appropriate amounts of heparin are given. Eur J Cardiothorac Surg 11:149, 1997
9. Ehrlich M, et al: Operations on the thoracic aorta and hypothermic circulatory arrest: Is aprotinin safe? J Thorac Cardiovasc Surg 115:220, 1998
10. Westaby S: Aprotinin in perspective. Ann Thorac Surg 55:1033, 1993
11. Murkin JM: A novel hemostatic agent: the potential role of recombinant activated factor VII (rFVIIa) in anesthetic practice. Can J Anaesth 49:S21, 2002
12. Stratmann G, Russell IA, Merrick SH: Use of recombinant factor VIIa as a rescue treatment for intractable bleeding following repeat aortic arch repair. Ann Thorac Surg 76:2094, 2003
13. Potapov EV, Pasic M, Bauer M, Hetzer R: Activated recombinant factor VII for control of diffuse bleeding after implantation of ventricular assist device. Ann Thorac Surg 74:2182, 2002
14. Hendriks HG, van der Maaten JM, de Wolf J, et al: An effective treatment of severe intractable bleeding after valve repair by one single dose of activated recombinant factor VII. Anesth Analg 93:287, 2001
15. Guvakov DV, Cheung AT, Weiss SJ, et al: Effectiveness of forced air warming after pediatric cardiac surgery employing hypothermic circulatory arrest without cardiopulmonary bypass. J Clin Anesth 12:519, 2000
16. van den Berghe G, Wouters P, Weekers F, et al: Intensive insulin therapy in the critically ill patients. N Engl J Med 345:1359, 2001
17. Johnston KW, Rutherford RB, Tilson MD, et al: Suggested standards for reporting on arterial aneurysms. J Vasc Surg 13:444, 1991
18. Pressler V, McNamara JJ: Aneurysm of the thoracic aorta. Review of 260 cases. J Thorac Cardiovasc Surg 89:50, 1985
19. Ellis RP, Cooley DA, DeBakey ME: Clinical considerations and surgical treatment of annulo-aortic ectasia. J Thorac Cardiovasc Surg 42:363. 1961
20. DeBakey ME, McCollum CH, Graham JM: Surgical treatment of aneurysms of the descending thoracic aorta: Long-term results in 500 patients. J Thorac Cardiovasc Surg 19:571, 1978
21. Lee JS, Chandraratna PA: Peripheral embolism from an aortic-arch atheroma. N Engl J Med 349:e23, 2003
22. Hollier LH, Taylor LM, Ochsner J: Recommended indications for operative treatment of abdominal aortic aneurysms. Report of a subcommittee of the Joint Council of the Society for Vascular Surgery and of the North American Chapter of the International Society for Cardiovascular Surgery. J Vasc Surg 15:1046, 1992
23. Ernst CB: Abdominal aortic aneurysm. N Engl J Med 328:1167, 1993
24. Safirstein R, Andrade L, Vieira JM: Acetylcysteine and nephrotoxic effects of radiographic contrast agents: A new use for an old drug. N Engl J Med 343:210, 2000
25. Olin JW, Kaufman JA, Bluemke DA, et al: Atherosclerotic Vascular Disease Conference: Writing Group. IV: Imaging. Circulation 109:2626, 2004
26. Nienaber CA, Eagle KA: Aortic dissection: New frontiers in diagnosis and management: Part II: Therapeutic management and follow-up. Circulation 108:772, 2003
27. Elefteriades JA: Natural history of thoracic aortic aneurysms: Indications for surgery, and surgical versus nonsurgical risks. Ann Thorac Surg 74:S1877, 2002
28. Bickerstaff LK, Pairolero PC, Hollier LH, et al: Thoracic aortic aneurysms: A population based study. Surgery 92:1103, 1982
29. Crawford ES, DeNatale RW: Thoracoabdominal aortic aneurysm: Observations regarding the natural course of the disease. J Vasc Surg 3:578, 1986
30. Griepp RB, Stinson EB, Hollingsworth JF, et al: Prosthetic replacement of the aortic arch. J Thorac Cardiovasc Surg 70:1051, 1975
31. Séguin JR, Picard E, Frapier J-M, et al: Aortic valve repair with fibrin glue for type A acute aortic dissection. Ann Thorac Surg 58:304, 1994
32. Bachet J, Goudot B, Dreyfus G, et al: The proper use of glue: A 20-year experience with the GRF glue in acute aortic dissection. J Card Surg 12(suppl):243, 1997
33. Coselli JS, Bavaria JE, Fehrenbacher J, et al: Prospective randomized study of a protein-based tissue adhesive used as a hemostatic and structural adjunct in cardiac and vascular anastomotic repair procedures. J Am Coll Surg 197:243, 2003
34. Safi HJ, Miller CC, Iliopoulos DC, et al: Staged repair of extensive aortic aneurysm: Improved neurologic outcome. Ann Surg 226:599, 1997
35. Harrington DK, Bonser M, Moss A, et al: Neuropsychometric outcome following aortic arch surgery: A prospective randomized trial of retrograde cerebral perfusion. J Thorac Cardiovasc Surg 126:638, 2003
36. Svensson LG, Crawford ES, Hess KR, et al: Deep hypothermia with circulatory arrest. Determinants of stroke and early mortality in 656 patients. J Thorac Cardiovasc Surg 106:19, 1993
37. Ergin MA, Galla JD, Lansman SL, et al: Hypothermic circulatory arrest in operations on the thoracic aorta. Determinants of operative mortality and neurologic outcome. J Thorac Cardiovasc Surg 107:788, 1994
38. Reich D, Uysal S, Sliwinski M, et al: Neuropsychologic outcome after deep hypothermic circulatory arrest in adults. J Thorac Cardiovasc Surg 117:156, 1999
39. Welz A, Pogarell O, Tatsch K, et al: Surgery of the thoracic aorta using deep hypothermic total circulatory arrest. Are there neurological consequences other than frank cerebral defects? Eur J Cardiothorac Surg 11:650, 1997
40. Ott DA, Frazier OH, Cooley DA: Resection of the aortic arch using deep hypothermia and temporary circulatory arrest. Circulation 58(suppl I):I-227, 1978
41. Griepp RB, Stinson EB, Hollingsworth JF, et al: Prosthetic replacement of the aortic arch. J Thorac Cardiovasc Surg 70:1051, 1975

42. Woodcock TE, Murkin JM, Farrar JK, et al: Pharmacologic EEG suppression during cardiopulmonary bypass: Cerebral hemodynamic and metabolic effects of thiopental or isoflurane during hypothermia and normothermia. Anesthesiology 67:218, 1987
43. Croughwell N, Smith LR, Quill T, et al: The effect of temperature on cerebral metabolism and blood flow in adults during cardiopulmonary bypass. J Thorac Cardiovasc Surg 103:549, 1992
44. McCullough JN, Zhang N, Reich DL, et al: Cerebral metabolic suppression during hypothermic circulatory arrest in humans. Ann Thorac Surg 67:1895, 1999
45. Cheung AT, Bavaria JE, Pochettino A, et al: Oxygen delivery during retrograde cerebral perfusion in humans. Anesth Analg 88:8, 1999
46. Stecker MM, Cheung AT, Pochettino A, et al: Deep hypothermic circulatory arrest: I, Effects of cooling on electroencephalogram and evoked potentials. Ann Thorac Surg 71:14, 2001
47. Coselli JS, Crawford ES, Beall AC, et al: Determination of brain temperatures for safe circulatory arrest during cardiovascular operation. Ann Thorac Surg 45:638, 1988
48. Bavaria JE, Woo YJ, Hall RA, et al: Circulatory management with retrograde cerebral perfusion for acute type A aortic dissection. Circulation 94(suppl II), 1996
49. Ergin MA, Galla JA, Lansman SL, et al: Hypothermic circulatory arrest in operations on the thoracic aorta. Cardiovasc Surg 107:788, 1994
50. Pochettino A, Cheung AT: Pro: Retrograde cerebral perfusion is useful for deep hypothermic circulatory arrest. J Cardiothorac Vasc Anesth 17:764, 2003
51. Ergin MA, Uysal S, Reich DL, et al: Temporary neurological dysfunction after deep hypothermic circulatory arrest: A clinical marker of long-term functional deficit. Ann Thorac Surg 67:1999
52. Usui A, Abe T, Murase M: Early clinical results of retrograde cerebral perfusion for aortic arch operations in Japan. Ann Thorac Surg 62:94, 1996
53. Pagano D, Carey J, Patel R, et al: Retrograde cerebral perfusion: Clinical experience in emergency and elective aortic operations. Ann Thorac Surg 59:393, 1995
54. Cheung AT, Bavaria JE, Weiss SJ, et al: Neurophysiologic effects of retrograde cerebral perfusion used for aortic reconstruction. J Cardiothorac Vasc Anesth 12:252, 1998
55. Juvonen T, Weisz DJ, Wolfe D, et al: Can retrograde perfusion mitigate cerebral injury after particulate embolization? A study in a chronic porcine model. J Thorac Cardiovasc Surg 115:1142, 1998
56. Imamaki M, Koyanagi H, Hashimoto A, et al: Retrograde cerebral perfusion with hypothermic blood provides efficient protection of the brain: A neuropathological study. J Card Surg 10:325, 1995
57. Anttila V, Pokela M, Kiviluoma K, et al: Is maintained cranial hypothermia the only factor leading to improved outcome after retrograde cerebral perfusion? An experimental study with a chronic porcine model. J Thorac Cardiovasc Surg 119:1021, 2000
58. Bavaria JE, Woo YJ, Hall RA, et al: Retrograde cerebral and distal aortic perfusion during ascending and thoracoabdominal aortic operations. Ann Thorac Surg 60:345, 1995
59. Safi HJ, Letsou GV, Iliopoulos DC, et al: Impact of retrograde cerebral perfusion on ascending aortic and arch aneurysm repair. Ann Thorac Surg 63:1601, 1997
60. Coselli J, LeMaire S: Experience with retrograde cerebral perfusion during proximal aortic surgery in 290 patients. J Card Surg 12:322, 1997
61. Ehrlich MP, Fang WC, Grabenwoger M, et al: Impact of retrograde cerebral perfusion on aortic arch aneurysm repair. J Thorac Cardiovasc Surg 118:1026, 1999
62. Okita Y, Takamoto S, Ando M, et al: Mortality and cerebral outcome in patients who underwent aortic arch operations using deep hypothermic circulatory arrest with retrograde cerebral perfusion: No relation of early death, stroke, and delirium to the duration of circulatory arrest. J Thorac Cardiovasc Surg 115:129, 1998
63. Kitamura M, Hashimoto A, Akimoto T, et al: Operation for type A aortic dissection: introduction of retrograde cerebral perfusion. Ann Thorac Surg 59:1195, 1995
64. Reich DL, Uysal S: Con: Retrograde cerebral perfusion is not an optimal method of neuroprotection in thoracic aortic surgery. J Cardiothorac Vasc Anesth 17:768, 2003
65. Boeckxstaens CJ, Flameng WJ: Retrograde cerebral perfusion does not perfuse the brain in nonhuman primates. Ann Thorac Surg 60:319, 1995
66. Bonser RS, Wong CH, Harrington D, et al: Failure of retrograde cerebral perfusion to attenuate metabolic changes associated with hypothermic circulatory arrest. J Thorac Cardiovasc Surg 123:943, 2002
67. Moon M, Sundt TS: Influence of retrograde cerebral perfusion during aortic arch procedures. Ann Thorac Surg 74:426, 2002
68. Juvonen T, Zhang N, Wolfe D, et al: Retrograde cerebral perfusion enhances cerebral protection during prolonged hypothermic circulatory arrest: A study in a chronic porcine model. Ann Thorac Surg 66:38, 1998
69. Bachet J, Guilmet D, Goudot B, et al: Cold cerebroplegia. A new technique of cerebral protection during operations on the transverse aortic arch. J Thorac Cardiovasc Surg 102:85, 1991
70. Kazui T, Washiyama N, Muhammad BA, et al: Total arch replacement using aortic arch branched grafts with the aid of antegrade selective cerebral perfusion. Ann Thorac Surg 70:3, 2000
71. Kazui T, Washiyama N, Muhammad BAH, et al: Improved results of atherosclerotic arch aneurysm operations with a refined technique. J Thorac Cardiovasc Surg 121:491, 2001
72. Jacobs MJ, de Mol BA, Veldman DJ: Aortic arch and proximal supraaortic arterial repair under continuous antegrade cerebral perfusion and moderate hypothermia. Cardiovasc Surg 9:396, 2001
73. Swain JA, McDonald TJ Jr., Griffith PK, et al: Low-flow hypothermic cardiopulmonary bypass protects the brain. J Thorac Cardiovasc Sur 102:76, 1991
74. Barbut D, Lo YW, Gold JP, et al: Impact of embolization during coronary artery bypass grafting on outcome and length of stay. Ann Thorac Surg 63:998, 1997
75. Clark RE, Brillman J, Davis DA, et al: Microemboli during coronary artery bypass grafting. J Thorac Cardiovasc Surg 109:249, 1995
76. Pugsley W, Klinger L, Paschalis C, et al: The impact of microemboli during cardiopulmonary bypass on neuropsychological functioning. Stroke 25:1393, 1994
77. Andropoulos DB, Diaz LK, Fraser CD, et al: Is bilateral monitoring of cerebral oxygen saturation necessary during neonatal aortic arch reconstruction? Anesth Analg 98:1267, 2004
78. Nussmeier NA, Arlundd C, Slogoff S: Neuropsychiatric complications after cardiopulmonary bypass: cerebral protection by a barbiturate. Anesthesiology 64:165, 1986
79. Zaidan JR, Klochany A, Martin WM, et al: Effect of thiopental on neurologic outcome following coronary artery bypass grafting. Anesthesiology 74:406, 1991
80. Blanck TJ, Haile M, Xu F, et al: Isoflurane pretreatment ameliorates postischemic neurologic dysfunction and preserves hippocampal Ca2+/calmodulin-dependent protein kinase in a canine cardiac arrest model. Anesthesiology 93:1285, 2000
81. Altman DI, Young RSK, Yagel SK: Effects of dexamethasone in hypoxic ischemic brain injury in the neonatal rat. Biol Neonate 46:149, 1984
82. Langley SM, Chai PJ, Jaggers JJ, Ungerleider RM: Preoperative high dose methylprednisolone attenuates the cerebral response to deep hypothermic circulatory arrest. Eur J Cardio-Thoracic Surg 17:279, 2000
83. Shum-Tim D, Tchervenkov CI, Jamal AM, et al: Systemic steroid pretreatment improves cerebral protection after circulatory arrest. Ann Thorac Surg 72:1465, 2001
84. Cowan JA Jr., Dimick JB, Henke PK, et al: Surgical treatment of intact thoracoabdominal aortic aneurysms in the United States: hospital and surgeon volume-related outcomes. J Vasc Surg 37:1169, 2003
85. Safi HJ, Miller CC 3rd, Carr C, et al: Importance of intercostal artery reattachment during thoracoabdominal aortic aneurysm repair. J Vasc Surg 27:58, 1998
86. Cambria RP, Davison JK, Zannetti S, et al: Clinical experience with epidural cooling for spinal cord protection during thoracic and thoracoabdominal aneurysm repair. J Vasc Surg 25:234, 1997
87. Crawford ES: Thoraco-abdominal and abdominal aortic aneurysms involving renal, superior mesenteric, celiac arteries. Ann Surg 179:763, 1974
88. Livesay JJ, Cooley DA, Ventemiglia RA, et al: Surgical experience in descending thoracic aneurysmectomy with and without adjuncts to avoid ischemia. Ann Thorac Surg 39:37, 1985
89. Roizen MF, Beaupre PN, Alpert RA, et al: Monitoring with two-dimensional transesophageal echocardiography. Comparison of myocardial function in patients undergoing supraceliac, suprarenal-infraceliac, or infrarenal aortic occlusion. J Vasc Surg 1:300, 1984
90. Verdant A: 1988: Surgery of the descending thoracic aorta: spinal cord protection with the Gott shunt. Updated in 1995. Ann Thor Surg 60:1151, 1995
91. Livesay JJ, Cooley DA, Ventemiglia RA, et al: Surgical experience in descending thoracic aneurysmectomy with and without adjuncts to avoid ischemia. Ann Thorac Surg 39:37, 1985
92. Comerota AJ, White JV: Reducing morbidity of thoracoabdominal aneurysm repair by preliminary axillofemoral bypass. Am J Surg 170:218, 1995
93. Coselli JS, Lemaire SA, Koksoy C, et al: Cerebrospinal fluid drainage reduces paraplegia after thoracoabdominal aortic aneurysm repair: results of a randomized clinical trial. J Vasc Surg 35:631, 2002

94. Cheung AT, Weiss SJ, McGarvey ML, et al: Interventions for reversing delayed-onset postoperative paraplegia after thoracic aortic reconstruction. Ann Thorac Surg 74:413, 2002
95. Hess PJ, Howe HR Jr., Robicsek F, et al: Traumatic tears of the thoracic aorta: improved results using the Bio-Medicus pump. Ann Thorac Surg 48:6, 1989
96. Cheung AT, Pochettino A, Guvakov DV, et al: Safety of lumbar drains in thoracic aortic operations performed with extracorporeal circulation. Ann Thorac Surg 76:1190, 2003
97. Griepp RB, Ergin MA, Galla JD, et al: Looking for the artery of Adamkiewicz: a quest to minimize paraplegia after operations for aneurysm of the descending thoracic and thoracoabdominal aorta. J Thorac Cardiovasc Surg 112:1202, 1996
98. Safi HJ, Hess KR, Randel M, et al: Cerebrospinal fluid drainage and distal aortic perfusion: reducing neurologic complications in repair of thoracoabdominal aortic aneurysm types I and II. J Vasc Surg 23:223, 1996
99. Svensson LG: An approach to spinal cord protection during descending or thoracoabdominal aortic repairs. Ann Thorac Surg 67:1935, 1999
100. Safi HJ, Miller CC: Spinal cord protection in descending thoracic and thoracoabdominal aortic repair. Ann Thorac Surg 67:1937, 1999
101. Connolly JE: Prevention of spinal cord complications in aortic surgery. Am J Surg 176:92, 1998
102. Jacobs MJHM, Myhre HO, Norgren L: State of the art. Thoracoabdominal aortic surgery with special reference to spinal cord protection and perfusion techniques. Eur J Vasc Endovasc Surg 17:253, 1999
103. Estrera AL, Miller CC 3rd, Huynh TT, et al: Neurologic outcome after thoracic and thoracoabdominal aortic aneurysm repair. Ann Thorac Surg 72:1225, 2001
104. Kouchoukos NT, Daily BB, Rokkas CK, et al: Hypothermic bypass and circulatory arrest for operations on the descending thoracic and thoracoabdominal aorta. Ann Thorac Surg 60:67, 1995
105. Kouchoukos NT, Masetti P, Rokkas CK, et al: Hypothermic cardiopulmonary bypass and circulatory arrest for operations on the descending thoracic and thoracoabdominal aorta. Ann Thorac Surg 74:S1885, 2002
106. Buth J, Penn O, Tielbeek A, et al: Combined approach to stent-graft treatment of an aortic arch aneurysm. J Endovasc Surg 5:329, 1998
107. Dietl CA, Kasirajan K, Pett SB, et al: Off-pump management of aortic arch aneurysm by using an endovascular thoracic stent graft. J Thorac Cardiovasc Surg 126:1181, 2003
108. Czerny M, Fleck T, Zimpfer D, et al: Combined repair of an aortic arch aneurysm by sequential transposition of the supra-aortic branches and endovascular stent-graft placement. J Thorac Cardiovasc Surg 126:916, 2003
109. Chuter TA, Schneider DB, Reilly LM, et al: Modular branched stent graft for endovascular repair of aortic arch aneurysm and dissection. J Vasc Surg 38:859, 2003
110. Schneider DB, Curry TK, Reilly LM, et al: Branched endovascular repair of aortic arch aneurysm with a modular stent-graft system. J Vasc Surg 38:855, 2003
111. Nitta Y, Tsuru Y, Yamaya K, et al: Endovascular flexible stent grafting with arch vessel bypass for a case of aortic arch aneurysm. J Thorac Cardiovasc Surg 126:1186, 2003
112. Drenth DJ, Verhoeven EL, Prins TR, et al: Relocation of supra-aortic vessels to facilitate endovascular treatment of a ruptured aortic arch aneurysm. J Thorac Cardiovasc Surg 126:1184, 2003
113. Usui A, Tajima K, Nishikimi N, et al: Implantation of an endovascular covered stent-graft for distal aortic arch aneurysm via midsternotomy under pigtail catheter guidance. Eur J Cardiothorac Surg 16:356, 1999
114. Iguro Y, Arata K, Yamamoto H, et al: A new concept in distal arch aneurysm repair with a stent graft. J Thorac Cardiovasc Surg 123:378, 2002
115. Campos JH: An update on bronchial blockers during lung separation techniques in adults. Anesth Analg 97:1266, 2003
116. Svensson LG, Crawford ES, Hess KR, et al: Experience with 1509 patients undergoing thoracoabdominal aortic operations. J Vasc Surg 17:357, 1993
117. LeMaire SA, Miller CC 3rd, Conklin LD, et al: Estimating group mortality and paraplegia rates after thoracoabdominal aortic aneurysm repair. Ann Thorac Surg 75:508, 2003
118. Gloviczki P, Cross SA, Stanson AW, et al: Ischemic injury to the spinal cord or lumbosacral plexus after aorto-iliac reconstruction. Am J Surg 162:131, 1991
119. Weiss SJ, Hogan MS, McGarvey ML, et al: Successful treatment of delayed onset paraplegia after suprarenal abdominal aortic aneurysm repair. Anesthesiology 97:504, 2002
120. Singh U, Silver JR, Welply NC: Hypotensive infarction of the spinal cord. Paraplegia. 32:314, 1994
121. Crawford ES, Crawford JL, Safi HJ, et al: Thoracoabdominal aortic aneurysms: preoperative and intraoperative factors determining immediate and long-term results of operations in 605 patients. J Vasc Surg 3:389, 1986
122. Cambria RP, Davison JK, Carter C, et al: Epidural cooling for spinal cord protection during thoracoabdominal aneurysm repair: a five year experience. J Vasc Surg 31:1093, 2000
123. Ackerman LL, Traynelis VC: Treatment of delayed-onset neurological deficit after aortic surgery with lumbar cerebrospinal fluid drainage. Neurosurgery 51:1414, 2002
124. Blaisdell FW, Cooley DA: The mechanism of paraplegia after temporary occlusion and its relationship to spinal fluid pressure. Surgery 51:351, 1962
125. Hill AB, Kalman PG, Johnston KW, et al: Reversal of delayed-onset paraplegia after thoracic aortic surgery with cerebrospinal fluid drainage. J Vasc Surg 20:315, 1994
126. Safi HJ, Miller CC, Azizzadeh A, et al: Observations on delayed neurologic deficit after thoracoabdominal aortic aneurysm repair. J Vasc Surg 26:616, 1997
127. Widmann MD, DeLucia A, Sharp WJ, et al: Reversal of renal failure and paraplegia after thoracoabdominal aneurysm repair. Ann Thorac Surg 65:1153, 1998
128. Azizzadeh A, Huynh TT, Miller CC, et al: Reversal of twice-delayed neurologic deficits with cerebrospinal fluid drainage after thoracoabdominal aneurysm repair: A case report and plea for a national database collection. J Vasc Surg 31:592, 2000
129. Oberwalder PJ, Tiesenhausen K, Hausegger K, et al: Successful reversal of delayed paraplegia after endovascular stent grafting. J Thorac Cardiovascular Surg 124:1259, 2002
130. Killen DA, Weinstein CL, Reed WA: Reversal of spinal cord ischemia resulting from aortic dissection. J Thorac Cardiovasc Surg 119:1049, 2000
131. Ling E, Arellano R: Systematic overview of the evidence supporting the use of cerebrospinal fluid drainage in thoracoabdominal aneurysm surgery for prevention of paraplegia. Anesthesiology 93:1115, 2000
132. Weaver KD, Wiseman DB, Farber M, et al: Complications of lumbar drainage after thoracoabdominal aortic aneurysm repair. J Vasc Surg 34:623, 2001
133. Dardik A, Perler BA, Roseborough GS, et al: Subdural hematoma after thoracoabdominal aortic aneurysm repair: an underreported complication of spinal fluid drainage? J Vasc Surg 36:47, 2002
134. Coplin WM, Avellino AM, Kim DK, et al: Bacterial meningitis associated with lumbar drains: a retrospective cohort study. J Neurol Neurosurg Psych 67:468, 1999
135. Crawford ES, Svensson LG, Hess KR, et al: A prospective randomized study of cerebrospinal fluid drainage to prevent paraplegia after high-risk surgery on the thoracoabdominal aorta. J Vasc Surg 13:36, 1991
136. Crawford ES, Mizrahi EM, Hess KR, et al: The impact of distal aortic perfusion and somatosensory evoked potential monitoring on prevention of paraplegia after aortic aneurysm operation. J Thorac Cardiovasc Surg 95:357, 1988
137. Guerit JM, Witdoeckt C, Verhelst R, et al: Sensitivity, specificity, and surgical impact of somatosensory evoked potentials in descending aorta surgery. Ann Thorac Surg 67:1943, 1999
138. Galla JD, Ergin MA, Lansman SL, et al: Use of somatosensory evoked potentials for thoracic and thoracoabdominal aortic resections. Ann Thorac Surg 67:1947, 1999
139. Jacobs MJ, Elenbaas TW, Schurink GW, et al: Assessment of spinal cord integrity during thoracoabdominal aortic aneurysm repair. Ann Thorac Surg 74:1864, 2002
140. Mizrahi EM, Crawford ES: Somatosensory evoked potentials during reversible spinal cord ischemia in man. Electroencephalogr Clin Neurophysiol 58:120, 1984
141. Laschinger JC, Cunningham JN Jr, Baumann FG, et al: Monitoring of somatosensory evoked potentials during surgical procedures on the thoracoabdominal aorta. III, Intraoperative identification of vessels critical to spinal cord blood supply. J Thorac Cardiovasc Surg 94:271, 1987
142. de Haan P, Kalkman CJ, de Mol BA, et al: Efficacy of transcranial motor-evoked myogenic potentials to detect spinal cord ischemia during operations for thoracoabdominal aneurysms. J Thorac Cardiovasc Surg 113:87, 1997
143. Jacobs MJ, Meylaerts SA, de Haan P, et al: Strategies to prevent neurologic deficit based on motor-evoked potentials in type I and II thoracoabdominal aortic aneurysm repair. J Vasc Surg 29:48, 1999
144. Coselli JS, LeMaire SA: Left heart bypass reduces paraplegia rates after thoracoabdominal aortic aneurysm repair. Ann Thorac Surg 67:1931, 1999

145. Motoyoshi N, Takahashi G, Sakurai M, et al: Safety and efficacy of epidural cooling for regional spinal cord hypothermia during thoracoabdominal aneurysm repair. Eur J Cardio-Thorac Surg 25:139, 2004
146. Davison JK, Cambria RP, Vierra DJ, et al: Epidural cooling for regional spinal cord hypothermia during thoracoabdominal aneurysm repair. J Vasc Surg 20:304, 1994
147. Hollier LH, Money SR, Naslund TC, et al: Risk of spinal cord dysfunction in patients undergoing thoracoabdominal aortic replacement. Am J Surg 164:210, 1992
148. Svensson LG, Hess KR, D'Agostino RS, et al: Reduction of neurologic injury after high-risk thoracoabdominal aortic operation. Ann Thorac Surg 66:132, 1998
149. Acher CW, Wynn MM, Hoch JR, et al: Combined use of cerebral spinal fluid drainage and naloxone reduces the risk of paraplegia in thoracoabdominal aneurysm repair. J Vasc Surg 19:236, 1994
150. Acher CW, Wynn MM, Archibald J: Naloxone and spinal fluid drainage as adjuncts in the surgical treatment of thoracoabdominal and thoracic aneurysms. Surgery 108:755, 1990
151. Kavanagh BP, Katz J, Sandler AN: Pain control after thoracic surgery. A review of current techniques. Anesthesiology 81:737, 1994
152. Fitzgibbon DR, Glosten B, Wright I, et al: Paraplegia, epidural analgesia, and thoracic aneurysmectomy. Anesthesiology 83:1355, 1995
153. Horlocker TT, Wedel DJ, Benzon H, et al: Regional anesthesia in the anticoagulated patient: defining the risk. Reg Anesth Pain Med 29(suppl 1):1, 2004
154. Sandhu H, Morley-Forster P, Spadafora S: Epidural hematoma following epidural analgesia in a patient receiving unfractionated heparin for thromboprophylaxis. Reg Anesth Pain Med 25:72, 2000
155. Nienaber CA, Eagle KA: Aortic Dissection: New Frontiers in Diagnosis and Management: Part I: From Etiology to Diagnostic Strategies. Circulation 108:628, 2003
156. Kouchoukos NT, Dougenis D: Surgery of the thoracic aorta. N Engl J Med 336:1876, 1997
157. DeBakey ME, Beall AC, Cooley DA, et al: Dissecting aneurysms of the aorta. Surg Clin North Am 46:1045, 1966
158. Daily PO, Trueblood HW, Stinson EB, et al: Management of acute aortic dissections. Ann Thorac Surg 10:237, 1970
159. Hagan PG, Nienaber CA, Isselbacher EM, et al: The international registry of acute aortic dissection (IRAD): new insights into an old disease. JAMA 283:897, 2000
160. Ergin MA, Galla JD, Lansman S, et al: Acute dissections of the aorta. Current surgical treatment. Surg Clin North Am 65:721, 1985
161. Hirst AE, Johns VJ, Kime SW: Dissecting aneurysm of the aorta: a review of 505 cases. Medicine 37:217, 1958
162. Joao I, Duarte JA, Cotrim C, et al: Acute Type A aortic dissection involving the left main coronary artery and the aortic valve—a case report. Rev Port Cardiol 20:333, 2001
163. Appelbaum A, Karp RB, Kirklin JW: Ascending vs descending aortic dissections. Ann Surg 183:296, 1976
164. DeBakey ME, McCollum CH, Crawford ES, et al: Dissection and dissecting aneurysms of the aorta: twenty-year follow-up of five hundred twenty-seven patients treated surgically. Surgery 92:1118, 1982
165. Jex RK, Schaff HV, Piehler JM, et al: Early and late results following repair of dissections of the descending thoracic aorta. J Vasc Surg 3:226, 1986
166. Haverich A, Miller DC, Scott WC, et al: Acute and chronic aortic dissections—determinants of long-term outcome for operative survivors. Circulation 72(suppl II), 1985
167. Nienaber CA, Sievers HH: Intramural hematoma in acute aortic syndrome: more than one variant of dissection? Circulation 106:284, 2002
168. O'Gara PT, DeSanctis RW: Acute aortic dissection and its variants: toward a common diagnostic and therapeutic approach. Circulation 92:1376, 1995
169. von Kodolitsch Y, Csosz SK, Koschyk DH, et al: Intramural hematoma of the aorta: predictors of progression to dissection and rupture. Circulation 107:1158, 2003
170. Kaji S, Akasaka T, Horibata Y, et al: Long-term prognosis of patients with type a aortic intramural hematoma. Circulation 106(suppl I):I-248, 2002
171. Evangelista A, Dominguez R, Sebastia C, et al: Long-term follow-up of aortic intramural hematoma: predictors of outcome. Circulation 108:583, 2003
172. Muluk SC, Kaufman JA, Torchiana DF, et al: Diagnosis and treatment of thoracic aortic intramural hematoma. J Vasc Surg 24:1022, 1996
173. Hudak AM, Konstadt SN: Aortic intussusception: a rare complication of aortic dissection. Anesthesiology 82:1292, 1995
174. Neri E, Capannini G, Carone E, et al: The missing flap: considerations about a case of aortic intussusception. J Thorac Cardiovasc Surg 117:829, 1999
175. Spittell PC, Spittell JA Jr, Joyce JW, et al: Clinical features and differential diagnosis of aortic dissection: experience with 236 cases (1980 through 1990). Mayo Clin Proc 68:642, 1993
176. Bloch MJ, Trost DW, Sos TA: Type B aortic dissection complicating renal artery angioplasty and stent placement. J Vasc Interv Radiol 12:517, 2001
177. Bordeleau L, Cwinn A, Turek M, et al: Aortic dissection and Turner's syndrome: Case report and review of the literature. J Emerg Med 16:593, 1998
178. Liu G, Shupak R, Chiu BKY: Aortic dissection in giant-cell arteritis. Semin Arthritis Rheum 25:160, 1995
179. Om A, Porter T, Mohanty PK: Transesophageal echocardiographic diagnosis of acute aortic dissection complicating cocaine abuse. Am Heart J 123:532, 1992
180. Rashid J, Eisenberg MJ, Topol EJ: Cocaine-induced aortic dissection. Am Heart J 132:1301, 1996
181. Rogers FB, Osler TM, Shackford SR: Aortic dissection after trauma: case report and review of the literature. J Trauma 41:906, 1996
182. Ochi M, Yamauchi S, Yajima T, et al: Aortic dissection extending from the left coronary artery during percutaneous coronary angioplasty. Ann Thorac Surg 62:1180, 1996
183. Jacobs LE, Fraifeld M, Kotler MN, et al: Aortic dissection following intraaortic balloon insertion: recognition by transesophageal echocardiography. Am Heart J 124:536, 1992
184. Still RJ, Hilgenberg AD, Akins CW, et al: Intraoperative aortic dissection. Ann Thorac Surg 53:374, 1992
185. Albat B, Thevenet A: Dissecting aneurysms of the ascending aorta occurring late after aortic valve replacement. J Cardiovasc Surg 33:272, 1992
186. von Kodolitsch Y, Simic O, Schwartz A, et al: Predictors of proximal aortic dissection at the time of aortic valve replacement. Circulation 100(suppl II), 1999
187. Prenger K, Pieters F, Cheriex E: Aortic dissection after aortic valve replacement: Incidence and consequences for strategy. J Card Surg 9:495, 1994
188. Murphy DA, Craver JM, Jones EL, et al: Recognition and management of ascending aortic dissection complicating cardiac surgical operations. J Thorac Cardiovasc Surg 85:247, 1983
189. Madu EC, Shala B, Baugh D: Crack-cocaine-associated aortic dissection in early pregnancy. A case report. Angiology 50:163, 1999
190. Larson EW, Edwards WD: Risk factors for aortic dissection: a necropsy study of 161 cases. Am J Cardiol 53:849, 1984
191. Januzzi JL, Sabatine MS, Eagle KA, et al: International Registry of Aortic Dissection Investigators. Iatrogenic aortic dissection. Am J Cardiol 89:623, 2002
192. Armstrong WF, Bach DS, Carey LM, et al: Clinical and echocardiographic findings in patients with suspected acute aortic dissection. Am Heart J 136:1051, 1998
193. Demos TC, Posniak HV, Marsan RE: CT of aortic dissection. Semin Roentgenol 24:22, 1989
194. Slater EE, DeSanctis RW: The clinical recognition of dissecting aortic aneurysm. Am J Med 60:625, 1976
195. Najafi H: Thoracic aortic aneurysm: Evaluation and surgical management. Compr Ther 20:282, 1994
196. Nienaber CA, von Kodolitsch Y, Nicolas V, et al: The diagnosis of thoracic aortic dissection by noninvasive imaging procedures. N Engl J Med 328:1, 1993
197. Kazerooni EA, Bree RL, Willliams DM: Penetrating atherosclerotic ulcers of the descending thoracic aorta: evaluation with CT and distinction from aortic dissection. Radiology 183:759, 1992
198. Movsowitz HD, Lampert C, Jacobs LE, et al: Penetrating atherosclerotic aortic ulcers. Am Heart J 128:1210, 1994
199. Miller JS, LeMare SA, Coselli JS: Editorial. Evaluating aortic dissection: when is coronary angiography indicated? Heart 83:615 2000
200. Vilacosta I, San Roman JA, Ferreiros J, et al: Natural history and serial morphology of aortic intramural hematoma: a novel variant of aortic dissection. Am Heart J 134:495, 1997
201. Rizzo RJ, Aranki SF, Aklog L, et al: Rapid noninvasive diagnosis and surgical repair of acute ascending aortic dissection. Improved survival with less angiography. J Thorac Cardiovasc Surg 108:567, 1994
202. Isselbacher EM, Cigarroa JE, Eagle KA: Pericardial tamponade: cardiac tamponade complicating proximal aortic dissection: is pericardiocentesis harmful? Circulation 90:2375, 1994
203. Miller DC, Stinson EB, Oyer PE, et al: Operative treatment of aortic dissections. Experience with 125 patients over a sixteen-year period. J Thorac Cardiovasc Surg 78:365, 1979
204. Masuda Y, Yamada Z, Morooka N, et al: Prognosis of patients with medically treated aortic dissections. Circulation 84(suppl III):III, 1991

205. Elefteriades JA, Hartleroad J, Gusberg RJ, et al: Long-term experience with descending aortic dissection: The complication-specific approach. Ann Thorac Surg 53:11, 1992
206. Reber D, Aebert H, Manke M, et al: Percutaneous fenestration of the aortic dissection membrane in malperfusion syndrome. Eur J Cardiothorac Surg 15:91, 1999
207. Connell DA, Thomson KR, Gibson RN, et al: Stent placement in coeliac and superior mesenteric arteries to restore vascular perfusion following aortic dissection. Australas Radiol 39:68, 1995
208. Saito S, Arai H, Kim K, et al: Percutaneous fenestration of dissecting intima with a transseptal needle. A new therapeutic technique for visceral ischemia complicating acute aortic dissection. Cathet Cardiovasc Diagn 26:130, 1992
209. Slonim SM, Nyman UR, Semba CP, et al: True lumen obliteration in complicated aortic dissection: endovascular treatment. Radiology 201:161, 1996
210. Slonim SM, Nyman U, Semba CP, et al: Aortic dissection: percutaneous management of ischemic complications with endovascular stents and balloon fenestration. J Vasc Surg 23:241, 1996
211. Chang WT, Kao HL, Liau CS, et al: Aortic stenting on a Type B aortic dissection with visceral and limb ischemia. Cathet Cardiovasc Intervent 52:112, 2001
212. Ince H, Nienaber CA: The concept of interventional therapy in acute aortic syndrome. J Card Surg 17:135, 2002
213. Nienaber CA, Fattori R, Lund G, et al: Nonsurgical reconstruction of thoracic aortic dissection by stent-graft placement. N Engl J Med 340:1539, 1999
214. Dake MD, Kato N, Mitchell RS, et al: Endovascular stent-graft placement for the treatment of acute aortic dissection. N Engl J Med 340:1546, 1999
215. Bortone AS, Schena S, D'Agostino D, et al: Immediate versus delayed endovascular treatment of post-traumatic aortic pseudoaneurysms and type B dissections: retrospective analysis and premises to the upcoming European trial. Circulation 106(suppl I):I, 2002
216. Glower DD, Fann JI, Speier RH, et al: Comparison of medical and surgical therapy for uncomplicated descending aortic dissection. Circulation 82(suppl IV):IV, 1990
217. Ganaha F, Miller DC, Sugimoto K, et al: Prognosis of aortic intramural hematoma with and without penetrating atherosclerotic ulcer: a clinical and radiological analysis. Circulation 106:342, 2002
218. Benitez RM, Gurbel PA, Chong H, et al: Penetrating atherosclerotic ulcer of the aortic arch resulting in extensive and fatal dissection. Am Heart J 129:821, 1995
219. Harris JA, Bis KG, Glover JL, et al: Penetrating atherosclerotic ulcers of the aorta. J Vasc Surg 19:90, 1994
220. Stanson AW, Kazmier FJ, Hollier LH, et al: Penetrating atherosclerotic ulcers of the thoracic aorta: natural history and clinicopathological correlations. Ann Vasc Surg 1:15, 1986
221. Pretre R, Chilcott M: Blunt Trauma to the Heart and Great Vessels. N Engl J Med 336:626, 1997
222. Kodali S, Jamieson WR, Leia-Stephens M, et al: Traumatic rupture of the thoracic aorta. A 20-year review: 1969–1989. Circulation 84(suppl):III-40, 1991
223. Nocolosi AC, Almassi GH, Bousamra M 2nd, et al: Mortality and neurologic morbidity after repair of traumatic aortic disruption. Ann Thorac Surg 61:875, 1996
224. Parmley LF, Manion WC, Mattingly TW: Nonpenetrating traumatic injury of the heart. Circulation 18:371, 1958
225. Buckmaster MJ, Kearney PA, Johnson SB, et al: Further experience with transesophageal echocardiography in the evaluation of thoracic aortic injury. J Trauma 37:989, 1994
226. Goarin JP, Cluzel P, Gosgnach M, et al: Evaluation of transesophageal echocardiography for diagnosis of traumatic aortic injury. Anesthesiology 93:1373, 2000
227. Goarin JP, Catoire P, Jacquens Y, et al: Use of transesophageal echocardiography for diagnosis of traumatic aortic injury. Chest 112:71, 1997
228. Vignon P, Boncoeur MP, Francois B, et al: Comparison of multiplane transesophageal echocardiography and contrast-enhanced helical CT in the diagnosis of blunt traumatic cardiovascular injuries. Anesthesiology 94:615, 2001
229. Fabian TC, Richardson JD, Croce MA, et al: Prospective study of blunt aortic injury: Multicenter Trial of the American Association for the Surgery of Trauma. J Trauma 42:374, 1997
230. Tatou E, Steinmetz E, Jazayeri S, et al: Surgical outcome of traumatic rupture of the thoracic aorta. Ann Thorac Surg 69:70, 2000
231. Cardarelli MG, McLaughlin JS, Downing SW, et al: Management of traumatic aortic rupture: a 30-year experience. Ann Surg 236:465, 2002
232. Scheinert D, Krankenberg H, Schmidt A, et al: Endoluminal stent-graft placement for acute rupture of the descending thoracic aorta. Eur Heart J 25:694, 2004
233. Karalis DG, Chandraskeran K, Victor MF, et al: Recognition and embolic potential of intraaortic atherosclerotic debris. J Am Coll Cardiol 17:73, 1991
234. Mitusch R, Stierle U, Tepe C, et al: Systemic embolism in aortic arch atheromatosis. Eur Heart J 15:1373, 1994
235. Amarenco P, Cohen A, Tzourio C, et al: Atherosclerotic disease of the aortic arch and the risk of ischemic stroke. N Engl J Med 331:1474, 1994
236. Tunick PA, Culliford AT, Lamparello PJ, et al: Atheromatosis of the aortic arch as an occult source of multiple systemic emboli. Ann Intern Med 114:391, 1991
237. Tunick PA, Rosensweig BP, Katz ES, et al: High risk for vascular events in patients with protruding aortic atheromas: A prospective study. J Am Coll Cardiol 23:1085, 1994
238. Tunick PA, Kronzon I: Protruding atherosclerotic plaque in the aortic arch of patients with systemic embolization: a new finding seen by transesophageal echocardiography. Am Heart J 120:658, 1990
239. Tunick PA, Kronzon I: Atheromas of the thoracic aorta: clinical and therapeutic update. J Am Coll Cardiol 35:545, 2000
240. Amarenco P, Duyckaerts C, Tzourio C, et al: The prevalence of ulcerated plaques in the aortic arch in patients with stroke. N Engl J Med 326:221, 1992
241. Khatibzadeh M, Mitusch R, Stierle U, et al: Aortic atherosclerotic plaques as a source of systemic embolism. J Am Coll Cardiol 27:664, 1996
242. Mitusch R, Doherty C, Wucherpfennig H, et al: Vascular events during follow-up in patients with aortic arch atherosclerosis. Stroke 28:36, 1997
243. Davila-Roman VG, Murphy SF, Nickerson NJ, et al: Atherosclerosis of the ascending aorta is an independent predictor of long-term neurologic events and mortality. J Am Coll Cardiol 33:1308, 1999
244. Ehlermann P, Mirau W, Jahn J, et al: Predictive value of inflammatory and hemostatic parameters, atherosclerotic risk factors, and chest x-ray for aortic arch atheromatosis. Stroke 35:34, 2004
245. Wareing TH, Davila-Roman VG, Barzilai B, et al: Management of the severely atherosclerotic aorta during cardiac operations. A strategy for detection and treatment. J Thorac Cardiovasc Surg 103:453, 1992
246. Davila-Roman VG, Phillips KJ, Daily BB, et al: Intraoperative transesophageal echocardiography and epiaortic ultrasound for assessment of atherosclerosis of the thoracic aorta. J Am Coll Cardiol 28:942, 1996
247. Arend WP, Michel BA, Bloch DA, et al: The American College of Rheumatology 1990 criteria for the classification of Takayasu arteritis. Arthritis Rheum 33:1129, 1990
248. Ishikawa K, Maetani S: Long-term outcome for 120 Japanese patients with Takayasu's disease. Clinical and statistical analyses of related prognostic factors. Circulation 90:1855, 1994
249. Miyata T, Sato O, Koyama H, et al: Long-term survival after surgical treatment of patients with Takayasu's arteritis. Circulation 108:1474, 2003
250. Fawzy ME, Awad M, Hassan W, et al: Long-term outcome (up to 15 years) of balloon angioplasty of discrete native coarctation of the aorta in adolescents and adults. J Am Coll Cardiol 43:1062, 2004
251. Harrison DA, McLaughlin PR, Lazzam C, et al: Endovascular stents in the management of coarctation of the aorta in the adolescent and adult: one year follow up. Heart 85:561, 2001
252. Cohen M, Fuster V, Steele PM, et al: Coarctation of the aorta. Long-term follow-up and prediction of outcome after surgical correction. Circulation 80:840, 1989
253. Toro-Salazar OH, Steinberger J, Thomas W, et al: Long-term follow-up of patients after coarctation of the aorta repair. Am J Cardiol 89:541, 2002
254. Doroghazi RM, Slater EE, DeSanctis RW, et al: Long-term survival of patients with treated aortic dissection. J Am Coll Cardiol 3:1026, 1984
255. Kawahito K, Adachi H, Yamaguchi A, et al: Preoperative risk factors for hospital mortality in acute type A aortic dissection. Ann Thorac Surg 71:1239, 2001
256. Kawahito K, Adachi H, Yamaguchi A, et al: Early and late surgical outcomes of acute type A aortic dissections in patients aged 75 years and older. Ann Thorac Surg 70:1455, 2000
257. Sabik JF, Lytle BW, Blackstone EH, et al: Long-term effectiveness of operations for ascending aortic dissections. J Thorac Cardiovasc Surg 119:946, 2000
258. Fann JI, Smith JA, Miller DC, et al: Surgical management of aortic dissection during a 30-year period. Circulation 92[suppl II]:II, 1995
259. Ehrlich MP, Ergin A, McCullough JN, et al: Results of immediate surgical treatment of all acute type A dissections. Circulation 102[suppl III]:III, 2000
260. Ehrlich M, Schillinger M, Grabenwoger M, et al: Predictors of outcome and transient neurologic dysfunction following surgical treatment of acute type A dissections. Circulation 108(suppl II):II, 2003

Chapter 24
UNCOMMON CARDIAC DISEASES

William C. Oliver, Jr., MD • Gregory A. Nuttall, MD

KEY POINTS

1. Uncommon diseases and coexisting problems of patients undergoing cardiac surgery are covered with a general overview of the disease or condition followed by guidelines and considerations to facilitate anesthetic management.
2. Carcinoid heart disease is a very serious condition that requires cardiac surgery. Optimal anesthetic management continues to evolve.
3. In 1995, the World Health Organization/International Society of Cardiology redefined the cardiomyopathies; updates in the management of these conditions are provided.
4. The emergence of technology to better diagnose pulmonary embolism and of echocardiography to assess the risk of mortality during acute pulmonary embolism continues to improve the treatment and management from both medical and surgical aspects.
5. The introduction of intravenous epoprostenol (synthetic salt of prostacyclin) in the 1990s improved hemodynamics, functional capacity, and survival in patients with primary pulmonary hypertension, as have treatment options that include a new generation of drugs developed to address the pathologic arms of primary pulmonary hypertension.
6. The definitive approach to a patient with both carotid and coronary artery disease requires a large multicenter, randomized trial; however, the many approaches to the surgical management of combined procedures are described.
7. Heart disease continues to be the leading cause of maternal and fetal death during pregnancy; the important features of managing the pregnant patient who requires cardiopulmonary bypass and cardiac surgery are updated.
8. With newly developed therapies, the incubation time to develop AIDS after infection and life expectancy of those with HIV infection have been extended. Therefore, the likelihood of cardiac surgery is greater; the rates of exposure, types of procedures, and precautions of the individuals providing care are addressed.
9. Individuals with chronic renal failure, not necessarily dialysis dependent, are more frequently undergoing cardiac surgery and are likely to develop worsening renal function after cardiopulmonary bypass; identification of steps that may improve outcome is provided.
10. Anesthetic concerns for patients with hematologic problems who undergo cardiac surgery are further complicated by the stress that cardiopulmonary bypass places on coagulation and oxygen-carrying systems, and special considerations and techniques are required.

Uncommon diseases and coexisting problems of patients undergoing cardiac surgery are reviewed in this chapter. Each subsection includes a general overview of the disease or condition and emphasizes anesthetic management of the coexistent disease in the setting of cardiac surgery. It is important that the anesthesiologist understand the pathology and pathophysiology of coexisting diseases, how they are affected by anesthesia, and how they affect the underlying cardiac problem.

CARDIAC TUMORS

Cardiac tumors are increasingly diagnosed before autopsy due to advancements in imaging, especially metastatic tumors of the heart and pericardium, which account for a majority of cardiac tumors. Data pooled from 22 large autopsy series show the prevalence of adult primary cardiac tumors as only about 0.02%, yet they are responsible for significant morbidity and mortality.[1] Malignant tumors encompass about 20% of primary tumors in adults.[2,3] Diagnosis can be elusive as these tumors may be associated with nonspecific symptoms mimicking other disease entities. Two-dimensional echocardiography (echo) modalities and magnetic resonance imaging (MRI) have allowed earlier, more frequent, and more complete assessment of cardiac tumors.[4]

Primary cardiac tumors may originate from any cardiac tissue. Myxoma is the most common cardiac neoplasm, accounting for nearly 50% of tumors in adults (Table 24–1). Less frequently observed benign tumors that may require surgery include rhabdomyoma, fibroma, papillary fibroelastoma, lipoma, and angioma. In contrast, malignant primary cardiac tumors are rare, with sarcomas comprising 95% of these tumors, followed by lymphomas. Sarcomas include angiosarcoma, rhabdomyosarcoma, and acquired immunodeficiency syndrome (AIDS)–related sarcomas.[5] Rhabdomyosarcoma represents 20% of malignant neoplasms. Excision of these tumors is seldom curative, in part due to the delay in diagnosis caused by the nonspecific nature of the clinical symptoms. Surgery, radiation therapy, and chemotherapy may slow a tumor's encroachment on intracavitary spaces or relieve obstruction.

The incidence of metastatic cardiac tumors has increased from 0.2% to 10% as a result of improved survival.[6] Metastatic cardiac tumors are much more common than primary cardiac tumors. Adenocarcinomas of the lung and breast, lymphomas that are commonly associated with AIDS or transplant immunosuppression, and melanoma are the most frequent metastatic cardiac tumors.[7] Melanoma has a special tendency for metastasis to the heart and pericardium. However, metastasis of these tumors is rarely limited to the heart. The advent of arrhythmias or congestive heart failure (CHF) in patients with carcinomas suggests cardiac metastasis, but more than 90% of metastatic lesions to the heart are clinically silent.[2]

Transthoracic echocardiography is excellent for identifying intracavitary tumors because it is noninvasive, identifies

Table 24–1 **Benign Neoplasms of the Heart**

Neoplasm	Incidence in Adults (%)
Myxoma	45
Lipoma	20
Papillary fibroelastoma	15
Angioma	5
Fibroma	3
Hemangioma	5
Rhabdomyoma	1
Teratoma	<1

From Shapiro LM: Cardiac tumors: Diagnosis and management. Heart 85:218, 2001.

tumor type, and permits complete visualization of each cardiac chamber[8] (Fig. 24–1). It is the predominant imaging modality for screening.[3] Often performed intraoperatively prior to initiation of cardiopulmonary bypass (CPB), transesophageal echocardiography (TEE) increases the diagnostic potential as the nature of the tumor according to location, dimensions, number of masses, and echogenic pattern is better identified.[9] Echolucencies, which are caused by hemorrhage within the tumor, rarely occur, but they may be helpful in distinguishing thrombus from myxoma.

The most effective treatment of primary tumors is generally surgical resection, and recurrence is rare (<5%).[3] However, overall early mortality for primary cardiac tumors is 5%. Orthotopic cardiac transplantation has been recommended for unresectable tumors, but the benefit is indeterminate.[10] Although more infrequent, the surgical risk and outcome for malignant tumor resection compared with benign tumor resection are significantly worse.[3]

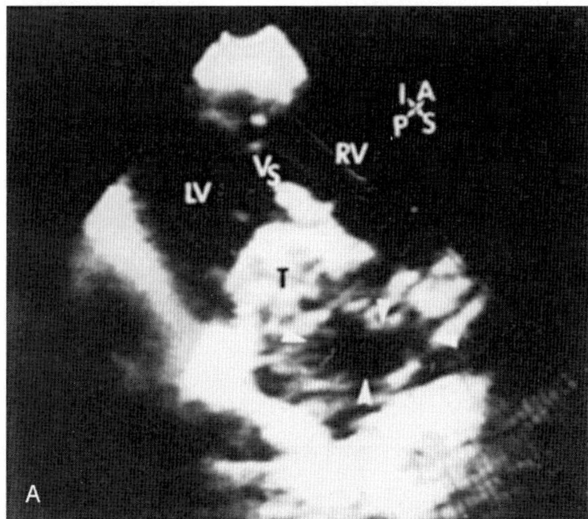

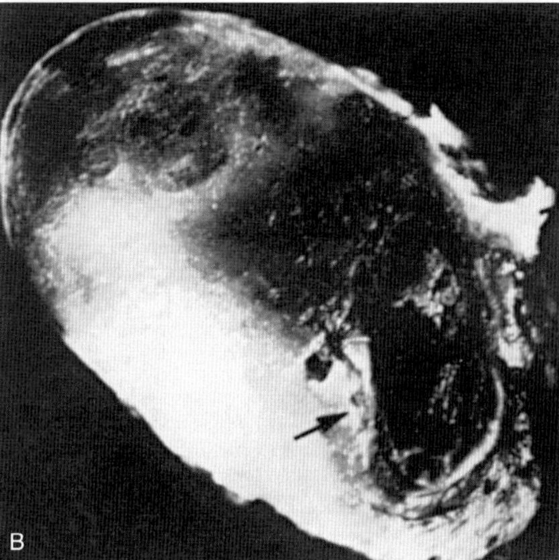

Figure 24–1 *(A)* Parasternal long-axis view of large, firm left atrial myxoma remaining impacted in left atrium. Tumor (T) contains a central region of echolucency *(arrowheads)* that corresponds to an area of liquefaction. LV = left ventricle; VS = ventricular septum; RV = right ventricle. *(B)* Cut section of gross specimen of myxoma. (Reprinted with permission from Fyke FE III, Seward JB, Edwards WD, et al: Primary cardiac tumors: Experience with 30 consecutive patients since the introduction of two-dimensional echocardiography. Reprinted with permission from the American College of Cardiology [Journal of the American College of Cardiology], 5:1465, 1985. Copyright 1985, with permission from The American College of Cardiology Foundation.)

Myxoma

Often a diagnostic challenge, myxoma, a benign, solitary neoplasm that is slowly and microscopically proliferating, resembles an organized clot, which often obscures its identity as a primary cardiac tumor. The pedunculated mass is believed to arise from undifferentiated cells in the fossa ovalis and adjoining endocardium, projecting into the left atrium (LA) and right atrium (RA) 75% and 20% of the time, respectively. However, myxomas appear in other locations of the heart, even occupying more than one chamber.[11] The undifferentiated cells of a myxoma develop along a variety of cell lines, accounting for the multiple presentations and pathologies observed.[12] Besides a variable amount of stroma, myxomas include hemorrhage, hemosiderin, thrombus, and calcium (see Fig. 24–1). Any age group can be affected. Myxomas predominate in the 30- to 60-year-old age range, with more than 75% of the affected patients being women.[13] Although most cases occur sporadically, 7% to 10% of atrial myxomas occur in a familial pattern, with an autosomal dominant transmission pattern.[14]

Rarely discovered by incidental echocardiography examination, myxomas may manifest a variety of symptoms. The classic triad includes embolism, intracardiac obstruction, and constitutional symptoms. Approximately 80% of individuals present with one component of the triad, yet up to 10% may be asymptomatic even with mitral myxomas, arising from both atrial and ventricular sides of the anterior mitral leaflet.[11,15] The most common initial symptom, dyspnea on exertion, reflects mitral valve obstruction usually present with LA myxomas (Fig. 24–2).[13] Because of the pedunculated nature of some myxomas, temporary obstruction of blood flow may cause hemolysis, hypotension, syncope, or sudden death. Other symptoms of mitral obstruction similar to mitral stenosis such as hemoptysis, systemic embolization, fever, and weight loss may also occur. The persistence of sinus rhythm in the presence of such symptoms may help distinguish atrial myxoma from mitral stenosis. Severe pulmonary hypertension without significant mitral valve involvement suggests obstruction of the tricuspid valve and recurrent pulmonary emboli known to occur with a myxoma in the RA or right ventricle (RV). Occasionally, right-sided tumors may appear as cyanotic congenital heart lesions due to intracardiac

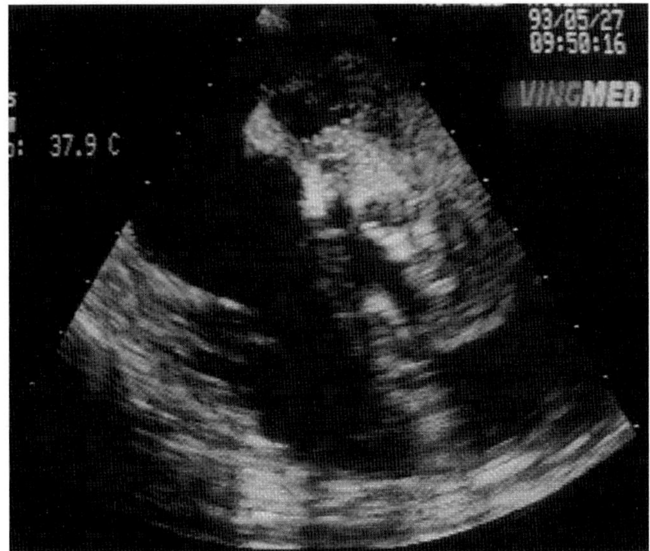

Figure 24–2 Transesophageal echocardiogram showing a left atrial myxoma prolapsing across and obstructing the mitral valve. (Reprinted with permission from Shapiro LM: General cardiology cardiac tumors: Diagnosis and management. Heart 85:219, 2001. Reproduced with permission from the BMJ Publishing Group.)

shunting.[16] Recurrent fragmentation and embolization of the gelatin-like tumor usually appear with systemic manifestations and are characteristic of myxoma. Cerebral aneurysms often exist in patients with recurrent systemic embolization from intracardiac myxoma probably secondary to damage by the systemic tumor emboli. The kidneys are also more susceptible to damage from myxoma emboli. Constitutional symptoms such as malaise, fever, and weight loss occur in about one third of patients, reflecting a possible autoimmune component but also delaying the diagnosis. Differential diagnosis includes endocarditis, connective tissue disorders, and malignancies. In general, the anatomic type of myxoma portends the clinical presentation. The solid, ovoid tumors are more often associated with CHF, whereas papillary myxomas present with cerebral embolization.[17] Tumor size does not correlate with symptoms.[13]

Findings on a chest roentgenogram of a myxoma may be absent in one third of persons. Calcification on the chest roentgenogram is more diagnostic of RA myxoma but is rarely present in LA myxoma. Before echocardiography, angiography was used to identify all myxomas, but now it is only useful to confirm the diagnosis or determine coronary anatomy if considered necessary.[3] TEE is 100% sensitive for diagnosis of myxoma. Specifically, it yields morphologic detail in the evaluation of cardiac tumors, including points of tumor attachment and degree of mobility. Computed tomography (CT) scanning and MRI can help delineate the extent of the tumor and its relationships to surrounding cardiac and thoracic structures.[18] MRI is especially valuable in the diagnosis of myxoma when masses are equivocal or suboptimal on echocardiography or if the tumor is atypical in presentation.[11] Difficulty may arise in differentiating thrombus from myxoma because both are so heterogeneous.

The first surgical resection of an atrial myxoma was performed in 1954. Subsequently, surgical resection has been recommended even if the myxoma is discovered incidentally, primarily because of the risk of embolization. Generally, the time interval between onset of symptoms and surgical resection is about 4 months, but surgery has been delayed for 10 years.[13] Surgery is associated with a mortality rate of 0% to 3%.[1]

Anesthetic Considerations for Myxoma

Tumor location has a strong influence on anesthetic management. LA myxomas most likely cause mitral valve obstruction, often in conjunction with pulmonary artery hypertension (PAH) and pulmonary venous hypertension. Anesthetic management closely resembles that for a patient with mitral stenosis. In contrast, RA myxomas may produce signs of right-sided heart failure corresponding to tricuspid valve obstruction. Positioning of the patient for surgery must be carefully performed to detect severe restriction of venous return that is often followed quickly by profound hypotension and arrhythmias. A large tumor increases the likelihood of hemodynamic instability. Perioperative arrhythmias, especially atrial fibrillation or flutter, may arise in 25% of these patients, requiring immediate treatment. Hemodynamic instability with low cardiac output (CO) and arrhythmias are common.

Intraoperative TEE monitoring can aid in recognizing and avoiding tumor embolization. Consideration for not placing a pulmonary artery catheter (PAC) as well as avoiding the RA completely should include the risk of tumor embolization. Evidence of postoperative neurologic injury should be carefully sought because of the likelihood of cerebral embolization and hemorrhage.

Median sternotomy is recommended for resection of atrial myxoma, although anterior thoracotomy and minimally invasive techniques may be possible in some benign tumors.[3] Femoral cannulation for initiation of CPB may minimize the risk of dislodgment or fragmentation of the tumor. Subsequently, a venous cannula can be placed high in the superior vena cava, because a biatrial approach to an atrial septal tumor is necessary. Moderate systemic hypothermia, deep topical cooling, and cardioplegic arrest are often used, while circulatory arrest is reserved for malignant tumors with significant extension.[3] To minimize systemic embolization of tumor fragments, the heart should not eject during CPB. Electrically induced ventricular fibrillation has been used to prevent ejection of blood after initiation of CPB. Wide excision of the septal base of the myxoma with Dacron or pericardial patching of the resulting defect is the preferred operation.[19] Mitral valve replacement may be necessary in large tumors, ventricular side tumors, or tumors with other manifestations besides a propensity to embolize.[15] Less-extensive operations risk a greater incidence of tumor recurrence because of incomplete tumor excision or a second tumor originating in susceptible atrial tissue. The recurrence rate after complete excision of a sporadic cardiac myxoma is low. Postoperatively, the most common complication is a 25% incidence of transient arrhythmias, mostly supraventricular in nature.

Other Benign Tumors

Papillomas (papillary fibroelastomas) are rare tumors but are the third most common primary cardiac tumor. Mostly singular, 1 to 4 cm in size, highly papillary, pedunculated, and avascular, papillomas are covered by a single layer of endothelium containing fine elastic fibrils in a hyaline stroma. Macroscopically, they resemble sea anemones. They originate most commonly from valvular endocardium, usually involving the ventricular surface of the aortic valve or the atrial surface of the mitral valve, infrequently rendering the involved valve incompetent.[20] They account for 75% of all primary cardiac valvular tumors.[21] Adults between the ages of 40 and 80 years are primarily affected. Most patients are asymptomatic, and the papilloma is discovered incidentally during echocardiography, catheterization, or even cardiac surgery. Symptoms are most common when the aortic valve is involved. Previously believed to be harmless, postmortem studies have shown a high incidence of embolization to the cerebral and coronary circulations.[2] Not surprisingly, symptoms are mostly related to embolization as in stroke or transient ischemic attack and myocardial infarction (MI). However, acute valvular dysfunction and even sudden death may occur.[20] Surgical resection is curative, rarely requiring valvular repair or replacement.

The incidence of cardiac lipomas is similar to that of papillary fibroelastoma.[2] They occur as intracavitary tumors, intramyocardial masses, and pericardial tumors. Histologically, they usually consist of encapsulated groups of mature fat cells. Patients with these tumors are often asymptomatic, but if they occur in an intracavitary location, they may resemble myxomas. An intramyocardial location may provoke arrhythmias and conduction abnormalities. Pericardial lipomas are associated with tamponade and cardiac compression.

Rhabdomyomas are primarily childhood tumors located intramyocardially that arise from all areas and at multiple locations of the heart. Tuberous sclerosis is often associated with these tumors. They represent 45% of all benign tumors of childhood but only 1% of benign adult primary cardiac tumors.[2] As pedunculated masses, rhabdomyomas usually originate in the ventricle leading to inflow and outflow ventricular obstruction. Symptoms are caused by the obstruction of blood flow and arrhythmias, but life-threatening complications are rare. Although surgical resection may be necessary in 25% of cases, these tumors may resolve spontaneously. Because of their space-occupying properties, rhabdomyomas may mimic other congenital defects such as left hypoplastic heart syndrome.

Fibromas are connective tissue tumors found primarily in children, making up 15% of pediatric benign primary cardiac tumors.[2] They are usually solitary, located in the wall of the heart, and often involve the apical or septal areas of the left ventricle (LV)[22] (Fig. 24–3, see Color Plates). These tumors frequently interfere with the conduction pathways. Ventricular arrhythmias are common and ventricular tachycardia with sudden death is not infrequent. The tumor may occlude or displace the coronary arteries. Patients may present with CHF or angina. Surgical resection is favored even for asymptomatic patients in view of the risk of fatal ventricular arrhythmias.[22] Cardiac transplantation has been advocated for septal tumors that are unresectable; however, a subtotal resection achieves excellent late survival.[22]

Two vascular tumors, angiomas and pheochromocytomas of the heart (paraganglioma), are very rare. Angiomas are found in the interventricular septum, and their vascular nature makes surgery difficult. Primary cardiac pheochromocytomas are located along the atrioventricular groove near the epicardial arteries.[23] Although cardiac pheochromocytomas become known based on symptoms related to catecholamine secretion, the symptoms are less dramatic than those of the corresponding adrenal tumors because norepinephrine is not converted to epinephrine in the cardiac tumors. Cardiac pheochromocytomas may go undiagnosed for years until patients undergo exploratory laparotomy and multiple diagnostic tests and a cardiac location is considered. Although surgical excision is curative, total excision may be difficult.

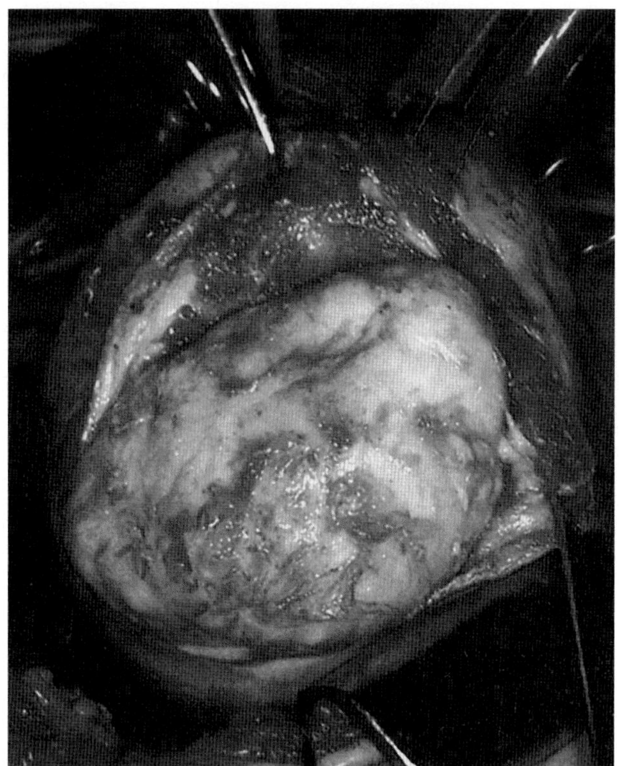

Figure 24–3 Dissection of ventricular fibroma (patient 12; patient's head is at top). (Reprinted with permission from Cho JM, Danielson GK, Puga FJ, et al: Surgical resection of ventricular cardiac fibromas: Early and late results. Ann Thorac Surg 76:1933, 2003. Copyright 2003, with permission from the Society of Thoracic Surgeons.) (See Color Plates.)

Severe intraoperative bleeding is known to occur with these tumors.[23]

Malignant Tumors

Approximately 95% of all primary malignant cardiac tumors are sarcomas. They are found primarily locally infiltrating the RA and causing cavitary obstruction. They usually occur between the ages of 30 and 50, rapidly progressing to death. Angiosarcomas, the most common sarcomas, are rapidly spreading vascular tumors that arise most often from the RA, appearing near the inferior vena cava with extension to the mediastinum.[2] Presenting symptoms include chest pain and dyspnea, progressive CHF, and bloody pericardial effusion.[5] Treatment is palliative and survival is less than 2 years. Rhabdomyosarcomas are aggressive tumors that have cellular elements that resemble striated muscle. They may originate in any chamber of the heart but, in contrast to angiosarcomas, rarely become diffusely involved with the pericardium. Resection may be possible but survival is poor.

Other primary malignant tumors of the heart include malignant fibrous histiocytoma, fibrosarcoma, osteosarcoma, leiomyosarcoma (the rarest malignant cardiac tumor), undifferentiated sarcoma, neurogenic sarcoma, and lymphoma. Primary cardiac lymphoma accounts for about 1% of primary cardiac tumors.[24] The prevalence of these tumors has been increasing in part due to AIDS and early detection from imaging advancements. Lymphomas are generally large masses with extensive infiltration into adjacent areas of the heart from the point of tumor origin. Treatment involves a combination of chemotherapy and radiation, extending survival up to 5 years. Malignant fibrous histiocytoma, in

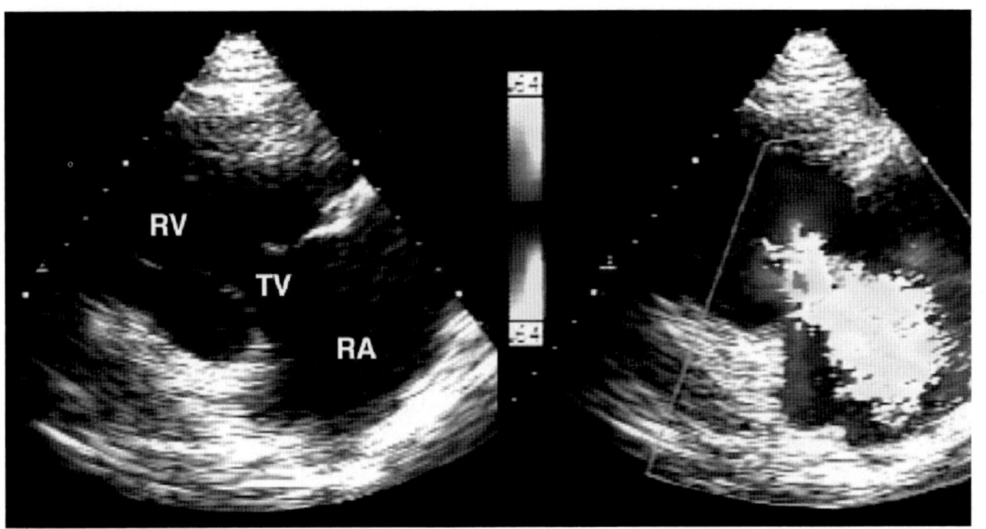

Figure 24–4 Echocardiogram of a patient with carcinoid heart disease displaying the right ventricle (RV), tricuspid valve (TV), and right atrium (RA) showing thickening and tethering of the TV due to carcinoid plaque (*left*) resulting in poor coaptation of the TV leaflets with severe tricuspid regurgitation demonstrated by the large color jet in the RA with ventricular systole (*right*). (Reprinted with permission from Oh JK, Seward JB, Tajik AJ: The Echo Manual, 2nd edition. Philadelphia, Lippincott Williams & Wilkins, 1999; © Mayo Foundation, Click RL, Olson LJ, Edwards WD, et al, Mayo Clinic, Department of Cardiovascular Diseases, Rochester, MN 55905: Echocardiography and systemic diseases. J Am Soc Echocardiogr 7:201, 1994, Fig. 13–7. Copyright 1994, with permission from The American Society of Echocardiography.) (See Color Plates.)

contrast to other sarcomas, is generally found in the LA. Despite resection, metastasis and local recurrence are common. Surgical excision may be useful to ameliorate symptoms but ultimately does not influence the poor survival.[25]

In general, malignant primary cardiac tumors may require a combination of surgery, radiation, and chemotherapy to simply limit cavitary obstruction to blood flow because of rapid growth and metastasis. Local recurrence is more likely than metastasis to cause death.[3] More aggressive approaches for malignant tumors with extensive local disease prior to metastasis include autotransplantation in which the heart is removed from the chest cavity and inverted to provide better exposure.[26] Its value is still indeterminate but no intraoperative deaths have occurred. Although still controversial, orthotopic heart transplantation may be considered for unresectable tumors that involve only the heart, but survival is not extended beyond 1 to 2 years.[3] The rate of intraoperative death with malignant tumor resection is seven times that of benign resection, and there is twice the morbidity rate.[3]

Most cardiac tumors are rarely associated with airway problems.[27] Rather, the large pericardial effusions create significant hemodynamic instability and deterioration. Manipulation of these tumors may also exacerbate hemodynamics. If a large pericardial effusion is present before induction of anesthesia, it should be drained. Beyond the standard monitoring used for a cardiac surgical patient, the overall physical status and risk of embolization must be evaluated. Femoral arterial and central venous monitoring are recommended for patients with RA tumors. Sudden right-sided tumor embolization may be recognized based on an increased end-tidal carbon dioxide gradient with the mass spectrometer. Left-sided embolization is more difficult to assess.

Tumors With Systemic Cardiac Manifestations

Carcinoid tumors are metastasizing tumors that arise primarily from the small bowel, occurring in 1 to 2 per 100,000 people in the population.[28] Fewer than 5% of individuals with carcinoid tumors develop carcinoid syndrome, which is characterized by vasomotor symptoms, bronchospasm, and right-sided heart disease attributed to the release of serotonin, histamine, bradykinins, and prostaglandins, often in response to manipulation or pharmacologic stimulation. Manifestations of carcinoid syndrome occur primarily in patients with liver metastasis that impairs the ability of the liver to inactivate large amounts of vasoactive substances.

Initially described in 1952, carcinoid heart disease develops in more than 50% of patients with carcinoid syndrome and may be the initial feature.[28] The prognosis has improved in the past 20 years for individuals with malignant carcinoid tumors, but carcinoid heart disease still causes considerable morbidity and mortality. Circulating serotonin levels have been found to be more than twice as high in persons with carcinoid syndrome who develop carcinoid heart disease.[29] Carcinoid heart disease characteristically involves tricuspid regurgitation and pulmonic stenosis, resulting in severe right-sided heart failure (Fig. 24–4, see Color Plates). Carcinoid plaques composed of myofibroblasts, collagen, and myxoid matrix are deposited primarily on the tricuspid and pulmonary valves, bringing about immobility and thickening of the valve leaflets, causing the distinctive valvular changes[30] (Fig. 24–5, see Color Plates). Following surgery, 80% of tricuspid valves are observed to be incompetent, with only 20% stenotic, whereas the affected pulmonary valves tend to be equally divided between incompetence and stenosis.[30] The left heart is usually spared involvement in carcinoid heart disease, possibly due to inactivation of serotonin in the lungs, but it may exist with the presence of a bronchial carcinoid or an interatrial shunt.[28]

Without treatment, survival with carcinoid heart disease rarely exceeds 3 years. Surgery to replace both tricuspid and pulmonary valves with either bioprosthetic or mechanical valves is the only viable therapeutic option.[31] The optimal timing to operate is uncertain, but consideration should be given to when signs of RV failure appear, in combination with steady follow-up.[31] Perioperative mortality has been reported as high as 35%, but more recent data suggest it is below 10%.[28,32] Despite surgery, RV dysfunction persists.[31]

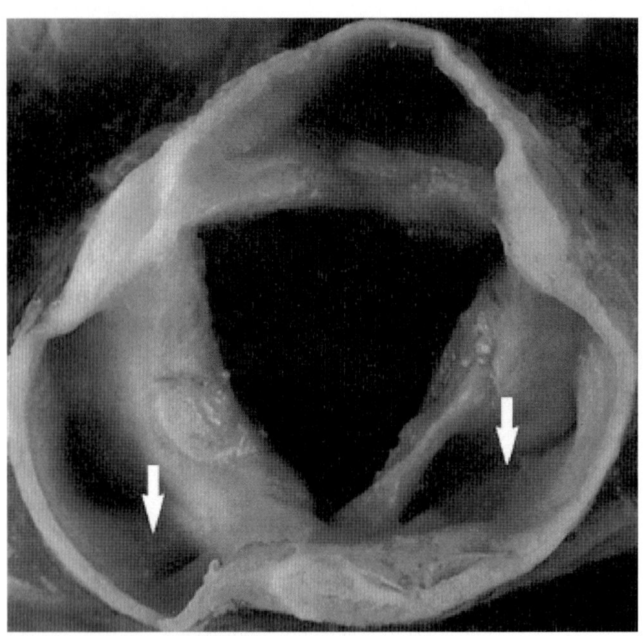

Figure 24–5 Photograph of a pulmonary valve excised from a patient with carcinoid heart disease showing carcinoid plaques that have caused cusp thickening and annular constriction (leading to stenosis) and cusp retraction with a fixed triangular orifice (leading to regurgitation). Carcinoid plaques in the pulmonary artery sinuses behind the cusps have produced irregular ridges that simulate coronary artery ostia *(arrows)*. (Reprinted with permission from Oh JK, Seward JB, Tajik AJ: The Echo Manual, 2nd edition. Philadelphia, Lippincott Williams & Wilkins, 1999; © Mayo Foundation, Click RL, Olson LJ, Edwards WD, et al, Mayo Clinic, Department of Cardiovascular Diseases, Rochester, MN 55905: Echocardiography and systemic diseases. J Am Soc Echocardiogr 7:201, 1994, Fig. 13-6. Copyright 1994, with permission from The American Society of Echocardiography.) (See Color Plates.)

Anesthetic Considerations

Patients who have carcinoid heart disease and require cardiac surgery pose an anesthetic challenge.[33-35] A carcinoid crisis with vasoactive mediator release can be provoked by stress, physical stimulation, or medications such as meperidine, morphine, or histamine-releasing muscle relaxants (atracurium). Preoperative control of carcinoid activity is a critical aspect of perioperative management, made considerably easier with the administration of octreotide, a synthetic analog of somatostatin that inhibits the vasoactive compounds that produce carcinoid syndrome. It reduces the occurrence of symptoms in more than 70% of patients. The longer half-life of octreotide than somatostatin allows subcutaneous injection of 150 μg three times daily to control symptoms. Intermittent intravenous doses of 50 to 200 μg or continuous infusions are given to stop severe hypotension and prevent further carcinoid symptoms.[34] Severe hyperglycemia may occur with octreotide due to its inhibition of insulin secretion.

Preoperative medication to reduce anxiety is strongly recommended for these patients.[34] Individuals with more active carcinoid disease experience greater reductions in systolic blood pressure with induction of anesthesia.[36] Sudden intraoperative hypotension should be regarded as a carcinoid crisis and intravenous octreotide administered until hemodynamic stability returns. Careful attention should be paid to physiologic parameters such as airway pressures as early warning signs of impending carcinoid crisis and treated before the onset of severe hypotension. Previously, certain catecholamines (epinephrine, norepinephrine, dopamine, and isoproterenol) were considered to provoke mediator release in carcinoid syndrome; consequently, phosphodiesterase-3 inhibitors became the preferred inotrope for cardiac surgery with carcinoid heart disease. More recently, 84 patients with carcinoid heart disease who underwent cardiac surgery did not display any deleterious effects or adverse outcomes with dopamine and epinephrine.[36] A test dose of epinephrine may still be prudent to ensure that carcinoid crisis will not occur, but the use of dopamine and epinephrine may be considered in patients with carcinoid heart disease.

The use of an antifibrinolytic is routine in many centers to reduce blood loss and transfusion requirements associated with CPB and cardiac surgery.[37] Because patients with carcinoid heart disease often require surgery involving several valves in association with liver metastasis, coagulopathy and excessive hemorrhage following CPB are more likely. Compared with other commonly used synthetic antifibrinolytic agents (tranexamic acid and aminocaproic acid), aprotinin has the dual properties of antifibrinolysis and anti-inflammation.[33] Consequently, the use of aprotinin in this group of patients may be especially advantageous. However, to achieve inhibition of bradykinin and kallikrein, sufficient dosing is necessary to achieve aprotinin levels of 250 KIU/mL.[38]

CARDIOMYOPATHY

Previously, the World Health Organization (WHO)/International Society of Cardiology (ISC) defined *cardiomyopathy* as "heart muscle disease of unknown cause, unlike heart muscle disease attributed to a specific cause or associated with a disease process."[39] With more knowledge concerning pathogenesis and etiology, the difference between cardiomyopathy and specific heart disease has become less distinct. Previously, cardiomyopathy was classified as dilated, hypertrophic, and restrictive. Over time, each classification has become a recognized clinical condition. In 1995, the WHO/ISC redefined the cardiomyopathies according to dominant pathophysiology or, if possible, by "etiological/pathogenetic factors."[39] Cardiomyopathies are now defined as "diseases of the myocardium associated with cardiac dysfunction."[39] The original cardiomyopathies classified as dilated cardiomyopathy (DCM), restrictive cardiomyopathy (RCM), and hypertrophic cardiomyopathy (HCM) were preserved, and arrhythmogenic RV cardiomyopathy (ARVC) was added.

The annual incidence of cardiomyopathy in adults is 8.7 cases per 100,000 person-years.[40] Underlying causes of cardiomyopathies vary and carry some prognostic significance.[41] General characteristics of all four cardiomyopathies are displayed in Table 24–2. Reviews of the clinical, pathophysiologic, and therapeutic aspects of these cardiomyopathies are available.[42-44] This section focuses on cardiomyopathy in relation to cardiac surgery, but it is relevant for the larger number of patients with a cardiomyopathy who undergo noncardiac surgery.

Dilated Cardiomyopathy

Formerly referred to as "congestive" cardiomyopathy or "idiopathic" cardiomyopathy, DCM is by far the most common of the four cardiomyopathies in adults (60%). The term *idiopathic* has become less applicable to cardiomyopathies as developments in molecular biology and genetics have provided better insight into the pathogenesis of DCM. In

Table 24–2 **Characteristics of Cardiomyopathies**

	Hypertrophic Cardiomyopathy	Dilated Cardiomyopathy	Arrhythmogenic Right Ventricular Cardiomyopathy	Restrictive Cardiomyopathy
Clinical				
Heart failure	Occasional (LV)	Frequent (LV or BV)	Frequent (RV)	Frequent (BV)
Arrhythmias	Atrial and ventricular arrhythmias	Atrial and ventricular arrhythmias, conduction defects	Ventricular tachycardia (RV), conduction defects	Atrial fibrillation
Sudden death	0.7% to 11% per year	Frequent (ND)	Frequent (ND)	1% to 5% per year
Hemodynamic				
Systolic function	Hyperdynamic, outflow tract obstruction (occasionally)	Reduced	Normal-reduced	Near normal
Diastolic function	Reduced	Reduced	Reduced	Severely reduced
Morphologic				
Cavity size				
Ventricle	Reduced (LV)	Enlarged (LV or BA)	Enlarged (RV)	Normal or reduced (BV)
Atrium	Normal-enlarged (LA)	Enlarged (LA or BA)	Enlarged (RV)	Enlarged (BA)
Wall thickness	Enlarged, asymmetric (LV)	Normal-reduced (LV or BV)	Normal-reduced (RV)	Normal (BV)

LV = left ventricle; BV = both ventricles; RV = right ventricle; ND = not determined; BA = both atria; LA = left atrium; RA = right atrium.
From Franz WM, Müller OJ, Katus HA: Cardiomyopathies: From genetics to the prospect of treatment. Lancet 358:1628, 2001.

Table 24–3 **Common Clinicopathologic Diagnoses in 1230 Patients With Initially Unexplained Cardiomyopathy**

Diagnosis	No. of Patients (%)
Idiopathic dilated cardiomyopathy	616 (50)
Myocarditis	111 (9)
Ischemic cardiomyopathy	91 (7)
Infiltrative disease	59 (5)
Peripartum cardiomyopathy	51 (4)
Hypertension	49 (4)
Human immunodeficiency virus infection	45 (4)
Connective tissue disease	39 (3)
Substance abuse	37 (3)
Doxyrubicin related	15 (1)
Other cases	111 (10)

From Wu LA, Lapeyre AC, Cooper LT: Current role of endomyocardial biopsy in the management of dilated cardiomyopathy and myocarditis. Mayo Clin Proc 76:1030, 2001.

the United States alone, nearly 550,000 individuals are newly diagnosed with CHF, whereas close to 4.6 million receive treatment for it. Even with current management, survival for adults at 1 and 5 years after diagnosis is 76% and 35%, respectively, representing a major health care concern.[45] Nonischemic causes comprise 25% to 35% of adult patients with LV dysfunction and CHF of which DCM is a major factor.[44]

DCM is a condition of diverse etiologies such as viral, inflammatory, toxic, or familial/genetic and is associated with many cardiac and systemic disorders that influence the prognosis. Approximately 1230 patients with cardiomyopathy were evaluated and grouped according to a specific cause in 50% of subjects (Table 24–3), yet 50% were characterized as idiopathic.[41] There is a greater appreciation for the role of genetic and familial factors in the etiology of DCM[46,47] (Fig. 24–6, see Color Plates). Between 10% and 35% of cases of DCM are familial with an autosomal dominant expression.[44] Similarities in clinical course that evoke a common set of molecular and cellular pathways may lead to better therapy in the future despite the many different etiologies of DCM.

DCM is characterized morphologically by enlargement of RV and LV cavities without an appropriate increase in the ventricular septal or free wall thickness, giving an almost spherical shape to the heart. The valve leaflets may be normal, yet dilation of the heart may cause a regurgitant lesion secondary to displacement of the papillary muscle. Histologic changes are nonspecific and not associated with positive immunohistochemical, ultrastructural, or microbiologic tests. Microscopically, instead of large losses of myocardium, there is patchy and diffuse loss of tissue with interstitial fibrosis and scarring, uncharacteristic of ischemic myocardium.[48]

With DCM, there is more impairment of systolic function even though diastolic function is affected. As contractile function diminishes, stroke volume is initially maintained by augmentation of end-diastolic volume. Despite a severely decreased ejection fraction, stroke volume may be almost normal. Eventually, increased wall stress due to marked LV dilation and normal or thin LV wall thickness, combined with probable valvular regurgitation, compromises the metabolic capabilities of heart muscle and produces overt circulatory failure.[44] Compensatory mechanisms may allow symptoms of myocardial dysfunction to go unnoticed for an extended period of time. The importance of corresponding neurohumoral influences, such as the renin-angiotensin system, on this pathologic process has only recently been appreciated as a major factor in the appearance of typical signs and symptoms of CHF and formation of therapeutic options[49,50] (Fig. 24–7). Additional evidence of cytokine activity and endothelium dysfunction provides a complex interplay of forces, leading to circulatory failure. The possibility of blocking this neurohumoral response of CHF pharmacologically has not been fully realized, as early trials have been disappointing.[51]

The clinical picture of DCM typically includes signs and symptoms of CHF often corresponding to months of fatigue, weakness, and reduced exercise tolerance prior to diagnosis.[42]

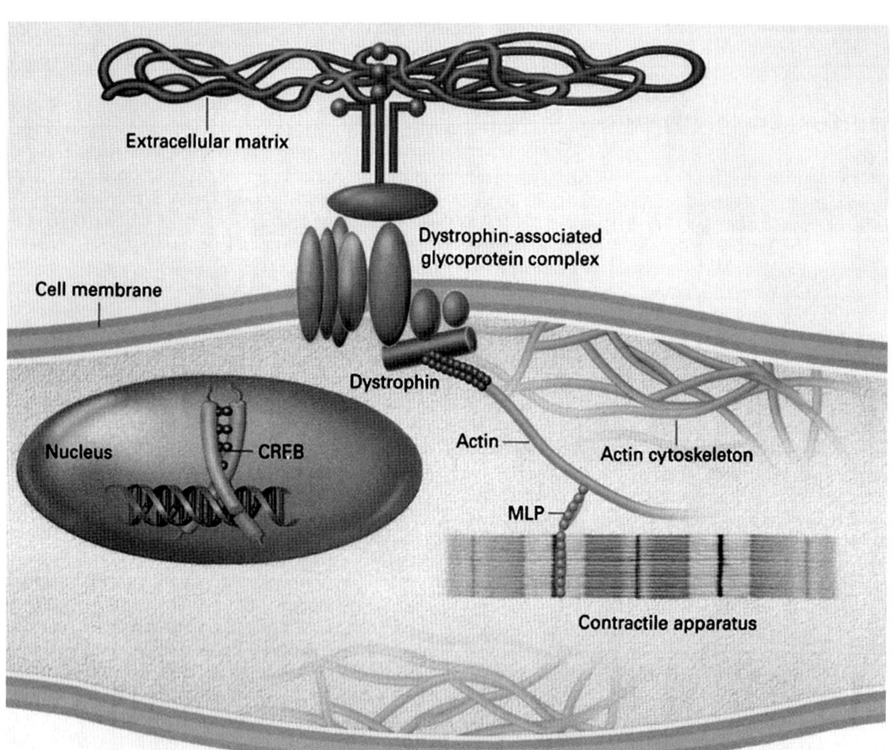

Figure 24–6 A cardiac myocyte and the molecules that have been implicated in dilated cardiomyopathy. (Reprinted with permission from Leiden JM: The genetics of dilated cardiomyopathy—Emerging clues to the puzzle. N Engl J Med 337;1080, 1997. Copyright © 1997 Massachusetts Medical Society. All rights reserved.) (See Color Plates.)

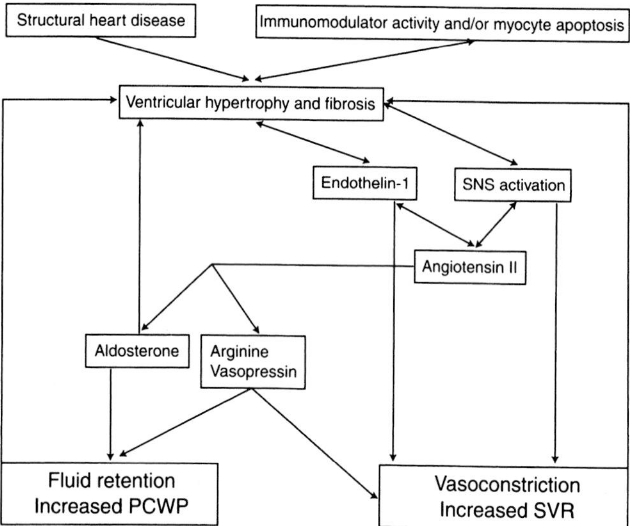

Figure 24–7 Impact of pathophysiologic mediators on hemodynamics in patients with heart failure. PCWP = pulmonary capillary wedge pressure; SNS = sympathetic nervous system; SVR = systemic vascular resistance. (Reprinted with permission from McBride BF, White CM: Acute decompensated heart failure: A contemporary approach to pharmacotherapeutic management. Pharmacotherapy 23:1002, 2003.)

One third of individuals complain of chest pain.[44] However, the first indication of DCM may be a stroke, arrhythmia, or even sudden death. Increasingly, individuals are presenting for routine medical screening, to be informed of cardiomegaly on a routine chest roentgenogram. Symptoms may appear insidiously over a period of years or evolve rapidly after an unrelated illness. Physical signs of DCM, depending on the disease's progression, include pulsus alternans, jugular venous distention, murmurs of atrioventricular valvular regurgitation, tachycardia, and gallop heart sounds.

A chest roentgenogram demonstrates varying degrees of cardiomegaly and pulmonary venous congestion (Fig. 24–8). An electrocardiogram (ECG) may be surprisingly normal or depict low QRS voltage, abnormal axis, nonspecific ST-segment abnormalities, LV hypertrophy, conduction defects, and evidence of atrial enlargement. Atrial fibrillation is common and about one fourth of patients have nonsustained ventricular tachycardia.[42] Two-dimensional echocardiography is instrumental in the diagnosis of DCM, nicely demonstrating the morphologic and physiologic aspects (Fig. 24–9). Although the LV is affected, the RV may be spared in some patients and has been associated with improved survival.[52] Coronary catheterization usually reveals normal coronary arteries, but coronary vasodilation may be impaired by elevated LV filling pressures.[44] Coronary angiography, which has therapeutic and prognostic implications, also distinguishes between ischemic and idiopathic DCM.[52] An endomyocardial biopsy is rarely valuable to identify the etiology of DCM; it is better identified by other means. The biopsy also has no prognostic value or correlation with ventricular function. It rarely influences treatment but may be obtained in a rapidly deteriorating patient in the hope that it may direct therapy.[53]

Management of acute decompensated CHF continues to evolve, but the onset of overt CHF is a poor prognostic indicator for patients with DCM.[50] Treatment revolves around management of symptoms and progression of DCM, while other measures are designed to prevent complications such as pulmonary thromboembolism and arrhythmias.[42] The mainstay of therapy for DCM is vasodilators combined with digoxin and diuretics.[42,54,55] All patients receive angiotensin-converting enzyme inhibitors (ACEIs) to reduce symptoms, improve exercise tolerance, and reduce cardiovascular mortality without a direct myocardial effect.[42,54,55] Perhaps more important than the hemodynamic effects, ACEIs suppress ventricular remodeling and endothelial dysfunction, accounting for the improvement in mortality noted with this med-

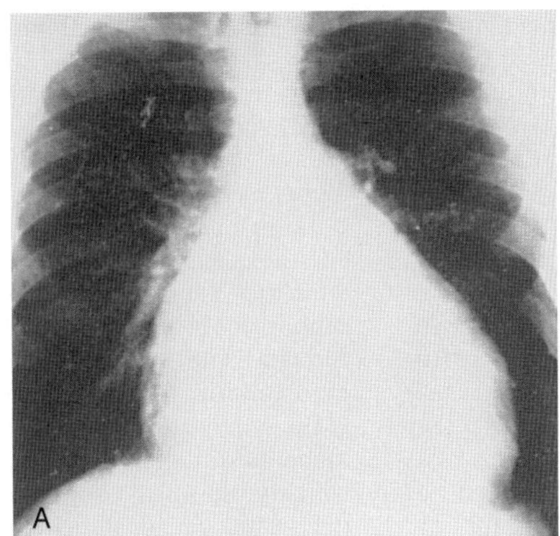

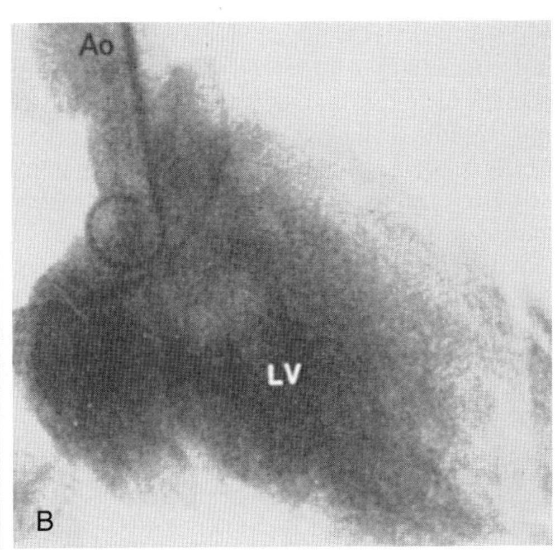

Figure 24–8 *(A)* Chest radiograph showing marked cardiomegaly in a 28-year-old man with idiopathic dilated cardiomyopathy. Pulmonary vascularity is within normal limits. *(B)* Left ventriculogram in systole shows marked dilatation. Ao = aorta; LV = left ventricle. (Reprinted with permission from Stevenson LW, Perloff JK: The dilated cardiomyopathies: Clinical aspects. Cardiol Clin 6:187, 1988.)

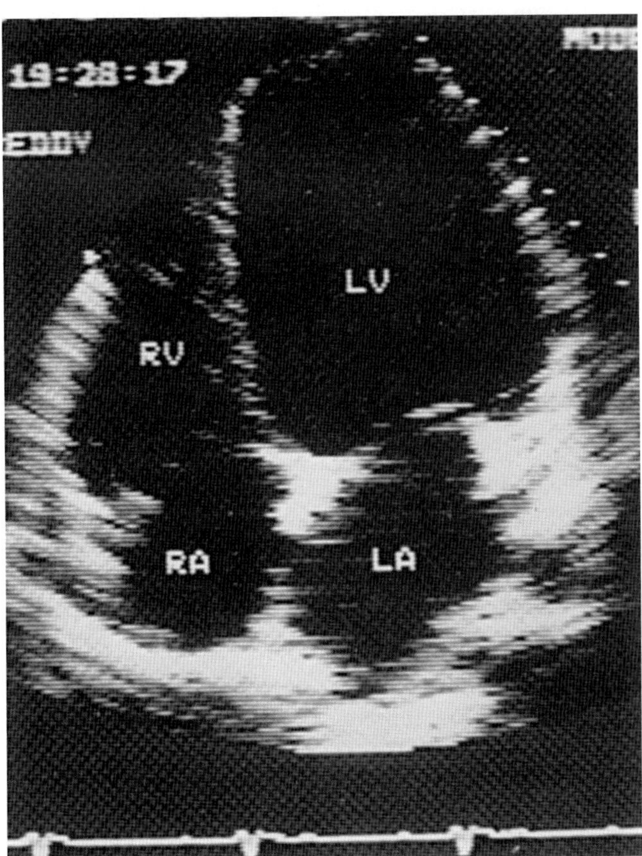

Figure 24–9 Four-chamber apical view of a patient with dilated cardiomyopathy. Both the right and left ventricles (RV and LV) were globally hypokinetic. The ejection fraction was 20%. The enlarged left ventricular chamber with severe hypocontractility results in the characteristic spherical appearance. RA = right atrium, LA = left atrium. (Reprinted with permission from Acquatella H, Rodriguez-Salas LA, Gomez-Mancebo JR: Doppler echocardiography in dilated and restrictive cardiomyopathies. Cardiol Clin 8:349, 1990.)

ication in DCM.[43] Other afterload-reducing agents, such as selective phosphodiesterase-3 inhibitors like milrinone, may improve quality of life but do not affect mortality, so they are rarely administered in chronic situations.[56] Spironolactone has assumed a greater role in treatment as mortality was reduced by 30% from all causes in patients receiving standard ACEIs for DCM with the addition of spironolactone in a large double-blind randomized trial.[57] Although aldosterone increases sodium retention and reduces potassium loss, it has also been shown to cause myocardial and vascular fibrosis, impair baroreceptor function, and prevent catecholamine reuptake by the myocardium (see Chapters 10 and 33).

Until recently, β-blockers were contraindicated in DCM. In 1982, Bristow et al[58] found a decreased catecholamine sensitivity and β-receptor density in the failing human myocardium, leading to loss of contractility. The association between excess sympathetic activity and the failing heart has been aptly demonstrated.[59] The use of β-blockers in DCM has provided not only symptomatic improvement but also substantial reductions in sudden death and progressive death in patients with New York Heart Association (NYHA) class II and III heart failure.[60] This is especially significant because almost 50% of deaths are sudden.[61]

High-grade ventricular arrhythmias are common with DCM.[42] Approximately 12% of all patients with DCM die suddenly, but overall prediction of sudden death in an individual with DCM is poor.[61,62] Electrophysiologic (EP) testing has a poor negative predictive value, limiting its usefulness.[62] The best predictor of sudden death remains the degree of LV dysfunction. Patients who have sustained ventricular tachycardia or out-of-hospital ventricular fibrillation are at increased risk for sudden death, but more than 70% of patients with DCM have nonsustained ventricular tachycardia during ambulatory monitoring.[54] Furthermore, the prognostic significance of ventricular arrhythmias and response to prophylactic antiarrhythmia therapy in patients with DCM are not well established. Antiarrhythmic medications are hazardous in patients with poor ventricular function due to their negative inotropic and sometimes proarrhythmic properties. Antiarrhythmic therapy may only be considered in DCM if inducible ventricular tachycardia or symptomatic arrhythmias are present. Class I agents are not indicated because they have clearly demonstrated increased mortality in patients with advanced heart failure.[42] Amiodarone is the preferred antiarrhythmic agent in DCM because its negative inotropic effect is less than that of other antiarrhythmic medications, and its proarrhythmic potential is lowest.[61,63] Counter to most trials of antiarrhythmic prophylaxis, results of a large multicenter trial of antiarrhythmic therapy in patients with CHF demonstrated that amiodarone was associated with a significantly lower mortality rate of 38% compared with 62% without therapy in patients with a higher resting heart rate.[63] Not withstanding these results, implantable defibrillators reduce the risk of sudden death as well as reducing mortality.[61,62] Evidence has indicated that with previous cardiac arrest or sustained ventricular tachycardia, more benefit was gained from use of an implantable defibrillator. This was based on a 27% reduction in the relative risk of death attributed to a 50% reduction in arrhythmia-related mortality compared with treatment with amiodarone[64] (see Chapters 10, 13, and 25).

Other treatments for DCM include digoxin, which has been reaffirmed as clinically beneficial in two large trials of adults.[52] The risk of thromboembolic complications is significant in DCM for adults.[44] Patients with moderate ventricular dilation and moderate-to-severe systolic dysfunction have intracavitary stasis and a decreased ejection of blood, so they are likely to receive anticoagulants if any history of stroke, atrial fibrillation, or evidence of intracardiac thrombus exists.

Patients who are resistant to pharmacologic therapy for CHF may derive benefit from dual-chamber pacing, cardiomyoplasty, or LV assist devices.[52] Placement of LV assist devices has improved patients sufficiently to avoid heart transplantation or enable later transplantation.[65] Transplantation can substantially prolong survival in patients with DCM, with a 5-year survival of 78% in adults[66] (see Chapters 13, 25 to 27).

Anesthetic Considerations

The most common cardiac procedures for patients with DCM are correction of atrioventricular valve insufficiency, placement of an implantable cardioverter/defibrillator (ICD) for refractory ventricular arrhythmias, and LV assist device placement or allograft transplantation. Anesthetic management is formulated on afterload reduction, optimal preload, and minimal myocardial depression.

Individuals with DCM are extremely sensitive to cardiodepressant anesthetic drugs. Intravenously administered anesthetic agents such as fentanyl (30 μg/kg) provide excellent anesthesia and hemodynamics in patients with ejection fractions less than 0.3, but contribute to prolonged respiratory depression, delaying extubation.[67] Shorter-acting narcotics such as remifentanil may be unsuitable for patients with poor LV function undergoing cardiac surgery due to a high incidence of bradycardia and severe hypotension.[68] A comparison of remifentanil-sevoflurane with fentanyl-etomidate-isoflurane found significantly greater reduction in mean arterial pressure and greater incidence of bradycardia with the remifentanil anesthetic.[69] Also, etomidate has been shown to have little effect on the contractility of the cardiac muscle in patients undergoing cardiac transplantation.[70] Ketamine has been recommended for induction in critically ill patients due to its cardiovascular actions attributed mainly to a sympathomimetic effect from the central nervous system.[71,72] Ketamine is a positive inotrope in the isolated rat papillary muscle and, more important, in a model of cardiomyopathic hamsters, did not display a negative inotropic effect.[73] This makes ketamine an excellent choice to use in combination with fentanyl for induction in patients with severe myocardial dysfunction secondary to cardiomyopathy. The use of propofol with cardiomyopathy may be a concern because cardiovascular depression has been observed, possibly due to inhibition of sympathetic activity and a vasodilatory property. However, in a cardiomyopathic hamster model, there was no direct effect on myocardial contractility with propofol.[74] Caution is still mandatory with propofol because of the indirect inhibitory effects of sympathetic activity that many patients with cardiomyopathy and reduced LV function may depend on for sustaining hemodynamic stability (see Chapter 9).

Volatile agents have long been a concern in patients with failing hearts because of the known depressant effects on myocardial contractility. The effect of currently used volatile anesthetics on intrinsic myocardial contractility is difficult to project clinically. Animal data indicate halogenated volatile agents may have more profound negative inotropic effects in cardiomyopathic muscle than in healthy cardiac muscle.[75] An anesthetic technique that minimizes myocardial depression is attractive. There is little from a cardiovascular standpoint to support the selection of sevoflurane over isoflurane in adults. Although the failing myocardium has been thought to be more sensitive to the depressant effects of volatile agents, there is no synergistic myocardial depression in the presence of moderate LV dysfunction and volatile agents.[76] Desflurane, which possesses the lowest blood–gas partition coefficient of the volatile agents allowing rapid induction and emergence, would appear to have some benefit for early extubation in patients undergoing cardiac surgery. In healthy hamster papillary muscles, desflurane did not appear to have a negative inotropic effect; however, in cardiomyopathic papillary muscles, there was a profound negative inotropic effect.[77] On the other hand, sevoflurane and desflurane were shown not to adversely affect the ability of the LV to respond to increased work in patients undergoing CPB and cardiac surgery despite their negative inotropic properties.[78] Even with the limitations of generalizing findings of in vitro experiments to clinical situations, this difference of inotropic effect regarding healthy versus cardiomyopathic myocardium is an important distinction not present in all halogenated anesthetics and should be taken into consideration in patients with cardiomyopathy.

Invasive hemodynamic monitoring is indispensable with volatile agents and DCM. Of particular pertinence for anesthesiologists is that physical signs and symptoms of DCM may not accurately reflect physiologic parameters. Eighty percent of patients with pulmonary capillary wedge pressures greater than 25 mm Hg have no detectable rales.[79] Patients receiving implantable defibrillators usually have severely depressed LV function but are routinely managed without a PAC.[80] Hemodynamic instability that may occur with DCM can be lessened with a low dose of an inotrope and a vasodilator. Acute administration of inotropes, such as dobutamine, improves hemodynamics temporarily, but tolerance begins in 3 to 4 days.[54] Phosphodiesterase 3 inhibitors are useful if combined with another β-adrenergic agonist for short-term hemodynamic support. Afterload reduction in DCM is important because it improves regional and global indices of ventricular relaxation and ejection fraction during anesthesia when myocardial depression may be significant. It may also reduce valvular regurgitation and atrial volumes.[81] Some patients with DCM may be taking amiodarone on a long-term basis, which has a negative inotropic effect that interacts with volatile agents to further reduce contractility and conduction, requiring careful titration of these anesthetic agents.[82] Arrhythmogenic factors such as hypokalemia, hypomagnesemia, and sympathetic activation should be monitored and corrected.[61]

Hypertrophic Cardiomyopathy

Referred to as *idiopathic hypertrophic subaortic stenosis*, *hypertrophic obstructive cardiomyopathy*, and *asymmetric septal hypertrophy*, among other names, the accepted name is now *hypertrophic cardiomyopathy*.[83] In the past 40 years, advancements regarding the hemodynamics, systolic and diastolic abnormalities, electrophysiology, genetics, and clinical care of

HCM have contributed to a greater understanding of this disease. HCM is the most common genetic cardiac disease, with marked heterogeneity in clinical expression, pathophysiology, and prognosis. The overall prevalence for adults in the general population is 0.2%, affecting men and women equally.[84]

HCM is a primary myocardial abnormality with sarcomeric disarray and asymmetric LV hypertrophy (Fig. 24–10). The extent of sarcomeric disarray distinguishes HCM from other conditions.[39] The hypertrophied muscle is composed of muscle cells with bizarre shapes and multiple intercellular connections arranged in a chaotic pattern.[84] Increased connective tissue combined with markedly disorganized and hypertrophied myocytes contributes to the diastolic abnormalities of HCM that manifest as increased chamber stiffness, impaired prolonged relaxation, and an unstable EP substrate that causes complex arrhythmias and sudden death. Diastolic abnormalities are more a function of impaired relaxation than of decreased compliance. Impaired relaxation produces a reduced rate of volume during rapid ventricular filling, with an increase in atrial systolic filling associated with atrial dilation. As the abnormal diastolic properties affect ventricular filling, the clinical manifestations of HCM become evident. In contrast to the diastolic function, systolic function in HCM is usually normal, with an increased ejection fraction that eventually diminishes in the later stages of the disease.

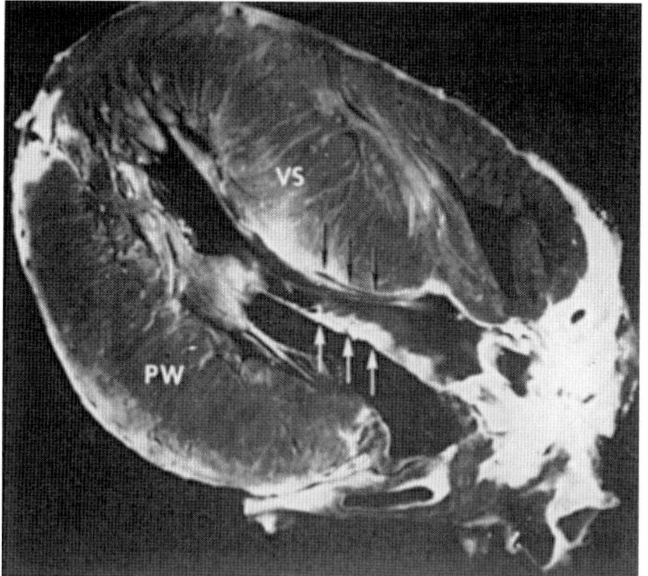

A

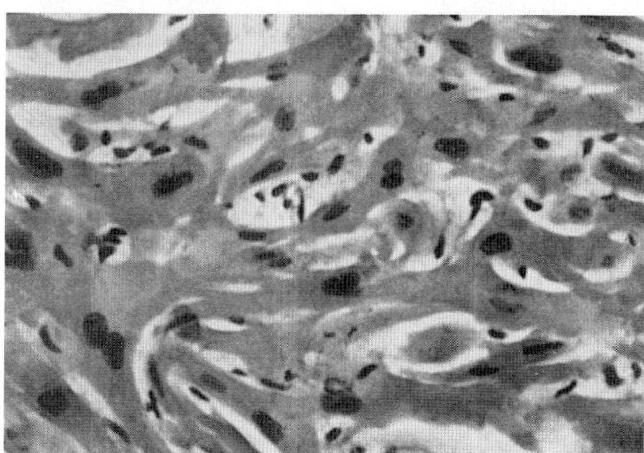

B

Figure 24–10 *(A)* Hypertrophic cardiomyopathy (HCM) from the long-axis view. Ventricular cavity is small and has pronounced septal and posterior wall thickening. *Arrows* indicate narrowing of the left ventricular outflow tract caused by the thickened ventricular septum and anterior leaflet of the mitral valve. VS = ventricular septum; PW = posterior wall of the left ventricle. (Reprinted with permission from Edwards WD, Zakheim R, Mattioli L: Asymmetric septal hypertrophy in childhood: Unreliability of histologic criteria for differentiation of obstructive and nonobstructive forms. Hum Pathol 8:277, 1977.) *(B)* Photomicrograph of the myocardium in HCM. There are pronounced disarray and hypertrophy of the individual muscle fibers, resulting in a "whorling" appearance of the muscle fiber (hematoxylin and eosin stain; original magnification ×165). (Photograph courtesy of William D. Edwards, MD. Reprinted with permission from Giuliani ER, Fuster V, Gersh BJ, et al: Cardiology: Fundamentals and Practice. St. Louis, Mosby, 1991. By permission of Mayo Foundation.)

Besides diastolic dysfunction, the other major abnormality and fundamental characteristic of HCM is myocardial hypertrophy unrelated to increased systemic vascular resistance (SVR). This nonuniform, asymmetric hypertrophy is marked in the basal anterior ventricular septum, with a disproportionate increase in the thickness of the ventricular wall relative to the posterior free wall (see Fig. 24–10*A*). The LV wall thickness is the most extensive of all cardiac conditions.[84] Heart size may be deceptive because it may vary from normal to more than 100% enlarged. However, chamber enlargement is not responsible for the increase in ventricular mass but rather increases in wall thickness.

HCM is the most common genetic cardiovascular disease inherited in an autosomal dominant manner.[39] It may be caused by mutations in any of 10 genes; however, three genes that encode proteins of the cardiac sarcomere predominate in frequency.[83] The similarity of the genes accounts for the many different expressions of HCM while resembling one disease entity. Patients without a family history of HCM may have sporadic gene mutations or simply a very mild form. DNA analysis of mutant genes is the most definitive method to establish the diagnosis.[83] The phenotype appears to depend not only on the mutation but also on other modifier genes and environmental factors.[83,85] Not all patients who possess a gene for HCM manifest clinical features of the disease reflecting incomplete genetic expression.[84] A preclinical diagnosis in a patient without symptoms is possible with gene testing, but it is not routinely performed now, and it cannot be used to establish a treatment strategy.

HCM is unique for its range of clinical presentations from infancy to 90 years of age. While major referral centers describe a disease with severe symptomatology, many elderly with mild-to-asymptomatic disease were unaccounted for, resulting in an actual annual mortality rate for HCM closer to 1% per year than the previously reported 3% to 6% per year.[84] Even LV outflow obstruction may be tolerated longer than initially believed. Most HCM patients are asymptomatic or have mild symptoms that progress slowly or not at all.[44] In contrast, children progress at a faster rate than adults with an annual mortality ranging from 2% to 6%.[84,86] However, as with adults, more children may be affected with milder forms of HCM than previously believed.[87] In one third of infants with HCM, myocardial hypertrophy resolves.

Symptoms of HCM are nonspecific and include chest pain, palpitations, dyspnea, and syncope. Dyspnea occurs in 90% of patients secondary to diastolic abnormalities that increase filling pressures, causing pulmonary congestion. Syncope occurs in only 20% of patients, but 50% may have presyncopal symptoms. The physical examination is usually unreliable because classic physical findings are associated with LV outflow obstruction that occurs in only 25% of patients with HCM. Symptoms usually appear in the second or third decade, but HCM is not a static disease and LV hypertrophy can occur at any age and increase or decrease dynamically throughout the patient's life.[84] The ECG is abnormal in most individuals, showing increased QRS voltage, ST-segment and T-wave abnormalities, QRS axis shift, and LV hypertrophy with strain pattern. There is little correlation between ECG voltages and LV hypertrophy.[84] A chest roentgenogram may show left atrial enlargement or be normal. Two-dimensional echocardiography establishes the diagnosis of HCM easily and reliably. Classic echocardiography features are thickening of the entire ventricular septum from base to apex disproportional to that of the posterior wall, poor septal motion, and anterior displacement of the mitral valve without LV dilation (Fig. 24–11). Echocardiography has reduced the need for invasive catheterization procedures, unless coronary artery disease (CAD) or severe mitral valve disease is suspected or diagnostic problems are present. MRI has been useful in cases in which echocardiography is technically inadequate.[84]

Angiography may show an LV pressure gradient, decreased ventricular volume, and increased LV end-diastolic pressure. CAD may be absent angiographically, but thallium redistribution scans demonstrate that HCM patients may experience myocardial ischemia often associated with atypical chest pain, not relieved with nitrates.[88] Thallium abnormalities may represent relatively underperfused myocardium with abnormal intramyocardial coronary arteries that are known to exist in patients with HCM. Abnormal coronary vasodilation in both nonhypertrophied and hypertrophied myocardium occurs in HCM.[89] This suggests that impaired coronary vasodilation has a major role in the pathogenesis of HCM and is not secondary to myocardial hypertrophy. However, a mismatch between

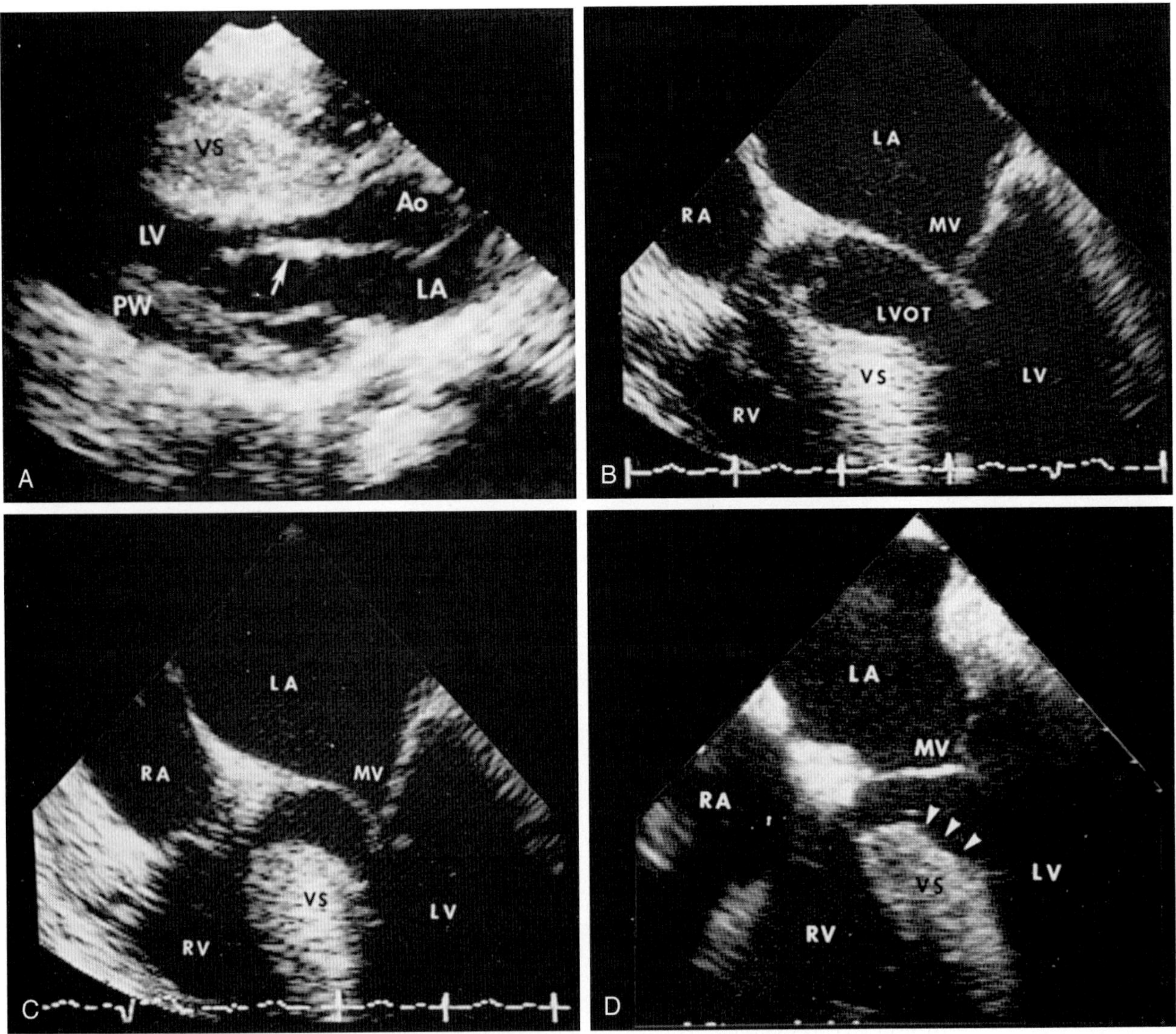

Figure 24–11 *(A)* Parasternal long-axis view of a patient with hypertrophic cardiomyopathy (HCM). There is increased thickness of the septum from the base to the apex as well as the anterior free wall. The left ventricular cavity size is normal here. (Reprinted with permission from Giuliani ER, Fuster V, Gersh BJ, et al: Cardiology: Fundamentals and Practice. St. Louis, Mosby 1991.) *(B)* Transesophageal echocardiography in a patient with HCM for myectomy-myotomy. Early systole, demonstrating septal hypertrophy and narrowing of the left ventricular outflow tract (LVOT). *(C)* Same patient in late systole. Systolic anterior motion of the mitral leaflets produced by a Venturi effect in the LVOT created by the high blood velocity. *(D)* Following myectomy-myotomy, the arrowheads point to the area of myocardium removed and the widened LVOT. LA = left atrium; RA = right atrium; LV = left ventricle; RV = right ventricle; VS = ventricular septum; MV = mitral valve; Ao = aorta; PW = posterior wall. (*B, C,* and *D* photographs courtesy of Martin D. Abel, MD, Mayo Clinic, Rochester, MN.)

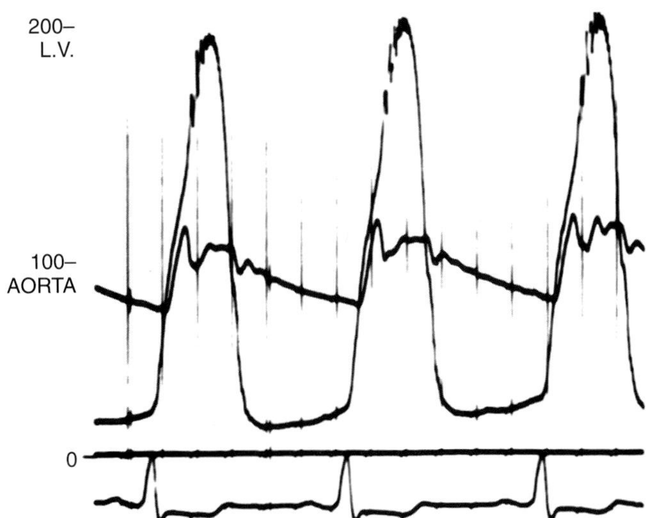

Figure 24–12 Simultaneous left ventricular (LV) and aortic pressure tracings from a patient with muscular subaortic stenosis (resting obstruction). (Reprinted with permission from Wigle ED, Sasson Z, Henderson MA, et al: Hypertrophic cardiomyopathy: The importance of the site and extent of hypertrophy: A review. Prog Cardiovasc Dis 28:1, 1985.)

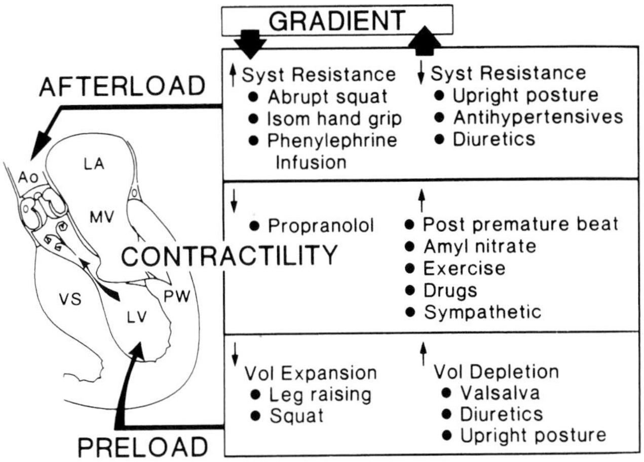

GRADIENT
AFTERLOAD
↑Syst Resistance
• Abrupt squat
• Isom hand grip
• Phenylephrine Infusion
↓Syst Resistance
• Upright posture
• Antihypertensives
• Diuretics
CONTRACTILITY
↓
• Propranolol
↑
• Post premature beat
• Amyl nitrate
• Exercise
• Drugs
• Sympathetic
PRELOAD
↓
Vol Expansion
• Leg raising
• Squat
↑
Vol Depletion
• Valsalva
• Diuretics
• Upright posture
Ao LA MV VS LV PW

Figure 24–13 Interventions that change the outflow gradient in hypertrophic cardiomyopathy (HCM), with resultant change in intensity of the systolic murmur in HCM. Outflow gradient is affected by changes in afterload, preload, and contractility. Ao = aorta; LA = left atrium; MV = mitral valve; VS = ventricular septum; LV = left ventricle; PW = posterior wall. (Reprinted with permission from Giuliani ER, Fuster V, Gersh BJ, et al: Cardiology: Fundamentals and Practice. St. Louis, Mosby, 1991. By permission of Mayo Foundation.)

myocardial oxygen demand resulting from systolic and diastolic abnormalities, and increased ventricular mass and coronary circulation, may exacerbate myocardial ischemia. Thus, myocardial death and scarring may serve as a substrate for ventricular tachycardia and fibrillation.[84]

Two thirds of individuals with LV outflow tract obstruction become severely symptomatic and 10% die within 4 years of diagnosis. The outflow tract is narrowed from septal hypertrophy and anterior displacement of the papillary muscles and mitral leaflets, creating a dynamic LV outflow obstruction (see Fig. 24–10). Elongation of the mitral leaflets results in coaptation of the body of the leaflets instead of the tips. The part of the anterior leaflet distal to the coaptation is subjected to strong Venturi forces that provoke systolic anterior motion (SAM), mitral septal contact, and ultimately LV outflow obstruction.[83] SAM of the anterior leaflet may also cause mitral regurgitation. The onset and duration of mitral leaflet–septal contact determine the magnitude of the gradient and the degree of mitral regurgitation. The pressure gradient between the aorta and LV (Fig. 24–12) is worsened by decreased end-diastolic volume, increased contractility, or decreased aortic outflow resistance[90] (Fig. 24–13). The cavity of the LV is often small in those with severe gradients (Fig. 24–14). Doppler echocardiography technology is generally used now to assess LV outflow tract gradients, greatly lessening the need for cardiac catheterization.

Dynamic LV outflow obstruction is not limited to HCM but may occur in cardiac tamponade or acute MI.[90] Importantly, dynamic pressure gradients do not necessarily correlate with symptoms of HCM. Significant functional limitation, disability, and sudden death may all occur even if a gradient is absent. However, gradients exceeding 30 mm Hg are usually

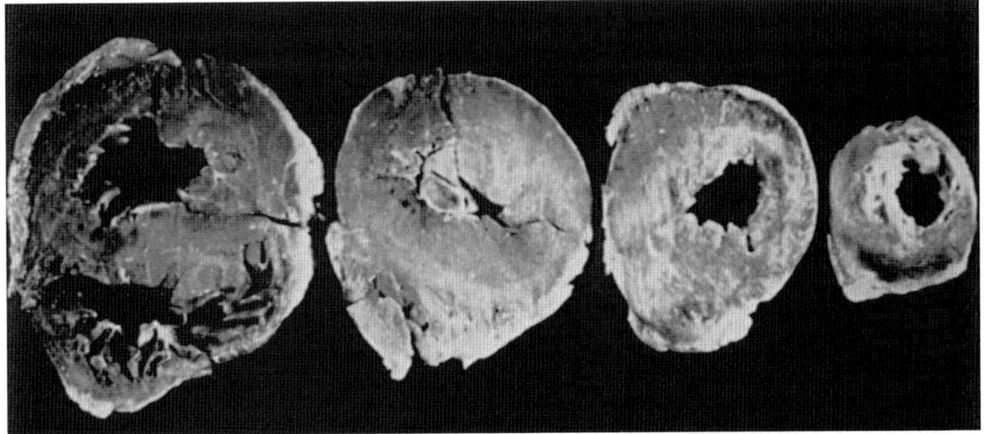

Figure 24–14 Midventricular hypertrophy. Cross-sectional slices of the heart from a patient who was shown, by hemodynamic, angiographic, and echocardiographic techniques, to have midventricular obstruction. The site of the obstruction was at the level of the papillary muscles, where there was massive hypertrophy (second slice from *left*). The slice at the *left* is from the base of the heart, and the two slices at the *right* are from the apex. The apex of the left ventricle was the site of extensive myocardial infarction and aneurysm formation that was evidenced in life by a dyskinetic apical chamber on angiography and by persistent ST-segment elevation in leads V_4 to V_6 on the electrocardiogram. The coronary arteries revealed no significant luminal narrowings. The patient died of intractable ventricular arrhythmias. (Reprinted with permission from Wigle ED, Rakowski H, Kimball BP, et al: Hypertrophic cardiomyopathy. Clinical spectrum and treatment. Circulation 92:1680, 1995.)

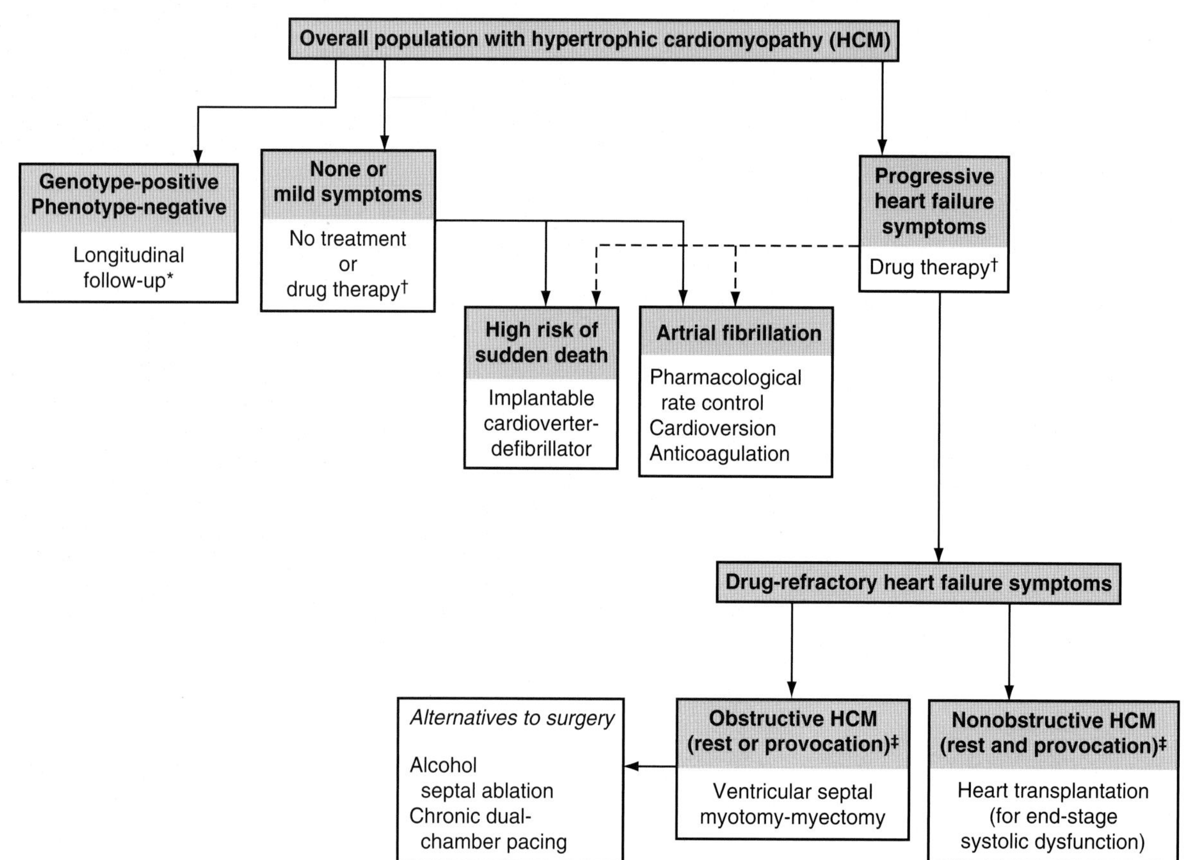

Figure 24–15 Hypertrophic cardiomyopathy (HCM) clinical subgroups are not necessarily mutually exclusive; overlap or progression from one subgroup to another may occur (*thin solid and dashed arrows*). Most patients with HCM who are at high risk of sudden death or who develop atrial fibrillation are initially in the "None or Mild Symptoms" clinical subgroup.

*Patients with a positive genotype and negative phenotype may subsequently show morphologic conversion to the HCM phenotype with left ventricular hypertrophy (usually in adolescence, but also in mid-life or later).

†Drug therapy may include β-blockers, calcium channel blockers (particularly verapamil), disopyramide, and diuretic agents.

‡For major interventions, obstructive HCM is generally regarded as a left ventricular outflow gradient of approximately 50 mm Hg at rest or with provocative maneuvers; in this context, nonobstructive HCM is regarded as a left ventricular outflow gradient of less than approximately 30 to 50 mm Hg at rest as well as with provocative maneuvers. Width of the arrows from the overall HCM population represents the approximate relative proportion of patients with HCM within each major clinical subgroup. (Originally adapted from Spirto et al: The management of hypertrophic cardiomyopathy. N Engl J Med 336:775, 1997, with permission of the Massachusetts Medical Society. Reprinted with permission from Maron BJ: Hypertrophic cardiomyopathy: A systematic review. JAMA 287:1313, 2002. Copyright © 1997 Massachusetts Medical Society. All rights reserved.)

of physiologic and prognostic importance in HCM patients.[83] The severity of symptoms is not worse once a gradient exceeds 30 mm Hg.[91] Outflow obstruction is an independent predictor of death in HCM. Because outflow obstruction is likely to be associated with increased wall stress, myocardial ischemia, cell death, and eventual fibrosis, treatment to relieve outflow obstruction is desirable.

The clinical course and treatment of HCM are best approached in relation to subgroups: sudden death, CHF, and atrial fibrillation with embolic stroke (Fig. 24–15). Sudden death increases the annual mortality from 1% to 5% overall.[84] Often these patients are asymptomatic or mildly symptomatic and constitute a very small part of the HCM population. Sudden death is not age restricted but occurs more commonly in younger individuals, frequently in association with physical exertion. HCM is the most common cause of sudden death in otherwise healthy young individuals.[92] Risk stratification for sudden death is useful now that it has been found that ventricular tachycardia or ventricular fibrillation is primarily responsible.[93,94] High-risk individuals have these characteristics: younger than 30 years of age at diagnosis, prior cardiac arrest, symptomatic ventricular tachycardia on Holter monitor, and family history of sudden death or syncope.[44] Additional risk factors include identification of a high-risk mutant gene, unexplained syncope, and abnormal blood pressure with exercise.[83] Two or more risk factors are associated with a risk of sudden death of 4% to 5% per year. A National Institutes of Health study found that the two most significant independent predictors of sudden death in HCM are the occurrence of EP-induced sustained ventricular tachycardia and previous syncope or cardiac arrest.[95]

The value of EP testing as it relates to prediction of sudden death is mixed.[83,92,94] Routine risk stratification with EP testing was abandoned in HCM patients.[83] Extreme LV wall thickness has been associated with greater incidence of spontaneous ventricular arrhythmias and sudden death.[83,84] Myocardial ischemia also appears to be related to sudden death in younger patients.[96] In the future, genotyping may be able to reliably define the risk of sudden death. The only effective modality to prevent sudden death associated with HCM is the ICD. Pharmacologic therapy for prevention has been abandoned. Symptomatic patients or those with a positive EP test appear to benefit from ICD placement. A retrospective study found that 25% of high-risk cohorts required termination of lethal ventricular arrhythmias and 60% experienced some type of intervention with an ICD.[93] ICD has been shown in a randomized prospective trial to be superior to drug therapy.[97] Amiodarone is no longer the first line of antiarrhythmic therapy for patients at risk for sudden death, as previous studies were nonrandomized case studies[44] (see Chapters 10, 13, and 25).

Another subgroup, patients with CHF, develop progressive symptoms with preserved systolic function but quickly advance to end-stage CHF with impaired systolic function.[83] Symptoms are primarily attributed to the diastolic abnormality, so symptomatic relief is achieved by improving ventricular relaxation. Medications with negative inotropic effect are generally successful in relieving symptoms of exercise intolerance and dyspnea associated with CHF. In general, β-blockers have been a mainstay of therapy for years in adults and are preferred over calcium channel blockers. Verapamil may be given if β-blockers are not tolerated or ineffective. The combination of β-blockers and calcium channel blockers has not proved to be beneficial. β-Blockers relieve symptoms of angina and dyspnea and improve exercise tolerance by limiting the gradient associated with exercise. The gradient is not reduced at rest by these medications.[83] Other beneficial effects of β-blockers include heart rate reduction, lower myocardial oxygen demand, and longer diastolic filling times, but diastolic function is not improved or long-term survival prolonged. Verapamil improves diastolic function and ventricular relaxation, causing improved filling and decreased obstructive features in 50% of HCM patients. Patients with obstructive symptoms may worsen with calcium channel blockers that contain strong vasodilator properties. Disopyramide, a negative inotrope that alters calcium kinetics and produces a vasoconstrictor effect, has been recommended instead of calcium channel blockers in obstructive HCM.[83] It is the most effective agent to reduce LV outflow obstruction and gradient as well as relieving symptoms.[98] Combined with β-blockers, disopyramide prolongs exercise times more successfully than verapamil.

Surgical correction of HCM is directed primarily at relieving symptoms of LV obstruction in the 5% of patients who are refractory to medication.[83] In general, these are individuals with subaortic gradients more than 50 mm Hg and frequently associated with severe CHF.[44,84] A myotomy-myectomy through a transaortic approach relieves the obstruction (Fig. 24–16). The muscle is excised from the proximal septum extending just beyond the mitral valve leaflets to widen the LV outflow tract. This is a technically challenging operation due to the limited exposure and precise area to excise the muscle. It is usually reserved for centers with considerable experience.[98] When myectomy is successful, the outflow tract of the LV is widened and SAM, mitral regurgitation and outflow gradient are all decreased (see Fig. 24–11*D*). A more detailed description of myotomy-myectomy is available.[98] Mitral valve repair or replacement has accompanied myectomy, although there is disagreement as to its value. Echocardiography is very helpful during the operation.

Surgery provides persistent, long-lasting relief from symptoms that exceeds any form of current medical treatment.[83] Five years after myectomy, 85% of patients have improved enough to advance one NYHA functional class.[99] The concomitant reduction in left atrial size may partially account for the lower incidence of atrial fibrillation after myectomy.[83] Myectomy is associated with a mortality rate of 1% to 3% in centers that commonly perform it.[100] This low mortality rate is even more noteworthy because surgical patients usually have more severe disease than those treated medically. The cumulative survival rate of 519 patients who underwent myectomy 10 years after surgery was 88%.[101] Complications of myectomy such as complete heart block or septal perforation (0% to 2%) are rare.[98] Similarly, recurrence of LV outflow tract gradient or SAM is rare.[83]

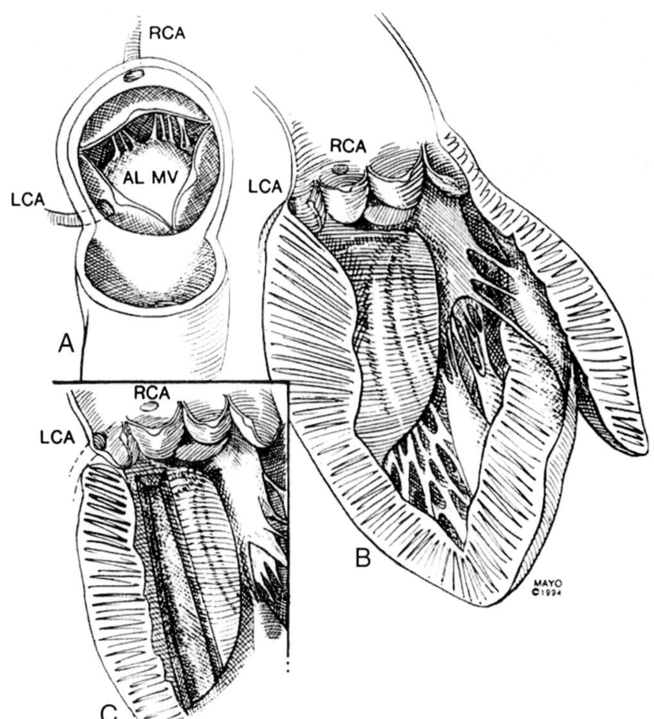

Figure 24–16 Anatomic characteristics of hypertrophic obstructive cardiomyopathy. *(A)* Surgeon's view through transverse aortotomy. Right coronary cusp is located anteriorly and left cusp is located posteriorly and to left. Gentle retraction of aortic cusps, combined with posterior displacement of left ventricle as needed, exposes ventricular septum and anterior leaflet of mitral valve (AL MV). *(B)* Sagittal view through opened left ventricle showing membranous septum below commissure between right and noncoronary cusps, distribution of left bundle branches, septal hypertrophy, and anterior leaflet of mitral valve with its subvalvular apparatus. *(C)* Extent of initial septal resection is shown. Resection is then extended leftward to anterior leaflet of mitral valve and apically to relieve all midventricular obstruction. RCA = right coronary artery; LCA = left coronary artery. (Reprinted with permission from Theodoro DA, Danielson GK, Feldt RH, Anderson BJ: Hypertrophic obstructive cardiomyopathy in pediatric patients: Results of surgical treatment. J Thorac Cardiovasc Surg 112:1589, 1996. Copyright 1996, with permission from the American Association for Thoracic Surgery.)

Surgery is not recommended for HCM without an obstructive component or if the individual is asymptomatic to mildly symptomatic because (1) better survival with surgery versus medical therapy is not established, (2) operative mortality may exceed the risk of HCM in mildly affected patients, (3) LV outflow obstruction may be compatible with longevity in selected individuals, and (4) there is no evidence that surgery halts the progression of HCM to end stage.[83] Medical treatment for asymptomatic HCM patients is not clearly indicated.[83]

Possible alternatives to surgery have included dual-chamber pacing and percutaneous alcohol septal ablation. Previously, atrioventricular sequential pacing had been shown to decrease subaortic gradients, so it was considered a possible treatment even though the mechanism was not apparent. However, symptoms may actually worsen with pacing despite gradient reductions; long-term improvement was not realized in most patients and is now rarely recommended.[44,102] Septal ablation with alcohol is a nonsurgical myocardial reduction first attempted in 1994 based on interruption of blood supply to the interventricular septum with resolution of symptoms in HCM.[103] Alcohol is administered through an angioplasty balloon to the first major septal perforator of the left anterior descending coronary artery. The success rate has been high with a low complication rate.[104] Although a number of favorable effects have been reported, the risk of arrhythmias is a concern.[83] The procedure continues to evolve as the proper patient selection and long-term effects are evaluated.

Anesthetic Considerations

Anesthetic management of individuals with HCM is based on similar principles for those having cardiac or noncardiac surgery. The characteristic diastolic dysfunction makes the heart sensitive to changes in volume, contractility, and SVR. Because of this diastolic dysfunction, an acute rise in the pulmonary artery pressure (PAP) may warn of the rapid onset of pulmonary congestion and edema. If the patient has LV outflow obstruction, anesthetic management should minimize or prevent any exacerbation of obstruction and the corresponding increase in the intraventricular gradient that will affect systolic blood pressure.[105] Induction of anesthesia is a hazardous period because the preoperative fast reduces preload combined with a rapid fall in the venous tone, provoking an increase in LV outflow obstruction. Central venous pressure (CVP) monitoring is recommended to optimize and maintain preload.[105] Hypotension may be treated temporarily with positioning (Trendelenburg), volume replacement, and/or vasoconstriction. Vasoconstrictors rather than inotropes are preferred to maintain SVR.[106] Following induction of anesthesia and intubation, TEE can complement CVP monitoring to guide intraoperative volume status. Intravenously administered agents, such as narcotics, have been used successfully in HCM for induction of anesthesia. For shorter surgical procedures, propofol is popular, but its effect on hemodynamics has not been fully established. The systolic blood pressure often decreases significantly with propofol during induction of anesthesia. The mechanism of this fall in blood pressure is unknown, but it is likely an interaction of baroreflex activity, direct peripheral vasodilation, blunting of the sympathetic nervous outflow, and possibly a decrease in the myocardial contractility.[107] In an experimental hamster with HCM that received propofol, the myocardium was found to be unaffected compared with the healthy muscle.[74] Additionally, continuous propofol infusion has been used successfully in a patient with HCM for mitral valve replacement and myectomy.[106]

For anesthesia maintenance, the volatile agent halothane is advantageous because it decreases contractility and heart rate, but it is rarely used today.[108] Halothane, in comparison with enflurane and isoflurane, has the least effect on SVR and heart rate.[108,109] The potential for severe myocardial depression with volatile agents in these patients has been shown to be less likely than once believed. There is continuing evidence in hamster models with HCM that the negative inotropic effect in the affected myocardium compared with healthy myocardium is more severe with desflurane than either isoflurane or sevoflurane.[75,77] Volatile agents also increase the risk of atrioventricular block and depressed cardiac function in patients chronically receiving verapamil.[110] Vecuronium is the preferred muscle relaxant because it does not have histamine-releasing properties or hemodynamic effects.

Arrhythmias may complicate the anesthetic management of individuals with HCM. Ninety percent of adults with HCM have complex ventricular arrhythmias on Holter monitoring regardless of whether HCM is obstructive or nonobstructive.[83] Nonsustained ventricular tachycardia occurs in 25% to 33% of patients, whereas sustained monomorphic ventricular tachycardia is rare.[111] Asymptomatic, nonsustained ventricular tachycardia tends to be benign.[93] Patients who have sustained ventricular tachycardia that is refractory to medical therapy or continue to have serious problems with syncope often have received an ICD that will need to be temporarily suspended before use of cautery in the operating room[93] (see Chapter 25).

Besides ventricular arrhythmias, there is a 30% to 50% incidence of paroxysmal supraventricular tachycardia in patients with HCM.[111] Atrial fibrillation is the most common supraventricular tachycardia, occurring in 25% of individuals.[44,84] Its onset may quickly lead to CHF, so prompt cardioversion may be necessary.[84,112] Junctional rhythms are also poorly tolerated in HCM, due to the loss of the atrial kick. Chronic atrial fibrillation can be controlled with β-blockers and verapamil, although this combination may be deleterious to some individuals with severe outflow obstruction and CHF.[84] Amiodarone is particularly effective in restoring normal sinus rhythm in HCM and reducing recurrences.[84]

Studies determining the risk of anesthesia with an uncommon disease such as HCM are rare. Haering et al[113] retrospectively reviewed 77 patients, half of whom had major and the other half minor noncardiac surgery with HCM defined by M-mode echocardiography. Based on the authors' definition of an adverse cardiac event, 40% of all patients had at least one adverse cardiac event. Among the patients who had major surgery, 57% had an adverse cardiac event. The type of surgery (major versus minor) and length of the surgery were predictors of adverse outcome but not indices of LV outflow obstruction. This study concluded that HCM patients with or without LV outflow obstruction are at increased risk for adverse cardiac outcomes defined as arrhythmias, CHF, hypotension, and myocardial ischemia. This is in contrast to Thompson et al,[109] who found no increased risk associated with anesthesia and HCM 20 years ago in noncardiac patients. The incidences of death and MI were low in this study, but only subjects undergoing noncardiac surgery were reviewed.[113]

Restrictive Cardiomyopathy

Restrictive cardiomyopathy (RCM) has included such entities as amyloidosis and eosinophilic endomyocardial disease. The 1995 WHO guidelines defined RCM as "restrictive filling and reduced diastolic volume of either or both ventricles with normal or near-normal systolic function and wall thickness."[39] Instead of being classified according to morphologic criteria, as are HCM and DCM, RCM is characterized by function. It may appear in the final stages of other cardiac conditions. Although a clinically challenging diagnosis to make, it is important to distinguish "restrictive" physiology from "constrictive" because management and treatment are decidedly different. Restrictive/constrictive physiology is not solely limited to RCM, but occurs in mitral stenosis, tricuspid stenosis, aortic stenosis, and other conditions.

RCM may be classified as myocardial (infiltrative, noninfiltrative, and storage) or endomyocardial (Box 24–1) according to etiology. RCM may be associated with another disease entity except pericardial disease. Restrictive myocardial disorders are characteristically atypical in presentation and hemodynamics at times, complicating perioperative management.

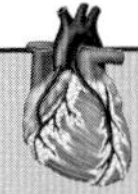

BOX 24–1 ***Classification of Types of Restrictive Cardiomyopathy According to Cause***

Myocardial

Noninfiltrative
- Idiopathic cardiomyopathy*
- Familial cardiomyopathy
- Hypertrophic cardiomyopathy
- Scleroderma
- Pseudoxanthoma elasticum
- Diabetic cardiomyopathy

Infiltrative
- Amyloidosis*
- Sarcoidosis*
- Gaucher's disease
- Hurler's disease
- Fatty infiltration

Storage diseases
- Hemochromatosis
- Fabry's disease
- Glycogen storage disease

Endomyocardial
- Endomyocardial fibrosis*
- Hypereosinophilic syndrome
- Carcinoid heart disease
- Metastatic cancers
- Radiation*
- Toxic effects of anthracycline*
- Drugs causing fibrous endocarditis (serotonin, methysergide, ergotamine, mercurial agents, busulfan)

*This condition is more likely than the others to be encountered in clinical practice.
From Kushwaha SS, Fallon JT, Fuster V: Medical progress: Restrictive cardiomyopathy. N Engl J Med 336:268, 1997.

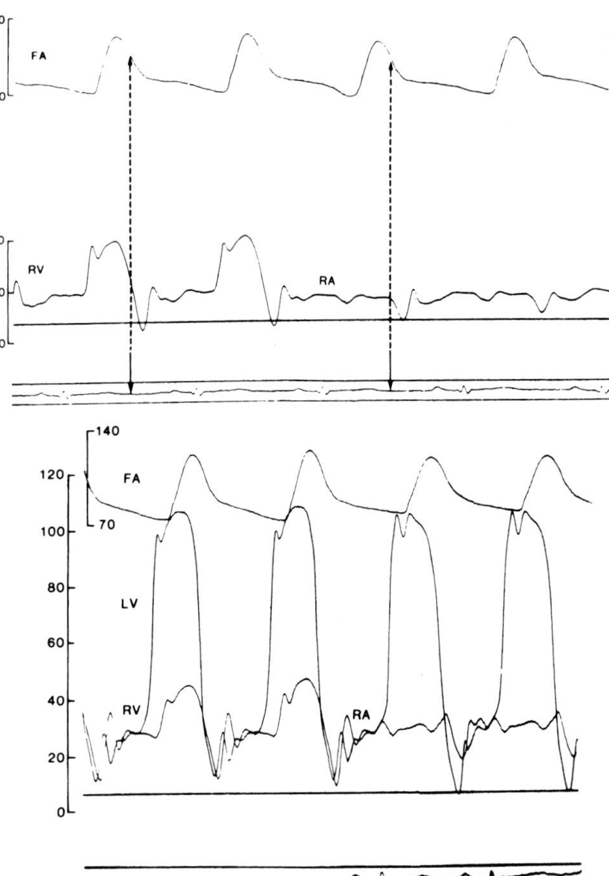

Figure 24–17 Intracardiac pressure tracings from a patient with idiopathic primary restrictive cardiomyopathy. *(Top)* Right ventricular (RV) and right atrial (RA) tracings with a typical diastolic square root configuration in the RV tracing and a prominent Y-descent in the early diastolic period of the RA tracing. FA = femoral artery. *(Bottom)* Simultaneous left ventricular (LV)–RV pressures and LV–RA pressures, showing a square root configuration in the LV tracing and equalization of pressures during diastole in the three chambers. FA = femoral artery. (Reprinted with permission from Giuliani ER, Fuster V, Gersh BJ, et al: Cardiology: Fundamentals and Practice. St. Louis, Mosby, 1991. By permission of Mayo Foundation.)

With idiopathic RCM, the cause is entirely unknown and lacks any identifiable histopathologic distinctiveness. Its occurrence is quite rare with few actual series in adults.[114] Reviews of the many types of RCM are available.[114-117]

Systolic function is minimally affected in RCM. Diastolic dysfunction is evident by abnormalities of ventricular relaxation and compliance. Impaired ventricular relaxation occurs before abnormal compliance. Poor compliance of the ventricle causes rapid filling in early diastole and the characteristic ventricular diastolic waveform of dip-and-plateau (square root sign) (Fig. 24–17). However, the characteristic dip-and-plateau pattern may be absent in 50% of individuals with RCM because it depends on the degree of impaired ventricular relaxation and the level of atrial driving pressure.[116] The atrial pressure waveform has the appearance of an "M" or a "W" pattern because of the rapid y-descent combined with a slightly greater x-descent. The rapid y-descent is due to the rapid early decline of the atrial pressure corresponding to the early diastolic ventricular filling. Filling early in diastole is accentuated and impeded during the rest of diastole due to reduced ventricular distensibility. Pressure in the ventricle rises precipitously in response to small volume. Once ventricular filling is restricted, the prognosis is much worse. Both ventricles appear thick with small cavities in contrast to the corresponding dilated atria despite normal LV volumes. Cardiomegaly or ventricular dilation should not exist. The left-sided pulmonary venous pressures usually exceed the right-sided venous pressures by 5 mm Hg. The pulmonary artery systolic pressure may also be elevated to 50 mm Hg.

Because one or both ventricles may be involved, symptoms may predominate as right- or left-sided. The elevated filling pressures that occur in early diastole of both ventricles lead to symptoms of right-sided failure manifested by elevated venous pressures and peripheral edema and ascites or of left-sided failure manifested by CHF and progressive dyspnea and orthopnea. Both groups of symptoms may occur separately or together. Insidious onset of fatigue and exertional dyspnea are common with RCM. These symptoms and signs should be present without evidence of cardiomegaly. The jugular venous pulse fails to fall during inspiration and may even rise (Kussmaul's sign).[115] Pulsus paradoxus is infrequent and nonspecific. The liver may be enlarged and actually pulsatile. The chest roentgenogram is nondiagnostic. Pulmonary congestion and normal or smaller-than-anticipated heart size are suggestive of RCM for adults. In contrast, most pediatric patients have cardiomegaly and severe atrial enlargement on chest roentgenogram and echocardiography (Fig. 24–18). The ECG may reflect abnormalities of depolarization such as bundle-branch block, low voltage, and QR or QS complexes, but these are not specific to RCM and rarely useful to distinguish RCM from constrictive pericarditis.

It is important to distinguish between RCM and constrictive pericarditis as the management of the two conditions varies greatly. Important distinguishing features of constrictive pericarditis and RCM are listed in Table 24–4. Both conditions have rapid and early diastolic filling with elevated filling pressures and normal filling volumes. In RCM, the impediment to filling is usually an infiltrative process involving the myocardium rather than the pericardium. Although not an absolute sign, the RV and LV end-diastolic pressures are elevated and equal with constrictive physiology, whereas end-diastolic pressure is usually 5 mm Hg higher on the left than on the right side in RCM because of the unequal compliance between the two ventricles in RCM.[114,118] However, symptoms and physical signs do not reliably differentiate between RCM and constrictive pericarditis.

Advances in echocardiography and other noninvasive methods have been used to try to reliably discriminate between pericardial disease and RCM. Classic Doppler findings are described in Table 24–5. Doppler findings may indicate the severity of RCM once the diagnosis is certain. Because the pericardium is responsible for constrictive pericarditis and a noncompliant ventricle for RCM, some differences exist between RCM and constrictive pericarditis regarding M-mode, two-dimensional, and Doppler examinations.[119] A pericardial thickness of 3 mm measured by echocardiography is highly suggestive of constrictive pericarditis. But overall, Doppler and echocardiography have insufficient sensitivity and specificity to provide a *clinically* significant differentiation between RCM and constrictive pericarditis. Consequently, cardiac catheterization is commonly performed and shows increased left and right venous pressures with large A and V waves in RCM (see Fig. 24–17). RA pressures of 15 to 20 mm Hg are not uncommon. The ventricular pressure curve has a diastolic dip-and-plateau pattern (square root sign) as described previously.

Endomyocardial biopsy may differentiate RCM from constrictive pericarditis. The biopsy in RCM is rarely normal

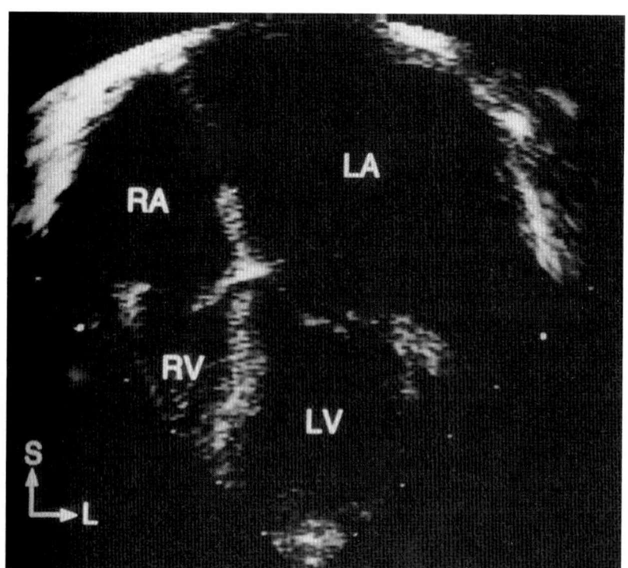

Figure 24–18 Two-dimensional echocardiogram, apical four-chamber projection, showing massive left atrial enlargement (left atrial dimension equals 29 mm) in 1-year-old girl with idiopathic restrictive cardiomyopathy. L = left; LA = left atrium; LV = left ventricle; RA = right atrium; RV = right ventricle; S = superior. (Reprinted with permission from Cetta F, O'Leary PW, Seward JB, Driscoll DJ: Idiopathic restrictive cardiomyopathy in childhood: Diagnostic features and clinical course. Mayo Clin Proc 70:634, 1995.)

Table 24–4 Differentiation of Pericardial Constriction Versus Myocardial Restriction

Characteristic	Constrictive Pericarditis	Restrictive Cardiomyopathy
Jugular venous waveform	Elevated with less rapid Y-descent	Elevated with more rapid Y-descent Large A waves
LAP > RAP	Absent	Almost always
Auscultation	Early S_3 high pitched; no S_4	Late S_3 low pitched; S_4 in some cases
Mitral or tricuspid regurgitation	Frequently absent	Frequently present
Chest roentgenogram	Calcification of pericardium (20% to 30%)	Pericardial calcification rare
Heart size	Normal to increased	Normal to increased
Electrocardiogram	Conduction abnormalities rare	Conduction abnormalities common
Echocardiogram	Slight enlargement of atria	Major enlargement of atria
Right ventricular pressure waveform	Square root pattern	Square root pattern; dip and plateau often less prominent
Right and left heart diastolic pressures (mm Hg)	Within 5 of each other in almost all cases	Seldom within 5 of each other
Peak right ventricular systolic pressure (mg Hg)	Almost always <60, sometimes <40	Usually >40 sometimes <60
Discordant respiratory variation of peak ventricular systolic pressures	Right and left are out of phase with respiration	In phase
Paradoxical pulse	Often present	Rare
CT/MRI imaging	Thickened pericardium	Rarely thickened pericardium
Endomyocardial biopsy	Normal or nonspecific changes	Nonspecific abnormalities

LAP = left atrial pressure; RAP = right atrial pressure; MRI = magnetic resonance imaging; CT = computerized axial tomography.
From Hancock EW: Cardiomyopathy: Differential diagnosis of restrictive cardiomyopathy and constrictive pericarditis. Heart 86:343, 2001; and Chatterjee K, Alpert J: Constrictive pericarditis and restrictive cardiomyopathy: Similarities and differences. Heart Failure Monit 3:118, 2003.

Table 24–5 **Doppler and Echocardiographic Features Differentiating Restrictive Cardiomyopathy and Constrictive Pericarditis**

Modality	Restrictive Cardiomyopathy	Constrictive Pericarditis
M-mode	No septal notch	Septal notch
Two-dimensional echocardiography	No septal shudder	Septal shudder
Pulsed wave mitral and tricuspid inflow	Less variation	Prominent respiratory variation (>10%) Significant decrease in IVRT from inspiration to expiration (usually noted in the first beat after expiration)
Pulsed wave pulmonary vein	Less variation S/D ratio <0.4	Significant increase (>18%) in peak diastolic velocity from inspiration to expiration S/D ratio ≥0.65 in inspiration
Pulsed wave hepatic veins		>25% reduction in diastolic forward flow Prominent late diastolic flow reversal after the onset of expiration
RVSP	>40 mm Hg	<40 mm Hg
Tricuspid regurgitation		Market inspiratory increase in peak velocity, time-velocity integral, and duration of jet
Tissue Doppler mitral annulus	E′ < 8 cm/s E/E′ >15	E′ ≥ 8 cm/s E/E′ <15
Color M-mode	Vp <45 cm/s	Vp ≥100 cm/s

IVRT, isovolumic relation time; S/D, systolic/diastolic; RVSP, right ventricular systolic pressure; E′, early peak velocity; Vp, propagation velocity.
From Tam JW, Shaikh N, Sutherland E: Echocardiographic assessment of patients with hypertrophic and restrictive cardiomyopathy: imaging and echocardiography. Curr Opin Cardiol 17:474, 2002.

compared with constrictive pericarditis. Although a biopsy may identify specific causes of restrictive myocardial physiology, more often only patchy endocardial and interstitial fibrosis with some myofibril hypertrophy is found.[114,118] If biopsy or tests such as radionuclide angiography, Doppler, or echocardiography do not identify either RCM or pericardial disease, exploratory surgery may be required. Although surgery is the most definitive method of differentiating RCM from constrictive pericarditis, the patient with RCM may not tolerate anesthesia and surgery well.[120]

There is no specific treatment for RCM. Various regimens have been developed based on the specific etiology of RCM[121] (Table 24–6). Diuretics are often administered to reduce pulmonary and venous congestion, but low CO with severe hypoperfusion is a risk. With the limited stroke volume, heart rate contributes significantly to CO. Atrial contraction is also important to maintain CO in these individuals. Anticoagulation with warfarin is important in view of the risk of thrombin formation with the large atria (Fig. 24–18). Surgical treatment for RCM is rare with the exception of endomyocardial fibrosis with eosinophilic cardiomyopathy. The fibrotic endocardium may be excised and the mitral or tricuspid valve replaced.

Survival with RCM depends largely on the etiology. True idiopathic RCM has a 5-year overall survival of 64%, but if increasing signs of pulmonary venous congestion appear, the prognosis worsens.[114] Transplantation is not always an option for adults with idiopathic RCM or other forms of RCM, because the conditions that led to RCM will affect the newly transplanted heart.

Anesthetic Considerations

Adults with RCM rarely require cardiac surgery for reasons other than transplantation or mitral or tricuspid valve replacement.[122] Occasionally, anesthesia is administered for a scheduled pericardiectomy only to find RCM instead of constrictive pericarditis. Despite essentially normal ventricular systolic function, diastolic dysfunction and filling abnormalities result in a poor CO and systemic perfusion.[118] Aggressive preoperative diuretic therapy may contribute to the difficulty of maintaining adequate circulating blood volume. Elevated airway pressures from pulmonary congestion may further impair oxygen delivery to the tissues.

For induction of anesthesia, medications associated with decreased venous return, bradycardia, or myocardial depression should be avoided. Fentanyl (30 μg/kg) or sufentanil (5 μg/kg) provides stable hemodynamics for induction and maintenance in patients with poor myocardial function.[67] These anesthetics maintain stable hemodynamics in patients undergoing cardiac surgery for valvular disease who have severely impaired preexisting volume or pressure loads on the heart and induce minimal hemodynamic fluctuation. Etomidate is an excellent alternative to fentanyl as an induction agent because it has minimal effect on contractility of the cardiac muscle, as demonstrated in patients undergoing cardiac transplantation.[70] Similarly, ketamine has been advocated for induction in patients with cardiac tamponade or constrictive pericarditis because sympathetic activity is preserved. Ketamine is an excellent choice to use with fentanyl for induction in patients with severe myocardial dysfunction due to cardiomyopathy. Concerns of exacerbating PAH with ketamine are unfounded if ventilation is maintained. Shorter-acting narcotics such as remifentanil may be unsuitable for patients with RCM due to a greater incidence of bradycardia and severe hypotension.[68] Fentanyl/etomidate/isoflurane has been shown to be superior to remifentanil/sevoflurane for maintenance of arterial pressure and heart rate.[69] Propofol may have no direct myocardial depression, but indirect inhibition of sympathetic activity and a vasodilatory property may cause hemodynamic instability in patients with RCM. The use of sevoflurane and desflurane have also been shown not to adversely affect the ability of the LV to respond to increased

Table 24–6 **Treatment Strategies in Restrictive Cardiomyopathy**

Etiology	Specific Symptom	Treatment
Idiopathic	To relieve congestion	Diuretics
	Control of heart rate	β-blockers, amiodarone, heart-rate-regulating CCB
	Atrial fibrillation: to maintain sinus rhythm paroxysmal or persistent	Amiodarone, dofetilide Long-term anticoagulation
	To control ventricular rate	β-Blockers, heart-rate-regulating calcium channel blockers, amiodarone, digoxin, atrioventricular node ablation, and pacemaker
	Atrioventricular block	Dual-chamber pacing
	To enhance myocardial relaxation	Calcium channel blockers (unproven), angiotensin inhibition (unproven)
	Refractory heart failure	Cardiac transplantation
Amyloidosis		Melphalan, prednisone, and colchicine; stem cell implant (under investigation); heart and liver transplant (in rare instances)
Hemochromatosis		Phlebotomy, desferrioxamine
Carcinoid heart disease		Somatostatin analogs; serotonin antagonists; valvuloplasty for severe tricuspid and pulmonary stenosis; valve replacement for severe tricuspid and pulmonary regurgitation
Sarcoidosis		Corticosteroids; pacemaker for heart block; implantable cardioverter-defibrillator for ventricular arrhythmia; cardiac transplant for refractory heart failure
Eosinophilic endocarditis		Initial stage: corticosteroids, hydroxyurea, vincristine
Endomyocardial fibrosis		Endocardiectomy with repair or replacement of tricuspid and mitral valves

CCB = Calcium channel blocker.
From Chatterjee K, Alpert J: Constrictive pericarditis and restrictive cardiomyopathy: Similarities and differences. Heart Failure Mont 3:125, 2003.

work despite their negative inotropic properties in patients undergoing CPB and cardiac surgery, making them attractive agents for maintenance of anesthesia in this population.[78]

Invasive hemodynamic monitoring and TEE are important because both left- and right-sided filling pressures do not accurately reflect ventricular volumes, so small volume shifts may greatly affect CO. Inotropic support is beneficial to maintain hemodynamics in these patients because of their risk of death from low CO. Despite chronic CHF, diuretics and vasodilators may be deleterious because higher filling pressures are needed to maintain CO. Some individuals may be sensitive to β-blockers and cardiac glycosides.[118] Patients may be chronically taking amiodarone, which has a negative inotropic effect that interacts with volatile agents to further reduce contractility and conduction, requiring careful titration of these anesthetic agents.[82]

Arrhythmogenic Right Ventricular Cardiomyopathy (ARVC)

Formerly called arrhythmogenic right ventricular dysplasia, ARVC is defined by the 1995 WHO as "progressive fibrofatty replacement of RV myocardium, initially with typical regional and later global RV and some LV involvement, with relative sparing of the septum."[39] Evidence of a more progressive involvement of not only the RV but also the LV with long-term follow-up convinced the WHO to classify ARVC as a "disease of the myocardium" that incorporates the many different clinical presentations and aspects of this condition.

ARVC is familial in at least 30% of people with primarily autosomal dominant inheritance.[44] The incidence and prevalence are uncertain, but it usually appears during adolescence, although it may occur in younger individuals. It presents with the onset of arrhythmias ranging from premature ventricular contractions to ventricular fibrillation originating from the RV. Diagnosis has been rare in the early stages but not at autopsy.[123,124] Identifying symptoms are absent even though structural changes exist in the myocardium. Postmortem examination reveals diffuse or segmental loss of myocardium, primarily in the RV, replaced with fat and fibrous tissue (Fig. 24–19, see Color Plates). These changes are believed to occur via three possible mechanisms: myoblasts differentiate to adipoblasts, apoptosis, or inflammation.[123] An inflammatory process is noticeable within the myocardial tissue. The replacement of myocardium with fat and fibrous tissue creates an excellent environment for a fatal arrhythmia, possibly the first sign of ARVC.[123] Sudden death occurs in up to 75% of patients, although it is difficult to accurately state in view of the extent of missed diagnosis. Sudden death occurs most often during sports-related exercise, primarily from ventricular tachycardia/fibrillation.[124] Twenty percent of patients die as a result of CHF.

The electrical instability characteristic of ARVC is not solely responsible for the natural history of the disease. Clinical presentation may range from asymptomatic myopathic involvement to overt clinical disease with diffuse biventricular involvement.[125] Progressive RV and LV dysfunction can be appreciated with serial echocardiography examinations. Myocardial loss with progressive ventricular dysfunction progresses ultimately to CHF. At end stage, ARVC may be difficult to distinguish from DCM because of the LV involvement that was discovered to be more common than previously believed. Diagnosis is based on the presence of criteria including ECG, structure, genetic studies, and arrhythmias.[123] Char-

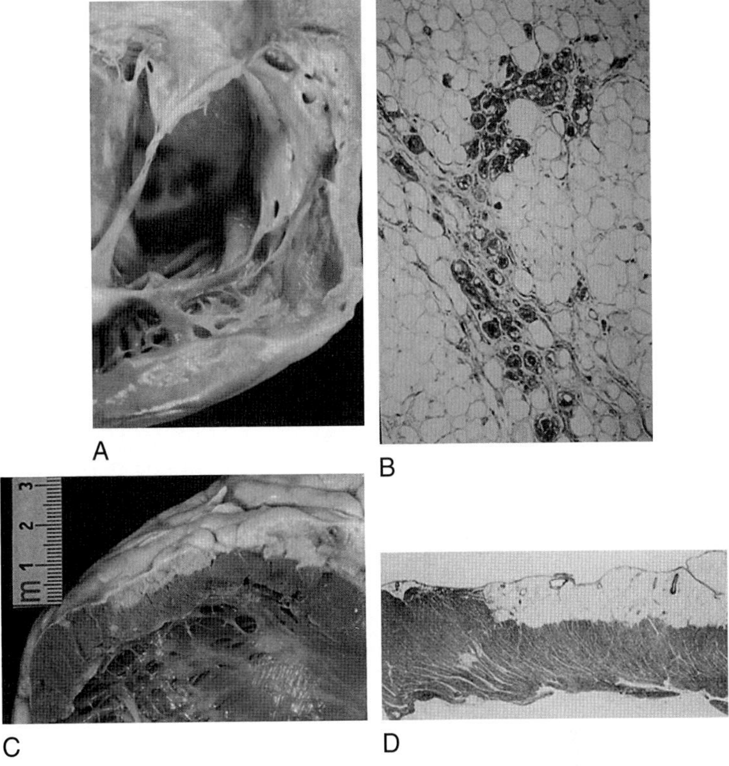

Figure 24–19 *(A)* Gross view of the RV outflow tract showing severe transmural loss of the RV free wall and an infundibular parchment-like aneurysm. *(B)* Histologic view at high magnification of surviving degenerated RV myocytes in the setting of extensive fatty replacement and tiny interstitial fibrosis. Gross *(C)* and histologic *(D)* sections of the anterior LV wall showing striking subepicardial fatty infiltration and fibrosis. (Reprinted with permission from Corrado D, Basso C, Thiene G, et al: Spectrum of clinicopathologic manifestations of arrhythmogenic right ventricular cardiomyopathy/dysplasia: A multicenter study. J Am Coll Cardiol 30:1517, 1997. Copyright 1997, with permission from The American College of Cardiology Foundation.) (See Color Plates.)

acteristics of the ECG include inverted T waves in the right precordial leads, QRS prolongation greater than 110 milliseconds, and extrasystoles with left bundle-branch block. Diagnosis may depend on endomyocardial biopsy to reveal the characteristic changes but may prove unrewarding because the biopsy sample is frequently obtained from the septal area of the myocardium where the characteristics of ARVC are often absent.[44]

Anesthetic Considerations

During the course of ARVC, arrhythmias may occur at any time. Presently, there are no guidelines for arrhythmia prevention. A family history of sudden death or syncope at an early age should heighten the awareness of ARVC.[123] With ARVC, arrhythmias are more likely in the perioperative period. During or after anesthesia, the patient should be carefully observed to avoid noxious stimuli, hypovolemia, hypercarbia, and light anesthesia. Acidosis may be especially detrimental due to its effect on arrhythmia generation and myocardial function. General anesthesia alone does not appear to be arrhythmogenic because reports describe multiple exposures to general anesthesia without arrhythmias. Houfani et al[124] reported that more than 200 patients with ARVC had undergone general anesthesia without a single cardiac arrest. Nonetheless, any family history of sudden death elicited during preoperative assessment merits further investigation. Anesthesia has been successfully conducted with propofol, midazolam, and alfentanil.[123] Amiodarone is the first line of antiarrhythmic medication during anesthesia.

Empiric administration of antiarrhythmic agents has been shown to be ineffective at preventing arrhythmias or sudden death in these patients.[125] Two adolescents undergoing routine procedures were reported to develop refractory arrhythmias and sudden death after general anesthesia.[124] Autopsy revealed typical features of ARVC. Sotalol appears to be the only antiarrhythmic that may reduce arrhythmias. Placement of an ICD is beneficial. Link et al[126] identified 12 patients with ARVC who had an ICD placed and determined 8 patients had appropriate discharges for ventricular tachycardia.

MITRAL VALVE PROLAPSE

Mitral valve prolapse (MVP), often referred to as Barlow's syndrome, is a structural and functional disorder affecting 2.5% to 5% of the population.[127] As the most commonly diagnosed cardiac valve abnormality, it occurs in adults who are otherwise healthy or in association with many pathologic conditions (Box 24–2). Women, representing two thirds of adults with MVP, are more frequently affected during the third, fourth, and fifth decades of life but account for a decreasing prevalence beyond the third decade.[128] The incidence of MVP in men is unrelated to age. MVP may be characterized as anatomic or functional (syndrome).[129] Anatomic MVP includes individuals with a broad range of valvular abnormalities corresponding to symptoms of progressive mitral valve regurgitation. MVP syndrome consists of MVP with various symptoms reflecting a neuroendocrine or an autonomic basis. Approximately 80% of patients with MVP experience MVP syndrome instead of anatomic MVP.

Anatomic MVP, inherited in an autosomal dominant manner, is believed to result from myxomatous degeneration of the mitral valve, elongation and thinning of the chordae tendineae, and the presence of redundant and excessive valve tissue.[128] The posterior leaflet is affected more frequently than the anterior leaflet. Changes are often observed at the site of chordal insertion, leading to rupture of the chordae and tethering of the valve leaflet. The degenerative changes of the mitral valve that are responsible for progression from an asymptomatic condition with murmurs and systolic clicks to

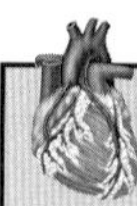

BOX 24–2 *Conditions Associated With Mitral Valve Prolapse*

Connective Tissue Disorders: Genetic

Mitral valve prolapse: isolated
The Marfan syndrome
Ehlers-Danlos syndrome: types I and II, IV
Pseudoxanthoma elasticum
Osteogenesis imperfecta
Polycystic kidneys

Other Genetic Disorders

Duchenne's muscular dystrophy
Myotonic dystrophy
Fragile X syndrome
Mucopolysaccharidoses

Acquired Collagen Vascular Disorders

Systemic lupus erythematosus
Relapsing polychondritis
Rheumatic endocarditis
Polyarteritis nodosa

Other Associated Disorders

Atrial septal defect, secundum
Hypertrophic obstructive cardiomyopathy
Wolff-Parkinson-White syndrome
Papillary muscle dysfunction
  Ischemic heart disease
  Myocarditis
Cardiac trauma
Post–mitral valve surgery
von Willebrand's disease

From Elsevier, O'Rourke RA (ed): Current Problems in Cardiology, May 1991, p 333.

dyspnea with severe mitral regurgitation occur over an average of 25 years.[130] With the onset of severe mitral regurgitation, PAH, left atrial enlargement, and atrial fibrillation frequently emerge. Subsequently, mitral valve repair or replacement is usually necessary within 1 year.

MVP syndrome is the more benign form of MVP in that the mitral valve annulus and LV size are essentially responsible for abnormal coaptation of the mitral leaflets during systole.[130] Mitral valve leaflets normally close just before ventricular systole, thus preventing regurgitation of blood into the LA (Fig. 24–20). Normal mitral valve leaflets may billow slightly with closure; but in MVP, redundant mitral leaflets prolapse into the LA during mid-to-late systole as the ventricle is emptied (see Fig. 24–20). Superior arching of the mitral leaflets above the level of the atrioventricular ring is diagnostic for MVP. Distortion or malfunction of any of the component structures of the mitral valve may cause prolapse and generate audible clicks or regurgitation associated with a murmur. If the chordae tendineae are lengthened, the valves may billow even more and progress to prolapse when valve leaflets fail to appose each other.

An array of symptoms has been associated with MVP syndrome, but most patients are asymptomatic. Altered autonomic function, catecholamine responsiveness, or possibly a combination of the two may account for symptoms of chest pain, fatigue, palpitations, dyspnea, dizziness, syncope, and panic attacks among others. However, controlled studies have identified palpitations as the only symptom linked to MVP.

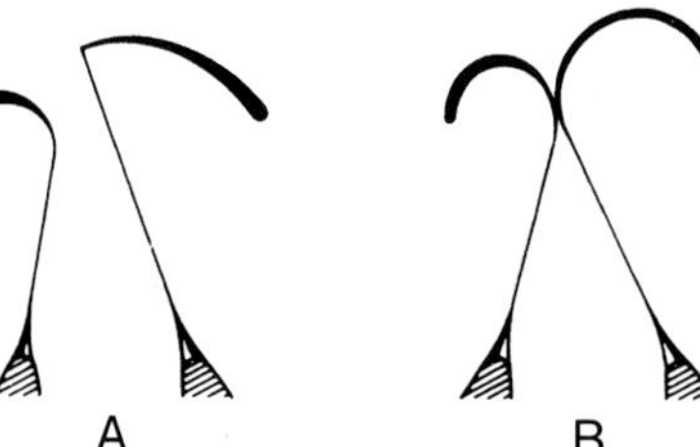

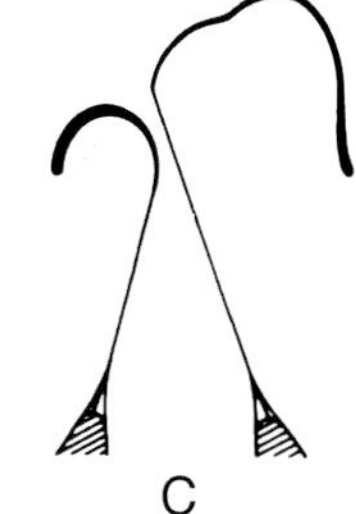

Figure 24–20 Diagrammatic representation of the functional pathology of the mitral valve mechanism. *(A)* Mitral valve prolapse. Regurgitation is present. *(B)* Billowing mitral valve without prolapse or regurgitation. *(C)* Billowing and prolapsed mitral leaflets with regurgitation. (Reprinted with permission from Barlow JB, Pocock WA: Mitral valve prolapse enigma—Two decades later. Mod Concepts Cardiovasc Dis 53:13, 1984. Copyright 1984, American Heart Association.)

Nearly 50% of patients describe palpitations.[128] Neuropsychiatric symptoms are no longer considered a part of MVP. Unique to MVP syndrome is the observation that symptoms may diminish or disappear over time.

There are no universal criteria for diagnosis of MVP. If auscultatory criteria are strictly applied, the diagnosis is reliable. Typical auscultatory features are mid-systolic click and late-systolic murmur. The click is related to deceleration of blood on the undersurface of the valve prolapsing into the LA. The murmur is late, with progressively increasing regurgitation that results in a crescendo systolic murmur. Although M-mode echocardiography is diagnostic, MVP is diagnosed more often now with two-dimensional echocardiography because recognition and assessment of the severity are superior.[128] Although a benign course is typical for many patients, serious complications such as severe mitral regurgitation, infective endocarditis, sudden death, and cerebral ischemia may occur.[131] The incidence of serious cardiovascular events in MVP was thought to be 2% to 4% per year, but data on 316 patients with MVP followed over 12 years demonstrated the incidence of cardiovascular morbidity and mortality to be just under 1% per year.[131,132]

Severe mitral regurgitation develops in approximately 2% to 4% of patients with MVP, two thirds of whom are male.[128] MVP is the most common cause of severe mitral regurgitation, and its onset signals the need for therapeutic intervention. Once dyspnea occurs secondary to mitral regurgitation, surgery is imminent. Mitral valve repair or replacement is effective and safe for mitral regurgitation due to MVP. Mitral valve repair is preferred for prolapse of a degenerative mitral posterior leaflet, but 10% of patients need mitral valve replacement instead. Mitral valve repair confers a significantly improved operative as well as 5- and 10-year survival compared with mitral valve replacement.[133] Early repair is recommended to preserve LV function and reduce the likelihood of atrial fibrillation. The Cox Maze procedure may be added safely to mitral valve repair with great effectiveness to reduce late complications of mitral valve disease.[134]

The association of arrhythmias and sudden death with MVP is a long-held observation. Premature atrial and ventricular beats, atrioventricular block, and supraventricular or ventricular tachyarrhythmias are common during ambulatory monitoring in adults with MVP.[135] Mechanisms that have been proposed for arrhythmias include ventricular enlargement, hyperadrenergic states, electrolyte imbalances, and mechanical irritation of the ventricle due to traction of the chordae tendineae.[135] Arrhythmias may be secondary to mitral regurgitation, not MVP. According to a study of individuals with nonischemic mitral regurgitation, complex arrhythmias were common and equally prevalent regardless of whether the patient had MVP.[136] Ventricular tachycardia occurred in 35% of those subjects with mitral regurgitation, in contrast to only 5% of participants with MVP alone. Similarly, the risk of sudden death for patients with MVP may be related to mitral regurgitation in view of a reduction in ventricular arrhythmias that occurred with mitral valve repair or replacement.

The occurrence of sudden death with MVP in adults has been argued for years.[137] Sudden death does occur within families of MVP patients.[135] The ECG is abnormal in approximately two thirds of patients with MVP. Nevertheless, EP testing has been unable to identify an arrhythmogenic focus or reliably identify those at increased risk. It is useful in the pharmacologic management of patients with ongoing complex sustainable arrhythmias.[135] Prophylaxis has not averted sudden death in high-risk patients with severe mitral regurgitation. An ICD is a consideration in patients with inducible ventricular tachycardia or ventricular fibrillation. In general, most patients do not require treatment for either their symptoms or prevention of sudden death.

MVP has been reported to be associated with cerebral ischemic events. Mitral cusp elongation and expansion that occur with MVP may generate thrombus, vegetation, and calcification of the mitral valve. Mobile masses have been found in conjunction with cerebral events. However, a population-based cohort study involving 1079 patients found no difference in the incidence of strokes in patients under 45 years of age with MVP unless another cardiac disease process was present.[138,139] Importantly, factors that were independently associated with stroke were advanced age, CAD, CHF, and diabetes.

Bacterial endocarditis is an infrequent complication of MVP, but its incidence is three to eight times greater in these individuals than in the general population.[128] Males are three times more likely to develop endocarditis. Guidelines from the American Heart Association are not specific concerning prophylaxis. Patients with isolated clicks probably do not benefit from antibiotic prophylaxis, nor is it cost effective.[128] Patients at higher risk of developing endocarditis (previous bacterial endocarditis, systolic murmurs, thickened leaflets, or mitral regurgitation) should receive antibiotics before undergoing procedures commonly associated with bacteremia. Patients with oral endotracheal intubation or fiberoptic bronchoscopy do not require antibiotic prophylaxis.[130]

Anesthetic Considerations

It is important to distinguish between MVP syndrome and anatomic MVP regarding anesthetic considerations. Most individuals with MVP have an uncomplicated general anesthetic because they have MVP syndrome. These patients are usually below 45 years of age with few risk factors for anesthesia. Invasive monitoring is usually unnecessary. Patients may be taking β-blockers. Preoperative sedation is useful to suppress an increased sensitivity to catecholamines. Painful stimuli may exacerbate the autonomic system, possibly causing arrhythmias. Significant decreases in LV end-diastolic volume and SVR, or increased contractility and tachycardia, should be avoided because MVP may be enhanced by decreasing CO and coronary perfusion. Intraoperative arrhythmias usually resolve spontaneously or respond to standard therapy. If an arrhythmia occurs, adequate oxygenation should be confirmed and other causes of intraoperative arrhythmias investigated. If β-blockers are required perioperatively, the use of esmolol avoids the potential for prolonged blockade that might cause hemodynamically significant bradycardia. Digoxin may worsen MVP.[130]

Anticholinergic preoperative medications are best avoided despite an increased vagal tone. A moderate anesthetic depth is desirable to minimize catecholamine levels and potential arrhythmias. Ketamine or drugs that have sympathomimetic effects must be cautiously administered. Volatile anesthetics sensitize the heart to catecholamines and potentially promote arrhythmias. Isoflurane is probably less sensitizing than halothane, yet autonomic imbalance may actually be more important in arrhythmogenesis than any direct effect of volatile agents in patients with MVP. These patients with MVP syndrome have been shown to possess good LV function if mitral regurgitation or CAD is absent; myocardial depression from volatile agents will be well tolerated.[140] Narcotics such as fentanyl block sympathetic responses and promote hemodynamic stability; however, prolonged postoperative respiratory depression is a disadvantage. Shorter-acting narcotics such as alfentanil and remifentanil, as well as other intravenous agents such as propofol, are available to facilitate rapid extubation.[141] Hypercapnia, hypoxia, and electrolyte disturbances increase ventricular excitability and should be corrected. If muscle relaxation is desired, vecuronium is an excellent choice because it does not cause tachycardia.

Patients with anatomic MVP warrant a different anesthetic approach compared with those with MVP syndrome. Patients with anatomic MVP are often in CHF and generally require cardiac surgery and CPB. The severity of mitral regurgitation strongly influences anesthetic decisions. Routine monitoring for patients undergoing cardiac surgery should be provided. TEE is placed after induction. Opioid agents provide excellent hemodynamic stability without depressing myocardial function.[67] Although avoidance of ketamine has been recommended by some for patients with MVP, it is an excellent choice to preserve hemodynamic stability in patients who are severely ill, especially when used in combination with opioids such as fentanyl, because ketamine better preserves sympathetic activity, which is important in the preservation of blood pressure in severe CHF. A more extensive review of anesthetic management of valvular disease is found in Chapter 20.

ACUTE PULMONARY EMBOLISM

Pulmonary embolism (PE) has an incidence in the United States of 1 per 1000 and a mortality rate of more than 15% at 3 months after diagnosis.[142] Approximately two thirds of deaths occur within the first hour of a PE, and many of the remaining occur within 4 to 6 hours.[143] Because 5% of patients present in cardiogenic shock, treatment involves not only prevention of a recurrence but also hemodynamic support.[144] Because a correct diagnosis can alter the outcome of PE measurably, it is unfortunate that 60% to 80% of cases of fatal PE in the hospital setting are clinically unsuspected.[145]

Formation of thrombus involves stasis, activation of coagulation, and vascular injury. Asymptomatic venous thrombus, originating primarily from proximal deep veins, is the source of pulmonary emboli in 80% of patients with documented PE.[146] The potent fibrinolytic capacity of the lung dissolves most emboli spontaneously, rendering them clinically silent. Although the likelihood of a genetic predisposition for venous thrombosis is now more evident, well-known risk factors for a clinically recognizable PE include advanced age, previous venous thromboembolism, prolonged immobility or paralysis, malignancy, CHF, use of oral contraceptives, obesity, prolonged mechanical ventilation, and surgery that involves extensive pelvic or abdominal dissection.[147] Compared with community residents, hospitalized individuals are 100 times more likely to develop venous thromboembolism and PE.[148] Immobility has been noted in more than 50% of patients within 3 months of a PE.[149] In most cases, immobility after surgery was less than 2 weeks.

A diagnosis of PE has always been problematic. In 1975, it was reported that only 29% of patients who survived 1 hour after PE were correctly diagnosed, and since then there has been little improvement.[147,150] A high index of suspicion is necessary to diagnose PE because symptoms are so nonspecific. Dyspnea, pleuritic chest pain, and hemoptysis are characteristic of a mild PE. Dyspnea is the most common symptom, occurring in 73% of patients with PE, followed by pleuritic chest pain (66%) and hemoptysis (13%).[149] Dyspnea, chest pain, or tachypnea occurs in 97% of documented cases.[151] However, symptoms or signs of venous thrombosis in the lower extremities appear in fewer than 25% of patients with documented PE.[152] Thirty percent of patients may be asymptomatic.[153] Even if classic signs and symptoms are present, a subsequent pulmonary angiogram may be negative. The multicenter study Prospective Investigation of Pulmonary Embolism Diagnosis (PIOPED) found that symptoms are as likely to be present in a patient with a negative angiogram as in a patient with a positive one.[147]

Objective testing is necessary to exclude or to establish a diagnosis of PE, but some tests are too insensitive and nonspecific. A large alveolar-to-arterial (A-a) oxygen gradient and respiratory alkalosis are common in PE, but an arterial oxygen pressure (PaO_2) greater than 80 mm Hg or a normal A-a oxygen gradient does not exclude PE.[142,149] A normal PaO_2 may occur in patients with PE who are able to hyperventilate. Similarly, a low PaO_2 is not diagnostic of PE; but in the PIOPED study, 74% of patients with PE had a PaO_2 of less than 80 mm Hg.[147] Arterial blood gas results may be more helpful in assessing the severity of a PE than in diagnosing it. A chest roentgenogram may show atelectasis or pulmonary parenchymal abnormalities in two thirds of these individuals and be normal in another 15%.[149,154] Its only value is to exclude other pulmonary conditions. Classic ECG findings of RV strain and $S_1Q_3T_3$ are uncommon except with a massive PE. Left-axis deviation occurs as often as right-axis deviation with PE. P pulmonale, RV hypertrophy, right-axis deviation, or right bundle-branch block was noted in only 6% of PIOPED patients.[147] Even in patients with echo-documented increased RV end-diastolic diameter and tricuspid regurgitation, there were three sets of specific ECG abnormalities.[155] The ECG is primarily useful to exclude conditions that may mimic PE such as MI or pericarditis. D-dimer enzyme-linked immunosorbent assay has been shown to have an excellent negative predictive value (99.6%) for acute PE.[156] Additionally, the D-dimer–to–fibrinogen ratio of greater than 103 is highly specific for acute PE.[157] These tests may someday reduce the number of CT and lung scans used to evaluate PE.

The most widely used technique to evaluate suspected PE is the technetium-xenon lung scan. As a cornerstone of diagnosis for PE, it is least affected by preexisting cardiac or pulmonary disease. A negative scan essentially eliminates a PE, and a high-probability scan has a positive predictability of 85%.[151] However, only 13% of patients suspected of PE had a high-probability scan and only 41% of suspected patients who had positive angiography had high-probability scans in the PIOPED study.[151] A corroborating clinical history increases the predictive ability of a lung scan.[154] A high-probability scan with low clinical suspicion was positive for PE in 56% of individuals. An intermediate scan was associated with a 30% likelihood of PE. Spiral CT scanning is gaining as the preferred imaging modality for acute PE.[142] It allows imaging of large areas of the chest, visualizing the pulmonary arteries with one large breath. It has a sensitivity and specificity of 90% and 90%, respectively, which give it a positive and negative predictive value of 93% and 94%, respectively.[154] Replication of the accuracy of these results may depend on the generation of scanner that is used. Spiral CT is also able to assist in the diagnosis if PE is not present, in contrast to the ventilation/perfusion ($\dot{V}/\dot{Q}$) scan. It may become the first test to obtain for moderate-to-high clinical suspicion of PE.[145] The need for anticoagulation in those at high risk for complications with anticoagulation may be better assessed by spiral CT.[158] In a retrospective review of 1500 consecutive patients suspected of acute PE, anticoagulation was withheld based on a negative spiral CT and the incidence of PE was very low.[159]

Echocardiography is not recommended to definitively diagnose PE.[160] There are some typical features of a large PE seen with echocardiography (Fig. 24–21). However, echocardiography has emerged as the principal tool to assess the risk of mortality during acute PE.[161] Patients fall into three categories—low risk (no RV dysfunction), submassive PE (RV dysfunction with preservation of systolic blood pressure), and massive PE (RV dysfunction and shock)—that carry an in-hospital mortality of less than 4%, 5% to 10%, and greater than 30%, respectively.[160] RV function is significant because it is an independent predictor of mortality.[162]

Pulmonary angiography is still the gold standard as it detects about 98% of all clinically significant PE.[147,163] It may actually be underused as fewer than 15% of patients with nondiagnostic $\dot{V}/\dot{Q}$ scans undergo angiography.[154] It is a contributing factor in the death of fewer than 0.5% of patients.[164] Most of those who die or have major nonfatal complications after angiography are in critical condition prior to angiography. Chronic PAH, respiratory failure, or RV failure heightens the risk of angiography. Complications such as tachyarrhythmias, myocardial injury, cardiac perforation, cardiac arrest, and hypersensitivity reactions to contrast media occur in 1% to 4% of patients.

A PE may occur in all operative settings, but recognition is difficult during general anesthesia.[165] The extensive pulmonary vascular network of the lung may be obliterated up to 50% by a clot, yet $\dot{V}/\dot{Q}$ match would be minimally affected. If additional pulmonary vasculature is removed physiologically, the pulmonary vascular resistance (PVR) increases and the RV dilates and fails because it cannot alter its stroke volume appreciably against increasing afterload. Abrupt hemodynamic changes may appear with the onset of a PE, but many factors may similarly influence intraoperative hemodynamics, not only PE. Meanwhile, other symptoms and signs of respiratory distress such as wheezing, cyanosis, hypoxemia, and hypocapnea may not occur during anesthesia. Capnography and pulse oximetry are nonspecific. Even if the patient is being monitored with a PAC, acute onset of PAH with a normal pulmonary capillary wedge pressure may also represent hypoxia, pneumothorax, pulmonary aspiration, vasoconstrictive medications, or air embolism.[166] Assessment of RV

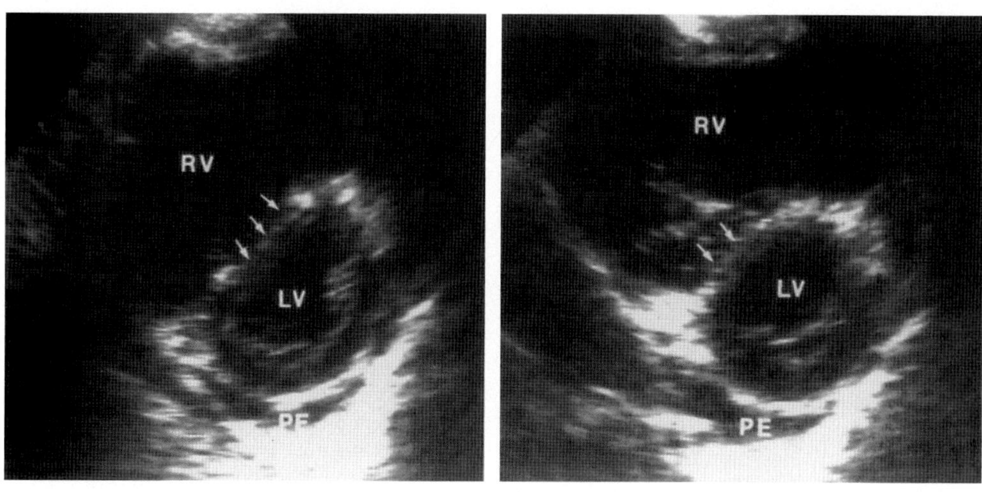

Figure 24–21 Typical findings on transthoracic echocardiography in patients with massive pulmonary embolism. In patients with pulmonary embolism, the transthoracic echocardiogram rarely shows thrombus; instead, findings suggestive of pulmonary embolism may be observed. Shown here are parasternal short-axis views of the right ventricle (RV) and left ventricle (LV) in diastole *(left)* and systole *(right)* in a patient with angiographically proved pulmonary embolism. There is diastolic and systolic bowing of the interventricular septum *(arrows)* into the left ventricle, a finding compatible with the presence of right ventricular volume overload and pressure overload, respectively. The left ventricle has assumed a classic D-shaped configuration, indicating impaired left ventricular relaxation. The right ventricle is appreciably dilated and markedly hypokinetic, with little change in the apparent right ventricular area from diastole to systole. There is a small pericardial effusion (PE). (Reprinted with permission from Goldhaber SZ: Echocardiography in the management of pulmonary embolism. Ann Intern Med 136:693, 2002.)

Figure 24–22 Pathophysiology of right ventricular dysfunction, ischemia, and infarction after acute pulmonary embolism. PA = pulmonary artery; RV = right ventricle; LV = left ventricle; O_2 = oxygen. (Reprinted with permission from Lualdi JC, Goldhaber SZ: Right ventricular dysfunction after acute pulmonary embolism: Pathophysiologic factors, detection, and therapeutic implications. Am Heart J 130:1276, 1995.)

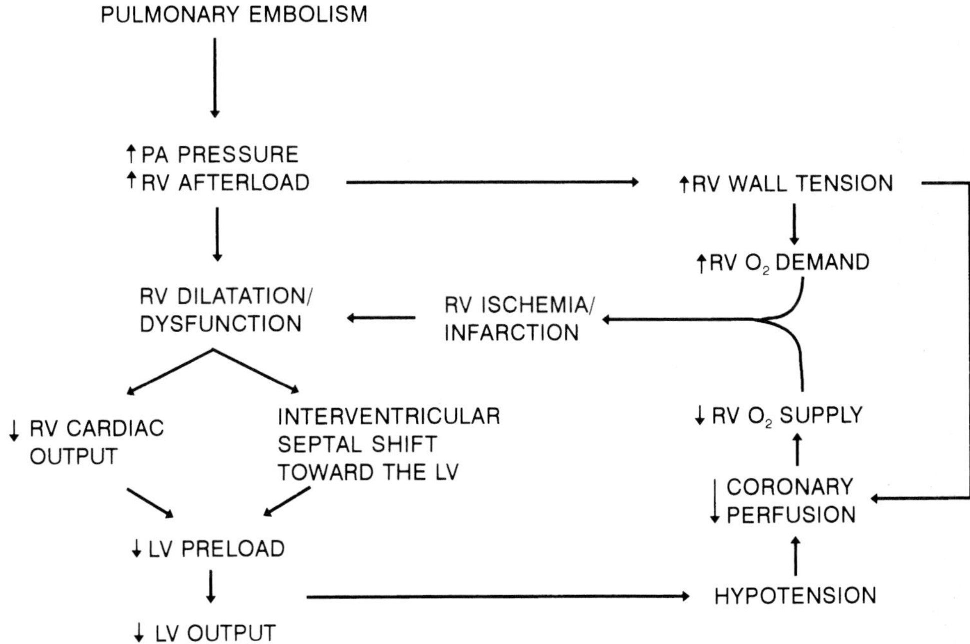

dysfunction with TEE better delineates PE as well as assesses and guides therapeutic measures.[160]

Massive PE represents 5% of cardiac arrests with more than 60% of those noted to be pulseless electrical activity.[160] Symptoms include severe dyspnea, cyanosis, tachycardia, and elevated central venous pressure. Massive PE is defined as 50% obstruction of pulmonary blood flow that usually leads to RV failure. Upon mechanical obstruction, humoral mediators are released, augmenting pulmonary vasoconstriction and PAH. This sudden increase in RV afterload results in RV dilation and dysfunction that displaces the interventricular septum, causing underfilling of the LV (Fig. 24–22). Low CO and severe hypotension follow, ultimately leading to circulatory collapse and death.[160,167] Increased RV pressure also compresses the right coronary artery, causing RV ischemia and contributing to RV failure.[168] Mortality is 40% to 80% within 2 hours of the onset of a PE.

Massive PE should be considered with the onset of unexplainable severe and sudden hypoxia and hypotension. The diagnosis is strengthened if LV function is relatively maintained in the midst of profound RV dysfunction.[160] The differential diagnosis is cardiac tamponade, MI, aortic dissection, and severe mitral regurgitation.[169] Interventions that improve RV function should receive priority as they may greatly benefit the patient.[168] Excessive fluid administration to correct hypotension must be avoided to prevent further RV dilation. Hemodynamic management after massive PE is often derived from case reports and animal studies.[170] Norepinephrine

(epinephrine) is the vasoactive agent of choice to achieve hemodynamic stability. Although isoproterenol is appealing due to its β-adrenergic properties and pulmonary vasodilation, RV perfusion pressure may fall, worsening RV ischemia.[169]

A major goal of treating PE is the prevention of new thrombi and death. Recurrence of PE is a major risk and is associated with a very high mortality. Frequently, the initial clot of a PE is small and symptoms are few or nonspecific, but a subsequent clot may significantly increase PVR and compromise hemodynamics without a clear warning. Prevention of recurrence may include one or more of the following: anticoagulation, thrombolysis, mechanical interruption (vena caval filters), and embolectomy.

Anticoagulation lessens morbidity, mortality, and recurrence of PE by addressing venous thromboembolism.[146] In general, if a patient has a high-probability $\dot{V}/\dot{Q}$ scan and there is strong clinical suspicion, anticoagulation is begun. Anticoagulation is initiated with a heparin bolus of 10,000 to 20,000 U, immediately followed by a heparin infusion to maintain the activated partial thromboplastin time at 1.5 to 2 times control.[171] There is no recognized benefit to the use of low-molecular-weight heparin versus unfractionated heparin (see Chapter 29). Subsequently, an oral anticoagulant is continued for *at least* 3 months. Clot is present in most patients 1 to 4 weeks after treatment with anticoagulation alone. If PE recurs during anticoagulation, a continuing predisposition to PE exists, or there is a contraindication to anticoagulation, a Greenfield filter is placed transvenously in the inferior vena cava in order to prevent a fatal embolus. It is effective in 98% of cases but does not provide absolute protection.[143]

With the advent of fibrinolytic agents that convert circulating plasminogen to plasmin, clots in the pulmonary arteries can be lysed, thus removing or decreasing mechanical obstruction to pulmonary blood flow. This is referred to as thrombolytic therapy. There is no absolute indication for it with PE, but consideration is given if pulmonary blood flow is reduced by 40% to 50% with severe hypoxia or right-sided failure and/or deteriorating hemodynamics are present.[172] Successful thrombolysis may reverse right-sided heart failure. Although no large randomized trials have been performed, combining the results of previous thrombolytic trials demonstrated a 50% reduction in the overall mortality of PE with thrombolytic therapy compared with heparin anticoagulation alone.[169] Thrombolytic agents are now recognized as superior to heparin therapy alone for correcting defects found on angiographic and perfusion scans and for correcting hemodynamic abnormalities including RV dysfunction.[160] Fewer complications and more rapid improvement occur with thrombolytic therapy than with heparin alone.[167,173] There is also a reduced incidence of recurrent PE compared with heparin therapy, in part due to a resolution of the probable underlying venous thrombus and less RV hypokinesis.[160] Nonetheless, anticoagulation with heparin should be started simultaneously with thrombolytic therapy. Based on RV dysfunction identified on echocardiography and impending right-sided heart failure, thrombolysis and anticoagulation together provide better results than anticoagulation alone.[144]

Streptokinase and urokinase are the most commonly used fibrinolytic agents. Because they are not fibrin specific, there is an increased risk of severe bleeding compared with heparin alone (22% versus 7.8%, respectively).[167] The development of more specific thrombolytic agents, such as recombinant tissue-type plasminogen activator (rt-PA), that preferentially activate plasminogen in the presence of fibrin should lessen severe bleeding. Direct comparisons of rt-PA and urokinase in two separate trials, however, found no statistically significant differences between the two fibrinolytic agents.[174]

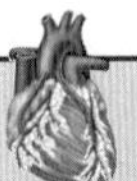

BOX 24–3 *Contraindications to Thrombolytic Therapy*

Absolute Contraindications

- Active internal bleeding
- Recent (within 2 months) cerebrovascular accident or other active intracranial processes

Relative Contraindications

- Recent (<10 days) major surgery
- Recent obstetric delivery
- Recent organ biopsy
- Gastrointestinal bleeding within 10 days
- Recent previous puncture of noncompressible vessels
- Recent serious trauma within 15 days
- Neurosurgery or ophthalmologic surgery within a month
- Severe hypertension (systolic >180 mm Hg, diastolic >110 mm Hg)
- Bacterial endocarditis
- Recent minor trauma including cardiopulmonary resuscitation
- High likelihood of left heart thrombus (eg, mitral stenosis with atrial fibrillation)
- Pregnancy
- Diabetic hemorrhagic retinopathy
- Platelet count <100,000/mm^3, prothrombin time less than 50%

From Raskob GE, Hull RD: Diagnosis and management of pulmonary thromboembolism. Q J Med 76:787, 1990.

There are contraindications to thrombolysis (Box 24–3). Bleeding is the major concern, and a neurologic event within 3 months of potential thrombolysis is a relative contraindication.[167,172] Bleeding complications are more likely with thrombolysis than with heparin alone, particularly if the patient has undergone pulmonary angiography. Specific thrombolytic agents, such as rt-PA, reduce bleeding complications. It is paramount to detect any neurologic deterioration in a patient receiving thrombolysis. Intracranial bleeding, the most feared complication, occurs in 1.9% of patients receiving thrombolysis.[144] It is a medical emergency. Bleeding can be treated with immediate transfusion of 10 units of cryoprecipitate and 2 units of fresh frozen plasma.

Beyond thrombolysis, pulmonary embolectomy remains an option for massive PE if pharmacologic thrombolysis has been unsuccessful. Echocardiography is particularly valuable in the triage of patients to either thrombolysis, catheter embolectomy, or surgical embolectomy.[169,175] As previously noted, RV function after PE is a major determinant of outcome, so aggressive efforts to reverse RV dysfunction should be pursued early after the onset of PE. Multiple percutaneous techniques are available to treat massive PE that include local catheter-directed thrombolytic therapy, thrombus aspiration with mechanical fragmentation techniques, and percutaneous mechanical thrombectomy.[170] The rationale for proximal clot dissolution is that the significantly greater cross-sectional area of the peripheral pulmonary arterioles than the central pulmonary arteries will permit the clot to travel distally and be tolerated far better hemodynamically than central pulmonary artery obstruction. Catheter embolectomy reduces embolic load with suction of clot in the pulmonary artery through a venotomy site, but mortality may reach 32%.[170] Percutaneous mechanical thrombectomy uses a combination of devices to fragment the thrombus.[176]

Anesthesia Considerations for Pulmonary Embolectomy and Pulmonary Embolism

The first surgical embolectomy without CPB was described by Trendelenburg in 1908, and the first with CPB was described by Cooley in 1961. Its frequency has decreased, partly due to the success of thrombolytic measures for massive PE; however, thrombolysis is unsuccessful in 15% to 30% of cases.[177] Of 3000 patients with documented PE over a 20-year period, 3% underwent pulmonary embolectomy.[177] In general, it has been reserved for patients with PE and refractory circulatory compromise, failed medical management, or contraindications to thrombolysis.[163] Contraindication to thrombolysis accounts for more than one third of embolectomies.[173] Opinions vary, but some clinicians deny an indication for embolectomy, arguing that those who survive embolectomy would have survived with medical therapy alone as well. Yet, 25% of patients deteriorate hemodynamically 24 to 48 hours after a major PE, signifying that the risk of death after PE does not decrease with time. The overall mortality of pulmonary embolectomy varies between 20% and 90%.[163,178] Most patients awaiting embolectomy are in sustained, acute shock; up to two thirds require closed-chest massage.[72,177] The patient's preoperative status is predictive of survival.[72] Preoperative cardiac arrest increases operative mortality by more than 50%. Age greater than 60 years and a long history of dyspnea also increase the mortality of embolectomy. Echocardiography has greatly decreased the time to surgery by enabling a rapid and reliable diagnosis to be made without angiography.[160] This has improved not only initial survival rate of embolectomy but also long-term survival.

Induction of anesthesia is a very hazardous period in the presence of PE and RV dysfunction that has precipitated cardiac arrest.[72] Intraoperative monitoring should include an arterial catheter, ECG, pulse oximeter, capnograph, and CVP catheter or PAC. An inotrope may also be needed prior to induction.[173] Individuals with massive PE have more of a "fixed" CO, which makes them extremely susceptible to decreases in volume and SVR.[72,179] Cannulation of the femoral vessels under local anesthetic in order to initiate CPB may be advisable if the administration of anesthesia is judged too hazardous. Once the cannula is in place, positioning, skin cleansing, and draping should proceed while the patient is awake and breathing oxygen. After the patient is placed in a slightly head-down position to prevent venous pooling, an intravenous induction is performed. Anesthetic agents that increase PVR must be used cautiously in this setting. Ketamine is well known as an anesthetic agent for use in critically ill patients to maintain hemodynamics.[71,72] In an animal model of septic shock, ketamine preserved hemodynamics and hypoxic tissues better than halothane, isoflurane, and alfentanil.[180] Concerns about ketamine and increased PVR are unfounded if ventilation is maintained.

Embolectomy via right or left thoracotomy may be performed without CPB through venous inflow occlusion while clamping the proximal portion of the involved pulmonary artery to allow clot removal. Rapid institution of CPB by femoral cannulation percutaneously may be lifesaving in patients with cardiovascular collapse.[181] If embolectomy is performed on CPB, the patient remains normothermic, the aorta is not cross-clamped, and cardioplegia is not administered.[163,177] Maintenance of higher perfusion pressures reduces RV stunning. The CPB time is usually less than 30 minutes for embolectomy. Reperfusion bleeding may occur when reestablishment of pulmonary blood flow causes severely damaged capillaries of the pulmonary parenchyma to rupture. Large amounts of blood may be aspirated from the endotracheal tube (ETT). Large-bore intravenous catheters are necessary for embolectomy because rapid and massive blood loss can occur through reperfusion pulmonary hemorrhage.[182]

The hemodynamics of the patient primarily depend on the degree of pulmonary vascular obstruction. The inotrope of choice for patients with RV dysfunction is norepinephrine. It improves RV function with a direct inotropic effect and maintains RV perfusion. When titrated to maintain a moderate blood pressure, ventricular performance improved while PVR did not increase significantly.[183] Dobutamine and epinephrine are also effective, but isoproterenol should be avoided.[167] Isoproterenol decreases PVR and is associated with arrhythmias, hypotension, and a worse outcome.[183] If severe hypotension is present during PE, isoproterenol likely worsens it and reduces survival, based on an experimental animal model of PE; in contrast, norepinephrine increased survival in this model.[184] The use of a pure α-agonist to increase the blood pressure during PE is not recommended because RV function may worsen. With acute RV failure, gentle preload reduction may improve the congested pulmonary circulation. An RA pressure of 15 to 20 mm Hg is usually adequate; however, the RA pressure may be too unreliable in RV failure. In this setting, it is important to avoid RV distention that inevitably worsens hemodynamics.[183]

It is also extremely important to implement measures to decrease PVR, such as treating acidosis and maintaining hypocapnea, without excessively increasing airway pressure.[165] None of the currently used intravenous agents for PAH demonstrate ideal selectivity for the pulmonary vasculature (see Pulmonary Arterial Hypertension). During the past 10 years, the effects of nitric oxide (NO) during PE have been studied.[185,186] PAP was noted to fall 10% to 20% while PVR fell 20% to 30%. Animal models of PE have demonstrated modest reductions in PAP and PVR with NO without significantly affecting systemic hemodynamics. Furthermore, NO inhibits platelet function, possibly lessening subsequent episodes of thrombosis and release of vasoactive substances that cause pulmonary vasoconstriction. Platelet inhibition with NO is rapidly reversible. The benefit of NO in PE has not been adequately investigated and requires well-designed prospective randomized trials to establish its role in PE, but it appears promising.

PULMONARY ARTERIAL HYPERTENSION (PAH)

PAH, according to the 2004 WHO classification, is defined as a group of diseases characterized by virtually identical obstructive pathologic changes of the pulmonary microcirculation and by a favorable response to the long-term administration of prostacyclin.[187] The WHO classifies PAH into the following groups: I—primary PAH and PAH associated with such conditions as collagen vascular disease, portal hypertension, and left-to-right shunting; II—pulmonary venous hypertension; III—pulmonary disease with hypoxemia; IV—thromboembolic disease; and V—miscellaneous.[188] When no demonstrable cause for a sustained increase in PAP can be identified, the diagnosis is primary PAH. Regardless of the primary pathologic mechanisms, once PAH exists, the effects on the right heart and pulmonary arteries are similar.[189]

Primary Pulmonary Hypertension

The essential characteristic of primary PAH is increased PVR that results in increased PAP, hypoxemia, elevated RV pressure, right heart failure, and death. The National Institutes of Health registry's criteria for primary PAH include a PAP of more than 25 mm Hg at rest or more than 30 mm Hg with exercise and exclusion of the causes of secondary PAH.[190] It is a rare disorder, occurring in one or two individuals per 1 million people per year, primarily women in their third decade. The diagnosis is often delayed an average of 2 years due to the nonspecific nature of the symptoms. Previously, even an early diagnosis yielded a median survival of 2.8 years.[191] The introduction of intravenous epoprostenol (synthetic salt of prostacyclin) in the 1990s improved hemodynamics, functional capacity, and survival in patients with primary PAH in New York Heart Association functional class III or IV.[192] Treatment options have expanded as a new generation of drugs is being developed to address the pathologic arms of primary PAH.

The pulmonary vasculature is a low-pressure, high-flow circuit balancing vasodilation and constriction, tilting toward vasodilation. The endothelium modulates vascular smooth muscle cell activity through the production of various vasodilators (prostacyclin and NO) and vasoconstrictors (thromboxane A_2 and endothelin). The endothelium of the lung is markedly different from endothelium of the systemic vasculature.[193] Although the stimuli that trigger primary PAH may differ, an undefined injury to the endothelium occurs that causes increased coagulation, proliferation, and vasoconstriction that are instrumental to the development of PAH[193] (Fig. 24–23). The endothelium releases thromboxane A_2, a potent vasoconstrictor, cell proliferator, and powerful platelet activator, in addition to prostacyclin, a potent vasodilator and potent inhibitor of platelet aggregation.[187] Mediator imbalance results in pulmonary vasoconstriction that leads to the disordered endothelial cell proliferation in combination with proliferation of intimal cells that forms the characteristic plexiform lesions (Fig. 24–24). However, there is no specific histopathologic lesion that defines primary PAH. Evidence of proliferative and obliterative intimal lesions composed of myofibroblasts is found in the pulmonary arteries and arterioles from increased production of endothelial mediators. Additionally, thickened arterial smooth muscle (isolated medial hypertrophy), destruction and fibrosis of vessel walls, and in situ thrombosis (see Fig. 24–24) lead to stiffening of the arteries, contributing to greater vasoconstriction. Eventually, the endothelial mediators that maintain the low-pressure, high-flow pulmonary circulation (NO, endothelium-derived hyperpolarizing factor, natriuretic peptides, adrenomedullin, and β_2-agonists) are lost and PAP increases at rest and exercise. Regardless of the primary pathophysiologic pathways to PAH, a similar end-point is reached.

Gradual onset of shortness of breath is the earliest symptom of PAH. Right-sided chest pain, syncope, fatigue, and peripheral edema may be present. Physical examination often focuses on identifying conditions frequently associated with PAH. Multiple risk factors contribute to PAH (Fig. 24–25). Figure 24–26 outlines an algorithm for the evaluation of PAH. Cardiac catheterization is required to assess the left and right cardiac hemodynamics. There is no cure for primary PAH.

Therapy for primary PAH is evolving but mostly remains empiric and nonspecific. Conventional therapy includes restricted activity, diuretics, anticoagulation, digoxin, and pulmonary vasodilators. For years, calcium channel blockers have

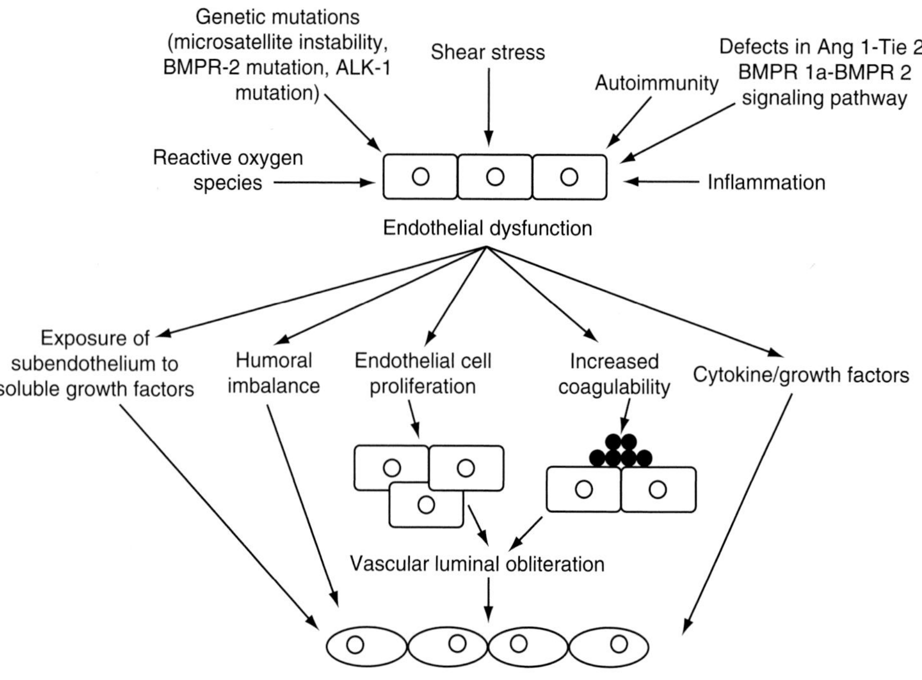

Figure 24–23 Mechanistic role of endothelial dysfunction in pulmonary hypertension and pulmonary vascular remodeling. *Squares* indicate endothelial cells; *ovals,* smooth muscle cells; and *closed circles*, platelets. (Reprinted with permission from Budhiraja R, Tuder RM, Hassoun PM: Endothelial dysfunction in pulmonary hypertension. Circulation 109:160, 2004.)

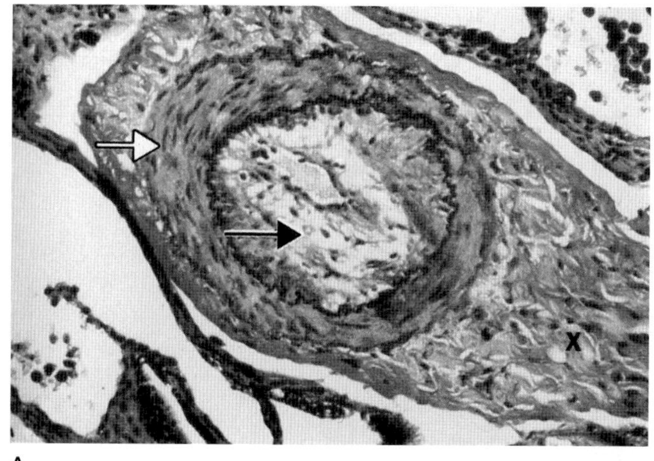

A

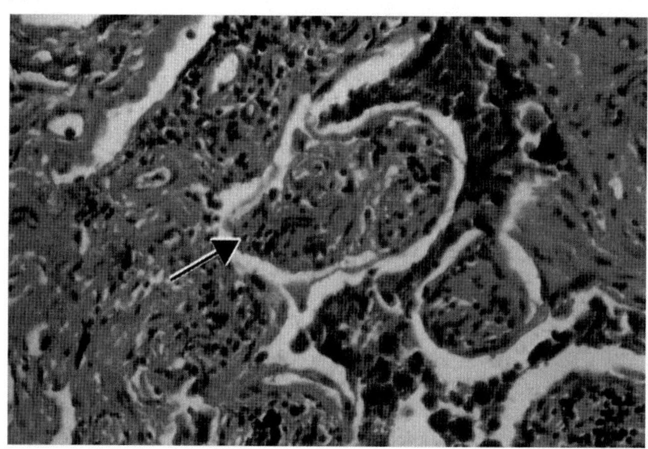

B

Figure 24–24 Characteristic lung pathology in primary pulmonary hypertension. *(A)* Muscular pulmonary artery from a patient with primary pulmonary hypertension and medial hypertrophy *(white arrow)*, luminal narrowing by intimal proliferation *(black arrow)*, and proliferation of adventitia *(X)*. *(B)* Characteristic plexiform lesion from an obstructed muscular pulmonary artery *(arrow)*. (Reprinted with permission from Gaine SP, Rubin LJ: Primary pulmonary hypertension. Lancet 352:721, 1998.)

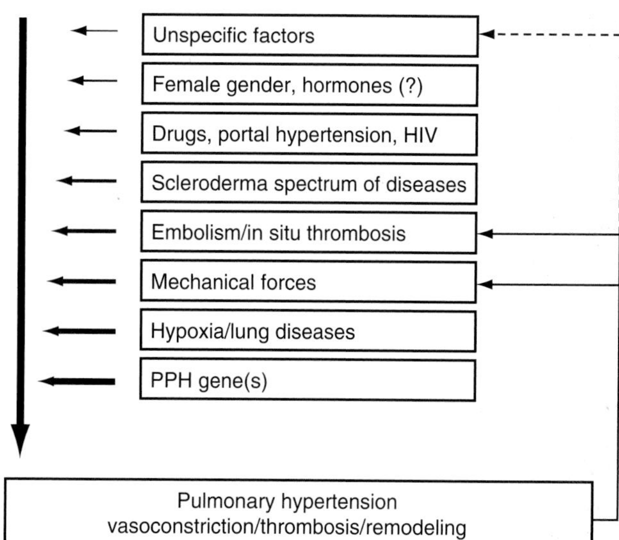

Figure 24–25 Multifactorial development of pulmonary hypertension. This graph illustrates the hypothesis that a variety of risk factors can add up to induce pulmonary hypertension. The size of the *arrows* represents the probability by which a risk factor induces pulmonary hypertension. Some of these factors may be strong enough to induce pulmonary hypertension per se, but the addition of other factors will increase the probability of disease manifestation. The figure also shows vicious circles induced by pulmonary hypertension. Among unspecific factors, autoimmune phenomena (e.g., lupus anticoagulant) could play a major role and could also be activated by pulmonary hypertension. (Reprinted with permission from Olschewski H, Rose F, Grünig E, et al: Cellular pathophysiology and therapy of pulmonary hypertension. J Lab Clin Med 138:368, 2001.)

been useful to lower PAP 10% to 20% if vasoreactivity testing was positive.[187] Otherwise, they may precipitate right-heart failure and even death in those with primary PAH. Pulmonary vasodilators are administered to decrease PVR, PAP, and RV afterload. Many pulmonary vasodilators have been tried, with unreliable and short-term benefit. Continuous prostaglandin therapy was found to improve hemodynamics and exercise to tolerance and to prolong survival.[192] Because prostaglandin therapy requires continuous intravenous administration to be efficacious, alternate forms have been created: oral (beraprost), subcutaneous (treprostinil), and inhaled (iloprost).[187,194] The full measure of their clinical effect has not been determined. Prostaglandin therapy contains valuable anti-inflammatory properties that represent treatment for PAH directed at the various pathologic mechanisms considered responsible for PAH besides pulmonary vasodilation. Newer agents targeting thromboxane inhibition (terbogrel) and endothelin-receptor antagonism (bosentan, sitaxsentan, and ambrisentan) have been developed.[195] A new pulmonary vasodilator, sildenafil, may act synergistically with other vasodilators by inactivating the phosphodiesterase enzymes that inactivate the second messengers for the vasodilating signals, cyclic adenosine monophosphate and cyclic guanosine monophosphate in lung tissues.[195] However, the long-term effect is still unknown.[196]

An important aspect of endothelial function that may suffer during PAH is the ability to inhibit in situ thrombosis. A prothrombotic state, with increased levels of tissue plasminogen activator inhibitor-1 and decreased tissue factor pathway inhibitor, has been found in those with primary PAH.[197] Thrombi have been found in small pulmonary vessels in many patients who have died of primary PAH. Even smaller thrombi that may not threaten most individuals may have catastrophic consequences if PAH is present. Consequently, anticoagulation is recommended to prolong survival.[198]

If right-sided heart failure does not respond to diuretic therapy in primary PAH, atrial septostomy may be performed in the catheterization laboratory. It decompresses the right heart by allowing greater filling of the left heart through a right-to-left shunt; thus preserving left-sided CO at the expense of systemic arterial desaturation. Heart-lung transplantation was introduced in 1981 and is effective therapy for certain individuals with primary PAH. Single- and double-lung transplantation have become popular in the management of PPH due to the marked improvement in right-sided heart function after lung transplantation and the shortage of suitable heart-lung donors. Double-lung transplantation improves right-sided heart function and graft survival more than does single-lung transplantation[199] (see Chapter 26).

Secondary Pulmonary Hypertension

In most patients, PAH is secondary to cardiac or pulmonary disease. The term "secondary" PAH is being used less because of the many therapies for PAH regardless of etiology.

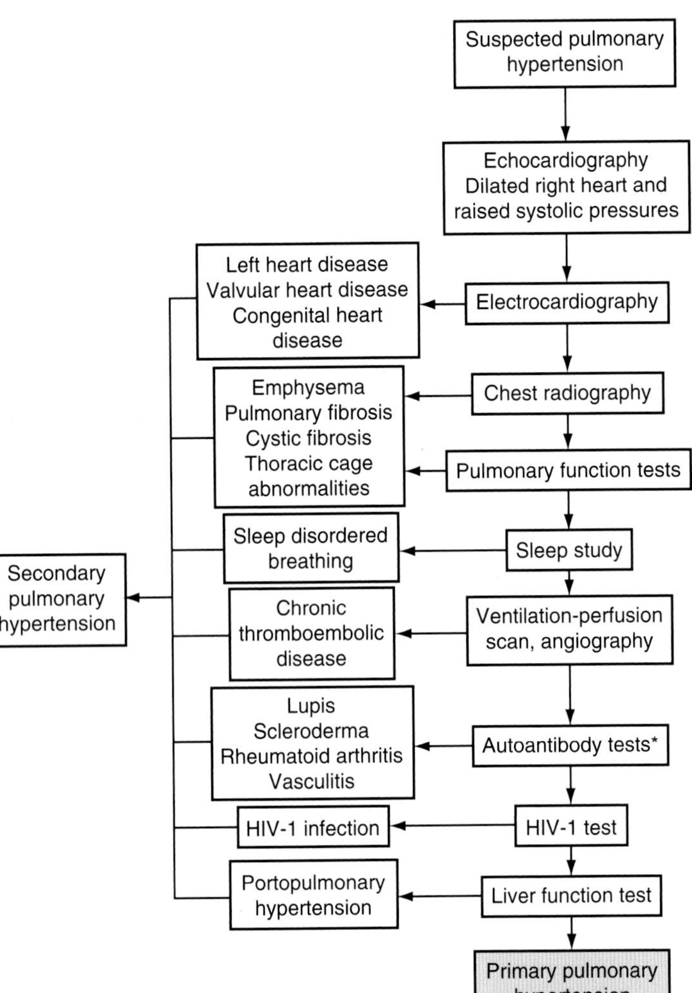

Figure 24–26 Algorithm for investigation of suspected pulmonary hypertension. *Antinuclear antibody, antineutrophilic cytoplasmic antibody, rheumatoid factor. (Reprinted with permission from Gaine SP, Rubin LJ: Primary pulmonary hypertension. Lancet 352:720, 1998.)

Table 24–7 Occurrence of Pulmonary Hypertension During Anesthesia

• Thromboembolism	Thrombectomy of deep veins, pregnancy, childbirth
• CO_2 embolism	Laparoscopy
• Air embolism	Surgery with patient in sitting position (e.g., neurosurgery)
• Bone cement (Pallacos)	Orthopedics
• Protamine	Cardiac surgery
• Extracorporeal circulation	Cardiac surgery
• Ischemia-reperfusion syndrome	Clamping/declamping of the aorta
• Loss of lung vessels	Pneumonectomy

From Fischer LG, Van Aken H, Bürkle H: Management of pulmonary hypertension: Physiological and pharmacological considerations for anesthesiologists. Anesth Analg 96:1607, 2003.

Secondary PAH is more common than primary PAH. Often, the underlying disease overshadows the clinical manifestations of PAH. The natural history, prognosis, and appropriate treatment of patients with secondary PAH depend on the underlying condition. Secondary PAH may be reversible. Once the etiology of PAH is identified, treatment should begin immediately because it is most effective if instituted before the onset of right-heart failure. Unfortunately, at the time of diagnosis, PAH has often progressed to the point that the value of any treatment is limited to palliation of incapacitating symptoms.

Anesthetic management of individuals with PAH is challenging because perioperative increases in PVR readily occur and may provoke right-sided heart failure, resulting in death (Table 24–7). The tolerance of the RV is a major concern. The RV is acutely sensitive to increases in PVR (afterload). Factors that increase PVR, such as hypoxia, acidosis, hypercapnea,

Table 24–8 **Causes of Massive Hemoptysis**

Tracheobronchial Disorders	**Localized Parenchymal Diseases**
Amyloidosis	Amebiasis
Bronchial adenoma	Aspergilloma*
Bronchiectasis*	Atypical mycobacterial infection*
Bronchogenic carcinoma	Coccidiomycosis
Broncholithiasis	Lung abscess
Bronchovascular fistula	Mucormycosis
Cystic fibrosis	Pulmonary tuberculosis*
Foreign body aspiration	**Diffuse Parenchymal Diseases**
Tracheobronchial trauma	Goodpasture's syndrome
Cardiovascular Disorders	Idiopathic pulmonary hemosiderosis
Congenital heart disease	Polyarteritis nodosa
Mitral stenosis	Systemic lupus erythematosus
Pulmonary arteriovenous fistula	Wegener's granulomatosis
Septic pulmonary emboli	**Other**
Ruptured thoracic aneurysm	Pulmonary artery rupture from a pulmonary artery catheter
Arteriovenous-malformation	Iatrogenic (e.g., bronchoscopy, cardiac catheterization) Pulmonary hypertension Pulmonary edema Pulmonary infarction

*Most common causes.

From Thompson AB, Tescheler H, Rennard SI: Pathogenesis, evaluation, and therapy for massive hemoptysis. Clin Chest Med 13:69, 1992.

hypothermia, and α-adrenergic stimulation, should be minimized. Furthermore, a decrease in blood pressure or increase in RV pressure impairs coronary perfusion of the right heart.[200] A PAC allows perioperative detection and monitoring of PVR and therapy, enabling hyperventilation to reduce PVR. In general, intravenous anesthetics have less effect on hypoxic pulmonary vasoconstriction, PVR, and oxygenation than do volatile agents.[200] Nitrous oxide has been reported to increase PVR, but it is not contraindicated in these patients.[200] Isoflurane may be beneficial by decreasing PAP and has been frequently used during noncardiac procedures. Fentanyl may be given as an adjunct or a primary anesthetic agent in these patients because it causes little myocardial depression and excellent circulatory stability.

Pulmonary endarterectomy (PEA) is the accepted treatment today for chronic thromboembolic pulmonary hypertension. The operation is not an embolectomy but rather a true endarterectomy, removing the fibrosis obstructive tissue from the pulmonary arteries.[201] Extracorporeal circulation and periods of circulatory arrest under deep hypothermia are essential for successful endarterectomy. The details of surgical and anesthetic management have been described by Jamieson et al[202] and Manecke et al,[203] respectively.

PULMONARY HEMORRHAGE

Pulmonary hemorrhage occurs in about 1.5% of patients with hemoptysis, but mortality may reach 85%.[204] The definition of massive hemoptysis varies but is commonly characterized as more than 600 mL of expectorated blood over 24 hours. Four hundred milliliters of blood in the alveolar space seriously impairs oxygenation. Pulmonary hemorrhage may stabilize only to worsen again without an obvious explanation, reflecting its unpredictable nature. Notably, death is not attributable to hemodynamic instability with hemorrhage but excessive blood in the alveoli that causes hypoventilation and refractory hypoxia. Moreover, one clot may obstruct an entire lobe of the lungs. Mortality is related to the amount of bleeding that occurs over time. If more than 600 mL of blood is lost over 16 hours, mortality is 45%; it is only 5% if blood loss totals 600 mL over 48 hours. A delay in initiating treatment because of difficulty in isolating the location of bleeding contributes greatly to the high mortality of pulmonary hemorrhage.

Hemoptysis may occur with various diseases and circumstances (Table 24–8). In the United States, chronic inflammatory lung disease and bronchogenic carcinoma are the most common causes of hemoptysis. Of these causes, bronchitis (26%), lung cancer (23%), pneumonia (10%), and tuberculosis (8%) are most frequent. Pulmonary hemorrhage may result from vigorous suctioning of the lungs, surgical procedures, and improper positioning of a PAC.[205] Massive hemoptysis is usually an emergency because the underlying pulmonary disorder gives the patient little reserve to tolerate it. Treatment may be medically or surgically directed. Pulmonary hemorrhage rarely occurs during cardiac surgery; however, when it does, it is life threatening because of the severity of cardiovascular disease and necessity for anticoagulation during CPB, which predisposes to coagulation abnormalities and excessive bleeding.[206]

To understand the pathogenesis of pulmonary hemorrhage, it is helpful to appreciate the anatomy of the pulmonary circulation. The lungs have a dual blood supply. The pulmonary arterial circuit is a high-flow, low-pressure circuit. The nutritive supply of the pulmonary structures is the bronchial arteries, which originate from the aorta. Bronchial arteries extend into many areas around the lymph nodes, esophagus, and lungs, ultimately penetrating the bronchial wall to supply the bronchial mucosa. The bronchial and pulmonary circulations anastomose at several locations. Massive pulmonary hemorrhage usually involves bleeding due to disruption of the high-pressure bronchial circulation. These high-pressure, tortuous bronchial arteries become dilated and rupture, or erode, or feed into the lower pressure pulmonary veins that can easily rupture. The bronchial circulation is also important because these arteries are widespread in the thoracic cage and account for 98% of pulmonary hemorrhage; whereas the pulmonary circulation accounts for the rest.[204]

A rare but often fatal cause of pulmonary hemorrhage in patients undergoing cardiac surgery is rupture of the pulmonary artery by a PAC.[205] Introduction of the PAC in 1970 enabled physicians to obtain CO, SVR, and estimates of LV performance and to detect early myocardial ischemia perioperatively. Subsequently, there was a dramatic increase in their use. The incidence of pulmonary artery rupture with a PAC ranges from 0.06% to 0.2% of cases, with a corresponding mortality of 45% to 64% and significant morbidity.[207] In cardiac surgical patients, death may occur within minutes of pulmonary artery rupture or over a period of 1 to 14 days postoperatively.[208] The diagnosis may be initially missed because patients may be asymptomatic or only mildly symptomatic. A small amount of hemoptysis may herald the onset of severe pulmonary hemorrhage.[208,209] If a patient is anticoagulated, bleeding may be profuse immediately. Other signs of pulmonary artery rupture are hypotension, decreased arterial oxygenation, bronchospasm, pleural effusion, hemothorax, and pneumothorax.

Certain factors predispose patients to pulmonary artery rupture such as age (older than 60 years), anticoagulation, and distal migration of a PAC.[205] Although PAH is often present with pulmonary artery rupture, it is not a risk factor but may simply promote distal migration of the PAC.[208] Chronic PAH weakens the pulmonary artery and veins; thus, a patient's susceptibility to rupture is increased. The mechanism of pulmonary artery rupture is multifactorial, but the catheter balloon is instrumental.[210] Maximal pressures for balloon inflation are approximately 1700 mm Hg and easily reach 1000 mm Hg with the start of inflation. PACs that reside distally lower the inflation pressures necessary to rupture the pulmonary artery, particularly in the elderly. Distal migration of the PAC also occurs more easily in patients undergoing hypothermic CPB because hypothermia stiffens the PAC. Eccentric inflation of the PAC balloon contributes to pulmonary artery rupture, as evidenced in both cadavers and patients.[211] Inflation that distorts the balloon drives the catheter tip through the vessel wall (Fig. 24–27). Manipulation of the heart may also perforate the pulmonary artery.

Diagnosis of hemoptysis requires a few simple tests. Visual inspection can usually distinguish gastrointestinal bleeding from pulmonary hemorrhage. Hemoptysis is often bright red with some sputum. Hemoptysis due to pulmonary artery rupture is usually copious (200 to 2000 mL).[205] Identification of the bleeding site is critical. A chest roentgenogram may reveal an infiltrate, but neither chest roentgenogram nor physical examination has been reliable to localize the affected lung. Flexible bronchoscopy may be limited by severe bleeding that obscures the view. Rigid bronchoscopy is better suited for massive hemoptysis but has a limited view of the upper lobes and requires general anesthesia. Instillation of epinephrine in the bronchi may facilitate better visualization by slowing the bleeding. Ultimately, angiography of the pulmonary and bronchial arteries may be required to localize the source of the bleeding. Subsequently, bronchial artery embolization may stop the bleeding 75% to 98% of the time, but 16% to 20% of patients rebleed in the following year.[212,213]

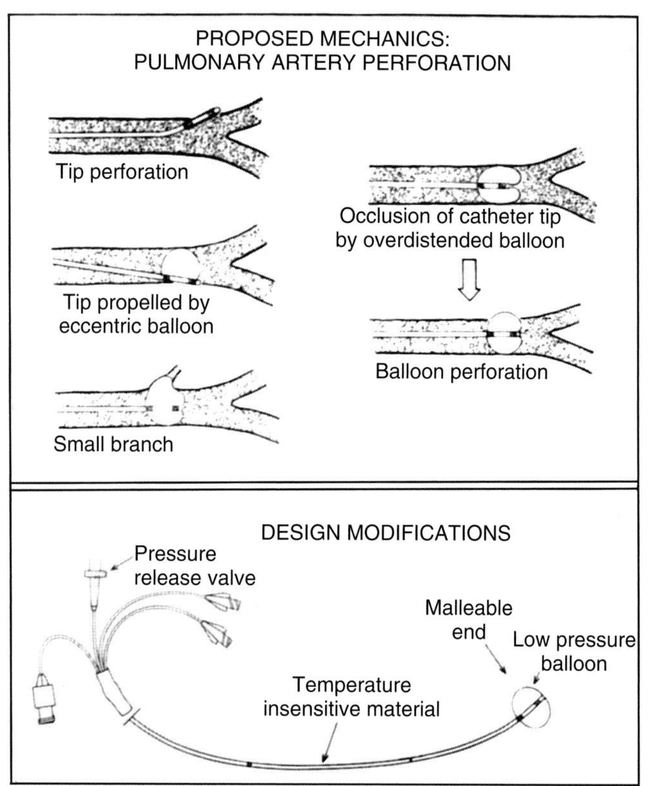

Figure 24–27 The possible mechanisms of pulmonary artery perforation with balloon-tipped flow-guided catheters. These problems require modifications in catheter design. (Reprinted with permission from Barash PG, Nardi D, Hammond G, et al: Catheter-induced pulmonary artery perforation: Mechanisms, management, and modifications. J Thorac Cardiovasc Surg 82:5, 1981.)

The extent of bleeding after pulmonary artery rupture will determine treatment. If rupture occurs during CPB, then CPB should be maintained to ensure adequate oxygenation and identify the site of rupture under controlled conditions. Mild bleeding may require positive end-expiratory pressure once anticoagulation is neutralized.[208,214] If bleeding is significant, a double-lumen ETT is beneficial to isolate the bleeding from the unaffected lung, although placement may prove difficult in the midst of active bleeding. Misplacement of double-lumen tubes in these situations has been identified in 45% of patients after the initial attempt and 54% after patient positioning.[215] Airway manipulation in an anticoagulated patient in connection with double-lumen tube placement may incite further mucosal damage and bleeding. A Fogarty catheter, as described by Larsen and Gasior,[216] passed within the existing ETT to the affected bronchus, may minimize additional trauma to the airway caused by reintubation and protects the uninvolved lung. The Univent ETT is an alternative to a double-lumen tube, but requires exchanging the existing ETT for the Univent ETT. A single-lumen ETT should not be advanced into the right main bronchus if bleeding is believed to be in the right lung, due to the proximal location of the right upper lobe bronchus. A Fogarty catheter may be used to tamponade a bleeding site with bronchoscopic guidance. Similarly, the balloon of a PAC may tamponade a bleeding site in the bronchus. These measures are only meant to be temporary until specific treatment is instituted.

If bleeding continues unabated, exsanguination may be unavoidable. If anticoagulation has been neutralized, blood loss of 1000 mL or more over 24 hours should merit consideration for early surgical intervention if the patient has the respiratory reserve to tolerate it. Surgery is the definitive treatment as it removes the bleeding site. Postoperative mortality rate varies widely from 1% to 50%.[204] A localized site of bleeding and sufficient lung function are essential to know before surgery as the resection may extend to a pneumonectomy. Alternatively, temporary unilateral occlusion of the designated pulmonary artery with a band for 48 hours has been successful in controlling massive hemorrhage without permanent sequelae.[217] Mortality rate varies between 1% and 25%.[204] Although this may appear high, an individual may not be a candidate for medical therapy so the surgical candidate by definition is the higher-risk patient. Surgery is contraindicated in those with lung carcinoma invading the trachea, mediastinum, heart, or great vessels; terminal malignancy; or progressive pulmonary fibrosis.

To reduce the possibility of pulmonary artery rupture, placement or migration of a PAC distally in the pulmonary artery should be guarded against. It is not advisable to advance the PAC more than 4 to 5 cm beyond the pulmonary valve. The balloon should not be inflated against increased resistance, particularly if the patient is anticoagulated or after separation from CPB. The pulmonary artery waveform should always be carefully observed with inflation and deflation of the balloon. Retracting the PAC into the RV upon the initiation of CPB or withdrawing the PAC 5 cm immediately before CPB has been recommended.

PERICARDIAL HEART DISEASE

The pericardium encloses the heart and the great vessels. Its inner layer is a serous membrane (visceral pericardium) covering the surface of the heart. Its outer layer is a fibrinous sac (parietal pericardium), which is attached to the great vessels, diaphragm, and sternum. The space between the two layers is the pericardial space. The two layers are joined at the level of the great vessels and at the central tendon of the diaphragm caudally, and a serous layer extends past these junctions to line the inside of the fibrinous sac (parietal pericardium). The pericardial space normally contains up to 50 mL of clear fluid that is an ultrafiltrate of plasma. The vagus nerve, left recurrent laryngeal nerve, and esophageal plexus innervate the pericardium, along with sympathetic contributions from the stellate ganglion, first dorsal ganglion, and other ganglia. The lateral course of the phrenic nerve on either side of the heart is an important anatomic relationship because this nerve is encapsulated in the pericardium and thus can easily be damaged during pericardiectomy (Fig. 24–28). The pericardium is not essential for life and pericardiectomy causes no apparent disability. The parietal pericardium is a stiff

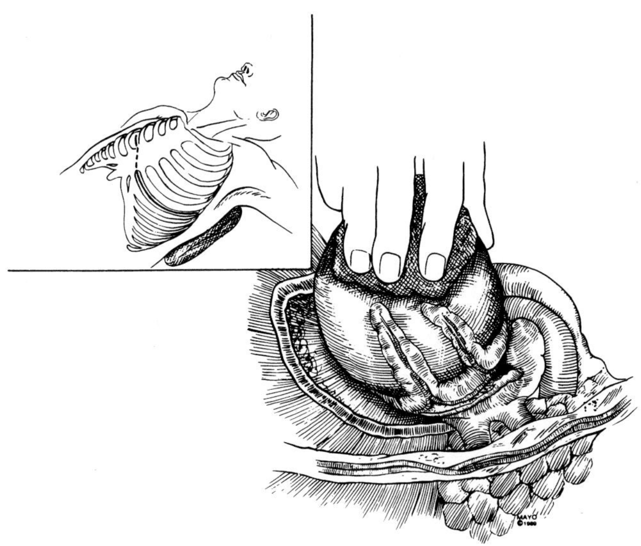

Figure 24–28 Approach for pericardiectomy through a fifth left intercostal space for anterolateral thoracotomy. The phrenic nerves are preserved on pedicles. The lateral course of the phrenic nerves and the pericardial attachment make the phrenic nerves easily damaged during removal of the pericardium. (Reprinted with permission from Tuna IC, Danielson GK: Surgical management of pericardial disease. Cardiol Clin 8:683, 1990.)

collagenous membrane that resists acute expansion, but it can gradually dilate to accept large volumes of fluid if slowly accumulated. Rapid accumulation of pericardial fluid causes cardiac tamponade.

Acute Pericarditis

Acute pericarditis is common but the actual incidence is unknown as it often goes unrecognized. It is generally self-limited, lasting 6 weeks. Acute pericarditis has many causes (Box 24–4)—the most common of which is viral (30% to 50%).[218] Only 25% of cases have a defined etiology, although this is improving.[219] Acute pericarditis resembles many other

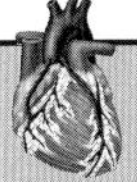

BOX 24–4 *Causes of Acute Pericarditis*

- Idiopathic
- Infectious
  - Viral
  - Bacterial
  - Fungal
  - Parasitic
- Immunologic
  - Post–myocardial infarction (Dressler's syndrome)
  - Post–cardiotomy syndrome
  - Still's disease
  - Rheumatoid arthritis
  - Systemic lupus erythematosus
  - Polyarteritis
- Neoplastic
- Radiation
- Traumatic
- Renal failure
- Drug induced

From Oakley CM: Myocarditis, pericarditis and other pericardial diseases. Heart 84:449, 2000.

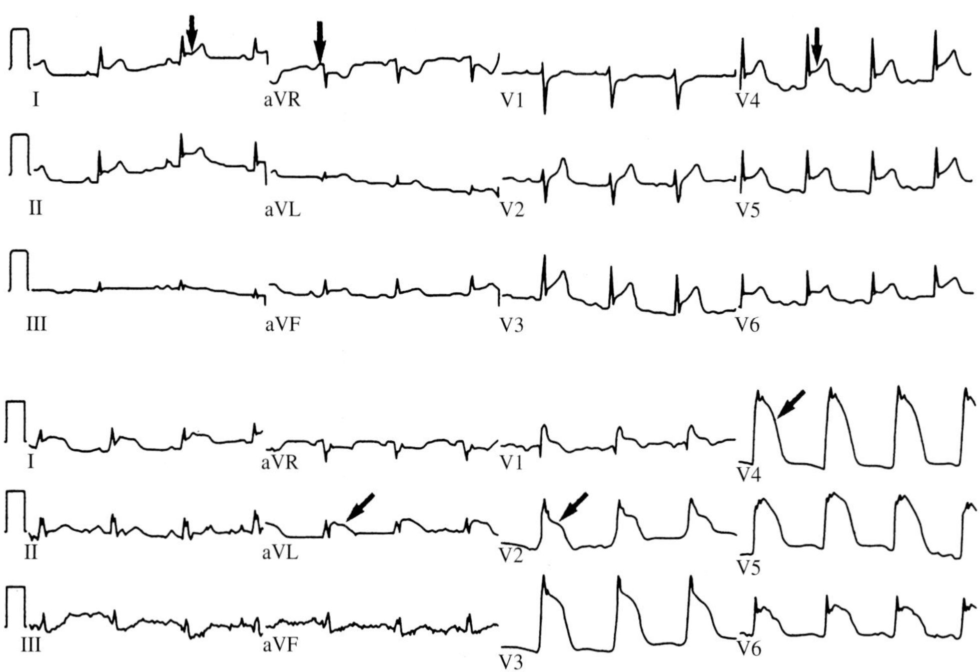

Figure 24–29 Acute pericarditis: Note the upward-concavity ST elevations in limb leads I, II, aVF, and aVL and in precordial leads V_3, V_4, V_5, and V_6 and the PR-segment elevation in aVR. Acute myocardial infarction: Note the concavity-downward ST elevation in leads I, aVL, V_1, V_2, V_3, V_4, V_5, and V_6, indicating a large anterior myocardial infarction. (Aikat S, Ghaffari S: A review of pericardial diseases: Clinical, ECG and hemodynamic features and management. Cleve Clin J Med 67:907, 2000.)

conditions. Anesthesiologists encounter patients with acute pericarditis in situations of malignancy, MI, postcardiotomy syndrome, uremia, or infection when surgery is required because symptoms are incapacitating and medical therapy has failed.

Acute pericarditis is characterized by fibrin deposits localized on the pericardial surface. A serous effusion may accompany the fibrinous inflammation. Consequently, the mesothelial cell layer is replaced by a fibrin membrane that has white blood cells scattered throughout it. Pericardial fluid may suggest a bacterial, neoplastic, or viral and inflammatory etiology.[218] Pericarditis occurs in about 20% of patients who sustain an MI, primarily within the first week.[220] A distinction is made between pericarditis that occurs during the first week and Dressler's syndrome, which usually appears 2 to 3 months after an MI. With acute pericarditis, pleuritic chest pain is described in the center of the chest radiating to the back and left trapezius muscle. This pain is more continuous than the pain of myocardial ischemia, which is intermittent. Some degree of dyspnea may be present with acute pericarditis. Occasionally, pericarditis may present as right-sided heart failure because large and rapid accumulations of pericardial fluid increase intrapericardial pressure sufficiently to obstruct RV filling through the superior and inferior vena cava, resulting in tamponade. Atrial arrhythmias may also occur.

In general, acute pericarditis can be differentiated from MI by measurement of serum cardiac enzymes, but myocardial enzymes are sometimes found in the serum of patients with pericarditis. It is also common to see the early onset of a low-grade fever that lasts for days to weeks and the presence of a friction rub after the onset of chest pain. Pericardial friction rub is pathognomonic of pericarditis but may be heard only intermittently. Early ECG changes typical of pericarditis are ST-segment elevation in two or three standard limb leads and in most of the precordial leads. ST-T wave elevation is often present but may be confused with MI (Fig. 24–29). Acute pericarditis generally results in diffuse ST-T changes, whereas MI usually is associated with more localized ST-T changes. T-wave inversions follow the acute ST-segment abnormalities as pericarditis enters the subacute phase. Q waves usually do not appear during progression of ECG changes. Echocardiography may effectively delineate the cause of the ST-T changes by identifying wall motion abnormalities[221] and pericardial effusions.[221] The chest roentgenogram may reveal a slightly enlarged cardiac silhouette with a pericardial effusion that indicates the effusion is at least 250 mL. A rapid accumulation of pericardial fluid may cause tamponade. On the other hand, if it accumulates slowly, 1 liter or more of pericardial fluid may collect without symptoms of cardiac tamponade. Pericardial fluid may also be found with CHF, valvular disease, or endocarditis. Pericardiocentesis is performed in acute pericarditis, either to confirm the diagnosis or to relieve tamponade. It may be associated with serious complications, even cardiovascular collapse and shock. Ventricular contractile function should be evaluated by echocardiography prior to pericardiocentesis. If repeated aspirations are required for relief of tamponade, pericardiectomy may be necessary.

Detection of myocardially directed serum antibodies in Dressler's syndrome and in postpericardiotomy syndrome suggests that these syndromes are immune-related responses. Postpericardiotomy syndrome consists of acute nonspecific pericarditis that usually begins between 10 days and 3 months after cardiac surgery or trauma. In a prospective study of 944 adult patients who underwent cardiac surgery, the incidence of postpericardiotomy syndrome was 17.8%.[222]

Treatment of acute pericarditis consists of symptomatic relief and treating the underlying systemic illness. Symptomatic relief involves support, bed rest, and nonsteroidal anti-inflammatory agents for analgesia. Left stellate ganglion block has been used to relieve unremitting pain.

Table 24–9 **Causes of Constrictive Pericarditis**

Cause	Percentage
Idiopathic pericarditis	40
Post-CABG	30
Tuberculosis	10
Radiation induced	5
Collagen vascular disease	5
Others (malignancy, uremia, purulent)	5

CABG = Coronary artery bypass grafting.
From Kabbani SS, LeWinter MM: Diastolic heart failure: Constrictive, restrictive and pericardial. Cardiol Clin 18:505, 2000.

Constrictive Pericarditis

Whatever the cause, the end result is a dense fibrosis of the parietal and visceral pericardium that limits diastolic filling of the heart and causes constrictive pericarditis. The changes in the pericardium can be due to scarring induced by a single episode of acute pericarditis or by a prolonged exposure to a recurrent or chronic inflammatory process. Constrictive pericarditis is a progressive disease. Tuberculosis was a major cause of constrictive pericarditis, but currently most cases (33%) are idiopathic.[223] Table 24–9 lists some of the causes of chronic constrictive pericarditis. Idiopathic, neoplastic, postirradiation, or uremic pericarditis accounts for most cases of constrictive pericarditis that require surgery. Eighteen percent of pericardiectomies were attributed to previous cardiac surgery, which may explain the increase in the number of cases of constrictive pericarditis.[223,224]

The most frequent physical signs of chronic constrictive pericarditis are jugular venous distention and hepatomegaly. The normal filling phases of the jugular venous pulse are shown in Figure 24–30. Venous pressure waves in pericardial constriction are characterized by a prominent Y descent. Kussmaul's sign (a paradoxic increase in venous pressure with inspiration) may be present. Systemic venous congestion accounts for some of the classic symptoms of constrictive pericarditis such as hepatic congestion and peripheral edema.[116] A significant paradoxic pulse occurs in only one third of patients with chronic constrictive pericarditis. Characteristic ECG changes are P mitrale (broadened P wave), low QRS voltage, and T-wave inversion.[224] One fourth of patients have atrial fibrillation. Cardiomegaly on chest roentgenogram is nonspecific. Pericardial calcification is sometimes apparent in lateral chest roentgenograms. Although calcification is very specific for constrictive pericarditis, it is not very sensitive. CT scanning and MRI may demonstrate the typically thickened pericardium of constrictive pericarditis. Characteristic findings on Doppler examination include a decrease in LV filling with inspiration (mitral inflow greater during expiration than inspiration) and limitation of RV filling with expiration (hepatic vein diastolic flow reversal during expiration). Doppler features in constrictive pericarditis have been reviewed.[116,225] Even with the Doppler echocardiogram, the clinician must be aware of the loading conditions and respiratory effort of the patient during the Doppler examination. Right and left cardiac catheterization are necessary to confirm hemodynamic abnormalities in cases that are unclear.[116,224]

Limitation of RV diastolic filling occurs when the cardiac volume approximates the pericardial volume, usually in mid and late diastole, characterized by the square root or dip-and-plateau sign (Fig. 24–31). Filling is limited by the noncompliant pericardium. The square root sign occurs because the constricting pericardium is essentially part of the ventricular wall. When the ventricle contracts, the pericardium is deformed like a spring. As diastole begins, the spring is released and the ventricle fills rapidly, decreasing the ventricular pressure and creating the dip of the dip-and-plateau wave. As cardiac filling approaches the limit set by the fixed pericardium, the plateau of the ventricular filling curve arrives. There are marked elevations of right and left atrial and ventricular filling pressures. Pulmonary artery diastolic pressure, pulmonary capillary wedge pressure, and RA pressure are equal and elevated ("pressure plateau") in constrictive pericarditis due to the limitation of the pericardium. Pulmonary artery systolic and RV systolic pressures range from 35 to 45 mm Hg, although PAH is rare. Most important, the myocardium is unaffected in constrictive pericarditis. The systolic and early diastolic functions are normal.[224] Differences between constrictive pericarditis and RCM have been reviewed previously.[224]

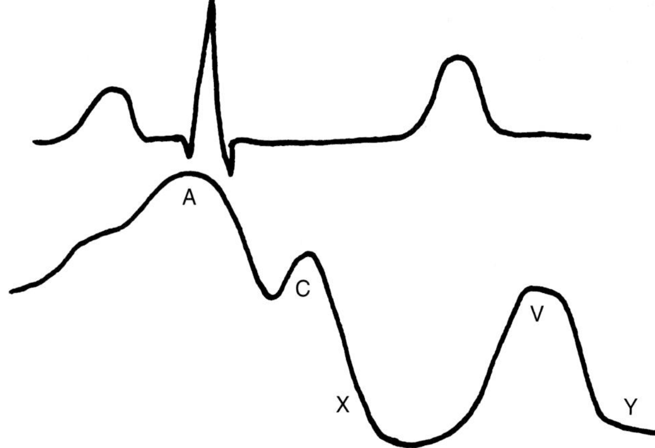

Figure 24–30 Schematic depiction of normal jugular venous pressure waves in relation to the electrocardiogram (ECG). The A wave is a result of atrial contraction; the prominent negative X-descent occurs during ventricular systole and is a result of downward displacement of the base of the heart and tricuspid valve as well as continued atrial relaxation. The small C wave, which interrupts the X-descent, is probably due to the bulging of the tricuspid valve into the right atrium. The V wave represents right atrial filling while the tricuspid valve is closed. Finally, the Y-descent occurs after opening of the tricuspid valve and during rapid inflow of blood from the right atrium into the ventricle. (Reprinted with permission from Legler D: Uncommon diseases and cardiac anesthesia. *In* Kaplan JA [ed]: Cardiac Anesthesia, 2nd edition. Philadelphia, WB Saunders Company, 1987, p 785.)

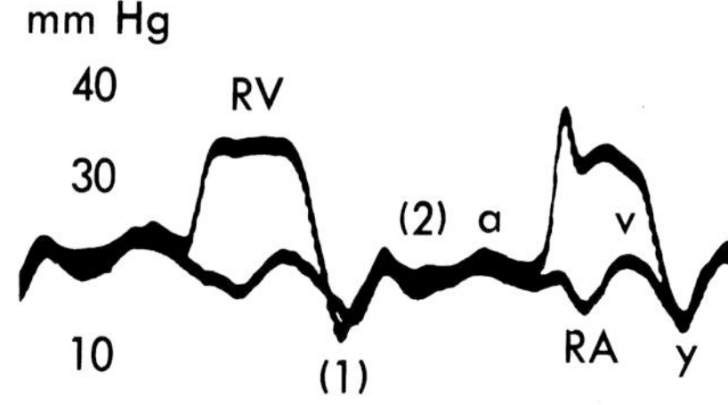

Figure 24–31 Right ventricular (RV) and right atrial (RA) pressure tracings recorded with a fluid-filled system from a patient with chronic constrictive pericarditis. (Reprinted with permission from Shabetai R: Pathophysiology and differential diagnosis of restrictive cardiomyopathy. Cardiovasc Clin 19:123, 1988.)

Anesthetic Considerations for Pericardial Disease

Pericardiectomy is performed for recurrent pericardial effusion and constrictive pericarditis. Pericardial dissection for effusive pericarditis is straightforward; however, pericardiectomy for constrictive pericarditis is a surgical challenge with a mortality of 5% to 15% and 5-year survival of 78%.[116,120,226] Persistent low CO immediately after pericardiectomy is the primary cause of morbidity and mortality.[226] In contrast to patients with cardiac tamponade, who usually improve clinically once the pericardium is opened, improvement is not always apparent initially after pericardiectomy. Instead, noticeable improvement in cardiac function may take weeks. Yet, 90% of patients ultimately experience relief of symptoms with surgery.[223]

Median sternotomy provides excellent exposure and access for pericardiectomy, but thoracotomy in the left anterolateral position is also used. Opinions vary regarding the extent of pericardial resection for alleviation of cardiac constriction and the use of CPB. Good results have been obtained with and without CPB. Removal of adherent and scarred pericardium to release both the RV and LV involves extensive manipulation of the heart. Some have advocated routine CPB for pericardiectomy because a more complete pericardial excision and hemodynamic stability were thought possible. Yet, heparinization and CPB may exacerbate blood loss from exposed cardiac surfaces. Furthermore, prolonged CPB in debilitated patients contributes to early mortality associated with pericardiectomy.

Anesthetic goals for managing patients with constrictive pericarditis who require pericardiectomy include minimizing bradycardia and myocardial depression and minimizing decreases in afterload or preload. Monitoring considerations include arterial and central venous pressures. A dorsalis pedis or femoral arterial catheter in patients with uremic pericarditis may preserve future potential arteriovenous fistula sites in the upper extremities. One groin site should be reserved in case femoral cannulation is necessary to emergently initiate CPB. PAC monitoring is recommended due to the occurrence of postoperative low CO syndrome. Low CO, hypotension, and arrhythmias (atrial and ventricular) are common during chest dissection. Due to limited ventricular diastolic filling, CO is rate dependent. If myocardial function or heart rate is depressed, β-agonists or pacing improve CO. Lidocaine infusion may partially suppress arrhythmias during dissection. Catastrophic hemorrhage can occur suddenly if the atrium or ventricle is perforated, so sufficient venous access is necessary. Damage to coronary arteries may also occur during dissection; careful monitoring of the ECG for signs of ischemia is prudent. Pericardiectomy via left anterior thoracotomy requires close monitoring of oxygenation because the left lung is severely compressed during dissection. Anesthetic technique is based on achieving early extubation; however, patients who undergo pericardiectomy for constrictive pericarditis benefit from remaining intubated for at least 6 to 12 hours to assess bleeding and CO.

Cardiac Tamponade

Cardiac tamponade occurs in a variety of clinical situations but most often with malignancies in medical patients and after pericardiocentesis.[227] Subacute effusions requiring drainage and, ultimately, pericardiectomy are not infrequent in patients with idiopathic pericarditis and uremic pericarditis. Hemorrhagic tamponade in patients who are excessively bleeding following CPB and cardiac surgery is increasingly common and may be fatal.

Tamponade exists when fluid accumulation in the pericardial sac limits filling of the heart. Hemodynamic manifestations are mainly due to atrial rather than ventricular compression. Initially, with mild tamponade, diastolic filling is limited, causing reduced stroke volume that stimulates sympathetic reflexes to increase heart rate and contractility to maintain CO.[224] The rising RA pressure reflexly stimulates tachycardia and peripheral vasoconstriction. Blood pressure is supported by vasoconstriction, but CO begins to fall as pericardial fluid continues to increase. Subsequently, diastolic filling begins to disappear so the jugular venous pulse has no prominent Y-descent but a prominent X-descent. Eventually, the pericardial pressure-volume curve becomes almost vertical so any additional fluid greatly restricts cardiac filling and reduces diastolic compliance.[228] Ultimately, the RA pressure, pulmonary artery diastolic pressure, and pulmonary capillary wedge pressure equilibrate (Fig. 24–32). Equilibration of pressures (within 5 mm Hg of each other) merits immediate action to rule out acute tamponade. The major hemodynamic changes and compensatory mechanisms of tamponade are outlined in Figure 24–33. Once the blood pressure begins to fall, it is a precipitous drop that reduces coronary artery blood flow, leading to ischemia, especially subendocardially.[228]

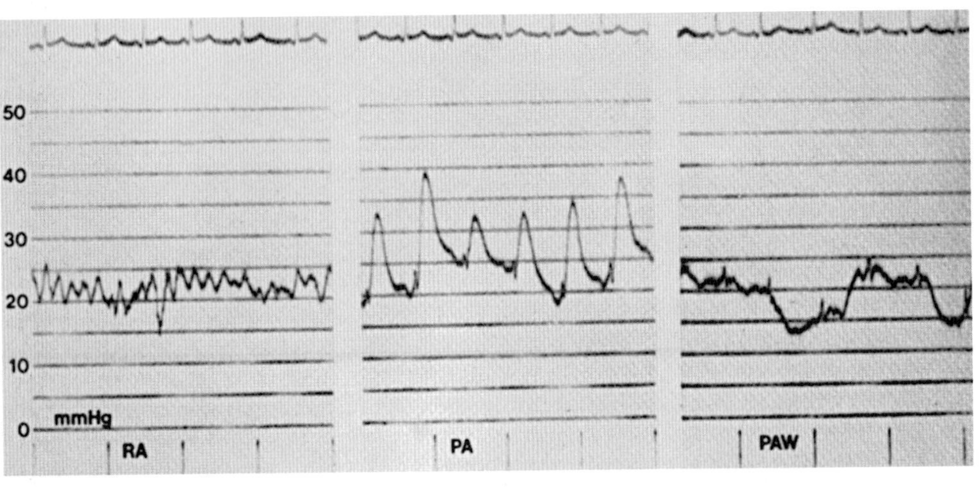

Figure 24–32 Hemodynamic changes in cardiac tamponade. Equilibration of right atrial (RA), pulmonary artery (PA) diastolic, and pulmonary artery wedge (PAW) pressures are demonstrated. (Reprinted with permission from Temkin LP, Ewy GA: Cardiac catheterization. *In* Conahan TJ III [ed]: Cardiac Anesthesia. Menlo Park, CA, Addison-Wesley, 1982, p 1.)

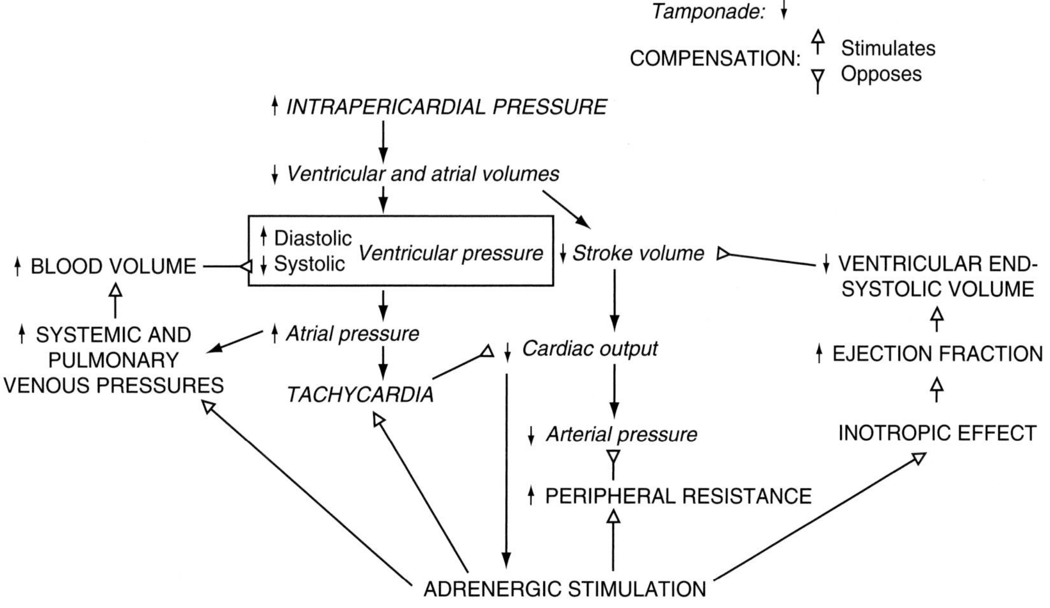

Figure 24–33 Cardiac tamponade: Relationships among major hemodynamic events and major compensatory mechanisms. *Simple arrows* = tamponade sequences; *pointed arrowheads* = stimulatory compensatory action; *blunt arrowheads* = oppositional compensatory actions. (Reprinted with permission from Spodick DH: Pathophysiology of cardiac tamponade. Chest 113:1374, 1998. Originally modified from Spodick DH [ed]: The Pericardium: A Comprehensive Textbook. New York, Dekker, 1997, p 182.)

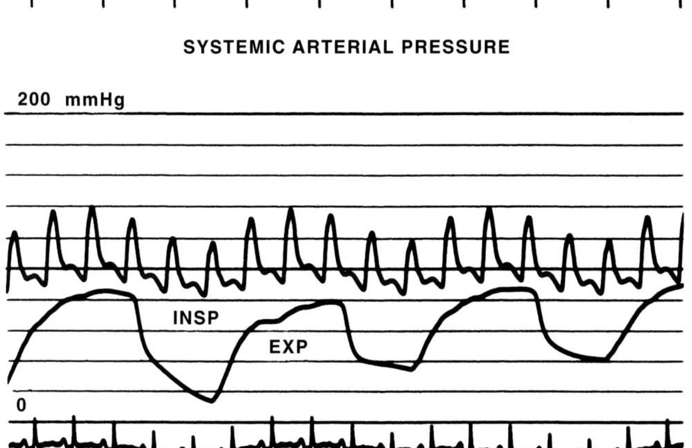

Figure 24–34 Pulsus paradoxus. During inspiration, arterial systolic pressure falls by more than 12 mm Hg. INSP = inspiration; EXP = expiration. (Reprinted with permission from Reddy PS, Curtiss EI: Card Clin 8:628, 1990.)

The classic diagnostic triad of acute tamponade consists of (1) decreasing arterial pressure, (2) increasing venous pressure, and (3) a small, quiet heart. Pulsus paradoxus may be present (Fig. 24–34); this is a fall in systolic blood pressure of more than 12 mm Hg during inspiration caused by reduced LV stroke volume generated by increased filling of the right heart during inspiration. It is not specific for tamponade, because it may be present in patients with obstructive pulmonary disease, RV infarction, or constrictive pericarditis. It may be absent if there is LV dysfunction, positive-pressure breathing, atrial septal defect, or severe aortic regurgitation. ECG changes with tamponade include low-voltage QRS complex, electrical alternans (Fig. 24–35), and T-wave abnormalities.[229] Sinus rhythm is usually present in tamponade. Echocardiography is the most reliable noninvasive method to detect pericardial effusion and exclude tamponade; echocardiography usually reveals an exaggerated motion of the heart within the pericardial sac in conjunction with atrial and ventricular collapse (Fig. 24–36). Echocardiographic features of tamponade

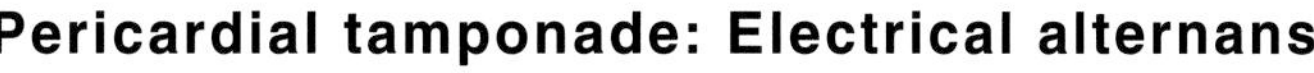

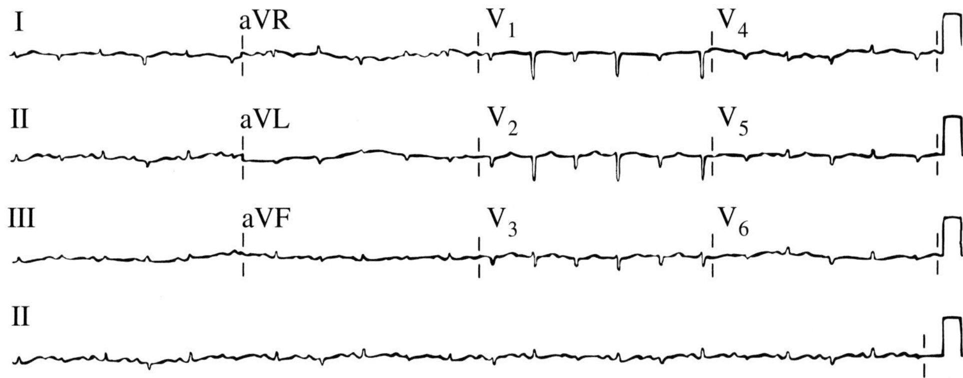

Figure 24–35 Electrical alternans in pericardial tamponade due to the swinging of the heart within the pericardial space. (Reprinted with permission from Aikat S, Ghaffari S: A review of pericardial diseases: Clinical, ECG and hemodynamic features and management. Cleve Clin J Med 67:909, 2000. Originally modified from Longo MJ, Jaffe CC: Images in clinical medicine electrical alternans. N Engl J Med 341:2060, 1999. Copyright © 1999 Massachusetts Medical Society. All rights reserved.)

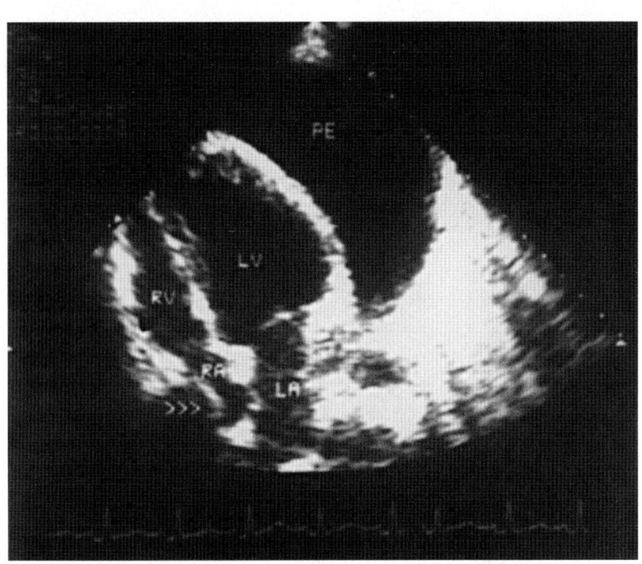

Figure 24–36 Example (four-chamber view) of an echocardiogram in a patient with a large posterolateral pericardial effusion (PE). Acute cardiac tamponade: Marked right atrial wall collapse *(arrowheads)*. (Reprinted with permission from Susini G, Pepi M, Sisillo E, et al: Percutaneous pericardiocentesis versus subxiphoid pericardiotomy in cardiac tamponade due to postoperative pericardial effusion. J Cardiothorac Vasc Anesth 7:178, 1993.)

have been reviewed.[224] Additionally, echocardiography is used to guide needle or catheter aspiration of pericardial effusion.

After cardiac surgery, tamponade due to hemorrhage requires immediate mediastinal exploration to determine bleeding site and stabilize hemodynamics. The numerous causes of hypotension in the postoperative cardiac surgical patient make tamponade more difficult to diagnose. Persistent poor CO with increased and equalized RA and LA pressures strongly suggest tamponade, but classic signs are often missing in the postoperative cardiac surgical patient. Arterial hypotension, pulsus paradoxus, and raised jugular venous pressures were absent in one series of cardiac surgical patients by 30%, 40%, and 50%, respectively.[230] Although echocardiography is capable of identifying the size of pericardial effusions postoperatively, it does not necessarily reflect its likelihood to cause tamponade.[230] Late cardiac tamponade occurs in 0.1% to 6% of patients after cardiac surgery. A delay in diagnosis contributes greatly to mortality in late cardiac tamponade.

Pericardiocentesis is indicated for life-threatening cardiac tamponade in conjunction with a fluid infusion to maintain filling pressures. Hemodynamics improves immediately after pericardiocentesis. Although it does provide immediate relief of the symptoms of tamponade, definitive therapy requires drainage of the pericardial space. Major complications of pericardiocentesis include coronary laceration, cardiac puncture, and pneumothorax. Surgical management of pericardial tamponade includes subxiphoid pericardiotomy, pericardial window through a left anterior thoracotomy, and pericardiectomy.[231]

Anesthesia Considerations for Cardiac Tamponade

Severe hypotension or cardiac arrest has followed induction of general anesthesia in patients with tamponade. The causes include further myocardial depression, sympatholysis, decreased venous return, and changes in heart rate. Resuscitation requires immediate drainage of pericardial fluid. Pericardiotomy via a subxiphoid incision with only local anesthetic infiltration or light sedation is an option. If intrapericardial injury is confirmed, general anesthesia can be induced after decompression of the pericardial space.[232] Ketamine (0.5 mg/kg) and 100% oxygen have been used with local anesthetic infiltration of the preexisting sternotomy to drain severe pericardial tamponade.[233] Spontaneous respiration instead of positive-pressure ventilation supports CO more effectively until tamponade is relieved. Volume expansion and correction of metabolic acidosis are mandatory. Catecholamine infusions or pacing may be used to avoid bradycardia. In a canine model of pericardial tamponade, dobutamine infusion delayed the onset of lactic acidosis by maintaining CO and tissue oxygen delivery.[234]

COMBINED CAROTID AND CORONARY ARTERY DISEASE

Patients with concomitant symptomatic coronary and carotid disease are known to be a much higher risk group than either group of patients with carotid or coronary disease alone.[235-237] In a staged approach to surgery, myocardial morbidity is as high as 20% if carotid endarterectomy is performed first, whereas the risk of stroke may reach 14% if coronary artery bypass grafting (CABG) is performed first.[235] A combined approach to carotid endarterectomy and CABG was first proposed by Bernhard et al in 1972.[238] Subsequently, many centers have opted to perform concomitant CABG and carotid endarterectomy, with conflicting outcomes and recommendations.[235]

The frequency of stroke with cardiac surgery is 2% to 6%.[239,240] Studies have better clarified neurologic injury associated with CPB as largely embolic in nature.[241] These cerebral emboli are largely derived from aortic cannulation, release of the aortic cross-clamp, and cardiac manipulation according to transcranial Doppler ultrasonography. Air or particulate emboli in connection with aortic cannulation or after valve replacement or repair may also cause perioperative stroke. Preoperative risk factors for stroke in patients undergoing CABG and CPB include carotid stenosis of 80% or more, carotid occlusion, prior stroke or transient ischemic attack, peripheral vascular disease, postinfarction angina, and prolonged duration of CPB.[242]

Carotid artery disease should be considered in all individuals with CAD. The patient with coexisting carotid disease is frequently older and has more severe CAD, an increased incidence of left main CAD, and greater LV dysfunction.[237] The incidence of hemodynamically significant carotid stenosis in patients needing CABG varies between 2% and 16%, but detecting it by auscultation for carotid bruits is unreliable. Carotid bruits may be audible with minimal carotid stenosis and silent with a carotid lumen of 1 to 2 mm in diameter.[243] Reed et al[244] found a mild increased risk of stroke when cervical carotid bruits were present, but others have not. Ultrasound with pulsed Doppler or duplex scans are appropriate noninvasive tests to assess the need for carotid angiography, the gold standard for evaluating carotid stenosis.[245] Faggioli et al[246] found carotid stenosis greater than 75% in 11% of patients more than 60 years of age scheduled for CABG. Additionally, between 3% and 12% of patients had more than 70% stenosis of their internal carotid artery prior to CABG.[242]

Severe carotid disease is a risk factor for hemispheric stroke during cardiac surgery with CPB, even if the patient is asymptomatic.[235,247] The stroke rate for the combined carotid endarterectomy and CABG is approximately twice the stroke rate of each operation alone.[235] This may be related to the overall severity of the atherosclerotic disease and likelihood of embolic plaque in the aorta in this population with multisystemic involvement. Similarly, individuals who undergo combined surgery appear to have a decreased long-term survival in comparison to patients who underwent CABG alone.[235] However, a comparative analysis of studies that included 50 patients or more who underwent CABG with unoperated major carotid disease found the risk of stroke averaged 5.5% for patients with unoperated carotid disease and CABG versus 3.1% for patients who underwent combined procedures.[235] There is also evidence from a retrospective analysis that patients older than 70 years may experience perioperative stroke and mortality at twice the rate of patients less than 70 years of age who undergo combined operations; but the differences were not statistically significant.[248]

Although MI is the major nonneurologic complication associated with carotid endarterectomy, CAD is often not detected until perioperative stress arises. Surgically uncorrectable CAD may exist in more than 40% of those presenting for carotid endarterectomy.[249] Carotid endarterectomy in patients with severe, symptomatic CAD has been associated with a 17% and 20% incidence of MI and mortality, respectively. Twenty percent of the MIs accounted for 60% of deaths.[242] On the contrary, there were no MIs in association with the combined approach to carotid disease with CAD, even with diffuse CAD. The combined approach not only may benefit the patient with CAD who has carotid disease but, even more important, also may influence outcome in the patient with severe carotid disease with CAD.

The optimal approach to a patient with both carotid and CAD requires a large multicenter, randomized trial; however, many approaches to the surgical management of combined procedures have been described. Schwartz et al[250] found no difference in outcome when carotid endarterectomy was performed immediately before initiation of CPB or during hypothermic CPB. Kouchoukos et al[251] performed carotid endarterectomy during hypothermic circulatory arrest in 50 patients undergoing CABG, with or without aortic or mitral valve replacement. The 30-day mortality was 6%. No patient sustained detectable neurologic injury. Comparisons between one versus two surgical teams performing the carotid endarterectomy and CABG simultaneously or sequentially during the same period of anesthesia were not conclusive regarding the best approach.[252]

Although there is no prospective, multicenter trial comparing various operative approaches, safety and efficacy have been demonstrated.[235,242,253] Daily et al[253] advocated the combined procedure as a way of decreasing surgical and hospital costs because morbidity and mortality were similar in their study with either sequential surgeries or combined surgeries. Trachiotis and Pfister[242] reported a median intensive care unit and hospital duration of 1 and 9 days, respectively, with a 30-day survival of 96.6%. However, those patients with an ejection fraction of less than 50% in particular experienced a worse 5-year survival (Fig. 24–37).

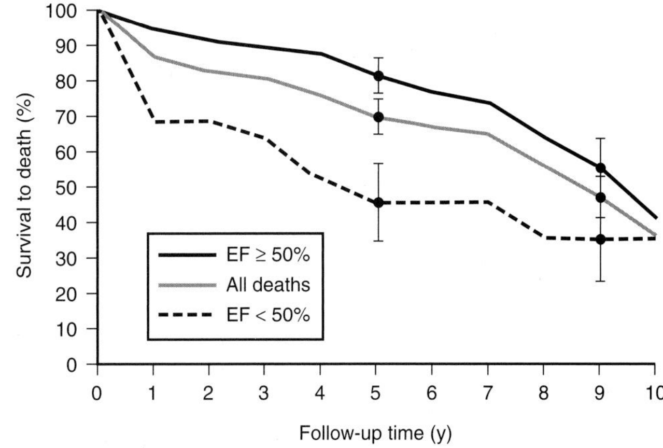

Figure 24–37 Actuarial survival to perioperative or late death in the carotid endarterectomy/coronary artery bypass grafting group for all patients and those with ejection fraction (EF) = 0.50 (50%) and <0.50. A significant difference in survival was observed between patients with preserved and depressed EF ($P < 0.003$). (Reprinted with permission from Rizzo RJ, Whittemore AD, Couper GS, et al: Combined carotid and coronary revascularization: The preferred approach to the severe vasculopathy. Ann Thorac Surg 54:1103, 1992. Copyright 1992, with permission from the Society of Thoracic Surgeons.)

Anesthetic Considerations

Anesthetic management of patients with both carotid artery disease and CAD must provide optimal conditions for the brain and myocardium. Beyond routine monitoring for cardiac surgery, electroencephalography or other modalities to assess neurophysiologic integrity are useful. Mean arterial pressure should be maintained in the middle to upper-normal range without large increases in afterload or heart rate. Normocapnia is recommended. Techniques often used during anesthesia for cerebral protection such as barbiturates, inhalation anesthetics, benzodiazepines, or propofol to decrease cerebral metabolic rate have not been proved beneficial in clinical trials. Attempts to provide cerebral protection should not be at the expense of myocardial perfusion and function.

Early extubation is desirable to allow earlier neurologic evaluation in combined cases. The safety of fast-track anesthetic management to achieve early extubation has been demonstrated with a propofol-based anesthetic and reduced opioids (fentanyl 10 to 15 µg/kg), forming an excellent anesthetic template for those undergoing combined operations.[254] Prompt tracheal extubation following cardiac surgery with CPB may be accomplished with various anesthetic agents.[255] Shorter-acting opioids have been characterized as achieving more rapid extubation than fentanyl;[256] Engoren et al[255] found no difference in the time to extubation with sufentanil or remifentanil compared with fentanyl, with the median time to extubation of 4.75 hours, 3.90 hours, and 2.78 hours, respectively. The combination of remifentanil and propofol was associated with mean extubation time of 163 minutes following arrival in the intensive care unit[257] (see Chapters 9, 32, 34, and 35).

Extubation in the operating room is possible with high-thoracic epidural, but early risks of hypothermia, bleeding, and hemodynamic instability may outweigh any benefit of prompt neurologic examination.[258] Aggressive vasoactive management is frequently required to treat hypertension and tachycardia resulting from reduced opioids. Shorter-acting muscle relaxants than pancuronium have also been considered to shorten the duration of intubation; however, a large multicenter trial of more than 1100 patients undergoing CABG did not demonstrate a difference in the duration of mechanical ventilation with either vecuronium or pancuronium and a fast-track anesthetic regimen.[256] Postoperatively, hypertension should be aggressively treated to avoid hyperperfusion syndromes leading to transient seizures or intracerebral hemorrhage and avoid exacerbation of bleeding at the site of the carotid endarterectomy.

CORONARY ARTERIOVENOUS FISTULA

Coronary arteriovenous fistula is an abnormal communication between a coronary artery and a venous structure. Common sites include coronary sinus, cardiac vein, pulmonary artery, superior vena cava, pulmonary vein, or one of the cardiac chambers. Coronary artery fistula is the most common significant coronary artery anomaly and occurs in 0.18% of patients undergoing angiography.[259,260] Most congenital arteriovenous fistulas (60%) involve the right coronary artery, are small, and have no clinical significance. However, larger fistulas result in significant left-to-right shunts, CHF, angina, infectious endocarditis, and aneurysmal dilation of the involved vessel. Intervention should be considered for all symptomatic arteriovenous fistulas. A continuous murmur with diastolic accentuation suggests an arteriovenous fistula. Angiography is useful to differentiate this condition from other causes of continuous murmurs, such as patent ductus arteriosus, ventricular septal defect, and atrial septal defect. Transesophageal echocardiography is useful to identify drainage sites of a coronary arteriovenous fistula.[261]

Coronary arteriovenous fistulas can occur after penetrating injury to the chest and present as pericardial tamponade. Rarely, iatrogenic arteriovenous fistulas are created by placement of a saphenous vein from the aorta to a coronary vein or internal mammary graft to a coronary vein.[262] Discovery of a continuous murmur along the upper left sternal border after CABG is an indication for angiography to verify proper placement of a saphenous vein graft into a coronary artery. Coronary arteriovenous fistulas cause angina pectoris by stealing blood from the normal coronary circulation. Symptomatic patients require surgery to eliminate the fistulous tract, which involves closing the distal end of the fistula from within the recipient cavity during CPB.[259] Selected fistulas may be ligated without CPB. Intraoperative TEE can localize fistulas, verify complete repair, and monitor ventricular function to avoid ischemic complication of ligation.[263]

Anesthetic Considerations

Anesthetic management of arteriovenous fistula is similar to anesthetic management for CABG. ECG monitoring for detection of ischemic changes is invaluable for ligation of coronary arteriovenous fistula. In selected patients, percutaneous transcatheter closure of coronary arteriovenous fistula is an alternative to surgical intervention.[264]

CARDIAC SURGERY DURING PREGNANCY

The incidence of maternal cardiac disease in North America has decreased by nearly 50% in the past 25 years to 1.5% to 2%.[265,266] Rheumatic heart disease accounts for nearly three fourths of it. Native valve disease and prosthetic valve dysfunction comprise most of the operations during pregnancy in addition to dissecting or traumatic rupture of the aorta, pulmonary embolism, closure of foramen ovale, and cardiac tumors representing only a small percentage of cases.[267] Heart disease is the leading cause of maternal and fetal death during pregnancy. Nonpregnant women with well-compensated cardiac disease may acutely or gradually decompensate as cardiac demands increase during pregnancy. Delaying surgery until after delivery carries a higher maternal mortality than does proceeding with the operation.[267] Extensive exposure to radiation may also limit therapeutic invasive catheterization procedures. If nonsurgical therapy is not possible or conflicts with fetal interests, cardiac surgery with CPB is the only option. Since 1958 when Leyse et al described the first cardiac operation requiring CPB in a pregnant patient, maternal morbidity has fallen from 5% to less than 1.0%.[267-269] Remarkably, pregnancy does not increase the risk of complications or mortality from cardiac surgical procedures for the mother, but fetal mortality is high, ranging from 16% to 33%.[266-268] CPB exposes the fetus to many undesirable effects that may have unpredictable consequences. Anesthetic management demands an appreciation for the cardiovascular changes of pregnancy and their impact on the corresponding heart disease and well-being of the fetus.

A number of physiologic changes of pregnancy affect the female with heart disease. Normally, heart rate and stroke volume are each increased by 25% at the end of the second trimester. Early in the third trimester, intravascular volume has expanded by nearly 50%.[270] These three changes result in a 50% increase in CO. Individuals with valvular heart disease do not tolerate such increases in blood volume and CO well. The corresponding increase in myocardial oxygen demand further worsens myocardial ischemia, exacerbating CHF. Decompensation from CHF, most commonly in association with mitral stenosis, is one of the most frequent indications for immediate cardiac surgery during pregnancy.[268] New onset of atrial fibrillation with mitral stenosis is not uncommon and can be imminently life threatening to the mother and fetus because of severe hypotension and decreased CO. The decrease in SVR that occurs with pregnancy may also compromise maternal coronary perfusion and pulmonary blood flow, or alter shunt physiology.

The nonphysiologic nature of CPB combines with the changes of pregnancy for an unpredictable response and tolerance by mother and fetus. Initiation of CPB activates a whole-body inflammatory response, with multiple effects on coagulation, autoregulation, release of vasoactive substances, hemodilution, and other physiologic processes that may adversely affect the fetus and mother.[271] Maternal blood pressure may fall immediately after or within 5 minutes of initiation of CPB, lowering placental perfusion secondary to low SVR, hemodilution, and release of vasoactive agents.[268] Fetal heart rate variability is often lost and fetal bradycardia (<80 bpm) also may occur at this time.[265] Because uterine blood flow is not autoregulated and relies on maternal blood flow, decreases in maternal blood pressure cause fetal hypoxia and bradycardia. Increasing CPB flows (>2.5 L/min/m^2) or perfusion pressure (>70 mm Hg) will raise maternal blood flow and usually returns the heart rate to 120 bpm.[272] A compensatory catecholamine-driven tachycardia (170 bpm) may ensue that suggests an oxygen debt existed.[265] Nonetheless, increasing CPB flow and mean arterial pressure does not always correct fetal bradycardia; if not, other causes must be considered. Problems with venous return or other mechanical aspects of extracorporeal circulation may also limit systemic flow, causing reduced placental perfusion. If acidosis persists throughout CPB, other factors may be responsible for it, such as maternal hypothermia, uterine contractions, or medications that are transferable to the fetus, rather than low maternal blood pressure. Monitoring the fetal heart rate is important to assess fetal viability and subsequent therapeutic initiatives. It partially reduces fetal mortality by early recognition of problems.[268]

Hypothermia has been used for years in cardiac surgery. There are reports of fetal survival with maternal core temperatures of 23° to 25°C, and fetal survival is even documented after 37 minutes of hypothermic (19°C) circulatory arrest.[273,274] However, when hypothermic versus normothermic CPB was examined retrospectively in 69 cases of cardiac surgery in pregnant patients during the period from 1958 to 1992, hypothermia was associated with an embryo-fetal mortality of 24% compared with 0% for normothermia (Table 24–10). Maternal mortality was not influenced by differences in CPB temperature. Consequently, hypothermic CPB is no longer advocated.[266] The fetus appears to maintain autoregulation of the heart rate with mild hypothermia, but most functions are reduced with severe hypothermia.[265] Beyond the effect of hypothermia on acid-base status, coagulation, and arrhythmias, it may precipitate uterine contractions that limit placental perfusion and risk fetal ischemia. The explanation for hypothermia-induced contractions may be related to the severe dilution of CPB that lowers progesterone levels, thus activating uterine contractions. Contractions are more likely to occur at greater gestational age of the fetus.[266,275] Accordingly, uterine monitoring is strongly recommended if CPB is required during pregnancy.

If uterine contractions should begin during CPB, it is vitally important for fetal survival to stop them. Treatment includes ethanol infusion, magnesium sulfate, terbutaline, or ritodrine. Many of these tocolytic agents have potential side effects and toxicities that can be especially detrimental to patients with heart disease,[276] but tocolytic agents may be necessary if the contractions are associated with marked fetal decelerations indicative of severe oxygen deficit. Infants have died from protracted contractions.[277] Prophylactic measures to prevent contractions, such as progesterone, have been of indeterminate benefit. Some have recommended pulsatile CPB to lessen the risk of contractions. Fewer premature contractions have been noted, although the mechanism is unclear.[278]

Approximately 30 to 60 minutes after separation from CPB, the fetus develops a severe and progressive respiratory acidosis.[265] Although correctable, hours later, a more severe metabolic acidosis ensues with the potential for fetal death. It has been postulated that catecholamines and the fetal stress response may be responsible for poor CO secondary to significant vasoconstriction, reflected by a persistent acidosis.[266] The effects of vasopressors and inotropic agents on uterine blood flow in pregnant patients with cardiac disease are indeterminate. Current guidelines are based on animal data, not the intact human maternal-fetal unit. Uterine blood flow is directly proportional to mean perfusion pressure and inversely proportional to uterine vascular resistance. The uterine vascular bed is maximally dilated during pregnancy. Stimulation of α-adrenergic receptors increases uterine vascular resistance and potentially decreases uterine blood flow. However, improvements in maternal CO, blood pressure, and uterine blood flow by certain vasopressors may outweigh any detrimental effect on uterine vascular resistance. Ephedrine has been the vasopressor of choice for maternal hypotension for years.[279] Ephedrine and phenylephrine are safe when treating maternal hypotension during cesarean section following spinal or epidural anesthesia.[280,281] In pregnant ewes, the effect of dopamine on uterine blood flow is mixed. Epinephrine has been associated with decreased uterine blood flow, although in one clinical report an infusion of epinephrine improved maternal hemodynamics after CPB and resolved fetal bradycardia.[282] Overall, the use of these agents during CPB appears to have few negative effects.[265]

Anesthesia Considerations

Medications for anesthesia must be considered in the context of the maternal heart disease, influence of CPB, and effect on the fetus. Maternal safety must be ensured as well as optimal fetal outcome. It is important to be aware of the safety of the more commonly used drugs in cardiac anesthesia during pregnancy. The risk of teratogenesis with the myriad medications and exposures of the fetus during cardiac surgery and CPB is present, but most infants have successfully avoided these effects.[274,275] No anesthetic agent has been shown to be teratogenic in humans. Fetal teratogenicity is always a concern of anesthetic management, especially during the first trimester when fetal organogenesis occurs. Commonly used induction agents and sedatives, such as thiopental, ketamine, etomidate, propofol, midazolam, and diazepam, rapidly cross the placental barrier to the fetal circulation.[283-286] Animal studies show that halothane, enflurane, isoflurane, and sevoflurane appear to be safe anesthetics and lack teratogenic effects.[287,288] Despite concerns about the action of nitrous oxide on DNA synthesis, human and animal studies indicate that it is safe to use nitrous

Table 24–10 Fetal and Maternal Mortality and Morbidity After Cardiopulmonary Bypass

Variable	Patients	Embryofetal Mortality	Maternal Mortality	Embryofetal Morbidity	Maternal Morbidity
Total cases	69	14 (20.2%)	2 (2.9%)	5 (7.2%)	3 (4.3%)
1958 to 1974	29	9 (31.0%)	2 (6.9%)	1 (3.4%)	0
1975 to 1991	40	5 (12.5%)	0	4 (10.0%)	3 (7.5%)
<15 Weeks	24	3 (12.5%)	1 (4.2%)	4 (16.6%)	1 (4.2%)
≥16 Weeks	41	9 (21.9%)	0	1 (2.4%)	2 (4.9%)
Hypothermia (<35°C)	25	6 (24.0%)	0	4 (16.0%)	1 (4.0%)
Normothermia (≥36°C)	13	0	0	0	2 (15.3%)

From Pomini F, Mercogliano D, Cavalletti C, et al: Cardiopulmonary bypass in pregnancy. Ann Thorac Surg 61:265, 1996.

oxide for anesthesia during pregnancy. Fentanyl and sufentanil decrease beat-to-beat variability and may mask fetal distress but do not produce teratogenic effects. Both depolarizing and nondepolarizing muscle relaxants cross the placenta to varying degrees. Pancuronium, atracurium, and pipecuronium have been administered either intramuscularly or intravenously directly to the human fetus in utero without apparent adverse sequelae.

There are many medications administered during cardiac anesthesia that do not provide anesthesia. β-Blockers such as propranolol, esmolol, and labetalol cross the placenta but appear safe for acute and chronic use.[289] Nitroprusside, nitroglycerin, and hydralazine appear to be safe for treating maternal hypertension. Nitroprusside rapidly crosses the placental membrane in pregnant ewes, but infusion rates of less than 2 μg/kg/min do not generate toxic levels of cyanide in fetal lambs.[290] Mannitol and furosemide cross the placenta and induce fetal diuresis but have no apparent adverse fetal consequences. Anticoagulation during pregnancy has been extensively reviewed.[291] Heparin is a large, polyionic compound that does not cross the placenta. Consequently, a cesarean section has been advised by some for neonates with a gestational age of more than 28 weeks immediately after heparinization and cannulation but prior to commencement of CPB.[266] This time period is recommended because at 24 to 28 weeks, organogenesis is complete and neonates appear to do well. If avoidance of CPB with the fetus is not possible, it has not been firmly established with prospective randomized trials the appropriate management to achieve optimal outcome for the mother and fetus. Regional anesthesia carries considerable risk in view of the degree of anticoagulation necessary for CPB, although it has been used successfully. Consequently, heparin and protamine should be administered as deemed appropriate for cardiac surgery. A team approach with anesthesiologist, surgeon, neonatologist, and obstetrician is critical for the care of mother and fetus, especially if optimal management for the mother does not necessarily coincide with fetal interests. The decision to operate needs to be made in the context of the potential survivability of the fetus outside the uterus should delivery of the baby become probable.

RISKS OF HUMAN IMMUNODEFICIENCY VIRUS TRANSMISSION

Concern exists among health care workers about the risk of infection with human immunodeficiency virus (HIV). About 100 cases of occupational HIV infection in health care workers worldwide have been documented, with another 170 cases suspected but not confirmed.[292] Cardiac surgery is one of the highest risk settings for occupational HIV transmission in medicine by reason of the considerable blood exposure that often occurs with CPB and excessive bleeding experienced by these patients. This risk is not expected to improve in the foreseeable future in cardiac surgery and may likely worsen. However, the pattern of HIV transmission is changing to include more heterosexual and progressively older individuals. With newly developed therapies, the incubation time to develop AIDS after infection and life expectancy of those with HIV have been extended.[293,294] As patients with HIV infection live longer and reach ages when the likelihood of cardiac surgery is greater, it will become more difficult to identify HIV-positive patients based on a set of common characteristics.

The risk of exposure to HIV for the health care worker continues to evolve. Earlier studies show transmission risks from patients are, overall, minimal. Henderson et al[295] prospectively studied 1344 health care workers over a 6-year period to assess the risk of HIV transmission during occupational activities. The authors combined data from multiple sources and stated "the risk for HIV-1 transmission associated with percutaneous exposure to blood from an HIV-1 infected patient is approximately 0.3% per exposure."[295] The risk after mucous membrane and cutaneous exposure to an HIV-infected patient is 0.09%. The Centers for Disease Control and Prevention prospective surveillance project found a 0.36% HIV seroconversion rate in health care workers who sustained percutaneous exposure to HIV-contaminated blood.[296] No seroconversions occurred in health care workers who had mucous membrane or cutaneous exposure to HIV-infected blood.

Rates of exposure are subject to the study methods, types of procedures, and precautions of the individuals involved; consequently, the stated risk of transmission with a single exposure may be greater than initially suspected. Factors that have been identified to alter rate of conversion are a deep injury contact, injury by a device visibly contaminated with a patient's blood, or injury by a device placed in the artery or vein. These factors are associated with a higher titer of viral exposure so the rate of conversion is greater than the rate of 0.5% noted previously.[297] Rates of conversion in surgical settings are known to vary widely.[298] The specific occupational risk of blood-borne infections in the health care setting primarily depends on three factors: (1) the prevalence of infected patients within the patient population, (2) the probability of acquiring a specific infection following a single occupational exposure, and (3) the frequency of at-risk exposures.[294] In a study that examined the risk of transmission of HIV by surgical subspecialties and occupation, cardiothoracic surgery had the highest rate.[294] The rate of mucocutaneous contamination by blood splashing during surgery has been estimated to be higher, approximately 50% for cardiothoracic surgery. It appears that almost 60% of exposures in cardiac surgery occur in the operating room, with suturing representing one third of the contacts. However, HIV infection accounts for only 5% of these exposures compared with 78% for hepatitis C. Blood-to-hand contacts represent many of the exposures in the operating room for the cardiac surgical setting.[298] Contact of blood with the body increases the risk of infection dramatically as blood loss exceeds 500 mL.

The best way to prevent occupationally related HIV infection is to prevent exposure to HIV-contaminated bodily fluids, most notably blood. Greene et al,[299] using data restricted to anesthesia personnel and obtained in 1991 to 1993, found that the majority of percutaneous injuries were from contaminated needles, usually hollow bore. The majority of these injuries were preventable. Hollow-bore needles that have been used in venous or arterial puncture appear to have a higher incidence of HIV transmission than do solid needles.[297] Needleless or protected needle infusion devices and revised anesthesia practice protocols may lower the incidence of percutaneous injuries. All anesthesia personnel should routinely wear face shields or eye protection and gloves to prevent cutaneous and mucous membrane contamination.

Studies have confirmed the safety of blood transfusion regarding infection.[300] All donated blood undergoes HIV antibody screening, but a "window period" of approximately 22 days exists when antigens may exist in a donor's blood without antibodies. As of 1995, there are only 29 documented cases of AIDS attributed to the receipt of HIV-seronegative blood, although the actual number may be higher.[300] Lackritz et al[301] evaluated the American Red Cross blood system and estimated that 1 in 360,000 blood donations occurred during the "window period" and that 15% to 42% of this blood was discarded because of other laboratory abnormalities. They also estimated that 1 in 2,600,000 donations was HIV positive but was missed due to laboratory error. The American Red Cross stated the risk for the administration of HIV-infected blood was 1 in 450,000 to 660,000 donations. Extrapolating their data nationwide to all 12 million annual donations, approximately 18 to 27 HIV-infected donations are available for transfusion. Schreiber et al[302] estimated that 1 in 493,000 donated units of blood would result in HIV transmission. They also estimated the risks of transmitting human T-cell lymphotropic virus, hepatitis C virus, and hepatitis B virus to be 1 in 641,000, 1 in 103,000, and 1 in 63,000, respectively. Despite the appropriate concern about HIV transmission during blood transfusion, attention should also be directed toward the transmission of hepatitis B and C viruses.

The effectiveness of postexposure prophylaxis has been difficult to prove in view of the lack of exposures in order to adequately statistically analyze the rate of seroconversion following contact. In case-control trials, zidovudine is the only drug that has been shown to reduce the rate of seroconversion.[293] Table 24–11 outlines the recommendations of the U.S. Public Health Service for postexposure prophylaxis. Postexposure chemoprophylaxis with zidovudine may be indicated when health care workers have significant risk for acquiring HIV via percutaneous exposure, according to recommendations from the Centers for Disease Control and Prevention.[297] If exposure is significant, a 4-week course of zidovudine-lamivudine is recommended, and the addition of a protease inhibitor is indicated if the risk is thought to be even higher. Therapy should begin as soon as possible because there is a "window" before the systemic infection occurs. Earlier exposure to the antiretroviral therapy permits a better chance to preserve immune function and alter the course of the disease. Regardless, all patients at any stage of infection with HIV, even during the "window of opportunity," are a risk for transmission.[292] Follow-up is required for at least 6 months after exposure. Zidovudine has potential complications, so it should be carefully considered because most exposures to HIV do not result in seroconversion. Additionally, zidovudine has been associated with several failures.[298]

Because new therapies for HIV have become more widespread, patients undergoing cardiac surgery may be receiving these newer medications. Triple-drug therapy is now the standard of care[293] (Table 24–12). The complexity of medications that these patients may receive certainly increases the possibility of drug interactions. The nucleoside analog reverse

Table 24–11 Provisional Public Health Service Recommendations for Chemoprophylaxis After Occupational Exposure to Human Immunodeficiency Virus (HIV)

Type of Exposure	Source Material*	Antiretroviral Prophylaxis†	Antiretroviral Regimen‡
Percutaneous	Blood§		
	Highest risk	Recommend	ZDV plus 3TC plus IDV¶
	Increased risk	Recommend	ZDV plus 3TC, ± IDV‖
	No increased risk	Offer	ZDV plus 3TC
	Fluid containing visible blood, other potentially infectious fluid¶, or tissue	Offer	ZDV plus 3TC
	Other body fluid (e.g., urine)	Not offer	
Mucous membrane	Blood	Offer	ZDV plus 3TC, ± ID‖
	Fluid containing visible blood, other potentially infectious fluid¶, or tissue	Offer	ZDV ± 3TC
	Other body fluid (e.g., urine)	Not offer	
Skin	Blood	Offer	ZDV plus 3TC, ± IDV¶
Increased risk**	Fluid containing visible blood, other potentially infectious fluid¶, or tissue	Offer	ZDV ± 3TC
	Other body fluid (e.g., urine)	Not offer	

*Any exposure to concentrated HIV (e.g., in a research laboratory or production facility) is treated as percutaneous exposure to blood with highest risk.

†Recommend = postexposure prophylaxis (PEP) should be recommended to the exposed worker with counseling; Offer = PEP should be offered to the exposed worker with counseling; Not offer = PEP should not be offered because these are not occupational exposures to HIV.

‡Regimens: zidovudine (ZDV) 200 mg three times a day; lamivudine (3TC) 150 mg twice daily; indinavir (IDV) 800 mg three times a day (if IDV is not available, saquinavir may be used, 600 mg three times a day). Prophylaxis is given for 4 weeks. For full prescribing information, see package inserts.

§Highest risk = both larger volume of blood (e.g., deep injury with large-diameter hollow needle previously in source patient's vein or artery, especially involving an injection of source patient's blood) and blood containing high titer of HIV (e.g., source with acute retroviral illness or end-stage AIDS; viral load measurement may be considered, but its use in relation to PEP has not been evaluated). Increased risk = either exposure to larger volume of blood or blood with high titer of HIV. No increased risk = neither exposure to larger volume of blood nor blood with high titer of HIV (e.g., solid suture needle injury from source patient with asymptomatic HIV infection).

‖Possible toxicity of additional drug may not be warranted.

¶Includes semen; vaginal secretions; or cerebrospinal, synovial, pleural, peritoneal, pericardial, and amniotic fluids.

**For skin, risk is increased for exposures involving high titer of HIV; prolonged contact, and extensive area, or an area in which skin integrity is visibly compromised. For skin exposures without increased risk, the risk of drug toxicity outweighs the benefit of PEP.

From Cardo DM, Bell DM: Bloodborne pathogen transmission in health care workers. Infect Dis Clin North Am 11:341 1997 (from Centers for Disease Control and Prevention: Update: Provisional public health service recommendations for chemoprophylaxis after occupational exposure to HIV. MMWR Morb Mortal Wkly Rep 45:468, 1996).

Table 24–12 Drugs Used in the Treatment of HIV Infection

Generic Drug Name	Trade Name
Nucleoside Analog Reverse Transcriptase Inhibitors	
Zidovudine (AZT)	Retrovir
Didanosine (ddI)	Videx
Zalcitabine (ddC)	Hivid
Stavudine (d4T)	Zerit
Lamivudine (3TC)	Epivir
Zidovudine plus lamivudine	Combivir
Abacavir	Ziagen
Nonnucleoside Reverse Transcriptase Inhibitors	
Nevirapine	Viramune
Delavirdine	Rescriptor
Efavirenz	Sustiva
Protease Inhibitors	
Saquinavir	
Hard gel	Invirase
Soft gel	Fortovase
Ritonavir	Norvir
Indinavir	Crixivan
Nelfinavir	Viracept

From Hovanessian HC: New developments in the treatment of HIV disease: An overview. Ann Emerg Med 33:547, 1999.

transcriptase inhibitors are primarily secreted by the kidneys, so fewer drug interactions are possible. However, the nonnucleoside analog reverse transcriptase inhibitors and protease inhibitors are metabolized by the liver with the cytochrome P450 mechanism so that many drug interactions are possible, especially with anesthetic agents.[293] Ritonavir, a potent protease inhibitor, can increase the blood concentration levels of amiodarone, midazolam, diazepam, and meperidine, to name a few. Drug interactions should be considered if a patient is taking these medications and requires cardiac surgery.

RENAL INSUFFICIENCY AND CARDIAC SURGERY

The number of individuals with chronic renal failure (CRF) undergoing cardiac surgery has increased to 2% to 3% of the cardiac surgical population.[303] These patients with CRF may not necessarily be dialysis dependent prior to surgery but are more likely to develop worsening renal function after CPB than are those with normal preoperative renal function.[304] Morbidity and mortality are especially high in long-term dialysis patients undergoing cardiac surgery and CPB, ranging from 17% to 77% and 8% to 31%, respectively.[305] Because CRF accelerates the development of atherosclerosis, myocardial revascularization is often necessary and provides longer-term benefit than percutaneous transluminal angioplasty.[306] Regardless of whether the CRF patient is dialysis dependent, the patient is a significant anesthetic challenge, especially in regard to fluid management, electrolyte status, and hemostasis. The capacity to avoid dialysis in the non–dialysis-dependent CRF patient is even more important in regard to long-term mortality. A collaborative effort by cardiac surgeon, anesthesiologist, nephrologist, and cardiologist is instrumental in the care of these patients. Unfortunately, long-term survival is still appreciably diminished even with minimal perioperative morbidity.

Patients with CRF are more prone to fluid overload, hyponatremia, hyperkalemia, and metabolic acidosis. Optimal hemodynamic and fluid status prior to surgery is important. Hemodialysis should be strongly considered the day before surgery, especially in those who are strictly dialysis dependent. Chronic dialysis patients tend to arrive for surgery with worsened LV function, possibly from inefficient waste and toxin removal. CHF can occur as a result of hypervolemia and poor cardiac function, manifesting as pulmonary edema and respiratory distress. Dialysis and medical therapy directed at improving cardiac function may be required to correct this prior to surgery. Chronic medications should be carefully reviewed to ensure that antihypertensive agents were given. The importance of preoperative preparation for patients with CRF is evident by the significantly higher mortality associated with urgent surgery.[303]

Beyond the increased perioperative mortality of patients with CRF undergoing cardiac surgery, several factors further increase mortality. A preoperative creatinine of 2.5 mg/dL increases the mortality even in those patients with non-dialysis-dependent CRF.[305] Late mortality may range from 8.3% to 55% if dialysis is ongoing for more than 60 months.[303] Pulmonary dysfunction also increases the perioperative mortality of CRF patients.

Patients with CRF differ from those with normal renal function in a variety of ways that influence anesthesia management. A normochromic, normocytic anemia is common, primarily due to decreased or absent erythropoietin secretion, because the kidney is the predominant source of erythropoietin. Anemia is now treated with recombinant human erythropoietin therapy instead of blood. The cardiovascular benefits are especially noticeable with correction of anemia.[307] However, treatment is costly and requires multiple injections weeks before surgery, which may not be possible in many cases.

Anesthesia Considerations

CRF affects dosing of medications that have a large volume of distribution. Decreased serum protein concentration diminishes plasma binding, leading to higher levels of free drug to bind with receptors. Many patients with CRF are hypoalbuminemic. In general, anesthetic induction agents and benzodiazepines are safe to use in patients with CRF. A common induction agent, thiopental, is highly protein bound so the dose should be reduced accordingly. Medications that rely totally on renal excretion have a limited role. Fentanyl and sufentanil may be more effective for pain management because excretion is not as renally dependent as morphine sulfate. Currently used volatile anesthetic agents rarely cause any additional renal dysfunction even with underlying CRF unless severely prolonged duration of anesthesia occurs. Muscle relaxants and agents for antagonism of muscle paralysis have varying degrees of renal excretion (Table 24–13).

A rapid-sequence induction with cricoid pressure is recommended in those with CRF in response to the likelihood of delayed gastric emptying. Significant extracellular volume

Relaxant	Acceptable	Renal Excretion
Atracurium	Yes	<5%
Curare	Yes, with caution	60%
Cisatracurium	Yes	<10%
Doxacurium	Yes, with caution	70%
Gallamine	No	100%
Metocurine	Yes	50%
Pancuronium	Yes, with caution	70%
Pipecuronium	Yes, with caution	70%
Vecuronium	Yes	30%
Rocuronium	Yes	9%†
Mivacurium	Yes	7%‡
Succinylcholine	Yes, with normokalemia	0%

†Khuenl-Brady K, Castagnoli KP, Canfell PC, et al: The neuromuscular blocking effects and pharmacokinetics of ORG 9426 and ORG 9616 in the cat. Anesthesiology 72:669, 1990.

‡Cook DR, Freeman JA, Lai AA, et al: Pharmacokinetics of mivacurium in normal patients and in those with hepatic or renal failure. Br J Anaesth 69:580, 1992.

Adapted from Barash PG, et al: Clinical Anesthesia. Philadelphia, JB Lippincott Company, 1989; and Miller RD, et al: Pharmacology of muscle relaxants and their antagonists. *In* Miller RD (ed): Anesthesia. New York, Churchill Livingstone Inc, 1990, pp 389–436, with permission.

contraction may also be present prior to induction of anesthesia due to a 6- to 8-hour fast prior to surgery and dialysis within 24 hours of surgery that may lead to hypotension on induction. Because fluid requirements are usually significant with CPB, a PAC is especially useful to manage fluid requirements. Transesophageal echocardiography may complement fluid management by assessment of LV volume and function. Prior to the initiation of CPB, fluid administration should be limited, especially if the patient is dialysis dependent. Otherwise, fluid should be given to maintain adequate urine output but avoid excessive cardiovascular filling pressures risking pulmonary edema. However, restricting fluids too aggressively in these patients may lead to acute renal failure superimposed on CRF. Low-dose dopamine has been recommended for patients with CRF, but its value is indeterminate. Fenoldopam, a new dopamine$_1$-receptor agonist, may reduce the incidence of renal dysfunction in patients with multiple risk factors for renal failure undergoing CPB. Patients with preoperative creatinine levels above 1.5 mg/dL were given renal-dose dopamine or fenoldopam perioperatively.[308] Postoperative parameters were only improved in those receiving fenoldopam, suggesting a renal protective effect, but additional studies are needed.

In general, CRF worsens after CPB in part due to a combination of nonpulsatile flow, low renal perfusion, and hypothermia.[305] Renal perfusion is lowered as CPB is initiated, increasing the chance for ischemia of the renal cortex. Mean arterial pressure should be kept above 80 mm Hg. The stress of surgery and hypothermia may impair autoregulation so that renal vasoconstriction reduces renal blood flow. The fluid required to initiate CPB may significantly reduce the hemoglobin (Hb) and oxygen-carrying capacity in view of the preexisting anemia of CRF without the addition of red blood cells (RBCs) to the priming volume or immediately upon initiation of CPB. A hematocrit of 25% should be maintained during CPB.[305] Washed RBCs are recommended for RBC transfusion to lessen excessive potassium and glucose levels intraoperatively. Potassium plasma levels should be checked periodically. Mannitol and furosemide may prevent early oliguric renal failure.[309] Patients with CRF often have glucose intolerance from an abnormal insulin response, so more frequent determination of serum glucose levels is advisable.

The anephric patient poorly tolerates post-CPB hypervolemia that often follows prolonged duration of CPB. Dialysis can be performed during CPB and is technically easy and effective because small molecules (uremic solutes, electrolytes) are removed.[310] Instead of dialysis during CPB, hemofiltration (ultrafiltration) is more frequently performed, effectively clearing excess water without the hemodynamic instability of dialysis. Circulating blood passes through the hollow fibers of the hemoconcentrators that have a smaller pore size than albumin (55,000 Da), which remove water and solutes. These midsize molecules (inflammatory molecules) are small enough to pass through the pores to concentrate the blood. Potassium is eliminated, helping reduce excessive potassium concentration commonly associated with cardioplegia administration. Hemofiltration during CPB may not achieve a net reduction in the overall total fluid balance of the patient, in part because a minimum volume of fluid must be maintained in the venous reservoir of the extracorporeal circuit.

Excessive bleeding following CPB is not uncommon in those with CRF, in part due to preoperative platelet dysfunction. Antifibrinolytic medications are pharmacologic measures used to successfully reduce excessive bleeding and transfusion requirements associated with cardiac surgery.[37] Tranexamic acid, an inexpensive, synthetic antifibrinolytic, is excreted primarily through the kidneys, so a dose reduction is required based on the preoperative creatinine level. Aprotinin, a serine protease inhibitor with anti-inflammatory as well as antifibrinolytic properties, is concentrated in the proximal renal tubules but rarely leads to a clinically important increase in the postoperative creatinine levels. If the patient is dialysis dependent, then aprotinin is recommended to reduce bleeding and transfusions.[311] On the contrary, if renal insufficiency without dialysis dependence is present with a corresponding serum creatinine level greater than 2.5 mg/dL, aprotinin should be discouraged or aprotinin dosing altered.[312]

The likelihood of dialysis is greater if the preoperative serum creatinine is above 2.5 mg/dL in patients undergoing cardiac surgery. Postoperatively, if dialysis is required in patients with end-stage renal disease, the likelihood of dialysis dependence is greatly increased.[309] If the patient is dialysis dependent preoperatively, dialysis is usually resumed within 48 hours of surgery and then implemented according to the patient's preoperative routine to optimize fluid, electrolyte, and metabolic status. Hemodialysis primarily corrects electrolyte imbalances and removes organic acids to correct metabolic acidosis. Dialysis may lessen the platelet dysfunction associated with uremia to minimize hemostatic abnormalities and excessive hemorrhage. Dialysis may be needed soon after return from the operating room if mobilization of fluids into the intravascular space causes CHF. Peritoneal dialysis may be preferable if the postoperative hemodynamic status of the patient is unstable. Peritoneal dialysis, compared with hemodialysis, is more convenient to administer and does not require the immediate support of a nephrologist.

Alternatively, continuous renal replacement therapy can be instituted intraoperatively and postoperatively in cardiac patients following CPB to manage acute renal failure with volume overload and metabolic instability.[313]

Patients with CRF are at high risk for morbidity and mortality with cardiac surgery involving CPB. Attention to the following steps may improve outcome: (1) assess conditions associated with CRF that lead to complications such as platelet function, lung function, and anemia; (2) provide adequate RBC mass; (3) carefully administer fluid and electrolyte, particularly after CPB; (4) use hemofiltration; (5) institute blood conservation techniques and treatment of coagulopathy; (6) provide judicious use of dialysis; and (7) scrutinize for infections to which patients with CRF are more susceptible.

HEMATOLOGIC PROBLEMS IN PATIENTS UNDERGOING CARDIAC SURGERY

Anesthetic concerns for patients with hematologic problems who undergo cardiac surgery are further complicated by the stress CPB places on coagulation and oxygen-carrying systems. Hemophilia, cold agglutinins, sickle cell disease, antithrombin deficiency, and von Willebrand's disease are a few of the hematologic disorders that may require special consideration if CPB is needed (see Chapters 18 and 29).

Hemophilia

In the 1940s and 1950s, the coagulation factors that separated hemophilia A (factor VIII deficiency) from hemophilia B (factor IX deficiency) were identified.[314] Prior to that discovery, hemophilia was a debilitating disease with a life expectancy of less than 20 years. The arrival of intermediate purity factor concentrates provided individuals with hemophilia autonomy and prolonged their life beyond 50 years. Patients were even able to successfully undergo cardiac surgery.[315] Early coagulation factor concentrates were not virally safe, so 60% to 95% of individuals with hemophilia beyond 8 years of age were infected with hepatitis C virus.[314] Likewise, more than 60% to 70% of individuals with hemophilia became infected with HIV.[316] AIDS reduced the life expectancy of those with hemophilia to 40 years.[317] New recombinant factor replacements may again improve life expectancy, as viral transmission becomes rare.

Hemophilia A is the third most common X-linked disorder, occurring in 1 in 5000 male births.[314] Hemophilia B, also known as Christmas disease, is also an X-linked disorder with one fourth the incidence of hemophilia A. Factor VIII is instrumental in a normally functioning clotting cascade. With a half-life of only 8 to 12 hours, factors VIII and IXa accelerate activation of factor X. Hemophilia is characterized by spontaneous bleeding in joints and muscles in its severe form.[318] Milder cases may only be associated with bleeding after surgery. Hemophilia A and B are very similar in presentation, course, and treatment. Gene mutations for both hemophilia A and B are better understood today; hemophilia may be the most likely disease to be cured by gene therapy.[316]

Treatment of hemophilia A and B primarily depends on replacement of factor VIII or IX, respectively. Preparations of recombinant factor VIII were developed in the 1990s, which effectively control 80% of bleeding episodes with a single dose.[316] Viral contamination has been essentially negated so the incidence of inhibitors is no more likely than plasma-derived factors. A new recombinant factor VIII, in clinical trial, is devoid of exposure to human or animal protein except the murine monoclonal antibodies necessary to create the product. Success with plasma-derived products depends on the virus inactivation procedures and screening processes and availability. Plasma-derived products are much less expensive and more available than are recombinant products. Furthermore, they are less likely to be associated with prolonged product shortages.

It is important during the perioperative assessment to estimate the severity of the patient's hemophilia because perioperative bleeding is related to the degree of factor deficiency. Factor deficiency in hemophilia may range from factor levels of 6% to 30% with occasional symptoms to a factor level below 1% with easy bleeding. A factor level near 50% of normal is regarded as adequate to achieve surgical hemostasis; however, most patients present for surgery with factor VIII or factor IX activity of less than 5%. Slightly lower levels have been maintained intraoperatively without excessive blood loss or significant hemostatic abnormalities; however, oozing may occur postoperatively.[319] Preoperatively, factor VIII activity should be 80% to 100%. Bleeding will be severe if factor VIII activity is less than 1%. The amount of factor replacement is estimated from the total fluid volume of the extracorporeal circuit (pump prime), plasma volume, and the desired factor activity. Because adequate levels of factor VIII or IX should be present prior to CPB, it is helpful to know factor VIII and IX levels prior to CPB. Severe hemodilution may necessitate the addition of factor VIII or IX replacements in the extracorporeal circuit.[315] However, the minimal acceptable factor activity during surgery requiring CPB is not established. Postoperatively, factor VIII activity should be maintained at 30% to 50%.[320] After blood product transfusion, factor VIII levels may be helpful to guide future transfusions. Factor VIII levels vary significantly because no treatment provides a sustained factor VIII level.

With newer recombinant factor replacements, there is less likelihood of allogeneic blood exposure for individuals with hemophilia. Because shortages do occur, some familiarity with component therapy is necessary. One milliliter of fresh frozen plasma (FFP) has 1 unit of factor VIII activity. A unit of cryoprecipitate contains 100 to 120 units of factor VIII activity. Several thousand plasma units are used to prepare each factor VIII or IX concentrate. For hemophilia B, factor IX is available only in FFP and factor concentrates and recombinant form.

1-Desamino-8-D-arginine vasopressin (DDAVP), a vasopressin analog, has been used successfully in mild-to-moderate hemophilia A to decrease intraoperative transfusion requirements.[314,321,322] A rapid increase in all components of factor VIII occurs after DDAVP administration, but factor VIII level falls by 50% in 10 hours. The response of DDAVP depends on the resting factor VIII level and hemostatic demand. If the patient with hemophilia possesses 5% to 20% procoagulant activity, he is more likely to respond to DDAVP, in contrast to those with severe factor VIII deficiencies who do not respond to DDAVP.[322] The peak effect occurs 1 hour after an intravenous dose of 0.3 μg/kg is given. DDAVP can be given at 12- to 24-hour intervals, but tachyphylaxis is possible after multiple doses.

Therapy for hemophilia B has changed significantly with the availability of a concentrated purified recombinant factor IX. Recombinant factor IX is not exposed to human or animal protein. Previously, individuals with hemophilia B were treated with plasma-derived products called prothrombin complex concentrates that contain factors IX, X, II, and VII. These active complexes have resulted in fatal thrombotic reactions because they are not normally generated or regulated by the coagulation pathway. Circulating factor IX levels do not increase as much as factor VIII after transfusion because factor IX is distributed in both intravascular and extravascular spaces, unlike factor VIII. Factor IX activity of approximately 50% is adequate to achieve hemostasis yet minimize the risk of thrombotic complications.[315]

Antifibrinolytic therapy has been used in patients with hemophilia to inhibit the normal clot-lysing process. Antifibrinolytic agents, aprotinin, tranexamic acid, and ε-aminocaproic acid are used prophylactically to reduce blood loss and transfusion requirements in cardiac surgery involving CPB.[37] Other methods and techniques for blood conservation should be considered to reduce the risk of bleeding and transfusion with hemophilia.

Antibodies to factor VIII or IX may occur in patients with hemophilia who have received replacement therapy. The incidence of factor VIII or IX inhibitors is 18% to 52% and 2% to 16% of the hemophilia population, respectively.[318,323,324] Inhibitors occur more often in patients receiving the purest replacement factors, which is a major concern for future replacement therapy with purer products.[325] The strength of the immune response is instrumental in the development of inhibitors. For example, HIV-positive patients with hemophilia do not develop factor VIII inhibitors.[317] The inhibitor titer characterizes the patients as mild or high responders. High responders are at great risk because the anamnestic response may generate very high antibody titers that can render factor replacement therapy totally ineffective hemostatically.[326] The problem with patients who develop inhibitors and require surgery is the inability to predict hemostasis at any point of the hospitalization.

Cardiac operations require more intense hemostasis than most other surgical and nonsurgical situations. Cardiac surgery has been successfully performed in patients with factor VIII inhibitors.[327] Patients with low antibody titers often tolerate conventional concentrate infusion but require higher and more frequent dosages for efficacy.[314] To achieve hemostasis in the presence of factor VIII and factor IX inhibitors, the defect in the intrinsic coagulation pathway must be bypassed and prothrombin complex concentrates given that contain activated forms of factors VII, IX, and X, which are largely successful in achieving hemostasis.[316] A new recombinant factor VIIa (FVIIa) has become available.[328] Factor VII appears to bind to tissue factor on the surface of the activated platelet to cause hemostasis. It is infused as a bolus of 90 to 120 μg/kg and repeated at 3-hour intervals to a maximum of 4 times. In more than 1900 surgical and nonsurgical bleeding episodes in more than 400 patients with hemophilia A or B, factor VIIa has been shown to be safe in major operations with excellent results in 80% of cases.[329] However, randomized controlled trials have not been performed. Newer approaches to inhibitors are presently being studied.

Particular caution must be taken in managing the airway in patients with hemophilia to avoid any trauma-induced bleeding. Nonsteroidal pain medications may be counterproductive in these patients due to the effect on platelet function. Strict asepsis must be maintained because the immune systems of these patients may be very weak and extremely susceptible to bacterial and viral infections.

von Willebrand's Disease

von Willebrand's disease (vWD) is the most commonly inherited hemostatic abnormality, with a prevalence in the general population of 0.8%.[330] It is an autosomal dominant bleeding disorder caused by a deficiency and/or abnormality of von Willebrand factor (vWF). An acquired form of vWD is associated with various disease states and medications.[331] The nomenclature of vWF and factor VIII complex has been standardized to resolve past confusion (Table 24–14).

vWF is a large, adhesive glycoprotein that is produced by vascular endothelial cells and megakaryocytes. It is found in platelet α-granules, plasma, and subendothelium. It circulates in blood as an array of multimers of various sizes. Large multimers have more binding sites for platelets, thereby augmenting platelet adhesion and aggregation. Each vWF subunit has a site for a platelet receptor to bind and the extracellular matrix component of the vessel wall to attach.[332] vWF has two major hemostatic functions: (1) a carrier protein and stabilizer for factor VIII and (2) mediation of platelet adhesion to injured sites.[333] It plays a crucial role in mediating platelet adhesion, platelet aggregation, and clotting during high shear conditions.[334] Patients with vWD have an abnormality of both vWF and factor VIII. vWD is classified into three major types and four subtypes: I, II, and III[335] (Table 24–15). Individuals with type 1 vWD and type 2 vWD comprise 70% and 20% of people with vWD, respectively.[336] Type 3 vWD represents only 10% of individuals and is autosomal recessive. Type 3 vWD individuals are severely affected and present in a similar manner to individuals with hemophilia who have a very low factor VIII activity (1% to 4%).

Erik von Willebrand identified the abnormal bleeding time (BT) that characterized vWD. The laboratory diagnosis of vWD is complex due to the broad phenotypes that exist. No single laboratory test is diagnostic for vWD. The BT is sensitive for vWD, but it is prolonged in only 50% of individuals with type 1 vWD. It is markedly prolonged in type 3 vWD. The activated partial thromboplastin time (aPTT) is usually prolonged, but it is not a good screening test for vWD because factor VIII activity, which affects the aPTT, varies greatly in vWD. The ristocetin cofactor assay, also known as the vWF activity, is the most sensitive and specific test for vWD and the

Table 24–14 Recommended Nomenclature of Factor VIII/V and von Willebrand Factor (vWF) Complex

Factor VIII	
Protein	VIII
Antigen	VIII:Ag
Function	VIII:C
vWF	
Protein	vWF
Antigen	vWF:Ag
Function	vWF:RCo*

*Although not measuring "true" vWF activity, ristocetin cofactor activity is used as a surrogate test for vWF activity in vitro. This activity depends on both vWF level and multimeric structure.

From Castaman G, Rodeghiero F: Current management of von Willebrand's disease. Drugs 50:602, 1995.

Table 24–15 Classification of von Willebrand's Disease

New	Old	Characteristics
1	I platelet normal, I platelet low, 1A, I-1, I-2, I-3	Partial quantitative deficiency of vWF
2A		Qualitative variants with decreased platelet-dependent function that is associated with the absence of high-molecular-weight vWF multimers
2B		Qualitative variants with increased affinity for platelet GPIb
2M		Qualitative variants with decreased platelet-dependent function that is not caused by the absence of high-molecular-weight vWF multimers
2N		Qualitative variants with markedly decreased affinity for factor VIII
3		Virtually a complete deficiency of vWF

vWF = von Willebrand factor; GPIb = glycoprotein receptor Ib.
From Castaman G and Rodeghiero F: Current management of von Willebrand's disease. Drugs 50:602, 1995.

Table 24–16 Patterns of von Willebrand's Disease

Type	RIPA	Ristocetin Cofactor	vWF Antigen	Factor VIII
1	D	D	D	D
2A	D	D or DD	D or N	N or D
2B	I	D	D or N	N or D
2M	D	D or DD	D	N or D
2N	D	D or DD	D	N or D
3	DD	DD	DD	DD

D = decreased; I = increased; N = normal; RIPA = ristocetin-induced platelet aggregation; vWF = von Willebrand factor.

single best test to identify vWD[336] (Table 24–16). It measures the ability of vWF to bind to glycoprotein Ib platelet receptors. The vWF antigen test measures the quantity of vWF protein, not functional activity. vWF multimers can be visualized by electrophoresis and establish the type of vWD by their presence or absence. Factor VIII activity is frequently low in vWD. In mild cases of vWD, aPTT, factor VIII, and BT may be normal with only a slight decrease in the ristocetin cofactor assay and vWF antigen.[337] Factors such as age, estrogen levels, adrenergic stimulus, and inflammation can directly affect vWF levels and complicate laboratory evidence of vWD. Consequently, several determinations of aPTT and BT may be required to correctly diagnose vWD.

A complete medical history is important to complement laboratory testing. Family history is a sensitive indicator of vWD. Individuals with vWD frequently describe bleeding that is more mucosal in origin (epistaxis) compared with people with hemophilia. Medical history is important because routine laboratory screening may fail to detect vWD. Unlike hemophilia, patients with mild vWD may go unnoticed for years with unremarkable bleeding patterns. Variant forms of vWD add to the possibility of misdiagnosis. If undiagnosed, surgical bleeding may be severe, particularly if combined with ingestion of antiplatelet medications.[338] Aspirin and anti-inflammatory medications should be identified preoperatively. It is important to question the patient individually to determine the severity of bleeding, because even within a family with similar laboratory tests, there can be significant differences in the bleeding tendency.[337]

Bleeding does not correlate closely with any specific level of vWF. Therapy is aimed at increasing factor VIII level and vWF to about 50% of normal as well as correcting an elevated BT. If the BT has been corrected, it is assumed that 50% of factors are present although a normal BT may not be essential for surgical hemostasis.[338] Correction of vWF deficiency may be accomplished by one of three methods: increase synthesis, facilitate release from storage sites, or administer exogenous components. Each type of vWD requires a different therapeutic approach.

DDAVP is the first choice for treatment in vWD, but not all types of vWD respond to it. It is effective in type 1 vWD, but the BT will be only temporarily corrected.[339] It is ill advised in type 2B vWD because thrombocytopenia may result. It is useless in type 3 vWD because there are no stores of vWF to release.[340] If cryoprecipitate is also given, DDAVP may be effective in type 3 vWD. DDAVP does not directly cause release of factor VIII/vWF from the endothelial cell but stimulates monocytes to produce a substance that releases vWF. A response to DDAVP should occur in 30 minutes, with threefold to eightfold increases in factor VIII and vWF that may persist 8 to 10 hours.[339] Hemostasis may require one or two doses of DDAVP at least 12 hours apart. It is readily available and inexpensive and has minimal risk for patients. DDAVP is effective given in an intravenous, intranasal, or subcutaneous manner, but the intranasal preparation lacks the predictability and strength of the intravenous preparation.[336] Intravenous dosing (0.3 μg/kg) requires 20 to 30 minutes to avoid a fall in mean arterial pressure of 15% to 20%. Tachyphylaxis may occur with a 30% decrease in the effectiveness of the second dose if DDAVP is given more than once in each 24-hour period.[339] For a majority of patients with mild vWD, DDAVP is effective and avoids exposure to plasma products. Side effects of DDAVP include facial flushing, headache, and fluid retention with hyponatremia. Reports of increased thrombosis with DDAVP are anecdotal.

Blood products should not be administered to patients with vWD unless other treatment is ineffective or contraindicated. Apart from DDAVP, controversy continues to exist regarding the optimal treatment of vWD. In the past, treatment for vWD included administration of cryoprecipitate and even FFP. The belief that a full complement of high-molecular-weight multimers is required to control bleeding is not totally correct.[341] It is still unclear as to the amount of vWF or factor VIII that is required to control bleeding. Treatment of vWD may require replacement therapy in type 3 and type 2B vWD. FFP contains the clotting factors to correct the deficiency of vWD, but the volume may be excessive. Cryoprecipitate contains 5 to 10 times more factor VIII, vWF, and fibrinogen than FFP in a smaller volume than FFP, but viral transmission is more likely. Cryoprecipitate given every 12 to 24 hours normalizes factor VIII levels and improves platelet function abnormalities. The role of factor VIII concentrates in vWD has been expanded. For many years, factor VIII concentrates were not effective in vWD because ristocetin cofactor activity was low and many of the hemostatically active vWF multimers were absent.[342] Factor VIII levels were adequately replenished with these concentrates, but the BT was not consistently corrected. Currently, virus-inactivated factor VIII/vWF concentrates are the blood product of choice in vWD.[339] A chromatography-purified concentrate rich with vWF but low in factor VIII called very-high-purity vWF has emerged.[339] Despite an extremely low factor VIII concentration, the product is effective.[341] The dose of 2454 IU/kg (0.21/IU factor VIII) followed by 2639 IU vWF:RCO/kg every 12 hours resulted in hemostasis.[341]

For pretreatment of patients about to undergo surgery with no vWF stores, such as in type 3 vWD, a dosage of 40 to 60 IU VIII:C/kg of a concentrate containing factor VIII and native vWF is recommended.[335] Because factor VIII level increases slowly, factor VIII may be given 1 day prior to surgery. Concentrates should be administered twice daily. There is no consensus regarding the best parameter for monitoring replacement therapy. For surgery, factor VIII levels should be obtained every 12 hours intraoperatively and then once per day postoperatively. vWF levels fall upon initiation of CPB, but subsequently rise as vWF is released from storage pools.[334] A BT is not necessary for management of most vWD patients. Further experience with factor VIII/vWF concentrates in surgical patients suggests a benefit. Platelet infusions should be considered in patients with type 3 vWD after failure to correct the BT with cryoprecipitate or factor VIII concentrates or if bleeding persists.[336] Antifibrinolytic agents should also be considered in patients with vWD to reduce clot lysis. As in hemophilia, inhibitors can occur in vWD, causing life-threatening bleeding. Prothrombin complex concentrates may be useful in these circumstances.

Antithrombin

Antithrombin (AT) and protein C are two primary inhibitors of coagulation. A delicate balance exists between the procoagulant system and the inhibitors of coagulation (Table 24–17).

Table 24–17 Balance That Normally Exists Between Prothrombotic and Antithrombotic Forces Within the Circulation

Prothrombotic Factors	Antithrombotic Factors
Thrombin	Antithrombin
Factor Xa	Protein C
Factor VIIa	Protein S
Tissue factor	Heparin cofactor II
Activated platelets	TFPI
Perturbed endothelial cells	Thrombomodulin
Others	APC cofactor 2
	Others

TFPI = tissue factor protein inhibitor; APC = activated protein C.
From Blajchman MA: An overview of the mechanism of action of antithrombin and its inherited deficiency states. Blood Coagul Fibrinolysis 5(suppl 1):S5, 1994.

AT is the most abundant and important of the coagulation pathway inhibitors. Deficiencies of AT increase the risk of thromboembolism and impact patients requiring CPB.

AT is an α_2-globulin that is produced primarily in the liver. It binds thrombin, as well as other serine proteases, factors IX, X, XI, and XII, kallikrein, and plasmin, irreversibly, which neutralizes their activity. However, only inhibition of thrombin and factor Xa by AT has physiologic and clinical significance.[343] AT activity of less than 50% is clinically important.[344] AT deficiency may occur as a congenital deficiency or as an acquired deficiency secondary to increased AT consumption, loss of AT from the intravascular compartment (renal failure, nephrotic syndrome), or liver disease (cirrhosis). Acquired deficiency is often associated with trauma, sepsis, and shock. Although AT deficiency may be acquired, cause and effect are difficult to prove because many factors may exist simultaneously to account for abnormal clotting.

Congenital deficiency of AT is the prototypical, hypercoagulable state produced by an imbalance of coagulation and fibrinolytic factors (see Table 24–17). The prevalence is 1 in 2000 to 5000 patients.[345] Congenital AT deficiency is separated into four types (I, II, III, and IV) based on the quantitative and qualitative defects of the AT molecule. It is transmitted in an autosomal dominant pattern with affected individuals typically maintaining 50% AT activity. If the levels fall below 50% of normal, the risk of thrombosis is significant.[346] The only abnormal coagulation test in this situation is the assay for AT activity, which is diagnostic. Affected individuals may experience a thromboembolic event at an early age, but arterial thrombosis is encountered in fewer than 1% of persons.[347] The advisability of long-term anticoagulation is indeterminate in these individuals. Anticoagulation prophylaxis is recommended in cases in which the risk of thrombosis is temporarily increased, such as surgery.[348] The risk of thrombosis is higher in congenital forms than in acquired forms of AT deficiency[345,349] (see Chapter 29).

Anticoagulation for CPB depends on AT to inhibit clotting as heparin alone has no effect on coagulation. Heparin catalyzes AT inhibition of thrombin by binding to a lysine residue on AT and altering its conformation. Thrombin actually attacks AT, disabling it, but in the process attaches AT to thrombin, forming the AT and thrombin complex. This complex has no activity and is rapidly removed.[343] Thirty

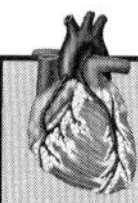

BOX 24–5 *Diseases or Situations Causing Increased Heparin Resistance*

- Infective endocarditis
- Intra-aortic balloon counterpulsation
- Hypereosinophilic syndrome
- Oral contraceptives
- Shock
- Low-grade intravascular coagulation
- Previous heparin therapy
- Previous streptokinase
- Presence of a clot within the body
- Congenital antithrombin deficiency
- Pregnancy
- Neonatal respiratory distress syndrome
- Increased platelet levels
- Increased factor VIII levels
- Secondary decrease in antithrombin levels
- Ongoing clotting and utilization of heparin

From Anderson EF: Heparin resistance prior to cardiopulmonary bypass. Anesthesiology 64:504, 1986.

percent of AT is consumed during this process, so AT levels are reduced. AT deficiency may occur with cardiac and non-cardiac operations. The "adequacy" of anticoagulation with heparin may be monitored with the activated coagulation time (ACT). If an individual has a reduced response to heparin, it is referred to as heparin resistance, which can lead to thrombus formation and serious complications. The many causes of heparin resistance are listed in Box 24–5 (see Chapters 18 and 29).

Heparin exposure prior to CPB is increasingly common in cardiac surgical practice today, resulting in more cases of heparin resistance. The incidence varies among hospitals, but in 2270 cardiac cases, 3.7% were identified as heparin resistant.[350] Although 50% more heparin may be required with heparin resistance, 30% of patients do not reach adequate ACT values despite having received 800 U/kg of heparin. Heparin anticoagulation for CPB causes further lowering of AT levels that were most likely low prior to surgery. AT activity falls an additional 25% to 50% with initiation of CPB, in part due to dilution and elimination of the AT and thrombin complex.[345,349] Unfortunately, AT levels are not routinely obtained prior to cardiac surgery, but if AT deficiency is suspected, a bedside determination of heparin resistance can be performed. A small volume of FFP is obtained and placed in one sample for an ACT while another ACT sample obtained at the same time is undisturbed. A large increase in the ACT value in the sample that received FFP makes the diagnosis of AT deficiency probable.[351] AT-deficient patients are at risk for major thrombosis if exposed to CPB, and clotting has been reported.[352] Neonates have very serious thrombotic complications with AT deficiency. Therefore, AT-deficient patients who require CPB should be treated aggressively. Once AT levels reach more than 80%, thrombosis is less likely. Paradoxically, because patients with congenital AT deficiency may be receiving warfarin, dipyridamole, aspirin, or any combination of medications to increase AT activity and because low AT levels lead to clotting factor and platelet consumption during CPB, hemostasis may be profoundly impaired during cardiac surgery. Postoperatively, AT levels continue to decline at a rate dependent on the extent of tissue disruption and hemorrhage.

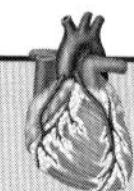

BOX 24–6 *Indications for Antithrombin Replacement Therapy*

Approved Indications (Clinical Data Suggest Efficacy)

- Congenital AT deficiency
  - Perioperative
  - Postsurgical prophylaxis for deep vein thrombosis
  - Acute thromboembolism
  - Pregnancy: delivery and abortion
  - Neonates with congenital AT deficiency*

Probable Indications (Data Suggest Improvement in Laboratory And Clinical Measures)

- Neonates born to mothers with congenital AT deficiency or with strong family history of thrombosis
- DIC due to sepsis, trauma, burns, associated with pregnancy
- Heparin resistance associated with low AT
- Extracorporeal circulation (cardiopulmonary bypass, hemodialysis)
- Hepatic artery thrombosis after OLT

Possible Indications (Data Suggest Improvement in Laboratory Values Without Proven Clinical Efficacy)

- VOD
- OLT
- LeVeen peritoneovenous shunt
- Chronic hepatic insufficiency

Investigational Use

- Nephrotic syndrome
- AT deficiency due to gastrointestinal loss (inflammatory bowel disease, protein-losing enteropathy)
- Pregnancy: preeclampsia, gestational hypertension, and acute fatty liver of pregnancy
- Neonatal respiratory distress syndrome

AT = antithrombin; DIC = disseminated intravascular coagulation; OLT = orthotopic liver transplant; VOD = veno-occlusive disease.
From Bucur SZ, Levy JH, Despotis GJ, et al: Uses of antithrombin III concentrate in congenital and acquired deficiency states. Transfusion 38:482, 1998.

The nadir occurs on the third day and preoperative levels return by the fifth day.[345] A summary of trials that evaluated the value of AT concentrate for prophylaxis regarding surgery in AT-deficient patients strongly recommended the administration of AT concentrates.[345] Other indications for AT are listed in Box 24–6.

Various blood products had been tried as an alternative to FFP to rapidly raise the AT level. Cryoprecipitate and FFP have similar amounts of AT, but the infectious risk is greater for cryoprecipitate. In 1974, AT was isolated from human plasma and AT concentrates were discovered.[347] AT concentrate preparations are derived from human plasma pools but are subjected to fractionation procedures and heating to inactivate viral contaminants. This process does not reduce biologic activity and viral transmission has not been reported.[347,349] One bottle of AT contains approximately 500 units or the equivalent of 2 units of FFP and can be safely administered over 10 to 20 minutes.[353] The baseline AT activity of the heparin-resistant patients was 56 ± 25%, which improved to 75 ± 31% after administration of AT concentrate.[350]

Recombinant AT concentrates have been used in cardiac surgical patients, but there is no consensus about their efficacy as few randomized trials have been performed.[354]

Recommendations are primarily derived from case reports, so the dose of AT concentrates to suppress thrombin generation in adults undergoing CPB is indeterminate.[349] Concentrates have been effective in suppressing activation of the coagulation cascade, particularly in the most susceptible group of patients—pediatric patients.[355] AT concentrates appear to be beneficial in both hereditary and acquired AT deficiency.[345,347] Hereditary AT-deficient patients who require heparin and those who need postoperative and postdelivery thrombosis prophylaxis, as well as hereditary AT-deficient neonates, have benefited from the administration of AT concentrates.[345,356] Improvement in AT activity has been shown to improve biochemical markers of hemostatic activation but not always clinical markers of improvement such as mediastinal chest tube drainage and transfusion requirements.[349,350,357] AT concentrate is expensive, but side effects are minimal.

Cold Agglutinins

Cold agglutinins (CAs) are common but rarely clinically important. Often associated with lymphoreticular neoplasms, *Mycoplasma* pneumonia, and infectious mononucleosis, they are IgM class autoantibodies directed against the RBC I-antigen or related antigens.[358] CAs form a complement antigen-antibody reaction on the surface of the RBC membrane that causes lysis. The degree of hemolysis is related to the circulating titer and thermal amplitude of the CAs.[359] Thermal amplitude, the blood temperature below which the CAs react, is the key factor influencing clinical relevance. The titer and thermal amplitude are determined at various temperatures in the serum by an indirect hemagglutination test. Most people have cold autoantibodies that react at 4°C but in very low titers. Accelerated destruction of RBCs primarily occurs if the thermal amplitude is above 30°C. The higher is the thermal amplitude of the CAs, the more pathologic. Pathologic cold autoantibodies also have much higher titers at 30°C. However, thermal amplitude is more important than titer. With pathologic CAs, vascular occlusion occurs due to RBC clumping, injuring the myocardium, liver, and kidney.[360] Microscopic RBC clumping may erroneously be attributed to other causes during hypothermic CPB unless agglutination is observed. Increasing temperature rapidly inactivates CAs.[361]

Blood banks routinely screen for the presence of autoantibodies at 37°C, but cold antibodies, only reactive at lower temperatures, are not detected. The significance of CAs is determined by evaluating agglutination of RBCs in 20°C saline and 30°C albumin. If there is no agglutination, significant hemolysis is unlikely.[362] Prior to initiation of CPB, the titer and thermal amplitude of CAs must be determined to avoid a temperature during CPB that would cause hemolysis. Intraoperatively, low-thermal-amplitude CAs can be determined by mixing cold cardioplegia with some of the patient's blood to check for separation of cells. If there is concern about CAs after routine testing, the sample can also be diluted to simulate CPB, cooled, and inspected for RBC agglutination. The hemodilution commonly associated with CPB may weaken agglutination and hemolysis in a patient with high reactivity and titer of CAs exposed to hypothermia.[359]

The actions of CA may be difficult to diagnose because there are many other causes for hemolysis with CPB, so some cardiac surgeons avoid hypothermia if CAs are suspected or identified preoperatively. Despite normothermic CPB, cold cardioplegia may cause RBC agglutination in small myocardial vessels.[363] Nevertheless, hypothermic myocardial protection has been used successfully in patients with CAs. A review of 832 patients scheduled to undergo surgery and CPB identified only seven cases of CAs that were strongly positive at 4°C.[361] The authors concluded that asymptomatic patients with nonspecific, low-titer, and low-thermal-amplitude CAs may undergo hypothermia and CPB without serious detectable sequelae. However, the possibility of subtle end-organ damage exists.

If hypothermic CPB is necessary despite the presence of CAs, the choices are preoperative plasmapheresis, standard hemodilution, and maintenance of CPB temperature above the CA thermal amplitude[359,364] (Fig. 24–38). Cold cardioplegia may be used without first undergoing plasmapheresis if normothermic CPB is used and 37°C cardioplegic solution is injected prior to administration of 4°C cardioplegic solution, clearing all potentially reactive cells. The risk of hemolysis is still high in patients with high-thermal-amplitude CAs. If CAs are particularly malignant, all of the patient's blood from the venous reservoir is drained and discarded. It is replaced entirely by donor blood, unfortunately exposing the patient to allogeneic blood products.[365] Today, normothermic CPB and antegrade or retrograde warm blood cardioplegia may be the best option.[366] If CAs should go undetected, postoperative end-organ damage or low CO may occur. Subsequently, plasma exchange, steroids, elevated urine output, and maintenance of a good CO are the best treatments.[367]

All participants in the care of the patient should be acutely aware that the patient has CAs. The patient must not be unnecessarily exposed to hypothermia. Anesthetic gases, intravenous fluids, blood, and plasma should be heated before administration to the patients. Operating room temperature should be warm. Washed RBCs may also be useful if transfusions of fresh components are necessary.[360]

Sickle Cell Disease

Sickle cell disease (SCD) is a heterogeneous group of inherited disorders involving the sickle β-globin gene. Survival in SCD has greatly improved due to early diagnosis, antibiotics, and supportive care; however, it still is an important health threat, particularly if major surgery is contemplated.[368] Preparation and meticulous intraoperative care are imperative for the best results.

The β-globin gene has worldwide distribution but is found most often in west central Africa. HbA and HbS genes have codominant expression, which allows both genes to be represented in the Hb molecule. One in 10 American blacks is a heterozygous carrier of the β-globin gene, referred to as sickle cell trait (AS); the homozygous state, sickle cell anemia (SS), occurs in 1 of 400 blacks. The prevalence of SCD in blacks is 0.2%. Hemoglobin C disease (SC) occurs in approximately 2% of American blacks. SS accounts for 60% to 70% of SCD in the United States. The β-globin gene has a mutation in the DNA that results in a substitution of the amino acid valine for glutamic acid in the β-globin chain that is responsible for normal Hb polymerization upon deoxygenation. The mutated Hb molecule is less negatively charged than the normal Hb, so as oxygen saturation approaches 85%, Hb tends to polymerize.[369] As the HbS comes out of solution and gels intracellularly, it causes the RBC to sickle (Fig. 24–39). Sickling is a reversible change in the RBC shape. Desaturation is the primary stimulus for sickling. Besides oxygen saturation, the likelihood of sickling is based on the amount of HbS in the RBC. AS patients do not sickle until the oxygen saturation

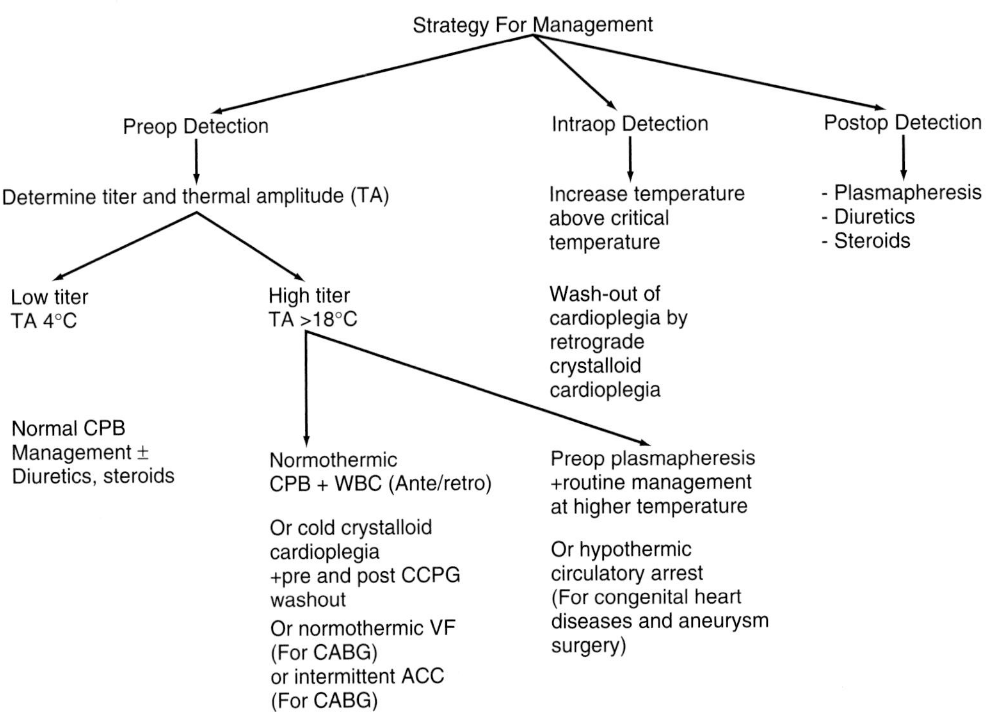

Figure 24–38 Algorithm for management. ACC = aortic cross-clamp; CABG = coronary artery bypass grafting; CCPG = cold crystalloid cardioplegia; CPB = cardiopulmonary bypass; Intraop = intraoperative; Postop = postoperative; Preop = preoperative; VF = ventricular fibrillation; WBC = warm blood cardioplegia; Ante = antegrade; Retro = retrograde. (The Annals of Thoracic Surgeons, 60:1143, 1995. Copyright 1995, with permission from the Society of Thoracic Surgeons.)

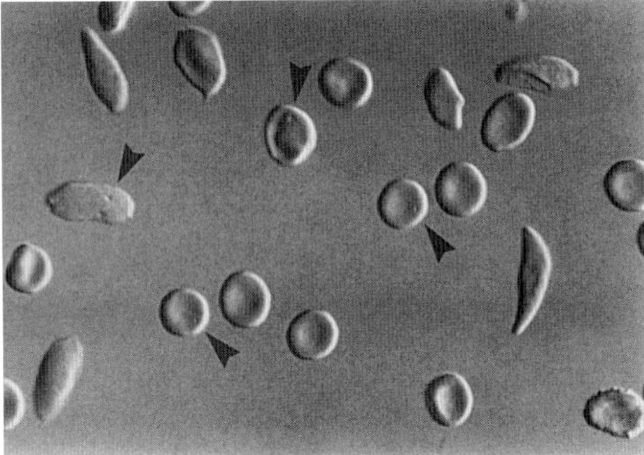

Figure 24–39 Use of the red cell pit count to assess splenic reticuloendothelial function. Erythrocytes from a child with sickle cell anemia were fixed in isotonic buffered glutaraldehyde and viewed with Nomarski differential interference contrast microscopy. The increased percentage of red cells with large endocytic vacuoles (pitted or pocked cells, *arrowheads*) indicates functional asplenia. (Reprinted with permission from Lane PA: Pediatric hematology. *In* Buchanan GR [ed]: Pediatric Clinics of North America. Philadelphia, WB Saunders Company 43:639, 1996.)

is below 40%, because their ratio of HbS to total Hb is low. Because SS and SC patients have significantly more HbS, they sickle at a saturation of 85%, which is normally the venous saturation. It is HbS that is responsible for the major hallmarks of SCD: sickling, hemolytic anemia, and vaso-occlusive events.[368,370] Vaso-occlusive events are more likely because sickled RBCs have an increased affinity for the endothelial surface of blood vessels and sickled RBCs greatly increase blood viscosity and stasis.[369,371] During a vaso-occlusive episode, the endothelium produces activators such as endothelin that alter the endothelial surface and cause vasoconstriction, leading to injury.

The clinical severity of SS, SC, and AS varies as a function of both inherited (thalassemia or fetal Hb) and acquired factors.[371] AS patients are asymptomatic unless they become profoundly hypoxic, acidotic, or hypothermic.[372] On the contrary, individuals with either SS or SC are chronically ill with a life-threatening illness. However, survival for individuals with SS is 95% at 20 years and even longer with SC disease.[373] Individuals with SS are usually undersized and skeletally deformed due to bone marrow hyperplasia and may be slightly jaundiced. They are chronically anemic with an Hb concentration often below 8 g/dL. The RBCs are more fragile, with an RBC viability of 10% of normal accounting for chronic anemia. As a major site of sickling, the spleen eventually becomes nonfunctional; consequently, individuals with SS are extremely susceptible to infections, especially bacterial infections. Strict asepsis is important.

Three critical conditions may occur in those with SCD: painful crisis, aplastic crisis, and crisis affecting major organs. The painful crisis (sickle cell crisis) is a vaso-occlusive, infarctive process, resulting in tissue anoxia exemplified by pulmonary infarctions. Diagnosis is often one of exclusion. Vaso-occlusive crises primarily affect males 15 to 25 years of age. They are initiated by exertion, infection, dehydration, cold, acidosis, hypoxia, or vascular stasis.[374] The rheologic properties of the sickle RBCs combine with the tendency for adherence to the vessel wall, causing poor microvascular perfusion. Hydration with D_5W is important during a crisis so that free water may enter the cells and lower the Hb concentration. Blood transfusion is not helpful in this situation.[369] Aplastic crisis is much less common than painful crisis but is the most feared hematologic complication of SS. It is characterized by a precipitous fall in Hb secondary to hemolysis without the expected bone marrow response. In contrast to vaso-occlusive crisis, transfusion is required. Aplastic crisis lasts 7 to 10 days. Finally, various major organ systems such as the lungs (acute chest syndrome), spleen (splenic infarcts), kidneys, heart (myocardial dysfunction), and the central nervous system (stroke) may be inadequately perfused, resulting in permanent injury. Stroke is secondary to an intimal injury and thrombosis within the artery. Stroke occurs in about 8% of individuals with SS and children are more likely affected. The lifetime chance of neurologic complications in those with SCD is 25%. Two thirds will have a subsequent stroke within 36 months. Coronary artery occlusions are rare.

Not all individuals with SCD have been identified before general anesthesia, and death has been the first manifestation of the disease.[375] Hb electrophoresis is the most accurate diagnostic test, whereas peripheral blood smears are not diagnostic. Hematologic consultation should be obtained in any person suspected to have SCD who is scheduled for any type of surgery or anesthesia. Patients with SS have been considered at increased risk for surgery, general anesthesia, and postoperative complications. Results from the Cooperative Study of SCD that included 3765 SCD patients in 23 clinical centers across the United States determined the overall mortality rate was 0.3% with only three deaths related to anesthesia or surgery.[376] No deaths occurred in children under 14 years of age. Postoperative complications were variable and primarily related to the operative procedure. Despite many different surgical procedures and anesthetics in this large multicenter study, there was a low mortality rate accompanied by few complications. Modern techniques and monitoring capabilities have enabled patients with SCD to receive improved care and outcome.[368] Therefore, surgery has become a more viable option for those with SCD.

Preoperatively, complete assessment of the cardiovascular system, specifically looking for myocardial ischemia, PAH, and CHF in the patient having cardiac surgery, is important. Renal function is also likely to be abnormal.[377] Folic acid administration and careful intravenous hydration in the preoperative period aid in avoiding dehydration, hyperosmolality, and low urine output.[378] An increased incidence of pulmonary dysfunction in patients with SS increases the risk of hypoxia so that preoperative sedation must be carefully titrated along with careful patient observation. The value of prophylactic antibiotics is indeterminate.

The role of preoperative transfusion in the management of SS patients has been debated for years. The recommendation for preoperative RBC transfusion in SS patients is based on a reduction in circulating concentration of HbS in an effort to improve oxygen-carrying capacity, suppress the erythropoietic drive, and shift the P_{50} to the left; nevertheless, the possibility of sickling is not eliminated.[371] An HbS below 30% has been traditionally regarded as necessary for individuals to undergo surgery. In order to verify this, a multicenter randomized trial of 551 patients with SCD undergoing various noncardiac operations was undertaken. Preoperative transfusion was designed with either a conservative or an aggressive strategy to be evaluated according to the incidence of perioperative complications.[379] The percentage of HbS in the patients managed conservatively was 60% compared with 30% for the aggressive strategy. The conservative strategy was associated with half as many transfusion-associated complications. Furthermore, maintaining HbS at 50% instead of 30% was found to be as effective in reducing the risk of stroke in nonsurgical situations.[380] For noncardiac surgery, there is growing evidence that dilution of sickle cells should be limited and intraoperative transfusion should reflect standard transfusion guidelines.[368,376] Blood for transfusion should be less than 7 days old and warmed.

For initiation of CPB, 5% HbS is often recommended, although a HbS of 30% appears suitable.[381,382] Presently, alternatives to allogeneic transfusion are few for CPB and cardiac surgery. Exchange transfusion has been used successfully to correct anemia preoperatively with less risk of volume overload than simple transfusion.[383] RBC transfusion alone increases blood viscosity more than exchange transfusion because a significant amount of HbS remains, possibly temporarily negating an improvement in oxygen delivery corresponding to the presence of more RBCs.[368,384] The lower blood viscosity and increased oxygen delivery to the tissues derived from the exchange transfusion are likely more efficient. Exchange transfusion has become routine prior to major surgery, but no prospective trials of exchange transfusion have been conducted to establish its value in these situations.[384]

Anesthetic management of individuals with SCD has been reviewed.[372,378] The availability of blood must be established prior to any surgery due to the possibility of alloimmunization. The incidence of antibodies may approach 50%, with more than two thirds being Kell or Rh in SCD.[384] Antibodies may delay availability of blood and increase the chance of a delayed hemolytic transfusion reaction that can mimic a painful crisis. Therefore, any donor blood must be typed to ensure compatibility for ABO, Rh, and Kell antigens. Before induction of anesthesia, preoxygenation is essential. Maintenance of oxygenation throughout the operation is critical but in no way guarantees an uncomplicated course. Volatile agents are associated with less sickling.[371] Maintenance of perfusion to the major organs and periphery is very important to maintain normal acid-base status. The occurrence of hypotension is best treated initially with fluid administration to optimize volume status and avoid vasopressors. Renal dysfunction causes SCD patients to concentrate urine poorly, so volume status is very dynamic. Efforts should be made to keep the patient normothermic. Intraoperative sickle crisis occurs sometimes despite the best care but poses a problem to diagnose during anesthesia. Signs of an intraoperative crisis include seizure, change in respiratory pattern, hypotension, or hematuria but are unfortunately nonspecific and unreliable. Laboratory tests are not helpful either. Nothing pharmacologic can reduce the tendency to sickle as alkalinization of the blood and administration of urea have aptly demonstrated.[371]

CPB has been associated with significant morbidity and mortality in adults and children with SCD, so there are many considerations to minimize the risk.[385] CPB imposes severe physiologic stresses such as low-flow states, circulatory arrest, aortic cross-clamping, mechanical destruction of blood elements, and protein denaturation that predispose to a sickling crisis. There are no set guidelines for temperature, cardioplegia, priming solution, and transfusion practice during CPB.[386] The effect and safety of systemic and regional hypothermia (cardioplegia) in patients with SCD are indeterminate. In vitro, the solubility of deoxygenated HbS increases as the body temperature is decreased, which reduces sickling. However, decreased temperature increases blood viscosity. Viscosity increases by 30% when body temperature falls to 30°C.[378] The harmful effects of hypothermia may be primarily related to vasoconstriction and vascular stasis. Hypothermia may be tolerated if peripheral perfusion and oxygenation are adequate. Today, many patients undergo normothermic instead of hypothermic CPB because of advantages related to postoperative myocardial function.[387] Patients with either AS or SS have been cooled to 26°C or less without a sickling crisis, but partial or total exchange transfusion with a final HbS of 10% was performed in some of the patients.[386] Speculation is that because oxygenation during CPB is excellent during moderate hypothermia, sickling may be less common even without partial or full exchange transfusion.[370]

A reduction in HbS has been recommended before initiation of CPB.[371] This can be accomplished by dilution with a nonsanguineous priming solution, a blood priming solution, cardioplegia, intravenous fluid, simple transfusion, or blood component sequestration. These measures decrease the percentage of HbS, but a significant number of RBCs remain at risk for sickling. Only a form of exchange transfusion removes sickled cells.[370] Exchange transfusions are advisable if deliberate hypothermia is planned.[386] Automated RBC exchange can be done in the operating room or in the preoperative area. Intraoperative exchange can be performed more safely with the benefit of intraoperative monitoring to guide transfusion and avoid volume overload and possible cardiac decompensation in patients with serious cardiac conditions. In addition, with CPB, it is possible to drain blood from the CPB circuit. Another novel approach involves partial RBC removal with the autotransfusion device prior to CPB to decrease the percentage of HbS, followed by an acute one-volume whole blood exchange during the initiation of CPB. The advantage is the procurement of a platelet-pheresed product with both techniques.[382]

Another option is to use primarily allogeneic blood in the priming volume where, upon initiation of CPB, venous blood is diverted to other reservoirs and the warmed blood in the priming volume reaches the patient, resulting in an HbS concentration under 5%. The diverted blood may have the RBCs separated from the plasma and platelets and discarded while the remaining non-RBC components are subsequently infused. This process decreases blood product exposure and allows transfusion of normal donor blood. These techniques of blood component sequestration may eliminate the need for a hemapheresis procedure.[382] They can also be used in patients with severe SCD who have a history of sickle crisis. On the contrary, Metras et al[388] described 15 patients with SCD (13 with AS) who underwent cardiac surgery. None of the patients received preoperative exchange transfusions despite use of moderate hypothermia, aortic cross-clamping, and cold cardioplegia. There was no evidence of sickling or increased postoperative complications. The authors concluded that as long as hypoxia, acidosis, and dehydration are avoided, preoperative exchange transfusions or blood transfusions are not mandatory; however, they did not study the most severe cases of SCD.

The advisability of cell salvage techniques in SCD is questionable. Intraoperative autotransfusion (IAT) has been condemned by those who claim an adverse effect on sickling but is supported by others.[389] The patient's percentage of HbS may influence how well IAT is tolerated. Patients with AS do not require RBC exchange because their transfusion risk is greater than the risk of crisis, but the conservative treatment options are to approach each AS patient as having SS. If IAT is used, recommendations are (1) exchange or transfuse to an HbS less than 40%, (2) increase hematocrit to greater than 30%, (3) heparinize until harvesting, and (4) provide solutions at a physiologic pH.[371]

Early extubation following CABG is not without undue risk (Box 24–7). Patients who return to the operating room for any reason may be at increased risk for postoperative pneumonia. Acute chest syndrome may appear as pneumonia or mask true pneumonia. Acute chest syndrome has resulted in fatalities.[371] Patients with AS are not at increased risk for postoperative complications.

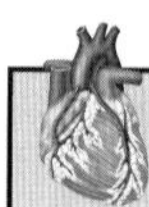

BOX 24–7 *Proposed Guidelines for Perioperative Management of Patients With Sickle Cell Disorders Undergoing Coronary Artery Bypass Graft Surgery*

Preoperative Period

- Hb electrophoretic studies
- Correction of any coexisting infection
- Partial or complete exchange transfusions for patients with HbSS
- Light benzodiazepine premedication
- Supplemental oxygen to avoid a decrease in oxygen saturation

Intraoperative Period

- Preoxygenation for 3 to 5 minutes in all cases
- Small dose of opioid and hypnotic induction
- Inhaled or intravenous maintenance of anesthesia
- Tepid or warm cardiopulmonary bypass
- Mean pump flow >50 mL/kg/min, perfusion pressure ≥60 mm Hg
- Blood transfusion if hematocrit <20%
- Retransfusion of pump blood is not advisable

Postoperative Period

- Early extubation within 2 to 6 hours
- Maintenance of intravascular volume and body temperature
- Avoidance of vasopressors is desirable
- Early incentive spirometry
- Multimodal approach to pain relief (opioids, NSAIDs, acetaminophen)
- Warming blankets to maintain temperature ≥37°C
- Shivering: meperidine 10 to 25 mg IV
- Routine antibiotic coverage for 2 days
- Blood transfusion: Hb <7.5 g/dL for those ≤70 years old; Hb <8.5 g/dL
- Close monitoring of oxygenation, perfusion, and acid-base indices for 12 to 24 hours

NSAIDs = nonsteroidal anti-inflammatory drugs, Hb = hemoglobin.
From Djaiani GN, Cheng DCH, Carroll JA, et al: Fast-track cardiac anesthesia in patients with sickle cell abnormalities. Anesth Analg 89:601, 1999.

Acknowledgments

This chapter is dedicated to the memory of Dwight C. Legler, MD, who first authored this chapter. He is still sadly missed by all members of the Cardiovascular Division of the Department of Anesthesiology at the Mayo Clinic. Many thanks to Maria A. de Castro, MD, and Robert A. Strickland, MD, for their previous excellent contributions to this chapter.

REFERENCES

1. Reynen K: Frequency of primary tumors of the heart. Am J Cardiol 77:107, 1996
2. Shapiro LM: Cardiac tumours: Diagnosis and management. Heart (British Cardiac Society) 85:218, 2001
3. Bakaeen FG, Reardon MJ, Coselli JS, et al: Surgical outcome in 85 patients with primary cardiac tumors. Am J Surg 186:641, 2003

4. Borges AC, Witt C, Bartel T, et al: Preoperative two- and three-dimensional transesophageal echocardiographic assessment of heart tumors. Ann Thorac Surg 61:1163, 1996
5. Raaf HN, Raaf JH: Sarcomas related to the heart and vasculature. Semin Surg Oncol 10: 374, 1994
6. Wee JO, Sepic JD, Mihaljevic T, et al: Metastatic carcinoid tumor of the heart. Ann Thorac Surg 76:1721, 2003
7. Klatt EC, Heitz DR: Cardiac metastases. Cancer 65:1456, 1990
8. Fyke FE 3rd, Seward JB, Edwards WD, et al: Primary cardiac tumors: Experience with 30 consecutive patients since the introduction of two-dimensional echocardiography. J Am Coll Cardiol 5:1465, 1985
9. Padalino MA, Basso C, Moreolo GS, et al: Left atrial myxoma in a child: Case report and review of the literature. Cardiovasc Pathol 12:233, 2003
10. Gowdamarajan A, Michler RE: Therapy for primary cardiac tumors: Is there a role for heart transplantation? Curr Opin Cardiol 15:121, 2000
11. Grebenc ML, Rosado-de-Christenson ML, Green CE, et al: Cardiac myxoma: Imaging features in 83 patients. Radiographics 22:673, 2002
12. Amano J, Kono T, Wada Y, et al: Cardiac myxoma: Its origin and tumor characteristics. Ann Thorac Cardiovasc Surg 9:215, 2003
13. Pinede L, Duhaut P, Loire R: Clinical presentation of left atrial cardiac myxoma. A series of 112 consecutive cases. Medicine 80:159, 2001
14. Percell RL Jr, Henning RJ, Siddique Patel M: Atrial myxoma: Case report and a review of the literature. Heart Dis 5:224, 2003
15. Choi BW, Ryu SJ, Chang BC, et al: Myxoma attached to both atrial and ventricular sides of the mitral valve: Report of a case and review of 31 cases of mitral myxoma. Int J Card Imaging 17:411, 2001
16. De Carli S, Sechi LA, Ciani R, et al: Right atrial myxoma with pulmonary embolism. Cardiology 84:368, 1994
17. Shimono T, Makino S, Kanamori Y, et al: Left atrial myxomas: Using gross anatomic tumor types to determine clinical features and coronary angiographic findings. Chest 107:674, 1995
18. Freedberg RS, Kronzon I, Rumancik WM, et al: The contribution of magnetic resonance imaging to the evaluation of intracardiac tumors diagnosed by echocardiography. Circulation 77:96, 1988
19. Cooley DA: Surgical treatment of cardiac neoplasms: 32-Year experience. Thorac Cardiovasc Surg 38(suppl 2): 176, 1990
20. Koolbergen DR, Voigt P, Kolowca M, et al: Elective surgery for fibroelastoma of the aortic valve. Ann Thorac Surg 77:725, 2004
21. Gowda RM, Khan IA, Nair CK, et al: Cardiac papillary fibroelastoma: A comprehensive analysis of 725 cases. Am Heart J 146:404, 2003
22. Cho JM, Danielson GK, Puga FJ, et al: Surgical resection of ventricular cardiac fibromas: Early and late results. Ann Thorac Surg 76:1929, 2003
23. Osranek M, Bursi F, Gura GM, et al: Echocardiographic features of pheochromocytoma of the heart. Am J Cardiol 91:640, 2003
24. Gowda RM, Khan IA: Clinical perspectives of primary cardiac lymphoma. Angiology 54:599, 2003
25. Okamoto K, Kato S, Katsuki S, et al: Malignant fibrous histiocytoma of the heart: Case report and review of 46 cases in the literature. Intern Med 40: 1222, 2001
26. Reardon MJ, DeFelice CA, Sheinbaum R, et al: Cardiac autotransplant for surgical treatment of a malignant neoplasm. Ann Thorac Surg 67:1793, 1999
27. Kussman BD, Devavaram P, Hansen DD, et al: Anesthetic implications of primary cardiac tumors in infants and children. J Cardiothorac Vasc Anesth 16:582, 2002
28. Connolly HM: Carcinoid heart disease: Medical and surgical considerations. Cancer Control 8:454, 2001
29. Robiolio PA, Rigolin VH, Wilson JS, et al: Carcinoid heart disease. Correlation of high serotonin levels with valvular abnormalities detected by cardiac catheterization and echocardiography. Circulation 92:790, 1995
30. Simula DV, Edwards WD, Tazelaar HD, et al: Surgical pathology of carcinoid heart disease: A study of 139 valves from 75 patients spanning 20 years. Mayo Clin Proc 77:139, 2002
31. Connolly HM, Schaff HV, Mullany CJ, et al: Carcinoid heart disease: Impact of pulmonary valve replacement in right ventricular function and remodeling. Circulation 106(suppl I):I-51, 2002
32. Connolly HM, Nishimura RA, Smith HC, et al: Outcome of cardiac surgery for carcinoid heart disease. J Am Coll Cardiol 25:410, 1995
33. Propst JW, Siegel LC, Stover EP: Anesthetic considerations for valve replacement surgery in a patient with carcinoid syndrome. J Cardiothorac Vasc Anesth 8:209, 1994
34. Botero M, Fuchs R, Paulus DA, et al: Carcinoid heart disease: A case report and literature review. J Clin Anesth 14:57, 2002
35. Neustein SM, Cohen E: Anesthesia for aortic and mitral valve replacement in a patient with carcinoid heart disease. Anesthesiology 82:1067, 1995
36. Weingarten TN, Abel MD, Connolly HM, et al: Anesthetic management for cardiac surgery in carcinoid heart disease—A review of 84 patients. Anesth Analg 96:SCA 138, 2003
37. Ereth MH, Oliver WC Jr, Santrach PJ: Perioperative interventions to decrease transfusion of allogeneic blood products. Mayo Clin Proc 69:575, 1994
38. Nuttall GA, Fass DN, Oyen LJ, et al: A study of a weight-adjusted aprotinin dosing schedule during cardiac surgery. Anesth Analg 94:283, 2002
39. Richardson P, McKenna W, Bristow M, et al: Report of the 1995 World Health Organization/International Society and Federation of Cardiology Task Force on the Definition and Classification of Cardiomyopathies. Circulation 93:841, 1996
40. Codd MB, Sugrue DD, Gersh BJ, et al: Epidemiology of idiopathic, dilated and hypertrophic cardiomyopathy. A population-based study in Olmsted County, Minnesota, 1975-1984. Circulation 80:564, 1989
41. Felker GM, Thompson RE, Hare JM, et al: Underlying causes and long-term survival in patients with initially unexplained cardiomyopathy. N Engl J Med 342:1077, 2000
42. Elliott P: Cardiomyopathy. Diagnosis and management of dilated cardiomyopathy. Heart 84:106, 2000
43. De Keulenaer GW, Brutsaert DL: Dilated cardiomyopathy: Changing pathophysiological concepts and mechanisms of dysfunction. J Card Surg 14:64, 1999
44. Franz WM, Muller OJ, Katus HA: Cardiomyopathies: From genetics to the prospect of treatment. Lancet 358:1627, 2001
45. Givertz MM: Underlying causes and survival in patients with heart failure. N Engl J Med 342:1120, 2000
46. Leiden JM: The genetics of dilated cardiomyopathy-emerging clues to the puzzle. N Engl J Med 337:1080, 1997
47. Bachinski LL, Roberts R: New theories. Causes of dilated cardiomyopathy. Cardiol Clin 16:603, vii, 1998
48. Haber RH, LeJemtel T, Sonnenblick EH: The pathophysiologic profile of congestive heart failure. Cardiovasc Drugs Ther 2(suppl 1):397, 1988
49. Patterson JH, Adams KF Jr: Pathophysiology of heart failure: Changing perceptions. Pharmacotherapy 16:27S, 1996
50. McBride BF, White CM: Acute decompensated heart failure: A contemporary approach to pharmacotherapeutic management. Pharmacotherapy 23:997, 2003
51. Tang WH, Francis GS: Novel pharmacological treatments for heart failure. Exp Opin Investig Drugs 12:1791, 2003
52. Siu SC, Sole MJ: Dilated cardiomyopathy. Curr Opin Cardiol 9:337, 1994
53. Wu LA, Lapeyre AC III, Cooper LT: Current role of endomyocardial biopsy in the management of dilated cardiomyopathy and myocarditis. Mayo Clin Proc 76:1030, 2001
54. O'Connell JB, Moore CK, Waterer HC: Treatment of end-stage dilated cardiomyopathy. Br Heart J 72(suppl):S52, 1994
55. Koga Y, Toshima H, Tanaka M, et al: Therapeutic management of dilated cardiomyopathy. Cardiovasc Drugs Ther 8:83, 1994
56. Packer M, Carver JR, Rodeheffer RJ, et al: Effect of oral milrinone on mortality in severe chronic heart failure. The PROMISE Study Research Group. N Engl J Med 325:1468, 1991
57. Pitt B, Zannad F, Remme WJ, et al: The effect of spironolactone on morbidity and mortality in patients with severe heart failure. Randomized Aldactone Evaluation Study Investigators. N Engl J Med 341:709, 1999
58. Bristow MR, Ginsburg R, Minobe W, et al: Decreased catecholamine sensitivity and β-adrenergic receptor density in failing human hearts. N Engl J Med 307:205, 1982
59. Waagstein F: The role of beta-blockers in dilated cardiomyopathy. Curr Opin Cardiol 10:322, 1995
60. Metoprolol CR/XL Randomised Intervention Trial in Congestive Heart Failure (MERIT-HF): Effect of metoprolol CR/XL in chronic heart failure. Lancet 353:2001, 1999
61. Borggrefe M, Block M, Breithardt G: Identification and management of the high-risk patient with dilated cardiomyopathy. Br Heart J 72(suppl):S42, 1994
62. Brachmann J, Hilbel T, Grunig E, et al: Ventricular arrhythmias in dilated cardiomyopathy. Pacing Clin Electrophysiol 20:2714, 1997
63. Nul DR, Doval HC, Grancelli HO, et al: Heart rate is a marker of amiodarone mortality reduction in severe heart failure. J Am Coll Cardiol 29:1199, 1997
64. Connolly SJ, Hallstrom AP, Cappato R, et al: Meta-analysis of the implantable cardioverter/defibrillator secondary prevention trials. Eur Heart J 21:2071, 2000
65. Tayama E, Nose Y: Can we treat dilated cardiomyopathy using a left ventricular assist device? Artif Organs 20:197, 1996
66. Kaye MP: The registry of the International Society for Heart Transplantation: Fourth official report. J Heart Transplant 6:63, 1987

67. Wynands JE, Wong P, Whalley DG, et al: Oxygen-fentanyl anesthesia in patients with poor left ventricular function: Hemodynamics and plasma fentanyl concentrations. Anesth Analg 62:476, 1983
68. Elliott P, O'Hare R, Bill KM, et al: Severe cardiovascular depression with remifentanil. Anesth Analg 91:58, 2000
69. Wang JY, Winship SM, Thomas SD, et al: Induction of anaesthesia in patients with coronary artery disease: A comparison between sevoflurane-remifentanil and fentanyl-etomidate. Anaesth Intensive Care 27:363, 1999
70. Sprung J, Ogletree-Hughes ML, Moravec CS: The effects of etomidate on the contractility of failing and nonfailing human heart muscle. Anesth Analg 91:68, 2000
71. Syed MA, Masters RW, Zsigmond EK: Haemodynamic stability with midazolam-ketamine-sufentanil analgesia in cardiac surgical patients. Can J Anaesth 36:617, 1989
72. Stulz P, Schlapfer R, Feer R, et al: Decision making in the surgical treatment of massive pulmonary embolism. Eur J Cardiothorac Surg 8:188, 1994
73. Riou B, Viars P, Lecarpentier Y: Effects of ketamine on the cardiac papillary muscle of normal hamsters and those with cardiomyopathy. Anesthesiology 73:910, 1990
74. Riou B, Lejay M, Lecarpentier Y, et al: Myocardial effects of propofol in hamsters with hypertrophic cardiomyopathy. Anesthesiology 82:566, 1995
75. Vivien B, Hanouz JL, Gueugniaud PY, et al: Myocardial effects of halothane and isoflurane in hamsters with hypertrophic cardiomyopathy. Anesthesiology 87:1406, 1997
76. Pagel PS, Lowe D, Hettrick DA, et al: Isoflurane, but not halothane improves indices of diastolic performance in dogs with rapid ventricular, pacing-induced cardiomyopathy. Anesthesiology 85:644, 1996
77. Vivien B, Hanouz JL, Gueugniaud PY, et al: Myocardial effects of desflurane in hamsters with hypertrophic cardiomyopathy. Anesthesiology 89:1191, 1998
78. De Hert SG, Van der Linden PJ, ten Broecke PW, et al: Effects of desflurane and sevoflurane on length-dependent regulation of myocardial function in coronary surgery patients. Anesthesiology 95:357, 2001
79. Stevenson LW, Perloff JK: The dilated cardiomyopathies: Clinical aspects. Cardiol Clin 6:187, 1988
80. Gaba DM, Wyner J, Fish KJ: Anesthesia and the automatic implantable cardioverter/defibrillator. Anesthesiology 62:786, 1985
81. Hamilton MA, Stevenson LW, Child JS, et al: Sustained reduction in valvular regurgitation and atrial volumes with tailored vasodilator therapy in advanced congestive heart failure secondary to dilated (ischemic or idiopathic) cardiomyopathy. Am J Cardiol 67:259, 1991
82. Rooney RT, Marijic J, Stommel KA, et al: Additive cardiac depression by volatile anesthetics in isolated hearts after chronic amiodarone treatment. Anesth Analg 80:917, 1995
83. Maron BJ, McKenna WJ, Danielson GK, et al: American College of Cardiology/European Society of Cardiology clinical expert consensus document on hypertrophic cardiomyopathy. A report of the American College of Cardiology Foundation Task Force on Clinical Expert Consensus Documents and the European Society of Cardiology Committee for Practice Guidelines. J Am Coll Cardiol 42:1687, 2003
84. Maron BJ: Hypertrophic cardiomyopathy: A systematic review. JAMA 287:1308, 2002
85. Roberts R, Sigwart U: New concepts in hypertrophic cardiomyopathies, part I. Circulation 104:2113, 2001
86. Theodoro DA, Danielson GK, Feldt RH, et al: Hypertrophic obstructive cardiomyopathy in pediatric patients: Results of surgical treatment. J Thorac Cardiovasc Surg 112:1589; discussion 1597, 1996
87. Skinner JR, Manzoor A, Hayes AM, et al: A regional study of presentation and outcome of hypertrophic cardiomyopathy in infants. Heart 77:229, 1997
88. Cannon RO 3rd, Dilsizian V, O'Gara PT, et al: Myocardial metabolic, hemodynamic, and electrocardiographic significance of reversible thallium-201 abnormalities in hypertrophic cardiomyopathy. Circulation 83:1660, 1991
89. Camici P, Chiriatti G, Lorenzoni R, et al: Coronary vasodilation is impaired in both hypertrophied and nonhypertrophied myocardium of patients with hypertrophic cardiomyopathy: A study with nitrogen-13 ammonia and positron emission tomography. J Am Coll Cardiol 17:879, 1991
90. Kern MJ, Deligonul U: Interpretation of cardiac pathophysiology from pressure waveform analysis: III. Intraventricular pressure gradients. Cathet Cardiovasc Diagn 22:145, 1991
91. Maron MS, Olivotto I, Betocchi S, et al: Effect of left ventricular outflow tract obstruction on clinical outcome in hypertrophic cardiomyopathy. N Engl J Med 348:295, 2003
92. Chang AC, McAreavey D, Fananapazir L: Identification of patients with hypertrophic cardiomyopathy at high risk for sudden death. Curr Opin Cardiol 10:9, 1995
93. Maron BJ, Shen WK, Link MS, et al: Efficacy of implantable cardioverter-defibrillators for the prevention of sudden death in patients with hypertrophic cardiomyopathy. N Engl J Med 342:365, 2000
94. Maron BJ: Risk stratification and prevention of sudden death in hypertrophic cardiomyopathy. Cardiol Rev 10:173, 2002
95. Fananapazir L, Chang AC, Epstein SE, et al: Prognostic determinants in hypertrophic cardiomyopathy. Prospective evaluation of a therapeutic strategy based on clinical, Holter, hemodynamic, and electrophysiological findings. Circulation 86:730, 1992
96. Dilsizian V, Bonow RO, Epstein SE, et al: Myocardial ischemia detected by thallium scintigraphy is frequently related to cardiac arrest and syncope in young patients with hypertrophic cardiomyopathy. J Am Coll Cardiol 22:796, 1993
97. The Antiarrhythmics versus Implantable Defibrillators (AVID) Investigators: A comparison of antiarrhythmic-drug therapy with implantable defibrillators in patients resuscitated from near-fatal ventricular arrhythmias. N Engl J Med 337:1576, 1997
98. Sherrid MV, Chaudhry FA, Swistel DG: Obstructive hypertrophic cardiomyopathy: Echocardiography, pathophysiology, and the continuing evolution of surgery for obstruction. Ann Thorac Surg 75:620, 2003
99. Louie EK, Edwards LC III: Hypertrophic cardiomyopathy. Prog Cardiovasc Dis 36:275, 1994
100. Mohr R, Schaff HV, Danielson GK, et al: The outcome of surgical treatment of hypertrophic obstructive cardiomyopathy. Experience over 15 years. J Thorac Cardiovasc Surg 97:666, 1989
101. Schulte HD, Borisov K, Gams E, et al: Management of symptomatic hypertrophic obstructive cardiomyopathy—Long-term results after surgical therapy. Thorac Cardiovasc Surg 47:213, 1999
102. Nishimura RA, Trusty JM, Hayes DL, et al: Dual-chamber pacing for hypertrophic cardiomyopathy: A randomized, double-blind, crossover trial. J Am Coll Cardiol 29:435, 1997
103. Sigwart U: Nonsurgical myocardial reduction for hypertrophic obstructive cardiomyopathy. Lancet 346:211, 1995
104. Roberts R, Sigwart U: New concepts in hypertrophic cardiomyopathies, part II. Circulation 104:2249, 2001
105. Tessler MJ, Hudson R, Naugler-Colville M, et al: Pulmonary oedema in two parturients with hypertrophic obstructive cardiomyopathy (HOCM). Can J Anaesth 37:469, 1990
106. Bell MD, Goodchild CS: Hypertrophic obstructive cardiomyopathy in combination with a prolapsing mitral valve. Anaesthesia for surgical correction with propofol. Anaesthesia 44:409, 1989
107. Searle NR, Sahab P: Propofol in patients with cardiac disease. Can J Anaesth 40:730, 1993
108. Loubser P, Suh K, Cohen S: Adverse effects of spinal anesthesia in a patient with idiopathic hypertrophic subaortic stenosis. Anesthesiology 60:228, 1984
109. Thompson RC, Liberthson RR, Lowenstein E: Perioperative anesthetic risk of noncardiac surgery in hypertrophic obstructive cardiomyopathy. JAMA 254:2419, 1985
110. Marijic J, Bosnjak ZJ, Stowe DF, et al: Effects and interaction of verapamil and volatile anesthetics on the isolated perfused guinea pig heart. Anesthesiology 69:914, 1988
111. Stewart JT, McKenna WJ: Management of arrhythmias in hypertrophic cardiomyopathy. Cardiovasc Drugs Ther 8:95, 1994
112. Wigle ED, Rakowski H, Kimball BP, et al: Hypertrophic cardiomyopathy. Clinical spectrum and treatment. Circulation 92:1680, 1995
113. Haering JM, Communale ME, Parker RA, et al: Cardiac risk of noncardiac surgery in patients with asymmetric septal hypertrophy. Anesthesiology 85:254, 1996
114. Ammash NM, Seward JB, Bailey KR, et al: Clinical profile and outcome of idiopathic restrictive cardiomyopathy. Circulation 101:2490, 2000
115. Kushwaha SS, Fallon JT, Fuster V: Restrictive cardiomyopathy. N Engl J Med 336:267, 1997
116. Kabbani SS, LeWinter MM: Diastolic heart failure. Constrictive, restrictive, and pericardial. Cardiol Clin 18:501, 2000
117. Denfield SW: Sudden death in children with restrictive cardiomyopathy. Cardiac Electrophysiol Rev 6:163, 2002
118. Wilmshurst PT, Katritsis D: Restrictive cardiomyopathy. Br Heart J 63:323, 1990
119. Tam JW, Shaikh N, Sutherland E: Echocardiographic assessment of patients with hypertrophic and restrictive cardiomyopathy: Imaging and echocardiography. Curr Opin Cardiol 17:470, 2002
120. Seifert FC, Miller DC, Oesterle SN, et al: Surgical treatment of constrictive pericarditis: Analysis of outcome diagnostic error. Circulation 72(suppl II):II-264, 1985

121. Chatterjee K, Alpert J: Constrictive pericarditis and restrictive cardiomyopathy: Similarities and differences. Heart Failure Monit 3:118, 2003
122. Metras D, Coulibaly AO, Ouattara K: Surgical treatment of endomyocardial fibrosis: results in 55 patients. Circulation 72(suppl II):II-274, 1985
123. Fontaine G, Gallais Y, Fornes P, et al: Arrhythmogenic right ventricular dysplasia/cardiomyopathy. Anesthesiology 95:250, 2001
124. Houfani B, Meyer P, Merckx J, et al: Postoperative sudden death in two adolescents with myelomeningocele and unrecognized arrhythmogenic right ventricular dysplasia. Anesthesiology 95:257, 2001
125. Corrado D, Basso C, Thiene G, et al: Spectrum of clinicopathologic manifestations of arrhythmogenic right ventricular cardiomyopathy/dysplasia: A multicenter study. J Am Coll Cardiol 30:1512, 1997
126. Link MS, Wang PJ, Haugh CJ, et al: Arrhythmogenic right ventricular dysplasia: Clinical results with implantable cardioverter/defibrillators. J Interv Card Electrophysiol 1:41, 1997
127. Stoddard MF, Prince CR, Dillon S, et al: Exercise-induced mitral regurgitation is a predictor of morbid events in subjects with mitral valve prolapse. J Am Coll Cardiol 25:693, 1995
128. Devereux RB: Recent developments in the diagnosis and management of mitral valve prolapse. Curr Opin Cardiol 10:107, 1995
129. Fontana ME, Sparks EA, Boudoulas H, et al: Mitral valve prolapse and the mitral valve prolapse syndrome. Curr Prob Cardiol 16:309, 1991
130. Hanson EW, Neerhut RK, Lynch C 3rd: Mitral valve prolapse. Anesthesiology 85:178, 1996
131. Zuppiroli A, Rinaldi M, Kramer-Fox R, et al: Natural history of mitral valve prolapse. Am J Cardiol 75:1028, 1995
132. Nishimura RA, McGoon MD, Shub C, et al: Echocardiographically documented mitral-valve prolapse. Long-term follow-up of 237 patients. N Engl J Med 313:1305, 1985
133. Enriquez-Sarano M, Schaff HV, Orszulak TA, et al: Valve repair improves the outcome of surgery for mitral regurgitation. A multivariate analysis. Circulation 91:1022, 1995
134. Handa N, Schaff HV, Morris JJ, et al: Outcome of valve repair and the Cox maze procedure for mitral regurgitation and associated atrial fibrillation. J Thorac Cardiovasc Surg 118:628, 1999
135. Levy S: Arrhythmias in the mitral valve prolapse syndrome: Clinical significance and management. Pacing Clin Electrophysiol 15:1080, 1992
136. Kligfield P, Hochreiter C, Kramer H, et al: Complex arrhythmias in mitral regurgitation with and without mitral valve prolapse: Contrast to arrhythmias in mitral valve prolapse without mitral regurgitation. Am J Cardiol 55:1545, 1985
137. Dollar AL, Roberts WC: Morphologic comparison of patients with mitral valve prolapse who died suddenly with patients who died from severe valvular dysfunction or other conditions. J Am Coll Cardiol 17:921, 1991
138. Orencia AJ, Petty GW, Khandheria BK, et al: Risk of stroke with mitral valve prolapse in population-based cohort study. Stroke 26:7, 1995
139. Petty GW, Orencia AJ, Khandheria BK, et al: A population-based study of stroke in the setting of mitral valve prolapse: Risk factors and infarct subtype classification. Mayo Clin Proc 69:632, 1994
140. Vavuranakis M, Kolibash AJ, Wooley CF, et al: Mitral valve prolapse: Left ventricular hemodynamics in patients with chest pain, dyspnea or both. J Heart Valve Dis 2:544, 1993
141. Bacon R, Chandrasekan V, Haigh A, et al: Early extubation after open-heart surgery with total intravenous anaesthetic technique. Lancet 345:133, 1995
142. Goldhaber SZ, Elliott CG: Acute pulmonary embolism: Part I: epidemiology, pathophysiology, and diagnosis. Circulation 108:2726, 2003
143. McCowan TC, Eidt JF, Ferris EJ: Interventions in pulmonary embolism. J Thorac Imaging 4:67, 1989
144. Goldhaber SZ: A contemporary approach to thrombolytic therapy for pulmonary embolism. Vasc Med 5:115, 2000
145. Ryu JH, Swensen SJ, Olson EJ, et al: Diagnosis of pulmonary embolism with use of computed tomographic angiography. Mayo Clin Proc 76:59, 2001
146. Hirsh J: Treatment of pulmonary embolism. Annu Rev Med 38:91, 1987
147. Hampson NB: Pulmonary embolism: Difficulties in the clinical diagnosis. Semin Respir Infect 10:123, 1995
148. Heit JA, Melton LJ 3rd, Lohse CM, et al: Incidence of venous thromboembolism in hospitalized patients vs community residents. Mayo Clin Proc 76:1102, 2001
149. Stein PD: Acute pulmonary embolism. Dis Mon 40:467, 1994
150. Dalen JE, Alpert JS: Natural history of pulmonary embolism. Prog Cardiovasc Dis 17:259, 1975
151. The PIOPED Investigators: Value of the ventilation/perfusion scan in acute pulmonary embolism. Results of the Prospective Investigation of Pulmonary Embolism Diagnosis (PIOPED). JAMA 263:2753, 1990
152. Kearon C, Hirsh J: The diagnosis of pulmonary embolism. Haemostasis 25:72, 1995
153. Ryu JH, Olson EJ, Pellikka PA: Clinical recognition of pulmonary embolism: Problem of unrecognized and asymptomatic cases. Mayo Clin Proc 73:873, 1998
154. Powell T, Muller NL: Imaging of acute pulmonary thromboembolism: Should spiral computed tomography replace the ventilation-perfusion scan? Clin Chest Med 24:29, 2003
155. Sreeram N, Cheriex EC, Smeets JL, et al: Value of the 12-lead electrocardiogram at hospital admission in the diagnosis of pulmonary embolism. Am J Cardiol 73:298, 1994
156. Dunn KL, Wolf JP, Dorfman DM, et al: Normal D-dimer levels in emergency department patients suspected of acute pulmonary embolism. J Am Coll Cardiol 40:1475, 2002
157. Kucher N, Kohler HP, Dornhofer T, et al: Accuracy of D-dimer/fibrinogen ratio to predict pulmonary embolism: A prospective diagnostic study. J Thromb Haemost 1:708, 2003
158. Kanne JP, Gotway MB, Thoongsuwan N, et al: Six cases of acute central pulmonary embolism revealed on unenhanced multidetector CT of the chest. AJR Am J Roentgenol 180:1661, 2003
159. Swensen SJ, Sheedy PF 2nd, Ryu JH, et al: Outcomes after withholding anticoagulation from patients with suspected acute pulmonary embolism and negative computed tomographic findings: A cohort study. Mayo Clin Proc 77:130, 2002
160. Goldhaber SZ: Echocardiography in the management of pulmonary embolism. Ann Intern Med 136:691, 2002
161. Kucher N, Goldhaber SZ: Cardiac biomarkers for risk stratification of patients with acute pulmonary embolism. Circulation 108:2191, 2003
162. Goldhaber SZ: Unsolved issues in the treatment of pulmonary embolism. Thromb Res 103:V245, 2001
163. Task Force on Pulmonary Embolism, European Society of Cardiology: Guidelines on diagnosis and management of acute pulmonary embolism. Eur Heart J 21:1301, 2000
164. Goldhaber SZ: Recent advances in the diagnosis and lytic therapy of pulmonary embolism. Chest 99:173S, 1991
165. Dehring DJ, Arens JF: Pulmonary thromboembolism: Disease recognition and patient management. Anesthesiology 73:146, 1990
166. Mangano DT: Immediate hemodynamic and pulmonary changes following pulmonary thromboembolism. Anesthesiology 52:173, 1980
167. Levine MN: Thrombolytic therapy for venous thromboembolism. Complications and contraindications. Clin Chest Med 16:321, 1995
168. Lualdi JC, Goldhaber SZ: Right ventricular dysfunction after acute pulmonary embolism: Pathophysiologic factors, detection, and therapeutic implications. Am Heart J 130:1276, 1995
169. Gossage JR: Early intervention in massive pulmonary embolism. A guide to diagnosis and triage for the critical first hour. Postgrad Med 111:27, 33, 39-40 passim, 2002
170. Tapson VF, Witty LA: Massive pulmonary embolism. Diagnostic and therapeutic strategies. Clin Chest Med 16:329, 1995
171. Hull RD, Pineo GF: Current concepts of anticoagulation therapy. Clin Chest Med 16:269, 1995
172. Kelley MA, Abbuhl S: Massive pulmonary embolism. Clin Chest Med 15:547, 1994
173. Gray HH, Miller GA, Paneth M: Pulmonary embolectomy: Its place in the management of pulmonary embolism. Lancet 1:1441, 1988
174. Goldhaber SZ, Kessler CM, Heit JA, et al: Recombinant tissue type plasminogen activator versus a novel dosing regimen of urokinase in acute pulmonary embolism: A randomized controlled multicenter trial. J Am Coll Cardiol 20:24, 1992
175. Tsai SK, Wang MJ, Ko WJ, et al: Emergent bedside transesophageal echocardiography in the resuscitation of sudden cardiac arrest after tricuspid inflow obstruction and pulmonary embolism. Anesth Analg 89:1406, 1999
176. Fava M, Loyola S: Applications of percutaneous mechanical thrombectomy in pulmonary embolism. Techn Vasc Interv Radiol 6:53, 2003
177. Meyer G, Tamisier D, Sors H, et al: Pulmonary embolectomy: A 20-year experience at one center. Ann Thorac Surg 51:232, 1991
178. Aklog L, Williams CS, Byrne JG, et al: Acute pulmonary embolectomy: A contemporary approach. Circulation 105:1416, 2002
179. Splinter WM, Dwane PD, Wigle RD, et al: Anaesthetic management of emergency caesarean section followed by pulmonary embolectomy. Can J Anaesth 36:689, 1989
180. Van der Linden P, Gilbart E, Engelman E, et al: Comparison of halothane, isoflurane, alfentanil, and ketamine in experimental septic shock. Anesth Analg 70:608, 1990

181. Ohteki H, Norita H, Sakai M, et al: Emergency pulmonary embolectomy with percutaneous cardiopulmonary bypass. Ann Thorac Surg 63:1584, 1997
182. Shimokawa S, Uehara K, Toyohira H, et al: Massive endobronchial hemorrhage after pulmonary embolectomy. Ann Thorac Surg 61:1241, 1996
183. Layish DT, Tapson VF: Pharmacologic hemodynamic support in massive pulmonary embolism. Chest 111:218, 1997
184. Molloy DW, Lee KY, Jones D, et al: Effects of noradrenaline and isoproterenol on cardiopulmonary function in a canine model of acute pulmonary hypertension. Chest 88:432, 1985
185. Bottiger BW, Motsch J, Dorsam J, et al: Inhaled nitric oxide selectively decreases pulmonary artery pressure and pulmonary vascular resistance following acute massive pulmonary microembolism in piglets. Chest 110:1041, 1996
186. Gries A, Bottiger BW, Dorsam J, et al: Inhaled nitric oxide inhibits platelet aggregation after pulmonary embolism in pigs. Anesthesiology 86:387, 1997
187. Galie N, Manes A, Branzi A: The new clinical trials on pharmacological treatment in pulmonary arterial hypertension. Eur Respir J 20:1037, 2002
188. Simonneau G, Galie N, Rubin LJ, et al: Clinical classification of pulmonary hypertension. J Am Coll Cardiol 43(suppl S):55, 2004
189. Rich S, Dantzker DR, Ayres SM, et al: Primary pulmonary hypertension. A national prospective study. Ann Intern Med 107:216, 1987
190. Farber HW, Loscalzo J: Pulmonary arterial hypertension. N Engl J Med 351:1655, 2004
191. Sitbon O, Humbert M, Simonneau G: Primary pulmonary hypertension: Current therapy. Prog Cardiovasc Dis 45:115, 2002
192. Sitbon O, Humbert M, Nunes H, et al: Long-term intravenous epoprostenol infusion in primary pulmonary hypertension: Prognostic factors and survival. J Am Coll Cardiol 40:780, 2002
193. Budhiraja R, Tuder RM, Hassoun PM: Endothelial dysfunction in pulmonary hypertension. Circulation 109:159, 2004
194. Olschewski H, Simonneau G, Galie N, et al: Inhaled iloprost for severe pulmonary hypertension. N Engl J Med 347:322, 2002
195. Humbert M, Sitbord O, Simonneau G: Treatment of pulmonary arterial hypertension. N Engl J Med 351:1425, 2004
196. Bhatia S, Frantz RP, Severson CJ, et al: Immediate and long-term hemodynamic and clinical effects of sildenafil in patients with pulmonary arterial hypertension receiving vasodilator therapy. Mayo Clin Proc 78:1207, 2003
197. Altman R, Scazziota A, Rouvier J, et al: Coagulation and fibrinolytic parameters in patients with pulmonary hypertension. Clin Cardiol 19:549, 1996
198. Gaine SP, Rubin LJ: Primary pulmonary hypertension. Lancet 352:719, 1998
199. Bando K, Armitage JM, Paradis IL, et al: Indications for and results of single, bilateral, and heart-lung transplantation for pulmonary hypertension. J Thorac Cardiovasc Surg 108:1056, 1994
200. Fischer LG, Van Aken H, Burkle H: Management of pulmonary hypertension: Physiological and pharmacological considerations for anesthesiologists. Anesth Analg 96:1603, 2003
201. Klepetko W, Mayer E, Sandoval J, et al: Interventional and surgical modalities of treatment for pulmonary arterial hypertension. J Am Cell Cardiol 43(suppl S):735, 2004
202. Jamieson SW, Kapelanski DP, Sakakibara N, et al: Pulmonary thromboendarterectomy. Ann Thorac Surg 76:1457, 2003
203. Manecke GR, Wilson W, Auger WR, et al: Anesthesia for pulmonary thromboendarterectomy. Semin Cardiothorac Vasc Anesth 9:189-204, 2005
204. Cahill BC, Ingbar DH: Massive hemoptysis. Assessment and management. Clin Chest Med 15:147, 1994
205. Sekkal S, Cornu E, Christides C, et al: Swan-Ganz catheter-induced pulmonary artery perforation during cardiac surgery concerning two cases. J Cardiovasc Surg (Torino) 37:313, 1996
206. Nuttall GA, Oliver WC, Santrach PJ, et al: Efficacy of a simple intraoperative transfusion algorithm for nonerythrocyte component utilization after cardiopulmonary bypass. Anesthesiology 94:773, 2001
207. Kearney TJ, Shabot MM: Pulmonary artery rupture associated with Swan-Ganz catheter. Chest 108:1349, 1995
208. Muller BJ, Gallucci A: Pulmonary artery catheter-induced pulmonary artery rupture in patients undergoing cardiac surgery. Can Anaesth Soc J 32:258, 1985
209. Rosenbaum L, Rosenbaum SH, Askanazi J, et al: Small amounts of hemoptysis as an early warning sign of pulmonary artery rupture by a pulmonary arterial catheter. Crit Care Med 9:319, 1981
210. Hardy J-F, Morissette M, Taillefer J, et al: Pathophysiology of rupture of the pulmonary artery by pulmonary artery balloon-tipped catheters. Anesth Analg 62:925, 1983
211. Barash PG, Nardi D, Hammond G, et al: Catheter-induced pulmonary artery perforation: Mechanisms, management, and modifications. J Thorac Cardiovasc Surg 82:5, 1981
212. Tan RT, McGahan JP, Link DP, et al: Bronchial artery embolisation in management of haemoptysis. J Intervent Radiol 6:67, 1991
213. Cremaschi P, Nascimbene C, Vitulo P, et al: Therapeutic embolization of bronchial artery: A successful treatment in 209 cases of relapse hemoptysis. Angiology 44:295, 1993
214. Hasnain JU, Moulton AL: Life-threatening pulmonary artery perforation during cardiopulmonary bypass. Crit Care Med 14:748, 1986
215. Klein U, Karzai W, Bloos F, et al: Role of fiberoptic bronchoscopy in conjunction with the use of double-lumen tubes for thoracic anesthesia: A prospective study. Anesthesiology 88:346, 1998
216. Larson CE, Gasior TA: A device for endobronchial blocker placement during one-lung anesthesia. Anesth Analg 71:311, 1990
217. Stone JG, Faltas AN, Khambatta HJ, et al: Temporary unilateral pulmonary artery occlusion: A method for controlling Swan-Ganz catheter-induced hemoptysis. Ann Thorac Surg 37:508, 1984
218. Maisch B, Ristic AD: The classification of pericardial disease in the age of modern medicine. Curr Cardiol Rep 4:13, 2002
219. Aikat S, Ghaffari S: A review of pericardial diseases: Clinical, ECG and hemodynamic features and management. Clev Clin J Med 67:903, 2000
220. Spodick DH: Pericarditis, pericardial effusion, cardiac tamponade, and constriction. Crit Care Clin 5:455, 1989
221. Oakley CM: Myocarditis, pericarditis and other pericardial diseases. Heart (Br Card Soc) 84:449, 2000
222. Miller RH, Horneffer PJ, Gardner TJ, et al: The epidemiology of the postpericardiotomy syndrome: A common complication of cardiac surgery. Am Heart J 116:1323, 1988
223. Ling LH, Oh JK, Schaff HV, et al: Constrictive pericarditis in the modern era: Evolving clinical spectrum and impact on outcome after pericardiectomy. Circulation 100:1380, 1999
224. Asher CR, Klein AL: Diastolic heart failure: Restrictive cardiomyopathy, constrictive pericarditis, and cardiac tamponade: Clinical and echocardiographic evaluation. Cardiol Rev 10:218, 2002
225. Oh JK, Hatle LK, Seward JB, et al: Diagnostic role of Doppler echocardiography in constrictive pericarditis. J Am Coll Cardiol 23:154, 1994
226. Tuna IC, Danielson GK: Surgical management of pericardial disease. Cardiol Clin 8:683, 1990
227. Laham RJ, Cohen DJ, Kuntz RE, et al: Pericardial effusion in patients with cancer: Outcome with contemporary management strategies. Heart 75:67, 1996
228. Spodick DH: Pathophysiology of cardiac tamponade. Chest 113:1372, 1998
229. Shabetai R: Diseases of the pericardium. *In* Hurst JW (ed): The Heart, Arteries and Veins. New York, McGraw-Hill Information Services Co, 1990, pp 1348–1374
230. Ball JB, Morrison WL: Experience with cardiac tamponade following open heart surgery. Heart Vessels 11:39, 1996
231. Ziskind AA, Pearce AC, Lemmon CC, et al: Percutaneous balloon pericardiotomy for the treatment of cardiac tamponade and large pericardial effusions: Description of technique and report of the first 50 cases. J Am Coll Cardiol 21:1, 1993
232. Johnson SB, Nielsen JL, Sako EY, et al: Penetrating intrapericardial wounds: Clinical experience with a surgical protocol. Ann Thorac Surg 60:117, 1995
233. Kaplan JA, Bland JW Jr, Dunbar RW: The perioperative management of pericardial tamponade. South Med J 69:417, 1976.
234. Zhang H, Spapen H, Vincent JL: Effects of dobutamine and norepinephrine on oxygen availability in tamponade-induced stagnant hypoxia: A prospective, randomized, controlled study. Crit Care Med 22:299, 1994
235. Rizzo RJ, Whittemore AD, Couper GS, et al: Combined carotid and coronary revascularization: The preferred approach to the severe vasculopathy. Ann Thorac Surg 54:1099, 1992
236. Mackey WC, O'Donnell TF Jr, Callow AD: Cardiac risk in patients undergoing carotid endarterectomy: Impact on perioperative and long-term mortality. J Vasc Surg 11:226, 1990
237. Hertzer NR, Loop FD, Beven EG, et al: Surgical staging for simultaneous coronary and carotid disease: A study including prospective randomization. J Vasc Surg 9:455, 1989
238. Bernhard VM, Johnson WD, Peterson JJ: Carotid artery stenosis. Association with surgery for coronary artery disease. Arch Surg 105:837, 1972
239. Frye RL, Kronmal R, Schaff HV, et al: Stroke in coronary artery bypass graft surgery: An analysis of the CASS experience. The participants in the Coronary Artery Surgery Study. Int J Cardiol 36:213, 1992

240. Redmond JM, Greene PS, Goldsborough MA, et al: Neurologic injury in cardiac surgical patients with a history of stroke. Ann Thorac Surg 61:42, 1996
241. Clark RE, Brillman J, Davis DA, et al: Microemboli during coronary artery bypass grafting: Genesis and effect on outcome. J Thorac Cardiovasc Surg 109:249, 1995
242. Trachiotis GD, Pfister AJ: Management strategy for simultaneous carotid endarterectomy and coronary revascularization. Ann Thorac Surg 64:1013, 1997
243. Balderman SC, Gutierrez IZ, Makula P, et al: Noninvasive screening for asymptomatic carotid artery disease prior to cardiac operations: Experience with 500 patients. J Thorac Cardiovasc Surg 85:427, 1983
244. Reed GL 3rd, Singer DE, Picard EH, et al: Stroke following coronary artery bypass surgery. A case-control estimate of the risk from carotid bruits. N Engl J Med 319:1246, 1988
245. Moore WS, Barnett HJ, Beebe HG, et al: Guidelines for carotid endarterectomy. A multidisciplinary consensus statement from the Ad Hoc Committee, American Heart Association. Circulation 91:566, 1995
246. Faggioli GL, Curl GR, Ricotta JJ: The role of carotid screening before coronary artery bypass. J Vasc Surg 12:724, 1990
247. Schwartz LB, Bridgman AH, Kieffer RW, et al: Asymptomatic carotid artery stenosis and stroke in patients undergoing cardiopulmonary bypass. J Vasc Surg 21:146, 1995
248. Busch T, Sirbu H, Aleksic I, et al: Combined approach for internal carotid artery stenosis and cardiovascular disease in septuagenarians: A comparative study. Eur J Cardiothorac Surg 16:602, 1999
249. Hertzer NR, Young JR, Beven EG, et al: Coronary angiography in 506 patients with extracranial cerebrovascular disease. Arch Intern Med 145:849, 1985
250. Schwartz RL, Garrett JR, Karp RB, et al: Simultaneous myocardial revascularization and carotid endarterectomy. Circulation 66(suppl I):I-97, 1982
251. Kouchoukos N, Daily BB, Wareing TH, et al: Hypothermic circulatory arrest for cerebral protection during combined carotid and cardiac surgery in patients with bilateral carotid artery disease. Ann Surg 219:699, 1994
252. Korompai FL, Hayward RH, Knight WL: Noncardiac operations combined with coronary artery bypass. Surg Clin N Am 62:215, 1982
253. Daily PO, Freeman RK, Dembitsky WP, et al: Cost reduction by combined carotid endarterectomy and coronary artery bypass grafting. J Thorac Cardiovasc Surg 111:1185, 1996
254. Cheng DC, Karski J, Peniston C, et al: Morbidity outcome in early versus conventional tracheal extubation after coronary artery bypass grafting: A prospective, randomized, controlled trial. J Thorac Cardiovasc Surg 112:755, 1996
255. Engoren M, Luther G, Fenn-Buderer N: A comparison of fentanyl, sufentanil, and remifentanil for fast-track cardiac anesthesia. Anesth Analg 93:859, 2001
256. Butterworth J, James R, Prielipp RC, et al: Do shorter-acting neuromuscular blocking drugs or opioids associate with reduced intensive care unit or hospital lengths of stay after coronary artery bypass grafting? CABG Clinical Benchmarking Data Base Participants. Anesthesiology 88:1437, 1998
257. Olivier P, Sirieix D, Dassier P, et al: Continuous infusion of remifentanil and target-controlled infusion of propofol for patients undergoing cardiac surgery: A new approach for scheduled early extubation. J Cardiothorac Vasc Anesth 14:29, 2000
258. Royse CF, Royse AG, Soeding PF: Routine immediate extubation after cardiac operation: A review of our first 100 patients. Ann Thorac Surg 68:1326, 1999
259. Fernandes ED, Kadivar H, Hallman GL, et al: Congenital malformations of the coronary arteries: The Texas Heart Institute experience. Ann Thorac Surg 54:732, 1992
260. Yamanaka O, Hobbs RE: Coronary artery anomalies in 126,595 patients undergoing coronary arteriography. Cathet Cardiovasc Diagn 21:28, 1990
261. Giannoccaro PJ, Sochowski RA, Morton BC, et al: Complementary role of transoesophageal echocardiography to coronary angiography in the assessment of coronary artery anomalies. Br Heart J 70:70, 1993
262. Calkins JB Jr, Talley JD, Kim NH: Iatrogenic aortocoronary venous fistula: A complication of coronary artery bypass surgery: Patient report and review of the literature. Cathet Cardiovasc Diagn 37:55, 1996
263. Stevenson JG, Sorensen GK, Stamm SJ, et al: Intraoperative transesophageal echocardiography of coronary artery fistulas. Ann Thorac Surg 57:1217, 1994
264. Harris WO, Andrews JC, Nichols DA, et al: Percutaneous transcatheter embolization of coronary arteriovenous fistulas. Mayo Clin Proc 71:37, 1996
265. Pomini F, Mercogliano D, Cavalletti C, et al: Cardiopulmonary bypass in pregnancy. Ann Thorac Surg 61:259, 1996
266. Parry AJ, Westaby S: Cardiopulmonary bypass during pregnancy. Ann Thorac Surg 61:1865, 1996
267. Weiss BM, von Segesser LK, Alon E, et al: Outcome of cardiovascular surgery and pregnancy: A systematic review of the period 1984-1996. Am J Obstet Gynecol 179:1643, 1998
268. Mahli A, Izdes S, Coskun D: Cardiac operations during pregnancy: Review of factors influencing fetal outcome. Ann Thorac Surg 69:1622, 2000
269. Gopal K, Hudson IM, Ludmir J, et al: Homograft aortic root replacement during pregnancy. Ann Thorac Surg 74:243, 2002
270. Conklin KA: Physiologic changes of pregnancy. *In* Chestnut DH (ed): Obstetric Anesthesia. Principles and Practice. St. Louis, Mosby, 1994, pp 17–42
271. Wan S, LeClerc JL, Vincent JL: Inflammatory response to cardiopulmonary bypass: Mechanisms involved and possible therapeutic strategies. Chest 112:676, 1997
272. Lamb MP, Ross K, Johnstone AM, et al: Fetal heart monitoring during open heart surgery. Two case reports. Br J Obstet Gynaecol 88:669, 1981
273. Buffolo E, Palma JH, Gomes WJ, et al: Successful use of deep hypothermic circulatory arrest in pregnancy. Ann Thorac Surg 58:1532, 1994
274. Strickland RA, Oliver WC Jr, Chantigian RC, et al: Anesthesia, cardiopulmonary bypass, and the pregnant patient. Mayo Clin Proc 66:411, 1991
275. Becker RM: Intracardiac surgery in pregnant women. Ann Thorac Surg 36:453, 1983
276. Chambers CE, Clark SL: Cardiac surgery during pregnancy. Clin Obstet Gynecol 37:316, 1994
277. Izquierdo LA, Kushnir O, Knieriem K, et al: Effect of mitral valve prosthetic surgery on the outcome of a growth-retarded fetus. A case report. Am J Obstet Gynecol 163:584, 1990
278. Jahangiri M, Clarke J, Prefumo F, et al: Cardiac surgery during pregnancy: Pulsatile or nonpulsatile perfusion? J Thorac Cardiovasc Surg 126:894, 2003
279. Ralston DH, Shnider SM, DeLorimier AA: Effects of equipotent ephedrine, metaraminol, mephentermine, and methoxamine on uterine blood flow in the pregnant ewe. Anesthesiology 40:354, 1974
280. Ramanathan S, Grant GJ: Vasopressor therapy for hypotension due to epidural anesthesia for cesarean section. Acta Anaesthesiol Scand 32:559, 1988
281. Moran DH, Perillo M, LaPorta RF, et al: Phenylephrine in the prevention of hypotension following spinal anesthesia for cesarean delivery. J Clin Anesth 3:301, 1991
282. Hood DD, Dewan DM, James FM III: Maternal and fetal effects of epinephrine in gravid ewes. Anesthesiology 64:610, 1986
283. Bakke OM, Haram K, Lygre T, et al: Comparison of the placental transfer of thiopental and diazepam in caesarean section. Eur J Clin Pharmacol 21:221, 1981
284. Ellingson A, Haram K, Sagen N, et al: Transplacental passage of ketamine after intravenous administration. Acta Anaesth Scand 21:41, 1977
285. Dailland P, Cockshott ID, Lirzin JD, et al: Intravenous propofol during Cesarean section: Placental transfer, concentrations in breast milk, and neonatal effects. A preliminary study. Anesthesiology 71:827, 1989
286. Bach V, Carl P, Ravlo O, et al: A randomized comparison between midazolam and thiopental for elective cesarean section anesthesia: III. Placental transfer and elimination in neonates. Anesth Analg 68:238, 1989
287. Mazze RI, Fujinaga M, Rice SA, et al: Reproductive and teratogenic effects of nitrous oxide, halothane, isoflurane, and enflurane in Sprague-Dawley rats. Anesthesiology 64:339, 1986
288. O'Leary G, Bacon CL, Odumeru O, et al: Antiproliferative actions of inhalational anesthetics: Comparisons to the valproate teratogen. Int J Dev Neurosci 18:39, 2000
289. Lowe SA, Rubin PC: The pharmacological management of hypertension in pregnancy. J Hypertens 10:201, 1992
290. Ellis SC, Wheeler AS, James FM III, et al: Fetal and maternal effects of sodium nitroprusside used to counteract hypertension in gravid ewes. Am J Obstet Gynecol 143:766, 1982
291. Oakley CM: Anticoagulation and pregnancy. Eur Heart J 16:1317, 1995
292. Ippolito G, Puro V, Heptonstall J, et al: Occupational human immunodeficiency virus infection in health care workers: Worldwide cases through September 1997. Clin Infect Dis 28:365, 1999
293. Hovanessian HC: New developments in the treatment of HIV disease: An overview. Ann Emerg Med 33:546, 1999
294. Puro V, De Carli G, Scognamiglio P, et al: Risk of HIV and other blood-borne infections in the cardiac setting: Patient-to-provider and provider-to-patient transmission. Ann N Y Acad Sci 946:291, 2001

295. Henderson DK, Fahey BJ, Willy M, et al: Risk for occupational transmission of human immunodeficiency virus type 1 (HIV-1) associated with clinical exposures. A prospective evaluation. Ann Intern Med 113:740, 1990
296. Tokars JI, Bell DM, Culver DH, et al: Percutaneous injuries during surgical procedures. JAMA 267:2899, 1992
297. Anonymous: Update: provisional Public Health Service recommendations for chemoprophylaxis after occupational exposure to HIV. MMWR Morb Mortal Wkly Rep 45:468, 1996
298. Cardo DM, Bell DM: Bloodborne pathogen transmission in health care workers. Risks and prevention strategies. Infect Dis Clin North Am 11:331, 1997
299. Greene ES, Berry AJ, Arnold WP 3rd, et al: Percutaneous injuries in anesthesia personnel. Anesth Analg 83:273, 1996
300. Sloand EM, Pitt E, Klein HG: Safety of the blood supply. JAMA 274:1368, 1995
301. Lackritz EM, Satten GA, Aberle-Grasse J, et al: Estimated risk of transmission of the human immunodeficiency virus by screened blood in the United States. N Engl J Med 333:1721, 1995
302. Schreiber GB, Busch MP, Kleinman SH, et al: The risk of transfusion-transmitted viral infections. N Engl J Med 334:1685, 1996
303. Gelsomino S, Morocutti G, Masullo G, et al: Open heart surgery in patients with dialysis-dependent renal insufficiency. J Card Surg 16:400, 2001
304. Provenchere S, Plantefeve G, Hufnagel G, et al: Renal dysfunction after cardiac surgery with normothermic cardiopulmonary bypass: Incidence, risk factors, and effect on clinical outcome. Anesth Analg 96:1258, 2003
305. Durmaz I, Buket S, Atay Y, et al: Cardiac surgery with cardiopulmonary bypass in patients with chronic renal failure. J Thorac Cardiovasc Surg 118:306, 1999
306. Koyanagi T, Nishida H, Kitamura M, et al: Comparison of clinical outcomes of coronary artery bypass grafting and percutaneous transluminal coronary angioplasty in renal dialysis patients. Ann Thorac Surg 61:1793, 1996
307. Mayer G, Horl WH: Cardiovascular effects of increasing hemoglobin in chronic renal failure. Am J Nephr 16:263, 1996
308. Caimmi PP, Pagani L, Micalizzi E, et al: Fenoldopam for renal protection in patients undergoing cardiopulmonary bypass. J Cardiothorac Vasc Anesth 17:491, 2003
309. Sutton RG: Renal considerations, dialysis, and ultrafiltration during cardiopulmonary bypass. Int Anesthesiol Clin 34:165, 1996
310. Kubota T, Miyata A, Maeda A, et al: Continuous haemodiafiltration during and after cardiopulmonary bypass in renal failure patients. Can J Anaesth 44:1182, 1997
311. Lemmer JH Jr, Metzdorff MT, Krause AH, et al: Aprotinin use in patients with dialysis-dependent renal failure undergoing cardiac operations. J Thorac Cardiovasc Surg 112:192, 1996
312. O'Connor CJ, Brown DV, Avramov M, et al: The impact of renal dysfunction on aprotinin pharmacokinetics during cardiopulmonary bypass. Anesth Analg 89:1101, 1999
313. Petroni KC, Cohen NH: Continuous renal replacement therapy: Anesthetic implications. Anesth Analg 94:1288, 2002
314. DiMichele D: Hemophilia 1996: New approach to an old disease. Pediatr Clin North Am 43:709, 1996
315. Roskos RR, Gilchrist GS, Kazmier FJ, et al: Management of hemophilia A and B during surgical correction of transposition of great arteries. Mayo Clin Proc 58:182, 1983
316. Mannucci PM: Hemophilia and related bleeding disorders: A story of dismay and success (lectures). Hematology 1, 2002
317. Evatt BL: AIDS and hemophilia-current issues. Thromb Haemost 74:36, 1995
318. Aledort LM: Hemophilia: Yesterday, today, and tomorrow. Mt Sinai J Med 63:225, 1996
319. Sampson JF, Hamstra R, Aldrete JA: Management of hemophiliac patients undergoing surgical procedures. Anesth Analg 58:133, 1979
320. McIntyre AJ: Blood transfusion and haemostatic management in the perioperative period. Can J Anaesth 39:R101, 1992
321. Mannucci PM, Cattaneo M: Desmopressin: A nontransfusional treatment of hemophilia and von Willebrand disease. Haemostasis 22:276, 1992
322. Warrier AI, Lusher JM: DDAVP: A useful alternative to blood components in moderate hemophilia A and von Willebrand disease. J Pedriatr 102:228, 1983
323. Mannucci PM: Modern treatment of hemophilia: From the shadows towards the light. Thromb Haemost 70:17, 1993
324. Nilsson IM: The management of hemophilia patients with inhibitors. Transfus Med Rev 6:285, 1992
325. Seremetis SV, Aledort LM: Congenital bleeding disorders. Rational treatment options. Drugs 45:541, 1993
326. DiMichele DM, Lasak ME, Miller CH: A study of in vitro factor VIII recovery during the delivery of four ultra-pure factor VIII concentrate by continuous infusion. Am J Hematol 51:99, 1996
327. Leggett PL, Doyle D, Smith WB, et al: Elective cardiac operation in a patient with severe hemophilia and acquired factor VIII antibodies. J Thorac Cardiovasc Surg 87:556, 1984
328. Tagariello G, De Biasi E, Gajo GB, et al: Recombinant FVIIa (NovoSeven) continuous infusion and total hip replacement in patients with haemophilia and high titre of inhibitors to FVIII: Experience of two cases. Haemophilia 6:581, 2000
329. Lusher J, Ingerslev J, Roberts H, et al: Clinical experience with recombinant factor VIIa. Blood Coagul Fibrinolysis 9:119, 1998
330. Rodeghiero F, Castaman G, Dini E: Epidemiological investigation of the prevalence of von Willebrand's disease. Blood 69:454, 1987
331. Rick ME: Diagnosis and management of von Willebrand's syndrome. Med Clin North Am 78:609, 1994
332. Oliver WC Jr, Nuttall GA: The effect of cardiopulmonary bypass on platelet function. *In* Pifarre R (ed): Philadelphia, Hanley and Belfus, 1997, pp 59–81. New Anticoagulants for the Cardiovascular Patient.
333. Sadler JE, Matsushita T, Dong Z, et al: Molecular mechanism and classification of von Willebrand disease. Thromb Haemost 74:161, 1995
334. Perrin EJ, Ray MJ, Hawson GA: The role of von Willebrand factor in haemostasis and blood loss during and after cardiopulmonary bypass surgery. Blood Coagul Fibrinolysis 6:650, 1995
335. Berntorp E: Plasma product treatment in various types of von Willebrand's disease. Haemostasis 24:289, 1994
336. Castaman G, Rodeghiero F: Current management of von Willebrand's disease. Drugs 50:602, 1995
337. Rick ME: Laboratory diagnosis of von Willebrand's disease. Clin Lab Med 14:781, 1994
338. Aledort LM: Treatment of von Willebrand's disease. Mayo Clin Proc 66:841, 1991
339. Batlle J, Noya MS, Giangrande P, et al: Advances in the therapy of von Willebrand disease. Haemophilia 8:301, 2002
340. Logan LJ: Treatment of von Willebrand's disease. Hematol Oncol Clin North Am 6:1079, 1992
341. Menache D, Aronson DL: New treatments of von Willebrand disease: Plasma-derived von Willebrand factor concentrates. Thromb Haemost 78:566, 1997
342. Mannucci PM: Biochemical characteristics of therapeutic plasma concentrates used in the treatment of von Willebrand disease. Haemostasis 24:285, 1994
343. Blajchman MA: An overview of the mechanism of action of antithrombin and its inherited deficiency states. Blood Coagul Fibrinolysis 5(suppl I):S5, 1994
344. Bick RL: Clinical relevance of antithrombin III. Semin Thromb Hemost 8:276, 1982
345. Bucur SZ, Levy JH, Despotis GJ, et al: Uses of antithrombin III concentrate in congenital and acquired deficiency states. Transfusion 38:481, 1998
346. Marciniak E, Farley CH, DeSimone PA: Familial thrombosis due to antithrombin III deficiency. Blood 43:219, 1974
347. Hellstern P, Moberg U, Ekblad M, et al: In vitro characterization of antithrombin III concentrates—A single-blind study. Haemostasis 25:193, 1995
348. Demers C, Ginsberg JS, Hirsh J, et al: Thrombosis in antithrombin-III-deficient persons. Report of a large kindred and literature review. Ann Intern Med 116:754, 1992
349. Slaughter TF, Mark JB, El-Moalem H, et al: Hemostatic effects of antithrombin III supplementation during cardiac surgery: Results of a prospective randomized investigation. Blood Coagul Fibrinolysis 12:25, 2001
350. Williams MR, D'Ambra AB, Beck JR, et al: A randomized trial of antithrombin concentrate for treatment of heparin resistance. Ann Thorac Surg 70:873, 2000
351. Soloway HB, Christiansen TW: Heparin anticoagulation during cardiopulmonary bypass in an antithrombin-III deficient patient. Implications relative to the etiology of heparin rebound. Am J Clin Pathol 73:723, 1980
352. Jackson MR, Olsen SB, Gomez ER, et al: Use of antithrombin III concentrates to correct antithrombin III deficiency during vascular surgery. J Vasc Surg 22:804, 1995
353. Lemmer JH Jr, Despotis GJ: Antithrombin III concentrate to treat heparin resistance in patients undergoing cardiac surgery. J Thorac Cardiovasc Surg 123:213, 2002

354. Levy JH, Despotis GJ, Szlam F, et al: Recombinant human transgenic antithrombin in cardiac surgery: A dose-finding study. Anesthesiology 96:1095, 2002
355. Hashimoto K, Yamagishi M, Sasaki T, et al: Heparin and antithrombin III levels during cardiopulmonary bypass: Correlation with subclinical plasma coagulation. Ann Thorac Surg 58:799, 1994
356. Lechner K, Kyrle PA: Antithrombin III concentrates—Are they clinically useful? Thromb Haemost 73:340, 1995
357. Koster A, Chew D, Kuebler W, et al: High antithrombin III levels attenuate hemostatic activation and leukocyte activation during cardiopulmonary bypass. J Thorac Cardiovasc Surg 126:906, 2003
358. Williams AC: Cold agglutinins. Cause for concern? Anaesthesia 35:887, 1980
359. Landymore R, Isom W, Barlam B: Management of patients with cold agglutinins who require open-heart surgery. Can J Surg 26:79, 1983
360. Shahian DM, Wallach SR, Bern MM: Open heart surgery in patients with cold-reactive proteins. Surg Clin North Am 65:315, 1985
361. Moore RA, Geller EA, Mathews ES, et al: The effect of hypothermic cardiopulmonary bypass on patients with low-titer, nonspecific cold agglutinins. Ann Thorac Surg 37:233, 1984
362. Leach AB, Van Hasselt GL, Edwards JC: Cold agglutinins and deep hypothermia. Anaesthesia 38:140, 1983
363. Dake SB, Johnston MF, Brueggeman P, et al: Detection of cold hemagglutination in a blood cardioplegia unit before systemic cooling of a patient with unsuspected cold agglutinin disease. Ann Thorac Surg 47:914, 1989
364. Klein HG, Faltz LL, McIntosh CL, et al: Surgical hypothermia in a patient with a cold agglutinin: Management by plasma exchange. Transfusion 20:354, 1980
365. Lee MC, Chang CH, Hsieh MJ: Use of a total wash-out method in an open heart operation. Ann Thorac Surg 47:57, 1989
366. Aoki A, Kay GL, Zubiate P, et al: Cardiac operation without hypothermia for the patient with cold agglutinin. Chest 104:1627, 1993
367. Agarwal SK, Ghosh PK, Gupta D: Cardiac surgery and cold-reactive proteins. Ann Thorac Surg 60:1143, 1995
368. Wayne AS, Kevy SV, Nathan DG: Transfusion management of sickle cell disease. Blood 81:1109, 1993
369. Steingart R: Management of patients with sickle cell disease. Med Clin North Am 76:669, 1992
370. Kingsley CP, Chronister T, Cohen DJ, et al: Anesthetic management of a patient with hemoglobin SS disease and mitral insufficiency for mitral valve repair. J Cardiothorac Vasc Anesth 10:419, 1996
371. Scott-Conner CEH, Brunson CD: The pathophysiology of the sickle hemoglobinopathies and implications for perioperative management. Am J Surg 168:268, 1994
372. Esseltine DW, Baxter MR, Bevan JC: Sickle cell states and the anaesthetist. Can J Anaesth 35:385, 1988
373. Lane PA: Sickle cell disease. Pediatr Clin North Am 43:639, 1996
374. Dorn-Beineke A, Frietsch T: Sickle cell disease—Pathophysiology, clinical and diagnostic implications. Clin Chem Lab Med 40:1075, 2002
375. Kalhan S, DeBoer G: Preoperative screening for sickle cell trait. JAMA 259:3558, 1988
376. Koshy M, Weiner SJ, Miller ST, et al: Surgery and anesthesia in sickle cell disease. Cooperative Study of Sickle Cell Diseases. Blood 86:3676, 1995
377. Gyasi HK, Zarroug AW, Matthew M, et al: Anaesthesia for renal transplantation in sickle cell disease. Can J Anaesth 37:778, 1990
378. Dobson MB: Anesthesia for patients with hemoglobinopathies. Int Anesthesiol Clin 23:197, 1985
379. Vichinsky EP, Haberkern CM, Neumayr L, et al: A comparison of conservative and aggressive transfusion regimens in the perioperative management of sickle cell disease. The Preoperative Transfusion in Sickle Cell Disease Study Group. N Engl J Med 333:206, 1995
380. Cohen AR, Martin MB, Silber JH, et al: A modified transfusion program for prevention of stroke in sickle cell disease. Blood 79:1657, 1992
381. Pagani FD, Polito RJ, Bolling SF: Mitral valve reconstruction in sickle cell disease. Ann Thorac Surg 61:1841, 1996
382. Shulman G, McQuitty C, Vertrees RA, et al: Acute normovolemic red cell exchange for cardiopulmonary bypass in sickle cell disease. Ann Thorac Surg 65:1444, 1998
383. Riethmuller R, Grundy EM, Radley-Smith R: Open heart surgery in a patient with homozygous sickle cell disease. Anaesthesia 37:324, 1982
384. Davies SC, Olatunji PO: Blood transfusion in sickle cell disease. Vox Sang 68:145, 1995
385. Baxter MR, Bevan JC, Esseltine DW, et al: The management of two pediatric patients with sickle cell trait and sickle cell disease during cardiopulmonary bypass. J Cardiothoracic Anesth 3:477, 1989
386. Balasundaram S, Duran CG, al-Halees Z, et al: Cardiopulmonary bypass in sickle cell anaemia. Report of five cases. J Cardiovasc Surg (Torino) 32:271, 1991
387. Lichtenstein SV, Ashe KA, el Dalati H, et al: Warm heart surgery. Ann Thorac Surg 101:269, 1991
388. Metras D, Coulibaly AO, Ouattara K, et al: Open-heart surgery in sickle-cell haemoglobinopathies: Report of 15 cases. Thorax 37:486, 1982
389. Brajtbord D, Johnson D, Ramay M: Use of the cell saver in patients with sickle cell trait. Anesthesiology 70:878, 1989

Chapter 25

CARDIAC PACING AND DEFIBRILLATION

Marc A. Rozner, PhD, MD • Mark Trankina, MD

KEY POINTS

Preoperative

1. Have any implanted pacemaker or defibrillator interrogated by a competent authority shortly before the procedure.
2. Obtain a copy of this interrogation. Ensure that the device will pace the heart.
3. Consider replacing any device near its elective replacement period in a patient scheduled to undergo either a major operation or surgery within 15 cm of the generator.
4. Determine the patient's underlying rhythm, rate, and pacemaker dependency to determine the need for backup pacing support.
5. If magnet use is planned, ensure that a magnet mode exists and verify its rate and pacing mode.
6. Program rate responsiveness off, if present.
7. Program rate enhancements off, if present.
8. Consider increasing the pacing rate to optimize oxygen delivery to tissues for major operations.
9. Disable antitachycardia therapy, if present.

Intraoperative

10. Monitor cardiac rhythm/peripheral pulse with pulse oximeter (plethysmography) or arterial waveform.
11. Disable the "artifact filter" on the electrocardiograph monitor.
12. Avoid use of the monopolar electrosurgical unit (ESU).
13. Use bipolar ESU if possible; if not possible, then pure cut (monopolar ESU) is better than "blend" or "coag."
14. Place the ESU current return pad in such a way to prevent electricity from crossing the generator-heart circuit, even if the pad must be placed on the distal forearm and the wire covered with sterile drape.
15. If the ESU causes ventricular oversensing and pacer quiescence, limit the period(s) of asystole.
16. Temporary pacing might be needed and consideration should be given to the possibility of pacemaker or defibrillator failure.

Postoperative

17. Have the device interrogated by a competent authority postoperatively. Some rate enhancements can be reinitiated, and optimum heart rate and pacing parameters should be determined. The ICD patient must be monitored until the antitachycardia therapy is restored.

PACEMAKERS

Battery-operated, implantable pacing devices were first introduced in 1958, just 4 years after the invention of the transistor. The complexity, calculation, and data storage abilities of these devices have grown in a manner similar to that seen within the computer industry. The natural progression of pacemaker developments led to the invention of the implanted cardioverter-defibrillator (ICD) around 1980. As this technology has advanced, the divisions between these devices have become less clear. For example, every ICD currently implanted has antibradycardia pacing capability, and patients, news media, and even physicians often misidentify an implanted defibrillator as a pacemaker. The consequence of mistaking an ICD for a conventional pacemaker can lead to patient harm, either due to electromagnetic interference (EMI) issues resulting in inappropriate ICD therapy or the unintentional disabling of ICD therapies in some ICDs that can be permanently disabled by magnet placement.[1] Figure 25–1 shows a three-lead defibrillation system and identifies the right ventricular shock coil, which differentiates an ICD system from a conventional pacemaking system. The complexity of cardiac pulse generators, as well as the multitude of programmable parameters, limits the number of sweeping generalizations that can be made about the perioperative care of the patient with an implanted pulse generator. Population aging, continued enhancements in implantable technology, and new indications for implantation will lead to growing numbers of patients with these devices in the new millennium. Both the American College of Cardiology (ACC) and the North American Society for Pacing and Electrophysiology—The Heart Rhythm Society (HRS-NASPE)* have taken note of these issues, and guidelines have been published regarding the care of the perioperative patient with such a device.[2,3] Pinski and Trohman[4,5] also have reviewed this subject, and they have published similar recommendations. Additional reviews have been published, and the American Society of Anesthesiology (ASA) has issued a practice advisory.[6-8]

Pacemaker Overview

Pacemaker manufacturers report that 26 companies have produced nearly 2000 models to date. More than 220,000 adults and children in the United States undergo new pacemaker placement each year, and nearly 3 million patients have pacemakers today. Many factors lead to confusion regarding the behavior of a device and the perioperative care of a patient with a device, especially because case reports, textbooks, and literature reviews have not kept pace with technological developments, and many of these reviews contain incorrect statements.[9] The patient with a pacemaker often has significant comorbid disease. The care of these patients requires attention to both their medical and psychological problems. Additionally, an understanding of pulse generators and their likely idiosyncrasies in the operating or procedure room is needed. Whether the patient with a pacemaker is at increased perioperative risk remains unknown, but two reports suggest that

*The North American Society of Pacing and Electrophysiology changed their name to the Heart Rhythm Society. In order to avoid confusion in this Chapter, the abbreviation HRS-NASPE is used.

these patients deserve extra perioperative attention. In 1995, Badrinath et al[10] retrospectively reviewed ophthalmic surgery cases in one hospital in Madras, India, from 1979 through 1988 (14,787 cases) and wrote that the presence of a pacemaker significantly increased the probability of a mortal event within 6 weeks postoperatively, regardless of the anesthetic technique. In abstract form, Samain et al[11] reported that 3 of 73 pacemaker patients (4.1%) undergoing significant surgery (not including cardiac surgery) died postoperatively of cardiac causes, although a timeframe was not specified.

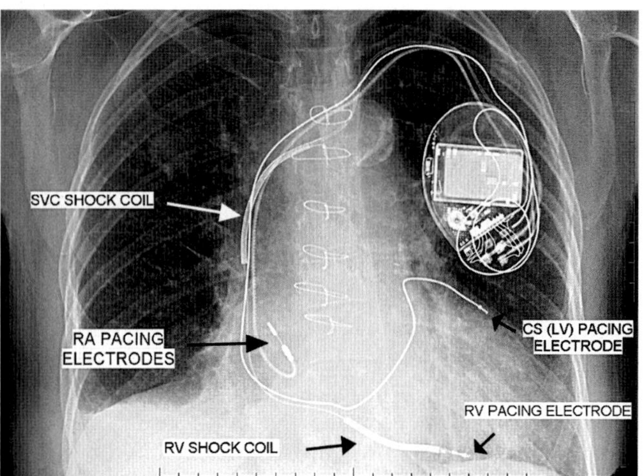

Figure 25–1 A defibrillator system with biventricular (BiV) antibradycardia pacemaker capability. Note that three leads are placed: a conventional, bipolar lead to the right atrium, a tripolar lead to the right ventricle (RV), and a unipolar lead to the coronary sinus (CS). This system is designed to provide "resynchronization biventricular-pacing therapy" in the setting of a dilated cardiomyopathy with a prolonged QRS (and frequently with a prolonged PR interval as well). The bipolar lead in the right atrium performs both sensing and pacing function. In the RV, the tip electrode functions as the cathode for pacing and sensing functions. The presence of a "shock" conductor (termed "shock coil") on the RV lead in the RV distinguishes a defibrillation system from a conventional pacemaking system. In this particular patient, the RV shock coil also functions as the pacing and sensing anode (this is called an integrated bipolar defibrillator lead; true bipolar leads have a ring electrode between the tip electrode and the shock coil). The lead in the CS depolarizes the left ventricle, and the typical current pathway includes the anode in the right ventricle. Because of the typically wide QRS complex in a left bundle-branch pattern, failure to capture the left ventricle can lead to ventricular oversensing (and inappropriate antitachycardia therapy) in an implanted cardioverter-defibrillator (ICD) system. Many defibrillation systems also have a shock coil in the superior vena cava, which is electrically identical to the defibrillator case (called the "can"). When the defibrillation circuit includes the ICD case, it is called "active can configuration." Incidental findings on this chest radiograph include the presence of sternal wires from prior sternotomy and the lung carcinoma seen in the right upper lobe.

No discussion of pacemakers can take place without an understanding of the generic pacemaker code, which has been published by the HRS-NASPE and The British Pacing and Electrophysiology Group (BPEG). This code, initially published in 1983, was revised in February 2002.[12] Shown in Table 25–1, the code (NBG) describes the basic behavior of the pacing device. Pacemakers also come with a variety of terms generally unfamiliar to the anesthesiologist, many of which are given elsewhere.

Pacemaker Indications

Indications for permanent pacing are shown in Box 25–1 and are reviewed in detail elsewhere.[13] Devices have also been approved by the U.S. Food and Drug Administration (FDA) for three-chamber pacing (right atrium, both ventricles) to treat dilated cardiomyopathy (DCM) (also called biventricular pacing [Bi-V] or cardiac resynchronization therapy [CRT]).[14,15] Also, specially programmed devices are used to treat hypertrophic obstructive cardiomyopathy (HOCM) in both adults and children.[16] Bi-V and HOCM indications require careful attention to pacemaker programming, because effective pacing in these patients often requires a pacing rate greater than native sinus or junctional escape rate (often accomplished with drugs) and an atrioventricular (AV) delay shorter than the native PR interval so that the ventricle is paced 100% of the time.[17] Inhibition or loss of pacing (e.g., from native conduction, atrial irregularity, ventricular irregularity, development of junctional rhythm, or EMI) can lead to deteriorating hemodynamics in these patients. Bi-V pacing can lengthen the QT interval in some patients, producing torsades de pointes.[18] Multisite atrial pacing to prevent or treat atrial arrhythmias is also on the clinical horizon.[19]

Pacemaker Magnets

Despite oft-repeated folklore, most pacemaker manufacturers warn that magnets were never intended to treat pacemaker emergencies or prevent EMI effects. Rather, magnet-activated

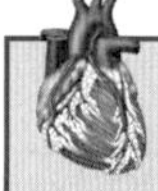

BOX 25–1 *Pacemaker Indications*

- Symptomatic sinus node disease
- Symptomatic atrioventricular node disease
- Long QT syndrome
- Hypertrophic obstructive cardiomyopathy*
- Dilated cardiomyopathy*

*See text and Pacemaker Programming for special precautions.

Table 25–1 **NASPE/BPEG Revised (2002) Generic Pacemaker Code (NBG)**

Position I Pacing Chamber(s)	Position II Sensing Chamber(s)	Position III Response(s) to Sensing	Position IV Programmability	Position V Multisite Pacing
O = None	O = None	O = None	O = None	O = None
A = Atrium	A = Atrium	I = Inhibited	R = Rate Modulation	A = Atrium
V = Ventricle	V = Ventricle	T = Triggered		V = Ventricle
D = Dual (A + V)	D = Dual (A + V)	D = Dual (T + I)		D = Dual (A + V)

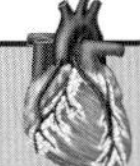

BOX 25–2 *Pacemaker Magnet Behavior**

- No apparent rhythm or rate change
- No magnet sensor (some pre-1985 Cordis, Telectronics models)
- Magnet mode disabled (possible with CPI, Pacesetter, Telectronics, Vitatron models)
- EGM mode enabled (CPI, others)
- Program rate pacing in already paced patient (many CPI, Intermedics, Telectronics, Vitatron, others)
- Improper monitor settings (pace filter on)
- Brief (10 to 100 beats) asynchronous pacing, then return to program values (most Intermedics, some Biotronik models)
- Continuous or transient loss of pacing
- Discharged battery (some pre-1990 devices)
- Pacer enters diagnostic "Threshold Test Mode" (some Siemens, Intermedics, Medtronic, others)
- Asynchronous pacing without rate responsiveness using parameters possibly not in patient's best interest

*Also see Appendix 25–1.

reed switches were incorporated to produce pacing behavior that demonstrates remaining battery life and, sometimes, pacing threshold safety factors. Some pacemakers also demonstrate the detection of a problem during a telephone check, which should result in a call from the telephone center to the patient's pacemaker physician.

Placement of a magnet over a generator might produce no change in pacing because NOT ALL PACEMAKERS SWITCH TO A CONTINUOUS ASYNCHRONOUS MODE WHEN A MAGNET IS PLACED. Also, not all models from a given company behave the same way. Only about 60% of pacemakers have "high-rate (80 to 100 bpm)" asynchronous pacing with a magnet. About 25% switch to asynchronous pacing at program rate, and 15% respond with a brief (60 to 100 bpm) asynchronous pacing event. Possible effects of magnet placement are shown in Box 25–2.[20-22] In some devices, magnet behavior can be altered via programming. Also, any pacemaker from CPI-Guidant ignores magnet placement after any electrical reset, which is a possibility in the presence of strong EMI. Appendix 25–1 lists pacemakers by manufacturer and provides a complete listing of magnet behaviors. For all generators, calling the manufacturer remains the most reliable method for determining magnet response and using this response to predict remaining battery life. A list of telephone numbers is shown in Appendix 25–2. For generators with programmable magnet behavior (Biotronik, CPI—Guidant, Pacesetter, and St. Jude Medical), only an interrogation with a programmer can reveal current settings. Most manufacturers publish a reference guide, although not all of these guides list all magnet idiosyncrasies. A telephone call can also alert the clinician to any recalls or alerts, which are not uncommon with these devices.

PREANESTHETIC EVALUATION AND PACEMAKER REPROGRAMMING

Preoperative management of the patient with a pacemaker includes evaluation and optimization of coexisting disease(s). No special laboratory tests or radiographs (chest films are remarkably insensitive for determination of lead problems) are needed for the patient with a pacemaker. Such testing should be dictated by the patient's underlying disease(s), medication(s), and planned intervention. For programmable devices, interrogation with a programmer remains the only reliable method for evaluating lead performance and obtaining current program information. A chest film might be useful to document the position of the coronary sinus (CS) lead in a patient with a Bi-V pacemaker or defibrillator, especially if central venous catheter placement is planned, because spontaneous CS lead dislodgment was found in more than 11% of patients in early studies.[23,24] A chest radiograph is certainly indicated for the patient with a device problem discovered during their pacemaker evaluation.

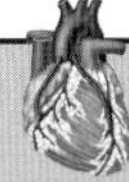

BOX 25–3 *Preanesthetic Pulse Generator (Pacemaker, Implanted Cardioverter-Defibrillator) Evaluation*

- Determine the indication for and date of initial device placement
- Identify the number and types of leads
- Determine the last generator test date and battery status
- Obtain a history of generator events (if any)
- Obtain the current program information (device interrogation)
- Ensure that pacing discharges become mechanical systoles with adequate safety margins
- Ensure that magnet detection is enabled
- Determine whether the pacing mode should be reprogrammed
- Determine if any recalls or alerts have been published

The prudent anesthesiologist reviews the patient's pacemaker history and follow-up schedule. Under the name NASPE, the HRS has published a consensus statement suggesting that pacemakers should be routinely evaluated with telephone checks for battery condition at least every 3 months. NASPE also recommends a comprehensive evaluation (interrogation) at least once per year. There are additional checks for devices implanted less than 6 or more than 48 (dual-chamber) or 72 (single-chamber) months.[25] Rozner et al[26] reported (in abstract form) a 2-year retrospective review of follow-up intervals in patients who presented for an anesthetic, and they found that more than 32% of 172 patients presenting for an anesthetic at their hospital did not meet the HRS-NASPE guideline for comprehensive evaluation. They also reported that 5% of the patients presented for their anesthetic with a pacemaker in need of replacement for battery depletion, and nearly 10% of patients had less-than-optimal pacing settings. Note that a recent, preoperative interrogation is now part of the ASA Pacemaker Advisory and the ACC guidelines.[2,8]

Important features of the preanesthetic device evaluation are shown in Box 25–3. Determining dependency on the pacemaker function might require temporary reprogramming to a VVI mode with a low rate. In patients from countries where pacemakers might be reused, battery performance might not be related to length of implantation in the current patient.[27,28] It should also be noted that in a registry of 345 pacemaker generator failures, 7% of failures were not related to battery depletion.[29]

Appropriate reprogramming (Box 25–4) might be the safest way to avoid intraoperative problems, especially if monopolar "Bovie" electrocautery will be used. For lithotripsy, consideration should be given to programming the pacing function from an atrial-paced mode, as some lithotriptors are designed to fire on the R wave, and the atrial pacing stimulus could be misinterpreted as the contraction of the ventricle.[30] All of

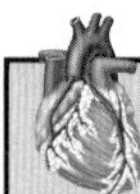

BOX 25–4 ***Pacemaker Reprogramming Probably Needed***

- Any rate-responsive device—see text (problems are well known,[134,135] problems have been misinterpreted with potential for patient injury,[20,35,37,136] and the Food and Drug Administration has issued an alert regarding devices with minute ventilation sensors[42] (see Box 25–5)
- Special pacing indication (hypertrophic obstructive cardiomyopathy, dilated cardiomyopathy, pediatric patient)
- Pacemaker-dependent patient
- Major procedure in the chest or abdomen
- Special procedures (see Box 25–6)

the manufacturers stand ready to assist with this task (see Appendix 25–2 for company telephone numbers). Reprogramming a pacemaker to asynchronous pacing at a rate greater than the patient's underlying rate usually ensures that no oversensing or undersensing during EMI will take place, thus protecting the patient. Reprogramming a device **will not** protect it from internal damage or reset caused by EMI.

Experts do not agree on the appropriate reprogramming for the pacemaker-dependent patient. Setting a device to asynchronous mode to prevent inappropriate oversensing and ventricular output suppression can cause the pacemaker to ignore premature atrial or ventricular systoles, which could have the potential to create a malignant rhythm in the patient with significant structural compromise of the myocardium.[31] Reviews by Stone and McPherson,[6] as well as Rozner,[32] demonstrate inappropriate R-on-T pacing with the development of a malignant ventricular rhythm. Hayes and Strathmore[33] suggest the VVT mode for the pacemaker-dependent patient, because EMI generally increases the pacing rate rather than inhibiting the pacing output. However, they do not consider the upper pacing rate for this mode. Although some pacemakers limit VVT pacing rates to the maximum tracking rate (e.g., CPI-Guidant), others will pace to the lower of the runaway pacing rate (typically around 200 bpm) or the minimum V-V interval defined by the ventricular refractory period (e.g., Medtronic), which is typically 200 milliseconds (representing 300 bpm). There are two other caveats for this mode: for the patient with a dual-chamber device and in need of AV synchrony to sustain cardiac output, hemodynamics might be compromised during VVT operation, because ventricular pacing takes place without regard to atrial activity. Additionally, in the VVT mode without rate-smoothing enabled, considerable increases and decreases in the paced rate could result during EMI. If VVT reprogramming is to be considered, the manufacturer should be contacted regarding programming for the upper rate.

In general, rate responsiveness and other "enhancements" (hysteresis, sleep rate, AV search, etc.) should be disabled by programming[2,34,35] (Fig. 25–2). Note that for many CPI devices, the Guidant Corporation recommends increasing the pacing voltage to "5 volts or higher" in any case in which the monopolar electrosurgical (ESU) unit will be used. In 1986, Levine et al[36] noted an increase in the amount of energy required to pace the ventricle (i.e., a pacing threshold increase) in the setting of intrathoracic surgery and monopolar ESU use. Rozner et al[26] reported increases in both atrial and ventricular thresholds in 6 of 141 consecutive operations involving pacemaker (but not ICD) cases in which the monopolar

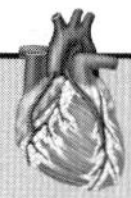

BOX 25–5 ***Pacemakers With Minute Ventilation (Bioimpedance) Sensors***

- ELA Medical—Symphony (new), Brio (212, 220, 222), Chorus RM (7034, 7134), Opus RM (4534), Talent (130, 213, 223)
- Guidant/CPI—Pulsar, Pulsar Max I and II (1170, 1171, 1172, 1180, 1181, 1270, 1272, 1280), Insignia (1190, 1194, 1290, 1291, 1297, 1298)
- Medtronic—Kappa (KDR401, KDR403, KSR401, KSR403)
- Telectronics/St. Jude—Meta (1202, 1204, 1206, 1230, 1250, 1254, 1256), Tempo (1102, 1902, 2102, 2902)

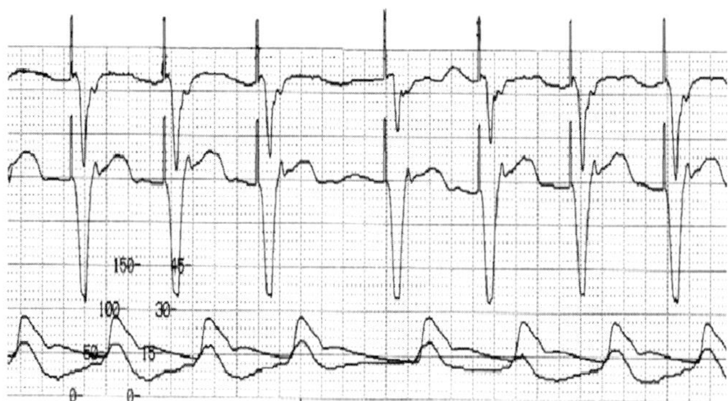

Figure 25–2 The feature "search hysteresis" mimics pacemaker malfunction. This patient has a single-chamber VVI pacemaker set to a lower rate of 70/min. It was placed for complete atrioventricular block. This programmable feature causes the pacemaker to delay pacing every 256th event for 1400 milliseconds (equal to a rate of 50/min). This delay in pacing is shown between the third and fourth QRS complexes. From top to bottom, the tracings are lead II, lead V_5, the invasive arterial pressure, and the central venous pressure. Hysteresis (where the pacemaker delays pacing after an intrinsic event) and search hysteresis often confuse caregivers regarding pacemaker malfunction (called pseudomalfunction). This electrocardiographic tracing could also result from ventricular oversensing, usually related to the T wave.

ESU was used, large volume and blood shifts were observed, or both. Although many of the operations were thoracic explorations, no pacing threshold changes were noted for these cases. No cardiopulmonary bypass cases were included in this cohort. Special attention must be given to any device with a minute ventilation (bioimpedance) sensor (Box 25–5), because inappropriate tachycardia has been observed secondary to mechanical ventilation,[37,38] monopolar "Bovie" ESU,[37,39,40] and connection to an electrocardiographic (ECG) monitor with respiratory rate monitoring.[41,42]

Intraoperative (or Procedure) Management

No special monitoring or anesthetic technique is required for the patient with a pacemaker. However, ECG monitoring of the patient must include the ability to detect pacemaker discharges. Often, noise filtering on the ECG monitor must be changed to permit demonstration of the pacemaker pulse, and devices like a nerve stimulator can interfere with detection and display of the pacemaker pulses.[43]

In addition, patient monitoring must include the ability to ensure that myocardial electrical activity is converted to mechanical systoles. Mechanical systoles are best evaluated by pulse oximetry, plethysmography, or arterial waveform display. Some patients might need an increased pacing rate during the perioperative period to meet an increased oxygen demand. A pulmonary artery catheter, an esophageal Doppler monitor, or a transesophageal echocardiogram can be used to evaluate pacing frequency and its relationship to cardiac output. In addition to blood pressure and systemic vascular resistance, the monitoring of acid-base status might be needed to determine adequacy of cardiac output.

With respect to anesthetic technique, no studies have championed one over another. Nevertheless, a number of reports of prolongation of the QT interval with the use of isoflurane, desflurane, or sevoflurane have been published, whereas halothane appears to reduce this interval.[44-48] No interactions have been reported for enflurane.

Monopolar "Bovie" electrocautery (ESU) use remains the principal intraoperative issue for the patient with a pacemaker. Between 1984 and 1997, the U.S. FDA was notified of 456 adverse events with pulse generators, 255 from electrocautery, and a "significant number" of device failures.[49] Monopolar ESU is more likely to cause problems than is bipolar ESU, and patients with unipolar electrode configuration are more sensitive to EMI than are those with bipolar configurations. Coagulation ESU will likely cause more problems than nonblended "cutting" ESU.[50] Magnet placement during electrocautery might allow reprogramming of an older (pre-1990) generator; however, newer generators are relatively immune to such effects. In fact, most devices from CPI-Guidant as well as St. Jude cannot be reprogrammed in the presence of a magnet. Note, however, that strong EMI can produce an electrical reset or a detection of battery depletion, which might change the programming mode, rate, or both. If monopolar electrocautery is to be used, then the current return pad should be placed to ensure that the electrocautery current path does not cross the pacemaking system. For cases such as head and neck surgery, the pad might be best placed on the shoulder contralateral to the implanted device. For breast and axillary cases, the pad might need to be placed on the ipsilateral arm with the wire prepped into the field by sterile plastic cover. Procedures with special pacing ramifications are shown in Box 25–6.

The use of an ultrasonic cutting device, commonly called a "harmonic scalpel," has been championed to prevent EMI while providing the surgeon with the ability to both cut and coagulate tissue. There are a number of case reports demonstrating successful surgery without EMI issues in these patients.[51-54]

At this time, magnetic resonance imaging (MRI) deserves special mention. In general, MRI has been contraindicated in pacemaker and ICD patients.[55,56] However, reports suggests that MRI is probably safe for some patients with newer devices, as well as any patient who will be wide awake in the MRI tunnel, who is not dependent upon his or her pacemaker for heart rhythm or survival, who will not need medication to undergo the MRI, and who can communicate regularly with the MRI care team.[57,58] Nevertheless, not all MRI sequences and energy levels have been studied, and caution is advised.[59]

BOX 25–6 *Special Procedures in Patients With Implantable Generators*

- Lithotripsy—acceptable with precautions to protect the generator and, possibly, programming out of an atrial pacing mode[30]
- Transurethral resection (bladder, prostate), and uterine hysteroscopy—procedures using monopolar electrocautery that can be easily accomplished after device reprogramming
- Magnetic resonance imaging (MRI)—absolutely contraindicated by most generator manufacturers, and deaths have been reported.[55] However, a report suggests that appropriate patients can safely undergo MRI[58] but not without appropriate precautions[59]
- Electroconvulsive therapy—requires asynchronous (nonsensing) mode[137]
- Nerve stimulator testing/therapy—inappropriate detection of transcutaneous electrical nerve stimulation, neuromuscular, and chiropractic electrical muscle stimulation as ventricular tachycardia or fibrillation has been reported[138,139]

Pacemaker Failure

Pacemaker failure has three etiologies: (1) failure of capture, (2) lead failure, and (3) generator failure. Failure of capture owing to a defect at the level of the myocardium (i.e., the generator continues to fire but no myocardial depolarization takes place) remains the most difficult problem to treat. Myocardial changes that result in noncapture include myocardial ischemia/infarction, acid-base disturbance, electrolyte abnormalities, or abnormal levels of antiarrhythmic drug(s). Temporary pacing (transvenous, transcutaneous, transthoracic, or transesophageal) might inhibit pacemaker output at voltages that will not produce myocardial capture.[60] Sympathomimetic drugs generally lower pacing threshold. Outright generator or lead failure is rare.

TEMPORARY PACEMAKERS

There are several techniques available to the anesthesiologist to establish reliable temporary pacing during the perioperative period or in the intensive care unit.[61] Cardiovascular anesthesiologists are more likely than generalists to routinely use temporary transvenous or epicardial pacing in their practices. Temporary cardiac pacing can serve as definitive therapy for transient bradyarrhythmias or as a bridge to permanent generator placement.

The various forms of temporary pacing include many transvenous catheter systems, transcutaneous pads, transthoracic wires, and esophageal pacing techniques. This section reviews the indications for temporary cardiac pacing and discusses the techniques available to the anesthesiologist. Many of the references in this section are old, because temporary pacing is an old technique and not many advances have taken place in the past 10 to 15 years. Table 25–2 summarizes these techniques.

Indications for Temporary Pacing

Temporary pacemakers are commonly used postoperatively following cardiac surgery, in the treatment of drug toxicity resulting in arrhythmias, with certain arrhythmias complicating myocardial infarction, and for intraoperative bradycardia due to β-blocker use.[62] The placement of a temporary pacing system can assist in the hemodynamic management in the perioperative period. Abnormal electrolytes, preoperative β-blocker use, and many of the intraoperative drugs have the potential to aggravate bradycardia and bradycardia-dependent arrhythmias.[63] Because drugs used to treat bradyarrhythmias have a number of important disadvantages compared with temporary pacing, hemodynamically unstable

Table 25–2 Comparison of Temporary Pacing Techniques

Temporary Pacing Method	Time to Initiate	Chambers Paced	Advantages	Disadvantages	Uses
Transcutaneous	1 to 2 minutes	Right ventricle	Simple, rapid, safe	Variable capture, chest wall movement, patient discomfort	Arrest, intraoperative, prophylactic
Transesophageal	Minutes	Left atrium	Reliable atrial capture, safe, simple	Requires special generator	Prophylactic atrial pacing, overdrive pacing for SVT, monitoring atrial electrogram
Transvenous semirigid	3 to 20 minutes	Atrium and/or ventricle	Most reliable, well tolerated	Invasive, time-consuming, potential complications	Arrest, prophylactic, maintenance
Transvenous flow directed	3 to 20 minutes	Right ventricle	Simple, does not require fluoroscopy	Invasive, stability questions, less readily available	Arrest, intraoperative, prophylactic, maintenance
Pacing pulmonary artery catheter (PAC)	Minutes (if PAC in place)	Atrium and/or ventricle	Reliable ventricular capture, well tolerated	Requires specific PAC, which must be placed first	Arrest, intraoperative, prophylactic, maintenance
Epicardial pacing wires	<1 minute	Atrium and/or ventricle	Reliable short term	Postoperative only, early lead failure	Arrest, prophylactic, maintenance
Transthoracic	10 to 60 seconds	Ventricle	Rapid and simple	Many potential complications	Arrest only

Table 25–3 Temporary Pacing Indications

Patient Condition	Event Requiring Temporary Pacing
AMI	Symptomatic bradycardia, medically refractory New bundle-branch block with transient complete heart block Complete heart block Postoperative complete heart block Symptomatic congenital heart block Mobitz II with AMI New bifascicular block Bilateral bundle-branch block and first-degree AV block Symptomatic alternating Wenckebach block Symptomatic alternating bundle-branch block
Tachycardia treatment or prevention	Bradycardia-dependent VT Torsades de pointes Long QT syndrome Treatment of recurrent SVT or VT
Prophylactic	Pulmonary artery catheter placement with left bundle-branch block (controversial) New AV block or bundle-branch block in acute endocarditis Cardioversion with sick sinus syndrome Post–defibrillation bradycardia Counteract perioperative pharmacologic treatment causing hemodynamically significant bradycardia AF prophylaxis post–cardiac surgery Post–orthotopic heart transplantation

AF = atrial fibrillation; AMI = anterior myocardial infarction; AV = atrioventricular; SVT = supraventricular tachycardia; VT = ventricular tachycardia.

perioperative bradyarrhythmias should be considered an indication for temporary pacing (Table 25–3). If the patient already has epicardial wires or a pacing catheter or wires, or transesophageal pacing is feasible, pacing is preferred to pharmacologic therapy. However, transcutaneous and ventricular-only transvenous pacing, even if feasible, may exacerbate hemodynamic problems in patients with heart disease because these pacing modalities do not preserve AV synchrony (i.e., produces ventricular or global activation).

Nearly every indication for a permanent pacemaker is an indication for temporary pacing in patients without a pacemaker who, due to circumstances (e.g., emergency surgery, critical illness), cannot have elective permanent pacemaker implantation. Temporary pacing may also be needed before implantation of a permanent pacemaker to stabilize patients with hemodynamically significant bradycardia.

Temporary pacing is also indicated if a patient with a myocardial infarction complicated by second- or third-degree heart block is scheduled for emergency surgery. Bifascicular block in an asymptomatic patient is not reason enough for temporary pacing preoperatively.[64] Bellocci et al[65] reported no occurrence of complete heart block in 98 patients with preoperative bifascicular block undergoing general anesthesia, despite 14% having prolonged conduction through their His-Purkinje system. The development of a new bifascicular block immediately postoperatively, though, suggests perioperative myocardial ischemia or infarction, and temporary pacing might be required. Surgical resection of neck and carotid sinus tumors may give rise to bradyarrhythmias requiring temporary cardiac pacing during surgical manipulation. Neurosurgical procedures involving the brainstem may also be associated with significant bradycardia.

Temporary antitachycardia pacing is most commonly used after cardiac surgery.[66] With increased availability of effective noninvasive pacing technology, antitachycardia pacing might be offered to other perioperative patients as well. Even when used properly, these techniques can induce more dangerous arrhythmias, and proper resuscitation equipment should be available.

AV junctional tachycardia (AVJT) can occur following cardiopulmonary bypass, where it could be a manifestation of reperfusion injury or possibly inadequate myocardial protection during bypass. AVJT does not respond well to most drug therapy, although its rate (≤120 bpm in adults) may be slowed by β-adrenergic blockers or edrophonium. AVJT is best managed by atrial or AV-sequential overdrive pacing, because both of these modalities preserve AV synchrony. Frequently, there is resumption of sinus rhythm upon withdrawal of temporary pacing.

Most sudden-onset paroxysmal supraventricular tachycardias (PSVTs) are initiated by a premature beat, which could be of atrial, AV junctional, or ventricular origin. PSVT may be terminated by competitive, atrial underdrive pacing (paced rate < PSVT rate) if, by chance, an atrial capture beat interferes with the circulating wavefront perpetuating the tachycardia. In contrast, with overdrive pacing, PSVT is paced at a rate 10% to 15% in excess of the tachycardia rate until there is evidence of 1:1 capture with paced beats. Pacing is continued at this rate for 20 to 30 seconds, then gradually slowed to some predetermined rate, and finally terminated. As with all pacing modalities, a gradual reduction in pacing rate is recommended in patients known to have sinus node dysfunction in order to reduce the risk of prolonged asystole when pacing is terminated. If pacing fails to terminate PSVT, or PSVT produces circulatory collapse, immediate DC cardioversion is recommended.

Type I atrial flutter (flutter rate <320 to 340 bpm) is pace terminable, but type II flutter (>340 bpm) is not. Type I flutter is treated by atrial overdrive pacing at a rate 15 to 20 beats more than the flutter rate, which is increased by 10- to 20-bpm increments if the first attempt is not successful. Once atrial capture is evident, pacing is continued for 20 to 30 seconds and then slowed as for PSVT. Usually, type I atrial flutter can be terminated by overdrive pacing, with prompt restoration of normal sinus rhythm.

Relative contraindications to transvenous ventricular pacing include digitalis toxicity with ventricular tachycardia (VT), tricuspid valve prostheses, or the presence of a coagulopathy. Pacing in the setting of severe hypothermia might induce ventricular fibrillation (VF) or alter the normal compensatory physiologic mechanisms to the hypothermia, although one prospective study in dogs using transcutaneous pacing suggests that pacing decreases rewarming time.[67] Atrial fibrillation, multifocal atrial tachycardia, and significant AV conduction system disease are relative contraindications to transvenous *atrial* pacing.

Transvenous Temporary Pacing

Transvenous cardiac pacing provides the most reliable means of temporary pacing. Temporary transvenous pacing is dependable and well tolerated by patients. With a device that can provide both atrial and ventricular pacing, transvenous pacing can maintain AV synchrony and improve cardiac output. Disadvantages include the need for practitioner experience, time to appropriately place the wire(s) to provide capture, the potential complications of catheter placement and manipulation, and the need for fluoroscopy in many cases. Three different types of typical transvenous leads are shown in Figure 25–3.

Rapid catheter position is most easily obtained by using the right internal jugular vein, even without fluoroscopy.[68] The left subclavian is also easily used in emergent situations. Other sites are often impassable without fluoroscopy. In addition, brachial and femoral routes can increase the frequency of lead dislodgment during motion of the extremities.

Once central access is obtained, the lead is guided into position using hemodynamic data (not possible with the simple bipolar lead) or by fluoroscopic guidance. ECG guidance is less desirable. The right atrial appendage and right ventricular apex provide the most stable catheter positions. Techniques for placement into these positions are part of cardiology training and likely are foreign to most anesthesiologists. When fluoroscopy is unavailable or in emergency situations, a flow-directed catheter can be attempted using ECG and pressure guidance. Once the right ventricle is entered, the balloon is deflated, if used, and the catheter gently advanced until electrical capture is noted. Flow-directed catheters and a right internal jugular approach afford the shortest insertion times.[69] The reported incidence of successful capture in urgent situations without fluoroscopy ranges from 30% to 90%.[68,70,71]

Once catheters are positioned, pacing is initiated using the distal electrode as the cathode and the proximal electrode as the anode. Ideally, the capture thresholds should be less than 1 mA and generator output should be maintained at three times threshold as a safety margin. In dual-chamber pacing, AV delays of between 100 and 200 milliseconds are used. Many patients are sensitive to this parameter. Cardiac output optimization with echocardiography and/or mixed venous oxygen saturation can be used to maximize hemodynamics by adjusting AV delay.[72] AV sequential pacing is clearly beneficial in many patients, but it should be remembered that emergency pacing starts with ventricular capture alone.[72-76] There is a potential risk of interference of external pacemaker generators by walkie-talkies and digital cellular phones.[77,78] Clinicians should also be aware of all complications related to transvenous lead placement.[79]

Pacing Pulmonary Artery Catheters

The pulmonary artery AV pacing thermodilution (TD) catheter (Fig. 25–3C) was described by Zaidan in 1983.[80] It allows for AV sequential pacing via electrodes attached to the outside of the catheter, as well as routine pulmonary artery catheter functions. Combination of the two functions into one catheter eliminates the need for separate insertion of tempo-

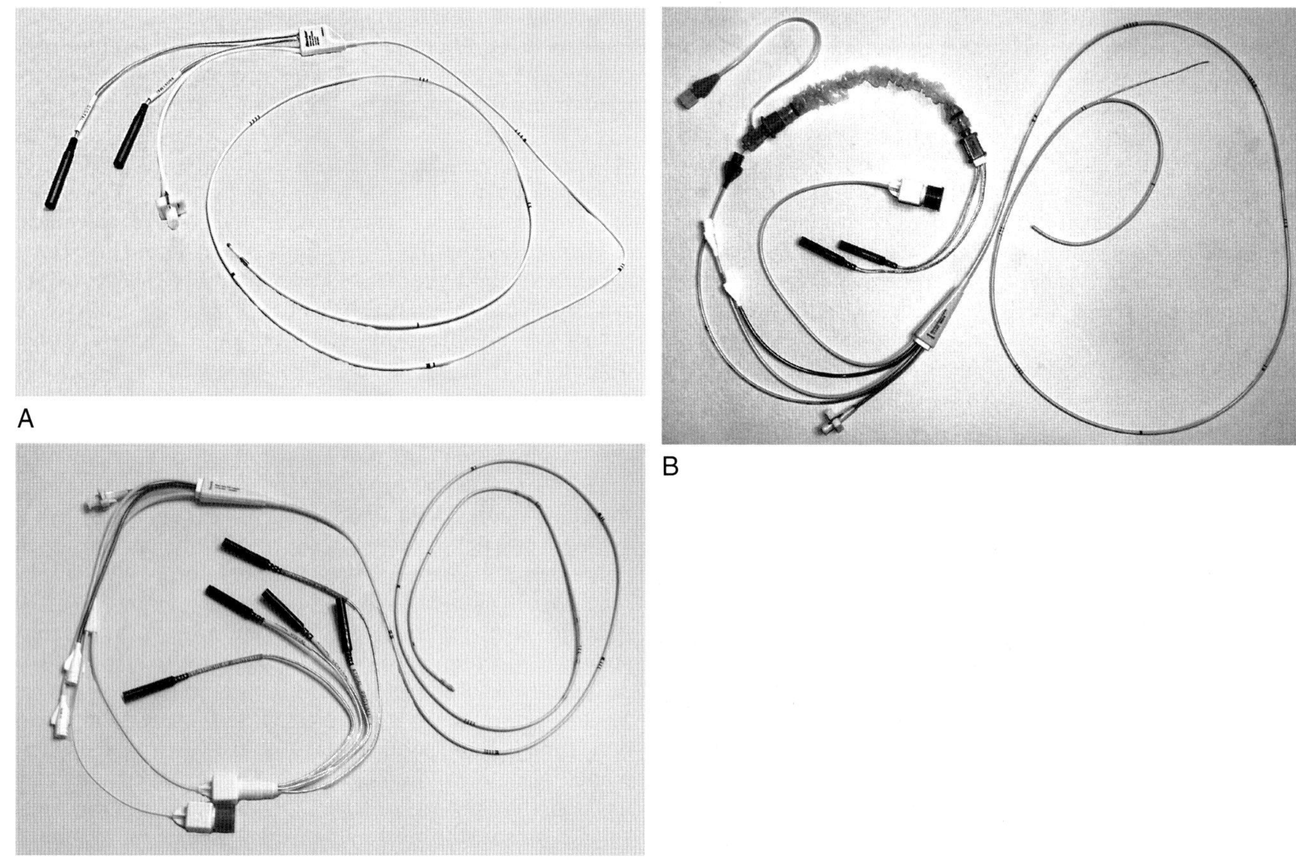

Figure 25–3 A variety of transvenous pacing leads are shown. (*A*) Simple, flow-directed, bipolar pacing wire. This lead is placed through a 6F introducer sheath, and it is advanced (usually under fluoroscopy) into the atrium or ventricle until mechanical systoles result from the electrical pacing event (called pacing capture). The principal disadvantage of this lead is the lack of hemodynamic measurements to guide placement. (*B*) Specially adapted pulmonary artery catheter with a channel for a bipolar, ventricular pacing wire. The bipolar pacing wire, sideport adapter, and condom are packaged separately from the pulmonary artery catheter. Note that the electrode is shown protruding from its orifice just distal to the 20-cm mark on the pulmonary artery catheter. (*C*) Atrioventricular (AV)-capable, pacing pulmonary artery (PA) catheter. Five electrodes are present: two for ventricular pacing and three for atrial pacing. This catheter is positioned to provide adequate ventricular capture, after which atrial pacing is attempted using two of the three atrial electrodes. Sometimes, the entire PA catheter must be repositioned to obtain atrial capture. In the setting of a functioning AV node, atrial capture can be determined by the presence of a narrow complex QRS following the atrial pace. In the setting of a significant AV block, atrial capture can be difficult to assess.

rary transvenous pacing electrodes. However, several potential disadvantages exist with this catheter, including (1) varying success in initiating and maintaining capture, (2) external electrode displacement from the catheter, and (3) relatively high cost compared to standard pacing pulmonary artery catheters (PACs).[80,81] The Paceport PAC (Fig. 25–3*B*) provides ventricular pacing with a separate bipolar pacing lead (Chandler probe), which allows for more stable ventricular pacing as well as hemodynamic measurements.[82] This catheter has been used for successful resuscitation after cardiac arrest during closed-chest cardiac massage when attempts to capture with transcutaneous and transvenous flow-directed bipolar pacing catheters had failed. However, this unit does not provide the potential advantages associated with atrial pacing capability. The newer pulmonary artery A-V Paceport adds a sixth lumen to the older Paceport to allow placement of an atrial J-wire, flexible-tip bipolar pacing lead. Both of these Paceport catheters are placed by transducing the right ventricular pressure port to ensure correct positioning of the port 1 to 2 cm distal to the tricuspid valve. This position usually guides the ventricular wire (Chandler probe) to the apex where adequate capture should occur with minimal current requirements. Although ventricular capture is easily obtained, atrial capture can be more difficult and less reliable.[72] This catheter has been used successfully after cardiac surgery.[72,83] The atrial wire can be used to diagnose supraventricular tachyarrhythmias (SVTs) by atrial electrograms and to overdrive atrial flutter and reentrant SVT.[84]

Transcutaneous Pacing

Transcutaneous pacing, first described by Zoll,[85] is readily available and can be rapidly implemented in emergency situations. Capture rate is variable and the technique may cause pain in awake patients, but usually it is tolerated until temporary transvenous pacing can be instituted. It may be effective even when endocardial pacing fails.[86] It is now considered by many to be the method of choice for prophylactic and emergent applications.[87]

The large patches typically are placed anteriorly (negative electrode or cathode) over the palpable cardiac apex (or V_3 lead location) and posteriorly (positive electrode or anode) at the inferior aspect of the scapula. The anode has also been placed on the anterior right chest with success in healthy volunteers.[88] The skin should be cleaned with alcohol (but not abraded) to reduce capture threshold and improve patient comfort. Abraded skin can cause more discomfort. Typical thresholds are 20 to 120 mA, but pacing may require up to 200 mA at long pulse durations of 20 to 40 milliseconds.[89] Transcutaneous pacing appears to capture the right ventricle followed by near-simultaneous activation of the entire left ventricle. The hemodynamic response is similar to that of right ventricular endocardial pacing. Both methods can cause reductions in left ventricular systolic pressure, a decrease in stroke volume, and an increase in right-sided pressures due to AV dyssynchrony. Capture should be confirmed by palpation or display of a peripheral pulse. Maintenance current is set 5 to 10 mA above threshold as tolerated by the patient. Success rates appear to be highest when the system is used prophylactically or early after arrest—upward of 90%.[90,91] When used in emergent situations, successful capture rates are usually lower but range from 10% to 93%.[92-94] A 3-year study of out-of-hospital asystolic arrest showed no difference in survival for the group that received early transcutaneous pacing compared with the group that received basic CPR without pacing.[95] Similarly, early use during in-hospital arrests may not alter long-term survival.[96] This technique has also been used to terminate VT, AV nodal reentrant tachycardia, and AV reciprocating tachycardia.[94,97]

Coughing and discomfort from cutaneous stimulation are the most frequent problems. The technique poses no electrical threat to medical personnel and complications are rare. There have been no reports of significant damage to myocardium, skeletal muscle, skin, or lungs in humans despite continuous pacing up to 108 hours and intermittent pacing up to 17 days.[85,90,98] Several commercially available defibrillators include transcutaneous pacing generators as standard equipment.

Esophageal Pacing

The newest technique available to anesthesiologists is esophageal pacing, and it has been shown to be quite reliable.[98-101] Significant bradycardia, secondary to underlying pathology or pharmacologic effects, can occur during anesthesia. The response to pharmacologic therapy for significant bradycardia with vagolytic drugs can be unpredictable and difficult to sustain accurately.[102] Chronotropic drugs may have little effect and can lead to tachyarrhythmias and/or myocardial ischemia. Esophageal pacing is relatively noninvasive and well tolerated even in the majority of awake patients, and it appears to be devoid of serious complications. This modality is useful for heart rate support of cardiac output, for overdrive suppression of reentrant SVT, and for diagnostic atrial electrograms. Ventricular capture must be excluded before attempts at rapid atrial pacing for overdrive suppression to prevent potential VT or VF. Some surgical positions (e.g., three-quarter prone) can increase the chance of unintentional ventricular capture, and esophageal atrial pacing should only be instituted after careful assessment.[103]

Problems with esophageal pacing include (1) the necessity for special generators that must provide 20 to 30 mA of current with wide pulse widths of 10 to 20 milliseconds and (2) the ability to pace only the left atrium reliably and not the left ventricle, which can be a significant problem in emergency situations.[99] By comparison, typical temporary generators designed for endocardial pacing have a maximum output of 20 mA with pulse width durations of only 1 to 2 milliseconds.

A typical transesophageal pacing generator and lead are shown in Figure 25–4. The pacing stimulus is delivered

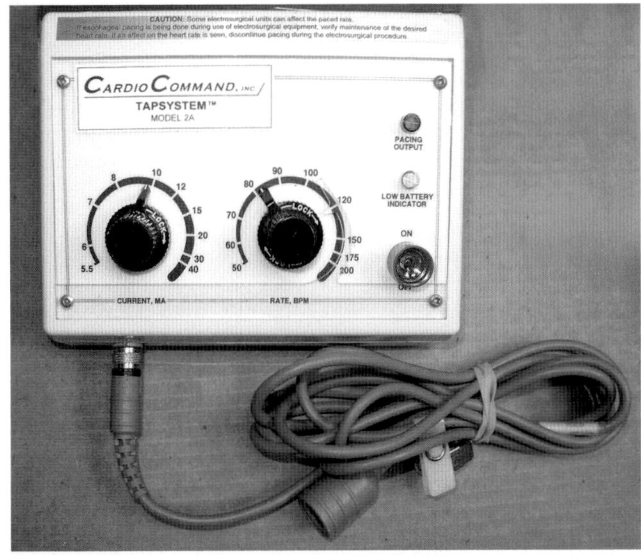

A

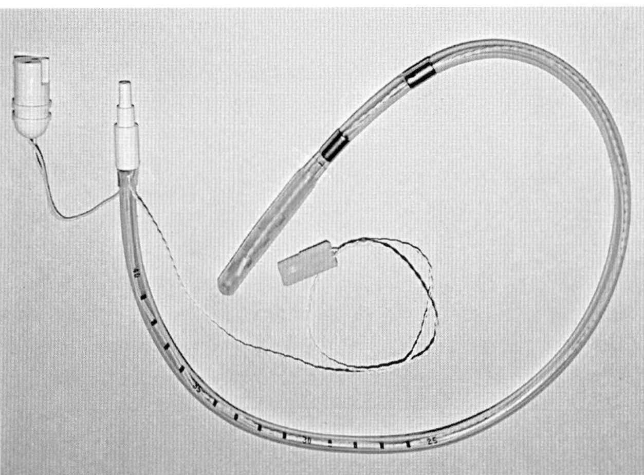
B

Figure 25–4 A typical transesophageal pacing generator (*A*) and esophageal stethoscope with bipolar electrodes (*B*) are shown. The esophageal stethoscope is placed to between 30 and 40 cm from the teeth, and pacing is initiated at a rate greater than the patient's native heart rate using an output setting of at least 20 mA. Atrial capture is determined by an increase in peripheral pulse rate. Detection of capture using only electrocardiographic monitoring can be difficult to discern, as the pacing impulse from these generators produces a large artifact and often distorts the surface electrocardiogram.

through a modified esophageal stethoscope. Pacing is initiated by connecting the system and placing the esophageal stethoscope to a depth of 30 to 40 cm from the teeth. Capture should be confirmed using the peripheral pulse (i.e., from the pulse oximeter plethysmogram or an invasive hemodynamic monitor), because the pacing stimulus often is large relative to the QRS and frequently fools the ECG counting algorithm on the monitor (Fig. 25–5). Atrial capture is obtained in virtually all patients using outputs of 8 to 20 mA, and the output should be set to two to three times the threshold for capture. Thresholds are not influenced by weight, age, atrial size, or previous cardiac surgery.[101] Because there is no sensing element involved, esophageal pacing is AOO mode pacing.

Transesophageal *ventricular* pacing is generally unreliable, yet the optimal site appears to be 2 to 4 cm distal to the atrial site. The esophageal stethoscope can also be used (with a special adapter) to record the intra-atrial electrogram. No long-term complications with this modality have been described. Induction of ventricular tachyarrhythmias during rapid atrial pacing has been noted. No significant esophageal trauma has been reported despite long-term therapy of up to 60 hours.[104] However, phrenic nerve stimulation has been described.[100]

Transthoracic Pacing

This technique has been used for more than 35 years and involves the direct introduction of a pacing wire or needle through the thorax into the ventricular cavity. Several commercial kits are available; even the use of a spinal needle has been described. The technique is rapid and simple and does not require venous access or fluoroscopy. In contrast to other temporary pacing modalities, there is a large potential for problems and no study demonstrates any benefit in survival. Transcutaneous techniques have supplanted this procedure in essentially all situations.

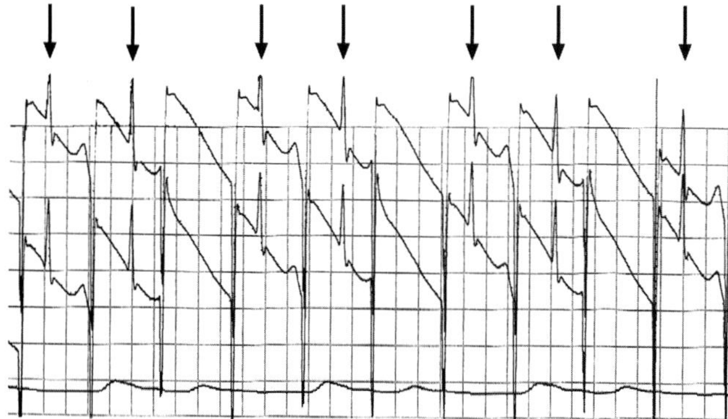

Figure 25–5 An electrocardiographic strip from a patient with a transesophageal pacemaker demonstrating atrial capture and Wenckebach second-degree atrioventricular nodal block. An 84-year-old man with coronary artery disease and taking atenolol developed a sinus bradycardia (rate 37/min) with hypotension during a general anesthetic procedure for transurethral bladder resection. An esophageal pacemaker was placed and the rate was set to 85 bpm (this is AOO pacing mode). The top two tracings are electrocardiographic leads II and V_5. The downward depolarization artifacts are the pacing stimuli from the esophageal pacemaker (15-mA output). The upward depolarization events are the QRS inscriptions, which are highlighted by the downward arrows. Atrial P waves can be found shortly after the esophageal pulse. Note the lengthening PR interval with the dropped ventricular depolarizations. Also note how distorted the electrocardiographic signal becomes in the setting of an esophageal pacemaker. The third tracing is the pulse oximeter plethysmographic waveform.

POSTANESTHESIA PACEMAKER EVALUATION

Any pacemaker that was reprogrammed for the perioperative period should be reset appropriately. For nonreprogrammed devices, most manufacturers recommend interrogation to ensure proper functioning and remaining battery life if any electrocautery was used. In their retrospective review, Trankina et al[105] reported 6% of 169 patients showed a problem during postoperative checks of pacemakers. In an editorial, Senthuran et al[106] suggest that failure to perform a postoperative pacemaker check led to an unexpected postoperative death in Great Britain. ACC guidelines now recommend a postprocedure interrogation.[2]

IMPLANTED CARDIOVERTER-DEFIBRILLATORS

The development of an implantable, battery-powered device able to deliver sufficient energy to terminate VT or VF has represented a major medical breakthrough for patients with a history of ventricular tachyarrhythmias. These devices prevent death in the setting of malignant ventricular tachyarrhythmias, and they clearly remain superior to antiarrhythmic drug therapy.[107-109] Initially approved by the U.S. FDA in 1985, more than 80,000 devices will be placed this year, and industry sources report that more than 240,000 patients have these devices today (see Chapter 13).

A significant number of technologic advances have occurred since the first ICD was placed, including considerable miniaturization (pectoral pocket placement with transvenous leads is the norm) and battery improvements that permit permanent pacing with these devices. Thus, a pectoral ICD could easily be confused with a pacemaker. Like pacemakers, ICDs have a generic code to indicate lead placement and function,[110] which is shown in Table 25–4. The most robust form of identification, called the "label form," expands the fourth character into its component generic pacemaker code (NBG—see Table 25–1).

Newer ICDs (since 1993) have many programmable features, but essentially they measure each cardiac R-R interval and categorize the rate as normal, too fast (short R-R interval), or too slow (long R-R interval). When the device detects a sufficient number of short R-R intervals within a period of time (all programmable), it begins an antitachycardia event. The internal computer decides to choose antitachycardia pacing (less energy use, better tolerated by patient) or shock,

Table 25–4 North American Society for Pacing and Electrophysiology/The British Pacing and Electrophysiology Group Generic Defibrillator Code (NBD)

Position I Shock Chambers(s)	Position II Antitachycardia Pacing Chamber(s)	Position III Tachycardia Detection	Position IV Antibradycardia Pacing Chamber(s)
O = None	O = None	E = Electrogram	O = None
A = Atrium	A = Atrium	H = Hemodynamic	A = Atrium
V = Ventricle	V = Ventricle		V = Ventricle
D = Dual (A + V)	D = Dual (A + V)		D = Dual (A + V)

depending on the presentation and device programming. If shock is chosen, an internal capacitor is charged. Most newer devices are programmed to reconfirm VT or VF after charging in order to prevent inappropriate shock therapy. Typically, ICDs have six therapies available for each type of event (VT, fast VT, VF), and some of these therapies can be repeated before moving to the next higher energy sequence. Thus, ICDs can deliver 6 to 18 shocks per event. In an ICD with antitachycardia pacing, once a shock is delivered, no further antitachycardia pacing can take place.

Approximately 20% to 40% of shocks are for rhythms other than VT or VF despite reconfirmation.[111-114] SVT remains the most common etiology of inappropriate shock therapy, and causes of inappropriate shock have been reviewed elsewhere.[114-116] Advances in ICDs to include dual-chamber detection might be able to lower the inappropriate shock rate, although it is still reported as high as 17%.[117,118] Whether inappropriate shocks injure patients remains a subject of considerable debate, but it was suggested that a significant number of patients who receive an inappropriate shock demonstrate elevated troponin levels in the absence of an ischemic event.[119]

Programmable features in current ICDs to differentiate VT from a tachycardia of supraventricular origin (SVT) include the following[120]:

1. Onset criteria—in general, onset of VT is abrupt, whereas onset of SVT has sequentially shortening R-R intervals.
2. Stability criteria—in general, the R-R interval of VT is relatively constant, whereas the R-R interval of atrial fibrillation with rapid ventricular response is quite variable.
3. QRS width criteria—in general, the QRS width in SVT is narrow (<110 milliseconds), whereas the QRS width in VT is wide (>120 milliseconds).
4. "Intelligence" in dual-chamber devices attempts to associate atrial activity with ventricular activity.
5. Morphology waveform analysis with comparison to stored historic templates

Note that once the R-R interval becomes sufficiently short for VF detection, the ICD begins a shock sequence. As noted, once the device delivers any shock therapy, no further antitachycardia pacing takes place. An ICD with antibradycardia pacing capability will begin pacing when the R-R interval is too long. In July 1997, the U.S. FDA approved devices with sophisticated dual-chamber pacing modes and rate-responsive behavior for ICD patients who need permanent pacing (about 20% of ICD patients).

Implanted Cardioverter-Defibrillator Indications

Initially, ICDs were placed for hemodynamically significant VT or VF. Newer indications associated with sudden death include long Q-T syndrome, Brugada syndrome (right bundle-branch block, ST-segment elevation in leads V_1 to V_3), and arrhythmogenic right ventricular dysplasia.[121] Studies suggest that ICDs can be used for primary prevention of sudden death (i.e., before the first episode of VT or VF) in young patients with hypertrophic cardiomyopathy, and data from the second Multicenter Automatic Defibrillator Intervention Trial (MADIT II) suggest that any post-MI patient with an ejection fraction less than 30% should undergo prophylactic implantation of an ICD.[122,123]

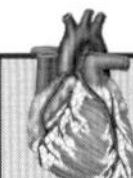

BOX 25–7 *Implanted Cardioverter-Defibrillator Indications*

- Ventricular tachycardia
- Ventricular fibrillation
- Brugada syndrome (right bundle-branch block, ST elevation V_1 to V_3)
- Arrhythmogenic right ventricular dysplasia
- Long QT syndrome
- Hypertrophic cardiomyopathy
- Prophylactic use post–myocardial infarction, ejection fraction < 30%

Trials are under way for the cardiomyopathy patient with nonischemic cardiomyopathy as well. The Sudden Cardiac Death—Heart Failure Trial (SCD-HeFT) results and the previously published Defibrillators In Non-Ischemic Cardiomyopathy Treatment Evaluation (DEFINITE) study suggest that ICD placement will result in lower mortality in any patient with an ejection fraction less than 35% regardless of the etiology of the cardiomyopathy. The DEFINITE results are important, as the patients in this study were randomized only after initiation of β-blockade and angiotensin-converting enzyme inhibitor therapy, which form the backbone of medical therapy for cardiomyopathy. The SCD-HeFT results showed ICDs reduced mortality by 23%. Based on these results, Medicare expanded its ICD coverage.[124-126]

Three-chamber (leads placed in atrium, right ventricle, and coronary sinus) ICDs (Fig. 25–1) for Bi-V have been FDA approved for patients with DCM and prolonged QRS intervals. Two-chamber (leads placed in atrium and right ventricle) ICDs are in clinical trial for patients with HOCM who have experienced VT or VF. Box 25–7 reviews ICD indications.

Dilated Cardiomyopathy

With the advent of Bi-V pacing for the patient with a DCM and prolonged QRS interval, and the approval of ICDs with Bi-V capability (currently named InSync [Medtronic Corporation]; Contak CD or Renewal [Guidant Corporation]; and Epic HF or Atlas + HF [St. Jude Medical]), the presence of a defibrillator with Bi-V pacing will become more common.[127] About 550,000 new diagnoses of congestive heart failure are made in the United States every year, and the prevalence of this disease includes nearly 5 million patients. Significant risk factors for the development of congestive heart failure include ischemic heart disease and/or hypertension. These data, combined with the results from SCD-HeFT and MADIT II trials (ICD is indicated in any patient with cardiomyopathy and ejection fraction <30% to 35%), suggest that the number of patients eligible to receive a defibrillator to include Bi-V pacing will increase dramatically. Whether any country's economy can absorb this economic burden remains to be seen. At present, Bi-V pacing without defibrillation capability improves functional status and quality of life and was shown to reduce mortality.[15,128]

Implanted Cardioverter-Defibrillator Magnets

Like pacemakers, magnet behavior in ICDs can be altered by programming. Most devices suspend tachyarrhythmia detection (and therefore therapy) when a magnet is appropriately placed to activate the reed switch. Some devices from Angeion, CPI, Pacesetter, and St. Jude Medical can be programmed to ignore magnet placement. **Antitachycardia therapy in some CPI devices can be permanently disabled by magnet placement for 30 seconds.**[1] In general, magnets will not affect antibradycardia pacing mode or rate (except ELA [rate change] and Telectronics Guardian 4202/4203* [disabled]). Interrogating the device and calling the manufacturer remain the most reliable methods for determining magnet response. Magnet effects on ICDs are shown in Appendix 25–3.

Note that confirmation of appropriate magnet placement, and therefore suspension of antitachyarrhythmic therapy, is present only in CPI-Guidant devices and ELA devices if the patient's native heart rate is less than 80 bpm. Medtronic markets a Smart-Magnet device that houses a magnet and electronics to show appropriate disablement of the ICD functions in their device. When using a Smart-Magnet, the "FOUND" light is often extinguished during EMI from the electrosurgical cautery, even though the magnet remains in place. Despite these features in Medtronic and CPI-Guidant devices, numerous anecdotal reports exist of inappropriate shock therapy during electrocautery, most often a result of movement of the magnet during patient repositioning.

Preanesthetic Evaluation and Implanted Cardioverter-Defibrillator Reprogramming

ALL ICDs should have their antitachycardia therapy disabled prior to the induction of anesthesia and commencement of the procedure (see ACC Guidelines[2]). The comments in the pacing section (and Boxes 25–3 through 25–6 also apply for any ICD with antibradycardia pacing. Guidelines from HRS-NASPE and the ASA Advisory suggest that every patient with an ICD have an in-office comprehensive evaluation every 1 to 4 months.[8,129] Devices with Bi-V pacing must have a sufficiently short AV delay for sensed events to ensure that all ventricular activity is paced. Failure of ventricular pacing (either right or left) owing to native AV conduction or threshold issues has been associated with inappropriate antitachycardia therapy (i.e., shock).[130]

Intraoperative or Procedure Management

At this time, no special monitoring (owing to the ICD) is required for the patient with an ICD. ECG monitoring and the ability to deliver external cardioversion or defibrillation must be present during the time of ICD disablement. Although many recommendations exist for defibrillator pad placement to protect the ICD, it must be remembered that the patient, not the ICD, is being treated.

*These two-device families were implanted during clinical trials only. Thus, the likelihood of encountering these devices is low; they are included for completeness.

Furthermore, no special anesthetic techniques have been advocated for the patient with an ICD. Most of these patients will have severely depressed systolic function, dilated ventricular cavities, and significant valvular regurgitation, and the choice of anesthetic technique should be dictated by the underlying physiologic derangements that are present. Conflicting data have been published regarding the choice of anesthetic agent(s) and changes to defibrillation threshold (DFT). In 1993, Gill et al[131] examined DFT in dogs and concluded that neither halothane nor isoflurane changed DFT in open-chest defibrillation compared with a pentobarbital infusion. However, Weinbroum et al[132] evaluated DFTs in humans during ICD implantation and found that halothane, isoflurane, and fentanyl increased DFT. Even with these causes, though, the increased DFTs found were still substantially lower than the maximum energy generally available in ICDs, and these increases would not have been noted under usual ICD testing conditions. As noted earlier, isoflurane, desflurane, and sevoflurane have been reported to lengthen the QT interval, which could increase the risk of torsades de pointes in certain patients.

Caution should be observed when placing a central venous catheter in any patient with an ICD. In the patient with an integrated bipolar ventricular sensing configuration, an inappropriate 30-J shock was delivered due to noise artifact created by the guidewire on the ventricular shock coil (which was serving as the heart rate sensor). The output of the ICD was short-circuited due to the presence of a shock coil in the superior vena cava, and the ICD was unknowingly rendered ineffective. Only after failure to deliver subsequent therapy was this problem noted, and the patient subsequently died.[133] It is important to note that some ICDs are configured to the "integrated bipolar sensing configuration" even in the presence of a true bipolar right ventricular lead.

Postanesthesia Implanted Cardioverter-Defibrillator Evaluation

The ICD must be reinterrogated and reenabled. All events should be reviewed and counters should be cleared, because the next device evaluator might not receive information about the EMI experience of the patient and might make erroneous conclusions regarding the patient's arrhythmia events.

SUMMARY

Electronic miniaturization has permitted the design and use of sophisticated electronics in patients who have need for artificial pacing or automated cardioversion/defibrillation of their heart, or both. Both the aging of the population and the ability to care for patients with increasingly complex disease suggest that many more patients with these devices will require subsequent surgery. Safe and efficient clinical management of these patients depends on an understanding of implantable systems, indications for their use, and the perioperative needs that they create.

Appendix 25–1 PACEMAKER RESPONSE TO MAGNET PLACEMENT

Pacemaker Company		Magnet Mode Designation	Explanation
Biotronik		AUTO	10 asynchronous events at 90 bpm if battery okay, 80 bpm at ERI (single-step then returns to original programmed mode, without rate responsiveness). Pacing is at LRL if okay or 11% below LRL if at ERI.
		ASYNCH	Asynchronous pacing at 90 bpm if battery okay, 80 bpm at ERI (single-step change).
		SYNCH	Pacing in the programmed mode at LRL (no change for ERI) without rate responsiveness.
ELA Medical			Asynchronous pacing at 96 bpm gradually declining to 80 bpm at ERI. ELA pacemakers take 8 additional asynchronous pacing cycles (the final 2 cycles are at LRL with long atrioventricular delay) upon magnet removal.
Guidant Medical (also CPI)		ASYNCH	Asynchronous pacing at 100 bpm if okay, 85 bpm at ERI (single step change). The Insignia model has an intermediate step at 90 bpm at IFI. For Triumph and Prelude models, see Medtronic pacemakers, below.
		OFF	No change, magnet is ignored. OFF is the magnet mode after a "power on reset," which can occur secondary to EMI.
		EGM mode	No change in pacing. Magnet application initiates data collection.
Intermedics			5 asynchronous events at 90 bpm (regardless of battery voltage), then 60 additional asynchronous events at LRL if battery okay, 90 bpm if ERI, and 80 bpm if EOL. The 5th paced event is emitted at 50% of the originally programmed pulse width; ventricular noncapture suggests an inadequate pacing safety margin. After the 65th asynchronous event, the magnet is ignored.
Medtronic			Asynchronous pacing at 85 bpm if okay, 65 SSI regardless of original programming if ERI (single-step change). Most Medtronic pacemakers emit one or more ventricular pulses during the first 3 to 7 asynchronous events (which might be at a rate of 100 bpm) at a reduced pulse width or voltage to demonstrate adequacy of ventricular pacing output. Also, Medtronic pacemakers default to SSI pacing at 65 bpm, without rate responsiveness, upon detection of ERI, whether a magnet is present or not.
St. Jude Medical	"SJM" x-ray logo	Battery Test	Asynchronous pacing at 98.6 bpm gradually decreasing to 86.3 bpm at ERI.
		OFF	No magnet response.
		Event snapshots	No change in pacing. Magnet application causes pacemaker to collect data. Identity and Entity models lack this feature.
		Event snapshots + Battery Test	For a magnet placed 2 seconds, pacing mode and rate are unchanged and the device stores an electrogram. If the magnet is placed ≥5 seconds, the Battery Test mode (see above) is activated. Identity and Entity models lack this feature.
	Pacesetter x-ray logo (ψ)	Battery Test	Asynchronous pacing, and the rate depends upon specific model. In general, a pacing rate of <90 bpm should prompt further evaluation.
		OFF	No magnet response.
		VARIO mode (present in some models)	VARIO results in a series of 32 asynchronous pacing events. The rate of the first 16 paces reflects battery voltage, gradually declining from 100 bpm to 85 bpm at ERI. The next 15 paces are used to document ventricular pacing capture safety margin. The rate will be 119 bpm with gradually declining pacing voltage. The 16th pace of this group is at no output. The next pace restarts the 32-event sequence. The 32-event sequence repeats as long as the magnet remains in place.
Telectronics	Meta 1202		Asynchronous pacing at 99 bpm gradually declining to <93 at ERI.
	Meta 1204 1206 1256		Asynchronous pacing at 100 bpm gradually declining to <82.5 bpm at ERI.
	Meta 1230 1250 1254		Asynchronous VOO pacing (regardless of original programming) at >85 bpm gradually declining to <78 bpm at ERI.
	Tempo		Asynchronous pacing at 100 bpm gradually declining to 80 bpm at ERI.
	Other models		Contact St. Jude Medical.

The effect(s) of appropriately placing a magnet over a pacemaker are shown. Column 1 shows the pacemaker manufacturer. If the magnet response is programmable, then column 2 shows the various programmable modes available. The first mode shown for a company is the default mode. Column 3 shows the effect on pacing therapy for the magnet mode shown in column 2. Unless otherwise specified, asynchronous pacing takes place, without rate responsiveness, in the chambers originally programmed. Thus, a dual chamber program would result in DOO pacing, and a single chamber program would result in VOO (unless an atrial device, which would be AOO) pacing, and a biventricular, dual chamber device would be DOOOV.

EOL = end of life. The device should be replaced immediately.

ERI = elective replacement indicator. The device should be replaced promptly.

IFI = intensified follow-up interval. The device needs monthly battery checks.

LRL = lower rate limit. The programmed lower rate, or set point, of the pacemaker.

SSI = single chamber, inhibited mode. If implanted for ventricular pacing, then SSI = VVI. For an atrial pacemaker, SSI = AAI.

Appendix 25–2 COMPANY TELEPHONE NUMBERS

AM Pacemaker Corp (Guidant Medical)	800-227-3422	Edwards Pacemaker Systems (Medtronic)	800-325-2518
Angeion	**800-264-2466**	**ELA Medical**	**800-352-6466**
Arco Medical (Guidant Medical)	800-227-3422	**Guidant Medical**	**800-227-3422**
Biotronik	**800-547-0394**	**Intermedics (Guidant Medical)**	**800-227-3422**
Cardiac Control Systems	*Unavailable*	**Medtronic**	**800-505-4636**
Cardio Pace Medical, Inc (Novacon)	*Unavailable*	**Pacesetter (St. Jude Medical)**	**800-722-3774**
Cardiac Pacemakers, Inc—CPI (Guidant Medical)	**800-227-3422**	Siemans—Elema (St. Jude Medical)	800-722-3774
Cook Pacemaker Corp	800-245-4715	**Telectronics Pacing (St. Jude Medical)**	**800-722-3774**
Coratomic (Biocontrol Technology)	unavailable	**Ventritex (St. Jude Medical)**	**800-722-3774**
Cordis Corporation (St. Jude Medical)	800-722-3774	Vitatron (Medtronic)	800-328-2518
Diag/Medcor (St. Jude Medical)	800-722-3774		

Companies in bold market defibrillators. Companies in *italics* are no longer available.

Appendix 25–3 IMPLANTED CARDIOVERTER-DEFIBRILLATOR (ICD) RESPONSE TO MAGNET PLACEMENT

ICD Manufacturer	Magnet Mode Designation	Effect on Tachy Therapy	Effect on Brady Therapy (regular pacing)	Magnet Mode Confirmation
Angeion	ENABLE DISABLE	Disables No effect	No effect No effect	None
Biotronik		Disables	No effect	None
ELA Medical		Disables	The pacing rate, but not mode, changes to 80 to 90 bpm. 80 bpm indicates elective replacement time.	None
Guidant Medical (also CPI)	ON	Disables	No effect	Short beep with each detected heartbeat or constant tone*
	OFF	No effect	No effect	None
Medtronic AT-500† All others		Disables Disables	No effect No effect	None‡
Pacesetter and St. Jude Medical	NORMAL IGNORE	Disables No effect	No effect No effect	None

The effect(s) of appropriately placing a magnet over an ICD are shown. Column 1 shows the manufacturer. If the magnet response is programmable, then column 2 shows the various modes available. The first mode shown is the default mode. Column 3 shows the effect on antitachycardia therapy (defibrillation, cardioversion, and antitachycardia pacing) for the magnet mode shown in column 2. Only ICDs from ELA Medical alter their antibradycardia pacing rate upon magnet placement (column 4), and this pacing rate can be used to predict remaining battery life provided that the patient's native heart rate is less than the magnet rate. Only ICDs from CPI/Guidant produce reliable audio feedback for confirmation of magnet placement (column 5). For devices from Angeion, Pacesetter, and St. Jude Medical, a device interrogation is required to determine the magnet mode.

*For CPI/Guidant ICDs, if magnet mode is programmed to "ON," appropriate magnet placement immediately disables tachy detection and therapy, and tachy therapies remain disabled for as long as the magnet remains appropriately applied. If each heartbeat produces a "beep," then the device will be enabled for tachy therapy upon magnet removal. If the device emits a constant tone, then tachy therapy is disabled whether or not a magnet is present.

If the "Change Tachy Mode with Magnet" feature also is programmed "ON," after 30 seconds of continuous magnet application the tachy mode changes; that is, it will switch from enabled (in absence of magnet, beeping) to permanently disabled (constant tone) or vice versa. Any CPI/Guidant ICD that does not emit sound when a magnet is applied should undergo an immediate device interrogation.

†The Medtronic AT-500 series defibrillators provide antitachycardia pacing and defibrillation shocks in the atrium ONLY, and usually after a delay often exceeding 1 minute. They do not have any shock coils on any lead and are very difficult to distinguish from a conventional two-chamber pacemaker. They have NO apparent magnet response.

‡Some Medtronic ICDs will emit a tone for 15 to 20 seconds when a magnet is placed on the device. However, this tone will not be interrupted with immediate magnet removal, and, as a result, the tone cannot be used for confirmation of appropriate magnet.

REFERENCES

1. Rasmussen MJ, Friedman PA, Hammill SC, Rea RF: Unintentional deactivation of implantable cardioverter-defibrillators in health care settings. Mayo Clin Proc 77:855, 2002
2. Eagle KA, Berger P B, Caulkins H, et al: ACC/AHA guideline update for perioperative cardiovascular evaluation for noncardiac surgery. January 2002. Available at: http://www.acc.org/clinical/guidelines/perio/update/pdf/perio_update.pdf. Accessed August 12, 2003
3. Goldschlager N, Epstein A, Friedman P, Gang E, et al: Environmental and drug effects on patients with pacemakers and implantable cardioverter/defibrillators: A practical guide to patient treatment. Arch Intern Med 161:649, 2001
4. Pinski SL, Trohman RG: Interference in implanted cardiac devices, part I. Pacing Clin Electrophysiol 25:1367, 2002
5. Pinski SL, Trohman RG: Interference in implanted cardiac devices, part II. Pacing Clin Electrophysiol 25:1496, 2002
6. Stone KR, McPherson CA: Assessment and management of patients with pacemakers and implantable cardioverter defibrillators. Crit Care Med 32(4 suppl):S155, 2004
7. Salukhe TV, Dob D, Sutton R: Pacemakers and defibrillators: Anaesthetic implications. Br J Anaesth 93:95, 2004
8. American Society of Anesthesiology Practice Advisory for the Perioperative Management of Patients with Rhythm Management Devices: Pacemakers and implantable cardioverter-defibrillators. Anesthesiology 103:186, 2005
9. Rozner M: Pacemaker misinformation in the perioperative period: Programming around the problem. Anesth Analg 99:1582, 2004
10. Badrinath SS, Bhaskaran S, Sundararaj I, et al: Mortality and morbidity associated with ophthalmic surgery. Ophthalmic Surg Lasers 26:535, 1995
11. Samain E, Schauveliege F, Henry C, Marty J: Outcome in patients with a cardiac pacemaker undergoing noncardiac surgery. Anesthesiology 95:A142, 2001
12. Bernstein AD, Daubert JC, Fletcher RD, et al: The revised NASPE/BPEG generic code for antibradycardia, adaptive-rate, and multisite pacing. North American Society of Pacing and Electrophysiology/British Pacing and Electrophysiology Group. Pacing Clin Electrophysiol 25:260, 2002
13. Gregorato SG, Abrams J, Epstein AE, et al: ACC/AHA/NASPE 2002 guidelines update for implantation of cardiac pacemakers and antiarrhythmia devices: Summary article. Circulation 106:2145, 2002
14. Auricchio A, Stellbrink C, Sack S, et al: The Pacing Therapies for Congestive Heart Failure (PATH-CHF) study: Rationale, design, and endpoints of a prospective randomized multicenter study. Am J Cardiol 83:130D, 1999
15. Bristow MR, Saxon LA, Boehmer J, et al: Cardiac-resynchronization therapy with or without an implantable defibrillator in advanced chronic heart failure. N Engl J Med 350:2140, 2004
16. Hayes DL: Evolving indications for permanent pacing. Am J Cardiol 83:161D, 1999
17. Gras D, Mabo P, Tang T, et al: Multisite pacing as a supplemental treatment of congestive heart failure: Preliminary results of the Medtronic Inc. InSync Study. Pacing Clin Electrophysiol 21(11 pt 2): 2249, 1998
18. Medina-Ravell VA, Lankipalli RS, Yan GX, et al: Effect of epicardial or biventricular pacing to prolong QT interval and increase transmural dispersion of repolarization: Does resynchronization therapy pose a risk for patients predisposed to long QT or torsade de pointes? Circulation 107:740, 2003
19. Delfaut P, Saksena S: Electrophysiologic assessment in selecting patients for multisite atrial pacing. J Interv Card Electrophysiol 4(suppl 1):81, 2000
20. Rozner MA, Nishman RJ: Pacemaker-driven tachycardia revisited. Anesth Analg 88:965, 1999
21. Purday JP, Towey RM: Apparent pacemaker failure caused by activation of ventricular threshold test by a magnetic instrument mat during general anaesthesia. Br J Anaesth 69:645, 1992
22. Bourke ME: The patient with a pacemaker or related device. Can J Anaesth 43:24, 1996
23. Valls-Bertault V, Mansourati J, Gilard M, et al: Adverse events with transvenous left ventricular pacing in patients with severe heart failure: Early experience from a single centre. Europace 3:60, 2001
24. Alonso C, Leclercq C, d'Allonnes FR, et al: Six year experience of transvenous left ventricular lead implantation for permanent biventricular pacing in patients with advanced heart failure: Technical aspects. Heart 86:405, 2001
25. Bernstein AD, Irwin ME, Parsonnet V, et al: Report of the NASPE Policy Conference on antibradycardia pacemaker follow-up: Effectiveness, needs, and resources. North American Society of Pacing and Electrophysiology. Pacing Clin Electrophysiol 17(11 pt 1):1714, 1994
26. Rozner MA, Roberson JC, Nguyen AD: Unexpected high incidence of serious pacemaker problems detected by pre-and postoperative interrogations: A two-year experience. J Am Coll Cardiol 43:113A, 2004
27. Sethi KK, Bhargava M, Pandit N, et al: Experience with recycled cardiac pacemakers. Indian Heart J 44:91, 1992
28. Panja M, Sarkar CN, Kumar S, et al: Reuse of pacemaker. Indian Heart J 48:677, 1996
29. Hauser R, Hayes D, Parsonnet V, et al: Feasibility and initial results of an Internet-based pacemaker and ICD pulse generator and lead registry. Pacing Clin Electrophysiol 24:82, 2001
30. Kato Y, Hou K, Hori J, et al: [Extracorporeal shock wave lithotripsy for ureteral stone in patient with implanted cardiac pacemaker: A case report]. Nippon Hinyokika Gakkai Zasshi 94:626, 2003
31. Preisman S, Cheng DC: Life-threatening ventricular arrhythmias with inadvertent asynchronous temporary pacing after cardiac surgery. Anesthesiology 91:880, 1999
32. Rozner MA: Implantable cardiac pulse generators: Pacemakers and cardioverter-defibrillators. *In* Miller RD, Fleisher L, Johns R, et al (eds): Anesthesia, 6th edition. New York, Churchill Livingstone, 2004
33. Hayes DL, Strathmore NF: Electromagnetic interference with implantable devices. *In* Ellenbogen KA, Kay GN, Wilkoff BL (eds): Clinical Cardiac Pacing and Defibrillation, 2nd edition. Philadelphia, WB Saunders, 2000, p 939
34. Andersen C, Madsen GM: Rate-responsive pacemakers and anaesthesia. A consideration of possible implications. Anaesthesia 45:472, 1990
35. Levine PA: Response to "Rate-adaptive cardiac pacing: Implications of environmental noise during craniotomy." Anesthesiology 87:1261, 1997
36. Levine PA, Balady GJ, Lazar HL, et al: Electrocautery and pacemakers: Management of the paced patient subject to electrocautery. Ann Thorac Surg 41:313, 1986
37. Madsen GM, Andersen C: Pacemaker-induced tachycardia during general anaesthesia: A case report. Br J Anaesth 63:360, 1989
38. von Knobelsdorff G, Goerig M, Nagele H, Scholz J: [Interaction of frequency-adaptive pacemakers and anesthetic management. Discussion of current literature and two case reports]. Anaesthesist 45:856, 1996
39. Van Hemel NM, Hamerlijnck RP, Pronk KJ, Van der Veen EP: Upper limit ventricular stimulation in respiratory rate responsive pacing due to electrocautery. Pacing Clin Electrophysiol 12:1720, 1989
40. Wong DT, Middleton W: Electrocautery-induced tachycardia in a rate-responsive pacemaker. Anesthesiology 94:710, 2001
41. Wallden J, Gupta A, Carlsen HO: Supraventricular tachycardia induced by Datex patient monitoring system. Anesth Analg 86:1339, 1998
42. Center for Devices and Radiologic Health: Interaction between minute ventilation rate-adaptive pacemakers and cardiac monitoring and diagnostic equipment. Published October 14, 1998. Available at: http://www.fda.gov/cdrh/safety/minutevent.html. Accessed December 1, 2002
43. Rozner MA: Peripheral nerve stimulators can inhibit monitor display of pacemaker pulses. J Clin Anesth 16:117, 2004
44. Michaloudis D, Fraidakis O, Lefaki T, et al: Anaesthesia and the QT interval in humans. The effects of isoflurane and halothane. Anaesthesia 51:219, 1996
45. Yildirim H, Adanair T, Atay A, et al: The effects of sevoflurane, isoflurane, and desflurane on QT interval of the Ecg. Eur J Anaesthesiol 21:566, 2004
46. Paventi S, Santevecchi A, Ranieri R: Effects of sevoflurane versus propofol on QT interval. Minerva Anestesiol 67:637, 2001
47. Gallagher JD, Weindling SN, Anderson G, Fillinger MP: Effects of sevoflurane on QT interval in a patient with congenital long QT syndrome. Anesthesiology 89:1569, 1998
48. Michaloudis D, Fraidakis O, Lefaki T, et al: Anaesthesia and the QT interval in humans: Effects of halothane and isoflurane in premedicated children. Eur J Anaesthesiol 15:623, 1998
49. Pressly N: Review of MDR Reports reinforces concern about EMI. FDA User Facility Reporting No. 20. Published 1997. Available at: http://www.fda.gov/cdrh/fuse20.pdf. Accessed December 1, 2002
50. Rozner MA: Letter to the editor. Pacing Clin Electrophysiol 26(4 pt 1):923, 2003
51. Nandalan SP, Vanner RG: Use of the harmonic scalpel in a patient with a permanent pacemaker. Anaesthesia 59:621, 2004
52. Epstein MR, Mayer JE Jr, Duncan BW: Use of an ultrasonic scalpel as an alternative to electrocautery in patients with pacemakers. Ann Thorac Surg 65:1802, 1998
53. Ozeren M, Dogan OV, Duzgun C, Yucel E: Use of an ultrasonic scalpel in the open-heart reoperation of a patient with pacemaker. Eur J Cardiothorac Surg 21:761, 2002

54. Erdman S, Levinsky L, Strasberg B, et al: Use of the Shaw scalpel in pacemaker operations. J Thorac Cardiovasc Surg 89:304, 1985
55. Gimbel JR, Johnson D, Levine PA, Wilkoff BL: Safe performance of magnetic resonance imaging on five patients with permanent cardiac pacemakers. Pacing Clin Electrophysiol 19:913, 1996
56. Gimbel JR, Kanal E: Can patients with implantable pacemakers safely undergo magnetic resonance imaging? J Am Coll Cardiol 43:1325, 2004
57. Roguin A, Zviman MM, Meininger GR et al: Modern pacemaker and implantable cardioverter/defibrillator systems can be magnetic resonance imaging safe: In vitro and in vivo assessment of safety and function at 1.5 T. Circulation 110:475, 2004
58. Martin ET, Coman JA, Shellock FG, et al: Magnetic resonance imaging and cardiac pacemaker safety at 1.5-Tesla. J Am Coll Cardiol 43:1315, 2004
59. Rozner MA: MRI in the patient with a pacemaker: Caution is indicated. J Am Coll Cardiol 2004
60. Mychaskiw G, Eichhorn JH: Interaction of an implanted pacemaker with a transesophageal atrial pacemaker: Report of a case. J Clin Anesth 11:669, 1999
61. Kaushik V, Leon AR, Forrester JS Jr, Trohman RG: Bradyarrhythmias, temporary and permanent pacing. Crit Care Med 28(10 suppl):N121, 2000
62. Kashima I, Shin H, Yozu R, Kawada S: Optimal positioning of temporary epicardial atrial pacing leads after cardiac surgery. Jpn J Thorac Cardiovasc Surg 49:307, 2001
63. Atlee JL III, Pattison CZ, Mathews EL, et al: Evaluation of transesophageal atrial pacing stethoscope in adult surgical patients under general anesthesia. Pacing Clin Electrophysiol 15(10 pt 1):1515, 1992
64. Zaidan JR: Pacemakers. Anesthesiology 60:319, 1984
65. Bellocci F, Santarelli P, Di Gennaro M, et al: The risk of cardiac complications in surgical patients with bifascicular block. A clinical and electrophysiologic study in 98 patients. Chest 77:343, 1980
66. Del Nido P, Goldman BS: Temporary epicardial pacing after open heart surgery: Complications and prevention. J Card Surg 4:99, 1989
67. Dixon RG, Dougherty JM, White LJ, et al: Transcutaneous pacing in a hypothermic-dog model. Ann Emerg Med 29:602, 1997
68. Syverud SA, Dalsey WC, Hedges JR, Hanslits ML: Radiologic assessment of transvenous pacemaker placement during CPR. Ann Emerg Med 15:131, 1986
69. Lang R, David D, Klein HO, et al: The use of the balloon-tipped floating catheter in temporary transvenous cardiac pacing. Pacing Clin Electrophysiol 4:491, 1981
70. Hazard PB, Benton C, Milnor JP: Transvenous cardiac pacing in cardiopulmonary resuscitation. Crit Care Med 9:666, 1981
71. Phillips SJ, Butner AN: Percutaneous transvenous cardiac pacing initiated at bedside: Results in 40 cases. J Thorac Cardiovasc Surg 59:855, 1970
72. Trankina MF, White RD: Perioperative cardiac pacing using an atrioventricular pacing pulmonary artery catheter. J Cardiothorac Anesth 3:154, 1989
73. Befeler B, Hildner FJ, Javier RP, et al: Cardiovascular dynamics during coronary sinus, right atrial, and right ventricular pacing. Am Heart J 81:372, 1971
74. Benchimol A, Ellis JG, Dimond EG: Hemodynamic consequences of atrial and ventricular pacing in patients with normal and abnormal hearts. Effect of exercise at a fixed atrial and ventricular rate. Am J Med 39:911, 1965
75. Hartzler GO, Maloney JD, Curtis JJ, Barnhorst DA: Hemodynamic benefits of atrioventricular sequential pacing after cardiac surgery. Am J Cardiol 40:232, 1977
76. Curtis J, Walls J, Boley T, et al: Influence of atrioventricular synchrony on hemodynamics in patients with normal and low ejection fractions following open heart surgery. Am Surg 52:93, 1986
77. Trigano AJ, Azoulay A, Rochdi M, Campillo A: Electromagnetic interference of external pacemakers by walkie-talkies and digital cellular phones: Experimental study. Pacing Clin Electrophysiol 22:588, 1999
78. Betts TR, Simpson IA: Inhibition of temporary pacing by a mobile phone. Heart 87:130, 2002
79. Cooper JP, Swanton RH: Complications of transvenous temporary pacemaker insertion. Br J Hosp Med 53:155, 1995
80. Zaidan JR, Freniere S: Use of a pacing pulmonary artery catheter during cardiac surgery. Ann Thorac Surg 35:633, 1983
81. Heiselman DE, Maxwell JS, Petno V: Electrode displacement from a multipurpose Swan-Ganz catheter. Pacing Clin Electrophysiol 9(1 pt 1):134, 1986
82. Colardyn F, Vandenbogaerde J, De Niel C, Jordaens L: Ventricular pacing via a Swan Ganz catheter: A new mode of pacemaker therapy. Acta Cardiol 41:23, 1986
83. Lumb PD: Atrioventricular sequential pacing with transluminal atrial and ventricular pacing probes inserted via a pulmonary artery catheter: A preliminary comparison with epicardial wires. J Clin Anesth 1:292, 1989
84. Trankina MF: Pacemakers and automatic implantable cardiac defibrillators. Semin Anesth 12:165, 1993
85. Zoll PM: Resuscitation of the heart in ventricular standstill by external electric stimulation. N Engl J Med 247:768, 1952
86. Estes NA III, Deering TF, Manolis AS, et al: External cardiac programmed stimulation for noninvasive termination of sustained supraventricular and ventricular tachycardia. Am J Cardiol 63:177, 1989
87. Zoll PM: Noninvasive cardiac stimulation revisited. Pacing Clin Electrophysiol 13(12 pt 2):2014, 1990
88. Falk RH, Ngai ST: External cardiac pacing: Influence of electrode placement on pacing threshold. Crit Care Med 14:931, 1986
89. Gauss A, Hubner C, Meierhenrich R, et al: Perioperative transcutaneous pacemaker in patients with chronic bifascicular block or left bundle branch block and additional first-degree atrioventricular block. Acta Anaesthesiol Scand 43:731, 1999
90. Zoll PM, Zoll RH, Falk RH, et al: External noninvasive temporary cardiac pacing: Clinical trials. Circulation 71:937, 1985
91. Madsen JK, Meibom J, Videbak R, et al: Transcutaneous pacing: experience with the Zoll noninvasive temporary pacemaker. Am Heart J 116:7, 1988
92. Falk RH, Ngai ST, Kumaki DJ, Rubinstein JA: Cardiac activation during external cardiac pacing. Pacing Clin Electrophysiol 10(3 pt 1): 503, 1987
93. Kelly JS, Royster RL: Noninvasive transcutaneous cardiac pacing. Anesth Analg 69:229, 1989
94. Altamura G, Bianconi L, Boccadamo R, Pistolese M: Treatment of ventricular and supraventricular tachyarrhythmias by transcutaneous cardiac pacing. Pacing Clin Electrophysiol 12:331, 1989
95. Cummins RO, Graves JR, Larsen MP, et al: Out-of-hospital transcutaneous pacing by emergency medical technicians in patients with asystolic cardiac arrest. N Engl J Med 328:1377, 1993
96. Knowlton AA, Falk RH: External cardiac pacing during in-hospital cardiac arrest. Am J Cardiol 57:1295, 1986
97. Altamura G, Bianconi L, Toscano S, et al: Transcutaneous cardiac pacing for termination of tachyarrhythmias. Pacing Clin Electrophysiol 13: 2026, 1990
98. Luck JC, Markel ML: Clinical applications of external pacing: A renaissance? Pacing Clin Electrophysiol 14:1299, 1991
99. Pattison CZ, Atlee JL III, Mathews EL, et al: Atrial pacing thresholds measured in anesthetized patients with the use of an esophageal stethoscope modified for pacing. Anesthesiology 74:854, 1991
100. Backofen JE, Schauble JF, Rogers MC: Transesophageal pacing for bradycardia. Anesthesiology 61:777, 1984
101. Atlee JL III, Pattison CZ, Mathews EL, Hedman AG: Transesophageal atrial pacing for intraoperative sinus bradycardia or AV junctional rhythm: Feasibility as prophylaxis in 200 anesthetized adults and hemodynamic effects of treatment. J Cardiothorac Vasc Anesth 7:436, 1993
102. Smith I, Monk TG, White PF: Comparison of transesophageal atrial pacing with anticholinergic drugs for the treatment of intraoperative bradycardia. Anesth Analg 78:245, 1994
103. Trankina MF, Black S, Mahla ME: Cardiac pacing using a pacing esophageal stethoscope in patients undergoing posterior fossa craniotomy in the three quarter prone position. J Neurosurg Anesth 6:340, 1994
104. Burack B, Furman S: Transesophageal cardiac pacing. Am J Cardiol 23:469, 1969
105. Trankina MF, Black S, Gibby G: Pacemakers: Perioperative evaluation, management and complications. Anesthesiology 93:A1193, 2000
106. Senthuran S, Toff WD, Vuylsteke A, et al: Editorial III—Implanted cardiac pacemakers and defibrillators in anaesthetic practice. Br J Anaesth 88:627, 2002
107. Moss AJ, Hall WJ, Cannom DS, et al: Improved survival with an implanted defibrillator in patients with coronary disease at high risk for ventricular arrhythmia. Multicenter Automatic Defibrillator Implantation Trial Investigators. N Engl J Med 335:1933, 1996
108. AVID Investigators: A comparison of antiarrhythmic-drug therapy with implantable defibrillators in patients resuscitated from near-fatal ventricular arrhythmias. The Antiarrhythmics versus Implantable Defibrillators (AVID) Investigators. N Engl J Med 337:1576, 1997
109. Buxton AE, Lee KL, Fisher JD, et al: A randomized study of the prevention of sudden death in patients with coronary artery disease. Multi-

center Unsustained Tachycardia Trial Investigators. N Engl J Med 341:1882, 1999
110. Bernstein AD, Camm AJ, Fisher JD, et al: North American Society of Pacing and Electrophysiology policy statement. The NASPE/BPEG defibrillator code. Pacing Clin Electrophysiol 16:1776, 1993
111. Grimm W, Flores BF, Marchlinski FE: Electrocardiographically documented unnecessary, spontaneous shocks in 241 patients with implantable cardioverter defibrillators. Pacing Clin Electrophysiol 15(11 pt 1):1667, 1992
112. Hurst TM, Krieglstein H, Tillmanns H, Waldecker B: Inappropriate management of self-terminating ventricular arrhythmias by implantable cardioverter defibrillators despite a specific reconfirmation algorithm: A report of two cases. Pacing Clin Electrophysiol 20(5 pt 1):1328, 1997
113. Begley DA, Mohiddin SA, Tripodi D, et al: Efficacy of implantable cardioverter defibrillator therapy for primary and secondary prevention of sudden cardiac death in hypertrophic cardiomyopathy. Pacing Clin Electrophysiol 26:1887, 2003
114. Prasad K, Kishore AG, Anderson MH, et al: Inappropriate shocks in patients receiving internal cardioverter-defibrillators for malignant ventricular arrhythmias. Indian Heart J 49:403, 1997
115. Schumacher B, Tebbenjohanns J, Jung W, et al: Radiofrequency catheter ablation of atrial flutter that elicits inappropriate implantable cardioverter defibrillator discharge. Pacing Clin Electrophysiol 20(1 pt 1):125, 1997
116. Rozner MA: The patient with an implantable cardioverter-defibrillator. Progr Anesthesiol 13:43, 1999
117. Hintringer F, Schwarzacher S, Eibl G, Pachinger O: Inappropriate detection of supraventricular arrhythmias by implantable dual chamber defibrillators: A comparison of four different algorithms. Pacing Clin Electrophysiol 24:835, 2001
118. Niehaus M, de Sousa M, Klein G, et al: Chronic experiences with a single lead dual chamber implantable cardioverter defibrillator system. Pacing Clin Electrophysiol 26:1937, 2003
119. Hasdemir C, Shah N, Rao AP, et al: Analysis of troponin I levels after spontaneous implantable cardioverter defibrillator shocks. J Cardiovasc Electrophysiol 13:144, 2002
120. Swerdlow CD: Supraventricular tachycardia-ventricular tachycardia discrimination algorithms in implantable cardioverter defibrillators: State-of-the-art review. J Cardiovasc Electrophysiol 12:606, 2001
121. Brugada P, Geelen P: Some electrocardiographic patterns predicting sudden cardiac death that every doctor should recognize. Acta Cardiol 52:473, 1997
122. Maron BJ, Shen WK, Link MS, et al: Efficacy of implantable cardioverter-defibrillators for the prevention of sudden death in patients with hypertrophic cardiomyopathy. N Engl J Med 342:365, 2000
123. Moss AJ, Zareba W, Hall WJ, et al: Prophylactic implantation of a defibrillator in patients with myocardial infarction and reduced ejection fraction. N Engl J Med 346:877, 2002
124. Kadish A, Dyer A, Daubert JP, et al: Prophylactic defibrillator implantation in patients with nonischemic dilated cardiomyopathy. N Engl J Med 350:2151, 2004
125. Bardy GH, Lee KL, Mark DB, et al: Amiodarone or an implantable cardioverter-defibrillator for congestive heart failure. N Engl J Med 352:225, 2005
126. McClellan M, Tunis S: Medicare coverage of ICDs. N Engl J Med 352: 222, 2005
127. Peters RW, Gold MR: Pacing for patients with congestive heart failure and dilated cardiomyopathy. Cardiol Clin 18:55, 2000
128. Gras D, Leclercq C, Tang AS, et al: Cardiac resynchronization therapy in advanced heart failure: The multicenter InSync clinical study. Eur J Heart Fail 4:311, 2002
129. Winters SL, Packer DL, Marchlinski FE, et al: Consensus statement on indications, guidelines for use, and recommendations for follow-up of implantable cardioverter defibrillators. North American Society of Electrophysiology and Pacing. Pacing Clin Electrophysiol 24:262, 2001
130. Garcia-Moran E, Mont L, Brugada J: Inappropriate tachycardia detection by a biventricular implantable cardioverter defibrillator. Pacing Clin Electrophysiol 25:123, 2002
131. Gill RM, Sweeney RJ, Reid PR: The defibrillation threshold: A comparison of anesthetics and measurement methods. Pacing Clin Electrophysiol 16:708, 1993
132. Weinbroum AA, Glick A, Copperman Y, et al: Halothane, isoflurane, and fentanyl increase the minimally effective defibrillation threshold of an implantable cardioverter defibrillator: first report in humans. Anesth Analg 95:1147, 2002
133. Varma N, Cunningham D, Falk R: Central venous access resulting in selective failure of ICD defibrillation capacity. Pacing Clin Electrophysiol 24:394, 2001
134. Schwartzenburg CF, Wass CT, Strickland RA, Hayes DL: Rate-adaptive cardiac pacing: Implications of environmental noise during craniotomy. Anesthesiology 87:1252, 1997
135. Aldrete JA, Brown C, Daily J, Buerke V: Pacemaker malfunction due to microcurrent injection from a bioimpedance noninvasive cardiac output monitor. J Clin Monit 11:131, 1995
136. Rozner MA, Nishman RJ: Electrocautery-induced pacemaker tachycardia: Why does this error continue? Anesthesiology 96:773, 2002
137. Alexopoulos GS, Frances RJ: ECT and cardiac patients with pacemakers. Am J Psychiatry 137:1111, 1980
138. Philbin DM, Marieb MA, Aithal KH, Schoenfeld MH: Inappropriate shocks delivered by an ICD as a result of sensed potentials from a transcutaneous electronic nerve stimulation unit. Pacing Clin Electrophysiol 21:2010, 1998
139. Vlay SC: Electromagnetic interference and ICD discharge related to chiropractic treatment. Pacing Clin Electrophysiol 21:2009, 1998

Chapter 26

ANESTHESIA FOR HEART, LUNG, AND HEART-LUNG TRANSPLANTATION

Joseph J. Quinlan, MD • Andrew W. Murray, MD • Alfonso Casta, MD

KEY POINTS

1. The key factor limiting the number of cardiac transplants is a shortage of donors.
2. The 1-year survival is 79% with subsequent mortality of about 4% per year.
3. Potential recipients have end-stage heart disease, New York Heart Association class IV symptoms, ejection fraction less than 20%, and a physiologic age less than 60 years.
4. Orthotopic heart transplantation is carried out via a median sternotomy, and the general approach is similar to that used for myocardial revascularization or valve replacement.
5. Candidates for transplantation are frequently treated with diuretics, vasodilators, and β-blockers. End-stage patients may require inotropic drugs, intra-aortic balloon pump, or ventricular assist devices.
6. After transplantation, the patient has a denervated heart, and heart rate increases only gradually with stress due to circulating catecholamines.
7. Denervation means direct-acting cardiovascular drugs must be used to obtain a response, because indirect-acting drugs have a minimal or unpredictable response.
8. Allograft-acquired coronary artery disease is the greatest threat to long-term survival of the patient after heart transplantation.
9. Increased experience with lung transplantation has been accompanied by a decrease in both operative and long-term mortality.
10. Surgical complications are uncommon immediately after lung transplantation but may be associated with high mortality. Pneumothorax and infection are constant concerns. The most common cause of death in the perioperative period is graft dysfunction from reperfusion injury.

HEART TRANSPLANTATION

The history of heart transplantation spans almost a century. Canine heterotopic cardiac transplantation was first reported in 1905,[1] but such efforts were doomed by ignorance of the workings of the immune system (Box 26–1). Further research in the late 1950s and early 1960s set the stage for the first human cardiac transplant by Barnard in 1966.[2] However, there were few long-term survivors in this era, due to continued deficiency in understanding and in modulating the human immune system, and the procedure fell into general disfavor. Continued research at selected centers (such as Stanford University) and lessons learned from renal transplantation led to greater understanding of the technical issues and immunology required, and by the early 1980s cardiac transplantation gained widespread acceptance as a realistic option for patients with end-stage cardiomyopathy.

Heart transplantation experienced explosive growth in the mid to late 1980s, but the annual number of heart transplants worldwide plateaued by the early 1990s at approximately 3500 per year.[3] The factor limiting continued growth has been a shortage of suitable donors. As of early May 2004, there were approximately 3500 patients on the United Network for Organ Sharing cardiac transplant waiting list (includes all U.S. candidates), whereas only 2055 heart transplantations were performed in the United States during the 2003 calendar year. The median waiting time for a cardiac graft varies widely according to blood type (approximately 39 days for type AB recipients but up to 303 days for type O recipients listed for the period 2001 through 2003). In aggregate, more than 48% of those patients on the heart transplant list had spent more than 2 years waiting for a transplant at year end 2002.[4] The most frequent recipient indications for adult heart transplantation remain either idiopathic or ischemic cardiomyopathy. Other less common diagnoses include viral cardiomyopathy, systemic diseases such as amyloidosis, and complex congenital heart disease.

The 1-year survival after heart transplantation has been reported to be 79%, with a subsequent mortality rate of approximately 4% per year.[3] There has been little change in the survival statistics over the past decade; the Organ Procurement and Transplant Network reports that the 1- and 3-year survivals after heart transplantation for those transplanted in the United States during the period 1999 through 2001 were approximately 85% and 77%, respectively. One-year survival after repeat heart transplantation more than 6 months after the original procedure is slightly lower (63%) but substantially worse if performed within 6 months of the original grafting (39%).[3] Risk factors for increased mortality have been associated with recipient factors (prior transplantation, poor human histocompatability leukocyte antigen

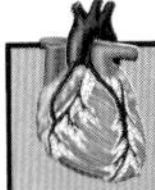

BOX 26–1 *Heart Transplantation*

- Frequency of transplantation remains limited by donor supply.
- Pathophysiology prior to transplantation is primarily that of end-stage ventricular failure.
- Pathophysiology after transplantation reflects the effects of denervation.
- Allograft coronary vasculopathy is a frequent long-term complication.

[HLA] matching, ventilator dependence, age, and race), medical center factors (volume of heart transplants performed, ischemic time), and donor factors (race, gender, age). Early deaths are most frequently due to graft failure, whereas intermediate-term deaths are caused by acute rejection or infection. Late deaths after heart transplantation are most frequently due to allograft vasculopathy, posttransplant lymphoproliferative disease or other malignancy, and chronic rejection.

Recipient Selection

Potential candidates for heart transplantation generally undergo a multidisciplinary evaluation including a complete history and physical examination, routine hematology, chemistries (to assess renal and hepatic function), viral serology, electrocardiography, chest radiography, pulmonary function tests, and right- and left-side heart catheterization. Ambulatory electrocardiography, echocardiography, and nuclear gated scans are performed if necessary. The goals of this evaluation are to confirm a diagnosis of end-stage heart disease that is not amenable to other therapies and that will likely lead to death within 1 to 2 years (see Chapter 27) and to exclude extracardiac organ dysfunction that could lead to death soon after heart transplantation. Patients typically have New York Heart Association (NYHA) class IV symptoms and a left ventricular ejection fraction (LVEF) of less than 20%. Although most centers eschew a strict age cutoff, the candidate should have a "physiologic" age of less than 60 years. Detecting pulmonary hypertension, and determining whether it is due to a fixed elevation of pulmonary vascular resistance (PVR), is crucial; early mortality due to graft failure is threefold higher in patients with elevated PVR (transpulmonary gradient >15 mm Hg or PVR >5 dynes/sec/cm^{-5}).[5] If elevated PVR is detected, a larger donor heart, a heterotopic heart transplant, or a heart-lung transplant may be more appropriate. Active infection and recent pulmonary thromboembolism with pulmonary infarction are additional contraindications to heart transplantation. The results of this extensive evaluation should be tabulated and available to the anesthesia team at all times, because heart transplantation is an emergency procedure.

Donor Selection and Graft Harvest

Once a brain-dead donor has been identified, the accepting transplant center must further evaluate the suitability of the allograft. Centers generally prefer donors to be previously free of cardiac illness and less than 35 years of age, because the incidence of coronary artery disease markedly increases at older ages. However, the relative shortage of suitable cardiac donors has forced many transplant centers to consider older donors without risk factors and symptoms of coronary artery disease. If it is necessary and the services are available at the donor hospital, the heart can be further evaluated by echocardiography (for regional wall motion abnormalities) or coronary angiography to complement standard palpation of the coronaries in the operating room. The absence of sepsis, prolonged cardiac arrest, severe chest trauma, and a high inotrope requirement are also important. The donor is matched to the prospective recipient for ABO blood-type compatibility and size (within 20%, especially if the recipient has high PVR); a cross-match is performed only if the recipient's preformed antibody screen is positive.

Donors can exhibit major hemodynamic and metabolic derangements that can adversely affect organ retrieval.[6] The vast majority of brain-dead donors will be hemodynamically unstable.[7,8] Reasons for such instability include hypovolemia (secondary to diuretics or diabetes insipidus), myocardial injury (possibly a result of "catecholamine storm" during periods of increased intracranial pressure), and inadequate sympathetic tone due to brainstem infarction. Donors often also have abnormalities of neuroendocrine function such as low T_3 and T_4 levels. Administration of T_3 to brain-dead animals improves ventricular function after transplantation; T_3 administration has enabled decreases in inotropic support in some, but not all, human studies.[9-11] Donor volume status should be assiduously monitored, and inotropic and vasopressor therapy should be guided by data from invasive monitors.

Donor cardiectomy is performed through a median sternotomy and usually simultaneous with recovery of other organs such as lungs, kidneys, and liver. Just prior to cardiac harvesting, the donor is heparinized and an intravenous cannula is placed in the ascending aorta for administration of conventional cardioplegia. The superior vena cava (SVC) is ligated, and the inferior vena cava (IVC) is transected to decompress the heart, simultaneous with the administration of cold hyperkalemic cardioplegia into the aortic root. The aorta is cross-clamped when the heart ceases to eject. The heart is also topically cooled with ice-cold saline. After arrest has been achieved, the pulmonary veins are severed, the SVC is transected, the ascending aorta is divided just proximal to the innominate artery, and the pulmonary artery (PA) transected at its bifurcation. The heart is then prepared for transport by placing it in a sterile plastic bag that is placed in turn in another bag filled with ice-cold saline, all of which are carried in an ice chest. Of all the regimens tested, conventional cardioplegia has proved most effective in maintaining cardiac performance.[12] The upper time limit for ex vivo storage of human hearts appears to be approximately 6 hours.[13]

SURGICAL PROCEDURES

Orthotopic Heart Transplantation

Orthotopic heart transplantation is carried out via a median sternotomy, and the general approach is similar to that used for coronary revascularization or valve replacement. Patients will frequently have undergone a prior median sternotomy; repeat sternotomy is cautiously performed using an oscillating saw. The groin should be prepped and draped to provide a rapid route for cannulation for cardiopulmonary bypass (CPB) if necessary. After the pericardium is opened, the aorta is cannulated as distally as possible, and the IVC and SVC are individually cannulated via the high right atrium (RA). Manipulation of the heart prior to institution of CPB is limited if thrombus is detected in the heart with transesophageal echocardiography (TEE) (Fig. 26–1). After initiation of CPB and cross-clamping of the aorta, the heart is arrested and excised (Fig. 26–2). The aorta and PA are separated and divided just above the level of their respective valves, and the atria are transected at their grooves. A variant of this classic approach totally excises both atria, mandating bicaval anastomoses. This technique may reduce the incidence of atrial arrhythmias, better preserve atrial function by avoiding tricuspid regurgitation, and enhance cardiac output (CO) after transplantation.[14,15]

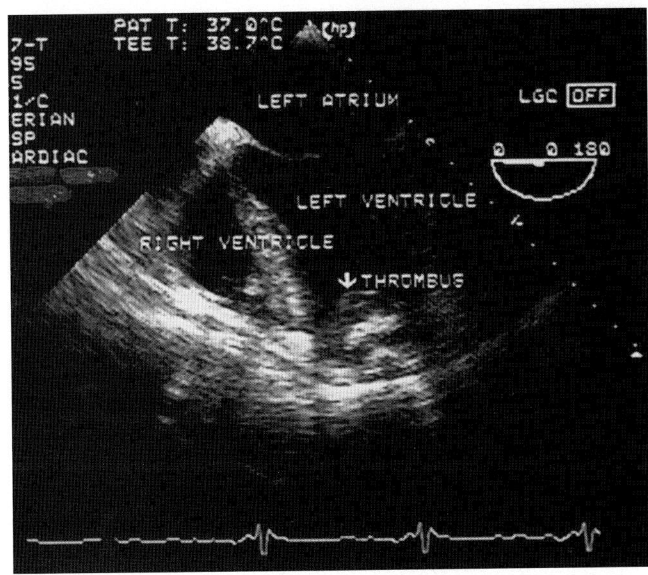

Figure 26–1 Transesophageal echocardiography image of laminated intraventricular thrombus in the native left ventricular apex. If intracavitary thrombus is found, great caution is warranted during dissection prior to cardiopulmonary bypass to avoid systemic embolization.

The donor graft is then implanted with every effort to maintain a cold tissue temperature, beginning with the left atrial (LA) anastomosis. If the foramen ovale is patent, it is sutured closed. The donor RA is opened by incising it from the IVC to the base of the RA appendage (to preserve the donor sinoatrial node), and the RA anastomosis constructed. Alternatively, if the bicaval technique is used, individual IVC and SVC anastomoses are sewn. The donor and recipient PAs are then brought together in an end-to-end manner, followed by the anastomosis of the donor to the recipient aorta. After removal of the aortic cross-clamp, the heart is de-aired via a vent in the ascending aorta. Just prior to weaning from CPB, one of the venous cannulas is withdrawn into the RA and the other removed. The patient is then weaned from CPB in the usual manner. After hemostasis is achieved, mediastinal tubes are placed for drainage, the pericardium is left open, and the wound is closed in the standard fashion.

Heterotopic Heart Transplantation

Although orthotopic placement of the cardiac graft is optimal for most patients, certain recipients are not candidates for the orthotopic operation, and instead the graft is placed in the right chest and connected to the circulation in parallel with the recipient heart. The two primary indications for heterotopic placement are significant irreversible pulmonary hypertension and gross size mismatch between the donor and recipient. Heterotopic placement may avoid the development of acute right ventricular (RV) failure in the unconditioned donor heart in the face of acutely elevated RV afterload.

Donor harvesting for heterotopic placement is performed in the previously described manner, except that the azygos vein is ligated and divided to increase the length of the donor SVC; the PA is extensively dissected to provide the longest possible main and right PA; and the donor IVC and right pulmonary veins are oversewn, with the left pulmonary veins incised to create a single large orifice. The operation is performed via a median sternotomy in the recipient, but the right

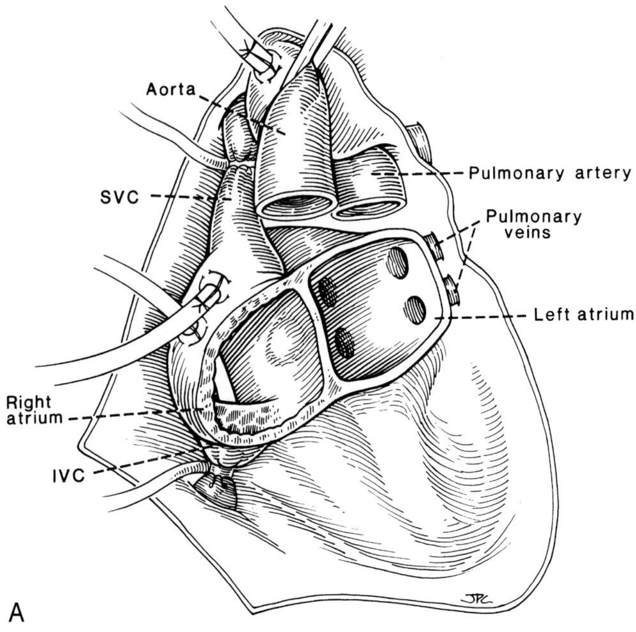

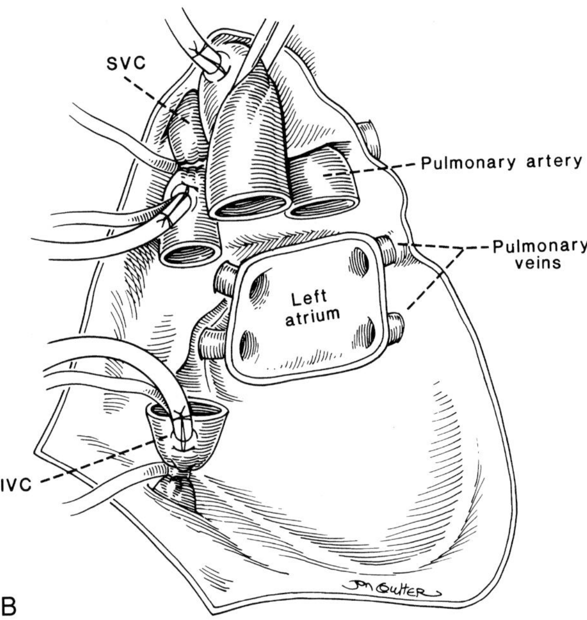

Figure 26–2 Mediastinum after excision of the heart but prior to allograft placement. Venous cannulas are present in the superior and inferior vena cava, and the arterial cannula is present in the ascending aorta. *(A)* Classic orthotopic technique. *(B)* Bicaval anastomotic technique.

pleura is entered and excised. The recipient SVC is cannulated via the RA appendage, and the IVC via the lower RA. After arrest of the recipient heart, the LA anastomosis is constructed by incising the recipient LA near the right superior pulmonary vein and extending this incision inferiorly, and then anastomosing the respective LA. The recipient RA-SVC is then incised and anastomosed to the donor RA-SVC, following which the donor aorta is joined to the recipient aorta in an end-to-side manner. Finally, the donor PA is anastomosed to the recipient main PA in an end-to-side manner if it is sufficiently long; otherwise, they are joined via an interposed vascular graft (Fig. 26–3).

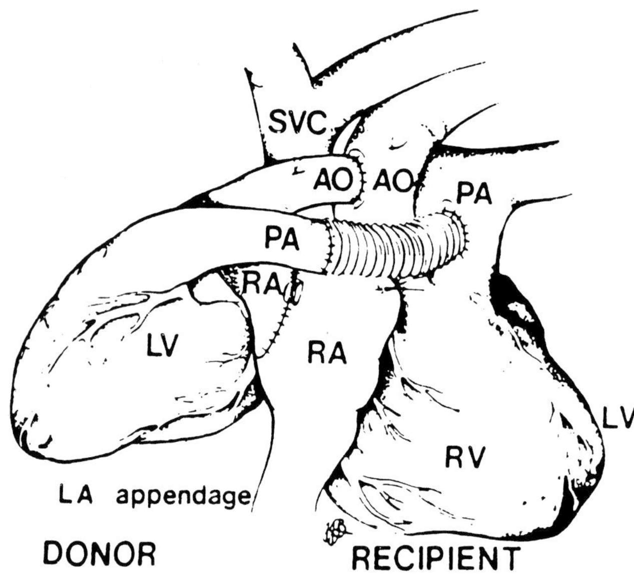

Figure 26–3 Placement of heterotopic graft in the right chest, with anastomoses to the corresponding native left and right atria, ascending aorta, and an interposition graft to the native pulmonary artery. (From Cooper DKC, Lanza LP: Heart Transplantation: The Present Status of Orthotopic and Heterotopic Heart Transplantation. Lancaster, UK, MTP Press, 1984.)

Special Situations

Mechanical ventricular assist devices (see Chapter 27) have been successfully used to "bridge" patients who would otherwise die of acute heart failure awaiting transplantation.[16] The technique of transplantation is virtually identical in such patients to that for ordinary orthotopic transplantation. However, repeat sternotomy is obligatory, and patients will often have been exposed to aprotinin during the assist device placement, increasing the probability of an anaphylactic response to the second aprotinin exposure. Although the incidence of anaphylaxis seems to be low,[17] the team should be in a position to expeditiously initiate CPB before administering aprotinin in this setting. Placement of large-bore intravenous access is prudent because excessive hemorrhage can occur during the transplant procedure.

Rarely, patients will present for cardiac transplantation combined with transplantation of the liver.[18] The cardiac allograft is usually implanted first to better enable the patient to survive potential hemodynamic instability associated with reperfusion of the hepatic allograft. Large-bore intravenous access is mandatory. Conventional full heparinization protocols plus aprotinin or low-dose heparin with heparin-bonded circuits may be used. A venous cannula can be left in the RA at the completion of the heart transplant procedure to serve as a return site for subsequent veno-veno bypass during liver transplantation.

Pathophysiology Before Transplantation

The pathophysiology of heart transplant candidates is predominantly end-stage cardiomyopathy. Such patients normally have both systolic dysfunction (characterized by decreased stroke volume and increased end-diastolic volume) and diastolic dysfunction, characterized by an elevated intracardiac diastolic pressure. As compensatory mechanisms to maintain CO fail, the elevated LV pressures lead to increases in pulmonary venous pressures and development of pulmonary vascular congestion and edema. A similar process occurs if RV failure also occurs. Autonomic sympathetic tone is increased in patients with heart failure, leading to generalized vasoconstriction as well as salt and water retention. Vasoconstriction and ventricular dilation combine to substantially increase myocardial wall tension. Over time, the high levels of catecholamines lead to a decrease in the sensitivity of the heart and vasculature to these agents via a decrease in receptor density (i.e., "down-regulation") and a decrease in myocardial norepinephrine stores.[19]

Therapy of heart failure seeks to reverse or antagonize these processes (see Chapters 10, 31, and 33). Almost all candidates will be maintained on diuretics; hypokalemia and hypomagnesemia secondary to urinary losses are likely, and the anesthesiologist must be alert to the possibility that a patient is hypovolemic from excessive diuresis. Another mainstay of therapy is vasodilators (such as nitrates, hydralazine, and angiotensin-converting enzyme inhibitors), which decrease the impedance to LV emptying and improve cardiac function and survival in patients with end-stage heart failure.[20,21] Paradoxically, slow incremental β-blockade with agents such as the β_1-antagonist metoprolol can also improve hemodynamics and exercise tolerance in some patients awaiting heart transplantation.[22] Patients who are symptomatic despite these measures often require inotropic therapy. Digoxin is an effective but weak inotrope, and its use is limited by toxic side effects. Phosphodiesterase inhibitors such as amrinone, milrinone, and enoximone are efficacious, but chronic therapy is restricted by concerns about increased mortality in those receiving these agents.[23,24] Therefore, inotrope-dependent patients are often treated with intravenous infusions of β-adrenergic agonists such as dopamine or dobutamine. Patients refractory to even these measures may be supported with intra-aortic balloon counterpulsation, but its use is fraught with significant vascular complications and essentially immobilizes the patient. Many patients with low CO are maintained on anticoagulants such as warfarin to prevent pulmonary or systemic embolization, especially if they have atrial fibrillation.

Pathophysiology After Transplantation

The physiology of patients after heart transplantation is of interest not only to anesthesiologists in cardiac transplant centers but also to the anesthesiology community at large because a substantial portion of these patients return for subsequent surgical procedures.[25,26]

Cardiac denervation is an unavoidable consequence of heart transplantation. Many long-term studies indicate that reinnervation is absent or at best partial or incomplete in humans.[27-29] Denervation does not significantly change baseline cardiac function, but it does substantially alter the cardiac response to demands for increased CO.[30,31] Normally, increases in heart rate can rapidly increase CO, but this mechanism is not available to the transplanted heart. Heart rate increases only gradually with exercise, and this effect is mediated by circulating catecholamines.[27] Increases in CO in response to exercise are instead mostly mediated via an increase in stroke volume.[32] Therefore, maintenance of adequate preload in cardiac transplant recipients is crucial. Lack of parasympathetic innervation is probably responsible for the gradual decrease in heart rate after exercise seen in transplant recipients, rather than the usual sharp drop.

Denervation has important implications in the choice of pharmacologic agents used after cardiac transplantation. Drugs that act indirectly on the heart via either the sympathetic (ephedrine) or parasympathetic (atropine, pancuronium, edrophonium) nervous systems will generally be ineffective. Drugs with a mixture of direct and indirect effects will exhibit only their direct effects (leading to the absence of the normal increase in refractory period of the atrioventricular node with digoxin,[33] tachycardia with norepinephrine infusion, and bradycardia with neostigmine).[34] Thus, agents with direct cardiac effects (such as epinephrine or isoproterenol) are the drugs of choice for altering cardiac physiology after transplantation. However, the chronically high catecholamine levels found in cardiac transplant recipients may blunt the effect of α-adrenergic agents, as opposed to normal responses to β-adrenergic agents.[35]

Allograft coronary vasculopathy remains the greatest threat to long-term survival after heart transplantation. Allografts are prone to the accelerated development of an unusual form of coronary atherosclerosis that is characterized by circumferential, diffuse involvement of entire coronary arterial segments, as opposed to the conventional form of coronary atherosclerosis with focal plaques often found in eccentric positions in proximal coronary arteries.[36] The pathophysiologic basis of this process remains elusive, but it is likely due to an immune cell-mediated activation of vascular endothelial cells to up-regulate the production of smooth muscle cell growth factors.[37] More than half of all heart transplant recipients have evidence of concentric atherosclerosis 3 years after transplant, and more than 80% at 5 years.[38] Because afferent cardiac reinnervation is rare, a substantial portion of recipients with accelerated vasculopathy have silent ischemia.[39] Noninvasive methods of detecting coronary atherosclerosis are insensitive for detecting allograft vasculopathy.[40] Furthermore, coronary angiography often underestimates the severity of allograft atherosclerosis[41]; other diagnostic regimens such as intravascular ultrasound and dobutamine stress echocardiography may detect morphologic abnormalities or functional ischemia, respectively, in the absence of angiographically significant lesions.[36,41,42] Therefore, the anesthesiologist should assume that there is a substantial risk of coronary vasculopathy in any heart transplant recipient beyond the first 2 years, regardless of symptoms, the results of noninvasive testing, and even angiography.

Anesthetic Management

Preoperative Evaluation and Preparation

The preoperative period is often marked by severe time constraints due to the impending arrival of the donor heart. Nevertheless, a rapid history should screen for last oral intake, recent anticoagulant use, intercurrent deterioration of ventricular function, or change in anginal pattern; a physical examination should evaluate present volume status, and a laboratory review (if available) and a chest radiograph should detect the presence of renal, hepatic, or pulmonary dysfunction. Many hospitalized patients will be supported with inotropic infusions and/or an intra-aortic balloon pump, and the infusion rates and timing of the latter should be reviewed.

Equipment and drugs similar to those usually used for routine cases requiring CPB should be prepared. A β-agonist such as epinephrine should be readily available both in bolus form and as an infusion to rapidly treat ventricular failure; and an α-agonist such as phenylephrine or norepinephrine is useful to compensate for the vasodilatory effects of anesthetics, because even small decreases in preload and afterload can lead to catastrophic changes in CO and coronary perfusion in these patients.

Placement of invasive monitoring prior to induction will facilitate rapid and accurate response to hemodynamic events during induction. In addition to standard noninvasive monitoring, an arterial catheter and a PA catheter (with a long sterile sheath to allow partial removal during graft implantation) are placed after judicious use of sedation and local anesthetics. Placing the arterial catheter in a central site rather than the radial artery will avoid the discrepancy between radial and central arterial pressure often seen after CPB, but it may also be necessary to cannulate a femoral artery for arterial inflow for CPB if there has been a prior sternotomy. Floating the PA catheter into correct position may be difficult due to cardiac chamber dilation and severe tricuspid regurgitation. Large-bore intravenous access is mandatory, especially if a sternotomy has been previously performed, in which case external defibrillator/pacing patches may also be useful. The overall hemodynamic "picture" should be evaluated and optimized insofar as possible just prior to induction. If the hemodynamics seem tenuous, then starting or increasing an inotrope infusion may be advisable.

Induction

Most patients presenting for heart transplantation will not be in a fasting state and should be considered to have a "full stomach." Therefore, the induction technique should aim to rapidly achieve control of the airway to prevent aspiration while avoiding myocardial depression. A regimen combining a short-acting hypnotic with minimal myocardial depression (etomidate, 0.3 mg/kg), a moderate dose of narcotic to blunt the tachycardia response to laryngoscopy and intubation (fentanyl, 10 μg/kg), and succinylcholine (1.5 mg/kg) is popular[43]; high-dose narcotic techniques with or without benzodiazepines have also been advocated.[44,45] Vasodilation should be countered with an α-agonist. Anesthesia can be maintained with additional narcotic and sedatives (benzodiazepines or scopolamine).[45,46]

Intraoperative Management

Following induction, the stomach can be decompressed with an orogastric tube and a TEE probe introduced while the bladder is catheterized. A complete TEE examination often reveals useful information not immediately available from other sources, such as the presence of cardiac thrombi (see Fig. 26–1), ventricular volume and contractility, and atherosclerosis of the ascending aorta and aortic arch. Cross-matched blood should be immediately available once surgery commences, especially if the patient has had a previous sternotomy; patients not previously exposed to cytomegalovirus should receive blood from donors who are likewise cytomegalovirus negative. Sternotomy and cannulation for CPB are performed as indicated earlier. The period prior to CPB is often uneventful, apart from arrhythmias and slow recovery of coronary perfusion due to manipulation of the heart during dissection and cannulation. The PA catheter should be withdrawn from the right heart prior to completion of bicaval cannulation.

Once CPB is initiated, ventilation is discontinued and the absence of a thrill in the carotid arteries is documented. Most patients will have an excess of intravascular volume, and administration of a diuretic and/or the use of hemofiltration via the pump may be beneficial for increasing the hemoglobin concentration. A dose of glucocorticoid (methylprednisolone, 500 mg) is administered as the last anastomosis is being completed prior to release of the aortic cross-clamp to attenuate any hyperacute immune response. During the period of reperfusion an infusion of an inotrope is begun for both inotropy and chronotropy. TEE is used to monitor whether the cardiac chambers are adequately de-aired prior to weaning from CPB.

Weaning from bypass begins after ventilation is resumed and the cannula in the SVC is removed (see Chapter 31). The donor heart should be paced if bradycardia is present despite the inotropic infusion. Once the patient is separated from bypass, the PA catheter can be advanced into position. Patients with elevated PVR are at risk for acute RV failure and may benefit from a pulmonary vasodilator such as prostaglandin E_1 (0.05 to 0.15 μg/kg/min).[47] Rarely, such patients require support with a RV assist device.[48] TEE often provides additional useful information about right and left heart function and volume and documents normal flow dynamics through the anastomoses.

Protamine is then given to reverse heparin's effect after satisfactorily weaning from CPB. Continued coagulopathy despite adequate protamine is common after heart transplantation, especially if there has been a prior sternotomy. Treatment is similar to that used for other postbypass coagulopathies: meticulous attention to surgical hemostasis, empiric administration of platelets, and subsequent addition of fresh frozen plasma and cryoprecipitate guided by subsequent coagulation studies (see Chapters 18 and 29). High-dose aprotinin infusion decreases blood loss, transfusion of red blood cells and clotting factors such as platelets, fresh frozen plasma, and cryoprecipitate, and blood donor exposures after heart transplant via "redo" sternotomy.[49,50] After adequate hemostasis is achieved, the wound is closed in standard fashion and the patient transported to the intensive care unit (ICU).

Postoperative Management and Complications

Management in the ICU after the conclusion of the procedure is essentially a continuation of the anesthetic management after CPB.[51] The electrocardiogram; arterial, central venous, and/or PA pressures; and arterial oxygen saturation are monitored continuously. Cardiac recipients will continue to require β-adrenergic infusions for chronotropy and inotropy for up to 3 to 4 days. Vasodilators may be necessary to control arterial hypertension and decrease impedance to LV ejection. Patients can be weaned from ventilatory support and extubated when the hemodynamics are stable and hemorrhage has ceased. The immunosuppressive regimen of choice (typically consisting of cyclosporine, azathioprine, and prednisone, or tacrolimus and prednisone) should be started after arrival in the ICU. Invasive monitoring can be withdrawn as the inotropic support is weaned, and mediastinal tubes removed after drainage subsides (usually after 24 hours). Patients can usually be discharged from the ICU after 2 or 3 days (see Chapters 32 through 34).

Early complications after heart transplantation include acute and hyperacute rejection, cardiac failure, systemic and pulmonary hypertension, cardiac arrhythmias, renal failure, and infection. Hyperacute rejection is an extremely rare but devastating syndrome mediated by preformed recipient cytotoxic antibodies against donor heart antigens. The donor heart immediately becomes cyanotic from microvascular thrombosis and ultimately ceases to contract.[52] This syndrome is lethal unless the patient can be supported mechanically until a suitable heart is found. Acute rejection is a constant threat in the early postoperative period and may present in many forms (e.g., low CO, arrhythmias). Acute rejection occurs most frequently during the initial 6 months after transplantation, so its presence is monitored by serial endomyocardial biopsies, with additional biopsies to evaluate any acute changes in clinical status. Detection of rejection mandates an aggressive increase in the level of immunosuppression, usually including pulses of glucocorticoid or a change from cyclosporine to tacrolimus. Low CO after transplantation may reflect a number of etiologies: hypovolemia, inadequate adrenergic stimulation, myocardial injury during harvesting, acute rejection, tamponade, or sepsis. Therapy should be guided by invasive monitoring, TEE, and endomyocardial biopsy. Systemic hypertension may be due to pain, so adequate analgesia should be obtained before treating blood pressure with a vasodilator. Because fixed pulmonary hypertension will have been excluded during the recipient evaluation, pulmonary hypertension after heart transplantation is usually transient and responsive to vasodilators such as prostaglandin E_1, nitrates, or hydralazine after either orthotopic or heterotopic placement.[53,54] Atrial and ventricular tachyarrhythmias are common after heart transplantation[55]; once rejection has been ruled out as a cause, antiarrhythmics are used for conversion or control (except those acting via indirect mechanisms such as digoxin, or those with negative inotropic properties such as β-blockers and calcium channel blockers). Almost all recipients will require either β-adrenergic agonists or pacing to increase heart rate in the immediate perioperative period, but 10% to 25% of recipients will also require permanent pacing.[56,57] Renal function often improves immediately after transplantation, but immunosuppressives such as cyclosporine and tacrolimus may impair renal function.[58,59] Finally, infection is a constant threat to immunosuppressed recipients. Bacterial pneumonia is frequent early in the postoperative period, with opportunistic viral and fungal infections becoming more common after the first several weeks (see Chapter 36).

Pediatric Considerations

In the pediatric population, dilated cardiomyopathy and complex congenital heart defects (CHDs) are the primary indications for heart transplantation. Although the number of donors and recipients has remained stable in recent years, the overall survival has improved in children undergoing heart transplantation. Factors contributing to this trend are enhanced preservation of the donor heart, improved selection of recipients and donors, and refinements in surgical techniques and immunosuppressive therapy.[60]

Cardiac transplantation is recommended when the child's expected survival is less than 1 year. In some centers, this therapy is offered as the primary intervention to the infant born with hypoplastic left heart syndrome (HLHS). The perioperative and intraoperative management of these infants undergoing heart transplant have been extensively reviewed.[61]

The preoperative assessment for heart transplantation in the patient with complex CHD might be more extensive depending on the heart defect and previous corrective or palliative procedures. Similar to the child with dilated cardiomyopathy, assessment of the indexed pulmonary vascular resistance (PVRI) is essential.[60] In adults, a PVRI greater than 5 units and a transpulmonary gradient greater than 15 mm Hg are contraindications for transplantation. In children, the acceptable PVRI is less than 10 units, but it is not unusual for a pediatric heart transplant candidate to have a PVRI greater than 10 units. In one pediatric cardiac center, 20% of the transplanted patients had PVRI greater than 6 units. However, in the 6- to 10-unit range, the child is at risk for acute RV failure because the donor's RV is thin walled and the myocardium has been ischemic. If the PVRI decreases significantly in the catheterization laboratory, with a trial of vasodilator testing, hyperventilation, 100% O_2, and nitric oxide, the candidate is acceptable for transplantation. If the PVRI remains borderline, the candidate is admitted to the hospital for a 1- or 2-week trial with milrinone and dobutamine. If the PVRI then falls, transplantation is offered. These patients might benefit from pulmonary vasodilation therapy during weaning from CPB and in the ICU.

Another aspect to be emphasized in the pretransplant evaluation of these patients with complex CHD is the need for a detailed anatomical evaluation. It is not uncommon for this group of patients to have branch PA stenosis or discontinuous PAs. Anomalies of systemic and pulmonary veins are associated with atrial isomerism, and different surgical techniques are needed to address these issues during transplantation. High output failure may develop in the recipient with large aortopulmonary collaterals in the postoperative period. Although the donor ischemic time, ICU days, and total hospital days are prolonged in these patients, the outcome is comparable to the patient with dilated cardiomyopathy after heart transplantation.

Cardiac transplantation is also offered to patients with the so-called failed Fontan for physiologic repair of cardiac defects with single ventricle. They present with protein losing enteropathy, chronic liver disease, and pulmonary arteriovenous malformations. These malformations may complicate the postoperative course. If they are large enough, moderate to severe hypoxemia may lead to primary graft failure. Small malformations may regress with time.

In some recipients, the circulation is supported by extracorporeal membrane oxygenation (ECMO) or a ventricular assist device prior to transplantation. Prolonged support is associated with bleeding, sepsis, and multiorgan dysfunction. It is not uncommon to list an infant for heart transplantation who is on ECMO after a failed Norwood procedure. Transportation of this infant to the operating room can be quite complicated.

Besides determining the blood type (ABO), it is important to assess for the presence of antibodies against HLA.[62] Antibodies against HLA may have developed in the recipient who was exposed to blood products during palliation for complex CHD. Hyperacute rejection may lead to graft loss in the operating room in this setting. The risk of primary graft failure is higher if more than mild systolic dysfunction was present in the donor heart before transplantation. In pediatrics, the donor-recipient heart size matching in weight ranges between 80-300%. At surgery the bi-caval technique is preferred.

As in adults, sedation prior to surgery is provided with benzodiazepines or scopolamine. Full stomach precautions are generally taken. Induction of anesthesia is accomplished with etomidate (0.2-0.3 mg/kg), fentanyl, and a muscle relaxant (succinylcholine or a non-depolarizer). Titration to vital signs is important. Frequently, the groin vessels are exposed for urgent cannulation before sternotomy and during this procedure less narcotics are required. If hemodynamics are adequate, a volatile agent can be used. An opioid with a benzodiazepine is used for maintenance of anesthesia. Recall of operative events has been documented in young adolescents. A PA catheter is useful in the older child but often just a RV catheter can be used when there are concerns about pulmonary hypertension. Aprotinin is commonly used in patients requiring redo sternotomies.

LUNG TRANSPLANTATION

History and Epidemiology

Although the first human lung transplant was performed in 1963, surgical technical problems and inadequate preservation and immunosuppression regimens prevented widespread acceptance of this procedure until the mid 1980s (Box 26–2). Advances in these areas have since made lung transplantation a viable option for many patients with end-stage lung disease. For the period January 1, 1985, to December 31, 1995, a total of 3194 single- and 1845 double-lung transplants were reported to the Registry of the International Society for Heart and Lung Transplantation.[3] The frequency of both single- and double-lung transplants increased exponentially during the period up until 1993, with the sharpest growth in unilateral transplants. According to data collected by UNOS between 2000 and 2002, the annual frequency of lung transplantation has remained stagnant, with the total number still averaging in the vicinity of 1000. This is unchanged from the time between 1993 and 1995 when the numbers first leveled off. Further growth in lung transplantation is constrained by a shortage of donor organs, with demand for organs still vastly exceeding supply. It is estimated that in excess of a million individuals with end-stage lung disease are potential recipients of lung transplants.[63] Some had hoped that non–heart-beating donors would provide an alternative source of organs, but this has not been the case. The Organ Procurement and Transplantation Network currently registers approximately 4000 patients for lung transplantation. This number does not accurately reflect the number of organs required as some patients will require bilateral lung transplantation. Average time to transplant increased to as much as 451 days in 1999, but now about one quarter of patients are transplanted within 251 days. Most of this improvement has been seen with recipients who are 50 years old and greater. One explanation for this may be increasing leniency in organ selection criteria. This seems to have not been associated with increasing mortality

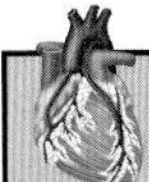

BOX 26–2 ***Lung Transplantation***

- Broader donor criteria have decreased the time from listing to transplantation.
- Nitric oxide minimizes reperfusion injury.
- Donor lungs should be ventilated with a protective strategy (low inspired oxygen, low tidal volume/inspired pressure) after transplantation.

rates. Mortality for patients on the waiting list has also continued to decline, from a 1993 high of close to 250 per 1000 patient years to approximately 140 in 2002. Although some of this improvement may be ascribed to better medical management of patients on the waiting list, it is also likely due to broadened criteria for acceptance for transplantation and subsequent inclusion of patients with less severe illness.

Increased experience with lung transplantation has been accompanied by a decrease in both operative and long-term mortality. For example, 30-day mortality for double-lung transplantation decreased from 44% in 1988 to 13.6% in 1991, whereas that for single-lung transplantation decreased from 22.7% to 12.6%.[64] As of the end of 1995, 3-year actuarial survival for recipients of both single- and double-lung transplants performed in the era 1992 to 1995 was approximately 60%, 10% better than for recipients transplanted in the previous 3-year interval.[3] Even better survival data have been reported from centers with extensive experience with these procedures (1-year survival rates of 82% for double-lung recipients and 90% for single-lung recipients).[65] Infection is the most frequent cause of death in the first year after transplant, but this is superceded in later years by bronchiolitis obliterans.[3]

Some of the most challenging patients are those with cystic fibrosis. The 1-year survival of 79% and 5-year survival of 57% after lung transplantation have shown that despite the high incidence of poor nutrition and the almost ubiquitous colonization by multidrug-resistant organisms, these patients can still successfully undergo lung transplantation with acceptable outcome data.[66]

It is a sign of the maturity of lung transplantation procedures that survival data for "redo" lung transplantation are also becoming available. A late 1991 survey of centers reported that actuarial survival after redo transplantation was significantly worse than that of first-time recipients (e.g., 35% versus greater than 75% at 1 year),[67] and subsequent data have confirmed this observation.[3] Infection and multiorgan failure prior to repeat transplant are associated with an almost uniformly fatal outcome.

Recipient Selection

Because donor lungs are scarce, it is important to select as recipients those most likely to benefit from lung transplantation. In general, candidates should be terminally ill with end-stage lung disease (NYHA class III or IV, with a life expectancy of approximately 2 years), be psychologically stable, and be devoid of serious medical illness (especially extrapulmonary infection) compromising other organ systems. Patients already requiring mechanical ventilation are poor candidates, although lung transplantation can be successful in such a setting. Other factors such as advanced age, previous thoracic surgery or deformity, and steroid dependence may be regarded as relative contraindications by individual transplant centers. Hepatic disease due solely to right heart dysfunction should not preclude candidacy.

Potential recipients undergo a multidisciplinary assessment of their suitability, including pulmonary spirometry, radiography (plain film and chest CT scan), and echocardiography or multiple gated image acquisition (MUGA) scan. Patients older than 40 years of age and those with pulmonary hypertension usually undergo left heart catheterization to exclude significant coronary atherosclerosis or an intracardiac shunt. TEE may yield data (e.g., unanticipated atrial septal defect) that will alter subsequent surgical approach in approximately one quarter of patients with severe pulmonary hypertension.[68] Candidates who are accepted are often placed on a physical conditioning regimen to reverse muscle atrophy and debilitation and to keep them within 20% of their ideal body weight. Because lung transplantation is an emergency procedure (limited by a lung preservation time of 6 to 8 hours),[69] results of this comprehensive evaluation should be readily available to the anesthesia team at all times.

Donor Selection and Graft Harvest

The ongoing shortage of suitable donor organs has led to a liberalization of selection criteria. Prospective lung donors who were cigarette smokers are no longer rejected simply based on a pack-year history. CT has been used to assess the structural integrity of the lung, particularly in donors who have sustained traumatic chest injury. Lungs that have contusion limited to less than 30% of a single lobe can be considered adequate.[70] Greater use has also been made of organs from older but otherwise healthy donors (55 to 60 years old) especially when the ischemic period will be short.[71] A clear chest radiograph, normal blood gas results, unremarkable findings on bronchoscopy and sputum stain, and direct intraoperative evaluation confirm satisfactory lung function. The lungs are matched to the recipient for ABO blood type and size (oversized lungs can result in severe atelectasis and compromise of venous return in the recipient, especially after double-lung transplantation). Donor serology and tracheal cultures guide subsequent antibacterial and antiviral therapy in the recipient.

Most lung grafts are recovered during a multivisceral donor harvest procedure. The heart is removed as described for heart transplantation, using inflow occlusion and cardioplegic arrest, with division of the IVC and SVC, the aorta, and the main PA. Immediately following cross-clamping, the pulmonary vasculature is flushed with ice-cold preservative solution, which often contains prostaglandin E_1. This is believed to promote pulmonary vasodilation, which aids homogeneous distribution of the preserving solution. Other additives that have been included are nitroglycerin and low-potassium 5% Dextran. The LA is divided so as to leave an adequate LA cuff for both the heart graft and lung graft(s) with the pulmonary veins. After explanation, the lung may also be flushed to clear all pulmonary veins of any clots. After the lung is inflated, the trachea (or bronchus for an isolated lung) is clamped, divided, and stapled closed. Inflating the lung has been shown to increase cold ischemia tolerance of the donor organ. The lung graft is removed, bagged, and immersed in ice-cold saline for transport.

Surgical Procedures

Because of the relative shortage of lung donors and the finding that recipients can gain significant exercise tolerance even with only one transplanted lung,[72] single-lung transplantation is the procedure of choice for all lung transplant candidates, except when leaving one of the recipient's lungs in place would predispose to complications. For example, the presence of lung disease associated with chronic infection (cystic fibrosis and severe bronchiectasis) mandates double-lung transplantation to prevent the recipient lung from acting as a reservoir of infection and subsequently cross-contaminating the allograft. Patients with severe air trapping may require double-lung transplantation if uncontrollable ventilation/perfusion mismatching will be likely after transplantation. Lobar transplantation into children and young adults from living-related donors is discussed separately.

Single-Lung Transplant

The choice of which lung to transplant is usually based on multiple factors, including avoidance of a prior operative site, preference for removing the native lung with the worst ventilation/perfusion ratio, and donor lung availability. The recipient is positioned for a posterolateral thoracotomy, with the ipsilateral groin prepped and exposed in case CPB becomes necessary. With the lung deflated, a pneumonectomy is performed, with special care to preserve as long a PA segment as possible. After removal of the diseased native lung, the allograft is positioned in the chest with precautions to maintain its cold tissue temperature. The bronchial anastomosis is performed first. A "telescoping" anastomosis is used if there is significant discrepancy in size between the donor and the recipient. The object of the technique is to minimize the chance of dehiscence. Although it was once common to wrap bronchial anastomoses with omentum, wrapping produces no added benefit when a telescoping anastomosis is performed. The PA is anastomosed next, and finally the pericardium is opened and the allograft LA cuff containing the pulmonary venous orifices is anastomosed to the native LA. The pulmonary circuit is then flushed with blood and de-aired. The initial flush solution is usually cold (4°C) but is followed by a warm (37°C) flush. The warm flush is usually performed during final completion of the vascular anastomoses. The goal of the flushing is to achieve a controlled reperfusion.[73] The contents of this solution are listed in Box 26–3. After glucocorticoid administration, the vascular clamps are removed, reperfusion is begun, and the lung reinflated with a series of ventilations to full functional residual capacity. After achieving adequate hemostasis and satisfactory blood gases, chest tubes are placed, the wound is closed, and the patient is transported to the ICU.

Double-Lung Transplant

Early attempts at double-lung transplantation using an en bloc technique via a median sternotomy were plagued by frequent postoperative airway dehiscence due to poor vascular supply of the tracheal anastomosis; by hemorrhage due to extensive mediastinal dissection (which also resulted in cardiac denervation); by the requirement for complete CPB and cardioplegic arrest (to facilitate pulmonary arterial and venous anastomoses); and by poor access to the posterior mediastinum. The subsequent development of the bilateral sequential lung transplant technique via a "clamshell" thoracosternotomy (essentially two single-lung transplants performed in sequence) has avoided many of the problems inherent in the en bloc technique.[74,75] An alternative to using a clamshell incision in slender patients is an approach through two individual anterolateral thoracotomies. This results in a particularly pleasing cosmetic result in female patients because the scar falls in the breast crease. Use of CPB is optional, exposure of the posterior mediastinum is enhanced (improving hemostasis), and cardiac denervation can usually be avoided. Pleural scarring is usually extensive in patients with cystic fibrosis, and postoperative hemorrhage and coagulopathy are the rule if CPB is required.

Transplantation of both lungs is performed in the supine position. The groins are prepped and exposed in case CPB is required. If a clamshell incision is used, the arms are padded and suspended over the head on an ether screen (Fig. 26–4). In the slender patient whose anteroposterior chest dimensions are normal, the arms may be tucked at the patient's sides. Recipient pneumonectomy and implantation of the donor lung are performed sequentially on both lungs in essentially the same manner as described above for a single-lung transplant. The native lung with the worst function should be transplanted first. In patients whose indication for transplantation is suppurative disease, the pleural cavity is pulse-lavaged with antibiotic-containing solution that has been tailored to that patient's antimicrobial sensitivity profile. In addition to this, the anesthesiologist irrigates the trachea and bronchi with diluted iodophore solution prior to the donor lung being brought onto the surgical field.

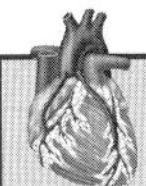

BOX 26–3 ***Warm Pulmonoplegia***

- Hematocrit 18 to 20, leukocyte depleted
- L-Glutamate
- L-Aspartate
- Adenosine
- Lidocaine
- Nitroglycerin
- Verapamil
- Dextrose
- Insulin

Pathophysiology Before Transplantation

Patients with highly compliant lungs and obstruction of expiratory airflow cannot completely exhale the delivered tidal volume, resulting in positive intrapleural pressure throughout the respiratory cycle ("auto-PEEP" [positive end-expiratory

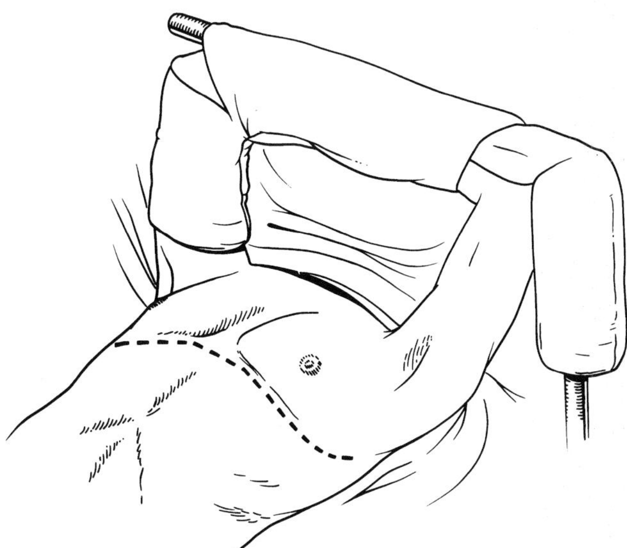

Figure 26–4 Patient positioning for "clamshell" thoracosternotomy. The arms are padded and suspended from an ether screen above the head of the patient. Path of surgical incision is shown with dotted line. (From Firestone LL, Firestone S: Organ transplantation. *In* Miller RD [ed]: Anesthesia, 4th edition. New York, Churchill Livingstone, 1994, p 1981.)

pressure] or "intrinsic PEEP"), which decreases venous return and causes hypotension.[76] The presence of auto-PEEP is highly negatively correlated with FEV_1 (percent predicted) and highly positively correlated with pulmonary flow resistance and resting hypercarbia.[77] Hyperinflation is a frequent complication of single-lung ventilation during lung transplantation in patients with obstructive lung disease. Hyperinflation-induced hemodynamic instability can be diagnosed by turning off the ventilator for 30 seconds and opening the breathing circuit to the atmosphere. If the blood pressure returns to its baseline value, hyperinflation is the underlying cause. Hyperinflation can be ameliorated with deliberate hypoventilation (decreasing both the tidal volume and/or rate).[78] Although this may result in profound hypercarbia, high carbon dioxide tensions are well tolerated in the absence of hypoxemia. PEEP may also decrease air trapping because it decreases expiratory resistance during controlled mechanical ventilation.[79] However, the application of PEEP requires close monitoring, because if the level of extrinsic PEEP applied exceeds the level of auto-PEEP, further air trapping may result.

RV failure is frequently encountered in lung transplant recipients with pulmonary hypertension due to chronically elevated RV afterload. The response of the RV to a chronic increase in afterload is to hypertrophy, but eventually this adaptive response is insufficient. As a result, RV volume decreases and chamber dilation results. The following should be kept in mind when caring for patients with severe RV dysfunction (Box 26–4). First, increases in intrathoracic pressure may markedly increase PVR,[80] leading to frank RV failure in patients with chronic RV dysfunction. Changes in RV function may occur immediately after adding PEEP, increasing tidal volume or decreasing expiratory time, and can have devastating consequences. In addition, although intravascular volume expansion in the presence of normal PVR increases CO, overzealous infusion in patients with elevated PVR increases RV end-diastolic pressure and RV wall stress, decreasing CO.[81] Inotropes with vasodilating properties (such as dobutamine or milrinone) are often a better choice than volume for augmenting CO in the setting of elevated PVR. Furthermore, the RV has a higher metabolic demand yet a lower coronary perfusion pressure than normal. RV performance can be augmented by improving RV coronary perfusion pressure with α-adrenergic agents, provided these vasoconstrictors do not disproportionately elevate PVR. This can sometimes be a better choice than augmenting the perfusion pressure with β-adrenergic agents because the oxygen supply is increased without a large increase in oxygen demand. Finally, vasodilators such as nitroprusside or prostaglandin E_1 may be effective in decreasing PVR and improving RV dysfunction early in the disease process, when only mild to moderate pulmonary hypertension is present. However, they are of notably limited value in the presence of severe, end-stage pulmonary hypertension. Systemic vasodilation and exacerbation of shunting often limit their use. Inhaled nitric oxide has shown promise as a means of acutely decreasing PVR without altering systemic hemodynamics both during the explanation phase and after lung transplantation.[82,83] Nitric oxide decreases both PA pressure and intrapulmonary shunting. Further, the combination of inhaled nitric oxide and aerosolized prostacyclin had a synergistic effect, without causing deleterious effects on the systemic perfusion pressure. The use of nitric oxide with or without inhaled prostacyclin may be helpful in avoiding CPB in patients having lung transplantation.

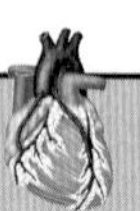

BOX 26–4 *Treatment of Intraoperative Right Ventricular Failure*

- Avoid large increases in intrathoracic pressure from:
  - Positive end-expiratory pressure (PEEP)
  - Large tidal volumes
  - Inadequate expiratory time
- Intravascular volume
  - Increase preload if pulmonary vascular resistance is normal.
  - Rely on inotropes (dobutamine) if pulmonary vascular resistance is increased.
- Maintain right ventricular coronary perfusion pressure with α-adrenergic agonists.
- Cautious administration of pulmonary vasodilators (avoid systemic and gas exchange effects)
  - Prostaglandin E_1 (0.05 to 0.15 μg/kg/min)
  - Inhaled nitric oxide (20 to 40 ppm)

Pathophysiology After Lung Transplantation

The implantation of the donor lung(s) causes marked alterations in recipient respiratory physiology. In single-lung recipients, the pattern of ventilation/perfusion matching depends on the original disease process. For example, with pulmonary fibrosis, blood flow and ventilation gradually divert to the transplanted lung, whereas in patients transplanted for diseases associated with pulmonary hypertension, blood flow is almost exclusively diverted to the transplanted lung, which still receives only half of the total ventilation.[84] In such patients the native lung represents mostly dead space ventilation. Transplantation results in obligatory sympathetic and parasympathetic denervation of the donor lung and therefore alters the physiologic responses of airway smooth muscle. Exaggerated bronchoconstrictive responses to the muscarinic agonist methacholine have been noted in some (but not all) studies of denervated lung recipients.[85,86] The mechanism of hyperresponsiveness may involve cholinergic synapses, inasmuch as they are the main mediators of bronchoconstriction. For example, electrical stimulation of transplanted bronchi (which activates cholinergic nerves) produces a hypercontractile response.[87] This suggests either enhanced release of acetylcholine from cholinergic nerve endings due to an increased responsiveness of parasympathetic nerves, or else loss of inhibitory innervation. Such effects are unlikely to be postsynaptic in origin because the number and affinity of muscarinic cholinergic receptors on transplanted human bronchi are similar to controls.[88] Reinnervation during subsequent weeks to months has been demonstrated in several animal models,[89,90] but there is no definitive evidence concerning reinnervation of transplanted human lungs. Mucociliary function is transiently severely impaired after lung transplantation and remains depressed for up to 1 year after the procedure.[91] Thus, transplant recipients require particularly aggressive endotracheal suctioning to remove airway secretions.

Lung transplantation also profoundly alters the vascular system. The ischemia and reperfusion that are an obligatory part of the transplantation process damage endothelia. Cold ischemia alone decreases β-adrenergic cyclic adenosine monophosphate (cAMP)-mediated vascular relaxation by approximately 40%, and subsequent reperfusion produces even greater decreases in both cyclic guanosine monophosphate (cGMP)-mediated and β-adrenergic cAMP-mediated pulmonary vascular smooth muscle relaxation.[92] Endothelial damage in the pulmonary allograft also results in "leaky" alveolar capillaries and the development of pulmonary edema. Pulmonary endothelial permeability is approximately three times greater in donor lungs than in healthy volunteers.[93] Regulation of pulmonary vasomotor tone solely by circulating humoral factors is another side effect of denervation. Changes in either the levels of circulating mediators or in the responsiveness of the pulmonary vasculature to such mediators may result in dramatic effects on the pulmonary vasculature. An example of the former is the finding that the potent vasoconstrictor endothelin is present at markedly elevated levels (two to three times normal) immediately after transplantation and remains elevated for up to 1 week thereafter.[94] Alterations in the response of denervated pulmonary vasculature to α_1-adrenergic agents[95] and prostaglandin E_1,[96] as well as a reduction in nitric oxide activity, have also been demonstrated in acutely denervated lung.[95] Dysfunctional responses to mediators may be exaggerated if CPB is required.[95] Pulmonary vascular resistance can be substantially decreased with the administration of inhaled nitric oxide after reperfusion. It remains unclear whether nitric oxide also ameliorates reperfusion injury. Several studies suggest that nitric oxide prevents or modulates reperfusion injury as measured by decreased lung water, lipid peroxidase activity, and neutrophil aggregation in the graft.[97-99] However, there are a number of studies that suggest that although nitric oxide has an effect on pulmonary hemodynamics, it does not ameliorate reperfusion injury.[100,101]

Aerosolized inhaled prostacyclin also decreases PVR after reperfusion and improves oxygenation without the added theoretical risk of worsening reperfusion injury.[102] Inhaled prostacyclin has approximately the same effectiveness as nitric oxide in treating lungs damaged by reperfusion injury and offers the added benefit of being cheaper.[103]

There are a number of other agents that have shown promise in decreasing postreperfusion injury in animal studies. Tetrahydrobiopterin, an essential co-factor in the nitric oxide synthase pathway, decreased the intracellular water, pyeloperoxidase activity, and lipid peroxidation and increased cGMP levels when given during reperfusion.[104] The administration of surfactant into the donor lung prior to harvest also appeared to ameliorate ischemia–reperfusion injury in pigs. There was a decrease in the PVR, less inflammatory cellular infiltrate, and an increase in nitric oxide levels in the group that received surfactant.[105]

Given these pathophysiologic derangements, it is not surprising that PVR increases in the transplanted lung.[106,107] However, what the clinician observes in the lung transplant patient will depend on the severity of pulmonary vascular dysfunction present preoperatively. PA pressures decrease dramatically during lung transplantation in patients who had pulmonary hypertension prior to transplantation,[108] and remain so for weeks to months thereafter.[108-114] Concomitant with the decrease in PA pressure, there is an immediate decrease in RV size after lung transplantation in those patients with preexisting pulmonary hypertension, as well as a return to a more normal geometry of the interventricular septum.[108] Both of these effects are sustained over several weeks to months.[108-114] Although echocardiographic indices of RV function (RV fractional area change) have not shown a consistent improvement in the immediate posttransplant period,[108] several other studies have documented improvement in RV function during the first several months after lung transplantation.[108-114] One striking finding was that persistent depression of RV function (defined as baseline RV fractional area change of less than 30% with failure to increase after transplant by at least 5% or by 20% of baseline) was statistically associated with death in the immediate perioperative period.[108]

Anesthetic Management

Preoperative Evaluation and Preparation

Immediate pretransplant reevaluation pertinent to intraoperative management includes a history and physical examination to screen for intercurrent deterioration or additional abnormalities that affect anesthetic management. Particular attention should be given to recent physical status, especially when the transplant evaluation was performed more than 9 to 12 months previously. A decrease in the maximal level of physical activity from that at the time of initial evaluation can be a sign of progressive pulmonary disease or worsening RV function. Most patients are maintained on supplemental nasal oxygen, yet are mildly hypoxemic. Patients who are bedridden, or who must pause between phrases or words while speaking, possess little functional reserve and are likely to exhibit hemodynamic instability during induction. The time and nature of the last oral intake should be determined to aid in deciding the appropriate method of securing the airway. The physical examination should focus on evaluation of the airway for ease of laryngoscopy and intubation; the presence of any reversible pulmonary dysfunction such as bronchospasm; and signs of cardiac failure. New laboratory data are often not available prior to the beginning of anesthesia care, but special attention should be directed to evaluation of the chest radiograph for signs of pneumothorax, effusion, or hyperinflation because they may affect subsequent management.

Equipment necessary for this procedure is analogous to that used in any procedure where CPB and cardiac arrest are real possibilities. Special mandatory pieces of equipment include some method to isolate the ventilation to each lung. Although bronchial blockers have their advocates, double-lumen endobronchial tubes offer the advantages of easy switching of the ventilated lung, suctioning of the nonventilated lung, and facile independent lung ventilation postoperatively. A left-sided double-lumen endobronchial tube is suitable for virtually all lung transplant cases (even left lung transplants) (Fig. 26–5). Regardless of whether a bronchial blocker or double-lumen tube is used, a fiberoptic bronchoscope is absolutely required to rapidly and unambiguously verify correct tube positioning, evaluate bronchial anastomoses, and clear airway secretions. An adult-sized bronchoscope offers better field of vision and superior suctioning capability but can be used only with 41 or 39 Fr double-lumen tubes. A ventilator with low internal compliance is necessary to adequately ventilate the noncompliant lungs of recipients with restrictive lung disease or donor lungs with reperfusion injury. The added capability of the ventilator to deliver pressure-controlled ventilation is also important, especially for the patients who have pulmonary fibrotic disease or reperfusion injury. Single-lung recipients with highly compliant lungs may require independent lung ventilation with a second

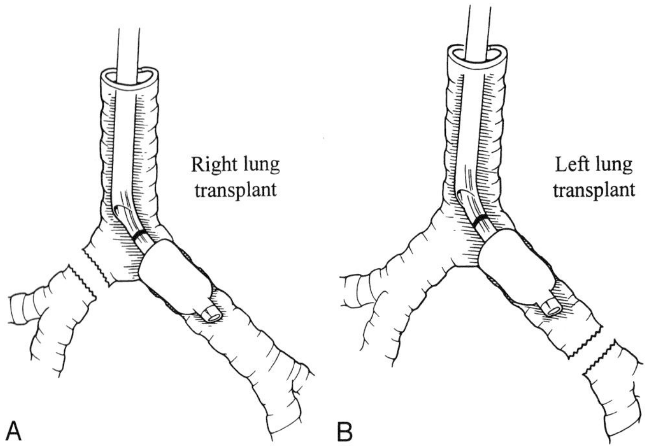

Figure 26–5 Left endobronchial tube during right and left lung transplantation. When the endobronchial tube is correctly positioned, either bronchus may be opened for anastomosis of the donor lung without compromising the surgical field or interfering with isolated lung ventilation.

ventilator after transplantation (discussed in detail later). A PA catheter capable of estimating RV ejection fraction (RVEF) can be useful in diagnosing RV failure and its response to inotropes and vasodilators, as well as the response of the RV to clamping of the PA. However, RVEF catheters are not accurate in the presence of significant tricuspid regurgitation or when malpositioned. Continuous mixed venous oximetry is beneficial in evaluating tissue oxygen delivery in patients subject to sudden, severe cardiac decompensation in the course of the operation, as well as the responses to therapy (see Chapter 14). A rapid infusion system can be lifesaving in patients in whom major hemorrhage occurs due to anastomotic leaks, inadequate surgical ligation of mediastinal collateral vessels, chest wall adhesions, or coagulopathy after CPB.

Induction of Anesthesia

Patients presenting for lung transplantation frequently arrive in the operating room area without premedication. Indeed, many are admitted directly to the operating room from home. Due to the nature of the procedure planned, and many months on the transplant waiting list, these patients are often extremely anxious. Considering the risk of respiratory depression from sedatives in patients who are chronically hypoxic and/or hypercapnic, only the most judicious use of intravenous benzodiazepines or narcotics is warranted. Assiduous administration of adequate local anesthesia during placement of invasive monitoring will also considerably improve conditions for both the patient and anesthesiologist. The standard noninvasive monitoring typical of cardiovascular procedures (two electrocardiogram [ECG] leads including a precordial lead, blood pressure cuff, pulse oximetry, capnography, and temperature measurement) is used. Intravenous access sufficient to rapidly administer large volumes of fluid is required. Generally, two large-bore (16- or, preferably, 14-gauge catheters, or a 9 Fr introducer sheath) intravenous catheters are placed. Patients for bilateral sequential lung transplantation who will receive a "clamshell" thoracosternotomy should have intravenous catheters placed in the internal or external jugular veins, because peripherally placed intravenous catheters are often unreliable when the arms are bent at the elbow and suspended from the ether screen. An intra-arterial catheter is an absolute requirement for blood pressure monitoring and for obtaining specimens for arterial blood gases. Continuous monitoring via a fiberoptic electrode placed in the arterial catheter may occasionally be useful if this technology is available. The femoral artery should be avoided if possible because the groin may be needed as a site for cannulation for CPB. Although the radial or brachial artery may be used in single-lung transplantation patients, these sites are not optimal in those who will require CPB (e.g., en bloc double-lung transplants or patients with severe pulmonary hypertension) because the transduced pressure may inaccurately reflect central aortic pressure during and after CPB, as well as in patients undergoing a clamshell thoracosternotomy, because of the positioning of the arms. An axillary arterial catheter may be useful in the latter situations because it provides a more accurate measure of central aortic pressure and allows sampling blood closer to that perfusing the brain. This may be important if partial CPB with a femoral arterial cannula is used because differential perfusion of the upper and lower half of the body may result. A PA catheter is inserted via the internal or external jugular veins. A TEE probe is placed after the airway is secured (see Chapters 14 and 15). PA pressure monitoring is most useful in patients who have preexisting pulmonary hypertension, especially during induction and during initial one-lung ventilation and PA clamping. Position of the PA catheter can be verified by TEE to ensure that it is residing in the main PA.

If the procedure is planned without CPB, care should be taken to ensure that the patient would be kept at ideal physiologic temperature to minimize coagulopathy and increases in the $M\dot{V}O_2$. This can be achieved with a warming blanket on the bed, on the patient's head and arms, and on the legs below the knees. A fluid warmer is also useful in this regard.

Three main principles should guide the formulation of a plan for induction: (1) protection of the airway; (2) avoidance of myocardial depression and increases in RV afterload in patients with RV dysfunction; and (3) avoidance and recognition of lung hyperinflation in patients with increased lung compliance and expiratory airflow obstruction (Box 26–5). All lung transplants are done on an emergency basis, and the majority of patients will have recently had oral intake and must be considered to have "full stomachs." Since aspiration during induction would be catastrophic, every measure must be taken to protect the airway. Patients with known or suspected abnormalities of airway anatomy should be intubated awake after topical anesthesia is applied to the airway. Although a conventional rapid-sequence intravenous (IV) induction with a short-acting hypnotic (e.g., etomidate 0.2 to 0.3 mg/kg), a small amount of narcotic (e.g., up to 10 μg/kg of fentanyl), and succinylcholine will usually be tolerated, patients with severe RV dysfunction may exhibit profound hemodynamic instability in response to this induction

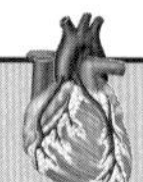

BOX 26–5 ***Key Principles of Anesthetic Induction for Lung Transplantation***

- Secure the airway
  - Intravenous rapid sequence induction versus gradual narcotic induction with continuous cricoid pressure
- Avoid myocardial depression and increases in right ventricular afterload
- Avoid lung hyperinflation

regimen. For such patients, a more gradual induction is recommended, with greater reliance on high doses of narcotics and ventilation with continuous application of cricoid pressure. Patients with bullous disease or fibrotic lungs requiring high inflation pressures may develop a pneumothorax during initiation of positive-pressure ventilation. Acute reductions in SaO_2 accompanied by difficulty in ventilating the lungs and refractory hypotension should generate strong suspicions that a tension pneumothorax has developed. RV function can be impaired during induction by drug-induced myocardial depression, increases in afterload, or by ischemia secondary to acute RV dilation. Agents that act as myocardial depressants (such as thiopental) should be avoided in such patients. Increases in RV afterload can result from inadequate anesthesia, exacerbation of chronic hypoxemia and hypercarbia and metabolic acidosis, as well as increases in intrathoracic pressure due to positive-pressure ventilation. Systemic hypotension is poorly tolerated because increased RV end-diastolic pressure will diminish net RV coronary perfusion pressure. In addition, chronic elevation of RV afterload increases the metabolic requirements of RV myocardium. Once the trachea is intubated and positive-pressure ventilation initiated, the avoidance of hyperinflation in patients with increased pulmonary compliance or bullous disease is crucial. Small tidal volumes and low respiratory rates and inspiratory/expiratory (I/E) ratios should be used ("permissive hypercapnia"). If hemodynamic instability does occur with positive-pressure ventilation, the ventilator should be disconnected from the patient. If hyperinflation is the cause of hypotension, blood pressure will increase within 10 to 30 seconds of the onset of apnea. Ventilation can then be resumed at a tidal volume and/or rate compatible with hemodynamic stability.

Anesthesia can be maintained using a variety of techniques. A moderate dose of narcotic (5 to 15 μg/kg of fentanyl or the equivalent), combined with low doses of a potent inhalation anesthetic, offers the advantages of stable hemodynamics, a high inspired oxygen concentration, a rapidly titratable depth of anesthesia, and the possibility of extubation in the early postoperative period. Patients with severe RV dysfunction who cannot tolerate even low concentrations of inhalation anesthetics may require a pure narcotic technique. Nitrous oxide is generally not used, because of the requirement for a high inspired oxygen concentration throughout the procedure, and its possible deleterious effects if gaseous emboli or an occult pneumothorax is present.

Intraoperative Management

Institution of one-lung ventilation (OLV) occurs prior to hilar dissection and may compromise hemodynamics and/or gas exchange (Box 26–6). Patients with diminished lung compliance can often tolerate OLV with normal tidal volumes and little change in hemodynamics. In contrast, patients with increased lung compliance and airway obstruction will often exhibit marked hemodynamic instability, unless the tidal volume is decreased and the expiratory time is increased. The magnitude of hypoxemia generally peaks about 20 minutes after beginning OLV. Hypoxemia during OLV may be treated with continuous positive airway pressure (CPAP) applied to the nonventilated lung,[115] PEEP to the ventilated lung, or both. CPAP attempts to oxygenate the shunt fraction but may interfere with surgical exposure. PEEP attempts to minimize atelectasis in the ventilated lung but may concomitantly increase shunt through the nonventilated lung. Definitive treatment of shunt in the nonventilated lung is provided by

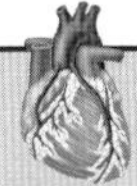

BOX 26–6 ***Management Principles for One-Lung Ventilation During Lung Transplantation***

- Tidal volume and respiratory rate
  - Maintain in patients with normal or decreased lung compliance (i.e., primary pulmonary hypertension, fibrosis)
  - Decrease both tidal volume and rate in patients with increased compliance (e.g., obstructive lung disease) to avoid hyperinflation ("permissive hypercapnia")
- Maintain oxygenation by
  - 100% Inspired oxygen
  - Applying CPAP (5 to 10 cm) to nonventilated lung
  - Adding PEEP (5 to 10 cm) to ventilated lung
  - Intermittent lung reinflation if necessary
  - Surgical ligation of the pulmonary artery of the nonventilated lung
- Be alert for development of pneumothorax on nonoperative side
  - Sharp drop in oxygen saturation, end-tidal carbon dioxide
  - Sharp rise in peak airway pressures
  - Increased risk with bullous lung disease
- Therapy
  - Relieve tension
  - Resume ventilation
  - Emergency cardiopulmonary bypass

PEEP = positive end-expiratory pressure; CPAP = continuous positive airway pressure.

rapid isolation and clamping of the PA of the nonventilated lung. Pneumothorax on the nonoperative side may result during OLV if a large tidal volume is used.

PA clamping is usually well tolerated, except in the face of pulmonary hypertension with diminished RV reserve. If the degree of RV compromise is uncertain, a 5- to 10-minute trial of PA clamping is attempted, then the RV is evaluated by serial CO, RVEF measurements, and TEE. A significant decrease in CO may predict patients who will require extracorporeal support.[116] Other indications for CPB in lung transplantation are listed in Box 26–7.[117]

Patients with severe pulmonary hypertension (greater than two thirds of systemic pressure) will generally be placed on CPB prior to PA clamping. The intraoperative use of nitric oxide (20 to 40 ppm) may allow some procedures to proceed without the use of CPB.[118]

Lung transplantation can usually be performed without the aid of CPB; even during bilateral sequential lung transplantation, experienced teams use CPB for only about one quarter of patients.[119,120] Although CPB may provide very stable hemodynamics, it is associated with an increased transfusion requirement.[78] In addition, graft function (as reflected by alveolar-arterial oxygen gradient) may be compromised,[121] endothelium-dependent cGMP- and β-adrenergic cAMP-mediated pulmonary vascular relaxation may be impaired to a greater degree,[122] and a longer period of mechanical ventilation may be necessary.[119] Several exceptional circumstances require CPB: the presence of severe pulmonary hypertension, because clamping of the PA will likely result in acute RV failure and "flooding" of the nonclamped lung; the repair of associated cardiac anomalies (e.g., patent foramen ovale, atrial or ventricular septal defects); treatment of severe hemodynamic or gas exchange instabilities; and living-related lobar

BOX 26–7 *Indications for Cardiopulmonary Bypass During Lung Transplantation*

Cardiac index	<2 L/min/m^2
Svo_2	<60%
Mean arterial pressure	<50 to 60 mm Hg
Sao_2	<85% to 90%
pH	<7.00

transplantation. Hypercarbia is generally well tolerated and should not be considered a requirement for CPB per se.[78] Thus, the frequency of CPB will depend on recipient population factors such as prevalence of end-stage pulmonary vascular disease and associated cardiac anomalies.[123]

The use of femoral venous and arterial cannulas for CPB during lung transplantation may lead to poor venous drainage and/or "differential perfusion" of the lower and upper body. Moreover, native pulmonary blood flow continues and may act as an intrapulmonary shunt during CPB. In this case, the cerebral vessels receive this desaturated blood, while the lower body is perfused with fully oxygenated blood from the CPB circuit. This effect is detectable by blood gas analysis of samples drawn from suitable arteries, or appropriately located pulse oximeter probes. Treatment includes conventional measures to increase venous return and augment bypass flow, or placing a venous cannula in the RA if this is feasible. The anesthesiologist should also maximize the inspired oxygen concentration and add PEEP to decrease intrapulmonary shunt. If all other measures fail, ventricular fibrillation can be induced using alternating current.[124]

Extracorporeal membrane oxygenation (ECMO) has also been suggested as an alternative method of CPB during lung transplantation. It has been suggested that the use of ECMO with heparin-bonded circuits might improve the outcome of both single- and double-lung transplants by lessening the amount of pulmonary edema especially in those patients who need CPB due to hemodynamic instability or with primary pulmonary hypertension. An added benefit of this technique is also that it clears the operative field of bypass cannulas making left-sided transplant as unimpeded as right-sided transplant. There is no apparent increase in transfusion requirement.[125] Another added benefit of using ECMO in situ is that reperfusion of the lungs can be more easily controlled since the CO transiting the newly transplanted lung can be precisely controlled. This is especially the case for patients with advanced pulmonary hypertension.[126]

If CPB is used, weaning from circulatory support occurs when the graft anastomoses are complete. Ventilation is resumed with a lung protection strategy similar to that used in the Acute Respiratory Distress Syndrome Network trial. This demonstrated that patients with decreased compliance related to acute respiratory distress syndrome had a 22% decrease in mortality when applying tidal volumes of 6 mL/kg and a plateau pressure less than 30 cm H_2O.[71] Minimizing the inspired fraction of O_2 may help prevent generation of oxygen free-radicals and modulate reperfusion injury. Fio_2 can be decreased to the minimum necessary to maintain the Spo_2 at greater than 90%. Special attention should be directed to assessing and supporting RV function during this period, inasmuch as RV failure is the most frequent reason for failure to wean. Although the RV can often be seen in the surgical field, TEE is more valuable for visualizing this structure's functional properties at this juncture. Inotropic support with dobutamine or epinephrine as well as pulmonary vasodilation with nitroglycerin, nitroprusside, milrinone, or nitric oxide may be necessary if RV dysfunction is evident. Milrinone has the advantage of providing both inotropic and vasodilatory effects; however, its administration can be complicated by significant systemic hypotension necessitating the concomitant use of epinephrine or norepinephrine.

Coagulopathy after weaning from CPB is common. The severity of coagulopathy may be worse after double- than single-lung transplantation, probably due to the more extensive dissection, presence of collaterals and scarring, and the longer duration of CPB. Factors under the anesthesiologist's control include incomplete reversal of heparin's effects, which should be assayed by the activated coagulation time. Similarly, preexisting deliberate anticoagulation (e.g., due to warfarin) should be aggressively corrected with fresh frozen plasma. Because platelet dysfunction is common after CPB, empiric administration is justified if coagulopathy persists. The thrombotic and fibrinolytic systems are activated during lung transplantation, especially if CPB is used, and aprotinin can reduce this activation and perhaps reduce perioperative hemorrhage.[49,127,128] The efficacy of ε-aminocaproic acid, tranexamic acid, and desmopressin (DDAVP) in this setting remains unknown.

Reperfusion without CPB is often accompanied by a mild to moderate decrease in systemic blood pressure, and occasionally is complicated by severe hypotension. This is usually the result of profound systemic vasodilation. The etiology is unknown but may be due to ionic loads such as potassium or additives such as prostaglandin E_1 in preservation solutions or vasoactive substances generated during ischemia and reperfusion. This hypotension generally responds well to large doses of α-adrenergic agents and fortunately is short-lived. Agents of greatest use in this setting are norepinephrine and vasopressin. Ventilation is resumed with a lung protection strategy identical to that used when weaning from CPB.

Patients with preexisting increased lung compliance as found in chronic obstructive pulmonary disease can manifest great disparity in lung compliance after single-lung transplant. The donor lung usually exhibits normal to decreased compliance, depending on the presence of reperfusion injury. This will result in relative hyperinflation of the native lung, and underinflation with loss of functional residual capacity in the donor lung. Hyperinflation of the native lung may cause hemodynamic instability due to mediastinal shift, especially if PEEP is applied. Therefore, patients exhibiting signs of hyperinflation during OLV, which improves with deliberate hypoventilation, should be treated with independent lung ventilation after reperfusion. To accomplish this, the patient's postoperative ventilator is brought to the operating room while the donor lung is being implanted. When all anastomoses are completed, the donor lung is ventilated with a normal tidal volume (8 to 10 mL/kg) and rate, with PEEP initially applied at 10 cm H_2O. These settings can be adjusted according to blood gases analysis. The vast majority of gas exchange will take place in the donor lung. The native lung is ventilated with a low tidal volume (2 to 3 mL/kg) and a low rate (2 to 4/min) without PEEP. The objective is to prevent this lung from overinflating or developing a large shunt. Carbon dioxide exchange occurs predominantly in the donor lung.

Although some degree of pulmonary edema is commonly detected by chest radiography postoperatively, it is uncommon to encounter severe pulmonary edema in the operating room immediately after reperfusion of the graft. However, when it does occur, postreperfusion pulmonary edema can be dramatic and life-threatening. Copious pink frothy secretions may require almost constant suctioning to maintain a patent airway and be accompanied by severe gas exchange and compliance abnormalities. Treatment includes high levels of PEEP using selective lung ventilation, diuresis, and volume restriction. Occasionally, patients may require support with ECMO for several days until reperfusion injury resolves; a high percentage of patients so treated ultimately survive.[129,130]

Adequate analgesia is crucial for these patients to facilitate the earliest possible extubation, ambulation, and participation in spirometric exercises to enhance or preserve pulmonary function. Lumbar or thoracic epidural narcotic analgesia provides excellent analgesia while minimizing sedation. Epidural catheters can be placed prior to the procedure if time permits or after conclusion of the procedure. Placement of epidural catheters in cases where a high expectation exists for the necessity of CPB still remains a controversial topic. If CPB has been used or coagulopathy has developed, placement should be deferred until coagulation tests have normalized (see Chapter 37).

Postoperative Management and Complications

Routine postoperative management of the lung transplant recipient continues many of the monitoring modes and therapies begun in the operating room. Positive-pressure ventilation is continued for at least several hours; if differential lung ventilation was used intraoperatively, this is continued in the early postoperative period. Because the lung graft is prone to the development of pulmonary edema due to preservation/reperfusion and the loss of lymphatic drainage, fluid administration is minimized and diuresis encouraged when appropriate. When hemorrhage has ceased, the chest radiograph is clear, and the patient meets conventional extubation criteria, the endotracheal tube can be removed. Prophylactic antibacterial, antifungal, and antiviral therapy, as well as the immunosuppressive regimen of choice, is begun after arrival in the ICU.

Surgical technical complications are uncommon immediately after lung transplantation but may be associated with high morbidity.[131] Pulmonary venous obstruction usually presents as acute, persistent pulmonary edema of the transplanted lung.[132] Color-flow and Doppler TEE will show narrowed pulmonary venous orifices with turbulent, high-velocity flow and loss of the normal phasic waveform. PA anastomotic obstruction should be suspected if PA pressures fail to decrease after reperfusion of the lung graft. If the right PA is obstructed, this is usually evident on a TEE examination in the same way as for pulmonary venous obstruction; it is usually much more difficult to adequately inspect the left PA anastomosis with TEE, although some centers have reported a high success rate.[133] The diagnosis can be definitively made by measuring the pressure gradient across the anastomosis either by inserting needles on both sides of the anastomosis to transduce the respective pressures, or by advancing the PA catheter across it. However, care should be taken not to measure this gradient while the contralateral PA is clamped, because the shunting of the entire CO through one lung will exaggerate the gradient present.[134] Angiography and perfusion scanning are also useful for making this diagnosis, but are not immediately available in the operating room. Bronchial dehiscence or obstruction is extremely rare in the immediate perioperative period, and can be evaluated by fiberoptic bronchoscopy.

Pneumothorax must be a constant concern for the anesthesiologist, especially involving the nonoperative side. Diagnosis of pneumothorax on the nonoperative side during a thoracotomy is extremely difficult. A sudden increase in inflation pressures with deterioration of gas exchange and possibly hypotension are characteristic. However, these same findings are possible with hyperinflation, mucous plugging, or malpositioning of the endobronchial tube. Transient cessation of ventilation and immediate fiberoptic bronchoscopy may rule out the former explanations, and the observation of an upward shift of the mediastinum in the surgical field may be observed in the presence of tension pneumothorax. If this diagnosis is strongly suspected, needle thoracostomy on the field may be lifesaving. Alternatively, the surgeon may be able to directly dissect across the mediastinum and decompress the nonoperative thorax, facilitating reinflation.

Tension pneumopericardium and postoperative hemothorax with complete ventilation/perfusion mismatch are other rare complications that have been reported after lung transplantation.[135,136] Patients with pulmonary hypertension and RV hypertrophy may occasionally develop dynamic RV outflow obstruction when transplantation acutely decreases RV afterload; the diagnosis can be confirmed using TEE.[137] Hyperacute rejection of a kind similar to that seen with heart transplantation has not been noted with lung transplantation.

The most common cause of death in the immediate perioperative period is graft dysfunction from reperfusion injury, which usually presents with hypoxemia, pulmonary infiltrates, poor lung compliance, pulmonary hypertension, and RV failure. If there are no technical reasons to account for pulmonary hypertension and RV failure, then graft dysfunction must be suspected. Unfortunately, few treatments will specifically ameliorate graft dysfunction, and therapy is largely supportive. Vasodilator therapy to directly decrease PVR and therefore RV afterload may improve hemodynamics, and in some cases may improve gas exchange. Both prostaglandin E_1 and nitrates can reverse severe hypoxemia and pulmonary hypertension after lung transplantation, and the latter attenuate the increase in transcription of vasoconstrictor genes (such as for endothelin and platelet-derived growth factor) induced by hypoxia.[138] Indeed, a “prophylactic” low-dose infusion of prostaglandin E_1 has been reported to preserve arterial oxygen tension without altering pulmonary hemodynamics in dogs after single-lung transplantation.[139] Improvement in pulmonary hemodynamics and gas exchange in patients with graft dysfunction has also been reported with the administration of nitric oxide.[82,140,141] Compared with historical control patients who developed graft dysfunction prior to the advent of nitric oxide, inhalation of nitric oxide decreased the duration of mechanical ventilation, frequency of airway complications, and mortality.[141] Improved hemodynamics and gas exchange may reflect the ability of nitric oxide to compensate for the decrease in endothelium-derived relaxant factor activity after transplantation. If nitric oxide has been used to control pulmonary hypertension post-operatively it should be weaned gradually to avoid any rebound pulmonary vasoconstriction.[142] Finally, extracorporeal membrane oxygenation may be employed to support the patient until there is adequate recovery of pulmonary function.[129,130]

Infection is a constant threat in these immunosuppressed patients. Prophylactic antibiotic coverage is aimed at agents commonly causing nosocomial and aspiration pneumonias because these are common in donors. Coverage can be modified once culture results from the donor trachea are available. Patients with cystic fibrosis should receive antibiotics targeted at bacteria found in the native lungs prior to transplantation. Infection should be suspected as the etiology of any infiltrate found on chest radiograph, especially if fever or leukocytosis develops, but distinguishing infection from reperfusion injury and rejection may be very difficult. Diagnostic bronchoscopy and bronchoalveolar lavage are useful in defining therapy and differentiating infection from rejection,[143,144] but open lung biopsy is occasionally necessary for definitive diagnosis. Patients who are seronegative to viral agents to which the donor was seropositive (e.g., cytomegalovirus) will require prophylactic antiviral therapy.

Rejection episodes are common and may occur as early as several days after transplantation. Rejection often presents as new infiltrates on chest radiograph in the setting of deteriorating gas exchange. Bronchoscopy with transbronchial biopsy helps to rule out other causes of deterioration and document acute changes consistent with rejection. Therapy for acute lung rejection consists of large pulses of steroids such as methylprednisolone, or changing the immunosuppressive agents (cyclosporine to tacrolimus or vice versa). Expired nitric oxide has been shown to be an indicator of chronic rejection in post-lung transplant patients. Measurements of expired nitric oxide have been shown to fall with the switch of cyclosporine to tacrolimus reflecting a decrease in the inflammation in the pulmonary mucosa.[145] Expired nitric oxide may be a useful tool to follow patients for the presence or change in chronic graft rejection.[146]

One of the most serious complications of lung transplantation occurs late. Bronchiolitis obliterans is a syndrome characterized by alloimmune injury leading to obstruction of small airways with fibrous scar.[147] Patients with bronchiolitis obliterans present with cough, progressive dyspnea, obstruction on flow spirometry, and interstitial infiltrates on chest radiograph. Therapy for this syndrome includes augmentation of immunosuppression,[148] cytolytic agents (which have been used with varying degrees of success),[149,150] or retransplantation in refractory cases.

Living-Related Lung Transplantation

The scarcity of suitable donor lungs has resulted in waiting times on transplant lists in excess of 2 years, during which as many as 30% of candidates succumb to their illness.[151] Living-related lung transplantation programs have developed to address the needs of lung transplant candidates with acute deterioration expected to preclude survival. Successful grafting of a single lobe for children with bronchopulmonary dysplasia or Eisenmenger's syndrome, or two lobes for children and young adults with cystic fibrosis, has encouraged several centers to consider such procedures.[73,152] The anesthetic management issues related to such undertakings have been recently reviewed.[66,153] Donor candidates will have undergone a rigorous evaluation to ensure that there are no contraindications to lobe donation, and that the donation is not being coerced. Donor lobectomy is performed via a standard posterolateral thoracotomy.[83] Of special note to the anesthesiologist during such procedures is the requirement for OLV to optimize surgical exposure, the continuous infusion of prostaglandin E_1 to promote pulmonary vasodilation, and the administration of heparin and steroids just prior to lobe harvest. Anesthetic management of the recipient is identical to that for a standard lung transplant, except that the use of CPB is mandatory for bilateral lobar transplant.

Pediatric Considerations

The number of pediatric lung transplants has decreased since the late 1990s. Cystic fibrosis, congenital heart disease, and primary pulmonary hypertension are the main indications for lung transplantation in children.[154] In infants, congenital heart disease is the most common indication for lung transplantation, while cystic fibrosis is the most common indication in adolescents. Because of the underlying pulmonary vascular disease or infectious process in these children, bilateral single-lung transplantation (BSLT) is the operation of choice. Single-lung transplantation is less commonly performed in this age group. Transplantation is recommended when the life expectancy of the child is 2 years or less.

BSLT operation is performed via a bilateral anterior thoracotomy with transverse division of the sternum ("clamshell" incision) while the patient is lying supine.[155] Size disparities between the donor and recipient are not uncommon due to the limited donor pool. Accommodation of a large donor lung is achieved by parenchymal reduction. Placement of a small donor lung is facilitated by intraoperative and postoperative pulmonary arterial vasodilation with nitric oxide.

The average experience in pediatric lung transplantation is two or three patients per center per year.[156] The majority of these patients are scheduled as emergencies the day of transplantation. The family and patient are usually very anxious. Judicious premedication is given to the recipient before general anesthesia. Morbidity during induction of anesthesia is increased by hypoxemia, hypercapnea, and systemic hypotension in these critically ill patients.

After placement of routine monitors, anesthesia is induced with a hypnotic agent (e.g., etomidate), an opioid, and titration of an inhalation agent. A muscle relaxant is added to facilitate tracheal intubation. Cardiac arrest and circulatory collapse may occur after induction of anesthesia in the recipient with primary pulmonary hypertension and congenital heart disease with pulmonary hypertension.[157] An inhalation agent, additional opioid, benzodiazepines, and muscle relaxants are used throughout the procedure. A thickened hypertrophic RV requires additional volume administration. Frequent endotracheal tube suctioning is usually required in the recipient with cystic fibrosis intraoperatively prior to transplantation.

In contrast to the adult population, CPB is frequently used during lung transplantation in children, and thus aprotinin will frequently be required. Bronchial anastomosis is assessed by fiberoptic bronchoscopy. A PA catheter is advanced after unclamping of the PA.

Weaning from CPB is challenging and may be complicated by bleeding, reperfusion injury, pulmonary hypertension, and pulmonary edema. During weaning from bypass, the FIO_2 is decreased to prevent reperfusion injury. Moderate levels of positive end-expiratory pressure are used to treat pulmonary edema. The patient is kept sedated and the trachea intubated. A thoracic epidural facilitates weaning from mechanical ventilation and extubation in the intensive care unit. Low dose dopamine enhances renal blood flow after CPB.[158]

The immediate postoperative course can be complicated by graft failure or dysfunction and/or infection. After the first year, morbidity is increased by bronchiolitis obliterans, systemic hypertension, renal dysfunction, and diabetes mellitus.

HEART-LUNG TRANSPLANTATION

History and Epidemiology

The diminished frequency of heart-lung transplantation over the past decade reflects that it is being supplanted by lung transplantation. The number of heart-lung transplants worldwide peaked at 241 in 1989, and there has been a continual decline in subsequent years to approximately half that number.[3] Approximately only 173 heart-lung transplant candidates were registered with the United Network for Organ Sharing as of early March 2005, less than 5% of the number on the lung transplant list. The most common recipient indications remain primary pulmonary hypertension, congenital heart disease (including Eisenmenger's syndrome), and cystic fibrosis.

One-year survival after heart-lung transplantation is 60%, significantly lower than that for isolated heart or lung transplantation.[3] Mortality in subsequent years is approximately 4% per year, similar to that for heart transplantation. Risk factors for increased mortality after heart-lung transplant are recipient ventilator dependence, male recipient gender, and a donor age greater than 40 years.[3] Early deaths are most often due to graft failure or hemorrhage, while midterm and late deaths are primarily due to infection and bronchiolitis obliterans, respectively. Repeat heart-lung transplant is a rare procedure and likely to remain so because the 1-year survival after repeat heart-lung transplant is dismal (28%).[3]

Recipient Selection

Candidates undergo an evaluation similar to that for lung transplant candidates. As more patients with pulmonary hypertension and cystic fibrosis are treated with isolated lung transplantation, it is likely that the indications for heart-lung transplantation will be limited to congenital heart disease with irreversible pulmonary hypertension that is not amenable to repair during simultaneous lung transplantation or diseases with both pulmonary hypertension and concomitant severe left ventricular dysfunction.

Donor Selection and Graft Harvest

Potential heart-lung donors must meet not only the criteria for heart donors but also those for lung donation, both described earlier in this chapter. Graft harvesting is carried out in a manner similar to that previously described for heart transplantation. After mobilization of the major vessels and trachea, cardiac arrest is induced with inflow occlusion and infusion of cold cardioplegia into the aortic root. After arrest, the pulmonary artery is flushed with a cold preservative solution often containing prostaglandin E_1. The ascending aorta, superior vena cava, and trachea are transected, and the heart-lung bloc removed after it is dissected free of the esophagus. The trachea is clamped and the graft immersed in cold solution prior to being bagged for transport.

Surgical Procedures

The operation is generally performed through a median sternotomy, but a clamshell thoracosternotomy is also an acceptable approach. Both pleurae are incised. Any pulmonary adhesions are taken down prior to anticoagulation for bypass. Cannulas for cardiopulmonary bypass are placed in a manner similar to that for heart transplantation. After the aorta is cross-clamped, the heart is excised in a manner similar to that for orthotopic heart transplant. Each lung is then individually removed, including its pulmonary veins. The airways are divided at the level of the respective main bronchi for bibronchial anastomoses. For a tracheal anastomosis, the trachea is freed to the level of the carina without stripping its blood supply, and an anastomosis is constructed just above the level of the carina. The atrial anastomosis is performed in a manner similar to that for orthotopic heart transplantation, and finally the aorta is joined to the recipient aorta. After de-airing and reperfusion, the patient is weaned from cardiopulmonary bypass, hemostasis is achieved, and the wound is closed.

Pathophysiology Before Transplantation

The pathophysiology of heart-lung transplant recipients combines the elements discussed earlier in this chapter. Patients usually have end-stage biventricular failure with severe pulmonary hypertension. The cardiac anatomy may be characterized by complex congenital malformations. If obstruction of pulmonary airflow is present, there is a danger of hyperinflation after application of positive-pressure ventilation.

Pathophysiology After Transplantation

Like isolated heart recipients, heart-lung transplant recipients' physiology is characterized by cardiac denervation; transient cardiac ischemic insult during graft harvest, transport, and implantation; and long-term susceptibility to accelerated allograft vasculopathy and rejection. As is the case for lung recipients, heart-lung recipients have denervated pulmonary vascular and airway smooth muscle responses, transient pulmonary ischemic insult, altered pulmonary lymphatic drainage, and impaired mucociliary clearance.

Anesthetic Management

The anesthetic management of heart-lung transplantation more closely resembles that of heart than lung transplantation, because the use of cardiopulmonary bypass is mandatory. After placement of invasive and noninvasive monitoring similar to that used for heart transplantation, anesthesia can be induced with any of the techniques previously described for heart and lung transplantation. Similar to lung transplantation, avoidance of myocardial depression as well as protection and control of the airway are paramount. Although a double-lumen endotracheal tube is not mandatory, it aids in exposure of the posterior mediastinum for hemostasis after weaning from cardiopulmonary bypass. Otherwise, anesthetic management prior to cardiopulmonary bypass is similar to that for heart transplantation.

A bolus of glucocorticoid (e.g., methylprednisolone, 500 mg) is given when the aortic cross-clamp is removed. After a period of reperfusion, an inotrope infusion is started, and the heart is inspected for adequate de-airing with TEE. Ventilation is resumed with normal tidal volume and rate and the addition of PEEP (5 to 10 cm) prior to weaning from cardiopulmonary bypass. After successful weaning from cardiopulmonary bypass, the pulmonary artery catheter can be advanced into the pulmonary artery again. Protamine is then administered to reverse heparin-induced anticoagulation. The inspired oxygen concentration can often be decreased to less toxic levels based on blood gas analysis.

Problems encountered after weaning from cardiopulmonary bypass are similar to those encountered after isolated heart or lung transplantation. Lung reperfusion injury and dysfunction may compromise gas exchange, so administration of crystalloid should be minimized. Occasionally, postreperfusion pulmonary edema may require support with high levels of PEEP and inspired oxygen in the operating room. Ventricular failure usually responds to an increase in β-adrenergic support. Unlike isolated heart or lung transplantation, frank right ventricular failure is uncommon immediately after heart-lung transplantation unless lung preservation was grossly inadequate. Coagulopathy is often present after heart-lung transplant, and should be aggressively treated with additional protamine (if indicated), platelets, and fresh frozen plasma. Aprotinin can dramatically decrease hemorrhage after heart-lung transplant and reduce transfusion of red blood cells and platelets, and it is associated with a lower alveolar-arterial gradient for oxygen after transplantation.[49,102]

Postoperative Management and Complications

The principles of the immediate postoperative care of heart-lung transplant recipients are a combination of those for isolated heart and lung recipients. Invasive and noninvasive monitoring done in the operating room is continued. Inotropic support is continued in a manner similar to that for heart transplantation. Ventilatory support is similar to that after lung transplantation; the lowest acceptable inspired oxygen concentration is used to avoid oxygen toxicity, and the patient is weaned from the ventilator after hemodynamics have been stable for several hours, hemorrhage has ceased, and satisfactory gas exchange is present. Diuresis is encouraged. Finally, the immunosuppressive regimen of choice is begun. Barring any complications, the patient can be discharged from the intensive care unit after several days.

Infection is a more frequent and serious complication in heart-lung recipients than in isolated heart recipients. Bacterial and fungal infections are especially common in the first month after transplantation, with viral and other pathogens (*Pneumocystis carinii* and *Nocardia*) occurring in subsequent months.[159]

Similar to isolated heart or lung transplants, rejection episodes are common early after heart-lung transplantation. Rejection may occur independently in either the heart or lung.[103] Therapy is similar to that for rejection of isolated heart or lung grafts.

Heart grafts in heart-lung blocks are prone to accelerated coronary vasculopathy in a manner similar to those of isolated heart grafts. As with lung transplantation, a feared late complication of heart-lung transplantation is bronchiolitis obliterans. Clinical presentation is similar to that seen with lung transplant patients. Approximately one third of heart-lung recipients develop this process. Anecdotal reports indicate that most affected patients also have accelerated coronary vasculopathy.

Pediatric Considerations

Although combined heart-lung transplant has been a rarely performed procedure, it saw substantial application in the pediatric population during its early history. Of the 49 cases performed in the United States in 1992, more than half were in children.[160] Since that time the number of pediatric heart-lung transplantations has continued to decrease.[161] Only 10 pediatric heart-lung transplants were performed in 2001 worldwide. In this group of patients, cystic fibrosis and congenital heart disease are the main indications. The overall decline has been attributed to earlier referral for isolated lung transplantation, before cor pulmonale becomes irreversible. Only 20% of recipients are alive 10 years after transplantation. Early mortality is caused by graft failure, while more than 1 year after transplantation the cause is often bronchiolitis obliterans. The lack of survival improvement in these patients calls for re-assessment of combined heart-lung transplantation in children.

REFERENCES

1. Carrel A, Guthrie CC: The transplantation of veins and organs. Am J Med 1:1101, 1905
2. Barnard CN: The operation. S Afr Med J 1271, 1967
3. Hosenpud JD, Novick RJ, Bennett LE, et al: The Registry of the International Society for Heart and Lung Transplantation: Thirteenth official report. J Heart Lung Transplant 15:655, 1996
4. Organ Procurement and Transplantation Network: OPTN 2003 Annual Report. Available at www.optn.org
5. Murali S, Kormos RL, Uretsky BF, et al: Preoperative pulmonary hemodynamics and early mortality after orthotopic cardiac transplantation: The Pittsburgh experience. Am Heart J 126:896, 1993
6. Darby JM, Stein K, Grenvik A, et al: Approach to management of the heartbeating brain dead organ donor. JAMA 261:2222, 1989
7. Nygaard CE, Townsend RN, Diamond DL: Organ donor management and organ outcome: A 6 year review from a level 1 trauma center. J Trauma 30:728, 1990
8. Wood KE, Becker BN, McCartney JG, et al: Care of the potential organ donor. N Engl J Med 351:2730, 2004
9. Votapka TV, Canvasser DA, Pennington DG, et al: Effect of triiodothyronine on graft function in a model of heart transplantation. Ann Thoracic Surg 62:78, 1996
10. Novitzky D, Cooper DKC, Reichart B: Hemodynamic and metabolic responses to hormonal therapy in brain-dead potential organ donors. Transplantation 43:852, 1987
11. Randell TT, Hockerstedt KA: Triiodothyronine treatment in brain-dead multiorgan donors: A controlled study. Transplantation 54:736, 1992
12. Hardesty RL, Griffith BP, Deep GM, et al: Improved cardiac function using cardioplegia during procurement and transplantation. Transplant Proc 15:1253, 1983
13. Watson DC, Reitz BA, Baumgartner WA: Distant heart procurement for transplantation. Surgery 86:56, 1979
14. Grant SCD, Khan MA, Yonan N, et al: Technique of anastomosis and incidence of atrial tachyarrhythmias following heart transplantation. Br Heart J 71:40, 1994
15. El-Gamel A, Deiraniya AK, Rahman AN, et al: Orthotopic heart transplantation hemodynamics: Does atrial preservation improve cardiac output after transplantation? J Heart Lung Transplant 15:564, 1996
16. Mehta SM, Aufiero TX, Pae WE: Combined Registry for the Clinical Use of Mechanical Ventricular Assist Pumps and the Total Artificial Heart in Conjunction with Heart Transplantation: Sixth official report. J Heart Lung Transplant 14:585, 1994
17. Goldstein DJ, Oz MC, Smith CR, et al: Safety of repeat aprotinin administration for LVAD recipients undergoing cardiac transplantation. Ann Thorac Surg 61:692, 1996
18. Shaw BW Jr, Bahnson HT, Hardesty RL, et al: Combined transplantation of the heart and liver. Ann Surg 202:667, 1985
19. Bristow MR, Ginsburg R, Minobe W, et al: Decreased catecholamine sensitivity and beta adrenergic receptor density in failing human hearts. N Engl J Med 307:205, 1982
20. Cohn JN, Archibald DG, Ziesche S, et al: Effect of vasodilator therapy on mortality in chronic congestive heart failure. N Engl J Med 314:1547, 1986

21. Anonymous: Effects of enalapril on mortality in severe congestive heart failure. Results of Cooperative North Scandinavian Enalapril Survival Study (Consensus). N Engl J Med 316:1429, 1987
22. Kalman J, Buchholz C, Steinmetz M, et al: Safety and efficacy of beta-blockade in patients with chronic congestive heart failure awaiting transplantation. J Heart Lung Transplant 14:1212, 1995
23. Remme WJ: Inodilator Therapy for heart failure. Early, late or not at all? Circulation 87:IV, 1993
24. Packer M, Carver JR, Rodeheffer RJ, et al: Effect of oral milrinone on mortality in severe chronic heart failure. N Engl J Med 325:1468, 1991
25. Steed DL, Brown B, Reilly JJ, et al: General surgical complications in heart and heart-lung transplantation. Surgery 98:739, 1985
26. Isono SS, Woolson ST, Schurman DJ: Total joint arthroplasty for steroid-induced osteonecrosis in cardiac transplant patients. Clin Orthop 217: 201, 1987
27. Stinson EB, Griepp RB, Schroeder JS: Hemodynamic observations one and two years after cardiac transplantation in man. Circulation 45:1183, 1972
28. Rowan RA, Billingham ME: Myocardial innervation in long-term heart transplant survivors: A quantitative ultrastructural survey. J Heart Transplant 7:448, 1988
29. Wilson RF, Christensen BV, Olivari MT, et al: Evidence for structural sympathetic reinnervation after orthotopic cardiac transplantation in humans. Circulation 83:1210, 1991
30. Stinson EB, Griepp RB, Clark DA, et al: Cardiac transplantation in man. VIII. Survival and function. J Heart Transplant 7:145, 1970
31. Verani MS, George SE, Leon CA, et al: Systolic and diastolic ventricular performance at rest and during exercise in heart transplantation recipients. J Heart Transplant 7:145, 1988
32. Kent KM, Cooper T: The denervated heart: A model for studying autonomic control of the heart. N Engl J Med 291:1017, 1974
33. Goodman DJ, Rossen RM, Cannom DS, et al: Effect of digoxin on atrioventricular conduction. Studies in patients with and without cardiac autonomic innervation. Circulation 51:251, 1975
34. Backman SB, Ralley FE, Fox GS: Neostigmine produces bradycardia in a heart transplant recipient. Anesthesiology 78:777, 1993
35. Borow KM, Neumann A, Arensman FW, et al: Cardiac and peripheral vascular responses to adrenoceptor stimulation and blockade after cardiac transplantation. J Am Coll Cardiol 14:1229, 1989
36. Tuzcu EM, DeFranco AC, Hobbs R, et al: Prevalence and distribution of transplant coronary artery disease. J Heart Lung Transplant 14:S202, 1995
37. Hosenpud JD, Morris TE, Shipley GD, et al: Cardiac allograft vasculopathy transplantation. Transplantation 61:939, 1996
38. Gao SZ, Hunt SA, Schroeder JS, et al: Early development of accelerated graft coronary artery disease: Risk factors and course. J Am Coll Cardiol 28:673, 1996
39. Stark RP, McGinn AL, Wilson RF: Chest pain in cardiac-transplant recipients. N Engl J Med 324:1791, 1991
40. Smart FW, Ballantyne CM, Cocanougher B, et al: Insensitivity of non-invasive test to detect coronary artery vasculopathy after heart transplant. Am J Cardiol 67:243, 1991
41. St Goar FG, Pinto FJ, Alderman EL, et al: Intracoronary ultrasound in cardiac transplant recipients: In vivo evidence of angiographically silent intimal thickening. Circulation 85:979, 1992
42. Akosah KO, Mohanty PK, Funai JT, et al: Noninvasive detection of transplant coronary artery disease by dobutamine stress echocardiography. J Heart Lung Transplant 13:1024, 1994
43. Waterman PM, Bjerke R: Rapid-sequence induction technique in patients with severe ventricular dysfunction. J Cardiothorac Anesth 2:602, 1988
44. Murkin JM, Moldenhauer CC, Hug CC Jr: High-dose fentanyl for rapid induction of anaesthesia in patients with coronary artery disease. Can Anaesth Soc J 32:320, 1985
45. Hensley FA, Martin DE, Larach DR, et al: Anesthetic management for cardiac transplantation in North America. J Cardiothorac Anesth 1:429, 1987
46. Berberich JJ, Fabian JA: A retrospective analysis of fentanyl and sufentanil for cardiac transplantation. J Cardiothorac Anesth 1:200, 1987
47. Armitage JM, Hardesty RL, Griffith BP: An effective treatment of right heart failure after orthotopic heart transplantation. J Heart Transplant 6:348, 1987
48. Fonger JD, Borkon AM, Baumgartner WA: Acute right ventricular failure following heart transplantation: Improvement with PGE1 and right ventricular assist. J Heart Transplant 5:317, 1986
49. Royston D: Aprotinin therapy in heart and heart-lung transplantation. J Heart Lung Transplant 12:S19, 1993
50. Propost JW, Siegel LC, Feeley TW: Effect of aprotinin on transfusion requirements during repeat sternotomy for cardiac transplantation surgery. Transplant Proc 26:3719, 1994
51. Stein KL, Armitage JM, Martich GD: Intensive care of the cardiac transplant recipient. *In* Ayres SM, Grenvik A, Holbrook PR, Shoemaker WC (eds): Textbook of Critical Care, 3rd edition. Philadelphia, WB Saunders, 1995, p 1649
52. Weil R III, Clarke DR, Iwaki Y, et al: Hyperacute rejection of a transplanted human heart. Transplantation 32:71, 1981
53. Bhatia SJS, Kirshenbaum JM, Shemin RJ, et al: Time course of resolution of pulmonary hypertension and right ventricular remodeling after orthotopic cardiac transplantation. Circulation 76:819, 1987
54. Villanueva FS, Murali S, Uretsky BF, et al: Resolution of severe pulmonary hypertension after heterotopic cardiac transplantation. J Am Coll Cardiol 14:1239, 1989
55. Jacquet L, Ziady G, Stein K, et al: Cardiac rhythm disturbances early after orthotopic heart transplantation: Prevalence and clinical importance of the observed abnormalities. J Am Coll Cardiol 16:832, 1990
56. Scott CD, Omar I, McComb JM, et al: Long-term pacing in heart transplant recipients is usually unnecessary. PACE Pacing Clin Electrophysiol 14:1792, 1991
57. Romhilt DW, Doyle M, Sagar KB, et al: Prevalence and significance of arrhythmias in long-term survivors of cardiac transplantation. Circulation 66:I, 1982
58. Chomette G, Auriol M, Beaufil H, et al: Morphology of cyclosporine nephrotoxicity in human heart transplant recipients. J Heart Transplant 5:273, 1986
59. Platz KP, Mueller AR, Blumhardt G, et al: Nephrotoxicity following orthotopic liver transplantation. A comparison between cyclosporine and FK506. Transplantation 58:170, 1994
60. Burch M: Current status of paediatric heart, lung, and heart-lung transplantation. Arch Dis Child 89:386, 2004
61. Lillehei CW, Mayer JE Jr, Shamberger RC, et al: Pediatric lung transplantation and "lessons from green surgery." Ann Thorac Surg 68:S25, 1999
62. Spray TL, Bridges ND: Lung transplantation for pediatric pulmonary hypertension. Prog Pediatr Cardiol 12:319, 2001
63. Olson CM (ed): Diagnostic and therapeutic technology assessment: Lung transplantation. JAMA 269:931, 1993
64. Kaye MP: The Registry of the International Society for Heart and Lung Transplantation: Ninth official report. J Heart Lung Transplant 11:599, 1992
65. Trulock EP, Cooper JD, Kaiser LR, et al: The Washington University-Barnes Hospital experience with lung transplantation. JAMA 266:1943, 1991
66. Quinlan JJ, Gasior TA, Firestone S, et al: Anesthesia for living-related (lobar) lung transplantation. J Cardiothorac Vasc Anesth 1996:391, 1996
67. Novick RJ, Kaye MP, Patterson GA, et al: Redo lung transplantation: A North American-European experience. J Heart Lung Transplant 12:5, 1993
68. Gorcsan J III, Edward TD, Ziady GM, et al: Transesophageal echocardiography to evaluate patients with severe pulmonary hypertension for lung transplantation. Ann Thorac Surg 59:717, 1995
69. Hardesty RL, Aeba R, Armitage JM, et al: A clinical trial of University of Wisconsin solution for pulmonary preservation. J Thorac Cardiovasc Surg 105:660, 1993
70. Gilbert S, Dauber J, Hattler B, et al: Lung and heart-lung transplantation at the University of Pittsburgh 1982-2002. Clin Transplants 253, 2002
71. Brower RG, Matthay MA, Morris A, et al: Ventilation with lower tidal volumes as compared with traditional tidal volumes for acute lung injury and the acute respiratory distress syndrome. The Acute Respiratory Distress Syndrome Network. N Engl J Med 342:1301, 2000
72. Low DE, Trulock EP, Kaiser LR, et al: Morbidity, mortality, and early results of single versus bilateral lung transplantation for emphysema. J Thorac Cardiovasc Surg 103:1119, 1992
73. Starnes VA, Barr ML, Cohen RG: Lobar transplantation: Indications, technique and outcome. J Thorac Cardiovasc Surg 108:403, 1994
74. Kaiser LR, Pasque MK, Trulock EP, et al: Bilateral sequential lung transplantation: The procedure of choice for double-lung replacement. Ann Thorac Surg 52:438, 1991
75. Bisson A, Bonnette P: A new technique for double-lung transplantation. J Thorac Cardiovasc Surg 103:40, 1992
76. Pepe PE, Marini JJ: Occult positive end-expiratory pressure in mechanically ventilated patients with airflow obstruction. The auto-PEEP effect. Am Rev Respir Dis 126:166, 1982

77. Haluszka J, Chartrand DA, Grassino AE, et al: Intrinsic PEEP and arterial PCO2 in stable patients with chronic obstructive pulmonary disease. Am Rev Respir Dis 1990:1194, 1990
78. Quinlan JJ, Buffington CW: Deliberate hypoventilation in a patient with air trapping during lung transplantation. Anesthesiology 78:1177, 1993
79. Smith TC, Marini JJ: Impact of PEEP on lung mechanics and work of breathing in severe airflow obstruction. J Appl Physiol 65:1488, 1988
80. Biondi JW, Hines RL, Matthay RA: Comparative Right ventricular function during assist control, intermittent mandatory and spontaneous ventilation. Anesthes Analg 65:S18, 1986
81. Prewitt R, Ghignone M: Treatment of right ventricular dysfunction in acute respiratory failure. Crit Care Med 5:346, 1983
82. Adatia I, Lillehei C, Arnold JH, et al: Inhaled nitric oxide in the treatment of postoperative graft dysfunction after lung transplantation. Ann Thorac Surg 57:1311, 1994
83. Cohen RG, Barr ML, Schenkel FA, et al: Living-related donor lobectomy for bilateral lobar transplantation in patients with cystic fibrosis. Ann Thorac Surg 1994:1423, 1994
84. Kramer MR, Marshall SE, McDougall IR, et al: The distribution of ventilation and perfusion after single-lung transplantation in patients with pulmonary fibrosis and pulmonary hypertension. Transplant Proc 23:1215, 1991
85. Maurer JR, McLean PA, Cooper JD, et al: Airway hyperractivity in patients undergoing lung and heart/lung transplantation. Am Rev Respir Dis 139:1038, 1989
86. Herve P, Picard N, Le Roy Ladurie M, et al: Lack of bronchial hyperresponsiveness to methacholine and to isocapnic dry air hyperventilation in heart/lung and double-lung transplant recipients with normal lung histology. Am Rev Respir Dis 145:1503, 1992
87. Tavakoli R, Buvry A, Le Gall G, et al: In vitro bronchial hyperresponsiveness after lung transplantation in the rat. Am J Physiol 262:L322, 1992
88. Stretton CD, Mak JCW, Belvisi MG, et al: Cholinergic control of human airways in vitro following extrinsic denervation of the human respiratory tract by heart-lung transplantation. Am Rev Respir Dis 142:1030, 1990
89. Takichi T, Maeda M, Shirakusa T, et al: Sympathetic reinnervation of unilaterally denervated rat lung. Acta Physiol Scand 154:43, 1995
90. Clifford PS, Coon RL, Von Colditz JH, et al: Pulmonary denervation in the dog. J Appl Physiol 54:1451, 1983
91. Dolovich M, Rossman C, Chambers C: Muco-ciliary function in patients following single lung or lung/heart transplantation. Am Rev Respir Dis 135:A363, 1987
92. Fullerton DA, Mitchell MB, McIntyre RC, et al: Cold ischemia and reperfusion each produce pulmonary vasomotor dysfunction in the transplanted lung. J Thorac Cardiovasc Surg 106:1213, 1993
93. Hunter DN, Morgan CJ, Yacoub M, et al: Pulmonary endothelial permeability following lung transplantation. Chest 102:417, 1992
94. Shennib H, Serrick C, Saleh D, et al: Plasma endothelin-1 levels in human lung transplant recipients. J Cardiovasc Pharmacol 26(suppl 3):S516, 1995
95. Flavahan NA, Aleskowitch TD, Murray PA: Endothelial and vascular smooth muscle responses are altered after left lung autotransplantation. Am J Physiol 266:H2026, 1994
96. Kukkonen S, Heikkila L, Verkkala K, et al: Pulmonary vasodilatory properties of prostaglandin E1 are blunted after experimental single-lung transplantation. J Heart Lung Transplant 14:280, 1995
97. Ueda K, Date H, Fujita T, et al: Effects of Inhaled nitric oxide in a canine living-donor lobar lung transplant model. Jpn J Thorac Cardiovasc Surg 48:693, 2000
98. Lang JD Jr, Leill W: Pro: Inhaled nitric oxide should be used routinely in patients undergoing lung transplantation. J Cardiothorac Vasc Anesth 15:7859, 2001
99. Karamasetty M, Klinger J: NO: More than just a vasodilator in lung transplantation. Am J Respir Cell Mol Biol 26:1, 2002
100. Meade MO, Granton J, Matte-Martyn A, et al: A randomized trial of inhaled nitric oxide to prevent ischemia reperfusion injury after lung transplantation. Am J Respir Crit Care Med 167:1483, 2003
101. Ardehali A, Laks H, Levine M, et al: A prospective trial of inhaled nitric oxide in clinical lung transplantation. Transplantation 72:112, 2001
102. Royston D: High-dose aprotinin therapy: A review of the first five years' experience. J Cardiothorac Vasc Anesth 6:76, 1992
103. Griffith BP, Hardesty RL, Trento A, et al: Asynchronous rejection of heart and lungs following cardiopulmonary transplantation. Ann Thorac Surg 40:488, 1985
104. Smyth RL, Scott JP, Whitehead B: Heart-lung transplantation in children. Transplant Proc 22:1470, 1990
105. Starnes VA, Marshall SE, Lewiston NJ, et al: Heart-lung transplantation in infants, children and adolescents. J Pediatr Surg 26:434, 1991
106. Corris PA, Odom NJ, Jackson G, et al: Reimplantation injury after lung transplantation in a rat model. J Heart Transplant 6:234, 1987
107. Jones MT, Hsieh C, Yoshikawa K, et al: A new model for assessment of lung preservation. J Thorac Cardiovasc Surg 96:608, 1988
108. Katz WE, Gasior TA, Quinlan JJ, et al: Immediate effects of lung transplantation on right ventricular morphology and function in patients with variable degrees of pulmonary hypertension. J Am Coll Cardiol 27:384, 1996
109. Yeoh TK, Kramer MR, Marshall S, et al: Changes in cardiac morphology and function following single-lung transplantation. Transplant Proc 23:1226, 1991
110. Frist WH, Lorenz CH, Walker ES, et al: MRI complements standard assessment of right ventricular function after lung transplantation. Ann Thorac Surg 60:268, 1995
111. Carere R, Patterson GA, Liu PP, et al: Right and left ventricular performance after single and double-lung transplantation. J Thorac Cardiovasc Surg 102:115, 1991
112. Ritchie M, Waggoner AD, Davila-Roman VG, et al: Echocardiographic characterization of the improvement in right ventricular function in patients with severe pulmonary hypertension after single-lung transplantation. J Am Coll Cardiol 22:1170, 1993
113. Scuderi LJ, Bailey SR, Calhoon JH, et al: Echocardiographic assessment of right and left ventricular function after single-lung transplantation. Am Heart J 127:636, 1994
114. Kramer MR, Valatine HA, Marshall SE, et al: Recovery of the right ventricle after single-lung transplantation in pulmonary hypertension. Am J Cardiol 73:494, 1994
115. Triantafillow AN, Benumof JL, Lecamwasam HS: Physiology of the lateral decubitus position, the open chest, and one lung ventilation. *In* Kaplan JA, Slinger PD (eds): Thoracic Anesthesia, 3rd edition. Philadelphia, Churchill Livingstone, 2003, pp 71–94
116. Hirt SW, Haverich A, Wahlers T, et al: Predictive criteria for the need of extracorporeal circulation in single-lung transplantation. Ann Thorac Surg 54:676, 1992
117. Chetham P: Anesthesia for heart or single or double lung transplantation. J Card Surg 15:167, 2000
118. Myles PS, Venama H: Avoidance of cardiopulmonary bypass during bilateral sequential lung transplantation using inhaled nitric oxide. J Cardiothorac Vasc Anesth 9:571, 1995
119. Myles PS, Weeks AM, Buckland MR, et al: Anesthesia for bilateral sequential lung transplantation: Experience of 64 cases. J Cardiothorac Vasc Anesth 11:177, 1997
120. Triantafillou AN, Pasque MK, Huddleston CB, et al: Predictors, frequency, and indications for cardiopulmonary bypass during lung transplantation in adults. Ann Thorac Surg 57:1248, 1994
121. Aeba R, Griffith BP, Kormos RL, et al: Effect of cardiopulmonary bypass on early graft dysfunction in clinical lung transplantation. Ann Thorac Surg 1994:715, 1994
122. Fullerton DA, McIntyre RC, Mitchell MB, et al: Lung transplantation with cardiopulmonary bypass exaggerates pulmonary vasomotor dysfunction in the transplanted lung. J Thorac Cardiovasc Surg 109:212, 1995
123. Firestone L, Carrera J, Firestone S, et al: Single-lung transplants: Who needs bypass? Anesthesiology 79:A46, 1993
124. Sekela ME, Noon GP, Holland VA, et al: Differential perfusion: Potential complication of femoral-femoral bypass during single lung transplantation. J Heart Lung Transplant 10:322, 1991
125. Ko WJ, Chen YS: Replacing cardiopulmonary bypass with extracorporeal membrane oxygenation in lung transplantation operations. Artif Organs 25:607, 2001
126. Pereszlenyi A, Lang G, Steltzer H, et al: Bilateral lung transplantation with intra and postoperatively prolonged ECMO support in patients with pulmonary hypertension. Eur J Cardiothorac Surg 21:858, 2002
127. Gu YJ, de Haan J, Brenken UP, et al: Clotting and fibrinolytic disturbance during lung transplantation: Effect of low-dose aprotinin. J Thorac Cardiovasc Surg 112:599, 1996
128. Jaquiss RD, Huddleston CB, Spray TL: Use of aprotinin in pediatric lung transplantation. J Heart Lung Transplant 14:302, 1995
129. Zenati M, Pham SM, Keenan RJ, et al: Extracorporeal membrane oxygenation for lung transplant recipients with primary severe donor lung dysfunction. Transplant Int 9:227, 1996
130. Glassman LR, Keenan RJ, Fabrizio MC, et al: Extracorporeal membrane oxygenation as an adjunct treatment for primary graft failure in adult lung transplant recipients. J Thorac Cardiovasc Surg 110:723, 1995
131. Leibowitz DW, Smith CR, Michler RE, et al: Incidence of pulmonary vein complications after lung transplantation: A prospective

transesophageal echocardiographic study. J Am Coll Cardiol 24:671, 1994
132. Malden ES, Kaiser LR, Gutierrez FR: Pulmonary vein obstruction following single-lung transplantation. Chest 102:671, 1992
133. Hausmann D, Daniel WG, Mugge A, et al: Imaging of pulmonary artery and vein anastomoses by transesophageal echocardiography after lung transplantation. Circulation 86:II, 1992
134. Despotis GJ, Karanikolas M, Triantafillou AN, et al: Pressure gradient across the pulmonary artery anastomosis during lung transplantation. Ann Thorac Surg 60:630, 1995
135. Cohrane LJ, Mitchell ME, Raju S, et al: Tension pneumopericardium as a complication of single-lung transplantation. Ann Thoracic Surg 50:808, 1990
136. Jellinek H, Klepetko W, Hiesmayr M: Komplettes Ventilations/Perfusions Mibverhaltnis Nachy Einseitiger Lungentransplantation und Postoperativem Hamatothorax. Anaesthetist 41:134, 1992
137. Gorcsan J III, Reddy SC, Armitage JM, et al: Acquired right ventricular outflow tract obstruction after lung transplantation: Diagnosis by transesophageal echocardiography. Am Soc Echocardiogr 6:324, 1993
138. Mentzer SJ, Reilly JJ, DeCamp M, et al: Potential mechanism of vasomotor dysregulation after lung transplantation for primary pulmonary hypertension. J Heart Lung Transplant 14:387, 1995
139. Aoe M, Trachiotis GD, Okabayashi K, et al: Administration of prostaglandin E1 after lung transplantation improves early graft function. Ann Thoracic Surg 58:655, 1994
140. MacDonald P, Mundy J, Rogers P, et al: Successful treatment of life-threatening acute reperfusion injury after lung transplantation with inhaled nitric oxide. J Thorac Cardiovasc Surg 110:861, 1995
141. Date H, Triantafillou AN, Trulock EP, et al: Inhaled nitric oxide reduced human lung allograft dysfunction. J Thorac Cardiovasc Surg 111:913, 1996
142. Lindberg L, Sjoberg T, Ingemansson R, et al: Inhalation of nitric oxide after lung transplantation. Ann Thorac Surg 61:956, 1996
143. Scott JP, Fradet G, Smyth RL, et al: Prospective study of transbronchial biopsies in the management of heart-lung and single lung transplant patients. J Heart Lung Transplant 10:626, 1991
144. Higgenbottam T, Stewart S, Penketh A, et al: Transbronchial lung biopsy for the diagnosis of rejection in heart-lung transplant patients. Transplantation 46:532, 1988
145. Verleden G, Dupont L, Raemdonck DV, et al: Effect of switching from cyclosporine to tacrolimus on exhaled nitric oxide and pulmonary function in patients with chronic rejection after lung transplantation. J Heart Lung Transpl 22:9083, 2002
146. Gabbay E, Walters EH, Orsida B, et al: Post-lung transplant bronchiolitis obliterans syndrome (BOS) is characterized by increased exhaled nitric oxide levels and epithelial inducible nitric oxide synthetase. Am J Respir Crit Care Med 162:2182, 2000
147. Reichenspurner H, Girgis RE, Robbins RC, et al: Obliterative bronchiolitis after lung and heart-lung transplantation. Ann Thorac Surg 60:1845, 1995
148. Allen MD, Burke CM, McGregor CGA, et al: Steroid-responsive bronchiolitis after human heart-lung transplantation. J Thorac Cardiovasc Surg 92:449, 1986
149. Snell GI, Esmore DS, Williams TJ: Cytolytic therapy for the bronchiolitis obliterans syndrome complicating lung transplantation. Chest 109:874, 1996
150. Kesten S, Rajagopalan N, Maurer J: Cytolytic therapy for the treatment of bronchiolitis obliterans syndrome following lung transplantation. Transplantation 61:427, 1996
151. Paradis I, Manzetti J, Foust D: When to refer for lung transplantation? Characteristics of candidates who die vs. those who survive to receive a transplant. Am Rev Respir Dis 147:A597, 1993
152. Starnes VA, Lewiston NJ, Luikart H, et al: Current trends in lung transplantation: Lobar transplantation and expanded use of single lungs. J Thorac Cardiovasc Surg 104:1060, 1992
153. Veeken C, Palmer SM, Davis RD, Gricknik KP: Living-related lobar lung transplantation. J Cardiothorac Vasc Anesth 18:506, 2004
154. Webber SA: The current state of, and future prospects for, cardiac transplantation in children. Cardiol Young 13:64, 2003
155. Quinlan JJ, Firestone S, Firestone LL: Anesthesia for heart, lung, and heart-lung transplantation
156. Brawn WJ, Barron DJ: Management and outcome in hypoplastic left heart syndrome. Curr Paediatr 14:26, 2004
157. Reddy SC, Webber SA: Pediatric heart and lung transplantation. Ind J Pediatr 70:19, 2003
158. Myles PS: Pulmonary transplantation. *In* Kaplan JA, Slinger PB (eds): Thoracic Anesthesia, 3rd edition. Philadelphia, Churchill Livingstone, 2003, pp 295–314
159. Kramer MR, Marshall SE, Starnes VA, et al: Infectious complications in heart-lung transplantation. Arch Int Med 153, 2010, 1993
160. Bailey LL: Heart transplantation techniques in complex congenital heart disease. J Heart Lung Transplant 12:S168, 1993
161. Boucek MM, Edwards LB, Keck BM, et al: The registry of the International Society for Heart and Lung Transplantation: Sixth official pediatric report-2003. J Heart Lung Transplant 22:636, 2003

Chapter 27

NEW APPROACHES TO THE SURGICAL TREATMENT OF END-STAGE HEART FAILURE

Marc E. Stone, MD • Gregory W. Fischer, MD

KEY POINTS

1. Congestive heart failure (CHF) is a chronic progressive disease of epidemic proportion that costs billions of dollars annually.
2. Current medical management alone is incapable of preventing the progression of CHF to the advanced stages of the disease.
3. Surgical options for the management of CHF exist and are being increasingly used at an earlier stage in the course of the disease. Implantation of a mechanical circulatory assist device remains an attractive management option for advanced cardiac failure because the underlying problem is mechanical pump failure. Currently available pulsatile devices have been shown to be effective but have a high incidence of complications. The next generation of continuous-flow devices (currently in human clinical trials) promises increased device durability and fewer complications.
4. Electrophysiologic maneuvers (e.g., biventricular pacing) can often improve cardiac output and decrease mortality in patients with advanced CHF.
5. New therapies (e.g., transplantation of skeletal myoblasts, stem cells, gene therapies) that can potentially reverse the adverse ventricular remodeling accompanying CHF and improve ventricular function are under development and in various stages of human clinical trials but are years away from routine clinical applicability.
6. The anesthetic management of patients presenting for "heart failure surgery" can be challenging due to the severely depressed cardiac function and the often debilitated state of the patient.
7. Patients with end-stage heart failure often present with significant co-morbidities that must be identified preoperatively.
8. The intraoperative management of the patient with advanced heart failure requires a careful titration of anesthetic agents and continuous optimization of hemodynamics. Such optimization generally requires meticulous management of preload, afterload, heart rate, heart rhythm, and contractility, as well as judicious manipulation of systemic and pulmonary vascular resistances where necessary.
9. Attention to postoperative pain management is critical in this population if exacerbations of hemodynamic instability are to be avoided.

EPIDEMIOLOGY, PATHOPHYSIOLOGY, AND LIMITATIONS OF CURRENT MANAGEMENT

Scope of the Problem

According to the American Heart Association, there are approximately 5 million people in the United States with congestive heart failure (CHF). Available statistics indicate that the incidence of CHF in the population approaches 10 per 1000 after age 65, with 550,000 new cases each year.[1] Heart failure (HF) is the leading cause of hospitalization in patients over age 65,[2] with a reported associated cost of $24 to $50 billion annually.[1-4] On a global scale, CHF reportedly affects 0.4% to 2.0% of the adult population.[5]

Despite great advances in the understanding of the pathophysiology of HF and the development of medications that can potentially attenuate the progression of that pathophysiology, morbidity and mortality from this disease remain very high. The incidence of hospitalization for HF rose by 70% during the 1990s,[2] and patients with New York Heart Association (NYHA) class IV symptoms currently have a reported 1-year mortality rate of 30% to 50%.[6] By comparison, the corresponding rates for NYHA class I-II patients and class II-III patients are 5% and 10% to 15%, respectively (Table 27–1 defines the NYHA symptomatic classes).[7] Thus, one of the major goals in the management of CHF is the prevention of progression to advanced stages.

While many patients successfully achieve temporary relief of CHF *symptoms* with medical management, the underlying pathophysiology inevitably progresses, and pharmacologic interventions alone will eventually become inadequate in the vast majority. A variety of surgical procedures can be performed to improve cardiac function and potentially arrest (or even reverse) the progression to severe dysfunction, but until very recently, surgical intervention (short of transplantation or placement of a ventricular assist device) was considered contraindicated in patients with advanced HF. Surprisingly good outcomes with "corrective" interventions, however, have now resulted in patients presenting for surgical treatment of their HF on a regular basis. This chapter describes the procedures typically performed in this population and the anesthetic considerations for patients with advanced HF.

Brief Review of the Pathophysiology

The current understanding of the pathophysiology of chronic HF maintains that initial increases in end-diastolic ventricular volume and pressure trigger the release of endogenous natriuretic peptides that promote diuresis.[8-10] Concurrent activation of the sympathetic nervous system causes peripheral vasoconstriction and increases the inotropic state of the myocardium. Initially, these mechanisms act to decrease excessive preload (which restores wall tension to normal) and maintain cardiac output (CO) and arterial blood pressure (BP) in the face of mildly depressed ventricular function. Eventually, however, the carotid, ventricular, and aortic arch baroreceptors are activated by the relative hypovolemia, which

Table 27–1 The New York Heart Association (NYHA) Functional Capacity[7]

Functional Capacity	Objective Assessment
Class I. Patients with cardiac disease but without resulting limitation of physical activity. Ordinary physical activity does not cause undue fatigue, palpitation, dyspnea, or anginal pain.	**A.** No objective evidence of cardiovascular disease.
Class II. Patients with cardiac disease resulting in slight limitation of physical activity. They are comfortable at rest. Ordinary physical activity results in fatigue, palpitation, dyspnea, or anginal pain.	**B.** Objective evidence of minimal cardiovascular disease.
Class III. Patients with cardiac disease resulting in marked limitation of physical activity. They are comfortable at rest. Less than ordinary activity causes fatigue, palpitation, dyspnea, or anginal pain.	**C.** Objective evidence of moderately severe cardiovascular disease.
Class IV. Patients with cardiac disease resulting in inability to carry on any physical activity without discomfort. Symptoms of heart failure or the anginal syndrome may be present even at rest. If any physical activity is undertaken, discomfort is increased.	**D.** Objective evidence of severe cardiovascular disease.

leads to further activation of the sympathetic nervous system (via the medullary vasomotor regulatory center) as well as the renin-angiotensin-aldosterone axis, and the release of vasopressin. The resultant peripheral vasoconstriction, mild fluid retention, and further increases in heart rate and inotropy will again compensate for the failing heart. Ultimately, however, chronic sympathetic stimulation causes myocardial β_1-adrenergic receptors to downregulate, and as ventricular function deteriorates, left ventricular (LV) end-diastolic volumes and pressures again increase, resulting in increased ventricular wall tension. During this time, increased levels of angiotensin II result in adverse myocardial remodeling. Remodeling is a key event in the progression of HF and refers to changes not only in ventricular geometry (e.g., dilation) but also in myocardial composition (e.g., myocyte hypertrophy, lengthening, hyperplasia, and fibrosis). Additionally, increased circulating levels of angiotensin II may enhance myocyte apoptosis (programmed cell death) via a protein kinase C–mediated increase in cytosolic calcium levels.[11]

Alterations in chamber geometry (dilation) and myocardial remodeling lead to progressively decreased forward CO, perpetuating the vicious cycle of adverse neurohumoral activation and transient, tenuous compensation. Myocardial oxygen demand increases while oxygen supply potentially decreases due to shortened diastolic periods and increased diastolic wall tension. This developing diastolic dysfunction (ventricular "stiffness") leads to increased left atrial (LA) and pulmonary pressures, functional mitral regurgitation, pulmonary congestion, and increased right ventricular (RV) afterload. This may eventually progress to signs and symptoms of right-sided HF.

Modern medical management of chronic CHF therefore uses agents that have been shown to decelerate the progression to severe failure, reduce adverse myocardial remodeling, and enhance survival (e.g., angiotensin-converting enzyme inhibitors,[12-14] β-blockers,[15-18] and aldosterone antagonists[19,20]) in combination with other agents that improve the symptoms but have not been shown to improve long-term survival alone (e.g., diuretics and digoxin).

Limitations of Current Medical Management

Given that there are presently between 300,000 and 800,000 patients in the United States who have progressed to NYHA class III and IV status despite modern medical management,[21] it appears that current treatment strategies have significant limitations. Part of the failure of medical management alone to control the progression of the disease may be that treatment has traditionally focused on systolic dysfunction. Four classic stages of HF have been described: (1) an initial cardiac injury or insult, (2) activation of specific neurohormonal axes with resultant cardiac remodeling, (3) compensatory fluid retention and peripheral vasoconstriction, and (4) ultimate contractile failure.[22] In contrast to this traditional conception, it is now known that diastolic dysfunction (decreased lusitropic function) is the primary problem in an estimated 30% to 40% of HF patients. Pharmacologic interventions aimed at improving diastolic dysfunction and attenuating (if not reversing) remodeling are currently the subject of randomized trials worldwide.

SURGICAL OPTIONS FOR HEART FAILURE

A growing number of surgical procedures exist (or have been developed) to relieve CHF symptoms and arrest the progression of the disease through correction of abnormal myocardial depolarization, enhancement of myocardial blood supply, improvement in ventricular loading conditions, and restoration of more normal ventricular geometry. Box 27–1 provides a list of current surgical interventions for CHF.

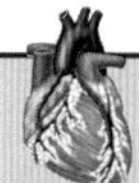

BOX 27–1 ***Surgical Options for the Management of Congestive Heart Failure***

- Cardiac resynchronization therapy with biventricular pacing
- Revascularization (coronary artery bypass grafting or percutaneous coronary artery stenting)
- Mitral valve repair or replacement
- Left ventricular reconstruction (e.g., with the Dor procedure or the Batista procedure)
- Dynamic cardiomyoplasty
- Extrinsic compression devices (e.g., the CorCap)
- Implantation of a left ventricular assist device (LVAD)
- Cardiac transplantation
- New therapies for congestive heart failure in various stages of development include transplantation of skeletal myoblasts and stem cells, "gene" therapy, and xenotransplantation

Cumulative worldwide experience with such interventions thus far suggests that these procedures not only relieve symptoms but may also attenuate or possibly arrest the progressive myocardial remodeling that accompanies chronic HF.[23-27] In some cases, partial reversal of the adverse myocardial remodeling has been demonstrated, and combination therapy (surgical intervention with targeted pharmacologic treatment) intended to enhance reverse remodeling is actively being investigated.[28]

Thus, interventions previously considered contraindicated by low ejection fraction (EF) are now being used precisely for that indication. It remains to be determined, however, which procedures will ultimately benefit which subpopulations of HF patients. Despite the common final pathway that leads to dilated pathophysiology seen in the majority of these patients, an individual's initial underlying etiology may again become an important consideration as these procedures are used earlier and earlier in the course of deterioration as a treatment intended to halt the progression of the disease.

REVASCULARIZATION

Coronary artery disease has become the most common etiology of HF.[29] Of those patients currently listed for heart transplantation, 42.3% carry a primary diagnosis of ischemic heart disease (OPTN data). Commonly used terms describing the extent of myocardial injury are defined in Table 27–2.

Where viable myocardium and feasible targets exist, revascularization of chronically ischemic, hibernating myocardium can improve ventricular function, downgrade NYHA functional class, and improve prognosis.[30,31] While the primary benefit of revascularization appears to be functional improvement of the LV, reducing ischemic substrate for arrhythmias and retarding adverse myocardial remodeling are important secondary benefits.[24]

Despite an increased perioperative risk of morbidity and mortality in this population, the world's literature reports current survival between 57% and 75% at 5 years with in-hospital mortality between 1.7% and 11%.[31] A recent review reported an 83.5% survival at 2 years following revascularization compared with only 57.2% survival in CHF patients who were not revascularized.[30] In general, morbidity and mortality tend to correlate inversely with EF and directly with NYHA functional class. Additional factors predisposing patients to higher morbidity and mortality include advanced age, female sex, hypertension, diabetes, and emergent operations.[32] The decreases in morbidity and mortality following revascularization in this high-risk population in recent years are at least partially attributable to improvements in surgical technique and myocardial protection, but the concurrent performance of mitral valve repair and ventricular reshaping address the adverse ventricular loading conditions present and may also contribute to improved outcomes. The results of ongoing clinical trials evaluating combinations of surgical procedures (e.g., revascularization plus ventricular reshaping versus revascularization alone) are eagerly awaited.

The importance of determining the viability of myocardium in the area to be revascularized cannot be understated because the potential for recovery of function depends on residual contractile reserve, integrity of the sarcolemma, and metabolically preserved cellular function.[31] Methods to detect viable myocardium include dobutamine echocardiography, single-photon emission computed tomography (SPECT), and positron-emission tomography (PET). While dobutamine stress echocardiography has often been shown to have the highest predictive accuracy,[33] there are important limitations that need to be taken into account. Dobutamine stress echocardiography, for example, can have false-negative results if there is loss of contractile proteins in the presence of preserved function of the muscle fiber membrane[31] (see Chapters 4, 6, 11, 12, 15, and 19). Some centers report using only the intraoperative assessment of myocardial wall thickness and contractility to determine potential viability with revascularization of the target region.[34] Regardless of the specific method used, the important point is that there needs to be viable tissue to revascularize, and the best results will be obtained in properly selected individuals. Overwhelmingly, encouraging results worldwide suggest that, when feasible, revascularization is of benefit and provides survival advantage to patients with significant ventricular dysfunction.

Table 27–2 Commonly Used Terms Describing the Extent of Myocardial Injury and the Potential for Recovery

Term	Definition
Ischemic	Insufficient oxygen supply to meet myocardial oxygen demand
Stunned	Acute myocardial dysfunction following an ischemic event with potential for full recovery
Hibernating	Chronically ischemic, dysfunctional myocardium with potential for full recovery
Maimed	Dysfunctional myocardium on the basis of ischemia that does not fully recover
Infarcted	Myocardial necrosis due to ischemia with no potential for recovery

CORRECTION OF MITRAL REGURGITATION

The mitral valve is a complex apparatus consisting of the anterior and posterior leaflets, the mitral annulus, the chordae tendineae, the papillary muscles, and the wall of the LV. The posterior portion of the annulus is flexible due to the fact that the fibrous skeleton is very thin in this area. This leads to the ability of the annulus to change its shape during the cardiac cycle. During systole, an elliptical shape is assumed that facilitates coaptation of the leaflets. During diastole, a more circular form increases orifice dimensions, decreasing resistance to LV inflow.[35] The LV free wall, papillary muscles, and chordae play an important role in the competence of the valve, as well as in LV function during systole.

Mitral regurgitation (MR) may result from several different pathophysiologic states (e.g., leaflet prolapse, annular dilation, leaflet perforation), but the MR seen in patients with CHF is most often functional, due primarily to restriction of leaflet motion with subsequent limitation of leaflet coaptation because the papillary muscles are tethered by the dilated LV.

Historically, many physicians considered MR advantageous for the failing LV. It was believed that a low-pressure atrial "pop off" allowed the failing ventricle to protect itself from the high afterload of the systemic circulation and gave the illusion that the heart had a better overall contractile state than really existed. This misconception was "supported" by the fact that surgical replacement of the mitral valve was associated with a very high mortality rate in patients with depressed LV function.[36] It is now known, however, that mitral valve replacement or repair can improve overall cardiac performance by eliminating the increased myocardial oxygen demand that accompanies the progressive pressure and volume overload due to MR.

Despite the slightly increased operative risk, the current literature supports mitral valve repair or replacement as beneficial to patients with severely depressed LV function, CHF, and MR. In a recent series, Romano and Bolling reported operative mortality of 5% with 1- and 2-year survival rates of 80% and 70%, respectively.[37] Not only was long-term mortality reduced, but the increase in LV systolic function (on average by 10%) enabled a downgrading of NYHA class and resulted in an improved quality of life. Rothenburger et al[38] showed 1-, 2-, and 5-year survival rates of 91%, 84%, and 77%, respectively, in 33 patients with LVEF less than 30%, and Bishay et al[39] demonstrated similar results in 44 patients with an LVEF less than 35%. In addition, Bishay et al demonstrated that the rate of re-hospitalization for CHF was decreased during the period of follow-up compared with a cohort that did not receive a mitral repair. Thus, both medical and economic benefits may result from mitral valve repair in this population (see Chapters 4, 12, and 20).

While the majority of end-stage HF patients will exhibit functional MR (as discussed earlier), there may be additional concurrent valvular pathology present in a given patient. An intraoperative transesophageal echocardiography (TEE) evaluation of the valvular anatomy, the mechanism of the MR, and direct surgical inspection will determine the feasibility of repair. It is generally believed that valve repair is preferable to valve replacement, because there are demonstrated hemodynamic advantages associated with preservation of the subvalvular apparatus,[40] and long-term anticoagulation is not required. When used for mitral prolapse, valve repair is associated with improved long-term survival rates compared with valve replacement,[41] but this finding has not always been reproduced in studies examining patients with the functional MR accompanying end-stage dilated cardiomyopathy or when the mechanism of MR is "complex." A series from the Cleveland Clinic examined 482 patients with ischemic MR who underwent either valve repair or replacement.[42] The multivariate analyses in this study suggested that the answer to the issue of repair versus replacement is not a simple one. The predictors of improved outcome included the complexity of the mechanism of MR, whether an internal mammary artery was used to revascularize the myocardium, the urgency of the procedure, and overall patient condition. The authors concluded that survival after repair and replacement is similar in complex and high-risk settings, although repair confers a survival advantage for most patients with ischemic MR.

Depending on the mechanism of MR identified, simple types of valve repair may include annuloplasty with ring insertion, commisurotomy, triangular or quadrangular leaflet resections, and the Alfieri technique. More complex types of repairs include chordal transposition, shortening, or fenestration, implantation of artificial chordae, and specific leaflet repairs. Following the procedure, TEE is used to assess the adequacy of the repair and potential improvement of overall cardiac function. Often, hemodynamic improvement is not immediately apparent, and TEE is used to optimize preload and guide pharmacologic interventions (see Chapters 14 through 16, 31, and 33).

LEFT VENTRICULAR RESHAPING: THE BATISTA PROCEDURE AND THE DOR PROCEDURE

In 1996, Batista et al[43] introduced the concept of surgically reshaping the dilated and failing LV of NYHA class IV patients to improve systolic performance. In the Batista procedure, resection of a wedge of normal myocardium from the LV apex to the base (laterally, between the papillary muscles) restored more normal ventricular geometry and decreased wall tension. Functional mitral regurgitation was also addressed during the Batista procedure by a valve replacement or repair. While many patients did benefit initially from this procedure (reduction of NYHA functional class to NYHA I in 57% and NYHA II in 33.3%),[44] perioperative mortality was high (>20% in both Batista's own series and in the large Cleveland Clinic experience).[44,45] Additionally, the experience of several centers was that many patients required rescue mechanical circulatory assistance following the procedure, and many patients experienced a redilation of their LV resulting in a return to NYHA class IV status.[46-48] Thus, despite a short-lived period of initial enthusiasm in the mid to late 1990s, the Batista procedure has essentially been abandoned. The concept of ventricular reshaping, however, remains of interest.

The modified Dor procedure (endoventricular circular patch plasty) is successfully used to reshape the dilated, spherical LV of patients who have had an anterior wall myocardial infarction with resulting aneurysm and akinesis/dyskinesis. Essentially, a Dacron patch is placed within the LV cavity so as to exclude the large akinetic/dyskinetic area of the anterior wall. This restores LV geometry to a more normal elliptical shape and improves systolic function. When performed concurrently with coronary artery bypass grafting (CABG), significant early and late improvements in both NYHA functional class and EF have been demonstrated with an in-hospital mortality rate of 12%.[49,50] A trial of 439 patients undergoing this procedure found an improved in-hospital mortality of 6.6% and an 18-month survival of 89.2%. In this series, CABG was performed concurrently in 89%; mitral valve repair in 22%; and mitral valve replacement in 4%.[51] As with the original Batista procedure, the intent of the modified Dor procedure is to reshape the dilated ventricle, reducing wall stress and therefore myocardial oxygen demand. Restoration of a more normal elliptical shape is predicted to improve systolic performance as well.

PROCEDURES TO ARREST THE DILATION OF THE FAILING VENTRICLE: EXTRINSIC CONSTRAINT WITH THE DYNAMIC CARDIOMYOPLASTY AND THE ACORN CORCAP

The intent of extrinsic constraint is to arrest the progressive dilation of the failing ventricle. As discussed above, decreasing the radius of the LV will reduce wall tension (law of Laplace), which will decrease myocardial oxygen demand. The law of Laplace is stated as

$$T = (P \times R)/2h$$

where T is surface tension, P is pressure gradient, R is radius, and h is wall thickness (see Chapter 5).

In addition, this may result in improved systolic and diastolic function, as well as subjective improvements in functional capacity. This type of ventricular reshaping can be accomplished with biological tissues and devices applied to the external surface of the heart.

Dynamic Cardiomyoplasty

Decades in development, this procedure was introduced into clinical practice in 1985 by Carpentier and Chachques.[52] In dynamic cardiomyoplasty, an electrically stimulated flap of skeletal muscle (e.g., latissimus dorsi) was wrapped around the heart in an attempt to augment systolic function. Between 1985 and 1991, approximately 185 dynamic cardiomyoplasties were performed worldwide in 17 countries.[53] While subjective improvement was widely reported by patients who had undergone the procedure, objective measurements of significant functional improvement were inconsistent. In one multicenter trial of 68 patients with NYHA class III symptoms, small but significant increases in EF (23% to 26%) and stroke volume (SV) (48 mL to 57 mL) were observed at 1 year following the procedure; however, there were no significant changes in pulmonary capillary wedge pressure or peak exercise performance.[53] In retrospect, the true benefit of this largely abandoned procedure most likely resided in the girdling effect of the wrap, which acted to prevent further dilation of the failing heart.

Acorn CorCap Cardiac Support Device

The CorCap Cardiac Support Device (Acorn Cardiovascular, Inc., Minneapolis, MN) is an investigational mesh fabric that is surgically wrapped around the heart (Fig. 27–1) in an attempt to prevent further dilation. This device has been shown in animal models to reduce wall stress, myocyte hypertrophy, and myocardial fibrosis.[54] A global multicenter study by Oz et al[55] showed promising results. There were significant reductions in LV end-diastolic dimensions, MR grade, and NYHA classification in patients 12 months after CorCap implantation. At the same time, a significant improvement was seen in LVEF and quality of life. Ongoing randomized clinical trials in Europe and the United States will further address the safety of implantation of the CorCap device and ultimate outcomes.

CARDIAC RESYNCHRONIZATION THERAPY AND IMPLANTABLE CARDIOVERTER-DEFIBRILLATORS

The progression of disease resulting in advanced cardiac failure is typically accompanied by conduction defects and arrhythmias, and pacemakers and implantable cardioverter-defibrillators (ICDs) are common in this population. In addition to the well-known defects in sinus or atrioventricular node function, intraventricular conduction defects delay the onset of RV or LV systole in 30% to 50% of patients with advanced HF.[56,57] This lack of coordination of LV and RV contractions further impairs CO[58-61] and has been reported to

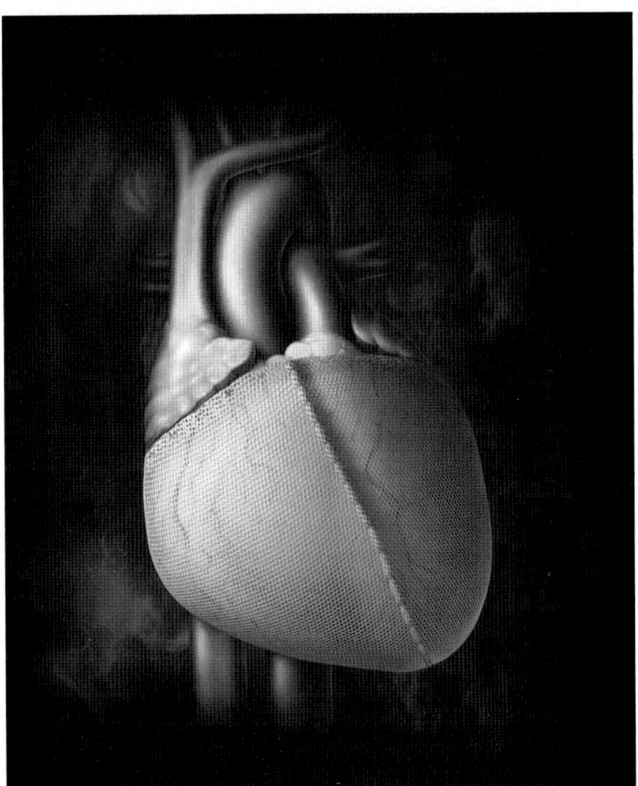

Figure 27–1 The Acorn CorCap cardiac support device. (Reproduced with permission from Acorn Cardiovascular, Inc.)

increase the risk of death in this population[62,63] (see Chapters 4, 13, and 25).

Cardiac resynchronization therapy (CRT) entails biventricular pacing (not to be confused with dual-chamber atrioventricular sequential pacing) to optimize the timing of RV and LV contractions. The right atrium (RA) is paced by a lead in the RA, the RV by a lead in the RV, and the LV by a lead in a coronary vein (accessed via the coronary sinus). While CRT is more an interventional cardiology procedure than a surgical procedure per se, anesthesiologists are frequently asked to provide sedation (if not general anesthesia) for these sometimes lengthy implantation procedures (see Chapters 4, 10, 13, and 25).

Studies have shown that atrial-synchronized biventricular pacing (pacing the LV and RV in a carefully timed manner) can "resynchronize" RV and LV contraction, improving CO and overall hemodynamics. This enhances these patients' ability to exercise (which improves their NYHA functional class) and decreases the length and frequency of their hospitalizations, which improves their quality of life.[64-68]

Sudden death from ventricular fibrillation (VF) accounts for approximately 250,000 deaths annually in the United States.[1] Patients with advanced HF experience VF with a frequency 6 to 9 times that of the general population,[1] and VF causes 40% of all deaths in this population even in the absence of apparent disease progression based on symptoms.[69] Thus, ICDs are commonly indicated for patients with advanced cardiac failure. An ICD is a device capable of arrhythmia detection and automatic defibrillation. ICDs successfully terminate VF in greater than 98% of episodes, and studies have demonstrated that an ICD increases survival and decreases the risk of sudden death in patients with ischemic cardiomyopathy and decreased LV function[70-72] (see Chapters 10, 13, and 25).

The Comparison of Medical Therapy, Pacing, and Defibrillation in Heart Failure (COMPANION) trial studied 1500 patients at 128 U.S. centers. In this recently completed trial, compared with optimal pharmacologic therapy alone, CRT decreased the risk of the combined endpoint of death from or hospitalization for HF by 34%. The combination of CRT and ICD implantation reduced these risks by 40%.[73] While many studies are ongoing, it is clear that CRT and ICDs significantly reduce morbidity and mortality in patients with advanced HF.

Pacemakers and ICDs are typically implanted in the electrophysiology suite by cardiologists using local anesthesia. Anesthesiologists are commonly asked to sedate or briefly induce anesthesia during these procedures so that proper functioning of the device(s) can be ascertained with patient amnesia during arrhythmia induction and therapy. Clinicians must consider all the same anesthetic issues and concerns when sedating/inducing one of these patients for device testing as one would for a surgical procedure in the operating room. Propofol is commonly used in small dosages (0.25-mg/kg increments); etomidate (0.05 to 0.1 mg/kg) is an alternative for patients with baseline hypotension. Many cardiologists use midazolam in this circumstance when an anesthesiologist cannot be present. Anesthesiologists may also choose a lighter plane of sedation if the risk of airway difficulty or gastric regurgitation is elevated (see Chapters 4, 9, 10, and 13).

VENTRICULAR ASSIST DEVICES

When cardiac failure is refractory to pharmacologic manipulations, mechanical circulatory assist devices are used as a temporary bridge-to-recovery, as a bridge-to-transplantation, or, in selected patients, as a final "destination therapy." While a thorough treatment of all mechanical circulatory assist devices is beyond the scope of this chapter, the following paragraphs introduce and briefly describe the most commonly used, currently available, Food and Drug Administration–approved ventricular assist devices (VADs), as well as the next generation of miniaturized, totally implantable continuous-flow VADs, and the AbioCor total artificial heart (Abiomed, Danvers, MA) now in human clinical trials. The societal importance of "destination therapy" is also discussed. See Chapter 31 for information on weaning off CPB using intraaortic balloon counterpulsation (pump) (IABP).

Currently Available Ventricular Assist Devices: Indications and the Basic Strategy of Their Use

Mechanical circulatory assistance with a VAD has become common management of intractable cardiogenic shock that follows cardiac surgery, myocardial infarction (MI), or severe viral myocarditis, as well as in the patient with end-stage cardiomyopathy awaiting transplantation. All currently available VADs are pumps that collect blood returning to the heart and eject it downstream of the failing ventricle. Effectively, they take over the pumping function of the failing ventricle and can provide adequate systemic perfusion to prevent the devastating sequelae of cardiogenic shock (e.g., multisystem organ failure). With the potential exception of centrifugal pumps, currently approved VADs do not provide oxygenation or removal of waste from the blood—they simply act as pumps that can maintain perfusion of the body in the place of a failing ventricle.

While the VAD is acting to maintain the circulation, decompression of the failing ventricle will decrease ventricular wall tension and therefore myocardial oxygen demand. In order to decompress the failing ventricle, cannulas must be placed in the heart to divert blood to the pump, and all currently approved devices use essentially the same cannulation strategies within the heart and great vessels. For LV support, blood is drained from the LA or, more commonly, the LV apex and returned to the ascending aorta. For RV support, blood is drained from the RA or RV and returned to the main pulmonary artery. These cannulation strategies are common to all VADs currently approved for clinical use and are demonstrated in Figure 27–2.

Temporary Ventricular Assist Device Use: Bridge-to-Recovery

In patients in whom there has been an acute myocardial insult resulting in refractory cardiogenic shock but myocardial recovery *is* expected, a short-term VAD (e.g., the Abiomed BVS5000; Abiomed, Danvers, MA), an intermediate-term VAD (e.g., the Thoratec VAD system; Thoratec Laboratories, Pleasanton, CA, or the AB5000 ventricle; Abiomed, Danvers, MA), or standard centrifugal devices can support the circulation as a "bridge-to-recovery." The Abiomed BVS5000 (Fig. 27–3), the Thoratec (Fig. 27–4), and the newly approved AB5000 ventricle (Fig. 27–5) are paracorporeal, pneumatically driven devices capable of providing pulsatile support for the LV (LVAD), the RV (RVAD), or both ventricles (BiVAD) as needed. With all these devices, the paracorporeal pump heads are connected to inflow and outflow cannulas anastomosed to the heart and great vessels (see Fig. 27–3). Table 27–3 summarizes the basic characteristics of these devices. The artificial blood contacting surfaces, unidirectional valves, and pulsatile nature of the pumping mechanism in these devices require

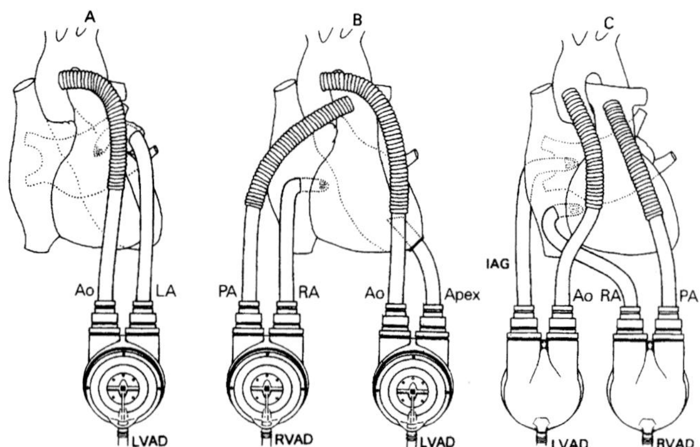

Figure 27–2 The Thoratec ventricular assist device and three cannulation approaches for univentricular left heart support (*A*) and biventricular support (*B* and *C*). This figure illustrates the currently used cannulation strategies for all currently available ventricular assist devices. As described in the text, cannulas are placed in the heart and great vessels to divert blood returning to the failing side of the heart to the pump. The blood collected in the VAD blood chamber is then ejected into the arterial circulation immediately downstream of the failing ventricle. Ao = aorta; LA = left atrial appendage; PA = pulmonary artery; RA = right atrium; Apex = left ventricular apex; IAG = cannula inserted via the interatrial groove and directed toward the LA roof. (Graphic reprinted with permission from Thoratec Corporation.)

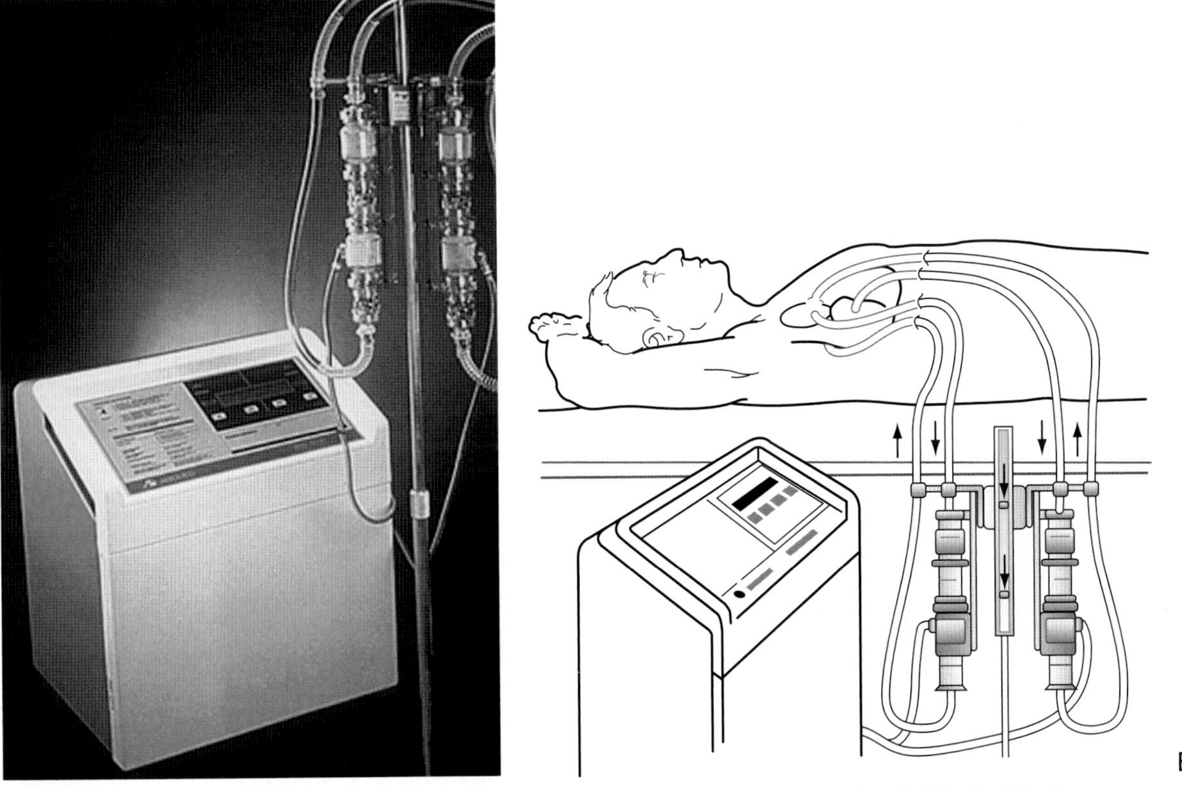

Figure 27–3 (*A*) The Abiomed BVS5000. (*B*) Biventricular support with the Abiomed BVS5000. As described in detail in the text, cannulas are placed in the heart and great vessels so as to divert blood to the extracorporeal BVS5000 pumps. Blood collected in the pumps is ejected into the ascending aorta (LVAD) and main pulmonary artery (RVAD). Note that the pumps fill by gravity drainage, and are therefore generally mounted below the level of the heart. Adjustments can be made to pump height to optimize filling and pump ejection. For example, lowering a pump can augment device filling, but will increase the afterload against which the device must eject. Conversely, raising a pump can facilitate pump emptying, but will decrease filling of the device. RVAD = right ventricular assist device; LVAD = left ventricular assist device. (*A* and *B* reprinted with permission from Abiomed Corporation.)

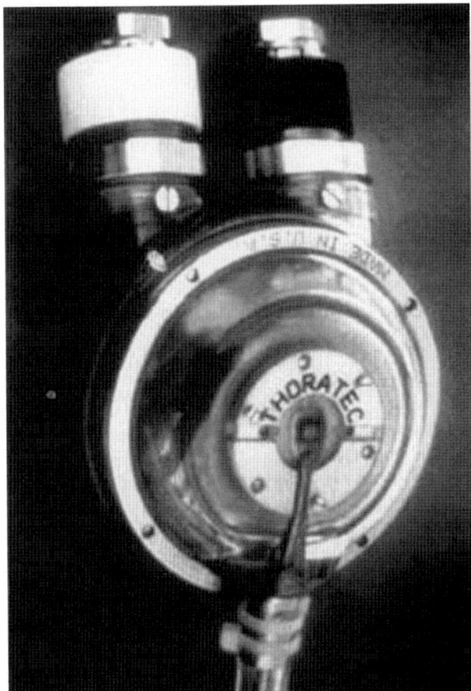

Figure 27–4 The Thoratec pump head. The blood chamber is contained within the clear plastic housing. Hookups for the inflow and outflow cannulas are at the *top* of the photograph. The driveline, which alternately provides vacuum to assist filling and compressed air to accomplish ejection is at the *bottom*. (Photograph reproduced with permission from Thoratec Laboratories.)

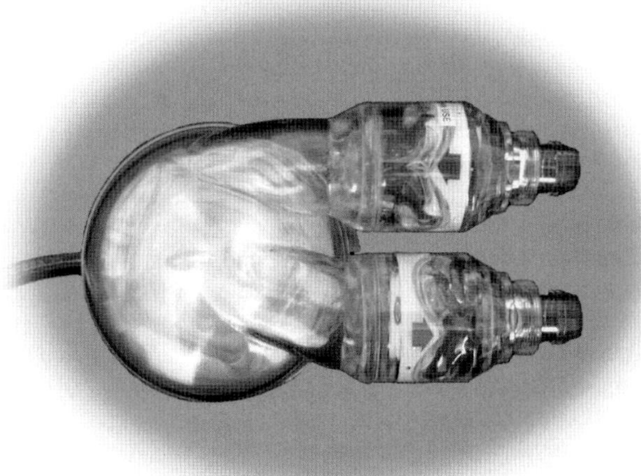

Figure 27–5 The Abiomed AB5000 ventricle. Hookups for the inflow and outflow cannulas are at the right of the photograph. While the *arrows* indicate the direction of flow, they also serendipitously point at the artificial unidirectional valves that mandate anticoagulation during support with this device. The drive line, which alternately provides vacuum to assist filling and compressed air to accomplish ejection, is at the *left*. (Photograph reproduced with permission from Abiomed Corporation.)

Table 27–3 **Basic Characteristics of the Devices Currently Used as a Bridge to Recovery**

Device	Fill Mechanism	Drive Mechanism	System Control and Output
Abiomed BVS5000	Gravity drainage	Pneumatic compression of blood chamber	Automatically adjusts rate of pumping to provide up to 5 L/min of outflow (output depends on intravascular volume status and downstream vascular resistances)
Thoratec	Vacuum assisted	Pneumatic compression of blood chamber	Depending on the mode of operation, user-defined settings determine the output (intravascular volume status is important)
Abiomed AB5000 ventricle	Vacuum assisted	Pneumatic compression of blood chamber	Automatically adjusts rate of pumping to provide up to 6 L/min of outflow (output depends on intravascular volume status and downstream vascular resistances)
Centrifugal pumps	Gravity drainage assisted by vortex	Centrifugal force drives blood	Output is dependent on user-defined speed of impeller rotation

that the patient be anticoagulated during support. While patients supported by an Abiomed BVS5000 are generally confined to bed, those supported by a Thoratec or an AB5000 ventricle can potentially be allowed to ambulate with assistance once they have been stabilized for a period of time.

Both the Abiomed BVS5000 and the AB5000 ventricles will automatically adjust their rate of pumping in response to intravascular volume status and downstream vascular resistances (systemic vascular resistance [SVR] in the case of an LVAD, pulmonary vascular resistance in the case of an RVAD) in an attempt to maintain approximately 5 L/min of pulsatile outflow (up to 6 L/min for the AB5000 ventricle). In contrast to the highly automated Abiomed control algorithm, the Thoratec has three different modes of operation. Depending on which mode is in use, the operator must manually set and make occasional adjustments to the device settings (e.g., in the "volume mode": the percentage of the pump cycle spent in systolic ejection, the drive pressure, and the fill vacuum pressure) in order to optimize pump outputs. While this can make operation of a Thoratec initially appear complicated, it actually imparts great versatility to the device in that a wide range of patients can be supported.

In general, intravascular volume status is the key determinant of the output from all these devices. With the Thoratec, the ability to adjust the vacuum-assisted filling pressure, the pneumatic drive pressure, and the amount of the pump cycle spent filling/ejecting enable a temporary compensation for relative hypovolemia. Despite the automated algorithm of the Abiomed BVS5000, relative underfilling of the intravascular tree will usually result in decreased pump output because pump filling depends on gravity drainage. The AB5000 ventricle provides the advantages of both devices; it has the automatic control algorithm of the Abiomed BVS5000 with the vacuum-assisted filling of the Thoratec, so partial compensation for hypovolemia is possible. With all these devices, it is desirable to maintain normal or slightly decreased downstream vascular resistance to allow for optimal pump output.

Nonpulsatile flow from standard centrifugal pumps (various manufacturers) is also commonly used to support the circulation as a bridge-to-recovery and to provide extracorporeal membrane oxygenation (ECMO), especially in the pediatric population. The ability to limit flows with the nonpulsatile centrifugal pumps makes these devices the only currently available source of mechanical circulatory assistance for neonates, infants, and small children.

Regardless of the device used as a bridge-to-recovery, the patient may potentially be weaned from mechanical support as the ventricle recovers from the acute stunning it has sustained. Unfortunately, complications are frequent (see discussion later) and recovery is not always assured. It would be an understatement to say that reported rates of successful bridge-to-recovery with these short-term devices are often disappointing. Appropriate patient selection for this application of VADs is critical. In general, the best outcomes are obtained when rescue mechanical circulatory assistance is initiated as soon as the severity of the myocardial insult is recognized and truly appreciated.

According to the Abiomed operation manual,[74] the best outcomes occur when

- Support is commenced to correct marginal hemodynamics within 30 to 45 minutes of attempted pharmacologic treatment (with or without an IABP).
- The time between the first attempt to wean from CPB and BVS implant is less than 6 hours.
- The BVS implant occurs as part of the initial operation.
- Due consideration is given to whether the patient requires univentricular or biventricular support.
- Hemostasis is ensured before leaving the operating room.

Poor outcomes occur when

- Signs of other end-organ failure are present.
- The patient is older than 75 years.
- The patient is brought back to the operating room for implantation following a period of time.

Intermediate- to Long-Term Ventricular Assist Device Use: Bridge-to-Transplantation

In cases when no myocardial recovery is expected (e.g., end-stage cardiomyopathy) or when an acutely stunned LV fails to recover despite support with a short-term VAD, an intermediate- to long-term paracorporeal VAD (e.g., the Thoratec VAD system; see Figs. 27–3 and 27–5) or a long-term "implantable" LVAD (e.g., the Novacor LVAS; World Heart, Ottawa, Canada, or the HeartMate LVAS; Thoratec Corporation, Woburn, MA) is commonly used as a "bridge-to-transplantation." By providing effective CO in place of the failed native heart, this technology can stave off the end-organ damage resulting from a rapidly deteriorating CO and allows

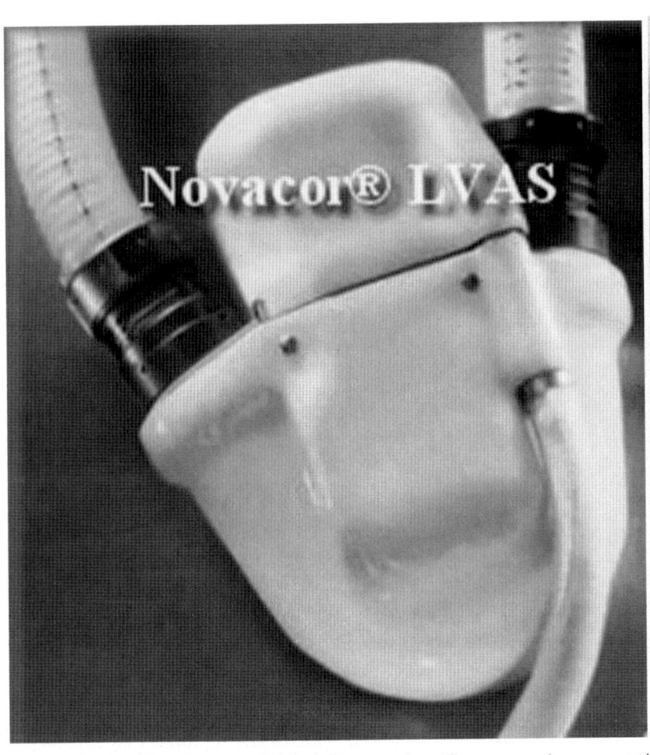

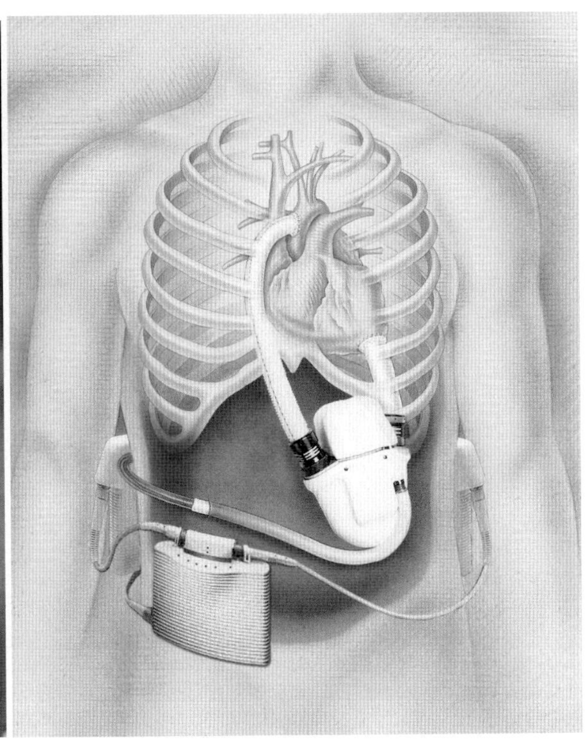

Figure 27–6 (*A*) The Novacor LVAS. Inflow and outflow cannulas are at the top, and the drive line, which provides electrical power and system control, can be seen at the *bottom right*. (Photograph reproduced with permission from WorldHeart, Inc.) (*B*) The appearance of an implanted Novacor LVAS. Blood is drained from the LV apex to the pump and ejected into the ascending aorta. The pump head is completely implanted in the preperitoneal space of the abdomen. The current model requires that a cable from the device be tunneled through the abdominal wall to connect to the external system controller and power supply. (Graphic reproduced with permission from WorldHeart, Inc.)

severely decompensated transplant-eligible patients to potentially survive long enough to receive a donor heart. An additional benefit of this application of VADs is an improved quality of life, often as an outpatient, while awaiting a new heart (see Chapter 26).

The Novacor (Fig. 27–6) and the HeartMate (World Heart, Inc., Oakland, CA) (Fig. 27–7) are the most commonly used bridge-to-transplantation devices for patients with advanced LV failure. Patients with biventricular failure are typically bridged with the Thoratec. While there are new and promising devices currently in clinical trials (see discussion later), the Thoratec is presently the only widely available mechanical circulatory support device capable of providing intermediate to long-term support of the native heart as a bridge-to-transplantation for patients who require biventricular support. According to the most recent voluntary Novacor, HeartMate, and Thoratec registries, more than 1300 patients have been implanted with the Novacor, more than 3500 with the HeartMate, and more than 1400 with the Thoratec worldwide. Of those implanted with the Thoratec for bridge-to-transplantation, 56% required biventricular assistance. Rates of successful bridging-to-transplantation with these devices are reportedly on the order of 51% to 78%.[75-78]

An implanted Novacor is shown in Figure 27–6, and a HeartMate in Figure 27–7. As depicted, the pump heads of these devices are implanted in a surgically created pocket in the preperitoneal space. Inflow and outflow conduits are connected to the heart and great vessels as shown (see Figs. 27–6B and 27–7B). Blood is drained to the implanted pump head from the LV apex and is ejected in a pulsatile fashion into the ascending aorta. Again, adequate intravascular volume status is a critical factor in optimizing pump outputs.

Current versions of these devices require a percutaneous cable to connect the implanted pump heads to an external source of power and system control, potentially increasing the incidence of infection. Additional common complications of long-term VAD use include a high incidence of perioperative bleeding and subsequent potential for cerebral thromboembolism (see discussion of complications of VAD use earlier).

The Novacor ultimately requires formal anticoagulation with warfarin (target INR 2.5 to 3 times normal) because its blood chamber is composed of smooth polyurethane. In contrast, the blood chamber of the HeartMate has an antithrombogenic lining composed of sintered titanium microspheres that encourages the ingrowth and development of a neointima. For this reason, patients supported by a HeartMate do not require formal anticoagulation and are generally maintained only on aspirin (perhaps in combination with dipyridamole) depending on the preferences of the implanting center.

The CardioWest total artificial heart (SynCardia Systems, Tucson, AZ; Fig. 27–8) is also available as a bridge-to-transplantation for patients with biventricular failure. This device is a pneumatically powered biventricular pump that is implanted orthotopically (the native heart is removed and replaced by this device, see Fig. 27–8). Since 1993, approximately 225 of these devices have been implanted clinically,[79] although if the Jarvik-7 total artificial heart (on which the CardioWest device is largely based) is included, over 430 patients have been implanted worldwide with this type of device.[80] A prospective study of 130 patients bridged-to-transplantation with the CardioWest total artificial heart (TAH) reported a successful bridge-to-transplantation rate of 79%.[81] When compared with the implantable LVADs, a

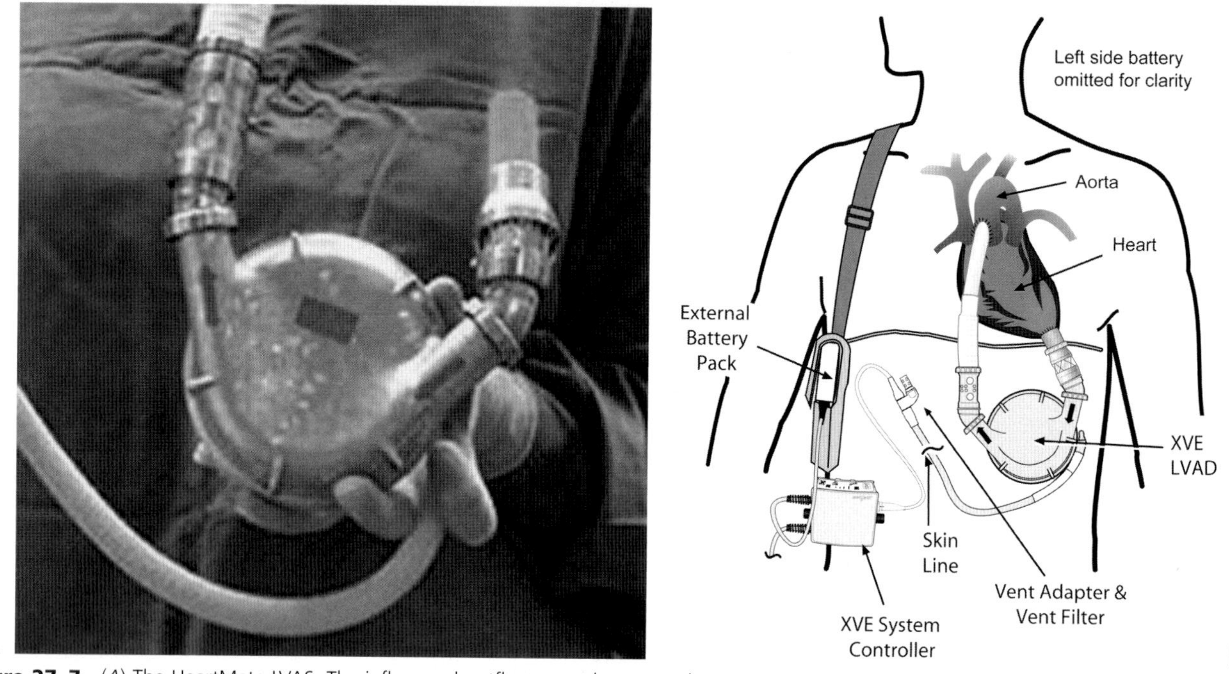

Figure 27–7 (*A*) The HeartMate LVAS. The inflow and outflow cannulas are at the *top*, and the drive line to bring power and system control is at the *bottom*. (Photograph reproduced with permission from Thoratec Laboratories, Inc.) (*B*) The appearance of an implanted HeartMate XVE LVAD. Blood is drained from the left ventricular apex to the pump and ejected into the ascending aorta. The pump head is completely implanted in the preperitoneal space of the abdomen. The current model requires that a cable from the device be tunneled through the abdominal wall to connect to the external system controller and power supply. (Graphic reproduced with permission from Thoratec Laboratories, Inc.)

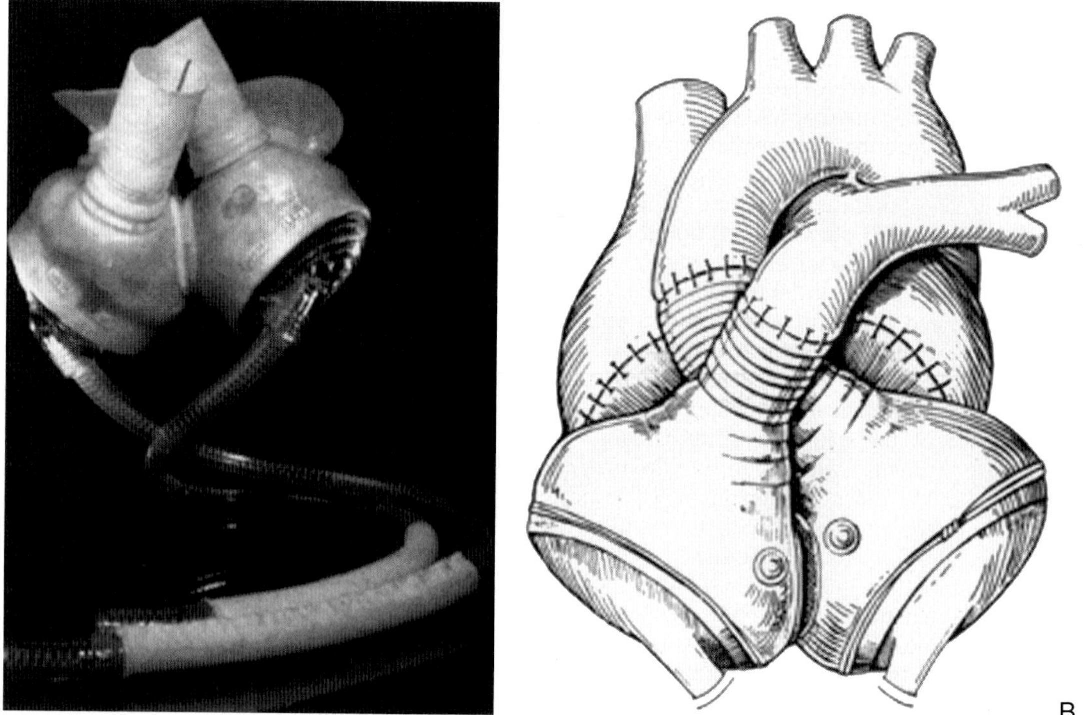

Figure 27–8 (*A*) The CardioWest Total Artificial Heart (TAH). (*B*) Orthotopic implantation of the CardioWest Total Artificial Heart. As described in the text, the failed native heart is removed and the CardioWest TAH is implanted orthotopically, anastomosed to cuffs of native atria and the great vessels. (Reproduced with permission from SynCardia Systems.)

potential disadvantage of the CardioWest device as a bridge-to-transplantation is a lack of portability, significantly limiting potential for physical rehabilitation and outpatient use, although a smaller and more portable driver is planned.

Permanent Ventricular Assist Device Use: Destination Therapy

A new indication for long-term VAD use is "destination therapy." Destination therapy refers to the intentionally permanent implantation of an LVAD in a nontransplant eligible patient as a permanent management solution for end-stage cardiac failure. While destination therapy is now said to be a "new indication," ironically, this was the original conception and intended use of VADs. The availability of this indication is a great advance in the treatment of HF because while cardiac transplantation remains the ultimate intervention for advanced HF, the number of donor organs is severely limited in comparison with the number of those who would benefit, and the vast majority of patients with end-stage cardiac disease cannot realistically expect to be transplanted. Effectively, the intentionally permanent implantation of a mechanical assist device may be the best option available if the vast numbers of patients in the population with advanced HF are to survive.

Based on the encouraging results of the REMATCH trial,[82] the HeartMate LVAS is now FDA-approved for use as "destination therapy" in the United States. Briefly, REMATCH (Randomized Evaluation of Mechanical Assistance for the Treatment of Congestive Heart Failure) was conducted to determine if the HeartMate could be effective as an alternative therapy for patients with end-stage cardiac failure who are not eligible to receive a transplant. In addition to patient survival, the study collected data on the implanted patient's quality of life, the cost of their care, and any adverse events that occurred during the treatment. In essence, the REMATCH study demonstrated that the use of a left-sided VAD was not only an effective tool to treat patients with advanced HF but also resulted in more than twice the survival rate and an improved quality of life in comparison to optimal medical management. This was especially the case if the patient was younger than 60 years. Summarized results of the REMATCH trial appear in Table 27–4.

A similar trial intended to establish the ability of the Novacor LVAS to provide destination therapy (INTREPID [Investigation of Non-Transplant-Eligible Patients who are Inotrope Dependent]) ended, but the results have not been published as of the time of this writing. A human clinical trial called RELIANT (Randomized Evaluation of the Novacor LVAS in a Non-Transplant Population) randomizes patients to receive the Novacor LVAS or the HeartMate XVE LVAS as treatment. The objective of the RELIANT trial is to demonstrate that use of the Novacor LVAS is superior to optimal medical therapy by demonstrating equivalence to HeartMate XVE LVAS, which has already been approved for destination therapy.

Table 27–4 **Summarized Results of the REMATCH Trial**

	HeartMate	Medical Treatment
1-Year survival (patients <60 years)	52% (74%)	25% (33%)
2-Year survival	23%	8%
Median survival	408 days	150 days

Ventricular Assist Device Use and the Potential for Myocardial Recovery

In cases of acute ventricular failure, removal of the sudden volume and pressure overload and improvement in the balance of myocardial oxygen supply and demand may allow for myocardial recovery and weaning from mechanical support. Clinical experience has shown that if recovery from an acute insult is going to occur, it generally does so over the course of 1 to 2 weeks. In cases of long-standing progressive failure, decompression of the dilated and chronically failing LV by an LVAD may also allow for some degree of recovery over time.

While echocardiographic and histiologic support for this general premise has been available for nearly a decade, the underlying biochemical mechanisms of remodeling (and its reversal) are only now being elucidated. Patten et al[83] showed that therapy with VAD normalizes inducible nitric oxide synthase expression in association with decreased cardiomyocyte apoptosis. Decompression of the LV by an LVAD has been reported to allow for normalization of LV geometry, regression of myocyte hypertrophy,[84] favorable changes in LV collagen content,[85] and normalized expression of genes controlling excitation-contraction coupling and the calcium content of the sarcoplasmic reticulum.[86] It has been reported that maximum structural reverse remodeling is complete after around 40 days of LV decompression, with reversal of some of the molecular aspects of remodeling by 20 days.[87] It should be appreciated, however, that while a great deal of knowledge regarding myocardial remodeling (and its reversal) has been elucidated, long-lasting ventricular recovery following chronic HF is a relatively infrequent event, reportedly occurring primarily in patients with dilated cardiomyopathy, and the actual number of patients who recover sufficiently to have their long-term VAD explanted is small. Worldwide efforts to understand the nature of adverse ventricular remodeling and its reversal are ongoing, and the relevant literature is rapidly burgeoning.

Complications of Currently Available Ventricular Assist Devices

Regardless of which short- or long-term device is in use, the major complications of VAD use include coagulopathic bleeding in the perioperative period, potential for thromboembolism during support, and infection. Additional complications of VAD use include RV failure while on isolated LV assistance (on the order of 30% due to the induced changes in RV geometry),[88,89] potential device malfunction, and progressive multisystem organ failure despite VAD support.

Perioperative Bleeding

Initial hemostatic abnormalities derive primarily from the implantation procedure itself with the attendant coagulopathy resulting from cardiopulmonary bypass (CPB) and continued extracorporeal circulation through the device. Large series have reported that approximately 50% of VAD-implanted patients experience significant perioperative bleeding requiring treatment.[75,81] It is during this period of sometimes massive transfusion of blood, platelets, and coagulation factors that LV dysfunction often becomes manifest. In the experience of most centers, on the order of 50% to 75% of these patients require reexploration for bleeding or evacuation of mediastinal hematoma.

Thromboembolism

Paradoxically, once the perioperative coagulopathy is controlled, a major concern is the prevention of thromboembolic events. With the exception of the HeartMate (which theoretically requires no formal anticoagulation due to the presence of an antithrombogenic lining in its blood chamber), all currently available devices require full anticoagulation with heparin and/or warfarin. However, despite anticoagulation, thromboembolism is a major problem with all currently available short- and long-term devices and results from exposure of blood to the foreign surfaces of the VAD. A review of 228 bridge-to-transplantation patients on long-term support with the Thoratec, Novacor, and HeartMate reported cerebral embolism in 24%, 39%, and 16%, respectively, despite appropriate anticoagulation.[75] The rate of successful bridge-to-transplantation in this series, however, was similar with all three devices (61% with the Thoratec, 54% with the Novacor, and 51% with the HeartMate). These numbers are somewhat lower than those reported from other large centers, where the successful rate of bridge-to-transplantation is reportedly on the order of 75%.

While the anticipated rate of thromboembolic events is lower with the HeartMate, differences do exist between manufacturers in the definitions and terms (e.g., neurologic dysfunction, thromboembolic event, embolism to the central nervous system versus the periphery) used to report such adverse events. For this reason, statistics may not always be directly comparable between devices from study to study. An interesting in-depth review and discussion of this issue were published.[78] Nevertheless, despite the reportedly higher rates of thromboembolism and overall neurologic dysfunction associated with the Novacor, it should be appreciated that the rates of successful bridge-to-transplantation with the Novacor and the HeartMate have never been shown to differ significantly. In fact, the rate has generally been reported to be slightly higher with the Novacor compared with the HeartMate.[75,78]

Infection

Infections are common with all current circulatory assist devices. Infection is largely a problem due to the current necessity for percutaneous components to provide power and system control (as in the Novacor and HeartMate). In one large series, rates of infection of the percutaneous driveline were reported to be 26% with the Novacor and 18% with the HeartMate, while pocket infection was reported to occur in 11% with the Novacor and 24% with the HeartMate.[75] Despite a reported incidence of percutaneous conduit infection of only 2% with the Thoratec in that same large series, sepsis occurred in 26%, compared with 24% supported by a Novacor and 11% supported by a HeartMate.[75] A large series reviewing bridge-to-transplantation with the HeartMate reported that 45% of patients developed "infection," with 72% of the observed infections at the exit site of the percutaneous driveline.[77] Given the long duration of hospitalization with indwelling bladder catheters, invasive hemodynamic monitoring catheters, and occasionally prolonged tracheal intubation in the setting of debilitated patients (often with poor nutritional status), other commonly seen infectious complications in VAD-supported patients include urinary tract infections, catheter sepsis, and pneumonia. Thus, while it is anticipated that some level of infection will exist in all patients supported by current incarnations of long-term support devices, the etiologies are likely multifactorial and may not be directly comparable between devices from study to study. The advent of transcutaneous energy transfer (TET) technology is a major advance that eliminates the need for percutaneous cables in these devices and may decrease the rate of infectious complications in the future.

Multisystem Organ Failure

Multisystem organ failure is a known complication of mechanical circulatory assistance, but it does not always reflect a problem with a VAD per se. It must be remembered that the population of patients requiring VAD support had acute refractory cardiogenic shock (in the case of short-term VADs) or a chronic low CO state prior to implantation of a long-term VAD, and it is this condition that most likely set the stage for organ insufficiency. By and large, patient selection is critical to the success of mechanical circulatory assistance.

Next Generation of Ventricular Assist Devices: Miniaturized, Totally Implantable Continuous-Flow Devices

While current long-term "implantable" pulsatile devices are effective, controversy regarding the superiority of pulsatile versus nonpulsatile outflow has continued for decades, and ongoing inherent problems related to the engineering required to produce pulsatile outflow suggest that the currently available long-term pulsatile LVADs are not likely to be the future of mechanical circulatory assistance. The following paragraphs briefly describe "the problem with pulsatility" and introduce the philosophy behind the radically different design of the next generation of VADs.

First, to create effective pulsatile flow, the device must be large because the blood chamber must accommodate a large stroke volume. This tends to disqualify small adults and pediatric patients from support with currently available long-term devices (body surface area must be greater than 1.5 m^2 to be eligible for a Novacor or HeartMate).

Second, the engineering required to create pulsatile outflow requires a "back-and-forth" motion of a diaphragm (HeartMate) or pusher-plates (Novacor) as well as unidirectional valves to prevent retrograde flow during pump systole. These create trauma to blood elements, require anticoagulation, and may also result in hemolysis.

Third, a reliable and durable pulsatile mechanism requires fairly complex engineering with several moving parts. The more complex a mechanical device, the more inherently inefficient it will be from an engineering standpoint, and the multiple moving parts will be subject to eventual mechanical failure, resulting in a life span too short to provide "destination therapy." In the midst of the enthusiasm for the availability of this indication, there has been expert speculation as well as editorials and articles published in the relevant literature expressing the opinion that the currently available long-term, implantable LVADs are not capable of providing the 10 or 15 years desired to constitute "destination therapy." Based on anecdotal reports and the published worldwide in vivo experience to date, a reasonable estimate of the average life span of a single Novacor device is on the order of 3½ to 4 years, and that of a single HeartMate device is around 2 years (although the HeartMate XVE that is currently available may have an increased longevity). Actual in vitro testing of these devices by their respective manufacturers supports these generalizations.[90-92] The reported "reliability" of the HeartMate at 2 months and 1 year is reportedly 93.5% and 84.7%, respectively. In contrast, that of the Novacor is greater than 99.9% at both of these timepoints. Additionally, the reported "reliability" of the Novacor at 2 and 3 years is 98.3% and 85.9%, respectively. Information about the reliability of the HeartMate at these later timepoints is not available.

A large series of LVAD support for bridge-to-transplantation at a single center in Germany reported that 9% of patients supported by a HeartMate experienced mechanical problems with their device (compared with no mechanical problems observed with the Novacor).[75] While only 1% of HeartMate-supported patients in a large multicenter series in the United States experienced "mechanical failure,"[77] there were 435 "confirmed device malfunctions" of one sort or another in the 280 supported patients, and 9% of the supported patients needed to use "backup components" because of "cable or controller malfunction" or "pump stoppage."

While the manufacturers work to solve many of these inherent mechanical problems and improve the mechanical durability of existing devices, others are focusing on new devices with a miniaturized impeller that rotates at high speed (on the order of 10,000 to 15,000 rpm) producing continuous, laminar flow as blood is smoothly entrained along the spiral vanes of the impeller, and propelled forward. Such an impeller is similar in design to an Archimedes screw. Another new design uses a miniaturized magnetically levitated centrifugal pump to create nonpulsatile blood flow.

Such designs have several potential advantages over currently available pulsatile VADs. First, there is essentially only one moving part, which, from a mechanical standpoint is simple, efficient, and likely to be much more durable than a pulsatile mechanism. Second, there is no "on/off" or "back and forth" motion to create stasis or cause trauma to blood elements that mandates formal anticoagulation. Third, because the flow is continuous, artificial unidirectional valves are not required, obviating the need for formal anticoagulation. In addition, it has been shown that there is the potential for less hemolysis with the newly designed continuous-flow devices than with pulsatile flow.[93] Last, these devices can be miniaturized and still produce a high flow rate, making them suitable for adult or pediatric use.

One of the main reasons that the currently available devices produce pulsatile flow is the belief that pulsatile flow is superior to continuous flow in terms of its ability to maintain normal homeostasis and physiology. Until fairly recently, the accepted dogma was that nonpulsatile flow caused

1. Stagnation in capillary beds leading to tissue edema and increased arteriovenous shunting, resulting in decreased oxygen extraction and impaired lactate clearance[94]
2. Redistribution of intrarenal and intrahepatic blood flow, resulting in renal and hepatic insufficiency[95,96]
3. Impairment of carotid baroreceptor function resulting in increased mean arterial pressure and total peripheral resistance[97]
4. Adverse alterations of catecholamines, prostaglandins, and cytokine levels[96]
5. Electrolyte imbalance, fluid overload, and anemia.[98,99]

Human and animal studies have shown, however, that the body can adapt to nonpulsatile flow if that flow is maintained at somewhat supranormal levels,[93] and it has been demonstrated that the abnormal physiology tends to correct itself after approximately 2 weeks if at least 20% or 30% higher flows than pulsatile support is used. While pulsatile flow does appear to better maintain physiologic homeostasis and allows more efficient oxygen metabolism at lower flow rates (especially in elderly patients with noncompliant blood vessels), many of the differences appear to be attenuated as the rate of nonpulsatile flow increases on a mL/kg/min basis, with no demonstrable differences as nonpulsatile flow rates approach 100 mL/kg/min (7 liters per minute for a 70-kg person).[94] As a conventional point of reference, the typical flow rates used during the routine conduct of nonpulsatile CPB are in the range of 50 to 60 mL/kg/min.

This information, along with technological advances over the past decade in the areas of biocompatible materials, computer chips, and miniaturization technology, has allowed for the design and development of the next generation of axial flow VADs now in human clinical trials and the subsequent generation of magnetically levitated, miniaturized, implantable centrifugal pumps. Because these devices are still in their clinical trials at the time of this writing, available information is limited to descriptions, technical specifications, and some interim details about their clinical performance thus far. Figures 27–9 to 27–15 show the appearance of selected new VADs, and the figure legends provide selected references in which details of these new devices can be found. It should be noted, however, that there are many new VADs under development globally, and those presented herein comprise only a small sampling of what may one day be available.

TOTAL ARTIFICIAL HEART

From the original pneumatically driven devices with their massive external control consoles to the totally implantable computer-controlled AbioCor Implantable Replacement Heart (Abiomed, Danvers, MA) now in clinical trials, the mechanical TAH has been the subject of intensive research and development for decades.

The first TAH was a pneumatically driven biventricular pump developed by Dr. Domingo Liotta and colleagues in the 1960s. This device (the Liotta TAH) was implanted in a 47-year-old patient with severe HF by Dr. Denton Cooley on April 4, 1969, and was used for 64 hours as a bridge-to-heart transplantation.[100] The patient died of *Pseudomonas* pneumonia 32 hours after his transplantation, but the Liotta heart proved that a mechanical device could be successfully used clinically to sustain a patient.

The second human implantation of a TAH was also performed by Dr. Cooley. In July 1981, the Akutsu III TAH was successfully used for 55 hours as bridge-to-transplantation in a 36-year-old patient with end-stage HF.[101] The Jarvik-7 TAH was first implanted as a permanent replacement heart in August 1985 in a 61-year-old man with primary cardiomyopathy and chronic obstructive pulmonary disease.[102] Although the patient survived only 112 days, the duration of his survival was encouraging. Since 1991, the Jarvik-7 has been known as the CardioWest TAH. As discussed, this device is still in use today as a bridge-to-human heart transplantation in selected centers in the United States, France, and Canada.

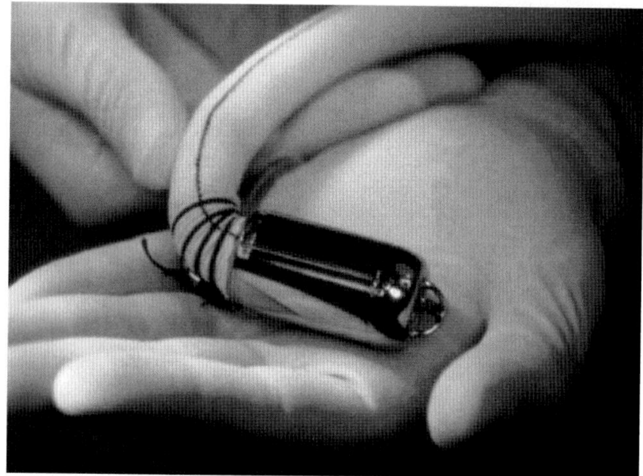

A

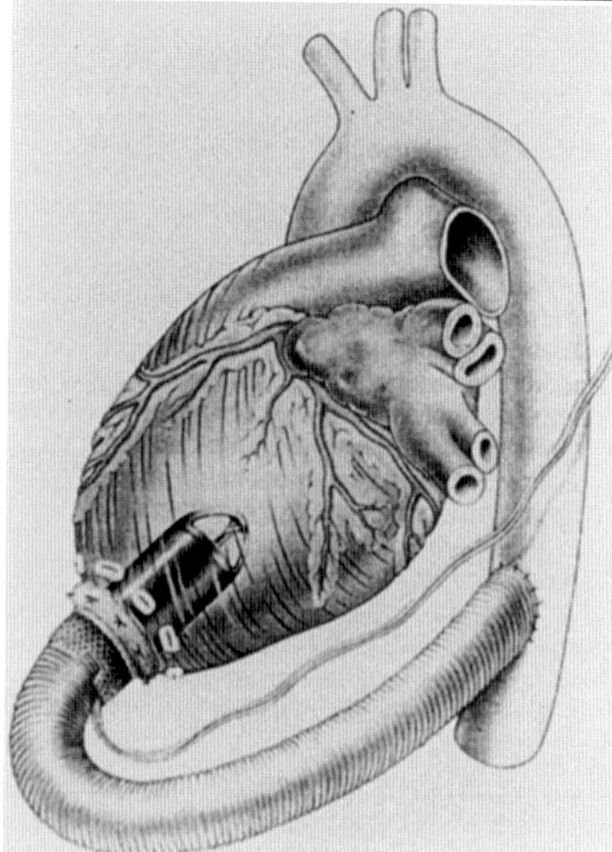

B

Figure 27–9 (*A*) The Jarvik 2000 LVAS. The Jarvik 2000 LVAS (Jarvik Heart, Inc., New York, NY) is an axial flow pump in clinical trials that has been implanted in more than 50 patients in the United States and Europe.[118-120] Those implantations in the United States are being evaluated as a bridge-to-transplantation, while those in Europe are being evaluated as both a bridge-to-transplantation and as destination therapy. (For the latest information, visit www.texasheart.org/j2000html. Photograph reproduced with permission from Jarvik Heart, Inc.) (*B*) Intraventricular position of the Jarvik 2000 LVAS. Unlike many of the other new axial flow devices, the Jarvik 2000 LVAS is implanted within the left ventricle and directs blood flow to the descending aorta. (Graphic reproduced with permission from The Artificial Heart Fund, UK.)

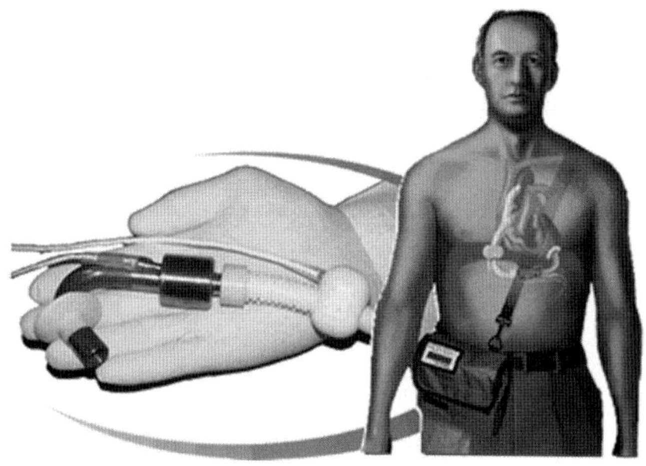

Figure 27–10 The MicroMed DeBakey VAD. The DeBakey VAD (MicroMed Technologies, Inc., Houston, TX) is an axial flow device in clinical trials that has been implanted in over 250 patients in Europe and the United States.[120-123] Like many of the new axial flow LVADs, the DeBakey VAD draws blood from the left ventricular apex and propels it into the ascending aorta. In addition to clinical trials in adults, the DeBakey has been further miniaturized and is being evaluated for use in the pediatric population. (For the latest information, visit www.micromedtech.com. Graphic reproduced with permission from Micromed Technologies, Inc.)

The Abiocor Implantable Replacement Heart (Fig. 27–16) represents a major advance in artificial heart technology because it is truly totally implantable; there are no percutaneous cables, conduits, or wires. The device is motor driven, so a source of compressed air to drive the pumping action is not required, allowing patients complete mobility. The device itself weighs approximately 2 pounds and is orthotopically implanted as illustrated in Figure 27–16.

Transcutaneous energy transfer is used (in lieu of a percutaneous cable) to supply the motor-driven hydraulic pumping of the artificial ventricles with power and system control. Artificial unidirectional valves within the device mandate anticoagulation during support.

The Abiocor TAH is currently in human clinical trials. Candidates for the clinical trial must be ineligible for cardiac transplantation, with biventricular HF and a high probability of dying within 30 days. The first and most successful implantation was performed by Gray and Dowling at the University of Louisville. Long-term survival of over 1 year has been achieved.

CARDIAC TRANSPLANTATION

Cardiac transplantation remains the ultimate surgical intervention for advanced HF and greatly impacts the lives of those patients who receive a new heart, but considering the massive scope of this public health issue, this management strategy is epidemiologically and biostatistically small due to the extremely limited number of donor organs available each year. While it is estimated that at least 100,000 patients could meet the transplant criteria at any given time,[21] only 3520 are currently listed to potentially receive one.[103] Further, it is appar-

Table 27–5 Number of Cardiac Transplantations Performed in the United States, 1998 through 2002

Cardiac transplants by year
1998: 2340 transplants
1999: 2184 transplants
2000: 2198 transplants
2001: 2202 transplants
2002: 2155 transplants

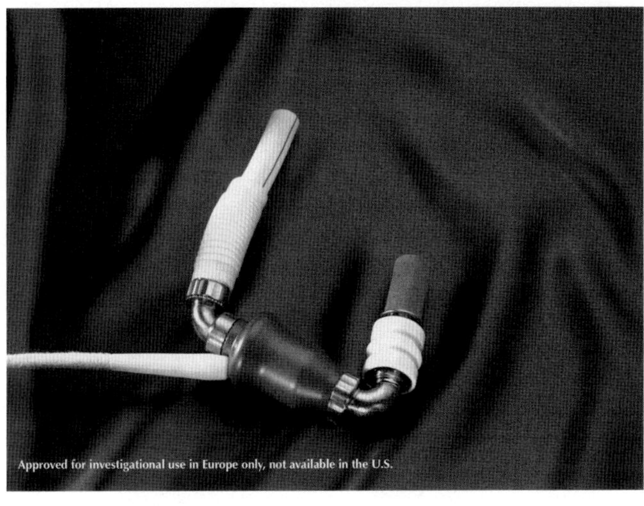

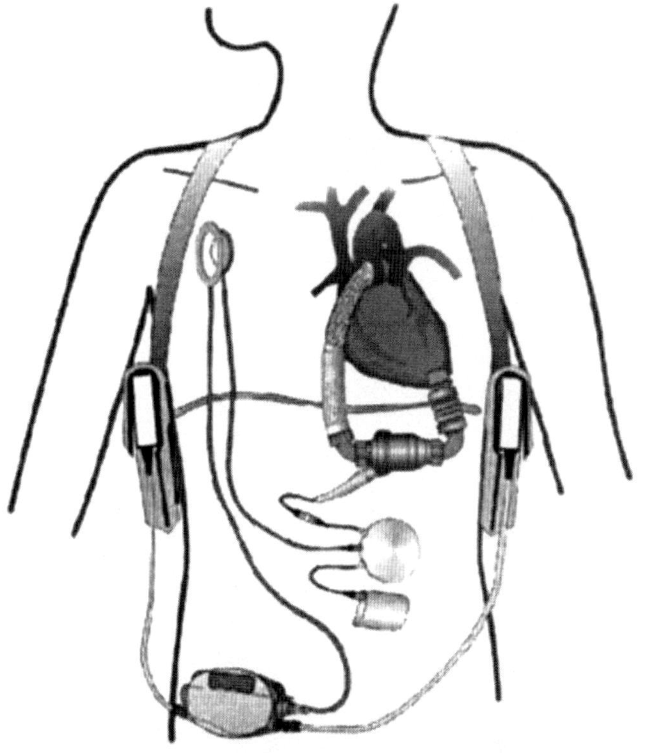

Figure 27–11 The HeartMate II Left Ventricular Assist System. The HeartMate II is an axial flow device in clinical trials in the United States and Europe. This new device occupies approximately one-eighth the volume of the pulsatile HeartMate I but can reportedly generate flows up to 10 L/min to meet the changing flow demands of the body.[124,125] Note the transcutaneous energy transmission (TET) system (upper right chest area in the schematic). This configuration obviates the need for a percutaneous line to deliver power and system control to the device, and may decrease the incidence of infection with long-term support. (For more information, visit www.thoratec.com. Graphics reproduced with permission from Thoratec Corporation.)

ent from the figures presented in Table 27–5 that the number of available donor hearts is limited to approximately 2200 each year in the United States. Thus, transplantation is simply not a realistic expectation for the majority of patients with advanced end-stage HF. Patients fortunate enough to get a donor organ can currently expect a 1-year survival rate of 86%, a 3-year survival rate of 77%, and a 5-year survival rate of 71%[1] (see Chapter 26).

NEW THERAPIES

Cellular Transplantation Into the Myocardium

A novel approach to treating severe systolic dysfunction is the injection of harvested autologous skeletal muscle cells into the failing myocardium. This procedure can be performed either surgically at the end of a revascularization procedure or percutaneously in the catheterization laboratory.

The use of cell transplantation is not a novel approach to treating disease. Skin and bone marrow transplantations were the first replacement therapies described. These were followed by embryologic neuron transplantation in patients with Parkinson's disease and islet cell transplantation for the treatment of diabetes mellitus.[104]

The basic understanding of the remodeling process is that viable and contractile cardiomyocytes undergo apotosis and become replaced by noncontractile tissue. This in turn leads to systolic and diastolic dysfunction. In an attempt to restore functionality, contractile cells are injected into this region. In clinical practice, myoblasts from the patient's quadriceps muscle have been used. Using the patient's own tissue has several advantages. First, the complications of pharmacologic immunosuppression are avoided. Second, there are no ethical problems in contrast to those frequently observed when fetal cells are used. Finally, the ease of harvest and processing makes this tissue ideal for this purpose.

Skeletal muscle cells, however, are histologically different from native cardiomyocytes. Adhesion molecules, which are found in native cardiomyocytes, are not found in skeletal myocytes (N-cadherin and connexin-43).[104] These adhesion molecules are important for adhesion to the extracellular matrix and for intercellular communication.

Clinically, a Phase I study from Poland, the POZNAN trial,[105] showed that myoblasts can be implanted safely via a percutaneous route, into a scarred region of the LV. There were only ten patients enrolled into this study. Nine were transplanted. One could not be transplanted due to technical reasons. Six patients of the nine were followed up. An improvement of NYHA class and EF was observed in all of them. Similar results were seen by Menasche et al.[104] A frequently encountered occurrence in the phase I studies was the fact that many patients had episodes of ventricular tachycardia after the procedure. They were successfully treated with amiodarone or electric cardioversion. Phase II studies are now in progress in the United States and Europe. Many other cell types are now being experimentally injected into the myocardium or given intravenously in an attempt to regrow cardiac myocytes.[106-108] These cells include adult bone marrow stem cells, embryonic stem cells, and cardiac progenitor cells found mainly in the atrium. They have been injected alone or with multiple growth factors such as granulocyte-macrophage

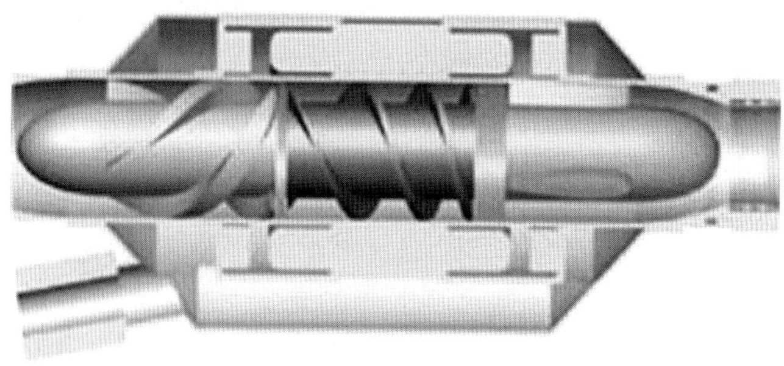

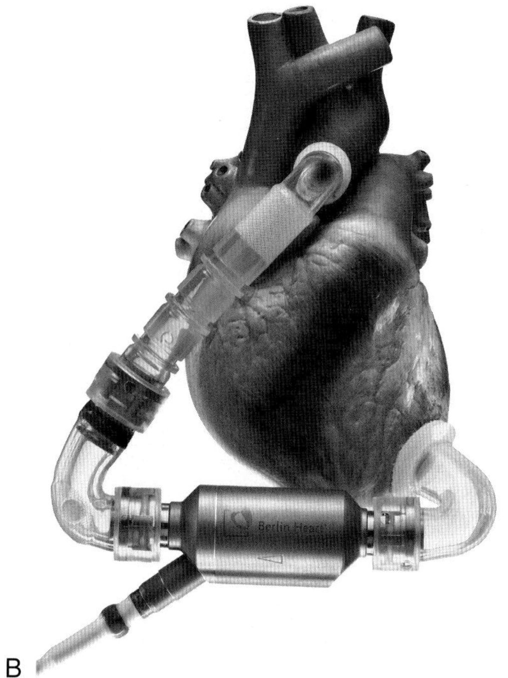

Figure 27–12 The Berlin Heart INCOR. The Berlin Heart INCOR (Berlin Heart AG, Berlin, Germany) is an axial flow LVAD in clinical trials in Europe and China.[120,126] This device has been implanted in both adult and pediatric patients. (For the latest information, visit www.berlinheart.com/products/incor. Graphics reproduced with permission from Berlin Heart AG.)

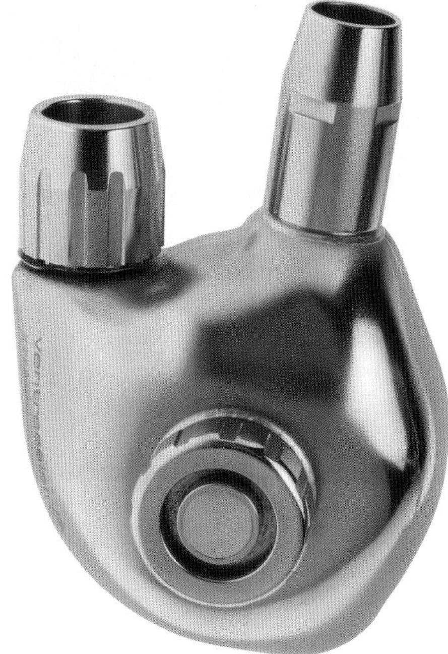

Figure 27–13 The VentrAssist LVAS. The VentrAssist LVAS (Ventracor Ltd., Sydney, Australia) is a miniaturized, implantable centrifugal pump in clinical trials in Australia, Great Britain, and New Zealand. The impeller of this third generation assist device is hydrodynamically suspended.[127,128] (For the latest information, visit www.ventracor.com. Photograph reproduced with permission from Ventracor Ltd.)

colony-stimulating factor (GM-CSF), vasoactive endothelial growth factor (VEGF), and angiopoietan-1, which mobilize progenitor cells and induce new cell growth. The transplanted cells may morph into new cardiac muscle cells or they may improve cardiac function by boosting the growth of new blood vessels, or releasing other growth factors that encourage cell proliferation and survival. Any of these effects could explain some of the early positive results seen to date.

Gene Transfer in Cardiac Myocytes

Gene therapy has received much interest by the media during the past decade. Multiple research groups are trying to cure or at least alleviate symptoms brought on by CHF through gene therapy. In order to change the genetic programming of a cell it is necessary to inoculate the cell with DNA. In order to achieve this goal vectors are being used. Vectors commonly used range from plasmid DNA to different virus types (e.g., adenovirus, herpesvirus). The two cellular pathways that are being targeted are the sarcoplasma reticulum and the β-adrenergic pathway.[109] The targets of gene therapy are to increase β-adrenergic function, adenylyl cyclase, the V_2 vasopressin receptor, and sarcoplasmic reticulum Ca^{++} ATPase (*SERCA2a*), while also decreasing phospholambam and β-adrenoreceptor kinase (*BARK 1*). All of these new therapies hold great promise and many trials are under way.[110]

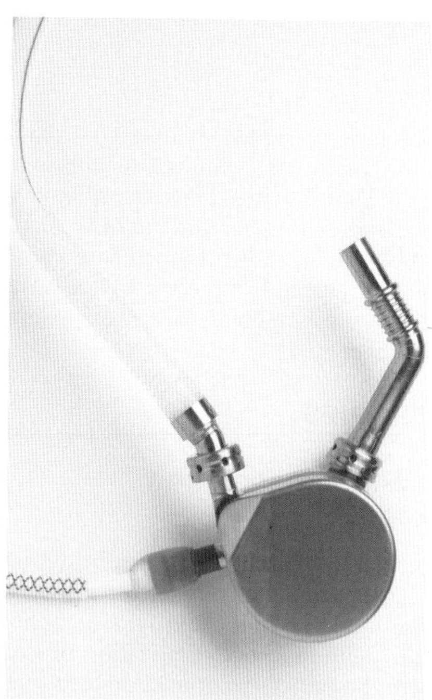

Figure 27–14 The Terumo DuraHeart LVAS. The Terumo DuraHeart LVAS (Terumo Heart, Inc., Ann Arbor, MI), an investigational device, is an implantable, miniaturized centrifugal pump in clinical trials in Europe.[129,130] The impeller of this device is magnetically levitated. Lack of bearings (or other points of contact) will likely result in increased longevity. (Photograph reproduced with permission from Terumo Heart, Inc.)

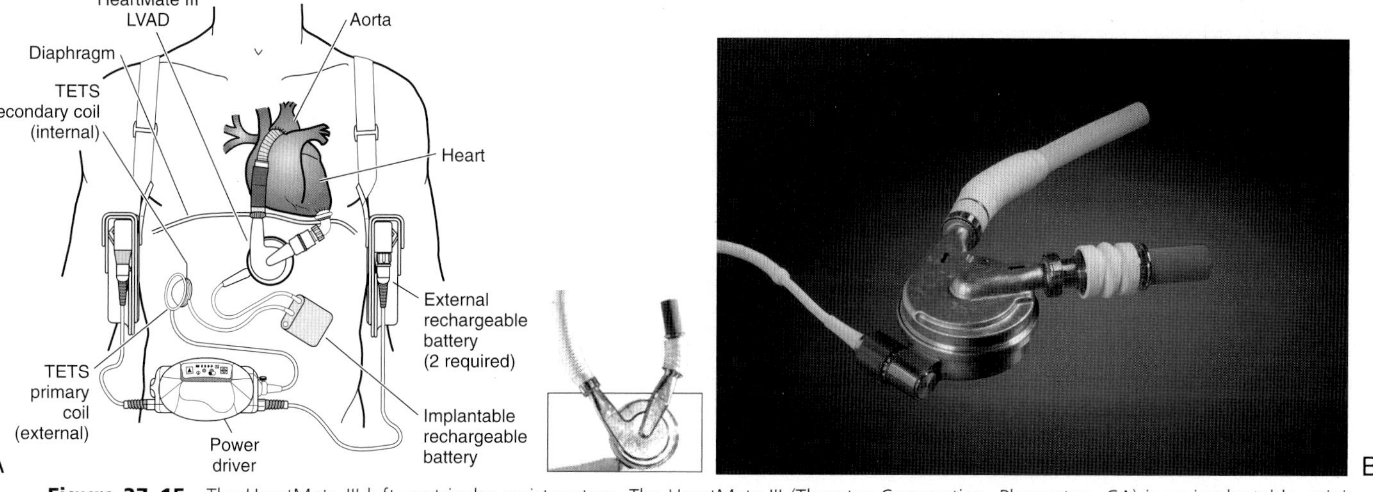

Figure 27–15 The HeartMate III left ventricular assist system. The HeartMate III (Thoratec Corporation, Pleasanton, CA) is an implantable, miniaturized, centrifugal flow device with a magnetically levitated impeller.[131] The HeartMate III is not yet in human clinical trials. (Reproduced with permission from Thoratec Corporation.)

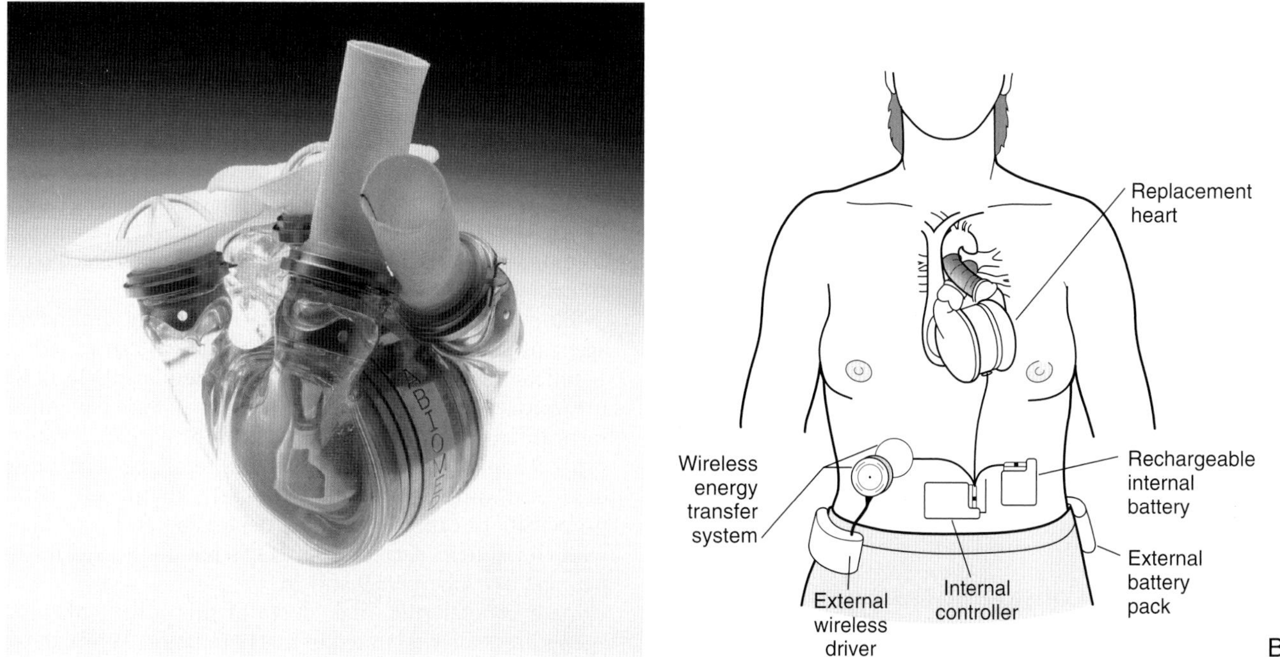

Figure 27–16 (*A*) The AbioCor Implantable Replacement Heart. (*B*) Orthotopic implantation of the AbioCor Implantable Replacement Heart. As discussed in the text, the native failed heart is removed, and the AbioCor is implanted orthotopically, anastomosed to cuffs of native atria and the great vessels. Transcutaneous energy transfer technology eliminates the need for percutaneous wires. Human clinical trials with this promising new device are ongoing.[132] (For the latest information, visit www.abiomed.com. Reproduced with permission from Abiomed, Inc.)

ANESTHETIC CONSIDERATIONS IN THE PATIENT WITH SEVERELY IMPAIRED CARDIAC FUNCTION

Essential Considerations

Cardiac failure can be the common outcome of a variety of underlying etiologies, and patients may therefore present with widely varying clinical status. Some may appear quite compromised while others may appear surprisingly well compensated despite significant underlying pathophysiology. Regardless of what is planned surgically, achieving hemodynamic stability during the induction and maintenance of anesthesia requires a preoperative knowledge of the status of the coronary arteries (including prior bypass grafts or stents), the extent of any valvular regurgitation and/or stenosis that may be present, and whether or not there is significant pulmonary hypertension. Additionally, all patients with significant ventricular dysfunction require a thorough preoperative evaluation of the major organ systems (particularly the renal, hepatic, and central nervous systems) for impairment. The anesthetic plan can then take any existing organ dysfunction into consideration.

Preoperative Optimization

Patients with cardiac failure are medically optimized by pharmacologic manipulations of SVR (afterload reduction), β-blockade, and diuresis. Most medications should be continued throughout the perioperative period, but the decision as to whether or not to withhold angiotensin-converting enzyme inhibitors and diuretics should be made on an individual basis.

Patients with HF often require preinduction optimization of intravascular volume status, pharmacologic manipulations of inotropy and afterload, adjustments to pacemaker settings (where present), and, on occasion, elective placement of an IABP (see Chapters 10 through 13, 25, and 31).

It is prudent to provide supplemental oxygen and monitor vital signs during the preoperative period. This is especially important if anxiolytic medications are given because this population will not tolerate sudden decreases in sympathetic tone, hypoxemia, nor the potentially increased pulmonary vascular resistance that may accompany a respiratory acidosis if hypoventilation results from anxiolysis.

Intraoperative Considerations

Most procedures intended to improve cardiac function will require CPB, but the potential availability of bypass cannot be taken for granted because the function of even a severely depressed ventricle can still get worse, and it is well known that having to emergently institute CPB significantly increases morbidity and mortality. In the prebypass period, further depression of cardiac function and significant increases in ventricular afterload must be avoided, which will increase myocardial oxygen demand, and may cause ischemia. Preload, afterload, heart rate, and contractility must be continuously optimized for each patient at all times.

Where CPB will be used, it is generally prudent to consider employing an antifibrinolytic agent (e.g., ε-aminocaproic acid, aprotinin, or tranexamic acid) in an attempt to decrease bleeding in the postbypass period. In some patients, CPB may not be needed to insert an LVAD.

Anesthetic Agents and Technique

While the usual sedative and hypnotic agents may be tolerated in patients with mild cardiac failure, the failing heart is chronically compensated by a heightened adrenergic state, and removal of that sympathetic tone may lead to rapid decompensation with cardiovascular collapse during anesthetic induction. Patients with severely decreased ventricular function tend to decompensate quickly from physiologic and hemodynamic aberrations (e.g., hypercarbia, hypoxemia, hypotension, brady/tachycardia, sudden alterations in volume status, loss of sinus rhythm), and agents should be chosen and used in a manner likely to maintain hemodynamic stability. Additionally, agent selection should take into account any coexisting renal or hepatic insufficiency. Intravascular volume status needs to be carefully considered and continuously optimized for each individual patient. Inotropic and vasoactive agents, including ephedrine, phenylephrine, dopamine, epinephrine, milrinone, vasopressin, nitroglycerin, and nitroprusside should be available and judiciously used at the first sign of refractory hemodynamic instability.

Unfortunately, there can be no cookbook approach to these patients. Despite the perceived similarity of one patient with cardiac failure to another, each individual's underlying pathophysiology must be carefully considered and then anesthetic agents chosen that will best maintain the hemodynamic goals for that patient.

Traditionally, a technique based on high-dose opioid (e.g., total fentanyl dose 50 to 100 μg/kg, or total sufentanil dose 5 to 10 μg/kg) together with a neuromuscular blocking agent has been used for patients with severely depressed cardiac function. While such a technique will likely result in many hours of hemodynamic stability, potential disadvantages of this technique are that amnesia may not be adequate, and the bradycardia and initial chest wall rigidity that typically accompany such an induction must be pharmacologically countered.

Etomidate (0.2 to 0.3 mg/kg IV) is usually the induction agent of choice in these patients because it causes neither a significant reduction in SVR nor a significant decrease in myocardial contractility. The decreases in vascular tone and myocardial contractility that accompany induction with propofol make this drug unsuitable for those with severely depressed cardiac function. Similarly, thiopental, with its propensity to cause myocardial depression and venodilation, with consequent decreases in CO, is not often used for these patients (see Chapters 9 and 26).

As a general rule, high doses of the potent inhalational agents are poorly tolerated in this population. While all of the inhalational agents (including nitrous oxide) are myocardial depressants to varying extents, enflurane and halothane are particularly potent in this regard and are generally avoided in patients with depressed ventricular function. Isoflurane, sevoflurane, and desflurane are more likely to be compatible with hemodynamic stability in the well-optimized patient, although isoflurane and desflurane must be used cautiously due to their particular tendency to decrease SVR. In comparison with the other currently available agents, sevoflurane appears to cause less myocardial depression and decrease in SVR. In addition to direct myocardial depression and vasodilation, the inhaled anesthetic agents may also affect myocardial automaticity, impulse conduction, and refractoriness, potentially resulting in reentry phenomena and arrhythmias.

Table 27–6 Carpentier Classification of Mitral Regurgitation[113]

Carpentier Class	Leaflet Motion	Typical Pathology
Type I	Normal leaflet motion	Annular dilation, leaflet perforation
Type II	Excessive leaflet motion	Leaflet prolapse or flail, chordal rupture or elongation
Type IIIa	Restricted leaflet motion	Rheumatic leaflet(s), thickened or fused leaflets or chordae
Type IIIb	Restricted leaflet motion	Papillary muscle displacement/dysfunction (dilated cardiomyopathy or ischemic)

Although its use in adults has decreased dramatically in recent years, ketamine remains an extremely useful agent in patients with severely decreased ventricular function. A ketamine induction (1 to 2.5 mg/kg IV or 2.5 to 5 mg/kg IM) followed by a maintenance infusion (50 to 100 μg/kg/min) will usually provide excellent hemodynamic stability while assuring adequate analgesia and amnesia. Where feasible, midazolam is generally provided prior to giving ketamine in an attempt to lessen the potential postemergence psychiatric side effects that may occur in some patients. Additional small doses (1 to 2 mg every 2 to 3 hours) or an infusion of midazolam (0.5 μg/kg/min) are often provided where a ketamine infusion is in use. For adults and older pediatric patients, a small dose of glycopyrrolate (e.g., 0.2 mg IV) is generally provided to act as an antisialogog. Atropine (10 μg/kg) is used for this purpose in neonates and infants. Once on CPB, the ketamine infusion can be stopped, and moderate-to-high doses of narcotics administered.

Central venous access and pulmonary artery catheterization (PAC) are extremely useful (if not mandatory) in this patient population for several reasons. First, pharmacologic interventions are frequently necessary, and potent inotropic and vasoactive agents are preferably administered to the circulation through a central route. Second, despite recent controversy regarding the usefulness and potentially increased morbidity and mortality with a PAC in critically ill patients, the ability to follow and optimize trends of CO and other hemodynamic indices, as well as the ability to assess the efficacy of pharmacologic interventions to manipulate pulmonary vascular resistance, cannot be overlooked.[111] The studies critical of routine PAC use do not directly address the cardiac surgical population, and so cannot reasonably be used to exclude this patient population from their use. Third, an extraordinarily useful monitor for evaluating the adequacy of oxygen delivery is measurement of mixed venous oxygen saturation. It might be argued that a central venous catheter alone can be used to estimate central filling pressures, and Mangano et al[112] demonstrated the ability to assess LV filling pressures using a central venous catheter, but only if the EF was greater than 40%. The population in question, however, will (by definition) present to the operating room with severely depressed LV function, justifying the use of a PAC in the majority of cases.

TEE is now considered one of the main monitoring devices used by a cardiac anesthesiologist. In addition to all the other two-dimensional and Doppler information obtainable, the main advantage of TEE over a PAC lies in the ability to directly visualize and optimize filling volumes. When using a PAC, the clinician assumes a certain filling volume by measuring filling pressures. However, this assumed correlation is accurate only when the pressure-volume curve is known, and this is rarely the case in clinical practice. This patient population with severe CHF, usually presenting with concurrent diastolic dysfunction, will have pathologic compliance curves, requiring higher-than-normal filling pressures to obtain normal filling volumes. In addition, the Doppler capabilities of modern day TEE systems can give the clinician a wealth of knowledge to help fine-tune pharmacologic interventions. There are, however, certain limitations to employing TEE. In addition to the fact that initial acquisition cost and maintenance of equipment are considerable, TEE *is* an invasive monitoring technique, and injuries to the pharynx and esophagus are well known (though uncommon) complications. Perhaps the biggest limiting factor in using TEE as a routine monitoring device, however, is the fact that interpretation of ultrasound images can be complex and requires an experienced echocardiographer (see Chapters 15 and 16).

Nowhere is TEE a more invaluable intraoperative tool than during surgical procedures intended to improve cardiac function, as the success of many of these procedures depends on specific information provided by the echocardiographer. For example, TEE visualization of the precise mechanism and location of mitral regurgitation often determines the feasibility of valve repair. TEE is used to assess the anatomy of the valve overall, as well as to specifically evaluate the leaflets for abnormal thickening, calcification, mobility, and points of coaptation with respect to the annular plane. Doppler analyses and color-flow mapping complement the two-dimensional evaluation and may provide additional information. The use of a mechanistic classification of MR greatly facilitates communication with the surgeon. The Carpentier classification of MR (Table 27–6) is often used because it mechanistically distinguishes valves with normal leaflet motion (type I), excessive leaflet motion (type II), and restricted leaflet motion (type III) (see Chapters 12, 15, 16, and 20).

Transesophageal Echocardiography and Ventricular Assist Devices

The role of TEE where mechanical ventricular assist devices are concerned really begins prior to placement of the device, with a TEE evaluation focused on detecting or ruling out specific anatomic pathologies which may prevent the device from functioning as intended, or lead to preventable complications, and often must be surgically addressed prior to starting support by the device.

In order to know what to look for, it is important to understand the basics of the device, including where the device or its components reside during support, how they are placed there, and the principles by which the device functions to assist the ventricle and support the circulation. As described above, the goal of such assist devices is twofold: (1) to decompress, or to empty, the failing ventricle by diverting blood from the failed side of the heart into the pump, and (2) once the pump is full, the stroke volume in the pump must be ejected into the arterial circulation immediately downstream of the failing ventricle to provide effective forward CO.

Regardless of the specific manufacturer's device attached to the inflow and outflow cannulas, TEE is an invaluable tool prior to, during, and following the placement of VADs.

Pre-LVAD placement, TEE is used to detect specific anatomic pathologies which will:

- Impair LVAD filling (e.g., mitral stenosis, severe tricuspid regurgitation, severe RV dysfunction)
- Decrease efficacy of LVAD ejection and LV decompression (e.g., aortic regurgitation)
- Cause complications once the LVAD is functioning (e.g., patent foramen ovale, atrial septal defect, intracardiac thrombus, ascending aortic atherosclerosis, mobile plaques)

During LVAD placement, TEE is used to:

- Ensure proper inflow cannula position in center of LV (pointing toward mitral valve)
- Ensure adequate deairing of device prior to startup

Post-LVAD placement, TEE is used to:

- Ensure adequate LV decompression (but not complete obliteration of the LV cavity)
- Ensure RV function does not deteriorate
- Ensure tricuspid regurgitation does not worsen (or assess the need for a tricuspid valve annuloplasty)
- Reevaluate for patent foramen ovale (must be closed if detected)

For a more detailed description of the utility of TEE prior to and during VAD placement and in the perioperative period, the interested reader is referred to the many published reviews available in the literature and major textbooks of echocardiography.[114-117]

Postoperative Considerations

By and large, improvements in ventricular function will not be immediately apparent in this population following the majority of surgical procedures described in this chapter. In fact, ventricular function is often worse following a major cardiotomy as there has often been some degree of myocardial stunning during CPB despite the best of myocardial protective techniques with modern cardioplegia. Generally, it will be necessary to optimize intravascular volume status and employ pharmacologic manipulations of afterload and contractility. Temporary pacing with epicardial wires placed during surgery is often used to optimize heart rate. In addition, meticulous management of electrolytes, coagulation status and red blood cell mass is necessary.

One area that is often neglected in this population with sometimes tenuous hemodynamics is postoperative pain management. Patients with severely decreased ventricular function will not tolerate the stress response and tachycardia that accompany postoperative pain due to the increased myocardial oxygen demand (potentially leading to ischemia) and decreased diastolic filling time (potentially leading to decreased stroke volume). This combination is especially deleterious in patients with poor ventricular function and will exacerbate hemodynamic instability.

Most often, postoperative pain management in this population is with intermittent boluses of opioids delivered by a nurse or via patient-controlled analgesia (PCA) pumps. Regional techniques (e.g., continuous epidural infusions and single-shot intrathecal opioids) are becoming popular, though concern for central neuraxial hematomas in light of intraoperative heparinization and the coagulopathy that results from CPB still limits their use in the adult population in many centers (see Chapter 37).

Placement of preservative-free morphine in the subarachnoid space (7.5 to 10 μg/kg) or the epidural space (75 to 100 μg/kg) will generally be well tolerated and can provide adequate analgesia for approximately 16 to 24 hours following cardiac surgical procedures. The main side effects of this technique are itching (usually controllable by a low-dose infusion of naloxone, 0.5 to 1 μg/kg/hr, titrated to effect) and sedation with potential late respiratory depression.

CONCLUSIONS

The preceding sections have summarized the advances made in surgical therapy of CHF. As one of the fastest growing segments of the population of patients with heart disease, CHF patients will be the subject of many ongoing investigations. As the biotechnology industry and practitioners make further advances, the interested reader must pay close attention to the medical literature to remain current on this subject.[133]

REFERENCES

1. American Heart Association: Heart Disease and Stroke Statistics–2003 Update. Dallas, American Heart Association, 2002
2. Lloyd-Jones DM: The risk of congestive heart failure: Sobering lessons from the Framingham Heart Study. Curr Cardiol Rep 3:184, 2001
3. O'Connell JB, Bristow MR: Economic impact of heart failure in the United States: Time for a different approach. J Heart Lung Transplant 13(suppl):S107, 1994
4. Zeltsman D, Acker MA: Surgical management of heart failure: An overview. Annu Rev Med 53:383, 2002
5. Vitali E, Colombo T, Fratto P, et al: Surgical therapy in advanced heart failure. Am J Cardiol 91(suppl):88F, 2003
6. Dec GW: Management of heart failure: Crossing boundary over to the surgical country. Surg Clin N Am 84:1, 2004
7. The Criteria Committee of the New York Heart Association: Nomenclature and Criteria for Diagnosis of Diseases of the Heart and Great Vessels, 9th edition. Boston, Little, Brown & Co, 1994, pp 253–256
8. Francis GS, Tang WH, Sonnenblick EH: Pathophysiology of heart failure. *In* Furster V, Alexander RW, O'Rourke RA, et al (ed): Hurst's The Heart, 11th edition. New York, McGraw-Hill, 2004, pp 697–722
9. Massie BM: Pathophysiology of heart failure. *In* Goldman L, Ausiello D (eds): Cecil Textbook of Medicine, 22nd edition. Philadelphia, WB Saunders, 2005, pp 291–299
10. Colucci WS, Braunwald E: Pathophysiology of heart failure. *In* Braunwald E: Heart Disease: A Textbook of Cardiovascular Medicine, 7th edition. Philadelphia, WB Saunders, 2005, pp 509–538
11. Kajstura J, Cigola E, Malhotra A, et al: Angiotensin II induces apoptosis of adult ventricular myocytes in-vitro. J Mol Cell Cardiol 29:859, 1997
12. The CONSENSUS Trial Study Group: Effects of enalapril on mortality in severe congestive heart failure. Results of the Cooperative North Scandinavian Enalapril Survival Study (CONSENSUS). N Engl J Med 316:1429, 1987
13. The SOLVD Investigators: Effect of enalapril on survival in patients with reduced left ventricular ejection fractions and congestive heart failure. N Engl J Med 325:293, 1991
14. Pfeffer MA, Braunwald E, Moye LA, et al, on behalf of the SAVE Investigators: Effect of captopril on mortality and morbidity in patients with left ventricular dysfunction after myocardial infarction. Results of the Survival and Ventricular Enlargement Trial. N Engl J Med 327:669, 1992
15. Packer M, Bristow MR, Cohn JN, et al, for the US Carvedilol Heart Failure Study Group: The effect of carvedilol on mortality and morbidity in patients with chronic heart failure. N Engl J Med 334:1349, 1996
16. Leizorovicz A, Lechat P, Cucherat M, et al: Bisoprolol for the treatment of chronic heart failure: A meta-analysis on individual data of two placebo-controlled studies—CIBIS and CIBIS II. Am Heart J 143:301, 2002
17. McGavin JK, Keating GM: Bisoprolol: A review of its use in chronic heart failure. Drugs 62: 2677, 2002

18. Wikstrand J, Hjalmarson A, Waagstein F, et al: Dose of metoprolol CR/XL and clinical outcome in patients with heart failure. Analysis of the experience in metoprolol CR/XL randomized intervention trial in chronic heart failure. J Am Coll Cardiol 40:491, 2002
19. Pitt B, Zannad F, Remme WJ, et al, for the Randomized Aldactone Evaluation Study Investigators: The effect of spironolactone on morbidity and mortality in patients with severe heart failure. N Engl J Med 341:709, 1999
20. Farquharson CAJ, Struthers AD: Spironolactone increases nitric oxide bioactivity, improves endothelial vasodilator dysfunction, and suppresses angiotensin I/angiotensin II conversion in patients with chronic heart failure. Circulation 101:594, 2000
21. Westaby S, Narula J: Preface: Surgical options in heart failure. Surg Clin N Am 84:15, 2004
22. Packer M: Management of heart failure. *In* Goldman L, Ausiello D (eds): Cecil Textbook of Medicine, 22nd edition. Philadelphia, WB Saunders, 2005, pp 300–310
23. Mickleborough L, Merchant N, Ivanov J, et al: Left ventricular reconstruction: Early and late results. J Thorac Cardiovasc Surg 128:27, 2004
24. Kumpati GS, McCarthy PM, Hoercher KJ: Surgical treatments for heart failure. Cardiol Clin 19:669, 2001
25. Elefteriades J, Edwards R: Coronary bypass in left heart failure. Semin Thorac Cardiovasc Surg 14:125, 2002
26. Bolling SF: Mitral reconstruction in cardiomyopathy. J Heart Valve Dis 11(suppl 1):S26, 2002
27. Tolis GA Jr, Korkolis DP, Kopf GS, et al: Revascularization alone (without mitral valve repair) suffices in patients with advanced ischemic cardiomyopathy and mild-moderate mitral regurgitation. Ann Thorac Surg 74:1476, 2002
28. Hon JKF, Yacoub MH: Bridge to recovery with the use of left ventricular assist device and clenbuterol. Ann Thorac Surg 75:S36, 2003
29. Miller WL, Tointon SK, Hodge DO, et al: Long-term outcome and the use of revascularization in patients with heart failure, suspected ischemic heart disease, and large reversible myocardial perfusion defects. Am Heart J 143:904, 2002
30. Liao L, Cabell CH, Jollis JG, et al: Usefulness of myocardial viability or ischemia in predicting long-term survival for patients with severe left ventricular dysfunction undergoing revascularization. Am J Cardiol 93:1275, 2004
31. Vitali E, Colombo T, Fratto P, et al: Surgical therapy in advanced heart failure. Am J Cardiol 91(suppl):88F, 2003
32. Trachiotis GD, Weintraub WS, Johnston T, et al: Coronary artery bypass grafting in patients with advanced left ventricular dysfunction. Ann Thorac Surg 66:1632, 1998
33. Carstensen S: Dobutamine-atropine stress echocardiography. Heart Drug 5:101, 2005
34. Mickleborough LL, Carson S, Tamariz M, Ivanov J: Results of revascularization in patients with severe left ventricular dysfunction. J Thorac Cardiovasc Surg 119:550, 2000
35. Geha AS, El-Zein C, Massad MG: Mitral valve surgery in patients with ischemic and nonischemic dilated cardiomyopathy. Cardiology 101:15, 2004
36. Phillips HR, Levine FH, Carter JE, et al: Mitral valve replacement for isolated mitral regurgitation: Analysis of clinical course and late postoperative left ventricular ejection fraction. Am J Cardiol 48:647, 1981.
37. Romano MA, Bolling SF: Mitral valve repair as an alternative treatment for heart failure patients. Heart Fail Monit 4:7, 2003
38. Rothenburger M, Rukosujew A, Hammel D, et al: Mitral valve surgery in patients with poor left ventricular function. Thorac Cardiovasc Surg 50: 351, 2002
39. Bishay ES, McCarthy PM, Cosgrove DM, et al: Mitral valve surgery in patients with severe left ventricular dysfunction. Eur J Cardiothorac Surg 17:213, 2000
40. Reese TB, Tribble CG, Ellman PI, et al: Mitral repair is superior to replacement when associated with coronary artery disease. Ann Surg 239:671–5, 2004
41. Mohty D, Orszulak TA, Schaff HV, et al: Very long-term survival and durability of mitral valve repair for mitral valve prolapse. Circulation 104(suppl I):I-1, 2001
42. Gillinov AM, Wierup PN, Blackstone EH, et al: Is repair preferable to replacement for ischemic mitral regurgitation? J Thorac Cardiovasc Surg 122:1125, 2001
43. Batista RJ, Santos JL, Takeshita N, et al: Partial left ventriculectomy to improve left ventricular function in end-stage heart disease. J Cardiac Surg 11:96, 1996
44. Batista RJV, Verde J, Nery P, et al: Partial left ventriculectomy to treat end-stage heart disease. Ann Thorac Surg 64:634, 1997
45. Franco-Cereceda A, McCarthy PM, Blackstone EH, et al: Partial left ventriculectomy for dilated cardiomyopathy: Is this an alternative to transplantation? J Thorac Cardiovasc Surg 121:879, 2001
46. McCarthy JF, McCarthy PM, Starling RC, et al: Partial left ventriculectomy and mitral valve repair for end-stage congestive heart failure. Eur J Cardiothorac Surg 13:337, 1998
47. Etoch SW, Koenig SC, Laureano MA, et al: Results after partial left ventriculectomy versus heart transplantation for idiopathic cardiomyopathy. J Thorac Cardiovasc Surg 117:952, 1999
48. Suma H, RESTORE Group: Left ventriculoplasty for nonischemic dilated cardiomyopathy. Semin Thorac Cardiovasc Surg 13:514, 2001
49. Dor V, Sabatier M, DiDonato M, et al: Efficacy of endoventricular patch plasty in large postinfarction akinetic scar and severe left ventricular dysfunction: Comparison with a series of large dyskinetic scars. J Thorac Cardiovasc Surg 116:47, 1998
50. DiDonato M, Sabatier M, Dor V, et al: Effects of the Dor procedure on left ventricular dimension and shape and geometric correlates of mitral regurgitation one year after surgery. J Thorac Cardiovasc Surg 121:91, 2001
51. Athanasuleas CL, Stanley AW Jr, Buckberg GD, et al: Surgical anterior ventricular endocardial restoration (SAVER) in the dilated remodeled ventricle after anterior myocardial infarction. RESTORE Group. Reconstructive Endoventricular Surgery, Returning Torsion Original Radius Elliptical Shape to the LV. J Am Coll Cardiol 37:1199, 2001
52. Carpentier A, Chachques JC: Myocardial substitution with a stimulated skeletal muscle: First successful case [letter]. Lancet 8440:1267, 1985.
53. Furnary AP, Jessup M, Moreira LF: Multicenter trial of dynamic cardiomyoplasty for chronic heart failure. J Am Coll Cardiol 28:1175, 1996
54. Mann DL, Acker MA, Jessup M, et al: Rationale, design, and methods for a pivotal randomized clinical trial for the assessment of a cardiac support device in patients with New York Heart Association Class III-IV heart failure. J Card Fail 10:185, 2004
55. Oz MC, Konerzt WF, Kleber FX, et al: Global surgical experience with the acorn cardiac support device. J Thorac Cardiovasc Surg 126:983, 2003
56. Kerwin WF, Botvinick EH, O'Connell JW, et al: Ventricular contraction abnormalities in dilated cardiomyopathy: Effect of biventricular pacing to correct interventricular dyssynchrony. J Am Coll Cardiol 35:1221, 2000
57. Jarcho J: Resynchronizing ventricular contraction in heart failure. N Engl J Med 352:1594, 2005
58. Shamin W, Francis DP, Yousufuddin M, et al: Intraventricular conduction delay: A prognostic marker in chronic heart failure. Int J Cardiol 70:171, 1999
59. Auricchio A, Stellbrink C, et al: The Pacing Therapies for Congestive Heart Failure Study: Rationale, design, and endpoint of a prospective randomized multicenter study. Am J Cardiol 83:130D, 1999
60. Cazeau S, Leclereq C, et al: The Multisite Stimulation in Cardiomyopathies Study Investigators. Effects of multisite biventricular pacing in patients with heart failure and intraventricular conduction delay. N Engl J Med 334:873, 2001
61. Abraham WT, Fisher WG, et al, for the multicenter Insync Randomized Clinical Evaluation Investigators and Coordinators: Double-blind, randomized, controlled trial of cardiac resynchronization in chronic heart failure. N Engl J Med 346:1845, 2002
62. Cleland J, Daubert J, Erdman E, et al: The effect of cardiac resynchronization on morbidity and mortality in heart failure. N Engl J Med 352:1539, 2005
63. Kass DA, Chen CH, Curry C, et al: Improved left ventricular mechanics from acute VDD pacing in patients with dilated cardiomyopathy and ventricular conduction delay. Circulation 99:1567, 1999
64. Auricchio A, Stellbrink C, Block M, et al: Effect of pacing chamber and atrioventricular delay on acute systolic function of paced patients with congestive heart failure. Circulation 99:2993, 1999
65. Gras D, Mabo P, Tang T, et al: Multisite pacing as a supplemental treatment of congestive heart failure: Preliminary results of the Medtronic Inc. InSync Study. Pacing Clin Electrophysiol 21:2249, 1998
66. Cazeau S, Leclercq C, Lavergne T, et al: Effects of multisite biventricular pacing in patients with heart failure and intraventricular conduction delay. N Engl J Med 344:873, 2001
67. Goldman S, Johnson G: for the V-HeFT VA Cooperative Studies Group: Mechanism of death in heart failure. The Vasodilator-Heart Failure Trials. Circulation 87(suppl VI):VI-24, 1993
68. Abraham WT, Fisher WG, Smith AL, for the MIRACLE Investigators and Coordinators. Multicenter InSync Randomized Clinical Evaluation (MIRACLE): Results of a randomized, double-blind, controlled trial to assess cardiac resynchronization therapy in heart failure patients [abstract]. Circulation 104:II, 2001

69. Hohnloser S, Kuck K, Dorlan P, et al: Prophylactic use of an implantable cardioverter-defibrillator after acute myocardial infarction. N Engl J Med 351:2481, 2004
70. Bardy E, Lee K, Mark D, et al: Amiodarone or an implanted cardioverter-defibrillator for congestive heart failure. N Engl J Med 352:225, 2005
71. Buxton AE, Lee KL, et al: A randomized study of the prevention of sudden death in patients with coronary artery disease. N Engl J Med 341:1882,1999
72. Moss AJ, Zareba W, et al: Prophylactic implantation of a defibrillator in patients with myocardial infarction and reduced ejection fraction. N Engl J Med 346:877, 2002
73. Bristow MR, Saxon LA, Boehmer J, et al: Cardiac-resynchronization therapy with or without an implantable defibrillator in advanced chronic heart failure. N Engl J Med 350:2140, 2004
74. BVS5000 Bi-ventricular Support Training Manual. Danvers, MA, Abiomed, Inc, July 1997
75. Minami K, El-Banayosy A, Sezai A, et al: Morbidity and outcome after mechanical support using Thoratec, Novacor, and HeartMate for bridging to heart transplantation. Artif Organs 24:421, 2000
76. Robbins RC, Kown MH, Portner PM, Oyer PE: The totally implantable Novacor left ventricular assist system. Ann Thorac Surg 71:S162, 2001
77. Frazier OH, Rose EA, Oz MC, et al: Multicenter clinical evaluation of the HeartMate vented electric left ventricular assist system in patients awaiting heart transplantation. J Thorac Cardiovasc Surg 122:1186, 2001
78. Pasque MK, Rogers JA: Adverse events in the use of HeartMate vented electric and Novacor left ventricular assist devices: Comparing apples and oranges. J Thorac Cardiovasc Surg 124:1063, 2002
79. Copeland JG, Arabia FA, Smith RG, et al: Mechanical assist device: The CardioWest total artificial heart. Transplant Proc 32:1523, 2000
80. Copeland JG, Arabia FA, Tsau PH, et al: Total artificial hearts: Bridge to transplantation. Cardiol Clin 21:101, 2003
81. Copeland JG, Smith RG, Arabia FA, et al: Cardiac replacement with a total artificial heart as a bridge to transplantation. N Engl J Med 351:859, 2004
82. Rose EA, Gelijns AC, Moskowitz AJ, et al: Long-term use of a left ventricular assist device for end-stage heart failure. N Engl J Med 345:1435, 2001
83. Patten R, DeNofrio D, El-Zaru M, et al: Ventricular assist device therapy normalizes inducible nitric oxide synthase expression and reduces cardiomyocyte apoptosis in the failing human heart. J Am Coll Cardiol 45:1419, 2005
84. Zafeirides A, Jeevanandam V, Houser SR, Margulies KB: Regression of cellular hypertrophy after left ventricular assist device support. Circulation 98:656, 1998
85. Kim S, Depre C, Vatner S: Novel Mechanisms of Stunned Myocardium. Heart Fail Rev 8:143, 2003
86. Terracciano CMN, Hardy J, Birks EJ, et al: Clinical recovery from end-stage heart failure using left ventricular assist device and pharmacological therapy correlates with increased sarcoplasmic reticulum calcium content but not with regression of cellular hypertrophy. Circulation 109:2263, 2004
87. Madigan JD, Barbone A, Choudhri AF, et al: Time course of reverse remodeling of the left ventricle during support with a left ventricular assist device. J Thorac Cardiovasc Surg 121:902, 2001
88. Santamore WP, Gray LA: Left ventricular contributions to right ventricular systolic function during LVAD support. Ann Thorac Surg 61:350, 1996
89. Horton S, Khodaverdian R, Powers A, et al: Left ventricular assist device malfunction: A systemic approach to diagnosis. J Am Coll Cardiol 43:1574, 2004
90. HeartMate sutures not applied vented electric (SNAP-VE) left ventricular assist system (LVAS): Directions for Use. Pleasanton, CA, Thoratec Corporation, Document 29123, revision B, April 25, 2001
91. Physician's Manual Novacor LVAS. Baxter Healthcare Corporation, Novacor Division, Technical Support Department, Deerfield, IL, Document GCP 9 105, revision B, 1998, pp 1-1–16-2
92. Lee J, Miller PJ, Chen H, Conley MG, et al: Reliability model from the in-vitro durability tests of a left ventricular assist system. ASAIO J 45:595, 1999
93. Allen GS, Murray KD, Olsen DB: The importance of pulsatile and nonpulsatile flow in the design of blood pumps. Artif Organs 21:922, 1997
94. Mavroudis C: To pulse or not to pulse. Ann Thorac Surg 25:259, 1978
95. Sezai A, Shiono M, Orime Y, Nakata K, et al: Major organ function under mechanical support: Comparative studies of pulsatile and nonpulsatile circulation. Artif Organs 23:280, 1999
96. Orime Y, Shiono M, Hata H, Yagi S, et al: Cytokine and endothelial damage in pulsatile and nonpulsatile cardiopulmonary bypass. Artif Organs 23:508, 1999
97. Shomura Y, Tanaka K, Takabayashi S, et al: Arterial baroreceptor afferent activity in nonpulsatile systemic circulation. Artif Organs 22:1056, 1998
98. Golding L, Murakami G, Harasaki H, et al: Chronic nonpulsatile flow. ASAIO Trans 28:81, 1982
99. Golding L: Centrifugal pumps. *In* Unger F (ed): Assisted Circulation 2. Berlin, Springer Verlag, 1984
100. Cooley DA, Liotta D, Hallman GL, et al: Orthotopic cardiac prosthesis for two staged cardiac replacement. Am J Cardiol 24:723, 1969
101. Cooley DA, Akutsu T, Norman JC, et al: Total artificial heart in two-stage cardiac transplantation. Cardiovasc Dis 8:305, 1981
102. DeVries WL, Anderson JL, Joyce LD, et al: Clinical use of the total artificial heart. N Engl J Med 310:273, 1984.
103. Organ Procurement and Transplant Network (OPTN) data www.OPTN.org/data, accessed 5/29/04
104. Menasche P: Cell transplantation in myocardium. Ann Thorac Surg 75:20, 2003
105. Siminiak T, Fiszer D, Jerzykowska O, et al: Percutaneous transvenous transplantation of autologous myoblasts in the treatment of postinfarction heart failure: The POZNAN trial. Presented at the American College of Cardiology, 53rd Annual Scientific Session, New Orleans, March 7, 2004
106. Len N: Mobilizing cells to the injured myocardium. J Am Coll Cardiol 44:1521, 2004
107. Rosenstrauch D, Poglajen G, Zidar N, Gregoric I: Stem cell therapy for ischemic heart failure. Tex Heart Inst J 32:339, 2005
108. Snakumar B, Harry L, Paleolog E: Modulating angiogenesis. JAMA 292:972, 2004
109. Chaudhri BB, del Monte F, Harding SE, et al: Gene transfer in cardiac myocytes. Surg Clin N Am: 84:141, 2004
110. Askuri A, Penn M: Targeted gene therapy for the treatment of cardiac dysfunction. Semin Thorac Cardiovasc Surg 14:167, 2002
111. Sandham JD, Hull RD, Brant RF, et al: A randomized, controlled trial of the use of pulmonary-artery catheters in high-risk surgical patients. N Engl J Med 348:5, 2003
112. Mangano DT: Monitoring pulmonary artery pressures in coronary artery disease. Anesth 53:364, 1980
113. Carpentier A, Chauvaud S, Fabiani JN, et al: Reconstructive surgery of mitral valve incompetence: Ten-year appraisal. J Thorac Cardiovasc Surg 79:338, 1980.
114. Horton S, Khodaverdian R, Chatelain P, et al: Left ventricular assist device malfunction: An approach to diagnosis by echocardiography. J Am Coll Cardiol 45:1435, 2005
115. Scalia GM, McCarthy PM, Savage RM, et al: Clinical utility of echocardiography in the management of implantable ventricular assist devices. J Am Soc Echocardiogr 13:754, 2000
116. Stone M: Transesophageal echocardiography and surgical devices: Cannulas, catheters, intraaortic balloon pumps, ventricular assist devices, and occluders. *In* Konstadt S, Shernan S, Oka Y (eds): Clinical Transesophageal Echocardiography: A Problem Oriented Approach, 2nd edition. Philadelphia, Lippincott Williams & Wilkins, 2003, Chapter 16
117. Mets B: Anesthesia for left ventricular assist device placement. J Cardiothorac Vasc Anesth 14:316, 2000
118. Frazier OH, Shah NA, Myers TJ, et al: Use of the Flowmaker (Jarvik 2000) left ventricular assist device for destination therapy and bridging to transplantation. Cardiology 101:111, 2004
119. Frazier OH, Myers TJ, Jarvik RK, et al: Research and development of an implantable, axial-flow left ventricular assist device: The Jarvik 2000 Heart. Ann Thorac Surg 71:S125, 2001
120. Song X, Throckmorton AL, Untaroiu A, et al: Axial flow blood pumps. ASAIO J 49:355, 2003
121. Potapov EV, Koster A, Loebe M, et al: The Micromed DeBakey VAD, Part I: The pump and the blood flow. J Extra Corp Technol 35:274, 2003
122. Goldstein DJ: Worldwide experience with the MicroMed DeBakey VAD as a bridge-to-transplantation. Circulation 9(suppl II):II-272, 2003
123. Vitali E, Lanfranconi M, Ribera E, et al: Successful experience in bridging patients to heart transplantation with the MicroMed DeBakey ventricular assist device. Ann Thorac Surg. 75:1200, 2003
124. Burke DJ, Burke E, Parsaie F, et al: The HeartMate II: Design and development of a fully sealed axial flow left ventricular assist system. Artif Organs 25:380, 2001
125. Griffith BP, Kormos RL, Borovetz HS, et al: HeartMate II left ventricular assist system: From concept to first clinical use. Ann Thorac Surg 71:S116, 2001

126. Berlin Heart: INCOR Berlin Heart AG Web Page, 2004. Available at: http://www.berlinheart.com/products/axial.html
127. Ventrassist: Ventracor Web Page, 2004. Available at: http://www.ventracor.com
128. Chung MKH, Zhang N, Tansley GD, et al: Impeller behavior and displacement of the VentrAssist implantable rotary blood pump. Artif Organs 28:287, 2004
129. DuraHeart: Terumo Heart Web Page, 2004. Available at: http://www.terumo.co.jp
130. Saito S, Westaby S, Piggott D, et al: Reliable long-term non-pulsatile circulatory support without anticoagulation. Eur J CardioThorac Surg 19:678, 2001
131. Loree HM II, Borque K, Gernes DB, et al: The HeartMate III: Design and in vivo studies of a Maglev centrifugal left ventricular assist device. Artif Organs 25:386, 2001
132. Dowling RD, Gray LA, Etoch SW, et al: The AbioCor implantable replacement heart. Ann Thorac Surg 75:S93, 2003
133. Jones RH: The year in cardiovascular surgery. J Am Coll Cardiol 45:1517, 2005

Part VI

EXTRACORPOREAL CIRCULATION

Chapter 28

CARDIOPULMONARY BYPASS AND THE ANESTHESIOLOGIST

Christina T. Mora-Mangano, MD • John L. Chow, MD •
Max Kanevsky, MD, PhD

KEY POINTS

1. Cardiopulmonary bypass (CPB) provides the extracorporeal maintenance of respiration and circulation at hypothermic and normothermic temperatures. CPB permits the surgeon to operate on a quiet—or nonbeating—heart at hypothermic temperatures, thus facilitating surgery in an ischemic environment.
2. CPB is associated with a number of profound physiological perturbations. The central nervous system, kidneys, gut, and heart are especially vulnerable to ischemic events associated with extracorporeal circulation.
3. Controversy regarding the optimal management of blood flow, pressure, and temperature during CPB remains. Perfusion should be adequate to support ongoing oxygen requirements; mean arterial pressures of more than 70 mm Hg may benefit patients with cerebral and/or diffuse arthrosclerosis. Arterial blood temperatures should never exceed 37.5°C.
4. The initiation and termination of CPB are key phases of a cardiac surgery procedure, but the anesthesiologist must remain vigilant throughout the entire bypass.
5. CPB is a complex system that is vulnerable to accidents. Careful and constant communication among the anesthesiologist, surgeon, perfusionist, and nurse is critical for patient safety.
6. Minimally invasive cardiac surgery can be performed with port-access bypass circuits. This approach adds considerable complexity to the procedure but is not as popular as minimally invasive off-pump techniques for coronary artery bypass grafting.
7. Bloodless cardiac surgery is possible, and numerous approaches including autotransfusion and hemodilution facilitate this goal.
8. Total CPB can be tailored to produce deep hypothermic, circulatory arrest or partial right-heart bypass. The special techniques require sophisticated monitoring and care.

An anesthesiologist-in-training posed the question, "Why is my presence necessary during cardiopulmonary bypass? The perfusionist has direct control of the patient's blood pressure and respiration. The inhalation anesthetic is attached to the bypass circuit. Drugs are administered into the venous reservoir. What is my role?" The resident's answer to her own question was incomplete but more robust than that argued by clinicians, who suggest that the presence of a member of the anesthesia care team (e.g., anesthesiologist, nurse anesthetist, physician assistant credentialed in the administration of anesthesia) during cardiopulmonary bypass (CPB) is not essential. The American Society of Anesthesiologists (ASA) states that the absence of anesthesia personnel during the conduct of a general anesthetic violates the first of the ASA Standards for Basic Anesthesia Monitoring.[1] The absence of a member of the anesthesia care team during CPB is below the accepted standard of care. Moreover, to bill for anesthesia care when an anesthesia provider is not physically present in the patient's operating room constitutes fraud.[2] At a minimum, the anesthesiologist's role during CPB is to maintain the anesthetic state—a more challenging task than the usual case when the patient's blood pressure, heart rate, and movement provide information regarding the depth of anesthesia. This chapter outlines the tasks, challenges, and responsibilities of the cardiovascular anesthesiologist beyond the maintenance of the anesthetic state.

HISTORICAL PERSPECTIVE ON CARDIOPULMONARY BYPASS

On May 6, 1953, John Gibbon, Jr., surgically treated a young woman suffering mitral stenosis using cardiopulmonary bypass (CPB), and the long-elusive goal of extracorporeal circulation was achieved (Fig. 28–1). This accomplishment was preceded by 15 years of work by Dr. Gibbon, Jr., and colleagues to develop a device that would provide extracorporeal circulation and support respiration. A young woman who died after a postpartum pulmonary embolism inspired Dr. Gibbon, Jr., then a surgical resident, to seek a way to provide temporary extracorporeal cardiopulmonary support to treat life-threatening disease. The fiftieth anniversary of the first successful use of cardiopulmonary bypass was celebrated in 2003. A number of insightful perspectives on this important medical landmark accompanied the anniversary of this achievement[3-6] (see Chapters 1 and 2).

Review of the history of CPB and cardiac surgery shows that the development of this lifesaving technology occurred in three distinct phases. In the 1950s, cardiac surgeons adopted extracorporeal circulation to care for patients suffering from previously untreatable congenital heart disease. At the conclusion of the decade, the backlog of patients with surgically correctable congenital heart disease had diminished, and a new frontier emerged: valvular heart disease. Through the early 1960s, Starr, Edwards, and other physicians described their success with prosthetic valves. Previously untreatable anatomic maladies of the heart could be corrected. As the population became more aged, the importance of coronary artery bypass with extracorporeal support increased. This third phase includes more than 1 million coronary artery bypass graft (CABG) patients annually. As observed by Pierre Galletti, during none of these phases was the next step in perfusion

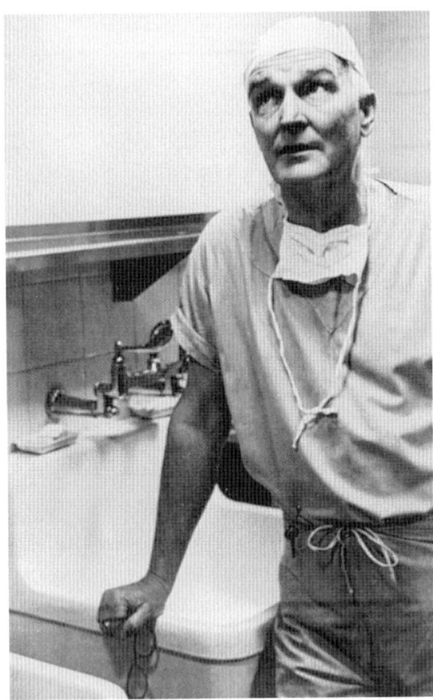

Figure 28–1 Dr. John Gibbon, Jr., before the first successful application of total extracorporeal circulation for cardiac surgery in humans. (Photograph courtesy of the Mütter Museum of the College of Physicians of Philadelphia, PA.)

quantitatively anticipated. It is difficult to predict how CPB will be used in the next millennium. Will human pregnancy become an ex vivo event? Will intravenous oxygenators replace lung allografts? Will bypass circuits become the product of genetic engineering, ensuring perfect biocompatibility?

This chapter briefly describes modern bypass circuits and highlights the many current controversies regarding the management of patients during CPB. The multiple pathophysiologic perturbations precipitated by the process of extracorporeal circulation and the putative effects of these phenomena on end-organ function are discussed in detail. Perfusion accidents can be life-threatening events. It is critical that all members of the heart surgery team anticipate and respond appropriately to mishaps during CPB. This chapter concludes with a synopsis of legal considerations in perfusion.

GOALS AND MECHANICS OF CARDIOPULMONARY BYPASS

The CPB circuit is designed to perform four major functions: oxygenation and carbon dioxide elimination, circulation of blood, systemic cooling and rewarming, and diversion of blood from the heart to provide a bloodless surgical field. Typically, venous blood is drained by gravity from the right side of the heart into a reservoir that serves as a large mixing chamber for all blood return, additional fluids, and drugs. Because (in most instances) negative pressure is not employed, the amount of venous drainage is determined by the central venous pressure, the column height between the patient and reservoir, and resistance to flow in the venous circuitry. Negative pressure (−0.5 cm H_2O) will enhance venous drainage and is used in some bypass approaches, including port-access CPB.

Venous return may be decreased deliberately (as is done when restoring the patient's blood volume before coming off bypass) by application of a venous clamp. From the reservoir, blood is pumped to an oxygenator and heat exchanger unit before passing through an arterial filter and returning to the patient. Additional components of the circuit generally include pumps and tubing for cardiotomy suction, venting, and cardioplegia delivery and recirculation, as well as in-line blood gas monitors, bubble detectors, pressure monitors and blood sampling ports. A schematic representation of a typical bypass circuit is depicted in Figure 28–2.

The cannulation sites and type of CPB circuit used are dependent on the type of operation planned.[7] Most cardiac procedures use full CPB, in which the blood is drained from

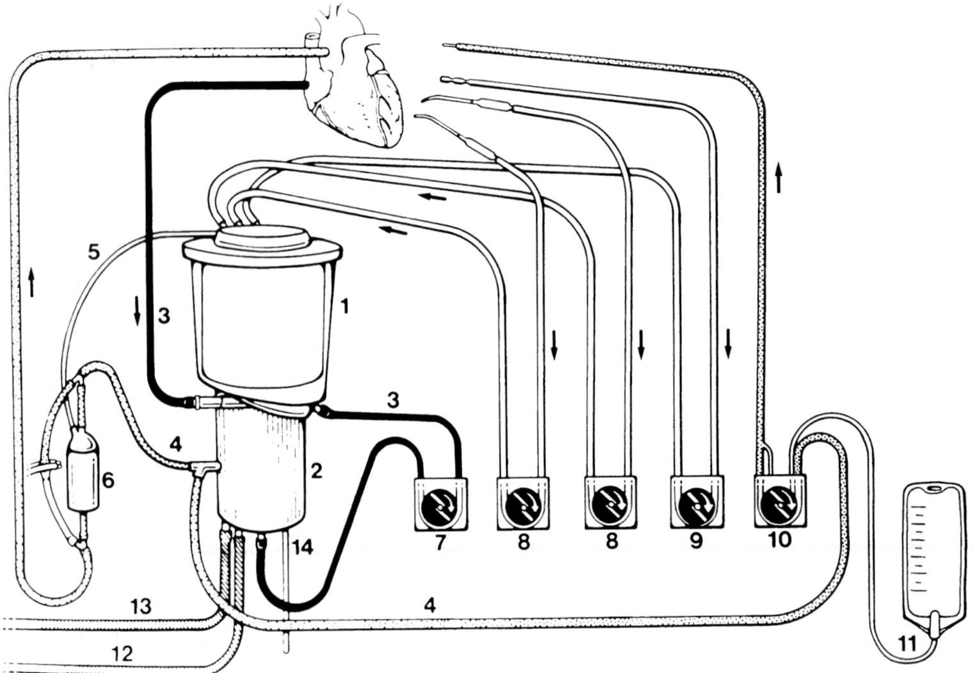

Figure 28–2 Components of the extracorporeal circuit: (1) integral cardiotomy reservoir; (2) membrane oxygenator bundle; (3) venous blood line; (4) arterial blood line; (5) arterial filter purge line; (6) arterial line filter; (7) venous blood pump (also called the arterial pump head; this pump forces venous blood through the membrane oxygenator and arterialized blood to the patient's aortic root); (8) cardiotomy suction pump; (9) ventricular vent pump; (10) cardioplegia pump; (11) crystalloid cardioplegia; (12) water inlet line; (13) water outlet line; and (14) gas inlet line. (From Davis RB, Kauffman JN, Cobbs TL, Mick SL: Cardiopulmonary Bypass. New York, Springer-Verlag, 1995, p 239.)

the right side of the heart and returned to the systemic circulation through the aorta. The CPB circuit performs the function of heart and lungs. Aortoatriocaval cannulation is the preferred method of cannulation for CPB, although femoral arteriovenous cannulation may be the technique of choice for emergency access, "redo" sternotomy, and other clinical settings in which aortic or atrial cannulation is not feasible. Procedures involving the thoracic aorta are often performed using partial bypass in which a portion of oxygenated blood is removed from the left side of the heart and returned to the femoral artery. Perfusion of the head and upper extremity vessels is performed by the beating heart, and distal perfusion is provided below the level of the cross-clamp by retrograde flow by the femoral artery (see Chapter 23). All blood passes through the pulmonary circulation, eliminating the need for an oxygenator.

PHYSIOLOGIC PARAMETERS OF CARDIOPULMONARY BYPASS

The primary objective of CPB is maintenance of systemic perfusion and respiration. Controversy arises with the question of whether systemic oxygenation and perfusion should be "optimal or maximal" or "adequate or sufficient." Remarkably, after more than one-half century of CPB, there is continued disagreement regarding the fundamental management of extracorporeal circulation. Clinicians and investigators disagree on what are the best strategies for arterial blood pressure goals, pump flow, hematocrit, temperature, blood gas management, or mode of perfusion (pulsatile versus nonpulsatile) (Box 28–1). Additional considerations of what is best relate to other goals of CPB: maintenance of homeostasis, facilitation of surgery, and avoidance of complications.

Perfusion Pressure during Cardiopulmonary Bypass

Selection of perfusion pressure during CPB is based on balancing the demands of surgical access (bloodless field) with patient outcome (adequate oxygen delivery). Lower flow and pressure during CPB may optimize visualization, whereas higher flow and pressure may minimize patient complications. Determining the optimum perfusion pressure has been extremely challenging because no single study can adequately address all the complexities of CPB. Because of the brain's poor tolerance of ischemia, neurologic outcome has been the most common outcome studied in relation to perfusion pressure. The complicated relationship between neurologic outcome and perfusion pressure is likely related to two causes of adverse neurologic outcomes: hypoperfusion and embolism.

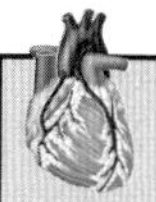

BOX 28–1 *Practice of Cardiopulmonary Bypass*

Best Practices Are Still Developing in Regard to

- Perfusion pressure
- Pump flow
- Temperature management
- Central nervous system monitoring
- Pulsatility

Between mean arterial pressures (MAP) of 50 and 150 mm Hg, cerebral autoregulation maintains a relatively constant blood flow and oxygen delivery. During hypothermic CPB, the lower limit of cerebral autoregulation may be as low as 20 to 30 mm Hg,[8,9] affording some additional protection against hypoperfusion. Increasing perfusion pressure to alleviate the risk of hypoperfusion may lead to greater embolic load and worse outcomes.[10-13] Ultimately, the selection of perfusion pressure during CPB will need to be based on clinical outcome studies (see Chapters 30 and 35).

The early studies highlighted an association between severe hypotension during CPB and adverse neurologic outcome (primarily stroke).[14-17] However, the observational nature of these studies and inconsistencies in the definition of hypotension do not allow a firm conclusion on the safe level of perfusion pressure during CPB. Stockard et al[18] proposed TM_{50}, the integral of perfusion pressure less than 50 mm Hg over time. They subsequently reported an increased incidence of adverse neurologic events (53% versus 10%) in patients who experienced an integrated hypotensive time of more than 100 mm Hg · minutes.[19] When these studies are coupled with knowledge of cerebral autoregulation, 50 mm Hg appears to be a safe lower limit for perfusion pressure during CPB.

However, TM_{50} and other measures of hypotension do not consistently predict postoperative neurologic deficits. For example, Slogoff et al,[20] in a prospective study of 204 patients, found perfusion pressures at 50 mm Hg or lower during CPB were not associated with an increase in the likelihood of postoperative cerebral dysfunction. In a subsequent study, neither the value of the lowest measured blood pressure nor integrated hypotension was predictive of postoperative neurologic dysfunction.[21] Other studies have also not found a relationship between intraoperative hypotension and neurologic dysfunction.[9,22-31] However, some have, and of these, only one is a randomized trial.[32-35] This trial reported fewer combined (cardiac and neurologic) adverse outcomes in the high (80 to 100 mm Hg) perfusion pressure group than the low (50 to 60 mm Hg) perfusion pressure group (4.8% versus 12.9%). However, the incidence of cardiac or neurologic adverse events did not differ significantly between the high or low perfusion pressure groups when considered independently. The suggested trend toward more cardiac complications in the low perfusion pressure group ($p = 0.3$) may be explained by the fact that this group suffered more preoperative cardiac dysfunction (greater nitrate use [$p = 0.007$] and incidence of angina [$p = 0.008$]). The trend ($p = 0.076$) toward a greater number of neurologic complications in the low (50 to 60 mm Hg) perfusion pressure group may have two explanations. First, a higher incidence of preexisting cerebrovascular disease was present in the low perfusion pressure group. Second, higher perfusion pressure is protective only in patients with more advanced cerebrovascular or aortic arch disease. Evidence for these explanations comes from a later publication by the same investigators reporting on atheroma grade in the descending aorta of 189 of the 248 study subjects, where atheroma in the descending aorta may be seen as a marker for severity of aortic arch or cerebrovascular disease.[36] Making comparisons among all of these studies (Tables 28–1 and 28–2) is difficult because they employ different clinical end-points (neurologic versus neuropsychologic), CPB management techniques have changed (e.g., pH-stat versus α-stat acid-base management, use of arterial filters), and the studies vary in design and power.

Table 28–1 Studies Supporting Relationship between Intraoperative Hypotension and Postoperative Neurologic Dysfunction

First Author	Year	Patients
Gilman[14]	1965	35
Javid[15]	1969	100
Tufo[16]	1970	100
Lee[17]	1971	71
Stockard[18]	1973	25
Stockard[19]	1974	75
Brainthwaite[34]	1975	538
Savageau[32]	1982	227
Gardner[33]	1985	168
Gold[35]	1995	248

Table 28–2 Studies Not Supporting Relationship between Intraoperative Hypotension and Postoperative Neurologic Dysfunction

First Author	Year	Patients
Kolka[29]	1980	204
Ellis[23]	1980	30
Sotaniemi[28]	1981	49
Slogoff[20]	1982	204
Govier[9]	1984	67
Nussmeier[27]	1986	182
Fish[26]	1987	100
Townes[25]	1989	90
Slogoff[21]	1990	504
Bashein[22]	1990	86
Stanley[30]	1990	19
Kramer[31]	1994	230
McKhann[24]	1997	456

What these studies have done is to identify some of the subgroups at increased risk for adverse outcomes that may benefit from higher perfusion pressure during CPB. These groups include patients with severe atheromatous disease (cerebrovascular or aortic arch), advanced age, systemic hypertension, and diabetes.[35-37]

Initially, it was thought that the elderly had impaired cerebral autoregulation and were more vulnerable to cerebral injury during bypass. However, Newman et al[38] found no effect of age on cerebral autoregulation (i.e., pressure-flow or metabolism-flow coupling), although elderly patients tended to have a greater difference in arterial and venous blood oxygen content. In a subsequent study, MAP less than 50 mm Hg and rapid rewarming were associated with a decline of cognitive function in one of five tests.[39] These two studies do not permit determination of whether the higher rate of cognitive dysfunction in the elderly results from hypoperfusion or a greater sensitivity to embolic load. In the first study, a positive correlation was found between cerebral arteriovenous blood oxygen content difference and five of nine tests for cognitive function.[38] Increased cerebral dysfunction in the elderly may be a result of slower vasodilatation of cerebral resistance vessels during periods of rewarming, and subsequent transient episodes of metabolism-flow mismatch with resultant ischemia. It is unknown what the effect of elevating perfusion pressure during rewarming would be on neurologic outcome.

Hypertensive patients are generally accepted to have intact pressure-flow autoregulation, with a rightward shift in the cerebral autoregulation curve such that pressure dependent flow patterns develop at higher perfusion pressures than in the normal population.[37] In hypertensive patients the use of higher perfusion pressure during CPB is common practice.

Patients with type I diabetes mellitus appear to have impaired metabolism-flow coupling during CPB.[40] They also have some loss of pressure-flow autoregulation, although it is unclear if this slightly positive slope is any different from that reported for nondiabetics.[10] Because of this, diabetics' primary risk for neurologic injury would likely come during periods of rapid rewarming or normothermia when cerebrovasodilation may not meet metabolic needs. The role of higher perfusion pressure during these periods—as in the case of bypass management for the elderly—is of uncertain but potential benefit.

Once the CPB team has selected target perfusion pressures during CPB, a few technical issues emerge. Throughout this discussion perfusion pressure and MAP have been used almost interchangeably. In general, cerebral perfusion pressure is what is of most concern. Cerebral perfusion pressure is determined by the difference between MAP and the higher of central venous pressure and intracranial pressure. The latter values are usually less than 5 mm Hg during CPB. However, in the presence of compromised cerebral venous drainage (malpositioned cannula, patient positioning), MAP will not accurately reflect cerebral perfusion pressure.

Measurement artifacts also play a role in perfusion pressure management. MAP may vary by as much as 20 mm Hg over 30 seconds while pump flow is constant. The mechanism of this oscillation and its relation to outcome are unclear, although it may be eliminated by droperidol.[41-43] A more common artifact is discordance between radial arterial and central arterial pressures during rewarming. This difference may be as great as 30% and is felt to occur from opening of arteriovenous shunts in the arm[44] (see Chapter 14).

After acknowledging the technical issues of pressure monitoring, the CPB team is left to maintain the selected perfusion pressure. To achieve these perfusion pressure goals the team has two general options: alterations of pump flow (discussed in the next section) or administration of vasoactive agents. Increasing pump flow may be used as a temporizing measure for hypotension if surgical demands allow it; however, this may come at the cost of dangerously reducing reservoir volume. Alternatively, phenylephrine and norepinephrine may be used to support perfusion pressure. In the case of hypertension, pump flow may be reduced, although this increases the potential for inadequate oxygen delivery; more commonly, a vasodilator, such as sodium nitroprusside or nitroglycerin, is employed. Isoflurane or another volatile anesthetic may be administered through the pump oxygenator, with careful attention paid to its use during weaning from CPB. Other less commonly used vasodilators include chlorpromazine, phentolamine, and trimethaphan. In any case, careful evaluation should precede management steps as alter-

Table 28–3 Comparison of Studies Investigating Pulsatile Flow during Cardiopulmonary Bypass

Proposed Effect of Pulsatile Flow	Yes*	No*
Reduced systemic vascular resistance	47, 48, 49, 50, 51, 52, 53	54, 55, 56, 57, 58, 59, 60, 61, 62
Changes in systemic blood flow distribution	47, 63	49, 54, 55, 60
Improved microcirculatory flow/aerobic metabolism	47, 48, 50, 62, 64, 65	49, 54, 55, 60, 61, 62
Attenuation of hormonal responses		
Catecholamines	66	48, 58
Renin/angiotensin	53, 58, 61	54, 55, 66, 67
ADH	52, 66	56
Cortisol		56, 67
Thromboxane/prostacyclin	59	
Improved renal blood flow or urine output	50, 52, 54, 63, 65	49, 55, 56, 57, 62, 68, 75
Improved pancreatic blood flow	63, 68	
Improved cerebral blood flow, metabolism, or outcome	51, 64, 69, 70, 71	76

*Numbers refer to references listed at end of chapter.

ations in pressure may be the first sign of more ominous problems (cannula malposition, arterial dissection).

Nonpulsatile versus Pulsatile Perfusion

A large volume of literature has accumulated comparing the physiology of pulsatile with nonpulsatile perfusion.[45,46] Nevertheless, it remains uncertain whether pulsatile CPB has shown substantive clinical improvement in any outcome measure compared with standard, nonpulsatile CPB. Table 28–3, although by no means complete, represents this highly contradictory body of literature.[47-76] Claims of advantages to pulsatile flow are effectively offset by conflicting studies of similar design.

A review by Hickey et al,[46] published in 1983, offers important criticism and insight into this controversy and remains germane to recent reports. A fundamental difference between pulsatile and nonpulsatile flow is that additional hydraulic energy is required and applied to move blood when pulsatile flow is used. This extra kinetic energy is known to improve red blood cell transit, increase capillary perfusion, and aid lymphatic function.[72] The hydraulic power of pulsatile flow is the sum over time of the product of instantaneous pressure and instantaneous flow. Cardiopulmonary bypass may influence many of the properties of the blood (viscosity) and the vasculature itself (arterial tone, size, and geometry) as a result of hemodilution, hypothermia, alteration of red blood cell deformability, and redistribution of flow. As a result of these changes, generation of what appears to be a normal pulsatile *pressure* waveform may not result in a normal pulsatile *flow* waveform. Simply reproducing pulsatile pressure is not sufficient to assure reproduction of pulsatile flow, nor does it allow quantification of energetics.

Virtually no study has quantified the energetics of the pulsatile or nonpulsatile perfusion used. Few studies report representative pressure waveforms.[47-52] Even fewer give *flow* waveforms.[73,74] When pulsatile flow is not quantified, critical features such as vascular impedance and the hydraulic power delivered cannot be evaluated (i.e., whether the pulsatile perfusion used in a particular study was really delivering more hydraulic power than the nonpulsatile perfusion with which it is compared). Grossi et al[74] developed two indices of pulsatility: the pulsatility index (PI), which quantitates the relative sharpness of a given waveform with respect to its mean flow, and the pulse power index (PPI), which quantifies the power of a pulsatile waveform compared with nonpulsatile equal flow. They found that despite use of a computer-controlled pulsatile pump, in every case PI or PPI was considerably less than control (non-bypass pulsatility). Only with specific combinations of pulse rate and pulsatile flow contours (which had high PI or PPI) was lactate production lower than the nonpulsatile perfusion at the same minute flow during pulsatile CPB. This study indicates that not all pulsatile perfusion is the same and that pulsatile modes are not necessarily capable of improved perfusion relative to nonpulsatile systems.

It is therefore not surprising that such a wide disparity of results should occur. The authors are unaware of any human study in which pulsatility has been quantitated in terms other than pulse pressures. Consequently, whether the generated pressure waveform is a sine wave or some other pattern cannot be ascertained.[52,53,56,58-62,65-67] The comparatively small size of the arterial inflow cannula can effectively filter out a large component of the pulsatile kinetic energy. Consequently, as achieved clinically, pulsatile flow may actually be quite similar energetically to nonpulsatile flow.

This potentially unrecognized lack of difference in types of flow may partly explain the failure of pulsatile perfusion to alter hormone levels and clinical outcome in many human studies. Lindberg et al[62] randomized 20 patients who were undergoing CABG to pulsatile or nonpulsatile perfusion groups. Postoperatively, the groups were indistinguishable by every measure of cardiac, pulmonary, metabolic, and renal status. In a study of 100 patients undergoing CPB, Badner et al[75] found no differences in any measure of renal function between patients receiving pulsatile flow versus those receiving nonpulsatile flow. In a large, prospective study of neurologic complications after cardiac surgery, Shaw et al[76] found that pulsatile perfusion had no effect on neurologic outcome.

It is believed, however, that under specific conditions pulsatile flow can improve tissue perfusion and better preserve endocrine and autonomic status compared with nonpulsatile flow. What remains to be determined are the necessary critical features of pulse contour and frequency and whether these improvements can be achieved clinically.

Pump Flow during Bypass

Like perfusion pressure, pump flow during CPB represents a careful balance between the conflicting demands of surgical visualization and adequate oxygen delivery. Two theoretical approaches exist. The first is to maintain oxygen delivery during bypass at normal levels for a given core temperature. Although this may limit hypoperfusion, it does increase the delivered embolic load. The second approach is to use the lowest flows that do not result in end-organ injury. This approach offers the potential advantage of less embolic delivery as well as potential improved myocardial protection and surgical visualization.[77,78] However, some of these advantages are not seen when the left ventricle is vented during CPB.[79]

During CPB, pump flow and pressure are related through overall arterial impedance, a product of hemodilution, temperature, and arterial cross-sectional area. This is important because the first two factors, hemodilution and temperature, are critical determinants of pump flow requirements. Pump flows of 1.2 L/min/m^2 perfuse most of the microcirculation when the hematocrit is near 22% and hypothermic CPB is being employed.[80] However, at lower hematocrits or periods of higher oxygen consumption these flows become inadequate.[81-83] Because of changes in oxygen demand with temperature and the plateauing of oxygen consumption with increasing flow, a series of nomograms have been developed for pump flow selection (Fig. 28–3).

In addition to use of these nomograms, most perfusion teams also monitor mixed venous saturation, targeting levels of 70% or greater. Unfortunately, this level does not guarantee adequate perfusion of all tissue beds, because some (muscle, subcutaneous fat) may be functionally removed from circulation during CPB.[83] Hypothermic venous saturation may overestimate end-organ reserves.[84] Slater et al[85] characterized the hierarchy of regional blood flows during CPB at 27°C. Animals were perfused at pump blood flows of 1.9, 1.6, 1.3, and 1.0 L/min/m^2. Regional perfusion of various end-organs (brain, kidney, small intestine, pancreas, and muscle) was quantified with a fluorescent microsphere technique. Cerebral blood flow was unchanged at the three greatest pump flows. Renal perfusion was maintained at flows of 1.9 and 1.6 L/min/m^2. Perfusion to the pancreas was constant at all flows studied, and small bowel perfusion varied linearly with pump flow. Muscle bed flows were decreased at all flows. This study confirmed previous work regarding end-organ perfusion during CPB and highlighted the vulnerability of the kidneys to reduced flows at moderate hypothermia.

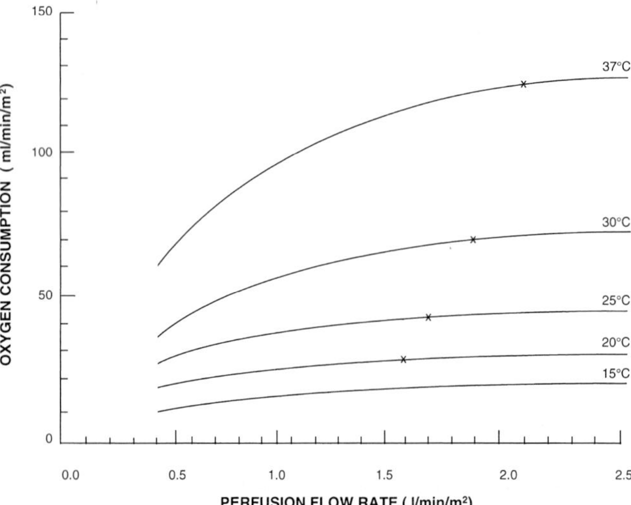

Figure 28–3 Nomogram depicting the relationship of oxygen consumption (V_{O_2}) to perfusion flow rate and temperature. The x on the curves represents common clinically used flow rates at the various temperatures. (From Kirklin JW, Barratt-Boyes BG: Cardiac Surgery. New York, Wiley, 1986, p 35.)

During CPB, most of the outcomes studied in relation to pump flow are those related to the organs at high risk for ischemic injury (i.e., kidney and brain). Much work has been applied to examining the relationship between renal dysfunction and pump flow.[21,86-88] Preexisting renal disease is a consistent predictor of postoperative renal dysfunction, the incidence of which ranges between 3% and 5%. Renal function appears unaltered when pump flows greater than 1.6 L/min/m^2 are employed,[21] but whether this management will affect outcomes in patients with preexisting renal dysfunction is less clear.[88] Because of autoregulation, most studies,[9,89] but not all,[90] suggest that cerebral blood flow is unaltered by variation in pump flow. At low-flow states, cerebral blood flow is probably more dependent on perfusion pressure.[11,12,91]

Bypass Temperature Management Strategy

Although hypothermic temperatures have been employed since the advent of extracorporeal circulation, the importance of reduced temperatures during bypass was challenged in the early 1990s. This section reviews the basis of hypothermic protection during bypass; and outlines the studies assessing the impact of warm bypass on the central nervous system.

Effects on Central Nervous System

The brain is arguably the organ most vulnerable to ischemic damage during CPB. Cerebral hypoperfusion and embolic phenomena are likely to occur in every patient undergoing bypass, resulting in ischemic events. It is believed that hypothermia provides protection from ischemic phenomena and resultant infarction by decreasing cerebral oxygen demands, maintaining energy (ATP, phosphocreatine) stores. The relationship between temperature and metabolic activity is expressed as Q_{10}. This measure is the ratio of two metabolic rates at temperatures separated by 10°C, and is the multiple by which global metabolism decreases for each 10°C reduction in temperature. The relationship between temperature and cerebral metabolic rate is controversial, but most published values range between 2.0 and 3.0. The most recent studies in humans undergoing hypothermic CPB report a Q_{10} at or above 2.8 for cerebral metabolism.[92] Every organ and every biochemical reaction, has a unique Q_{10} ratio. Although the effect of reduced temperatures on metabolism is of importance, there is increasing evidence that the most important salutary effects of hypothermia on cerebral ischemia are not related to the reduction in metabolism but rather to the attenuation of the excitotoxic cascade.[93-95] Busto et al[95] and Natale and D'Alecy[96] demonstrated that even mild reductions in temperature (34°C) reduce the amount of glutamate release after an ischemic insult and have a palliative effect on the perturbation in calcium metabolism inherent in ischemic damage (see Chapters 30 and 35).

Several groups of investigators have assessed the effect of normothermic temperatures during bypass on perioperative CNS events in cardiac surgery patients.[97-102] Given the disparity in study designs among the various reports, it is not surprising that these investigators report conflicting results regarding the effect of normothermia on CNS outcomes. These studies and factors that likely influenced the results of

Table 28–4 Warm Cardiopulmonary Bypass and Central Nervous System Outcome Studies

Investigator	No. of Patients	Pre- and Post-Op CNS Exams	% New Postoperative CNS Adverse Outcomes (Warm/Cold)	Reported Temperature during CPB*	Temperature Monitoring Site	Active Warming during Bypass	Probable Cerebral Temperature
Singh[103]	2817	–	1/1	36–37°C	Bladder	+	>37–38°C
Martin[100]	1001	–	4.5/1.4†	35–37°C	Bladder	+	>37–38°C
Warm Heart Investigators[98]	1732	–	1.6/1.5	33–37°C	Bypass circuit venous line	±	33–38°C
McLean[99]	155	+	2.6/5.2	34.4 (1.2)°C‡	Bypass circuit venous line	±	33–38°C
Mora[97]	138	+	10.4/0.0†	35–37°C	Bladder	+	>37–38°C
Engelman[102]	130	+	4.7/8.1/0.0§	20°C‡	Rectum/nasopharynx	+	>37–39°C¶
Birdi[101]	300	?	1/0/1§	37°C	Nasopharynx	+	?
Heyer[410]	99	+	N/A	34°C	Nasopharynx	–	~34°C
Nathan[411]	194	+	62/48	37°C**	Nasopharynx	+	37°C

*In warm group.
†*P* ≤ 0.05% new postoperative CNS adverse outcome in warm versus cold bypass patients.
‡Mean ± standard deviation.
§Warm/cold/tepid.
¶Patients in cold treatment group.
**At end of rewarming.
CPB = cardiopulmonary bypass.

Table 28–5 Morbidity and Mortality Rates in Hypothermic versus Normothermic Bypass Patients

Variable	Hypothermic Group (*n* = 1605)	Normothermic Group (*n* = 2585)	*P* Value
Perioperative myocardial infarction	41 (2.6%)	41 (1.6%)	0.037
Postoperative bleeding	17 (1.0%)	36 (1.4%)	NS
Renal insufficiency	25 (1.6%)	28 (1.1%)	NS
Intra-aortic balloon pump	53 (3.3%)	0 (0%)	0.0001
Mediastinal infection	21 (1.3%)	25 (1.0%)	NS
Low cardiac output	127 (7.9%)	145 (5.6%)	0.004
Stroke	21 (1.3%)	25 (1.0%)	NS
Operative deaths	33 (2.1%)	25 (1.0%)	0.005

NS = not significant.
Adapted and reprinted with permission from the Society of Thoracic Surgeons (The Annals of Thoracic Surgery, 59:86, 1995).

each study are outlined in Tables 28–4 and 28–5. Summary of the data reported in these studies suggests that mild hypothermia provides some magnitude of cerebral protection during CPB (likely through attenuation of the excitotoxic cascade), whereas mildly hyperthermic temperatures (>37°C) exacerbate and amplify the ischemic injury associated with CPB. Chapters 30 and 35 provide additional information on this important topic. Briefly, studies that provided for some degree of hypothermia in the "warm" treatment groups demonstrated no difference between warm and cold treatment groups.[98,99] In contrast, studies in which hyperthermic temperatures were most likely employed demonstrated an increase of cerebral damage in patients treated with a normothermic temperature management strategy during bypass.[97,100] Engleman[102] reported that the greatest incidence of adverse CNS events occurred in the hypothermic treatment group, and suggested that hypothermic temperatures (compared with the normothermic or tepid values) increase the risk of cerebral injury in cardiac surgery patients. Of interest is the fact that the hypothermic group was the only treatment group subjected to temperatures above 37°C at any time during the bypass run. In the studies by Singh et al[103] and Birdi et al,[101] the lack of rigorous preoperative and postoperative neurologic examinations precluded their ability to determine true adverse CNS event rates in their treatment groups. Both groups of investigators report an overall stroke rate of 1% or less. This low incidence most likely reflects the lack of careful preoperative neurologic testing.[104,105]

Temperature Monitoring

Because the brain is vulnerable to hyperthermic temperatures, it is important to use the temperature-monitoring site most likely to reflect cerebral temperature. The most commonly used sites in cardiac surgery patients include esophageal, nasopharyngeal, tympanic, pulmonary arterial, rectal, urinary bladder, subcutaneous (or muscle), and cutaneous sites. Unfortunately, none of these monitoring locations has been demonstrated to reflect cerebral temperature reliably. Stone et al[106] addressed the question of surrogate monitoring sites for cerebral temperature in their study of patients undergoing

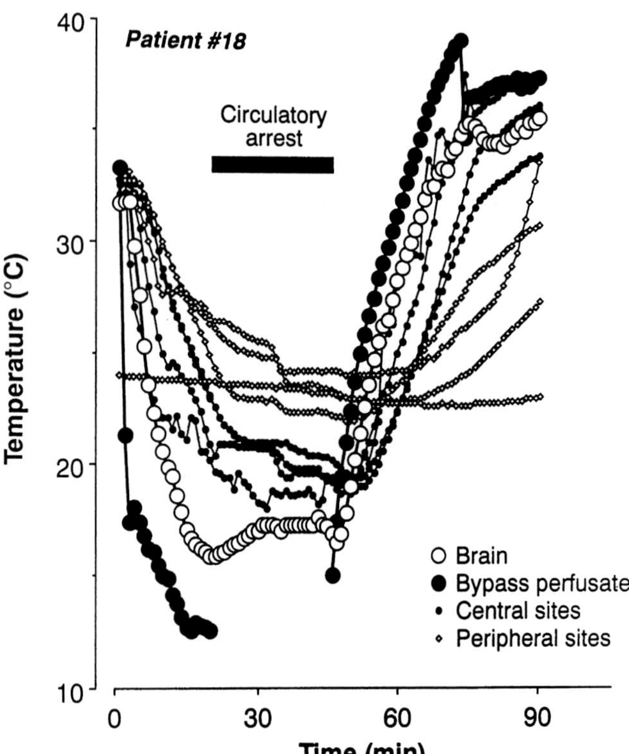

Figure 28–4 Graphic depiction of temperature-time relationship during cardiopulmonary bypass and deep hypothermic circulatory arrest. Temperatures are plotted every minute. Central sites are the nasopharynx, tympanic membrane, esophagus, and pulmonary artery. Peripheral sites are the bladder, rectum, axilla, and sole of the foot. The two slowest cooling central sites were tympanic membrane and esophagus. (From Stone JG, Young WL, Smith CR, et al: Do standard monitoring sites reflect true brain temperature when profound hypothermia is rapidly induced and reversed? Anesthesiology 82:344, 1995.)

CPB and deep hypothermic circulatory arrest (DHCA) for repair of cerebral vascular malformations. In this study, with exposure of the brain, investigators placed a thermocouple directly in the cerebral cortex. Brain temperature was compared with values obtained from sensors in eight locations. Investigators found a poor concordance between cerebral temperature and values obtained at the other monitoring sites. Locations hypothesized to best reflect core temperature—tympanic membrane, esophagus, nasopharynx, pulmonary artery—sometimes overestimated cerebral temperature or underestimated brain temperature. Because of the substantial variability noted in central temperature readings (Fig. 28–4) and lack of the concordance of central temperature measures in every study patient, the investigators recommended the use of at least three measures of central or core temperature. Stone et al[106] concluded that this redundancy was necessary to enhance the likelihood of accurately predicting brain temperature. In their study of 26 patients undergoing circulatory arrest or normothermic CPB, Kaukuntla et al[107] similarly reported a poor correlation among surrogate measures of cerebral temperature and peripheral monitoring sites.

Acid-Base Strategy

The management of acid-base status during hypothermic CPB has been a long-standing source of debate. Understanding of the physiologic responses to hypothermia, and the influences of P_{CO_2} have led to shifts in clinical practice over the past decades. Two strategies exist for managing acid-base balance during periods of hypothermia: α-stat and pH-stat. The term α-stat was first proposed to describe the theory that acid-base regulation in vertebrate animals functioned during temperature fluctuation to maintain a constant ratio (α) of dissociated to undissociated forms of the imidazole ring on histidine.[108] It is this protein charge state that is important in regulating pH-dependent cellular processes. Hypothermia increases the solubility of oxygen and carbon dioxide in the blood, leading to a decrease in P_{CO_2} and an increase in pH at lower temperatures. With α-stat blood gas management, the uncorrected (37°) pH is kept at 7.40 with the P_{CO_2} at 40 mm Hg, creating a relative alkalosis at the patient's actual body temperature. This strategy is considered to be physiologic because the ionization state of histidine is unchanged over all temperature ranges, and protein structure and function are preserved.

The pH-stat approach to acid-base balance maintains a pH of 7.40 and P_{CO_2} of 40 mm Hg when corrected for body temperature, typically requiring the addition of CO_2 during hypothermic CPB. This method of blood gas management was generally favored until the mid-1980s because it was felt that the potent vasodilatory effects of CO_2 would provide increased cerebral blood flow and thereby minimize the risk of cerebral ischemia during CPB. It is now recognized that pH-stat management during hypothermia produces passive cerebral vasodilation, impairs autoregulatory responses to blood pressure changes and metabolic demands in the brain, and does not improve overall oxygen balance.[8,109,110] In contrast, α-stat management preserves autoregulation and the relationship between cerebral blood flow and metabolism.[8,9] Neither blood gas strategy has any significant effect on hypothermic cerebral metabolism.[109] The increased CBF seen with pH-stat may also increase the risk of cerebral embolization[111] or produce a steal phenomenon.[112]

Despite the theoretical mechanisms by which acid-base management during hypothermic CPB may affect the risk of cerebral injury, reports of neurologic outcomes related to blood gas management are conflicting. Bashein et al[22] found no difference in neuropsychologic outcome between patients undergoing cardiac surgery randomized to α-stat or pH-stat management, whereas Stephan et al[109] reported that neurologic disorders in patients undergoing CABG surgery were significantly greater in the group assigned to pH-stat. Differences in blood pressure management, type of oxygenator used (bubble versus membrane), and type of surgical procedure (intracardiac versus coronary artery) may account for the conflicting conclusions in these two studies. In a large, randomized study of 316 patients undergoing CABG surgery, Murkin et al[113] found that α-stat management resulted in less cognitive impairment in patients undergoing prolonged CPB. The effects of acid-base management on the heart have been investigated, but because the heart is not exposed to the systemic circulation during cross-clamping, many of these effects may have little significance. Management with α-stat leads to preserved protein structure and function.[108] It has been observed that myocardial function and electrical stability are maintained better in α-stat than in pH-stat animals.[114,115] In their study of anesthetized pigs on CPB, Willford et al[116] reported significantly lower whole-body and myocardial oxygen consumption in α-stat versus pH-stat animals. Although this would not be predicted based on the known effects of hypothermia and alkalosis on the oxygen-hemoglobin dissociation curve (i.e., greater hemoglobin affinity for O_2 and less tissue O_2 availability),[117] the investigators speculated that pH-stat led to activation of the sympathetic nervous system, with increases in norepinephrine levels and the oxygen consumption rate.[118] In direct contrast, Baraka et al[119] were not able to demonstrate any significant differences in whole-body oxygen consumption in human subjects undergoing hypothermic CPB. In Murkin's clinical trial of 316 patients undergoing CABG, no significant differences in cardiovascular morbidity related to acid-base management were observed.[113] These differences may be related to the exclusion of the myocardium from the systemic circulation in the patients studied.

Fluid Management

The choice of fluid for priming the extracorporeal circuit in CPB remains controversial. The idea of using nonblood prime was first introduced by Panico and Neptune in 1959.[120] This technique of hemodilution was found to be safe when combined with hypothermia to reduce oxygen consumption and demand. The use of nonblood primes and moderate hemodilution for CPB has become routine in most centers. Although this practice is desirable because it reduces the need for blood transfusions and associated complications, another effect related to hemodilution is important in the management of extracorporeal support.

Blood viscosity (η) increases with increasing hematocrit and decreasing temperature. During systemic cooling, increasing blood viscosity increases systemic vascular resistance (SVR) according to the equation:

$$\mathrm{SVR} = \eta \times \mathrm{SVH}$$

in which SVH represents inherent systemic vascular hindrance and is assumed to remain constant. Remembering the relationship

$$\mathrm{CO} = \mathrm{MAP} \div \mathrm{SVR}$$

in which CO is cardiac output, the necessary driving pressure (MAP) to maintain constant flow (CO) during hypothermia increases if the hematocrit remains constant, and may become excessive, leading to increased risk of inflow line disruption or arterial dissection. Hemodilution produces desirable effects by reducing blood viscosity and resistance to flow during hypothermia. Data published by Rand et al[121] demonstrate that a reduction in hematocrit from 40% to 20% allows cooling to 22°C without an increase in blood viscosity or required driving pressure. Hematocrit reduction may be achieved before bypass by means of acute normovolemic hemodilution in the hope of reinfusing patient's own heparin-free blood, rather than allogeneic red blood cells, after CPB; however, this technique failed to lower the likelihood of transfusion in a controlled trial.[122]

Several studies have investigated the differences between colloid and crystalloid priming solutions. In general, crystalloid solutions lead to decreased colloid osmotic pressure with a resultant increase in extracellular water retention, irrespective of the osmolarity of the pump prime. Scott et al[123] compared albumin, polygeline, and crystalloid priming solutions and found no hematologic or hemodynamic advantage in using colloid-based prime solution over a purely crystalloid solution despite greater fluid retention in the crystalloid group. Jenkins and Curtis[124] did a study comparing lactated Ringer's (LR) solution with albumin and mannitol in the pump prime, and also found that despite increased positive fluid balance in the LR group, there were no differences between groups with respect to measured indices of oxygenation or time to extubation. This is in direct contrast to Sade et al,[125] who documented significant increases in body weight and pulmonary shunt fraction in the crystalloid group when compared with the groups receiving hydroxyethyl starch or albumin pump prime. Albumin, unlike a pure crystalloid prime, can decrease the interaction of blood components with the bypass circuit by coating the fluid pathway surfaces. In their meta-analysis of 21 controlled trials enrolling 1346 patients, Russell et al[126] showed a notably smaller drop in on-bypass platelet counts in patients treated with albumin in the pump prime. The effects of various colloid solutions with respect to coagulation parameters and transfusion requirements have been evaluated, although no significant differences were observed.[127] Although there are conflicting data, most studies suggest that the observed increases in tissue edema, extravascular lung water, and increased pulmonary shunt fraction are due to low colloid oncotic pressure. There is no evidence that low oncotic pressure adversely affects cardiac performance or hemodynamic variables.[128]

Ultrafiltration during bypass can be used as a means of reducing excess water accumulation. Modified ultrafiltration describes the process of hemofiltration immediately after the cessation of bypass. This process results in a more consistent reduction in total body water with significant increases in hematocrit, myocardial contractility, cardiac index, and improved pulmonary compliance.[129] Peri-bypass modified ultrafiltration is an area of current research. Studies in the pediatric cardiac surgery population suggest that post-bypass ultrafiltration may remove some of the inflammatory mediators produced during extracorporeal circulation.

Perfluorocarbons have gained interest as priming solutions because of their ability to preserve oxygen-carrying capacity under conditions of extreme hemodilution. In their study evaluating perfluorocarbon-based versus LR-based priming solution in goats undergoing normothermic, nonpulsatile CPB, Briceno et al[130] reported increased cerebral blood flow and brain tissue $\mathrm{PO_2}$ in the perfluorocarbon group. Vocelka et al[131] compared cerebral blood flow and electroencephalographic (EEG) data in pigs receiving crystalloid or crystalloid plus perfluorocarbon prime. They concluded that the perfluorocarbon group had more stable arterial blood pressure, an increased cerebral blood flow, and an earlier recovery of the EEG power. Perfluorocarbons may be important blood substrate products and may help reduce the risk of infection, blood trauma, and the incidence of complications after CPB.

END-ORGAN EFFECTS OF CARDIOPULMONARY BYPASS

Myocardial Injury

Most coronary revascularization procedures are completed with the assistance of CPB. Although the completion of coronary anastomoses is facilitated by CPB (i.e., the surgeon can operate on a quiet, nonbeating heart), the heart is subjected to a series of events leading to ischemic myocardium during extracorporeal circulation. The operation, which is designed to preserve and improve myocardial function, is sometimes associated with myocardial damage (Box 28–2). The extent and incidence of this injury are dependent on the sensitivity and specificity of the diagnostic methods being used. However, most patients who undergo cardiac operations sustain some degree of myocardial injury. Although patients

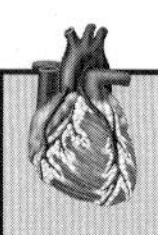

BOX 28–2 ***End Organs That Can Be Adversely Affected by Cardiopulmonary Bypass***

- Heart
- Brain
- Kidneys
- Gastrointestinal tract
- Endocrine system

Table 28–6 Factors Associated with Myocardial Injury during Cardiopulmonary Bypass

1. Abnormal perfusate composition
2. Persistent ventricular fibrillation
3. Inadequate myocardial perfusion
4. Ventricular distention
5. Ventricular collapse
6. Coronary embolism
7. Catecholamines
8. Aortic cross-clamping
9. Reperfusion

with normal ventricular function may tolerate these minor amounts of injury without detectable sequelae, those with impaired ventricular function preoperatively may not be able to tolerate the slightest injury. As the patient population for CPB continues to become older and have greater degrees of concomitant illness, understanding the physiology of and developing effective preventive strategies for myocardial injury during CPB are increasingly important. Because myocardial damage influences early and long-term results, the identification and control of factors associated with myocardial injury are critical to ensuring good outcomes. Although injury may be linked to anesthetic and surgical management, myocardial injury usually is thought to occur from inadequate myocardial protection during CPB (see Chapters 19 and 30).

Mechanisms

The underlying mechanism for most types of myocardial injury during CPB is ischemia. Ischemia develops when oxygen demand outstrips its supply in the heart. This process involves a complex cascade of events that compromise high-energy phosphate and calcium homeostasis. Many reports confirm the role of high-energy phosphate depletion and intracellular calcium accumulation in the pathogenesis of myocardial damage during ischemia and subsequent reperfusion. Oxidative phosphorylation ceases when the tissue PO_2 falls below 5 to 10 mm Hg. Then creatine phosphate (CP) and anaerobic production become the main sources of high-energy phosphate. These mechanisms are unfortunately limited. Creatine kinase (CK)-mediated transfer of high-energy phosphate from CP to adenosine diphosphate (ADP) provides an immediate source of energy; the amount of adenosine triphosphate (ATP) produced by transfer is limited initially by substrate availability and subsequently by lactate inhibition. Anaerobic production is inefficient and self-limiting because of accumulation of metabolites (i.e., lactate, pyruvate, and hydrogen ions) with inhibition of enzyme systems. As high-energy phosphate stores become depleted, the cardiac cells are no longer able to maintain normal transport of calcium out of the cell. Energy-dependent mechanisms that lower intracellular ionized calcium concentration and terminate the contractile process fail because of a lack of high-energy phosphate. The cytosolic concentration of ionized calcium remains high, and energy use persists with the formation of rigor bonds between the contractile proteins. Continued energy use with calcium and proton-activated release of destructive lipoprotein lipase eventually leads to loss of cell integrity and function.

Certain specific events during CPB are associated with myocardial ischemia and injury (Table 28–6). These events lead to ischemia by increasing oxygen demands, decreasing oxygen supply, or a combination of both. When these factors are present together they potentiate myocardial damage. For example, the distended, fibrillating ventricle with a low perfusion pressure is particularly susceptible to damage (see Chapters 6, 19, 30, 31, and 33).

Perfusate composition may lead to myocardial damage through its increasing titers of free fatty acids, denatured plasma proteins, and vasoactive substances. Alternatively, the potential for sludging and microemboli during CPB may cause impaired flow and ischemia. Ventricular fibrillation (VF) during CPB increases myocardial wall tension and myocardial oxygen consumption and impairs subendocardial blood flow. The occurrence of fibrillation may be limited by minimizing manipulation of the heart and avoiding rapid myocardial cooling. If fibrillation occurs, the duration should be kept to a minimum. This may be accomplished through timely cross-clamping and infusion of cardioplegia, cardioversion with minimum energy settings (5 to 10 J), or antiarrhythmics (after CPB).

Myocardial perfusion during CPB may be inadequate to meet myocardial oxygen demands for multiple reasons. Aortic root or direct coronary cannulation can lead to variable or nonpulsatile perfusion pressure. Coronary vascular resistance may be elevated (coronary artery disease, emboli, altered lymph flow, and myocardial edema), flow may be nonuniform (VF, distention or collapse, technical problems), and autoregulation may be lost (hypothermia). Ventricular distention is particularly problematic because balance between oxygen supply and demand is upset by the increased myocardial oxygen consumption (increased wall tension) and decreased delivery (lower perfusion pressure from raised intracavitary pressure). Ventricular distention during CPB may occur for multiple reasons (inadequate venous drainage, aortic insufficiency, VF, infusion of cardioplegia, pulmonary venous flow, and noncoronary collateral flow). Detection occurs through atrial pressure monitoring and palpation, and decompression may be obtained mechanically (e.g., venous drainage, cross-clamping, defibrillation, altered cardioplegia infusion, vent) or pharmacologically.

Ventricular collapse (beating heart) also predisposes the ventricle to damage through changes in compressive forces and ventricular geometry. These effects are most pronounced in patients with small, hypertrophic ventricles. Appropriate management of venous drainage and vents should prevent collapse. Coronary embolism, however, is more difficult to completely eliminate. Use of filters, venting of vein grafts, and evacuation of intracardiac air are the current mainstays of prevention.

The use of inotropic agents during weaning from CPB may cause a disproportionate increase in myocardial oxygen demand relative to supply. Optimization of heart rate, preload, and afterload should be ascertained before resorting to the use of inotropic drugs. Consideration should be given to the use of mechanical support if CO remains low (see Chapter 31).

Aortic Cross-Clamping

Aortic cross-clamping, potentially a major cause of myocardial injury during CPB, was a product of evolution. Initially, continuous aortic or direct coronary artery perfusion of the empty, beating heart was used to "protect" the myocardium during cardiac repairs. Ventricular fibrillation was frequently induced and maintained to "quiet" the heart and thereby improve exposure and prevent air embolism. Despite continuous perfusion, myocardial damage commonly occurred for many of the reasons discussed previously. Although myocardial protection improved with the addition of moderate cardiac hypothermia (28° to 32°C), operating conditions did not. Most surgeons found it difficult to perform precise repairs on the firm, bleeding, beating, or fibrillating heart. To improve exposure and minimize the complications associated with direct coronary cannulation for aortic valve replacement (AVR), myocardial ischemia was induced by aortic cross-clamping. Sapsford et al,[132] in a randomized study comparing coronary perfusion with cold ischemic arrest, found the latter technique to be equally effective, yet simpler. However, the technique of normothermic or moderate hypothermic ischemic arrest is not without problems. First, the heart continues to beat for some time after application of the aortic cross-clamp, thereby compromising the anticipated improvement in operating conditions. Persistent electrical and mechanical activity during much of the ischemic period needlessly depletes high-energy phosphate and compromises post-repair ventricular performance. Second, few surgeons can complete a complex repair quickly enough to prevent significant myocardial damage in the unprotected heart. Third, the use of intermittent cross-clamping with periods of reperfusion does little to improve operating conditions or prevent necrosis. Reactive hyperemia after release of the aortic clamp continues to obscure the operative field. Multiple short periods of reperfusion, particularly in the presence of VF, may potentiate rather than prevent ischemic damage. Defibrillation to improve reperfusion reintroduces the problem of systemic air embolism during open repairs. Akins and Carroll,[133] however, reported good clinical results using hypothermic fibrillatory arrest.

In summary, rapid cessation of electrical and mechanical activity immediately after aortic cross-clamping is desirable to potentiate surgical exposure and myocardial preservation. The extent of necrosis in unprotected myocardium is directly related to the duration of aortic cross-clamping. The ischemic time should be minimized. Variability among patients in terms of myocardial vulnerability makes it difficult to accurately predict safe periods of interval ischemia. Prolonged surgical time demands direct interventions to protect the myocardium. These focus along the lines of maximizing high-energy phosphate production while minimizing high-energy phosphate use and intracellular calcium accumulation during the ischemic period. Specific interventions include hypothermia, cardioplegia, β-adrenergic and calcium channel blockade, and adenosine-regulating compounds. Uninterrupted periods of ischemia provide the best operating conditions while minimizing the risk of reperfusion injury and air embolism.

Table 28–7 Abnormalities Encountered during Reperfusion

Class	Type	Reference*
Structural	Myocardial edema	376, 379–381
	Platelet deposition	382, 383
	Neutrophil activation	403–407
	Vascular injury	384
	Vascular compression	385, 386
Biochemical	Acidosis	370, 375
	Decreased oxygen use	377, 378, 387
	Decreased high-energy phosphate production	388–392
	Increased catecholamines	372–374
	Complement activation	401, 402
	Increased intracellular calcium	393–395, 408, 409
	Increased free radicals	396–399
Electrical	Arrhythmias	371
Mechanical	Impaired systolic or diastolic function	400

*Numbers refer to references listed at end of chapter.

Reperfusion

Before reperfusion, the myocardium is made up of a heterogeneous population of cells that can be classified as irreversibly damaged, minimally damaged, and stunned myocardium. The outcome of the latter group is dependent on reperfusion management. The proper use of supplemental reperfusion methods in vulnerable patients can mean the difference between a small rise in the postoperative CK level and inability to wean from bypass (see Chapter 31).

The many changes associated with reperfusion are interrelated (Table 28–7). They are the same as previously described for ischemia but also include the triggering of acute inflammatory responses in the body. This otherwise normal physiologic process in the setting of CPB unfortunately leads to increasing cell damage (see Chapter 8). Together, these anatomic, biochemical, electrical, and mechanical abnormalities occur during reperfusion. For most patients, these abnormalities normalize with time, and minimal intervention is needed. For a few vulnerable patients exposed to prolonged periods of ischemia or with inadequate protection, reperfusion can result in extension of damage.

Myocardial Protection

During the initiation of CPB, the anesthesiologist must renew vigilance to ensure the maintenance of physiologic conditions that will prevent perioperative organ damage. Several organs—especially the brain, heart, and kidney—are susceptible to ischemic damage during CPB. Although the surgical team is best positioned to administer cardioplegia, it is important for the anesthesiologist to monitor myocardial protection during bypass; the magnitude of sustained ischemic injury will greatly influence the strategy to discontinue bypass support. An outline of various strategies to attenuate myocardial damage during CPB is presented here and in Chapter 30.

Myocardial protection strategies can be summarized with four basic concepts:

1. Myocardial protection begins with preparation of the heart before arrest
2. Metabolic requirements should be reduced during the arrest interval
3. A favorable metabolic milieu during arrest helps provide a margin of safety with reduced metabolism
4. Reperfusion modification after an ischemic insult can minimize structural and functional damage to the myocardium

The first concept includes phenomena under the direct control of the anesthesiologist. In the pre-bypass period, the heart should be prepared for ischemic arrest by optimizing myocardial metabolism and providing hemodynamic conditions that optimize myocardial oxygen supply-demand ratios.

Patients coming to cardiac surgery (especially in this era of same-day admissions) are frequently dehydrated and hypoglycemic. The anesthesiologist should rehydrate the patient and administer sufficient glucose to improve the heart's ability to tolerate ischemic arrest.[134,135] Because the initiation of bypass is frequently accompanied by hypotension, the anesthesiologist should be prepared to administer vasoconstrictive drugs (e.g., phenylephrine) to maintain coronary perfusion pressure. Similarly, ventricular distention must be avoided (especially before fibrillatory arrest) because increases in left ventricular end-diastolic pressure decrease coronary perfusion pressures and greatly compromise subendocardial oxygen delivery. The anesthesiologist should monitor intraventricular volume with a transesophageal echocardiography (TEE) probe after the initiation of bypass. The surgeon can prevent ventricular distention by placing a hole in the left atrium, left ventricle, or pulmonary artery or by placing a vent in the left ventricle. Although negative pressure venting enhances the risk of intracavitary air entrapment, many surgeons prefer active venting to passive methods. Several pharmacologic interventions administered to patients or added to the cardioplegic solution may enhance myocardial protection. β-Receptor antagonists (e.g., propranolol, esmolol) provide myocardial protection by decreasing heart rate and myocardial metabolism.[136] The heart rate should be maintained at less than 80 beats per minute in patients with ischemic heart disease in the pre-bypass period. Even in the absence of tachycardia, β-blockers should be administered at the beginning of bypass, especially in patients with hypertrophic myocardium. Schwinn and others have demonstrated that β-receptor down-regulation occurs during CPB as a result of the greatly increased circulating catecholamines that occur during bypass.[137] β-Blockade may attenuate this down-regulation and permit enhanced response to post-bypass β-agonists.

Brain Injury

The brain is highly susceptible to injury during CPB. Many clinicians believe that cerebral injuries after cardiac surgery are the most devastating adverse outcomes associated with CPB. A study of 2400 elective CABG surgery patients from 24 U.S. centers reported that 6.1% of patients suffer adverse postoperative gross neurologic or psychiatric CNS events. These patients remain in the ICU and hospital for greater periods of time, and one in every three surviving patients does not return home, but requires continued long-term care and rehabilitation.[138] Chapters 30 and 35 provide information on the important issue of perioperative adverse CNS events in the cardiac surgery patient.

Renal Dysfunction

The effects of CPB on the renal system have significant health and economic impacts; however, despite intensive investigation into the pathogenesis and prevention of renal failure, there remains limited progress in the development of effective protective strategies in recent decades.[139-149] As intravascular volume depletion and hypoperfusion can lead to exacerbation of renal ischemia and accentuate the risk for postoperative ARF, avoidance of nephrotoxic agents and close attention to intravascular volume, blood pressure and CO are central in the effort to reduce the occurrence of ARF after cardiac surgery. Chapters 30 and 36 discuss acute renal injuries after CPB.

Gastrointestinal Effects

The effects of CPB on the gastrointestinal system are complex and not fully elucidated. Although most patients undergoing cardiac surgery do not suffer adverse changes in gastrointestinal function, subclinical perturbations including transient elevations in hepatocellular enzymes and hyperamylasemia have been observed after CPB. Although the incidence of gastrointestinal complications after CPB is low (range, 0.3% to 3.7%), they are associated with significant morbidity and remarkably high mortality (range, 11% to 67%) compared with cardiac surgery patients without postoperative gastrointestinal compromise. The frequently reported adverse gastrointestinal outcomes include gastroesophagitis, upper and lower gastrointestinal hemorrhage, hyperbilirubinemia, hepatic and splenic ischemia, colitis, pancreatitis, cholecystitis, diverticulitis, mesenteric ischemia, as well as intestinal obstruction, infarction, and perforation[150-164] (see Chapters 30 and 36).

Although the pathophysiology of gastrointestinal complications after cardiac surgery is likely multifactorial, a unifying mechanism is splanchnic hypoperfusion.[153-158] The gastrointestinal system is particularly vulnerable for ischemia due to the lack of autoregulation and to the preferential shunting of blood away from the gastrointestinal circulation during periods of hypotension. Hypothermia and nonpulsatile flow during CPB may be detrimental to mucosal perfusion. However, hypothermia has little effect on hepatic arterial blood flow, and may actually increase portal flow. There is no significant difference in hepatic blood flow between pulsatile and nonpulsatile perfusion at high flow rates (2.4 L/min/m^2) during hypothermia. Perhaps more important to the development of inadequate gastrointestinal perfusion is the significant increase in total body oxygen consumption in the immediate hours after CPB. Visceral hypotension is the most significant factor in the development of gastrointestinal complications after cardiac surgery. Gut ischemia of sufficient duration impairs gastrointestinal tract barrier function. Studies evaluating gut permeability have shown that CPB is associated with an increase in mucosal permeability and systemic endotoxin concentration.[159,160]

Endocrine and Inflammatory Responses

Endocrine Response. Cardiopulmonary bypass provokes a marked stress response, which has been quantified by measurements of hormones and vasoactive substances in plasma. Hypothermia, hemodilution, nonpulsatile flow, as well as insulin, prostaglandin, and renin release are common during CPB, and are all potent stimuli for catecholamine release. Replogle et al[165] reported a 200% increase in plasma norepinephrine and a 1500% increase in plasma epinephrine during bypass. As summarized by Reves,[139] epinephrine levels increase throughout CPB with a ninefold increase that peaks during rewarming, after aortic cross-clamp release. Philbin et al[66] and Landymore et al[58] found that epinephrine and norepinephrine continued to increase well into the post-bypass period. Although striking, the magnitude of the catecholamine responses is comparable to that after syncope, myocardial infarction, strenuous exercise, or caffeine ingestion. Even more dramatic responses have been observed in infants and children during CPB.[166,167] It is likely that increased plasma catecholamine concentrations are in part due to decreased clearance. The heart and lungs, which serve as primary clearance organs for these substances, are partially or completely excluded from the circulation during much of CPB. Hypothermia slows all enzymatic processes responsible for metabolism.

Many other hormones increase in concentration during CPB. Cortisol does not peak during CPB, but on the first postoperative day. Vasopressin increases up to 20 times baseline levels during CPB.[52,66] Prostaglandin metabolism is altered by CPB.[168] For example, thromboxane, which induces vasoconstriction and platelet aggregation, progressively increases during CPB,[59] especially in children.[169] Some investigators suggest that vasopressin[52] and angiotensin II[53,61] are responsible for the elevations in SVR observed during CPB, and this may explain why vasopressin can be a useful drug to increase SVR on CPB in patients who are extremely vasodilated.[170]

There is some evidence for a greater incidence of postoperative complications in adult patients who experience increased hormonal and metabolic responses.[171] There are also indications that morbidity and mortality rates are increased in ICU patients with heightened stress responses.[172] Investigators have reported anesthetic techniques that attenuate the stress response to surgical stimulus, particularly through use of high-dose narcotics.[173] The effectiveness of this attenuation has been questioned by some clinicians.[174,175] No outcome studies have proved specific benefits of stress response attenuation in CPB patients (see Chapter 9).

There seems to be greater evidence that lessening the stress response in young children undergoing cardiac surgery is of benefit. The response of newborns in particular to the stress of cardiac surgery is greater than that of adults.[166] Similar results were reported by Firmin et al[167] in slightly older children (6 months); the most prominent hormonal response was marked intraoperative catecholamine elevation. A later study comparing preterm infants undergoing patent ductus ligation with nitrous oxide, curare, and no fentanyl and those with fentanyl supplementation found lower hormonal levels with narcotic supplementation.[176] Anand and Hickey[177] suggested that neonates undergoing CPB who receive "deep anesthesia" (i.e., high doses of sufentanil and postoperative infusions of narcotics for 24 hours after surgery) show reduced hormonal responses compared with those given halothane and morphine.

A lack of agreement existed among clinicians regarding the management of hyperglycemia in diabetic and nondiabetic cardiovascular surgery patients.[178,179] Data from both clinical and laboratory investigators now conclusively demonstrate the untoward affects of hyperglycemia in cardiac surgery.[180-186] Van den Berghe et al randomized 1548 ICU subjects (including 970 postoperative cardiac surgery patients) to either conventional (target glucose values 180–200 mg/dL) or intensive (target glucose values 80–110 mg/dL) glucose management.[180] Patients in the intensive group were more likely to survive in the early hospitalization and after discharge at 30 days. In the first 5 postoperative days, the death rate was 5.1% and 2.1% in the conventional and intensive groups, respectively. Patients targeted to glucose values of 80 to 110 mg/dL were less likely to remain in the ICU for more than 5 days, require prolonged ventilatory support, undergo dialysis, or suffer septicemia. Work by Furnary et al,[181] confirmed the importance of perioperative glucose control in cardiac surgery patients, especially those suffering Type 1 diabetes mellitus. They analyzed their practice's mortality rates in diabetics between 1994 and 2004 and compared their rates with those reported in the STS database. The study group was increasingly aggressive in reducing the tolerance for perioperative hyperglycemia. In 2005, protocol called for maintaining perioperative glucose values less than 120 mg/dL. Operative mortality in Type 1 diabetics was 0.8% compared with the 3.6% reported by the STS. The findings are consistent with the report by Lazar et al.[182] This group randomized 141 Type 1 diabetics scheduled for cardiac surgery to tight glycemic control (glucose values 125 to 200 mg/dL) or conventional treatment (glucose less than 250 mg/dL). Diabetics in the "tight control" group were treated with glucose-insulin-potassium and had a reduced duration of hospitalization, fewer episodes of recurrent wound infection, and less myocardial ischemia in the 2 years after surgery. Aggressive control of perioperative glucose values represents the standard of care in cardiac surgery. Glucose values should not be maintained at levels less than 200 mg/dL. Lower values (blood glucose 80 to 120 mg/dL) are likely superior to values of glucose more than 120 mg/dL. A protocol for management of glucose in cardiac surgery patients is outlined in Table 28-8.

Virtually every organ system is affected in some manner by thyroid hormones. With respect to the cardiovascular system,

Table 28-8 Stanford University Adult Cardiac Anesthesia Continuous Insulin Infusion Protocol

- *Bolus and start infusion as follows*

Blood glucose	Insulin bolus units	Units/hr
<125	0	0
125–175	5	1
175–225	10	2
>225	15	3

*Blood glucose measurements **every 30 minutes** intraoperatively!*

Insulin titration

Blood glucose	*Treatment*
<75	Stop insulin; D5W and recheck in 30 min; when >150, restart at 50% of previous rate
75–100	Stop insulin; recheck in 30 min; restart at 50% of previous rate (unless <0.25 u/hr)
101–125	If <10% lower than last value, decrease by 0.5 u/hr If >10% lower than last value, decrease by 50% If neither, continue current rate
126–175	Continue current rate
176–225	If lower than last value continue current rate If higher than last value increase by 0.5 u/hr
>225	If >10% lower than last value continue current rate If <10% lower or greater than last value increase by 1 u/hr If >225 and not decreased after 3 adjustments double current rate

thyroid hormones increase heart rate and force of contraction by increasing the responsiveness of the heart to circulating catecholamines. The heat load generated by the metabolic effects of thyroid hormones results in vasodilation and a reduction in peripheral vascular resistance. These effects are mediated by the two primary hormones secreted by the thyroid gland, tetraiodothyronine (T_4) or thyroxine, and triiodothyronine (T_3). T_3 has a biologic potency several times greater than T_4. Approximately 80% of T_3 is formed by extrathyroidal metabolism of T_4. In critical illness, a condition known as *euthyroid sick syndrome* occurs in which T_4 is metabolized to reverse T_3 (rT_3), which has virtually no biologic activity. Patients with thyroid hormone deficiency may have significant cardiovascular abnormalities including decreased CO, increased SVR, and rhythm disturbances.

The effects of CPB on thyroid hormone levels and function have been described. Similar to the changes seen in euthyroid sick syndrome, reverse T_3 levels are increased and T_3 levels are decreased. Holland et al[187] studied the effects of CPB on thyroid hormone extensively. They found a 75% decrease in T_3 levels and a 300% increase in rT_3 levels beginning in the first few hours after CPB and persisting at least 24 hours. Total T_4 and TSH remain in the low-normal range throughout CPB. Heparin decreases cellular binding of thyroxine, increasing free T_4 levels.[188-190] Decreases in TSH may be secondary to negative feedback from the elevated free T_4 levels. The thyroid-stimulating hormone (TSH) response to thyrotropin-releasing hormone (TRH) is markedly blunted by nonpulsatile flow during CPB, although no difference in patient outcome has been attributed to this effect.[191] The normal TSH response to low T_3 levels is absent in patients after CPB.[187]

The use of exogenously administered T_3 to correct the low levels seen after CPB has been evaluated in a number of experimental and clinical studies. In their initial experiments, Novitsky et al[192] found that there was no significant difference between T_3 treatment and placebo groups in baboons undergoing 3 hours of hypothermic CPB. There was an increase in myocardial high-energy phosphates and a decrease in myocardial lactate levels in those animals receiving a bolus of T_3 at aortic cross-clamp removal. Subsequent studies in pigs undergoing hypothermic CPB demonstrated that T_3 repletion improved postischemic ventricular function and CO.[193,194] Administration of T_3 to normal isolated, perfused rabbit hearts did not enhance ventricular function, but the same experiment performed in injured, isolated, perfused hearts demonstrated improved ventricular recovery over a wide dose range.[195,196] In vitro aortic ring experiments have shown that T_3 pretreatment decreased the force of norepinephrine-induced contraction.[197] It was hoped that the improved postischemic ventricular function and decreased norepinephrine-induced vasoconstriction in experimental studies would be consistent in clinical trials of patients undergoing cardiac surgery. In a number of small clinical studies, patients undergoing CABG who received T_3 had increased CO after surgery, but there were no significant changes in outcome or postoperative therapy.[193,198-200] Despite promising experimental evidence, clinical trials have not demonstrated a benefit to T_3 repletion in patients undergoing CABG surgery. Although routine administration of T_3 to patients after CPB cannot be recommended, some investigators suggest that anecdotal experience supports the use of T_3 as a rescue agent to safely improve CO in patients who are difficult to wean from CPB support[197] (see Chapter 31).

Immunologic Inflammatory Response. The physiologic insult of CPB results in a myriad of exaggerated, complex, and mostly pathologic immunologic events. The passage of blood through the extracorporeal circuit causes activation of complement, platelets, neutrophils, and proinflammatory kinins. At the conclusion of bypass, blood perturbed by the process of extracorporeal circulation reperfuses ischemic organs, exacerbating the local inflammatory responses in end-organs including the brain, kidney, heart, and lung. These phenomena result in whole-body inflammatory response and represent the collective effect of activation of the complement, fibrinolytic, kallikrein, and coagulation systems. These systems are discussed here and in Chapters 8, 18, and 29.

The complement system, composed of at least 20 plasma proteins, normally acts as the body's defense against a wide variety of traumatic, infectious, and immunologic challenges. The result of complement activation centers on cell membranes and includes histamine release from basophil and mast cells, cell lysis, smooth muscle contraction, increased vascular permeability, and activation of phagocytic cells. The complement system is also closely linked with the coagulation, kinin, and fibrinolytic systems.

The complement system is formed by two interconnected cascades: the classical and the alternative pathways. The elements of the classical pathway are C1, C4, and C2, with subunits and fragments of these elements developing as the cascade progresses. The classical pathway is thought to be normally triggered by antigen-antibody complexes. The alternative pathway, bypassing C1, C4, and C2 to activate C3, is triggered by complex polysaccharides, lipopolysaccharides, IgA and IgD, and exposure of blood to foreign surfaces. The two pathways converge at C3 and lead to activation of the terminal components, C5 to C9. The fragments C3a and C5a are known anaphylatoxins (see Chapter 8).

With initiation of CPB, complement is thought to be activated through the alternative pathway.[201-203] Exposure of blood to the CPB circuit initiates activation of the coagulation cascade by means of the Hageman factor (XII). Although the coagulation cascade is initiated, it is not completed because of the presence of heparin (see Chapters 18 and 29). Activated factor XII (XIIa) results in plasmin generation. Plasmin activates complement by C1 (classical pathway), cleaves C3 (alternative pathway), and cleaves factor XII, which activates the kallikrein-kinin systems. Complement activation can also occur through the classical pathway by heparin-protamine complexes.[204] Complement activation leads to direct membrane injury by complement subunits, neutrophil activation, enhancement of phagocytosis due to interaction of complement components and phagocytic cells, and release of lysosomal enzymes. The complement fragments are stimulants that induce changes in neutrophil behavior, causing neutrophil activation and migration, and the promotion of adhesive and secretory events. These phenomena contribute to the reperfusion injury observed in cardiac surgery patients. Activated neutrophils attach to the endothelium, causing translocation of P-selectin from intracellular vesicles to the cell membrane and platelet-activating factor (PAF) synthesis. Endothelial membrane-bound PAF leads to increased neutrophil adhesion and activation, and neutrophil adhesion protein (CD11/CD18) expression (Fig. 28–5). Ultimately, increases in adhesion molecule emission in the endothelium and other tissue cell types (e.g., myocytes, alveolar cells, glomerular or renal tubular epithelium) result in transmigration of neu-

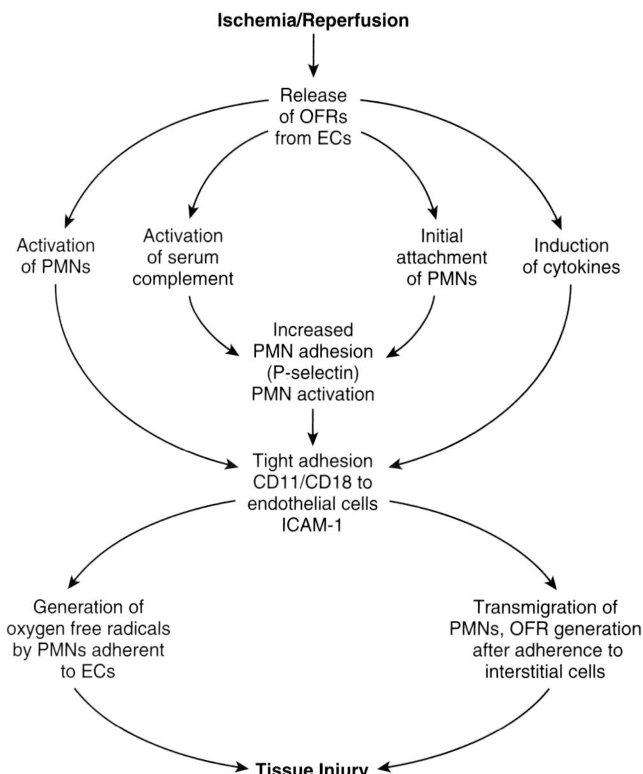

Figure 28–5 A schematic representation of the interactive components of the immune response that likely occurs during the postischemic inflammatory state after cardiopulmonary bypass. EC = endothelial cells; ICAM = intercellular adhesion molecules; OFR = oxygen free radicals; PMN = neutrophil. (From Herskowitz A, Mangano DT: Inflammatory cascade: A final common pathway for perioperative injury? Anesthesiology 85:957, 1996.)

trophils into the interstitial space, and release of large amounts of free radicals. These phenomena are schematically presented in Figure 28–6.[205]

Although complement has been recognized as a significant factor in the development of the physiologic disturbances seen after cardiac surgery, endotoxins released into the bloodstream during CPB are also felt to play a significant role in the inflammatory cascade.[160] Endotoxin binds to lipopolysaccharide-binding protein normally present in serum. This complex binds to specific receptors on macrophages with subsequent production of cytokines. The collective result of these cellular and humoral responses may be manifest by cardiovascular instability, pulmonary dysfunction, renal insufficiency, alterations in hemostasis, fever, and excess extravascular fluid retention.

Cytokines are small proteins produced in a variety of cells in response to different immune-mediated signals. The cytokines known as interleukin-1 (IL-1) through IL-16 have been identified. They have a number of physiologic effects that are characteristic of the systemic inflammatory response including fever, hypotension, altered mental status, and increased production of acute-phase proteins. Cytokines are important intercellular regulators of cellular immune function. They stimulate proliferation and terminal differentiation of T cells, differentiation and secretion of immunoglobulins from B cells, and neutrophil chemotaxis and transendothelial migration.

One of the early mediators of the inflammatory cascade is tumor necrosis factor (TNF-α), which is synthesized after binding of LBP-endotoxin complex to the macrophage CD14 receptor. In addition to its physiologic effects, it stimulates the production and release of other cytokines involved in the inflammatory cascade: IL-1, IL-6, and IL-8. IL-2 is involved in cell-mediated immune responses and is produced in helper T cells. Reduced numbers of helper T cells and impaired ability

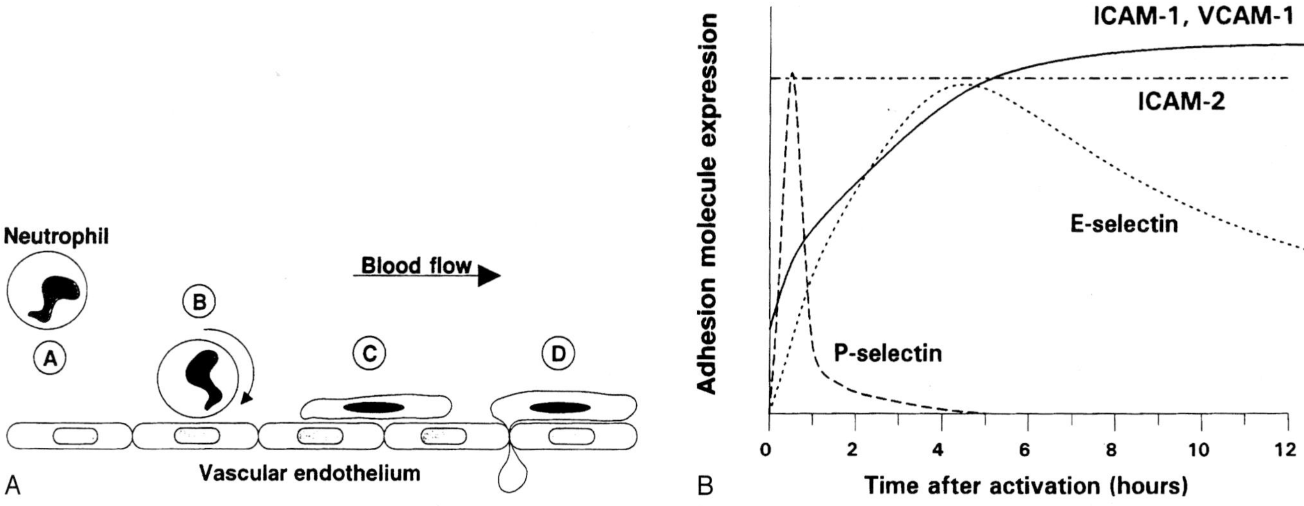

Figure 28–6 General mechanism for neutrophil adherence and extravasation. *(A)* After activation of the endothelium, neutrophils, which were previously free in the circulation (A), start to roll (B) on endothelium that has been activated, a process controlled through the interaction of members of the selectin family with carbohydrate ligands. After subsequent activation of the neutrophils (e.g., interleukin-8, C5a, platelet-activating factor), there is activation of integrin molecules (e.g., leukocyte function–associated antigen-1) on the surface of the cells that causes their firm adherence (C) through interaction with receptors that belong to the Ig superfamily (e.g., intercellular adhesion molecules [ICAMs]). The molecules extravasate through the endothelial layer (D) into the tissue. *(B)* Activation of the endothelium is associated with expression of a range of adhesion molecules, including members of the selectin family (P- and E-selectin) and the Ig superfamily (i.e., ICAM-1, ICAM-2, ICAM-3, and vascular cell adhesion molecule-1 [VCAM-1]). Each molecule has its own particular kinetics of expression, ranging from P-selectin, which is rapidly expressed following activation (through release of preformed molecules), to VCAM-1 and ICAM-1, which have slower kinetics of expression. Many of the molecules are not expressed on the resting endothelium, although some are expressed at low level. (From Hornick H, George A: Blood contact activation: Pathophysiological effects and therapeutic approaches. Perfusion 11:3, 1996.)

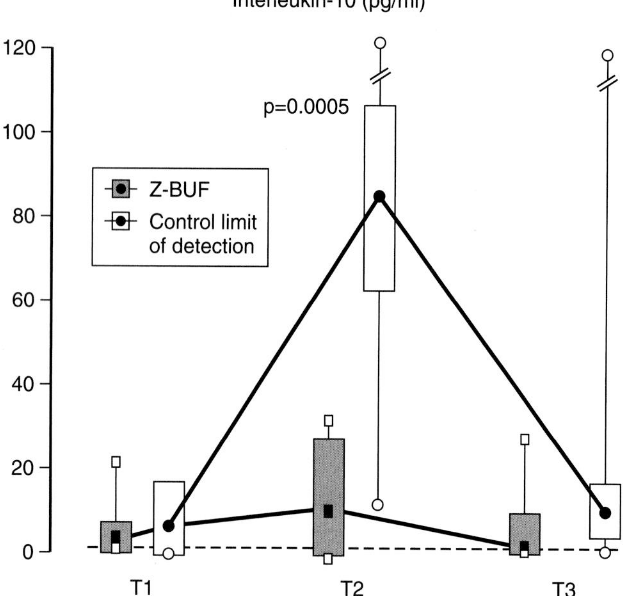

Figure 28–7 Comparative changes in plasma interleukin-10 concentration over time (Mann-Whitney test). Data are expressed as the median, 25th and 7th percentiles, minimum, and maximum. (From Journois D, Israel-Biet D, Pouard P, et al: High-volume, zero-balanced hemofiltration to reduce delayed inflammatory response to cardiopulmonary bypass in children. Anesthesiology 85:965, 1996.)

to synthesize IL-2 after cardiac surgery may be responsible for the altered cell-mediated immune function observed after cardiac surgery.[206,207] TNF-α is responsible for stimulating production of an anti-inflammatory cytokine, IL-10. It exerts its effects by inhibiting the synthesis of the inflammatory cytokines, and may represent an endogenous negative feedback system to limit the inflammatory response.[208]

Interventions aimed at reducing morbidity associated with the systemic inflammatory response seen after CPB may be directed at preventing or minimizing the activation of the various systems contributing to the response, or at blocking the physiologic effects once activation occurs. Studies evaluating membrane versus bubble oxygenators have reported conflicting data regarding the degree of complement activation or clinical outcome.[209-211] For example, although Cavarocchi et al[212] and Tamiya et al[213] found bubble oxygenators increased complement activation compared with membrane oxygenators, Hammerschmidt et al[214] found the opposite. Jones et al[215] found no discernible difference between the two oxygenator types. Bonded extracorporeal circuits have been shown to reduce neutrophil activation compared with conventional circuits, but outcome studies and cost-benefit analysis are lacking.[216-218] Hemofiltration is known to reduce levels of circulating inflammatory mediators and improve outcomes, particularly in the pediatric population.[219-222]

Journois et al[220] assessed the effectiveness of ultrafiltration (hemofiltration) immediately after the discontinuation of bypass support on inflammatory mediator removal and postoperative alveolar-arterial (A-a) oxygen gradients, time to extubation, systemic temperature, and blood loss. Children randomized to undergo ultrafiltration were found to have a significant reduction of tumor necrosis factor, IL-10, and myeloperoxidase immediately after ultrafiltration. Twenty-four hours after surgery, levels of IL-1, IL-6, IL-8, and myeloperoxidase were decreased. The reduction of IL-10 in the ultrafiltration group warrants attention (Fig. 28–7). IL-10 is a potent anti-inflammatory and is thought to play an important role during profound inflammatory events. Removal of this moiety therefore may have important deleterious effects. Although A-a gradients, time to extubation, and blood loss were improved in the ultrafiltration treatment group, a cause-and-effect relationship could not be proved.[221,222]

Corticosteroids may play an important role in minimizing the inflammatory response by reducing complement activation, decreasing production of cytokines, and interfering with neutrophil adherence and migration. Most clinical trials have reported a beneficial effect on markers of inflammation (e.g., cytokine and complement levels, histamine release, leukocyte counts, endothelial activation).[223-228] Boscoe et al[229] reported that methylprednisolone (two doses of 30 mg/kg at induction and immediately before CPB) modified bypass-related complement activation. Cavarocchi's group reported that methylprednisolone reduced anaphylatoxin levels during their oxygenator studies.[212] One large-scale trial of glucocorticoid use in the treatment of the systemic inflammatory response in septic shock, on the other hand, showed no beneficial effect on outcome.[228] Jones et al[215] also found steroids ineffective.

The use of aprotinin or other protease inhibitors has been shown to produce a dose-dependent reduction in complement activation, cytokine release and neutrophil activation during cardiac surgery.[230,231] Indomethacin may restore cell-mediated immunity by decreasing synthesis of prostaglandin E_2, which acts to reduce production of IL-2.[232,233]

Of interest is the concept of plasmapheresis for conservation of platelets and leukocytes before CPB. Davies et al[234] attempted to decrease platelet activation by the CPB circuit by harvesting platelet- and leukocyte-rich plasma. They removed approximately 850 mL of platelet-rich plasma per patient, which was reinfused after separation from CPB and protamine administration. Mediastinal chest tube drainage was reduced by nearly 50%, fewer units of allogeneic blood products were transfused, and arterial oxygen tension on extubation was higher.

A prospective, randomized study of 4000 CABG patients assessed pexelizumab, a C5 complement inhibitor, on the incidence of death and MI. The primary endpoints were not achieved, and this agent appears to have little value during cardiac surgery.[234,235]

MANAGEMENT BEFORE BYPASS

An important objective of this phase is to prepare the patient for CPB (Box 28–3). This phase invariably involves two key steps: anticoagulation and vascular cannulation. Heparin is still the only anticoagulant clinically used for CPB. Dose, method of administration, and opinions as to what constitutes adequate anticoagulation vary. Heparin must be administered

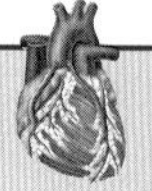

BOX 28–3 *Management before Cardiopulmonary Bypass*

- Anticoagulation
- Cannulation of the heart
- Careful monitoring
- Protection of the heart
- Preparation for cardiopulmonary bypass

before cannulation for CPB, even if cannulation must be done emergently. Failure to do so is to risk thrombosis in the patient and extracorporeal circuit. Chapters 18 and 29 offer a complete discussion of hemostasis management for the cardiac surgery patient. After heparin has been administered, a period of 3 to 5 minutes is customarily allowed for systemic circulation and onset of effect. Various confirmatory tests of actual achievement of anticoagulation are performed if time permits.

Vascular Cannulation

The next major step in the pre-bypass phase is vascular cannulation. The goal of vascular cannulation is to provide access whereby the CPB pump may divert all systemic venous blood to the pump oxygenator at the lowest possible venous pressures and deliver oxygenated blood to the arterial circulation at pressure and flow sufficient to maintain systemic homeostasis.

Arterial Cannulation

Arterial cannulation is generally established before venous cannulation to allow volume resuscitation of the patient, should it be necessary. The ascending aorta is the preferred site for aortic cannulation because it is easily accessible, does not require an additional incision, accommodates a larger cannula to provide greater flow at a reduced pressure, and carries a lower risk of aortic dissection compared with other arterial cannulation sites (femoral or iliac arteries). Because hypertension increases the risk of aortic dissection during cannulation, the aortic pressure may be temporarily lowered (MAP < 80 mm Hg during aortotomy and cannula insertion). Several potential complications are associated with aortic cannulation including embolization of air or atheromatous debris, inadvertent cannulation of aortic arch vessels, aortic dissection, and other vessel wall injury.[236-241]

Reviews and clinical reports emphasize the importance of embolization as the major mechanism of focal cerebral injury in cardiac surgery patients. Barzilai et al[242] and Wareing et al[237] reported intraoperative use of two-dimensional ultrasound to image the ascending aorta as a guide to selection of cross-clamping and cannulation sites. In 24% and 33% of the patients in the Barzilai and Wareing studies, respectively, ultrasonic findings led to selection of alternate cannulation sites (see Chapters 15, 17, 30, and 35). A femoral artery, rather than the ascending aorta, can be cannulated for systemic perfusion. Femoral cannulation is used when ascending aortic cannulation is considered relatively contraindicated, as in severe aortic atherosclerosis, aortic aneurysm or dissection, or known cystic medical necrosis.[7,57,243,244] The anesthesiologist should seek evidence of cannula malposition by looking for unilateral blanching of the face, gently palpating carotid pulses and checking for new unilateral diminution, and by measuring blood pressure in both arms and checking for new asymmetries.

Venous Cannulation

Venous cannulation can be achieved using a single atrial cannula that is inserted into the right atrium and directed inferiorly (Fig. 28–8). Drainage holes are located in the inferior vena cava (IVC) and right atrium to drain blood returning from the lower extremities and the superior vena cava (SVC) and coronary sinus, respectively. This technique has the advantage of being simpler, faster and requiring only one incision; however, the quality of drainage can be easily compromised when the heart is lifted for surgical exposure.[245] The bicaval cannulation technique, required in cases in which right atrial (RA) access is needed, involves cannulating the SVC and IVC (Fig. 28–9). Loops placed around the vessels can be tightened to divert all caval blood flow away from the heart. Blood returning to the right atrium from the coronary sinus will not be drained using this technique, so an additional vent or atriotomy is necessary.

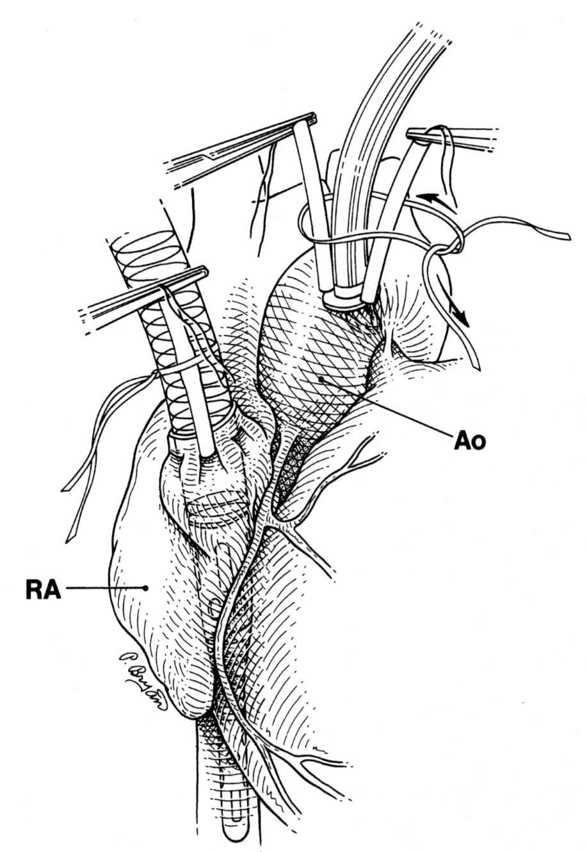

Figure 28–8 Aortic (Ao) and single, double-staged, right atrial (RA) cannulation. Notice the drainage holes of venous cannula in right atrium and inferior vena cava. (From Connolly MW: Cardiopulmonary Bypass. New York, Springer-Verlag, 1995, p 59.)

During CPB, blood will continue to return to the left ventricle from a variety of sources, including the bronchial and thebesian veins, as well as blood that traverses the pulmonary circulation. Abnormal sources of venous blood include a persistent left SVC, systemic-to-pulmonary shunts, and aortic regurgitation. It is important to avoid left ventricular (LV) filling and distention during CPB to prevent myocardial rewarming and to minimize LV wall tension and limit myocardial oxygen demand.[246] This can be accomplished with the use of a vent placed in the pulmonary artery, aortic root, or left ventricle, depending on the likely source of LV blood return.

Venous cannulas, using a two-stage or bicaval cannula, are large and can impair venous return from the IVC or SVC. Superior vena caval obstruction is detected by venous engorgement of the head and neck, conjunctival edema, and elevated SVC pressure. Inferior vena caval obstruction is far more insidious, presenting only as decreased filling pressures because of lowered venous return.

Femoral venous cannulation is sometimes used to permit partial CPB without, or before, sternotomy or RA cannulation (e.g., redos, ascending aortic aneurysms). Because of their

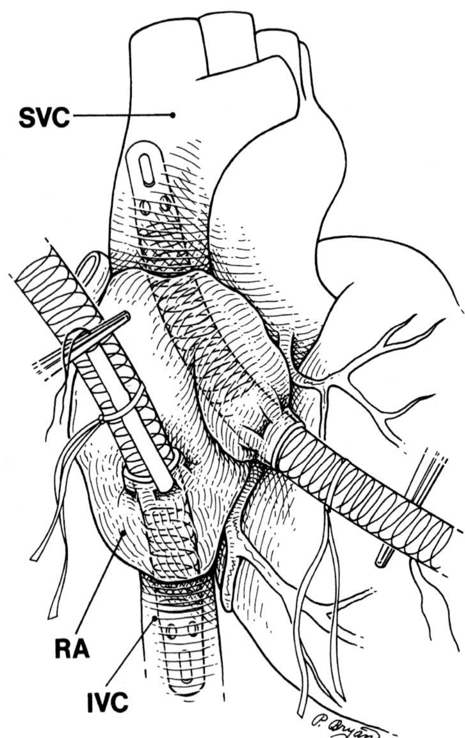

Figure 28–9 Position of two-vessel cannulation of right atrium (RA) with placement of drainage holes into superior vena cava (SVC) and inferior vena cava (IVC). The aortic cannula is not shown. (From Connolly MW: Cardiopulmonary Bypass. New York, Springer-Verlag, 1995, p 59.)

comparatively small size and placement in the distal IVC, femoral venous cannulas do not permit complete drainage of systemic venous blood, and only partial CPB may be achieved. A long cannula with multiple fenestrations can be inserted through the femoral vein and passed to the level of the IVC-RA junction to enhance venous return.

Other Preparations

Once anticoagulation and cannulation are complete, CPB can be instituted. Because there is redundant pulmonary artery catheter (PAC) length in the right ventricle, and the heart is manipulated during CPB, there is a tendency for distal migration of the catheter into pulmonary artery branches.[247] This distal migration of the catheter increases the risks of "autowedging" and pulmonary artery perforation. During the pre-bypass phase it is advisable to withdraw the PAC 3 to 5 cm to decrease the likelihood of these untoward events. It is also advisable to check the integrity of all vascular access and monitoring devices. A PAC placed through an external jugular[248,249] or subclavian vein[250] can become kinked or occluded on full opening of the sternal retractor. If TEE is being used, the probe should be placed in the "freeze" mode and the tip of the scope placed in the neutral and unlocked position. Leaving the electronic scanning emitter on during hypothermic CPB adds heat to the posterior wall of the ventricle (see Chapter 15).

Before initiating CPB, the anesthesiologist should assess the depth of anesthesia and muscle relaxation. It is important to maintain paralysis to prevent patient movement that could result in dislodgment of bypass-circuit cannulas and prevent shivering as hypothermia is induced (with the attendant increases in oxygen consumption).[251] It is difficult to determine the depth of anesthesia during the various stages of CPB.

Table 28–9 Preparation for Bypass: Pre-bypass Checklist

1. Anticoagulation
   a. Heparin administered
   b. Desired level of anticoagulation achieved
2. Arterial cannulation
   a. Absence of bubbles in arterial line
   b. Evidence of dissection or malposition?
3. Venous cannulation
   a. Evidence of superior vena cava obstruction?
   b. Evidence of inferior vena cava obstruction?
4. Pulmonary artery catheter (if used) pulled back
5. Are all monitoring/access catheters functional?
6. Transesophageal echocardiograph (if used)
   a. In "freeze" mode
   b. Scope in neutral/unlocked position
7. Supplemental medications
   a. Neuromuscular blockers
   b. Anesthetics, analgesics, amnestics
8. Inspection of head and neck
   a. Color
   b. Symmetry
   c. Venous drainage
   d. Pupils

Because blood pressure, heart rate, pupil diameter, and the autonomic nervous system are profoundly affected by extracorporeal circulation (e.g., the heart is asystolic; blood pressure is greatly influenced by circuit blood flow; sweating occurs with rewarming), these variables do not reliably reflect the anesthetic state. Although hypothermia decreases anesthetic requirements, it is necessary to provide analgesia, unconsciousness, and muscle relaxation during CPB. With the initiation of bypass and hemodilution, blood levels of anesthetics and muscle relaxants will acutely decrease. However, plasma protein concentrations also decrease, which increases the free-fraction and active drug concentrations. Every drug has a specific kinetic profile during CPB, and kinetics and pharmacodynamics during CPB will vary greatly among patients. Many clinicians administer additional muscle relaxants and opioids at the initiation of CPB. A vaporizer for potent inhalation drugs may be included in the bypass circuit. Chapter 9 and Hall et al[252] offer extended discussions of pharmacokinetics and bypass. A final inspection of the head and neck for color, symmetry, adequacy of venous drainage (neck vein and conjunctiva engorgement), and pupil equality is reasonable to serve as a baseline for the anesthetic state. A summary of preparatory steps to be accomplished during the pre-bypass phase is given in Table 28–9 and Chapter 31.

INITIATION AND DISCONTINUATION OF BYPASS SUPPORT: AN OVERVIEW

Initiation of Cardiopulmonary Bypass

Uncomplicated Initiation

Once all preparatory steps have been taken, the perfusionist progressively increases delivery of oxygenated blood to the patient's arterial system, as systemic venous blood is diverted from the patient's right side of the heart, maintaining the

Table 28–10 Checklist for Bypass Procedure

1. Assess arterial inflow
   - Is arterial perfusate oxygenated?
   - Is direction of arterial inflow appropriate?
   - Evidence of arterial dissection?
     - Patient's arterial pressure persistently low?
     - Inflow line pressure high?
     - Pump/oxygenator reservoir level falling?
     - Evidence of atrial cannula malposition?
     - Patient's arterial pressure persistently high or low?
     - Unilateral facial swelling, discoloration?
2. Assess venous outflow
   - Is blood draining to the pump/oxygenator's venous reservoir?
     - Evidence of SVC obstruction?
     - Facial venous engorgement or congestion, CVP elevated?
3. Is bypass complete?
   - High CVP/low PA pressure?
   - Impaired venous drainage?
   - Low CVP/high PA pressure?
   - Large bronchial venous blood flow?
   - Aortic insufficiency?
   - Arterial and PA pressure nonpulsatile?
   - Desired pump flow established?
4. Discontinue drug and fluid administration
5. Discontinue ventilation and inhalation drugs to patient's lungs

CVP = central venous pressure; PA = pulmonary artery; SVC = superior vena cava.

Table 28–11 Preparation for Separation-from-Bypass Checklist

1. Air clearance maneuvers completed
2. Rewarming completed
   a. Nasopharyngeal temperature 36–37°C
   b. Rectal/bladder temperature ≥35°C, but ≤37°C
3. Address issue of adequacy of anesthesia and muscle relaxation
4. Obtain stable cardiac rate and rhythm (use pacing if necessary)
5. Pump flow and systemic arterial pressure
   a. Pump flow to maintain mixed venous saturation ≥70%
   b. Systemic pressure restored to normothermic levels
6. Metabolic parameters
   a. Arterial pH, P_{O_2}, P_{CO_2} within normal limits
   b. Hct: 20–25%
   c. K^+: 4.0–5.0 mEq/L
   d. *Possibly* ionized calcium
7. Are all monitoring/access catheters functional?
   a. Transducers re-zeroed
   b. TEE (if used) out of freeze mode
8. Respiratory management
   a. Atelectasis cleared/lungs reexpanded
   b. Evidence of pneumothorax?
   c. Residual fluid in thoracic cavities drained
   d. Ventilation reinstituted
9. Intravenous fluids restarted
10. Inotropes/vasopressors/vasodilators prepared

Hct = hematocrit; TEE = transesophageal echocardiography.

pump's venous reservoir volume. After full flow is achieved, all systemic venous blood is (ideally) draining from the patient to the pump reservoir. The central venous pressure (CVP) and pulmonary arterial pressure (PAP) should decrease to near zero (2 to 5 mm Hg), whereas systemic flow, arterial pressure, and oxygenation are maintained at desired values. Table 28–10 outlines tasks to be completed within 5 minutes of initiating CPB.

Hypotension with Onset of Bypass

Systemic arterial hypotension (MAP = 30 to 40 mm Hg) is relatively common on initiation of CPB. Gordon et al[253] proposed that much of this could be explained by the acute reduction of blood viscosity that results from hemodilution with nonblood priming solutions. These investigators proposed systemic vascular resistance (SVR = MAP − CVP/CO) to be the product of blood viscosity (η) and inherent systemic vascular hindrance: SVR = $\eta \cdot$ SVH. MAP increases with initiation of hypothermia-induced vasoconstriction, along with levels of endogenous catecholamines and angiotensin. Treatment with α-agonists is *usually* not necessary. Of concern is the potential for myocardial and cerebral ischemia because hypothermia has not yet been achieved.

Until the aortic cross-clamp is applied, the coronary arteries are perfused with hemodiluted, nonpulsatile blood. Schaff et al[254] showed that subendocardial ischemia occurred in the distribution of critical coronary stenosis when MAP was less than 80 mm Hg in the normothermic empty beating heart. If placement of the aortic cross-clamp is delayed, MAP should be maintained in the range of 60 to 80 mm Hg to support myocardial perfusion, especially in the presence of known coronary stenosis or ventricular hypertrophy. This arterial pressure is likely adequate to maintain cerebral blood flow until hypothermia is induced.

Unless pulsatile perfusion is used, once at full flow, the arterial pressure waveform should be nonpulsatile except for small (5 to 10 mm Hg) deflections created by the roller pump heads. Continued pulsatile arterial pressure indicates that the left ventricle is receiving blood from some source. Chapter 30 provides a discussion of organ protection during CPB.

Preparation for Separation

Before discontinuation of CPB, conditions that optimize cardiac and pulmonary function must be restored. To a great extent this is achieved by reversing the processes and techniques used to initiate and maintain CPB (Table 28–11) (see Chapter 31).

Potential for Patient Awareness

It is not uncommon for patients to sweat during rewarming. This is almost certainly caused by perfusion of the hypothalamus (i.e., the thermoregulatory site) with blood that is warmer than the latter organ's set-point (37°C). The brain is a high-flow organ and can be assumed to equilibrate fairly quickly (15 to 20 minutes) with cerebral perfusate temperature (i.e., nasopharyngeal temperature). A less likely but more disturbing possibility is that restoration of brain normothermia with decreased anesthetic concentration may result in inadequate depth of anesthesia and the potential for awareness. It is estimated that awareness occurs during cardiac surgery in 1% of patients.[255]

The following suggestions are made to attempt to limit the possibility and sequelae of awareness during cardiac surgery with CPB. During the preoperative evaluation, the possibility of awareness and why it could occur should be discussed with the patient. Use of volatile agents for their amnestic properties should be considered. During the postoperative visit, a mechanism whereby the patient can freely communicate perioperative experiences should be provided. Necessary support, including counseling, to minimize potential long-term psychologic problems should awareness be reported should be provided.

Patient movement before discontinuation of CPB is, at the least, extremely disruptive and may be genuinely life-threatening if it results in cannula dislodgment or disruption of the procedure. Additional muscle relaxant should be administered. If awareness is suspected, supplemental amnestics or anesthetics should be administered during rewarming. Because sweating stops almost immediately on discontinuation of bypass, continued sweating after emergence from CPB may be a sign of awareness. Neurologic monitors such as the Bispectral Index are being used by some clinicians to help judge the depth of anesthesia during and after weaning from CPB[256] (see Chapter 17).

Rewarming

When systemic hypothermia is used, body temperature is restored to normothermia by gradually increasing perfusate temperature with the heat exchanger. Time required for rewarming (i.e., heat transfer) varies with arterial perfusate temperature, patient temperature, and systemic flow. Excessive perfusate heating is not advisable for at least three key reasons: possible denaturation of plasma proteins, possible cerebral hyperthermia, and the fact that dissolved gas can condense into bubbles if the temperature gradient is too great. Because small increases (0.5°C) in cerebral temperature exacerbate ischemic injury in the brain, it is critical to perfuse the patient with blood temperatures at or below 37°C. Although this will increase the duration of rewarming, the risk of hyperthermic brain injury is greatly increased with hyperthermic blood temperatures. Many centers employ mild hypothermia (i.e., systemic temperature = 31° to 34°C) instead of moderate hypothermia (26° to 28°C), reducing the amount of heat transfer to achieve normothermia.

Rewarming may be enhanced by increasing pump flow, which thereby increases heat input. At levels of hypothermia routinely used (25° to 30°C), the patient behaves as if vasoconstricted (calculated SVR is relatively high). Increasing pump flow in this setting may result in unacceptable hypertension. There are two approaches to this problem: wait out the vasoconstriction or pharmacologically induce patient vasodilation. When rectal or bladder temperature approaches 30° to 32°C, patients appear to rapidly vasodilate. This is probably the result of decreasing blood viscosity or relaxation of cold-induced vasoconstriction with warming. Increasing pump flow at this point serves several purposes: increased heat transfer, support of systemic arterial pressure, and increased oxygen delivery in the face of increasing oxygen consumption. Often, waiting for the patient to spontaneously "vasodilate" is sufficient, and with subsequent increased pump flows, rewarming will be adequate at separation from bypass support. Circumstances in which more aggressive rewarming may be needed include profound hypothermia with a large hypoperfused "heat sink" and late initiation of warming by accident or design.

Skeletal muscle and subcutaneous fat are relatively hypoperfused during CPB. These tissues cool slowly and are also slow to warm. Temperatures at high-flow regions (e.g., esophagus, nasopharynx) do not reflect the temperature of these tissues. Davis et al[257] reported that restoration of normothermia (as monitored at high-flow sites) led to a net heat deficit after CPB, with subsequent recooling after emergence (i.e., after-drop). Pharmacologic vasodilation allows an earlier increase in pump flow and delivery of warmed arterial blood to low-flow beds, making the rewarming process more uniform. Noback and Tinker[258] used sodium nitroprusside (3.5 ± 0.8 μg/kg/min) to permit increased pump flows during warming, from 4.0 to 4.5 L/min, keeping MAP at approximately 70 mm Hg. Compared with a group who were warmed without sodium nitroprusside for an equivalent period of time, the sodium nitroprusside group had much greater peripheral warming and a much smaller decline in postbypass temperature. Arteriolar vasodilators (e.g., sodium nitroprusside, hydralazine) are much more likely to be effective in this process than venodilators (e.g., nitroglycerin). Other aids to warming during or after CPB are heating blankets, warmed fluids,[259] heated humidified gases,[260] and increased room temperature. Sterile forced-air rewarming devices and servoregulated systems are also available.[261]

Unfortunately, there is a very narrow range for acceptable systemic temperatures at the end of CPB. Just as temperatures that are "too hot" increase the risk of cerebral injury, those that are "too cool" may lead to inadequate rewarming and the problem of shivering, increased oxygen consumption and carbon dioxide production, and coagulopathies. It is imperative to prevent cerebral hyperthermia in patients undergoing CPB. Additional heat may be added to the patient *after* discontinuation of bypass support with the use of external heating devices. This approach can prevent the complications of hypothermia without the use of hyperthermic blood.

Targets for rectal or bladder temperature before separation from CPB vary among institutions; some centers simply assess whether the shoulders "feel warm" as an index of muscle (deltoid) temperature. Nathan and Polis[262] surveyed 28 Canadian centers regarding temperature monitoring practices during cardiac surgery and found the use of a variety of monitoring sites (Fig. 28–10). Many centers failed to use monitors likely to reflect cerebral temperatures routinely—not one center studied routinely monitored tympanic membrane temperature, and only slightly more than one half monitored nasopharyngeal temperature. The investigators were unable to discern any uniformity of practice regarding monitors or rewarming temperature end-points. In general, temperatures measured at highly perfused tissues exceeded 37°C in most centers at the end of bypass.

Cook et al[263] reported that cerebral hyperthermia occurs with rewarming. They studied 10 cardiac surgery patients requiring hypothermic CPB and measured nasopharyngeal and cerebral venous temperature (monitored at the jugular bulb). Ten minutes after the onset of rewarming from 27°C, cerebral venous temperature was 37°C, but nasopharyngeal temperature was only 34 ± 2.9°C. After 18 minutes of rewarming, nasopharyngeal temperature reached 37°C and cerebral venous temperature was 38.2 ± 1.1°C. Peak central venous temperature exceeded 39°C for an average of 15 minutes in all 10 patients before the termination of CPB.

Nathan and Polis[262] found a substantial difference between tympanic membrane and urinary bladder temperature in 11 patients rewarmed after hypothermic CPB (Fig. 28–11). The peak temperature for each patient was aligned at minute 0; temperatures were displayed for 30 minutes before (−30 to 0 minutes) and after (0 to 30 min) the peak temperature. There was a smooth increase in bladder temperature from 31.4° to

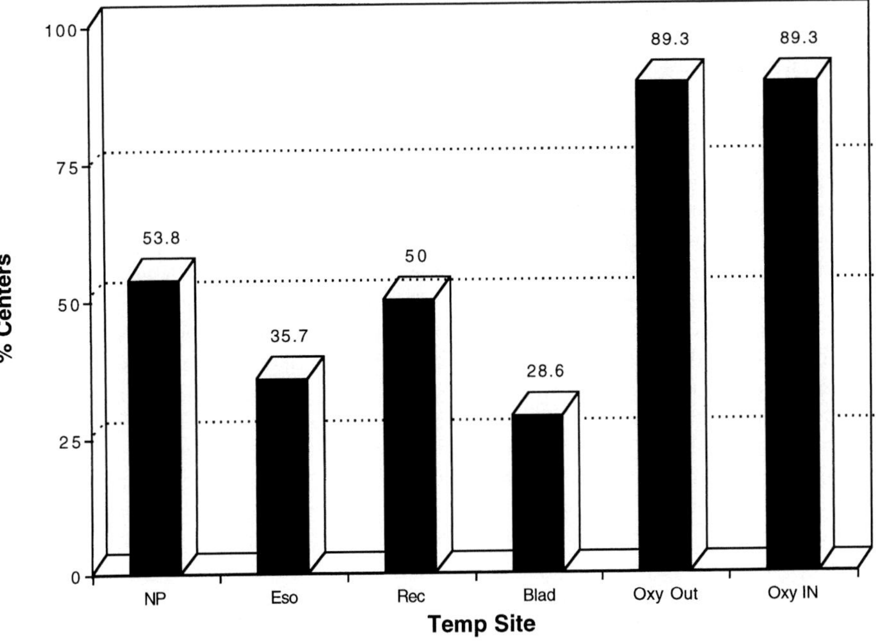

Figure 28–10 Temperature monitoring sites in 30 adult cardiac surgery centers in Canada. Blad = bladder; Eso = esophageal; NP = nasopharyngeal; Oxy Out = oxygenator outlet; Oxy In = oxygenator inlet; Rec = rectal. (From Nathan HJ, Polis T: The management of temperature during hypothermic cardiopulmonary bypass. I. Canadian Survey. Can J Anaesth 42:672, 1995.)

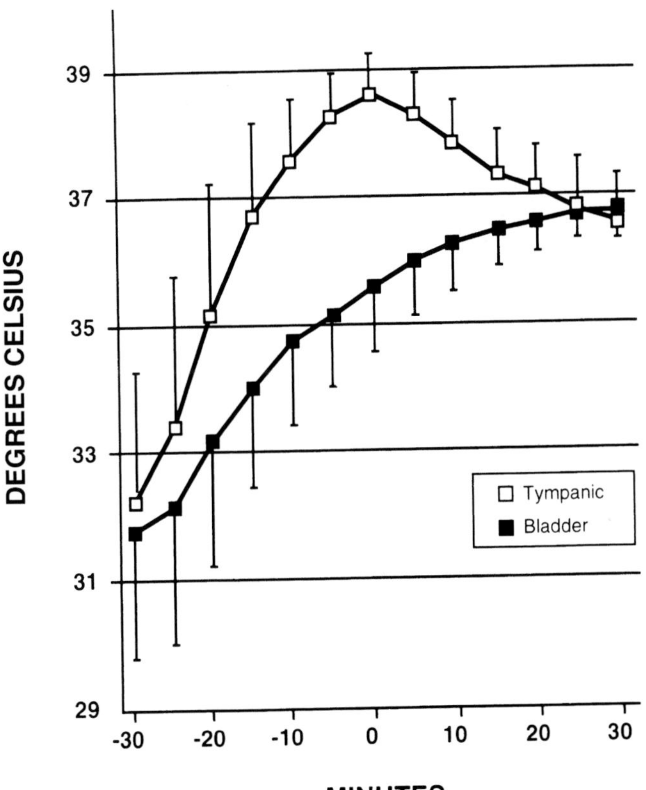

Figure 28–11 Tympanic and bladder temperatures during rewarming. Time 0 = maximum temperature achieved. Mean ± SD are shown. (From Nathan JH, Polis T: The management of temperature during hypothermic cardiopulmonary bypass. I. Canadian Survey. Can J Anaesth 42:672, 1995.)

36°C, but an "overshoot" in peak tympanic membrane temperature to a mean of 38.6°C (range 37.7° to 39.7°C). Because tympanic membrane temperature better reflects cerebral temperature than bladder temperature, it is likely that all 11 patients were exposed to hyperthermic cerebral temperatures.

Restoration of Systemic Arterial Pressure to Normothermic Value

After aortic cross-clamp release, the heart is again perfused through the native coronary arteries. Until the proximal anastomoses are made, myocardial perfusion may be compromised in the presence of a low MAP. Consequently, it is advisable to gradually increase MAP during rewarming to levels approximately 70 to 80 mm Hg.

With discontinuation of CPB, a marked discrepancy often exists between blood pressure readings measured from the radial artery and the central aorta. Radial arterial catheters may underestimate central aortic systolic pressures by 10 to 40 mm Hg. Discrepancies in MAP tend to be of a lesser magnitude (5 to 15 mm Hg). Such a discrepancy is not present before CPB, nor is it present after CPB in all patients. Mechanisms are undefined, but evidence supports vasodilatory and arteriovenous shunting phenomena in the forearm and hand.[264] Gravlee et al[265] found that systolic pressure differences after CPB were not significantly influenced by duration of CPB, use of sodium nitroprusside or phenylephrine during the final 15 minutes of CPB, SVR, minimum CPB temperature, CPB separation temperature, or duration of rewarming. Blood pressure readings from brachial or femoral arterial catheters tend to more accurately reflect central aortic pressure. It is unknown at what point during CPB radial artery-central aortic blood pressure discrepancies develop, but most investigators report their resolution 20 to 90 minutes after discontinuation of CPB (see Chapter 14).

If measured radial arterial pressure is suspected to be low in relation to central aortic pressure, several actions can be taken. Have the surgeon estimate central aortic pressure by palpation of the ascending aorta, ask the surgeon to place a small needle in the aortic lumen or use an aortic cannula to allow temporary monitoring of aortic pressure, or place a femoral arterial catheter.

Removal of Intracardiac Air

At the end of the procedure, intracardiac air is present in virtually all cases that require opening the heart (i.e., valve repair or replacement, aneurysmectomy, septal defect repair, repair of congenital lesions).[266] In such cases, it is important to remove as much air as possible before resumption of ejection. Surgical techniques differ. With the aortic cross-clamp still applied, the surgeon or perfusionist can partially limit venous return and LV vent flow, causing the left atrium and left ventricle to fill with blood. Through a transventricular approach, the left ventricle then can be aspirated. The left atrium and left ventricle are ballotted to dislodge bubbles, and the cycle is repeated. The operating table can be rotated from side to side and the lungs ventilated to promote clearance of air from the pulmonary veins. Rather than transventricular aspiration, some surgeons vent air through the cardioplegia cannula or a needle vent in the ascending aorta. Before removal of the aortic cross-clamp, the patient is placed head down, so that bubbles will float away from the dependent carotid arteries. Some surgeons favor temporary manual carotid occlusion before cross-clamp removal, but safety and efficacy of this potentially dangerous maneuver are undocumented. A venting cannula is often left in the aorta at a location that should allow air pickup after resumption of ejection. The aortic cross-clamp can be temporarily reapplied for additional air-clearing maneuvers.

Oka et al,[266] using TEE, have shown that routine air clearance techniques are not completely effective. Transcranial Doppler studies document a high incidence of intracranial gas emboli on release of the aortic cross-clamp or resumption of ejection. Oka et al[266] described three essential elements of air removal: mobilization of air by positive chamber filling, stretching of the atrial wall and repeated chamber ballottement; removal of mobilized air by continuous ascending aortic venting; and proof of elimination by TEE. The investigators contended that using these techniques could completely eliminate intracardiac air. Carbon dioxide gas insufflated by gravity into open cardiac chambers during CPB helps replace nitrogen in the bubbles with a more soluble gas. Accordingly, the persistence of gas bubbles observed by TEE after release of the aortic cross-clamp was lower in patients exposed to CO_2 in the chest wound than in the controls. However, CO_2 insufflation should be used in addition to, rather than instead of, other de-airing maneuvers.[267]

Intracardiac air may be present in 10% to 30% of closed cardiac cases as well (e.g., CABG).[266] Robicsek and Duncan[268] demonstrated that during aortic cross-clamping, air may enter the aorta and left ventricle retrograde through native coronary arteries opened in the course of CABG surgery, particularly when suction is applied to vent the left side of the heart or aortic root. They suggest that efforts to expel air from the left ventricle and aortic root should be routine before unclamping the aorta. It is unclear to what extent gas emboli originating from the heart and aorta contribute to neurologic injury. Oka et al[266] found most patients in whom LV microbubbles were detected to be free of major neurologic injury. This result is in agreement with the findings of several investigators who detected left ventricular and cerebral microbubbles for various periods after CPB without apparent neurologic sequelae. However, microembolic load correlates with magnitude of cognitive dysfunction[269] (see Chapter 35). Other studies report that air ejected from the left ventricle can also travel to the coronary arteries, resulting in sudden and sometimes extreme myocardial ischemia and failure after separation from bypass.

Defibrillation

Before discontinuation of CPB, the heart must have an organized rhythm that is spontaneous or pacer induced. Ventricular fibrillation (VF), common after cross-clamp release and warming, will often spontaneously convert to some other rhythm. Prolonged VF is undesirable during rewarming for at least three reasons: Subendocardial perfusion is compromised in the presence of normothermic VF; myocardial oxygen consumption is greater with VF compared with a beating heart at normothermia; and if the left ventricle receives a large amount of blood (aortic insufficiency or bronchial return) in the absence of mechanical contraction, the left ventricle may distend. LV distention increases wall tension and further compromises subendocardial perfusion. On the other hand, early resumption of mechanical contraction may make some surgical procedures difficult (e.g., modification of distal anastomoses).

Defibrillation, when necessary, is accomplished with internal paddles at much lower energies than would be used for external cardioversion. In the adult, starting energies of 5 to 10 J are routine. Defibrillation is less effective when the heart has not fully rewarmed, and it is rarely successful if myocardial (perfusate) temperature is less than 30°C.[270] Repeated attempts at defibrillation, particularly with escalating energy levels, can lead to myocardial injury. If defibrillation is not successful after two to four attempts, options include further warming, correction of blood gas and electrolyte abnormalities if present (high P_{O_2} and high normal serum potassium [K^+] seem favorable), increased MAP, and antiarrhythmic therapy. Bolus administration of 100 mg of lidocaine before the release of the cross-clamp significantly lowers the incidence of reperfusion ventricular fibrillation.[271] Increasing coronary perfusion by increased MAP is believed to result in myocardial reperfusion and recovery of the energy state. Larger loading doses of antiarrhythmics will be needed to achieve therapeutic concentrations, because of the larger CPB volume of distribution.

Restoration of Ventilation

With discontinuation of CPB, the venous outflow line is gradually occluded and pulmonary arterial blood flow restored. Studies disagree as to the nature and magnitude of pulmonary dysfunction after CPB, and various aspects of this problem were discussed earlier. Some studies have found evidence of increased dead space/tidal volume ratio (V_D/V_T) after CPB, whereas others have not.[272] Increased V_D/V_T would result in less effective alveolar ventilation than pre-bypass, which would result in elevated Pa_{CO_2}. Other studies report modest increases in pulmonary shunt fraction after CPB, which leads to less effective oxygenation and decreased Pa_{O_2}. Catastrophic bypass-induced pulmonary injury with severe hypoxemia immediately on discontinuation of CPB is exceedingly uncommon in adults.

Before discontinuation of CPB, the lungs must be reinflated. Positive pressure (20 to 40 cm H_2O) is repeatedly applied until all areas of atelectasis are visually reinflated. Attention is specifically directed at the left lower lobe, which seems more difficult to reexpand. Fluid that has collected in the thoracic cavities during CPB is removed by the surgeon, and if the pleural cavity has not been opened, evidence of pneumothorax is also sought. The tidal volume or ventilatory rate is increased 10% to 20% above pre-bypass values to compensate for increased V_D/V_T if present. Ventilation is resumed with 100% oxygen and subsequent adjustments in F_{IO_2} are made based on arterial blood gas analysis and pulse oximetry. Many investigators have expressed the theoretical concern that nitrous oxide, by enlarging gas emboli, might be deleterious if administered after bypass. Although evidence that nitrous oxide is harmful in this setting is scant, most anesthesiologists avoid nitrous oxide entirely after bypass.

Correction of Metabolic Abnormalities and Arterial Oxygen Saturation

When rewarming is nearly complete and separation from CPB is anticipated to occur in 10 to 20 minutes, an arterial blood sample is taken and analyzed for acid-base status, PO_2, PCO_2, hemoglobin or hematocrit, potassium, and in some centers, ionized calcium.

Before discontinuation of CPB, many surgeons slightly impede venous outflow to the pump or oxygenator, giving the heart some blood to eject. If the lungs are not yet being ventilated, deoxygenated venous blood may traverse the pulmonary vascular bed and enter the systemic circulation, mixing with the well-oxygenated perfusate of the pump. If this blood flow is large, arterial desaturation could result. Most of the time this is not a problem, but with resumption of ejection, pulse oximetry should be reestablished to permit monitoring of arterial saturation.

OXYGEN-CARRYING CAPACITY

Generally, a hematocrit of at least 20% to 25% is sought before discontinuation of bypass. The primary compensatory mechanism to assure adequate systemic oxygen delivery in the presence of normovolemic anemia is increased CO. Increased CO results in an increased myocardial oxygen need, which is met by increased coronary oxygen delivery by coronary vasodilation. The lower limit of the hematocrit, below which increased CO can no longer support systemic oxygen needs, is reported to be 17% to 20% in dogs with *completely healthy hearts.*[273] With increases in systemic VO_2, such as occur with exercise, fever, or shivering, higher values of the hematocrit are required. Patients with good ventricular function and good coronary reserve (or good revascularization) might be expected to tolerate hematocrit values in the 20s. When ventricular function is impaired or revascularization is incomplete, hematocrit above 25% may aid in support of the systemic circulation and concomitantly lower myocardial oxygen requirements on discontinuation of bypass.

When pump or oxygenator reservoir volume is in excess, the hematocrit can be increased by use of hemofiltration. As described by Kleinberg et al,[274] application of a hydrostatic pressure gradient across a porous membrane results in transport of water and low-molecular-weight solutes (MW of 20,000 to 60,000). Ultrafiltrate composition is similar to glomerular filtrate with solute concentrations identical to that of plasma water.

ARTERIAL PH

Considerable debate has centered on the extent to which acidemia affects myocardial performance and whether correction of arterial pH with sodium bicarbonate is advantageous or deleterious to the heart.[275] Studies have challenged long-held beliefs that acidemia impairs myocardial performance. Nevertheless, most in vivo and clinical studies have found metabolic acidosis impairs contractility and alters responses to exogenous catecholamines.[276] Hemodynamic deterioration is usually mild above pH 7.2 because of compensatory increases in sympathetic nervous system activity.[276] Attenuation of sympathetic nervous system responses by β-blockade or ganglionic blockade increases the detrimental effect of acidosis. The ischemic or hypoxic myocardium has been found to be particularly vulnerable to detrimental effects of acidosis. Patients with poor contractile function or reduction of myocardial sympathetic responsiveness (e.g., chronic left ventricular failure), those treated with β-blockers, or those with myocardial ischemia are especially susceptible to the adverse effects of acidosis. For these reasons arterial pH is corrected to near-normal levels before discontinuation of CPB, using sodium bicarbonate. Concerns regarding carbon dioxide generation and acidification of the intracellular space can be obviated by slow administration and appropriate adjustment of ventilation, both of which are easily achieved during CPB.

ELECTROLYTES

Electrolytes most commonly of concern before discontinuation of CPB are potassium and calcium. Serum potassium concentration may be acutely low because of hemodilution with nonpotassium priming solutions or large-volume diuresis during CPB. More commonly, potassium concentration is elevated as a result of systemic uptake of potassium-containing cardioplegic solution; values exceeding 6 mEq/L are not uncommon. Other potential causes of hyperkalemia that must be considered are hemolysis, tissue ischemia or necrosis, and acidemia. Hypokalemia can be rapidly corrected during CPB with *relative* safety because the heart and systemic circulation are supported. Increments of 5 to 10 mEq of KCl over 1- to 2-minute intervals can be given directly into the pump or oxygenator by the perfusionist, and potassium subsequently is rechecked. Depending on severity and urgency of correction, elevated potassium can be treated or reduced by any of several standard means: alkali therapy, diuresis, calcium administration, or insulin and glucose. Alternatively, hemofiltration can be used to lower serum potassium. While still on CPB, potassium-containing extracellular fluid is removed from the patient and replaced with fluid not containing potassium.

Ionized calcium is involved in the maintenance of normal excitation-contraction coupling and therefore in maintaining cardiac contractility and peripheral vascular tone. Low concentrations of ionized calcium lead to impaired cardiac contractility and lowered vascular tone. Concerns have been raised about the contribution of calcium administration to myocardial reperfusion injury and to the action of various inotropes.[277] Some investigators argue in favor of measuring ionized calcium before discontinuation of CPB and to administer calcium in patients with low concentrations to optimize cardiac performance.[278] Although they routinely measure ionized calcium before discontinuation of bypass, calcium salts are not routinely administered. When confronted with poor myocardial or peripheral vascular responsiveness to inotropes or vasopressors after bypass *in the presence of a low level of ionized calcium,* calcium salts should be administered to restore ionized calcium to normal (not elevated) levels in the hope of restoring responsiveness. The same strategy can be used for measuring and administering magnesium.

Other Final Preparations

Before separating from CPB, all monitoring and access catheters should be checked and calibrated. The zero-pressure calibration points of the pressure transducers are routinely checked. Not uncommonly, finger pulse oximeter probes do not have a good signal after CPB. In those cases, a nasal or ear probe is placed to obtain reliable oximetry. Intravenous infusions are restarted before separation from CPB, and their flow characteristics are assessed for evidence of obstruction or disconnection.

During warming and preparation for separation, an assessment should be made of the functional status of the heart and peripheral vasculature based on visual inspection, hemodynamic indices, and metabolic parameters. Based on this assessment, inotropes, vasodilators, and vasopressors thought likely to be necessary for successful separation from bypass should be prepared and readied for administration.

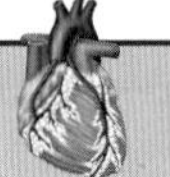

BOX 28–4 ***Perfusion Emergencies***

- Arterial cannula malposition
- Aortic dissection
- Massive air embolism
- Venous air lock
- Reversed cannulation

Separation from Bypass

After all preparatory steps are taken (see Table 28–11), CPB can be discontinued. Venous outflow to the pump or oxygenator is impeded by slowly clamping the venous line, and the patient's intravascular volume and ventricular loading conditions are restored by transfusion of perfusate through the aortic inflow line. When loading conditions are optimal, the aortic inflow line is clamped, and the patient is separated from CPB.

At this juncture it must be determined whether oxygenation, ventilation, and more commonly myocardial performance (systemic perfusion) are adequate. A discussion of these issues no longer involves CPB per se, but rather applied cardiopulmonary physiology. Consequently, a discussion of this extremely important topic is detailed in Chapters 31 and 33. Should separation fail for any reason, CPB can simply be reinstituted by unclamping the venous outflow and arterial inflow lines and restoring pump flow. This allows for support of systemic oxygenation and perfusion while steps are taken to diagnose and treat those problems that precluded successful separation.

PERFUSION EMERGENCIES

Accidents or mishaps occurring during CPB can quickly evolve into life-threatening emergencies (Box 28–4). Many of the necessary conditions of bypass (cardiac arrest, hypothermia, volume depletion) preclude the ability to resume normal cardiorespiratory function if an accident threatens the integrity of the extracorporeal circuit. Fortunately, major perfusion accidents occur infrequently and are rarely associated with permanent injury or death (Table 28–12). However, all members of the cardiac surgery team must be able to respond to perfusion emergencies to limit the likelihood of perfusion-related disasters. Some of the most common emergencies are discussed in the subsequent sections.

Arterial Cannula Malposition

Ascending aortic cannulas can be malpositioned such that the outflow jet is directed primarily into the innominate artery,[279-281] the left common carotid artery (rare),[282,283] or the left subclavian artery (rare).[284] In the first two circumstances, unilateral cerebral *hyperperfusion*, usually with systemic hypoperfusion, occurs, whereas flow directed to the subclavian artery results in global cerebral *hypoperfusion*. Despite the fact that not all combinations of arterial pressure monitoring site and cannula malposition produce systemic hypotension, it is commonly regarded as a cardinal sign of cannula malposition. For example, right arm blood pressure monitor and innominate artery cannulation,[279] or left arm monitor and left subclavian artery cannulation[284] may result in *high* arterial pressure on initiation of bypass. With other positioning and monitoring combinations, investigators report persistently low systemic arterial pressure (MAP = 25 to 35 mm Hg), which is poorly responsive to increasing pump flow or vasoconstrictors. Over time (minutes), signs of systemic hypoperfusion (e.g., acidemia, oliguria) develop.[282] Because a variable period

Table 28–12 Comparison of the Five Most Common Accidents from the Three Perfusion Surveys

	Stoney 1972–1977		Wheeldon 1974–1979		Kurusz 1982–1985	
Complication*	***Incidents***	***PI/D***	***Incidents***	***PI/D***	***Incidents***	***PI/D***
Air embolism	(2) 1.14	0.41	(2) 0.79	0.18	(6) 0.80	0.12
Coagulopathy	(1) 1.26	0.51	(6) 0.26	0.09	(8) 0.21	0.05
Electrical failure	(3) 0.67	0.01	(1) 1.00	0.06	(4) 0.84	0.003
Mechanical failure	(4) 0.38	0.02	(5) 0.27	0	(7) 0.30	0.007
Inadequate oxygenation	(5) 0.33	0.02	(3) 0.59	0	(3) 0.88	0.07
Hypoperfusion	—	—	(4) 0.30	0.18	(2) 0.96	0.15
Protamine reaction	—	—	—	—	(1) 2.80	0.22
Drug error	—	—	—	—	(5) 0.82	0.08

*The five most common complications for each study are listed as incidence per 1000 perfusions and the number of permanent injuries and mortalities as incidence per 1000 perfusions. The numbers in parentheses are the rank of each complication from most to least.

PI/D = permanent injury or death.

Data from Stoney WS, Alford WC Jr, Burrus GR, et al: Air embolism and other accidents using pump oxygenators. Ann Thorac Surg 29:336, 1980; Wheeldon DR: Can cardiopulmonary bypass be a safe procedure? *In* Longmore DB (ed): Towards Safer Cardiac Surgery. Lancaster, London, MTP, 1981, pp 427–446; Kurusz M, Conti VR, Arens JF, et al: Perfusion accident survey. Proc Am Acad Cardiovasc Perf 7:57, 1986.

of systemic hypotension with CPB initiation is nearly always seen with hemodilution, hypotension alone is not significant evidence to establish a diagnosis of arterial cannula malposition. Ross et al[282] described a case of accidental left common carotid cannulation with unilateral facial and conjunctival edema accompanied by rhinorrhea, otorrhea, and signs of systemic hypoperfusion. In a similar case, Sudhaman[283] found left facial congestion, whereas the right side was pale. Watson[279] described a case of innominate artery cannulation. On initiation of CPB, the skin over the carotid vessels on the right was colder than on the left. Three cases of innominate cannulation produced dramatic unilateral facial blanching with onset of CPB due to perfusion with nonblood-containing priming solution.[280,281] On initiation of CPB and periodically thereafter, it is advisable to inspect the face for color change and edema, rhinorrhea, or otorrhea and to palpate the neck with onset of cooling for temperature asymmetry. EEG monitoring has been advocated as a method of detecting cannula malposition. In one study, cannula malposition, detected by EEG asymmetry, occurred in 3 (3.5%) of 84 patients[285] (see Chapter 17).

Two other arterial cannula malpositions are possible: abutment of the cannula tip against the aortic intima, which results in high line pressure, poor perfusion, or even acute dissection when bypass is initiated, and the cannula tip directed caudally toward the aortic valve. This may result in acute aortic insufficiency, with sudden left ventricular distention and systemic hypoperfusion on bypass. If the aortic inflow cannula is soft, aortic cross-clamping will occlude the arterial perfusion line, which can rupture the aortic inflow line. Suspicion of any cannula malposition must immediately be brought to the attention of the surgeon.

Aortic or Arterial Dissection

Signs of arterial dissection, often similar to those of cannula malposition, must also be sought continuously, especially on initiation of CPB. Dissection may originate at the cannulation site, aortic cross-clamp site, proximal vein graft anastomotic site, or partial occlusion (side-biting) clamp site. Dissections are due to intimal disruption, or more distally to fracture of atherosclerotic plaque. In either case, some systemic arterial blood flow becomes extraluminal, being forced into the arterial wall. The dissection propagates mostly in the direction of the systemic flow, but not exclusively. Extraluminal blood compresses the luminal origins (take-offs) of major arterial branches such that vital organs (heart, brain, kidney, intestinal tract, spinal cord) may become ischemic. Because systemic perfusion may be low, and origins of the innominate and subclavian arteries may be compressed, probably the best sign of arterial dissection is persistently low systemic arterial pressure.[286] Venous drainage to the pump decreases (blood is sequestered), and arterial inflow "line pressure" is usually inappropriately high. The surgeon may see the dissection if it involves the anterior or lateral ascending aorta (bluish discoloration), or both.[286,287] It is possible the surgeon may *not* see any sign of dissection, because the dissection is out of view (e.g., posterior ascending aorta, aortic arch, descending aorta). Dissection can occur at any time before, during, or after CPB. As with cannula malposition, a suspicion of arterial dissection must be brought to the attention of the surgeon. The anesthesiologist must not assume that something is suddenly wrong with the arterial pressure transducer but should "think dissection."

After a dissection of the ascending aorta is diagnosed, immediate steps to minimize propagation must be taken. If it has occurred before CPB, the anesthesiologist should take steps to reduce MAP and the rate of rise of aortic pressure (dP/dt) (see Chapter 23). If it occurs during CPB, pump flow and MAP are reduced to the lowest acceptable levels. Arterial perfusate is frequently cooled to profound levels (14° to 19°C) as rapidly as possible to decrease metabolic demand and protect vital organs.[287] A different arterial cannulation site is prepared (e.g., the femoral artery is cannulated or the true aortic lumen is cannulated at a site more distal on the aortic arch). Arterial inflow is shifted to that new site in hopes that perfusing the true aortic lumen will reperfuse vital organs.[287] The ascending aorta is cross-clamped just below the innominate artery, and cardioplegia is administered (into the coronary ostia or coronary sinus). The aorta is opened to expose the site of disruption, which is then resected and replaced. Reimplantation of the coronary arteries or aortic valve replacement, or both, may be necessary. The false lumina at both ends of the aorta are obliterated with Teflon buttresses, and the graft is inserted by end-to-end suture.[243] With small dissections it is sometimes possible to avoid open repair by application of a partial occlusion clamp with plication of the dissection and exclusion of the intimal disruption.[287] Troianos et al[288] described three cases of arterial dissection during CPB in which TEE was found useful. Although provisional diagnoses were made on the basis of traditional signs, TEE allowed assessment of the origin and extent of dissection. Diagnosis of arterial dissection has also been assisted by presence of EEG asymmetry.[289]

Arterial dissections originating from femoral cannulation also necessitate reductions in arterial pressure, systemic flow, and temperature. If the operation is near completion, the heart may be transfused and CPB discontinued; otherwise, the aortic arch must be cannulated and adequate systemic perfusion restored to allow completion of the operation.[286]

Massive Arterial Gas Embolus

Macroscopic gas embolus is a rare but disastrous CPB complication. Two independent studies in 1980 reported incidences of recognized massive arterial gas embolism of 0.1% to 0.2%.[290,291] The current incidence is probably lower because of the widespread use of reservoir level alarms and bubble detection devices. Between 20% and 30% of affected patients died immediately, with another 30% having transient or nondebilitating neurologic deficits, or both. Circumstances that most commonly contributed to these events were inattention to oxygenator blood level, reversal of left ventricular vent flow, or unexpected resumption of cardiac ejection in a previously opened heart. Rupture of a pulsatile assist device[292] or intra-aortic balloon pump[293] may also introduce large volumes of gas into the arterial circulation.

The pathophysiology of cerebral gas embolism (macroscopic and microscopic) is not well understood. Tissue damage after gas embolization is initiated from simple mechanical blockage of blood vessels by bubbles.[294,295] Although gas emboli may be absorbed or pass through the circulation within 1 to 5 minutes,[294-297] the local reaction of platelets and proteins to the blood gas interface or endothelial damage is thought to potentiate microvascular stasis,[297-302] prolonging cerebral ischemia to the point of infarction. Areas of marginal perfusion, such as arterial boundary zones, do not clear gas emboli as rapidly as well-perfused zones,[294] producing patterns of ischemia or infarction difficult to distinguish from those due to hypotension or particulate emboli.

Recommended treatment for massive arterial gas embolism includes immediate cessation of CPB with aspiration of as much gas as possible from the aorta and heart, assumption of steep Trendelenburg position, and clearance of air from the arterial perfusion line. After resumption of CPB, treatment continues with implementation or deepening of hypothermia (18° to 27°C) during completion of the operation, clearance of gas from the coronary circulation before emergence from CPB, and administration of glucocorticoids in an attempt to minimize cerebral edema.[291,292,303,304] In many reports of patients suffering massive arterial gas embolus, seizures occurred postoperatively and were treated with anticonvulsants.[65,304-306] Because seizures after ischemic insults are associated with poor outcomes, due perhaps to hypermetabolic effects, prophylactic phenytoin seems reasonable. Hypotension has been shown to lengthen the residence time of cerebral air emboli and worsen the severity of resulting ischemia.[307] Maintenance of moderate hypertension therefore is reasonable and clinically attainable to hasten clearance of emboli from the circulation and, hopefully, improve neurologic outcome.

Many clinicians have reported dramatic neurologic recovery when hyperbaric therapy is used for arterial gas embolism, even if delayed up to 26 hours after the event.[292,302,303,308] Spontaneous recovery from air emboli has also been reported,[299,304,306,308] and no prospective study of hyperbaric therapy in the cardiac surgery setting has been performed.[309] Few institutions that do cardiac surgery have an appropriately equipped and staffed compression chamber to allow expeditious and safe initiation of hyperbaric therapy. Nonetheless, immediate transfer by air is often possible and should seriously be considered. It seems reasonable to expect that institutions that do cardiac surgery should have policies regarding catastrophic air embolism.

In 1980, Mills and Ochsner[291] suggested venoarterial perfusion as an alternative to hyperbaric therapy. Retrograde perfusion through the SVC cannula at 1.2L/min at 20°C for 1 to 2 minutes was used in five of their eight patients with massive gas embolism. The goal was to flush air from the cerebral arterial circulation. None of the patients so treated had evidence of neurologic injury. Other reports using this technique have followed.[310,311] Hendricks et al,[312] in a porcine model of venoarterial perfusion, found that only 50% of injected gas (nitrogen) could be recovered from the aorta. Ninety-eight percent of the removable gas was collected from the aorta in the first 7 to 10 minutes of retrograde perfusion. Although no animal (clinically or pathologically) appeared to sustain neurologic injury, the investigators concluded that venoarterial perfusion did not adequately remove embolized gas, and hyperbaric therapy remained the treatment of choice.

Venous Air Lock

Air entering the venous outflow line can result in complete cessation of flow to the venous reservoir, and this is called *air lock*. Loss of venous outflow necessitates immediate slowing, even cessation of pump flow, to prevent emptying the reservoir and subsequent delivery of air to the patient's arterial circulation. After an air lock is recognized, a search for the source of venous outflow line air must be undertaken (e.g., loose atrial purse string, atrial tear, open intravenous access), and repaired before reestablishing full bypass.

Reversed Cannulation

In this case, the venous outflow limb of the CPB circuit is incorrectly connected to the arterial inflow cannula and the arterial perfusion limb of the circuit is attached to the venous cannula. On initiation of CPB, blood is removed from the arterial circulation and returned to the venous circulation at high pressure. Arterial pressure is found to be extremely low by palpation and arterial pressure monitoring. Very low arterial pressures can also (more commonly) be due to dissection in the arterial tree. In the latter case, the perfusionist will rapidly lose volume, whereas with reversed cannulation, the perfusionist will have an immediate gross excess of volume. If high pump flow is established, venous or atrial rupture may occur. The CVP will be dramatically elevated, with evidence of facial venous engorgement.

Line pressure is the pressure in the arterial limb of the CPB circuit. Because arterial cannulas are much smaller than the aorta, there is always a pressure drop across the aortic cannula. Arterial inflow line pressure will always be considerably higher than systemic (patient) arterial pressure. The magnitude of the pressure drop depends on cannula size and systemic flow; small cannulas and higher flows result in greater gradients. The CPB pump must generate a pressure that overcomes this gradient to provide adequate systemic arterial pressure. For a typical adult (i.e., MAP of about 60 mm Hg, systemic flow of about 2.4 L/min/m^2, and a 24 Fr aortic cannula), line pressure in an uncomplicated case usually ranges from 150 to 250 mm Hg. The fittings on the arterial inflow line are plastic; the fittings and the line itself can rupture. Perfusionists typically do not want a line pressure in excess of 300 mm Hg.

CPB must be discontinued and the cannula disconnected and inspected for air. If air is found in the arterial circulation, an air embolus protocol is initiated. Once arterial air is cleared, the circuit is correctly reconnected and CPB restarted. In adults, the venous outflow limb of the CPB circuit is a larger-diameter tubing than the arterial inflow tubing, precisely to eliminate reversed cannulation. This is why reversed cannulation is rare in adults—but it has happened. In pediatric cases, the arterial inflow and venous outflow limbs of the CPB circuit are close or equal in size.

SPECIAL PATIENT POPULATIONS

Care of the Gravid Patient during Bypass

Studies assessing the effects of cardiac surgery and CPB on obstetric physiology and fetal well-being are lacking. However, several reviews and many case reports describe individual experience in caring for the gravid patient and fetus during cardiac surgery and extracorporeal circulation.[313-318] These surveys and anecdotal reports, along with an understanding of the well-documented physiology of pregnancy and the effects of cardiac therapeutics on fetal physiology, can serve as a basis for a rational approach to care for the pregnant patient and fetus during cardiac surgery (Box 28–5).

Six groups have published reports detailing their individual experiences or survey data on maternal and fetal outcomes After cardiac surgery and CPB.[313-318] Jacobs et al[314] reported their experience with three first-trimester gravid patients. All recovered from their operative procedures and delivered normal term infants. The first survey data on pregnancy and cardiac surgery were reported in 1969 by Zitnik et al[315] from the Mayo Clinic. Among the 20 patients, there was only one

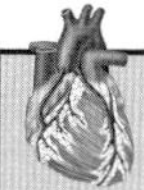

BOX 28–5 ***Special Patients Who May Need Cardiopulmonary Bypass***

- Pregnant women
- Heparin-resistant patients
- Accidental hypothermia victims
- Neurosurgical patient with an intracranial aneurysm

maternal death, but seven fetuses died before term. The study authors concluded that cardiac surgery does not increase the likelihood of death in the pregnant patient with heart disease, but is associated with substantial fetal mortality. Lapiedra et al[317] and Becker[316] individually published reports in the 1980s on gravid patients undergoing heart surgery. Lapiedra et al[317] reviewed their own experiences and found only one fetal death and no instance of maternal death in their review of 23 cases. Becker[316] surveyed members of the Society of Thoracic Surgeons on their experiences with pregnant patients requiring cardiac surgery. Of the 600 surgeons responding, 119 reported on a total of 169 gravid patients undergoing cardiac surgery, 68 of whom were managed with CPB. Pomini et al[318] reviewed 69 case reports of gravid patients undergoing cardiac procedures and CPB. Overall, the embryo-fetal mortality rate was 20.2%, but fetal loss was reduced to 12.5% in the last 40 cases. The reported experience on maternal and fetal outcomes after cardiac procedures with CPB suggests that cardiac surgery is well tolerated by the mother, but poses a significant risk to the fetus.

Although most physicians advocate providing perioperative care that can ensure maternal well-being, appropriate investigation would enable clinicians to care optimally for mother and fetus. This section outlines recommendations for perioperative management of the gravid patient requiring cardiac surgery and CPB. The basic principles for the perioperative management of the gravid patient requiring any type of surgery are outlined by Levinson and Shnider[319]: maternal safety, avoidance of teratogenic drugs, avoidance of intrauterine asphyxia, and prevention of preterm labor.

Considerations before Bypass

PREMEDICATION AND PATIENT POSITIONING

Premedication should be appropriate for the specific cardiac lesion and physical status of the patient. Teratogenic drugs should be avoided, especially in the first trimester of pregnancy. After the thirty-fourth week of gestation, stomach emptying is delayed and patients are at increased risk for pulmonary aspiration. Although it is not possible to ensure gastric emptying before anesthesia induction, sodium citrate and an H_2-receptor antagonist may provide some protection against aspiration pneumonia. The gravid uterus obstructs aortic flow and inferior vena cava blood return to the heart. Gravid patients should never be supine; they must be positioned with left uterine displacement throughout the perioperative period.

MATERNAL AND FETAL MONITOR INFORMATION

The pregnant patient undergoing cardiac surgery requires the usual monitors employed during cardiac surgery, as well as monitors that can assess fetal well-being. Monitors that help assess the adequacy of maternal cardiovascular performance and oxygen delivery to the fetus are of paramount importance. Little is known about the effects of cardiovascular drugs and other therapeutic measures on the pregnant cardiac patient undergoing CPB. Appropriate monitors permit the assessment of an individual therapy on maternal and fetal oxygen delivery.

Monitors for cardiac surgery and CPB are discussed in detail in Chapters 14 to 18. A two-lead (II, V_5) electrocardiogram (ECG), peripheral pulse oximeter, and blood pressure cuff should be placed first. These monitors provide information concerning cardiorespiratory function as other, more invasive monitors are placed. Before the induction of anesthesia, radial artery and thermodilution pulmonary artery catheters (PAC) should be placed. These monitors provide beat-to-beat systemic and pulmonary artery blood pressure information and the ability to measure CO and arterial and mixed-venous blood gases. An oximetry PAC provides continuous information on venous oxygen saturation-an indirect, approximate measure of the adequacy of maternal tissue oxygen delivery.

Uterine activity should be monitored with a tocodynamometer applied to the maternal abdomen. This monitor transduces the tightening of the abdomen during uterine contractions. As is the case with other types of major surgery, the tocodynamometer should not interfere with the conduct of cardiac surgery; if necessary, the monitor may be intermittently displaced by the operating surgeon. The use of an intra-amniotic catheter to monitor uterine activity and pressure may be inadvisable in a patient who will be fully heparinized. Intraoperative uterine contractions may have a deleterious effect on fetal oxygen delivery (by causing an increase in uterine venous pressure and decrease in uterine blood flow) and signal the onset of preterm labor. Use of the tocodynamometer is imperative, as it will provide important information about the state of the uterus and allow intervention if necessary. Various case reports have documented the common occurrence of uterine contractions during cardiac surgery and CPB. Uterine contractions may appear at any time during the perioperative period, but occur most frequently immediately after the discontinuation of CPB and in the early ICU period.[320] It is therefore important to leave the tocodynamometer in place after the completion of surgery. Although uterine contractions occur frequently in the perioperative course, they usually are effectively treated with magnesium sulfate, ritodrine, or ethanol infusions, and they do not result in preterm labor and fetal demise.[321,322]

Fetal heart rate (FHR) monitors should be employed in all gravid patients after 16 weeks' gestation, as one of the primary perioperative goals is to avoid fetal loss. Use of an FHR monitor permits recognition of fetal distress and allows the clinician to institute measures to improve fetal oxygen delivery. The FHR monitor recognizes and records the FHR, FHR variability, and uterine contractions. A spinal electrode placed in the fetal scalp gives the most reliable fetal ECG and therefore the best FHR information. However, this method may be undesirable in the presence of maternal anticoagulation. External FHR monitoring—using ultrasound, phonocardiography, or external abdominal ECG—is less exact but preferable in this clinical setting.

The cardiac surgeon and perfusionist may not be familiar with uterine and FHR monitors; the anesthesiologist is accustomed to caring for these patients during labor and delivery and can assess uterine and FHR tracings. However, in some clinical circumstances, such as preoperative fetal distress, or anticipated need for emergency cesarean section during

Table 28–13 Recommendations for the Conduct of Extracorporeal Circulation in the Gravid Patient

Variable	Recommended Value/Characteristic	Rationale
Blood flow	3.0 L/min/m²	Cardiac index normally is increased during pregnancy.
Blood pressure (MAP)	60–70 mm Hg	Uterine blood flow depends on maternal MAP.
Temperature	32–34°C	Mild hypothermia decreases fetal oxygen requirements and is less likely to cause fetal arrhythmia.
Oxygenator type	Membrane	Membrane oxygenators are associated with fewer embolic phenomena than bubblers.
Hematocrit	25–27%	The quantity of oxygen carried in maternal blood (and therefore the oxygen available to the fetus) greatly depends on hemoglobin concentration.
Duration of perfusion	Minimized (?)	The duration of bypass is dictated by the complexity of the operative procedure.
Cardioplegia	?	
Pulsatile perfusion	?	

MAP = mean arterial pressure.

cardiac surgery, having a perinatologist or an obstetrician present during cardiac surgery may be desirable.

FHR is usually normal in the pre-bypass period but decreases precipitously with the initiation of CPB and remains below normal for the entire bypass period. There are many potential causes of this observed decrease in FHR. Persistent fetal bradycardia is a classic sign of acute fetal hypoxia. However, in the CPB setting, especially when hypothermia is employed, it is difficult to ascribe fetal bradycardia to hypoxia or to decreased fetal oxygen demand. Fetal tachycardia typically occurs after the discontinuation of bypass support. This tachycardia may represent a compensatory mechanism for the oxygen debt incurred during CPB. The FHR usually returns to normal by the end of the operative period.

Interventions optimizing maternal blood oxygen content, correcting any acid-base imbalance, and replenishing fetal glycogen stores may alleviate signs of fetal hypoxia. Some clinicians recommend an increase in CPB pump flow to improve fetal oxygen delivery.[316,318]

After anesthesia induction, a urinary bladder catheter with a temperature probe and TEE probe should be placed. The former provides information on fluid balance and core temperature. Transesophageal echocardiography is especially important in the patient undergoing valvular or congenital heart surgery, because it can document pathologic change and help assess the adequacy of repair. The author reported a case of a gravid patient requiring replacement of aortic and mitral porcine prosthetic valves in 1987.[321] The patient was thought to have cardiac disease limited to her aortic valve; however, after an unsuccessful attempt to wean from CPB, mitral valve dysfunction was diagnosed and a second period of CPB was required to replace the mitral valve. Pre-bypass TEE would have identified mitral valve dysfunction before extracorporeal circulation, and obviated the need for two separate periods of CPB.

Conducting the Bypass Procedure

The conditions of extracorporeal circulation—nonpulsatile blood flow, hypothermia, anemia, and requisite anticoagulation—will likely have a negative impact on fetal well-being during CPB. There are no studies that recommend a CPB management strategy in gravid patients. Recommendations are summarized (Table 28–13) for the management of bypass in pregnant patients, based on the survey and anecdotal reports in the literature (Table 28–14).

Table 28–14 Prevalence of Maternal and Fetal Mortality Following Cardiac Surgery and Cardiopulmonary Bypass in Gravid Patients

Study	Maternal Death	Fetal Death
Jacobs/Cooley (1965)	0/3 (0%)	0/3 (0%)
Zitnik (1968)	1/20 (5%)	7/20 (35%)
Becker (1983)	1/68 (1.5%)	11/68 (16%)
Lapiedra (1986)	0/23 (0%)	1/23 (4.3%)
Pomini (1996)*	2/69 (2.9%)	8/69 (20.2%)
Pomini (1996)†	0/40 (0%)	5/40 (12.5%)
Arnoni (2003)	5/58 (8.6%)	11/58 (18.6%)

*All patients from 1958 to 1992.
†Last 40 patients in series only.

BLOOD FLOW

The optimal extracorporeal circuit blood flow in the *non-gravid* patient is controversial. Some clinicians recommend that blood flow be maintained at relatively normal values (i.e., cardiac index ≥ 2.3 L/min/m²), but others believe that lower blood flows, especially with hypothermia, are desirable, and may decrease the morbidity associated with CPB and embolization of particulate matter.

Optimal CPB blood flow in the gravid patient is unknown. However, the increase in CO associated with pregnancy is well defined, and it might be argued that high blood flows during CPB are more physiologic in the gravid patient. Becker[316] suggested that flow during CPB in the pregnant patient be maintained at a minimum of 3.0 L/min/m². A few reports demonstrate that increasing CPB circuit blood flow improves FHR, suggesting improvement in fetal oxygen delivery. In a report by Koh et al,[323] FHR improved when pump flow was increased from 3100 to 3600 mL/min. Similarly, Werch and Lambert[324] reported an improvement in FHR when blood flow was increased from 2800 to 4600 mL/min. However, another report, describing two separate cases of perfusion in which fetal monitors were used, suggested that increasing pump flow did not consistently improve FHR. In one case, flow was increased from 2.3 to 2.9 L/min/m^2, with a brief, unsustained apparent improvement in fetal oxygen delivery.[324]

BLOOD PRESSURE

Under normal conditions, uterine blood flow is determined solely by maternal blood pressure, as the placental vasculature is maximally dilated. However, it is not known what factors determine uterine blood flow during the very abnormal condition of CPB. For example, catecholamine levels increase by several times during CPB; therefore, uterine vascular resistance may increase during extracorporeal circulation in response to increased levels of norepinephrine and epinephrine. However, regardless of the state of uterine vascular resistance during CPB, maternal blood pressure will be an important determinant of uterine blood flow and fetal oxygen delivery. Moderately high pressure (mean arterial pressure ≥65 mm Hg) should be employed during perfusion in the gravid patient.[316]

There are no reports demonstrating that increasing blood pressure during CPB improves FHR or fetal oxygen delivery. Most case reports on CPB in the gravid patient do not include information on blood pressure during CPB. The few blood pressure values reported in gravid perfusion cases ranged from 55 to 95 mm Hg.[321,325]

In theory, the use of short-acting vasodilators, such as nitroglycerin or sodium nitroprusside, may counteract the effects of CPB, and norepinephrine- or epinephrine-induced increases in uterine vasculature resistance. If maternal blood pressure is maintained by increasing extracorporeal circuit pump flow, uterine blood flow and fetal oxygen delivery may be increased with vasodilators. Monitoring should be conducted to assess the effect of a given therapeutic on fetal oxygen delivery during CPB.

TEMPERATURE

Although hypothermic CPB has been the standard of care in the last 15 years or more, several groups have advocated the use of normothermic bypass and warm blood cardioplegia to improve myocardial protection. However, the effects of warm versus cold cardioplegia on myocardial protection are controversial, and one group has reported an increase in adverse neurologic sequelae in patients treated with normothermic perfusion.[97] Controversy exists regarding temperature management during CPB in the *non*gravid patient, although most perfusions are conducted under hypothermic conditions. Similarly, there are few data and no consensus regarding temperature management in the gravid patient undergoing CPB.

There are theoretical advantages and disadvantages for normothermic and hypothermic CPB in the gravid patient. Hypothermia can cause fetal bradycardia and may lead to fetal ventricular arrhythmias resulting in fetal wastage. Rewarming after hypothermic bypass may precipitate uterine contractions and preterm labor.[316] However, others reported the onset of uterine contractions at the time of discontinuation of bypass support in spite of normothermic perfusion. Uterine contractions also occur at various times in the post-bypass and postoperative periods. The association of uterine contractions with rewarming after hypothermic bypass is unclear.

Hypothermia may be protective to the fetus during extracorporeal circulation by decreasing fetal oxygen requirements. Asali and colleagues[326] demonstrated that hypothermia to 28°C in gravid dogs causes an increase in uterine vascular resistance but does not result in a decrease in uterine blood flow. Hypothermia did not affect fetal survival. Pardi et al,[327] using a fetal lamb model, reported. Temperatures above 18°C were well tolerated. More profound hypothermia caused irreversible fetal acidosis and hypoxia. Several reports discuss the effects of deliberately induced and septicemia-associated hypothermia in gravid patients. The investigators observed that the FHR decreased with maternal hypothermia but improved with maternal rewarming.[328]

Perfusion temperatures of 25° to 37°C have been used in gravid patients undergoing CPB.[316,321,322,325] Because Pomini et al[318] found an apparent decrease in fetal loss when CPB temperatures were maintained at or above 36°C, they recommend normothermic temperatures during bypass. However, they acknowledge the lack of follow-up in many of the case reports they reviewed. The authors reported a case in which hypothermic bypass at 25°C was required for 2 hours 40 minutes, and in which the patient underwent two periods of rewarming. Uterine contractions occurring in the early postoperative period were successfully treated with magnesium sulfate. Despite the magnitude and duration of hypothermia and two periods of rewarming, a normal infant was delivered 10 days postoperatively.[321]

In conclusion, the optimal gravida temperature during CPB has not been established. There are no data that suggest hypothermia is harmful to the mother or fetus undergoing bypass. Normothermic CPB may increase the likelihood of untoward neurologic sequelae in the mother, an event that would be catastrophic in a woman with young children.

Accidental Hypothermia

In the early 1950s Bigelow and colleagues demonstrated a direct relationship between metabolic rate and temperature and postulated that deep hypothermia with circulatory arrest (DHCA) could facilitate cardiac surgery.[329] Although extracorporeal circulation was not used in these early cardiac cases (a tub of ice and warming coils were used to induce hypothermia and rewarm the patient), the notion that a patient could survive hypothermic arrest was established. With the introduction of CPB in the mid-1950s,[330] the induction of profound hypothermia with circulatory arrest, followed by resuscitation, was greatly facilitated by the extracorporeal circuit. It was a short leap to consider the use of CPB to resuscitate the victim suffering accidental hypothermia.

This section outlines the care of a subgroup of accidental hypothermia patients. Patients with core temperatures below 32°C, and without a perfusing cardiac rhythm, are best managed with some type of extracorporeal support.[331] Passive external rewarming, with or without active core warming strategies (airway warming, warm fluid resuscitation, peritoneal lavage, pleural irrigation), can be employed in hypothermic patients maintaining cardiac function.[332] This section discusses the management of hypothermic patients who are optimally managed with CPB for rewarming. The excellent review by Danzl and Prozus[332] outlines treatment algorithms for hypothermic patients who do not necessarily require extracorporeal circulation for resuscitation (e.g., patients with preserved circulation and suffering only moderate hypothermia [temperature ≥ 32°C]).

Patient Selection

Clinicians lack a consensus regarding the absolute indications or contraindications for the use of CPB in the treatment of accidental deep hypothermia.[333] However, there are theoretical considerations, and some data to help guide the decision-making process regarding the rewarming of accidental hypothermia patients. Phenomena that greatly limit the likelihood of successful resuscitation (that leads to an acceptable patient outcome) include the presence of asphyxia before the initiation of hypothermia. (This occurs commonly in avalanche and drowning victims.) Similarly, patients with severe traumatic injury, or extremely elevated potassium levels (≥10 mmol/L) are unlikely to benefit from resuscitative efforts.

One report suggests that several factors may increase the likelihood of a desirable patient outcome after accidental hypothermia managed with CPB.[334] Victims suffering profound hypothermia (without prior asphyxia), as opposed to moderate hypothermia, benefit from the substantial slowing of metabolic processes, and are less likely to have severe end-organ (brain, heart) damage. Young patients in good health are more likely to survive resuscitative efforts than older, debilitated victims. Patients who are malnourished (the homeless, alcoholics) or have multiple preexisting medical problems are less likely to have a desirable outcome. Initial rescue treatment algorithms may influence the likelihood of surviving profound hypothermia. The maintenance of profound hypothermia in the rescued patient before the initiation of extracorporeal warming may greatly enhance the likelihood of successful recovery. Rewarming with CPB is the most efficient method to resuscitate the hypothermic patient. Tissue perfusion is enhanced by hemodilution, and metabolic perturbations can be easily corrected.

Caring for the Accidental Hypothermia Victim

After the decision is made to resuscitate an accidental hypothermia victim, the patient should be maintained at the hypothermic temperature and rapidly transferred to a facility that can provide extracorporeal rewarming. In the operating room, various vascular sites may be cannulated to initiate rewarming. Groin vessels or mediastinal vasculature may serve as conduits for rewarming. Because the ventricle is noncompliant at temperatures below 32°C, sternotomy or thoracotomy may be preferable to facilitate direct cardiac massage and defibrillation. Although hypothermia reduces anesthetic requirements, the prudent use of anesthetics, analgesics, sedative-hypnotics, and volatile drugs is recommended. These agents should be administered through the extracorporeal circuit.

To treat an asystolic patient, the extracorporeal circuit must include a pump, oxygenator, and heat exchange waterbath. At flow rates of 2 to 3 L/min, with the waterbath at 38° to 40°C, the patient's core temperature will increase 1° to 2°C every 3 to 5 minutes. Slowly, the flow rate can be increased to 7 L/min. Given the data regarding the adverse effects of mildly hyperthermic blood on ischemic cerebral damage, the accidental hypothermia patient should not be perfused with blood warmed to temperatures in excess of 37°C. If the victim has a perfusing cardiac rhythm, venovenous rewarming may be used.

One study suggests that under certain circumstances (e.g., profound hypothermia before asphyxia; young, healthy patients; maintenance of hypothermia before bypass-supported rewarming) accidental hypothermia patients have an almost even chance of surviving and not suffering significant end-organ (including cerebral) deficits. Walpoth and colleagues[334] reviewed the hospital records of 234 patients suffering accidental hypothermia. Forty-six of these patients had core temperatures below 28°C and had circulatory arrest. Of the 32 patients rewarmed with CPB support, 15 were long-term survivors. These 15 patients were reexamined and studied an average of 7 years after their resuscitation from accidental hypothermia. The survivors were uniformly young (25.2 ± 9.9 years) and were resuscitated with CPB 141 ± 15 minutes after discovery. Although neurologic and neuropsychologic deficits were observed in all the victims in the early postresuscitation period, all patients had fully or almost completely recovered at the long-term follow-up. The investigators concluded that otherwise healthy individuals can survive accidental deep hypothermia with a preserved good quality of life.

Table 28–15 Typical Anesthetic and Operative Sequence for Intracranial Surgery Employing Deep Hypothermic Circulatory Arrest

Preoperative medication
Peripheral IV access, arterial catheter placement in holding area
To operating room
Induction of anesthesia, endotracheal intubation
Central venous pressure or pulmonary artery catheter, second IV or arterial catheter to remove autologous blood
Place TEE probe, EEG monitors
Final positioning, external defibrillation pads
Head holder on
Prep and drape
Normovolemic hemodilution
Craniotomy, initial dissection, surface cooling, IV mannitol
Heparinization, cannulation
Burst suppression with thiopental
On CPB—cool to 15°C
Circulatory arrest
Restart pump at low flow once lesion controlled
Rewarm if repair acceptable (with nitroprusside), defibrillate if needed
Separate from CPB at 36°C
Protamine after decannulation
Platelets; fresh frozen plasma or cryoprecipitate if needed
Wound closure
To intensive care unit

CPB, cardiopulmonary bypass; EEG = electroencephalographic; IV = intravenous; TEE = transesophageal echocardiography.

Intracranial Aneurysm

Surgery for intracranial aneurysm represents a major challenge for the surgeon and anesthesiologist. For a small number of these cases, DHCA has been applied to improve surgical access and cerebral protection. Like many areas, significant evolution in technique and application has occurred over time. Initial enthusiasm for DHCA in intracranial aneurysm surgery was tempered by the unfortunate occurrence of coagulopathies. Its use was further restricted by advances in neurosurgical microscopic technique (aneurysm wrapping, parent vessel ligation, and use of temporary clips). Improvements in perioperative monitoring and neuroanesthesia have reserved a use for DHCA in the approach to giant aneurysms that might otherwise be inoperable.

DHCA for intracranial aneurysm requires precise integration of a remarkably large and diverse team, which includes anesthesiologists, nurses, perfusionists, electroencephalographers, cardiac surgeons, and neurosurgeons. All components and demands of the operation should be thoroughly familiar to all participants (Table 28–15). The anesthesiologist is primarily occupied by five areas. The first area is patient selection and consent, which needs to include a careful assessment for preexisting coagulation problems or contraindication to TEE. The second area entails careful premedication and induction. This is undertaken to blunt hemodynamic response to invasive monitor placement and intubation, and avoid respiratory depression in that subgroup of patients with elevated intracranial pressure. The third area of focus for the anesthesiologist is maintenance and monitoring. This often includes TEE, electroencephalography, end-tidal N_2 monitoring, and placement of defibrillator pads in addition to the routine anesthetic monitors. Next, the anesthesiologist prepares for initiation of CPB and arrest. This stage involves isovolemic hemodilution to a target hematocrit of 20%, mannitol administration, burst suppression with thiopental or fixed-dose (25 mg/kg) administration of thiopental, surface cooling, and heparinization. The anesthesiologist manages rewarming, resumption of native circulation, and correction of coagulation abnormalities. Depending on the length of arrest and adequacy of cardiac protection, these steps may proceed smoothly or be complicated by significant hemodynamic embarrassment.

DHCA has been used for intracranial aneurysm surgery with good success at a number of centers.[335-340] The high percentage of patients surviving is probably the best indicator of the value of this technique, although the relatively small number of cases performed on an annual basis make controlled outcome trials difficult to complete. Silverberg et al[335] reported nine operative cases with no operative deaths, although six modest perioperative complications occurred (i.e., small stroke, transient cranial nerve palsy, frontal lobe hematoma, and pulmonary embolus). Baumgartner et al[336] also had no reported deaths in their series, and all patients went on to live independently. Like Silverberg's series, a fair number of patients experienced modest perioperative complications (i.e., four thromboembolic episodes, three strokes, three transient neurologic palsies). The other reported series[337-340] were similar in the respect that most patients went on to live independently and modest perioperative complications were in the range of 50%. Given the small numbers involved, it is very difficult to develop precise estimates for morbidity and mortality rates. However, given that DHCA in intracranial aneurysm surgery has been reserved for only the most difficult cases, the results seen are encouraging.

Heparin Resistance

Anticoagulation must be instituted before initiation of CPB to prevent massive clotting within the extracorporeal circuit (see Chapters 18 and 29). The nonendothelialized surface of the circuit activates the intrinsic coagulation cascade by factor XII, high-molecular-weight kininogen, and prekallikrein (contact factors) and causes direct platelet activation. Heparin is the standard anticoagulant used to prevent coagulation during CPB. It is a negatively charged proteoglycan that combines with antithrombin III to inhibit activated coagulation factors in the distal intrinsic and common pathway. Heparin also binds to platelets, interfering with normal platelet function. Reductions in antithrombin III levels, as may occur in patients receiving heparin therapy or with intravascular clotting, may lead to apparent heparin resistance.[341-343] Administration of fresh frozen plasma[344] or antithrombin III concentrates[345] may be necessary to boost antithrombin III levels to achieve the desired anticoagulant effect. The two adverse effects of greatest concern with the use of heparin include bleeding and heparin-induced thrombocytopenia. Several studies have been published evaluating the use of heparin-coated circuits and reduced intravenous heparin doses for CPB and the effect on postoperative bleeding and transfusion requirements.[346-349] In general, these studies suggest that heparin-coated circuits and low-dose systemic heparin appear to provide adequate anticoagulation for CPB with reduced postoperative bleeding and need for allogeneic blood transfusion.

Heparin-induced thrombocytopenia is an important immunohematologic problem characterized by the presence of heparin-dependent IgG antibodies directed against platelets or heparin-platelet complexes.[350] After antibody-platelet binding occurs, subsequent platelet activation or aggregation occurs, leading to platelet consumption and fibrin formation. Thrombocytopenia generally develops in 2% to 5% of patients after 5 or more days of heparin therapy, with venous and arterial thrombosis occurring in approximately 0.4%.[351] Patients diagnosed with heparin-induced thrombocytopenia should not receive heparin, and platelet transfusions are contraindicated because of the risk of thrombosis.

To avoid these life-threatening complications of standard heparin therapy, alternatives during CPB have been sought. Substitution of porcine heparin for bovine heparin, and the use of a prostacyclin analog to elevate platelet cAMP levels to prevent platelet aggregation have been tried.[352] Low-molecular-weight heparins (LMWH) have been developed that are less immunogenic and have a lower incidence of thrombocytopenia and potential for thrombosis.[353] A few case reports have been published on LMWH as an anticoagulant during CPB in patients with history of heparin-induced thrombocytopenia.[354-356] Alternative anticoagulants (e.g., bivalirudin) have been developed and used as heparin substitutes during CPB[357-362] (see Chapter 29).

MINIMALLY INVASIVE SURGERY AND CARDIOPULMONARY BYPASS

In the mid-1990s, interest in minimally invasive techniques for cardiac surgery emerged as a greater number of various surgical procedures (e.g., cholecystectomy, herniorrhaphy) were completed with so-called noninvasive techniques. Today, coronary revascularization with arterial conduits is being performed in many centers with minimally invasive approaches. This approach avoids the pathophysiologic events associated with extracorporeal circulation, but it demands surgical expertise that permits completion of anastomoses on a "beating" heart. The substantial amount of safety afforded by CPB and hypothermia is not available. The proponents of port-access surgery suggest that endoclamp bypass permits minimally invasive cardiac surgery while providing the support of extracorporeal circulation. This section describes the current technology and expertise with port-access CPB. Minimally invasive procedures and off-pump cardiac surgery are discussed further in Chapters 21 and 19, respectively.

Port-Access Bypass Circuit

The port-access system consists of a series of catheters that are introduced through various puncture sites, including the femoral artery and vein, and threaded through the aorta and venous system to the heart. An inflatable balloon on the end of the endoaortic clamp (EAC) (Cardiovations, Somerset, NJ) catheter arrests the blood flow in the aorta, and other catheters

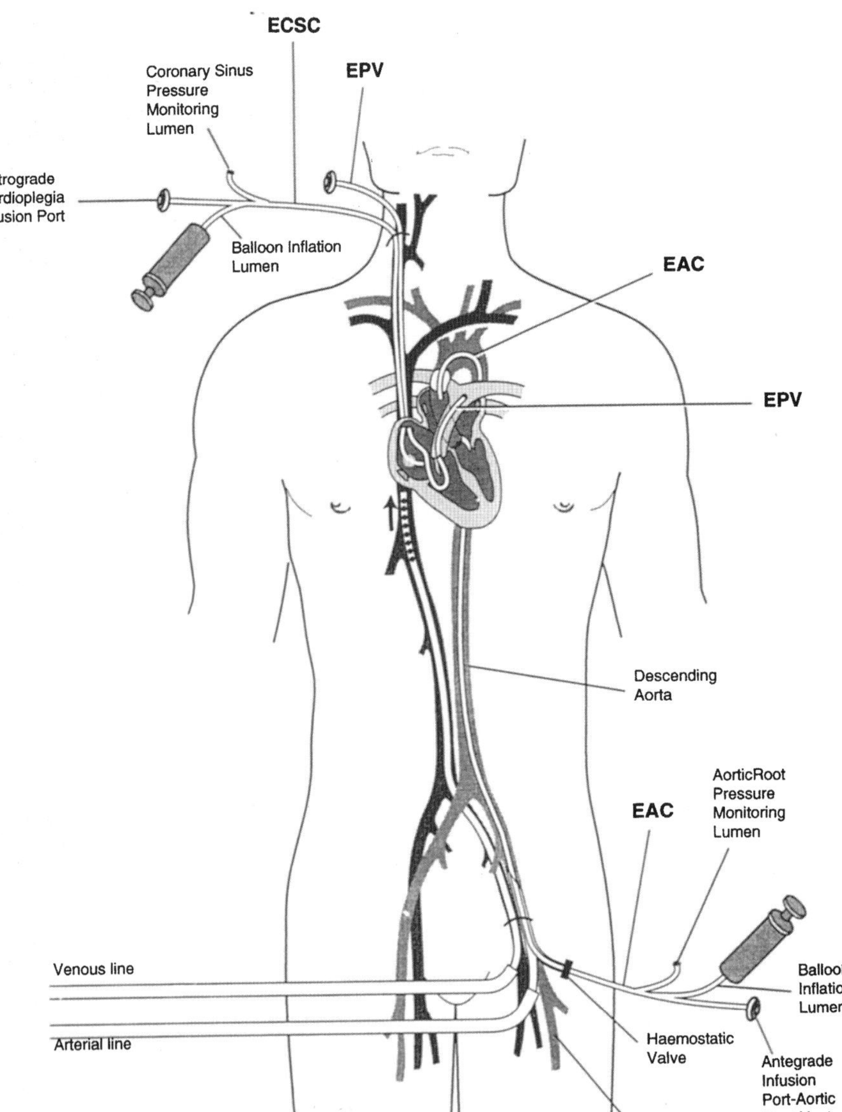

Figure 28–12 Positioning of endovascular catheters. The femoral venous drainage catheter tip is positioned at the right atrium–superior vena cava junction by fluoroscopy and transesophageal echocardiography. EAC = endoaortic clamp; ECSC = endocoronary sinus catheter; EPV = cardiopulmonary vent. (From Toomasian JM, Peters SP, Siegel LC, Stevens JH: Extracorporeal circulation for port-access cardiac surgery. Perfusion 12:83, 1997.)

help drain and reroute the blood flow to the heart-lung machine. Through two of the catheters, cardioplegia solution can be administered to the heart (Fig. 28–12).[363,364]

The endoaortic clamp is an occlusion balloon that functions as an aortic cross-clamp and permits antegrade cardioplegia infusion into the aortic root and coronary arteries. The lumen used to administer cardioplegia can also function as an aortic root-venting catheter (Fig. 28–13).

Retrograde cardioplegia can be delivered through an endocoronary sinus catheter that is placed with a percutaneous approach (Fig. 28–14). Blood returns to the extracorporeal circuit through the femoral venous catheter that is advanced to the level of the IVC-right atrial junction. Because extrathoracic gravity drainage is usually insufficient in providing adequate blood flow for complete CPB support, kinetic assisted venous drainage, with controlled suction, is used to augment the drainage of blood to the heart-lung machine.

Port-access CPB demands an expanded role of the anesthesiologist during CPB. The anesthesiologist is responsible for inserting the endopulmonary vent (EPV) and endocoronary sinus catheters through introducer sheaths placed in the

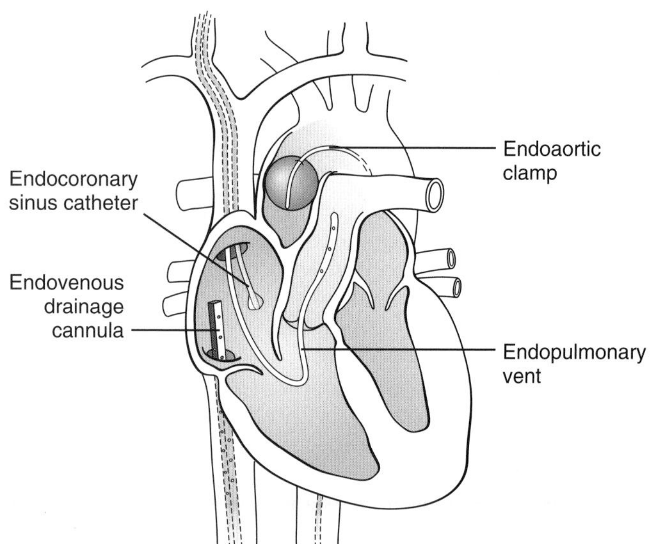

Figure 28–13 Correct positions of endocoronary sinus catheter, endoaortic clamp, endovenous drainage cannula, and endopulmonary vent for port-access cardiopulmonary bypass.

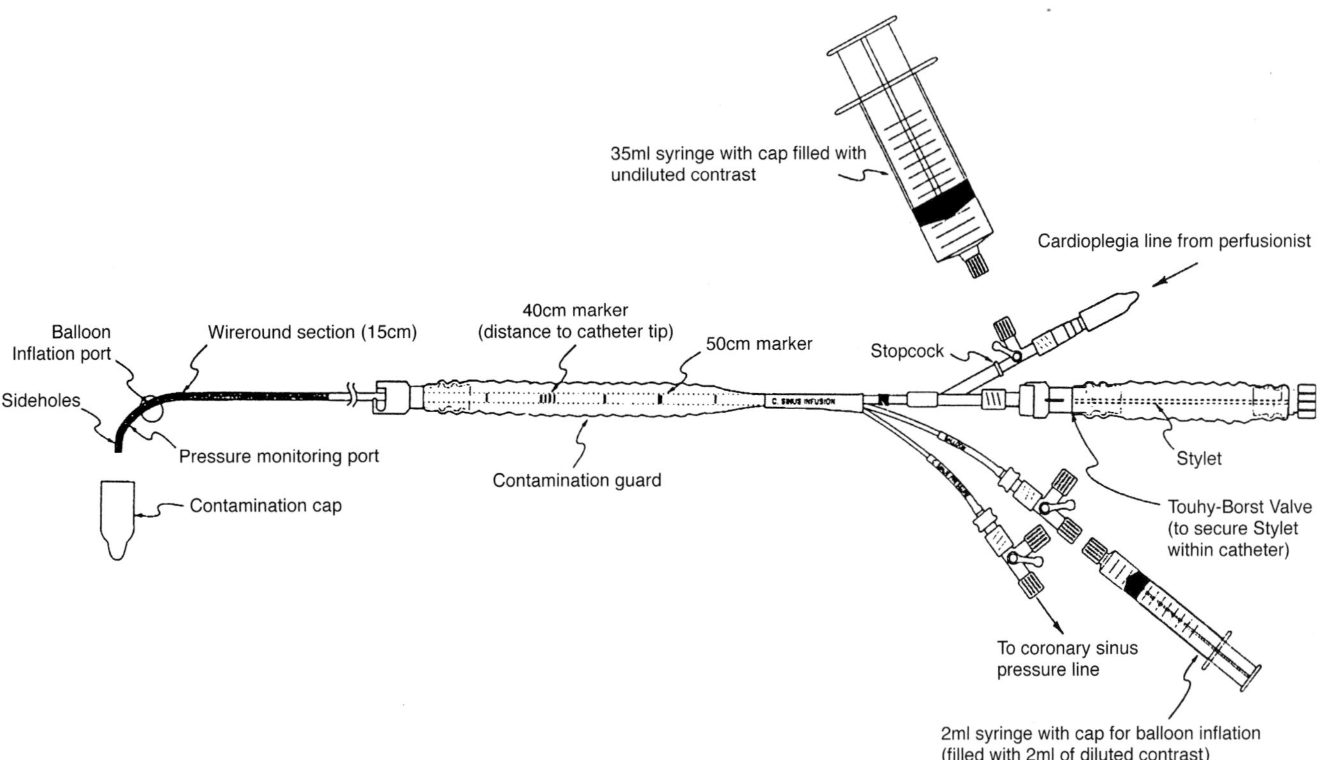

Figure 28–14 Diagrammatic representation of components of endocoronary sinus catheter. (Courtesy of Cardiovations, Somerset, NJ.)

internal jugular vein. The endocoronary sinus catheter should be placed first with the assistance of both fluoroscopy and TEE. However, some centers rely on TEE only for catheter placement. The EPV catheter is evolving in design. To assist EPV catheter placement, a balloon at the tip of the flow-directed catheter is inflated so that it floats into the pulmonary artery. The EPV is subsequently advanced over the flow-directed catheter until the tip is seated within the pulmonary artery. The balloon-tipped catheter is then withdrawn. In addition to fluoroscopy and TEE, distal catheter pressures facilitate positioning of the catheter. As with any new procedure or technology, the anesthesiologist should expect a learning curve regarding the skill of placing an endocoronary sinus catheter and a pulmonary artery vent. A side benefit of port-access bypass is the necessity of increased communication among members of the health care team. It is hoped that this phenomenon will spill over to all CPB cases and decrease the likelihood of perfusion mishaps.

Monitoring for Endovascular Clamp Bypass

To ensure safe and adequate bypass and myocardial protection, measures of venous drainage, the arterial blood flow, ventricular venting, cardioplegic delivery, regional perfusion, and aortic occlusion must be carefully monitored. Although the surgical staff is positioned to assess cardioplegia delivery and left ventricular venting and the perfusionist monitors arterial flow and venous drainage to and from the bypass circuit, the anesthesiologist is responsible for determining the proper placement of the endovascular clamp and adequacy of cerebral blood flow.[365]

Because cephalad migration of the endovascular aortic root clamp may compromise cerebral blood flow, it is imperative to monitor endovascular clamp position continuously. There are several proposed methods to achieve this essential goal (Table 28–16). TEE and color-flow Doppler aid in visualizing the placement of the EAC balloon in the ascending aorta and in detecting any leakage of blood around the balloon. Right radial artery pressure will decrease acutely if the endoaortic balloon migrates and obstructs the brachiocephalic artery. Some clinicians choose to measure blood pressure in the left and right radial arteries. The occurrence of acute difference in radial artery pressures may indicate cephalad migration of the endovascular clamp. Pulse-wave Doppler of the right carotid artery can verify cerebral perfusion, but is frequently difficult to assess under the conditions of nonpulsatile blood flow. The ability of transcranial Doppler monitoring of the middle cerebral artery and cerebral oximetry techniques to determine the adequacy of cerebral blood flow requires further evaluation. Nuttall et al[366] found that transcranial Doppler measurements of the middle cerebral artery blood flow velocity correlated poorly with cerebral blood flow during nonpulsatile, hypothermic CPB. The TEE probe may be useful in visualizing the ascending aorta and location of the balloon; however, many clinicians report the inadequacy of this technique.

Port-Access Cardiac Surgery Outcome Data

Early advocates of port-access cardiac surgery hoped that this new approach provided the benefits of minimally invasive surgery with the advantage of extracorporeal support and myocardial preservation during procedures on the heart. The anticipated benefits of port-access surgery have proved to be less than expected. A relatively steep learning curve exists, and multiple, unexpected complications have been reported (e.g., inadequate de-airing of the ventricle before discontinuation of bypass support, aortic or femoral artery dissection, malposition of the endovascular clamp).

Table 28–16 Potential Strategies to Monitor Cerebral Blood Flow during Port-Access Bypass

Monitor	Limitations	Observation with Cephalad Migration of Endoaortic Clamp*
Fluoroscopy	1. Must interrupt surgery to use monitor	EAC occluding great vessels
Transesophageal echocardiography	1. May be difficult to visualize EAC position during cardiopulmonary bypass	EAC in area of great vessels
Carotid ultrasound	1. Difficult to monitor signal continuously—depends on index of suspicion 2. Difficult to obtain signal with nonpulsatile blood flow	Sudden loss of blood flow signal
Transcranial Doppler	1. Difficult to monitor MCA blood flow continuously—depends on index of suspicion 2. Difficult to insonate MCA during nonpulsatile blood flow 3. Poor sensitivity/specificity	1. Loss of MCA blood flow velocity signal 2. Change in ratio of RMCA vs. LMCA blood flow velocity 3. ? Change in RMCA or LMCA blood flow direction
Cerebral venous blood oximetry (R vs. L signal)	1. Sensitivity/specificity?	Decrease in cerebral venous blood oxygen saturation; change in R vs. L signal†
Electroencephalography	1. Hypothermia, anesthetics and roller pump artifacts limit interpretation of EEG signals	EEG slowing/change in right vs. left EEG signal
Right and left radial arterial pressures	1. Requires cannulation of both radial arteries; increased risk of hand ischemia 2. Left radial arterial free graft conduit not possible	Change in the ratio of right and left radial arteries measured MAP

*Hypothetical observation; the sensitivity and specificity of these monitors in this clinical setting have not been evaluated.
†The rate and magnitude of change depend on many factors, including the patient's cerebral temperature, magnitude of obstruction, and collateral blood flow.
EAC = endoaortic clamp; MAP = mean arterial pressure; MCA = middle cerebral artery; r = right; l = left.

Mohr et al[367] reported a 9.8% mortality rate in their series of 51 patients undergoing elective mitral valve replacement or repair. Two patients suffered femoral artery dissections (requiring conversion to conventional techniques), and three patients required second operations for repair of postoperative perivalvular leaks. Patients in the port-access group reported the same amount of pain as those undergoing sternal splitting (as measured by a visual analog pain scale), challenging the hypothesis that minimally invasive procedures result in less pain than conventional approaches (see Chapter 21).

LEGAL CONSIDERATIONS OF CARDIOPULMONARY BYPASS

The complex interactions required to initiate, maintain, and discontinue extracorporeal support predispose CPB to unexpected, undesirable events. A system is considered susceptible to accidents if "tight coupling" is required to avoid mishaps. That is to say, a slight perturbation in one part of the system may lead to major dysfunction within the entire system. Because tight coupling of complex interactions is required for successful CPB, it is often difficult to discern who or what event precipitated a given adverse outcome.

As described by Gaba et al,[368] there are three types of complexities—intrinsic complexity, proliferation, and uncertainty—that make a system vulnerable to adverse events. This type of system analysis is readily applied to CPB. Many complex interactions must be integrated carefully for successful bypass (intrinsic complexity), and health professionals from various backgrounds (e.g., perfusionists, surgeons, nurses, anesthesiologists) must communicate effectively (proliferation). The problem of uncertainty persists in CPB because it is difficult to judge the adequacy of organ perfusion. Medicolegal issues regarding CPB in the area of tort law are always difficult and complex. It is difficult to discern who or what series of events was responsible for an adverse event or outcome occurring in connection with CPB. The following hypothetical case is an example of the potential difficulty encountered in determining liability for an adverse outcome after CPB.

An essentially healthy 48-year-old man with ischemic heart disease undergoes triple-vessel CABG for the treatment of crescendo angina. After an apparently uneventful operation, he fails to awaken. Review of anesthesia and perfusion records reveals a period of profound hypertension (MAP ≥ 95 mm Hg) followed by 10 minutes of profound hypotension (MAP < 15 mm Hg). The perfusionist, without direction from the anesthesiologist (who was not in the operating room) or surgeon, attempted to control the blood pressure with 5% isoflurane. When the anesthesiologist returned to the operating room, he recalibrated the arterial pressure transducer and determined that it was malfunctioning. The pressure transducer initially suggested that the patient's MAP was 95 mm Hg, although the MAP was below 15 mm Hg. The operating surgeon was aware of all these events.

Who is responsible—the manufacturer of the transducer, the absent anesthesiologist, the perfusionist, the surgeon? The health care personnel in this case failed to coordinate the many interactions required to use the complex system of CPB successfully. This case is hypothetical, but it includes many events encountered in malpractice suits. Some of the principles applied for determining liability are outlined in the following section.

Negligence, Vicarious Liability, and Strict Liability

Depending on the circumstances of a case, damages are awarded on the basis of strict liability or medical malpractice (i.e., negligence). Malpractice damages are awarded if health care personnel are shown to be negligent. Four phenomena must be present to prove negligence:

1. *Duty*: The physician or health care professional owed the patient a duty to act given a particular situation and circumstances in conformity with patient care standards established by the profession
2. *Breach-of-duty*: An act of commission or omission on the part of the physician violated the established patient care standards.
3. *Proximate cause*: The act of omission by the physician resulted in injury to the patient.
4. *Damages*: The patient suffered loss or damage as a result of the injury.

Many medical professional societies have specific, published standards of care. For example, the American Society of Anesthesiologists has an accepted standard of care regarding the minimal monitoring requirements during the administration of anesthesia. Similarly, the American Society of Perfusion Technology sets minimal standards for patients during CPB. More broadly, the *standard of care* is defined as the care ordinarily used by well-qualified physicians or other clinicians practicing under similar circumstances. However, in the arena of CPB, it is frequently unclear who determines or is responsible for a specific clinical decision (e.g., what is an appropriate rate of rewarming?) If the anesthesiologist is charged with administering the heparin and measuring its effect with an activated coagulation time, and fails to do so, the occurrence of circuit and patient thrombosis with the initiation of bypass would be the fault of the anesthesiologist. Similarly, transection of the aorta and hemorrhage resulting from use of the sternal saw would be the responsibility of the operating surgeon. But who is responsible for life-threatening end-organ damage? Who is responsible for the other personnel intimately involved with managing CPB (e.g., the perfusionist)? (See Chapters 39 to 41.)

Because perfusionists practice under a variety of circumstances—some are self-employed and carry their own malpractice insurance, others are employees of the hospital, surgeons, or anesthesiologists—liability for perfusionists' mishaps varies. Individuals other than the perfusionist can be held responsible for perfusion mishaps on the basis of several legal doctrines that allow for *vicarious liability*. Although party A may be innocent of any fault, this party may be held accountable for actions of B. If the perfusionist is employed by a surgeon, anesthesiologist, or hospital, the doctrine of *respondant superior* (i.e., let the master respond) may be used to hold the employer liable for the actions of the employee. Similarly, vicarious liability may occur under the doctrine of the so-called borrowed servant. In this case, an employee of one master is "borrowed" by another for a specific purpose. The surgeon or anesthesiologist may temporarily assume control or responsibility for the perfusionist, despite the fact they are not direct employers.

Strict Liability

If a device or product that is part of the extracorporeal circuit or apparatus used to conduct CPB is found to be unreasonably dangerous or defective, the doctrine of strict liability may be applied. In most instances, injury or dysfunction resulting from apparent product failure or malfunction is directed against the manufacturers. However, in some cases, hospitals and doctors have been held liable under the doctrine of strict liability. Some courts have suggested that the physician and hospital are in the best position to identify defective products.

SUMMARY

The complex nature of CPB predisposes this system to mishaps and serious accidents. Unfortunately, perfusion accidents can result in significant patient morbidity and in some cases death. Perhaps it is intuitively apparent that it is unsafe to redirect the blood from its normal course to the heart and lungs into a complex system of tubes, pumps, and connectors. Kirklin et al[369] suggested that "the conclusion that cardiopulmonary bypass is safe has not been vigorously supported. Some damage is manifested in most patients." The problem of CPB-induced patient morbidity persists. The current litigious nature of American culture increases the likelihood of malpractice suits directed at those caring for cardiac surgery patients. Close communication among members of the health care team managing patients during CPB is necessary. The well-being of the patient depends on the surgical team avoiding perfusion accidents.

REFERENCES

1. American Society of Anesthesiologists: Standards for basic anesthetic monitoring. Available at: http://www.asahq.org/publicationsAndServices/standards/02.pdf. Accessed September 23, 2005
2. American Society of Anesthesiologists: Compliance with Medicare and Other Payor Billing Requirements. Park Ridge, IL, ASA, 1997
3. Braunwalk E: The Simon Dack lecture. Cardiology: The past, the present, and the future. J Am Coll Cardiol 42:2031, 2003
4. Edmunds LH: Cardiopulmonary bypass after 50 years. N Engl J Med 351:1603, 2004
5. Cohn LH: Fifty years of open heart surgery. Circulation 107:2168, 2003.
6. Mora CT: Cardiopulmonary Bypass. New York, Springer-Verlag, 1995.
7. Taylor PC, Effler DB: Management of cannulation for cardiopulmonary bypass in patients with adult-acquired heart disease. Surg Clin North Am 55:1205, 1975
8. Murkin JM, Farrar JK, Tweed WA, et al: Cerebral autoregulation and flow/metabolism coupling during cardiopulmonary bypass: The influence of Pa_{CO_2}. Anesth Analg 66:825, 1987
9. Govier AV, Reves JG, McKay RD, et al: Factors and their influence on regional cerebral blood flow during nonpulsatile cardiopulmonary bypass. Ann Thorac Surg 38:592, 1984
10. Newman MF, Croughwell ND, White WD, et al: Effect of perfusion pressure on cerebral blood flow during normothermic cardiopulmonary bypass. Circulation 94:II353, 1996
11. Michler RE, Sandhu AA, Young WL, Schwartz AE: Low-flow cardiopulmonary bypass: Importance of blood pressure in maintaining cerebral blood flow. Ann Thorac Surg 60:S525, 1995
12. Schwartz AE, Sandhu AA, Kaplon RJ, et al: Cerebral blood flow is determined by arterial pressure and not cardiopulmonary bypass flow rate. Ann Thorac Surg 60:165, 1995
13. Murkin J: Stroke and the elderly: Aortis atheroma and CNS outcome after cardiac surgery. Cardiovasc Rev Rep 22:397, 2001
14. Gilman S: Cerebral disorders after open-heart operations. N Engl J Med 272:489, 1965
15. Javid H, Tufo HM, Najafi H, et al: Neurologic abnormalities following open heart surgery. J Thorac Cardiovasc Surg 58:502, 1969
16. Tufo HM, Ostfeld AM, Shekelle R: Central nervous system dysfunction following open heart surgery. JAMA 212:1333, 1970
17. Lee LW Jr, Brady MP, Rowe JM, Miller WC Jr: Effects of extracorporeal circulation upon behavior, personality, and brain function. II. Hemodynamic, metabolic, and psychometric correlations. Ann Surg 173:1013, 1971

18. Stockard JJ, Bickford RG, Schauble JF: Pressure-dependent cerebral ischemia during cardiopulmonary bypass. Neurology 23:521, 1973
19. Stockard JJ, Bickford RG, Myers RR, et al: Hypotension-induced changes in cerebral function during cardiac surgery. Stroke 5:730, 1974
20. Slogoff S, Girgis KZ, Keats AS: Etiologic factors in neuropsychiatric complications associated with cardiopulmonary bypass. Anesth Analg 61:903, 1982
21. Slogoff S, Reul GJ, Keats AS, et al: Role of perfusion pressure and flow in major organ dysfunction after cardiopulmonary bypass. Ann Thorac Surg 50:911, 1990
22. Bashein G, Townes BD, Nessly ML, et al: A randomized study of carbon dioxide management during hypothermic cardiopulmonary bypass. Anesthesiology 72:7, 1990
23. Ellis RJ, Wigniewski A, Potts R, et al: Reduction of flow rate and arterial pressure at moderate hypothermia does not result in cerebral dysfunction. J Thorac Cardiovasc Surg 79:173, 1980
24. McKhann GM, Goldsborough MA, Borowicz LM Jr, et al: Predictors of stroke risk in coronary artery bypass patients. Ann Thorac Surg 63:516, 1997
25. Townes BD, Bashein G, Hornbein TF, et al: Neurobehavioral outcomes in cardiac operations. A prospective controlled study. J Thorac Cardiovasc Surg 98:774, 1989
26. Fish KJ, Helms KN, Sernquist FH, et al: A prospective, randomized study of the effects of prostacyclin on neuropsychologic dysfunction after coronary artery operation. J Thorac Cardiovasc Surg 93:609, 1987
27. Nussmeier NA, Arlund C, Slogoff S: Neuropsychiatric complications after cardiopulmonary bypass: Cerebral protection by a barbiturate. Anesthesiology 64:165, 1986
28. Sotaniemi KA, Juolasmas A, Hokkanen ET: Neuropsychologic outcome after open-heart surgery. Arch Neurol 38:2, 1981
29. Kolkka R, Hilbermann M: Neurologic dysfunction following cardiac operation with low-flow, low-pressure cardiopulmonary bypass. J Thorac Cardiovasc Surg 79:432, 1980
30. Stanley TE, Smith LR, White WD, et al: Effect of cerebral perfusion pressure during cardiopulmonary bypass on neuropsychiatric outcome following coronary artery bypass grafting. Anesthesiology 73:A93, 1990
31. Kramer DC, Stanley TE, Sanderson I: Failure to demonstrate relationship between mean arterial pressure during cardiopulmonary bypass and postoperative cognitive function. Presented at the Society of Cardiovascular Anesthesiologists, Montreal, 1994, p 211
32. Savageau JA, Stanton B, Jenkins CD, Klein MD: Neuropsychological dysfunction following elective cardiac operation. I. Early assessment. J Thorac Cardiovasc Surg 84:585, 1982
33. Gardner TJ, Horneffer PJ, Manolio TA, et al: Stroke following coronary artery bypass grafting: A ten-year study. Ann Thorac Surg 40:574, 1985
34. Branthwaite MA: Prevention of neurological damage during open heart surgery. Thorax 30:258, 1975
35. Gold JP, Charlson ME, Williams-Russo P, et al: Improvement of outcomes after coronary artery bypass: A randomized trial comparing intraoperative high versus low mean arterial pressure. J Thorac Cardiovasc Surg 110:1302, 1995
36. Hartman GS, Yao FS, Bruefach M 3rd, et al: Severity of aortic atheromatous disease diagnosed by transesophageal echocardiography predicts stroke and other outcomes associated with coronary artery surgery: A prospective study. Anesth Analg 83:701, 1996
37. Schell RM, Kern FH, Greeley WJ, et al: Cerebral blood flow and metabolism during cardiopulmonary bypass. Anesth Analg 76:849, 1993
38. Newman MF, Croughwell ND, Blumenthal JA, et al: Effect of aging on cerebral autoregulation during cardiopulmonary bypass. Association with postoperative cognitive dysfunction. Circulation 90:II, 1994
39. Newman MF, Kramer D, Croughwell ND, et al: Differential age effects of mean arterial pressure and rewarming on cognitive dysfunction after cardiac surgery. Anesth Analg 81:236, 1995
40. Croughwell N, Lyth M, Quill TJ, et al: Diabetic patients have abnormal cerebral autoregulation during cardiopulmonary bypass. Circulation 82:IV, 1990
41. Vainionpaa V, Timisjarvi J, Tarkka M: Spontaneous oscillation of systemic arterial pressure during cardiopulmonary bypass in the dog. Basic Res Cardiol 84:160, 1989
42. Suwa K, Asahara H: Vasomotor waves during cardiopulmonary bypass in the dog. Tohoku J Exp Med 125:45, 1978
43. Gilston A: Cyclic variations in blood pressure (letter). Crit Care Med 12:925, 1984
44. Stern DH, Gerson JI, Allen FB, Parker FB: Can we trust the radial artery pressure immediately after cardiopulmonary bypass? Anesthesiology 62:557, 1985
45. Edmunds LH: Pulseless cardiopulmonary bypass. J Thorac Cardiovasc Surg 84:800, 1982
46. Hickey PR, Buckley MJ, Philbin DM: Pulsatile and nonpulsatile cardiopulmonary bypass: Review of a counterproductive controversy. Ann Thorac Surg 36:720, 1983
47. Nakayama K, Tamiya T, Yamamoto K: High-amplitude pulsatile pump in extracorporeal circulation with particular reference to hemodynamics. Surgery 54:798, 1963
48. Shephard RB, Kirklin JW: Relation of pulsatile flow to oxygen consumption and other variables during cardiopulmonary bypass. J Thorac Cardiovasc Surg 58:694, 1969
49. Dunn J, Kirsh NM, Harness J: Hemodynamic, metabolic, and hematologic effects of pulsatile cardiopulmonary bypass. J Thorac Cardiovasc Surg 68:138, 1974
50. Jacobs LA, Klopp EH, Seamone W: Improved organ function during cardiac bypass with a roller pump modified to deliver pulsatile flow. J Thorac Cardiovasc Surg 58:703, 1969
51. Dernevik L, Arvidsson S, William-Olsson G: Cerebral perfusion in dogs during pulsatile and nonpulsatile extracorporeal circulation. J Cardiovasc Surg 26:32, 1985
52. Philbin DM, Levine PH, Emerson CW: Plasma vasopressin levels and urinary flow in patients during cardiopulmonary bypass in patients with valvular heart disease. J Thorac Cardiovasc Surg 7:779, 1979
53. Taylor KM, Bain WH, Russell M: Peripheral vascular resistance and angiotensin II levels during pulsatile and nonpulsatile cardiopulmonary bypass. Thorax 34:594, 1979
54. Boucher JK, Rudy LW, Edmunds LH: Organ blood flow during pulsatile cardiopulmonary bypass. J Appl Physiol 36:86, 1974
55. Singh RKK, Barratt-Boyes BG, Harris EA: Does pulsatile flow improve perfusion during hypothermic cardiopulmonary bypass? J Thorac Cardiovasc Surg 79:827, 1980
56. Frater RWM, Wakayama S, Oka Y: Pulsatile cardiopulmonary bypass: Failure to influence hemodynamics or hormones. Circulation 62:1, 1980
57. Salerno TA, Henderson M, Keith FM, Charrett EJP: Hypertension after coronary operation. Can it be prevented by pulsatile perfusion? J Thorac Cardiovasc Surg 81:396, 1981
58. Landymore RW, Murphy DA, Kinley CE: Does pulsatile flow influence the incidence of postoperative hypertension? Ann Thorac Surg 28:261, 1978
59. Watkins WD, Peterson MB, Kong DL: Thromboxane and prostacyclin changes during cardiopulmonary bypass with and without pulsatile flow. J Thorac Cardiovasc Surg 84:250, 1982
60. Nieminen M-T, Philbin DM, Rosow CE: Temperature gradients and rewarming time during hypothermic cardiopulmonary bypass with and without pulsatile flow. Ann Thorac Surg 35:488, 1983
61. Nagaoka H, Innami R, Arai H: Effects of pulsatile cardiopulmonary bypass on the renin-angiotensin-aldosterone system following open-heart surgery. Jpn J Surg 18:390, 1988
62. Lindberg H, Svennevig JL, Lilleaasen P, Vatne K: Pulsatile vs. non-pulsatile flow during cardiopulmonary bypass. Scand J Thorac Cardiovasc Surg 18:195, 1984
63. Mori A, Watanabe K, Onoe M: Regional blood flow in the liver, pancreas and kidney during cardiopulmonary bypass. Arch Surg 124:458, 1988
64. Matsumoto T, Wolferth CC, Perlman MH: Effects of pulsatile and non-pulsatile perfusion upon cerebral and conjunctival microcirculation in dogs. Am Surg 37:61, 1971
65. Williams GD, Seifen AB, Lawson NW: Pulsatile perfusion versus conventional high-flow non-pulsatile perfusion for rapid core cooling and rewarming of infants for circulatory arrest in cardiac operation. J Thorac Cardiac Surg 78:667, 1979
66. Philbin DM, Levine FH, Kono K: Attenuation of the stress response to cardiopulmonary bypass by the addition of pulsatile flow. Circulation 64:808, 1981
67. Kono K, Philbin DM, Coggins CH: Adrenocortical hormone levels during cardiopulmonary bypass with and without pulsatile flow. J Thorac Cardiovasc Surg 85:129, 1983
68. Murray WR, Mittra S, Mittra D: The amylase-creatinine clearance ratio following cardiopulmonary bypass. J Thorac Cardiovasc Surg 82:248, 1981
69. Andersen K, Waaben J, Husum B: Nonpulsatile cardiopulmonary bypass disrupts the flow-metabolism couple in the brain. J Thorac Cardiovasc Surg 90:570, 1985
70. Sanderson JM, Wright G, Sims FW: Brain damage in dogs immediately following pulsatile and non-pulsatile blood flow in extracorporeal circulation. Thorax 27:275, 1972
71. Tranmer BI, Gross CE, Kindt GW, Adey GR: Pulsatile versus non-pulsatile blood flow in the treatment of acute cerebral ischemia. Neurosurgery 19:724, 1986

72. Mavroudis C: To pulse or not to pulse. Ann Thorac Surg 25:259, 1978
73. Evans PJD, Ruyjrok P, Seelye ER, Harris EA: Does sodium nitroprusside improve tissue oxygenation during cardiopulmonary bypass? Br J Anaesth 49:799, 1977
74. Grossi EA, Connolly MW, Krieger KH: Quantification of pulsatile flow during cardiopulmonary bypass to permit direct comparison of the effectiveness of various types of "pulsatile" and "non-pulsatile" flow. Surgery 98:547, 1985
75. Badner NH, Murkin JM, Lok P: Difference in pH management and pulsatile/nonpulsatile perfusion during cardiopulmonary bypass do not influence renal function. Anesth Analg 75:696, 1992
76. Shaw PJ, Bates D, Cartlige NEF: An analysis of factors predisposing to neurological injury in patients undergoing coronary bypass operations. Q J Med 72:633, 1989
77. Brazier J, Hottenrott C, Burkberg G: Noncoronary collateral myocardial blood flow. Ann Thorac Surg 19:426, 1975
78. Lajos TZ, Glicken D: Metabolic measurements in the human heart-lung preparation during hypothermic cardioplegia. Thorac Cardiovasc Surg 28:34, 1980
79. Olinger GN, Bonchek LI, Geiss DM: Noncoronary collateral distribution in coronary artery disease. Ann Thorac Surg 32:554, 1981
80. Fox LS, Blackstone EH, Kirklin JW: Relationship of whole-body oxygen consumption to perfusion flow rate during hypothermic cardiopulmonary bypass. J Thorac Cardiovasc Surg 83:239, 1982
81. Hirsch DM, Hadidian C, Neville WE: Oxygen consumption during cardiopulmonary bypass with large volume hemodilution. J Thorac Cardiovasc Surg 56:197, 1968
82. Kawamura M, Minamikawa O, Yokochi H: Safe limit of hemodilution in cardiopulmonary bypass-comparative analysis between cyanotic and acyanotic congenital heart disease. Jpn J Surg 10:206, 1980
83. Niinikoski J, Laaksonen V, Meretoja O: Oxygen transport to tissue under normovolemic moderate and extreme hemodilution during coronary artery bypass operation. Ann Thorac Surg 31:134, 1981
84. Dexter F, Hindman BJ: Theoretical analysis of cerebral venous blood hemoglobin oxygen saturation as an index of cerebral oxygenation during hypothermic cardiopulmonary bypass. Anesthesiology 83:405, 1995
85. Slater JM, Orszulak TA, Cook DJ: Distribution and hierarchy of regional blood flow during hypothermic cardiopulmonary bypass. Ann Thorac Surg 72:542, 2001
86. Hilberman M, Myers BD, Carrie BJ, et al: Acute renal failure following cardiac surgery. J Thorac Cardiovasc Surg 77:880, 1979
87. Abel RM, Buckley MJ, Austen WG, et al: Etiology, incidence, and prognosis of renal failure following cardiac operations. J Thorac Vasc Surg 71:323, 1976
88. Koning HM, Koning AJ, Defauw JJAM: Optimal perfusion during extracorporeal circulation. J Thorac Cardiovasc Surg 21:207, 1987
89. Rogers AT, Prough DS, Roy RC: Cerebrovascular and cerebral metabolic effects of alterations in perfusion flow rate during hypothermic cardiopulmonary bypass in man. J Thorac Cardiovasc Surg 103:363, 1992
90. Soma Y, Hirotani T, Yozu R: A clinical study of cerebral circulation during extracorporeal circulation. J Thorac Cardiovasc Surg 97:187, 1989
91. Schwartz AE, Kaplon RJ, Young WL, et al: Cerebral blood flow during low-flow hypothermic cardiopulmonary bypass in baboons. Anesthesiology 81:959, 1994
92. Croughwell N, Smith LR, Quill T, et al: The effect of temperature on cerebral metabolism and blood flow in adults during cardiopulmonary bypass. J Thorac Cardiovasc Surg 103:549, 1992
93. Astrup J, Siesjo BK, Symon L: Thresholds in cerebral ischemia: The ischemic penumbra. Stroke 12:723, 1981
94. Baba S, Ozawa H, Nakamoto Y, et al: Enhanced blood pressure response to regular daily stress in urban hypertensive men. J Hypertens 8:647, 1990
95. Busto R, Globus MY-T, Dietrich WD, et al: Effect of mild hypothermia on ischemia-induced release of neurotransmitters and free fatty acids in rat brain. Stroke 20:904, 1989
96. Natale JA, D'Alecy LG: Protection from cerebral ischemia by brain cooling without reduced lactate accumulation in dogs. Stroke 20:770, 1989
97. Mora CT, Henson MB, Weintraub WS et al: The effect of temperature management during cardiopulmonary bypass on neurological and neuropsychological outcomes in coronary revascularization patients. J Thorac Cardiovasc Surg 112:514, 1996
98. Warm Heart Investigators: Randomised trial of normothermic versus hypothermic coronary bypass surgery. Lancet 343:559, 1994
99. McLean RF, Wong BI, Naylor CD, et al: Cardiopulmonary bypass, temperature, and central nervous system dysfunction. Circulation 90 (Pt 2):II250, 1994
100. Martin TC, Craver JM, Gott JP, et al: Prospective, randomized trial of retrograde warm-blood cardioplegia: Myocardial benefit and neurologic threat. Ann Thorac Surg 57:298, 1994
101. Birdi I, Regragui I, Izzat MB, et al: Influence of normothermic systemic perfusion during coronary artery bypass operations: A randomized prospective study. J Thorac Cardiovasc Surg 114:475, 1997
102. Engelman RM: Mechanisms to reduce hospital stays. Ann Thorac Surg 61:S26, 1996
103. Singh AK, Feng WC, Bert AA, Rostenberg FA: Warm body, cold heart surgery: Clinical experience in 2817 patients. Eur J Cardiothorac Surg 7:225, 1993
104. Bert AA, Singh AK: Right ventricular function after normothermic versus hypothermic cardiopulmonary bypass. J Thorac Cardiovasc Surg 106:988, 1993
105. Singh AK, Bert AA, Feng WC, Rotenberg FA: Stroke during coronary artery bypass grafting using hypothermic versus normothermic perfusion. Ann Thorac Surg 59:84, 1995
106. Stone JG, Young WL, Smith CR, et al: Do standard monitoring sites reflect true brain temperature when profound hypothermia is rapidly induced and reversed? Anesthesiology 82:344, 1995
107. Kaukuntla H, Harrington D, Bilkoo I, et al: Temperature monitoring during cardiopulmonary bypass—do we undercool or overheat the brain? Eur J Cardiothorac Surg 26:580, 2004
108. Reeves RB: An imidazole alpha-stat hypothesis for vertebrate acid-base regulation: Tissue carbon dioxide content and body temperature in bullfrogs. Respir Physiol 14:219, 1972
109. Stephan H, Weyland A, Kazmaier S, et al: Acid-base management during hypothermic cardiopulmonary bypass does not affect cerebral metabolism but does affect blood flow and neurological outcome. Br J Anaesth 69:1, 1992
110. Kiziltan HT, Baltali M, Bilen A, et al: Comparison of alpha-stat and pH-stat cardiopulmonary bypass in relation to jugular venous oxygen saturation and cerebral glucose-oxygen utilization. Anesth Analg 96:644, 2003
111. Henriksen L: Brain luxury perfusion during cardiopulmonary bypass in humans: A study of the cerebral blood flow response to changes in CO_2, O_2 and blood pressure. J Cereb Blood Flow Metab 6:366, 1986
112. Prough DS, Stump DA, Roy RC, et al: Response of cerebral blood flow to changes in carbon dioxide tension during hypothermic cardiopulmonary bypass. Anesthesiology 64:576, 1986
113. Murkin JM, Martzke JS, Buchan AM, et al: A randomized study of the influence of perfusion technique and pH management strategy in 316 patients undergoing coronary artery bypass surgery. J Thorac Cardiovasc Surg 110:349, 1995
114. Kroncke GM, Nichols RD, Mendenhall JT, et al: Ectothermic philosophy of acid-base balance to prevent fibrillation during hypothermia. Arch Surg 121:303, 1986
115. Swain JA, White FN, Peters RM: The effect of pH on the hypothermic ventricular fibrillation threshold. J Thorac Cardiovasc Surg 87:445, 1984
116. Willford DC, Moores WY, Ji SY, et al: Importance of acid-base strategy in reducing myocardial and whole body oxygen consumption during perfusion hypothermia. J Thorac Cardiovasc Surg 100:699, 1990
117. Willford DC, Hill EP, White FC, Moores WY: Decreased critical mixed venous oxygen tension and critical oxygen transport during induced hypothermia in pigs. J Clin Monit 2:155, 1986
118. Willford DC, Schaffartzik W, Bain R, Ziegler MG: Elevated norepinephrine level and oxygen consumption rate (VO_2) with pH-stat acid-base management during hypothermia. Physiologist 32:203, 1989
119. Baraka AS, Baroody MA, Haroun ST, et al: Effect of alpha-stat versus pH-stat strategy on oxyhemoglobin dissociation and whole-body oxygen consumption during hypothermic cardiopulmonary bypass. Anesth Analg 74:32, 1992
120. Panico FG, Neptune LS, et al: A mechanism to eliminate the donor blood prime from the pump oxygenator. Surg Forum 10:605, 1959
121. Rand PW, Lacombe E, Hunt HE, Austin WH: Viscosity of normal human blood under normothermic and hypothermic conditions. J Appl Physiol 19:117, 1964
122. Hohn L, Schweitzer A, Licker M, et al: Absence of beneficial effect of acute normovolemic hemodilution combined with aprotinin on allogeneic blood transfusion requirements in cardiac surgery. Anesthesiology 96:276, 2002.
123. Scott DA, Hore PJ, Cannata J, et al: A comparison of albumin polygeline and crystalloid priming solutions for cardiopulmonary bypass in patients having coronary artery bypass graft surgery. Perfusion 10:415, 1995

124. Jenkins IR, Curtis AP: The combination of mannitol and albumin in the priming solution reduces positive intraoperative fluid balance during cardiopulmonary bypass. Perfusion 10:301, 1995
125. Sade RM, Stroud MR, Crawford FA: A prospective, randomized study of hydroxyethyl starch, albumin, and lactated Ringer's solution as priming fluid for cardiopulmonary bypass. J Thorac Cardiovasc Surg 89:713, 1985
126. Russell JA, Navickis RJ, Wilkes MM: Albumin versus crystalloid for pump priming in cardiac surgery: meta-analysis of controlled trials. J Cardiothorac Vasc Anesth 18:429, 2004
127. Brutocao D, Bratton SL, Thomas JR, et al: Comparison of hetastarch with albumin for postoperative volume expansion in children after cardiopulmonary bypass. J Cardiothorac Vasc Anesth 10:348, 1996
128. Hall TS: The pathophysiology of cardiopulmonary bypass. The risks and benefits of hemodilution. Chest 107:1125, 1995
129. Kiziltepe U, Uysalel A, Corapcioglu T, et al: Effects of combined conventional and modified ultrafiltration in adult patients. Ann Thorac Surg 71:684, 2001
130. Briceno JC, Runge TM, McGinity JW, et al: Changes in brain pH, pO_2, pCO_2, cerebral blood flow, and blood gases induced by a hyperosmolar oxyreplete hemsubstitute during cardiopulmonary bypass. ASAIO J 43:13, 1997
131. Vocelka C, et al: A perfluorocarbon emulsion prime additive improves the electroencephalogram and cerebral blood flow at the initiation of cardiopulmonary bypass. J Extracorpor Technol 27:6, 1995
132. Sapsford RN, Blackstone EH, Kirklin JW, et al: Coronary perfusion versus cold ischemic arrest during aortic valve surgery. A randomized study. Circulation 49:1190, 1974
133. Akins CW, Carroll DL: Event-free survival following non-emergency myocardial revascularization during hypothermic fibrillatory arrest. Ann Thorac Surg 43:628, 1987
134. Lolley DM, Ray JF III, Myers WO, et al: Importance of preoperative myocardial glycogen levels in human cardiac preservation. J Thorac Cardiovasc Surg 78:678, 1979
135. Salerno TA, Wasan SM, Charrette EJP: Glucose substrate in myocardial protection. J Thorac Cardiovasc Surg 79:59, 1980
136. Komai H, Yamamoto F, Tanaka K, et al: Harmful effects of inotropic agents on myocardial protection. Ann Thorac Surg 52:927, 1991
137. Schwinn DA, Leone BJ, Spahn DR, et al: Desensitization of myocardial beta-adrenergic receptors during cardiopulmonary bypass. Evidence for early uncoupling and late down regulation. Circulation 84:2559, 1991
138. Roach GW, Kanchuger M, Mora Mangano CT, et al: Adverse cerebral outcomes after coronary bypass surgery. N Engl J Med 335:1857, 1996
139. Reves JG, Karp RB, Buttner EE, et al: Neuronal and adrenomedullary catecholamine release in response to cardiopulmonary bypass in man. Circulation 66:49, 1982
140. Donohoe JF, Ventatachalam MA, Bernard DB, Levinsky NG: Tubular leakage and obstruction after renal ischemia: Structural functional correlations. Kidney Int 13:208, 1978
141. Ramsay JG: The respiratory, renal, and hepatic systems: Effects of cardiac surgery and cardiopulmonary bypass. *In* Mora C (ed): Cardiopulmonary Bypass. New York, Springer-Verlag, 1995, p 147
142. Yeboah ED, Petrie A, Peak JL: Acute renal failure and open heart surgery. Br Med J 1:415, 1972
143. McLeish KR, Loft FC, Kleit SA: Factors affecting prognosis in acute renal failure following cardiac operations. Surg Gynecol Obstet 145:28, 1977
144. Bhat JG, Gluck MC, Lowenstein J, Baldwin DS: Renal failure after open heart surgery. Ann Intern Med 84:677, 1976
145. Gailiunas P Jr, Chawla R, Lazarus JM, et al: Acute renal failure following cardiac operations. J Thorac Cardiovasc Surg 79:241, 1980
146. Lange HW, Aeppli DM, Brown DC: Survival of patients with acute renal failure requiring dialysis after open heart surgery: Early prognostic indicators. Am Heart J 113:1138, 1986
147. Corwin HL, Sprague SM, DeLaria GA, Norusis MJ: Acute renal failure associated with cardiac operations. Thorac Cardiovasc Surg 98:1107, 1989
148. Zanardo G, Michielon P, Paccagnella A, et al: Acute renal failure in the patient undergoing cardiac operation. J Thorac Cardiovasc Surg 107:1489, 1994
149. Mora Mangano CT, Diamondstone LS, Ramsay JG, et al: Renal dysfunction following myocardial revascularization: Risk factors, adverse outcomes and hospital resource utilization. Ann Intern Med 128:194, 1998
150. Perugini RA, Orr RK, Porter D, et al: Gastrointestinal complications following cardiac surgery: An analysis of 1477 cardiac surgery patients. Arch Surg 132:352, 1997
151. Yilmaz AT, Arslan M, Demirkilc U, et al: Gastrointestinal complications after cardiac surgery. Eur J Cardiothorac Surg 10:763, 1996
152. Mercado PD, Farid H, O'Connell TX, et al: Gastrointestinal complications associated with cardiopulmonary bypass procedures. Am Surg 60:789, 1994
153. Gaer JA, Shaw AD, Wild R, et al: Effect of cardiopulmonary bypass on gastrointestinal perfusion and function. Ann Thorac Surg 57:371, 1994
154. Ohri SK, Bowles CW, Mathie RT, et al: Effect of cardiopulmonary bypass perfusion protocols on gut tissue oxygenation and blood flow. Ann Thorac Surg 64:163, 1997
155. Mathie RT: Hepatic blood flow during cardiopulmonary bypass. Crit Care Med 21:S72, 1993
156. Christenson JT, Schmuziger M, Maurice J, et al: Postoperative visceral hypotension-the common cause for gastrointestinal complications after cardiac surgery. Thorac Cardiovasc Surg 42:152, 1994
157. Kumon K, Tanaka K, Hirata T, et al: Organ failures due to low cardiac output syndrome following open heart surgery. Jpn Circ J 50:329, 1986
158. Landow L, Andersen LW: Splanchnic ischaemia and its role in multiple organ failure. Acta Anaesthesiol Scand 38:626, 1994
159. Ohri SK, Bjarnason I, Pathi V, et al: Cardiopulmonary bypass impairs small intestinal transport and increases gut permeability. Ann Thorac Surg 55:1080, 1993
160. Andersen LW, Landow L, Baek L, et al: Association between gastric intramucosal pH and splanchnic endotoxin, antibody to endotoxin, and tumor necrosis factor-alpha concentrations in patients undergoing cardiopulmonary bypass. Crit Care Med 21:210, 1993
161. Collins JD, Bassendine MF, Ferner R, et al: Incidence and prognostic importance of jaundice after cardiopulmonary bypass surgery. Lancet 1:1119, 1983
162. Kazmierczak SC, Van Lente F: Incidence and source of hyperamylasemia after cardiac surgery. Clin Chem 34:916, 1988
163. Rattner DW, Gu ZY, Vlahakes GJ, Warshaw AL: Hyperamylasemia after cardiac surgery. Incidence, significance and management. Ann Surg 209:279, 1989
164. Svensson LG, Deckner G, Kinsley RB: A prospective study of hyperamylasemia and pancreatitis after cardiopulmonary bypass. Ann Thorac Surg 39:409, 1985
165. Replogle R, Levy M, DeWall RA, Lillehei RC: Catecholamine and serotonin response to cardiopulmonary bypass. J Thorac Cardiovasc Surg 44:638, 1962
166. Anand KJS, Phil D, Hansen DD, Hickey PR: Hormonal-metabolic stress responses in neonates undergoing cardiac surgery. Anesthesiology 73:661, 1990
167. Firmin RK, Bouloux P, Alan P: Sympathoadrenal function during cardiac operation in infants with the technique of surface cooling, limited cardiopulmonary bypass, circulatory arrest. J Thorac Cardiovasc Surg 90:729, 1985
168. Faymonville ME, Deby-DuPont G, Larbuisson R: Prostaglandin E_2, prostacyclin, and thromboxane changes during non-pulsatile cardiopulmonary bypass in humans. J Thorac Cardiovasc Surg 91:858, 1986
169. Greeley WJ, Bushman GA, Kong DL: Effects of cardiopulmonary bypass on eicosanoid metabolism during pediatric cardiac surgery. J Thorac Cardiovasc Surg 95:842, 1988
170. Holmes C, Landry D, Granton J: Vasopressin and the cardiovascular system. Crit Care 8:15, 2004
171. Yeager MP, Glass DD, Neff RK, Brinck-Johnsen T: Epidural anesthesia and analgesia in high-risk surgical patients. Anesthesiology 66:729, 1987
172. Moyer E, Cerra F, Chenier R: Multiple systems organ failure. IV. Death predictors in the trauma-septic state: The most critical determinants. J Trauma 21:862, 1981
173. Stanley TH, Berman L, Green O, Robertson D: Plasma catecholamine and cortisol response to fentanyl-oxygen anesthesia for coronary operations. Anesthesiology 53:250, 1980
174. Hug CC Jr, Hall RI, Angert KC: Alfentanil plasma concentrations v. effect relationships in cardiac surgical patients. Br J Anaesth 61:435, 1988
175. Philbin DM, Rosow CE, Schneider RC: Fentanyl and sufentanil anesthesia revisited: How much is enough? Anesthesiology 73:5, 1990
176. Anand KJS, Sippell WG, Anysley-Green A: Randomized trial of fentanyl anesthesia in preterm babies undergoing surgery: Effects on stress-response. Lancet 1:62, 1987
177. Anand KJS, Hickey PR: Halothane-morphine compared with high-dose sufentanil for anesthesia and postoperative analgesia in neonatal cardiac surgery. N Engl J Med 326:1, 1992
178. Metz S, Keats AS: Benefits of a glucose-containing priming solution for cardiopulmonary bypass. Anesth Analg 72:428, 1991
179. Lanier WL: Glucose management during cardiopulmonary bypass: Cardiovascular and neurologic implications. Anesth Analg 72:423, 1991
180. van den Berghe G, Wouters P, Weekers F, et al: Intensive insulin therapy in the critically ill patients. N Engl J Med 345:1359, 2001

181. Furnary AP, Gao G, Grunkemeier GL, et al: Continuous insulin infusion reduces mortality in patients with diabetes undergoing coronary artery bypass grafting. J Thorac Cardiovasc Surg 125:1007, 2003
182. Lazar HL, Chipkin SR, Fitzgerald CA, et al: Tight glycemic control in diabetic coronary artery bypass graft patients improves perioperative outcomes and decreases recurrent ischemic events. Circulation 109:1497, 2004
183. Ahmed Z, Lockhart CH, Weiner M, Klingensmith G: Advances in diabetic management: implications for anesthesia. Anesth Analg 100:666, 2005
184. Coursin DB, Connery LE, Ketzler JT: Perioperative diabetic and hyperglycemic management issues. Crit Care Med 32:S116, 2004
185. Finney SJ, Zekveld C, Elia A, Evans TW: Glucose control and mortality in critically ill patients. JAMA 290:2041, 2003
186. Gu W, Pagel PS, Warltier DC, Kersten JR: Modifying cardiovascular risk in diabetes mellitus. Anesthesiology 98:774, 2003
187. Holland FW, Brown PS Jr, Weintraub BD, Clark RE: Cardiopulmonary bypass and thyroid function: A "euthyroid sick syndrome." Ann Thorac Surg 52:46, 1991
188. Schwartz HL, Schadlow AR, Faierman D, et al: Heparin administration appears to decrease cellular binding of thyroxine. J Clin Endocrinol Metab 36:598, 1973
189. Saeed-uz-Zafar M, Miller JM, Breneman GM, Mansour J: Observations on the effect of heparin on free and total thyroxine. J Clin Endocrinol Metab 32:633, 1971
190. Herschman JM, Jones CM, Bailey AL: Reciprocal changes in serum thyrotropin and free thyroxine produced by heparin. J Clin Endocrinol Metab 34:574, 1972
191. Taylor KM, Wright GS, Bain WH, et al: Comparative studies of pulsatile and nonpulsatile flow during cardiopulmonary bypass. III. Response of anterior pituitary gland to thyrotropin-releasing hormone. J Thorac Cardiovasc Surg 75:579, 1978
192. Novitzky D, Human PA, Cooper DK: Effect of triiodothyronine (T_3) on myocardial high energy phosphates and lactate after ischemia and cardiopulmonary bypass. An experimental study in baboons. J Thorac Cardiovasc Surg 96:600, 1988
193. Novitzky D, Human PA, Cooper DK: Inotropic effect of triiodothyronine following myocardial ischemia and cardiopulmonary bypass: An experimental study in pigs. Ann Thorac Surg 45:50, 1988
194. Dyke CM, Ding M, Abd-Elfattah AS, et al: Effects of triiodothyronine supplementation after myocardial ischemia. Ann Thorac Surg 56:215, 1993
195. Kadletz M, Mullen PG, Ding M, et al: Effect of triiodothyronine on postischemic myocardial function in the isolated heart. Ann Thorac Surg 57:657, 1994
196. Dyke CM, Yeh T Jr, Lehman JD, et al: Triiodothyronine-enhanced left ventricular function after ischemic injury. Ann Thorac Surg 52:14, 1991
197. Broderick TJ, Wechsler AS: Triiodothyronine in cardiac surgery. Thyroid 7:133, 1997
198. Novitzky D, Cooper DK, Barton CI, et al: Triiodothyronine as an inotropic agent after open heart surgery. J Thorac Cardiovasc Surg 98:972, 1989
199. Teiger E, Menasche P, Mansier P, et al: Triiodothyronine therapy in open-heart surgery: From hope to disappointment. Eur Heart J 14:629, 1993
200. Klemperer JD, Klein I, Gomez M, et al: Thyroid hormone treatment after coronary-artery bypass surgery. N Engl J Med 333:1522, 1995
201. Chenoweth DE, Cooper SW, Hugli TE, et al: Complement activation during cardiopulmonary bypass: Evidence for generation of C3a and C5a anaphylatoxins. N Engl J Med 304:497, 1981
202. Kirklin JK, Chenoweth DE, Naftel DC, et al: Effects of protamine administration after cardiopulmonary bypass on complement, blood elements, and the hemodynamic state. Ann Thorac Surg 41:193, 1986
203. Best N, Sinosich MJ, Teinser B: Complement activation during cardiopulmonary bypass by heparin-protamine interaction. Br J Anaesth 56:339, 1984
204. Best N, Teisner B, Grudzinskas JG, Fisher MM: Classical pathway activation during an adverse response to protamine sulfate. Br J Anaesth 55:1149, 1983
205. Dreyer WJ, Smith CW, Entman ML: Neutrophil activation during cardiopulmonary bypass [invited letter concerning]. J Thorac Cardiovasc Surg 102:318, 1991
206. Markewitz A, Faist E, Lang S, et al: An imbalance in T-helper cell subsets alters immune response after cardiac surgery. Eur J Cardiothorac Surg 10:61, 1996
207. Markewitz A, Faist E, Weinhold C, et al: Alterations of cell-mediated immune response following cardiac surgery. Eur J Cardiothorac Surg 7:193, 1993
208. De Waal, Malefyt R, Abrams J, et al: Interleukin 10 (IL-10) inhibits cytokine synthesis by human monocytes: An autoregulatory role of IL-10 produced by monocytes. J Exp Med 174:1209, 1991
209. Nilsson L, Nilsson V, Venge P, et al: Inflammatory system activation during cardiopulmonary bypass as an indicator of biocompatibility: A randomized comparison of bubble and membrane oxygenators. Scand J Thorac Cardiovasc Surg 24:53, 1990
210. Videm V, Fosse E, Mollnes TE, et al: Complement activation with bubble and membrane oxygenators in aortocoronary bypass grafting. Ann Thorac Surg 50:387, 1990
211. Butler J, Chong GL, Baigrie RJ, et al: Cytokine responses to cardiopulmonary bypass with membrane and bubble oxygenation. Ann Thorac Surg 53:833, 1992
212. Cavarocchi NC, Pluth JR, Schaff HB: Complement activation during cardiopulmonary bypass. Comparison of bubble and membrane oxygenators. J Thorac Cardiovasc Surg 91:252, 1986
213. Tamiya T, Yamasaki M, Yoshinobu M: Complement activation in cardiopulmonary bypass with special reference to anaphylatoxin production in membrane and bubble oxygenators. Ann Thorac Surg 46:47, 1988
214. Hammerschmidt DE, Stroncek DF, Bowers TK, et al: Complement activation and neutropenia occurring during cardiopulmonary bypass. J Thorac Cardiovasc Surg 81:370, 1981
215. Jones HM, Matthews N, Vaughn RS: Cardiopulmonary bypass and complement activation: Involvement and classical and alternative pathways. Anaesthesia 37:629, 1982
216. Fosse E, Moen D, Johnson E, et al: Reduced complement and granulocyte activation with heparin-coated cardiopulmonary bypass. Ann Thorac Surg 58:472, 1994
217. Gu YJ, van Deveren W, Akkerman C, et al: Heparin-coated circuits reduce the inflammatory response to cardiopulmonary bypass. Ann Thorac Surg 55:917, 1993
218. Videm V, Svennevig JL, Fosse E, et al: Reduced complement activation with heparin-coated oxygenator and tubings in coronary bypass operations. J Thorac Cardiovasc Surg 103:806, 1992
219. Millar AB, Armstrong L, vander Linden J, et al: Cytokine production and hemofiltration in children undergoing cardiopulmonary bypass. Ann Thorac Surg 56:1499, 1993
220. Journois D, Israel-Biet D, Pouard P, et al: High-volume zero-balanced hemofiltration to reduce delayed inflammatory response to cardiopulmonary bypass in children. Anesthesiology 85:965, 1996
221. Journois D, Pouard P, Rolland B, et al: Ultrafiltration allows to reduce cytokine plasma concentrations during pediatric cardiopulmonary bypass. Contrib Nephrol 116:86, 1995
222. Journois D, Pouard P, Greeley WJ, et al: Hemofiltration during cardiopulmonary bypass in pediatric cardiac surgery. Effects on hemostasis, cytokines and complement components. Anesthesiology 81:1181, 1994
223. Jorens PG, De Jongh R, De Backer W, et al: Interleukin-8 production in patients undergoing cardiopulmonary bypass. The influence of pretreatment with methylprednisolone. Am Rev Respir Dis 148:1993
224. Hill GE, Alonso A, Thiele GM, et al: Glucocorticoids blunt neutrophil CD11b surface glycoprotein upregulation during cardiopulmonary bypass in humans. Anesth Analg 79:23, 1994
225. Engelman RM, Rousou JA, Flack JE 3rd, et al: Influence of steroids on complement and cytokine generation after cardiopulmonary bypass. Ann Thorac Surg 60:801, 1995
226. van Overveld FJ, et al: Pretreatment with methylprednisolone in coronary artery bypass grafting influences the levels of histamine and tryptase in serum but not in bronchoalveolar lavage fluid. Clin Sci 86:49, 1994
227. Tabardel Y, Duchateau J, Schmartz D, et al: Corticosteroids increase blood interleukin-10 levels during cardiopulmonary bypass in men. Surgery 119:76, 1996
228. Parrillo JE: Pathogenetic mechanisms of septic shock. N Engl J Med 328:1471, 1993
229. Boscoe MJ, Yeudall VMA, Thompson MA: Complement activation during cardiopulmonary bypass: Quantitative study of effects of methylprednisolone and pulsatile flow. Br Med J 287:1747, 1983
230. Hill GE, Pohorecki R, Alonso A, et al: Aprotonin reduces interleukin-8 production and lung neutrophil accumulation after cardiopulmonary bypass. Anesth Analg 83:696, 1996
231. Ashraf S, Tian Y, Cowan D, et al: "Low-dose" aprotinin modifies hemostasis but not proinflammatory cytokine release. Ann Thorac Surg 63:68, 1997
232. Markewitz A, Faist E, Lang S, et al: Successful restoration of cell-mediated immune response after cardiopulmonary bypass by immunomodulation. J Thorac Cardiovasc Surg 105:15, 1993

233. Davies GG, Wells DG, Mabee TM: Platelet-leukocyte plasmapheresis attenuates the deleterious effects of cardiopulmonary bypass. Ann Thorac Surg 53:274, 1992
234. Verrier ED, Shernan SK, Taylor KM, et al: Terminal complement blockade with pexelizumab during coronary artery bypass graft surgery requiring cardiopulmonary bypass. JAMA 291:2319, 2004
235. Jones RH: The year in cardiovascular surgery. J Am Coll Cardiol 45:1517, 2005
236. Mills NL, Everson CT: Atherosclerosis of the ascending aorta and coronary artery bypass. Pathology, clinical correlates, and operative management. J Thorac Cardiovasc Surg 102:546, 1991
237. Wareing TH, Davila-Roman VG, Barzilai B, et al: Management of the severely atherosclerotic ascending aorta during cardiac operations: A strategy for detection and treatment. J Thorac Cardiovasc Surg 103:453, 1992
238. Ohteki H, Itoh T, Natsuaki M, et al: Intraoperative ultrasonic imaging of the ascending aorta in ischemic heart disease. Ann Thorac Surg 50:539, 1990
239. Magilligan DJ Jr, Eastland MW, Lell WA, et al: Decreased carotid flow with ascending aortic cannulation. Circulation 45:130, 1972
240. Benedict JS, Buhl TL, Henney RP: Acute aortic dissection during cardiopulmonary bypass. Successful treatment of three patients. Arch Surg 108:810, 1974
241. Still RJ, Hilgenberg AD, Atkins CW, et al: Intraoperative aortic dissection. Ann Thorac Surg 53:374, 1992
242. Barzilai B, Marshall WG, Saffitz JE, Kouchoukos N: Avoidance of embolic complications by ultrasonic characterization of the ascending aorta. Circulation 80:1, 1989
243. Coselli JS, Crawford ES: Aortic valve replacement in the patient with extensive calcification of the ascending aorta (a porcelain aorta). J Thorac Cardiovasc Surg 91:184, 1986
244. Pillai R, Venn G, Lennox S, Paneth M: Elective femoro-femoral bypass for operations on the heart and great vessels. J Thorac Cardiovasc Surg 88:635, 1984
245. Bennett EV Jr, Fewel JG, Ybarra J, et al: Comparison of flow differences among venous cannulas. Ann Thorac Surg 36:59, 1983
246. Rosenfeldt FL, Watson DA: Interference with local myocardial cooling by heat gain during aortic cross-clamping. Ann Thorac Surg 27:13, 1979
247. Johnston WE, Royster RL, Choplin RH: Pulmonary artery catheter migration during cardiac surgery. Anesthesiology 64:258, 1986
248. Bromley JJ, Moorthy SS: Acute angulation of a pulmonary artery catheter (letter). Anesthesiology 59:367, 1983
249. Campbell FW, Schwartz AJ: Pulmonary artery catheter malfunction? Anesthesiology 65:13, 1984
250. Mantia AM, Robinson JN, Lolley DM: Sternal retraction and pulmonary artery catheter compromise. J Cardiothorac Vasc Anesth 2:430, 1988
251. Baraka A, Darwish R, Mora Mangano CT: Drastic mixed venous hemoglobin desaturation in a patient during hypothermic cardiopulmonary bypass. J Cardiothorac Vasc Anesth 9:764, 1995
252. Hall RI, Thomas BL, Hug CC Jr: Pharmacokinetics and pharmacodynamics during cardiac surgery and cardiopulmonary bypass. *In* Mora C (ed): Cardiopulmonary Bypass: Principles and Techniques of Extracorporeal Circulation. New York, Springer-Verlag, 1995, p 55
253. Gordon RJ, Ravin M, Rawitscher RE, Daicoff GR: Changes in arterial pressure, viscosity, and resistance during cardiopulmonary bypass. J Thorac Cardiovasc Surg 69:552, 1975
254. Schaff HV, Ciardullo RC, Flaherty JT, Gott VL: Development of regional myocardial ischemia distal to a critical coronary stenosis during cardiopulmonary bypass: Comparison of the fibrillating vs. the beating nonworking states. Surgery 83:57, 1978
255. Mark JB, Greenberg LM: Intraoperative awareness and hypertensive crisis during high-dose fentanyl-diazepam-oxygen anesthesia. Anesth Analg 62:698, 1983
256. Liu E, Dhara S: Monitoring oxygenator expiratory isoflurane concentrations and the bispectral index to guide isoflurane requirements during cardiopulmonary bypass. J Cardiothorac Vasc Anesth 19:485, 2005
257. Davis FM, Parimelazhagan KN, Harris EA: Thermal balance during cardiopulmonary bypass with moderate hypothermia in man. Br J Anaesth 49:1127, 1977
258. Noback CR, Tinker JH: Hypothermia after cardiopulmonary bypass in man: Amelioration by nitroprusside-induced vasodilation during rewarming. Anesthesiology 53:277, 1980
259. Jani K, Carli F, Bidstrup BP: Changes in body temperature following cardiopulmonary bypass procedures: The effects of active rewarming. Life Support Syst 4:269, 1986
260. Ralley FE, Ramsay JG, Wynands JE: Effect of heated humidified gases on temperature drop after cardiopulmonary bypass. Anesth Analg 63:1106, 1984
261. Clark J, Bar-Yosef S, Anderson A, et al: Postoperative hyperthermia following off-pump versus on-pump coronary artery bypass surgery. J Cardiothorac Vasc Anesth 19:426, 2005
262. Nathan HJ, Polis T: The management of temperature during hypothermic cardiopulmonary bypass: II. Effect of prolonged hypothermia. Can J Anaesth 42:672, 1995
263. Cook DJ, Orszulak TA, Buda DA, et al: Cerebral hyperthermia during cardiopulmonary bypass in adults. J Thorac Cardiovasc Surg 111:269, 1996
264. Mohr R, Lavee J, Goor DA: Inaccuracy of radial artery pressure measurement after cardiac operations. J Thorac Cardiovasc Surg 94:286, 1987
265. Gravlee GP, Wong AB, Adkins TG: A comparison of radial, brachial, and aortic pressures after cardiopulmonary bypass. J Cardiothorac Vasc Anesth 3:20, 1989
266. Oka Y, Inoue T, Hong Y, et al: Retained intracardiac air. Transesophageal echocardiography for definition of incidence and monitoring removal by improved techniques. J Thorac Cardiovasc Surg 91:329, 1986
267. Persson M, Svenarud P, van der Linden J: What is the optimal device for carbon dioxide deairing of the cardiothoracic wound and how should it be positioned? J Cardiothorac Vasc Anesth 18:180, 2004
268. Robicsek P, Duncan GD: Retrograde air embolization in coronary operations. J Thorac Cardiovasc Surg 94:110, 1987
269. Clark RE, Brillman J, Davis DA, et al: Microemboli during coronary artery bypass grafting: Genesis and effect on outcome. J Thorac Cardiovasc Surg 109:249, 1995
270. Lake CL, Sellers TD, Nolan SP: Energy dose and other variables possibly affecting ventricular fibrillation during cardiac surgery. Anesth Analg 63:743, 1984
271. Baraka A, Kawkabani N, Dabbous A, Nawfal M: Lidocaine for prevention of reperfusion ventricular fibrillation after release of aortic cross-clamping. J Cardiothorac Vasc Anesth 14:531, 2000
272. Fletcher R, Veintemilla F: Changes in the arterial to end-tidal P_{CO_2} differences during coronary artery bypass grafting. Acta Anaesthesiol Scand 33:656, 1989
273. Crystal GJ, Ruiz JR, Rooney MW, Salem MR: Regional hemodynamics and oxygen supply during isovolemic hemodilution in the absence and presence of high-grade beta-adrenergic blockade. J Cardiothorac Vasc Anesth 2:772, 1988
274. Kleinberg PL, Kam CA, Johnson DC: Hematocrit and blood volume control during cardiopulmonary bypass with the use of hemofiltration. Anesthesiology 60:478, 1984
275. Hindman BJ: Sodium bicarbonate in the treatment of subtypes of acute lactic acidosis: Physiologic considerations. Anesthesiology 72:1064, 1990
276. Kaplan JA, Guffin AB, Yin A: The effects of metabolic acidosis and alkalosis on the response to sympathomimetic drugs in dogs. J Cardiothorac Vasc Anesth 2:481, 1988
277. Robertie PG, Butterworth JF, Royster RL: Normal parathyroid hormone response to hypocalcemia during cardiopulmonary bypass. Anesthesiology 73:43, 1991
278. Hosking MP: Should calcium be administered prior to separation from cardiopulmonary bypass (letter)? Anesthesiology 75:1121, 1991
279. Watson BG: Unilateral cold neck. A new sign of misplacement of the aortic cannula during cardiopulmonary bypass. Anaesthesia 38:659, 1983
280. Dalal BG, Patel KD: Another sign of inadvertent carotid cannulation (letter). Anesthesiology 55:1981
281. Chapin JW, Nance P, Yarbrough JW: Facial paleness (letter). Anesth Analg 61:745, 1982
282. Ross WT, Lake CL, Wellons HA: Cardiopulmonary bypass complicated by inadvertent carotid cannulation. Anesthesiology 54:85, 1981
283. Sudhaman DA: Accidental hyperperfusion of the left carotid artery during CPB (letter). J Cardiothorac Vasc Anesth 5:100, 1991
284. McLeskey CH, Cheney PW: A correctable complication of cardiopulmonary bypass. Anesthesiology 56:214, 1982
285. Salerno TA, Lince DP, White DN: Arch versus femoral artery perfusion during cardiopulmonary bypass. J Thorac Cardiovasc Surg 76:681, 1978
286. Carey JS, Skow JR, Scott C: Retrograde aortic dissection during cardiopulmonary bypass: "Nonoperative management." Ann Thorac Surg 24:44, 1977
287. Murphy DA, Craver JM, Jones EL: Recognition and management of ascending aortic dissection complicating cardiac surgical operations. J Thorac Cardiovasc Surg 85:247, 1983
288. Troianos CA, Savino JS, Weiss RL: Transesophageal echocardiographic diagnosis of aortic dissection during cardiac surgery. Anesthesiology 75:149, 1991

289. Michaels I, Sheehan J: EEG changes due to unsuspected aortic dissection during cardiopulmonary bypass. Anesth Analg 63:946, 1984
290. Stoney WS, Alford WC, Burrus GR: Air embolism and other accidents using pump oxygenators. Ann Thorac Surg 29:336, 1980
291. Mills NL, Ochsner JL: Massive air embolism during cardiopulmonary bypass. Causes, prevention, and management. J Thorac Cardiovasc Surg 80:708, 1980
292. Tomatis L, Nemiroff M, Riahi M: Massive arterial air embolism due to rupture of pulsatile assist device: Successful treatment in the hyperbaric chamber. Ann Thorac Surg 32:604, 1981
293. Hayal HA, Wang AM: CT diagnosis of delayed cerebral air embolism following intraaortic balloon pump catheter insertion. Comput Radiol 10:307, 1986
294. Fritz H, Hossmann KA: Arterial air embolism in the cat brain. Stroke 10:581, 1979
295. Kort A, Kronzon I: Microbubble formation: In vitro and in vivo observation. J Clin Ultrasound 10:117, 1982
296. Feinstein SB, Shah PM, Bing RJ: Microbubble dynamics visualized in the intact capillary circulation. J Am Coll Cardiol 4:595, 1984
297. Helps SC, Meyer-Witting M, Reilly PL, Gorman DF: Increasing doses of intracarotid air and cerebral blood flow in rabbits. Stroke 21:1340, 1990
298. Hekmatpanah J: Cerebral microvascular alterations in arterial air embolism. Adv Neurol 20:245, 1978
299. Menkin M, Schwartzman RJ: Cerebral air embolism. Arch Neurol 34:168, 1977
300. Warren BA, Philp RB, Inwood MJ: The ultrastructural morphology of air embolism: Platelet adhesion to the interface and endothelial damage. Br J Exp Pathol 54:163, 1973
301. Butler BD, Kurusz M: Gaseous microemboli: A review. Perfusion 5:81, 1990
302. Armon C, Deschamps C, Adkinson C: Hyperbaric treatment of cerebral air embolism sustained during an open-heart surgical procedure. Mayo Clin Proc 66:565, 1991
303. Steward D, Williams WG, Freedom R: Hypothermia in conjunction with hyperbaric oxygenation in the treatment of massive air embolism during cardiopulmonary bypass. Ann Thorac Surg 24:591, 1977
304. Bayindir O, Paker T, Akpinar B: Case Conference: Massive air embolism during cardiopulmonary bypass. J Cardiothorac Vasc Anesth 5:627, 1991
305. Bojar RM, Najafi H, DeLaria GA: Neurological complications of coronary revascularization. Ann Thorac Surg 36:427, 1983
306. Voorhies RM, Fraser RAR: Cerebral air embolism occurring at angiography and diagnosed by computerized tomography. J Neurosurg 60:177, 1984
307. Furlow TW: Experimental air embolism of the brain: An analysis of the technique in the rat. Stroke 13:847, 1982
308. Pierce EC: Specific therapy for air embolism. Ann Thorac Surg 29:800, 1980
309. Layton AJ: Hyperbaric oxygen treatment for cerebral air embolism-where are the data (editorial)? Mayo Clin Proc 66:641, 1991
310. Stark J, Hough J: Air in the aorta: Treatment by reversed perfusion. Ann Thorac Surg 41:337, 1986
311. Brown JW, Dierdorf SF, Moorthy SS, Halpin M: Venoarterial cerebral perfusion for treatment of massive arterial air embolism. Anesth Analg 66:673, 1987
312. Hendricks FFA, Bogers AJJC, de la Riviere AB: The effectiveness of venoarterial perfusion in treatment of arterial air embolism during cardiopulmonary bypass. Ann Thorac Surg 36:433, 1983
313. Arnoni RT, Arnoni AS, Bonini RC, et al: Risk factors associated with cardiac surgery during pregnancy. Ann Thorac Surg 75:1605, 2003
314. Jacobs WM, Cooley D, Goen GP: Cardiac surgery with extracorporeal circulation. Report of 3 cases. Obstet Gynecol 25:167, 1965
315. Zitnik RS, Brandenburg RO, Sheldon R: Pregnancy and open heart surgery. Circulation 39(suppl):125, 1969
316. Becker RM: Intracardiac surgery in pregnant women. Ann Thorac Surg 36:453, 1983
317. Lapiedra OJ, Bernal JM, Ninot S: Open heart surgery for thrombosis of a prosthetic mitral valve during pregnancy: Fetal hydrocephalus. J Cardiovasc Surg (Torino) 27:217, 1986
318. Pomini F, Mercogliano D, Cavalletti C, et al: Cardiopulmonary bypass in pregnancy. Ann Thorac Surg 61:259, 1996
319. Levinson G, Shnider SM: Anesthesia for surgery during pregnancy. *In* Shnider S, Levinson G (eds): Anesthesia for Obstetrics. Baltimore, Williams & Wilkins, 1987, p 188
320. Bahary CM, Ninio A, Gorodesky IG, Neri A: Tococardiography in pregnancy during extracorporeal bypass for mitral valve replacement. Isr J Med Sci 16:395, 1980
321. Mora CT, Grunewald KE: Preoperative aortic and mitral prosthetic valve replacement in the third trimester of pregnancy. J Cardiothorac Anesth 1:313, 1987
322. Lamb MP, Manners JM: Fetal heart monitoring during open heart surgery. Br J Obstet Gynaecol 88:669, 1981
323. Koh KS, Friesen RM, Livingston RA: Fetal monitoring during maternal cardiac surgery with cardiopulmonary. Can Med Assoc J 112:1102, 1975
324. Werch A, Lambert HM: Fetal monitoring and maternal open heart surgery. South Med J 70:1024, 1977
325. Trimakas AP, Maxwell KD, Berkay S, et al: Fetal monitoring during cardiopulmonary bypass for removal of a left atrial myxoma during pregnancy. Johns Hopkins Med J 144:156, 1979
326. Asali NS, Westin B: Effects of hypothermia on uterine circulation in the fetus. Proc Soc Exp Biol Med 109:485, 1962
327. Pardi G, Ferrari MM, Iorio F, et al: The effect of maternal hypothermic cardiopulmonary bypass on fetal lamb temperature, hemodynamics, oxygenation, and acid-base balance. J Thorac Cardiovasc Surg 127:1728, 2004
328. Jadhon ME, Main EK: Fetal bradycardia associated with maternal hypothermia. Obstet Gynecol 72:496, 1988
329. Bigelow WG, Lindsay WK, Greenwood WF: Hypothermia: Its possible role in cardiac surgery. Ann Surg 132:849, 1950
330. Gibbon JH Jr, Dobell AR, Voigt GB, et al: The closure of interventricular septal defects on dogs during open cardiotomy with the maintenance of the cardiorespiratory functions by a pump oxygenator. J Thorac Surg 28:235, 1954
331. Splittgerber FH, Talbert JG, Sweezer WP, Wilson RF: Partial cardiopulmonary bypass for core rewarming in profound accidental hypothermia. Am Surg 52:407, 1986
332. Danzl DF, Prozos RS: Accidental hypothermia. A review article. N Engl J Med 331:1756, 1994
333. Walpoth BH, Locher T, Leupi F, et al: Accidental deep hypothermia with cardiopulmonary arrest: Extracorporeal blood rewarming in 11 patients. Eur J Cardiothorac Surg 4:390, 1990
334. Walpoth BH, Walpoth-Aslan BN, Mattle HP, et al: Outcome of survivors of accidental deep hypothermia and circulatory arrest treated with extracorporeal blood warming. N Engl J Med 337:1500, 1997
335. Silverberg GD, Reitz BA, Ream AK: Hypothermia and cardiac arrest in the treatment of giant aneurysms of the cerebral circulation and hemangioblastoma of the medulla. J Neurosurg 55:337, 1981
336. Baumgartner WA, Silverberg GD, Ream AK: Reappraisal of cardiopulmonary bypass with deep hypothermia and circulatory arrest for complex neurosurgical operations. J Surg 242:242, 1983
337. Richards PG, Marath A, Rice-Edwards JM: Management of difficult intracranial aneurysms by deep hypothermia and elective cardiac arrest using cardiopulmonary bypass. Br J Neurosurg 1:261, 1987
338. Spetzler RF, Hadley MN, Rigamonti D: Aneurysms of the basilar artery treated with circulatory arrest, hypothermia, and barbiturate cerebral protection. J Neurosurg 68:868, 1988
339. Williams MD, Ranier WG, Fieger HG: Cardiopulmonary bypass, profound hypothermia, and circulatory arrest for neurosurgery. Ann Thorac Surg 52:1069, 1991
340. Solomon RA, Smith CR, Raps EC: Deep hypothermic circulatory arrest for the management of complex anterior and posterior circulation aneurysms. Neurosurgery 29:732, 1991
341. Levy J: Heparin resistance and antithrombin: should it still be called heparin resistance? J Cardiothorac Vasc Anesth 18:129, 2004
342. Esposito RA, Culliford AT, Colvin SB, et al: Heparin resistance during cardiopulmonary bypass. The role of heparin pretreatment. J Thorac Cardiovasc Surg 85:346, 1983
343. Cloyd GM, D'Ambra MN, Akins CW: Diminished anticoagulant response to heparin in patients undergoing coronary artery bypass grafting. J Thorac Cardiovasc Surg 94:535, 1987
344. Sabbagh AH, Chung GK, Shuttleworth P, et al: Fresh frozen plasma: A solution to heparin resistance during cardiopulmonary bypass. Ann Thorac Surg 37:466, 1984
345. Levy J, Despotis G, Szlam F, et al: Recombinant human transgenic antithrombin in cardiac surgery: a dose-finding study. Anesthesiology 96:1095, 2002
346. Weiss BM, von Segesser LK, Turina MI, et al: Perioperative course and recovery after heparin-coated cardiopulmonary bypass: Low-dose versus high-dose heparin management. J Cardiothorac Vasc Anesth 10:464, 1996
347. von Segesser LK: Heparin-bonded surfaces in extracorporeal membrane oxygenation for cardiac support. Ann Thorac Surg 61:330, 1996
348. Jones DR, Hill RC, Vasilakis A, et al: Safe use of heparin-coated bypass circuits incorporating a pump-oxygenator. Ann Thorac Surg 57:815, 1994

349. Ovrum E, Holen EA, Tangen G, et al: Completely heparinized cardiopulmonary bypass and reduced systemic heparin: Clinical and hemostatic effects. Ann Thorac Surg 60:365, 1995
350. Warkentin TE: Heparin-induced thrombocytopenia: IgG-mediated platelet activation, platelet microparticle generation, and altered procoagulant/anticoagulant balance in the pathogenesis of thrombosis and venous limb gangrene complicating heparin-induced thrombocytopenia. Transfus Med Rev 10:249, 1996
351. King DJ, Kelton JG: Heparin-associated thrombocytopenia. Ann Intern Med 100:535, 1984
352. Kappa JR, Fischer CA, Todd B, et al: Intraoperative management of patients with heparin-induced thrombocytopenia. Ann Thorac Surg 49:714, 1990
353. Warkentin TE, Levine MN, Hirsh J, et al: Heparin-induced thrombocytopenia in patients treated with low-molecular-weight heparin or unfractionated heparin. N Engl J Med 332:1330, 1995
354. Gouault-Heilmann M, Huet Y, Contant G, et al: Cardiopulmonary bypass with a low-molecular-weight heparin fraction. Lancet 2:1374, 1983
355. Altes A, Martino R, Gari M, et al: Heparin-induced thrombocytopenia and heart operation: Management with tedelparin. Ann Thorac Surg 59:508, 1995
356. Robitaille D, Leclerc JR, Laberge R, et al: Cardiopulmonary bypass with a low-molecular-weight heparin fraction (enoxaparin) in a patient with a history of heparin-associated thrombocytopenia. J Thorac Cardiovasc Surg 103:597, 1992
357. Brister SJ, Ofosu FA, Heingenhauser GJ, et al: Is heparin the ideal anticoagulant for cardiopulmonary bypass? Dermatan sulphate may be an alternate choice. Thromb Haemost 71:468, 1994
358. Brister SJ, Buchanan MR: Heparinless cardiopulmonary bypass revisited: A newer strategy to avoid heparin-related bleeding using dermatan sulfate. J Cardiothorac Vasc Anesth 9:317, 1995
359. Koster A, Fischer T, Gruendel M, et al: Management of heparin resistance during cardiopulmonary bypass: The effect of five different anticoagulation strategies on hemostatic activation. J Cardiothorac Vasc Anesth 17:171, 2003
360. Riess FC, Löwer C, Seelig C, et al: Recombinant hirudin as a new anticoagulant during cardiac operations instead of heparin: Successful for aortic valve replacement in man. J Thorac Cardiovasc Surg 110:265, 1995
361. Koster A, Spiess B, Chew D, et al: Effectiveness of bivalirudin as a replacement for heparin during cardiopulmonary bypass in patients undergoing coronary artery bypass grafting. Am J Cardiol 93:356, 2004
362. Beijering RJ, ten Cate H, Nurmohamed MT, ten Cate JW: Anticoagulants and extracorporeal circuits. Semin Thromb Hemost 23:225, 1997
363. Stevens JH, Burdon TA, Peters WS, et al: Port-access coronary artery bypass grafting: A proposed surgical method. J Thorac Cardiovasc Surg 111:567, 1996
364. Schwartz DS, Ribakove GH, Grossi EA, et al: Single and multivessel port-access coronary artery bypass grafting with cardioplegic arrest: Technique and reproducibility. J Thorac Cardiovasc Surg 114:46, 1997
365. Siegel LC, St. Goar FG, Stevens JH, et al: Monitoring considerations for port-access cardiac surgery. Circulation 96:562, 1997
366. Nuttall GA, Cook DJ, Fulgham JR, et al: The relationship between cerebral blood flow and transcranial Doppler blood flow velocity during hypothermic cardiopulmonary bypass in adults. Anesth Analg 82:1146, 1996
367. Mohr FW, Falk V, Diegeler A, et al: Minimally invasive port-access mitral valve surgery. J Thorac Cardiovasc Surg 115:567, 1998
368. Gaba DM, Maxwell M, DeAnda A: Anesthetic mishaps: Breaking the chain of accident evolution. Anesthesiology 66:670, 1987
369. Kirklin JW, Barratt-Boyes BG: Cardiac Surgery. New York, Wiley, 1985
370. Pasque MK, Wechsler AS: Metabolic intervention to affect myocardial recovery following ischemia. Ann Surg 200:1, 1984
371. Lake CL, Sellers TD, Noland SP, et al: Determinants of reperfusion cardiac electrical activity after cold cardioplegic arrest during coronary bypass surgery. Am J Cardiol 54:519, 1984
372. Reves JG, Karp RB, Buttner EE, et al: Neuronal and adrenomedullary catecholamine release in response to cardiopulmonary bypass in man. Circulation 66:49, 1982
373. Lazar HL, Buckberg GD, Foglia RP, et al: Detrimental effects of premature use of inotropic drugs to discontinue cardiopulmonary bypass. J Thorac Cardiovasc Surg 82:18, 1981
374. Simons M, Downing SE: Coronary vasoconstriction and catecholamine cardiomyopathy. Am Heart J 109:297, 1985
375. Swan H: The importance of acid-base management for cardiac and cerebral preservation during open heart operations. Surg Gynecol Obstet 158:391, 1984
376. Foglia RP, Steed DL, Follette DM, et al: Iatrogenic myocardial edema with potassium cardioplegia. J Thorac Cardiovasc Surg 78:217, 1979
377. Engleman RM, Rousou JH, Lemeshow S, et al: The metabolic consequences of blood and crystalloid cardioplegia. Circulation 64:II-67, 1981
378. Buttner EE, Karp RB, Reves JG, et al: A randomized comparison of crystalloid and blood-containing cardioplegic solutions in 60 patients. Circulation 69:973, 1984
379. Kloner RA, Ganote CE, Whalen DA, et al: Effect of a transient period of ischemia on myocardial cells. Am J Pathol 74:399, 1974
380. Rosenblum HM, Haasler GB, Spotnitz WD, et al: Effects of simulated clinical cardiopulmonary bypass and cardioplegia on mass of the canine left ventricle. Ann Thorac Surg 39:139, 1985
381. Singh AK, Corwin RD, Teplitz C, et al: Consecutive repair of complex congenital heart diseases using hypothermic cardioplegia arrest—its results and ultrastructural study of the myocardium. J Thorac Cardiovasc Surg 32:23, 1984
382. Huddleston CB, Hammon JW Jr, Wareing TH, et al: Amelioration of the deleterious effects of platelets activated during cardiopulmonary bypass. Comparison of a thromboxane synthetase inhibitor and a prostacyclin analogue. J Thorac Cardiovasc Surg 89:190, 1985
383. Rosenbaum D, Levitsky S, Silverman N, et al: Cardioplegia does not prevent reperfusion injury induced by intracoronary platelet deposition. Circulation 68:II-102, 1983
384. McDonagh PF, Laks H: Use of cold blood cardioplegia to protect against coronary microcirculatory injury due to ischemia and reperfusion. J Thorac Cardiovasc Surg 84:609, 1982
385. Humphrey SM, Gavin JB, Herdson PB: The relationship of ischemic contracture to vascular reperfusion in the isolated rat heart. J Mol Cell Cardiol 12:1397, 1980
386. Lee BY, Wilson GJ, Domenech RJ, et al: Relative role of edema versus contracture in the myocardial postischemic "no-reflow" phenomenon. J Surg Res 29:50, 1980
387. Klooker P, Hilse B, Mittmann U, et al: Myocardial function, blood flow, and metabolism with different forms of myocardial protection. J Thorac Cardiovasc Surg 30:393, 1982
388. Bomfin V, Kaijser L, Bendz R, et al: Myocardial protection during aortic valve replacement. Cardiac metabolism and enzyme release following continuous blood cardioplegia. Scand J Thorac Cardiovasc Surg 15:141, 1981
389. Flameng W, Borgers M, Daenen W, et al: St. Thomas cardioplegia versus topical cooling: Ultrastructural and biochemical studies in humans. Ann Thorac Surg 31:339, 1981
390. Kaijser L, Jansson E, Schmidt W, et al: Myocardial energy depletion during profound hypothermic cardioplegia for cardiac operations. J Thorac Cardiovasc Surg 90:896, 1985
391. Silverman NA, Kohler J, Feinberg H, et al: Beneficial metabolic effect of nucleotide augmentation on reperfusion injury following cardioplegic arrest. Chest 83:787, 1983
392. Ward HB, St. Cry JA, Cogordan JA, et al: Recovery of adenine nucleotide levels after global myocardial ischemia in dogs. Surgery 96:248, 1984
393. Digerness SB, Tracy WG, Andrews NF, et al: Reversal of myocardial ischemic contracture and the relationship to functional recovery and tissue calcium. Circulation 68:II-34, 1983
394. Nayler WG: Protection of the myocardium against postischemic reperfusion damage. The combined effect of hypothermia and nifedipine. J Thorac Cardiovasc Surg 84:897, 1982
395. Nayler WG, Ferrari R, Williams A: Protective effect of pretreatment with verapamil, nifedipine and propranolol on mitochondrial function in the ischemic and reperfused myocardium. Am J Cardiol 46:242, 1980
396. Chambers DE, Parks DA, Patterson G, et al: Xanthine oxidase as a source of free radical damage in myocardial ischemia. J Mol Cell Cardiol 17:145, 1985
397. McCord JM: Oxygen-derived free radicals in postischemic tissue injury. N Engl J Med 312:159, 1985
398. Shlafer M, Kane PF, Kirsh MM: Superoxide dismutase plus catalase enhances the efficacy of hypothermic cardioplegia to protect the globally ischemic, reperfused heart. J Thorac Cardiovasc Surg 83:830, 1982
399. Thompson JA: The oxygen free radical system: A fundamental mechanism in the production of myocardial necrosis. Prog Cardiovasc Dis 28:449, 1986
400. Chitwood WR, Hill RC, Sink JD, et al: Diastolic ventricular properties in patients during coronary revascularization. J Thorac Cardiovasc Surg 85:595, 1983
401. Chenowith DE, Cooper SW, Hugli TE, Stewart RW, Blackstone EH, Kirklin JW. Complement activation during cardiopulmonary bypass: Evidence for generation of C3a and C5a anaphylatoxins. N Engl J Med 304:497, 1981

402. Videm V, Fosse E, Moflines TE, et al: Complement activation with bubble and membrane oxygenators in aortocoronary bypass grafting. Ann Thorac Surg 50:387, 1990
403. Faymonville ME, Pincemail J, Duchateau J, et al: Myeloperoxidase and elastase as markers of leukocyte activation during cardiopulmonary bypass in humans. J Thorac Cardiovasc Surg 102:309, 1991yy
404. Lucchesi BR, Mullane KM: Leukocytes and ischemia-induced myocardial injury. Annu Rev Pharmacol Toxicol 26:201, 1986
405. Lucchesi BR, Werns SW, Fantone JC: The role of the neutrophil and free radicals in ischemic myocardial injury. J Mol Cell Cardiol 21:1241, 1989
406. Engler RL: Free-radical and granulocyte-mediated injury during myocardial ischemia and reperfusion. Am J Cardiol 63:19E, 1989
407. Mullane K: Neutrophil and endothelial changes in reperfusion injury. Trends Cardiovasc Med 1:282, 1991
408. Shen AC, Jennings RB: Kinetics of calcium accumulation in acute myocardial ischemic injury. Am J Pathol 67:441, 1972
409. Walsh LG, Tormey JM: Subcellular electrolyte shifts during in vitro myocardial ischemia and reperfusion. Am J Physiol 255:H917, 1988
410. Heyer EJ, Adams DC, Delphin E, et al: Cerebral dysfunction after coronary artery bypass grafting done with mild or moderate hypothermia. J Thorac Cardiovasc Surg 114:270, 1997
411. Nathan HJ, Wells GA, Munson JL, Wozny D: Neuroprotective effect of mild hypothermia in patients undergoing coronary artery surgery with cardiopulmonary bypass: a randomized trial. Circulation 104:I85, 2001

Chapter 29

TRANSFUSION MEDICINE AND COAGULATION DISORDERS

Bruce D. Spiess, MD, FAHA • Jay Horrow, MD, FAHA • Joel A. Kaplan, MD

KEY POINTS

1. It is easiest to think of coagulation as a wave of biologic activity occurring at the site of tissue injury consisting of initiation, acceleration, control, and lysis.
2. Hemostasis is part of a larger body system, inflammation. The protein reactions in coagulation have important roles in signaling inflammation.
3. Thrombin is the most important coagulation modulator, interacting with multiple coagulation factors, platelets, tissue plasminogen activator, prostacyclin, nitric oxide, and various white blood cells.
4. The serine proteases that compose the coagulation pathway are balanced by serine protease inhibitors, termed serpins. Antithrombin is the most important inhibitor of blood coagulation.
5. Platelets are the most complex part of the coagulation process, and antiplatelet drugs are important therapeutic agents.
6. Heparin requires antithrombin to anticoagulate blood and is not an ideal anticoagulant for cardiopulmonary bypass. Newer anticoagulants are actively being sought to replace heparin.
7. Protamine can have many adverse effects. Ideally, a new anticoagulant will not require reversal with a toxic substance like protamine.
8. Antifibrinolytic drugs are now often given during cardiac surgery; these drugs include ε-aminocaproic acid, tranexamic acid, and aprotinin.
9. Recombinant factor VIIa is the latest drug to be studied as a "rescue agent" to stop bleeding during cardiac surgery. It appears to be very effective but has not been studied adequately to date.
10. Every effort should be made to avoid transfusion of banked blood products during routine cardiac surgery. In fact, bloodless surgery is a reality in many cases.

Coagulation and bleeding assume particular importance when operations are performed on the heart using extracorporeal circulation. This chapter provides an understanding of the depth and breadth of hemostasis relating to cardiac procedures, beginning with coagulation pathophysiology. The pharmacology of heparin and protamine follows. This background is then applied to treatment of the bleeding patient. Coagulation monitoring is covered in Chapter 18.

OVERVIEW OF HEMOSTASIS

Proper hemostasis requires the participation of innumerable biologic elements (Box 29–1). This section groups them into four topics to facilitate understanding: coagulation factors, platelet function, the endothelium, and fibrinolysis. The reader must realize this is for simplicity of learning and that in biology the activation creates many reactions and control mechanisms, all interacting simultaneously. The interaction of the platelets, endothelial cells, and proteins to either activate or deactivate coagulation is a highly buffered and controlled process. It is perhaps easiest to think of coagulation as a wave of biologic activity occurring at the site of tissue injury (Fig. 29–1).[1] Although there are subcomponents to coagulation itself the injury/control leading to hemostasis is a four-part event: initiation, acceleration, control, and lysis (recanalization/fibrinolysis). The initiation phase begins with tissue damage, which is really begun with endothelial cell destruction or dysfunction. This initiation phase leads to binding of platelets, as well as protein activations; both happen nearly simultaneously and each has feedbacks into the other. Platelets adhere and create an activation or acceleration phase that gathers many cells to the site of injury and creates a large number of biochemical protein cascade events. As the activation phase ramps up into an explosive set of reactions, counterreactions are spun off, leading to control proteins damping the reactions. It is easiest, conceptually, to think of these control mechanisms as analogous to a nuclear reactor. The activation phase would continue to grow and overcome the whole organism unless control rods were inserted (e.g., protein C and tissue plasminogen activator [t-PA]) to stop the spread of the reaction. The surrounding normal endothelium exerts control over the reactions. Eventually the control reactions overpower the acceleration reactions and lysis comes into play. The diagram in Figure 29–1 shows lysis as relatively quick, but it can take 24 hours to days to have its full effects. The other key concept is that hemostasis is part of a larger body system, inflammation. Most, if not all, of the protein reactions of coagulation control have importance in signaling inflammation and other healing mechanisms. Entire books have been written merely to examine these fascinating inter-

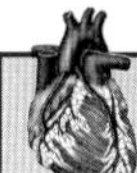

BOX 29–1 *Components of Hemostasis*

- Coagulation factor activation
- Platelet function
- Vascular endothelium
- Fibrinolysis and modulators of coagulation

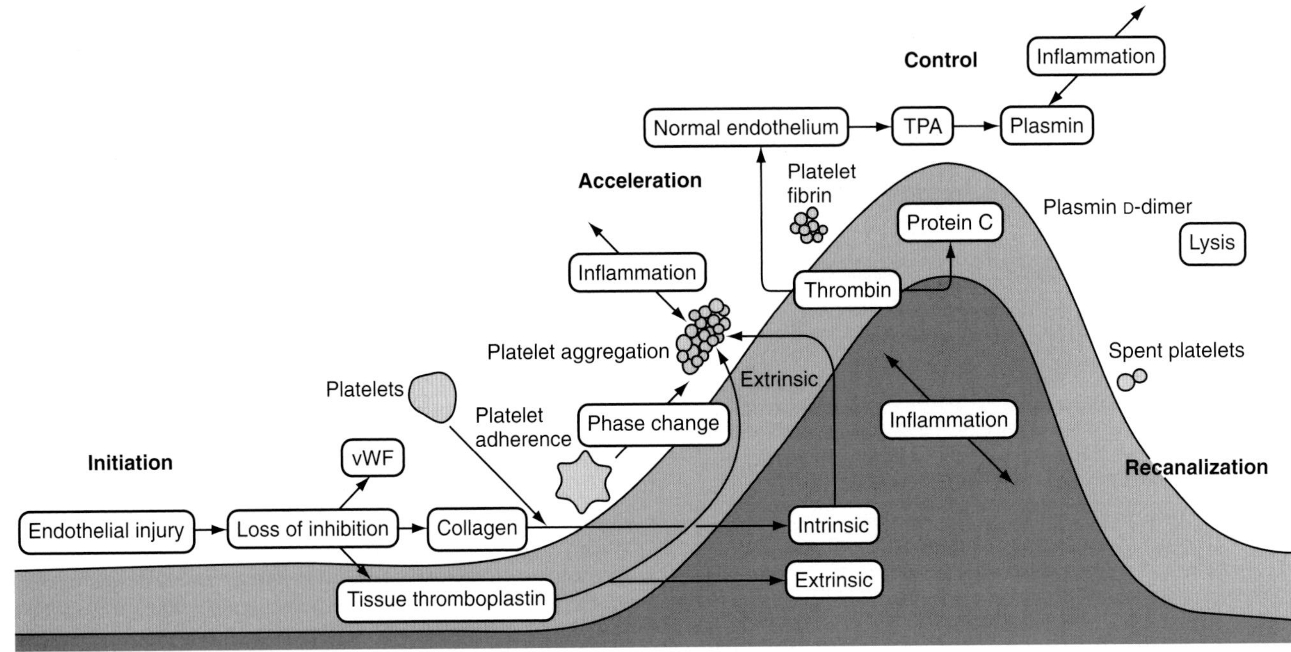

Figure 29–1 Coagulation is a sine wave of activity at the site of tissue injury. It goes through four stages: initiation, acceleration, control, and lysis/recanalization. (Redrawn with permission from Spiess BD: Coagulation function and monitoring. *In* Lichtor JL [ed]: Atlas of Clinical Anesthesia. Philadelphia, Current Medicine, 1996.)

actions. It is no wonder that cardiopulmonary bypass (CPB) has such profound inflammatory effects when it is considered that each of the activated coagulation proteins and cell lines then feeds into upregulation of inflammation.

During cardiac surgery, the endothelium is disturbed.[2] The coronary arteries are made either partially or fully ischemic for some period of time with cardioplegia (perfused bypass being relatively rare today). High concentrations of potassium are particularly insulting to endothelial cells, and ischemia–reperfusion injury is therefore the norm for every cardiac surgical case using CPB.[3] Systemic ischemia and reperfusion occur throughout every capillary bed as micro-air, thrombus, and fat emboli are byproducts of CPB[4] (see Chapters 28, 30, and 35).

The coagulation proteins and platelets are both hemodiluted and consumed. Platelets are activated and inhibited by different means. Coagulation dysfunction in cardiac surgery has been studied for more than 50 years, and relatively little is known when the extreme complexity of this system is appreciated.

Protein Coagulation Activations

Coagulation Pathways

The coagulation factors participate in a series of activating and feedback inhibition reactions, ending with the formation of an insoluble clot.[5] A *clot* is the sum total of platelet-to-platelet interactions leading to the formation of a platelet plug and then the cross-linking of platelets to each other by way of the final insoluble fibrin that leads to a stable clot. Clot is not simply the activation of proteins leading to more protein deposition. Clinicians have been shaped in their thinking about coagulation by the historic way that coagulation proteins were discovered and the resulting coagulation tests. This is not the way coagulation proceeds biologically.

With few exceptions, the coagulation factors are glycoproteins synthesized in the liver, which circulate as inactive molecules termed *zymogens.* Factor activation proceeds sequentially, each factor serving as substrate in an enzymatic reaction catalyzed by the previous factor in the sequence. Hence this has classically been termed a "cascade" or "waterfall" sequence. Cleavage of a polypeptide fragment changes an inactive zymogen to an active enzyme. The active form is termed a *serine protease* because the active site for its protein-splitting activity is a serine amino acid residue. Many reactions require the presence of calcium ion (Ca^{++}) and a phospholipid surface (platelet phosphotidylserine). The phospholipids occur most often either on the surface of an activated platelet or endothelial cell and occasionally on the surface of white cells. So anchored, their proximity to one another permits reaction rates profoundly accelerated (up to 300,000-fold) from those measured when the enzymes remain in solution. The factors form four interrelated arbitrary groups (Fig. 29–2): the contact activation, intrinsic, extrinsic, and common pathways. They are labeled by human need for order. In biology they are all highly interactive.

CONTACT ACTIVATION

Factor XII, high-molecular-weight kininogen (HMWK), prekallikrein (PK), and factor XI form the contact, or surface, activation group. The in vivo events that activate factor XII remain unconfirmed. Because factor XII autoactivates by undergoing a shape change in the presence of a negative charge, in vitro coagulation tests use glass, silica, kaolin, and other compounds with negative surface charge (see Chapter 18). One potential in vivo mechanism for factor XII activation is disruption of the endothelial cell layer, which exposes the underlying negatively charged collagen matrix. Activated platelets also provide negative charges on their membrane surfaces. HMWK anchors the other surface activation molecules,

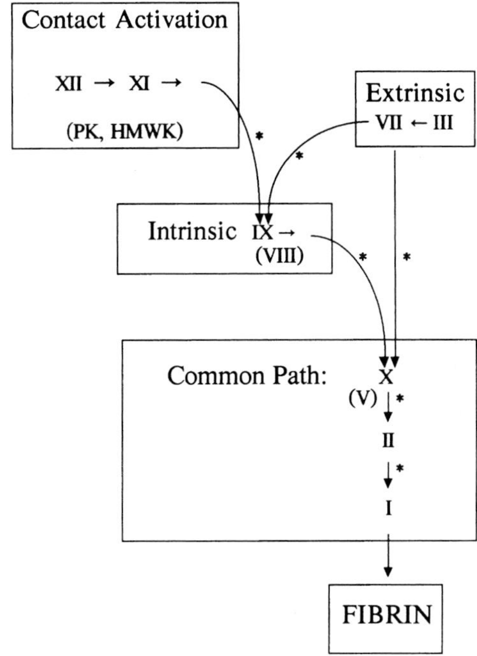

Figure 29–2 Depiction of coagulation protein activation sequence. Asterisks denote participation of calcium ion.

PK and factor XI, to damaged endothelium or activated platelets. Factor XIIa cleaves both factor XI, to form factor XIa, and PK, to form kallikrein. Figure 29–3 depicts the events of surface activation.

This system also interlinks to the complement cascade and fibrinolytic process as follows. Kallikrein converts HMWK to bradykinin, which activates the complement proteins. Kallikrein may also convert plasminogen to plasmin (see later). This latter function is quite weak, however, and of unknown significance in vivo.

It was rather tempting historically to attribute all coagulation abnormalities to activation of the contact system. This seemed like an obvious conclusion since the CPB circuit contained a negatively charged plastic surface that must therefore lead to contact activation. Today it is known that the effects of contact activation in the entire scheme of CPB coagulation dysfunction are quite small. Of note, patients with completely absent factor XII do just fine and do not bleed. Therefore, the presence or absence of factor XII in the evolution of mankind seems to not be critical.

INTRINSIC SYSTEM

Intrinsic activation forms factor XIa from the products of surface activation. Factor XIa splits factor IX to form factor IXa, with Ca^{++} required for this process. Then factor IXa activates factor X with help from Ca^{++}, a phospholipid surface (platelet), and a glycoprotein cofactor, factor VIIIa. Figure 29–4 displays a stylized version of factor X activation. The phospholipids and glycoprotein cofactors are on the surface of platelets.

EXTRINSIC SYSTEM

Activation of factor X can proceed independently of factor XII by substances classically thought to be extrinsic to the vasculature. This is of historic interest only since today it is known that the expression of tissue factor is actually a highly regulated event in endothelial cells. Any number of endothelial cell insults can lead to the production of tissue factor by the endothelial cell.[3-10] At rest, the endothelial cell is very antithrombotic. However, with ischemia, reperfusion, sepsis, or cytokines, the endothelial cell will stimulate its production of intracellular NFκb and send messages for the production

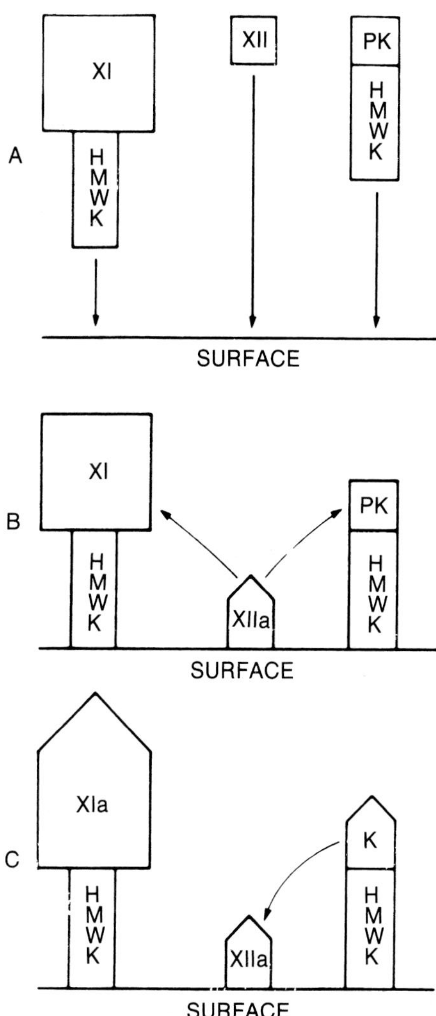

Figure 29–3 *(A-C)* Activation of the contact factors XII, XI, and prekallikrein (PK). The cofactor, high-molecular-weight kininogen (HMWK), binds factor XI and PK to the endothelial surface. Kallikrein (K) amplifies factor XII activation. (From Colman RW, Marder VJ, Salzman EW, Hirsh J: Overview of hemostasis. *In* Colman RW, Hirsh J, Marder VJ, Salzman EW [eds]: Hemostasis and Thrombosis, 3rd edition. Philadelphia, JB Lippincott, 1994, pp 3.)

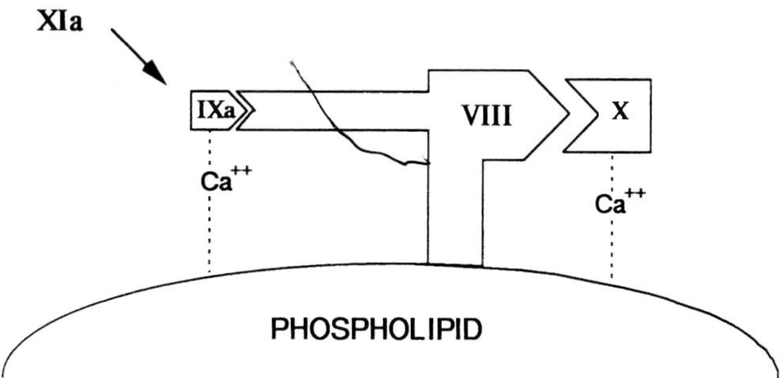

Figure 29–4 Factor VIII facilitates the activation of factor X by factor IXa. Calcium tethers the molecules to the phospholipid surface. (From Horrow JC: Desmopressin and antifibrinolytics. In Gravlee GP [ed]: Blood Conservation. Int Anesthesiol Clin 28:230, 1990.)

of messenger RNA for tissue factor production.[6] This can happen quickly and the resting endothelial cell can turn out large amounts of tissue factor. It is widely held today that the activation of tissue factor is what drives many of the abnormalities of coagulation after cardiac surgery, rather than contact activation.[7,8] Thromboplastin, also known as tissue factor, released from tissues into the vasculature, acts as a cofactor for initial activation of factor X by factor VII. Factors VII and X then activate one another with the help of platelet phospholipid and Ca^{++}, thus rapidly generating factor Xa. (Factor VIIa also activates factor IX, thus linking the extrinsic and intrinsic paths.)

Thromboplastin straddles the extravascular cell membrane, with its extracellular portion available to bind factor VIIa. Cytokines (particularly tumor necrosis factor [TNF]α and interleukin [IL]-6) and endotoxins can stimulate its expression on endothelium.[9,10] It anchors factor VIIa to the cell surface, thus facilitating activation of factor X. The amount of available factor Va seems also to be quite important for the adequate functioning of the normal coagulation cascades.

COMMON PATHWAY

Using membrane phospholipids (phosphotidylserine) as a catalyst site, Ca^{++} as a ligand, and factor Va as cofactor, factor Xa splits prothrombin (factor II) to thrombin (factor IIa). The combination of factors Xa, Va, and Ca^{++} is termed the prothrombinase complex. Factor Xa anchors to the membrane surface (of platelets) via Ca^{++}. Factor Va, assembling next to it, initiates a rearrangement of the complex, vastly accelerating binding of the substrate, prothrombin. Most likely, the factor Xa formed from the previous reaction is channeled along the membrane to this next reaction step without detaching from the membrane.

Figure 29–5 depicts the steps involved in formation of thrombin from its precursor, prothrombin. The byproduct, fragment F1.2, serves as a plasma marker of prothrombin activation. An alternative scheme generates a different species, meizathrombin, involved more specifically in activation of coagulation inhibitors.[11]

Thrombin cleaves the fibrinogen molecule to form soluble fibrin monomer and polypeptide fragments termed *fibrinopeptides A* and *B*. Fibrin monomers associate to form a soluble fibrin matrix. Factor XIII, activated by thrombin, cross-links these fibrin strands to form an insoluble clot. Patients with lower levels of factor XIII have been found to have more bleeding after cardiac surgery.

VITAMIN K

Those factors that require calcium (II, VII, IX, X) depend on vitamin K to add between 9 and 12 γ-carboxyl groups to glutamic acid residues near their amino termini. Calcium tethers the negatively charged carboxyl groups to the phospholipid surface (platelets), thus facilitating molecular interactions. Some inhibitory proteins also depend on vitamin K (proteins C and S).

Modulators of the Coagulation Pathway

Thrombin, the most important coagulation modulator, exerts a pervasive influence throughout the coagulation factor pathways. It activates factors V, VIII, and XIII; cleaves fibrinogen to fibrin; stimulates platelet recruitment and chemotaxis of leukocytes and monocytes; releases tissue plasminogen activator (t-PA), prostacyclin, and nitric oxide from endothelial cells; releases IL-1 from macrophages; and with thrombomodulin, activates protein C, a substance that then inactivates factors Va and VIIIa.[12] Note the negative feedback aspect of this last action (Figure 29–6). The latest thinking on coagulation function centers around the effects of thrombin. The platelets, tissue factor, and contact activation all are interactive and are activated by a rent in the surface of the endothelium or through the loss of endothelial coagulation control. Platelets adhere to a site of injury and in turn are activated, leading to sequestration of other platelets. It is the interaction of all of those factors together that eventually creates a critical mass. Once enough platelets are interacting together, with their attached surface concomitant serine protease reactions, then a thrombin burst is created. Only when enough thrombin activation has been encountered in a critical time point, then a threshold is exceeded, and the reactions become massive and much larger than the sum of the whole. It is thought that the concentration and ability of platelets to react fully affect the ability to have a critical thrombin burst. CPB may affect the ability to get that full thrombin burst due to its effects on platelet number, platelet-to-platelet interactions, and the decreased amounts of protein substrates.

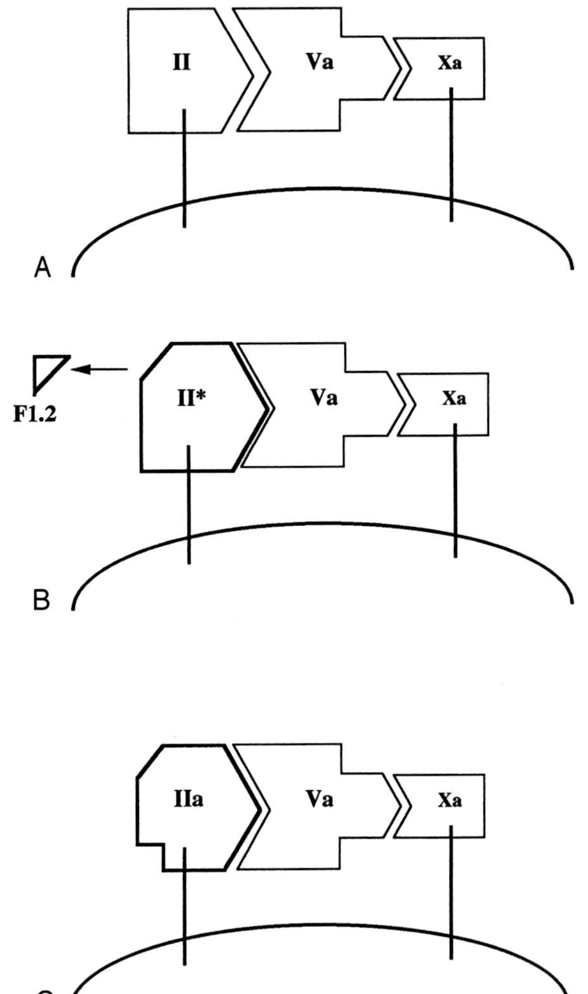

Figure 29–5 Activation of prothrombin by factor Xa proceeds in a multistep fashion. *(A)* On the phospholipid surface the prothrombinase complex consists of prothrombin (factor II), factor Xa, and factor Va. *(B)* The first activation step in which the prothrombin fragment F1.2 is split from prothrombin to form prethrombin (II*). *(C)* Molecular rearrangement of prethrombin yields thrombin.

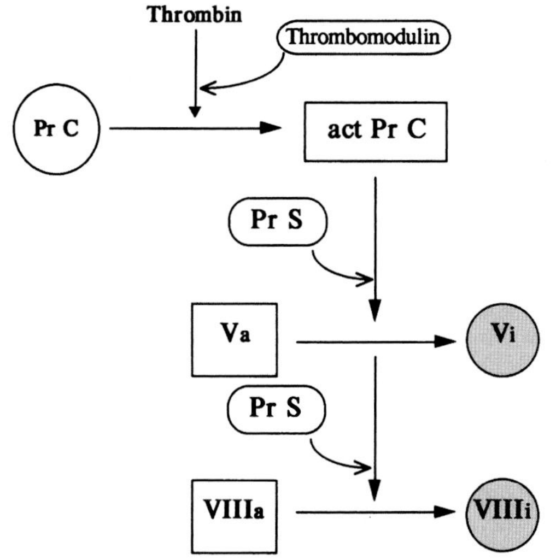

Figure 29–6 Modulating effects of protein C on coagulation. Thrombomodulin from endothelial cells accelerates thrombin activation of protein C (Pr C). In the presence of protein S (Pr S), activated protein C [(act Pr C)a] inactivates factors V and VIII. Protein C and protein S are vitamin K-dependent.

The many serine proteases that compose the coagulation pathways are balanced by serine protease inhibitors, termed *serpins.*[13] This biologic yin and yang leads to an excellent buffering capacity. It is only when the platelet driven thrombin burst so overwhelms the body's localized anticoagulation or inhibitors that clot proceeds forward. Serpins include α_1-antitrypsin, α_2-macroglobulin, heparin cofactor II, α_2-antiplasmin, antithrombin (also termed antithrombin III), and others.

Antithrombin (ATIII) constitutes the most important inhibitor of blood coagulation. It binds to the active site (serine) of thrombin, thus inhibiting thrombin's action. It also inhibits, to a much lesser extent, the activity of factors XIIa, XIa, IXa, and Xa; kallikrein; and the fibrinolytic molecule, plasmin. Thrombin bound to fibrin is protected from the action of antithrombin, thus explaining the poor efficacy of heparin in treating established thrombosis. ATIII is a relatively inactive zymogen. To be most effective antithrombin must bind to a unique pentasaccharide sequence contained on the wall of endothelial cells in the glycosaminoglycan surface known as heparan; the same active sequence is present in the drug heparin. An important note is that activated ATIII is active only against free thrombin.[14] Most thrombin in its active form is either bound to glycoprotein binding sites of platelets or in fibrin matrices. When blood is put into a test tube and clot begins to form (such as in an activated coagulation time [ACT]), 96% of thrombin production is yet to come. The vast majority of thrombin generation is on the surface of platelets and on clot-held fibrinogen. Platelets through their glycoprotein binding sites and phospholipid folds protect activated thrombin from attack by ATIII. Therefore, the biologic role of ATIII is to create an anticoagulant surface on endothelial cells. It is not present biologically to sit and wait for a dose of heparin before CPB.

CPB dilutes ATIII substantially and the further consumption of ATIII during CPB (thrombin generation) leads in some patients to profoundly low levels of this important inhibitor.[15] Research work adding ATIII back to the CPB circuit has shown promise in that by doing so there is better preservation of serine protease proteins and platelets. Unfortunately, no pharmaceutical company has decided to pursue this line of research to the point that it would be either commonplace or economically feasible to add large amounts of ATIII to CPB and therefore avoid consumptive coagulopathies. Congenital ATIII deficiency can lead to in utero fetal destruction if the fetus is homozygous for the abnormal ATIII. However, patients who are heterozygous for ATIII abnormalities have about 40% to 60% of normal ATIII activity. They have a particularly high risk for deep vein thrombosis. Low ATIII levels have been described during extracorporeal membrane oxygenation (ECMO) and the addition of ATIII to the ECMO circuit has been effective in improving outcome and decreasing bleeding in some circumstances.[16] It is not known how useful it would be in all patients on CPB because only small trials have been performed, but these have been encouraging.[17,18]

Heparin cofactor II also inhibits thrombin, once it is activated. While large doses of heparin activate heparin cofactor II, dermatans on endothelial cell surfaces activate it far more effectively, suggesting dermatans as alternative drugs to heparin.[19] Dermatan sulfates are not available for use today in the United States.

Another serpin, *protein C,* degrades factors Va and VIIIa. Like other vitamin K-dependent factors, it requires Ca^{++} to bind to phospholipid. Its cofactor, termed *protein S,* also exhibits vitamin K dependence. Genetic variants of protein C are less active and lead to increased risk for deep vein thrombosis and pulmonary embolism. When endothelial cells release thrombomodulin, thrombin then accelerates by 20,000-fold its activation of protein C[20] (Fig. 29–6). Activated protein C also promotes fibrinolysis.[21]

Regulation of the extrinsic limb of the coagulation pathway occurs via tissue factor pathway inhibitor (TFPI), a glycosylated protein that associates with lipoproteins in plasma.[22] TFPI is not a serpin. It impairs the catalytic properties of the factor VIIa–tissue factor complex on factor X activation. Both vascular endothelium and platelets appear to produce TFPI.[23,24] Heparin releases TFPI from endothelium, increasing TFPI plasma concentrations by as much as six-fold, which should be viewed as a biologic indicator of how poor heparin is as an anticoagulant. TFPI is not tested for in routine coagulation testing. It may be that some individuals with certain types of TFPI or who have very large amounts of circulating TFPI could be at risk for severe adverse bleeding after cardiac surgery.[25-30] This area is just beginning to be examined today both in terms of whether TFPI is responsible for abnormal bleeding and whether its genetic variants have abnormal bleeding or thrombosis.

von Willebrand factor (vWF), a massive molecule composed of disulfide-linked glycosylated peptides, associates with factor VIII in plasma, protecting it from proteolytic enzymes. It circulates in the plasma in its coiled inactive form.[31] Disruption of the endothelium either allows for binding of vWF from the plasma or allows for expression of vWF from tissue and from endothelial cells. Once bound, vWF uncoils to its full length and exposes a hitherto cryptic domain in the molecule. This A-1 domain has a very high affinity for platelet glycoproteins. Initially, vWF attaches to the GPIα platelet receptor, which slows platelet shear forces. This is not enough to bind the platelet, but it creates a membrane signal that allows for early shape change and expression of other glycoproteins, GPIb and GPIIb/IIIa. Then, secondary GPIb binding connects to other vWF nearby, binding the platelet and beginning the activation sequence. It bridges normal platelets to damaged subendothelium by attaching to the GPIb platelet receptor. An ensuing platelet shape change then releases thromboxane, β-thromboglobulin, and serotonin and exposes GPIIb/IIIa, which binds fibrinogen.

Deficiency States

Decreased amounts of coagulation proteins may be inherited or acquired. Deficiencies of each part of the coagulation pathway are considered in turn. Table 29–1 summarizes the coagulation factors, their activation sequences, and vehicles for factor replacement when deficient.

CONTACT ACTIVATION

Although decreased amounts of factor XII, PK, and HMWK can occur, these defects do not have clinical sequelae. The autosomal dominant deficiency of factor XI is very rare. However, its incidence among Ashkenazi Jews is as high as 0.1% to 0.3%.[32] Most of these patients require factor replacement for surgery with fresh frozen plasma (FFP). Spontaneous bleeding does not occur. Factor XI concentrations do not correlate with bleeding after trauma or surgery. An FFP dose of 10 mL/kg will yield target concentrations of 20% activity.

INTRINSIC

Hemophilia occurs worldwide, with a prevalence of 1 in 10,000. Hemophilia A, which constitutes about 80% to 85% of cases, originates from decreased activity of factor VIII. Because platelet function remains normal, minor cuts and abrasions do not bleed excessively. Joint and muscle hemorrhages ensue from minor trauma or, seemingly, spontaneously. Airway issues include epistaxis and obstruction from bleeding into the tongue. The bleeding time and prothrombin time (PT) remain normal, while the activated partial thromboplastin time (aPTT) is prolonged.[33] Desmopressin, a synthetic analog of vasopressin, will increase factor VIII activity by releasing vWF from endothelial cells, except in patients with severe hemophilia A, who have too little functional factor VIII available for vWF.[34] Major surgery requires replenishment of factor VIII functional activity to greater than 80% of normal with FFP, cryoprecipitate, or factor VIII concentrate.[35] After surgery, factor VIII concentrations should be maintained above 30% for 2 weeks with repeat doses. Current plasma-derived concentrates are solvent detergent and heat-treated to remove lipid-coated viruses (HIV, hepatitis B, HTLV). However, this was not historically the case and in Europe during the early parts of the HIV/AIDS crisis most hemophiliacs contracted HIV/AIDS from contaminated products. A recombinant product also is now available, but costs about three times that of the plasma-derived one.

Factor IX deficiency manifests as hemophilia B, constituting 15% to 20% of all hemophilia cases. Patients present with symptoms identical to those with hemophilia A. No study demonstrates a salutary effect of desmopressin. Prothrombin complex concentrates will replenish levels, but consumptive coagulopathy remains a possible complication, stemming from the presence of activated coagulation factors, principally factor VIIa, in the preparation.[36] Purified factor IX concentrate, a plasma-derived, solvent detergent and heat-treated product, currently constitutes the replacement vehicle of choice for patients with hemophilia B.[37] Recombinant pure factor IX concentrate will be available, but at considerable expense (factor VIIa is now available as well). Consultation with an experienced hematologist aids in the care of hemophiliacs undergoing surgery.

EXTRINSIC

Inheritance of factor VII deficiency follows an autosomal recessive pattern with a prevalence of 1 in 500,000. Although factor VII deficiency may mimic hemophilia in presentation,

Table 29–1 The Coagulation Pathway Proteins, Minimal Amounts Needed for Surgery, and Replacement Sources*

Factor	Activated By	Acts On	Minimal Amount Needed	Replacement Source	Alternate Name and Comments
XIII	IIa	Fibrin	<5%	FFP, CRYO	Fibrin-stabilizing factor; not a serine protease, but an enzyme
XII	Endothelium	XI	None	Not needed	Hagemann factor; activation enhanced by XIIa
XI	XIIa	IX	15% to 25%	FFP	Plasma thromboplastin antecedent
X	VIIa or IXa	II	10% to 20%	FFP, 9C	Stuart-Prower factor; vitamin K dependent
IX	VIIa or XIa	X	25% to 30%	FFP, 9C, PCC	Christmas factor; vitamin K dependent
VIII	IIa	X	>30%	CRYO, 8C, FFP	Antihemophilic factor; a cofactor; RES synthesis
VII	Xa	X	10% to 20%	FFP, PCC	Serum prothrombin conversion accelerator; vitamin K dependent
V	IIa	II	<25%	FFP	Proaccelerin; a cofactor; RES and liver synthesis
IV	—	—	—	—	Calcium ion; binds II, VII, IX, X to phospholipid
III	—	X	—	—	Thromboplastin/tissue factor; a cofactor
II	Xa	I	20% to 40%	FFP, PCC	Prothrombin; vitamin K-dependent
I	IIa	—	1 g/L	CRYO, FFP	Fibrinogen; activated product is soluble fibrin
vWF	—	VIII	See VIII	CRYO, FFP	von Willebrand factor; endothelial cell synthesis

*Unless otherwise specified, all coagulation proteins are synthesized in the liver. Note that there is no factor VI. For von Willebrand factor, cryoprecipitate or FFP is administered to obtain a factor VIII coagulant activity >30%.

RES = reticuloendothelial system; FFP = fresh frozen plasma; CRYO = cryoprecipitate; 8C = factor VIII concentrate; 9C = purified factor IX complex concentrate; PCC = prothrombin complex concentrate.

most often clinical bleeding is absent, and surgery is well tolerated without replacement. The PT is elevated, while the PTT is normal. When necessary, replacement of factor VII levels to 10% to 20% of normal with FFP suffices.

COMMON PATHWAY

Deficiency of either factor V or factor X, both extremely rare autosomal recessive disorders, elevates both the PT and PTT. The bleeding time is normal in factor X deficiency but prolonged in one third of patients with factor V deficiency. The bleeding time prolongation arises from the role of factor V in platelet function.[38] Prothrombin complex concentrate or FFP supplies prothrombin, factor V, and factor X. Numerous inherited abnormalities of prothrombin and fibrinogen occur, with varying characteristics. Cryoprecipitate, which contains 250 mg of fibrinogen and 100 U of factor VIII per 10-mL bag, as well as vWF and factor XIII, treats inherited or acquired disorders of fibrinogen.

LIVER DISEASE

Hepatic compromise decreases the circulating amounts of factors II, VII, and X, but the level of factor IX is often normal. Decreases in factor V are variable. Factor VIII levels, in contrast, can reach as much as five times normal in acute hepatitis. Factors XIII, XII, and XI, HMWK, and PK suffer mild decreases. Administration of FFP restores these factors to normal levels. Liver disease also leads to decreases in the production of ATIII and protein S. Therefore the buffering capacity of coagulation is thrown off. A small change in activation could therefore lead to a large and diffuse, whole body event such as consumptive coagulopathy.

WARFARIN

Administration of this vitamin K antagonist affects plasma levels of factors II, VII, IX, and X and proteins C and S.[39] Protein C has the shortest half-life, followed by factors VII (6 hours), IX (24 hours), X (2 days), and II (3 days).[36] Substantial PT prolongations and some PTT prolongation accompany warfarin therapy. For immediate restoration of clotting function, FFP is given. Otherwise, parenteral vitamin K or cessation of warfarin (Coumadin) suffices. Clinicians should be extremely careful in administering these compounds if a patient is suspected of having heparin-induced thrombocytopenia.

INHERITED THROMBOTIC DISORDERS

A number of genetic abnormalities lead to thrombosis. The most prevalent (2% to 5%) in European-derived populations is factor V Leiden, in which a point mutation at residue 1691 on factor V renders it resistant to inactivation by activated protein C.[40] Venous thromboembolism risk increases sevenfold in heterozygotes and 80-fold in homozygotes, but episodes are less severe than in other thrombotic disorders. Pregnancy and/oral contraceptives greatly exacerbate the thrombotic tendency.[41]

ATIII deficiency causes venous thromboembolism and heparin resistance. This autosomal dominant disorder involves three types: absence of antithrombin (type I); dysfunctional antithrombin (type II); and antithrombin with dysfunction limited to a reduced response to heparin (type III). Clinical presentation begins at age 15 or later, with venous thrombosis occurring with surgery, pregnancy, or bed rest. Replacement antithrombin III is now available for use in the United States.

Protein C or S deficiencies, if homozygous, present at birth as neonatal purpura fulminans. Protein C deficiency heterozygotes demonstrate 40% to 60% protein C activity and present with venous thrombosis beginning in adolescence. The role of reduced concentrations of protein S in causing thrombosis has come into question.[41] Together, deficiencies of antithrombin, protein C, and protein S account for 10% to 15% of inherited thrombosis.[42]

Deficiency of heparin cofactor II is rare. Its role in thrombosis is uncertain. Other conditions that cause thrombosis are dysfibrinogenemia with lysis-resistant fibrinogen, plasminogen deficiency, t-PA deficiency, excess PAI-1 (plasminogen activator inhibitor) activity (PAI-1 inhibits t-PA), and homocysteinemia.

Homocysteinemia is the mild heterozygous state of cystathione beta-synthetase deficiency, known as homocysteinuria in its more serious homozygous form. Increased plasma concentrations of homocysteine induce endothelial cell tissue factor activity, stimulate factor V activation, and impair protein C activation, all of which contribute to thrombosis. Folic acid and vitamins B_6 and B_{12} reduce homocysteine plasma concentrations.[43]

Platelet Function

Most clinicians think first of the coagulation proteins when considering hemostasis. Although no one element of the many that participate in hemostasis assumes dominance, platelets may be the most complex.[44] Without platelets, there is no coagulation and no hemostasis. Without the proteins, there is hemostasis, but it lasts only about 10 to 15 minutes as the platelet plug is inherently unstable and breaks apart under the shear stress of the vasculature. Platelets provide phospholipid for coagulation factor reactions; contain their own microskeletal system and coagulation factors; secrete active substances affecting themselves, other platelets, the endothelium, and other coagulation factors; and alter shape to expose membrane glycoproteins essential to hemostasis. Their cell signaling has been intensively studied for more than a decade. Platelets have perhaps as many as 30 to 50 different types of cell receptors.

The initial response to vascular injury is formation of a platelet plug. Good hemostatic response depends on proper functioning of platelet adhesion, activation, and aggregation (Fig. 29–7). This section first discusses these aspects, and then follows with the effects of platelet disorders and platelet-inhibiting pharmaceuticals.

Platelet Adhesion

Capillary blood exhibits laminar flow, which maximizes the likelihood of interaction of platelets with the vessel wall. Red cells and white cells stream near the center of the vessels and marginate platelets. However, turbulence causes reactions in endothelium that leads to the secretion of vWF, adhesive molecules, and tissue factor. Shear stress is high as fast-moving platelets interact with the endothelium. When the vascular endothelium becomes denuded or injured, the platelet has the opportunity to contact vWF, which is bound to the exposed collagen of the subendothelium. A platelet membrane component, glycoprotein (GP)Ib, attaches to vWF, thus anchoring the platelet to the vessel wall. Independently, platelet membrane GPIa and GPIIa and IX may attach directly to exposed collagen, furthering the adhesion stage.[44-46]

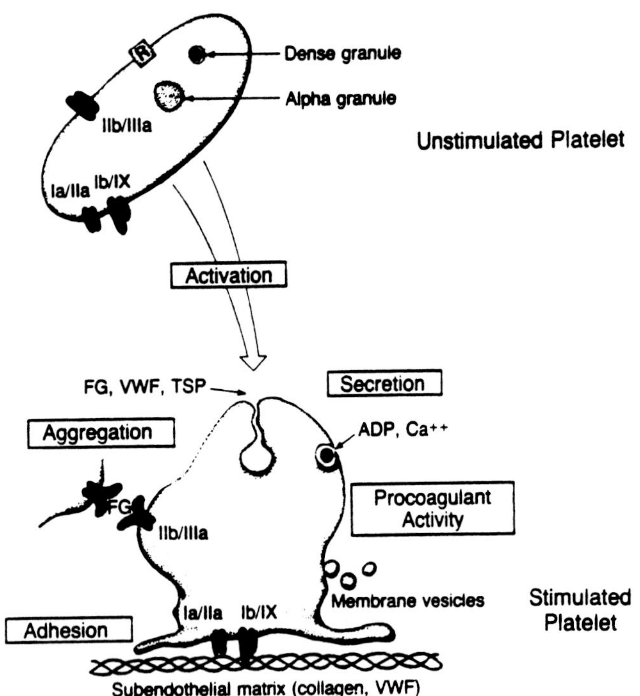

Figure 29–7 Platelet function in hemostasis. Glycoproteins Ib and IX and von Willebrand factor (vWF) mediate adhesion to the vessel wall. Glycoproteins IIb and IIIa and integrin molecules (FG [fibrinogen], TSP [thrombospondin]) mediate platelet aggregation. (From George J, Shattil SJ: The clinical importance of acquired abnormalities of platelet function. N Engl J Med 324:27, 1991.)

Following activation (see later), additional adhesive mechanisms come into play. Release of selectin glycoproteins from α granules allows their membrane expression, thus promoting platelet–leukocyte adhesion. This interaction may ultimately allow expression of tissue factor on monocytes, thus amplifying coagulation.[47]

The integrin glycoproteins form diverse types of membrane receptors from combinations of 20 α and 8 β subunits.[48] One such combination is GPIIb/IIIa, a platelet membrane component that initially participates in platelet adhesion. Platelet activation causes a conformational change in GPIIb/IIIa, which results in its aggregator activity.

Platelet adhesion begins rapidly—within 1 minute of endothelial injury—and completely covers exposed subendothelium within 20 minutes.[45] It begins with decreased platelet velocity when GPIb/IX and vWF mediate adhesion, followed by platelet activation, GPIIb/IIIa conformational change, then vWF binding and platelet arrest on the endothelium at these vWF ligand sites.[44,46]

Adhesion requires margination of platelets: high hematocrits concentrate red blood cells in the central regions of a vessel, promoting marginal placement of platelets. Dilute hematocrit (e.g., post-CPB) impairs this effect, thus adversely affecting platelet adhesion. For this reason, red blood cell transfusion alone may improve hemostasis. However, transfusion should not be used primarily to achieve this goal since red cell concentrates carry a high concentration of cytokines and platelet-activating factor (PAF), which may contribute to platelet dysfunction or consumptive coagulopathy.

Platelet Activation and Aggregation

Platelet activation results after contact with collagen, when adenosine diphosphate (ADP), thrombin, or thromboxane A_2 binds to membrane receptors, or from certain platelet-to-platelet interactions. Platelets then release the contents of their dense (δ) granules and α granules. Dense granules contain serotonin, ADP, and Ca^{++}; α granules contain platelet factor V (previously termed platelet factor 1), β-thromboglobulin, platelet factor 4, P-selectin, and various integrin proteins (vWF, fibrinogen, vitronectin, and fibronectin). Simultaneously, platelets employ their microskeletal system to change shape from a disk to a sphere, which changes platelet membrane GPIIb/IIIa exposure. Released ADP recruits additional platelets to the site of injury and stimulates platelet G protein, which in turn activates membrane phospholipase. This results in the formation of arachidonate, which platelet cyclooxygenase converts to thromboxane A_2. Other platelet agonists besides ADP and collagen include serotonin, a weak agonist, and thrombin and thromboxane A_2, both potent agonists. Thrombin is by far the most potent platelet agonist, and it can overcome all other platelet antagonists as well as inhibitors. In total, there are more than 70 agonists that can produce platelet activation and aggregation.

Agonists induce a shape change, increase platelet intracellular Ca^{++} concentration, and stimulate platelet G protein. In addition, serotonin and thromboxane A_2 are potent vasoconstrictors.[49] The presence of sufficient agonist material results in platelet aggregation. Aggregation occurs when the integrin proteins (mostly fibrinogen) released from α granules form molecular bridges between the GPIIb/IIIa receptors of adjacent platelets (the final common platelet pathway).

Platelet Disorders

Dysfunctional vWF produces von Willebrand disease (vWD), an autosomal dominant disorder of variable expressivity.[34] With an incidence of 1.4 to 5 cases per 1000 population, vWD is the most common inherited coagulopathy. Patients present with mucocutaneous hemorrhages rather than hemarthroses. Common symptoms include epistaxis, ecchymoses, and excessive bleeding after trauma, with surgery, or during menses. Because vWF concentrations vary greatly with time, symptoms have variable expressivity. Desmopressin reverses the prolonged bleeding time in patients with mild vWD.[50] As with hemophilia A, severe cases of vWD do not benefit from desmopressin therapy. In one rare class of vWD (type IIB, 3% to 5% of vWD), desmopressin aggregates platelets, inducing thrombocytopenia and worsening rather than helping hemostasis. Table 29–2 summarizes features of the more common types of vWD. When blood products are needed, cryoprecipitate constitutes the replacement vehicle of choice in vWD, although recent factor VIII concentrates retain vWF activity and have been used successfully during cardiac surgery.[51]

The addition of agonist (ADP or collagen) to platelets allows measurement of platelet aggregation in vitro. In Glanzmann's thrombasthenia, the GPIIb/IIIa receptor is absent, preventing aggregation. However, ristocetin, a cationic antibiotic similar to vancomycin, can agglutinate platelets directly via GPIb receptors and vWF. Absence of the GPIb receptor, Bernard-Soulier syndrome, prevents adhesion and agglutination with ristocetin, but aggregation to ADP is normal, since the GPIIb/IIIa receptor is intact. Patients with vWD also exhibit impaired platelet adhesion and normal aggregation. Decreased amounts of vWF antigen distinguish it from the Bernard-Soulier syndrome. In platelet storage pool deficiency, impairment of dense granule secretion yields no ADP upon adhesion. In vitro addition of collagen will not aggregate platelets because of absence of ADP release, while added ADP

Table 29–2 **Major Types of von Willebrand Disease**

Classification	Prevalence	vWf:Ag	R:Co	Molecular Pathology
I (Classic)	70% to 80%	Decreased	Decreased	Normal multimers; decreased quantity
IIA	10% to 12%	Decreased	Decreased	Intermediate and large multimers decreased
IIB	3% to 5%	Decreased	Near normal	Abnormal, large multimers that bind platelets
III	1% to 3%	None	None	No vWF present
Platelet-type	0% to 1%	Decreased	Decreased	Normal vWF; platelet GP Ib receptors bind large multimers

vWF:Ag = von Willebrand factor antigen measurement; R:Co = ristocetin cofactor activity measurement.
Data from Montgomery RR, Colier BS: von Willebrand disease. *In* Colman RW, Hirsh J, Marder VJ, Salzman EW (eds): Hemostasis and Thrombosis, 3rd edition. Philadelphia, JB Lippincott, 1994, pp 134–168.

Table 29–3 **Diagnosis of Some Inherited Platelet Disorders**

Disorder	Deficiency	Platelet Adhesion	Platelet Aggregation	Ristocetin Agglutination	vWF:Ag Level
Glanzmann's thrombasthenia	GPIIb/IIIa	Normal	Absent	Occurs	Normal
Bernard-Soulier syndrome	GPIb	Absent	Normal	Absent	Normal
Storage pool deficiency	Dense granule secretion	Normal	Impaired	Occurs	Normal
von Willebrand disease	VWF	Absent	Normal	Absent or decreased	Low

GP = glycoprotein receptor; vWF = von Willebrand factor; vWF:Ag = von Willebrand factor antigen.

will initiate some aggregation. Table 29–3 summarizes these diagnostic findings. Uremia impairs the secretory and aggregating functions of platelets, resulting in an elevated bleeding time. However, the most common effect of renal dysfunction is hypercoagulability. It is only with severe uremia that the platelets are poisoned. It is therefore a common misconception in the operating room that a patient with mild to moderate renal failure will be at increased risk for bleeding. The utilization of thromboelastography (TEG) can help in deciding whether the extent of renal failure is causing hypocoagulability. The etiology and clinical significance remain poorly defined (see Chapter 18).

Prostaglandins and Aspirin

Endothelial cell cyclooxygenase synthesizes prostacyclin, which inhibits aggregation and dilates vessels. Platelet cyclooxygenase forms thromboxane A_2, a potent aggregating agent and vasoconstrictor. Aspirin irreversibly acetylates cyclooxygenase, rendering it inactive. Low doses of aspirin, 80 to 100 mg, easily overcome the finite amount of cyclooxygenase available in the nucleus-free platelets. However, endothelial cells can synthesize new cyclooxygenase. Thus, with low doses of aspirin, prostacyclin synthesis continues while thromboxane synthesis ceases, decreasing platelet activation and aggregation. High doses of aspirin inhibit the enzyme at both cyclooxygenase sites.[49]

Reversible platelet aggregation is blocked by aspirin, as the platelet cyclooxygenase is inhibited. However, the more powerful agonists that yield the calcium release response can still aggregate and activate platelets, because cyclooxygenase is not required for those pathways (Fig. 29–8).

In many centers, a majority of the patients presenting for coronary artery bypass grafting (CABG) will have received aspirin within 7 days of surgery in hopes of preventing coronary thrombosis.[52] Aspirin is a drug for which an increased risk of bleeding often has been demonstrated.[53] Although most early research studies said that aspirin leads to increased bleeding, since the mid 1990s, that early impression has not been upheld. Today, it is probably more likely that in some patients a mild-to-moderate increased risk of bleeding is possible.

Unfortunately, most of the early studies of aspirin were not blinded, and it may be that the pervading belief that aspirin caused increased bleeding was actually self-fulfilling. Since the early 1990s, there have been a number of therapeutic changes including use of lower doses and greater use of aprotinin and lysine analog antifibrinolytics. These changes alone may have decreased the overall risk of bleeding from aspirin. Follow-up prospective studies have thus yielded varied results. In the largest cohort of 772 men, aspirin increased bleeding after CABG by 33%,[54] and a group of 101 aspirin-taking patients bled 25% to 56% more than a control group.[55] In another study, the need to explore the mediastinum for excessive bleeding nearly doubled (factor of 1.82) in patients taking aspirin.[56] However, many other studies have not shown increased bleeding with aspirin.[57-62] Although a single aspirin can irreversibly inhibit platelet cyclooxygenase for the life of the platelet, aspirin-related bleeding after surgery usually requires more extensive exposure to the drug.

Drug-Induced Platelet Abnormalities

Many other agents inhibit platelet function. β-Lactam antibiotics coat the platelet membrane, while the cephalosporins are rather profound but short-term platelet inhibitors.[63] Many cardiac surgeons may not realize that their standard drug regimen for antibiotics may be far more of a bleeding risk than aspirin. Hundreds of drugs can inhibit platelet function. Calcium channel blockers, nitrates, and β-blockers are ones

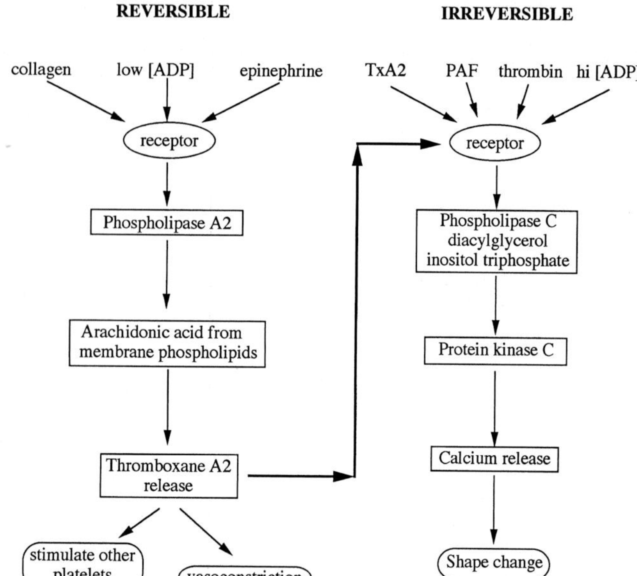

Figure 29–8 Pathways for reversible (left column) and irreversible (right column) platelet aggregation. Note the different agents that activate distinct receptors. Aspirin inhibits reversible platelet aggregation via the phospholipase A_2 pathway by affecting the arachidonic acid enzyme cyclooxygenase, but does not prevent more powerful agonists from aggregating platelets by directly stimulating phospholipase C pathway receptors. (Adapted from Kroll MH, Schafer A: Biochemical mechanisms of platelet activation. Blood 74:1181, 1989.)

commonly utilized in cardiac surgery. Nitrates are effective antiplatelet agents and that may be part of why they are of such benefit in angina, not just for their vasorelaxing effect upon large blood vessels. Nonsteroidal anti-inflammatory drugs (NSAIDs) reversibly inhibit both endothelial cell and platelet cyclooxygenase. In addition, anecdotal reports of platelet inhibition, without clear confirmatory studies, exist for many pharmaceuticals including dextran, and for innumerable foods (e.g., onion, garlic, alcohol) and spices (e.g., ginger, tumeric, cloves).[24]

Rofecoxib (Vioxx), a cyclooxygenase 2 (COX-2) inhibitor, was withdrawn from the United States market due to its cardiovascular risk profile (a small increase in associated acute myocardial infarctions).[64] This COX-2 inhibitor has the highest selectivity for COX-2 versus COX-1 and thus leads to an imbalance between thromboxane A_2 (TxA_2) and prostacyclin production. The other COX-2 inhibitors are now also undergoing cardiovascular investigation.

In addition to the partial inhibitory effects of aspirin and the other drugs mentioned above, new therapies have been developed that inhibit platelet function in a more specific manner. These drugs include platelet adhesion inhibitor agents, platelet-ADP-receptor antagonists, and GPIIb/IIIa receptor inhibitors (Table 29–4).[65]

ADHESION INHIBITORS

Dipyridamole (Persantine) and cilostazol (Pletal) alter platelet adhesion by various mechanisms including cyclic AMP, phosphodiesterase III, and TxA_2 inhibition. Dipyridamole has been used with warfarin in some patients with artificial valves and with aspirin in patients with peripheral vascular disease.

ADP RECEPTOR ANTAGONISTS

Clopidogrel (Plavix) and ticlopidine (Ticlid) are thienopyridine derivatives that inhibit the ADP receptor pathway to platelet activation. They have a slow onset of action since they must be converted to active drugs, and their potent effects last the lifetime of the platelets affected (5 to 10 days). Clopidogrel is the preferred drug since it has a better safety record than ticlopidine. It is administered orally once daily to inhibit platelet function and is quite effective in decreasing myocardial infarctions after percutaneous coronary interventions (PCIs) (see Chapter 12). The combination of aspirin and clopidogrel has led to increased bleeding, but is sometimes used in an effort to keep vessels and stents open. The TEG with ADP added can be used to determine the degree of inhibition due to these drugs (see Chapter 18). In addition, aprotinin may be able to partially reverse the drug's effects (see later).

Table 29–4 Antiplatelet Therapy

Drug Type	Composition	Mechanism	Indications	Route	Half-life	Metabolism
Aspirin	Acetylsalicylic acid	Irreversible COX inhibition	CAD, AMI, PVD, PCI, ACS	Oral	10 days	Liver, kidney
NSAIDs	Multiple	Reversible COX inhibition	Pain	Oral	2 days	Liver, kidney
Adhesion inhibitors (e.g., dipyridamole)	Multiple	Block adhesion to vessels	VHD, PVD	Oral	12 hr	Liver
ADP receptor antagonists (e.g., clopidogrel)	Thienopyridines	Irreversible inhibition of ADP binding	AMI, CVA, PVD, ACS, PCI	Oral	5 days	Liver
GPIIb/IIIa receptor inhibitors						
Abciximab (ReoPro)	Monoclonal antibody	Nonspecific—binds to other receptors	PCI, ACS	IV	12 to 18 hr	Plasma proteinase
Eptifibatide (Integrilin)	Peptide	Reversible—specific to GPIIb/IIIa	PCI, ACS	IV	2 to 4 hr	Kidney
Tirofiban (Aggrastat)	Nonpeptide-tyrosine derivative	Reversible—specific to GPIIb/IIIa	PCI, ACS	IV	2 to 4 hr	Kidney

CAD = coronary artery disease; AMI = acute myocardial infarction; PVD = peripheral vascular disease; PCI = percutaneous coronary intervention; ACS = acute coronary syndrome; VHD = valvular heart disease; CVA = cerebrovascular disease; IV = intravenous.

GPIIB/IIIA RECEPTOR INHIBITORS

These are the most potent (>90% platelet inhibition) and important platelet inhibitors since they act at the final common pathway of platelet aggregation with fibrinogen, no matter which agonist began the process. All of the drugs mentioned above work at earlier phases of activation of platelet function. These drugs are all administered by intravenous infusion and they do not work orally. The GPIIb/IIIa inhibitors are often used in patients taking aspirin since they do not block TxA_2 production. The dose of heparin is usually reduced when used with these drugs (i.e., PCI to avoid bleeding at the vascular puncture sites). Platelet activity can be monitored to determine the extent of blockade. Excessive bleeding requires allowing the short-acting drugs to wear off, while possibly administering platelets to patients receiving the long-acting drug abciximab (see Table 29–4). Most studies have found increased bleeding in patients receiving these drugs who required emergency CABG.

Vascular Endothelium

The cells that form the intima of vessels provide an excellent nonthrombogenic surface. Characteristics of this surface, which may account for its nonthrombogenicity, include negative charge; incorporation of heparan sulfate in the grid substance; the release of prostacyclin, nitric oxide, adenosine, and protease inhibitors by endothelial cells; binding and clearance of activated coagulation factors both directly, as occurs with thrombin, and indirectly, as evidenced by the action of thrombomodulin to inactivate factors Va and VIIIa via protein C; and stimulation of fibrinolysis.

Nitric oxide vasodilates blood vessels and inhibits platelets. Its mechanism involves activation of guanylate cyclase with eventual uptake of calcium into intracellular storage sites. Prostacyclin (PGI_2) possesses powerful vasodilator and antiplatelet properties. Endothelium-derived prostacyclin opposes the vasoconstrictor effects of platelet-produced TxA_2. Prostacyclin also inhibits platelet aggregation, disaggregates clumped platelets, and, at high concentrations, inhibits platelet adhesion. Prostacyclin increases intracellular concentrations of cyclic adenosine monophosphate (cAMP), which inhibits aggregation. Thromboxane acts in an opposite manner. The mechanism of prostacyclin action is stimulation of adenylyl cyclase, leading to reduced intracellular calcium concentrations. Some vascular beds (e.g., lung) and atherosclerotic vessels secrete thromboxane, endothelins, and angiotensin, all vasoconstrictors, as well as prostacyclin. Activation of platelets releases endoperoxides and arachidonate. These substances, utilized by nearby damaged endothelial cells, provide substrate for prostacyclin production.[5]

The endothelial cell also participates in coagulation factor activation. Playing a role similar to that of platelet phospholipid, the endothelial surface facilitates activation of factor IX. Thrombospondin, a substance formed in endothelial cells and platelets, helps complete platelet aggregation and binds plasminogen. The latter effect decreases the amount of locally available plasmin, thus inhibiting fibrin breakdown.

Fibrinolysis

Fibrin breakdown, a normal hematologic activity, is localized to the vicinity of a clot. It remodels formed clot and removes thrombus when endothelium heals. Like clot formation, clot breakdown may occur by intrinsic and extrinsic pathways. As with clot formation, the extrinsic pathway plays the dominant role in clot breakdown. Each pathway activates plasminogen, a serine protease synthesized by the liver, which circulates in zymogen form. Cleavage of plasminogen by the proper serine protease forms plasmin. Plasmin splits fibrinogen or fibrin at specific sites. Plasmin is the principal enzyme of fibrinolysis, just as thrombin is principal to clot formation. Plasma normally contains no circulating plasmin, since a scavenging protein, α_2-antiplasmin, quickly consumes any plasmin formed from localized fibrinolysis. Thus, localized fibrinolysis, not systemic fibrinogenolysis, accompanies normal hemostasis.

Extrinsic Fibrinolysis

Endothelial cells synthesize and release t-PA. Both t-PA and a related substance, urokinase plasminogen activator (u-PA), are serine proteases that split plasminogen to form plasmin. The activity of t-PA magnifies upon binding to fibrin. In this manner also, plasmin formation remains localized to sites of clot formation. Epinephrine, bradykinin, thrombin, and factor Xa cause endothelium to release t-PA, as do venous occlusion and CPB.[66] Fibrinolysis during and after CPB is discussed later.

Intrinsic Fibrinolysis

Factor XIIa, formed during the contact phase of coagulation, cleaves plasminogen to plasmin. The plasmin so formed then facilitates additional cleavage of plasminogen by factor XIIa, forming a positive feedback loop. Also, kallikrein can activate plasminogen. The physiologic importance of this pathway for fibrin breakdown has not been established.

Exogenous Activators

Streptokinase (made by bacteria) and urokinase (found in human urine) both cleave plasminogen to plasmin, but do so with low fibrin affinity. Thus, systemic plasminemia and fibrinogenolysis as well as fibrinolysis ensue. Acetylated streptokinase plasminogen activator complex (ASPAC) provides an active site, which is not available until deacetylation occurs in blood. Its systemic lytic activity lies intermediate to those of t-PA and streptokinase. Recombinant t-PA (rt-PA; Alteplase) is a second-generation agent that is made by recombinant DNA technology and is relatively fibrin specific (see Chapter 12).

Clinical Applications

Figure 29–9 illustrates the fibrinolytic pathway, with activators and inhibitors. Streptokinase, ASPAC, and t-PA find application in the lysis of thrombi associated with myocardial infarction. These intravenous agents "dissolve" clots that form on atheromatous plaque. Clinically significant bleeding may result from administration of any of these exogenous activators or streptokinase.[67]

Fibrinolysis also accompanies CPB. This undesirable breakdown of clot after surgery may contribute to postoperative hemorrhage and the need to administer allogeneic blood products. Regardless of how they are formed, the breakdown products of fibrin intercalate into sheets of normally forming fibrin monomers, thus preventing cross-linking. In this way, extensive fibrinolysis exerts an antihemostatic action.

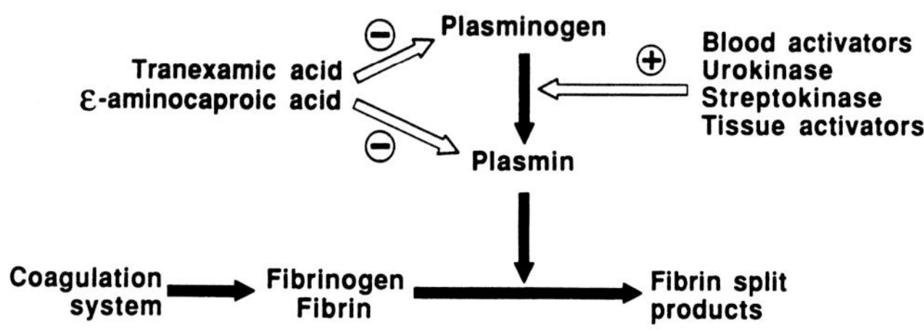

Figure 29–9 The fibrinolytic pathway. Antifibrinolytic drugs inhibit fibrinolysis by binding to both plasminogen and plasmin. Intrinsic blood activators (factor XIIa), extrinsic tissue activators (t-PA, u-PA), and exogenous activators (streptokinase, ASPAC) split plasminogen to form plasmin. (From Horrow JC, Hlavacek J, Strong MD, et al: Prophylactic tranexamic acid decreases bleeding after cardiac operations. J Thorac Cardiovasc Surg 99:70, 1990.)

HEPARIN

In 1916, in the course of experiments to determine if the phospholipid component of cephalin caused clotting, a second-year medical student, Jay McLean, instead discovered a substance derived from liver that prolonged coagulation.[68] His mentor, William Howell, named this substance heparin. Heparin has been used almost exclusively as the anticoagulant for CPB for more than 50 years.

Pharmacology

Chemical Structure

In the 1920s, Howell's group isolated heparin and identified it as a carbohydrate containing glucuronic acid residues. In the 1930s, Jorpes demonstrated a hexosamine component to heparin (glucosamine, in particular) present in a ratio of 1:1 with the glucuronic acid. Of greater importance, he discovered that heparin contains many sulfate groups—two per uronic acid residue—making it one of the strongest acids found in living things. In the 1950s, Jorpes' group identified the sulfate groups at the N-position on glucosamine, where solely acetyl groups were previously thought to reside. In the 1960s they corrected identification of the uronic acid as L-iduronic acid, an epimer of D-glucuronic acid, and refined its structural detail.[69]

The *N*-sulfated-D-glucosamine and L-iduronic acid residues of heparin alternate in copolymer fashion to form chains of varying length (Fig. 29–10). As a linear anionic polyelectrolyte, the negative charges being supplied by sulfate groups, heparin demonstrates a wide spectrum of activity with enzymes, hormones, biogenic amines, and plasma proteins. A pentasaccharide segment binds to antithrombin.[70] Heparin is a heterogeneous compound: the carbohydrates vary in both length and side chain composition, yielding a range of molecular weights from 5000 to 30,000, with most chains between 12,000 and 19,000.[71] Today, the standard heparin is called unfractionated heparin (UFH).

HEPARIN VERSUS HEPARAN

Heparan, a glycosaminoglycan found in the connective tissue and the coating of the endothelial surfaces of nearly all species, can be distinguished from heparin by (1) a predominance of glucuronic acid over iduronic acid and (2) *N*-acetylation, rather than *N*-sulfation, of more than 20% of glucosamine residues. Bound to cellular proteins, heparan resides inside cells, on cell surfaces, and in the extracellular matrix.[69-73]

Source and Biologic Role

Heparin is found mostly in the lungs, intestines, and liver of mammals, with skin, lymph nodes, and thymus providing less plentiful sources.[73] Abundance of heparin in tissues rich in mast cells suggests these as the source of the compound. Its presence in tissues with environmental contact suggests a biologic role relating to immune function. Heparin may assist white blood cell movements in the interstitium after an immunologic response has been triggered. Mollusks have no coagulation system, yet possess heparin, arguing against a biologic role in hemostasis. It is clear that heparin, per se, was never intended biologically to be circulating in large dosages throughout the vascular tree.

Most commercial preparations of heparin now use pig intestine, 40,000 pounds of which yield 5 kg of heparin.[69] Prevention of postoperative thrombosis constituted the initial clinical use of heparin in 1935 by Best, Jaques, and colleagues in Toronto, and by Crafoord in Stockholm.[69]

Potency

Heparin potency is determined by comparing the test specimen against a known standard's ability to prolong coagulation.[74] Current United States Pharmacopeia (USP) and British Pharmacopoeia (BP) assays use a PT-like method on pooled sheep's plasma obtained from slaughterhouses. The plasma is commonly contaminated with tissue extracts or other hemostatically active substances. The European Pharmacopoeia's

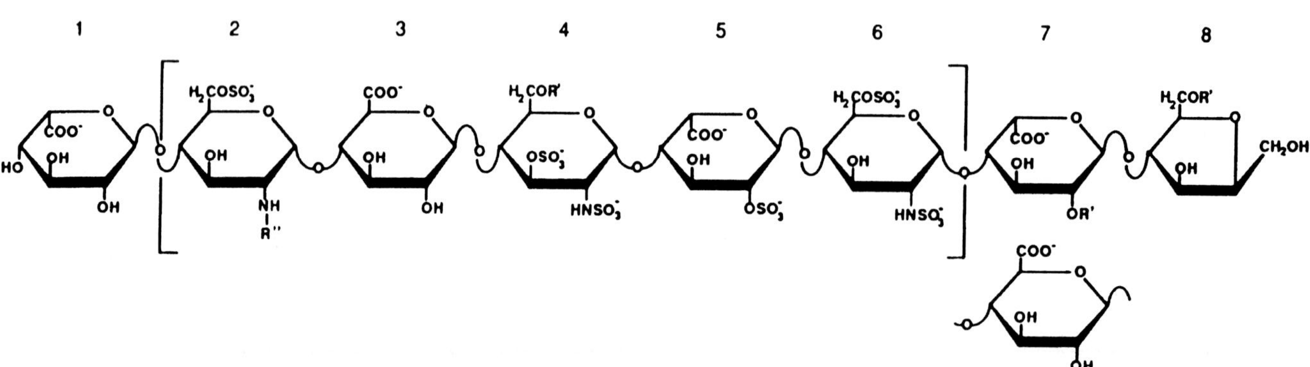

Figure 29–10 An octasaccharide fragment of heparin, a substituted alternating copolymer of iduronic acid and glucosamine. The leftmost sugar is iduronic acid. Note the numerous sulfate groups and the acetyl substitution on the second sugar. Variations in sugar substitutions and in chain length produce molecular heterogeneity. Brackets indicate the pentasaccharide sequence that binds to antithrombin. (From Rodén L: Highlights in the history of heparin. *In* Lane DA, Lindahl U [eds]: Heparin. Boca Raton, FL, CRC Press, 1989, pp 1.)

method, an activated PTT (aPTT) on fresh sheep's plasma, is superior to that of the USP.[75] Modern research assays employ human FFP, an aPTT-like method, and require linear log versus log plots of standard and test samples.[74]

UFH dose should not be specified by weight (milligrams) because of the diversity of anticoagulant activity expected from so heterogeneous a compound. Unfortunately, because of the flawed USP assay, even units of activity often do not reflect clinical effects. As originally defined, 1 unit of heparin prolongs the clotting of cat's blood for only 24 hours at 0°C.[76] Milligram usage, introduced in 1937 as a Swedish standard, was superseded by the first international standard, in which 130 units of activity corresponded to 1 mg. The fourth international standard uses a porcine mucosal preparation.[74]

One USP unit of heparin activity is the quantity that prevents 1.0 mL of citrated sheep's plasma from clotting for 1 hour after addition of calcium.[77] Units cannot be cross-compared among heparins of different sources, such as mucosal versus lung, or low-molecular-weight heparin (LMWH) versus UFH, or even lot to lot, because the assay used may or may not reflect actual differences in biologic activity. None of these measures has anything to do with the effect of a unit upon anticoagulation effect for human cardiac surgery.

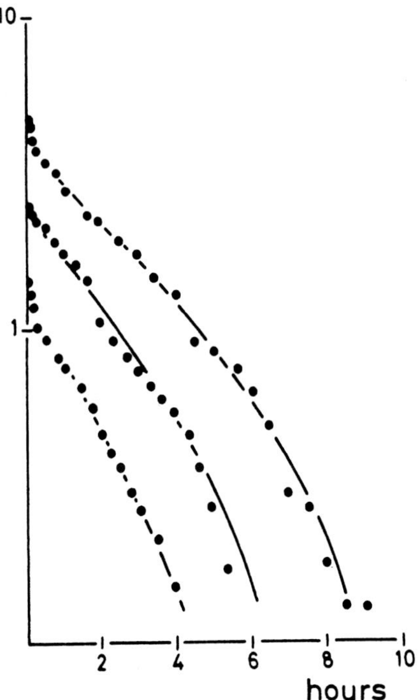

Figure 29–11 Decay of heparin anticoagulant activity (U/mL on a logarithmic scale) after injections of 75, 150, and 250 U/kg to a single volunteer. Note the rapid initial decline in all curves and nonlinearity at higher doses. (From deSwart CAM, Nijmeyer B, Roelofs JMM, Sixma JJ: Kinetics of intravenously administered heparin in normal humans. Blood 60:1251, 1982.)

Pharmacokinetics and Pharmacodynamics

The heterogeneity of UFH molecules produces variability in the relationship of dose administered to plasma level of drug. In addition, the relationship of plasma level to biologic effect varies with the test system. A three-compartment model describes heparin kinetics in healthy humans: rapid initial disappearance, saturable clearance observed in the lower dose range, and exponential first-order decay at higher doses[78,79] (Fig. 29–11). The rapid initial disappearance may arise from endothelial cell uptake.[80,81] The reticuloendothelial system, with its endoglycosidases and endosulfatases, and uptake into monocytes, may represent the saturable phase of heparin kinetics. Finally, renal clearance via active tubular secretion of heparin, much of it desulfated, explains heparin's exponential clearance.

Male gender and cigarette smoking are associated with more rapid heparin clearance.[82] The resistance of patients with deep vein thrombosis or pulmonary embolism to heparin therapy may be due to the release from thrombi of platelet factor 4 (PF4), a known heparin antagonist.[83,84] Chronic renal failure prolongs elimination of high, but not low, heparin doses.[82] Chronic liver disease does not change elimination.[85]

Loading doses for CPB (200 to 400 units/kg) are substantially higher than those used to treat venous thrombosis (70 to 150 units/kg). Plasma heparin levels, determined fluorometrically, vary widely (2 to 4 units/mL) following doses of heparin administered to patients about to undergo CPB.[86] The ACT response to these doses of heparin displays even greater dispersion. Gravlee et al[87] identified thrombocytosis and advanced age as causing a decreased ACT response to administered heparin. This effect may arise from alterations in pharmacokinetics, pharmacodynamics, or both. Interpatient variability in heparin response (pharmacodynamics) does affect the clotting time.[88,89] However, the clinical response to heparin administered to various patients is more consistent than suggested by in vitro measurements.

Although not substantiated formally, most clinicians would agree that hypothermia prolongs heparin's effect. Precise documentation remains impeded by inability to warm the patient's blood immediately to 37°C for standardized measurement of its ACT. Delayed metabolism or excretion or both most likely account for the prolongation of heparin presence during systemic hypothermia, while prolongation of the ACT more likely relates to decreased activity of coagulation enzymatic processes (see later).

Actions and Interactions

Heparin exerts its anticoagulant activity via ATIII, one of the many circulating serine protein inhibitors (serpins), which counter the effects of circulating proteases.[90] The major inhibitor of thrombin and factors IXa and Xa is ATIII; that of the contact activation factors XIIa and XIa is α_1-proteinase inhibitor; kallikrein inhibition arises mostly from C1 inhibitor. Antithrombin activity is greatly decreased at a site of vascular damage, underscoring its primary role as a scavenger for clotting enzymes that escape into the general circulation.

Antithrombin inhibits serine proteases even without heparin. The extent to which heparin accelerates antithrombin inhibition depends on the substrate enzyme: UFH accelerates the formation of the thrombin–antithrombin complex by 2000-fold, but accelerates formation of the factor Xa–antithrombin complex by only 1200-fold[91] (Table 29–5). In contrast, LMWH fragments preferentially inhibit factor Xa. Enzyme inhibition proceeds by formation of a ternary complex consisting of heparin, antithrombin, and the proteinase to be inhibited (e.g., thrombin, factor Xa). For UFH, inhibition of thrombin occurs only upon simultaneous binding to both antithrombin and thrombin. This condition requires a heparin fragment of at least 18 residues.[90,92] A pentasaccharide sequence binds to antithrombin (see Fig. 29–10).

Table 29–5 Some Coagulation Factor Inhibitors and the Effects of Heparin

Factor	Major Inhibitor	Acceleration of Antithrombin Activity by Heparin
Kallikrein	C1 inhibitor	—
XIIa	α_1-Proteinase inhibitor	—
XIa	α_1-Proteinase inhibitor	40-fold
Xa	Antithrombin	1200-fold
IXa	Antithrombin	10,000-fold
IIa	Antithrombin	2000-fold

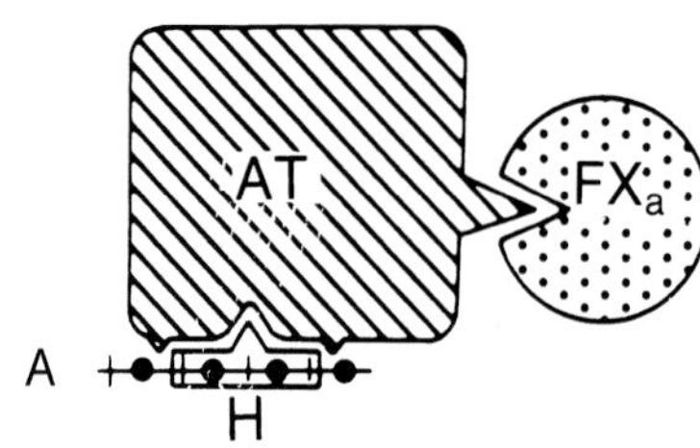

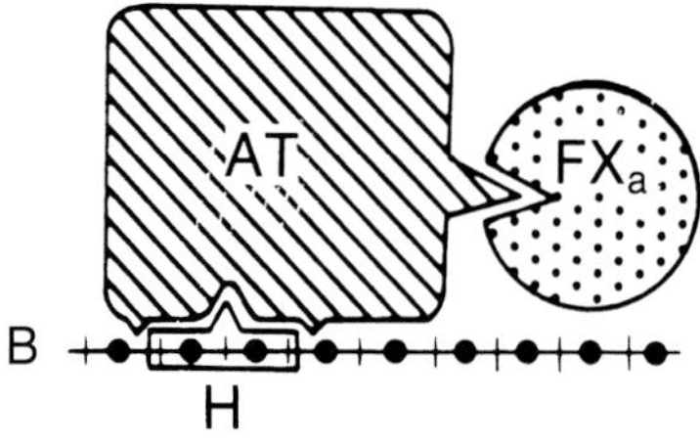

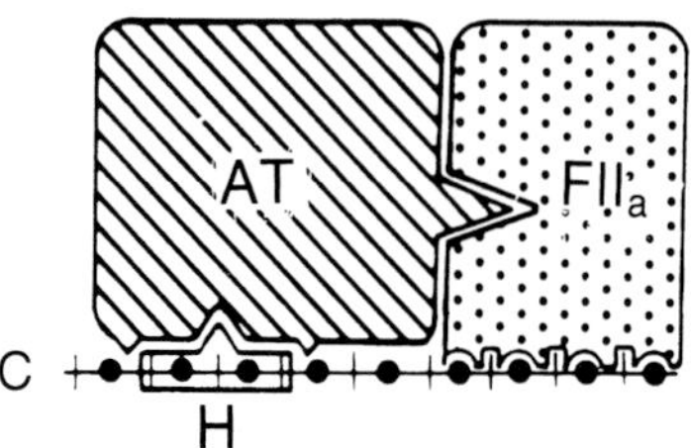

Figure 29–12 Antithrombin interaction with factor Xa may occur with either low-molecular-weight heparin (panel A) or standard unfractionated heparin (panel B). Inhibition of thrombin (factor IIa), however, requires simultaneous binding of the heparin molecule to both antithrombin and thrombin (panel C). (From Holmer E, Soderberg K, Bergqvist D, Lindahl U: Heparin and its low-molecular-weight derivatives. Anticoagulant and antithrombotic properties. Haemostasis 16[suppl 2]:1, 1986.)

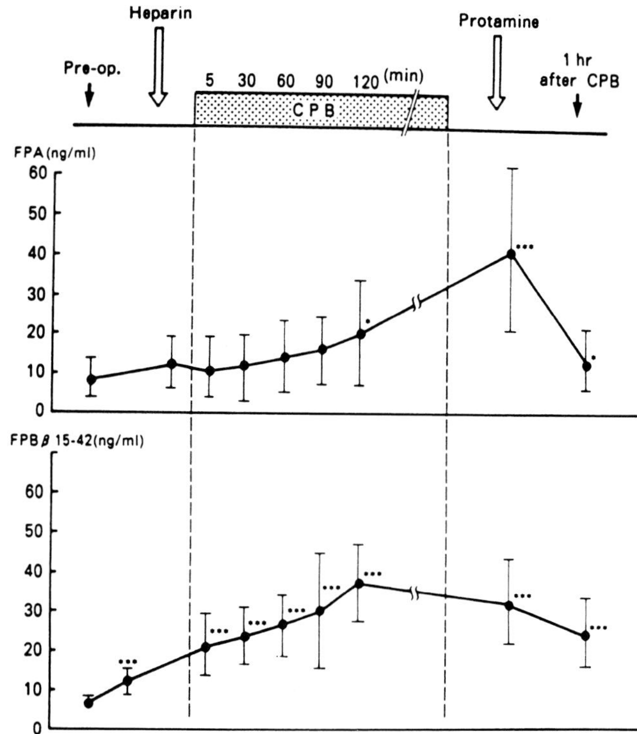

Figure 29–13 Serial measurements of fibrinopeptides A (upper panel) and B (lower panel) during cardiopulmonary bypass in 20 patients. Asterisks denote statistically significant changes compared with the preoperative measurement. Note continued presence of these markers of thrombin activity despite heparin administration. (From Tanaka K, Takao M, Yada I, et al: Alterations in coagulation and fibrinolysis associated with cardiopulmonary bypass during open heart surgery. J Cardiothorac Anesth 3:181, 1989.)

LMWHs, consisting of chains 8 to 16 units long, preferentially inhibit factor Xa. In this case, the heparin fragment activates antithrombin, which then sequentially inactivates factor Xa; heparin and factor Xa do not directly interact (Fig. 29–12).[93,94]

Several investigators have demonstrated continued formation of fibrinopeptides A[95-96] and B[97] (Fig. 29–13), and prothrombin fragment F1.2 and thrombin–antithrombin complexes,[98] despite clearly acceptable anticoagulation for CPB by many criteria. These substances indicate thrombin activity. The clinical significance of this ongoing thrombin activity has had limited study. The ACT must be more prolonged to prevent fibrin formation during cardiac surgery compared with during extracorporeal circulation without surgery, since surgery itself incites coagulation. UFH in conjunction with antithrombin appears to work in plasma only on free thrombin. When considering what is known today about thrombin burst and thrombin activity, heparin appears to be relatively inefficient, because there is not much free thrombin. Thrombin is held on the surface of activated platelets at various glycoprotein binding sites including the GPIIb/IIIa site. Most thrombin is fibrin bound, and heparin–antithrombin complexes do not bind at all to this thrombin unless the level of heparin is pushed far above what is used routinely for CPB. The idea behind using heparin for CPB is that by creating a large circulating concentration of activated antithrombin, whenever a thrombin molecule is produced, an available antithrombin molecule will be there to immediately bind to it before it can have any further activating effect. Clearly, that is unrealistic with the knowledge that thrombin exerts its main activity by binding to the surface of platelets.

Bovine Versus Porcine Preparations

Bovine lung heparin contains greater amounts of iduronic acid and sulfamino groups than pork mucosal heparin. Because endothelial endoglycosidases degrade heparin at sulfamino groups, elimination of beef lung heparin proceeds more quickly than that of pork mucosal heparin. Its ATIII affinity and anticoagulant activity are less than those of porcine heparin. Either preparation can establish suitable

BOX 29–2 *Problems With Heparin as an Anticoagulant for Cardiopulmonary Bypass*

- Heparin resistance
- Heparin-induced thrombocytopenia
- Heparin rebound
- Heparin's heterogeneity and variable potency

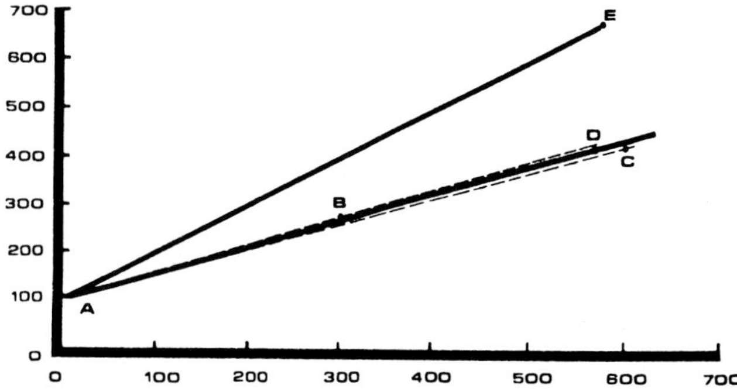

Figure 29–14 ACT response in seconds (vertical axis) to heparin administered in U/kg (horizontal axis) to a single patient. *(A)* baseline measurement; *(B)* after 300 U/kg; *(C)* after an additional 300 U/kg; *(D)* soon after C; *(E)* following 2 units of fresh frozen plasma. (From Sabbagh AH, Chung GKT, Shuttleworth P, et al: Fresh frozen plasma: A solution to heparin resistance during cardiopulmonary bypass. Ann Thorac Surg 37:466, 1984.)

anticoagulation for CPB. Beef lung heparin may be more amenable to protamine neutralization than the pork mucosal preparation because it exerts less anti–factor Xa activity.[99] Heparin-induced thrombocytopenia is less common with pork heparin (see later). This information may be of historic value only because bovine heparin is no longer available in the United States.

Heparin Resistance

In the course of continuous infusions of UFH to treat venous thrombosis, some patients develop tachyphylaxis, requiring increasing amounts of heparin to maintain the laboratory measurement of anticoagulation, the aPTT, at its designated therapeutic level. Likewise, patients receiving UFH infusions exhibit a much diminished ACT response to full anticoagulating doses of UFH for CPB (200 to 400 units/kg). With widespread use of heparin infusions to treat myocardial ischemia and infarction, heparin resistance or, more appropriately, "altered heparin responsiveness" has become more problematic during cardiac surgery (Box 29-2).[100,101]

Mechanism

Although several observations suggest that decreased levels of ATIII mediate heparin resistance, these observations lack sufficient evidence to establish this relationship.[101] First, a patient with congenital ATIII deficiency displayed heparin resistance.[102] This hardly proves that all heparin resistance stems from ATIII deficiency. Second, of six patients with venous thrombosis, three receiving heparin infusions displayed a 25% shorter half-life for ATIII compared with the three untreated patients.[103] Accelerated ATIII consumption could have resulted from the thrombotic process rather than the heparin infusion. Third, plasma levels of ATIII decreased by 17% to 33% during heparin administration by intravenous or subcutaneous routes.[104-109] Might this measurement result merely from formation of heparin–antithrombin complexes? Perhaps accelerated elimination of ATIII indeed arises from some modification of the protein during or following its interaction with heparin.[108]

Hemodilution accompanying CPB decreases antithrombin levels to about half of normal levels.[86] There are, however, outlier patients who have profoundly low antithrombin levels. It is possible to see ATIII levels as low as 20% of normal, and these levels correspond to levels seen in septic shock and diffuse intravascular coagulation.[15] However, supplemental antithrombin may not prolong the ACT, which means that the heparin available has been bound to sufficient or available antithrombin. The only way that the ACT would be prolonged is if there is excess heparin beyond available antithrombin. Reports of heparin resistance for CPB ascribe its occurrence variously to the use of autotransfusion,[109] previous heparin therapy,[110-113] infection,[114,115] and ventricular aneurysm with thrombus.[112,114] The differential diagnosis also includes hypereosinophilia, oral contraceptive therapy, consumptive coagulopathy, thrombocytosis, and congenital antithrombin deficiency.[112] Heparin resistance might also occur in patients with subclinical thrombotic processes releasing platelet factor 4.

The individual anticoagulant response to heparin varies tremendously.[116] Some presumed cases of heparin resistance may represent nothing more than this normal variation. Regardless of cause, measurement of each individual's anticoagulant response to heparin therapy for CPB is warranted.[117] Heparin resistance helps focus the debate regarding whether anticoagulation monitoring should measure heparin concentrations or heparin effect: the goal of anticoagulation is not to achieve heparin presence in plasma but to inhibit the action of thrombin on fibrinogen, platelets, and endothelial cells (see Chapter 18). Therefore, heparin effect is usually measured.

Treatment

Most commonly, additional heparin prolongs the ACT sufficiently for the conduct of CPB. Amounts up to 800 units/kg may be necessary to obtain an ACT of 400 to 480 seconds or longer. While administration of FFP, which contains antithrombin,[118] should correct antithrombin depletion (Fig. 29–14) and suitably prolong the ACT,[119] such exposure to transfusion-borne infectious diseases should be avoided whenever possible. This modality is reserved for the rare refractory case. Rather than administer FFP, centers normally accepting only ACTs of 480 seconds or longer for CPB might consider accepting 400 seconds or less, or administering ATIII concentrate.[119,120]

Antithrombin concentrate specifically addresses antithrombin deficiency.[15-18,118] It is a solvent detergent treated and heat-inactivated product providing greater protection against infectious disease transmission than that provided by FFP. The literature supports its success in treating heparin resistance during cardiac surgery[101,121] (see Chapter 24). A multicenter study on the efficacy of using a recombinant human antithrombin (rhAT) in heparin-resistant patients undergoing CPB was published.[122] The patients received 75 units/kg of rhAT, which was effective in restoring heparin responsiveness in most patients. However, some patients still required

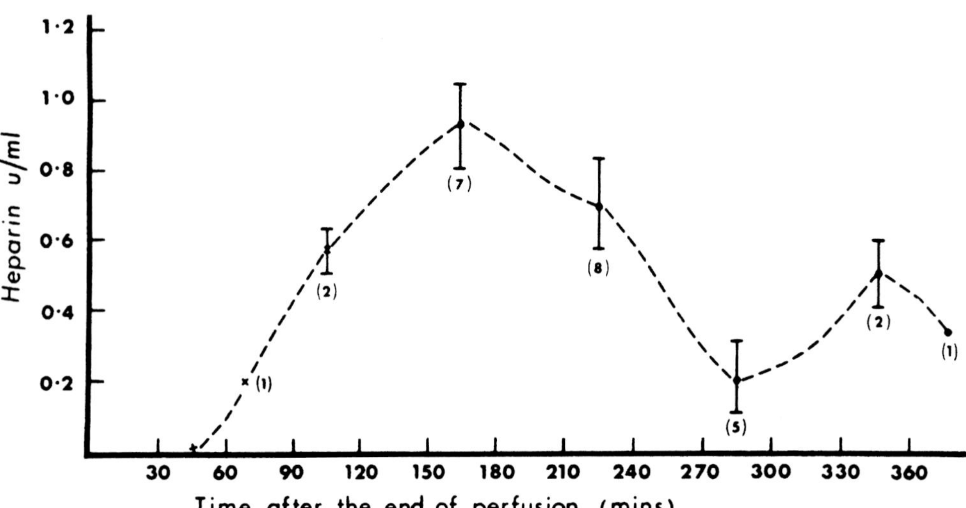

Figure 29–15 Heparin rebound measured by protamine titration in 10 of 24 patients given heparin by a fixed-time protocol. Parentheses denote number of patients. (From Kaul TK, Crow MJ, Rajah SM, et al: Heparin administration during extracorporeal circulation. J Thorac Cardiovasc Surg 78:95, 1979.)

FFP and the patients bled more than did a control group postoperatively.

Heparin Rebound

Several hours after protamine neutralization for cardiac surgery, some patients develop clinical bleeding associated with prolongation of coagulation times. This phenomenon is often attributed to reappearance of circulating heparin. Theories accounting for "heparin rebound" include late release of heparin sequestered in tissues, delayed return of heparin to the circulation from the extracellular space via lymphatics, clearance of an unrecognized endogenous heparin antagonist, and more rapid clearance of protamine in relation to heparin.[123,124] Studies demonstrating uptake of heparin into endothelial cells suggest that these cells may slowly release the drug into the circulation once plasma levels decline with protamine neutralization.[81] It is doubtful how much heparin rebound contributes to actual bleeding. This phenomenon may be caused by TFPI release from the surface of endothelial cells or other causes of bleeding.

Incidence and Timing

Although initial reports placed the incidence of heparin rebound after cardiac surgery at about 50%, modifications in the timing and amount of protamine administration decreased the incidence.[125,126] Heparin rebound can occur as soon as 1 hour after protamine neutralization.[126] When present, prolonged coagulation times or more direct evidence of circulating heparin may persist for 6 or more hours.[86,126-129]

Treatment and Prevention

Although still debated by a few, most clinicians accept heparin rebound as a real phenomenon. However, clinical bleeding does not always accompany heparin rebound. When it does, administration of supplemental protamine will neutralize the remaining heparin (Box 29–3). Can the initial protamine dose be adjusted to prevent heparin rebound? Available studies yield conflicting results. All of six patients who received protamine based on the estimated amount of *remaining* heparin developed heparin rebound, compared with none of six who received protamine based on the total administered dose of heparin.[126] However, 42% of patients receiving large, fixed doses of both drugs experienced heparin rebound and increased bleeding compared with patients whose doses were titrated to clotting assays[127] (Fig. 29–15). Likewise, patients receiving smaller doses of protamine bled less than those receiving protamine doses based on the total amount of heparin administered.[129] In contrast, a fourth study recommended that the ratio of protamine given to heparin remaining be as much as 1.6 mg/100 units.[86]

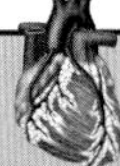

BOX 29–3 ***Considerations in Determining the Proper Dose of Protamine to Reverse Heparin***

- The proper dose is very broad and difficult to know exactly.
- The dose should be determined by a measurement of coagulation.
- The dose should be administered over at least 10 minutes.

It should be noted that in vitro work shows that as little as one third the heparin dose is all the protamine that is actually required to reverse the heparin in a test tube. It is still difficult to know exactly what the best heparin reversal dose is by protamine. Some effort at titration with a heparin dose-response curve, seems worthwhile.

While larger initial doses of protamine may decrease the likelihood of heparin rebound, two potential complications of protamine overdosage must be considered: adverse cardiovascular sequelae of protamine administration and the anticoagulant effects of protamine itself. Although protamine is an in vitro anticoagulant, doses up to 6 mg/kg in volunteers, in the absence of heparin, do not prolong the clotting time.[130] However, doses 4 times in excess of a neutralizing dose doubled the ACT in dogs.[131] The dose after CPB that causes anticoagulation in patients remains unknown. Clinical studies comparing fixed-ratio protamine doses to protocols that gauge protamine dose to remaining heparin activity and protamine drug lot potency demonstrated decreased doses of protamine, decreased chest tube drainage after surgery, and fewer transfusions.[132,133]

Heparin Effects Other Than Anticoagulation

UFH was never biologically intended to circulate freely in plasma.[134,135] As such it has a number of underappreciated and untoward effects. All too often the effects of CPB have been asserted as causing a coagulopathy; however, the effect of heparin contributing to this has not been widely studied. That is because there has not been an alternative anticoagulant to compare with heparin until now. In the future, there may be better anticoagulants to use during cardiac surgery (see later).

Heparin exerts its anticoagulant activity by activating a binding site on ATIII, and without antithrombin, heparin has no intrinsic anticoagulation effect. Antithrombin does have anticoagulant effects of its own, but its ability to bind to thrombin is increased 100- to 2000-fold by the presence of the pentasaccharide sequence of heparin. Less than one third of all mucopolysaccharides present in a dose of heparin contain the active pentasaccharide sequence. The other molecules may have a number of adverse properties.

Heparin binds ATIII during CPB, and through ongoing thrombin generation, the ATIII levels are decreased over time, as well as via hemodilution. Thus, the ATIII levels may become quite low, in the range seen during DIC, septic shock, and eclampsia.[15,136-138] ATIII is not able to be constitutively increased by production. Therefore, the level at the beginning of a CPB case is all that is available. The liver will slowly manufacture more ATIII, but it may take 1 to 3 days to return to normal after cessation of CPB. In at least one study in which ATIII was repleted to normal, the levels of coagulation proteins were much improved after CPB in patients who received exogenous ATIII.[15,118]

UFH chelates calcium.[139] When a large bolus dose of heparin is given, there is a slow and steady decline in blood pressure, probably due to decreased vascular resistance and decreased preload. Both arterial and venous vessels are dilated by the decrease in the calcium level. The heparin is given while patients are being prepared for CPB, and there are numerous mechanical events (i.e., catheters being inserted into the right atrium and vena cava and arrhythmias) that can be blamed for the hypotension, rather than the heparin itself.

Heparin, even in very small doses, partially and reversibly activates platelets and forces them to express many if not all of their glycoprotein binding sites.[140-142] This fact alone makes clinicians wonder if there is not a better anticoagulant that might not do this. Heparan, the endothelial analog of heparin, does not break off freely into the circulation, and if it does, it is immediately neutralized by platelets through expression of PF4 and adsorption. Thus, it makes sense that platelets seeing loose heparin would suspect a site of tissue injury nearby and, therefore, an evolutionary advantage would be created by making these cells react and get ready to create a thrombus. Every coagulation activation is also an inflammatory signal. The fact that platelets take this reactive step means that they are now primed to either become highly reactive and contribute to the inflammatory events or have their receptors targeted by other subsequent events. After CPB, platelets have many of their membrane glycoproteins either destroyed or competitively occupied by a number of products of inflammation produced during CPB. The expression of binding sites in response to heparin, therefore, is important and probably has profound implications.

Heparin causes the competitive release of some heparan from endothelial cells and the release of tissue factor pathway inhibitor (TFPI).[25,26] Endothelial cells all over the body change from being anticoagulant producing to rapidly producing tissue factor. What role large doses of heparin have in this whole-body event is hard to say, but it is known that heparin also causes the release of single-chain urokinase from endothelial cells.[143] The amount of fibrinolysis caused by heparin infusion is not as great as the release of t-PA, which is probably mediated by cytokines as a result of the inflammatory reactions. When released from mast cells, heparin promotes leukocyte chemotaxis and movement through the interstitium.[134,135] However, it is unclear whether heparin upregulates or decreases white cell activations.[135]

Heparin is important for a number of angiogenesis and repair activities of tissue,[135] and these effects may have something to do with its antineoplastic effect.[135] Heparin also affects lipid, sodium and potassium, and acid-base metabolism. These effects are not usually seen acutely but come into play when patients have been on heparin infusions for days in the ICU.

The immunologic effects of heparin are profound. The next section discusses heparin-induced thrombocytopenia, but recent work shows that 30% to 50% of cardiac surgery patients have heparin antibodies present in their blood by the time of hospital discharge.[144] The clinical implications of these prevalent antibodies remain unknown and are the subject of investigation.

Heparin-Induced Thrombocytopenia

Heparin normally binds to platelet membranes at GPIb and other sites, and aggregates normal platelets by releasing ADP.[144,145] A moderate, reversible, heparin-induced thrombocytopenia (HIT), now termed type I, has been known for half a century.[146] The fact that heparin actually triggers an acute drop in platelet count should be considered a biologic event, since heparin, even in trace amounts, triggers the expression of many different platelet glycoproteins. Some have termed this activation of platelets, but it is not total activation. Heparin's prolongation of the bleeding time is probably related to both activation of the platelets as well as heparin binding to the GPIb surface. It may be that a number of platelets adhere to endothelial cells simply due to their expression of these glycoprotein binding sites. Margination, particularly within the pulmonary vasculature, may be an event of HIT type I.

In contrast to these predictable effects of heparin, occasional patients develop progressive and severe thrombocytopenia ($<100{,}000/mm^3$), sometimes accompanied by a debilitating or fatal thrombosis. This syndrome is termed type II heparin-induced thrombocytopenia (HIT II). A platelet count in excess of $100{,}000/mm^3$ does not mean that HIT-II is not present. A drop in platelet count in excess of 30% to 50% over several days in a patient who is receiving or who has just finished receiving heparin is probably HIT II.

Mechanism

These patients demonstrate a heparin-dependent antibody, usually IgG, although others are described, which aggregates platelets in the presence of heparin.[143,144] During heparin therapy, measured antibody titers remain low owing to antibody binding to platelets. Titers rise after heparin therapy ceases; but paradoxically, antibody may be undetectable a few

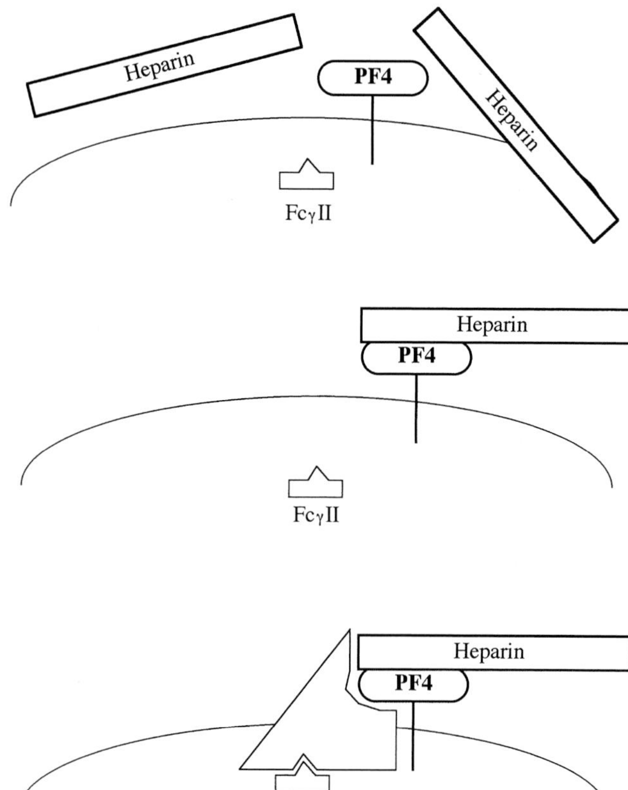

Figure 29–16 Presumed mechanism of the interaction among heparin, platelets, and antibody in heparin-induced thrombocytopenia. Top, PF4 released from platelet granules is bound to the platelet surface. Middle, heparin and PF4 complexes form. Bottom, the antibody binds to the PF4-heparin complex and activates platelet FcγII receptors.

months later.[147] Two other features are unexpected: first, the antibody does not aggregate platelets in the presence of excess heparin; and second, not all reexposed patients develop thrombocytopenia.[148-150]

The platelet surface contains complexes of heparin and PF4. Affected patients have antibody to this complex. Antibody binding activates platelets via their FcγII receptors and activates endothelium[151-153] (Fig. 29–16). The activation of the platelet surface triggers a secondary thrombin release. Platelets can attach to each other creating what is known as a white clot syndrome. But if secondary thrombin generation is created through antibody activation of the platelets then a fibrin clot can be the result. In the absence of heparin, the heparin-PF4 antigen cannot form. However, there seems to be some sort of continuum between idiopathic thrombocytopenia (ITP) and HIT.

In the absence of an endothelial defect, the only responses to the antibody-antigen interaction are platelet consumption and thrombocytopenia. Atheroma rupture, endovascular interventions such as balloon angioplasty, vascular surgery, and other procedures that disrupt endothelium can provide a nidus for platelet adhesion and subsequent activation. PF4, released with platelet activation, binds to heparin locally, thus not only removing the inhibition of coagulation but also generating additional antigenic material (Fig. 29–17). Clumps of aggregated platelets thrombose vessels, resulting in organ and limb infarction. Amputation and/or death often occur with established HIT with thrombosis (HITT). The presence of heparin-PF4 antibodies has recently been associated with other adverse effects. It appears that if a patient undergoes cardiac surgery with positive antibodies, the risk of mortality and/or myocardial infarction may at least double.

Incidence and Diagnosis

Estimates of the true incidence of this syndrome are confounded by different diagnostic thresholds for platelet count, varying efforts to detect other causes, and incomplete reports.[154,155] After 7 days of therapy with UFH, probably 1% of patients develop HIT; after 14 days of therapy the prevalence is 3%.[153] Using a platelet count of 100,000/mm^3, multiple reports comprising more than 1200 patients revealed an overall incidence of HIT of 5.5% with bovine heparin and 1.0% with porcine heparin.[144] Other recent research has found the preoperative incidence of ELISA-positive patients to be between 6.5% to 10%. This means that antibodies are present and that may not mean that thrombocytopenia is occurring. Of great interest is that many more patients develop positive tests for ELISA antibodies by days 7 to 30 after cardiac surgery. Somewhere between 25% and 50% of patients develop these antibodies.[144] Unfortunately, direct comparative studies of the two heparin sources contain too few patients for meaningful interpretation; this is moot today because bovine heparin is no longer used in the United States. Some particular lots of heparin may be more likely to cause HIT than others.[156]

Heparin-induced thrombocytopenia can occur not only during therapeutic heparin administration but also with low prophylactic doses, although the incidence is dose related. Even heparin flush solution or heparin-bonded intravascular catheters can incite HIT.[157-160] Cases of platelet-to-platelet adhesion creating a "white clot" in otherwise normal patients have been observed in the oxygenator and the reservoir of CPB machines. The fact that such events have been reported even when all other tests appeared normal signals the unpredictable nature of the heparin-PF4 antibody as well as the biologic activity of UFH.

Although HIT usually begins 3 to 15 days (median, 10 days) after heparin infusions commence, it can occur within hours in a patient previously exposed to heparin. Platelet count steadily decreases to a nadir between 20,000 and 150,000/mm^3. Absolute thrombocytopenia is not necessary; only a significant decrease in platelet count matters, as witnessed by patients with thrombocytosis who develop thrombosis with normal platelet counts after prolonged exposure to heparin. Occasionally, thrombocytopenia resolves spontaneously despite continuation of heparin infusion.[161]

Clinical diagnosis of HIT requires a new decrease in platelet count during heparin infusion. Laboratory confirmation is obtained from several available tests. In the serotonin release assay, patient plasma, donor platelets, and heparin are combined. The donor platelets contain radio-labeled serotonin, which is released when donor platelets are activated by the antigen–antibody complex. Measurement of serotonin release during platelet aggregation at both low and high heparin concentrations provides excellent sensitivity and specificity.[148]

A second assay measures more traditional markers of platelet degranulation in a mixture of heparin, patient plasma, and donor platelets.[162] The most specific test is an enzyme-linked immunosorbent assay (ELISA) for antibodies to the heparin–PF4 complex.[142,143,163,164]

The type, source, and lot of heparin used affects the outcome of these tests. The heterogeneous nature of heparin demands that a lot-specific drug be employed in serotonin release assays, especially when used to determine suitability of future administration. For example, if LMWH administration is planned for a patient who developed HIT II with UFH, testing of patient plasma with the lot of LMWH to be given should precede its administration.

Measurement of platelet-associated IgG is poorly specific for HIT, because of numerous other causes of antiplatelet IgG. This test should not be used in the diagnosis of HIT.

Heparin-Induced Thrombocytopenia with Thrombosis

The incidence of HITT is 1.7% with bovine heparin and 0.3% with porcine heparin; thus, thrombosis accompanies more than one in five cases of HIT.[143,144] It is clear that the longer patients are on heparin the more likely it is that they will develop antibody, and with the knowledge that today close to 50% of cardiac patients develop antibodies, it is possible that a significant number of long-term or early mortalities might be due to undiagnosed HITT.[144] In several studies in the catheterization laboratory, it has been shown that if HITT antibodies are present prior to the performance of angioplasty, the mortality and combined morbidity are greatly increased, perhaps double or more.[165,166] One study has been carried out in almost 500 patients undergoing CABG surgery looking for the presence of antibodies and outcome. The incidence of antibody-positive patients was approximately 15%, and their length of stay in the hospital and mortality were more than doubled. Occasional rare situations in which the CPB circuit suddenly clots or when there are early graft thrombosis or whole-body clotting may all be variants of HITT, but none of these cases can be readily studied since they are so rare.[165] If such an occurrence does happen, HITT should be in the differential diagnosis. The occurrence of thrombosis at first seems paradoxical. However, HITT has as its hallmark a huge thrombin burst that can occur all over the body. With such massive thrombin generation the triggering of thrombosis is natural. Thrombosis may then activate the fibrinolytic system to produce a picture of consumptive coagulopathy.[157]

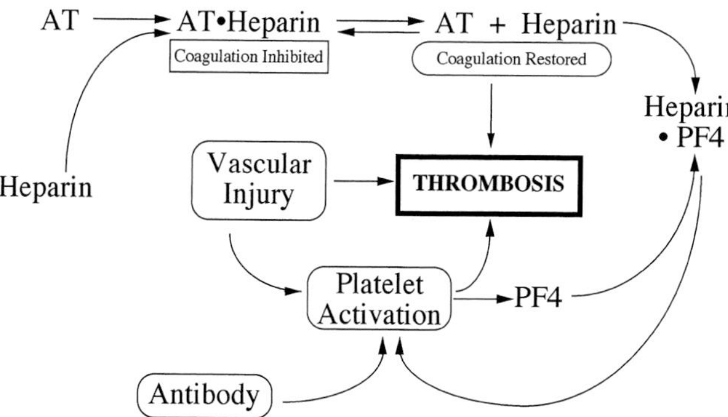

Figure 29–17 Mechanism of thrombosis accompanying heparin-induced thrombocytopenia. Normally, heparin and antithrombin form a complex that inhibits coagulation. Platelet factor 4 (PF4), released from platelets upon activation, binds heparin and drives the dissociation reaction of the antithrombin-heparin complex to the right, restoring coagulation locally. Restored coagulation mechanisms and activated platelets form thrombus in the presence of vascular injury. (Adapted from Parmet JL, Horrow JC: Hematologic diseases. *In* Benumof J [ed]: Anesthesia and Uncommon Diseases, 3rd edition. Philadelphia, WB Saunders Company, 1997.)

From 15% to 30% of patients who develop HIT with thrombosis will develop severe neurologic complications, require amputation of a limb, or die. Lower limb ischemia constitutes the most frequent presentation. Venous clots occur probably as frequently as arterial ones, but are not detected as often. Unfortunately, no test predicts the thrombosis component of HIT; thrombosis should be anticipated in the presence of vascular injury, such as puncture sites for catheterization.

Treatment and Prevention

In the absence of surgery, bleeding from thrombocytopenia with HIT is rare. In contrast to other drug-induced thrombocytopenias, in which severe thrombocytopenia commonly occurs, more moderate platelet count nadirs characterize HIT. Platelet transfusions are not indicated and may incite or worsen thrombosis. Heparin infusions must be discontinued, and an alternative anticoagulant should be instituted. LMWHs can be tested in the laboratory using serotonin release prior to patient administration. Although thrombosis may be treated with fibrinolytic therapy,[167] surgery is often indicated. No heparin should be given for vascular surgery. Monitoring catheters should be purged of heparin flush, and heparin-bonded catheters should not be placed. Antiplatelet agents, such as aspirin, triclopidine, or dipyridamole, which block adhesion and activation and, thus, PF4 release, provide ancillary help (see Table 29–4).

The patient presenting for cardiac surgery who has sustained HIT in the past presents a therapeutic dilemma. Antibodies may have regressed; if so, a negative serotonin release assay using the heparin planned for surgery will predict that transient exposure during surgery will be harmless. However, no heparin should be given at catheterization or in flush solutions after surgery.[144,145]

Patients with HIT who require urgent surgery may receive heparin once platelet activation has been blocked with aspirin and dipyridamole[138-170] or, in the past, the prostacyclin analog iloprost.[171-174] Unfortunately, iloprost is no longer available. The problem with this strategy is obtaining sufficient blockade of platelet activity.

Another alternative, delaying surgery to wait for antibodies to regress, may fail because of the variable offset of antibody presence and the unpredictable nature of platelet response to heparin rechallenge. Plasmapheresis may successfully eliminate antibodies and allow benign heparin administration.[175] Finally, methods of instituting anticoagulation without heparin may be chosen (see below). Of these, the alternative thrombin antagonists pose the greatest risk of uncontrolled bleeding, while LMWHs and heparinoids carry the greatest chance of success.[176,177]

LMWH heparin, as an alternative to UFH, has been used for urgent surgery.[178-180] While LMWHs can also induce thrombocytopenia,[181-183] by displaying different antigenic determinants, they may prove acceptable alternatives for patients who develop HIT from UFH. Table 29–6 summarizes the therapeutic options available for urgent cardiac surgery in patients with HIT. For additional information on HIT, see the following reviews.[144,145,184]

New Modes of Anticoagulation

The hemostatic goal during CPB is complete inhibition of the coagulation system. Unfortunately, even large doses of heparin

Table 29–6 Therapeutic Options for Anticoagulation for Bypass in Patients With Heparin-Induced Thrombocytopenia*

1. Ancrod
2. Low-molecular-weight heparin or heparinoid (test first!)
3. Alternative thrombin inhibitor (hirudin, bivalirudin, argatroban)
4. Use a single dose of heparin, promptly neutralize with protamine, *and*
   a. Delay surgery so antibodies can regress; *or*
   b. Employ plasmapheresis to decrease antibody levels; *or*
   c. Inhibit platelets with iloprost, aspirin and persantine, abciximab, or RGD blockers

In all cases

1. No heparin in flush solutions
2. No heparin-bonded catheters
3. No heparin lock intravenous ports

*No agent is indicated for anticoagulation in CPB at the time of this writing.

do not provide this, as evidenced by formation of fibrinopeptides during surgery.[95-97] Despite being far from the ideal anticoagulant, heparin still performs better than its alternatives. Heparans, dermatans, and other glycosaminoglycans with minimal antihemostatic properties may replace heparin in the future. If the discovery of heparin was an accident, what could be found by actually looking? Current substitutes for heparin include ancrod, a proteinase obtained from snake venom that destroys fibrinogen; heparin fragments, which provide less thrombin inhibition than the parent, unfractionated molecule; direct factor Xa inhibitors; and direct thrombin inhibitors (Box 29–4).

Ancrod

Ancrod abnormally cleaves fibrinogen, resulting in its rapid clearance by the reticuloendothelial system. Thrombin, thus, has no substrate on which to act. Proper patient preparation for CPB (plasma fibrinogen, 0.4 to 0.8 g/L) requires more than 12 hours. Figure 29–18 demonstrates the extent of fibrinogen depletion (from normal value of 1.5 to 4.5 g/L) and repletion for cardiac surgery using ancrod.[185] Replenishment of fibrinogen via hepatic synthesis is slow; cryoprecipitate and/or FFP administration will speed restoration of coagulation. Patients anticoagulated in this fashion bleed more and require more cryoprecipitate and FFP compared with heparin-anticoagulated patients.[185] One case was done with ancrod in which the coagulation activation was carefully studied.[186] Unbridled thrombin production led to massive platelet activation with a secondary precipitous decline in platelet count. No clot formed but a grey slime of platelets adhered to the wall of the oxygenator and the reservoir. The platelet count fell below 1000/mm^3. However, transfusion with platelet concentrates and cryoprecipitate reestablished normal coagulation and the patient had less than 500 mL of blood loss for the first 24 hours. No neurological deficits occurred. Ancrod is not commercially available in the United States.[186]

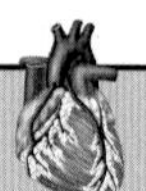

BOX 29–4 *Potential Replacements as an Anticoagulant for Cardiopulmonary Bypass*

- Ancrod
- Low-molecular-weight heparins
- Factor Xa inhibitors
- Bivalirudin or other direct thrombin inhibitors
- Platelet receptor inhibitors

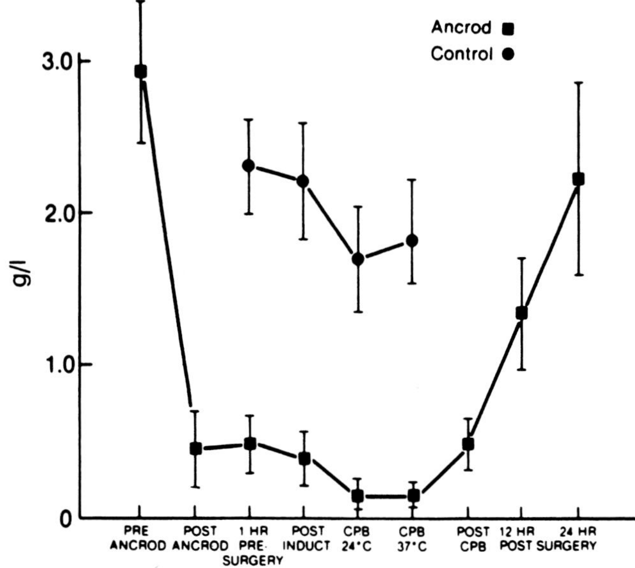

Figure 29–18 Plasma fibrinogen concentrations (normal, 1.5 to 4.5 g/L) in 20 patients who received snake venom (Ancrod) and 20 patients who received heparin (control) for anticoagulation during cardiopulmonary bypass. Note the slow return of plasma fibrinogen, despite administration of 9.3 ± 16.3 SD units of cryoprecipitate and 5.6 ± 3.1 units of fresh frozen plasma to the Ancrod group. (From Zulys VJ, Teasdale SJ, Michel ER, et al: Ancrod [Arvin] as an alternative to heparin anticoagulation for cardiopulmonary bypass. Anesthesiology 71:870, 1989.)

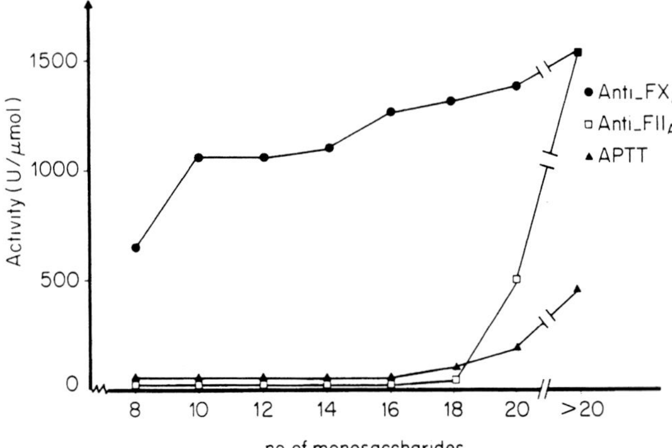

Figure 29–19 Heparin activity as a function of chain length. Oligosaccharides containing 8 to 16 units exhibit strong anti-factor Xa activity, whereas anti-IIa activity requires 20 or more units. Note that prolongation of the aPTT tracks anti-factor IIa activity. (From Holmer E, Soderberg K, Bergqvist D, Lindahl U: Heparin and its low-molecular-weight derivatives. Anticoagulant and antithrombotic properties. Haemostasis 16[suppl 2]:1, 1986.)

Low-Molecular-Weight Heparins

Figure 29–19 displays the effect of polysaccharide chain length on the inhibition of thrombin and factor Xa. Note that thrombin inhibition requires chains longer than 18 saccharide units and that aPTT activity follows anti–factor IIa activity more closely than it does anti–factor Xa activity.[92] Thrombin must

Table 29–7 **Properties of Unfractionated Heparin**
1. Anti*thrombotic**—Prevents thrombus formation in vivo
2. Anti*coagulant**—Prolongs clotting time in vitro
3. Anti*hemostatic*—Promotes bleeding
4. Anti*platelet*—Activates platelets

*Properties of an ideal agent.

bind to a portion of the heparin chain in order for antithrombin to inhibit it. In contrast, factor Xa inhibition by antithrombin does not require interaction of factor Xa with the heparin molecule. Only about 1% to 2% of standard heparin consists of low-molecular-weight (MW 6000 to 7000) fragments.[82] Short polysaccharide chains of heparin can be synthesized, or extracted from standard heparin, but both processes cost much more than depolymerization of standard heparin utilizing nitric acid, peroxides, or the enzyme heparinase. Preparations of LMWH formed by these methods include fraxiparin, dalteparin, and enoxaparin.

Standard heparin can inhibit thrombus formation in vivo (antithrombotic activity) and prolong in vitro clotting tests (anticoagulant activity). It also leads to clinical bleeding (antihemostatic activity). Table 29–7 highlights these definitions. LMWHs may dissociate these activities, displaying greater antithrombotic activity and less antihemostatic activity.[82] Unfortunately, coagulation tests sensitive to thrombin inhibition and insensitive to inhibition of factor Xa, namely the aPTT and ACT (see Fig. 29–19), do not adequately monitor the antithrombotic effects of LMWHs. For additional information regarding LMWHs, there are several good reviews.[187-189]

LMWHs have undergone clinical trials for antithrombosis following orthopedic procedures, and for prevention of deep-vein thrombosis.[190-192] The traditional LMWHs, such as enoxaparin, have not been used for CPB cases because of a limited ability of protamine to neutralize them.[193,194]

Heparinoids

Danapariod (Orgaran), a mixture of LMWHs and dermatans, can adequately provide anticoagulation for CPB, but lack of readily available monitoring and sure neutralization limit its application to cases in which UFH is clearly contraindicated.[194,195] Dermatans alone might prove suitable, but much more investigative work must first occur.[7,195] Case reports of these agents have shown severe bleeding and in some cases death from hemorrhage after cardiac surgery. It appears at this point that dermatan sulfate will not be used for cardiac surgery, and danaparoid was removed from the U.S. market.

Fondaparinux (Arixtra) is a synthetic pentasaccharide identical to that in heparin. It is a primary factor Xa inhibitor that requires ATIII, which does not affect thrombin, platelets, or fibrinolytic activity. It is being used for prophylaxis of deep vein thrombosis following surgery, but it does not alter routine coagulation tests (requires a factor Xa assay).[196] There is no direct antidote, but patients may respond to factor VIIa (see later).

Direct Thrombin Inhibitors

Hirudin, a single-chain polypeptide containing 65 amino acids with a molecular weight of 7000 and produced by the medicinal leech *Hirudo medicinalis,* binds directly to thrombin without need of a cofactor or enzyme, inhibiting all the proteolytic functions of thrombin. This inhibition includes actions on fibrinogen; factors V, VIII, and XIII; and platelets.

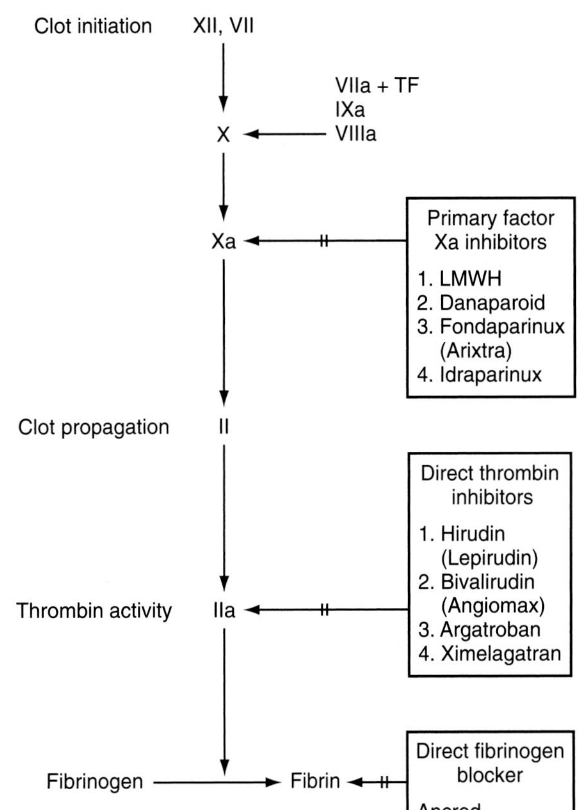

Figure 29–20 Alternatives to heparin. New modes of anticoagulation are shown in the boxes on the right side of the figure where they inhibit either factor Xa, thrombin, or fibrinogen.

Modifications of hirudin include hirugen, a synthetic peptide containing residues 53–64 of the native hirudin, and hirulog, formed by attaching the amino acid sequence d-phe-pro-arg-pro-(gly) to the amino-terminal end of hirugen. Hirugen inhibits thrombin's action on fibrinogen, but not on factor V. Hirulog has full inhibitory properties, but is slowly cleaved by thrombin itself to a hirugen-like molecule.

Hirudin depends on renal excretion; renal failure prolongs its elimination half-life of 0.6 to 2.0 hours. Although there are no known direct neutralizing agents for these drugs, administration of prothrombin complex may partially restore coagulation by enhancing thrombin generation. Clinical trials of hirudin compounds have yielded mixed results. It has been used for patients with HITT but the longer half-life of approximately 90 minutes means that many of these patients bleed after cardiac surgery.[197] Hirudin is highly antigenic and will lead to immune complexes being created to itself in about 40% of patients. If it is used a second time, the overall incidence of anaphylaxis may be as high as 10% of all patients who have received it before.[197]

New direct thrombin inhibitors are now available (Fig. 29–20). These include argatroban and bivalirudin. Argatroban is a derivative of arginine and is a relatively small molecule.[198,199] It binds at the active cleavage site of thrombin and stops thrombin's action on serine proteases. It is completely hepatically cleared and has a half-life of 45 to 55 minutes with prolongation when liver function is depressed or liver blood flow is decreased. There is no reversal agent for argatroban. It has been FDA approved for anticoagulation in the face of HITT, but there has not been, to date, a large-scale prospective randomized trial for cardiac surgery or any type of comparison to heparin/protamine. Some case reports do exist of successful usage of argatroban in HITT patients with acceptable amounts of postoperative bleeding. It has been more commonly utilized in the ICU for patients with hypercoagulable syndromes and HITT.[200,201]

Bivalirudin is a synthetic peptide based on the structure of hirudin (previously called hirulog).[202-209] Pharmacologists have taken the active amino acids at either end of the hirudin molecule and biosynthesized them. One active site competitively binds to the fibrinogen-binding site of thrombin, and the other 20-amino-acid sequence binds to the active serine cleavage site of thrombin. The two sequences of amino acids are connected together by a tetraglycine spacer. This fully manufactured molecule is highly specific for thrombin and has the unique property that it binds to both clot-bound and free thrombin. Heparin binds only to free plasma thrombin. Bivalirudin has a shorter half-life than argatroban and hirudin; the $t_{1/2}$ is approximately 20 to 25 minutes. Like the other direct thrombin inhibitors, it also has no reversal agent analogous to protamine. So when it is used, it must wear off. Bivalirudin undergoes destruction by the molecule to which it binds and deactivates, thrombin; it spontaneously is destroyed by thrombin (proteolytic cleavage). The more thrombin activation that is present (i.e., the less bivalirudin that is present), the shorter is the half-life. Only about 20% of the molecular activity is eliminated by renal clearance.[203] In mild to moderate renal failure, the effect on bivalirudin clearance is fairly small.

Several clinical trials of bivalirudin for cardiology procedures or cardiac surgery have been completed and published.[203-209] Other ongoing and pivotal trials aiming for FDA approval are under way comparing bivalirudin to heparin/protamine for both on- and off-pump CABG cases as well as for patients with HITT. Bivalirudin has been FDA approved as a primary anticoagulant for angioplasty. In trials comparing bivalirudin to either heparin/protamine alone or heparin plus the use of a IIb/IIIa inhibitor, bivalirudin was found to have at least equal or better safety and less bleeding than either of the other therapies. When compared to heparin/protamine alone in PCI, bivalirudin was found to be superior, not just in bleeding, but also in terms of morbidity and mortality (as a combined endpoint).[208] In a trial of 100 off-pump CABG patients randomized to receive either bivalirudin or heparin/protamine, bleeding and outcome were equal between the groups.[203] These patients underwent recatheterization at 3 months, and it was found that the bivalirudin patients had overall better flow down their grafts than did the patients who had received heparin/protamine. A phase I/II safety trial of bivalirudin in 30 on-pump CABG patients has also shown good safety, but no comparison was carried out to look at advantages against heparin/protamine. At this time, considerable research is ongoing and whether bivalirudin will prove superior to heparin/protamine for routine CABG is yet to be seen. When used, the doses for CPB have been a 0.75-mg/kg bolus followed by an infusion at 1.75 mg/kg/hr titrated to the ACT (target, 2.5 times baseline). The CPB system is also primed with 50 mg and no stasis can be allowed in the CPB circuit due to metabolism of bivalirudin during CPB. The infusion is stopped about 15 to 30 minutes before CPB is discontinued, and patients bleed for up to 4 to 6 hours. OPCAB cases have used similar doses to ACT targets of 350 to 450 seconds.[203]

In the face of HITT syndrome, case reports continue to show effectiveness and utility of bivalirudin.[205,206,209] This is an off-label use of the drug as it has not been FDA approved. In animal studies, bivalirudin does not activate platelets, and those animals who have received the drug for CPB have a better platelet count at the end of surgery. Other inflammatory mediators such as cytokines may also be decreased with bivalirudin administration as compared to heparin/protamine administration. Heparin, even in small doses, activates platelets to express their binding sites, while bivalirudin seems to leave the platelets quiescent. It also has no cross reactivity with any immunoglobulin that is present to heparin/PF4 and does not produce an immune response of its own, which can be seen with hirudin.

The latest direct thrombin inhibitors being developed are for long-term oral use. Ximelagatran is in active phase III clinical trials at the present time. This is a prodrug that is rapidly biotransformed into the active drug melagatran. The drug produces a predictable anticoagulant response and no laboratory monitoring is required. This drug may be able to replace warfarin, which is a very difficult drug to manage. Unfortunately, the FDA turned down ximelagatran in 2004 due to elevated ALT levels in 6% of patients. It is approved in Europe for short-term use and the FDA will reevaluate it after further clinical trials.[210-213]

Nonthrombogenic Surface

Considered the "Holy Grail" of extracorporeal circulation, an artificial surface that does not incite thrombus formation remains undiscovered. The endothelial surface, which the artificial one should mimic, performs a host of biochemical functions related to antithrombosis. Two that appear crucial are (1) secretion of substances that inhibit both platelet activation and aggregation and (2) surface and matrix adsorption of heparin and heparan, which may locally potentiate antithrombin.[214]

Heparin may be immobilized onto surfaces by ionic bonding onto cationic surfactants. Unfortunately, both heparin and surfactant leach off the coated surface upon exposure to blood. Covalent binding or surface grafting of heparin provides a more stable preparation. A properly heparin-bonded surface should bind antithrombin sufficiently to prevent fibrinogen-induced platelet adhesion. Heparin-coated CPB tubing reduces the need for systemic heparin, but has not been sufficiently effective to replace systemic anticoagulation.[215-217] Other approaches include increasing surface hydrophilicity with polyethylene oxide and sequestration of the thrombogenic surface by endothelialization, albumin activation, or phospholipid mimicking.[218] New materials might permit cardiac surgery with minimal doses of heparin or even without it.

PROTAMINE

Pharmacology

Protamine neutralizes heparin-induced anticoagulation. This section considers the history, pharmacology, and clinical use of protamine during cardiovascular surgery, including toxic and idiosyncratic adverse effects. Alternatives to protamine complete the discussion.

History

Miescher, investigating cell nuclei in 1868, discovered and named protamine, a nitrogenous alkaline substance in sperm heads of salmon.[219] Composed of nearly two-thirds arginine, protamines contain many positive charges (Fig. 29–21). Their biologic role is to associate with the negatively charged phosphate groups of nucleic acids[220] (Fig. 29–22).

In 1936, Hagedorn and colleagues used protamine to delay the absorption of insulin administered subcutaneously. They (correctly) chose protamine, hoping that its alkaline pH would maintain insulin in an ionized, slowly absorbed state. When others attempted to mix protamine with heparin to make a long-acting subcutaneous preparation for thrombosis prophylaxis, they obtained a white precipitate instead of a useful mixture.[221] Chargaff and Olson[222] recognized that this precipitate represented the salt of polycationic protamine and polyanionic heparin. They established protamine as the neutralizing drug for heparin's anticoagulant effect. Jaques developed the in vitro protamine titration test for blood heparin levels and documented adverse circulatory effects from protamine.[223,224]

HOOC - Gln - **Arg** - Thr - Cys - **Arg**
| Ile |
Gly - **Arg** - **Arg** - **Arg** - **Arg** - **Arg** - **Arg** - Val - Cys - Tyr - Thr - Val
| Phe |
Arg Ala - **Arg** - Tyr - **Arg** - Cys - Cys - Leu - Thr - His - Ser - Gly
Arg H_2N Ser
Arg **Arg**
Arg - **Arg** - **Arg** - Cys - **Arg** - **Arg** - **Arg** - **Arg** - **Arg** - **Arg** - **Arg** - Cys

Figure 29–21 The complete amino acid sequence of protamine from steer. Note the abundance of arginine residues (50% for this species). (Modified from Coelingh JP, Monfoort CH, Rozijn TH, et al: The complete amino acid sequence of the basic nuclear protein of bull spermatozoa. Biochim Biophys Acta 285:1, 1972.)

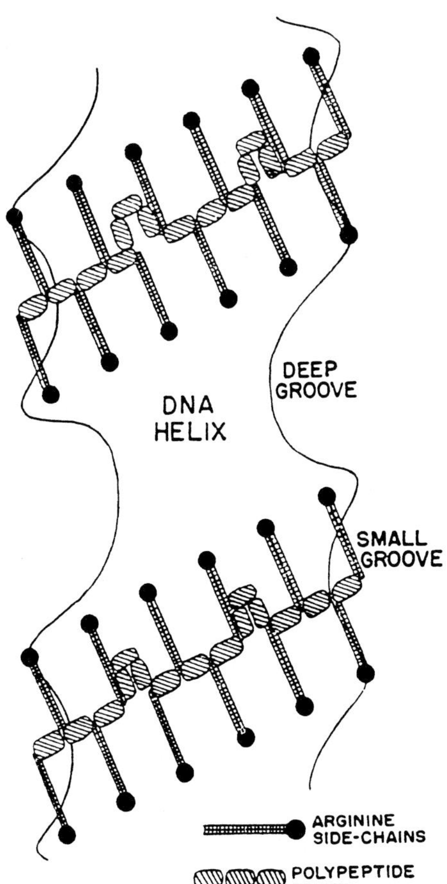

Figure 29–22 The polypeptide chain of protamine with its arginine residues seen residing in the small groove of the DNA helix. (From Wilkins MHF: Physical studies of the molecular structure of deoxyribonucleic acid and nucleoprotein. Cold Spring Harbor Symp Quant Biol 21:83, 1956.)

Source and Preparation

Most vertebrate species synthesize a protamine residing in the heads of sperm. Human protamine closely resembles that of other species.[225] Salmon milt provides the pharmaceutical source of protamine. The crushed gonads of male salmon undergo a crude extraction and filtration process using salt and alcohol. The final product, a dried powder, is commonly reconstituted as a 10 mg/mL solution. Like insulin and some other protein products, it is stable without refrigeration for several weeks. Protamine is available as sulfate and chloride salts. Protamine chloride may have a more rapid onset compared with protamine sulfate.[226] Nevertheless, clinical study reveals no superiority of one preparation over the other.[227]

Uses and Actions

Two long-acting insulin preparations contain protamine. Protamine-zinc insulin contains 10 to 15 μg of protamine per unit of insulin, while NPH (neutral protamine Hagedorn) insulin contains 3 to 6 μg/unit. The former compound, with more protamine, exhibits a 36-hour duration, compared with 24 hours for the NPH insulin. Both heparin and protamine alter cell division and influence angiogenesis and tumor size.[228,229] However, these effects have not yet developed into therapeutic modalities. In addition, both protamine and its substitute polycation, hexadimethrine, possess broad antimicrobial activity, suggesting application as a topical antibiotic.[230]

Neutralization of heparin-induced anticoagulation remains the primary use of protamine. Formation of complexes with the sulfate groups of heparin forms the basis for this "antidote" effect. Protamine neutralizes the antithrombin effect of heparin far better than its anti–factor Xa effect.[99] This distinction may arise from the need for thrombin, but not factor Xa, to remain complexed to heparin for antithrombin to exert its inhibitory effect. Since porcine mucosal heparin has more potent anti–factor Xa activity than bovine lung heparin,[231] today's available heparin may prove to be more difficult to neutralize with protamine. Protamine's poor efficacy in neutralizing anti–factor Xa activity limits the utility of LMWH compounds as anticoagulants for CPB.

Protamine exhibits antihemostatic properties by affecting platelets and by releasing t-PA from endothelial cells.[99] Thrombocytopenia follows protamine administration in dogs[224,232] and in humans.[233] Heparin–protamine complexes inhibit thrombin-induced platelet aggregation.[234-236] In addition, protamine appears to bind to thrombin, inhibiting its ability to convert fibrinogen to fibrin.[237] Initial attempts to document an in vivo antihemostatic effect of protamine proved unsuccessful.[130] Rapid degradation of protamine by circulating proteases may account for this discrepancy.

Administration, Distribution, and Fate

Neutralization of heparin occurs by intravenous injection of protamine. Subcutaneous administration is limited to pro-

Table 29–8 Basis for Variability in Protamine Dose

Ratio of protamine to heparin
Amount of heparin to neutralize
Heparin rebound
Protamine overdose

longation of insulin absorption. Presumably, these highly charged polycations distribute only to the extracellular space.

In the presence of circulating heparin, protamine forms large complexes with heparin.[238] Excess protamine creates larger complexes. The reticuloendothelial system may then dispose of these particles by endocytosis. Although this action has not been proved, macrophages in the lung may constitute the site for elimination of these complexes, since intravenous administration of protamine permits formation of heparin–protamine complexes in the pulmonary circulation first. Protamine may also bind to circulating plasma proteins, the significance of which remains unclear.[239] Proteolytic degradation of the protamine complexed to heparin conceivably results in free heparin. Protamine degradation in vivo proceeds by the action of circulating proteases, among them carboxypeptidase N, an enzyme that also clears anaphylatoxins and kinin pathway products.[240] The time course of protamine disappearance from plasma in patients remains poorly investigated.

Dosage

The recommended dose of protamine to neutralize heparin varies widely. Table 29–8 lists factors accounting for this variability. First, what is the proper ratio of protamine to heparin? Reports of the optimal ratio of milligrams of protamine to units of heparin cite values as low as zero (i.e., they do not neutralize heparin)[241] to as much as 4 mg/100 units.[140] This variability has been accounted for by differences in timing, temperature, and other environmental factors; choices for coagulation tests and outcome variables; and speculation and unproven assumptions. Second, what forms the basis for calculating protamine dose: the total amount of heparin given or the amount remaining in the patient? Protamine titration tests at the conclusion of CPB can determine the amount of heparin remaining in the patient. With automated versions of this test and simple assumptions regarding the volume of distribution of heparin, the amount needed to neutralize the heparin detected in the patient's vasculature can easily be calculated. However, this technique may invite heparin rebound, the third concern (see Chapter 18).

An alternative scheme splits a 1 mg/100 units calculated dose of protamine into two separate doses: an initial dose (75% of the total) following CPB, with the remainder following reinfusion of blood from the bypass circuit. This scheme prevented increased plasma heparin levels and prolongation of the aPTT, compared with a control group.[242] The ACT remained unchanged, perhaps a reflection of its insensitivity to small amounts of circulating heparin. Protamine chloride did not prove superior to protamine sulfate in preventing the occurrence of heparin rebound.[227]

A system utilizing coagulation test tubes that contain lyophilized heparin and protamine matched by lot to that administered to the patient permits calculation of dosages to account for variations arising from patient and pharmaceutical factors. It results in increased doses of heparin and decreased doses of protamine compared with those calculated by weight alone. Nevertheless, decreased bleeding and less use of allogeneic blood products result.[132]

Finally, lest fear of heparin rebound prompt the clinician to administer protamine in large excess, gross overdosage may likely anticoagulate patients. Dogs given excess protamine exhibited a dose-dependent prolongation of the ACT, with the ACT nearly doubling following a protamine dose four times that needed to neutralize heparin. At a 10-fold dose, the aPTT prolonged and thrombocytopenia developed[131] (Fig. 29–23). Without prior heparin, the coagulation test abnormalities occurred at lower protamine doses. The cautious clinician realizes that the protease enzyme system that degrades protamine can be saturated. Prolongation of coagulation times may conceivably result from protamine overdose as well as from un-neutralized heparin. Fortunately, the safe range of protamine dose regarding neutralization of anticoagulation is large; therefore, the prudent clinician will not hesitate to administer a small additional dose of protamine should incomplete neutralization or heparin rebound be suspected, while limiting administration so as not to overwhelm the proteases that degrade protamine.

Adverse Reactions

The potential for a deleterious response to protamine administration raises serious questions and difficult choices in clinical care before, during, and after cardiac operations. This section presents the spectrum of adverse reactions, the presumed mechanism for each, and treatment options. These adverse events can become rare with proper clinical technique. Thus, a clinical perspective at the end of this section discusses preventive measures to guard against untoward responses. The causes of hypotension following protamine (rapid administration, anaphylactic reaction, and pulmonary vasoconstriction) are considered in turn.

Rapid Administration

PERIPHERAL CARDIOVASCULAR CHANGES

Jaques initially identified that systemic hypotension from protamine administered to dogs required a rapid (15-second) injection. Subsequent study confirmed that hypotension accompanies intravenous protamine.[224,243-250] However, repeat doses are benign when given slowly or rapidly within 4 to 6 hours of an initial reaction unless heparin is given prior to the second dose.[244,251] Pulmonary arterial pressures (PAPs) also rise.[244,252] While increased PAP and pulmonary vascular resistance (PVR) follow protamine predictably in dogs, pigs, and sheep, humans respond in a more idiosyncratic fashion. Decreased systemic vascular resistance (SVR) accompanies the systemic hypotension,[232,247,248] while venous return and cardiac filling pressures decrease.[247,248] Rapid volume administration may, in fact, avert systemic hypotension in both dogs and man.[247,253]

What constitutes slow administration? A neutralizing dose given over 5 minutes or longer will rarely engender cardiovascular changes.[254] Systemic hypotension from rapid injection in humans has been ascribed to pharmacologic displacement of histamine from mast cells by the highly alkaline protamine, similar to the mechanism by which curare, morphine, and alkaline antibiotics (e.g., vancomycin and clindamycin) cause hypotension. However, protamine alone, in

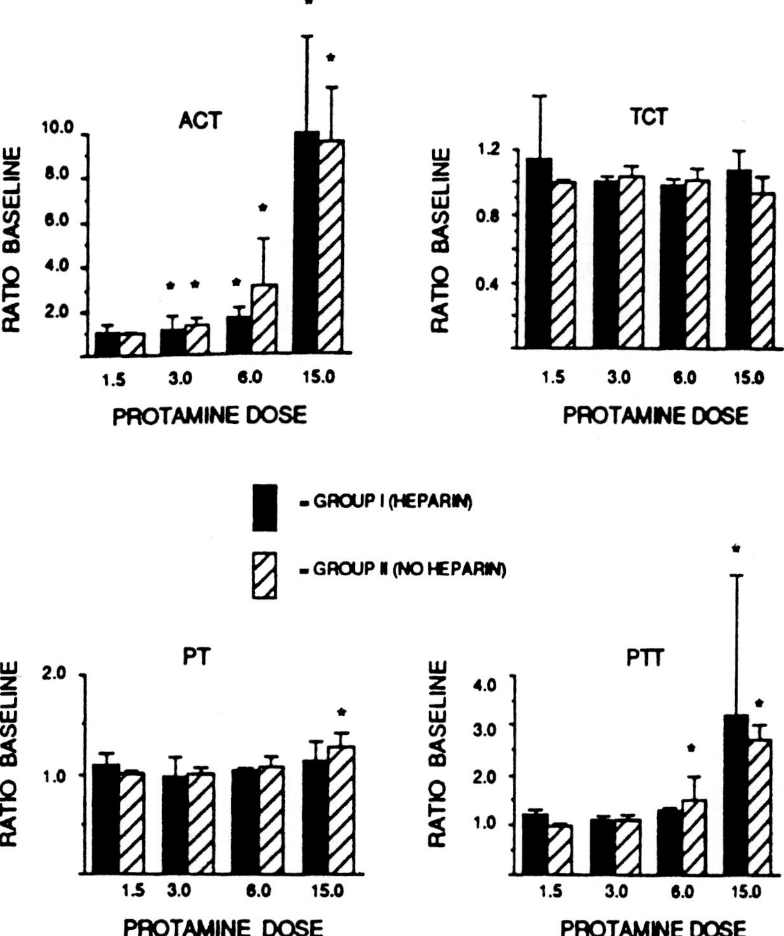

Figure 29–23 Effect on the ACT, thrombin clotting time (TCT), PT, and aPTT of protamine dose (in mg/kg) given to dogs 10 minutes after 150 U/kg of heparin (black bars) or without prior heparin (hatched bars). Error bars represent standard deviation (SD). Asterisks denote statistical significance compared with baseline values. (From Kresowik TF, Wakefield TW, Fessler RD, Stanley JC: Anticoagulant effects of protamine sulfate in a canine model. J Surg Res 45:8, 1988.)

concentrations similar to those expected in vivo, fails to release histamine from minced animal lung tissue,[255] or from dispersed human mast cells.[256] More recent investigations link hypotension to the release of nitric oxide from endothelium.[257]

EFFECTS ON CARDIAC INOTROPY

Cardiac output (CO) predictably decreases following rapid administration to animals when preload is allowed to decrease.[232,243,245,246,250,252] Most human studies document no change in CO with rapid[258,260] or slow administration.[261-265] When volume infusion accompanies protamine, CO rises.[253] However, protamine's effects on CO do not assess its impact on inotropy, which constitutes only one of many determinants of CO.

Initial reports indicated a myocardial depressant effect.[243,245,246,248] Studies using strips of myocardium bathed in concentrated protamine solutions produced similar results.[266-269] Clinically relevant bath concentrations yielded conflicting results as regards depressed myocardial mechanics.[270,271] One study suggested that only concentrated noncomplex protamine would compromise patients clinically.[269] Another suggested that patients with established ventricular compromise might suffer further degradation of contractile performance upon exposure to unbound protamine.[272] The mechanism may relate to altered membrane ion conductances that increase intracellular calcium.[273] Well-conducted studies in intact organisms revealed no effect of protamine on contractility in animals[249,274] or humans[244,274-280] (Fig. 29–24).

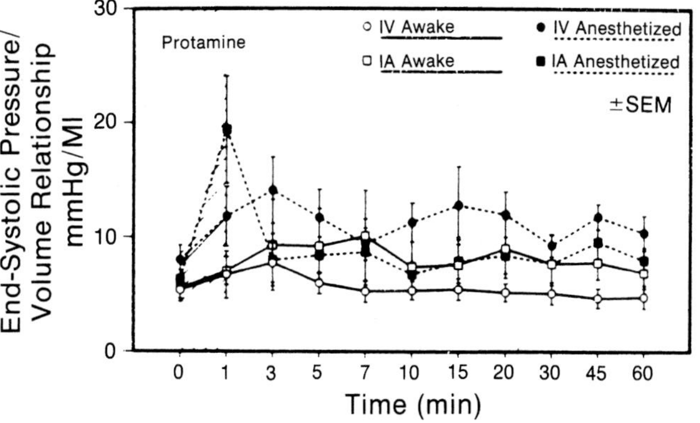

Figure 29–24 Effect of protamine infusion to dogs on a measure of inotropic state, the end-systolic pressure-volume relationship. Neither route of administration (IA = intraaortic, IV = intravenous) nor the presence of anesthesia modified the absence of an effect of protamine on inotropic state. (From Taylor RL, Little WC, Freeman GL, et al: Comparison of the cardiovascular effects of intravenous and intraaortic protamine in the conscious and anesthetized dog. Ann Thorac Surg 42:22, 1986.)

LEFT-SIDED INJECTION

Based on early reports claiming protection from adverse responses, injection of protamine directly into the left side of the circulation (left atrium or aortic root) became popular.[277,278] Some subsequent animal investigations confirmed a left-sided advantage;[279,280] others demonstrated no advantage[274,281] or more compromised hemodynamics[274] compared with a control right-sided group. Left-sided injection provides no protection from pulmonary hypertension.[282] In humans, the published evidence weighs against left-sided injection; three separate investigations in a total of 130 patients demonstrated more hypotension from left-sided than right-sided injection.[260,283,284] The clinician must consider that left-sided injection also increases the risk for systemic particulate and air embolization.

Platelet Reactions

The most underappreciated reaction to protamine is thrombocytopenia. The heparin–protamine complex activates the microcirculation. For a quick graphic example the reader should merely mix heparin and protamine in a well or syringe. A milky precipitate is observed that grows into larger beads of precipitate. It is clear that when protamine is administered, it binds heparin wherever it comes into contact with it. It may find heparin attached to the surface of platelets and then coat the surface of the platelets with heparin–protamine complexes. It is also possible that heparin and protamine could form cross-links between platelets since the protamine is polycationic and can bind a number of heparin molecules. The end result is a decrease in platelet count within 10 to 15 minutes of administration of protamine. The usual is roughly a 10% drop in platelet count, but it can be larger, when normalization of coagulation is expected. It appears that the platelets are sequestered by the reticuloendothelium and particularly the pulmonary vasculature. It is unclear if those patients with the largest drop in platelets develop the worst bleeding or if they are at the highest risk of pulmonary vasoconstriction and pulmonary hypertension secondary to thromboxane release. The sequestered platelets come back into the circulation over the next few hours, and by 1 to 4 hours the platelet count returns toward normal.

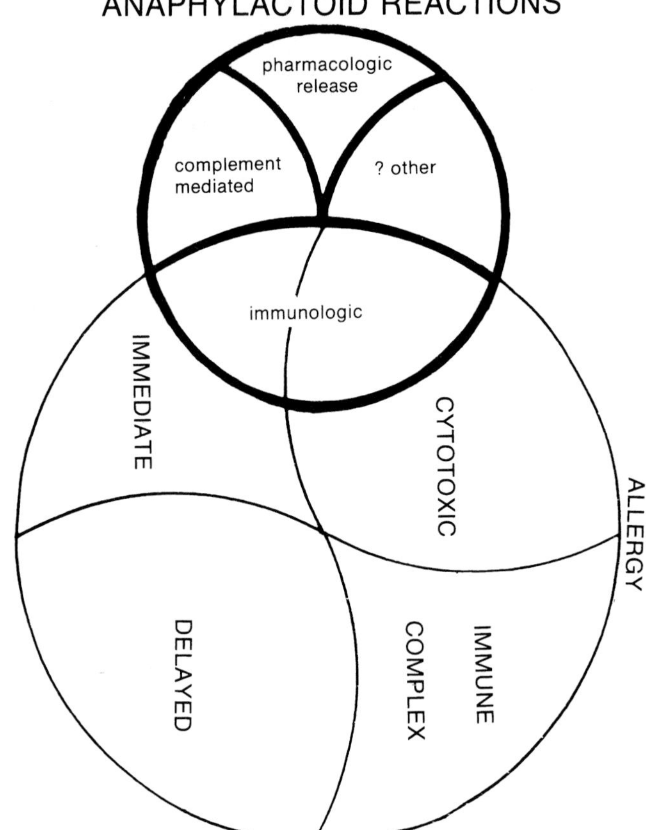

Figure 29–25 Venn diagram depicting the spectrum of allergy and of anaphylactoid reactions. Anaphylaxis to protamine is an immunologic-type anaphylactoid reaction classified as an immediate allergic reaction. (From Horrow JC: Protamine allergy. J Cardiothorac Vasc Anesth 2:225, 1988.)

Anaphylactoid Reaction

ALLERGY, ANAPHYLAXIS, AND ADVERSE RESPONSES

Not all adverse responses to protamine are allergic reactions. Rapid protamine injection decreases blood pressure just as morphine induces nausea; neither side effect is allergic. Immediate hypersensitivity allergic reactions involve release of vasoactive mediators resulting from antigen-antibody interaction. The broader term anaphylactoid reactions includes not only severe immediate hypersensitivity allergy, termed anaphylaxis, but also other life-threatening idiosyncratic responses of nonimmunologic origin[285,286] (Fig. 29–25). The initial classification of protamine reactions split the anaphylactoid category (type II) into three subsets: anaphylaxis (IIA), nonimmunologic anaphylactoid reaction (IIB), and delayed noncardiogenic pulmonary edema (IIC).[287] The last two are poorly defined phenomena. Complement-mediated nonimmunologic effects do occur, but are not discussed here.[288] This section deals mainly with allergic responses and polycation lung injury.[287-289]

DIABETES MELLITUS

Patients receiving protamine-containing insulin develop antibodies to protamine. Between 38% and 91% of these patients demonstrate an antiprotamine IgG[290-292]; far fewer patients develop an antiprotamine IgE. Do these antibodies cause adverse responses to protamine administration? Few patients with diabetes actually develop hemodynamic compromise from protamine.[292] The numerous case reports of diabetic patients who developed adverse responses to protamine reflect either a truly increased incidence of adverse response in this population or merely a reporting bias, because cases in nondiabetics are not published.[293-304] Retrospective attempts to determine the risk of protamine reaction in diabetic patients yield diverse results.[305,306] A case-control study found a 95-fold increase in risk relative to patients taking NPH insulin,[307] while prospective studies[292,308] demonstrated no increased risk. Table 29–9 displays these data. If risk is increased, it still remains quite small (0.6%).[292]

PRIOR EXPOSURE TO PROTAMINE

Previous protamine exposure may occur at catheterization,[295,309] at prior vascular surgery,[293,296] at dialysis,[310] or during blood component donation (pheresis),[311] although modern techniques for the latter two procedures no longer use heparin and protamine. Multiple exposures at intervals of about 2 weeks maximize the chance of an allergic response.[312]

A single intravenous exposure to protamine will engender an IgG or IgE antibody response in 28% of patients.[313] Nevertheless, many thousands of patients each year receive protamine at both catheterization and then later at surgery without sequelae. They offer evidence of the safety of this sequence and the rarity of intravenous exposure to protamine generating clinically significant antibodies.

FISH ALLERGY

Salmon is a vertebrate, or true fish (also known as "fin" fish), as opposed to shellfish, which are invertebrates. Patients aller-

Table 29–9 Studies on the Incidence of Protamine Reactions (Type Unspecified)

Authors	Type	Size	Situation	Nondiabetics	Diabetics, No Insulin	Diabetics-NPH
Stewart et al[305]	Retrospective	651	Catheterization	0.50%	0.0%	27.0% (4/15)
Gottschlich et al[306]	Retrospective	2996	Catheterization	0.07%	—	2.9% (2/68)
Levy et al[292]	Prospective	3245	Surgery	0.06%	—	0.6% (1/160)
Weiss et al[307]	Case control	27	Various	25 × (IgG)*	—	95 × (IgE)†

*Nondiabetics who sustained an adverse response to protamine were 25 times more likely to demonstrate an antiprotamine IgG than nondiabetics who did not suffer an adverse protamine response.

†Diabetics taking NPH insulin who sustained an adverse response to protamine were 95 times more likely to demonstrate an antiprotamine IgE than NPH-taking diabetics who did not suffer an adverse protamine response.

gic to fin fish can respond to protamine with anaphylaxis. Several case reports support this statement.[314,315] As with diabetic patients, fish allergy patients followed prospectively do not exhibit an adverse response to protamine challenge.[292] One of the authors (JH) has documented negative skin tests in several patients with fish allergy in whom subsequent protamine administration was benign, and a positive skin test in one patient who did not receive protamine (unpublished data). Since skin tests have high sensitivity and poor specificity, negative results suggest lack of allergy. No data link shellfish and protamine allergies.

VASECTOMY

Within 1 year of vasectomy, 22% of men develop cytotoxic (IgG) antibody to human protamine, which may cross-react with salmon protamine due to similarity among protamines.[316] These autoantibodies exist in weak titers, however. Prospective studies demonstrate that patients with prior vasectomy receive protamine during cardiac surgery without adverse response.[316,317] Case reports of vasectomy-related protamine allergy[318] display insufficient evidence to demonstrate a causal relationship.[287,319] Vasectomy remains only a theoretical risk for protamine allergy.

NONCARDIOGENIC PULMONARY EDEMA

Systemic hypotension accompanied by massive pulmonary capillary leak, accumulation of alveolar fluid, decreased pulmonary compliance, wheezing, and pulmonary edema can occur after CPB. Originally attributed to protamine, these rare responses occur sporadically at least 20 minutes following protamine administration.[299,320-323] Others have attributed the problem to administration of banked blood products[324,325] or other substances.[326] CPB itself activates complement via the alternate pathway, which can (but usually does not) result in leukocyte aggregation, free radical formation, and lung injury.[285,327]

Many polycations, including protamine, hexadimethrine, and polylysine, can directly induce delayed pulmonary vascular damage.[327] Verapamil may attenuate polycation injury via its inhibitory effects on calcium channels.[328] The delayed noncardiogenic pulmonary edema seen clinically might arise from protamine, from administration of leukocytes that accompany banked blood products,[325] or from CPB.[329,330] Perhaps the marked decrease in occurrence of this phenomenon in the last decade arises from less frequent use of FFP, more widespread administration of calcium channel blockers perioperatively, or both.

Pulmonary Vasoconstriction

CLINICAL FEATURES

Several years after pulmonary artery catheters (PACs) achieved common usage and case reports sensitized clinicians to adverse responses to protamine, Lowenstein et al reported a series of cases in which protamine caused systemic hypotension, decreased left atrial pressure, elevated rather than decreased PAP, and right ventricular distention and failure.[331] This syndrome resembles the predictable response seen in certain laboratory animals.[331-335] Unlike in anaphylaxis, plasma histamine levels do not change during this idiosyncratic, catastrophic pulmonary vasoconstriction,[333] thus justifying a separate classification for this unusual response.[334]

The duration of pulmonary hypertension may vary substantially from brief episodes[335] (Fig. 29–26) to those requiring reinstitution of CPB.[331,335,336] Rechallenge with protamine immediately following recovery from this type III reaction can be benign,[335] similar to the results in laboratory animals.[224] However, because rechallenge could also induce repeat pulmonary vasoconstriction, it is best avoided whenever possible.

PROPOSED MECHANISM

Animal models of type III protamine responses demonstrate that heparin must precede the protamine,[213,337] that heparin–protamine complexes activate the complement pathway,[338] and that blockade of complement activation attenuates pulmonary damage.[339] Furthermore, leukocytes respond to complement activation by forming free radicals, which stimulate the arachidonate pathway.[328,340] Blockade of this pathway mitigates the pulmonary response,[341,342] while antihistamines do not.[282,333]

Unlike the immediate pulmonary damage induced by heparin–protamine complexes, polycations alone (for example, poly-L-lysine) induce pulmonary damage in a more delayed fashion. Polycation-induced injury probably involves pulmonary macrophages and arachidonate metabolites.[328,338,343-346] Heparin–protamine complex size varies with the molar ratios of heparin and protamine present[229]; an excess of protamine forms larger complexes.[238] Rapid protamine administration in humans may not predictably cause pulmonary hypertension because, unlike those of the pig and sheep, human lungs do not contain large numbers of macrophages.[299,328] Polycations can block nitric oxide syn-

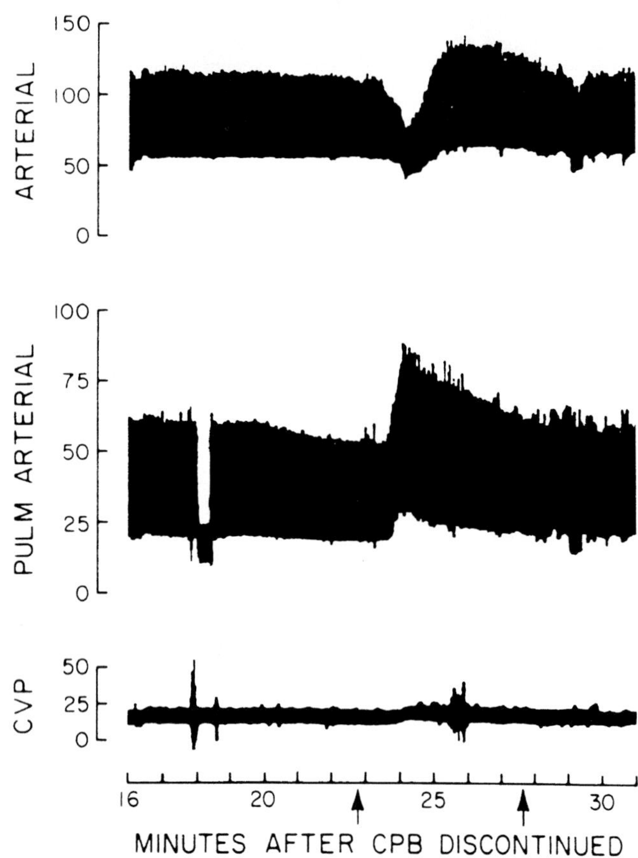

Figure 29–26 Example of a type III protamine reaction of brief duration. Compressed waveforms of radial arterial, pulmonary arterial, and central venous pressures (all in mm Hg) demonstrate sudden systemic hypotension and pulmonary hypertension soon after administration of 10 mg of protamine sulfate (arrow at 23 min after bypass). Note lack of adverse response to an additional 10 mg of protamine sulfate 5 minutes later. (From Horrow JC: Thrombocytopenia accompanying a reaction to protamine sulfate. Can Anesth Soc J 32:49, 1985.)

thetase, leading to speculation that this pathway also participates in the development of pulmonary vasoconstriction. Figure 29–27 summarizes the speculative mechanisms of various adverse responses to protamine.

TREATMENT AND PREVENTION

Theoretically, slow administration should limit type III reactions, because large heparin–protamine complexes would less likely form. Slow dilute infusion (see below) has decreased this adverse response to protamine.

Some have suggested routine administration of antihistamines to prevent protamine-induced circulatory changes. For type III reactions, in which histamine has no mechanistic role, such a plan should fail. Indeed, antihistamines confer no advantage in general.[347] Hydrocortisone or aminophylline prophylaxis may lessen any circulatory changes with protamine administration, but for nonspecific reasons.[348,349]

Upon detection of sudden pulmonary hypertension and systemic hypotension, protamine infusion should cease, as should administration of any cardiovascular depressant. Administration of a heparin bolus should be considered in an attempt to reduce heparin–protamine complex size.[336] Excess heparin would theoretically attract protamine away from large complexes to yield a larger number of smaller size particles. If hemodynamics have not deteriorated sufficiently to warrant immediate reinstitution of CPB, 70 units/kg of heparin should be tried first, then 300 units/kg if that fails. Inotropic support should be selected so as not to worsen the pulmonary hypertension; isoproterenol (0.1 to 0.2 μg/kg bolus followed by 0.1 to 0.3 μg/kg/min) or milrinone appear best suited for this purpose. Milder cases may revert without intervention,[335] merely by halting protamine administration,[350] a highly desirable outcome insofar as the treatments outlined above all extract a price, whether it be arrhythmias from inotropes or bleeding from heparin. Rechallenge with protamine should be avoided.

Guidelines for Clinical Use

The most important principle in avoiding adverse responses to protamine is to administer the drug slowly. Dilution aids this goal by limiting the impact of an undetected rapid administration. A neutralizing dose (3 mg/kg, or 21 mL on average of 10 mg/mL solution) can be added to 50 mL of clear fluid; then the diluted drug can be administered into a central vein by a small drop infusion (60 drops/mL) over 10 to 15 minutes. It is important to provide a carrier flow when administering by peripheral vein, so that the long tubing does not slowly fill with drug rather than the drug enter the patient. Additional doses of undiluted protamine are given from small syringes (5 mL) at a maximum rate of 20 mg/min to adults. Proper choice of materials (small syringes, small drop administration sets, and use of diluent) helps protect against too-rapid drug delivery.

Slow administration should decrease the likelihood of a type I and a type III adverse response. However, anaphylactic response (type IIA) may occur at any delivery rate. Preparation for groups at risk to receive protamine is discussed in the following sections.

DIABETIC PATIENTS

No screening test predicts an adverse response to protamine. Serum IgE levels are nonspecific. Skin tests do not correlate with antiprotamine antibody measurements.[351,352] Using too concentrated a protamine solution in performing skin tests may produce false-positive results.[353,354] Antiprotamine antibody determinations, available by radioallergosorbent test (RAST) or enzyme-linked immunosorbent assay (ELISA), appear equally nonspecific and are expensive.[351,352] Although most diabetic patients have antiprotamine immunoglobulin (38% to 91%), most receive protamine without adverse sequelae (>99.4%).

VASECTOMY AND FISH ALLERGY PATIENTS

Like diabetic patients, vasectomy patients demonstrate antibodies but show a benign response to protamine. All skin tests on vasectomy patients by these authors have displayed negative results and benign responses to protamine after CPB, including one who demonstrated an anaphylactoid reaction at catheterization, probably arising from radiocontrast administration.

Patients with strong evidence by history or laboratory tests of allergy to fin fish are uncommon. After CPB, these patients receive 1 mg of protamine diluted in 50 mL of intravenous fluid over 10 minutes. If hemodynamics do not deteriorate, the neutralizing dose is administered as previously outlined. Otherwise, protamine is withheld. Skin testing may predict this allergy, but would not change the approach, since false-positive skin tests are common, and too few reported cases of protamine–fin fish cross-allergy exist to warrant more aggressive drug administration to those demonstrating negative skin

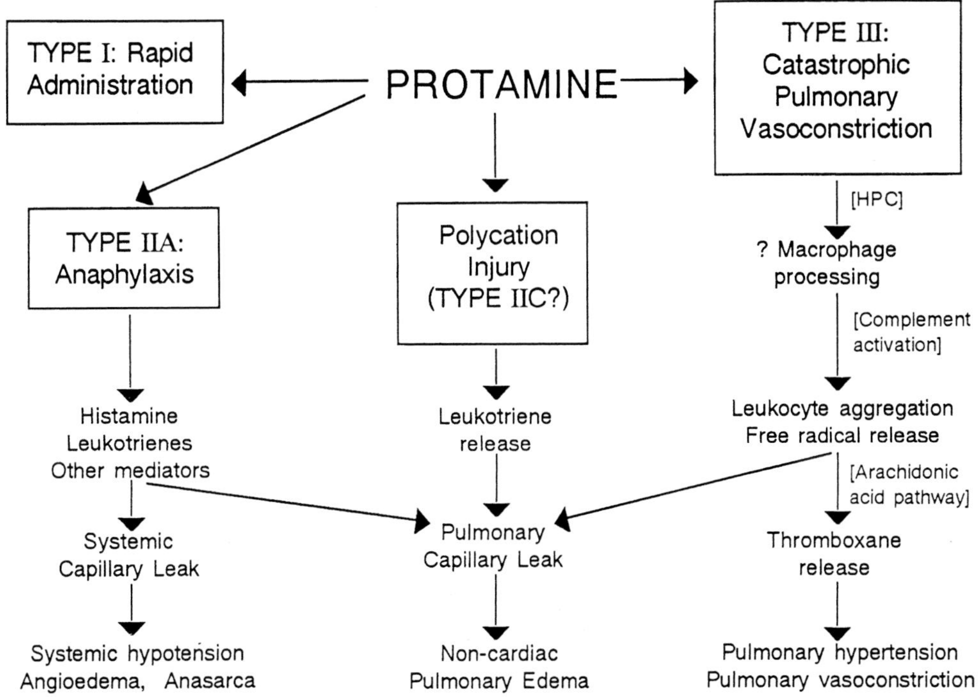

Figure 29–27 Speculative mechanisms of some protamine reactions HPC, heparin-protamine complex. (From Horrow JC: Heparin reversal of protamine toxicity: Have we come full circle? J Cardiothorac Vasc Anesth 4:539, 1990.)

tests. Heparin has been successfully neutralized in a patient with a history of fin fish anaphylaxis and positive skin tests to protamine by using the enzyme heparinase I (Neutralase). This case is unpublished.

PRIOR REACTION TO PROTAMINE

For these patients, skin testing, RAST, and ELISA are appropriate, because negative responses provide greater comfort in attempting a rechallenge. If the historical or laboratory evidence for protamine sensitivity is poor, then a challenge as described for fish allergy patients may be attempted. Otherwise, an alternative to protamine should be chosen. Availability of a safe alternative would save the cost of these tests and any prolonged hospitalization that accompanies them.

Alternatives to Protamine

This section discusses techniques for neutralizing heparin other than administration of protamine. Substitutes for protamine in long-acting insulin preparations are not considered.

Hexadimethrine

This synthetic polycation (Fig. 29–28) is 1.1 to 2.0 times more potent than protamine.[355,356] Hexadimethrine (Polybrene) engenders the same biologic responses as protamine when administered rapidly: systemic hypotension, decreased SVR, and rapid disappearance from plasma.[356,357] Pulmonary hypertension occurs after hexadimethrine neutralization of UFH.[358] Patients allergic to protamine have received hexadimethrine without adverse effects.[295] The small group of patients with true anaphylaxis, as demonstrated by clinical history and antiprotamine IgE, may benefit from hexadimethrine insofar as this protamine substitute may not cross-react with the antibodies present.

Following reports of renal toxicity, hexadimethrine was withdrawn from clinical use in the United States.[359,360] Animal studies confirm glomerular injury from hexadimethrine. Urinary excretion of lactic dehydrogenase, aspartase aminotransferase, and other enzymes occurs.[361] Binding of the polycation to the carboxyl groups of proteoglycans in the glomerular basement membrane probably mediates this injury.[362] Although protamine also causes renal toxicity, larger doses are required.[363,364] Hexadimethrine appears unlikely to replace protamine for routine clinical use.[365]

Platelet Factor 4

Platelets contain this potent antiheparin compound. An early attempt to neutralize heparin by platelet concentrate transfusion in two patients produced poor results, however. Despite 18 units of platelets and 400 mL of FFP, one patient bled 4 L, while 12 units of platelets and 1100 mL of FFP accompanied more than 2 L of blood loss in another.[301]

Rather than bind to heparin electrostatically, like protamine, PF4 utilizes lysine residues at its C termini to neutralize heparin. Both native and recombinant PF4 effectively neutralize heparin in rats without adverse effects at one-fifth the potency of protamine, i.e., 5 mg/100 U of heparin.[83] In heparinized human blood, recombinant PF4 was half as potent as protamine in restoring the ACT and whole blood clotting time.[366] Doses of 2.5 and 5.0 mg/kg of recombinant PF4 neutralized the 5000 U of heparin given for cardiac catheterization.[367] Doses of 5 mg/kg of recombinant PF4 to

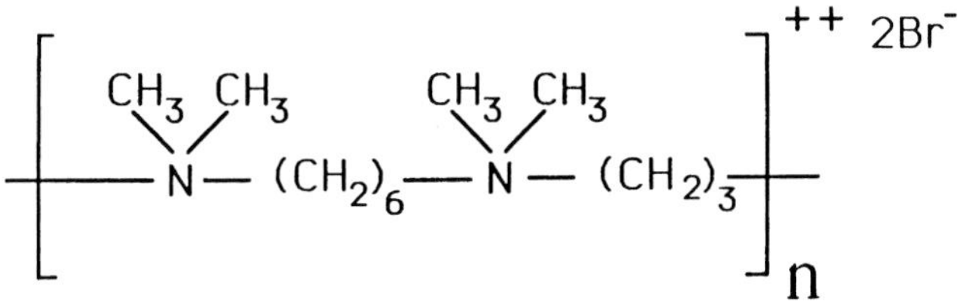

$$\left[-\overset{CH_3\ CH_3}{\underset{}{N}}-(CH_2)_6-\overset{CH_3\ CH_3}{N}-(CH_2)_3- \right]_n^{++}\ 2Br^-$$

Figure 29–28 Hexadimethrine, a synthetic polycationic polymer. (From Horrow JC: Protamine. A necessary evil. *In* Ellison N, Jobes DR [eds]: Effective Hemostasis in Cardiac Surgery. Philadelphia, WB Saunders Company 1988, pp 15.)

a small number of patients successfully neutralized the 300 U/kg of heparin given for CPB.[368]

Does PF4 avoid the adverse effects of protamine? Kurrek et al[369] demonstrated pulmonary hypertension in lambs when neutralizing heparin with PF4. The lamb, like the dog, responds predictably to protamine with increased pulmonary pressures, and thus serves as a model for predicting the idiosyncratic effects of protamine in humans. Those patients likely to respond to protamine with pulmonary hypertension might respond likewise to PF4.[369] Another less likely explanation is that PF4 constitutes a foreign protein to the lamb, thus engendering the adverse pulmonary hemodynamic response.[370] Further clinical work on PF4 as a protamine substitute appears to have slowed.

Interposed Filters

The enzyme heparinase, bonded to an exit filter of an experimental bypass circuit and interposed at the conclusion of CPB, decreased blood heparin levels within two passes.[371] Current filters achieve 90% heparin removal with a single pass.

A modification of this concept uses a hollow-fiber filter to which protamine has been immobilized. While not a true alternative to protamine, the protamine filter traps heparin extracorporeally, limiting tissue interaction with heparin–protamine complexes.[372,373] This "protamine filter" attenuates both thrombocytopenia and leucopenia. The clinical efficacy and safety of this technique are not yet clearly demonstrated. Heparin removal proceeds much too slowly, requiring 10 minutes to remove half of circulating heparin: the potential for clot formation in the circuit from return of unheparinized blood for successive passes through the filter remains an unresolved problem.

Methylene Blue

This positively charged chemical dye binds to heparin in an electrostatic fashion similar to that of protamine. Sloand et al[374] administered 2 mg/kg to a patient who had sustained a severe reaction to protamine, successfully restoring the ACT and aPTT and decreasing chest tube output. Follow-up work ex vivo confirmed a potential benefit.[375] However, more rigorous laboratory testing[376] and a clinical trial of ascending doses of methylene blue to neutralize heparin administered for elective CPB demonstrated no efficacy whatsoever in restoring the ACT to normal.[377] Furthermore, doses above 6 mg/kg resulted in moderate-to-severe pulmonary hypertension, necessitating administration of inotropic support.[378] Methylene blue, an inhibitor of nitric oxide synthetase, predictably increases pulmonary and systemic vascular resistance at higher doses. Methylene blue should not be used to neutralize heparin.

Omit Neutralization

Heparin activity will decay spontaneously with time, owing to drug elimination. Castaneda omitted heparin neutralization in 92 patients.[241] Despite lower doses of heparin and meticulous hemostasis, most of those patients bled excessively. Another patient in whom heparin was not neutralized bled 5 L over 13 hours and required more than 15 units of blood products.[378] Although this option avoids exposure to protamine, hemodynamic instability and consumptive coagulopathy may likely result from massive hemorrhage. Substantial exposure to transfusion-related viral disease also creates serious concern for the clinician.

Heparinase

Systemic administration of the enzyme heparinase I, produced by *Flavobacterium*, results in a return of the ACT to normal in an ex vivo model,[379] animal models of CPB,[379] and human volunteers.[380] Initial investigation in patients undergoing elective coronary artery bypass grafting operations confirms the utility of heparinase in neutralizing heparin-induced anticoagulation.[381]

Because the enzyme remains in the vasculature for some time after administration (the half-life is 12 minutes in healthy subjects), should an immediate need arise to reinstitute CPB, patients would require not only repeat doses of heparin, but also an infusion of heparin to counter the lingering effects of the enzyme. All work on the development of heparinase has stopped after failure of initial clinical trials.

Designer Polycations

If protamine's action is derived from its polycationic structure, could artificial polycations be developed to retain the heparin-neutralizing property while minimizing or eliminating adverse effects? Wakefield and colleagues have generated a series of designed molecules with this purpose in mind.[382,383]

Unfortunately, adverse effects appear to correlate with ability to neutralize UFH. However, some of the polycations developed can neutralize LMWH species without adverse sequelae, suggesting replacement of both UFH and protamine with a doubly superior regimen for achieving anticoagulation for CPB.[383] Much more investigation must precede clinical trials. The future may be in using the new direct thrombin inhibitors and completely avoiding the need for protamine.

BLEEDING PATIENT

Following cardiac surgery, some patients bleed excessively. Prompt diagnostic and therapeutic action will avoid impaired hemodynamics from hemorrhage, decreased oxygen-carrying capacity from anemia, and impaired hemostasis from depletion of endogenous hemostatic resources. The surgical act creates the potential for hemorrhage, sometimes aided by preoperative attempts to lyse intracoronary thromboses. Beyond that, however, many factors govern whether a particular patient will experience excessive bleeding after cardiac surgery. This section details the causes, prevention, and management of the bleeding patient.

Although many different criteria can define excessive bleeding, a chest tube drainage of more than 10 mL/kg in the first hour after operation or a total of more than 20 mL/kg over the first 3 hours after operation for patients weighing above 10 kg is considered significant. Also, any sudden increase of 300 mL/hr or greater following minimal initial drainage in an adult usually indicates anatomic disruption warranting surgical intervention.[384]

Patient Factors

The medical history can reveal information relevant to hemostasis. Any patient with a personal or family history of abnormal bleeding following surgery deserves specific coagulation testing for an inherited disorder. Routine PT, aPTT, and bleeding times probably offer little as screening tests.[385,386] The bleeding time has been investigated in a meta-analysis of over

800 published articles, and it was concluded that it has no correlation with postoperative coagulopathic bleeding.[387] The other routine tests have less than a 50% accuracy for predicting who will bleed and who will have normal chest tube outputs.

The thromboelastograph has been extensively tested both alone and in conjunction with a number of other tests including PT, platelet count, and fibrinogen. The TEG has been shown to have the best predictive accuracy for postoperative bleeding.[388-396] In work using an algorithm based upon the TEG and other tests, blood product utilization was cut considerably.[395] Chest tube bleeding was not different but the TEG did predict which patients might bleed abnormally. Work with TEG monitoring has shown that it can detect both hypocoagulable states as well as hypercoagulable states. New additives to the testing make it sensitive to the ADP receptor platelet antagonists as well as the IIb/IIIa inhibitors (see Chapter 18).

Concurrent systemic disease affects hemostasis during surgery as well. Uremia from renal failure results in platelet dysfunction. Severe hepatic compromise impairs every aspect of hemostasis: prekallikrein and most coagulation factors circulate in decreased concentration; additional sialic acid residues on fibrinogen and other coagulation factors impair clotting function; splenomegaly induces thrombocytopenia; maldistribution of vWF multimers impairs platelet adhesiveness and aggregation; impaired clearance of endogenous plasminogen activators accentuates fibrinolysis; and decreased levels of coagulation inhibitors induce a consumptive coagulopathy.[397]

Medications significantly affect surgical bleeding. Many patients taking aspirin or other platelet-inhibiting drugs regularly cannot halt that therapy within 7 days of surgery. No antidote can correct the platelet defect. Fortunately, most patients taking aspirin within 7 days of surgery do not exhibit excessive bleeding. The new antiplatelet drugs can all lead to postoperative bleeding (see Table 29–4).

Patients taking warfarin require 2 to 5 days without therapy for correction of the INR. Patients for urgent surgery may receive parenteral vitamin K or FFP, which corrects the warfarin defect more quickly. Some patients may receive thrombolytic therapy for acute ischemic events just prior to surgery. Systemic fibrinogenolysis resulting from use of nonspecific thrombolytic agents such as streptokinase should respond to antifibrinolytic therapy with ε-aminocaproic acid (EACA) or tranexamic acid.

Insult of Cardiopulmonary Bypass

More so than patient factors, CPB itself acts to impair hemostasis. Bypass activates fibrinolysis, impairs platelets, and affects coagulation factors. Hypothermia, employed in most centers during CPB, adversely affects hemostasis as well.

Fibrinolysis

Numerous investigations support the notion that CPB activates the fibrinolytic pathway.[398-400] Why might this occur? Despite clinically adequate doses and blood concentrations of heparin, coagulation pathway activity persists. Formation of prothrombin and fibrinopeptide fragments and thrombin–antithrombin complexes document continued thrombin activity in this setting (see Fig. 29–13). The site of thrombin activity probably resides in the extracorporeal circuit, which contains a large surface of thrombogenic material. Thrombin activation results in fibrinolytic activity. Activation of fibrinolysis may be localized to those external sites of fibrin formation. Plasminogen activator concentrations rise during CPB, while levels of its inhibitor PAI-1 remain unchanged. This scenario is consistent with activation of fibrinolysis during CPB. Neither of the labels "primary" or "secondary" applies to the fibrinolysis peculiar to bypass.

Does fibrin formation during CPB constitute a consumptive coagulopathy? It is not a systemic event. Presuming that plasminogen activation occurs only where fibrin is formed (extracorporeally), a systemic fibrinogenolytic state should not ensue. Should α_2-antiplasmin become overwhelmed by plasmin formation, however, systemic manifestations may result. Previous generations of oxygenators may have engendered systemic fibrinogenolysis more easily due to their more thrombogenic designs. In these (now more uncommon) instances of fibrinolysis, the TEG may demonstrate clot lysis. Even when fibrinolysis remains limited to the sites of extravascular fibrin formation, the fibrin degradation products so formed might impair hemostasis. In many cases, the mild fibrinolytic state engendered during CPB resolves spontaneously with little clinical impact.

Platelet Dysfunction

Thrombocytopenia occurs during CPB as a result of hemodilution, heparin, hypothermia-induced splenic sequestration of platelets, and platelet destruction from the blood–gas and blood–tissue interfaces created by cardiotomy suction, filters, and bubble oxygenators.[401-403] Platelet count rarely dips below 50,000/mm^3, however.

Not only does the number of platelets decrease during CPB, but remaining platelets become impaired by partial activation. Fibrinogen and fibrin, which adhere to artificial surfaces of the extracorporeal circuit, form a nidus for platelet adhesion and aggregation. A reduced content of platelet α granules constitutes the evidence for partial activation.[404] Nearly one-third of circulating platelets undergo α-granule release during CPB.[405] Bypass also depletes platelet glycoprotein receptors Ib and IIb/IIIa.[405,406] These platelets cannot respond fully when subsequent hemostatic stimuli call for release of granule contents. Use of frequent cardiotomy suction and bubble oxygenators aggravates the extent of platelet activation.

Activation of the fibrinolytic system may contribute to platelet dysfunction. Local formation of plasmin affects platelet membrane receptors.[406] Antifibrinolytic medications preserve platelet function and prevent some platelet abnormalities that occur during bypass[407-410] (Fig. 29–29).

Clotting Factors

Denaturation of plasma proteins, including the coagulation factors, occurs at blood–air interfaces. Liberal use of cardiotomy suction and prolonged use of bubble oxygenators potentially impair coagulation by decreasing coagulation factor availability. Hemodilution also decreases factor concentrations. However, rarely do coagulation factor levels fall below the thresholds for adequate formation of fibrin in adult surgery. In infants, however, the smallest achievable pump priming volumes can dilute factors to below 30% of normal levels.

Hypothermia

Hypothermia potentially affects hemostasis in many ways. First, the splanchnic circulation responds to hypothermia with sequestration of platelets.[411-413] After warming, the accompa-

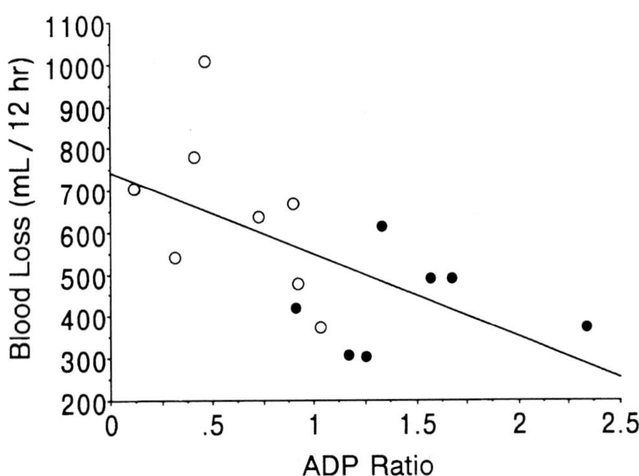

Figure 29–29 Antifibrinolytics may aid hemostasis by platelet preservation. Here, blood loss appears as a function of platelet ADP, expressed as a ratio (after bypass: before bypass). Solid circles represent patients who received prophylactic tranexamic acid. Placebo-treated patients appear as open circles. Note that the antifibrinolytic afforded less bleeding after operation and higher platelet ADP. (From Soslau G, Horrow JC, Brodsky I: The effect of tranexamic acid on platelet ADP during extracorporeal circulation. Am J Hematol 38:113, 1991.)

nying thrombocytopenia reverses over 1 hour. Second, transient platelet dysfunction occurs, evidenced by a platelet shape change, increased adhesiveness, inhibition of ADP-induced aggregation, and decreased synthesis of both thromboxane and prostacyclin.[411,412] Third, a specific heparin-like inhibitor of factor Xa becomes more active.[413] Protamine cannot neutralize this factor, which might be heparan.

Fourth, hypothermia slows the enzymatic cleavage upon which activation of coagulation factors depends. Many biologic phenomena display a 7% attenuation of activity for each decrease of 1°C in temperature.[414] While coagulation factor structure remains unaltered, formation of fibrin may be sluggish when the patient is cold. Fifth, hypothermia accentuates fibrinolysis.[415] The fibrin degradation products so formed then impair subsequent fibrin polymerization. Cold-induced injury of vascular endothelium can release thromboplastin, which then incites fibrin formation and activates fibrinolysis. Table 29–10 summarizes these effects.

Table 29–10 Antihemostatic Effects of Hypothermia

Hemostatic Component	Effect of Hypothermia
Factors	Increased Anti-Xa Activity; Heparan? Slows enzymes of the coagulation cascade
Platelets	Splanchnic sequestration Partial activation
Fibrinolysis	Enhanced
Endothelium	Tissue factor release

Prevention of Bleeding

The possible transmission of serious viral illness during transfusion of blood products and impairment of immune function may generate great concern among clinicians and patients. Many techniques attempt to limit viral exposure, including donation of autologous blood or directed blood, blood scavenging during and after surgery, and efforts to limit perioperative hemorrhage (Table 29–11). Advances in blood banking have decreased infectious disease transmission.[416] Blood sterilization techniques may render such concerns moot.[417]

Preoperative Factors

What can be done prior to surgery to minimize the extent of bleeding during and after surgery? First, existing disorders of hemostasis must be identified and treated. The bleeding diathesis of uremia responds to hemodialysis, red blood cell transfusion, and administration of desmopressin.[418,419] Because impaired hemostasis from hepatic failure may respond to intravenous desmopressin, preoperative verification of an appropriate response will permit proper administration of this drug following protamine neutralization of heparin after bypass.[420] Likewise, patients with hematologic disorders potentially amenable to desmopressin therapy, such as hemophilia and vWD, should receive desmopressin prior to surgery to determine the extent of response, if any.[421] When specific factor replacement is indicated, withholding it until after neutralization of heparin will provide less extensive exposure to allogeneic blood products.

Administration of platelet-inhibiting drugs should cease prior to operation. Two to 3 days should elapse for nonsteroidal anti-inflammatory medications, which cause reversible inhibition of cyclooxygenase. Seven to 10 days are required for regeneration of platelets following administration of aspirin, which irreversibly acetylates cyclooxygenase and some other platelet inhibitors (see Table 29–4).

Physical Factors

Hypothermia still forms an essential component of organ protection during CPB in many centers. Sufficient rewarming with adequate distribution of heat from central to intermedi-

Table 29–11 Ways to Prevent* Excessive Bleeding in Decreasing Order of Importance

Intervention†	Purpose
Ligatures	Repair all vascular trespass
Neutralize	Heparin fully neutralized
Blood pressure	Avoid hypertension after aortotomy
Suctions	Limit cardiotomy suction
Drugs	Cease platelet-inhibiting drugs in advance
Preoperative	Diagnose and treat first
Oxygenator	Membrane oxygenators for long cases
EACA	Antifibrinolytic prophylaxis
Temperature	Rewarm sufficiently
Go	Act with deliberate speed (tardiness begets bleeding)
Intravenous	Limit fluids, hemoconcentrate, and diurese
Extracorporeal circuit	Minimize volume

*These maneuvers do not all apply to the treatment of excessive bleeding after operation.
†The entries in this column form a mnemonic device: the initial letters of each entry, when rearranged, form the words STOP BLEEDING.

ate and peripheral zones should help prevent hypothermia-induced impairment of hemostasis.

Incomplete surgical hemostasis may occur from a slipped ligature, unclipped vessel branch, loose anastomosis, unattended open vessel at the wound edge, or sternal wire placed through the internal mammary artery. Because few fresh aortic suture lines fail to leak at high systemic pressures (systolic pressure >180 mm Hg or mean pressure >120 mm Hg), control of hypertension following CPB promotes hemostasis (see Chapter 33).

Limiting the intensity and frequency of use of the cardiotomy suction fosters platelet preservation during CPB and improves hemostasis after operation.[422] Selection of a membrane rather than a bubble-type oxygenator for cases involving prolonged CPB limits platelet destruction and fibrinolysis, thus aiding hemostasis.[423]

A small priming volume of the extracorporeal circuit restricts the extent of hemodilution. Hemodilution engenders bleeding not only by providing decreased concentrations of clotting factors and platelets; it also decreases margination of platelets, making them less available for adhesion and aggregation. Other measures that help include regulating cardioplegia volumes, restricting intravenous fluids, administering mannitol or loop diuretics, and providing hemoconcentration with filtration devices during CPB.

Removal of platelet-rich plasma at the induction of anesthesia for return to the patient following CPB by plasmapheresis supplies autologous, functional thrombocytes when they are most needed.[424-429] Previously, some centers collected autologous whole blood from patients at the beginning of surgery, reinfusing it following CPB, with controversial benefit.

Speed of surgery receives less attention now than in the past, when the therapeutic index of available anesthetics was less favorable. However, patients undergoing quick surgery enjoy several advantages. Shorter CPB duration preserves platelet function and limits the coagulant stimulus for subsequent fibrinolysis. More rapid closure after CPB limits tissue exposure to the hypothermic operating room environment.

Pharmacologic Factors

HEPARIN AND PROTAMINE

The prudent clinician's admonition to administer no drug to excess applies well to this pair of essential drugs. Too little heparin invites active fibrin formation during CPB with consumption of clotting factors and platelets and excessive activation of the fibrinolytic system. Too much heparin risks postoperative heparin rebound. With too little protamine, the remaining unneutralized heparin impairs hemostasis by its anticoagulant action. Doses of protamine excessive enough to overwhelm the endogenous proteases may exert an anticoagulant effect, as well as invite polycation-induced lung injury and pulmonary vasoconstriction. The optimal approach utilizes coagulation testing to estimate the appropriate heparin and protamine doses, and confirm both adequate anticoagulation and its neutralization.

DESMOPRESSIN

This analog of vasopressin (Fig. 29–30) provides more potent and longer lasting antidiuretic activity than vasopressin, with little vasoconstriction (Box 29–5). Like the parent compound and like epinephrine and insulin, desmopressin releases coagulation system mediators from vascular endothelium. Factor VIII coagulant activity increases 2- to 20-fold and is maximal about 30 to 90 minutes after injection.[419,430-450] Factor XII levels also increase.[430] In response to desmopressin, endothelium releases the larger multimers of vWF, as well as t-PA and prostacyclin.[431] The latter two compounds potentially thwart clot formation and stability. Nevertheless, the overall effect of desmopressin is procoagulant, perhaps because of the impact of factor VIII and vWF.

The optimal dose of desmopressin is 0.3 μg/kg. Intravenous, subcutaneous, and intranasal routes are all acceptable. Following plasma redistribution with an 8-minute half-life,

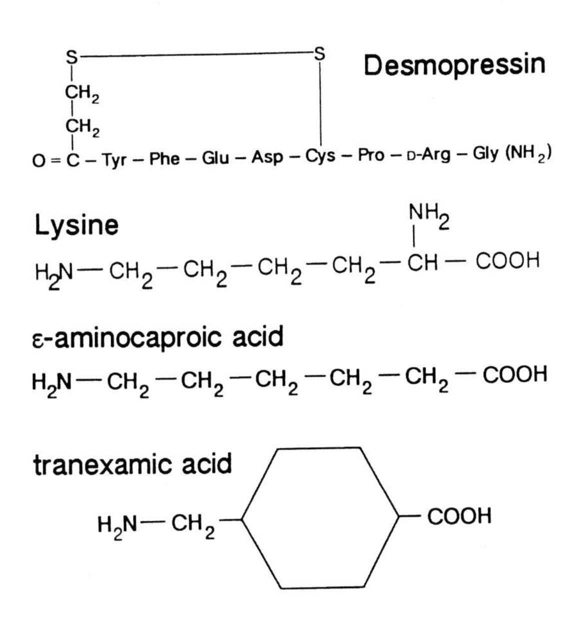

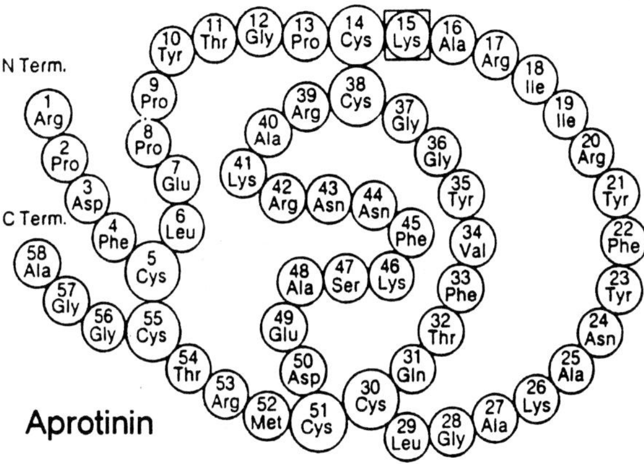

Figure 29–30 Molecular configurations of drugs used to decrease surgical bleeding. For comparison, the amino acid lysine is also depicted. (Modified from Horrow JC: Desmopressin and antifibrinolytics. Int Anesthesiol Clin 28:230, 1990, and Fritz H, Wunderer G: Biochemistry and applications of aprotinin, the kallikrein inhibitor from bovine organs. Drug Res 33:479, 1983.)

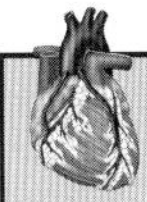

BOX 29–5 ***Useful Drugs to Reduce Bleeding During Cardiac Surgery***

- Aprotinin
- Tranexamic acid or epsilon aminocaproic acid
- Recombinant factor VIIa
- Desmopressin

metabolism in liver and kidney and urinary excretion yield a plasma half-life of 2.5 to 4 hours.[419] Levels of factor VIII persist in plasma long after desmopressin excretion due to the release of vWF. Depletion of vWF stores in endothelial cells accounts for the drug's tachyphylaxis. Rapid intravenous administration decreases systemic blood pressure and SVR, possibly by prostacyclin release or stimulation of extra renal vasopressin V_2 receptors.[433-437] The drug's antidiuretic action poses no problem in the absence of excessive free water administration.[438]

Specific applications of desmopressin's hemostatic benefit include uremia, cirrhosis, aspirin therapy, and surgery of various types. Correction of prolonged bleeding times in uremic patients follows desmopressin administration, making desmopressin the treatment of choice for bleeding emergencies in uremia.[419] Administration of desmopressin to cirrhotic patients also shortens prolonged bleeding times.[421] Desmopressin corrected the aspirin-induced prolongation in bleeding time in two patients and 10 volunteers.[439] It is also effective in some rare platelet disorders.[430] Evidence of a hemostatic effect during surgery is varied. Early success in adolescents undergoing Harrington rod placement was not confirmed with subsequent studies.[440]

Initial reports of a hemostatic effect during cardiac surgery were largely unsubstantiated by subsequent investigations.[441-450] von Willebrand factor activity increased in both control and desmopressin-treated patient groups, thus explaining the absence of a salutary effect of desmopressin on blood loss[446] (Fig. 29–31). Does desmopressin-induced release of t-PA overcome its hemostatic action during cardiac surgery? No, because antifibrinolytic therapy fails to uncover an additional hemostatic effect of desmopressin.[448]

Which subgroups of patients undergoing cardiac surgery might benefit from desmopressin? Certainly, those with uremia or cirrhosis. Those who display decreased maximum amplitude (MA) on TEG for whatever reason constitute a third group.[450] The heparinase-augmented TEG permits timely identification of patients in this subgroup.

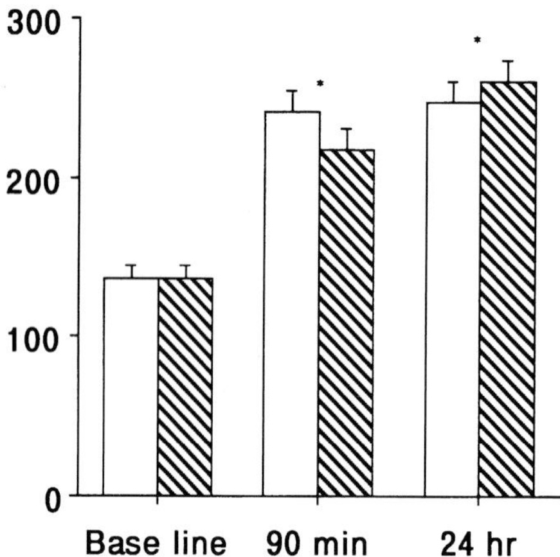

Figure 29–31 At 90 minutes and 24 hours after receiving desmopressin (hatched bars), ristocetin cofactor (von Willebrand factor) activity was not different from a placebo-treated group (open bars). However, in each group ristocetin cofactor activity increased (asterisks) from baseline values, possibly from surgical stress. Blood loss did not differ in the two groups. Error bars denote SEM. (Modified from Hackmann T, Gascoyne RD, Naiman SC, et al: A trial of desmopressin [1-desamino, 8-D-arginine vasopressin] to reduce blood loss in uncomplicated cardiac surgery. N Engl J Med 321:1437, 1989.)

Desmopressin afforded no hemostatic benefit to patients taking aspirin prior to cardiac surgery,[447,448] and the bulk of evidence currently points away from desmopressin as a prophylactic hemostatic agent for patients undergoing elective cardiac surgery.[388]

SYNTHETIC ANTIFIBRINOLYTICS

These simple molecules (see Fig. 29–30), analogs of the amino acid lysine, bind to plasminogen and plasmin, thus inhibiting binding of plasminogen at the lysine residues of fibrinogen. Antifibrinolytics may be administered intravenously or orally, and undergo renal concentration and excretion with a plasma half-life of about 80 minutes. Effective fibrinolysis inhibition requires an intravenous loading dose of 10 mg/kg for tranexamic acid followed by 1 mg/kg/hr or 50 mg/kg of EACA followed by infusions of 25 mg/kg/hr.[451,452] Infusion rates require downward adjustment when serum creatinine is elevated. Plasma concentrations of tranexamic acid achieve higher values with decreasing glomerular function. The author's practice is to administer only a loading dose to patients with serum creatinine concentrations in excess of 2.0 mg/dL. Antifibrinolytics are not given to patients with significant upper urinary tract bleeding or consumptive coagulopathy, as they prevent the clot lysis needed for continued patency of the ureters or circulatory system, respectively. However, they can also halt ongoing consumption.[453]

Pharmacokinetic studies demonstrate a need to readminister a bolus of EACA upon institution of CPB.[452,454] This may not apply to tranexamic acid,[455] perhaps because of a larger volume of distribution of this drug, although definitive data are still lacking.

Antifibrinolytics aid clotting in hemophiliacs and patients with vWD by blocking lysis of whatever clot can form.[456,457] Spontaneous bleeding after chemotherapy is decreased with oral tranexamic acid.[458] Prostate surgery, well known for excessive bleeding from release of t-PA, responds beneficially to antifibrinolytic therapy.[459] Fibrinolysis contributes to bleeding during the anhepatic phase of liver transplantation; antifibrinolytic therapy proves useful in this setting.

Ongoing thrombin activity with varied activation of fibrinolysis plagues cardiac surgery. Figure 29–13 demonstrates thrombin activity as reflected in continuing formation of fibrinopeptides despite adequate heparin anticoagulation. For decades, antifibrinolytics have been proposed as potential hemostatic agents during cardiac surgery. Initial investigations of the efficacy of synthetic antifibrinolytics as hemostatic agents during or following cardiac surgery lacked blinding, randomization, and control groups.[460-468] Most subsequent studies administered EACA after CPB. One study demonstrated a salutary effect in cyanotic children, but not in acyanotic children.[463]

Several investigations, using prophylactic antifibrinolytics, document a savings in blood loss, as well as in blood transfused in a general population of cardiac surgery patients[448,466-468] (Fig. 29–32). By commencing administration of tranexamic acid prior to CPB, chest tube drainage in the first 12 hours following operation decreased by 30%, and the likelihood of receiving banked blood within 5 days of operation decreased from 41% to 22%.[448] Prophylactic antifibrinolytics may spare platelet function by inhibiting the deleterious effects of plasmin.[469] Administration of very large doses of antifibrinolytics appears to offer no greater savings.[470]

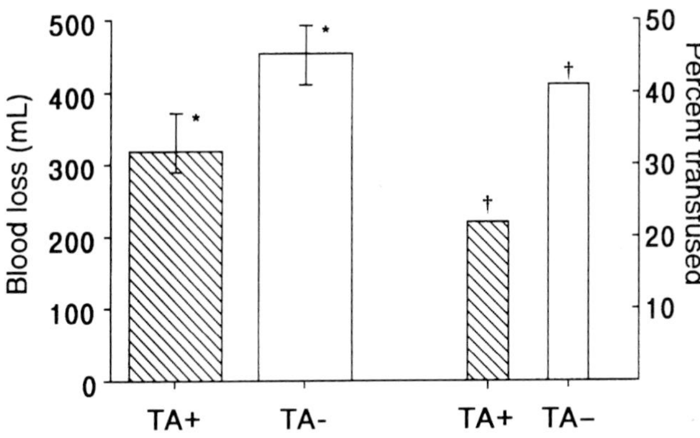

Figure 29–32 The effect of prophylactic tranexamic acid on blood loss (left vertical axis) and on the percent of patients receiving homologous red blood cell transfusion within 5 days of operation (right vertical axis). Hatched bars denote patients who received tranexamic acid, open bars denote those not receiving tranexamic acid. *$P < 0.0001$. †$P = 0.011$. (From Horrow JC, Van Riper DF, Strong MD, et al: The hemostatic effects of tranexamic acid and desmopressin during cardiac surgery. Circulation 84:2063, 1991.)

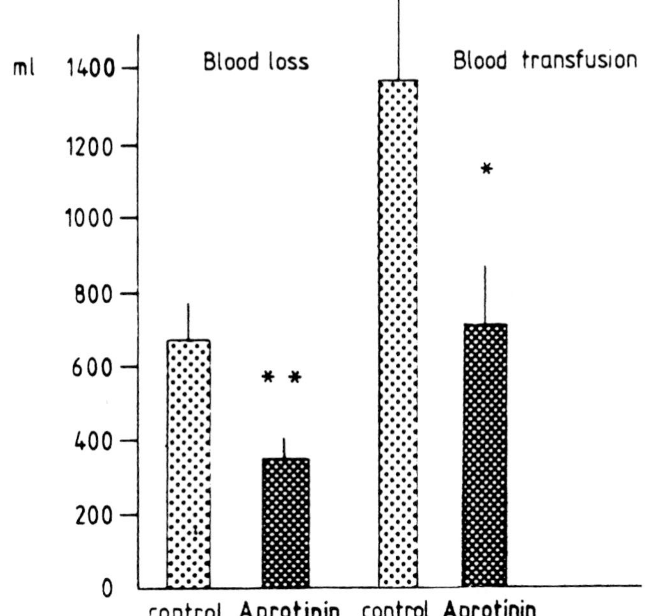

Figure 29–34 Savings in blood loss and blood transfused with aprotinin in a representative study of 22 patients. Asterisks denote statistical significance. (From van Oeveren W, Jansen NJG, Bidstrup BP, et al: Effects of aprotinin on hemostatic mechanisms during cardiopulmonary bypass. Ann Thorac Surg 44:640, 1987.)

Cardiac surgery patients undergoing repeat operation may benefit particularly from prophylactic antifibrinolytic administration.[471]

APROTININ

Bovine lung provides the source of this 58-residue polypeptide serine protease inhibitor[472] (see Fig. 29–30). Aprotinin inhibits a host of proteases, including trypsin, plasmin, kallikrein, and factor XIIa activation of complement[473] (Fig. 29–33). The adult intravenous dose for surgical hemostasis is 2 million kallikrein inhibitor units (KIU) for both patient and bypass pump, followed by 600,000 KIU/hr.[474,475] The elimination half-life of aprotinin, 7 hours, is considerably longer than that of the synthetic antifibrinolytics; after 6 days, aprotinin continues to be excreted in the urine. Volume-loaded rats respond to aprotinin with decreases in glomerular filtration rate, renal plasma flow, and sodium and potassium excretion; however, no significant renal impairment follows routine clinical use.[476]

Decades ago, several investigations failed to show decreased bleeding after cardiac operations with moderate doses of aprotinin.[477,478] After the serendipitous discovery of unusually dry surgical fields while investigating high-dose aprotinin for respiratory distress syndrome, Royston et al documented more than a fourfold reduction in blood loss during repeat cardiac surgery.[479] Subsequent studies using high-dose aprotinin confirmed conservation of blood products and a reduction in bleeding, ranging from 29% to 50%.[480-486] Figure 29–34 demonstrates the efficacy of aprotinin in this regard. Although studies clearly demonstrate decreased fibrinolysis in aprotinin-treated patient groups, preservation of platelet GPIb or blockade of a plasmin-mediated platelet defect may better explain the hemostatic mechanism of aprotinin.[400,407,408,484]

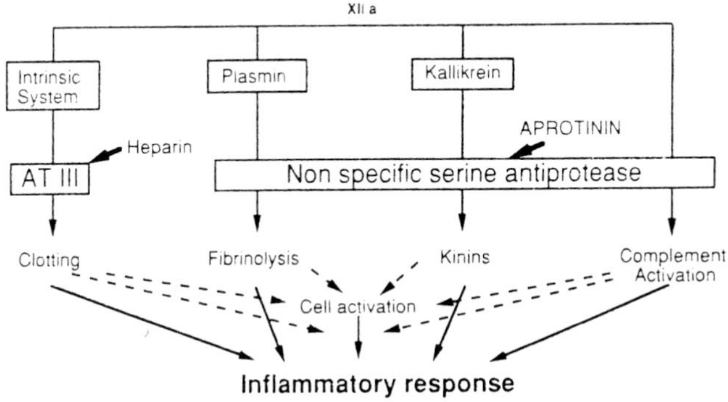

Figure 29–33 Actions of aprotinin on the contact coagulation system, fibrinolytic pathway, and complement activation. (From Royston D: The serine antiprotease aprotinin [Trasylol]: A novel approach to reducing postoperative bleeding. Blood Coag Fibrin 1:55, 1990.)

High-dose aprotinin alone prolongs the celite ACT, leading some investigators to limit use of heparin during CPB.[486] Reports of clot formation during CPB, however, mandate continued use of heparin despite administration of aprotinin. Most investigators today simply avoid the cellite ACT and use kaolin ACT. The kaolin ACT adsorbs about 98% of aprotinin and any intrinsic antithrombin effect that aprotinin has is therefore mitigated. It is recommended to use the kaolin ACT and keep the length of ACT time the same as if aprotinin was not being used.[487-490] An animal protein, aprotinin can cause anaphylaxis, although uncommon (<1 in 1000).[484,491] Aprotinin costs significantly more than equivalent doses of synthetic antifibrinolytics drugs.[492] The discussion and argument about cost effectiveness of aprotinin versus other antifibrinolytics has been ongoing now for almost 10 years.[493] There have never been large safety trials nor have there ever been any trials looking at graft patency with either EACA or tranexamic acid. As blood products become increasingly expensive and as data gather regarding their severe adverse outcomes (prolonged length of stay, increased mortality, and increased infection rate in patients with blood transfusion), the old arguments about aprotinin cost are no longer pertinent. The group at Duke University took a look at overall cost effectiveness of aprotinin therapy and found it highly cost effective.[494] That is in light of its effects upon stroke and blood transfusion utilization alone.[495]

Management of the Bleeding Patient

The initial approach to perioperative bleeding violates the medical paradigm of treatment based on diagnosis. The clinician must simultaneously initiate diagnostic tests, begin treating a presumed cause, and replace lost hemostatic resources. The latter two actions influence all three. The all-encompassing ("shotgun") approach to bleeding after operation should be shunned. Avoiding it will simplify patient management and yield superior results.

Determine the Cause

The complexity of human hemostasis, augmented by unexpected behavior of coagulation tests, can lead to confusion in the diagnosis of bleeding after cardiac surgery. For example, warfarin (Coumadin) inhibits the vitamin K–dependent factors II, VII, IX, and X; yet the aPTT, which involves factors II, IX, and X, typically is not markedly prolonged with warfarin therapy. Likewise, heparin inhibits factors II, IX, X, and XI, yet the PT, which tests factors II and X, remains normal with heparin plasma concentrations below 1.5 units/mL. As a third example, the thrombin time tests only the ability of activated factor II to convert fibrinogen to fibrin; why should it be much more sensitive to heparin than the ACT or aPTT, which also depend on other heparin-inhibited factors? These examples underscore to the clinician the importance of seeking expert consultation in hemostasis instead of using inference and theory to diagnose postoperative hemorrhage.

Anatomic sources of bleeding frequently present once systemic blood pressure achieves sufficient magnitude. Some clinicians prefer to identify these sources prior to chest closure with a provocative test, i.e., allowing brief periods of hypertension. Generous chest tube drainage early after operation suggests an anatomic source. Retained mediastinal clot may engender a consumptive coagulopathy. A widened mediastinum on chest radiograph suggests the need for surgical drainage.

Nonsurgical causes of bleeding (platelets, coagulation factors, and fibrinolysis) usually manifest as a generalized ooze. Inspection of vascular access puncture sites aids in this diagnosis. Bleeding from other areas not manipulated during surgery (stomach, bladder) may also occur.

Coagulation tests aid diagnosis. Since the PT and aPTT are usually prolonged by several seconds after CPB, only values more than 1.5 times control suggest factor deficiency. Elevation of the ACT should first suggest unneutralized heparin, then factor deficiency.

A decreased platelet count, usually denoting hemodilution or consumption, requires correction with exogenous platelets in any bleeding patient. However, bleeding patients with insufficient functional platelets may demonstrate normal platelet counts early after operation. For this reason, clinicians have sought rapid diagnostic tests of platelet function and attempted correlation with bleeding after CPB[493,496] (see Chapter 18).

Low plasma fibrinogen occurs from excessive hemodilution or factor consumption, and is corrected with cryoprecipitate or FFP. The thrombin time is useful here. Most clinical laboratories can perform this test with rapid turnaround. A prolonged thrombin time denotes unneutralized heparin, insufficient fibrinogen, or high concentrations of fibrin degradation products. Finally, direct measurement of fibrin degradation products denotes fibrinolytic activity. In the absence of a cause for a consumptive coagulopathy, antifibrinolytic therapy may be useful.

Table 29–12 lists a treatment plan for excessive bleeding after cardiac surgery. Interventions appear not in order of likelihood, but rather by priority of consideration. Thus, surgical causes should be ruled out prior to seizing upon the diagnosis of a consumptive coagulopathy. The priority will also vary among institutions, depending upon the availability and cost of resources. This table provides a simple algorithm for treating postoperative bleeding. More complete schemes present a daunting level of complexity that deter implementation (Fig. 29–35). The material presented in this chapter is intended to assist the clinician in developing, refining, and implementing a personal approach to this problem.

Adjunctive Therapy

WARMING

Bleeding patients with core or intermediate zone temperatures below 35°C will benefit from warming efforts, both passive

Table 29–12 **A Treatment Plan for Excessive Bleeding After Cardiac Surgery**

Action	Amount	Indication
Rule out surgical cause	—	No oozing at puncture sites; chest radiograph
More protamine	0.5 to 1 mg/kg	ACT >150 sec or aPTT >1.5 times control
Warm the patient	—	"Core" temperature <35°C
Apply PEEP*	5 to 10 cm H_2O	—
Desmopressin	0.3 μg/kg IV	Prolonged bleeding time
Aminocaproic acid	50 mg/kg, then 25 mg/kg/hr	Elevated D-dimer or teardrop shaped TEG tracing
Tranexamic acid	10 mg/kg, then 1 mg/kg/hr	Elevated D-dimer or teardrop shaped TEG tracing
Platelet transfusion	1 unit/10 kg	Platelet count <100,000/mm^3
Fresh frozen plasma	15 mL/kg	PT or aPTT >1.5 times control
Cryoprecipitate	1 unit/4 kg	Fibrinogen <1 g/L or 100 mg/dL

*Positive end-expiratory pressure (PEEP) is contraindicated in hypovolemia.

(warm ambient temperature, adequate body coverings, low ventilator fresh gas flows, airway heat and humidity exchangers) and active (heated humidifiers, warmed intravenous fluids, forced air convective warming blankets). All too often, in the effort to maintain intravascular volume, intensive care unit personnel administer liters of room-temperature (≤20°C) or refrigerated (0° to 4°C) fluids, which render patients hypothermic. Ready availability of fluid warmers reduces the possibility of the treatment of hemorrhage becoming its continuing cause.

POSITIVE END-EXPIRATORY PRESSURE

One popular method to limit bleeding after cardiac surgery is application of positive end-expiratory pressure (PEEP) (5 to 10 cm H_2O).[497,498] A tamponade effect in the mediastinum may explain this salutary effect. Unfortunately, controlled studies have not confirmed this benefit.[499,500] Also, excessive pressure impedes venous return, worsening hemodynamics in the hypovolemic patient.

BLOOD PRESSURE

Maintenance of systemic blood pressure in the low-normal range promotes tissue perfusion while limiting leakage around suture lines. Adequate depth of anesthesia during surgery and sufficient postoperative analgesia and sedation should be verified prior to initiating vasodilator therapy.

Blood Products

The bleeding patient becomes subject to additional hemostatic derangements. The need to maintain intravascular blood volume arises in nearly all cases prior to identification of the cause of bleeding. Protracted hypovolemia can lead to shock. Consumptive coagulopathy accompanies prolonged shock,[501] and failure to treat hypovolemia from bleeding may induce this second hemostatic abnormality. Clear fluid or colloid will replenish intravascular volume. However, red blood cells, platelets, and coagulation factors become diluted when continued bleeding is treated with such replacement. Also, packed red blood cells and banked whole blood do not provide platelets or sufficient factor V or factor VIII to maintain hemostasis. Although routine prophylactic administration of FFP or platelets plays no role in modern cardiac surgical care,[502] demonstration of a platelet count below 100,000/mm^3 or prolongation of the PT or aPTT despite adequate heparin neutralization *in a patient actively bleeding* is an indication for platelet or plasma replacement.[502]

Banked blood should be infused to maintain a hemoglobin concentration that allows appropriate oxygen delivery to tissues. In the absence of coagulation tests to guide therapy, when reconstituted red blood cells adequately replace blood lost, platelets should be given after 15 units of red blood cells to patients undergoing noncardiac surgery.[502,503] Since patients undergoing cardiac surgery also experience the hemodiluting and antihemostatic effects of CPB, the prudent clinician will commence platelet and factor replenishment earlier in the course of hemorrhage while awaiting laboratory confirmation. Each unit of platelet concentrate supplies about 10^{11} platelets, which increases platelet count by about 20,000/mm^3 in the adult. Enough plasma accompanies platelet concentrates to supply the equivalent of 1.0 to 1.5 units of plasma for each 6 units of platelets.[502]

Shed mediastinal blood can be collected and given back to patients using a closed drainage system. The drainage fluid, often collected in citrate, contains little fibrinogen. Presence of tissue and other debris in this fluid suggests the need for filtration before reinfusion. Shed mediastinal fluid supplies red blood cells without risk of viral transmission via allogeneic blood products.[503]

Drugs

Desmopressin often fails in the treatment of established bleeding,[504] despite initial uncontrolled studies to the contrary.[443,505] Desmopressin's efficacy in treating surgical hemorrhage associated with aspirin therapy also remains anecdotal.[506] Of course, desmopressin administration carries no risk of viral disease transmission, and, therefore, its substitution for otherwise unneeded, prophylactic FFP or platelets prevents potential patient harm.

Although antifibrinolytic therapy initiated prior to CPB decreases bleeding after operation, its efficacy after CPB or once bleeding is established remains controversial. Two studies of adult patients undergoing CABG yielded opposite conclusions regarding a savings of blood shed.[464,465] Lack of sufficient antifibrinolytic dose (only 4 or 5 g of aminocaproic acid loading) confounds both investigations. In the control of postoperative hemorrhage, antifibrinolytic therapy is suggested by any of the following: a TEG demonstrating clot lysis; fibrin degradation products of 40 μg/mL or more; or elevated thrombin time coexisting with normal fibrinogen and known absence of heparin.

Recombinant factor VIIa (rFVIIa NovoSeven) has been approved for use in hemophiliacs who are resistant to factor VIII concentrates. When rFVIIa is administered, it binds to tissue factor and activates factor X leading to thrombin and fibrin formation. These then activate platelets. Thrombin generation and clotting take place on the surface of platelets and at sites of injury.[507-510] Numerous reports have been published of the off-label use of this "rescue agent" to stop bleeding in surgical patients, including cardiac surgical patients after CPB.

In hemophiliacs, the recommended dose is 90 μg/kg. However, reports in cardiac surgical patients have suggested doses of 30 μg/kg, while continuing ongoing component therapy and monitoring the PT/INR. The half-life is about 2 hours and the dose may have to be repeated if bleeding continues. Most of the anecdotal reports have been positive with a marked decrease in bleeding taking place.[511-513] This treatment should not be used in the presence of disseminated intravascular coagulation or sepsis. Other potential indications for it include warfarin reversal, thrombocytopenia, factor XI deficiency, hepatic failure, von Willebrand disease, reversal of fondaparinux, and in cardiac surgery following deep hypothermic circulatory arrest or after use of direct thrombin inhibitors. Further studies are needed to determine dosing, safety, and efficacy for these potential uses.

Perspective on Bleeding After Cardiac Surgery

The differential diagnosis of bleeding after cardiac surgery derives from the elements of hemostasis outlined in the first section of this chapter. After initiating action to determine the cause, the prudent clinician ensures continued adequacy of circulating volume and, when indicated, of platelets and coagulation factors. Above all, it is important to avoid embracing one possibility, no matter how obvious, as the cause of bleeding until confirmatory evidence becomes available. In this way, the actual cause will not go undisclosed.

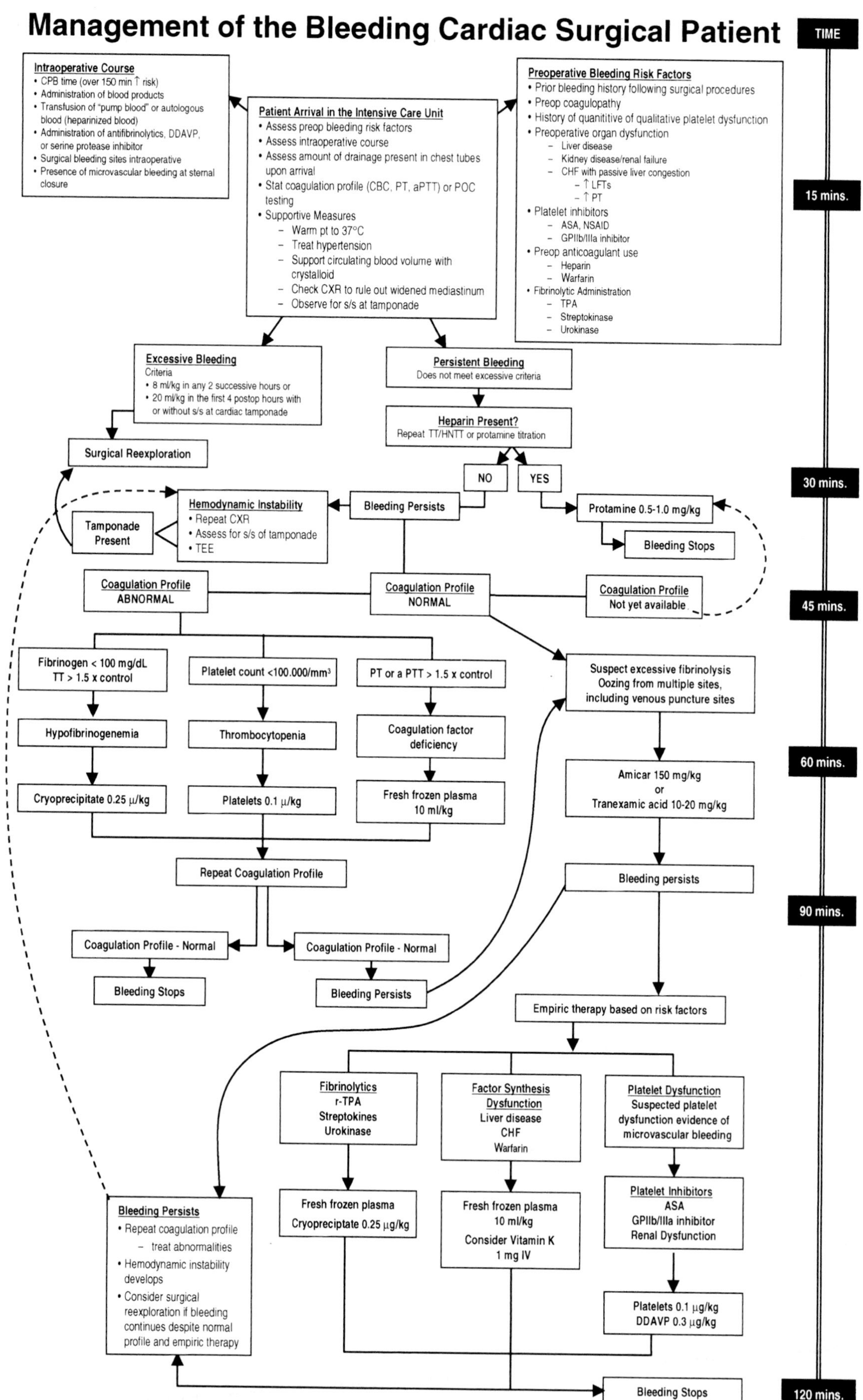

Figure 29–35 Example of a scheme for treating excessive bleeding. (From Milas B, Johes D, Gorman R: Management of bleeding and coagulopathy after heart surgery. Semin Thorac Cardiovasc Surg 12:326, 2000.)

CONCLUSIONS

The basic science and clinical knowledge of coagulation, hemostasis, and thrombosis have evolved dramatically in the past 30 years. Continued insights and advances in understanding pathophysiology and in developing pharmaceutical preparations will continue to have significant impact on clinical practice in the next decade. Perhaps the future will hold great strides in genetics and other realms. Of particular interest is a new focus upon short and long term outcomes after CABG surgery. Genetics is just now beginning to be studied in the coagulation field, and although there are a number of genetic polymorphisms that have been discovered, it is not known which ones are the most important. It is also not known yet what the implications are if a particular patient has one or more of these genetic polymorphisms. Some genetic abnormalities make patients more likely to thrombose or have early graft atherosclerosis, while others may affect drug metabolism or the way in which patients react with inflammation. The future may also involve genetic engineering and correction of defects.[515-517]

REFERENCES

1. Spiess BD: Coagulation function and monitoring. *In* Lichtor JL (ed): Atlas of Clinical Anesthesia. Philadelphia, Current Medicine, 1996
2. Spiess BD: The Relationships Between Coagulation, Inflammation and Endothelium—A Pyramid Towards Outcome. Baltimore, Lippincott, Williams & Wilkins, 2002, SCA monograph
3. Boyle EM Jr, Morgan EN, Verrier ED: The endothelium disturbed: The procoagulant response. *In* Spiess BD (ed): The Relationship Between Coagulation, Inflammation and Endothelium—A Pyramid Towards Outcome. Baltimore, Lippincott, Williams and Wilkins, 2002, p 79, SCA Monograph
4. Boyle EM Jr, Verrier ED, Spiess BD: Endothelial cell injury in cardiovascular surgery: The procoagulant response. Ann Thorac Surg 62:1549, 1996
5. Colman RW, Marder VJ, Salzman EW, Hirsh J: Overview of hemostasis. *In* Colman RW, Hirsh J, Marder VJ, Salzman EW (eds): Hemostasis and Thrombosis, 3rd edition. Philadelphia, JB Lippincott, 1994, p 3
6. Mackman N: Regulation of tissue factor gene expression in human monocytic and endothelial cells. Haemostasis 26(suppl 1):17, 1996
7. Edmunds LH Jr: Blood-surface interactions during cardiopulmonary bypass. J Card Surg 8:404, 1993
8. Boisclair MD, Lane DA Philippau H, et al: Mechanisms of thrombin generation during surgery and cardiopulmonary bypass. Blood 82:3350, 1993
9. Almus FE, Rao LV, Rapaport SI: Decreased inducibility of tissue factor activity on human umbilical vein endothelial cells cultured with endothelial cell growth factor and heparin. Thromb Res 50:339, 1988
10. Rao LV, Rapaport SI, Lorenzi M: Enhancement by human umbilical vein endothelial cells of factor Xa-catalyzed activation of factor VII. Blood 71:791, 1988
11. Krishnaswamy S, Mann KG, Nesheim ME: The prothrombinase-catalyzed activation of prothrombin proceeds through the intermediate meizathrombin in an ordered, sequential reaction. J Biol Chem 261:8977, 1986
12. Jones A, Geczy CL: Thrombin and factor Xa enhance the production of interleukin. Immunology 71:236, 1990
13. Salvesen G, Pizzo SV: Proteinase inhibitors: Alpha-macroglobulins, serpins, and kinins. *In* Colman RW, Hirsh J, Marder VJ, Salzman EW (eds): Hemostasis and Thrombosis, 3rd edition. Philadelphia, JB Lippincott, 1994, p 241
14. Spiess BD: Heparin: Beyond an anticoagulant. *In* Spiess BD (ed): The Relationship Between Coagulation, Inflammation and Endothelium—A Pyramid Towards Outcome. Baltimore, Lippincott, Williams and Wilkins, 2002, p 169
15. Van Norman GA, Gernsheimer T, Chandler WL, et al: Indicators of fibrinolysis during cardiopulmonary bypass after exogenous antithrombin III administration for antithrombin deficiency. J Cardiothorac Vasc Anesth 11:760, 1997
16. Hashimoto Y, Yamgishi M, Sasaki T, et al: Heparin and antithrombin III levels during cardiopulmonary bypass: Correlation with subclinical plasma coagulation. Ann Thorac Surg 58:799, 1994
17. Despotis GJ, Levine V, Joist JH, et al: Antithrombin III during cardiac surgery: Effect on response of activated clotting time to heparin and relationship to markers of hemostatic activation. Anesth Analg 85:498, 1997
18. Levy JH, Despotis GJ, Szlam F, et al: Recombinant human transgenic antithrombin in cardiac surgery: A dose finding study. Anesthesiology 96: 1095, 2002
19. Brister SJ, Buchanan MR: Heparinless cardiopulmonary bypass revisited: A newer strategy to avoid heparin-related bleeding using dermatan sulfate. J Thorac Cardiovasc Anesth 9:317, 1995
20. Esmon CT, Owen WG: Identification of an endothelial cell cofactor for thrombin-catalyzed activation of protein C. Proc Natl Acad Sci U S A 78:2249, 1981
21. DeFouw NJ, van Hinsbergh VW, deJong YF, et al: The interaction of activated protein C and thrombin with the plasminogen activator inhibitor released from human endothelial cells. Thromb Haemost 57:176, 1987
22. Novotny WF, Girard TJ, Miletich JP, Broze GJ: Purification and characterization of the lipoprotein-associated coagulation inhibitor from human plasma. J Biol Chem 264:18832, 1989
23. Bajaj MS, Kuppuswamy MN, Saito H, et al: Cultured normal human hepatocytes do not synthesize lipoprotein-associated coagulation inhibitor: Evidence that endothelium is the principal site of its synthesis. Proc Natl Acad Sci U S A 87:8869, 1990
24. Novotny WF, Girard TJ, Miletich JP, Broze GJ: Platelets secrete a coagulation inhibitor functionally and antigenically similar to the lipoprotein-associated coagulation inhibitor. Blood 72:2020, 1988
25. Hansen JB, Sarset PM: Differential effects of low molecular weight heparin and unfractionated heparin on circulating levels of antithrombin and tissue factor pathway inhibitor (TFPI): A possible mechanism for difference in therapeutic efficacy. Thromb Res 91:177, 1998
26. Soejima H, Ogawa H, Yasue H, et al: Plasma tissue factor pathway inhibitor and tissue factor antigen levels after administration of heparin in patients with angina pectoris. Thromb Res 93:17, 1999
27. Jeske W, Hoppensteadt D, Callas D, et al: Pharmacologic profiling of recombinant tissue factor pathway inhibitor. Semin Thromb Hemost 22:213, 1996
28. Kojima T, Gando S, Kemmotsu O, et al: Another point of view on the mechanism of thrombin generation during cardiopulmonary bypass: Role of tissue factor inhibitor. J Cardiothorac Vasc Anesth 15:60, 2001
29. Adams MJ, Cardigan RA, Marchant WA, et al: Tissue factor pathway inhibitor antigen and activity in 96 patients receiving heparin for cardiopulmonary bypass. J Cardiothoracic Vasc Anesth 16:59, 2002
30. Fischer R, Kuppe H, Koster A: Impact of heparin management on release of tissue factor pathway inhibitor during cardiopulmonary bypass. Anesthesiology 100:1040, 2004
31. Tsai H, Sussman I, Nagel R: Shear stress enhances the proteolysis of von Willebrand factor in normal plasma. Blood 83:2171, 1994
32. Asakai R, Chung DW, Davie EW, Seligsohn U: Factor XI deficiency in Ashkenazi Jews in Israel. N Engl J Med 325:153, 1991
33. Brettler DB, Levine PH: Clinical manifestations and therapy of inherited coagulation factor deficiencies. *In* Colman RW, Hirsh J, Marder VJ, Salzman EW (eds): Hemostasis and Thrombosis, 3rd edition. Philadelphia, JB Lippincott, 1994, p 169
34. Mannucci PM: Desmopressin: A nontransfusional form of treatment for congenital and acquired bleeding disorders. Blood 72:1449, 1988
35. Blajchman MA, Hirst R, Perrault RA: Blood component therapy in anaesthetic practice. Can Anaesth Soc J 30:382, 1983
36. Van Aken WG: Preparation of plasma derivatives. *In* Rossi EC, Simon TL, Moss GS, Gould SA (eds): Principles of Transfusion Medicine, 2nd edition. Baltimore, Williams & Wilkins, 1996, p 403
37. Palenzo DA, Sadr FS: Coronary artery bypass grafting in a patient with haemophilia B. Perfusion 10:265, 1995
38. Flier JS, Underhill LH: Molecular and cellular biology of blood coagulation. N Engl J Med 326:800, 1992
39. Bertina RM, Koeleman BPC, Koster T, et al: Mutation in blood coagulation factor V associated with resistance to activated protein C. Nature 369:64, 1994
40. Florell SR, Rodgers GM: Inherited thrombotic disorders. An update. Am J Hematol 54:53, 1997
41. Koster T, Rosendaal FR, Briet E, et al: Protein C deficiency in a controlled series of unselected outpatients: An infrequent but clear risk for venous thrombosis. Blood 85:2756, 1995
42. Rodgers GM, Chandler WL: Laboratory and clinical aspects of inherited thrombotic disorders. Am J Hematol 41:113, 1992

43. Mayer O, Filipovsky J, Hromadka M, et al: Treatment of hyperhomocysteinemia with folic acid. J Cardiovasc Pharmacol 39:851, 2002
44. Rinder CS: Platelet and their interactions. *In* Spiess BD (ed): The Relationship Between Coagulation, Inflammation and Endothelium—A Pyramid Towards Outcome. Baltimore, Lippincott, Williams and Wilkins, 2002, p 107
45. Kroll MH, Schafer A: Biochemical mechanisms of platelet activation. Blood 74:1181, 1989
46. Savage B, Saldivar E, Ruggeri ZM: Initiation of platelet adhesion by arrest onto fibrinogen or translocation on von Willebrand factor. Cell 84:289, 1996
47. Celi A, Pellegrini G, Lorenzet R, et al: P-selectin induces the expression of tissue factor on monocytes. Proc Natl Acad Sci U S A 91:8767, 1994
48. Hynes RO: Integrins: Versatility, modulation, and signaling in cell adhesion. Cell 69:11, 1992
49. Kessler CM: The pharmacology of aspirin, heparin, coumarin, and thrombolytic agents. Chest 99:97S, 1991
50. Montgomery RR, Coller BS: von Willebrand disease. *In* Colman RW, Hirsh J, Marder VJ, Salzman EW (eds): Hemostasis and Thrombosis, 3rd edition. Philadelphia, JB Lippincott, 1994, p 134
51. Slaughter TF, Mody EA, Oldham HN Jr, et al: Management of a patient with type IIC von Willebrand's disease during coronary artery bypass graft surgery. Anesthesiology 78:195, 1993
52. Steering Committee of the Physicians' Health Study Research Group: Final report on the aspirin component of the ongoing Physicians' Health Study. N Engl J Med 321:129, 1989
53. George J, Shattil SJ: The clinical importance of acquired abnormalities of platelet function. N Engl J Med 324:27, 1991
54. Goldman S, Copeland J, Moritz T, et al: Improvement in early saphenous vein graft patency after coronary artery bypass surgery with antiplatelet therapy: Results of a Veterans Administration cooperative study. Circulation 77:1324, 1988
55. Taggart DP, Siddiqui A, Wheatley DJ: Low-dose preoperative aspirin therapy, postoperative blood loss and transfusion requirements. Ann Thorac Surg 50:425, 1990
56. Bashein G, Nessly ML, Rice AL, et al: Preoperative aspirin therapy and reoperation for bleeding after coronary artery bypass surgery. Arch Intern Med 151:89, 1991
57. Weksler BB, Pett SB, Aloso D, et al: Differential inhibition by aspirin of vascular and platelet prostaglandin synthesis in atherosclerotic patients. N Engl J Med 308:800, 1983
58. Rajah SM, Salter MCP, Donaldson DR: Acetylsalicylic acid and dipyridamole improve the early patency of aorta-coronary bypass grafts. J Thorac Cardiovasc Surg 90:373, 1985
59. Karwande S, Weksler BB, Gay WA, Subramanian VA: Effect of preoperative antiplatelet drugs on vascular prostacyclin synthesis. Ann Thorac Surg 43:318, 1987
60. Rawitscher RE, Jones JW, McCoy TA, Lindsley DA: A prospective study of aspirin effect on red blood cell loss in cardiac surgery. J Cardiovasc Surg 32:1, 1991
61. Tuman KJ, McCarthy RJ, O'Connor CJ, et al: Aspirin does not increase allogeneic blood transfusion in reoperative coronary artery surgery. Anesth Analg 83:1178, 1996
62. Reich DL, Patel GC, Vela-Cantos F, et al: Aspirin does not increase homologous blood requirements in elective coronary bypass surgery. Anesth Analg 79:4, 1994
63. Baeuerle JJ, Mongan PD, Hosking MP: An assessment of the duration of cephapirin-induced coagulation abnormalities as measured by thromboelastography. J Cardiothorac Vasc Anesth 7:422, 1993
64. Juni P, Nartey L, Reichenbach S et al: Risk of cardiovascular events and rofecoxib: Cumulative meta-analysis. Lancet 364:2021, 2004
65. Lange RA, Hillis LD: Antiplatelet therapy for ischemic heart disease. N Engl J Med 350:277, 2004
66. Teufelsbauer H, Proidl S, Havel M, Vukovich T: Early activation of hemostasis during cardiopulmonary bypass. Evidence for thrombin-mediated hyperfibrinolysis. Thromb Haemost 68:250, 1992
67. Goldberg M, Colonna-Romano P, Babins N: Emergency coronary artery bypass surgery following intracoronary streptokinase. Anesthesiology 61:601, 1984
68. McLean J: The discovery of heparin. Circulation 19:75, 1959
69. Rodén L: Highlights in the history of heparin. *In* Lane DA, Lindahl U (eds): Heparin. Boca Raton, FL, CRC Press, 1989, p 1
70. Casu B: Structure of heparin and heparin fragments. *In* Ofosu FA, Danishefsky I, Hirsh J (eds): Heparin and Related Polysaccharides. New York, New York Academy of Sciences, 1989, p 1
71. Holmer E: Low-molecular-weight heparin. *In* Lane DA, Lindahl U (eds): Heparin. Boca Raton, FL, CRC Press, 1989, p 575
72. Freedman JE, Loscalzo J: New antithrombitic strategies. *In* Loscalzo J, Schafer AI (eds): Thrombosis and hemorrhage, 3rd edition. Philadelphia, Lippincott Williams and Wilkins, 2003, pp 978–995
73. Nader HB, Dietrich CP: Natural occurrence and possible biological role of heparin. *In* Lane DA, Lindahl U (eds): Heparin. Boca Raton, FL, CRC Press, 1989, p 81
74. Barrowcliffe TW: Heparin assays and standardization. *In* Lane DA, Lindahl U (eds): Heparin. Boca Raton, FL, CRC Press, 1989, p 393
75. Coyne E, Outschoorn AS: Some thoughts on a new USP heparin assay—Aren't we ready for an upgrade? Pharmacopeial Forum Jan-Feb:1492, 1991
76. Howell WH: Heparin, an anticoagulant. Am J Physiol 631:434, 1922
77. Majerus PW, Broze GJ, Miletich JP, Tollefsen DM: Anticoagulant, thrombolytic, and antiplatelet drugs. *In* Hardman JG, Limbird LE, Molinoff PB, et al (eds): Goodman & Gilman's The Pharmacological Basis of Therapeutics, 9th edition. New York, McGraw-Hill, 1996, p 1341
78. Albada H, Nieuwenhuis HK, Sixma JJ: Pharmacokinetics of standard and low-molecular-weight heparin. *In* Lane DA, Lindahl U (eds): Heparin. Boca Raton, FL, CRC Press, 1989, p 417
79. deSwart CAM, Nijmeyer B, Roelofs JMM, Sixma JJ: Kinetics of intravenously administered heparin in normal humans. Blood 60:1251, 1982
80. Mahadoo J, Heibert L, Jaques LB: Vascular sequestration of heparin. Thromb Res 12:79, 1978
81. Glimelius B, Busch C: Binding of heparin on the surface of cultured human endothelial cells. Thromb Res 12:773, 1978
82. Cipolle RJ, Seifert RD, Neilan BA, et al: Heparin kinetics: Variables related to disposition and dosage. Clin Pharmacol Ther 29:387, 1981
83. Cook JJ, Niewiarowski S, Yan Z, et al: Platelet factor 4 efficiently reverses heparin anticoagulation in the rat without adverse effects of the heparin-protamine complexes. Circulation 85:1102, 1992
84. Okuno T, Crockatt D: Platelet factor, activity and thromboembolic episodes. Am J Clin Pathol 67:351, 1977
85. Sette H, Hughes RD, Langley PG, et al: Heparin response and clearance in acute and chronic liver disease. Thromb Haemost 54:591, 1985
86. Kesteven PJ, Ahred A, Aps C, et al: Protamine sulphate and rebound following open heart surgery. J Cardiovasc Surg 27:600, 1986
87. Gravlee GP, Brauer SD, Roy RC, et al: Predicting the pharmacodynamics of heparin: A clinical evaluation of the Hepcon System 4. J Cardiothorac Anesth 1:379, 1987
88. Estes JW: Kinetics of the anticoagulant effect of heparin. JAMA 212:1492, 1970
89. Seifert R, Borchert W, Letendre P, et al: Heparin kinetics during hemodialysis: Variation in sensitivity, distribution volume, and dosage. Ther Drug Monit 8:32, 1986
90. Ofosu FA: Antithrombotic mechanisms of heparin and related compounds. *In* Lane DA, Lindahl U (eds): Heparin. Boca Raton, FL, CRC Press, 1989, p 433
91. Jordan RE, Oosta GM, Gardner WT, Rosenberg RD: The kinetics of hemostatic enzyme-antithrombin interactions in the presence of low-molecular-weight heparin. J Biol Chem 225:10,081, 1980
92. Barrowcliffe TW, Thomas DP: Anticoagulant activities of heparin and fragments. *In* Ofosu FA, Danishefsky I, Hirsh J (eds): Heparin and Related Polysaccharides. New York, New York Academy of Sciences, 1989, p 132
93. Bjork I, Olson ST, Shore JD: Molecular mechanisms of the accelerating effect of heparin on the reactions between antithrombin and clotting proteinases. *In* Lane DA, Lindahl U (eds): Heparin. Boca Raton, FL, CRC Press, 1989, p 229
94. Holmer E, Soderberg K, Berggvist D, Lindahl U: Heparin and its low-molecular-weight derivatives: Anticoagulant and antithrombotic properties. Haemostasis 16(suppl 2):1, 1986
95. Gravlee GP, Haddon WS, Rothberger HK, et al: Heparin dosing and monitoring for cardiopulmonary bypass. J Thorac Cardiovasc Surg 99:518, 1990
96. Tanaka K, Takao M, Yada I, et al: Alterations in coagulation and fibrinolysis associated with cardiopulmonary bypass during open heart surgery. J Cardiothorac Anesth 3:181, 1989
97. Davies GC, Sobel M, Salzman EW: Elevated plasma fibrinopeptide A and thromboxane B2 levels during cardiopulmonary bypass. Circulation 61:808, 1980
98. Slaughter TF, LeBleu TH, Douglas JM Jr, et al: Characterization of prothrombin activation during cardiac surgery by hemostatic molecular markers. Anesthesiology 80:520, 1994
99. Racanelli A, Fareed J, Walenga JM, Coyne E: Biochemical and pharmacologic studies on the protamine interactions with heparin, its fractions and fragments. Semin Thromb Hemost 11:176, 1985
100. Levy JH: Heparin resistance and antithrombin: Should it still be called heparin resistance? J Cardiothorac Vasc Anesth 18:129, 2004

101. Koster A, Fischer T, Grunendel M, et al: Management of heparin: Resistance and cardiopulmonary bypass: The effect of 5 different anticoagulation strategies on hemostatic activation. J Cardiothorac Vasc Anesth 18:131, 2004
102. Soloway HB, Christansen TW: Heparin anticoagulation during cardiopulmonary bypass in an antithrombin III-deficient patient. Implications relative to the etiology of heparin. Am J Clin Pathol 73:723, 1980
103. Collen D, Schetz J, deCock F, et al: Metabolism of antithrombin III (heparin cofactor) in man: Effects of venous thrombosis and of heparin administration. Eur J Clin Invest 7:27, 1977
104. Linden MD, Schneider M, Baker S, Erber WN: Decreased concentrations of antithrombin after preoperative therapeutic heparin does not cause heparin resistance during cardiopulmonary bypass. J Cardiothorac Vasc Anesth 2004
105. Andersson G, Fagrell B, Holngren K, et al: Antithrombin III in patients with acute deep vein thrombosis during heparin treatment (subcutaneous and intravenous) and during and after treatment with oral coumarins. Thromb Res 34:333, 1984
106. Holm HA, Kalvenes S, Abidgaard U: Changes in plasma antithrombin (heparin cofactor activity) during intravenous heparin therapy: Observations in 198 patients with deep venous thrombosis. Scand J Haematol 35:564, 1985
107. Marciniak E, Gockerman JP: Heparin-induced decrease in circulating antithrombin III. Lancet 1:581, 1977
108. deSwart CA, Nijmeyer B, Andersson LO, et al: Elimination of intravenously administered radiolabeled antithrombin III and heparin in humans. Thromb Haemost 52:66, 1984
109. Mummaneni N, Istanbouli M, Pifarri R, El-Etr AA: Increased heparin requirements with autotransfusion. J Thorac Cardiovasc Surg 86:446, 1983
110. Hicks GL: Heparin resistance during cardiopulmonary bypass (letter). J Thorac Cardiovasc Surg 86:633, 1983
111. Esposito RA, Culliford AT, Colvin SB, et al: Heparin resistance during cardiopulmonary bypass. J Thorac Cardiovasc Surg 85:346, 1983
112. Anderson EF: Heparin resistance prior to cardiopulmonary bypass. Anesthesiology 64:504, 1986
113. Rivard DC, Thompson SJ, Cameron D: The role of antithrombin III in heparin resistance. Proc 28th Internatl Conf Amer Soc Extracorporeal Tech, Dallas, TX, 1990, p 66
114. Chung F, David TE, Watt J: Excessive requirement for heparin during cardiac surgery. Can Anaesth Soc J 28:280, 1981
115. Mabry CD, Read RC, Thompson BW, et al: Identification of heparin resistance during cardiac and vascular surgery. Arch Surg 114:129, 1979
116. Young JA, Kisker T, Doty DB: Adequate anticoagulation during cardiopulmonary bypass determined by activated clotting time and the appearance of fibrin monomer. Ann Thorac Surg 26:231, 1978
117. Jobes DR: Tight control of anticoagulation, not empiric management, improves outcome from cardiopulmonary bypass. J Cardiothorac Anesth 3:655, 1989
118. Jackson MR, Olsen SB, Gomez ER, Alving BM: Use of antithrombin III concentrates to correct antithrombin III deficiency during vascular surgery. J Vasc Surg 22:804, 1995
119. Sabbagh AH, Chung GKT, Shuttleworth P, et al: Fresh frozen plasma: A solution to heparin resistance during cardiopulmonary bypass. Ann Thorac Surg 37:466, 1984
120. Metz S, Keats AS: Low activated coagulation time during cardiopulmonary bypass does not increase postoperative bleeding. Ann Thorac Surg 49:440, 1990
121. Lemmer JH, Despotis GJ: Antithrombin III concentrate to treat heparin resistance in patients undergoing cardiac surgery. J Thorac Cardiovasc Surg 123:213, 2002
122. Avidan M, Levy J, Scholz J, et al: A phase III, double blind, placebo-controlled, multicenter study on the efficacy of recombinant human antithrombin in heparin-resistant patients scheduled to undergo cardiac surgery necessitating cardiopulmonary bypass. Anesthesiology 102:276, 2005
123. Milas B, Jobes D, Gorman R: Management of bleeding and coagulopathy after heart surgery. Semin Thorac Cardiovasc Surg 12:326, 2000
124. Frick PG, Brogli H: The mechanism of heparin rebound after extracorporeal circulation for open cardiac surgery. Surgery 59:721, 1966
125. Gollub S: Heparin rebound in open heart surgery. Surg Gynecol Obstet 124:337, 1967
126. Ellison N, Beatty P, Blake DR, et al: Heparin rebound. J Thorac Cardiovasc Surg 67:723, 1974
127. Kaul TK, Crow MJ, Rajah SM, et al: Heparin administration during extracorporeal circulation. J Thorac Cardiovasc Surg 78:95, 1979
128. Fiser WP, Read RC, Wright FE, Vecchio TJ: A randomized study of beef lung and pork mucosal heparin in cardiac surgery. Ann Thorac Surg 35:615, 1983
129. Guffin AV, Dunbar RW, Kaplan JA, Bland JW: Successful use of a reduced dose of protamine after cardiopulmonary bypass. Anesth Analg 55:110, 1976
130. Ellison N, Ominsky AJ, Wollman H: Is protamine a clinically important anticoagulant? Anesthesiology 35:621, 1971
131. Kresowik TF, Wakefield TW, Fessler RD, Stanley JC: Anticoagulant effects of protamine sulfate in a canine model. J Surg Res 45:8, 1988
132. Jobes DR, Aitken GL, Shaffer GW: Increased accuracy and precision of heparin and protamine dosing reduces blood loss and transfusion in patients undergoing primary cardiac operations. J Thorac Cardiovasc Surg 110:36, 1995
133. DeLaria GA, Tyner JJ, Hayes CL, Armstrong BW: Heparin-protamine mismatch. A controllable factor in bleeding after open heart surgery. Arch Surg 129:944, 1994
134. Spiess BD: Heparin: Beyond an anticoagulant. *In* Spiess BD (ed): The Relationship Between Coagulation, Inflammation and Endothelium—A Pyramid Towards Outcome. Baltimore, Lippincott, Williams and Wilkins, 2002, p 169
135. Day JRS, Landis RC, Taylor KM: Heparin is more than just an anticoagulant. J Cardiothorac Vasc Anesth 18:93, 2004
136. Chang CH, Chang FM, Chen CP, et al: Antithrombin III activity in normal and toxemic preganancies. J Formosa Med Assoc 91:680, 1992
137. Saveliega GM, Efinov VS, Grislin VL, et al: Blood coagulation changes in pregnant women at risk of developing preeclampsia. Int J Gynaecol Obstet 48:3, 1995
138. Fourrier F, Chopin C, Hwart JJ, et al: Double blind placebo-controlled trial of antithrombin III concentrate in septic shock with disseminated intravascular coagulation. Chest 104:882, 1993
139. Urban P, Scheidegger D, Buchmann B, Skarvan K: The hemodynamic effects of heparin and their relation to ionized calcium levels. J Thorac Cardiovasc Surg 91:303, 1986
140. Thomson C, Forkes CD, Prentice CR: Potentiation of platelet aggregation and adhesion by heparin both in vitro and in vivo. Clin Sci Mol Med 33:63, 1973
141. Schneider DJ, Tracy PB, Mann KG, Sobel BE: Differential effects of anticoagulants on the activation of platelets ex vivo. Circulation 96:2877, 1997
142. Warkentin TE, Kelton JG: Heparin and platelets. Hematol Oncol Clin North Am 4:243, 1990
143. Fareed J, Walenga JM, Hoppensteadt DA, Messmore HL: Studies on the profibrinolytic actions of heparin and its factors. Semin Thromb Hemost 11:199, 1985
144. Warkentin TE, Greinacher A: Heparin induced thrombocytopenia and cardiac surgery. Ann Thorac Surg 18:2121, 2003
145. Godal HC: Heparin-induced thrombocytopenia. *In* Lane DA, Lindahl U (eds): Heparin. Boca Raton, FL, CRC Press, 1989, p 533
146. Fidlar E, Jaques LB: The effects of commercial heparin on the platelet count. J Lab Clin Med 33:1410, 1948
147. Sandler RM, Seifer DB, Morgan K, et al: Heparin-induced thrombocytopenia and thrombosis. Detection and specificity of a platelet-aggregating IgG. Am J Clin Pathol 83:760, 1985
148. Sheridan D, Carter C, Kelton JC: A diagnostic test for heparin-induced thrombocytopenia. Blood 67:27, 1986
149. Rhodes GR, Dixon RH, Silver D: Heparin-induced thrombocytopenia with thrombotic and hemorrhagic manifestations. Surg Gynecol Obstet 136:409, 1973
150. Eika C, Godal AC, Laake K, Hamborg T: Low incidence of thrombocytopenia during treatment with hog mucosa and beef lung heparin. Scand J Haematol 25:19, 1980
151. Kelton JG, Smith JW, Warkentin TE, et al: Immunoglobulin G from patients with heparin-induced thrombocytopenia binds to a complex of heparin and platelet factor 4. Blood 83:3232, 1994
152. Amiral J, Bridey F, Dreyfus M: Platelet factor 4 complexed to heparin is the target for antibodies generated in heparin-induced thrombocytopenia (letter). Thromb Haemost 68:95, 1992
153. Hirsh J, Raschke R, Warkentin TE, et al: Heparin: Mechanism of action, pharmacokinetics, dosing considerations, monitoring, efficacy, and safety. Chest 108:258S, 1995
154. Chong BH, Castaldi PA: Heparin-induced thrombocytopenia: Further studies of the effects of heparin-dependent antibodies on platelets. Br J Haematol 64:347, 1986
155. Schwartz KA, Roger G, Kaufman DB, Penner JA: Complications of heparin administration in normal individuals. Am J Hematol 19:355, 1985

156. Stead RB, Schafer AI, Rosenberg RD, et al: Heterogeneity of heparin lots associated with thrombocytopenia and thromboembolism. Am J Med 77:185, 1984
157. Godal HC: Thrombocytopenia and heparin. Thromb Haemost 43:222, 1980
158. Rizzoni WE, Miller K, Rick M, Lotze MT: Heparin-induced thrombocytopenia and thromboembolism in the postoperative period. Surgery 103:470, 1988
159. Moberg PQ, Geary VM, Sheich FM: Heparin-induced thrombocytopenia: A possible complication of heparin-coated pulmonary artery catheters. J Cardiothorac Anesth 4:226, 1990
160. Laster J, Silver D: Heparin-coated catheters and heparin-induced thrombocytopenia. J Vasc Surg 7:667, 1988
161. Ansell J, Slepchuk N Jr, Kumar R, et al: Heparin-induced thrombocytopenia: A prospective study. Thromb Haemost 43:61, 1980
162. Kelton JG, Sheridan D, Brain M: Clinical usefulness of testing for a heparin-dependent platelet-aggregating factor in patients with suspected heparin-induced thrombocytopenia. J Lab Clin Med 103:6062, 1984
163. Arepally G, Reynolds C, Tomaski A, et al: Comparison of PF4/heparin ELISA with the 14C-serotonin release assay in the diagnosis of heparin-induced thrombocytopenia. Am J Clin Pathol 104:648, 1995
164. Nelson JC, Lerner RG, Goldstein R, Cagin NA: Heparin-induced thrombocytopenia. Arch Intern Med 138:548, 1978.
165. Taylor-Williams R, Damaraju LV, Mascelli MA, et al: Antiplatelet factor 4/heparin antibodies. Circulation 107:2307, 2003
166. Mattioli AV, Bonetti L, Sternieri S, Mattioli G: Heparin-induced thrombocytopenia in patients treated with unfractionated heparin: Prevalence of thrombosis in a 1 year follow-up. Ital Heart J 1:39, 2000
167. Mehta DP, Yoder EL, Appel J, Bergsman KL: Heparin-induced thrombocytopenia and thrombosis. Am J Hematol 36:275, 1991
168. Kappa JR, Cottrell ED, Berkowitz HD, et al: Carotid endarterectomy in patients with heparin-induced platelet activation: Comparative efficacy of aspirin and Iloprost (ZK36374). J Vasc Surg 5:693, 1987
169. Makhoul RG, McCann RL, Austin EH, et al: Management of patients with heparin-associated thrombocytopenia and thrombosis requiring cardiac surgery. Ann Thorac Surg 43:617, 1987
170. Smith JP, Walls JT, Muscato MS, et al: Extracorporeal circulation in a patient with heparin-induced thrombocytopenia. Anesthesiology 62:363, 1985
171. Addonizio VP, Fisher CA, Kappa JR, Ellison N: Prevention of heparin-induced thrombocytopenia during open heart surgery with iloprost (ZK36374). Surgery 102:796, 1987
172. Kappa JR, Horn D, McIntosh CL, et al: Iloprost (ZK36374): A new prostacyclin analogue permits open cardiac operation in patients with heparin-induced thrombocytopenia. Surg Forum 36:285, 1985
173. Kraezler EJ, Starr NJ: Heparin-associated thrombocytopenia: Management of patients for open heart surgery. Anesthesiology 69:964, 1988
174. Ellison N, Kappa JR, Fisher CA, Addonizio VP: Extracorporeal circulation in a patient with heparin-induced thrombocytopenia. Anesthesiology 63:336, 1985
175. Vender JS, Matthew EB, Silverman IM, et al: Heparin-associated thrombocytopenia: Alternative managements. Anesth Analg 65:520, 1986
176. Magnani HN: Heparin-induced thrombocytopenia (HIT). An overview of 230 patients treated with Orgaran (ORG 10172). Thromb Haemost 70:554, 1993
177. Bretelle C, Leude E, Quilici J, Vaillant A: Utilisation de l'Orgaran pour une circulation extra-corporelle chez une patiente allergique à l'héparine. Presse Méd 25:1846, 1996
178. Gouault-Heilmann M, Huet Y, Contant G, et al: Cardiopulmonary bypass with a low-molecular-weight heparin fraction. Lancet 2:1374, 1983
179. Roussi JH, Houbouyan LL, Goguel AF: Use of low-molecular-weight heparin in heparin-induced thrombocytopenia with thrombotic complications. Lancet 1:1183, 1984
180. Rowlings PA, Mansberg R, Rozenberg MC, et al: The use of a low-molecular-weight heparinoid (Org 10172) for extracorporeal procedures in patients with heparin-dependent thrombocytopenia and thrombosis. Aust NZ J Med 21:52, 1991
181. Roynard JL, Pourriat JL, LeRoux G, et al: Hyperaggrabilité plaquettaire induit par une héparine de bas poids molculaire au cours d'un syndrome de détresse respiratoire de l'adulte. Ann Fr Anesth Reanim 10:70, 1991
182. Lecompte T, Luo S, Stieltjes N, et al: Thrombocytopenia associated with low-molecular-weight heparin. Lancet 338:1217, 1991
183. Leroy J, Leclerc MH, Delahousse B, et al: Treatment of heparin-associated thrombocytopenia and thrombosis with low-molecular-weight heparin (CY 216). Semin Thromb Hemost 11:326, 1985
184. Chong BH: Heparin-induced thrombocytopenia. Br J Haematol 89:431, 1995
185. Zulys VJ, Teasdale SJ, Michel ER, et al: Ancrod (Arvin) as an alternative to heparin anticoagulation for cardiopulmonary bypass. Anesthesiology 71:870, 1989
186. Spiess BD, Gernsheimer T, Vocelka C, et al: Hematologic changes with ancrod anticoagulated cardiopulmonary bypass: A case report. J Cardiothorac Vasc Anesth 10:918, 1996.
187. Samama MM, Bara L, Gouin-Thibault I: New data on the pharmacology of heparin and low-molecular-weight heparins. Drugs 52(suppl)7:8, 1996
188. Bergqvist D: Low-molecular-weight heparins. J Intern Med 240: 63, 1996
189. Weitz JI: Low-molecular-weight heparin(s). N Engl J Med 337:688, 1997
190. Planes A, Vochelle N, Fagola M, et al: Efficacy and safety of a perioperative enoxaparin regimen in total hip replacement under various anesthesia. Am J Surg 161:525, 1991
191. Turpie AG: Efficacy of a postoperative regimen of enoxaparin in deep vein thrombosis prophylaxis. Am J Surg 161:532, 1991
192. Hirsh J: Rationale for development of low-molecular-weight heparin and their clinical potential in the prevention of postoperative venous thrombosis. Am J Surg 161:512, 1991
193. Van Ryn-McKenna J, Cai L, Ofosu FA, et al: Neutralization of enoxaparin-induced bleeding by protamine sulfate. Thromb Haemost 63:271, 1990
194. Massonnet-Castel S, Pelissier E, Bara L, et al: Partial reversal of low-molecular-weight heparin (PK10169) anti-Xa activity by protamine sulfate: In vitro and in vivo study during cardiac surgery with extracorporeal circulation. Haemostasis 16:139, 1986
195. Gravlee GP: Dermatan sulfate anticoagulation: Future replacement for heparin (editorial)? J Cardiothorac Vasc Anesth 9:237, 1995
196. Bauer KA, Ericksson BI, Lassen MR, et al: Fondaparinux compared with enoxaparin for the prevention of venous thromboembolism after elective major knee surgery. N Engl J Med 345:1305, 2001
197. Koster A, Hansen R, Kuppe H, et al: Recombinant hirudin as an alternative for anticoagulation during cardiopulmonary bypass with HIT II. J Cardiothorac Vasc Anesth 14:243, 2000
198. Dinisio M, Middeldorp S, Buller H: Direct thrombin inhibitors. N Engl J Med 353:1028, 2005
199. Lewis BE, Wallis DE, Berkowitz SD, et al: Argatroban anticoagulant therapy in patients with heparin-induced thrombocytopenia. Circulation 103:1838, 2002
200. Lewis BE, Walenga JM, Wallis DE: Anticoagulation with Novastatin (argatroban) in patients with heparin induced thrombocytopenia and heparin-induced thrombocytopenia and thrombosis syndrome. Semin Thromb Haemost 23:197, 1997
201. McKeage K, Plosker GL: Argatroban. Drugs 61:515, 2001
202. Koster A, Chew D, Grundel M, et al: An assessment of different filter systems for extracorporeal elimination of bivalirudin: An in vitro study. Anesth Analg 96:1316, 2003
203. Merry AF, Raudkivi P, White HD, et al: Anticoagulation with bivalirudin (a direct thrombin inhibitor) vs heparin. A randomized trial in OPCAB graft surgery. Ann Thorac Surg 77:925, 2004
204. Koster A, Spiess BD, Chew DP, et al: Effectiveness of bivalirudin as a replacement for heparin during cardiopulmonary bypass in patients undergoing coronary artery bypass grafting. Am J Cardiology 93:356, 2004
205. Koster A, Chew D, Grundel M, et al: Bivalirudin monitored with the ecarin clotting time for anticoagulation during cardiopulmonary bypass. Anesth Analg 96:383, 2003
206. Vasquez JC, Vichiendilokkul A, Mahmood S, Baciewicz FA Jr: Anticoagulation with bivalirudin during cardiopulmonary bypass in cardiac surgery. Ann Thorac Surg 74:2177, 2002
207. Gurm H, Sarembock I, Kereiakes D, et al: Use of Bivalirudin during percutaneous coronary intervention in patients with diabetes mellitus. J Am Coll Cardiol 45:1932, 2005
208. Lincoff M, Bittle J, Harrington R, et al: Bivalirudin and provisional gycoprotein IIb/IIIa blockade compared to heparin and GIIb/IIIa inhibition during PCI: replace-2. JAMA 289:853, 2003
209. Spiess B, Deanda A, McCarthy H, et al: Off Pump CABG Surgery anticoagocation with bivalirudin. J Cardiothorac Vasc Anesth In press
210. Francis CW, Davidson BL, Berkowitz SD, et al: Ximalagatran versus warfarin for the prevention of venous thromboembolism after total knee arthroplasty. Ann Intern Med 137:548, 2002
211. Eriksson H, Wahlander K, Gustafsson D, et al: Randomized, controlled, dose-guiding study of the oral direct thrombin ximelagatran compared with standard therapy for treatment of acute deep venous thrombosis. J Thromb Haemost 1:41, 2002

212. Heit JA, Colwell CW, Francis CA, et al: Comparison of ximelagatran with enoxaparin as prophylaxis against venous thromboembolism. Arch Intern Med 161:2215, 2001
213. Schulman S, Wahlander K, Lundstrom T, et al: Secondary prevention of venous thromboembolism with the oral direct thrombin inhibitor ximelagatran. N Engl J Med 349:1713, 2003
214. Larm O, Larsson R, Olsson P: Surface-immobilized heparin. *In* Lane DA, Lindahl U (eds): Heparin. Boca Raton, FL, CRC Press, 1989, p 597
215. Von Segesser LK, Weiss BM, Garcia E, et al: Reduction and elimination of systemic heparinization during cardiopulmonary bypass. J Thorac Cardiovasc Surg 103:790, 1992
216. Videm V, Svennevig JL, Fosse E, et al: Reduced complement activation with heparin-coated oxygenator and tubings in coronary bypass operations. J Thorac Cardiovasc Surg 103:806, 1992
217. Gravlee GP: Heparin-coated cardiopulmonary bypass circuits (review). J Cardiothoracic Vasc Anesth 8:213, 1994
218. Engbers GH, Feijen J: Current techniques to improve the blood compatibility of biomaterial surfaces (editorial). Int J Artif Organs 14:199, 1991
219. Ando T, Yamasaki M, Suzuki K: Protamines. *In* Kleinzeller A, Springer GF, Wittmann HG (eds): Molecular Biology, Biochemistry and Biophysics, Vol 12. Berlin, Springer-Verlag, 1973, p 1
220. Wilkins MHF: Physical studies of the molecular structure of deoxyribonucleic acid and nucleoprotein. Cold Spring Harbor Symp Quant Biol 21:83, 1956
221. Jaques LB: Personal communication to the author. February 14, 1986
222. Chargaff E, Olson KB: Studies on the chemistry of blood coagulation, part VI. J Biol Chem 122:153, 1937
223. Jaques LB: Protamine-antagonist to heparin. J Can Med Assoc 108:1291, 1973
224. Jaques LB: A study of the toxicity of the protamine, salmine. Br J Pharmacol 4:135, 1949
225. Samuel T, Kolk A: Auto-antigenicity of human protamines. *In* Lepow IH, Crozier R (eds): Vasectomy. Immunologic and Pathophysiologic Effects in Animals and Man. New York, Academic Press, 1979, p 203
226. Moriou M, Masure R, Hurlet A, et al: Haemostasis disorders in open heart surgery with extracorporeal circulation. Vox Sang 32:41, 1977
227. Kuitunen AH, Salmenpera MT, Heinonen J, et al: Heparin rebound: A comparative study of protamine chloride and protamine sulfate in patients undergoing coronary artery bypass surgery. J Cardiothorac Vasc Anesth 5:221, 1991
228. Folkman J, Langer R, Linhardt RJ, et al: Angiogenesis inhibition and tumor regression caused by heparin or a heparin fragment in the presence of cortisone. Science 221:719, 1983
229. Taylor S, Folkman J: Protamine is an inhibitor of angiogenesis. Nature 297:307, 1982
230. Mulholland B, Mellersh AR: The antimicrobial activity of protamine and polybrene. J Hosp Infect 10:305, 1987
231. O'Reilly RA: Anticoagulant, antithrombotic and thrombolytic drugs. *In* Gilman AG, Goodman LS, Rall TW, Murad F (eds): The Pharmacological Basis of Therapeutics, 7th edition. New York, Macmillan, 1985, p 1340
232. Radegran K, McAshlan C: Circulatory and ventilatory effects of induced platelet aggregation and their inhibition by acetylsalicylic acid. Acta Anaesthesiol Scand 16:76, 1972
233. Bjoraker DG, Ketcham TR: In vivo platelet response to clinical protamine sulfate infusion. Anesthesiology 57:A7, 1982
234. Ellison N, Edmunds LH, Colman RW: Platelet aggregation following heparin and protamine administration. Anesthesiology 48:65, 1978
235. Lindblad B, Wakefield TW, Whitehouse WM, Stanley JC: The effect of protamine sulfate on platelet function. Scand J Thorac Cardiovasc Surg 22:55, 1988
236. Eika C: On the mechanism of platelet aggregation induced by heparin, protamine and polybrene. Scand J Haematol 9:248, 1972
237. Cobel-Geard RJ, Hassouna HI: Interaction of protamine sulfate with thrombin. Am J Hematol 14:227, 1983
238. Shanberge JN, Murato M, Quattrociocchi-Longe T, et al: Heparin-protamine complexes in the production of heparin rebound and other complications of extracorporeal bypass procedures. Am J Clin Pathol 87:210, 1987
239. DePaulis R, Mohammed SF, Chiariello L, et al: The role of plasma proteins in formation of obstructive protamine complexes. J Cardiothorac Vasc Anesth 5:227, 1991
240. Tan F, Jackman H, Skidgel RA, et al: Protamine inhibits plasma carboxypeptidase N, the inactivator of anaphylatoxins and kinins. Anesthesiology 70:267, 1989
241. Castaneda AR: Must heparin be neutralized following open-heart operations? J Thorac Cardiovasc Surg 52:716, 1966
242. Arn C, Feddersen K, Radegran K: Comparison of two protocols for heparin neutralization by protamine after cardiopulmonary bypass. J Thorac Cardiovasc Surg 94:539, 1987
243. Welsby I, Newman M, Phillips-Bute B, et al: Hemodynamic changes after protamine administration. Anesthesiology 102:308, 2005
244. Radegran K, Taylor GA, Olsson P: Mode of action of protamine in regard to its circulatory and respiratory side effects. Eur Surg Res 3:139, 1971
245. Fadali MA, Ledbetter M, Papacostas CA, et al: Mechanism responsible for the cardiovascular depressant effect of protamine sulfate. Ann Surg 180:232, 1974
246. Marin-Neto JA, Sykes MK, Marin JLB, et al: Effect of heparin and protamine on left ventricular performance in the dog. Cardiovasc Res 13:254, 1979
247. Gourin A, Streisand RL, Greineder JK, Stuckey JH: Protamine sulfate administration and the cardiovascular system. J Thorac Cardiovasc Surg 62:193, 1971
248. Gourin A, Streisand RL, Stuckey JH: Total cardiopulmonary bypass, myocardial contractility, and the administration of protamine sulfate. J Thorac Cardiovasc Surg 61:160, 1971
249. Greene CE, Higgins CB, Kelley MI, et al: Cardiovascular effects of protamine sulfate. Invest Radiol 16:324, 1981
250. Jones MM, Hill AB, Nahrwold ML, Tait AR: Effect of protamine on plasma ionized calcium in the dog. Can Anaesth Soc J 29:65, 1982
251. Komatsu H, Enzan K: Repeated administration of protamine attenuates protamine-induced systemic hypotension [in Japanese]. Masui Jpn J Anesth 45:1319, 1996
252. Stefaniszyn HJ, Novick RJ, Salerno TA: Toward a better understanding of the hemodynamic effects of protamine and heparin interaction. J Thorac Cardiovasc Surg 87:678, 1984
253. Pauca AL, Graham JE, Hudspeth AS: Hemodynamic effects of intraaortic administration of protamine. Ann Thorac Surg 35:637, 1983
254. Wakefield TW, Hantler CB, Wrobleski SK, et al: Effects of differing rates of protamine reversal of heparin anticoagulation. Surgery 119:123, 1996
255. Levy JH, Faraj BA, Zaidan JR, Camp VM: Effects of protamine on histamine release from human lung. Agents Actions 28:70, 1989
256. Sauder RA, Hirshman CA: Protamine-induced histamine release in human skin mast cells. Anesthesiology 73:165, 1990
257. Raikar GV, Hisamochi K, Raikar BL, Schaff HV: Nitric oxide inhibition attenuates systemic hypotension produced by protamine. J Thorac Cardiovasc Surg 111:1240, 1996
258. Frater RWM, Oka Y, Hong Y, et al: Protamine-induced circulatory changes. J Thorac Cardiovasc Surg 87:687, 1984
259. Masone R, Oka Y, Hong YW, et al: Cardiovascular effects of right atrial injection of protamine sulfate as compared to left atrial injection. Anesthesiology 57:A6, 1982
260. Milne B, Rogers K, Cervenko F, et al: The haemodynamic effects of intraaortic versus intravenous administration of protamine for reversal of heparin in man. Can Anaesth Soc J 30:347, 1983
261. Jastrzebski J, Sykes MK, Woods DG: Cardiorespiratory effects of protamine after cardiopulmonary bypass in man. Thorax 29:534, 1974
262. Conahan TJ, Andrews RW, MacVaugh H: Cardiovascular effects of protamine sulfate in man. Anesth Analg 60:33, 1981
263. Sethna DH, Moffitt E, Gray RJ, et al: Effects of protamine sulfate on myocardial oxygen supply and demand in patients following cardiopulmonary bypass. Anesth Analg 61:247, 1982
264. Michaels IA, Barash PG: Hemodynamic changes during protamine administration. Anesth Analg 62:831, 1983
265. Hanowell ST, Jones M, Pierce E, et al: Protamine titration: What degree of precision is necessary? Anesthesiology 59:A91, 1983
266. Iwatsuki N, Matsukawa S, Iwatsuki K: A weak negative inotropic effect of protamine sulfate upon the isolated canine heart muscle. Anesth Analg 59:100, 1980
267. Caplan RA, Su JY: Differences in threshold for protamine toxicity in isolated atrial and ventricular tissue. Anesth Analg 63:1111, 1984
268. Hendry PJ, Taichman GC, Keon WJ: The myocardial contractile responses to protamine sulfate and heparin. Ann Thorac Surg 44:263, 1987
269. Wakefield TW, Bies LE, Wrobleski SK, et al: Impaired myocardial function and oxygen utilization due to protamine sulfate in an isolated rabbit heart preparation. Ann Surg 212:387, 1990
270. Housmans PR, Ferguson DM: Inotropic effects of protamine sulfate on isolated mammalian cardiac muscles: Mechanisms of action. Anesthesiology 67:A24, 1987
271. Hird RB, Wakefield TW, Mukherjee R, et al: Direct effects of protamine sulfate on myocyte contractile processes. Cellular and molecular mechanisms. Circulation 92(suppl II):II-433, 1995

272. Hird RB, Crawford FA, Spinale FG: Differential effects of protamine sulfate on myocyte contractile function with left ventricular failure. J Am Coll Cardiol 25:773, 1995
273. Park WK, Pancrazio JJ, Lynch C 3rd: Mechanical and electrophysiological effects of protamine on isolated ventricular myocardium. Evidence for calcium overload. Cardiovasc Res 28:505, 1994
274. Taylor RL, Little WC, Freeman GL, et al: Comparison of the cardiovascular effects of intravenous and intraaortic protamine in the conscious and anesthetized dog. Ann Thorac Surg 42:22, 1986
275. Humphrey LS, Topol EJ, Casella ES, et al: Absence of direct myocardial depression by protamine. Anesthesiology 61:A50, 1984
276. Oe M, Asou T, Morita S, et al: Protamine-induced hypotension in heart operations. Application of the concept of ventricular-arterial coupling. J Thorac Cardiovasc Surg 112:462, 1996
277. Aris A, Solanes H, Bonnin JO, et al: Intraaortic administration of protamine: Method for heparin neutralization after cardiopulmonary bypass. Cardiovasc Dis Bull Texas Heart Inst 8:23, 1981
278. Iida Y, Tsuchiya K, Sakakibara N, et al: Intraaortic administration of protamine. Kyobu Geka 35:704, 1982
279. Wakefield TW, Whitehouse WM, Stanley JC: Depressed cardiovascular function and altered platelet kinetics following protamine sulfate reversal of heparin activity. J Vasc Surg 1:346, 1984
280. Casthely PA, Goodman K, Fyman PN, et al: Hemodynamic changes after the administration of protamine. Anesth Analg 65:78, 1986
281. Rogers K, Milne B, Salerno TA: The hemodynamic effects of intraaortic versus intravenous administration of protamine for reversal of heparin in pigs. J Thorac Cardiovasc Surg 85:851, 1983
282. Habezettl H, Conzen PF, Vollmar B: Pulmonary hypertension after heparin-protamine: Roles of left-sided infusion, histamine, and platelet-activating factor. Anesth Analg 71:637, 1990
283. Cherry DA, Chiu RCJ, Wynands JE, et al: Intraaortic vs intravenous administration of protamine: A prospective randomized clinical study. Surg Forum 36:238, 1985
284. Procaccini B, Clementi G, Bersanetti L, et al: Cardiopulmonary effects of protamine sulfate in man: Intraaortic vs intra-right atrial rapid administration after cardiopulmonary bypass. J Cardiovasc Surg 28:112, 1987
285. Levy JH: Anaphylactic Reactions in Anesthesia and Intensive Care. Boston, Butterworth's, 1986, p 39
286. Dockhorn RJ: Diagnostic tests for allergic disease. *In* Korenblat PE, Wedner HJ (eds): Allergy: Theory and Practice. Philadelphia, Grune & Stratton, 1984, p 57
287. Horrow JC: Protamine allergy. J Cardiothorac Vasc Anesth 2:225, 1988
288. Kirklin JK, Chenoweth DE, Naftel DC: Effects of protamine administration after cardiopulmonary bypass on complement, blood elements, and the hemodynamic state. Ann Thorac Surg 41:193, 1986
289. Horrow JC: Heparin reversal of protamine toxicity: Have we come full circle? J Cardiothorac Vasc Anesth 4:539, 1990
290. Kurtz AB, Gray RS, Markanday S, Nabarro JD: Circulating IgG antibodies to protamine in patients treated with protamine-insulins. Diabetologia 25:322, 1983
291. Nell LJ, Thomas JW: Frequency and specificity of protamine antibodies in diabetic and control subjects. Diabetes 37:172, 1988
292. Levy JH, Schwieger IA, Zaidan JR, et al: Evaluation of patients at risk for protamine reactions. J Thorac Cardiovasc Surg 98:200, 1989
293. Jackson DR: Sustained hypotension secondary to protamine sulfate. Angiology 21:295, 1970
294. Moorthy SS, Pond W, Rowland RG: Severe circulatory shock following protamine (an anaphylactic reaction). Anesth Analg 59:77, 1980
295. Doolan L, McKenzie I, Kratchek J, et al: Protamine sulfate hypersensitivity. Anaesth Intensive Care 9:147, 1981
296. Cobb CA, Fung DL: Shock due to protamine hypersensitivity. Surg Neurol 17:245, 1981
297. Vontz FK, Puestow EC, Cahill DJ: Anaphylactic shock following protamine administration. Ann Surg 48:549, 1982
298. Vierthaler LD, Becker KE Jr: Protamine anaphylaxis. Protocols for therapy in acute reactions. J Kans Med Soc 84:454, 1983
299. Holland CL, Singh AK, McMaster PRB, et al: Adverse reactions to protamine sulfate following cardiac surgery. Clin Cardiol 7:157, 1984
300. Chung F, Miles J: Cardiac arrest following protamine administration. Can Anaesth Soc J 31:314, 1984
301. Walker WS, Reid KG, Hider CF, et al: Successful cardiopulmonary bypass in diabetics with anaphylactoid reactions to protamine. Br Heart J 52:112, 1984
302. Grant JA, Cooper JR, Albyn KC, et al: Anaphylactic reactions to protamine in insulin-dependent diabetics during cardiovascular procedures (abstract). J Allergy Clin Immunol 73:180, 1984
303. Sharath MD, Metzger WJ, Richerson HB, et al: Protamine-induced fatal anaphylaxis: Prevalence of antiprotamine immunoglobulin E antibody. J Thorac Cardiovasc Surg 90:86, 1985
304. Menk EJ: Cardiac arrest following protamine sulfate infusion during regional anesthesia. Milit Med 151:318, 1986
305. Stewart WJ, McSweeney SM, Kellett MA, et al: Increased risk of severe protamine reactions in NPH insulin-dependent diabetics undergoing cardiac catheterization. Circulation 70:788, 1984
306. Gottschlich G, Gravlee GP, Georgitis JW: Adverse reactions to protamine sulfate during cardiac surgery in diabetic and non-diabetic patients. Ann Allergy 61:277, 1988
307. Weiss ME, Nyhan D, Peng Z, et al: Association of protamine IgE and IgG antibodies with life-threatening reactions to intravenous protamine. N Engl J Med 320:886, 1989
308. Reed DC, Gascho JA: The safety of protamine sulfate in diabetics undergoing cardiac catheterization. Cathet Cardiovasc Diagn 144:19, 1988
309. Best N, Teisner B, Grudzinskas JG, et al: Classical pathway activation during an adverse response to protamine sulfate. Br J Anaesth 55:1149, 1983
310. Andersen JM, Johnson TA: Hypertension associated with protamine sulfate administration. Am J Hosp Pharm 38:701, 1981
311. Lakin JD, Blocker TJ, Strong DM, et al: Anaphylaxis to protamine sulfate by a complement-dependent IgG antibody. J Allergy Clin Immunol 61:102, 1978
312. Stoelting RK: Allergic reactions during anesthesia. Anesth Analg 63:341, 1983
313. Nyhan DP, Shampaine EL, Hirshman CA, et al: Single doses of intravenous protamine result in the formation of protamine-specific IgE and IgG antibodies. J Allergy Clin Immunol 97:991, 1996
314. Knape JTA, Schuller JL, de Haan P, et al: An anaphylactic reaction to protamine in a patient allergic to fish. Anesthesiology 55:324, 1981
315. Caplan SN, Berkman EM: Protamine sulfate and fish allergy (letter). N Engl J Med 295:172, 1976
316. Samuel T, Kolk AHJ, Rumke P, et al: Autoimmunity to sperm antigens in vasectomized men. Clin Exp Immunol 21:65, 1975
317. Sheridan P, Blain R, Vezina D, Bleau G: Prospective evaluation of the safety of heparin reversal with protamine in vasectomized patients after cardiopulmonary bypass. Proceedings of the 10th Annual Meeting of the Society of Cardiovascular Anesthesiologists, 1988, p 140
318. Watson RA, Ansbacher R, Barry M, et al: Allergic reaction to protamine: A late complication of elective vasectomy? Urology 22:493, 1983
319. Metz S: Prior vasectomy and anaphylaxis following protamine. No cause and effect (letter). Anesthesiology 79:617, 1993
320. Olinger GN, Becker RM, Bonchek LI: Noncardiac pulmonary edema and peripheral vascular collapse following cardiopulmonary bypass: Rare protamine reaction? Ann Thorac Surg 29:20, 1980
321. Baimbridge MV: Fulminating noncardiogenic pulmonary edema (discussion). J Thorac Cardiovasc Surg 80:868, 1980
322. Just-Viera JO, Fischer CR, Gago O, et al: Acute reaction to protamine its importance to surgeons. Am Surg 50:52, 1984
323. Pajuelo A, Otero C, Jiminez D, et al: Edema pulmonary no cardiogenico tras circulacion extracorporea: Implicaciones del sulfato de protamina. Rev Espanola Anest Rean 33:187, 1986
324. Culliford AT, Thomas S, Spencer FC: Fulminating noncardiogenic pulmonary edema. J Thorac Cardiovasc Surg 80:868, 1980
325. Hashim SW, Kay HR, Hammond GL, et al: Noncardiogenic pulmonary edema after cardiopulmonary bypass: An anaphylactic reaction to fresh frozen plasma. Am J Surg 147:560, 1984
326. Frater RWM: Fulminating noncardiogenic pulmonary edema (discussion). J Thorac Cardiovasc Surg 80:868, 1980
327. Chang S-W, Voelkel NF: Charge-related lung microvascular injury. Am Rev Resp Dis 139:534, 1989
328. Toyofuku T, Koyama S, Kobayashi T, et al: Effects of polycations on pulmonary vascular permeability in conscious sheep. J Clin Invest 83:2063, 1989
329. Iglesias A, Nuez L: Pulmonary edema (letter). Ann Thorac Surg 33:304, 1982
330. Kirklin JK: Prospects for understanding and eliminating deleterious effects of cardiopulmonary bypass. Ann Thorac Surg 51:529, 1991
331. Lowenstein E, Johnston WE, Lappas DG, et al: Catastrophic pulmonary vasoconstriction associated with protamine reversal of heparin. Anesthesiology 59:470, 1983
332. Jastrzebski J, Hilgard P, Sykes MK: Pulmonary vasoconstriction produced by protamine and protamine-heparin complex in the isolated cat lung perfused with blood or dextran. Cardiovasc Res 9:691, 1975
333. Morel DR, Zapol WM, Thomas SJ, et al: C5a and thromboxane generation associated with pulmonary vaso- and bronchoconstriction during protamine reversal of heparin. Anesthesiology 66:597, 1987

334. Horrow JC: Protamine—A review of its toxicity. Anesth Analg 64:348, 1985
335. Horrow JC: Thrombocytopenia accompanying a reaction to protamine sulfate. Can Anaesth Soc J 32:49, 1985
336. Lock R, Hessel EA: Probable reversal of protamine reactions by heparin administration. J Cardiothorac Vasc Anesth 4:604, 1990
337. Fiser WP, Fewell JE, Hill DE, et al: Cardiovascular effects of protamine sulfate are dependent on the presence and type of circulation heparin. J Thorac Cardiovasc Surg 89:63, 1985
338. Rent R, Ertel N, Eisenstein R, et al: Complement activation by interaction of polyanions and polycations: I. Heparin-protamine-induced consumption of complement. J Immunol 114:120, 1975
339. Kreil E, Montalescot G, Greene E, et al: Nafamstat mesilate attenuates pulmonary hypertension in heparin-protamine reactions. J Appl Physiol 67:1463, 1989
340. Colman RW: Humoral mediators of catastrophic reactions associated with protamine neutralization. Anesthesiology 66:595, 1987
341. Hobbhahn J, Conzen PF, Zenker B, et al: Beneficial effect of cyclooxygenase inhibition on adverse hemodynamic responses after protamine. Anesth Analg 67:253, 1988
342. Conzen PF, Habazettl H, Gutman R, et al: Thromboxane mediation of pulmonary hemodynamic responses after neutralization of heparin by protamine in pigs. Anesth Analg 68:25, 1989
343. Nuttall GA, Murray MJ, Bowie EJW: Protamine-heparin-induced pulmonary hypertension in pigs: Effects of treatment with a thromboxane receptor antagonist on hemodynamics and coagulation. Anesthesiology 74:138, 1991
344. Schumacher WA, Heran CL, Ogletree ML: Protamine-induced pulmonary hypertension in heparinized monkeys and pigs is inhibited by the thromboxane receptor antagonist SQ 30,741. Eicosanoids 3:87, 1990
345. Wakefield TW, Wrobleski SK, Stanley JC: Reversal of depressed oxygen consumption accompanying in vivo protamine sulphate-heparin interactions by the prostacyclin analogue, iloprost. Eur J Vasc Surg 4:25, 1990
346. Degges RD, Foster ME, Dang AQ, Read RC: Pulmonary hypertensive effect of heparin and protamine interaction: Evidence for thromboxane B2 release from the lung. Am J Surg 154:696, 1987
347. Kanbak M, Kahraman S, Celebioglu B, et al: Prophylactic administration of histamine, and/or histamine-receptor blockers in the prevention of heparin- and protamine-related haemodynamic effects. Anaesth Intensive Care 24:559, 1996
348. Baraka A, Choueiry P, Taha S, et al: Hydrocortisone pretreatment for attenuation of protamine-induced adverse hemodynamic reactions (letter). J Cardiothorac Vasc Anesth 9:481, 1995
349. Katircioglu SF, Kucukaksu DS, Buzdayi M, et al: The beneficial effects of aminophylline administration on heparin reversal with protamine. Surg Today 24:99, 1994
350. Van der Starre PJA, Solinas C: Ketanserin in the treatment of protamine-induced pulmonary hypertension. Texas Heart Inst J 23:301, 1996
351. Horrow JC, Pharo G, Levit LS, Freeland C: Neither skin tests nor serum enzyme-linked immunosorbent assay tests provide specificity for protamine allergy. Anesth Analg 82:386, 1996
352. Weiler JM, Gellhaus MA, Carter JG, et al: A prospective study of the risk of an immediate adverse reaction to protamine sulfate during cardiopulmonary bypass surgery. J Allerg Clin Immunol 85:713, 1990
353. Kindler CH, Bircher AJ: Anaphylactoid reactions to protamine (letter). Anesthesiology 85:1209, 1996
354. Fisher M: Intradermal testing after anaphylactoid reaction to anaesthetic drugs: Practical aspects of performance and interpretation. Anaesth Intensive Care 12:115, 1984
355. Wright JS, Osborn JJ, Perkins HA, Gerbode F: Heparin levels during and after hypothermic perfusion. J Cardiovasc Surg 5:244, 1964
356. Godal HC: A comparison of two heparin-neutralizing agents: Protamine and polybrene. Scand J Clin Lab Invest 12:446, 1960
357. Egerton WS, Robinson CLN: The anti-heparin, anticoagulant and hypotensive properties of hexadimethrine and protamine. Lancet 2:635, 1961
358. Montalescot G, Zapol WM, Carvalho A, et al: Neutralization of low-molecular-weight heparin by polybrene prevents thromboxane release and severe pulmonary hypertension in awake sheep. Circulation 82:1754, 1990
359. Haller JA, Ransdell HT, Stowens D, Rubel WF: Renal toxicity of polybrene in open heart surgery. J Thorac Cardiovasc Surg 44:486, 1962
360. Ransdell HT, Haller JA, Stowens D, Barton PB: Renal toxicity of polybrene (hexadimethrine bromide). J Surg Res 5:195, 1965
361. Ohata H, Momose K, Takahashi A, Omori Y: Urinalysis for detection of chemically induced renal damage-changes in urinary excretions of enzymes and various components caused by p-aminophenol, puromycin aminonucleoside and hexadimethrine. J Toxicol Sci 12:357, 1987
362. Bertolatus JA, Hunsicker LG: Polycation binding to glomerular basement membrane. Lab Invest 56:170, 1987
363. Messina A, Davies DJ, Ryan GB: Protamine sulfate-induced proteinuria: The roles of glomerular injury and depletion of polyanion. J Pathol 158:147, 1989
364. Saito T, Sumithran E, Glasgow EF, Atkins C: The enhancement of aminonucleoside nephrosis by the co-administration of protamine. Kidney Int 32:691, 1987
365. Schapira M, Christman BW: Neutralization of heparin by protamine. Circulation 82:1877, 1990
366. Levy JH, Cormack JG, Morales A: Heparin neutralization by recombinant platelet factor 4 and protamine. Anesth Analg 81:35, 1995
367. Dehmer GJ, Fisher M, Tate DA, et al: Reversal of heparin anticoagulation by recombinant platelet factor 4 in humans. Circulation 91:2188, 1995
368. Giesecke M, Cooper J, Keats A, Austin J: Recombinant platelet factor r (rPF4) neutralizes heparin in patients undergoing coronary artery bypass. Anesth Analg 80:SCA131, 1995
369. Kurrek MM, Winkler M, Robinson DR, Zapol WM: Platelet factor 4 injection produces acute pulmonary hypertension in the awake lamb. Anesthesiology 82:183, 1995
370. Giesecke M, Alexander A: rPF4 does not cause pulmonary hypertension in humans (letter). Anesthesiology 83:644, 1995
371. Bernstein H, Yang BC, Cooney CL, et al: Immobilized heparin lysis system for blood deheparinization. Methods Enzymol 137:515, 1988
372. Kim J-S, Vincent C, Teng C-LC, et al: A novel approach to anticoagulation control. ASAIO Trans 35:644, 1989
373. Yang VC, Port FK, Kim J-S, et al: The use of immobilized protamine in removing heparin and preventing protamine-induced complications during extracorporeal blood circulation. Anesthesiology 75:288, 1991
374. Sloand EM, Kessler CM, McIntosh CL, et al: Methylene blue for neutralization of heparin. Thromb Res 54:677, 1989
375. Kikura M, Lee MK, Levy JH: What is the concentration of hexadimethrine and methylene blue required for neutralization of heparin following cardiopulmonary bypass (abstract)? Anesthesiology 81:A177, 1994
376. Kikura M, Lee MK, Levy JH: Heparin neutralization with methylene blue, hexadimethrine, or vancomycin after cardiopulmonary bypass. Anesth Analg 83:223, 1996
377. Metz S, Horrow JC, Goel IP, et al: Methylene blue does not neutralize heparin after cardiopulmonary bypass. J Cardiothorac Vasc Anesth 10:474, 1996
378. Campbell FW, Goldstein MF, Atkins PC: Management of the patient with protamine hypersensitivity for cardiac surgery. Anesthesiology 61:761, 1984
379. Michelsen LG, Kikura M, Levy JH, et al: Heparinase I (Neutralase) reversal of systemic anticoagulation. Anesthesiology 85:339, 1996
380. Zimmerman J, McIntosh C, Clementi W, et al: Heparin reversal with Neutralase (heparinase I) in adult male volunteers. Anesth Analg 82:SCA93, 1996
381. Van Riper DF, Heres E, Bennett JA, et al: Neutralase 7 mcg/kg reverses heparin-induced prolongation of ACT better than 5 mcg/kg in patients undergoing CABG (abstract). Anesthesiology 87:A95, 1997
382. DeLucia A 3rd, Wakefield TW, Andrews PC, et al: Efficacy and toxicity of differently charged polycationic protamine-like peptides for heparin anticoagulation reversal. J Vasc Surg 18:49, 1993
383. Wakefield TW, Andrews PC, Wrobleski SK, et al: Effective and less toxic reversal of low-molecular-weight heparin anticoagulation by a designer variant of protamine. J Vasc Surg 21:839, 1995
384. Kirklin JW, Barratt-Boyes BG: Postoperative care. *In* Cardiac Surgery. New York, Churchill Livingstone, 1986, p 139
385. Erban SB, Kinman JL, Schwartz S: Routine use of the prothrombin and partial thromboplastin times. JAMA 262:2428, 1989
386. Ratnatunga CP, Rees GM, Kovacs IB: Preoperative hemostatic activity and excessive bleeding after cardiopulmonary bypass. Ann Thorac Surg 52:250, 1991
387. Rodgers RP, Levin J: Bleeding time revisited. Blood 79:2495, 1992
388. Horrow JC: Desmopressin and antifibrinolytics. *In* Gravlee GP(ed): Blood Conservation. Int Anesthesiol Clin 28:230, 1990
389. Spiess BD, Wall MH, Gillies BS, et al: A comparison of thromboelastography with heparinase or protamine sulfate added in-vitro during heparinized cardiopulmonary bypass. Thromb Haemost 78:820, 1997
390. Spiess BD: Thromboelastogram and postoperative hemorrhage. Ann Thorac Surg 54:810, 1992

391. Ostrowsky J, Foes J, Warchol M, et al: Plateletworks platelet function test compared to the Thrombelastograph for prediction of postoperative outcomes. J Extracor Technol 36:149, 2004
392. Cammerer U, Dietrich W, Rampf T, et al: The predictive value of modified computerized thromboelastography and platelet function analysis for postoperative blood loss in routine cardiac surgery. Anesth Analg 96:51, 2003
393. Royston D, von Kier S: Reduced haemostatic factor transfusion using heparinase-modified thromboelastography during cardiopulmonary bypass. Br J Anaesth 86:575, 2001
394. Shore-Lesserson L, Manspeizer HE, DePerio M, et al: Thromboelastography-guided transfusion algorithm reduces transfusions in complex cardiac surgery. Anesth Analg 88:312, 1999
395. Tuman KJ, McCarthy RJ, Djuric M, et al: Evaluation of coagulation during cardiopulmonary bypass with a heparinase modified thromboelstographic assay. J Cardiothorac Vasc Anesth 8:144, 1994
396. Essell JH, Martin TJ, Salinas J, et al: Comparison of thromboelastography to bleeding time and standard coagulation tests in patients after cardiopulmonary bypass. J Cardiothoracic Vasc Anesth 7:410, 1993
397. Marengo-Rowe AJ, Leveson JE: Fibrinolysis: A frequent cause of bleeding. *In* Ellison N, Jobes DR (eds): Effective Hemostasis in Cardiac Surgery. Philadelphia, WB Saunders, 1988, p 41
398. Umlas J: Fibrinolysis and disseminated intravascular coagulation in open heart surgery. Transfusion 16:460, 1976
399. Stibbe J, Kluft C, Brommer EJ, et al: Enhanced fibrinolytic activity during cardiopulmonary bypass in open-heart surgery in man is caused by extrinsic (tissue-type) plasminogen activator. Eur J Invest 14:375, 1984
400. Havel M, Teufelsbauer H, Knöbl P, et al: Effect of intraoperative aprotinin administration on postoperative bleeding in patients undergoing cardiopulmonary bypass operation. J Thorac Cardiovasc Surg 101:968, 1991
401. Villalobos TJ, Aderson E, Barila TG: Hematologic changes in hypothermic dogs. Proc Soc Exp Biol Med 89:192, 1985
402. Hessell EA, Schmer G, Dillard DH: Platelet kinetics during deep hypothermia. J Surg Res 28:23, 1980
403. Harker LA, Malpass TW, Branson HE: Mechanism of abnormal bleeding in patients undergoing cardiopulmonary bypass: Acquired transient platelet dysfunction associated with selective α-granule release. Blood 56:824, 1980
404. Rinder CS, Bohnert J, Rinder H, et al: Platelet activation and aggregation during cardiopulmonary bypass. Anesthesiology 75:388, 1991
405. Rinder CS, Mathew JP, Rinder HM, et al: Modulation of platelet surface adhesion receptors during cardiopulmonary bypass. Anesthesiology 75:563, 1991
406. Adelman B, Rizk A, Hanners E: Plasminogen interactions with platelets in plasma. Blood 72:1530, 1988
407. van Oeveren W, Eijsman L, Roozendaal KJ, Wildevuur CRH: Platelet preservation by aprotinin during cardiopulmonary bypass. Lancet 1:644, 1988
408. van Oeveren W, Harder MP, Roozendaal KJ, et al: Aprotinin protects platelets against the initial effect of cardiopulmonary bypass. J Thorac Cardiovasc Surg 99:788, 1990
409. Soslau G, Horrow J, Brodsky I: The effect of tranexamic acid on platelet ADP during extracorporeal circulation. Am J Hematol 38:113, 1991
410. Khuri SF, Wolfe JA, Josa M, et al: Hematologic changes during and after bypass. J Thorac Cardiovasc Surg 104:94, 1992
411. Valeri CR, Khabbaz K, Khuri SF, et al: Effect of skin temperature on platelet function in patients undergoing bypass. J Thorac Cardiovasc Surg 104:108, 1992
412. Paul J, Cornillon B, Baguet J, et al: In vivo release of a heparin-like factor in dogs during profound hypothermia. J Thorac Cardiovasc Surg 82:45, 1981
413. Cornillon B, Mazzorana M, Dureau G, et al: Characterization of a heparin-like activity released in dogs during deep hypothermia. Eur J Clin Invest 18:460, 1988
414. Michenfelder JD, Theye RA: Hypothermia: Effects on canine brain and whole-body metabolism. Anesthesiology 29:1107, 1968
415. Yoshihara H, Yamamoto T, Mihara H: Changes in coagulation and fibrinolysis occurring in dogs during hypothermia. Thromb Res 37:503, 1985
416. Lackritz EM, Satten GA, Aberle-Grasse J, et al: Estimated risk of the transmission of the human immunodeficiency virus by screened blood in the United States. N Engl J Med 333:1721, 1995
417. Corash L: Photochemical decontamination of cellular blood components. *In* Horrow JC: Pharmacology of blood and haemostasis. Anaesth Pharmacol Rev 3(2):138, 1995
418. Castaldi PA, Gorman DJ: Disordered platelet function in renal disease. *In* Colman RW, Hirsh J, Marder VJ, Salzman EW (eds): Hemostasis and Thrombosis, 2nd edition. Philadelphia, JB Lippincott, 1987, p 960
419. Mannucci PM, Remuzzi G, Pusineri F, et al: Deamino, 8-D-arginine vasopressin shortens the bleeding time in uremia. N Engl J Med 308:8, 1983
420. Mannucci PM, Vicente V, Vianello L, et al: Controlled trial of desmopressin in liver cirrhosis and other conditions associated with a prolonged bleeding time. Blood 67:1148, 1986
421. Mannucci PM: Desmopressin: A nontransfusional form of treatment for congenital and acquired bleeding disorders. Blood 72:1449, 1988
422. Boonstra PW, van Imhoff GW, Eysman L, et al: Reduced platelet activation and improved hemostasis after controlled cardiotomy suction during clinical membrane oxygenator perfusions. J Thorac Cardiovasc Surg 89:900, 1985
423. van den Dungen JJ, Karliczek GF, Brenken U, et al: Clinical study of blood trauma during perfusion with membrane and bubble oxygenators. J Thorac Cardiovasc Surg 83:108, 1982
424. Giordano GF, Rivers SL, Chung GK, et al: Autologous platelet-rich plasma in cardiac surgery: Effect on intraoperative and postoperative transfusion requirements. Ann Thorac Surg 46:416, 1988
425. Giordano GF Sr, Giordano GF Jr, Rivers SL, et al: Determinants of homologous blood usage utilizing autologous platelet-rich plasma in cardiac operations. Ann Thorac Surg 47:897, 1989
426. Boldt J, Von Bormann B, Kling D, et al: Preoperative plasmapheresis in patients undergoing cardiac surgery procedures. Anesthesiology 72:282, 1990
427. Pliam MB, McGoon DC, Tarhan S: Failure of transfusion of autologous whole blood to reduce banked-blood requirements in open heart surgical patients. J Thorac Cardiovasc Surg 70:338, 1975
428. Silver H: Banked and fresh autologous blood in cardiopulmonary bypass surgery. Transfusion 15:600, 1975
429. Ereth MH, Oliver WC Jr, Beynen FM, et al: Autologous platelet-rich plasma does not reduce transfusion of homologous blood products in patients undergoing repeat valvular surgery. Anesthesiology 79:540, 1993
430. DiMichele DM, Hathaway WE: Use of DDAVP in inherited and acquired platelet dysfunction. Am J Hematol 33:39, 1990
431. MacGregor IR, Roberts EN, Provose CV, et al: Fibrinolytic and haemostatic responses to desamino-D-arginine vasopressin (DDAVP) administered by intravenous and subcutaneous routes in healthy subjects. Thromb Haemost 59:34, 1988
432. Williams TD, Dunger DB, Lyon CC, et al: Antidiuretic effect and pharmacokinetics of oral 1-desamino, 8-D-arginine vasopressin. 1. Studies in adults and children. J Clin Endocrinol Metab 63:129, 1986
433. D'Alauro FS, Johns RA: Hypotension related to desmopressin administration following cardiopulmonary bypass. Anesthesiology 69:962, 1988
434. Salmenpera M, Kuitunen A, Hynynen M, Heinonen H: Hemodynamic responses to desmopressin acetate after CABG: A double-blind trial. J Cardiothorac Vasc Anesth 5:146, 1991
435. Jahr JS, Marquez J, Cottington E, Cook RD: Hemodynamic performance and histamine levels after desmopressin acetate administration following cardiopulmonary bypass in adult patients. J Cardiothorac Vasc Anesth 5:139, 1991
436. Reich DL, Hammerschlag BC, Rand JH, et al: Desmopressin acetate is a mild vasodilator that does not reduce blood loss in uncomplicated cardiac surgical procedures. J Cardiothorac Vasc Anesth 5:142, 1991
437. Bichet DG, Razi M, Lonergan M, et al: Hemodynamic and coagulation responses to 1-desamino (8-D-arginine) vasopressin in patients with congenital nephrogenic diabetes insipidus. N Engl J Med 318:881, 1988
438. Weinstein RE, Bona RD, Althman AJ, et al: Severe hyponatremia after repeated intravenous administration of desmopressin. Am J Hematol 32:258, 1989
439. Kobrinsky NL, Gerrard JM, Watson CM, et al: Shortening of bleeding time by 1-desamino, 8-D-arginine vasopressin in various bleeding disorders. Lancet 1:1145, 1984
440. Guay J, Reinberg C, Poitras B, et al: A trial of desmopressin to reduce blood loss in patients undergoing spinal fusion for idiopathic scoliosis. Anesth Analg 75:405, 1992
441. Salzman EW, Weinstein MJ, Weintraub RM, et al: Treatment with desmopressin acetate to reduce blood loss after cardiac surgery. N Engl J Med 314:1402, 1986
442. Czer LSC, Bateman TM, Gray RJ, et al: Treatment of severe platelet dysfunction and hemorrhage after cardiopulmonary bypass: Reduction in blood product usage with desmopressin. J Am Coll Cardiol 9:1139, 1987
443. Seear MD, Wadsworth LD, Rogers PC, et al: The effect of desmopressin acetate (DDAVP) on postoperative blood loss after cardiac operations in children. J Thorac Cardiovasc Surg 98:217, 1989

444. Rocha E, Llorens R, Paramo JA, et al: Does desmopressin acetate reduce blood loss after surgery in patients on cardiopulmonary bypass? Circulation 77:1319, 1988
445. Andersson TLG, Solem JO, Tengborn L, Vinge E: Effects of desmopressin acetate on platelet aggregation, von Willebrand factor, and blood loss after cardiac surgery with extracorporeal circulation. Circulation 81:872, 1990
446. Hackmann T, Gascoyne RD, Naiman SC, et al: A trial of desmopressin (1-desamino, 8-D-arginine vasopressin) to reduce blood loss in uncomplicated cardiac surgery. N Engl J Med 321:1437, 1989
447. Lazenby WD, Russo I, et al: Treatment with desmopressin acetate in routine coronary artery bypass surgery to improve postoperative hemostasis. Circulation 82(suppl IV):IV-413, 1990
448. Horrow JC, Van Riper DF, Strong MD, et al: The hemostatic effects of tranexamic acid and desmopressin during cardiac surgery. Circulation 84:2063, 1991
449. Reynolds LM, Nicolson SC, Jobes DR, et al: Desmopressin does not decrease bleeding after cardiac operation in young children. J Thorac Cardiovasc Surg 106:954, 1993
450. Mongan PD, Hosking MP: The role of desmopressin acetate in patients undergoing coronary artery bypass surgery. Anesthesiology 77:38, 1992
451. Verstraete M: Clinical application of inhibitors of fibrinolysis. Drugs 29:236, 1985
452. Butterworth J, James R, Lin Y, et al: Pharmacokinetics of episilon aminocaproic acid in patients undergoing coronary artery bypass surgery. Anesthesiology 90:1624, 1999
453. Takada A, Takada Y, Mori T, Sakaguchi S: Prevention of severe bleeding by tranexamic acid in a patient with disseminated intravascular coagulation. Thromb Res 58:101, 1990
454. Butterworth JF, James RL, Kennedy DJ, et al: Pharmacokinetics of ε-aminocaproic acid in adult patients undergoing coronary artery surgery. Anesthesiology 85:A151, 1996
455. Horrow JC, DiGregorio GJ, Ruch E: The dose-plasma concentration relationship of tranexamic acid during surgery. Am J Ther 1:206, 1994
456. Williamson R, Eggleston DJ: DDAVP and EACA used for minor oral surgery in von Willebrand disease. Aust Dent J 33:32, 1988
457. Blomback M, Johansson G, Johnsson H, et al: Surgery in patients with von Willebrand disease. Br J Surg 76:398, 1989
458. Avvisati G, Büller HR, ten Cate JW, Mandelli F: Tranexamic acid for control of haemorrhage in acute promyelocytic leukaemia. Lancet 2:122, 1989
459. Sharifi R, Lee M, Ray P, et al: Safety and efficacy of intravesical aminocaproic acid for bleeding after transurethral resection of prostate. Urology 27:214, 1986
460. Sterns LP, Lillehei CW: Effect of epsilon aminocaproic acid upon blood loss following open heart surgery: An analysis of 340 patients. Can J Surg 10:304, 1967
461. Gomes MMR, McGoon DC: Bleeding patterns after open heart surgery. J Thorac Cardiovasc Surg 60:87, 1970
462. Midell AI, Hallman GL, Bloodwell RD, et al: Epsilon-aminocaproic acid for bleeding after cardiopulmonary bypass. Ann Thorac Surg 11:577, 1971
463. McClure PD, Izsak J: The use of epsilon-aminocaproic acid to reduce bleeding during cardiac bypass in children with congenital heart disease. Anesthesiology 40:604, 1974
464. Saussine M, Delpech S, Allien M, et al: Saignement apres circulation extracorporelle et acide epsilon amino-caproque. Ann Fr Anesth Reanim 4:403, 1985
465. Vander Salm T, Ansell JE, Okike ON, et al: The role of epsilon-aminocaproic acid in reducing bleeding after cardiac operation: A double-blind randomized study. J Thorac Cardiovasc Surg 95:538, 1988
466. Del Rossi AJ, Cernaianu AC, Botros S, et al: Prophylactic treatment of postperfusion bleeding using EACA. Chest 96:27, 1989
467. Horrow JC, Hlavacek J, Strong MD, et al: Prophylactic tranexamic acid decreases bleeding after cardiac operations. J Thorac Cardiovasc Surg 99:70, 1990
468. Isetta C, Samat C, Kotaiche M, et al: Low-dose aprotinin or tranexamic acid treatment in cardiac surgery (abstract). Anesthesiology 75:A80, 1991
469. Karski JM, Teasdale SJ, Norman P, et al: Prevention of bleeding after cardiopulmonary bypass with high-dose tranexamic acid. J Thorac Cardiovasc Surg 110:835, 1995
470. Horrow JC, Van Riper DF, Strong MD, et al: The dose-response relationship of tranexamic acid. Anesthesiology 82:383, 1995
471. Shore-Lesserson L, Reich DL, Vela-Cantos F, et al: Tranexamic acid reduces transfusions and mediastinal drainage in repeat cardiac surgery. Anesth Analg 83:18, 1996
472. Fritz H, Wunderer G: Biochemistry and applications of aprotinin, the kallikrein inhibitor from bovine organs. Drug Res 33:479, 1983
473. Royston D: The serine antiprotease aprotinin (Trasylol): A novel approach to reducing postoperative bleeding. Blood Coag Fibrin 1:55, 1990
474. Royston D: High-dose aprotinin therapy: A review of the first five years experience. J Cardiothorac Vasc Anesth 6:76, 1992
475. D'Ambra MN, Risk SC: Aprotinin, erythropoietin, and blood substitutes. *In* Gravlee GP (ed): Blood Conservation. Int Anesthesiol Clin 28:237, 1990
476. Lemmer JH, Stanford W, Bonney SL, et al: Aprotinin for coronary artery bypass grafting: Effect on postoperative renal function. Ann Thorac Surg 59:132, 1995
477. Tice DA, Woeth MH, Clauss RH, Reed GE: The inhibition of Trasylol of fibrinolytic activity associated with cardiovascular operations. Surg Gynecol Obstet 119:71, 1964
478. Mammen EF: Natural proteinase inhibitors in extracorporeal circulation. Ann NY Acad Sci 146:754, 1968
479. Royston D, Taylor KM, Bidstrup BP, Sapsford RN: Effect of aprotinin on need for blood transfusion after repeat open heart surgery. Lancet 2:1289, 1987
480. van Oeveren W, Jansen NJG, Bidstrup BP, et al: Effects of aprotinin on hemostatic mechanisms during cardiopulmonary bypass. Ann Thorac Surg 44:640, 1987
481. Bidstrup BP, Royston D, Sapsford RN, Taylor KM: Reduction in blood loss and use after cardiopulmonary bypass with high-dose aprotinin (Trasylol). J Thorac Cardiovasc Surg 97:364, 1989
482. Dietrich W, Barankay A, Dilthey G, et al: Reduction of homologous blood requirements in cardiac surgery by intraoperative aprotinin application-clinical experience in 152 cardiac surgical patients. Thorac Cardiovasc Surg 37:92, 1989
483. Royston D: Aprotinin versus lysine analogues: The debate continues. Ann Thorac Surg 65:59, 1998
484. Blauhut B, Gross C, Necek S, et al: Effects of high-dose aprotinin on blood loss, platelet function, fibrinolysis, complement, and renal function after cardiopulmonary bypass. J Thorac Cardiovasc Surg 101:958, 1991
485. Edmunds LH, Niewiarowski S, Colman RW: Aprotinin (letter). J Thorac Cardiovasc Surg 101:1103, 1991
486. deSmet AAEA, Joen MCN, van Oeveren W, et al: Increased anticoagulation during cardiopulmonary bypass by aprotinin. J Thorac Cardiovasc Surg 100:520, 1990
487. Dietrich W, Dilthey G, Spannagl M, et al: Influence of high-dose aprotinin on anticoagulation, heparin requirement, and celite- and kaolin-activated clotting time in heparin-pretreated patients undergoing open heart surgery. A double-blind, placebo-controlled study. Anesthesiology 83:679, 1995
488. Wang J, Lin C, Hung W, Karp RB: Monitoring of heparin-induced anticoagulation with kaolin-activated clotting time in cardiac surgical patients treated with aprotinin. Anesthesiology 77:1080, 1992
489. Dietrich W, Jochum M: Effect of celite and kaolin on activated clotting time in the presence of aprotinin: Activated clotting time is reduced by binding of aprotinin to kaolin. J Thorac Cardiovasc Surg 109:177, 1995
490. Huyzen RJ, Harder MP, Huet RC, et al: Alternative perioperative anticoagulation monitoring during cardiopulmonary bypass in aprotinin-treated patients. J Cardiothorac Vasc Anesth 8:153, 1994
491. Bohrer H, Bach A, Fleischer F, Lang J: Adverse haemodynamic effects of high-dose aprotinin in a paediatric cardiac surgical patient. Anaesthesia 45:853, 1990
492. Harmon DE: Cost/benefit analysis of pharmacologic hemostasis. Ann Thorac Surg 61(2 suppl):S21, 1996
493. Greilich PE, Carr ME Jr, Carr SL, Chang AS: Reductions in platelet force development by cardiopulmonary bypass are associated with hemorrhage. Anesth Analg 80:459, 1995
494. Smith PK, Datta SK, Muhlbaier LH, et al: Cost analysis of aprotinin for coronary artery bypass patients: Analysis of the randomized trials. Ann Thorac Surg 2004 77:635,
495. Smith PK, Shah AS: The role of aprotinin in a blood-conservation program J Cardiothoracic Vasc Anesth 18(suppl):S24, 2004
496. Despotis GJ, Levine V, Filos KS, et al: Evaluation of a new point-of-care test that measures PAF-mediated acceleration of coagulation in cardiac surgical patients. Anesthesiology 85:1311, 1996
497. Thomson DS: Effect of positive end-expiratory pressure on postoperative bleeding (letter). J Thorac Cardiovasc Surg 88:457, 1984
498. Ilabaca PA, Ochsner JL, Mills NL: Positive end-expiratory pressure in the management of the patient with a postoperative bleeding heart. Ann Thorac Surg 30:281, 1980

499. Murphy DA, Finlayson DC, Craver JM, et al: Effect of positive end-expiratory pressure on excessive mediastinal bleeding after cardiac operations. J Thorac Cardiovasc Surg 85:864, 1983
500. Zurick AM, Urzua J, Ghattas M, et al: Failure of positive end-expiratory pressure to decrease postoperative bleeding after cardiac surgery. Ann Thorac Surg 34:608, 1982
501. Marder VJ, Feinstein DI, Francis CW, Colman RW: Consumptive thrombohemorrhagic disorders. *In* Colman RW, Hirsh J, Marder VJ, Salzman EW (eds): Hemostasis and Thrombosis, 3rd edition. Philadelphia, JB Lippincott, 1994, p 1023
502. Gravlee GP: Optimal use of blood components. *In* Gravlee GP (ed): Blood Conservation. Int Anesthiol Clin 28:216, 1990
503. Murray DJ, Olson J, Strauss R, Tinker JH: Coagulation changes during packed red cell replacement of major blood loss. Anesthesiology 69:839, 1988
504. de Prost D, Barbier-Boehm G, Hazebroucq J, et al: Desmopressin has no beneficial effect on excessive postoperative bleeding or blood product requirements associated with cardiopulmonary bypass. Thromb Haemost 68:106, 1992
505. Shiffrin JS, Glass DD: Desmopressin is of value in the treatment of post-cardiopulmonary bypass bleeding. J Cardiothorac Vasc Anesth 5:285, 1991
506. Chard RB, Kam CA, Nunn GR, et al: Use of desmopressin in the management of aspirin-related and intractable hemorrhage after cardiopulmonary bypass. Aust NZ J Surg 60:125, 1990
507. Erhardtsen E: Pharmacokinetics of recombinant activated factor VII. Semin Thromb Hemost 26:385, 2000
508. Roberts H, Monroe D, Hoffman M: Safety profile of recombinant factor VIIa. Semin Hematol 41(suppl 1):101, 2004
509. O'Connell N, Perry D, Hudgson A, et al: Recombinant FVIIa in the management of uncontrolled hemorrhage. Transfusion 43:1711, 2003
510. Key N: Recombinant FVIIa for intractable hemorrhage: More questions than answers. Transfusion 43:1649, 2003
511. Tanaka K, Waly A, Cooper W, Levy J: Treatment of excessive bleeding in Jehovah's Witness patients after cardiac surgery with recombinant factor VIIa. Anesthesiology 98:1513, 2003
512. Zietkiewicz M, Garlicki M, Domagala J, et al: Successful use of activated recombinant factor VII to control bleeding abnormalities in a patient with left ventricular assist device. J Thorac Cardiovasc Surg 123:384, 2002
513. Hendricks H, van der Maaten, de Wolf J, et al: An effective treatment of severe intractable bleeding after valve repair by one single dose of activated recombinant factor VII. Anesth Analg 93:287, 2001
514. Milas B, Jobes D, Gorman R: Management of bleeding and coagulopathy after heart surgery. Semin Thorac Cardiovasc Surg 12:326, 2000
515. Body SC, Shernan SK: Genetic basis of cardiovascular disease and perioperative pain. *In* Van Aken H (ed): Clinical Anesthesiology. London, Baillière Tindall, 2001
516. Ginsburg G, Donahue M, Newby L: Prospects for personalized cardiovascular medicine. J Am Coll Cardiol 46:1615, 2005
517. Podgoreanu M, Schwinn D: New paradigms in cardiovascular medicine. J Am Coll Cardiol 46:1965, 2005

Chapter 30

ORGAN PROTECTION DURING CARDIOPULMONARY BYPASS

Hilary P. Grocott, MD, FRCPC • Mark Stafford-Smith, MD, CM, FRCPC

KEY POINTS

1. Understanding organ dysfunction produced by cardiopulmonary bypass (CPB) and organ protection strategies is important.
2. Central nervous system injury from CPB ranges from neurocognitive deficits in 25% to 80% of patients to stroke in 1% to 5% of patients.
3. Advanced age is the most important risk factor for stroke and neurocognitive dysfunction after CPB.
4. Acute renal injury from CPB can contribute directly to poor outcomes.
5. Drugs such as dopamine and diuretics do not prevent renal failure after CPB.
6. Myocardial stunning represents injury caused by short periods of myocardial ischemia that can occur with CPB.
7. Blood cardioplegia has the potential advantage of delivering oxygen to ischemic myocardium, whereas crystalloid cardioplegia does not carry much oxygen.
8. Gastrointestinal complications after CPB include pancreatitis, gastrointestinal bleeding, bowel infarction, and cholecystitis.
9. Pulmonary complications such as atelectasis and pleural effusions are common after cardiac surgery with CPB.
10. Organ dysfunction cannot definitively be prevented with off-pump cardiac surgery.

Modern cardiac surgery, heralded by the advent of cardiopulmonary bypass (CPB) more than 5 decades ago, continues to be challenged by the risk of organ dysfunction and the morbidity and mortality that accompanies it. Catastrophic organ system failure was common in the early days of CPB, but advances in perfusion, anesthesia, and surgical techniques have allowed most patients to undergo surgery without major morbidity or mortality. However, organ dysfunction ranging in severity from the most subtle to the most severe still occurs, manifesting most frequently in patients with decreased functional reserves or extensive co-morbidities. With more than 1,000,000 patients worldwide undergoing various cardiac operations annually, understanding organ dysfunction and developing perioperative organ protective strategies are of paramount importance.

A number of injurious common pathways may account for the organ dysfunction typically associated with cardiac surgery. CPB itself initiates a whole-body inflammatory response with the release of various injurious inflammatory mediators (see Chapter 8). Add to this the various preexisting patient co-morbidities and the potential for organ ischemic injury due to embolization and hypoperfusion, and it becomes clear why organ injury can occur. Most cardiac surgery, due to its very nature, causes some degree of myocardial injury. Other body systems can be affected by the perioperative insults associated with cardiac surgery (particularly CPB), including the kidneys, lungs, gastrointestinal tract, and central nervous system.

Understanding the fundamentals of organ dysfunction, including the incidence, significance, associated risk factors, causes, and pathophysiology, provides a framework for discussing various organ-specific protective strategies. This chapter describes the various organ dysfunction syndromes that can occur in the cardiac surgical patient, with particular emphasis directed at strategies for reducing these injuries.

CENTRAL NERVOUS SYSTEM INJURY

Incidence and Significance of Injury

Central nervous system dysfunction after CPB represents deficits ranging from neurocognitive deficits, occurring in approximately 25% to 80% of patients, to overt stroke, occurring in 1% to 5% of patients.[1-4] The significant disparity between studies in the incidence of these adverse cerebral outcomes relates in part to their definition and to numerous methodologic differences in the determination of neurologic and neurocognitive outcome. Retrospective versus prospective assessments of neurologic deficits account for a significant portion of this inconsistency, as does the experience and expertise of the examiner. The timing of postoperative testing also affects determinations of outcome. For example, the rate of cognitive deficits is as high as 80% for patients at discharge, between 10% and 35% at 6 weeks or longer after coronary artery bypass grafting (CABG), and 10% to 15% more than a year after surgery. Higher rates of cognitive deficits recurs 5 years after surgery, when as many as 43% of patients have documented deficits[2] (see Chapter 35).

Although the incidence of this dysfunction varies greatly, the significance of these injuries cannot be overemphasized. Cerebral injury is a most disturbing outcome of cardiac surgery. To have a patient's heart successfully treated by the planned operation but discover that the patient no longer functions as well cognitively or is immobilized from a stroke can be devastating. There are enormous personal, family, and financial consequences of extending a patient's life with surgery, only to have the quality of the life significantly diminished.[4,5] Mortality after CABG, although having reached relatively low levels in the past decade (approximately 1% overall), is increasingly attributable to cerebral injury.[4]

Risk Factors for Central Nervous System Injury

Successful strategies for perioperative cerebral and other organ protection begin with a thorough understanding of the risk factors, causes, and pathophysiology. Risk factors for central nervous system injury can be considered from several different perspectives. Most studies outlining risk factors take into account only stroke. Few describe risk factors for neurocognitive dysfunction. Although it is often assumed that their respective risk factors are similar, few studies have consistently reported the preoperative risks of cognitive loss after cardiac surgery. Factors such as a poor baseline (preoperative) cognitive state, years of education (i.e., more advanced education is protective), age, diabetes, and CPB time are frequently described.[6,7]

Stroke is better characterized with respect to risk factors. Although studies differ somewhat as to all the risk factors, certain patient characteristics consistently correlate with an increased risk for cardiac surgery–associated neurologic injury. In a study of 2108 patients from 24 centers in a study conducted by the Multicenter Study of Perioperative Ischemia, incidence of adverse cerebral outcome after CABG surgery was determined and the risk factors analyzed. Two types of adverse cerebral outcomes were defined. Type I included nonfatal stroke, transient ischemic attack (TIA), stupor or coma at time of discharge, and death caused by stroke or hypoxic encephalopathy. Type II included new deterioration in intellectual function, confusion, agitation, disorientation, and memory deficit without evidence of focal injury. A total of 129 (6.1%) of the 2108 patients had an adverse cerebral outcome in the perioperative period. Type I outcomes occurred in 66 (3.1%) of 2108 patients, with type II outcomes occurring in 63 (3.0%) of 2108 patients. Stepwise logistic regression analysis identified eight independent predictors of type I outcomes and seven independent predictors of type II outcomes (Table 30–1).

In a subsequent analysis of the same study database, a stroke risk index using preoperative factors was developed (Fig. 30–1). This risk index allowed for the preoperative calculation of the stroke risk based on the weighted combination of the preoperative factors, including age, unstable angina, diabetes mellitus, neurologic disease, prior coronary artery or other cardiac surgery, vascular disease, and pulmonary disease.[8] Of all the factors in the Multicenter Study of Perioperative Ischemia analysis and in multiple other analyses,[4,9-12] age appears to be the most overwhelmingly robust predictor of stroke and of neurocognitive dysfunction after cardiac surgery.[1,2] Tuman et al[12] described that age has a greater impact on neurologic outcome than it does on perioperative myocardial infarction or low cardiac output states after cardiac surgery (Fig. 30–2).

The influence of gender on adverse perioperative cerebral outcomes after cardiac surgery has been evaluated. Women appear to be at higher risk for stroke after cardiac surgery than men.[13] Hogue et al[14] found that women appear more likely to suffer deficits in the visuospatial cognitive domain after cardiac surgery, although the frequency of cognitive dysfunction after cardiac surgery is similar for women and men.

Another consistent risk factor for stroke after cardiac surgery is the presence of cerebrovascular disease and atheromatous disease of the aorta. With respect to cerebrovascular disease, patients who have had a prior stroke or TIA are more likely to suffer a perioperative stroke.[13,15-17] Even in the absence of symptomatic cerebrovascular disease, such as the presence of a carotid bruit, the risk of stroke increases with the severity of the carotid disease. Breslau et al[18] reported that Doppler-detected carotid disease increased the risk of stroke after

Table 30–1 Risk Factors for Adverse Cerebral Outcomes after Cardiac Surgery

Risk Factor	Type I Outcomes	Type II Outcomes
Proximal aortic atherosclerosis	4.52 [2.52 to 8.09]*	
History of neurologic disease	3.19 [1.65 to 6.15]	
Use of IABP	2.60 [1.21 to 5.58]	
Diabetes mellitus	2.59 [1.46 to 4.60]	
History of hypertension	2.31 [1.20 to 4.47]	
History of pulmonary disease	2.09 [1.14 to 3.85]	2.37 [1.34 to 4.18]
History of unstable angina	1.83 [1.03 to 3.27]	
Age (per additional decade)	1.75 [1.27 to 2.43]	2.20 [1.60 to 3.02]
Admission systolic BP > 180 mm Hg		3.47 [1.41 to 8.55]
History of excessive alcohol intake		2.64 [1.27 to 5.47]
History of CABG		2.18 [1.14 to 4.17]
Arrhythmia on day of surgery		1.97 [1.12 to 3.46]
Antihypertensive therapy		1.78 [1.02 to 3.10]

*Adjusted odds ratio [95% confidence intervals] for type I and type II cerebral outcomes associated with selected risk factors from the Multicenter Study of Perioperative Ischemia.

BP = blood pressure; CABG = coronary artery bypass graft surgery; IABP = intra-aortic balloon pump.

From Arrowsmith JE, Grocott HP, Reves JG, et al: Central nervous system complications of cardiac surgery. Br J Anaesth 84:378, 2000.

Risk factor	Score
Age	(Age −25) × 1.43
Unstable angina	14
Diabetes mellitus	17
Neurological disease	18
Prior CABS	15
Vascular disease	18
Pulmonary disease	15

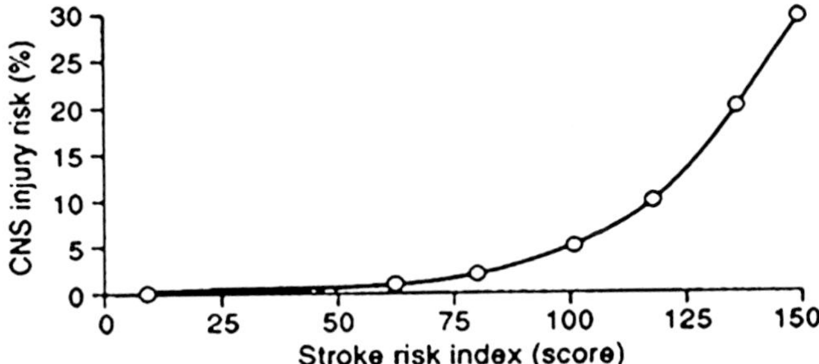

Figure 30–1 Preoperative stroke risk for patients undergoing coronary artery bypass graft surgery. The individual patient's stroke risk can be determined from the corresponding cumulative risk index score in the nomogram. (From Arrowsmith JE, Grocott HP, Reves JG, et al: Central nervous system complications of cardiac surgery. Br J Anaesth 84:378, 2000.)

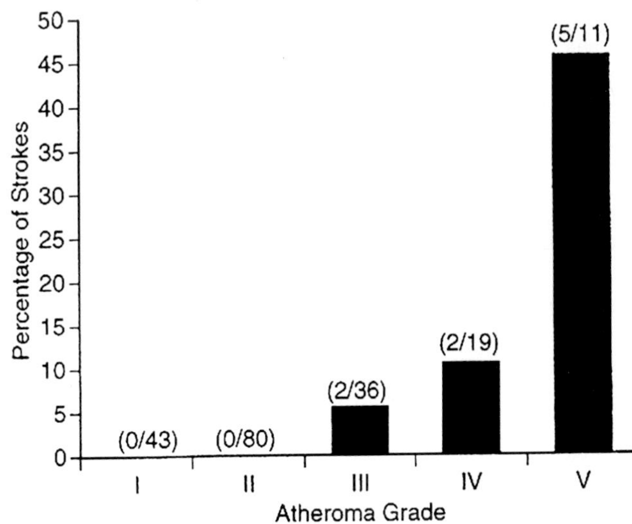

Figure 30–3 Stroke rate 1 week after cardiac surgery as a function of atheroma severity. Atheroma was graded by transesophageal echocardiography as follows: I, normal; II, intimal thickening; III, plaque < 5 mm thick; IV, plaque > 5 mm thick; V, any plaque with a mobile segment. (From Hartman GS, Yao FS, Bruefach M 3rd, et al: Severity of aortic atheromatous disease diagnosed by transesophageal echocardiography predicts stroke and other outcomes associated with coronary artery surgery: A prospective study. Anesth Analg 83:701, 1996.)

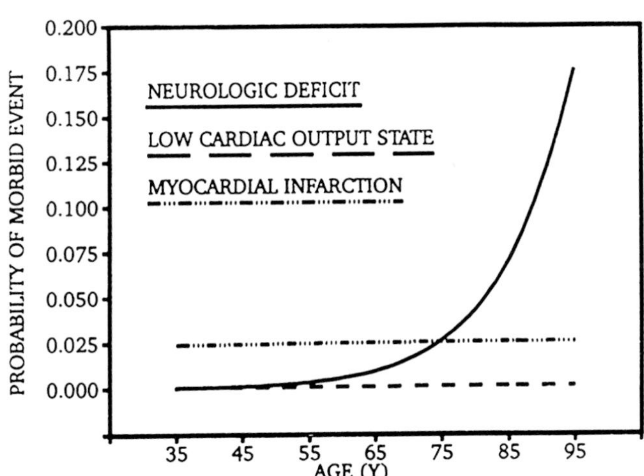

Figure 30–2 The relative effect of age on the predicted probability of neurologic and cardiac morbidity after cardiac surgery. (From Tuman KJ, McCarthy RJ, Najafi H, et al: Differential effects of advanced age on neurologic and cardiac risks of coronary artery operations. J Thorac Cardiovasc Surg 104:1510, 1992.)

cardiac surgery by threefold. Similarly, Brener et al[19] described that a carotid stenosis greater than 50%, increased the risk of stroke from 1.9% to 6.3%.

Although the presence of cerebrovascular disease is a risk factor for perioperative stroke, it does not always correlate well with the presence of significant aortic atherosclerosis.[20] Atheromatous disease of the ascending, arch, and descending thoracic aorta has been consistently implicated as a risk factor for stroke in cardiac surgical patients.[21-24] The increased use of transesophageal echocardiography (TEE) and epiaortic ultrasonography has added new dimensions to the detection of aortic atheromatous disease and the understanding of its relation to stroke risk (see Chapters 15 and 16). These imaging modalities have allowed the diagnosis of atheromatous disease to be made in a more sensitive and detailed manner, contributing greatly to the information regarding potential stroke risk. The risk of cerebral embolism from aortic atheroma was described early in the history of cardiac surgery[25] and has repeatedly been described in detail since then.[4,26-28] For example, Katz et al[29] found that the incidence of stroke was 25% in patients with a mobile atheromatous plaque in the aortic arch, compared with a stroke rate of 2% in those with limited atheromatous disease. Studies have consistently reported higher stroke rates for patients with increasing atheromatous aortic involvement (particularly the ascending and arch segments).[30] This relationship is outlined in Figure 30–3.

Cause of Perioperative Central Nervous System Injury

Because central nervous system dysfunction represents a wide range of injuries, differentiating the individual causes of these different types of injuries becomes somewhat difficult (Box 30–1). They are frequently grouped together and superficially discussed as representing different severities on a continuum of similar injury. This likely misrepresents the different causes

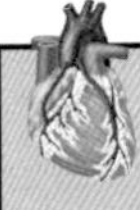

BOX 30–1 ***Causes of Central Nervous System Complications after Cardiopulmonary Bypass***

- Cerebral emboli
- Global hypoperfusion
- Inflammation
- Cerebral edema
- Blood-brain barrier dysfunction

Table 30–2 Causes of Cognitive Dysfunction after Cardiac Surgery

Cause	Possible Settings
Cerebral microemboli	Generated during cardiopulmonary bypass (CPB); mobilization of atheromatous material or entrainment of air from the operative field; gas injections into the venous reservoir of the CPB apparatus
Global cerebral hypoperfusion	Hypotension, occlusion by an atheromatous embolus leading to stroke
Inflammation (systemic and cerebral)	Injurious effects of CPB, such as blood interacting with the foreign surfaces of pump-oxygenator; up-regulation of proinflammatory cyclooxygenase mRNA
Cerebral hyperthermia	Hypothermia during CPB; hyperthermia during and after cardiac surgery, such as aggressive rewarming
Cerebral edema	Edema from global cerebral hypoperfusion or from hyponatremia; increased cerebral venous pressure from cannula misplacement
Blood-brain barrier dysfunction	Diffuse cerebral inflammation; ischemia from cerebral microembolization or increased intracranial pressure
Pharmacologic influences	Anesthetic-related cognitive damage; necrosis of neonatal brains; proteomic changes
Genetic influences	Effects of single nucleotide polymorphisms on risk for Alzheimer's disease or for acute coronary syndromes and other thrombotic disorders

of these injuries. The following section addresses stroke and cognitive injury (Table 30–2), and their respective causes are differentiated when appropriate (see Chapters 28 and 35).

Cerebral Embolization

Macroemboli (e.g., atheromatous plaque) and microemboli (i.e., gaseous and particulate) are generated during CPB, and many emboli find their way to the cerebral vasculature.[31] Macroemboli are responsible for stroke, and microemboli are fundamental to the development of neurocognitive dysfunction. Sources for the microemboli are numerous and include those generated de novo from the interactions of blood within the CPB apparatus (e.g., platelet-fibrin aggregates) and those generated within the body by the production and mobilization of atheromatous material or entrainment of air from the operative field. Other sources for emboli include lipid-laden debris that can be added by cardiotomy suction.[32] Other gaseous emboli may be generated though injections into the venous reservoir of the CPB apparatus itself.[33,34]

Numerous studies outline the relationship between emboli and cognitive decline after cardiac surgery.[35-37] However, one of the major limitations in understanding this relationship has been the relative inability to discern between gaseous and particulate microemboli. Typically, Doppler ultrasonography has been used to measure cerebral embolic signals, but Doppler cannot reliably distinguish between gaseous and particulate emboli.[38] In addition to using Doppler evidence, Moody et al[31] performed histologic analyses on brains from cardiac surgical patients and described the presence of millions of cerebral emboli represented as small capillary arteriolar dilations (SCADs).

The impact of aortic atheroma on cognitive decline is incompletely understood. It is widely known from nonsurgical and cardiac surgical studies that there is a clear relationship between aortic atheroma and stroke,[21,39-41] but the relationship between cognitive outcome and cerebral atheroma is much less uncertain. Several studies describe different results.[42,43] Whereas some data suggest that cerebral emboli are more likely with a higher degree of atheroma in the ascending aorta,[44] there is a relative failure demonstrating that these atheroma correspond to cognitive decline.[42] Part of the discordance between these two findings may reflect the limitation of Doppler technology to discriminate between gaseous and particulate emboli, thereby possibly misrepresenting somewhat the actual cerebral embolic load.[45]

Global Cerebral Hypoperfusion

The concept that global cerebral hypoperfusion during CPB may lead to neurologic and neurocognitive complications originates from the earliest days of cardiac surgery, when significant (in degree and time) systemic hypotension was a relatively common event. Although making intuitive sense (i.e., that hypotension would lead to global cerebral hypoperfusion), studies that have examined the relationship between mean arterial pressure (MAP) and cognitive decline after cardiac surgery have generally failed to show any significant relationship.[7,46,47]

This is not the case for stroke, for which Hartman et al[28] and Gold et al[48] demonstrated a link between hypotension and the presence of a significantly atheromatous aorta with increased stroke (see Fig. 30–3). This is not a clear relationship, however, and likely represents an interaction between macroembolism and global cerebral hypoperfusion. It is likely, for example, that if one area of the brain that is being perfused by a cerebral vessel becomes occluded by an atheromatous embolus, it may be more susceptible to hypoperfusion if collateral perfusion is compromised by concomitant systemic hypotension.[49] Other evidence for global cerebral hypoperfusion comes from Mutch et al,[50] who examined magnetic resonance imaging (MRI) assessments of cerebral blood flow (CBF) showing progressive decreases in CBF during the course of experimental CPB in pigs. Additional supportive data come from a magnetic resonance spectroscopy (MRS) study demonstrating that there are MRS characteristics consistent with global cerebral ischemia after CPB and that the signals that are associated with cognitive decline return to normal when the cognitive function returns to normal.[51]

Temperature-Related Factors

The impact of CPB temperature (i.e., hypothermia) on outcome is addressed further in this section. However, with the various trials of hypothermia during CPB and with detailed temperature monitoring, the observation has been made that *hyperthermia* can occur during certain periods during and after cardiac surgery. During rewarming from hypothermic CPB, there can be an overshoot in cerebral temperature due to aggressive rewarming generally aimed at decreasing time on CPB and overall operating room time. This cerebral hyperthermia may well be responsible for some of the injury that occurs in the brain.[52]

The postoperative period is also a critical time in which hyperthermia can contribute to brain injury.[53,54] Grocott et al[53] demonstrated that the peak temperature in the postoperative period (24 hours after surgery) was related to cognitive decline 6 weeks after cardiac surgery. It is not clear whether this hyperthermia causes de novo injury or it exacerbates injury that has already occurred (e.g., injury that might be induced by cerebral microembolization or global cerebral hypoperfusion). It is necessary to be cautious in concluding whether these relationships are temporal or causal. However, it is assumed that the brain is injured during CPB, and because experimental brain injury is known to cause hyperthermia (resulting from hypothalamic injury[55]), the hyperthermia that is demonstrated in the postoperative period may be caused by the occurrence or extent of brain injury. However, if hyperthermia results from the inflammatory response to bypass, the hyperthermia itself may induce or exacerbate cerebral injury.

Inflammation

Although it is well known that blood interacts with the foreign surfaces of the pump-oxygenator to stimulate a profound inflammatory response,[56] the systemic end-organ effects of this inflammatory response are less clearly defined. Much of the data relating organ dysfunction in the central nervous system to the inflammatory response in the cardiac surgical patient has focused on indirect experimental and clinical evidence. It is not clear whether a cerebral inflammatory response occurs as a result of CPB in humans. Hindman et al[57] reported that cyclooxygenase mRNA was up-regulated after CPB, suggesting that on the molecular biologic level, CPB induces overexpression of this proinflammatory gene in the brain. What is not clear was whether this was a primary event (i.e., as a direct result of the proinflammatory effects of CPB) or a secondary event as a result of other injurious effects of CPB (e.g., microembolization). In settings other than cardiac surgery, inflammation has been demonstrated to directly injure the brain (e.g., sepsis-mediated encephalopathy),[58] but it is also known to result as a response to various cerebral injuries (e.g., ischemic stroke).[59]

There is no direct evidence that inflammation causes cardiac surgery-associated adverse cerebral outcome; however, there is some supportive indirect evidence. For example, Mathew et al[60] demonstrated a relationship between poor cognitive outcome and an impaired immune response to circulating endotoxin, which inevitably translocates from the gut into the bloodstream due to alterations in splanchnic blood flow during CPB. Having a low antibody response to circulating endotoxin is paradoxically associated with an overstimulated inflammatory response,[61] thus demonstrating that the relationship between low endotoxin antibodies and poor cognitive outcome may be mediated by an augmented inflammatory response. There are no other direct data linking cognitive dysfunction with inflammation after cardiac surgery.

Cerebral Edema

Cerebral edema after CPB has been reported in several studies.[62,63] The explanation for why cerebral edema may occur early in the postbypass period is not clear. It may be caused by cytotoxic edema resulting from global cerebral hypoperfusion or possibly by hyponatremia-induced cerebral edema. Generalized cerebral edema due to increases in cerebral venous pressure caused by cannula misplacement, which frequently occurs during CPB, is another reason.[64] Specifically, use of a dual-stage venous cannula can often lead to cerebral venous congestion with vertical displacement of the heart during access to the posterior epicardial coronary arteries. It is not clear from these studies whether the edema results because of injury that occurs during CPB, leading to cognitive decline, or whether the edema itself directly causes the injury by consequent increases in intracranial pressure with global or regional decreases in CBF and resulting ischemia.

Blood-Brain Barrier Dysfunction

The function of the blood-brain barrier (BBB) is to aid in maintaining the homeostasis of the extracellular cerebral milieu protecting the brain against fluctuations in various ion concentrations, neurotransmitters, and growth factors that are present in the serum.[65] The impact of CPB on the function and integrity of the BBB is not clearly known. Gillinov et al[66] were unable to show any changes in BBB dysfunction 2 hours after CPB in piglets as assessed using carbon 14–aminoisobutyric acid tracer techniques in postbypass brain homogenates. However, Cavaglia et al,[67] measuring the leakage of fluorescent albumin from blood vessels in brain slices after CPB, were able to demonstrate significant breaches in the BBB. Both studies looked at a single time point (i.e., immediately after CPB), and it is not known whether there are temporal changes in the BBB integrity.

It is difficult to determine whether the changes in BBB integrity, if present at all, are a primary cause of brain dysfunction or simply a result of other initiating events such as ischemia (i.e., from cerebral microembolization) or a diffuse cerebral inflammatory event. Changes in the BBB could cause some of the cerebral edema that has been demonstrated, or it could result from cerebral edema if the edema resulted in ischemic injury (from increases in intracranial pressure).[63]

Possible Pharmacologic Influences

Anesthetics have been demonstrated to affect cognitive loss after surgery. Experimental studies of cognitive outcome in rats exposed to anesthetics have demonstrated that relatively brief (several hours) exposure to isoflurane can lead to long-term cognitive changes in the animals.[68] Coupled with the demonstration in other experimental models of necrosis in neonatal brains exposed to certain anesthetic agents (e.g., isoflurane, midazolam, nitrous oxide),[69] this added to the data suggesting that corresponding proteomic changes can occur in the brain after exposure to anesthetics[70] and highlighted this as a potential area for further research.

Genetic Influences

Genetics may play a role in modifying the degree of central nervous system injury or in the ability of the brain to recover after an injury has occurred. Several investigations have assessed the genetic influences on cerebral outcome after CPB. The most commonly explored gene variant, or single nucleotide polymorphism (SNP), has been the ε4 allele of the apolipoprotein gene. This gene has been reported to be responsible for increasing the risk of sporadic and late-onset Alzheimer's disease (as well as complicating outcome after a variety of other head injuries).[71] Although early reports suggest that this may be an important influence,[72] later reports shed some doubt on how robust this effect is.[73] A second SNP examined relates to the PLA2 receptor polymorphism. This platelet integrin receptor polymorphism is important in the cause of acute coronary syndromes and other thrombotic disorders.[74,75] A small study in cardiac surgery patients demonstrated worse impairments in the mini-mental status examination in the PLA2-positive patients compared with PLA2-negative patients.[76] There are probably many other genes involved in the complex injuries after cardiac surgery.

Neuroprotective Strategies

Emboli Reduction

There are multiple sources of particulate and gaseous emboli during cardiac surgery. Within the CPB circuit itself, particulate emboli in the form of platelet-fibrin aggregates and other debris are generated. Gaseous emboli can be created in the circuit or augmented if already present by factors such as turbulence-related cavitation and potentially even by vacuum-assisted venous drainage.[77] Air in the venous return tubing is variably handled by the bypass circuit (i.e., reservoir, oxygenator, and arterial filters). The ability of the circuit to prevent the transit of gaseous emboli through the oxygenator varies considerably between manufacturers and remains a significant source of emboli. The impact of perfusionist interventions on cerebral embolic load has also been studied. Borger et al[34] found that after drug injections into the venous reservoir, gaseous emboli can make a rapid passage through to the arterial outflow. Reducing these perfusionist interventions reduced emboli generation and neurocognitive impairment.

Significant quantities of air can be entrained from the surgical field into the heart itself; flooding the field with carbon dioxide has been proposed as being effective in reducing this embolic source.[78] Its ability to specifically reduce cerebral injury has not been rigorously evaluated although it has been demonstrated to significantly reduce the amount of TEE detectable bubbles in the heart after cardiac surgery.[79] Even with the use of carbon dioxide in the surgical field, significant amounts of entrained air can be present. Although the oxygenator–venous reservoir design attempts to purge this air before reaching the inflow cannula, the arterial line filter handles a great deal of what is left. The capacity of the arterial filter to remove all sources of emboli (gaseous or particulate) has significant limitations and despite its use, emboli can easily pass through and on into the aortic root.

The aortic cannula may be very important to reduce cerebral emboli production. Placement of the cannula into an area of the aorta with a large atheroma burden may cause the direct generation of emboli from the "sandblasting" of atherosclerotic material in the aorta. The use a of distal aortic cannula, where the tip of the cannula lies beyond the origin of the cerebral vessels has also been found to reduce emboli load.[80] The type of cannula itself may be an important factor. Various designs have allowed the reduction of various sandblasting-type jets emanating from the aortic cannula. Baffled cannulas and cannulas that allow the incorporation of regional brain hypothermia and diversion of emboli away from the cerebral vessels have been used.[81] A cannula that has a basket-like extension that can be inserted just before cross-clamp removal has been studied.[82] In a large (n = 1289) study, this Embol-X cannula was unable to reduce the incidence of central nervous system dysfunction.[83] A smaller (n = 24) study showed an increase in embolic signals with its deployment in the aorta.[84] Few other emboli-reducing strategies, besides arterial line filtration and reducing perfusion interventions itself,[34,37] have been studied sufficiently to determine their impact on cognitive loss after cardiac surgery. The safety of introducing new techniques also has not been thoroughly studied; the additional risk assumed when significantly altering a standard of practice to use a new device must be considered (see Chapter 40).

Blood that is returned from the surgical field though the use of the cardiotomy suction may significantly contribute to the particulate load in the CPB circuit and subsequently in the brain. The use of cell-salvage devices to process shed blood before returning it to the venous reservoir may minimize the amount of particulate- or lipid-laden material that contributes to embolization.[32,33] Most of this material is small enough or so significantly deformable (due to its high lipid content) that it can pass through standard 40-µm arterial filters. There are several issues with the cell saver, however. One is the cost that is incurred with its use, and the other is its side effects of reducing platelet and coagulation factors through its intrinsic washing processes. Modest use of cell salvage up to a certain, although as yet undefined, volume of blood is likely prudent.

Management of Aortic Atherosclerosis

Although the previous section dealt with issues related to reduction of emboli, many of which are likely spawned from atheromatous plaque in the aorta, further specific management of the atheromatous aorta, particularly as it relates to stroke risk, requires special attention. The widespread use of TEE and complementary (and preferably routine) epiaortic scanning has had a tremendous impact on the understanding of the risks involved in the patient with a severely atheromatous aorta. There is indisputable evidence linking stroke to atheroma.[21,39-41] However, the strength of association between atheroma and cognitive decline seen after cardiac surgery is less clear. There is insufficient evidence to say without doubt that there is a relationship between atheroma and cognitive decline. Regardless of whether atheromas cause cognitive dysfunction, their contribution to cardiac surgery–associated stroke is enough to warrant specific strategies for its management.

A small study used a combination of epiaortic scanning and atheroma avoidance techniques (with respect to cannulation, clamping, and vein graft anastomosis placement) to attempt to reduce neurocognitive deficits.[43] In that study, the incidence of cognitive decline was lower in patients who had an avoidance technique guided by epiaortic scanning compared with no epiaortic scanning. It was limited by its small size, but it identified an area that requires more investigation. We have examined this issue and found the relationship between cognitive decline and atheroma to be much less clear.[85]

One of the difficulties in interpreting studies that have evaluated atheroma avoidance strategies is the absence of any form of blinding of the investigators. For the most part, a strategy is chosen based on the presence of known atheroma, and the results of these patients are compared with historical controls. What constitutes the best strategy is unclear. Multiple techniques can be used to minimize atheromatous material liberated from the aortic wall from getting into the cerebral circulation. These range from optimizing placement of the aortic cannula in the aorta up to an area relatively devoid of plaque to the use of specialized cannulas that reduce the sandblasting of the aortic wall. Alternative aortic cannulas and using different locations possess the ability to decrease embolization of atheromatous plaque. The avoidance of partial occlusion clamping for proximal vein graft anastomosis using a single-step automated anastomotic device and the use of alternatives to cross-clamping all possess the ability to mitigate injury due to embolization. Specialized cannulas that contain filtering technologies[82] and other means to deflect emboli to more distal sites have been developed and are being studied.[86] Technology is advancing rapidly, and proximal (and distal) coronary artery anastomotic devices are becoming increasingly available and focus on minimizing manipulation of the ascending aorta. None of these aortic manipulations has yet yielded significant neuroprotective results in large, prospective, randomized trials, but the potential holds great promise.

Pulsatile Perfusion

Nonpulsatile CPB is the most commonly practiced form of artificial perfusion. As intuitive as it may seem that this type of nonphysiologic, nonpulsatile pump flow could be injurious, there is an overall lack of data to suggest that pulsatile flow during clinical CPB is beneficial. In a large (n = 316), double-blind, randomized investigation by Murkin et al[87] examining the effect of pulsatile versus nonpulsatile CPB on neurologic and neuropsychologic outcome, no significant benefit was demonstrated. A significant limitation to most pulsatility studies is that, because of technical reasons, true "physiologic" pulsatility is almost never accomplished. Instead, variations of sinusoidal pulse waveforms are produced that do not replicate the kinetics and hydrodynamics of normal physiologic pulsation. One study of balloon pump–induced pulsatile perfusion during CPB failed to show any improvements in jugular venous oxygen saturation of regional brain oxygenation.[88]

Newer pulsatile technologies may better reproduce the normal biologic state of cardiac pulsatility. Computer technologies that allow creating a more physiologic pulsatile perfusion pattern have, at least experimentally, demonstrated preservation of cerebral oxygenation. This approach showed some promise in a pig model of CPB in which pulsatile flow controlled by a computer to replicate the normal biologic variability in pulsatility was associated with significantly lower jugular venous oxygen desaturation during rewarming after hypothermic CPB.[89] However, most studies do not present convincing evidence to suggest that routine pulsatile flow during CPB, as can be achieved by widely available technology, is warranted.

Acid-Base Management: Alpha-Stat versus pH-Stat

Optimal acid-base management during CPB has long been debated. Theoretically, alpha-stat management maintains normal CBF autoregulation with the coupling of cerebral metabolism ($CMRO_2$) to CBF, allowing adequate oxygen delivery while minimizing the potential for emboli. Although early studies[87] were unable to document a difference in neurologic or neuropsychologic outcome between the two techniques, later studies showed reductions in cognitive performance when pH-stat management was used, particularly in cases with prolonged CPB times.[90] pH-stat management (i.e., CO_2 is added to the fresh oxygenator gas flow) results in a higher CBF than is needed for the brain's metabolic requirements. This luxury perfusion risks excessive delivery of emboli to the brain. Except for congenital heart surgery, for which most outcome data support the use of pH-stat management[91,92] due to its improvement in homogenous brain cooling before circulatory arrest, adult outcome data support the use of alpha-stat management.

Temperature and Rewarming Strategies

The use of hypothermia remains a mainstay of perioperative management in the cardiac surgical patient. Its widespread use relates to its putative, although not definitively proved, global organ protective effects. Although hypothermia has a measurable effect on suppressing cerebral metabolism (approximately 6% to 7% decline per 1°C),[93] it is likely that its other neuroprotective effects may be mediated by nonmetabolic actions. In the ischemic brain, for example, moderate hypothermia has multimodal effects, including blocking the release of glutamate,[94] reducing calcium influx,[95] hastening recovery of protein synthesis,[96] diminishing membrane-bound protein kinase C activity,[97] slowing of the time to onset of depolarization,[98] reducing formation of reactive oxygen species (ROS),[99] and suppressing nitric oxide synthase activity.[100] Some or all of these effects in combination may convey some of the neuroprotective effects of hypothermia. Although experimental demonstrations of this are abundant, clinical examples of hypothermia neuroprotection have been elusive until recently.[101-104]

Some of the most meaningful data on CPB temperature and cerebral outcome came from work that had its origins in the late 1980s and early 1990s. It was at that time the judicious use of warm CPB was used because of its putative myocardial salvaging effects when used with continuous warm cardioplegia.[105-108] However, because CPB was being carried out at higher temperatures than what were considered conventional, the implications on the brain were also studied. Several large studies have been undertaken to elucidate the effects of temperature management on cerebral outcome after cardiac surgery. The Warm Heart Investigators trial,[105] a trial performed at Emory University,[109] and a later trial at Duke University,[110] although having several methodologic differences, had very similar results with respect to neurocognitive outcome[111,112] but some very divergent results with respect to stroke. None of the studies demonstrated any neuroprotective effect of hypothermia on neurocognitive outcome after cardiac surgery. However, the Emory trial did demonstrate an apparent injurious effect (as manifest by a worse stroke outcome) of what was most likely mild degrees of hyperthermia during CPB. Neither the Warm Heart Investigators trial nor the Duke trial showed any effect of temperature on stroke per se. These data suggest that active warming to maintain temperatures at (or greater) than 37°C may pose an unnecessary risk of stroke.

Just as hypothermia has some likely protective effects on the brain, hyperthermia, in an opposite and disproportionate fashion, has some injurious effects. Although the studies referred to previously[105,109,110] demonstrated no neuroprotective effect, there is emerging evidence that if some degree of neuroprotection is afforded by hypothermia, it may be negated by the obligatory rewarming period that must ensue.[52]

Grigore et al[52] demonstrated in a prospective trial that compared with conventional "fast" rewarming, slower rewarming resulted in a lower incidence of neurocognitive dysfunction 6 weeks after cardiac surgery. These lower rewarming rates led to lower peak cerebral temperatures during rewarming, consistent with past observations that rapid rewarming can lead to an overshoot in cerebral temperature resulting in inadvertent cerebral hyperthermia.[113] By reducing this rewarming rate, it reduces the overshoot in temperature and prevents the negative effects of cerebral hyperthermia. Consistent with the concept that preventing some of the rewarming may be protective was a study by Nathan et al[114] that demonstrated a neurocognitive benefit for patients who were maintained between 34°C and 36°C for a prolonged (12 hours) period postoperatively. That trial may have had its beneficial effect by the avoidance of cerebral hyperthermia during rewarming rather than the prolonged hypothermia.[114]

Although there are numerous sites for monitoring temperature during cardiac surgery, several warrant special consideration. One of the lessons learned from the three warm versus cold trials, as well as from other information regarding temperature gradients between the CPB circuit, nasopharynx, and brain,[113] is that it is important to monitor (and use as a target) a temperature site relevant to the organ of interest. If it is the body, a core temperature measured in the bladder, rectum, pulmonary artery, or esophagus is appropriate. However, if the temperature of the brain is desired, barring implantation of a thermistor directly into the brain (which has been done),[115] it is important to look at surrogates of brain temperatures. These include nasopharyngeal temperature and tympanic membrane temperature. More invasive surrogates of brain temperature have been obtained using a jugular bulb thermistor.[113,116] Testing these different temperature sites has demonstrated that vast temperature gradients appear across the body and across the brain. It is likely that during periods of rapid flux (e.g., during rewarming), these temperature gradients are maximal (see Chapter 28).

Mean Arterial Pressure Management during Cardiopulmonary Bypass

The relationship between pressure during CPB and CBF is pertinent to understanding whether MAP can be optimized to prevent neurologic injury. Plochl et al[117] examined the threshold of the autoregulatory curve in dogs whereby lowering blood pressure further would result in inadequate CBF and oxygen delivery during CPB. In that study, the brain became perfusion pressure dependent below 50 mm Hg. The investigators also demonstrated that hypothermia did not shift this threshold leftward. Clinically, the available data suggest that in an otherwise normal patient, CBF during nonpulsatile hypothermic CPB using alpha-stat blood gas management is largely independent of MAP as long as that MAP is within or near the autoregulatory range for the patient (i.e., 50 to 100 mm Hg).[118] Although the autoregulatory curve is traditionally considered a horizontal plateau, this plateau has a slightly positive slope, but this slight upward slope is unlikely to have a significant clinically meaningful effect. For example, Newman et al[7] demonstrated that under hypothermic conditions, CBF changes only 0.86 mL/100g/min for every 10-mm Hg change in MAP. Although this change (1.78 mL/100 g/min) was greater with normothermia,[119] these changes represent a relatively small fraction of the normal CBF of approximately 50 mL/100 g/min. Underlying essential hypertension as a comorbidity, however, likely is the effect of a rightward shift in the autoregulatory curve. The degree to which this rightward shift occurs, is not clear, but it would be reasonable to expect that it is at least 10 mm Hg, suggesting that the lower range of autoregulatory blood flow is more likely to be 60 than 50 mm Hg.[120]

Although the data associating MAP with neurologic and neurocognitive outcome after CABG surgery are inconclusive, most data suggest that MAP during CPB is not a primary predictor of cognitive decline or stroke after cardiac surgery. However, with increasing age, MAP during CPB may play a role in improving cerebral collateral perfusion to regions embolized, improving neurologic and cognitive outcome.[7]

Gold et al[48] added significantly to the understanding of the influence of perfusion pressure on outcome after cardiac surgery in a study of 248 patients randomized to low (50 to 60 mm Hg) or high (80 to 100 mm Hg) MAP during CPB. Although a difference was demonstrated in their composite end-point of combined adverse cardiac and neurologic outcome (4.8% high versus 12.9% low, $p = 0.026$), when the individual outcomes were compared, there were similar trends but no statistical differences. A secondary analysis of the same data performed by Hartman et al[28] found interesting interactions among pressure, aortic atheroma, and stroke; patients who were at risk of cerebral embolic stroke (from having severely atheromatous aortas) were more likely to manifest a stroke if MAP was maintained in the lower range than in the higher range. Intuitively, this is logical. Some experimental data in the noncardiac surgical setting suggest that collateral perfusion to penumbral areas of brain suffering from ischemic injury are relatively protected by higher perfusion pressure.[49] Overall, it appears that MAP (in the normal range) has little effect on cognitive outcome, but in those with significant aortic atheroma, it may be prudent to modestly increase blood pressure.

Glucose Management

Hyperglycemia is a common occurrence during the course of cardiac surgery. Administration of cardioplegia containing glucose and stress response-induced alterations in insulin secretion and resistance increase the potential for significant hyperglycemia.[121] Hyperglycemia has been repeatedly demonstrated to impair neurologic outcome after experimental focal and global cerebral ischemia.[122-124] The explanation for this adverse effect likely relates to the effects that hyperglycemia have on anaerobic conversion of glucose to lactate which ultimately cause intracellular acidosis and impair intracellular homeostasis and metabolism.[125] A second injurious mechanism relates to an increase in the release of excitotoxic amino acids in response to hyperglycemia in the setting of cerebral ischemia.[123] If hyperglycemia is injurious to the brain, the threshold for making injuries worse appears to be 180 to 200 mg/dL.[126,127]

Despite much experimental data, the role of glucose management on cerebral outcome after clinical CPB is not clear. Although Hindman et al[128] caution about the use of glucose-containing prime for CPB, Metz et al[129] did not find a difference in neurologic outcome in patients undergoing CPB with a glucose prime (blood glucose during CPB of 600 to 800 mg/dL) versus no glucose prime (blood glucose level of 200 to 300 mg/dL). This finding was supported by Nussmeier et al,[130] who reported that use of a glucose-containing prime was not a risk factor for cerebral injury in nondiabetic or diabetic patients having CABG procedures. In the largest retrospective review, outcome data from 2862 CABG patients showed no association between the intraoperative maximum glucose concentration and major adverse neurologic outcome or in-hospital mortality.[131,132]

The appropriate type of perioperative serum glucose management and whether it adversely affects neurologic outcome in patients undergoing CPB remain unclear. The major difficulty in hyperglycemia treatment is the relative ineffectiveness of insulin therapy. Using excessive amounts of insulin during hypothermic periods may lead to rebound hypoglycemia after CPB. Chaney et al[133] attempted to maintain normoglycemia during cardiac surgery with the use of an insulin protocol and came to the conclusion that even with aggressive insulin treatment, hyperglycemia is often resistant and may actually predispose to postoperative hypoglycemia. Attempting to mediate injury may actually predispose to additional injury.

Off-Pump Cardiac Surgery

Off-pump coronary artery bypass (OPCAB) surgery is frequently used for the operative treatment of coronary artery disease (see Chapter 19). Although its ability to optimally treat coronary disease (through the demonstration of long-term graft patency) has not yet been shown in a long-term, prospective, randomized, controlled fashion, it is clear that OPCAB and similar operations (e.g., MIDCAB) will continue to be mainstays of cardiac surgery, although in an evolving fashion. Their impact on adverse cerebral outcomes after cardiac surgery has been variably reported.[134]

Some preliminary data suggest less cognitive decline after OPCAB procedures, but most studies have not seen it eliminated altogether (see Chapter 19). The reasons for this are unclear but likely reflect on the complex pathophysiology involved. For example, if inflammatory processes play a role in initiating or propagating cerebral injury, OPCAB, with its continued use of sternotomy, heparin administration, and wide hemodynamic swings, all of which may contribute to a stress and inflammatory response, may be a significant reason why cognitive dysfunction is still seen. Ascending aortic manipulation, with its ensuing particulate embolization, is also still commonly used.

The results of the largest OPCAB study by Van Djik et al[135] to examine cognitive dysfunction showed that although there was a reduction in cognitive decline in the early months after surgery, by 1 year, there were no differences between groups. Although it was the largest trial ($n = 281$), it was still not large enough to determine subtle differences between groups, and it is likely that the failure to see a difference at 1 year was related to a lack of power.[136] The effects of OPCAB on stroke risk have not been sufficiently analyzed, but one meta-analysis showed no beneficial effect on the incidence of stroke.[137]

Pharmacologic Neuroprotection

In addition to the improvements in CPB technology, knowledge of the molecular workings of the brain has improved significantly, revealing potential pharmacologic neuroprotective targets. The oversimplified concept that depletion of high-energy phosphates and destruction of brain tissue rapidly follows ischemia has been replaced by a considerably more complex temporal, topographic, and biochemical picture. Advanced imaging techniques have discovered spatial gradations of residual CBF in the downstream territory of an occluded cerebral vessel producing an ischemic penumbra, where CBF is critically reduced but still sufficient to prevent immediate cell death. There is a marked difference in the temporal association between the ischemic insult and eventual cell

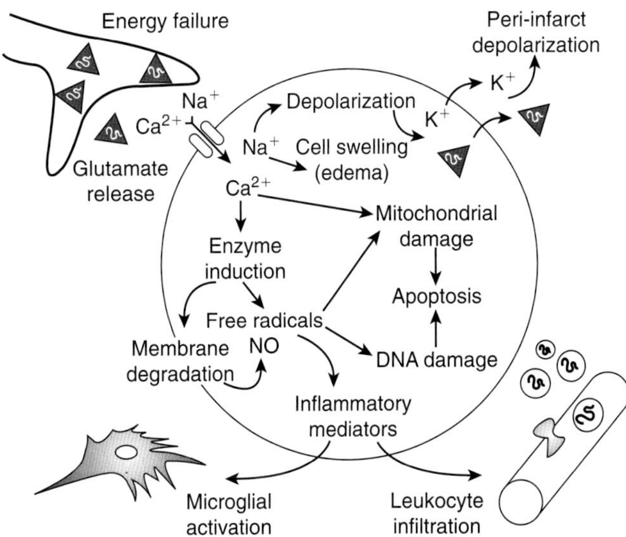

Figure 30–4 Cerebral ischemic cascade. A simplified overview of central nervous system events that occur after energy failure in the ischemic brain. (From Dirnagl U, Iadecola C, Moskowitz M: Pathobiology of ischemic stroke: An integrated review. Trends Neurosci 22:391, 1999.)

death, resulting in a therapeutic window in which intervention (particularly pharmacologic) may attenuate infarct size. This window differs between the profoundly ischemic core and the penumbra. In the ischemic core, restoration of oxygen and glucose supplies is essential where high-energy phosphates have been severely depleted. In contrast, in the penumbra, the decrease in oxygen and glucose delivery is insufficient to kill cells directly. In these regions, pharmacologic agents with little or no ability to modify CBF have been shown experimentally to effectively reduce cerebral infarct volume, even if administered after the onset of permanent focal ischemia.

The central nervous system ischemic cascade (Fig. 30–4) is triggered by reductions in CBF, globally or regionally, to the point at which the demands of cerebral metabolism can no longer be met.[138] This depletion in cerebral energy stores leads to membrane ionic pump failure resulting in a number of injurious events mediated by the influx of sodium, the opening of voltage-dependent calcium gates, a release of stored intracellular calcium, and overall membrane depolarization. Membrane depolarization results in the release of excitatory amino acids (e.g., glutamate, aspartate), with subsequent dramatic increases in intracellular calcium. This increase in cytoplasmic calcium propagates the cascade through the activation of a number of calcium-dependent enzymes, including endonucleases, nitric oxide synthase, various proteases, protein kinases, and phospholipases. If left unabated, these enzymes will result in neuronal death.

Although some of these events are potentially reversible if reperfusion is quickly reestablished, reperfusion itself initiates a number of other destructive pathways. The reestablishment of oxygen delivery provides substrate for the production of reactive oxygen species, so-called free radicals. Reperfusion initiates a number of other damaging extracellular events, including BBB breakdown, endothelial swelling, and localized thrombosis that together may culminate in microvascular occlusion and further ischemia. Each of these pathways in the ischemic cascade represents discrete groups of potential targets for neuroprotection. The ischemic cascade has formed the basis for the initiation of pharmacologic neuroprotective

Table 30–3 Agents Studied as Pharmacologic Neuroprotectants During Cardiac Surgery

Agent	Study Reference
Thiopental	46
Propofol	143
Acadesine	148
Aprotinin	152, 153
Nimodipine	158–160
GM_1 ganglioside	161
Dextromethorphan	163
Remacemide	163
Lidocaine	168
β-Blockers	170
Pegorgotein	172
C5 complement inhibitor (Pexelizumab)	174
Lexiphant (platelet-activating factor antagonist)	176
Clomethiazole	181
Ketamine	188

strategies in the setting of overt stroke and of cardiac surgery-related cerebral injury.

There are no pharmacologic therapies approved by the U.S. Food and Drug Administration or foreign regulatory agencies for the prevention or treatment of cardiac surgery–associated cerebral injury, despite numerous previous investigations of specific pharmacologic agents in this setting (Table 30–3). This has not stopped progress, however, with multiple clinical trials ongoing. The most relevant cardiac surgery pharmacologic neuroprotection strategies, past and present, are reviewed here.

THIOPENTAL

Thiopental was one of the first agents investigated as a potential neuroprotective agent for cardiac surgery. In a study by Nussmeier et al,[46] thiopental was administered (until electroencephalographic [EEG] isoelectricity was obtained) before cannulation and continued until separation from CPB. In this study, neurologic complications on postoperative day 10 were significantly reduced in the thiopental group versus controls. Based on the encouraging results of this trial, high-dose thiopental was frequently used for valvular and other open ventricular procedures. The mechanism of this effect related to the suppressive effects of barbiturates on cerebral metabolism. This mechanism, along with experimental data reporting the beneficial effects of the barbiturates,[139] made it a logical choice for cardiac surgery. However, results of additional investigations of the use of thiopental were not as positive. A study by Pascoe et al[140] and one by Zaidan et al[141] failed to support a beneficial effect of thiopental on neurologic outcome after cardiac surgery. These negative trials and the side effects of prolonged sedation with barbiturates served to quell the optimism for barbiturates. Retrospectively examining the initial Nussmeier study, the beneficial effects of the thiopental might not have been related to a direct neuroprotective effect but to an indirect effect on reducing emboli-containing CBF. The well-known cerebral vasoconstricting effects of thiopental (matching CBF with a barbiturate-induced reduction in $CMRO_2$) may have resulted in a reduction in embolic load to the brain during CPB and as a result, a beneficial effect on neurologic outcome. It has subsequently been shown that isoelectricity itself is not necessary to incur a neuroprotective benefit from barbiturates.[142] Evaluations of sub-isoelectric doses of thiopental have not been performed (see Chapter 9).

PROPOFOL

Propofol has effects similar to those of thiopental on $CMRO_2$ and CBF and has some antioxidant and calcium channel antagonist properties.[143] Along with supportive data from experimental cerebral ischemia studies,[144-146] propofol has been evaluated as a neuroprotectant in the setting of cardiac surgery. A prospective, randomized clinical trial was conducted to determine whether propofol-induced EEG burst suppression would reduce the incidence or severity of cerebral injury during valvular surgery.[147] In 109 of 215 patients randomized to receive burst-suppression doses of propofol, there was no beneficial effect on cognitive outcome at 2 months. The investigators concluded that EEG burst-suppression doses of propofol provided no neuroprotection during valvular cardiac surgery. No other studies in nonvalve cardiac surgery have assessed the effects of propofol on the brain.

ACADESINE

The adenosine-regulating agent, acadesine, was studied in the early 1990s with the aim of improving myocardial outcome; stroke was examined as a secondary outcome.[148] Compared with placebo, high- and low-dose infusions of acadesine resulted in a lower stroke rate ($p = 0.016$). Other adenosine-like agents have provided neuroprotection in preclinical experimental settings.[149,150] Despite this positive, albeit indirect, clinical data and supportive experimental data, no further clinical neuroprotection indication for acadesine has been pursued.[151]

APROTININ

Aprotinin is a nonspecific serine protease inhibitor that was first used in the 1950s for the treatment of pancreatitis. Its current indication in cardiac surgery is for the prevention of blood loss and transfusion (see Chapter 29). In a large, multicenter trial of aprotinin for primary or redo CABG and valvular surgery evaluating its blood loss–reducing effects, the high-dose aprotinin group also had a lower stroke rate compared with placebo ($p = 0.032$).[152,153] Similarly, Frumento et al[154] retrospectively examined patients at high risk for stroke (due to the presence of significant aortic atheroma), and those who received aprotinin had a significantly lower stroke rate. In a small ($n = 36$) study examining the effect of aprotinin on cognitive deficit after CABG surgery, the incidence of cognitive deficit was reduced in the aprotinin group (58%, aprotinin versus 94% placebo, $p = 0.01$).[155] However, the high rate in the placebo group, the small size of the study, and methodologic concerns limit the applicability of these results to broader populations.[156] Animal investigations in the setting of cerebral ischemia failed to show any direct benefit on functional or neurohistologic outcome after cerebral ischemia.[157]

There has been considerable investigation of the potential mechanism for aprotinin-derived neuroprotection. Initial enthusiasm focused on its anti-inflammatory effects potentially preventing some of the adverse inflammatory sequelae of cerebral ischemia. However, aprotinin may have beneficial effects independent of any direct neuroprotective effect through an indirect effect of modulating cerebral emboli. Brooker et al[32] identified the cardiotomy suction as a major source of cerebral emboli during CPB. By extrapolation, if a drug reduces the amount of particulate-containing blood returning from the operative field to the cardiotomy reservoir (by decreasing overall blood loss), cerebral emboli and the resulting neurologic consequences may also be decreased.

NIMODIPINE

Calcium plays a central role in propagating cerebral ischemic injury. For this reason, as well as a demonstrated beneficial effect of the calcium channel blocker nimodipine in subarachnoid hemorrhage and experimental cerebral ischemia, a randomized, double-blind, placebo-controlled, single-center trial was undertaken to assess the effect of nimodipine on neurologic, neuro-ophthalmologic, and neuropsychologic outcomes after valvular surgery.[158-160] The trial was not completed after safety concerns regarding an increased bleeding and death rate in the nimodipine group prompted an external review board to suspend the study after enrolling 150 of 400 patients planned to be studied. There was also no neuropsychologic deficit difference between the placebo or nimodipine groups at this interim review. As a result, the true effect of this drug or similar calcium trial blockers may never be fully known in this setting.

GM_1 GANGLIOSIDE

The monosialoganglioside, GM_1 ganglioside, has been investigated as a potential neuroprotectant during cardiac surgery.[161] In addition to the potential beneficial effects of this type of compound on preserving neuronal membranes, some data suggest that it has a potential beneficial effect on reducing excitatory amino acid transmission.[162] In a preliminary (but underpowered) cardiac surgery study, there was no beneficial effect demonstrated. However, the study authors used this pilot trial to describe useful statistical methodology needed to measure differences in neurocognitive outcome, thereby constituting a template for later trials. This trial highlights one of the biggest difficulties in this investigative field—the interpretation of negative but underpowered studies.

DEXTROMETHORPHAN

The *N*-methyl-D-aspartate (NMDA) receptor plays a major role in cerebral ischemic injury.[138] Although human stroke trials have been limited by distressing psychomimetic side effects, a wealth of experimental data points to NMDA receptor antagonists as being robust neuroprotective agents with a potential role in CPB-associated cerebral injury.[163] Dextromethorphan, known for its antitussive activity, has some nonspecific NMDA antagonistic properties. A small ($n = 12$) pilot study examined dextromethorphan in the setting of pediatric cardiac surgery using EEG and MRI end-points to determine a difference between treatment groups but saw no difference, probably because of the small size of the study.[164] There have been no other studies examining NMDA receptor antagonism in the setting of pediatric cardiac surgery.

REMACEMIDE

A second NMDA receptor antagonist that has been evaluated for neuroprotection during CABG surgery is remacemide. In a well-designed and well-executed study by Arrowsmith et al,[163] remacemide was given orally for 4 days before CABG. A neurocognitive battery was performed 1 week before and 8 weeks after CABG. A deficit was defined as a decrease in one standard deviation in 2 or more of the 12 tests within the neurocognitive battery. The patients were evaluated for their learning ability by subtracting the postoperative neurocognitive score from the preoperative score (formulating a Z score). Although there was no difference between groups with respect to the dichotomous outcome of cognitive deficit ($p = 0.6$), examination of a continuous measure of learning ability showed there was a beneficial cognitive effect in the patients who received remacemide ($p = 0.028$). Despite these apparently beneficial results, due to the length of time that it took to perform this single center trial, initial nonbeneficial preliminary results, and a prolonged period of data analysis and review for publication, this drug was not further pursued for this indication. It has, however, highlighted the potential utility of this class of drugs for this indication and ongoing investigations examining other NMDA receptor antagonists continue.[165-167]

LIDOCAINE

Intravenous lidocaine, because of its properties as a sodium channel blocking agent and potential anti-inflammatory effects, has been investigated as a neuroprotectant in cardiac surgery. In a study of 55 patients undergoing valvular surgery, a lidocaine infusion (in an antiarrhythmic dose of 1 mg/min) was begun preinduction and maintained for 48 hours after surgery.[168] Neurocognitive testing was performed preoperatively and 8 days, 2 months, and 6 months postoperatively. Compared with placebo, neurocognitive outcome 8 days after surgery was significantly better in the lidocaine group ($p = 0.025$). However, a much larger double-blind, randomized trial in cardiac surgery failed to replicate the finding.[169] Lidocaine cannot be recommended as a clinical neuroprotective agent in cardiac surgery.

β-BLOCKERS

Although the use of β-blockers in patients with cardiac disease has been predominantly directed toward the prevention of adverse myocardial events, in a study of neurologic outcomes after cardiac surgery, β-blockers were demonstrated to be associated with an improvement in neurologic outcome.[170] In this retrospective study of almost 3000 patients, stroke and encephalopathy were studied. Patients receiving β-blocker therapy had a significantly lower incidence of neurologic deficit versus those not receiving β-blockers. Although the reasons for this potential benefit are not clear, there are several potential reasons why β-blockers may be efficacious, including the modulation of cerebrovascular tone and CPB-related inflammatory events. Support for the potential neuroprotective effects from β-blockers has come from a study of carvedilol, which is known to have mixed adrenergic antagonist effects, as well as acting as an antioxidant and inhibitor of apoptosis[171] (see Chapter 10).

PEGORGOTEIN

The generation of ROS is a well-described pathophysiologic mechanism of ischemic reperfusion injury. Combined with the whole-body inflammatory response associated with CPB and its own generation of ROS, this mechanism has opened the field of neuroprotection and cardiac surgery to antioxidant therapies. Superoxide dismutase is involved in the catabolism of free radicals, and its mimetics have had beneficial results in the setting of experimental ischemia. Pegorgotein, a monomethyoxy-polyethyleneglycol covalently linked to superoxide dismutase, is protective against reperfusion-mediated cardiac and neuronal injury in animal studies.[172] One study was initiated to examine whether pegorgotein would be associated with a reduced number of neurocognitive deficits after cardiac surgery.[173] In this study of 67 patients undergoing primary elective CABG surgery (n = 22 to 23 in each of three groups: placebo, 200 IU/kg of pegorgotein, or 5000 IU/kg of pegorgotein), no difference in neurocognitive outcome was found.

C5 COMPLEMENT INHIBITOR: PEXELIZUMAB

The activation of complement is central to the inflammatory response seen as a response to CPB.[174] In a small (n = 18) study using a simple assessment of cognitive function, patients receiving an inhibitor to C5 (h5G1.1-scFv, pexelizumab), demonstrated fewer visuospatial deficits at hospital discharge.[175] Additional large-scale (phase III) investigations of this compound to more adequately delineate any potential longer-term neuroprotective effects from this drug in this setting have been performed. Mathew et al[175] assessed pexelizumab in a 914-patient study aimed at evaluating its effect on myocardial outcome and mortality. A secondary end-point of neurocognitive outcome demonstrated that pexelizumab, although having no effect on global measures of cognition, appeared to have a benefit with respect to the visuospatial domain.

PLATELET-ACTIVATING FACTOR ANTAGONIST: LEXIPHANT

Platelet-activating factor (PAF) antagonists have demonstrated neuroprotective effects in experimental models of cerebral ischemia.[176] PAF is thought to modulate postischemic injury by the release of cerebral cellular lipids and free fatty acids that may result in cellular injury and cerebral edema.[177] In an investigation of 150 cardiac surgery patients receiving placebo or one of two different doses of lexiphant, no protective effects were found in neurocognitive outcome 3 months after cardiac surgery. This study was significantly underpowered, which is a recurring and troublesome feature of many studies in this field.[178]

CLOMETHIAZOLE

Clomethiazole, which enhances γ-aminobutyric acid (GABA) receptor activity, has been evaluated in CABG surgery. GABA has repeatedly been shown to be an important neuroprotective target in focal and global experimental ischemia.[179,180] However, in a relatively large, well-designed, and well-conducted study, it failed to decrease neurocognitive dysfunction after cardiac surgery.[181]

STEROIDS

Corticosteroids have long been considered as potential cerebroprotective agents in part due to their ability to reduce the inflammatory response. Inflammation is considered an important factor in propagating ischemia mediated brain injury.[182,183] However, with the exception of spinal cord injury,[184] they have never been demonstrated to possess any significant clinical neuroprotective properties. Furthermore, the administration of steroids has actually worsened cerebral outcome in a large trial (n = 10,000). The Corticosteroid Randomization after Significant Head Injury (CRASH) trial demonstrated an increased relative risk of death (1.18 [95% CI, 1.09–1.27]; p = 0.0001) in those receiving high-dose steroids within 8 hours of injury.[185,186] Part of their lack of effect may result from the hyperglycemia that generally follows their administration. Hyperglycemia in animal models and several human studies of cerebral injury has been associated with worsened neurologic outcome.[126,187] The administration of steroids with the intent of conferring some degree of neuroprotection during cardiac surgery cannot be recommended.

KETAMINE

The neuroprotective effects of $S(+)$-ketamine, a frequently used anesthetic that is also an NMDA-receptor antagonist, was evaluated in a small (n = 106) study enrolling cardiac surgery patients.[188] The incidence of neurocognitive dysfunction 10 weeks after surgery trended toward being lower in the ketamine group (20% for ketamine versus 25% for controls, p = 0.54), but because the study was underpowered, it was not a significant change. There are no other published trials evaluating ketamine for neuroprotection in this setting.

DEXANABINOL

Dexanabinol is another synthetic noncompetitive NMDA receptor antagonist. It also possesses some tumor necrosis factor-α antagonist properties. Its neuroprotective potential has been evaluated extensively in various models of cerebral ischemia.[189,190] It is being evaluated in early-phase clinical trials of CABG for the prevention of neurocognitive dysfunction.

ACUTE RENAL INJURY

Despite the recognition, made more than 40 years ago, of acute renal injury as a serious complication of cardiac surgery,[191-194] postoperative renal dysfunction persists today as an independent predictor of postoperative mortality.[195] Even during procedures where there is no evidence of acute renal injury as reflected by a rise in serum creatinine, more subtle markers have demonstrated renal tubular injury.[196] Patients with increasing degrees of acute renal injury after cardiac surgery require disproportionately more short- and long-term resources and have increasingly poorer outcome and greater costs.[192,197-200] The association of acute renal dysfunction with mortality and major morbidity may reflect its role as a marker of, rather than as a contributor to, the insult of cardiac surgery; however, there is compelling evidence that acute renal injury itself also contributes directly to adverse outcome.[201-206] Accumulation of "uremic toxins" and release of inflammatory mediators from the injured kidney also appear to contribute significantly to remote organ dysfunction[201,202] (see Chapter 36).

Evidence that acute renal injury itself has a primary role in influencing outcome, even when dialysis is avoided, continues to fuel the search for therapeutic strategies directed to protect the kidney. This search has been somewhat disappointing, with no single effective therapeutic intervention available; given the diversity of the mechanisms by which the kidney can be damaged, this is not surprising. Difficulties in accurately assessing renal dysfunction during the perioperative period have made research in this area challenging. For example, reported renal end-points have varied from significant change in creatinine from baseline (despite still being an otherwise normal range) to including only those with dialysis-dependent renal failure.

Incidence and Significance

Definitions and the incidence of renal injury vary, with approximately 8% to 15% of cardiac surgery patients sustaining a moderate renal injury (defined by a peak rise in the serum creatinine level of more than 1.0 mg/dL) and 1% to 5% requiring dialysis.[192,197,207] Each type of cardiac surgical procedure has its own specific pattern of renal injury.[208-210] As a result, surgical procedure type is an important variable when examining the incidence and severity of postoperative acute renal injury. For example, elevation of the serum creatinine level, a common marker of acute renal injury, typically peaks on the second day after CABG with CPB and, in most cases, returns to baseline by postoperative day 4 or 5.[211,212] Evidence of minor, arguably clinically insignificant, renal injury (representing a reduced renal reserve) can be demonstrated in almost all patients.[196,213]

The most common intermediate end-points used to reflect kidney injury include the greatest reduction in creatinine clearance and the peak rise in serum creatinine after surgery; these markers correlate with renal functional impairment (i.e., reductions in glomerular filtration rate) and have been validated by strong associations with overall outcome in numerous large series of cardiac surgical patients.[192,193,197,207,214-217] Markers other than creatinine have been used less frequently to assess renal risk and in smaller populations. Subtle proximal tubular injury impairs reuptake of small proteins; elevated urine levels of these proteins are sometimes used as markers of renal dysfunction (e.g., α_1- and β_2-microglobulin, albumin, lysozyme, ribonuclease, retinol binding protein).[218] However, the use of antifibrinolytic drugs (commonly used in cardiac surgery) interact with these transport mechanisms, making tubular proteinuria an unreliable marker whenever they are used.[219] In contrast, urine protein markers that reflect tubular cell leakage (e.g., *N*-acetyl-β-D-glucosaminidase [NAG]) are not affected by antifibrinolytic use.[218]

In-hospital mortality rates for CABG range from less than 1% for patients with subclinical renal injury to 20% for those with moderate renal injury, and rates exceed 60% when dialysis is required.[192,193,197,207,214-216] Survivors of significant postoperative renal injury have higher in-hospital resource use. In addition to the direct relationship with renal injury of morbidity, mortality, and perioperative cost, intensive care unit stays are up to five to six times longer and overall hospital length of stay increases approximately three times.[197,198] In-hospital costs for CABG patients with escalating degrees of renal dysfunction ranged from $32,680 for uncomplicated cases to $100,593 if dialysis was required.[198] Patients with renal dysfunction are also more likely to be discharged to an extended-care facility, with its own associated costs. Accelerated long-term decline of renal function after cardiac surgery may lead to later end-stage renal disease.[220-225]

Risk Factors for Surgery-Related Acute Renal Injury

Numerous studies have characterized risk factors for nephropathy after cardiac surgery (Table 30–4). Preoperative variables are most useful for renal risk stratification with intraoperative and postoperative issues contributing to overall clinical management decisions. A considerable debate with regard to renal risk surrounds the relationship between preexisting renal impairment and renal injury after cardiac surgery. Up to 20% of individuals presenting for CABG have preexisting renal disease[226,227]; these patients are at especially high risk for postoperative complications.[227-229] Patients with preexisting renal dysfunction are clearly at greater risk for major complications,[227-229] including the requirement for dialysis,[192,193,197,207,216] but they *are not* at greater risk for renal injury relative to their baseline renal function.[200,214,215] However, equivalent renal injury for a patient with preoperative renal dysfunction does result in a greater rise in serum creatinine due to the nonlinear relationship between reductions in glomerular filtration rate (GFR) and creatinine rise. Even small amounts of additional renal impairment may lead to dialysis for a surgical patient with severe renal disease at baseline. Although the absolute risk of acute renal injury is not greater for those with preoperative renal dysfunction, these patients do have the most to gain from any effective renoprotective strategy.

Despite an increasing understanding of perioperative renal dysfunction, known risk factors account for only one third of the observed variability in creatinine rise after cardiac surgery.

Table 30–4 Risk Factors for Renal Injury

Important Factors	Probably Not Important
Preoperative Factors	
Advanced age	Gender
Obesity	Renal artery stenosis
Preexisting renal insufficiency	
Diabetes	
Hyperglycemia	
Hypertension	
Ascending aortic atherosclerosis	
Peripheral vascular disease	
IABP	
COPD	
Loop diuretic therapy	
Steroid therapy	
Nephrotoxins (radiocontrast dye, cyclosporin, aminoglycosides, cephalosporins, NSAIDs)	
Genetic variants	
Intraoperative Factors	
Loop diuretic (increased risk)	Low-dose dopamine
Transfusion	Mannitol
Hyperglycemia	Antifibrinolytic therapy (lysine analog or aprotinin)
Procedure type (CABG < valve < HCA)	
Emergency procedure	
Reoperation	
IABP	
CPB management	CPB management
Extended CPB duration	Hypothermia
Hemodilution	Blood pressure management
Postoperative Factors	
Low cardiac output	
Excessive inotrope use	
Prolonged ventilation	
Transfusion	
Sepsis	
CMV infection	

CABG = coronary artery bypass graft surgery; CPB = cardiopulmonary bypass; CMV = controlled mechanical ventilation; COPD = chronic obstructive pulmonary disease; HCA = hypothermic circulatory arrest; IABP = intra-aortic balloon pump; NSAIDs = nonsteroidal anti-inflammatory drugs.

Procedure-related risk factors include emergent and redo operations,[207,230] valvular procedures,[207,215,216] and operations requiring a period of circulatory arrest[230] or extended durations of CPB.[192,197,231,232] Infection and sepsis,[230,231,233] atrial fibrillation,[234] and indicators of low cardiac output states, including need for inotropic agents and insertion of an intra-aortic balloon pump (IABP) during surgery, also have been associated with renal impairment.[197,207,214,230,231,235]

Preoperative demographic risk factors identified include advanced age,[193,197,214,216,230] increased body weight,[192] African American ethnicity,[192,236] hypertension,[207,217] peripheral or carotid atherosclerotic disease,[207] diabetes or preoperative hyperglycemia,[192,197,217] reduced left ventricular function and obstructive pulmonary disease.[192,207,230-232] Other preoperative markers of renal risk have been identified that increase understanding of the pathophysiology of this disorder. Davilla-Roman et al[237] described a relationship between ascending aortic atherosclerosis, assessed using intraoperative epiaortic scanning and postoperative renal dysfunction. Sreeram et al[238] also found a direct relationship between arterial emboli count and aortic renal injury after cardiac procedures. However, Conlon et al[239] could not demonstrate a relationship between increasing degrees of renal artery stenosis and postoperative renal dysfunction.

A genetic predisposition to postoperative acute renal injury related to polymorphisms of the apolipoprotein E (ApoE) gene also exists; there is a lower risk of acute renal injury in patients with an ApoE4 phenotype compared with the E3 and E2 phenotypes.[240] Our investigative group also identified an interaction between ApoE phenotype and the degree of renal dysfunction after CABG related to a given severity of ascending aortic atherosclerosis.[241] Wider genetic profiling has identified several other SNPs in interaction with ethnic background that are partly responsible for cardiac surgery-related nephropathy, adding credence to the hypothesis that much of the variability in postoperative acute renal injury may result from genetic influences and may offer clues about potential renoprotective targets.[242] Six percent of whites possess a combination of variants associated with more than a doubling of serum creatinine levels, and similar variant combinations may also be important in African Americans.

Causes and Pathophysiology of Renal Injury

Ischemia-Reperfusion Injury

A long-standing assumption regarding the causes and pathophysiology of renal dysfunction after cardiac surgery is that hypoperfusion with resulting renal ischemia plays a central role (Box 30–2). This assumption is supported by an understanding of the precarious oxygen supply and demand physiology of the renal medulla (Fig. 30–5), particularly during CPB,[243] as well as the responsiveness of experimental acute renal injury to improved renal perfusion. However, clinically applied techniques directed at improving perfusion (e.g., including low-dose dopamine) and reducing oxygen consumption (e.g., loop diuretics) have been uniformly unsuccessful in cardiac surgical patients and in most other settings.[244-247] Other risk factors supporting the ischemia-reperfusion hypothesis of acute renal injury and nephropathy after cardiac surgery include episodes of circulatory arrest[230] and perioperative low cardiac output states,[214,230,231] and prolonged bypass duration.[192,197,231,232]

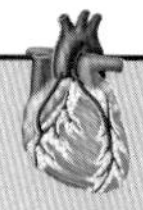

BOX 30–2 ***Causes of Renal Injury During Cardiopulmonary Bypass***

- Emboli
- Renal ischemia
- Reperfusion injury
- Pigments
- Contrast agents

Ischemia-reperfusion injury involves not only damage to the glomerulus and tubules, but also to the renal microvasculature.[248] Vessel damage by local oxidants, cytokines and proteases affects basic properties of vascular function; increased resting tone reduces the GFR, autoregulatory responsiveness is altered, and sensitivity to vasoconstrictor stimuli heightened, increasing vulnerability of the kidney to further injury. After ischemia-reperfusion injury, the kidney may be particularly susceptible to toxins that insult the renal vasculature, such as nonsteroidal anti-inflammatory agents, radiocontrast media, and cyclosporine. Additional factors that may contribute to renal injury in patients with low output states after cardiac surgery include interventions, such as the use of inotropic agents, and IABP use that may themselves contribute to renal injury though other pathophysiologies (discussed later).

Despite the initial, albeit superficial, argument for ischemia causing renal injury, lack of success with strategies aimed at improving renal blood flow and reducing ischemia, combined with accumulating evidence that nephropathy after cardiac surgery possesses characteristics of multiple types of acute renal injury, has resulted in a expansion in the understanding of its increasingly complex pathophysiology.

Contrast-Associated Nephropathy

Intravenous contrast is known to have nephrotoxic effects. Because most cardiac surgical patients have exposure to contrast in the preoperative period, it is logical to assume this may be a factor in cardiac surgery–related renal injury. Contrast-associated nephropathy (CAN) is usually heralded by a significant rise in serum creatinine within 5 days after intravascular contrast injection and occurs in approximately 2% to 7% of patients.[249,250] The pathophysiology is primarily results from vasoconstriction and direct renal tubular cell injury. Those at greatest risk typically have preprocedure renal impairment.[251] In a study of 27 CABG patients, Garwood et al[252] found indicators of tubular injury to be elevated in those presenting for surgery within 5 days of cardiac catheterization relative to those further separated from an intravenous contrast injection.

Use of low-osmolar contrast media and aggressive prestudy hydration have significantly reduced the risk of CAN for patients with diabetic nephropathy and other causes of chronic renal disease. Complicating the issue of CAN, a small but significant number of patients is believed to sustain a coincident atheroembolic renal injury during coronary angiography, making it difficult to ascertain the respective relative contributions to injury.[253,254] A common practice is to delay elective cardiac surgery if CAN has been diagnosed. Although little has been studied regarding the contribution of CAN to nephropathy after cardiac surgery, this pathophysiology must be considered for emergent cardiovascular surgical

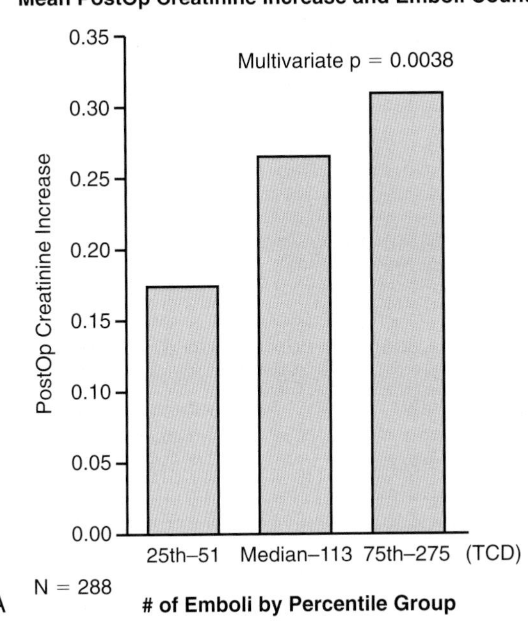

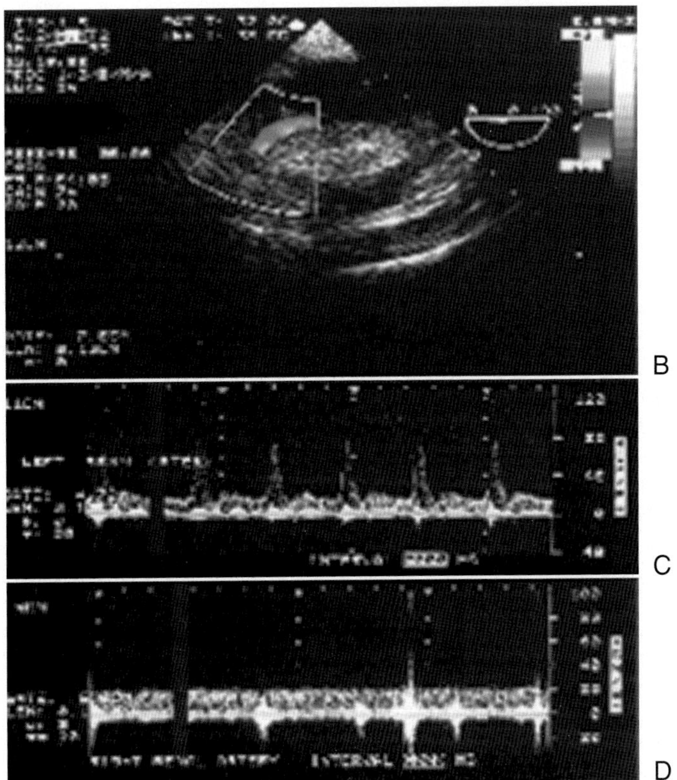

Figure 30–5 *(A)* Intraoperative arterial emboli counts, as estimated by transcranial Doppler scanning of the middle cerebral artery, are directly associated with a rise in the serum level of creatinine after coronary artery bypass surgery. *(B)* Intraoperative renal monitoring for emboli is possible by TEE imaging of the left renal artery. *(C)* Pulsed-wave Doppler renal artery monitoring before bypass demonstrates pulsatile flow and no evidence of emboli. *(D)* Doppler signals during bypass reveal nonpulsatile flow with intermittent emboli. See also Color Plates. (*A*, adapted from Sreeram GM, Grocott HP, White WD, et al: Transcranial Doppler emboli count predicts rise in creatinine after coronary artery bypass graft surgery. J Cardiothorac Vasc Anesth 18:548, 2004.)

patients, particularly those transferred directly from a cardiac catheterization laboratory for a surgical procedure.

Norepinephrine-Induced Nephropathy

Autonomic innervation of the kidney is important to the normal regulation of renal blood flow. Catecholamine-related effects include renal vasoconstriction, mediated through α_1-adrenergic receptors and dopaminergic and α_2-adrenergic agonist effects that mediate renal vasodilation. In animal models, high-dose infusions of norepinephrine, administered for even short periods, precipitate reproducible, long-lasting, severe reductions in the GFR.[255,256] In animals, α_1-mediated effects have shifted the autoregulatory threshold for renal perfusion 20 to 30 mm Hg higher.[257] This may partially explain the clinical observation that renal blood flow during CPB in humans does not appear to be autoregulated.[258] However, studies of renal blood flow autoregulation portray a complex picture that may be oversimplified by these observations.[259] There are numerous sources of α_1-adrenergic agonism during cardiac surgery, including the stress response to CPB,[260,261] and the use of exogenous vasopressors and inotropic agents. To distinguish between the adverse renal effects of α_1-adrenergic agents and nephropathy associated with the conditions they are used to treat is difficult. Whatever the exact nature of the relationship, use of inotropic agents is an independent predictor of nephropathy after cardiac surgery.[214,230,231]

Embolism Nephropathy

Embolic phenomena are common during cardiac procedures. Due to the organization of renal vasculature,[262] embolic arterial obstruction is poorly compensated for by collateral flow and affects related regions of cortex and medulla, resulting in wedge-shaped infarcts. The composition of these emboli varies considerably but includes atheroma, thrombi, lipid, air, and other particulate emboli.

Nephropathy related to dislodgement of atherosclerotic plaque is well described in settings other than cardiovascular surgery, and there is considerable evidence that it occurs in cardiac surgery.[263] Blauth et al[264] reported high rates of atheroembolism to one or more major organs in a study that included 221 autopsies after cardiac surgery; 10.4% of subjects had renal emboli. These authors also observed that organ-specific emboli were more common in those with a premortem history of dysfunction, and that severity of atherosclerosis of the ascending aorta was highly correlated with the overall likelihood of emboli.[264,265] Using an intra-aortic filter device deployed just before cross-clamp release, Reichenspurner et al[82] observed macroscopic atheromatous debris in the filter in 30 (39%) of 77 cardiac surgery patients. In a cadaveric study, Tierney et al[266] examined the effects of IABP counterpulsation on diseased aortas and concluded that ischemic complications were caused by interactions between the balloon and aortic wall during repeated inflation-deflation cycles, involving plaque disruption and embolus formation. Several later studies have found IABP use to be independently associated with renal impairment after CABG.[230,235] Using epiaortic ultrasonographic assessment of aortic atherosclerotic plaque and transcranial Doppler emboli counts, higher emboli counts in CABG patients with increased ascending aortic plaque scores and greater postoperative renal injury were correlated.[44,238] All evidence suggests that manipulation of diseased aortic regions during surgery can result in liberation of atheromatous material and downstream embolism[267]; this phenomenon is likely to be a common occurrence during most types of adult cardiovascular surgery[268] and is probably an important and in some cases dominant contributor to nephropathy after cardiovascular surgery.[269,270]

In addition to atheromatous emboli, thrombotic and lipid-containing emboli have been implicated in renal injury. Despite the increasing use of perioperative anticoagulant therapies in cardiovascular surgery patients, concern persists regarding the potential for perioperative thromboembolism and microthrombi.[271] In the study by Reichenspurner et al,[82] the use of intra-aortic filtration identified, in addition to atheromatous material, macroscopic platelet fibrin debris in 21% of patients and thrombus in 14% on filter removal. Lipid emboli have been identified as the cause of the SCADs observed in the brain after cardiac surgery.[36,272] Scavenged blood from the chest cavity, contaminated by sternal bone marrow, is thought to be the major source of these lipid emboli. Deal et al[273] reported renal SCADs. Observing the effect of lipid droplets on renal cortical vessels in an animal model, they identified vessel obstruction, spasm, steal, and even reversal of blood flow. These investigators advocate strategies to reduce or eliminate the return of lipid emboli to the circulation and have documented differences between scavenging strategies (e.g., cell savers) and perfusion technologies in their efficient clearance of these particles.[274] The overall value of reducing lipid microemboli to the kidney during cardiac surgery has not been studied sufficiently to speculate on the significance of this issue with regard to nephropathy after cardiac surgery.

Gaseous emboli also must be considered. Although massive air embolism is a catastrophic complication of cardiac surgery, the significance of commonly seen microbubbles and larger bubbles, particularly after open-chamber cardiac procedures, is less clearly known. Sreeram et al[238] described a relationship between transcranial Doppler–detected emboli and renal dysfunction manifested by increases in postoperative creatinine (Fig. 30–6).

Systemic Inflammatory Response Syndrome and Infection

Many cardiac surgery patients meet the criteria for systemic inflammatory response syndrome (SIRS) in the early postoperative period (see Chapter 8). Acute renal injury is a major consequence of SIRS.[275] Considerable evidence exists to suggest that the pathophysiology of renal injury related to SIRS involves microcirculatory-related ischemia mediated by endotoxemia and elevated levels of inflammatory cytokines. Systemic[276,277] and local renal[278,279] inflammatory responses are observed after cardiac surgery. In addition to inflammation initiated as a result of the blood-foreign surface interactions during CPB, endotoxin is a potent trigger and probably plays an important role in the inflammatory response of the kidney during cardiac surgery.[280,281] In a study of 461 cardiac surgical patients, low preoperative immunity to endotoxin, reflected by IgM EndoCAb levels less than 80 MU, was associated with a significantly greater occurrence of nephropathy after cardiac surgery.[282]

Infectious agents may cause or complicate acute renal injury in many settings.[283] When postoperative infection is present, up to a threefold increase in acute renal injury after otherwise uncomplicated CABG has been documented.[208]

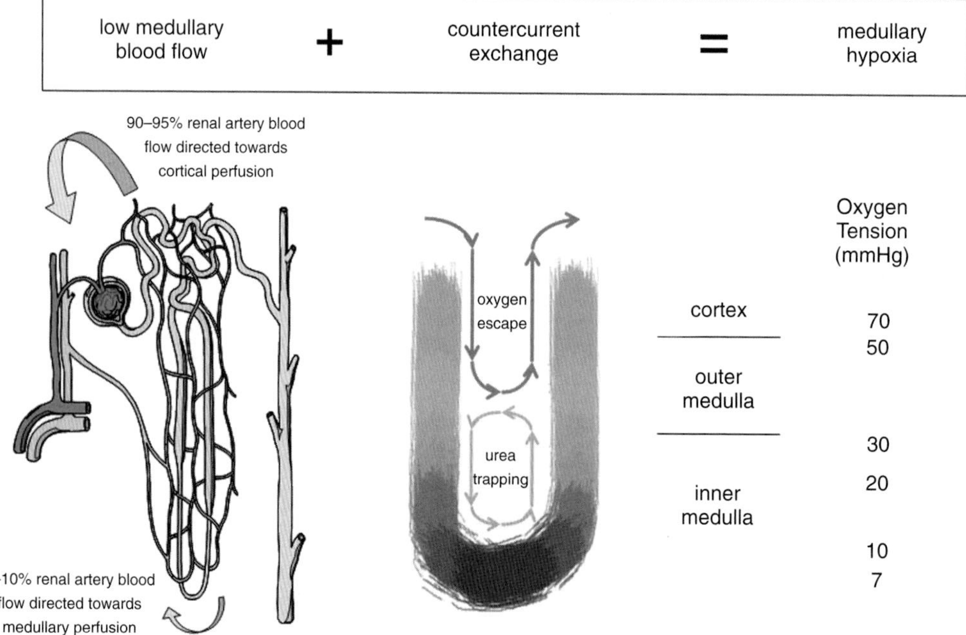

Figure 30–6 Normally sluggish blood flow in the renal medulla facilitates the countercurrent exchange mechanism that maintains the medullary urea gradient necessary for water reabsorption. However, this characteristic of the renal microcirculation also permits an oxygen diffusion shunt to occur, and combined with metabolic demands from active tubular reabsorption, it contributes to the precarious physiology of renal perfusion, including low medullary Po_2, also known as medullary hypoxia (7 to 10 mm Hg). Medullary hypoxia is exaggerated by hypovolemia or hemorrhage because reduced medullary blood flow, increased countercurrent exchange, and increased tubular solute reabsorption are associated with these conditions. See also Color Plates.

Even for patients whose only notable postoperative complication was a urinary tract infection, a study found a twofold increase in acute renal injury relative to uncomplicated patients.[208] A diagnosis of postoperative sepsis complicating cardiac surgery significantly increases renal risk.[230,231] Preexisting cytomegalovirus infection may further predispose postoperative cardiac patients with infectious complications to acute renal failure.[233]

Drug-Related Nephropathy

Several agent-specific nephrotoxicities are relevant to cardiac surgery. Cephalosporin-related renal injury to the proximal renal tubule has been reported.[284] Aminoglycoside antibiotics also have a potent nephrotoxic effect.[285] Nonsteroidal anti-inflammatory drug nephrotoxicity is thought to be related to renal vasoconstriction from inhibition of locally synthesized endogenous renal vasodilator prostaglandins.[286] Cyclosporin is well known for its long-term effects on renal function but can also cause acute renal injury.[287]

Concern continues regarding the use of antifibrinolytic agents during cardiac surgery. Benign proximal tubule effects of lysine analog agents cause "tubular proteinuria" in cardiac surgery patients[219]; however, no change in the incidence of acute renal injury has been documented in longitudinal studies examining institutional rates of renal injury before and after periods of ε-aminocaproic acid use.[288] Study of the renal consequences of epsilon aminocaproic acid use during cardiac surgery has been complicated by its apparently benign effects on renal reuptake of small proteins.[219] Aprotinin also interacts with the proximal renal tubule and is thought to saturate tubular transport mechanisms, resulting in tubular proteinuria.[219,289] Although aprotinin has been implicated in the presence of renal platelet-fibrin thrombi and postoperative renal dysfunction after hypothermic circulatory arrest,[290] this was likely confounded by inadequate anticoagulation, as other studies have not confirmed this observation with more adequate degrees of anticoagulation.[291,292] No link was identified in a review of controlled trials evaluating the relationship of aprotinin and renal failure.[293]

Pigment Nephropathy: Hemoglobinuria and Myoglobinuria

Severe intravascular hemolysis leading to release of hemoglobin in amounts sufficient to exceed the absorptive capacity of circulating haptoglobin and the normal renal metabolic reserve can lead to hemoglobinuria and acute renal injury. Myoglobinuria is seen in several situations, including as a consequence of crush syndrome related to major limb injuries.[294] It is thought that the mechanisms underlying myoglobin and hemoglobin-related acute renal injury are related.[295] The deterioration in kidney function appears to be the result of a combination of renal vasoconstriction, direct cytotoxicity, and tubular obstruction by casts.[296]

Although free hemoglobin is often seen in the urine during and after cardiac surgery, particularly after prolonged CPB, the significance of hemoglobinuria as a contributor to nephropathy after cardiac surgery is unknown. Myoglobinuria can occur after femoral artery cannulation for CPB or IABP insertion if ipsilateral leg ischemia develops. Myoglobinuric acute renal failure has been reported after cardiac surgery with femoral artery cannulation, particularly in children.[297,298] However, it is not clear that femoral artery cannulation is a concern for most patients. McCreath et al[299] found no difference in peak fractional creatinine level rise between port-access mitral valve surgery patients performed with femoral compared with ascending aortic arterial cannulation sites.

Strategies for Renal Protection

Cardiopulmonary Bypass Management

Basic issues in the management of CPB that relate to the kidney involve the balance between oxygen supply and oxygen demand, particularly to the renal medulla. Perfusion pressure (i.e., MAP during CPB) and oxygen-carrying capacity (as related to hemodilution and transfusion) address the supply issues, with the use of hypothermia being directed at modulating renal oxygen demand.

Profound hypothermia is a highly effective component of the protective strategy used during renal transplantation. Mild hypothermia during CPB would therefore seem to be a logical component of a perioperative renal protective strategy.[300] However, three separate studies have not found any protective benefit of mild hypothermia during CPB.[301-303] In the largest study, including 298 elective CABG patients who were randomly assigned to normothermic (35.5° to 36.5°C) or hypothermic (28° to 30°C) CPB, there was no association between normothermic (as compared with hypothermic) bypass and increased renal dysfunction after cardiac surgery.[303]

Studies addressing the role of CPB perfusion pressure have not been able to demonstrate an association with nephropathy after cardiac surgery.[193,236,304,305] Low perfusion pressure during CPB typically is not associated with low flow. It should be differentiated from the hypoperfusion with hemorrhagic shock or low cardiac output states that are associated with acute renal injury. In the largest study, 1404 CABG patients in a retrospective, multivariable analysis, using minute-to-minute MAP data to generate a degree-duration integral index of MAP below 50 mm Hg, demonstrated no relationship between low MAP during CPB and nephropathy after cardiac surgery[306] (see Chapter 28).

Moderate hemodilution is thought to reduce the risk of kidney injury during heart surgery through blood viscosity–related improvement in regional blood flow.[307,308] However, the practice of extreme hemodilution (hematocrit < 20%) during CPB has been linked to adverse renal outcome after cardiac surgery.[309-311] Accounting for perfusion pressure, in the same study of 1404 CABG patients,[306] an independent association was found between lowest hematocrit during CPB and postoperative creatinine rise. In a subsequent multivariable analysis, accounting for blood transfusion, the lowest hematocrit during CPB remained significantly associated with postoperative creatinine rise. Because blood transfusion was also independently associated with creatinine rise in this study, guidelines for an optimal CPB hematocrit target that include the potential risk of transfusion are difficult to define. In a prospective, randomized study including three different target hematocrit values during CPB, no major differences in postoperative renal dysfunction were observed.[312] Renal oxygen demand resulting from increased active transport of solutes (e.g., electrolytes, glucose) also may be important (discussed later).

Pharmacologic Intervention

Dopamine. Mesenteric dopamine$_1$ (D_1) receptor agonists increase renal blood flow, decrease renal vascular resistance, and enhance natriuresis and diuresis. Despite the absence of clinical evidence of renoprotection, this rationale has been used to justify the use of low-dose ("renal-dose") dopamine (<5 μg/kg/min) for decades. However, numerous double-blind, randomized studies in several surgical and nonsurgical settings have failed to demonstrate any renal benefits.[313-315] Dopamine in cardiac surgery is not benign and concerns have been raised regarding documented impairment of hepatosplanchnic metabolism despite an increase in regional perfusion[316] and increased postoperative arrhythmias.[317] Despite the lack of benefit and accumulating concerns regarding the use of low-dose dopamine,[318] continued use of this agent for renoprotection is prevalent (see Chapters 10, 31, and 33).

FENOLDOPAM

Fenoldopam mesylate, a derivative of benzazepine, is a selective D_1-receptor agonist. Although first approved as an antihypertensive agent, fenoldopam has shown promise in the prevention of contrast-induced nephropathy.[319-321] There is, however, very little in the way of randomized, controlled studies to evaluate the agent as a therapy for postoperative renal dysfunction. In one prospective, randomized study involving 160 patients with preoperative renal dysfunction, improved renal function with fenoldopam versus placebo was reported after cardiac surgery; however, no long-term benefit was evaluated.[322] Other prospective, randomized, double-blind studies enrolling patients with established postoperative renal injury have proved inconclusive or even indicated possible adverse outcomes in diabetic patients.[323] More systematic study is needed before this agent can be recommended for renoprotection in cardiac surgery.

DIURETIC AGENTS

Diuretics increase urine generation by reducing reuptake of tubular contents. This can be achieved by numerous mechanisms, including inhibiting active mechanisms that lead to solute reuptake (e.g., loop diuretics), altering the osmotic gradient in the tubular contents to favor solute remaining in the tubule (e.g., mannitol), or hormonal influences that affect the balance of activities of the tubule to increase urine generation (e.g., atrial natriuretic peptide). The general renoprotective principle of diuretic agents is that increasing tubular solute flow through injured renal tubules will maintain tubular patency, avoiding some of the adverse consequences of tubular obstruction, including oliguria or anuria and possibly the need for dialysis. Other agent-specific properties (e.g., antioxidant effects, reduced active transport) have also been proposed to have beneficial effects in the setting of ischemic renal injury. However, reduced solute transport in one segment of the renal tubule results in obligate increased solute load and oxygen demand in downstream tubular segments.

Loop diuretics, such as furosemide, produce renal cortical vasodilation and inhibit reabsorptive transport in the medullary thick ascending limb, causing more solute to remain in the renal tubule and increasing urine generation. In animal models, administration of furosemide and other loop diuretics has been shown to raise oxygen levels in the renal medulla,[324] presumably by reducing oxygen consumption by tubular active transport, but it also results in distal tubular hypertrophy.[325] In experimental models, loop diuretics have provided protection from renal tubular damage after ischemia-reperfusion and nephrotoxic injuries.[326-328] In contrast to evidence from animal experiments, several clinical studies have shown no benefit and possibly even harm from perioperative diuretic therapy in cardiac surgery patients.[329-332] In a double-blind, randomized, controlled trial comparing infusions of furosemide, low-dose dopamine, or placebo administered during and for 48 hours after surgery in 126 cardiac surgery patients, Lassnigg et al[333] found no benefit of dopamine and a greater postoperative rise in serum creatinine in the group receiving furosemide. Although they may facilitate avoidance of dialysis in responsive patients by maintaining fluid balance in selected patients, there is insufficient evidence to support the routine use of loop diuretics as specific renoprotective agents. However, in situations of severe hemoglobinuria, they may facilitate urine production and tubular clearance of this nephrotoxin.

Mannitol, an osmotic diuretic, has been evaluated in several studies of cardiac surgical patients.[301,334,335] Although an increased diuresis has been documented, very few studies have carefully assessed postoperative renal dysfunction in these patients. In an animal model of thoracic aortic clamping, mannitol did not provide evidence of improved renal function after unclamping.[336] In addition to the lack of beneficial effect on the kidney, several studies have identified a nephrotoxic potential of high-dose mannitol, especially in patients with preexisting renal insufficiency.[337]

Atrial Natriuretic Peptide. Atrial natriuretic peptide (ANP, Anaritide), a hormone synthesized by the cardiac atria, increases the glomerular filtration rate by constricting efferent arterioles and dilating afferent arterioles. ANP improves glomerular filtration, urinary output, and renal histopathology in experimental models of acute renal dysfunction. In a small (n = 14), randomized, double-blind clinical trial in patients suffering from impending acute renal failure after cardiac surgery, ANP demonstrated a reduced incidence of acute renal failure requiring dialysis.[338] In a separate randomized, placebo-controlled, double-blind study of 24 patients after heart transplantation, an ANP infusion of 40 ng/kg/min for 6 days did not reduce the need for dialysis, but it was associated with a reduced duration of hemofiltration and frequency of hemodialysis compared with the placebo group.[339]

***N*-acetylcysteine.** *N*-acetylcysteine is an antioxidant that enhances the endogenous glutathione scavenging system and has shown promise as a renoprotective agent by attenuating intravenous contrast-induced nephropathy. Although several studies have demonstrated evidence of renoprotection, two meta-analyses concluded that research on *N*-acetylcysteine and the incidence of contrast nephropathy are too inconsistent to warrant any definitive conclusion on efficacy or a recommendation for its routine use.[340,341] Only preliminary data are available on the role of *N*-acetylcysteine as a renoprotective agent in surgical patients. A study comparing *N*-acetylcysteine with mannitol or placebo in 30 abdominal aortic surgery patients suggested benefit.[342] However, a prospective, double-blind, placebo-controlled investigation comparing *N*-acetylcysteine with placebo in 128 patients did not demonstrate a benefit in reducing nephropathy after cardiac surgery.[343]

ASPIRIN

Although there is little evidence or rationale for the use of aspirin as a renoprotective agent, Mangano et al[344] reported that early reinstitution (<48 hours postoperatively) of aspirin therapy was associated with a 74% reduction in the incidence of renal failure (0.9% versus 3.4%, $p < 0.001$) after CABG. However, this type of association study makes it difficult to understand any cause and effect relationship that might be useful in making therapeutic recommendations.

OMAPATRILAT

Omapatrilat is a vasopeptidase inhibitor that preserves natriuretic peptides and inhibits the renin-angiotensin-aldosterone system by simultaneously inhibiting angiotensin-converting enzyme and neutral endopeptidase. In animal studies, it increased effective renal blood flow and single-nephron plasma flow associated with reduced glomerular arteriolar resistances.[345] Although omapatrilat has not been studied for renoprotection in humans undergoing cardiac surgery, studies of this agent as an antihypertensive therapy in large populations suggest that it has an acceptable safety profile.[346]

ADRENERGIC AGONISTS

The α_1- and α_2-adrenergic receptors in the kidney respectively modulate vasoconstrictor and vasodilatory effects. Agents that attenuate renal vasoconstriction may have potential as renal protective drugs because vasoconstriction most likely contributes to the pathophysiology of acute renal injury. Clonidine, an α_2-agonist, has been shown experimentally to inhibit renin release and cause a diuresis, and it has been evaluated in an experimental acute renal injury model confirming its potential as a renoprotective agent.[347-351] Similarly, two clinical trials have demonstrated some promise. A prospective, double-blind, randomized, placebo-controlled clinical trial evaluating preoperative clonidine in 48 CABG patients found that creatinine clearance decreased over the first postoperative night from 98 ± 18 (preoperatively) to 68 ± 19 mL/min ($p < 0.05$) in the placebo-treated group, but it remained unchanged in clonidine-treated patients (90 ± 19 [preoperatively] to 92 ± 17 mL/min, $p < 0.05$).[352] The effect was transient, however, with creatinine clearance in both groups being no different at postoperative day 3. Despite being positively supported in a second trial,[353] clonidine has not gained popular acceptance as a renoprotective agent.

CALCIUM CHANNEL BLOCKERS

The calcium channel blocker diltiazem has been evaluated as a renoprotective agent in cardiac surgery, with its ability to antagonize vasoconstricting signals that have been reported to exert beneficial effects in experimental models of toxic and ischemic acute renal failure.[354,355] Zanardo et al[356] randomized 35 cardiac surgery patients into three groups: control or 36-hour perioperative infusions of diltiazem at 1 or 2 mg/kg/min. They found that the GFR was significantly elevated in the high-dose diltiazem group compared with controls; tubular function, however, was not influenced by diltiazem.[356] In a prospective, randomized, placebo-controlled, double-blind study of a 24-hour perioperative diltiazem infusion in 24 cardiac surgery patients with preoperatively elevated serum creatinine levels, Bergman et al[357] found no differences in serum creatinine levels on postoperative days 1, 3, and 5 or at 3 weeks postoperatively. The overall inconclusive evidence from these trials requires reassessment in a larger study before diltiazem could be recommended in this setting.

ANGIOTENSIN-CONVERTING ENZYME INHIBITOR AND ANGIOTENSIN-1 RECEPTOR BLOCKERS

The renin-angiotensin system (RAS) mediates vasoconstriction and is important in the paracrine regulation of the renal microcirculation. Angiotensin-converting enzyme (ACE) inhibitor and angiotensin-1 receptor blocker (ARB) agents act by inhibiting steps in activation of the RAS. Although ACE inhibitor and ARB agents have demonstrated effects at slowing the progression of most chronic renal diseases,[358] their role in acute renal injury has not been well studied.[359,360] In a study of 249 aortic surgery patients, Cittanova et al[361] reported an increased risk of postoperative renal dysfunction in patients receiving preoperative ACE inhibitor therapy. Animal studies suggest that both groups of drugs have protective properties in experimental acute renal injury.[362] In a small (n = 18), double-blind, placebo-controlled clinical trial enrolling CABG patients, preservation of renal plasma flow intraoperatively in patients receiving the ACE inhibitor captopril relative to placebo was demonstrated.[363] A similar study assessing perioperative enalaprilat (an ARB) therapy in 14 CABG patients demonstrated greater renal plasma flow in the enalaprilat group before CPB and on postoperative day 7, as well as greater creatinine clearance after CPB[364] (see Chapter 10).

INSULIN

In experimental models of diabetes mellitus, renal oxygen consumption is elevated by approximately one third,[365] presumably reflecting the active transport demands imposed by increased glucose reuptake in the proximal convoluted tubule. Hyperglycemia is common during cardiac surgery; increased serum glucose before surgery and CPB have been independently associated with acute renal injury after surgery.[197,209] Although no rigorous clinical evaluation of insulin as a renoprotective therapy has been performed in humans, ischemia-reperfusion models in rats demonstrate significant benefit of insulin when it is given before (but not after) a renal insult.[366]

MYOCARDIAL INJURY

From the earliest days of modern cardiac surgery, perioperative myocardial dysfunction, with its associated morbidity and mortality, has been reported.[367] Evidence, including substantial subendocardial cellular necrosis, led to the conclusion that this injury resulted from an inadequate substrate supply to the metabolically active myocardium.[368] Optimizing myocardial protection during cardiac surgery involves several compromises inherent in allowing surgery to be performed in a relatively immobile, bloodless field while preserving postoperative myocardial function. The fundamental tenets of this protection center on the judicious use of hypothermia along with the induction and maintenance of chemically induced electromechanical diastolic cardiac arrest. Bigelow et al[369] were the first to describe the use of hypothermia for this purpose, and this was complemented by subsequent work by Melrose et al,[370] who first reported the electromechanical arrest of the heart by the administration of potassium-containing cardioplegia. Despite continued efforts directed at myocardial protection, it is clear that myocardial injury, although reduced, still remains a problem, and with it, the representative phenotype of myocardial dysfunction (see Chapters 1, 2, 5, 6, 10, 31, and 33).

Incidence and Significance of Myocardial Dysfunction after Cardiopulmonary Bypass

Unlike other organs at risk of damage during cardiac surgery, it is assumed, due to the very nature of the target of the operation being performed, that all patients having cardiac surgery suffer some degree of myocardial injury. Although the injury can be subclinical, represented only by otherwise asymptomatic elevations in cardiac enzymes (e.g., myocardial creatine kinase isoenzyme [CK-MB]), it frequently manifests more overtly. The degree to which these enzymes are released by injured myocardium, frequently to levels sufficiently high to satisfy criteria for myocardial infarction, have been related to perioperative outcome after cardiac surgery.[371-373] Chaitman et al[372] reported CK-MB results from the Guard During Ischemia Against Necrosis (GUARDIAN) trial in 11,950 patients with acute coronary syndromes or undergoing high-risk percutaneous intervention or CABG surgery. CK-MB values more than 10 times the upper limit of normal during the initial 48 hours after CABG were significantly associated with 6-month mortality ($p < 0.001$).[372]

Risk Factors for Myocardial Injury

With an increasingly sicker cohort of patients presenting for cardiac surgery,[374] many with acute ischemic syndromes (e.g., often with evolving myocardial infarction) or significant left ventricular dysfunction, the need has never been greater for optimizing myocardial protection to minimize the myocardial dysfunction consequent to aortic cross-clamping and cardioplegia.[375] The continued increase in cardiac transplantation and other complex surgeries in the heart failure patient has served to fuel the search for better myocardial protection strategies.

Pathophysiology of Myocardial Injury

Myocardial stunning represents the myocardial dysfunction that follows a brief ischemic event. It is differentiated from the reversible dysfunction associated with chronic ischemia, which is called *hibernation*.[376] Myocardial stunning typically resolves over the 48 to 72 hours after the ischemic event, and is frequently observed after aortic cross-clamping with cardioplegic arrest.[377,378] Important factors that contribute to stunning include not only the metabolic consequences of oxygen deprivation, but also the premorbid condition of the myocardium, reperfusion injury, acute alterations in signal transduction systems, and the effects of circulating inflammatory mediators (see Chapters 6, 8, 10, 27, 28, and 31).

The metabolic consequences of oxygen deprivation become apparent within seconds of coronary artery occlusion. With the rapid depletion of high-energy phosphates, accumulation of lactate and intracellular acidosis in the myocytes soon follows, with the subsequent development of contractile dysfunction. When myocyte ATP levels decline to a critical level, the subsequent inability to maintain electrolyte gradients requiring active transport (e.g., Na^+, K^+, Ca^{++}) leads to cellular edema, intracellular Ca^{++} overload, and loss of membrane integrity.

Predictably with the release of the aortic cross-clamp and the restoration of blood flow, myocardial reperfusion occurs. With reperfusion the paradox, represented by the balance of substrate delivery restoration needed for normal metabolism that also can serve as the substrate for injurious free radical production, becomes a significant issue for consideration. Reperfusion causes a rapid increase in free radical production within minutes, and it plays a major role initiating myocardial stunning. Bolli et al[379] identified the importance of this effect by demonstrating that antioxidants administered just before reperfusion significantly diminished myocardial stunning, an effect not observed if the same substance were introduced after reperfusion. Sun and colleagues[380,381] subsequently demonstrated the significance of the free radical effect by demonstrating that up to 80% of myocardial stunning could be avoided with an appropriately timed regimen of free radical scavengers.

Free radical insults during myocardial reperfusion result in the near immediate dysfunction of proteins involved in ion transport and excitation-contraction coupling, as well as injury to membranes through damage mediated through lipid peroxidation.[382] Free radical–mediated myocardial dysfunction is related to a myofilament defect manifest by an impairment in Ca^{++}-activated excitation-contraction coupling.[382] Although free radicals can directly injure these myofilament components, injury to other proteins related to ion transport and membrane integrity serve to increase intracellular calcium. Several mechanisms have been proposed to explain this impairment of myofilament function, although the most likely explanation includes physiologic down-regulation of excitation-contraction coupling in response to cellular Ca^{++} overload. The mechanisms underlying Ca^{++} overload are not well understood, but they are thought to involve free radical–related and free radical–independent abnormalities in Ca^{++} homeostasis. Whatever the cause, the rapid calcium influx during myocardial reperfusion can quickly overload the myocyte with Ca^{++}.[383] The importance of Ca^{++} overload is demonstrated by the substantial protection from reperfusion injury obtained by pretreatment with traditional Ca^{++} blocking agents.[384]

A free radical–independent mechanism for Ca^{++} overload involves activation of the Na^+/H^+ exchanger during reperfusion in an attempt by the cell to correct intracellular pH.[385] The resultant increase in intracellular Na^+ from activation of the Na^+/H^+ exchanger further activates the Na^+/Ca^{++} exchanger, increasing Ca^{++} influx.[386] Evidence for the activation of Na^+/H^+ exchangers being responsible for some of the harmful effects of reperfusion is shown by the benefits that Na^+/H^+ exchanger inhibitors have had on myocardial stunning with reductions in arrhythmias, improvement in systolic and diastolic function, and reductions in myocyte injury.[387] In addition to its role in Ca^{++} overload, activation of the Na^+/H^+ exchanger has been linked to increased phospholipase activity, generation of prostaglandins and other eicosanoids, and activation of platelets and neutrophils—all potentially injurious processes.[385,387]

In addition to free radical up-regulation, myocardial reperfusion associated with acute myocardial ischemic injury induces inflammation mediated by neutrophils and an array of humoral inflammatory components.[385,388,389] Several studies using novel neutrophil inhibitors have demonstrated a cardioprotective effect in models of myocardial stunning.[389,390] Prostaglandins are also generated during reperfusion. The adverse effects of prostaglandins appear to be synergistic with increases in intracellular calcium. The relationship of leukotriene and cytokine release to reperfusion injury is less clear.[385,388] Consistent with a role for prostaglandins in this injury is the demonstration that inhibition of prostaglandins by nonsteroidal anti-inflammatory agents can significantly diminish myocardial stunning.[391]

A potential additional mechanism for myocardial dysfunction specific to the setting of CPB relates to proposed acute alterations in β-adrenergic signal transduction.[392] Acute desensitization and down-regulation of myocardial β-adrenergic receptors during CPB has been demonstrated after cardiac surgery.[393,394] Although the role of the large elevations in circulating catecholamines seen with CPB on β-adrenergic malfunction is unclear, it has been proposed that an increased incidence of post-CPB low cardiac output states and reduced responsiveness to inotropic agents may in part be attributed to this effect.[261,395]

Myocardial Protection During Cardiac Surgery: Cardioplegia

Optimizing the metabolic state of the myocardium is fundamental to preserving its integrity. The major effects of temperature and functional activity (i.e., contractile and electrical work) on the metabolic rate of myocardium have been extensively described.[368,396,397] With the institution of CPB, the emptying of the heart significantly reduces contractile work and myocardial oxygen consumption ($M\dot{V}O_2$). Nullifying this cardiac work reduces the $M\dot{V}O_2$ by 30% to 60%. With subsequent reductions in temperature, the $M\dot{V}O_2$ further decreases, and with induction of cardiac arrest and hypothermia, 90% of the metabolic requirements of the heart can be reduced (Fig. 30–7). Temperature reductions diminish metabolic rate for all electromechanical states (i.e., beating or fibrillating) of the myocardium (Table 30–5) (see Chapter 28).

Although cardiac surgery on the empty beating heart or under conditions of hypothermic fibrillation (both with the support of CPB) is sometimes performed, aortic cross-clamping with cardioplegic arrest remains the most prevalent method of myocardial preservation (Box 30–3). Based on the principle of reducing metabolic requirements, the introduction of selective myocardial hypothermia and cardioplegia (i.e., diastolic arrest) marked a major clinical advance in myocardial protection.[398,399] With the various additives in cardioplegia solutions (designed to optimize the myocardium during arrest and attenuate reperfusion injury) and the use of warm cardioplegia, the idea of delivering metabolic substrates (as opposed to solely reducing metabolic requirements) is also commonplace. Several effective approaches to chemical cardioplegia are employed. The clinical success of a cardioplegia strategy may be judged by its ability to achieve and maintain prompt continuous arrest in all regions of the myocardium, early return of function after cross-clamp removal, and minimal inotropic requirements for successful separation from CPB. Composition, temperature, and route of delivery constitute the fundamentals of cardioplegia-derived myocardial protection.

Table 30–5 Influence of Temperature on Myocardial Oxygen Consumption for Different Work and Electrical Conditions

	Myocardial Oxygen Consumption (mL/100 mg/min)			
Cardiac Conditions	37°C	32°C	28°C	22°C
Beating, empty	5.5	5.0	4.0	2.9
Fibrillating, empty	6.5	3.8	3.0	2.0
K^+ cardioplegia	1.8	0.8	0.6	0.3
Beating, full	9.0	—	—	—

Data from references 368 and 396.

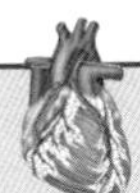

BOX 30–3 *Uses for Retrograde Cardioplegia*

- Along with anterograde cardioplegia
- In the presence of aortic insufficiency
- For aortic valve surgery
- To perfuse severely diseased coronary arteries

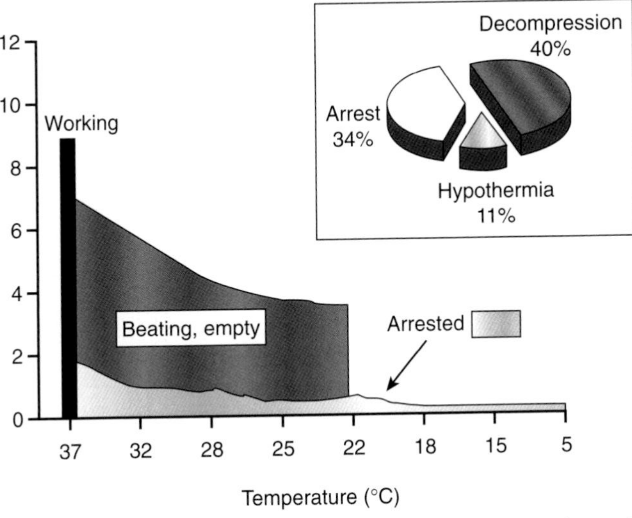

Figure 30–7 Myocardial oxygen uptake (reflecting oxygen demand) versus temperature. Compared with the oxygen uptake of a normally beating heart, eliminating cardiac work by venting the beating heart during bypass reduces oxygen demand by 30% to 60%. Arresting the heart reduces demands by another 50%, producing a total reduction of approximately 90%. Hypothermia extends the reductions in oxygen demand. (From Vinten-Johansen J, Thourani VH: Myocardial protection: An overview. J Extra Corpor Technol 32:38, 2000.)

Composition of Cardioplegia Solutions

The composition of the various cardioplegia solutions used during cardiac surgery varies as much between institutions as it does between individual surgeons. In very general terms, cardioplegia can be classified into blood-containing and non-blood-containing (i.e., crystalloid) solutions. Crystalloid cardioplegia has fallen out of favor, with blood cardioplegia in various combinations of temperatures and routes of delivery being the most used solution. However, even within the category of blood cardioplegia, the individual chemical constituents of the solution vary considerably with respect to the addition of numerous additives. Table 30–6 outlines the various additives to cardioplegia solutions along with their corresponding rationale for use. Although all cardioplegia solutions contain higher than physiologic levels of potassium, solutions used for the induction of diastolic arrest contain the highest concentrations of potassium as opposed to solutions used for the maintenance of cardioplegia. In addition to adjustment of electrolytes, manipulation of buffers (e.g., bicarbonate, tromethamine), osmotic agents (e.g., glucose, mannitol, potassium), and metabolic substrates (e.g., glucose, glutamate and aspartate) constitutes the commonest variations in cardioplegia content. Oxygenation of crystalloid cardioplegia before infusion is aimed at increasing aerobic

Table 30–6 **Strategies for the Reduction of Ischemic Injury with Cardioplegia**

Principle	Mechanism	Component
Reduce O_2 demand	Hypothermia Perfusion Topical/lavage Asystole	Blood, crystalloid, ice slush, lavage KCl, adenosine (?), hyperpolarizing agents
Substrate supply and use	Oxygen Glucose Amino acids Buffer acidosis Buffers Optimize metabolism	Blood, perfluorocarbons, crystalloid(?) Blood, glucose, citrate-phosphate-dextrose Glutamate, aspartate Hypothermia (Rosenthal factor), intermittent infusions Blood, tromethamine, histidine, bicarbonate, phosphate Warm induction (37°C), warm reperfusion
Reduce Ca^{++} overload	Hypocalcemia	Citrate, Ca^{++} channel blockers, K channel openers (?)
Reduce edema	Hyperosmolarity Moderate infusion pressure	Glucose, KCl, mannitol 50 mm Hg

From Vinten-Johansen J, Thourani VH: Myocardial protection: An overview. J Extra Corpor Technol 32:38, 2000.

metabolism, but the limited oxygen-carrying capacity of crystalloid makes a rapid decline in metabolic rate through immediate and sustained diastolic arrest critical to effective cardioprotection with this technique.

Blood cardioplegia has the potential advantage of delivering sufficient oxygen to ischemic myocardium to sustain basal metabolism or even augment high-energy phosphate stores, as well as possessing free radical scavenging properties.[400] The introduction of blood cardioplegia in the late 1970s followed recognition of the clinical utility of this technique.[401] Although low-risk cardiac surgical patients appear to do equally well with crystalloid or blood cardioplegic protection, evidence is compelling that more critically ill patients, including those with "energy-depleted" hearts (e.g., cardiogenic shock, acute myocardial infarction before CPB), have improved outcomes using blood cardioplegia.[402,403] Patients at high risk also appear to have better recovery employing a combination of antegrade and retrograde blood cardioplegia delivery, when compared with antegrade administration alone.[403]

Because an infusion of oxygenated blood cardioplegia is in many ways similar to myocardial reperfusion, it is not surprising that the composition of blood cardioplegia is based on reperfusate parameters known to minimize myocardial stunning.[404,405] These parameters include maintenance of Ca^{++} at 1.0 mEq/L (by chelating Ca^{++} from perfusate blood) to diminish myocyte Ca^{++} uptake; pH between 7.6 and 7.8 (the pH of water in the hypothermic temperature range used); osmolality between 340 and 360 mOsm to minimize edema-related myocardial dysfunction after reperfusion; and hyperkalemia between 10 and 25 mEq/L to safely sustain electromechanical arrest. To create blood cardioplegia with these characteristics, blood is mixed in a ratio of 4:1 with a prepared crystalloid solution.

Infusion of a single, warm (37°C) reperfusion dose of cardioplegia (so-called hot shot) containing metabolic substrates (i.e., glucose, glutamate, and aspartate) just before aortic cross-clamp removal is preferred by some clinicians. The rational for this is evidence that normothermia maximally enhances myocardial aerobic metabolism and recovery after an ischemic period. Although, some have advocated continuous infusion of hyperkalemic warm cardioplegia throughout the period of aortic cross-clamping,[406] this technique has not gained wide popularity for CABG because of the technical challenges of grafting vessels perfused in this way and the threat of ischemia to nonperfused (warm) myocardium during grafting.

Numerous other cardioplegia additives continue to be assessed involving various buffers, osmotic agents, metabolites, ATP and precursors, enzymes controlling ATP synthesis and catabolism, oxygen radical scavengers and antioxidants. Protection of myocardial β-adrenergic receptor function using intracoronary administration of esmolol appears to hold promise as an alternate cardioprotective method.[407] Alternative cardioplegia strategies potentially extending safe ischemic periods for heart transplantation to up to 24 hours are also being evaluated.[408-410]

Cardioplegia Temperature

The composition of cardioplegia solutions varies considerably; in contrast, myocardial temperature during cardioplegia is almost uniformly reduced to between 10° and 15°C or less by the infusion of refrigerated cardioplegia and external topical cooling with ice slush. However, the introduction of warm cardioplegia has challenged this once universally considered necessity of hypothermia for successful myocardial protection.[105] Although hypothermic cardioplegia is the most commonly used temperature, numerous investigations have examined tepid (27° to 30°C) and warm (37° to 38°C) temperature ranges for the administration of cardioplegia. Much of the work aimed at determining the optimum temperature of the cardioplegia solution centered on the fact that although hypothermia clearly offered some advantages to the myocardium in suppressing metabolism (particularly when intermittent cardioplegia was delivered), it may have some detrimental effects.

The deleterious effects of hypothermia include the increased risk of myocardial edema (through ion pump activity inhibition) and the impaired function of various membrane receptors on which some pharmacologic therapy depends (such as the various additives to the cardioplegia solutions). The other disadvantages of hypothermic cardioplegia, in addition to the production of the metabolic inhibition in the myocardium, are an increase in plasma viscosity and a decrease in red blood cell deformability.[106,397,411] As a result, investigations aimed at using warmer cardioplegia temperatures have been explored.[105,412] During the initial phase of cardioplegia delivery, hypothermic temperatures, in addition to inhibiting some of the needed drug-receptor interactions, fail to optimize the metabolic rate in the myocardium. Hypothermia results in a leftward shift in the oxygen hemoglobin dissociation curve, inhibiting the release of oxygen into tissues. The myocardium is relatively ischemic during this initial induction phase of cardioplegia, with the uptake of the oxygen to this tissue being low and, as a result, significant oxygen debt occurring.

The adverse effects of hypothermia spawned interest in using warm cardioplegia. With the warm induction of cardiac arrest, metabolic activity is maintained, ion exchanges through cellular membranes are maintained, intracellular acidosis occurring with hypothermia is eliminated, oxygen delivery is optimized by maintaining a near normal hemoglobin-oxygen dissociation curve, hypothermia-induced changes in viscosity and blood rheology are avoided, and red blood cell deformability and resulting flow through the myocardial microvasculature are maintained. The principal differences in cold versus warm cardioplegia result from the timing and route of delivery. If the myocardium is maintained at normothermic temperature, continuous cardioplegia must be delivered to adequately supply substrate to the metabolically active myocardium. In most cases, this is done using continuous retrograde cardioplegia (discussed later).

A compromise temperature (tepid, 27° to 30°C) has also been proposed.[412] Ikonomidis et al[412] compared outcomes for patients receiving warm, tepid, or cold cardioplegia. Although numerous differences were found between the various groups, the recovery of left ventricular stroke work at 1 and 4 hours after surgery was optimal in the tepid group. The researchers concluded that tepid cardioplegia provided better overall protection with superior functional recovery.[413] Hayashida et al[413] conducted a randomized trial comparing the effects of cold (9°C), tepid (29°C), and warm (37°C) cardioplegia in 42 patients undergoing CABG surgery. Overall, the investigators found that $M\dot{V}O_2$ and lactate production were greatest in the warm, intermediate in the tepid group, and least in the cold cardioplegia. However, early postoperative left ventricular function was optimized in the tepid cardioplegia group.[413]

Cardioplegia Delivery Routes

If using tepid or warm cardioplegia administration, the continuous administration of this cardioplegia needs to be ensured. Retrograde cardioplegia, where a cardioplegia catheter is introduced into the coronary sinus, allows for almost continuous cardioplegia administration. Retrograde delivery is also useful in settings where antegrade cardioplegia is problematic such as with severe aortic insufficiency or during aortic root or aortic valve surgery. It also allows the distribution of cardioplegia to areas of myocardium supplied by significantly stenosed coronary vessels. Retrograde cardioplegia has proved safe and effective for cardioplegia in patients with coronary artery disease and in those undergoing valve surgery.[414,415] With the administration of retrograde cardioplegia, certain provisos should be considered. The acceptable perfusion pressure to limit perivascular edema and hemorrhage needs to be limited to less than 40 mm Hg.[416]

Two trials added information about cardioplegia routes of delivery. The CABG patch trial[417] enrolled high-risk coronary artery disease patients with impaired left ventricular function and demonstrated the superiority of the combined antegrade and retrograde delivery of blood cardioplegia compared with antegrade cardioplegia alone. The limitation of this trial was that the antegrade group received crystalloid cardioplegia (as opposed to blood cardioplegia in the antegrade-retrograde group), raising questions about whether the differences in the groups were seen because of the route of administration or the constituents of the cardioplegia itself. A second trial failed to demonstrate any differences when the administration of intermittent antegrade cold blood cardioplegia was compared with a group receiving antegrade cold blood cardioplegia induction followed by retrograde cold blood maintenance valve surgery.[418] They did find that the antegrade-retrograde approach was technically more convenient, allowing for shorter aortic cross-clamp times.

Retrograde cardioplegia does have some limitations. Although the retrograde approach has been shown to effectively deliver cardioplegia adequately to the left ventricle, because of shunting and blood flowing into the atrium and ventricles by the thebesian veins (i.e., venae cordis minimae) and various arteriosinusoidal connections, the right ventricle and septum frequently receive inadequate delivery of cardioplegia. Difficulties with retrograde delivery can also occur if the coronary sinus catheter is placed beyond the great cardiac vein, or if anatomic variants occur which communicate with systemic veins, such as a persistent left superior vena cava.[416,419,420] Because retrograde cardioplegia is inefficient in producing arrest of the beating heart, induction of arrest with this technique must be achieved by a single antegrade infusion of cardioplegia before its institution.

Ischemic Preconditioning

Myocardial stunning during cardiac surgery is affected by several parameters. The preischemic state of the myocardium can influence the degree of stunning which follows an ischemic event. Ischemic preconditioning (IPC) is endogenous myocardial protection triggered by exposure to brief (5 to 15 minutes) ischemia. Ischemic preconditioning is a natural defense mechanism that permits the heart to better tolerate myocardial ischemia. Although brief ischemic episodes in themselves result in stunning, they also build up a temporary resistance to the adverse effects of subsequent more prolonged ischemia.[421,422] Ischemic preconditioning has been well described experimentally.[423-425] Several proposed mechanisms are responsible for IPC, including the activation of several myocardial G protein–coupled receptors, most notably A_1 adenosine and α_1-adrenergic receptors.[426] Protein kinase C (PKC) appears to be a key cellular mediator of IPC, in part through activation of ATP-sensitive potassium channels.[427]

Myocardial protection strategies continue to be an active area of investigation, including assessment of IPC. Attempts to induce IPC by brief ischemia or pharmacologic means before CPB have been assessed in human cardiac surgical patients. Sevoflurane, a frequently used volatile anesthetic, has been demonstrated to pharmacologically replicate IPC[428] (see Chapters 9 and 19). Administration of adenosine, before bypass or in cardioplegic solutions, has been studied as a pharmacologic means to induce IPC. It has been associated with reduced postoperative myocardial injury, reduced inotropic requirements, and improved myocardial recovery.[429,430] The potential for myocardial stunning after beating heart CABG without CPB (OPCAB) has not been fully assessed. Intermittent coronary occlusion before beating heart OPCAB to induce IPC, although unclear as to its effect, is also undergoing clinical assessment.[431]

GASTROINTESTINAL COMPLICATIONS

Incidence and Significance

Gastrointestinal complications after cardiac surgery, although occurring relatively infrequently (0.5% to 5.5%), portend a significantly increased incidence of overall adverse patient outcome. The variability in the reported incidence of gastrointestinal complications is partly a reflection of how they are defined and the variable patient and operative risk factors in the studied cohorts.[432-440] Although the most commonly considered gastrointestinal complications include pancreatitis gastrointestinal bleeding, cholecystitis, and bowel perforation or infarction, hyperbilirubinemia (total bilirubinemia > 3.0 mL/dL) has also been described as an important complication after cardiac surgery. In one of the largest prospective studies examining these complications after CPB, McSweeney et al[440] studied 2417 patients undergoing CABG (with or without concurrent intracardiac procedures) in a multicenter study in the United States. The overall incidence of gastrointestinal complications in this study was 5.5%, ranging from 3.7% for hyperbilirubinemia to 0.1% for major bowel perforation or infarction (Table 30–7).

In addition to their association with other morbid events, adverse gastrointestinal complications are significantly associated with increased mortality after cardiac surgery.[440-443] The average mortality among subtypes of gastrointestinal complications in the study by McSweeney was 19.6%, and in other reports, the mortality rate ranges from 13% to 87%, with an overall average mortality of 33%. Even the seemingly insignificant complication of having an increased laboratory measurement of total bilirubin was associated with an odds ratio of death of 6.6 in the McSweeney study, compared with a death odds ratio of 8.4 for all adverse gastrointestinal outcomes combined. Apart from the significant effect on mortality, the occurrence of an adverse gastrointestinal outcome also significantly increases the incidence of perioperative myocardial infarction, renal failure, and stroke, as well as significantly prolonging intensive care unit and hospital length of stay.[440]

Risk Factors

A long list of preoperative, intraoperative, and postoperative risk factors for gastrointestinal complications have been identified in a number of studies.[438,440,444-449] As many factors are associated with one another, it is only when these risk factors are examined in multivariable analyses that a more accurate understanding of what the most significant risk factors for visceral complications after cardiac surgery are. Table 30–8 represents the most consistently reported risk factors for gastrointestinal complications after cardiac surgery. Preoperatively, age (>75 years), history of congestive heart failure, presence of hyperbilirubinemia (>1.2 mg/dL), combined cardiac procedures (e.g., CABG plus valve), repeat cardiac operation, preoperative ejection fraction less than 40%, preoperative elevations in partial thromboplastin time, emergency operations; intraoperatively, prolonged CPB, use of TEE, and blood transfusion; and postoperatively, requirements for prolonged inotropic vasopressor support, IABP use for the treatment of low cardiac output; and prolonged ventilatory support are all risk factors. These factors identify patients at high risk, and they lend some credence to the overall pathophysiology and suspected causes of these adverse events. If there is a common link between all these risks, it is that many of these factors would be associated with impairment in oxygen delivery to the splanchnic bed.

Pathophysiology and Etiology

Impairments in splanchnic perfusion commonly occur during even the normal conduct of cardiac surgery. When this is superimposed on an already depressed preoperative cardiac output or is associated with prolonged postoperative low cardiac output, the impairment in splanchnic blood flow is further perpetuated. The systemic inflammatory response to CPB itself can be initiated by splanchnic hypoperfusion by means of translocation of endotoxin from the gut into the circulation. De novo splanchnic hypoperfusion can be a result of the humoral vasoactive substances that are released by inflammation remote from the gut.[450-452] Another etiologic factor for

Table 30–7 Adverse Gastrointestinal Outcomes

	No. of Patients	Percent of Patients with a Gastrointestinal Event (n = 133)	Percent of Total Patients (n = 2417)
Hyperbilirubinemia, total*	90	67.7	3.7
3.1–5.0 mg/dL	54	40.6	2.2
5.1–9.0 mg/dL	19	14.2	0.8
>9.0 (mg/dL)	17	12.8	0.7
Gastrointestinal bleeding	28	21.0	1.2
Pancreatitis	19	14.3	0.8
Cholecystitis	7	5.3	0.3
Bowel perforation	2	1.5	0.1
Bowel infarction	2	1.5	0.1

*Hyperbilirubinemia was defined as maximum total bilirubin after surgery of 3.0 mg/dL.

From McSweeney ME, Garwood S, Levin J, et al: Adverse gastrointestinal complications after cardiopulmonary bypass: Can outcome be predicted from preoperative risk factors? Anesth Analg 98:1610, 2004.

Table 30–8 **Commonly Identified Risk Factors for Visceral Complications after Cardiac Surgery**

Preoperative Risk Factors	Type of Cardiac Surgery	Cardiopulmonary Bypass Factors	Postoperative Risk Factors
Age	Emergency surgery	Duration of CPB	Low cardiac output, use of inotropes, vasopressors, or IABP
History of CHF or low EF	Reoperations	Cross-clamp duration	Reoperation for bleeding
Renal insufficiency	Valve or combined procedures		Loss of normal sinus rhythm
Peptic ulcer disease, chronic lung disease, recent acute myocardial infarction, diabetes mellitus, peripheral vascular disease, use of IABP*	Cardiac transplantation		Renal failure
			Ventilation > 24 hours ICU stay > 1 day Increased bilirubin or lactate level, mediastinitis*

*Less commonly mentioned risk factors.
CHF = congestive heart failure; CPB = cardiopulmonary bypass; EF = ejection fraction; IABP = intra-aortic balloon bump; ICU = intensive care unit.
From Hessel EA 2nd: Abdominal organ injury after cardiac surgery. Semin Cardiothorac Vasc Anesth 8:243, 2004.

gastrointestinal complications directly related to splanchnic hypoperfusion is atheroembolism. Several studies have directly attributed atheroembolism to splanchnic hypoperfusion and gut infarction.[444,448,453] Prolonged ventilator support is another etiologic factor for gastrointestinal complications. Several lines of investigation have described a relationship between prolonged ventilation and gastrointestinal adverse events; this likely results from a direct effect of positive pressure ventilation impairing cardiac output and subsequently splanchnic perfusion.[436,438,447,454] Lung volume reduction surgery and lung transplantation also produce (approximately 9%) gastrointestinal complications.[455,456]

Protecting the Gastrointestinal Tract during Cardiac Surgery

As with other aspects of organ protection, critical etiologic factors need to be addressed with specific targeted therapies (Box 30–4). Unfortunately, as with most other organ-protective strategies, the major limitation in making definitive recommendations is an overall lack of large, well-controlled, prospectively randomized studies to provide supportive data for any one particular technique. However, some recommendations can be made, and attention can be focused on a number of other less well-studied but potentially valid strategies.

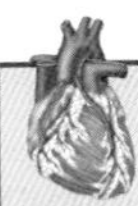

BOX 30–4 ***Protecting the Gastrointestinal Tract during Cardiopulmonary Bypass***

- Avoiding use of profound vasopressors
- Decontaminating the gastrointestinal tract
- Maintaining a high perfusion flow
- Reducing emboli-producing maneuvers

Cardiopulmonary Bypass Management

Because CPB itself has been shown to impair splanchnic blood flow, modifications in how it is conducted may have some salutary effects on gastrointestinal tract integrity. Several studies have focused on the issue of the relative importance of pressure versus flow during CPB, demonstrating that it is likely more beneficial to maintain an adequate bypass flow rate than only maintaining pressure during bypass.[457-459] The addition of significant vasoconstrictors to artificially maintain an adequate MAP in the presence of inadequate flow on CPB may lead to further compromise of splanchnic blood flow. Few definitive data offer guidance about pulsatility. Some studies have shown improvements with pulsatility by indirect measurements (i.e., gastric mucosal pHi), but no studies have found definitive differences in clinical outcomes. Similarly, the optimal bypass temperature to protect the gut is also unknown. Just as aggressive rewarming can be injurious to the brain,[52] there is some evidence that rewarming can cause increases in visceral metabolism, making any overshoot in temperature suspect by adversely altering the balance of gut oxygen consumption and delivery[460] (see Chapter 28).

Emboli Reduction

Whereas microembolization and macroembolization to the splanchnic bed clearly occur during CPB and possibly even during the postbypass period, there are few data to determine whether emboli reduction strategies can alter gastrointestinal outcome. Mythen et al[461] found a relationship between transcranial Doppler–detected emboli (used as a surrogate for overall microembolic load within the body) and adverse changes in gastric mucosal pHi. However, with respect to microembolization, a trial that used an intra-aortic filter to reduce atheroemboli failed to have any influence on the rate of gastrointestinal complications.[83] It remains prudent to avoid maneuvers (i.e., aortic cannulation and cross-clamping) in areas of high atheroma burden, which is an overall tenet of cardiac surgery for the prevention of all other complications.

Drugs

A range of vasoactive drugs has been used to enhance splanchnic blood flow during CPB. It is likely that most of these drugs, such as the phosphodiesterase III inhibitors, dobutamine, and other inotropic agents, maintain or enhance splanchnic blood flow not because of a direct effect on the vasculature but by the inherent enhancement in cardiac output. Dobutamine and dopamine have had a paradoxical detrimental effect on the splanchnic vasculature, with some evidence that they cause further mucosal ischemia.[462,463] Dopexamine has also been studied in a small group that did show an improvement in mucosal blood flow (using laser Doppler flowmetry), but there was no beneficial effect on gastric mucosal pHi.[464] An increasingly common drug in the setting of cardiac surgery is vasopressin. Although vasopressin can clearly augment systemic MAP, it does so at the cost of severe impairments to splanchnic blood flow.[465] Although there are always trade-offs when choosing which vasoactive agent to use, if having a very low MAP is going to be detrimental to other organ systems, the choice to use vasopressin should at least be made with the knowledge that it can have an adverse effect on splanchnic blood flow.

Selective Gastrointestinal Decontamination

Addressing the concept that gut translocation of endotoxin plays a role in inflammation and other organ injuries, one interesting therapy that has been tried in the setting of cardiac surgery involves the administration of oral antibiotics to selectively decontaminate the gastrointestinal tract preoperatively.[466] Although examined in a small ($n = 100$) study, a combination of oral polymyxin, tobramycin, and amphotericin preoperatively for 3 days reduced the degree of endotoxemia; it was not associated with a beneficial effect on patient outcomes. One possible explanation is that there is such an overwhelmingly large depot of gram-negative organisms in the gastrointestinal tract that the elimination of even a large population of these by oral antibiotics still leaves significant repositories of endotoxin in the gut. Killing these bacteria may in itself cause the release of the endotoxin, which can then be absorbed into the systemic circulation by impairment of mucosal blood flow inherent in the unphysiologic flow during CPB.

Off-Pump Cardiac Surgery

There is little evidence that the use of off-pump cardiac surgery is in any way beneficial to the gastrointestinal tract. Three retrospective studies[440,445,467] have shown no differences in gastrointestinal complications. One reason for this lack of apparent difference between on-pump and off-pump cardiac surgery may again be related to the common denominator of splanchnic perfusion. OPCAB surgery is fraught with hemodynamic compromise that may lead to prolonged periods of splanchnic hypoperfusion by itself or as a result of the concurrent administration of vasopressors to maintain normal hemodynamics during the frequent manipulations of the heart.

Anti-inflammatory Therapies

Although the inflammatory response to CPB has been implicated as an etiologic factor in gastrointestinal complications after cardiac surgery, few data are available to assess the ability of various anti-inflammatory therapies (e.g., corticosteroids, aprotinin, complement inhibitors) to reduce these types of complications.

LUNG INJURY DURING CARDIAC SURGERY

Incidence and Significance

Pulmonary dysfunction was one of the earliest recognized complications of cardiac surgery employing CPB.[468] However, as improvements in operative technique and CPB perfusion technologies occurred, the overall frequency and severity of this complication decreased. Juxtaposed to the improvements in cardiac surgery, which led to an overall reduction in complications, is an evolving patient population that now comprises a higher-risk group with a higher degree of pulmonary co-morbidities, increasing their risks of postoperative pulmonary dysfunction. With the advent of fast-track techniques,[469] even minor degrees of pulmonary dysfunction have reemerged as significant contributors to patient morbidity and the potential need for extended postoperative ventilation. As with most postoperative organ dysfunction, there is a range of dysfunction severity. Arguably, some degree of pulmonary dysfunction occurs in most patients after cardiac surgery; however, it manifests clinically only when the degree of dysfunction is particularly severe or the pulmonary reserve is significantly impaired. As a result, even minor CPB-related pulmonary dysfunction can cause significant problems in some patients.

The full range of reported pulmonary complications includes simple atelectasis, pleural effusions, pneumonia, cardiogenic pulmonary edema, pulmonary embolism, and various degrees of acute lung injury ranging from the mild to the most severe (i.e., acute respiratory distress syndrome [ARDS]). Although the final common pathway in all these forms of pulmonary dysfunction complications is the occurrence of hypoxemia, these complications vary widely in their incidence, cause, and clinical significance. Understanding that the changes that occur after CPB represent a continuum, it becomes necessary to define what constitutes pulmonary dysfunction and injury.

Definitions have varied. One commonly accepted definition that was used in a large study (n = 1461 patients) performed in the setting of cardiac surgery defined acute pulmonary dysfunction as a patient requiring mechanical ventilation with a PaO_2/FIO_2 ratio of less than 150, irrespective of positive end-expiratory pressure (PEEP), coupled with a chest radiograph that indicated the development of bilateral pulmonary infiltrates, assuming that other causes of a hypoxia such as pneumothorax could be excluded. Using this definition, approximately 12% of patients on admission to the cardiovascular intensive unit after cardiac surgery met the criteria of early acute pulmonary dysfunction.[470,471] Early acute pulmonary dysfunction should be differentiated from the more severe but less common ARDS that occurs in 1% to 2% of patients.[470,472] Although these two forms likely represent similar processes with different degrees of severity, ARDS differs particularly in its timing. The definition of ARDS in the setting of cardiac surgery generally requires the presence of refractory hypoxemia, diffuse bilateral pulmonary infiltrates on chest radiograph, the requirement for mechanical ventilation with an FIO_2 of more than 0.40, and most importantly, duration of at least 3 days (as opposed to on admission to the intensive care unit). This must be in the presence of a low pulmonary artery wedge pressure (PCWP < 18 mm Hg). In a study by Welsby et al[473] of 2609 consecutive adult cardiac surgery patients, 7.5% of whom had pulmonary complications, the overall mortality rate was 21%, with 64% of these patients remaining in the hospital more than 10 days. In another study, the most significantly affected patients (i.e., those with ARDS) had a mortality rate upward of 80%.[474] These significant morbidity and mortality rates lend credence to pulmonary complications remaining as significant and relevant a complication today as in the early days of cardiac surgery (see Chapter 34).

Atelectasis and pleural effusions are the most common pulmonary abnormalities seen after cardiac surgery presenting in more than 60% of patients.[475,476] Atelectasis is commonly attributed to a number of intraoperative and postoperative events. With the induction of general anesthesia, physical compression of the left lower lobe to aid exposure of the heart and facilitate in the dissection of the internal mammary artery and the apnea occurring during the conduct of CPB itself have been implicated.[477,478] Postoperative causes include the poor respiratory efforts by patients with impaired coughing, lack of deep inspirations, and pleural effusions.[479] Despite a high incidence of these radiographically recognized complications, the clinical significance is relatively low.[480,481]

Similar to atelectasis, pleural effusions, despite occurring commonly after cardiac surgery (40% to 50%), rarely cause significant perioperative morbidity. More common in the left thorax, likely as a consequence of the bleeding from the dissection of the internal mammary artery, other causes of pleural effusions relate to continued postoperative bleeding, pulmonary edema from cardiogenic and noncardiogenic causes, and pneumonia. Surgical trauma can also disrupt the normal pleural lymphatic flow through the thorax and, very rarely, direct damage to the internal thoracic duct can lead to the development of a chylothorax. Small effusions tend to resolve over time (a few months postoperatively) and rarely require any specific treatment. However, large pleural effusions that compromise the underlying lung respond well to thoracentesis and temporary chest tube placement, but if persistent, they may require decortication.

Pneumonia after cardiac surgery also has a variable incidence but a much higher significance to overall patient outcome. Reported rates of pneumonia range widely from 2% to 22%.[482-485] Pneumonia occurring early after cardiac surgery portends a very poor outcome, illustrated in one study by a mortality rate of 27%.[486] A number of factors increase the risk for postoperative pneumonia, including smoking, the presence of chronic obstructive pulmonary disease (COPD), other pulmonary complications requiring prolonged intubation, significant cardiac failure itself, and the transfusion of large volumes of blood products.

Risk Factors for Pulmonary Dysfunction

Rady et al[470] defined preoperative, operative, and postoperative variables that represent risk factors for early pulmonary dysfunction after cardiac surgery. Although it is not entirely clear whether any of these risk factors can be modified, identifying their presence raises the level of vigilance for the subsequent development of pulmonary dysfunction. The risk factors for the most severe ARDS syndrome as defined by Christenson et al[472] include hypertension, current smoking, emergency surgery, congestive heart failure (New York Heart Association class III and IV), low postoperative cardiac output, and a left ventricular ejection fraction of less than 40%.

Pathophysiology and Etiology

Studies have demonstrated bypass-induced changes in the mechanical properties (i.e., elastance or compliance and resistance) of the pulmonary apparatus (particularly the lung as opposed to the chest wall) and changes in pulmonary capillary permeability. Impairment in gas exchange has been demonstrated to be a result of atelectasis with concomitant overall loss of lung volume.[468,487-491] Most research has focused on the development of increases in pulmonary vascular permeability (leading to various degrees of pulmonary edema) as the principal cause of the impaired gas exchange that occurs during cardiac surgery and results in a high alveolar-arteriolar gradient (A-a DO_2).

The cause of pulmonary dysfunction and ARDS after cardiac surgery is complex but largely revolves around the CPB-induced systemic inflammatory response with its associated increase in pulmonary endothelial permeability.[277,492] A central etiologic theme is a significant up-regulation in the inflammation induced because of the interaction between the blood and foreign surfaces of the heart-lung machine or the inflammation related to the consequences of splanchnic hypoperfusion with the subsequent translocation of significant amounts of endotoxin into the circulation. Endotoxin is proinflammatory, and it has direct effects on the pulmonary vasculature.[493] Clinical studies have demonstrated an increase in circulating intracellular adhesion molecules after CPB in patients with development of acute lung injury.[494] Pathologic examination of the lungs of patients manifesting ARDS has shown extensive injury to the tissue, including swelling and necrosis of endothelial cells and type I and II pneumocytes.[495] In addition to CPB-mediated inflammation, inflammation mediated by endotoxemia has been reported. Several studies have identified transfusion of packed red blood cells (>4 units) as a risk factor for ARDS in the cardiac surgical patient.[496,497] Transfusion-related ARDS has been repeatedly recorded in noncardiac surgical settings.

Pulmonary Thromboembolism

Although not an injury to the lungs occurring as a direct result of CPB itself, deep vein thrombosis (DVT) and pulmonary embolism occur with regular frequency in the cardiac surgical population. The incidence of pulmonary embolism after cardiac surgery ranges from 0.3% to 9.5%, with a mortality rate approaching 20%.[271,498,499] The incidence of pulmonary embolism appears to be lower after valve surgery compared with CABG, which may be due to the anticoagulation that is started soon after valve surgery.[499,500]

The incidence of DVT is 17% to 46%, and most cases are asymptomatic.[271,499] The higher incidences were reported from series that used lower extremity ultrasound to examine entire populations.[271] DVT has been reported for the leg from which the saphenous vein grafts were harvested and for the contralateral leg.[499,501] In a study of post-CABG patients ($n = 270$) admitted to a rehabilitation unit who underwent lower extremity ultrasound examinations, DVT was detected in 17%, with two patients subsequently developing pulmonary emboli.[502] In a postmortem study in 147 patients after cardiac surgery, pulmonary embolism was the cause of death for 4%.

The recommendations for DVT prophylaxis in cardiac surgery are aspirin and elastic gradient compression stockings in patients who ambulate within 2 to 3 days after surgery and low-molecular-weight heparin and sequential compression stockings in nonambulatory patients.[271] These recommendations are based on a randomized trial in which prophylaxis with sequential pneumatic compression stockings provided no added protection against DVT in ambulating CABG patients treated with aspirin and elastic gradient-compression stockings.[503]

Pulmonary Protection

Ventilatory Strategies

Several studies have examined the use of continuous positive airway pressure (CPAP) during CPB as a means to minimize some of the changes in the A-a Do_2 gradient that occur after surgery. In a small study by Gilbert et al,[504] the effect of CPAP was examined in a randomized trial of 18 patients undergoing CABG surgery with CPB. Continuous positive airway pressure did not appear to make any difference with respect to changes in measured lung resistance and elastance. In a larger ($n = 61$) study by Berry et al,[505] CPAP did appear to have some transient beneficial effects on A-a Do_2; however, these minor differences dissipated 4 hours after bypass. Overall, it is unlikely that CPAP plays any major role in preventing or treating the pulmonary dysfunction that occurs in the setting of cardiac surgery.

The inspired oxygen content of the gases that the lungs see during the period of apnea during CPB may have an effect on the A-a Do_2 gradient, probably because of the enhanced effect of higher Fio_2 on the ability of atelectasis (so-called absorption atelectasis) on these gradients. With these findings in mind, it would be prudent to reduce the Fio_2 to room air levels during CPB. Several simple therapies can be introduced before separation from CPB, including adequate tracheobronchial toilet and the delivery of several vital capacity breaths that may reduce the amount of atelectasis that has occurred during bypass (Box 30–5).

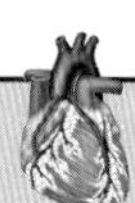

BOX 30–5 *Strategies to Protect the Lungs*

- Reduced Fio_2 during bypass
- Low postop tidal volume
- Steroid avoidance
- Aprotinin (?)
- Nitric oxide (?)

Ventilatory support of patients with acute lung injury (including ARDS) has undergone changes.[506,507] Although not studied specifically in the setting of cardiac surgery, a study authored by the Acute Respiratory Distress Syndrome network highlighted the avoidance of ventilator-associated pulmonary mechanotrauma.[507] Delivery of repeated large tidal volumes may damage the alveoli and other small lung structures, and these mechanical stresses may activate a pulmonary inflammatory response with a local release of cytokines, further enhancing injury to the lungs. As a result, these groups of investigators randomized patients to small (approximately 6 mL/kg) or traditional tidal volumes (12 mL/kg). They demonstrated in this multicenter trial that the low tidal volume ventilation strategy could reduce mortality in patients with ARDS by up to 25%. Although this has not been specifically studied in the setting of cardiac surgery, it would be prudent to employ this beneficial ventilator strategy in the cardiac surgical patient presenting with significant acute lung injury.

Pharmacologic Pulmonary Protection

STEROIDS

Anti-inflammatory therapies may play a role in moderating the effects of the more significant forms of pulmonary dysfunction that occur after cardiac surgery and that have inflammation as a central etiologic factor. However, with the exception of aprotinin and corticosteroids, few anti-inflammatory therapies are available for routine use. Corticosteroid use can reduce the amount of systemic inflammation as measured by circulating cytokines.[508-510] However, this has not been coupled with a reduction in pulmonary dysfunction. Chaney et al, in two separate studies,[133,511] demonstrated that methylprednisolone actually had a detrimental effect on post-CPB pulmonary function. Both studies demonstrated no improvement or worsening in lung compliance, shunt, A-a Do_2, and delays in extubation. It was speculated that the A-a Do_2 deterioration and delayed pulmonary extubation associated with steroid administration was attributable to steroid-induced sodium retention and vasodilation resulting in increased shunt and increased lung water content with pulmonary edema. Steroid administration led to significant hyperglycemia, which is difficult to treat during CPB.[511] In a similar study by Oliver et al[510] comparing placebo to steroids or hemofiltration, the steroid-treated patients had larger increases in postoperative A-a Do_2 gradients. Using a preset mechanical ventilation protocol to guide ventilation weaning, steroids again failed to reduce the time to tracheal extubation (519 ± 293 versus 618 ± 405 min, $p = 0.21$), confirming the findings of Chaney et al.[511]

APROTININ

The nonspecific serum protease inhibitor aprotinin is used selectively to reduce blood loss and transfusion after cardiac surgery, and it has reduced CPB-related systemic inflammation.[512-514] Aprotinin was first investigated for use in the setting of cardiac surgery as a means to protect the lungs from the whole-body inflammatory response initiated as a result of the contact activation of blood with the foreign surfaces of the CPB apparatus.[515,516] These studies serendipitously discovered aprotinin's salutary effect on preventing blood loss and transfusion in cardiac surgery.[517] After these studies, aprotinin was extensively evaluated for its blood loss and transfusion-sparing effects, with little further work focused on the pulmonary effects. Despite being a robust inhibitor of CPB-related inflammatory response, any ability to prevent the pulmonary complications of CPB has not yet been demonstrated.

NITRIC OXIDE

One of the consistent sequelae of pulmonary dysfunction is the development of elevated pulmonary vascular resistance (PVR) and pulmonary hypertension. As a result, several pulmonary vasodilators have been used, most notably inhaled nitric oxide, in an attempt to reduce the pulmonary artery pressures and with it the workload of the right ventricle.[518-520]

Nitric oxide has been used in cardiac surgery and in heart and lung transplantation as a selective pulmonary vasodilator.[521] However, there are no trials demonstrating any beneficial use for its prophylactic administration in the setting of cardiac surgery. Although it has statistically significantly reduced pulmonary artery pressures in cardiac surgery, it is unclear whether these reductions are reflected in improvements in overall outcome.

REFERENCES

1. Wolman RL, Nussmeier NA, Aggarwal A, et al: Cerebral injury after cardiac surgery: Identification of a group at extraordinary risk. Stroke 30:514, 1999
2. Newman MF, Kirchner JL, Phillips-Bute B, et al: Longitudinal assessment of neurocognitive function after coronary artery bypass surgery. N Engl J Med 344:395, 2001
3. Nussmeier N: Adverse neurologic events: Risks of intracardiac versus extracardiac surgery. J Cardiothorac Vasc Anesth 10:31, 1996
4. Roach GW, Kanchuger M, Mangano CM, et al: Adverse cerebral outcomes after coronary bypass surgery. N Engl J Med 335:1857, 1996
5. Newman MF, Grocott HP, Mathew JP, et al: Report of the substudy assessing the impact of neurocognitive function on quality of life 5 years after cardiac surgery. Stroke 32:2874, 2001
6. Arrowsmith JE, Grocott HP, Reves JG, et al: Central nervous system complications of cardiac surgery. Br J Anaesth 84:378, 2000
7. Newman MF, Croughwell ND, Blumenthal JA, et al: Effect of aging on cerebral autoregulation during cardiopulmonary bypass. Association with postoperative cognitive dysfunction. Circulation 90(Pt 2):II243, 1994
8. Aoki M, Nomura F, Stromski ME, et al: Effects of pH on brain energetics after hypothermic circulatory arrest. Ann Thorac Surg 55:1093, 1993
9. Cosgrove D, Loop F, Lytle B, et al: Primary myocardial revascularizations. J Thorac Cardiovasc Surg 88:673, 1984
10. Gardner TJ, Horneffer PJ, Gott VL, et al: Coronary artery bypass grafting in women. A ten-year perspective. Ann Surg 201:780, 1985
11. Newman M, Kramer D, Croughwell N, et al: Differential age effects of mean arterial pressure and rewarming on cognitive dysfunction after cardiac surgery. Anesth Analg 81:236, 1995
12. Tuman KJ, McCarthy RJ, Najafi H, et al: Differential effects of advanced age on neurologic and cardiac risks of coronary artery operations. J Thorac Cardiovasc Surg 104:1510, 1992
13. Hogue CW Jr, De Wet CJ, Schechtman KB, et al: The importance of prior stroke for the adjusted risk of neurologic injury after cardiac surgery for women and men. Anesthesiology 98:823, 2003
14. Hogue CW, Lillie R, Hershey T, et al: Gender influence on cognitive function after cardiac operation. Ann Thorac Surg 76:1119, 2003
15. Martin WR, Hashimoto SA: Stroke in coronary bypass surgery. Can J Neurol Sci 9:21, 1982
16. Sotaniemi K: Brain damage and neurological outcome after open-heart surgery. J Neurol Neurosurg Psychiatry 43:127, 1980
17. Turnipseed WD, Berkoff HA, Belzer FO: Postoperative stroke in cardiac and peripheral vascular disease. Ann Surg 192:365, 1980
18. Breslau PJ, Fell G, Ivey TD, et al: Carotid arterial disease in patients undergoing coronary artery bypass operations. J Thorac Cardiovasc Surg 82:765, 1981
19. Brener BJ, Brief DK, Alpert J, et al: The risk of stroke in patients with asymptomatic carotid stenosis undergoing cardiac surgery: A follow-up study. J Vasc Surg 5:269, 1987
20. Amarenco P, Duyckaerts C, Tzourio C, et al: The prevalence of ulcerated plaques in the aortic arch in patients with stroke. N Engl J Med 1992:221, 1992
21. Blauth CI, Cosgrove DM, Webb BW, et al: Atheroembolism from the ascending aorta. An emerging problem in cardiac surgery. J Thorac Cardiovasc Surg 103:1104, 1992
22. Blumenthal J, Mahanna E, Madden D, et al: Methodological issues in the assessment of neuropsychologic function after cardiac surgery. Ann Thorac Surg 59:1345, 1995
23. Borowicz L, Goldsborough M, Selenes O, et al: Neuropsychological changes after cardiac surgery: A critical review. J Cardiothorac Vasc Anesth 10:105, 1996
24. Branthwaite MA: Neurological damage related to open-heart surgery. A clinical survey. Thorax 27:748, 1972
25. Harris LS, Kennedy JH: Atheromatous cerebral embolism. A complication of surgery of the thoracic aorta. Ann Thorac Surg 4:319, 1967
26. Barbut D, Lo YW, Hartman GS, et al: Aortic atheroma is related to outcome but not numbers of emboli during coronary bypass. Ann Thorac Surg 64:454, 1997
27. Davila-Roman VG, Barzilai B, Wareing TH, et al: Intraoperative ultrasonographic evaluation of the ascending aorta in 100 consecutive patients undergoing cardiac surgery. Circulation 84(suppl):III-47, 1991
28. Hartman GS, Yao FS, Bruefach M 3rd, et al: Severity of aortic atheromatous disease diagnosed by transesophageal echocardiography predicts stroke and other outcomes associated with coronary artery surgery: A prospective study. Anesth Analg 83:701, 1996
29. Katz ES, Tunick PA, Rusinek H, et al: Protruding aortic atheromas predict stroke in elderly patients undergoing cardiopulmonary bypass: Experience with intraoperative transesophageal echocardiography. J Am Coll Cardiol 20:70, 1992
30. Cheng MA, Theard MA, Tempelhoff R: Intravenous agents and intraoperative neuroprotection. Beyond barbiturates. Crit Care Clin 13:185, 1997
31. Moody DM, Brown WR, Challa VR, et al: Brain microemboli associated with cardiopulmonary bypass: A histologic and magnetic resonance imaging study. Ann Thorac Surg 59:1304, 1995
32. Brooker RF, Brown WR, Moody DM, et al: Cardiotomy suction: A major source of brain lipid emboli during cardiopulmonary bypass. Ann Thorac Surg 65:1651, 1998
33. Aldea GS, Soltow LO, Chandler WL, et al: Limitation of thrombin generation, platelet activation, and inflammation by elimination of cardiotomy suction in patients undergoing coronary artery bypass grafting treated with heparin-bonded circuits. J Thorac Cardiovasc Surg 123:742, 2000
34. Borger MA, Peniston CM, Weisel RD, et al: Neuropsychologic impairment after coronary bypass surgery: Effect of gaseous microemboli during perfusionist interventions. J Thorac Cardiovasc Surg 121:743, 2001
35. Stump D, Rogers A, Hammon J, et al: Cerebral emboli and cognitive outcome after cardiac Surgery. J Cardiothorac Vasc Anesth 10:113, 1996
36. Stump DA, Kon NA, Rogers AT, et al: Emboli and neuropsychological outcome following cardiopulmonary bypass. Echocardiography 13:555, 1996
37. Pugsley W, Klinger L, Paschalis C, et al: Microemboli and cerebral impairment during cardiac surgery. Vasc Surg 24:34, 1990
38. Tegeler CH, Babikian VL, Gomez CR: Neurosonology. St. Louis, Mosby; 1996
39. Djaiani G, Fedorko L, Borger M, et al: Mild to moderate atheromatous disease of the thoracic aorta and new ischemic brain lesions after conventional coronary artery bypass graft surgery. Stroke 35:e356, 2004
40. Davila-Roman VG, Murphy SF, Nickerson NJ, et al: Atherosclerosis of the ascending aorta is an independent predictor of long-term neurologic events and mortality. J Am Coll Cardiol 33:1308, 1999
41. Amarenco P, Cohen A, Tzourio C, et al: Atherosclerotic disease of the aortic arch and the risk of ischemic stroke. N Engl J Med 331:1474, 1994
42. Bar-Yosef S, Mathew JP, Newman MF, et al: Prevention of cerebral hyperthermia during cardiac surgery by limiting on-bypass rewarming in combination with post-bypass body surface warming: A feasibility study. Ann Thorac Surg 99:641, 2004
43. Royse AG, Royse CF, Ajani AE, et al: Reduced neuropsychological dysfunction using epiaortic echocardiography and the exclusive Y graft. Ann Thorac Surg 69:1431, 2000
44. Mackensen GB, Ti LK, Phillips-Bute BG, et al: Cerebral embolization during cardiac surgery: Impact of aortic atheroma burden. Br J Anaesth 91:656, 2003
45. Grocott HP, Homi HM, Puskas F: Cognitive dysfunction after cardiac surgery: Revisiting etiology. Semin Cardiothorac Vasc Anesth 9:123, 2005
46. Nussmeier N, Arlund A, Slogoff S: Neuropsychiatric complications after cardiopulmonary bypass: Cerebral protection by a barbiturate. Anesthesiology 64:165, 1986
47. Newman M, Murkin J, Roach G, et al: Cerebral physiologic effects of burst suppression doses of propofol during nonpulsatile cardiopulmonary bypass. Anesth Analg 81:452, 1995
48. Gold JP, Charlson ME, Williams-Russo P, et al: Improvement of outcomes after coronary artery bypass. J Thorac Cardiovasc Surg 110:1302, 1995
49. Sillesen H, Nedergaard M, Schroeder T, et al: Middle cerebral artery occlusion in presence of low perfusion pressure increases infarct size in rats. Neurol Res 10:61, 1988
50. Mutch WA, Ryner LN, Kozlowski P, et al: Cerebral hypoxia during cardiopulmonary bypass: A magnetic resonance imaging study. Ann Thorac Surg 64:695, 1997
51. Bendszus M, Reents W, Franke D, et al: Brain damage after coronary artery bypass grafting. Arch Neurol 59:1090, 2002
52. Grigore AM, Grocott HP, Mathew JP, et al: The rewarming rate and increased peak temperature alter neurocognitive outcome after cardiac surgery. Anesth Analg 94:4, 2002

53. Grocott HP, Mackensen GB, Grigore AM, et al: Postoperative hyperthermia is associated with cognitive dysfunction after coronary artery bypass graft surgery. Stroke 33:537, 2002
54. Thong WY, Strickler AG, Li S, et al: Hyperthermia in the forty-eight hours after cardiopulmonary bypass. Anesth Analg 95:1489, 2002
55. Gerriets T, Stolz E, Walberer M, et al: Neuroprotective effects of MK-801 in different rat stroke models for permanent middle cerebral artery occlusion: Adverse effects of hypothalamic damage and strategies for its avoidance. Stroke 34:2234, 2003
56. Pintar T, Collard CD: The systemic inflammatory response to cardiopulmonary bypass. Anesthesiol Clin North Am 21:453, 2003
57. Hindman BJ, Moore SA, Cutkomp J, et al: Brain expression of inducible cyclooxygenase 2 messenger RNA in rats undergoing cardiopulmonary bypass. Anesthesiology 95:1380, 2001
58. Bogdanski R, Blobner M, Becker I, et al: Cerebral histopathology following portal venous infusion of bacteria in a chronic porcine model. Anesthesiology 93:793, 2000
59. Chamorro A: Role of inflammation in stroke and atherothrombosis. Cerebrovasc Dis 17(suppl 3):1, 2004
60. Mathew JP, Grocott HP, Phillips-Bute B, et al: Lower endotoxin immunity predicts increased cognitive dysfunction in elderly patients after cardiac surgery. Stroke 34:508, 2003
61. Hamilton-Davies C, Barclay GR, Cardigan RA, et al: Relationship between preoperative endotoxin immune status, gut perfusion, and outcome from cardiac valve replacement surgery. Chest 112:1189, 1997
62. Harris D, Oatridge A, Dob D, et al: Cerebral swelling after normothermic cardiopulmonary bypass. Anesthesiology 88:340, 1998
63. Harris D, Bailey S, Smith P, et al: Brain swelling in first hour after coronary artery bypass surgery. Lancet 342:586, 1993
64. Murkin JM, Stump DA: Conference on cardiac and vascular surgery: Neurobehavioral assessment, physiological monitoring and cerebral protective strategies. Ann Thorac Surg 70:1767, 2000
65. Kandel ER, Schwartz JH, Jessell TM: Principles of Neural Science, 3rd edition. Norwalk, CT, Appleton & Lange, 1991
66. Gillinov A, Davis E, Curtis W, et al: Cardiopulmonary bypass and the blood brain barrier. An experimental study. J Thorac Cardiovasc Surg 104:1110, 1992
67. Cavaglia M, Seshadri SG, Marchand JE, et al: Increased transcription factor expression and permeability of the blood brain barrier associated with cardiopulmonary bypass in lambs. Ann Thorac Surg 78:1418, 2004
68. Culley DJ, Baxter M, Yukhananov R, et al: The memory effects of general anesthesia persist for weeks in young and aged rats. Anesth Analg 96:1004, 2003
69. Jevtovic-Todorovic V, Beals J, Benshoff N, et al: Prolonged exposure to inhalational anesthetic nitrous oxide kills neurons in adult rat brain. Neuroscience 122:609, 2003
70. Futterer CD, Maurer MH, Schmitt A, et al: Alterations in rat brain proteins after desflurane anesthesia. Anesthesiology 100:302, 2004
71. Saunders A, Strittmatter W, Schmechel D, et al: Association of apolipoprotein E allele epsilon 4 with late-onset familial and sporadic Alzheimer's disease. Neurology 43:1467, 1993
72. Tardiff BE, Newman MF, Saunders AM, et al: Preliminary report of a genetic basis for cognitive decline after cardiac operations. Ann Thorac Surg 64:715, 1997
73. Gaynor JW, Gerdes M, Zackai EH, et al: Apolipoprotein E genotype and neurodevelopmental sequelae of infant cardiac surgery. J Thorac Cardiovasc Surg 126:1736, 2003
74. Barakat K, Kennon S, Hitman GA, et al: Interaction between smoking and the glycoprotein IIIa P1(A2) polymorphism in non-ST-elevation acute coronary syndromes. J Am Coll Cardiol 38:1639, 2001
75. Kenny D, Muckian C, Fitzgerald DJ, et al: Platelet glycoprotein Ib alpha receptor polymorphisms and recurrent ischaemic events in acute coronary syndrome patients. J Thromb Thrombolysis 13:13, 2002
76. Mathew JP, Rinder CS, Howe JG, et al: Platelet PlA2 polymorphism enhances risk of neurocognitive decline after cardiopulmonary bypass. Multicenter Study of Perioperative Ischemia (McSPI) Research Group. Ann Thorac Surg 71:663, 2001
77. Lapietra A, Grossi EA, Pua BB, et al: Assisted venous drainage presents the risk of undetected air microembolism. J Thorac Cardiovasc Surg 120:856, 2000
78. Webb WR, Harrison LH Jr, Helmcke FR, et al: Carbon dioxide field flooding minimizes residual intracardiac air after open heart operations. Ann Thorac Surg 64:1489, 1997
79. Svenarud P, Persson M, van der Linden J: Effect of CO2 insufflation on the number and behavior of air microemboli in open-heart surgery: A randomized clinical trial. Circulation 109:1127, 2004
80. Borger MA, Taylor RL, Weisel RD, et al: Decreased cerebral emboli during distal aortic arch cannulation: A randomized clinical trial. J Thorac Cardiovasc Surg 118:740, 1999
81. Cook DJ, Zehr KJ, Orszulak TA, et al: Profound reduction in brain embolization using an endoaortic baffle during bypass in swine. Ann Thorac Surg 73:198, 2002
82. Reichenspurner H, Navia JA, Berry G, et al: Particulate emboli capture by an intra-aortic filter device during cardiac surgery. J Thorac Cardiovasc Surg 119:233, 2000
83. Banbury MK, Kouchoukos NT, Allen KB, et al: Emboli capture using the Embol-X intraaortic filter in cardiac surgery: A multicentered randomized trial of 1,289 patients. Ann Thorac Surg 76:508, 2003
84. Eifert S, Reichenspurner H, Pfefferkorn T, et al: Neurological and neuropsychological examination and outcome after use of an intra-aortic filter device during cardiac surgery. Perfusion 18(suppl 1):55, 2003
85. Bar-Yosef S, Anders M, Mackensen GB, et al: Aortic atheroma burden and cognitive dysfunction after coronary artery bypass graft surgery. Ann Thorac Surg 78:1556, 2004
86. Cook DJ, Orszulak TA, Zehr KJ, et al: Effectiveness of the Cobra aortic catheter for dual-temperature management during adult cardiac surgery. J Thorac Cardiovasc Surg 125:378, 2003
87. Murkin J, Martzke J, Buchan A, et al: A randomized study of the influence of perfusion technique and pH management strategy in 316 patients undergoing coronary artery bypass surgery. J Thorac Cardiovasc Surg 110:349, 1995
88. Kawahara F, Kadoi Y, Saito S, et al: Balloon pump-induced pulsatile perfusion during cardiopulmonary bypass does not improve brain oxygenation. J Thorac Cardiovasc Surg 118:361, 1999
89. Mutch W, Lefevre G, Thiessen D, et al: Computer-controlled cardiopulmonary bypass increases jugular venous oxygen saturation during rewarming. Ann Thorac Surg 65:59, 1998
90. Patel RL, Turtle MR, Chambers DJ, et al: Alpha-stat acid-base regulation during cardiopulmonary bypass improves neuropsychologic outcome in patients undergoing coronary artery bypass grafting. J Thorac Cardiovasc Surg 111:1267, 1996
91. Duebener LF, Hagino I, Sakamoto T, et al: Effects of pH management during deep hypothermic bypass on cerebral microcirculation: Alpha-stat versus pH-stat. Circulation 106(suppl 1):I103, 2002
92. Laussen PC: Optimal blood gas management during deep hypothermic paediatric cardiac surgery: Alpha-stat is easy, but pH-stat may be preferable. Paediatr Anaesth 12:199, 2002
93. Michenfelder J, Milde J: The relationship among canine brain temperature, metabolism, and function during hypothermia. Anesthesiology 75:130, 1991
94. Busto R, Globus M, Dietrich W, et al: Effect of mild hypothermia on ischemia-induced release of neurotransmitters and free fatty acids in rat brain. Stroke 20:904, 1989
95. Bickler PE, Buck LT, Hansen BM: Effects of isoflurane and hypothermia on glutamate receptor-mediated calcium influx in brain slices. Anesthesiology 81:1461, 1994
96. Widmann R, Miyazawa T, Hossmann K: Protective effect of hypothermia on hippocampal injury after 30 minutes of forebrain ischemia in rats is mediated by postischemic recovery of protein synthesis. J Neurochem 61:200, 1993
97. Busto R, Globus M, Neary J, et al: Regional alterations of protein kinase C activity following transient cerebral ischemia: Effects of intraischemic brain temperature modulation. J Neurochem 63:1095, 1994
98. Nakashima K, Todd MM, Warner DS: The relation between cerebral metabolic rate and ischemic depolarization. A comparison of the effects of hypothermia, pentobarbital, and isoflurane. Anesthesiology 82:1199, 1995
99. Globus M, Busto R, Lin B, et al: Detection of free radical activity during transient global ischemia and recirculation: Effects of intraischemic brain temperature modulation. J Neurochem 65:1250, 1995
100. Kader A, Frazzini V, Baker C, et al: Effect of mild hypothermia on nitric oxide synthesis during focal cerebral ischemia. Neurosurgery 35:272, 1994
101. Bernard SA, Gray TW, Buist MD, et al: Treatment of comatose survivors of out-of-hospital cardiac arrest with induced hypothermia. N Engl J Med 346:557, 2002
102. Mild therapeutic hypothermia to improve the neurologic outcome after cardiac arrest. N Engl J Med 346:549, 2002
103. Clifton GL, Miller ER, Choi SC, et al: Lack of effect of induction of hypothermia after acute brain injury. N Engl J Med 344:556, 2001
104. Todd MM, Hindman BJ, Clarke WR, et al: Mild intraoperative hypothermia during surgery for intracranial aneurysm. N Engl J Med 352:135, 2005

105. The Warm Heart Investigators: Randomized trial of normothermic versus hypothermic coronary bypass surgery. Lancet 343:559, 1994
106. Gaillard D, Bical O, Paumier D, et al: A review of myocardial normothermia: Its theoretical basis and the potential clinical benefits in cardiac surgery. Cardiovasc Surg 8:198, 2000
107. Nicolini F, Beghi C, Muscari C, et al: Myocardial protection in adult cardiac surgery: Current options and future challenges. Eur J Cardiothorac Surg 24:986, 2003
108. Panos AL, Deslauriers R, Birnbaum PL, et al: Perspectives on myocardial protection: Warm heart surgery. Perfusion 8:287, 1993
109. Martin T, Craver J, Gott J, et al: Prospective, randomized trial of retrograde warm blood cardioplegia: Myocardial benefit and neurologic threat. Ann Thorac Surg 57:298, 1994
110. Grigore AM, Mathew J, Grocott HP, et al: Prospective randomized trial of normothermic versus hypothermic cardiopulmonary bypass on cognitive function after coronary artery bypass graft surgery. Anesthesiology 95:1110, 2001
111. Mora C, Henson M, Weintraub W, et al: The effect of temperature management during cardiopulmonary bypass on neurologic and neuropsychologic outcomes in patients undergoing coronary revascularization. J Thorac Cardiovasc Surg 112:514, 1996
112. McLean RF, Wong BI, Naylor CD, et al: Cardiopulmonary bypass, temperature, and central nervous system dysfunction. Circulation 90(Pt 2):II-250, 1994
113. Grocott HP, Newman MF, Croughwell ND, et al: Continuous jugular venous versus nasopharyngeal temperature monitoring during hypothermic cardiopulmonary bypass for cardiac surgery. J Clin Anesth 9:312, 1997
114. Nathan HJ, Wells GA, Munson JL, et al: Neuroprotective effect of mild hypothermia in patients undergoing coronary artery surgery with cardiopulmonary bypass: A randomized trial. Circulation 104(suppl 1):I85, 2001
115. Stone JG, Young WL, Smith CR, et al: Do standard monitoring sites reflect true brain temperature when profound hypothermia is rapidly induced and reversed? Anesthesiology 82:344, 1995
116. Cook DJ, Oliver WC Jr, Orszulak TA, et al: A prospective, randomized comparison of cerebral venous oxygen saturation during normothermic and hypothermic cardiopulmonary bypass. J Thorac Cardiovasc Surg 107:1020, 1994
117. Plochl W, Liam BL, Cook DJ, Orszulak TA: Cerebral response to haemodilution during cardiopulmonary bypass in dogs: The role of nitric oxide synthase. Br J Anaesth 82:237, 1999
118. Govier AV, Reves JG, McKay RD, et al: Factors and their influence on regional cerebral blood flow during nonpulsatile cardiopulmonary bypass. Ann Thorac Surg 38:592, 1984
119. Newman MF, Croughwell ND, White WD, et al: Effect of perfusion pressure on cerebral blood flow during normothermic cardiopulmonary bypass. Circulation 94(suppl):II353, 1996
120. Barry DI, Strandgaard S, Graham DI, et al: Cerebral blood flow in rats with renal and spontaneous hypertension: Resetting of the lower limit of autoregulation. J Cereb Blood Flow Metab 2:347, 1982
121. Lanier WL: Glucose management during cardiopulmonary bypass: Cardiovascular and neurologic implications. Anesth Analg 72:423, 1991
122. Dietrich WD, Alonso O, Busto R: Moderate hyperglycemia worsens acute blood-brain barrier injury after forebrain ischemia in rats. Stroke 24:111, 1993
123. Siesjö B: Acidosis and ischemic brain damage. Neurochem Pathol 9:31, 1988
124. Warner DS, Gionet TX, Todd MM, et al: Insulin-induced normoglycemia improves ischemic outcome in hyperglycemic rats. Stroke 22:1775, 1992
125. Feerick AE, Johnston WE, Jenkins LW, et al: Hyperglycemia during hypothermic canine cardiopulmonary bypass increases cerebral lactate. Anesthesiology 82:512, 1995
126. Lam A, Winn H, Cullen B, et al: Hyperglycemia and neurological outcome in patients with head injury. J Neurosurg 75:545, 1991
127. Li PA, Shuaib A, Miyashita H, et al: Hyperglycemia enhances extracellular glutamate accumulation in rats subjected to forebrain ischemia. Stroke 31:183, 2000
128. Hindman B: Con: Glucose priming solutions should not be used for cardiopulmonary bypass. J Cardiothorac Vasc Anesth 9:605, 1995
129. Metz S, Keats AS: Benefits of a glucose-containing priming solution for cardiopulmonary bypass. Anesth Analg 72:428, 1991
130. Nussmeier N, Marino M, Cooper J, et al: Use of glucose-containing prime is not a risk factor for cerebral injury or infection in nondiabetic or diabetic patients having CABG procedures. Anesthesiology 91:A122, 1999
131. Hill SE, van Wermeskerken GK, Lardenoye JW, et al: Intraoperative physiologic variables and outcome in cardiac surgery. Part I. In-hospital mortality. Ann Thorac Surg 69:1070, 2000
132. van Wermeskerken GK, Lardenoye JW, Hill SE, et al: Intraoperative physiologic variables and outcome in cardiac surgery. Part II. Neurologic outcome. Ann Thorac Surg 69:1077, 2000
133. Chaney MA, Nikolov MP, Blakeman BP, et al: Attempting to maintain normoglycemia during cardiopulmonary bypass with insulin may initiate postoperative hypoglycemia. Anesth Analg 89:1091, 1999
134. Bainbridge D, Martin J, Cheng D: Off pump coronary artery bypass graft surgery versus conventional coronary artery bypass graft surgery: A systematic review of the literature. Semin Cardiothorac Vasc Anesth 9:105, 2005
135. Van Dijk D, Jansen EW, Hijman R, et al: Cognitive outcome after off-pump and on-pump coronary artery bypass graft surgery: A randomized trial. JAMA 287:1405, 2002
136. Mark DB, Newman MF: Protecting the brain in coronary artery bypass graft surgery. JAMA 287:1448, 2002
137. Bainbridge D, Cheng DCH, Martin JE, et al: Off-pump versus on-pump coronary artery bypass surgery: A meta-analysis of clinical outcomes from randomized controlled trials. Anesth Analg 96:SCA100, 2003
138. Dirnagl U, Iadecola C, Moskowitz M: Pathobiology of ischemic stroke: An integrated review. Trends Neurosci 22:391, 1999
139. Michenfelder J, Theye R: Cerebral protection by thiopental during hypoxia. Anesthesiology 39:510, 1973
140. Pascoe E, Hudson R, Anderson B, et al: High-dose thiopentone for open-chamber cardiac surgery: A retrospective review. Can J Anaesth 43:575, 1996
141. Zaidan J, Klochany A, Martin W: Effect of thiopental on neurologic outcome following coronary artery bypass grafting. Anesthesiology 74:406, 1991
142. Warner D, Takaoka S, Wu B, et al: Electroencephalographic burst suppression is not required to elicit maximal neuroprotection from pentobarbital in a rat model of focal cerebral ischemia. Anesthesiology 84:1475, 1996
143. Zhou W, Fontenot HJ, Liu S, et al: Modulation of cardiac calcium channels by propofol. Anesthesiology 86:670, 1997
144. Pittman JE, Sheng HX, Pearlstein R, et al: Comparison of the effects of propofol and pentobarbital on neurologic outcome and cerebral infarct size after temporary focal ischemia in the rat. Anesthesiology 87:1139, 1997
145. Young Y, Menon DK, Tisavipat N, et al: Propofol neuroprotection in a rat model of ischaemia reperfusion injury. Eur J Anaesthesiol 14:320, 1997
146. Wang J, Yang X, Camporesi CV, et al: Propofol reduces infarct size and striatal dopamine accumulation following transient middle cerebral artery occlusion: A microdialysis study. Eur J Pharmacol 452:303, 2002
147. Roach GW, Newman MF, Murkin JM, et al: Ineffectiveness of burst suppression therapy in mitigating perioperative cerebrovascular dysfunction. Multicenter Study of Perioperative Ischemia (McSPI) Research Group. Anesthesiology 90:1255, 1999
148. Mangano D: Effects of acadesine on the incidence of myocardial infarction and adverse cardiac outcomes after coronary artery bypass graft surgery. Anesthesiology 83:658, 1995
149. MacGregor DG, Miller WJ, Stone TW: Mediation of the neuroprotective action of R-phenylisopropyl-adenosine through a centrally located adenosine A1 receptor. Br J Pharmacol 110:470, 1993
150. Perez-Pinzon MA, Mumford PL, Rosenthal M, et al: Anoxic preconditioning in hippocampal slices: Role of adenosine. Neuroscience 75:687, 1996
151. Grocott HP, Nussmeier NA: Neuroprotection in cardiac surgery. Anesthesiol Clin North Am 21:487, 2003
152. Levy J, Ramsay J, Murkin J: Aprotinin reduces the incidence of strokes following cardiac surgery. Circulation 94(suppl):I-535, 1996
153. Levy JH, Pifarre R, Schaff HV, et al: A multicenter, double-blind, placebo-controlled trial of aprotinin for reducing blood loss and the requirement for donor-blood transfusion in patients undergoing repeat coronary artery bypass grafting. Circulation 92:2236, 1995
154. Frumento RJ, O'Malley CM, Bennett-Guerrero E: Stroke after cardiac surgery: A retrospective analysis of the effect of aprotinin dosing regimens. Ann Thorac Surg 75:479, 2003
155. Harmon DC, Ghori KG, Eustace NP, et al: Aprotinin decreases the incidence of cognitive deficit following CABG and cardiopulmonary bypass: A pilot randomized controlled study: [L'aprotinine reduit l'incidence de deficit cognitif a la suite d'un PAC et de la circulation extracorporelle: Une etude pilote randomisee et controlee]. Can J Anaesth 51:1002, 2004
156. Murkin JM: Postoperative cognitive dysfunction: Aprotinin, bleeding and cognitive testing. Can J Anaesth 51:957, 2004

157. Grocott HP, Sheng H, Miura Y, et al: The effects of aprotinin on outcome from cerebral ischemia in the rat. Anesth Analg 88:1, 1999
158. Forsman M, Olsnes BT, Semb G, Steen PA: Effects of nimodipine on cerebral blood flow and neuropsychological outcome after cardiac surgery. Br J Anaesth 65:514, 1990
159. Gelmers H, Gorter K, de Weerdt C, et al: A controlled trial of nimodipine in acute ischemic stroke. N Engl J Med 318:203, 1988
160. Legault C, Furberg C, Wagenknecht L, et al: Nimodipine neuroprotection in cardiac valve replacement. Report of an early terminated trial. Stroke 27:593, 1996
161. Grieco G, d'Hollosy M, Culliford A, et al: Evaluating neuroprotective agents for clinical anti-ischemic benefit using neurological changes after cardiac surgery under cardiopulmonary bypass. Stroke 27:858, 1996
162. Leon A, Lipartiti M, Seren MS, et al: Hypoxic-ischemic damage and the neuroprotective effects of GM1 ganglioside. Stroke 21(suppl):III-95, 1990
163. Arrowsmith J, Harrison M, Newman S, et al: Neuroprotection of the brain during cardiopulmonary bypass. A randomized trial of remacemide during coronary artery bypass in 171 patients. Stroke 29:2357, 1998
164. Schmitt B, Bauersfeld U, Fanconi S, et al: The effect of the *N*-methyl-D-aspartate receptor antagonist dextromethorphan on perioperative brain injury in children undergoing cardiac surgery with cardiopulmonary bypass: Results of a pilot study. Neuropediatrics 28:191, 1997
165. Ma D, Yang H, Lynch J, et al: Xenon attenuates cardiopulmonary bypass-induced neurologic and neurocognitive dysfunction in the rat. Anesthesiology 98:690, 2003
166. Homi HM, Yokoo N, Ma D, et al: The neuroprotective effect of xenon administration during transient middle cerebral artery occlusion in mice. Anesthesiology 99:876, 2003
167. Homi HM, Yokoo N, Venkatakrishnan K, et al: Neuroprotection by antagonism of the *N*-methyl-D-aspartate receptor NR2B subtype in a rat model of cardiopulmonary bypass. Anesthesiology 101:A878, 2004
168. Mitchell SJ, Pellett O, Gorman DF: Cerebral protection by lidocaine during cardiac operations. Ann Thorac Surg 67:1117, 1999
169. Mathew JP, Grocott HP, Phillips-Bute B, et al: Lidocaine does not prevent cognitive dysfunction after cardiac surgery. Anesth Analg 98:SCA 13, 2004
170. Amory DW, Grigore A, Amory JK, et al: Neuroprotection is associated with beta-adrenergic receptor antagonists during cardiac surgery: Evidence from 2,575 patients. J Cardiothorac Vasc Anesth 16:270, 2002
171. Savitz SI, Erhardt JA, Anthony JV, et al: The novel beta-blocker, carvedilol, provides neuroprotection in transient focal stroke. J Cereb Blood Flow Metab 20:1197, 2000
172. Liu TH, Beckman JS, Freeman BA, et al: Polyethylene glycol-conjugated superoxide dismutase and catalase reduce ischemic brain injury. Am J Physiol 256(Pt 2):H589, 1989
173. Butterworth J, Legault C, Stump DA, et al: A randomized, blinded trial of the antioxidant pegorgotein: No reduction in neuropsychological deficits, inotropic drug support, or myocardial ischemia after coronary artery bypass surgery. J Cardiothorac Vasc Anesth 13:690, 1999
174. Levy JH, Tanaka KA: Inflammatory response to cardiopulmonary bypass. Ann Thorac Surg 75:S715, 2003
175. Mathew JP, Shernan SK, White WD, et al: Preliminary report of the effects of complement suppression with pexelizumab on neurocognitive decline after coronary artery bypass graft surgery. Stroke 35:2335, 2004
176. Hofer RE, Christopherson TJ, Scheithauer BW, et al: The effect of a platelet activating factor antagonist (BN 52021) on neurologic outcome and histopathology in a canine model of complete cerebral ischemia. Anesthesiology 79:347, 1993
177. Panetta T, Marcheselli VL, Braquet P, et al: Effects of a platelet activating factor antagonist (BN 52021) on free fatty acids, diacylglycerols, polyphosphoinositides and blood flow in the gerbil brain: Inhibition of ischemia-reperfusion induced cerebral injury. Biochem Biophys Res Commun 149:580, 1987
178. Taggart D, Browne S, Wade D, et al: Neuroprotection during cardiac surgery: A randomized trial of a platelet activating factor antagonist. Heart 89:897, 2003
179. Sethy VH, Wu H, Oostveen JA, et al: Neuroprotective effects of the GABA(A) receptor partial agonist U-101017 in 3-acetylpyridine-treated rats. Neurosci Lett 228:45, 1997
180. Yang Y, Shuaib A, Li Q, et al: Neuroprotection by delayed administration of topiramate in a rat model of middle cerebral artery embolization. Brain Res 804:169, 1998
181. Kong R, Butterworth J, Aveling W, et al: Clinical trial of the neuroprotectant clomethiazole in coronary artery bypass graft surgery. Anesthesiology 97:585, 2002
182. Clark RK, Lee EV, White RF, et al: Reperfusion following focal stroke hastens inflammation and resolution of ischemic injured tissue. Brain Res Bull 35:387, 1994
183. Chopp M, Zhang RL, Chen H, et al: Postischemic administration of an anti-Mac-1 antibody reduces ischemic cell damage after transient middle cerebral artery occlusion in rats. Stroke 25:869, 1994
184. Bracken MB, Shepard MJ, Collins WF, et al: A randomized, controlled trial of methylprednisolone or naloxone in the treatment of acute spinal-cord injury. Results of the Second National Acute Spinal Cord Injury Study. N Engl J Med 322:1405, 1990
185. Roberts I, Yates D, Sandercock P, et al: Effect of intravenous corticosteroids on death within 14 days in 10008 adults with clinically significant head injury (MRC CRASH trial): Randomised placebo-controlled trial. Lancet 364:1321, 2004
186. Wass CT, Lanier WL: Glucose Modulation of Ischemic Brain Injury: Review and Clinical Recommendations. Mayo Clin Proc 71:801, 1996
187. Li P, Kristian T, Shamloo M, et al: Effects of preischemic hyperglycemia on brain damage incurred by rats subjected to 2.5 or 5 minutes of forebrain ischemia. Stroke 27:1592, 1996
188. Nagels W, Demeyere R, Van Hemelrijck J, et al: Evaluation of the neuroprotective effects of *S*(+)-ketamine during open-heart surgery. Anesth Analg 98:1595, 2004
189. Lavie G, Teichner A, Shohami E, et al: Long term cerebroprotective effects of dexanabinol in a model of focal cerebral ischemia. Brain Res 901:195, 2001
190. Leker RR, Shohami E, Abramsky O, et al: Dexanabinol: A novel neuroprotective drug in experimental focal cerebral ischemia. J Neurol Sci 162:114, 1999
191. Doberneck R, Reiser M, Lillehei C: Acute renal failure after open-heart surgery utilizing extracorporeal circulation and total body perfusion. J Thor Cardiovasc Surg 43:441, 1962
192. Conlon PJ, Stafford-Smith M, White WD, et al: Acute renal failure following cardiac surgery. Nephrol Dial Transplant 14:1158, 1999
193. Abel RM, Buckley MJ, Austen WG, et al: Etiology, incidence, and prognosis of renal failure following cardiac operations. Results of a prospective analysis of 500 consecutive patients. J Thorac Cardiovasc Surg 71:323, 1976
194. Yeh T, Brackney E, Hall D, et al: Renal complications of open-heart surgery: predisposing factors, prevention and management. J Thor Cardiovasc Surg 47:79, 1964
195. Chertow GM, Levy EM, Hammermeister KE, et al: Independent association between acute renal failure and mortality following cardiac surgery. Am J Med 104:343, 1998
196. Mazzarella V, Gallucci MT, Tozzo C, et al: Renal function in patients undergoing cardiopulmonary bypass operations. J Thorac Cardiovasc Surg 104:1625, 1992
197. Mora-Mangano C, Diamondstone LS, Ramsay JG, et al: Renal dysfunction after myocardial revascularization: Risk factors, adverse outcomes, and hospital resource utilization. The Multicenter Study of Perioperative Ischemia Research Group. Ann Intern Med 128:194, 1998
198. Page US, Washburn T: Using tracking data to find complications that physicians miss: The case of renal failure in cardiac surgery. Jt Comm J Qual Improv 23:511, 1997
199. Mora-Mangano C, Boisvert D, Zhou S, et al: Small reductions in renal function following CABG independently predict hospitalization. Anesth Analg 90:SCA 35, 2000
200. Stafford-Smith M, Phillips-Bute B, Reddan DN, et al: The association of postoperative peak and fractional change in serum creatinine with mortality after coronary bypass surgery. Anesthesiology 93:A240, 2000
201. Kelly KJ: Distant effects of experimental renal ischemia/reperfusion injury. J Am Soc Nephrol 14:1549, 2003
202. Rabb H, Wang Z, Nemoto T, et al: Acute renal failure leads to dysregulation of lung salt and water channels. Kidney Int 63:600, 2003
203. Deng J, Hu X, Yuen PS, et al: Alpha-melanocyte-stimulating hormone inhibits lung injury after renal ischemia/reperfusion. Am J Respir Crit Care Med 169:749, 2004
204. Kramer AA, Postler G, Salhab KF, et al: Renal ischemia/reperfusion leads to macrophage-mediated increase in pulmonary vascular permeability. Kidney Int 55:2362, 1999
205. Serteser M, Koken T, Kahraman A, et al: Changes in hepatic TNF-alpha levels, antioxidant status, and oxidation products after renal ischemia/reperfusion injury in mice. J Surg Res 107:234, 2002
206. Meldrum KK, Meldrum DR, Meng X, et al: TNF-alpha-dependent bilateral renal injury is induced by unilateral renal ischemia-reperfusion. Am J Physiol Heart Circ Physiol 282:H540, 2002
207. Chertow GM, Lazarus JM, Christiansen CL, et al: Preoperative renal risk stratification. Circulation 95:878, 1997

208. Stafford-Smith M, Swaminathan M, McCreath BJ, et al: Morbidity-related serum creatinine patterns after coronary bypass surgery. Anesth Analg 92:SCA123, 2001
209. Swaminathan M, Phillips-Bute BG, Conlon PJ, et al: The association of lowest hematocrit during cardiopulmonary bypass with acute renal injury after coronary bypass surgery. Ann Thorac Surg 76:784, 2003
210. Swaminathan M, Albahrani M, Phillips-Bute B, et al: Postoperative creatinine rise: Does MIDCAB surgery make a difference? Anesthesiology 95:A124, 2001
211. Brown R, Babcock R, Talbert J, et al: Renal function in critically ill postoperative patients: Sequential assessment of creatinine osmolar and free water clearance. Crit Care Med 8:68, 1980
212. Holper K, Struck E, Sebening F: The diagnosis of acute renal failure (ARF) following cardiac surgery with cardio-pulmonary bypass. Thorac Cardiovasc Surg 27:231, 1979
213. Myers BD, Hilberman M, Spencer RJ, et al: Glomerular and tubular function in non-oliguric acute renal failure. Am J Med 72:642, 1982
214. Andersson LG, Ekroth R, Bratteby LE, et al: Acute renal failure after coronary surgery—a study of incidence and risk factors in 2009 consecutive patients. Thorac Cardiovasc Surg 41:237, 1993
215. Mangos GJ, Brown MA, Chan WY, et al: Acute renal failure following cardiac surgery: Incidence, outcomes and risk factors. Aust N Z J Med 25:284, 1995
216. Corwin HL, Sprague SM, DeLaria GA, et al: Acute renal failure associated with cardiac operations. A case-control study. J Thorac Cardiovasc Surg 98:1107, 1989
217. Ostermann ME, Taube D, Morgan CJ, et al: Acute renal failure following cardiopulmonary bypass: A changing picture. Intensive Care Med 26:565, 2000
218. Porter GA: Urinary biomarkers and nephrotoxicity. Miner Electrolyte Metab 20:181, 1994
219. Stafford-Smith M: Antifibrinolytic agents make alpha1- and beta2-microglobulinuria poor markers of post cardiac surgery renal dysfunction. Anesthesiology 90:928, 1999
220. Schrier RW, Harris DC, Chan L, et al: Tubular hypermetabolism as a factor in the progression of chronic renal failure. Am J Kidney Dis 12:243, 1988
221. Whitworth JA, Ihle BU, Becker GJ, et al: Preservation of renal function in chronic renal failure. Tohoku J Exp Med 166:165, 1992
222. Small G, Watson AR, Evans JH, et al: Hemolytic uremic syndrome: Defining the need for long-term follow-up. Clin Nephrol 52:352, 1999
223. Kikuchi Y, Koga H, Yasutomo Y, et al: Patients with renal hypouricemia with exercise-induced acute renal failure and chronic renal dysfunction. Clin Nephrol 53:467, 2000
224. Schweda F, Blumberg FC, Schweda A, et al: Effects of chronic hypoxia on renal renin gene expression in rats. Nephrol Dial Transplant 15:11, 2000
225. Bach PH: Detection of chemically induced renal injury: The cascade of degenerative morphological and functional changes that follow the primary nephrotoxic insult and evaluation of these changes by in-vitro methods. Toxicol Lett 46:237, 1989
226. Stafford-Smith M, Phillips-Bute B, Black JD, et al: Association of ε-aminocaproic acid with acute renal dysfunction following coronary bypass surgery in 1334 patients. Anesthesiology 91:A87 1999
227. Anderson RJ, O'Brien M, MaWhinney S, et al: Renal failure predisposes patients to adverse outcome after coronary artery bypass surgery. VA Cooperative Study #5. Kidney Int 55:1057, 1999
228. Rao V, Weisel RD, Buth KJ, et al: Coronary artery bypass grafting in patients with non-dialysis-dependent renal insufficiency. Circulation 96(suppl):II-38, 1997
229. Anderson RJ, O'Brien M, MaWhinney S, et al: Mild renal failure is associated with adverse outcome after cardiac valve surgery. Am J Kidney Dis 35:1127, 2000
230. Zanardo G, Michielon P, Paccagnella A, et al: Acute renal failure in the patient undergoing cardiac operation. Prevalence, mortality rate, and main risk factors. J Thorac Cardiovasc Surg 107:1489, 1994
231. Llopart T, Lombardi R, Forselledo M, et al: Acute renal failure in open heart surgery. Ren Fail19:319, 1997
232. Hilberman M, Myers BD, Carrie BJ, et al: Acute renal failure following cardiac surgery. J Thorac Cardiovasc Surg 77:880, 1979
233. Domart Y, Trouillet JL, Fagon JY, et al: Incidence and morbidity of cytomegaloviral infection in patients with mediastinitis following cardiac surgery. Chest 97:18, 1990
234. Albahrani MJ, Swaminathan M, Phillips-Bute B, et al: Postcardiac surgery complications: Association of acute renal dysfunction and atrial fibrillation. Anesth Analg 96:637, 2003
235. Brenner RM, Chertow GM: The rise and fall of atrial natriuretic peptide for acute renal failure. Curr Opin Nephrol Hypertens 6:474, 1997
236. Stafford-Smith M, Conlon PJ, White WD, et al: Low hematocrit but not perfusion pressure during CPB is predictive for renal failure following CABG surgery. Anesth Analg 86:SCA102, 1998
237. Davila-Roman VG, Kouchoukos NT, Schechtman KB, et al: Atherosclerosis of the ascending aorta is a predictor of renal dysfunction after cardiac operations. J Thorac Cardiovasc Surg 117:111, 1999
238. Sreeram GM, Grocott HP, White WD, et al: Transcranial Doppler emboli count predicts rise in creatinine after coronary artery bypass graft surgery. J Cardiothorac Vasc Anesth 18:548, 2004
239. Conlon PJ, Crowley J, Stack R, et al: Renal artery stenosis is not associated with the development of acute renal failure following coronary artery bypass grafting. Ren Fail 27:81, 2005
240. Chew ST, Newman MF, White WD, et al: Preliminary report on the association of apolipoprotein E polymorphisms, with postoperative peak serum creatinine concentrations in cardiac surgical patients. Anesthesiology 93:325, 2000
241. Mackensen GB, Swaminathan M, Ti LK, et al: Preliminary report on the interaction of apolipoprotein E polymorphism with aortic atherosclerosis and acute nephropathy after CABG surgery. Ann Thorac Surg 78:520, 2004
242. Stafford-Smith M, Podgoreanu M, Swaminathan M, et al: Association of genetic polymorphisms with risk of renal injury after coronary after bypass graft surgery. Am J Kidney Dis 45:519, 2005
243. Stafford-Smith M, Grocott HP: Renal medullary hypoxia during experimental cardiopulmonary bypass: A pilot study. Perfusion 20:53, 2005
244. Conger JD: Interventions in clinical acute renal failure: What are the data? Am J Kidney Dis 26:565, 1995
245. Vijayan A, Miller SB: Acute renal failure: Prevention and nondialytic therapy. Semin Nephrol 18:523, 1998
246. Galley HF: Renal-dose dopamine: Will the message now get through? Lancet 356:2112, 2000
247. Bellomo R, Chapman M, Finfer S, et al: Low-dose dopamine in patients with early renal dysfunction: A placebo-controlled randomised trial. Australian and New Zealand Intensive Care Society (ANZICS) Clinical Trials Group. Lancet 356:2139, 2000
248. Conger J: Hemodynamic factors in acute renal failure. Adv Ren Replace Ther 4(suppl 1):25, 1997
249. Porter GA: Contrast-associated nephropathy: Presentation, pathophysiology and management. Miner Electrolyte Metab 20:232, 1994
250. Kahn JK, Rutherford BD, McConahay DR, et al: High-dose contrast agent administration during complex coronary angioplasty. Am Heart J 120:533, 1990
251. Gussenhoven MJ, Ravensbergen J, van Bockel JH, et al: Renal dysfunction after angiography; a risk factor analysis in patients with peripheral vascular disease. J Cardiovasc Surg (Torino) 32:81, 1991
252. Garwood S, Mathew J, Hines R: Renal function and cardiopulmonary bypass: Does time since catheterization impact renal performance? Anesthesiology 87:A90, 1997
253. Saklayen MG, Gupta S, Suryaprasad A, et al: Incidence of atheroembolic renal failure after coronary angiography. A prospective study. Angiology 48:609, 1997
254. Thadhani RI, Camargo CA Jr, Xavier RJ, et al: Atheroembolic renal failure after invasive procedures. Natural history based on 52 histologically proven cases. Medicine (Baltimore) 74:350, 1995
255. Taguma Y, Sasaki Y, Kyogoku Y, et al: Morphological changes in an early phase of norepinephrine-induced acute renal failure in unilaterally nephrectomized dogs. J Lab Clin Med 96:616, 1980
256. Baehler RW, Williams RH, Work J, et al: Studies on the natural history of the norepinephrine model of acute renal failure in the dog. Nephron 26:266, 1980
257. Persson PB, Ehmke H, Nafz B, et al: Resetting of renal autoregulation in conscious dogs: Angiotensin II and alpha1-adrenoceptors. Pflugers Arch 417:42, 1990
258. Andersson LG, Bratteby LE, Ekroth R, et al: Renal function during cardiopulmonary bypass: Influence of pump flow and systemic blood pressure. Eur J Cardiothorac Surg 8:597, 1994
259. Pallone TL, Silldorff EP, Turner MR: Intrarenal blood flow: Microvascular anatomy and the regulation of medullary perfusion. Clin Exp Pharmacol Physiol 25:383, 1998
260. Reves JG: Adrenergic response to cardiopulmonary bypass. Mt Sinai J Med 52:511, 1985
261. Reves JG, Buttner E, Karp RB, et al: Elevated catecholamines during cardiac surgery: Consequences of reperfusion of the postarrested heart. Am J Cardiol 53:722, 1984
262. Bookstein JJ, Clark RL (eds): Renal Microvascular Disease: Angiographic-Microangiographic Correlates. Boston, Little, Brown, 1980

263. Tunick PA, Culliford AT, Lamparello PJ, et al: Atheromatosis of the aortic arch as an occult source of multiple systemic emboli. Ann Intern Med 114:391, 1991
264. Blauth CI, Cosgrove DM, Webb BW, et al: Atheroembolism from the ascending aorta. An emerging problem in cardiac surgery. J Thorac Cardiovasc Surg 103:1104, 1992
265. Blauth J: Macroemboli and microemboli during cardiopulmonary bypass. Ann Thorac Surg 59:1300, 1995
266. Tierney G, Parissis H, Baker M, et al: An experimental study of intra aortic balloon pumping within the intact human aorta. Eur J Cardiothorac Surg 12:486, 1997
267. Ura M, Sakata R, Nakayama Y, et al: Ultrasonographic demonstration of manipulation-related aortic injuries after cardiac surgery. J Am Coll Cardiol 35:1303, 2000
268. Kolh PH, Torchiana DF, Buckley MJ: Atheroembolization in cardiac surgery. The need for preoperative diagnosis. J Cardiovasc Surg (Torino) 40:77, 1999
269. Fernandez S, Garcia A, Quintela B, et al: Multiple cholesterol atheroembolisms after resection of an abdominal aortic aneurysm. Rev Esp Anestesiol Reanim 47:485, 2000
270. Nakamoto S, Kaneda T, Inoue T, et al: Disseminated cholesterol embolism after coronary artery bypass grafting. J Card Surg 16:410, 2001
271. Shammas NW: Pulmonary embolus after coronary artery bypass surgery: A review of the literature. Clin Cardiol 23:637, 2000
272. Moody D, Bell M, Challa V, et al: Brain microemboli during cardiac surgery or aortography. Ann Neurol 28:477, 1990
273. Deal DD, Jones TJ, Vernon JC, et al: Real time OPS imaging of embolic injury of the renal micro-circulation during cardiopulmonary bypass. Anesth Analg 92:S23, 2001
274. Kincaid EH, Jones TJ, Stump DA, et al: Processing scavenged blood with a cell saver reduces cerebral lipid microembolization. Ann Thorac Surg 70:1296, 2000
275. Rangel-Frausto MS, Pittet D, Costigan M, et al: The natural history of the systemic inflammatory response syndrome (SIRS). A prospective study. JAMA 273:117, 1995
276. Hall R, Stafford-Smith M, Rocker G: The systemic inflammatory response to cardiopulmonary bypass: Pathophysiological, therapeutic, and pharmacological considerations. Anesth Analg 85:766, 1997
277. Laffey JG, Boylan JF, Cheng DC: The systemic inflammatory response to cardiac surgery: Implications for the anesthesiologist. Anesthesiology 97:215, 2002
278. Gormley SM, McBride WT, Armstrong MA, et al: Plasma and urinary cytokine homeostasis and renal function during cardiac surgery without cardiopulmonary bypass. Cytokine 17:61, 2002
279. Gormley SM, McBride WT, Armstrong MA, et al: Plasma and urinary cytokine homeostasis and renal dysfunction during cardiac surgery. Anesthesiology 93:1210, 2000
280. Boelke E, Storck M, Buttenschoen K, et al: Endotoxemia and mediator release during cardiac surgery. Angiology 51:743, 2000
281. Fouqueray B, Philippe C, Herbelin A, et al: Cytokine formation within rat glomeruli during experimental endotoxemia. J Am Soc Nephrol 3:1783, 1993
282. Stafford-Smith M, Phillips-Bute B, Swaminathan M, et al: Relationship of preoperative antiendotoxin core antibodies and acute renal injury following cardiac surgery. Anesthesiology 95:A404, 2001
283. Wiecek A, Zeier M, Ritz E: Role of infection in the genesis of acute renal failure. Nephrol Dial Transplant 9(suppl 4):40, 1994
284. Tune B: Renal tubular transport and nephrotoxicity of beta lactam antibiotics: Structure activity relationships. Miner Electrolyte Metab 20:221, 1994
285. Bennett WM, Luft F, Porter GA: Pathogenesis of renal failure due to aminoglycosides and contrast media used in roentgenography. Am J Med 69:767, 1980
286. Baisac J, Henrich W: Nephrotoxicity of nonsteroidal anti-inflammatory drugs. Miner Electrolyte Metab 20:187, 1994
287. Olyaei AJ, de Mattos AM, Bennett WM: Immunosuppressant-induced nephropathy: Pathophysiology, incidence and management. Drug Saf 21:471, 1999
288. Stafford-Smith M, Phillips-Bute B, Reddan DN, et al: The association of epsilon-aminocaproic acid with postoperative decrease in creatinine clearance in 1502 coronary bypass patients. Anesth Analg 91:1085, 2000
289. Feindt PR, Walcher S, Volkmer I, et al: Effects of high-dose aprotinin on renal function in aortocoronary bypass grafting. Ann Thorac Surg 60:1076, 1995
290. Sundt TM 3rd, Kouchoukos NT, Saffitz JE, et al: Renal dysfunction and intravascular coagulation with aprotinin and hypothermic circulatory arrest. Ann Thorac Surg 55:1418, 1993
291. Mora-Mangano CT, Neville MJ, Hsu PH, et al: Aprotinin, blood loss, and renal dysfunction in deep hypothermic circulatory arrest. Circulation 104(suppl 1):I-276, 2001
292. Ehrlich M, Grabenwoger M, Cartes-Zumelzu F, et al: Operations on the thoracic aorta and hypothermic circulatory arrest: Is aprotinin safe? J Thorac Cardiovasc Surg 115:220, 1998
293. Henry DA, Moxey AJ, Carless PA, et al: Anti-fibrinolytic use for minimising perioperative allogeneic blood transfusion. Cochrane Database Syst Rev 2:CD001886, 2001
294. Luft FC, Vinicor F: Recurrent acute renal failure with idiopathic paroxysmal myoglobinuria. JAMA 233:349, 1975
295. Corwin HL, Schreiber MJ, Fang LS: Low fractional excretion of sodium. Occurrence with hemoglobinuric- and myoglobinuric-induced acute renal failure. Arch Intern Med 144:981, 1984
296. Heyman SN, Rosen S, Fuchs S, et al: Myoglobinuric acute renal failure in the rat: A role for medullary hypoperfusion, hypoxia, and tubular obstruction. J Am Soc Nephrol 7:1066, 1996
297. Maccario M, Fumagalli C, Dottori V, et al: Rhabdomyolytic acute renal failure in cardiac surgery. A clinical case. Minerva Anestesiol. 61:397, 1995
298. Kugimiya T, Shirabe J, Kusaba E, et al: Myonephropathic-metabolic syndrome as a complication of cardiopulmonary bypass. Jpn J Surg 13:431, 1983
299. McCreath BJ, Swaminathan M, Booth JV, et al: Mitral valve surgery and acute renal injury: Port access versus median sternotomy. Ann Thorac Surg 75:812, 2003
300. Lieberthal W, Rennke H, Sandock K, et al: Ischemia in the isolated erythrocyte-perfused rat kidney. Protective effect of hypothermia. Ren Physiol Biochem 11:60, 1988
301. Ip-Yam PC, Murphy S, Baines M, et al: Renal function and proteinuria after cardiopulmonary bypass: The effects of temperature and mannitol. Anesth Analg 78:842, 1994
302. Regragui IA, Izzat MB, Birdi I, et al: Cardiopulmonary bypass perfusion temperature does not influence perioperative renal function. Ann Thorac Surg 60:160, 1995
303. Swaminathan M, East C, Phillips-Bute B, et al: Report of a substudy on warm versus cold cardiopulmonary bypass: Changes in creatinine clearance. Ann Thorac Surg 72:1603, 2001
304. Bhat JG, Gluck MC, Lowenstein J, et al: Renal failure after open heart surgery. Ann Intern Med 84:677, 1976
305. Urzua J, Troncoso S, Bugedo G, et al: Renal function and cardiopulmonary bypass: Effect of perfusion pressure. J Cardiothorac Vasc Anesth 6:299, 1992
306. Swaminathan M, Knauth K, Phillips-Bute B, et al: Lowest CPB Hematocrit is inversely associated with creatinine rise after coronary bypass surgery. Anesth Analg 94:S70, 2002
307. Shah D, Corson J, Karmody A, et al: Effects of isovolemic hemodilution on abdominal aortic aneurysmectomy in high risk patients. Ann Vasc Surg 1:50, 1986
308. Messmer K: Hemodilution. Surg Clin North Am 55:659, 1975
309. DeFoe G, Ross C, Olmstead E, et al: Lowest hematocrit on bypass and adverse outcomes associated with coronary artery bypass grafting. Ann Thor Surg 71:769, 2001
310. Fang WC, Helm RE, Krieger KH, et al: Impact of minimum hematocrit during cardiopulmonary bypass on mortality in patients undergoing coronary artery surgery. Circulation 96(suppl):II-194, 1997
311. Ranucci M, Pavesi M, Mazza E, et al: Risk factors for renal dysfunction after coronary surgery: The role of cardiopulmonary bypass technique. Perfusion 9:319, 1994
312. Barbeito A, Phillips-Bute B, Mathew JP, et al: Hemodilution and acute renal injury: The relationship of three different target CPB hematocrit strategies with post-cardiac surgery renal dysfunction. Anesth Analg 100:18, 2005
313. Marik PE: Low-dose dopamine: A systematic review. Intensive Care Med 28:877, 2002
314. Kellum JA, Decker MJ: Use of dopamine in acute renal failure: A meta-analysis. Crit Care Med 29:1526, 2001
315. Prins I, Plotz FB, Uiterwaal CS, et al: Low-dose dopamine in neonatal and pediatric intensive care: A systematic review. Intensive Care Med 27:206, 2001
316. Jakob SM, Ruokonen E, Takala J: Effects of dopamine on systemic and regional blood flow and metabolism in septic and cardiac surgery patients. Shock 18:8, 2002
317. Hoffman TM, Bush DM, Wernovsky G, et al: Postoperative junctional ectopic tachycardia in children: Incidence, risk factors, and treatment. Ann Thorac Surg 74:1607, 2002
318. Duke GJ, Bersten AD: Dopamine and renal salvage in the critically ill patient. Anaesth Intensive Care 20:277, 1992

319. Stone GW, McCullough PA, Tumlin JA, et al: Fenoldopam mesylate for the prevention of contrast-induced nephropathy: A randomized controlled trial. JAMA 290:2284, 2003
320. Kini AS, Mitre CA, Kim M, et al: A protocol for prevention of radiographic contrast nephropathy during percutaneous coronary intervention: Effect of selective dopamine receptor agonist fenoldopam. Catheter Cardiovasc Interv 55:169, 2002
321. Stone GW, Tumlin JA, Madyoon H, et al: Design and rationale of CONTRAST—a prospective, randomized, placebo-controlled trial of fenoldopam mesylate for the prevention of radiocontrast nephropathy. Rev Cardiovasc Med 2(suppl 1):S31, 2001
322. Caimmi PP, Pagani L, Micalizzi E, et al: Fenoldopam for renal protection in patients undergoing cardiopulmonary bypass. J Cardiothorac Vasc Anesth 17:491, 2003
323. Tumlin J, Finckle K, Murray P, et al: Dopamine receptor 1 agonists in early acute tubular necrosis: A prospective, randomized, double blind, placebo-controlled trial of fenoldopam mesylate. J Am Soc Nephrol 14:PUB001, 2003
324. Brezis M, Agmon Y, Epstein FH: Determinants of intrarenal oxygenation. I. Effects of diuretics. Am J Physiol 267(Pt 2):F1059, 1994
325. Ellison DH, Velazquez H, Wright FS: Adaptation of the distal convoluted tubule of the rat. Structural and functional effects of dietary salt intake and chronic diuretic infusion. J Clin Invest 83:113, 1989
326. Liss P: Effects of contrast media on renal microcirculation and oxygen tension. An experimental study in the rat. Acta Radiol Suppl 409:1, 1997
327. Lindner A, Cutler R, Goodman W: Synergism of dopamine plus furosemide in preventing acute renal failure in the dog. Kidney Int 16:158, 1979
328. Heyman SN, Rosen S, Epstein FH, et al: Loop diuretics reduce hypoxic damage to proximal tubules of the isolated perfused rat kidney. Kidney Int 45:981, 1994
329. Hager B, Betschart M, Krapf R: Effect of postoperative intravenous loop diuretic on renal function after major surgery. Schweiz Med Wochenschr 126:666, 1996
330. Shilliday IR, Quinn KJ, Allison ME: Loop diuretics in the management of acute renal failure: A prospective, double-blind, placebo-controlled, randomized study. Nephrol Dial Transplant 12:2592, 1997
331. Nuutinen L, Hollmen A: The effect of prophylactic use of furosemide on renal function during open heart surgery. Ann Chir Gynaecol 65:258, 1976
332. Charlson M, Krieger KH, Peterson JC, et al: Predictors and outcomes of cardiac complications following elective coronary bypass grafting. Proc Assoc Am Physicians 111:622, 1999
333. Lassnigg A, Donner E, Grubhofer G, et al: Lack of renoprotective effects of dopamine and furosemide during cardiac surgery. J Am Soc Nephrol 11:97, 2000
334. Fisher AR, Jones P, Barlow P, et al: The influence of mannitol on renal function during and after open-heart surgery. Perfusion 13:181, 1998
335. Nishimura O, Tokutsu S, Sakurai T, et al: Effects of hypertonic mannitol on renal function in open heart surgery. Jpn Heart J 24:245, 1983
336. Pass LJ, Eberhart RC, Brown JC, et al: The effect of mannitol and dopamine on the renal response to thoracic aortic cross-clamping. J Thorac Cardiovasc Surg 95:608, 1988
337. Visweswaran P, Massin EK, Dubose TD Jr: Mannitol-induced acute renal failure. J Am Soc Nephrol 8:1028, 1997
338. Meyer M, Wiebe K, Wahlers T, et al: Urodilatin (INN:ularitide) as a new drug for the therapy of acute renal failure following cardiac surgery. Clin Exp Pharmacol Physiol 24:374, 1997
339. Brenner P, Meyer M, Reichenspurner H, et al: Significance of prophylactic urodilatin (INN: ularitide) infusion for the prevention of acute renal failure in patients after heart transplantation. Eur J Med Res 1:137, 1995
340. Kshirsagar AV, Poole C, Mottl A, et al: *N*-acetylcysteine for the prevention of radiocontrast induced nephropathy: A meta-analysis of prospective controlled trials. J Am Soc Nephrol 15:761, 2004
341. Pannu N, Manns B, Lee HH, et al: Systematic review of the impact of *N*-acetylcysteine n contrast nephropathy. Kidney Int 65:1366, 2004
342. Kretzschmar M, Klein U, Palutke M, et al: Reduction of ischemia-reperfusion syndrome after abdominal aortic aneurysmectomy by *N*-acetylcysteine but not mannitol. Acta Anaesthesiol Scand. 40:657, 1996
343. Cote G, Denault A, Belisle S, et al: *N*-acetylcysteine in the preservation of renal function in patients undergoing cardiac surgery. ASA Annual Meeting Abstracts 99(3A):A420, 2003
344. Mangano DT: Aspirin and mortality from coronary bypass surgery. N Engl J Med 347:1309, 2002
345. Zhou X, Ono H, Ono Y, et al: Renoprotective effects of omapatrilat are mediated partially by bradykinin. Am J Nephrol 23:214, 2003
346. Kostis JB, Packer M, Black HR, et al: Omapatrilat and enalapril in patients with hypertension: The Omapatrilat Cardiovascular Treatment vs. Enalapril (OCTAVE) trial. Am J Hypertens 17:103, 2004
347. Solez K, Ideura T, Silvia CB, et al: Clonidine after renal ischemia to lessen acute renal failure and microvascular damage. Kidney Int 18:309, 1980
348. Ideura T, Solez K, Heptinstall RH: The effect of clonidine on tubular obstruction in postischemic acute renal failure in the rabbit demonstrated by microradiography and microdissection. Am J Pathol 98:123, 1980
349. Eknoyan G, Dobyan DC, Senekjian HO, et al: Protective effect of oral clonidine in the prophylaxis and therapy of mercuric chloride–induced acute renal failure in the rat. J Lab Clin Med 102:699, 1983
350. Eknoyan G, Bulger RE, Dobyan DC: Mercuric chloride-induced acute renal failure in the rat. I. Correlation of functional and morphologic changes and their modification by clonidine. Lab Invest 46:613, 1982
351. Zou AP, Cowley AW Jr: Alpha(2)-adrenergic receptor-mediated increase in NO production buffers renal medullary vasoconstriction. Am J Physiol Regul Integr Comp Physiol 279:R769, 2000
352. Kulka PJ, Tryba M, Zenz M: Preoperative alpha2-adrenergic receptor agonists prevent the deterioration of renal function after cardiac surgery: Results of a randomized, controlled trial. Crit Care Med 24:947, 1996
353. Myles PS, Hunt JO, Holdgaard HO, et al: Clonidine and cardiac surgery: Haemodynamic and metabolic effects, myocardial ischaemia and recovery. Anaesth Intensive Care 27:137, 1999
354. Schramm L, Heidbreder E, Kartenbender K, et al: Effects of urodilatin and diltiazem on renal function in ischemic acute renal failure in the rat. Am J Nephrol 15:418, 1995
355. Schramm L, Heidbreder E, Lukes M, et al: Endotoxin-induced acute renal failure in the rat: Effects of urodilatin and diltiazem on renal function. Clin Nephrol 46:117, 1996
356. Zanardo G, Michielon P, Rosi P, et al: Effects of a continuous diltiazem infusion on renal function during cardiac surgery. J Cardiothorac Vasc Anesth 7:711, 1993
357. Bergman AS, Odar-Cederlof I, Westman L, et al: Diltiazem infusion for renal protection in cardiac surgical patients with preexisting renal dysfunction. J Cardiothorac Vasc Anesth 16:294, 2002
358. Kitagawa S, Komatsu Y, Futatsuyama M, et al: Renoprotection of ace inhibitor and angiotensin II receptor blocker for the patients with severe renal insufficiency. Nephrology 8(suppl):A26, 2003
359. Rady MY, Ryan T: The effects of preoperative therapy with angiotensin-converting enzyme inhibitors on clinical outcome after cardiovascular surgery. Chest 114:487, 1998
360. Gamoso MG, Phillips-Bute B, Landolfo KP, et al: Off-pump versus On-pump coronary artery bypass surgery and postoperative renal dysfunction. Anesth Analg 91:1080, 2000
361. Cittanova ML, Zubicki A, Savu C, et al: The chronic inhibition of angiotensin-converting enzyme impairs postoperative renal function. Anesth Analg 93:1111, 2001
362. Welch WJ, Wilcox CS: AT1 receptor antagonist combats oxidative stress and restores nitric oxide signaling in the SHR. Kidney Int 59:1257, 2001
363. Colson P, Ribstein J, Mimran A, et al: Effect of angiotensin converting enzyme inhibition on blood pressure and renal function during open heart surgery. Anesthesiology 72:23, 1990
364. Ryckwaert F, Colson P, Ribstein J, et al: Haemodynamic and renal effects of intravenous enalaprilat during coronary artery bypass graft surgery in patients with ischaemic heart dysfunction. Br J Anaesth 86:169, 2001
365. Baines A, Ho P: Glucose stimulates O2 consumption, NOS, and Na/H exchange in diabetic rat proximal tubules. Am J Physiol Renal Physiol 283:F286, 2002
366. Melin J, Hellberg O, Larsson E, et al: Protective effect of insulin on ischemic renal injury in diabetes mellitus. Kidney Int 61:1383, 2002
367. Najafi H, Henson D, Dye WS, et al: Left ventricular hemorrhagic necrosis. Ann Thorac Surg 7:550, 1969
368. Buckberg GD: Left ventricular subendocardial necrosis. Ann Thorac Surg 24:379, 1977
369. Bigelow WG, Lindsay WK, Greenwood WF: Hypothermia; its possible role in cardiac surgery: An investigation of factors governing survival in dogs at low body temperatures. Ann Surg 132:849, 1950
370. Melrose DG, Dreyer B, Bentall HH, et al: Elective cardiac arrest. Lancet 269:21, 1955
371. Erhardt LR: GUARD during Ischemia Against Necrosis (GUARDIAN) trial in acute coronary syndromes. Am J Cardiol 83:23G, 1999
372. Chaitman BR: A review of the GUARDIAN trial results: Clinical implications and the significance of elevated perioperative CK-MB on 6-month survival. J Card Surg 18(suppl 1):13, 2003
373. Theroux P, Chaitman BR, Danchin N, et al: Inhibition of the sodium-hydrogen exchanger with cariporide to prevent myocardial infarction in

high-risk ischemic situations. Main results of the GUARDIAN trial. GUARD during Ischemia Against Necrosis (GUARDIAN) Investigators. Circulation 102:3032, 2000

374. Ferguson TB Jr, Hammill BG, Peterson ED, et al: A decade of change—risk profiles and outcomes for isolated coronary artery bypass grafting procedures, 1990–1999: A report from the STS National Database Committee and the Duke Clinical Research Institute. Society of Thoracic Surgeons. Ann Thorac Surg 73:480, 2002
375. Ovize M: Still looking for the ultimate mechanism of myocardial stunning. Basic Res Cardiol 92(suppl 2):16, 1997
376. Braunwald E, Kloner RA: The stunned myocardium: Prolonged, postischemic ventricular dysfunction. Circulation 66:1146, 1982
377. Gray R, Maddahi J, Berman D, et al: Scintigraphic and hemodynamic demonstration of transient left ventricular dysfunction immediately after uncomplicated coronary artery bypass grafting. J Thorac Cardiovasc Surg 77:504, 1979
378. Kloner RA, Przyklenk K, Kay GL: Clinical evidence for stunned myocardium after coronary artery bypass surgery. J Card Surg 9(suppl): 397, 1994
379. Bolli R: Mechanism of myocardial "stunning." Circulation 82:723, 1990
380. Sun JZ, Kaur H, Halliwell B, et al: Use of aromatic hydroxylation of phenylalanine to measure production of hydroxyl radicals after myocardial ischemia in vivo. Direct evidence for a pathogenetic role of the hydroxyl radical in myocardial stunning. Circ Res 73:534, 1993
381. Sekili S, McCay PB, Li XY, et al: Direct evidence that the hydroxyl radical plays a pathogenetic role in myocardial "stunning" in the conscious dog and demonstration that stunning can be markedly attenuated without subsequent adverse effects. Circ Res 73:705, 1993
382. Shattock MJ: Myocardial stunning: Do we know the mechanism? Basic Res Cardiol 92(suppl 2):18, 1997
383. Shen AC, Jennings RB: Kinetics of calcium accumulation in acute myocardial ischemic injury. Am J Pathol 67:441, 1972
384. Clark RE, Magovern GJ, Christlieb IY, et al: Nifedipine cardioplegia experience: Results of a 3-year cooperative clinical study. Ann Thorac Surg 36:654, 1983
385. Karmazyn M: The 1990 Merck Frosst Award. Ischemic and reperfusion injury in the heart. Cellular mechanisms and pharmacological interventions. Can J Physiol Pharmacol 69:719, 1991
386. Karmazyn M, Moffat MP: Role of Na+/H+ exchange in cardiac physiology and pathophysiology: Mediation of myocardial reperfusion injury by the pH paradox. Cardiovasc Res 27:915, 1993
387. Karmazyn M: The sodium-hydrogen exchange system in the heart: Its role in ischemic and reperfusion injury and therapeutic implications. Can J Cardiol 12:1074, 1996
388. Kawamura T, Wakusawa R, Okada K, et al: Elevation of cytokines during open heart surgery with cardiopulmonary bypass: Participation of interleukin 8 and 6 in reperfusion injury. Can J Anaesth 40:1016, 1993
389. Hansen PR: Myocardial reperfusion injury: Experimental evidence and clinical relevance. Eur Heart J 16:734, 1995
390. Kofsky ER, Julia PL, Buckberg GD, et al: Studies of controlled reperfusion after ischemia. XXII. Reperfusate composition: Effects of leukocyte depletion of blood and blood cardioplegic reperfusates after acute coronary occlusion. J Thorac Cardiovasc Surg 101:350, 1991
391. Karmazyn M: Synthesis and relevance of cardiac eicosanoids with particular emphasis on ischemia and reperfusion. Can J Physiol Pharmacol 67:912, 1989
392. Schwinn D, Liggett S, McRae R, et al: Desensitization of myocardial beta-adrenergic receptors during cardiopulmonary bypass. Evidence for early uncoupling and late downregulation. Circulation 84:2559, 1991
393. Schwinn DA, Leone BJ, Spahn DR, et al: Desensitization of myocardial beta-adrenergic receptors during cardiopulmonary bypass. Evidence for early uncoupling and late downregulation. Circulation 84:2559, 1991
394. Smiley RM, Kwatra MM, Schwinn DA: New developments in cardiovascular adrenergic receptor pharmacology: Molecular mechanisms and clinical relevance. J Cardiothorac Vasc Anesth 12:80, 1998
395. Reves JG, Karp RB, Buttner EE, et al: Neuronal and adrenomedullary catecholamine release in response to cardiopulmonary bypass in man. Circulation 66:49, 1982
396. Sarnoff S, Braunwald E, Welch G: Hemodynamic determinants of oxygen consumption of the heart with special reference to the tension time index. Am J Physiol 192:148, 1958
397. Vinten-Johansen J, Thourani VH: Myocardial protection: An overview. J Extra Corpor Technol 32:38, 2000
398. Gay WA Jr: Potassium-induced cardioplegia. Ann Thorac Surg 20:95, 1975
399. Gay WA Jr, Ebert PA: Functional, metabolic, and morphologic effects of potassium-induced cardioplegia. Surgery 74:284, 1973
400. Julia PL, Buckberg GD, Acar C, et al: Studies of controlled reperfusion after ischemia. XXI. Reperfusate composition: Superiority of blood cardioplegia over crystalloid cardioplegia in limiting reperfusion damage—importance of endogenous oxygen free radical scavengers in red blood cells. J Thorac Cardiovasc Surg 101:303, 1991
401. Follette DM, Mulder DG, Maloney JV, et al: Advantages of blood cardioplegia over continuous coronary perfusion or intermittent ischemia. Experimental and clinical study. J Thorac Cardiovasc Surg 76:604, 1978
402. Fremes SE, Christakis GT, Weisel RD, et al: A clinical trial of blood and crystalloid cardioplegia. J Thorac Cardiovasc Surg 88(Pt 1):726, 1984
403. Loop FD, Higgins TL, Panda R, et al: Myocardial protection during cardiac operations. Decreased morbidity and lower cost with blood cardioplegia and coronary sinus perfusion. J Thorac Cardiovasc Surg 104:608, 1992
404. Follette DM, Fey K, Buckberg GD, et al: Reducing postischemic damage by temporary modification of reperfusate calcium, potassium, pH, and osmolarity. J Thorac Cardiovasc Surg 82:221, 1981
405. Follette D, Fey K, Mulder D, et al: Prolonged safe aortic clamping by combining membrane stabilization, multidose cardioplegia, and appropriate pH reperfusion. J Thorac Cardiovasc Surg 74:682, 1977
406. Salerno TA, Houck JP, Barrozo CA, et al: Retrograde continuous warm blood cardioplegia: A new concept in myocardial protection (see comments). Ann Thorac Surg 51:245, 1991
407. Mehlhorn U: Improved myocardial protection using continuous coronary perfusion with normothermic blood and beta-blockade with esmolol. Thorac Cardiovasc Surg 45:224, 1997
408. Segel LD, Follette DM: Cardiac function and glycogen content after twenty-four-hour preservation with various metabolic substrates. J Heart Lung Transplant 17:299, 1998
409. Segel LD, Follette DM, Baker JM, et al: Recovery of sheep hearts after perfusion preservation or static storage with crystalloid media. J Heart Lung Transplant 17:211, 1998
410. Smolens IA, Follette DM, Berkoff HA, et al: Incomplete recovery of working heart function after twenty-four-hour preservation with a modified University of Wisconsin solution. J Heart Lung Transplant 14:906, 1995
411. Mauney MC, Kron IL: The physiologic basis of warm cardioplegia. Ann Thorac Surg 60:819, 1995
412. Ikonomidis JS, Rao V, Weisel RD, et al: Myocardial protection for coronary bypass grafting: The Toronto Hospital perspective. Ann Thorac Surg 60:824, 1995
413. Hayashida N, Weisel RD, Shirai T, et al: Tepid antegrade and retrograde cardioplegia. Ann Thorac Surg 59:723, 1995
414. Menasche P, Subayi JB, Veyssie L, et al: Efficacy of coronary sinus cardioplegia in patients with complete coronary artery occlusions. Ann Thorac Surg 51:418, 1991
415. Menasche P, Subayi JB, Piwnica A: Retrograde coronary sinus cardioplegia for aortic valve operations: A clinical report on 500 patients. Ann Thorac Surg 49:556, 1990
416. Hammond GL, Davies AL, Austen WG: Retrograde coronary sinus perfusion: A method of myocardial protection in the dog during left coronary artery occlusion. Ann Surg 166:39, 1967
417. Flack JE 3rd, Cook JR, May SJ, et al: Does cardioplegia type affect outcome and survival in patients with advanced left ventricular dysfunction? Results from the CABG Patch Trial. Circulation 102(suppl 3):III-84, 2000
418. Dagenais F, Pelletier LC, Carrier M: Antegrade/retrograde cardioplegia for valve replacement: A prospective study. Ann Thorac Surg 68:1681, 1999
419. Shahian DM: Retrograde coronary sinus cardioplegia in the presence of persistent left superior vena cava. Ann Thorac Surg 54:1214, 1992
420. Roberts W, Risher W, Schwarz K: Transesophageal echocardiographic identification of persistent left superior vene cava: Retrograde administration of cardioplegia during cardiac surgery. Anesthesiology 81:760, 1994
421. Murry CE, Jennings RB, Reimer KA: Preconditioning with ischemia: A delay of lethal cell injury in ischemic myocardium. Circulation 74:1124, 1986
422. Ikonomidis JS, Weisel RD, Mickle DA: Ischemic preconditioning: Cardioprotection for cardiac surgery. J Card Surg 9(suppl):526, 1994
423. Finegan BA, Lopaschuk GD, Gandhi M, et al: Ischemic preconditioning inhibits glycolysis and proton production in isolated working rat hearts. Am J Physiol 269(Pt 2):H1767, 1995
424. Hagar JM, Hale SL, Kloner RA: Effect of preconditioning ischemia on reperfusion arrhythmias after coronary artery occlusion and reperfusion in the rat. Circ Res 68:61, 1991

425. Liu GS, Thornton J, Van Winkle DM, et al: Protection against infarction afforded by preconditioning is mediated by A1 adenosine receptors in rabbit heart. Circulation 84:350, 1991
426. Perrault LP, Menasche P: Role of preconditioning in cardiac surgery. Basic Res Cardiol 92(suppl 2):54, 1997
427. Speechly-Dick M, Grover G, Yellon D: Does ischemic preconditioning in the human involve protein kinase C and the ATP-dependent K+ channel? Studies of contractile function after simulated ischemia in an atrial in vitro model. Circ Res 77:1030, 1995
428. De Hert S, Vermeyen K, Adriensen H: Influence of thiopental, etomidate and propofol on regional myocardial function in the normal and acute ischemic heart segments. Anesth Analg 70:600, 1990
429. Mentzer RM Jr, Rahko PS, Molina-Viamonte V, et al: Safety, tolerance, and efficacy of adenosine as an additive to blood cardioplegia in humans during coronary artery bypass surgery. Am J Cardiol 79:38, 1997
430. Lee HT, LaFaro RJ, Reed GE: Pretreatment of human myocardium with adenosine during open heart surgery. J Card Surg 10:665, 1995
431. Finegan B, Cohen M: Myocardial protection: Is there anything better than ice? Can J Anaesth 45:R32, 1998
432. Lawhorne TWJ, Davis JL, Smith GW: General surgical complications after cardiac surgery. Am J Surg 136:254, 1976
433. Lucas A, Max MH: Emergency laparotomy immediately after coronary bypass. JAMA 244:1829, 1980
434. Reath DB, Maull KI, Wolfgang TC: General surgical complications following cardiac surgery. Am Surg 49:11, 1983
435. Aranha GV, Pickleman J, Pifarre R, et al: The reasons for gastrointestinal consultation after cardiac surgery. Am Surg 50:301, 1984
436. Ohri SK, Desai JB, Gaer JA, et al: Intraabdominal complications after cardiopulmonary bypass. Ann Thorac Surg 52:826, 1991
437. Rosemurgy AS, McAllister E, Karl RC: The acute surgical abdomen after cardiac surgery involving extracorporeal circulation. Ann Surg 207:323, 1988
438. D'Ancona G, Baillot R, Poirier B, et al: Determinants of gastrointestinal complications in cardiac surgery. Tex Heart Inst J 30:280, 2003
439. Fitzgerald T, Kim D, Karakozis S, et al: Visceral ischemia after cardiopulmonary bypass. Am Surg 66:623, 2000
440. McSweeney ME, Garwood S, Levin J, et al: Adverse gastrointestinal complications after cardiopulmonary bypass: Can outcome be predicted from preoperative risk factors? Anesth Analg 98:1610, 2004
441. Halm MA: Acute gastrointestinal complications after cardiac surgery. Am J Crit Care 5:109, 1996
442. Sakorafas GH, Tsiotos GG: Intra-abdominal complications after cardiac surgery. Eur J Surg Sep 165:820, 1999
443. Hessel EA 2nd: Abdominal organ injury after cardiac surgery. Semin Cardiothorac Vasc Anesth 8:243, 2004
444. Christenson JT, Schmuziger M, Maurice J, et al: Gastrointestinal complications after coronary artery bypass grafting. J Thorac Cardiovasc Surg 108:899, 1994
445. Musleh GS, Patel NC, Grayson AD, et al: Off-pump coronary artery bypass surgery does not reduce gastrointestinal complications. Eur J Cardiothorac Surg 23:170, 2003
446. Perugini RA, Orr RK, Porter D, et al: Gastrointestinal complications following cardiac surgery. An analysis of 1477 cardiac surgery patients. Arch Surg 132:352, 1997
447. Spotnitz WD, Sanders RP, Hanks JB, et al: General surgical complications can be predicted after cardiopulmonary bypass. Ann Surg 221:489, 1995
448. Zacharias A, Schwann TA, Parenteau GL, et al: Predictors of gastrointestinal complications in cardiac surgery. Tex Heart Inst J 27:93, 2000
449. Sanisoglu I, Guden M, Bayramoglu Z, et al: Does off-pump CABG reduce gastrointestinal complications? Ann Thorac Surg 77:619, 2004
450. Lennon MJ, Gibbs NM, Weightman WM, et al: Transesophageal echocardiography-related gastrointestinal complications in cardiac surgical patients. J Cardiothorac Vasc Anesth 19:141, 2005
451. Bolke E, Jehle PM, Orth K, et al: Changes of gut barrier function during anesthesia and cardiac surgery. Angiology 52:477, 2001
452. Sack FU, Hagl S: Extracorporeal circulation and intestinal microcirculation: Pathophysiology and therapeutical options. An intravital microscopic study in a large animal model. Eur Surg Res 34:129, 2002
453. Doty JR, Wilentz RE, Salazar JD, et al: Atheroembolism in cardiac surgery. Ann Thorac Surg 75:1221, 2003
454. Simic O, Strathausen S, Hess W, et al: Incidence and prognosis of abdominal complications after cardiopulmonary bypass. Cardiovasc Surg 7:419, 1999
455. Cetindag IB, Boley TM, Magee MJ, et al: Postoperative gastrointestinal complications after lung volume reduction operations. Ann Thorac Surg 68:1029, 1999
456. Smith PC, Slaughter MS, Petty MG, et al: Abdominal complications after lung transplantation. J Heart Lung Transplant 14(Pt 1):44, 1995
457. Bastien O, Piriou V, Aouifi A, et al: Relative importance of flow versus pressure in splanchnic perfusion during cardiopulmonary bypass in rabbits. Anesthesiology 92:457, 2000
458. Boston US, Slater JM, Orszulak TA, et al: Hierarchy of regional oxygen delivery during cardiopulmonary bypass. Ann Thorac Surg 71:260, 2001
459. Slater JM, Orszulak TA, Cook DJ: Distribution and hierarchy of regional blood flow during hypothermic cardiopulmonary bypass. Ann Thorac Surg Aug 72:542, 2001
460. Landow L: Splanchnic lactate production in cardiac surgery patients. Crit Care Med 21(suppl):S84, 1993
461. Mythen MG, Webb AR: Perioperative plasma volume expansion reduces the incidence of gut mucosal hypoperfusion during cardiac surgery. Arch Surg 130:423, 1995
462. Debaveye YA, Van den Berghe GH: Is there still a place for dopamine in the modern intensive care unit? Anesth Analg 98:461, 2004
463. Parviainen I, Ruokonen E, Takala J: Dobutamine-induced dissociation between changes in splanchnic blood flow and gastric intramucosal pH after cardiac surgery. Br J Anaesth 74:277, 1995
464. Gardeback M, Settergren G: Dopexamine and dopamine in the prevention of low gastric mucosal pH following cardiopulmonary by-pass. Acta Anaesthesiol Scand 39:1066, 1995
465. Westphal M, Freise H, Kehrel BE, et al: Arginine vasopressin compromises gut mucosal microcirculation in septic rats. Crit Care Med 32:194, 2004
466. Martinez-Pellus AE, Merino P, Bru M, et al: Endogenous endotoxemia of intestinal origin during cardiopulmonary bypass. Role of type of flow and protective effect of selective digestive decontamination. Intensive Care Med 23:1251, 1997
467. Matheson PJ, Wilson MA, Garrison RN: Regulation of intestinal blood flow. J Surg Res 93:182, 2000
468. Rea HH, Harris EA, Seelye ER, et al: The effects of cardiopulmonary bypass upon pulmonary gas exchange. J Thorac Cardiovasc Surg 75:104, 1978
469. Cheng DC: Fast track cardiac surgery pathways: Early extubation, process of care, and cost containment. Anesthesiology 88:1429, 1998
470. Rady MY, Ryan T, Starr NJ: Early onset of acute pulmonary dysfunction after cardiovascular surgery: Risk factors and clinical outcome. Crit Care Med 25:1831, 1997
471. Bernard GR, Artigas A, Brigham KL, et al: Report of the American-European consensus conference on ARDS: Definitions, mechanisms, relevant outcomes and clinical trial coordination. The Consensus Committee. Intensive Care Med 20:225, 1994
472. Christenson JT, Aeberhard JM, Badel P, et al: Adult respiratory distress syndrome after cardiac surgery. Cardiovasc Surg 4:15, 1996
473. Welsby IJ, Bennett-Guerrero E, Atwell D, et al: The association of complication type with mortality and prolonged stay after cardiac surgery with cardiopulmonary bypass. Anesth Analg 94:1072, 2002
474. Ng CS, Wan S, Yim AP, et al: Pulmonary dysfunction after cardiac surgery. Chest 121:1269, 2002
475. Jindani A, Aps C, Neville E, et al: Postoperative cardiac surgical care: An alternative approach. Br Heart J 69:59, 1993
476. Jain U, Rao TL, Kumar P, et al: Radiographic pulmonary abnormalities after different types of cardiac surgery. J Cardiothorac Vasc Anesth 5:592, 1991
477. Magnusson L, Zemgulis V, Wicky S, et al: Atelectasis is a major cause of hypoxemia and shunt after cardiopulmonary bypass: An experimental study. Anesthesiology 87:1153, 1997
478. Magnusson L, Zemgulis V, Tenling A, et al: Use of a vital capacity maneuver to prevent atelectasis after cardiopulmonary bypass: An experimental study. Anesthesiology 88:134, 1998
479. Daganou M, Dimopoulou I, Michalopoulos N, et al: Respiratory complications after coronary artery bypass surgery with unilateral or bilateral internal mammary artery grafting. Chest 113:1285, 1998
480. Johnson D, Kelm C, Thomson D, et al: The effect of physical therapy on respiratory complications following cardiac valve surgery. Chest 109:638, 1996
481. Lim E, Callaghan C, Motalleb-Zadeh R, et al: A prospective study on clinical outcome following pleurotomy during cardiac surgery. Thorac Cardiovasc Surg 50:287, 2002
482. Lainez RM, Losada M, Nieto E, et al: Pneumonia in patients undergoing heart surgery [in Spanish]. Enferm Infec Microbiol Clin 12:4, 1994
483. Bouza E, Perez A, Munoz P, et al: Ventilator-associated pneumonia after heart surgery: A prospective analysis and the value of surveillance. Crit Care Med 31:1964, 2003

484. Kollef MH, Sharpless L, Vlasnik J, et al: The impact of nosocomial infections on patient outcomes following cardiac surgery. Chest 112:666, 1997
485. Leal-Noval SR, Marquez-Vacaro JA, Garcia-Curiel A, et al: Nosocomial pneumonia in patients undergoing heart surgery. Crit Care Med 28:935, 2000
486. Gaynes R, Bizek B, Mowry-Hanley J, et al: Risk factors for nosocomial pneumonia after coronary artery bypass graft operations. Ann Thorac Surg 51:215, 1991
487. Auler JO Jr, Zin WA, Caldeira MP, et al: Pre- and postoperative inspiratory mechanics in ischemic and valvular heart disease. Chest 92:984, 1987
488. Barnas GM, Watson RJ, Green MD, et al: Lung and chest wall mechanical properties before and after cardiac surgery with cardiopulmonary bypass. J Appl Physiol 76:166, 1994
489. Hachenberg T, Brussel T, Roos N, et al: Gas exchange impairment and pulmonary densities after cardiac surgery. Acta Anaesthesiol Scand 36:800, 1992
490. Raijmakers PG, Groeneveld AB, Schneider AJ, et al: Transvascular transport of 67Ga in the lungs after cardiopulmonary bypass surgery. Chest 104:1825, 1993
491. Messent M, Sinclair DG, Quinlan GJ, et al: Pulmonary vascular permeability after cardiopulmonary bypass and its relationship to oxidative stress. Crit Care Med 25:425, 1997
492. Sinclair DG, Haslam PL, Quinlan GJ, et al: The effect of cardiopulmonary bypass on intestinal and pulmonary endothelial permeability. Chest 108:718, 1995
493. Baue AE: The role of the gut in the development of multiple organ dysfunction in cardiothoracic patients. Ann Thorac Surg 55:822, 1993
494. Gorlach G, Sroka J, Heidt M, et al: Intracellular adhesion molecule-1 in patients developing pulmonary insufficiency after cardiopulmonary bypass. Thorac Cardiovasc Surg 51:138, 2003
495. Wasowicz M, Sobczynski P, Biczysko W, et al: Ultrastructural changes in the lung alveoli after cardiac surgical operations with the use of cardiopulmonary bypass (CPB). Pol J Pathol 50:189, 1999
496. Milot J, Perron J, Lacasse Y, et al: Incidence and predictors of ARDS after cardiac surgery. Chest 119:884, 2001
497. Asimakopoulos G, Taylor KM, Smith PL, et al: Prevalence of acute respiratory distress syndrome after cardiac surgery. J Thorac Cardiovasc Surg 117:620, 1999
498. Gillinov AM, Davis EA, Alberg AJ, et al: Pulmonary embolism in the cardiac surgical patient. Ann Thorac Surg 53:988, 1992
499. Josa M, Siouffi SY, Silverman AB, et al: Pulmonary embolism after cardiac surgery. J Am Coll Cardiol 21:990, 1993
500. Weissman C: Pulmonary complications after cardiac surgery. Semin Cardiothorac Vasc Anesth 8:185, 2004
501. DeLaria GA, Hunter JA: Deep venous thrombosis. Implications after open heart surgery. Chest 99:284, 1991
502. Ambrosetti M, Salerno M, Zambelli M, et al: Deep vein thrombosis among patients entering cardiac rehabilitation after coronary artery bypass surgery. Chest 125:191, 2004
503. Goldhaber SZ, Hirsch DR, MacDougall RC, et al: Prevention of venous thrombosis after coronary artery bypass surgery (a randomized trial comparing two mechanical prophylaxis strategies). Am J Cardiol 76:993, 1995
504. Gilbert TB, Barnas GM, Sequeira AJ: Impact of pleurotomy, continuous positive airway pressure, and fluid balance during cardiopulmonary bypass on lung mechanics and oxygenation. J Cardiothorac Vasc Anesth 10:844, 1996
505. Berry CB, Butler PJ, Myles PS: Lung management during cardiopulmonary bypass: Is continuous positive airways pressure beneficial? Br J Anaesth 71:864, 1993
506. Lee AH, Gallagher PJ: Post-mortem examination after cardiac surgery. Histopathology 33:399, 1998
507. Ventilation with lower tidal volumes as compared with traditional tidal volumes for acute lung injury and the acute respiratory distress syndrome. The Acute Respiratory Distress Syndrome Network. N Engl J Med 342:1301, 2000
508. Hill G, Alonso A, Thiele G, et al: Glucocorticoids blunt neutrophil CD11b surface glycoprotein upregulation during cardiopulmonary bypass in humans. Anesth Analg 79:23, 1994
509. Kilger E, Weis F, Briegel J, et al: Stress doses of hydrocortisone reduce severe systemic inflammatory response syndrome and improve early outcome in a risk group of patients after cardiac surgery. Crit Care Med 31:1068, 2003
510. Oliver WC Jr, Nuttall GA, Orszulak TA, et al: Hemofiltration but not steroids results in earlier tracheal extubation following cardiopulmonary bypass: A prospective, randomized double-blind trial. Anesthesiology 101:327, 2004
511. Chaney MA, Nikolov MP, Blakeman B, et al: Pulmonary effects of methylprednisolone in patients undergoing coronary artery bypass grafting and early tracheal extubation. Anesth Analg 87:27, 1998
512. Bidstrup B, Royston D, Sapsford R, et al: Reduction in blood loss and blood use after cardiopulmonary bypass with high dose aprotinin (Trasylol). J Thorac Cardiovasc Surg 97:364, 1989
513. Hill GE, Alonso A, Spurzem JR, et al: Aprotinin and methylprednisolone equally blunt cardiopulmonary bypass-induced inflammation in humans. J Thorac Cardiovasc Surg 110:1658, 1995
514. Royston D, Bidstrup BP, Taylor KM, et al: Effect of aprotinin on need for blood transfusion after repeat open-heart surgery. Lancet 2:1289, 1987
515. Royston D: High dose aprotinin therapy: A review of the first five years' experience. J Cardiothorac Vasc Anesth 6:76, 1992
516. Royston D: Aprotinin therapy. Br J Anaesth 73:734, 1994
517. van Oeveren W, Jansen N, Bidstrup B, et al: Effects of aprotinin on hemostatic mechanisms during cardiopulmonary bypass. Ann Thorac Surg 44:640, 1987
518. Wessel DL, Adatia I, Giglia TM, et al: Use of inhaled nitric oxide and acetylcholine in the evaluation of pulmonary hypertension and endothelial function after cardiopulmonary bypass. Circulation 88(Pt 1):2128, 1993
519. Rich GF, Murphy GD Jr, Roos CM, et al: Inhaled nitric oxide. Selective pulmonary vasodilation in cardiac surgical patients. Anesthesiology 78:1028, 1993
520. Fullerton DA, Jones SD, Jaggers J, et al: Effective control of pulmonary vascular resistance with inhaled nitric oxide after cardiac operation. J Thorac Cardiovasc Surg 111:753, 1996
521. Bacha EA, Head CA: Use of inhaled nitric oxide for lung transplantation and cardiac surgery. Respir Care Clin North Am 3:521, 1997
522. Newman MF, Wolman R, Kanchuger M, et al: Multicenter preoperative stroke risk index for patients undergoing coronary artery bypass graft surgery. Circulation 94(suppl):II-74, 1996

Chapter 31

DISCONTINUING CARDIOPULMONARY BYPASS

Jack S. Shanewise, MD • Roberta L. Hines, MD • Joel A. Kaplan, MD

KEY POINTS

1. The key to success in weaning from cardiopulmonary bypass (CPB) is proper preparation.
2. After rewarming the patient, correcting any abnormal blood gases, and inflating the lungs, be sure to turn on the ventilator!
3. To prepare the heart for discontinuing CPB, optimize the cardiac rhythm, heart rate, myocardial contractility, preload, and afterload.
4. The worse the heart's condition, the more gradually CPB should be weaned. If hemodynamic values are not adequate, immediately return to CPB. Assess the problem, and choose an appropriate pharmacologic intervention before trying to terminate CPB again.
5. Perioperative ventricular dysfunction usually is caused by myocardial stunning and is a temporary state of contractile dysfunction that should respond to positive inotropic drugs.
6. In addition to left ventricular dysfunction, right ventricular failure is a possible source of morbidity and mortality after cardiac surgery.
7. Epinephrine is frequently the inotropic drug of choice when terminating CPB because of its mixed α- and β-adrenergic stimulation.
8. Milrinone is an excellent inodilator drug that can be used alone or combined with other drugs such as epinephrine for discontinuing CPB in patients with poor ventricular function.
9. In patients with high preloads, vasodilators such as nitroglycerin or nitroprusside may markedly improve ventricular function.
10. Intra-aortic balloon pump counterpulsation increases coronary blood flow during diastole and unloads the left ventricle during systole. These effects can help in weaning patients with poor left ventricular function and severe myocardial ischemia.

Cardiopulmonary bypass (CPB) has been used since the 1950s to facilitate surgery on the heart and great vessels, and even with the increased interest in off-pump coronary artery bypass grafting (CABG), CPB remains a critical part of most cardiac operations. Managing patients with CPB remains one of the defining characteristics of cardiac surgery and cardiac anesthesiology (see Chapters 1, 2, and 28). Discontinuing CPB is a necessary part of every operation involving extracorporeal circulation. Through this process, the support of the circulation by the bypass pump and oxygenator is transferred back to the patient's heart and lungs. This chapter reviews important considerations involved with discontinuing CPB and presents an approach to managing this critical component of a cardiac operation, which may be routine and easy or extremely complex and difficult. The key to success in discontinuing CPB is proper preparation. The period during and immediately after weaning from CPB is usually very busy for the anesthesiologist, and having to do things that could have been accomplished earlier in the operation is not helpful. The preparations for bringing a patient off CPB may be organized into several parts: general preparations, preparing the lungs, preparing the heart, and final preparations.

GENERAL PREPARATIONS

Temperature

Because at least moderate hypothermia is used during CPB in most cardiac surgery cases, it is important that the patient is sufficiently rewarmed before attempting to wean from CPB (Table 31–1).[1] Initiation of rewarming is a good time to consider whether additional drugs need to be given to keep the patient anesthetized. Anesthetic vaporizers need to be off for 20 to 30 minutes before coming off CPB to clear the agent from the patient if so desired.[2] Monitoring the temperature of a highly perfused tissue such as the nasopharynx is useful to help prevent overheating the brain during rewarming, but these temperatures may rise more rapidly than others, such as bladder, rectum, or axilla temperatures, leading to inadequate rewarming and temperature drop-off after CPB as the heat continues to distribute throughout the body.[3] Different institutions have various protocols for rewarming, but the important point is to warm gradually, avoiding hyperthermia of the central nervous system while getting enough heat into the patient to prevent significant drop-off after CPB[4] (see Chapters 28 and 30). After CPB, there is a tendency for the patient to lose heat, and measures to keep the patient warm such as fluid warmers, a circuit heater-humidifier, and forced-air warmers should be set up and turned on before weaning from CPB. The temperature of the operating room may need to be increased as well; this is probably an effective measure to keep a patient warm after CPB, but it may make the scrubbed and gowned personnel uncomfortable.

Laboratory Results

An arterial blood gas should be measured before weaning from CPB and any abnormalities corrected. Severe metabolic acidosis depresses the myocardium and should be treated with $NaHCO_3$ or THAM.[5-8] The optimal hematocrit for weaning

Table 31–1 General Preparations for Discontinuing Cardiopulmonary Bypass

Temperature	Laboratory Results
Adequately rewarm before weaning from CPB	Correct metabolic acidosis
Avoid overheating the brain	Optimize hematocrit
Start measures to keep patient warm after CPB	Normalize K^+
Use fluid warmer, forced air warmer	Consider giving Mg^{++} or checking Mg^{++} level
Warm operating room	Check Ca^{++} level and correct deficiencies

CPB, cardiopulmonary bypass.

from CPB is controversial and probably varies from patient to patient.[9,10] It makes sense that sicker patients with lower cardiovascular reserve may benefit from a higher hematocrit, but the risks and adverse consequences of transfusion need to be considered as well. Suffice it to say that the hematocrit should be measured and optimized before weaning from CPB (see Chapter 29). Serum potassium level should be measured before weaning from CPB and may be high due to cardioplegia or low, especially in patients receiving loop diuretics. Hyperkalemia may make establishing an effective cardiac rhythm difficult and can be treated with $NaHCO_3$, $CaCl_2$, or insulin, but the levels usually decrease quickly after cardioplegia has been stopped. Low serum potassium levels should probably be corrected before coming off CPB, especially if arrhythmias are present. Administration of magnesium (Mg^{++}) to patients on CPB decreases postoperative arrhythmias and may improve cardiac function, and many centers routinely give all CPB patients magnesium sulfate.[11] Theoretical disadvantages include aggravation of vasodilation and inhibition of platelet function.[12] If Mg^{++} is not given routinely, the level should be checked before weaning from CPB and deficiencies corrected. The ionized calcium level should be measured and significant deficiencies corrected before discontinuing CPB. Many centers give all patients a bolus of calcium chloride just before coming off CPB because it transiently increases contractility and systemic vascular resistance.[13] However, it has been argued that this practice is to be avoided because Ca^{++} may interfere with catecholamine action and aggravate reperfusion injury.[14]

PREPARING THE LUNGS

As the patient is weaned from CPB and the patient's heart starts to support the circulation, the lungs again become the site of gas exchange, delivering oxygen and eliminating carbon dioxide. Before weaning from CPB, the lung function must be restored (Table 31–2). The trachea should be suctioned and, if necessary, lavaged with saline to clear secretions. If the abdomen appears to be distended, the stomach should be suctioned so that gastric distention does not impair ventilation after CPB. The lungs are reinflated by hand gently and gradually, with sighs using up to 30 cm H_2O pressure, and then mechanically ventilated with 100% oxygen. Care should be taken not to allow the left lung to injure an in situ internal mammary artery graft as the lung is reinflated. The compliance of the lungs can be judged by their feel with hand ventilation, with stiff lungs suggesting more difficulty with oxygenation or ventilation after CPB. If visible, both lungs should be inspected for residual atelectasis, and they should be rising and falling with each breath. Ventilation alarms and monitors should be activated. If prolonged expiration or wheezing is detected, bronchodilators should be given. The surgeon should inspect both pleural spaces for pneumothorax, which should be treated with chest tubes. Any fluid present in the pleural spaces should be removed before attempting to wean the patient from CPB. In its most severe form, pulmonary dysfunction after CPB may require positive end-expiratory pressure, an intensive care unit–type ventilator, or nitric oxide (see Chapters 33 and 34). If needed, this equipment should be obtained before attempting to wean the patient from CPB.

Table 31–2 Preparing the Lungs for Discontinuing Cardiopulmonary Bypass

Suction trachea and endotracheal tube.
Inflate lungs gently by hand.
Ventilate with 100% oxygen.
Treat bronchospasm with bronchodilators.
Check for pneumothorax and pleural fluid.
Consider need for positive end-expiratory pressure, intensive care unit ventilator, and nitric oxide.

PREPARING THE HEART

Preparing the heart to resume its function pumping blood involves optimizing the five hemodynamic parameters that can be controlled: rhythm, rate, contractility, afterload, and preload (Table 31–3).

Rhythm

There must be an organized, effective, and stable cardiac rhythm before attempting to wean from CPB. This can occur spontaneously after removal of the aortic cross-clamp, but the heart may resume electrical activity with ventricular fibrillation. If the blood temperature is greater than 30°C, the heart may be defibrillated with internal paddles applied directly to the heart using 10 to 20 J. Defibrillation at lower temperatures may be unsuccessful because extreme hypothermia can cause ventricular fibrillation.[15-17] If ventricular fibrillation persists or recurs repeatedly, antiarrhythmic drugs such as lidocaine or amiodarone may be administered to help achieve a stable rhythm. It is not unusual for the rhythm to remain unstable for several minutes immediately after cross-clamp removal, but persistent or recurrent ventricular fibrillation should prompt concern about impaired coronary blood flow. Because it provides an atrial contribution to ventricular filling and a normal, synchronized contraction of the ventricles, normal sinus rhythm is the ideal cardiac rhythm for weaning from CPB.[18,19] Atrial flutter or fibrillation, even if present before CPB, can often be converted to normal sinus rhythm with synchronized cardioversion, especially if antiarrhythmic drugs are administered. It is often helpful to look directly at the heart

Table 31–3 **Preparing the Heart for Discontinuing Cardiopulmonary Bypass**

Hemodynamic Parameters	Preparation
Rhythm	Normal sinus rhythm is ideal. Defibrillate if necessary when temperature >30°C. Consider antiarrhythmic drugs if ventricular fibrillation persists more than a few minutes. Try synchronized cardioversion for atrial fibrillation or flutter. Look at the heart to diagnose atrial rhythm. Try atrial pacing if AV conduction exists. Try AV pacing for heart block.
Heart rate	Rate should be between 75 and 95 beats per minute in most cases. Treat slow rates with electrical pacing. Treat underlying causes of fast heart rates. Heart rate may decrease as the heart fills. Control fast supraventricular rates with drugs and then pace as needed. Always have pacing available during heart surgery.
Contractility	Inotropic support is more likely needed with depressed cardiac function before CPB, advanced age, long bypass or clamp time, poor preservation, or incomplete revascularization. Look for the vigorous "snap" of a heartbeat with good contractility. If depressed contractility is likely, begin inotropic drugs before weaning from CPB. Severely impaired function may require mechanical support.
Afterload	Systemic vascular resistance is a major component of afterload. Keep MAP between 60 and 80 mm Hg at full CPB flow. Consider a vasoconstrictor if the MAP is low and a vasodilator if the MAP is high.
Preload	End-diastolic volume is the best measure of preload and can be seen with TEE. Filling pressures provide a less direct measure of preload. Consider baseline filling pressures. Assess RV volume and function with direct inspection. Assess LV volume and function with TEE. Cardiac distention may cause MR and TR.

AV = atrioventricular; CPB = cardiopulmonary bypass; LV = left ventricular; MAP = mean arterial pressure; MR = mitral regurgitation; RV = right ventricular; TEE = transesophageal echocardiography; TR, tricuspid regurgitation.

when there is any question about the cardiac rhythm. Atrial contraction, flutter, and fibrillation are easily seen on CPB. Ventricular arrhythmias should be treated by correcting underlying causes such as potassium or magnesium deficits and, if necessary, with antiarrhythmic drugs such as amiodarone.[20] If asystole or complete heart block occurs after cross-clamp removal, electrical pacing with temporary epicardial pacing wires may be needed to achieve an effective rhythm before weaning from CPB. If atrioventricular conduction is present, atrial pacing should be attempted because, as with normal sinus rhythm, it provides atrial augmentation to filling and synchronized ventricular contraction. Atrioventricular sequential pacing is used when there is heart block, which is frequently present for 30 to 60 minutes as the myocardium recovers after cross-clamp removal. Ventricular pacing remains the only option if no organized atrial rhythm is present, but this sacrifices the atrial "kick" to ventricular filling and the more efficient synchronized ventricular contraction of the normal conduction system[21,22] (see Table 33–1 in Chapter 33).

Rate

In most situations for adult patients, the heart rate (HR) should be between 75 and 95 beats per minute (bpm) for weaning from CPB. Lower rates may theoretically be desirable for hearts with residual ischemia or incomplete revascularization. Higher HRs may be needed for hearts with limited stroke volume such as after ventricular aneurysmectomy. Slow HRs are best treated with electrical pacing, but β-agonist or vagolytic drugs also may be used to increase the HR. Tachycardia before weaning from CPB is more worrisome and difficult to deal with, and treatable causes such as inadequate anesthesia, hypercarbia, and ischemia should be identified and corrected. The HR often decreases as the heart is filled in the weaning process, and electrical pacing should always be immediately available during cardiac surgery. Supraventricular tachycardias should be electrically cardioverted if possible, but drugs such as β-antagonists or calcium channel antagonists may be needed to control the ventricular rate if they persist, most typically occurring in patients with chronic atrial fibrillation. If drug therapy lowers the rate too much, pacing may be used.

Contractility

The contractile state of the myocardium should be considered before attempting to wean from CPB. The likelihood of decreased contractility requiring inotropic support after CPB is greater with preexisting ventricular impairment (e.g., low ejection fraction, high left ventricular end-diastolic pressure [LVEDP] preoperatively or before CPB), advanced age, long CPB time, long aortic cross-clamp time, inadequate myocardial preservation, and incomplete revascularization.[23] A heart with good contractility often has a vigorous snap with contraction that can be seen while on CPB, in contrast to the weak contractions of a heart with impaired contractility, but it may be difficult to assess global ventricular function while the heart is empty and on CPB. If significant depression of contractility is likely, inotropic support can be started before attempt-

Table 31–4 **Final Preparations for Discontinuing Cardiopulmonary Bypass**

Anesthesiologist's Preparations	Surgeon's Preparations
Level operating table	Remove macroscopic collections of air from the heart
Re-zero transducers	Control major sites of bleeding
Activate monitors	CABG lying nicely without kinks
Check drug infusions	Cardiac vents off or removed
Have resuscitation drugs and fluid volume at hand	Clamps off the heart and great vessels
Reestablish TEE/PAC monitoring	Tourniquets around caval cannulas loose

CABG = coronary artery bypass graft; TEE = transesophageal echocardiography; PAC, pulmonary artery catheter.

ing to wean the patient from CPB. If depressed myocardial contractility becomes evident during weaning, the safest approach is to prevent cardiac distention by resuming CPB, resting the heart for 10 to 20 minutes while inotropic therapy with a catecholamine or phosphodiesterase inhibitor drug is started. Extreme depression of contractile function of the myocardium may require mechanical support with an intra-aortic balloon pump (IABP) or ventricular assist device (VAD) (see Ventricular Dysfunction below, and Chapter 27).

Afterload

Afterload is the tension developed within the ventricular muscle during contraction. An important component of afterload in patients is the systemic vascular resistance (SVR) (see Chapters 5, 14, and 33).[24] While on CPB at full flow, usually about 2.2 L/min/m^2, mean arterial pressure (MAP) is directly related to SVR and indicates whether the SVR is appropriate, too high, or too low. Low SVR after CPB can cause inadequate systemic arterial perfusion pressure, and high SVR can significantly impair cardiac performance, especially in patients with poor ventricular function. SVR is usually within a reasonable range when the arterial pressure is between 60 and 80 mm Hg at full pump flow. If below that range, infusion of a vasopressor may be needed to increase SVR before attempting to wean from CPB. If the MAP is high while on CPB, vasodilator therapy may be needed.

Preload

Preload is the amount of stretch on the myocardial muscle fibers just before contraction. In the intact heart, the best measure of preload is end-diastolic volume. Less direct clinical measures of preload include left atrial pressure (LAP), pulmonary artery occlusion pressure (PAOP), and pulmonary artery diastolic pressure, but there may be a poor relationship between end-diastolic pressure and volume during cardiac surgery[25,26] (see Chapters 5, 14, and 33). Transesophageal echocardiography (TEE) is a useful tool for weaning from CPB because it provides direct visualization of the end-diastolic volume and contractility of the left ventricle[27-29] (see Chapters 15 and 16). The process of weaning a patient from CPB involves increasing the preload (i.e., filling the heart from its empty state on CPB) until an appropriate end-diastolic volume is achieved. When preparing to discontinue CPB, some thought should be given to the appropriate range of preload for the particular patient at hand. The filling pressures before CPB may indicate what they need to be after CPB; a heart with high filling pressures before CPB may require high filling pressures after CPB to achieve an adequate preload.

FINAL PREPARATIONS

The final preparations before discontinuing CPB include leveling the operating table, rezeroing the pressure transducers, ensuring the proper function of all monitoring devices, confirming that the patient is receiving only intended drug infusions, ensuring the immediate availability of resuscitation drugs and appropriate fluid volume, and verifying that the lungs are being ventilated with 100% oxygen (Table 31–4).

The surgeon must confirm that he or she has completed the necessary preparations in the surgical field before discontinuing CPB. Macroscopic collections of air in the heart should be evacuated before starting to wean from CPB. These are most easily detected with TEE, which can also be helpful in monitoring and directing the deairing process.[30] Major sites of bleeding should be controlled, cardiac vent suction should be off, all clamps on the heart and great vessels should be removed, coronary artery bypass grafts should be checked for kinks and bleeding, and tourniquets around the caval cannulas should be loosened or removed before starting to wean a patient from CPB.

ROUTINE WEANING FROM CARDIOPULMONARY BYPASS

There should be close and clear communication among the perfusionist, the surgeon, and the anesthesiologist while weaning a patient from CPB, and the surgeon or the anesthesiologist should be in charge of the process. The anesthesiologist should be positioned at the head of the table, able to readily see the CPB pump and perfusionist, the heart and the surgeon, and the anesthesia monitor display. If present, the TEE display should also be easily in view. Weaning a patient from CPB is accomplished by diverting blood back into the patient's heart by occluding the venous drainage to the CPB pump. The arterial pump flow is decreased simultaneously as the pump reservoir volume empties into the patient and the heart's contribution to systemic flow increases. This can be accomplished most abruptly by simply clamping the venous return cannula and transfusing blood from the pump until the heart fills and the preload appears to be adequate. Some patients will tolerate this method of discontinuing CPB, but many will not, and a more gradual transfer from the pump to the heart is usually desirable. The worse the function of the heart, the slower the transition from full CPB to off CPB needs to be.

Before beginning to wean the patient from CPB, the perfusionist should communicate to the physicians involved three important parameters: the current flow rate of the pump, the volume in the pump reservoir, and the oxygen saturation of venous blood returning to the pump from the patient. The current flow rate of the pump indicates the stage of weaning as it is decreased. Weaning is just beginning at full flow, is well underway when down to 2 or 3 L/min in adults, and is almost finished at less than 2 L/min. The reservoir volume indicates how much blood is available for transfusion to fill the heart and lungs as CPB is discontinued. If the volume is low, less than 400 to 500 mL in adults, more fluid may need to be added to the reservoir before weaning from CPB. The oxygen saturation of the venous return (SvO_2) gives an indication of the adequacy of peripheral perfusion during CPB. If the SvO_2 is greater than 60%, oxygen delivery during CPB is adequate; if less than 50%, oxygen delivery is inadequate, and measures to improve delivery (e.g., increase pump flow or hematocrit) or decrease consumption (e.g., give more anesthetic agents or neuromuscular blocking drugs) need to be taken before coming off CPB. An SvO_2 between 50% and 60% is marginal and must be followed closely. As the patient is weaned from CPB, a rising SvO_2 suggests that the net flow to the body is increasing and that the heart and lungs will support the circulation; a falling SvO_2 indicates that tissue perfusion is decreasing and that further intervention to improve cardiac performance will be needed before coming off CPB.

The actual process of weaning from CPB begins with partially occluding the venous return cannula with a clamp (Fig. 31–1). This may be done in the field by the surgeon or at the pump by the perfusionist. This causes blood to flow into the right ventricle. As the right ventricle fills and begins to pump blood through the lungs, the left heart will begin to fill. When this occurs, the left ventricle will begin to eject, and the arterial waveform will become pulsatile. Next, the perfusionist will gradually decrease the pump flow rate. As more of the venous return goes through the heart and less to the pump reservoir, it becomes necessary to gradually decrease the pump flow to avoid emptying the pump reservoir. One approach to weaning from CPB is to bring the filling pressure being monitored (e.g., central venous pressure [CVP], PAOP, LAP) to a specific, predetermined level somewhat lower than may be necessary and then assess the hemodynamics. Volume (preload) of the heart may also be judged by direct observation of its size or with TEE. Further filling is done in small increments (50 to 100 mL) while closely monitoring the preload until the hemodynamics appear satisfactory as judged by the arterial pressure, the appearance of the heart, and the trend of the SvO_2. It is typically easy to see the right-heart volume and function directly in the surgical field and the left heart with TEE, and combining the two observations is a useful approach for weaning from CPB. Overfilling and distention of the heart should be avoided because it may stretch the myofibrils beyond the most efficient length and dilate the annuli of the mitral and tricuspid valves, rendering them incompetent, which is easily detected with TEE. If the patient has two venous cannulas, the smaller of the two may be removed when the pump flow is one half of the full flow rate to improve movement of blood from the great veins into the right atrium. When the pump flow has been decreased to 1 L/min or less in an adult and the hemodynamics are satisfactory, the venous cannula may be completely clamped and the pump flow turned off. At this point, the patient is "off bypass" (Fig. 31–2).

This is a critical juncture in the operation. The anesthesiologist should pause a moment to make a brief scan of the patient and monitors to confirm that the lungs are being ventilated with oxygen, the hemodynamic status is acceptable and stable, the electrocardiogram shows no new signs of ischemia, the heart does not appear to be distending, and the drug infusions are functioning as desired. Further fine-tuning of the preload is accomplished by transfusing 50- to 100-mL boluses from the pump reservoir through the arterial cannula and observing the effect on hemodynamics. If there is acute failure of the circulation as evidenced by unstable rhythm, falling arterial and rising filling pressures, or visible distention of the heart, the patient is put back on CPB by unclamping the venous return cannula and turning on the arterial pump flow. Once back on CPB, an assessment of the cause of failure to wean is made and appropriate interventions undertaken before attempting to wean again. When the hemodynamics appear to be stable and adequate, the surgeon may remove the venous cannula from the heart.

The next step in discontinuing CPB is to transfuse as much as possible of the blood remaining in the pump reservoir into the patient before removal of the arterial cannula. This is

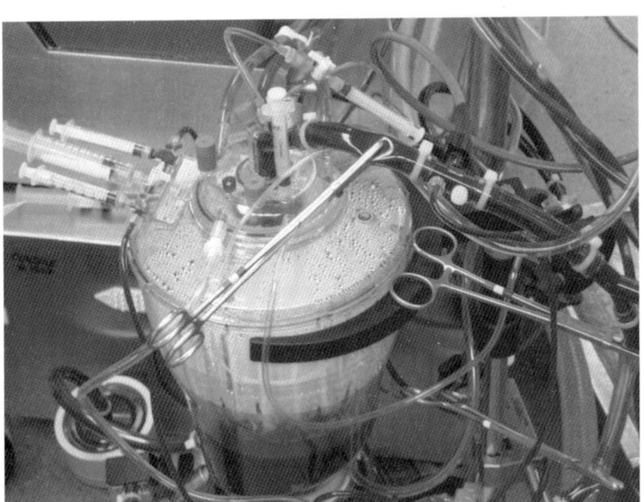

Figure 31–1 The process of weaning from cardiopulmonary bypass is started by partially occluding the venous return cannula with a clamp.

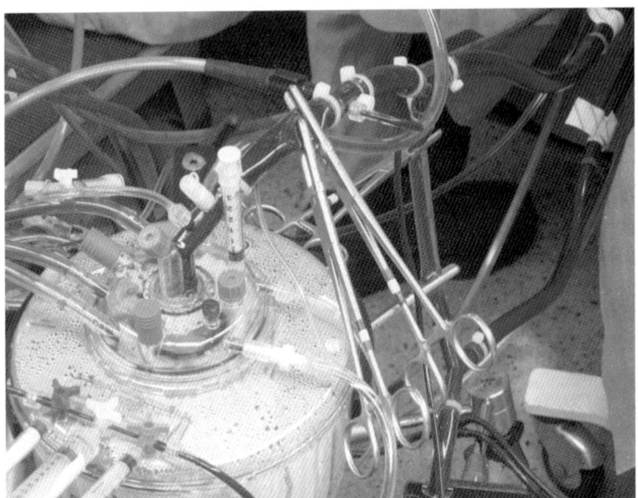

Figure 31–2 When the venous return cannula is completely clamped, the patient is "off bypass."

usually easier and quicker than transfusing through the intravenous infusions after decannulation. The blood in the venous cannula and tubing (usually about 500 mL) may be drained into the reservoir for transfusion. The patient's venous capacitance can be increased by raising the head of the bed (i.e., reverse Trendelenburg position) or giving nitroglycerin, being more cautious with these maneuvers in patients with impaired cardiac function. Filling the vascular space with the head up and while infusing nitroglycerin increases the ability to cope with volume loss after decannulation by allowing rapid augmentation of the central vascular volume by leveling the bed and decreasing the nitroglycerin infusion rate.

After discontinuing CPB, the anticoagulation by heparin is reversed with protamine. Depending on institutional preference, protamine may be administered before or after removal of the arterial cannula. Giving it before removal allows for continued transfusion from the pump and easier return to CPB if there is a severe protamine reaction (see Chapter 29). Giving protamine after removal of the arterial cannula probably decreases the risk of thrombus formation and systemic embolization. After the infusion of protamine is started, pump suction return to the reservoir should be stopped to keep protamine out of the pump circuit in case subsequent return to CPB becomes necessary. Protamine should be given slowly through a peripheral intravenous catheter over 7 to 15 minutes while watching for systemic hypotension and pulmonary hypertension, which may indicate that an untoward (allergic) reaction to protamine is occurring.[31-33] Technically flawed coronary artery bypass grafts may thrombose after protamine administration, causing acute ischemia mimicking a protamine reaction.

When transfusion of the pump reservoir blood is completed, a thorough assessment of the patient's condition should be made before removing the arterial cannula, because after this is done, returning to CPB becomes much more difficult. The cardiac rhythm should be stable. Cardiac function is assessed by evaluating pressures, cardiac output, and TEE. Hemodynamics should be satisfactory and stable. Adequate oxygenation and ventilation should be confirmed by arterial blood gas or pulse oximetry and capnography. Bleeding from the heart should be at a manageable level before removal of the arterial cannula. The perfusionist should not have to transfuse significant amounts of blood through the arterial cannula before removing it, because it may be difficult to keep up with the blood loss through intravenous infusions alone. Bleeding sites behind the heart may have to be repaired on CPB if the patient cannot tolerate lifting the heart to expose the problem area. At the time of arterial decannulation, the systolic pressure should be between 85 and 105 mm Hg to minimize the risk of dissection or tearing of the aorta.[34] The head of the bed may be raised, or small boluses of a short-acting vasodilator (e.g., nitroglycerin, nitroprusside) may be given to lower the systemic blood pressure as necessary. Tight control of the arterial blood pressure may be needed for a few minutes until the cannulation site is secure.

When the arterial cannula has been removed, the heparin effects are reversed with protamine, and the hemodynamic status remains stable, the routine process of discontinuing CPB is complete. However, in patients with poor ventricular function after CPB, multiple drugs or even mechanical assist devices may be required throughout the rest of the operation and continued in the intensive care unit.

PHARMACOLOGIC MANAGEMENT OF VENTRICULAR DYSFUNCTION

Perioperative ventricular dysfunction is usually a transient state of contractile impairment that may require temporary support with positive inotropic agents. In a subset of patients, contractility may be significantly depressed such that combination therapy with positive inotropes and vasodilator agents is needed to effectively improve cardiac output and tissue perfusion. The use of mechanical assist devices is reserved for conditions of overt or evolving cardiogenic shock.

Severe ventricular dysfunction, specifically the low-cardiac-output syndrome (LCOS), occurring after CPB and cardiac surgery differs from chronic congestive heart failure (CHF) (Box 31–1). Patients emerging from CPB have hemodilution, moderate hypocalcemia, hypomagnesemia, and altered potassium levels. Depending on temperature and depth of anesthesia, these individuals may demonstrate low, normal, or high SVR. Increasing age, female sex, decreased LVEF, and increased duration of CPB are associated with a greater likelihood that inotropic support will be needed after CABG surgery[23] (Table 31–5).

Contractile dysfunction during or after cardiac surgery can result from preexisting impairment in contractility or be a new-onset condition. Abnormal contraction, especially in the setting of coronary artery disease (CAD), usually is caused by myocardial injury resulting in ischemia or infarction. The magnitude of contractile dysfunction corresponds to the extent and duration of injury. Brief periods of myocardial oxygen deprivation (<10 minutes) produce regional contractile dysfunction, which can be rapidly reversed by reperfusion. Extension of the ischemia to 15 to 20 minutes is also associated with restoration of cardiac function with reperfusion; however, this process is very slow and can take hours to days. This condition of postischemic reversible myocardial dysfunction in the presence of normal flow is referred to as *myocardial stunning*.[35-37] Irreversible cell injury will occur with longer periods of ischemia, producing a myocardial infarction characterized by release of intracellular enzymes, disruption of cell membranes, influx of calcium, persistent contractile dysfunction, and eventual cellular swelling and necrosis.[38]

In addition to the previously described factors, right ventricular (RV) dysfunction and failure are potential sources of morbidity and mortality after cardiac surgery. Numerous factors may predispose patients to the development of perioperative RV dysfunction, including CAD, RV hypertrophy, previous cardiac surgery, and operative considerations such as inadequate revascularization or hypothermic protection. Technical and operative difficulties are associated with various cardiac surgical procedures (e.g., right ventriculotomy), RV trauma, rhythm and conduction abnormalities, injury to the

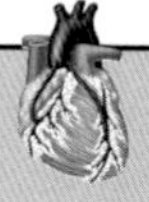

BOX 31–1 *Risk Factors for the Low-Cardiac-Output Syndrome after Cardiopulmonary Bypass*

- Preoperative ventricular dysfunction
- Myocardial ischemia
- Poor myocardial preservation
- Reperfusion injury
- Inadequate cardiac surgical repair or revascularization

Table 31–5 Patient Characteristics Associated with the Use of Inotropic Drug Support

Variable	No Inotropic Drug Support* (*n* = 58)	Inotropic Drug Support* (*n* = 70)	*p*
Age (yr)	57 ± 8	62 ± 8	0.005
Sex			
Female (%)	10	26	0.027
Male (%)	90	74	
Collateral circulation (%)	64	73	0.271
WMA (%)	78	84	0.334
Patients demonstrating cardiac enlargement (%)	7	21	0.021
Baseline LVEDP (mm Hg)	14 ± 7	16 ± 6	0.044
Postcontrast LVEDP (mm Hg)	21 ± 8	24 ± 7	0.054
Change in LVEDP (mm Hg)	7 ± 6	7 ± 7	0.534
EF (%)	61 ± 11	54 ± 13	0.002
PT (min)	106 ± 30	125 ± 37	0.004
IT (min)	42 ± 15	50 ± 19	0.009

*All values except for sex, collateral circulation, WMA, and patients demonstrating cardiac enlargement are expressed as mean ± SD. From Royster RL, Butterworth JF, Prough DS, et al: Preoperative and intraoperative predictors of inotropic support and long-term outcome in patients having coronary bypass grafting. Anesth Analg 72:729, 1991.
WMA = wall motion abnormalities identified during preoperative radiographic-contrast ventriculography; LVEDP = left ventricular end-diastolic pressure; EF = preoperative ejection fraction calculated from end-diastolic and end-systolic measurements from radiograph-contrast ventriculography; PT = total duration of cardiopulmonary bypass (pump time); IT = duration of aortic cross-clamping (ischemic time).

Table 31–6 Management of Cardiac Dysfunction

Physiologic Variable	Management
Heart rate and rhythm	Maintain normal sinus rhythm, avoid tachycardia; for tachycardia or bradycardia, consider pacing or chronotropic agents (atropine, isoproterenol, epinephrine), correct acid-base, electrolytes, and review of current medications
Preload	Reduce increased preload with diuretics or venodilators (nitroglycerin or sodium nitroprusside); monitor CVP, PCWP, and SV; obtain echocardiogram to rule out ischemia, valvular lesions, tamponade, and intracardiac shunts; consider using inotropes, IABP, or both
Afterload	Avoid increased afterload (increased wall tension), use vasodilators (sodium nitroprusside); avoid hypotension; maintain coronary perfusion pressure; consider IABP, inotropes devoid of α_1-adrenergic effects (dobutamine or milrinone), or both IABP and inotropes
Contractility	Assess hemodynamics, rule out ischemia/infarction, assess rate/rhythm, preload, and afterload, use inotropes; if uncertain, obtain echocardiogram to assess cardiac function. Consider combination therapy with inotropes and vasodilators and/or assist devices (IABP/LVAD/RVAD)
Oxygen delivery	Increase FIO_2 and CO; check ABGs and chest radiograph; mechanical ventilation if indicated; correct acid-base disturbances

FIO_2 = inspired oxygen concentration; ABGs = arterial blood gas; CO = cardiac output; CVP = central venous pressure; IABP = intraaortic balloon pump; PCWP = pulmonary capillary wedge pressure; SV = stroke volume.

right ventricle during cessation of CPB, or protamine reaction (see Chapter 29).

The following discussion provides an overview of the pharmacologic approach to management of perioperative ventricular dysfunction in the setting of cardiac surgery. Management goals are described in Table 31–6.[39] These are extensions of the routine preparations made for discontinuing CPB shown in Table 31–3.

Sympathomimetic Amines

Sympathomimetic drugs (i.e., catecholamines) are pharmacologic agents capable of providing inotropic and vasoactive effects (Box 31–2). Catecholamines exert positive inotropic action by stimulation of the β_1-receptor. The predominant hemodynamic effect of a specific catecholamine depends on the degree to which the various α-, β-, and dopaminergic receptors are stimulated (Tables 31–7 and 31–8).

The physiologic effect of an adrenergic agent is determined by the sum of its actions on α-, β-, and dopaminergic receptors. The effectiveness of any adrenergic agent will be influenced by the availability and responsiveness of adrenergic receptors. Chronically elevated levels of plasma catecholamines (e.g., chronic CHF and long CPB time) cause downregulation of the number and sensitivity of β-receptors.[40] Maintenance of normal acid-base status, normothermia, and electrolytes also improve the responsiveness to adrenergic-receptor stimulation.

The selection of a drug to treat ventricular dysfunction is influenced by pathophysiologic abnormalities as well as by the physician's preference. If LV performance is decreased primarily as a result of diminished contractility, the drug chosen should increase contractility. Although β-agonists improve contractility and tissue perfusion, their effects may increase myocardial oxygen consumption ($M\dot{V}O_2$) and reduce coronary perfusion pressure (CPP). However, if the factor most responsible for decreased cardiac function is hypotension with concomitantly reduced CPP, use of an α-adrenergic agonist

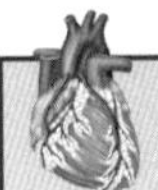

BOX 31–2 *Pharmacologic Approaches to Ventricular Dysfunction*

- Inotropic drugs
- Phosphodiesterase inhibitors
- Vasodilators
- Vasopressors
- Metabolic supplements

Table 31–7 Sympathomimetics

Drug	Dosage: *Intravenous*	Dosage: *Infusion*	Site of Action: α	Site of Action: β	*Mechanism of Action*
Methoxamine	2–10 mg	—	++++		Direct
Phenylephrine	50–500 μg	10 mg/500 mL 20 μg/mL 10–50 μg/min	++++	±	Direct
Norepinephrine	—	8 mg/500 mL 16 μg/mL 2–16 μg/min	++++	+++	Direct
Metaraminol	100 μg	20–200 mg/500 mL 40–400 μg/mL 40–500 μg/min	++++	+	Direct and indirect
Epinephrine	2–16 μg	4 mg/500 mL 8 μg/mL 2–10 μg/min	+++	+++	Direct
Ephedrine	5–25 mg	—	+	++	Direct and indirect
Dopamine	—	400 mg/500 mL 800 μg/mL 2–30 μg/kg/min	++	+++	Direct and indirect
Dobutamine	—	250 mg/500 mL 500 μg/mL 2–20 μg/kg/min	+	++++	Direct
Dopexamine	—	0.5–4 μg/kg/min		++	Direct
Isoproterenol	1–4 μg	2 mg/500 mL 4 μg/mL 1–5 μg/min		++++	Direct

Table 31–8 Hemodynamic Effects of Catecholamines and Phosphodiesterase Inhibitors

Durg	CO	dp/dt	HR	SVR	PVR	PCWP	MVO_2
Dobutamine 2–12 μg/kg/min*	⇑⇑⇑	⇑	⇑⇑	⇓	⇓	⇓ or ⇔	⇑
Dopamine							
0–3 μg/kg/min	⇑	⇑	⇑	⇓	⇓	⇑	⇑
3–8 μg/kg/min	⇑⇑	⇑	⇑	⇓	⇓	⇑	⇑
>8 μg/kg/min	⇑⇑	⇑	⇑⇑	⇑	⇔ (⇑)	⇑ or ⇔	⇑⇑
Isoproterenol 0.5–10 μg/min	⇑⇑	⇑⇑	⇑⇑	⇓⇓	⇓	⇓	⇑⇑
Epinephrine 0.01–0.4 μg/kg/min	⇑⇑	⇑	⇑	⇑ (⇓)	(⇑)	⇑ or ⇔	⇑⇑
Norepinephrine 0.01–0.3 μg/kg/min	⇑	⇑	⇔ (⇑⇓)	⇑⇑	⇔	⇔	⇑
PDE inhibitors†	⇑⇑	⇑	⇑	⇓⇓	⇓⇓	⇓⇓	⇓

*The indicated doses represent the most common dose ranges. For the individual patient, a deviation from these recommended doses might be indicated.

†PDE inhibitors are usually given as a loading dose followed by a continuous infusion: amrinone: 0.5–1.5 mg/kg loading dose, 10–30 μg/kg/min continuous infusion; milrinone: 50 μg/kg loading dose, 0.375–0.75 μg/kg/min continuous infusion.

CO = cardiac output; dp/dt = myocardial contractility; HR = heart rate; SVR = systemic vascular resistance; PVR = pulmonary vascular resistance; PCWP = pulmonary capillary wedge pressure; MVO_2 = myocardial oxygen consumption; PDE inhibitors = phosphodiesterase inhibitors.

Modified from Lehmann A, Boldt J: New pharmacologic approaches for the perioperative treatment of ischemic cardiogenic shock. J Cardiothorac Vasc Anesth 19:97–108, 2005.

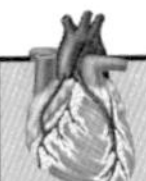

BOX 31–3 *Inotropic Drugs*

- Epinephrine
- Norepinephrine
- Dopamine
- Dobutamine
- Isoproterenol

can increase blood pressure and improve diastolic coronary perfusion.

Catecholamines are also effective for treating primary RV contractile dysfunction, with all of the β_1-adrenergic agonists augmenting RV contractility. Studies have documented the efficacy of epinephrine, norepinephrine, dobutamine, isoproterenol, dopamine, and phosphodiesterase-III (PDE-III) inhibitors in managing RV contractile dysfunction. When decreased RV contractility is combined with increased afterload, agents that exert vasodilator and positive inotropic effects should be used, including epinephrine, isoproterenol, dobutamine, and the PDE-III inhibitors.[41-44]

Epinephrine

Epinephrine stimulates α- and β-adrenergic receptors in a dose-dependent fashion. It is frequently the inotrope of choice after CPB (Box 31–3). Doses of 10, 20, and 40 ng/kg/min increased stroke volume by 2%, 12%, and 22%, respectively, and increased cardiac index (CI) by 0.1, 0.7, and 1.2 L/min/m^2. The HR also increased, but by no more than 10 bpm at any dose.[45] Epinephrine is frequently used after cardiac surgery to support the function of the "stunned" reperfused heart. During emergence from CPB, Butterworth et al[46] showed epinephrine (30 ng/kg/min) increased CI and stroke volume by 14% without increasing HR. In cardiac surgical patients, epinephrine infusion (0.01 to 0.4 µg/kg/min) effectively increases cardiac output, minimally increases HR, and has acceptable side effects (see Table 31–8) (see Chapters 10 and 33).

Dobutamine

Dobutamine is a synthetic catecholamine that generally produces dose-dependent increases in cardiac output and reductions in diastolic filling pressures. The effects of epinephrine (30 ng/kg/min) were compared with dobutamine (5 µg/kg/min) in 52 patients recovering from CABG surgery.[46] Both drugs significantly and similarly increased stroke volume index, but epinephrine increased the HR by only 2 bpm, whereas dobutamine increased the HR by 16 bpm.

In addition to increasing contractility, dobutamine may have favorable metabolic effects on ischemic myocardium. Intravenous and intracoronary injections of dobutamine increase coronary blood flow in animal studies.[47] In paced cardiac surgical patients, dopamine increased oxygen demand without increasing oxygen supply, whereas dobutamine increased myocardial oxygen uptake and coronary blood flow. However, because increases in HR are a major determinant of $\dot{M}VO_2$, these favorable effects of dobutamine could be lost if dobutamine induces tachycardia. During dobutamine stress-echocardiography, segmental wall motion abnormalities suggestive of myocardial ischemia can occur as a result of tachycardia and increases in $\dot{M}VO_2$.[48]

Dopamine

Dopamine is an endogenous catecholamine and an immediate precursor of norepinephrine and epinephrine. Its actions are mediated by stimulation of adrenergic receptors and specific postjunctional dopaminergic receptors (D_1-receptors) in the renal, mesenteric, and coronary arterial beds.[49] In low doses (0.5 to 3.0 µg/kg/min), dopamine predominantly stimulates the dopaminergic receptors; at doses ranging from 3 to 7 µg/kg/min, it activates most adrenergic receptors in a nonselective fashion; and at higher doses (>10 µg/kg/min), dopamine behaves as a vasoconstrictor. The dose-dependent effects of dopamine are not very specific and can be influenced by multiple factors such as receptor regulation, concomitant drug use, and interindividual and intra-individual variability.

Dopamine is unique in comparison with other endogenous catecholamines because of its effects on the kidneys. It has been shown to increase renal artery blood flow by 20% to 40% by causing direct vasodilation of the afferent arteries and indirect vasoconstriction of the efferent arteries.[50] This results in an increase in glomerular filtration rate and in oxygen delivery to the juxtamedullary nephrons.

Despite favorable effects, dopamine has several undesirable features that may limit its use. Its propensity to raise HR and cause tachyarrhythmias can result in demand-related myocardial ischemia. After cardiac surgery, dopamine causes more frequent and less predictable degrees of tachycardia than dobutamine or epinephrine at doses that produce comparable improvement in contractile function.[51]

Norepinephrine

Norepinephrine is used primarily to treat vasodilated patients after CPB. Meadows et al[52] treated 10 patients with severe sepsis and hypotension unresponsive to volume expansion, dopamine, and dobutamine. Norepinephrine infusion (0.03 to 0.89 µg/kg/min) alone improved arterial blood pressure, left ventricular stroke work index (LVSWI), urine output, and in most cases, CI. Desjars et al[53] studied the renal effects of prolonged norepinephrine infusion in hypotensive patients with sepsis. Norepinephrine (0.5 to 1.5 µg/kg/min) plus low-dose dopamine improved urine flow and renal function compared with dopamine alone.[53] The α-adrenergic agonists benefit certain patients with circulatory failure refractory to inotropic and fluid therapy. Phenylephrine, norepinephrine, or vasopressin may be used to restore MAP in patients with a low SVR after CPB (i.e., vasoplegia syndrome).[54] When RV dysfunction primarily is a result of decreased CPP, vasoconstrictors can be used to optimize RV performance.[55]

Isoproterenol

Isoproterenol is a potent, nonselective β-adrenergic agonist, devoid of α-adrenergic agonist activity. Isoproterenol dilates skeletal, renal, and mesenteric vascular beds and decreases diastolic blood pressure. The potent chronotropic action of isoproterenol, combined with its propensity to decrease CPP, limits its usefulness in patients with CAD. Applications include treatment of bradycardia (especially after orthotopic heart transplantation), pulmonary hypertension, and heart failure after congenital cardiac surgery.[55] Isoproterenol remains the inotrope of choice for stimulation of cardiac pacemaker cells in the management of acute bradyarrhythmias or atrioventricular heart block. It reduces refractoriness to conduction and increases automaticity in myocardial tissues. The tachycardia seen with isoproterenol is a result of

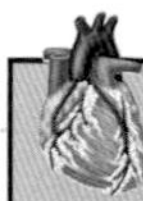

BOX 31–4 *Inodilator Drugs*

- Inamrinone
- Milrinone
- Dobutamine
- Epinephrine plus nitroprusside ("epipride")

direct effects of the drug on the sinoatrial and atrioventricular nodes and reflex effects caused by peripheral vasodilation. It is routinely used in the setting of cardiac transplantation for increasing automaticity and inotropy and for its vasodilatory effect on the pulmonary arteries (see Chapter 26).

Phosphodiesterase Inhibitors

The PDE-III inhibitors amrinone (inamrinone) and milrinone increase cAMP, calcium flux, and calcium sensitivity of contractile proteins. These drugs have a similar mode of action because they are noncatecholamine and nonadrenergic agents. They do not rely on β-receptor stimulation for their positive inotropic activity. As a result, the effectiveness of the PDE-III inhibitors is not altered by previous β-blockade, nor is it reduced in patients who may experience β-receptor downregulation.[40] In addition to their positive inotropic effects, these agents produce systemic and pulmonary vasodilation. As a result of this combination of hemodynamic effects (i.e., positive inotropic support and vasodilation), the term *inodilator* has been used to describe these drugs (Box 31–4).

Amrinone is more effective than dobutamine for weaning from CPB, with increases in stroke volume and cardiac output and decreases in SVR and pulmonary vascular resistance (PVR).[56,57] Because these agents exert their hemodynamic effects by a nonadrenergic mechanism of action, when used in combination with β-agonists, they have an additive effect on myocardial performance. Gage et al[58] reported that when amrinone was used in combination with dobutamine, cardiac output was significantly increased compared with therapy with dobutamine alone. Since this initial report, other investigators have demonstrated the clinical application of combination therapy using PDE-III inhibitors and dopamine, phenylephrine, epinephrine, and nitroglycerin.[59]

A second-generation PDE-III inhibitor, milrinone has a similar hemodynamic profile to amrinone; however, its positive inotropic action is approximately 15 to 30 times that of amrinone. Thrombocytopenia has been a potential clinical concern with the administration of PDE-III inhibitors, particularly amrinone. However, George et al were unable to demonstrate any significant reduction in platelet count after 48 hours of milrinone infusion in cardiac surgical patients.[60] Intravenous milrinone has been studied extensively and demonstrates a favorable short-term effect in CHF and ventricular dysfunction after CPB[61] (see Chapters 10 and 33).

Milrinone, like other PDE-III inhibitors, appears to increase cardiac output without increasing overall $M\dot{V}O_2$. Monrad et al[62] administered milrinone to patients with CHF, increasing CI by 45%, but overall $M\dot{V}O_2$ did not change. Data also suggest that milrinone may improve myocardial diastolic relaxation (i.e., positive "lusitropic" effect) and augment coronary perfusion. The proposed mechanism for this effect on diastolic performance is that by decreasing LV wall tension, ventricular filling is enhanced, and myocardial blood flow and oxygen delivery are optimized (see Table 31–8).

The ability of short-term administration of milrinone to augment ventricular performance in patients undergoing cardiac surgery was shown in the results from the European Milrinone Multicentre Trial Group.[63] In this prospective study, intravenous milrinone was studied in patients after CPB. All patients received a bolus infusion of milrinone at 50 μg/kg over 10 minutes, followed by a maintenance infusion of 0.375, 0.5, or 0.75 μg/kg/min for 12 hours. Significant increases in stroke volume and CI were observed. In addition, significant decreases in pulmonary capillary wedge pressure (PCWP), CVP, PAP, MAP, and SVR were seen. Eighteen patients (14%) had arrhythmias; most occurred in the group receiving 0.75 μg/kg/min. Two arrhythmic events were deemed serious; both were bouts of rapid atrial fibrillation occurring with the higher dose.

Bailey et al[64] showed that after CPB, a loading dose of milrinone at 50 μg/kg, followed by a continuous infusion of 0.5 μg/kg/min, resulted in a significant increase in cardiac output. Butterworth et al[65] also studied the pharmacokinetics and pharmacodynamics of milrinone in adult patients undergoing cardiac surgery; milrinone (25, 50, or 75 μg/kg) was given if the CI was less than 3.0 L/min/m² after separation from CPB. All three doses of milrinone significantly increased CI. The 50- and 75-μg/kg doses produced significantly greater increases in CI than the 25-μg/kg dose. The 75-μg/kg dose produced increases in CI comparable with the 50-μg/kg dose, but it was associated with more hypotension, despite administration of intravenous fluid, blood, and a phenylephrine infusion. The initial redistribution half-lives were 4.6, 4.3, and 6.9 minutes, and the terminal elimination half-lives were 63, 82, and 99 minutes for the 25-, 50-, and 75-μg/kg doses, respectively. The results of these investigations suggest that for optimizing hemodynamic performance (while minimizing any potential for arrhythmias), the middle dose range (i.e., loading dose of 50 μg/kg) of milrinone may be most efficacious with a continuous infusion of 0.5 μg/kg/min, leading to a plasma concentration of more than 100 mg/mL. In patients with poor LV function, the loading dose should be given during CPB to avoid a decrease in MAP and to minimize the need for other inotropes on discontinuing CPB.[66]

Vasodilators

The indications for using vasodilators such as nitroglycerin or nitroprusside in cardiac surgery include management of perioperative systemic or pulmonary hypertension, myocardial ischemia, and ventricular dysfunction complicated by excessive pressure or volume overload[67] (Box 31–5). In most conditions, nitroglycerin or nitroprusside may be used. Both share

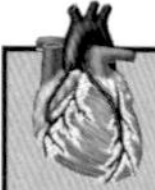

BOX 31–5 *Vasodilator Mechanisms Helpful in Discontinuing Cardiopulmonary Bypass*

- Decreased right and left ventricular wall stress (afterload)
- Decreased venous return (preload)
- Improved lusitropy
- Improved coronary blood flow

common features such as rapid onset, ultra-short half-lives (several minutes), and easy titratability. Nevertheless, there are important pharmacologic differences between nitroglycerin and nitroprusside. In the setting of ischemia, nitroglycerin is preferred because it selectively vasodilates coronary arteries without producing a coronary "steal" (see Chapters 6, 10, and 19). Likewise, in the management of ventricular volume overload or RV pressure overload, nitroglycerin may offer some advantage over nitroprusside. It has a predominant influence on the venous bed such that preload can be reduced without significantly compromising systemic arterial pressure. The benefits of nitroglycerin are improvement in stroke volume, reduction in wall tension and $M\dot{V}O_2$, increased perfusion to the subendocardium as a result of a lower LVEDP, and maintenance of CPP. Nitroprusside is a more potent arterial vasodilator and may potentiate myocardial ischemia due to a coronary steal phenomenon or a reduction in coronary perfusion pressure. Its greater potency, however, makes nitroprusside the vasodilator of choice for management of perioperative hypertensive disorders and for afterload reduction during or after surgery for regurgitant valvular lesions (see Chapter 20).

Additional uses of vasodilators include management of RV dysfunction. Sodium nitroprusside can augment cardiac output by decreasing RV afterload and PVR.[68] Similarly, nitroglycerin has been shown to decrease PVR, transpulmonary pressure, and mean PAP and to increase cardiac output in patients with elevated PVR resulting from mitral valve disease.[69] Although nitroglycerin and nitroprusside decrease the impedance to RV ejection and increase the RV ejection fraction by reducing afterload, they are nonspecific pulmonary vasodilators. As a result, new studies have focused on the ability of agents such as prostaglandins (particularly prostaglandin E_1), nitric oxide, and the PDE-III inhibitors to more specifically decrease PVR (see Chapters 10 and 33).

Despite proven benefits of vasodilator therapy in the management of CHF, they can be difficult drugs to use in treatment of perioperative ventricular dysfunction. This is most evident in cases of the LCOS when impaired pump function is complicated by inadequate perfusion pressure. In these situations, multidrug therapy with vasoactive and cardioactive agents is warranted (i.e., nitroglycerin or nitroprusside plus epinephrine or milrinone and norepinephrine). Combination therapy enables greater selectivity of effect. The unwanted side effects of one drug can be avoided while supplementing the desired effects with another agent.[70,71] To maximize the desired effects of any particular combination of agents, frequent assessment of cardiac performance with a PAC and TEE is needed. This allows the Starling curve and the pressure-volume loops to be visualized as they are shifted up and to the left with therapy (see Chapter 5).

Additional Pharmacologic Therapy

Following the steps outlined in Tables 31–3 and 31–6, most patients can be weaned off of CPB. However, a small percentage will be difficult to safely remove from CPB because of their chronic end-stage CHF or an acute insult during cardiac surgery producing cardiogenic shock. These patients will probably require mechanical circulatory support (i.e., IABP) as discussed subsequently or in Chapter 27 (i.e., VAD). However, while instituting these further steps, some clinicians try additional pharmacologic therapy.

Controversial Older Treatments

Some studies suggest that a reduction in plasma thyroid hormone concentration may be the cause of decreased myocardial function after CPB.[72,73] Some patients exhibit signs of hypothyroidism, including decreases in HR, CI, and myocardial and systemic oxygen consumption and increases in arteriovenous oxygen difference and SVR. Multiple investigators have documented declines in the circulating triiodothyronine (T_3) concentration during and after CPB, and the most dramatic decreases in T_3 are seen at the end of CPB and during the first few hours after CPB.[72,73] The reduced thyroid hormone concentrations after CPB may exacerbate myocardial stunning and the LCOS encountered in the post-CPB period. Thyroid hormone in the form of an intravenous T_3 infusion (2 µg/hr to a total dose of 0.5 µg/kg) has been used during cardiac surgery. This therapy has resulted in increases in the MAP and HR, and reductions in LAP and CVP in patients who initially could not be weaned from CPB. Some of these patients have been successfully weaned from CPB and have required lower doses of dobutamine and other cardiac drug support after the treatment with thyroid hormone.[74-76]

The administration of glucose-insulin-potassium (GIK) or just glucose and insulin has been found to be useful for metabolic support of the heart after CPB. The trauma of cardiac surgery produces insulin resistance, which restricts the availability of carbohydrates to the heart. The increased level of catecholamines during CPB may also put further strain on the energy metabolism of the heart, whereas insulin may improve this situation.[77-79] The administration of high-dose insulin has been compared with dopamine in patients undergoing CABG surgery. The infusion of dopamine (7 µg/kg/min) alone induced metabolic changes unfavorable to the myocardium, whereas dopamine plus insulin increased carbohydrate use with cessation of cardiac uptake of free fatty acids.[80] Gradinac et al[81] studied GIK in patients with refractory CHF after CPB. All of the patients started with a low CI and were receiving cardiac support with an inotropic drug and an IABP. There was a significant increase in CI in the GIK patients at 12 and 24 hours, the need for inotropic and IABP support was decreased, and the 30-day survival rate was increased.[81]

New Treatments for Heart Failure and Cardiogenic Shock

Levosimendan is a new positive inotropic drug belonging to the class of calcium sensitizers. The drug stabilizes the calcium-induced conformational change in cardiac troponin C and prolongs the effective cross-bridging time. In contrast to other positive inotropic drugs, levosimendan does not increase intracellular calcium. The drug has vasodilating and anti-ischemic properties produced by opening K^+-ATP channels[82-84] (Table 31–9) (see Chapter 33).

Levosimendan is recommended by the European Society of Cardiology for treatment of acute worsening of heart failure and for acute heart failure after myocardial infarction.[85] It has also been found to enhance contractile function of stunned myocardium in patients with acute coronary syndromes.[86] It is available clinically in Europe and is undergoing evaluation in the United States. The use of levosimendan has been reported in cardiac surgical patients with high perioperative risk, compromised LV function, difficulties in weaning from CPB, and severe RV failure after mitral valve replacement.[87,88] The doses used were 12 µg/kg as a 10-minute loading dose, followed by an infusion of 0.1 µg/kg/min. It has been used pre-

Table 31–9 Emerging Drugs for Heart Failure and Cardiogenic Shock

Drug*	CO	PCWP	AP	HR	Arrhyth.	Onset	Offset	Diur.	Shock
Toborinone	⇑⇑⇑	⇓⇓	⇑ or ⇓	⇔	⇑⇑⇑	Short	Moderate	⇔	No
L-Simendan	⇑⇑	⇓	⇓	⇑	⇔	Short	Very long	⇔	Yes
Tezosentan	⇑⇑	⇓	⇓	⇔	⇔	Short	Short	⇔	No
Nesiritide	⇑	⇓⇓	⇓	⇔	⇔	Short	Long	⇑⇑	No
L-NAME	⇓	⇑⇑	⇑⇑⇑	(⇓)	?	Short	Moderate	⇑	Yes

*Positive inotropic drugs: toborinone: phosphodiesterase inhibitor. L-Simendan: levosimendan, calcium sensitizer. Vasodilating drugs: tezosentan: endothelin antagonist. Nesiritide: natriuretic peptide. Vasoconstricting drug: L-NAME: N^G-nitro-L-arginine-methyl ester, inhibitor of nitric oxide synthase.
CO = cardiac output; PCWP = pulmonary capillary wedge pressure; AP = arterial pressure; HR = heart rate; Arrhyth. = arrhythmogenic potential; Diur. = diuresis; Shock = cardiogenic shock; No = not yet used in patients with cardiogenic shock; Yes = already used in patients with cardiogenic shock.
Modified from Lehman A, Boldt J: New pharmacologic approaches for the perioperative treatment of ischemic cardiogenic shock. J Cardiothorac Vasc Anesth 19:97, 2005.

operatively, during emergence from CPB, and in the postoperative period for up to 28 days. The potential for levosimendan to produce increased contractility, decreased resistance, minimal metabolic cost, and no arrhythmias makes it a potentially useful addition to the treatments for patients with the LCOS or RV failure.

Nesiritide is a recombinant human brain-type natriuretic peptide with vasodilatory and diuretic effects. In patients with heart failure, intravenous nesiritide acts as a vasodilator and reduces preload; SVR is decreased, and CI subsequently increases.[89-91] The drug has no positive inotropic effects (see Chapter 10). Compared with nitroglycerin and dobutamine, nesiritide had a greater effect on decreasing preload than nitroglycerin, and it did not cause as many arrhythmias as dobutamine.[92,93] Its ultimate role in the treatment of acute heart failure is uncertain, but it may augment the vasodilators or diuretics.

Numerous other drugs are being studied for their uses in patients with acute decompensated heart failure and cardiogenic shock. These drugs include positive inotropic agents such as toborinone (a PDE-III inhibitor), vasodilators such as tezosentan (a specific and potent dual endothelin-receptor antagonist), and vasopressors such as L-NAME (a nitric oxide inhibitor) (Table 31–9).[82] These various drugs may prove useful for certain types of cardiovascular problems in the future.

INTRA-AORTIC BALLOON PUMP COUNTERPULSATION

The IABP is a device that is designed to augment myocardial perfusion by increasing coronary blood flow during diastole and unloading the left ventricle during systole. This is accomplished by mass displacement of a volume of blood (usually 30 to 50 mL) by alternately inflating and deflating a balloon positioned in the proximal segment of the descending aorta. The gas used for this purpose is carbon dioxide (because of its great solubility in blood) or helium (because of its inertial properties and rapid diffusion coefficients). Inflation and deflation are synchronized to the cardiac cycle by the electronics of the balloon console producing counterpulsations. The results of effective use of the IABP are often quite dramatic. Improvements in cardiac output, ejection fraction, coronary blood flow, and MAP are frequently seen, as well as decreases in aortic and ventricular systolic pressures, LVEDP, PCWP, LAP, HR, frequency of premature ventricular contractions, and suppression of atrial arrhythmias.

Table 31–10 Intra-aortic Balloon Pump Counterpulsation Indications and Contraindications

Indications	Contraindications
1. Cardiogenic shock a. Myocardial infarction b. Myocarditis c. Cardiomyopathy	1. Aortic valvular insufficiency 2. Aortic disease a. Aortic dissection b. Aortic aneurysm
2. Failure to separate from CPB	3. Severe peripheral vascular disease
3. Stabilization of preoperative patient a. Ventricular septal defect b. Mitral regurgitation 4. Stabilization of noncardiac surgical preoperative patient	4. Severe noncardiac systemic disease 5. Massive trauma 6. Patients with "do not resuscitate" instructions
5. Procedural support during coronary angiography	
6. Bridge to transplantation	

Indications and Contraindications

Since its introduction, the indications for the IABP have grown (Table 31–10). The most common use of the IABP is for treatment of cardiogenic shock. This may occur after CPB or after cardiac surgery in patients with shock preoperatively with acute postinfarction ventricular septal defects or mitral regurgitation, those who require stabilization before surgery, or patients who decompensate hemodynamically during cardiac catheterization. Patients with myocardial ischemia refractory to coronary vasodilation and afterload reduction are stabilized with an IABP before cardiac catheterization, and some patients with severe CAD will prophylactically have an IABP inserted before undergoing CABG or off-pump coronary artery bypass surgery.[94-98]

Contraindications to IABP use are relatively few (see Table 31–10). The presence of severe aortic regurgitation or aortic dissection is listed as an absolute contraindication for the IABP, although successful reports of its use in patients with aortic insufficiency or acute trauma to the descending thoracic aorta have appeared. Other relative contraindications are listed; use of the IABP in these instances is at the discretion of the physician.

Insertion Techniques

In the initial development of the IABP, insertion was by surgical access to the femoral vessels. In the late 1970s, refinements in IABP design allowed the development of percutaneous insertion techniques. Now the technique most commonly used, percutaneous IABP insertion is rapidly performed with commercially available kits.

The femoral vessel with the greater pulse is sought by careful palpation. The length of the balloon to be inserted is estimated by laying the balloon tip on the patient's chest at Louis' angle and appropriately marking the distal point corresponding to the femoral artery. Care must be taken when removing the balloon from its package to follow the manufacturer's procedures exactly so as not to cause perforation of the balloon before insertion. Available balloons come wrapped and need only be appropriately deflated before removal from the package. The femoral artery is entered with the supplied needle, a J-tipped guidewire is inserted to the level of the aortic arch, and the needle is removed. The arterial puncture site is enlarged with the successive placement of an 8 Fr dilator and then a 10.5 or 12 Fr dilator and sheath combination (Fig. 31–3). In the adult-sized (30- to 50-mL) balloons, only the dilator needs to be removed, leaving the sheath and guidewire in the artery. The balloon is threaded over the guidewire into the central aorta and into the previously estimated correct position in the proximal segment of the descending aorta. The sheath is gently pulled back to connect with the leak-proof cuff on the balloon hub, ideally so that the entire sheath is out of the arterial lumen to minimize risk of ischemic complications to the distal extremity. Alternatively, the sheath may be stripped off the balloon shaft much like a peel-away pacemaker lead introducer, thereby entirely removing the sheath from the insertion site. At least one manufacturer offers a "sheathless" balloon for insertion.

If fluoroscopy is available during the procedure, correct placement is verified before fixing the balloon securely to the skin. Position may also be checked by radiography or echocardiography after insertion. If an indwelling left radial arterial catheter is functioning at the time of insertion, a reasonable estimate of position may be made by watching balloon-mediated alteration of the arterial pulse waveform (Fig. 31–4). After appropriate positioning and timing of the balloon, 1:1 counterpulsation may be initiated. The entire external balloon assembly should be covered in sterile dressings.

Removal of a percutaneously inserted IABP may be by the open (surgical removal) or closed technique. If a closed technique is chosen, the artery should be allowed to bleed for several seconds while pressure is maintained on the distal artery after balloon removal to flush any accumulated clot from the central lumen. This maneuver helps prevent distal embolization of clot. Pressure is then applied for 20 to 30 minutes on the puncture site for hemostasis. If surgical removal is chosen, embolectomy catheters may be passed antegrade and retrograde before suture closure of the artery.

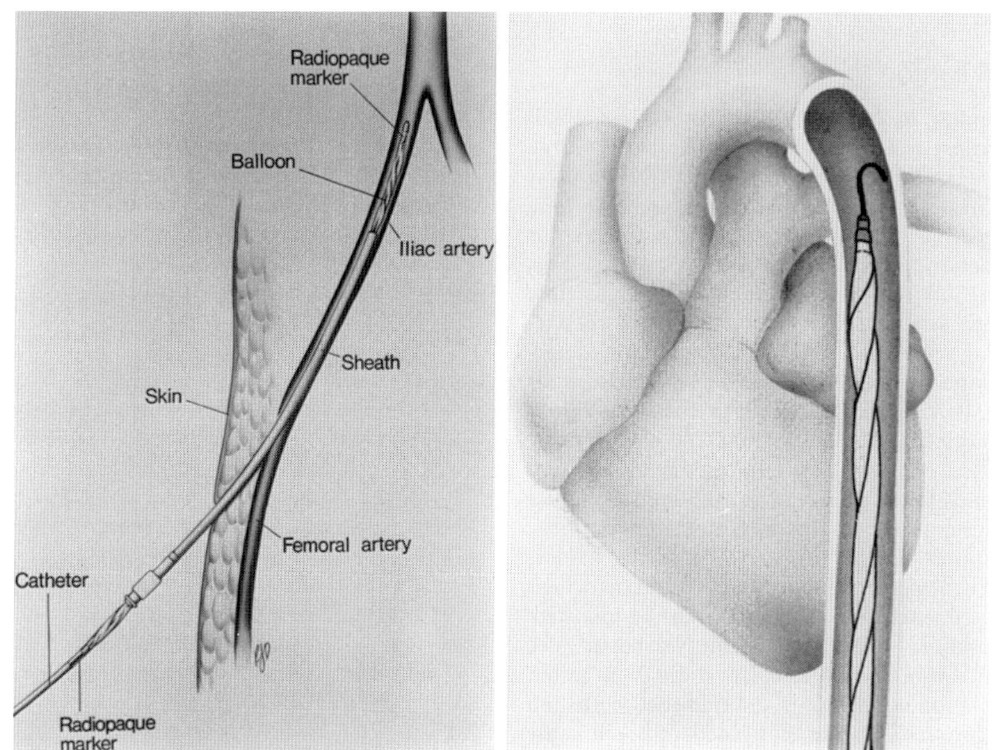

Figure 31–3 Diagram of intra-aortic balloon pump (IABP) insertion. *(A)* Cannulation and insertion of the balloon through the femoral artery. Notice the tightly wrapped balloon as it traverses the sheath. A guidewire is not visible in this drawing. *(B)* Correct positioning of balloon in proximal descending aorta. The J-tipped guidewire is seen exiting from the balloon's central lumen. (*A*, Courtesy of Datascope Corporation; *B*, Courtesy of Kontron, Inc.)

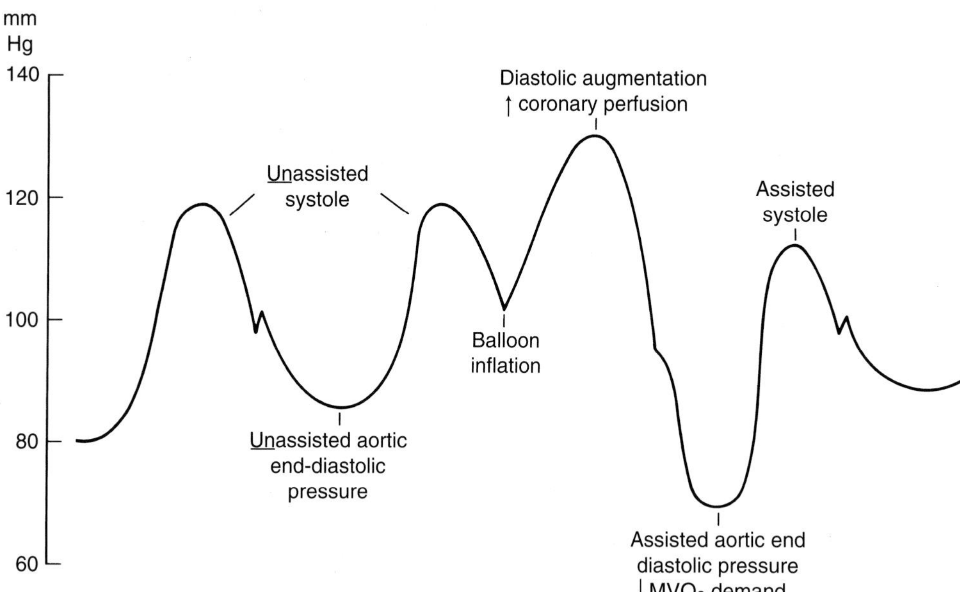

Figure 31–4 Arterial waveforms seen during intra-aortic balloon pump (IABP) assist. The first two waveforms are unassisted, and the last is assisted. Notice the decreased end-systolic and end-diastolic pressures and augmented diastolic pressures caused by IABP augmentation and the (correct) point at which balloon inflation occurs. These are waveforms generated by a correctly positioned and timed balloon. (Courtesy of Datascope Corporation.)

Alternate routes of IABP insertion exist. The balloon may be placed surgically through the femoral artery. This is now performed without the use of an end-to-side vascular conduit, although this placement still requires a second surgical procedure for removal. In patients in whom extreme peripheral vascular disease exists or in pediatric patients in whom the peripheral vasculature is too small, the ascending aorta or aortic arch may be entered for balloon insertion. These approaches necessitate median sternotomy for insertion and usually require reexploration for removal. Other routes of access include the abdominal aorta and the subclavian, axillary, and iliac arteries. The iliac approach may be especially useful for pediatric cases.

Timing and Weaning

There are a number of different manufacturers of IABP systems commercially available (Fig. 31–5). The basic console design includes electrocardiographic and arterial blood pressure waveform monitoring and printing, balloon volume monitoring, triggering selection switches, adjustments for inflation and deflation timing, battery backup power sources, and gas reservoir. Some of these systems have become quite sophisticated, with advanced computer microprocessor circuits allowing triggering based on pacemaker signals or detection of and compensation for aberrant rhythms such as atrial fibrillation. Portable models exist for transportation of patients by ground, helicopter, or air ambulances.

For optimal effect of the IABP, inflation and deflation need to be correctly timed to the cardiac cycle. Although a number of variables, including positioning of the balloon within the aorta, balloon volume (Fig. 31–6), and the patient's cardiac rhythm, can affect the performance of the IABP, basic principles regarding the function of the balloon must be followed. Balloon inflation should be timed to coincide with aortic valve closure, or aortic insufficiency and LV strain will result. Similarly, late inflation will result in a diminished perfusion pressure to the coronary arteries. Early deflation will cause inappropriate loss of afterload reduction, and late deflation will increase LV work by causing increased afterload, if only transiently. These errors and correct timing diagrams are illustrated in Figures 31–4 and 31–7.

As the patient's cardiac performance improves, the IABP support must be removed in stages rather than abruptly. Judicious application and dosing of vasodilator and inotropic medications can assist this procedure. The balloon augmentation may be reduced in steps from 1:1 counterpulsation to 1:2 and then to 1:4, with appropriate intervals at each stage to assess hemodynamic and neurologic stability, cardiac output, and mixed venous oxygen saturation changes. After appropriate observation at 1:4 or 1:8 counterpulsation, balloon assistance can be safely discontinued, and the device can be removed by one of the methods discussed. If percutaneous removal is chosen, an appropriate interval for reversal of anticoagulation (if employed) before removal of the balloon should be allowed.

Complications

Several complications have been associated with IABP use (Table 31–11). The most frequently seen complications are vascular injuries, balloon malfunction, and infection.[95,98]

Table 31–11 Intra-aortic Balloon Pump Counterpulsation Complications

Vascular	Miscellaneous	Balloon
Arterial injury (perforation, dissection)	Hemolysis	Perforation (preinsertion)
Aortic perforation	Thrombocytopenia	Tear (during insertion)
Aortic dissection	Infection	Incorrect positioning
Femoral artery thrombosis	Claudication (postremoval)	Gas embolization
Peripheral embolization	Hemorrhage	Inadvertent removal
Femoral vein cannulation	Paraplegia	
Pseudoaneurysm of femoral vessels	Entrapment	
Lower extremity ischemia	Spinal cord necrosis	
Compartment syndrome	Left internal mammary artery occlusion	
Visceral ischemia		

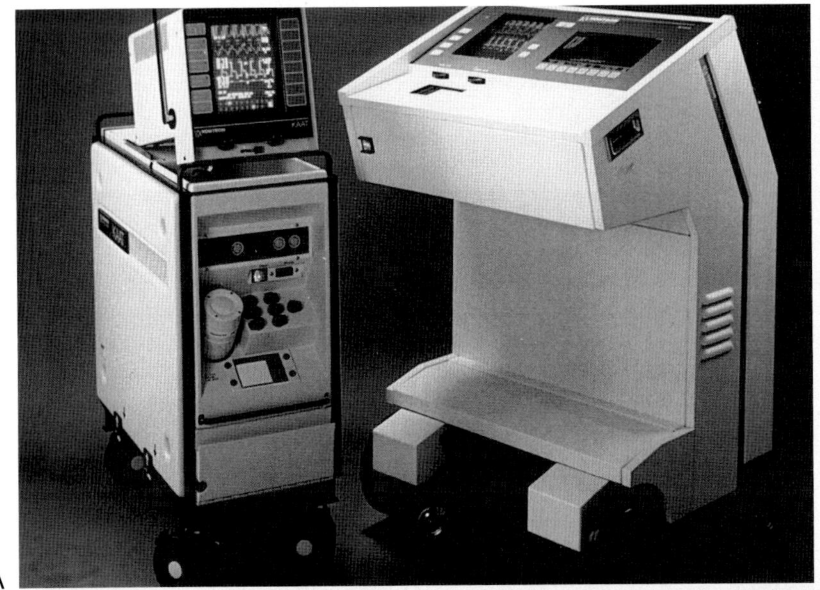
A

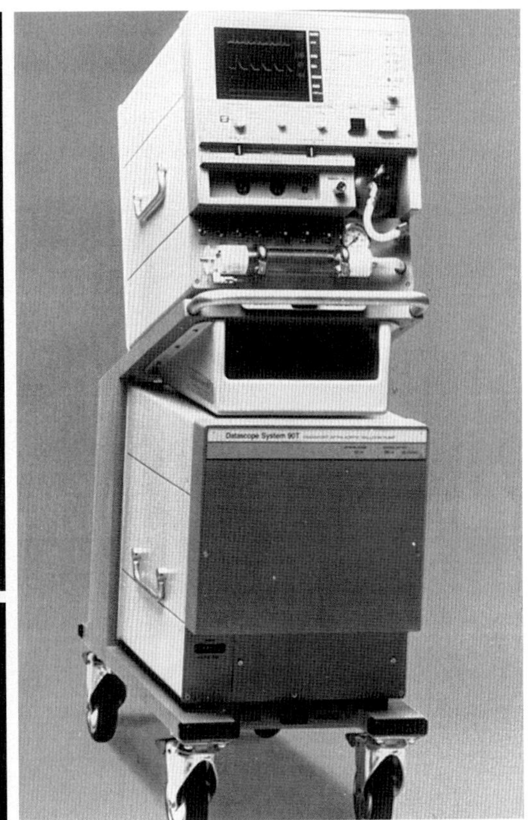

B

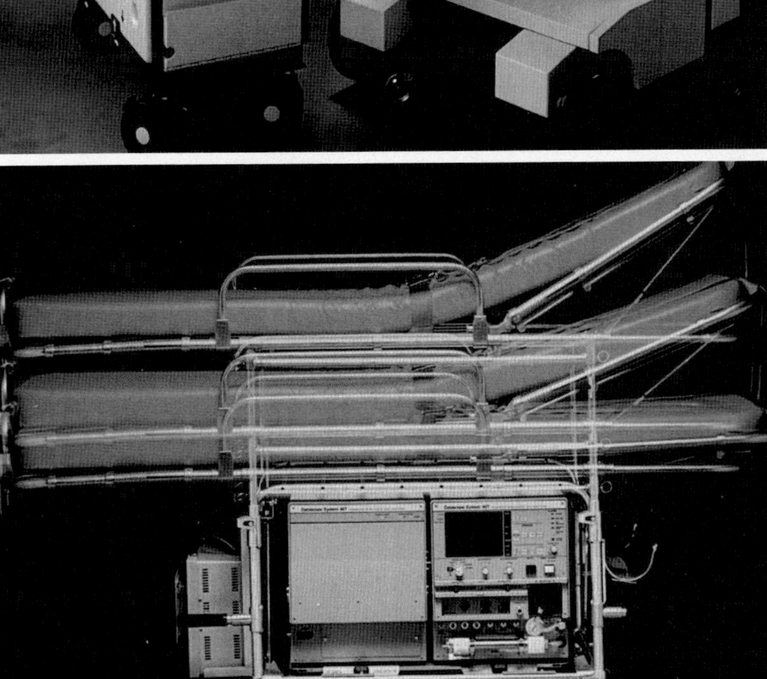
C

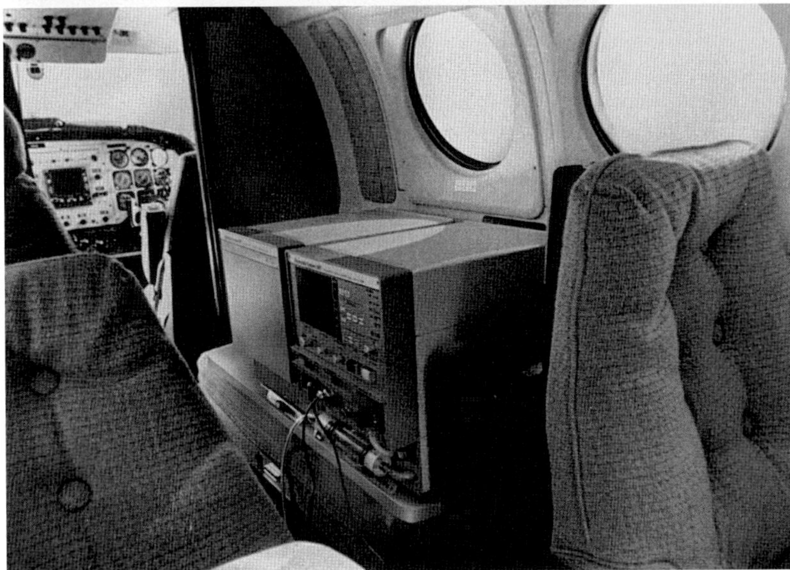
D

Figure 31–5 Models of intra-aortic balloon pump (IABP) consoles. *(A)* The Kontron models K2000 *(right)* and KAAT *(left)*. The KAAT can be separated into its two components *(top and bottom)* for increased maneuverability. *(B)* The Datascope model 90T. Like the KAAT, this IABP console can be split into two segments for flexibility in transport. *(C)* The model 90T on a stretcher mount. *(D)* The model 90T in a jet ambulance. (*B–D,* Courtesy of Datascope Corporation.)

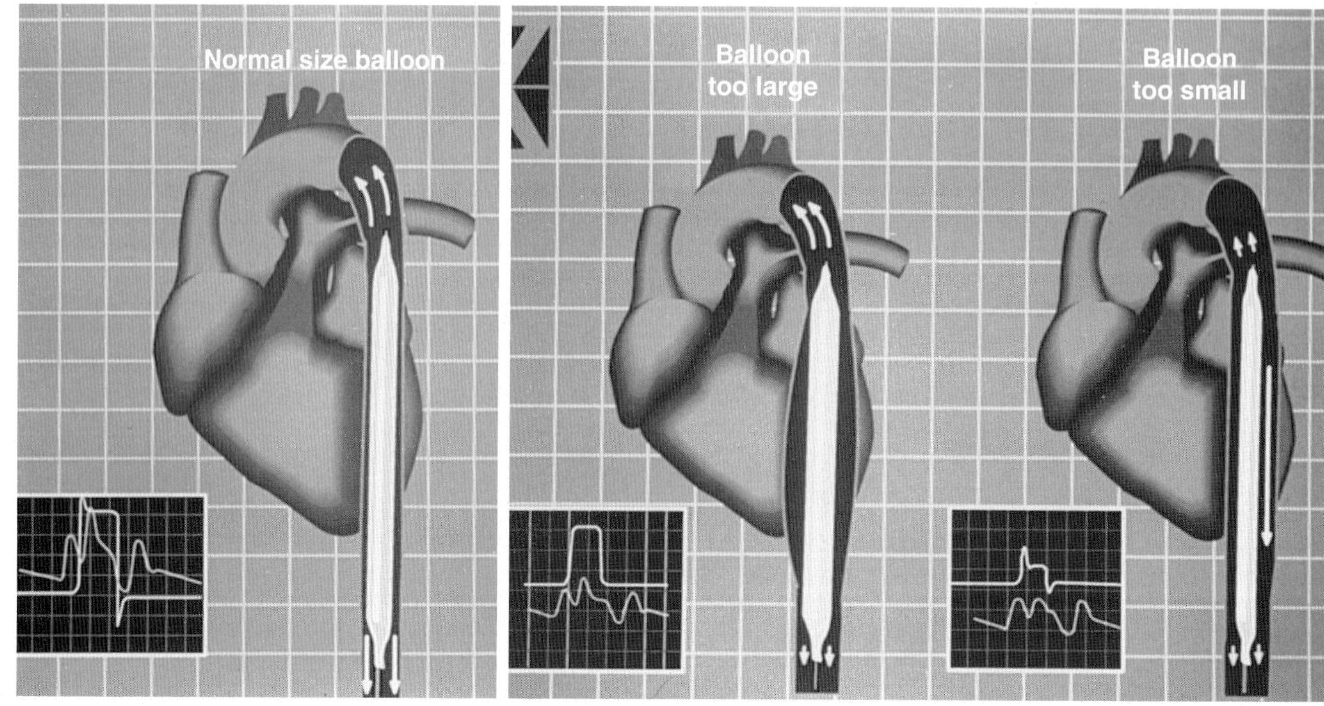

Figure 31–6 Variations in waveform caused by incorrect balloon size. *(A)* The balloon is correctly positioned and appropriately sized for the aorta. Notice the arterial waveform diagram in lower left corner. *(B)* Examples of too large *(left)* or too small *(right)* balloon sizes with their correspondingly altered arterial waveforms. A similar effect can result from overinflation and underinflation of balloon. Compare waveforms in *B* with the ideal waveform in *A*. (Courtesy of Kontron, Inc.)

Premature deflation of the IAB during the diastolic phase

Waveform Characteristics:
- Deflation of IAB is seen as a sharp drop following diastolic augmentation
- Suboptimal diastolic augmentation
- Assisted aortic end diastolic pressure may be equal to or greater than the unassisted aortic end diastolic pressure
- Assisted systolic pressure may rise

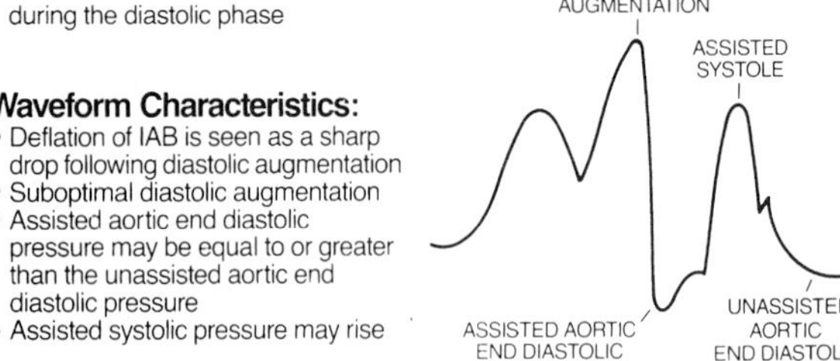

Physiologic Effects:
- Sub-optimal coronary perfusion
- Potential for retrograde coronary and carotid blood flow
- Angina may occur as a result of retrograde coronary blood flow
- Sub-optimal afterload reduction
- Increased MVO_2 demand

A

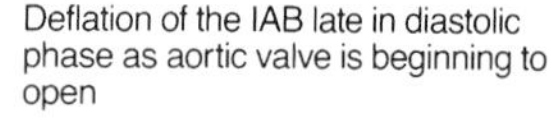

Deflation of the IAB late in diastolic phase as aortic valve is beginning to open

Waveform Characteristics:
- Assisted aortic end-diastolic pressure may be equal to the unassisted aortic end diastolic pressure
- Rate of rise of assisted systole is prolonged
- Diastolic augmentation may appear widened

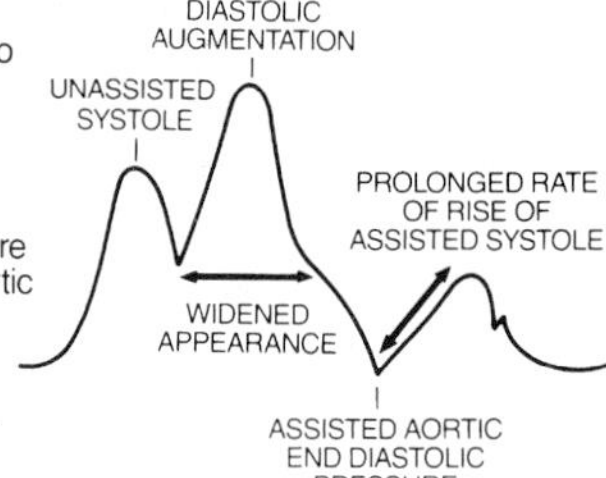

Physiologic Effects:
- Afterload reduction is essentially absent
- Increased MVO_2 consumption due to the left ventricle ejecting against a greater resistance and a prolonged isovolumetric contraction phase
- IAB may impede left ventricular ejection and increase the afterload

B

Inflation of the IAB prior to aortic valve closure

Waveform Characteristics:
- Inflation of IAB prior to dicrotic notch.
- Diastolic augmentation encroaches onto systole (may be unable to distinguish)

DIASTOLIC AUGMENTATION
UNASSISTED SYSTOLE
ASSISTED SYSTOLE
ASSISTED AORTIC END DIASTOLIC PRESSURE

Physiologic Effects:
- Potential premature closure of aortic valve
- Potential increased in LVEDV and LVEDP or PCWP
- Increased left ventricular wall stress or afterload
- Aortic Regurgitation
- Increased MVO_2 demand

C

Inflation of the IAB markedly after closure of the aortic valve

Waveform Characteristics:
- Inflation of the IAB after the dicrotic notch.
- Absence of sharp V
- Sub-optimal diastolic augmentation

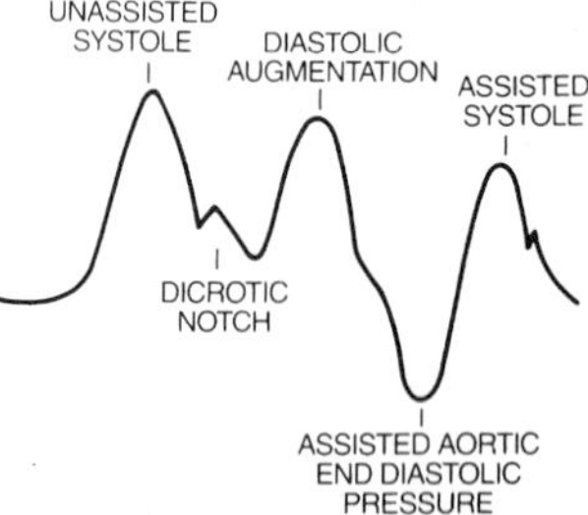

Physiologic Effects:
- Sub-optimal coronary artery perfusion

D

Figure 31–7 Alterations in arterial waveform tracings caused by errors in timing of intra-aortic balloon pump (IABP). *(A)* The balloon was deflated too early. *(B)* The balloon was deflated too late. *(C)* The balloon was inflated too early. *(D)* The balloon was inflated too late. (Courtesy of Datascope Corporation.)

Treatment for these respective problems is straightforward. Flaps, dissections, perforations, embolic events, and pseudoaneurysms should be dealt with directly by surgical intervention and repair. Steal syndromes or ischemia, if not severe, may be dealt with expectantly, but if severe extremity compromise is observed, the balloon should be moved to another site. An alternative means of treatment is a femoral-to-femoral crossover graft placed surgically to help alleviate the affected extremity.

Problems associated with the balloon are managed directly by removal or replacement or, if necessary, repositioning. Gas embolization, although rare, has been successfully treated with hyperbaric oxygen.

Infections usually require removal or replacement of the balloon in an alternate site. Appropriate antibiotic coverage should be instituted and adjusted as culture results become available. Prosthetic materials should be removed if present and debridement of the insertion site conducted as necessary. Septicemia can occur and have detrimental effects if not aggressively treated.

SUMMARY

Because of multiple improvements in medical and anesthetic management, myocardial preservation (see Chapters 28 and 30), and surgical techniques, most patients can be safely weaned off CPB after successful surgery. However, perioperative heart failure and the LCOS still occur in high-risk patients who require complex pharmacologic support to discontinue CPB. Other patients may require treatment of arrhythmias with drugs or pacemakers. Patients with the most severe ventricular dysfunction will require mechanical support (e.g., IABP, LVAD, RVAD) and possibly an artificial heart (e.g., AbioCor, Abiomed, Danvers, MA) or heart transplantation (see Chapters 26 and 27).

REFERENCES

1. Cook DJ: Changing temperature management for cardiopulmonary bypass. Anesth Analg 88:1254, 1999
2. Nussmeier NA, Moskowitz GJ, Weiskopf RB, et al: In vitro anesthetic washin and washout via bubble oxygenators. Anesth Analg 67:982, 1988
3. Stone JG, Young WL, Smith CR, et al: Do standard monitoring sites reflect true brain temperature when profound hypothermia is rapidly induced and reversed? Anesthesiology 82:344, 1995
4. Grigore AM, Grocott HP, Mathew JP, et al: Neurologic Outcome Research Group of the Duke Heart Center. The rewarming rate and increased peak temperature alter neurocognitive outcome after cardiac surgery. Anesth Analg 94:4, 2002
5. Gerst PH, Fleming WH, Malm JR: Increased susceptibility of the heart to ventricular fibrillation during metabolic acidosis. Circ Res 19:63, 1966
6. Cingolani HE, Mattiazzi AR, Blesa ES, Gonzalez NC: Contractility in isolated mammalian heart muscle after acid-base changes. Circ Res 26:269, 1970
7. Kassirer JP: Serious acid-base disorders. N Engl J Med 291:773, 1974
8. Bleich HL, Schwartz WB: TRIS buffer (THAM). N Engl J Med 274:782, 1966
9. Jonas RA: Optimal hematocrit for adult cardiopulmonary bypass. J Cardiothorac Vasc Anesth 15:672, 2001
10. Spiess BD: Blood transfusion for cardiopulmonary bypass: The need to answer a basic question. J Cardiothorac Vasc Anesth 16:535, 2002
11. Boyd WC, Thomas SJ: Pro: Magnesium should be administered to all coronary artery bypass graft surgery patients undergoing cardiopulmonary bypass. J Cardiothorac Vasc Anesth 14:339, 2000
12. Grigore AM, Mathew JP: Con: Magnesium should not be administered to all coronary artery bypass graft surgery patients undergoing cardiopulmonary bypass. J Cardiothorac Vasc Anesth 14:344, 2000
13. DiNardo JA: Pro: Calcium is routinely indicated during separation from cardiopulmonary bypass. J Cardiothorac Vasc Anesth 11:905, 1997
14. Prielipp R, Butterworth J: Con: Calcium is not routinely indicated during separation from cardiopulmonary bypass. J Cardiothorac Vasc Anesth 11:908, 1997
15. Tofler OB: Electrocardiographic changes during profound hypothermia. Br Heart J 24:265, 1962
16. Schwab RH, Lewis DW, Killough JH, Templeton JY: Electrocardiographic changes occurring in rapidly induced deep hypothermia. Am J Med Sci 248:290, 1964
17. Trevino A, Razi B, Beller BM: The characteristic electrocardiogram of accidental hypothermia. Arch Intern Med 127:470, 1971
18. Braunwald E: The hemodynamic significance of atrial systole. Am J Med 37:665, 1964
19. Konstadt SN, Reich DL, Thys DM, et al: Importance of atrial systole to ventricular filling predicted by transesophageal echocardiography. Anesthesiology 72:971, 1990
20. England MR, Gordon G, Salem M, Chernow B: Magnesium administration and dysrhythmias after cardiac surgery. JAMA 268:2395, 1992
21. Abraham WT, Hayes DL: Cardiac resynchronization therapy for heart failure. Circulation 108:2596, 2003
22. Dubin AM, Feinstein JA, Reddy VM, et al: Electrical resynchronization: A novel therapy for the failing right ventricle. Circulation 107:2287, 2003
23. Royster RL, Butterworth JF, Prough DS, et al: Preoperative and intraoperative predictors of inotropic support and long-term outcome in patients having coronary artery bypass grafting. Anesth Analg 72:729, 1991
24. Evans GL, Smulyan H, Eich RH: Role of peripheral resistance in the control of cardiac output. Am J Cardiol 20:216, 1967
25. Hansen RM, Viquerat CE, Matthay MA, et al: Poor correlation between pulmonary arterial wedge pressure and left ventricular end-diastolic volume after coronary artery bypass graft surgery. Anesthesiology 64:764, 1986
26. Entress JJ, Dhamee S, Olund T, et al: Pulmonary artery occlusion pressure is not accurate immediately after cardiopulmonary bypass. J Cardiothorac Anesth 4:558, 1990
27. Cheung AT, Savino JS, Weiss SJ, et al: Echocardiographic and hemodynamic indexes of left ventricular preload in patients with normal and abnormal ventricular function. Anesthesiology 81:376, 1994
28. Konstadt SN, Thys D, Mindich BP, et al: Validation of quantitative intraoperative transesophageal echocardiography. Anesthesiology 65:418, 1986
29. Abel MD, Nishimura RA, Callahan MJ, et al: Evaluation of Intraoperative transesophageal echocardiography. Anesthesiology 66:64, 1987
30. Hoka S, Okamoto H, Yamaura K, et al: Removal of retained air during cardiac surgery with transesophageal echocardiography and capnography. J Clin Anesth 9:457, 1997
31. Park KW: Protamine and protamine reactions. Int Anesthesiol Clin 42:135, 2004
32. Horrow JC: Protamine: A review of its toxicity. Anesth Analg 64:348, 1985
33. Kimmel SE, Sekeres M, Berlin JA, Ellison N: Mortality and adverse events after protamine administration in patients undergoing cardiopulmonary bypass. Anesth Analg 94:1402, 2002
34. Murphy DA, Craver JM, Jones EL, et al: Recognition and management of ascending aortic dissection complicating cardiac surgical operations. J Thorac Cardiovasc Surg 85:247, 1983
35. Branwald E, Kloner RA: The stunned myocardium: Prolonged postischemic ventricular dysfunction. Circulation 66:1146, 1982
36. Bolli R: Mechanism of myocardial "stunning." Circulation 82:723, 1990
37. Bolli R: Myocardial 'stunning' in man. Circulation 86:1671, 1992
38. Ferrari R, Ceconi C, Cerullo S, et al: Myocardial damage during ischaemia and reperfusion. Eur Heart J 14:25, 1993
39. Fontes ML, Hines RL: Pharmacologic management of perioperative left and right ventricular dysfunction. *In* Kaplan JA (ed): Cardiac Anesthesia. Philadelphia, WB Saunders Company, 1999, pp 1155–1191
40. Bristow MR, Ginsburg R, Minobe W, et al: Decreased catecholamine sensitivity and beta-adrenergic-receptor density in failing human hearts. N Engl J Med 307:205, 1982
41. Givertz M, Hare J, Loh E, et al: Effect of milrinone on hemodynamics and pulmonary vascular resistance. J Am Coll Cardiol 28:1775, 1986
42. Mentzer RM, Alegre C, Nolan SP: The effects of dopamine and isoproterenol on the pulmonary circulation. J Thorac Cardiovasc Surg 71:807, 1976
43. Cuffe MS, Califf RM, Adams KF Jr, et al: Short-term intravenous milrinone for acute exacerbation of chronic heart failure: A randomized controlled trial. JAMA 287:1541, 2002
44. Stevenson LW: Inotropic therapy for heart failure. N Engl J Med 339:1848, 1998

45. Leenen FH, Chan YK, Smith DL, Reeves RA: Epinephrine and left ventricular function in humans: Effects of beta-1 vs nonselective beta-blockade. Clin Pharmacol Ther 43:519, 1988
46. Butterworth JF 4th, Prielipp RC, Royster RL, et al: Dobutamine increases heart rate more than epinephrine in patients recovering from aortocoronary bypass surgery. J Cardiothorac Vasc Anesth 6:535, 1992
47. Miura T, Yoshida S, Iimura O, Downey JM: Dobutamine modifies myocardial infarct size through supply-demand balance. Am J Physiol 254(Pt 2):H855, 1988
48. Kertai MD, Poldermans D: The utility of dobutamine stress echocardiography for perioperative and long-term cardiac risk assessment. J Cardiothorac Vasc Anesth 19:520, 2005
49. Frishman WH, Hotchkiss H: Selective and nonselective dopamine receptor agonists: An innovative approach to cardiovascular disease treatment. Am Heart J 132:861, 1996
50. Richer M, Robert S, Lebel M: Renal hemodynamics during norepinephrine and low-dose dopamine infusions in man. Crit Care Med 24:1150, 1996
51. Steen PA, Tinker JH, Pluth JR, et al: Efficacy of dopamine, dobutamine, and epinephrine during emergence from cardiopulmonary bypass in man. Circulation 57:378, 1978
52. Meadows D, Edwards JD, Wilkins RG, Nightingale P: Reversal of intractable septic shock with norepinephrine therapy. Crit Care Med 16:663, 1988
53. Desjars P, Pinaud M, Potel G, et al: A reappraisal of norepinephrine therapy in human septic shock. Crit Care Med 15:134, 1987
54. Kristof AS, Magder S: Low systemic vascular resistance state in patients undergoing cardiopulmonary bypass. Crit Care Med 27:1121, 1999
55. Molloy DW, Lee KY, Jones D, et al: Effects of noradrenaline and isoproterenol on cardiopulmonary function in a canine model of acute pulmonary hypertension. Chest 88:432, 1985
56. Dupuis JY, Bondy R, Cattran C, et al: Amrinone and dobutamine as primary treatment of low-cardiac-output syndrome following coronary artery surgery: A comparison of their effects on hemodynamics and outcome. J Cardiothorac Vasc Anesth 6:542, 1992
57. Butterworth JF, Royster RL, Prielipp RC, et al: Amrinone in cardiac surgical patients with left ventricular dysfunction. A prospective, randomized placebo-controlled trial. Chest 104:1660, 1993
58. Gage J, Rutman H, Lucido E, LeJemtel TH: Additive effects of dobutamine and amrinone on myocardial contractility and ventricular performance in patients with severe heart failure. Circulation 74:367, 1986
59. Royster RL, Butterworth JF 4th, Prielipp RC, et al: Combined inotropic effects of amrinone and epinephrine after cardiopulmonary bypass in humans. Anesth Analg 77:662, 1993
60. George M, Lehot JJ, Estanove S: Haemodynamic and biological effects of intravenous milrinone in patients with a low-cardiac-output syndrome following cardiac surgery: Multicentre study. Eur J Anaesthesiol Suppl 5:31, 1992
61. Levy JH, Bailey JM, Deeb JM: Intravenous milrinone in cardiac surgery. Ann Thorac Surg 73:325, 2002
62. Monrad ES, Baim DS, Smith HS, et al: Effects of milrinone on coronary hemodynamics and myocardial energetics in patients with congestive heart failure. Circulation 71:972, 1985
63. Feneck RO: Intravenous milrinone following cardiac surgery. I. Effects of bolus infusion followed by variable dose maintenance infusion. The European Milrinone Multicentre Trial Group. J Cardiothorac Vasc Anesth 6:554, 1992
64. Bailey JM, Levy JH, Kikura M, et al: Pharmacokinetics of intravenous milrinone in patients undergoing cardiac surgery. Anesthesiology 81:616, 1994
65. Butterworth JF 4th, Hines RL, Royster RL, James RL: A pharmacokinetic and pharmacodynamic evaluation of milrinone in adults undergoing cardiac surgery. Anesth Analg 81:783, 1995
66. Kikura M, Sato S: The efficacy of preemptive milrinone or amrinone therapy in patients undergoing coronary artery bypass grafting. Anesth Analg 94:22, 2002
67. Leien CV, Banbach D, Thompson MJ, et al: Central and regional hemodynamic effects of intravenous isosorbide dinitrate, nitroglycerin, and nitroprusside in patients with congestive heart failure. Am J Cardiol 48:115, 1981
68. Lee KY: Effects of hydralazine and nitroprusside on cardiopulmonary function when cardiac output is acutely reduced by pulmonary vascular resistance. Circulation 69:1299, 1983
69. Ziskind Z, Pohoryles L, Mohr R, et al: The effect of low-dose intravenous nitroglycerin on pulmonary hypertension immediately after replacement of a stenotic mitral valve. Circulation 72:164, 1985
70. Felker JM: Inotropic therapy for heart failure: An evidence-based approach. Am Heart J 142:393, 2001
71. Stevenson LW, Massie BM, Francis GS, et al: Optimizing therapy for complex or refractory heart failure. Am Heat J 135:5293, 1998
72. Holland FW 2nd, Brown PS, Weintraub BD, Clark RE: Cardiopulmonary bypass and thyroid function: A "euthyroid sick syndrome." Ann Thorac Surg 52:46, 1991
73. Chu SH, Huang TS, Hsu RB, et al: Thyroid hormone changes after cardiovascular surgery and clinical implications. Ann Thorac Surg 52:791, 1991
74. Salter DR, Dyke CM, Wechsler CS: Triiodothyronine (T_3) and cardiovascular therapeutics: A review. J Card Surg 7:363, 1991
75. Gomberg-Maitland M, Frishman W: Thyroid hormone and cardiovascular disease. Am Heart J 135:187, 1998
76. Novitzky D, Cooper DK, Swanepoel A: Ionotropic effect of triiodothyronine (T_3) in low cardiac output following cardioplegic arrest and cardiopulmonary bypass: An initial experience in patients undergoing open heart surgery. Eur J Cardiothorac Surg 3:140, 1989
77. Smith A, Grattan A, Harper M, et al: Coronary revascularization: A procedure in transition from on-pump to off-pump? The role of glucose-insulin-potassium revisited in a randomized, placebo-controlled study. J Cardiothorac Vasc Anesth 16:413, 2002
78. Van den Berghe G, Wouters P, Weekers F, et al: Intensive insulin therapy and critically ill patients. N Engl J Med 245:1359, 2001
79. Wallin M, Barr G, Owall A, et al: The influence of glucose-insulin-potassium on GH/IGF-1/IGFBP-1 axis during elective coronary artery bypass surgery. J Cardiothorac Vasc Anesth 17:470, 2003
80. Svedjeholm R, Hallhagen S, Ekroth R, et al: Dopamine and high-dose glucose-insulin-potassium after a cardiac operation: Effects on myocardial metabolism. Ann Thorac Surg 51:262, 1991
81. Gradinac S, Coleman G, Taegtmeyer H, et al: Improved cardiac function with glucose-insulin-potassium after aortocoronary artery bypass grafting. Ann Thorac Surg 48:484, 1989
82. Lehmann A, Boldt J: New pharmacologic approaches for the perioperative treatment of ischemic cardiogenic shock. J Cardiothorac Vasc Anesth 19:97, 2005
83. Haikala H, Pollesello P: Calcium sensitivity enhancers. Drugs 3:1199, 2000
84. Lehmann A, Boldt J, Kirchner J: The role of calcium sensitizers for the treatment of heart failure. Curr Opin Crit Care 9:337, 2003
85. Remme W, Swedberg K, and the Task Force for the Diagnosis and Treatment of Heart Failure, European Society of Cardiology: Guidelines for the diagnosis and treatment of chronic heart failure. Eur Heart J 22:1527, 2001
86. Sonntag S, Sundberg S, Lehtonen L, et al: The calcium sensitizer levosimendan improves the function of stunned myocardium after percutaneous transluminal coronary angioplasty and acute myocardial ischemia. J Am Coll Cardiol 43:2177, 2004
87. Morais R: Levosimendan in severe right ventricular failure following mitral valve replacement. J Cardiothorac Vasc Anesth in press
88. Siirila-Waris K, Suojaranta-Ylinen R, Harjola VP: Levosimendan in cardiac surgery. J Cardiothorac Vasc Anesth 19:345, 2005
89. Mills R, Hobbs R: Nesiritide in perspective: Evolving approaches to the management of acute decompensated heart failure. Drugs Today 39:767, 2003
90. Keating G, Goa K: Nesiritide: A review of its use in acute decompensated heart failure. Drugs 63:47, 2003
91. Zineh I, Schofield R, Johnson J: the evolving role of nesiritide in advanced decompensated heart failure. Pharmacotherapy 23:1266, 2003
92. Publications Committee for the VMAC Investigators: Intravenous nesiritide versus nitroglycerin for treatment of decompensated congestive heart failure: A randomized, controlled trial. JAMA 287:1531, 2002
93. Burger A, Horten D, LeJemel T, et al: the effect of nesiritide and dobutamine on ventricular arrhythmias in the treatment of patients with acutely decompensated heart failure. A Heart J 144:1102, 2002
94. Goldstein D, Oz M: Mechanical support for postcardiotomy cardiogenic shock. Semin Thorac Cardiovasc Surg 12:220, 2000
95. Stone G, Ohman E, Miller M, et al: Contemporary utilization and outcomes of intra-aortic balloon counterpulsation in acute myocardial infarction: The Benchmark Registry. J Am Coll Cardiol 41:1940, 2003
96. Craver J, Murrah C: Elective intra-aortic balloon counterpulsation for high-risk off-pump coronary artery bypass operations. Ann Thorac Surg 71:1220, 2001
97. Babatasi G, Massetti M, Bruno P, et al: Preoperative balloon counterpulsation and off-pump coronary artery surgery for high-risk patients. Cardiovasc Surg 11:145, 2003
98. Ferguson J, Cohen M, Freedan R, et al: The current practice of intra-aortic balloon counterpulsation: Results from the Benchmark Registry. J Am Coll Cardiol 38:1456, 2001

Part VII

POSTOPERATIVE CARE

Chapter 32

POSTOPERATIVE CARDIAC RECOVERY AND OUTCOMES

Davy C. H. Cheng, MD, MSc, FRCPC •
Daniel Bainbridge, MD, FRCPC

KEY POINTS

1. Cardiac anesthesia has fundamentally shifted from a high-dose narcotic technique to a more balanced approach using moderate-dose narcotics, shorter-acting muscle relaxants, and volatile anesthetics.
2. This new paradigm has also led to renewed interest in perioperative pain management involving multimodal techniques that facilitate rapid tracheal extubation such as regional blocks, intrathecal morphine, and supplementary nonsteroidal anti-inflammatory drugs.
3. This has prompted a shift from the classic model of recovering patients in the traditional intensive care unit manner, with weaning protocols and intensive observation, to management more in keeping with the recovery room practice of early extubation and rapid discharge, which has shifted the care of cardiac patients to more specialized postcardiac surgical recovery units.
4. Fast track cardiac anesthesia appears to be safe in comparison to conventional high-dose narcotic anesthesia, but if complications occur that would prevent early tracheal extubation, then the management strategy should be modified accordingly.
5. The goal of a postcardiac surgery recovery model is a postoperative unit that allows variable levels of monitoring and care based on patient needs.
6. The initial management in the postoperative care of fast track cardiac surgical patients consists of ensuring an efficient transfer of care from operating room staff to cardiac recovery area staff while at the same time maintaining stable patient vital signs.
7. It is important to know risk factors associated with cardiac surgery and to review treatment options for patients with specific reference to outcomes, all placed within the context of cost and resource utilization, especially as medicine increasingly involves economic realities.
8. There are many risk assessment models for cardiac surgery, but one primary drawback of scoring systems is the geographic variability that occurs among institutions, especially ones that are geographically and/or politically distinct and may not have the same risk factors for their cardiac surgery programs.

Care of the cardiac surgical patient has become increasingly specialized as the volume of cases has increased and patient care has become more complicated. Not only are clinical outcomes important, reflected in mortality and morbidity statistics, but also the costs associated with delivering patient care are playing an increasingly greater role in determining clinical practice.

Cardiac anesthesia itself has fundamentally shifted from a high-dose narcotic technique to a more balanced approach using moderate-dose narcotics, shorter-acting muscle relaxants, and volatile anesthetics. This has primarily been driven by a realization that high-dose narcotics delay extubation and recovery following surgery. This new paradigm has also led to renewed interest in perioperative pain management involving multimodal techniques that facilitate rapid tracheal extubation such as regional blocks, intrathecal morphine, and supplementary nonsteroidal anti-inflammatory drugs (NSAIDs). In addition to changes in anesthetic practice, the type of patients presenting for cardiac surgery is changing. Patients are now older and have more associated comorbidities (stroke, myocardial infarction [MI], renal failure). Treatment options for coronary artery disease have expanded, ranging from medical therapy only to percutaneous interventions and surgery. Surgical options, however, have also expanded and include conventional coronary artery bypass graft surgery (CABG), off-pump coronary artery bypass surgery (OPCAB), minimally direct invasive coronary artery bypass (MIDCAB), and robotically assisted coronary artery bypass (RACAB) techniques. Change has also taken place in the recovery of cardiac patients. While cardiac surgical procedures were often associated with a high mortality and long intensive care unit (ICU) stays, the use of moderate doses of narcotics has allowed for rapid ventilator weaning and discharge from the ICU within 24 hours. This has prompted a shift from the classic model of recovering patients in the traditional ICU manner, with weaning protocols and intensive observation, to management more in keeping with the recovery room practice of early extubation and rapid discharge. This, in turn, has shifted the care of cardiac patients to more specialized postcardiac surgical recovery units.

Finally, hard clinical outcomes have driven change in the ongoing management of cardiac patients and are increasingly the focus of research. Intraoperative management now exists within the continuum of preoperative assessment and postoperative care. The outcomes of a patient within the hospital setting are only one small aspect of success. Long-term mortality, morbidity, and quality-of-life indicators are becoming the gold standard in determining benefit or harm interventions.

This chapter reviews fast track cardiac anesthesia (FTCA) and its impact on cardiac recovery. The initial perioperative care of routine cardiac surgical cases, including postoperative pain management techniques such as regional blockade and intrathecal morphine, are discussed, followed by specific management issues of commonly occurring problems in the cardiac ICU. Finally, important cardiac outcomes are reviewed, focusing on the different treatment options available to patients with coronary artery disease and discussing available evidence for their implementation.

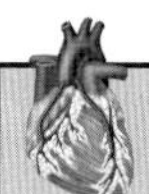

BOX 32–1 ***Benefits of Fast Track Cardiac Anesthesia***

- Decreased duration of intubation
- Decreased length of intensive care unit stay
- Decreased cost

FAST TRACK CARDIAC SURGERY CARE

Anesthetic Techniques

There have been few trials comparing inhalation agents for FTCA. A single trial comparing sevoflurane and isoflurane in patients undergoing valve surgery was unable to demonstrate reductions in tracheal extubation times.[1] There have been several studies examining the effectiveness of propofol versus inhalation agent, which demonstrated reductions in myocardial enzyme release (CK-MB, troponin I) and preservation of myocardial function in patients receiving inhalation agents.[2-5] While this endpoint is a surrogate for myocardial damage and does not show improved outcome per se, CK-MB release post-CABG may be associated with poor outcome[6] (see Box 32–1).

The choice of muscle relaxant in FTCA is important to reduce the incidence of muscle weakness in the cardiac recovery area (CRA), which may delay tracheal extubation.[7] Several randomized trials have compared rocuronium (0.5 to 1 mg/kg) versus pancuronium (0.1 mg/kg) and found significant differences in residual paralysis in the ICU.[8-11] Two studies found statistically significant delays in the time to extubation in the pancuronium group.[9,10] None of the trials used reversal agents, so the use of pancuronium appears acceptable so long as neostigmine or edrophonium is administered to patients with residual neuromuscular weakness.

There have been several trials examining the use of different short-acting narcotic agents during FTCA. In these trials, fentanyl, remifentanil, and sufentanil were all found to be efficacious for early tracheal extubation. The anesthetic drugs and their suggested dosages are given in Table 32–1.

Table 32–1 Suggested Dosages for Fast Track Cardiac Anesthesia

Induction
Narcotic
Fentanyl 5 to 10 μg/kg
Sufentanil 1 to 3 μg/kg
Remifentanil infusions of 0.5 μg/kg/min to 1.0 μg/kg/min
Muscle relaxant
Rocuronium 0.5 to 1 mg/kg
Vecuronium 1 to 1.5 mg/kg
Hypnotic
Midazolam 0.05 to 0.1 mg/kg
Propofol 0.5 to 1.5 mg/kg
Maintenance
Narcotic
Fentanyl 1 to 5 μg/kg
Sufentanil 1 to 1.5 μg/kg
Remifentanil infusions of 0.5 μg/kg/min to 1.0 μg/kg/min
Hypnotic
Inhalational 0.5 to 1 MAC
Propofol 50 to 100 μg/kg/min
Transfer to CRA
Narcotic
Morphine 0.1 to 0.2 mg/kg
Hypnotic
Propofol 25 to 75 μg/kg/min

MAC = minimal alveolar concentration; CRA = cardiac recovery area.
From Mollhoff T, Herregods L, Moerman A, et al: Comparative efficacy and safety of remifentanil and fentanyl in 'fast track' coronary artery bypass graft surgery: A randomized, double-blind study. Br J Anaesth 87: 718, 2001; Engoren M, Luther G, Fenn-Buderer N: A comparison of fentanyl, sufentanil, and remifentanil for fast-track cardiac anesthesia. Anesth Analg 93: 859, 2001; and Cheng DC, Newman MF, Duke P, et al: The efficacy and resource utilization of remifentanil and fentanyl in fast-tract coronary artery bypass graft surgery: A prospective randomized, double-blinded controlled, multi-center trial. Anesth Analg 92:1094, 2001.

Evidence Supporting Fast Track Cardiac Recovery

There are several randomized trials and one meta-analysis of randomized trials that have addressed the question of safety of FTCA.[12-18] None of the trials was able to demonstrate differences in outcomes between the fast track group and the conventional anesthesia group (Fig. 32–1). The meta-analysis of randomized trials demonstrated a reduction in the duration of intubation by 8 hours (Fig. 32–2) and the ICU length of stay (ICU LOS) by 5 hours in favor of the fast track group. However, the length of hospital stay was not statistically different.

One concern with FTCA is the potential for an increase in the incidence of adverse events, notably awareness. Awareness in patients undergoing FTCA was systematically investigated in a single trial, a prospective observational study of 617 FTCA patients. The reported incidence of explicit intraoperative awareness was 0.3% (2 of 608).[19] This is comparable to the reported incidence during conventional cardiac surgery.[20] This suggests that FTCA does not increase the incidence of awareness compared with conventional cardiac surgery.

FTCA appears safe in comparison to conventional high-dose narcotic anesthesia. It reduces the duration of ventilation and ICU LOS considerably without increasing the incidence of awareness or other adverse events.[17,18] It appears effective at reducing costs and resource utilization.[21] As such, it is becoming the standard of care in many cardiac centers. The usual practice at many institutions is to treat all patients as fast track candidates with the goal of allowing early tracheal extubation for every patient. However, if complications occur that would prevent early tracheal extubation, then the management strategy is modified accordingly. It has been demonstrated that the risk factors for delayed tracheal extubation (>10 hours) are increased age, female gender, postoperative use of intra-aortic balloon pump (IABP), inotropes, bleeding, and atrial arrhythmia. The risk factors for prolonged ICU LOS (>48 hours) are those of delayed tracheal extubation plus preoperative MI and postoperative renal insufficiency.[22] Care should be taken to avoid excess bleeding (antifibrinolytics) and to treat arrhythmias either prophylactically or on occurrence (β-blockers, amiodarone).

Postcardiac Surgical Recovery Models

The failure of many randomized FTCA trials to show reductions in resource utilization likely stems from the traditional

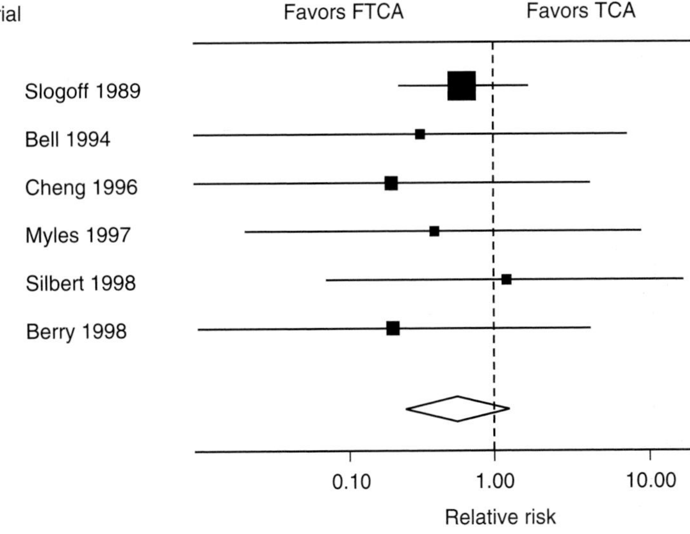

Figure 32–1 Forrest plot of mortality indicating no difference when FTCA was compared with conventional high-dose narcotic anesthesia. FTCA = fast track cardiac anesthesia, TCA = traditional cardiac anesthesia.

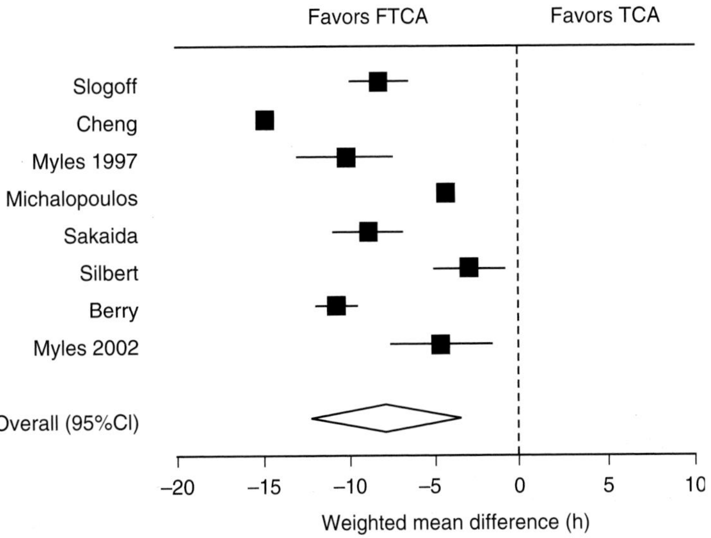

Figure 32–2 Forrest plot showing the weighted mean difference in extubation times. The overall effect was a 8.1 hour reduction in extubation times. FTCA = fast track cardiac anesthesia, TCA = traditional cardiac anesthesia.

ICU models used by these centers during the study period. Even when trials were combined in a meta-analysis, the ICU LOS was reduced only by 5 hours despite patients being extubated a mean of 8 hours earlier.[18] Typically, patients who are extubated within the first 24 hours of ICU admission are transferred to the ward on postoperative day 1 in the morning or early afternoon. This allows the following daytime cardiac cases to have available ICU beds but prevents patient transfers during nighttime hours. Two models have been proposed to deal with this issue: the parallel model and the integrated model (Fig. 32–3). In the parallel model, patients are admitted directly to a CRA, where they are monitored with 1:1 nursing care until tracheal extubation. Following this, the level of care is reduced to reflect reduced nursing requirements with ratios of 1:2 or 1:3. Any patients requiring overnight ventilation are transferred to the ICU for continuation of care. The primary drawback with the parallel model is the physical separation of the CRA and ICU, which leads to two separate units, and thus does not eliminate the requirement to transfer patients. The integrated model overcomes these limitations because all patients are admitted to the same physical area, but postoperative management such as nursing-to-patient ratio is

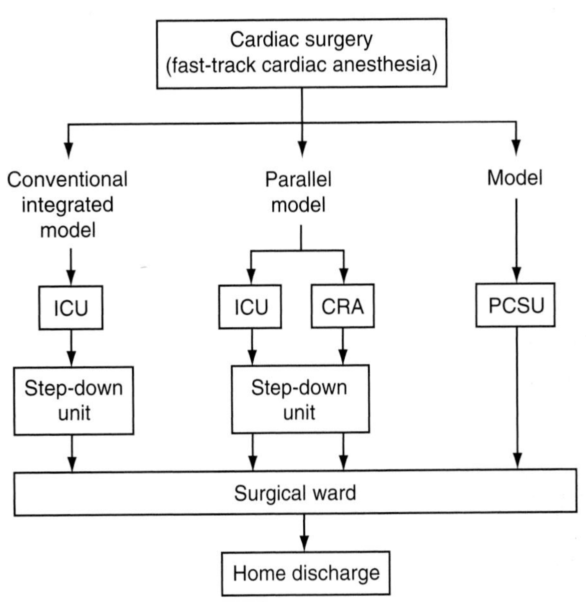

Figure 32–3 Postcardiac surgical recovery models. ICU = intensive care unit; CRA = cardiac recovery area; PCSU = postcardiac surgical unit.

Table 32–2 Suggested Initial Laboratory Work in Routine Cases, With Additional Laboratory Work to be Ordered Where Indicated

Routine
CBC
Electrolytes
BUN/creatinine
aPTT/INR
ABGs
As indicated
Fibrinogen
LFTs (AST/ALT)
Calcium
Magnesium
Cardiac enzymes (CK-MB, CK, troponin I)

CBC = complete blood count; BUN = blood urea nitrogen; aPTT = activated partial thromboplastin time; INR = international normalized ratio; ABGs = arterial blood gases; LFTs = liver function tests; AST = aspartate aminotransferase; ALT = alanine aminotransferase; CK-MB = creatine kinase myocardium band; CK = creatine kinase.

variable based on patient requirements.[23-25] As nursing care accounts for 45% to 50% of ICU costs, reducing the nursing requirements where possible creates the greatest saving. Other cost savings from reductions in arterial blood gases measurement, use of sedative drugs, and ventilator maintenance are small. The goal is a postoperative unit that allows variable levels of monitoring and care based on patient need.[25] Furthermore, FTCA has been demonstrated to be a safe and cost-effective practice that decreases resource utilization after patient discharge from the index hospitalization up to 1-year follow-up.[26]

INITIAL MANAGEMENT OF FAST TRACK CARDIAC ANESTHESIA PATIENTS: THE FIRST 24 HOURS

Upon arrival in the CRA, initial management of cardiac patients consists of ensuring an efficient transfer of care from operating room staff to CRA staff while at the same time maintaining stable patient vital signs. The anesthesiologist should relay important clinical parameters to the CRA team. To accomplish this, many centers have devised hand-off sheets to aid in the transfer of care. Initial laboratory work should be sent (Table 32–2). An electrocardiogram should be ordered, but a chest radiograph is required only in certain circumstances (Table 32–3). The patient's temperature should be recorded, and if low, active rewarming measures should be initiated with the goal of rewarming the patient to 36.5°C. Shivering may be treated with low doses of meperidine (12.5 to 25 mg IV). Hyperthermia, however, is common within the first 24 hours following cardiac surgery and may be associated with an increase in neurocognitive dysfunction, possibly a result of hyperthermia exacerbating cardiopulmonary bypass (CPB)–induced neurologic injury[27,28] (Box 32–2).

Ventilation Management: Admission to Tracheal Extubation

Ventilatory requirements should be managed with the goal of early tracheal extubation in patients (Table 32–4). Arterial blood gases (ABGs) are initially drawn within 1/2 hour after admission and then repeated as necessary. Patients should be awake and cooperative, be hemodynamically stable, and have no active bleeding with coagulopathy. Respiratory strength should be assessed by hand grip or head lift to ensure complete reversal of neuromuscular blockade. The patient's temperature should be above 36°C, preferably normothermic. When these conditions are met and ABG results are within the normal range, tracheal extubation may take place. ABGs should be drawn about 30 minutes after tracheal extubation to ensure adequate ventilation with maintenance of PaO_2 and $PaCO_2$. Inability to extubate patients as a result of respiratory failure, hemodynamic instability, or large amounts of medi-

Table 32–3 Suggested Indications for Ordering a Chest Radiograph

Respiratory
PaO_2/FIO_2 ratio >200
Peak pressure >30 cm H_2O
Asymmetric air entry
Circulatory
Uncertainty of pulmonary artery catheter position (poor trace, unable to wedge)
Hypotension resistant to treatment
Excessive bleeding
Gastrointestinal
Nasogastric/orogastric tube feeding

Table 32–4 Ventilation Management Goals During the Initial Trial of Weaning From Extubation

Initial ventilation parameters
A/C at 10 to 12 bpm
TV 8 to 10 mL/kg
PEEP 5 cm H_2O
Maintain ABGs
pH 7.35 to 7.45
$PaCO_2$ 35 to 45
PaO_2 >90
Saturations >95%
Extubation criteria
ABGs as above
Awake and alert
Hemodynamically stable
No active bleeding (<400 mL/2 hr)
Temperature >36°C
Return of muscle strength (>5 seconds, head lift/strong hand grip)

A/C = assist-controlled ventilation, TV = tidal volume, PEEP = positive end-expiratory pressure.

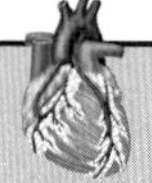

BOX 32–2 *Initial Management of the Fast Track Cardiac Anesthesia Patient*

- Normothermia
- Hemoglobin >70 mg/dL
- $PaCO_2$ 35 to 45 mm Hg
- SaO_2 >95%
- Mean blood pressure >50 to 70 mm Hg
- Potassium 3.5 to 5.0
- Blood sugar <10.0 mmol/L (<200 mg/dL)

astinal drainage will necessitate more complex weaning strategies (see Chapter 34). Some patients may arrive following extubation in the operating room. Careful attention should be paid to these patients as they may subsequently develop respiratory failure. The patient's respiratory rate should be monitored every 5 minutes during the first several hours. An ABG should be drawn on admission and 30 minutes later to ensure the patient is not retaining carbon dioxide. If the patient's respirations become compromised, ventilatory support should be provided. Simple measures such as reminders to breathe may be effective in the narcotized/anesthetized patient. Low doses of naloxone (0.04 mg IV) may also be beneficial. Trials of continuous positive airway pressure (CPAP) or bilevel positive airway pressure (BiPAP) may provide enough support to allow adequate ventilation. Reintubation should be avoided as it may delay recovery; however, it may become necessary if the above-mentioned measures fail, resulting in hypoxemia, hypercarbia, and a declining level of consciousness.

Regulation of Hemoglobin Level

Anemia is common during and after cardiac surgery as a result of both dilutional changes and bleeding. While a hemoglobin transfusion threshold of 10 g% was once common, increasing evidence suggests that a threshold of 7 g% is reasonably safe.[29] However, in the post-CPB period, patients with incomplete revascularization or with poor target vessels may require a higher transfusion threshold.[29] As a result, blood transfusions should be individualized for each patient but should certainly be used to maintain a minimal hemoglobin level of 7 g%.

Management of Bleeding

Chest tube drainage should be checked every 15 minutes after ICU admission to assess a patient's coagulation status. While blood loss is commonly divided into two types, surgical or medical, determining the cause of bleeding is often difficult. When bleeding exceeds 400 mL/hr during the first hour, 200 mL/hr for each of the first 2 hours, or 100 mL/hr over the first four hours, returning to the operating room for chest reexploration should be considered. The clinical situation must be individualized for each patient, however, and in the face of a known coagulopathy, more liberal blood loss prior to chest reexploration may be acceptable. There are numerous medical causes for bleeding following cardiac surgery. Platelet dysfunction following cardiac surgery is common. The CPB circuit itself leads to contact activation and degranulation of platelets, resulting in their dysfunction. Residual heparinization is common post–cardiac surgery and frequently occurs when either heparinized pump blood is transfused following CPB or insufficient protamine is administered. Fibrinolysis is also very common after CPB, predominantly caused by a host of activated inflammatory and coagulation pathways. Coagulation factors may decrease from activation at air–blood interfaces or from dilution with the CPB pump priming solution. Hypothermia may also aggravate the coagulation cascade and lead to further bleeding. Conventional coagulation tests are helpful to identify the coagulation abnormality contributing to the bleeding. Common laboratory testing includes aPTT, INR, platelet count, fibrinogen level, and D-dimers. Unfortunately, most conventional measures take 20 to 40 minutes before results are available. This has led to the development of new methods to help guide treatment. These bedside point-of-care tests are providing more rapid, clinically relevant results compared with laboratory testing. The use of point-of-care testing such as thromboelastography has been demonstrated to reduce transfusion requirements without increasing blood loss and is commonly used, especially following difficult cardiac cases[30,31] (see Chapters 18 and 29).

Initial medical treatment of excessive blood loss consists of 50 to 100 mg of IV protamine to ensure complete heparin reversal. This may need to be repeated if heparinized CPB pump blood has been administered after protamine reversal. While the reinfusion of chest tube blood was common to avoid exposure to donor packed red blood cells, it is no longer used routinely in practice as this blood is known to contain activated coagulation and inflammatory mediators that may predispose to an increased risk of infection.[32]

Fresh frozen plasma is usually given in the setting of an elevated INR (>1.5). Platelet levels of less than 100,000/mm^3 may warrant platelet transfusion, but caution must be exercised when considering this course. Platelet transfusions carry the greatest risk of transfusion-related complications of any blood component, typically sepsis from bacterial contamination. Platelets should only be used when platelet counts are low or the patient has a known platelet dysfunction, secondary to the use of ASA, glycoprotein (GP) IIb/IIIa inhibitors, or clopidogrel.[33] Certain physical measures should be instituted, including warming of the hypothermic patient. The benefit of PEEP on postoperative bleeding is equivocal and likely has little benefit in the face of surgical bleeding or in patients who are coagulopathic.[34,35] The use of antifibrinolytics following cardiac surgery is likely of little benefit as several randomized trials were unable to demonstrate the efficacy of antifibrinolytics used postoperatively[36,37] (Box 32–3).

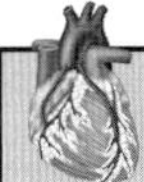

BOX 32–3 ***Management of the Bleeding Patient***

- Review ACT, PT, INR, platelet count
- Protamine if due to excess heparin (reinfusion of pump blood)
- Treat medical cause: platelets, fresh frozen plasma, cryoprecipitate if 2° to decreased fibrinogen
- Treat surgical cause: reexploration

Electrolyte Management

Hypokalemia is common following cardiac surgery, especially if diuretics were given intraoperatively. Hypokalemia contributes to increased automaticity and may lead to ventricular arrhythmias, ventricular tachycardia, or ventricular fibrillation. Treatment consists of potassium infusions (20 mEq of potassium in 50 mL of D_5W infused over 1 hour) until the potassium exceeds 3.5 mEq/mL. In patients with frequent premature ventricular contractions caused by increased automaticity, a potassium of 5.0 mEq/mL may be desirable. Hypomagnesemia contributes to ventricular preexcitation and may contribute to atrial fibrillation (AF). It is common in malnourished and sick patients, a frequent occurrence in the cardiac surgical setting. Management consists of intermittent boluses of magnesium—1 to 2 grams over 15 minutes. Hypocalcemia is also frequent during cardiac surgery and may reduce cardiac contractility. Intermittent boluses of calcium chloride or calcium gluconate (1 gram) may be required (Table 32–5).

Table 32–5 **Common Electrolyte Abnormalities and Possible Treatment Options**

Hypokalemia (K^+<3.5 mmol/L) SSx: muscle weakness, ST-segment depression, "u" wave, T wave flat, ventricular preexcitation Rx: IV KCl at 10 to 20 mEq/hr via central catheter
Hyperkalemia (K^+ >5.2 mmol/L) SSx: muscle weakness, peaked T wave, loss of P wave, prolonged PR/QRS Rx: $CaCl_2$ 1 g, insulin/glucose, HCO_3^-, diuretics, hyperventilation, dialysis
Hypocalcemia (ionized Ca^{++} <1.1 mmol/L) SSx: hypotension, heart failure, prolonged QT interval Rx: $CaCl_2$ or Ca gluconate
Hypercalcemia (Ionized Ca^{++} >1.3 mmol/L) SSx: altered mental state, coma, ileus Rx: dialysis, diuretics, mithramycin, calcitonin
Hypermagnesemia (Mg^{++} >0.7 mmol/L) SSx: weakness, absent reflexes Rx: stop Mg infusion, diuresis
Hypomagnesemia (Mg^{++} <0.5 mmol/L) SSx: arrhythmia, prolonged PR and QT intervals Rx: Mg infusion 1 to 2 g

SSx = signs and symptoms, Rx = treatment.

Table 32–6 **Pain Management Options Following Cardiac Surgery**

Patient-Controlled Analgesia May be of benefit in a stepdown unit Reduced 24-hour morphine consumption demonstrated in 2 of 7 randomized trials
Intrathecal Morphine Doses studied: 500 μg to 4 mg May be of benefit to reduce IV morphine use May be of benefit in reducing VAS pain scores *Potential for respiratory depression Ideal dosing not ascertained; range from 250 to 400 μg
Thoracic Epidurals Common dosages from literature Ropivacaine 1% with 5 μg/mL fentanyl at 3 to 5 mL/hr Bupivacaine 0.5% with 25 μg/mL morphine at 3 to 10 mL/hr Bupivacaine 0.5% to 0.75% at 2 to 5 mL/hr Reduced pain scores Shorter duration of intubation *Risk of epidural hematoma difficult to quantify
Nonsteroidal Anti-inflammatory Drugs Common dosages from literature Indomethacin 50 mg to 100 mg PR BID Diclofenac 50 to 75 mg PO/PR q8h Ketorolac 10 to 30 mg IM/IV q8h Reduces narcotic utilization Many different drugs studied; difficult to determine superiority of a given agent *May increase serious adverse events (one trial using COX-2–specific inhibitors)

Glucose Management

Diabetes is a common comorbidity (up to 30%) and is a known risk factor for adverse outcome in patients presenting for cardiac surgery.[38-40] Hyperglycemia itself is common during CPB. The risk factors for hyperglycemia include diabetes, administration of steroids prior to CPB, volume of glucose-containing solutions administered, and use of epinephrine infusions.[41] Poor perioperative glucose control is associated with increases in mortality and morbidity, including an increased risk of infection and a prolonged duration of ventilation.[42-46] In a large prospective, randomized, controlled trial of tight glucose control (blood glucose levels of 4.1 to 6.5 mmol/L) during postoperative ICU stay, reductions in mortality were shown by the authors compared with more liberal glucose control (blood glucose levels of 12 mmol/L). This trial enrolled both diabetic and nondiabetic hyperglycemic patients who underwent cardiothoracic surgery and demonstrates that tight management of glucose is beneficial in the CRA. Given all the associated risks of hyperglycemia, attempts should be made to maintain euglycemia throughout the perioperative setting in all patients presenting for surgery.

Pain Control

Pain control following cardiac surgery has become a concern as narcotic doses have been reduced to facilitate fast track protocols. Intravenous morphine is still the mainstay of treatment for post–cardiac surgery patients. The most common approach is patient-demanded, nurse-delivered intravenous morphine, and this treatment remains popular because of 1:1 to 1:2 nursing typically provided during cardiac recovery. However, with a change to more flexible nurse coverage and, therefore, higher nurse-to-patient ratios, patient-controlled analgesia (PCA) morphine is becoming increasingly popular. Several studies have examined PCA morphine use in patients following cardiac surgery.[47-53] While most of these trials showed no difference in pain scores, two studies did show improved pain scores in the PCA group during the first 2 days, and one trial showed reduced VAS pain scores in the PCA morphine group at 3 days[51-53] (Table 32–6) (see Chapter 37).

Regional Analgesia Techniques

INTRATHECAL MORPHINE

Intrathecal morphine (ITM) has been investigated, in randomized trials, as an adjuvant for pain control in cardiac patients, with doses ranging from 500 μg to 4 mg.[54-63] Several of these studies found decreased 24-hour morphine requirements or improved VAS pain scores.[54-59,61] However, several trials were unable to find a difference in pain scores[55,56,60,61] or morphine requirements postoperatively.[55,56,60-63] Of the studies reviewed, three showed prolonged ventilatory support in patients undergoing FTCA with doses ranging from 2 to 20 μg/kg.[56,61,63] The remaining studies found no difference or, in some cases, decreased duration of ventilation with doses up to 4 mg. Two of these trials had ventilation times greater than 18 hours in both ITM and placebo groups and are therefore not applicable to FTCA protocols.[54,59] Caution is advised when using intrathecal morphine because an accurate or optimal dose-response relationship has not yet been established. Intrathecal morphine offers the advantage of good pain control but with the risk of delayed extubation or the necessity for reintubation as the result of respiratory depression.

THORACIC EPIDURAL ANALGESIA

Thoracic epidural analgesia has gained some popularity as a method of providing intraoperative and postoperative pain control in cardiac surgery (see Table 32–6). There have been several randomized studies conducted to assess the benefits of this technique.[64-69] These trials overall were mixed with regard to findings. Tracheal extubation times were reduced in some trials but were no different in another.[64,66,68] One study showed benefit in pulmonary mechanics, but again others showed no difference.[64,65,67] Pain scores were improved in one study but showed no difference in others.[65,66,68] There were no reported complications as a result of epidural insertion, specifically epidural hematoma; however, all trials were inadequately powered to detect this complication. Attempts have been made to calculate the risk of epidural hematoma using available published series with estimates of maximum risk ranging from 1:1000 to 1:3500 depending on the confidence limits chosen (99% versus 95%).[70] A large retrospective review reported no epidural hematomas in 727 patients undergoing cardiac surgery with CPB receiving thoracic epidural analgesia the day of surgery (on entrance into the operating room).[71] At least 1 hour elapsed between the insertion of the epidural catheter and heparin administration. There were nine failed catheter insertions and four failed analgesia blocks with 11 bloody taps in this study.[71] Unfortunately, the population of cardiac surgical patients is increasingly on antiplatelet medication, such as GP IIIa/IIb inhibitors, which increase the risk of epidural hematoma.[72] The risk of epidural hematoma and with the potential delay of surgery from a bloody tap have limited the widespread adoption of thoracic epidural analgesia for cardiac surgery.

Nonsteroidal Anti-inflammatory Drugs

The use of NSAIDs has gained popularity in a multimodal approach, allowing reductions in both pain levels and narcotic side effects (see Table 32–6). The conventional NSAIDs, which nonselectively block the cyclooxygenase (COX)-2 isoenzyme, reduce inflammation, fever, and pain and also block the COX-1 isoenzyme resulting in the side effects of gastrointestinal toxicity and platelet dysfunction.[73] There are numerous randomized trials examining the benefit of NSAID use for postoperative pain control.[74-85] Most trials demonstrated reduced narcotic requirements with few adverse events, but one large study on COX-2 selective NSAIDs observed a higher rate of adverse events, including an increase in postoperative wound infection.[85] Whether this was a class effect of COX-2 inhibition or is generalizable to all NSAIDs is difficult to determine. Studies examining the nonspecific NSAIDs were small, and few adverse events were reported in these trials. In addition to wound infection, there is some concern regarding the effect of NSAIDs on bone healing and the potential for interaction with aspirin, reducing platelet inhibition.[86-88] Although NSAIDs have theoretical side effects, the benefit in reduced narcotic consumption and improved VAS pain scores is well demonstrated; many centers continue to use nonselective NSAIDs as analgesia adjuvants in cardiac surgery.[89-91] However, NSAIDs should be avoided in patients with renal insufficiency, a history of gastritis, or peptic ulcer disease. Adjuvant ranitidine treatment should be considered to prevent gastric irritation.

Medications for Risk Reduction After Coronary Artery Bypass Graft Surgery

CABG surgery itself reduces the risk of mortality and angina recurrence, but several medical management issues may help maintain the long-term benefit following CABG surgery. Specifically, the use of aspirin, β-blockers, and lipid-lowering agents has been demonstrated to prolong survival and/or reduce graft restenosis (Box 32–4).

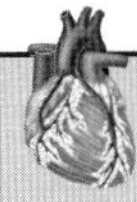

BOX 32–4 *Medications for Risk Reduction After Coronary Artery Bypass Graft Surgery*

- Aspirin: all patients after bypass grafting
- Clopidogrel: patients who have contraindication to aspirin (may have superior efficacy compared with aspirin)
- β-Blockers: especially with perioperative myocardial infarction
- Lipid-lowering agents

Aspirin

Several studies have demonstrated the efficacy of aspirin (ASA) use on graft patency and reductions in MI and mortality after CABG surgery.[92-96] A large observational study showed a reduction in mortality of nearly 3% and a reduction in MI rate of 48% with the early use of aspirin postoperatively (within 48 hours).[96] ASA dosages have ranged from 100 mg OD to 325 mg TID orally or by suppository up to 48 hours following ICU admission. There was no additional benefit from the use of aspirin prior to surgery.[97] The beneficial effect on saphenous vein graft patency appears to be lost after 1 year, with prolonged use of aspirin having no further benefit.[98] However, as aspirin, in doses of 75 mg to 325 mg per day, reduces mortality and morbidity in patients at risk for cardiovascular disease; its continued long-term use is clearly warranted.[99] Both ticlopidine and clopidogrel may be suitable alternatives in patients who are allergic to aspirin. Clopidogrel, through reductions in all-cause mortality, stroke, and MI, may be superior to ASA in patients who return with recurrent ischemic events following cardiac surgery.[100] Ticlopidine, however, should be used with caution as it may cause neutropenia (necessitating white blood cell counts to be monitored during initial use). Clopidogrel has a lower incidence of adverse reactions compared with ticlopidine and is therefore preferred as a second-line agent when aspirin is contraindicated.

β-Blockers

The use of β-blockers in patients following CABG surgery has not been shown to improve mortality.[101] It has also failed to reduce myocardial ischemia rate, unlike the angiotensin-converting enzyme inhibitor quinapril, which has, in a single study, demonstrated efficacy at reducing ischemic events following CABG.[102,103] However, patients who receive β-blockers following perioperative MI had reductions in mortality at 1 year.[104] Patients with a previous history of MI should be continued on β-blocker therapy.

Lipid-Lowering Agents

Aggressive lowering of low-density lipoprotein (LDL) cholesterol levels to 60 to 85 mg/dL (1.6 to 2.2 mmol/L) is associated with reduced rates of saphenous vein graft lesions following CABG surgery.[105] Unfortunately, this trial found no reductions in mortality or MI. There was also no improvement in vein graft patency from the use of low-dose warfarin.

Anticoagulation for Valve Surgery

Anticoagulation should be started in the early postoperative period for patients who have undergone valve replacement with either a mechanical or bioprosthesis and should also be considered when AF complicates the postoperative course.[106]

Table 32–7 Suggested Antithrombotic Therapy for Heart Valve Prophylaxis

		Class
1. First 3 months after valve replacement	Warfarin, INR 2.5 to 3.5	I
2. ≥3 months after valve replacement		
A. Mechanical valve		
AVR and no risk factor*		
Bileaflet valve or Medtronic Hall valve	Warfarin, INR 2 to 3	I
Other disk valves or Starr-Edwards valve	Warfarin, INR 2.5 to 3.5	I
AVR + risk factor*	Warfarin INR 2.5 to 3.5	I
MVR	Warfarin INR 2.5 to 3.5	I
B. Bioprosthesis		
AVR and no risk factor*	Aspirin, 80 to 100 mg/d	I
AVR and risk factor*	Warfarin, INR 2 to 3	I
MVR and no risk factor*	Aspirin, 80 to 100 mg/d	I
MVR and risk factor*	Warfarin, INR 2.5 to 3.5	I
3. Addition of aspirin, 80 to 100 mg once daily if not on aspirin		IIa
4. Warfarin, INR 3.5 to 4.5 in high-risk patients when aspirin cannot be used		IIa
5. Warfarin, INR 2.0 to 3.0 in patients with Starr-Edwards AVR and no risk factor		IIb
6. Mechanical valve, no warfarin therapy		III
7. Mechanical valve, aspirin therapy only		III
8. Bioprosthesis, no warfarin and no aspirin therapy		III

AVR = aortic valve replacement, MVR = mitral valve replacement.
Modified from Task Force on Practice Guidelines (Committee on Management of Patients with Valvular Heart Disease): ACC/AHA guidelines for the management of patients with valvular heart disease. A report of the American College of Cardiology/American Heart Association. J Am Coll Cardiol 32:1486-1588, 1998.
*Risk factors—atrial fibrillation, LV dysfunction, previous thromboembolism.

The recommended prophylactic regimens for patients with both mechanical and bioprosthetic heart valves are shown in Table 32–7. AF management is discussed in the following section.

MANAGEMENT OF COMPLICATIONS

Complications are frequent following cardiac surgery. While many are short-lived, some complications, like stroke, are long-term catastrophic events that seriously affect a patient's functional status (see Chapter 36). The incidence and predisposing risk factors are well studied for many of the complications (Table 32–8). Many of these complications have specific management issues, which may improve recovery following surgery (Box 32–5).

Table 32–8 Common Complications Following Heart Surgery

Complication	Incidence	Risk Factors
Stroke	2% to 4%	Age Previous stroke/TIA PVD Diabetes Unstable angina
Delirium	8% to 15%	Age Previous stroke Duration of surgery Duration of aortic cross-clamp A Fib Blood transfusion
Atrial fibrillation	Up to 35%	Age Male gender Previous A Fib Mitral valve surgery Previous CHF
Renal failure	1%	Low postoperative CO Repeat cardiac surgery Valve surgery Age Diabetes

TIA = transient ischemic attack; PVD = peripheral vascular disease; A Fib = atrial fibrillation; CO = cardiac output.

Stroke

Stroke following cardiac surgery occurs in 2% to 4% of patients and carries a very high 1-year mortality rate of 15% to 30%.[39,107-109] Known risk factors for stroke include age, diabetes, previous history of stroke or transient ischemic attack, peripheral vascular disease, and unstable angina.[39,107] The most common cause is emboli sheared off the aorta during aortic manipulation (proximal anastomosis of the vein grafts, clamping and unclamping of the aorta). However, hemorrhagic and watershed infarcts do occur secondary to the use of large doses of heparin and the frequent occurrence of hypotension during surgery, respectively. AF in the postoperative period also appears to be an important cause of strokes in cardiac patients.[110] Resource utilization is increased in patients who sustained a stroke, with prolonged ICU and hospital stays.[107] There are numerous proposed methods of preventing neurologic injury during the intraoperative period including epiaortic scanning, alpha-stat pH management during CABG with CPB, and OPCAB surgery with no-touch surgical techniques.[111-115] Prevention of postoperative neurologic injury may be possible with the aggressive treatment of

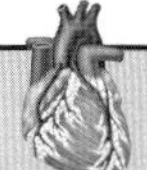

BOX 32–5 ***Treatment for Complications After Bypass Surgery***

Stroke

- Supportive treatment
- Avoid potential aggravating factors such as hyperglycemia, hyperthermia, and severe anemia (<70 mg/dL)

Delirium

- Usually self-limited
- Requires close observation
- May require sedatives (midazolam, lorazepam)

Atrial Fibrillation

- Rate control: calcium channel blockers, β-blockers, digoxin
- Rhythm control: amiodarone, sotalol, procainamide
- Thromboembolic prophylaxis: for atrial fibrillation >48 hours

Left Ventricular Dysfunction

- Volume
- Inotropes: epinephrine, milrinone, norepinephrine
- Mechanical support: intra-aortic balloon pump

Renal Failure

- Remove the causative agent (nonsteroidal anti-inflammatory drugs, antibiotics)
- Hemodynamic support if necessary
- Supportive care

AF (antiarrhythmics, anticoagulants, early cardioversion) to prevent thromboembolism (see Atrial Fibrillation later). Patients who sustain an intraoperative stroke should be managed with the goal of preventing further brain injury. Hyperglycemia should be avoided, as it is associated with poor outcome in brain injury patients.[116-118] Hyperthermia is also known to exacerbate brain injury and should also be avoided.[119] Hemoglobin concentrations should certainly be maintained above 7 g%. Whether there is benefit to maintaining hemoglobin levels greater than 10 g% is uncertain, but this may be prudent in patients with perioperative stroke.

Delirium

Delirium is defined generally as an acute transient neurologic condition with impairment of cognitive function, attention abnormalities, and altered psychomotor activity. It often includes a disorder with the sleep-wake cycle. It is fairly common following cardiac surgery with a prevalence of 8% to 15%.[120,121] Risk factors associated with delirium include age, previous history of stroke, duration of surgery, duration of aortic cross-clamp, AF, and blood transfusion.[120-123] Interestingly, delirium is self-limited and does not adversely affect patient outcome or hospital LOS.[122,123] Treatment is supportive, involving close observation of patients, and sedatives (midazolam, diazepam) or antipsychotics (haloperidol) as required.

Atrial Fibrillation

AF following cardiac surgery is common and occurs in up to 35% of patients.[124] While the cause of AF is not completely understood, it is associated with an increase in mortality, stroke, and prolonged hospital stay.[107,110,125] Known risk factors include age, male gender, previous AF, mitral valve surgery, and a history of congestive heart failure.[107,126] Prevention and treatment of AF can be achieved effectively with amiodarone, sotalol, magnesium, or β-blockers.[127] Biatrial pacing may also be effective prophylaxis.[127,128] Management of AF consists of rate control with conversion to sinus rhythm or anticoagulation. Several studies conducted to determine which strategy was superior were unable to find a difference between treatment strategies (AFFIRM and RACE trials).[129-131]

Rate control may be achieved with a β-blocker or a calcium channel blocker. Digoxin may also be effective, but it is difficult to achieve therapeutic levels quickly. An observational review of the AFFIRM trial suggests that β-blockers are superior to either calcium channel blockers or digoxin for rate control in AF.[132] Conversion to sinus rhythm in the stable patient may be achieved with amiodarone, sotalol, or procainamide. Amiodarone is more commonly used in acute management of postoperative AF (150 to 300 mg IV) than other antiarrhythmics, particularly in patients with compromised ventricular function, as it causes little cardiac depression. Finally, persistent AF over 48 to 72 hours requires thromboembolic prophylaxis. Warfarin is recommended for patients at high risk of thromboembolic complications (previous stroke, congestive heart failure, diabetes mellitus, age), with an INR between 2 and 3 considered therapeutic. In a meta-analysis of randomized trials, warfarin reduced the risk of stroke by 67% and 32% compared with placebo or ASA, respectively. However, the incidence of hemorrhagic complications was also higher with warfarin (0.3% absolute risk increase per year).[133] Aspirin, 325 mg OD, may be sufficient for patients with a low thromboembolic risk[134,135] (Table 32–9).

Left Ventricular Dysfunction

Patients with poor left ventricular function commonly require inotropes or mechanical support following cardiac surgery. Preoperative factors that predict inotrope use in patients undergoing cardiac surgery include age, underlying left ventricular function, and female gender.[136,137] The significance of inotrope use on postoperative outcome is uncertain, as some centers routinely use these drugs following CPB.[136] While pulmonary artery catheters are useful for monitoring trends in cardiac function, transesophageal echocardiography (TEE) provides more detailed information for diagnosing the cause of acute hypotensive episodes and cardiac function. TEE is commonly used in the ICU to assess patients following cardiac surgery and has demonstrated efficacy for diagnosing cardiac tamponade, cardiac ischemia, and valve dysfunction, resulting in improvements in the postoperative course for these patients.[138-141] TEE also provides more accurate information on the filling volumes following CPB than does use of the pulmonary artery catheter.[142-144]

Patients who have an unstable intraoperative course should have pulmonary artery filling pressures correlated to TEE findings and the results then passed to the recovery unit to allow for optimal initial management in the recovery unit. If the patient remains unstable in the ICU, then TEE is used and cardiac function is reassessed. When hypovolemia is thought to be the underlying cause of hypotension/low cardiac output, then colloids (Pentaspan, Hestarch) are initially used to optimize filling, as third spacing of fluids is common following CPB. The intravascular hypovolemia is best treated with the use of small intermittent boluses of colloid with continuous

Table 32–9 **Suggested Atrial Fibrillation (AF) Thromboembolic Prophylaxis**

Patient Features	Antithrombotic Therapy	Recommendation
Age <60 years, no heart disease (lone AF)	Aspirin (325 mg/day) or no therapy	I
Age <60 years, heart disease but no risk factors*	Aspirin (325 mg/day)	I
Age ≥60 years, no risk factors*	Aspirin (325 mg/day)	I
Age ≥60 years, with diabetes mellitus or CAD	Oral anticoagulation (INR 2.0 to 3.0) Addition of aspirin, 81 to 162 mg/day is optional	I IIb
Age ≥75 years, especially women	Oral anticoagulation (INR ≈2.0)	I
HF	Oral anticoagulation (INR 2.0 to 3.0)	
LV ejection fraction ≤0.35		I
Thyrotoxicosis and hypertension		
Rheumatic heart disease (mitral stenosis)	(INR 2.5 to 3.5 or higher may be appropriate)	I
Prosthetic heart valves		
Prior thromboembolism		
Persistent atrial thrombus on TEE		

AF = atrial fibrillation; CAD = coronary artery disease; HF = heart failure; INR = international normalized ratio; LV = left ventricular; TEE = transesophageal echocardiography.
*Risk factors are heart failure, LV ejection fraction <0.35, and a history of hypertension.
Modified from Fuster V, Ryden LE, Asinger RW, et al: ACC/AHA/ESC guidelines for the management of patients with atrial fibrillation: executive summary. A Report of the American College of Cardiology/ American Heart Association Task Force on Practice Guidelines and the European Society of Cardiology Committee for Practice Guidelines and Policy Conferences (Committee to Develop Guidelines for the Management of Patients With Atrial Fibrillation): developed in Collaboration With the North American Society of Pacing and Electrophysiology. J Am Coll Cardiol 38:1231-1266, 2001.

reassessment of central venous pressure, pulmonary artery pressure, wedge pressure, systemic pressures, or left ventricular end-diastolic area.[142]

If ventricular dysfunction is the main cause of hypotension/low cardiac output state, then inotropes and vasopressors should be added (see Chapter 33). Unfortunately, few articles have been published looking at the superiority of one inotrope over another. Epinephrine (0.02 to 0.04 μg/kg/min) or dopamine (3 to 5 μg/kg/min) is commonly used to support patients coming off CPB and is usually continued into the ICU. If systolic pressure remains low, then the epinephrine infusion is usually increased to allow for greater α-receptor action (vasoconstriction). For patients with a low cardiac output or poor myocardial function on TEE, milrinone is commonly used (with or without a full loading dose). Milrinone, a cAMP phosphodiesterase inhibitor, has the advantage of bypassing β-adrenergic receptors, which are downregulated following cardiac surgery.[145] Phosphodiesterase inhibitors appear to improve myocardial performance even with the concomitant use of epinephrine.[146] If despite this blood pressure remains low, then a vasopressin infusion is typically started with doses ranging from 1 U/hr to 10 U/hr. When volume and medical strategies are insufficient, especially in the presence of ischemic heart disease, mechanical support is used (see Chapters 27 and 31). IABPs are used in approximately 3% of cardiac surgical patients. The IABP is commonly placed preoperatively in patients with unstable angina unresponsive to medical treatment, intraoperatively in high-risk patients (redo sternotomy with poor left ventricular function), in patients who fail to wean from CPB, or in patients on maximal inotropic support after bypass.

For patients who fail to wean from CPB, one retrospective study found 85% success in weaning with the institution of an IABP; however, the overall mortality was 35%.[147] Several studies have looked at the timing of IABP insertion and found reductions in mortality in patients who received the IABP prior to initiation of CPB.[148-151] Complications from the use of IABP are numerous and include wound site infections, leg ischemia, and renal dysfunction. Several retrospective reviews have examined the outcomes following IABP insertion; again, mortality rates were high in patients who received an IABP in the operating room or recovery unit (35%).[152,153] Finally, in patients who require long-term inotropic support and use of an IABP, angiotensin-converting enzyme inhibitors may help to reduce mortality. One small trial investigated the use of captopril in patients who required more than two inotropes and/or IABP placement and showed reductions in mortality in patients randomized to receive captopril.[154]

Renal Insufficiency

Renal failure in the postoperative period is rare, occurring in approximately 1% of patients following cardiac surgery. Not surprisingly, when it does occur, it prolongs CRA LOS and hospital LOS and increases mortality.[40,155] Unfortunately, no clear definition exists as to what constitutes renal impairment or failure following CPB. While the need for dialysis is a straightforward and easily measured outcome, it unfortunately ignores patients who have reductions in creatinine clearance but do not require dialysis.[40,155] Change in calculated creatinine clearance, which is predictive of need for dialysis, prolonged hospitalization, and mortality, may be a more suitable outcome measurement of renal failure.[156] There are several risk factors for postoperative renal failure, including postoperative low cardiac output, repeat cardiac surgery, valve surgery, age greater than 65, and diabetes.[40,155,157] Management of these patients consists of supportive treatment, determining the primary cause, and then directing specific treatment as necessary. Supportive treatment consists of ensuring adequate cardiac output, perfusion pressure, and intravascular volume. The cause of renal failure is broadly defined as prerenal, renal, or postrenal failure. Prerenal causes are commonly related to poor cardiac output or low systemic pressure and also may be associated with the use of angiotensin-converting enzyme inhibitors and NSAIDs. Renal causes include acute tubular necrosis (ATN) from an ischemic insult or interstitial nephritis caused by a host of medications including NSAIDs and antibiotics.

Although uncommon in the face of bladder catheterization, the potential for postrenal obstruction is also possible. Management of renal failure usually requires correction of the underlying problem, which may include improving renal blood flow (volume, inotropes) or discontinuing the offending agent (NSAIDs, antibiotic). To date there is no specific treatment to prevent ATN. While dopamine and diuretics were once both thought to be renoprotective, neither has demonstrated efficacy to prevent renal failure.[158] There is a suggestion that diuretics may be potentially harmful in patients developing renal failure.[159] If patients do require dialysis, continuous dialysis may be better than intermittent dialysis.[160] *N*-Acetylcysteine (NAC) has demonstrated efficacy in preventing further renal failure, in patients with chronic renal insufficiency, from radiocontrast agent.[161] This may translate to cardiac surgery, especially if angiograms are performed just prior to surgery. Unfortunately, results of prophylactic NAC have been mixed, with some trials showing benefit and others no difference.[162-164]

POSTOPERATIVE RISK AND OUTCOME

One question that every patient asks and every anesthesiologist answers concerns the risks from this operation and the recovery course. While seemingly a straightforward question, it gets to the heart of current medical practice, namely, assessing risk, weighing potential treatment options, determining best evidence for each patient, and then prescribing a course of treatment with the ultimate goal of providing the best possible care. It is important to know risk factors associated with cardiac surgery and to review treatment options for patients with specific reference to outcomes. This should all be placed within the context of cost and resource utilization, especially as medicine increasingly involves economic realities.

Risk Assessment

There are many risk assessment models for cardiac surgery published in the literature, including the Higgins score, Ontario score, French, Bayes, Parsonnet, and Euroscore.[165-169] One of the most well known is the Parsonnet score[168] (Table 32–10). In Europe, the Euroscore has been popularized and validated for the prediction of mortality[169] (Table 32–11). All of the above scoring systems define preoperative variables associated with postoperative mortality either in hospital or at 30 days postoperatively.

To determine how well an individual test predicts outcome, a receiver operating characteristics (ROC) curve is created. It is simply a graphic plot of sensitivity versus specificity. An ROC of 1.0 indicates accurate prediction each time and 0.5 indicates random chance alone. ROC scores of 0.65 to 0.75 indicate moderate prediction and are typically the range for most risk assessment scores.[170,171] Risk scoring systems have allowed a greater appreciation of the factors that contribute to adverse events in cardiac surgery. They have allowed the comparison of different patient groups over time and between centers. In addition, they have been used to adjust for direct comparisons of outcome and resource utilization between institutions. Unfortunately, risk scoring has some inherent limitations, which may lead to the inappropriate use of risk scoring and to drawing erroneous conclusions.

Table 32–10 The Original Parsonnet Score

Risk Factor	Assigned Weight
Female gender	1
Morbid obesity (≥1.5 × ideal weight)	3
Diabetes (unspecified type)	3
Hypertension (systolic BP > 140 mm Hg)	3
Age (yr)	
70 to 74	7
75 to 79	12
≥80	20
Reoperation	
First	5
Second	10
Preoperative IABP	2
Left ventricular aneurysm	5
Emergency surgery following PTCA or catheterization complications	10
Dialysis dependency (PD or hemodialysis)	10
Catastrophic states (e.g., acute structural defect, cardiogenic shock, acute renal failure)	10 to 50
Other rare circumstances (e.g., paraplegia, pacemaker dependency, congenital HD in adult, severe asthma)	2 to 10
Valve surgery	
Mitral	5
PA pressure ≥60 mm Hg	8
Aortic	5
Pressure gradient >120 mm Hg	7
CABG at the time of valve surgery	2

IABP = intra-aortic balloon pump, PTCA = percutaneous transluminal coronary angioplasty, PD = peritoneal dialysis, HD = heart disease, PA = pulmonary artery, CABG = coronary artery bypass grafting.

Modified from Parsonnet V, Dean D, Bernstein AD: A method of uniform stratification of risk for evaluating the results of surgery in acquired adult heart disease. Circulation 79:I-3-I-12, 1989.

Limitations of Risk Scoring

One primary drawback of scoring systems is the geographic variability that occurs among institutions, especially ones that are geographically and/or politically distinct and may not have the same risk factors for their cardiac surgery programs. Indeed, the poor applicability of the Parsonnet score in France led to the development of the French score system.[167,172] Numerous scoring systems have slight differences in included variables and weightings, which suggests subtle differences between centers. Another consideration is the time point used to determine mortality. While Parsonnet and Higgins both use 30-day mortality, the French score uses in-hospital mortality. These two estimates begin to diverge at the onset of hospital

Table 32–11 EuroScore

Factor	Definition	Score
Patient-Related Factors		
Age	Per 5 years or part thereof over 60 years	1
Sex	Female	1
Chronic pulmonary disease	Long-term use of bronchodilators or steroids for lung disease	1
Extracardiac arteriopathy	Any one or more of the following: claudication, carotid occlusion or >50% stenosis, previous or planned intervention on the abdominal aorta, limb arteries, or carotids	2
Neurologic dysfunction	Disease severely affecting ambulation or day-to-day functioning	2
Previous cardiac surgery	Requiring opening of the pericardium	3
Serum creatinine	>200 μmol/L preoperatively	2
Active endocarditis	Patient still under antibiotic treatment for endocarditis at the time of surgery	3
Critical preoperative state	Any one of more of the following: Ventricular tachycardia or fibrillation or aborted sudden death, preoperative cardiac massage, preoperative ventilation before arrival in the anesthetic room, preoperative inotropic support, intra-aortic balloon counterpulsation or preoperative acute renal failure (anuria or oliguria <10 mL/hr)	3
Cardiac-Related Factors		
Unstable angina	Rest angina requiring IV nitrates until arrival in the anesthetic room	2
LV dysfunction	Moderate or LVEF 30% to 50%	1
	Poor or LVEF <30	3
Recent myocardial infarct	(<90 days)	2
Pulmonary hypertension	Systolic PA pressure >60 mm Hg	2
Operation-Related Factors		
Emergency	Carried out on referral before the beginning of the next working day	2
Other than isolated CABG	Major cardiac procedure other than or in addition to CABG	2
Surgery on thoracic aorta	For disorder of ascending arch or descending aorta	3
Postinfarct septal rupture		4

LV = left ventricular, LVEF = left ventricular ejection fraction, PA = pulmonary artery, CABG = coronary artery bypass grafting.
Modified from Nashef SA, Roques F, Michel P, et al: European system for cardiac operative risk evaluation (EuroSCORE). Eur J Cardiothorac Surg 16:9–13, 1999.

discharge and may be substantially different by 30 days.[173] In-hospital mortality is, however, much easier to record and avoids follow-up of discharged patients. For CABG patients, mortality may remain elevated for up to 3 months following surgery and therefore 3-month mortality may be a better measure of outcome than an arbitrary cutoff at 30 days. The complexity of some systems makes them difficult to apply clinically or makes data collection for research cumbersome. This has led to simpler systems that are clinically more intuitive[174] (Box 32–6).

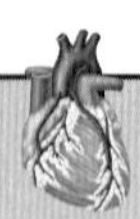

BOX 32–6 ***Limitations of Risk Scoring Systems***

- Geographic variability
- Temporal variability
- Endpoints used
- Complexity of some systems

Postoperative Outcomes—Treatment Options for Coronary Artery Disease

Until the advent of CABG surgery, medical management was the only treatment option for patients with CAD. Today, treatment can be broadly categorized as medical or invasive management, with invasive management divided geographically into interventions performed in the cardiac catheterization laboratory or in the operating room. Catheterization procedures commonly performed include balloon angioplasty, cardiac stenting, and drug-eluting stents, which release drugs capable of preventing restenosis (see Chapter 12). Operating room procedures include conventional CABG (with the use of the CPB machine) and OPCAB (without the use of the CPB machine). OPCAB surgery may include full sternotomy, thoracotomy (MIDCAB), or robotically assisted thoracotomy (RAOPCAB) surgery. With the ever-increasing number of available options, it becomes crucial to establish which option is superior with regard to angina recurrence, graft patency, and long-term survival with the least morbidity (MI, stroke, AF) at the lowest costs (hospital LOS, ICU LOS, blood transfusions).

Medical Treatment Versus Surgical Management

Several large randomized trials have examined the efficacy of medical versus surgical management in patients with symptomatic coronary artery disease (Table 32–12). Most trials were conducted between 1974 and 1984. A meta-analysis was published in 1994 that incorporated seven trials addressing medical versus surgical management with a 10-year follow-up.[175] While surgical and medical management have advanced since then (i.e., only 9% of patients received IMA grafts), the findings clearly support the benefits of surgery in high-risk patients. This study reviewed 2600 patients and observed an absolute risk reduction in mortality for patients undergoing CABG of 5.6% at 5 years, 5.9% at 7 years, and 4.1% at 10 years. This improvement was most marked in patients with left main disease, proximal left anterior descending coronary artery disease, or triple-vessel disease. The results tended to underestimate the benefits of surgical treatment, as 37.4% of medically treated patients eventually underwent surgery.

Table 32–12 **Treatment Options and Outcomes for Coronary Artery Disease**

Comparison	Outcome	Revascularization
Medical versus surgical management	Absolute risk reduction in mortality 5.6% at 5 years 5.9% at 7 years 4.1% at 10 years Benefit of surgery greatest in LM, 3-vessel disease	37% of medically treated patients converted to surgery
Angioplasty versus surgical management	Absolute risk reduction in mortality 1.9% at 5 years Rates of in hospital MI and stroke significantly lower in angioplasty group Benefit of surgery greatest in diabetics, multivessel revascularization	50% rate of revascularization at 5 years in angioplasty group
Stent versus surgical management	Mortality mixed results, relative reduction ranged from a 50% reduction in favor of CABG to a 75% reduction in favor of stenting. MI rates at 1-year equivalent	15% to 25% rate of revascularization in stent group
OPCAB versus conventional surgical management	No difference in mortality No difference for in-hospital stroke No difference for in-hospital MI	Most OPCAB patients received fewer grafts than CCAB group (0.2 fewer grafts per patient)

OPCAB = off-pump coronary artery bypass; LM = left main disease; MI = myocardial infarction.

CABG surgery reduces mortality significantly compared with medical management alone. This benefit is significantly improved beyond 10 years. In addition, many patients initially treated medically eventually require surgical revascularization.

Balloon Angioplasty Versus Conventional Coronary Artery Bypass Graft Surgery

A number of randomized trials comparing PTCA to CABG have been performed (see Chapters 12, 19, and 21). One of the largest trials was the Bypass Angioplasty Revascularization Investigation (BARI), which enrolled 1829 patients who were randomized to undergo either percutaneous transluminal coronary angioplasty (PTCA) or CABG.[176] It found no significant differences in survival at both 1 year and 5 years, with the 5-year survival rates of 89.3% in the CABG group and 86.3% in PTCA group. The rates of in-hospital MI and stroke were higher in the CABG patients compared with the PTCA group (4.6% and 2.1% for Q-wave MI, $P < 0.01$; 0.8% and 0.2% for stroke). For diabetic patients, 5-year survival was 80.6% in the CABG group compared with 65.5% in the PTCA group ($P = 0.003$). The need for repeated revascularization after initial intervention was also higher in the PTCA group; at 5 years, only 8% of the patients assigned to CABG had undergone additional revascularization procedures, compared with 54% of those assigned to PTCA (31% of PTCA patients eventually underwent CABG). Several smaller randomized trials found similar results.[177,178]

A meta-analysis of randomized trials has recently been published comparing PTCA with CABG for the management of symptomatic CAD. A total of 13 trials involving 7964 patients were included.[179] They reported a 1.9% absolute survival advantage favoring CABG over PTCA at 5 years ($P < 0.02$). There was no significant difference at 1, 3, or 8 years. In subgroup analysis of patients with multivessel disease, CABG provided a significant survival advantage at both 5 and 8 years. Patients randomized to PTCA had more repeat revascularizations at all time points. This meta-analysis included some coronary stent trials, in which angina recurrence was reduced by 50% at 1 and 3 years, and the stent cohort had a significant decrease in nonfatal MI at 3 years compared with CABG.

The above trials focused primarily on patients with multivessel disease. In patients with single-vessel left anterior descending coronary artery disease, few randomized trials have been conducted. One trial enrolled 134 patients randomized to PTCA or CABG. After 5 years, 6 patients (9%) had died in the PTCA group versus 2 (3%) in the CABG group (NS). MI was more frequent after PTCA (15% versus 4%, $P = 0.0001$), but there were no differences in the rates of Q-wave infarction (6% in the PTCA group versus 3% in the CABG group, NS). Repeat revascularization was required in significantly more patients assigned to the PTCA group, 38% versus 9% ($P = 0.0001$).[180]

When compared with coronary angioplasty, CABG surgery reduces mortality at 5 years. It also reduces the need for additional revascularization procedures. This benefit is greatest in patients with multivessel disease.

Stenting Versus Conventional Coronary Artery Bypass Graft Surgery

Surprisingly similar results have been seen when stent implantation (bare metal stents) is compared with CABG surgery[181-183] (see Chapter 12). Two trials found no difference in the mortality rate at 1 year.[182,183] One trial found a higher mortality rate in the percutaneous coronary intervention (PCI) patients (5% PCI versus 2% CABG, $P = 0.01$), whereas another trial found reduced mortality in the PCI group (0.9% versus 5.7%, $P < 0.013$).[181,184] For Q-wave MI, the studies demonstrated equivalent or slightly higher rates with CABG at 1 year. The requirement for repeat revascularizations was still high in all the stent trials, ranging from approximately 15% to 25% (over 1 to 2 years). The costs associated with both PTCA and PCI stents are lower than the cost of CABG. The greatest cost difference is seen at 1 year and decreases after this, due to the high rate of repeat revascularization in the PCI and PTCA groups. While drug-eluting stents offer the promise of reductions in restenosis, too few trials are published to make a meaningful comment on the effect of this new technology.

Coronary stenting with bare metal stents demonstrates a similar rate of mortality compared with surgical bypass. The benefit of stenting is a reduction in morbidity outcomes in the short term (MI). However, patients are less likely to be symptom free following stenting and the need for further revascularization procedures is higher.

Off-Pump Coronary Artery Bypass Surgery Versus Coronary Artery Bypass Graft Surgery

The use of OPCAB techniques has increased in popularity and its greatest benefit will likely be in patients at highest risk of stroke (elderly, patients with high-grade aortic atheromatous disease).[185-187] A number of randomized trials have investigated the benefits of OPCAB surgery.[188-191] A comprehensive meta-analysis of randomized trials was published demonstrating that OPCAB reduces the rate of blood transfusion, AF, infections, and resource utilization (hospital LOS, ICU LOS, and ventilation time). OPCAB surgery may also minimize midterm cognitive dysfunction compared with CABG.[192] OPCAB should be considered a safe alternative to CABG with respect to risk of mortality. However, most trials to date have focused on relatively healthy patients and have been underpowered to determine benefits in the high-risk cohort group purported to benefit the most by OPCAB surgery.[185-187]

In addition, the number of coronary vessels bypassed was usually lower in the OPCAB group. Whether this will translate into worsened outcomes at 1 or 5 years is unknown. Finally, concern has been raised over graft patency.[191] Reports on graft patency following OPCAB are conflicting, with some studies suggesting reduced patency and others suggesting no difference.[193] With appropriate use of modern stabilizers, heart positioning devices, and adequate surgeon experience, similar completeness of revascularization and graft patency should be achievable with OPCAB. Ultimately, long-term outcomes are needed to assess whether important direct outcomes like mortality, angina recurrence, MI, and reoperation differ in patients undergoing OPCAB versus CABG. In healthy patients, OPCAB has similar rates of mortality and major morbidity compared with CABG while reducing the rate of AF, blood transfusion, and the LOS in both the ICU and hospital.

REFERENCES

1. Bennett SR, Griffin SC: Sevoflurane versus isoflurane in patients undergoing valvular cardiac surgery. J Cardiothorac Vasc Anesth 15:175, 2001
2. De Hert SG, Cromheecke S, ten Broecke PW, et al: Effects of propofol, desflurane, and sevoflurane on recovery of myocardial function after coronary surgery in elderly high-risk patients. Anesthesiology 99:314, 2003
3. De Hert SG, ten Broecke PW, Mertens E, et al: Sevoflurane but not propofol preserves myocardial function in coronary surgery patients. Anesthesiology 97:42, 2002
4. Julier K, Da Silva R, Garcia C, et al: Preconditioning by sevoflurane decreases biochemical markers for myocardial and renal dysfunction in coronary artery bypass graft surgery: A double-blinded, placebo-controlled, multicenter study. Anesthesiology 98:1315, 2003
5. Belhomme D, Peynet J, Louzy M, et al: Evidence for preconditioning by isoflurane in coronary artery bypass graft surgery. Circulation 100:II-340, 1999
6. Boyce SW, Bartels C, Bolli R, et al: Impact of sodium-hydrogen exchange inhibition by cariporide on death or myocardial infarction in high-risk CABG surgery patients: Results of the CABG surgery cohort of the GUARDIAN study. J Thorac Cardiovasc Surg 126:420, 2003
7. Van Oldenbeek C, Knowles P, Harper NJ: Residual neuromuscular block caused by pancuronium after cardiac surgery. Br J Anaesth 83:338, 1999
8. McEwin L, Merrick PM, Bevan DR: Residual neuromuscular blockade after cardiac surgery: Pancuronium vs rocuronium. Can J Anaesth 44:891, 1997
9. Murphy GS, Szokol JW, Marymont JH, et al: Impact of shorter-acting neuromuscular blocking agents on fast-track recovery of the cardiac surgical patient. Anesthesiology 96:600, 2002
10. Thomas R, Smith D, Strike P: Prospective randomised double-blind comparative study of rocuronium and pancuronium in adult patients scheduled for elective 'fast-track' cardiac surgery involving hypothermic cardiopulmonary bypass. Anaesthesia 58:265, 2003
11. Murphy GS, Szokol JW, Marymont JH, et al: Recovery of neuromuscular function after cardiac surgery: pancuronium versus rocuronium. Anesth Analg 96:1301, 2003
12. Quasha AL, Loeber N, Feeley TW, et al: Postoperative respiratory care: A controlled trial of early and late extubation following coronary artery bypass grafting. Anesthesiology 52:135, 1980
13. Cheng DC, Karski J, Peniston C, et al: Morbidity outcome in early versus conventional tracheal extubation after coronary artery bypass grafting: A prospective randomized controlled trial. J Thorac Cardiovasc Surg 112:755, 1996
14. Berry PD, Thomas SD, Mahon SP, et al: Myocardial ischaemia after coronary artery bypass grafting: Early vs late extubation. Br J Anaesth 80:20, 1998
15. Silbert BS, Santamaria JD, O'Brien JL, et al: Early extubation following coronary artery bypass surgery: A prospective randomized controlled trial. The Fast Track Cardiac Care Team. Chest 113:1481, 1998
16. Ovrum E, Tangen G, Schiott C, et al: Rapid recovery protocol applied to 5,658 consecutive "on-pump" coronary bypass patients. Ann Thorac Surg 70:2008, 2000
17. Meade MO, Guyatt G, Butler R, et al: Trials comparing early vs late extubation following cardiovascular surgery. Chest 120:445S-453S, 2001
18. Myles PS, Daly DJ, Djaiani G, et al: A systematic review of the safety and effectiveness of fast-track cardiac anesthesia. Anesthesiology 99:982, 2003
19. Dowd NP, Cheng DC, Karski JM, et al: Intraoperative awareness in fast-track cardiac anesthesia. Anesthesiology 89:1068-1073, 1998
20. Liu WH, Thorp TA, Graham SG, et al: Incidence of awareness with recall during general anaesthesia. Anaesthesia 46:435, 1991
21. Cheng DC, Karski J, Peniston C, et al: Early tracheal extubation after coronary artery bypass graft surgery reduces costs and improves resource use. A prospective, randomized, controlled trial. Anesthesiology 85:1300, 1996
22. Wong DT, Cheng DC, Kustra R, et al: Risk factors of delayed extubation, prolonged length of stay in the intensive care unit, and mortality in patients undergoing coronary artery bypass graft with fast-track cardiac anesthesia: A new cardiac risk score. Anesthesiology 91:936, 1999
23. Brown MM: Implementation strategy: One-stop recovery for cardiac surgical patients. AACN Clin Issues 11:412, 2000
24. Joyce L, Pandolph P: One stop postop cardiac surgery recovery—a proven success. J Cardiovasc Manag 12:16, 2001
25. Cheng DC, Byrick RJ, Knobel E: Structural models for intermediate care areas. Crit Care Med 27:2266, 1999
26. Cheng DC, Wall C, Djaiani G, et al: Randomized assessment of resource use in fast-track cardiac surgery 1 year after hospital discharge. Anesthesiology 98:651, 2003
27. Grocott HP, Mackensen GB, Grigore AM, et al: Postoperative hyperthermia is associated with cognitive dysfunction after coronary artery bypass graft surgery. Stroke 33:537, 2002
28. Nathan HJ, Wells GA, Munson JL, et al: Neuroprotective effect of mild hypothermia in patients undergoing coronary artery surgery with cardiopulmonary bypass: A randomized trial. Circulation 104:I85, 2001
29. Hebert PC: Transfusion requirements in critical care (TRICC): A multicentre, randomized, controlled clinical study. Transfusion Requirements in Critical Care Investigators and the Canadian Critical Care Trials Group. Br J Anaesth 81(suppl 1):25, 1998
30. Shore-Lesserson L, Manspeizer HE, DePerio M, et al: Thromboelastography-guided transfusion algorithm reduces transfusions in complex cardiac surgery. Anesth Analg 88:312, 1999
31. Spiess BD, Gillies BS, Chandler W, et al: Changes in transfusion therapy and reexploration rate after institution of a blood management program in cardiac surgical patients. J Cardiothorac Vasc Anesth 9:168, 1995
32. Body SC, Birmingham J, Parks R, et al: Safety and efficacy of shed mediastinal blood transfusion after cardiac surgery: A multicenter observational study. Multicenter Study of Perioperative Ischemia Research Group. J Cardiothorac Vasc Anesth 13:410, 1999
33. Hillyer CD, Josephson CD, Blajchman MA, et al: Bacterial contamination of blood components: Risks, strategies, and regulation: Joint ASH and AABB educational session in transfusion medicine. Hematology (Am Soc Hematol Educ Program):575, 2003

34. Zurick AM, Urzua J, Ghattas M, et al: Failure of positive end-expiratory pressure to decrease postoperative bleeding after cardiac surgery. Ann Thorac Surg 34:608, 1982
35. Collier B, Kolff J, Devineni R, et al: Prophylactic positive end-expiratory pressure and reduction of postoperative blood loss in open-heart surgery. Ann Thorac Surg 74:1191, 2002
36. Forestier F, Belisle S, Robitaille D, et al: Low-dose aprotinin is ineffective to treat excessive bleeding after cardiopulmonary bypass. Ann Thorac Surg 69:452, 2000
37. Ray MJ, Hales MM, Brown L, et al: Postoperatively administered aprotinin or epsilon aminocaproic acid after cardiopulmonary bypass has limited benefit. Ann Thorac Surg 72:521, 2001
38. BARI: Seven-year outcome in the Bypass Angioplasty Revascularization Investigation (BARI) by treatment and diabetic status. J Am Coll Cardiol 35:1122, 2000
39. Newman MF, Wolman R, Kanchuger M, et al: Multicenter preoperative stroke risk index for patients undergoing coronary artery bypass graft surgery. Multicenter Study of Perioperative Ischemia (McSPI) Research Group. Circulation 94:II74, 1996
40. Conlon PJ, Stafford-Smith M, White WD, et al: Acute renal failure following cardiac surgery. Nephrol Dial Transplant 14:1158, 1999
41. London MJ, Grunwald GK, Shroyer AL, et al: Association of fast-track cardiac management and low-dose to moderate-dose glucocorticoid administration with perioperative hyperglycemia. J Cardiothorac Vasc Anesth 14:631, 2000
42. van den Berghe G, Wouters P, Weekers F, et al: Intensive insulin therapy in the critically ill patients. N Engl J Med 345:1359, 2001
43. Goldberg PA, Sakharova OV, Barrett PW, et al: Improving glycemic control in the cardiothoracic intensive care unit: Clinical experience in two hospital settings. J Cardiothorac Vasc Anesth 18:690, 2004
44. Guvener M, Pasaoglu I, Demircin M, et al: Perioperative hyperglycemia is a strong correlate of postoperative infection in type II diabetic patients after coronary artery bypass grafting. Endocr J 49:531, 2002
45. McAlister FA, Man J, Bistritz L, et al: Diabetes and coronary artery bypass surgery: An examination of perioperative glycemic control and outcomes. Diabetes Care 26:1518, 2003
46. Latham R, Lancaster AD, Covington JF, et al: The association of diabetes and glucose control with surgical-site infections among cardiothoracic surgery patients. Infect Control Hosp Epidemiol 22:607, 2001
47. Munro AJ, Long GT, Sleigh JW: Nurse-administered subcutaneous morphine is a satisfactory alternative to intravenous patient-controlled analgesia morphine after cardiac surgery. Anesth Analg 87:11, 1998
48. Tsang J, Brush B: Patient-controlled analgesia in postoperative cardiac surgery. Anaesth Intensive Care 27:464, 1999
49. O'Halloran P, Brown R: Patient-controlled analgesia compared with nurse-controlled infusion analgesia after heart surgery. Intensive Crit Care Nurs 13:126, 1997
50. Myles PS, Buckland MR, Cannon GB, et al: Comparison of patient-controlled analgesia and nurse-controlled infusion analgesia after cardiac surgery. Anaesth Intensive Care 22:672, 1994
51. Searle NR, Roy M, Bergeron G, et al: Hydromorphone patient-controlled analgesia (PCA) after coronary artery bypass surgery. Can J Anaesth 41:198, 1994
52. Boldt J, Thaler E, Lehmann A, et al: Pain management in cardiac surgery patients: Comparison between standard therapy and patient-controlled analgesia regimen. J Cardiothorac Vasc Anesth 12:654, 1998
53. Gust R, Pecher S, Gust A, et al: Effect of patient-controlled analgesia on pulmonary complications after coronary artery bypass grafting. Crit Care Med 27:2218, 1999
54. Chaney MA, Smith KR, Barclay JC, et al: Large-dose intrathecal morphine for coronary artery bypass grafting. Anesth Analg 83:215, 1996
55. Bettex DA, Schmidlin D, Chassot PG, et al: Intrathecal sufentanil-morphine shortens the duration of intubation and improves analgesia in fast-track cardiac surgery. Can J Anaesth 49:711, 2002
56. Boulanger A, Perreault S, Choiniere M, et al: Intrathecal morphine after cardiac surgery. Ann Pharmacother 36:1337, 2002
57. Zarate E, Latham P, White PF, et al: Fast-track cardiac anesthesia: Use of remifentanil combined with intrathecal morphine as an alternative to sufentanil during desflurane anesthesia. Anesth Analg 91:283, 2000
58. Fitzpatrick GJ, Moriarty DC: Intrathecal morphine in the management of pain following cardiac surgery. A comparison with morphine IV. Br J Anaesth 60:639, 1988
59. Aun C, Thomas D, St John-Jones L, et al: Intrathecal morphine in cardiac surgery. Eur J Anaesthesiol 2:419, 1985
60. Shroff A, Rooke GA, Bishop MJ: Effects of intrathecal opioid on extubation time, analgesia, and intensive care unit stay following coronary artery bypass grafting. J Clin Anesth 9:415, 1997
61. Lena P, Balarac N, Arnulf JJ, et al: Intrathecal morphine and clonidine for coronary artery bypass grafting. Br J Anaesth 90:300, 2003
62. Chaney MA, Nikolov MP, Blakeman BP, et al: Intrathecal morphine for coronary artery bypass graft procedure and early extubation revisited. J Cardiothorac Vasc Anesth 13:574, 1999
63. Chaney MA, Furry PA, Fluder EM, et al: Intrathecal morphine for coronary artery bypass grafting and early extubation. Anesth Analg 84:241, 1997
64. Stenseth R, Bjella L, Berg EM, et al: Effects of thoracic epidural analgesia on pulmonary function after coronary artery bypass surgery. Eur J Cardiothorac Surg 10:859-865; discussion 866, 1996
65. Priestley MC, Cope L, Halliwell R, et al: Thoracic epidural anesthesia for cardiac surgery: the effects on tracheal intubation time and length of hospital stay. Anesth Analg 94:275, table of contents, 2002
66. Fillinger MP, Yeager MP, Dodds TM, et al: Epidural anesthesia and analgesia: Effects on recovery from cardiac surgery. J Cardiothorac Vasc Anesth 16:15, 2002
67. Tenling A, Joachimsson PO, Tyden H, et al: Thoracic epidural analgesia as an adjunct to general anaesthesia for cardiac surgery. Effects on pulmonary mechanics. Acta Anaesthesiol Scand 44:1071, 2000
68. Loick HM, Schmidt C, Van Aken H, et al: High thoracic epidural anesthesia, but not clonidine, attenuates the perioperative stress response via sympatholysis and reduces the release of troponin T in patients undergoing coronary artery bypass grafting. Anesth Analg 88:701, 1999
69. Yung MC, Chang Y, Lai ST, et al: Improved postoperative pain relief via pre-emptive analgesia in relation to heart rate variability for coronary artery bypass grafting: A preliminary report. Zhonghua Yi Xue Za Zhi (Taipei) 60:28, 1997
70. Ho AM, Chung DC, Joynt GM: Neuraxial blockade and hematoma in cardiac surgery: Estimating the risk of a rare adverse event that has not (yet) occurred. Chest 117:551, 2000
71. Pastor MC, Sanchez MJ, Casas MA, et al: Thoracic epidural analgesia in coronary artery bypass graft surgery: Seven years' experience. J Cardiothorac Vasc Anesth 17:154, 2003
72. Horlocker TT, Wedel DJ, Benzon H, et al: Regional anesthesia in the anticoagulated patient: Defining the risks. Reg Anesth Pain Med 29:1, 2004
73. Lipsky PE: Defining COX-2 inhibitors. J Rheumatol Suppl 60:13, 2000
74. Bigler D, Moller J, Kamp-Jensen M, et al: Effect of piroxicam in addition to continuous thoracic epidural bupivacaine and morphine on postoperative pain and lung function after thoracotomy. Acta Anaesthesiol Scand 36:647, 1992
75. Carretta A, Zannini P, Chiesa G, et al: Efficacy of ketorolac tromethamine and extrapleural intercostal nerve block on post-thoracotomy pain. A prospective, randomized study. Int Surg 81:224, 1996
76. Fayaz K, Abel R, Pugh S, et al: Opioid sparing and side effect profile of three different analgesic techniques for cardiac surgery. Eur J Anesth 20:A6, 2003
77. Gust R, Pecher S, Gust A, et al: Effect of patient-controlled analgesia on pulmonary complications after coronary artery bypass grafting. Crit Care Med 27:2218, 1999
78. Hynninen MS, Cheng DC, Hossain I, et al: Nonsteroidal anti-inflammatory drugs in treatment of postoperative pain after cardiac surgery. Can J Anaesth 47:1182, 2000
79. Immer FF, Immer-Bansi AS, Trachsel N, et al: Pain treatment with a COX-2 inhibitor after coronary artery bypass operation: A randomized trial. Ann Thorac Surg 75:490, 2003
80. Jones RM, Cashman JN, Foster JM, et al: Comparison of infusions of morphine and lysine acetyl salicylate for the relief of pain following thoracic surgery. Br J Anaesth 57:259, 1985
81. Kavanagh BP, Katz J, Sandler AN, et al: Multimodal analgesia before thoracic surgery does not reduce postoperative pain. Br J Anaesth 73:184, 1994
82. Keenan DJ, Cave K, Langdon L, et al: Comparative trial of rectal indomethacin and cryoanalgesia for control of early postthoracotomy pain. Br Med J (Clin Res Ed) 287:1335, 1983
83. McCrory C, Diviney D, Moriarty J, et al: Comparison between repeat bolus intrathecal morphine and an epidurally delivered bupivacaine and fentanyl combination in the management of post-thoracotomy pain with or without cyclooxygenase inhibition. J Cardiothorac Vasc Anesth 16:607, 2002
84. Merry AF, Wardall GJ, Cameron RJ, et al: Prospective, controlled, double-blind study of IV tenoxicam for analgesia after thoracotomy. Br J Anaesth 69:92, 1992
85. Ott E, Nussmeier NA, Duke PC, et al: Efficacy and safety of the cyclooxygenase 2 inhibitors parecoxib and valdecoxib in patients undergoing coronary artery bypass surgery. J Thorac Cardiovasc Surg 125:1481, 2003

86. Gajraj NM: The effect of cyclo-oxygenase-2 inhibitors on bone healing. Reg Anesth Pain Med 28:456, 2003
87. Glassman SD, Rose SM, Dimar JR, et al: The effect of postoperative nonsteroidal anti-inflammatory drug administration on spinal fusion. Spine 23:834, 1998
88. Patrono C, Ciabattoni G, Patrignani P, et al: Clinical pharmacology of platelet cyclooxygenase inhibition. Circulation 72:1177, 1985
89. Reuben SS, Connelly NR: Postoperative analgesic effects of celecoxib or rofecoxib after spinal fusion surgery. Anesth Analg 91:1221, 2000
90. Reuben SS, Bhopatkar S, Maciolek H, et al: The preemptive analgesic effect of rofecoxib after ambulatory arthroscopic knee surgery. Anesth Analg 94:55, 2002
91. Camu F, Beecher T, Recker DP, et al: Valdecoxib, a COX-2-specific inhibitor, is an efficacious, opioid-sparing analgesic in patients undergoing hip arthroplasty. Am J Ther 9:43, 2002
92. Antiplatelet Trialists' Collaboration: Collaborative overview of randomised trials of antiplatelet therapy—II: Maintenance of vascular graft or arterial patency by antiplatelet therapy. BMJ 308:159, 1994
93. Weber M, von Schacky C, Lorenz R, et al: [Low-dose acetylsalicylic acid (100 mg/day) following aortocoronary bypass operation]. Klin Wochenschr 62:458, 1984
94. Goldman S, Copeland J, Moritz T, et al: Starting aspirin therapy after operation. Effects on early graft patency. Department of Veterans Affairs Cooperative Study Group. Circulation 84:520, 1991
95. Goldman S, Copeland J, Moritz T, et al: Saphenous vein graft patency 1 year after coronary artery bypass surgery and effects of antiplatelet therapy. Results of a Veterans Administration Cooperative Study. Circulation 80:1190, 1989
96. Mangano DT: Aspirin and mortality from coronary bypass surgery. N Engl J Med 347:1309, 2002
97. Sethi GK, Copeland JG, Goldman S, et al: Implications of preoperative administration of aspirin in patients undergoing coronary artery bypass grafting. Department of Veterans Affairs Cooperative Study on Antiplatelet Therapy. J Am Coll Cardiol 15:15, 1990
98. Goldman S, Zadina K, Krasnicka B, et al: Predictors of graft patency 3 years after coronary artery bypass graft surgery. Department of Veterans Affairs Cooperative Study Group No. 297. J Am Coll Cardiol 29:1563, 1997
99. Antiplatelet Trialists' Collaboration: Collaborative overview of randomised trials of antiplatelet therapy—I: Prevention of death, myocardial infarction, and stroke by prolonged antiplatelet therapy in various categories of patients. BMJ 308:81, 1994
100. Bhatt DL, Chew DP, Hirsch AT, et al: Superiority of clopidogrel versus aspirin in patients with prior cardiac surgery. Circulation 103:363, 2001
101. The MACB Study Group: Effect of metoprolol on death and cardiac events during a 2-year period after coronary artery bypass grafting. Eur Heart J 16:1825, 1995
102. Sjoland H, Caidahl K, Lurje L, et al: Metoprolol treatment for two years after coronary bypass grafting: Effects on exercise capacity and signs of myocardial ischaemia. Br Heart J 74:235, 1995
103. Oosterga M, Voors AA, Pinto YM, et al: Effects of quinapril on clinical outcome after coronary artery bypass grafting (the QUO VADIS Study). QUinapril on Vascular ACE and Determinants of Ischemia. Am J Cardiol 87:542, 2001
104. Chen J, Radford MJ, Wang Y, et al: Are beta-blockers effective in elderly patients who undergo coronary revascularization after acute myocardial infarction? Arch Intern Med 160:947, 2000
105. The Post Coronary Artery Bypass Graft Trial Investigators: The effect of aggressive lowering of low-density lipoprotein cholesterol levels and low-dose anticoagulation on obstructive changes in saphenous-vein coronary-artery bypass grafts. N Engl J Med 336:153, 1997
106. Task Force on Practice Guidelines (Committee on Management of Patients with Valvular Heart Disease): ACC/AHA guidelines for the management of patients with valvular heart disease. A report of the American College of Cardiology/American Heart Association. J Am Coll Cardiol 32:1486, 1998
107. Stamou SC, Hill PC, Dangas G, et al: Stroke after coronary artery bypass: Incidence, predictors, and clinical outcome. Stroke 32:1508, 2001
108. Naylor AR, Mehta Z, Rothwell PM, et al: Carotid artery disease and stroke during coronary artery bypass: A critical review of the literature. Eur J Vasc Endovasc Surg 23:283, 2002
109. Salazar JD, Wityk RJ, Grega MA, et al: Stroke after cardiac surgery: Short- and long-term outcomes. Ann Thorac Surg 72:1195-1201; discussion 1201, 2001
110. Lahtinen J, Biancari F, Salmela E, et al: Postoperative atrial fibrillation is a major cause of stroke after on-pump coronary artery bypass surgery. Ann Thorac Surg 77:1241, 2004
111. Murkin JM, Martzke JS, Buchan AM, et al: A randomized study of the influence of perfusion technique and pH management strategy in 316 patients undergoing coronary artery bypass surgery. II. Neurologic and cognitive outcomes. J Thorac Cardiovasc Surg 110:349, 1995
112. Murkin JM: Attenuation of neurologic injury during cardiac surgery. Ann Thorac Surg 72:S1838, 2001
113. Royse AG, Royse CF, Ajani AE, et al: Reduced neuropsychological dysfunction using epiaortic echocardiography and the exclusive Y graft. Ann Thorac Surg 69:1431, 2000
114. Sharony R, Bizekis CS, Kanchuger M, et al: Off-pump coronary artery bypass grafting reduces mortality and stroke in patients with atheromatous aortas: A case control study. Circulation 108(suppl 1):II-15, 2003
115. Leacche M, Carrier M, Bouchard D, et al: Improving neurologic outcome in off-pump surgery: The "no touch" technique. Heart Surg Forum 6:169, 2003
116. Bruno A, Levine SR, Frankel MR, et al: Admission glucose level and clinical outcomes in the NINDS rt-PA Stroke Trial. Neurology 59:669, 2002
117. Williams LS, Rotich J, Qi R, et al: Effects of admission hyperglycemia on mortality and costs in acute ischemic stroke. Neurology 59:67, 2002
118. Quast MJ, Wei J, Huang NC, et al: Perfusion deficit parallels exacerbation of cerebral ischemia/reperfusion injury in hyperglycemic rats. J Cereb Blood Flow Metab 17:553, 1997
119. Dietrich WD, Busto R, Valdes I, et al: Effects of normothermic versus mild hyperthermic forebrain ischemia in rats. Stroke 21:1318, 1990
120. Bucerius J, Gummert JF, Borger MA, et al: Predictors of delirium after cardiac surgery delirium: Effect of beating-heart (off-pump) surgery. J Thorac Cardiovasc Surg 127:57, 2004
121. van der Mast RC, van den Broek WW, Fekkes D, et al: Incidence of and preoperative predictors for delirium after cardiac surgery. J Psychosom Res 46:479, 1999
122. Gokgoz L, Gunaydin S, Sinci V, et al: Psychiatric complications of cardiac surgery postoperative delirium syndrome. Scand Cardiovasc J 31:217, 1997
123. Rolfson DB, McElhaney JE, Rockwood K, et al: Incidence and risk factors for delirium and other adverse outcomes in older adults after coronary artery bypass graft surgery. Can J Cardiol 15:771, 1999
124. Ommen SR, Odell JA, Stanton MS: Atrial arrhythmias after cardiothoracic surgery. N Engl J Med 336:1429, 1997
125. Zimmer J, Pezzullo J, Choucair W, et al: Meta-analysis of antiarrhythmic therapy in the prevention of postoperative atrial fibrillation and the effect on hospital length of stay, costs, cerebrovascular accidents, and mortality in patients undergoing cardiac surgery. Am J Cardiol 91:1137, 2003
126. Mathew JP, Fontes ML, Tudor IC, et al: A multicenter risk index for atrial fibrillation after cardiac surgery. JAMA 291:1720, 2004
127. Crystal E, Connolly SJ, Sleik K, et al: Interventions on prevention of postoperative atrial fibrillation in patients undergoing heart surgery: A meta-analysis. Circulation 106:75, 2002
128. Toraman F, Karabulut EH, Alhan HC, et al: Magnesium infusion dramatically decreases the incidence of atrial fibrillation after coronary artery bypass grafting. Ann Thorac Surg 72:1256-1261; discussion 1261, 2001
129. Blackshear JL, Safford RE: AFFIRM and RACE trials: Implications for the management of atrial fibrillation. Card Electrophysiol Rev 7:366, 2003
130. Wyse DG, Waldo AL, DiMarco JP, et al: A comparison of rate control and rhythm control in patients with atrial fibrillation. N Engl J Med 347:1825, 2002
131. Hagens VE, Ranchor AV, Van Sonderen E, et al: Effect of rate or rhythm control on quality of life in persistent atrial fibrillation. Results from the Rate Control Versus Electrical Cardioversion (RACE) Study. J Am Coll Cardiol 43:241, 2004
132. Olshansky B, Rosenfeld LE, Warner AL, et al: The Atrial Fibrillation Follow-up Investigation of Rhythm Management (AFFIRM) study: Approaches to control rate in atrial fibrillation. J Am Coll Cardiol 43:1201, 2004
133. Hart RG, Benavente O, McBride R, et al: Antithrombotic therapy to prevent stroke in patients with atrial fibrillation: A meta-analysis. Ann Intern Med 131:492, 1999
134. Prystowsky EN, Benson DW Jr, Fuster V, et al: Management of patients with atrial fibrillation. A statement for healthcare professionals. From the Subcommittee on Electrocardiography and Electrophysiology, American Heart Association. Circulation 93:1262, 1996
135. Fuster V, Ryden LE, Asinger RW, et al: ACC/AHA/ESC guidelines for the management of patients with atrial fibrillation: executive summary. A Report of the American College of Cardiology/American Heart Association Task Force on Practice Guidelines and the European Society of Cardiology Committee for Practice Guidelines and Policy Conferences

(Committee to Develop Guidelines for the Management of Patients With Atrial Fibrillation): Developed in collaboration with the North American Society of Pacing and Electrophysiology. J Am Coll Cardiol 38:1231, 2001

136. Butterworth JF 4th, Legault C, Royster RL, et al: Factors that predict the use of positive inotropic drug support after cardiac valve surgery. Anesth Analg 86:461, 1998
137. Royster RL, Butterworth JF 4th, Prough DS, et al: Preoperative and intraoperative predictors of inotropic support and long-term outcome in patients having coronary artery bypass grafting. Anesth Analg 72:729, 1991
138. Krivec B, Voga G, Zuran I, et al: Diagnosis and treatment of shock due to massive pulmonary embolism: Approach with transesophageal echocardiography and intrapulmonary thrombolysis. Chest 112:1310, 1997
139. van der Wouw PA, Koster RW, Delemarre BJ, et al: Diagnostic accuracy of transesophageal echocardiography during cardiopulmonary resuscitation. J Am Coll Cardiol 30:780, 1997
140. Cicek S, Demirilic U, Kuralay E, et al: Transesophageal echocardiography in cardiac surgical emergencies. J Card Surg 10:236, 1995
141. Wake PJ, Ali M, Carroll J, et al: Clinical and echocardiographic diagnoses disagree in patients with unexplained hemodynamic instability after cardiac surgery. Can J Anaesth 48:778, 2001
142. Tousignant CP, Walsh F, Mazer CD: The use of transesophageal echocardiography for preload assessment in critically ill patients. Anesth Analg 90:351, 2000
143. Swenson JD, Bull D, Stringham J: Subjective assessment of left ventricular preload using transesophageal echocardiography: Corresponding pulmonary artery occlusion pressures. J Cardiothorac Vasc Anesth 15:580, 2001
144. Fontes ML, Bellows W, Ngo L, et al: Assessment of ventricular function in critically ill patients: Limitations of pulmonary artery catheterization. Institutions of the McSPI Research Group. J Cardiothorac Vasc Anesth 13:521, 1999
145. Schwinn DA, Leone BJ, Spahn DR, et al: Desensitization of myocardial beta-adrenergic receptors during cardiopulmonary bypass. Evidence for early uncoupling and late downregulation. Circulation 84:2559, 1991
146. Royster RL, Butterworth JF 4th, Prielipp RC, et al: Combined inotropic effects of amrinone and epinephrine after cardiopulmonary bypass in humans. Anesth Analg 77:662, 1993
147. Tokmakoglu H, Farsak B, Gunaydin S, et al: Effectiveness of intraaortic balloon pumping in patients who were not able to be weaned from cardiopulmonary bypass after coronary artery bypass surgery and mortality predictors in the perioperative and early postoperative period. Anadolu Kardiyol Derg 3:124, 2003
148. Marra C, De Santo LS, Amarelli C, et al: Coronary artery bypass grafting in patients with severe left ventricular dysfunction: A prospective randomized study on the timing of perioperative intraaortic balloon pump support. Int J Artif Organs 25:141, 2002
149. Christenson JT, Badel P, Simonet F, et al: Preoperative intraaortic balloon pump enhances cardiac performance and improves the outcome of redo CABG. Ann Thorac Surg 64:1237, 1997
150. Christenson JT, Simonet F, Badel P, et al: Optimal timing of preoperative intraaortic balloon pump support in high-risk coronary patients. Ann Thorac Surg 68:934, 1999
151. Christenson JT, Schmuziger M, Simonet F: Effective surgical management of high-risk coronary patients using preoperative intra-aortic balloon counterpulsation therapy. Cardiovasc Surg 9:383, 2001
152. Torchiana DF, Hirsch G, Buckley MJ, et al: Intraaortic balloon pumping for cardiac support: Trends in practice and outcome, 1968 to 1995. J Thorac Cardiovasc Surg 113:758-764; discussion 764, 1997
153. Castelli P, Condemi A, Munari M, et al: Intra-aortic balloon counterpulsation: Outcome in cardiac surgical patients. J Cardiothorac Vasc Anesth 15:700, 2001
154. Sirivella S, Gielchinsky I, Parsonnet V: Angiotensin-converting enzyme inhibitor therapy in severe postcardiotomy dysfunction: A prospective randomized study. J Card Surg 13:11, 1998
155. Abrahamov D, Tamariz M, Fremes S, et al: Renal dysfunction after cardiac surgery. Can J Cardiol 17:565, 2001
156. Wijeysundera DN, Rao V, Beattie WS, et al: Evaluating surrogate measures of renal dysfunction after cardiac surgery. Anesth Analg 96:1265, 2003
157. Wang F, Dupuis JY, Nathan H, et al: An analysis of the association between preoperative renal dysfunction and outcome in cardiac surgery: Estimated creatinine clearance or plasma creatinine level as measures of renal function. Chest 124:1852, 2003
158. Kellum JA: The use of diuretics and dopamine in acute renal failure: A systematic review of the evidence. Crit Care 1:53, 1997
159. Mehta RL, Pascual MT, Soroko S, et al: Diuretics, mortality, and nonrecovery of renal function in acute renal failure. JAMA 288:2547, 2002
160. Kellum JA, Angus DC, Johnson JP, et al: Continuous versus intermittent renal replacement therapy: A meta-analysis. Intensive Care Med 28:29, 2002
161. Alonso A, Lau J, Jaber BL, et al: Prevention of radiocontrast nephropathy with N-acetylcysteine in patients with chronic kidney disease: A meta-analysis of randomized, controlled trials. Am J Kidney Dis 43:1, 2004
162. Baker CS, Wragg A, Kumar S, et al: A rapid protocol for the prevention of contrast-induced renal dysfunction: The RAPPID study. J Am Coll Cardiol 41:2114, 2003
163. Vallero A, Cesano G, Pozzato M, et al: [Contrast nephropathy in cardiac procedures: No advantages with prophylactic use of N-acetylcysteine (NAC)]. G Ital Nefrol 19:529, 2002
164. Durham JD, Caputo C, Dokko J, et al: A randomized controlled trial of N-acetylcysteine to prevent contrast nephropathy in cardiac angiography. Kidney Int 62:2202, 2002
165. Tu JV, Naylor CD: Coronary artery bypass mortality rates in Ontario. A Canadian approach to quality assurance in cardiac surgery. Steering Committee of the Provincial Adult Cardiac Care Network of Ontario. Circulation 94:2429, 1996
166. Higgins TL, Estafanous FG, Loop FD, et al: Stratification of morbidity and mortality outcome by preoperative risk factors in coronary artery bypass patients. A clinical severity score. JAMA 267:2344, 1992
167. Roques F, Gabrielle F, Michel P, et al: Quality of care in adult heart surgery: Proposal for a self-assessment approach based on a French multicenter study. Eur J Cardiothorac Surg 9:433, 1995
168. Parsonnet V, Dean D, Bernstein AD: A method of uniform stratification of risk for evaluating the results of surgery in acquired adult heart disease. Circulation 79:I-3, 1989
169. Nashef SA, Roques F, Michel P, et al: European system for cardiac operative risk evaluation (EuroSCORE). Eur J Cardiothorac Surg 16:9, 1999
170. Weightman WM, Gibbs NM, Sheminant MR, et al: Risk prediction in coronary artery surgery: A comparison of four risk scores. Med J Aust 166:408, 1997
171. Immer F, Habicht J, Nessensohn K, et al: Prospective evaluation of 3 risk stratification scores in cardiac surgery. Thorac Cardiovasc Surg 48:134, 2000
172. Gabrielle F, Roques F, Michel P, et al: Is the Parsonnet's score a good predictive score of mortality in adult cardiac surgery: Assessment by a French multicentre study. Eur J Cardiothorac Surg 11:406, 1997
173. Osswald BR, Tochtermann U, Schweiger P, et al: Target, application, and interpretation of scores and alternative methods for risk assessment in cardiac surgery. Thorac Cardiovasc Surg 48:72, 2000
174. Dupuis JY, Wang F, Nathan H, et al: The cardiac anesthesia risk evaluation score: A clinically useful predictor of mortality and morbidity after cardiac surgery. Anesthesiology 94:194, 2001
175. Yusuf S, Zucker D, Peduzzi P, et al: Effect of coronary artery bypass graft surgery on survival: Overview of 10-year results from randomised trials by the Coronary Artery Bypass Graft Surgery Trialists Collaboration. Lancet 344:563, 1994
176. BARI: Comparison of coronary bypass surgery with angioplasty in patients with multivessel disease. The Bypass Angioplasty Revascularization Investigation (BARI) Investigators. N Engl J Med 335:217, 1996
177. Carrie D, Elbaz M, Puel J, et al: Five-year outcome after coronary angioplasty versus bypass surgery in multivessel coronary artery disease: Results from the French Monocentric Study. Circulation 96:II-1, 1997
178. Hamm CW, Reimers J, Ischinger T, et al: A randomized study of coronary angioplasty compared with bypass surgery in patients with symptomatic multivessel coronary disease. German Angioplasty Bypass Surgery Investigation (GABI). N Engl J Med 331:1037, 1994
179. Hoffman SN, TenBrook JA, Wolf MP, et al: A meta-analysis of randomized controlled trials comparing coronary artery bypass graft with percutaneous transluminal coronary angioplasty: One- to eight-year outcomes. J Am Coll Cardiol 41:1293, 2003
180. Goy JJ, Eeckhout E, Moret C, et al: Five-year outcome in patients with isolated proximal left anterior descending coronary artery stenosis treated by angioplasty or left internal mammary artery grafting. A prospective trial. Circulation 99:3255, 1999
181. Rodriguez A, Bernardi V, Navia J, et al: Argentine Randomized Study: Coronary Angioplasty with Stenting versus Coronary Bypass Surgery in patients with Multiple-Vessel Disease (ERACI II): 30-Day and one-year follow-up results. ERACI II Investigators. J Am Coll Cardiol 37:51, 2001
182. Serruys PW, Unger F, Sousa JE, et al: Comparison of coronary artery bypass surgery and stenting for the treatment of multivessel disease. N Engl J Med 344:1117, 2001

183. Legrand VM, Serruys PW, Unger F, et al: Three-year outcome after coronary stenting versus bypass surgery for the treatment of multivessel disease. Circulation 109:1114, 2004
184. SOS: Coronary artery bypass surgery versus percutaneous coronary intervention with stent implantation in patients with multivessel coronary artery disease (the Stent or Surgery Trial): A randomised controlled trial. Lancet 360:965, 2002
185. D'Ancona G, Karamanoukian H, Kawaguchi AT, et al: Myocardial revascularization of the beating heart in high-risk patients. J Card Surg 16:132, 2001
186. Hoff SJ, Ball SK, Coltharp WH, et al: Coronary artery bypass in patients 80 years and over: Is off-pump the operation of choice? Ann Thorac Surg 74:S1340, 2002
187. Yokoyama T, Baumgartner FJ, Gheissari A, et al: Off-pump versus on-pump coronary bypass in high-risk subgroups. Ann Thorac Surg 70:1546, 2000
188. Lee JD, Lee SJ, Tsushima WT, et al: Benefits of off-pump bypass on neurologic and clinical morbidity: A prospective randomized trial. Ann Thorac Surg 76:18, 2003
189. Puskas J, Sharoni E, Williams W, et al: Is routine use of temporary epicardial pacing wires necessary after either OPCAB or conventional CABG/CPB? Heart Surg Forum 6 (suppl 1):s47, 2003
190. Angelini GD, Taylor FC, Reeves BC, et al: Early and midterm outcome after off-pump and on-pump surgery in Beating Heart Against Cardioplegic Arrest Studies (BHACAS 1 and 2): A pooled analysis of two randomised controlled trials. Lancet 359:1194, 2002
191. Khan NE, De Souza A, Mister R, et al: A randomized comparison of off-pump and on-pump multivessel coronary artery bypass surgery. N Engl J Med 350:21, 2004
192. Cheng D, Bainbridge D, Martin J, et al: Does off-pump coronary artery bypass reduce mortality, morbidity and resource utilization when compared to conventional coronary artery bypass? A meta-analysis of randomized trials. Anesthesiology 102:188, 2005
193. Puskas JD, Williams WH, Mahoney EM, et al: Off-pump vs conventional coronary artery bypass grafting: Early and 1-year graft patency, cost, and quality-of-life outcomes: A randomized trial. JAMA 291:1841, 2004

Chapter 33

POSTOPERATIVE CARDIOVASCULAR MANAGEMENT

Jerrold H. Levy, MD • Kenichi Tanaka, MD •
James M. Bailey, MD, PhD • James G. Ramsay, MD

KEY POINTS

1. Maintaining oxygen transport and oxygen delivery appropriately to meet the tissue metabolic requirements is the goal of postoperative circulatory control.
2. Multiple parameters of cardiac function worsen after cardiac surgery. Therapeutic approaches to reversing this dysfunction are important.
3. Myocardial ischemia often occurs postoperatively, and it is associated with adverse cardiac outcomes. Multiple strategies have been studied to reduce this complication.
4. Therapeutic interventions for postoperative biventricular dysfunction include the standard concerns of managing low cardiac output states by controlling the heart rate and rhythm, providing an acceptable preload, and adjusting afterload and contractility. In most patients, pharmacologic interventions can be rapidly weaned or stopped within the first 24 hours after surgery.
5. In the postoperative period, supraventricular tachyarrhythmias become a major problem, with atrial fibrillation predominating. Multiple therapeutic strategies have been employed to prevent or treat the problem.
6. Postoperative hypertension has been a common complication of cardiac surgery, and newer therapeutic interventions, including the dihydropyridine calcium channel blockers, have an expanding role in the treatment.
7. Multiple drugs that increase contractility, including catecholamines, phosphodiesterase inhibitors, and levosimendan, have been studied for treating biventricular dysfunction.
8. Many drugs are important for producing vasodilation in systemic, pulmonary, and other vascular beds. Phosphodiesterase inhibitors and levosimendan have clinical effects as inodilators. Novel agents, including the natriuretic peptides (nesiritide), also have an expanding role. Vasoactive therapies often are required after cardiac surgery and are useful in understanding vasodilatory shock. Vasopressin has an expanding role in the treatment of this problem.
9. Right ventricular dysfunction is an important complication of cardiac surgery that warrants specific vasodilator therapy for reducing right ventricular afterload.
10. Mechanical positive-pressure ventilation has multiple effects on the cardiovascular system, with complex interactions that should be considered in patients after cardiac surgery.

Postoperative cardiovascular dysfunction is increasingly common as older and potentially more critically ill patients undergo cardiac surgery. Biventricular dysfunction and circulatory changes occur after cardiopulmonary bypass (CPB) but can also occur in patients undergoing off-pump surgery. Pharmacologic therapy with appropriate monitoring and mechanical support may be needed for patients in the postoperative period until ventricular or circulatory dysfunction improves. This chapter reviews management considerations of postoperative circulatory failure.

OXYGEN TRANSPORT

Maintaining oxygen transport (i.e., oxygen delivery [DO_2]) satisfactory to meet the tissue metabolic requirements is the goal of postoperative circulatory control. Oxygen transport is the product of cardiac output (CO) times arterial content of oxygen (CaO_2) (i.e., hemoglobin concentration $\times$ 1.34 mL of oxygen per 1 g of hemoglobin $\times$ oxygen saturation), and it can be affected in many ways by the cardiovascular and respiratory systems, as shown in Figure 33–1. Low CO, anemia from blood loss, and pulmonary disease can decrease DO_2. Before altering the determinants of CO, including the inotropic state of the ventricles, an acceptable hemoglobin concentration and adequate oxygen saturation (SaO_2) should be provided, enabling increases in CO to provide the maximum available DO_2. As hemoglobin concentration increases, so does blood viscosity and therefore the work of the heart to eject the blood. In normal hearts (e.g., athletes), increasing hemoglobin levels to supranormal will increase performance, suggesting that in this setting the increased viscosity is less important than the increase in oxygen-carrying capacity.[1] This has not been examined in patients with cardiac disease. Model analysis of data from animal investigations suggests that maintenance of the hematocrit between 30% and 33% provides the best balance between oxygen-carrying capacity and viscosity.[2] This analysis also suggests that in ischemic states a hematocrit in this range may result in increased tissue DO_2, compared with that seen with higher hematocrits. Patients needing inotropic or mechanical support of ventricular function should be transfused to a hematocrit in this range. Blood transfusion is associated with diminished organ function and increased mortality in critically ill patients, and a randomized trial suggested a transfusion threshold of 7 g, rather than 9 g, was associated with at least equivalent outcomes in critically ill patients who did not have acute myocardial infarction (MI) or unstable angina.[3-5] Neither of these studies identified cohorts of patients who had undergone cardiac surgery. Wu et al[5] found transfusion for a hematocrit of 30% or lower in elderly patients with acute MI was associated with better outcome. This is probably the most appropriate transfusion trigger in elderly cardiac surgery patients or those experiencing a complicated course.

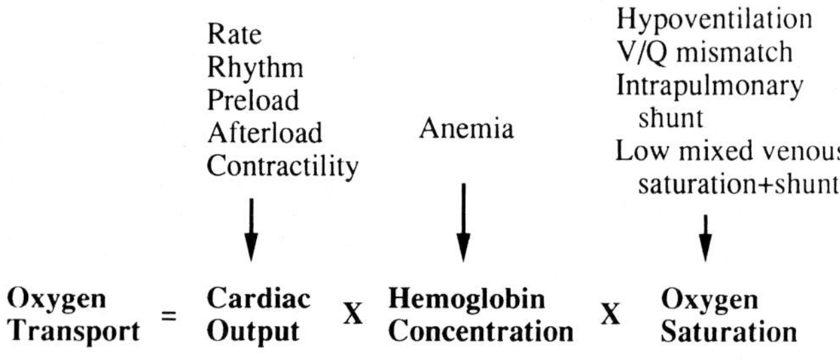

Figure 33–1 Important factors that contribute to abnormal oxygen transport.

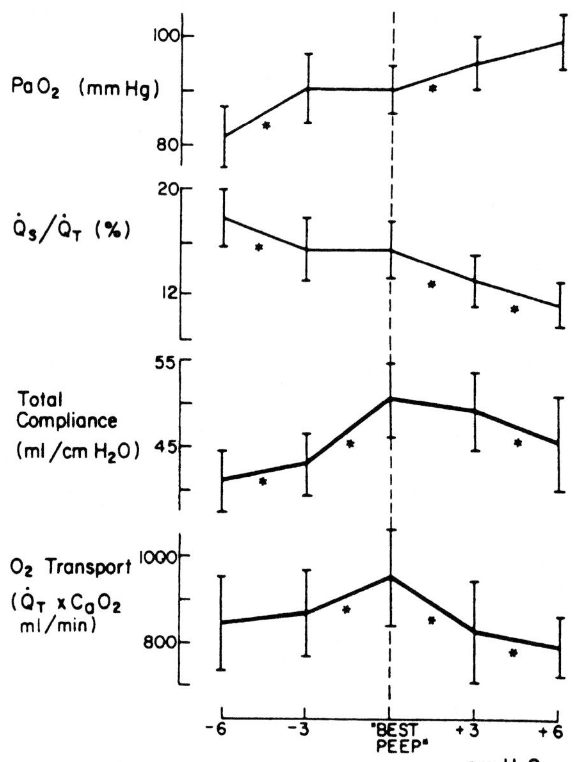

Figure 33–2 Mean values ± SEM of arterial oxygen tension (PaO_2), intrapulmonary shunt ($\dot{Q}_S/\dot{Q}_T$), total static compliance, and oxygen transport, measured at the level of positive end-expiratory pressure (PEEP), resulting in maximum oxygen transport ("best PEEP") compared with values obtained at 3 and 6 cm H_2O of PEEP above and below that level in 15 patients with acute respiratory failure. The *asterisk* indicates $p < 5.005$ versus the value at best PEEP. (From Suter PM, Fairley HB, Isenbery MD: Optimum end-expiratory pressure in patients with acute pulmonary failure. N Engl J Med 292:284, 1975.)

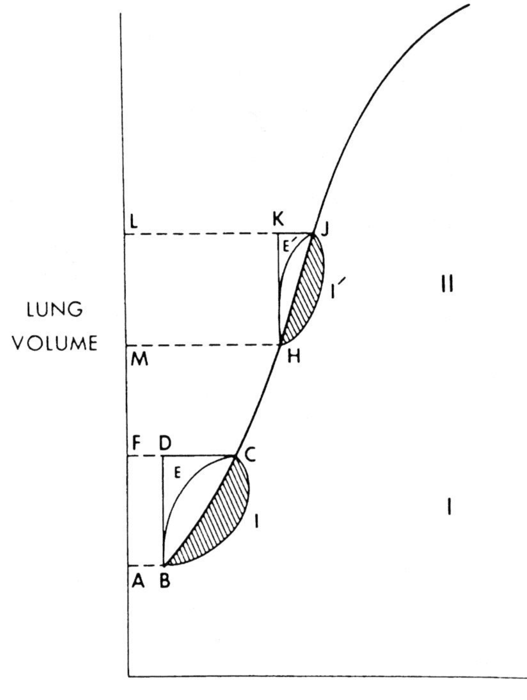

Figure 33–3 Pressure-volume diagram of elastic and resistive (nonelastic) work done on noncompliant lungs. Breathing at ambient airway pressure and low lung volume (by T tube) (I) versus breathing with continuous positive airway pressure (CPAP) at increased lung volume (II). *Solid line* BCHJ is the elastic pressure-volume curve for the lung, determined by measuring transpulmonary pressures at the instant of zero flow. *Hatched areas* represent nonelastic work (BIC and HI'J), whereas elastic work is represented by BCD and HJK. With CPAP, both types of work are reduced. Without CPAP, the area ABDF is additional elastic work partly done by the patient and partly by elastic recoil of the chest wall, whereas with CPAP, the additional work represented by MHKL is mostly done by the CPAP system. (From Katz JA, Marks JD: Inspiratory work with and without continuous positive airway pressure in patients with acute respiratory failure. Anesthesiology 63:598, 1985.)

Hypoxemia from any cause reduces DO_2, and acceptable arterial oxygenation (PaO_2) may be achieved with the use of an elevated inspired oxygen concentration (FIO_2) or positive end-expiratory pressure (PEEP) in the ventilated patient. Use of PEEP or continuous positive airway pressure (CPAP) in the spontaneously breathing patient may improve PaO_2 by reducing intrapulmonary shunt; however, venous return may be reduced, causing a decrease in CO, with DO_2 decreased despite an increased PaO_2 (Fig. 33–2).[6] It is important to measure CO as PEEP is applied. Intravascular volume expansion may be used to offset this damaging effect of PEEP[7] (see Chapter 34).

In patients with marginal arterial oxygenation, pulmonary function must be closely monitored to allow prompt therapy to be undertaken for abnormalities. Measurements of airway resistance and respiratory system compliance should be made. When resistance is increased, treatment of bronchospasm may improve the PaO_2 and CO, because decreases in intrathoracic pressure improve venous return. Treatment of lung overinflation may decrease pulmonary vascular resistance (PVR), benefiting right ventricular (RV) function.[8] If compliance is decreased, application of PEEP or CPAP may help promote reexpansion of atelectatic areas and move the tidal volume to a more compliant section of the pressure-volume relation of the respiratory system[9] (Fig. 33–3). This will reduce the work expended by the patient during spontaneous efforts and may reduce PVR[10] (see Chapter 34).

Unexplained hypoxemia may be caused by right-to-left intracardiac shunting, most commonly by a patent foramen ovale. This is most likely to occur when right-sided pressures are abnormally elevated; an example is the use of high levels of PEEP.[11] If suspected, echocardiography should be performed, and therapy to reduce right-sided pressures should be initiated.

Patients with pulmonary disease may experience dramatic worsening of oxygenation when vasodilator therapy is started, because of release of hypoxic vasoconstriction in areas of diseased lung.[12] Although CO may be increased, the worsening in CaO_2 will result in a decrease in DO_2. Reduced dosage of direct-acting vasodilators or trials of different agents may be indicated.

When DO_2 cannot be increased to an acceptable level as judged by decreased organ function or development of lactic acidemia, measures to decrease oxygen consumption ($\dot{V}O_2$) may be taken while awaiting improvement in cardiac or pulmonary function. For example, sedation and paralysis may buy time to allow reversible postoperative myocardial dysfunction to improve.

TEMPERATURE

Patients are often admitted to the intensive care unit (ICU) after cardiac surgery with core temperatures below 35°C, especially after off-pump cardiac surgery. The typical pattern of temperature change during and after cardiac surgery and the hemodynamic outcomes are illustrated in Figure 33–4. Decreases in temperature after CPB occur in part because of redistribution of heat within the body and because of heat loss. Noback and Tinker[13] found that administration of nitroprusside and the use of high flows (>2.2 L/min/m^2) during rewarming on CPB could improve the uniformity of rewarming and reduce this afterdrop from 4°C to about 2°C. Monitoring of body sites other than the blood and brain (e.g., urinary bladder, tympanic membrane temperatures) can help provide more complete rewarming, but the body temperature usually falls after bypass, especially when difficulties are encountered and the chest remains open for an extended period, and some degree of hypothermia is an almost unavoidable result.[14,15] Newer external heating devices are effective at reducing postoperative hypothermia but are more costly than traditional forced-air systems and mattress warmers.[16]

The normal thermoregulatory and metabolic responses to hypothermia remain intact after cardiac surgery, resulting in peripheral vasoconstriction that contributes to the hypertension commonly seen early in the ICU.[17] As temperature decreases, CO is decreased because of bradycardia, whereas oxygen consumed per beat is actually increased.[18] Coagulation, platelet, and immune functions are also impaired by hypothermia to potentiate postoperative bleeding and infection.[19-21] Other adverse outcomes of postoperative hypothermia during rewarming include large increases in VO_2 and CO_2 production during this process.[22] When patients cannot increase CO (i.e., O_2 delivery), the effects of this large increase in VO_2 include mixed venous desaturation and metabolic acidosis. Unless end-tidal carbon dioxide is monitored or arterial blood gases are analyzed frequently to show the increased CO_2 production and guide increases in ventilation, hypercarbia will occur, causing catecholamine release, tachycardia, and pulmonary hypertension.[23] These effects of rewarming are most intense when patients shiver.[24] Shivering may be effectively treated with meperidine, which lowers the threshold for shivering. Muscle relaxation may provide more stable hemodynamics than meperidine but needs accompanying sedation to avoid having an awake and paralyzed patient.[25,26]

As the temperature rises, usually to about 36°C, the vasoconstriction and hypertension are replaced by vasodilation, tachycardia, and hypotension, even without hypercarbia. Often, over minutes, a patient who needs vasodilators for hypertension transforms into one requiring vasopressors or large volumes of fluid for hypotension. Volume loading during the rewarming period can help to reduce the rapid swings in blood pressure (BP) that may occur. It is important to recognize when these changes result from changes in body temperature to avoid attributing them to other processes that may call for different therapy.

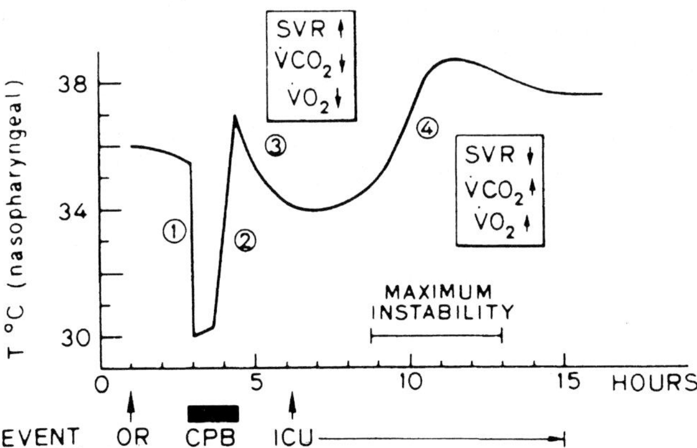

Figure 33–4 Nasopharyngeal temperature during and after cardiac surgery. *(1)* Core (i.e., blood) cooling on cardiopulmonary bypass (CPB). *(2)* Core warming on CPB. *(3)* Afterdrop in temperature (T) after separation from CPB. *(4)* Rewarming after admission to the intensive care unit (ICU). Systemic vascular resistance (SVR) is increased, and carbon dioxide production ($\dot{V}CO_2$) and oxygen consumption ($\dot{V}O_2$) are decreased on admission to the ICU because of residual hypothermia. During rapid rewarming, SVR decreases and $\dot{V}CO_2$ and $\dot{V}O_2$ increase, which can cause marked cardiac and ventilatory instability. OR = operating room. (From Sladen RN: Management of the adult cardiac patient in the intensive care unit. *In* Ream AK, Fogdall RP [eds]: Acute Cardiovascular Management: Anesthesia and Intensive Care. Philadelphia, JB Lippincott, 1982, p 495.)

ASSESSMENT OF THE CIRCULATION

Physical Examination

Surgical dressings, chest tubes attached to suction, fluid in the mediastinum and pleural spaces, peripheral edema, and temperature gradients can distort or mask information obtained by the classic techniques of inspection, palpation, and auscultation in the postoperative period. However, the physician should not be deterred from applying these basic techniques in view of the potential benefit. Physical examination may be of great value in diagnosing gross or acute pathology, such as pneumothorax, hemothorax, or acute valvular insufficiency, but it is of limited value in diagnosing and managing ventricular failure. For example, in the critical care setting, experienced clinicians (e.g., internists) using only physical findings often misjudge cardiac filling pressures by a large margin.[27] Low CO in particular is not consistently recognized by clinical signs, and systemic BP does not correlate with CO after cardiac surgery. Oliguria and metabolic acidosis, classic indicators of a low CO, are not always reliable because of the polyuria induced by hypothermia, oxygen debts induced during CPB causing acidosis, and medications or fluids given during or immediately after bypass.[28]

Although clinicians are taught that the adequacy of CO can be assessed by the quality of the pulses, capillary refill, and peripheral temperature, there is no relationship between these indicators of peripheral perfusion and CO or calculated systemic vascular resistance (SVR) in the postoperative period.[29] By the first postoperative day, there is a crude correlation between peripheral temperature and cardiac index (CI) ($r = -0.60$). Many patients arrive in the ICU in a hypothermic state, and residual anesthetic agents can decrease the threshold for peripheral vasoconstriction in response to this condition.[30] A patient's extremities may therefore remain warm despite a hypothermic core or a decreasing CO. Even after temperature stabilization on the first postoperative day, the relationship between peripheral perfusion and CO is too crude to be used for hemodynamic management.

Invasive Monitoring

The routine use of pulmonary artery catheters (PACs) in all patients undergoing cardiac surgery has been questioned, because there is no convincing evidence that use of PACs improves outcome.[31,32] If the patient develops problems such as oliguria, hypotension, or acidosis in the postoperative period, a central venous pressure (CVP) catheter can be changed to a PAC. Placing a PAC in this situation is simplified if the patient's CVP is being monitored with a central catheter through an 8.5- or 9.0-Fr introducer.

Despite the lack of a proven benefit with PAC use, most patients in North America continue to have this monitor placed for cardiac surgery. This reflects a desire to have the information regarding myocardial performance readily at hand, and the potential difficulty in changing to a PAC in an emergency requiring resuscitation. Many cardiac anesthesiologists believe that the lack of evidence regarding the PAC may reflect the lack of a well-designed randomized trial. There can be little doubt that management of acute heart failure is facilitated by measures of filling pressures and CO. Postoperatively, many cardiac surgical centers do not have in-house physicians, and surgeons believe they can obtain more objective data over the telephone if a PAC is in place.

Beyond the standard PAC, which permits measurement of pressures, CO, and mixed venous blood sampling, newer PACs provide more sophisticated and continuous monitoring modalities. Use of the fiberoptic PAC to continuously monitor mixed venous oxygen saturation (SvO_2) helps evaluate the adequacy of DO_2 and allows continuous assessment of the response to therapy, which may affect DO_2 or VO_2 (e.g., PEEP therapy). The trend in the SvO_2 may function as an early warning signal of worsening in the oxygen supply-demand relationship as DO_2 falls or VO_2 increases. In the postoperative period, the SvO_2 does not correlate with CO, because the latter is only one of the factors in the oxygen supply-demand relationship.[33] Catheters that continuously measure the CO are also available. A wire coil on the catheter warms the blood passing by it at time intervals determined by an algorithm, and the measured changes in temperature at the tip of the catheter are used to provide a continuous display of the CO. Although the CO displayed needs gathering of information over several minutes and is therefore not as quick as conventional thermodilution, it avoids having to give injected volumes to the patient (which can add up to a significant amount every 24 hours) and provides trends that may give earlier warning than intermittent injections. A volumetric PAC-computer system (REF-1, Edwards Lifesciences, Irvine, CA) is also available, providing accurate right-sided volumes[34] (see Chapter 14).

Echocardiography

There can be little doubt that echocardiography is the technique of choice for acute assessment of cardiac function. Just as transesophageal echocardiography (TEE) has become essential for intraoperative management in a variety of conditions, several studies document its utility in the postoperative period in the presence and absence of the PAC.[35-38] It provides information that may lead to urgent surgery or prevent unnecessary surgery, gives important information about cardiac preload, and can detect acute structural and functional abnormalities. Although transthoracic echocardiography (TTE) can be performed more rapidly in this setting, adequate images can be obtained only in about 50% of patients in the ICU[39] (see Chapters 15 and 16).

POSTOPERATIVE MYOCARDIAL DYSFUNCTION

Studies using hemodynamic, nuclear scanning, and metabolic techniques have documented worsening in cardiac function after coronary artery bypass grafting (CABG) surgery.[40-53] Although improvements in myocardial protection, surgical techniques, and operative care have been reported, similar incidences of early biventricular dysfunction (90%) were reported between 1979 and 1990. All of these studies showed significant declines in left ventricular (LV) or biventricular (when measured) function in the first postoperative hours, with gradual return to preoperative values by 8 to 24 hours. In one study, this decline was evident only in one half the patients,[44] but in the other studies, more than 90% of patients showed at least a transient decrease in function. Decreased ventricular performance at normal or elevated filling pressures occurs, suggesting decreased contractility. Similarly, "flattening" of the ventricular function curves is usually obvious, suggesting that preload augmentation much above 10 mm Hg for CVP or 12 mm Hg for pulmonary capillary wedge pressure (PCWP) is of little benefit. In the classic study by Mangano,[45] patients with a left ventricular ejection fraction (LVEF) of less than 0.45 or ventricular dyssynergy showed more marked and prolonged dysfunction than did those patients with normal ventricles.

Satisfactory myocardial protection is important to prevent postoperative dysfunction. In off-pump surgery, the idea is to preserve coronary perfusion, but during mechanical manipulation, changes in CO and BP can occur. For CABG with CPB, most surgeons use some combination of hypothermia and crystalloid or blood cardioplegia to arrest the heart and reduce its metabolism. Although there is little consensus that any one technique is preferable in all circumstances, cold intermittent crystalloid cardioplegia with systemic hypothermia is the most widely used technique clinically and in the reported studies. Salerno et al[54] recommended continuous, warm, retrograde blood cardioplegia without systemic hypothermia. Mullen et al[50] suggested that blood cardioplegia had at least short-term benefit with less myocardial damage and better function; however, other studies of blood cardioplegia have showed mixed results[47-52] (see Chapters 28 and 30).

Other proposed factors that contribute to postoperative ventricular dysfunction include myocardial ischemia,[55] residual hypothermia,[46,47] preoperative medications such as β-adrenergic antagonists,[53] and ischemia-reperfusion injury (Box 33–1). Inflammatory cell activation from cytokine generation, upregulation of neutrophil adhesion molecules with neutrophil activation, oxygen free radical formation, and lipoperoxidation after ischemia-reperfusion injury may be important pathways accounting for the dysfunction. Multiple

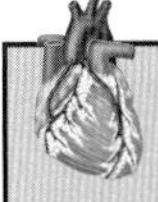

BOX 33–1 *Risk Factors for Low Cardiac Output Syndrome after Cardiopulmonary Bypass*

- Preoperative left ventricular dysfunction
- Valvular heart disease requiring repair or replacement
- Long aortic cross-clamp time and total cardiopulmonary bypass time
- Inadequate cardiac surgical repair
- Myocardial ischemia and reperfusion
- Residual effects of cardioplegia solution
- Poor myocardial preservation
- Reperfusion injury and inflammatory changes

studies have showed the importance of limiting myocardial ischemia-reperfusion injury.[56,57] Briesblatt et al[40] observed the timing of ventricular dysfunction, and recovery after CPB for CABG was similar to what had been suggested in animal models of reperfusion injury.[58-60] This nadir at 4 hours corresponds to the peak in cytokine levels. Cytokines can release nitric oxide from endothelium, which produces myocardial depression. Data evaluating complement inhibition with pexelizumab in improving outcomes represent a novel strategy[61] (see Chapter 8).

POSTOPERATIVE MYOCARDIAL ISCHEMIA

Although intraoperative myocardial ischemia has often been a focus, studies have demonstrated that ischemia often occurs postoperatively and is associated with adverse cardiac outcomes. Leung et al[55] found the electrocardiographic (ECG) and segmental wall motion abnormality (SWMA) evidence of ischemia early postoperatively in up to 40% of patients undergoing CABG surgery. Postbypass SWMAs were significantly associated with adverse outcomes (e.g., MI, death) (Fig. 33–5). Surprisingly, these abnormalities most often appeared in the regions of the heart that had been revascularized. Hemodynamic changes rarely preceded ischemia; however, postoperative heart rates (HRs) were, as reported in other studies, significantly higher than intraoperative or preoperative values. Jain et al[62] found major ECG changes in the 8 hours after cross-clamp release in 58% of CABG patients, and these changes were independent predictors of perioperative MI. Whether such changes occur because of surgery-reperfusion or events after CPB is not known. These findings do suggest that monitoring for ischemia must continue after revascularization. It may be that early recognition and treatment of ischemia or prophylactic medication can help prevent or reduce myocardial ischemia and dysfunction occurring after CABG surgery (see Chapters 6, 10, 12, 15, and 19).

Early recovery, or fast-tracking, of the cardiac surgical patient has led to some concern that ischemia will occur as patients awaken early after surgery in pain, especially because Mangano et al[63] showed that sedation with a sufentanil infusion could reduce ischemia in this period. A randomized study by Cheng et al[64] appears to dispel this concern, because awakening and extubation within 6 hours of CABG were not associated with more CK-MB (isoenzyme of creatine kinase with muscle and brain subunits) release or ECG changes than overnight ventilation. Wahr et al[65] showed that even with the use of propofol sedation, hemodynamic episodes (significant changes in HR and BP) are common in the 12 hours after surgery, and ST-segment changes occur in 12% to 13% of patients.

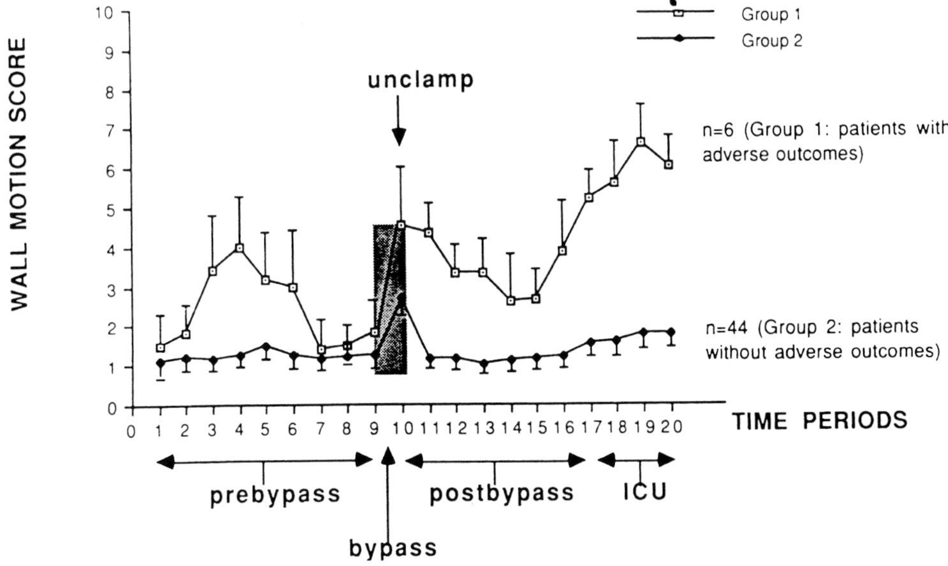

Figure 33–5 Sequential changes in wall motion score, as measured by transesophageal echocardiography, in patients undergoing elective coronary artery bypass grafting. Score is defined as follows: 0 = normal; 1 = mild hypokinesis; 2 = severe hypokinesis with myocardial thickening; 3 = akinesis; and 4 = dyskinesis. Adverse outcomes were myocardial infarction, death, or congestive heart failure. The time periods were as follows: 1 = after tracheal intubation; 2 = before incision; 3 = after incision; 4 = before sternotomy; 5 = after sternotomy; 6 and 7 = internal mammary dissection; 8 = after pericardiotomy; 9 = immediately before bypass; 10 = unclamping of aortic side-clamp; 11 to14 = off bypass; 15 = after chest closure; 16 = skin closure; 17 to 20 = intensive care unit for the first 4 hours. The *shaded area* indicates the bypass period. (From Leung JM, O'Kelly B, Browner WS, et al: Prognostic importance of postbypass regional wall motion abnormalities in patients undergoing coronary artery bypass graft surgery. Anesthesiology 71:16, 1989.)

THERAPEUTIC INTERVENTIONS

Therapeutic interventions for postoperative biventricular dysfunction include the standard concerns of managing low cardiac output states (LCOS) by controlling the HR and rhythm, providing an acceptable preload, and adjusting afterload and contractility. In most patients, pharmacologic interventions can be rapidly weaned or stopped within the first 24 hours after surgery.

Postoperative Arrhythmias

Patients with preoperative or newly acquired noncompliant ventricles need a correctly timed atrial contraction to provide satisfactory ventricular filling, especially when they are in sinus rhythm preoperatively (see Chapters 10, 13, 20, and 25). Although atrial contraction provides approximately 15% to 20% of ventricular filling, this may be more important in postoperative patients, when ventricular dysfunction and reduced compliance may be present. For example, in medical patients with acute MI, atrial systole contributed 35% of the stroke volume (SV).[66] The SV is often relatively fixed in patients with ventricular dysfunction, and the HR is an important determinant of CO. Rate and rhythm disorders need to be corrected when possible, using epicardial pacing wires. Approaches to postoperative rate and rhythm disturbances are shown in Table 33–1. The use of a PAC with atrial or ventricular pacing electrodes or use of lumens for pacing wires can facilitate temporary pacing if epicardial wires are not functioning. Failing that, temporary transvenous pacing wires can be placed (see Chapters 13 and 25).

Later in the postoperative period (days 1 through 3), supraventricular tachyarrhythmias become a major problem, with atrial fibrillation (AF) predominating. The overall incidence is between 30% and 40%, but with increasing age and valvular surgery, the incidence may be in excess of 60%.[67] There are probably many reasons for this, including genetic factors, inadequate atrial protection during surgery, electrolyte abnormalities, change in atrial size with fluid shifts, epicardial inflammation, stress, and irritation.[68] Randomized trials of off-pump coronary artery bypass (OPCAB) have found a similar incidence of postoperative AF compared with on-pump CABG.[69,70]

Advanced age, a history of AF, and valvular heart operations are the most consistently identified risk factors for AF.[68] Because efforts to terminate AF after its initiation are problematic, and its occurrence is associated with other complications, as well as increased duration and cost of hospitalization, there is a great interest in finding effective prophylactic therapy.[67] Many studies have demonstrated that β-blockade significantly reduces the incidence of postoperative AF and that withdrawal of β-blockers in patients receiving them preoperatively is an important risk factor. Guidelines published by the American Heart Association, American College of Cardiology, and the North American Society of Pacing and Electrophysiology recommend administration of β-blockers to prevent postoperative AF if there are no contraindications.[71] The reduction in incidence with β-blockade is modest; probably the most effective agent is sotalol, which also has some class III actions.[72] This drug is not available in the intravenous form in North America, and it is a potent, long-acting nonselective β-antagonist. The limitations of such a drug in the acute postoperative setting should be readily apparent (see Chapters 10 and 13).

Several studies have examined the use of amiodarone for prophylaxis, with encouraging results. Until recently, this was an expensive option, with an intravenous form of the loading dose costing more than $1000. The cost is much lower now because the patent period has expired. Clinicians may be confused by the different studies that have evaluated oral versus intravenous amiodarone; the use of intravenous amiodarone has continued to increase in clinical practice because "acute" loading with oral therapy is often not feasible. Two pivotal studies of amiodarone deserve mention. Daoud et al[73] assessed preoperative prophylaxis in 124 patients who were given oral amiodarone (64 patients) or placebo (60 patients) for a minimum of 7 days before elective cardiac surgery. Therapy consisted of 600 mg of amiodarone per day for 7 days and then 200 mg per day until the day of discharge from the hospital. The preoperative total dose of amiodarone was 4.8 ± 0.96 g over a period of 13 ± 7 days. Postoperative AF occurred in 16 (25%) of the 64 patients in the amiodarone group and 32 (53%) of the 60 patients in the placebo group. Patients in the amiodarone group were hospitalized for significantly fewer days than were patients in the placebo group (6.5 ± 2.6 versus 7.9 ± 4.3 days, $p = 0.04$). Total hospitalization costs were sig-

Table 33–1 Postoperative Rate and Rhythm Disturbances

Disturbance	Usual Causes	Treatments
Sinus bradycardia	Pre/intraoperative β-blockade	Atrial pacing β-Agonist Anticholinergic
Heart block (first, second, and third degree)	Ischemia Surgical trauma	Atrioventricular sequential pacing Catecholamines
Sinus tachycardia	Agitation/pain Hypovolemia Catecholamines	Sedation/analgesia Volume administration Change or stop drug
Atrial tachyarrhythmias	Catecholamines Chamber distention Electrolyte disorder (hypokalemia, hypomagnesemia)	Change or stop drug Treat underlying cause (e.g., vasodilator, diuresis, give K^+/Mg^{++}) May require synchronized cardioversion or pharmacotherapy
Ventricular tachycardia or fibrillation	Ischemia Catecholamines	Cardioversion Treat ischemia, may require pharmacotherapy Change or stop drug

nificantly less for the amiodarone group than for the placebo group (\$18,375 ± \$13,863 versus \$26,491 ± \$23,837, $p = 0.03$). Guarnieri et al[74] evaluated 300 patients randomized in a double-blind fashion to intravenous amiodarone (1 g/day for 2 days) or to placebo immediately after open heart surgery. The primary end-points of the trial were incidence of AF and length of hospital stay. AF occurred in 67 (47%) of 142 patients on placebo versus 56 (35%) of 158 on amiodarone ($p = 0.01$). Length of hospital stay for the placebo group was 8.2 ± 6.2 days, and 7.6 ± 5.9 days for the amiodarone group.

After AF or other supraventricular arrhythmias develop, treatment is often urgently required for symptomatic relief or hemodynamic benefit. The longer a patient remains in AF, the more difficult it may be to convert, and the greater the risk for thrombus formation and embolization.[68,72] Treatable underlying conditions such as electrolyte disturbances or pain should be corrected, while specific pharmacologic therapy is being instituted. Paroxysmal supraventricular tachycardia (uncommon in this setting) can be abolished or converted by intravenous adenosine, and atrial flutter can sometimes be converted by overdrive atrial pacing by temporary wires placed at the time of surgery. Electrical cardioversion may be required if hypotension is caused by the rapid rate; however, atrial arrhythmias tend to recur in this setting.[67] Rate control for AF or flutter can be achieved with a variety of atrioventricular nodal blocking drugs, and conversion is facilitated by many of these drugs as well. Table 33–2 summarizes the various treatment modalities for supraventricular arrhythmias. If conversion to sinus rhythm does not occur, electrical cardioversion in the presence of antiarrhythmic drug therapy should be attempted, or anticoagulation with Coumadin instituted (see Chapters 10, 13, and 25).

In summary, AF is a frequent complication of cardiac surgery, but the incidence can be significantly reduced with appropriate prophylactic therapy. β-Adrenergic blockers should be administered to patients without contraindication, and prophylactic amiodarone can be considered for patients at high risk for postoperative AF. Patients who are poor candidates for β-blockade may not tolerate sotalol, whereas amiodarone does not have this limitation. Additional studies need to be performed to better assess the role of prophylactic therapy in off-pump cardiac surgery. After AF occurs, there is a high incidence of recurrence so treatment with specific ongoing pharmacologic therapy is usually necessary.

Preload

The Frank-Starling law states that myocardial work increases as the resting length of the myocardial fiber increases.[75] In vivo, this implies that SV will increase with increasing end-

Table 33–2 Treatment Modalities for Supraventricular Arrhythmias

Treatment	Specifics*	Indications
Overdrive pacing by atrial wires†	Requires rapid pacer (up to 800/min); start above arrhythmia rate and slowly decrease	PAT, atrial flutter
Adenosine	Bolus dose of 6–12 mg; may cause 10 sec of complete heart block	AV nodal tachycardia Bypass-tract arrhythmia Atrial arrhythmia diagnosis
Amiodarone	150 mg IV over 10 min, followed by infusion	Rate control/conversion to NSR in atrial fibrillation/flutter
β-Blockade	Esmolol, up to 0.5 mg/kg load over 1 min, followed by infusion if tolerated Metoprolol, 0.5–5 mg, repeat effective dose q4–6 hr Propranolol, 0.25–1 mg; repeat effective dose q4 hr‡ Labetolol, 2.5–10 mg; repeat effective dose q4 hr‡ Sotalol, 40–80 mg PO q12 hr	Rate control/conversion to NSR in atrial fibrillation/flutter Rate control/conversion to NSR in atrial fibrillation/flutter Conversion of atrial fibrillation/flutter to NSR Conversion of PAT to NSR
Ibutilide Verapamil	1 mg over 10 min; may repeat after 10 min 2.5–5 mg IV, repeated PRN‡	Rate control/conversion to NSR in atrial fibrillation/flutter
Diltiazem	0.2 mg/kg over 2 min, followed by 10–15 mg/hr‖	Rate control/conversion to NSR in atrial fibrillation/flutter
Procainamide	50 mg/min up to 1 g, followed by 1–4 mg/min	Rate control/conversion to NSR in atrial fibrillation/flutter Prevention of recurrence of arrhythmias Treatment of wide-complex tachycardias¶
**Digoxin	Load of 1 mg in divided doses over 4–24 hr§; may give additional 0.125-mg doses 2 hr apart (3–4 doses)	Rate control/conversion to NSR in atrial fibrillation/flutter
Synchronized cardioversion	50–300 J (external); most effective with anterior-posterior patches	Acute tachyarrhythmia with hemodynamic compromise (usually atrial fibrillation or flutter)

*See specific drug monographs for full description of indications, contraindications, and dosage. Doses are for intravenous administration; use lowest dose and administer slowly in patients with hemodynamic compromise.
†Verify pacer is not capturing ventricle.
‡Infusion may provide better control. This drug is less useful than diltiazem due to myocardial depression.
§Rate of administration depending on urgency of rate control.
‖Limited experience; may cause less hypotension than verapamil.
¶When diagnosis is unclear (ventricular versus supraventricular) and there is no acute hemodynamic compromise (i.e., cardioversion not indicated).
**Less useful than other drugs due to slow onset and modest effect.
AV = atrioventricular; NSR = normal sinus rhythm; PAT = paroxysmal atrial tachycardia; SVT = supraventricular tachycardia.

diastolic volume, although there is a limit at which SV reaches a plateau (and possibly decreases) with further increases in end-diastolic volume due to excessive muscle stretch. In the normal myocardium, the Frank-Starling mechanism is the most important mechanism for increasing CO, and hypovolemia is a common cause of decreased CO and hypotension in the perioperative period. Assessment of preload is probably the single most important clinical skill for the management of hemodynamic instability. Preload rapidly changes in the postoperative period because of bleeding, spontaneous diuresis, vasodilation during warming, the effects of positive-pressure ventilation and PEEP on venous return, capillary leak, and other causes.

Direct assessment of preload is clinically feasible using echocardiography. Several studies have demonstrated a fair-to-good correlation between echocardiographic and radionuclide measures of end-diastolic volume, and there is a good correlation between end-diastolic area by TEE and SV.[76-79] Although the use of echocardiography to assess preload must always be tempered by the realization that the clinician is viewing a two-dimensional image of a three-dimensional object, this is the most direct technique clinically available. Increased awareness of the value of TEE in the ICU and increased availability of echocardiography in general have made this modality a first choice in acute assessment of preload in the setting of unexplained or refractory hypotension. In the absence of echocardiography, pressure measurements are used as surrogates for volume measurements. For example, in the absence of mitral valve disease, left atrial pressure (LAP) is almost equal to left ventricular end-diastolic pressure (LVEDP), and pulmonary artery occlusion pressure (PAOP) is virtually equivalent to these two pressures. In patients without LAP catheters, the PAOP or, when shown to be equivalent to this latter number, the pulmonary artery diastolic (PA_d) pressure is used (see Chapters 5 and 14).

The use of PAOP as a measure of preload may be misleading in a variety of settings, including after cardiac surgery, when changes in pressure may not accurately reflect changes in ventricular end-diastolic volume. Studies by Ellis et al[80] and Calvin et al[81] suggest that fluid therapy in postoperative patients could cause a substantial increase in left ventricular end-diastolic volume (LVEDV), with minimal or no change in PAOP. Mangano et al[45,82] reported that fluid loading after CPB can uncover LV dysfunction and have also shown that there is little benefit to be derived from exceeding a PAOP of approximately 12 mm Hg. Whether this is secondary to an open pericardium, which permits overdistention of the left ventricle, the use of PEEP causing RV distention, or other factors is unclear. Briesblatt et al[83] evaluated changes in ventricular pressure-volume relationships after CABG surgery while maintaining a low-to-normal PAOP (10 to 15 mm Hg). The increase seen in LVEDV was not significant enough to explain the degree of ventricular dysfunction they observed. Bouchard et al[84] compared ventricular performance assessments from the PAC (i.e., left ventricular stroke work index [LVSWI]) with fractional area change and regional wall motion score index from TEE in 60 patients during and after cardiac surgery. They found no correlation between LVSWI and fractional area change and postulated that changes in ventricular compliance, loading conditions, and ventricular function alter the pressure-volume relationship of the left ventricle in a manner that leads to discordant interpretations between the two techniques.

When ventricular compliance is normal and the ventricle is not distended, small changes in end-diastolic volume are usually accompanied by small changes in end-diastolic pressure. In patients with noncompliant ventricles from preexisting congestive heart failure (CHF), chronic hypertrophy resulting from hypertension or valvular disease, postoperative MI, or ventricular dysfunction, small increases in ventricular volume may produce rapid increases in end-diastolic pressure, requiring therapeutic intervention.[83-89] Increased intraventricular pressure will increase myocardial oxygen demand ($M\dot{V}O_2$) and decrease subendocardial coronary blood flow.[90] Myocardial ischemia may be the result. Elevations in LVEDP are transmitted to the pulmonary circulation, causing congestion and possibly hydrostatic pulmonary edema. Although PAOP or LAP may not always indicate true preload, there are still good reasons to monitor them. The periods when patients are at particular risk for elevations in end-diastolic pressure include awakening, endotracheal suctioning, and rapid-volume resuscitation. If myocardial ischemia or acute CHF occurs, sudden increases in the end-diastolic pressure may result.

Many drugs may be used to reduce cardiac preload. Direct-acting vasodilators, especially nitroglycerin, increase venous capacitance, decreasing end-diastolic volume and pressure.[89-91] Intravenous furosemide, in addition to its diuretic effect, increases venous capacitance.[92] Diuretics are important to help remove the fluid that is mobilized in the days after surgery. In patients who may not tolerate the acute volume loss that is induced by the loop diuretics, a furosemide infusion allows a more gradual diuresis. Such infusions have been shown to be effective in patients with renal dysfunction.[93,94] In a patient who appears refractory to diuresis, it is important to evaluate the circulatory state. Such refractoriness may indicate that a renal insult has been suffered, but it may also suggest underperfusion of the kidneys. In the latter case, the preload must be maintained at the upper range of normal and CO augmented.

A new agent used in treatment of acute decompensated left-heart failure is recombinant B-type natriuretic peptide (nesiritide). The mechanism of action occurs by means of specific cell-surface receptors, stimulation of which increases levels of intracellular cyclic guanosine monophosphate (cGMP). The physiologic effects are predominantly vasodilation, natriuresis, and renin inhibition. The result is balanced vasodilation, reducing preload and afterload while simultaneously increasing SV and CO and promoting diuresis.[95] Nesiritide has not been widely studied in the cardiac surgery population, but it has been used anecdotally in patients with poor ventricular function and elevated filling pressures, pulmonary hypertension, or right ventricular failure.[96] A related drug, human atrial natriuretic peptide, was shown in a small, randomized trial to reduce the need for dialysis and to improve dialysis-free survival after complicated heart surgery.[97]

Angiotensin-converting enzyme (ACE) inhibitors can also cause venodilation and reduce preload. Alternatively, opioids or benzodiazepines, or both, used to reduce endogenous catecholamine release, should be considered in the patient who needs mechanical ventilation. Morphine causes histamine release, which directly induces venodilation. In the patient with oliguria and renal failure who is fluid overloaded, peritoneal dialysis, hemodialysis, or continuous hemofiltration or dialysis may be needed.[98,99]

Contractility

Contractility is a well-defined concept in vitro, where it can be measured in terms of the velocity of shortening of isolated muscle strips. However, it has been more difficult to quantify the contractility of the intact heart because it has been difficult to find a variable to measure contractility that is also independent of preload and afterload. The pioneering work of Suga and Sagawa has shown that contractility can be measured by the end-systolic elastance of the ventricle, defined as

$$E_{ES} = P_{ES} / (V_{ES} - V_0)$$

in which P_{ES} is the end-systolic pressure, V_{ES} is the end-systolic volume, and V_0 is a deadspace term.[100,101] E_{ES} is strictly determined by evaluating ventricular pressure-volume loops for different preloads or afterloads and by defining end-systole as the point in time at which the time-varying elastance is maximal.[102] The slope of the line connecting the points at end-systole is E_{ES}. This parameter varies with changes in inotropic state but is *approximately* independent of preload and afterload. Routine measurement of end-systolic elastance is not clinically feasible. However, consideration of the above definition underscores the utility of TEE for the qualitative evaluation of contractility in the clinical setting. A decrease in contractility is manifested as some combination of a decrease in pressure or an increase in V_{ES} (i.e., a decrease in SV). End-systolic volume can be estimated using TEE. A large V_{ES} (implying a low ejection fraction) with a low or normal BP suggests a low value for E_{ES} and poor contractility. If BP is high, a large value of V_{ES} may be seen even if contractility is normal. By interpreting end-diastolic volume, end-systolic volume, and ejection fraction in the context of BP, an assessment of contractility is possible with TEE (see Chapters 5, 14, and 15).

An alternative measure of contractility is the preload-recruitable stroke work, which is the slope of the line relating stroke work to preload.[103] In the operating room or ICU, it is often estimated by the extent of the increase in CO that accompanies an increase in preload and is not dependent on the availability of TEE. If preload is increased by a change in patient position, BP can be a surrogate for CO because it is unlikely that SVR will change in the short time needed for the position change. A change in BP, therefore, is proportional to the change in CO.

Therapy for decreased contractility should be directed toward correcting any reversible causes, such as myocardial depressants, metabolic abnormalities, or myocardial ischemia. If the cause of depressed myocardial contractility is irreversible, positive inotropic agents may be necessary to maintain a CO adequate to support organ function (see Chapters 5, 10, 28, 30, and 31).

Afterload

Afterload is a concept that is well defined in vitro, where it refers to the added tension imposed on isolated muscle strips with contraction, but it is harder to define in vivo. In analogy with in vitro studies, afterload can be equated with ventricular wall stress, expressed as the product of cavity radius times transmural pressure divided by wall thickness, as described by the law of Laplace. However, many investigators find this definition unsatisfactory because it implies the heart generates its own afterload and because afterload would be viewed as changing during the cardiac cycle.[104] If afterload is viewed as the external forces opposing ejection, possibly the best definition is the aortic input impedance, the complex ratio of pressure to flow, expressed in terms of magnitude, and the phase angle between flow and pressure for any given frequency. However, it has been difficult to quantitatively analyze the impact of impedance on overall cardiac performance (see Chapter 5). Sunagawa et al[105] proposed a simplified theory of ventricular-vascular coupling within the framework of the end-systolic pressure-volume relationship. Using the definition of end-systolic elastance produces the following:

$$E_{ES} = P_{ES} / (V_{ES} - V_0)$$

Equating SV with $V_E - V_{ES}$ (ignoring the difference between end-ejection and end-systole), it is a matter of algebra to show that

$$P_{ES} = E_{ES}\,(V_{ED} - V_0) - E_{ES} \cdot SV$$

This means that an increase in SV implies a decrease in P_{ES}. The interpretation of this from the heart's perspective is that the work that can be done is finite and that a greater SV can only be achieved by lowering the end-systolic pressure, if contractility (E_{ES}) is fixed. At the same time, it is known that from the perspective of the vasculature, if the SV increases, BP increases when vascular tone does not change.

The application of an electrical law describing constant voltages and flows to the circulation, in which pulsatile flow is generated by a pump, has resulted in estimates of afterload that are questionable.[104] Although SVR is a component of impedance, it cannot be equated with it. The correct downstream pressure is probably not the CVP.[106] There is instead a critical opening pressure that should be used in calculating SVR that is not measurable in routine clinical care.[106] Clinical use of such calculated resistances is made complex by the relation of CO to body size; the normal resistance of a small patient is much higher than that of a large one. The use of a resistance index (i.e., using CI instead of CO) partly overcomes this problem, but it is not widely used.

Calculated SVR continues to be widely used in guiding therapy or drawing conclusions about the state of the circulation. This should only be done cautiously, if at all. SVR is not a complete indicator of afterload. Even if SVR were an accurate measure of impedance, the response to vasoactive agents depends on the coupling of ventricular-vascular function, not on impedance alone. Hemodynamic therapy should be guided based on the primary variables, BP and CO. If preload is appropriate, low BP and low CO are treated with an inotropic drug. If BP is acceptable (and preload appropriate) but CO is low, a vasodilator alone or in combination with an inotropic drug is used. If the patient is hypertensive (with low CO), vasodilators are indicated; if the patient is vasodilated (low BP and high CO), vasoconstrictors are employed (Box 33–2).

BOX 33–2 ***Hemodynamic Therapy Guidelines***

Blood Pressure	Cardiac Output	Treatment
Low	Low	Inotrope
Normal	Low	Vasodilator ± inotrope
High	Low	Vasodilator
Low	High	Vasopressor

POSTOPERATIVE HYPERTENSION

Hypertension has been a common complication of cardiac surgery, reported to occur in 30% to 80% of patients.[107-109] The current population of older, sicker patients appears to have fewer problems with hypertension than with low-output syndromes or vasodilation. Although hypertension most commonly occurs in patients with normal preoperative ventricular function or a prior history, any patient may develop hypertension. Multiple factors contribute to postoperative hypertension, including awakening from general anesthesia, increases in endogenous catecholamines, activation of the plasma renin-angiotensin system, neural reflexes (e.g., heart, coronary arteries, great vessels), and hypothermia.[110] Arterial vasoconstriction with various degrees of intravascular hypovolemia is the hallmark.

The hazards of untreated postoperative hypertension include depressed LV performance, increased $M\dot{V}O_2$, cerebrovascular accidents, suture line disruption, MI, rhythm disturbances, and increased bleeding.[108,111,112] Historically, pharmacologic therapy for hypertension in this setting has often been with sodium nitroprusside because of its rapid onset and short duration of action.[113,114] With the introduction of alternative vasodilators, sodium nitroprusside is no longer the drug of choice for a number of reasons. Nitroprusside has a potent effect on venous capacitance (decreasing preload) and on the arterial vasculature, often leading to precipitous decreases in BP and a hyperdynamic cardiac state. Sodium nitroprusside can cause coronary arteriolar dilation with the potential for a steal phenomenon, resulting in myocardial ischemia.[115,116] In patients with renal failure, the elimination of sodium nitroprusside is reduced, potentially leading to toxic effects of its metabolites cyanide or thiocyanate. This can occur if large doses are given to patients with normal renal function.

There are many alternative drugs to sodium nitroprusside for the treatment of hypertension after cardiac surgery, including nitroglycerin,[117] adrenergic-blocking agents such as phentolamine,[113] β-adrenergic blockers,[115,118] and the mixed α- and β-adrenergic blocker labetalol.[119] Direct-acting vasodilators, dihydropyridine calcium channel blockers (e.g., nifedipine,[120,121] diltiazem, nicardipine,[122] isradipine,[123] clevidipine[124]), ACE inhibitors,[113] and fenoldopam (a dopamine$_1$ [D_1] receptor agonist)[125,126] have also been used. Novel therapeutic approaches are listed in Table 33–3.

Dihydropyridine calcium channel blockers relax arterial resistance vessels without negative inotropic actions or effects on atrioventricular nodal conduction and are important therapeutic options. Dihydropyridines are artery-specific vasodilators of peripheral resistance arteries, resulting in a generalized vasodilation, including the renal, cerebral, intestinal, and coronary vascular beds. In doses that effectively reduce BP, the dihydropyridines have little or no direct negative effect on cardiac contractility or conduction. Although the dihydropyridines may be considered more vasoselective than verapamil and diltiazem, there are also differences between dihydropyridines in this respect. Nifedipine is the least vasoselective of the dihydropyridines, isradipine and clevidipine are the most selective, and nicardipine and nimodipine are intermediately selective.[127] Nicardipine is available for intravenous administration and is an important therapeutic agent to consider because of its lack of effects on vascular capacitance vessels and preload in patients after cardiac surgery.[127] The pharmacokinetic profile of nicardipine suggests that effective administration requires variable rate infusions when trying to treat hypertension because of the half-life of 40 minutes. If even more rapid control is essential, a dosing strategy consisting of a loading bolus or rapid infusion dose with a constant-rate infusion may be more efficient. The effect of nicardipine may persist even though the infusion is stopped. Clevidipine, a new ultra-short-acting dihydropyridine, is in phase III studies, has a half-life of only minutes, and may represent a potential alternative to sodium nitroprusside in the future.[124]

Table 33–3 Novel Vasodilators

Drug	Mechanism of Action	Half-Life
Nicardipine	Calcium channel blocker	Intermediate
Clevidipine	Calcium channel blocker	Ultra-short
Fenoldopam	Dopamine$_1$ agonist	Ultra-short
Nesiritide	β-Natriuretic agonist	Short
Levosimendan	K^+-ATP channel modulator	Intermediate

Fenoldopam is a short-acting, dopamine agonist that causes arterial-specific vasodilation by stimulation of D_1-receptors approved for short-term intravenous therapy. Unlike sodium nitroprusside, D_1-receptor stimulation also increases renal blood flow to produce diuresis and natriuresis. Fenoldopam and sodium nitroprusside were similarly effective in reducing BP in patients who developed hypertension after CABG surgery.[125] Fenoldopam often needs higher doses for severe hypertension that may be associated with increases in HR.

The ACE inhibitors are used in treating chronic hypertension and ventricular dysfunction. Enalaprilat is the intravenous preparation used for administration in the postoperative setting.[128] These drugs are indirect vasodilators that function by inhibiting angiotensin II formation and breakdown of bradykinin. Intravenous enalaprilat has an unpredictable effect and may be long acting. A suitable role is for replacing intravenous ACE inhibitors in a patient being weaned from short-acting agents or with heart failure (see Chapter 10).

POSTOPERATIVE VASODILATION

Vasodilation and a need for vasoconstrictor support are relatively frequent complications of cardiac surgery with and without CPB. The reported incidence is 4% to 44%, but this wide range largely results from lack of a common definition.[129,130] Vasodilation alone should be associated with a hyperdynamic circulatory state presenting as systemic hypotension in association with an increased CO (and a low calculated SVR). More commonly after cardiac surgery, a combination of vasodilation and myocardial dysfunction occurs, requiring vasoconstrictor and inotropic therapy. Gomez et al[131-133] coined the term *vasoplegic syndrome* for the condition that requires very high doses of vasoconstrictors, and they reported its occurrence after off-pump and on-pump surgery.

Multiple humoral and inflammatory cascades are activated by surgery alone and by CPB, aortic cross-clamping, and reperfusion, generating complement anaphylatoxins, kinins, and cytokines, many of which cause vasodilation by direct and indirect vascular mechanisms.[134-136] Another potential cause of systemic vasodilation is splanchnic circulatory insufficiency resulting in endotoxemia, and this, too, has been observed after off-pump surgery[137,138] (see Chapter 8). The cellular mechanisms and pathogenesis of vasodilatory shock were summarized by Landry and Olivier.[135] Although the most common clinical context of vasodilatory shock is sepsis, the similarity in the cytokine response and clinical syndrome seen in sepsis with the vasodilated state seen after cardiac surgery is striking. As described by Landry and Olivier,[135] the stimuli of cytokines and increased tissue lactate lead to increased nitric oxide synthase and the generation of vasodilating guanosine monophosphate. Nitric oxide and metabolic acidosis activate potassium channels, which hyperpolarize the cell membrane, making it refractory to calcium entry and thereby refractory to norepinephrine and angiotensin II action. At this time, plasma vasopressin levels are low due to central depletion. Reports of profound vasodilatory shock after CPB responsive to vasopressin, appeared when this pathophysiology was being actively investigated.[139] The ability of vasopressin to block the potassium channels and interfere with nitric oxide signaling makes it an important therapy for this syndrome. Provided there is an adequate CO, vasopressin is a valuable agent for treating vasodilation after cardiac surgery, significantly reducing the dose requirement for norepinephrine. Systemic vasodilation also can result from hyperthermia caused by excessive warming during CPB (see Chapters 8, 28, and 30) and during warming in the ICU.

When patients develop acute systemic vasodilation after administration of drugs or blood products, an anaphylactic reaction should be considered. Acute anaphylaxis caused by immunoglobulin E–mediated responses can present with systemic vasodilation and increased CO.[140] Alternatively, complement-mediated transfusion reactions to any blood product can present with hypotension produced by systemic vasodilation or by thromboxane-mediated acute pulmonary vasoconstriction and RV dysfunction. Antibodies in the donor blood called leukoagglutinins, when directed against recipient white cell antigens, can actively produce white cell aggregation and thromboxane generation. These reactions have been called *transfusion-related acute lung injury,* which can manifest with hypotension, RV failure, and noncardiogenic pulmonary edema.[140] Monitoring of RV function may therefore help to identify these transfusion reactions.

While underlying causes are being sought and treated, the therapeutic approach to systemic vasodilation includes intravascular volume expansion, α-adrenergic agents, and vasopressin. Administration of vasoconstrictors for more than a brief period must be guided by measures of cardiac performance, because restoration of BP may camouflage a low-output state. There are no established guidelines for initiation of vasoconstrictor therapy; autoregulation in vital organs is lost at arterial mean pressures below 60 mm Hg, and it is reasonable to attempt to achieve this pressure in normotensive patients (possibly higher in hypertensive patients). A study in septic shock patients was unable to demonstrate a benefit from mean arterial pressures greater than 65 mm Hg.[141]

Clinicians are often concerned about the potential for constricting supply vessels or the microcirculation to vital beds (e.g., brain, kidney); although not fully evaluated in the postoperative setting, giving vasoconstrictors in septic states does not appear to have such harmful effects.[142] Use of relatively low doses of vasopressin to restore responsiveness to catecholamines is physiologically sensible, but there is no clear evidence to suggest that use of vasopressin in addition to or instead of norepinephrine is associated with better outcome.

CORONARY ARTERY SPASM

Coronary artery or internal mammary artery (IMA) vasospasm can occur postoperatively. Mechanical manipulation and underlying atherosclerosis of the native coronary circulation and the IMA have the potential to produce transient endothelial dysfunction. The endothelium is responsible for releasing endothelium-derived relaxing factor (EDRF), which is nitric oxide, a potent endogenous vasodilator substance that maintains normal endogenous vasodilation (see Chapters 6 to 8). Thromboxane can be liberated as a result of heparin-protamine interactions, CPB, platelet activation, or anaphylactic reactions to produce coronary vasoconstriction.[143-145] Calcium administration, increased α-adrenergic tone from vasoconstrictor administration (especially in bolus doses), platelet thromboxane liberation, and calcium channel blocker withdrawal represent additional factors that may put the cardiac surgical patient at risk for spasm of native coronary vessels and arterial grafts. Engelman et al[145] reported four patients who developed coronary artery spasm after discontinuation of their calcium channel blockers 8 to 18 hours before surgery. In three of these patients, spasm was identified by the ECG pattern and documented as the cause of ischemia in the distribution of a nondiseased right coronary artery, with the fourth patient developing spasm in a bypassed native vessel. In two of the patients, the problem was recognized retrospectively; MIs developed, and one patient died. In the other two patients, spasm was recognized, and intravenous nitroglycerin was given (1 to 3 μg/kg/min) in combination with nifedipine, 10 mg sublingually every 5 to 6 hours, to reverse the ischemic process. The therapy of choice remains empirical. Nitroglycerin is a first-line drug, but nitrate tolerance can occur. Phosphodiesterase (PDE) inhibitors represent novel approaches to this problem and have been reported to be effective in vascular models of spasm.[146] Intravenous dihydropyridine calcium channel blockers are also important therapeutic considerations.[147]

Reports of successful use of the radial artery as a bypass conduit have rekindled interest in this vessel.[148-150] In the early days of CABG surgery, this conduit was abandoned because of its propensity to spasm. In later reports, techniques developed in the use of the IMA have been applied to the radial artery, as well as prophylactic use of diltiazem infusions.[148,150] Which components of this approach are responsible for the reported success are not known, but use of a calcium channel blocking drug is recommended by many surgeons. The arterial selectivity of the dihydropyridine drugs (e.g., nicardipine) should be an advantage in this setting. However, addition of a vasodilator drug to prevent spasm of the radial artery in a patient requiring a vasopressor for systemic vasodilation makes no pharmacologic sense.

DECREASED CONTRACTILITY

Drugs that increase contractility all result in increased calcium mobilization from intracellular sites to and from the contractile proteins, or sensitize these proteins to calcium. Although calcium chloride has been used to increase inotropy, evidence suggests that after CPB, its principal action is peripheral vasoconstriction.[151] The same group of investigators has showed that exogenously administered calcium chloride attenuates the response to catecholamines in this setting.[152] The administration of calcium salts will improve myocardial performance if there is severe hypocalcemia or hyperkalemia, and may be indicated during rapid transfusion of citrated blood.[153]

Catecholamines, through β_1-receptor stimulation in the myocardium, increase intracellular cyclic adenosine monophosphate (cAMP). This second messenger increases intracellular calcium, causing an improvement in myocardial contraction.[154] Inhibition of the breakdown of cAMP by PDE inhibitors increases intracellular cAMP independent of the β-receptor.[155] Intracellular calcium availability can be increased by inhibiting Na^+/K^+-ATPase with digitalis glycosides, promoting transmembranous Na^+/Ca^{++} exchange. However, the use of digoxin to increase myocardial contractility for postoperative ventricular dysfunction is limited by its slow onset, low potency, and narrow therapeutic safety margin. The "calcium sensitizers" constitute a new class of inotropic agents. One drug in this class, levosimendan, is being evaluated in clinical trials (Box 33–3).

Catecholamines

The catecholamines used postoperatively include dopamine, dobutamine, epinephrine, norepinephrine, and isoproterenol (Box 33–4). These drugs have various effects on α- and β-receptors and therefore various effects on HR, rhythm, and myocardial metabolism (see Chapter 31). Dosing recommendations for the catecholamines are provided in Table 33–4.

Isoproterenol

Isoproterenol is the most potent β-agonist in the heart (β_1) and in the periphery (β_2). Its positive inotropic effect is accompanied by an increase in HR and a propensity for arrhythmias. In patients with coronary artery disease, tachycardia and associated peripheral vasodilation increase $M\dot{V}O_2$ and decrease coronary perfusion pressure (CPP). In patients with bradycardias in whom pacing is not an immediate or practical option or in those in whom an elevated HR is desirable (e.g., cardiac transplant recipients, patients with regurgitant valvular lesions), isoproterenol may be used cautiously bearing in mind its rather narrow therapeutic window. Although used for its β_2 effects in the pulmonary vasculature, it is a weak pulmonary vasodilator.

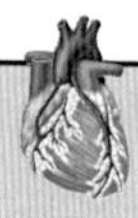

BOX 33–3 ***Pharmacologic Approaches for Perioperative Ventricular Dysfunction***

- Inotropic agents
  - Catecholamines
  - Phosphodiesterase inhibitors
  - Levosimendan
- Vasodilator therapy
- Pulmonary vasodilators
  - Phosphodiesterase inhibitors
  - Inhaled nitric oxide
  - Prostaglandins

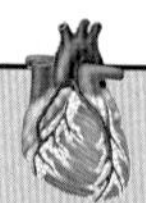

BOX 33–4 ***Disadvantages of Catecholamines***

- Increased myocardial oxygen consumption
- Tachycardia
- Arrhythmias
- Excessive peripheral vasoconstriction
- Coronary vasoconstriction
- β-receptor downregulation and decreased drug efficacy

Table 33–4 Catecholamines Used Postoperatively

Drug	Infusion Dose (μg/kg/min)
Dopamine*,†	2–10
Dobutamine†	2–10
Epinephrine‡	0.03–0.20
Norepinephrine‡	0.03–0.20
Isoproterenol‡	0.02–0.10

*Less than 2 μg/kg/min predominantly "dopaminergic" (renal and mesenteric artery dilatation).
†If 10 μg/kg/min is ineffective; change to epinephrine or norepinephrine.
‡Dose to effect; may require higher dose than indicated.

Epinephrine

Epinephrine is a potent adrenergic agonist with the desirable feature that, in low doses (<3 μg/min), β_1 and β_2 effects predominate. As the dose is increased, α effects (e.g., vasoconstriction) and tachycardia occur. However, in the acutely failing heart postoperatively, only drugs such as epinephrine or norepinephrine provide positive inotropy and perfusion pressure. These features and its low cost make it a common first-line drug in the postoperative setting. Despite what is often stated in older literature, epinephrine causes less tachycardia than dopamine[156] or dobutamine[157] at equivalent inotropic doses.[158] Epinephrine is a first-line therapy for anaphylaxis and when titrated does not produce ventricular arrhythmias. Because of the metabolic actions of β_2 stimulation, epinephrine infusion can cause hyperglycemia and increased serum lactate levels.[159]

Norepinephrine

Norepinephrine, which has potent β_1- and α-receptor effects, preserves CPP while not increasing HR, actions that are favorable to the ischemic, reperfused heart. When norepinephrine is used alone without a vasodilator or PDE inhibitor, the potent β_1 effects may have variable effects on CO. Ventricular filling pressures usually increase when this drug is given, because of constriction of the capacitance vessels. Administration of a vasodilator, including the PDE inhibitors, with norepinephrine may partially oppose the vasoconstriction.[160] Clinicians may express concern for the renal blood flow when norepinephrine is given for hypotension; however, when a dose of this drug as high as 1 μg/kg/min was administered into the left atrium to maintain BP during infusion of prostaglandin E_1, there was no evidence of renal dysfunction and urine output ranged from 1 to 6 mL/kg/hr.[161] End-organ ischemia would appear to be unlikely if CO can be preserved at normal levels when norepinephrine is given. PDE inhibitors in combination with norepinephrine attenuate the arterial vasoconstrictive effects.[146]

Dopamine

A precursor of norepinephrine, dopamine probably achieves its therapeutic effects by releasing myocardial norepinephrine or preventing its reuptake, especially when administered in high doses.[162] This indirect action may result in reduced effectiveness when given to patients with chronic CHF or shock states, because the myocardium becomes depleted of norepinephrine stores.[163] In contrast to dobutamine, the α-agonist properties of dopamine cause increases in pulmonary artery pressure (PAP), PVR, and LV filling pressure.[164-166] At low doses (<2 μg/kg/min), dopamine stimulates renal dopaminergic receptors to increase renal perfusion more than can be explained by an increase in CO.[167] Despite this action, a multicenter study in New Zealand and Australia clearly demonstrated that use of low-dose dopamine in critically ill patients confers no protection from renal dysfunction.[168] One review suggests there is no justification for low-dose dopamine in the ICU and that it is "bad medicine."[169] At doses higher than 10 μg/kg/min, tachycardia and vasoconstriction become the predominant actions of this drug.

Dobutamine

In contrast to dopamine, dobutamine exhibits mainly β_1-agonist properties, with decreases in diastolic BP and sometimes systemic BP being observed.[170,171] Dobutamine is functionally similar to isoproterenol, with less tendency to induce tachycardia in the postoperative setting.[172] However, Romson et al[173] demonstrated that after CPB, the principal effect of dobutamine is a dose-related increase in HR. A very modest effect on SV was observed in patients with poor ventricular function. Salomon et al[174] demonstrated that dobutamine increased $\dot{M}VO_2$, which was matched by an increase in coronary blood flow, whereas dopamine increased $\dot{M}VO_2$ but failed to increase coronary blood flow. However, the favorable actions of dobutamine may be limited if a tachycardia develops, and, like dopamine, its inotropic potency is modest in comparison with that of epinephrine or norepinephrine.[174]

Phosphodiesterase Inhibitors

The PDE inhibitors are nonglycosidic, nonsympathomimetic drugs that have positive inotropic effects independent of the β_1-adrenergic receptor and unique vasodilatory actions independent of endothelial function or nitrovasodilators.[154,155] Patients with CHF have downregulation of the β_1-receptor, with a decrease in receptor density and altered responses to catecholamine administration.[154,175] Milrinone, amrinone, and enoximone bypass the β_1-receptor, causing increases in intracellular cAMP by selective inhibition of PDE fraction III (i.e., fraction IV), a cAMP-specific PDE enzyme.[155,176] In vascular smooth muscle, these agents cause vasodilation in the arterial and capacitance beds.[177,178] PDE inhibitors increase CO, decrease PCWP, and decrease SVR and PVR in patients with biventricular dysfunction, and they are important therapeutic approaches in postoperative cardiac surgical patients.

Effects on Vascular Responses

Any drug that increases cyclic nucleotides (e.g., cAMP, cGMP) in vascular smooth muscle will produce vasodilation.[176-178] The concentration of cGMP can be increased by the release of nitric oxide generated by nitroglycerin, sodium nitroprusside, and inhaled nitric oxide, and cAMP can be increased by stimulation of the β_2-adrenergic receptor, prostaglandin E_1 or I_2, or by inhibiting its breakdown by PDE inhibition. Increasing cAMP in vascular smooth muscle promotes calcium uptake by the sarcoplasmic reticulum, decreasing calcium available for contraction. The net effect of increasing calcium uptake is smooth muscle relaxation. This effect can also occur through stimulation by drugs that inhibit the breakdown of cGMP (e.g., nonspecific PDE inhibitor). Sildenafil and its congeners are type V PDE inhibitors that were originally developed for nitrate tolerance but are currently marketed for erectile dysfunction.

PDE III inhibitors have a clinical effect as inodilators; they produce dilation of arterial and venous beds, decreasing the mean arterial pressure and central filling pressures. Increases in CO are induced by multiple mechanisms, including afterload reduction and positive inotropy, but not by increasing HR.[179-189] The net effect is a decrease in myocardial wall tension, representing an important contrast to most sympathomimetic agents.[181] Catecholamine administration often needs the simultaneous administration of vasodilators to reduce ventricular wall tension. Milrinone and other PDE inhibitors also have unique mechanisms of vasodilation that may be favorable for coronary artery and IMA flow[146] (Box 33–5).

Combination Therapy: Catecholamines and Phosphodiesterase Inhibitors

Catecholamine therapy depends on the myocardial cell's capacity to respond to β_1-agonist activity. In patients with preoperative CHF, the number of effective β_1-receptors decreases because of downregulation, which refers to reduced density or uncoupling, such that fewer receptors are available for binding with the β-agonist.[154,175] When postoperative ventricular dysfunction is treated, a pharmacologic ceiling effect may occur with increasing doses of a single β_1-agonist or even when other catecholamines are added.[176] Combining PDE inhibitors with a catecholamine may significantly increase cAMP levels in patients with β_1-receptor downregulation, such as patients after cardiac surgery.[190] The two forms of therapy may attenuate each other's adverse effects. Catecholamine stimulation of vascular α-receptors induces vasoconstriction, which is attenuated by PDE inhibitors.[146] Catecholamines with potent α-agonist effects may be needed to prevent hypotension when PDE inhibitors are given postoperatively; or, alternatively, when an α agent is needed to obtain an acceptable perfusion pressure, PDE inhibitors may be administered to augment CO. The additive improvement in hemodynamic effects of catecholamines plus amrinone, milrinone, or enoximone has also been described.[187,191-195] Combined therapy may theoretically avoid dose-related adverse

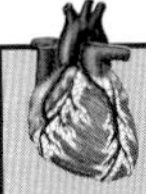

BOX 33–5 ***Advantages of Preemptive Phosphodiesterase Inhibitor Administration***

- Increased myocardial contractility (left and right ventricles)
- Pulmonary vasodilation
- Resolution and prevention of ischemia
- Minimal drug side effects while on cardiopulmonary bypass
- Dilation of internal mammary artery
- Avoidance of mechanical intervention
- Prevention of a "failed wean"

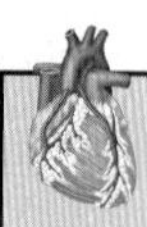

BOX 33–6 *Acute Heart Failure: Therapeutic Goals and Treatment Summary*

Goals	Treatment
Reduce impedance to ventricular ejection	Vasodilator
Reduce wall stress	Vasodilator
Reduce filling pressures	Diuretics, venodilators
Increase contractility	Inotropic agents, phosphodiesterase inhibitors

Table 33–5 Dosing for Phosphodiesterase Inhibitors (cAMP-Specific) Used Postoperatively

Drug	Loading Dose*	Infusion Rate
Amrinone	1.5–2.0 mg/kg	5–20 μg/kg/min
Milrinone	50 μg/kg	0.375–0.75 μg/kg/min
Enoximone	0.5–1.0 mg/kg	5–10 μg/kg/min

*Loading doses should be administered over 5 to 10 minutes to avoid excessive vasodilation.

effects of high doses of each individual agent and is useful in RV failure[196] (Box 33–6) (see Chapter 10).

Dosage and Administration

Suggested dosing is provided in Table 33–5. Available drugs are reviewed in the following sections.

Amrinone

Amrinone, the first bipyridine studied in cardiac surgery, has the longest half-life of almost 3.5 hours.[197-201] In 14 patients with CHF, an intravenous loading dose of 1.5 mg/kg and an infusion of 10 μg/kg/min resulted in a plasma concentration of 1.7 μg/mL and produced a 30% increase in CI.[197] Recommended dosing includes a bolus dose of 0.75 mg/kg given intravenously over 2 to 3 minutes, followed by a maintenance infusion of 5 to 10 μg/kg/min. This dose regimen produces subtherapeutic concentrations after 5 to 10 minutes, and it failed to demonstrate any hemodynamic effect after it was given 10 minutes before termination of CPB.[201,202] A loading dose of 1.5 to 2.0 mg/kg of this drug during CPB will produce therapeutic concentrations for 30 to 60 minutes, after which an infusion is required to keep therapeutic blood levels. With prolonged administration, amrinone will produce thrombocytopenia. Goenen et al[182] reported 15 patients with low postoperative COs given amrinone infusions over 12 hours. In 10 patients, CI increased by 31%, whereas LV and RV filling pressures decreased by 26% and 28%, respectively. The remaining five patients were in cardiogenic shock refractory to catecholamines and intra-aortic balloon pump (IABP) counterpulsation. In these patients, amrinone in doses up to 20 μg/kg/min increased CO significantly (up to 60%), while decreasing the PCWP (by up to 29%). There was no significant change in HR or BP.

Milrinone

Milrinone, an analog of amrinone, is a bipyridine derivative with an inotropic activity that is almost 20 times more potent than that of amrinone, and it has a shorter half-life.[183] Milrinone is an effective inodilator for patients with decompensated CHF and low CO after cardiac surgery. Suggested dosing for milrinone is a loading dose of 50 μg/kg over 10 minutes, followed by an infusion of 0.5 μg/kg/min (0.375 to 0.75 μg/kg/min). By loading the patient with milrinone over a longer period, high peak concentrations can be prevented, and the vasodilation that is observed with rapid loading can be attenuated. Bailey et al[183] demonstrated this to be effective when administered to 25 patients just before or immediately after separation from CPB, with infusions continuing into the ICU. A milrinone loading dose of 50 μg/kg in conjunction with an infusion of 0.5 μg/kg/min consistently maintained plasma concentrations more than 100 ng/mL. Clearance was 3.8 ± 1.7 mL/kg/min, volume of distribution was 465 ± 159 mL/kg, and terminal elimination half-time was 107 ± 77 minutes (values expressed as mean ± SD).[183] Pharmacokinetic parameters were independent of dose. The relationship between plasma concentration and pharmacodynamic effects produced about a 30% improvement in CI with plasma levels of 100 ng/mL, and there was a curvilinear relationship between plasma levels and improvement in CI. Bailey et al[183] observed that a dose of 50 μg/kg with an infusion rate of 0.5 μg/kg/min can maintain plasma concentrations near the threshold of its therapeutic effects. Compared with amrinone, milrinone appears to offer the pharmacokinetic advantage of shorter half-times after administration is stopped without adverse effects on platelet function.[189]

Kikura et al[194] reported the effects of milrinone on hemodynamics and LV function in cardiac surgical patients who were already treated with catecholamines. After emergence from CPB, patients were randomly assigned to a control group ($n = 10$) or to one of the milrinone dosing groups: intravenous milrinone at 50 μg/kg ($n = 8$), 50 μg/kg + 0.5 μg/kg/min ($n = 10$), or 75 μg/kg + 0.75 μg/kg/min ($n = 9$). Hemodynamics and TEE were recorded while constant filling pressures were maintained by volume reinfusion. In all three milrinone groups, CI and velocity of circumferential fiber shortening (Vcfc) significantly increased from the baseline, and both were significantly higher at 5 and 10 minutes than those in the control group. The plasma concentration of milrinone with one half of the maximal increase in Vcfc was 139 ng/mL on the dose-response curve. Milrinone improves hemodynamics and LV function when constant loading conditions are maintained.[194]

Feneck et al[203] studied 99 adult patients with a low CO after elective cardiac surgery. Milrinone was administered as a loading dose of 50 μg/kg over a 10-minute period, followed by a continuous infusion of 0.375, 0.5, or 0.75 μg/kg/min (low-, middle-, and high-dose groups, respectively) for a minimum of 12 hours. They observed that milrinone therapy was associated with a rapid and well-sustained increase in CO, and a decrease in PAOP in all groups. They found the increase in CI was associated with increases in SV and HR (Table 33–6).

Enoximone

Enoximone, an imidazolone derivative, is eliminated mostly by sulfoxidation, is solubilized in propylene glycol, and cannot be diluted when administered intravenously. The loading dose is 0.5 to 1.0 mg/kg, followed by an infusion of 5 to 10 μg/kg/min. Gonzalez et al[187] reported using enoximone in managing a CI of less than 2.2 L/min/m^2 despite a PCWP of 15 mm Hg, catecholamine administration (e.g., dobutamine,

Table 33–6 Hemodynamic Effect of Milrinone after Cardiac Surgery§

Parameter	% Change (Mean ± SEM)			
	15 Min	60 Min	12 Hr	Post
CI (L/min/m²)				
Low	+40* (4.2)	+42* (4.9)	+58* (8.8)	+44* (6.3)
Mid	+30* (4.5)	+34* (4.5)	+49* (5.1)	+27* (3.8)
High	+36* (4.9)	+44* (4.7)	+66* (6.5)	+47* (6.6)
PCWP (mm Hg)				
Low	−30* (4.7)	−20* (4.7)	−15† (7.2)	+22‡ (6.3)
Mid	−34* (4.5)	−25* (4.1)	−20* (4.3)	−3 (6.7)
High	−35* (4.0)	−22* (4.3)	−15† (6.0)	−6‡ (6.3)

*$p < .001$ versus control.
†$p < .05$ versus control.
‡$p < .01$ versus control.
§Loading dose of 50 μg/kg/min over 10 minutes, then 0.375 (low, n = 34); 0.5 (mid, n = 34); and 0.75 (high, n = 31) μg/kg/min.
CI = cardiac index; PCWP = pulmonary capillary wedge pressure.
From Feneck RO: Effects of variable dose milrinone in patients with low cardiac output after cardiac surgery. Am Heart J 121(suppl 2):1995, 1991.

dopamine) or IABP counterpulsation after cardiac surgery. Enoximone was administered as a 1-mg/kg loading dose over 10 minutes after a minimum of 4 hours of unsuccessful conventional therapy. An additional dose (0.5 mg/kg) was given if the increase in CO was less than 20%. A continuous infusion of the drug was administered at 3 to 10 μg/kg/min and continued for at least 8 hours. In all patients, significant increases in CI and a significant decrease in PCWP occurred. Naeije et al[204] also reported variable effects on BP, HR, and CO of enoximone in a dose of 0.5 mg/kg after cardiac surgery. Boldt et al[193] demonstrated potentiating effects of enoximone, 0.5 mg/kg, with epinephrine in a dose of 0.1 μg/kg/min.

Levosimendan

Levosimendan is a calcium-sensitizing drug that exerts positive inotropic effects through sensitization of myofilaments to calcium and vasodilation through opening of ATP-dependent potassium channels on vascular smooth muscle. These effects occur without increasing intracellular cAMP or calcium and without an increase in $M\dot{V}O_2$ at therapeutic doses. As would be expected with an inodilator, the hemodynamic effects include a reduction in PAOP in association with an increase in CO. β-Blockade does not block the hemodynamic effects of this drug. Levosimendan itself has a short elimination half-life, but it has active metabolites with elimination half-lives up to 80 hours. A study in patients with decompensated CHF found hemodynamic improvements at 48 hours were similar whether patients received the drug for 24 hours or 48 hours. Increasing plasma levels of the active metabolite were found for 24 hours after the drug infusion was stopped.[205] Levosimendan is in phase III clinical studies in the United States and Europe, and it has been granted fast-track status by the U.S. Food and Drug Administration.

A randomized study enrolling 203 low-output heart failure patients found that levosimendan improved hemodynamics more effectively than dobutamine and that it was associated with a lower 6-month mortality rate.[206] However, the latter finding may be caused more by adverse effects related to dobutamine than by a positive effect of levosimendan. Another study in 504 patients with LV dysfunction after acute MI demonstrated better 6-month survival with levosimendan, this time compared with placebo.[207] In a small study after cardiac surgery, patients were given levosimendan; of 11 patients with severely impaired CO and hemodynamic compromise, 8 patients (73%) showed evidence of hemodynamic improvement within 3 hours after the start of levosimendan infusion. Specifically, CI and SV were significantly increased, whereas the mean arterial pressure, indexed SVR, mean pulmonary artery pressure, right atrial pressure, and PAOP were significantly lowered.[208] Clinical studies continue to evaluate the potential role for this new positive inotropic agent in patients with heart failure.

RIGHT-HEART FAILURE

Heart failure after cardiac surgery usually results from LV impairment. Although an isolated right-sided MI can occur perioperatively, most perioperative inferior MIs show variable involvement of the right ventricle.[209] The myocardial preservation techniques that are best for the left ventricle may not offer ideal RV protection because the right ventricle is thin walled and more exposed to body and atmospheric temperature. Cardioplegic solution given through the coronary sinus (retrograde) may not reach parts of the right ventricle because of positioning of the cardioplegia cannula in relation to the venous outflow from this chamber and because the thebesian veins do not drain into the coronary sinus.[210] Impairment of RV function postoperatively is more severe and persistent when preoperative right coronary artery (RCA) stenosis is present.[211] Although depression of the ejection fraction is compensated by preload augmentation, right ventricular ejection fraction (RVEF) cannot be preserved if CPP is reduced or impedance to ejection is increased.

Certain aspects of the physiology of the right ventricle make it different from the left. Normally, the RV free wall receives its blood flow during systole and diastole; however, systemic hypotension or increased RV systolic and diastolic pressures may cause supply-dependent depression of contractility when $M\dot{V}O_2$ is increased while CPP is decreased.[212] The normal thin-walled right ventricle is at least twice as sensitive to increases in afterload as is the left ventricle[213] (Fig. 33–6). Relatively modest increases in outflow impedance from multiple causes in the postoperative period can exhaust preload reserve, causing a decrease in RVEF with ventricular dilation. RV pressure overload may be complicated by volume overload caused by functional tricuspid regurgitation.[214] Decreases in RV SV will diminish LV filling, and dilation of the right ventricle can cause a leftward shift of the interventricular septum, interfering with diastolic filling of the left ventricle (i.e., ventricular interaction) (Fig. 33–7). A distended right ventricle limited by the pericardial cavity further decreases LV filling. RV failure has the potential to affect LV performance by decreasing pulmonary venous blood flow, decreasing diastolic distending pressure, and decreasing LV diastolic compliance. The resulting decrease in LV output will further impair RV pump function. The mechanical outcomes of RV failure in

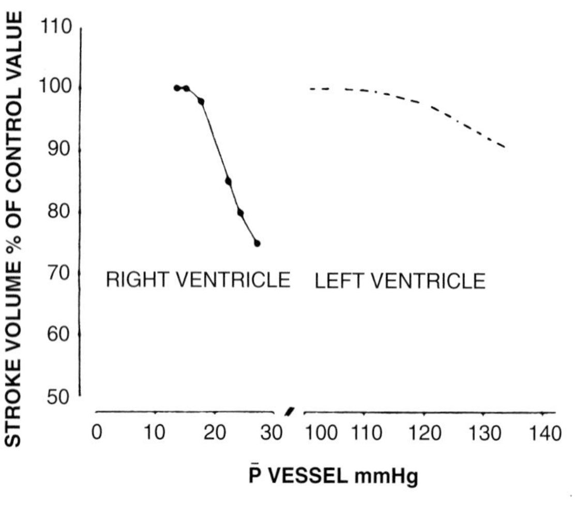

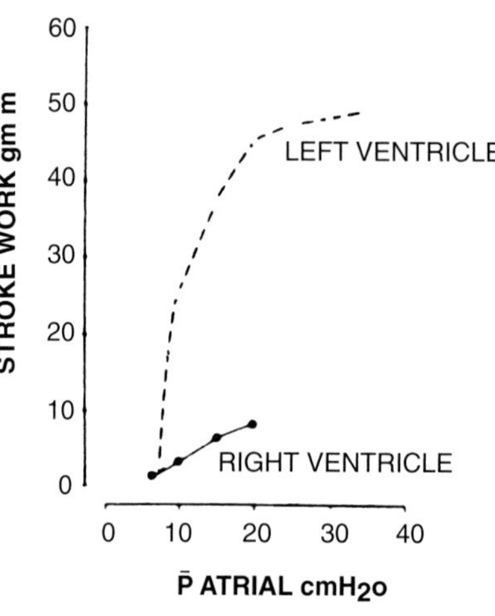

Figure 33–6 Various effects of afterload and preload seen in ventricular function curves from the right and left ventricle. The right ventricular output is more afterload dependent and less preload dependent than the left ventricular output. (From McFadden ER, Braunwald E: Cor pulmonale and pulmonary thromboembolism. *In* Braunwald E (ed): Textbook of Cardiovascular Medicine. Philadelphia, WB Saunders Company, 1980, pp 1643–1680.)

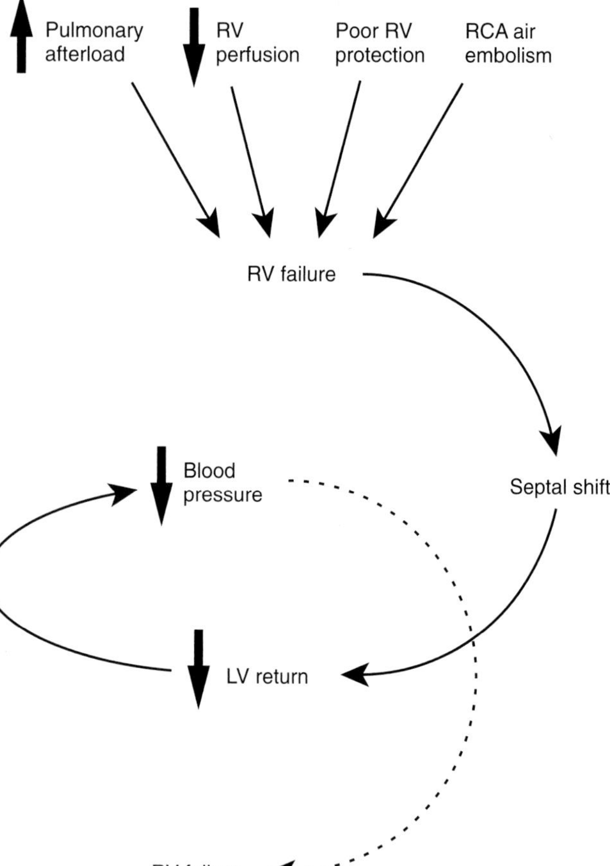

Figure 33–7 Sequence inducing right ventricular failure and causing a downward spiral of events. RCA = right coronary artery; RV = right ventricle.

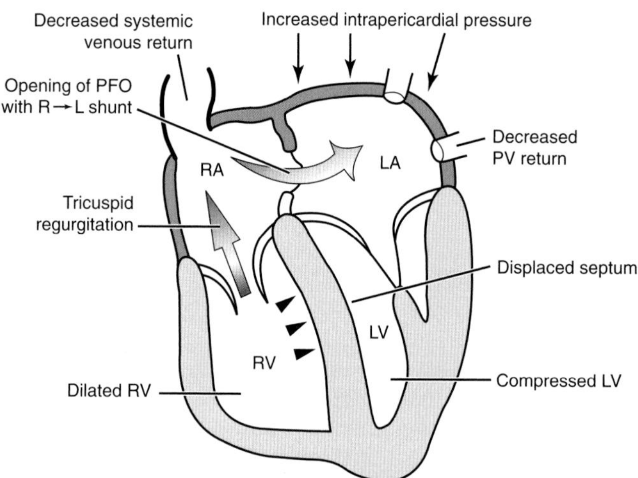

Figure 33–8 Mechanical changes produced by acute right ventricular failure. LA = left atrium; LV = left ventricle; PFO = patent foramen ovale; PV = pulmonary veins; RA = right atrium; R→L = right to left; RV = right ventricle.

postoperative cardiac surgical patients are depicted in Figure 33–8. It can therefore be appreciated how, once established, RV failure is self-propagating, and aggressive treatment interventions may be needed to interrupt the vicious cycle.

Although not consistently proved, PVR has been shown to be reversibly increased immediately after CPB and for several hours into the postoperative period.[215,216] The possible mechanisms include extravascular compression by increased lung water,[216] endocrine-mediated or autonomic nervous system–mediated increases in pulmonary vascular tone,[217] vasoactive substances released from activated platelets and leukocytes,[218] and leukocytes or platelet aggregates obstructing pulmonary vascular beds.[219] Hypoxic pulmonary vasoconstriction may result in increased PVR; more commonly, hypercarbia causes an important increase in PAP.[220,221] The pulmonary vascular bed has been shown to be more sensitive to the vasoconstrictor influences of respiratory acidosis after CPB as compared with the preoperative situation.[222] Moderate respiratory acidosis was shown to cause depression of the RVEF and increased right ventricular end-diastolic volume, and these changes were immediately reversed when normocarbia was reinstituted.[223]

Diagnosis

In the postoperative cardiac surgical patient, a low CI with right atrial pressure increased disproportionately compared with changes in left-sided filling pressures is highly suggestive of RV failure. The PAOP may also increase because of ventricular interaction, but the relationship of right atrial pressure to PAOP stays close to or higher than 1.0. The absence of a step-up in pressure in going from the RA to the pulmonary artery (mean), provided PVR is low, suggests that RV failure is severe and the right side of the heart is acting only as a conduit. This hemodynamic presentation is typical of cardiogenic shock associated with RV infarction. The venous waveforms are accentuated with a prominent Y descent similar to constrictive pericarditis, suggesting reduced RV compliance.[224] Large V waves may also be discernible and may relate to tricuspid regurgitation.

The use of a volumetric PAC to calculate right-sided volumes and ejection fraction could potentially guide management in the setting of RV failure, because increased end-diastolic volume in association with a decreased RVEF indicates decompensation. This catheter-computer system has been validated in comparison to radionuclear and ventriculographic measures, but it may not be accurate when there is tricuspid regurgitation[34,225,226] (see Chapter 14). Unfortunately, tricuspid regurgitation is a common finding with RV dilatation.

Echocardiography allows a qualitative interpretation of RV size, contractility, and configuration of the interventricular septum, and can provide a definitive diagnosis of RV dysfunction or failure. Because of the crescent shape of the right ventricle, volume determination is not easy but the qualitative examination and assessment for tricuspid regurgitation are very valuable. TEE is also useful to determine if the increased right atrial pressures open a patent foramen ovale, producing a right-to-left shunt (see Chapters 15, 16, and 22). This is important because traditional methods to treat hypoxemia such as PEEP and larger tidal volumes in this setting will only increase the afterload of the right ventricle and potentially increase the shunt and hypoxemia.

Table 33–7 Treatment Approaches in Postoperative Right-Heart Failure

Preload Augmentation
Volume, vasopressors, or leg elevation (CVP/PCWP < 1)
Decrease juxtacardiac pressures (pericardium and/or chest open)
Establish atrial kick (sinus rhythm, atrial pacing)
Afterload Reduction (pulmonary vasodilation)
Nitroglycerin, isosorbide dinitrate nesiritide
cAMP-specific phosphodiesterase inhibitors, β_2-adrenergic agonists
Inhaled nitric oxide
Nebulized PGI_2
Intravenous PGE_1 (+ left atrial norepinephrine)
Inotropic Support
cAMP-specific phosphodiesterase inhibitors, isoproterenol, dobutamine
Norepinephrine
Levosimedan
Ventilatory Management
Lower intrathoracic pressures (tidal volume < 7 mL/kg, low PEEP)
Attenuation of hypoxic vasoconstriction (high FIO_2)
Avoidance of respiratory acidosis ($PaCO_2$ 30–35 mm Hg, metabolic control with meperidine or relaxants)
Mechanical Support
Intra-aortic counterpulsation
Pulmonary artery counterpulsation
Right ventricular assist devices

CVP/PCWP = central venous pressure/pulmonary capillary wedge pressure; cAMP = cyclic adenosine monophosphate; PGI_2 = prostaglandin I_2; PGE_1 = prostaglandin E_1; PEEPs = positive end-expiratory pressures.

Treatment

Treatment approaches in postoperative RV failure may differ from those used in LV failure, and they are affected by the presence of pulmonary hypertension (Table 33–7). In all cases, preload should be increased to the upper range of normal; however, the Frank-Starling relationship is flat in RV failure, and to avoid ventricular dilation, the CO response to an increasing CVP should be determined. Volume loading should be stopped when the CVP exceeds 10 mm Hg and CO does not increase despite increases in this pressure.[227,228] If a volumetric PAC is in use, an increase in the end-diastolic volume with unchanged or declining RVEF suggests there will be no advantage to further volume loading. The CVP should not be permitted to exceed the PAOP, because if these pressures equalize, any increase obtained in pulmonary blood flow will be offset by decreased diastolic filling of the left ventricle by means of ventricular interdependence.[229] The atrial contribution to RV filling is important when the ventricle is dilated and noncompliant. Maintenance of sinus rhythm and use of atrial pacing are important components of treating postoperative RV failure (see Chapters 5, 10, 13, 20, and 25).

Although vasodilators may lead to cardiovascular collapse in RV infarction (as a result of decreases in RV filling and coronary perfusion), postoperative RV failure is often associated with increased PVR and pulmonary hypertension. In this context, attempts to decrease RV outflow impedance may be worthwhile. Intravenous vasodilators invariably reduce systemic BP, mandating the simultaneous administration of a vasoconstrictor. One way to reduce the pulmonary effects of the required vasoconstrictor is to administer the vasoconstrictor through a left atrial catheter. In 1985, D'Ambra et al[161] successfully treated RV dysfunction after mitral valve replacement with intravenous prostaglandin E_1 and left atrial norepinephrine. The PDE inhibitors are commonly used for their effect on the pulmonary vasculature and RV function,[230] but this also usually requires systemic norepinephrine. In recent years, there has been an increased interest in and availability of aerosolized pulmonary vasodilators. This route of administration reduces or even abolishes the undesirable systemic vasodilation. Delivery of the drug directly to the alveoli improves pulmonary blood flow to these alveoli, potentially improving oxygenation by better matching blood flow to ventilation. Three drugs have been used: nitric oxide, prostaglandin I_2 (i.e., epoprostenol or prostacyclin), and milrinone.

Nitric oxide is an important signaling molecule throughout the body. In the lung, it rapidly diffuses across the alveolar-capillary membrane and activates soluble guanylate cyclase, leading to smooth muscle relaxation by several mechanisms.[231] Inhaled nitric oxide is given through a specialized delivery system in a concentration of 5 to 80 parts per million. It is commercially available in the United States, but it is costly. It has been used successfully to treat RV dysfunction associated with pulmonary hypertension after congenital heart surgery,[232] mitral valve replacement,[233] cardiac transplantation,[234] and placement of LV assist devices.[235] Although it is widely used to treat the same problem in lung transplantation, a randomized trial of prophylactic inhaled nitric oxide in this population failed to demonstrate a benefit.[236] This finding should not prevent its use should RV dysfunction occur in the lung transplant recipient. Potential adverse effects of inhaled nitric oxide include toxicity from the formation of nitrogen dioxide (NO_2) and methemoglobin, rebound pulmonary hypertension from abrupt disconnection or withdrawal, and pulmonary vascular congestion due to increased pulmonary blood flow in patients with poor LV function. If administered at the recommended dosage, toxicity should not be observed; patients should have the drug gradually withdrawn, and those with poor ventricular function should be closely monitored for increases in left-sided filling pressures.

A less expensive alternative to inhaled nitric oxide is aerosolized epoprostenol (i.e., prostacyclin or prostaglandin I_2 [PGI_2]). This compound binds to cell-surface prostaglandin receptors, activating adenylate cyclase, which activates protein kinase A to cause a decrease in cytosolic free calcium. It also stimulates endothelial release of nitric oxide. It is a profound vasodilator and inhibitor of platelet aggregation. Similar to inhaled nitric oxide, its delivery to ventilated alveoli can improve oxygenation by augmenting blood flow to these alveoli. Aerosolized PGI_2 has been successfully used to treat pulmonary hypertension after cardiac surgery[237] and pulmonary embolism[238] and to treat hypoxemia in patients with lung injury.[239,240] Its use requires collaboration with pharmacy and respiratory therapy, and appropriate care and monitoring of the nebulizer device. Adverse effects include the possibility of vagus-mediated bradycardia at low doses and risks similar to those of inhaled nitric oxide with respect to abrupt withdrawal or left-sided heart failure.

Haraldsen et al[241] investigated the use of inhaled (i.e., aerosolized) milrinone in patients with mild pulmonary hypertension after CPB. They found that when delivered by this route milrinone was an effective pulmonary vasodilator without causing systemic hypotension and that the pulmonary vasodilation was additive to that caused by inhaled PGI_2.

Even a moderate increase in arterial carbon dioxide tension ($PaCO_2$) should be avoided in patients with RV failure. Although induced hypocarbia is of proven benefit in controlling low PVR in neonates, the evidence in adults does not warrant this as a standard therapy because mechanical ventilation-induced changes in intrathoracic pressure have important therapeutic implications[242,243] (see Chapter 34). IABP may be of substantial benefit, even in patients in whom the right ventricle is mainly responsible for circulatory decompensation. This beneficial effect is mediated by increased coronary perfusion. Right-heart assist devices have a place as temporizing measures in severe intractable failure. Pulmonary artery counterpulsation is experimental, and its clinical role is uncertain.[244] In cases of severe RV failure it may be necessary to leave the sternum open or to reopen the chest if it has been closed. This decreases the tamponade-like compression of the left ventricle by the distended right ventricle, right atrium, and edematous mediastinal tissues.

Effects of Mechanical Ventilation in Heart Failure

CHF at the time of surgery has been identified as a significant predictor of postoperative respiratory complications.[245] Maintenance of gas exchange in these situations usually mandates prolonged ventilatory support. Besides improving PaO_2, mechanical ventilation can influence DO_2 through its effects on CO. Suppression of spontaneous respiratory efforts may substantially decrease the work of breathing and improve the oxygen supply-demand relationship (see Chapter 34). Traditionally, the influence of mechanical ventilation on hemodynamics has been viewed as negative. The inevitable rise in intrathoracic pressure caused by positive-pressure ventilation or PEEP is associated with a decreased CO.[246] However, in the presence of CHF or myocardial ischemia, raised intrathoracic pressure has the potential to favorably affect the determinants of global cardiac performance. Understanding these heart-lung interactions is essential for the integrated management of the ventilated patient with CHF after cardiac surgery. The effects of ventilation on RV and LV failure need to receive independent consideration.

Systemic venous return is proportional to the pressure gradient between the systemic veins and the right atrium. Changes in intrathoracic pressure imposed by positive-pressure ventilation or PEEP are transmitted to the compliant right atrium, causing an increase in right atrial pressure. This decreases the driving pressure for venous return, with a decrease in RV preload as the clinically most important mechanism of the decrease in RV SV caused by ventilatory support.[247] The effects of mechanical ventilation on RV preload may be accentuated by hypovolemia or by an increase in venous capacitance caused by vasodilator administration.[248] The effects of raised intrathoracic pressure can be overcome by fluid administration, leg elevation, or even vasopressors to raise the systemic venous pressure. Preload augmentation must be done cautiously if there is RV failure.

Two other factors related to raised intrathoracic pressure potentially impede the diastolic filling of the left ventricle. If positive-pressure ventilation or PEEP causes an increase in PVR, RV systolic emptying may be impaired, and the right ventricle will dilate. This may cause leftward displacement of the interventricular septum and decrease LV compliance.[229] Independent of ventricular interaction, increased lung volume also raises juxtacardiac pressures, decreasing the transmural distending pressure.[249]

The end-diastolic volume and systolic BP are directly proportional to systolic wall stress or ventricular afterload. Because ventricles and the outflow vessels are surrounded by intrathoracic pressure, increases in this pressure by positive-pressure ventilation decrease the transmural pressure load (aortic or PAP relative to intrathoracic pressure) of each ventricle.[250] On the right side of the heart, the hemodynamic consequences of ventilatory support usually result from changes in PVR. To the extent that PEEP increases lung volume above functional residual capacity, PVR may decrease from reduced compression of extra-alveolar vessels.[251] Beyond that, large tidal volumes and high levels of PEEP increase PVR.[252] The increase in PVR may be conspicuous even with normal tidal volumes in airflow-limited diseases. The consequences of increased PVR in RV failure are decreased CO and further dilation.

Raised intrathoracic pressure may significantly improve LV performance as a result of the reduced transmural pressure required to generate an adequate systemic BP.[253] This can be viewed as afterload reduction, a beneficial effect separate from the resistance to venous return that may also help such patients. Clinically significant improvements in cardiac function have been documented in patients ventilated for cardiogenic respiratory failure produced by myocardial ischemia and after CABG surgery.[254,255] High LV filling pressures may help identify a subgroup benefiting from reduced afterload with increased intrathoracic pressure.[256]

Raised intrathoracic pressure and PEEP have also been suggested to affect the inotropic state of the ventricles. Dilation of the right ventricle in response to an increase in afterload raises the RV distending pressure, which can reduce the pressure gradient for subendocardial coronary blood flow. Diminished RV contractility related to a decreased coronary blood flow has been described with high levels of PEEP in an animal model with critical RCA obstruction[212] and in patients with significant RCA disease.[256] Left ventricular contractility does not seem to be affected by this mechanism.[257] Raised intrathoracic pressure and lung distention may also modulate contractility by stimulating vagal afferents[258] and releasing prostaglandins.[259] The impairment of contractility by these mechanisms appears to be minimal.

The circulatory responses to changes in ventilation should always be assessed in patients with cardiac disease; the goal of improving or maintaining DO_2 must be kept in mind. This usually requires measurement of arterial oxygenation and CO. In right and biventricular failure the increase in the airway pressure caused by ventilatory support should be kept at a minimum compatible with adequate gas exchange. This means avoidance of high levels of PEEP and trials of decreased inspiratory times, flow rates, and tidal volumes. Breathing modes that emphasize spontaneous efforts such as intermittent mandatory ventilation, pressure support, or CPAP should be considered. Alternatively, if isolated LV failure is the reason for ventilatory therapy, improvements in cardiac performance may be achieved by the use of positive-pressure ventilation with PEEP. In particular, patients with elevated LV filling pressures, mitral regurgitation, and reversible ischemic dysfunction may improve from afterload reduction related to increased airway and intrathoracic pressures. Newer modes of ventilatory support that decrease mean airway pressure, such as cardiac cycle–specific, high-frequency jet ventilation[260] and airway pressure release ventilation,[261] and their roles in supporting heart function, are discussed in Chapter 34.

Effects of Ventilatory Weaning on Heart Failure

Traditional criteria for weaning of ventilatory support assess the adequacy of gas exchange and peak respiratory muscle strength.[262] In the patient with CHF, the response of global hemodynamics to spontaneous respirations must also be considered. The changes of the loading conditions of the heart brought about by the resumption of spontaneous ventilation can induce a vicious cycle resulting in hypoxemia and pulmonary edema.

Pulmonary congestion, often present in patients with LV dysfunction, decreases pulmonary compliance. Consequently, large decreases in inspiratory intrathoracic pressure are needed to cause adequate lung inflation. These negative swings of intrathoracic pressure increase venous return.[263] Increased diaphragmatic movements may increase intra-abdominal pressure, further increasing the pressure gradient for venous return.[264] Decreased intrathoracic pressure also raises the ventricular transmural pressures, raising the impedance to ventricular emptying. The increased afterload causes further increases in preload, with these changes jeopardizing the myocardial oxygen balance. Accordingly, worsening of myocardial ischemia as evidenced by ST-segment deviations was demonstrated when ventilatory support was removed in patients ventilated after MI.[265] Spontaneous ventilation episodes also precipitated ischemic dysfunction, causing LV dilation and altered thallium 201 uptake, in ventilator-dependent patients after lung injury caused by infection or complications of surgery.[266]

In the patient with severe ventricular dysfunction, one of the main methods of improving cardiac performance to allow separation from CPB and to maintain function in the postoperative period is to augment preload with fluid therapy. The inevitable consequence is a positive fluid balance and a weight gain of several kilograms, even after uncomplicated surgery. Diuretic therapy to reduce this hypervolemia, and vasodilator therapy to reduce ventricular wall stress, should be considered before these patients are exposed to the afterload stress of ventilatory weaning.[263,267]

CARDIAC TAMPONADE

Cardiac tamponade is an important cause of the LCOS after cardiac surgery and occurs when the heart is compressed by an external agent, most commonly blood accumulated in the mediastinum. Hemodynamic compromise, to some degree attributable to the constraining effect of blood accumulating within the chest, is often observed in the 3% to 6% of patients needing multiple blood transfusions for hemorrhage after cardiac surgery.[268] Postoperative cardiac tamponade usually manifests acutely during the first 24 hours after surgery, but delayed tamponade may develop 10 to 14 days after surgery, and it has been associated with postpericardiotomy syndrome or postoperative anticoagulation.[269-271]

The mechanism of hemodynamic deterioration during tamponade is discussed in Chapter 24 and primarily is the result of impaired filling of one or more of the cardiac chambers. As the external pressure on the heart increases, the distending or transmural pressure (external-intracavitary pressure) is decreased. The intracavitary pressure increases in compensation lead to impaired venous return and elevation of the venous pressure. If the external pressure is high enough to exceed the ventricular pressure during diastole, diastolic ventricular collapse occurs. These changes have been documented in the right and the left hearts after cardiac surgery.[272] As the end-diastolic volume and end-systolic volume decrease, there is a concomitant decrease in SV. In the most severe form of cardiac tamponade, ventricular filling occurs only during atrial systole. Adrenergic and endocrine mechanisms are activated in an effort to maintain venous return and perfusion pressure.[273,274] Intense sympathoadrenergic activation increases venous return by constricting venous capacitance vessels. Tachycardia helps to maintain CO in the face of a reduced SV. Adrenergic mechanisms may also explain decreased urinary output and sodium excretion, but these phenomena may also be caused by reduced CO or a reduction in atrial natriuretic factor from decreased distending pressure of the atria.[237]

The diagnosis of cardiac tamponade depends on a high degree of suspicion. Tamponade after heart surgery is a clinical entity distinct from the tamponade typically seen in medical patients in whom the pericardium is intact and the heart is surrounded by a compressing fluid. In the setting of cardiac surgery, the pericardial space is often left open and in communication with one or both of the pleural spaces, and the compressing blood is at least in part in a clotted, nonfluid state and able to cause localized compression of the heart. Serious consideration should be given to the possibility of tamponade after cardiac surgery in any patient with inadequate or deteriorating hemodynamics, as evidenced by hypotension, tachycardia, increased filling pressures, or low CO, especially when there has been excessive chest tube drainage. A more subtle presentation of postoperative tamponade is gradually increasing requirements for inotropic and pressor support. Many of the classic signs of tamponade may not be present in these patients, partly because they are usually sedated and ventilated, but also because the pericardium is usually left open, resulting in a more gradual increase in the restraining effects of blood accumulation. There may be localized accumulations that affect one chamber more than another.[275] The classic findings of elevated CVP or equalization of CVP, PA_d, and PAOP may not occur.[276,277] It may therefore be difficult in the face of a declining CO and elevated filling pressures to distinguish tamponade from biventricular failure. A useful clue may be pronounced respiratory variation in BP with mechanical ventilation in association with high filling pressures and low CO, because the additional external pressure applied to the heart by positive-pressure ventilation may further impair the already compromised ventricular filling in the presence of tamponade.

Echocardiography may provide strong evidence for the diagnosis of tamponade.[277-280] Echolucent crescents between the RV wall and the pericardium or the posterior LV wall and the pericardium are discernible with transthoracic imaging or TEE. Echogenicity of grossly bloody pericardial effusions, especially when clots have been formed, may sometimes make delineation of the borders of the pericardium and the ventricular wall difficult, compromising the sensitivity of this technique. A classic echocardiographic sign of tamponade is diastolic collapse of the right atrium or right ventricle, with the duration of collapse bearing a relationship to the severity of the hemodynamic alteration, but such findings are frequently absent in the postcardiac surgery patient.[277,281,282] In many cases, transthoracic imaging is difficult because of mechanical ventilation, and TEE is required for adequate visualization (see Chapters 15 and 16).

The definitive treatment of tamponade is surgical exploration with evacuation of hematoma. The chest may have to be opened in the ICU if tamponade proceeds to hemodynamic collapse. In the case of delayed tamponade, pericardiocentesis may be adequate. Medical palliation in anticipation of reexploration consists of reinforcing the physiologic responses that are already occurring while preparing for definitive treatment. Venous return can be increased by volume administration and leg elevation. The lowest tidal volume and PEEP compatible with adequate gas exchange should be used.[283] Epinephrine in high doses gives the needed chronotropic and inotropic boost to the ventricle and increases systemic venous pressures. Sedatives and opioids should be given cautiously because they may interfere with adrenergic discharge and precipitate abrupt hemodynamic collapse. Occasionally, patients develop significant cardiac tamponade without accumulation of blood in the chest. Edema of the heart, lungs, and other tissues in the chest after CPB may not permit chest closure at the initial operation and necessitate staged chest closure after the edema has subsided.[285] Similarly, it was found that some patients with inadequate hemodynamics after cardiac surgery despite maximum support in the ICU improve with opening of the chest because of relief of this tamponade effect. Reclosure of the chest in the operating room is often possible after a few days of continued cardiovascular support and diuresis.

TRANSPLANTED HEART

Postoperative circulatory control in the heart transplant recipient differs from that of the nontransplant population in three major respects. The transplanted heart is noncompliant with a relatively fixed SV, acute rejection must be considered when cardiac performance is poor or suddenly deteriorates, and these patients are at risk for acute RV failure if pulmonary hypertension develops.[285]

The fixed SV combined with denervation of the donor heart means that maintenance of CO is often dependent on therapy to maintain an elevated HR (110 to 120 bpm). The drug most commonly used is isoproterenol, because it is a potent inotropic agent and because it causes a dose-related increase in HR. Its vasodilating β_2 effect on the pulmonary vasculature may be of benefit if PVR is above normal. Alternatively, atrial pacing may be used to maintain HR if contractility appears normal. Pacing is often used to allow the withdrawal of isoproterenol in the first postoperative days. Parasympatholytic drugs, such as atropine, do not have any effect on the transplanted heart (see Chapter 26).

Major concerns in monitoring and therapy for the transplant recipient are the potential for infection and rejection. Immunosuppressive therapy regimens include cyclosporine and usually steroids or azathioprine, or both. These drugs also suppress the patient's response to infection, and steroid therapy may induce elevations in the white blood cell count, further confusing the issue. Protocols for postoperative care stress strict aseptic technique and frequent careful clinical evaluations for infection.

The adequacy of immunosuppression is monitored by percutaneous myocardial biopsy, usually performed at weekly intervals in the first month. Less-invasive techniques, such as echocardiographic evaluation of diastolic function and sophisticated ECG analysis, are being evaluated.[286] Although acute rejection is diagnosed histologically, if suspected clinically (i.e., acute deterioration in cardiac function), it must be treated with intense immunosuppressive therapy. The agents and doses used vary from institution to institution, but they usually include high-dose steroids and monoclonal antibody to T_3 lymphocytes (OKT3).[287] Pharmacologic management and sometimes mechanical support of biventricular function are required because severe impairment of contractility, ventricular dilation, and even cardiovascular collapse may occur (see Chapter 27).

Preoperative evaluation helps screen patients with fixed pulmonary hypertension, because the normal donor RV may acutely fail if presented with an elevated PAP in the recipient.[285] However, patients may have progression of disease between the time of evaluation and surgery, or the right ventricle may be inadequately protected during harvest or transport. When separation from CPB is attempted, acute RV dilation and failure occur, and such patients may emerge from the operating room on multiple drug therapy, including the inhaled agents nitric oxide and prostacyclin, as described above. Gradual withdrawal of these drugs occurs in the first postoperative days, with close monitoring of PAPs and oxygenation.

There is a heightened concern for fluid balance in the perioperative period because transplant recipients are often fluid overloaded as a result of chronic biventricular failure, and because of the potential for edema in the donor heart. It is not unusual for vigorous diuretic therapy to be initiated within 24 hours of surgery, with the goals of negative fluid balance and a PAOP less than 12 mm Hg. Inotropic agents rather than preload augmentation are used to keep CO at an acceptable level while this is being done. Electrolyte abnormalities induced by this therapy and the use of cyclosporine (which causes potassium and magnesium wasting) are common in this period.

REFERENCES

1. Jones M, Tunstall-Pedow DS: Blood doping—a literature review. Br J Sports Med 23:84, 1989
2. Mirhashemi S, Ertefai S, Merrmer K, Intaglietta M: Model analysis of the enhancement of tissue oxygenation by hemodilution due to increased microvascular flow velocity. Microvasc Res 34:290, 1987
3. Vincent JL, Baron JF, Reinhart K, et al: Anemia and blood transfusion in critically ill patients. JAMA 288:1499, 2002
4. Hebert PC, Wells G, Blajchman MA, et al: A multicenter, randomized, controlled clinical trial of transfusion requirements in critical care. N Engl J Med 340:409, 1999
5. Wu WC, Rathore SS, Wang Y, et al: Blood transfusions in elderly patients with acute myocardial infarction. N Engl J Med 345:1230, 2001
6. Suter PM, Fairley HB, Isenbery MD: Optimum end-expiratory pressure in patients with acute pulmonary failure. N Engl J Med 292:284, 1975
7. Dhainaut JF, Devaux JY, Monsallier JE, et al: Mechanisms of decreased left ventricular preload during continuous positive-pressure ventilation in ARDS. Chest 90:74, 1986
8. Robotham JL, Scharf SM: Effects of positive and negative pressure ventilation on cardiac performance. Clin Chest Med 4:161, 1983
9. Katz JA, Marks JD: Inspiratory work with and without continuous positive airway pressure in patients with acute respiratory failure. Anesthesiology 63:598, 1985
10. Rasanen J, Vaisanen IT, Heikkil J, et al: Acute myocardial infarction complicated by left ventricular dysfunction and respiratory failure. The effects of continuous airway pressure. Chest 87:158, 1987
11. Sukernik MR, Mets B, Bennett-Guerrero E: Patent foramen ovale and its significance in the perioperative period. Anesth Analg 93:137, 2001
12. Radermacher P, Santak B, Becker H, et al: Prostaglandin E_1 and nitroglycerin reduce pulmonary capillary pressure but worsen Va/Q distribution in patients with ARDS. Anesthesiology 70:601, 1989
13. Noback CR, Tinker JH: Hypothermia after cardiopulmonary bypass in man; amelioration by nitroprusside-induced vasodilation during rewarming. Anesthesiology 53:277, 1980
14. Ramsay JG, Ralley FE, Whalley DG, et al: Site of temperature monitoring and prediction of afterdrop after open heart surgery. Can Anaesth Soc J 32:607, 1985
15. Pujol A, Fusciardi J, Ingrand P, et al: Afterdrop after hypothermic cardiopulmonary bypass: The value of tympanic membrane temperature monitoring. J Cardiothorac Vasc Anesth 10:336, 1996
16. Grocott HP, Mathew JP, Carver EH, et al: A randomized controlled trial of the Arctic Sun temperature management system versus conventional methods for preventing hypothermia during off-pump cardiac surgery. Anesth Analg 98:298, 2004
17. Licker M, Schweizer A, Ralley FE: Thermoregulatory and metabolic responses following cardiac surgery. Eur J Anaesthesiol 13:502, 1996
18. Buckberg GD, Brazier JR, Nelson RL, et al: Studies of the effects of hypothermia on regional myocardial blood flow and metabolism during cardiopulmonary bypass. 1. The adequately perfused beating, fibrillating, and arrested heart. J Thorac Cardiovasc Surg 73:87, 1977
19. Reed LR II, Bracey AW Jr, Hudson JD, et al: Hypothermia and blood coagulation: Dissociation between enzyme activity and clotting factor levels. Circ Shock 32:141, 1990
20. Valeri CR, Khabbaz K, Khuri SF, et al: Effect of skin temperature on platelet function in patients undergoing extracorporeal bypass. J Thorac Cardiovasc Surg 104:108, 1992
21. Valeri CR, Feingold H, Cassidy G, et al: Hypothermia-induced reversible platelet dysfunction. Ann Surg 205:175, 1987
22. Donati F, Maille JG, Blain R, et al: End-tidal carbon dioxide tension and temperature changes after coronary artery bypass surgery. Can Anaesth Soc J 32:272, 1985
23. Sladen RN: Temperature and ventilation after hypothermic cardiopulmonary bypass. Anesth Analg 64:816, 1985
24. Ralley FE, Wynands JE, Ramsay JG, et al: The effects of shivering on oxygen consumption and carbon dioxide production in patients rewarming from hypothermic cardiopulmonary bypass. Can J Anaesth 35:332, 1988
25. Kurz A, Ikeda T, Sessler DI, et al: Meperidine decreases the shivering threshold twice as much as the vasoconstriction threshold. Anesthesiology 86:1046, 1997
26. Sladen RN, Berend JZ, Fassero JS, Zehnder EB: Comparison of vecuronium and meperidine on the clinical and metabolic effects of shivering after hypothermic cardiopulmonary bypass. J Cardiothorac Vasc Anesth 9:147, 1995
27. Connors AF, McCaffree DR, Gray BA: Evaluation of right heart catheterization in the critically ill patient with acute myocardial infarction. N Engl J Med 308:263, 1983
28. Ariza M, Gothard JW, Macnaughton P, et al: Blood lactate and mixed venous-arterial P_{CO_2} gradient as indices of poor peripheral perfusion following cardiopulmonary bypass surgery. Intensive Care Med 17:320, 1991
29. Bailey JM, Levy JH, Kopel MA, et al: Relationship between clinical evaluation of peripheral perfusion and global hemodynamics in adults after cardiac surgery. Crit Care Med 18:1353, 1990
30. Sessler D: Mild perioperative hypothermia. N Engl J Med 336:1730, 1997
31. Tuman KJ, McCarthy RJ, Spiess BD, et al: Effect of pulmonary artery catheterization on outcome in patients undergoing coronary artery surgery. Anesthesiology 70:199, 1989
32. Tuman KJ, Roizen MF: Outcome assessment and pulmonary artery catheterization: Why does the debate continue? Anesth Analg 84:1, 1997
33. Magilligan DJ, Teasdall R, Eisinminger R, Peterson E: Mixed venous oxygen saturation as a predictor of cardiac output in the postoperative cardiac surgical patient. Ann Thorac Surg 44:260, 1987
34. Spinale FG, Smith AC, Crawford FA: Right ventricular function using thermodilution. Surg Forum 39:242, 1988
35. Reichert CLA, Visser CA, Doolen JJ, et al: Transesophageal echocardiography in hypotensive patients after cardiac operations. Comparison with hemodynamic parameters. J Thorac Cardiovasc Surg 104:321, 1992
36. Kochar GS, Jacobs LE, Kotler MN: Right atrial compression in postoperative cardiac patients: Detection by transesophageal echocardiography. J Am Coll Cardiol 16:511, 1990
37. Chan K-L: Transesophageal echocardiography for assessing cause of hypotension after cardiac surgery. Am J Cardiol 62:1142, 1988
38. Costachescu T, Denault A, Guimond JG, et al: The hemodynamically unstable patient in the intensive care unit: Hemodynamic vs TEE monitoring. Crit Care Med 30:1214, 2002
39. Hwang JJ, Shyu KG, Chen JJ, et al: Usefulness of transesophageal echocardiography in the treatment of critically ill patients. Chest 104:861, 1993
40. Breisblatt WM, Stein KL, Wolfe CJ, et al: Acute myocardial dysfunction and recovery: A common occurrence after cardiopulmonary bypass surgery. J Am Coll Cardiol 15:1261, 1990
41. Roberts AJ, Spies M, Meyers SN, et al: Early and long-term improvement in left ventricular performance following coronary bypass surgery. Surgery 88:467, 1980
42. Roberts AJ, Spies M, Sanders JH, et al: Serial assessment of left ventricular performance following coronary artery bypass grafting. J Thorac Cardiovasc Surg 81:69, 1981
43. Gray R, Maddahi J, Berman D, et al: Scintigraphic and hemodynamic demonstration of transient left ventricular dysfunction immediately after uncomplicated coronary artery bypass grafting. J Thorac Cardiovasc Surg 77:504, 1979
44. Reduto LA, Lawrie GM, Reid JW, et al: Sequential postoperative assessment of left ventricular performance with gated cardiac blood pool imaging following aortocoronary bypass surgery. Am Heart J 101:59, 1981
45. Mangano DT: Biventricular function after myocardial revascularization in humans: Deterioration and recovery patterns during the first 24 hours. Anesthesiology 62:571, 1985
46. Czer L, Hamer A, Murthey F, et al: Transient hemodynamic dysfunction after myocardial revascularization. J Thorac Cardiovasc Surg 86:226, 1983
47. Fremes SE, Weisel RD, Mickle DG, et al: Myocardial metabolism and ventricular function following cold potassium cardioplegia. J Thorac Cardiovasc Surg 89:531, 1985
48. Codd JE, Barner HB, Pennington DG, et al: Intraoperative myocardial protection: Comparison of blood and asanguineous cardioplegia. Ann Thorac Surg 39:125, 1985
49. Roberts AJ, Woodhall DD, Knauf DG, Alexander JA: Coronary artery bypass graft surgery: Clinical comparison of cold blood potassium cardioplegia, warm cardioplegic induction, and secondary cardioplegia. Ann Thorac Surg 40:483, 1985
50. Mullen JC, Christakis GT, Weisel RD, et al: Late postoperative ventricular function after blood and crystalloid cardioplegia. Circulation 74(suppl III):89, 1986
51. Rousou JA, Engleman RM, Breyer RH, et al: The effect of temperature and hematocrit level of oxygenated cardioplegic solutions of myocardial preservation. J Thorac Cardiovasc Surg 95:625, 1988

52. Khuri SF, Warner KG, Josa M, et al: The superiority of continuous cold blood cardioplegia in the metabolic protection of the hypertrophied human heart. J Thorac Cardiovasc Surg 95:442, 1988
53. Phillips HR, Carter JE, Okada RD, et al: Serial changes in left ventricular ejection in the early hours after aortocoronary bypass grafting. Chest 83:28, 1983
54. Salerno TA, Houck JP, Barrozo CAM, et al: Retrograde continuous warm blood cardioplegia: A new concept in myocardial protection. Ann Thorac Surg 51:245, 1991
55. Leung JM, O'Kelly B, Browner WS, et al: Prognostic importance of postbypass regional wall-motion abnormalities in patients undergoing coronary artery bypass graft surgery. Anesthesiology 71:16, 1989
56. Shernan SK: Perioperative myocardial ischemia reperfusion injury. Anesthesiol Clin North Am 21:465, 2003
57. Verrier ED, Shernan SK, Taylor KM: Terminal complement blockade with pexelizumab during coronary artery bypass graft surgery requiring cardiopulmonary bypass: A randomized trial. JAMA 291:2319, 2004
58. Bolli R: Oxygen-derived free radicals and postischemic myocardial dysfunction. J Am Coll Cardiol 12:239, 1988
59. Entman M, Michael M, Rossen R, et al: Inflammation in the course of early myocardial ischemia. FASEB J 5:2529, 1991
60. Maxwell S, Lip G: Reperfusion injury: A review of the pathophysiology, clinical manifestations and therapeutic options. Int J Cardiol 58:95, 1997
61. Shernan SK, Fitch JC, Nussmeier NA, et al: Impact of pexelizumab, an anti-C5 complement antibody, on total mortality and adverse cardiovascular outcomes in cardiac surgical patients undergoing cardiopulmonary bypass. Ann Thorac Surg 77:942, 2004
62. Jain U, Laflamme CJA, Aggarwal A, et al: Electrocardiographic and hemodynamic changes and their association with myocardial infarction during coronary artery bypass surgery. Anesthesiology 86:576, 1997
63. Mangano DT, Siciliano D, Hollenberg M, et al: Postoperative myocardial ischemia. Therapeutic trials using intensive analgesia following surgery. Anesthesiology 76:342, 1992
64. Cheng DCH, Karski J, Peniston C, et al: Morbidity outcome in early versus conventional tracheal extubation after coronary artery bypass grafting: A prospective randomized controlled trial. J Thorac Cardiovasc Surg 112:755, 1996
65. Wahr JA, Plunkett JJ, Ramsay JG, et al: Cardiovascular responses during sedation after coronary revascularization. Anesthesiology 84:1350, 1996
66. Rahimtoola SH, Ehsani A, Sinno MZ, et al: Left atrial transport function in myocardial infarction: Importance of its booster function. Am J Med 59:686, 1975
67. Mathew JP, Fontes ML, Tudor IC, et al: A multicenter risk index for atrial fibrillation after cardiac surgery. JAMA 291:1720, 2004
68. Hill LL, Kattapuram M, Hogue CW: Management of atrial fibrillation after cardiac surgery. Part 1. Pathophysiology and risks. J Cardiothorac Vasc Anesth 16:483, 2002
69. Van Dijk D, Nierich AP, Jansen EWL, et al: Early outcome after off-pump versus on-pump coronary bypass surgery. Circulation 104:1761, 2001
70. Puskas JD, Williams WH, Mahoney EM, et al: Off-pump versus conventional coronary artery bypass grafting: Early and 1-year graft patency, cost, and quality of life outcomes. JAMA 291:1841, 2004
71. Fuster V, Ryden LE, Asinger RW, et al: ACC/AHA/ECC guidelines for the management of patients with atrial fibrillation (executive summary). J Am Coll Cardiol 38:1231, 2001
72. Hill LL, De Wet C, Hogue CW: Management of atrial fibrillation after cardiac surgery. Part II. Prevention and treatment. J Cardiothorac Vasc Anesth 16:626, 2002
73. Daoud E, Strickberber S, Man K, et al: Preoperative amiodarone as prophylaxis against atrial fibrillation after heart surgery. N Engl J Med 337:1785, 1997
74. Guarnieri T, Nolan S, Gottlieb SO, et al: Intravenous amiodarone for the prevention of atrial fibrillation after open heart surgery: The Amiodarone Reduction in Coronary Heart (ARCH) trial. J Am Coll Cardiol 34:343, 1999
75. Sarnoff ST, Berglund E: Ventricular function. I. Starling's law of the heart studied by means of simultaneous right and left ventricular function curves in the dog. Circulation 9:706, 1954
76. Urbanowicz JH, Shaaban MJ, Cohen NH, et al: Comparison of transesophageal echocardiographic and scintigraphic estimates of left ventricular end-diastolic volume index and ejection fraction in patients following coronary artery bypass grafting. Anesthesiology 72:607, 1990
77. Harpole DH, Clements FM, Quill T, et al: Right and left ventricular performance during and after abdominal aortic aneurysm repair. Ann Surg 209:356, 1989
78. Thys DM, Hillel Z, Goldman ME, et al: A comparison of hemodynamic indices derived by invasive monitoring and two-dimensional echocardiography. Anesthesiology 67:630, 1987
79. Smith MD, MacPhail B, Harrison MR, et al: Value and limitations of transesophageal echocardiography in determination of left ventricular volumes and ejection fraction. J Am Coll Cardiol 19:1213, 1992
80. Ellis RJ, Mangano DT, Van Dyke DC: Relationship of wedge pressure to end-diastolic volume in patients undergoing myocardial revascularization. J Thorac Cardiovasc Surg 78:605, 1974
81. Calvin JE, Driedger AA, Sibbald WJ: Does the pulmonary capillary wedge pressure predict left ventricular preload in critically ill patients? Crit Care Med 9:437, 1981
82. Mangano DT, Van Dyke DC, Ellis RJ: The effect of increasing preload on ventricular output and ejection in man. Circulation 62:535, 1980
83. Breisblatt WM, Vita N, Armuchastegui M, et al: Usefulness of serial radionuclide monitoring during graded nitroglycerin infusion for unstable angina pectoris for determining left ventricular function and individualized therapeutic dose. Am J Cardiol 61:685, 1988
84. Bouchard MJ, Denault A, Couture P, et al: Poor correlation between hemodynamic and echocardiographic indexes of left ventricular performance in the operating room and intensive care unit. Crit Care Med 32:644, 2004
85. Breisblatt WM, Navratil DL, Burns MJ, Spaccavento LJ: Comparable effects of intravenous nitroglycerin and intravenous nitroprusside in acute ischemia. Am Heart J 116:465, 1988
86. Ghani MF, Parker BM, Smith JR: Recognition of myocardial infarction after cardiac surgery and its relation to cardiopulmonary bypass. Am Heart J 88:18, 1974
87. Chiarello M, Gold WK, Leinbach RC, et al: Comparison between the effects of nitroprusside and nitroglycerin on ischemic injury during acute myocardial infarction. Circulation 54:766, 1976
88. Marchionni N, Schneeweiss A, Di Bari M, et al: Age-related hemodynamic effects of intravenous nitroglycerin for acute myocardial infarction and left ventricular failure. Am J Cardiol 61:81E, 1988
89. Natarajan D, Khurana TR, Karnade V, et al: Sustained hemodynamic effects with therapeutic doses of intravenous nitroglycerin in congestive heart failure. Am J Cardiol 62:319, 1988
90. Katz AM: Cardiomyopathy of overload: A major determinant of prognosis in congestive heart failure. N Engl J Med 322:100, 1990
91. Muir AL, Nolan J: Modulation of venous tone in heart failure. Am Heart J 6:1948, 1991
92. Dikshit K, Vyden JK, Forrester JS, et al: Renal and extrarenal hemodynamic effects of furosemide in congestive heart failure after acute myocardial infarction. N Engl J Med 288:1087, 1973
93. Copeland JG, Campbell DW, Plachetka JR, et al: Diuresis with continuous infusion of furosemide after cardiac surgery. Am J Surg 146:796, 1983
94. Krasna MJ, Scott GE, Scholz PM, et al: Postoperative enhancement of urinary output in patients with acute renal failure using continuous furosemide therapy. Chest 89:294, 1986
95. Adams KF, Mathur VS, Gheorghiade M: B-type natriuretic peptide: From bench to bedside. Am Heart J 145:S34, 2003
96. Moazami N, Damiano DJ, Bailey MS, et al: Nesiritide (BNP) in the management of postoperative cardiac patients. Ann Thorac Surg 75:1974, 2003
97. Sward K, Valsson F, Odencrants P, et al: Recombinant human atrial natriuretic peptide in ischemic acute renal failure: A randomized placebo-controlled trial. Crit Care Med 32:1310, 2004
98. Caver A, Saccaggi A, Ronco C, et al: Continuous arteriovenous hemofiltration in the critically ill patient. Clinical use and operational characteristics. Ann Intern Med 99:455, 1983
99. Lamer C, Valleaux T, Plaisance P, et al: Continuous arteriovenous hemodialysis for acute renal failure after cardiac operations (letter). J Thorac Cardiovasc Surg 99:175, 1990
100. Sagawa K: The end-systolic pressure-volume relation of the ventricle: Definition, modifications, and clinical use. Circulation 63:1223, 1981
101. Suga H, Sagawa K, Shoukas AA: Load independence of the instantaneous pressure-volume ratio of the canine left ventricle and effects of epinephrine and heart rate on the ratio. Circ Res 32:314, 1973
102. Kass DA, Maughan WL: From "Emax" to pressure-volume relations: A broader view. Circulation 77:1203, 1988
103. Glower DD, Spratt JA, Snow ND, et al: Linearity of the Frank-Starling relationship in the intact heart: The concept of preload recruitable stroke work. Circulation 71:994, 1985
104. Hettrick DA, Warltier DC: Ventriculoarterial coupling. *In* Warltier DC (ed): Ventricular Function. Baltimore, Williams & Wilkins, 1995, pp 153–179
105. Sunagawa K, Maughan WL, Sagawa K: Optimal arterial resistance for the maximal stroke work studied in isolated canine left ventricle. Circ Res 56:586, 1985

106. Urzua J, Meneses G, Fajardo C, et al: Arterial pressure-flow relationships in patients undergoing cardiopulmonary bypass. Anesth Analg 84:958, 1997
107. Estafanous FG, Tarazi RC: Systemic arterial hypertension associated with cardiac surgery. Am J Cardiol 46:685,1980
108. Roberts AJ, Niarchos AP, Subramanian VA, et al: Systemic hypertension associated with coronary artery bypass surgery. Predisposing factors, hemodynamic characteristics, humoral profile, and treatment. J Thorac Cardiovasc Surg 74:846, 1977
109. Vuylsteke A, Feneck RO, Jolin-Mellgard A, et al: Perioperative blood pressure control: A prospective survey of patient management in cardiac surgery. J Cardiothorac Vasc Anesth 14:269, 2000
110. Wallach R, Karp RB, Reves JG, et al: Pathogenesis of paroxysmal hypertension developing during and after coronary bypass surgery: A study of hemodynamic and humoral factors. Am J Cardiol 46:559, 1980
111. Stinson EB, Holloway EL, Derby GC, et al: Control of myocardial performance early after open-heart operations by vasodilator treatment. J Thorac Cardiovasc Surg 73:523, 1977
112. Aronson S, Boisvert D, Lapp W: Isolated systolic hypertension is associated with adverse outcomes from coronary artery bypass grafting surgery. Anesth Analg 94:1079, 2002
113. Roberts AJ, Niarchos AP, Subramanian VA, et al: Hypertension following coronary artery bypass surgery. Comparison of hemodynamic responses to nitroprusside, phentolamine and converting enzyme inhibitor. Circulation 58(suppl I):49, 1978
114. Fremes SE, Weisel RD, Baird RJ, et al: Effect of postoperative hypertension and its treatment. J Thorac Cardiovasc Surg 86:47, 1983
115. Mann T, Cohn PF, Holman BL, et al: Comparison of esmolol and nitroprusside for acute postcardiac surgical hypertension. Am J Cardiol 57:732, 1978
116. Becker LC: Conditions of vasodilator-induced coronary steal in experimental myocardial ischemia. Circulation 57:1103, 1978
117. Flaherty JT, MaGee PA, Gardner TL, et al: Comparison of intravenous nitroglycerin and sodium nitroprusside for treatment of acute hypertension developing after coronary artery bypass surgery. Circulation 65:1072, 1982
118. Gray RJ, Bateman JM, Czer LSC, et al: Comparison of esmolol and nitroprusside for acute postcardiac surgical hypertension. Am J Cardiol 59:887, 1987
119. Morel DR, Forster A, Suter PM: IV labetalol in the treatment of hypertension following coronary artery surgery. Br J Anaesth 54:1191, 1982
120. Nordlander M, Abrahamsson T, Åkerblom B, Thalén P: Vascular versus myocardial selectivity of dihydropyridine calcium antagonists as studied in vivo and in vitro. Pharmacol Toxicol 75:56, 1995
121. Hess W, Schulte-Sasse U, Tarnow J: Nifedipine versus nitroprusside for controlling hypertensive episodes during coronary artery bypass surgery. Eur Heart J 5:140, 1984
122. David D, Dubois C, Loria Y: Comparison of nicardipine and sodium nitroprusside in the treatment of paroxysmal hypertension following aortocoronary bypass surgery. J Cardiothorac Vasc Anesth 5:357, 1991
123. Leslie J, Brister NW, Levy JH, et al: Treatment of postoperative hypertension following coronary artery bypass surgery: Double-blind comparison of intravenous isradipine and sodium nitroprusside. Circulation 90(suppl II):256, 1994
124. Bailey JM, Lu W, Levy JH, et al: Clevidipine in adult cardiac surgical patients: A dose-finding study. Anesthesiology 96:1086, 2002
125. Hill AJ, Feneck RO, Walesby RK: A comparison of fenoldopam and nitroprusside in the control of hypertension following coronary artery surgery. J Cardiothorac Vasc Anesth 7:279, 1993
126. Goldberg ME, Cantillo J, Nemiroff MS, et al: Fenoldopam infusion for the treatment of postoperative hypertension. J Clin Anesth 5:386, 1993
127. Levy JH, Huraux C, Nordlander M: Treatment of perioperative hypertension. *In* Epstein M (ed): Calcium Antagonists in Clinical Medicine. Philadelphia, Hanley & Belfus, 1997
128. Demarco T, Daly PA, Liv N, et al: Enalaprilat, a new parenteral angiotensin-converting enzyme inhibitor: Rapid changes in systemic and coronary hemodynamics and humoral profile in chronic heart failure. J Am Coll Cardiol 9:1131, 1987
129. Tuman KJ, McCarthy RJ, O'Connor CJ, et al: Angiotensin-converting enzyme inhibitors increase vasoconstrictor requirements after cardiopulmonary bypass. Anesth Analg 80:473, 1995
130. Kristoff AS, Magder S: Low systemic vascular resistance state in patients undergoing cardiopulmonary bypass. Crit Care Med 27:1121, 1999
131. Gomez WJ, Erlichman MR, Batista-Filho ML, et al: Vasoplegic syndrome after off-pump coronary artery bypass surgery. Eur J Cardiothorac Surg 23:165, 2003
132. Biglioli P, Cannata A, Alamanni F, et al: Biological effects of off pump vs on pump coronary artery surgery: Focus on inflammation, hemostasis and oxidative stress. Eur J Cardiothorac Surg 24:260, 2003
133. Gomez WJ, Carvalho AC, Palma JH, et al: Vasoplegic syndrome: A new dilemma. J Thorac Cardiovasc Surg 107:942, 1994
134. Chenoweth DE, Cooper SW, Hugli TE, et al: Complement activation during cardiopulmonary bypass: Evidence of generation of C3a and C5a anaphylatoxins. N Engl J Med 304:497, 1981
135. Landry DW, Oliver JA: The pathogenesis of vasodilatory shock. N Engl J Med 345:588, 2001
136. Haeffner-Cavaillon N, Roussellier N, Ponzio O, et al: Induction of interleukin-1 production in patients undergoing cardiopulmonary bypass. J Thorac Cardiovasc Surg 98:1100, 1989
137. Bennett-Guerrero E, Barclay GR, Weng PL, et al: Endotoxin-neutralizing capacity of serum from cardiac surgical patients. J Cardiothorac Vasc Anesth 15:451, 2001
138. Aydin NB, Gercekoglu H, Aksu B, et al: Endotoxemia in coronary artery bypass surgery: A comparison of the off-pump technique and conventional cardiopulmonary bypass. J Thorac Cardiovasc Surg 125:843, 2003
139. Argenziano M, Chen JM, Choudhri AF, et al: Management of vasodilatory shock after cardiac surgery: Indentification of predisposing factors and use of a novel pressor agent. J Thorac Cardiovasc Surg 116:973, 1998
140. Levy JH: Anaphylactic Reactions in Anesthesia and Intensive Care, 2nd edition. Boston, Butterworth-Heinemann, 1992
141. LeDoux D, Astiz ME, Carpati CM, et al: Effects of perfusion pressure on tissue perfusion in septic shock. Crit Care Med 28:2729, 2000
142. Desjars P, Pinaud M, Potel G, et al: A reappraisal of norepinephrine therapy in human septic shock. Crit Care Med 15:134, 1987
143. Levy JH, Tanaka KA: Inflammatory response to cardiopulmonary bypass. Ann Thorac Surg 75:S715, 2003
144. Addonizio VP, Smith JB, Strauss JF, et al: Thromboxane synthesis and platelet secretion during cardiopulmonary bypass with bubble oxygenator. J Thorac Cardiovasc Surg 79:91, 1980
145. Engelman RM, Harji-Rovsov I, Breyer RH, et al: Rebound vasospasm after coronary revascularization. Ann Thorac Surg 37:469, 1984
146. Salmenpera MT, Levy JH: Effects of phosphodiesterase inhibitors on the human internal mammary artery. Anesth Analg 82:954, 1996
147. Huraux C, Makita T, Szlam F, et al: Vasodilator effects of clevidipine on human internal mammary artery. Anesth Analg 85:1000, 1997
148. Acar C, Jebara VA, Portoghese M, et al: Revival of the radial artery for coronary artery bypass grafting. Ann Thorac Surg 54:652, 1992
149. da Costa FDA, da Costa IA, Poffo R, et al: Myocardial revascularization with the radial artery: A clinical and angiographic study. Ann Thorac Surg 62:475, 1996
150. Dietl CA, Benoit CH: Radial artery graft for coronary revascularization: Technical considerations. Ann Thorac Surg 60:102, 1995
151. Royster RL, Butterworth JF IV, Prielipp RC, et al: A randomized, blinded, placebo-controlled evaluation of calcium chloride and epinephrine for inotropic support after emergence from cardiopulmonary bypass. Anesth Analg 74:3, 1992
152. Zaloga GP, Strickland RA, Butterworth JF IV, et al: Calcium attenuated epinephrine's beta-adrenergic effects in postoperative heart surgery patients. Circulation 81:196, 1991
153. Drop LJ: Ionized calcium, the heart, and hemodynamic function. Anesth Analg 64:432, 1985
154. Bristow MR, Ginsburg R, Umans V, et al: β_1- and β_2-adrenergic receptor subpopulations in normal and failing human ventricular myocardium. Coupling of both receptor subtypes to muscle contraction and selective β_1-receptor down-regulation in heart failure. Circ Res 59:297, 1986
155. Levy JH, Bailey JM, Deeb M: Intravenous milrinone in cardiac surgery. Ann Thorac Surg 73:325, 2002
156. Stephenson LW, Blackstone EH, Kouchoukos NT: Dopamine vs. epinephrine in patients following cardiac surgery: Randomized study. Surg Forum 27:272, 1976
157. Butterworth JF, Prielipp RC, Zaloga GP, et al: Is dobutamine less chronotropic than epinephrine after coronary bypass surgery? Anesthesiology 73(suppl 3A): A61, 1990
158. Sung BH, Robinson C, Thadani U, et al: Effects of L-epinephrine on hemodynamics and cardiac function in coronary disease: Dose-response studies. Clin Pharmacol Ther 43:308, 1988
159. Totaro RJ, Raper RF: Epinephrine-induced lactic acidosis following cardiopulmonary bypass. Crit Care Med 25:1693, 1997
160. Levy JH: Pharmacologic and mechanical methods of discontinuing extracorporeal circulation. J Cardiothorac Vasc Anesth 7(suppl 1):12, 1993

161. D'Ambra MN, LaRaia PJ, Philbin DM, et al: Prostaglandin E_1—a new therapy for refractory right heart failure and pulmonary hypertension after mitral valve replacement. J Thorac Cardiovasc Surg 89:567, 1985
162. Leier CV, Heran PT, Huss P, et al: Comparative systemic and regional hemodynamic effects of dopamine and dobutamine in patients with cardiomyopathic heart failure. Circulation 58:466, 1978
163. Port JD, Gilbert EM, Larrabee P, et al: Neurotransmitter depletion compromises the ability of indirect acting amines to provide inotropic support in the failing human heart. Circulation 81:929, 1990
164. Lehmann A, Boldt J: New pharmacologic approaches for the perioperative treatment of ischemic cardiogenic shock. J Cardiothorac Vasc Anesth 19:97, 2005
165. DiSesa V, Gold J, Shemin R, et al: Comparison of dopamine and dobutamine in patients requiring postoperative circulatory support. Clin Cardiol 9:253, 1986
166. Royster RL: Intraoperative administration of inotropes in cardiac surgery patients. J Cardiothorac Anesth 4:17, 1990
167. Davis RF, Cappas DG, Kirklin JK, et al: Acute oliguria after cardiopulmonary bypass: Renal functional improvement with low-dose dopamine infusion. Crit Care Med 10:852, 1982
168. Bellomo R, Chapman M, Finfer S, et al: Low-dose dopamine in patients with early renal dysfunction: A placebo-controlled randomized trial: Australian and New Zealand Intensive Care Society (ANZICS) Clinical Trials Group. Lancet 356:2139, 2000
169. Holmes C, Walley KR: Bad medicine: Low-dose dopamine in the ICU. Crit Care Med 123:1266, 2003
170. Ward HB, Einzig S, Wang T, et al: Enhanced cardiac efficiency with dobutamine after global ischemia. J Surg Res 33:32, 1982
171. Stephens J, Ead H, Spurrell R: Haemodynamic effects of dobutamine with special reference to myocardial blood flow: A comparison with dopamine and isoprenaline. Br Heart J 42:269, 1981
172. Fowler MB, Alderman EL, Oesterle SN, et al: Dobutamine and dopamine after cardiac surgery: Greater augmentation of myocardial blood flow with dobutamine. Circulation 70(suppl I):103, 1984
173. Romson JL, Leung JM, Bellows WH, et al: Effects of dobutamine on hemodynamics and left ventricular performance after cardiopulmonary bypass in cardiac surgical patients. Anesthesiology 91:1318, 1999
174. Salomon NW, Plachetka JR, Copeland JG: Comparison of dopamine and dobutamine following coronary artery bypass grafting. Ann Thorac Surg 33:48, 1982
175. Bristow MR, Ginsburg R, Minobe W, et al: Decreased catecholamine sensitivity and beta-adrenergic receptor density in failing human hearts. N Engl J Med 307:205, 1982
176. Gain KR, Appleman MM: Distribution and regulation of the phosphodiesterases of muscle tissues. Adv Cyclic Nucleotide Res 10:221, 1978
177. Weishaar RE, Burrows SD, Kobylarz DC, et al: Multiple molecular forms of cyclic nucleotide phosphodiesterase in cardiac and smooth muscle and in platelets. Isolation, characterization, and effects of various reference phosphodiesterase inhibitors and cardiotonic agents. Biochem Pharmacol 35:787, 1986
178. Kukovetz WR, Poch G, Holzmann S: Cyclic nucleotides and relaxation of vascular smooth muscle. *In* Vanhoutte PM, Leusen I (eds): Vasodilatation. New York, Raven Press, 1981, pp 339–353
179. Benotti JR, Grossman W, Braunwald E, et al: Hemodynamic assessment of amrinone. N Engl J Med 299:1373, 1987
180. Levy JL, Bailey JM: Amrinone: Its effects on vascular resistance and capacitance in human subjects. Chest 105:62, 1994
181. Benotti JR, Grossman W, Braunwald E, et al: Effects of amrinone on myocardial energy metabolism and hemodynamics in patients with severe congestive heart failure due to coronary artery disease. Circulation 62:28, 1980
182. Goenen M, Pedemonte O, Baele P, et al: Amrinone in the management of low cardiac output after open heart surgery. Am J Cardiol 56:33B, 1985
183. Bailey JM, Levy JH, Kikura M, et al: Pharmacokinetics of milrinone during cardiac surgery. Anesthesiology 81:616, 1994
184. Konstam MA, Cohen SR, Weiland DS, et al: Relative contribution of inotropic and vasodilator effects to amrinone-induced hemodynamic improvement in congestive heart failure. Am J Cardiol 57:242, 1986
185. Firth BG, Ratner AV, Grassman ED, et al: Assessment of the inotropic and vasodilator effects of amrinone versus isoproterenol. Am J Cardiol 54:1331, 1984
186. Baim DS, McDowell AV, Cherniles J, et al: Evaluation of a new bipyridine inotropic agent—Milrinone—in patients with severe congestive heart failure. N Engl J Med 309:748, 1983
187. Gonzalez M, Desager J-P, Jacquemart J-L, et al: Efficacy of enoximone in the management of refractory low-output states following cardiac surgery. J Cardiothorac Anesth 2:409, 1988
188. Boldt J, Kling D, Zickmann B, et al: Efficacy of the phosphodiesterase inhibitor enoximone in complicated cardiac surgery. Chest 98:53, 1990
189. Kikura M, Lee MK, Safon R, et al: Effect of milrinone on platelets in patients undergoing cardiac surgery. Anesth Analg 81:44, 1995
190. Gilbert EM, Mealey P, Volkman K, et al: Combination therapy with enoximone and dobutamine is superior to nitroprusside and dobutamine in heart failure. Circulation 78:109, 1988
191. Gage J, Rutman H, Lucido D, et al: Additive effects of dobutamine and amrinone on myocardial contractility and ventricular performance in patients with severe heart failure. Circulation 74:367, 1986
192. Prielipp RC, MacGregor DA, Butterworth JF, et al: Pharmacodynamics and pharmacokinetics of milrinone administration to increase oxygen delivery in critically ill patients. Chest 109:1291, 1996
193. Boldt J, Kling D, Moosdorf R, Hempelmann G: Enoximone treatment of impaired myocardial function during cardiac surgery: Combined effects with epinephrine. J Cardiothorac Anesth 4:462, 1990
194. Kikura M, Levy JH, Bailey JM, et al: Effects of milrinone on ventricular function after emergence from cardiopulmonary bypass. Anesth Analg 85:16, 1997
195. Kikura M, Levy JH, Bailey JM, et al: A bolus dose of 1.5 mg/kg amrinone effectively improves low cardiac output state following separation from cardiopulmonary bypass in cardiac surgical patients. Acta Anaesthesiol Scand 42:825, 1998
196. Bondy R, Ramsay JG: Reversal of refractory right ventricular failure with amrinone. J Cardiothorac Anesth 5:255, 1991
197. Edelson J, LeJemtel TH, Alousi AA, et al: Relationship between amrinone plasma concentration and cardiac index. Clin Pharmacol Ther 29:723, 1981
198. Park GB, Kershner RP, Angelotti J, et al: Oral bioavailability and intravenous pharmacokinetics of amrinone in humans. J Pharm Sci 72:817, 1983
199. Kikura M, Levy JH: New cardiac drugs. Int Anesthesiol Clin 33:21, 1995
200. Rocci ML, Wilson H, Likoff M, et al: Amrinone pharmacokinetics after single and steady-state doses in patients with chronic cardiac failure. Clin Pharmacol Ther 33:260, 1983
201. Bailey JM, Levy JH, Rogers G, et al: Pharmacokinetics of amrinone during cardiac surgery. Anesthesiology 75:961, 1991
202. Ramsay JG, DeJesus JM, Wynands JE, et al: Amrinone before termination of cardiopulmonary bypass: Hemodynamic variables and oxygen utilization in the postbypass period. Can J Anaesth 39:342, 1992
203. Feneck RO: Effects of variable dose milrinone in patients with low cardiac output after cardiac surgery. Am Heart J 121(suppl 2):1995, 1991
204. Naeije R, Carlier E, DeSmet JM, et al: Enoximone in low-output states following cardiac surgery. J Crit Care 4:112, 1989
205. Kivikko M, Lehtonen L, Colucci WS, et al: Sustained hemodynamic effects of intravenous levosimendan. Circulation 107:81, 2003
206. Follath F, Cleland JG, Just H, et al: Efficacy and safety of intravenous levosimendan compared with dobutamine in severe low-output heart failure (the LIDO study): A randomized double-blind trial. Lancet 360:196, 2002
207. Moiseyev VS, Poder P, Anderjevs N, et al: Safety and efficacy of a novel calcium sensitizer, levosimendan, in patients with left ventricular failure due to an acute myocardial infarction. A randomized, placebo-controlled, double-blind study (RUSSLAN). Eur Heart J 23:1422, 2002
208. Labriola C, Siro-Brigiani M, Carrata F, et al: Hemodynamic effects of levosimendan in patients with low-output heart failure after cardiac surgery. Int J Clin Pharmacol Ther 42:204, 2004
209. Jacobs A, Leopold J, Bates E, et al: Cardiogenic shock caused by right ventricular infarction: A report from the SHOCK registry. J Am Coll Cardiol 41:1273, 2003
210. Hayashida N, Ikonomidis JS, Weisel RD, et al: Adequate distribution of warm cardioplegic solution. J Thorac Cardiovasc Surg 110:800, 1995
211. Boldt J, Kling D, Thiel A, et al: Revascularization of the right coronary artery: Influence on thermodilution right ventricular ejection fraction. J Cardiothorac Anesth 2:140, 1988
212. Schulman DS, Biondi JW, Zohgbi S, et al: Coronary flow and right ventricular performance during positive end-expiratory pressure. Am Rev Respir Dis 141:1531, 1990
213. Matthay RA, Ellis JH, Steele PP: Methoxamine-induced increase in afterload. Effect on left ventricular performance in chronic obstructive pulmonary disease. Am Rev Respir Dis 117:871, 1978
214. Mikami T, Kudo T, Sakurai N, et al: Mechanisms for development of functional tricuspid regurgitation determined by pulsed Doppler and two-dimensional echocardiography. Am J Cardiol 53:160, 1984
215. Heinonen J, Salmenpera M, Takkunen O: Increased pulmonary artery diastolic-pulmonary wedge pressure gradient after cardiopulmonary bypass. Can Anaesth Soc J 32:165, 1985

216. Byrick RJ, Kay JC, Noble WH: Extravascular lung water accumulation in patients following coronary artery surgery. Can Anaesth Soc J 24:332, 1977
217. Chernow B, Rainey TG, Lake CR: Endogenous and exogenous catecholamines in critical care medicine. Crit Care Med 10:407, 1982
218. Colman RW: Platelet and neutrophil activation in cardiopulmonary bypass. Ann Thorac Surg 49:32, 1990
219. Chenoweth DE, Cooper SW, Hugli TE, et al: Complement activation during cardiopulmonary bypass. Evidence for generation of C3a and C5a anaphylatoxins. N Engl J Med 304:497, 1991
220. Anjoyu-Lindskog E, Broman L, Broman M, Holmgren A: Effects of oxygen on central hemodynamics and VA/Q distribution after coronary bypass surgery. Acta Anaesthesiol Scand 27:378, 1983
221. Salmenpera M, Heinonen J: Pulmonary vascular responses to moderate changes in $Pa{CO_2}$ after cardiopulmonary bypass. Anesthesiology 64:311, 1986
222. Viitanen A, Salmenpera M, Hynynen M, Heinonen J: Pulmonary vascular resistance before and after cardiopulmonary bypass. The effect of $Pa{CO_2}$. Chest 95:773, 1989
223. Viitanen A, Salmenpera M, Heinonen J: Right ventricular response to hypercarbia after cardiac surgery. Anesthesiology 73:393, 1990
224. Lloyd EA, Gersh BJ, Kennelly BM: Hemodynamic spectrum of "dominant" right ventricular infarction in 19 patients. Am J Cardiol 48:1016, 1981
225. Kay H, Afshari M, Barash P, et al: Measurement of ejection fraction by thermal dilution techniques. J Surg Res 34:337, 1983
226. Spinale FG, Smith AC, Carabello BA, Crawford FA: Right ventricular function computed by thermodilution and ventriculography; a comparison of methods. J Thorac Cardiovasc Surg 99:141, 1990
227. Dell'Italia LJ, Starling MR, Blumhardt R, et al: Comparative effects of volume loading, dobutamine, and nitroprusside in patients with predominant right ventricular infarction. Circulation 72:1327, 1985
228. Berisha S, Kastrati A, Goda A, Popa Y: Optimal value of filling pressure in the right side of the heart in acute myocardial infarction. Br Heart J 63:98, 1990
229. Brinker JA, Weiss JL, Lapp DL, et al: Leftward septal displacement during right ventricular loading in man. Circulation 61:626, 1980
230. Hess W, Arnold B, Veit S: The haemodynamic effects of amrinone in patients with mitral stenosis and pulmonary hypertension. Eur Heart J 7:800, 1986
231. Ichinose F, Roberts JD, Zapol WM: Inhaled nitric oxide: A selective pulmonary vasodilator; current uses and therapeutic potential. Circulation 109:3106, 2004
232. Shime N: Contemporary trends in postoperative intensive care for pediatric cardiac surgery. J Cardiothorac Vasc Anesth 18:218, 2004
233. Girard C, Lehot J-J, Pannetier J-C, et al: Inhaled nitric oxide after mitral valve replacement in patients with chronic pulmonary artery hypertension. Anesthesiology 77:880, 1992
234. Ardehali A, Hughes K, Sadeghi A, et al: Inhaled nitric oxide for pulmonary hypertension after cardiac transplantation. Transplantation 72:638, 2001
235. Argenziano M, Choudhri AF, Moazami N, et al: Randomized, double-blind trial of inhaled nitric oxide in LVAD recipients with pulmonary hypertension. Ann Thorac Surg 65:340, 1998
236. Meade MO, Granton JT, Matte-Martyn A et al: A randomized trial of inhaled nitric oxide to prevent ischemia-reperfusion injury after lung transplantation. Am J Respir Crit Care Med 167:1483, 2003
237. Haraldsson A, Kieler-Jensen N, Ricksten S-E: Inhaled prostacyclin for treatment of pulmonary hypertension after cardiac surgery or heart transplantation: A pharmacodynamic study. J Cardiothorac Vasc Anesth 10:864, 1996
238. Webb SA, Scott S, van Heerden PV: The use of inhaled aerosolized prostacyclin (IAP) in the treatment of pulmonary hypertension secondary to pulmonary embolism. Intensive Care Med 22:353, 1996
239. Heerden PV, Barden A, Michalopoulos N, et al: Dose-response to inhaled aerosolized prostacyclin for hypoxemia due to ARDS. Chest 117:819, 2000
240. Domenighetti G, Stricker H, Waldispuehl B: Nebulized prostacyclin (PGI_2) in acute respiratory distress syndrome: Impact of primary (pulmonary injury) and secondary (extrapulmonary injury) on gas exchange response. Crit Care Med 29:57, 2001
241. Haraldsson A, Kieler-Jensen N, Ricksten SE: The additive pulmonary vasodilatory effects of inhaled prostacyclin and inhaled milrinone in postcardiac surgical patients with pulmonary hypertension. Anesth Analg 93:1439, 2001
242. Drummond WH, Gregory GA, Heyman MA, Phibbs RA: The independent effects of hyperventilation, tolazoline, and dopamine on infants with persistent pulmonary hypertension. J Pediatr 98:603, 1981
243. Mahdi M, Salem MR, Joseph NJ, et al: Influence of moderate hypocapnia on pulmonary vascular tone following mitral valve replacement. Anesthesiology 75:A166, 1991
244. Miller DC, Moreno-Cabral RJ, Stinson EB, et al: Pulmonary artery balloon counterpulsation for acute right ventricular infarction. J Thorac Cardiovasc Surg 80:760, 1980
245. Higgins TL, Yared JP, Paranandi L, et al: Risk factors for respiratory complications after cardiac surgery. Anesthesiology 75:A258, 1991
246. Vuori A, Jalonen J, Laaksonen V: Continuous positive airway pressure during mechanical ventilation and spontaneous ventilation: Effects on central hemodynamics and oxygen transport. Acta Anaesthesiol Scand 23:453, 1979
247. Morgan BC, Abel FL, Mullins GL, Guntheroth WG: Flow patterns in cavae, pulmonary artery, pulmonary vein and aorta in intact dogs. Am J Physiol 210:903, 1966
248. Harken HA, Brennan MF, Smith B, Barsamian EM: The hemodynamic response to positive end-expiratory pressure ventilation in hypovolemic patients. Surgery 76:786, 1974
249. Wallis TW, Robotham JL, Compean R, Kindred MK: Mechanical heart-lung interaction with positive end-expiratory pressure. J Appl Physiol 54:1039, 1983
250. Pinsky MR, Matuschak GM, Klain M: Determinants of cardiac augmentation by elevations in intrathoracic pressure. J Appl Physiol 58:1189, 1985
251. Canada E, Benumof JL, Tousdale FR: Pulmonary vascular resistance correlates in intact normal and abnormal canine lungs. Crit Care Med 10:719, 1982
252. Permutt S, Howell JBL, Proctor DF, Riley RL: Effect of lung inflation on static pressure-volume characteristics of pulmonary vessels. J Appl Physiol 16:64, 1961
253. McGregor M: Pulsus paradoxus. N Engl J Med 301:480, 1979
254. Grace MP, Greenbaum DM: Cardiac performance in response to PEEP in patients with cardiac dysfunction. Crit Care Med 10:358, 1982
255. Mathru M, Rao TLK, El-Etr AA, Pifarre R: Hemodynamic response to changes in ventilatory patterns in patients with normal and poor left ventricular reserve. Crit Care Med 10:423, 1982
256. Schulman DS, Biondi JW, Matthay RA, et al: Effect of positive end-expiratory pressure on right ventricular performance-importance of baseline right ventricular function. Am J Med 84:57, 1988
257. Calvin JE, Driedger AA, Sibbald WJ: Positive end-expiratory pressure (PEEP) does not depress left ventricular function in patients with pulmonary edema. Am Rev Respir Dis 124:121, 1981
258. Glick G, Wechsler AS, Epstein SE: Reflex cardiovascular depression produced by stimulation of pulmonary stretch receptors in the dog. J Clin Invest 48:467, 1979
259. Dunham BM, Grindlinger GA, Utsunomiya T, et al: Role of prostaglandins in positive end-expiratory pressure-induced negative inotropism. Am J Physiol 241:783, 1981
260. Pinsky MR, Marquez J, Martin D, Klain M: Ventricular assist by cardiac cycle–specific increases in intrathoracic pressure. Chest 91:709, 1987
261. Garner W, Downs JB, Stock MC, Rasanen J: Airway pressure release ventilation (APRV)—a human trial. Chest 94:779, 1988
262. Cane RD, Shapiro BA: Ventilator discontinuance and weaning. Anesth Clin North Am 5:749, 1987
263. Lemaire F, Teboul J-L, Cinotti L, et al: Acute left ventricular dysfunction during unsuccessful weaning from mechanical ventilation. Anesthesiology 69:171, 1988
264. Permutt S: Circulatory effects of weaning from mechanical ventilation: The importance of transdiaphragmatic pressure. Anesthesiology 69:157, 1988
265. Rasanen J, Nikki P, Heikkila J: Acute myocardial infarction complicated by respiratory failure. The effects of mechanical ventilation. Chest 85:21, 1984
266. Hurford WE, Lynch KE, Strauss W, et al: Myocardial perfusion as assessed by thallium 201 scintigraphy during the discontinuation of mechanical ventilation in ventilator-dependent patients. Anesthesiology 74:1007, 1991
267. Tahvanainen J, Salmenpera M, Nikki P: Extubation criteria after weaning from intermittent mandatory ventilation and continuous positive airway pressure. Crit Care Med 11:702, 1983
268. Russo A, O'Connor W, Waxman H: Atypical presentations and echocardiographic findings in patients with cardiac tamponade occurring early and late after cardiac surgery. Chest 104:71, 1993
269. Yilmaz AT, Arslan M, Demirklic U, et al: Late posterior cardiac tamponade after open heart surgery. J Cardiovasc Surg 37:615, 1996
270. Borkon AM, Schaff HV, Gardner TJ, et al: Diagnosis and management of postoperative pericardial effusions and late cardiac tamponade following open heart surgery. Ann Thorac Surg 31:512, 1981

271. King TE, Stelzner TJ, Steven A, Sahn SA: Cardiac tamponade complicating the postpericardiotomy syndrome. Chest 83:500, 1983
272. Chuttani K, Pandian NG, Mohanty PK, et al: Left ventricular diastolic collapse. An echocardiographic sign of regional cardiac tamponade. Circulation 83:1999, 1991
273. Fowler NO: Physiology of cardiac tamponade and pulsus paradoxus. Physiological, circulatory, and pharmacologic responses in cardiac tamponade. Mod Concepts Cardiovasc Dis 47:115, 1978
274. Hynynen M, Salmenpera M, Harjula ALJ, et al: Atrial pressure and hormonal and renal responses to acute cardiac tamponade. Ann Thorac Surg 49:632, 1990
275. Kochar GS, Jacobs LE, Kotler MN: Right atrial compression in postoperative cardiac patients: Detection by transesophageal echocardiography. J Am Coll Cardiol 16:511, 1990
276. Bommer WJ, Follette D, Pollock M, et al: Tamponade in patients undergoing cardiac surgery: A clinical-echocardiographic diagnosis. Am Heart J 130:1216, 1995
277. Chuttani K, Tischler MD, Pandian NG, et al: Diagnosis of cardiac tamponade after cardiac surgery: Relative value of clinical, echocardiographic, and hemodynamic signs. Am Heart J 127:913, 1994
278. D'Cruz IA, Kensey K, Campbell C, et al: Two-dimensional echocardiography in cardiac tamponade occurring after cardiac surgery. J Am Coll Cardiol 5:1250, 1985
279. Reichert CL, Visser CA, Koolen JJ, et al: Transesophageal echocardiography in hypotensive patients after cardiac operations. Comparison with hemodynamic parameters. J Thorac Cardiovasc Surg 104:321, 1992
280. Settle HP, Adolph RJ, Fowler NO, et al: Echocardiographic study of cardiac tamponade. Circulation 56:951, 1977
281. Singh SM, Wann LS, Schuchard GH, et al: Right ventricular and right atrial collapse in patients with cardiac tamponade-a combined echocardiographic and hemodynamic study. Circulation 70:966, 1984
282. Russo AM, O'Connor WH, Waxman HL: Atypical presentations and echocardiographic findings in patients with cardiac tamponade occurring early and late after cardiac surgery. Chest 104:71, 1993
283. Mattila I, Takkunen O, Mattila P, et al: Cardiac tamponade and different modes of artificial ventilation. Acta Anaesthesiol Scand 23:236, 1984
284. Ziemer G, Karck M, Muller H, Luhmer I: Staged chest closure in pediatric cardiac surgery preventing typical and atypical cardiac tamponade. Eur J Cardiothorac Surg 6:91, 1992
285. Addonizio LJ, Gersony WM, Robbins RC, et al: Elevated pulmonary vascular resistance and cardiac transplantation. Circulation 76(suppl V): 52, 1987
286. Valantine HA, Schroeder JS: Cardiac transplantation. Intensive Care Med 15:283, 1989
287. O'Connell JB, Renlund DG, Bristow MR: Murine monoclonal CD3 antibody (OKT3) in cardiac transplantation: Three-year experience. Transplant Proc 21(suppl 2): 31, 1989

Chapter 34

POSTOPERATIVE RESPIRATORY CARE

Thomas L. Higgins, MD • Jean-Pierre Yared, MD

KEY POINTS

1. Pulmonary complications following cardiopulmonary bypass are relatively common, with up to 12% of patients experiencing acute lung injury and about 1.5% requiring tracheostomy for long-term ventilation.
2. Risk factors for postoperative respiratory insufficiency include advanced age, presence of diabetes or renal failure, chronic obstructive lung disease, peripheral vascular disease, prior cardiac surgery, and emergency or unstable status.
3. Patients with preexisting chronic obstructive lung disease have higher rates of pulmonary complications, atrial fibrillation, and death.
4. Operating room events that increase risk include reoperation, blood transfusion, prolonged cardiopulmonary bypass time, and low cardiac output states, particularly if a mechanical support device is required.
5. Hospital-acquired infections are an important cause of postoperative morbidity and nosocomial pneumonia. Strategies to reduce the incidence of ventilator-associated pneumonia include early removal of gastric and tracheal tubes, formal infection control programs, handwashing, semirecumbent positioning of the patient, and scheduled drainage of condensate from ventilated circuits.
6. Patients at risk for acute lung injury and those developing acute respiratory distress syndrome should be switched to a lung-protective ventilation strategy, which involves maintaining peak inspiratory pulmonary pressure less than 35 cm H_2O and restricting tidal volumes to 6 mL/kg of ideal body weight.
7. Permissive hypercapnia may be necessary to accomplish lung-protective ventilatory strategy.
8. Impediments to weaning and extubation include delirium, unstable hemodynamics, respiratory muscle dysfunction, renal failure with fluid overload, and sepsis.
9. Short-term weaning success can be achieved with any variety of ventilation modes. The long-term patient requires an individualized approach, which may encompass pressure-support ventilation, synchronized intermittent mandatory ventilation weaning, or T-piece trials.
10. While a number of parameters exist to assess respiratory strength and endurance, the single best parameter is the frequency–to–tidal volume ratio.
11. Long-term administration of neuromuscular blocking agents is associated with persistent muscle weakness. Possible causes include accumulation of drug metabolites, critical illness polyneuropathy, or neurogenic atrophy.
12. A very small percentage of patients will not be able to be weaned from ventilation support. Characteristics of these patients include persistent low-output state with multisystem organ failure. Long-term weaning may be best accomplished in a specialized unit rather than an acute cardiovascular recovery area.

Patients undergoing cardiac surgery experience physiologic stresses from anesthesia, thoracotomy, surgical manipulation, and cardiopulmonary bypass (CPB). Each of these interventions can create transient deleterious effects on pulmonary function even with normal lungs; the effects may be exaggerated in the presence of preexisting pulmonary pathology. Important pulmonary changes after cardiac surgery include diminished functional residual capacity (FRC) following general anesthesia and muscle relaxants, transient 50% to 75% reduction in vital capacity (VC) following median sternotomy and intrathoracic manipulation, atelectasis, and increased intravascular lung water.[1-3] Acute FRC reduction results in arterial hypoxemia due to mismatch between ventilation and perfusion, and diminished lung compliance with increased work of breathing (WOB). This additional WOB, which increases oxygen consumption by up to 20% in spontaneously breathing patients, also increases myocardial work at a time when myocardial reserves may be limited.[4] Changes in spirometric measurements and respiratory muscle strength can last up to 8 weeks postoperatively.[5]

Thus, a sizeable proportion of cardiac surgical patients can be expected to have respiratory complications. In recent experience, about a quarter of cardiac surgical patients were extubated in the operating room or within 4 hours of intensive care unit (ICU) arrival, and about half within 8 hours of ICU arrival (Fig. 34–1). Median postprocedure intubation time was 7.6 hours. About 8% of patients experienced prolonged mechanical ventilation (defined as >72 hours following ICU arrival), and about 7% required reintubation of the trachea either shortly after initial extubation or because of delayed respiratory failure. Acute lung injury (ALI), sometimes progressing to acute respiratory distress syndrome (ARDS), can occur in up to 12% of postoperative cardiac patients.[6] Tracheostomy was performed in 1.4% of post-CPB patients to facilitate recovery and weaning from ventilatory support. While these figures represent the experience of one referral center, others have reported similar results (Table 34–1).

RISK FACTORS FOR RESPIRATORY INSUFFICIENCY

The lung is especially vulnerable as disturbances may affect it directly (atelectasis, effusions, pneumonia) or indirectly (via fluid overload in heart failure, as the result of mediator release during CPB, shock states, or infection, or via changes in respiratory pump function as with phrenic nerve injury). Postoperative status will be determined in part by the patient's preoperative pulmonary reserve, as well as by the level of stress imposed by the procedure. Thus, a patient with reduced VC due to restrictive lung disease, undergoing minimally invasive surgery, may have fewer postoperative pulmonary issues than a relatively healthy patient undergoing simultaneous coronary artery bypass grafting and valve replacement with its accompanying longer operative/anesthetic and CPB times. Respiratory muscle weakness contributes to postoperative pulmonary

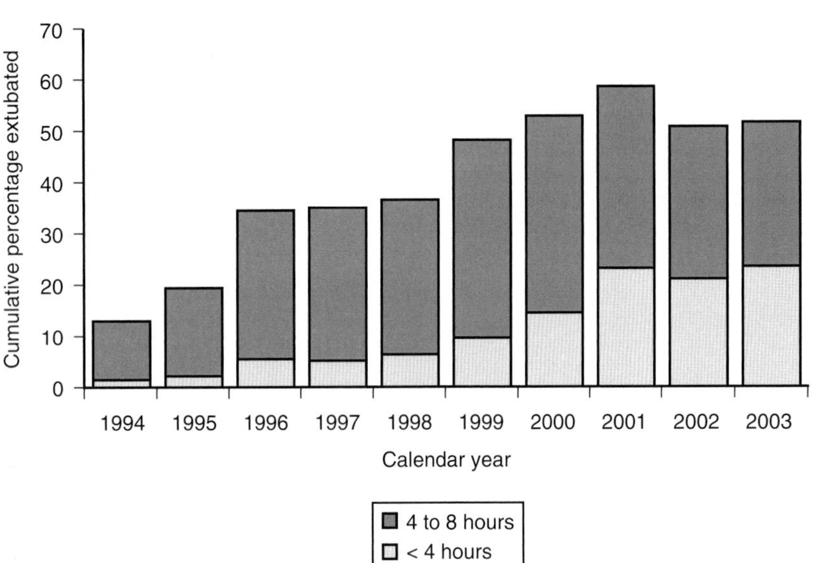

Figure 34–1 A decade of process improvement with fast-track recovery from cardiac anesthesia is demonstrated. Most recently, about one quarter of patients are extubated within 4 hours of arrival and another quarter within the first 8 hours at the Cleveland Clinic.

Table 34–1 **Pulmonary Complications**

Reference	No. of Patients	Median Time to Extubation (days)	Prolonged Mechanical Ventilation	Reintubation	Tracheostomy	In-Hospital Mortality
Spivack et al, Chest 1996;109:1222, 1991 to 1992	513	0.83 (0.2 to 36)	8.3% (>48 hr)	NR	NR	2.0%
Rady et al, Crit Care Med 1999;27:340, 1993 to 1996	11,330	2.2	NR	6.6%	NR	3.5%
Branca et al, Chest 2001;119:537, 1996 to 1997	4,863	2 (1 to 105)	5.9% (>72 hr)	3.2%	0.8%	1.95%
Recent Cleveland Clinic experience 1998 to 2001 (unpublished)	13,191	0.32 day	4% to 11%	7%	1.4%	NR

NR = not reported.

dysfunction, and prophylactic inspiratory muscle training has been shown to improve respiratory muscle function, pulmonary function tests, and gas exchange. Training reduces the percentage of patients requiring more than 24 hours of postoperative ventilation support from 26% to 5%.[7]

Assessing Risk Based on Preoperative Status

A number of robust models are available to stratify mortality outcome by preoperative risk factors in patients undergoing cardiac surgery.[8] The independent (predictive) variables and their weighting vary somewhat from model to model, and vary between models predicting mortality versus those predicting morbidity or length-of-stay outcomes, but the commonalities are greater than the differences.[9] The Society of Thoracic Surgeons National Adult Cardiac Surgery Database is widely used and offers, in addition to mortality model, a model customized to predict prolonged ventilation.[10,11] Factors common to outcome risk-adjustment models include age, gender, body surface area, presence of diabetes or renal failure, chronic lung disease, peripheral vascular disease, cerebrovascular disease, prior cardiac operation, and emergency or unstable status. Chronic obstructive pulmonary disease (COPD) might be expected to be a major risk for postoperative morbidity and mortality and appears as a factor in many models. However, hospital mortality with mild-to-moderate COPD is not especially high; it is the minority of patients with severe COPD, especially those over the age of 75 years of age and receiving steroids, who are at highest risk.[12] Patients with preexisting COPD have higher rates of pulmonary complications (12%), atrial fibrillation (27%), and death (7%).[13] Obesity, defined by increased body mass index, does not appear to increase the risk of postoperative respiratory failure.[14] On the other hand, even modest elevations of serum creatinine (above 1.5 mg/dL) are independently associated with morbidity and mortality outcomes[9,15] (see Chapter 32).

At least four studies have used multivariate regression techniques to elucidate factors specifically associated with postoperative respiratory failure (Table 34–2). The studies differ in their endpoints for outcome and in their choice of preoperative versus operative versus postoperative variables. Spivack et al[16] examined 513 consecutive patients undergoing coronary artery bypass grafting and identified reduced left ventricular ejection fraction, preexisting congestive heart failure, angina, current smoking, and diabetes mellitus as predictors of mechanical ventilation support beyond 48 hours. In this study, pulmonary diagnosis, lung mechanics, and blood gas parameters were not independently useful in predicting outcome. The mortality rate predicted by the Society for

Table 34–2 **Factors Predicting Postoperative Respiratory Outcome**

	Spivack et al, Chest 1996;109:1222	Branca et al, Chest 2001;119:537	Rady et al, Crit Care Med 1999;27:340	Canver/Chandra, Ann Thorac Surg 2003;75:853
Endpoint	Mechanical Ventilation >48 hr	Mechanical Ventilation >72 hr	Extubation failure (reintubation after initial extubation)	Mechanical Ventilation >72 hr
Risk Factors	Reduced LVEF Preexisting CHF Angina Current smoking Diabetes	STS-predicted mortality estimate Mitral valve disease Advanced age Pressors/inotropes Renal failure Operative urgency Type of operation Preoperative ventilation Prior CABG Female gender MI within 30 days Previous stroke	Age ≥65 yr Inpatient Vascular disease COPD/asthma Pulmonary hypertension Reduced LVEF Cardiac shock Hct ≤34% BUN ≥24 mg/dL Serum albumin ≤4.0 mg/dL Do_2 ≤320 mL/mm/L^2 >1 prior CABG Thoracic aortic surgery ≥10 units of blood products Total CPB time >120/min	CPB time Sepsis and endocarditis GI bleeding Renal failure Deep sternal wound infection New CVA Bleeding requiring reoperation

LVEF = left ventricular ejection fraction; CHF = congestive heart failure; STS = Society of Thoracic Surgeons; CABG = coronary artery bypass grafting; MI = myocardial infarction; COPD = chronic obstructive pulmonary disease; BUN = blood urea nitrogen; mg/dL = milligrams per deciliter; Do_2 = systemic oxygen delivery; CPB = cardiopulmonary bypass; GI = gastrointestinal; Hct = hematocrit.

Thoracic Surgeons model was found to be the single best predictor of mechanical ventilation support for longer than 72 hours but also identified mitral valvular disease, age, vasopressor and inotrope use, renal failure, operative urgency, type of operation, preoperative ventilation, prior cardiac surgery, female gender, myocardial infarction within 30 days, and previous stroke as contributors.[10,17] Rady and Ryan[18] examined both preoperative and intraoperative factors and noted that transfusion of more than 10 units of blood products or total CPB time in excess of 120 minutes were important operative events in addition to the usual preoperative predictors of extubation failure. Canver and Chandra[19] looked only at operative and postoperative predictors versus the endpoint of mechanical ventilation for more than 72 hours; they found that prolonged CPB time, sepsis and endocarditis, gastrointestinal bleeding, renal failure, deep sternal wound infection, new stroke, and bleeding requiring reoperation were important predictors of prolonged ventilatory support. None of these models, general or specific for respiratory complications, is sufficiently sensitive or specific to prohibit consideration of surgery for an individual patient, but they do provide the clinician with early warning for patients at high risk.

Operating Room Events

Identification of the patient who is difficult to intubate is important for planning extubation at a time when sufficient personnel and equipment are available to deal with a potentially difficult reintubation. Opioids and neuromuscular blocking agents with long half-lives might be expected to influence extubation time, but it is not the specific duration of action of these drugs but rather the skill of the anesthesiologist in knowing how to use them well that influences extubation time. Reoperative patients are at risk, partly because of longer CPB time with reoperation, increased blood transfusion, and the additional likelihood of bleeding in this population.[18-20] CPB time is repeatedly identified as a risk, and a correlation between CPB time and inflammatory cytokine release has been demonstrated.[18-21] Low-cardiac-output (CO) states are important because prolonged periods of inadequate perfusion result in additional mediator release. Hemodynamic management when separating from CPB includes the use of vasopressors, inotropes, and potentially mechanical support (intra-aortic balloon pump [IABP], ventricular assist device [VAD]) to avoid multisystem organ failure as a consequence of persistent low CO. Patients maintained on an IABP or a VAD have borderline or insufficient CO ; it makes little sense to impose the additional WOB until the cardiac issues have resolved.[4] Cardiovascular collapse occasionally occurs at the time of chest closure secondary to severe distention or edema of the lungs. Physiologically, this acts much like cardiac tamponade, and the solution is to leave the chest open for 24 to 48 hours. An open chest delays early extubation and also has a potential to produce long-term ventilator dependency should infection or sternal osteomyelitis develop.

The prognostic and therapeutic implications of an IABP depend on the reasons for which the device was inserted (Fig. 34–2). Not surprisingly, mortality and ventilation-dependency rates are lowest in those not requiring any mechanical support. In patients in whom the IABP was placed preoperatively for unstable angina, definitive surgery should correct the problem and removal of the IABP and extubation need not be delayed. In all other scenarios, intubation and ventilatory support may be required beyond the time of removal of the IABP because of residual cardiac dysfunction, fluid overload, or associated organ injury. Patients whose IABP was placed for preoperative cardiogenic shock, as an assist to separating from CPB or for low-output states in the postoperative period, have a high mortality risk and frequently need prolonged ventilatory support.

Positive end-expiratory pressure (PEEP) while on CPB has been advocated as one method to prevent atelectasis. This turns out to be impractical in patients with obstructive lung disease because air trapping interferes with surgical exposure.

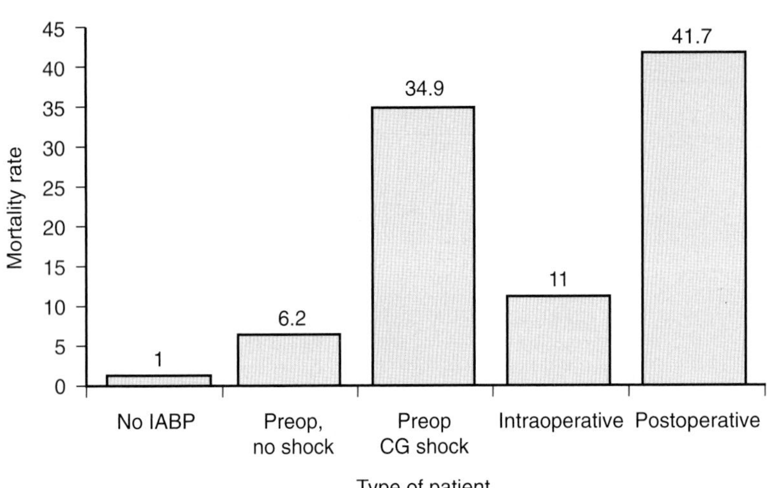

Figure 34–2 The prognostic implications of an intra-aortic balloon pump (IABP) depend on the timing and reason for insertion. In patients undergoing isolated coronary artery bypass grafting, the basal mortality rate is less than 1%. Patients who received a preoperative IABP for unstable angina have a 6.2% mortality rate. Preoperative insertion for cardiogenic shock has the worst prognosis, with nearly 35% mortality. Intraoperative insertion of a balloon pump, generally to facilitate separation from cardiopulmonary bypass, carries an 11% mortality rate. The worst prognosis is if a balloon pump is required postoperatively for any reason. Patients in the highest risk category are likely to require prolonged ventilatory support.

Recruitment maneuvers following CPB have variable impact on intubation time; most studies show it to be ineffective in reducing the need for long-term ventilatory support. There are no compelling data that fluid management choices or the use of steroids prior to CPB have substantial effects on intubation time or respiratory failure. A number of studies by Boldt and colleagues[22,23] suggest that infusion of small volumes of hypertonic saline prepared in a hydroxyethyl starch solution may reduce total fluid needs, improve cardiac index, and lessen the pulmonary gas exchange compromise; but studies have not examined whether these differences in the operating room translate to improved outcome or shorter length of stay.

Postoperative Events

The expected postoperative course is a short period of ventilation support while the patient is warmed, allowed to awaken, and observed for bleeding or hemodynamic instability. Preoperative risks, issues with difficult intubation, and operating room events should be communicated from the operating room team to the ICU team at the time of ICU admission. Box 34–1 outlines criteria to be met prior to routine extubation.

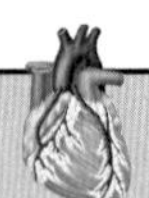

BOX 34–1 *Criteria to Be Met Before Early Postoperative Extubation*

- *Neurologic*: Awake, neuromuscular blockade fully dissipated; following instructions, able to cough and protect airway
- *Cardiac*: Stable without mechanical support; cardiac index ≥2.2 L/min/m^2; MAP ≥70 mm Hg, no serious arrhythmias
- *Respiratory*: Acceptable CXR and ABGs (pH ≥7.35); MIP at least 25 cm H_2O; minimal secretions, comfortable on CPAP or T-piece with spontaneous respiratory rate ≤20 breaths/minute
- *Renal*: Diuresing well; urine output >0.8 mL/kg/hr; not markedly fluid overloaded from operative/CPB fluid administration or SIRS
- *Hematologic*: Chest tube drainage minimal
- *Temperature*: Fully rewarmed; not actively shivering

MAP = mean arterial pressure; CXR = chest radiograph; ABG = arterial blood gas; MIP = maximal inspiratory pressure; CPAP = continuous positive airway pressure; CPB = cardiopulmonary bypass; SIRS = systemic immune response syndrome.

Aspiration of mouth flora or gastric contents is a major risk factor for later pulmonary compromise. Oral rather than nasal routes should be used for the endotracheal and gastric sump tubes, and these devices removed, at the earliest possible opportunity. Prior to extubation, a quick neurologic examination should be performed to rule out new cerebrovascular events, presence of excess opioids, or residual neuromuscular blocking agents. Knowledge that the WOB can consume up to 20% of CO should preclude extubation in the hemodynamically unstable patient. Although patients may be successfully extubated while on IABP, the need to lie flat after balloon and sheath removal may dictate continued temporary ventilator support.

Postoperative care of low-risk cardiac surgical patients has come to resemble a recovery room model, but high-risk patients benefit from postoperative involvement of anesthesiologists, cardiologists, and critical care specialists.[24,25] The presence of full-time ICU staff physicians improves outcome and is now recommended by the Leapfrog Group as a patient safety standard.[26-28]

Hospital-acquired infections are an important cause of postoperative morbidity and nosocomial pneumonia is common in patients receiving continuous mechanical ventilation. The actuarial risk of ventilator-associated pneumonia appears to be around 1% per day when diagnosed using protected specimen brush and quantitative culture techniques.[29] Strategies thought to be effective at reducing the incidence of ventilator-associated pneumonia include early removal of nasogastric or endotracheal tubes, formal infection control programs, handwashing, semirecumbent positioning of the patient, avoiding unnecessary reintubation, providing adequate nutritional support, avoiding gastric overdistention, use of the oral rather than the nasal route for intubation, scheduled drainage of condensate from ventilator circuits, and maintenance of adequate endotracheal tube cuff pressure.[30-32] The reader is referred to an excellent review by Kollef[33] on the prevention of ventilator-associated pneumonia. Strategies that are *not* considered effective include routine changes of the ventilator circuit, dedicated use of disposable suction catheters, routine changes of in-line suction catheters, daily changes of heat and moisture exchanges, and chest physiotherapy.[33] Postural changes, humidification, and use of protective gowns and gloves are recommended for clinical use but have not been adequately studied.[33] While continuous aspiration of subglottic secretions is recommended, it may only be

Table 34–3 Scoring Acute Lung Injury

Points	0	1	2	3	4
CXR No. of quadrants	No infiltration	One	Two	Three	All four
PaO_2/FIO_2	≥300	225 to 299	165 to 224	100 to 174	<100
PEEP cm H_2O	≤5	6 to 8	9 to 11	12 to 14	>15
C_{stat}	≥80	60 to 79	40 to 59	20 to 39	≤19

Final score = aggregate sum/No. of components assessed.
0 = No lung injury; 0.1 to 2.5 = acute lung injury; >2.5 = adult respiratory distress syndrome; C_{STAT} = static compliance.
Modified from Murray JF, Matthay MA, Luce JM, Flick MR: An expanded definition of the adult respiratory distress syndrome. Am Rev Respir Dis 138:720, 1988.

cost-effective in the specific subgroups of patients evaluated in the published study.[34]

DIAGNOSIS OF ACUTE LUNG INJURY AND ACUTE RESPIRATORY DISTRESS SYNDROME

ARDS may develop as a sequela of CPB, or, more commonly, in the postoperative patient with cardiogenic shock, sepsis, or multisystem organ failure. Components of ARDS include diffuse alveolar damage resulting from endothelial and type I epithelial cell necrosis, and noncardiogenic pulmonary edema due to breakdown of the endothelial barrier with subsequent vascular permeability. The exudative phase of ARDS occurs in the first 3 days after the precipitating event and is thought to be mediated by neutrophil activation and sequestration. Neutrophils release mediators, causing endothelial damage. Ultimately, the alveolar spaces fill up with fluid as a result of increased endothelial permeability.

Intravascular and intra-alveolar fibrin deposition is common. Procoagulant activity becomes enhanced in ARDS, and bronchoalveolar lavage reveals increased tissue factor levels.[35] The clinical presentation is typically an acute onset of severe arterial hypoxemia resistant to oxygen therapy, with a PaO_2- to-FIO_2 (P/F) ratio of less than 200 mm Hg. ARDS is classically diagnosed only in the absence of left ventricular failure, which complicates the issue in the postoperative cardiac patient who may also be in congestive heart failure (CHF). Other findings in ARDS include decreased lung compliance (<80 mL/cm H_2O) and bilateral infiltrates on chest x-ray.[36] Murray et al[37] created a Lung Injury Score (Table 34–3) that awards points for affected quadrants on chest x-ray, P/F ratio, amount of PEEP applied, and static compliance of the lung. Scores above zero but less than 2.5 are considered ALI, and scores greater than 2.5 meet the threshold for ARDS.

The proliferative phase of ARDS occurs on days 3 to 7 as inflammatory cells accumulate as a result of chemoattractants released by the neutrophils. At this stage, the normal repair process would remove debris and begin repair, but a disordered repair process may result in exuberant fibrosis, stiff lungs, and inefficient gas exchange. Evidence suggests that careful medical and ventilator management may affect this process. Any precipitating factors should be addressed (e.g., draining closed-space infections). Conventional ventilator support following cardiac surgery is to maintain large tidal volumes (typically 10 to 12 mL/kg) to reopen atelectatic but potentially functional alveoli. The problem is that the compromised lung is no longer homogenous and high pressures can further damage the remaining normal lung over time. Direct mechanical injury may occur as a result of overdistention (volutrauma), high pressures (barotrauma), or shear injury from repetitive opening and closing. "Biotrauma" may also occur as a result of inflammatory mediator release and impaired antibacterial barriers. Nahum et al[38] showed that dissemination of *Escherichia coli* via bacterial translocation from the lung was highest in dogs ventilated with a high-tidal-volume strategy. Thus, current clinical practice with known or suspected lung injury is to limit inflation pressures. The maximal "safe" inflation pressure is not known, but evidence favors keeping peak inspiratory pressures at less than 35 cm H_2O and restricting tidal volumes to less than 6 mL/kg of ideal body weight.[39] The landmark ARDSNet trial randomized patients to 6 mL/kg versus 12 mL/kg of ideal body weight and demonstrated a significant difference in 28-day survival with the low-tidal-volume group.[40] The same study showed significant decreases in interleukin 6 release when the low-tidal-volume strategy was used.

Additional Therapy for Acute Lung Injury/Acute Respiratory Distress Syndrome

A number of other factors may enter into the optimal treatment of the ALI patient, and trials are investigating the role of fluid management and the utility of pulmonary artery catheterization in this population.[41] Maintaining a lung-protective ventilatory strategy (LPVS) can involve permissive hypercapnea if normal PCO_2 levels cannot be achieved with low tidal volumes.[42] Prone positioning is useful in achieving oxygenation.[43] A short daily turn to prone position does not appear to improve outcome in ARDS, although one post hoc analysis found lower mortality in the very sickest patients.[44] Lower tidal volumes with increasing amounts of PEEP may increase alveolar recruitment and thus improve oxygenation.[45] Taken to an extreme, ALI patients may be ventilated with high-frequency oscillation (HFO), which is essentially high PEEP and tiny, frequently delivered tidal volumes. Other experimental techniques include extracorporeal CO_2 removal, extracorporeal membrane oxygenation, partial liquid ventilation, inhaled nitric oxide, and inhaled prostacyclin.[46-51] None of these modalities has yet been documented to improve outcome. Large prospective trials in the late 1980s demonstrated that high-dose corticosteroids had no effect when given at diagnosis or early in the course of ARDS. Miduri et al[52] gave prolonged lower dose methylprednisolone therapy in unresolving ARDS and were able to document improvements in P/F ratio with improved ICU survival and shortened duration of mechanical ventilation.

In the healthy cardiac surgical population, the use of PEEP is not usually necessary.[53,54] Increased levels of PEEP decrease CO, unless volume loading is used to maintain transmural filling pressures.[55] The effects of PEEP are most marked in the presence of abnormal right ventricular function, particularly if the right coronary artery is compromised.[56] PEEP neither protects against the development of ARDS nor reduces the amount of mediastinal bleeding after cardiac procedures involving CPB.[57,58] Most clinicians will routinely use 5 cm H_2O of PEEP in ventilated patients. However, higher levels of PEEP (often 8 to 15+ cm H_2O) are usually necessary to maintain adequate oxygenation with ALI or developing ARDS; application of PEEP in the postsurgical patient usually involves a tradeoff between cardiac and pulmonary goals.

Lung Recruitment

In laboratory and clinical models, an important component of a lung-protective ventilatory strategy (LPVS) is recruitment of the lung.[39] This is the closed-chest analogy to the open-chest recruitment maneuver typically done at the end of CPB to reexpand the collapsed lung. The goal of opening the lung is to allow ventilation to occur at a point on the pressure–volume curve that avoids repetitive atelectasis (by staying above a critical closing pressure) and at the same time avoids overinflation.[59] ARDSNet data suggest that the short-term effects of recruitment maneuvers are highly variable and that further study is needed to determine the role of recruitment maneuvers in the management of ALI/ARDS.[60] With anesthetic techniques geared to early extubation, suboptimal oxygenation in the early postoperative period appears to be more common today. In most instances, impaired oxygenation is due to atelectasis and responds quickly to brief recruitment maneuvers. These should be performed cautiously because of the adverse impact of increased airway pressure on venous return and CO. While the benefits of early application of the LPVS in the high-risk cardiac surgical patient have not been formally studied, the benefits of LPVS in other populations suggest that this strategy should be considered as soon as ALI is identified.

Permissive Hypercapnea

Conventional management is to maintain arterial $P\text{CO}_2$ ($Pa\text{CO}_2$) within a "normal" or eucapnic range, classically between 35 and 45 mm Hg. A patient who chronically retains CO_2 would be considered eucapnic at his or her higher baseline $Pa\text{CO}_2$. The traditional reason for maintaining eucapnia is primarily that acute deviation from a normal or acclimatized $Pa\text{CO}_2$ results in alkalemia or acidemia to which the kidneys respond by retaining or excreting bicarbonate ion. Normal kidneys can compensate for a $Pa\text{CO}_2$-induced pH change in 12 to 36 hours.[61] If high airway pressures would be required to maintain a "normal" $Pa\text{CO}_2$, arterial $P\text{CO}_2$ values up to 60 mm Hg are acceptable as long as cardiovascular stability is present and the pH remains above 7.30. It has been hypothesized that raised $Pa\text{CO}_2$ levels might even be protective and that low levels of $Pa\text{CO}_2$ could play a role in organ injury.[62]

Cardiopulmonary Interactions

Understanding cardiopulmonary interactions associated with mechanical ventilation is essential. Hemodynamic changes may occur secondary to changes in lung volume and intrathoracic pressure even when tidal volume remains constant.[63] Pulmonary vascular resistance and mechanical heart–lung interactions play prominent roles in determining the hemodynamic response to mechanical ventilation. Because lung inflation alters pulmonary vascular resistance and right ventricular wall tension, there are limits to intrathoracic pressure that a damaged heart will tolerate. High lung volumes may also mechanically limit cardiac volumes. In patients with airflow obstruction, occult PEEP (auto-PEEP) may also contribute to hypotension and low CO.[64] Auto-PEEP can be detected by respiratory waveform monitoring or by pressure monitoring with the ventilator's expiratory port held closed at end-exhalation. Auto-PEEP often responds to bronchodilators and/or increased expiratory time to permit more complete exhalation.

GENERAL SUPPORT ISSUES

Patients requiring long-term ventilation support are prone to a number of complications including venous thromboembolism, central venous catheter–related bloodstream infections, surgical site infections, ventilator-associated pneumonia, pressure ulcers, nutritional depletion, delirium, and gastrointestinal bleeding. The Agency for Healthcare Research and Quality has identified a number of patient safety practices applicable to the ICU patient; at the top of the list are appropriate venothromboembolism (VTE) prophylaxis, use of perioperative β-blockers, use of maximum sterile barriers during catheter insertion, and appropriate use of antibiotic prophylaxis.[65] Standard practice in long-term patients includes prophylaxis against gastrointestinal bleeding with histamine blockers or proton pump inhibitors, unless the patient is receiving continuous gastric feedings; head of bed elevation to 30° or more in hemodynamically stable patients; a brief daily wake-up from sedation; use of in-line suction catheters; tight glucose control; and appropriate VTE prophylaxis.[30,66,67] Box 34–2 summarizes these risk-reduction efforts. Ensuring that each of these goals is met on each patient every day requires

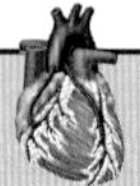

BOX 34–2 *Specific Ways to Reduce Intensive Care Unit–Associated Morbidity*

- Earliest possible removal of oral gastric and ETTs
- Use oral (not nasal) tubes
- Formal infection control program (handwashing, feedback to staff)
- Head of bed (HOB) elevation to 30° or more if hemodynamics permits
- In-line suction catheters to avoid circuit contamination with repeated opening
- Scheduled drainage of condensate
- Adequate ETT cuff pressure
- Avoid need for reintubation (adequate restraints, sedation)
- Glucose control protocol (insulin infusion)
- Early nutritional support, preferably via enteral route
- Stress ulcer prophylaxis
- Deep venous thrombosis (DVT) prophylaxis
- Brief daily wakeup from sedation
- Early tracheostomy if >14 days of predicted ventilator support
- Use of BiPAP (if used preoperatively) to avoid reintubation
- Swallowing evaluation before oral feeding if patient at risk for aspiration

extra work but can be accomplished with a daily goals form or with information technology.[68,69]

Impediments to Weaning and Extubation

Factors limiting the removal of mechanical ventilatory support include delirium, neurologic dysfunction, unstable hemodynamics, respiratory muscle dysfunction, renal failure with fluid overload, and sepsis. Figure 34–3 outlines one approach to identifying readiness to wean and possible alternative approaches to weaning.

Neurologic Complications

Delirium is common in long-stay ICU patients and is associated with higher costs in the ICU unit and for the entire hospital stay.[70] Transient postoperative delirium occurs in about 7% of patients, resolving spontaneously or with pharmacologic intervention in almost all patients by postoperative day 6.[71] Alcohol or benzodiazepine withdrawal should be considered in the differential diagnosis of delirium. Initial management of agitation consists of reassurance and orientation of the patient and control of pain with opioids. Agitation accompanied by disorientation may be worsened by benzodiazepines, which should be restricted to treatment of oriented but anxious patients or for prophylaxis of alcohol and benzodiazepine withdrawal. If the patient remains agitated and disoriented haloperidol is useful.[72] Promising newer agents such as rispiradone and olanzepine have not been well studied in the ICU setting.

Diaphragmatic paralysis may complicate any procedure, but it is more common in patients undergoing reoperation, owing to the difficulty in identifying the phrenic nerve in fibrotic pericardial tissue. In the authors' experience, permanent bilateral diaphragmatic paralysis occurs in less than 0.1% of patients after CPB, but temporary diaphragmatic weakness may occur in 4% or more. The diagnosis of diaphragmatic paralysis should be considered whenever a patient fails to wean from mechanical ventilation; it should be documented by observing paradoxical movement of the diaphragm during

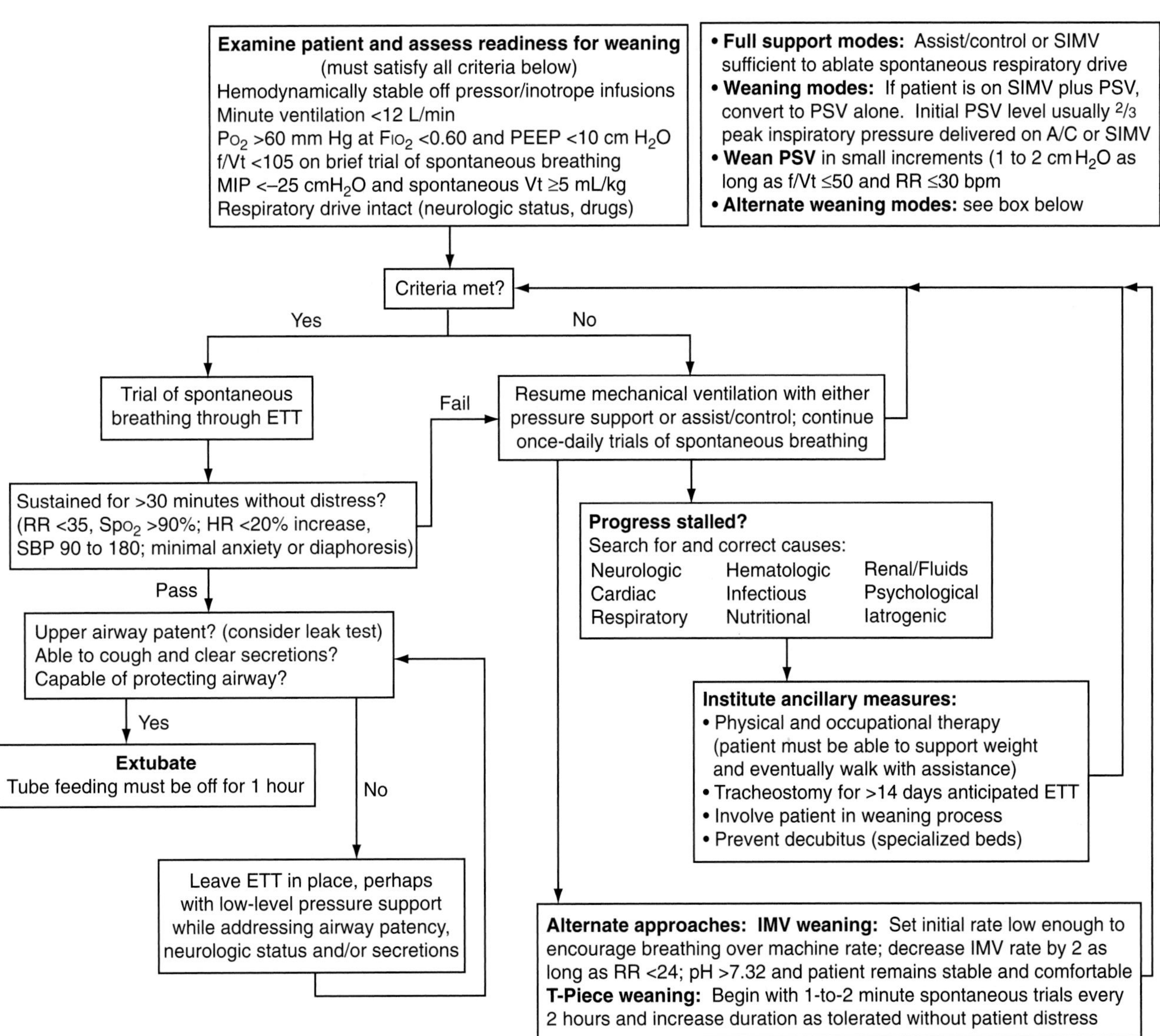

Figure 34–3 This flow chart addresses the broad categorization of patients, both short and long term, in the cardiothoracic intensive care unit. All patients require periodic assessment for readiness for weaning, and if they meet criteria are eligible for spontaneous trials leading to extubation. Patients who do not meet the criteria should have mechanical ventilation maintained until criteria are met. Pressure-support weaning may be possible; if not, alternative approaches include IMV weaning and TP weaning. Patients who stall in their weaning progress should have a comprehensive examination and an assessment of organ systems to search for correctable causes.

inspiration and by comparing vital capacity (VC) and tidal volume (V_T) in the supine and seated positions. Differences in supine and seated VC of more than 10% to 15% should prompt fluoroscopic examination of the diaphragm ("sniff" test). Bilateral paralysis may be missed by this test, because comparison of left and right diaphragmatic excursion has lower specificity when both diaphragms are involved. Transient diaphragmatic paralysis can occur secondary to cold injury to the phrenic nerve.[73] Less often, the phrenic nerve is injured or transected during dissection of the internal mammary arteries or during mobilization of the heart in patients undergoing reoperation.

Patients with respiratory failure and systemic inflammatory response syndrome (SIRS) frequently develop critical illness polyneuropathy, the first sign of which may be failure to wean from the ventilator.[74] Disuse atrophy and steroid administration also contribute to muscle weakness.[75,76] Severe COPD patients who are dependent on diaphragmatic breathing preoperatively are most likely to manifest diaphragmatic weakness as postoperative ventilator dependency. Full recovery of diaphragmatic function may take from 4 months to more than 2 years; partial recovery is apparent when the patient can lie flat without dyspnea.[77] Adjuncts to improving diaphragmatic strength include inspiratory muscle training, normalizing calcium and phosphate levels, and possible use of aminophylline.[7,78]

Cardiac Complications

Acute myocardial dysfunction occurs in almost all post-CPB patients, reaching a nadir about 4 hours (range, 2 to 6) after CPB. Patients with persistent low-output syndrome have an increased risk of cardiac death, as well as complications such as renal failure, respiratory failure, disseminated intravascular coagulation, gastrointestinal bleeding, and neurologic sequelae. Regional differences in blood flow can also occur even in the presence of an adequate overall CO, so a normal whole-body cardiac index does not guarantee adequate perfusion of individual organs. Multiorgan failure may be precipitated by a period of gut ischemia or hyperpermeability followed by translocation of gut bacteria and release of endotoxin and other vasoactive substances, leading to generalized inflammation and organ injury.[79]

Patients maintained on chronic amiodarone therapy are prone to postoperative respiratory failure, longer intubation times, and longer ICU stays, even with only subclinical evidence of pulmonary amiodarone toxicity.[80] Rarely, patients taking amiodarone develop life-threatening pulmonary complications, including ARDS. Histologic lung examination of these patients demonstrates marked interstitial fibrosis with enlarged air spaces ("honeycomb" appearance), and hyperplasia of type II pneumocytes.[81]

Acute left ventricular dysfunction may occur in patients with COPD during the shift from mechanical to spontaneous ventilation.[82] Attention to fluid balance and aggressive diuresis or use of ultrafiltration help with weaning. Although it is useful to compare the patient's current and preoperative body weights, catabolic states arising postoperatively, and especially during sepsis, reduce lean body weight. Patients may be "unweanable" until fluid removal reduces body weight to several kilograms below the preoperative value.

Patients with valvular disease have significantly higher respiratory system and lung elastances and resistances than those undergoing surgery for ischemic heart disease, but these may correct with successful surgery.[83] Thus, valve surgery patients have less WOB and improved respiratory function after correction of the valvular pathology, but coronary artery bypass grafting patients are less likely to show dramatic improvement postoperatively.

Renal Failure and Fluid Overload

Significant oliguria or anuric renal failure occurs after 1% to 4% of cardiac surgery procedures, and lesser degrees of renal dysfunction, marked by elevated serum creatinine, occur in up to 30%. Univariate predictors of serious acute renal failure include low CO at the end of CPB, advanced age, preoperative cardiac failure, and need for postoperative circulatory support, blood transfusions, and prolonged time on CPB.[84]

When renal failure occurs, it usually follows one of three well-defined patterns.[85] Abbreviated acute renal failure occurs after an isolated insult, results in a peak in serum creatinine around the fourth postevent day, and generally resolves if no other events occur. The second pattern initially resembles the first, except that the acute insult is accompanied by prolonged circulatory failure. This pattern runs a longer course, with recovery typically occurring in the second or third week after injury, in tandem with improvements in CO. In the third pattern, recovery is complicated by a second insult such as sepsis, massive gastrointestinal bleeding, or myocardial infarction, and permanent renal failure may result. Because fluid overload with renal failure may precipitate respiratory and cardiac failure, early application of continuous hemofiltration and related techniques to remove excess fluid can facilitate separation from ventilator support.[86]

Infectious Complications

Mediastinitis, sternal dehiscence, or both, are complications of coronary revascularization, with an incidence of about 1% and a mortality rate of about 13% and a tendency to prolong ventilator dependency. Predisposing factors for wound complications after cardiac surgery include diabetes, low CO, use of bilateral internal mammary grafts, and reoperation for control of bleeding.[87] Keeping blood glucose lower than 200 mg/dL in the perioperative period reduces the sternal wound infection rate from 2.4% to 1.5%.[88] Mediastinal infection manifests as unexplained fever, an unstable sternum and, sometimes, failure to wean. In addition to selective antibiotic therapy, surgical debridement and drainage of the wound are usually necessary. Polymicrobial isolates are associated with poor outcome. Additional management of mediastinitis may include primary or delayed sternal closure using pectoralis or omental flaps.

Pneumonia, tracheobronchitis, catheter sepsis, and urinary tract infections are frequent in the ventilator-dependent patient. Continuous lateral rotational therapy reduces the prevalence of pneumonia, but may not affect mortality or length of mechanical support.[89] The diagnosis of ventilator-associated pneumonia (VAP) can be difficult to confirm, as upper airway organisms can contaminate the sputum specimen.[90] Special suction catheters with a protected tip may be used for a "mini" bronchoalveolar lavage to improve the yield of sputum cultures. Because typical perioperative antibiotic prophylaxis consists of an anti-staphylococcal penicillin or cephalosporin, nosocomial pneumonia is likely to occur with organisms such as *Pseudomonas, Klebsiella, Serratia, Acinetobacter,* or methicillin-resistant *Staphylococcus aureus* (MRSA). Treatment of the secondary infection may be followed by a tertiary infection with more difficult organisms, such as *Candida, Torulopsis,* or other fungal species.

Gastrointestinal Complications

Gastrointestinal complications requiring intervention occur in 1% to 3% of patients.[91] Postoperative ileus can affect diaphragmatic excursion and increase WOB. Upper gastrointestinal bleeding is common. Pancreatitis, mesenteric ischemia, perforation, and bleeding elsewhere in the gastrointestinal tract are problems of any critically ill patient with multisystem failure. Mesenteric ischemia can be the result of low perfusion or embolic atheroma from large-vessel manipulation. Gut ischemia is a potential source of bacteremia and is especially problematic in patients with artificial valves. The risk of gastrointestinal bleeding can be minimized with antacid therapy, histamine blockers, or barrier protection agents. Enteral nutritional support also appears to protect the gastric mucosa.[92]

Diarrhea can occur as the result of mesenteric ischemia but is also frequently due to *Clostridium difficile* overgrowth in patients treated with antibiotics, especially later-generation cephalosporins. The rapid assay for *C. difficile* can miss certain strains; culture of stool is not as rapid but is more reliable. Treatment of *C. difficile* colitis can be accompanied by oral or intravenous metronidazole or enteral (*not* intravenous) vancomycin. Toxic megacolon is a surgical emergency requiring immediate attention. Nutrition depletion is common in long-term ventilation patients, and early enteral feeding should be implemented in high-risk patients unless there are specific contraindications such as ongoing bowel ischemia.

Nutritional Support and Weaning

Respiratory failure can be precipitated by high carbohydrate loads delivered during attempts to provide nutritional support, so the goal should be to institute support early before serious depletion occurs and to use an appropriate mix of fat and carbohydrate to maintain a respiratory quotient less than 1.0. Weekly monitoring of transferrin or prealbumin levels screen for changes in nutritional status; more sophisticated analysis, including metabolic monitoring and nitrogen balance, can identify issues with poor response to therapy.

The adequacy of nutritional support has a strong influence on the ability to wean from ventilation. Successful weaning occurs in about 93% of those with adequate nutritional support but only 50% of those with inadequate nutrition.[93] Increases in albumin and transferrin level with parenteral nutrition predict eventual ability to wean.[94]

MODES OF VENTILATOR SUPPORT

Positive-pressure ventilators employed outside the operating room have a nonrebreathing circuit, may be volume- or pressure-limited, and may be triggered by changes in flow or changes in pressure. All modern ventilators contain multiple modes of ventilatory support that accommodate both mandatory and patient-triggered breaths. The most common modes of positive-pressure ventilation are assist control (A/C), synchronized intermittent mandatory ventilation (SIMV), and pressure-support ventilation (PSV). Volume-cycled support is still most common. With volume modes, the inspiratory flow rate, targeted volume, and inspiratory time are set by the clinician, and inspiratory peak pressure will vary depending on the patient's lung compliance and synchrony with the ventilator. Volume cycling ensures consistent delivery of a set tidal volume as long as the pressure limit is not exceeded. With

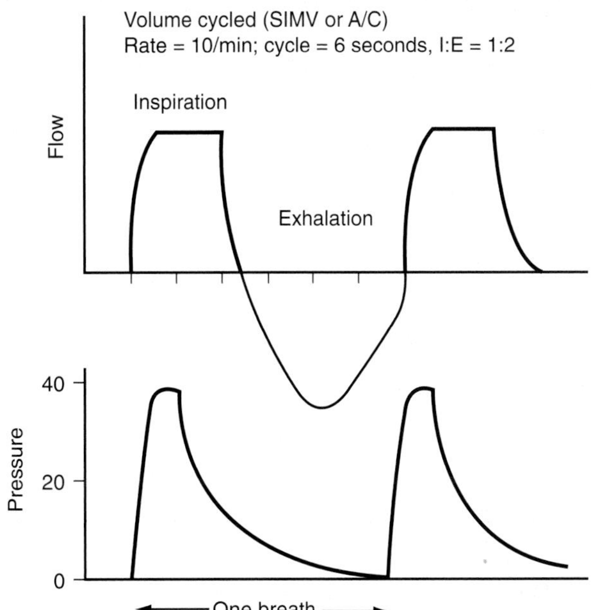

Figure 34–4 The top tracing shows the inspiratory flow, which is close to a square wave. Originally, this flow pattern was dictated by the function of mechanical valves, but may now be duplicated electronically. Note that the flow waveform becomes negative during the exhalation phase. The typical volume cycle breath with a square waveform results in a rapid rise to peak inspiratory pressure followed by a gradual decline. If the safety pressure limit is exceeded, the peak of the pressure waveform may be truncated.

nonhomogenous lung pathology, however, delivered volume tends to flow to the area of low resistance, which may result in overdistention of healthy segments of lung and underinflation of atelectatic segments and consequent VQ mismatching. Figure 34–4 demonstrates pressure and flow tracings with volume ventilation. Volume breaths may be triggered by a timer (control-mode ventilation) or by patient effort between the control-mode breaths (A/C ventilation). In either case, the tidal volume delivered will be determined by the ventilator settings. This can present a problem in a patient with tachypnea as a response to neurologic injury. If the patient breathes inappropriately in response to normal arterial levels of carbon dioxide, significant respiratory alkalosis will result. Assist-control mode is most appropriate for the patient whose respiratory drive is normal but muscles are weak, and when neuromuscular blockade is used, in which case A/C essentially becomes control-mode ventilation.

Intermittent mandatory ventilation (IMV) and then SIMV were developed to facilitate weaning from mechanical ventilatory support. With either IMV modality, a basal respiratory rate is set by the clinician, which may be supplemented by patient-initiated breaths. In contrast to assist-control ventilation, however, the tidal volume of the patient's spontaneous breaths will be determined by their own respiratory strength and lung compliance rather than delivered as a preset volume. SIMV mode is appropriate for patients with normal lungs recovering from opioid anesthesia. Weaning is accomplished by reducing the mandatory IMV rate and allowing the patient to assume more and more of the respiratory effort over time. SIMV mode has been used for weaning complex patients, but the weaning effort may stall at very low IMV rates if the patient cannot achieve spontaneous volumes sufficient to activate their pulmonary stretch receptors. Under these circumstances, the patient is likely to become tachypneic and fail

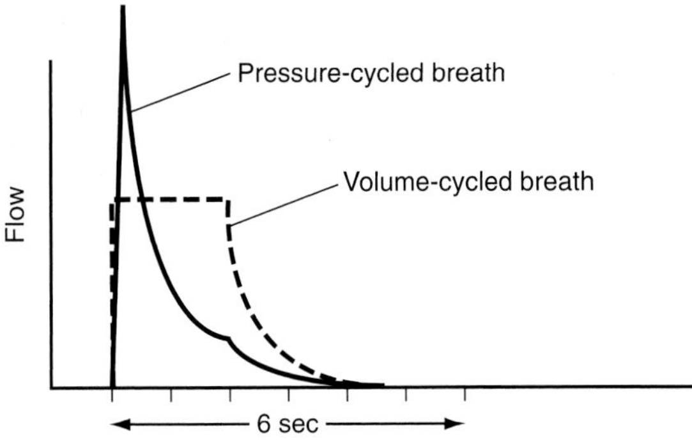

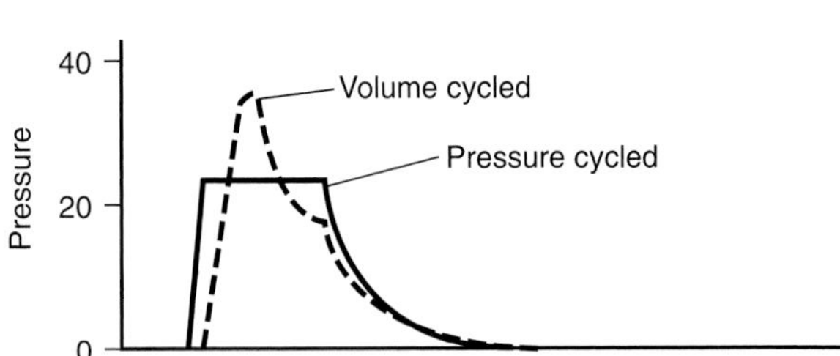

Figure 34–5 The difference between pressure-cycled breaths and volume-cycled breaths is demonstrated. With a pressure-cycled breath, the flow is titrated by a feedback mechanism to maintain a set inspiratory pressure. Thus, flow is very rapid at the beginning of the inspiratory cycle and rapidly tapers, in contrast to a volume-cycled breath in which the waveform is more or less consistent throughout the inspiratory cycle. The bottom section shows the difference in pressure tracings. As noted before, volume-cycled ventilation reaches a peak and then falls back. In contrast, pressure-cycled ventilation reaches a lower but sustained pressure limit and holds at that level for the inspiratory time. In the absence of significant pulmonary disease, either mode of ventilation results in a rapid decrease of pressure once exhalation occurs.

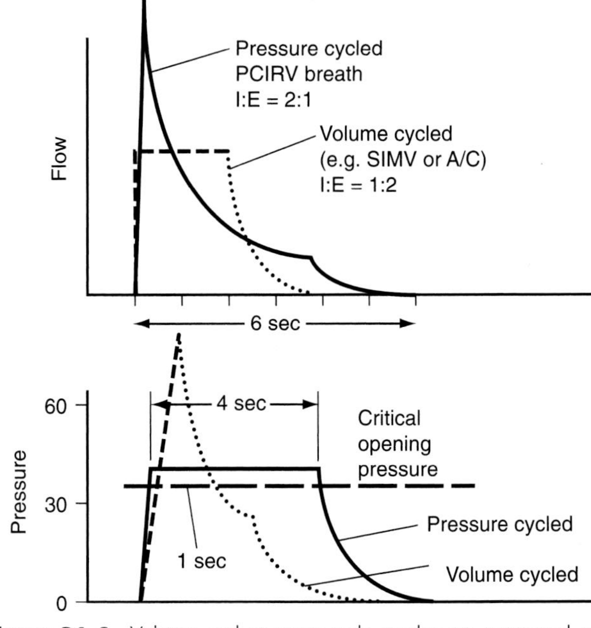

Figure 34–6 Volume and pressure cycle modes are compared as in Figure 34–5. If there is a critical opening pressure to recruit atelectatic lung segments, a pressure-controlled ventilation mode, particularly if the I:E ratio is inverted, is far more successful at maintaining an inspiratory pressure above the critical opening pressure for a greater length of time. Attempting to increase the volume-cycled flow would result in unacceptably high peak inspiratory pressures in an attempt to achieve more time above the critical opening pressure. But even in volume control, inspiratory pauses or changes to the flow rate in I:E ratio may be able to achieve longer sustained inspiratory pressures.

weaning attempts. Thus, other methods of weaning ventilatory support may need to be implemented.

Pressure-Controlled Ventilation

Pressure-controlled ventilation (PCV) is available on most newer ventilators and allows the clinician to specify a target inspiratory pressure; the ventilator then calculates and delivers the optimal flow rate to achieve the desired tidal volume and inspiratory-to-expiratory ratio. Figure 34–5 demonstrates the difference between pressure- and volume-controlled ventilation with regard to inspiratory flow. Pressure-controlled inverse-ratio ventilation (PC-IRV) is PCV with an inspiratory time that exceeds expiratory time (I:E ratio >1.0). Consider that opening alveoli with damaged lungs sometimes requires exceeding a critical opening pressure for an adequate amount of time (Fig. 34–6). With standard ventilation, this time above the critical pressure can only be lengthened by increasing the peak inspiratory pressure, which is generally undesirable with a damaged lung. With PC-IRV, the pressure waveform is optimized to allow a long inspiratory time above the critical opening pressure while avoiding high peak pressures. The disadvantage of PC-IRV is that the increased inspiratory time necessarily reduces exhalation time, which may lead to stacking of breaths or auto-PEEP in patients with abnormal lungs. Tharat et al[95] demonstrated that PC-IRV allowed a reduction in minute ventilation and reduced peak pressures while increasing mean airway pressures in patients with ARDS.

Changing a patient from conventional volume ventilation to pressure-control or PC-IRV can be accomplished by noting the existing tidal volume, inspiratory pressures, and inspiration-to-expiration (I:E) ratio and switching to PCV mode with similar inspiratory pressure, rate, and inspiratory time. The level of inspiratory pressure is then titrated to deliver a tidal volume similar to what the patient was receiving with volume-controlled ventilation. The inspiratory time can then be lengthened to achieve better oxygenation, or decreased to allow sufficient exhalation time if auto-PEEP is evident. In any patient with abnormal lungs, but particularly if an inverse-ratio ventilation mode is used, the patient must be monitored for the development of auto-PEEP, identified either by monitoring failure of the pressure waveform to return to baseline between breaths or by instituting an expiratory hold and noting the difference in pressure between the ventilator's pressure gauge and the level of PEEP that was specified. Sedation and often neuromuscular blockade are necessary if the I:E ratio is inverted. Adjusting the ventilator settings in pressure-control mode is not always intuitive. Increased rates may paradoxically decrease CO_2 elimination if tidal volumes decrease. Improvements in oxygenation may not occur until the patient is stabilized and given time to recruit atelectatic segments. Recruitment maneuvers when initiating PCV may help to open up atelectatic segments. The expectation is that these segments will remain open once recruited.

Pressure-Support Ventilation

Pressure-support ventilation (PSV), which is primarily a weaning tool, must be distinguished from pressure-control ventilation, which is generally used during the maintenance phase of ALI. PSV may be used in conjunction with continuous positive airway pressure (CPAP) or SIMV modes. Pressure support augments the patient's spontaneous inspiratory effort with a clinician-selected level of pressure. Putative advantages include improved patient comfort, reduced ventilatory work, and more rapid weaning. The volume delivered with each PSV breath depends on the pressure set for inspiratory assist as well as the patient's lung compliance. The utility of PSV in weaning from chronic ventilation support is that it allows the patient's ventilatory muscles to assume part of the workload while augmenting tidal volume, thus preventing atelectasis, sufficiently stretching lung receptors, and keeping the patient's spontaneous respiratory rate within a reasonable physiologic range. With some older ventilators, the inspiratory phase of PSV is terminated when flow falls to less than 25% of the initial value. In the presence of a cuff leak around the endotracheal tube, the flow rate may not fall to sufficiently low levels to terminate the breath, and the patient will struggle trying to exhale against the inspiratory flow. This problem is rare or nonexistent with the newer ventilators. Tidal volume will vary markedly with the patient's lung compliance, so close clinical observation is needed with the initiation of PSV. It is useful to monitor end-tidal CO_2 as well as pulse oximetry readings during the PSV weaning phase to limit phlebotomy for ABGs.

LIBERATION FROM MECHANICAL SUPPORT (WEANING)

An important concept to consider is that weaning from ventilator support is not synonymous with extubation. There are conditions when weaning is possible, but extubation is not; for example, upper airway edema or compression, glottic dysfunction with aspiration, neurologic dysfunction, or any other inability to protect the airway. A formal weaning process is not essential in a normal patient, although SIMV or PSV weaning may be convenient. In the absence of significant cardiopulmonary dysfunction, extubation depends more on a stable clinical condition, adequate warming, elimination and metabolism of anesthetics, and reversal of neuromuscular blockade. Weaning strategies are almost always required after more than 3 days of ventilation support.

When terminating mechanical ventilation, two phases of decision-making are involved. First, there should be resolution of the initial process for which mechanical ventilation was begun. The patient cannot be septic, hemodynamically unstable, or burdened with excessive respiratory secretions. If these general criteria are met, then specific weaning criteria can be examined. These include oxygenation (typically a $PaO_2 > 60$ mm Hg on 35% inspired oxygen and low levels of PEEP), adequate oxygen transport (measurable by O_2 extraction ratio or assumed if the cardiac index is adequate and lactic acidosis is not present), adequate respiratory mechanics (tidal volume, maximal inspiratory pressure) and adequate respiratory reserve (minute ventilation at rest of <10 L/min), and a low frequency–to–tidal volume ratio ($f/V_T < 100$) indicating adequate volume at a sustainable respiratory rate.

Objective Measures of Patient Strength and Endurance

While clinicians may use a variety of parameters to determine readiness for extubation, few have been examined carefully. Vital capacity, defined as the volume of gas exhaled after maximal inspiration, is normally greater than 70 mL/kg. A clinical readiness threshold of 10 to 15 mg/kg has been proposed but is neither sensitive nor specific. For short-term ventilated patients, VC is less reliable than the ability to maintain a pH > 7.35 while the IMV rate is decreased to CPAP.[96] Maximal inspiratory pressure (MIP) is often referred to as inspiratory force, negative inspiratory force (NIF), or peak negative pressure and quantifies inspiratory effort as a marker of respiratory muscle strength. The proper technique involves airway occlusion for up to 20 seconds starting at full exhalation using a one-way valve that allows the patient to exhale after attempted inspiration. Normal values of MIP should exceed 100 cm H_2O in males and 80 cm H_2O in females. Values are usually expressed as an absolute to avoid confusion with "less than" or "greater than" when referring to a negative number. The classic cutoff value of 20 to 30 cm H_2O is associated with a 26% false-positive and 100% false-negative rate. MIP is best used for serial evaluation of patients and is more a measure of strength than endurance.

Attempts have been made to predict endurance using the resting minute ventilation rate, but using the common value of 10 L/min as the cutoff results in a false-positive rate of 11% and a false negative rate of 75% in predicting successful extubation. Similarly, the ability to sustain maximum voluntary ventilation (MVV) twice the minute ventilation correctly predicts in only about 75% of the patients. More sophisticated measurement of endurance can be accomplished using a diaphragmatic or intercostal electromyograph (EMG) power spectrum, but these are not practical for routine clinical use. Yang and Tobin[97] attempted to develop a scoring system for weaning that integrated lung compliance, respiratory rate, oxygenation levels, and maximum inspiratory pressure to predict weaning success. While all of these elements and the total score have some predictive value, the best index turned out to be the f/V_T. An f/V_T greater than 105 has a predictive value of 89% for weaning failure. The tension-time index of the diaphragm (TT_{di}) integrates the inspiratory pressure with time and is a reliable measurement of endurance but difficult to perform in the clinical setting. If the percentage of inspiratory time over total time in a spontaneously breathing patient is greater than 15%, respiratory failure will eventually ensue, probably due to limitations of diaphragmatic blood flow, which only occurs during the expiratory phase.[98] The tension-time of the human diaphragm (TT_{di}) is calculated by plotting the inspiratory time on the y axis against the ratio of transdiaphragmatic pressure with normal and maximal effort on the *x* axis (Fig. 34–7). Fatigue is unlikely with values of TT_{di} less than 0.15; values above 0.18 define the fatigue zone.[99] Commercially available equipment such as the BiCor CP-100 pulmonary monitor can provide inspiratory time, f/V_T, and $P_{0.1}$, a marker of respiratory drive. Some newer ventilators also incorporate this technology. A problem with all measured respiratory parameters or scoring systems relying on pulmonary function is that they do not include the nonrespiratory parameters affecting weaning (Box 34–3).

Weaning: The Process

The actual process of weaning from mechanical ventilatory support must be individualized. There is no "one size fits all" method. While gradually lowering the rate in increments of two breaths per minute generally works for short-term

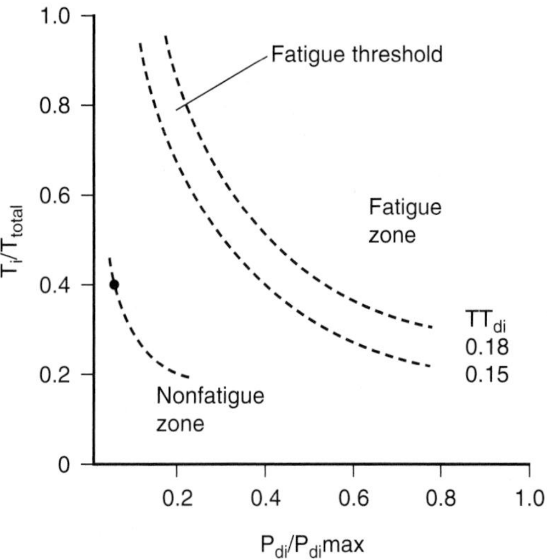

Work of breathing is the work expended by the ventilatory muscles in supporting breathing

Figure 34–7 The tension-time index for the human diaphragm is displayed. This graph is created by plotting the inspiratory cycle percentage (T_i/T_{total}) against transdiaphragmatic pressure during normal breathing as a fraction of the maximal transdiaphragmatic pressure (P_{di}/P_{dimax}). The fatigue threshold represents a tension time of the diaphragm that can be sustained for 1 hour or longer and typically ranges from 0.15 to 0.18 in healthy humans. Note that this threshold can be achieved with a variety of combinations of inspiratory time and inspiratory pressure. Grassino and colleagues demonstrated that patterns in the fatigue zone cause the patient to fail spontaneous ventilation within 1 hour, whereas patterns in the nonfatigue zone can be sustained more or less indefinitely. (From Grassino A, Bellemare F, Laporta D: Diaphragm fatigue and the strategy of breathing of COPD. Reproduced with permission from Chest 85:515, 1984.)

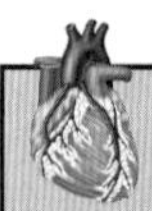

BOX 34–3 ***Nonrespiratory Factors Affecting Weaning***

- Nutrition status
- Renal function
- Fluid balance
- Sepsis/infection
- Hematologic status/anemia
- Metabolic disturbance
- Cardiac function
- Pharmacologic therapy
- Neurologic compromise
- Neuropsychiatric issues/delirium
- Sleep deprivation
- Endotracheal tube size
- Perception of breathing

ventilatory support, long-term patients often have difficulty making the transition from SIMV rates of 2 to CPAP. The time-honored method of weaning by maintaining a patient on full ventilatory support alternating with increasingly longer periods of spontaneous ventilation on a T-piece is effective, but time consuming since it requires setting up additional equipment and requires a nurse or respiratory therapist to be immediately available at bedside during each weaning attempt. Breath-to-breath monitoring, display of tidal volumes, and ventilator alarms will not be available during a T-piece trial. More commonly, pressure support is used as an adjunct to weaning either with IMV or CPAP while still connected to the ventilator and its alarm system. The preference is to use CPAP with pressure support alone (i.e., no additional IMV rate) since mechanical ventilation introduces one more variable into the evaluation of a patient's progress. Sufficient CPAP is applied to maintain open alveoli (generally 5 to 8 cm H_2O but often higher when recovering from ALI/ARDS) and then the pressure support level titrated to provide the patient with sufficient volume and a respiratory rate less than 24. As the patient's exercise tolerance improves, the pressure support level can be lowered in increments of 2 to 3 cm H_2O. It is usually necessary to address fluid overload, nutritional support, and other nonpulmonary factors in order to achieve the pressure support reduction.

Regardless of which weaning method is chosen, it is important to end each weaning trial with success rather than to stress the patient to the point of fatigue. Cohen et al identified the clinical sequence of inspiratory muscle fatigue.[100] The earliest sign of inspiratory muscle fatigue is a spectrum shift in the EMG power spectrum, which is impractical in the clinical setting. However, the next most sensitive sign was an increase in respiratory rate, which occurred before respiratory alternans, abdominal paradox, and increase in the $Pa{CO_2}$ level, or acidemia. Thus, respiratory rate can serve as a sensitive marker of weaning progress. Daily screening and spontaneous breathing trials using f/Vt less than 100 as a marker of readiness to extubate have not been validated in cardiac-only populations, but may be considered in patients with satisfactory hemodynamic stability.

Specific Impediments to Weaning

Weaning from ventilator support affects CO due to changes in pulmonary vascular resistance (PVR). Increased PVR can lead to septal shifts and consequent changes in the efficiency of right and left ventricular function. Thus, it makes little sense to attempt weaning in the hemodynamically unstable patient. The standard approach has been to keep these patients on full ventilator support with sedation and neuromuscular blockade if necessary until the acute cardiac problem is resolved.

Older ventilators with demand-valve systems impose an additional WOB, although it would be rare to see such ventilators (Bear I and II, Puritan Bennett MA-II) in clinical use today. Most newer ventilators employ computer-assisted demand valve technology to supply a variable flow rate, unlike older ventilators where a fixed low gas flow rate occasionally resulted in the inability to supply peak flow on demand. Nonetheless, if the patient is demonstrating apparent air hunger during the weaning process, a quick check of the inspiratory flow rates can often solve the problem. Pulmonary effusions and pneumothorax can develop in otherwise stable patients and may also present as stalled weaning. Stacking of breaths or auto-PEEP can occur if the expiratory time is too short for patients, particularly those with obstructive disease, to exhale fully before the next breath is delivered. Brown and Pierson[101] demonstrated that magnitude of auto-PEEP varied between 0 and 16 cm H_2O during routine ventilator checks.

Ventilator Dyssynchrony

Increases in intercostal muscle tone and increases in abdominal muscle tone, pressure, or contents decrease chest-cage compliance. During volume-cycled ventilation, a decrease in chest-cage compliance results in increased intrathoracic pressure that may reduce venous return to the right heart. A patient may also actively attempt to impede flow during the inspiratory cycle, a process referred to as "fighting," being "out of phase," or "breathing against" the ventilator. This should not be confused with a patient making ventilatory efforts during the ventilator's expiratory cycle, which has little, if any, detrimental effect.

The most common reasons for fighting the ventilator are (1) inadequate ventilation (hypercarbia), (2) acidemia, (3) inadequate oxygenation;,(4) central nervous system dysfunction, and (5) pain or anxiety. Assisting the patient with manual ventilation or switching to assist modes for a short time will allow the patient to settle down and return to synchrony with the ventilator. These maneuvers are temporizing during evaluation and treatment of the underlying cause for the patient/ventilator dyssynchrony. Endotracheal cuff leak, misplaced endotracheal tube, inadequate inspiratory flow rates, pneumothorax, abdominal distention, pain, and anxiety should all be considered in the differential.

Muscle Weakness and Critical Illness Polyneuropathy

Long-term administration of neuromuscular blocking agents, particularly those like vecuronium with a steroid structure, has been associated with persistent paralysis.[102] One explanation may be the accumulation of the metabolite 3-desacetylvecuronium, which is rarely seen in patients with normal renal function but is quite common in patients with delayed recovery.[102] However, prolonged paralysis can also be seen after treatment with other drugs such as pancuronium, metacurine, and cisatracurium, which do not necessarily share the same structure or have persistent metabolites. The suspicion is that neurogenic atrophy occurs with prolonged paralysis resulting in a flaccid quadriplegia or more localized weakness of respiratory muscles.

Prolonged ICU stay may also precipitate psychiatric problems even in normal patients, although the experience has been that these difficulties are more common in patients with an underlying psychiatric history. Light, noise, and lack of sleep can change a patient's perception of reality. Psychological dependency on the ventilator may also develop, although this is rare. While this issue has not been examined with controlled trials, careful attention to maintaining a normal day/night sleep cycle, assuring adequate sleep, creating quiet ICU environment, judicious use of pharmacologic agents such as haloperidol, and involving the patient and family as participants in the weaning process are all helpful when there are psychological impediments to weaning.

Tracheostomy

Prolonged endotracheal intubation results in damage to the respiratory epithelium and cilia, and may lead to vocal cord damage and airway stenosis.[103,104] If mechanical ventilation is anticipated for longer than 14 days, consideration should be given to early tracheostomy.[105,106] Other indications for tracheostomy include copious or tenacious secretions in debilitated patients who are unable to clear them spontaneously. Tracheostomy is relatively contraindicated with ongoing mediastinitis or local infection at the tracheostomy site because of the potential for mediastinal contamination with respiratory secretions. Tracheostomy is not a risk-free procedure and complications include pneumothorax, pneumomediastinum, subcutaneous emphysema, incisional hemorrhage, late tracheal stenosis or tracheomalacia, stomal infections, and rarely tracheoinnominate fistula. Early tracheostomy can be accomplished at the bedside with commercially available kits such as the Cook-Ciaglia or the "Rhino" device.[107,108] Swallowing dysfunction may occur following tracheostomy or after prolonged endotracheal intubation, introducing the risk of aspiration pneumonia or respiratory failure. A swallowing evaluation is indicated prior to allowing a tracheostomy patient to attempt oral feeding. This is usually accomplished with a formal speech pathology consult, but swallowing difficulty may also be noted by the nurses during attempted feedings.

Inability to Wean

A small percentage of patients will not be able to wean from ventilator support despite all efforts. Predictive models, however, are rarely useful for deciding which individuals will not benefit from further intensive care.[6,9,16,20,109]

The experience has been that it is rarely a single problem, but the interaction among multiple morbidities that creates a situation in which the patient may not separate from the ventilator. At this point, a frank discussion with the patient (if he or she has decisional capacity) or the health care proxy can be helpful in defining the benefits and burdens of further therapy and the patient's desires. Consultation from the hospital's ethics team may be very helpful.[110] Patients who remain in a low-cardiac-output state and who have sustained multiorgan failure rarely if ever end their dependence on high-technology support including ventilation and hemodialysis. On the other hand, malnutrition and deconditioning in the absence of ongoing sepsis and organ system failure sometimes respond to prolonged rehabilitation, which may be better handled by a long-term ventilation facility than an acute-care hospital.

CONCLUSIONS

Success in weaning from mechanical ventilation requires an individualized and holistic approach to the patient. Weaning should be the first priority for the day, and all other demands minimized if possible. If trips to the CT scanner or therapeutic intervention such as wound debridement are anticipated, weaning may not be possible for part of the day. Thus, interruptions should be minimized and grouped so as not to interrupt the weaning process. With that goal in mind, it is also essential to avoid disrupting the patient's nighttime sleep, so that the patient can be well rested and ready to participate in the weaning process. Detailed and full instructions need to be given to the patient, and it is frequently helpful to include family members in the discussion so that they can serve as adjunct respiratory coaches. Try to avoid pushing the patient to the point of exhaustion or panic and use a planned, conservative approach such that weaning always ends in a sense of accomplishment for the patient rather than failure. Windows of opportunity for weaning from mechanical support are few, and must often be created. Box 34–4 summarizes recommendations for the difficult-to-wean cardiac surgical patient.

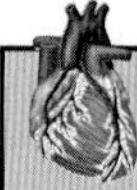

BOX 34–4 *The Difficult-to-Wean Patient*

- Recognize patients at risk based on preoperative and operating room events (see Table 34–2).
- Where possible, minimize risk (see Box 34–2).
- Prioritize organ system support; without adequate perfusion, all other systems will fail.
- Maintain full ventilator support during acute phase of respiratory insufficiency or circulatory failure.
- Adopt a lung-protective ventilation strategy for ALI/ARDS patients.
- Expect and defend against common problems (see Box 34–3).
- Pay attention to general support measures and safety issues including sedation holidays and infection control.
- Prepare patient and family for involvement in rehabilitation phase.
- Have a clear weaning plan or protocol and follow it.
- Recognize when the burdens of treatment are disproportionate, and initiate appropriate discussions with the patient or health care proxy.

REFERENCES

1. Westbrook RR, Stuvs SE, Sessler AD, et al: Effects of anesthesia and muscle paralysis on respiratory mechanisms in normal man. J Appl Physiol 34:81, 1973
2. Churchill E: The reduction in vital capacity following operation. Surg Gynecol Obstet 44:482, 1927
3. Sivak ED, Wiedemann HP: Clinical measurement of extravascular lung water. Crit Care Clin 2:511, 1986
4. Wilson RS, Sullivan SF, Malm JR, et al: The oxygen cost of breathing following anesthesia and cardiac surgery. Anesthesiology 99:387, 1973
5. Johnson D, Hurst T, Thompson D, et al: Respiratory function after cardiac surgery. J Cardiothorac Vasc Anesth 10:571, 1996
6. Rady MY, Ryan T, Starr NJ: Early onset of acute pulmonary dysfunction after cardiovascular surgery: Risk factors and clinical outcome. Crit Care Med 25:11, 1997
7. Weiner P, Zeidan F, Zamir D, et al: Prophylactic inspiratory muscle training in patients undergoing coronary artery bypass graft. World J Surg 22:427, 1998
8. Higgins TL: Quantifying risk in assessing outcome in cardiac surgery. J Cardiothorac Vasc Anesth 12:330, 1998
9. Higgins TL, Estafanous EG, Loop FD, et al: Stratification of morbidity and mortality outcome by preoperative risk factors in coronary artery bypass patients. A clinical severity score. JAMA 267:2344, 1992
10. Hatler BG, Armitage JM, Haristy RL, et al: Risk stratification using the Society of Thoracic Surgeons program. Ann Thorac Surg 58:1348, 1994
11. The Society of Thoracic Surgeons: 30-Day operative mortality and morbidity risk models. Ann Thorac Surg 75:1856, 2003
12. Samuels LE, Kaufman MS, Rohinton BA, et al: Coronary artery bypass grafting in patients with COPD. Chest 113:878, 1998
13. Samuels LE, Kaufman MS, Morris RJ, et al: Coronary artery bypass grafting in patients with COPD. Chest 113:878, 1998
14. Rockx MA, Fox SA, Stitt LW, et al: Is obesity a predictor of mortality, morbidity and readmission after cardiac surgery? Can J Surg 47:34, 2004
15. O'Brien MM, Gonzales R, Shroyer AL, et al: Modest serum creatinine elevation affects adverse outcome after general surgery. Kidney Int 62:585, 2002
16. Spivack SD, Shinozaki T, Albertini JJ, Deane R: Preoperative prediction of postoperative respiratory outcome. Coronary artery bypass grafting. Chest 109:1222, 1996
17. Branca P, McGaw P, Light RW, et al: Factors associated with prolonged mechanical ventilation following coronary artery bypass surgery. Chest 119:537, 2001
18. Rady MY, Ryan T: Perioperative predictors of extubation failure and the effect on clinical outcomes after cardiac surgery. Crit Care Med 27:340, 1999
19. Canver CC, Chanda J: Intraoperative and postoperative risk factors for respiratory failure after coronary bypass. Ann Thorac Surg 75:853, 2003
20. Higgins TL, Estafanous FG, Loop FD, et al: ICU admission score for predicting morbidity and mortality risk after coronary artery bypass grafting. Ann Thorac Surg 64:1050, 1997
21. Hall RI, Smith MS, Rocker G: The systemic inflammatory response to cardiopulmonary bypass—pathophysiological, therapeutic and pharmacological considerations. Anesth Analg 85:766, 1997
22. Boldt J, Kling D, Weidler B, et al: Acute preoperative hemodilution in cardiac surgery: volume replacement with a hypertonic saline-hydroxyethyl starch solution. J Cardiothorac Vasc Anesth 5:23, 1991
23. Boldt J, Zickmann B, Ballesteros M, et al: Cardiorespiratory responses to hypertonic saline solution in cardiac operations. Ann Thorac Surg 51:610, 1991
24. Lee A, Lum ME, O'Regan WJ, et al: Early postoperative emergencies requiring an intensive care team intervention: The role of ASA physical status and after-hours surgery. Anaesthesia 53:529, 1998
25. Jacobs MC, Hussain E, Hall MH, Cohn E: Stranger in a strange land: Internists in cardiothoracic intensive care. New Horizons 7:562, 1999
26. Reynolds HN, Haupt MT, Thill-Baharozian MC, et al: Impact of critical care physician staffing on patients with septic shock in a university hospital medical intensive care unit. JAMA 260:3446, 1988
27. Brown JJ, Sullivan G: Effect on ICU mortality of a full-time critical care specialist. Chest 96:127, 1989
28. www.leapfroggroup.org/factsheets/ICU_factsheet.pdf accessed on April 28, 2004
29. Fagon J-Y, Chastre J, Domart Y, et al: Nosocomial pneumonia in patients receiving continuous mechanical ventilation. Prospective analysis of 52 episodes with use of a protected specimen brush and quantitative culture techniques. Am Rev Respir Dis 139:877, 1989
30. Drakulovic MB, Torres A, Bauer TT, et al: Supine body position as a risk factor for nosocomial pneumonia in mechanically ventilated patients: A randomized trial. Lancet 354:1851, 1999
31. Craven DE, Goularte TA, Make BJ: Contaminated condensate in mechanical ventilator circuits: A risk factor for nosocomial pneumonia? Am Rev Respir Dis 129:625, 1984
32. Sonora R, Jubert P, Artigas A, et al: Pneumonia in intubated patients: Role of respiratory airway care. Am J Respir Crit Care Med 154:111, 1996
33. Kollef MH: The prevention of ventilator-associated pneumonia. N Engl J Med 340:627, 1999
34. Vallas J, Artigas A, Rello J, et al: Continuous aspiration of subglottic secretions in preventing ventilator-associated pneumonia. Ann Intern Med 122:179, 1995
35. Ware LB, Matthay MA: Protein C and thrombomodulin in human acute lung injury. Am J Physiol Lung Cell Mol Physiol 285:L514, 2003
36. Bernard GR, Artigas A, Brigham KL, et al: The American-European Consensus Conference on ARDS. Definitions, mechanisms, relevant outcomes, and clinical trial coordination. Am J Respir Crit Care Med 149:818, 1994
37. Murray JF, Matthay MA, Luce JM, Flick MR: An expanded definition of the adult respiratory distress syndrome. Am Rev Respir Dis 138:720, 1988
38. Nahum A, Hoyt J, Schmitz L, et al: Effect of mechanical ventilation strategy on dissemination of intrathecally instilled Escherichia coli in dogs. Crit Care Med 25:1733, 1997
39. Amato MB, Barbas CS, Medeiros DM, et al. Beneficial effects of the "open lung approach" with low distending pressures in acute respiratory distress syndrome: A prospective randomized study on mechanical ventilation. Am J Respir Crit Care Med 152:1835, 1995
40. The Acute Respiratory Distress Syndrome Network: Ventilation with lower tidal volumes as compared with traditional tidal volumes for acute lung injury and the acute respiratory distress syndrome. N Engl J Med 342:1301, 2000
41. Steinbrook R: How best to ventilate? Trial design and patient safety in studies of the acute respiratory distress syndrome. N Engl J Med 348:1393, 2003
42. Bidani A, Tzouanakis AE, Cardenas VJ, Zwischenberger JB: Permissive hypercapnea in acute respiratory failure. JAMA 272:957, 1994
43. Tidswell M: Prone ventilation. Clin Intens Care 12:193, 2001
44. Gattinoni L, Tognoni G, Pesenti A et al: Effect of prone positioning on the survival of patients with acute respiratory failure. N Engl J Med 345:568, 2001
45. Richard J-C, Brochard L, Vandelet P, et al: Respective effects of end-expiratory and end-inspiratory pressures on alveolar recruitment in acute lung injury. Crit Care Med 31:89, 2003
46. Morris AH, Wallace CJ, Menlove Rl, et al: Randomized clinical trial of pressure-controlled inverse ratio ventilation and extracorporeal CO2 removal for adult respiratory distress syndrome. Am J Respir Crit Care Med 149:295, 1994

47. Pranikoff T, Hirschl RB, Steimle CN, et al: Mortality is directly related to the duration of mechanical ventilation before the initiation of extracorporeal life support for severe respiratory failure. Crit Care Med 25:28, 1997
48. Hirschl RB, Pranikoff T, Wise C et al: Initial experience with partial liquid ventilation in adult patients with the acute respiratory distress syndrome. JAMA 275:383, 1996
49. Body SC, Shernan SK: The utility of nitric oxide in the postoperative period. Semin Cardiothorac Vasc Anesth 2:4, 1998
50. Ullrich R, Lorber C, Röder G, et al: Controlled airway pressure therapy, nitric oxide inhalation, prone position, and extracorporeal membrane oxygenation (ECMO) as components of an integrated approach to ARDS. Anesthesiology 91:1577, 1999
51. Walmrath D, Schneider T, Schermuly R, et al: Direct comparison of inhaled nitric oxide and aerosolized prostacyclin in acute respiratory distress syndrome. Am J Respir Crit Care Med 153:991, 1996
52. Miduri GU, Headley AS, Golden E, et al: Effect of prolonged methylprednisolone therapy in unresolving acute respiratory distress syndrome. JAMA 280:159, 1998
53. Michalopoulos A, Anthi A, Rellos K, Geroulanos S: Effects of positive end-expiratory pressure (PEEP) in cardiac surgery patients. Respir Med 92:858, 1998
54. Calzia E, Lindner KH, Radermacher P, Georgieff M: Effects of continuous positive airway pressure on respiratory mechanics and work of breathing after cardiac surgery. Clin Intens Care 9:105, 1998
55. Guyton RA, Chiavarelli M, Padgett CA, et al: The influence of positive end-expiratory pressure on intrapericardial pressure and cardiac function after coronary artery bypass surgery. J Cardiothorac Vasc Anesth 1:98, 1987
56. Boldt J, Kling D, Bormann BV, et al: Influence of PEEP ventilation immediately after cardiopulmonary bypass on right ventricular function. Chest 94:566, 1988
57. Pepe PE, Hudson LD, Carrico CJ: Early application of positive end-expiratory pressure in patients at risk for the adult respiratory distress syndrome. N Engl J Med 311:281, 1984
58. Zurick AM, Urzua J, Ghattas M, et al: Failure of positive end-expiratory pressure to decrease postoperative bleeding after cardiac surgery. Ann Thorac Surg 34:608, 1982
59. Rimensberger PC, Pristine G, Mullen BM, et al: Lung recruitment during small tidal volume ventilation allows minimal positive end-expiratory pressure without augmenting lung injury. Crit Care Med 27:1940, 1999
60. The ARDS Clinical Trials Network, National Heart, Lung and Blood Institute, National Institutes of Health: Effects of recruitment maneuvers in patients with acute lung injury and acute respiratory distress syndrome ventilated with high positive end-expiratory pressure. Crit Care Med 31:2592, 2003
61. Hood VL, Tannen RL: Protection of acid-base balance by pH regulation of acid production. N Engl J Med 339:819, 1998
62. Laffrey JG, Kavanagh BP: Carbon dioxide and the critically ill: Too little of a good thing? Lancet 354:1283, 1999
63. Steingrub JS, Tidswell MA, Higgins TL: Hemodynamic consequences of heart-lung interactions. J Intens Care Med 18:92, 2003
64. Pepe PE, Marini JJ: Occult positive end-expiratory pressure in mechanically ventilated patients with airflow obstruction. Am Rev Respir Dis 126:166, 1982
65. http://www.AHRQ.gov/clinic/ptsafety/addend.htm accessed May, 20, 2004
66. Kress JP, Pohlman AS, O'Connor MF, Hall JB: Daily interruption of sedative infusions in critically ill patients undergoing mechanical ventilation. N Engl J Med 342:1471, 2000
67. Van den Berghe G, Wouters P, Welkes F, et al: Intensive insulin therapy in the critically ill patient. N Engl J Med 345:1359, 2001
68. Pronovost P, Berenholtz S, Dorman T, et al: Improving communication in the ICU using daily goals. J Crit Care 18:71, 2003
69. Bates DW, Gawande AA: Improving safety with information technology. N Engl J Med 348:2526, 2003
70. Milbrandt EB, Deppen S, Harrison PL, et al: Costs associated with delirium in mechanically ventilated patients. Crit Care Med 31:955, 2004
71. Calabrese JR, Skwerer RG, Gulledge AD, et al: Incidence of postoperative delirium following myocardial revascularization. Cleve Clin J Med 54:29, 1987
72. Tesar GE, Murray GB, Cassem NH: Use of high-dose intravenous haloperidol in the treatment of agitated cardiac patients. J Clin Psychopharmacol 5:344, 1985
73. Wilcox P, Baile EM, Hards J, et al: Phrenic nerve function and its relationship to atelectasis after coronary artery bypass surgery. Chest 93:693, 1988
74. Lorin S, Sivak M, Nierman DM: Critical illness polyneuropathy: What to look for in at-risk patients. Diagnosis requires a high index of suspicion. J Crit Illness 13:608, 1998
75. Ibebunjo C, Martyn JAJA: Fiber atrophy, but not changes in acetylcholine receptor expression, contributes to the muscle dysfunction after immobilization. Crit Care Med 27:275, 1999
76. Van Balkom RHH, Dekhuijzen R, Folgering HTM, et al: Effects of long-term low-dose methylprednisone on rat diaphragm function and structure. Muscle Nerve 20:983, 1997
77. Abd AG, Braun NMT, Baskin MI, et al: Diaphragmatic dysfunction after open heart surgery; treatment with a rocking bed. Ann Intern Med 111:881, 1989
78. Aubier M, Detroyer A, Sampson M, et al: Aminophylline improves diaphragmatic contractility. N Engl J Med 305:249, 1981
79. Riddington DW, Venkatesh B, Boivin CM, et al: Intestinal permeability, gastric intramucosal pH and systemic endotoxemia in patients undergoing cardiopulmonary bypass. JAMA 275:1007, 1996
80. Tuzcu EM, Maloney JD, Sangani BH, et al: Cardiopulmonary effects of chronic amiodarone therapy in the early postoperative course of cardiac surgery patients. Cleve Clin J Med 54:491, 1987
81. Nalos PC, Kass RM, Gang ES, et al: Life-threatening postoperative pulmonary complications in patients with previous amiodarone pulmonary toxicity undergoing cardiothoracic operations. J Thorac Cardiovasc Surg 93:904, 1987
82. Manthous CA, Zarich S. Myocardial ischemia during weaning from mechanical ventilation. Semin Cardiothorac Vasc Anesth 2:78, 1998
83. Zin WA, Caldeira MPR, Cardoso WV, et al: Expiratory mechanics before and after uncomplicated heart surgery. Chest 1:21, 1989
84. Koning HM, Koning AJ, Leusink JA: Serious acute renal failure following open heart surgery. J Thorac Cardiovasc Surg 33:283, 1985
85. Myers BD, Moran SM: Hemodynamically mediated acute renal failure. N Engl J Med 314:97, 1987
86. Joy MS, Matske GR, Armstrong DK, et al: A primer on continuous renal replacement therapy for critically ill patients. Ann Pharmacother 32:362, 1998
87. Loop FD, Lytle BW, Cosgrove DM, et al: Sternal wound complications after isolated coronary artery bypass grafting: early and late mortality, morbidity, and cost of care. Ann Thorac Surg 49:179, 1990
88. Zerr KJ, Furnary AP, Grunkemeier GL, et al: Glucose control lowers the risk of wound infection in diabetics after open heart operations. Ann Thorac Surg 63:356, 1997
89. Kirschenbaum L, Azzi E, Sfeir T, et al: Effect of continuous lateral rotational therapy on the prevalence of ventilator-associated pneumonia in patients requiring long-term ventilatory care. Crit Care Med 30:1983, 2002
90. Chastre J, Fagon J-Y: Ventilator-associated pneumonia. Am J Respir Crit Care Med 165:867, 2002
91. Krasna MJ, Flanchbaum L, Trooskin ZS, et al. Gastrointestinal complications after cardiac surgery. Surgery 104:733, 1988
92. Ephgrave KS, Kleinman-Wexler RL, Adar CG: Enteral nutrients prevent stress ulceration and increase intragastric volume. Crit Care Med 18:621, 1990
93. Bassilli HR, Deitel M: Effect of nutritional support on weaning patients off mechanical ventilators. J Parenter Enteral Nutr 5:161, 1981
94. Larca L, Greenbaum DM: Effectiveness of intensive nutritional regimens in patients who fail to wean from mechanical ventilation. Crit Care Med 10:297, 1982
95. Tharratt RS, Allen RP, Albertson TE: Pressure-controlled inverse ratio ventilation in severe adult respiratory failure. CHEST 94:755, 1988
96. Millbern SM, Downs JB, Jumper LC, Modell JH: Evaluation of criteria for discontinuing mechanical ventilator. Arch Surg 113:1441, 1978
97. Yang KL, Tobin MJ: A prospective study of indexes predicting the outcome of trials of weaning from mechanical ventilation. N Engl J Med 324:1445, 1991
98. Bellemare F, Grassino A: Effect of pressure and timing of contraction on human diaphragm fatigue. J Appl Physiol 53:1190, 1982
99. Grassino A, Bellemare F, Laporta D: Diaphragm fatigue and the strategy of breathing in COPD. CHEST 85:515, 1984
100. Cohen CA, Zagelbaum G, Cross D, et al: Clinical manifestations of inspiratory muscle fatigue. Am J Med 73:308, 1982
101. Brown DG, Pierson DJ: Auto-PEEP is common in mechanically ventilated patients: A study of incidence, severity, and detection. Respir Care 31:1069, 1986
102. Segredo V, Caldwell JE, Matthay MA, et al: Persistent paralysis in critically ill patients after long-term administration of vecuronium. N Engl J Med 327:524, 1992

103. Kastanos N, Estopa R, Peez AM, et al: Laryngotracheal injury due to endotracheal intubation: Incidence, evolution, and predisposing factors. A prospective long-term study. Crit Care Med 11:362, 1983
104. Norwood S, Vallina VL, Short K, et al: Incidence of tracheal stenosis and other late complications after percutaneous tracheostomy. Ann Surg 232:233, 2000
105. Gibbons KJ: Tracheostomy: Timing is everything. Crit Care Med 28:1663, 2000
106. Brook AD, Sherman G, Malen J, et al: Early versus late tracheostomy in patients who require prolonged mechanical ventilation. Am J Crit Care 9:352, 2000
107. Westphal K, Byhahn C, Rinne T, et al: Tracheostomy in cardiosurgical patients: Surgical tracheostomy versus Ciaglia and Fantoni methods. Ann Thorac Surg 68:486, 1999
108. Freeman BD, Isabella K, Cobb P, et al: A prospective, randomized study comparing percutaneous with surgical tracheostomy in critically ill patients. Crit Care Med 29:926, 2001
109. Holmes L, Loughead K, Treasure T, Gallivan S: Which patients will not benefit from further intensive care after cardiac surgery? Lancet 344:1200, 1994
110. Baldyga AP: Ethical issues in the postoperative intensive care unit. Semin Cardiothoracic Vasc Anesth 2:90, 1998

Chapter 35

CENTRAL NERVOUS SYSTEM DYSFUNCTION AFTER CARDIOPULMONARY BYPASS

Ivan Iglesias, MD • John M. Murkin, MD, FRCPC

KEY POINTS

1. Notwithstanding a progressive decrease in cardiac surgical mortality over the past decades, the incidence of postoperative neurologic complications remains relatively unchanged.
2. Different studies have shown an association between advanced age and a higher incidence of neurologic events in cardiac surgical patients.
3. Neurologic events in cardiac surgical patients are associated with increased postoperative mortality, prolonged intensive care unit and hospital stay, decreased quality of life, and decreased long-term survival.
4. Neurologic complications range from coma, stroke, and visual field deficits to impairments of cognitive processes (e.g., impaired memory and attention, mood alterations, etc.).
5. Mechanisms for neurologic injury in cardiac surgery include some combination of cerebral embolism, hypoperfusion, and inflammation; associated vascular disease and altered cerebral autoregulation render the brain more susceptible to injury.
6. Perioperative risk factors for neurologic complications include diabetes mellitus, hypertension, prior cerebrovascular disease, aortic atheromatosis, manipulation of ascending aorta, complex surgical procedures, bypass time longer than 2 hours, hemodynamic instability during and after bypass, hyperglycemia, hyperthermia, and hypoxemia.
7. Routine epiaortic scanning before instrumentation of the ascending aorta is a sensitive and specific technique to detect nonpalpable aortic atheromatosis.
8. In patients with significant ascending aorta atheromatosis, avoidance of aortic manipulation ("no-touch technique") can decrease perioperative stroke.
9. Perioperative blood glucose concentration below 200 mg/dL may positively influence neurologic outcome.
10. Strategies to decrease the impact of cardiopulmonary bypass on embolization, inflammation, and coagulation will decrease neurologic complications.

Overt and subclinical perioperative cerebral injury remains an unresolved problem. As reported by Fersuson et al,[1] whereas overall mortality for patients undergoing coronary artery bypass grafting (CABG) has decreased by 23% over the past decade despite a projected risk-adjusted mortality predicting a 33% increase in mortality, the incidence of stroke has remained relatively unchanged.

AGE-ASSOCIATED RISK OF CENTRAL NERVOUS SYSTEM INJURY

In 1985, Gardner et al[2] reported a retrospective review of 3279 patients who underwent CABG between 1974 and 1983. They noted that despite an overall decrease in mortality, there was a corresponding increase in the incidence of stroke over that same decade.[2] They also observed a progressive increase in the average age of the patients and noted an elevated stroke rate of 7.1% in patients older than 75 years compared with an incidence of 0.42% in patients younger than 50 years. Of note is the fact that at that time, septuagenarians accounted for only 14.7% of their operative population. Approximately a decade later, Tuman et al[3] undertook a prospective study of 2000 patients undergoing CABG and also demonstrated a disproportionately increased risk of neurologic complications as compared with cardiac complications in elderly patients (Fig. 35–1). Neurologic events, defined as new sensory, motor, or reflex abnormalities, occurred with an overall frequency of 2.8%, having an incidence of 0.9% in those patients less than 65 years of age, 3.6% in those aged 65 to 74 years, and 8.9% in those patients over the age of 75. Of note, they observed that patients with a neurologic event had a nine-fold increase in mortality: 35.7% versus 4.0%.

Current data confirm a persistent association between increased age and cerebral injury after cardiac surgery.[4-12] In a review of 67,764 cardiac surgical patients, of whom there were 4743 octogenarians, and who underwent cardiac surgery at 22 centers in the National Cardiovascular Network, Alexander et al[12] reported that the incidence of type I cerebral injury, defined by Roach et al[13] as stroke, transient ischemic attack (TIA), or coma, was 10.2% in patients older than 80, versus 4.2% in patients less than 80 years old. Although global mortality for cardiac surgery in octogenarians was higher than in younger patients, the authors reported that when octogenarians without significant comorbidities were considered, their mortality rates were similar to those of younger patients.[12] In this respect, in addition to the age-related factor, reports from Europe and North America consistently describe previous cerebrovascular disease, diabetes mellitus, hypertension, peripheral vascular disease, aortic atherosclerosis, and intraoperative and postoperative complications as all being additional factors increasing the incidence of cerebral injury in cardiac surgical patients (Box 35–1). The presence of preoperative comorbidities further increases the age-associated risk of central nervous system (CNS) complications. For example, in a population of 149 patients older than 70 years who also had significant comorbidities including aortic atheroma, diabetes mellitus, history of previous CNS event, and who underwent cardiac surgery with cardiopulmonary bypass (CPB), Frumento et al[8] reported a stroke incidence of 16%.

The impact of age-associated cerebral injury in cardiac surgery is becoming more relevant due to the progressive

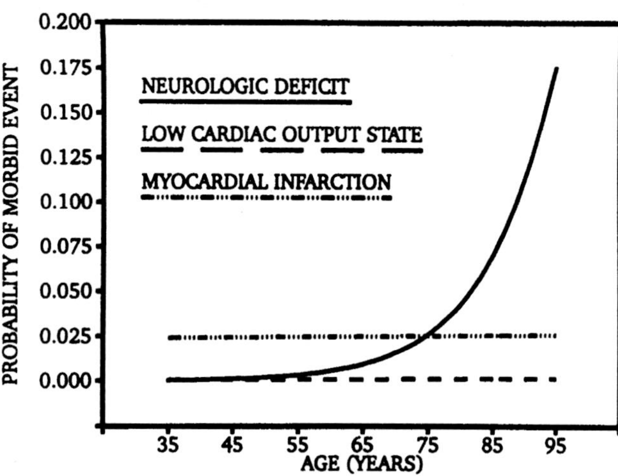

Figure 35–1 Effect of advanced age on the predicted probability of neurologic and cardiac morbidity. (From Tuman KJ, McCarthy RJ, Najafi H, et al: Differential effects of advanced age on neurologic and cardiac risks of coronary artery operations. J Thorac Cardiovasc Surg 104:1510, 1992.)

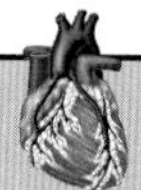

BOX 35–1 ***Factors Related to Cerebral Injury in Cardiac Surgery***

- Hemodynamic instability[4,5,26,100]
- Diabetes mellitus[4,8,25,191]
- Age[5,18,55,101,230,231]
- Combined/complex procedures[4,5]
- Prolonged cardiopulmonary bypass time[4,26,34,55]
- Prior stroke[5,7,25,55]
- Aorta atheromatosis[6,8,53-56]
- Peripheral vascular disease[6,34]

Risk factors are consistently reported for perioperative cerebral injury in cardiac surgery patients; see reference numbers and discussion in the text.

increase in the average age of the general population and, in particular, of the cardiac surgical population.[10,11,13-15] As overall survival and quality of life after cardiac surgery continue to improve in elderly patients, advanced age alone is no longer considered a deterrent when evaluating a patient for cardiac surgery.[10-12,16] The presence and extent of comorbidities should be considered as being of equal or greater importance than age itself as a risk factor for cerebral injury in cardiac surgical patients.

CENTRAL NERVOUS SYSTEM INJURY

Roach et al[13] classified cerebral injury in two broad categories: type I (focal injury, stupor, or coma at discharge) and type II (deterioration in intellectual function, memory deficit, or seizures). A similar classification was adopted by the American College of Cardiology/American Heart Association (ACC/AHA) guidelines for CABG.[17] Cerebral injury can also be broadly classified as stroke, delirium (encephalopathy), or cognitive dysfunction. *Stroke* is defined as any new and persistent focalized sensorimotor deficit, identified either on clinical grounds only, or ideally, as confirmed by magnetic resonance imaging (MRI), computed tomography (CT), or other form of brain imaging. *Delirium* is described as a transient global impairment of cognitive function, reduced level of consciousness, profound changes in sleep pattern, and attention abnormalities. Perioperative cognitive performance is assessed through the administration of a series of standardized psychometric tests, ideally administered preoperatively and postoperatively, with *cognitive dysfunction* being defined as a decrease in score falling below some predetermined threshold, such as a decrease in postoperative score of magnitude 1 standard deviation or more derived from the preoperative performance of the study group as a whole.

The incidence of stroke or type I injury after closed-chamber cardiac procedures is generally considered to be approximately 1% to 4%, increasing to about 8% to 9% in open-chamber (e.g., valvular surgery) or combined/complex procedures. The incidence of cognitive dysfunction (type II) is reported as ranging in incidence from 30% to 80% in the early postoperative period.[4,17-24] To some extent, there is a difference in the incidence of cerebral injury after cardiac surgery related to the type and complexity of the procedure, such as open chamber, combined valvular and CABG, etc.[4,19,25,26]

Overall, the increased length of stay (LOS) and increased mortality rates associated with any form of cerebral complication in cardiac surgical patients are especially striking findings.[14,17,19,20] Despite the relatively greater impact on mortality of stroke as opposed to cognitive dysfunction, type II injury is still associated with a five-fold increase in mortality. In their study, Roach et al[13] evaluated 2108 patients undergoing CABG at 24 U.S. institutions and recorded adverse cerebral outcomes in 6.1% of patients overall. Of these, 3.1% experienced type I focal injury, stupor, or coma and had an associated in-hospital mortality rate of 21%, whereas 3.0% of patients experienced deterioration of intellectual function or seizures and had a mortality rate of 10%. In contrast, a significantly lower overall mortality rate of 2% was seen in those patients without adverse cerebral outcomes. In addition, patients with neurologic complications had, on average, a 2-fold increase in hospital LOS and a 6-fold likelihood of discharge to a nursing home. Independent risk factors were identified for both type I and type II cerebral injury. Predictors of both types of cerebral complications included advanced age of greater than 70 years and a history or the presence of significant hypertension. Predictors of type I deficits included the presence of proximal aortic atherosclerosis as defined by the surgeon at the time of surgery, a history of prior neurologic disease, use of the intra-aortic balloon pump (IABP), diabetes, a history of hypertension, a history of unstable angina, and increasing age. Perioperative hypotension and the use of ventricular venting were also weakly associated with this type of outcome.[13]

An important caveat that must be borne in mind when interpreting the results of Roach et al is that type II injury as identified in their study is not necessarily equivalent to perioperative cognitive dysfunction as demonstrated in other studies. Type II injury was detected on clinical grounds alone rather than on the basis of a deterioration in performance on a predefined series of specific cognitive tests. The latter are a much more sensitive measure of performance and thus detect cognitive dysfunction with a considerably greater frequency, and as such potentially have a much different, although not necessarily benign, implication from the elevated

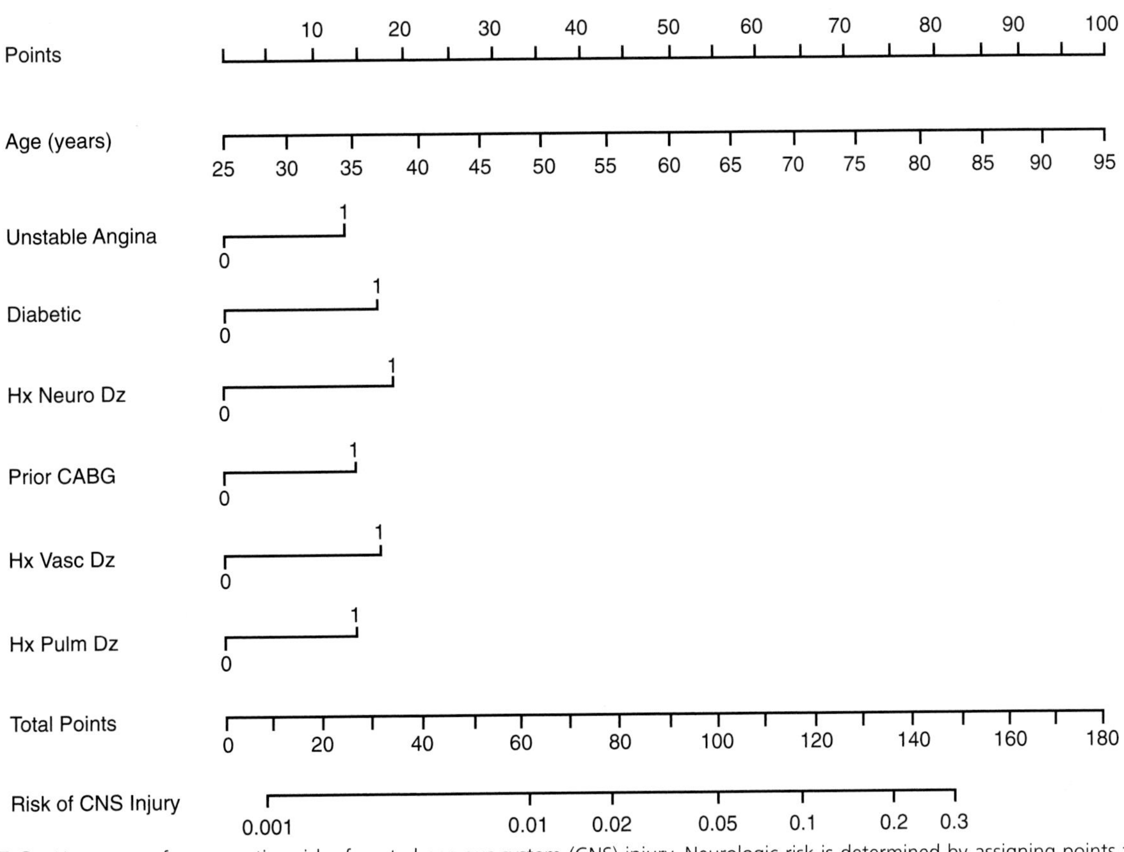

Figure 35–2 Nomogram for computing risk of central nervous system (CNS) injury. Neurologic risk is determined by assigning points for age and positive history of the predictors listed. Total points for each variable are read from the points line at the top of the nomogram. After the total points for an individual patient are computed, the risk of CNS injury can be determined by plotting the total points received against the risk score at the bottom of the nomogram. For example, 100 total points predict a risk of CNS injury of 5%. Hx Neuro Dz = history of symptomatic neurologic disease; Hx of Vasc Dz = history of atherosclerotic vascular disease or previous vascular surgery; Hx of Pulm Dz = history of emphysema, chronic bronchitis, asthma, or restrictive lung disease. (From Newman MF, Wolman R, Kanchuger M, et al: Multicenter preoperative stroke risk index for patients undergoing coronary artery bypass graft surgery. Multicenter Study of Perioperative Ischemia [McSPI] Research Group. *Circulation* 49[suppl II]:II-74, 1996.)

mortality associated with type II injury demonstrated by Roach et al.[13,27]

Using a risk stratification analysis of this same database, Newman et al developed a preoperative index predicting major perioperative neurologic events of which key predictors were age, history of neurologic disease, diabetes, previous CABG, unstable angina, and history of pulmonary disease[13,28] (Fig. 35–2). The Stroke Risk Index allows neurologic risk to be estimated for each patient, thus enabling the most appropriate perioperative therapy to be used, whether surgical modification, change in perfusion management, applied neuromonitoring, or administration of putative pharmacologic cerebroprotectants. It is also useful as a scale to compare risk indices and thus the efficacy of different interventions across clinical outcome studies.[8,20]

Retrospective Versus Prospective Neurologic Assessment

The detection of CNS injury depends critically on the methodology used, and retrospective studies have been deemed insensitive by different authors.[22,23,29,30] As was demonstrated by Sotaniemi,[30] a retrospective chart review is inadequate as an assessment of the overall incidence of postoperative neurologic dysfunction. In a study of 100 patients in whom a 37% incidence of neurologic dysfunction had been diagnosed by careful neurologic examination, the prevalence of cerebral abnormalities detected by retrospective analysis of the same patient pool was only 4%. The reasons for the inability of retrospective chart audit to detect the majority of patients with neurologic dysfunction are readily apparent and include incompleteness of records, a reluctance to document apparently minor complications, and, most important, an insensitivity to subtle neurologic dysfunction. Many of the types of neurologic impairment now being documented are subclinical and not readily detectable by a standard "foot-of-the-bed" assessment. The timing, thoroughness, and reproducibility (single examiner) of the neurologic examinations, as well as the incorporation of a preoperative assessment for comparison, all determine the sensitivity and accuracy with which postoperative CNS injury can be detected.[22,23,29,31]

Valvular Versus Coronary Artery Bypass Graft Surgery

It appears that increasing the complexity or undertaking open chamber–type procedures increases the risk of CNS injury. Ebert et al[32] prospectively studied 42 patients who underwent valve replacement surgery and 42 patients for CABG, with both groups matched post hoc for age, sex, and preoperative cognitive status. Patients were investigated preoperatively as well as 2 and 7 days postoperatively with a comprehensive neuropsychological and neuropsychiatric assessment. Valve replacement surgery patients exhibited more severe neuropsychological deficits and showed a slower recovery than patients who underwent CABG.[32] In a study by Alexander et al[12] of 64,467 patients who underwent CABG alone and 3297 patients who underwent CABG in conjunction with aortic valve replacement (CABG/AVR) or CABG in conjunction with mitral valve repair or replacement (CABG/MVR), the incidence of type I cerebral injury in patients younger than 80 years was 4.2% for CABG, 9.1% for CABG/AVR, and 11.2% for CABG/MVR. It should be noted that the total CPB time was 96 minutes for CABG, 148 minutes for CABG/AVR, and 161 minutes for CABG/MVR. It thus remains unclear whether it is the procedure itself, or the prolonged duration of CPB, either acting directly or as a marker of a greater surgical difficulty and thus perioperative hemodynamic instability, that is fundamentally causative.[33]

Wolman et al[19] prospectively studied 273 patients from 24 U.S. medical centers who underwent combined intracardiac surgery and CABG. Included were clinical, historic, specialized testing, neurologic outcome, and autopsy data, and measures of resource utilization. Adverse cerebral outcomes occurred in 16% of patients (43 of 273), being nearly equally divided between type I cerebral injury (8.4%; 5 cerebral deaths, 16 nonfatal strokes, and 2 new TIAs) and type II cerebral injury (7.3%; 17 new intellectual deteriorations persisting at hospital discharge and 3 newly diagnosed seizures), rates of injury 2- to 3-fold higher than demonstrated after CABG alone by this same group of investigators.[19] Associated resource utilization was significantly increased according to type of CNS injury: prolonging median intensive care unit (ICU) stay from 3 days (no adverse cerebral outcome) to 8 days associated with type I injury and from 3 to 6 days in those patients with type II injury. Significant risk factors for type I cerebral injury related primarily to embolic phenomena, including proximal aortic atherosclerosis, intracardiac thrombus, and intermittent clamping of the aorta during surgery. Risk factors for type II cerebral injury included proximal aortic atherosclerosis, as well as a preoperative history of endocarditis, alcohol abuse, perioperative arrhythmia, or poorly controlled hypertension, and the development of a low-output state after CPB.[19]

Interestingly, there is some evidence that the incidence of subtle neurologic dysfunction and cognitive abnormalities is similar in all adult patients undergoing surgical coronary artery revascularization, which some studies have related to the duration of CPB.[4,12,23,34-37] Increasing age has been repeatedly shown to be one of the major risk factors for stroke after CABG, likely related to the greater prevalence of severe aortic atherosclerosis in the elderly. This suggests that there may be different factors operative in the production of gross neurologic damage than in the genesis of cognitive dysfunction. While calcific or atheromatous macroembolic debris from the ascending aorta or aortic arch appears to be a prime factor in the production of clinical stroke syndromes and it was formerly thought that microembolic elements, either gaseous or particulate, produced cognitive dysfunction, studies from beating-heart surgery in which CPB is avoided, despite a much lower incidence of embolic events, appear to have a relatively similar incidence of cognitive dysfunction to CABG using conventional CPB.[38-40]

Aortic Atherosclerosis

Atheroembolism from an atheromatous ascending aorta and aortic arch is recognized as a major risk factor in the patient undergoing cardiac surgery and is a widespread problem.[41-47] In a study of 298 asymptomatic members from the Framingham cohort aged 60 ± 9 years and of whom 51% were women, subjects underwent thoracoabdominal aortic cardiovascular MRI and demonstrated aortic plaque of 1-mm radial thickness in 38% of the women and 41% of the men.[41] The Stroke Prevention: Assessment of Risk in the Community (SPARC) study used transesophageal echocardiography (TEE) in 581 people older than 44.[47] Atheroma was identified in 51.3% of patients, of whom 7.6% had severe atheroma (>4-mm thick, ulcerated or mobile). The prevalence of aortic arch atheroma increased with age, such that severe atheroma was seen in more than 20% of patients older than 74.[47]

Atheroembolism in cardiac surgery has a broad spectrum of clinical presentations, including devastating injuries and death, yet its true incidence is probably underestimated.[48-51] Thoracic aorta atheromatosis is associated with coronary artery disease and stroke in the general population.[42,43,45-47] In a review by Macleod et al,[42] the evidence shows that the risk of stroke is four times greater in patients with severe arch atheroma. Yahia et al[45] prospectively studied patients with diagnoses of TIA or stroke using TEE for assessment of aortic atheromatosis. Thoracic aortic atheromas were present in 141 of 237 patients (59%); mild plaque (<2 mm) was present in 5%, moderate plaque (2 to 4 mm) in 21%, severe plaque (≥4 mm) in 33%, and complex plaque in 27%. Plaques were more frequently present in the descending aorta and the arch of the aorta than in the ascending aorta.[45] Watanabe et al[46] investigated whether thoracic aorta calcification on computed tomography and coronary risk factors had any correlation with obstructive coronary artery disease on angiography. Two hundred twenty-five consecutive patients underwent both thoracic conventional helical computed tomography and coronary angiography. Thoracic aorta calcification was detected in 185 patients; 141 of 225 patients had significant obstructive coronary artery disease, all of the 13 patients without thoracic aorta calcification and no coronary risk factors had no coronary artery disease.[46] Overall, it can be seen that atherosclerosis of the ascending aorta is present in 20% to 40% of cardiac surgical patients, the percentage increasing with age (Fig. 35–3), and it is an independent risk factor for type I cerebral injury.[6-8,52-58]

Transesophageal Echocardiography Versus Epiaortic Scanning

The detection of ascending aorta atheromatosis is a cornerstone of strategies to decrease cerebral injury in cardiac surgery. Despite its widespread utilization, manual palpation of the aorta has a very low sensitivity for this purpose.[59,60] The association of severe thoracic aortic plaques (defined as 5-mm-thick focal hyperechogenic zones of the aortic intima and/or lumen irregularities with mobile structures or ulcerations) and coronary artery disease is well established.[57] Identifying severe aortic disease has important clinical implications because surgical technique, including surgical procedure and siting of cannulation and anastomotic sites for proximal grafts, may be altered to avoid producing emboli and stroke. Intraoperative epiaortic ultrasound scanning (EAS) has emerged as a most helpful tool for the diagnosis of ascending aortic atherosclerosis and has revealed major insights into the nature and distribution of this disease.

Djaiani et al[58] performed TEE and EAS to assess the severity of aortic atherosclerosis in the ascending aorta and the

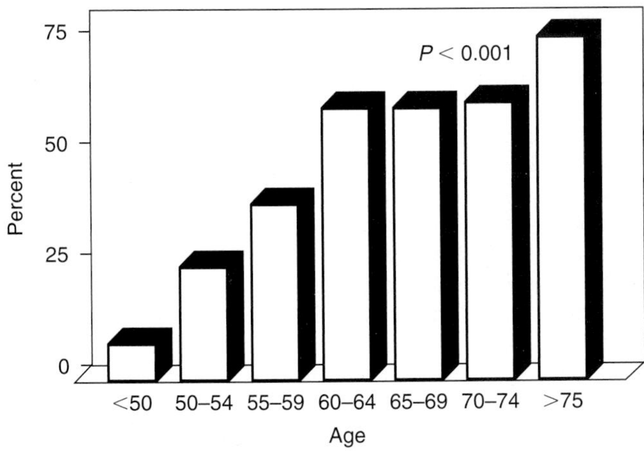

Figure 35–3 Prevalence of severe atherosclerosis of the ascending aorta at autopsy after operations for coronary and valvular heart disease, 1982 through 1989. (From Blauth CI, Cosgrove DM, Webb BW, et al: Atheroembolism from the ascending aorta. An emerging problem in cardiac surgery. J Thorac Cardiovasc Surg 103:1104, 1992.)

aortic arch. Patients were allocated to either low-risk or high-risk groups according to aorta intimal thickness. Transcranial Doppler was used to monitor the middle cerebral artery. Diffusion-weighted (DW)-MRI was performed 3 to 7 days after surgery. The NEECHAM Confusion Scale was used for assessment and monitoring patient consciousness level. In the high-risk group (intimal thickness >2 mm), confusion was present in six (16%) patients versus five (7%) patients in the low-risk group, and there was a three-fold increase in median embolic count, 223.5 versus 70.0 ($p = 0.0003$). DW-MRI–detected brain lesions were only present in patients from the high-risk group, 61.5% versus 0% ($p < 0.0001$). There was significant correlation between the NEECHAM scores and embolic count in the high-risk group.[58] Multiple studies have documented that most of the significant atherosclerotic lesions in the ascending aorta are missed by intraoperative palpation by the surgeon and intraoperative echocardiographic studies of the aorta have been recommended[21,54,56,58-64] (Fig. 35–4). However, the ability of TEE to reliably detect all ascending aorta and aortic arch lesions is limited.

The high acoustic reflectance attributable to the air–tissue interface resulting from overlying right main bronchus and trachea limits TEE assessment of the upper ascending aorta where cannulation is generally undertaken.[59,60,64,65] Intraoperative EAS has emerged as a most helpful tool for the diagnosis of ascending aortic atherosclerosis and has revealed major insights into the nature and distribution of this disease. Konstadt et al[61,65] investigated 81 patients (57 male and 24 female; aged 32 to 88 years, mean age 64 years) scheduled for elective cardiac surgery. A comprehensive examination of the entire thoracic aorta in both the longitudinal and transverse planes was performed by biplane TEE. After pericardiotomy, a sterile-draped 7-MHz probe was used to scan the entire ascending aorta in both long- and short-axis views. In both echocardiographic examinations, the presence and location of protruding plaques and intimal thickening greater than 3 mm were recorded. Fourteen (17%) of the 81 patients had significant atherosclerotic disease of the ascending aorta as diagnosed by EAS echocardiography. The sensitivity of TEE was 100%, the specificity was 60%, the positive predictive value was 34%, and the negative predictive value was 100%. According to the authors, if the complete biplane TEE examination is negative for plaque, it is highly unlikely that there is significant plaque in the ascending aorta. If the TEE examination is positive for plaque, there is a 34% chance that there is significant disease of the ascending aorta, and EAS should be considered. TEE is a very sensitive but only mildly specific method of determining whether ascending aortic atherosclerosis is present.[61-65]

The standard for aortic assessment prior to instrumentation continues to be visual inspection and palpation by the surgeon, despite the fact that this has been shown to identify atheromatous disease in only 25% to 50% of patients, and even then to significantly underestimate its severity.[59,60,66-68] Identification of ascending aorta atheromatous disease would prompt the surgical team for strategies to either modify, decrease, or avoid aortic manipulation. Management strategies for the diseased ascending aorta range from minimally invasive aortic "no-touch" techniques (NTTs) to maximally invasive procedures, including ascending aorta replacement with application of deep hypothermic circulatory arrest. Operative modifications in CABG include avoidance of aortic cross-clamping, alternative methods of aortic cross-clamping, and placement of all arterial in situ bypass conduits, Y-grafts, or extra-anatomic bypass grafts. Improvements in CNS outcome are likely to be associated with this approach (Fig. 35–5).

"No-Touch" Technique

Avoidance of instrumentation of the ascending aorta in patients with severe aortic atheromatosis has been advocated. Leacche et al[53] retrospectively reviewed data from 640 off-pump CABG (OPCAB) patients and identified 84 patients in whom they adopted an NTT. In these patients, revascularization was carried out with single or bilateral internal thoracic

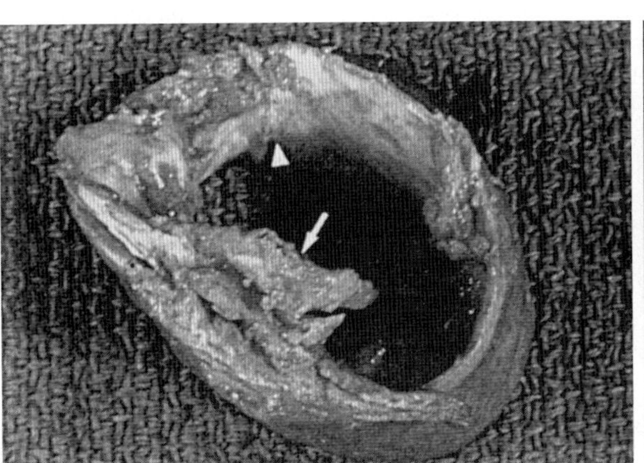
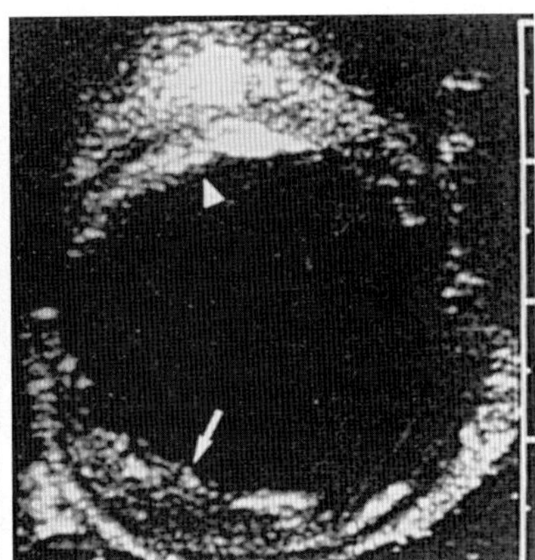

Figure 35–4 Transverse ultrasonic image of the ascending aorta and the corresponding segment of aorta in a patient with severe atherosclerosis. Note the calcification (*triangle*) and the projection of atheroma (*arrow*) into the lumen. (From Wareing TH, Davila-Roman VG, Barzilai B, et al: Management of the severely atherosclerotic ascending aorta during cardiac operations. A strategy for detection and treatment. J Thorac Cardiovasc Surg 103:453, 1992.)

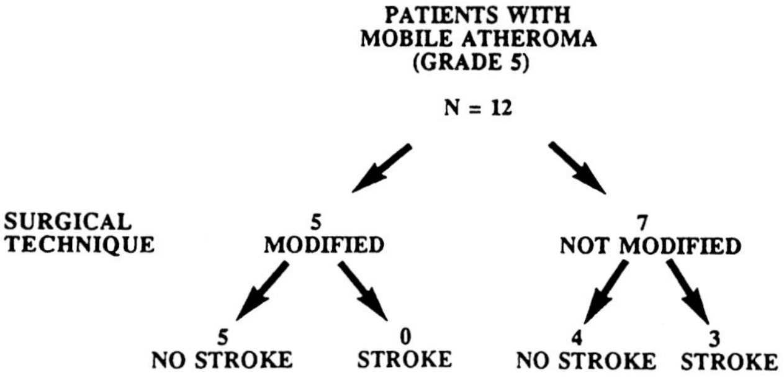

PATIENTS WITH MOBILE ATHEROMA (GRADE 5)

N = 12

SURGICAL TECHNIQUE	5 MODIFIED		7 NOT MODIFIED	
	5 NO STROKE	0 STROKE	4 NO STROKE	3 STROKE

Figure 35–5 Influence on neurologic outcome of altering operative technique on the basis of the finding of mobile aortic atheromas on transesophageal echocardiography. (Reprinted with permission from the American College of Cardiology [Journal of the American College of Cardiology 20:70-77, 1992]. Copyright 1992, with permission from the American College of Cardiology Foundation.)

arteries and by connecting additional coronary grafts (saphenous vein, radial artery) in a T or Y configuration. The right gastroepiploic artery was used as a conduit in two patients, while the brachiocephalic artery was used as an alternative inflow site for arterial cannulation in three reoperations. Age, sex, risk factors, functional class, and history of congestive heart failure were comparable in the two groups. In the NTT group, the frequencies were higher for severe atherosclerosis of the aorta (13% versus 0%), carotid disease (25% versus 16%), and history of previous cerebrovascular accidents (17% versus 8%). In the NTT group, weak trends toward a lower incidence of postoperative delirium (8% versus 15%; $p = 0.12$), a lower incidence of stroke (0% versus 1%; $p = 0.85$), and a shorter intensive care unit stay ($p = 0.07$) were observed.[53] In a review of 1993 beating-heart surgery patients, Calafiore et al[69] observed that in patients with evidence of peripheral vascular disease, use of aortic partial occlusion clamp was associated with a similar stroke rate as in patients in whom conventional CPB was used. They concluded that in patients with extracoronary vasculopathy, aortic manipulation must be avoided to reduce the incidence of stroke. Gaspar et al[64] used EAS and TEE in 22 patients considered to be at high risk of stroke in whom severe aortic atheroma (maximum aortic wall thickness >5 mm or mobile plaque) was detected, and with the use of aortic NTT and beating-heart surgery, no strokes occurred.

Royse et al[59] performed screening of the aorta for atheroma before aortic manipulation and used an exclusive Y-graft revascularization technique, which has no aortic coronary anastomoses. Aortic atheroma was detected using EAS and TEE. In the control group, aortic atheroma was assessed by manual palpation, while transcranial Doppler (TCD) of the right middle cerebral artery was used to detect cerebral microemboli. Neuropsychological dysfunction was assessed using a battery of 10 psychometric tests, and they demonstrated that at 60 days postoperatively, dysfunction in the control group was 38.1% while in the TEE/Y-graft group it was reduced to 3.8%. Microemboli detected by TCD during periods of aortic manipulation were greater for those with late dysfunction (5.2 ± 3.0 compared with 0.5 ± 0.2), consistent with an embolic etiology for cognitive dysfunction.[59]

NEUROPSYCHOLOGICAL DYSFUNCTION

Compared with stroke, cognitive dysfunction is a considerably more frequent sequela of cardiac surgery and has been demonstrated in up to 80% of patients early postoperatively.[23,70-73] The pathogenesis of cognitive dysfunction after cardiac surgery is still uncertain. Variables that have been postulated to explain the development of postoperative neurocognitive decline include advanced age, concomitant cerebrovascular disease and severity of cardiovascular disease, and intraoperative factors such as embolization, cerebral hypoperfusion or hypoxia, activation of inflammatory processes, aortic cross-clamp or CPB time, and possibly low mean arterial pressure in patients with impaired cerebrovascular autoregulation. In many instances, subtle signs of neuropsychological dysfunction are detectable only with sophisticated cognitive testing strategies. The fact that many of these abnormalities are difficult to properly assess on routine clinical work and their apparently transient nature have led to a tendency to minimize their clinical relevance. It should be recognized, however, that such reproducible and quantifiable dysfunction is an objective outcome measure and can, at the very least, act as a benchmark to assess various therapeutic interventions (e.g., the efficacy of putative cerebroprotectants, equipment modifications, and pH management strategies[74]).

In addition, such subclinical cognitive dysfunction may actually represent permanent neurologic damage, despite being apparently transient in nature. In a long-term follow-up study of 97 patients having undergone CABG an average of 39 months earlier, Murkin et al[71] demonstrated an incidence of neuropsychological dysfunction of 22%, and 18% of patients exhibited abnormal neurologic findings. The overall incidence of combined neurobehavioral dysfunction was 35%, similar to the incidence at 2 to 3 months postoperatively in this same group.[74] Knibb et al[70] prospectively investigated cerebral injury early and 3 months after CABG. Patients were studied at three points in time: before operation, early before discharge, and 3 months after operation using a well-validated battery of 13 standardized psychometric tests. Neurocognitive assessment early after surgery disclosed a significant decline in performance in 4 of the 11 psychometric tests compared with the preoperative status; while at the 3-month follow-up examination, three of the four tests disclosed early cognitive decline and both depression and mood scores had returned to their baseline values. However, the test score for verbal learning ability remained significantly lower at 3 months.[70] Newman et al[72] sought to determine the course of cognitive change 5 years after CABG and the effect of perioperative decline on long-term cognitive function. They performed neurocognitive tests in 261 patients who underwent CABG; tests were administered preoperatively (at baseline), before discharge, and 6 weeks, 6 months, and 5 years after CABG. Among the patients studied, the incidence of cognitive decline was 53% at discharge, 36% at 6 weeks, 24% at 6 months, and 42% at 5 years. Cognitive function at discharge was a significant predictor of long-term function. Their results confirmed the relatively high prevalence and persistence of cognitive decline after CABG and suggested a pattern of early improvement followed by a later decline that is predicted by the presence of early postoperative cognitive decline.[72] What is interesting is the apparent lack of association between cognitive dysfunction and aortic atherosclerosis, at least in one study. Of 162 CABG patients who had a perioperative neurocognitive evaluation and evaluable intraoperative TEE images, no significant relationship was found between cognitive dysfunction and atheroma burden in the ascending arch or descending aorta, suggesting that aortic atherosclerosis may not be the primary factor in the pathogenesis of post-CABG cognitive changes.[75]

In the systematic review and meta-analysis by van Dijk et al,[23] data from six highly comparable studies were pooled and demonstrated an incidence of cognitive deficit, defined as a decrease of at least 1 standard deviation in at least 2 of 9 or 10 neuropsychological tests, of 22.5% (95% confidence interval, 18.7% to 26.4%) in CABG patients at 2 months postoperatively. In a prospective study of 316 CABG patients, Murkin et al[74] reported a perioperative stroke rate of 2.8% and demonstrated that 33% of 239 patients assessed 2 months postoperatively evidenced cognitive dysfunction and that 45% experienced either neurologic or cognitive dysfunction, in comparison with their preoperative performance.

The mid and long-term impact of cognitive dysfunction on quality of life after cardiac surgery has been addressed by different studies.[72,76,77] Ahlgren et al[76] prospectively evaluated neurocognitive function and driving performance after CABG in 27 patients who underwent neuropsychological examination involving 12 cognitive tests, including a standardized on-road driving test and a test in an advanced driving simulator before and 4 to 6 weeks after surgery. Twenty patients who underwent percutaneous coronary interventions (PCIs) under local anesthesia served as a control group. After surgery, 48% of patients in the CABG group showed cognitive decline, whereas significantly fewer patients in the PCI group, only 10%, showed cognitive decline after intervention. Of particular relevance to functional quality of life, patients demonstrating cognitive decline also tended to drop in the on-road driving scores to a larger extent than did patients without a cognitive decline.[76] Di Carlo et al[77] administered a series of cognitive tests before and 6 months after the operation to 110 patients (mean age 64.1 years; 70.9% males) undergoing cardiac surgery. The degree of the impairment was determined by two independent neuropsychologists in relation to its impact on everyday life activities. At 6-month assessment, 10 patients (9.1%) were ranked as severely deteriorated, 22 (20%) as mildly or moderately deteriorated, and 78 (70.9%) as unchanged or improved.[77] At 5-year follow-up, Newman et al[27] also found a significant correlation between cognitive function and quality of life in patients after cardiac surgery. Lower overall cognitive function scores at 5 years were associated with lower general health and a less productive working status.

Neuropsychological Testing

As noted in the studies discussed, neuropsychological testing has been increasingly used in an attempt to discriminate the efficacy of various treatment modalities or as an index of cognitive functioning after CPB. In large measure, the sensitivity of this type of testing is such that very small decrements in performance can be assessed and quantified. It appears that a patient may have a consistent decrease in cognitive performance, with or without evidence of subtle neurologic abnormalities, yet may be apparently oblivious to it, whether because of denial or an absence of awareness. Commonly, such a patient's family may have noted some nonspecific alteration in mood or behavior, likely a manifestation of the same dysfunction as detected on cognitive testing.

Preoperative Cognitive Function

One of the earliest prospective reports of neurobehavioral sequelae of cardiac surgery appeared in 1954, and it focused on the acute and chronic stress responses manifested as psychobehavioral syndromes in patients undergoing valvular surgery.[78] As stated by Tufo et al,[79,80] this led to a tendency for some investigators to focus on postoperative emotional reactions, regarding them as primarily psychiatric syndromes, rather than systematically investigating cardiac patients for neurologic deficits. Millar et al[81] examined the effect of preexisting cognitive impairment on cognitive outcome in 81 patients undergoing CABG. Patients performed the Stroop Neuropsychological Screening Test and other psychometric assessments prior to and at 6 days and 6 months after CABG. Those with preexisting cognitive deficits were significantly more likely to display impairment at 6-day and 6-month follow-ups than were those without preexisting deficits, possibly reflecting underlying intrinsic pathology rather than specific intraoperative events. Rankin et al[82] used a 1-hour neuropsychological battery administered preoperatively to 43 patients before prospective randomization to either CABG or OPCAB and again to 34 of those patients 2 to 3 months postoperatively by an examiner blind to surgical condition. Neuropsychological status did not change 2.5 months postsurgically between either OPCAB or CABG groups. However, both groups showed dramatic presurgical cognitive deficits in multiple domains, particularly verbal memory and psychomotor speed. This corroborates previous research suggesting that patients requiring CABG may evidence significant presurgical cognitive deficits as a result of existing vascular disease. In a study by Di Carlo et al[77] of 110 patients undergoing cardiac surgery, the previous level of education was protective against cognitive decline (odds ratio per year of increment 0.53, 95% confidence interval 0.31 to 0.90). It is speculative whether this suggests that greater education reflects greater intellectual capacity and thus a better ability to compensate for perioperative stresses.

Neuropsychological Test Selection

Research examining cognitive functioning in patients undergoing CPB has frequently focused on the assessment of cognitive functioning within the domains of attention/concentration, psychomotor speed, motor dexterity, and verbal learning. Under the "best-case scenario," it might be desirable to use a complete battery of neuropsychological tests assessing the entire spectrum of cognitive functions. However, the cost of such a procedure and the time demands make such an approach unrealistic. This is especially the case if patients are to be assessed in the perioperative period, when practical time limitations or patient fatigue levels are likely to be prohibitive. A more practical approach is to use tests that can be administered relatively quickly and easily and that assess functions particularly dependent, for successful execution, on brain areas most vulnerable to insult (i.e., "watershed" areas).

An additional criterion in test selection is that tests chosen be sensitive to brain dysfunction, broadly defined. In perioperative cardiac surgical patients, the evaluation is necessarily limited by constraints of time and fatigue; thus, tests used should have good sensitivity to dysfunction, even if at the expense of specificity. Tests that can be administered quickly and reliably and are highly sensitive, particularly to dysfunction within cognitive domains localized to brain regions vulnerable to effects of microemboli or transient hypoxia, are those that should be selected.

Research suggests that among the tests most appropriate under these circumstances are tests of attention/concentration, psychomotor speed, motor dexterity, and verbal learning. Research as to the behavioral consequences of hypoxia (and other conditions associated with more diffuse brain damage) suggests these domains are likely to be compromised.[83,84] This presumption has also been supported by research to date examining behavioral consequences of CPB. Frequently, the Grooved Pegboard Test (motor dexterity), various subtests of the Wechsler Adult Intelligence Scale-Revised (Digit Symbol [psychomotor speed]), some of the seven subtests of the Wechsler Memory Scale (Mental Control [Attention], Digit Span [concentration], Paired Associates Verbal Learning [verbal learning]), as well as the Halstead Reitan Trail Making Test (Trails A and B), have been used in whole or in part for the assessment of cognitive impairment after CPB.[27,32,34,59,70,72,74,76,77,81,85-89]

Methodologic Issues in Neurobehavioral Assessment

The Statement of Consensus on assessment of neurobehavioral outcomes after cardiac surgery encouraged a more standardized and comparable methodology in assessment of cognitive injury, identifying several key issues of concern in perioperative cognitive testing.[31]

1. A spectrum of postoperative CNS dysfunction both acute and persistent occurs in a proportion of patients after cardiac surgery, including brain death, stroke, subtle neurologic signs, and neuropsychological impairment.
2. A number of patients presenting for cardiac surgery have preexisting CNS abnormalities. Patients' neurologic and neuropsychological states need to be assessed at a time prior to surgery in order to provide accurate baseline information.
3. The individual change in performance from baseline to a time after surgery is essential to any evaluation of the impact of surgery or any intervention associated with it.
4. When indicated, designs should incorporate the use of a control or comparison group.
5. Because of the time constraints and physical limitations of the patient in performing a neuropsychological assessment in the context of cardiac surgery, care must be taken to select appropriate tests. Selection of tests should take the following issues into consideration:
   - Cognitive domain of the test
   - Sensitivity and reliability of the test
   - Time taken to perform the test
   - Degree to which learning may occur in the test
   - Availability of parallel forms of the test
   - Physical effort required to perform the test
   - Overall balance of the cognitive domains assessed in the battery
6. Tests should be free from gender, race, and ethnic bias and be structured to avoid floor and ceiling effects.
7. Because of the multifocal nature of the potential lesion locations, no single test will always detect postoperative neurobehavioral dysfunction.
8. Care must be taken in performing the assessments as neurobehavioral performance can be influenced by environmental, psychiatric, physiologic, and pharmacologic factors.
9. As the performance of neuropsychological tests may be influenced by mood state and mood state variations, it is important that mood state assessments be performed concurrently with the neuropsychological assessments.
10. To ensure objectivity and reliability of the assessment, for each patient the testing should be performed by the same suitably qualified and trained individual and tests should minimize subjectivity and be performed in a standardized manner. The examiner should be blinded to any treatment.
11. A comprehensive and concise neurologic examination should be performed by a suitably qualified and trained individual.
12. As the incidence of postoperative neurobehavioral dysfunction is highest in the immediate postoperative period and then declines, care must be taken to perform at least one assessment when performance is more stable. Ideally, this should be at least 3 months postsurgery.
13. Investigators should be aware that new events may occur in the days postsurgery.
14. Cognitive testing may be associated with improvement in performance on repeated testing, recognized as "practice effect." This improvement needs to be taken into consideration in any analyses of the data. In addition, study design incorporating procedures to minimize practice effects (i.e., providing sufficient practice trials on each test at each assessment period) is encouraged.[26]

Based on the proceedings of these consensus conferences, the following cognitive tests were recommended as necessary but not sufficient components of any neuropsychological test battery *based on their availability in multiple languages, and availability of paper and pencil versions* for use in cardiac surgical patients:

Rey Auditory Verbal Learning Test
Trail Making A
Trail Making B
Grooved Pegboard

At a second consensus conference on methodologic issues related to data analysis in the assessment of neurobehavioral dysfunction occurring in the postoperative period after cardiac surgery, further recommendations were formulated and published.[90]

1. **Individual change scores represent the most sensitive means of detecting clinical factors impacting postoperative neurobehavioral change in cardiac surgical patients.** There is a need to identify *individuals* experiencing postoperative neurobehavioral change within various study groups in order to identify potential underlying etiologic mechanisms. This is further impetus for the development of a minimum decrement in performance, identified by change score results, definable as the threshold level for cognitive change. This threshold should be set to combine sufficient sensitivity with a high degree of specificity to avoid false-positive outcomes and can best be achieved by knowing how much change might be expected in an appropriate control group.
2. **Group mean score is influenced by the variable performance on test scores of the study group as a whole.** In a cardiac surgical population, certain individuals will be expected to score at an improved level as a conse-

quence of previous exposure to the testing techniques. Individuals experiencing postoperative neurobehavioral dysfunction will often score less well than their baseline measure. As a consequence, a group mean score will reflect both the individuals whose performance is enhanced as a consequence of practice and those whose performance is compromised due to postoperative neurobehavioral dysfunction. Accordingly, the net result may be no significant group differences from baseline score. Therefore, the group mean score does not necessarily detect a significant decline in a subset of individuals in the group.

3. **Consistency of setting for cognitive testing is a prerequisite for valid data collection.** Cognitive test performance can be affected by a variety of extraneous factors to influence test scores. The test-retest variability attributable to changes in test setting and examiner is not known but is likely to be test specific. To optimize reproducible results, subjects should ideally be tested by appropriately trained individuals in a quiet, neutral environment designed to minimize distractions and interruptions. For repeat testing, a similar setting, time of day, and same tester should ideally be used. The effect of significant variability in test setting between follow-ups is to reduce the likelihood of detecting a change between follow-ups where one exists.
4. **Scores on repeat cognitive testing may be influenced by the "practice effect."** Performance of the various tests used in a series of cognitive tests is influenced by previous experience and familiarity with tests of a similar nature, known as the "practice effect." As such, there is a small but quantifiable improvement in performance associated with repeat administration of cognitive tests independent of the use of parallel forms. The magnitude of the practice effect is test specific and depends on a number of factors, in particular, age and education. The effect of not correcting for test-retest practice effect is to reduce the likelihood of detecting a change between follow-ups where one in fact exists.[90]

MECHANISMS OF BRAIN INJURY

Determining which factor or, more likely, which combination of factors is responsible for postoperative neurologic or behavioral dysfunction in patients undergoing cardiac surgery using CPB is problematic (Box 35–2). From the few studies in which a surgical control group has been used, it appears that elements inherent to CPB are etiologic, particularly in dysfunction occurring in the immediate postoperative period.[74,91] How much of this dysfunction is as a direct result of exposure to CABG and CPB or occurs as a result of underlying comorbid disease, such as aortic and cerebrovascular atherosclerosis, hypertension, and diabetes, which predisposes such patients to CNS dysfunction as a result of nonspecific "stress" associated with major surgery independent of CABG, is an area of active ongoing investigation. Based on postmortem studies, as well as correlative analysis of intraoperative events with neurologic outcomes, two primary mechanisms appear to be responsible for brain injury in otherwise uncomplicated cardiac operations: cerebral hypoperfusion and cerebral emboli.

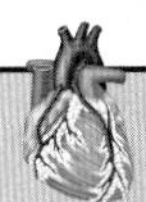

BOX 35–2 ***Risk Factors for Neurologic Complications in Cardiac Surgery***

- Hemodynamic instability
- Diabetes mellitus
- Advanced age
- Combined/complex procedures
- Prolonged CPB time
- Prior stroke
- Aortic atheromatosis
- Peripheral vascular disease

Intraoperative cerebral embolization of particulate and microgaseous elements has been demonstrated to have a significant role in the genesis of cerebral events in postoperative cardiac surgical patients.[36,49,51,73,92-99] Increasing attention is also being paid to the role of perioperative hypoperfusion, particularly in patients with intracranial and extracranial atherosclerosis, and to the effect of inflammatory processes triggered during exposure to surgery and CPB.[26,34,68,99-104]

In a prospective study of 151 consecutive Japanese patients (115 men and 36 women ranging in age from 41 to 82 years) scheduled for CABG, carotid and intracranial arteries were examined for occlusive lesions with MR angiography.[105] Cervical carotid artery stenoses of more than 50% narrowing were detected in 16.6% of the subjects, and intracranial artery stenoses of more than 50% narrowing were detected in 21.2% of the subjects.[105] In a similar study of 201 Korean patients presenting for CABG, more than 50% of patients had evidence of either extracranial or intracranial atherosclerotic disease (ECAD and ICAD, respectively), while 13% of patients had evidence of both.[106] In this series 25.4% of patients had single or multiple postoperative CNS complications, and ICAD was found to have a strong independent association with the development of CNS complications. The presence of both ECAD and ICAD was even more strongly associated with adverse perioperative CNS outcomes than was ICAD alone.[106]

In those studies in which a control group (subjected to a noncardiac procedure) was used, the incidence of both new neurologic signs and cognitive dysfunction was significantly higher in the patients undergoing CABG in the first several postoperative days compared with the surgical cohort.[74,76,107] Cognitive dysfunction after noncardiac surgery can also be persistent on long-term follow-up, although to a smaller extent compared with the incidence reported for cardiac surgery. Abildstrom et al[107] reported that 1% of patients showed persistent cognitive dysfunction 2 years after major noncardiac surgery. Several studies have also demonstrated the release of markers of cerebral injury and demonstrated a lesser but significant incidence of cognitive dysfunction after noncardiac surgery.[108,109] The occurrence of cerebral emboli during noncardiac surgery has also been demonstrated.[110-112] Accordingly, it appears as though some of the same mechanisms operative in CABG may also be culpable. Edmonds et al[110] recorded transcranial Doppler signals from the middle cerebral artery in 23 patients undergoing total hip arthroplasty and demonstrated that in 8 of 20 patients there were embolic signals ranging in number from 1 to 200. In all eight of these patients, signals were recorded during impaction of a cemented component or after relocation of the hip. In two patients there were 150 and 200 embolic signals, in both of whom mild respiratory symptoms developed; one patient also became overtly agitated during a flurry of emboli.

Neuropathologic Studies

In an early series from 1962 to 1970 that examined 206 patients dying after cardiac surgery or CABG and a group of 110 patients dying after non-CPB vascular surgery, Aguilar et al[113] reported that there was a high correlation between the use of CPB and the incidence of brain lesions. They reported that the most significant abnormalities found, in both severity and frequency of occurrence, were emboli in small cerebral vessels; acute petechial, perivascular, and focal subarachnoid hemorrhages; and acute ischemic neuronal damage (Box 35–3). They noted the virtual disappearance from the brain of nonfat emboli such as fibrin, platelet aggregates, polarizable crystalline material, xanthomatous debris, striated muscle, and calcium in cases examined after the introduction of arterial line filtration, whereas they reported that cerebral embolization of such debris was commonly observed in patients dying after CPB prior to the introduction of arterial line filtration.[113] Other early studies showed that measures taken to decrease the duration of CPB, as well as the introduction of arterial line filtration and filtration of the cardiotomy suction return, decreased overt neurologic dysfunction.[94,95,114]

A review of autopsy findings from 221 patients dying after CABG or valve surgery between 1982 and 1989 reported a direct correlation among age, severe atherosclerosis of the ascending aorta, and presence of atheroemboli. Atheroemboli were significantly more common in patients who underwent CABG versus valvular surgery, and there was a high correlation of atheroemboli with severe atherosclerosis of the ascending aorta, being present in 37.4% of patients with severe disease of the aorta versus only 2% of those without. Of all patients who had evidence of atheroemboli, 95.8% had severe atherosclerosis of the ascending aorta.[48] Doty et al[49] reviewed the records of 49,377 autopsies and surgical specimens from the Johns Hopkins Hospital between 1973 and 1995. Three hundred twenty-seven patients (0.7%) had an identifiable atheroembolism on histologic examination. Of these patients, 29 (0.2%) had undergone a cardiac surgical procedure within 30 days of autopsy or surgical resection. Six of the 29 patients (21%) had atheroembolism to the heart, 7 patients (24%) had embolism to the CNS, 19 patients (66%) had embolism to the gastrointestinal tract, 14 patients (48%) had embolism to one or both kidneys, and 5 patients (17%) had embolism to a lower extremity. Sixteen patients (55%) had atheroembolism in two or more areas. In six patients (21%), death was directly attributable to atheroembolism, including intraoperative cardiac failure from coronary embolism (three), massive stroke (two), and extensive gastrointestinal embolization (one).[49] Godwin et al[115] conducted a prospective consecutive postmortem data collection on 167 patients representing 84.4% of all in-hospital cardiac surgical deaths in a single institution, identifying stroke as a cause of death in 3.6%.

In a neuropathologic study of brains from 262 patients dying after having undergone CABG, valve replacement, or heart transplantation surgery, 49% of cases demonstrated evidence of circulatory disturbances identified as macrohemorrhages and microhemorrhages, infarcts, subarachnoid hemorrhages, or hypoxemic brain damage.[116] The infarcts were caused by local arteriosclerosis of cerebral arteries, fat emboli, arterial emboli from operative sites, or foreign body emboli. These authors concluded that histologically overt microemboli did not play a major role in their findings and that nonfatal white matter microhemorrhages were found with varying frequency, especially after valve operations. These observations are not inconsistent with the apparent lack of correlation seen in several beating-heart surgery studies between differing incidences of TCD-detected cerebral emboli and cognitive dysfunction.[38,39]

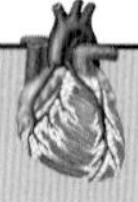

BOX 35–3 ***Mechanisms and Factors for Neurologic Lesions***

- Embolization
- Hypoperfusion
- Inflammation
- Influencing Factors
  - Aortic atheroma plaque
  - Cerebrovascular disease
  - Altered cerebral autoregulation
  - Hypotension
  - Intracardiac debris
  - Air
  - Venous obstruction on bypass
  - CPB circuit surface
  - Reinfusion of unprocessed shed blood
  - Cerebral hyperthemia
  - Hypoxia

Watershed Infarctions

Watershed, or boundary zone, infarcts are ischemic lesions that are situated along border zones between the territories of two major cerebral arteries (e.g., the middle and posterior, or the anterior and middle cerebral arteries) where terminal arteriolar anastomoses exist[117-119] (Fig. 35–6). In a series reported by Malone et al,[120] a correlation was made between the presence of intraoperative electroencephalographic (EEG) abnormalities (virtual or complete electrical silence) usually seen in

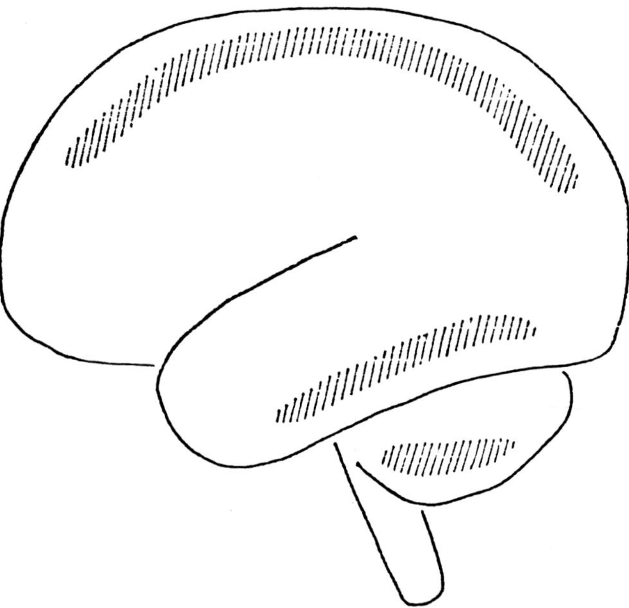

Figure 35–6 Hatched areas showing the most frequent locations of boundary area, or watershed zone infarcts in the brain, situated between the territories of major cerebral or cerebellar arteries. (From Torvik A: The pathogenesis of watershed infarcts in the brain. Stroke 2:221, 1984.)

conjunction with sustained hypotensive episodes and neuropathologic lesions found at necropsy. In all nine patients with clinical evidence of brain damage, cortical boundary zone (watershed) lesions were observed in the parieto-occipital areas. They suggest that this location is the most sensitive area for placement of recording EEG electrodes because it is where minimal boundary zone ischemic lesions occurred in the absence of other lesions, and it is also where ischemic lesions were found in their maximal severity and extent.

A profound reduction in systemic blood pressure is the most frequent cause of watershed infarcts. These areas are thought to be more susceptible to ischemia resulting from hypotension because of their critical dependence on a single blood supply. Wityk et al[121] studied the pattern of ischemic changes on diffusion- and perfusion-weighted magnetic resonance imaging (DWI and PW-MRI, respectively) in 14 patients with neurologic complications after cardiac surgery of whom eight patients presented with encephalopathy, which was associated with focal neurologic deficits in four, four with focal deficits alone, and two with either fluctuating symptoms or transient ischemic attacks. Acute ischemic lesions were classified as having a territorial, watershed, or lacunar pattern of infarction. Patients with multiple territorial infarcts in differing vascular distributions that were not explained by occlusive vascular lesions were classified as having multiple emboli. Acute infarcts were found in 10 of 14 patients by DWI. Among patients with encephalopathy, seven of eight had patterns of infarction suggestive of multiple emboli, including three of four patients with no focal neurologic deficits. Several patients had combined watershed and multiple embolic patterns of ischemia. Findings of MRPI studies were abnormal in two of four patients, showing diffusion-perfusion mismatch; both patients had either fluctuating deficits or transient ischemic attacks, and their conditions improved with blood pressure increase.[121]

By the same rationale, however, these areas are also highly susceptible to ischemia due to end-artery embolization, and it is also recognized that although severe hypotension is the most common cause, showers of microemboli may lodge preferentially in these areas and cause infarcts in the underlying brain.[121-124] As such, although they are commonly due to profoundly hypotensive episodes, watershed lesions are not pathognomonic of a hypotensive episode and may be the result of cerebral emboli. Embolization and hypoperfusion acting together play a synergistic role and either cause or magnify the brain damage of cardiac surgical patients. The negative influence of hemodynamic instability and hypoxia has been demonstrated by several authors, showing improved outcomes by an early and aggressive recognition and correction of hypoperfusion.[5,26,34,77,100,125-127]

Cerebral Perfusion Pressure

Intraoperative hypotension during cardiac surgery has been related to postoperative neurologic dysfunction.[4,5,20,26,36,128] Ridderstolpe et al[26] published a retrospective study of 3282 patients of mean age 65.6 years who underwent cardiac surgery in the period from July 1996 through June 2000. Standard CPB technique was used for most patients. Cerebral complications occurred in 107 patients (3.3%). Of these, 60 (1.8%) were early, and 33 (1.0%) were delayed, and in 14 (0.4%) patients the onset was unknown. Predictors of early cerebral complications were older age, preoperative hypertension, aortic aneurysm surgery, prolonged CPB time, hypotension at CPB completion and soon after CPB, and postoperative arrhythmia and supraventricular tachyarrhythmia. Predictors of delayed cerebral complications were female gender, diabetes, previous cerebrovascular disease, combined valve and CABG, postoperative supraventricular tachyarrhythmia, and prolonged ventilator support. Early cerebral complications seemed to be more serious, with more permanent deficits and a higher overall mortality (35.0% versus 18.2%). The results of this study suggest that aggressive antiarrhythmic treatment and blood pressure control may improve the cerebral outcome after cardiac surgery.[26]

EEG patterns consistent with ischemia—increased slow wave activity, diffuse slowing of EEG activity—have been reported to occur during CPB episodes thought to be associated with cerebral hypoperfusion.[129-131] Episodes of flow reduction during normothermia frequently produced ischemic changes, whereas similar decreases during stable hypothermia were not associated with EEG changes.[130] Ischemic EEG changes are also frequently seen in association with reductions in perfusion flow rate during the initiation of CPB[129,130] (see Chapters 5, 17, 28, and 30). Using computerized EEG to quantitate episodes of low-frequency power as an index of cerebrocortical ischemia in 96 patients undergoing CABG, a correlation was made among episodes of hypotension, focal increases in low-frequency EEG power, and the occurrence of postoperative disorientation.[132]

During the transition to CPB, the brain is particularly vulnerable to ischemia, inasmuch as cerebral metabolic rate for oxygen ($CMRO_2$) is apparently unchanged, yet the brain is initially perfused with an asanguinous prime, and even after equilibration during established CPB, hematocrit is generally maintained at a range between 20% and 30%. As a result, any further decreases in cerebral perfusion, in the absence of concomitant decreases in $CMRO_2$, are poorly tolerated. During hypothermic conditions, there is a profound decrease in $CMRO_2$, exceeding 50% for a 10°C reduction in temperature.[133] Without need to postulate an extension of the lower limit of cerebral autoregulation, it is clear that under anesthesia, and particularly during hypothermic CPB, cerebral blood flow (CBF) is maintained at very low levels of cerebral perfusion pressure (CPP). As discussed later, this was initially reported by Govier et al and further explored by Murkin et al and Prough et al.[133-135] As the average age and extent of disease in patients presenting for CABG continue to increase, however, the number of patients with concomitant cerebrovascular disease and thus potentially deranged cerebral autoregulation presents an increasingly important group.

Using radioisotope techniques for measurement of CBF, and incorporating a jugular venous catheter for calculation of $CMRO_2$, it was determined that there is a profound reduction in $CMRO_2$ during hypothermic CPB and that CBF is decreased proportionately, and will autoregulate down to a CPP of 20 mm Hg, in the presence of alpha-stat pH management.[133] Low arterial pressure during the hypothermic phase of CPB is, thus, unlikely to result in cerebral ischemia *in the absence of cerebrovascular disease.* In a study of high versus low arterial pressure management during CPB in 248 patients undergoing CABG, however, an apparently lower rate of postoperative complications was reported by Gold et al[136] for those patients in the high-pressure group. While specific CNS morbidity, cognitive and functional status outcomes, and mortality did not differ significantly between groups, the overall complication rate for combined cardiac and neurologic complications was significantly lower in the high-pressure group. This is not

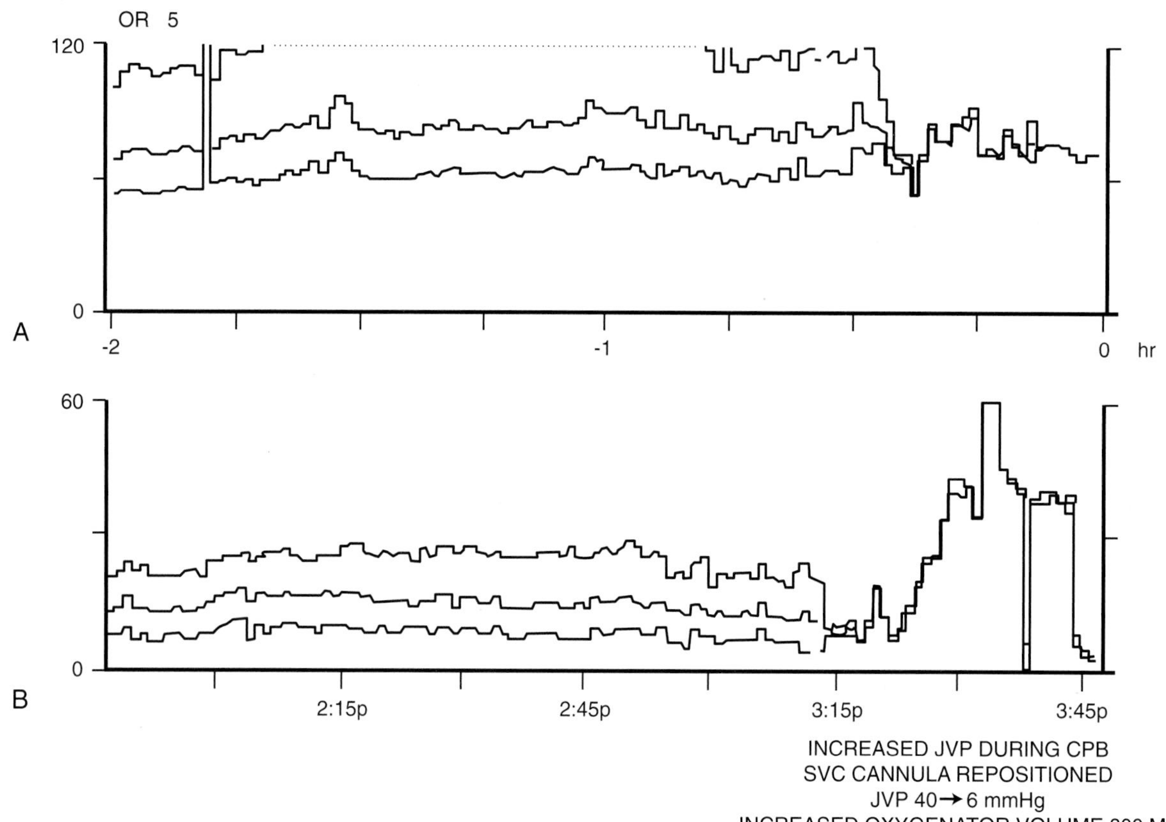

Figure 35–7 *A,* Systolic, mean, and diastolic arterial blood pressures, with commencement of cardiopulmonary bypass (CPB) indicated at 3:15 PM, after which mean arterial pressure (MAP) is shown. *B,* Pulmonary artery systolic, mean, and diastolic pressures with proximal jugular venous pressure (JVP) recorded at 3:15 PM, with commencement of CPB. A single two-stage venous cannula was used for CPB and, with rotation of the heart, venous return to the oxygenator decreased and JVP approached MAP values. (Modified from Murkin JM: Intraoperative management. *In* Estaphanous FG, Barash PG, Reves JG [eds]: Cardiac Anesthesia Principles and Clinical Practice. Philadelphia, Lippincott, 1994, p 326.)

inconsistent with data demonstrating a high incidence of cerebrovascular disease in coronary revascularization patients.[106]

It should also be appreciated that during CPB cerebral venous hypertension can result from partial obstruction of the superior vena cava (SVC) (Fig. 35–7), particularly in the presence of a single two-stage venous cannula, and may give rise to cerebral edema, as well as producing a disproportionate lowering of CPP relative to arterial pressure.[137] In a study by Avraamides, surgical dislocation of the heart during CPB produced increases in proximal SVC pressure and resulted in significant decreases in CBF velocity as measured with TCD, despite stable arterial pressure and pump flow rates.[138] This strongly suggests that cerebral venous hypertension, as can occur during CPB with myocardial dislocation and impaired drainage of SVC, may result in cerebral ischemia and necrosis if unrecognized and untreated. It is feasible that such unrecognized cerebral venous hypertension has resulted in some of the postoperative neurologic syndromes that have been reported.[139]

Although the association between hypotension during CPB and cerebral dysfunction remains contentious, there is some evidence that certain subsets of patients may be at particular risk. Newman et al[140] used preoperative and postoperative cognitive testing to assess the effects of mean arterial pressure (MAP) and rate of rewarming on cognitive decline in 237 patients. They demonstrated significant interactions between cognitive decline and MAP less than 50 mm Hg on one measure of cognitive performance and between rate of rewarming and age on another. They concluded that although MAP and rewarming were not primary determinants of cognitive decline, hypotension and rapid rewarming contributed significantly to cognitive dysfunction in the elderly. Again, because elderly patients comprise an increasing segment of the cardiac surgical population, these aspects are becoming increasingly important clinical management issues.

The interaction of emboli, perfusion pressure, and the particular conditions of the regional cerebral circulation (e.g., preexisting cerebral intravascular lesions) will determine the final expression of brain damage in the cardiac surgical patient. Ganushchak et al[141] tested with a retrospective study the hypothesis that combinations of hemodynamic events from apparently normal CPB procedures are related to the development of postoperative neurologic complications and affect the impact of common clinical risk factors. A multivariate statistical procedure (cluster analysis) was applied to a data set of automatically recorded perfusions from 1395 patients who underwent CABG. The following five parameters emerged for cluster analysis: MAP, dispersion of MAP, dispersion of systemic vascular resistance, dispersion of arterial pulse pressure, and the maximum value of mixed venous saturation. Using these parameters, they found four clusters that were significantly different by CPB performance (first cluster, 389 patients; second cluster, 431 patients; third cluster and fourth cluster, 229 patients each). Patients in the fourth cluster had the highest dispersion of MAP, that is, highest instability on CPB. The frequency of postoperative neurologic complications was 0.3% in the first cluster and increased to 3.9% in the fourth cluster. Importantly, the impact of common clinical risk factors for postoperative neurologic complications was affected by the performance of the CPB procedure. For example, the frequency of neurologic complications among patients with cerebrovascular disease in their medical history was 22% in the fourth cluster, whereas it was zero in the second cluster. Patients who underwent CPB procedures with large fluctuations in hemodynamic parameters particularly showed an increased risk for the development of postoperative neurologic complications.[141]

Cerebral Emboli and Outcome

Two different types of cerebral emboli appear to occur during CPB, composed of solid or gaseous matter, such as macroemboli (e.g., atherosclerotic debris) and microemboli (e.g., microgaseous bubbles, microparticulate matter). Overt and focal neurologic damage likely reflects the occurrence of cerebral macroemboli (e.g., calcific and atheromatous debris generated during valve tissue removal or instrumentation of an atheromatous aorta), whereas less focal neurologic dysfunction has been ascribed to cerebral microemboli.[13] Microemboli appear to have some role in diffuse, subtle neurologic and cognitive disturbances, whereas macroemboli likely produce clinically apparent catastrophic strokes. Whatever the nature of the cerebral insult, however, it seems that coexistent inflammatory processes can exacerbate the magnitude of injury.

In a study to assess the impact of surgical manipulation of the aorta and correlations with postoperative stroke, Ura et al[142] performed EAS before aortic cannulation and after decannulation in 472 patients undergoing cardiac surgery with CPB. A new lesion in the ascending aortal intima was identified in 16 patients (3.4%) after aortic decannulation, of whom 10 patients sustained neurologic complications. New lesions were severe, with mobile lesions or disruption of the intima in 10 patients. Six of the severe lesions were related to aortic clamping and the other four to aortic cannulation. Three patients in this group had postoperative stroke. The incidence of new lesions was directly related to extent of aortic atheroma, being 11.8% if the atheroma was approximately 3 to 4 mm thick and as high as 33.3% if the atheroma was greater than 4 mm, but only 0.8% when it was less than 3 mm.[142] Again, this underscores the need to reliably detect and ultimately to avoid disruption of aortic atherosclerotic plaque.

Sylivris et al[143] studied 41 consecutive patients undergoing CABG with TCD monitoring and preoperative and postoperative MRI brain scans. A subgroup of 32 patients underwent neuropsychological testing the day before and 5 to 6 days after the operation, of whom 27 had TCD data. Among the subgroup of patients with reliable TCD data and neuropsychological studies, early neuropsychological deficit after CABG was found in 17 (63%) of the 27 patients. On univariate analysis, the time duration on CPB, total microembolic load during bypass, and microembolic rates during bypass were all significantly higher in the group with neuropsychological decline. Actual rates of emboli detected per minute were highest during release of the aortic cross-clamp. Five patients had strokes, of whom four had a significant decline in neuropsychological functioning. Unlike the association between microembolic signals during bypass and neuropsychological deficits, there was no relationship between these factors and radiologic evidence of cerebral infarction. Not inconsistent with the findings of Ura et al described earlier, there was a significantly higher microembolic load at cannulation in patients with cerebral infarction, temporally suggestive of particulate emboli, which was not apparent in comparison with patients with neuropsychological deficits alone.[142,143]

A study with a newer generation of TCD, which uses two different frequencies for insonation and purportedly discriminates between gaseous and particulate emboli, compared the number and nature of intraoperative microemboli in patients undergoing on-pump and off-pump cardiac surgery procedures in 45 patients (15 OPCAB, 15 on-pump CABG, and 15 open cardiac procedures).[96] They demonstrated significantly fewer emboli in the OPCAB, versus on-pump CABG, and open procedure groups, averaging 40 (28 to 80), 275 (199 to 472), and 860 (393 to 1321) emboli, respectively ($p < 0.01$). Twelve percent of microemboli in the OPCAB group were defined as solid compared with 28% and 22% in the on-pump CABG and open procedure groups, respectively. In the on-pump groups, 24% of microembli occurred during CPB, and 56% occurred during aortic manipulation for cannulation, decannulation, application, and removal of cross-clamp or side-clamp, again underscoring the importance of minimizing aortic instrumentation.[38]

Gaseous emboli are not innocuous, however. It has been demonstrated that the effects of air emboli on the cerebral vasculature not only are due to bubble entrapment with direct blockage of cerebral vessels but also represent the effects that such bubbles have on vascular endothelial cells.[144] Ultrastructural examinations of pial vessels in rats exposed to cerebral air emboli demonstrated severe injury to endothelial plasmalemma, leading to loss of cellular integrity and endothelial cell swelling.[145] Such endothelial damage produces disruptions of vasoreactivity, as has been observed in cat pial vessels exposed to air emboli. In these capillary beds, the endothelial layer demonstrated ultrastructural abnormalities that included degradation of intercellular junctions, flattening of nuclei, and crenation of the plasmalemma. Air embolism also produces changes in blood elements leading to formation of a proteinaceous capsule around the bubbles, marked dilation of pial vessels, platelet sequestration, and damage to endothelial cells.[146-148] Air-induced mechanical trauma to the endothelium causes basement membrane disruption, thrombin production, release of P-selectin from intracellular vesicles, synthesis of platelet-activating factor (PAF), and a reperfusion-like injury with perturbations in inflammation and thrombotic processes. These phenomena likely impair nitric oxide (NO) production, giving rise to alterations in cerebral microvascular regulation.[149-151]

In a study by Moody et al, four of five patients dying after CPB, two patients dying after proximal aortography, and six dogs placed on CPB were all found to have small cerebral capillary and arteriolar dilations (SCADs), consistent with sites of gas bubbles or fat emboli[94] (Fig. 35–8). These microvascular anomalies were only found in conjunction with utilization of CPB or proximal aortic instrumentation. In a subsequent series of elegant studies by this same group, use of colored microspheres was able to "time-lock" the development of SCADs to the period associated with CPB[152] (Fig. 35–9). In further studies from this group, Challa et al[153] identified SCADs in thick colloidin sections of the brains of eight patients who died after cardiac surgery supported with a membrane oxygenator and in two dogs that underwent CPB with a bubble oxygenator. In SCADs of the eight patients who had cardiac surgery, both aluminum and silicone values were higher, and silicone values were also high in the two dogs in

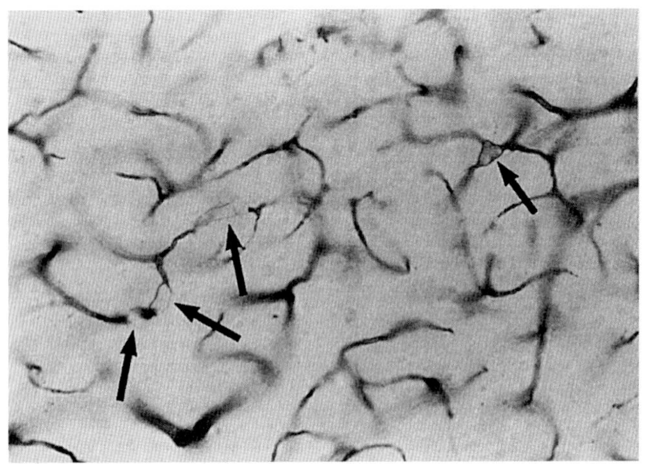

Figure 35–8 Microemboli or small capillary and arteriolar dilatations (SCADs) in arterioles of human brain 1 day after cardiopulmonary bypass. The afferent microvessels are black. The SCADs are dilated clear areas (*arrows*); the largest one here measures 25 μm in diameter. It is believed these represent the "footprints" of emboli that were almost completely removed by the reagents used in this histochemical staining method (alkaline phosphatase–stained 100-μm-thick celloidin section; magnification ×300 before 50% reduction). (Reprinted with permission from the Society of Thoracic Surgeons [The Annals of Thoracic Surgery 59:1304, 1995]. Copyright 1995, with permission from the Society of thoracic Surgeons.)

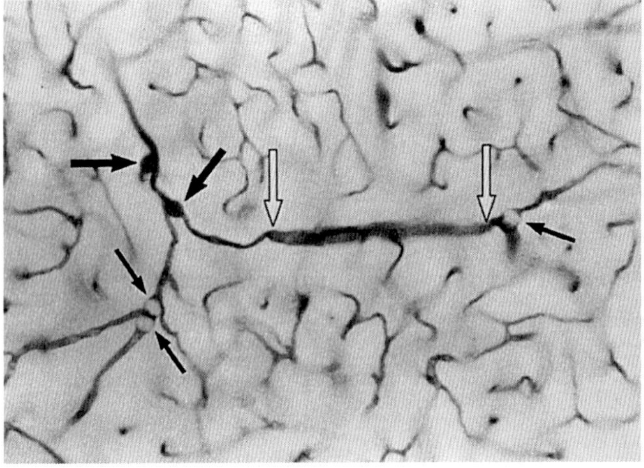

Figure 35–9 Microemboli (*white arrows*) "bracketed in time" by sequentially injected microspheres of different colors. Clear microspheres (*small black arrows*), and black microspheres (*large black arrows*) can be seen in distal to proximal order in a single arteriolar complex. In this experiment, clear spheres were injected into the carotid artery of a dog, followed in succession by injection of corn oil and then black spheres. Direction of blood flow in the arteriole is from top to bottom (alkaline phosphatase–stained 100-μm-thick celloidin section; microspheres = 15 μm). (Reprinted with permission from the Society of Thoracic Surgeons [The Annals of Thoracic Surgery 59:1304, 1995]. Copyright 1995, with permission from the Society of thoracic Surgeons.)

which a bubble oxygenator was used. Their results indicated that contamination with aluminum and silicone occurred during cardiac surgery assisted by CPB and that switching to membrane oxygenators from bubble oxygenators for CPB may have reduced silicone contamination of blood.[153] Kincaid et al[154] used a cell saver to process the cardiotomy blood in dogs who underwent hypothermic CPB. The brain tissue from two groups of dogs (group I, cardiotomy suction blood reinfused through arterial line filter; group II, cardiotomy suction blood collected and processed in a cell saver) was examined for the presence of SCADs. Mean SCADs density in the cell saver group was less than the arterial filter group (11 ± 3 versus 24 ± 5, $p = .02$). The authors concluded that using a cell saver to scavenge shed blood during CPB decreases cerebral lipid microembolization.[154]

CEREBRAL BLOOD FLOW

In the mid-1960s, Wollman et al used changes in the arterial and jugular venous oxygen content differences (A-V_{DO_2}) to estimate changes in CBF during alterations of MAP and arterial carbon dioxide tensions (Pa_{CO_2}) in patients undergoing CPB.[155] They observed a direct correlation between Pa_{CO_2} and A-V_{DO_2} (CBF), and no relationship between A-V_{DO_2} and MAP. Although the concepts of alpha-stat and pH-stat pH management had not been formulated at that time, these authors recommended maintaining temperature-corrected Pa_{CO_2} between 30 and 40 mm Hg during hypothermic CPB (see Chapters 28 and 30).

In 1968, a Japanese investigator, using the recently developed technique of radioisotope clearance, measured CBF and CMR_{O_2} during CPB.[156] In a series of 40 patients, krypton-85 clearance, with concomitant cannulation of the superior jugular bulb, was used to measure CBF and calculate CMR_{O_2} during CPB. The influence of nonpulsatile CPB on the cerebral vasculature was also directly observed using retinal photomicrography. Although critical data such as esophageal temperatures and hematocrits were not reported, the observed 35% decrease in CBF with institution of CPB, 63% decrease in CMR_{O_2} during hypothermia, 23% decrease in CMR_{O_2} during rewarming, and retinal venous engorgement during rewarming, are consistent with subsequent research findings. This report apparently also marked the first observations in humans of retinal microembolism occurring during CPB, markedly preceding the reports of Blauth and colleagues.[95]

There were few subsequent radioisotope CBF studies during CPB in humans reported for the next 15 years. Other investigators used indirect estimates of CBF (e.g., A-V_{DO_2}, TCD CBF velocities, or thermodilution techniques) to estimate CBF.[157]

pH Management and CBF

Relatively little new information regarding the cerebral circulation in human beings during CPB appeared until 1983, when Henriksen et al[158] reported evidence of cerebral hyperemia occurring during CPB. This report was followed in 1984 by a seminal paper from Govier et al,[134] who not only incited controversy with their observations of ischemic threshold levels of CBF during CPB, in direct contrast to the hyperperfusion reported by Henriksen, but also made preliminary observations on many of the other critical variables thought to influence CBF during CPB.

Without the measurement of concomitant cerebral metabolism, these apparently discordant observations of CBF could not be reconciled. Murkin et al subsequently reported their observations of both CBF and CMR_{O_2} during hypothermic CPB in humans, using a xenon-133 clearance technique for measurement of CBF, similar to techniques used by Kubota, Govier et al, and Henriksen et al, but with the addition of a jugular bulb catheter for sampling effluent cerebral venous blood for measurement of cerebral metabolic activity.[113,134,156,158] It was hypothesized that differences in pH management accounted for the divergent values previously reported for CBF during hypothermic CPB. Accordingly,

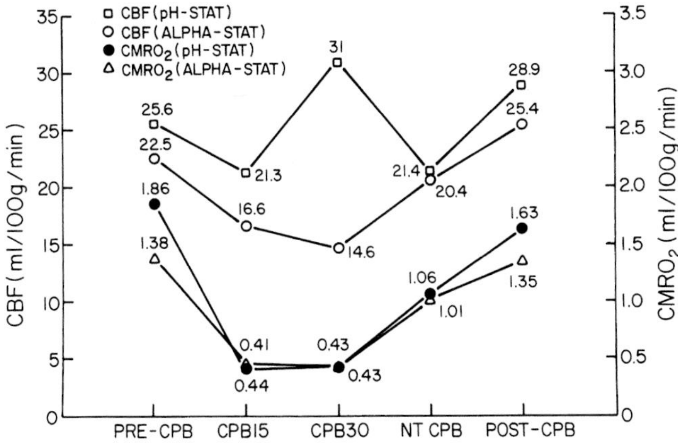

Figure 35–10 Cerebral blood flow (CBF) and cerebral metabolic rate for oxygen ($CMRO_2$) in the alpha-stat (non–temperature-corrected) and pH-stat (temperature-corrected) groups. Note the convergence of $CMRO_2$ and divergence of CBF between groups during the hypothermic phase of cardiopulmonary bypass (CPB). (From Murkin JM: Cerebral hyperperfusion during cardiopulmonary bypass: The influence of $PaCO_2$. *In* Mark Hilberman [ed]: Brain Injury and Protection During Heart Surgery. Boston, Martinus Nijhoff, 1988, p 57.)

patients were managed with either alpha-stat or pH-stat pH management during hypothermic CPB. A similar and pronounced reduction in $CMRO_2$ was observed in both groups during hypothermia (Fig. 35–10), and in the alpha-stat group, global cerebral flow/metabolism coupling was preserved in comparison with the group managed with pH-stat (Fig. 35–11). Decreases in CBF and $CMRO_2$, significantly lower than similar measures before and after CPB, were still evident after rewarming during normothermic nonpulsatile CPB. These low values for CBF and $CMRO_2$ were restored to control levels shortly after separation from CPB. Alpha-stat management preserved autoregulation and the relationship between CBF and metabolism.[159]

Temperature and Coronary Artery Bypass Grafting

How much does cerebral hyperthermia superimposed on a brain suffused with focal ischemic lesions contribute to postoperative CNS dysfunction?[152] It is known that the vulnerability of the normothermic brain to focal ischemic insult demonstrates a surprising variability in the presence of small gradations in temperature. Busto et al[160] demonstrated that at 33°C expression of cerebral ischemia was virtually eliminated compared with controls maintained at 36°C. In fact, a large measure of the apparent cerebroprotective efficacy of the glutamate-receptor antagonist MK-801 in global ischemia was demonstrated by Buchan and Pulsinelli[161] to be mediated by just such a small secondary decrease in brain temperature. Conversely, small increases in brain temperature, such as to 39°C increments as may occur during CABG (Fig. 35–12), have been shown to profoundly enhance the susceptibility of the brain to focal ischemic insult and result in ischemic lesions of much greater extent in comparison with controls at 37°C.[162]

The demonstration of apparently improved myocardial performance and shorter CPB and operating room times after normothermic CPB has prompted several outcome studies to assess the efficacy of this therapy, with particular focus now centered on CNS outcomes. Hypothermia reduces cerebral metabolic rate; thus, mild hypothermia might protect the brain by preferentially suppressing energy utilization to maintain cellular integrity.[163] In support of this are results from a subset of 138 patients randomized to normothermic or hypothermic CPB, in whom a detailed prospective neurologic examination and a series of cognitive tests were performed preoperatively, at postoperative days 1 to 3 and 7 to 10, and again at 1 month postoperatively.[164] Seven of 68 patients in the normothermic group were found to have a central neurologic deficit compared with none of the patients in the hypothermic group, a significantly greater incidence. In a separate study of 96 patients undergoing CABG and randomized to CPB at either 28°C, 32°C, or 37°C, patients managed at 37°C had a significantly greater incidence of deterioration on cognitive test scores than did those managed at either 28°C or 32°C. No additional benefit in terms of cognitive function was conferred by cooling to 28°C versus 32°C.[165] Nathan et al[166] reported on CABG patients operated under hypothermic (32°C) CPB and then randomly assigned to rewarming to 37°C (control) or 34°C (hypothermic), with no further intraoperative warming. Neurocognitive testing was performed 1 week and 3 months postoperatively. Eleven tests were combined into three cognitive domains: memory, attention, and psychomotor speed and dexterity. The incidence of cognitive deficits 1 week after surgery was 62% in the control group and 48% in the hypothermic group (relative risk 0.77, $p = 0.048$). In the hypothermic group, the magnitude of deterioration in attention and in speed and dexterity was reduced by 55.6% ($p = 0.038$) and 41.3% ($p = 0.042$), respectively. At 3 months, the hypothermic group still performed better on one test of speed and dexterity.[166]

Other studies have demonstrated apparently different results, however. Engelman et al[167] randomized a series of 291 patients undergoing coronary revascularization to either hypothermic or tepid/normothermic perfusion. Twelve intraoperative ischemic strokes occurred; six of these were in the group receiving hypothermic perfusion and six were in the group receiving the tepid/normothermic perfusion. Measuring the infarct volume documented that three of the strokes in each group resulted in minor or small infarcts and that three in each group were significant, major strokes. The volume of infarction, whether including all six patients in each group or only those with major strokes, was no different between the hypothermic and the tepid/normothermic groups. The authors observed no relationship between the size of a cerebral ischemic infarct and the perfusate temperature during coronary revascularization.[167] Similarly, Dworschak et al[168] found no difference in brain isoenzyme S-100 beta release pattern or in clinical neurologic complications between two groups of CABG patients randomly assigned to normothermic or hypothermic (32°C) CPB. In a large prospective study, Grigore et al[85] randomly assigned 300 patients undergoing elective CABG to tepid/normothermic (35.5° to 36.5°C) or hypothermic (28° to 30°C) CPB and used a battery of neurocognitive tests evaluating four distinct cognitive domains administered preoperatively and at 6 weeks after surgery. Again, there were no differences in neurologic or neurocognitive outcomes between normothermic and hypothermic groups in multivariable models. In a separate study, Grimm et al[169] actually found subclinical impairment of cognitive brain function to be more pronounced in CABG patients undergoing mildly hypothermic CPB compared with

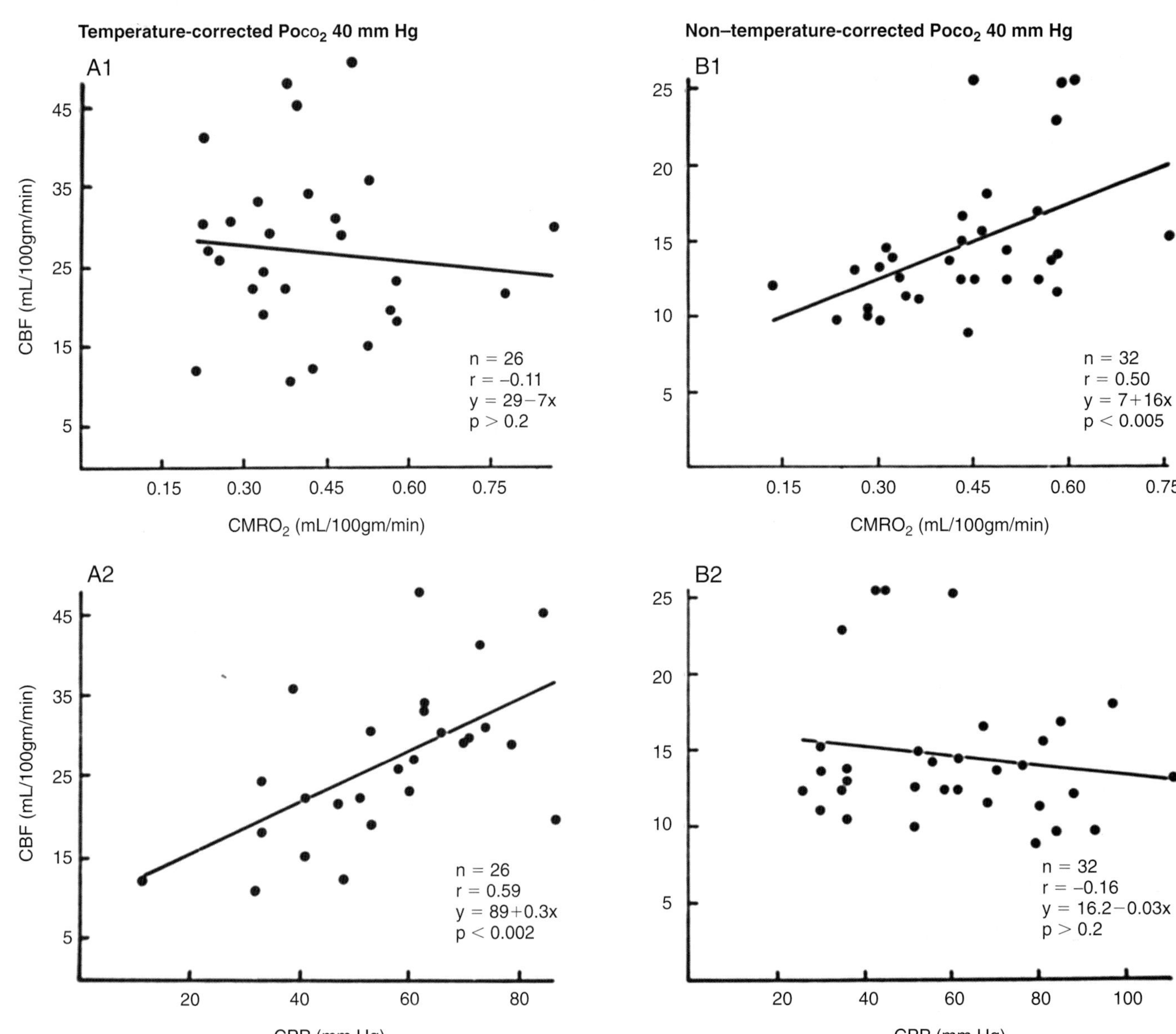

Figure 35–11 Simple linear regression of cerebral blood flow versus cerebral perfusion pressure or cerebral oxygen consumption for temperature-corrected and non–temperature-corrected groups. *Top,* There is no significant correlation between CBF and $CMRO_2$ in the temperature-corrected group (A1), whereas CBF significantly correlates with $CMRO_2$ in the non–temperature-corrected group (B1). *Bottom,* CBF is significantly correlated with CPP in the temperature-corrected group (A2), whereas CBF is independent of CPP in the non–temperature-corrected group (B2). CBF = cerebral blood flow; CPP = cerebral perfusion pressure; $CMRO_2$ = cerebral metabolic rate for oxygen. (From Murkin JM, Farrar JK, Tweed A, et al: Cerebral autoregulation and flow/metabolism coupling during cardiopulmonary bypass: The influence of $PaCO_2$. Anesth Analg 66:825, 1987.)

normothermic CPB. Accordingly, a protective effect of hypothermia on neurologic outcome in CABG has not been verified in most clinical trials, possibly because of too fast and/or excessive rewarming of patients or, more likely, because the impact of only transient cooling during CPB does not extend into the postoperative interval when cerebral hyperthermia has also been demonstrated and correlated with impaired cognitive performance at 6 weeks postoperatively.[20,170-174]

Cerebral hyperthermia during the rewarming phase of CPB can exacerbate a preexisting injury prior to rewarming and may be detrimental in itself. Hyperthermia can have a strong impact on cerebral oxygen transfer and neurologic outcome. Glutamate levels can increase during cerebral hyperthermia, leading to eventual cell death. Rapid rewarming decreases jugular venous hemoglobin saturation, creating a mismatch between cerebral oxygen consumption and delivery.[175,176] Okano et al assessed the effects of normothermia and mild hypothermia (32°C) during CPB on jugular oxygen saturation ($SjvO_2$) in 20 patients scheduled for elective CABG. The $SjvO_2$ in the normothermic group was decreased significantly at 20 and 40 minutes after the onset of CPB compared with pre-CPB, while there was no change in $SjvO_2$ in the mild hypothermic group during the study.[177] The authors concluded that cerebral oxygenation, as assessed by $SjvO_2$, was increased during mild hypothermic CPB compared with normothermic CPB. Kawahara et al examined the effect of rewarming rates on $SjvO_2$ in 100 patients scheduled for elective CABG and randomly divided into two groups: a control group and a slow rewarming group. Cerebral desaturation

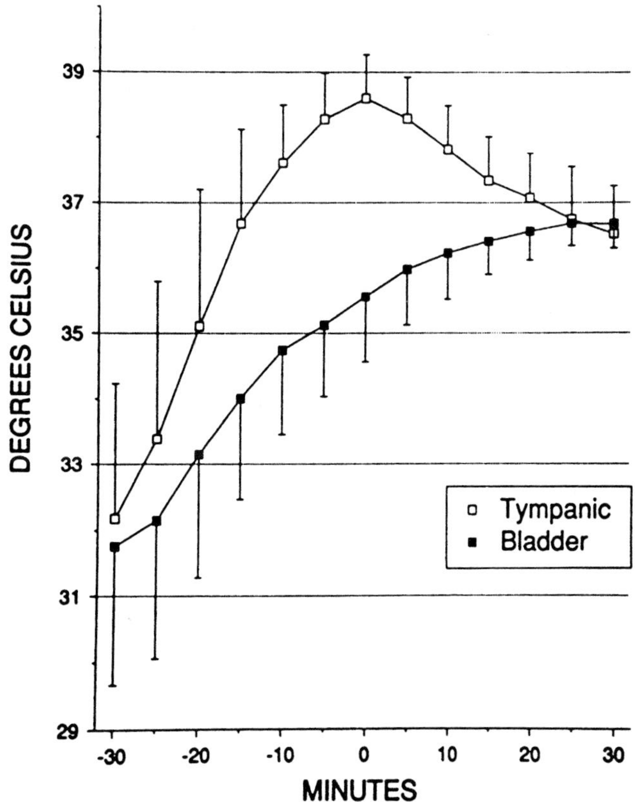

Figure 35–12 Tympanic and bladder temperatures during rewarming. Time 0 = maximal temperature achieved. Mean ± SD values are shown. (From Nathan JH, Lavallee G: The management of temperature during hypothermic cardiopulmonary bypass: I, Canadian survey. Can J Anaesth 42:669, 1995.)

(defined as an $SjvO_2$ value below 50%) during rewarming was more frequent in the control group than in the slow group.[176] Cerebral desaturation time was defined as duration when $SjvO_2$ was less than 50% and the ratio of the cerebral desaturation time to the total CPB time in the control group differed significantly from those in the slow group (control group: 17 ± 11 minutes, 12 ± 4%; slow group: 10 ± 8 minutes, 7 ± 4%, respectively; $p < 0.05$).[176] Consistent with this, in a study of the impact of rate of rewarming on cognitive outcomes in 165 CABG patients randomized to two differing rewarming strategies, Grigore et al[85] demonstrated a significant association between change in cognitive function and rate of rewarming.

Grocott et al[174] recorded hourly postoperative temperatures in 300 patients undergoing CABG on CPB and determined the degree of postoperative hyperthermia using the maximum temperature within the first 24 hours as well as by calculating the area under the curve for temperatures higher than 37°C. Patients underwent a battery of cognitive testing both before surgery and 6 weeks after surgery. The maximum temperature within the first 24 hours after CABG ranged from 37.2° to 39.3°C, and they demonstrated that the maximum postoperative temperature was independently associated with cognitive dysfunction at 6 weeks.[174] Accordingly, slower rewarming rate with lower peak temperatures during CPB may be an important factor in the prevention of neurocognitive decline after hypothermic CPB, and interventions to avoid postoperative hyperthermia may be warranted to improve cerebral outcome after cardiac surgery.

Cerebrovascular Disease

Relatively few studies have examined the cerebrovascular responses to CPB in patients with known cerebrovascular disease. Because of the vasodilatory effects of increased carbon dioxide in patients with cerebrovascular disease, pH-stat management could theoretically induce redistribution of regional CBF from marginally perfused to well-perfused regions (i.e., an intracerebral steal). Gravlee et al[178] investigated patients with cerebrovascular disease undergoing CABG and assessed the CBF responses to varying pH management, between alpha-stat and pH-stat. They confirmed the responsiveness of the cerebral vasculature to changes in $PaCO_2$ during hypothermic CPB but did not demonstrate evidence of intracerebral steal at higher $PaCO_2$ levels in any of these patients. In all patients, however, arterial perfusion pressure was greater than 65 mm Hg during CBF measurements, which may have offset any tendency for regional CBF inhomogeneities.

Using TCD monitoring of CBF velocity, 18 patients with severe carotid stenosis and 37 with no or mild stenosis were monitored during CPB.[179] Although not specified, it appears as though pH-stat management was used, because flow velocities correlated with $PaCO_2$ and arterial pressure. There were no significant differences detectable in flow velocity between patients with or without significant carotid stenosis. In a case report of a single patient with bilateral carotid stenoses, alpha-stat pH management was used and arterial pressure was varied from 35 to 85 mm Hg, while CBF was measured during hypothermic CPB.[180] The CBF values obtained from contralateral hemispheres were essentially equal and remained so throughout the range of different perfusion pressures used. These studies suggest that the cerebrovascular responses to CPB in patients with cerebrovascular disease do not differ significantly from those of normal patients with respect to gross measures of cerebrovascular responsiveness. This suggests that other factors, including associated aortic atherosclerosis, may be a more important factor.

Hogue et al[7] examined demographic and perioperative data prospectively collected from 2972 patients undergoing cardiac surgery. Carotid artery ultrasound examination was performed before surgery for patients aged 65 years or older or when there was a history of transient ischemic attacks or prior stroke. Epiaortic ultrasound was performed at the time of surgery in all patients to assess for atherosclerosis of the ascending aorta. Strokes occurred after surgery in 30 women and 18 men ($p < 0.0001$). A history of a stroke was the strongest predictor of new stroke for both women and men. A prior cerebrovascular event was a more important predictor of stroke for men than women.[7]

In a study by Bucerius et al[5] assessing CNS outcomes from 16,184 patients undergoing cardiac operations, the overall prevalence of postoperative delirium was 8.4%. Stepwise logistic regression revealed history of cerebrovascular disease, peripheral vascular disease, atrial fibrillation, diabetes mellitus, left ventricular ejection fraction of 30% or less, preoperative cardiogenic shock, urgent operation, intraoperative hemofiltration, operation time of 3 hours or more, and a high perioperative transfusion requirement as being independent predictors of delirium.

In the current cardiac surgical population, 17% to 22% of patients have a moderate carotid artery stenosis of 50% or more and 6% to 12% have a severe stenosis of 80% or more.[20] The risk of postoperative stroke is 10% in patients with moderate and 11% to 19% in patients with severe stenosis, while it remains 2% or less in patients with a stenosis of less than 50%. Although in patients presenting for cardiac surgery severe bilateral carotid artery disease is rare, the risk of perioperative stroke is as high as 20%.[20,181-183] It is not clear that carotid endarterectomy (CEA) decreases this rate, because in a meta-analysis, pooled data for stroke or death did not support CEA for risk reduction from asymptomatic carotid stenosis during CABG (relative risk 0.9, $p = 0.5$).[184] In a review, it was estimated that only about 40% of perioperative strokes (at most) could be directly attributable to ipsilateral carotid artery disease.[185] Accordingly, in a patient with asymptomatic carotid stenosis, unless the surgical team is very experienced in combined CEA/CABG procedures, concomitant CEA is unlikely to decrease a patient's stroke risk. Rather, carotid stenosis should be regarded as indicating a high likelihood of aortic and/or concomitant intracerebral disease, and there is increasing evidence that use of EAS with appropriate modification of surgical approach and, potentially, applied neuromonitoring can be of particular benefit in this high-risk group.

Diabetes Mellitus and Hyperglycemia

The presence of diabetes is recognized as a factor related to increased morbidity and mortality in cardiac surgical patients.[186-190] The incidence of diabetes mellitus increases with age, and its presence is known to accelerate the damage caused by atherosclerosis; thus, an increasingly greater percentage of patients coming for CABG have concomitant diabetes, currently estimated as a comorbidity in approximately 30% to 40% of CABG patients. Brucerius et al[191] found diabetes to be associated with increased incidence of stroke and delirium and prolonged intensive care unit and hospital stay. Mortasawi et al and Nussmeier describe diabetes mellitus as associated with increased incidences of stroke and mortality.[25,192] In a large study, McKahnn et al[18] prospectively collected data on 2711 CABG patients and identified diabetes mellitus as an independent risk factor for both stroke and encephalopathy. Part of the risk may involve cerebral hypoperfusion, because cerebral oxygen desaturation during CPB has been documented in diabetic patients, with insulin-dependent diabetics demonstrating the lowest values as measured via jugular oximetry and the poorest response to increases in mean arterial pressure.[193]

Studies identify normoglycemia as a desirable perioperative goal in cardiac surgical patients whether they are diabetics or not.[188,190] There is both experimental and clinical evidence that hyperglycemia is associated with exacerbation of neurologic injury.[194] Approaches to maintain serum glucose values under 150 mg/dL have shown favorable results. Furnary et al[186] reported on 3554 patients who underwent CABG from 1987 through 2001, demonstrating that the observed mortality in the group managed with tighter glucose values was lower and concluded that continuous intravenous insulin infusion added a protective effect against death. Carvalho et al[189] used an aggressive approach to maintain serum glucose values between 80 and 110 mg/dL and found that this is a safely attainable goal. One study positively correlated average blood glucose on the first postoperative day with a variety of adverse outcomes (stroke, myocardial infarction, septic complication, or death). For each 1-mmol/L increase above 6.1 mmol/L (1 mmol = 18 mg/dL), risk increased by 17%.[195] The ideal value of serum glucose in cardiac surgical patients is still unknown, but the evidence available suggests that maintenance of euglycemia is related to a better prognosis.

Hemodynamic Instability

Hemodynamic complications either preoperatively, intraoperatively, or postoperatively have been found to increase cerebral injury in cardiac surgical patients. In the report by Bucerius et al,[5] ejection fraction less than 30%, urgent operations, and preoperative cardiogenic shock were related to increased postoperative delirium. Riddelstope et al[26] found that hypotension and postoperative arrhythmias were related to cerebral complications, while Stanley et al[100] reported that postoperative atrial fibrillation was related to increased cognitive decline. Ganushchak et al[141] reported in a retrospective analysis of 1395 patients that the frequency of neurologic complications was 3.9% in the group of patients that experienced large fluctuations in hemodynamic parameters while on CPB, whereas in the group of patients with more stable values on CPB, the incidence of neurologic complications was 0.3%. These studies indicate an increased susceptibility of the brain in cardiac surgical patients to apparently "benign" hemodynamic alterations that either produce or enhance cerebral injury, probably through hypoperfusion of the brain tissue, particularly since it has been estimated that more than 50% of CABG patients have coexisting cerebrovascular disease.[106]

CEREBROPROTECTIVE STRATEGIES

Cardiopulmonary Bypass Equipment

Early studies demonstrated increased microemboli in patients undergoing CPB using bubble oxygenators, with a reduction in cerebral embolization with the use of membrane oxygenators and arterial line filtration[92,95,196-198] (Boxes 35–4 and 35–5). Using intraoperative fluorescein retinal angiography, Blauth et al[92] reported retinal microembolizations occurring during CPB with much greater frequency in patients in whom bubble versus membrane oxygenators were used. Using TCD for detection of cerebral emboli, Padayachee et al[197] demonstrated continuous generation of cerebral emboli in all patients managed using bubble oxygenators and none in patients in whom a membrane oxygenator was used. They also demonstrated the efficacy of arterial line filtration to significantly decrease cerebral embolic load.[198] It is apparent that emboli may be generated continuously during CPB, and that

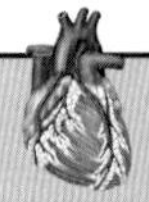

BOX 35–4 ***Clinical Strategies That May Decrease Neurologic Complications in Cardiac Surgery***

- Early and aggressive control of hemodynamic instability
- Perioperative glycemia <200 mg/dL
- Routine epiaortic scanning before manipulation of ascending aorta
- Avoidance of manipulation of ascending aorta in severe atheromatosis
- Maintenance of adequate cerebral perfusion pressure (neuromonitoring/cerebral oximetry?)
- Full-dose aprotinin in high-risk patients

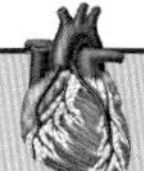

BOX 35–5 ***Strategies to Decrease Impact of CPB on Neurologic Complications***

- Avoidance of reinfusion of unprocessed shed blood
- Use of cell saver
- Monitoring of cerebral venous pressure via a proximal central venous pressure catheter or the introducer port of a pulmonary artery catheter
- Management of alpha-stat pH during moderate hypothermic CPB
- Avoidance of arterial inflow temperature >37°C
- Use of CPB circuitry incorporating membrane oxygenator and 40-micron arterial line filter
- Use of surface-modified and reduced-area CPB circuitry

equipment modification (e.g., arterial line microfiltration and preferential usage of membrane oxygenators) can decrease the generation of such emboli.[54] Membrane oxygenators are currently recommended for CPB.[128] It is equally evident that such equipment modifications, while decreasing the embolic load, cannot completely eliminate it.[62,199] Giorgiadis et al[200] used Doppler ultrasound and evaluated the percentage of microembolic signal (MES) reduction caused by the arterial filter and the proportion of MES actually reaching the brain by comparing the MES counts detected before the arterial filter, after the arterial filter, and in both middle cerebral arteries (MCAs). Eleven patients underwent surgery using normothermic CPB, alpha-stat, a membrane oxygenator, and a 40-μm arterial filter. Evaluation of MES was only performed during extracorporeal circulation and was initiated after cannulation and clamping of the ascending aorta and terminated shortly before the aortic clamp was removed. The arterial filter resulted in a 58.9% reduction of MES with only 4.4% (2624 of 59,132) of the MES detected after the arterial filter. The proportion of MES detected in the MCA corresponded to the total cerebral perfusion under CPB, estimated as 5% to 10% of the total perfusion volume.[200]

Schoenburg et al[201] used a dynamic bubble trap, incorporated in the arterial line after a 40-μm filter, to reduce the number of gaseous microemboli in 50 patients undergoing CABG. In 26 patients, a dynamic bubble trap was placed between the arterial filter and the aortic cannula (group 1), and in 24 patients, a placebo dynamic bubble trap was used (group 2) with TCD continuously measured on both sides during bypass, which was separated into four periods: phase 1, start of bypass until aortic clamping; phase 2, aortic clamping until rewarming; phase 3, rewarming until clamp removal; and phase 4, clamp removal until end of bypass. The bubble elimination rate during bypass was 77% in group 1 and 28% in group 2. The number of high-intensity signals was lower in group 1 during phase 1 (5.8 ± 7.3 versus 16 ± 15.4, $p < 0.05$ versus group 2) and phase 2 (6.9 ± 7.3 versus 24.2 ± 27.3, $p < 0.05$ versus group 2) but not during phases 3 and 4.[201] The authors found that the dynamic bubble trap can remove gaseous microemboli. Unfortunately, no psychometric studies were performed on either group of patients, but future research in this area might yield positive influence on neurologic outcome by decreasing gas microemboli. Other investigators have demonstrated that air within the venous line of the CPB circuit, resulting from air entrainment at the venous cannulation site, injection of drugs into the venous line, or use of cardiotomy suction, can pass through the oxygenator and appear as microemboli within the arterial line, even in the presence of a venous line defoamer and with use of a membrane oxygenator.[202,203] Giorgiadis et al[200] used tubing systems that included an arterial line 40-μm filter and demonstrated that the arterial filter resulted in a 58.9% reduction of microemboli signals with only 4.4% of the MESs detected after the arterial filter being actually detected in the MCA.

Modification of the inflammatory response to the CPB using modified surface CPB circuits and leukocyte-depleting filters has been explored. Hamada et al[102] examined the combined use of heparin coating of the CPB circuit and a leukocyte-depleting arterial line filter in 30 patients allocated randomly to equal groups with a conventional circuit and arterial line filter, a heparin-coated circuit with a conventional filter, or a heparin-coated circuit with a leukocyte-depleting arterial line filter. Plasma interleukin (IL)-6 and IL-8 concentrations in the heparin bonded with leukocyte-depleting filter group were lower than in the conventional circuit group. Although a decrease in inflammatory mediator release has been observed by using leukocyte-depleting filters, the impact of these types of filters on neurologic outcome is less clear. In a meta-analysis of 28 relevant clinical studies, Whitaker et al[204] concluded that conventional arterial line filtration had a definite effect in reducing neuropsychological deficit post-CPB. The results of studies using the leucocyte-depleting filter were less clear cut.

In an attempt to decrease emboli originating from the surgical field, cell savers have been used for processing cardiotomy suction blood before returning it to the CPB circuit. Jewell et al[205] reported on 20 patients prospectively randomized to either cell saver or cardiotomy suction and demonstrated that compared with cardiotomy suction, cell saver removed significantly more fat from shed blood, such that the percentage reduction in fat weight achieved by cell saver or cardiotomy suction was 87% compared with 45%. de Vries et al[206] published a study on patients randomly assigned to have a fat removal filter for the cardiotomy suction. The fat filter removed 40% fat, leukocytes, and platelets from cardiotomy suction blood during cardiac surgery compared with the control group without the filter.

In addition, various intraoperative manipulations, particularly instrumentation of the atherosclerotic aorta, are independent risks for the generation of cerebral emboli, and likely produce particulate or macrogaseous emboli, rather than oxygenator-generated microgaseous and microaggregate emboli.[48,52,207,208] Avoidance of manipulation of a diseased aorta seems to decrease embolization and cerebral injury.[59,64,209] An alternative approach, emboli reduction by capture using an intra-aortic filter inserted through a side chamber of a modified aortic cannula, was assessed (Fig. 35–13).

In a nonrandomized study, Schmitz et al examined the impact of intra-aortic filtration during CPB.[101] Three hundred four cardiac surgical patients had intra-aortic filtration using a 150-μm net deployed through the aortic cannula, while a further 278 patients formed the control group. Patients in the filter group experienced a lower incidence of adverse neurologic outcomes than patients in the control group (4.3% versus 11.9%) with significantly fewer TIAs (0% versus 1.4%), delirium (3.0% versus 6.5%), and memory deficit (1.3% versus 6.2%). There were also fewer strokes in the filter group

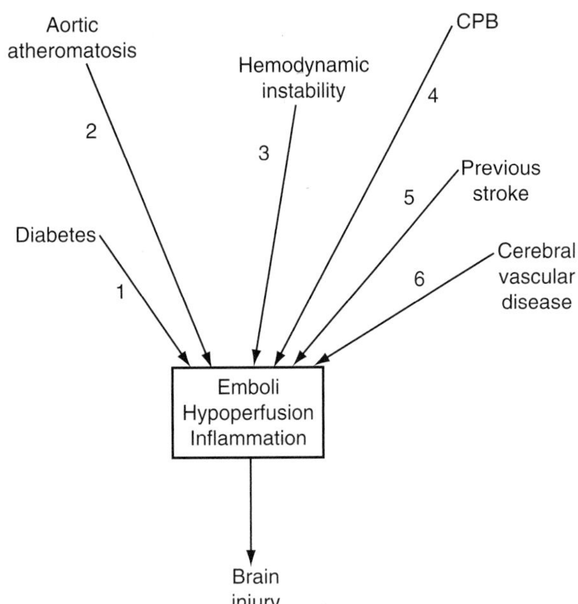

Figure 35–13 The "Brain Mileau" concept. Cerebral injury in cardiac surgery is the product of concurrent risk factors related to the surgical procedure and the patient's previous condition. This unique combination of embolic, perfusion, inflammatory, coagulation, and metabolic events yields a broad spectrum of neurologic manifestations. The graphic shows factors and potential interventions to decrease neurologic morbidity in cardiac surgery. These are numbered clockwise: *1,* tight perioperative control of glycemia; *2,* epiaortic scanning to detect severe atheromatosis of ascending aorta; modified surgical technique to decrease or avoid aortic manipulation; *3,* early pharmacologic and/or mechanical support to attain stable circulatory conditions; *4,* CPB circuitry of reduced and modified surface, use of arterial line 40-μm filters, alpha-stat CO_2 management, mild/moderate hypothermia, use of cell savers to process shed blood before reinfusing to CPB circuitry, arterial inflow temperature <37°C; and *5* and *6,* aprotinin full dose, intraoperative neurophysiologic monitoring (central venous pressure on CPB, brain oximetry [NIRS], retinal and transcranial Doppler, evoked potentials), and maintenance of cerebral perfusion pressure >60 mm Hg.

compared with the control group (0.7% versus 2.2%). Although the sample size was relatively small and the patients were not randomly assigned, the study findings suggest a protective effect of intra-aortic filters on CNS injury.[101] In a large multi-institutional prospective randomized trial of 1289 patients in whom intra-aortic filtration or conventional CPB cannula was used, emboli were identified in 598 (96.8%) of 618 filters successfully deployed and their post hoc analysis indicated a reduction in postoperative renal complications.[210] In other studies, intra-aortic emboli trapping devices have been used with varied results.[63,200] In a small study by Eifert et al[62] in 24 patients, the use of the intra-aortic filter device did not show any difference in neurologic, neuroradiographic, or neuropsychological outcomes, yet the intra-aortic filter was effective in capturing particulate material. Similar efficacy in capturing intraoperative material using intraaortic filters during CPB was reported by Reichenspurner et al.[211] It does appear as though intra-aortic filters can be safely deployed and that they do capture particulate emboli, the predominant origin of which is atheromatous. The overall impact of this device on neurologic outcomes in cardiac surgical patients has yet to be determined in a randomized prospective study.[62,209,211]

Applied Neuromonitoring

Intraoperative neurophysiologic monitoring may be of benefit to decrease CNS injury.[212] Brain oximetry studies using noninvasive near-infrared spectrophotometry (NIRS) have shown promising results.[213-216] In a large nonrandomized cohort study from Goldman,[217] NIRS was used to monitor cerebral oxygen saturation in 1034 cardiac surgical patients and compared with outcomes in 1245 patients who underwent cardiac surgery immediately before cerebral oximetry was incorporated. The study group had significantly more patients in New York Heart Association (NYHA) classes III and IV than the control group, but the study group overall had fewer permanent strokes (10 [0.97%] versus 25 [2.5%]; $p < 0.044$) and the proportion of patients requiring prolonged ventilation was significantly smaller in the study group, as was the length of hospital stay.[217] Murkin et al[218] reported a prospective, blinded, randomized study of NIRS cerebral oximetry in 199 cardiac surgical patients and demonstrated significantly fewer adverse clinical outcomes in NIRS versus control groups ($p = 0.027$).

Intraoperative TCD has been demonstrated to detect embolic events in real time and allows modification of perfusion and surgical techniques. It has been shown that the numbers of emboli generated by perfusionist interventions (e.g., drug injection, blood return), as well as episodes of entrainment of air from the surgical field, are rapidly identified and corrected by TCD detection of intraoperative emboli.[219] Even during beating-heart procedures, compromised cerebral perfusion can occur relatively frequently, and if unrecognized may account for the relative lack of difference in CNS outcomes between CABG and OPCAB surgery.[220] Combined EEG and cerebral oximetry identified episodes of cerebral ischemia in 15% of a series of 550 beating-heart patients; all were treated successfully by a combination of pharmacologically improved cardiac output, increased perfusion pressure, and cardiac repositioning.[221]

Pharmacologic Cerebral Protection

In general, pharmacologic protection from cerebral ischemia remains an elusive goal. Although there had been one clinical study in which a significant reduction in persistent neurologic defects following open-chamber cardiac surgery was reported after administration of high-dose thiopental, this was not confirmed in closed-chamber CABG procedures.[222,223] Other data have suggested that if there is any such thiopental-derived cerebroprotective effect, the mechanism may be due to a metabolically driven decrease in CBF, with a concomitant reduction in the delivery of emboli into the brain, rather than occurring primarily as a result of a decrease in $CMRO_2$.[224] However, a three-center study in 225 patients undergoing mitral or aortic valve surgery and randomized to high-dose propofol with induction of burst-suppression on EEG or a sufentanil control group was unable to detect any significant differences in neurologic or neuropsychological outcomes between groups.[225] These authors concluded that neither cerebral metabolic suppression nor reduction in CBF reliably provides neuroprotection in open-chamber cardiac surgery. A large trial of perioperative nimodipine in valve replacement surgery had to be terminated prematurely after enrollment of only 150 of 400 patients because of a significant increase in major bleeding and an increased mortality in the 6-month follow-up period.[226]

There are some interesting associations between certain drug therapies having anti-inflammatory properties and lowered incidences of stroke and adverse CNS events. In a retrospective review of 2575 CABG patients, Amory et al reported that patients who received perioperative β-blockers had a significantly lower incidence of severe neurologic outcomes versus those who did not receive these drugs, demonstrating a 1.9% incidence of stroke and coma versus 4.3%, respectively.[227] The serine protease inhibitor aprotinin has been shown to positively impact coagulation and inflammatory alterations triggered by CPB and has also been associated with decreased incidences of stroke and major CNS injury in cardiac surgical patients.[68,103,104] Aprotinin has also been demonstrated to have anti-inflammatory and antithrombotic effects.[228] Frumento et al[8] retrospectively analyzed stroke outcomes in 1524 patients undergoing cardiac surgery and identified a subset of 149 patients older than 70, history of hypertension, diabetes mellitus, stroke or transient ischemic attack, and presence of aortic atheroma who were deemed to be at similarly high risk of stroke. They reported that in this high-risk subset of patients, intraoperative administration of full-dose aprotinin, but not half-dose, was associated with a lower incidence of stroke. In an important prospective study of 5065 patients undergoing CABG conducted at 70 centers in 17 countries, the relation between early aspirin use and fatal and nonfatal outcomes was investigated.[229] Among patients who received aspirin within 48 hours after revascularization, subsequent mortality was 1.3% compared with 4% among those who did not receive aspirin during this period. Aspirin therapy was associated with a 48% reduction in the incidence of myocardial infarction (2.8% versus 5.4%, $p < 0.001$), a 50% reduction in the incidence of stroke (1.3% versus 2.6%, $p = 0.01$), a 74% reduction in the incidence of renal failure (0.9% versus 3.4%, $p < 0.001$), and a 62% reduction in the incidence of bowel infarction (0.3% versus 0.8%, $p = 0.01$). Taken together, these studies seem to indicate that therapies associated with decreased inflammatory and sympathetic responses appear to be associated with lowered incidence of stroke and adverse CNS events.

While these results suggest that there is as yet no pharmacologic "magic bullet" that can be used to reduce neurologic injury in patients undergoing cardiac surgery, there is a combination of technical and pharmacologic measures currently available that might positively affect the outcome of these patients.[128] In patients identified as being at risk for perioperative cerebral injury, preventive measures as outlined in Box 35–6 should be instituted with organ-targeted management to guide the whole intraoperative and postoperative period. The Best Practice Cardiopulmonary Bypass Group summarized these measures as the avoidance of embolic injury by means of intraoperative EAS prior to aortic instrumentation, the employment of arterial line filters, modified-surface and reduced-area CPB circuits and membrane oxygenators, the use of cell savers to process shed blood before reinfusion to the CPB circuit, the use of alpha-stat pH management during moderate hypothermic CPB, monitoring cerebral venous outflow pressure via proximal jugular venous pressure with maintenance of cerebral perfusion pressure above 60 mm Hg, the avoidance of cerebral hyperthermia during rewarming, aggressive control of glycemia, and the use of "tepid" rather than normothermic perfusion during CPB. As the age and incidence of comorbid disease in the cardiac surgical population continue to rise, the importance of these issues becomes ever more acute because primary prevention continues to be at present the only effective measure to decrease cerebral injury in cardiac surgical patients.

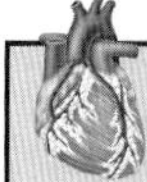

BOX 35–6 *Strategies to Improve Cardiopulmonary Bypass Influence on Outcome*

- Minimization of "blind" manipulation or clamping of the ascending aorta
- Avoidance of reinfusion of unprocessed shed blood (use of cell saver recommended)
- Monitoring of cerebral venous pressure via a proximal central venous pressure catheter or the introducer port of a pulmonary artery catheter
- Maintaining high cerebral perfusion pressure (>60 mm Hg)
- Alpha-stat pH management
- Avoidance of arterial inflow temperature >37°C
- Cardiopulmonary bypass circuitry incorporating membrane oxygenator and 40-μm arterial line filter
- Surface modified and reduced area cardiopulmonary bypass circuitry
- Perioperative blood glucose concentration below 200 mg/dL

The Best Practice Cardiopulmonary Bypass[128]

REFERENCES

1. Ferguson TB Jr, Hammill BG, Peterson ED, et al: A decade of change—Risk profiles and outcomes for isolated coronary artery bypass grafting procedures, 1990-1999: A report from the STS National Database Committee and the Duke Clinical Research Institute. Society of Thoracic Surgeons. Ann Thorac Surg 73:480, 2002
2. Gardner TJ, Horneffer PJ, Manolio TA, et al: Stroke following coronary artery bypass grafting: A ten-year study. Ann Thorac Surg 40:574, 1985
3. Tuman KJ, McCarthy RJ, Najafi H, Ivankovich AD: Differential effects of advanced age on neurologic and cardiac risks of coronary artery operations. J Thorac Cardiovasc Surg 104:1510, 1992
4. Bucerius J, Gummert JF, Borger MA, et al: Stroke after cardiac surgery: A risk factor analysis of 16,184 consecutive adult patients. Ann Thorac Surg 75:472, 2003
5. Bucerius J, Gummert JF, Borger MA, et al: Predictors of delirium after cardiac surgery: Effect of beating-heart (off-pump) surgery. J Thorac Cardiovasc Surg 127:57, 2004
6. Ricotta JJ, Char DJ, Cuadra SA, et al: Modeling stroke risk after coronary artery bypass and combined coronary artery bypass and carotid endarterectomy: Stroke 34:1212, 2003
7. Hogue CW Jr, De Wet CJ, Schechtman KB, Davila-Roman VG: The importance of prior stroke for the adjusted risk of neurologic injury after cardiac surgery for women and men. Anesthesiology 98:823, 2003
8. Frumento RJ, O'Malley CM, Bennett-Guerrero E: Stroke after cardiac surgery: A retrospective analysis of the effect of aprotinin dosing regimens. Ann Thorac Surg 75:479, 2003
9. Ridderstolpe L, Ahlgren E, Gill H, Rutberg H: Risk factor analysis of early and delayed cerebral complications after cardiac surgery. J Cardiothorac Vasc Anesth 16:278, 2002
10. D'Alfonso A, Mariani MA, Amerini A, et al: Off-pump coronary surgery improves in-hospital and early outcomes in octogenarians. Ital Heart J 5:197, 2004
11. Gerrah R, Izhar U, Elami A, et al: Cardiac surgery in octogenarians—A better prognosis in coronary artery disease. Isr Med Assoc J 510:713, 2003
12. Alexander KP, Anstrom KJ, Muhlbaier LH, et al: Outcomes of cardiac surgery in patients ≥80 years: Results from the National Cardiovascular Network. J Am Coll Cardiol 135:731, 2000
13. Roach GW, Kanchuger M, Mangano CM, et al: Adverse cerebral outcomes after coronary bypass surgery. Multicenter Study of Perioperative Ischemia Research Group and the Ischemia Research and Education Foundation Investigators. N Engl J Med 525:1857, 1996

14. Blacker DJ, Flemming KD, Link MJ, Brown RD Jr: The preoperative cerebrovascular consultation: Common cerebrovascular questions before general or cardiac surgery. Mayo Clin Proc 79:223, 2004
15. Naylor AR, Mehta Z, Rothwell PM, Bell PR: Carotid artery disease and stroke during coronary artery bypass: A critical review of the literature. Eur J Vasc Endovasc Surg 23:283, 2002
16. Hewitt TD, Santa Maria PL, Alvarez JM: Cardiac surgery in Australian octogenarians: 1996-2001. ANZ J Surg 73:749, 2003
17. Eagle KA, Guyton RA, Davidoff R, et al: ACC/AHA Guidelines for Coronary Artery Bypass Graft Surgery: A Report of the American College of Cardiology/American Heart Association Task Force on Practice Guidelines Committee to Revise the 1991 Guidelines for Coronary Artery Bypass Graft Surgery. American College of Cardiology/American Heart Association. J Am Coll Cardiol 34:1262, 1999
18. McKhann GM, Grega MA, Borowicz LM Jr, et al: Encephalopathy and stroke after coronary artery bypass grafting: Incidence, consequences, and prediction. Arch Neurol 59:1422, 2002
19. Wolman RL, Nussmeier NA, Aggarwal A, et al: Cerebral injury after cardiac surgery: identification of a group at extraordinary risk. Multicenter Study of Perioperative Ischemia Research Group (McSPI) and the Ischemia Research Education Foundation (IREF) Investigators. Stroke 30:514, 1999
20. Ahonen J, Salmenpera M: Brain injury after adult cardiac surgery. Acta Anaesthesiol Scand 48:4, 2004
21. Arrowsmith JE, Grocott HP, Reves JG, Newman MF: Central nervous system complications of cardiac surgery. Br J Anaesth 84:378, 2000
22. Baker RA, Andrew MJ, Knight JL: Evaluation of neurologic assessment and outcomes in cardiac surgical patients. Semin Thorac Cardiovasc Surg 13:149, 2001
23. van Dijk D, Keizer AM, Diephuis JC, et al: Neurocognitive dysfunction after coronary artery bypass surgery: A systematic review. J Thorac Cardiovasc Surg 120:632, 2000
24. Hogue CW Jr, Barzilai B, Pieper KS, et al: Sex differences in neurological outcomes and mortality after cardiac surgery: A Society of Thoracic Surgery National Database report. Circulation 12:133, 2001
25. Nussmeier NA: A review of risk factors for adverse neurologic outcome after cardiac surgery. J Extracorp Technol 34:4, 2002
26. Ridderstolpe L, Ahlgren E, Gill H, Rutberg H: Risk factor analysis of early and delayed cerebral complications after cardiac surgery. J Cardiothorac Vasc Anesth 16:278, 2002
27. Newman MF, Grocott HP, Mathew JP, et al: Report of the substudy assessing the impact of neurocognitive function on quality of life 5 years after cardiac surgery. Stroke 1:2874, 2001
28. Newman MF, Wolman R, Kanchuger M, et al: Multicenter preoperative stroke risk index for patients undergoing coronary artery bypass graft surgery. Multicenter Study of Perioperative Ischemia (McSPI) Research Group. Circulation 1949(suppl II):II-74, 1996
29. Maruff P, Silbert B, Evered L: Cognitive decline following cardiac surgery. Br J Anaesth 87:518, 2001
30. Sotaniemi KA: Cerebral outcome after extracorporeal circulation. Comparison between prospective and retrospective evaluations. Arch Neurol 40:75, 1983
31. Murkin JM, Newman SP, Stump DA, Blumenthal JA: Statement of consensus on assessment of neurobehavioral outcomes after cardiac surgery. Ann Thorac Surg 59:1289, 1995
32. Ebert AD, Walzer TA, Huth C, Herrmann M: Early neurobehavioral disorders after cardiac surgery: A comparative analysis of coronary artery bypass graft surgery and valve replacement. J Cardiothorac Vasc Anesth 15:15, 2001
33. Murkin JM: Neurologic dysfunction after CAB or valvular surgery: Is the medium the miscreant? Anesth Analg 76:213, 1993
34. Ho PM, Arciniegas DB, Grigsby J, et al: Predictors of cognitive decline following coronary artery bypass graft surgery. Ann Thorac Surg 77:597, 2004
35. Arrowsmith JE, Grocott HP, Newman MF: Neurologic risk assessment, monitoring and outcome in cardiac surgery. J Cardiothorac Vasc Anesth 13:736, 1999
36. Fearn SJ, Pole R, Wesnes K, Faragher EB, et al: Cerebral injury during cardiopulmonary bypass: Emboli impair memory. J Thorac Cardiovasc Surg 121:1150, 2001
37. Almassi GH, Sommers T, Moritz TE, et al: Stroke in cardiac surgical patients: Determinants and outcome. Ann Thorac Surg 68:391, 1999
38. Omar Y, Balacumaraswami L, Pigott DW, et al: Solid and gaseous cerebral microembolization during off-pump, on-pump, and open cardiac surgery procedures. J Thorac Cardiovasc Surg 127:1759, 2004
39. Watters MP, Cohen AM, Monk CR, et al: Reduced cerebral embolic signals in beating heart coronary surgery detected by transcranial Doppler ultrasound. Br J Anaesth 84:629, 2000
40. van DD, Jansen EW, Hijman R, et al: Cognitive outcome after off-pump and on-pump coronary artery bypass graft surgery: A randomized trial. JAMA 2028711:1405, 2002
41. Jaffer FA, O'Donnell CJ, Larson MG, et al: Age and sex distribution of subclinical aortic atherosclerosis: A magnetic resonance imaging examination of the Framingham Heart Study. Arterioscler Thromb Vasc Biol 122:849, 2002
42. Macleod MR, Amarenco P, Davis SM, Donnan GA: Atheroma of the aortic arch: An important and poorly recognised factor in the aetiology of stroke. Lancet Neurol 3:408, 2004
43. Macleod MR, Donnan GA: Atheroma of the aortic arch: The missing link in the secondary prevention of stroke? Expert Rev Cardiovasc Ther 1:487, 2003
44. Li AE, Kamel I, Rando F, et al: Using MRI to assess aortic wall thickness in the multiethnic study of atherosclerosis: Distribution by race, sex, and age. AJR Am J Roentgenol 182:593, 2004
45. Yahia AM, Kirmani JF, Xavier AR, et al: Characteristics and predictors of aortic plaques in patients with transient ischemic attacks and strokes. J Neuroimaging 14:16, 2004
46. Watanabe K, Hiroki T, Koga N: Relation of thoracic aorta calcification on computed tomography and coronary risk factors to obstructive coronary artery disease on angiography. Angiology 54:433, 2003
47. Agmon Y, Khandheria BK, Meissner I, et al: Relation of coronary artery disease and cerebrovascular disease with atherosclerosis of the thoracic aorta in the general population. Am J Cardiol 189:262, 2002
48. Blauth CI, Cosgrove DM, Webb BW, et al: Atheroembolism from the ascending aorta. An emerging problem in cardiac surgery. J Thorac Cardiovasc Surg 103:1104, 1992
49. Doty JR, Wilentz RE, Salazar JD, et al: Atheroembolism in cardiac surgery. Ann Thorac Surg 75:1221, 2003
50. Goodwin AT, Goddard M, Taylor GJ, Ritchie AJ: Clinical versus actual outcome in cardiac surgery: A postmortem study. Eur J Cardiothorac Surg 17:747, 2000
51. Mackensen GB, Swaminathan M, Ti LK, et al: Preliminary report on the interaction of apolipoprotein E polymorphism with aortic atherosclerosis and acute nephropathy after CABG. Ann Thorac Surg 78:520, 2004
52. Davila-Roman VG, Barzilai B, Wareing TH, et al: Atherosclerosis of the ascending aorta. Prevalence and role as an independent predictor of cerebrovascular events in cardiac patients. Stroke 2510:2010, 1994
53. Leacche M, Carrier M, Bouchard D, et al: Improving neurologic outcome in off-pump surgery: the "no touch" technique. Heart Surg Forum 6:169, 2003
54. Mackensen GB, Ti LK, Phillips-Bute BG, et al: Cerebral embolization during cardiac surgery: Impact of aortic atheroma burden. Br J Anaesth 91:656, 2003
55. Sharony R, Bizekis CS, Kanchuger M, et al: Off-pump coronary artery bypass grafting reduces mortality and stroke in patients with atheromatous aortas: A case control study. Circulation 9(suppl I):II-15, 2003
56. Wareing TH, Davila-Roman VG, Daily BB, et al: Strategy for the reduction of stroke incidence in cardiac surgical patients. Ann Thorac Surg 55:1400, 1993
57. Sekoranja L, Vuille C, Bianchi-Demicheli F, et al: Thoracic aortic plaques, transoesophageal echocardiography and coronary artery disease. Swiss Med Wkly 71345-6:75, 2004
58. Djaiani G, Fedorko L, Borger M, et al: Mild to moderate atheromatous disease of the thoracic aorta and new ischemic brain lesions after conventional coronary artery bypass graft surgery. Stroke 29, 2004
59. Royse AG, Royse CF, Ajani AE, et al: Reduced neuropsychological dysfunction using epiaortic echocardiography and the exclusive Y graft. Ann Thorac Surg 69:1431, 2000
60. St Amand MA, Murkin JM, Menkis AH, Downey DB: Aortic atherosclerotic plaque identified by epiaortic scanning predicts cerebral embolic load in cardiac surgery. Can J Anaesth 44:A7, 1997
61. Konstadt SN, Reich DL, Kahn R, Viggiani RF: Transesophageal echocardiography can be used to screen for ascending aortic atherosclerosis. Anesth Analg 81:225, 1995
62. Eifert S, Reichenspurner H, Pfefferkorn T, et al: Neurological and neuropsychological examination and outcome after use of an intra-aortic filter device during cardiac surgery. Perfusion 18(suppl 1):55, 2003
63. Bonatti J: Ascending aortic atherosclerosis—A complex and challenging problem for the cardiac surgeon. Heart Surg Forum 2:125, 1999
64. Gaspar M, Laufer G, Bonatti J, et al: Epiaortic ultrasound and intraoperative transesophageal echocardiography for the thoracic aorta atherosclerosis assessment in patient undergoing CABG. Surgical technique modification to avoid cerebral stroke. Chirurgia (Bucur) 97:529, 2002

65. Konstadt SN, Reich DL, Quintana C, Levy M: The ascending aorta: How much does transesophageal echocardiography see? Anesth Analg 78:240, 1994
66. Wareing TH, Davila-Roman VG, Barzilai B, et al: Management of the severely atherosclerotic ascending aorta during cardiac operations. A strategy for detection and treatment. J Thorac Cardiovasc Surg 103:453, 1992
67. Ohteki H, Itoh T, Natsuaki M, et al: Intraoperative ultrasonic imaging of the ascending aorta in ischemic heart disease. Ann Thorac Surg 50:539, 1990
68. Murkin JM: Attenuation of neurologic injury during cardiac surgery. Ann Thorac Surg 72:S1838, 2001
69. Calafiore AM, Di MM, Teodori G, et al: Impact of aortic manipulation on incidence of cerebrovascular accidents after surgical myocardial revascularization. Ann Thorac Surg 73:1387, 2002
70. Knipp SC, Matatko N, Wilhelm H, et al: Evaluation of brain injury after coronary artery bypass grafting. A prospective study using neuropsychological assessment and diffusion-weighted magnetic resonance imaging. Eur J Cardiothorac Surg 25:791, 2004
71. Murkin JM: Long-term neurological and neuropsychological outcome 3 years after coronary artery bypass surgery. Anesth Analg 82, S328, 1996
72. Newman MF, Kirchner JL, Phillips-Bute B, et al: Longitudinal assessment of neurocognitive function after coronary-artery bypass surgery. N Engl J Med 8344:395, 2001
73. Taggart DP, Westaby S: Neurological and cognitive disorders after coronary artery bypass grafting. Curr Opin Cardiol 16:271, 2001
74. Murkin JM, Martzke JS, Buchan AM, et al: A randomized study of the influence of perfusion technique and pH management strategy in 316 patients undergoing coronary artery bypass surgery. II. Neurologic and cognitive outcomes. J Thorac Cardiovasc Surg 110:349, 1995
75. Bar-Yosef S, Anders M, Mackensen GB, et al: Aortic atheroma burden and cognitive dysfunction after coronary artery bypass graft surgery. Ann Thorac Surg 78:1556, 2005
76. Ahlgren E, Lundqvist A, Nordlund A, et al: Neurocognitive impairment and driving performance after coronary artery bypass surgery. Eur J Cardiothorac Surg 23:334, 2003
77. Di Carlo CA, Perna AM, Pantoni L, et al: Clinically relevant cognitive impairment after cardiac surgery: A 6-month follow-up study. J Neurol Sci 85, 2001
78. Fox HM, Rizzo ND, Gifford S: Psychological observations of patients undergoing mitral surgery: A study of stress. Psychosom Med 16:186, 1954
79. Tufo HM, Ostfeld AM, Shekelle R: Central nervous system dysfunction following open-heart surgery. JAMA 25212:1333, 1970
80. Kornfeld DS, Heller SS, Frank KA, et al: Delirium after coronary artery bypass surgery. J Thorac Cardiovasc Surg 76:93, 1978
81. Millar K, Asbury AJ, Murray GD: Pre-existing cognitive impairment as a factor influencing outcome after cardiac surgery. Br J Anaesth 86:63, 2001
82. Rankin KP, Kochamba GS, Boone KB, et al: Presurgical cognitive deficits in patients receiving coronary artery bypass graft surgery. J Int Neuropsychol Soc 9:913, 2003
83. Muramoto O, Kuru Y, Sugishita M, Toyokura Y: Pure memory loss with hippocampal lesions: A pneumoencephalographic study. Arch Neurol 36:54, 1979
84. Grant I: Neuropsychological findings in hypoxemic chronic obstructive pulmonary disease. Proceedings of the 10th Annual Meeting of the International Neuropsychology Society, Pittsburgh, 1982
85. Grigore AM, Grocott HP, Mathew JP, et al: The rewarming rate and increased peak temperature alter neurocognitive outcome after cardiac surgery. Anesth Analg 94:4, 2002
86. Harrington DK, Bonser M, Moss A, et al: Neuropsychometric outcome following aortic arch surgery: A prospective randomized trial of retrograde cerebral perfusion. J Thorac Cardiovasc Surg 126:638, 2003
87. Rasmussen LS, Sperling B, Abildstrom HH, Moller JT: Neuron loss after coronary artery bypass detected by SPECT estimation of benzodiazepine receptors. Ann Thorac Surg 74:1576, 2002
88. Wang D, Wu X, Li J, et al: The effect of lidocaine on early postoperative cognitive dysfunction after coronary artery bypass surgery. Anesth Analg 1134, 2002
89. Basile AM, Fusi C, Conti AA, et al: S-100 protein and neuron-specific enolase as markers of subclinical cerebral damage after cardiac surgery: Preliminary observation of a 6-month follow-up study. Eur Neurol 45:151, 2001
90. Murkin JM, Stump DA, Blumenthal JA, McKhann G: Defining dysfunction: Group means versus incidence analysis—A statement of consensus. Ann Thorac Surg 64:904, 1997
91. Shaw PJ, Bates D, Cartlidge NE, et al: Neurologic and neuropsychological morbidity following major surgery: Comparison of coronary artery bypass and peripheral vascular surgery. Stroke 18:700, 1987
92. Blauth CI, Smith PL, Arnold JV, et al: Influence of oxygenator type on the prevalence and extent of microembolic retinal ischemia during cardiopulmonary bypass. Assessment by digital image analysis. J Thorac Cardiovasc Surg 99:61, 1990
93. Harrison MJ, Pugsley W, Newman S, et al: Detection of middle cerebral emboli during coronary artery bypass surgery using transcranial Doppler sonography. Stroke 2110:1512, 1990
94. Moody DM, Bell MA, Challa VR, et al: Brain microemboli during cardiac surgery or aortography. Ann Neurol 28:477, 1990
95. Blauth C, Arnold J, Kohner EM, Taylor KM: Retinal microembolism during cardiopulmonary bypass demonstrated by fluorescein angiography. Lancet 2:837, 1986
96. bu-Omar Y, Balacumaraswami L, Pigott DW, et al: Solid and gaseous cerebral microembolization during off-pump, on-pump, and open cardiac surgery procedures. J Thorac Cardiovasc Surg 127:1759, 2004
97. Motallebzadeh R, Kanagasabay R, Bland M, et al: S100 protein and its relation to cerebral microemboli in on-pump and off-pump coronary artery bypass surgery. Eur J Cardiothorac Surg 25:409, 2004
98. Wimmer-Greinecker G: Reduction of neurologic complications by intra-aortic filtration in patients undergoing combined intracardiac and CABG procedures. Eur J Cardiothorac Surg 23:159, 2003
99. Hindman BJ: Emboli, inflammation, and CNS impairment: An overview. Heart Surg Forum 5:249, 2002
100. Stanley TO, Mackensen GB, Grocott HP, et al: The impact of postoperative atrial fibrillation on neurocognitive outcome after coronary artery bypass graft surgery. Anesth Analg 94:290, 2002
101. Schmitz C, Weinreich S, White J, et al: Can particulate extraction from the ascending aorta reduce neurologic injury in cardiac surgery? J Thorac Cardiovasc Surg 126:1829, 2003
102. Hamada Y, Kawachi K, Nakata T, et al: Antiinflammatory effect of heparin-coated circuits with leukocyte-depleting filters in coronary bypass surgery. Artif Organs 2512:1004, 2001
103. Greilich PE, Brouse CF, Whitten CW, et al: Antifibrinolytic therapy during cardiopulmonary bypass reduces proinflammatory cytokine levels: A randomized, double-blind, placebo-controlled study of epsilon-aminocaproic acid and aprotinin. J Thorac Cardiovasc Surg 126:1498, 2003
104. Murkin JM: Inflammatory responses and CNS injury: Implications, prophylaxis, and treatment. Heart Surg Forum 6:193, 2003
105. Uehara T, Tabuchi M, Kozawa S, Mori E: MR angiographic evaluation of carotid and intracranial arteries in Japanese patients scheduled for coronary artery bypass grafting. Cerebrovasc Dis 11:341, 2001
106. Yoon BW, Bae HJ, Kang DW, et al: Intracranial cerebral artery disease as a risk factor for central nervous system complications of coronary artery bypass graft surgery. Stroke 32:94, 2001
107. Abildstrom H, Rasmussen LS, Rentowl P, et al: Cognitive dysfunction 1-2 years after noncardiac surgery in the elderly. ISPOCD group. International Study of Post-Operative Cognitive Dysfunction. Acta Anaesthesiol Scand 4410:1246, 2000
108. Linstedt U, Meyer O, Kropp P, et al: Serum concentration of S-100 protein in assessment of cognitive dysfunction after general anesthesia in different types of surgery. Acta Anaesthesiol Scand 46:384, 2002
109. Connolly ES Jr, Winfree CJ, Rampersad A, et al: Serum S100B protein levels are correlated with subclinical neurocognitive declines after carotid endarterectomy. Neurosurgery 49:1076, 2001
110. Edmonds CR, Barbut D, Hager D, Sharrock NE: Intraoperative cerebral arterial embolization during total hip arthroplasty. Anesthesiology 93:315, 2000
111. Colonna DM, Kilgus D, Brown W, et al: Acute brain fat embolization occurring after total hip arthroplasty in the absence of a patent foramen ovale. Anesthesiology 96:1027, 2002
112. Kinoshita H, Iranami H, Fujii K, et al: The use of bone cement induces an increase in serum astroglial S-100B protein in patients undergoing total knee arthroplasty. Anesth Analg 97:1657, 2003
113. Aguilar MJ, Gerbode F, Hill JD: Neuropathologic complications of cardiac surgery. J Thorac Cardiovasc Surg 61:676, 1971
114. Aberg T, Kihlgren M: Cerebral protection during open-heart surgery. Thorax 32:525, 1977
115. Parolari A, Alamanni F, Cannata A, et al: Off-pump versus on-pump coronary artery bypass: Meta-analysis of currently available randomized trials. Ann Thorac Surg 76:37, 2003
116. Emmrich P, Hahn J, Ogunlade V, et al: [Neuropathological findings after cardiac surgery—retrospective study over 6 years]. Z Kardiol 9211:925, 2003

117. Torvik A: The pathogenesis of watershed infarcts in the brain. Stroke 15:221, 1984
118. Salazar JD, Wityk RJ, Grega MA, et al: Stroke after cardiac surgery: Short- and long-term outcomes. Ann Thorac Surg 72:1195, 2001
119. Koga M, Shimokawa S, Moriyama Y, et al: Watershed infarction after combined coronary and axillobifemoral bypass surgery. Jpn J Thorac Cardiovasc Surg 48:258, 2000
120. Malone M: Brain damage after cardiopulmonary bypass: Correlations between neurophysiological and neuropathological findings. J Neurol Neurosurg Psychiatry 44:924, 1981
121. Wityk RJ, Goldsborough MA, Hillis A, et al: Diffusion- and perfusion-weighted brain magnetic resonance imaging in patients with neurologic complications after cardiac surgery. Arch Neurol 58:571, 2001
122. Torvik A, Skullerud K: Watershed infarcts in the brain caused by microemboli. Clin Neuropathol 1:99, 1982
123. Boyajian RA, Otis SM: Embolic stroke syndrome underlies encephalopathy and coma following cardiac surgery. Arch Neurol 60:291, 2003
124. Boyajian RA, Otis SM, Tyner JJ, DeLaria GA: Study design validation for consolidating global with focal neurological events in cardiac surgery stroke risk factor analyses. Eur J Neurol 10:71, 2003
125. Browne SM, Halligan PW, Wade DT, Taggart DP: Postoperative hypoxia is a contributory factor to cognitive impairment after cardiac surgery. J Thorac Cardiovasc Surg 126:1061, 2003
126. Koga M, Shimokawa S, Moriyama Y, et al: Watershed infarction after combined coronary and axillobifemoral bypass surgery. Jpn J Thorac Cardiovasc Surg 48:258, 2000
127. Caplan LR, Hennerici M: Impaired clearance of emboli (washout) is an important link between hypoperfusion, embolism, and ischemic stroke. Arch Neurol 5511:1475, 1998
128. Shann KG, Likosky DS, Murkin JM, et al: An evidenced-based review of the practice of cardiopulmonary bypass in adults. J Thorac Cardiovasc Surg 2006. In press
129. Bolsin SN: Detection of neurological damage during cardiopulmonary bypass. Anaesthesia 41:61, 1986
130. Levy WJ: Electroencephalographic evidence of cerebral ischemia during acute extracorporeal hypoperfusion. J Cardiothorac Anesth 1:300, 1987
131. Russ W, Kling D, Sauerwein G, Hempelmann G: Spectral analysis of the EEG during hypothermic cardiopulmonary bypass. Acta Anaesthesiol Scand 31:111, 1987
132. Edmonds HL Jr, Griffiths LK, Slater AD, Shields CB: Quantitative electroencephalographic monitoring during myocardial revascularization predicts postoperative disorientation and improves outcome. J Thorac Cardiovasc Surg 103:555, 1992
133. Murkin JM, Farrar JK, Tweed WA, et al: Cerebral autoregulation and flow/metabolism coupling during cardiopulmonary bypass: The influence of $PaCO_2$. Anesth Analg 66:825, 1987
134. Govier AV, Reves JG, McKay RD, et al: Factors and their influence on regional cerebral blood flow during nonpulsatile cardiopulmonary bypass. Ann Thorac Surg 38:592, 1984
135. Prough DS, Stump DA, Roy RC, et al: Response of cerebral blood flow to changes in carbon dioxide tension during hypothermic cardiopulmonary bypass. Anesthesiology 64:576, 1986
136. Gold JP, Charlson ME, Williams-Russo P, et al: Improvement of outcomes after coronary artery bypass. A randomized trial comparing intraoperative high versus low mean arterial pressure. J Thorac Cardiovasc Surg 110:1302, 1995
137. Lundar T, Froysaker T, Lindegaard KF, et al: Some observations on cerebral perfusion during cardiopulmonary bypass. Ann Thorac Surg 39:318, 1985
138. Avraamides EJ: The effect of surgical dislocation of the heart on cerebral blood flow in the presence of a single, two-stage venous cannula during cardiopulmonary bypass. Can J Anaesth 43:A36, 1996
139. Russell RW, Bharucha N: The recognition and prevention of border zone cerebral ischaemia during cardiac surgery. Q J Med 47187:303, 1978
140. Newman MF, Kramer D, Croughwell ND, et al: Differential age effects of mean arterial pressure and rewarming on cognitive dysfunction after cardiac surgery. Anesth Analg 81:236, 1995
141. Ganushchak YM, Fransen EJ, Visser C, et al: Neurological complications after coronary artery bypass grafting related to the performance of cardiopulmonary bypass. Chest 125:2196, 2004
142. Ura M, Sakata R, Nakayama Y, Goto T: Ultrasonographic demonstration of manipulation-related aortic injuries after cardiac surgery. J Am Coll Cardiol 35:1303, 2000
143. Sylivris S, Levi C, Matalanis G, et al: Pattern and significance of cerebral microemboli during coronary artery bypass grafting. Ann Thorac Surg 66:1674, 1998
144. Eckmann DM, Armstead SC, Mardini F: Surfactants reduce platelet-bubble and platelet-platelet binding induced by in vitro air embolism. Anesthesiology 103:1204, 2005
145. Persson LI, Johansson BB, Hansson HA: Ultrastructural studies on blood-brain barrier dysfunction after cerebral air embolism in the rat. Acta Neuropathol (Berl) 1344:53, 1978
146. Philp RB, Inwood MJ, Warren BA: Interactions between gas bubbles and components of the blood: implications in decompression sickness. Aerospace Med 43:946, 1972
147. Warren BA, Philp RB, Inwood MJ: The ultrastructural morphology of air embolism: Platelet adhesion to the interface and endothelial damage. Br J Exp Pathol 54:163, 1973
148. Helps SC, Parsons DW, Reilly PL, Gorman DF: The effect of gas emboli on rabbit cerebral blood flow. Stroke 21:94, 1990
149. Haller C, Sercombe R, Verrecchia C, et al: Effect of the muscarinic agonist carbachol on pial arteries in vivo after endothelial damage by air embolism. J Cereb Blood Flow Metab 7:605, 1987
150. Mangano CM: Scuds, scads, and other air-borne hazards. Anesthesiology 87:476, 1997
151. Mitchell S, Gorman D: The pathophysiology of cerebral arterial gas embolism. J Extracorp Technol 34:18, 2002
152. Moody DM, Brown WR, Challa VR, et al: Brain microemboli associated with cardiopulmonary bypass: A histologic and magnetic resonance imaging study. Ann Thorac Surg 59:1304, 1995
153. Challa VR, Lovell MA, Moody DM, et al: Laser microprobe mass spectrometric study of aluminum and silicon in brain emboli related to cardiac surgery. J Neuropathol Exp Neurol 57:140, 1998
154. Kincaid EH, Jones TJ, Stump DA, et al: Processing scavenged blood with a cell saver reduces cerebral lipid microembolization. Ann Thorac Surg 70:1296, 2000
155. Wollman H, Stephen GW, Clement AJ, Danielson GK: Cerebral blood flow in man during extracorporeal circulation. J Thorac Cardiovasc Surg 52:558, 1966
156. Kubota Y: Clinical study of the cerebral hemodynamics during extracorporeal circulation. Nagoya J Med Sci 31:117, 1968
157. Branthwaite MA: Cerebral blood flow and metabolism during open-heart surgery. Thorax 29:633, 1974
158. Henriksen L, Hjelms E, Lindeburgh T: Brain hyperperfusion during cardiac operations. Cerebral blood flow measured in man by intra-arterial injection of xenon 133: Evidence suggestive of intraoperative microembolism. J Thorac Cardiovasc Surg 86:202, 1983
159. Taylor KM: Brain damage during cardiopulmonary bypass. Ann Thorac Surg 654(suppl):S20, 1998
160. Busto R, Dietrich WD, Globus MY, et al: The importance of brain temperature in cerebral ischemic injury. Stroke 20:1113, 1989
161. Buchan A, Pulsinelli W: Hypothermia but not the N-methyl-D-aspartate antagonist, MK801, attenuates neuronal damage in gerbils subjected to transient global ischemia. J Neurosci 10:311, 1990
162. Chopp M, Knight R, Tidwell CD, et al: The metabolic effects of mild hypothermia on global cerebral ischemia and recirculation in the cat: Comparison to normothermia and hyperthermia. J Cereb Blood Flow Metab 9:141, 1989
163. Nemoto EM, Klementavicius R, Melick JA, Yonas H: Suppression of cerebral metabolic rate for oxygen CMRO(2) by mild hypothermia compared with thiopental. J Neurosurg Anesthesiol 8:52, 1996
164. Mora CT, Henson MB, Weintraub WS, et al: The effect of temperature management during cardiopulmonary bypass on neurologic and neuropsychological outcomes in patients undergoing coronary revascularization. J Thorac Cardiovasc Surg 112:514, 1996
165. Murkin JM: Hypothermic cardiopulmonary bypass—Time for a more temperate approach. Can J Anaesth 42:663, 1995
166. Nathan HJ, Wells GA, Munson JL, Wozny D: Neuroprotective effect of mild hypothermia in patients undergoing coronary artery surgery with cardiopulmonary bypass: a randomized trial. Circulation 18(suppl I):I-85, 2001
167. Engelman RM, Pleet AB, Hicks R, et al: Is there a relationship between systemic perfusion temperature during coronary artery bypass grafting and extent of intraoperative ischemic central nervous system injury? J Thorac Cardiovasc Surg 119:230, 2000
168. Dworschak M, Lassnigg A, Tenze G, et al: Perfusion temperature during cardiopulmonary bypass does not affect serum S-100beta release. Thorac Cardiovasc Surg 52:29, 2004
169. Grimm M, Czerny M, Baumer H, et al: Normothermic cardiopulmonary bypass is beneficial for cognitive brain function after coronary artery bypass grafting—A prospective randomized trial. Eur J Cardiothorac Surg 18:270, 2000
170. Arrowsmith JE, Dunning JL: Normothermic cardiopulmonary bypass is beneficial for cognitive brain function after coronary artery bypass graft-

ing—A prospective randomized trial. Eur J Cardiothorac Surg 19:732, 2001
171. Engelman R, Pleet AB: Cardiopulmonary bypass temperature and extension of intraoperative brain damage: Controversies persist. J Thorac Cardiovasc Surg 120:1014, 2000
172. Gaudino M, Possati G: Cardiopulmonary bypass temperature and extension of intraoperative brain damage: Controversies persist. J Thorac Cardiovasc Surg 120:1013, 2000
173. Taylor KM: Brain damage during cardiopulmonary bypass. Ann Thorac Surg 654(suppl):S20, 1998
174. Grocott HP, Mackensen GB, Grigore AM, et al: Postoperative hyperthermia is associated with cognitive dysfunction after coronary artery bypass graft surgery. Stroke 33:537, 2002
175. Scheffer T, Sanders DB: The neurologic sequelae of cardiopulmonary bypass-induced cerebral hyperthermia and cerebroprotective strategies. J Extracorp Technol 35:317, 2003
176. Kawahara F, Kadoi Y, Saito S, et al: Slow rewarming improves jugular venous oxygen saturation during rewarming. Acta Anaesthesiol Scand 47:419, 2003
177. Okano N, Owada R, Fujita N, et al: Cerebral oxygenation is better during mild hypothermic than normothermic cardiopulmonary bypass. Can J Anaesth 47:131, 2000
178. Gravlee GP, Roy RC, Stump DA, et al: Regional cerebrovascular reactivity to carbon dioxide during cardiopulmonary bypass in patients with cerebrovascular disease. J Thorac Cardiovasc Surg 99:1022, 1990
179. von Reutern GM, Hetzel A, Birnbaum D, Schlosser V: Transcranial Doppler ultrasonography during cardiopulmonary bypass in patients with severe carotid stenosis or occlusion. Stroke 19:674, 1988
180. Brusino FG, Reves JG, Prough DS, Stump DA: Cerebral blood flow during cardiopulmonary bypass in a patient with occlusive cerebrovascular disease. J Cardiothorac Anesth 3:87, 1989
181. Berens ES, Kouchoukos NT, Murphy SF, Wareing TH: Preoperative carotid artery screening in elderly patients undergoing cardiac surgery. J Vasc Surg 15:313, 1992
182. Schwartz LB, Bridgman AH, Kieffer RW, et al: Asymptomatic carotid artery stenosis and stroke in patients undergoing cardiopulmonary bypass. J Vasc Surg 21:146, 1995
183. Salasidis GC, Latter DA, Steinmetz OK, et al: Carotid artery duplex scanning in preoperative assessment for coronary artery revascularization: The association between peripheral vascular disease, carotid artery stenosis, and stroke. J Vasc Surg 21:154, 1995
184. Palerme LP, Hill AB, Obrand D, Steinmetz OK: Is Canadian cardiac surgeons' management of asymptomatic carotid artery stenosis at coronary artery bypass supported by the literature? A survey and a critical appraisal of the literature. Can J Surg 43:93, 2000
185. Naylor AR: A critical review of the role of carotid disease and the outcomes of staged and synchronous carotid surgery. Semin Cardiothorac Vasc Anesth 8:37, 2004
186. Furnary AP, Gao G, Grunkemeier GL, et al: Continuous insulin infusion reduces mortality in patients with diabetes undergoing coronary artery bypass grafting. J Thorac Cardiovasc Surg 125:1007, 2003
187. Latham R, Lancaster AD, Covington JF, et al: The association of diabetes and glucose control with surgical-site infections among cardiothoracic surgery patients. Infect Control Hosp Epidemiol 2210:607, 2001
188. Coursin DB, Prielipp RC: The new anesthesia diet plan: Keeping perioperative carbs in check. Anesth Analg 99:316, 2004
189. Carvalho G, Moore A, Qizilbash B, et al: Maintenance of normoglycemia during cardiac surgery. Anesth Analg 99:319, 2004
190. Jessen ME: Glucose control during cardiac surgery: How sweet it is. J Thorac Cardiovasc Surg 125:985, 2003
191. Bucerius J, Gummert JF, Walther T, et al: Impact of diabetes mellitus on cardiac surgery outcome. Thorac Cardiovasc Surg 51:11, 2003
192. Mortasawi A, Arnrich B, Rosendahl U, et al: Is age an independent determinant of mortality in cardiac surgery as suggested by the EuroSCORE? BMC Surg 72:8, 2002
193. Kadoi Y, Saito S, Yoshikawa D, et al: Increasing mean arterial blood pressure has no effect on jugular venous oxygen saturation in insulin-dependent patients during tepid cardiopulmonary bypass. Anesth Analg 95:266, 2002
194. Murkin JM: Pro: Tight intraoperative glucose control improves outcome in cardiovascular surgery. J Cardiothorac Vasc Anesth 14:475, 2000
195. McAlister FA, Man J, Bistritz L, et al: Diabetes and coronary artery bypass surgery: An examination of perioperative glycemic control and outcomes. Diabetes Care 26:1518, 2003
196. Blauth CI, Arnold JV, Schulenberg WE, et al: Cerebral microembolism during cardiopulmonary bypass. Retinal microvascular studies in vivo with fluorescein angiography. J Thorac Cardiovasc Surg 95:668, 1988
197. Padayachee TS, Parsons S, Theobold R, et al: The detection of microemboli in the middle cerebral artery during cardiopulmonary bypass: A transcranial Doppler ultrasound investigation using membrane and bubble oxygenators. Ann Thorac Surg 44:298, 1987
198. Padayachee TS, Parsons S, Theobold R, et al: The effect of arterial filtration on reduction of gaseous microemboli in the middle cerebral artery during cardiopulmonary bypass. Ann Thorac Surg 45:647, 1988
199. Williams IM, Stephens JF, Richardson EP Jr, et al: Brain and retinal microemboli during cardiac surgery. Ann Neurol 30:736, 1991
200. Georgiadis D, Hempel A, Baumgartner RW, Zerkowski HR: Doppler microembolic signals during cardiac surgery: Comparison between arterial line and middle cerebral artery. J Thorac Cardiovasc Surg 126:1638, 2003
201. Schoenburg M, Kraus B, Muehling A, et al: The dynamic air bubble trap reduces cerebral microembolism during cardiopulmonary bypass. J Thorac Cardiovasc Surg 126:1455, 2003
202. Edmunds LH Jr: Advances in the heart-lung machine after John and Mary Gibbon. Ann Thorac Surg 76:S2220, 2003
203. Haworth WS: The development of the modern oxygenator. Ann Thorac Surg 76:S2216, 2003
204. Whitaker DC, Stygall JA, Newman SP, Harrison MJ. The use of leukocyte-depleting and conventional arterial line filters in cardiac surgery: A systematic review of clinical studies. Perfusion 16:433, 2001
205. Jewell AE, Akowuah EF, Suvarna SK, et al: A prospective randomised comparison of cardiotomy suction and cell saver for recycling shed blood during cardiac surgery. Eur J Cardiothorac Surg 23:633, 2003
206. de Vries AJ, Gu YJ, Douglas YL, et al: Clinical evaluation of a new fat removal filter during cardiac surgery. Eur J Cardiothorac Surg 25:261, 2004
207. Marschall K, Kanchuger M, Kessler K, et al: Superiority of transesophageal echocardiography in detecting aortic arch atheromatous disease: Identification of patients at increased risk of stroke during cardiac surgery. J Cardiothorac Vasc Anesth 8:5, 1994
208. Hosoda Y, Watanabe M, Hirooka Y, et al: Significance of atherosclerotic changes of the ascending aorta during coronary bypass surgery with intraoperative detection by echography. J Cardiovasc Surg (Torino) 32:301, 1991
209. Van Boven WJ, Berry G: Intra-aortic filtration captures particulate debris in OPCAB cases using anastomotic devices. Heart Surg Forum 5(suppl 4):S461, 2002
210. Banbury MK, Kouchoukos NT, Allen KB, et al: Emboli capture using the Embol-X intraaortic filter in cardiac surgery: A multicentered randomized trial of 1,289 patients. Ann Thorac Surg 76:508, 2003
211. Reichenspurner H, Navia JA, Berry G, et al: Particulate emboli capture by an intra-aortic filter device during cardiac surgery. J Thorac Cardiovasc Surg 119:233, 2000
212. Murkin JM: Perioperative multimodality neuromonitoring: An overview. Semin Cardiothorac Vasc Anesth 8:167, 2004
213. Bar-Yosef S, Sanders EG, Grocott HP: Asymmetric cerebral near-infrared oximetric measurements during cardiac surgery. J Cardiothorac Vasc Anesth 17:773, 2003
214. Daubeney PE, Smith DC, Pilkington SN, et al: Cerebral oxygenation during paediatric cardiac surgery: Identification of vulnerable periods using near-infrared spectroscopy. Eur J Cardiothorac Surg 13:370, 1998
215. Austin EH, III, Edmonds HL Jr, Auden SM, et al: Benefit of neurophysiologic monitoring for pediatric cardiac surgery. J Thorac Cardiovasc Surg 114:707, 1997
216. Chen CS, Leu BK, Liu K: Detection of cerebral desaturation during cardiopulmonary bypass by cerebral oximetry. Acta Anaesthesiol Sin 34:173, 1996
217. Goldman S: Optimizing intraoperative cerebral oxygen delivery using noninvasive cerebral oximetry decreases the incidence of stroke for cardiac surgical patients. Heart Surg Forum 7, 2004
218. Murkin JM, Adams SJ, Novick RJ, et al: Monitoring brain oxygen saturation during coronary bypass surgery: A randomized, prospective study. Anesth Analg 2006. In press
219. Borger MA, Djaiani G: Reduction of cerebral emboli during cardiac surgery: Influence of surgeon and perfusionist feedback. Heart Surg Forum 6:204, 2003
220. van Dkijk D, Moons KG, Keizer AM, et al: Association between early and three month cognitive outcome after off-pump and on-pump coronary bypass surgery. Heart 90:431, 2004
221. Novitzky D, Boswell BB: Total myocardial revascularization without cardiopulmonary bypass utilizing computer-processed monitoring to assess cerebral perfusion. Heart Surg Forum 3:198, 2000
222. Nussmeier NA, Arlund C, Slogoff S: Neuropsychiatric complications after cardiopulmonary bypass: cerebral protection by a barbiturate. Anesthesiology 64:165, 1986

223. Zaidan JR, Klochany A, Martin WM, et al: Effect of thiopental on neurologic outcome following coronary artery bypass grafting. Anesthesiology 74:406, 1991
224. Woodcock TE, Murkin JM, Farrar JK, et al: Pharmacologic EEG suppression during cardiopulmonary bypass: Cerebral hemodynamic and metabolic effects of thiopental or isoflurane during hypothermia and normothermia. Anesthesiology 67:218, 1987
225. Roach GW: Neurologic and neuropsychological function following cardiac valve surgery: Lack of a protective effect with burst suppression doses of propofol. Anesthesiology 1998
226. Legault C, Furberg CD, Wagenknecht LE, et al: Nimodipine neuroprotection in cardiac valve replacement: Report of an early terminated trial. Stroke 27:593, 1996
227. Amory DW, Grigore A, Amory JK, et al: Neuroprotection is associated with beta-adrenergic receptor antagonists during cardiac surgery: Evidence from 2,575 patients. J Cardiothorac Vasc Anesth 16:270, 2002
228. Landis RC, Asimakopoulos G, Poullis M, et al: The antithrombotic and antiinflammatory mechanisms of action of aprotinin. Ann Thorac Surg 72:2169, 2001
229. Mangano DT: Aspirin and mortality from coronary bypass surgery. N Engl J Med 2434:1309, 2002

Chapter 36

LONG-TERM COMPLICATIONS AND MANAGEMENT

Dean T. Giacobbe, MD • Michael J. Murray, MD, PhD

KEY POINTS

1. Cardiac surgical patients usually follow a fairly predictable postoperative course that involves physiologic derangements and treatments that are routine for cardiac anesthesiologists.
2. A small percentage of cardiac surgical patients have complicated postoperative courses and prolonged intensive care unit stays.
3. This small subset of patients dies primarily of noncardiac organ dysfunction.
4. The anesthesiologist/intensivist caring for this complex patient population must consider all organ systems when considering diagnosis and treatment.
5. Meticulous attention to detail and the application of recent evidence-based treatments will result in improved survival in this complicated group of patients.

In the modern era, the majority of cardiac surgical patients have brief stays in the intensive care unit (ICU) (<24 hours), and these stays follow a predictable pattern. During this time, most instability and morbidity are attributable to the cardiopulmonary organ systems, bleeding, hypothermia, and the emergence from anesthesia.[1] A small minority of patients, however, have prolonged ICU stays characterized by multisystem complications involving both the cardiac and noncardiac systems. This group of patients consumes a disproportionate number of ICU resources, generates enormous hospital costs, and ultimately has a much worse prognosis (both in-hospital and long term).[1-4] For example, Bashour and colleagues described a case series of 2618 cardiac surgical patients at one institution in 1993.[1] In their study, 5.4% of patients had an ICU length of stay (LOS) of longer than 10 days. In this prolonged LOS group, the in-hospital mortality was 33.1% (versus 1.5% in group with LOS <10 days). Of those with prolonged ICU LOS who survived to discharge, 46.8% died within 30 months.[1] Similarly, Williams and colleagues[2] described another single-institution case series of 1280 in 1998. In their cohort, only 3.8% of patients had ICU LOS of longer than 14 days. In this group, the hospital mortality was 25.8% (versus 5.3% in short LOS group), and only 62% of patients discharged were alive at 2 years. Welsby and colleagues[4] analyzed types of complications in a cohort of cardiac surgical patients with prolonged LOS and demonstrated that noncardiac complications are more deleterious than isolated cardiac complications.

These data highlight the fact that when caring for the unfortunate minority of cardiac surgical patients requiring prolonged stays in the ICU, a distinct shift in orientation of the health care providers must occur—from a "recovery room" mode, focusing primarily on the cardiovascular organ system, to a true intensive care mode, focusing on preventing and treating dysfunction in multiple organ systems. At the same time, the physician's decision to continue aggressive treatment must be tempered with a realistic view of the patient's prognosis and an assessment of the "cost" of that treatment to the patient, family, and society.

SEDATION IN THE INTENSIVE CARE UNIT

The major goals of sedation in the ICU are to provide anxiolysis and to improve the patient's perceptual experience during this physiologically and emotionally stressful period[5] (Box 36–1). Secondarily, sedation reduces the physiologic stress response and attendant cardiovascular work, may facilitate the maintenance of circadian rhythms, and lessens delirium and agitation.[6] These goals are distinct from those associated with analgesia, which are the alleviation of pain through non-pharmacologic and pharmacologic means, and to facilitate diagnostic and therapeutic procedures.[5] While sedation and analgesia are separate therapeutic goals usually provided by individual drugs, there is often synergism between anxiolytic and analgesic drugs, and some newer agents provide elements of both analgesia and anxiolysis, thus blurring the distinction in clinical practice (see Chapter 37).

In 1995, the Society of Critical Care Medicine (SCCM) published guidelines for sedation,[7] revised the guidelines in 2002,[8] and recently decided the guidelines do not require revision (personal communication, Michael J. Murray, MD, PhD, October, 2004). The guidelines emphasize the need for the goal-directed delivery of psychoactive medications. Goal-directed sedation is supported by an increasing body of literature that shows that daily interruption of sedation, intermittent sedation, and sedation protocols all reduce the

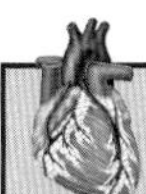

BOX 36–1 ***Sedation***

- Use specific agents targeted to therapeutic goals (e.g., sedatives for agitation; opioids for analgesia).
- Use goal-directed sedation therapy titrated to objective scoring system.
- Wean sedatives daily to assess the patient and re-evaluate need for sedation.

Table 36–1 Range of Sedation and Agitation for 138 Patient Assessments

Patient Category	SAS (%)	Ramsey (%)	Harris A (%)
Agitated	62 (45)	67 (49)	74 (54)
Calm	36 (26)	30 (22)	23 (17)
Sedated	40 (29)	41 (30)	41 (30)

SAS = Sedation-Agitation Scale.
Reprinted with permission from Riker RR, Picard JT, Fraser GL: Prospective evaluation of the Sedation-Agitation Scale for adult critically ill patients. Crit Care Med 27:1325, 1999.

Table 36–2 The Ramsey Sedation Scale

Awake levels	1 Patient anxious and agitated or restless or both 2 Patient cooperative, oriented and tranquil 3 Patient responds to commands only
Asleep levels	4 Brisk response to a light glabellar tap or loud auditory stimulus 5 Sluggish response to a light glabellar tap or loud auditory stimulus 6 No response to a light glabellar tap or loud auditory stimulus

Reprinted with permission from Young C, Knudsen N, Hilton A, Reves JG: Sedation in the intensive care unit. Crit Care Med 28:854, 2000.

duration of mechanical ventilation and in some instances decrease ICU LOS.[9-12]

There are several scoring systems available to assess a patient's degree of sedation in the ICU and facilitate goal-directed therapy (Table 36–1). The Riker Sedation-Agitation Scale (SAS) was the first scale proved to be reliable and valid in critically ill adults.[13] The SAS score is assigned by choosing a score from a seven-item scale that best matches a patient's behavior. Another scale, the Motor Activity Assessment Scale (MAAS), has seven categories to describe patients' behavior in response to stimulation. Like the SAS, it has been validated in critically ill adults.[14] Most comparative clinical studies of sedation in critically ill patients have used the Ramsey scale.[15] This scale is a six-point scale of motor activity that ranges from 1 ("patient anxious, agitated or restless, or both") to 6 ("no response to light glabellar tap or loud auditory stimulus")[6] (Table 36–2). This scale was originally designed as a research tool but has been used for decades in clinical practice.[16] While no scientific consensus exists about which level of sedation using the Ramsey scale is optimal, recent literature frequently cites sedation goals of Ramsey 2 to 4, reflecting more realistic levels of sedation as part of goal-directed therapy.[17] Other sedation scales that have been validated in critically ill adults include the Vancouver Interaction and Calmness Scale (VICS), the COMFORT Scale, and the Richmond Agitation-Sedation Scale (RASS).[16] The SCCM's guidelines do not advocate one specific scoring system. Instead, they advocate defining a specific sedation goal or end-point for each patient and then regularly assessing and documenting the patient's level of sedation in response to therapy.[8]

More objective parameters to assess sedation are being pursued. The Bispectral Index (BIS) is a monitor that measures a simple, three-lead, frontal montage electroencephalogram (EEG) and then through proprietary software converts the EEG activity to a digital scale from 1 to 100.[17] For specific agents such as midazolam, propofol, and, most recently, dexmedetomidine, the BIS may correlate with level of sedation in the ICU.[18-22]

Sedative Agents

Benzodiazepines

Many drugs are available for sedating patients in the cardiothoracic ICU. The most frequently used agents for sedation include benzodiazepines (midazolam, lorazepam), propofol, and the new α_2-agonist, dexmedetomidine. While there are multiple medications that can be used to allay anxiety, the traditional approach has been to use benzodiazepines. These drugs act by binding to benzodiazepine receptors (subunits of the $GABA_A$ [γ-aminobutyric acid] receptors, in the limbic area of the brain).[23] This binding enhances the effects of GABA in a dose-dependent fashion. Benzodiazepines can be titrated to effect; the effect ranging from light sedation to coma.[15] Side effects such as respiratory depression are also dose dependent and are more likely to appear in patients with comorbid conditions such as chronic obstructive pulmonary disease (COPD), at the extremes of age, and in patients receiving drugs with synergistic properties, such as opioids.

Midazolam is a short-acting benzodiazepine that can only be given parenterally. It is water soluble,[24] its intravenous administration causes no pain or venous irritation (and therefore thrombosis), and its potency is two to four times that of diazepam. Midazolam is readily redistributed in tissues and is rapidly cleared by the liver and kidneys. It is enzymatically degraded in the liver to alpha-hydroxy-midazolam, which has minimal, if any, clinical sedative or hypnotic effects. The clinical effects of midazolam are short lived due to an elimination half-life of 1.5 to 3.5 hours. These properties make midazolam ideal as an anxiolytic benzodiazepine for short-term use in the ICU.[25] Depending on the situation, intermittent boluses of midazolam can be given or a continuous infusion of 0.5 to 5.0 mg/hr can be used. Higher doses may be required, and infusions of up to 20 mg/hr have been safely used in mechanically ventilated patients.[26]

In patients whose condition deteriorates while in the ICU, such as the patient who develops sepsis or multiple organ dysfunction syndrome (MODS), midazolam elimination may be decreased, and its clinical effect prolonged.[27,28] This prolongation of effect may be due to the increased volume of distribution that occurs in patients with MODS whose renal clearance is decreased.

Lorazepam is a long-acting agent with sedative effects that last 6 to 8 hours following a single dose. Lorazepam has minimal effect on cardiovascular and respiratory function and can be given orally or parenterally.[29] Because its potency is two to four times that of midazolam, the dose must be adjusted accordingly. Due to its long half-life and despite the fact that its onset is considerably longer than that of midazolam, it is preferred to midazolam for patients requiring long-term sedation.[30] Because of different volumes of distribution, elimination half-lives, etc., especially in patients with MODS and in critically ill patients who require benzodiazepines for longer than 24 hours, lorazepam has a clinical half-life similar to midazolam.[31]

Diazepam, the most well-known benzodiazepine, can be given orally or intravenously. It is considered a long-acting benzodiazepine because of its prolonged elimination half-life (up to 50 hours with active metabolites that also have hypnotic effects). After an intravenous bolus, diazepam is rapidly redistributed in body tissues; therefore, its initial sedative effect quickly diminishes. However, drug clearance becomes dependent on hepatic metabolism when tissues become saturated during prolonged use. This saturation causes a prolongation of clinical effect even in patients with normal liver function. Because diazepam is not water soluble and because its diluent is ethyl alcohol, propylene glycol, and sodium benzoate, with a pH of 6.6, it is irritating to veins and frequently causes pain on administration. However, a new formulation of diazepam, in a lipid emulsion, should decrease this latter side effect.[32]

The usual dose of diazepam is 2 to 5 mg given by slow intravenous injection every 1 to 4 hours and is titrated to achieve the desired effect. Very high doses may be required in some patients, especially those with a history of ethanol abuse.

If a benzodiazepine is used to manage patients in the ICU, the antagonist of the benzodiazepines, flumazenil, should be readily available.[33] Flumazenil is a highly specific benzodiazepine antagonist that reverses all known central nervous system effects of the benzodiazepines. It reaches maximum concentration in the brain within 5 to 10 minutes after intravenous administration. The mean terminal half-life of flumazenil is approximately 1 hour. It is completely metabolized to free carboxylic acid and glucuronide, both of which are inactive metabolites and renally excreted.

Propofol

Propofol is an intravenous alkylphenol anesthetic agent that is chemically unrelated to other anesthetics.[34] It has been used to provide sedation for patients in ICUs and is the preferred drug for "fast tracking" patients. Because it is so hydrophobic, it is formulated in a lipid emulsion (10% Intralipid), which must be taken into account when it is administered to patients.[35] It is short-acting and rapidly redistributed and metabolized, making it very suitable for continuous infusion. Because of its rapid recovery and favorable side effect profile, it is an appealing drug not only to sedate patients, but for certain procedures, such as cardioversions, chest tube insertions or discontinuations, pleurodesis, etc.

Several studies have shown that propofol, compared with midazolam, allows for more rapid weaning of patients from mechanical ventilation, and it is because of this property that it is more commonly used for "fast tracking" cardiac surgical patients.[36] When used for sedation, an initial dose of 0.5 to 1.0 mg/kg should be used followed by an infusion of approximately 25 to 50 µg/kg/min. Because of case reports of mortality in patients who receive excessively high doses of propofol, the maximum dose should probably be 100 µg/kg/min.[37,38] This propofol infusion syndrome has been reported in patients who have received propofol for a very short period of time, indicating that this may be an idiosyncratic reaction.[39]

When given in bolus administration, propofol may cause a decrease in mean arterial pressure due to peripheral vasodilation and not to direct myocardial depression. There have been reports of death from metabolic acidosis in patients with neurologic/neurosurgical conditions and in children with upper respiratory tract infections.[37,38] Myoclonic activity versus frank seizures has been reported in patients receiving propofol,[40] and there are isolated case reports of patients becoming chemically dependent to propofol infusion.[41] These side effects, however, are rare (with the exception of the hypotension following bolus infusion) and should not limit the use of propofol in patients following cardiac surgical procedures, as it is particularly effective in those patients undergoing a "fast track" protocol. A limited number of studies specifically address sedation in patients following cardiac surgery. Most of the studies have compared midazolam with propofol and in general have shown no specific advantage of one agent over another.[42,43]

Dexmedetomidine

Herr and colleagues conducted a multicenter trial comparing dexmedetomidine and propofol for sedation following coronary artery bypass grafting (CABG).[44] In their trial, there was no significant difference in time to extubation between groups, but the dexmedetomidine patients had significantly reduced use of supplemental analgesics, antiemetics, epinephrine, and diuretics.

After examining the literature applying to all critical care patients, not just those following cardiac surgery, the SCCM's guidelines made the following recommendations (these recommendations predate the introduction of dexmedetomidine)[8]:

1. Midazolam or diazepam should be used for rapid sedation of acutely agitated patients.
2. Propofol is the preferred sedative when rapid awakening is important. Triglyceride concentrations should be monitored after 2 days of propofol infusion, and total caloric intake from lipids should be included in the nutritional assessment.
3. Midazolam is recommended for short-term use only as it produces unpredictable awakening and time to extubation when infusions continue longer than 48 to 72 hours.
4. Lorazepam is recommended for the sedation of most patients via either intermittent intravenous administration or continuous infusion.
5. Dexmedetomidine can be used for chemically dependent patients and for patients who have failed any of the above, but should not be used for longer than 24 to 48 hours, as there is a high incidence of withdrawal-hypertensive crisis if dexmedetomidine is used for longer than 48 hours and abruptly discontinued.

Neuromuscular Blocking Agents

Occasionally, some patients are so critically ill that they cannot be adequately sedated to receive appropriate care. This most commonly happens in an agitated patient requiring mechanical ventilation in whom the level of sedation would mimic a general anesthetic and whose hemodynamic status does not tolerate this degree of deep sedation. In these circumstances, neuromuscular blocking agents (NMBAs) are used.

An NMBA is a drug that binds the nicotinic acetylcholine receptor (nAChR) on the muscle membrane, thus inhibiting the receptor from binding to two molecules of acetylcholine, which would open the sodium channel, allowing the influx of sodium and other electrolytes with activation of actin and myosin and muscle contraction. There are two classes of NMBAs—polarizing and nondepolarizing. Succinylcholine is a classic depolarizing NMBA, which structurally resembles acetylcholine, and when it binds to the nAChR, results in depolarization of the membrane and a muscle fasciculation.

Table 36–3 **Selected Neuromuscular Blocking Agents* for Intensive Care Unit Use**

	Benzylisoquinolinium		
Variable	**Cisatracurium (Nimbex)**	**Atracurium (Tracrium)**	**Doxacurium (Nuromax)**
Introduced (yr)	1995	1983	1991
ED_{95} dose (mg/kg)	0.05	0.25	0.025 to 0.03
Initial dose (mg/kg)	0.1 to 0.2	0.4 to 0.5	0.025 to 0.05
Duration (min)	45 to 60	25 to 35	120 to 150
Infusion described	Yes	Yes	Yes
Infusion dose (μg/kg/min)	2.5 to 3.0	4 to 12	0.3 to 0.5
Recovery (min)	90	40 to 60	120 to 180
% Renal excretion	Hofmann elimination	5 to 10 (uses Hofmann elimination)	70
Renal failure	No change	No change	Increased duration
% Biliary excretion	Hofmann elimination	Minimal (uses Hofmann elimination)	Insufficient data
Hepatic failure	Minimal to no change	Minimal to no change	—
Active metabolites	No	No, but can accumulate laudanosine	—
Histamine release hypotension	No	Minimal but dose-dependent	No
Vagal block tachycardia	No	No	No
Ganglionic blockade hypotension	No	Minimal to none	No
Prolonged ICU block	Rare	Rare	Insufficient data

*Drugs for use in a 70-kg man.
ED_{95} = effective dose for 95% of patients studied.
Modified with permission from Prielipp RC, Coursin DB: Applied pharmacology of common neuromuscular blocking agents in critical care. New Horizons 2:34, 1994.

Depolarizing NMBAs are rarely used outside the operating room.

Nondepolarizing NMBAs are divided into two classes of medications—benzylisoquinolinium compounds and the aminosteroidal compounds. Both classes of drugs can be used to chemically paralyze a patient in the ICU. Occasionally this is done to intubate a patient's trachea who has developed acute respiratory failure[45] (Table 36–3). The majority of patients in the ICU receiving NMBAs are on mechanical ventilation, typically patients with acute lung injury or acute respiratory distress syndrome (ARDS) in whom mechanical ventilation cannot be appropriately managed without the use of an NMBA.[46]

If these medications are used, it cannot be overemphasized that the patient must be adequately sedated prior to the initiation of the NMBA—it has been several decades since reports appeared of chemically paralyzed awake patients,[47] but it is a situation that all individuals working in an ICU must strive to avoid. Once an adequate degree of sedation (usually to include an analgesic medication such as an opioid) is achieved, the patient is administered a bolus and then a continuous infusion of an NMBA. Although there are several drugs available, the drugs most commonly used in the ICU are the aminosteroidal compounds (pancuronium, vecuronium, and rocuronium) and the benzylisoquinolinium compounds (doxacurium, atracurium, and cisatracurium). Pancuronium and doxacurium are long-acting NMBAs, whereas rocuronium and vecuronium are intermediate-duration medications, and atracurium and cisatracurium are short-acting medications, at least when given by bolus. Because these drugs are infused continuously, this attribute is not as important, but it does become important when the medication is discontinued and the physician is assessing the return of the patient's neuromuscular function. When infusing these medications, a twitch monitor should be used, and the physician should strive to achieve a train-of-four of one or two twitches.[48] If there are no twitches observed, then the patient may be overdosed and may be at risk for development of acute quadriplegic myopathy syndrome (AQMS), a situation that develops in patients receiving NMBAs in which, when the medication is discontinued, the patient remains flaccid for much longer than would be predicted simply based on pharmacokinetics of the medications that were infused.[49] The etiology of this syndrome is unknown but is most likely secondary to the destruction of myosin by the NMBA or one of its metabolites. Often-times, it is difficult to differentiate between AQMS and critical illness polyneuropathy, but in the latter, profound muscle necrosis as is seen with AQMS would not be expected to occur.

Another way to minimize the likelihood of this syndrome is to institute a daily drug holiday. Not only is this beneficial in decreasing the incidence of AQMS, but in patients receiving opioids and benzodiazepines, the incidence of drug withdrawal also decreases with the discontinuation of the medication. When using NMBAs in the ICU, the algorithm as listed in Figure 36–1 is recommended.[48]

INFECTIONS IN THE INTENSIVE CARE UNIT

Microbiologic infections are some of the most common and frequently serious secondary complications that plague patients in the ICU.[50] The following is a brief review of the

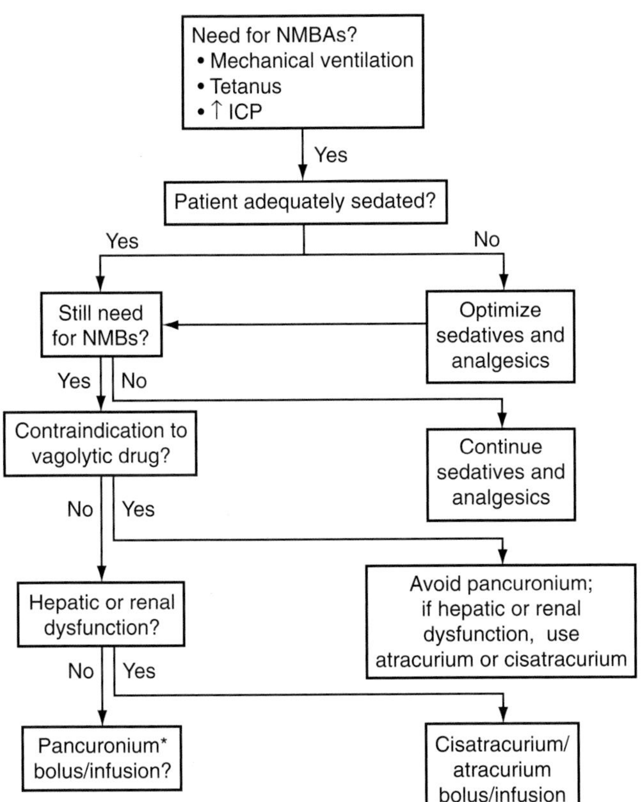

Figure 36–1 Use of neuromuscular blocking agents (NMBAs) in the intensive care unit. Monitor train-of-four ratio, protect eyes, position patient to protect pressure points, and address deep venous thrombosis prophylaxis. Reassess every 12 to 24 hours for continued NMBA indication. ICP = intracranial pressure. (Redrawn from Murray MJ, Cowen J, DeBlock H, et al: Clinical practice guidelines for sustained neuromuscular blockade in the adult critically ill patient. Crit Care Med 30:142, 2002.)

most frequent infectious complications occurring in critically ill, cardiothoracic surgical patients (pneumonia and ARDS are reviewed in Chapter 34).

Intravascular Device–Related Infections

Virtually all adult patients having cardiac surgery are monitored with invasive intravascular devices (IVDs) such as arterial, central venous, and pulmonary artery catheters (see Chapter 14). Unfortunately, these IVDs are frequently associated with bloodstream infections (BSIs). IVD-related BSIs are associated with an attributable mortality of 12% to 15%, prolonged hospitalization (mean of 7 days), and increased hospital cost of approximately $35,000.[51,52]

Approximately 90% of all vascular catheter–related BSIs occur with use of short-term central venous catheters (CVCs).[53] CVCs that are present for a short term are most commonly colonized from the skin surrounding the insertion site.[54,55] Organisms migrate along the external surface of the catheter and then the intercutaneous and subcutaneous segments, leading to colonization of the intravascular segment.[56] Once colonized, it is difficult to eradicate organisms from the intravascular segment without catheter removal because the microbes adhere to and are covered by either a biofilm layer they produce or the thrombin layer the host forms on the device.[57] Because the skin is the most common site of colonization, coagulase-negative staphylococci and *Staphylococcus aureus* from the host's skin and the hands of hospital personnel caring for the patient are the most common infecting pathogens.[58] However, with long-term catheters, contamination of the catheter hub also contributes to intraluminal colonization.[56]

Several factors have been associated with a risk of CVC-related bacteremia. These include site of insertion (femoral > internal jugular > subclavian), number of lumens (multiple > single), duration of catheter in situ, established infection elsewhere in body, bacteremia, and experience of personnel placing the catheter.

In an effort to reduce IVD-related BSIs, a Centers for Disease Control and Prevention advisory committee has formulated evidence-based guidelines pertaining to the prevention of IVD-related BSIs. These guidelines can be summarized as follows[51] (Box 36–2):

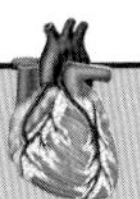

BOX 36–2 *Central Catheter Management*

- Central catheters should only be placed by practitioners with documented competency.
- Place under maximal sterile barrier precautions.
  - 2% Chlorhexidine is skin preparation of choice.
  - Use chlorhexidine-impregnated sponge dressings.
  - Use antibiotic-impregnated catheters in high-risk patients.
- Do not "routinely" replace catheters.
- Remove as soon as clinically feasible.

1. CVCs should be placed by designated individuals with documented competence in insertion. Provide adequate supervision of those learning central vascular access.
2. Use maximal sterile barrier precautions when inserting catheters (gowns, sterile gloves, mask, maximal draping).
3. Two percent chlorhexidine is the agent of choice to prevent bacterial colonization of catheters and BSI (alcohol tinctures of iodine, 10% povidone-iodine combination, and alcohol alone are acceptable but secondary).
4. Chlorhexidine-impregnated sponge dressings are associated with 60% reduction in IVD-related BSI.
5. Sulfadizine- and chlorhexidine- or minocycline-rifampin–impregnated catheters are associated with a reduction in BSI in short-term CVCs. There is no evidence of an increase in bacterial resistance in studies to date. Guidelines recommend using these catheters in high-risk patients if institutional IVD-related BSI rates are unacceptable after instituting other prevention strategies (Box 36–3).

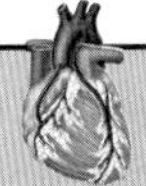

BOX 36–3 *Latent Sources of Infection in the Cardiothoracic Intensive Care Unit*

- Intravascular device-related bloodstream infections
- Sternal wound infections
- Prosthetic valve endocarditis
- Sepsis
- Urinary tract infection
- *C. difficile* enterocolitis
- Sinusitis

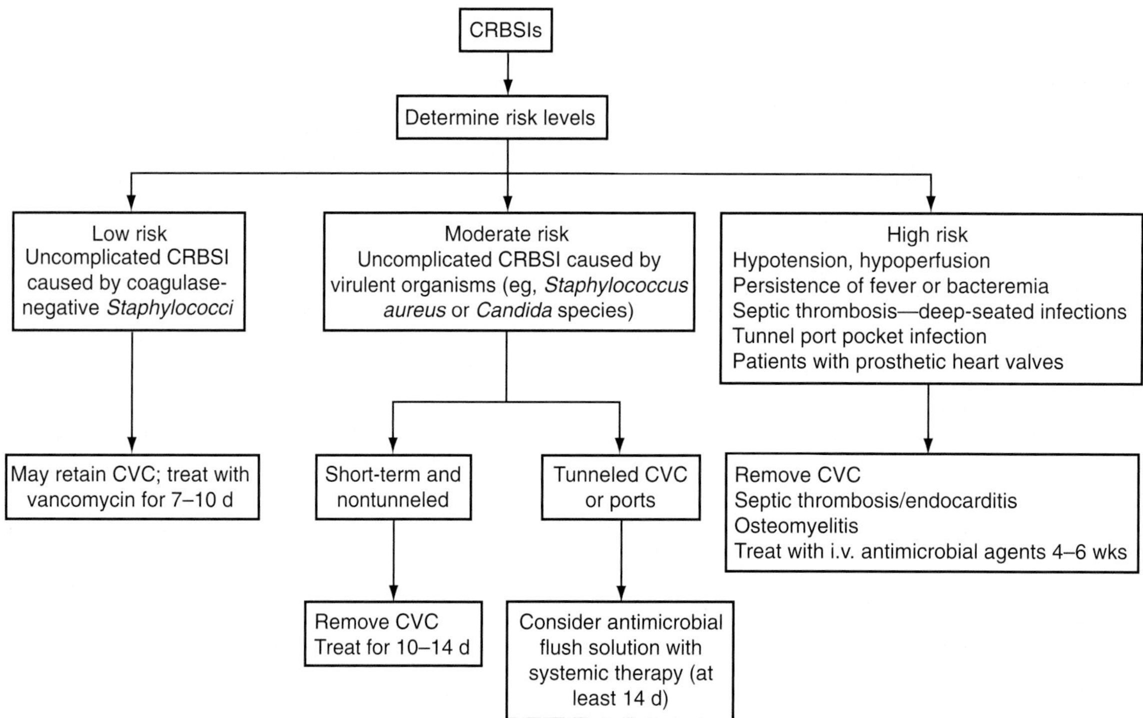

Figure 36–2 Algorithm for the management of catheter-related bloodstream infections (CRBSIs). A prelude to appropriate management involves confirming the diagnosis of a CRBSI through simultaneous blood cultures (5:1 of colony-forming units from blood cultures drawn through the catheter compared with the peripheral vein or differential time to positivity of 2 hours) or colonization of the catheter demonstrated through semiquantitative or quantitative catheter cultures with the same organism isolated from the peripheral blood culture. CVC = central venous catheter, i.v. = intravenous. (Redrawn from Raad II, Hanna HA: Intravascular catheter-related infections. New horizons and recent advances. Arch Intern Med 162:871, 2002.)

6. Do not routinely replace CVCs to prevent infection.
7. Change gauze dressings every 2 days and transparent dressings every 7 days. Replace sooner if the dressing becomes soiled or contaminated or a site inspection is required.
8. No advice is given on sutureless securement devices.
9. Catheters do not need to be replaced in bacteremic or febrile patients if the catheter is not suspected as the source of infection.
10. If there is evidence of an exit site infection or if the patient is bacteremic with a suspected CVC BSI, the catheter should be removed and placed at a new site. Changing catheters over a wire is not recommended.

The diagnosis of central catheter infection can be challenging. The diagnosis should be suspected in patients with evidence of infection (fever, leukocytosis, positive blood cultures, etc.) when another source is not evident. Careful inspection of the catheter site is warranted, as exit site erythema or purulence strongly supports the diagnosis. If there are no visible signs of infection, then clinical suspicion and supporting data must be used to guide therapy. The most commonly used technique to culture CVCs is the semiquantitative roll-plate technique. With this technique, the most common threshold to define colonization is the growth of a colony count greater than 15.[57,59] A meta-analysis by Siegman-Igra and colleagues[58] showed that quantitative culture of sonicated catheters is superior to the roll-plate technique. However, because both of these techniques require catheter removal, novel techniques for in vivo catheter culture are being investigated.[57] These include the following:

- Simultaneously collecting quantitative blood cultures from both the catheter and a peripheral site, with a positive result showing a 5-fold greater number of organisms from the catheter culture
- Simultaneously collecting qualitative cultures from the catheter and a peripheral source, with a positive response showing growth two hours earlier in the catheter culture
- Culture from an endoluminal brushing of the catheter and staining with an acridine orange leukocyte cytospin test

The first clinical decision to make when managing a suspected CVC-related BSI is whether to remove the catheter. This decision is influenced by whether the risk of CVC-related BSI is low, intermediate, or high. Risk, in turn, is determined by the infecting organism and whether the CVC-related BSI is complicated or uncomplicated. Complicated infections are those associated with shock, persistence of positive blood cultures for longer than 48 hours after appropriate antibiotics, CVC-related BSIs associated with septic thrombosis, septic emboli, or deep-seated infections (e.g., endocarditis), or a tunnel or port-pocket infection[56] (Fig. 36–2).

- A low-risk CVC-related BSI is caused by organisms of low virulence (e.g., coagulase-negative *staphylococci*) that are uncomplicated.
- A moderate-risk CVC-related BSI is characterized by uncomplicated infections with moderate to highly virulent organisms (*S. aureus*, *Candida* species).
- High risk is a complicated CVC-related BSI.

Low-risk CVC-related BSIs can be treated without catheter removal.[60,61] However, catheters should be removed in low-risk patients with prosthetic heart valves. In intermediate-risk patients, the catheters should be removed and the patients treated with a 10- to 14-day course of antibiotics. In high-risk patients, catheters should be removed and duration of antibiotic use based upon the nature of the complication. In deep-seated infections such as septic thrombosis or endocarditis, antimicrobials should be administered for 4 to 6 weeks.[62]

Sternal Wound Infections

Deep and superficial surgical site infections are infrequent but morbid complications following cardiac surgery, with an incidence of approximately 1% to 4%.[63] Deep sternal infections are defined as those infections involving muscle and fascial layers or any other organ spaces manipulated during the operation or organ involvement.[64] They are associated with a 250% higher mortality than for matched individuals without infection, and postoperative wound infections double the length of hospitalization.[65] A host of preoperative, intraoperative, and postoperative risk factors have been identified for chest wall infections. These include the following[62-64,66-68]:

- *Host factors:* obesity, diabetes mellitus, hyperglycemia, use of internal mammary artery grafts (especially bilateral), advanced age, male gender, COPD, smoking, prolonged mechanical ventilation, steroids, preoperative hospital stay longer than 5 days
- *Surgical factors:* duration of surgery and bypass, use of intra-aortic balloon pump, postoperative bleeding, reoperation, sternal rewiring, extensive electrocautery, shaving with razors, and use of bone wax
- *Postoperative factors:* postoperative bleeding, prolonged ventilation, chest reexploration, blood transfusion, and use of intra-aortic balloon pump

The diagnosis of sternal infections is based on wound tenderness, drainage, cellulitis, fever, leukocytosis, and sternal instability.[66] *S. aureus* and coagulase-negative staphylococci account for approximately 50% of the organisms associated with post-CABG sternal wound infections.[64] Several preventive strategies have been proposed to reduce cardiac surgical site infection rates. Martorell and colleagues[69] reported a reduction in chest wall infections from greater than 8% to less than 2% following an intensive surveillance and intervention program that included nasal mupirocin and preoperative chlorhexidine showering. Other variables that are being investigated to reduce infection rates include perioperative antibiotics, adequacy of glycemic control, perioperative temperature control, and conservative transfusion protocols.[70] The treatment of mediastinitis involves the prompt institution of antibiotics (empirically cover *staphylococci* species prior to culture results), debridement, open packing, and frequent dressing changes. Upon resolution, the chest is closed by primary closure or flap transposition in cases with large chest wall defects.[66]

Prosthetic Valve Endocarditis

Prosthetic valve endocarditis (PVE), the infection of a prosthetic heart valve and/or the surrounding cardiac tissues, is a rare but serious source of infection in postoperative cardiac surgical patients.[70] The incidence of PVE is between 0.3% and 0.8% following valve replacement surgery.[71-75] PVE cases can be clustered into two groups according to the time of infection. In early PVE (within 2 months of valve implantation), the valve and sewing ring have not yet endothelialized and hence microorganisms frequently invade the surrounding tissue planes, causing perivalvular abscess and perivalvular leak. In early PVE, the responsible micro-organisms are nosocomial pathogens such as staphylococci, gram-negative bacilli, and *Candida* species that are introduced at the time of surgery or are hematogenously seeded in the immediate postoperative period. The pathophysiology of late PVE probably resembles that of native valve endocarditis; that is, platelet-fibrin thrombi form on the valve leaflet and are then hematogenously seeded during episodes of transient bacteremia. In late PVE, the infecting organisms are usually streptococci, *S. aureus,* enterococci, and fastidious gram-negatives (the HACEK group).[76-80] Infection appears to occur with equal frequency in both the mitral and aortic position and is exceedingly rare in tricuspid prosthesis (excluding intravenous drug abusers).[71]

In the ICU, cases of early PVE present more dramatically than the often-subtle presentation of either native valve endocarditis or late PVE. The clinical signs that suggest PVE include new or changing murmurs, congestive heart failure, new electrocardiographic conduction disturbances, and systemic emboli. In fact, 40% of patients have clinically apparent central nervous system emboli.[81-84] The diagnosis is confirmed by positive blood cultures and transesophageal echocardiography (TEE). If blood cultures are obtained prior to antibiotic therapy, more than 90% will be positive. TEE is the diagnostic imaging modality of choice because it has a sensitivity of 82% to 96% versus 17% to 36% with transthoracic echocardiography.[85-87] TEE also allows the detection of abscesses, fistulas, and perivalvular leaks.[88] The treatment of early PVE involves antibiotics directed at the cultured organism and prompt surgical intervention in cases of complicated PVE[89] (Table 36–4). In complicated PVE, survival is improved with both medical and surgical therapy versus with medical therapy alone.[83,90-93]

Table 36–4 Indications for Cardiac Surgery in Patients With Prosthetic Valve Endocarditis (PVE)

Moderate-to-severe congestive heart failure due to valve dysfunction (regurgitant or stenotic)
Unstable prosthesis
Paravalvular extension of infection
Uncontrolled infection (persistent bacteremia) on optimal antimicrobial therapy
PVE caused by selected microorganisms Fungi *Pseudomonas aeruginosa* *Staphylococcus aureus* Enterococci in the absence of bactericidal therapy Other gram-negative bacilli and microorganisms that usually require surgery when infecting native valves, e.g., *Brucella* spp., *Coxiella burnetii*
Relapse after optimal therapy
Large (>10-mm) hypermobile vegetations
Culture-negative PVE with unexplained persistent (≥10 days) fever

Reprinted with permission from Karchmur AW: Infections of prosthetic valves and intravascular devices. *In* Mandell GL, Bennett JE, Dolin R (eds): Principles and Practice of Infectious Disease, 5th edition, Vol 1. Philadelphia, Churchill Livingstone, 1999, pp 903–917.

Systemic Inflammatory Response Syndrome and Sepsis

Despite somewhat confusing nomenclature, systemic inflammatory response syndrome (SIRS) and sepsis are part of a spectrum of disorders that produce dysfunction in a variety of organ systems and arise from a combination of tissue injury and the host's response to that injury. In 1991, 1997, and 2001, a consensus statement was published by the American College of Chest Physicians, the SCCM, the European Society of Intensive Care Medicine, the American Thoracic Society, and the Surgical Infection Society to clarify the definitions used to describe this spectrum.[94] In 1991, the consensus statement introduced the now widely used term "SIRS" to describe a syndrome with multiple, clinically evident organ system effects (e.g., fever, oliguria, mental status changes) that occurred as the result of the body's inflammatory response activated by a variety of causes.[95] Historically it had been thought that infection, particularly gram-negative infection, was the sole source of this clinical phenomenon.[96,97] It is now accepted that any major tissue injury (burns, sterile pancreatitis, major trauma) can precipitate such a dramatic inflammatory response with or without the presence of infection.[96,97] However, in the most recent consensus statement, the authors acknowledge that while this syndrome exists, it is too broad and lacks the specificity to make it a useful, working "diagnosis" at the present time.[98]

Sepsis is defined as the clinical syndrome that occurs as the result of an infection (or suspected infection) and an inflammatory response[96,98] (Table 36–5). Severe sepsis is sepsis that is associated with organ dysfunction, hypoperfusion, or hypotension. Septic shock is sepsis-induced hypotension and organ perfusion abnormalities that persist despite fluid resuscitation.[95] A detailed description of the current understanding of the pathophysiology of SIRS and sepsis is beyond the scope of this chapter, and the reader is referred to reviews of this topic.[99,100]

Sepsis is the leading cause for admission to surgical ICUs and, despite recent advances in therapy, remains the leading cause of mortality in ICUs.[95,96,99] The mortality rate increases across the inflammatory spectrum from SIRS to septic shock[101] (Table 36–6).

Because of the unacceptably high mortality rate associated with sepsis and the inflammatory disorders, an international group of experts in sepsis convened in 2003 and launched the

Table 36–5 Diagnostic Criteria for Sepsis

Infection,* documented or suspected, and some of the following†:

General variables
- Fever (core temperature >38.3°C)
- Hypothermia (core temperature <36°C)
- Heart rate >90/min or >2 SDs above the normal value for age
- Tachypnea
- Altered mental status
- Significant edema or positive fluid balance (>20 mL/kg over 24 hr)
- Hyperglycemia (plasma glucose >120 mg/dL or 7.7 mmol/L) in the absence of diabetes

Inflammatory variables
- Leukocytosis (WBC count >12,000/μL)
- Leukopenia (WBC count <4000/μL)
- Normal WBC count with >10% immature forms
- Plasma C-reactive protein >2 SDs above the normal value
- Plasma procalcitonin >2 SDs above the normal value

Hemodynamic variables
- Arterial hypotension† (SBP <90 mm Hg, MAP <70, or an SBP decrease >40 mm Hg in adults or <2 SDs below normal for age)
- $S\bar{v}O_2$ >70%†
- Cardiac index >3.5 L/min/m^2

Organ dysfunction variables
- Arterial hypoxemia (PaO_2/FIO_2 <300)
- Acute oliguria (urine output <0.5 mL/kg/hr)
- Creatinine increase >0.5 mg/dL
- Coagulation abnormalities (INR >1.5 or aPTT >60 sec)
- Ileus (absent bowel sounds)
- Thrombocytopenia (platelet count <100,000/μL)
- Hyperbilirubinemia (plasma total bilirubin >4 mg/dL or 70 mmol/L)

Tissue perfusion variables
- Hyperlactatemia (>1 mmol/L)
- Decreased capillary refill or mottling

*Infection defined as a pathologic process induced by a microorganism.
†$S\bar{v}O_2$ saturation >70% is normal in children (normal, 75% to 80%), and CI 3.5 to 5.5 is normal in children.
WBC = white blood cell; SBP = systolic blood pressure; MAP = mean arterial blood pressure; $S\bar{v}O_2$ = mixed venous oxygen saturation; INR = international normalized ratio; aPTT = activated partial thromboplastin time.
Reprinted with permission from Levy MM, Fink MP, Marshall JC, et al: 2001 SCCM/ESICM/ACCP/ATS/SIS International Sepsis Definitions Conference. Crit Care Med 31:1250, 2001.

Table 36–6 Mortality of SIRS, Sepsis, Severe Sepsis, and Septic Shock

Reference	SIRS (%)	Sepsis (%)	Severe Sepsis (%)	Septic Shock (%)
Rangel-Frausto et al: JAMA 273:117–123, 1995	7	16	20	46
Pittet et al: Intensive Care Med 21:302–309, 1995	6	0	35	58
Salvo et al: Intensive Care Med 21:S244–S249, 1995	27	36	52	82
Saez-Llorens et al: Pediatr Infect Dis J 14:557–561, 1995	—	16	40	62
Jones et al: Q J Med 89:515–522, 1996	23	—	38	56
Muchart et al: Crit Care Med 25:1789–1795, 1997	8	10	18	53
Bossink et al: Chest 113:1533-1541, 1998	6	13	—	—

SIRS = systemic inflammatory response syndrome.
Reprinted with permission from Matot I, Sprung C: Definition of sepsis. Intensive Care Med 27:S3, 2001.

"surviving sepsis campaign" with the goal of producing treatment recommendations that could be used to reduce the mortality from sepsis.[102] These recommendations were formulated from an evidence-based review of the medical literature, and expert opinion when high-level evidence was absent. They reflect the current "state of the art" in the management of critically ill, septic patients. They can be summarized as follows:

1. Initial Resuscitation (first 6 hours)

Resuscitation should begin as soon as possible (do not delay for ICU admission). The goals of resuscitation should be the following:

- CVP 8 to 12 mm Hg (12 to 15 in mechanically ventilated patients, or if high abdominal pressure).
- MAP greater than 65 mm Hg.
- Urine output greater than 0.5 mL/kg/hr.
- Central venous or mixed venous oxygen saturation greater than 70%.
- If unable to increase central venous/mixed venous saturation above 70%, then transfuse to hematocrit greater than 30% and/or administer dobutamine (to maximum dose of 20 μg/kg/min) to achieve this goal.

2. Diagnosis
   - Appropriate cultures should always be obtained prior to initiating antibiotics.
   - At least two blood cultures—one from peripheral and one from each vascular access device.
   - Culture other sites as clinically indicated (cerebrospinal fluid, wounds, urine, respiratory secretions, other body fluids).
   - Diagnostic and imaging studies should be performed promptly to identify the source of infection.
3. Antibiotic Therapy
   - Intravenous antibiotic therapy should be started within the first hour of recognition of severe sepsis (after cultures).
   - Empiric antibiotics should include one with activity against the most likely pathogen and that can penetrate the likely source.
   - Empiric antibiotics should be broad spectrum until the causative organism is identified.
   - The antibiotic regimen should be reassessed after 48 to 72 hours on the basis of clinical and microbiological data. The goal is to use a narrow-spectrum antibiotic to limit toxicity, cost, and development of superinfection and microbial resistance.
   - Once the causative organism is identified, use monotherapy for 7 to 10 days (some experts prefer combination therapy for *Pseudomonas* infections).
   - Most experts use combination therapy for neutropenic patients and treat for the duration of neutropenia.
4. Source Control
   - Every patient should be evaluated for the presence of a focus of infection that is amenable to source control measures (drainage of abscess, removal of infected vascular access device, etc.).
   - Risks versus benefits of source control procedures must be weighed. Source control with the least physiologic insult is generally best (e.g., percutaneous rather than surgical drainage of abscess).
   - Source control measures should be instituted as soon as possible following initial resuscitation.
5. Fluid Therapy
   - Fluid challenge with crystalloids or colloids in cases of suspected hypovolemia.
   - Repeat boluses based on response (increase in blood pressure and urine output) and tolerance (evidence of intravascular volume overload).
   - No evidence to support preference of crystalloid or colloid.
6. Vasopressors
   - Following fluid resuscitation, a vasopressor should be started to restore blood pressure.
   - In life-threatening hypotension, a vasopressor and fluid resuscitation may need to be simultaneously started.
   - Dopamine and norepinephrine are the vasopressors of choice.
   - All patients requiring vasopressors should be monitored with an arterial catheter.
   - Vasopressin may be considered in hypotension refractory to conventional vasopressors.
7. Inotropic Therapy
   - In patients with low cardiac output despite fluid resuscitation, dobutamine is the agent of choice to increase cardiac output.
   - A vasopressor can be added to raise blood pressure, once cardiac output is normalized.
8. Steroids
   - Intravenous corticosteroids (hydrocortisone 200 to 300 mg/day for 7 days in three or four divided doses or by continuous infusion) can be used for patients with septic shock who require vasopressor therapy despite adequate fluid resuscitation.
   - Some experts recommend using a 250-μg adrenocorticotropic hormone (ACTH) stimulation test to identify responders (>9 μg/dL increase in cortisol after 30 to 60 minutes), and recommend only treating nonresponders.
   - Dose should not exceed 300 mg hydrocortisone daily.
   - Some experts add 50 μg of fludrocortisone orally (controversial because hydrocortisone has mineralocorticoid activity).
   - No evidence to recommend fixed-duration therapy over taper or clinically guided regimen.
9. Recombinant Human Activated Protein C (rhAPC)
   - rhAPC is recommended in patients with high risk of death (APACHE II score >25, sepsis-induced MODS, septic shock, or sepsis-induced ARDS) without any contraindications.
   - Contraindications:
     Active internal bleeding
     Recent (within 3 months) hemorrhagic stroke
     Recent (within 2 months) intracranial, intraspinal surgery or severe head trauma
     Trauma with increased risk of life-threatening bleeding
     Presence of epidural catheter
     Intracranial neoplasm, mass lesion, or cerebral herniation
10. Blood Product Administration
    - Once tissue hypoperfusion has resolved, red blood cell transfusion should only occur when hemoglobin decreases to less than 7.0 g/dL and to target a hemoglobin of 7.0 to 9.0 g/dL.

- Erythropoietin is not recommended to treat anemia of sepsis (may use if other coexisting conditions merit treatment with erythropoietin, e.g., renal failure).
- Fresh frozen plasma should not be administered to correct laboratory abnormalities in the absence of bleeding or planned invasive procedures.
- Antithrombin administration is not recommended to treat severe sepsis or septic shock.
- Platelet transfusion:
  Administer if counts less than $5000/mm^3$
  Consider when counts 5000 to $30{,}000/mm^3$ and there is significant risk of bleeding
  Counts greater than $50{,}000/mm^3$ are typically required for surgery or invasive procedures

11. Mechanical Ventilation of Sepsis-Induced Acute Lung Injury/ARDS (see Chapter 34)
    - Use low tidal volumes (6 mL/kg) with goal of plateau pressure less than 30 cm H_2O.
    - Permissive hypercapnia is tolerated to minimize plateau pressures and tidal volumes.
    - A minimum amount of positive end-expiratory pressure (PEEP) should be set to minimize lung collapse at end-expiration.
    - Prone positioning may be considered in patients requiring potentially injurious levels of plateau pressure or FIO_2 who are not at high risk for adverse consequences of prone positioning.
    - Unless contraindicated, mechanically ventilated patients should be maintained with the head of the bed raised to 45 degrees to prevent the development of ventilator-associated pneumonia.
    - A weaning protocol should be in place.
    - When stable, patients should undergo daily, spontaneous-breathing trials (T-piece or 5 cm H_2O continuous positive airway pressure [CPAP]).
    - If spontaneous breathing trials are successful, consideration should be given to extubation.
12. Sedation, Analgesia, and Neuromuscular Blockade
    - Sedation protocols should be used that include the use of a sedation goal, measured by a standardized subjective sedation scale.
    - Use either continuous infusion or intermittent bolus to achieve predetermined end-points.
    - Sedation should be interrupted/lightened daily to evaluate patients.
    - Neuromuscular blocking agents should be avoided if possible. When used, train-of-four monitoring of depth of blockade should be used.
13. Glucose Control
    - Maintain blood glucose levels less than 150 mg/dL with the use of insulin infusion.
    - Blood glucose should be monitored every 30 minutes initially, and then regularly (every 4 hours) once glucose concentration has stabilized.
    - Glycemic control should include the use of a nutrition protocol that favors enteral feeding.
14. Renal Replacement
    - In acute renal failure (ARF), continuous venovenous hemofiltration and intermittent hemodialysis are equivalent.
    - Venovenous hemofiltration may be tolerated better in hemodynamically unstable patients.
    - There is no evidence to support hemofiltration in sepsis independent of renal replacement needs.
15. Bicarbonate Therapy
    - No evidence to support the use of bicarbonate therapy for treatment of hypoperfusion-induced lactic acidemia.
16. Deep Vein Thrombosis Prophylaxis
    - Severe sepsis patients should receive deep vein thrombosis (DVT) prophylaxis with low-dose unfractionated heparin or low-molecular-weight heparin.
    - Mechanical prophylaxis should be used in patients with contraindications to heparin.
    - In extremely high-risk patients (history of DVT), a combination of pharmacologic and mechanical therapy is recommended.
17. Stress Ulcer Prophylaxis
    - All septic patients should receive stress ulcer prophylaxis.
    - H_2-receptor antagonists are more efficacious than sucralfate.
    - No studies have directly compared the use of proton-pump inhibitors with H_2-receptor antagonists, so their efficacy is unknown.
18. Consideration of Limitation of Support
    - Advance care planning, including the communication of likely outcomes and realistic treatment goals, should be discussed with patients and their families.
    - Less aggressive therapy and withdrawal of therapy may be in the patient's best interest.

Urinary Tract Infection

Urinary tract infections (UTIs) are the most common hospital-acquired infections,[103] and are thought to represent 25% to 50% of ICU-acquired infections.[104] Traditionally, hospital-acquired UTIs have been defined as greater than 10^5 colony-forming units (cfu)/mL of urine in patients during bladder catheterization. In the early 1980s, Platt and colleagues[105] showed that hospitalized patients meeting this definition of nosocomial UTI had a 2.8-fold increase in mortality. However, more data suggest that many of these cases may represent asymptomatic bacteriuria rather than invasive infection and perhaps do not merit treatment.[104] Stark and Maki have demonstrated that in catheterized patients, colonic bacteria rapidly proliferated in the urinary system and exceeded 10^5 cfu/mL.[106] In fact, up to 30% of catheterized, hospitalized patients demonstrated greater than 10^5 cfu/mL of urine.[107] Additionally, pyuria is not helpful in differentiating between infection and colonization since most catheter-associated bacteriurias have accompanying pyuria.[108] The rate of UTI-associated bacteremia is quite low (Box 36–4). A recent, large

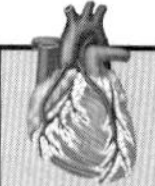

BOX 36–4 ***Nosocomial Urinary Tract Infections***

- Traditional diagnostic criteria (pyuria, $>10^5$ cfu) are misleading because both are common in hospitalized patients with bladder catheters.
- Only treat when signs are present, patient has signs/symptoms of infection and *no other obvious source of infection.*
- Treat with 10 to 14 days of culture-directed antimicrobial treatment.

Canadian case series demonstrated an ICU UTI rate of 9% with only a 0.4% incidence of bacteremic UTI.[103]

Bladder irrigation with antibiotic solutions does not reduce the likelihood of catheter-related UTI,[109] nor does prophylactic, systemic antibiotics.[110] Antimicrobial agent–impregnated urinary catheters do appear to reduce infection rates. A randomized, controlled trial demonstrated that silver-alloy hydrogel-coated catheters resulted in a 30% reduction in nosocomial UTI and, despite a 2.5 times greater acquisition cost, was still economically beneficial because of the increased cost associated with the infections.[111]

In light of the clinical uncertainty in the diagnosis of nosocomial, catheter-related UTI discussed previously, patients with asymptomatic catheter-related bacteriuria should not be treated. However, symptomatic patients or patients with signs of infection and urine cultures demonstrating greater than 10^5 cfu/mL and no other obvious source merit 10 to 14 days of antimicrobial treatment.

Clostridium difficile *Enterocolitis*

The anaerobic, gram-positive rod *Clostridium difficile* was first described in 1935 by Hall and O'Toole.[112] It was not until 1978, however, that its two toxogenic exotoxins (toxin A and toxin B) were identified to be the cause of antibiotic-associated pseudomembranous enterocolitis.[113,114] While it is part of the normal fecal flora in 50% of newborns, it is not found in adults until the normal microbial barrier is altered by antibiotic therapy.[112,114] *C. difficile* colonization occurs via the fecal-oral route and can follow exposure to any antibiotic. It is unclear why only a small percentage of patients exposed to a given antibiotic become colonized and of those colonized why only some develop symptomatic infection.[114,115] There is some speculation that antibody titers to the toxins may play a role.[116,117]

C. difficile diarrhea is the most common enteric infection in hospitalized patients, infecting approximately 10% of individuals admitted for longer than 2 days.[118] The organism enters the hospital environment via asymptomatic carriers and is then transmitted from patient to patient primarily via contact from hospital personnel. The risk factors that predispose a patient to *C. difficile* colonization include the severity of illness at admission, multiple antibiotic exposures, gastrointestinal surgery, enteral feeding, an infected roommate, and the use of proton-pump inhibitors.[119,120] Once colonized, clinical infection occurs following the secretion and adherence of toxin to receptors on the host's colonocyte brush border. The bound toxins cause necrosis of the epithelial cells, an intense inflammatory response, and exudative secretion into the bowel lumen. Clinically this cellular response is visible on endoscopy as "volcano" or "summit" lesions and pseudomembranes.[121] Hospital and unit epidemics of *C. difficile* are common, are often attributable to a single strain (despite multiple strains being present in the environment) and are associated with the use of clindamycin.[122,123]

C. difficile diarrhea produces a spectrum of clinical disease. The typical presentation includes low-grade fever, leukocytosis, frequent watery bowel movements (10 to 15 per day) and abdominal pain following the administration of antibiotics. However, at its most severe, the disease results in fulminant illness with "toxic megacolon."[124] It is important to note that the majority of antibiotic-associated diarrhea results from an osmotic diarrhea and not from *C. difficile* infection. In osmotic diarrhea, antibiotics inhibit the intestinal flora from metabolizing carbohydrates, which results in increased intraluminal osmotic pressure, the translocation of water into the bowel lumen, and diarrhea.[125] The diagnosis of *C. difficile* infection is suggested by fecal leukocytosis (not present in osmotic diarrhea), systemic toxicity (fever, leukocytosis) and the persistence despite the discontinuation of enteral feeding (will decrease carbohydrate source in osmotic diarrhea). The diagnosis is confirmed by bioassay of *C. difficile* cytotoxins.[126] Endoscopy is reserved for suspected cases in which diagnosis is not confirmed by toxin assay or when a diagnosis must be made before assay results are available. In these instances, colonoscopy is superior to sigmoidoscopy (lesions are often proximal in the colon) and the presence of pseudomembranes in a patient with antibiotic-associated diarrhea is pathopneumonic of *C. difficile* diarrhea.[127,128]

The treatment of *C. difficile* diarrhea is with oral metronidazole (500 mg, three times daily) or oral vancomycin (125 mg, four times daily) for 10 to 14 days. Metronidazole is considered first choice because of similar efficacy but a lower price.[129] In severely ill patients, oral vancomycin (up to 500 mg, four times daily) is supplemented with intravenous metronidazole.[130] Relapse occurs in 10% to 25% of patients, is not from antibiotic resistance (not described to date), and should be treated by repeating the same therapy for another 10 to 14 days.

Sinusitis

Sinusitis is a frequent and clinically silent source of infection in intubated patients.[104] Sinusitis is particularly common following nasal intubation, with an incidence of up to 85% following 1 week of intubation.[104,131-134] The diagnosis is suggested by the presence of air-fluid levels or total opacification of the sinuses on computed tomography scan.[133] However, opacification of the sinuses is common following intubation. In one series, 96% of nasotracheally intubated and 23% of orotracheally intubated patients with previously clear sinuses had new sinus opacification following 1 week of intubation.[133] The diagnosis can be confirmed by the presence of pus and high quantitative cultures that can be obtained either via transnasal puncture of the maxillary sinus or open ethmoidectomy/sphenoidectomy.[104,131] Several case series have reported a resolution of fever and leukocytosis following the treatment of sinusitis.[131,133] Treatment consists of removal of all nasal tubes, drainage of the maxillary sinuses, and broad-spectrum antibiotics.

HEMATOLOGY

Transfusion

Blood products are frequently transfused into critically ill patients. In a general ICU population, patients receive an average of 0.2 U/day, and this incidence is increased to 1.3 U/day in cardiothoracic ICUs.[135,136] While transfusion is often necessary to either improve oxygen delivery or restore the coagulation system, there is a growing body of literature that suggests that transfusion carries substantial risk for postoperative cardiac surgical patients.

Several large studies have identified transfusion as increasing the risk of infection following cardiac surgery (Box 36–5). In fact, in a review of 19 retrospective studies, in 17 transfusion was found to be a significant factor and frequently the best predictor of postoperative infection.[135,137] Transfusion has

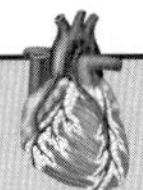

BOX 36–5 *Transfusion Strategy in Cardiothoracic Intensive Care Unit*

- Transfusion is associated with increased morbidity and mortality.
- During first 24 to 48 hours, transfuse to target oxygen delivery and resolution of coagulopathy/bleeding.
- Long-term ICU patients have lower morbidity and mortality when conservative transfusion strategy used.

been cited as a risk factor for mediastinitis,[63-65] early bacteremia,[138] pneumonia,[139] increased mortality rate, and LOS following cardiac surgery.[140] A randomized, controlled trial identified nosocomial pneumonia as the most frequent infection after cardiac surgery, and that it only occurred in patients transfused more than 4 units of blood components.[141] In 2001, Leal-Noval and colleagues[135] published a large cohort study that identified transfusion as a risk factor for severe postoperative infections. In their series of 738 cardiac surgical patients at a large Spanish teaching hospital, a transfusion of more than 4 units of blood components was associated with a statistically significant increased risk of pneumonia, mediastinitis, mortality, and longer ICU LOS (Fig. 36–3).

In 1999, Hebert and colleagues[142] published a landmark study that has fundamentally altered the approach to transfusion in critically ill patients. Their large, multicenter, randomized, prospective trial of 838 patients admitted to Canadian ICUs found no difference in 30-day mortality between patients assigned to a liberal (hemoglobin 10 to 12 g/dL) and conservative red blood cell transfusion protocol (hemoglobin 7 to 9 g/dL). In fact, mortality was lower in less ill patients (APACHE II score ≤20) and in younger patients (≤55 years of age). Also, the restrictive strategy resulted in a 54% reduction in red blood cell transfusions. Prior to this study, red blood cell transfusion had been extensively investigated as a component of the now dated paradigm that supranormal oxygen delivery was associated with increased survival in critically ill patients.[135] Hebert et al's study showed that a conservative strategy was not only associated with no increase in mortality, but that it halved the number of transfused units with its attendant decrease in infectious risk, immunomodulation, and cost. Two similar, small trials in cardiac surgical patients have also shown no difference in outcome between conservative and liberal transfusion strategies.[141,143]

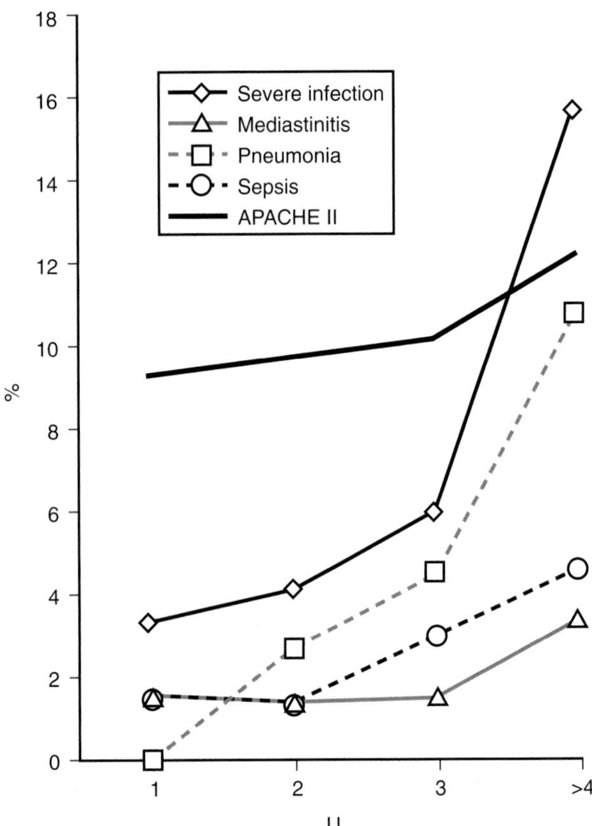

Figure 36–3 Relationship between the units of blood transfused and the percentage of infections. (Redrawn from Leal-Noval SR, Rincon-Ferrari MD, Carcia-Curiel A, et al: Transfusion of blood components and postoperative infection in patients undergoing cardiac surgery. Chest 119:1461, 2001.)

These data, combined with the evidence supporting the use of early "goal-directed" therapy in sepsis, are what has led to the recommendations for transfusion cited in the Surviving Sepsis Campaign Guidelines noted previously. While no consensus guidelines exist for transfusion practices following cardiac surgery, an extrapolation of these recommendations for postoperative cardiac patients seems prudent at the present time. That is, in the initial 24 to 48 hours of "resuscitation," a more liberal transfusion strategy targeting oxygen delivery (with objective end-points, e.g., lactate levels, mixed venous oxygen saturation) and resolution of coagulopathy/bleeding seems appropriate. Once stabilized, long-term cardiothoracic ICU patients should probably be subjected to a conservative (hemoglobin 7 to 9 g/dL) transfusion strategy. However, a multicenter, retrospective review of patients following myocardial infarction suggested that a more liberal goal of transfusing to achieve a hemoglobin of 10 g/dL is associated with increased mortality.[144] While not directly applicable to a cardiothoracic ICU setting, it does suggest that improving oxygen delivery in patients with coronary artery disease by transfusing red blood cells to a hemoglobin of 10 g/dL is not the panacea clinicians once thought.

Acute Renal Failure (ARF)

ARF, like many of the clinical syndromes frequently encountered in the ICU, has been difficult to precisely define.[145] If it is agreed that the principal functions of the kidney are to create urine and excrete water-soluble waste products of metabolism, then ARF is the sudden loss of these functions.[146]

Renal solute excretion is a function of glomerular filtration. Glomerular filtration rate (GFR) is a convenient and time-honored way of quantifying renal function. It must be appreciated, however, that GFR varies considerably under normal circumstances as a function of protein intake.[145] A normal GFR for men is 120 ± 25 mL/min, and it is 95 ± 20 mL/min for women. Creatinine is the most frequently used surrogate of GFR and hence solute excretion. When measured in the *steady state* and analyzed in the context of age, gender, and race, it loosely reflects renal function. In fact, when baseline serum creatinine is unknown, standardized tables allow the estimation of baseline creatinine that can then be compared with actual serum creatinine levels to estimate decremental changes in renal function[145] (Table 36–7).

Table 36–7 **Estimated Baseline Creatinine**

Age (yr)	African-American Men, mg/dL (μmol/L)	Caucasian Men, mg/dL (μmol/L)	African-American Women, mg/dL (μmol/L)	Caucasian Women, mg/dL (μmol/L)
20 to 24	1.5 (133)	1.3 (115)	1.2 (106)	1.0 (88)
25 to 29	1.5 (133)	1.2 (106)	1.1 (97)	1.0 (88)
30 to 39	1.4 (124)	1.2 (106)	1.1 (97)	0.9 (80)
40 to 54	1.3 (115)	1.1 (97)	1.0 (88)	0.9 (80)
55 to 65	1.3 (115)	1.1 (97)	1.0 (88)	0.8 (71)
>65	1.2 (106)	1.0 (88)	0.9 (80)	0.8 (71)

Estimated glomerular filtration rate = 75 (mL/min per 1.73 m^2) = 186 × (Scr) − 1.154 × (age) − 0.203 × (0.742 if woman) × (1.210 if African-American) = exp (5.228 − 1.154 × ln [Scr] − 0.203 × ln [age] − [0.299 if female] + [0.192 if African-American]).

Reprinted with permission from Bellomo R, Kellum JA, Ronco C: Defining acute renal failure: physiologic principles. Intensive Care Med 30:33, 2004.

Creatinine is much less accurate in estimating renal function in non–steady state conditions (e.g., ARF in the critically ill). Creatinine is formed from nonenzymatic dehydration of creatine (98% muscular in origin) in the liver. Because critical illness affects liver function, muscle mass, tubular excretion of creatinine, and the volume of distribution of creatinine, its limitations as a useful marker of renal function become apparent.[145] Nonetheless, changes in serum creatinine and the rate of change in creatinine remain the most convenient and frequently used surrogates of renal dysfunction.

Urine output is the other frequently measured parameter of renal function in the ICU. Oliguria is defined by a urine output of less than 0.5 mL/kg/hr.[145] Under a wide range of normal physiologic conditions, urine output primarily reflects changes in renal hemodynamics and volume status rather than representing renal parenchymal function and reserve. Hence, it is very nonspecific for renal dysfunction unless urine output is severely reduced or absent.[145] And, while oliguric renal failure has a higher mortality rate than nonoliguric renal failure, no data demonstrate that the pharmacologic creation of urine in patients with renal failure reduces mortality.[147]

The incidence of ARF following cardiovascular surgery is high and is associated with a "formidable" mortality rate.[148] A cohort study from Duke University described a 0.7% incidence of dialysis-dependent ARF that was associated with an increase in mortality from 1.8% to 28%.[149] Another cohort described an incidence of dialysis-dependent ARF of 1.1% following cardiac surgery that was associated with a mortality rate of 63.7%.[148] In critically ill patients (noncardiac), the mortality for ARF is 50% to 80% and has not declined significantly since the advent of acute dialysis therapy.[147]

The pathogenesis of ARF following cardiac surgery is thought to primarily result from hypoperfusion and ischemia.[149] Other contributing factors include nephrotoxins, nonpulsatile flow during cardiopulmonary bypass, and aortic emboli. The two most important determinants of ARF following cardiopulmonary bypass are preexisting renal insufficiency and postoperative low cardiac output states.[150,151]

Several strategies for preventing perioperative renal failure have been evaluated in cardiac surgical patients. "Renal-dose" dopamine has been shown to have no effect on either renal function or mortality following both cardiac and vascular surgery.[152-154] Similarly, the diuretics furosemide and mannitol have demonstrated no renal-protective effects. In fact, a small study demonstrated a significantly worse renal outcome in patients treated with prophylactic furosemide infusion versus controls.[154] Results with pulsatile perfusion during cardiopulmonary bypass have been similarly disappointing.[146]

The new recombinant brain atrial natriuretic peptide (B-ANP) nesiritide has demonstrated some initial promise in treating perioperative renal failure in patients following cardiac surgery. In a randomized, prospective, double-blinded trial in two cardiothoracic ICUs in Sweden, patients with an increase in serum creatinine more than 50% above baseline had improved renal excretion, decreased need for hemodialysis, and improved survival following treatment with ANP, compared with controls.[155] Nesiritide works via a cGMP-coupled receptor (NPR-A) in vascular smooth muscle cells. Physiologically it produces arterial and venous vasodilation, inhibition of aldosterone production, and increases urine volume and sodium excretion.[156] Further trials are under way to more clearly define this promising agent's role in cardiac surgical patients (see Chapters 10, 31, and 33).

Treatment and Renal Replacement Therapies

Just as the diagnosis and prevention of ARF remain enigmatic, so too does the treatment of ARF. In the critically ill patient developing ARF, the initial treatment strategy is to create an optimal "environment" for the kidney to heal, that is, to maximize oxygen delivery to the renal parenchyma via the manipulation of hemodynamics and volume status, while simultaneously avoiding nephrotoxins (e.g., contrast, aminoglycosides, etc.) and ensuring no postrenal obstruction exists. If provided this optimization and the kidney does not recover, the clinician must provide renal replacement therapy (RRT).

Many of the classic indications for RRT are noncontroversial and include the following[157]:

- Uremic symptoms (anorexia, nausea, vomiting).
- Uremic signs (uremic pericarditis, bleeding, encephalopathy)
- Hyperkalemia refractory to medical therapy
- Volume overload unresponsive to restriction and diuretics
- Metabolic acidosis
- Dialyzable intoxications (e.g., lithium, toxic alcohols, salicylate)
- Some cases of hypocalcemia/hypercalcemia, hyperphosphatemia

In the absence of these indications, the decision to initiate RRT in critically ill patients is a matter of clinical judgment. Typical laboratory parameters that suggest the need for RRT include a blood urea nitrogen above 100 mg/dL or a creatinine above 4.5 mg/dL.[152]

Once the decision to initiate RRT has been made, the mode of replacement must be chosen. In broad terms, RRT can be divided into intermittent hemodialysis or continuous RRT. The latter comes in a wide variety of forms, each associated with its own unique acronym (slow continuous ultrafiltration [SCUF], slow low-efficiency daily dialysis [SLEDD], continuous venovenous hemofiltration [CVVH], continuous venovenous hemofiltration-dialysis [CVVH-D], etc.). The differences between these different forms of continuous RRT lie in the membrane used, the mechanism of solute transport, the presence or absence of a dialysis solution and the type of vascular access.[152,157,158] In the United States, the majority of patients with ARF are treated with hemodialysis, but the trend is toward the increased use of continuous RRT, while in other countries, continuous RRT predominates.[152,159-161] At present, there are no studies supporting the use of one modality over another, but most intensivists prefer continuous RRT in hemodynamically unstable patients or in whom the hypotension associated with hemodialysis would be adverse.[152,157] A trial of weaning of continuous RRT should be considered when the following criteria have been met[157]:

- Criteria to initiate have resolved.
- Urine output averages 1 mL/kg/hr over 24 hours.
- Fluid balance can be maintained with present urine output.
- Complications of continuous RRT outweigh benefits.

NUTRITION SUPPORT

Any patient who is going to be in the ICU for an extended period of time (longer than 2 to 3 days) will require nutrition assessment, and if the patient is malnourished or if the patient will remain *non per os* (NPO) without parenteral nutrition, they should be examined and assessment made whether they should receive enteral or parenteral nutrition support. In the 1970s, there were several articles in the nutrition literature that concluded that anywhere from 40% to 70% of patients in the hospital, and by extension in the ICU, were malnourished.[162] Three decades of aggressive intervention have not yet changed that assessment—because of chronic illness and because of the sequelae of acute illness, many patients remain cachectic and hypermetabolic, and even aggressive nutrition support will not completely reverse the sequelae.[163,164]

The stress response that many, if not all, critically ill patients have is responsible for this ongoing altered metabolic state. With any form of injury or acute illness, a number of hormones and cytokines are released that affect metabolism, including catecholamines, glucagons, tumor necrosis factor, etc. These hormones create a state in which metabolic rate is increased, protein synthetic rate is decreased, and glycolysis and lipolysis are increased. Patients who remain NPO and have an ongoing critical illness such that the stress response does not abate as it normally would after a surgical procedure require a nutritional assessment, and afterward a decision must be made whether the patient should be fed.

Nutritional Assessment

The nutritional assessment of anyone in the ICU begins by a history of the patient's eating habits, weight loss or gain, medications, alcohol use, and symptoms that would be compatible with a nutrient or vitamin deficiency. A history of an unplanned weight loss of 10% in the preceding 6 months places patients at increased risk of perioperative complications, and such patients should receive further evaluation, additional tests, and perhaps earlier intervention from a nutrition standpoint. Patients who have increased alcohol intake, alcoholics, and patients with malabsorption are at risk of nutrient deficiency and for the sequelae associated with it. In addition, while making the initial nutrition assessment, the integrity of the gastrointestinal tract should be assessed as to whether the patient might be a candidate for enteral feeding if nutrition support is indicated or, if not, potential intravenous access sites.

As part of the nutrition assessment, the patient warrants a thorough physical examination, first assessing the patient's general appearance and overall condition, a brief neurologic examination specifically looking at ability to swallow and protect the airway, muscle stores (in the temporal fossa), fat stores (usually in the triceps area), evidence of jaundice, glossitis, edema, and cheilosis. Clinicians are often able to complete what is known as a subjective global assessment (SGA), a tool developed by Jeejeebhoy and colleagues to grade a patient's overall nutritional status with C being the worst, B being moderate, and those patients given an A have a mild nutrient deficiency.[165] In the validating study, two observers had concordant views with the patient's nutritional status, a view that correlated with a bank of laboratory tests of the patient's immunity and nutrient status. Because of the ease of facility of conducting such a study, this is rapidly becoming the gold standard by which patients are assessed.

For the final part of the nutrition assessment, laboratory tests should be obtained. Many nutritionists rely on a serum albumin, but because of the half-life, others prefer a serum pre-albumin. Often, any of the plasma proteins will be decreased, but they do serve as a marker for adequacy of anabolism that can be measured at baseline and weekly thereafter to assess the efficacy of nutrition interventions. Other laboratory tests that should be assessed on a regular basis include acid-base status; electrolytes, to include phosphorus, magnesium, and calcium; and measures of renal and liver function. Finally, all patients on nutrition assessment should have a blood sugar measured on a regular basis. As indicated earlier, every attempt should be made to keep the blood sugar below 150 mg/dL, using an insulin infusion if necessary. Caloric support should not be decreased merely to meet this goal, but any patient receiving nutrition intervention should have blood glucose tests monitored.

Measuring resting energy expenditure is a test that is used for the extremely obese patient and the profoundly anorexic patient to help guide support. Otherwise, using a simple measure such as a Harris-Benedict equation allows an estimation of the number of calories patients require:

$$\text{For men: RMR} = 66.4 + 13.8 \times W + 5 \times H - 6.8 \times A$$
$$\text{For women: RMR} = 655 + 9.6 \times W + 1.8 \times H - 4.7 \times A$$

where RMR is resting metabolic rate, W is weight (kg), H is height (cm), and A is age (years).

After the initial nutrition assessment, the patient is classified as having mild, moderate, or severe malnutrition. Patients who are moderately to severely malnourished should have more attention paid to their nutrition support. If the patient is going to remain NPO for several days, many intensivists and nutrition support personnel would implement nutrition support early in the hospital course, within the first 3 days. The data for this recommendation are lacking except in trauma patients in whom there are studies that justify early nutrition support.[166] As long as there are no side effects, there should be no danger to early intervention using a tube placed through the pylorus to aliment the patient.

Depending on the institution, enteral feeding tubes are placed fluoroscopically by radiologists, endoscopically by a gastroenterologist, or at the bedside by an intensivist using several different techniques and approaches. There are several complications from enteral nutrition including placement of the feeding tube past the tracheal tube and into the trachea, remaining in the stomach and not passing through the pylorus, etc. Bloating is one of the more frequent side effects of enteral nutrition and if there is significant ileus with gastric residuals, it increases the risk of aspiration of gastric contents. In addition, distention of the large or small intestine can increase intra-abdominal pressure, displacing the diaphragm in a cephalad direction and interfering with weaning from mechanical ventilation if the patient is mechanically ventilated. Another frequent side effect of enteral nutrition is diarrhea, which can be secondary to bacterial overgrowth, the osmolality of the nutritional formula, the administration through the enteral feeding tube of medications containing sorbitol or glycerol, and because of *C. difficile* infection.

Although enteral nutrition is preferred and has been reported to decrease the incidence of infectious complications in some patient populations, occasionally some patients cannot be fed enterally and must be fed parenterally. Enteral formulas in use that are commercially available are listed in Table 36–8. If the parenteral route is chosen, then placement of the central venous access line using a sterile technique[167] is critical. If the incidence of catheter-related infection at an institution is less than 1%, then there is likely little difference between enteral and parenteral feeding when it comes to catheter-related infectious complications. Furthermore, if blood glucose levels are kept below or equal to 150 mg/dL, this also decreases the incidence of catheter-related infections and pneumonia.[168] If there are protocols in the ICU for how the alimentation intravascular device should be placed, then in most circumstances, parenteral nutrition is an acceptable alternative to enteral nutrition.

Formulas

Protein

Most authorities currently recommend 1.0 to 1.5 g of protein/kg/day based on patient's average weight including the admission weight, current weight, and ideal body weight. Unless the patient has renal insufficiency and is not on dialysis or unless the patient has hepatic encephalopathy that responds to administration of branch-chain amino acids, there are no unique protein formulas that should be used to feed enterally or parenterally.

Lipids and Carbohydrates

The majority of a patient's energy needs should be met with a combination of carbohydrate (glucose) and lipids (lipid emulsion). The amount of glucose that a critically ill patient can oxidize is limited to 6 g of glucose/kg/day or 4 mg/kg/min. Patients who receive more than this are at increased risk of development of complications such as hyperglycemia, diuresis, increased carbon dioxide production (which in some circumstances may keep the patient mechanically ventilated), and development of a fatty liver.

Lipids are the other mainstay for supplying calories to a critically ill patient. They are not adequately oxidized if more than 1.0 to 1.5 g of lipid emulsion/kg/day is administered to the patient. When using lipids as part of a parenteral nutrition regimen, serum triglycerides should be checked on a regular basis to ensure that the patient does not develop hypertriglyceridemia, with its attendant side effects and toxicity.

Electrolytes

Electrolyte abnormalities are common to patients in the ICU. In patients fed parenterally who have renal failure, there are formulas that have low levels of potassium, phosphate, etc. In patients receiving parenteral nutrition, it is relatively easy to manipulate the concentration of deficient or excessive electrolytes in the total parenteral nutrition formula.

Vitamins

Most enteral products contain 100% of the recommended daily dose of nutrients (RDA), but some patients may require supplementation of vitamins. Patients who are alcoholic should receive supplemental thiamin, a patient with short-bowel syndrome who is deficient in fat-soluble vitamins may benefit from the administration of them, and unless patients are on anticoagulants, they need to be supplemented with vitamin K. Fluid balance in patients fed enterally and parenterally also must be monitored and occasionally formulas for both enteral and parenteral nutrition may need to be changed to accommodate fluid excess or dehydration.

Finally, there are a number of immune-enhancing compounds that could be administered to critically ill patients, including glutamine, arginine, essential omega-3 fatty acids, nucleotides, and structured lipids. Unfortunately, several studies have failed to show benefit of any of the immune-enhancing diets, although many investigators remain optimistic that such diets will in the future be demonstrated to be beneficial.[169,170]

ELECTROLYTE ABNORMALITIES

Fluid and electrolyte abnormalities are common following cardiac surgery. Diagnosis and treatment algorithms are shown in Figures 36–4 and 36–5 for hypernatremia and hyponatremia, Figure 36–6 and Table 36–9 for hyperkalemia, Figure 36–7 for hypokalemia, and Table 36–10 for hypercalcemia. Hypomagnesemia is common and the underlying cause should be identified, if possible, and then treated with an intravenous infusion of 0.1 to 0.2 mEq/kg/day or via the oral route at 0.4 mEq/kg/day. Close monitoring is necessary with treatment of any electrolyte disorder.

Table 36–8 **Nutrient Analysis Enteral Tube Feeding Formulas: Nutrients / 1000 mL**

Product	kcal/mL	Vol (RDI)	Water (mL)	mOsm	Protein (g/%)	Fat (g/%)	CHO (g/%)	Na (mEq)	K (mEq)	Ca (mg)	Phos (mg)	Mg (mg)	Fiber	Comments
Jevity	1.06	1321	829	300	44.3/16.7	34.7/29	154.7/54.3	40.4	40.2	910	760	305	14.4	Isotonic, with fiber
Jevity 1.5	1.5	1000	760	525	63.8/17	49.8/29.4	215.7/53.6	60.9	47.4	1200	1200	400	22	Calorically dense, with fiber
Nepro	2	947	699	665	70/14	95.6/43	223/43	36.7	27.1	1370	695	215	15.6	Low electrolyte, renal failure
Osmolite	1.06	1887	841	300	37.1/14	34.7/29	151.1/57	27.8	26.1	535	535	215	0	Isotonic, moderate protein
Osmolite 1.2 cal	1.2	1000	820	360	55.5/18.5	39.3/29	15.7/52.5	61.7	49.7	1200	1200	400	0	Calorically dense
Subdue (unflavored)	1	1000	840	330	50/20	34/30	130/50	48	41	1100	1050	360	0	Elemental
Promote	1	1000	837	340	62.5/25	26/23	130/52	43.5	50.8	1200	1200	400	0	High protein, wound healing
Twocal HN	2	948	701	725	83.5/16.7	90.5/40.1	218/43.2	63	62.6	1050	1050	425	5	Calorically dense, high protein
Modular														
Proteinex (30 mL)					15	0								Liquid protein supplement
MCT oil (15 mL)	115/15 mL				0	14	0							For fat malabsorption

Oral Supplements: Per Serving

Product	kcal	Pro	Fat	CHO	Na	K	Ca	Phos	Mg	Fiber	Flavors
Boost	240/8 oz	10	4	41	5.7	10.2	325	312	105	0	Strawberry, vanilla, chocolate
Ceralyte 90					90						Chicken
Carnation Instant Breakfast	130/pkg	4.5	1	28	4.3	8.9	300	250	80	0–1	Strawberry, vanilla, chocolate
Sugar-free CIB	70/pkg	4.5	1	12	4	8.9	300	250	80	0–1	Strawberry, vanilla, chocolate
Enlive	300/8 oz	10	0	65	2.8		60	20	8	0	Apple, peach
Ensure Plus	355/8 oz	13	11.4	50.1	10.4	11.3	200	200	100	0	Strawberry, vanilla, chocolate
Glucerna Shake	220/8 oz	10	8.5	29	210	9.5	250	250	100	3	Vanilla, chocolate
Nepro	475/8 oz	16.7	22.7	52.8	8.7	6.4	325	165	50	3.7	Vanilla
Twocal HN	475/8 oz	19.9	21.5	51.8	15	14.8	250	250	100	1.2	Vanilla
Subdue (flavored)	240/8 oz	11.8	8	30	11.3	9.7	260	250	84	0	Chocolate, orange

Hypernatremia
Fluid volume status assessed by physical exam
Hypovolemic hypernatremia
Loss of H_2O >Na^+ loss
Check urine Na^+
>20 mEq/L
<10 mEq/L
Renal loss
Diuretic
Glycosuria
Renal failure
External loss
GI–vomiting
GI–diarrhea
Excess sweating
Respiratory loss
Treatment
Saline then hypotonic solutions
Isovolemic hypernatremia
Loss of H_2O
Check urine Na^+
Renal loss
Diabetes insipidus
Central
Nephrogenic
External loss
Insensible losses
Skin
Respiration
Treatment
Water replacement
D5W at 1–2 mEq/L/hr
± vasopressin for central DI
Hypervolemic hypernatremia
Gain of H_2O and Na^+
Check urine Na^+
>20 mEq/L
Iatrogenic
Hypertonic $NaHCO_3$
NaCl tablets
Hypertonic solutions
Mineralocorticoid
1° Hyperaldosteronism
Cushing's disease
Adrenal
Hypertonic dialysis
Hemodialysis
Peritoneal dialysis
Treatment
Diuretic ± dialysis

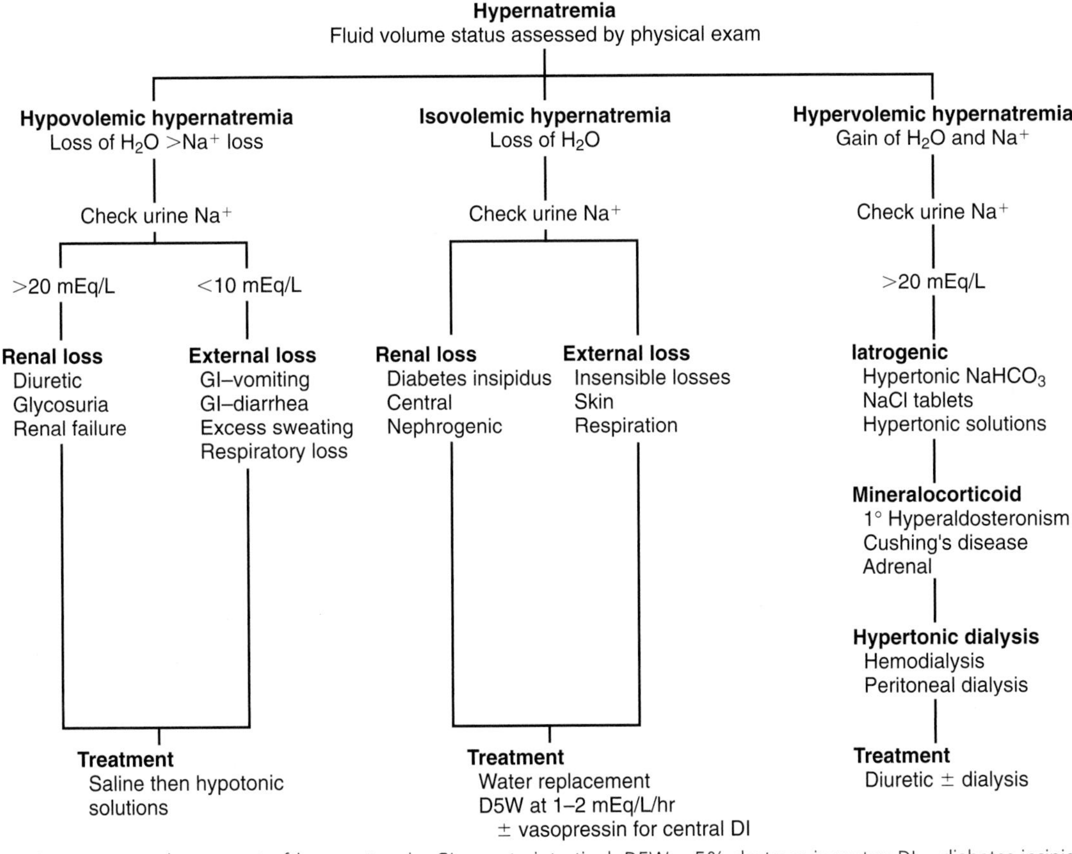

Figure 36–4 Assessment and treatment of hypernatremia. GI = gastrointestinal; D5W = 5% dextrose in water; DI = diabetes insipidus. (Modified from Torres N: Electrolyte abnormalities: Sodium. *In* Faust RJ [ed]: Anesthesiology Review, 2nd edition. New York, Churchill Livingstone, 1994, p 34; with permission of Mayo Foundation.)

Hyponatremia
Serum osmolality
Normal
(250–285 mOsm/L)
Low
(<250 mOsm/L)
High
(>285 mOsm/L)
Isosmotic hyponatremia
1) Pseudohyponatremia
Hyperlipidemia
Hyperproteinemia
2) Isotonic infusions
Glucose Glycerol
Mannitol Sorbitol
Glycine Ethanol
Hyperosmotic hyponatremia
1) Hypernatremia
2) Hypertonic infusions
Glucose Glycerol
Mannitol Sorbitol
Glycine Ethanol
Assess extracellular fluid volume state
Hypovolemic Hypo-osmotic Hyponatremia
Urine Na^+
<10 mEq/L
Extrarenal
GI–vomiting
GI–diarrhea
Pancreatitis
Skin losses
Lung losses
<20 mEq/L
Renal
Diuretic
Obstruction
Renal damage
Renal tubular acidosis
Adrenal insufficiency
Treatment
Isotonic saline (asymptomatic patient)
Hypertonic saline (symptomatic patient)
Isovolemic Hypo-osmotic Hyponatremia
Urine Na^+
<10 mEq/L
H_2O intoxication
<20 mEq/L
Renal failure
Hypothyroid
Pain
SIADH
Emotion
Adrenal insufficiency
Treatment
Water restriction (no symptoms)
Isotonic saline (no symptoms)
Hypertonic saline (symptoms)
Furosemide diuresis (symptoms)
Hypervolemic Hypo-osmotic Hyponatremia
Urine Na^+
<10 mEq/L
Cirrhosis
Heart failure
Renal failure
<20 mEq/L
Acute/chronic renal failure
Treatment
Isotonic saline (asymptomatic patient)
Hypertonic saline (symptomatic patient)

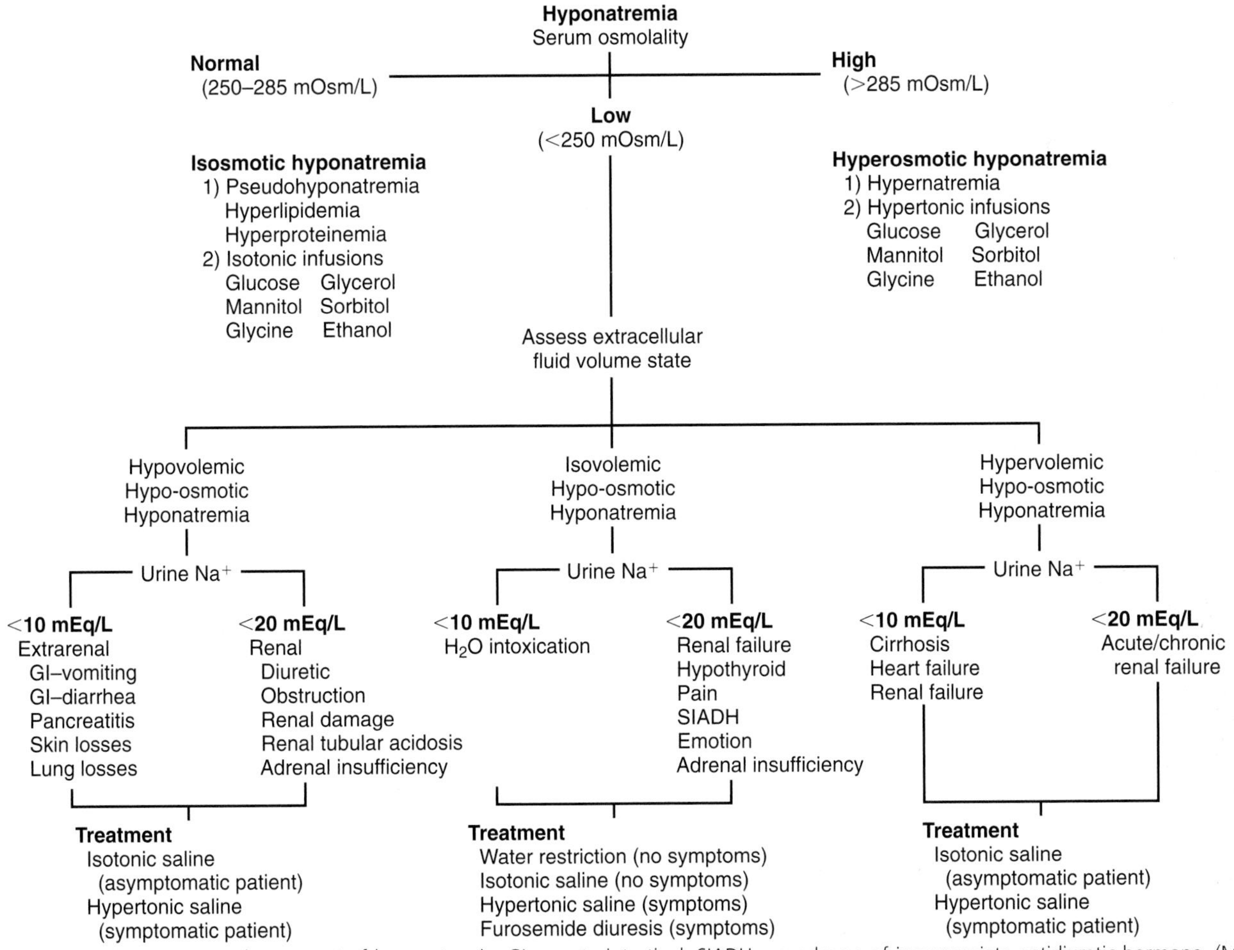

Figure 36–5 Assessment and treatment of hyponatremia. GI = gastrointestinal; SIADH = syndrome of inappropriate antidiuretic hormone. (Modified from Torres N: Electrolyte abnormalities: Sodium. *In* Faust RJ [ed]: Anesthesiology Review, 2nd edition. New York, Churchill Livingstone, 1994, p 35; with permission of Mayo Foundation.)

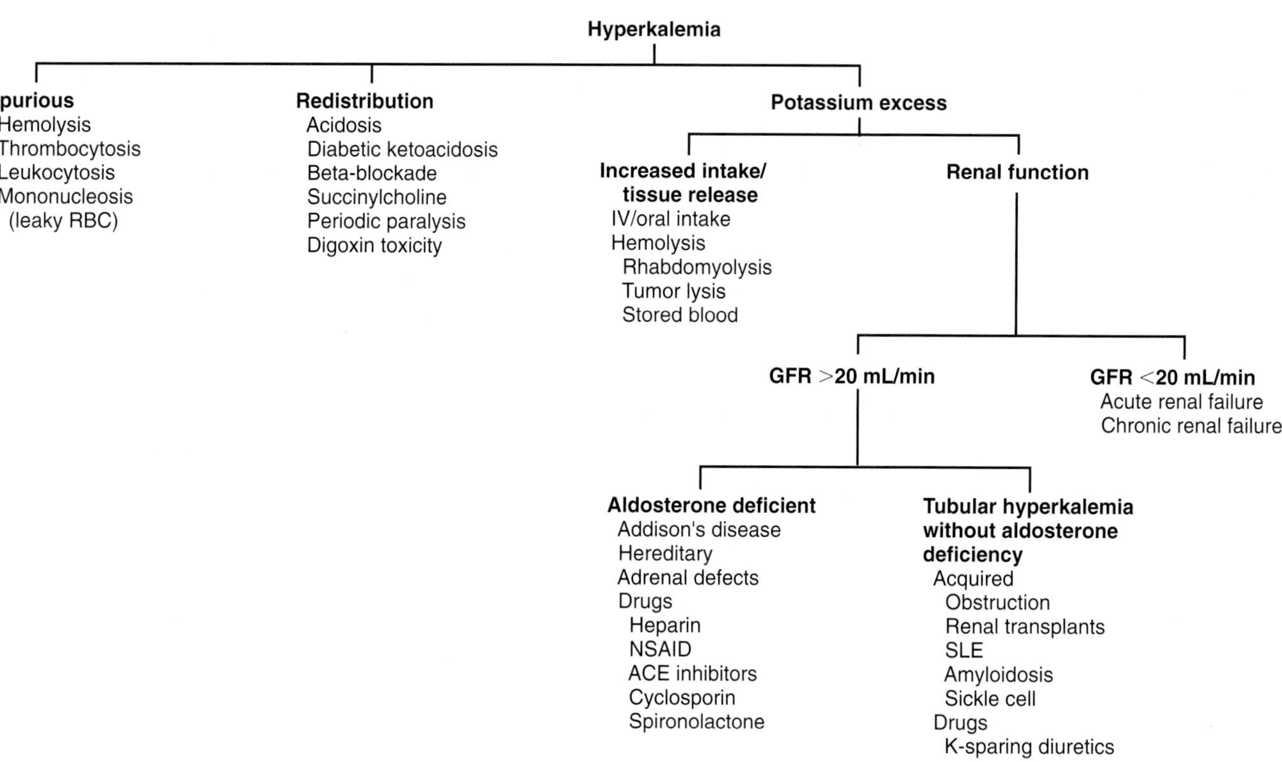

Figure 36–6 Causes of hypernatremia. (Modified from Torres N: Electrolyte abnormalities: Sodium. *In* Faust RJ [ed]: Anesthesiology Review, 2nd edition. New York, Churchill Livingstone, 1994, p 37; with permission of Mayo Foundation.)

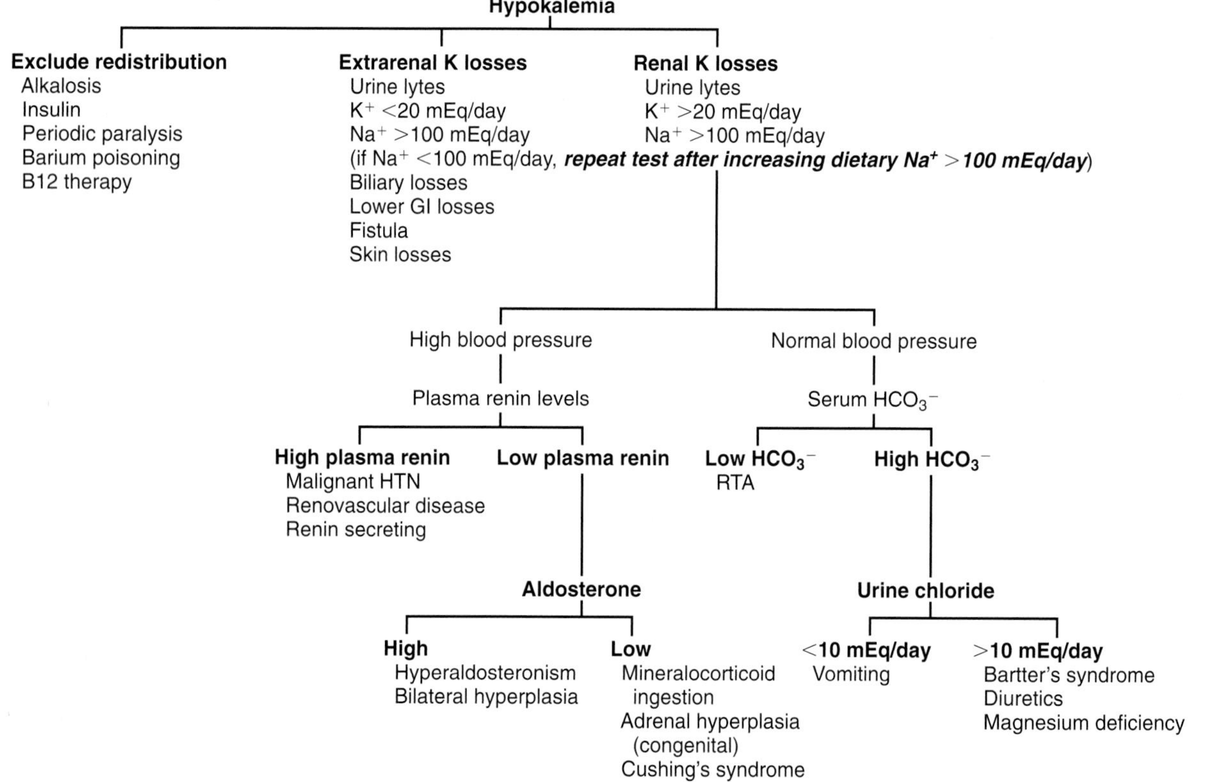

Figure 36–7 Algorithmic approach to hypokalemia. GI = gastrointestinal; RTA = renal tubular acidosis. (Modified from Torres N: Electrolyte abnormalities: Sodium. *In* Faust RJ [ed]: Anesthesiology Review, 2nd edition. New York, Churchill Livingstone, 1994, p 38; with permission of Mayo Foundation.)

Table 36–9 Treatment of Hyperkalemia

Treatment	Dose	Mechanism	Onset	Duration
1. Calcium chloride	7 to 14 mg/kg	Direct antagonism	Instantly	15 to 30 min
2. Sodium bicarbonate	0.7 to 1.4 mEq/kg	Direct antagonism Redistribution	15 to 30 min	3 to 6 hr
3. Glucose + insulin	25 g + 10 to 15 units	Redistribution	15 to 30 min	3 to 6 hr
4. Kayexalate	30 g PO/PR	Elimination of K^+	1 to 3 hr	
5. Peritoneal dialysis		Elimination of K^+	1 to 3 hr	
6. Hemodialysis		Elimination of K^+	Rapid	

Table 36–10 Features of Hypercalcemia and Its Treatment

Calcium level, mg/dL	>13.0 <11.5	Symptoms: anorexia, nausea, vomiting, lethargy, dehydration, coma, death Asymptomatic			
Treatment	**Onset of Action**	**Duration of Action**	**% Normalization**	**Advantages**	**Disadvantages**
Saline (200 to 500 mL/hr) (increases urine calcium and excretion)	Hours	During infusion	0 to 10	Rehydration	Cardiac failure, electrolyte changes, hypokalemia, hypomagnesemia, intensive monitoring
Saline + loop diuretics (furosemide 40 to 80 mg every 2 hrs)	Hours	During treatment (saline infusion rate = urine flow rate)	0 to 10	Enhanced calcium elimination	As above
Zoledronate (most potent biphosphonate available, administer 4 mg IV over 15 min)	1 to 2 days	32 to 39 days	60 to 80	Potency efficacy	Increase phosphate, 3-day infusion
Calcitonin (4 units/kg SQ or IM every 12 hr) (inhibits osteoclasts and stimulates calciuresis)	Hours	2 to 3 days	10 to 20 rapid onset	Nontoxic	Only decrease calcium by 2 to 3 mg/dL, tachyphylaxis
Gallium nitrate (200 mg/m²/day in 1 L normal saline over 5 days)	2 to 3 days	10 to 14 days	70 to 80	Potent	Long infusion time, cannot use in renal failure

IM = intramuscular; IV = intravenous; SQ = subcutaneous.

REFERENCES

1. Bashour CA, Yared J-P, Ryan TA, et al: Long-term survival and functional capacity in cardiac surgery patients after prolonged intensive care. Crit Care Med 28:3847, 2000
2. Williams MR, Wellner RB, Hartnett EA, et al: Long-term survival and quality of life in cardiac surgical patients with prolonged intensive care unit length of stay. Ann Thorac Surg 73:1472, 2002
3. Treasure T, Holmes L, Loughead K, Gallivan S: Survival and quality of life in patients with protracted recovery from cardiac surgery. Can we predict poor outcome? Eur J Cardiothorac Surg 9:426, 1995
4. Welsby IJ, Bennett-Guerrero E, Atwell D, et al: The association of complication type with mortality and prolonged stay after cardiac surgery with cardiopulmonary bypass. Anesth Analg 94:1072, 2002
5. Maze M, Scarfini C, Cavaliere F: New agents for sedation in the intensive care unit. Crit Care Clin 17:881, 2001
6. Young C, Knudsen N, Hilton A, Reves JG: Sedation in the intensive care unit. Crit Care Med 28:854, 2000
7. Shapiro BA, Warren J, Egol A, et al: Practice parameters for intravenous analgesia and sedation for adult patients in the intensive care unit: An executive summary. Crit Care Med 23:1596, 1995
8. Nasraway SA, Jacobi J, Murray MJ, Lumb PD: Sedation, analgesia, and neuromuscular blockade of the critically ill adult: Revised clinical practice guidelines for 2002. Crit Care Med 30:117, 2002
9. Murdoch S, Cohen A: Intensive care sedation: A review of current British practice. Intensive Care Med 26:922, 2000
10. Kollef MH, Levy NT, Ahrens TS, et al: The use of continuous i.v. sedation is associated with prolongation of mechanical ventilation. Chest 114:541, 1998
11. Kress JP, Pohlman AS, O'Conner MF, Hall JB: Daily interruption of sedative infusions in critically ill patients undergoing mechanical ventilation. N Engl J Med 342:1471, 2000
12. Brook AD, Ahrens TS, Schaiff R, et al: Effect of a nursing-implemented sedation protocol on the duration of mechanical ventilation. Crit Care Med 27:2609, 1999
13. Riker RR, Picard JT, Fraser GL: Prospective evaluation of the Sedation-Agitation Scale for adult critically ill patients. Crit Care Med 27:1325, 1999
14. Devlin JW, Boleski G, Mlynarek M, et al: Motor Activity Assessment Scale: A valid and reliable sedation scale for use with mechanically ventilated patients in the adult surgical intensive care unit. Crit Care Med 27:1271, 1999
15. Ramsey MA, Savege TM, Simpson BR, Goodwin R: Controlled sedation with alphaxalone-alphadolone. BMJ 2:656, 1974
16. Ely EW, Truman B, Shintani A, et al: Monitoring sedation status over time in ICU patients: Reliability and validity of the Richmond Agitation-Sedation Scale (RASS). JAMA 289:2983, 2003

17. Rosow C, Manberg PJ: Bispectral index monitoring. Anesthesiol Clin North Am 19:947, 2001
18. Triltsch AE, Welte M, von Homeyer P, et al: Bispectral index-guided sedation with dexmedetomidine in intensive care: A prospective, randomized, double-blind, placebo-controlled phase II study. Crit Care Med 30:1007, 2002
19. De Deyne C, Struys M, Decruyenaere J, et al: Use of continuous bispectral EEG monitoring to assess depth of sedation in ICU patients. Intensive Care Med 24:1294, 1998
20. Simmons LE, Riker RR, Prato BS, Fraser GL: Assessing sedation during intensive care unit mechanical ventilation with the bispectral index and the Sedation-Agitation Scale. Crit Care Med 27:1499, 1999
21. Shapiro BA: Bispectral Index: Better information for sedation in the intensive care unit? Crit Care Med 27:1663, 1999
22. Ostermann ME, Keenan SP, Seiferling RA, Sibbald WJ: Sedation in the intensive care unit: A systematic review. JAMA 283:1451, 2000
23. Tanelian DL, Kosek P, Mody I, MacIver MB: The role of the $GABA_A$ receptor/chloride channel complex in anesthesia. Anesthesiology 78:757, 1993
24. Greenblatt DJ, Shader RI, Divoll M, Harmatz JS: Benzodiazepines: A summary of pharmacokinetic properties. Br J Clin Pharmacol 11:11S, 1981
25. Dundee J, Halliday N, Fee JP: Midazolam in intensive care (letter). BMJ 289:1540, 1984
26. Woo E, Greenblatt DJ: Massive benzodiazepine requirements during acute alcohol withdrawal. Am J Psychiatry 136:821, 1979
27. Shelly MP, Sultan MA, Bodenham A, Park GR: Midazolam infusions in critically ill patients. Eur J Anaesthesiol 8:21, 1991
28. Bauer TM, Ritz R, Haberthür C, et al: Prolonged sedation due to accumulation of conjugated metabolites of midazolam. Lancet 346:145, 1995
29. Deppe SA, Sipperly ME, Sargent AI, et al: Intravenous lorazepam as an amnestic and anxiolytic agent in the intensive care unit: A prospective study. Crit Care Med 22:1248, 1994
30. Shapiro BA, Warren J, Egol AB, et al: Practice parameters for intravenous analgesia and sedation for adult patients in the intensive care unit: An executive summary. Crit Care Med 23:1596, 1995
31. Pohlman AS, Simpson KP, Hall JB: Continuous intravenous infusions of lorazepam versus midazolam for sedation during mechanical ventilatory support: A prospective, randomized study. Crit Care Med 22:1241, 1994
32. Te Wierik GH, Eissens AC, Lerk CF: Preparation, characterization, and pharmaceutical application of linear dextrins. III. Drug release from fatty suppository bases containing amylodextrin. Pharmaceut Res 11:108, 1994
33. Park GR, Navapurkar V, Ferenci P: The role of flumazenil in the critically ill. Acta Anaesthesiol Scand Suppl 108:23, 1995
34. Sebel PS, Lowdon JD: Propofol: A new intravenous anesthetic. Anesthesiology 71:260, 1989
35. Glen JB, Hunter SC: Pharmacology of an emulsion formulation of ICI 35 868. Br J Anaesth 56:617, 1984
36. Myles PS, Buckland MR, Weeks AM, et al: Hemodynamic effects, myocardial ischemia, and timing of tracheal extubation with propofol-based anesthesia for cardiac surgery. Anesth Analg 84:12, 1997
37. Parke TJ, Stevens JE, Rice AS, et al: Metabolic acidosis and fatal myocardial failure after propofol infusion in children: Five case reports. BMJ 305:613, 1992
38. Strickland RA, Murray MJ: Fatal metabolic acidosis in a pediatric patient receiving an infusion of propofol in the intensive care unit: Is there a relationship? Crit Care Med 23:405, 1995
39. Burow B, Johnson ME, Packer DL: Metabolic acidosis associated with propofol in the absence of other causative factors. Anesthesiology 101:239, 2004
40. Drummond JC, Iragui-Madoz VJ, Alksne JF, Kalkman CJ: Masking of epileptiform activity by propofol during seizure surgery. Anesthesiology 76:652, 1992
41. Au J, Walker WS, Scott DH: Withdrawal syndrome after propofol infusion. Anaesthesia 45:741, 1990
42. Sherry KM, McNamara J, Brown JS, Drummond M: An economic evaluation of propofol/fentanyl compared with midazolam/fentanyl on recovery in the ICU following cardiac surgery. Anaesthesia 51:312, 1996
43. Searle NR, Cote S, Taillefer J, et al: Propofol or midazolam for sedation and early extubation following cardiac surgery. Can J Anaesth 44:629, 1997
44. Herr DL, Sum-Ping ST, England M: ICU sedation after coronary artery bypass graft surgery: Dexmedetomidine-based versus propofol-based sedation regimens. J Cardiothorac Vasc Anesth 17:576, 2003
45. Murray MJ, Strickland RA, Weiler C: The use of neuromuscular blocking drugs in the intensive care unit: A U.S. perspective. Intensive Care Med 19:S40, 1993
46. Klessig HT, Geiger HJ, Murray MJ, Coursin DB: A national survey on the practice patterns of anesthesiologist intensivists in the use of muscle relaxants. Crit Care Med 20:1341, 1992
47. Shovelton DS: Reflections on an intensive therapy unit. BMJ 1:737, 1979
48. Murray MJ, Cowen J, DeBlock H, et al: Clinical practice guidelines for sustained neuromuscular blockade in the adult critically ill patient. Crit Care Med 30:142, 2002
49. Hund E: Myopathy in critically ill patients. Crit Care Med 27:2544, 1999
50. Alberti C, Brun-Buisson C, Burchardi H, et al: Epidemiology of sepsis and infection in ICU patients from an international multicentre cohort study. Intensive Care Med 28:108, 2002
51. Garland JS, Henrickson K, Maki DG: The 2002 Hospital Infection Control Practices Advisory Committee Centers for Disease Control and Prevention Guideline for Prevention of Intravascular Device-Related Infection. Pediatrics 110:1009, 2002
52. Maki DG, Weise CE, Sarafin HW: A semiquantitative culture method for identifying intravenous-catheter-related infection. N Engl J Med 296:1305, 1977
53. Maki DG: Yes, Virginia, aseptic technique is very important: Maximal barrier precautions during insertion reduce the risk of central venous catheter-related bacteremia. Infect Control Hosp Epidemiol 15:227, 1994
54. Linaraes J, Sitges-Serra A, Garau J, et al: Pathogenesis of catheter sepsis: A prospective study with quantitative and semiquantitative cultures of catheter hub and segments. J Clin Microbiol 21:357, 1985
55. Mermel LA, McCormick RD, Springman SR, Maki DG: The pathogenesis and epidemiology of catheter-related infection with pulmonary artery Swan-Ganz catheters: A prospective study utilizing molecular subtyping. Am J Med 91:197S, 1991
56. Raad II, Hanna HA: Intravascular catheter-related infections. New horizons and recent advances. Arch Intern Med 162:871, 2002
57. Sitges-Serra A, Puig P, Liñares J, et al: Hub colonization as the initial step in an outbreak of catheter-related sepsis due to coagulase negative Staphylococci during parenteral nutrition. JPEN 8:668, 1984
58. Siegman-Ingra Y, Anlim AM, Shapiro DE, et al: Diagnosis of vascular catheter-related bloodstream infection: A meta-analysis. J Clin Microbiol 35:928, 1997
59. Fidalgo S, Vazquez F, Mendoza MC, et al: Bacteremia due to Staphylococcus epidermidis: Microbiologic, epidemiologic, clinical, and prognostic features. Rev Inf Dis 12:520, 1990
60. Raad I, Davis S, Khan A, et al: Impact of central venous catheter removal on the recurrence of catheter-related coagulase-negative staphylococcal bacteremia. Infect Control Hosp Epidemiol 13:215, 1992
61. Raad I, Narro J, Khan A, et al: Serious complications of vascular catheter-related Staphylococcus aureus bacteremia in cancer patients. Eur J Clin Microbiol Infect Dis 11:675, 1992
62. Zacharias A, Habib RH: Factors predisposing to median sternotomy complications. Deep vs. superficial infection. Chest 110:1173, 1996
63. Roy MC: Surgical-site infections after coronary artery bypass graft surgery: Discriminating site-specific risk factors to improve prevention efforts. Infect Control Hosp Epidemiol 19:229, 1998
64. Mekontso-Dessap A, Kirsch M, Brun-Buisson C, Loisance D: Poststernotomy mediastinitis due to Staphylococcus aureus: Comparison of methicillin-resistant and methicillin-susceptible cases. Clin Infect Dis 32:877, 2001
65. Parisian Mediastinitis Group: Risk factors for deep sternal wound infections after sternotomy: A prospective, multicenter trial. J Thorac Cardiovasc Surg 111:1200, 1996
66. Hollenbeak CS, Murphy DM, Koenig S, et al: The clinical and economic impact of deep chest surgical site infections following coronary artery bypass graft surgery. Chest 118:397, 2000
67. Lazar HL, Fitzgerald C, Gross S, et al: Determinants of length of stay after coronary artery bypass graft surgery. Circulation 92:1120, 1995
68. Centers for Disease Control and Prevention: Nosocomial infection surveillance, 1980-1982. CDC Surveillance Summaries 32:1, 1983
69. Martorell C, Engelman R, Corl A, Brown RB: Surgical site infections in cardiac surgery: An 11-year perspective. Am J Infect Control 32:63, 2004
70. Edwards MB, Ratnatunga CP, Dore CJ, Taylor KM: Thirty-day mortality and long-term survival following surgery for prosthetic endocarditis: A study from the UK heart valve registry. Eur J Cardiothorac Surg 14:156, 1998
71. de Gevigney G, Pop C, Delahaye JP: The risk of infective endocarditis after cardiac surgical and interventional procedures. Eur Heart J 16:7, 1995
72. Grover FL, Cohen DJ, Oprian C, et al: Determinants of the occurrence of and survival from prosthetic valve endocarditis. J Thorac Cardiovasc Surg 108:207, 1994

73. Kuyvenhoven JP, Van Rijk-Zwikker GL, Hermans J, et al: Prosthetic valve endocarditis: Analysis of risk factors for mortality. Eur J Cardiothorac Surg 8:420, 1994
74. Vlessis AA, Khaki A, Grunkenmeuer GL, et al: Risk and diagnosis and management of prosthetic valve endocarditis: A review. J Heart Valve Dis 6:443, 1997
75. Arvay A, Lengyel M: Incidence and risk factors of prosthetic valve endocarditis. Eur J Cardiothorac Surg 2:340, 1988
76. Calderwood SB, Swinski LA, Waternaux CM, et al: Risk factors for the development of prosthetic valve endocarditis. Circulation 72:31, 1985
77. Rutledge R, Kim BJ, Applebaum RE: Actuarial analysis of the risk of prosthetic valve endocarditis in 1,598 patients with mechanical and bioprosthetic valves. Arch Surg 120:469, 1985
78. Ivert TS, Dismukes WE, Cobbs CG, et al: Prosthetic valve endocarditis. Circulation 69:223, 1984
79. Horstkotte D, Piper C, Niehues R, et al: Late prosthetic valve endocarditis. Eur Heart J 16:39, 1995
80. Agnihotri AK, McGiffin DC, Galbraith AJ, O'Brien MF: The prevalence of infective endocarditis after aortic valve replacement. J Thorac Cardiovasc Surg 110:1708, 1995
81. Ben Ismail M, Hannachi N, Abid F, et al: Prosthetic valve endocarditis. A survey. Br Heart J 58:72, 1987
82. Masur H, Johnson WD Jr: Prosthetic valve endocarditis. J Thorac Cardiovasc Surg 80:31, 1980
83. Tornos P, Sanz E, Permanyer-Miralda G, et al: Late prosthetic valve endocarditis. Immediate and long-term prognosis. Chest 101:37, 1992
84. Keyser DL, Biller J, Coffman TT, Adams HP Jr: Neurologic complications of late prosthetic valve endocarditis. Stroke 21:472, 1990
85. Vered Z, Mossinson D, Peleg E, et al: Echocardiographic assessment of prosthetic valve endocarditis. Eur Heart J 16:63, 1995
86. Daniel WG, Mugge A, Grote J, et al: Comparison of transthoracic and transesophageal echocardiography for detection of abnormalities of prosthetic and bioprosthetic valves in the mitral and aortic positions. Am J Cardiol 71:210, 1993
87. Morguet AJ, Werner GS, Andreas S, Kreuzer H: Diagnostic value of transesophageal compared with transthoracic echocardiography in suspected prosthetic valve endocarditis. Herz 20:390, 1995
88. Daniel WG, Mugge A, Martin RP, et al: Improvement in the diagnosis of abscesses associated with endocarditis by transesophageal echocardiography. N Engl J Med 324:795, 1991
89. Karchmur AW: Infections of prosthetic valves and intravascular devices. *In* Mandell GL, Bennett JE, Dolin R (eds): Principles and Practice of Infectious Disease, 5th edition, Vol 1. Philadelphia, Churchill Livingstone, 1999, pp 903–917
90. Calderwood SB, Swinski LA, Karchmer AW, et al: Prosthetic valve endocarditis: Analysis of factors affecting outcome of therapy. J Thorac Cardiovasc Surg 92:776, 1986
91. Yu VL, Fang GD, Keys TF, et al: Prosthetic valve endocarditis: Superiority of surgical valve replacement versus medical therapy only. Ann Thorac Surg 58:1073, 1994
92. Saffle JR, Gardner P, Schoenbaum SC, Wild W: Prosthetic valve endocarditis. The case for prompt valve replacement. J Thorac Cardiovasc Surg 73:416, 1977
93. Gordon SM, Serkey JM, Longworth DL, et al: Early onset prosthetic valve endocarditis: The Cleveland Clinic experience 1992-1997. Ann Thorac Surg 69:1388, 2000
94. Muckart DJ, Bhagwanjee S: American College of Chest Physicians/ Society of Critical Care Medicine Consensus Conference: Definition of the systemic inflammatory response syndrome and allied disorders in relation to critically injured patients. Crit Care Med 25:1789, 1997
95. Bone RC, Balk RA, Cerra FB, et al: Definitions for sepsis and organ failure and guidelines for the use of innovative therapies in sepsis. American College of Chest Physicians Society of Critical Care Medicine Consensus Conference Committee. Chest 101:1644, 1992
96. Orbach S, Weiss Y, Deutschman CS. The Patient with Sepsis or the Systemic Inflammatory Response Syndrome. *In* Murray MJ, Coursin DB, Pearl RG, Prough DS (eds): Critical Care Medicine. Perioperative Management, 2nd edition. Philadelphia, Lippincott Williams and Wilkins, 2002, pp 601–615
97. Natanson C: Selected treatment strategies for septic shock based on proposed mechanisms of pathogenesis. Ann Intern Med 271:226, 1994
98. Levy MM, Fink MP, Marshall JC, et al: 2001 SCCM/ESICM/ACCP/ ATS/SIS International Sepsis Definitions Conference. Crit Care Med 31:1250, 2003
99. Hotchkiss RS, Karl IE: The pathophysiology and treatment of sepsis. N Engl J Med 348:138, 2003
100. Landry DW, Oliver JA: The pathogenesis of vasodilatory shock. N Engl J Med 345:588, 2001
101. Matot I, Sprung CL: Definition of sepsis. Intensive Care Med 27:S3-S9, 2001
102. Dellinger RP, Carlet JM, Masur H, et al: Surviving sepsis campaign guidelines for the management of severe sepsis and septic shock. Crit Care Med 32:858, 2004
103. Laupland KB, Zygun DA, Davies HD, et al: Incidence and risk factors for acquiring nosocomial urinary tract infection in the critically ill. J Crit Care 17:50, 2002
104. Marik PE: Fever in the ICU. Chest 117:855, 2000
105. Platt R, Polk BF, Murdock B, Rosner B: Mortality associated with nosocomial urinary-tract infection. N Engl J Med 307:637, 1982
106. Stark RP, Maki DG: Bacteriuria in the catheterized patient. What quantitative level of bacteriuria is relevant? N Engl J Med 311:560, 1984
107. Brown DF, Warren RE: Effect of sample volume on yield of positive blood cultures from adult patients with hematological malignancy. J Clin Pathol 43:777, 1990
108. Warren JW: Catheter-associated urinary tract infections. Infect Dis Clin North Am 11:609, 1997
109. Warren JW, Platt R, Thomas RJ, et al: Antibiotic irrigation and catheter-associated urinary-tract infections. N Engl J Med 299:570, 1978
110. Sandock DS, Gothe BG, Bodner DR: Trimethoprim-sulfamethoxazole prophylaxis against urinary tract infection in the chronic spinal cord injury patient. Paraplegia 33:156, 1995
111. Karchmer TB, Giannetta ER, Muto CA, et al: A randomized crossover study of silver-coated urinary catheters in hospitalized patients. Arch Intern Med 160:3294, 2000
112. Hall IC, O'Toole E: Intestinal flora in newborn infants with a description of a new pathogenic anaerobe Bacillus difficilis. Am J Dis Child 49:390, 1935
113. George RH, Symonds JM, Dimock F, et al: Identification of Clostridium difficile as a cause of pseudomembranous colitis. Br Med J 1:695, 1978
114. Bartlett JG, Moon N, Chang TW, et al: Role of Clostridium difficile in antibiotic-associated pseudomembranous colitis. Gastroenterology 75:778, 1978
115. Thomas C, Stevenson M, Riley TV: Antibiotics and hospital-acquired Clostridium difficile-associated diarrhoea: A systematic review. J Antimicrob Chemother 51:1339, 2003
116. Kyne L, Warny M, Qamar A, Kelly CP: Asymptomatic carriage of Clostridium difficile and serum levels of IgG antibody against toxin A. N Engl J Med 342:390, 2000
117. Kyne L, Warny M, Qamar A, Kelly CP: Association between antibody response to toxin A and protection against recurrent Clostridium difficile diarrhoea. Lancet 357:189, 2001
118. McFarland LV, Mulligan ME, Kwok RY, Stamm WE: Nosocomial acquisition of Clostridium difficile infection. N Engl J Med 320:204, 1989
119. Cunningham R, Dale B, Undy B, Gaunt N: Proton pump inhibitors as a risk factor for Clostridium difficile diarrhoea. J Hosp Infect 54:243, 2003
120. Kyne L, Sougioultzis S, McFarland LV, Kelly CP: Underlying disease severity as a major risk factor for nosocomial Clostridium difficile diarrhea. Infect Control Hosp Epidemiol 23:653, 2002
121. Riegler M, Sedivy R, Pothoulakis C, et al: Clostridium difficile toxin B is more potent than toxin A in damaging human colonic epithelium in vitro. J Clin Invest 95:2004, 1995
122. Samore MH, Venkataraman L, DeGirolami PC, et al: Clinical and molecular epidemiology of sporadic and clustered cases of nosocomial Clostridium difficile diarrhea. Am J Med 100:32, 1996
123. Johnson S, Samore MH, Farrow KA, et al: Epidemics of diarrhea caused by a clindamycin-resistant strain of Clostridium difficile in four hospitals. N Engl J Med 341:1645, 1999
124. Kelly CP, Pothoulakis C, LaMont JT: Clostridium difficile colitis. N Engl J Med 330:257, 1994
125. Rao SS, Edwards CA, Austen CJ, et al: Impaired colonic fermentation of carbohydrate after ampicillin. Gastroenterology 94:928, 1988
126. Bartlett JG: Clinical practice. Antibiotic-associated diarrhea. N Engl J Med 346:334, 2002
127. Tedesco FJ: Antibiotic associated pseudomembranous colitis with negative proctosigmoidoscopy examination. Gastroenterology 77:295, 1979
128. Triadafilopoulos G, Hallstone AE: Acute abdomen as the first presentation of pseudomembranous colitis. Gastroenterology 101:685, 1991
129. Wenisch C, Parschalk B, Hasenhundl M, et al: Comparison of vancomycin, teicoplanin, metronidazole, and fusidic acid for the treatment of Clostridium difficile-associated diarrhea. Clin Infect Dis 22:813, 1996
130. Bolton RP, Culshaw MA: Faecal metronidazole concentrations during oral and intravenous therapy for antibiotic associated colitis due to Clostridium difficile. Gut 27:1169, 1986

131. Grindlinger GA, Niehoff J, Hughes L, et al: Acute paranasal sinusitis related to nasotracheal intubation of head-injured patients. Crit Care Med 15:214, 1987
132. Deutschman CS, Wilton P, Sinow J, et al: Paranasal sinusitis associated with nasotracheal intubation: A frequently unrecognized and treatable source of sepsis. Crit Care Med 14:111, 1986
133. Rouby JJ, Laurent P, Gosnach M, et al: Risk factors and clinical relevance of nosocomial maxillary sinusitis in the critically ill. Am J Respir Crit Care Med 150:776, 1994
134. Fassoulaki A, Pamouktsoglou P: Prolonged nasotracheal intubation and its association with inflammation of paranasal sinuses. Anesth Analg 69:50, 1989
135. Leal-Noval SR, Rincón-Ferrari MD, García-Curiel A, et al: Transfusion of blood components and postoperative infection in patients undergoing cardiac surgery. Chest 119:1461, 2001
136. Mezrow CK, Bergstein I, Tartter PI: Postoperative infections after autologous and homologous blood transfusions. Transfusion 32:27, 1992
137. Gu YJ, de Vries AJ, Boonstra PW, van Oeveren W: Leukocyte depletion results in improved lung function and reduced inflammatory response after cardiac surgery. J Thorac Cardiovasc Surg 112:494, 1996
138. Goodnough LT, Despotis GJ, Hogue CW Jr, Ferguson TB Jr: On the need for improved transfusion indicators in cardiac surgery. Ann Thorac Surg 60:473, 1995
139. van de Watering LM, Hermans J, Houbiers JG, et al: Beneficial effects of leukocyte depletion of transfused blood on postoperative complications in patients undergoing cardiac surgery: A randomized clinical trial. Circulation 97:562, 1998
140. Blumberg N, Heal J: Transfusion and recipient immune function. Arch Pathol Lab Med 113:246, 1989
141. Weisel RD, Charlesworth DC, Mickleborough LL, et al: Limitations of blood conservation. J Thorac Cardiovasc Surg 88:26, 1984
142. Hebert PC, Wells G, Blajchman MA, et al: A multicenter, randomized, controlled clinical trial of transfusion requirements in critical care. Transfusion Requirements in Critical Care Investigators: Canadian Critical Care Trials Group. N Engl J Med 340:409, 1999
143. Johnson RG, Thurer RL, Kruskall MS, et al: Comparison of two transfusion strategies after elective operations for myocardial revascularization. J Thorac Cardiovasc Surg 104:307, 1992
144. Rao SV, Jollis JG, Harrington RA, et al: Relationship of blood transfusion and clinical outcomes in patients with acute coronary syndromes. JAMA 292:1555, 2004
145. Bellomo R, Kellum JA, Ronco C: Defining acute renal failure: Physiologic principles. Intensive Care Med 30:33, 2004
146. Lee HT, Sladen RN: Perioperative renal protection. *In* Murray MJ, Coursin DB, Pearl RG, Prough DS (eds): Critical Care Medicine. Perioperative Management, 2nd edition. Philadelphia, Lippincott Williams and Wilkins, 2002, pp 501–520
147. Block CA, Manning HL: Prevention of acute renal failure in the critically ill. Am J Resp Crit Care Med 165:320, 2002
148. Chertow GM, Levy EM, Hammermeister KE, et al: Independent association between acute renal failure and mortality following cardiac surgery. Am J Med 104:343, 1998
149. Conlon PJ, Stafford-Smith M, White WD, et al: Acute renal failure following cardiac surgery. Nephrol Dial Transplant 14:1158, 1999
150. Higgins TL, Estafanous FG, Loop FD, et al: Stratification of morbidity and mortality outcome by preoperative risk factors in coronary bypass patients. A clinical severity score. JAMA 267:2344, 1992
151. Hilberman M, Derby GC, Spencer RJ, et al: Sequential pathophysiological changes characterizing the progression from renal dysfunction to acute renal failure following cardiac operation. J Thorac Cardiovasc Surg 79:838, 1980
152. Murray P, Hall J: Renal replacement therapy for acute renal failure. Am J Respir Crit Care Med 162:777, 2000
153. Baldwin L, Henderson A, Hickman P: Effect of postoperative low-dose dopamine on renal function after elective major vascular surgery. Ann Intern Med 120:744, 1994
154. Lassnigg A, Donner E, Grubhofer G, et al: Lack of renoprotective effects of dopamine and furosemide during cardiac surgery. J Am Soc Nephrol 11:97, 2000
155. Sward K, Valsson F, Odencrants P, et al: Recombinant human atrial natriuretic peptide in ischemic acute renal failure: A randomized placebo-controlled trial. Crit Care Med 32:1310, 2004
156. de Denus S, Pharand C, Williamson DR: Brain natriuretic peptide in the management of heart failure: the versatile neurohormone. Chest 125:652, 2004
157. Bellomo R, Ronco C: Continuous renal replacement therapy in the intensive care unit. Intensive Care Med 25:781, 1999
158. Forni LG, Hilton PJ: Continuous hemofiltration in the treatment of acute renal failure. N Engl J Med 336:1303, 1997
159. Silvester W: Outcome studies of continuous renal replacement therapies in the intensive care unit. Kidney Int 53:S138-S141, 1998
160. Lewis J, Chertow GM, Paganini EP, et al: A multicenter survey of patient characteristics, practice patterns, and outcomes in critically ill patients with ARF (abstract). J Am Soc Nephrol 8:A0673, 2000
161. Mehta RL, Letteri JM: Current status of renal replacement therapy for acute renal failure: A survey of US nephrologists. The Kidney Foundation Council on Dialysis. Am J Nephrol 19:377, 1999
162. Butterworth CE Jr: Malnutrition in the hospital (editorial). JAMA 230:879, 1974
163. The Scientific Committee, Malnutrition Conference: The skeleton in the hospital closet—20 Years later: Malnutrition in patients with GI disease, cancer, and AIDS—Diagnosis, frequency, treatment and outcome (editorial). Nutrition 9:558, 1993
164. Blackburn GL, Ahmad A: Skeleton in the hospital closet—Then and now. Nutrition 11:193, 1995
165. Hirsch S, de Obaldia N, Petermann M, et al: Subjective global assessment of nutritional status: Further validation. Nutrition 7:35, 1991
166. Kompan L, Kremzar B, Gadzijev E, Prosek M: Effects of early enteral nutrition on intestinal permeability and the development of multiple organ failure after multiple injury. Intensive Care Med 25:157, 1999
167. O'Grady NP, Alexander M, Dellinger EP, et al: Guidelines for the prevention of intravascular catheter-related infections. CDC Morbidity and Mortality Weekly Report, Vol 51; August 9, 2002. Available at http://www.cdc.gov/mmwr/PDF/RR/RR5110.pdf
168. Murray MJ, Brull SJ, Coursin DB: Strict blood glucose control in the ICU: Panacea or Pandora's box? (editorial) Cardiothorac Vasc Anesth 2004
169. Wilmore D: Enteral and parenteral arginine supplementation to improve medical outcomes in hospitalized patients. J Nutr 134:2863S-2867S, 2004
170. Bistrian BR: Practical recommendations for immune-enhancing diets. J Nutr 134:2868S, 2004

Chapter 37

PAIN MANAGEMENT FOR THE POSTOPERATIVE CARDIAC PATIENT

Mark A. Chaney, MD

KEY POINTS

1. Inadequate postoperative analgesia and/or an uninhibited perioperative surgical stress response has the potential to initiate pathophysiologic changes in all major organ systems, including the cardiovascular, pulmonary, gastrointestinal, renal, endocrine, immunologic, and/or central nervous systems, all of which may lead to substantial postoperative morbidity. Adequate postoperative analgesia prevents unnecessary patient discomfort, may decrease morbidity, may decrease postoperative hospital length of stay, and thus may decrease cost.
2. Pain following cardiac surgery may be intense and originates from many sources, including the incision (sternotomy or thoracotomy), intraoperative tissue retraction and dissection, vascular cannulation sites, vein-harvesting sites, and chest tubes, among others. Achieving optimal pain relief following cardiac surgery is often difficult, yet may be attained via a wide variety of techniques, including local anesthetic infiltration, nerve blocks, intravenous agents, intrathecal techniques, and epidural techniques.
3. Traditionally, analgesia following cardiac surgery has been obtained with intravenous opioids (specifically morphine). However, intravenous opioid use is associated with definite detrimental side effects (nausea/vomiting, pruritus, urinary retention, respiratory depression) and longer-acting opioids such as morphine may delay tracheal extubation during the immediate postoperative period via excessive sedation and/or respiratory depression. Thus, in the current era of early extubation ("fast-tracking"), cardiac anesthesiologists are exploring unique options other than traditional intravenous opioids for control of postoperative pain in patients following cardiac surgery.
4. While patient-controlled analgesia is a well-established technique (used for more than two decades) and offers potential unique benefits (reliable analgesic effect, improved patient autonomy, flexible adjustment to individual needs, etc.), whether it truly offers significant clinical advantages (compared with traditional nurse-administrated analgesic techniques) to patients immediately following cardiac surgery remains to be determined.
5. Cyclooxygenase (COX)-2 inhibitors possess analgesic (opioid-sparing) effects and lack deleterious effects on coagulation (in contrast to nonselective nonsteroidal anti-inflammatory drugs [NSAIDs]). However, current evidence does not suggest that COX-2 inhibitors provide major advantages over traditional NSAIDs. Furthermore, potential links between this class of drugs and cardiovascular complications, sternal wound infections, and thromboembolic complications need to be fully evaluated.
6. Administration of intrathecal morphine to patients initiates reliable postoperative analgesia following cardiac surgery. Intrathecal opioids or local anesthetics cannot reliably attenuate the perioperative stress response associated with cardiac surgery that persists during the immediate postoperative period. Although intrathecal local anesthetics (not opioids) may induce perioperative thoracic cardiac sympathectomy, the hemodynamic changes associated with a "total spinal" make the technique unpalatable in patients with cardiac disease.
7. Administration of thoracic epidural opioids or local anesthetics to patients initiates reliable postoperative analgesia following cardiac surgery. The quality of analgesia obtained with thoracic epidural anesthetic techniques is sufficient to allow cardiac surgery to be performed in "awake" patients (without general endotracheal anesthesia). Administration of thoracic epidural local anesthetics (not opioids) can both reliably attenuate the perioperative stress response associated with cardiac surgery that persists during the immediate postoperative period and induce perioperative thoracic cardiac sympathectomy.
8. Use of intrathecal and epidural techniques in patients undergoing cardiac surgery, while seemingly increasing in popularity, remains extremely controversial. Concerns regarding hematoma risk and the fact that the numerous clinical investigations regarding this topic are suboptimally designed and utilize a wide array of disparate techniques have prevented clinically useful conclusions.
9. As a general rule, it is best to avoid intense, single-modality therapy for the treatment of acute postoperative pain. The administration of two analgesic agents that act by different mechanisms ("multimodal" or "balanced" analgesia) provides superior analgesic efficacy with equivalent or reduced adverse effects. Analgesic therapies should be used only after thoughtful consideration of the risks and benefits for each individual patient. The therapy (or therapies) selected should reflect the individual anesthesiologist's expertise, as well as the capacity for safe application of the chosen modality in each practice setting. The choice of medication, dose, route, and duration of therapy should always be individualized.

Adequate postoperative analgesia prevents unnecessary patient discomfort, may decrease morbidity, may decrease postoperative hospital length of stay, and thus may decrease cost. Because postoperative pain management has been deemed important, the American Society of Anesthesiologists has published practice guidelines regarding this topic.[1] Furthermore, in recognition of the need for improved pain management, the Joint Commission on Accreditation of Healthcare Organizations has developed new standards for the assessment and management of pain in accredited hospitals and other health care settings.[2] Patient satisfaction (no doubt linked to adequacy of postoperative analgesia) has become an essential element that influences clinical activity of not only anesthesiologists but also all health care professionals.

Achieving optimal pain relief following cardiac surgery is often difficult. Pain may be associated with many interventions, including sternotomy, thoracotomy, leg vein harvesting, pericardiotomy, and/or chest tube insertion, among others. Inadequate analgesia and/or an uninhibited stress response during the postoperative period may increase morbidity by

Table 37–1 **Techniques Available for Postoperative Analgesia**
• Local anesthetic infiltration
• Nerve blocks
• Opioids
• Nonsteroidal anti-inflammatory agents
• α-Adrenergic agents
• Intrathecal techniques
• Epidural techniques
• Multimodal analgesia

causing adverse hemodynamic, metabolic, immunologic, and hemostatic alterations.[3-5] Aggressive control of postoperative pain, associated with an attenuated stress response, may decrease morbidity and mortality in high-risk patients following noncardiac surgery[6,7] and may also decrease morbidity and mortality in patients following cardiac surgery.[8,9] Adequate postoperative analgesia may be attained via a wide variety of techniques (Table 37–1). Traditionally, analgesia following cardiac surgery has been obtained with intravenous opioids (specifically morphine). However, intravenous opioid use is associated with definite detrimental side effects (nausea/vomiting, pruritus, urinary retention, respiratory depression), and longer-acting opioids such as morphine may delay tracheal extubation during the immediate postoperative period via excessive sedation and/or respiratory depression. Thus, in the current era of early extubation ("fast-tracking"), cardiac anesthesiologists are exploring unique options other than traditional intravenous opioids for control of postoperative pain in patients following cardiac surgery.[10,11] No single technique is clearly superior; each possesses distinct advantages and disadvantages. It is becoming increasingly clear that a multimodal approach/combined analgesic regimen (utilizing a variety of techniques) is likely the best way to approach postoperative pain (in all patients following surgery) in order to maximize analgesia and minimize side effects. When addressing postoperative analgesia in cardiac surgical patients, choice of technique (or techniques) is made only after a thorough analysis of the risk/benefit ratio of each technique in the specific patient in whom analgesia is desired.

PAIN AND CARDIAC SURGERY

Surgical or traumatic injury initiates changes in the peripheral and central nervous systems that must be addressed therapeutically in order to promote postoperative analgesia and,

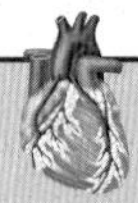

BOX 37–1 ***Pain and Cardiac Surgery***

- Originates from many sources
- Most commonly originates from chest wall
- Preoperative expectations influence postoperative satisfaction
- Quality of postoperative analgesia may influence morbidity/mortality

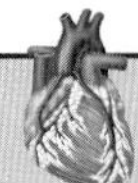

BOX 37–2 ***Potential Clinical Benefits of Adequate Postoperative Analgesia***

- Hemodynamic stability
- Metabolic stability
- Immunologic stability
- Hemostatic stability
- Stress response attenuation
- Decreased morbidity/mortality

it is hoped, positively influence clinical outcome (Boxes 37–1 and 37–2). The physical processes of incision, traction, and cutting of tissues stimulate free nerve endings and a wide variety of specific nociceptors. Receptor activation and activity are further modified by the local release of chemical mediators of inflammation and sympathetic amines released via the perioperative surgical stress response. The perioperative surgical stress response peaks during the immediate postoperative period and exerts major effects on many physiologic processes. The potential clinical benefits of attenuating the perioperative surgical stress response (above and beyond simply attaining adequate clinical analgesia) have received much attention during the past decade and remain fairly controversial.[12] However, it is clear that inadequate postoperative analgesia and/or an uninhibited perioperative surgical stress response has the potential to initiate pathophysiologic changes in all major organ systems, including the cardiovascular, pulmonary, gastrointestinal, renal, endocrine, immunologic, and/or central nervous systems, all of which may lead to substantial postoperative morbidity.

Pain following cardiac surgery may be intense and originates from many sources, including the incision (sternotomy, thoracotomy, etc.), intraoperative tissue retraction and dissection, vascular cannulation sites, vein-harvesting sites, and chest tubes, among others.[13,14] Patients in whom an internal mammary artery is surgically exposed and used as a bypass graft may have substantially more postoperative pain.[15]

A prospective clinical investigation involving 200 consecutive patients undergoing cardiac surgery via median sternotomy assessed the location, distribution, and intensity of postoperative pain.[13] All patients received 25 to 50 μg/kg of intraoperative intravenous fentanyl, were subjected to routine cardiopulmonary bypass (CPB), had their arms positioned along their body on the operating table, had their sternum closed with five peristernal wires, and received mediastinal and thoracic drains passed through the rectus abdominis muscle just below the xiphoid. A subgroup (127 patients) also underwent long saphenous vein harvesting either from the calf (men) or thigh (women). All patients were extubated before the first postoperative morning. Postoperative analgesic management was standardized and included intravenous morphine, oral paracetamol, oral tramadol, and subcutaneous morphine. Pain location, distribution, and intensity were documented in the morning on the first, second, third, and seventh postoperative days using a standardized picture dividing the body into 32 anatomic areas. A numerical rating scale of 0 to 10 (with 0 representing no pain and 10 representing worst possible pain) was used to assess maximal pain intensity.

These investigators found that maximal pain intensity was highest on the first postoperative day and lowest on the third postoperative day. However, maximal pain intensity was only graded as "moderate" (mean pain score was approximately 3.8) and did not diminish during the first two postoperative days yet started to decline between postoperative days 2 and 3. Pain distribution did not appear to vary throughout the postoperative period, yet location did (more shoulder pain observed on the seventh postoperative day). As time from operation increased, pain usually moved from primarily incisional/epigastric to osteoarticular. Another source of postoperative pain in patients following cardiac surgery is thoracic cage rib fractures, which may be common.[16,17] Furthermore, sternal retraction, causing posterior rib fracture, may lead to brachial plexus injury. In these patients, routine chest radiographs may be normal despite the presence of fracture. Thus, bone scans (better at detecting rib fractures than chest radiographs) are recommended whenever there is unexplained postoperative nonincisional pain in a patient who has undergone sternal retraction.[17] Other studies have indicated that the most common source of pain in patients following cardiac surgery is the chest wall. Age also appears to impact pain intensity; patients younger than 60 often have higher pain intensity than patients older than 60. While maximal pain intensity following cardiac surgery is usually only moderate, there remains ample room for clinical improvement in analgesic control to minimize pain intensity, especially during the first few postoperative days.

Persistent pain following cardiac surgery, while rare, can be problematic.[18-20] The cause of persistent pain following sternotomy is multifactorial, yet tissue destruction, intercostal nerve trauma, scar formation, rib fractures, sternal infection, stainless-steel wire sutures, and/or costochondral separation may all play roles. Such chronic pain is often localized to the arms, shoulders, or legs. Postoperative brachial plexus neuropathies may also occur and have been attributed to rib fracture fragments, internal mammary artery dissection, suboptimal positioning of patients during surgery, and/or central venous catheter placement. Postoperative neuralgia of the saphenous nerve has also been reported following harvesting of saphenous veins for coronary artery bypass grafting (CABG). Younger patients appear to be at higher risk for developing chronic, long-lasting pain. The correlation of severity of acute postoperative pain and development of chronic pain syndromes has been suggested (patients requiring more postoperative analgesics may be more likely to develop chronic pain), yet the causative relationship is still vague.

Ho and associates[18] assessed via survey 244 patients following cardiac surgery and median sternotomy and found that persistent pain (defined as pain still present 2 or more months following surgery) was reported in almost 30% of patients. The incidence of persistent pain at any site was 29% (71 patients), and for sternotomy was 25% (61 patients). Other common locations of persistent pain reported to these investigators were the shoulders (17.4%), back (15.9%), and neck (5.8%). However, such persistent pain was usually reported as mild, with only 7% of patients reporting interference with daily living. The most common words used to describe the persistent pain were "annoying" (57%), "nagging" (33%), "dull" (30%), "sharp" (25%), "tiring" (22%), "tender" (22%), and "tight" (22%). The temporal nature of this pain was mostly reported as being brief/transient and periodic/intermittent. Twenty patients (8%) also described symptoms of numbness, burning pain, and tenderness over the internal mammary artery–harvesting site, symptoms suggestive of internal mammary artery syndrome. Thus, Ho and associates conclude that mild persistent pain following cardiac surgery and median sternotomy is common yet only infrequently substantially interferes with daily life.

While the most common source of pain in patients following cardiac surgery remains the chest wall, leg pain from vein graft harvesting can be problematic as well. Such pain may not become apparent until the late postoperative period, which may be related to the progression of patient mobilization as well as the decreasing impact of sternotomy pain (unmasking leg incisional pain). The recent utilization of minimally invasive vein graft harvesting techniques (endoscopic vein graft harvesting) decreases postoperative leg pain intensity and duration compared with conventional open techniques.[21] While initial harvest times may be prolonged, harvest times become equivalent between the two techniques (endoscopic versus conventional) once a short learning curve is overcome. Furthermore, leg morbidity (infection, dehiscence, etc.) may be less in patients undergoing endoscopic vein harvest compared with patients undergoing conventional open techniques because of different incisional lengths.

Patient satisfaction with quality of postoperative analgesia is as much related to the comparison between anticipated and experienced pain as it is to the actual level of pain experienced. Satisfaction is related to a situation that is better than predicted, dissatisfaction to one that is worse than expected. Patients undergoing cardiac surgery remain concerned regarding the adequacy of postoperative pain relief and tend to preoperatively expect a greater amount of postoperative pain than that which is actually experienced.[14] Because of these unique preoperative expectations, patients following cardiac surgery who receive only moderate analgesia postoperatively will likely still be satisfied with their pain control. Thus, patients may experience pain of moderate intensity after cardiac surgery yet still express very high satisfaction levels.[14,15]

Scientific advances have allowed a better understanding of how and why pain occurs, leading to unique, and possibly clinically beneficial, pain management strategies. Clinicians now know that noxious input from acute injury may trigger a state of central nervous system sensitization, called "wind-up." In essence, dorsal horn neurotransmitter release via nociceptive input conditions the central nervous system such that there is enhanced responsiveness (secondary hyperalgesia). While experimental evidence exists indicating that enhanced responsiveness outlasts the initial provocative insult (induced sensitivity outlasts stimulus), the exact clinical relevance remains to be determined. Advances regarding spinal cord neuropharmacology have led to research aimed at modifying or blocking *N*-methyl-D-aspartate (NMDA) receptors to influence pain control and to the concept of preemptive analgesia. The concept of preemptive analgesia is predicated on addressing pain before it initiates peripheral and central sensitization. However, given the redundancy in the neurotransmitter–receptor systems in the central nervous system, it is unlikely that blocking only one component will result in clear clinical benefits. While the use of NMDA-receptor antagonists and the concept of preemptive analgesia are intriguing and certain clinical investigations appear to support their utility, clear and definite clinical benefits in humans remain to be determined. Debate continues over the potential benefits of NMDA-receptor antagonists and the utility of preemptive analgesic treatment as well as direction in which research and conceptual development in this exciting field need to proceed.

POTENTIAL CLINICAL BENEFITS OF ADEQUATE POSTOPERATIVE ANALGESIA

Inadequate analgesia (coupled with an uninhibited stress response) during the postoperative period may lead to many adverse hemodynamic (tachycardia, hypertension, vasoconstriction), metabolic (increased catabolism), immunologic (impaired immune response), and hemostatic (platelet activation) alterations. In patients undergoing cardiac surgery, perioperative myocardial ischemia (diagnosed by electrocardiography and/or transesophageal echocardiography) is most commonly observed during the immediate postoperative period and appears to be related to outcome.[22,23] Intraoperatively, initiation of CPB causes substantial increases in stress response hormones (norepinephrine, epinephrine, etc.) that persist into the immediate postoperative period and may contribute to myocardial ischemia observed during this time.[24-26] Furthermore, postoperative myocardial ischemia may be aggravated by cardiac sympathetic nerve activation, which disrupts the balance between coronary blood flow and myocardial oxygen demand.[27] Thus, during the pivotal immediate postoperative period after cardiac surgery, adequate analgesia (coupled with stress-response attenuation) may potentially decrease morbidity and enhance health-related quality of life.[27,28]

Evidence exists indicating that aggressive control of postoperative pain in patients following noncardiac surgery may beneficially affect outcome.[6,7] In 1987, Yeager and associates[7] in a small (n = 53 patients) randomized, controlled clinical trial involving patients undergoing major thoracic/vascular surgery revealed that patients who were managed to receive more intense perioperative anesthesia and analgesia demonstrated decreased postoperative morbidity and improved operative outcome. In 1991, Tuman and associates[6] in another small (n = 80 patients) randomized, controlled clinical trial involving patients undergoing lower extremity revascularization revealed that patients who were managed to receive more intense perioperative anesthesia and analgesia demonstrated improved outcome compared with patients receiving routine on-demand narcotic analgesia.

Evidence also exists that aggressive control of postoperative pain in patients following cardiac surgery may beneficially affect outcome. Two intriguing clinical investigations published in 1992 hint at such possibilities.[8,9] Mangano and associates[8] prospectively randomized 106 adult patients undergoing elective CABG to receive either standard postoperative analgesia or intensive analgesia during the immediate postoperative period. Standard care patients received low-dose intermittent intravenous morphine for the first 18 postoperative hours, whereas intensive analgesia patients received a continuous intravenous sufentanil infusion during the same time period. Patients receiving sufentanil demonstrated a lesser severity of myocardial ischemia episodes (detected by continuous electrocardiographic monitoring) during the immediate postoperative period. The authors postulate that the administration of intensive analgesia during the immediate postoperative period may have more completely suppressed sympathetic nervous system activation, thereby having numerous beneficial clinical effects, including beneficial alterations in sensitivity of platelets to epinephrine, beneficial alterations in fibrinolysis, enhanced regional left ventricular function, and decreased coronary artery vasoconstriction, all potentially leading to a reduced incidence/severity of myocardial ischemia. Anand and Hickey[9] prospectively randomized 45 neonates undergoing elective cardiac surgery (mixed procedures) to receive either standard perioperative care or deep opioid anesthesia. Standard care patients received a halothane/ketamine/morphine anesthetic with intermittent intravenous morphine for the first 24 postoperative hours, whereas deep opioid patients received an intravenous sufentanil anesthetic with a continuous infusion of either intravenous fentanyl or intravenous sufentanil during the same postoperative time period. Neonates receiving continuous postoperative opioid infusions demonstrated a reduced perioperative stress response (assessed via multiple blood mediators), less perioperative morbidity (hyperglycemia, lactic acidemia, sepsis, metabolic acidosis, disseminated intravascular coagulation), and significantly fewer deaths than the control group (0 of 30 versus 4 of 15, respectively; $p < 0.01$).

The accompanying editorial accurately summarizes this clinical investigation: "What Anand and Hickey have shown is that this reluctance to treat pain adequately is not a necessary evil. It markedly contributes to a bad outcome."[29] Unfortunately, aggressive control of postoperative pain in patients following cardiac surgery with relatively large amounts of intravenous opioids in this manner does not allow tracheal extubation in the immediate postoperative period (a goal of current practice).

TECHNIQUES AVAILABLE FOR POSTOPERATIVE ANALGESIA

While the mechanisms of postoperative pain and the pharmacology of analgesic drugs are relatively well understood, the delivery of effective postoperative analgesia remains far from universal. Many techniques are available (see Table 37–1). In general, the American Society of Anesthesiologists Task Force on Acute Pain Management in the Perioperative Setting reports that the existing literature supports the efficacy and safety of three techniques used by anesthesiologists for perioperative pain control: regional analgesic techniques (including but not limited to intercostal blocks, plexus blocks, and local anesthetic infiltration of incisions), patient-controlled analgesia (PCA) with systemic opioids, and intrathecal/epidural opioid analgesia.[1] Regarding regional analgesic techniques, the existing literature supports the analgesic efficacy of peripheral nerve blocks and postincisional infiltration with local anesthetics for postoperative analgesia yet is equivocal regarding the analgesic benefits of preincisional infiltration. Regarding PCA with systemic opioids, the existing literature supports its efficacy (compared with intramuscular techniques) for postoperative pain management yet the existing literature is equivocal regarding the efficacy of PCA techniques compared with nurse- or staff-administered intravenous analgesia. In addition, the existing literature is equivocal regarding the comparative efficacy of epidural PCA versus intravenous PCA techniques.

When background opioid infusions are included with PCA techniques, patients report better analgesia and higher morphine consumption without increased incidence of nausea, vomiting, pruritus, or sedation. Although higher morphine consumption during PCA with continuous background infusion might predispose patients to respiratory depression, the existing literature is insufficient to reveal this potential adverse effect. Last, regarding intrathecal and epidural opioid analgesia, the existing literature supports the efficacy of epidural

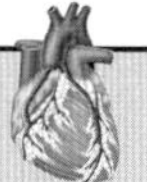

BOX 37–3 *Local Anesthetic Infiltration*

- Advantage: Simple, reliable analgesia
- Disadvantage: Tissue necrosis?

morphine and fentanyl for perioperative analgesia but is insufficient to characterize the spectrum of risks and benefits associated with the use of other specific opioids given by these routes. Pruritus and urinary retention occur more frequently when morphine is given intrathecally or epidurally compared with systemic (intravenous or intramuscular) administration. Furthermore, epidural morphine provides more effective pain relief than intramuscular morphine. Similarly, epidural fentanyl provides more effective postoperative analgesia than intravenous fentanyl. The existing literature is insufficient to evaluate the effects of epidural techniques administered at different times (preincisional, postincisional, postoperative).

LOCAL ANESTHETIC INFILTRATION

Pain following cardiac surgery is often related to median sternotomy (peaking during the first 2 postoperative days). Because of problems associated with traditional intravenous opioid analgesia (nausea and vomiting, pruritus, urinary retention, respiratory depression) and the more recently introduced nonsteroidal anti-inflammatory drugs (NSAIDs) and cyclooxygenase (COX) inhibitors (gastrointestinal bleeding, renal dysfunction), alternative methods of achieving postoperative analgesia in cardiac surgical patients have been sought. One such alternative method that may hold promise is continuous infusion of local anesthetic (Box 37–3). In a prospective, randomized, placebo-controlled, double-blind clinical trial, White and associates[30] studied 36 patients undergoing cardiac surgery. Intraoperative management was standardized. All patients had two indwelling infusion catheters placed at the median sternotomy incision site at the end of surgery (one in the subfascial plane above the sternum, one above the fascia in the subcutaneous tissue). Patients received 0.25% bupivacaine (n = 12), 0.5% bupivacaine (n = 12), or normal saline (n = 12) via a constant rate, infusion through the catheter (4 mL/hr) for 48 hours following surgery. Average times to tracheal extubation were similar in the three groups (approximately 5 to 6 hours). Compared with the control group (normal saline), there was a statistically significant reduction in verbal rating scale pain scores and intravenous PCA morphine use in the 0.5% bupivacaine group. Patient satisfaction with their pain management was also improved in the 0.5% bupivacaine group (versus control). However, there were no significant differences in PCA morphine use between the 0.25% bupivacaine and control groups. Although tracheal extubation time and the duration of the intensive care unit (ICU) stay (30 hours versus 34 hours, respectively) were not significantly altered, time to ambulation (1 day versus 2 days, respectively) and duration of hospital stay (4.2 days versus 5.7 days, respectively) were lower in the 0.5% bupivacaine group than in the control group.

Serum bupivacaine concentrations in patients were reasonable, yet one complication related to the local anesthetic delivery system was encountered when a catheter tip was inadvertently broken off during its removal from the incision site, which required surgical reexploration of the wound under local anesthesia. The authors conclude that continuous infusion of 0.5% bupivacaine at 4 mL/hr is effective for decreasing postoperative pain and the need for postoperative supplemental opioid analgesic medication as well as for improving patient satisfaction (earlier ambulation, reduced length of hospital stay) with pain management after cardiac surgery.

Another clinical investigation reveals the potential benefits of using a continuous infusion of local anesthetic in patients following cardiac surgery.[31] In this prospective, randomized, placebo-controlled, double-blind clinical trial, Dowling and associates[31] studied 35 healthy patients undergoing cardiac surgery. Patients undergoing elective CABG via median sternotomy were randomized to either "ropivacaine" or "placebo" groups. At the end of the operation, prior to wound closure, bilateral intercostal nerve injections from T1 to T12 were performed using 20 mL of either 0.2% ropivacaine or normal saline. After sternal reapproximation with wires, two catheters with multiple side openings were placed anterior to the sternum (Fig. 37–1). These catheters were connected to a pressurized elastomeric pump containing a flow regulator, which allowed for delivery of 0.2% ropivacaine or normal saline at approximately 4 mL/hr. The intraoperative anesthetic technique was standardized (short-acting anesthetics were used to minimize the presence of residual anesthetic agents in the postoperative period), as was postoperative pain management via intravenous PCA morphine (for 72 hours).

Both groups exhibited similar postoperative extubation times (approximately 8 hours). The sternal catheters were

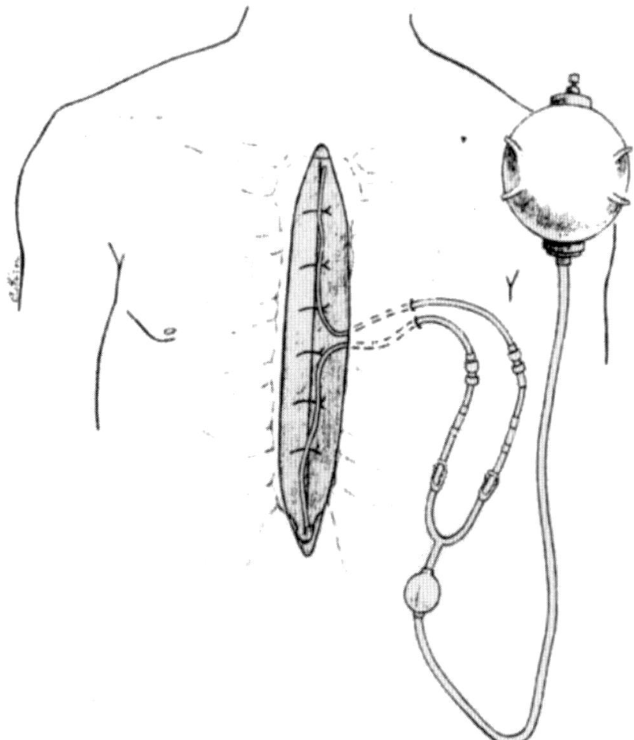

Figure 37–1 Intraoperative placement of the pressurized elastomeric pump and catheters. (From Dowling R, Thielmeier K, Ghaly A, et al: Improved pain control after cardiac surgery: Results of a randomized, double-blind, clinical trial. J Thorac Cardiovasc Surg 126:1271, 2003.)

removed in both groups after 48 hours. Total mean PCA morphine consumption during the immediate postoperative period (72 hours) was significantly decreased in the ropivacaine group compared with the placebo group (47.3 mg versus 78.7 mg, respectively; $p = 0.038$). Mean overall pain scores (scale ranging from 0 for no pain to 10 for maximum pain imaginable) were also significantly decreased in the ropivacaine group compared with the placebo group (1.6 versus 2.6, respectively; $p = 0.005$). Most interestingly, patients receiving ropivacaine had a mean hospital length of stay of 5.2 days ± 1.3 days compared with 8.2 days ± 7.9 days for patients receiving normal saline, a difference that was statistically significant ($p = 0.001$). One patient in the placebo group had an extremely long postoperative hospitalization (39 days). However, the difference between the two groups regarding length of hospital stay remained statistically significant even if this outlier was removed (5.2 ± 1.3 days versus 6.3 ± 2.8 days, respectively; $p < 0.01$). Despite differences in postoperative analgesia, postoperative pulmonary function (assessed via forced expiratory volume in 1 second and peak expiratory flow) was similar between the two groups. There was no difference in wound infections or wound healing between the two groups during hospitalization or after hospital discharge. No complications related to placement of the sternal wound catheters or performance of the intercostal nerve blocks were encountered.

The authors conclude that their analgesic technique significantly improves postoperative pain control while decreasing the amount of opioid analgesia required in patients subjected to standard median sternotomy. The significant decrease in hospital length of stay observed by the investigators is intriguing, may result in substantial cost reductions, and deserves further study.

The management of postoperative pain with continuous direct infusion of local anesthetic into the surgical wound has been described following a wide variety of surgeries other than cardiac (inguinal hernia repair, upper abdominal surgery, laparoscopic nephrectomy, cholecystectomy, knee arthroplasty, shoulder surgery, and gynecologic operative laparoscopy).[32] The infusion pump systems used for anesthetic wound perfusion are regulated by the U.S. Food and Drug Administration (FDA) as medical devices. Thus, adverse events involving these infusion pump systems during direct local anesthetic infusion into surgical wounds are reported to this organization.

Complications encountered with these infusion pump systems reported to the FDA include tissue necrosis, surgical wound infection, and cellulitis following orthopedic, gastrointestinal, podiatric, and other surgeries. None of these reported adverse events have involved patients undergoing cardiac surgery. The most commonly reported complication is tissue necrosis, an adverse event almost never seen following normal surgical procedures. Furthermore, consequences of these reported adverse events were typically severe and required intervention and additional medical and/or surgical treatment. While these initial reports may be isolated incidents, they may also represent an early warning that is representative of a problem that is widespread. Nevertheless, these reports provide a potentially important signal, suggesting the need for further investigation into the relationship between use of these infusion pumps for direct continuous infusion of local anesthetics and other drugs into surgical wounds and tissue necrosis, serious infections, or cellulitis. Neither of the two clinical investigations involving local anesthetic infusion in patients following cardiac surgery with median sternotomy reported such wound complications.[30,31] Regardless, these safety issues merit careful consideration because of the importance of sternal wound complications in this setting.

NERVE BLOCKS

With the increasing popularity of minimally invasive cardiac surgery, which utilizes nonsternotomy incisions (minithoracotomy), the use of nerve blocks for the management of postoperative pain has increased as well[33-38] (Box 37–4). Thoracotomy incisions (transverse anterolateral minithoracotomy, vertical anterolateral minithoracotomy), owing to costal cartilage trauma tissue damage to ribs, muscles, or peripheral nerves, may induce more intense postoperative pain than that resulting from median sternotomy. Adequate analgesia following thoracotomy is important because pain is a key component in alteration of lung function following thoracic surgery. Uncontrolled pain causes a reduction in respiratory mechanics, reduced mobility, and increases in hormonal and metabolic activity. Perioperative deterioration in respiratory mechanics may lead to pulmonary complications and hypoxemia, which may in turn lead to myocardial ischemia/infarction, cerebrovascular accidents, thromboembolism, and delayed wound healing, leading to increased morbidity and prolonged hospital stay. Various analgesic techniques have been developed to treat postoperative thoracotomy pain. The most commonly used techniques include intercostal nerve blocks, intrapleural administration of local anesthetics, and thoracic paravertebral blocks. Intrathecal techniques and epidural techniques are also very effective in controlling postthoracotomy pain and are covered in detail later in this chapter.

Intercostal nerve block has been used extensively for analgesia following thoracic surgery.[33,35] Intercostal nerve blocks can be performed either intraoperatively or postoperatively and usually provide sufficient analgesia lasting approximately 6 to 12 hours (depending on amount and type of local anesthetic used) and may need to be repeated if additional analgesia is required. Local anesthetics may be administered as a single treatment under direct vision, before chest closure, as a single preoperative percutaneous injection, as multiple percutaneous serial injections, or via an indwelling intercostal catheter. Blockade of intercostal nerves interrupts C-fiber afferent transmission of impulses to the spinal cord. A single intercostal injection of a long-acting local anesthetic can provide pain relief and improve pulmonary function in patients following thoracic surgery for up to 6 hours. To achieve longer duration of analgesia, a continuous extrapleural intercostal nerve block technique may be used in which a catheter is placed percutaneously into an extrapleural pocket by the surgeon. A continuous intercostal catheter allows frequent dosing or infusions of local anesthetic agents and avoids multiple needle injections. Various clinical studies have confirmed the analgesic efficacy of this technique, and

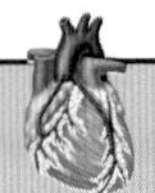

BOX 37–4 ***Nerve Blocks***

- Advantage: Simple, long-lasting analgesia
- Disadvantage: Unreliable?

the technique compares favorably with thoracic epidural analgesic techniques.[33] A major concern associated with intercostal nerve block is the potentially high amount of local anesthetic systemic absorption, yet multiple clinical studies involving patients undergoing thoracic surgery have documented safe blood levels with standard techniques. Clinical investigations involving patients undergoing thoracic surgery indicate that intercostal nerve blockade by intermittent or continuous infusion of 0.5% bupivacaine with epinephrine is an effective method, as is continuous infusion of 0.25% bupivacaine through indwelling intercostal catheters for supplementing systemic intravenous opioid analgesia for postthoracotomy pain. The value of single preclosure injections remains doubtful.

Intrapleural administration of local anesthetics initiates analgesia via mechanisms that remain incompletely understood. However, the mechanism of action of extrapleural regional anesthesia seems to depend primarily on diffusion of the local anesthetic into the paravertebral region. Local anesthetic agents then affect not only the ventral nerve root but also afferent fibers of the posterior primary ramus. Posterior ligaments of the posterior primary ramus innervate posterior spinal muscles and skin and are traumatized during posterolateral thoracotomy. Intrapleural administration of local anesthetic agent to this region through a catheter inserted in the extrapleural space thus creates an anesthetic region in the skin. The depth and width of the anesthetic region depend on diffusion of the local anesthetic agent in the extrapleural space. With this technique, local anesthetics may be administered via an indwelling intrapleural catheter placed between the parietal and visceral pleura by intermittent or continuous infusion regimens. Concerns regarding systemic absorption of local anesthetic and toxicity are always a concern with this technique yet have not been substantiated in clinical studies that assayed plasma levels. A handful of clinical investigations involving patients undergoing thoracic surgery via thoracotomy incision suggests that 0.25% to 0.5% bupivacaine may improve analgesia in patients following thoracic surgery yet its true efficacy as a postoperative analgesic in this patient population remains somewhat controversial.[36] The analgesic benefits are of short duration and there does not appear to be a significant overall opioid-sparing effect. Furthermore, the optimum concentration and duration regimen remains to be defined. However, a prospective, randomized clinical study involving 50 patients undergoing minimally invasive direct CABG (via minithoracotomy) indicates that an intrapleural analgesic technique (with 0.25% bupivacaine) is safe and effective and compares favorably (provided superior postoperative analgesia) to a conventional thoracic epidural technique.[37] These investigators noted, however, that careful catheter positioning, chest tube clamping, and anchoring of the catheter are mandatory for postoperative intrapleural analgesia to be effective. A major factor implicated in lack of efficacy regarding intrapleural techniques is loss of local anesthetic solution through intercostal chest drainage tubes. While clamping the chest tubes during the postoperative period will increase analgesic efficacy, it may not be safe to clamp chest tubes because they provide important drainage of hemorrhage and air and allow for enhanced lung patency and expansion. Apart from proper catheter positioning (insertion of catheter under direct vision and anchoring catheter to skin are essential), effective analgesia with this technique also appears to depend on whether lung surgery was performed or whether the pleural anatomy and physiology are relatively intact.

Thoracic paravertebral block involves injection of local anesthetic adjacent to the thoracic vertebrae close to where the spinal nerves emerge from the intervertebral foramina (Fig. 37–2). Thoracic paravertebral block, compared with thoracic epidural analgesic techniques, appears to provide equivalent analgesia, is technically easier, and may harbor less risk. Several different techniques exist for successful thoracic paravertebral block and have recently been extensively reviewed.[34] The classic technique, most commonly used, involves eliciting loss of resistance. Injection of local anesthetic results in ipsilateral somatic and sympathetic nerve blockade in multiple contiguous thoracic dermatomes above and below the site of injection (along with possible suppression of the neuroendocrine stress response to surgery). These blocks may be effective in alleviating acute and chronic pain of unilateral origin from the chest and/or abdomen. Bilateral use of thoracic paravertebral block has also been described. Continuous thoracic paravertebral infusion of local anesthetic via a catheter placed under direct vision at thoracotomy is also a safe, simple, and effective method of providing analgesia following thoracotomy. It is usually used in conjunction with adjunct intravenous medications (opioid or other analgesics) to provide optimum relief following thoracotomy.

Although supplemental intravenous analgesics are usually required, opioid requirements are substantially reduced. Unilateral paravertebral block is useful for attaining postthoracotomy analgesia because pain following lateral thoracotomy is essentially always unilateral. The role of bilateral thoracic paravertebral block remains to be defined. The benefits of unilateral paravertebral blockade are a lesser incidence of adverse events (hypotension, urinary retention) and a decreased risk of systemic local anesthetic toxicity because less local anesthetic is used. The clinical investigations involving unilateral paravertebral block in patients undergoing thoracic surgery are few. Therefore, it is not possible to determine from the available literature whether the technique of paravertebral blockade (single injection) is truly useful in the postoperative analgesic management of patients following thoracotomy. However, continuous thoracic paravertebral block, as part of a balanced analgesic regimen, may provide effective pain relief with very few side effects following thoracotomy and appears to be comparable to thoracic epidural analgesia.[34]

Intercostal nerve blocks, intrapleural administration of local anesthetics, and thoracic paravertebral blocks offer the advantages of simplicity and efficacy in controlling postoperative pain in patients following thoracic surgery. However, while analgesic efficacy of these techniques sometimes is comparable to intrathecal techniques and epidural techniques, these techniques appear to work best as a part of a multimodal analgesic regimen (supplementing other analgesic techniques). Complications associated with infiltrations of large quantities of local anesthetic (often required) are always a concern when utilizing these analgesic techniques.

OPIOIDS

Beginning in the 1960s (and continuing for essentially 30 years), large doses of intravenous opioids (starting with morphine) have been administered to patients undergoing cardiac surgery[39,40] (Box 37–5). Because even very large amounts of intravenous opioids do not initiate "complete anesthesia" (unconsciousness, muscle relaxation, suppression of reflex responses to noxious surgical stimuli), other intravenous/

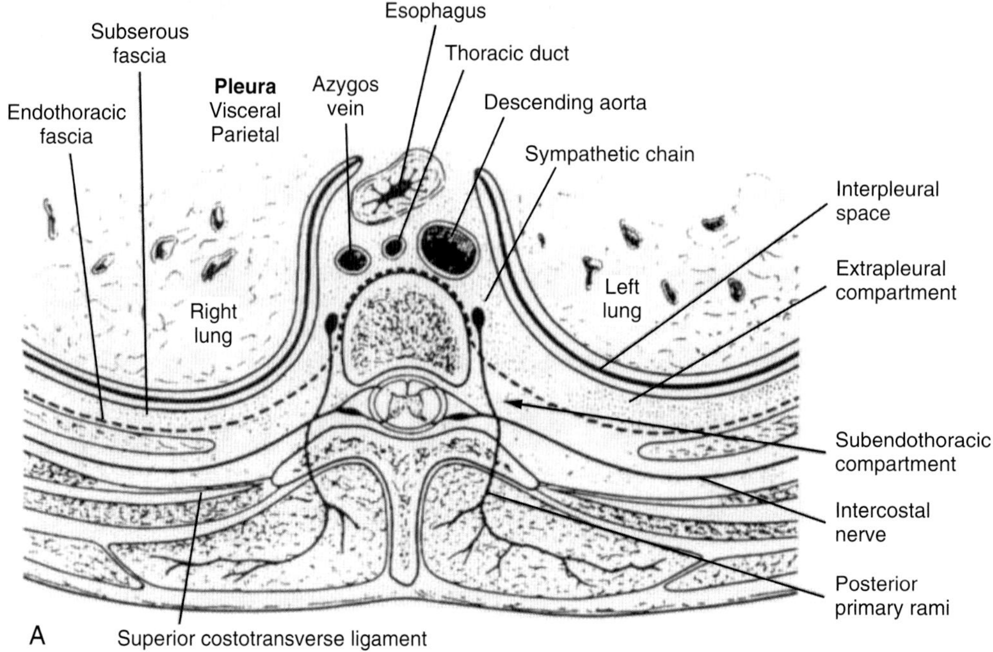

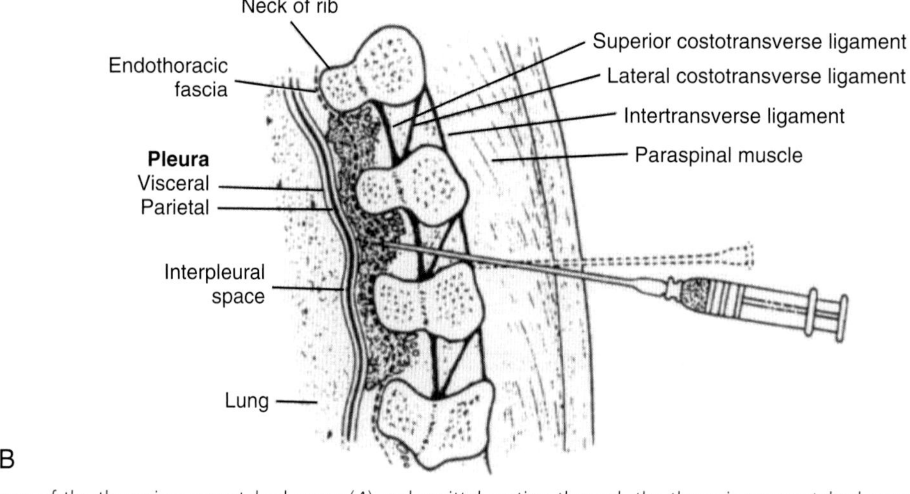

Figure 37–2 Anatomy of the thoracic paravertebral space (*A*) and sagittal section through the thoracic paravertebral space showing a needle that has been advanced above the transverse process (*B*). (From Karmakar MK: Thoracic paravertebral block [review article]. Anesthesiology 95:771, 2001.)

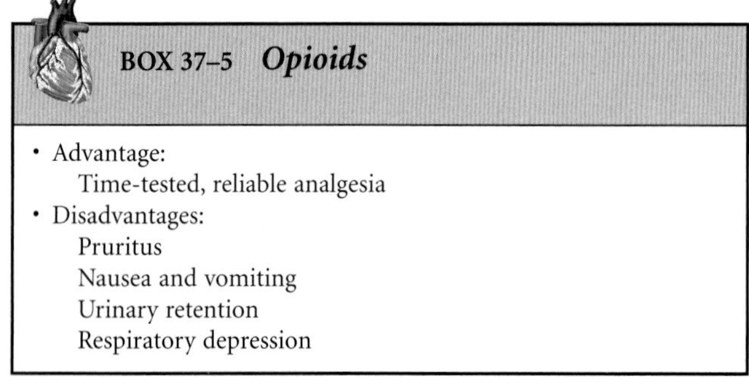

BOX 37–5 ***Opioids***

- Advantage:
  - Time-tested, reliable analgesia
- Disadvantages:
  - Pruritus
  - Nausea and vomiting
  - Urinary retention
  - Respiratory depression

inhalation agents must be administered during the intraoperative period.[41] Analgesia is the best known and most extensively investigated opioid effect, yet opioids are also involved in a diverse array of other physiologic functions, including control of pituitary and adrenal medulla hormone release and activity, control of cardiovascular and gastrointestinal function, and in the regulation of respiration, mood, appetite, thirst, cell growth, and the immune system.[42] A number of well-known and potential side effects of opioids (nausea and vomiting, pruritus, urinary retention, respiratory depression) may limit postoperative recovery when they are used for postoperative analgesia.

Opioids interact with specific receptors that are widely distributed within the central nervous system to produce a variety of pharmacologic effects. Currently, three distinct opioid receptor types are recognized: μ, κ, and δ. The μ-receptor has two subtypes, a high-affinity μ_1-receptor and a low-affinity μ_2-receptor. The supraspinal mechanisms of analgesia are thought to involve μ_1-receptors, whereas spinal analgesia, respiratory depression, and gastrointestinal effects are associated with the μ_2-receptor. Other subtypes of the μ-receptor have been isolated yet their clinical relevance remains to be elucidated. Likewise, subtypes of the κ-receptor and δ-receptor have also been isolated. Selective κ agonists may have therapeutic potential as analgesics, lacking the adverse side effects produced by the current μ-receptor agonists. δ_1-Receptors appear to mediate spinal analgesia whereas δ_2-receptors appear to mediate supraspinal analgesia. Unfortunately, despite extensive pharmacologic and functional studies of the wide variety of opioid receptors, understanding of the structural basis of their actions remains quite limited.

The classic pharmacologic effect of opioids is analgesia, and these drugs have traditionally been the initial choice when a potent postoperative analgesic is required. Two anatomically distinct sites exist for opioid receptor–mediated analgesia: supraspinal and spinal. Systemically administered opioids produce analgesia at both sites. Supraspinally, the μ_1-receptor is primarily involved in analgesia whereas the μ_2-receptor is the one predominantly involved in the spinal modulation of nociceptive processing. κ-Receptors are important in mediating spinal and supraspinal analgesia as well. δ-Ligands may have a modulatory rather than a primary analgesic role. All three types of opioid receptors (μ, κ, and δ) have been demonstrated in peripheral terminals of sensory nerves. Activation of these receptors seems to require an inflammatory reaction because locally applied opioids do not produce analgesia in healthy tissue. The inflammatory process may also activate previously inactive opioid receptors.

While nausea and vomiting, pruritus, and urinary retention are more commonly encountered, respiratory depression remains the most feared complication associated with use of opioids. All μ-receptor agonist opioids produce dose-related respiratory depression, which appears to be mediated via μ_2-receptors. Pure κ agonists have little effect on respiration, and the role of δ-receptors in respiratory control remains to be elucidated. The primary respiratory effect of opioids is a reduction in the sensitivity of the respiratory center to carbon dioxide (along with depression of both medullary and peripheral chemoreceptors). Initially, respiratory rate is affected more than tidal volume, which may even increase. With increasing doses of opioids, respiratory rhythmicity is disturbed, resulting in the irregular gasping breathing characteristic of opioid overdose. In addition to retention of carbon dioxide, respiratory depression may also result in hypoxia (the hypoxic drive to ventilation is depressed by the opioids as well). Elderly patients seem to be more sensitive to the respiratory depressant effects of opioids than younger patients and the dose used needs to be adjusted accordingly. It is also important to keep in mind that all other central nervous system depressants, such as benzodiazepines, barbiturates, and/or inhalation anesthetics will potentiate the respiratory depressant effects of the opioids. Furthermore, in addition to the parent opioid drug, metabolites may in some circumstances contribute to respiratory depression. For instance, metabolites of morphine (morphine-6-β-glucuronide) may occur in substantial quantities following intravenous administration and may be responsible for a considerable proportion of the clinical effects of intravenous morphine.

Morphine is the prototype opioid agonist with which all opioids are compared. Morphine is perhaps the most popular analgesic used in patients following cardiac surgery. Many semisynthetic derivatives are made by simple modifications of the morphine molecule. Morphine is poorly lipid soluble and binds approximately 35% to plasma proteins, particularly albumin. Morphine is primarily metabolized in the liver, principally by conjugation to water-soluble glucuronides. The liver is the predominant site for morphine biotransformation although extrahepatic metabolism also occurs in the kidney, brain, and possibly gut. Extrahepatic clearance accounts for approximately 30% of the total body clearance. The terminal elimination half-life of morphine is on the order of 2 to 3 hours. In patients with liver cirrhosis, morphine pharmacokinetics are variable, probably reflecting the variability of liver disease in patients. Morphine's terminal elimination half-life in patients with renal disease is comparable to that of normal patients. While morphine is perhaps the most popular intravenous analgesic used in patients following cardiac surgery, other synthetically derived opioids have been developed and may be utilized as well. These include fentanyl, alfentanil, sufentanil, and remifentanil.

Fentanyl is considerably more potent (60 to 80 times) than morphine. However, at the opioid receptor, the intrinsic affinities of fentanyl and morphine differ by only a factor of two to three. The differences between receptor affinities and clinical potency ratios arise from differing physiochemical and pharmacokinetic properties of the drugs (in particular, the differences in lipid solubility). Fentanyl is highly lipid soluble, which influences rate of entry and exit to and from organs and tissues, especially the central nervous system, which has a high lipid content.

Fentanyl is rapidly transferred across the blood-brain barrier, resulting in a rapid onset of action after intravenous injection. The relative potential for entering the central nervous system is approximately 150 times greater for fentanyl than for morphine. However, the large quantities of fentanyl taken up by adipose tissues may act as a reservoir (depending on dosage amounts) that slowly releases fentanyl back into the circulation when plasma concentrations fall below that in fat. This slow reentry may serve to maintain the plasma concentration and is one factor in the relatively long plasma terminal elimination half-life of fentanyl. Fentanyl is rapidly and extensively metabolized by the liver to inactive metabolites. After bolus intravenous injection, plasma fentanyl concentrations decrease rapidly due to distribution from the plasma to tissues, so that after moderate (10 μg/kg) doses, fentanyl has a short duration of action.

However, larger doses convert fentanyl from a short-acting to a long-acting drug. With increased doses, the distribution phase is completed before the fentanyl concentration declines to threshold levels, so duration of action becomes dependent on the decrease in concentration during the much slower elimination phase. Thus, to avoid accumulation of fentanyl, successive doses at regular intervals should be progressively reduced in amount, or the interval between doses of the same size should be progressively lengthened. When fentanyl is given by continuous intravenous infusion, the rate of decline of fentanyl plasma concentration is markedly dependent on the duration of the infusion. Fentanyl undergoes substantial first-pass uptake in the lungs (approximately 80% of the injected dose). Hepatic extraction of fentanyl is also high, making its clearance dependent on liver blood flow. Thus, factors that reduce liver blood flow will also decrease fentanyl clearance. It is likely that fentanyl metabolites accumulate in patients with impaired renal function yet this is unlikely to have clinical consequences since they are pharmacologically inactive. Because the liver is the principal organ for fentanyl biotransformation, decreases in hepatic function due to liver disease will be expected to alter fentanyl pharmacokinetics.

Fentanyl's popularity as an intraoperative analgesic agent relates directly to the cardiovascular stability it provides, even in critically ill patients. Also, its analgesic efficacy relative to the intensity of side effects has prompted much interest in its use as an analgesic postoperatively and/or in critically ill patients.[43] Fentanyl (as well as any opioid) can be administered intravenously for postoperative analgesia in many ways: using a loading dose with a continuous fixed or variable infusion, a fixed background infusion with PCA, or PCA alone. An intravenous bolus of 1 to 2 µg/kg usually is administered before initiating an infusion. If variable, the infusion rate is usually 1 to 2 µg/kg/hr and may be adjusted upward or downward as required by fluctuations in analgesic requirements or appearance of side effects. Before the infusion rate is increased, small intravenous bolus doses of fentanyl may be administered. Infusion rates of 1.5 to 2.5 µg/kg/hr usually provide good-to-excellent postoperative analgesia. At rest, the quality of analgesia remains stable; however, with movement, analgesia may not be sufficient, even with higher infusion rates.

A background low-dose intravenous infusion of fentanyl may be combined with PCA to provide satisfactory analgesia with potentially fewer side effects. Patient-controlled analgesia bolus doses typically range from 5 to 50 µg, and background infusion rates may be fixed (ranging from 5 to 50 µg/hr) or be variable (adjusted up and down according to clinical criteria). Generally, the larger the background infusion rate, the smaller is the PCA bolus dose. Lockout intervals (minimum time period between doses) range from "on demand" (no lockout) to 15 minutes, the most common interval being 1 to 5 minutes. The technique of using a background infusion plus PCA produces excellent postoperative analgesia. Fentanyl is rarely used alone for PCA because of its brief duration of action. The most commonly administered opioid used in this manner (PCA alone) remains morphine. Transdermal delivery of fentanyl has also been investigated extensively. This modality is simple, noninvasive, and allows continuous release of fentanyl into the systemic circulation. However, the steady release of fentanyl in such a manner does not allow flexibility in dose adjustment, which may result in inadequate treatment of postoperative pain during rapidly changing intensity. Thus, intravenous opioids are often necessary to supplement analgesia when transdermal fentanyl is used to manage acute postoperative pain.

Alfentanil is about 5 to 10 times less potent than fentanyl. The drug acts rapidly; peak effect being reached within minutes following intravenous administration. Its duration of action following bolus administration is also shorter than fentanyl. Alfentanil is highly lipid soluble (about 100 times more lipid soluble than morphine) and rapidly crosses the blood-brain barrier. Alfentanil pharmacokinetics are minimally affected by renal disease, and hepatic extraction is more a function of intrinsic hepatic enzyme capacity and protein binding than liver blood flow.

The performance of a patient-demand, target-controlled alfentanil infusion system has compared favorably to traditional morphine PCA in patients following cardiac surgery.[44] Checketts and associates[44] prospectively randomized 120 patients undergoing elective cardiac surgery to receive either morphine PCA or alfentanil PCA for postoperative analgesia (nonblinded). All patients received a similar standardized intraoperative anesthetic technique and were extubated during the immediate postoperative period. Overall median visual analog pain scores were significantly lower in patients receiving alfentanil yet both alfentanil and morphine delivered high-quality postoperative analgesia (Fig. 37–3). While the clinical impression by these investigators was that alfentanil patients were less sedated in the immediate postoperative period, this clinical observation was not substantiated following statistical analysis of sedation scores. The two groups did not differ with respect to overall sedation scores, frequency of nausea and vomiting, hemodynamic instability, myocardial ischemia, or hypoxemia during the immediate postoperative period.

Sufentanil is approximately ten times more potent than fentanyl. The drug is extremely lipid soluble and highly bound to plasma proteins. Because of its high potency, conventional clinical doses of sufentanil result in plasma concentrations that rapidly fall below the sensitivity of most assay methods, making it difficult to determine accurate pharmacokinetic parameters. However, sufentanil pharmacokinetics appear not to be altered in patients with renal disease. Because hepatic sufentanil clearance approaches liver blood flow, it is expected that the drug's pharmacokinetics would change with hepatic disease yet the clinical relevance remains undetermined. Sufentanil undergoes substantial (approximately 60%) first-pass uptake in the lungs.

Remifentanil has a very fast onset and an ultrashort duration of action and is unique in that it is readily susceptible to rapid hydrolysis by nonspecific esterases in the blood and tissues. Remifentanil is moderately lipophilic and is half as potent as fentanyl when blood concentrations causing equivalent analgesia are compared. Remifentanil has an elimination half-life of ten to twenty minutes. The time required for a 50% reduction in blood concentration after discontinuation of an infusion that has attained steady state is about 3 minutes and

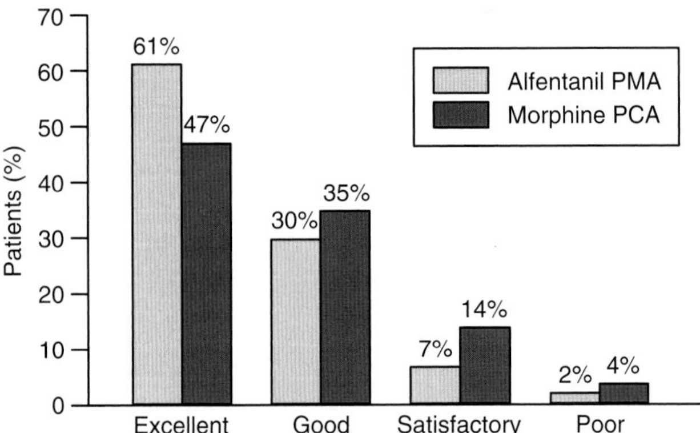

Figure 37–3 Overall patient satisfaction with postoperative analgesia. Ninety-one percent of patients using alfentanil rated their postoperative analgesia as excellent or good, whereas 82% of patients using morphine rated their postoperative analgesia similarly (differences not statistically significant). (From Checketts MR, Gilhooly CJ, Kenny GNC: Patient-maintained analgesia with target-controlled alfentanil infusion after cardiac surgery: A comparison with morphine PCA. Br J Anaesth 80:748, 1998 © The Board of Management and Trustees of the British Journal of Anaesthesia. Reproduced by permission of Oxford University Press/British Journal of Anaesthesia.)

does not increase with duration of infusion. Available evidence suggests that neither pharmacokinetics or pharmacodynamics of remifentanil is significantly altered in patients with severe hepatic or renal disease. These properties should confer ease of titration to changing analgesic conditions. However, the quick offset of action, while desirable, may result in inadequate postoperative analgesia. Because of the rapid offset of effect of remifentanil, the continued requirement for postoperative analgesia needs to be considered before the remifentanil is discontinued. A transition must be made from remifentanil to some other longer-acting analgesic for substantial postoperative pain. Although the transition to postoperative pain management can be made using a remifentanil infusion alone, this appears to be associated with a high incidence of adverse respiratory effects.

In 1996, Bowdle and associates[45] evaluated the use of a remifentanil infusion to provide postoperative analgesia during recovery from total intravenous anesthesia with remifentanil and propofol from a wide variety of noncardiac surgeries (abdominal, spine, joint replacement, thoracic surgery). This multi-institutional study involving 157 patients had a detailed protocol that specified doses and method of administration of all anesthetic drugs. In essence, total intraoperative intravenous anesthesia consisted of midazolam (premedication only), remifentanil, propofol, and vecuronium. Propofol was stopped immediately prior to intraoperative extubation and the remifentanil infusion was continued for postoperative analgesia. During the immediate postoperative period, intravenous morphine was administered during tapering of remifentanil infusion. Adverse respiratory events (oxygen saturation via pulse oximetry less than 90%, respiratory rate less than 12 per minute, apnea) affected 45 patients (29%, two required naloxone). Apnea occurred in 11 patients (7%, treated with mask ventilation and downward titration of remifentanil infusion, one required naloxone). The administration of a bolus of remifentanil preceded the onset of adverse respiratory events in 19 of 45 cases and in 9 of 11 cases of apnea.

These data suggest that remifentanil boluses plus an infusion are particularly likely to produce clinically significant adverse respiratory events. The authors of this open, dose-ranging study conclude that while remifentanil certainly initiates analgesia, its use in the immediate postoperative period may pose dangers. Additional studies are needed to investigate the transition from remifentanil to longer-lasting analgesics and to refine strategies that minimize respiratory depression while optimizing pain control. The administration of a potent, rapidly acting opioid such as remifentanil by continuous infusion for postoperative analgesia must be performed with meticulous attention to detail and constant vigilance. Extreme caution should be exercised in the postoperative administration of bolus doses of remifentanil as substantial respiratory depression (including apnea) may develop. Furthermore, the remifentanil infusion should be inserted into the intravenous line as close as possible to the patient in order to minimize deadspace, and the rate of the main intravenous infusion should be controlled at a rate that is high enough to continuously flush remifentanil from the tubing. A more dilute remifentanil solution that would run at higher rates (on a volume per time basis) would help to minimize the effect of variations in flow rate of the main intravenous tubing on delivery of remifentanil to the patient. Remifentanil may also possess detrimental cardiovascular effects via bradycardia and decreases in systemic vascular resistance, leading to decreased cardiac output and hypotension.[46] Such changes may occur during clinically utilized doses for cardiac surgery (0.1 to 1.0 μg/kg/min), inducing significant cardiovascular disturbances that are potentially deleterious to patients with cardiac disease.[46]

PATIENT-CONTROLLED ANALGESIA

When intravenous opioids are used for controlling postoperative pain (most commonly morphine and fentanyl), PCA technology is generally used. Essentials in the successful use of PCA technology include "loading" the patient with intravenous opioids to the point of patient comfort prior to initiating PCA, ensuring that the patient wants to control analgesic treatment, using an appropriate PCA dose and lockout interval, and considering the use of a basal rate infusion. Focused guidance of PCA dosing by a dedicated acute pain service, compared with surgeon-directed PCA, may result in more effective analgesia with fewer side effects. Patient-controlled epidural analgesic techniques, with opioids and/or local anesthetics, have also been proved reliable, effective, and safe.[47,48]

While PCA is a well-established technique (used for more than two decades) and offers potential unique benefits (reliable analgesic effect, improved patient autonomy, flexible adjustment to individual needs, etc.), whether it truly offers significant clinical advantages (compared with traditional nurse-administrated analgesic techniques) to patients immediately following cardiac surgery remains to be determined.[49-54] A clinical investigation by Gust and associates indicates that PCA techniques provide a higher quality of postoperative analgesia, which may lead to a reduction in postoperative respiratory complications.[50] In this prospective, randomized, clinical investigation involving 120 healthy patients after extubation following elective CABG, patients received either intravenous PCA piritramide, intravenous PCA piritramide plus rectal indomethacin, or conventional nurse-controlled analgesia with intravenous piritramide and/or rectal indomethacin for 3 days. Postoperative assessment included daily visual analog pain scoring and chest radiographs graded for the extent of atelectasis by a radiologist blinded as to treatment. Perioperative management (surgical treatment, intraoperative anesthetic management) was standardized. While chest radiography atelectasis scores and visual analog pain score values were similar among the three groups on the first and second postoperative days, on the third postoperative day chest radiography atelectasis scores and visual analog pain score values were significantly better in the two PCA groups compared with the control (nurse-controlled analgesia) group.

At the end of the study, all patients retrospectively graded their postoperative pain management on average as good, but significantly more patients in the two PCA groups assessed their pain management as excellent compared with the control group. These investigators conclude that treatment with PCA may reduce respiratory complications in patients following CABG. However, no difference was observed regarding perioperative oxygenation values among the three groups during the entire study period and not a single patient in any group met prospectively defined criteria for diagnosis of pneumonia. Other clinical investigations have indicated that PCA techniques, compared with standard nurse-based pain therapy, may provide higher quality analgesia leading to

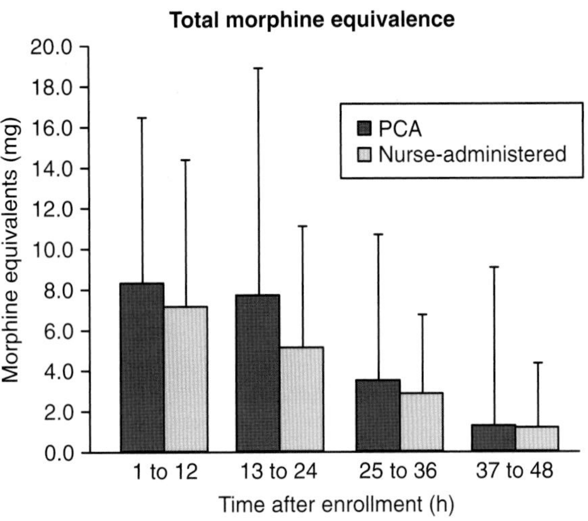

Figure 37–4 Total morphine equivalents. Dosages of morphine equivalents in the PCA nurse-administered groups during each observation period. No differences existed between the two groups at any observation period. (From Tsang J, Brush B: Patient-controlled analgesia in postoperative cardiac surgery. Anaesth Intens Care 27:464, 1999.)

reduced cardiopulmonary morbidity following cardiac surgery.[51,54]

Despite the popularity of PCA techniques and the results of the above-quoted studies, other clinical investigations reveal no major benefits offered.[49,52,53] Tsang and Brush[49] prospectively evaluated 69 patients following cardiac surgery via median sternotomy. Thirty-nine were randomized to receive PCA morphine postoperatively, while 30 were randomized to receive nurse-administered morphine postoperatively. Perioperative care was standardized, visual analog pain scores were used for pain assessment, and pulmonary function tests were performed preoperatively and every 6 hours after surgery until discharge from the ICU. These clinical investigators found no difference between the two groups regarding postoperative morphine consumption (Fig. 37–4), postoperative visual analog pain scores, postoperative sedation scores, and postoperative pulmonary function (Fig. 37–5). These investigators conclude that there are no significant advantages achieved when using PCA routinely in patients following cardiac surgery. Interestingly, in this study, opinions expressed by the nursing staff on the use of PCA were not as positive as expected (repetition of PCA instruction to patients was often required during the study period). Potential reasons for required repeated instructions on PCA include poor retention of preoperative learning because of anxiety following hospital admission, incomplete recovery of higher cognitive function after prolonged general anesthesia and CPB, and/or ICU-induced disorientation.

These results suggest that there may be additional patient limitations to the effective use of PCA immediately after cardiac surgery even though patients can obey simple commands and acknowledge discomfort. Munro and associates, when comparing intravenous PCA morphine and nurse-administered subcutaneous morphine, detail similar findings.[52] They prospectively randomized 92 patients undergoing elective cardiac surgery to receive either intravenous PCA morphine or nurse-administered subcutaneous morphine during the postoperative period. They found no differences between the two groups regarding many postoperative variables, including total postoperative morphine requirements, postoperative visual analog pain scores at rest and with movement, daily verbal pain relief scores, side effect profiles, and physiotherapist's evaluation of effectiveness of analgesia for chest physiotherapy. Subcutaneous techniques are attractive because they have low equipment and disposable costs, eliminate the need for bulky pumps in ambulating patients, and may be more effective for the elderly or mildly confused postoperative patient.

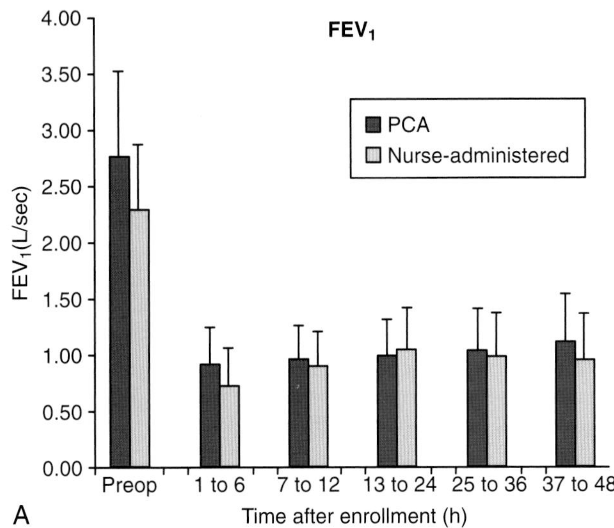

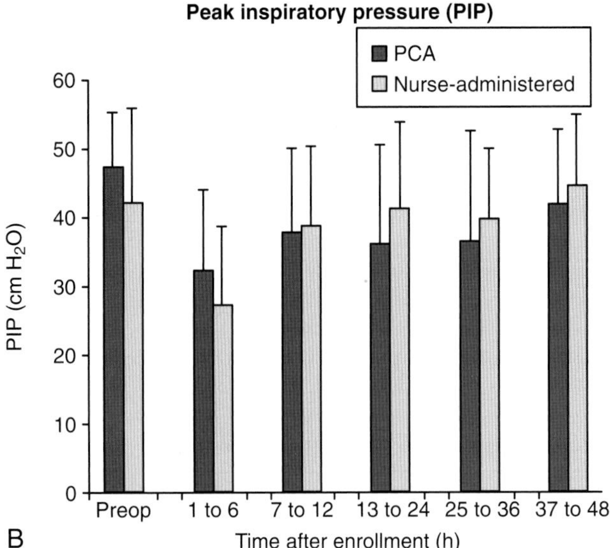

Figure 37–5 Postoperative pulmonary function. Postoperative pulmonary function tests in the PCA and nurse-administered groups during each observation period. A significant decrease in FEV_1 in both groups was observed immediately after surgery (and lasting 48 hours). No differences existed between the two groups at any observation period. (From Tsang J, Brush B: Patient-controlled analgesia in postoperative cardiac surgery. Anaesth Intens Care 27:464, 1999.)

Myles and associates[53] were also unable to find any specific clinical benefits during use of PCA techniques in patients following cardiac surgery. In their prospective clinical investigation, 72 patients undergoing elective cardiac surgery were randomized to receive either intravenous PCA morphine or intravenous nurse-titrated morphine during the immediate postoperative period. They found no differences between the two groups regarding many postoperative variables, including postoperative morphine consumption, postoperative pain scores, postoperative nausea scores, and postoperative serum cortisol levels (Fig. 37–6). Much like Munro and associates, they noted that patients also had variable ability and understanding of the requirements of PCA, particularly in the early postoperative period when they were confused or too weak to operate the demand button. These investigators also noted that overall pain management in their patients was optimized by receiving experienced one-to-one nursing care (other studies evaluating PCA have also found that nurse-administered techniques may provide the highest quality analgesia). It could therefore be argued that these studies support increased staff education and involvement to optimize postoperative analgesia. The nurses in these clinical investigations all raised concerns regarding the time required for PCA set-up and the inability of patients to cope with the demands of PCA in the early stages of their recovery, particularly if elderly and/or confused. However, PCA was well received later in the recovery process and was found to be less demanding on nursing time.

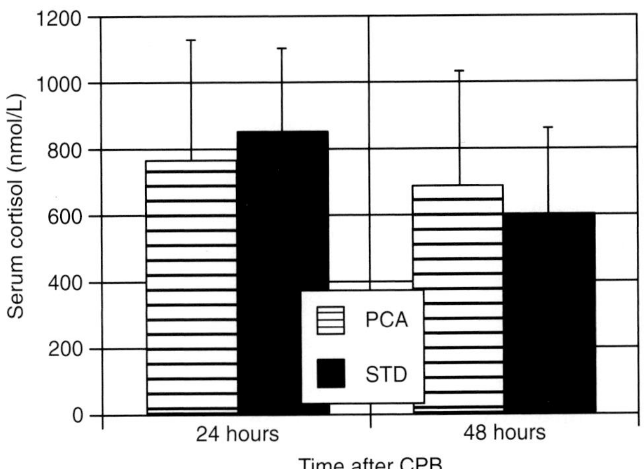

Figure 37–6 Postoperative serum cortisol. Mean serum cortisol level at 24 hours and 48 hours following CPB for patients receiving intravenous PCA morphine (PCA) or intravenous nurse-titrated morphine (STD). (From Myles PS, Buckland MR, Cannon GB, et al: Comparison of patient-controlled analgesia and nurse-controlled infusion analgesia after cardiac surgery. Anaesth Intens Care 22:672, 1994.)

NONSTEROIDAL ANTI-INFLAMMATORY AGENTS

NSAIDs, in contrast to the opioids' central nervous system mechanism of action, mainly exert their analgesic, antipyretic, and anti-inflammatory effects peripherally by interfering with prostaglandin synthesis following tissue injury[55,56] (Box 37–6). NSAIDs inhibit COX, the enzyme responsible for the conversion of arachidonic acid to prostaglandin (Fig. 37–7). Com-

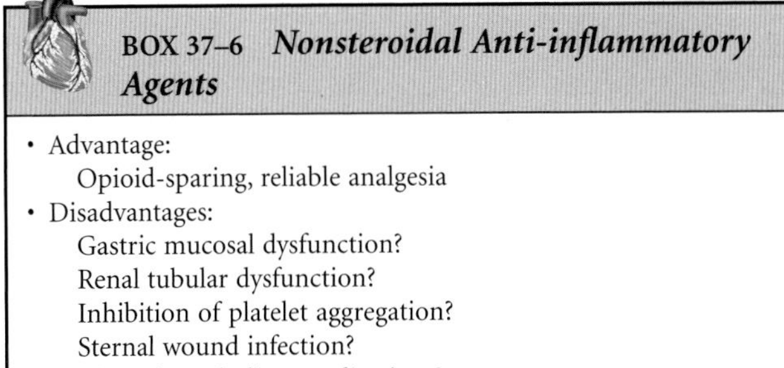

BOX 37–6 ***Nonsteroidal Anti-inflammatory Agents***

- Advantage:
  - Opioid-sparing, reliable analgesia
- Disadvantages:
  - Gastric mucosal dysfunction?
  - Renal tubular dysfunction?
  - Inhibition of platelet aggregation?
  - Sternal wound infection?
  - Thromboembolic complications?

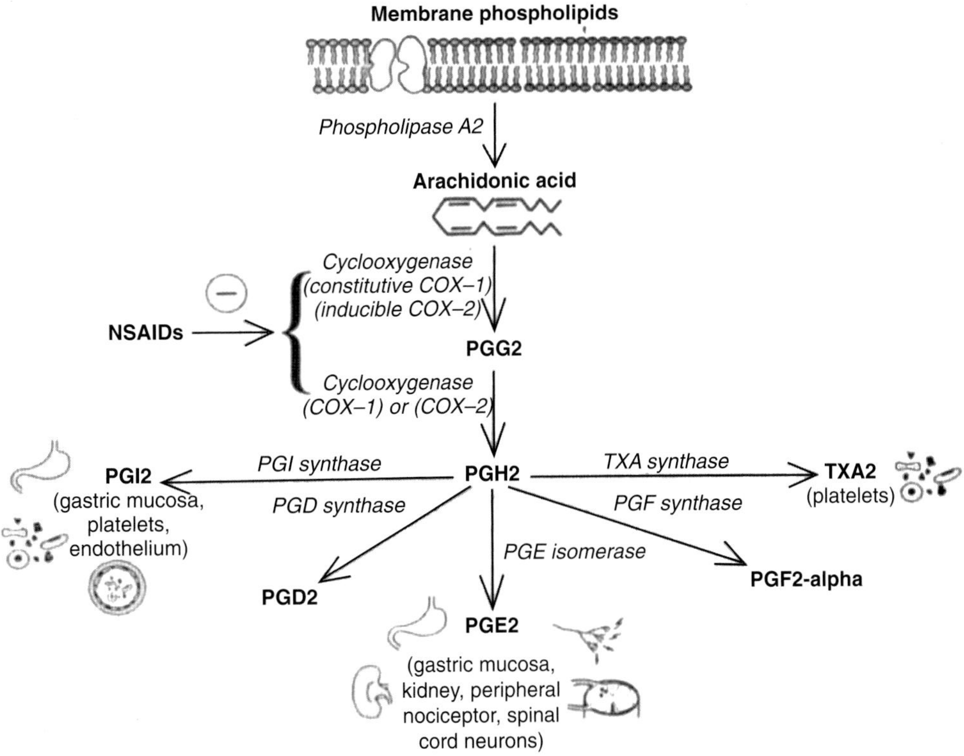

Figure 37–7 The role of cyclooxygenase in prostaglandin synthesis. Prostaglandin and thromboxanes, which are important in inflammation and homeostasis, are products of a biochemical cascade by which membrane phospholipids are converted to arachidonic acid, then to intermediate prostaglandins by cyclooxygenase, and to their final products by a series of synthases. (From Gilron I, Milne B, Hong M: Cyclooxygenase-2 inhibitors in postoperative pain management: Current evidence and future directions [review article]. Anesthesiology 99:1198, 2003.)

bining NSAIDs with traditional intravenous opioids may allow a patient to achieve an adequate level of analgesia with fewer side effects than if a similar level of analgesia was obtained with intravenous opioids alone. Numerous clinical investigations reveal the potential value (opioid-sparing effects) of NSAIDs when combined with traditional intravenous opioids during the postoperative period following noncardiac surgery. In fact, the administration of NSAIDs is one of the most common nonopioid analgesic techniques currently used for postoperative pain management. The efficacy of NSAIDs for postoperative pain has been repeatedly demonstrated in many analgesic clinical trials. Unlike opioids, which preferentially reduce spontaneous postoperative pain, NSAIDs have comparable efficacy for both spontaneous and movement-evoked pain, the latter of which may be more important in causing postoperative physiologic impairment. Certainly, NSAIDs reduce postoperative opioid consumption and accelerate postoperative recovery and represent an integral component of balanced postoperative analgesic regimens following noncardiac surgery. However, little is known regarding NSAID use in the management of pain following cardiac surgery. It is likely that concerns regarding NSAID side effects, including alterations in the gastric mucosal barrier, renal tubular function, and inhibition of platelet aggregation, have made clinicians reluctant to use NSAIDs in patients undergoing cardiac surgery. Other rare side effects of NSAIDs (from COX inhibition) include hepatocellular injury, asthma exacerbation, anaphylactoid reactions, tinnitus, and urticaria. Despite these fears, a small number of clinical investigations seem to indicate that NSAIDs may provide analgesia in patients following cardiac surgery without untoward effects (gastrointestinal ulceration, renal dysfunction, excessive bleeding). Although NSAIDs have been associated with reports of increased postoperative blood loss, other studies have failed to corroborate this.

NSAIDs are not a homogenous group and vary considerably in analgesic efficacy as a result of differences in pharmacodynamic and pharmacokinetic parameters. NSAIDs are nonspecific inhibitors of COX, which is the rate-limiting enzyme involved in the synthesis of prostaglandins. A major scientific discovery revealed that COX exists in multiple forms. Most important, a constitutive form is present in normal conditions in healthy cells (COX-1) and an inducible form (COX-2) exists, which is the major isozyme induced by and associated with inflammation. Simplistically, COX-1 is ubiquitously and constitutively expressed and has a homeostatic role in platelet aggregation, gastrointestinal mucosal integrity, and renal function, whereas COX-2 is inducible and expressed mainly at sites of injury (and kidney and brain) and mediates pain and inflammation. NSAIDs are nonspecific inhibitors of both forms of COX yet vary in their ratio of COX-1 to COX-2 inhibition. Recent molecular studies distinguishing between constitutive COX-1 and inflammation-inducible COX-2 enzymes have led to the exciting hypothesis that the therapeutic and adverse effects of NSAIDs could be uncoupled[57-62] (Fig. 37–8). Subsequently, over the past few years, clinicians have witnessed an exponential increase in publications and the growing use of COX-2 inhibitors in the perioperative period following noncardiac surgery. A compelling body of evidence now exists that COX-2 inhibitors, like their predecessors the nonselective NSAIDs in general, provide postoperative analgesia, decrease intravenous opioid requirements, and provide greater patient satisfaction compared with placebo. There is also some evidence that opioid-

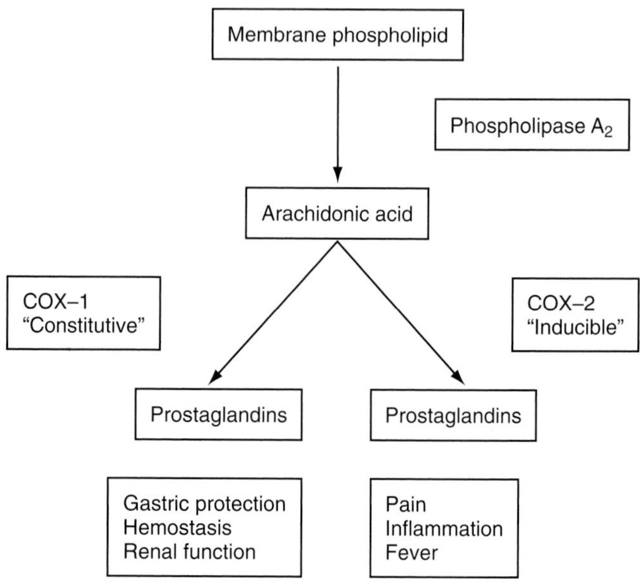

Figure 37–8 Cyclooxygenase pathways. Recent molecular studies distinguishing between COX-1 and COX-2 enzymes have led to the exciting hypothesis that the therapeutic and adverse effects of the nonspecific inhibitors (NSAIDs) could be uncoupled. (From Gajraj NM: Cyclooxygenase-2 inhibitors [review article]. Anesth Analg 96:1720, 2003.)

sparing by COX-2 inhibitors also spares opioid side effects. The primary advantage of COX-2 inhibitors, compared with NSAIDs, is their lack of effect on platelet function and bleeding, hence the opportunity for perioperative administration.

Only a handful of clinical studies have investigated the potential of NSAIDs in the management of postoperative pain following cardiac surgery.[63-66] One well-designed clinical investigation reveals that a combination of NSAID and intravenous opioid may provide superior analgesia following cardiac surgery without untoward effects. Rapanos and associates prospectively randomized 57 patients to receive either indomethacin suppositories or placebo suppositories in a double-blinded fashion during the immediate postoperative period following elective CABG.[65] Patients receiving indomethacin suppositories demonstrated significantly less ($p = 0.019$) morphine consumption (assessed via PCA morphine) and significantly lower ($p = 0.006$) pain scores (assessed via visual analog pain scores) during the immediate postoperative period compared with controls. Postoperative morphine use during the first 24 postoperative hours was 22.40 ± 12.55 mg in the indomethacin group and 35.99 ± 25.84 mg in the placebo group. There was no difference between groups regarding tracheal extubation time or postoperative blood loss (assessed via chest tube output). None of the study subjects (either group) developed postoperative renal dysfunction. In fact, a moderate reduction in serum creatinine concentration was observed in both groups. These investigators conclude that the combination of indomethacin suppositories with morphine following cardiac surgery results in reduced postoperative pain scores and opioid consumption without an increase in side effects.

However, two well-designed clinical investigations reveal that the use of NSAIDs or NSAID-like drugs (acetaminophen) in patients following cardiac surgery may not offer any substantial clinical benefits.[63,66] Hynninen and associates, in a prospective, double-blind, placebo-controlled study, randomized patients to receive either diclofenac (n = 28 patients), ketoprofen (n = 28 patients), indomethacin (n = 27 patients), or placebo (n = 31 patients) for postoperative analgesia following elective CABG via a median sternotomy.[63] All patients received standardized fast-track cardiac anesthesia and standardized postoperative analgesia treatment. Mean morphine consumption in the immediate postoperative period was significantly reduced only in the diclofenac group when compared with placebo (12.4 mg versus 19.0 mg, respectively; $p < 0.05$). Total analgesic consumption calculated as morphine equivalents was also significantly lower only in the diclofenac group compared with placebo (18.1 mg versus 26.5 mg, respectively; $p \leq 0.05$). No additional important differences were observed when doses of other analgesics were compared. The visual analog pain scores at rest were comparable among the four groups at all times. Also, there were no postoperative differences among the four groups regarding creatinine concentration, percentage of patients with 20% and above increases in creatinine level postoperatively, and 24-hour blood loss. These findings indicate that while some NSAIDs may offer opioid-sparing effects, others may not.

Lahtinen and associates,[66] in a prospective, double-blind, placebo-controlled study, randomized patients to receive either propacetamol, a prodrug of acetaminophen (n = 40 patients), or placebo (n = 39 patients) for postoperative analgesia following elective CABG via a median sternotomy. Acetaminophen (not an NSAID) might be a safer nonopioid analgesic in cardiac surgery because it does not depress platelet function or renal function as much as traditional NSAIDs. The mechanism behind the analgesic action of acetaminophen remains unclear. Acetaminophen has only a weak inhibitory influence on peripheral COXs and has no substantial anti-inflammatory activity. Acetaminophen-induced analgesia may be partially centrally mediated, and the peak cerebrospinal fluid concentrations may reflect analgesic actions. Intravenous propacetamol is quickly hydrolyzed to acetaminophen in the blood stream. In the clinical investigation by Lahtinen and associates, a standardized intraoperative anesthetic technique was used for all patients and extubation times were identical between the two groups (approximately 5.3 hours). From the time of extubation, all patients had access to PCA oxycodone using a standardized protocol. The variation of oxycodone consumption was large in both groups and while postoperative cumulative oxycodone consumption (combined amount administered via PCA and given as rescue doses) was less in the propacetamol group compared with the placebo group, the difference was not statistically significant (123.5 ± 51.3 mg versus 141.8 ± 57.5 mg, respectively; $p = 0.15$). Postoperative visual analog pain scores (obtained at rest and during a deep breath) were similar, as well as patient's satisfaction with analgesia, between the two groups. Furthermore, no differences existed between the two groups regarding postoperative pulmonary function tests (forced expiratory volume in 1 second, peak expiratory volume, forced vital capacity), blood gas analysis, bleeding, renal function tests, and liver function tests. Postoperative nausea and vomiting were the most common adverse events, which occurred with identical frequency in both groups. These investigators concluded that propacetamol neither enhances postoperative opioid-based analgesia in patients following CABG, nor does it decrease cumulative opioid consumption or reduce adverse effects.

One prospective, randomized clinical study investigated the potential advantages and disadvantages of using COX inhibitors in patients following cardiac surgery.[67] Immer and associates prospectively randomized 69 patients scheduled for elective CABG with conventional sternotomy to receive either a COX-2 inhibitor (etodolac), a nonselective COX inhibitor (diclofenac), or a weak opioid (tramadol) for postoperative analgesia.[67] Postoperative pain was assessed via a visual analog scale, perioperative blood samples were obtained for serum creatinine and urea levels, and creatinine clearance was determined on the first postoperative day (prior to starting study medication) and on the fourth postoperative day (after receiving study medication). In patients with insufficient postoperative analgesia (defined via predetermined visual analog scale score), supplemental subcutaneous morphine was administered. Total morphine consumption and occurrence of nausea were recorded daily. At the doses analyzed by these investigators, etodolac and diclofenac produced slightly better postoperative analgesia (assessed via visual analog scale scores and morphine consumption) with fewer side effects (assessed via antiemetic therapy) than tramadol. However, a short-lasting impairment of renal function was found in patients treated with etodolac and diclofenac (assessed via serum creatinine and urea levels; Figs. 37–9 and 37–10). However, at hospital discharge, no significant differences existed among the three groups regarding serum creatinine and urea levels (see Figs. 37–9 and 37–10). Furthermore, all three groups experienced similar decreases in postoperative creatinine clearance.

Another clinical investigation in CABG patients suggested a proportionately, but not significantly, greater incidence of cardiac and cerebrovascular serious adverse events in patients taking COX-2 inhibitors.[68] In this multicenter (58 institutions), prospective, randomized, double-blind, parallel-group trial performed by Ott and associates, 462 patients undergoing CABG were allocated at a ratio of 2:1 to parecoxib/valdecoxib (311 patients) or standard care (151 patients; control) groups, respectively.[68] Patients in the parecoxib/valdecoxib group required significantly less morphine or morphine equivalents than patients in the control group during the postoperative period (up to 6 days). Both patients and physicians evaluated the study medication (parecoxib/valdecoxib) as significantly better than control therapy. Pain questionnaires detected significant improvements in the parecoxib/valdecoxib group beginning on day 4 and continuing for at least

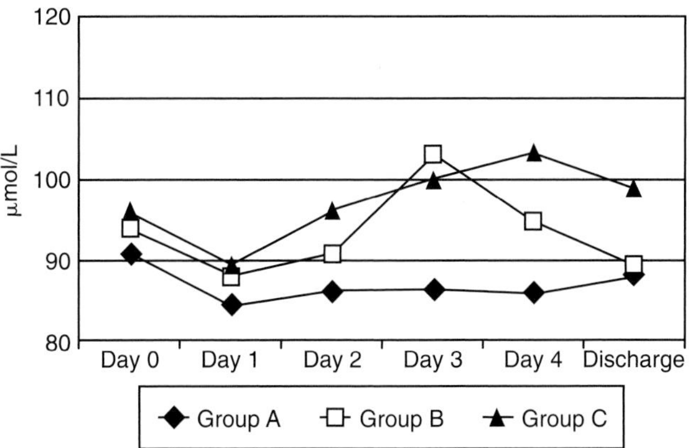

Figure 37–9 Serum creatinine values. Serum creatinine values for groups A (tramadol), B (diclofenac), and C (etodolac) on postoperative days 1 to 4 and at discharge. Results are displayed as mean values. Serum creatinine levels were significantly higher on postoperative days 3 and 4 in groups B and C compared with group A ($p < 0.05$). However, at discharge, no significant differences were found among the three groups. (From Immer FF, Immer-Bansi AS, Trachsel N, et al: Pain treatment with a COX-2 inhibitor after coronary artery bypass operation: A randomized trial. Ann Thorac Surg 75:490, 2003.)

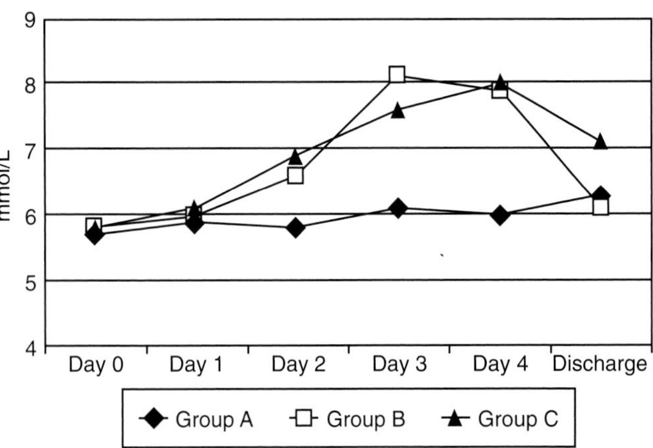

Figure 37–10 Serum urea values. Serum urea values for groups A (tramadol), B (diclofenac), and C (etodolac) on postoperative days 1 to 4 and at discharge. Results are displayed as mean values. Serum urea levels were significantly higher on postoperative days 3 and 4 in groups B and C compared with group A ($p < 0.05$). However, at discharge no significant differences were found among the three groups. (From Immer FF, Immer-Bansi AS, Trachsel N, et al: Pain treatment with a COX-2 inhibitor after coronary artery bypass operation: A randomized trial. Ann Thorac Surg 75:490, 2003.)

4 days. However, although there were no differences between the groups in overall adverse events, serious adverse events occurred twice as frequently in parecoxib/valdecoxib-treated patients than in control patients (19.0% versus 9.9%, respectively; $p = 0.015$).

Regarding individual serious adverse events, a greater incidence in sternal wound infection was found in the parecoxib/valdecoxib patients (3.2%) versus control patients (0.0%) ($p = 0.035$). The effects of NSAIDs on sternal wound complications had not been previously reported. The COX-2 enzyme enables prostaglandin release and the inflammatory response; inhibition of this enzyme by nonspecific COX inhibitors (NSAIDs) as well as specific COX-2 inhibitors might impede reparative inflammatory responses and increase susceptibility to sternal wound infections. An alternative hypothesis is that reduced fever and tachycardia in NSAID/COX-2 inhibitor–treated patients may delay detection of infection, resulting in further progression and greater consequence. Regardless of the mechanism, these safety issues merit careful consideration because of the importance of sternal wound complications in this setting. The incidence of other individual serious adverse events, including cerebrovascular complications, myocardial infarction, and renal dysfunction, were proportionally greater in the parecoxib/valdecoxib patients but not significantly different between the two groups. Specifically, when the groups were compared, more patients in the treatment group (parecoxib/valdecoxib) experienced cerebrovascular disorders (2.9% versus 0.7%, $p = 0.177$), myocardial infarction (1.6% versus 0.7%, $p = 0.669$), and renal dysfunction (1.9% versus 0.0%, $p = 0.184$) compared with control patients.

Such thrombosis-mediated complications also merit careful consideration. In cardiac surgery patients exposed to CPB, the delicate balance among platelets, endothelial cells, and serum clotting factors is disturbed, with consequent thrombosis and clot lysis occurring disparately and unpredictably throughout the vascular system. Given that COX-2 inhibitors are platelet sparing, they might tip the balance toward thrombosis during periods of platelet activation. In addition, because COX-1 is unaffected, consequent release of thromboxane A_2 may further promote platelet activation and thrombosis. Of note, some analyses addressing these issues in chronically treated patients with arthritis indicate a potential association between COX-2 inhibition and thrombogenic events (myocardial infarction, stroke, vascular death).[69] Ott and associates conclude that in patients undergoing CABG, the COX-2 inhibitor combination of parecoxib/valdecoxib is effective in controlling postoperative analgesia. However, the treatment regimen may be associated with an increased incidence of serious adverse events overall and sternal wound infections in particular. Their study, therefore, raises important concerns requiring a comprehensive evaluation of the potential link between this class of drugs and perioperative complications in a large-scale clinical trial before the COX-2 inhibitors are routinely used in patients undergoing cardiac surgery.

Over the next decade, much more will be learned about COX-2 inhibitors. Their analgesic (opioid-sparing) effects and lack of deleterious effects on coagulation (in contrast to nonselective NSAIDs) certainly are desirable. The evidence to date does not suggest that COX-2 inhibitors provide major advantages over traditional NSAIDs. It is possible that their continued development will lead to specific drugs with a superior therapeutic profile. Many important questions regarding their safety remain to be answered, such as effects on central nervous system sensitization, perioperative renal function, preemptive analgesia, clinically significant blood loss, the gastrointestinal system, the cardiovascular system, chronic postsurgical pain, bone/wound healing, blood pressure, and peripheral edema, among others. Specifically regarding patients undergoing cardiac surgery, the potential links between this class of drugs and sternal wound infections and thromboembolic complications need to be fully evaluated.

α_2-ADRENERGIC AGONISTS

The α_2-adrenergic agonists provide analgesia, sedation, and sympatholysis (Box 37–7). The initial impetus for the use of α_2-agonists in anesthesia resulted from astute clinical observations made in patients during intraoperative anesthesia who were receiving clonidine therapy. Soon thereafter, investigators revealed that clonidine substantially reduced anesthetic requirements (minimal alveolar concentration). More recently, dexmedetomidine has undergone extensive clinical evaluation for perioperative use. Dexmedetomidine exerts profound effects on cardiovascular parameters and thus appears to effect its own pharmacokinetics. At high doses, there is marked vasoconstriction, which probably reduces the drug's volume of distribution. The elimination half-life of dexmedetomidine is two to three hours.

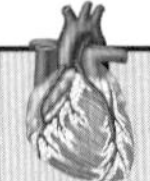

BOX 37–7 ***α_2-Adrenergic Agonists***

- Advantage:
  - Cardiovascular stability?
- Disadvantages:
  - Sedation
  - Hypotension

α_2-Adrenergic agonists produce clinically sedative effects via stimulation of α_2-receptors in the locus ceruleus and clinically analgesic effects via stimulation of α_2-receptors within the locus ceruleus and the spinal cord.[70] Evidence exists indicating that α_2-agonists enhance the analgesic effects of the opioids via an unknown mechanism of action. Several mechanisms of action have been postulated for the analgesia noted with α_2-adrenergic agonists, including supraspinal, ganglionic, spinal, and peripheral mechanisms. Clinically, systemic administration of these agents produces antinociception and sedation, whereas intrathecal administration usually produces only antinociception. Like other adrenergic receptors, the α_2-adrenergic agonists demonstrate tolerance following prolonged administration.

As with all clinically used analgesics, the α_2-adrenergic agonists possess clinically important side effects that may limit their usefulness. Dexmedetomidine's effects on the respiratory system include a decrease in tidal volume, minimal changes in respiratory rate, and a rightward shift and depression of slope of the carbon dioxide response curve (all of which may cause hypercarbia). However, respiratory depression associated with the drug is usually clinically unimportant even during profound levels of sedation. Dexmedetomidine's effects on the cardiovascular system are many, and in contrast to the respiratory effects, may become clinically important. Physiologic changes include decreased heart rate, decreased systemic vascular resistance, and possibly indirectly decreased myocardial contractility, all potentially leading to decreased cardiac output and decreased blood pressure in susceptible patients. By developing more highly selective α_2-adrenergic agonists, it is hoped that these detrimental cardiovascular effects will be minimized while maximizing desired analgesic and sedative properties. At the present time, the clinical role of these drugs includes preoperative sedation, an intraoperative adjuvant during anesthesia to reduce sedative and analgesic requirements, and postoperative sedation and analgesia. The potential ability of the α_2-adrenergic agonists to reduce and/or prevent perioperative myocardial ischemia, while intriguing, remains to be determined.[71]

The potential perioperative analgesic benefits of α_2-agonists, when administered to patients undergoing cardiac surgery, were demonstrated almost 20 years ago.[72] In 1987, Flacke and associates,[72] in prospective, nonblinded fashion, randomized patients undergoing elective CABG to receive either perioperative oral clonidine supplementation (10 patients) or serve as controls (10 patients). Outside of oral clonidine supplementation, management of the two study groups was identical. Patients receiving oral clonidine required significantly less preinduction diazepam and significantly less intraoperative sufentanil (Fig. 37–11) and isoflurane to maintain intraoperative normotension (clearly establishing clonidine's sedative/analgesic properties). Furthermore, patients receiving oral clonidine were extubated earlier during the postoperative period compared with control patients (approximately 11 hours versus 16 hours, respectively; $p < 0.05$). However, 4 of 10 patients receiving oral clonidine required atropine for treatment of intraoperative bradycardia. Unfortunately, postoperative analgesia was not assessed in this clinical investigation.

While the analgesic properties of α_2-adrenergic agonists are undisputed,[73] most of the clinical investigations regarding perioperative use of this class of drugs remain focused on exploiting the sedative effects and beneficial cardiovascular effects (decreasing hypertension and tachycardia) associated with their use.[74-76] α_2-Adrenergic agonists have been used perioperatively in patients undergoing cardiac surgery yet the focus of such clinical investigations has been on the intraoperative period and the potential for enhanced postoperative hemodynamic stability, potentially leading to reduced postoperative myocardial ischemia (not specifically at enhanced postoperative analgesia).[77-80] Taken together, these clinical investigations indicate that perioperative administration of α_2-adrenergic agonists to patients undergoing cardiac surgery decreases intraoperative anesthetic requirements, may enhance perioperative hemodynamic stability, and may decrease perioperative myocardial ischemia yet may cause excessive postoperative sedation and aggravate postoperative hemodynamic instability via bradycardia and/or decreased systemic vascular resistance (leading to hypotension and increased pacing requirements in susceptible patients). The potential ability of this class of drugs to initiate reliable postoperative analgesia awaits definitive investigation.

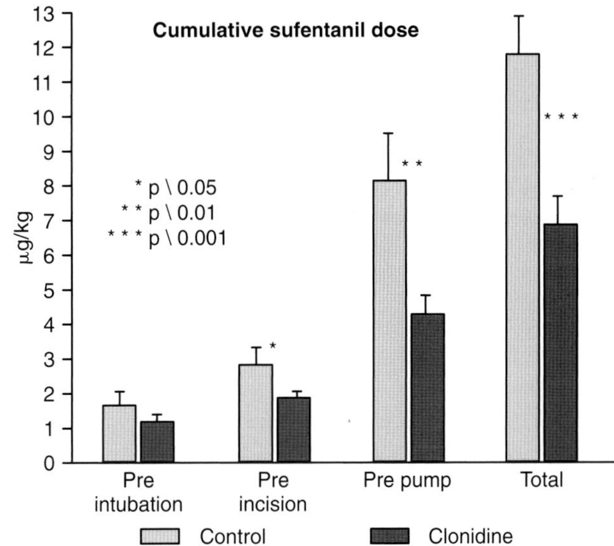

Figure 37–11 Cumulative sufentanil dose. Mean cumulative sufentanil doses are shown for the periods prior to intubation, prior to incision, prior to CPB, and for the entire anesthetic period. (From Flacke JW, Bloor BC, Flacke WE, et al: Reduced narcotic requirement by clonidine with improved hemodynamic and adrenergic stability in patients undergoing coronary bypass surgery. Anesthesiology 67:11, 1987.)

INTRATHECAL AND EPIDURAL TECHNIQUES

It is clear from numerous clinical investigations that intrathecal and/or epidural techniques (using opioids and/or local anesthetics) initiate reliable postoperative analgesia in patients following cardiac surgery[81] (Boxes 37–8 and 37–9). Additional potential advantages of using intrathecal and/or epidural techniques in patients undergoing cardiac surgery include stress-response attenuation and thoracic cardiac sympathectomy.

An uninhibited stress response during the postoperative period may lead to many adverse hemodynamic (tachycardia, hypertension, vasoconstriction), metabolic (increased catabolism), immunologic (impaired immune response), and hemostatic (platelet activation) alterations. Intrathecal or epidural anesthesia and analgesia (with local anesthetics or opioids)

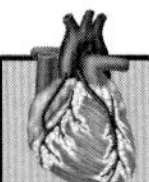

BOX 37–8 *Intrathecal Techniques*

- Advantages:
  - Simple, reliable analgesia
  - Stress-response attenuation
  - Less hematoma risk than epidural techniques
- Disadvantages:
  - No cardiac sympathectomy
  - Hematoma risk increased
  - Side effects of intrathecal opioids

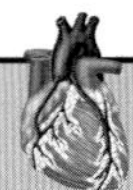

BOX 37–9 *Epidural Techniques*

- Advantages:
  - Reliable analgesia
  - Stress-response attenuation
  - Cardiac sympathectomy
- Disadvantages:
  - Labor intensive
  - Hematoma risk increased
  - Side effects of epidural opioids

can effectively inhibit the stress response associated with surgical procedures.[27] Local anesthetics appear to possess greater efficacy than opioids in perioperative stress response attenuation, perhaps because of their unique mechanism of action. Although still a matter of some debate, perioperative stress response attenuation with epidural local anesthetics and/or opioids in high-risk patients after major noncardiac surgery may decrease morbidity and mortality.[6,7,27] In patients undergoing cardiac surgery, initiation of CPB causes significant increases in stress response hormones that persist into the immediate postoperative period.[24-26] Attenuation of this component of the perioperative stress response with intravenous opioids may also decrease morbidity and mortality in these patients.[8,9] Unfortunately, perioperative stress response attenuation in patients undergoing cardiac surgery with intravenous opioids in this manner does not allow tracheal extubation to occur in the immediate postoperative period. Intrathecal or epidural anesthesia and analgesia techniques (particularly with local anesthetics) are attractive alternatives to intravenous opioids in this setting for their potential to attenuate the perioperative stress response yet still allow tracheal extubation to occur in the immediate postoperative period.

The myocardium and coronary vasculature are densely innervated by sympathetic nerve fibers that arise from T1 to T5 and profoundly influence total coronary blood flow and distribution.[82] Cardiac sympathetic nerve activation initiates coronary artery vasoconstriction[83] and paradoxical coronary vasoconstriction in response to intrinsic vasodilators.[84] In patients with coronary artery disease, cardiac sympathetic nerve activation disrupts the normal matching of coronary blood flow and myocardial oxygen demand.[85,86] Animal models have revealed an intense poststenotic coronary vasoconstrictive mechanism mediated by cardiac sympathetic nerve activation that attenuates local metabolic coronary vasodilation in response to myocardial ischemia.[87,88] Furthermore, myocardial ischemia initiates a cardiocardiac reflex mediated by sympathetic nerve fibers, which augments the ischemic process.[89] Cardiac sympathetic nerve activation likely plays a central role in initiating postoperative myocardial ischemia by decreasing myocardial oxygen supply via the mechanisms listed above.[27,90]

Thoracic epidural anesthesia with local anesthetics effectively blocks cardiac sympathetic nerve afferent and efferent fibers.[27] Opioids, administered similarly, are unable to effectively block such cardiac sympathetic nerve activity.[27] Patients with symptomatic coronary artery disease benefit clinically from cardiac sympathectomy, and the application of thoracic sympathetic blockade in the management of angina pectoris was described as early as 1965.[91] Thoracic epidural anesthesia with local anesthetics increases the diameter of stenotic epicardial coronary artery segments without causing dilation of coronary arterioles,[85] decreases determinants of myocardial oxygen demand,[86] improves left ventricular function,[92] and decreases anginal symptoms.[86,93] Furthermore, cardiac sympathectomy increases the endocardial-to-epicardial blood flow ratio,[94,95] beneficially affects collateral blood flow during myocardial ischemia,[95] decreases poststenotic coronary vasoconstriction,[88] and attenuates the myocardial ischemia-induced cardiocardiac reflex.[88] In an animal model, thoracic epidural anesthesia with local anesthetics actually decreased myocardial infarct size following coronary artery occlusion.[94] Of note, these beneficial effects are not caused by systemic absorption of the local anesthetic.[94] In short, thoracic epidural anesthesia with local anesthetics may benefit patients undergoing cardiac surgery by effectively blocking cardiac sympathetic nerve activity and improving the myocardial oxygen supply-demand balance.

INTRATHECAL TECHNIQUES

Application of intrathecal analgesia to patients undergoing cardiac surgery was initially reported by Mathews and Abrams in 1980.[96] They described the administration of intrathecal morphine (1.5 to 4.0 mg) to 40 adults after the induction of general anesthesia for cardiac surgery. Somewhat remarkably, all 40 patients awakened pain free at the end of surgery (prior to leaving the operating room) and 36 patients were tracheally extubated prior to transfer to the intensive care unit. Postoperatively, all 40 patients were entirely pain-free for the first 27.5 postoperative hours and 17 did not require any supplemental analgesics prior to discharge from the hospital. Of the 17 patients who received 4.0 mg of intrathecal morphine, 11 did not require any postoperative analgesic drugs. Mathews and Abrams summarize: "The benefits of recovering from surgery free from pain have been impressive. This has been particularly appreciated by patients who have had previous operations with conventional anesthesia and postoperative analgesic drugs. The patients have been remarkably comfortable, able to move more easily in bed, and more cooperative, thus greatly helping their nursing care."[96] After this impressive clinical display, other investigators have subsequently applied intrathecal anesthesia and analgesia techniques to patients undergoing cardiac surgery.[97-122]

Most clinical investigators have used intrathecal morphine in hopes of providing prolonged postoperative analgesia. Some clinical investigators have used intrathecal fentanyl, sufentanil, and/or local anesthetics for intraoperative anesthesia and analgesia (with stress response attenuation) and/or thoracic cardiac sympathectomy. An anonymous survey of members of the Society of Cardiovascular Anesthesiologists indicates that almost 8% of practicing anesthesiologists incorporate intrathecal techniques into their anesthetic management of adults undergoing cardiac surgery.[123] Of these anesthesiologists, 75% practice in the United States, 72% perform the intrathecal injection prior to induction of anesthesia, 97% use morphine, 13% use fentanyl, 2% use sufentanil, 10% use lidocaine, and 3% use tetracaine.[123]

Two randomized, blinded, placebo-controlled clinical studies revealed the ability of intrathecal morphine to induce significant postoperative analgesia following cardiac surgery.[109,116] In 1988, Vanstrum and associates[116] prospectively randomized 30 patients to receive either intrathecal morphine (0.5 mg) or intrathecal placebo prior to induction of anesthesia. Intraoperative anesthetic management was standardized, and postoperatively all patients received only intravenous morphine administered by a nurse who attempted to keep the linear analog pain score at less than 4 (a score of 1 represented no pain, 10 represented the worst pain imaginable; the scale was 25 cm long). Although pain scores between groups were not significantly different at any postoperative time interval tested, patients who received intrathecal morphine required significantly less intravenous morphine than placebo controls (2.4 mg versus 8.3 mg, respectively; $p < 0.02$) during the initial 30 hours following intrathecal injection (Fig. 37–12). Associated with this enhanced analgesia in patients receiving intrathecal morphine was a substantially decreased need for antihypertensive medications (sodium nitroprusside, nitroglycerin, hydralazine) during the immediate postoperative period. Time to tracheal extubation (approximately 20 hours) and postoperative arterial blood gas tensions following anesthesia were not significantly affected by the use of intrathecal morphine. In 1996, Chaney and associates prospectively randomized 60 patients to receive either intrathecal morphine (4.0 mg) or intrathecal placebo prior to induction of anesthesia for elective CABG.[109] Intraoperative anesthetic management was standardized and after tracheal extubation all patients received intravenous morphine via PCA exclusively. The mean time from ICU arrival to tracheal extubation was similar in all patients (approximately 20 hours). However, patients who received intrathecal morphine required significantly less intravenous morphine than placebo controls (33.2 mg versus 51.1 mg, respectively; $p < 0.05$) during the initial postoperative period (Table 37–2). Despite enhanced analgesia, no clinical differences between groups existed regarding postoperative morbidity (pruritus, nausea, vomiting, urinary retention, prolonged somnolence, atrial fibrillation, ventricular tachycardia, myocardial infarction, cerebral infarction), mortality, or duration of postoperative hospital stay (approximately 9 days in each group).

The mid 1990s saw the emergence of fast-track cardiac surgery, with the goal being tracheal extubation in the immediate postoperative period. Chaney and associates in 1997[108] were the first to study the potential clinical benefits of intrathecal morphine when used in patients undergoing cardiac surgery and early tracheal extubation. They prospectively randomized 40 patients to receive either intrathecal morphine (10 μg/kg) or intrathecal placebo prior to induction of anesthesia for elective CABG. Intraoperative anesthetic management was standardized (intravenous fentanyl, 20 μg/kg, and intravenous midazolam, 10 mg) and postoperatively all patients received intravenous morphine via PCA exclusively. Of the patients who were tracheally extubated during the immediate postoperative period, the mean time from ICU arrival to tracheal extubation was significantly ($p = 0.02$) prolonged in patients who received intrathecal morphine (10.9

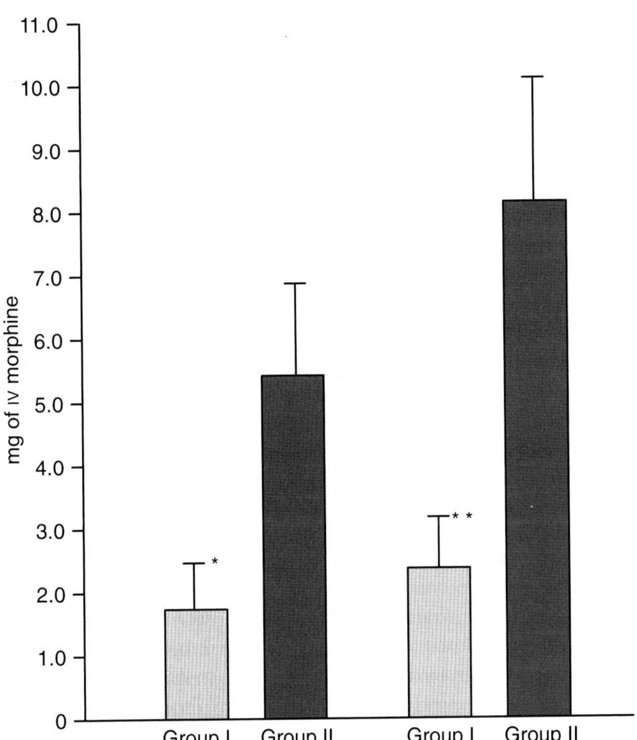

Figure 37–12 Postoperative supplemental intravenous morphine requirements. Patients receiving intrathecal morphine (Group I) required significantly less supplemental intravenous morphine during the initial 24 postoperative hours (*left*, $p < 0.048$) and during the initial 30 postoperative hours (*right*, $p < 0.02$) compared with patients receiving intrathecal placebo (Group II). (From Vanstrum GS, Bjornson KM, Ilko R: Postoperative effects of intrathecal morphine in coronary artery bypass surgery. Anesth Analg 67:261, 1988.)

Table 37–2 **Postoperative Supplemental Intravenous Midazolam and Morphine Requirements**

	Group MS (n = 27)	Group NS (n = 29)
Midazolam use from ICU arrival to extubation, mg (range)	8.7 ± 15.8 (0 to 80)	8.3 ± 15.4 (0 to 66)
Morphine use from ICU arrival to 8:00 AM POD 2, mg (range)	33.2 ± 15.8 (4 to 74)	51.1 ± 45.7 (4 to 254)
Morphine use from 8:00 AM POD 2 to 8:00 AM POD 3, mg (range)	14.2 ± 16.4 (0 to 68)	12.1 ± 12.6 (0 to 42)

Patients receiving intrathecal morphine (group MS) required significantly less supplemental intravenous morphine during the immediate postoperative period compared with patients receiving intrathecal placebo (group NS) (33.2 mg versus 51.1 mg, respectively; $p < 0.05$). POD = postoperative day.

From Chaney MA, Smith KR, Barclay JC, Slogoff S: Large-dose intrathecal morphine for coronery artery bypass grafting. Anesth Analg 83:215, 1996.

hours ± 4.4 hours) compared with placebo controls (7.6 hours ± 2.5 hours). Three patients who received intrathecal morphine had tracheal extubation substantially delayed (12 to 24 hours) because of prolonged ventilatory depression (likely secondary to intrathecal morphine). Although the mean postoperative intravenous morphine use for 48 hours was less in patients who received intrathecal morphine (42.8 mg) compared with patients who received intrathecal placebo (55.0 mg), the difference between groups was not statistically significant. No clinical differences existed between groups regarding postoperative morbidity, mortality, or duration of postoperative hospital stay (approximately 9 days in each group).

These somewhat discouraging findings (absence of enhanced analgesia, prolongation of tracheal extubation time) stimulated the same group of investigators in 1999 to try again, this time decreasing the amount of intraoperative intravenous fentanyl patients received (hoping to decrease fentanyl's effect on augmenting postoperative respiratory depression associated with intrathecal morphine).[106] Forty patients were prospectively randomized to receive either intrathecal morphine (10 μg/kg) or intrathecal placebo prior to induction of anesthesia for elective CABG. Intraoperative anesthetic management was standardized (intravenous fentanyl, 10 μg/kg, and intravenous midazolam, 200 μg/kg) and all patients postoperatively received intravenous morphine exclusively via PCA. Of the patients tracheally extubated during the immediate postoperative period, mean time to tracheal extubation was similar in patients who received intrathecal morphine (6.8 hours ± 2.8 hours) compared with intrathecal placebo patients (6.5 hours ± 3.2 hours). However, once again, four patients who received intrathecal morphine had tracheal extubation substantially delayed (14 hours, 14 hours, 18 hours, and 19 hours) because of prolonged respiratory depression (likely secondary to intrathecal morphine). The mean postoperative intravenous morphine use during the immediate postoperative period was actually higher in patients receiving intrathecal morphine (49.8 mg) compared with patients receiving intrathecal placebo (36.2 mg), yet the difference between groups was not statistically significant. No clinical differences existed between groups regarding postoperative morbidity, mortality, or duration of postoperative hospital stay (approximately 6 days in each group). Thus, Chaney and associates, from their three prospective, randomized, double-blind, placebo-controlled clinical investigations in the late 1990s involving 140 healthy adults undergoing elective CABG, concluded that although intrathecal morphine certainly can initiate reliable postoperative analgesia, its use in the setting of fast-track cardiac surgery and early tracheal extubation may be detrimental by potentially delaying tracheal extubation in the immediate postoperative period.

Since this time, however, other clinical investigators have revealed that certain combinations of intraoperative anesthetic techniques, coupled with appropriate doses of intrathecal morphine, will allow both tracheal extubation following cardiac surgery within the immediate postoperative period along with enhanced analgesia. Alhashemi and associates[98] prospectively randomized 50 adults undergoing elective CABG to receive either one of two doses of intrathecal morphine (250 μg or 500 μg) or intrathecal placebo. Intraoperative anesthetic management was standardized (fentanyl, midazolam) and all patients received intermittent morphine by a blinded practitioner during the postoperative period. Tracheal extubation times were similar in the placebo group, 250 μg intrathecal morphine group, and 500 μg intrathecal morphine group (7.3 hours, 5.4 hours, and 6.8 hours, respectively; $p = 0.270$). However, postoperative morphine requirements in the placebo group (21.3 mg ± 6.2 mg), 250 μg intrathecal morphine group (13.6 mg ± 7.8 mg), and the 500 μg intrathecal morphine group (11.7 mg ± 7.4 mg) were substantially different. There was at least a 36% reduction in postoperative intravenous morphine requirements among those patients who received intrathecal morphine. While there were no differences in postoperative intravenous morphine requirements between patients randomized to receive either 250 μg or 500 μg of intrathecal morphine, both groups required significantly less intravenous morphine during the immediate postoperative period compared with control patients ($p = 0.001$). However, despite enhanced analgesia, there were no differences among the study groups in regard to midazolam, nitroglycerin, and sodium nitroprusside requirements in the postoperative period (Table 37–3). Furthermore, postextubation blood gas analysis, use of supplemental inspired oxygen, and ICU length of stay (approximately 22 hours in all groups) were comparable among the three groups.

These investigators, as well as others, reveal that the use of intrathecal morphine in patients undergoing fast-track cardiac surgery and early tracheal extubation may (if used appropriately) provide enhanced postoperative analgesia without delaying tracheal extubation. The authors also interestingly postulate that limiting the amounts of intraoperative intravenous opioids and intravenous sedatives and the application of a postoperative tracheal extubation protocol may be more important in achieving the goal of early tracheal extubation following cardiac surgery than adequate pain control during the immediate postoperative period.

Table 37–3 Analysis of Outcome Measures in Patients Receiving Either Placebo, 250 μg Intrathecal Morphine, or 500 μg Intrathecal Morphine

	Placebo (n = 19)	250 μg (n = 16)	500 μg (n = 15)	*p* Value
Ventilatory time (min)	441 ± 207	325 ± 187	409 ± 245	0.270
Morphine (mg)	21.3 ± 6.2	13.6 ± 7.8	11.7 ± 7.4	0.001
Midazolam (mg)	2.3 ± 3.5	0.9 ± 1.8	1.5 ± 2.7	0.346
Nitroglycerin (mg)	52.5 ± 37.6	55.0 ± 38.4	52.8 ± 43.0	0.982
Nitroprusside (mg)	7.9 ± 22.7	0.1 ± 0.4	1.4 ± 4.0	0.230

From Alhashemi JA, Sharpe MD, Harris CL, et al: Effect of subarachnoid morphine administration on extubation time after coronary artery bypass graft surgery. J Cardiothorac Vasc Anesth 14:639, 2000.

Many other suboptimally designed clinical investigations (retrospective, observational, etc.) attest to the ability of intrathecal morphine to induce substantial postoperative analgesia in patients following cardiac surgery (Table 37–4). Intrathecal doses of 0.5 to 10.0 mg administered prior to CPB initiate reliable postoperative analgesia, the quality of which depends not only on the intrathecal dose administered but also on the type and amount of intravenous analgesics and sedatives used for the intraoperative baseline anesthetic. The optimal dose of intrathecal morphine for achieving the maximum postoperative analgesia with minimum undesirable drug effects is uncertain. Naturally, when larger doses of intrathecal morphine are used, more intense and prolonged postoperative analgesia is obtained at the expense of more undesirable drug effects (nausea and vomiting, pruritus, urinary retention, respiratory depression).

Because of morphine's low lipid solubility, analgesic effects following intrathecal injection are delayed. Thus, even large doses of intrathecal morphine administered to patients prior to cardiac surgery will not initiate reliable intraoperative analgesia[116-118,121] and therefore would not be expected to potentially attenuate the intraoperative stress response associated with CPB. Only an extremely large dose of intrathecal morphine (10.0 mg) may initiate reliable intraoperative analgesia in this setting.[120] Only one clinical investigation has examined the ability of intrathecal morphine to potentially attenuate the intraoperative stress response associated with CPB as measured by blood catecholamine levels.[109] In this clinical investigation by Chaney and associates, patients were prospectively randomized to receive either intrathecal morphine (4.0 mg) or intrathecal placebo prior to induction of anesthesia for elective CABG with CPB. Intraoperative anesthetic management was standardized, and multiple arterial blood samples were obtained perioperatively to ascertain norepinephrine and epinephrine levels. Patients who were administered intrathecal morphine experienced similar perioperative increases in blood catecholamine levels when compared with placebo controls. Thus, it appears that intrathecal morphine (even in relatively large doses) is unable to reliably attenuate the perioperative stress response associated with cardiac surgery and CPB.

Although unable to reliably attenuate the perioperative stress response associated with CPB, intrathecal morphine (by initiating postoperative analgesia) may potentially attenuate the stress response during the immediate postoperative period.[116] Vanstrum and associates revealed that patients who were administered 0.5 mg of intrathecal morphine prior to the induction of anesthesia not only required significantly less intravenous morphine postoperatively compared with placebo controls but also required significantly less intravenous nitroprusside (58.1 mg versus 89.1 mg, respectively; $p < 0.05$) during the initial 24 postoperative hours to control hypertension, which suggests partial postoperative stress response attenuation.

Some clinical investigators have used intrathecal fentanyl, sufentanil, and/or local anesthetics for patients undergoing cardiac surgery, hoping to provide intraoperative anesthesia and analgesia (and stress response attenuation), with mixed results (see Table 37–4). Administration of intrathecal local anesthetics to patients after the induction of anesthesia for cardiac surgery may help promote intraoperative hemodynamic stability,[110,112] whereas intrathecal sufentanil (50 μg) administered prior to the induction of anesthesia for cardiac surgery can reduce volatile anesthetic requirements during mediastinal dissection but is unable to reliably block intraoperative hemodynamic responses to laryngoscopy and intubation.[113]

Most clinical attempts at inducing thoracic cardiac sympathectomy in patients undergoing cardiac surgery have used thoracic epidural anesthesia with local anesthetics. However, a small number of clinical investigators have attempted cardiac sympathectomy in this setting with an intrathecal injection of local anesthetic. In 1994, as reviewed retrospectively, 18 adult patients were administered lumbar intrathecal hyperbaric bupivacaine (23 to 30 mg) and/or hyperbaric lidocaine (150 mg) mixed with morphine (0.5 to 1.0 mg) following the induction of anesthesia.[112] In an attempt to produce a "total spinal" and, thus, thoracic cardiac sympathectomy, Trendelenburg position was maintained for at least 10 minutes following intrathecal injection. Heart rate decreased significantly (baseline mean 67 bpm to postinjection mean 52 bpm) after the intrathecal injection (indicating cardiac sympathectomy was obtained) and not a single patient exhibited electrocardiographic evidence of myocardial ischemia prior to CPB. Although these authors report that the technique provided stable perioperative hemodynamics, 17 of 18 patients required intravenous phenylephrine at some time intraoperatively to increase blood pressure. In 1996, the same group of investigators reported similar hemodynamic changes in a case report involving a 10-year-old child with Kawasaki disease who underwent CABG and receiving intrathecal hyperbaric bupivacaine mixed with morphine via a lumbar puncture following induction of anesthesia.[110] While Kowalewski's group reports that these patients experienced enhanced postoperative analgesia, definite conclusions cannot be reached regarding this technique because of study design formats (retrospective review, case report).

A small (n = 38 patients), prospective, randomized, blinded clinical investigation reveals that large doses of intrathecal bupivacaine (37.5 mg) administered to patients immediately prior to induction of general anesthesia (19 patients received intrathecal bupivacaine, 19 patients served as controls) for elective CABG may potentially initiate intraoperative stress response attenuation (assessed via serum mediator levels, hemodynamics, and qualitative/quantitative alterations in myocardial β-receptors).[124] However, no effect on real clinical outcome parameters (tracheal extubation times, respiratory function, perioperative spirometry, etc.) was observed. Mean tracheal extubation times (measured from the time of sternotomy dressing application) were extremely short in both groups (11 to 19 minutes). Specifically regarding postoperative analgesia, postoperative pain scores and morphine use via PCA did not differ between the two groups. Not surprisingly, phenylephrine use was more common in patients who received intrathecal bupivacaine compared with control patients.

The many clinical investigations involving the use of intrathecal analgesic techniques in patients undergoing cardiac surgery indicate that the administration of intrathecal morphine to patients prior to CPB initiates reliable postoperative analgesia following cardiac surgery. Intrathecal opioids or local anesthetics cannot reliably attenuate the perioperative stress response associated with CPB that persists during the immediate postoperative period. Although intrathecal local anesthetics (not opioids) may induce perioperative thoracic cardiac sympathectomy, the hemodynamic changes associated with a "total spinal" make the technique unpalatable in patients with cardiac disease.

Table 37–4 **Reports of Intrathecal Anesthesia and Analgesia for Cardiac Surgery**

First Author	Year	Study Design	Total Patients	Drugs: Dose	Intraoperative Management	Remarks
Lee	2003	Prospective, randomized blind, placebo-controlled	38	Bupivacaine: 37.5 mg	Standardized	Potential stress-response attenuation
Bowler	2002	Prospective, randomized	24	Morphine: 2.0 mg	Not standardized	No benefit
Bettex	2002	Prospective, randomized	24	Morphine: 0.5 mg Sufentanil: 50 μg	Not standardized	Reliable postoperative analgesia. Facilitated early extubation
Alhashemi	2000	Prospective, randomized, blind, placebo-controlled	50	Morphine: 250 μg or 500 μg	Standardized	Significant postoperative analgesia
Latham	2000	Prospective, randomized	40	Morphine: 8 μg/kg	Standardized	No benefit
Zarate	2000	Prospective, randomized	40	Morphine: 8 μg/kg	Standardized	Reliable postoperative analgesia
Peterson	2000	Retrospective	18	Morphine: 5 to 10 μg/kg Tetracaine: 1 to 2 mg/kg	Not standardized	No benefit
Hammer	2000	Retrospective	25	Morphine: 7 to 10 μg/kg Tetracaine: 0.5 to 2 mg/kg	Not standardized	No benefit
Chaney	1999	Prospective, randomized, blind, placebo-controlled	40	Morphine: 10 μg/kg	Standardized	No benefit
Shroff	1997	Prospective, randomized	21	Morphine: 10 μg/kg Fentanyl: 25 μg	Not standardized	Reliable postoperative analgesia, facilitated early extubation
Chaney	1997	Prospective, randomized, blind, placebo-controlled	40	Morphine: 10 μg/kg	Standardized	Hindered early extubation
Chaney	1996	Prospective, randomized, blind, placebo-controlled	60	Morphine: 4.0 mg	Standardized	Significant postoperative analgesia, no stress-response attenuation
Taylor	1996	Retrospective	152	Morphine: 30 μg/kg	Not standardized	Reliable postoperative analgesia
Kowalewski	1994	Retrospective	18	Morphine: 0.5 to 1.0 mg Bupivacaine: 23 to 30 mg Lidocaine: 150 mg	Not standardized	Reliable postoperative analgesia, possible thoracic cardiac sympathectomy
Swenson	1994	Retrospective	10	Morphine: 0.5 mg Sufentanil: 50 μg	Not standardized	Reliable postoperative analgesia, facilitated early extubation
Fitzpatrick	1988	Prospective, randomized	44	Morphine: 1.0 to 2.0 mg	Not standardized	Significant postoperative analgesia
Vanstrum	1988	Prospective, randomized, blind, placebo-controlled	30	Morphine: 0.5 mg	Standardized	Significant postoperative analgesia, possible stress-response attenuation
Casey	1987	Prospective, randomized, blind, placebo-controlled	40	Morphine: 20 μg/kg	Standardized	No benefit
Cheun	1987	Prospective, observational	180	Morphine: 0.1 mg/kg Meperidine: 1.5 mg/kg	Not standardized	Reliable postoperative analgesia
Aun	1985	Prospective, randomized	60	Morphine: 2.0 to 4.0 mg	Not standardized	Significant postoperative analgesia
Jones	1984	Prospective, observational	56	Morphine: 20 to 30 μg/kg	Not standardized	Reliable postoperative analgesia
Mathews	1980	Retrospective	40	Morphine: 1.5 to 4.0 mg	Not standardized	Reliable postoperative analgesia

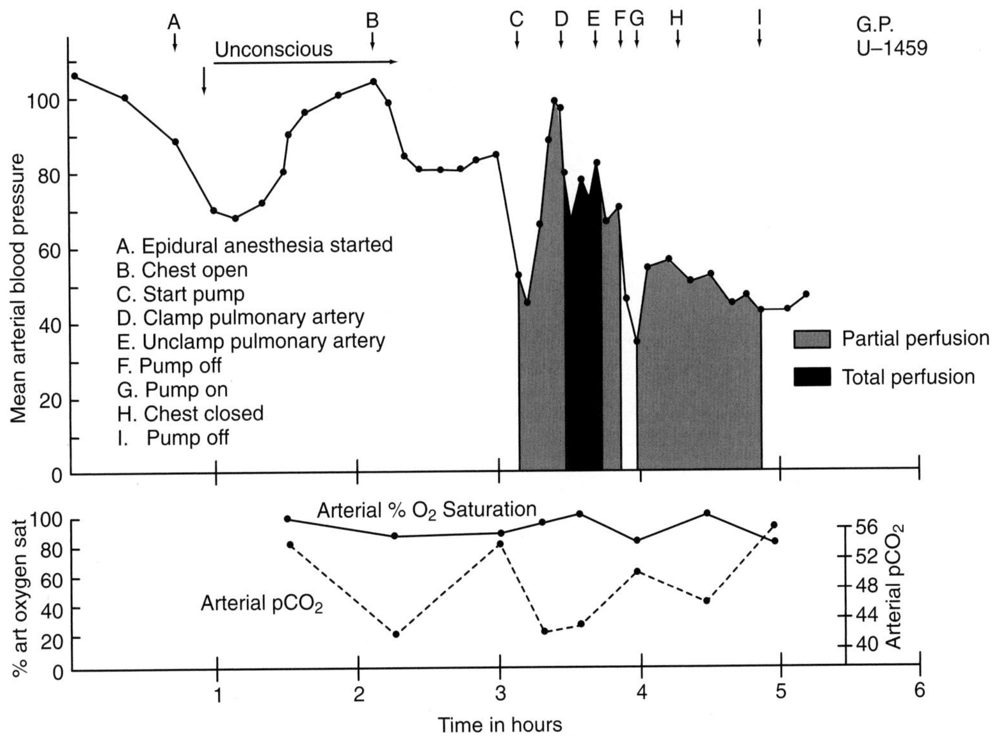

Figure 37–13 Graph of clinical course of initial cardiac patient receiving presurgical epidural anesthesia in 1954. (From Clowes GHA, Neville WE, Hopkins A, et al: Factors contributing to success or failure in the use of a pump oxygenator for complete by-pass of the heart and lung: Experimental and clinical. Surgery 36:557, 1954.)

EPIDURAL TECHNIQUES

The initial description of thoracic epidural anesthesia and analgesia applied to a cardiac surgical patient occurred in 1954, during the formative years of CPB.[125] Clowes and associates[125] describe their presurgical anesthetic technique in a 55-year-old man with severe cardiac failure: "An endotracheal tube was passed with topical anesthesia. Under extradural block of the upper thorax, hypotension developed but responded to the administration of a vasopressor drug. At this time the patient became comatose" (Fig. 37–13). The patient eventually died. Application of thoracic epidural anesthesia and analgesia to patients undergoing cardiac surgery during the modern surgical era was initially reported by Hoar and associates in 1976.[126] They described the intraoperative insertion of thoracic epidural catheters in 12 patients following CABG (after intravenous protamine, prior to transfer to ICU). The epidural catheters were injected with lidocaine and bupivacaine during the immediate postoperative period to promote analgesia and effectively control hypertension. Administration of epidural local anesthetics to these patients significantly decreased postoperative blood pressure in hypertensive and normotensive patients and not a single patient required cardiac or peripheral vascular stimulants during the immediate postoperative study period. The 1987 report by El-Baz and Goldin[127] was the first to describe the insertion of thoracic epidural catheters in patients prior to performance of cardiac surgery. In prospective, randomized fashion, patients undergoing elective CABG received either routine treatment for postoperative pain (n = 30 patients, intravenous morphine) or a continuous infusion of morphine (0.1 mg/hr) via a thoracic epidural catheter (n = 30 patients). Thoracic epidural catheters were inserted at T3-4 immediately prior to induction of anesthesia on the day of surgery. Intraoperative anesthetic technique was standardized and mean postoperative tracheal extubation time was significantly shorter in patients receiving thoracic epidural anesthesia compared with control patients (9 ± 3 hours versus 18 ± 5 hours, respectively; $p < 0.01$).

Continuous thoracic epidural infusion of morphine also achieved better postoperative pain relief in patients than intravenous morphine (significantly better pain scores, significantly less supplemental intravenous morphine). Furthermore, in a subgroup of 20 patients (10 per group), postoperative "stress" was assessed via serum cortisol and beta-endorphin levels. Patients receiving thoracic epidural anesthesia had significantly lower postoperative levels of these mediators compared with control patients, indicating potential postoperative stress response attenuation. Continuous thoracic epidural infusion of morphine (compared with controls) was also associated with a lower incidence of opioid-related side effects during the immediate postoperative period. The insertion of the thoracic epidural catheter immediately prior to systemic heparin administration was not associated with any neurological problems. Since this initial impressive display of potential benefits (reliable postoperative analgesia, stress response attenuation, facilitation of early tracheal extubation), other clinical investigators have subsequently applied thoracic epidural anesthesia and analgesia to patients undergoing cardiac surgery.[128-163] Most clinical investigators have used thoracic epidural local anesthetics in hopes of providing perioperative stress response attenuation and/or perioperative thoracic cardiac sympathectomy. Some clinical investigators have used thoracic epidural opioids to provide intraoperative and/or postoperative analgesia. An anonymous survey of members of the Society of Cardiovascular Anesthesiologists indicates that 7% of practicing anesthesiologists incorporate thoracic epidural techniques into their anesthetic management of adults undergoing cardiac surgery.[123] Of these anesthesiologists, 58% practice in the United States. Regarding the timing of epidural instrumentation, 40% perform instrumentation before induction of general anesthesia, 12% perform instrumentation following induction of general anesthesia, 33% perform instrumentation at the end of surgery, and 15% perform instrumentation on the first postoperative day.[123]

Thoracic epidural anesthesia and analgesia with local anesthetics and/or opioids induce significant postoperative analgesia in patients following cardiac surgery. Patients randomized to receive a continuous thoracic epidural morphine infusion (0.1 mg/hr) following cardiac surgery required significantly less postoperative supplemental intravenous morphine compared with patients without thoracic epidural catheters (5 mg/day versus 18 mg/day per patient, respectively; $p < 0.05$) during the initial 3 postoperative days.[127] Children (aged 2 to 12 years) randomized to receive caudal epidural morphine (75 μg/kg) intraoperatively following cardiac surgery required significantly less postoperative supplemental intravenous morphine compared with patients who did not receive epidural morphine (0.32 mg/kg versus 0.71 mg/kg, respectively; $p < 0.01$) during the initial 24 postoperative hours.[147] Numerous additional clinical studies further attest to the ability of thoracic epidural anesthesia and analgesia with local anesthetics and/or opioids to induce substantial postoperative analgesia in patients following cardiac surgery (Table 37–5).

One unique clinical investigation directly compared thoracic epidural anesthesia and intravenous clonidine in patients undergoing cardiac surgery.[131] Loick and associates[131] prospectively randomized 70 patients undergoing elective CABG to receive thoracic epidural anesthesia supplementation (bupivacaine, sufentanil continuous infusion) perioperatively to general anesthesia (n = 25 patients), to receive intravenous clonidine supplementation (continuous infusion) perioperatively to general anesthesia (n = 24 patients), or to receive only general anesthesia (n = 21 patients, controls). Hemodynamics, plasma epinephrine and norepinephrine levels, plasma cortisol levels, the myocardium-specific contractile protein troponin T levels, and other plasma cardiac enzymes were assessed perioperatively. Both the thoracic epidural anesthesia and intravenous clonidine groups experienced postoperative decreases in heart rate compared with the control group (without jeopardizing cardiac output or perfusion pressure). The effects on stress response mediators were unpredictable and variable. Electrocardiographic evidence of ischemia (ST-segment elevation, ST-segment depression) occurred in 70% of control patients, 50% of thoracic epidural anesthesia patients, and 40% of intravenous clonidine patients. The release of troponin T was attenuated (compared with controls) in the thoracic epidural anesthesia group only (no effect in the intravenous clonidine group). Interestingly enough, the highest quality of postoperative analgesia was found in the patients receiving intravenous clonidine. In the intravenous clonidine group, visual analog pain scores were nearly halved when compared with the two other groups. Sedation scores were similar among the three groups, with the exception of the 24-hour value in the intravenous clonidine group, which was higher than that in the thoracic epidural anesthesia group. The postoperative comfort scores (rated between excellent and good) did not differ among the three groups.

Many clinical investigations have proven that thoracic epidural anesthesia with local anesthetics also significantly attenuates the perioperative stress response in patients undergoing cardiac surgery. Patients randomized to receive intermittent boluses of thoracic epidural bupivacaine intraoperatively followed by continuous infusion postoperatively exhibited significantly decreased blood levels of norepinephrine and epinephrine perioperatively when compared with patients managed similarly without thoracic epidural catheters.[141] Furthermore, increased blood catecholamine levels in these patients were associated with increased systemic vascular resistance.[141] Patients randomized to receive continuous thoracic epidural bupivacaine infusion perioperatively exhibited significantly decreased blood levels of norepinephrine and cortisol perioperatively when compared with patients managed similarly without thoracic epidural catheters.[138] Patients randomized to receive a continuous thoracic epidural bupivacaine and sufentanil infusion perioperatively exhibited significantly decreased blood levels of norepinephrine following sternotomy when compared with patients managed similarly without thoracic epidural catheters.[144]

Other clinical studies further attest to the ability of thoracic epidural anesthesia with local anesthetics to promote perioperative hemodynamic stability in patients undergoing cardiac surgery, which suggests perioperative stress response attenuation.[126,140,141,144] While most clinical attempts at stress response attenuation involve thoracic epidural administration of local anesthetics, one investigation indicates that thoracic epidural analgesia with opioids may significantly attenuate the perioperative stress response in patients undergoing cardiac surgery.[127] In this clinical investigation, patients randomized to receive a continuous thoracic epidural morphine infusion postoperatively exhibited significantly decreased blood levels of cortisol and β-endorphin postoperatively when compared with patients managed similarly without thoracic epidural catheters.[127]

Two provocative clinical studies demonstrate the ability of thoracic epidural anesthesia to induce significant thoracic cardiac sympathectomy in patients undergoing cardiac surgery.[139,140] In the first study, patients undergoing CABG were evaluated with reverse thermodilution catheters that had been inserted into the mid-coronary sinus under fluoroscopic guidance prior to the induction of anesthesia.[139] Intraoperative anesthetic management was standardized. Coronary sinus blood flow was measured by a constant infusion technique and coronary vascular resistance was calculated using coronary perfusion pressure (arterial diastolic pressure minus pulmonary capillary wedge pressure) and coronary sinus blood flow. Patients who had been randomized to receive intermittent boluses of thoracic epidural bupivacaine intraoperatively followed by a continuous infusion postoperatively exhibited significant decreases in coronary vascular resistance post-CPB when compared with pre-CPB values, whereas patients managed similarly without thoracic epidural catheters exhibited significant increases in coronary vascular resistance post-CPB. In the second study, patients undergoing CABG were evaluated with catheters that had been inserted into the coronary sinus under fluoroscopic guidance and continuous pressure monitoring prior to the induction of anesthesia.[140] Intraoperative anesthetic management was standardized and all patients received a continuous intravenous infusion of tritiated norepinephrine (allowed assessment of cardiac norepinephrine spillover to plasma via isotope dilution technique). To assess cardiac sympathetic activity, blood samples were obtained from the coronary sinus and radial artery and the rate of norepinephrine spillover from the heart was calculated according to the Fick principle.

Table 37–5 **Reports of Epidural Anesthesia and Analgesia for Cardiac Surgery**

First Author	Year	Study Design	Total Patients	Drugs: Dosage Method	Intraoperative Management	Remarks
Royse	2003	Prospective, randomized	80	Ropivacaine, fentanyl infusion	Not standardized	Reliable postoperative analgesia
Pastor	2003	Prospective, observational	714	Bupivacaine or ropivacaine boluses plus infusion	Not standardized	No hematoma formation
Priestley	2002	Prospective, randomized	100	Ropivacaine, fentanyl infusion	Not standardized	Reliable postoperative analgesia
de Vries	2002	Prospective, randomized	90	Bupivacaine: bolus plus infusion Sufentanil: bolus plus infusion	Standardized	Reliable postoperative analgesia Facilitated early extubation Possible decreased hospital stay
Canto	2002	Prospective, observational	305	Ropivacaine: bolus plus infusion	Not standardized	No hematoma formation
Fillinger	2002	Prospective, randomized	60	Bupivacaine: bolus plus infusion Morphine: bolus plus infusion	Not standardized	No benefit
Jideus	2001	Prospective, randomized	41	Bupivacaine: bolus plus infusion Sufentanil: infusion	Not standardized	Stress response attenuation Thoracic cardiac sympathectomy
Scott	2001	Prospective, randomized	206	Bupivacaine: bolus plus infusion Clonidine: infusion	Standardized	Decreased postoperative arrhythmias Improved postoperative pulmonary function Decreased postoperative renal failure Decreased postoperative confusion
Dhole	2001	Prospective, randomized	41	Bupivacaine: bolus plus infusion	Not standardized	No benefit
Djaiani	2001	Retrospective	37	Bupivacaine: bolus plus infusion	Not standardized	Facilitated early extubation
Warters	2000	Retrospective	278	Not specified	Not standardized	No hematoma formation
Loick	1999	Prospective, randomized	25	Bupivacaine: bolus plus infusion Sufentanil: bolus plus infusion	Standardized	Stress response attenuation Thoracic cardiac sympathectomy Facilitated early extubation
Tenling	1999	Prospective, randomized	14	Bupivacaine: bolus plus infusion	Not standardized	Reliable postoperative analgesia Facilitated early extubation
Sanchez	1998	Prospective, observational	571	Bupivacaine: boluses	Not standardized	No hematoma formation
Fawcett	1997	Prospective, randomized	16	Bupivacaine: bolus plus infusion	Standardized	Reliable postoperative analgesia Improved pulmonary function Stress response attenuation
Turfrey	1997	Retrospective	218	Bupivacaine: bolus plus infusion Clonidine: infusion	Not standardized	Facilitated early extubation Possible thoracic cardiac sympathectomy

Table continued on following page

Table 37–5 Reports of Epidural Anesthesia and Analgesia for Cardiac Surgery—(Continued)

First Author	Year	Study Design	Total Patients	Drugs: Dosage, Method	Intraoperative Management	Remarks
Shayevitz	1996	Retrospective	54	Morphine: bolus plus infusion	Not standardized	Reliable postoperative analgesia Facilitated early extubation
Stenseth	1996	Prospective, randomized	54	Bupivacaine: bolus plus infusion	Not standardized	Facilitated early extubation Possible thoracic cardiac sympathectomy
Moore	1995	Prospective, randomized	17	Bupivacaine: bolus plus infusion	Standardized	Stress response attenuation Possible thoracic cardiac sympathectomy
Stenseth	1995	Prospective, randomized	30	Bupivacaine: bolus plus infusion	Standardized	Thoracic cardiac sympathectomy
Kirno	1994	Prospective, randomized	20	Mepivacaine: bolus	Standardized	Stress response attenuation Thoracic cardiac sympathectomy
Stenseth	1994	Prospective, randomized	30	Bupivacaine: bolus plus infusion	Standardized	Stress response attenuation Possible thoracic cardiac sympathectomy
Liem	1992	Prospective, randomized	54	Bupivacaine: bolus plus infusion Sufentanil: bolus plus infusion	Not standardized	Reliable postoperative analgesia Stress response attenuation Possible thoracic cardiac sympathectomy
Rosen	1989	Prospective, randomized	32	Morphine: bolus	Not standardized	Reliable postoperative analgesia Facilitated early extubation
Joachimsson	1989	Observational	28	Bupivacaine: boluses	Not standardized	Reliable postoperative analgesia
El-Baz	1987	Prospective, randomized	60	Morphine: infusion	Standardized	Reliable postoperative analgesia Stress response attenuation Facilitated early extubation
Robinson	1986	Prospective, observational	10	Meperidine: bolus	Standardized	Reliable postoperative analgesia
Hoar	1976	Prospective, observational	12	Lidocaine: boluses Bupivacaine: boluses	Not standardized	Reliable postoperative analgesia Possible stress response attenuation

Patients randomized to receive a single bolus of thoracic epidural mepivacaine immediately following induction of anesthesia exhibited significantly decreased cardiac norepinephrine spillover after sternotomy when compared with patients managed similarly without thoracic epidural catheters. Furthermore, 20% of patients managed without thoracic epidural catheters exhibited electrocardiographic evidence of myocardial ischemia following sternotomy, whereas no patient managed with a thoracic epidural catheter exhibited myocardial ischemia during this time.

Perioperative cardiac sympathectomy induced via thoracic epidural anesthesia with local anesthetics may clinically benefit patients undergoing cardiac surgery by increasing myocardial oxygen supply.[85,94,95] However, such a cardiac sympathectomy may offer additional benefits to patients undergoing cardiac surgery. Multiple clinical studies demonstrate that thoracic epidural anesthesia with local anesthetics significantly decreases heart rate before[144] and after[138,144] initiation of CPB and significantly decreases the need to administer β-blockers following CPB.[141] Multiple clinical studies also demonstrate that thoracic epidural anesthesia with local anesthetics significantly decreases systemic vascular resistance before[140,141] and after[144,148] initiation of CPB. Furthermore, patients undergoing cardiac surgery who receive thoracic epidural anesthesia with local anesthetics not only exhibit significant decreases in postoperative heart rate and systemic vascular resistance but also exhibit significant decreases in postoperative electrocardiographic evidence of myocardial ischemia when compared with patients managed similarly without thoracic epidural catheters.[144]

A relatively large clinical investigation highlights the potential clinical benefits of thoracic epidural anesthesia in cardiac surgical patients.[129] Scott and associates[129] prospectively randomized (nonblinded) 420 patients undergoing elective CABG to receive either thoracic epidural anesthesia (bupivacaine/clonidine) and general anesthesia or general anesthesia alone (control group). The two groups received similar intraoperative anesthetic techniques. In thoracic epidural anesthesia patients, the thoracic epidural infusion was continued for 96 hours following surgery (titrated according to need). In control patients, target-controlled infusion alfentanil was used for the first 24 postoperative hours, then followed by PCA morphine for the next 48 hours. Postoperatively, striking clinical differences were observed between the two groups (Table 37–6). Postoperative incidence of supraventricular arrhythmia, lower respiratory tract infection, renal failure, and acute confusion were all significantly lower in patients receiving thoracic epidural anesthesia compared with control patients. However, data from this clinical investigation must be viewed with caution. The clinical protocol dictated that β-adrenergic blocker therapy could not be used intraoperatively or postoperatively for the 5 days of the study period (except in those patients who developed a new arrhythmia requiring additional therapy). Since approximately 90% of this study's patients were taking β-adrenergic blockers preoperatively, this unique perioperative management clouds interpretation of postoperative supraventricular arrhythmia data.

Despite prospective randomization, substantially fewer patients receiving thoracic epidural anesthesia were current active smokers preoperatively compared with controls (5.8% versus 13.4%, respectively), which clouds interpretation of postoperative lower respiratory tract infection data. These investigators also found that postoperative preextubation maximal expiratory lung volumes were increased in thoracic epidural anesthesia patients (compared with controls), and postoperative tracheal extubation was facilitated via thoracic epidural anesthesia as well (yet thoracic epidural anesthesia patients and control patients were managed somewhat differently during the immediate postoperative period). While postoperative analgesia was not definitively assessed in this clinical investigation, 11.9% of control patients were converted to thoracic epidural anesthesia during the first 24 postoperative hours because of suboptimal postoperative analgesia, whereas only 2.9% of thoracic epidural anesthesia patients were converted to target-controlled infusion alfentanil or PCA morphine because of suboptimal postoperative analgesia. The results of this clinical investigation are certainly intriguing, but definitive conclusions regarding the use of thoracic epidural techniques in patients undergoing cardiac surgery cannot be drawn because of the study's substantial limitations, highlighted by an accompanying editorial[164] and three subsequent letters to the editor.[165-167]

Table 37–6 Various Outcomes of Patients

Outcome	TEA (n = 206) n (%)	GA (n = 202) n (%)
Supraventricular arrhythmia	21 (10.2)	45 (22.3)
Lower respiratory tract infection	31 (15.3)	59 (29.2)
Renal failure	4 (2.0)	14 (6.9)
Cerebrovascular accident	2 (1.0)	6 (3.0)
Acute confusion	3 (1.5)	11 (5.5)
Significant bleeding	35	23
Any complications	84	108

Significant (unadjusted) differences existed between groups regarding supraventricular arrhythmia ($p = 0.0012$), lower respiratory tract infection ($p = 0.0007$), renal failure ($p = 0.016$), acute confusion ($p = 0.031$), and any complications ($p = 0.011$). TEA = thoracic epidural analgesia; GA = general anesthesia.

From Scott NB, Turfrey DJ, Ray DAA, et al: A prospective randomized study of the potential benefits of thoracic epidural anesthesia and analgesia in patients undergoing coronary artery bypass grafting. Anesth Analg 93:528, 2001.

In contrast to the encouraging findings of the clinical investigation by Scott and associates, two prospective, randomized, nonblinded clinical investigations reveal that using thoracic epidural anesthesia techniques in patients undergoing cardiac surgery may not offer substantial clinical benefits.[168,169] In 2002, Priestley and associates[169] prospectively randomized 100 patients undergoing elective CABG to receive either thoracic epidural anesthesia (ropivacaine/fentanyl) and general anesthesia or general anesthesia alone (control group). The two groups received quite different intraoperative anesthetic techniques. Postoperatively, thoracic epidural anesthesia patients received epidural ropivacaine/fentanyl for 48 hours (supplemental analgesics available if needed), while control patients received nurse-administered intravenous morphine, followed by PCA morphine. Patients receiving thoracic epidural anesthesia were extubated sooner than controls (3.2 hours versus 6.7 hours, respectively; $p < 0.001$), yet this difference may have been secondary to the different amounts of intraoperative intravenous opioid administered to the two groups (intraoperative intravenous anesthetic technique not standardized).

Postoperative pain scores at rest were significantly lower in patients receiving thoracic epidural anesthesia only on postoperative days 0 and 1 (equivalent on days 2 and 3). Postoperative pain scores during coughing were significantly lower in patients receiving thoracic epidural anesthesia only on postoperative day 0 (equivalent on days 1, 2, and 3) (Fig. 37–14). There were no significant differences between the two groups in postoperative oxygen saturation on room air, chest radiograph changes, or spirometry (Table 37–7). Furthermore, no clinical differences were detected between the two groups regarding postoperative mobilization goals, atrial fibrillation, postoperative hospital discharge eligibility, or actual postoperative hospital discharge. In short, this clinical investigation revealed that thoracic epidural anesthesia may provide enhanced postoperative analgesia (though brief) and enhance early postoperative tracheal extubation, yet has no effect on important clinical parameters (morbidity, hospital length of stay, etc.). In 2003, Royse and associates[168] prospectively randomized 80 patients undergoing elective CABG to receive either thoracic epidural anesthesia (ropivacaine/fentanyl) and general anesthesia or general anesthesia alone (control group).

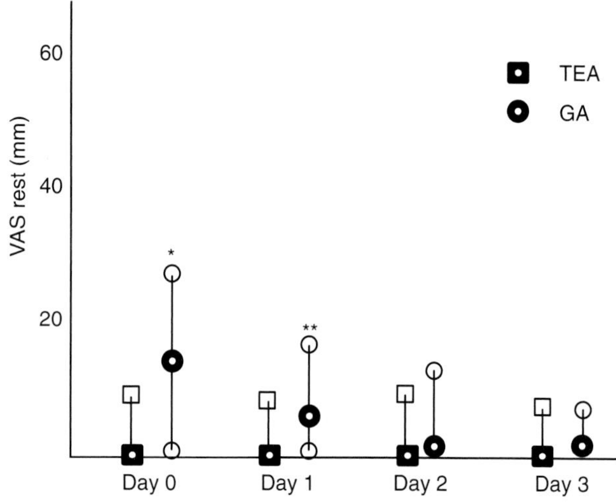

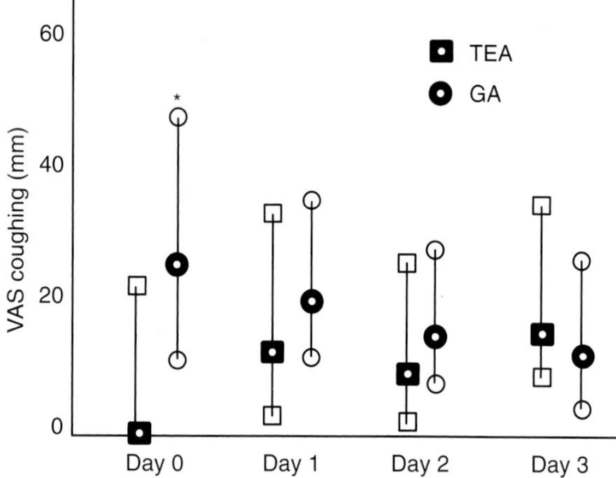

Figure 37–14 Visual analog scale (VAS) scores. Visual analog scale scores for pain at rest (*top*) and with coughing (*bottom*) on the day of surgery and the first 3 postoperative days. Significant differences ($p <$ 0.03) existed between the two groups only on day 0 (rest and coughing) and on day 1 (rest only). TEA = thoracic epidural analgesia; GA = general anesthesia. (From Priestley MC, Cope L, Halliwell R, et al: Thoracic epidural anesthesia for cardiac surgery: The effects on tracheal intubation time and length of hospital stay. Anesth Analg 94:275, 2002.)

Table 37–7 Spirometry Results

Variable	FEV_1 (TEA) (L)	FEV_1 (GA) (L)	FVC (TEA) (L)	FVC (GA) (L)
Predicted	2.9 (0.4)	2.9 (0.5)	3.9 (0.5)	3.9 (0.6)
Preoperative	2.5 (0.4)	2.6 (0.8)	3.3 (0.8)	3.4 (0.9)
Postoperative day 1	1.0 (0.3)	1.0 (0.4)	1.2 (0.4)	1.4 (0.5)
Postoperative day 2	1.1 (0.3)	1.1 (0.4)	1.4 (0.4)	1.5 (0.5)
Postoperative day 4	1.4 (0.4)	1.3 (0.5)	1.8 (0.6)	1.7 (0.6)

No significant differences existed between patients receiving thoracic epidural analgesia (TEA) and control (general anesthesia [GA]) patients. Values are given as mean (SD). FEV_1 = forced expiratory volume in 1 second; FVC = forced vital capacity.

From Priestley MC, Cope L, Halliwell R, et al: Thoracic epidural anesthesia for cardiac surgery: The effects on tracheal intubation time and length of hospital stay. Anesth Analg 94:275, 2002.

Table 37–8 Visual Analog Scale Scores

Pain Score	High Thoracic Epidural Analgesia (mean ± SD)	Control (mean ± SD)
Rest day 1	0.02 ± 0.2	0.8 ± 1.8
Cough day 1	1.2 ± 1.7	4.4 ± 3.1
Rest day 2	0.1 ± 0.4	1.2 ± 2.7
Cough day 2	1.5 ± 2.0	3.6 ± 3.1
Rest day 3	0.2 ± 1.0	0.3 ± 1.1
Cough day 3	1.7 ± 2.3	2.7 ± 3.0

Mean pain scores at rest and with cough for days 1, 2, and 3. Significant differences ($p < 0.05$) existed between groups on days 1 and 2 (at rest and with cough) yet not on day 3.

From Royse C, Royse A, Soeding P, et al: Prospective randomized trial of high thoracic epidural analgesia for coronary artery bypass surgery. Ann Thorac Surg 75:93, 2003.

The two groups received quite different intraoperative anesthetic techniques. Postoperatively, thoracic epidural anesthesia patients received epidural ropivacaine/fentanyl until the third postoperative day, while control patients received nurse-administered intravenous morphine followed by PCA morphine. Patients receiving thoracic epidural anesthesia were tracheally extubated sooner during the immediate postoperative period than controls (2.6 hours versus 5.4 hours, respectively; $p < 0.001$); yet this difference may have been secondary to the different amounts of intraoperative intravenous anesthetics administered (intraoperative anesthetic technique not standardized). Postoperative pain scores at rest and with cough were significantly lower in patients receiving thoracic epidural anesthesia on postoperative days 1 and 2 only (equivalent on postoperative day 3) (Table 37–8). Much like the Priestley et al[169] investigation, there were no substantial differences between the two groups regarding important postoperative clinical parameters (respiratory function, renal function, atrial fibrillation, ICU length of stay, hospital length of stay).

Despite enhanced postoperative analgesia offered via thoracic epidural techniques, such analgesia does not appear to decrease the incidence of persistent pain following cardiac surgery. Ho and associates[18] assessed via survey 244 patients following cardiac surgery via median sternotomy. One hundred fifty patients received perioperative supplementation of general anesthesia with thoracic epidural anesthesia (ropivacaine/fentanyl infusion initiated prior to induction of anesthesia and continued postoperatively for 2 to 3 days), and 94 patients received general anesthesia and routine postoperative nurse-controlled intravenous morphine infusion for analgesia (along with intraoperative wound infiltration with ropivacaine at chest wall closure). Persistent pain (defined as pain still present 2 or more months following surgery) was similar in the two cohorts (reported in almost 30% of patients). However, persistent pain reported by these patients was mild in most cases, infrequently interfering with daily life.

The quality of analgesia obtained with thoracic epidural anesthetic techniques is sufficient to allow cardiac surgery to be performed in awake patients without general endotracheal anesthesia. The initial report of awake cardiac surgery was published in the *Annals of Thoracic Surgery* in 2000. Karagoz and associates,[170] from Turkey, described the perioperative course of five patients who underwent elective off-pump single-vessel CABG via minithoracotomy with only thoracic epidural anesthesia (spontaneous ventilation throughout). All five patients did well and none had to be converted to general endotracheal anesthesia. Soon thereafter, a group of investigators from Germany described the perioperative course of 12 patients who underwent elective off-pump multivessel CABG via complete sternotomy with only thoracic epidural anesthesia.[171] All patients did well yet two patients required conversion to general endotracheal anesthesia (one for incomplete analgesia, one for pneumothorax). Also in 2002, investigators from Brazil revealed that "outpatient" CABG was possible (discharge to home within 24 hours of hospital admission) in a small (n = 20) group of patients undergoing cardiac surgery solely via thoracic epidural anesthesia.[172] Since these initial small clinical reports appeared, larger series of patients have been published, demonstrating that "awake" cardiac surgery is feasible and safe.[173-183] In 2003, the first case report of awake cardiac surgery requiring CPB was published.[184] In this astonishing case report from Austria, a 70-year-old man with aortic stenosis underwent aortic valve replacement with assistance of normothermic CPB (total time 123 minutes, cross-clamp time 82 minutes) solely via thoracic epidural anesthesia. Verbal communication with the patient was possible on demand throughout CPB. The patient did well and experienced an unremarkable postoperative course.

The many clinical investigations involving the use of epidural analgesic techniques in patients undergoing cardiac surgery indicate that administration of thoracic epidural opioids or local anesthetics before and/or after CPB initiates reliable postoperative analgesia following cardiac surgery. Administration of thoracic epidural local anesthetics (not opioids) can both reliably attenuate the perioperative stress response associated with CPB (that persists during the immediate postoperative period) and induce perioperative thoracic cardiac sympathectomy. Enhanced postoperative analgesia likely facilitates early tracheal extubation following cardiac surgery yet patients may be extubated following cardiac surgery (with or without CPB) in the operating room without assistance of thoracic epidural techniques.[185]

All clinical reports involving utilization of intrathecal and thoracic epidural anesthesia and analgesia techniques for cardiac surgery involve small numbers of patients and few (if any) are well designed (see Tables 37–4 and 37–5). Only a handful of clinical studies involving intrathecal analgesia are prospective, randomized, blinded, and placebo-controlled (see Table 37–4). There are no blinded, placebo-controlled clinical studies involving thoracic epidural anesthesia and analgesia (see Table 37–5). Furthermore, none of the existing clinical studies involving intrathecal and thoracic epidural anesthesia and analgesia techniques for cardiac surgery use clinical outcome as a primary end-point. Thus, there are clear deficiencies in the literature that prohibit definitive analysis of the risk/benefit ratio of intrathecal and thoracic epidural anesthesia and analgesia techniques as applied to patients undergoing cardiac surgery.

A 2004 meta-analysis by Liu and associates[186] assessed effects of perioperative central neuraxial analgesia on outcome after CABG. These authors, via MEDLINE and other databases, searched for randomized controlled trials in patients undergoing CABG with CPB. Fifteen trials enrolling 1178 patients were included for thoracic epidural anesthesia analysis, and 17 trials enrolling 668 patients were included for intrathecal analysis. Thoracic epidural techniques did not affect the incidences of mortality or myocardial infarction yet reduced risk of arrhythmias (atrial fibrillation and tachycardia), reduced risk of pulmonary complications (pneumonia and atelectasis), reduced time to tracheal extubation, and reduced analog pain scores. Intrathecal techniques did not affect incidences of mortality, myocardial infarction, arrhythmias, or time to tracheal extubation and only modestly decreased systemic morphine utilization and pain scores (while increasing incidence of pruritus). These authors conclude that central neuraxial analgesia does not affect rates of mortality or myocardial infarction following CABG yet is associated with improvements in faster time to tracheal extubation, decreased pulmonary complications and cardiac arrhythmias, and reduced pain scores. However, the authors also note that the majority of potential clinical benefits offered by central neuraxial analgesia (earlier extubation, decreased arrhythmias, enhanced analgesia) may be reduced and/or eliminated with changing cardiac anesthesia practice using fast-track techniques, use of β-adrenergic blockers or amiodarone, and/or use of NSAIDs or COX-2 inhibitors. These authors also note that the risk of spinal hematoma (addressed later in this chapter) due to central neuraxial analgesia in patients undergoing full anticoagulation for CPB remains uncertain.

The use of intrathecal and/or epidural techniques in patients undergoing thoracotomy incisions (rare during cardiac surgery, yet sometimes used in certain circumstances) deserves brief mention.[187] Many factors are involved in the occurrence of pulmonary dysfunction following thoracotomy. Postoperative changes in pulmonary function result from lung resection, atelectasis, and/or volume loss due to pneumothorax and inspiratory muscle dysfunction. Pain following thoracotomy can be intense, which may produce pulmonary complications following surgery. Somewhat surprisingly, patients undergoing a "clamshell" incision (transverse thoracosternotomy) for bilateral lung transplantation do not experience more postoperative pain than patients undergoing a standard thoracotomy for single-lung transplantation and lung transplant recipients undergoing thoracotomy have a lower incidence of adequate pain relief than patients undergoing thoracotomy for other indications.[188] These clinical observations emphasize that the condition of the patient may play a major role (along with type of incision) regarding adequacy of postoperative pain control.[188] Clearly, compared with standard thoracotomy incisions, patients receiving minithoracotomy incisions experience less postoperative pain and consume fewer supplemental analgesics during the immediate postoperative period. Furthermore, up to half of all patients undergoing thoracotomy incision will develop chronic pain related to the surgical site.

Evidence exists that indicates adequate postoperative pain control following thoracotomy may help prevent the development of chronic postoperative thoracotomy pain. Therefore, an effective postoperative analgesic plan must be developed for these patients. In contrast to median sternotomy incisions and minithoracotomy incisions, there appears to be some clinical evidence indicating that use of regional anesthetic techniques may decrease postoperative complications following thoracotomy incisions. Specifically, Ballantyne and associates[189] and Licker and associates[190] provide ample evidence that postoperative pain control with epidural techniques following thoracotomy incision may reduce pulmonary morbidity and overall patient mortality. However, while ample evidence exists suggesting that thoracic epidural analgesia (superiority of thoracic over lumbar routes has been recently called into question) offers superior postoperative analgesia, not all clinical studies have shown that such techniques truly improve postoperative pulmonary function and reduce postoperative pulmonary complications.

SIDE EFFECTS OF INTRATHECAL AND EPIDURAL LOCAL ANESTHETICS

The most troubling and undesirable drug effect of intrathecal and epidural local anesthetics is hypotension. Spinal anesthesia to upper thoracic dermatomes produces a decrease in mean arterial blood pressure that is accompanied by a parallel decrease in coronary blood flow.[191,192] Exactly what percentage of blood pressure decrease is acceptable remains speculative, especially in patients with coronary artery disease. Disturbances in myocardial oxygenation appear to occur in patients with coronary artery disease if coronary perfusion pressure is allowed to decrease by more than 50% during induction of thoracic epidural anesthesia with local anesthetics.[193] Furthermore, if α-adrenergic agonists are used to increase blood pressure during this time, there may be detrimental effects (vasoconstriction) on the native coronary arteries and bypass grafts.[194,195] Of the 19 patients who received intrathecal local anesthetics to produce a "total spinal" for cardiac surgery, 18 required intravenous phenylephrine intraoperatively to increase blood pressure, indicating that hypotension is a substantial problem with this technique.[110,112] Hypotension also appears to be relatively common when thoracic epidural local anesthetics are used in this setting. Volume replacement, β-adrenergic agonists, and/or α-adrenergic agonists are required in a fair proportion of patients, and coronary perfusion pressure may decrease in susceptible patients following CPB.

Following epidural administration, local anesthetics can produce blood concentrations of drug that may initiate detrimental cardiac electrophysiologic effects and myocardial depression.[196] In fact, myocardial depression has been detected in patients receiving thoracic epidural anesthesia with bupivacaine, a clinical effect at least partially caused by increased blood concentrations of the drug.[197] Concomitant use of β-adrenergic blockers may further decrease myocardial contractility in this setting.[198,199] Patients undergoing cardiac surgery who were randomized to receive intermittent boluses of thoracic epidural bupivacaine intraoperatively followed by continuous infusion postoperatively exhibited significantly increased pulmonary capillary wedge pressures following CPB when compared with patients managed similarly without epidural catheters (10.8 versus 6.4 mm Hg, respectively; $p < 0.001$), which suggests myocardial depression.[141]

Two case reports also indicate that the use of epidural anesthesia and analgesia may either mask myocardial ischemia or initiate myocardial ischemia.[200,201] Oden and Karagianes[201] describe the perioperative course of an elderly patient who had a history of exertional angina and underwent uneventful cholecystectomy. Postoperatively, analgesia was achieved with continuous lumbar epidural fentanyl. On the second postoperative day, with continuous lumbar epidural fentanyl being administered, ST-segment depression was noted on the electrocardiogram. The patient was awake, alert, and did not experience angina. Initiation of intravenous nitroglycerin at this time resulted in normalization of ischemic electrocardiographic changes. It was thought by these authors that epidural fentanyl-induced analgesia masked the patient's typical anginal pain. Easley and associates describe the perioperative course of a middle-aged patient without cardiovascular symptoms ("borderline" hypertension) who was scheduled for exploratory laparotomy.[200] Prior to surgery, a low thoracic epidural catheter was inserted and local anesthetic was administered (sensory level peaked by pinprick at T2). The patient at this time began complaining of left-sided jaw pain and substantial (2.7-mm) ST-segment depression was noted on the electrocardiogram. Surgery was cancelled and the patient was treated with aspirin and nitroglycerin. The electrocardiogram normalized, yet based on electrocardiographic changes, troponin levels, and creatine kinase–MB fractions, the patient was diagnosed with a non–Q-wave myocardial infarction. Coronary angiography on the following day was unremarkable and a presumptive diagnosis of coronary artery spasm was made. It was thought by these authors that low thoracic epidural-induced sympathectomy led to alterations in the sympathetic–parasympathetic balance (i.e., vasoconstriction above level of block) leading to coronary artery spasm.

SIDE EFFECTS OF INTRATHECAL AND EPIDURAL OPIOIDS

Although many have been described, the four clinically relevant undesirable drug effects of intrathecal and epidural opioids are pruritus, nausea and vomiting, urinary retention, and respiratory depression.[202] Following administration of intrathecal or epidural opioids, the most common side effect is pruritus. The incidence varies widely (from 0% to 100%) and is often identified only after direct questioning of patients. Severe pruritus is rare, occurring in only approximately 1% of patients. The incidence of nausea and vomiting is approximately 30%. The incidence of urinary retention varies widely (from 0% to 80%) and occurs most frequently in young male patients. When intrathecal or epidural opioids are used in patients undergoing cardiac surgery, the incidence of pruritus, nausea and vomiting, and urinary retention is similar to that described above. Of note, if a large dose (4.0 mg) of intrathecal morphine is administered, prolonged postoperative urinary retention may occur.[109]

The most important undesirable drug effect of intrathecal and epidural opioids is respiratory depression. Only four months after the initial use of intrathecal[203] and epidural[204] opioids in humans, life-threatening respiratory depression was reported.[205-207] The incidence of respiratory depression that requires intervention after conventional doses of intrathecal and epidural opioids is approximately 1%, the same as that after conventional doses of intramuscular and intravenous opioids. Early respiratory depression occurs within minutes of opioid injection and is associated with administration of intrathecal or epidural fentanyl or sufentanil. Delayed respiratory depression occurs hours after opioid injection and is associated with administration of intrathecal or epidural morphine. Delayed respiratory depression results from cephalad migration of morphine in cerebrospinal fluid and the subsequent stimulation of opioid receptors located in the ventral medulla.[208] Factors that increase the risk of respiratory depression include large and/or repeated doses of opioids, intrathecal utilization, advanced age, and concomitant use of intravenous sedatives.[202] The magnitude of postoperative respiratory depression is profoundly influenced by the dose of intrathecal or epidural morphine administered and the type and amount of intravenous analgesics and amnestics used for the intraoperative baseline anesthetic. Prolonged postoperative respiratory depression may delay tracheal extubation and naloxone may be required in some patients.

Children may be more susceptible to developing postoperative respiratory depression when intrathecal morphine is used in this setting. Of 56 children (aged 1 to 17 years) administered either 20 or 30 μg/kg intrathecal morphine prior to surgical incision for cardiac surgery, 3 of 29 who received 20 μg/kg and 6 of 27 receiving 30 μg/kg required naloxone postoperatively for respiratory depression.[121]

One clinical study indicates that administration of intrathecal morphine to patients undergoing cardiac surgery may be contraindicated if early extubation is planned.[108] Patients were randomized to receive either intrathecal morphine (10 μg/kg) or intrathecal placebo prior to the induction of anesthesia. Intraoperative anesthetic management was standardized and consisted of intravenous fentanyl (20 μg/kg) and intravenous midazolam (10 mg total) along with inhaled isoflurane and/or intravenous nitroglycerin, if required. Regarding patients extubated during the immediate postoperative period, the mean time from ICU arrival to extubation was significantly increased in those who received intrathecal morphine compared with those who received intrathecal placebo (10.9 versus 7.6 hours, respectively; $p = 0.02$). However, other clinical studies indicate that intrathecal or epidural morphine may yet prove to be a useful adjunct for cardiac surgery and early extubation. The optimal dose of intrathecal or epidural morphine in this setting, along with the optimal intraoperative baseline anesthetic that will provide significant postoperative analgesia yet not delay tracheal extubation in the immediate postoperative period, remains to be elucidated. In contrast to intrathecal and epidural opioids, epidural local anesthetics (which initiate no respiratory depression) should not delay tracheal extubation in the immediate postoperative period.

RISK OF HEMATOMA FORMATION

Intrathecal or epidural instrumentation entails risk, the most feared complication being epidural hematoma formation. The estimated incidence of hematoma formation is approximately 1:220,000 following intrathecal instrumentation.[209] Hematoma formation is more common (approximately 1:150,000) following epidural instrumentation because larger needles are used, catheters are inserted, and the venous plexus in the epidural space is prominent.[209] Furthermore, hematoma formation does not occur exclusively during epidural catheter insertion; almost half of all cases develop following catheter removal.[209]

Although spontaneous hematomas can occur in the absence of intrathecal or epidural instrumentation,[210] most occur when instrumentation is performed in a patient with a coagulopathy (from any cause) or when instrumentation is difficult or traumatic.[209] Paradoxically, intrathecal or epidural instrumentation has been performed safely in patients with known clinical coagulopathy.[211,212] Of 1000 epidural catheterizations performed in 950 patients receiving oral anticoagulants at time of catheter insertion, none developed signs or symptoms of hematoma formation.[212] Of 336 epidural injections performed in 36 patients with chronic cancer pain either fully anticoagulated (oral anticoagulants or intravenous heparin) or profoundly thrombocytopenic (platelet count $<50{,}000/mm^3$) at the time of instrumentation, none developed signs or symptoms of hematoma formation.[211]

Risk is increased when intrathecal or epidural instrumentation is performed prior to systemic heparinization, and hematoma formation has occurred in patients when diagnostic or therapeutic lumbar puncture has been followed by systemic heparinization.[213-216] When lumbar puncture is followed by systemic heparinization, concurrent use of aspirin, difficult or traumatic instrumentation, and administration of intravenous heparin within 1 hour of instrumentation increase the risk of hematoma formation.[215] However, by observing certain precautions, intrathecal or epidural instrumentation can be performed safely in patients who will subsequently receive intravenous heparin.[217,218] By delaying surgery 24 hours in the event of a traumatic tap, by delaying heparinization 60 minutes after catheter insertion, and by maintaining tight perioperative control of anticoagulation, more than 4000 intrathecal or epidural catheterizations were performed safely in patients undergoing peripheral vascular surgery who received intravenous heparin following catheter insertion.[218] A retrospective review involving 912 patients further indicates that epidural catheterization prior to systemic heparinization for peripheral vascular surgery is safe.[217] However, the magnitude of anticoagulation in these two studies (activated partial thromboplastin time of approximately 100 seconds[217] and activated clotting time approximately twice the baseline value[218]) involving patients undergoing peripheral vascular surgery was substantially less than the degree of anticoagulation required in patients subjected to CPB.

Most clinical studies investigating the use of intrathecal or epidural anesthesia and analgesia techniques in patients undergoing cardiac surgery include precautions to decrease risk of hematoma formation. Some used the technique only after the demonstration of laboratory evidence of normal coagulation parameters, delayed surgery 24 hours in the event of traumatic tap, or required that the time from instrumentation to systemic heparinization exceed 60 minutes. While most clinicians investigating use of epidural anesthesia and analgesia techniques in patients undergoing cardiac surgery insert catheters the day before scheduled surgery, investigators have performed instrumentation on the same day of surgery. Institutional practice (same-day admit surgery) may eliminate the option of epidural catheter insertion on the day before scheduled surgery. An alternative is to perform epidural instrumentation postoperatively (prior to or after tracheal extubation), following the demonstration via laboratory evidence of normal coagulation parameters.

Although most investigators agree that risk of hematoma is likely increased when intrathecal or epidural instrumentation is performed in patients prior to systemic heparinization required for CPB, the absolute degree of increased risk is somewhat controversial; some believe the risk may be as high as 0.35%.[213] An extensive mathematical analysis by Ho and associates[219] of the approximately 10,840 intrathecal injections in patients subjected to systemic heparinization required for CPB (without a single episode of hematoma formation) reported in the literature as of the year 2000 estimated that the minimum risk of hematoma formation was 1:220,000 and the maximum risk of hematoma formation was 1:3600 (95% confidence level); however, the maximum risk may be as high as 1:2400 (99% confidence level). Similarly, of the approximately 4583 epidural instrumentations in patients subjected to systemic heparinization required for CPB (without a single episode of hematoma formation) reported in the literature as of the year 2000, the minimum risk of hematoma formation was 1:150,000 and the maximum risk of hematoma formation was 1:1500 (95% confidence level);

however, the maximum risk may be as high as 1:1000 (99% confidence level).[219]

Certain precautions, however, may decrease the risk.[209,213] The technique should not be used in a patient with known coagulopathy from any cause. Surgery should be delayed 24 hours in the event of a traumatic tap, and time from instrumentation to systemic heparinization should exceed 60 minutes. Additionally, systemic heparin effect and reversal should be tightly controlled (smallest amount of heparin used for the shortest duration compatible with therapeutic objectives) and patients should be closely monitored postoperatively for signs and symptoms of hematoma formation. An obvious economic disadvantage of intrathecal or epidural instrumentation in patients prior to cardiac surgery is the possible delay in surgery in the event of a traumatic tap. However, one study involving more than 4000 intrathecal or epidural catheterizations via a 17-gauge Touhy needle indicates that the incidence of traumatic tap (blood freely aspirated) is rare (<0.10%).[218]

In 2004, the first case report of an epidural hematoma associated with a thoracic epidural catheter inserted in a patient prior to cardiac surgery was published.[220] This 18-year-old man had a thoracic (T9-10) epidural catheter uneventfully inserted following induction of general anesthesia (the patient had intense fear of needles) immediately prior to initiation of CPB for aortic valve replacement surgery. Three hours elapsed from instrumentation to systemic heparinization. The entire intraoperative course and immediate postoperative course were uneventful (tracheally extubated soon after surgery, ambulating without difficulty on the first postoperative day). At 49 hours following surgery, intravenous heparin therapy was initiated (prosthetic valve thromboprophylaxis). At 53 hours following surgery, alteplase (thrombolytic drug) was used to flush a dysfunctional intravenous catheter. Within 2 hours of intravenous alteplase administration, the patient reported intense back pain while ambulating. At this point, the epidural catheter was removed. The activated partial thromboplastin time assessed at this time (during catheter removal) was 87.4 seconds (normal range, 24.8 to 37.3 seconds). The patient was also thrombocytopenic at this time. Upon catheter removal, the patient experienced sudden onset of numbness and weakness distal to T9. Intravenous heparin was discontinued, a computed tomographic scan was inconclusive, requiring a magnetic resonance imaging scan, which revealed an epidural hematoma. Five hours from the onset of neurologic symptoms, the patient underwent surgical evacuation of the hematoma (which extended from the T8 to T11 levels). Intraoperatively, intravenous methylprednisolone (30 mg/kg) was administered, followed by an infusion (5.4 mg/kg/hr), which was continued for 72 hours. Twenty-four hours post laminectomy, the patient demonstrated mild residual lower extremity motor and sensory deficits. Six weeks later, his neurologic examination had returned to normal. The authors note the factors affecting coagulation in this patient (heparin, alteplase, thrombocytopenia) that likely led to hematoma formation and theorize that removing the catheter may have increased bleeding, further compounding the problem.

Use of regional anesthetic techniques in patients undergoing cardiac surgery, while seemingly increasing in popularity, remains extremely controversial, prompting numerous editorials by recognized experts in the field of cardiac anesthesia.[221-224] One of the main reasons such controversy exists (and likely will continue for some time) is that the numerous clinical investigations regarding this topic are suboptimally designed and use a wide array of disparate techniques, preventing clinically useful conclusions on which all can agree.[225,226]

MULTIMODAL ANALGESIA

The possibility of synergism between analgesic drugs is a concept that is nearly a century old.[227,228] While subsequent research has revealed the difference between additivity and synergy, the fundamental strategy behind such combinations ("multimodal" or "balanced" analgesia) remains unchanged: enhanced analgesia with minimization of adverse physiological effects. Use of analgesic combinations during the postoperative period, specifically the combination of traditional intravenous opioids with other analgesics (NSAIDs, COX-2 inhibitors, ketamine, etc.), has been proved clinically effective in noncardiac patients for decades. Early clinical investigations simply reported analgesic efficacy, whereas more recent clinical investigations have additionally evaluated and described specific opioid-sparing effects (which should lead to a reduction in side effects). For example, in the late 1980s, initial clinical studies involving ketorolac (the first parenteral NSAID available in the United States) revealed significant opioid-sparing effects (analgesia) along with a reduction in respiratory depression. Subsequently, substantial clinical research has clearly established the perioperative analgesic efficacy and opioid-sparing effects of NSAIDs (along with reduction of side effects).

The American Society of Anesthesiologists Task Force on Acute Pain Management in the Perioperative Setting reports that the literature supports the administration of two analgesic agents that act by different mechanisms via a single route for providing superior analgesic efficacy with equivalent or reduced adverse effects.[1] Potential examples include epidural opioids administered in combination with epidural local anesthetics or clonidine, and intravenous opioids in combination with ketorolac or ketamine. Dose-dependent adverse effects reported with administration of a medication occur whether it is given alone or in combination with other medications (opioids may cause nausea, vomiting, pruritus, or urinary retention, and local anesthetics may produce motor block). The literature is insufficient to evaluate the postoperative analgesic effects of oral opioids combined with NSAIDs, COX-2 inhibitors, or acetaminophen compared with oral opioids alone. The Task Force believes that NSAIDs, COX-2 inhibitors, or acetaminophen administration has a dose-sparing effect for systemically administered opioids. The literature also suggests that two routes of administration, when compared with a single route, may be more effective in providing perioperative analgesia. Examples include intrathecal or epidural opioids combined with intravenous, intramuscular, oral, transdermal, or subcutaneous analgesics versus intrathecal or epidural opioids alone. Another example is intravenous opioids combined with oral NSAIDs, COX-2 inhibitors, or acetaminophen versus intravenous opioids alone. The literature is insufficient to evaluate the efficacy of pharmacologic pain management combined with nonpharmacologic, alternative, or complementary pain management compared with pharmacologic pain management alone.

CONCLUSIONS

Multiple factors are important during the perioperative period that potentially affect outcome and quality of life fol-

Table 37–9 Factors Affecting Outcome Following Cardiac Surgery

• Type and quality of surgical intervention
• Extent of postoperative neurologic dysfunction
• Extent of postoperative myocardial dysfunction
• Extent of postoperative pulmonary dysfunction
• Extent of postoperative renal dysfunction
• Extent of postoperative coagulation abnormalities
• Quality of postoperative analgesia
• Extent of systemic inflammatory response

lowing cardiac surgery, including type and quality of surgical intervention, extent of postoperative neurologic dysfunction, myocardial dysfunction, pulmonary dysfunction, renal dysfunction, coagulation abnormalities, quality of postoperative analgesia and/or extent of systemic inflammatory response, among others[229] (Table 37–9). This list of factors is presented in no particular order; obviously, depending on specific clinical situations (surgical procedure, patient comorbidity, etc.), certain factors will be more important than others. It is extremely difficult (if not impossible) to determine exactly how important attaining adequate postoperative analgesia truly is in relation to all of these clinical factors surrounding a patient undergoing cardiac surgery. A clear link between "adequate" or "high-quality" postoperative analgesia and outcome in patients following cardiac surgery has yet to be established.[230-232]

However, despite the absence of substantiating scientific evidence, most clinicians intuitively believe that attaining high-quality postoperative analgesia is important because it may prevent adverse hemodynamic, metabolic, immunologic, and hemostatic alterations, all of which may potentially increase postoperative morbidity. While many analgesic techniques are available, intravenous systemic opioids form the cornerstone of post–cardiac surgery analgesia. Opioids have been used for many years in the treatment of postoperative pain in patients following cardiac surgery with good results. While NSAIDs (specifically COX-2 inhibitors) have received much recent attention, very important clinical issues regarding their safety (gastrointestinal effects, renal effects, hemostatic effects, immunologic effects) need to be resolved. While PCA techniques are commonly used, their clear superiority over traditional nurse-controlled analgesic techniques remains unproved. As a general rule, it is likely best to avoid intense, single-modality therapy for the treatment of acute postoperative pain. Clinicians should strive for an approach that uses a number of different therapies (multimodal therapy), each counteracting pain via different mechanisms. Preemptive analgesia, while intriguing, needs further study in order to determine its role in affecting postoperative analgesia and outcome.[233-236]

Finally, the American Society of Anesthesiologists Task Force on Acute Pain Management in the Perioperative Setting offers sound advice.[1] It recommends that anesthesiologists who manage perioperative pain use analgesic therapeutic options only after thoughtfully considering the risks and benefits for the individual patient. The therapy (or therapies) selected should reflect the individual anesthesiologist's expertise, as well as the capacity for safe application of the chosen modality in each practice setting. This includes the ability to recognize and treat adverse effects that emerge after initiation of therapy. Whenever possible, anesthesiologists should employ multimodal pain management therapy. Dosing regimens should be administered to optimize efficacy while minimizing the risk of adverse events. The choice of medication, dose, route, and duration of therapy should always be individualized.

REFERENCES

1. American Society of Anesthesiologists Task Force on Acute Pain Management: Practice guidelines for acute pain management in the perioperative setting: An updated report by the American Society of Anesthesiologists Task Force on Acute Pain Management. Anesthesiology 100:1573, 2004
2. Joint Commission on Accreditation of Healthcare Organizations: Pain assessment and management—An organizational approach. 2000. Available at http://www.jcaho.org. Accessed October 15, 2005
3. Weissman C: The metabolic response to stress: An overview and update. Anesthesiology 73:308, 1990
4. Kehlet H: Surgical stress: The role of pain and analgesia. Br J Anaesth 63:189, 1989
5. Roizen MF: Should we all have a sympathectomy at birth? Or at least preoperatively? (editorial). Anesthesiology 68:482, 1988
6. Tuman KJ, McCarthy RJ, March RJ, et al: Effects of epidural anesthesia and analgesia on coagulation and outcome after major vascular surgery. Anesth Analg 73:696, 1991
7. Yeager MP, Glass DD, Neff RK, Brinck-Johnsen T: Epidural anesthesia and analgesia in high-risk surgical patients. Anesthesiology 66:729, 1987
8. Mangano DT, Siliciano D, Hollenberg M, et al: Postoperative myocardial ischemia: therapeutic trials using intensive analgesia following surgery. Anesthesiology 76:342, 1992
9. Anand KJS, Hickey PR: Halothane-morphine compared with high-dose sufentanil for anesthesia and postoperative analgesia in neonatal cardiac surgery. N Engl J Med 326:1, 1992
10. Wallace AW: Is it time to get on the fast track or stay on the slow track? (editorial) Anesthesiology 99:774, 2003
11. Myles PS, Daly DJ, Djaiani G, et al: A systematic review of the safety and effectiveness of fast-track cardiac anesthesia. Anesthesiology 99:982, 2003
12. Royston D, Kovesi T, Marczin N: The unwanted response to cardiac surgery: Time for a reappraisal? (editorial) J Thorac Cardiovasc Surg 125:32, 2003
13. Mueller XM, Tinguely F, Tevaearai HT, et al: Pain location, distribution, and intensity after cardiac surgery. Chest 118:391, 2000
14. Nay PG, Elliott SM, Harrop-Griffiths AW: Postoperative pain. Expectation and experience after coronary artery bypass grafting. Anaesthesia 51:741, 1996
15. Meehan DA, McRae ME, Rourke DA, et al: Analgesic administration, pain intensity, and patient satisfaction in cardiac surgical patients. Am J Crit Care 4:435, 1995
16. Moore R, Follette DM, Berkoff HA: Poststernotomy fractures and pain management in open cardiac surgery. Chest 106:1339, 1994
17. Greenwald LV, Baisden CE, Symbas PN: Rib fractures in coronary bypass patients: Radionuclide detection. Radiology 148:553, 1983
18. Ho SC, Royse CF, Royse AG, et al: Persistent pain after cardiac surgery: An audit of high thoracic epidural and primary opioid analgesia therapies. Anesth Analg 95:820, 2002
19. Kalso E, Mennander S, Tasmuth T, Nilsson E: Chronic post-sternotomy pain. Acta Anaesth Scand 45:935, 2001
20. Chaney MA, Morales M, Bakhos M: Severe incisional pain and long thoracic nerve injury after port-access minimally invasive mitral valve surgery. Anesth Analg 91:288, 2000
21. Davis Z, Jacobs HK, Zhang M, Castellanos Y: Endoscopic vein harvest for coronary artery bypass grafting: Technique and outcomes. J Thorac Cardiovasc Surg 116:228, 1998
22. Smith RC, Leung JM, Mangano DT, SPI Research Group: Postoperative myocardial ischemia in patients undergoing coronary artery bypass graft surgery. Anesthesiology 74:464, 1991
23. Leung JM, O'Kelly B, Browner WS, et al: Prognostic importance of post-bypass regional wall-motion abnormalities in patients undergoing coronary artery bypass graft surgery. Anesthesiology 71:16, 1989

24. Philbin DM, Rosow CE, Schneider RC, et al: Fentanyl and sufentanil anesthesia revisited: How much is enough? Anesthesiology 73:5, 1990
25. Reves JG, Karp RB, Buttner EE, et al: Neuronal and adrenomedullary catecholamine release in response to CPB in man. Circulation 66:49, 1982
26. Roberts AJ, Niarchos AP, Subramanian VA, et al: Systemic hypertension associated with coronary artery bypass surgery: Predisposing factors, hemodynamic characteristics, humoral profile, and treatment. J Thorac Cardiovasc Surg 74:846, 1977
27. Liu S, Carpenter RL, Neal MJ: Epidural anesthesia and analgesia: their role in postoperative outcome. Anesthesiology 82:1474, 1995
28. Wu CL, Naqibuddin M, Rowlingson AJ, et al: The effect of pain on health-related quality of life in the immediate postoperative period. Anesth Analg 97:1078, 2003
29. Rogers MC: Do the right thing. Pain relief in infants and children (editorial). N Engl J Med 326:55, 1992
30. White PF, Rawal S, Latham P, et al: Use of a continuous local anesthetic infusion for pain management after median sternotomy. Anesthesiology 99:918, 2003
31. Dowling R, Thielmeier K, Ghaly A, et al: Improved pain control after cardiac surgery: Results of a randomized, double-blind, clinical trial. J Thorac Cardiovasc Surg 126:1271, 2003
32. Brown SL, Morrison AE: Local anesthetic infusion pump systems adverse events reported to the Food and Drug Administration. Anesthesiology 100:1305, 2004
33. Soto RG, Fu ES: Acute pain management for patients undergoing thoracotomy. Ann Thorac Surg 75:1349, 2003
34. Karmakar MK: Thoracic paravertebral block. Anesthesiology 95:771, 2001
35. Kavanagh BP, Katz J, Sandler AN: Pain control after thoracic surgery. A review of current techniques. Anesthesiology 81:737–759, 1994
36. Bilgin M, Akcali Y, Oguzkaya F: Extrapleural regional versus systemic analgesia for relieving postthoracotomy pain: A clinical study of bupivacaine compared with metamizol. J Thorac Cardiovasc Surg 126:1580, 2003
37. Mehta Y, Swaminathan M, Mishra Y, Trehan N: A comparative evaluation of intrapleural and thoracic epidural analgesia for postoperative pain relief after minimally invasive direct coronary artery bypass surgery. J Cardiothorac Vasc Anesth 12:162, 1998
38. Riedel BJ: Regional anesthesia for major cardiac and noncardiac surgery: More than just a strategy for effective analgesia? (editorial) J Cardiothorac Vasc Anesth 15:279, 2001
39. Raja SN, Lowenstein E: The birth of opioid anesthesia (classic papers revisited). Anesthesiology 100:1013, 2004
40. Bovill JG, Sebel PS, Stanley TH: Opioid analgesics in anesthesia: With special reference to their use in cardiovascular anesthesia. Anesthesiology 61:731, 1984
41. Hug CC: Does opioid "anesthesia" exist? (editorial) Anesthesiology 73:1, 1990
42. Kehlet H, Rung GW, Callesen T: Postoperative opioid analgesia: Time for a reconsideration? J Clin Anesth 8:441, 1996
43. Peng PWH, Sandler AN: A review of the use of fentanyl analgesia in the management of acute pain in adults. Anesthesiology 90:576, 1999
44. Checketts MR, Gilhooly CJ, Kenny GNC: Patient-maintained analgesia with target-controlled alfentanil infusion after cardiac surgery: A comparison with morphine PCA. Br J Anaesth 80:748, 1998
45. Bowdle TA, Camporesi EM, Maysick L, et al: A multicenter evaluation of remifentanil for early postoperative analgesia. Anesth Analg 83:1292, 1996
46. Ouattara A, Boccara G, Kockler U, et al: Remifentanil induces systemic arterial vasodilation in humans with a total artificial heart. Anesthesiology 100:602, 2004
47. Liu SS, Allen HW, Olsson GL: Patient-controlled epidural analgesia with bupivacaine and fentanyl on hospital wards: Prospective experience with 1,030 surgical patients. Anesthesiology 88:688, 1998
48. Boylan JF, Katz J, Kavanagh BP, et al: Epidural bupivacaine-morphine analgesia versus patient-controlled analgesia following abdominal aortic surgery: Analgesic, respiratory, and myocardial effects. Anesthesiology 89:585, 1998
49. Tsang J, Brush B: Patient-controlled analgesia in postoperative cardiac surgery. Anaesth Intens Care 27:464, 1999
50. Gust R, Pecher S, Gust A, et al: Effect of patient-controlled analgesia on pulmonary complications after coronary artery bypass grafting. Crit Care Med 27:2218, 1999
51. Boldt J, Thaler E, Lehmann A, et al: Pain management in cardiac surgery patients: Comparison between standard therapy and patient-controlled analgesia regimen. J Cardiothorac Vasc Anesth 12:654, 1998
52. Munro AJ, Long GT, Sleigh JW: Nurse-administered subcutaneous morphine is a satisfactory alternative to intravenous patient-controlled analgesia morphine after cardiac surgery. Anesth Analg 87:11, 1998
53. Myles PS, Buckland MR, Cannon GB, et al: Comparison of patient-controlled analgesia and nurse-controlled infusion analgesia after cardiac surgery. Anaesth Intens Care 22:672, 1994
54. Searle NR, Roy M, Bergeron G, et al: Hydromorphone patient-controlled analgesia (PCA) after coronary artery bypass surgery. Can J Anaesth 41:198, 1994
55. Ralley FE, Day FJ, Cheng DCH: Pro: Nonsteroidal anti-inflammatory drugs should be routinely administered for postoperative analgesia after cardiac surgery. J Cardiothorac Vasc Anesth 14:731, 2000
56. Griffin M: Con: Nonsteroidal anti-inflammatory drugs should not be routinely administered for postoperative analgesia after cardiac surgery. J Cardiothorac Vasc Anesth 14:735, 2000
57. Kharasch ED: Perioperative COX-2 inhibitors: Knowledge and challenges (editorial). Anesth Analg 98:1, 2004
58. Gilron I, Milne B, Hong M: Cyclooxygenase-2 inhibitors in postoperative pain management: Current evidence and future directions. Anesthesiology 99:1198, 2003
59. Gajraj NM: Cyclooxygenase-2 inhibitors. Anesth Analg 96:1720, 2003
60. McCrory CR, Lindahl SGE: Cyclooxygenase inhibition for postoperative analgesia. Anesth Analg 95:169, 2002
61. FitzGerald GA, Patrono C: The coxibs, selective inhibitors of cyclooxygenase-2. N Engl J Med 345:433, 2001
62. Crofford LJ: Rational use of analgesic and antiinflammatory drugs (editorial). N Engl J Med 345:1844, 2001
63. Hynninen MS, Cheng DCH, Hossain I, et al: Non-steroidal antiinflammatory drugs in treatment of postoperative pain after cardiac surgery. Can J Anesth 47:1182, 2000
64. Lin JC, Szwerc MF, Magovern JA: Nonsteroidal anti-inflammatory drug-based pain control for minimally invasive direct coronary artery bypass surgery. Heart Surg Forum 2:169, 1999
65. Rapanos T, Murphy P, Szalai JP, et al: Rectal indomethacin reduces postoperative pain and morphine use after cardiac surgery. Can J Anesth 46:725, 1999
66. Lahtinen P, Kokki H, Hendolin H, et al: Propacetamol as adjunctive treatment for postoperative pain after cardiac surgery. Anesth Analg 95:813, 2002
67. Immer FF, Immer-Bansi AS, Trachsel N, et al: Pain treatment with a COX-2 inhibitor after coronary artery bypass operation: A randomized trial. Ann Thorac Surg 75:490, 2003
68. Ott E, Nussmeier NA, Duke PC, et al: Efficacy and safety of the cyclooxygenase 2 inhibitors parecoxib and valdecoxib in patients undergoing coronary artery bypass surgery. J Thorac Cardiovasc Surg 125:1481, 2003
69. Mukherjee D, Nissen SE, Topol EJ: Risk of cardiovascular events associated with selective COX-2 inhibitors. JAMA 286:954, 2001
70. Guo TZ, Jiang JY, Buttermann AE, Maze M: Dexmedetomidine injection into the locus ceruleus produces antinociception. Anesthesiology 84:873, 1996
71. Nishina K, Mikawa K, Uesugi T, et al: Efficacy of clonidine for prevention of perioperative myocardial ischemia: A critical appraisal and meta-analysis of the literature. Anesthesiology 96:323, 2002
72. Flacke JW, Bloor BC, Flacke WE, et al: Reduced narcotic requirement by clonidine with improved hemodynamic and adrenergic stability in patients undergoing coronary bypass surgery. Anesthesiology 67:11, 1987
73. Ebert TJ, Hall JE, Barney JA, et al: The effects of increasing plasma concentrations of dexmedetomidine in humans. Anesthesiology 93:382, 2000
74. Multz AS: Prolonged dexmedetomidine infusion as an adjunct in treating sedation-induced withdrawal. Anesth Analg 96:1054, 2003
75. Arain SR, Ebert TJ: The efficacy, side effects, and recovery characteristics of dexmedetomidine versus propofol when used for intraoperative sedation. Anesth Analg 95:461, 2002
76. Triltsch AE, Welte M, von Homeyer P, et al: Bispectral index-guided sedation with dexmedetomidine in intensive care: A prospective, randomized, double-blind, placebo-controlled phase II study. Crit Care Med 30:1007, 2002
77. Myles PS, Hunt JO, Holdgaard HO, et al: Clonidine and cardiac surgery: Haemodynamic and metabolic effects, myocardial ischaemia and recovery. Anaesth Intens Care 27:137–147, 1999
78. Boldt J, Rothe G, Schindler E, et al: Can clonidine, enoximone, and enalaprilat help to protect the myocardium against ischaemia in cardiac surgery? Heart 76:207, 1996
79. Abi-Jaoude F, Brusset A, Ceddaha A, et al: Clonidine premedication for coronary artery bypass grafting under high-dose alfentanil anesthesia:

Intraoperative and postoperative hemodynamic study. J Cardiothorac Vasc Anesth 7:35, 1993
80. Dorman BH, Zucker JR, Verrier ED, et al: Clonidine improves perioperative myocardial ischemia, reduces anesthetic requirement, and alters hemodynamic parameters in patients undergoing coronary artery bypass surgery. J Cardiothorac Vasc Anesth 7:386, 1993
81. Chaney MA: Intrathecal and epidural anesthesia and analgesia for cardiac surgery. Anesth Analg 84:1211, 1997
82. Feigl E: Coronary physiology. Physiol Rev 63:1, 1983
83. Lee DDP, Kimura S, DeQuattro V: Noradrenergic activity and silent ischaemia in hypertensive patients with stable angina: Effect of metoprolol. Lancet 1:403, 1989
84. Vanhoutte PM, Shimokawa H: Endothelium-derived relaxing factor and coronary vasospasm. Circulation 80:1, 1989
85. Blomberg S, Emanuelsson H, Kvist H, et al: Effects of thoracic epidural anesthesia on coronary arteries and arterioles in patients with coronary artery disease. Anesthesiology 73:840, 1990
86. Blomberg S, Curelaru I, Emanuelsson H, et al: Thoracic epidural anaesthesia in patients with unstable angina pectoris. Eur Heart J 10:437–444, 1989
87. Heusch G, Deussen A, Thamer V: Cardiac sympathetic nerve activity and progressive vasoconstriction distal to coronary stenosis: Feed-back aggravation of myocardial ischemia. J Auton Nerv Syst 13:311, 1985
88. Heusch G, Deussen A: The effects of cardiac sympathetic nerve stimulation on perfusion of stenotic coronary arteries in the dog. Circ Res 53:8, 1983
89. Uchida Y, Murao S: Excitation of afferent cardiac sympathetic nerve fibers during coronary occlusion. Am J Physiol 226:1094, 1974
90. Mangano DT: Perioperative cardiac morbidity. Anesthesiology 72:153, 1990
91. Birkett DA, Apthorp GH, Chamberlain DA, et al: Bilateral upper thoracic sympathectomy in angina pectoris: Results in 52 cases. Br Med J 2:187, 1965
92. Kock M, Blomberg S, Emanuelsson H, et al: Thoracic epidural anesthesia improves global and regional left ventricular function during stress-induced myocardial ischemia in patients with coronary artery disease. Anesth Analg 71:625, 1990
93. Blomberg SG: Long-term home self-treatment with high thoracic epidural anesthesia in patients with severe coronary artery disease. Anesth Analg 79:413, 1994
94. Davis RF, DeBoer LWV, Maroko PR: Thoracic epidural anesthesia reduces myocardial infarct size after coronary artery occlusion in dogs. Anesth Analg 65:711, 1986
95. Klassen GA, Bramwell RS, Bromage PR, Zborowska-Sluis DT: Effect of acute sympathectomy by epidural anesthesia on the canine coronary circulation. Anesthesiology 52:8, 1980
96. Mathews ET, Abrams LD: Intrathecal morphine in open heart surgery (correspondence). Lancet 2:543, 1980
97. Bowler I, Djaiani G, Abel R, et al: A combination of intrathecal morphine and remifentanil anesthesia for fast-track cardiac anesthesia and surgery. J Cardiothorac Vasc Anesth 16:709, 2002
98. Alhashemi JA, Sharpe MD, Harris CL, et al: Effect of subarachnoid morphine administration on extubation time after coronary artery bypass graft surgery. J Cardiothorac Vasc Anesth 14:639, 2000
99. Latham P, Zarate E, White PF, et al: Fast-track cardiac anesthesia: A comparison of remifentanil plus intrathecal morphine with sufentanil in a desflurane-based anesthetic. J Cardiothorac Vasc Anesth 14:645, 2000
100. Zarate E, Latham P, White PF, et al: Fast-track cardiac anesthesia: Use of remifentanil combined with intrathecal morphine as an alternative to sufentanil during desflurane anesthesia. Anesth Analg 91:283, 2000
101. Bowler I, Djaiani G, Hall J, et al: Intravenous remifentanil combined with intrathecal morphine decreases extubation times after elective coronary artery bypass graft (CABG) surgery (abstract). Anesth Analg 90:S33, 2000
102. Lee TWR, Jacobsohn E, Maniate JM, et al: High spinal anesthesia in cardiac surgery: Effects on hemodynamics, perioperative stress response, and atrial β-receptor function (abstract). Anesth Analg 90: SCA90, 2000
103. Peterson KL, DeCampli WM, Pike NA, et al: A report of two hundred twenty cases of regional anesthesia in pediatric cardiac surgery. Anesth Analg 90:1014, 2000
104. Hammer GB, Ngo K, Macario A: A retrospective examination of regional plus general anesthesia in children undergoing open heart surgery. Anesth Analg 90:1020, 2000
105. Djaiani G, Bowler I, Hall J, et al: A combination of remifentanil and intrathecal morphine improves pulmonary function following CABG surgery (abstract). Anesth Analg 90:SCA64, 2000
106. Chaney MA, Nikolov MP, Blakeman BP, Bakhos M: Intrathecal morphine for coronary artery bypass graft procedure and early extubation revisited. J Cardiothorac Vasc Anesth 13:574, 1999
107. Shroff A, Rooke GA, Bishop MJ: Effects of intrathecal opioid on extubation time, analgesia, and ICU stay following coronary artery bypass grafting. J Clin Anesth 9:415, 1997
108. Chaney MA, Furry PA, Fluder EM, Slogoff S: Intrathecal morphine for coronary artery bypass grafting and early extubation. Anesth Analg 84:241, 1997
109. Chaney MA, Smith KR, Barclay JC, Slogoff S: Large-dose intrathecal morphine for coronary artery bypass grafting. Anesth Analg 83:215, 1996
110. Kowalewski R, MacAdams C, Froelich J, et al: Anesthesia supplemented with subarachnoid bupivacaine and morphine for coronary artery bypass surgery in a child with Kawasaki disease. J Cardiothorac Vasc Anesth 10:243, 1996
111. Taylor A, Healy M, McCarroll M, Moriarty DC: Intrathecal morphine: One year's experience in cardiac surgical patients. J Cardiothorac Vasc Anesth 10:225, 1996
112. Kowalewski RJ, MacAdams CL, Eagle CJ, et al: Anaesthesia for coronary artery bypass surgery supplemented with subarachnoid bupivacaine and morphine: A report of 18 cases. Can J Anaesth 41:1189, 1994
113. Swenson JD, Hullander RM, Wingler K, Leivers D: Early extubation after cardiac surgery using combined intrathecal sufentanil and morphine. J Cardiothorac Vasc Anesth 8:509, 1994
114. Shroff AB, Bishop MJ: Intrathecal morphine analgesia speeds extubation and shortens ICU stay following coronary artery bypass grafting (CABG) (abstract)). Anesthesiology 81:A129, 1994
115. Fitzpatrick GJ, Moriarty DC: Intrathecal morphine in the management of pain following cardiac surgery. A comparison with morphine i.v. Br J Anaesth 60:639, 1988
116. Vanstrum GS, Bjornson KM, Ilko R: Postoperative effects of intrathecal morphine in coronary artery bypass surgery. Anesth Analg 67:261, 1988
117. Casey WF, Wynands JE, Ralley FE, et al: The role of intrathecal morphine in the anesthetic management of patients undergoing coronary artery bypass surgery. J Cardiothorac Vasc Anesth 1:510, 1987
118. Cheun JK: Intraspinal narcotic anesthesia in open heart surgery. J Kor Med Sci 2:225, 1987
119. Aun C, Thomas D, St. John-Jones L, et al: Intrathecal morphine in cardiac surgery. Eur J Anaesth 2:419, 1985
120. Vincenty C, Malone B, Mathru M, Bahman V: Comparison of intrathecal and intravenous morphine in post coronary bypass surgery (abstract). Crit Care Med 13:308, 1985
121. Jones SEF, Beasley JM, Macfarlane DWR, et al: Intrathecal morphine for postoperative pain relief in children. Br J Anaesth 56:137, 1984
122. Bettex DA, Schmidlin D, Chassot PG, Schmid ER: Intrathecal sufentanil-morphine shortens the duration of intubation and improves analgesia in fast-track cardiac surgery. Can J Anesth 49:711, 2002
123. Goldstein S, Dean D, Kim SJ, et al: A survey of spinal and epidural techniques in adult cardiac surgery. J Cardiothorac Vasc Anesth 15:158, 2001
124. Lee TWR, Grocott HP, Schwinn D, et al: High spinal anesthesia for cardiac surgery: Effects on β-adrenergic receptor function, stress response, and hemodynamics. Anesthesiology 98:499, 2003
125. Clowes GHA, Neville WE, Hopkins A, et al: Factors contributing to success or failure in the use of a pump oxygenator for complete by-pass of the heart and lung, experimental and clinical. Surgery 36:557, 1954
126. Hoar PF, Hickey RF, Ullyot DJ: Systemic hypertension following myocardial revascularization. A method of treatment using epidural anesthesia. J Thorac Cardiovasc Surg 71:859, 1976
127. El-Baz N, Goldin M: Continuous epidural infusion of morphine for pain relief after cardiac operations. J Thorac Cardiovasc Surg 93:878, 1987
128. Jideus L, Joachimsson PO, Stridsberg M, et al: Thoracic epidural anesthesia does not influence the occurrence of postoperative sustained atrial fibrillation. Ann Thorac Surg 72:65, 2001
129. Scott NB, Turfrey DJ, Ray DAA, et al: A prospective randomized study of the potential benefits of thoracic epidural anesthesia and analgesia in patients undergoing coronary artery bypass grafting. Anesth Analg 93:528, 2001
130. Warters D, Knight W, Koch SM, Luehr S: Thoracic epidurals in coronary artery bypass surgery. Anesth Analg 90:767, 2000
131. Loick HM, Schmidt C, Van Aken H, et al: High thoracic epidural anesthesia, but not clonidine, attenuates the perioperative stress response via sympatholysis and reduces the release of troponin T in patients undergoing coronary artery bypass grafting. Anesth Analg 88:701, 1999
132. Tenling A, Joachimsson PO, Tyden H, et al: Thoracic epidural anesthesia as an adjunct to general anesthesia for cardiac surgery: Effects on ventilation-perfusion relationships. J Cardiothorac Vasc Anesth 13:258, 1999

133. Sanchez R, Nygard E: Epidural anesthesia in cardiac surgery: Is there an increased risk? J Cardiothorac Vasc Anesth 12:170, 1998
134. Loick HM, Mollhoff T, Erren M, et al: Thoracic epidural anesthesia lowers catecholamine and TNFa release after CABG in humans (abstract). Anesth Analg 86:S81, 1998
135. Warters RD, Koch SM, Luehr SL, Katz J: Thoracic epidural anesthesia in CABG surgery (abstract). Anesth Analg 86:S116, 1998
136. Shayevitz JR, Merkel S, O'Kelly SW, et al: Lumbar epidural morphine infusions for children undergoing cardiac surgery. J Cardiothorac Vasc Anesth 10:217, 1996
137. Frank RS, Boltz MG, Sentivany SK, Krane EJ: Combined epidural-general anesthesia for the repair of atrial septal defects in children results in shorter ICU stays (abstract). Anesthesiology 83:A1176, 1995
138. Moore CM, Cross MH, Desborough JP, et al: Hormonal effects of thoracic extradural analgesia for cardiac surgery. Br J Anaesth 75:387, 1995
139. Stenseth R, Berg EM, Bjella L, et al: Effects of thoracic epidural analgesia on coronary hemodynamics and myocardial metabolism in coronary artery bypass surgery. J Cardiothorac Vasc Anesth 9:503, 1995
140. Kirno K, Friberg P, Grzegorczyk A, et al: Thoracic epidural anesthesia during coronary artery bypass surgery: Effects on cardiac sympathetic activity, myocardial blood flow and metabolism, and central hemodynamics. Anesth Analg 79:1075, 1994
141. Stenseth R, Bjella L, Berg EM, et al: Thoracic epidural analgesia in aortocoronary bypass surgery, I: Haemodynamic effects. Acta Anaesthesiol Scand 38:826, 1994
142. Stenseth R, Bjella L, Berg EM, et al: Thoracic epidural analgesia in aortocoronary bypass surgery, II: Effects on the endocrine metabolic response. Acta Anaesthesiol Scand 38:834, 1994
143. Shapiro JH, Wolman RL, Lofland GK: Epidural morphine as an adjunct for early extubation following congenital cardiac surgery (abstract). Anesth Analg 78: S385, 1994
144. Liem TH, Booij LHDJ, Hasenbos MAWM, Gielen MJM: Coronary artery bypass grafting using two different anesthetic techniques: Part I: Hemodynamic results. J Cardiothorac Vasc Anesth 6:148, 1992
145. Liem TH, Hasenbos MAWM, Booij LHDJ, Gielen MJM: Coronary artery bypass grafting using two different anesthetic techniques: Part 2: Postoperative outcome. J Cardiothorac Vasc Anesth 6:156, 1992
146. Liem TH, Booij LH, Gielen MJ, et al: Coronary artery bypass grafting using two different anesthetic techniques: Part 3: Adrenergic responses. J Cardiothorac Vasc Anesth 6:162, 1992
147. Rosen KR, Rosen DA: Caudal epidural morphine for control of pain following open heart surgery in children. Anesthesiology 70:418, 1989
148. Joachimsson PO, Nystrom SO, Tyden H: Early extubation after coronary artery surgery in efficiently rewarmed patients: A postoperative comparison of opioid anesthesia versus inhalational anesthesia and thoracic epidural analgesia. J Cardiothorac Anesth 3:444, 1989
149. Robinson RJS, Brister S, Jones E, Quigly M: Epidural meperidine analgesia after cardiac surgery. Can Anaesth Soc J 33:550, 1986
150. Pastor MC, Sanchez MJ, Casas MA, et al: Thoracic epidural analgesia in coronary artery bypass graft surgery: Seven years' experience. J Cardiothorac Vasc Anesth 17:154, 2003
151. Vlachtsis H, Vohra A: High thoracic epidural with general anesthesia for combined off-pump coronary artery and aortic aneurysm surgery. J Cardiothorac Vasc Anesth 17:226, 2003
152. Sisillo E, Salvi L, Juliano G, et al: Thoracic epidural anesthesia as a bridge to redo coronary artery bypass graft surgery. J Cardiothorac Vasc Anesth 17:629, 2003
153. Varadarajan B, Whitaker DK, Vohra A, Stafford Smith M: Case 2-2002. Thoracic epidural anesthesia in patients with ankylosing spondylitis undergoing coronary artery surgery. J Cardiothorac Vasc Anesth 16:240, 2002
154. de Vries AJ, Mariani MA, van der Maaten JM, et al: To ventilate or not after minimally invasive direct coronary artery bypass surgery: The role of epidural anesthesia. J Cardiothorac Vasc Anesth 16:21, 2002
155. Canto M, Casas A, Sanchez MJ, et al: Thoracic epidurals in heart valve surgery: Neurologic risk evaluation. J Cardiothorac Vasc Anesth 16:723, 2002
156. Fillinger MP, Yeager MP, Dodds TM, et al: Epidural anesthesia and analgesia: Effects on recovery from cardiac surgery. J Cardiothorac Vasc Anesth 16:15, 2002
157. Dhole S, Mehta Y, Saxena H, et al: Comparison of continuous thoracic epidural and paravertebral blocks for postoperative analgesia after minimally invasive direct coronary artery bypass surgery. J Cardiothorac Vasc Anesth 15:288, 2001
158. Djaiani GN, Ali M, Heinrich L, et al: Ultra-fast-track anesthetic technique facilitates operating room extubation in patients undergoing off-pump coronary revascularization surgery. J Cardiothorac Vasc Anesth 15:152, 2001
159. Visser WA, Liem TH, Brouwer RM: High thoracic epidural anesthesia for coronary artery bypass graft surgery in a patient with severe obstructive lung disease. J Cardiothorac Vasc Anesth 15:758, 2001
160. Liem TH, Williams JP, Hensens AG, Singh SK: Minimally invasive direct coronary artery bypass procedure using a high thoracic epidural plus general anesthetic technique. J Cardiothorac Vasc Anesth 12:668, 1998
161. Fawcett WJ, Edwards RE, Quinn AC, et al: Thoracic epidural analgesia started after CPB. adrenergic, cardiovascular and respiratory sequelae. Anaesthesia 52:294, 1997
162. Turfrey DJ, Ray DAA, Sutcliffe NP, et al: Thoracic epidural anaesthesia for coronary artery bypass graft surgery. Effects on postoperative complications. Anaesthesia 52:1090, 1997
163. Stenseth R, Bjella L, Berg EM, et al: Effects of thoracic epidural analgesia on pulmonary function after coronary artery bypass surgery. Eur J Cardiothorac Surg 10:859-865, 1996
164. O'Connor CJ, Tuman KJ: Epidural anesthesia and analgesia for coronary artery bypass graft surgery: Still forbidden territory? (editorial) Anesth Analg 93:523, 2001
165. Amar D: Beta-adrenergic blocker withdrawal confounds the benefits of epidural analgesia with sympathectomy on supraventricular arrhythmias after cardiac surgery (correspondence). Anesth Analg 95:1119, 2002
166. Riedel BJ, Shaw AD: Thoracic epidural anesthesia and analgesia in patients undergoing coronary artery bypass surgery (correspondence). Anesth Analg 94:1365, 2002
167. Alston RP: Thoracic epidurals and coronary artery bypass grafting surgery (correspondence). Anesth Analg 94:1365, 2002
168. Royse C, Royse A, Soeding P, et al: Prospective randomized trial of high thoracic epidural analgesia for coronary artery bypass surgery. Ann Thorac Surg 75:93, 2003
169. Priestley MC, Cope L, Halliwell R, et al: Thoracic epidural anesthesia for cardiac surgery: The effects on tracheal intubation time and length of hospital stay. Anesth Analg 94:275, 2002
170. Karagoz HY, Sonmez B, Bakkaloglu B, et al: Coronary artery bypass grafting in the conscious patient without endotracheal general anesthesia. Ann Thorac Surg 70:91, 2000
171. Aybek T, Dogan S, Neidhart G, et al: Coronary artery bypass grafting through complete sternotomy in conscious patients. Heart Surgery Forum 5:17, 2002
172. Souto GLL, Junior CSC, de Souza JBS, et al: Coronary artery bypass in the ambulatory patient. J Thorac Cardiovasc Surg 123:1008, 2002
173. Aybek T, Kessler P, Dogan S, et al: Awake coronary artery bypass grafting: Utopia or reality? Ann Thorac Surg 75:1165, 2003
174. Aybek T, Kessler P, Khan MF, et al: Operative techniques in awake coronary artery bypass grafting. J Thorac Cardiovasc Surg 125:1394, 2003
175. Karagoz HY, Kurtoglu M, Bakkaloglu B, et al: Coronary artery bypass grafting in the awake patient: Three years' experience in 137 patients. J Thorac Cardiovasc Surg 125:1401, 2003
176. Chakravarthy M, Jawali V, Patil TA, et al: High thoracic epidural anesthesia as the sole anesthetic for redo off-pump coronary artery bypass surgery. J Cardiothorac Vasc Anesth 17:84, 2003
177. Chakravarthy MR, Jawali V, Patil TA, et al: High thoracic epidural anaesthesia as the sole anaesthetic technique for minimally invasive direct coronary artery bypass in a high-risk patient. Ann Cardiac Anaesth 6:62, 2003
178. Kessler P, Neidhart G, Bremerich DH, et al: High thoracic epidural anesthesia for coronary artery bypass grafting using two different surgical approaches in conscious patients. Anesth Analg 95:791, 2002
179. Vanek T, Straka Z, Brucek P, Widimsky P: Thoracic epidural anesthesia for off-pump coronary artery bypass without intubation. Eur J Cardiothorac Surg 20:858, 2001
180. Anderson MB, Kwong KF, Furst AJ, Salerno TA: Thoracic epidural anesthesia for coronary bypass via left anterior thoracotomy in the conscious patient. Eur J Cardiothorac Surg 20:415, 2001
181. Paiste J, Bjerke RJ, Williams JP, et al: Minimally invasive direct coronary artery bypass surgery under high thoracic epidural. Anesth Analg 93:1486, 2001
182. Zenati MA, Paiste J, Williams JP, et al: Minimally invasive coronary bypass without general endotracheal anesthesia. Ann Thorac Surg 72:1380, 2001
183. Chakravarthy M, Jawali V, Patil TA, et al: High thoracic epidural anesthesia as the sole anesthetic for performing multiple grafts in off-pump coronary artery bypass surgery. J Cardiothorac Vasc Anesth 17:160, 2003
184. Schachner T, Bonatti J, Balogh D, et al: Aortic valve replacement in the conscious patient under regional anesthesia without endotracheal intubation. J Thorac Cardiovasc Surg 125:1526, 2003

185. Straka Z, Brucek P, Vanek T, et al: Routine immediate extubation for off-pump coronary artery bypass grafting without thoracic epidural analgesia. Ann Thorac Surg 74:1544, 2002
186. Liu SS, Block BM, Wu CL: Effects of perioperative central neuraxial analgesia on outcome after coronary aftery bypass surgery: A meta-analysis. Anesthesiology 101:153, 2004
187. Ochroch EA, Gottschalk A, Augostides J, et al: Long-term pain and activity during recovery from major thoracotomy using thoracic epidural analgesia. Anesthesiology 97:1234, 2002
188. Richard C, Girard F, Ferraro P, et al: Acute postoperative pain in lung transplant recipients. Ann Thorac Surg 77:1951–1955, 2004
189. Ballantyne JC, Carr DB, deFerranti S, et al: The comparative effects of postoperative analgesic therapies on pulmonary outcome: Cumulative meta-analyses of randomized, controlled trials. Anesth Analg 86:598, 1998
190. Licker M, de Perrot M, Hohn L, et al: Perioperative mortality and major cardiopulmonary complications after lung surgery for non-small-cell carcinoma. Eur J Cardiothorac Surg 15:314, 1999
191. Sivarajan M, Amory DW, Lindbloom LE, Schuettmann RS: Systemic and regional blood-flow changes during spinal anesthesia in the rhesus monkey. Anesthesiology 43:78, 1975
192. Hackel DB, Sancetta SM, Kleinerman J: Effect of hypotension due to spinal anesthesia on coronary blood flow and myocardial metabolism in man. Circulation 13:92, 1956
193. Reiz S, Nath S, Rais O: Effects of thoracic epidural block and prenalterol on coronary vascular resistance and myocardial metabolism in patients with coronary artery disease. Acta Anaesth Scand 24:11, 1980
194. DiNardo JA, Bert A, Schwartz MJ, et al: Effects of vasoactive drugs on flows through left internal mammary artery and saphenous vein grafts in man. J Thorac Cardiovasc Surg 102:730, 1991
195. Heusch G: α-Adrenergic mechanisms in myocardial ischemia. Circulation 81:1, 1990
196. Reiz S, Nath S: Cardiotoxicity of local anaesthetic agents. Br J Anaesth 58:736, 1986
197. Wattwil M, Sundberg A, Arvill A, Lennquist C: Circulatory changes during high thoracic epidural anaesthesia—influence of sympathetic block and of systemic effect of the local anaesthetic. Acta Anaesth Scand 29:849, 1985
198. Blomberg S, Ricksten SE: Effects of thoracic epidural anaesthesia on central haemodynamics compared to cardiac beta-adrenoceptor blockade in conscious rats with acute myocardial infarction. Acta Anaesth Scand 34:1, 1990
199. Hotvedt R, Refsum H, Platou ES: Cardiac electrophysiological and hemodynamic effects of β-adrenoceptor blockade and thoracic epidural analgesia in the dog. Anesth Analg 63:817, 1984
200. Easley RB, Rosen RE, Lindeman KS: Coronary artery spasm during initiation of epidural anesthesia. Anesthesiology 99:1015, 2003
201. Oden RV, Karagianes TG: Postoperative myocardial ischemia possibly masked by epidural fentanyl analgesia. Anesthesiology 74:941, 1991
202. Chaney MA: Side effects of intrathecal and epidural opioids. Can J Anaesth 42:891, 1995
203. Wang JK, Nauss LA, Thomas JE: Pain relief by intrathecally applied morphine in man. Anesthesiology 50:149, 1979
204. Behar M, Magora F, Olshwang D, Davidson JT: Epidural morphine in treatment of pain. Lancet 1:527, 1979
205. Glynn CJ, Mather LE, Cousins MJ, et al: Spinal narcotics and respiratory depression (correspondence). Lancet 2:356, 1979
206. Liolios A, Andersen FH: Selective spinal analgesia (correspondence). Lancet 2:357, 1979
207. Scott DB, McClure J: Selective epidural analgesia (correspondence). Lancet 1:1410, 1979
208. Shook JE, Watkins WD, Camporesi EM: Differential roles of opioid receptors in respiration, respiratory disease, and opiate-induced respiratory depression. Am Rev Respir Dis 142:895, 1990
209. Vandermeulen EP, Van Aken H, Vermylen J: Anticoagulants and spinal-epidural anesthesia. Anesth Analg 79:1165, 1994
210. Markham JW, Lynge HN, Stahlman EB: The syndrome of spontaneous spinal epidural hematoma. Report of three cases. J Neurosurg 26:334, 1967
211. Waldman SD, Feldstein GS, Waldman HJ, et al: Caudal administration of morphine sulfate in anticoagulated and thrombocytopenic patients. Anesth Analg 66:267, 1987
212. Odoom JA, Sih IL: Epidural analgesia and anticoagulant therapy. Experience with one thousand cases of continuous epidurals. Anaesthesia 38:254, 1983
213. Owens EL, Kasten GW, Hessel EA: Spinal subarachnoid hematoma after lumbar puncture and heparinization: A case report, review of the literature, and discussion of anesthetic implications. Anesth Analg 65:1201, 1986
214. Brem SS, Hafler DA, Van Uitert RL, et al: Spinal subarachnoid hematoma: A hazard of lumbar puncture resulting in reversible paraplegia. N Engl J Med 303:1020, 1981
215. Ruff RL, Dougherty JH: Complications of lumbar puncture followed by anticoagulation. Stroke 12:879, 1981
216. Varkey GP, Brindle GF: Peridural anaesthesia and anticoagulant therapy. Can Anaesth Soc J 21:106, 1974
217. Baron HC, LaRaja RD, Rossi G, Atkinson D: Continuous epidural analgesia in the heparinized vascular surgical patient: A retrospective review of 912 patients. J Vasc Surg 6:144, 1987
218. Rao TLK, El-Etr AA: Anticoagulation following placement of epidural and subarachnoid catheters: An evaluation of neurologic sequelae. Anesthesiology 55:618, 1981
219. Ho AMH, Chung DC, Joynt GM: Neuraxial blockade and hematoma in cardiac surgery: Estimating the risk of a rare adverse event that has not (yet) occurred. Chest 117:551, 2000
220. Rosen DA, Hawkinberry DW, Rosen KR, et al: An epidural hematoma in an adolescent patient after cardiac surgery. Anesth Analg 98:966, 2004
221. Mora Mangano CT: Risky business (editorial). J Thorac Cardiovasc Surg 125:1204, 2003
222. Castellano JM, Durbin CG: Epidural analgesia and cardiac surgery: Worth the risk? (editorial). Chest 117:305, 2000
223. Schwann NM, Chaney MA: No pain, much gain? (editorial) J Thorac Cardiovasc Surg 126:1261, 2003
224. Gravlee GP: Epidural analgesia and coronary artery bypass grafting: The controversy continues (editorial). J Cardiothorac Vasc Anesth 17:151, 2003
225. de Leon-Casasola OA: When it comes to outcome, we need to define what a perioperative epidural technique is (editorial). Anesth Analg 96:315, 2003
226. Rosenquist RW, Birnbach DJ: Epidural insertion in anesthetized adults: will your patients thank you? (editorial). Anesth Analg 96:1545, 2003
227. White PF: The role of non-opioid analgesic techniques in the management of pain after ambulatory surgery. Anesth Analg 94:577, 2002
228. Kehlet H, Dahl JB: The value of "multimodal" or "balanced analgesia" in postoperative pain treatment. Anesth Analg 77:1048, 1993
229. Myles PS, Hunt JO, Fletcher H, et al: Relation between quality of recovery in hospital and quality of life at 3 months after cardiac surgery. Anesthesiology 95:862, 2001
230. Fleron MH, Weiskopf RB, Bertrand M, et al: A comparison of intrathecal opioid and intravenous analgesia for the incidence of cardiovascular, respiratory, and renal complications after abdominal aortic surgery. Anesth Analg 97:2, 2003
231. Beattie WS, Badner NH, Choi P: Epidural analgesia reduces postoperative myocardial infarction: A meta-analysis. Anesth Analg 93:853, 2001
232. Wu CL, Raja SN: Optimizing postoperative analgesia: The use of global outcome measures (editorial). Anesthesiology 97:533, 2002
233. Gottschalk A, Ochroch EA: Preemptive analgesia: What do we do now? (correspondence) Anesthesiology 98:280, 2003
234. Hogan QH: No preemptive analgesia: Is that so bad? (editorial) Anesthesiology 96:526, 2002
235. Moiniche S, Kehlet H, Dahl JB: A qualitative and quantitative systematic review of preemptive analgesia for postoperative pain relief: The role of timing of analgesia. Anesthesiology 96:725, 2002
236. Katz J, Cohen L, Schmid R, et al: Postoperative morphine use and hyperalgesia are reduced by preoperative but not intraoperative epidural analgesia: Implications for preemptive analgesia and the prevention of central sensitization. Anesthesiology 98:1449, 2003

Part VIII

PRACTICE MANAGEMENT

Chapter 38

FINANCIAL ASPECTS OF PATIENT CARE

James R. Zaidan, MD, MBA

KEY POINTS

1. Traditional costing leads to incorrect interpretation of the true costs of running a practice.
2. Activity-based costing applies overhead so that practice managers will realize true costs of specific service lines.
3. Physicians can no longer assume that caring for patients will automatically provide an income.
4. Anesthesiologists must find ways to demonstrate their value to the enterprise they serve.
5. Hospital personnel understand the business aspects of patient care. They do not understand exactly how an anesthesiology department works; therefore, anesthesiologists must provide very precise reasons why the practice should receive their support now, when in years past, the practice did not require their financial backing.

Cardiac anesthesiologists have played important roles in managing cardiac surgical patients since the 1970s. Anesthesiologists assumed vital roles in patient care, both in operating rooms and in intensive care units, having learned the physiology of cardiac function, and developed an in-depth understanding of the pathophysiology of coronary arterial, valvular, and congenital heart diseases. Cardiac anesthesiologists became masters at interpreting numerical data, analyzing waveforms from pulmonary arterial catheters, and discussing the clinical findings of transesophageal echocardiograms. Cardiac anesthesiologists were part of and continue to be part of a larger team consisting of surgeons, perfusionists, and nurses that added financial value to their institutions. Like all other areas of anesthesiology, cardiac anesthesiologists experience increased costs, decreased reimbursements, and inability to maintain compensation levels based on revenues.

This chapter reviews the past, but it also looks to the future from a viewpoint of labor markets, finances, and marketing.

CURRENT MARKET

In essentially any other market, a buyer who cannot afford an item or a service simply does not receive that item or service. The health care market does not behave like a free market. Third-party payers negotiate with health care providers and influence the market. The final buyer of the service, the patient, has little to do with the process and simply expects the best of care unrelated to the ability to pay. Patients pay only through premiums, co-pays, and deductibles, and for the greater good through taxes.

The development of a federal, third-party payer system started in the early 1900s with the establishment of the Public Health Service; proceeded through multiple laws, several administrations, including Roosevelt, Truman, Johnson, and Bush, and health care provider networks; and ended with onerous federal and state laws, fraud hotlines for patients to report substandard care,[1] threatened incarceration, and incredibly increased costs.

After reviewing readily available data about global statistics, it becomes obvious that the United States spends more of its gross domestic product (GDP), approximately $11 trillion, on health care than any other nation.[2,3] The staggering amount is approximately 13% of the GDP. The average life expectancy in the United States is 77.1 years. In contrast, the country of Taiwan spends 0.4% of its GDP on health care, and the average life expectancy is only slightly lower at 76.7 years. American society begins to wonder why.

Observing the consumer price index and reviewing its composition, compared with 1994 (=100), the city average index for all items for October 2004 was 312.2 for total medical care. The index for the same month for medical care commodities was 271.2, and for medical services, 324.8.[4] It is obvious that despite the measures taken by government and big business to curtail costs of health care, their efforts have not been successful.

The United States spends more than $1 trillion a year on health care, health care–related expenses are escalating at enormous rates, and American life expectancy is not the best in the world. It is with these concepts that American health care exists. Cardiac anesthesiology must exist within a subset of these issues. The subspecialty is clearly under the influence of federal and state governments, payers and patients, new technology and new pharmaceuticals, and cardiac anesthesiologists compelled to find new ways to remain financially viable and scientifically sound.

COST ACCOUNTING SYSTEMS

In the past, health care systems and physicians' practices did not have a need to determine precise costs, because payer systems reimbursed a percentage of the physician's bill. Costs obviously did not matter when third-party payers were willing to pay the bills. The concept of managed care ended more traditional ways of determining costs when it placed caps on reimbursements, thereby forcing health care systems to precisely define costs of service lines and procedures. By defining costs, it is possible to determine areas of financial improvement; therefore, physicians quickly entered the world of

Table 38–1 Costing Methodologies

Type of Costing	Concept	Methodology	Comment
Traditional	The cost object consumes resources.	Trace direct costs and use a single factor to evenly allocate overhead costs to each service line.	Overestimates costs of least complex service lines; underestimates costs of most complex service lines
Activity based	Cost object consumes activities and activities consume resources.	Trace direct costs. Determine activities required to provide a service and apply a cost driver to link the activity to the resource.	Expensive to initiate; time required to interview personnel; correctly allocates overhead to a service line

business through activity-based costing and activity-based management.

A traditional costing system traces direct costs and direct labor to a product or service and then applies overhead based on a single measure of volume. The concept is that services consume resources. Unfortunately, traditional systems incorrectly develop internal cross-subsidies so that a patient care service line that is inexpensive to manage could be presented as very expensive because of applied overhead. In this situation, if it were to overestimate the costs, the practice would inadvertently run a deficit on paper when, in fact, it is earning a profit.

Health care systems have used several types of traditional costing. A ratio of cost to charges (RCC) is a costing method that was commonly used in the past to determine the cost of a single test or service line. To determine the cost of a procedure using the RCC, find the total costs and the total charges of the department and then multiply this ratio by the charge for the procedure. For example, if a department incurs $17 million in total costs and $20 million in charges, then the RCC is 0.85. If a charge for a procedure is $500, then the cost is reported as $425. The problem with this method is the assumption that costs and charges are linked in some constructive way. With an RCC methodology, service line cost estimates obviously decrease when charges increase, costs are evenly allocated to all procedures, and the ratio has no predictive value concerning budgeted revenue. Relative value units (RVUs), another traditional system, also apply costs to direct labor, direct supplies, and overhead. These cost components are weighted and then multiplied by a factor of dollars per RVU. Medicare uses this system with a multiplier based on region. Like the RCC, an RVU system evenly allocates overhead to every procedure.

Activity-based costing, on the other hand, allocates overhead costs based on the concept that services consume activities and those activities consume resources. By using this method of cost analysis, the practice is able to determine rather precisely the cost of a procedure by avoiding average overhead costs. The first step is to define the cost object, or the service, and to trace direct labor and direct costs to the service in a process similar to that of traditional costing; then the individual activities that must occur in order to deliver the service are described. Finally, the resources are applied to each activity through cost drivers. The problem with activity-based costing is that it takes time and is expensive. However, once completed, precise allocation of overhead will result in correct costing of the service. Armed with these data, a practice can approach hospital administration to ask for financial support for the correct services based on correct costs.

In academic institutions, overhead costs are applied to the department from the university and the school of medicine. Committees are appointed to allocate these costs to each department, but departments have no control over the absolute amount of these costs. The department in turn allocates these costs to service lines such as cardiac anesthesia. The question that practice administrators should ask is, How did these costs get allocated to this department? This allocation must never be based on a percent of revenues. University and school of medicine overhead allocation should be based on activities linked through cost drivers to the service provided. If "carve-outs" occur that allow individual departments or service lines to avoid overhead, then the driver of the activity is incorrect. A department might not incur overhead, but this avoidance should be based on the fact that the correct driver indicates that the activity was not used. In similar fashion, the department must determine the activities that should be assigned to service lines to properly allocate the overhead assigned to the department. A brief review of traditional and activity-based costing is given in Table 38–1.

COMMONLY USED TERMS

Terms commonly used in business circles are now well known to anesthesiologists who manage their practices. Several of these terms are briefly defined in Box 38–1. *Charge capture* assumes that a practice has a mechanism to know how many cases were performed. Surgeons' offices commonly perform *financial clearance* procedures. *Payment variances* are very prevalent and are difficult to discover. Several commercial software products are available to find payment variances. *Denials* occur usually through insufficient or incorrect information populating the claim form. *Accounts receivable* are important numbers in that they define potential revenue by payer mix. A large portion of self-pay becomes bad debt that the practice writes off after a period of time. Generally, state insurance commissioners require that third-party payers pay the claim within a short period of time after receiving the invoice. Third-party payers, in return, require a *clean claim.* Payers can hold back payment without a clean claim; therefore, much of the front-end work of the business office is spent on producing a clean claim.

BUSINESS FACTORS IMPORTANT TO A PRACTICE

Practice administrators constantly review factors that influence revenue streams into their practices. The factors are payer mix, or the percentage of revenue that derives directly from patients, from third-party payers such as Medicare, Medicaid,

BOX 38–1 *Definitions of Commonly Used Terms*

Term	Definition
Charge capture	The percent of charges posted to total cases performed. This number should be 100%.
Financial clearance	A process by which the business office ensures that patients have received precertifications for their procedures.
Payment variance	The managed care contract defines the amount of the payment for each procedure. Payment variance implies a difference between the contracted amount and the amount received.
Denial	A denial is a disallowed charge. Usually the third-party payer requires additional information, imagined or real.
Accounts receivable (AR)	AR is the amount billed to the patient minus adjustments that the business office expects but has not yet received.
Clean claim	A claim in which all electronic fields are populated and all data are correct. A clean claim seldom enters a third-party payer's office.

and other federal insurance, from commercial insurance, and from managed care; efficient operating room management including items such as room turnover, time involved in each case, and number of rooms per surgeon; the total number of cases; and business office functions such as contract negotiation, charge capture, coding, financial clearance, denials, payment variances, and accounts receivable management. As a business, cardiac anesthesia can control business office functions and possibly some elements of operating room efficiency. It is difficult to control efficiency, however, when surgeons' referral patterns are inconsistent and not in their control, cases are of long duration, and most operating rooms are filled. Anesthesiologists cannot control case mix and payer mix, and they certainly cannot control technologic advances in cardiology that destabilize surgical caseload.

FUNDING DEPARTMENTAL DEFICITS

Business office affairs and financial reports were at one time important only to accountants as they assured that physicians received reasonable compensation and retirement packages. Now, anesthesiologists must understand concepts of payer mix, malpractice costs, charge capture, coding, financial clearance, denials, payment variance, and accounts receivable. Armed with these data, group practices that are running deficits can develop templates for contracts with third-party payers and negotiate with hospitals to cover the shortfalls in revenue. In two articles in the *ASA Newsletter*, Bierstein[5,6] outlined several of the issues that anesthesiologists and hospital administrators face when negotiating with each other. Points of view differ between anesthesiologists and administrators, because hospital administrators do not understand the world of anesthesia management, have other basic concerns, and make decisions differently from anesthesiologists.[5]

Hospital administrators need information on which to base their decisions. Key elements in gaining desired endpoints in negotiations with hospitals are (1) presenting concise data, (2) showing hospital administrators why the practice is disadvantaged by working at that hospital, and (3) developing a highly organized, data-focused request for support from the hospital.[6] Rather than demanding money, show how costs other than physician compensation have increased, and describe why revenues have decreased and accounts receivable has increased despite front office management of denials and payment variances. The practice also must show that its physicians, despite being disadvantaged by working there, are essential in maintaining revenue streams of the enterprise. The practice must demonstrate its value rather than simply demanding financial support. As an example, it would be inappropriate to state that cardiac anesthesiologists should earn stable incomes. Rather, remind the chief financial officer of the hospital, for instance, that 10% of the charges and 20% of the hospital's revenue are derived from performing cardiac cases. This revenue is based on the presence of cardiac anesthesiologists who lose money because of unfavorable payer mix and malpractice costs.

LABOR MARKET AND ITS EFFECT ON SUBSPECIALTY ADVANCEMENT AND COMPENSATION

Anesthesiologists work in a labor market that is currently understaffed and likely will be understaffed in the foreseeable future.[7,8] National politics of the early 1990s helped lead U.S. medical graduates out of the specialty of anesthesiology and into primary care areas. As shown by Figure 38–1, the ploy was highly successful.[9-11] Although the good news is that the number and academic standing of students entering anesthesiology are increasing, the deficit created in the 1990s will be around for years. A shortage in the general labor market conceptually creates shortages in specialty areas. The labor market responds by increasing compensation packages and benefits, and practitioners respond with a diminishing sense of loyalty to the employer. As compensation is bid up by the shortage, graduates do not enter subspecialties such as cardiothoracic anesthesiology, because residency graduates are well paid without fellowships. In the meantime, there is a shortage of transesophageal echocardiography–trained cardiac anesthesiologists.

Anesthesiologists are somewhat protected from marketing attacks that cardiologists experienced in the 1990s regarding the value of their procedures. Like any service industry, specialty care physicians occasionally must verify that their procedures are aiding humanity. Remember that life expectancy in the United States is not the best in the world, and society continues to ask what it is receiving for the trillion-dollar expenditure. Cardiologists responded to these challenges with outcome studies.[12] For instance, a study by McGlynn et al[13] reviewed the appropriate and inappropriate incidences of coronary artery bypass graft surgery and angiography in the state of New York and compared the results with those of two provinces in Canada, where government monitors health care delivery. The authors found no significant differences among the sites of clinical care.

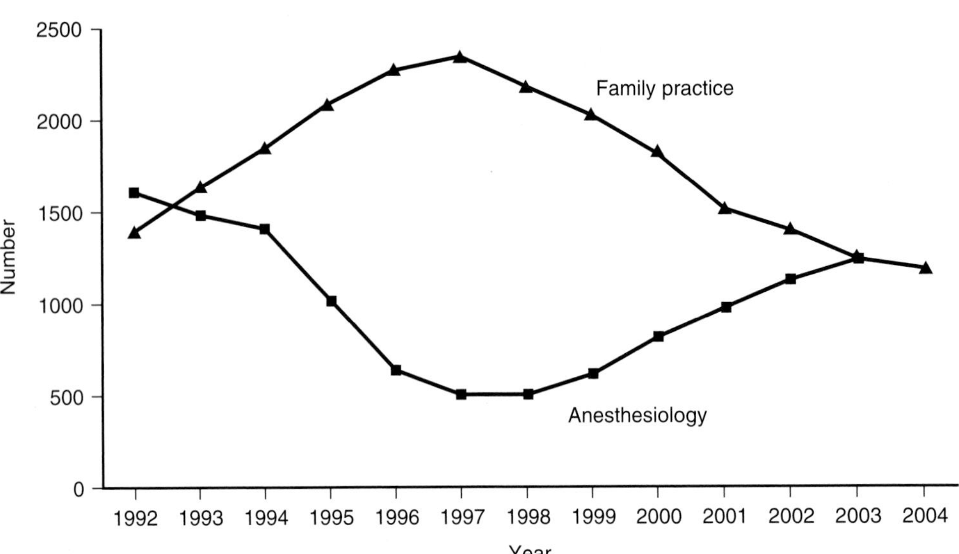

Figure 38–1 Number of U.S. medical graduates entering the specialties of family practice at the postgraduate year 1 level and anesthesiology at the postgraduate year 2 level between 1992 and 2004.

A study by Hilborne et al[14] revealed that the incidence of inappropriate use of coronary angioplasty in 15 randomly selected hospitals involving 1306 patients was only 4%. Jollis et al[15] reviewed mortality according to the specialty of the admitting physician in more than 8000 Medicare patients. After statistical adjustments, the authors found that additional training in cardiology was linked with an important reduction in mortality in patients who had experienced acute coronary events. Selby et al[16] studied patients with acute myocardial infarctions admitted to hospitals that offered coronary angiography versus hospitals that did not offer this service. After statistical corrections, the authors found that patients who were admitted to hospitals that had a higher rate of angiography, implying the presence of cardiologists, also had a lower risk of death. A study by Ayanian et al[17] revealed very similar results in that cardiologists were significantly more likely to prescribe up-to-date therapy than were primary care physicians. Cardiologists defended their position and continued to develop essentially unimpeded, even newer procedures that surgeons performed in the past. Cardiologists have shown third-party payers their value in patient care. Anesthesiologists have minimal data regarding these types of outcome studies to prove their value.

It is difficult to imagine that another specialty could take over a cardiac anesthesiology practice; however, anesthesiologists are not protected from other specialty physicians who work in other areas of the hospital such as critical care units and interventional cardiology laboratories. A labor market that includes possible outflanking maneuvers by specialties that are looking for procedures to increase revenues should be of concern. When sufficient numbers of anesthesiologists were not being trained, some of the services could not be provided. Other specialties assumed control of these services. For example, pediatric intensivists currently provide "sedation services" for patients in pediatric intensive care units, pulmonary critical care physicians offer the same care as anesthesiologists who work in adult units, and hospitalists are becoming "sedationists." These individuals do not earn the same level of compensation as anesthesiologists. Hospitals underwrite the compensation for the surgical work, but they refuse to hire additional anesthesiologists to cover patient care in these other areas. Hospital administrators are simply asking why they should pay anesthesiologists additional amounts to accomplish the same care. Physicians in other specialties perform the work and earn revenue at essentially no additional cost.

THIRD-PARTY PAYERS

Indemnity

This type of insurance is the most lucrative to all physicians in that it pays cost plus. Patients pay very high monthly premiums and co-pays depending on the chosen plan. Companies pay physicians depending on internal policies, but usually the amount is 80% of the allowable charge. Business offices balance-bill patients to the allowable charge. Depending on the area of the country and the type of hospital, indemnity insurance generally represents a minor portion of a practice's total revenue.

Managed Care

Contracts with managed care organizations result in negotiated payment for services. Items that departmental administrators must negotiate include, but are not limited to, number of minutes per unit; method of charging for fractions of time units; modifiers such as ASA classification, age, and position; monitors considered beyond ASA standard monitoring; and allocations among the hospital, the anesthesiologists, and other physicians.

Managed care originated from the viewpoint of the insurance companies; however, billion dollar industries have banded together and are now driving a different force in health care coverage. Industry is controlling its own costs by reversing nonmarket influences and by responding to the recurrence of double-digit health care inflation. The basic idea is to return to a consumer-driven, competitive health care system so that the patient buys only the highest possible value.[18] Competition should exist not only among providers of health care but also among third-party payers.[19] Physicians and hospitals theoretically will respond by providing higher quality care at lower cost. One method of returning to a consumer-driven, competitive state is to define contributions to a plan in which patients receive specific employer contributions for health care for which the patient pays higher premiums, co-pays, and deductibles. Other processes include elimination of free insurance coverage for the employee, increased premiums for family coverage, and tiered benefits for pharmaceuticals and hospital care. The consumer, therefore, will shop for the lowest cost and the highest quality care, or the highest possible value.[20]

The Business Roundtable, started in 1972, is an association of chief executive officers from 150 corporations that now represent approximately 10 million workers in the United States. The Business Roundtable, through its desire to encourage national and global economic growth, developed an initiative called "Leapfrog" in 2000.[21] The concept behind the Leapfrog initiative is that American health care is below obtainable levels of basic safety and overall customer value and that the health care industry would improve more rapidly if purchasers better recognized and rewarded superior safety and overall value.[21,22] Cardiac anesthesiologists are involved by default, because two of the procedures specifically monitored by Leapfrog are coronary artery bypass graft surgical procedures and percutaneous coronary interventions. Leapfrog also sets standards in other areas including intensive care unit staffing and computerized drug ordering. The implications are obvious for everyone in health care. Clinicians are beginning to work in a competitive model that must meet patient satisfaction and quality-of-care standards or patients and third-party payers will eventually close the doors of the hospitals that do not meet Leapfrog's standards.

In attempting to increase their revenues in response to managed care, primary care physicians have developed luxury primary care.[23] Patients who pay the premium for this personal attention in return receive benefits, such as their own physician day or night, the physician's private telephone number, personal attention whenever desired, and longer lengths of time per appointment. Physicians, in turn, care for fewer patients and receive greater revenue. In other words, by increasing the price, volume has decreased, but because the practice is inelastic, revenue increases. Is there such a market in anesthesiology? Could cardiac anesthesiologists present themselves in such a way to charge a premium for personal services that would include no transfer of care during the day and immediate postoperative care? Because the vast majority of patients are adults with Medicare or children with Medicaid, this option remains very remote. It could be considered, however, if the group practice has such a plan for internists. As noted with commercial insurance, managed care contracts represent a variable and expanding percentage of total revenue depending on the area of the country and the type of hospital.

Medicare

Congress enacted Medicare in 1965 as Title 18 of the Social Security Act and originally intended this law to extend from care for the elderly to universal coverage.[24] If one reviews the Federal Register and simply types in "Medicare," thousands of pages of information appear. Most every sentence is cross-referenced to every other sentence. Buried in this information are basic guidelines of how to bill the agency for services. Methods of financing this federal insurance program include mandatory contributions by employees and employers, general tax revenues, premiums paid by beneficiaries, and deductibles and co-payments.[25]

Medicare likely represents the majority of a cardiac practice's revenue. In fact, national figures show that in 1970, Medicare provided 11.8% of physicians' income. In 2000, physicians counted on Medicare to provide 20.8% of their revenue.[26] Medicare initially paid physicians based on actual or prevailing and customary fees. With this scheme, annual physicians' payments grew in double-digit figures.[26]

The Omnibus Budget Reconciliation Act of 1989 changed the method of Medicare's payments to physicians from charge-based, practice expense RVUs to resources needed to provide the service. This act also restricted physicians' ability to balance-bill the patients. These changes, found in Section 121 of the Social Security Act Amendments of 1994, were phased in between 1999 and 2001 and became fully functional in 2002. As physicians provide patient care, they also consume resources. Iglehart[26] best outlined the resources developed by Medicare: "The first is work—the time, skill and training required of a physician to provide the service. The second is cost of operating a practice—expenditures for rent, utilities, equipment, supplies, and salaries of staff. The third is the cost of professional liability insurance." These components are summed to develop a total number of units in the resource-based relative value scale (RBRVS). The number of units assigned to an individual patient's care, that is, the resources consumed, is multiplied by Medicare's geographically and annually determined multiplier and then by the conversion factor, changing RVUs to dollars. In round numbers, the conversion factor is currently approximately $37 per RVU. Anesthesiologists do not fall under the RBRVS system except with certain intraoperative modifiers, with echocardiography, and with intensive care, of the anesthesiology time-based system. Anesthesiologists receive approximately $17 per 15-minute time unit in addition to the basic units assigned to a case based on the 1988 ASA Relative Value Guide.

Anesthesiologists also must follow other Medicare guidelines in order to receive reimbursement for their services. Anesthesia for surgical procedures is provided by personally performing, medically directing, or medically supervising the service. Box 38–2 outlines the differences among these three methods of performing a case.[27]

Reimbursement implications are such that performing a case alone or alone with one resident allows 100% payment for services at the Medicare rate.[28] Medicare splits the reimbursement between the anesthetist and the anesthesiologist

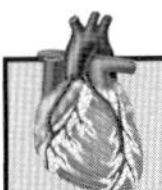

BOX 38–2 *Definitions of Levels of Care Provision by the Anesthesiologist*

Personally performed	Case performed alone
	Establishes an attending physician relationship and a teaching physician relationship with a resident or an intern
	Performs a single case with a CRNA or an AA and the services of each are medically necessary
	Continuously involved in a single case with a student nurse anesthetist
Medically directed	Physician meets the criteria listed in 42CFR415.110
	Physician directs qualified individuals in two, three, or four cases
Medically supervised	Physician supervises more than four concurrent anesthesia services

under medical direction. If the anesthetists are working for the department, then both portions of the revenue return to the department. On the contrary, if the attending works with multiple residents, then the attending receives 50% of the reimbursement; however, because the resident is paid under Part A, the department does not receive the other portion of the revenue. Working alone, therefore, results in 100% payment for services, while working with two residents results in 50% reimbursement. Medical supervision implies that one anesthesiologist is concurrently supervising more than four anesthetists. In this case, Medicare pays 50% of the reimbursement under the anesthetist's name, and the anesthesiologist receives three units for preanesthesia services. In reviewing these three methods of payment for services, performing patient care alone results in the highest reimbursement. Medical direction is the most common method for anesthesiologists to receive their reimbursements from Medicare but results in lost revenue in locations that educate residents. Medical supervision results in the lowest reimbursement for the anesthesiologist unless the procedures are extremely short.

Medicare applies other rules to reimbursements that commonly affect cardiac anesthesiology.[27] If the surgeon performs multiple procedures in an individual patient, then the anesthesiologist is reimbursed for the procedure receiving the highest number of base units plus the total time for all procedures. For instance, if a patient undergoes an aortic valve replacement, then the anesthesiologist would bill 20 base and 16 time units for a 4-hour procedure. If the patient undergoes an AVR-CABG in 6 hours, then the anesthesiologist would bill 20 base and 24 time units. The additional time units calculate to approximately $140. Anesthesiologists must follow rules regarding medical direction in order to receive reimbursement.[29] These rules are outlined in Box 38–3.

BOX 38–3 *Conditions for Payment of Medically Directed Anesthesia Services*

Payment rules	Perform a preanesthetic examination and evaluation Prescribe the anesthetic plan Personally participate in the most demanding aspect of the plan Ensure that a qualified individual performs procedures that the anesthesiologist does not perform Frequently monitor the course of the anesthetic administration Remain physically present and available Provide indicated postanesthesia care Direct no more than four concurrent services
Documentation	Specifically document that he or she performed the preanesthetic examination and evaluation, provided indicated postanesthetic care, and was present during the most demanding procedures

Medicaid

Title 19 of the Social Security Act describes this federal and state jointly sponsored program. Medicaid differs from Medicare in that Medicaid is a means-driven system; however, both programs are legal entitlements. The federal government funds Medicaid by formulas depending on state revenue. It is open-ended in that the more that a state pays for patient care, the greater is the formula-based revenue that the federal government transfers to the state. Medicaid is larger than Medicare in terms of dollars and variety of programs provided for patient care.[30] Financially, Medicaid suffers because economic downturns secondarily increase Medicaid enrollment as citizens lose both their jobs and their health care insurance just at a time when state tax revenues decrease. While private insurers are able to protect themselves against financial risk, Medicaid assumes the financial risk in the worst economic times.[31] If a state has a balanced budget amendment, Medicaid funding could suffer as revenue is diverted to other areas of the state government. For instance, in the state of Georgia, documents related to the General Appropriations Act present the House of Representatives funding guidelines for state agencies, the offices of the governor and the secretary of state, and bond issues. Medicaid is included, but it is not necessarily fully funded until the supplemental budget appropriates additional funds for the previous fiscal year. This procedure led to insufficient state Medicaid funds in the spring of 2004 and emergency funding by the legislature. Medicaid tries to control financial risk by redefining financial entry criteria. In Georgia, Medicaid benefits will now begin only when family income is less than 200% of the federal poverty level. Also, Medicaid implemented a sliding scale for premiums for PeachCare for Kids based on income and then reduced payments for ambulatory surgery.

Implications for anesthesiologists are that patients could be eligible for Medicaid but not know it, or could have had procedures performed under Medicaid but become ineligible because of changes in entry criteria. Because of its size and chronic underfunding, Medicaid pays an abysmally low rate. Added to this issue is that if the hospital directly pays the practice's anesthetists, then a large portion of the revenue stream related to Medicaid flows to the hospital with a smaller portion going to the practice.

Self-Pay

Self-pay does not necessarily indicate that the patent is unemployed. In many instances, these patients are working adults who cannot afford health care insurance and who fall below Medicaid financial enrollment guidelines. Self-pay patients can make up 3% to 4% of some hospitals' patient populations or up to 45% of those in larger city- or county-run hospitals. Anesthesia groups must underwrite the costs of these patients including the cost of attempting to recover the potential revenue. Revenue collections might approach up to 20% in some populations. Some practices outsource working these accounts and write them off after approximately 120 days. When outsourcing these accounts, clinicians must ensure that the contract includes the definition of "touching" the account; otherwise, the consultant will collect a portion of the practice's insurance revenue.

MALPRACTICE INSURANCE

The following quote from an anonymous lawyer that appeared in the *Medical Association of Georgia Journal* in 2004 emphasizes the opinion of the "opposition" in the issue of tort reform.[32]

Not only is there no factual basis to justify passing tort reform laws, the doctors who are complaining have no reason to complain. U.S. Labor Department statistics show that doctors are the richest people in the country, occupying eight of the ten top-paying jobs in America! Contact your legislators and tell them to protect patients' rights and vote "No" on tort reform, a scam being perpetrated by the richest people in America to line their fat pockets at the expense of the constitutional and legal rights of their dead, wounded, and permanently disabled patients.

This statement describes the misunderstanding that many have regarding malpractice insurance. The point is that tort reform, in particular a cap on damages, does not reduce the number or severity of medical errors. Defensive medicine forces an increase in the cost of medical care. Eighteen states have severe difficulty obtaining and paying for insurance, and another 26 states are experiencing skyrocketing malpractice premiums.[33]

As described by Studdert et al,[34] two other medical malpractice crises have occurred since the 1980s. The first crisis occurred in the 1980s and was characterized by inability to afford the insurance premiums. In the 1980s, physicians could pass the additional costs to patients. The current crisis appears to be related to both issues. The problems are multifactorial and there appears to be no single answer. Studdert et al also suggest that conventional tort reform could include three basic categories to relieve the current malpractice crisis. The first category establishes processes to limit access to court. A second category modifies liability rules and therefore limits the number of claims. A final category reforms payouts secondary to damages. The authors also describe system reforms that could reduce overall payouts and reduce the number of suits. These reforms include alternative mechanisms for dispute resolution, alternatives to the negligence standard, and relocation of legal responsibility. Placing a cap on noneconomic damages as a sole solution to the malpractice problems will not settle the situation that is now faced. If only economic damages were recoverable, then only high wage earners could benefit from a lawsuit. Because physicians are unable to respond to the increases in malpractice premiums by passing the cost to patients and other payers, this single area of cost could force individual previously financially viable practices to approach hospitals for support.[35]

EVALUATION AND MANAGEMENT CODES

Physicians working in critical care units receive Medicare payments for service under evaluation and management CPT codes 99291 and 99292. In order to receive payment for services, pursuant to 42 CFR 415.170, a physician must personally perform the service and must be present during critical or key portions of the service that a resident performs. The physician must document time in which he or she was personally involved with the case. Time that the resident spends with the patient before the services of the teaching physician begin does not count for payment.

TRANSESOPHAGEAL ECHOCARDIOGRAPHY

Echocardiography has become an integral part of cardiac anesthesiology. Some senior members of cardiac anesthesia groups might not have transesophageal echocardiography (TEE) boards and should receive backup coverage for interpretation of echocardiographic results. Revenue derived from TEE does not fully cover the costs associated with its use if a cardiac anesthesia group practice develops a service line to perform TEE. A review of the CPT code 93312.26 for insertion of the probe, interpretation, and reporting of the findings reveals that the number of RVUs totals 3.09. Using $37 as an approximate conversion factor, each complete TEE exam in a Medicare patient collects 80% of $114, or $91. Figuring in direct labor costs and overhead will lead to a cost higher than this reimbursement even if the hospital owns the capital expenditure for the equipment. In the academic setting, formal evaluations must be performed in the presence of a faculty member and are not billed after the first evaluation. If multiple examinations are performed per case and multiple simultaneous cases are occurring, then the practice loses even more revenue.

COST SAVINGS

It is not easy to reduce costs in cardiac surgical procedures when caring for increasingly older and sicker patients.[36] Despite this fact, it remains imperative that cardiac anesthesiologists fully support cost savings initiatives of the hospital. In 1994, Hamilton et al[37] analyzed cost reduction steps in cardiac surgery. The authors reported a 24% reduction in costs by managing all activities associated with cardiac surgery. Critical care medicine costs are also very expensive and run second only to cardiac surgery.[38] Also, it is important to understand the effect of patient demographics, because less than 4% of the patients who have an intensive care unit stay greater than 2 weeks consume 40% of patient bed days and a major share of total costs.[39] Efficiency is important; however, it is very difficult to become more efficient when cases last for 4 to 6 hours and to-follow cases almost always result in overtime pay. Everyone in cardiac anesthesiology is already providing fast-track and early extubations. Given that the costs of personnel in an anesthesiology department are likely around 75% of total costs, practices must find other ways to reduce their costs. Malpractice cost moderation will be an important step in reducing overall costs. Salary moderation could occur in the future.

SUMMARY

Cardiac anesthesiology continues to thrive from the academic viewpoint, and adding TEE to patients' care has added value to anesthesiologists' position within the enterprise. The financial picture, however, is vastly different from that of the 1980s and 1990s. In fact, relationships among physicians, third-party payers, hospitals, lawyers, and federal and state governments border on hostility. As expressed by Bartlett and Steele in *Time* magazine[40], "This is the picture of health care in America. We spend more money than anyone else in the world—and yet have less to show for it than other developed countries. That's one reason we don't live as long."

Politics and payment systems have grossly altered physicians' thinking. If they do not take care of business, they will not have practice locations and patients will suffer in the long run. They must understand the importance of and the methods of cost accounting so that when they approach hospitals for financial support, they will understand why anesthesiologists' clinical and academic skills drive the system. Likewise, it is imperative to aid hospitals with cost-saving initiatives to help them increase profit margins. Anesthesiologists must be important players in reform of malpractice issues, and they must visit their state legislators and travel to Washington, DC, to carry a message of their value. There is much work to do, and not all of this work is located within the operating room setting.

REFERENCES

1. Medicare Fraud Overview. Available at: http://www.medicare.gov/Fraud-Abuse/Overview.asp. Accessed: July 26, 2005
2. The World Factbook. Available at: http://www.cia.gov/cia/publications/factbook/geos/us.html#Econ. Accessed: July 26, 2005
3. The World in Figures, 2004 Edition. The Economist 212–213, 2004
4. U.S. Department of Labor, Bureau of Labor Statistics. Washington, DC, Series CUUR 0000SA0, Series CUUR 0000SAM, Series CUUR 0000SAM2: http://www.bls.gov
5. Bierstein K: Negotiation with hospital administrators. ASA Newsletter January 2004. Available at: http://www.asahq.org/Newsletters/2004/01_04/pracMgmt01_04.html. Accessed: July 26, 2005
6. Bierstein K: Negotiation with hospital administrators, part II: Conducting an effective negotiation. ASA Newsletter March 2004. Available at: http://www.asahq.org/Newsletters/2004/03_04/pracMgmt03_04.html. Accessed: July 26, 2005
7. Schubert A, Eckhout G, Tremper K: An updated view of the national anesthesia personnel shortage. Anesth Analg 96:207, 2003
8. Schubert A, Eckhout G, Cooperider T, Kuhel A: Evidence of a current and lasting national anesthesia personnel shortfall: Scope and implications. Mayo Clin Proc 76:995, 2001
9. Grogono AW: Resident numbers and total graduating from residencies and nurse anesthesia schools in 2003: Continuing shortages expected. ASA Newsletter 67:16, 2003
10. National Resident Matching Program, 2004 Match Data, Tables 1 and 12. Available at: http://www.aafp.org/match. Accessed: July 26, 2005
11. Brotherton SE, Rockey PH, Etzel SI: U.S. graduate medical education, 2003–2004. JAMA 292:1032, 2004
12. Goldman L: The value of cardiology. N Engl J Med 335:1917, 1996
13. McGlynn EA, Naylor CD, Anderson GM, et al: Comparison of the appropriateness of coronary angiography and coronary artery bypass graft surgery between Canada and New York State. JAMA 272:934, 1994
14. Hilborne LH, Leape LL, Bernstein SJ, et al: The appropriateness of use of percutaneous transluminal angioplasty in New York State. JAMA 269:761, 1993
15. Jollis JG, DeLong ER, Peterson ED, et al: Outcome of acute myocardial infarction according to the specialty of the admitting physician. N Engl J Med 335:1880, 1996
16. Selby JV, Fireman BH, Lundstrom RJ, et al: Variation among hospitals in coronary-angiography practices and outcomes after myocardial infarction in a large health maintenance organization. N Engl J Med 335:1888, 1996
17. Ayanian JZ, Hauptman PJ, Guadagnoli E, et al: Knowledge and practices of generalist and specialist physicians regarding drug therapy for acute myocardial infarction. N Engl J Med 331:1136, 1994
18. Galvin R, Milstein A: Large employers' new strategies in health care. N Engl J Med 347:939, 2003
19. Enthoven AC: Employment-based health insurance is failing: Now what? Health Affairs. Available at: http://www.leapfrog.org
20. Iglehart JK: Changing health insurance trends. N Engl J Med 347:956, 2003
21. Available at: http://www.businessroundtable.org/taskForces/taskforce/issue.aspx. Accessed: July 26, 2005
22. Epstein AM: Volume and outcome—It is time to move ahead. N Engl J Med 346:1161, 2002
23. Brennan TA: Innovation or threat to access? N Engl J Med 346:1165, 2002
24. Ball RM: What Medicare's architects had in mind. Health Aff (Millwood) 14:62, 1995
25. Iglehart JK: The American health care system: Medicare. N Engl J Med 340:327, 1999
26. Iglehart JK: Medicare's declining payments to physicians. N Engl J Med 346:1924, 2002
27. Code of Federal Regulations, revised as of October 1, 2003, 42CFR414.46
28. Code of Federal Regulations, revised as of October 1, 2003, 42CFR415.178
29. Code of Federal Regulation, revised as of October 1, 2003, 42CFR415.110
30. Inglhart JK: The dilemma of Medicaid. N Engl J Med 348:2140, 2003
31. Rosenbaum S: Medicaid. N Engl J Med 346:635, 2002
32. Brune DA: Tort reform: What happens next? Med Assoc Georgia J 2:3, 2004
33. Mello MM, Studdert DM, Brennan TA: The new medical malpractice crisis. N Engl J Med 248:2281, 2003
34. Studdert DM, Mello MM, Brennan TA: Medical malpractice. 350:283, 2004
35. Danzon PM, Pauly MV, Kington RS: The effects of malpractice litigation on physicians' fees and incomes. Am Econ Rev 80:22, 1990
36. Engoren M, Arslanian-Engoren C, Steckel D, et al: Cost, outcome and functional status in octogenarians and septuagenarians after cardiac surgery. Chest 122:1309, 2002
37. Hamilton A, Norris C, et al: Cost reduction in cardiac surgery. Cardiovasc Med 10:721, 1994
38. Krueger H, Concalves TL, Caruth FM, et al: Coronary artery bypass grafting: How much does it cost? Can Med Assoc J 146:163, 1992
39. Ryan TA, Rady MY, Bashour CA, et al: Predictors of outcome in cardiac surgical patients with prolonged intensive care stay. Chest 112:1035, 1997
40. Barlett DL, Steele JB: Health care can be cured: Here's how. Time, October 11, 2004

Chapter 39

EVALUATING QUALITY IN CARDIOVASCULAR SURGERY

Joseph S. Savino, MD • Michael J. Mercincavage, MAd

Baseball managers get paid for home runs other people hit.

Casey Stengel

KEY POINTS

1. The standard paradigm for evaluating quality in health care is based on the Donabedian methods: structure (input), process, and outcome (mortality).
2. Value equals quality divided by cost.
3. Quality and accountability are demanded by patients, patient advocates, third-party payers, medical peer groups, licensing agencies (e.g., Joint Commission on Accreditation of Hospitals Organization), the government (e.g., Center of Medicare and Medicaid), and the courts.
4. Quality metrics in cardiovascular surgery include patient satisfaction, quality of life, resolution of symptoms, freedom from disease recurrence, and mortality. Complication rates may not be a reliable marker of quality of care rendered.
5. The measurement of an outcome through the recording of an outcome measure is valid only in the assessment of quality of care if the outcome measure is a function of the actions of the provider.
6. Risk stratification and patient mix are critical in assessment of quality outcome.
7. The standards for assessment of regional outcome data emanate from New York State.
8. The relationship between volume and quality of care in cardiac surgery is equivocal.
9. National rankings of hospitals in cardiac surgery (e.g., in *U.S. News and World Report*) are often based on Medicare data and may include subjective variables such as a reputation score.
10. Quality assessment is most productive when used for quality improvement. Self-assessment and self-reporting permit identification of outcome metrics that are inferior to benchmarks and should be targeted in a clinical effectiveness quality improvement (CEQI) process. Outcomes that outperform benchmarks may contribute to the development of new benchmarks, which is how care for patients is improved.

QUALITY OF CARE: MEASURES AND PERTINENCE

Quality care is an inimitable attribute in human achievement. Quality is undeniable and distinguishable but difficult to measure and quantify. The relationship between quality of care and outcome in medicine is intuitive but poorly documented. An increasing national emphasis on improving quality of health care and safety has established a need for a systematic method to evaluate quality and safety. The method remains a "work in progress," albeit surrogates to quality and safety evaluation have been developed and applied in cardiovascular medicine and surgery.

The primary surrogate measures of quality care in cardiac surgery are based on the Donabedian three-element model for quality assessment: structure, process and outcome.[1] *Structure* is the input into health care and often is measured by facilities, supplies, physical plant, and staffing. Nurse-to-bed ratios, board certification of providers, availability of advanced technology, teaching programs, and case volumes are commonly used to measure structure-related quality. *Process* measures of quality are targeted at defining the practices to which patients are subjected and adherence to best practice protocols. *Best practice* is defined through evidence, expert opinion, or consensus. Best practices with data to support their implementation are few but include precautions to decrease hospital-acquired bloodstream infections, glycemic control, angiotensin-converting enzyme (ACE) inhibitors after acute myocardial infarction, prophylactic antibiotics, coronary artery grafting using arterial conduits, heart valve reparative versus replacement procedures, and blood conservation. Process measures advocated based on consensus include smoking cessation counseling, fast-tracking in the intensive care unit (ICU), and atrial fibrillation prophylaxis.

Inefficiency of health care decreases quality. Inefficiency of health care leads to the consumption of increased resources, which deprive other patients of treatment. Guidelines and practice protocols decrease the variability in the practices of providers. The "Get with the Guidelines Program" is an American Heart Association (AHA) initiative.[2] It is an algorithm to ensure that patients are cared for using agreed-on best practices based on the patient's admitting diagnosis. In this quality effort, patients who present with an acute myocardial infarction receive aspirin, β-blocker therapy, and smoking cessation counseling by protocol. Compliance with the protocol is monitored and data returned back to the users. The Veterans Administration system has described large differences in processes of care in performing coronary artery bypass grafting (CABG) surgery.[3-5] The study of variations in processes for cardiac surgery and their relation to risk-adjusted outcomes were aimed at defining the specific processes of care that produce better outcomes. Enormous variations in practice across hospitals were found: type of cardioplegia, blood versus crystalloid, myocardial temperature monitoring, personnel responsible for vein harvesting, blood conservation techniques, use of blood and blood products in the operating room, and cardiopulmonary bypass (CPB) and ischemic time, including specific type of anesthesia, type and dose of opioids, type of inhalation agent, type of hemodynamic monitoring, and use of intraoperative transesophageal echocardiography.[6,7]

Outcome measures commonly include mortality, complications such as myocardial infarction, and economic measures such as length of hospital stay. Less often cited but no less important are quality of life, patient satisfaction, freedom from complications, and ability to rescue.[8]

Quality matters, and although this may sound intuitive, from a strict business analysis, there have been few incentives for physicians and hospitals to focus on quality. Payers, including the Center for Medicare and Medicaid, pay for services and procedures. They do not pay for quality and safety. Complications often produce incremental revenue for hospitals and physician groups through a perverse system of rewarding providers whose care results in little or no benefit but the need for more care.[8]

How often are patients harmed by health care? The data are controversial, with hospital-acquired bloodstream infections producing relatively more robust data regarding the relationship between quality processes (e.g., hand washing, central venous catheter insertion with total-body draping) and decreased infection rates. The Institute of Medicine's (IOM) report of 1999, *To Err Is Human: Building a Safer Health System*, estimated the range of deaths annually in the United States due to medical errors in hospitals was between 44,000 and 98,000. The inference regarding deaths that result from preventable harm is that they are a result of poor quality.[9,10]

Errors are of two types: commission and omission. Errors of commission are mistakes of poor decisions or technical or procedural errors. Errors of commission are errors of action. Errors of omission are errors of inaction. The estimate of the preventable harm in medicine likely includes only errors of commission and does not include mistakes of omission. The estimate published by the IOM of preventable harm in American medicine is likely an underestimate.

Poor outcome with subsequent death or morbidity is typically attributed to patient condition or provider error. An undesirable outcome in high-risk patients undergoing complex procedures is often attributed to co-morbidity and patient characteristics. In essence, the patient is blamed. Providers are blamed when a poor outcome occurs in the setting of low preoperative risk. It is uncommon to attribute poor outcome to the system of decision making or the system of conducting procedures in response to an untoward event. Increasing evidence suggests the presence of dedicated intensivists in critical care units results in improved outcome.[11] Do physicians and hospitals disclose to patients admitted for high-risk cardiac surgery that their care in the ICU will or will not be supervised by an intensivist? Is the lack of intensivists in an ICU a contributor to preventable harm and an error of omission?

Formalized systems to assess "near misses" and poor outcomes have attracted unprecedented attention. The imperative to learn from mistakes through a formalized process of continuous quality improvement and root cause analysis has prompted the evolution of large quality-assurance divisions within medical centers. Self-reporting systems may not be as effective as a comprehensive systematic assessment of errors and poor outcomes. In most cases of mistakes, a common factor appears to be breach in communication. The "old school" system of a physician giving an order and a nurse taking the order without questioning is flawed in many circumstances. Other industries, such as aviation, nuclear energy, and submarine navigation, have attempted to address these deficiencies by empowering all members of the team, breaking down barriers, and designing redundancy in safety systems. Everyone from the captain to the baggage handler can terminate takeoff of an aircraft should a problem be detected. Although redundancy at first glance may seem inefficient and expensive, it is a necessary safety net when dealing with the fallibility of the human condition.

The U.S. healthcare system has experienced unprecedented growth over 2 decades at a rate several times the rate of growth of the general economy.[12] Metrics used to monitor growth vary and include cost expenditures, volume of activity, and advances in quality and access. Unfortunately, the growth in health care cost in the United States has not been accompanied by a corresponding reduction in the percent of the population that is uninsured, suggesting that increased access is not a major contributor to increased growth and cost.[13] Despite the increased dollars devoted to the health of the nation, metrics of health outcome, such as infant mortality rates, life expectancy, and quality of life indicators, have lagged behind other nations whose health care expenditures do not nearly match those of the United States.[14] The failure of much of the managed care revolution in the United States over the past decade can be attributed to the failure of health care to define its product, manage its product, and market its product on the basis of outcome and quality.[14]

The discrepancy between escalating costs without corresponding increases in access or health outcome suggests the value Americans receive in return for their health care dollars can be improved. The relationships among value, quality, and cost are represented by the following equation:

$$\text{Value} = \text{Quality}/\text{Cost}$$

Improvement in *value* is achieved through reductions in cost or enhancements in quality. In cardiovascular surgery, as many as 14% to 20% of surgical procedures in the treatment of carotid artery and coronary artery disease have been considered by some as "inappropriate."[15,16] Reduction in the amount of inappropriate care would produce an increase in quality accompanied by a significant decrease in cost. The geographic distribution of cardiovascular procedures in the United States appears to be linked to the geographic distribution of health care providers and hospital resources. Increased numbers of CABG procedures in a region are not reliably explained by differences in the incidence of coronary artery disease (CAD). Is it possible that more heart surgeons in a region equates to more heart operations, even in the absence of differences in underlying cardiovascular disease in the population?[17,18] Competitive behavior in health care is typically linked to the pursuit of profit.[14]

There is an increasing imperative for health care systems and health care providers to be accountable for what they do. Quality and accountability are demanded by patients, patient advocates, third-party payers, medical peer groups, licensing agencies (e.g., Joint Commission on Accreditation of Hospitals Organization), the government (e.g., Center for Medicare and Medicaid), and the courts. Physicians are held accountable for the quality of their work through assessment of their actions and outcomes and by the responses of their patients. Difficulties in evaluating and tracking quality stem from the lack of valid and reliable metrics.

Patients are the consumers of physician services and tools have been devised to ascertain *patient satisfaction, quality of life*, and *mortality rates* as indices to quality. The measurement of an outcome through the recording of a metric is only valid in the assessment of quality of care if the metric is a function of the actions of the provider. The outcome cannot be random; otherwise there is no basis for estimating quality of care. If the outcome has an expected frequency, deviations from this expected frequency may provide insight into quality of care.[19] The ideal outcome measure is strongly associated with provider actions and decision making and only weakly or not associated with severity of illness. Unfortunately, such an outcome measure in cardiovascular medicine does not exist, rendering risk stratification models an integral part of quality assessment.

Complication rates are often cited as a metric in the assessment of quality of care. However, complication rates in CABG may be associated with increased nurse staffing ratios, teaching status of the hospital, and increased levels of technology, all factors that may be associated with improved hospital quality of care, not an increased complication rate.[20] There is no clear correlation between hospital complication rate and hospital death rate after severity of risk adjustment.[19]

Measuring a quality indicator specific to a physician or hospital provides limited information regarding quality unless it can be compared with a benchmark. An overall 3% CABG mortality rate as a marker of quality could be an outstanding result or a poor one, depending on the patient mix. Mortality rates after cardiac surgery require comparison with large data sets with comparable patient cohorts. Mortality rate is a commonly used but nonetheless limited tool to assess quality in cardiovascular care (see Chapters 11, 16, 32, and 40).

QUALITY OF LIFE

Despite an emphasis on outcomes-based practice, clinical trials comparing surgical and medical therapy for CAD have documented improved survival with surgery for only select cohorts of patients. The Coronary Artery Surgery Study (CASS) suggested improved survival for CABG versus medical therapy in patients with left main and three-vessel disease.[21-23] Such an improved survival benefit is predicated on the assumption that the patient's life expectancy will be sufficiently long to realize any net benefit, considering the increased short-term morbidity and mortality of the surgical procedure. In the elderly population, CABG surgery is more likely aimed at relief of symptoms and improvement in quality of life, because demonstrating improved survival in these octogenarians is difficult since life expectancy is often limited by noncoronary causes. Survival benefits do not exist or are very difficult to discern for many cardiovascular procedures. If extending life is not achievable, the rationale for intervention is improving the quality of life. Quality-of-life assessment is an outcome metric in patients undergoing coronary revascularization and a variety of other cardiovascular procedures, including cardiac transplantation and valvular surgery. Health-related quality of life provides important information regarding the effects of interventions and the effect of the natural history of disease on patients' lives. Nonmedical measures of quality-of-life outcome have been available for many years in various fields of medicine, including functional assessment scores for cancer patients.[24] Functional scores have been developed by the New York Heart Association (NYHA) and the American Rheumatism Association.[25]

Models developed to describe quality of life were initially designed to define functional status. Schipper et al[26] proposed that five basic tenets contribute to understanding health-related quality of life: the psychologic approach, the time trade off utility concept, the community-centered concept, the reintegration concept, and the gap principle. Wenger et al[27] defined health related quality of life as "... those attributes valued by patients, including: resultant comfort or sense of well-being; the extent to which they were able to maintain reasonable physical, emotional, and intellectual function; and the degree to which they retained their ability to participate in valued activities within the family, in the workplace, and in the community." Health-related quality of life is multidimensional and difficult to quantify because much of the data are based on patient attitudes and beliefs and their perception of health. However, once established, the methods and metrics to describe health-related quality of life could be applied across medicine in cross-sectional assessments of health in a population or in longitudinal studies to assess the impact of interventions.

Measures of health-related quality of life include general questions asked of patients related to quality of life in multiple domains. A more disease-specific methodology would include the administration of system scales to patients with defined disease entities. Scales are commonly used in the assessment of interventions. The NYHA and Canadian Cardiovascular Classification for functional status of cardiovascular disease has been applied nearly worldwide in the assessment of patients undergoing cardiac surgery, angioplasty, and medical therapy.[25,28] Scales may be aimed at neurologic function, patient independence, and social interactions. In cardiovascular surgery, these scales are particularly applicable because of the high incidence of neurologic and psychometric changes after CPB and the supposition that newer techniques that avoid CPB may reduce these complications.[29,30]

The Cardiac Health Profile is a health related quality-of-life measuring tool designed to include cardiac surgery patients.[31] Despite the development of the Cardiac Health Profile, most scrutiny of quality of life after cardiac surgery uses more conventional instruments. The application of a generic quality-of-life measure, such as the Short Form 12 and 36, the Sickness Impact Profile, and the Nottingham Health Profile, allows for exploring a wide range of quality-of-life domains.

The most widely used and validated generic measure of health-related quality of life is the Short Form 36 (SF-36). SF-36 is a multipurpose survey of general health status, which was derived from work by the Rand Corporation.[32-35] Quality-of-life measures such as the SF-36 have been available in the United States for decades. However, they have been largely ignored as a means of defining, measuring, and managing health care quality.[14] The SF-36 is a short version of the 245-item health status assessment questionnaire developed for chronic medical and psychiatric conditions. The SF-36 questionnaire consists of 36 items evaluating eight domains of physical and mental health, including functional ability, limitations in performance of physical role requirements, bodily pain, anxiety and depression, sense of well-being, limitations of the fulfillment of emotional role requirements, social functioning, energy or fatigue levels, and perceived health status. It may be self-administered or used in personal or telephone interviews. SF-36 has been validated to discriminate changes in health status.[34,36] The scale contains 15 internal checks of consistency to identify respondents who enter internally inconsistent responses. The SF-12 is a condensed version of SF-36, with a smaller subset of items that encompasses the same eight dimensions, and it has been used when resources are limited.[37]

Although the SF-36 and SF-12 are commonly used in patients undergoing coronary revascularization procedures,[38] their validity and ability to discriminate changes have been poorly defined in the CABG population. Unfortunately, preoperative and postoperative (POD 3, 5, and 14) queries of cardiac surgery patients with SF-12 and a free-form interview with patient and spouse revealed significant patient concerns that were not adequately assessed with the SF-12 or SF-36.[39] These instruments may not fully discriminate changes in health related quality of life after coronary artery surgery.

The Sickness Impact Profile (SIP) is a tool designed to indicate changes in a person's behavior as a result of illness. It was intended for use in measuring the outcomes of care in program planning and policy formation and in monitoring patient progress. It consists of 136 items, which include an assessment of physical function with specific measures of ambulation, mobility, and body care; a psychosocial parameter with specific measures of social interactions and emotional behavior; and five independent categories regarding eating, work, home management, sleep, and recreations.[40,41] It has theoretical advantages for use in the cardiovascular population but requires greater resources for routine administration.

The Nottingham Health Profile (NHP) is a generic measure originally intended for use in primary care settings to give an indication of perceived physical, social, and emotional health problems, but it has also been used in clinical trials.[42] Part I is composed of 38 statements that convey limitations of activity or aspects of frustration in six dimensions: physical mobility, pain, energy, sleep, social isolation, and emotional reactions. Part II provides a brief indicator of handicap and contains seven items that record the effect of health problems. This form of assessment is thought to be a major predictor of future use of medical services and satisfaction with outcomes. The measure is scored by adding the weighting attached to each "yes" answer regarding a degree of disability. The NHP has been used in several studies to assess the impact of CABG surgery. Sjoland et al[43] studied 462 patients preoperatively and 578 patients postoperatively using the NHP. An increased NHP score (poorer quality of life) was found preoperatively compared with age-matched normal values. Improvement occurred postoperatively to a level similar to the normal values. The improvement was related to the severity of preoperative angina and was inversely related to preoperative exercise performance. The NHP also has been used to evaluate the influence of cardiac surgery on health-related quality of life in the elderly. A cohort of 130 patients (65 to 82 years old) were monitored preoperatively and at 3 months and 1 year postoperatively.[44] They demonstrated significant improvements in all of the domains of part I of the NHP at 3 months, with the improvements maintained or further enhanced after surgery. The percentage of patients who had problems in the seven activities of daily living in part II of the NHP also decreased significantly postoperatively.

The NHP is an established research tool to assess differences in quality of life in randomized clinical trials. In the Randomized Intervention Treatment of Angina (RITA) trial, CABG was compared with percutaneous transluminal coronary angioplasty (PTCA).[45] Both interventions demonstrated improvements in all health-related quality-of-life dimensions and all seven aspects of daily living, although the PTCA group had slightly greater impairment than the CABG patients at 2 years. Patients with angina at 2-year follow-up had more impairment of health-related quality of life compared with angina-free patients, which may account for the differences between the two groups because the PTCA cohort had a significantly greater chance of having angina.

A medical intervention or therapy may have small effects on overall health related quality of life but profound effects on very specific aspects of life. For cardiovascular patients, domains of importance include symptoms and functional capacity, psychologic and neurologic functioning, social functioning, and economic measures. Inadequate focus on the concerns that are not important to the cardiac patient may render the generic instrument unable to detect clinically important changes in quality of life.

Two of the most important outcomes after coronary revascularization are angina and functional capacity. Coronary revascularization improves symptoms regardless of age.[45] Improvements in exercise tolerance and physical activity with less activity limitation were reported with coronary revascularization in case series and randomized trials of different interventions.[43,46,47] Subjectively, patients report a decrease in fatigue and increases in stamina and energy levels.[48]

Activities of daily living scales permit better assessment of functional limitations related to cardiovascular disease than the simple assessment of symptoms. The Duke Activity Status Index (DASI) measures the ability to perform activities of daily living and has been correlated with maximal exercise capacity.[47] In the Bypass Angioplasty Revascularization Investigation (BARI), patients randomized to CABG reported significantly improved levels of activity on the DASI compared with those undergoing PTCA.[49] This difference was found despite similar improvements in other measures of quality of life. Patients appear to benefit from cardiac surgery in regards to psychosocial outcomes. Specific measures of the emotional and psychologic aspects of quality of life include satisfaction, mood, and levels of anxiety and depression.

Anxiety, depression, and irritability have been reported in approximately two thirds of patients in the early weeks after surgery.[46,48,50,51] Severe symptoms may persist, although most improve in the long term.[50] In many conditions, as symptoms increase in severity and activities become more limited, patients' expectations decrease as the potential for improvement decreases. Patients' expectations are an important consideration in addressing patient care. Perceptions of patients and their families represent their personal value systems regarding issues of general health status, life satisfaction, and well-being, and they appear to improve after cardiac surgery.[46,52,53]

The importance of determining risk aversion and individual perceptions of a particular health state is extremely relevant to the area of cardiac surgery. Nease et al[54] performed a utility assessment on 220 patients with chronic stable angina on medical therapy to assess their individual attitudes toward their angina using the rating scale, time trade-off, and standard gamble utility metrics. Reliability of measurements was evaluated by repeating the assessments 2 weeks later on a subset of individuals. Although the mean responses followed the expected patterns (those with more severe Canadian Cardiovascular Society scores chose lower utilities), attitudes toward symptoms varied substantially among patients with similarly severe angina. Considering surgery has a defined incidence of mortality for a given individual, there are many patients who should be considered for surgery because their perception of angina is such that they would risk a probability of death greater than the actual rate to relieve their symptoms. Similarly, some patients with severe anginal symptoms may be considered for CABG on symptomatic grounds, but based on the standard gamble assessment, their symptoms would not be considered severe enough to balance the risk of surgery.

Return to work is a quality-of-life indicator after CABG. Return to work has significant economic implications for the individual and society. The ability to perform productive work is an important component of an individual's well-being, self-esteem, and quality of life. Almost 90% of patients have little or no restriction of their functional capacity after coronary revascularization. However, only 60% or fewer of these patients actually are working 1 year after their cardiac procedure.[55] Predictors of returning to work after cardiac surgery are not solely related to cardiovascular or general medical condition. Age is an important factor because cardiac surgery patients are often near retirement age. Psychosocial factors are more predictive than physiologic factors for resumption of employment status after cardiac surgery. Predictors of return to work included preoperative employment status, age, preoperative perceptions, differences in financial status, and the presence of other forms of income.[56-59] Repeat CABG was associated with a rate of 14% for return to work compared with 61.2% after the first surgery.[60]

PATIENT SATISFACTION

Although patient satisfaction might be considered far removed from quality of care, the perceptions of patients are not falling on deaf ears and their satisfaction with the care they receive is being heard by hospitals and payers. Patients want attention, time devoted to their personal medical conditions, time spent with their doctors, and to be served with professionalism, efficiency, and understanding. Many of the tools used to assess patient satisfaction are limited. A five-point scale seems to provide discriminative ability.[61] Patient satisfaction may be linked more to medical outcome than services rendered. A good medical outcome may result in improved patient satisfaction despite inconveniences and poor service. Likewise, a poor medical outcome may produce patient dissatisfaction despite outstanding care and services provided.

Few reports address anesthesia-specific patient satisfaction. Many patients are unaware of the specific impact of their anesthesiologist. Anesthesiologists could improve patient satisfaction with anesthesia-related services through patient education. Outpatient surgical patients having received an anesthetic and a written discharge summary of the drugs and techniques used in their care seem to have an increased level of satisfaction, implying that patients do want to be informed about aspects of their anesthesia care.[62]

REPORTING OF CARDIOVASCULAR OUTCOMES: REGIONAL

Reporting systems have been developed in an effort to inform the public, payers, and health care providers of differences in quality across hospitals and physicians. Informing the public allows consumers to gauge their choice of providers based on outcome data. Payers pay for service rather than performance, but the trend is changing. Reimbursement for health care services is often not identical for all hospitals despite close geographic proximity. Differentials in payment are often negotiated based on differences in quantifiable quality measures, such as mortality rates. Teaching institutions are paid differently, usually more, than nonteaching institutions for similar procedures. More than 80 pay-for-performance initiatives exist in the United States involving a coalition of interests among Medicare, physician groups, and national and regional plans (BlueCross/BlueShield), along with the American Diabetes Association, AHA, and the American Stroke Association.[63] The intent is to reward performance based on outcome data. Informing providers permits self-assessment and quality improvement.

Generalized hospital-wide databases are cost efficient and provide uniform platforms for data entry and analysis for all patients across an institution. However, the lack of detail in information hinders their application in problem solving. Subspecialty-specific national databases for cardiovascular services include the Society of Thoracic Surgeons and the American College of Cardiology (ACC) databases.

Regional efforts to measure and report quality have been undertaken at the state level. The sentinel projects that addressed quality of cardiovascular intervention and cardiovascular surgery at the state level stem from the work done in New York State and Northern New England beginning in the 1990s.[64-67] The New York State Cardiac Surgery Reporting System (CSRS) made quality of care a high priority through reporting of physician-specific and hospital-specific observed and risk-adjusted mortality rates. It was the first statewide program to address outcomes for cardiac surgery in the United States and was begun in 1989. The discrimination and the calibration of New York's CABG surgery models with other models from other states have proved to be indicative of a good fit.[68-70]

An unanticipated finding of the National Halothane Study in the 1960s was an unexplained 24-fold variation in operative mortality across participating centers.[71-73] The Collaborative Study in Coronary Artery Surgery (CASS) reported variations in operative mortality among the 15 participating institutions involved in the large, National Institutes of Health–funded, randomized, controlled trial of CABG patients between 1975 and 1978. The mortality rates ranged from 0.3% to 6.6%.[74] A multivariate model defined by 20 clinical variables was used to predict operative mortality. For each patient, the model calculated an expected mortality rate. The ratio of the observed to the expected mortality rate for the sample population was defined as an index of quality of care: a mortality ratio of less than 1 suggested outcomes were better than expected and greater than one suggested the hospital CABG mortality was worse than predicted by the clinical model. The CASS data suggested a greater than 30-fold variability in mortality ratios across the participating centers. The differences in outcome were attributed to differences in "surgical expertise," presuming that patients were appropriately risk stratified.[74] Beginning with these early studies, CABG patients have been the most scrutinized population regarding surgical outcome.

The New York State CSRS represented the first statewide attempt to assess outcomes using specific data from hospitals and surgeons. A broadly constituted advisory body advised the New York Department of Health about issues concerning the quality of cardiac care, the prevention of CAD, and the establishment of new cardiac surgery, angioplasty, and catheterization programs. The intent of publishing mortality data was twofold: to inform the public about differences among hospitals and surgeons in operative death rate and to improve the quality of cardiac care in New York by stimulating local efforts by providing cardiac surgery programs for the first time with reliable and valid data on how their performance compared with that of their state peers.

New York State has a strict certificate-of-need (CON) program that explicitly limits the number of hospitals that are permitted to perform invasive cardiac procedures. Relatively few hospitals perform cardiac surgery in New York State, in contrast to other states that have abandoned the requirement for a CON program. The New York State program is guided by an evolving set of explicit criteria that were adopted by the state. The intent was to minimize the number of low-volume programs and to direct patients to high-volume institutions. New York State continues to regulate the capacity of health care systems by having a CON requirement. The effect of state regulation of cardiac surgery has limited the number of hospitals that perform cardiac surgery in New York State.[75] The intended consequence of the CON program is to foster large cardiac surgical programs and select high-quality hospitals. Between 1989 and 1998, contrasting health care systems have emerged in New York and California. In California, approximately 31% of the hospitals that performed cardiac surgery had annual volumes of fewer than 100 cases; in contrast, only 10% of New York hospitals doing cardiac surgery had such low volumes. The differences between New York and California hospitals continued to widen after 1989, with 73% of patients in New York having CABG surgery in high-volume hospitals and 27% of patients having CABG surgery in high-volume hospitals in California.[76-78]

Intuitively, increased volume of cardiac surgery equates with better quality and better results. Increased volume produces increased repetition, focused learning (cognitive and technical performance), and increased experience with uncommon complications, and it may improve rescue. However, the relationship between hospital volume and mortality after cardiac surgery is equivocal.[76,79-82] In 1979, the initial reports suggested an inverse relationship between the volume of CABG procedures performed at a hospital and risk-adjusted hospital mortality.[79] The link between low-volume cardiac surgery and increased mortality was supported by scattered reports in the 1980s and 1990s in the United States and Canada.[83,84] In 1996, a multicenter study in Ontario addressing adult CABG surgery over a 3-year period suggested that strict regionalization of cardiac surgery resulted in improved outcome. By maintaining an average annual CABG volume of more than 300 cases per year, the centers produced a significantly lower mortality rate compared with the lower-volume programs in the United States (3.01% versus 5.0%).[84] The argument of regionalization resulted in the funneling of adult patients to cardiac surgery centers, producing high-volume programs and high-volume surgeons. In a Medicare CABG population across multiple hospitals, mortality rates ranged from 5.6% for institutions performing fewer than 200 cases to 4.5% for institutions performing more than 849 cases annually.[85] Unfortunately, many of these reports lacked sophisticated risk stratification methodology to account for differences in patient mix. The studies tended to be retrospective and used databases designed for billing and administrative purposes rather than clinical data gathering and assessment of demographics and outcomes. These observational studies may not have accurately accounted for case mix. Later investigations more aggressively adjusting for risk suggested the relationship between volume of CABG and mortality was less than previously believed.[86] Are increased volume and increased quality independent variables? It is plausible that increased quality of care leads to increasing patient referrals, which produces increasing volume for a particular surgeon and for a specific institution. Volume therefore becomes a surrogate for quality, although this relationship has not been proved.

In 2004, two sentinel studies reexamined the relationship between hospital volume and outcomes in CABG surgery. The first trial used the Society of Thoracic Surgeons database that included almost two thirds of CABG patients in the United States spanning 2000 and 2001. The results suggested only a modest relationship between CABG mortality and procedural volume, with low-volume institutions having a mortality rate of 3.2%, compared with high-volume institutions with 2.5%.[87] The study concluded that the contribution of volume to outcome after CABG surgery was relatively weak. There was a suggestion that the highest mortality rate occurred for patients treated by low-volume surgeons, a finding that corroborated previous observations. The consequence of outcomes related to surgeon-specific volume was that New York State restricted privileges of low-volume surgeons with high mortality rates.[75,88]

The ACC and the AHA published a recommendation in 1991 stating that "all cardiac surgery hospitals (should) perform a yearly minimum of 200 to 300 open heart operations a year and that all cardiac surgeons (should) perform a yearly minimum of 100 to 150 open heart operations, the majority of which should be CABG operations."[84] These recommendations could not be sustained. In 2001, cardiac surgery programs in the United States performed an average of 253 surgeries per year.[87] There is even a lack of consensus regarding what defines a cardiac surgery program in the United States. In 2004, the ACC and the AHA revised the practice guidelines for CABG surgery, omitting a formal threshold for institution or surgeon volume, reflecting the growing controversy between volumes and outcomes.

The public reporting of physician-specific outcome data is not without the risk of changing medical practice in an unintended manner. A New York newspaper, *Newsday*, sued the New York Department of Health under the state's Freedom of Information Law in an effort to have the data pertaining to individual surgeon's mortality data released to the public. The Department opposed making data on surgeons public, because low annual volumes of operations per surgeon would lead to data on mortality rates that would be imprecise (with broad confidence intervals), highly variable from year to year, and subject to misinterpretation. The Department lost the lawsuit and was forced to give *Newsday* the data, which were published in December 1991.[89] In an effort to appease the physician leaders in the community, an agreement was reached in 1992 on a format for publishing surgeon-specific mortality data that included publishing physician-specific data only for the most recent 3 years combined. Physician data would be reported by name only for those who performed at least 200 cases during that 3-year period.[89-91]

Physician report cards are not passive tools. They have a significant influence on physician and hospital behavior by exerting their effect on clinical decision making. Physicians were more likely to withhold procedures from high-risk patients despite the likelihood that the procedure would be beneficial.[92] Physician report cards therefore could result in a potentially negative effect on physicians' decisions. An additional limitation of publishing physician specific outcome data is the risk of physicians "gaming" the system in an attempt to improve their risk adjustment patient mortality. The exaggeration of co-morbidities in an attempt to place patients in higher-risk categories is an indication that physicians lack the confidence in the risk stratification algorithm used in New York State.[92] Additional undesirable effects include the referral of high-risk patients to other cardiac care programs outside the state.[93-96] The effect is not limited to cardiac surgery. Interventional cardiologists in New York State did not have confidence in the risk adjustment models and were more reluctant to perform procedures on high-risk patients, even though they believed that the patients might benefit from them.[92] In the SHOCK trial (SHould we emergently revascularize Occlusive Coronaries for cardiogenic shocK), patients who presented with acute myocardial infarction and cardiogenic shock were randomized to early coronary revascularization or medical stabilization. The data suggest that early coronary revascularization by surgery or angioplasty was associated with a significant reduction in 6-month mortality compared with results for patients who underwent medical stabilization, which did not include early revascularization (50.3% mortality versus 63.1% mortality).[95] In this population of patients, the good-outcome cohort still had a 6-month mortality rate in excess of 50%. Cardiac surgeons confronted with this patient population may be reluctant to offer surgical coronary revascularization with such an expected high mortality rate, even though the alternative for the patient would be worse. Unfortunately, many of the publications that cite influences of public reporting on physician medical decision making are based on respondents of questionnaires. The respondents are presumed to represent the general population of physicians. However, the physicians who elect not to respond are likely to differ significantly from those who did respond, and their impact on the conclusions cannot be assessed.[92]

Improvements in CABG mortality occurred during the New York State program of hospital and surgeon reporting.[96] The state acted on the data and occasionally closed a cardiac surgery program until a recommended reorganization was completed. However, improvements in CABG mortality rates may occur in the absence of any public reporting systems, such as occurred in Massachusetts.[97] Likewise, between the years of 1987 and 1992, during the interval of aggressive regulation of cardiac surgery programs in New York State, there was a national secular trend toward improving mortality rates after CABG surgery.[75] The states of Maine, New Hampshire, and Vermont had comparable improvements in their results during the same period.

The advocates of the systems used in New York State suggest that the improvements in risk-adjusted mortality that occurred in New York State are attributable to individual hospitals and cardiac surgery programs making specific changes and improvements in the way they care for CABG patients. There is little or no evidence to suggest that patients actively avoided high-mortality hospitals, that managed care companies used the data to reward better-performing hospitals, or that other influence on market forces existed.[75]

The Leapfrog Group is based in Washington, DC. It is a hospital safety and quality advisory group. Leapfrog Group has released a set of evidence-based hospital referrals intended to affect the market share by guiding patients to high-volume centers for specific procedures. Leapfrog Group took into account institutional volume and released a recommendation to patients and payers to select hospitals with an annual CABG volume greater than 500 cases. The numbers published by Leapfrog in their 2004 report were unrealistic, because less than 15% of hospitals in the United States had an annual volume of greater than 500 CABG procedures.[98] With the decreasing number of CABG procedures being performed, this threshold became even more impractical.

The significant declines in observed and risk-adjusted mortality for CABG surgery in New York appear to have been largely a consequence of actions taken on the part of New York hospitals to improve outcomes and quality of care. These efforts are a mixture of general improvements in cardiac surgical care and specific activities initiated by data provided by the New York State Cardiac Surgery Reporting System. These efforts included the identification of groups of patients with significantly higher mortality rates than those observed throughout the state, and subsequent actions to improve processes of care for those groups; improvement in the postoperative monitoring of patients; reduction in the percentage of low-volume surgeons and the percentage of patients undergoing surgery performed by low-volume surgeons; and redistribution of high-risk patients to surgeons with outstanding risk-adjusted mortality rates and away from surgeons whose principal training and experience were in other specialties. The increasing proportion of patients receiving CABG surgery in very high-volume hospitals may also have played a role. Improvements in individual hospital performance and New York statewide mortality occurred without significant movement of patients away from hospitals with high mortality rates or toward hospitals with low rates.[99,100] Other factors contributing to improvements in operative mortality included improved surgical methods and techniques with internal mammary artery grafts and advances in cardioplegia. New York was not the only state in the United States with close scrutiny of CABG patients.[97] Massachusetts had a 42% decrease in risk-adjusted CABG mortality using an administrative database.

Mortality databases and reports often spawn a variety of specific actions aimed at improving quality. Perhaps the most promising development with respect to quality improvement was the use of the data by hospitals to identify specific processes of care that could be improved to decrease mortality. St. Peter's Hospital in Albany, New York, was one of three hospitals in 1991 with a risk-adjusted mortality rate that was statistically significantly above the state average. An initial concern about the accuracy of the coded data on risk factors was resolved by an internal review. When a standard review of morbidity and mortality failed to reveal any quality problems, physicians at St. Peter's Hospital began exploring the reasons for the hospital's increased mortality rate.[101] Close analysis of the data revealed that patients undergoing emergency CABG surgery had a 26% mortality rate, compared with the state average for this cohort of 7%. When a multidisciplinary group reviewed the care of these patients, it concluded patients at St. Peter's Hospital required more time to be stabilized before surgery, the intra-aortic balloon assist device was not being used as frequently as in other institutions, and hemodynamic parameters were often not stabilized before surgery. The hospital's response was not to discourage operations on these high-risk patients, but to address each of the identified processes individually. The improvement was dramatic. In 1992, 11 of 42 emergency CABG patients died. In 1993, none of the 54 emergency patients died. By 1994, St. Peter's Hospital had an observed mortality rate of 1.25%, the fourth lowest in the state, and a risk-adjusted rate of 1.4%, the third lowest in the state. Surgeons performing 50 or fewer cases per year had greater risk-adjusted mortality rates.[96,102] Hospitals may elect to restrict the privileges of surgeons with very low volumes. A response to such data resulted in the percentage of all surgeons performing CABG surgery in New York who performed 50 or fewer isolated CABG procedures decreasing from 31% in 1989 to 24% in 1992. The low-volume surgeons who discontinued CABG surgery in New York appear to be those with the poorest outcomes. The comparative performance data enables individual hospitals to discover that certain surgeons had unsatisfactory performance, even if they performed more than 50 cases per year. Other hospitals used the data to identify surgeons with especially superior performance, particularly for high-risk patients, and set up administrative processes to match these cases with these surgeons.

In 2005, Hannan et al[103] published data from the New York State cardiac registries, showing that for patients with two or more diseased coronary arteries, CABG was associated with higher adjusted rates of long-term survival than percutaneous coronary intervention with stenting. They compared 37,212 patients with multivessel CAD who underwent CABG (Cardiac Surgery Reporting System) with 22,102 patients after percutaneous coronary intervention with stenting (Percutaneous Coronary Intervention Reporting System) from 1997 to 2000 over a 3-year follow-up period. The patients were risk adjusted for ejection fraction, diabetes, congestive heart failure, chronic obstructive pulmonary disease, carotid artery disease, aortoiliac disease, shock, femoral or popliteal artery disease, renal failure, stroke, age, and sex. The risk-adjusted survival rates were significantly higher among the CABG patients in all of the anatomic subgroups studied. The 3-year rate of additional revascularization procedures was higher for the stented group. This is the first use of this type of data that compares interventional cardiology procedures with surgery since the introduction of stenting. However, the study did not include drug-eluting stents or advances in coronary artery surgery such as off-pump coronary artery bypass procedures.

REPORTING OF CARDIOVASCULAR OUTCOMES: NATIONAL

No single standard measure of hospital quality across specialties exists at the national level. In 1993, in response to this dilemma, the National Opinion Research Center (NORC) at the University of Chicago in collaboration with *U.S. News and World Report* (USNWR) developed a measure of quality for hospitals across the United States.[104] The report published annually in USNWR's July issue (entitled *America's Best Hospitals*) identifies and ranks 50 centers across 17 medical specialties from 6012 hospitals in the United States. The specialty that includes cardiovascular diagnosis-related groups (DRGs) is defined as *Heart and Heart Surgery*.

Donabedian methods for quality assessment are employed by USNWR and include structure or input, process, and outcome.[1] Structure was defined based on physical characteristics of the hospital. These data are obtained from the annual survey of the American Hospital Association. Outcomes were strictly defined by in-hospital risk-adjusted mortality rates. The weakest parameter was describing processes, which is not measured by USNWR. Instead of processes, the USNWR relied on a surrogate: a survey of board-certified physicians who were asked to nominate the five best hospitals in the specialty.

Structure defines the tools and environment available to care providers in the treatment of patients. For Heart and Heart Surgery, structure is measured by the following:

- AHA annual hospital survey results
- Technology indices: angioplasty, cardiac catheterization laboratory, cardiac ICU, computed tomography scanner, magnetic resonance imaging, open heart surgery, positron emission tomography scanner, single photon emission computed tomography, ultrasound
- Volume
- Registered nurses-to-beds ratio
- Trauma
- Patient and community services
- Geriatric services
- Hospice and palliative care
- Nurse magnet status

Process is the net effect of decision making. The process of the delivery of care is conceptualized as one that patients move through that produces results or outcomes. Because national measurements of process are extremely difficult to obtain, an alternate measure is used as a proxy. A physician (board certified) survey was used. It was assumed that when a qualified expert identifies a hospital as one of the best, that expert is endorsing the process choices made by the hospital. A reputation score was generated for each hospital based on the survey results, and it was used as a proxy measure of process of care. The use of reputation score as an index of hospital quality has significant limitations.[105]

Outcome is the comparison of actual mortality to risk-adjusted expected mortality, producing a mortality ratio and mortality index. The data for the calculation of expected mortality are based on the most current pooled 3 federal fiscal years of Medicare reimbursement claims made to the Center for Medicare Services (CMS) by hospitals. Hospitals that are included must meet at least one of the following criteria:

1. Council of Teaching Hospitals (COTH) membership
2. Medical school affiliation
3. A minimum score on the hospital-wide technology index

The DRG list for Heart and Heart Surgery is listed in Table 39–1.

The outcome measure (mortality ratio) is based on Medicare billing data submitted to CMS using the Universal Bill 92(UB92). UB92 is the technical component of a medical bill for services rendered from a hospital. It is designed for charge capture but contains primary and secondary diagnosis and procedure codes. It is submitted by the hospital to all payers (e.g., CMS, private payers, CHAMPUS). UB92 data submitted to private payers are not easily accessible and are not included in the analysis. CMS compiles the UB92 data into a global database called MEDPAR, sorted by hospital.

Calculations of the adjusted mortality rate for each hospital are based on predicted and observed mortality rates using the All Patient Refined-Diagnosis Related Group (APR-DRG) risk stratification algorithm, designed by 3M, Inc.[106] APR-DRG adjustments are based on severity of illness (SOI) and risk of mortality (ROM) estimates. Computation of SOI is based on the extent of physiologic decompensation or organ system loss of function. ROM relates to the likelihood of

Table 39–1 **Heart and Heart Surgery**

DRG Code	DRG Description
75	Major chest procedures
104	Cardiac valve and other major cardiothoracic procedures with CC
105	Cardiac valve and other major cardiothoracic procedures without CC
106	Coronary bypass with PTCA
107	Coronary bypass with CC
108	Other cardiothoracic procedures
109	Coronary bypass without CC
110	Major cardiovascular procedures with CC
111	Major cardiovascular procedures without CC
115	Permanent cardiovascular pacemaker implantation with AMI, heart failure or stroke, AICD lead
116	Other permanent cardiac pacemaker implantation
117	Cardiac pacemaker revision except device replacement
118	Cardiac pacemaker replacement
121	Circulatory disorders with AMI and major complications, discharged alive
122	Circulatory disorders with AMI without major complication, discharged alive
123	Circulatory disorders with AMI, expired
124	Circulatory disorders except AMI with CC and complex diagnosis
125	Circulatory disorders except AMI with CC without complex diagnosis
126	Acute and subacute endocarditis
127	Heart failure and shock
132	Atherosclerosis with CC
133	Atherosclerosis without CC
134	Hypertension
135	Cardiac congenital and valvular disorders, age > 17 years, with CC
136	Cardiac congenital and valvular disorders, age > 17 years, without CC
138	Cardiac arrhythmia and conduction disorders with CC
139	Cardiac arrhythmia and conduction disorders without CC
140	Angina pectoris
143	Chest pain
144	Other circulatory system diagnosis with CC
145	Other circulatory system diagnosis without CC
514	Cardiac defibrillator implantation with CC
515	Cardiac defibrillator implantation without CC
516	Percutaneous cardiovascular procedures with AMI
517	Percutaneous cardiovascular procedures with coronary stent without AMI
518	Percutaneous cardiovascular procedures without coronary stent or AMI

AICD = automatic implantable cardioverter-defibrillator; AMI = acute myocardial infarction; CC = cardiac catheter; DRG = diagnosis-related group; PTCA = percutaneous transluminal coronary angioplasty.
Data from the 2004 Index of Hospital Quality, NORC (National Organization for Research), Chicago, IL.

dying. Computation of both parameters is based on principal and secondary diagnoses.

A composite variable was calculated based on the equal weighting of structure, reputation, and mortality ratio. The composite variable was called the Index of Hospital Quality (IHQ). The hospitals are ranked based on the IHQ.

USNWR offers a global hospital rank and a rank by each specialty, including Heart and Heart Surgery. Does the ranking in USNWR *America's Best Hospitals* represent any meaningful difference in the quality of care rendered by these institutions? Does the applied methodology provide an opportunity to improve quality at a specific site? The rankings are reported in the medical literature and are widely recognized by hospitals, physicians, and consumers.[107,108] The USNWR rankings may have an association with decreased 30-day mortality in patients admitted with an acute myocardial infarction. In the comparison of mortality after acute myocardial infarction from 1995 to 1999, patients cared for at hospitals ranked by USNWR as America's best hospitals had a significantly lower mortality rate compared with other Medicare patients cared for in hospitals not in the top rankings.[109] The hospitals cited by USNWR had higher rates of aspirin and β-blocker therapy in patients with acute myocardial infarction.

Does the methodology developed for this analysis provide a window for improving quality? Let us consider the following vignette. A hospital ranked in the top 20 by USNWR for global score was not ranked in Heart and Heart Surgery. The initial step was to reconsider the evaluation: "Maybe we are not as good as we think we are!" A comprehensive review of hospital outcomes and process in cardiovascular care was in order. The hospital began a process to analyze and better understand the dynamics of the calculation of the IHQ. Of the three dimensions of health care quality defined by USNWR—structure, process, and outcome—only outcome was affected by actions in the short term. Structure was for the most part a static characteristic for an urban academic medical center with all of the structural components in the specialty present. Process, as measured by the random survey of physicians, could be affected by increased program visibility through increased media exposure, direct-to-consumer advertising, and broad-based continuous medical education programs. None of these was thought to be attainable short-term objectives in an effort to improve rankings among America's best hospitals.

It became abundantly clear that if an organization desired to improve quality and its respective IHQ, the Mortality Index was an important value on which to focus its efforts. The first step was to re-create as closely as possible the NORC-calculated Mortality Index for the organization. The hospital contracted with a third-party data supplier to provide the appropriate years of MEDPAR data. Based on the selection criteria defined by NORC, the resulting population of hospitals was verified against the published NORC results. Once the national population (i.e., cases and mortalities within specialty) and the hospital population were validated, it was necessary to re-create the calculation of actual and expected mortality for both populations.

In an attempt to mimic the NORC methodology and create a risk-adjusted Mortality Index, all the cases in the national population and in the site-specific population were risk adjusted using the 3M APR-DRG methodology. This was done only for Heart and Heart Surgery DRGs because it was the targeted sample. The APR-DRG methodology was calculated based on surgical procedure and diagnostic information, a patient-specific SOI and ROM score for all cases (including those who die). The resulting scores of 1 to 4 are assigned to each case, with 1 indicating the lowest severity and 4 indicating the highest severity of illness. Likewise, 1 indicated the lowest ROM, and 4 indicated the highest ROM. For computational purposes, any given population was compared with another like population by creating a 4 × 4 matrix of SOI and ROM scores. The results for the hospital analysis of Heart and Heart Surgery resulted in the matrices shown in Tables 39–2 to 39–7.

Hospital and physician practices can compare their performances with the Medicare population, and they can calculate their own mortality ratio. Are patients at a specific institution sicker than the rest of the nation, an argument posed by many centers as an explanation for increased mortality rates? The APR-DRG methodology provides a means of addressing this issue. The distribution of patients in the SOI/ROM matrix (see Table 39–5) allows calculation of the percentage of patients in high-risk groups and allows for comparisons to the nation. In the example previously cited, the percent of patients at the

Table 39–2 Heart and Heart Surgery National Population

	ROM				
SOI	*1*	*2*	*3*	*4*	*Total**
1	548,721	133,115	20,269	57	
2	825,145	1,016,443	279,777	4,606	
3	25,539	274,207	625,953	91,446	
4	328	2,391	52,956	231,273	
Total					4,132,226

*National population of 4,132,226 patients with Heart and Heart Surgery diagnosis-related groups distributed across 4 × 4 matrix of SOI (rows) and ROM (columns). Because severity of illness (SOI) and risk of mortality (ROM) have overlapping criteria, most of the patients fall in common cells (e.g., SOI1/ROM1 or SOI4/ROM4), and few patients are in severely discordant cells (SOI1/ROM4).

Table 39–3 Heart and Heart Surgery—National Population Deaths

	ROM				
SOI	*1*	*2*	*3*	*4*	*Total**
1	716	1,626	1,354	7	
2	1,546	9,331	10,702	2,180	
3	191	4,215	30,073	20,329	
4	15	118	6,376	86,963	
Total					175,742

* Deaths among the national population is 175,742. These patients are grouped by severity of illness (SOI) and risk of mortality (ROM) cell.

Table 39–4 Heart and Heart Surgery—National Population Risk-Adjusted Mortality Ratio

	ROM*			
SOI	*1*	*2*	*3*	*4*
1	0.00130485	0.01221500	0.06680152	0.12280702
2	0.00187361	0.00918005	0.03825189	0.47329570
3	0.00747876	0.01537160	0.04804354	0.22230606
4	0.04573171	0.04935174	0.12040184	0.37601882

*For the national population risk-adjusted mortality ratio, each cell has a calculated value = deaths in cell/population of cell. These patients are grouped by severity of illness (SOI) and risk of mortality (ROM). Notice that the risk-adjusted mortality ratio increases with increasing SOI and ROM. SOI1/ROM1 = 0.13%, and SOI4/ROM4 = 37%. The mortality rate computed from the national population for each cell serves as the expected risk-adjusted mortality rate for patients with similar SOI/ROM scores and can be used for comparison with individual institutions.

Table 39–5 **Heart and Heart Surgery—AAMC Hospital—Sample Population Distribution***

	Risk of Mortality				
Severity	*1*	*2*	*3*	*4*	*Total*
1	845	154	50	0	
2	980	1070	359	1	
3	59	319	733	76	
4	0	3	43	217	
					4909

* Association Academic Medical Centers hospital distribution of patients is based on severity of illness (SOI) and risk of mortality (ROM).

Table 39–6 **Heart and Heart Surgery—AAMC Hospital Risk-Adjusted Expected Number of Deaths**

	ROM*				
SOI	*1*	*2*	*3*	*4*	*Total*
1	1	2	3	0	
2	2	10	14	0	
3	0	5	35	17	
4	0	0	5	82	
Total					177

Association Academic Medical Centers hospital expected mortality is based on the national population percentages of death rates for each severity of illness (SOI) and risk of mortality (ROM) cell applied to the Table 39–5 data.

Table 39–7 **Heart and Heart Surgery—AAMC Hospital Actual Mortality**

	ROM				
SOI	*1*	*2*	*3*	*4*	*Total*
1	1	0	0	0	
2	1	8	5	0	
3	0	2	34	16	
4	0	0	6	88	
Total					161

Association Academic Medical Centers hospital actual mortality = 161. The matrix illustrates the distribution of deaths by severity of illness (SOI) and risk of mortality (ROM) index. The overall mortality ratio = 0.912 was favorable.

AAMC hospital in the lower right quartile (SOI3-4/ROM3-4) of the matrix was about 22%. The national data have a distribution of 24% for the high-risk patients (in the corresponding quartile). This suggests the percent of AAMC hospital high-risk patients does not differ significantly from the rest of the nation based on the risk stratification model applied.

In what DRG does an institution excel? In what DRG does an institution need to devote resources to improve performance? Because all 4909 patients in Heart and Heart Surgery are also grouped by DRG, it is possible to perform the same analysis by individual DRG. For this analysis, all patients in DRGs with fewer than 100 patients were excluded. Included were only DRG groups with *n* greater than 100 as a volume-based cutoff: group A (Table 39–8). Likewise defined were all DRG groups whose DRG-specific mortality ratio was more than 0.91, with the presumption that these groups of patients have relatively poorer outcomes compared with other patients in the same AAMC hospital (Table 39–9). Call them group B. Cross-reference of groups A and B represents the DRGs with sufficient numbers of patients and in whom it can be concluded that outcomes are less than the average Heart and Heart Surgery outcome for the institution (Table 39–10).

The methodology provides a systematic approach of identifying patient cohorts (defined by DRG grouping) whose care could be more closely monitored in an attempt to improve quality. The fallout of this process includes improved ranking on USNWR.

The self-assessment report card produced by these methods is directed to service chiefs and can be physician specific: individual cardiac surgeons, the number of cases performed, their patients stratified based on minor, moderate, major, and extreme risk of death and how many of them actually died. Disclosures to individual surgeons and service chiefs can guide quality-assurance efforts without public access to the physician-specific data. The USNWR analysis of American hospitals is fraught with *limitations*, including the use of a reputation score as a proxy for process. The reputation score is self-fulfilling and lacks objectivity. Institutions that rank highly in the report gain the notoriety and market influence that feeds future reputation scores. To a certain degree, high rankings are self-perpetuating. The data are limited to Medicare patients, and the quality assessment may not apply to different patient cohorts. Mortality is based on in-hospital mortality, with no information on other markers of quality, such as 30-day mortality, quality of life, relief of symptoms, freedom from rehospitalization, functional status, and patient satisfaction. Nonetheless, the USNWR approach introduces a methodology that can be applied to improve institutional and practice quality through the identification of patient cohorts and procedures whose risk-adjusted outcomes are below par. As an added bonus, improved rankings in the highly publicized USNWR list would result.

When a characteristic is difficult to quantify, multiple modalities of measurement evolve, each with advantages and disadvantages. Quality of care rendered to patients will continue to foster increased attention and accountability. Physicians and hospitals prepared to institute systematic processes to measure and improve quality will better serve their patients and society.

Acknowledgments

The authors would like to acknowledge L. A. Fleisher, MD, and W. Bernstein, MD, for their chapter (Quality of Life and Patient Satisfaction Surrounding Cardiovascular Surgery) and Mark R. Chassin, MD, MPP, MPH, Edward L. Hannan, PhD, and Frank C. Spencer, MD, for their chapter (Measuring and Improving the Outcomes of Coronary Artery Bypass Graft Surgery: New York's Experience), both of which appear in *Cardiac Anesthesia,* edited by Joel Kaplan and published by Elsevier. This chapter includes some of the work from these authors and their contributions to chapters from prior editions of this textbook.

Table 39–8 Heart and Heart Surgery Patients at AAMC Hospital: Group A

DRG	DRG Description	Comparison Group Cases	Comparison Group Mortalities	Cases	Risk-Adjusted Expected Mortality	Actual Mortality	Mortality Score	Incl/Not incl
111	Major cardiovascular procedures without CC	19,596	332	100	0.8	2	2.534	Incl
107	Coronary bypass with CC	246,702	9,050	128	3.5	6	1.698	Incl
105	Cardiac valve and other major cardiothoracic procedures without CC	86,024	4.899	252	12.6	16	1.271	Incl
110	Major cardiovascular procedures with CC	122,475	19,199	388	26.9	32	1.191	Incl
112	Percutaneous cardiovascular procedures	164,696	2,083	345	6	7	1.163	Incl
75	Major chest procedures	83,858	4,687	362	10.4	12	1.155	Incl
144	Other circulatory system diagnoses with CC	131,462	6,807	267	12.7	14	1.104	Incl
104	Cardiac valve and other major cardiothoracic procedures with CC	102,844	5,825	294	13.3	13	0.975	Incl
127	Heart failure and shock	833,465	42,691	769	32.2	25	0.775	Incl
116	Other permanent cardiac pacemaker implant	841,788	8,058	544	4.9	2	0.412	Incl
143	Chest pain	290,781	370	521	0.6	0	0	Incl
138	Cardiac arrhythmia and conduction disorders with CC	254,312	8,933	229	9.9	7	0.708	Incl
121	Circulatory disorders with AMI and major complications, discharged alive	194,600	0	125	10.9	0	0	Incl
139	Cardiac arrhythmia and conduction disorders without CC	110,688	375	112	0.2	0	0	Incl
115	Permanent cardiac pacemaker implant with AMI, heart failure or stroke, or AICD lead	28,634	970	87	1.6	1	0.619	Not incl

Table 39–8 Heart and Heart Surgery Patients at AAMC Hospital: Group A—(Continued)

DRG	DRG Description	Comparison Group		Cases	Risk-Adjusted Expected Mortality	Actual Mortality	Mortality Score	Incl/Not incl
		Cases	Mortalities					
132	Atherosclerosis with CC	151,848	1,713	77	0.5	1	1.894	Not incl
122	Circulatory disorders with AMI and major complications, discharged alive	82,871	0	66	1.2	0	0	Not incl
134	Hypertension	38,245	122	55	0.4	0	0	Not incl
108	Other cardiothoracic procedures	16,518	1,935	52	5.8	8	1.38	Not incl
145	Other circulatory system diagnoses without CC	10,010	74	36	0.2	0	0	Not incl
118	Cardiac pacemaker device replacement	14,383	55	27	0.1	0	0	Not incl
123	Circulatory disorders with AMI, died	54,573	54,344	24	24.2	24	0.993	Not incl
135	Cardiac congenital and valvular disorders, age >17 years, with CC	10,789	676	21	0.9	3	3.244	Not incl
140	Angina pectoris	44,950	268	21	0.1	0	0	Not incl
117	Cardiac pacemaker revision except device replacement	7,899	109	14	0.3	0	0	Not incl
126	Acute and subacute endocarditis	8,186	1,219	10	1.6	3	1.935	Not incl
106	Coronary bypass with PTCA	9,737	868	5	0.2	0	0	Not incl
136	Cardiac congenital and valvular disorders, age >17 years, without CC	1,695	11	5	0	0	0	Not incl
133	Atherosclerosis without CC	9,103	40	4	0	0	0	Not incl

AAMC = Association Academic Medical Centers; AICD = automatic implantable cardioverter-defibrillator; AMI = acute myocardial infarction; CC = cardiac catheter; DRG = diagnosis-related group; PTCA = percutaneous transluminal coronary angioplasty.

Table 39–9 Heart Surgery Patients at the AAMC Hospital by Diagnosis-Related Group: Group B

DRG	DRG Description	Comparison Group Cases	Comparison Group Mortalities	Cases	Risk-Adjusted Expected Mortality	Actual Mortality	Mortality Score
135	Cardiac congenital and valvular disorders age >17 years, with CC	10,789	676	21	0.9	3	3.244
111	Major cardiovascular procedures without CC	19,596	332	100	0.8	2	2.534
126	Acute and subacute endocarditis	8,186	1,219	10	1.6	3	1.935
132	Atherosclerosis with CC	151,848	1,713	77	0.5	1	1.894
107	Coronary bypass with CC	246,702	9,050	128	3.5	6	1.698
108	Other cardiothoracic procedures	16,518	1,935	52	5.8	8	1.38
105	Cardiac valve and other major cardiothoracic procedures without CC	86,024	4,899	252	12.6	16	1.271
110	Major cardiovascular procedures with CC	122,475	19,199	388	26.9	32	1.191
112	Percutaneous cardiovascular procedures	164,696	2,083	345	6	7	1.163
75	Major chest procedures	83,858	4,687	362	10.4	12	1.155
144	Other circulatory system diagnoses with CC	131,462	6,807	267	12.7	14	1.104
123	Circulatory disorders with AMI, died	54,573	54,344	24	24.2	24	0.993
104	Cardiac valve and other major cardiothoracic procedures with CC	102,844	5,825	294	13.3	13	0.975
127	Heart failure and shock	833,465	42,691	769	32.2	25	0.775
138	Cardiac arrhythmia and conduction disorders with CC	254,312	8,933	229	9.9	7	0.708
115	Permanent cardiac pacemaker implant with AMI, heart failure or shock, or AICD lead	28,634	970	87	1.6	1	0.619
116	Other permanent cardiac pacemaker implant	841,788	8,058	544	4.9	2	0.412
143	Chest pain	290,781	370	521	0.6	0	0
121	Circulatory disorders with AMI and major complications, discharged alive	194,600	0	125	10.9	0	0
139	Cardiac arrhythmia and conduction disorders without CC	110,688	375	112	0.2	0	0
122	Circulatory disorders with AMI without major complications, discharged alive	82,871	0	66	1.2	0	0
134	Hypertension	38,245	122	55	0.4	0	0
145	Other circulatory system diagnoses without CC	10,010	74	36	0.2	0	0
118	Cardiac pacemaker device replacement	14,383	55	27	0.1	0	0
140	Angina pectoris	44,950	268	21	0.1	0	0
117	Cardiac pacemaker revision except device replacement	7,899	109	14	0.3	0	0
106	Coronary bypass with PTCA	9,737	868	5	0.2	0	0
136	Cardiac congenital and valvular disorders, age >17 years, without CC	1,695	11	5	0	0	0
133	Atherosclerosis without CC	9,103	40	4	0	0	

AAMC = Association Academic Medical Centers; AICD = automatic implantable cardioverter-defibrillator; AMI = acute myocardial infarction; CC = cardiac catheter; DRG = diagnosis-related group; PTCA = percutaneous transluminal coronary angioplasty.

Table 39–10 **Heart and Heart Surgery Patients at AAMC Hospital: Areas to Improve Quality**

DRG	DRG Description	Comparison Group		Cases	Risk-Adjusted Expected Mortality	Actual Mortality	Mortality Score	Incl/Not incl
		Cases	Mortalities					
111	Major cardiovascular procedures without CC	19,596	332	100	0.8	2	2.534	Incl
107	Coronary bypass with CC	246,702	9,050	128	3.5	6	1.698	Incl
105	Cardiac valve and other major cardiothoracic procedures without CC	86,024	4.899	252	12.6	16	1.271	Incl
110	Major cardiovascular procedures with CC	122,475	19,199	388	26.9	32	1.191	Incl
112	Percutaneous cardiovascular procedures	164,696	2,083	345	6	7	1.163	Incl
75	Major chest procedures	83,858	4,687	362	10.4	12	1.155	Incl
144	Other circulatory system diagnoses with CC	131,462	6,807	267	12.7	14	1.104	Incl
104	Cardiac valve and other major cardiothoracic procedures with CC	102,844	5,825	294	13.3	13	0.975	Incl

AAMC = Association Academic Medical Centers; CC = cardiac catheter; DRG = diagnosis-related group.

REFERENCES

1. Donabedian A: The quality of care: How can it be assessed? JAMA 260: 1743, 1988
2. Smaha LA: American Heart Association. The American Heart Association Get with the Guidelines Program. Am Heart J 148:S46, 2004
3. Hammermeister KE, Shroyer L, Sethi GK, et al: Why it is important to demonstrate linkages between outcomes of care and processes and structures of care. Med Care 33:OS5, 1995
4. Shroyer AL, London MJ, Grover FL, et al: The processes, structures, and outcomes of care in cardiac surgery study: An overview. Med Care 33:OS1, 1995
5. Shroyer AL, London MJ, VillaNueva CB, et al: The processes, structures, and outcomes of care in cardiac surgery study protocol. Med Care 33:OS17, 1995
6. Tobler HG, Sethi GK, Grover FL, et al: Variations in processes and structures of cardiac surgery practice. Med Care 33:OS43, 1995
7. London MJ, Shroyer AL, Grover FL, et al: Evaluating anesthesia health care delivery for cardiac surgery: The role of process and structure variables. Med Care 33:OS66, 1995
8. Silber JH, Kennedy SK, Even-Shoshan O, et al: Anesthesiologist board certification and patient outcomes. Anesthesiology 96:1044, 2002
9. Institute of Medicine. Crossing the Quality Chasm: A new health system for the 21st century. Washington, DC, National Academy Press, 1999
10. Kohn LT, Corrigan JM, Donaldson MS (eds): To Err Is Human: Building a Safer Health System. Washington, DC, National Academy Press, 1999
11. Suarez JI, Zaidat OO, Suri MF, et al: Length of stay and mortality in neurocritically ill patients: Impact of specialized neurocritical care team. Crit Care Med 32:2311, 2004
12. Levit K, Smith C, Cowan C, et al: Health spending rebound continues in 2002. Health Affairs 23:147, 2004
13. Orkin FK: Application of outcomes research to clinical decision making in cardiovascular medicine. *In* Tumen K (ed): Outcome Measurements in Cardiovascular Medicine. Society of Cardiovascular Anesthesiologists Monograph. Philadelphia, Lippincott Williams & Wilkins, 1999, pp 39–66
14. Maynard A: Competition and quality: rhetoric and reality. Int J Q Health Care 10:379, 1998
15. Park RE, Fink A, Brook RH, et al: Physician ratings of appropriate indications for six medical and surgical procedures. Am J Pub Health 76:766, 1986
16. Leape LL, Hilborne LH, Park RH, et al: The appropriateness of use of coronary artery bypass graft surgery in New York State. JAMA 269:753, 1993
17. Wennberg JE, Freeman JL, Shelton RM, Bubolz TA: Hospital use and mortality among Medicare beneficiaries in Boston and New Haven. N Engl J Med 321:1168, 1989
18. Wennberg JE, Cooper MM (eds): Dartmouth Atlas of Health Care 1998. Chicago, American Hospital Publishing, 1998
19. Silber JH: Using outcomes analysis to assess quality of care: Applications for cardiovascular surgery. *In* Tumen K (ed): Outcome Measurements in Cardiovascular Medicine. Society of Cardiovascular Anesthesiologists Monograph. Philadelphia, Lippincott Williams & Wilkins, 1999, pp 1–22
20. Silbur JH, Rosenbaum PR, Schwartz JS, et al: Evaluation of the complication rate as a measure of quality of care in coronary artery bypass surgery. JAMA 274:317, 1995
21. Coronary Artery Surgery Study (CASS): A randomized trial of coronary artery bypass surgery. Quality of life in patients randomly assigned to treatment groups. Circulation 68:951, 1983
22. Caracciolo EA, Davis KB, Sopko G, et al: Comparison of surgical and medical group survival in patients with left main equivalent coronary artery disease. Long-term CASS experience. Circulation 91:2335, 1995
23. Davis KB, Chaitman B, Ryan T, et al: Comparison of 15-year survival for men and women after initial medical or surgical treatment for coronary artery disease: A CASS registry study. Coronary Artery Surgery Study. J Am Coll Cardiol 25:1000, 1995
24. Brundage MD, Davidson JR, Mackillop WJ: Trading treatment toxicity for survival in locally advanced non-small cell lung cancer. J Clin Oncol 15:330, 1997
25. The Criteria Committee of the New York Heart Association: Nomenclature and Criteria for Diagnosis, 9th edition. Boston, Little, Brown, 1994
26. Schipper H: Why measure quality of life? Can Med Assoc J 128:1367, 1983
27. Wenger NK, Mattson ME, Furberg CD, et al: Assessment of quality of life in clinical trials of cardiovascular therapies. Am J Cardiol 54:908, 1984
28. Campeau L: Grading of angina pectoris (letter). Circulation 54:522, 1976
29. Nussmeier NA: Adverse neurologic events: Risks of intracardiac versus extracardiac surgery. J Cardiothorac Vasc Anesth 10:31, 1996
30. Roach GW, Kanchuger M, Mangano CM, et al: Adverse cerebral outcomes after coronary bypass surgery. Multicenter Study of Perioperative Ischemia Research Group and the Ischemia Research and Education Foundation Investigators. N Engl J Med 335:1857, 1996
31. Wahrborg P, Emanuelsson H: The cardiac health profile: Content, reliability and validity of a new disease-specific quality of life questionnaire. Coron Artery Dis 7:823, 1996

32. Ware JE Jr, Sherbourne CD: The MOS 36-item short-form health survey (SF-36). I. Conceptual framework and item selection. Med Care 30:473, 1992
33. McHorney CA, Ware JE Jr, Raczek AE: The MOS 36-item short-form health survey (SF-36). II. Psychometric and clinical tests of validity in measuring physical and mental health constructs. Med Care 31:247, 1993
34. McHorney CA, Ware JE Jr, Lu JF, et al: The MOS 36-item short-form health survey (SF-36). III. Tests of data quality, scaling assumptions, and reliability across diverse patient groups. Med Care 32:40, 1994
35. Beusterien KM, Steinwald B, Ware JE Jr.: Usefulness of the SF-36 health survey in measuring health outcomes in the depressed elderly. J Geriatr Psychiatr Neurol 9:13, 1996
36. Ware JE, Jr., Kosinski M, Bayliss MS, et al: Comparison of methods for the scoring and statistical analysis of SF-36 health profile and summary measures: Summary of results from the Medical Outcomes Study. Med Care 33:AS264, 1995
37. Ware J Jr, Kosinski M, Keller SD: A 12-item short-form health survey: Construction of scales and preliminary tests of reliability and validity. Med Care 34:220, 1996
38. McCarthy MJ Jr, Shroyer AL, Sethi GK, et al: Self-report measures for assessing treatment outcomes in cardiac surgery patients. Med Care 33:OS76, 1995
39. Bernstein W, Fleisher LA, Wu A, et al: Assessment of quality of life after cardiac surgery: Determination of critical domains (abstract). Proceedings of the International Meeting on Quality of Life, Vienna, Austria, 1997
40. Bergner M, Bobbitt RA, Kressel S, et al: The sickness impact profile: Conceptual formulation and methodology for the development of a health status measure. Int J Health Serv 6:393, 1976
41. Carter WB, Bobbitt RA, Bergner M, et al: Validation of an interval scaling: The sickness impact profile. Health Serv Res 11:516, 1976
42. Hunt SM, McEwen J, McKenna SP: Measuring health status: A new tool for clinicians and epidemiologists. J R Coll Gen Pract 35:185, 1985
43. Sjoland H, Wiklund I, Caidahl K, et al: Improvement in quality of life and exercise capacity after coronary bypass surgery. Arch Intern Med 156:265, 1996
44. Caine N, Tait S, Wallwork J: Survival and health-related quality of life of elderly patients undergoing cardiac surgery. *In* Walter PJ (ed): Coronary Bypass Surgery in the Elderly. Dordrecht, Kluwer Academic Publishers, 1995, pp 155–166
45. Pocock SJ, Henderson RA, Seed P, et al: Quality of life, employment status, and anginal symptoms after coronary angioplasty or bypass surgery: 3-year follow-up in the Randomized Intervention Treatment of Angina (RITA) Trial. Circulation 94:135, 1996
46. Kornfeld DS, Heller SS, Frank KA, et al: Psychological and behavioral responses after coronary artery bypass surgery. Circulation 66:III-24, 1982
47. Alonso J, Permanyer-Miralda G, Cascant P, et al: Measuring functional status of chronic coronary patients. Reliability, validity and responsiveness to clinical change of the reduced version of the Duke Activity Status Index (DASI). Eur Heart J 18:414, 1997
48. Jenkins CD, Stanton BA, Savageau JA, et al: Coronary artery bypass surgery. Physical, psychological, social, and economic outcomes six months later. JAMA 250:782, 1983
49. Hlatky MA, Rogers WJ, Johnstone I, et al: Medical care costs and quality of life after randomization to coronary angioplasty or coronary bypass surgery. Bypass Angioplasty Revascularization Investigation (BARI) Investigators. N Engl J Med 336:92, 1997
50. Page SA, Verhoef MJ, Emes CG: Quality of life, bypass surgery and the elderly. Can J Cardiol 11:777, 1995
51. Fisher DC, Lake KD, Reutzel TJ, et al: Changes in health-related quality of life and depression in heart transplant recipients. J Heart Lung Transplant 14:373, 1995
52. Dierier E, Emmons RA, Larsen RJ, et al: The Satisfaction with Life Scale. J Pers Assess 49:71, 1985
53. Penckofer SH, Holm K: Early appraisal of coronary revascularization on quality of life. Nurs Res 33:60, 1984
54. Nease RF Jr, Kneeland T, O'Connor GT, et al: Variation in patient utilities for outcomes of the management of chronic stable angina. Implications for clinical practice guidelines. Ischemic Heart Disease Patient Outcomes Research Team. JAMA 273:1185, 1995
55. Siegel JE, Weinstein MC, Russell LB, et al: Recommendations for reporting cost-effectiveness analyses. Panel on Cost-Effectiveness in Health and Medicine. JAMA 276:1339, 1996
56. Walter PJ: Return to work after coronary artery bypass surgery. Eur Heart J 9:58, 1988
57. Oberman A, Finklea JF: Return to work after coronary artery bypass grafting (editorial). Ann Thorac Surg 34:353, 1982
58. Oberman A, Wayne JB, Kouchoukos NT, et al: Employment status after coronary artery bypass surgery. Circulation 65:115, 1982
59. Hammermeister KE, DeRouen TA, English MT, et al: Effect of surgical versus medical therapy on return to work in patients with coronary artery disease. Am J Cardiol 44:105, 1979
60. Dougenis D, Nail S, Brown AH: Is repeated coronary surgery for recurrent angina cost effective? Eur Heart J 14:623, 1992
61. Rubin HR: Patient evaluations of hospital care. A review of the literature. Med Care 28:S3, 1990
62. Klafta JM, Roizen MF: Current understanding of patients' attitudes toward and preparation for anesthesia: A review. Anesth Analg 83:1314, 1996
63. National Committee for Quality Assurance: Physicians, business, government, and industry embrace common strategy to improve health care: pay-for-performance. Available at: http://www.ncqa.org/Communications/News/BTE_P4P2005.htm. Accessed October 7, 2005
64. Hannan EL, Kilburn H, Racz M, et al: Improving the outcomes of coronary artery bypass surgery in New York State. JAMA 271:761, 1994
65. Altman L: Heart surgery death rates decline in New York. New York Times December 5, 1990
66. O'Connor GT, Plume SK, Olmstead EM, et al, for the Northern New England Cardiovascular Disease Study Group: A regional prospective study of in-hospital mortality associated with coronary artery bypass grafting. JAMA 266:803, 1991
67. O'Connor GT, Plume SK, Olmstead EM, et al: A regional intervention to improve the hospital mortality associated with coronary artery bypass graft surgery. JAMA 275:841, 1996
68. Tu JV, Jaglal SB, Naylor CD, et al: Multicenter validation of a risk index for mortality, intensive care unit stay, and overall hospital length of stay after cardiac surgery. Circulation 91:677, 1995
69. O'Connor GT, Plume SK, Olmstead EM, et al: Multivariate prediction of in-hospital mortality associated with coronary artery bypass graft surgery. Circulation 85:2110, 1992
70. Coronary Artery Bypass Graft Surgery: Technical Report, Vol 2. Harrisburg, PA, Pennsylvania Health Care Cost Containment Council, February 1994
71. Bunker JP, Forrest WH, Mosteller F, et al: The National Halothane Study. Washington, DC, US Government Printing Office, 1969
72. Moses LE, Mosteller F: Institutional differences in postoperative death rates: Commentary on some of the findings of the National Halothane Study. JAMA 203:492, 1968
73. Stanford Center for Health Care Research: Comparison of hospitals with regard to outcomes of surgery. Health Serv Res 11:112, 1976
74. Kennedy JW, Kaiser GC, Fisher LD, et al: Multivariate discriminant analysis of the clinical and angiographic predictors of operative mortality from the collaborative study in coronary artery surgery (CASS). J Thorac Cardiovasc Surg 80:876, 1980
75. Chassin MR: Achieving and sustaining improved quality: Lessons from New York State and cardiac surgery. Health Affairs 21:40, 2002
76. Grumbach K, Anderson GM, Luft HS, Roos LL, Brook R: Regionalization of cardiac surgery in the United States and Canada: Geographic access, choice, and outcomes. JAMA 274:1282, 1995
77. New York State Department of Health: Coronary Artery Bypass Graft Surgery in New York State 1996–1998. Albany, NY, State Department of Health, January 2001
78. Damberg CL, Chung RE, Steimle A: The California Report on Coronary Artery Bypass Graft Surgery: 1997–1998. Hospital Data, Technical Report. San Francisco, CA, Pacific Business Group on Health and California Office of Statewide Health Planning and Development, July 2001
79. Luft HS, Bunker JP, Enthoven AC: Should operations be regionalized? The empirical relation between surgical volume and mortality. N Engl J Med 301:1364, 1979
80. Hannan EL, O'Donnell JF, Kilburn H Jr, et al: Investigation of the relationship between volume and mortality for surgical procedures performed in New York State hospitals. JAMA 262:503, 1989
81. Savino JS, Ley C, Boisvert D, et al: Practice pattern variability for myocardial revascularization: Impact on resource use across 24 centers. J Cardiothorac Vasc Anesth 16:149, 2002
82. Shahian D: Improving cardiac surgery quality—volume, outcome, process? JAMA 291:246, 2004
83. Clark RE: Outcome as a function of annual coronary artery bypass graft volume. The Ad Hoc Committee on Cardiac Surgery Credentialing of The Society of Thoracic Surgeons. Ann Thorac Surg 61:21, 1996
84. Tu J, Naylor C: Coronary artery bypass mortality rates in Ontario: A Canadian approach to quality assurance in cardiac surgery. Circulation 94; 2430, 1996

85. Birkmeyer JD, Stukel TA, Siewers AE, et al: Surgeon volume and operative mortality in the United States. N Engl J Med 349:2117, 2003
86. Sowden AJ, Deeks JJ, Sheldon TA: Volume and outcome in coronary artery bypass graft surgery: True association or artefact? BMJ 311:151, 1995
87. Peterson ED, Coombs LP, DeLong ER, et al: Procedural volume as a marker of quality for CABG surgery. JAMA 29:195, 2004
88. Zinman D: Heart surgeons rated. Newsday, December 18, 1991, pp 3, 35, 37
89. Coronary Artery Bypass Surgery in New York State: 1991–1993. Albany, New York State Department of Health, June 1995
90. Coronary Artery Bypass Surgery in New York State: 1990–1992. Albany, New York State Department of Health, December 1993
91. Coronary Artery Bypass Surgery in New York State: 1989–1991. Albany, New York State Department of Health, December 1992
92. Narins CR, Dozier AM, Ling FS, Zareba W: The influence of public reporting of outcome data on medical decision making by physicians. Arch Intern Med 165; 83, 2005
93. Green J, Wintfeld N: Report cards on cardiac surgeons: Assessing New York's approach. N Engl J Med 332:1229, 1995
94. Omoigui NA, Miller DP, Brown KJ, et al: Outmigration for coronary bypass surgery in an era of public dissemination of clinical outcomes. Circulation 93:27, 1996
95. Hochman JS, Sleeper LA, Webb JG, et al, for the SHOCK Investigators: Early revascularization in acute myocardial infarction complicated by cardiogenic shock. Should we emergently revascularize occluded coronaries for cardiogenic shock? N Engl J Med 341:625, 1999
96. Hannan EL, Siu AL, Kumar D, et al: The decline in coronary artery bypass graft surgery mortality in New York State: The role of surgeon volume. JAMA 273:209, 1995
97. Ghali WA, Ash AS, Hall RE, Moskowitz MA: Statewide quality improvement initiatives and mortality after cardiac surgery. JAMA 277:379, 1997
98. Cardiovascular Roundtable: Cardiac Surgery Performance: Best Practices for Enhancing Margins and Clinical Outcomes, Vol 17. Washington, DC, The Advisory Board Company, 2004
99. Enthoven AC, Singer SJ: Market-based reform: What to regulate and by whom? Health Affairs 14:105, 1995
100. Zwanziger J, Melnick GA: Can managed care plans control health care costs? Health Affairs 15:185, 1996
101. Dziuban SW Jr, McIlduff JB, Miller SJ, et al: How a New York cardiac surgery program uses outcomes data. Ann Thorac Surg 58:1871, 1994
102. Hannan EL, O'Donnell JF, Kilburn H Jr, et al: Investigation of the relationship between volume and mortality for surgical procedures performed in New York State hospitals. JAMA 262:503, 1989
103. Hannan EL, Racz MJ, Walford G, et al: Long-term outcomes of coronary-artery bypass grafting versus stent implantation. N Engl J Med 352:2174, 2005
104. The National Opinion Research Center at the University of Chicago (NORC): Available at: http://norc.uchicago.edu. Accessed October 7, 2005.
105. Green J, Wintfeld N, Krasner M, Wells C: In search of America's Best Hospitals: The promise and reality of Quality Assessment. JAMA 277:1152, 1997
106. Averill R, Goldfield N, Hughes J, et al: What Are APR-DRGS? An Introduction to Severity of Illness and Risk of Mortality Adjustment Methodology. Salt Lake City, UT, 3M Health Information Systems, 2003 (www.3Mhis.com)
107. Roberts WC: The best hospitals in the USA for heart disease—1997. Am J Cardiol 80:1258, 1997
108. Rosenthal GE, Chren MM, Lasek RJ, Landefeld CS: The annual guide to "America's best hospitals": Evidence of influence among health care leaders. J Gen Intern Med 11:366, 1996
109. Chen J, Radford MJ, Wang Y, et al: Do "America's best hospitals" perform better for acute myocardial infarction? N Engl J Med 340:286, 1999

Chapter 40

REDUCING ERRORS IN CARDIAC ANESTHESIOLOGY

T. Andrew Bowdle, MD, PhD • Mark Edwards, MBChB, FANZCA • Karen B. Domino, MD, MPH

KEY POINTS

1. Evidence-based recommendations for reducing complications from central venous catheters include use of maximum sterile barriers, real-time ultrasound guidance during central venous catheter insertion, and selective use of antibiotic-impregnated central venous catheters.
2. Most cases of cardiac tamponade caused by central venous catheters should be preventable by taking a chest radiograph following placement to confirm that the position of the tip of the catheter is outside of the pericardial sac and parallel to the walls of the vena cava.
3. Evidence suggests that the most reliable method for avoiding inadvertent cannulation of an artery during central venous catheter insertion is measurement of the intravascular pressure by use of a transducer or manometry.
4. The reported risk of intraoperative awareness during cardiac surgery is around 0.4% to 1%, a 10-fold increase compared with the overall level of around 0.1% to 0.2%.
5. Evidence suggests that the use of processed electroencephalography to monitor the depth of anesthesia may significantly reduce the risk of intraoperative awareness.
6. Errors related to drug administration are common in anesthesia practice, with self-reporting studies finding a rate of error of approximately 0.75% of anesthetics.
7. Anecdotal evidence suggests that infusion pumps with advisory systems known as "error reduction systems" can significantly reduce drug administration errors resulting from incorrect manual entry of dosing information at the point of care; these pumps use predefined dosing limits and warn the practitioner if the dosing parameters that are entered at the point of care will result in an inappropriate dose.
8. Anecdotal evidence suggests that bar coding of patient identifiers, drugs, and infusion pumps at the point of care may significantly reduce the rate of errors related to drug administration.
9. Evidence suggests that fatigue may contribute significantly to errors, although specific studies in cardiac anesthesiology are lacking.
10. The American Society of Anesthesiologists Closed Claims Project database contains 250 claims related to cardiac anesthesia, with an increased proportion of claims for brain damage, stroke, and awareness during anesthesia and decreased proportion of claims for airway injury compared with 3813 other claims for other surgical procedures under general anesthesia.

Although the safety of anesthesiology has improved over recent years with an attributable mortality on the order of 1 in 79,000 anesthetic procedures,[1] errors still occur. Like other medical practitioners, anesthesiologists are prone to human error. The complex arena of cardiac anesthesia provides an opportunity for making just about any of the errors that can possibly be made by an anesthesiologist. It is just because of the complexity and the high stakes encountered in the cardiac anesthesia environment that cardiac anesthesiologists should be most interested in methods for reducing errors. This is particularly relevant now as regulatory agencies and the public in general have become acutely aware of medical errors since the publication of the Institute of Medicine's landmark report on the subject.[2] The purpose of this chapter is not to catalogue the errors that may be made in cardiac anesthesia but rather to point to specific areas where there are data in support of methods for significantly reducing errors. These specific areas are (1) errors involving the placement of central catheters, (2) errors in the assessment of anesthetic depth that may result in intraoperative awareness, (3) errors involving the process of administering drugs, such as giving the wrong drug (the principles also apply to errors in administering blood products), and (4) errors related to diminished vigilance due to fatigue.

In each of these categories of errors, there are methods that should enable clinicians to reduce error. Clinicians may also find previous descriptions of mechanisms of error in anesthesia useful.[3-5]

ERRORS INVOLVING THE PLACEMENT OF CENTRAL CATHETERS

Central catheters have long been regarded as dangerous by practitioners, manufacturers of central catheters, and the Food and Drug Administration (FDA). In 1993, the FDA, in cooperation with industry, produced and distributed a series of three educational videotapes designed to reduce the complications of central catheters. These videos are still available from the National Technical Information Service (http://www.ntis.gov/search/product.asp?ABBR=AVA18176VNB3&starDB=GRAHIST) and can be previewed on the FDA Web site (http://www.fda.gov/cdrh/ohip/dupsa/cvcvideo.html). Complications from central catheters were reviewed.[6-9]

Agency for Healthcare Research and Quality

The Agency for Healthcare Research and Quality (AHRQ) is an agency of the Public Health Service of the federal Department of Health and Human Services. The mission of the AHRQ is "to support research designed to improve the quality, safety, efficiency, and effectiveness of health care for all Americans." In 2001 AHRQ published a document entitled, "Making Health Care Safer: A Critical Analysis of Patient Safety Practices," an evidence-based review of practices intended to improve patient safety.[10] There were 11 practices that were most highly rated of 79 practices that were reviewed in detail based on the strength of evidence supporting their widespread implementation. These included three practices related to the management of central venous catheters (CVCs) (Box 40–1):

1. Use of maximum sterile barriers while placing central intravenous catheters to prevent infections
2. Use of real-time ultrasound guidance during central catheter insertion to prevent complications
3. Use of antibiotic-impregnated CVCs to prevent catheter-related infections

These recommendations clearly have implications for the practice of cardiac anesthesiology. Before examining these recommendations in more detail, this chapter takes a broader look at the complications from central catheters.

Central Catheter Complications and the American Society of Anesthesiologists Closed Claims Project Database

The American Society of Anesthesiologists (ASA) Closed Claims Project database is a standardized collection of case summaries of adverse anesthesia-related outcomes derived from closed liability claims collected from 35 insurance organizations. While it is impossible to know the true incidence of the adverse events that appear in the Closed Claims Project database (there is no "denominator" for the database), this relatively large set of cases may reveal patterns of events that contribute to patient injury and subsequent legal action, which would not be possible to discern by looking at individual cases.

This review of the Closed Claims Project database confirmed the hazards previously associated with central catheters.[11] Among the 6449 claims reported through December 2002, there were 110 claims for injuries related to central catheters (1.7%). Claims related to central catheters had a high degree of severity of patient injury degree of with an increased proportion of death (47%) compared with other claims in the database (29%, $p < 0.01$).

The main results of the review are shown in Table 40–1. Inspection of this table reveals that the most important injuries in terms of both numbers and death rate are cardiac tamponade and injuries to major arteries and veins, representing 15 in 110 and 35 in 110 cases, respectively, not including pulmonary artery (PA) injuries (the latter figure comes from combining "carotid artery puncture/cannulation," "hemothorax," and "miscellaneous other vessel injury"). This impression is reinforced when the injuries reported after 1990 are compared with those reported before 1990 (Fig. 40–1). Since 1990, the vast majority of injuries have been vascular injuries.

While a great deal of attention has been paid to PA injuries caused by PA catheters (PACs), it is interesting that this made up only 6 of 110 central catheter–related cases in the Closed Claims Project database.[11] In addition, the anecdotal literature suggests that injuries to PAs by PACs are sporadic and probably not related to specific errors or problems with technique. While highly lethal[12] and certainly to be feared, probably the main thing the practitioner can do to reduce the likelihood of

Table 40–1 Central Catheter–Related Injuries From the ASA Closed Claims Project Database

Type of Complication	n	Death, n (%)
Wire/catheter embolus	20	1 (5)*
Cardiac tamponade	15	12 (80)*
Carotid artery injury	14	5 (36)
Hemothorax	14	12 (92)*
Pneumothorax	12	2 (15)*
Miscellaneous vessel injury	7	2 (29)
Pulmonary artery rupture	6	6 (100)
Hydrothorax	5	2 (40)
Air embolism	4	3 (75)
Fluid extravasation in neck	4	2 (50)
Cardiac arrhythmia	1	0 (0)

*$p < 0.05$ compared with other complications.
Data from Domino KB, Bowdle TA, Posner KL, et al: Injuries and liability related to central vascular catheters. Anesthesiology 100:1411, 2004.

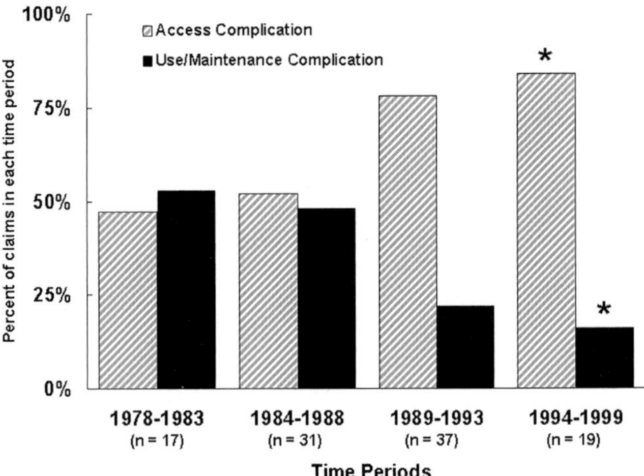

Figure 40–1 Central catheter–related claims or injuries from the ASA Closed Claims Project database. A greater proportion of claims from 1989 to 1999 involved complications related to access (mostly vascular injuries). *$p < 0.05$ 1994 through 1999 compared with other periods.

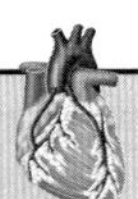

BOX 40–1 *Reducing Errors From Use of Central Venous Catheters*

- Sterile barrier precautions during catheter placement
- Ultrasound guidance for location of the internal jugular vein
- Pressure waveform monitoring or manometry to avoid cannulation of an artery
- Tip of a central venous catheter should be outside of the heart
- Chest radiograph to confirm a safe location of the tip of a central venous catheter
- Consider use of antibiotic-impregnated central venous catheters

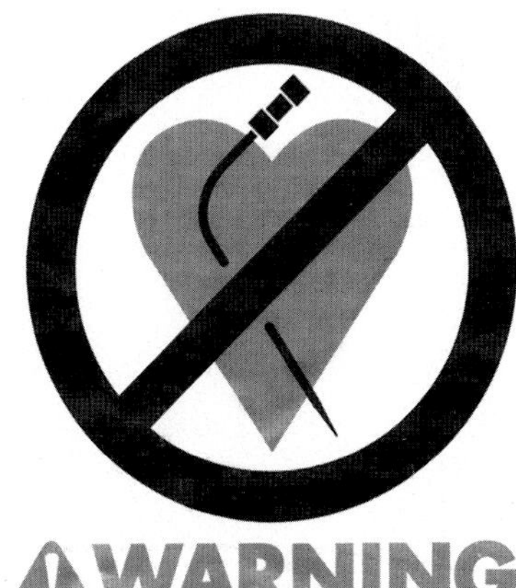
WARNING
DO NOT PLACE THE CATHETER INTO OR ALLOW IT TO REMAIN IN THE RIGHT ATRIUM OR RIGHT VENTRICLE. FAILURE TO FOLLOW THESE INSTRUCTIONS CAN RESULT IN SEVERE PATIENT INJURY OR DEATH.
READ INSTRUCTIONS

Figure 40–2 From the package insert of a central catheter kit.

PA injury is to avoid using a PAC in the first place. The appropriate use of PACs has been highly contentious,[13-24] and since the literature is not clear regarding the safety of PACs, they are not considered further here (see Chapter 14).

Preventing Cardiac Tamponade

Cardiac tamponade from a central catheter occurs when the tip of a CVC is allowed to remain in the right atrium, or up against the wall of the vena cava at an acute angle, resulting in perforation of the atrium or cava. This problem has been documented by numerous case reports[25-31] and accounted for 16 of 110 cases of central catheter-related claims in the ASA Closed Claims Project database; 13 of 16 of these cases resulted in death.[11] Perforation can occur immediately after placement or, more commonly, after hours to days. Package inserts in central catheter kits contain vigorous warnings against placing a CVC into the right atrium or with the CVC tip at an acute angle to the superior vena cava (Fig. 40–2). Most of the cases of cardiac tamponade from central catheters should be preventable by taking chest radiographs following placement, and adjusting the position of the tip of the CVC accordingly (Figs. 40–3 and 40–4).[32,33] The tip should be outside of the pericardial sac and parallel to the walls of the vena cava.[34] The carina is a useful structure for assessing the position of the catheter tip on the chest radiograph, since the vena cava is outside the pericardium at the level of the carina.[35,36] Locating the catheter tip at or above the level of the carina should ensure that the catheter tip lies outside of the pericardial sac. The carina may be a better landmark than the radiographic cardiac silhouette, since several centimeters of the superior vena cava may lie inside of the pericardium but outside of the radiographic cardiac silhouette.[35,36] Particular caution should be exercised when catheters are placed from the left side (left internal jugular or subclavian) to ensure that the catheter tip makes the turn into the superior vena cava, ending with the tip parallel to the cava and not abutting the wall of the cava at an acute or right angle. Most

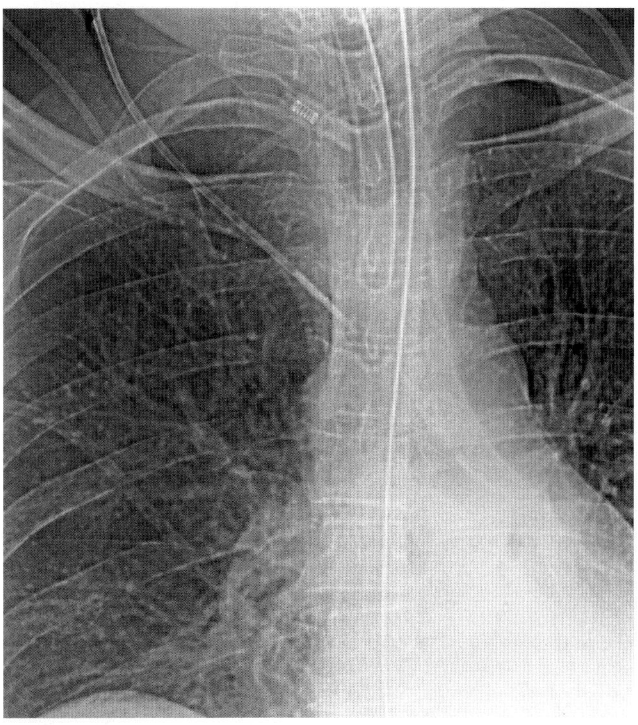

Figure 40–3 A routine chest radiograph taken in the recovery room showed the central venous catheter pointing toward the wall of the superior vena cava at an acute angle. Such positioning may increase the risk of perforation of the vena cava by the tip of the catheter. This catheter was repositioned as shown in Figure 40–4.

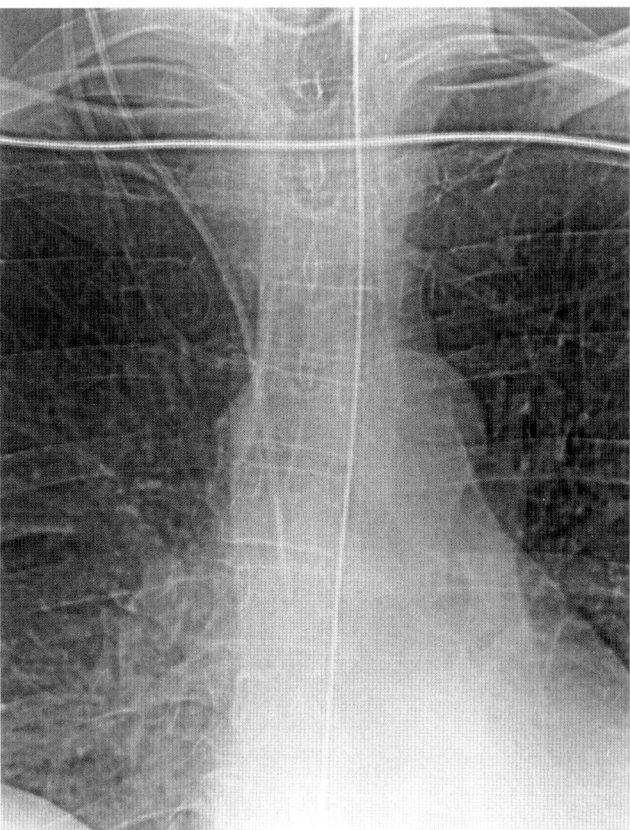

Figure 40–4 The central venous catheter shown in Figure 40–3 was repositioned so that the catheter is parallel to the walls of the superior vena cava. This position is thought to be safer than the original position shown in Figure 40–3 in which the catheter was pointed toward the wall of the vena cava at an acute angle.

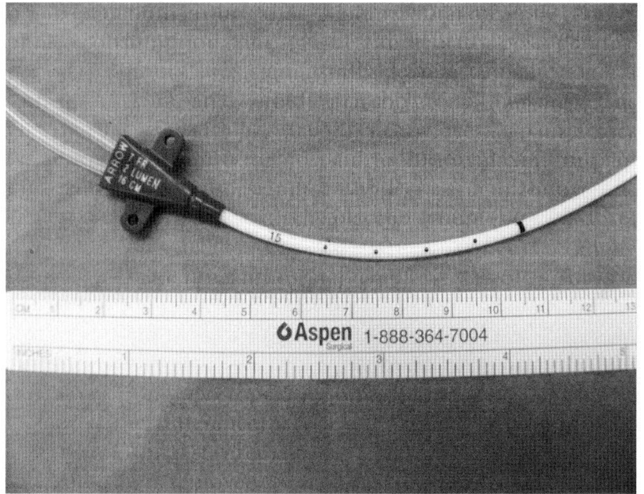

Figure 40–5 A central venous catheter is shown with markings to indicate the distance to the tip of the catheter. The dark band is 10 cm from the tip of the catheter. Inserting this catheter as far as possible will result in the tip being 16 cm from the skin puncture site. If this catheter were inserted 16 cm into the right internal jugular vein from a skin puncture site low in the neck, the tip of the catheter could easily be in the right atrium. Allowing the catheter tip to reside in the right atrium may result in perforation of the atrial wall. Prior to obtaining a chest radiograph to confirm the location of the catheter tip, limiting the insertion to 10 to 12 cm for the right internal jugular approach in a typical adult patient will usually avoid right atrial placement.

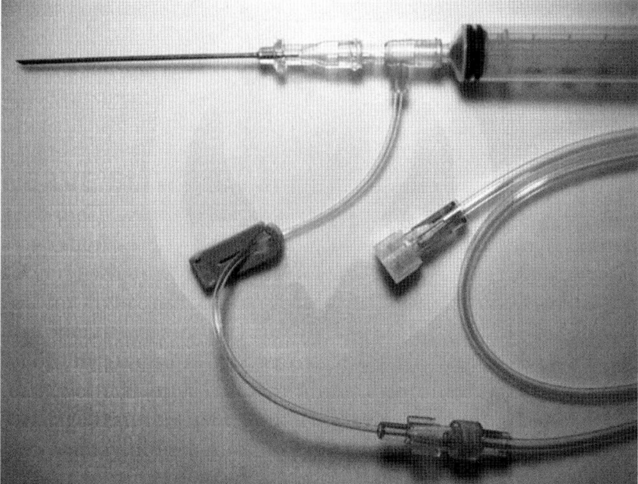

Figure 40–6 This setup is used by the authors for obtaining a pressure waveform during central catheter placement. The T-shaped adapter and a length of pressure tubing are added to a standard central catheter kit, and the device is assembled as shown using the needle and syringe found in the kit. The pressure tubing is handed off to the assistant, who connects it to a transducer and flushes the system. When blood is aspirated into the syringe, indicating entry into the blood vessel, inspection of the waveform on the monitor immediately allows differentiation between artery and vein. Once the presence of a venous waveform is confirmed, the syringe or T-adapter is removed and the wire is inserted.

anesthesiologists obtain the chest radiograph in the recovery room or intensive care unit following surgery, and this is a widely accepted practice. Nevertheless, it should be recognized that perforation can occur immediately after placement, and CVCs should be placed at an appropriate depth to avoid the right atrium. Many catheters can be inserted to a depth sufficient to reach the right atrium (Fig. 40–5), and this should be avoided by placing the CVC only to a depth of 10 to 12 cm from the right internal jugular vein approach in the typical adult. Because of anatomic variation the placement should be confirmed by chest radiograph.

Preventing Vascular Injury

Vascular injury related to central catheters is conveniently divided into injuries to arteries and injuries to veins. The mechanisms of injury and the methods of prevention are different in each category.

Preventing Injuries to Arteries

PRESSURE WAVEFORM MEASUREMENT

Because anesthesiologists usually use the internal jugular veins for central venous access, the most common injury to arteries is related to puncture or cannulation of the carotid artery. Puncturing the carotid artery with a small needle, although undesirable, does not generally produce any harm. However, if the arterial puncture is not recognized and a guidewire is placed into the artery and followed with a CVC or a PAC introducer sheath, there is the possibility of a major problem. More than 20 years ago, Jobes et al[37] reported on a retrospective study of 1021 attempts at internal jugular venous access in which there were 43 arterial punctures. Five of 43 arterial punctures were unrecognized, resulting in the placement of 8 Fr introducer sheaths into the carotid artery and one fatality from hemothorax. Subsequently, these investigators performed a prospective trial of 1284 attempts at internal jugular venous access in which they measured a pressure waveform from the vessel prior to inserting the guidewire. Prior to measuring the pressure waveform, a clinical assessment was made as to whether the needle was in an artery or a vein, based on the usual criteria of color and pulsatility. There were 51 arterial punctures, 10 of which were incorrectly identified as being venous based on color and pulsatility but were determined to be arterial from the pressure waveform. Thus, 10 inadvertent cannulations of the carotid artery were avoided by pressure waveform monitoring. Despite these findings and the anecdotal experiences of many anesthesiologists who have placed catheters and sheaths into carotid arteries, many anesthesiologists continue to rely on color and pulsatility of blood in the hub of a needle to differentiate arteries from veins.

The pressure waveform can be most conveniently measured using the setup shown in Figure 40–6. This setup has the advantage of giving the pressure waveform without the need to disconnect the syringe and connect monitoring tubing to the needle, with the risk of dislodging the needle from the vein. An alternative method used by many anesthesiologists involves manometry. The syringe is disconnected from the needle, and a length of tubing is connected, allowed to fill with blood, and then held vertically to identify the pressure from the height of the blood column. There are no data comparing these alternative methods of pressure measurement; however, the manometry technique requires an additional step to connect the manometry tubing.

ULTRASOUND GUIDANCE

The availability of relatively inexpensive, portable ultrasound equipment led to the application of two-dimensional ultrasound imaging to guide central catheter placement. Troianos et al[38] first reported the use of ultrasound-guided central vascular access in the anesthesia literature in 1991. Their prospective, randomized study of ultrasound guidance versus the traditional landmark method found a higher overall success rate, a higher success rate on the first attempt, and reduced rate of arterial puncture with ultrasound guidance. Numerous studies of ultrasound guidance have appeared subsequently, including two major meta-analyses. As noted, a review commissioned by the AHRQ strongly advocated the use of ultrasound guidance.[10]

The two major meta-analyses of ultrasound guidance concluded that ultrasound guidance was superior to landmarks for overall success rate, a higher success rate on the first attempt, and reduced complications from arterial puncture for the internal jugular vein approach.[38,39] The advantage of ultrasound guidance for the subclavian approach was less clear.

The authors examined central catheter complications from the ASA Closed Claims Project database in an attempt to determine whether the use of pressure waveform monitoring or ultrasound guidance would have prevented the complications. This is clearly inferential; nevertheless, it is interesting that nearly half (48 of 110) of the complications were judged to be possibly preventable by the use of (1) either pressure waveform monitoring or ultrasound guidance, (2) only ultrasound guidance, (3) only pressure waveform monitoring, or (4) chest radiography[11] (Table 40–2).

Table 40–2 Potential Effects of Ultrasound Guidance or Pressure Waveform Monitoring on Central Catheter–Related Injuries From the ASA Closed Claims Project Database

Possibly preventable by either ultrasound guidance or pressure waveform monitoring (n = 19)	
Carotid artery puncture/cannulation	16
Hemothorax	1
Wire/catheter embolus	1
Other miscellaneous vessel injury	1
Possibly preventable by pressure waveform monitoring only (n = 6)	
Other miscellaneous artery injury	5
Hemothorax	1
Possibly preventable by ultrasound guidance only (n = 9)	
Hemothorax	4
Pneumothorax	4
Other miscellaneous vessel injury	1
Possibly preventable by chest radiograph (n = 14)	
No chest radiograph taken (n = 7)	3
Carotid tamponade	2
Wire/catheter embolus	1
Pneumothorax	4
Misread, not read, or inappropriate action taken (n = 7)	
Cardiac tamponade	4
Wire/catheter embolus	3

The cases related to central lines from the ASA Closed Claims Project database were examined to determine whether the use of ultrasound guidance, pressure waveform monitoring, or chest radiograph (following placement) might have prevented the injuries. Of 110 injuries, 48 were thought to be potentially preventable by these means.

Data from Domino KB, Bowdle TA, Posner KL et al: Injuries and liability related to central vascular catheters. Anesthesiology 100:1411–1418, 2004.

An important caveat for the use of ultrasound guidance is that the needle and/or wire may not always be visualized in the vein, depending upon the type of ultrasound equipment used. If the needle and/or wire is not definitely visualized in the vein, measurement of a pressure waveform in conjunction with ultrasound guidance is strongly recommended by the authors. Anecdotal experience has shown that despite the use of ultrasound guidance and the appearance that the needle is pointed toward the vein, the needle may hit the artery, particularly when the artery is visualized inferior to the vein on the screen. In the authors' practice, ultrasound guidance and pressure waveform monitoring are used together routinely. Needles with a special echogenic surface are available that may enhance ultrasound visualization of the needle in the vein.

Given the abundance of data in favor of the use of ultrasound guidance, it appears that the use of ultrasound guidance should be the "preferred method of insertion."[40] At this time, many anesthesiologists who would like to use ultrasound guidance do not have equipment readily available. While a British economic modeling study has suggested that ultrasound guidance would be cost effective, saving $3249 per 1000 procedures,[41] the capital for purchase of the ultrasound equipment is not always available. However, it seems very likely that the use of ultrasound guidance will become more prevalent over time.

Preventing Injuries to Veins

Pressure waveform monitoring and ultrasound guidance are valuable primarily for avoiding injury to arteries, especially to the carotid artery during attempted internal jugular vein cannulation. There is another category of vascular injury that is not addressed by pressure waveform monitoring or ultrasound guidance, which is injury to intrathoracic veins, made clear from anecdotal reports and from the ASA Closed Claims Project database, which contains 15 cases of hemothorax, of which 14 were fatal. A large puncture or tear in a large intrathoracic vein can bleed profusely and may be very difficult to repair surgically in time to prevent exsanguination. While the mechanism of these injuries is not known in every case, certain mechanisms appear to be particularly likely.

Guidewires can take a circuitous route so that when devices are advanced over them, the device may trap the wire up against the wall of the vein, and if the device is stiff enough, perforation of the vein may occur[42] (Fig. 40–7). The inner dilators of PAC introducer sheaths are very stiff and may be particularly likely to cause this kind of perforation. The dilator is intended to create a passage through the skin and fascia but has no useful role once the device has entered the vein. Therefore, it is prudent to advance the dilator the minimum distance necessary to reach the vein and no farther. The introducer sheath may then be advanced over the dilator into the vein.

The left internal jugular approach may be particularly hazardous because the innominate (brachiocephalic) vein crosses the internal jugular vein at a right angle. It does not require much imagination to see that a device inserted into the left internal jugular vein could perforate the innominate vein, and anecdotal reports verify that this is indeed the case. The right internal jugular vein should be preferred to the left internal jugular vein primarily for this reason. If the left internal jugular vein is used, special care should be exercised not to advance the dilator of a PAC introducer beyond the internal

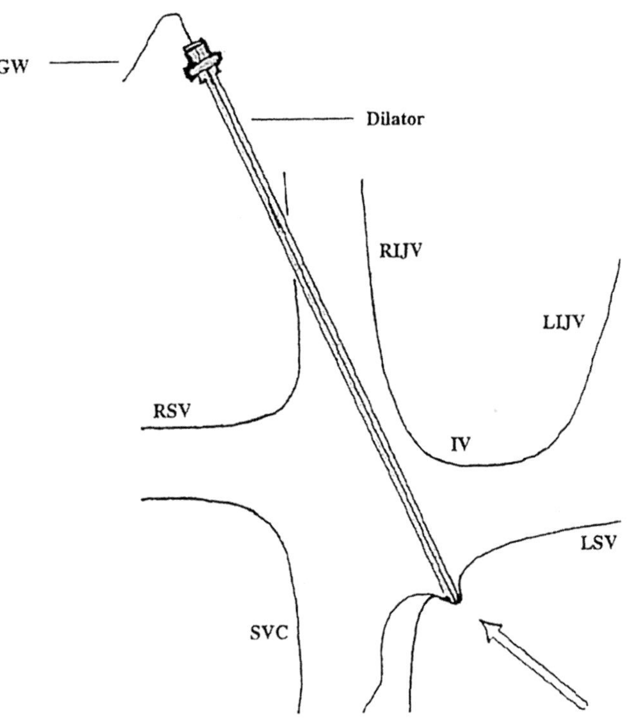

Figure 40–7 A hypothetical mechanism of perforation of a great vein inside the chest (in this case, the innominate vein–vena cava junction) by a dilator (the pulmonary artery catheter introducer sheath, normally loaded onto the dilator, is not shown for simplicity) is shown. The dilator traps the guidewire against the wall of the vein and then perforates the vein as it is advanced. There are numerous anecdotal reports of injuries that could be explained by this mechanism. Direct observation of the progress of the insertion of the wire and intravascular device under fluoroscopy may be useful for avoiding this potentially fatal complication. (GW, guidewire; RIJV, right internal jugular vein; LIJV, left internal jugular vein; LSV, left subclavian vein; RSV, right subclavian vein; SVC, superior vena cava; IV, innominate vein.) (From Oropello JM, Leibowitz AB, Manasia A, et al: Dilator-associated complications of central vein catheter insertion: Possible mechanisms of injury and suggestions for prevention. J Cardiothorac Vasc Anesth 10:634, 1996.)

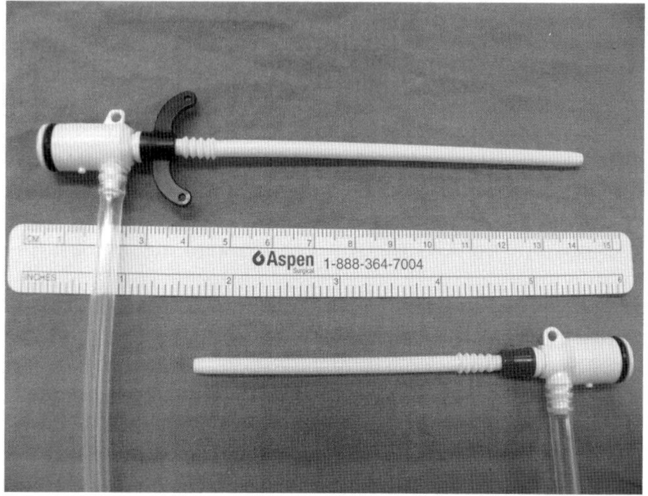

Figure 40–8 A "standard" pulmonary artery catheter introducer sheath (*top*) is compared with a shorter sheath (*bottom*). The authors prefer the shorter sheath for the left internal jugular approach with the intention to avoid having to push the longer sheath past the right angle junction between the left internal jugular vein and the innominate (brachiocephalic) vein. Perforation of the innominate vein is a potentially fatal complication of left internal jugular cannulation.

jugular vein. The authors prefer to use a shorter-than-normal introducer sheath in this situation (Fig. 40–8). Another potential problem with the left-sided approach is injury to the thoracic duct, which terminates variably in the left internal jugular vein, the left subclavian vein, or the left innominate vein. The duct may be perforated in the process of placing a CVC catheter, or, rarely, the duct may actually be cannulated. Chylothorax and chylopericardium may result, and infusion of fluids into the thoracic duct may produce cardiac tamponade or constrictive pericarditis by retrograde flow into the pericardial lymphatics.[43]

The use of fluoroscopy is an important consideration in avoiding injuries to veins. Fluoroscopy allows visualization of the guidewire and the intravascular device as it passes over the guidewire in real time. Fluoroscopy is used routinely by interventional radiologists, cardiologists, and surgeons (the latter when placing surgically implanted central catheters). Fluoroscopy is not often used in anesthesia, emergency medicine, or critical care medicine, but perhaps it should be. In the authors' opinion, anesthesiologists wishing to place central catheters in the safest possible manner should strongly consider the use of fluoroscopy, especially when there is difficulty passing wire or catheters into the central circulation. However, availability of fluoroscopy equipment and radiology technical support are significant obstacles to using fluoroscopy for most anesthesiologists.

Preventing Infections Related to Central Catheters

Infections from CVCs and PACs are related to the time that the catheter is in place and increase significantly after 3 days.[44,45] Because many central catheters placed by anesthesiologists for intraoperative monitoring are removed soon after surgery, the risk of infection is reduced. Nevertheless, anesthesiologists should use the evidence-based methods for preventing central catheter infections.[46] The most important of these is the use of maximum sterile barriers, including chlorhexidine preparation, gloves, gown, and a large sterile drape. As noted earlier, the use of maximum sterile barriers was strongly recommended by the AHRQ in the document, "Making Health Care Safer: A Critical Analysis of Patient Safety Practices."[10] For most anesthesiologists working in the operating room, the only change in practice that needs to be made to use maximum sterile barriers is to don a sterile gown for central catheter placement. There is substantial evidence that chlorhexidine is a more effective skin cleaning solution than povidone-iodine. Antibiotic ointments applied to the skin puncture site do not affect the risk of bloodstream infection and may actually increase the rate of colonization by fungi and promote antibiotic-resistant bacteria. The use of antimicrobial agent–impregnated catheters reduces the incidence of bloodstream infections related to central catheters and should be considered. As noted, antimicrobial agent–impregnated catheters are recommended in the AHRQ report on evidence-based safety measures. However, these catheters are more expensive and may not be cost-effective when the catheters are going to be removed soon after surgery. For catheters that are intended to remain in place or for high-risk patients (e.g., immunosuppressed patients), antibiotic-impregnated catheters should certainly be considered (see Chapter 14).

BOX 40–2 *Avoiding Intraoperative Awareness*

- Overall rate of intraoperative awareness is 0.1% to 0.2%.
- Intraoperative awareness during cardiac surgery is higher, 0.4% to 1%.
- Severity of intraoperative awareness experiences varies from mild to profound.
- Some patients experience posttraumatic stress disorder.
- Evidence suggests that the use of computerized EEG monitoring may help to reduce the incidence of intraoperative awareness.
- Limitation and artifacts encountered with computerized EEG monitoring must be understood by the user.

PREVENTING INTRAOPERATIVE AWARENESS

There are two large prospective multicenter studies of intraoperative awareness, one from Europe and one from the United States, which have reported similar overall rates of intraoperative awareness of around 0.1% to 0.2%.[47,48] An analysis of cases of awareness during anesthesia from the ASA Closed Claims Project was reported in 1999.[49]

Undergoing cardiac surgery increases the risk of intraoperative awareness from the overall level of around 0.1% to 0.2%[47,48] to around 0.4% to 1%,[48,50-54] an increased risk of up to 10-fold. Intraoperative awareness may be a minor or a major complication depending upon the severity of the episode of awareness and the response of the individual patient (Box 40–2). Intraoperative awareness may result in a significant psychiatric condition such as posttraumatic stress disorder.[55] The explanation for increased risk of intraoperative awareness during cardiac surgery is unknown. Possible causes include deliberately light anesthesia during periods of hemodynamic instability and gaps in anesthetic delivery during separation from cardiopulmonary bypass (CPB) when volatile anesthetic being administered into the CPB circuit is discontinued. While vasoactive drugs used during cardiac surgery may mask hemodynamic responses to light anesthesia, it is clear that intraoperative awareness often occurs in the absence of hemodynamic clues, rendering that explanation less likely. Whatever the cause may be, cardiac anesthesiologists should be concerned about the high incidence of intraoperative awareness during cardiac surgery. The Joint Commission on Accreditation of Healthcare Organizations (JCAHO) issued a "Sentinel Event Alert" regarding intraoperative awareness, which is likely to make intraoperative awareness the subject of further public scrutiny (http://www.jcaho.org/about+us/news+letters/sentinel+event+alert/sea_32.htm).

Some anesthesiologists are skeptical about an incidence of intraoperative awareness of 0.1% to 1%. This skepticism is usually based upon personal experience such that individual anesthesiologists believe that the rate of intraoperative awareness in their personal practice is much less than this. However, caution should be used in applying personal experience, because of observations in the literature showing that anesthesiologists may frequently miss cases of intraoperative awareness for a variety of reasons, not the least of which is that patients do not always have the opportunity to relate their experience to the anesthesiologist.[56] Several studies have shown that the patient may not report their awareness experience immediately after surgery.[47,48]

Electroencephalography (EEG) has been used extensively by neuropharmacologists to study the effects of anesthetic drugs since the 1960s. As the power of desktop computers increased, it became possible to process raw EEG using fast Fourier transforms and other mathematical methods in order to make the information contained in the raw EEG immediately accessible in the operating room to those without formal training in the interpretation of raw EEG. The original use of processed EEG in the operating room was for the detection of cerebral ischemia during carotid endarterectomy, and it has only been in recent years that attention has turned once again to the use of EEG to measure the effects of anesthetic drugs. The technological obstacles to reliably measuring the effects of anesthetic drugs in the operating room with EEG and providing clinically useful information to the anesthesiologist were daunting. Many individuals who were familiar with EEG technology believed that it would never be possible to measure "anesthetic depth" in real time, in the typical operating room setting. Nevertheless, the major obstacles have been overcome and there are now several commercial products available for this purpose. The processed EEG monitor known as BIS (Bispectral Index) is by far the most prevalent, and by far the best documented with more than 1500 abstracts and papers in its bibliography. Therefore, most of the information here will be concerned with BIS. However, it should be clearly understood that there are other commercial products that purport to provide similar data for clinical monitoring. BIS monitoring has been reviewed elsewhere[57] (see Chapter 17).

The result of EEG processing by the BIS monitor is a number ranging from 0 to 100, where 0 is an isoelectric (flat) EEG and 100 is "awake." Assuming that artifacts, interference, signal quality and other idiosyncrasies of EEG processing have been appropriately evaluated by the user (see later), a BIS value below 60 should be associated with an extremely low probability of awareness during anesthesia.[58,59] Clinicians might think that if BIS monitoring were used and BIS values kept below 60, the incidence of intraoperative awareness could be reduced to a very low level. However, an alternative notion has been proposed[60]—that the use of BIS monitoring might actually elevate the incidence of intraoperative awareness due to the well-documented tendency of anesthesiologists to administer lower doses of anesthetic drugs when BIS monitoring is used as a guide to anesthetic drug administration.[61,62]

Two studies have been published that support the hypothesis that the use of BIS monitoring can result in a lower incidence of intraoperative awareness. In a retrospective case-comparison study, 5057 consecutive BIS-monitored patients were compared with 7826 non-BIS monitored patients from the same institutions.[63] There were 2 cases of intraoperative awareness (during intubation; both had BIS values >60) in the BIS-monitored series compared with 14 in the non–BIS-monitored series ($p < 0.039$). In a prospective, randomized multicenter trial, 2503 "high-risk" (e.g., cardiac anesthesia, trauma, obstetrics) patients were randomized to BIS or non-BIS monitoring.[54] There were 2 cases of intraoperative awareness in the BIS-monitored group (in one case, the BIS was <60) compared with 11 in the non–BIS-monitored group (odds ratio, 0.18; 95% adjusted confidence interval, 0.02 to 0.84; $p = 0.022$). These studies suggest that BIS monitoring may be a useful tool for helping to reduce the incidence of intraoperative awareness.

While BIS monitoring for the reduction of intraoperative awareness remains controversial, the currently available evidence suggests that cardiac anesthesiologists should seriously consider the use of BIS or other similar processed EEG monitor, especially given the high rate of intraoperative awareness that has been consistently demonstrated in patients undergoing cardiac surgery.

While it is not the purpose of this chapter to review processed EEG monitoring, there are several important caveats for BIS or other processed EEG monitoring that should be familiar to clinicians (see also Chapter 17):

- The use of processed EEG to evaluate anesthetic depth depends upon certain fundamental similarities in the effects of anesthetic drugs on the EEG. Ketamine and nitrous oxide[64] have distinct EEG effects that are not taken into account by the BIS algorithm.
- EEG signals are of very low amplitude, and therefore electrical artifacts are a significant problem. Common sources of electrical artifact include cautery, electromyographic (EMG) activity, 60-Hz noise from electrical appliances, and high-frequency artifact from temporary external pacing devices (but usually not permanently implanted internal pacemakers). The latter is particularly relevant during cardiac surgery. All of these sources of high-frequency electrical noise tend to elevate the BIS, because their frequency spectrum overlaps the EEG spectrum (2 to 60 Hz) and high-frequency EEG is associated with wakefulness or light anesthesia and higher BIS values. The BIS monitor identifies the presence of high-frequency artifacts and notifies the user by lighting up an "EMG" signal strength bar on the display of the monitor. In the presence of high-frequency artifact, the BIS number cannot be interpreted in the usual manner. Small doses of muscle relaxant usually obliterate high-frequency artifact caused by muscle activity.
- Processing of the raw EEG and data smoothing occur over 15 or 30 seconds (user configurable). This means that the BIS number will lag slightly behind clinical events. This is particularly noticeable during induction, when the patient may be obviously unconscious before the BIS number begins to change.
- BIS numbers reflect the EEG state of the brain but do not reveal how the brain arrived at that state. For example, BIS declines during sleep,[65] yet clearly natural sleep is not the same as anesthesia. Moreover, a BIS number does not reveal what will happen in the future. For example, while BIS may be 45 at one moment, a change in surgical stimulus could result in a BIS of 75 moments later. The propensity of response to a surgical stimulus is more likely with volatile anesthetics and less likely with an anesthetic that includes a substantial amount of opioid[66]; however, the BIS number does not distinguish among the various possible combinations of opioid and hypnotic drugs.[67] BIS is an additional piece of information for use in conducting the anesthetic, but it definitely does not substitute for the conventional judgments that anesthesiologists make in the absence in BIS.

Drug Errors

Adverse drug events (ADEs) are a major cause of morbidity and mortality in hospitalized patients, affecting more than 770,000 patients per year in the United States. Hospital costs for treating patients who suffer ADEs are enormous, estimated at between $1.56 and $5.6 billion annually. Most ADEs in hospitalized patients are caused by errors of various kinds,[68] as brought to wide public attention in the Institute of Medicine's report, "To Err Is Human: Building a Safer Health System."[2] This is an international problem, as shown by a recent investigation that used "disguised observation" to discover that one or more errors occurred in the preparation and administration of 58 of 122 intravenous drug doses on the nursing wards of a German hospital. Many of the errors were minor, but there were three cases of a wrong dose, one omitted dose, and two "unauthorized" doses.[69]

A great deal of attention has been directed at errors that occur in the process of writing and transcribing physicians' orders for drugs. There is evidence that computerization of physician ordering (computerized physician order entry [CPOE]) along with computerized advice (clinical decision support system [CDSS]) can significantly reduce these types of errors.[70] The AHRQ review "Making Health Care Safer: A Critical Analysis of Patient Safety Practices" rated CPOE and CDSS as patient safety practices with medium strength of evidence.[10] The Leapfrog Group ("a coalition of more than 150 public and private organizations...created to help save lives and reduce preventable medical mistakes by mobilizing employer purchasing power to initiate breakthrough improvements in the safety of health care and by giving consumers information to make more informed hospital choices"), founded by the Business Roundtable, a national association of Fortune 500 CEOs, has made CPOE one of its "safety standards" (http://www.leapfroggroup.org).

Because anesthesiologists working in the operating room seldom write orders for drugs (with the possible exception of the recovery room), CPOE is of relatively little interest. What is of greater interest is errors involving the administration of drugs at the "point of care," such as giving the wrong drug or the wrong dose. There is substantial evidence that drug administration errors are common in anesthetic practice. In 1993, the Australian Incident Monitoring Study (AIMS) identified 144 instances of a wrong drug being given or nearly given to a patient among the first 2000 incidents reported to the study.[71] There was the potential for serious harm in 74% of reports, but no deaths occurred. In 1995, Merry and Peck reported on a survey of 75 anesthesiologists in New Zealand, 89% of whom indicated they had made at least one error of drug administration, with 12.5% indicating that they had harmed a patient by a drug-related error.[72] Subsequently, the Merry and Peck group performed a survey of 10,806 anesthetics in two hospitals in New Zealand. Anesthesiologists volunteered information about drug errors using a standardized reporting form.[73] The overall rate of drug error was 0.75%, or 1 in 133 anesthetic procedures. Drug errors resulted in 1 case of intraoperative awareness, 2 cases of prolonged neuromuscular blockade, and 47 cases of transient physiological effects, 5 of which required intervention. A similar survey of 687 anesthesiologists in Canada found that 85% of the respondents had made at least one drug error or "near miss."[74] Four deaths resulted from a total of 1038 reported errors. A report based on annual surveys conducted by the Japanese Society of Anesthesiologists between 1999 and 2002, reflecting 4,201,925 anesthetic procedures, found an incidence of "critical events" due to drug administration error of 0.02%. The incidence of death resulting from drug error was 0.00044%. Clearly, drug administration errors in anesthesia are relatively common and occur in diverse practice settings.

Table 40–3 Drug Errors in a University Anesthesia Practice

6705 Anesthetic procedures	
6066 Forms completed	
41 Errors (0.68%)	
Incorrect dose	18
Substitution	7
Insertion	6
Repetition	2
Incorrect route	2
Omission	3
Incorrect label	1
Unintended effects	31
<5 minutes	18
>5 minutes	13

A study of self-reported drug-related errors by anesthesiology attendings, residents, and certified registered nurse anesthetists (CRNAs) in a university medical center found the errors shown in the table. The overall rate of drug-related error was 0.68% of anesthetic procedures. There were no permanent injuries; however, in 31 of 41 cases, unintended drug effects occurred. One patient had possible intraoperative awareness associated with an empty vaporizer, and one patient had a longer-than-expected hospital stay due to inadvertent administration of neuraxial morphine.

Data from Bowdle A, Kruger C, Grieve R, et al: Anesthesia drug administration errors in a university hospital. Anesthesiology 99:A1358, 2003.

The incidence of drug administration errors in an academic practice in the United States appears to be similar to that reported from elsewhere in the world. In a study modeled after the New Zealand study cited earlier, anesthesiologists and nurse anesthetists at the University of Washington completed survey forms; 6066 forms were returned for 6709 anesthetics, for a response rate of 90%[75] (Table 40–3). There were 41 reports of errors (0.68%) and 23 reports of pre-errors (near misses) (0.38%). Drug administration errors resulted in transient unintended drug effects (<5 minutes) in 17 cases and prolonged unintended drug effects (>5 minutes) in 12 cases. Of these 29 cases of unintended drug effect, 14 were associated with drug infusions administered by a pump. One patient had possible intraoperative awareness associated with an empty vaporizer, and one patient had a longer-than-expected hospital stay due to inadvertent administration of neuraxial morphine. There were no cases of drug-related permanent physical injury.

Analysis of the ASA Closed Claims Project database also reveals interesting information about anesthetic drug administration errors in the United States.[76] In 2003, there were 205 drug errors, 4% of the database of 5803 cases. Drug errors were categorized into the following categories (after Webster[73]):

- Omission—drug not given
- Repetition—extra dose of an intended drug
- Substitution—incorrect drug instead of the desired drug; a swap
- Insertion—drug that was not intended to be given at a particular time or at any time
- Incorrect dose—wrong dose of an intended drug
- Incorrect route—wrong route of an intended drug
- Other—usually a more complex event not fitting the other categories

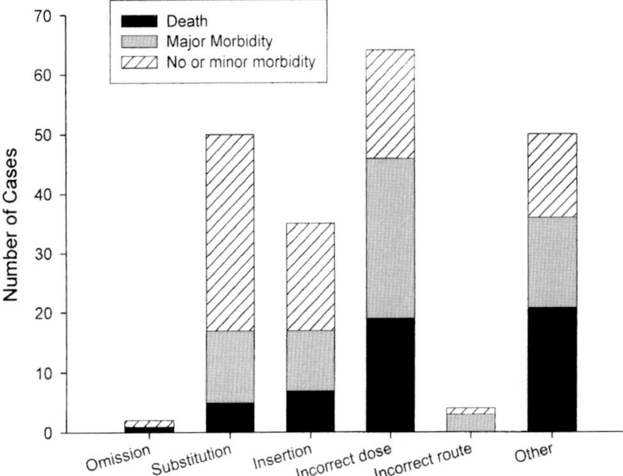

Figure 40–9 A review of claims related to drug errors in the ASA Closed Claims Project database found the mechanisms of error shown in the figure. (Data from Bowdle TA: Drug administration error from the ASA Closed Claims Project. Am Soc Anesthesiol Newsletter 67:11, 2003.)

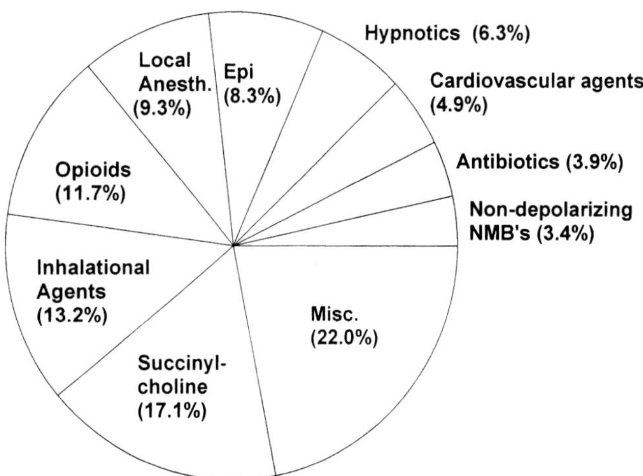

Figure 40–10 A review of claims related to drug errors in the ASA Closed Claims Project database identified the drugs shown. The two individual drugs implicated most frequently were epinephrine and succinylcholine. (Data from Bowdle TA: Drug administration error from the ASA Closed Claims Project. Am Soc Anesthesiol Newsletter 67:11, 2003.)

The numbers of cases in each category and the types of drugs involved are shown in Figures 40–9 and 40–10. The most common distinct mechanisms of drug administration error were substitution, insertion, and incorrect dose.

Drug errors were also a significant factor in claims that involved multiple problems in patient management ("other"). Two drugs in particular were most involved. Succinylcholine was involved in 35 cases (17%) and epinephrine was involved in 17 cases (8%). Twelve of the 35 cases involving succinylcholine resulted in patients being awake while paralyzed, due to succinylcholine boluses given prior to induction agents, or succinylcholine infusions that were started inadvertently in awake patients. Succinylcholine was administered to five patients with a previous history of definite or probable pseudocholinesterase deficiency, resulting in prolonged neuromuscular blockade. Hyperkalemic cardiac arrest occurred in two paraplegic patients and a patient with Guillain-Barre syndrome who received succinylcholine. Succinylcholine infusions were involved in 14 of the 35 succinylcholine-related cases. Drug administration errors involving epinephrine were particularly dangerous, with death or major morbidity resulting in 11 of the 17 epinephrine-related cases. Six of the 17 cases involving epinephrine were caused by ampule swaps. Drugs interchanged with epinephrine were ephedrine (two cases), Pitocin (three cases), and hydralazine (one case). An informative case report describing the nearly fatal results of inadvertent epinephrine administration due to an ampule swap has been published.[77]

There were 19 cases of intraoperative awareness (9%), 14 of which involved inadvertent administration of muscle relaxant to awake patients; a patient who received vecuronium instead of cefazolin developed posttraumatic stress disorder as a result of being paralyzed while awake. The remaining five cases of awareness were either unexplained (one case), related to omission of an induction agent (one case), or apparently related to inadequate doses of general anesthetic agents (three cases).

ASA Closed Claims Project reviewers judge the care to be "less than appropriate" in 84% of the drug error claims, compared with 35% in no drug error claims. Payments were made to plaintiffs in 72% of the drug error claims compared with 52% of the non–drug error claims.

Drug Errors by Perfusionists

Cardiac surgery requiring CPB presents the relatively unusual situation in which the anesthesiologist may not be the only person in the operating room administering drugs to the patient. Perfusionists frequently administer anesthetic drugs during CPB and may administer a variety of other drugs as well. Rarely, the perfusionist may also be an anesthesiologist (particularly in Australia). Whether the anesthesiologist supervises the perfusionist in the administration of drugs varies depending upon the particular practice setting. In some practice settings, the anesthesiologist may leave the operating room during some portion of the time on CPB. While the statement has been made that the anesthesiologist should not leave the operating room during CPB (http://www.asahq.org/Newsletters/2004/04_04/gravlee04_04.html), the practice of doing so is probably widespread, particularly outside of academic institutions. Apparently there are no studies documenting drug errors made by perfusionists, despite several general reports on error and incidents during CPB.[78-81] Any comprehensive effort to reduce drug errors during cardiac surgery should include the perfusionist. Common sense suggests that the perfusionist and anesthesiologist should work together as much as possible to ensure that the patient receives drugs appropriately during CPB.

Prevention of Drug Administration Errors—Bar Coding

While drug administration errors are clearly very important, relatively little is known about preventing these errors (Box 40–3). A review evaluated the evidence for various measures for reducing drug administration errors in anesthetic practice and made recommendations; however, most of the evidence available for review was anecdotal.[82] Recommendations included carefully reading the label on any ampule or syringe, optimizing legibility and contents of labels, labeling syringes,

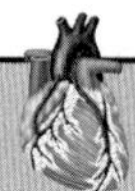

BOX 40–3 *Reducing Errors Related to Drug Administration*

- Drug administration errors are common in anesthetic practice.
- A multifaceted approach is required to reduce drug administration errors.
- Bar coding patient identifiers, drugs, infusion pumps, and blood products at the point of care may help to reduce errors.
- The FDA will require bar code labeling of most prescription drugs and blood products.
- "Error-reduction systems" for infusion pumps may reduce errors related to incorrect manual entry of dosing information at the point of care.
- Perfusionists administer drugs during cardiopulmonary bypass and should be included in error reduction strategies.

formal organization of drug drawers and workspaces, and double-checking drugs with another person or use of a device.

A bar code reader represents just such a device, and bar coding drugs at the point of care to verify the correctness of the drug and the dose is widely regarded as a technological solution that might improve the accuracy of drug administration. There is useful information about bar coding available on the Website of the Healthcare Information and Management Systems Society (HIMSS; http://www.himss.org/asp/issuesbytopic.asp?TopicID=17). The HIMSS has a position statement in support of bar coding in the health care environment for a variety of purposes. ECRI, the nonprofit health services research agency, has also published a review concerning the bar coding of medications.[83] The proceedings of the HIMSS from 2000, available on the Internet (http://himss.org/content/files/proceedings/2000/sessions/ses073.pdf, "Veterans Affairs: Eliminating Medication Errors Through Point-of-Care Devices), contains interesting anecdotal information about the experience of the Department of Veterans Affairs with bar coding. According to this report, wireless, point-of-care bar coding of patient wristbands and medications was used at the Comery-O'Neil Veterans Affairs Medical Center to deliver 5.7 million doses and in the process prevented 378,000 errors. The report claims that "no medication errors occurred when the technology was used as designed," although errors continued to occur when the technology was not properly used. Application of bar coding technology reduced wrong medication errors by 74%, wrong dose errors by 57%, wrong patient errors by 91%, wrong time errors by 92%, and omission errors by 70%. Clearly, these are promising results that should cause clinicians to look very carefully at the prospects for bar coding in the anesthesia environment. However, the authors are not aware of any peer-reviewed data from appropriately designed trials to confirm the efficacy of bar coding for prevention of drug errors. This is interesting considering the widespread support for the concept and the potentially large investments that might be made in equipment and software to widely implement bar coding of drugs in hospitals.

The Food and Drug Administration (FDA) issued a rule in February 2004 that requires bar codes on most prescription drugs, certain over-the-counter drugs, and blood products (http://www.fda.gov/cber/rules/barcodelabel.pdf). The FDA believes that bar codes would be used in the following manner:

- A patient is admitted to the hospital. The hospital gives the patient a bar-coded identification bracelet to link the patient to his or her computerized medical record.
- As required by the rule, most prescription drugs and certain over-the-counter drugs would have a bar code on their labels. The bar code would reflect the drug's NDC (national drug code) number.
- The hospital would have bar code scanners or readers that are linked to the hospital's computer system of electronic medical records.
- Before a health care worker administers a drug to the patient, the health care worker scans the patient's bar code. This allows the computer to pull up the patient's computerized medical record.
- The health care worker then scans the drug(s) that the hospital pharmacy has provided to be administered to the patient. This scan informs the computer which drug is being administered.
- The computer then compares the patient's medical record to the drug(s) being administered to ensure that they match. If there is a problem, the computer sends an error message, and the health care worker investigates the problem. The problem could be one of many things:
  Wrong patient
  Wrong dose of drug
  Wrong drug
  Wrong time to administer the drug
  Patient's chart has been updated and the prescribed medication has changed

The FDA has estimated that the scheme outlined above would result in a 50% reduction in medication errors, preventing 500,000 adverse events and transfusion errors while saving $93 billion over 20 years.

To the best of the authors' knowledge there are two commercially available systems designed specifically for bar coding drugs in the anesthesia clinical environment. One was designed by an anesthesiologist and marketed in the United States by DocuSys (http://www.docusys.net). Another was designed by an anesthesiologist and marketed in New Zealand by Safer Sleep Limited (http://www.safersleep.co.nz/).[84] Unfortunately there are no prospective, randomized data showing that the use of these devices affects outcome, although a study of user ratings of the New Zealand system gave results in favor of the bar coding system in comparison to the traditional system of drug administration.[85] Hypothetically, automated anesthesia record-keeping systems provided by other vendors could be adapted to bar coding of drugs, because bar code readers can be operated by most desktop computer systems.

Prevention of Drug Errors—Infusion Pumps

As noted, the study of drug errors at the University of Washington found that among 29 cases of unintended drug effect, 14 were associated with drug infusions administered by a pump.[75] Although there is no comprehensive assessment of the incidence and nature of errors related to infusion pumps, it is clear from anecdotal reports that programming errors are a significant source of error. Obviously infusion pumps play a major role in drug administration in cardiac surgery patients, so errors related to infusion pumps are of significant concern to cardiac anesthesiologists.

ECRI made recommendations concerning improvements in the safety of infusion pumps. Based on reports of pump-related problems and accident investigations, ECRI has found that pump incidents typically involve either unintentional free flow of a drug or the delivery of an incorrect dose due to a practitioner error in programming the pump.[86]

Pump sets that prevent free flow when the set is removed from the pump have been available for many years, but not all pumps in current use require the use of sets that prevent free flow, and unprotected sets continue to be available. ECRI recommends the use of pumps with tubing sets that prevent free flow when the set is removed from the pump and that only pumps that *require* the use of sets with free-flow prevention be purchased. They rate pumps that do not require set-based free-flow protection as "unacceptable."[86]

Some infusion pumps have advisory systems known as "error-reduction systems" that use predefined dosing limits and warn the practitioner if the dosing parameters that are entered at the point of care will result in a dose that is out of the predefined dosing limits. Such systems can also keep a computerized log that yields data regarding the incidence of "reprogramming" in response to an alert message; this is essentially the incidence of potential errors due to programming errors. Anecdotal information suggests that error-reduction systems may be very valuable for helping practitioners to recognize and avoid administering incorrect doses due to programming errors. A report of experience with 135 pumps with an error-reduction system installed in a community hospital found that 40,644 infusion starts generated 693 alert messages (1.7%), resulting in 158 programming changes. The 1400 bed hospital projected that if all of their pumps had error reduction systems, in a year more than 1 million infusion starts would result in 18,500 alert messages and 4000 programming changes. All pumps rated "preferred" or "acceptable" by ECRI include dose error-reduction systems, while pumps without such systems are rated "not recommended" for new purchase.[87]

An error programming the concentration of morphine in a patient-controlled analgesia (PCA) pump caused the death of a patient who received a 5-fold overdose of morphine because of the programming error. The authors of the case report made an estimate of the likely death rate from similar programming errors of the particular PCA pump involved in this incident, based on an FDA database and other reports, using a denominator supplied by the pump manufacturer. The estimate was adjusted to take the likely underreporting of incidents into account. Their estimate was a range of 1 death in 33,000 pump uses to 1 in 338,800, amounting to 65 to 667 deaths for 22,000,000 pump uses in the period 1988 through 2000.[88]

While error-reduction systems help to recognize programming errors that may result in an incorrect dose, they do not recognize that a wrong drug has been placed in the pump or that the drug is being administered to the wrong patient. Bar coding may be a solution to this problem. A bar code on a medication bag can be scanned, along with the patient's bar-coded identification, to electronically prompt the pump with the appropriate drug and drug concentration, preventing misidentification of the drug or the patient as well as preventing pump programming errors that can occur during manual entry. Furthermore, if the pump is connected to the electronic medical record (or automated anesthesia record in the operating room), all of the dosing information from the pump can be automatically documented in the record. Application of bar coding to infusion pumps is a relatively new and evolving technology.

Transfusion Safety

Although bar coding of drugs has received greater publicity, bar coding of blood units and the use of bar coding to ensure accurate matching of blood component to recipient are other promising avenues for application of bar coding technology to prevent error. ABO-mismatched transfusion because of administering the wrong blood to a patient is a classic example of a preventable medical error and is a significant cause for concern in the practice of cardiac anesthesia. A study of transfusion errors in New York state estimated the incidence of ABO-mismatched transfusion at 1:12,000 to 1:33,000.[89] A report from a hospital in Japan specializing in cardiovascular disease described a computer-assisted transfusion management system with bar coding at the bedside; 60,000 blood components were transfused without error, and one human error was prevented. The system also improved the efficiency of blood component management, reducing the outdate rate on red blood cells from 3.9% to 0.32%.[90] Bar coding blood components in the operating room could contribute to both efficiency and accuracy, especially if the data from the bar coding operation were automatically entered in a computerized anesthesia record. As noted, in anticipation of bar coding of blood components, the FDA has mandated bar codes on blood products, as well as drugs (http://www.fda.gov/cber/rules/barcodelabel.pdf).

FATIGUE AND ERROR IN CARDIAC ANESTHESIA

Anesthesia care requires maintenance of physiologic stability of the patient, often for prolonged periods of time, by constant synthesis of patient data and appropriate responses to surgical and patient-related events. Vigilance, or sustained attention, by the anesthesiologist is particularly important and is vulnerable to the effects of fatigue,[91] even in the form of a mildly disturbed night.[92] Fatigue has been implicated as a contributor to impaired performance, critical incidents, and errors in anesthesia.[93-95] Although no studies have specifically addressed cardiac anesthesia there is no reason to suspect that errors caused by or contributed to by fatigue are less common. In fact there are several reasons why they may occur more commonly. Cardiac anesthesia involves complex cognitive and psychomotor tasks with the routine use of invasive monitoring and transesophageal echocardiography (TEE) and arguably requires more vigilance than routine anesthesia. Some of the most complex work with the sickest patients (e.g., transplant recipients, urgent institution of mechanical circulatory devices, and patients with aortic dissection) often occurs at night when the anesthesia care team may have already been working all day. There is a requirement for good communication not only with the surgeon but also the perfusionist, who may be impaired by fatigue. In addition, cases are often prolonged, and there may be no other anesthesiologists available to give breaks during the case.

Long working hours and the effects of subsequent fatigue as a contributor to error have received attention in patient safety circles, and this has had implications for hospital workplace practices and policy in many countries.[96-98] This section briefly examines the effects of fatigue on humans and then looks at the effects of fatigue on anesthesia performance and error production. Some of the implications of the increasing recognition of fatigue as a problem in anesthesia are outlined, along with suggestions on limiting and mitigating the effects of fatigue. Finally, the effects of TEE on vigilance during cardiac anesthesia are briefly examined.

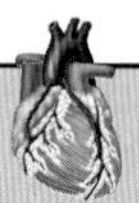

BOX 40–4 ***Reducing Errors Related to Fatigue and Distraction***

- Fatigue may contribute to critical incidents and errors.
- Sleep deprivation impairs psychomotor and cognitive performance.
- Anesthesiologists older than 50 may be more vulnerable to the effects of sleep deprivation and fatigue.
- Operating room logistics and scheduling of personnel should take the demonstrated effects of fatigue and sleep deprivation into account.
- TEE interpretation and monitoring may be a distraction from fundamental patient care.

Effects of Fatigue on Performance

Many effects of sleep deprivation and fatigue on humans have been characterized. According to a meta-analysis of 19 studies by Pilcher and Huffcutt,[99] sleep deprivation "strongly impairs human functioning" (Box 40–4). A single night of sleep loss can produce measurable performance decrements on psychomotor and cognitive tasks that have been described as equivalent to alcohol intoxication.[100] In their review, Howard et al[101] outline some of the effects of sleep deprivation; they include reduced vigilance, impaired decision-making, a progressive slowing in reaction times, impaired memory, impaired communication, the occurrence of "microsleeps" (when fatigued workers have a tendency to fall asleep even for as little as a few seconds at a time), and increased performance variability with cyclic reductions in alertness and performance. Fatigued workers may not be aware of their own performance impairment due in part to reduced alertness, especially if there is no performance feedback from their task.[102] Of particular importance to trainees, learning is impaired by fatigue and sleep debt.[103] Combinations of these factors can create situations where there is increased risk for the occurrence of errors, critical incidents, and accidents.

The effects of fatigue due to both acute and chronic sleep deprivation on performance have been studied in physicians. Most studies have investigated junior medical staff.[101,103-106] While results have shown performance impairment in laboratory or simulator-based performance tests and tasks, it has been difficult to prove a link between fatigue and an increase in medical error in a clinical setting. Most of the studies lack control groups, have small sample sizes with inadequate power, and do not directly examine effects on patient care and medical error. However, a randomized, prospective investigation has clearly documented the effects of fatigue on clinical performance.[107] Reducing weekly work hours and eliminating 24-hour shifts by introducing an extra intern to an intensive care unit roster resulted in a significant reduction in serious medical errors. This occurred despite concerns that continuity of care was impaired by the requirement for extra handovers.

Effects of Fatigue on Errors in Anesthesia

The work hours and schedules of anesthesiologists expose them to circadian disruption and both acute and chronic sleep deprivation, causing fatigue. The performance of anesthesiologists may be more susceptible to the effects of even mild sleep deprivation compared with other medical specialties due to the vigilance required to provide safe anesthesia care. However, study of the effects of fatigue on the clinical performance of anesthesiologists is difficult and to date no clinical studies have shown a definite link between fatigued anesthesiologists and errors.

In a well-designed, realistic, simulation-based trial, Howard et al[108] studied 12 residents who anesthetized a simulated patient for 4 hours in both a sleep-deprived state and a rested state. In the sleep-deprived group, there was a trend to poorer vigilance with slower response to vigilance probes during the simulation. In clinical tasks, the sleep-deprived group took longer to detect and correct abnormal clinical events, but this was not statistically significant. During the simulated anesthetic procedure, nearly one third of the sleep-deprived group fell asleep at some stage.

In an analysis of the first 5700 critical incidents reported to the AIMS database, 2.7% of incidents listed fatigue as a factor contributing to the incident.[94] Drug errors (syringe swaps/wrong drug, underdose, and overdose) were more frequent, and anesthesiologists reported that haste, distraction, inattention, failure to check equipment, fault of technique, and pressure to proceed with surgery were all more common in fatigue-related than in non–fatigue-related incidents. Experience and training did not render an anesthesiologist any less likely to make a fatigue-related error. A healthy patient and relief anesthesiologist/staff change were factors identified that tended to minimize the critical incident. In a survey of 301 anesthesiologists and trainees in New Zealand, 86% responded that they had at some time made an error in patient care related to fatigue[109]; 50% of trainees and 27% of anesthesiologists felt that their average work week exceeded what they believed they could do on an ongoing basis while maintaining patient safety. In addition, the anesthesiologists who exceeded their self-defined safety limits for continuous anesthesia administration (with breaks) or their weekly safe working hours were more likely to report a fatigue-related error in the 6 months prior to the survey compared with those who had not exceeded their limits. The conclusions from these two studies are limited because they are based on retrospective, self-reported data, but the majority of respondents consistently indicated that quality of care was compromised and attributed some errors to working while fatigued.

A Scottish study raised different issues. Flin et al[110] surveyed 222 anesthesiologists. When questioned about stress and fatigue, 83% agreed they were less effective when stressed or tired but 37% thought they performed effectively during the critical phases of operation even when tired. Eighty-four percent had made errors during patient care, but they did not attribute any causation to fatigue and did not list being rested or changing work schedules/reducing work hours as methods for reducing errors. The authors conclude "with regard to attitudes suggesting invulnerability to the effects of stress and fatigue, a significant number of anesthetists were found to show these beliefs" and this "suggests that anesthetists (like pilots) may benefit from additional training in human performance limitations, both in postgraduate education or for consultants through continuing professional development programs."

Sleep quality and quantity become impaired in those around age 50 and older.[111,112] There have been no formal studies assessing whether these changes affect the performance of older anesthesiologists. However, there is reduced tolerance of late-night and shift work with aging.[112] Thus, many of the fatigue-related performance impairments identified in residents are potentially worse in older anesthesiologists.

Changes in Work Practices: Implications and Potential Solutions

Despite the lack of direct evidence for fatigue causing errors in anesthesia practice, many anesthesia regulatory bodies, societies, and government agencies have recognized fatigue as a patient safety issue, and changes in anesthesia work practices have begun to occur. Both the Australian and New Zealand College of Anaesthetists[113] and the Association of Anaesthetists of Great Britain and Ireland[114] have published guidelines with suggestions for limiting the effects of fatigue for both individuals and anesthesia departments. Work hours have been reduced in many countries, with junior staff mostly affected to date. For example, in the United States, the Accreditation Council for Graduate Medical Education imposed limitations on resident work hours in July 2003. Although in many countries junior physicians currently receive the day off after a night of work, the same is not always true of most specialist anesthesiologists, who may be required to work after a disturbed night of sleep. There are implications of these changes at an individual level (e.g., training experience with fewer work hours, importance of handover of care at shift changes) and at a department level (rostering changes and medicolegal and compliance issues). Given the trend to reduced work hours, more staff may be required to staff rosters, with significant financial burdens for hospital anesthesia departments and health services.

Although working at night may contribute to error, the nature of anesthetic work makes it difficult to avoid at least some work during nighttime hours. Therefore, work patterns need to be designed to minimize the possibility of fatigue-related error. These designs should involve consideration of not only total individual work hours but also the importance of the effects of shift work on sleep and circadian rhythm. Useful overviews for individual practitioners on the impact of fatigue on learning and good sleep hygiene to mitigate the impact of fatigue and for departments on the impacts of different rostering systems are available.[101,114-117] Some areas to address to limit fatigue and fatigue-related error in anesthesia providers are shown in Table 40–4.

It is important to emphasize that studies of fatigue and its effects on patient care are needed in the complex domain of cardiac anesthesia. More investigation is also necessary to identify whether error is related to length of work without a break, shift length, or chronic work duration, in addition to the effects of aging and whether the quality of care is interrupted or enhanced by handover of care to another provider.

Effects of the Use of Transesophageal Echocardiography on Vigilance

The introduction and subsequent widespread use of TEE have brought about a major advance in cardiac surgery and anesthesia for both diagnosis and monitoring intraoperatively.

Table 40–4 Some Areas to Address to Limit Fatigue and Fatigue-Related Error in Anesthesia Providers

Individual
Length of time without break
Length of time for shifts
Length of break between shifts
Handover[114,120]
Sleep hygiene education
Education on effects of fatigue on performance and increased likelihood of errors
Naps
Pharmacologic aids (e.g., modafinil[121-124])
Tighten monitor alarm limits after hours
Department
Roster design to limit circadian rhythm disruption
Staffing levels
Stop after-hours or night work for older anesthesiologists
Sleep hygiene education
Use of written protocols/checklists, especially for complex cases after hours
Hospital
Lighting levels after hours
Nap rooms
Food and drink provision
Limit after-hours work to emergency cases

The topics in this table are intended as a starting point for consideration of possible ways in which errors related to fatigue might be reduced. See the text for additional details.

Anecdotally, the authors have noticed times when all attention in the operating room is focused on the TEE machine rather than the patient. This seems to be more noticeable during the phase of learning TEE than with those who are more experienced. The surgical team may also comment that the anesthesia providers are all looking at the TEE rather than the patient. The authors are aware of only one study that has addressed this issue. During a study on task distribution, workload, and vigilance during cardiac anesthesia, Weinger et al[118] found that there was a significant increase in response time to vigilance probes (a light was illuminated on the monitor screen) when the TEE was being manipulated and analyzed compared with times when it was not. The authors concluded that "the use of the TEE may decrease vigilance to changes in other clinical data." Several factors limit the applicability of this study—it involved anesthesia residents with limited cardiac anesthesia experience and limited TEE experience. The operating room setup had the TEE machine placed opposite to the anesthesia machine and monitor display (where the vigilance light was located) and the study involved only 20 cases. The findings of the study were questioned in a subsequent letter to the editor.[119]

This area needs further investigation before definite conclusions can be reached. However, an important factor may be the operating room setup. In particular, where the TEE machine is placed in relation to the patient and the other monitors may be important. To date, there are no studies that address operating room ergonomics with regard to optimizing TEE machine and anesthesia machine setup for ease of reviewing both patient monitors and the TEE machine. The anesthesiologist working alone may be more vulnerable to this problem given that there is only one place on which attention can be focused at a time.

Table 40–5 Influence of Type of Surgery on Severity of Injury*

Injury	Cardiac Surgery, n (%)	Other Surgery, n (%)
Major Category		
Death	75 (31)	1336 (35)
Brain damage	49 (20)†	497 (13)†
Nerve damage	39 (16)	576 (15)
Specific Complications		
Stroke	25 (10)‡	114 (3)‡
Airway injury	13 (5)‡	367 (10)‡
Awareness	15 (6)†	88 (2)†
Myocardial infarction	2 (1)	90 (2)

*American Society of Anesthesiologists Closed Claims database (total N = 6448); table contains only number for surgery under general anesthesia.
†$p < 0.05$ cardiac surgery versus other surgery by *Z*-test.
‡$p < 0.01$ cardiac surgery versus other surgery by *Z*-test.
Cases related to cardiac surgery from the ASA Closed Claims Project database were compared with non–cardiac surgery cases (only cases of general anesthesia were considered).

Table 40–6 Influence of Type of Surgery on Primary Damaging Event*

Damaging Event	Cardiac Surgery, n (%)	Other Surgery, n (%)
Respiratory	26 (11)‡	1189 (31)‡
Cardiovascular	37 (15)	563 (15)
Wrong blood administered	3 (1)	15 (0)
Equipment	75 (31)‡	431 (11)
Peripheral catheter	34 (14)‡	73 (2)‡
Central catheter	16 (7)†	69 (2)†
Adverse drug reaction/drug error	10 (5)	192 (5)
Surgical/patient condition	23 (10)‡	168 (4)‡

*American Society of Anesthesiologists Closed Claims database (total N = 6448); table contains only number for surgery under general anesthesia.
†$p < 0.05$ cardiac surgery versus other surgery by *Z*-test.
‡$p < 0.01$ cardiac surgery versus other surgery by *Z*-test.
Cases related to cardiac surgery from the ASA Closed Claims Project database were compared with non–cardiac surgery cases (only cases of general anesthesia were considered).

AMERICAN SOCIETY OF ANESTHESIOLOGISTS CLOSED CLAIMS PROJECT RESULTS FOR CARDIAC ANESTHESIA

It may be interesting to end this chapter with data describing the problems encountered by cardiac anesthesiologists that resulted in litigation. The American Society of Anesthesiologists Closed Claims Project database contains 250 claims related to cardiac anesthesia. When compared with 3813 other claims for other surgical procedures under general anesthesia, cardiac surgery claims had an increased proportion of claims for brain damage, stroke, and awareness during anesthesia and decreased proportion of claims for airway injury (Table 40–5). The primary damaging event, for example, the specific incident that led to the injury, was more often related to equipment problems, particularly with central or peripheral catheters (Table 40–6). In addition, a greater proportion of cardiac claims were related to surgical technique or patient condition than other surgical claims in the database (see Table 40–6). Approaches for avoiding problems with intraoperative awareness and central venous access have been reviewed in this chapter. Brain damage and stroke during cardiac anesthesia is a vast topic that is addressed elsewhere in this textbook (see Chapters 28, 30, and 35).

REFERENCES

1. Safety of Anaesthesia in Australia: A review of anaesthesia-related mortality 1997-1999. Australian and New Zealand College of Anaesthesia, 2004. Available at *http://www.anzca.edu.au/pdfdocs/mortality97.pdf*
2. Institute of Medicine: To Err Is Human. Building a Safer Health Care System. Washington, DC, National Academy Press, 2000
3. Arnstein F: Catalogue of human error. Br J Anaesth 79:645, 1997
4. Gaba DM, Fish KJ, Howard SK: Crisis Management in Anesthesiology. New York, Churchill Livingstone, 1994, pp 5–53
5. Reason J: Human error: Models and management. BMJ 320:768, 2000
6. McGee DC, Gould MK: Preventing complications of central venous catheterization. N Engl J Med 348:1123, 2003
7. Bowdle T: Complications of invasive monitoring. Anesthesiol Clin North Am 20:333, 2002
8. Polderman KH, Girbes ARJ: Central venous catheter use. Part 1: Mechanical complications. Intensive Care Med 1, 2002
9. Polderman KH, Girbes ARJ: Central venous catheter use. Part 2: Infectious complications. Intensive Care Med 28:18, 2002
10. AHRQ: Making Health Care Safer: A Critical Analysis of Patient Safety Practices. Evidence Report/Technology Assessment: Number 43. AHRQ, 2001, AHRQ Publication No. 01-E058
11. Domino KB, Bowdle TA, Posner KL, et al: Injuries and liability related to central vascular catheters. Anesthesiology 100:1411, 2004
12. Urschel JD, Myerowitz D: Catheter-induced pulmonary artery rupture in the setting of cardiopulmonary bypass. Ann Thorac Surg 56:585, 1993
13. Connors AF, Speroff T, Dawson NV, et al: The effectiveness of right heart catheterization in the initial care of critically ill patients. JAMA 276:889, 1996
14. Dalen JE, Bone RC: Is it time to pull the pulmonary catheter? JAMA 276:916, 1996
15. Isaacson IJ, Lowdon JD, Berry AJ, et al: The value of pulmonary artery and central venous monitoring in patients undergoing abdominal aortic reconstructive surgery: A comparative study of two selected, randomized groups. J Vasc Surg 12:754, 1990
16. Mimoz O, Rauss A, Rekik N, et al: Pulmonary artery catheterization in critically ill patients: A prospective analysis of outcome changes associated with catheter-prompted changes in therapy. Crit Care Med 22:573, 1994
17. Ramsey SD, Saint S, Sullivan SD, et al: Clinical and economic effects of pulmonary artery catheterization in non-emergent coronary artery bypass graft surgery. J Cardiothorac Vasc Anesth 14:113, 2000
18. Tuman KJ, McCarthy RJ, Spiess BD, et al: Effect of pulmonary artery catheterization on outcome in patients undergoing coronary artery surgery. Anesthesiology 70:199, 1989
19. Bashein G, Johnson PW, Davis KB, et al: Elective coronary bypass surgery without pulmonary artery catheter monitoring. Anesthesiology 63:451, 1985
20. Bender JS, Smith-Meek MA, Jones CE: Routine pulmonary artery catheterization does not reduce morbidity and mortality of elective vascular surgery: Results of a prospective, randomized trial. Ann Surg 226:229, 1997
21. Coles NA, Hibberd M, Russell M, et al: Potential impact of pulmonary artery catheter placement on short-term management decisions in the medical intensive care unit. Am Heart J 126:815, 1993
22. Mueller HS, Chatterjee K, Davis KB, et al: Present use of bedside right heart catheterization in patients with cardiac disease. JACC 32:840, 1998
23. Richard C, Warszawski J, Anguel N, et al: Early use of the pulmonary artery catheter and outcomes in patients with shock and acute respiratory distress syndrome: A randomized controlled trial. JAMA 290:2713, 2003
24. Sandham JD, Hull RD, Brant RF, et al: A randomized, controlled trial of the use of pulmonary-artery catheters in high-risk surgical patients. N Engl J Med 348:5, 2003
25. Bar-Joseph G, Galvis AG: Perforation of the heart by central venous catheters in infants: Guidelines to diagnosis and management. J Pediatr Surg 18:284, 1983
26. Brandt RL, Foley WJ, Fink GH, et al: Mechanism of perforation of the heart with production of hydropericardium by a venous catheter and its prevention. Am J Surg 119:311, 1970
27. Collier PE, Ryan JJ, Diamond DL: Cardiac tamponade from central venous catheters—A report of a case and review of English literature. Angiology 35:595, 1984
28. Jiha JG, Weinberg GL, Laurito CE: Intraoperative cardiac tamponade after central venous cannulation. Anesth Analg 82:664, 1996
29. Maschke SP, Rogove HJ: Cardiac tamponade associated with a multilumen central venous catheter. Crit Care Med 12:611, 1984
30. Scott WL: Complications associated with central venous catheters. Chest 94:1221 , 1988
31. Sheep RE, Guiney WB: Fatal cardiac tamponade: Occurrence with other complications after left internal jugular vein catheterization. JAMA 248:1632, 1982
32. Tocino IM, Watanabe A: Impending catheter perforation of superior vena cava: Radiographic recognition. AJR Am J Roentgenol 146:487, 1986
33. Trigaux JP, Goncette L, Van Beers B, et al: Radiologic findings of normal and compromised thoracic venous catheters. J Thorac Imaging 9:246, 1994
34. Fletcher SJ, Bodenham AR: Safe placement of central venous catheters: Where should the tip of the catheter lie? Br J Anaesth 85:188, 2000
35. Albrecht K, Nave H, Breitmeir D, et al: Applied anatomy of the superior vena cava—The carina as a landmark to guide central venous catheter placement. Br J Anaesth 92:75, 2004
36. Schuster M, Nave H, Piepenbrock S, et al: The carina as a landmark in central venous catheter placement. Br J Anaesth 85:192, 2000
37. Jobes DR, Schwartz AJ, Greenhow DE, et al: Safer jugular vein cannulation: Recognition of arterial puncture and preferential use of the external jugular route. Anesthesiology 59:353, 1983
38. Troianos CA, Kuwik R, Pasqual J, et al. Internal jugular vein and carotid artery anatomic relation as determined by ultrasonography. Anesthesiology 85:43, 1996
39. Randolph AG, Cook DJ, Gonzales CA, et al: Ultrasound guidance for placement of central venous catheters: A meta-analysis of the literature. Crit Care Med 24:2053, 1996
40. Hind D, Calvert N, McWilliams R, et al: Ultrasonic locating devices for central venous cannulation: Meta-analysis. BMJ 327:361, 2003
41. National Institute for Clinical Excellence: Guidance on the use of ultrasound locating devices for placing central venous catheters. National Institute for Clinical Excellence, 2005, Available at http://www.nice.org.uk/pdf/Ultrasound_49_GUIDANCE.pdf
42. Calvert N, Hind D, McWilliams RG, et al: The effectiveness and cost-effectiveness of ultrasound locating devices for central venous access: A systematic review. Health Technol Assess 7:2003
43. Oropello JM, Leibowitz AB, Manasia A, et al: Dilator-associated complications of central vein catheter insertion: Possible mechanisms of injury and suggestions for prevention. J Cardiothorac Vasc Anesth 10:634, 1996
44. Welliver MD, Masoud PJ: Thoracic duct cannulation during central venous catheterization: A case report. Am J Anesthesiol 28:199, 2001
45. Raad II, Bodey GP: Infectious complications of indwelling vascular catheters. Clin Infect Dis 15:197, 1992
46. Mermel LA, Maki DG: Infectious complications of Swan-Ganz pulmonary artery catheters. Pathogenesis, epidemiology, prevention and management. Am J Respir Crit Care Med 149:1020, 1994
47. Sandin RH, Enlund G, Samuelsson P, et al: Awareness during anaesthesia: A prospective case study. Lancet 355:707, 2000
48. Sebel PS, Bowdle TA, Ghoneim MM, et al: The incidence of awareness during anesthesia: A multicenter United States study. Anesth Analg 99:833, 2004
49. Domino KB, Posner KL, Caplan RA, et al: Awareness during anesthesia: A closed claims analysis. Anesthesiology 90:1053, 1999
50. Ranta SO-V, Hernanen P, Hynynen M: Patient's conscious recollections from cardiac anesthesia. J Cardiothorac Vasc Anesth 16:426, 2002
51. Ranta S, Jussila J, Hynynen M: Recall of awareness during cardiac anesthesia: Influence of feedback information to the anesthesiologist. Acta Anaesthesiol Scand 40:554, 1996
52. Dowd NP, Cheng DCH, Karski JM, et al: Intraoperative awareness in fast-track cardiac anesthesia. Anesthesiology 89:1068, 1998
53. Phillips AA, McLean RF, Devitt JH, et al: Recall of intraoperative events after general anaesthesia and cardiopulmonary bypass. Can J Anaesth 40:922, 1993

54. Myles PS, Leslie K, McNeil J, et al: Bispectral index monitoring to prevent awareness during anaesthesia: The B-Aware randomized controlled trial. Lancet 1757, 2004
55. Osterman JE, Hopper J, Heran WJ, et al: Awareness under anesthesia and the development of posttraumatic stress disorder. Gen Hosp Psychiatry 23:198, 2001
56. Moerman N, Bonke B, Oosting J: Awareness and recall during general anesthesia. Facts and feelings. Anesthesiology 79:454, 1993
57. Bowdle TA: The Bispectral Index (BIS): An update. Curr Rev Clin Anesth 25:17, 2004
58. Glass PS, Bloom M, Kearse L, et al: Bispectral analysis measures sedation and memory effects of propofol, midazolam, isoflurane, and alfentanil in healthy volunteers. Anesthesiology 86:836, 1997
59. Islein-Chaves IA, Flaishon R, Sebel PS, et al: The effect of the interaction of propofol and alfentanil on recall, loss of consciousness, and the bispectral index. 87:949, 1998
60. Kalkman CJ, Drummond J: Monitors of depth of anesthesia, quo vadis? Anesthesiology 96:784, 2002
61. Gan T, Glass P, Windsor A, et al: Bispectral index monitoring allows faster emergence and improved recovery from propofol, alfentanil and nitrous oxide anesthesia. Anesthesiology 87:808, 1997
62. Liu SS: Effects of bispectral index monitoring on ambulatory anesthesia. A meta-analysis of randomized controlled trials and a cost analysis. Anesthesiology 101:311, 2004
63. Ekman A, Lindholm M-L, Lennmarken C, et al: Reduction in the incidence of awareness using BIS monitoring. Acta Anaesthesiol Scand 48:20, 2004
64. Rampil IJ, Kim JS, Lenhardt R, et al: Bispectral EEG index during nitrous oxide administration. Anesthesiology 89:671, 1998
65. Nieuwenhuijs D, Coleman EL, Douglas NJ, et al: Bispectral index values and spectral edge frequency at different stages of physiologic sleep. Anesth Analg 94:125, 2002
66. Sebel PS, Lang E, Rampil IJ, et al: A multicenter study of bispectral electroencephalogram analysis for monitoring anesthetic effect. Anesth Analg 84:891, 1997
67. Bouillon TW, Bruhn J, Radulescu L, et al: Pharmacodynamic interaction between propofol and remifentanil regarding hypnosis, tolerance of laryngoscopy, bispectral index, and electroencephalographic approximate entropy. Anesthesiology 100:1353, 2004
68. Bates DW, Cullen DJ, Laird N, et al: Incidence of adverse drug events and potential adverse drug events: Implications for prevention. JAMA 274:29, 1995
69. Taxis K, Barber N: Incidence and severity of intravenous drug errors in a German hospital. Eur J Clin Pharmacol 59:815, 2004
70. Reducing and preventing adverse drug events to decrease hospital costs. Research in Action, Issue 1 AHRQ Publication No. 01, March 2001
71. Currie M, Mackay P, Morgan C, et al: The "wrong drug" problem in anaesthesia: An analysis of 2000 incident reports. Anaesth Intens Care 21:596, 1993
72. Merry AF, Peck DJ: Anaesthetists, errors in drug administration and the law. NZ Med J 108:185, 1995
73. Webster CS, Merry AF, Larsson L, et al: The frequency and nature of drug administration error during anaesthesia. Anaesth Intensive Care 29:494, 2001
74. Orser BA, Chen RJB, Yee DA: Medication errors in anesthetic practice: A survey of 687 practitioners. Can J Anesth 48:139, 2001
75. Bowdle A, Kruger C, Grieve R, et al: Anesthesia drug administration errors in a university hospital. Anesthesiology 99:A1358, 2003
76. Bowdle TA: Drug administration errors from the ASA Closed Claims Project. Am Soc Anesthes Newsletter 67:11, 2003
77. Orser BA, Oxorn DC: An anaesthetic drug error: Minimizing the risk. Can J Anaesth 41:120, 1994
78. Svenmarker S, Soren H, Jansson E, et al: Quality assurance in clinical perfusion. Eur J Cardiothorac Surg 14:409, 1998
79. Jenkins OF, Morris R, Simpson JM: Australasian perfusion incident survey. Perfusion 12:279, 1997
80. Mejak BL, Stammers A, Rauch E, et al: A retrospective study on perfusion incidents and safety devices. Perfusion 15:51, 2000
81. Stammers A, Mejak BL: An update on perfusion safety: Does the type of perfusion practice affect the rate of incidents related to cardiopulmonary bypass? Perfusion 16:189, 2001
82. Jensen LS, Merry AF, Webster CS, et al: Evidence-based strategies for preventing drug administration errors during anaesthesia. Anaesthesia 59:493, 2004
83. ECRI: Bar-coded medication administration (BCMA) systems: Future promise, present challenges. Health Devices 32:373, 2003
84. Merry AF, Webster CS, Mathew DJ: A new, safety-oriented, integrated drug administration and automated anesthesia record system. Anesth Analg 93:385, 2001
85. Webster CS, Merry AF, Gander PH, et al: A prospective, randomized clinical evaluation of a new safety-oriented injectable drug administration system in comparison with conventional methods. Anaesthesia 59:80, 2004
86. New perspectives on general-purpose infusion pumps. Advances in the technology, changes in our ratings. Health Devices 31:354, 2002
87. Eye on medical errors: Dose error reduction systems—A valuable tool for reducing IV medication errors. Health Devices 31:356, 2002
88. Vicente KJ, Kada-Bekhaled K, Hillel G, et al: Programming errors contribute to death from patient-controlled analgesia: Case report and estimate of probability. Can J Anesth 50:328, 2003
89. Linden JV, Paul B, Dressler KP: A report of 104 transfusion errors in New York State. Transfusion 32:601, 1992
90. Miyata S, Kawai T, Yamamoto S, et al: Network computer-assisted transfusion-management system for accurate blood component-recipient identification at the bedside. Transfusion 44:364, 2004
91. Denisco RA, Drummond JN, Gravenstein JS: The effect of fatigue on the performance of a simulated anesthetic monitoring task. J Clin Monit 3:22, 1987
92. Murray D, Dodds C: The effect of sleep disruption on performance of anaesthetists. A pilot study. Anaesthesia 58:520, 2003
93. Williamson JA, Webb RK, Sellen A, et al: The Australian Incident Monitoring Study. Human failure: An analysis of 2000 incident reports. Anaesth Intensive Care 21:678, 1993
94. Morris GP, Morris RW: Anaesthesia and fatigue: An analysis of the first 10 years of the Australian Incident Monitoring Study 1987-1997. Anaesth Intensive Care 28:300, 2000
95. Gravenstein JS, Cooper JB, Orkin FK: Work and rest cycles in anesthesia practice. Anesthesiology 72:737, 1990
96. Accreditation Council for Graduate Medical Education: Resident duty hours and the working environment. Accreditation Council for Graduate Medical Education, 2004. Available at http://www.acgme.org/acWebsite/dutyHours/dh_Lang703.pdf
97. Council of the European Union: Council Directive 93/104/EC of 23 November 1993 concerning certain aspects of the organization of working time. Council of the European Union, 1993. Available at http://europe.osha.eu.int/legislation/directives/leg2.php3?cat_id=3.1&ctab=cat_a
98. Australian Medical Association: National Code of Practice—Hours of Work, Shiftwork and Rostering for Hospital Doctors. Kingston, ACT, Australian Medical Association, 1999
99. Pilcher JJ, Huffcutt AI: Effects of sleep deprivation on performance: A meta-analysis. Sleep 19:318, 1996
100. Dawson D, Reid K: Fatigue, alcohol and performance impairment. Nature 388:235, 1997
101. Howard SK, Rosekind MR, Katz JD, et al: Fatigue in anesthesia: Implications and strategies for patient and provider safety. Anesthesiology 97:1281, 2002
102. Dorrian J, Lamond N, Holmes AL, et al: The ability to self-monitor performance during a week of simulated night shifts. Sleep 26:871, 2003
103. Buysse DJ, Barzansky B, Dinges D, et al: Sleep, fatigue, and medical training: Setting an agenda for optimal learning and patient care. Sleep 26:218, 2003
104. Gaba DM, Howard SK: Fatigue among clinicians and the safety of patients. N Engl J Med 347:1249, 2002
105. Fletcher KE, Davis SQ, Underwood W, et al: Systematic review: Effects of resident work hours on patient safety. Ann Intern Med 141:851, 2004
106. Owens JA, Veasey SC, Rosen RC: Physician, heal thyself: Sleep, fatigue, and medical education. Sleep 24:493, 2001
107. Landrigan CP, Rothschild JM, Cronin JW, et al: Effect of reducing interns' work hours on serious medical errors in intensive care units. N Engl J Med 351:1838, 2004
108. Howard SK, Gaba DM, Smith BE, et al: Simulation study of rested versus sleep-deprived anesthesiologists. Anesthesiology 98:1345; discussion 5A, 2003
109. Gander PH, Merry A, Millar MM, et al: Hours of work and fatigue-related error: A survey of New Zealand anaesthetists. Anaesth Intensive Care 28:178, 2000
110. Flin R, Fletcher G, McGeorge P, et al: Anaesthetists' attitudes to teamwork and safety. Anaesthesia 58:233, 2003
111. Kryger M, Monjan A, Bliwise D, et al: Sleep, health, and aging. Bridging the gap between science and clinical practice. Geriatrics 59:24, 29, 2004
112. Reilly T, Waterhouse J, Atkinson G: Aging, rhythms of physical performance, and adjustment to changes in the sleep-activity cycle. Occup Environ Med 54:812, 1997

113. Australian and New Zealand College of Anaesthetists: PS 43: Statement on fatigue and the anaesthetist. Australian and New Zealand College of Anaesthetists, 2001. Available at http://www.anzca.edu.au/pdfdocs/PS43_2001.pdf
114. Association of Anaesthetists of Great Britain and Ireland: Fatigue and anaesthetists: London, Association of Anaesthetists of Great Britain and Ireland, 2004. Available at http://www.aagbi.org/pdf/Fatigue.pdf
115. Anonymous: Shift work, the anaesthetist and Santayana's warning. Anaesthesia 59:735, 2004
116. Australian Medical Association: Best Practice Rostering: Training and Resource Kit. Practical Tools for Rostering Doctors. Kingston, ACT. Australian Medical Association, 2004. Available at http://www.ama.com.au/web.nsf/doc/WEEN-5QM2U4
117. Jha A, Duncan B, Bates D: Chapter 46. Fatigue, sleepiness and medical errors. Making health care safer: A critical analysis of patient safety practices. Evidence Report/Technology Assessment: No. 43. AHRQ Publication No. 01-E058. Agency for Healthcare Research and Quality, 2004. Available at http://www.ahrq.gov/clinic/ptsafety/
118. Weinger MB, Herndon OW, Gaba DM: The effect of electronic record keeping and transesophageal echocardiography on task distribution, workload, and vigilance during cardiac anesthesia. Anesthesiology 87:144, 1997
119. Aronson S, Cook R: Vigilance—A main component of clinical quality. Anesthesiology 88:1122, 1998
120. Australian and New Zealand College of Anaesthetists: PS 10: Guidelines on the handover of responsibility during an anaesthetic. Australian and New Zealand College of Anaesthetists, 2004. Available at http://www.anzca.edu.au/pdfdocs/PS10_2004.pdf
121. Batejat DM, Lagarde DP: Naps and modafinil as countermeasures for the effects of sleep deprivation on cognitive performance. Aviat Space Environ Med 70:493, 1999
122. Buguet A, Montmayeur A, Pigeau R, et al: Modafinil, d-amphetamine and placebo during 64 hours of sustained mental work. II. Effects on two nights of recovery sleep. J Sleep Res 4:229, 1995
123. Caldwell JA, Caldwell JL, Smith JK, et al: Modafinil's effects on simulator performance and mood in pilots during 37 hours without sleep. Aviat Space Environ Med 75:777, 2004
124. Caldwell JA Jr, Caldwell JL, Smythe NK, 3rd, et al: A double-blind, placebo-controlled investigation of the efficacy of modafinil for sustaining the alertness and performance of aviators: A helicopter simulator study. Psychopharmacology (Berl) 150:272, 2000

Chapter 41

CARDIAC ANESTHESIA: TRAINING, QUALIFICATIONS, TEACHING, AND LEARNING

Alan Jay Schwartz, MD, MSEd

KEY POINTS

1. Education is change in behavior based on experience. The fact that 64.4 million Americans present with one or more types of cardiovascular disease (CVD) and that an estimated 6,188,000 inpatient cardiovascular operations and procedures were performed in the United States in 2001 speaks directly to the point that anesthesiologists treating patients with CVD have vast experience that requires and results in considerable education.
2. The complexity of many cardiothoracic diseases requires that there be a cadre of specialty educated cardiothoracic anesthesiologists. Specialty educated cardiothoracic anesthesiologists care for the more complex patients and they are the individuals who educate residents about these special patients.
3. Essential ingredients of clinical cardiothoracic anesthesiology fellowship education are completion of a 3-year core residency in anesthesiology followed by an additional minimum 1-year clinical training program during which an exhaustive list of didactic topics for study is coupled with mastery of an inclusive set of psychomotor skills, including basic and advanced perioperative echocardiography.
4. Through concentrated full immersion in a minimum 1-year clinical fellowship devoted exclusively to cardiothoracic anesthesiology, an anesthesiologist will be able to gain sufficient and sophisticated knowledge and skill to be a subspecialist able to care for patients with very high acuity CVD. In similar fashion, it will only be through accredited fellowship education that subspecialists in cardiac anesthesiology will be on a par with the large number of fellowship-educated cardiologists, cardiothoracic surgeons, and all other medical, pediatric, surgical, and diagnostic subspecialists who care for patients with CVD.
5. Being a "qualified" cardiothoracic anesthesiologist implies having met standard criteria and complied with specified requirements. These requirements may include one, two, or all three of the following: (1) having successfully completed postgraduate medical education in an accredited training program, (2) having successfully completed a certification process (examination) when available, and (3) being credentialed and granted clinical privileges to practice within the scope of the subspecialty within a health care facility.
6. The ABA Oral Examination process is designed "to assess the candidate's ability to demonstrate the attributes of an ABA Diplomate [understand and apply complex cognitive functions] when managing patients presented in clinical scenarios. The attributes are sound judgment in decision-making and management of surgical and anesthetic complications, appropriate application of scientific principles to clinical problems, adaptability to unexpected changes in the clinical situations, and logical organization and effective presentation of information. The oral examination emphasizes the scientific rationale underlying clinical management decisions."[21]
7. Simulation is imitation of real-life clinical situations using stand-in devices that assume the patient role, providing learner experience while permitting teaching and learning in repetitive fashion with zero risk to both the provider and recipient of the simulated care.
8. Simulation adds sophisticated aspects to education that are not possible from traditional textbook learning, classroom lectures, or single-learner computer-based programs. These missing ingredients are teamwork and improved processes of care, including, among others, interpersonal communication, situational awareness, appropriate management of available patient care resources, fatigue management, adverse event recognition, team decision-making, and performance feedback.
9. Improved patient outcome from simulation education is intuitively obvious, yet scant evidence-based medicine exists to prove this.
10. Student evaluation will be meaningless without the ability to (1) provide the resident/fellow constructive feedback, on as frequent a basis as daily, and (2) have the faculty attest to the resident's/fellow's competence at the completion of the educational process.
11. Collection of data about an individual faculty member's "teaching abilities, commitment to the educational program, clinical knowledge, and scholarly activities"[2] arms the chair with ammunition for constructive suggestions for change of teaching techniques by the faculty member.
12. Resident performance on certification examinations and review of patient care data are prime educational assessment techniques for educational program evaluation. A department's and its institutional continuous quality improvement programs serve as effective analysis methods for documenting the success of the educational program and clinical care provided to patients by ongoing review of data showing that unacceptable morbidity and mortality are not present and that the educational program does not result in and in fact may improve these parameters.

Is cardiovascular disease (CVD) an issue that the anesthesiologist must be aware of, educated about, and qualified to deal with clinically? A very obvious and resounding "yes" is the answer to this question. Anesthesiologists are confronted with the patient care dilemmas posed by the presence of CVD as a primary or comorbid diagnosis in an enormous number of patients spanning all age groups. Consider the following CVD statistics for the United States, as compiled and published in the American Heart Association's Heart Disease and Stroke Statistics—2004 Update.[1]

I. PREVALENCE

Some 64.4 million Americans have one or more types of cardiovascular disease (CVD); 25.3 million are estimated to be age 65 and older; one in five has CVD.[1]

A. High blood pressure—50 million (defined as systolic pressure 140 mm Hg or greater and/or diastolic pressure 90 mm Hg or greater, or taking antihypertensive medication)
B. Coronary heart disease—13.2 million
Myocardial infarction (heart attack)—7.8 million
Angina pectoris (chest pain)—6.8 million
C. Congestive heart failure—5 million
D. Stroke—4.8 million
E. Congenital cardiovascular defects—1 million

II. INCIDENCE

A. The average annual rates of first major cardiovascular events rise from 7 per 1000 men at ages 35 to 44 to 68 per 1000 at ages 85 to 94.
B. The aging of the population will undoubtedly result in an increased incidence of chronic diseases, including coronary artery disease (CAD), heart failure, and stroke; the U.S. census estimates that there will be 40 million Americans aged 65 and older in 2010.
C. There has been an explosive increase in the prevalence of obesity and type 2 diabetes. Their related complications—hypertension, hyperlipidemia, and atherosclerotic vascular disease—also have increased.

III. MORTALITY

A. CVD accounted for 38.5% of all deaths, or 1 of every 2.6 deaths in the United States in 2001. CVD mortality was about 60% of "total mortality." This means that of over 2,400,000 deaths from all causes, CVD was listed as a primary or contributing cause on about 1,408,000 death certificates.
B. Since 1900, CVD has been the No. 1 killer in the United States every year except 1918. Nearly 2600 Americans die of CVD each day, an average of one death every 34 seconds. CVD claims more lives each year than the next five leading causes of death combined, which are cancer, chronic lower respiratory diseases, accidents, diabetes mellitus, and influenza and pneumonia.

IV. HOSPITAL/PHYSICIAN/NURSING HOME VISITS

A. From 1979 to 2001, the number of Americans discharged from short-stay hospitals with CVD as the first listed diagnosis increased 27%. In 2001, CVD ranked highest among all disease categories in hospital discharges.
B. In 2001, there were 4,214,000 visits to emergency departments with a primary diagnosis of CVD.

V. COST

A. In 2004, the estimated direct and indirect cost of CVD was $368.4 billion.[1]

VI. OPERATIONS AND PROCEDURES

A. In 2001, an estimated 6,188,000 inpatient cardiovascular operations and procedures were performed in the United States; 3.6 million were performed on males and 2.6 million were performed on females.[1]
B. If the focus is on CAD alone, the statistics highlight the same striking message. In 2001, an estimated 1,051,000 angioplasty procedures, 516,000 coronary artery bypass grafting (CABG) procedures, 1,314,000 diagnostic cardiac catheterizations, 46,000 implantable defibrillators, and 177,000 pacemaker procedures were performed in the United States.[1]
C. CVD is not only a geriatric phenomenon. Congenital heart disease (CHD) is a major issue for the pediatric anesthesiologist. In addition, an ever-increasing number of patients with CHD are living longer after surgical palliation or repair, forming an adult CHD population that presents for anesthetic care for surgical and nonsurgical therapeutic and diagnostic procedures.
D. Incidence of CHD is 9.0 defects per 1000 live births, or 36,000 babies per year in the United States. Of these, several studies suggest that 9200, or 2.3 per 1000 live births, require invasive treatment or result in death in the first year of life.[1]
E. In 2000, over 25,000 cardiovascular operations for CHD were performed on children less than 20 years of age.
F. In 2000, over 130,000 hospitalizations occurred in infants or children with congenital CVD; hospital charges were $6.5 billion.[1]

With statistics such as those listed, there is quite a compelling argument that being aware of, educated about, and qualified to deal with patients with CVD are essential for all anesthesiologists. *The complexity of many of the cardiothoracic diseases also requires that there be a cadre of specialty educated cardiothoracic anesthesiologists.* Specialty-educated cardiothoracic anesthesiologists care for the more complex patients and they are the individuals who educate residents about these special patients. The Anesthesiology Residency Review Committee (RRC) is quite clear about this in its statement defining *faculty* in the program requirements for graduate medical education (GME) in anesthesiology[2]:

> The faculty should have varying interests, capabilities, and backgrounds, and must include individuals who have specialized expertise in the subspecialties of anesthesiology, which includes but is not limited to . . . cardiothoracic anesthesia. . . . Didactic and clinical teaching must be provided by faculty with documented interests and expertise in the subspecialty involved. Fellowship training, several years of practice (primarily within a subspecialty), and membership and active participation in national organizations related to the subspecialty may signify expertise.[2]

It is these same specialists who conduct the basic science and clinical research that advances new knowledge and understanding of CVD and its anesthetic implications. What is the education available and required for cardiothoracic anesthesiologists?

FORMALIZED TRAINING OF CARDIOTHORACIC ANESTHESIOLOGISTS

The continuum of education in anesthesiology is defined by the Accreditation Council for Graduate Medical Education (ACGME)[2] and the American Board of Anesthesiology (ABA).[3] The continuum begins with an initial 4 years of post-graduate (post–medical school) education and constitutes the "core" anesthesiology residency.

Clinical Base Year

The first year is a clinical nonanesthesiology year. According to the ACGME, "the clinical base year should provide the resident with 12 months of broad education in medical disciplines relevant to the practice of anesthesiology."[2] According to the ABA, "The clinical base year must include at least ten months of patients with a variety of medical and surgical problems, of which at most one month may involve the administration of anesthesia. At most two months of the clinical base year may involve training in specialties or subspecialties that do not meet the aforementioned criteria."[3]

Clinical Anesthesia Years

The next 3 years are clinical anesthesiology years, providing ". . . training in basic and advanced anesthesia [to] encompass all aspects of perioperative care to include evaluation and management during the preoperative, intraoperative, and postoperative periods."[2] "The three-year clinical anesthesia curriculum (CA 1-3) consists of experience in basic anesthesia training, subspecialty anesthesia training, and advanced anesthesia training. It is a graded curriculum of increasing difficulty and learning that is progressively more challenging of the resident's intellect and technical skills."[3]

The ability to provide extensive specialized education in cardiac anesthesiology during the core residency is restricted primarily due to the time-limited nature of clinical anesthesia training, that is, a total of 36 months. Cardiac anesthesiology education commonly occurs during the CA-1 or CA-2 year and is similar in emphasis to all of the fundamental subspecialties:

> Anesthesiology encompasses the theoretical background and clinical practice of a variety of subspecialty disciplines. Exposure to these should occupy a minimum of 7 months [19% of the required 36 month clinical anesthesia education] . . . There must be [an] identifiable 1-month [rotation] [3% of the required 36 month clinical anesthesia education] . . . in . . . cardiothoracic anesthesia. Experiences in perioperative care must include a 2-month rotation in critical care. . . .[2]

The goals, timing, and *minimum required perioperative clinical experiences in cardiothoracic anesthesiology* include:

> A wide spectrum of disease processes and surgical procedures . . . available within the program to provide each resident with broad exposure to different types of anesthetic management. The following list represents the minimum clinical experience that should be obtained by each resident in the program. Although the minimum requirements are for the CA-1 through CA-3 years, the majority of these should be accomplished in the CA-1 and CA-2 years. . . .
>
> c) Anesthesia for 20 patients undergoing surgical procedures involving cardiopulmonary bypass.
>
> d) Twenty other major vascular cases (including endovascular cases). . . .
>
> e) Twenty intrathoracic (thoracotomy, thoracoscopy) noncardiac cases . . .
>
> n) Significant experience with certain specialized techniques for airway management (such as fiberoptic intubation, double lumen endotracheal tube placement . . .), central vein catheter placement, pulmonary artery catheter placement, peripheral artery cannulation, transesophageal echocardiography. . . .[2]

There is an opportunity for more extensive education about cardiac anesthesiology in the last year of core residency education:

> Clinical assignments in the CA-3 year must include difficult or complex anesthesia procedures and the care of seriously ill patients. Subspecialty rotations are encouraged, but none may be longer than 6 months. This curriculum must be distinct from the CA-1 and CA-2 years' subspecialty curricula, and must reflect increased responsibility and learning opportunities. These assignments must not compromise the learning opportunities for the CA-1 and CA-2 residents.[2]

More extensive education about cardiac anesthesiology in the CA-3 year would be most appropriate for those practitioners electing to subspecialize; however, the CA-3, 6-month subspecialty education option is out of vogue. In 1988–1989, the ABA extended the core anesthesiology residency to a compulsory CA-3 year. In 1989–1990, 56% (606 of 1084) of CA-3 residents elected more than 6 months of subspecialty training (all anesthesiology subspecialties are represented in this composite number).[4,5] By 1993–1994, only 29%, by 1995–1996, only 21%, and by 2000–2001, a mere 6% (66 of 1043) elected more than 6 months of subspecialty training in the CA-3 year.[4,5] At the same time that CA-3 subspecialty education was becoming rare, the absolute number and percentage of total CA-4 residents who electively enrolled in a 12-month postresidency fellowship program increased (1989–1990, 63 of 105 [60%]; 1998–1999, 523 of 605 [86%]; and 2000–2001, 383 of 525 [73%] CA-4 residents enrolled in a 12-month subspecialty fellowship).[4,5]

It is quite apparent from the residency curriculum outlined above that a graduating core resident will most likely be modestly educated as a specialist cardiac anesthesiologist. More complete subspecialty education is provided through a fellowship (minimum 1-year clinical Graduate Medical Education [GME] program) that follows the core residency. Over the years, an increasing number of individuals have elected CA-4 cardiac anesthesiology subspecialty fellowship education (in 2000–2001, 69 of 383 [18%] CA-4 residents selected cardiac anesthesiology as their fellowship track).[4] These data blend well with the fact that many other medical, surgical, and diagnostic disciplines offer accredited fellowship education to develop so-called subspecialists in their respective specialties. Accredited subspecialty graduate education programs of a year or more in duration exist in anesthesiology and medical, pediatric, surgical, and diagnostic disciplines related to cardiac anesthesiology[6,7] (Table 41–1).

At the same time that the number of CA-3 residents electing cardiac anesthesiology subspecialty education was dwindling and becoming almost nonexistent, and the number of CA-4 residents electing a full 1-year cardiac anesthesiology fellowship was increasing dramatically, standardized cardiothoracic anesthesiology fellowship education did not exist. Standardized and accredited anesthesiology fellowship subspecialty education in critical care, pain management, and pediatric anesthesiology exists. An Anesthesiology RRC–developed standardized curriculum in cardiac anesthesiology

Table 41–1 Number of Resident Physicians (Fellows) on Duty August 1, 2003,[6] in Selected ACGME-Accredited Subspecialty and Combined Specialty GME Programs Related to Cardiothoracic Anesthesiology (Anesthesiology Subspecialty Programs for Comparison)

Specialty/Subspecialty	No. of Programs	No. of Fellows
Internal medicine		
Cardiovascular disease	173	2061
Clinical cardiac electrophysiology	78	97
Critical care medicine	31	146
Pulmonary disease	30	97
Pulmonary disease and critical care medicine	122	1007
Pediatrics		
Pediatric cardiology	48	244
Pediatric critical care medicine	58	254
Pediatric pulmonary	46	100
Radiology-diagnostic		
Cardiothoracic radiology	1	0
Vascular and interventional radiology	103	118
Surgery		
Surgical critical care	82	90
Thoracic surgery	93	303
Subtotal	865	4,517
Anesthesiology		
Critical care medicine	50	43
Pediatric anesthesiology	43	119
Total*	8192	99,964

*Resident physicians (fellows) on duty in all ACGME-accredited and combined specialty GME programs August 1, 2003.[6]

has been resisted for many years. Reluctance to accredit specialty education in cardiac anesthesiology relates to a desire to avoid creating divisions in clinical practice among anesthesiologists. It has been reasoned that all anesthesiologists care for patients with CVD; therefore, all anesthesiologists need and gain, through core residency education, the requisite knowledge and skills. The data cited above negate this supposition.

The Society of Cardiovascular Anesthesiologists (SCA) has championed a different viewpoint.[8] The SCA reasoned that while it is true that all anesthesiologists care for patients with cardiac disease, there has developed, over the past 20 to 30 years, a highly sophisticated knowledge base (e.g., physiology of deep hypothermic circulatory arrest, clinical management of anticoagulation, anesthetic management of patients undergoing electrophysiologic diagnostic and therapeutic procedures, and physiologic management of mechanical assist devices bridging to heart and lung transplantation) and a technically demanding set of psychomotor skills (e.g., pulmonary artery catheterization, intra-aortic balloon counterpulsation, and transesophageal echocardiography) that enables the safe and effective care of patients with very high acuity CVD.

Cardiothoracic anesthesiology has blossomed into a subdiscipline that exists adjunctively to the core discipline of anesthesiology. More than 6500 anesthesiologists (approximately 18% of the total American Society of Anesthesiologists [ASA] membership) are SCA members identifying themselves as individuals who recognize that cardiac anesthesiology constitutes more than the basic discipline of anesthesiology. Scientific and educational meetings to disseminate this subspecialty knowledge and develop practice protocols and research programs and projects devoted specifically to cardiac anesthesiology exist to serve the needs of these subspecialists.[8]

SCA believes that only through concentrated full immersion in a minimum 1-year clinical fellowship devoted exclusively to cardiothoracic anesthesiology will an anesthesiologist be able to gain sufficient and sophisticated enough knowledge and skill to be a subspecialist able to care for patients with very high acuity CVD. In similar fashion, it will only be through accredited fellowship education that subspecialists in cardiac anesthesiology will be on a par with the large number of fellowship-educated cardiologists, cardiothoracic surgeons, and all other medical, pediatric, surgical, and diagnostic subspecialists who care for patients with CVD (see Table 41–1).

Draft program requirements for standardized cardiothoracic anesthesiology fellowship education have been recommended by the SCA[9] (Appendix 41–1). *The recommended essential ingredients of clinical cardiothoracic anesthesiology fellowship education are a minimum one-year time frame during which an exhaustive list of didactic topics for study is coupled with mastery of a much more inclusive set of psychomotor skills (including Basic and Advanced Perioperative Echocardiography* [Appendix 41–2]) *than that which is required for core resident education.*[9]

QUALIFICATIONS OF CARDIOTHORACIC ANESTHESIOLOGISTS

Being a "qualified" cardiothoracic anesthesiologist implies having met standard criteria and complied with specified requirements. The standard criteria and specified requirement(s) are "defined and regulated" by agencies vested with the authority to delineate and maintain the "qualified" status. *Qualified,* therefore, implies a minimum achievement that is accomplished and available for public review. Having met the qualifications ensures the public trust, as it defines for the public a "common yardstick" by which educational programs, physicians, and medical practice can be measured. For cardiothoracic anesthesiology, qualifications refer to (1) GME programs (accreditation), (2) physicians who have completed and subsequently demonstrated mastery of the proscribed GME (certification), and (3) physician practice settings where anesthesia patient care takes place (credentialing and clinical privileging).

Accreditation

The "ACGME is responsible for the accreditation of post-MD medical training programs within the United States. Accreditation is accomplished through a peer review process and is based upon established standards and guidelines."[10]

> The mission of the ACGME is to improve the quality of health in the United States by ensuring and improving the quality of graduate medical education experience for the physicians in training. The ACGME establishes national standards for graduate medical education by which it approves and continually assesses educational programs under its aegis. It uses the most effective methods available to evaluate the quality of graduate medical education programs. It strives to develop evaluation methods and processes that are valid, fair, open and ethical.[11]

GME programs voluntarily apply for accredited status and agree to meet the defined program requirements and undergo periodic scrutiny to document compliance. Accredited status brings with it public recognition and the benefits of being subject to specialty-specific and general institutional ACGME standards. As an example of such a benefit, common program requirements that provide a "level playing field" for all GME programs have been published by the ACGME.[12]

The Anesthesiology RRC of the ACGME does not accredit cardiothoracic anesthesiology GME. The Anesthesiology RRC and the ABA are currently weighing all of the issues surrounding accreditation of cardiothoracic anesthesiology GME as proposed by the SCA. Until cardiothoracic anesthesiology fellowship education is accredited, it is incumbent upon graduate trainees to thoroughly evaluate any fellowship program to which they wish to apply because wide variations may exist in the depth and breadth of education and training experience that are available.

Certification

A physician who successfully completes an accredited fellowship program may voluntarily apply to become identified as a board-certified specialist. Board certification is under the auspices of the American Board of Medical Specialties: "The American Board of Medical Specialties (ABMS) is an organization of 24 approved medical specialty boards. The intent of the certification of physicians is to provide assurance to the public that those certified by an ABMS Member Board have successfully completed an approved training program and an evaluation process assessing their ability to provide quality patient care in the specialty."[13] An increasing amount of scientific evidence exists that attests to the fact that board certification status relates directly to better patient outcome. Silber et al's studies particularly suggest that quality of patient care improves when anesthesiologists are board certified.[14-16] Brennan et al[17] provide considerable evidence making the case for considering certification status as an evidence-based quality measure.

> The ABMS serves to coordinate the activities of its Member Boards and to provide information to others concerning issues involving specialization and certification of medical specialists.[13] [The ABA is one of the ABMS Member Boards.]
>
> A Board certified anesthesiologist is a physician who provides medical management and consultation during the perioperative period, in pain medicine and in critical care medicine. A diplomate of the Board must possess knowledge, judgment, adaptability, clinical skills, technical facility and personal characteristics sufficient to carry out the entire scope of anesthesiology practice. An ABA diplomate must logically organize and effectively present rational diagnoses and appropriate treatment protocols to peers, patients, their families and others involved in the medical community. A diplomate of the Board can serve as an expert in matters related to anesthesiology, deliberate with others, and provide advice and defend opinions in all aspects of the specialty of anesthesiology. A Board certified anesthesiologist is able to function as the leader of the anesthesiology care team . . . [The Board will] establish and conduct those processes by which the Board may judge whether a physician who voluntarily applies should be issued a certificate indicating that the required standards for subspecialty certification or recertification in an ABA designated subdiscipline of anesthesiology have been met.[3]

Board certification in cardiac anesthesiology does not exist in the United States. The prerequisite training for cardiac anesthesiology board certification does not exist as accredited cardiac anesthesiology fellowships do not exist.

Credentialing and Clinical Privileges

Anesthesiologists may practice as cardiac subspecialists even though accredited fellowship education and board certification do not exist in the United States. Hospital medical staffs have the privilege and obligation to define what physicians can and cannot do with respect to patient care in their institution. This process is medical credentialing.

> To be awarded medical staff privileges in anesthesiology, a physician must fully meet certain required criteria. It is possible to make all the following criteria mandatory or to have a mixture of required and optional criteria. Organizations [Hospital Medical Staffs] should determine which criteria to include and whether to include additional criteria based on the institution's individual requirements and preferences. For example, some facilities may decide that certification by the [ABA] is a requirement for clinical privileges in anesthesiology, while others may deem board certification to be desirable but not essential. Similarly, some institutions may decide that subspecialty fellowship training is needed for certain clinical privileges, while others may not. Some organizations may wish to recognize residency training obtained or certification awarded outside the United States. Institutions granting subspecialty clinical privileges may wish to recognize experience as an alternative to formal training in a subspecialty of anesthesiology. Some institutions may wish to modify certain requirements for physicians who have recently completed their residency or fellowship training.[18]

The ASA has published guidelines for delineating clinical privileges in anesthesiology taking into consideration educational, licensure, performance improvement, personal qualification, and practice pattern criteria.[18] Many physicians are recognized as credentialed cardiac anesthesiologists and are granted specific clinical privileges defined by their practice group and hospital medical staff while at the same time they have not been educated in accredited fellowships and are not certified by the ABA. These cardiac anesthesiologists are "experts" in their subspecialty and clearly qualified to care for patients with CVD.

TEACHING AND LEARNING CARDIAC ANESTHESIOLOGY

Teachers and the Teaching/Learning Environment

Teaching and learning cardiac anesthesiology best take place in an environment conducive to the educational process with a set of goals and objectives to guide the endeavor. This has been defined by the Anesthesiology RRC in their program requirements for GME in anesthesiology[2] for the core residency, and this same perspective is quite applicable to teaching cardiothoracic anesthesiology:

> An accredited program in [cardiothoracic] anesthesiology must provide education, training, and experience in an atmosphere of mutual respect between instructor and residents so that residents will be stimulated and prepared to apply acquired knowledge and talents independently. The program must provide an environment that promotes the acquisition of the knowledge, skills, clinical judgment, and attitudes essential to the practice of anesthesiology.
>
> In addition to clinical skills, the program should emphasize interpersonal skills, effective communication, and professionalism. The residency [fellowship] program must work toward ensuring that its residents [fellows], by the time they graduate, assume responsibility and act responsibly and with integrity; demonstrate a

> commitment to excellence and ethical principles of clinical care, including confidentiality of patient information, informed consent, and business practices; demonstrate respect and regard for the needs of patients and society that supersede self-interest; and work effectively as members of a health-care team or other professional group. Further, residents [fellows] are expected to create and sustain a therapeutic relationship with patients, engage in active listening, provide information using appropriate language, ask clear questions, provide an opportunity for comments and questions, and demonstrate sensitivity and responsiveness to cultural differences, including awareness of their own and their patients' cultural perspectives.
>
> These objectives can be achieved only when the program leadership, faculty, supporting staff, and administration demonstrate a commitment to the educational program and provide appropriate resources and facilities. Service commitments must not compromise the achievement of educational goals and objectives.[2]

A key factor for successful education is the commitment of effective teachers. A description of the effective clinical teacher has been put forth that, while written about the internal medicine teaching setting, is applicable to all disciplines and certainly cardiothoracic anesthesiology.[19] Effective teachers demonstrate, among other traits, the characteristics outlined in Box 41–1.[19]

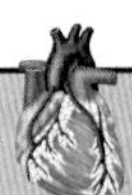

BOX 41–1 ***Characteristics of an Effective Clinical Teacher***[19]

- Allocates dedicated time for teaching
- Creates a trusting learning environment
- Demonstrates clinical credibility
- Provides an initial orientation and final evaluation for the teaching event
- Engages learners by expecting them to present cases, the pertinent details and educational benefit of which are managed by the teacher
- Enhances clinical case material with complementary didactic sessions
- Role models physician-patient relationships through bedside teaching
- Encourages student consideration of and interactive discussions about the psychosocial aspects of medical care
- Transfers the teaching responsibility to the students who are the future medical educators

Curriculum

There are three fundamental categories of curricular material for all educational topics that certainly apply to the curriculum for cardiothoracic anesthesiology: cognitive, psychomotor, and affective. The cognitive or knowledge base of cardiothoracic anesthesiology is readily recognized as the basic medical sciences applied clinically. Cardiac embryology, histology, and gross anatomy; cardiorespiratory physiology; and adrenergic, anticoagulation, and antiarrhythmic pharmacology and pathophysiology of cardiac valve disorders are examples of some of the required cognitive base of cardiothoracic anesthesiology. An expansive listing of the topical content of cardiothoracic anesthesiology is recommended in Appendix 41–1.[9] "The didactic curriculum . . . provided through lectures, conferences and workshops should supplement clinical experience as necessary for the subspecialty [fellow] to acquire the knowledge to care for cardiothoracic patients and conditions outlined in the guidelines for the minimum clinical experience for each [fellow]."[9]

Complete cognitive learning is a process whereby the facts are considered in a variety of ways that take them beyond simple uninterpreted and unapplied statements. Teaching in the content area requires attention to increasingly complex cognitive functions described by Bloom[20] (Box 41–2).

Bloom's taxonomy fits well with the ABA oral examination process that is designed "to assess the candidate's ability to demonstrate the attributes of an ABA Diplomate [understand and apply complex cognitive functions] when managing patients presented in clinical scenarios. The attributes are sound judgment in decision-making and management of surgical and anesthetic complications, appropriate application of scientific principles to clinical problems, adaptability to unexpected changes in the clinical situations, and logical organization and effective presentation of information. The oral examination emphasizes the scientific rationale underlying clinical management decisions"[21] (Box 41–3).

When confronted with a patient with an ascending aortic arch dissection, for example, the clear expectation for teaching and learning is more than to just know the anatomy; it is to understand the interrelationships of the aortic and coronary anatomy, the effect of the aortic dissection on coronary artery blood flow, ventricular function, and total body perfusion, and to be able to develop an anesthetic management plan that considers all of these co-dependent factors and selects anesthetic and cardiovascular medications and physiologic monitoring appropriate to the care of the specific patient in question.

While much of medical knowledge is broadly applicable to a wide variety of specialties, psychomotor learning is often quite specific to the specialty in question. Psychomotor skills

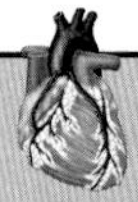

BOX 41–2 ***Bloom's Taxonomy of Cognitive Learning Outlining a Hierarchy From Simple (Knowledge) to Complex (Evaluation) Processes***[20]

- Knowledge—recall
- Comprehension—understanding
- Application—use of abstractions
- Analysis—break down; seeing the relationship of parts
- Synthesis—put together; creating a new entity
- Evaluation—judgment of value

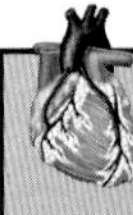

BOX 41–3 ***Attributes of an ABA Diplomate to Be Evaluated During the Oral Examination and Not by the Written Examination***[21]

- Sound judgment in decision-making and management of surgical and anesthetic complications
- Appropriate application of scientific principles to clinical problems
- Adaptability to unexpected changes in the clinical situations
- Logical organization and effective presentation of information

that must be learned by the cardiac anesthesiologist, for example, do not apply at all to the dermatologist. Bedside cardiac catheterization with the balloon flotation pulmonary artery catheter, administration of carefully titrated vasoactive infusions, manipulation of cardiac output using the intra-aortic balloon pump, and transesophageal echocardiography (TEE) are examples of the required psychomotor skills of cardiothoracic anesthesiology. TEE is a prime example of a set of psychomotor skills that, once learned, sets the cardiac anesthesiologist apart from all other anesthesiologists unskilled in this technique. Appendix 41–2 details both the cognitive and psychomotor learning necessary for mastery of perioperative TEE.[9]

The psychomotor skill lesson is vital to effective learning in cardiothoracic anesthesiology. Cardiac anesthesiology psychomotor techniques such as internal jugular catheterization and fiberoptic bronchoscopy are most effectively and efficiently taught with less potential harm to patients when using a systematically applied skill lesson plan.

Developing a psychomotor skill lesson is an example of how understanding instructional methodology can lead to effective teaching and learning. The old adage about teaching psychomotor skills in medicine is "see one, do one, teach one." The absurd nature of this approach has been highlighted in the following way: "This is akin to a piano instructor playing 'The Minute Waltz' for a beginner and then saying, 'Now, try it yourself.' "[22,23]

Rather than the repetitive trial-and-error approach to teaching/learning psychomotor skills, a systemic methodology can be used[23] (Box 41–4).

Affective teaching and learning are perhaps the least understood and appreciated of the categories of curricular material:

Affective teaching/learning deals with feelings or emotions. The taxonomy of affective learning addresses the following[22,24]: Receiving, Responding, Valuing, Organizing, Value complexing. While we actively and consciously teach in the cognitive and psychomotor areas, we are much less aware of our affective teaching. Even though we may not be aware of it, however, we are constantly teaching in the affective arena by the role modeling we perform . . . an example of how affective teaching and learning takes place [is] described.[22]

Picture the educational setting in which an anesthesiology resident [cardiothoracic anesthesiology fellow] is learning how to use epinephrine when weaning a patient from cardiopulmonary bypass. The knowledge and skills that must be learned include application of the pharmacologic principles of catecholamines to the pathophysiology of cardiovascular disease by turning on a mechanical infusion pump to deliver the indicated dose of a medication while technically monitoring for dose response and toxicity. Learning these facts and the skills sufficient to employ them is much different when done from a textbook or a preoperative conference with a staff preceptor than when done during the operating room interaction between the surgeon and anesthesiologist, where varied opinions may consider dopamine a more sound physiologic choice or intermittent boluses a better administration technique. The interposition of the concerned surgeon and real-time patient setting between the student and the knowledge and skills to be learned changes the learning environment and, hence, the educational experience for the resident [fellow]. More is learned than the facts and psychomotor skills. As the attitudes of both the anesthesiologist and the surgeon are displayed during the resolution of the questions about the "best" drug to use and the "right" way to give it, the resident [subspecialty fellow] learns how these two types of practitioners are supposed to relate to one another.[22]

In the real-life setting, the agg ressive, passive-aggressive, or passive posture of the anesthesiology teacher interacting with the surgeon provides a lasting lesson in the affective domain for the resident [fellow] anesthesiology learner.[22]

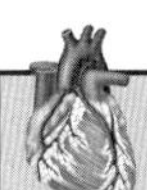

BOX 41–4 *Systematic Methodology for Psychomotor Skill Lessons*[22,23]

1. Analyze and separate the skills into component parts and determine which aspects of the skill are most difficult to perform
2. Provide students with a model of the skill they are expected to perform, demonstrated effectively in its entirety
3. Make provisions for students to practice until the expected behavior is mastered
4. Provide adequate supervision and an evaluation of the final performance

Simulation may be the educational solution to issues described in the psychomotor and affective learning scenarios (see later).

TEACHING PROCESS AND CONTENT RESOURCES

The actual teaching process may take the form of one of many time-tested methods available, including formal classroom didactic lectures, interactive teaching conferences, problem-based learning discussions, journal club review of the pertinent and current literature, bedside (in the operating room, intensive care unit, and preanesthesia evaluation clinic) patient interactive care/teaching, "surfing the Web," and simulation exercises.

Print materials (textbooks and journals) offering information about cardiothoracic anesthesiology and its related subjects are so numerous and constantly being updated and added to that it is impossible to have a current, complete, and comprehensive library. The Internet solves the problem of constantly being out-of-date with one's print library. The Internet has opened up the teaching environment to an enormous wealth of didactic and interactive teaching materials. Search engines, databases, and Internet links make an encyclopedic amount of up-to-date information available to the learner in cardiothoracic anesthesiology. Utilization of these Web resources gives the cardiothoracic anesthesiology fellow access to learning materials and teaching methods that she or he might never have known existed. In addition, using Web-based resources reduces the need for the cardiothoracic anesthesiology fellow to "reinvent the wheel" as she or he can take advantage of what others have already discovered and "published" on the Internet. Appendix III offers a catalogue of cardiothoracic anesthesiology Web-based resources. While it would be nice to state that this catalogue is all-inclusive, by its very nature, the Internet is never exhausted and more cardiothoracic anesthesiology Web-based resources exist and will be listed in the future. The cardiothoracic anesthesiology trainee and practitioner are encouraged to use the Web-based resource listing as a springboard to continually explore this vast educational reservoir as a lifelong learning exercise.

Simulation

Atul Gawande has made a critically important medical education dichotomy and dilemma transparent to the public in his book *Complications: A Surgeon's Notes on an Imperfect Science* in the chapter entitled, "Education of a Knife," writing that there is an ". . . imperative to give patients the best possible care and [at the same time] to provide novices with experience [education is a change in behavior based on experience]."[25] To accomplish these two conflicting imperatives in the past, learning clinical care (cardiac anesthesia, for example) was most often a process of application of knowledge and trial of techniques, both new to the student, on high acuity/low physiologic reserve patients in real-time patient care settings. This scenario was characterized by high anxiety for the student and significant risk of complications to the patient cared for by the novice. For the present and future, Gawande makes it clear that the traditional medical education paradigm is no longer acceptable: "By traditional ethics and public insistence (not to mention court rulings), a patient's right to the best care possible must trump the objective of training novices."[25]

The aviation industry long ago recognized this dilemma when teaching pilots. Acknowledging the high-stakes nature of flying, simulation technology was instituted to teach and evaluate a pilot's competence rather than allow him/her to fly a jumbo-jet and risk loss of hundreds of lives. Learning to apply the knowledge and perform the techniques before entering the "cockpit" reduces the risk of a "crash disaster." Medical care in general and anesthesia patient care in particular, especially of very high-risk patients with CVD, is analogous to the jumbo-jet situation and logically calls for a similar approach to education, that is, use of simulation.[26] The public is no longer willing to accept teaching on patients. In the cardiothoracic patient care arena, for example, education has moved to virtual reality training for cardiac operating room and catheterization procedures.[27]

Imitation of a real-life clinical situation using stand-in devices that assume the patient role provides learner experience while permitting teaching and learning in repetitive fashion with zero risk to both the provider and recipient of the simulated care.[28] An exponential growth of simulation devices has occurred in medicine over the past several decades, many of which are directly applicable to education of cardiothoracic anesthesiologists. Flat-screen computer and mannequin-based simulators have been developed to mimic many patient care settings. Examples of relatively high-fidelity high-technology simulators especially pertinent to learning cardiothoracic anesthesiology include "Harvey," the cardiology patient simulator,[29-31] multimedia computer-assisted cardiology simulation,[32] anesthesia simulators,[33-35] and bronchoscopy simulators.[36] Evidence has been accumulated that simulation results in a better educational outcome for the learner. Schwid and colleagues randomized anesthesiology residents and faculty into two learning groups (textbook reading versus computerized ACLS [Advanced Cardiac Life Support] simulation education) preparing for performance evaluation at an ACLS mock resuscitation.[37] Computer simulation–prepared learners were judged to perform better than textbook-prepared learners during standardized mega codes that required treatment protocols for clinical simulation of cardiovascular life-threatening scenarios with supraventricular tachycardia, ventricular fibrillation, and second-degree type II atrioventricular block.[37] Pulmonary artery catheterization and cardiovascular physiologic management can be effectively presented through a computer-based critical care training simulation.[38]

Simulation adds other more sophisticated aspects to education that are not possible from traditional textbook learning, classroom lectures, or single-learner computer-based programs. These missing ingredients are teamwork and improved processes of care. Multidiscipline teams working effectively together must develop if the best medical care is to be provided to patients. Aviation's crew resource management (CRM) concepts can be effectively taught through group simulation exercises.[39] The potential for CRM teaching to positively impact care of patients with CVD is enormous when the team of cardiac anesthesiologists is educated with others who care for the same patients, including cardiac surgeons, cardiologists, cardiac operating room nurses, perfusionists, and respiratory therapists. Holzman and colleagues[40] and Grogan and colleagues[39] have demonstrated that CRM (also called anesthesia crisis resource management [ACRM]) enhances (a) interpersonal communication, situational awareness, and appropriate management of available patient care resources[40] and (b) fatigue management, adverse event recognition, team decision-making, and performance feedback.[39] CRM is so timely a topic that an entire supplement issue of *Quality & Safety in Health Care* entitled "Simulation and Team Training" described the state of the art.[41]

While improved patient outcome from simulation education is intuitively obvious, scant evidence-based medicine exists to prove this. Sedlack and colleagues,[42] for example, have demonstrated that patients reported more comfort, a direct benefit to the patient, during gastrointestinal endoscopy provided by computer-based simulation trained endoscopists than when the same procedure was performed by patient-based trained endoscopists. Combing the literature for similar studies that document "direct patient benefit" and "improved patient outcome" related to simulation education of anesthesiologists results in virtually nothing of scientific significance. On the other hand, studies do document the educational benefit of simulation technology.[43] The clear challenge is to devise methods to scientifically prove that simulation education does benefit patients.

EVALUATION

Completion of the educational loop requires more than what has been described so far. In addition to providing a rationale for learning cardiothoracic anesthesiology, considering who the students and teachers are, describing the teaching/learning environment, defining the concepts of curricular development, and cataloguing teaching methodology, evaluation processes must be instituted to complete the educational circle of planning and implementing the teaching process. Evaluation of all aspects of the educational endeavor, including students, teachers, program, and patient outcome, is essential.

Resident/Fellow Evaluation

The Anesthesiology RRC and the ABA outline the process for evaluation of the resident and fellow.

The ACGME states:

1. Formative Evaluation

   The faculty must evaluate in a timely manner the residents whom they supervise. In addition, the residency program must demonstrate that it has an effective mechanism for assessing resident performance throughout the program, and for utilizing the results to improve resident performance.

a) Assessment should include the use of methods that produce an accurate assessment of residents' competence in patient care, medical knowledge, practice-based learning and improvement, interpersonal and communication skills, professionalism, and systems-based practice.
b) Assessment should include the regular and timely performance feedback to residents that includes at least semiannual written evaluations. Such evaluations are to be communicated to each resident in a timely manner and maintained in a record that is accessible to each resident.
c) Assessment should include the use of assessment results, including evaluation by faculty, patients, peers, self, and other professional staff, to achieve progressive improvements in residents' competence and performance.

2. Final Evaluation

The program director must provide a final evaluation for each resident who completes the program. This evaluation must include a review of the resident's performance during the final period of education and should verify that the resident has demonstrated sufficient professional ability to practice competently and independently. The final evaluation must be part of the resident's permanent record maintained by the institution.[2]

The ABA states:

D. Have on file in the [ABA] Board office evidence of having satisfactorily fulfilled all requirements of the continuum of education in anesthesiology before the date of examination and after receiving a medical or osteopathic degree acceptable to the ABA. Such evidence must include a satisfactory Certificate of Clinical Competence covering the final six months of Clinical Anesthesia training in each residency program. . . .[3]

Key components of student evaluation cited above include ". . . regular and timely performance feedback" and ". . . satisfactory Certificate of Clinical Competence. . . ." Without the ability to (1) provide the resident/fellow constructive feedback, on as frequent a basis as daily, and (2) have the faculty attest to the resident's/fellow's competence at the completion of the educational process, student evaluation will be meaningless.

Faculty Evaluation

The ACGME guides department chairs about evaluation of the faculty.

The performance of the faculty must be evaluated by the program no less frequently than at the midpoint of the accreditation cycle, and again prior to the next site visit. The evaluations should include a review of their teaching abilities, commitment to the educational program, clinical knowledge, and scholarly activities. This evaluation must include annual written confidential evaluations by residents.[2]

Collection of data about an individual faculty member's ". . . teaching abilities, commitment to the educational program, clinical knowledge, and scholarly activities . . ."[2] arms the chair with ammunition for constructive suggestions for change of teaching techniques by the faculty member.

Program Evaluation

Program evaluation is based upon the successful completion of the residency/fellowship by the trainees and their subsequent success at mastery of certifying examinations.[2]

The educational effectiveness of a program must be evaluated at least semiannually in a systematic manner:

1. Representative program personnel (i.e., at least the program director, representative faculty, and one resident) must be organized to review program goals and objectives, and the effectiveness with which they are achieved. This group must conduct a formal documented meeting at least annually for this purpose. In the evaluation process, the group must take into consideration written comments from the faculty, the most recent report of the GMEC of the sponsoring institution, and the residents' confidential written evaluations. If deficiencies are found, the group should prepare an explicit plan of action, which should be approved by the faculty and documented in the minutes of the meeting.
2. The program should use resident performance and outcome assessment in its evaluation of the educational effectiveness of the residency program. Performance of program graduates on the certification examination should be used as one measure of evaluating program effectiveness. The program should maintain a process for using assessment results together with other program evaluation results to improve the residency program.
3. As part of the overall evaluation of the program, the RRC will take into consideration the information provided by the ABA regarding resident performance on the certifying examinations over the most recent 5-year period. The RRC will also take into account noticeable improvements or declines during the period considered. Program graduates should take the certifying examination, and at least 70% of the program graduates should become certified.[2]

Review of patient care data is another prime educational assessment technique for program evaluation. A department's and its institutional CQI (continuous quality improvement) programs serve as effective analysis methods for documenting the success of the educational program and clinical care provided to patients by ongoing review of data showing that unacceptable morbidity and mortality are not present and that the educational program does not result in and in fact may improve these parameters. The CQI program serves as a basis for CME of the residents, fellows, and faculty.

LIFELONG LEARNING, CONTINUING MEDICAL EDUCATION, AND MAINTENANCE OF CERTIFICATION

As defined by the American Medical Association, "CME consists of educational activities that serve to maintain, develop, or increase the knowledge, skills, and professional performance and relationships a physician uses to provide services for patients, the public, or the profession. CME represents that body of knowledge and skills generally recognized and accepted by the profession as within the basic medical sciences, the discipline of clinical medicine, and the provision of health care to the public."[44] Continued physician licensure, hospital/medical staff appointment, and maintenance of board certification status require documentation of lifelong learning and participation in accredited CME activities. Since January 1, 2000, the ABA issues 10-year time-limited certificates. Anesthesiologists wishing to renew their board certification status will have to complete the 10-year Maintenance of Certification Process in Anesthesiology (MOCA).[45] The MOCA process serves as the formal mechanism for recertification of board certification status and its principles serve as a lifelong learning process for cardiothoracic anesthesiologists.

SUMMARY

The following practical advice on learning cardiothoracic anesthesia includes pearls to consider.[46]

Education is a change in behavior based upon experiences. The first and foremost perspective that the student of cardiothoracic anesthesiology must have is to engage in experiences related to this subspecialty.

Pearl 1: To gain experiences, immerse yourself in every conceivable clinical and didactic activity related to cardiothoracic anesthesiology.

Enhance every experience by raising its cognitive level. Full understanding of cardiothoracic anesthesiology can only come from questioning each scenario.[46]

Pearl 2: Seek the answer to the most important question related to learning—why?

In order to ensure that the resident [fellow] has had sufficient experiences from which to learn and has asked "why" to fully understand, insist that the resident [fellow] become a teacher.[46]

Pearl 3: Learn how to teach cardiothoracic anesthesiology to others, and you will ensure that you have learned it![46]

Pearl 4: Continue to learn the ever-changing landscape of cardiothoracic anesthesiology. Enroll in and maintain an interest and activity in lifelong learning CME.

Be a lifelong participant in cardiothoracic anesthesiology CME and a MOCA-like program even in the absence of accredited cardiothoracic residency/fellowship educational programs and board certification of the subspecialty of cardiothoracic anesthesiology.

CME consists of educational activities that serve to maintain, develop, or increase the knowledge, skills, and professional performance and relationships a physician uses to provide services for patients, the public, or the profession. CME represents that body of knowledge and skills generally recognized and accepted by the profession as within the basic medical sciences, the discipline of clinical medicine, and the provision of health care to the public.[44]

Appendix 41–1 PROGRAM REQUIREMENTS FOR RESIDENCY (FELLOWSHIP) EDUCATION IN CARDIOTHORACIC ANESTHESIOLOGY PROPOSAL–2004

I. Introduction

A. Definition and Scope of the Specialty

Cardiothoracic anesthesiology is the subspecialty of anesthesiology devoted to the preoperative, intraoperative and postoperative care of adult and pediatric patients undergoing cardiothoracic surgery and related invasive procedures.

B. Duration and Scope of Education

Subspecialty training in adult or pediatric cardiothoracic anesthesiology shall be a minimum of twelve months in duration, beginning after satisfactory completion of an Accreditation Council for Graduate Medical Education (ACGME) accredited residency program in anesthesiology, as required for entrance into the examination system of the American Board of Anesthesiology. Subspecialty training in adult or pediatric cardiothoracic anesthesiology is in addition to the minimum requirements described in the Program Requirements for the core program in anesthesiology. Because cardiothoracic anesthesiology education requires an intensive continuum of training, it should not be interrupted by frequent and/or prolonged periods of absence. The majority of the training in cardiothoracic anesthesiology must be spent in caring for patients in the operating room, other anesthetizing locations and intensive care units. The training will include experience in providing anesthesia for cardiac, non-cardiac thoracic and intrathoracic vascular surgical procedures. It may also include anesthesia for non-operative diagnostic and interventional cardiac and thoracic procedures outside of the operating room. Preanesthesia preparation and postanesthesia care, pain management and advanced cardiac life support will also be included.

C. Goals and Objectives

The subspecialty program in cardiothoracic anesthesiology must be structured to ensure optimal patient care while providing residents the opportunity to develop skills in clinical care and judgement, teaching, and research. The subspecialist in cardiothoracic anesthesiology should be proficient in providing anesthesia care for patients undergoing cardiac surgery with and without extracorporeal circulation and thoracic surgery including operations on the lung, esophagus and thoracic aorta. It will also include patients undergoing nonoperative diagnostic and interventional cardiac, thoracic and electrophysiological procedures. In addition, the subspecialist in cardiothoracic anesthesiology should develop skills in the conduct of preoperative patient evaluation and interpretation of cardiovascular and pulmonary diagnostic test data, hemodynamic and respiratory monitoring, advanced level perioperative transesophageal echocardiography (TEE), management of cardiopulmonary bypass (CPB), pharmacological and mechanical hemodynamic support, perioperative critical care including ventilatory support and perioperative pain management. To meet these goals, the program should provide exposure to the wide variety of clinical problems in cardiothoracic patients as outlined below in Section V.B. that are necessary for the development of these clinical skills.

II. Institutional Organization

A. Relationship to the Core Residency Program.

Accreditation of the subspecialty program in cardiothoracic anesthesiology will be granted only when the program is associated with a core residency program in anesthesiology that is accredited by the ACGME. Therefore, the subspecialty training in cardiothoracic anesthesiology can occur only in an institution related to a core program by a formal agreement. The director of the core anesthesiology residency program is responsible for the appointment of the director of the cardiothoracic anesthesiology subspecialty program and determines the activities of the appointee and the duration of the appointment. There must be close cooperation between the core program and the subspecialty-training program. The division of responsibilities between the residents in the core program and those in the subspecialty program must be clearly delineated. The presence of a cardiothoracic anesthesiology residency must not be permitted to compromise the clinical experience and number of cases available to the residents in a core program in anesthesiology.

B. Institutional Policy

There should be an institutional policy governing the educational resources committed to the cardiothoracic anesthesiology program.

III. Faculty Qualifications and Responsibilities

A. Program Director

1. Qualifications of the Program Director

The program director in cardiothoracic anesthesiology must be an anesthesiologist who is certified by the American Board of Anesthesiology or who has equivalent qualifications. The program director also must be licensed to practice medicine in the state where the institution that sponsors the program is located (in certain federal programs unrestricted medical licensure in any state may be accepted) and have an appointment in good standing to the medical staff of an institution participating in the program. She/he must have training and/or experience in providing anesthesia care for cardiothoracic surgical patients beyond the requirement for completion of a core anesthesiology residency. The program director should have training and experience that would generally meet or exceed that associated with the completion of a one-year cardiothoracic anesthesiology residency. The program director in cardiothoracic anesthesiology has responsibility for the training program subject to the approval of the program director of the core residency-training program in anesthesiology. She/he must devote sufficient time to provide substantial leadership to the program and supervision for the residents. The clinical director of the cardiothoracic anesthesiology service may be someone other than the program director.

2. Responsibilities of the Program Director

a. Preparation, periodic review and, if necessary, revision of a written outline of the educational goals of the program with respect to the knowledge, skills and other attributes of residents for each rotation or other aspect of the program assignment. This statement must be distributed to residents and members of the teaching staff. It should be readily available for review.

b. Selection of residents for appointment to the program in accordance with institutional and departmental policies and procedures.

c. Selection and supervision of the teaching staff and other program personnel.

d. Supervision of residents through explicit written descriptions of supervisory lines of responsibility for the care of patients. Such guidelines must be communicated to all members of the program staff. Residents must be provided with prompt, reliable systems for communication and interaction with supervisory physicians.

e. Implementation of fair procedures, as established by the sponsoring institution, regarding academic discipline and resident complaints or grievances.

f. Preparation of an accurate statistical and narrative description of the program, as requested by the Residency Review Committee (RRC).

B. Faculty

Although the number of faculty members involved in teaching residents in cardiothoracic anesthesiology will vary, it is recommended that at least three faculty members be involved and that these be equal to or greater than two full-time equivalents, including the program director. A ratio of no less than one full-time equivalent faculty member to one subspecialty resident shall be maintained. The RRC understands that full-time means that the faculty member devotes essentially all professional time to the program. There must be evidence of active participation by qualified physicians with training and/or expertise in cardiothoracic anesthesiology beyond the requirement for completion of a core anesthesiology residency. The faculty should have training and experience that would generally meet or exceed that associated with the completion of a one-year cardiothoracic anesthesiology residency. The faculty must possess expertise in the care of cardiothoracic patients and must have a continuous and meaningful role in the subspecialty-training program. The faculty must include at least one individual who has successfully completed advanced perioperative echocardiography education according to echocardiography training objectives of the American Society of Echocardiography and the Society of Cardiovascular Anesthesiologists "Guidelines for Training in Perioperative Echocardiography" and has successfully completed the certification examination of Special Competence in Advanced Perioperative Transesophageal Echocardiography. The program should include teaching in multidisciplinary conferences by faculty in cardiology, cardiothoracic surgery, pediatrics, intensive care and pulmonary medicine. The cardiothoracic anesthesiology program director and faculty responsible for teaching subspecialty residents in cardiothoracic anesthesiology must maintain an active role in scholarly pursuits pertaining to cardiothoracic anesthesiology, as evidenced by participation in continuing medical education as well as by involvement in research that pertains to the care of cardiothoracic patients.

IV. Clinical and Educational Facilities and Resources

The following resources and facilities are necessary to the program:

A. Intensive care units for both surgical and nonsurgical cardiothoracic patients.

B. An emergency department in which cardiothoracic patients are effectively managed 24 hours a day.

C. Operating rooms adequately designed and equipped for the management of cardiothoracic patients. A postanesthesia care area adequately designed and equipped for the management of cardiothoracic patients must be located near the operating room suite.

D. Cardiothoracic patients in sufficient volume and variety to provide a broad educational experience for the program. Physicians with special training and/or experience in cardiovascular disease, clinical cardiac electrophysiology, cardiac and noncardiac thoracic surgery, general vascular surgery, pediatrics and pulmonary diseases must be available.

E. Monitoring and advanced life support equipment representative of current levels of technology.

F. Allied health staff and other support personnel.

G. Facilities that are readily available at all times to provide prompt laboratory measurement pertinent to the care of cardiothoracic patients. These include but are not limited to measurement of blood chemistries, blood gas and acid base analysis, oxygen saturation, hematocrit/hemoglobin and coagulation function.

H. Facilities that are readily available at all times to provide prompt noninvasive and invasive diagnostic and therapeutic cardiothoracic procedures. These include but are not limited to echocardiography, cardiac stress testing, cardiac catheterization, electrophysiological testing and therapeutic intervention, cardiopulmonary scanning procedures and pulmonary function testing.

I. Conveniently located library facilities and space for research and teaching conferences in cardiothoracic anesthesiology.

V. Educational Program.

A. Goals and Objectives

The director and teaching staff must prepare and comply with written goals for the program. All educational components should be related to the program goals. The program design must be approved by the RRC as part of the regular review process. A written statement of the educational objectives must be given to each resident at the start of the program.

B. Clinical Components

The subspecialty resident in cardiothoracic anesthesiology should gain clinical experience in the following areas of care of patients with cardiothoracic diseases. The subspecialty resident in cardiothoracic anesthesiology should gain the majority of her/his clinical experience providing hands-on clinical care of patients. The subspecialty resident should also care for some patients while simultaneously supervising core residents in anesthesiology, both being ultimately supervised by a faculty anesthesiologist. It is the expectation that the subspecialty resident will have a significantly different and essential experience when simultaneously caring for a patient and functioning in the role of teacher and supervisor of a core resident. The goal of having subspecialty residents teach and supervise core residents while also caring for patients is to prepare subspecialty residents to become faculty supervisors and teachers. The following represents the guidelines for the minimum clinical experience for each resident:

1. Adult Cardiothoracic Anesthesiology Residency Track

a. Required Core

1. Six months operating room clinical activity providing a minimum of 90 surgical procedures involving adult patients and requiring CPB to include a minimum of 40 anesthetics involving valve repair or replacement and a minimum of 60 myocardial revascularization procedures with or without CPB. The resident should provide anesthetic management for patients undergoing minimally invasive cardiac surgery. The resident should provide anesthetic management for congenital cardiac procedures performed on adult patients. The resident must gain sufficient experience to independently manage intra-aortic balloon counterpulsation. The resident should be actively involved in the management of patients with left ventricular assist devices.

2. Additional required clinical experience within the full one-year residency should include at least one month or its equivalent of anesthetic management of patients undergoing noncardiac thoracic surgery and the anesthetic management of 10 adult patients undergoing surgery on the ascending or descending thoracic aorta requiring full CPB, left heart bypass and/or deep hypothermic circulatory arrest.

3. The resident is required to have experience in the anesthetic management of adult patients for cardiac pacemaker and automatic implantable cardiac defibrillator placement, surgical treatment of cardiac arrhythmias, cardiac catheterization and cardiac electrophysiologic diagnostic/therapeutic procedures.

4. Additional clinical experience within the full one-year residency must include successful completion of advanced perioperative echocardiography education according to the training objectives from the American Society of Echocardiography and the Society of Cardiovascular Anesthesiologists "Guidelines for Training in Perioperative Echocardiography." This will include the study of 300 complete perioperative echocardiographic examinations, at least 150 of which are comprehensive intraoperative TEE examinations personally performed, interpreted and reported by the trainee.

5. The resident is required to have a one-month experience managing adult cardiothoracic surgical patients in a critical care (ICU) setting. This experience may include the management of nonsurgical cardiothoracic patients.

b. Elective Rotations

1. Two months of elective rotations (none less than 2 weeks in duration) from the following categories: Inpatient or outpatient cardiology, invasive cardiology, inpatient or outpatient pulmonary medicine, medical or surgical critical care, extracorporeal perfusion technology and pediatric cardiothoracic anesthesia. One to two months devoted to a research project in cardiothoracic anesthesiology may be substituted for the two months of clinical elective rotations.

2. Pediatric Cardiothoracic Anesthesiology Residency Track

a. Required Core

1. Six months operating room clinical activity providing a minimum of 80 surgical procedures on pediatric patients requiring CPB and 60 patients undergoing cardiac surgical procedures not requiring the use of CPB. At least 25% of these patients should be neonates and 50% of all patients should be infants up to one year of age. The resident should be actively involved in the management of patients on extracorporeal membrane oxygenation (ECMO) and with left ventricular assist devices.

2. The resident is required to have experience in the management of pediatric patients for cardiac pacemaker and automatic implantable cardiac defibrillator placement, surgical treatment of cardiac arrhythmias, cardiac catheterization and cardiac electrophysiologic diagnostic/therapeutic procedures.

3. Three-months experience combining evaluation of pediatric patients utilizing echocardiography and cardiac catheterization. This will also include the anesthetic management of pediatric patients in the cardiac catheterization laboratory. Cardiac evaluation should also include cardiac MRI and exercise testing to evaluate a pediatric patient's functional capacity. Echocardiography, cardiac catheterization and other noninvasive cardiac evaluation training may be done in conjunction with operating room clinical activity or as independently designed rotations.

4. The resident is required to have a one-month experience managing pediatric cardiothoracic surgical patients in a critical care (ICU) setting. This experience may include the management of nonsurgical cardiothoracic patients.

b. Elective Rotations

1. Two months of elective rotations (none less than 2 weeks in duration) from the following pediatric categories: Inpatient or outpatient cardiology, invasive cardiology, inpatient or outpatient pulmonary medicine, medical or surgical

critical care and extracorporeal perfusion technology. The resident may care for adult cardiothoracic patients to fulfill this elective requirement.

C. The didactic curriculum (applicable to both tracks), provided through lectures, conferences and workshops should supplement clinical experience as necessary for the subspecialty resident to acquire the knowledge to care for cardiothoracic patients and conditions outlined in the guidelines for the minimum clinical experience for each resident. The didactic components should include the following areas, with emphasis on how cardiothoracic diseases affect the administration of anesthesia and life support to cardiothoracic patients. The didactic program for the adult and pediatric cardiothoracic anesthesiology residency tracks will focus primarily on topics pertinent to their respective patient populations. The following represents guidelines for the minimum didactic experience and academic project (see below) for each resident. *

1. Embryological development of the cardiothoracic structures
2. Pathophysiology, pharmacology and clinical management of patients with cardiac disease including cardiomyopathy, heart failure, cardiac tamponade, ischemic heart disease, acquired and congenital valvular heart disease, congenital heart disease, electrophysiologic disturbances and neoplastic and infectious cardiac diseases
3. Pathophysiology, pharmacology and clinical management of patients with respiratory disease including pleural, bronchopulmonary, neoplastic, infectious and inflammatory diseases
4. Pathophysiology, pharmacology and clinical management of patients with thoracic vascular, tracheal, esophageal and mediastinal diseases including infectious, neoplastic and inflammatory processes
5. Non-invasive cardiovascular evaluation: electrocardiography, transthoracic echocardiography, TEE, stress testing, cardiovascular imaging

   a. TEE education must be based upon the training objectives for advanced perioperative echocardiography of the American Society of Echocardiography and the Society of Cardiovascular Anesthesiologists outlined in "Guidelines for Training in Perioperative Echocardiography" (Appendix II).

6. Cardiac catheterization procedures and diagnostic interpretation; invasive cardiac catheterization procedures including angioplasty, stenting and transcatheter laser and mechanical ablations
7. Non-invasive pulmonary evaluation: pulmonary function tests, blood gas and acid-base analysis, oximetry, capnography, pulmonary imaging
8. Preanesthetic evaluation and preparation of cardiothoracic patients
9. Pharmacokinetics and pharmacodynamics of medications prescribed for medical management of cardiothoracic patients
10. Perianesthetic monitoring: non-invasive and invasive (intraarterial, central venous, pulmonary artery, mixed venous saturation, cardiac output)
11. Pharmacokinetics and pharmacodynamics of anesthetic medications prescribed for cardiothoracic patients
12. Extracorporeal circulation, including myocardial preservation, effects of CPB on pharmacokinetics and pharmacodynamics, cardiothoracic, respiratory, neurological, metabolic, endocrine, hematological, renal and thermoregulatory effects of CPB and coagulation/anticoagulation before, during and after CPB
13. Pharmacokinetics and pharmacodynamics of medications prescribed for management of hemodynamic instability: inotropes, chronotropes, vasoconstrictors, vasodilators
14. Circulatory assist devices: intra-aortic balloon counterpulsation, left and right ventricular assist devices and biventricular assist devices
15. Cardiac surgical procedures: adult and pediatric, minimally invasive, myocardial revascularization, valve repair and replacement, pericardial, neoplastic procedures and heart and/or lung transplantation
16. Thoracic aortic surgery: ascending, transverse and descending aortic surgery with circulatory arrest, CPB employing low flow and or retrograde perfusion
17. Esophageal surgery: varices, neoplastic, colon interposition, foreign body, stricture
18. Pulmonary surgery: thoracoscopic or open; lung reduction, bronchopulmonary lavage, one lung ventilation, lobectomy, pneumonectomy and bronchoscopy: fiberoptic, rigid, laser resection
19. Postanesthetic critical care of cardiothoracic surgical patients
20. Perioperative ventilator management: intraoperative anesthetic and critical care unit ventilators and techniques
21. Pain management of cardiothoracic surgical patients
22. Research methodology/statistical analysis
23. Quality assurance/improvement
24. Ethical and legal issues
25. Practice management

Cardiothoracic anesthesiology subspecialty conferences, including lectures, interactive conferences, hands-on workshops, morbidity and mortality conferences, cardiac catheterization and echocardiography conferences, cardiothoracic surgery case review conferences, journal reviews and research seminars should be regularly attended. Active participation of the cardiothoracic anesthesiology resident in the planning and production of these conferences is essential. However, the faculty should be the conference leaders in the majority of the sessions. Attendance by subspecialty residents at multidisciplinary conferences especially in cardiovascular medicine, pulmonary medicine, cardiothoracic surgery, vascular surgery and pediatrics relevant to cardiothoracic anesthesiology is encouraged.

The resident must complete a minimum of one academic assignment. Academic projects may include grand rounds presentations, preparation and publication of review articles, book chapters, and manuals for teaching or clinical practice, clinical research investigation or similar scholarly activities. A faculty supervisor must be in charge of each project.

VI. Evaluation

A. Faculty responsible for teaching subspecialty residents in cardiothoracic anesthesiology must provide critical evaluations of each resident's progress and competence to the cardiothoracic anesthesiology program director at the end of 6 and 12 months of training. These evaluations should include essential character attributes, acquired character attributes,

*Some of the topics listed constitute components of the Core Residency in Anesthesiology. They are included in the requirements for the Cardiothoracic Anesthesiology Residency to emphasize their importance to the foundation of the discipline of cardiothoracic anesthesiology and stress the need to reinforce and enrich them in the subspecialty residency educational program.

fund of knowledge, clinical judgment and clinical psychomotor skills, as well as specific tasks and skills for patient management and critical analysis of clinical situations. The program director or designee must inform each resident of the results of the evaluations at least every 6 months during training, advise the resident of areas needing improvement and document the communication. Subspecialty residents in cardiothoracic anesthesiology must obtain overall satisfactory evaluations at the completion of 12 months training to receive credit for training.

B. There must be a regular opportunity for residents to provide written, confidential evaluation of the faculty and program.

C. Periodic evaluation of patient care (quality assurance) is mandatory. Subspecialty residents in cardiothoracic anesthesiology should be involved in continuing quality improvement and risk management.

D. Periodic evaluation of subspecialty training objectives is encouraged. Cardiothoracic anesthesiology resident participation in this process is encouraged.

Appendix 41–2 AMERICAN SOCIETY OF ECHOCARDIOGRAPHY AND SOCIETY OF CARDIOVASCULAR ANESTHESIOLOGISTS TASK FORCE GUIDELINES FOR TRAINING IN PERIOPERATIVE ECHOCARDIOGRAPHY

Task Force Members: Michael Cahalan, MD (Chair) • Martin Abel, MD • Martin Goldman, MD • Alan Pearlman, MD • Pamela Sears-Rogan, MD • Isobel Russell, MD • Jack Shanewise, MD • William Stewart, MD • Christopher Troianos, MD

Introduction and Overview

When expertly utilized, perioperative echocardiography can lead to improved outcome in patients requiring cardiovascular surgery and in those suffering perioperative cardiovascular instability. However, prior publications have not specified the requisite training for perioperative echocardiography. Therefore, the American Society of Echocardiography (ASE) and the Society of Cardiovascular Anesthesiologists (SCA) appointed a joint task force to delineate guidelines for training in perioperative echocardiography including the prerequisite medical knowledge and training, echocardiographic knowledge and skills, training components and duration, training environment and supervision, and equivalence requirements for post graduate physicians already in practice. This document is the result of the task force's deliberations and recommendations.

For the purposes of these guidelines, perioperative echocardiography is defined as transesophageal echocardiography (TEE), epicardial echocardiography, or epiaortic ultrasonography performed in surgical patients immediately before, during, or after surgery. Although transthoracic echocardiography may be indicated and is often performed before and after surgery, it is rarely performed during surgery. Thus, these guidelines do not apply to perioperative transthoracic echocardiography, nor do they apply to transesophageal echocardiography performed in non-surgical patients.

Related Guidelines Previously Published

In 1987, the ASE recommended three levels of training in echocardiography for physicians.[1] In 1995, the American College of Cardiology task force on Training in Echocardiography reaffirmed these recommendations.[2] Level 1 requires three months of full-time echocardiography training in an approved fellowship and supervised participation in 150 transthoracic studies. This level of training does "not qualify the trainee to perform echocardiography or to interpret echocardiograms independently." Level 2 training requires an additional 3 months of full-time training and an additional 150 supervised studies. This level of training "should provide the knowledge and experience necessary to be capable fully of performing and interpreting an M-mode, two-dimensional and Doppler examination independently under the supervision of a laboratory director." Level 3 requires an additional 6 months of training (for a total of 1 year) and 450 additional examinations (total of 750) including experience in specialized techniques like TEE. This level of training qualifies the trainee to supervise an echocardiography laboratory and the training of others.

In 1992 the ASE Committee for Physician Training in Echocardiography published its guidelines for training in TEE.[3] They are based on the prior recommendations for training in transthoracic echocardiography (see above), and are directed at training for TEE in both operative and nonoperative applications. These guidelines require the trainee to attain at least level 2 training in echocardiography and also perform and interpret at least 50 supervised TEE examinations.

In 1996 a joint task force of the American Society of Anesthesiologists (ASA) and the SCA published guidelines for perioperative TEE, which defined two levels (basic and advanced) of perioperative TEE practice.[4] Anesthesiologists with basic training in perioperative TEE "should be able to use TEE for indications that lie within the customary practice of anesthesiology" and "must be able to recognize their limitations in this setting and request assistance, in a timely manner, from a physician with advanced training." Anesthesiologists with advanced training in perioperative TEE "should, in addition to the above, be able to exploit the full diagnostic potential of TEE in the perioperative period." Although these guidelines broadly defined the general principles for training in perioperative TEE, including cognitive and technical objectives, they provided no specific requirements.

General Principles

Practitioners from different specialties must attain comparable expertise in perioperative echocardiography. However, they will need different training to attain this goal. Thus, while these recommendations provide specific guidelines for training, they are designed to allow enough flexibility to ensure that individual circumstances are appropriately accommodated. Minimum numbers of cases are delineated; however, these numbers are less important than the depth and diversity of the clinical experience and quality of training. The goal of the training must be to provide exposure to the entire spectrum of perioperative echocardiography that a trainee will likely encounter in subsequent practice. While these guidelines should serve equally well for adult or pediatric practices, the delineated minimum requirements are not sufficient for training in both disciplines. The trainee who plans to practice both adult and pediatric perioperative echocardiography should complete appropriate curricula in both.

Like prior published guidelines, these guidelines recognize different levels of expertise in echocardiography and make level-specific recommendations for training. Specifically, these guidelines provide training recommendations for a basic level and an advanced level of perioperative echocardiography. Regardless of the level of expertise, all practitioners, even experts, must recognize that timely consultation during perioperative echocardiography may be necessary because of constraints of time or experience. Unlike prior guidelines, these guidelines do not specify the duration of training. Instead, these guidelines emphasize the goals of training and the number and diversity of cases required to meet those goals. The time required for perioperative training will vary markedly depending on the volume and diversity of the affiliated cardiac surgical program.

Prerequisite Medical Knowledge and Training

Trainees in perioperative echocardiography must be licensed physicians enrolled in, or having completed, an accredited residency.

Scope of Echocardiographic Knowledge and Skills

The 1996 ASA and SCA guidelines delineated training objectives for cognitive and technical skills for perioperative TEE.[4] For the current guidelines, these training objectives have been updated and modified to include epicardial echocardiography and epivascular ultrasonography (Table 1). Essentially, basic training in perioperative echocardiography should impart a detailed appreciation of when and how to perform perioperative echocardiography as well as the underlying principles of ultrasound. In addition to these cognitive skills, a basic practitioner should possess the technical skills to use TEE to recognize markedly abnormal cardiac structure and function, severe hypovolemia, large pericardial effusions, and the presence of intracardiac air. As defined in these guidelines, basic training does not prepare the practitioner to influence the surgical plan without the assistance of a physician with advanced training in perioperative echocardiography. Advanced training in perioperative echocardiography should impart the cognitive and technical skills necessary to employ independently the full diagnostic potential of perioperative echocardiography including the expertise to affect changes in cardiac surgical procedures.

Components of Training

Basic Training. The essential components of basic training include independent work, supervised activities, and assessment programs. Through a structured independent reading and study program, trainees must acquire an understanding of the principles of ultrasound and indications for perioperative echocardiography. This independent work should be supplemented by regularly scheduled didactics such as lectures and seminars designed to reinforce the most important aspects of perioperative echocardiography. Under appropriate supervision (see section on "Training Environment and Supervision") the trainee learns to place the TEE probe, operate the ultrasonograph, and perform a TEE examination. Subsequently, some clinical work should be performed with progressively more independence. However, a practitioner with advanced training must review every examination performed by the trainee with him/her. The trainee should be encouraged to master the comprehensive examination defined by the ASE and SCA.[5,6] Although not all components of this examination are needed for a basic examination, the basic practitioner should be able to acquire all 20 of the recommended cross sections in the event they are needed for remote consultation with an advanced practitioner. For basic training, the task force recommends study of 150 complete examinations under appropriate supervision (see next section for definition of appropriate supervision). These examinations must include the full spectrum of commonly encountered perioperative diagnoses, and at least 50 comprehensive intraoperative TEE examinations personally performed, interpreted, and reported by the trainee (Table 2). The trainee must be taught how to convey and document the results of his/her examination effectively. Periodic formal and informal evaluations of the trainee's progress should be conducted during training. Trainees should keep a log of examinations performed and reviewed to document the depth and breadth of their training.

Advanced Training. For advanced practice, the comprehensiveness of training is paramount. The essential components include independent work, supervised activities, and assessment programs. The task force recommends study of 300 complete examinations under appropriate supervision (see section on "Training Environment and Supervision"). These examinations must include a wide spectrum of cardiac diagnoses and at least 150 comprehensive intraoperative TEE examinations personally performed, interpreted, and reported by the trainee (see Table 2). The trainee must develop the skills to convey and document the results of his/her examinations effectively and independently. Periodic formal and informal evaluations of the trainee's progress should be conducted during training. The experience and case numbers acquired during basic training may be counted for advanced training provided the basic training was completed in an advanced training environment (see section on "Training Environment and Supervision"). The task force recognizes that trainees from different specialties should use their time in training somewhat differently depending on their varying backgrounds. A cardiologist with little operating room experience will need to spend more time in this environment than a cardiac anesthesiologist or surgeon to fully understand cardiac surgical techniques. A cardiac anesthesiologist or surgeon working in a center with a limited variety of cardiac surgery will need to spend more time in the echocardiographic laboratory than a cardiologist to fully understand the diagnostic

Table 1 **Recommended Training Objectives for Basic and Advanced Perioperative Echocardiography***

Basic Training

COGNITIVE SKILLS

1. Knowledge of the physical principles of echocardiographic image formation and blood velocity measurement
2. Knowledge of the operation of ultrasonographs including all controls that affect the quality of data displayed
3. Knowledge of the equipment handling, infection control, and electrical safety associated with the techniques of perioperative echocardiography
4. Knowledge of the indications, contraindications, and potential complications for perioperative echocardiography
5. Knowledge of the appropriate alternative diagnostic techniques
6. Knowledge of the normal tomographic anatomy as revealed by perioperative echocardiographic techniques
7. Knowledge of commonly encountered blood flow velocity profiles as measured by Doppler echocardiography
8. Knowledge of the echocardiographic manifestations of native valvular lesions and dysfunction
9. Knowledge of the echocardiographic manifestations of cardiac masses, thrombi, cardiomyopathies, pericardial effusions, and lesions of the great vessels
10. Detailed knowledge of the echocardiographic presentations of myocardial ischemia and infarction
11. Detailed knowledge of the echocardiographic presentations of normal and abnormal ventricular function
12. Detailed knowledge of the echocardiographic presentations of air embolization

TECHNICAL SKILLS

1. Ability to operate ultrasonographs including the primary controls affecting the quality of the displayed data
2. Ability to insert a TEE probe safely in the anesthetized, tracheally intubated patient
3. Ability to perform a comprehensive TEE examination and differentiate normal from markedly abnormal cardiac structures and function
4. Ability to recognize marked changes in segmental ventricular contraction indicative of myocardial ischemia or infarction
5. Ability to recognize marked changes in global ventricular filling and ejection
6. Ability to recognize air embolization
7. Ability to recognize gross valvular lesions and dysfunction
8. Ability to recognize large intracardiac masses and thrombi
9. Ability to detect large pericardial effusions
10. Ability to recognize common echocardiographic artifacts
11. Ability to communicate echocardiographic results effectively to health care professionals, the medical record, and patients
12. Ability to recognize complications of perioperative echocardiography

Advanced Training

COGNITIVE SKILLS

1. All the cognitive skills defined under basic training
2. Detailed knowledge of the principles and methodologies of qualitative and quantitative echocardiography
3. Detailed knowledge of native and prosthetic valvular function including valvular lesions and dysfunction
4. Knowledge of congenital heart disease (if congenital practice is planned then this knowledge must be detailed)
5. Detailed knowledge of all other diseases of the heart and great vessels that is relevant in the perioperative period (if pediatric practice is planned then this knowledge may be more general than detailed)
6. Detailed knowledge of the techniques, advantages, disadvantages, and potential complications of commonly used cardiac surgical procedures for treatment of acquired and congenital heart disease
7. Detailed knowledge of other diagnostic methods appropriate for correlation with perioperative echocardiography

TECHNICAL SKILLS

1. All the technical skills defined under basic training
2. Ability to acquire or direct the acquisition of all necessary echocardiographic data including epicardial and epiaortic imaging
3. Ability to recognize subtle changes in segmental ventricular contraction indicative of myocardial ischemia or infarction
4. Ability to quantify systolic and diastolic ventricular function and to estimate other relevant hemodynamic parameters
5. Ability to quantify normal and abnormal native and prosthetic valvular function
6. Ability to assess the appropriateness of cardiac surgical plans
7. Ability to identify inadequacies in cardiac surgical interventions and the underlying reasons for the inadequacies
8. Ability to aid in clinical decision making in the operating room

*Adapted from: Practice guidelines for perioperative transesophageal echocardiography. A report by the American Society of Anesthesiologists and the Society of Cardiovascular Anesthesiologists Task Force on Transesophageal Echocardiography. Anesthesiology 84:986, 1996.

techniques of echocardiography. Like basic trainees, advanced trainees should keep a log of examinations performed and reviewed to document the depth and breadth of their training.

Comparison with Previously Published Guidelines. Training guidelines in basic and advanced perioperative echocardiography are similar to the training guidelines for level I and level II in general echocardiography except that a greater number of personally performed cases (see above) and a specified number of months are required for training in general echocardiography.[1-3] The task force believes these differences are justified because the spectrum of cardiac diagnoses is more limited in perioperative echocardiography than in general echocardiography and because the volume and diversity of the supporting surgical program are more crucial for attaining training goals in perioperative echocardiography than the absolute duration of training.

Training Environment and Supervision

Basic Training. The director of the echocardiographic training program should be a physician with advanced training and demonstrated expertise in perioperative echocardiography or equivalent experience. At the start of training, the trainee must be supervised directly as he/she learns to place the TEE probe, operate the ultrasonograph, and perform a TEE examination. This direct supervision should continue until the trainee can introduce the TEE probe safely and con-

Table 2 Numbers of Examinations and Other Key Training Recommendations for Basic and Advanced Perioperative Echocardiography

	Basic*	Advanced*
Minimum number of examinations†	150	300
Minimum number personally performed‡	50	150

Program director qualifications: Basic = advanced perioperative echocardiography training; Advanced = advanced perioperative echocardiography training plus at least 150 additional perioperative TEE examinations.

Program qualifications: Basic = wide variety of perioperative applications of echocardiography; Advanced = full spectrum of perioperative applications of echocardiography.

*Totals for basic training may be counted toward advanced training provided the basic training was completed in an advanced training environment. See text for additional details and explanation of training environments and program director qualifications.

†Complete echocardiographic examinations interpreted and reported by the trainee under appropriate supervision. May include transthoracic studies recorded by qualified individuals other than the trainee.

‡Comprehensive intraoperative TEE examinations personally performed, interpreted, and reported by the trainee under appropriate supervision.[5,6]

sistently and perform an appropriate examination. The trainee should have access to a wide variety of surgery in which TEE is performed as an integral part of patient management. The perioperative echocardiography-training program should have an affiliation with an echocardiography laboratory so that basic trainees can gain regular and frequent exposure to teaching and clinical resources within that laboratory.

Advanced Training. Advanced training should take place in a training program specifically designed to accomplish comprehensive training in perioperative echocardiography. The director of the training program must be a physician with advanced training and demonstrated expertise in perioperative echocardiography who has performed at least 450 complete examinations including 300 personally performed intraoperative TEE examinations or equivalent experience. If the advanced trainee has not already accomplished basic training, then the same initial direct supervision should be provided for the advanced trainee as outlined above for the basic trainee. Subsequently, some clinical work may be performed with progressively more independence, but the immediate availability and direct involvement of an advanced practitioner are essential components of advanced training. The supporting surgical program must have the volume and diversity to ensure that the trainee will experience a wide spectrum of diagnostic challenges encountered in perioperative echocardiography. The task force wishes to emphasize the importance of case diversity by noting that practitioners with advanced training must be able to use TEE effectively in all its established perioperative applications.[4] The perioperative echocardiography-training program should have an affiliation with an echocardiography laboratory so that trainees can gain regular and frequent exposure to teaching and clinical resources within that laboratory.

Training within Specialty Fellowship Programs

Both accredited and non-accredited fellowship programs may wish to offer training in perioperative echocardiography. This may require revision of their current curricula to accomplish the training goals outlined in this document. Alternatively, the task force recommends the creation of fellowships solely devoted to advanced perioperative echocardiography and offered to graduates of qualifying training programs.

Training Equivalence for Specialists Already in Practice

Physicians already in practice can achieve appropriate training in perioperative echocardiography without enrolling in a formal training program. However, the same prerequisite medical knowledge, medical training, and goals for cognitive and technical skills (Table 1) apply to them as apply to physicians in formal training programs.

When a physician has already acquired extensive experience in perioperative echocardiography, then this physician should document his/her experience in detail and be able to demonstrate its equivalence in depth, diversity, and case numbers to the training levels delineated above. When a physician has no or little experience in perioperative echocardiography, then he/she should work with another physician who has advanced TEE training or equivalent experience to achieve the same training goals and case numbers as the training levels delineated above. In addition, the task force recommends that physicians seeking basic training via this pathway should have at least 20 hours of continuing medical education devoted to echocardiography. Physicians seeking advanced training via this pathway should have at least 50 hours of continuing medical education devoted to echocardiography. The continuing medical education in echocardiography should be obtained during the time the physician is acquiring the requisite clinical experience in TEE.

Acknowledgement

These data are available at http://www.scahq.org/sca3/tee_guidelines.pdf

REFERENCES

1. Pearlman AS, et al: Guidelines for optimal physician training in echocardiography. Recommendations of the American Society of Echocardiography Committee for Physician Training in Echocardiography. Am J Cardiol 60:158, 1987
2. Stewart WJ, et al: Guidelines for training in adult cardiovascular medicine. Core Cardiology Training Symposium (COCATS). Task Force 4: training in echocardiography. J Am Coll Cardiol 25:16, 1995
3. Pearlman AS, et al: Guidelines for physician training in transesophageal echocardiography: recommendations of the American Society of Echocardiography Committee for Physician Training in Echocardiography. J Am Soc Echocardiogr 5:187, 1992
4. Practice guidelines for perioperative transesophageal echocardiography. A report by the American Society of Anesthesiologists and the Society of Cardiovascular Anesthesiologists Task Force on Transesophageal Echocardiography. Anesthesiology 84:986, 1996
5. Shanewise JS, et al: ASE/SCA guidelines for performing a comprehensive intraoperative multiplane transesophageal echocardiography examination: recommendations of the American Society of Echocardiography Council for Intraoperative Echocardiography and the Society of Cardiovascular Anesthesiologists Task Force for Certification in Perioperative Transesophageal Echocardiography. Anesth Analg 89:870, 1999
6. Shanewise JS, et al: ASE/SCA guidelines for performing a comprehensive intraoperative multiplane transesophageal echocardiography examination: recommendations of the American Society of Echocardiography Council for Intraoperative Echocardiography and the Society of Cardiovascular Anesthesiologists Task Force for Certification in Perioperative Transesophageal Echocardiography. J Am Soc Echocardiogr 12:884, 1999

Appendix 41–3 DEPARTMENT OF ANESTHESIOLOGY AND CRITICAL CARE MEDICINE, CHILDREN'S HOSPITAL OF PHILADELPHIA, CARDIAC ANESTHESIOLOGY WEB-BASED RESOURCES

Organizations

www.acgme.org Accreditation Council for Graduate Medical Education
www.ahrq.gov Agency for Healthcare Research and Quality
www.aap.org American Academy of Pediatrics
www.aabb.org American Association of Blood Banks
www.aahp.org American Association of Health Plans
www.abanes.org American Board of Anesthesiology
www.abim.org American Board of Internal Medicine
www.abms.org American Board of Medical Specialties
www.abp.org American Board of Pediatrics
www.absurgery.org American Board of Surgery
www.americanheart.org American Heart Association
www.ama-assn.org American Medical Association
www.apsf.org Anesthesia Patient Safety Foundation
www.redcross.org American Red Cross
www.auahq.org Association of University Anesthesiologists
www.bma.org.uk/ap.nsf/content/splashpage British Medical Association
www.cdc.gov Centers for Disease Control and Prevention
www.fda.gov Food and Drug Administration
www.faer.org Foundation for Anesthesia Education & Research
www.jcaho.org Joint Commission on Accreditation of Healthcare Organizations
www.echoboards.org National Board of Echocardiography
www.nih.gov National Institutes of Health
www.resus.org.uk/siteindx.htm Resuscitation Council (UK)

Specialty Societies

www.acc.org American College of Cardiology
www.asahq.org American Society of Anesthesiologists
http://gasnet.med.yale.edu/ascca/ American Society of Critical Care Anesthesiologists
http://asecho.org/ American Society of Echocardiography
www.amsect.org American Society of Extra-Corporeal Technology
www.aspan.org American Society of PeriAnesthesia Nurses
www.asra.com American Society of Regional Anesthesia and Pain Medicine
www.acta.org.uk Association of Cardiothoracic Anaesthetists
www.aagbi.org Association of Anaesthetists of Great Britain and Ireland
www.apagbi.org.uk Association of Paediatric Anaesthetists of Great Britain and Ireland
www.asa.org.au Australian Society of Anaesthetists
www.bsecho.org British Society of Echocardiography
www.cas.ca Canadian Anesthesiologists' Society
www.eacta.org European Association of Cardiothoracic Anaesthesiologists
www.euroanesthesia.org European Society of Anaesthesiologists
www.esicm.org European Society of Intensive Care Medicine
www.iars.org International Anesthesia Research Society
www.ismics.org International Society for Minimally Invasive Cardiothoracic Surgery
www.rcoa.ac.uk Royal College of Anaesthetists
www.sambahq.org Society for Ambulatory Anesthesia
www.scahq.org Society of Cardiovascular Anesthesiologists
www.sccm.org Society of Critical Care Medicine
www.seahq.org Society for Education in Anesthesia
www.snacc.org Society of Neurosurgical Anesthesia and Critical Care
www.soap.org Society for Obstetric Anesthesia and Perinatology
www.pedsanesthesia.org Society for Pediatric Anesthesia
www.anestech.org Society for Technology in Anesthesia
www.sts.org Society of Thoracic Surgeons
www.hsforum.com The Heart Surgery Forum (Official Publication of the International Society for Minimally Invasive Cardiothoracic Surgery)
www.nda.ox.ac.uk/wfsa World Federation of Societies of Anaesthesiologists
www.world-critical-care.org World Federation of Societies of Intensive and Critical Care Medicine

Journals

www.anesthesia-analgesia.org Anesthesia and Analgesia
www.anesthesiology.org Anesthesiology
http://ats.ctsnetjournals.org/ Annals of Thoracic Surgery
www.asa-refresher.com American Society of Anesthesiologists Refresher Courses in Anesthesiology
www.bja.oupjournals.org British Journal of Anaesthesia
http://bmj.bmjjournals.com/ British Medical Journal
www.cja-jca.org Canadian Journal of Anesthesia
http://circ.ahajournals.org/ Circulation
http://circres.ahajournals.org/ Circulation Research
http://ctdigest.com/ CTdigest
www.cardiosource.com/jacc.html Journal of the American College of Cardiology
http://jama.ama-assn.org/ Journal of the American Medical Association
www.jcardioanesthesia.com Journal of Cardiothoracic and Vascular Anesthesia
www.journals.elsevierhealth.com/periodicals/JCA Journal of Clinical Anesthesia
www.ject.org Journal of Extracorporeal Technology
http://jtcs.ctsnetjournals.org/ Journal of Thoracic and Cardiovascular Surgery
www.nejm.org New England Journal of Medicine
www.blackwellpublishing.com/journal.asp?ref=1155-5645 Paediatric Anaesthesia
www.pediatrics.org Pediatrics
http://qhc.bmjjournals.com/ Quality & Safety in Health Care

Literature Search Sites

The Review Group
www.cochrane-anaesthesia.suite.dk Cochrane Anaesthesia Review Group

www.ncbi.nlm.nih.gov National Center for Biotechnology Information

www.nlm.nih.gov National Library of Medicine

www.pubmed.gov National Library of Medicine

http://medlineplus.gov/ Medline Plus

Educational Resource Sites

http://depts.washington.edu/asaccp/ American Society of Anesthesiologists Closed Claims Project

American Society of Anesthesiologists (ASA) Closed Claims Project—Home page links to:

http://depts.washington.edu/asaccp/ASA/index.shtml ASA Closed Claims Project

http://depts.washington.edu/asaccp/POCA/index.shtml Pediatric Perioperative Cardiac Arrest (POCA) Registry

http://depts.washington.edu/asaccp/eye/index.shtml The Postoperative Visual Loss Registry

http://depts.washington.edu/asaccp/prof/index.shtml The ASA Committee on Professional Liability

www.invivo.net/bg/index2.html Anesthesia, Critical Care Medicine and Emergency Medicine

http://gasnet.med.yale.edu Anesthesiology Discussion Group Site

www.ucsf.edu/teeecho/CardiacLinks/index.htm#Anchor-49575 Cardiac Web Links-Martin J London, MD, University of California San Francisco

www.ctsnet.org Cardiothoracic Surgery Network on the Internet

www.pediheart.org Congenital Heart Disease Information Site

www.theanswerpage.com Family of educational websites for the medical professional—Anesthesiology, pain management, hospital and CCM, newborn medicine and ob-gyn. Specialty sites feature Question of the Day with a peer-reviewed, referenced answer

www.healthfinder.gov Health Information Site

www.ucsf.edu/teeecho Intraoperative TEE: A Web Based Video Primer

www.medscape.com Medical information from WebMD

www.guideline.gov National Guideline Clearinghouse—a public resource for evidence-based clinical practice guidelines. NGC is sponsored by the Agency for Healthcare Research and Quality (formerly the Agency for Health Care Policy and Research) in partnership with the American Medical Association and the American Association of Health Plans

www.ncbi.nlm.nih.gov/omim/ Online Mendelian Inheritance in Man (database catalog of human genes and genetic disorders) (syndrome clinical synopsis)

www.sickkids.ca/Anaesthesia/pac_list.asp Paediatric Anaesthesia Conference—Discussion Group: Hospital for Sick Children, Toronto, Canada

www.picucourse.org Pediatric Critical Care Education Site

http://pedsccm.wustl.edu PedsCCM is a collaborative, independent, information resource and communication tool for professionals caring for critically ill and injured infants and children

http://pedsccm.wustl.edu/All-Net/english/mainpage/contents/cardanesth.html Pediatric Cardiac Anesthesia section of picuBOOK an on-line resource for pediatric critical care

www.perfusion.com The Perfusion Home Page

www.pacep.org Pulmonary Artery Catheter Education Project

Practice Guidelines and Advisories

www.asahq.org/practice/pulm/pulm_artery.html ASA PAC (Pulmonary Artery Catheterization) Practice Parameter

www.asahq.org/practice/tee/tee.html ASA Perioperative TEE (Transesophageal Echocardiography) Practice Parameter

www.asahq.org/publicationsAndServices/blood_component.html Practice Guidelines for Blood Component Therapy

www.asahq.org/publicationsAndServices/CRMDAdvisory.pdf Practice Advisory for the Perioperative Management of Patients with Cardiac Rhythm Management Devices: Pacemakers and Implantable Cardioverter-Defibrillators

Research Resource Sites

www.scs.uiuc.edu/suslick/seminaronseminars.html Collection of points on how to (and how not to) give a good research seminar

www.niaid.nih.gov/ncn/grants NIH tutorial on the Do's and Don'ts for grant writing

www.niaid.nih.gov/ncn Useful information on other sections of an application including human subjects, training grants, and budgets

Pharmacology Resource Sites

www.epocrates.com Medication information

www.pdr.net Physicians Desk Reference

General Search Engines

www.altavista.com Internet Search Engine

www.google.com Internet Search Engine

www.lycos.com Internet Search Engine

www.msn.com Internet Search Engine

www.yahoo.com Internet Search Engine

www.searchengineguide.com/searchengines.html Search Engine Guide

Computer-Palm Resource Sites

www.aether.com AetherPalm

www.handheldmed.com Handheld Med

www.palm.com/us Palm

http://avantgo.com/frontdoor/index/html Palm computer resource

http://dir.yahoo.com/Health/medicine/anesthesiology/ Yahoo Anesthesiology

REFERENCES

1. http://www.americanheart.org/downloadable/heart/1079736729696HDSStats2004UpdateREV3-19-04.pdf. Accessed 12/03/2004
2. ACGME program requirements. Available at http://www.acgme.org/acWebsite/downloads/RRC_progReq/040pr703_u804.pdf. Accessed 12/03/2004
3. American Board of Anesthesiology. Available at http://www.abanes.org/booklet/BOI-2004.pdf. Accessed 12/03/2004
4. Reves JG: Resident subspecialty training. ASA (Section on Representation, Park Ridge, IL, 60068), 2000–2001
5. Havidich JE, Haynes GR, Reves JG: The effect of lengthening anesthesiology residency on subspecialty education. Anesth Analg 99:844, 2004
6. Appendix II. Graduate medical education. JAMA 292:1099, 2004
7. Brotherton SE, Rockey PH, Etzel SI: US graduate medical education, 2003–2004. JAMA 292: 1032, 2004
8. Available at http://www.scahq.org/sca3/fellowships/Criteria_for_Recognition-2004.pdf. Accessed 12/07/2004

9. Available at http://www.scahq.org/sca3/fellowships/Program_Requirements_for_Residency_Education_in_CardiothoracicAnesthesiology-2004-final1.doc. Accessed 12/07/2004
10. Accreditation Council for Graduate Medical Education: Available at http://www.acgme.org/acWebsite/home/home.asp. Accessed 12/09/2004
11. Accreditation Council for Graduate Medical Education: Available at http://www.acgme.org/acWebsite/about/ab_purposeAccred.asp. Accessed 12/09/2004
12. Accreditation Council for Graduate Medical Education: Available at http://www.acgme.org/acWebsite/dutyHours/dh_dutyHoursCommonPR.pdf. Accessed 12/09/2004
13. American Board of Medical Specialties: Available at http://www.abms.org/. Accessed 12/09/2004
14. Silber JH, Williams SV, Krakauer H, Schwartz JS: Hospital and patient characteristics associated with death after surgery. A study of adverse occurrence and failure to rescue. Med Care 30:615, 1992
15. Silber JH, Kennedy SK, Even-Shoshan O, et al: Anesthesiologist direction and patient outcomes. Anesthesiology 93:152, 2000
16. Silber JH, Kennedy, SK, Even-Shoshan O, et al: Anesthesiologist board certification and patient outcomes. Anesthesiology 96:1044, 2002
17. Brennan TA, Horwitz RI, Duffy FD, et al: The role of physician specialty board certification status in the quality movement. JAMA 292:1038, 2004
18. Guidelines for delineation of clinical privileges in anesthesiology. Available at http://www.asahq.org/publicationsAndServices/standards/08.pdf. Accessed 12/09/2004
19. Mattern WD, Weinholtz D, Friedman CP: The attending physician as teacher. N Engl J Med 308:1129, 1983
20. Bloom BS (ed): Taxonomy of Educational Objectives. Handbook I: Cognitive Domain. New York, David McKay, 1956
21. American Board of Anesthesiology. Available at http://www.theaba.org/examination/exam_oral.html. Accessed 12/28/2004
22. Schwartz AJ: Teaching anesthesiology. In Miller RD (ed): Miller's Anesthesia, 6th edition. Philadelphia, Elsevier Churchill Livingstone, 2005, pp 3105–3117
23. Foley RP, Smilansky: Teaching Techniques. A Handbook for Health Professionals. New York, McGraw-Hill, 1980
24. Krathwohl DR, Bloom BS, Masia BB: Taxonomy of Educational Objectives. Handbook. II: Affective Domain. New York, David McKay, 1964
25. Gawande A: Complications: A Surgeon's Notes on an Imperfect Science. New York, Henry Holt and Company, 2002, pp 11–34
26. Issenberg SB, McGaghie WC, Hart IR, et al: Simulation technology for health care professional skills training and assessment. JAMA 282:861, 1999
27. Gallagher AG, Cates CU: Virtual reality for the operating room and cardiac catheterisation laboratory. Lancet 364:1538, 2004
28. Friedrich MJ: Practice makes perfect: Risk-free medical training with patient simulators. JAMA 288:2808, 2002
29. Gordon MS, Ewy GA, Felner JM, et al: Teaching bedside cardiologic examination skills using "Harvey," the cardiology patient simulator. Med Clin North Am 64:305, 1980
30. Sajid AW, Ewy GA, Felner JM, et al: Cardiology patient simulator and computer-assisted instruction technologies in bedside teaching. Med Educ 24:512, 1990
31. Jones JS, Hunt SJ, Carlson SA, Seamon JP: Assessing bedside cardiologic examination skills using "Harvey," a cardiology patient simulator. Acad Emerg Med 4:980, 1997
32. Waugh RA, Mayer JW, Ewy GA, et al: Multimedia computer-assisted instruction in cardiology. Arch Intern Med 155:197, 1995
33. Euliano T, Good ML: Simulator training in anesthesia growing rapidly. J Clin Monit 13:53, 1997
34. Good ML: Patient simulation for training basic and advanced clinical skills. Med Educ 37(suppl 1):14, 2003
35. Murray DJ, Boulet JR, Kras JF, et al: Acute care skills in anesthesia practice: A simulation-based resident performance assessment. Anesthesiology 101:1084, 2004
36. Blum MG, Powers TW, Sundaresan S: Bronchoscopy simulator effectively prepares junior residents to competently perform basic clinical bronchoscopy. Ann Thorac Surg 78:287, 2004
37. Schwid HA, Rooke GA, Ross BK, Sivarajan M: Use of a computerized advanced cardiac life support simulator improves retention of advanced cardiac life support guidelines better than a textbook review. Crit Care Med 27:821, 1999
38. Saliterman SS: A computerized simulator for critical-care training: New technology for medical education. Mayo Clin Proc 65:968, 1990
39. Grogan EL, Stiles RA, France DJ, et al: The impact of aviation-based teamwork training on the attitudes of health-care professionals. J Am Coll Surg 199:843, 2004
40. Holzman RS, Cooper JB, Gaba DM, et al: Anesthesia crisis resource management: Real-life simulation training in operating room crises. J Clin Anesth 7:675, 1995
41. Henriksen K: Simulation and team training. Qual Saf Health Care 13(suppl 1):i1, 2004
42. Sedlack RE, Kolars JC, Alexander JA: Computer simulation training enhances patient comfort during endoscopy. Clin Gastroenterol Hepatol 2:348, 2004
43. Schwid HA, Rooke A, Carline J, et al: Evaluation of anesthesia residents using mannequin-based simulation Anesthesiology 97:1434, 2002
44. The AMA definition of CME. Available at http://www.ama-assn.org/ama/pub/category/2937.html. Accessed 01/02/2005
45. Maintenance of certification frequently asked questions. Available at https://secure.abanes.org/portal/AboutMOC.asp. Accessed 01/02/2005
46. Schwartz AJ: Learning cardiothoracic anesthesia. *In* Thys DM (ed): Textbook of Cardiothoracic Anesthesiology. New York, McGraw-Hill, 2001, pp 11–23

SELECTED READINGS

Barrows HS: Simulated (Standardized) Patients and Other Human Simulations. Chapel Hill, NC, Health Sciences Consortium, 1987

Bunker JP (ed): Education in Anesthesiology. New York, Columbia University Press, 1967

Chin C, Schwartz AJ: Teaching Pediatric Cardiac Anesthesiology. *In* Lake CL, Booker PD (eds): Pediatric Cardiac Anesthesia. Philadelphia, Lippincott Williams & Wilkins, 2005, pp 755–765

Comroe JH: Exploring the heart. *In* Discoveries in Heart Disease and High Blood Pressure. New York, WW Norton, 1983

Jason H, Westberg J: Instructional Decision-Making Self-Study Modules for Teachers in the Health Professions (Preview Package). National Center for Faculty Development. Miami, University of Miami School of Medicine, 1980

Lear E (ed): Virtual reality in patient simulators. Am Soc Anesthesiol Newsletter 61(October), 1997

Lyman RA: Disaster in pedagogy. N Engl J Med 257:504, 1957

McCauley KM, Brest A: McGoon's Cardiac Surgery: An Interprofessional Approach to Patient Care. Philadelphia, FA Davis, 1985

Miller GE: Adventure in pedagogy. JAMA 162:1448, 1956

Miller GE: Educating Medical Teachers. Cambridge, MA, Harvard University Press, 1980

Schwartz AJ: Teaching and learning congenital cardiac anesthesia. *In* Andropoulos DB, Stayer SA, Russell LA (eds): Anesthesia for Congenital Heart Disease. Armonk, NY, Futura, 2005

INDEX

Note: Page numbers in *italic* refer to illustrations. Page numbers followed by b refer to boxes, and t to tables. Color plate numbers are in **boldface.**

A

B

D

E

H

I

Q

R

S

U

V

W

X

Z